Family-Centered Nursing Care of Children

Roxie L. Romness Foster, R.N. M.S.N., PH. D.
Research Fellow, University of Colorado
Health Sciences Center
School of Nursing
Denver, Colorado

Mabel Metzger Hunsberger, R.N., M.S.N.
Associate Professor, McMaster University
School of Nursing
Hamilton, Ontario

Jo Joyce Tackett Anderson, R.N., M.P.H.N.
Consultant in Health Care
Chandler, Arizona

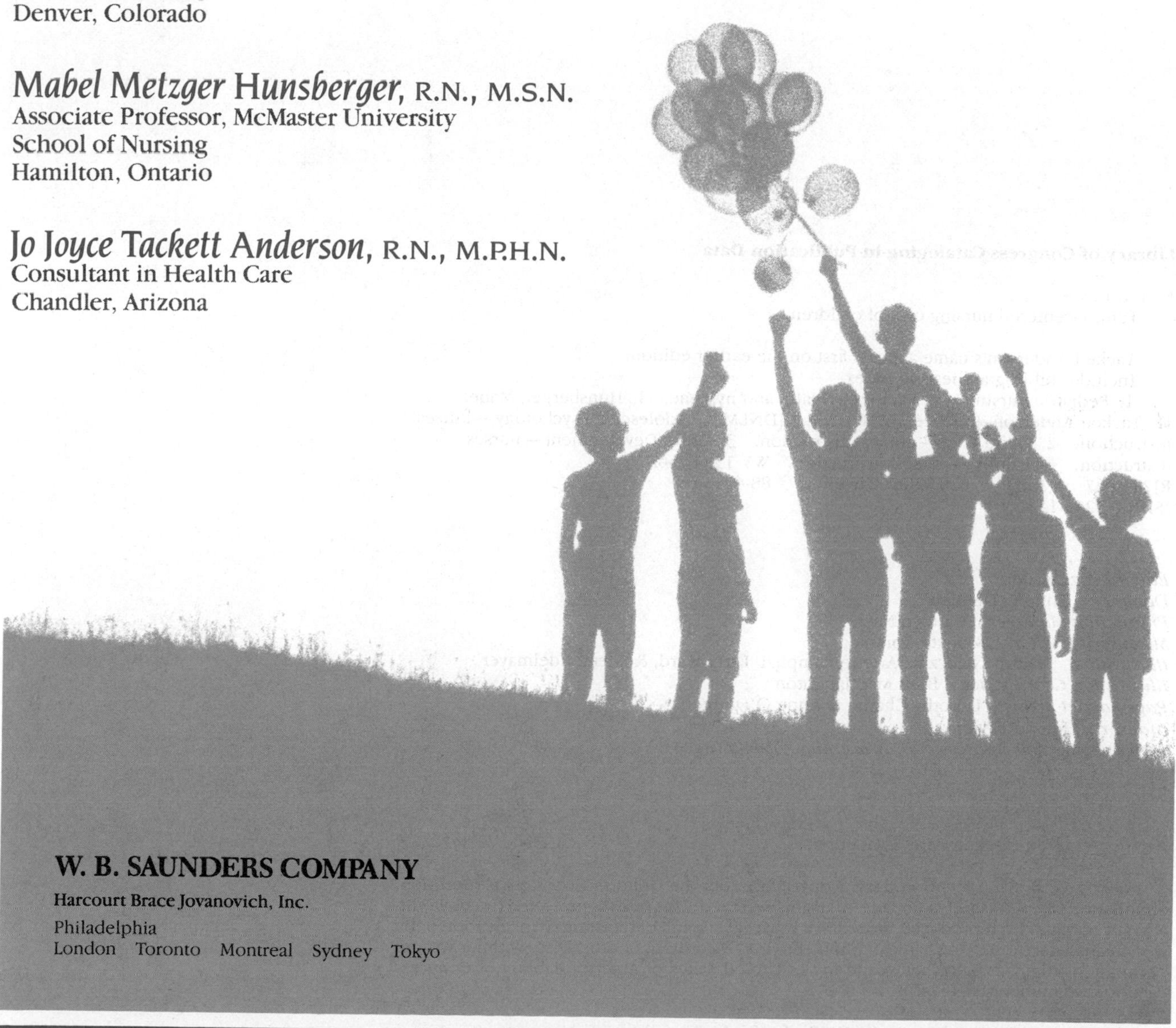

W. B. SAUNDERS COMPANY
Harcourt Brace Jovanovich, Inc.
Philadelphia
London Toronto Montreal Sydney Tokyo

W. B. SAUNDERS COMPANY
Harcourt Brace Jovanovich, Inc.

The Curtis Center
Independence Square West
Philadelphia, PA 19106

Library of Congress Cataloging-in-Publication Data

Foster, Roxie.
Family-centered nursing care of children.

Tackett-Anderson's name appears first on the earlier edition.
Includes bibliographies and index.
1. Pediatric nursing. 2. Family—Health and hygiene. I. Hunsberger, Mabel II. Tackett-Anderson, Jo Joyce. III. Title. [DNLM: 1. Adolescent Psychology—nurses' instruction. 2. Child Care—nurses' instruction. 3. Child Development—nurses' instruction. 4. Family—nurses' instruction. WY 159 F756f]
RJ245.F67 1989 618.92'00024613 88-4644
ISBN 0-7216-1222-9

Editor: Ilze Rader
Designer: Anne O'Donnell
Production Manager: Carolyn Naylor
Manuscript Editor: Wynette Kommer
Illustrators: Sharon Iwanczuk, Arlette Ramphal, Larry Ward, & Glenn Edelmayer
Illustration Coordinator: Brett MacNaughton
Page Layout Artists: Dorothy Chattin & Anne O'Donnell
Indexer: Helene Taylor
Cover photograph courtesy of H. Armstrong Roberts, Inc.

Family-Centered Nursing Care of Children ISBN 0-7216-1222-9

Last digit is the print number: 9 8 7 6 5 4 3

To my parents, Gudrun and Gordon Romness, to my husband, Ron, and our daughters, Kristen and Andrea, for their love, their faith, and their patience during this time when I have not always been family-centered.

RLF

To my parents and family for their encouragement and support. To my husband, Merrill, for his enduring patience and generous gift of time, and to our son, Jason, whose presence in my life has given me wisdom.

MMH

To the memory of my father, the loyalty of my mother, the love of my husband, the flexibility of my children, and the understanding of my coauthors.

JJA

About the Authors

Roxie L. Foster *received her M.S. in Parent-Child Nursing from the University of Colorado. She is a doctoral candidate in nursing at the University of Colorado Health Sciences Center with an emphasis in clinical research. She is associated with the C.U. Center for Nursing Research and currently manages a federally funded grant to explore nurses' clinical decision-making about children in pain. She was Assistant Professor of Nursing at Loretto Heights College in Denver, Colorado, and also taught nursing at Denver Auraria Community College and at Purdue University.*

Mabel Hunsberger *received her M.S.N. in Nursing of Children at the University of Pennsylvania. She is currently an Associate Professor in the School of Nursing at McMaster University and is in clinical practice at the McMaster University Medical Centre Growth and Development Clinic. She has had 20 years of experience in the care of children and taught parent-child nursing for 12 years at Albert Einstein Medical Center in Philadelphia; University of Michigan, Ann Arbor; and McMaster University in Hamilton, Ontario. At McMaster she developed and coordinates the Neonatal Advanced Clinical Practice component of the Master of Health Sciences Program and teaches in the Undergraduate Nursing Program.*

Jo Anderson *has a dual background in pediatric nursing and community health nursing, with an M.P.H. in Nursing from the University of North Carolina—Chapel Hill. She has had over 15 years of experience teaching nursing at the University of Evansville, Indiana; University of Michigan, Ann Arbor; and Blackhawk College and McKendree College, Illinois; and was Nursing Director and Associate Professor at Maryville College, St. Louis. She is currently with a private health care consulting firm in Arizona.*

Contributing Editors

Sandra Frick, RN, PhD
Associate Professor, Department of Developmental Nursing, University of South Carolina, College of Nursing, Columbia, South Carolina

Debra Hymovich, RN, PhD, FAAN
Postdoctoral Fellow, University of Pennsylvania, School of Nursing, Philadelphia, Pennsylvania

Contributors

Claudella Archambeau-Jones, RN
Executive Director, National Institute for Burn Medicine, Ann Arbor, Michigan

S. Elizabeth Baldwin, RNC, MSN, PNP
Doctoral Student, Columbia University School of Public Health, New York, New York

Kathleen Boggs, PhD, RN
Associate Professor, University of North Carolina School of Nursing, Charlotte, North Carolina

Carolyn M. Byrne, RN, MHSc
Assistant Professor, School of Nursing, McMaster University; Clinical Specialist, Community Mental Health, Hamilton Wentworth Department of Health Services, Hamilton, Ontario

Maureen H. Clark, RN, MS
Instructor, Ohio State University, College of Medicine, Department of Pediatrics; Genetics Nurse Associate, Children's Hospital, Columbus, Ohio

Deborah K. Coody, RN, MSN, PNP
Pediatric Nurse Practitioner, University of Texas Medical School, Houston, Texas

Margaret Crandall, RN, MSN
Nonsalaried Clinical Faculty at the University of California, San Francisco, Department of Family Health Care Nursing; Pediatric Clinical Nurse Specialist, Department of Nursing, University of California, Davis, Medical Center, California

Elaine Daberkow, RN, MSN
Pediatric Clinical Nurse Specialist and Director, Exercise Physiology Laboratory, Pediatric Cardiology; University of Colorado Health Services Center, Denver, Colorado

M. Corinne Devlin, MD, FRCS(C), FACOG, FSOGC
Professor of Obstetrics and Gynecology, Faculty of Health Sciences, McMaster University; Active Staff, McMaster University Medical Centre; Affiliate Staff, Hamilton Civic Hospitals and St. Joseph's Hospital, Hamilton, Ontario

Jennifer Disabato, RN, MS
Clinical Nurse Specialist, Neurosurgical Unit, The Children's Hospital, Denver, Colorado

Peggy J. Drapo, PhD, RN
Professor, Texas Woman's University College of Nursing, Denton, Texas

Irving Feller, MD
Professor of Surgery, University of Michigan Burn Center, Ann Arbor, Michigan

Janet S. Hadley, BSN, MSN, CPNP
Head Nurse, Pediatric Clinic, Denver General Hospital, Denver, Colorado

Ann Harkins, BSN, MSN
Doctoral Student, University of California, San Francisco; Nursing Supervisor, Children's Hospital at Stanford, Palo Alto, California

Ruth M. Heyn, MD
Professor Emeritus, Department of Pediatrics, University of Michigan, Ann Arbor, Michigan

Robert M. Issenman, MD
Associate Professor, Department of Pediatrics, McMaster University; Chief of Pediatric Gastroenterology, McMaster University Medical Centre, Hamilton, Ontario

Marcia Sosnowski Leonard, RN, PNP
Clinical Nurse IV, P.N.P./Oncology, Department of Pediatrics, Hematology/Oncology Section, University of Michigan, Ann Arbor, Michigan

Judith W. Maserang, MSN, RN
Doctoral Candidate in Family Development and Therapy, St. Louis University; Associate Director for the R.N. Completion Program and Associate Professor, Community Health, Maryville College, St. Louis, Missouri

Darlene E. McCown, PhD, MSN, PNP, RN
Associate Dean for Academic Affairs, University of Rochester, Rochester, New York

Alba Mitchell, RegN, MSc
Assistant Professor, School of Nursing, McMaster University, Hamilton, Ontario

Mary Lou Moore, PhD, RNC, FAAN
Research Instructor, Department of Obstetrics and Gynecology, Bowman Gray School of Medicine, Wake Forest University; Neonatal Intensive Care Nursery, North Carolina Baptist Hospital, Winston-Salem, North Carolina

Eleanor G. Pask, RN, RN(HON), BScN, MScN
Associate Professor, Faculty of Nursing, University of Toronto; Coordinator of Nursing Research, Hospital for Sick Children, Toronto, Ontario

Charlotte R. Patrick, MS, MEd, RN
Lecturer, Texas Woman's University, College of Nursing, Denton, Texas

Carolyn G. Pedigo, RN, MSN
Associate Professor and Director, Accelerated Option and Mobility in Nursing Education, University of Southwestern Louisiana, Lafayette, Louisiana

Janet Pinelli, RN, MScN
Associate Professor, McMaster University, School of Nursing; Clinical Nurse Specialist, Chedoke-McMaster Hospitals, McMaster University Medical Centre Division, Hamilton, Ontario

Lynn Rew, BSN, MSN, EdD, RN
Assistant Professor, School of Nursing, The University of Texas at Austin, Austin, Texas

Joan Meighan Rimar, RN, BSN, MSN
Head Nurse, Infant-Toddler Ward, Yale–New Haven Hospital, New Haven, Connecticut

Patricia Neel Scott, RN, MSN, CPNP
Pediatric Nurse Practitioner, Maternal and Child Health Services, Comprehensive School Health Services Program, Baltimore City Health Department, Baltimore, Maryland

Claire Smith, RN
Nurse in Gastroenterology Clinic, Hospital for Sick Children, Toronto, Ontario

Bonnie Stevens, RN, BScN, MScN
Assistant Professor, McMaster University School of Nursing; Clinical Nurse Specialist, Department of Pediatrics, Chedoke-McMaster Hospital, Hamilton, Ontario

B. Helen Thomas, RN, BNSc, MSc
Assistant Professor, School of Nursing, McMaster University, Hamilton, Ontario

Linda Upton, RN, MS
Director, Nursing Education/Research, Children's Hospital of Michigan, Detroit, Michigan

Susan N. Van Cleve, RN, MS, CPNP
Assistant Professor, Yale University School of Nursing; Pediatric Nurse Practitioner, Yale–New Haven Hospital, New Haven, Connecticut

Mary J. Waskerwitz, BSN, CPNP
Pediatric Nurse Practitioner, University of Michigan, Department of Pediatrics, Section of Hematology-Oncology, Ann Arbor, Michigan

Anna Frances Z. Wenger, RN, MSN, PhD
Director and Associate Professor, Division of Nursing, Goshen College, Goshen, Indiana

Ann Wiebmer, BSN, MSN
Visiting Fellow, Curtin University of Technology, Perth, Australia

Elizabeth Wonnacott, RN, BScN
Lecturer, School of Nursing, McMaster University, Hamilton, Ontario

Stephanie Wright, RN,C, MSN
Instructor, University of Maryland School of Nursing, College Park, Maryland

Judith Wulf, BSN, MN, CNRN
Clinical Nurse Specialist, Gillette Children's Hospital, St. Paul, Minnesota

Mary Jean Yablonky, CRNA, MA
Chief Nurse Anesthetist, employed at Horizon Surgery Center, Livonia, Michigan

Preface

Family-Centered Nursing Care of Children is a state-of-the-art textbook that details both the theoretical concepts and the specific nursing strategies necessary to today's nursing practice with children and their families. The text reflects the authors' professional experience in nursing education, nursing research, and clinical nursing practice. These experiences have given us an appreciation for and dedication to excellence in nursing practice, an empathy for nursing educators who bear the task of teaching the expanding knowledge of children's health care within an unyielding curricular time frame, and an empathy for the students who must comprehend and integrate this base of knowledge and skills. It reflects, as well, the pragmatism that comes from our personal experiences as parents and consumers of child health care. Additionally, the book is strengthened by the expertise of the contributors who are practicing specialists within the various clinical areas.

This text is designed to provide the comprehensive information vital to the practice of nursing care for children and families at a time when changes within society at large and within the health care profession are invoking changes in nursing practice and education. Poverty and the increasing prevalence of alternate family structures are influencing children's health care. Increased patient acuity and a shortage of staff nurses to provide this care affect the availability of clinical placements for nursing students and the amount of direct supervision required of clinical instructors. The need for expertise in discharge planning and care of the child in the community is being dictated by shorter hospital stays, and by the prevalence of day surgery and home care. Educators are being called upon to prepare students not only as beginning practitioners in acute care settings but as consultants to families in the community. The purpose of this text is to assist nursing educators in meeting these challenges.

Framework

The components of the framework for this text are:

- The nursing process (including nursing diagnosis)
- A conceptual approach
- Child and family development
- Nursing care across health care settings
- Research-based intervention strategies

The five-step nursing process is used as an organizing framework throughout the text and includes an emphasis on nursing diagnosis. The diagnostic stems that appear in the text are NANDA approved and include those adopted in 1988. The authors are committed, however, to providing examples of diagnoses that are most useful for clinical practice. For this reason every NANDA-approved diagnostic stem is followed by a specific etiology statement ("related to" clause) that explains the reason for the determined problem. These diagnoses help demonstrate that when the *analysis* of *assessment* data includes the reason(s) for the problem, the nursing and client goals *(plan)*, nursing strategies *(interventions)*, and *evaluation* criteria follow quite logically.

We believe this text is unprecedented in its comprehensive adaptation of NANDA diagnoses for nursing care of children and families. Nursing diagnoses pertinent to health promotion are included in each of the concept chapters in Unit Three. Illness-focused nursing diagnoses are provided for all the major illnesses discussed in the text.

Nursing process provides the format for each major childhood illness discussed. Assessment data (incidence, etiology, pathophysiology, and clinical manifestations) provide the basis for analysis and are followed by a list of the major nursing diagnoses for that illness. Nursing strategies sections contain both nursing goals pertaining to the identified diagnoses (highlighted as paragraph headings) and strategies for meeting the goals. The information presented provides the detail needed to formulate client goals and specific evaluation criteria for individual clients.

Nursing process is further demonstrated in Nursing Process Plans, so named because they lead the student through each step of the process: assessment pertinent to that illness or situation, analysis of the data (nursing diagnoses that include specific etiology and defining characteristics), client goals, nursing goals, nursing strategies, and identifiable criteria for evaluation.

A conceptual approach is emphasized throughout the text for three purposes: (1) to help the student build a strong theoretical base to support nursing judgments, (2) to address principles of nursing care that are common across many health and illness situations, and (3) to assist the student to learn essential principles for care of children and families from which care for individual clients can then be adapted. This method addresses the challenge of teaching and learning a wealth of content specific to child health care in what is often a very limited time frame. It is based on both sound educational principles and on techniques used by practicing nurses to maintain a standard of excellence in the care of clients with a variety of health care needs. The approach is evident in the use of specific concept chapters related to health promotion, stress and illness, illness management, and developmental-behavioral health concerns. It is emphasized as well in sections detailing developmental differences in structure and function of the body systems, and in comprehensive sections on pathophysiology and psychosocial care. Where appropriate, nursing process plans, although incorporating very specific information, are concept based and apply to children with a variety of illnesses. For example, Table 31-2, Nursing Process Plan: The Hospitalized Child, details the care common to children hospitalized with acute, chronic, or terminal illnesses regardless of diagnosis.

Child development and family development are presented throughout this text not as separate theoretical concepts, but as they actually occur—superimposed upon one another. This approach is designed to prepare the student to work with *actual* families and to anticipate the influences of family development upon an individual child.

Nursing care across health care settings is incorporated throughout the text, with strategies detailing care within the community (including the school) as well as in acute care facilities. *Knowledge deficit* diagnoses within nursing diagnosis sections for major diseases in Unit Seven guide discharge planning. In addition, the discussion of each major illness concludes with a section entitled *Strategies for Nursing Care in the Home or Clinic,* a section designed to guide nursing care in outpatient and home care settings. Chapter 32 describes the principles and strategies of home care and includes a nursing process plan for home care.

Research-based intervention strategies provide the reader with documented sources of information for both medical and nursing interventions. Nursing research is not presented as isolated highlights but is incorporated into the text to provide a rationale for strategies and a perspective on theoretical concepts.

Organization of Content

Unit One discusses *historical, social, cultural, economic,* and *genetic* influences on children and families, explores the role of the pediatric nurse, and presents theories of both child and family development. In-depth information on *alternative family structures* is included.

Unit Two focuses on the specific *developmental stages* of childhood and details the corresponding stages of family development. This unit is primarily oriented toward care of the well child with an emphasis on anticipatory guidance appropriate for children of various ages.

Unit Three presents the concepts that underlie *health promotion* strategies. Chapters in this unit provide more in-depth information about health promotion concepts, which appear as strong threads throughout the text. Included are chapters on such central issues as communicating with children and families, family assessment, parenting, and self-esteem.

Unit Four discusses the concepts of *stress, crisis, and coping* in relation to the reaction of children and their families to illness. The chapters detail nursing strategies to meet the needs specific to acute and chronic illnesses, and to death and dying.

Unit Five deals with *nursing principles and skills* as adapted to the care of children and families. It includes unique concept chapters on pediatric pharmacology and pain, and emphasizes developmental differences in teaching strategies and in preparation of children for procedures.

Unit Six consists of chapters pertaining to *developmental and behavioral health concerns.* These concepts are pertinent for anticipatory guidance of families. Chapter 37, strategies for care of the pregnant adolescent, provides a unique reference. Chapter 35 is devoted to an in-depth discussion of child abuse and failure-to-thrive.

Unit Seven deals with the various *alterations in physiologic function.* The body systems format is designed for ease of reference and class assignments, and to correspond with clinical experiences. The nursing process framework for these chapters was discussed previously. Recognizing the demands on modern clinical educators and the limited opportunities for one-on-one teaching at the bedside, nursing strategies in this text are detailed and specific, reflecting the experience of clinically expert authors. For example, after reading the textbook description of how to assess neurovascular status (page 1785), the student could be expected to perform the task quite adequately the first time. Each major illness is discussed in detail to provide the student with the conceptual base and specific strategies to perform competent nursing care. Nursing process plans throughout the textbook assist the student in establishing a standard of excellence in care for children and families.

Reflecting on this book, we realize that it is a product of our deep commitment to the profession of nursing—a product of our faith in and respect for the nurse. As practitioners we know personally the healing power of nursing care, as educators we facilitate the "becoming" of nurses prepared to deliver that care, as researchers we step back to observe and study the complexity of nurse-patient encounters, and as authors we attempt to convey all that we have learned. We hope this text reflects our humility in the face of this subject matter and our continuing awe of the wonder of childhood and of the unfolding of human potential. Nurses have a unique opportunity to influence the health and well-being of children and families; the purpose of this text will be fulfilled to the extent we can assist in that process.

ROXIE L. FOSTER
MABEL HUNSBERGER
JO JOYCE ANDERSON

Acknowledgments

We are grateful for the many people who have helped and supported us in the creation of this book. We want to thank friends and colleagues who listened daily to our recounting of the details of writing and editing; our editor, Ilze Rader, for her wisdom, professionalism, and unflagging support; Wynette Kommer, Carolyn Naylor, Pat Morrison, Karen O'Keefe, Brett MacNaughton, Marie Thomas, and the many others at W. B. Saunders for their commitment to this project; Gladys Brubacher, Joëlle Paulson, and Lee Ecker for their dedication and persistence in preparing this manuscript; Lynda Baker for her expert advice and assistance in searching the literature and nursing students Karrin Boche, Jennifer Robinson, Kathryn Gillow, and Shirley Yun for their help in retrieving vast numbers of articles from the library; and Dianna Webb for her clerical assistance.

We also are appreciative of the children and families who agreed to be photographed for this book; they included friends, members of our families, and children and families at Children's Hospital—Chedoke-McMaster Hospitals and St. Joseph's Hospital of Hamilton, Ontario, and at The Children's Hospital of Denver, Colorado. Our thanks to Merrill Hunsberger and Jim Tackett and to Ian Matheson of the audiovisual services at McMaster University, Tom Daly and the medical photography department at St. Joseph's Hospital, and all others who have taken photographs for this book.

We are grateful to the many reviewers, listed below, who took the time to give us thoughtful comments on the manuscript. Further, we thank our contributing editors, Sandra Frick, RN, PhD, and Debra Hymovich, RN, PhD, for sharing with us their time and their wealth of nursing knowledge. Thank you as well to our contributors, who dedicated countless hours to writing and revision and whose professional expertise has helped us convey the state of the art in clinical practice.

- Rosalie J. Benchot, RN, MSN, School of Nursing, Kent State University, Kent, Ohio
- Wendy Watson Berry, RN, MSN, National Jewish Center for Immunology and Respiratory Medicine, Denver, Colorado
- Joan E. Bowers, RN, EdD, College of Nursing, University of Nebraska, Omaha, Nebraska
- Susan Burke, MSN, RN, School of Nursing, Thomas Jefferson University, Philadelphia, Pennsylvania
- Patricia Clinton, RN, BSN, MA, College of Nursing, University of Iowa, Iowa City, Iowa
- Toni Clow, RN, MSN, PNP, College of Nursing, University of Iowa, Iowa City, Iowa
- Linda Evans, RN, MNSc, College of Nursing, University of Arizona, Tucson, Arizona
- Carol Flaugher, RN, MSN, College of Nursing, State University of New York, Buffalo, New York
- Beverly Foerder, PhD, RN, School of Nursing, Department of Parent and Child Nursing, University of Washington, Seattle, Washington
- Barbara Fuller, RN, PhD, Professor, School of Nursing, University of Colorado Health Sciences Center, Denver, Colorado
- Deeann A. Gerken, RN, MSN, Department Administrator, Kaiser Foundation Hospital, Fontana, California
- Joan Holter Gildea, RNC, MA, School of Nursing, New York University, New York, New York
- Ilene B. Gottesfeld, RN, MSN, Clinical Nurse Specialist, Pediatric Cardiology, Northshore University Hospital, Manhasset, New York
- Nancy Hester, RN, PhD, Assistant Professor of Nursing; Senior Faculty Associate for the Center for Nursing Research, School of Nursing, University of Colorado Health Sciences Center, Denver, Colorado
- Alice S. Hill, PhD, RN, School of Nursing, University of Texas Medical Branch, Galveston, Texas
- Rosemary Johnson, RN, PhD, Assistant Professor, School of Nursing, University of Southern Maine, Portland, Maine
- Lynn E. Kelly, RN, MSN, School of Nursing, Widener University, Chester, Pennsylvania

- Carole Kenner, RNC, DNS, Parent-Child Nursing, University of Cincinnati, Cincinnati, Ohio
- Juanita Lee, EdD, RN, College of Nursing, University of Southern California, Los Angeles, California
- Alice T. Mazur, RN, PNP, Patient Care Coordinator, Children's Hospital of Philadelphia, Philadelphia, Pennsylvania
- Joseph M. McMahon, EdD, RN, School of Nursing, University of Texas, Houston, Texas
- Margaret Miller, RN, MSN, College of Nursing and Health, University of Cincinnati, Cincinnati, Ohio
- Mary T. Munton, RN, MSN, Medical College of Virginia, Virginia Commonwealth University School of Nursing, Richmond, Virginia
- Beverly Nachem, RN, MS, School of Nursing, Humboldt State University, Arcata, California
- Audrey E. Nelson, RN, BSN, MSN, College of Nursing, University of Nebraska, Omaha, Nebraska
- Noreen Nicol, RN, MS, FNC, Dermatology Clinical Specialist, National Jewish Center for Immunology and Respiratory Medicine, Denver, Colorado
- Susan Ross, RN, MS, Division of Nursing, American International College, Springfield, Massachusetts
- Joyce M. Ruth, RN, MSN, School of Nursing, University of North Carolina, Charlotte, North Carolina
- Linda J. Scheetz, RN, MA, EdD, School of Nursing, Mount Saint Mary College, Newburgh, New York
- Janice Selekman, DNSc, RN, Baccalaureate Nursing Department, Thomas Jefferson University, Philadelphia, Pennsylvania
- Rosemary A. Simkins, RN, MN, National Jewish Center for Immunology and Respiratory Medicine, Denver, Colorado
- Valerie M. Siml, RN, MSN, National Jewish Center for Immunology and Respiratory Medicine, Denver, Colorado
- Perle Slavik, ADN, BSN, MA, PhD, College of Nursing, University of Iowa, Iowa City, Iowa
- Julie L. Townsend, RN, MSN, School of Nursing, Viterbo College, La Crosse, Wisconsin
- Ruth R. Voignier, RN, MS, MSN, School of Nursing, University of Louisville, Louisville, Kentucky
- Judith Ann Walker, RN, EdD, Department of Associate Degree Nursing, North Harris County College, Houston, Texas
- Jean M. Wills, RN, BSN, BSEd, MSN, School of Nursing, University of Pittsburgh, Pittsburgh, Pennsylvania
- Marilyn L. Winkelstein, RN, MS, School of Nursing, University of Maryland, Baltimore, Maryland

Brief Contents

Detailed Contents

Unit One

Introduction to Nursing Care of Children and Adolescents

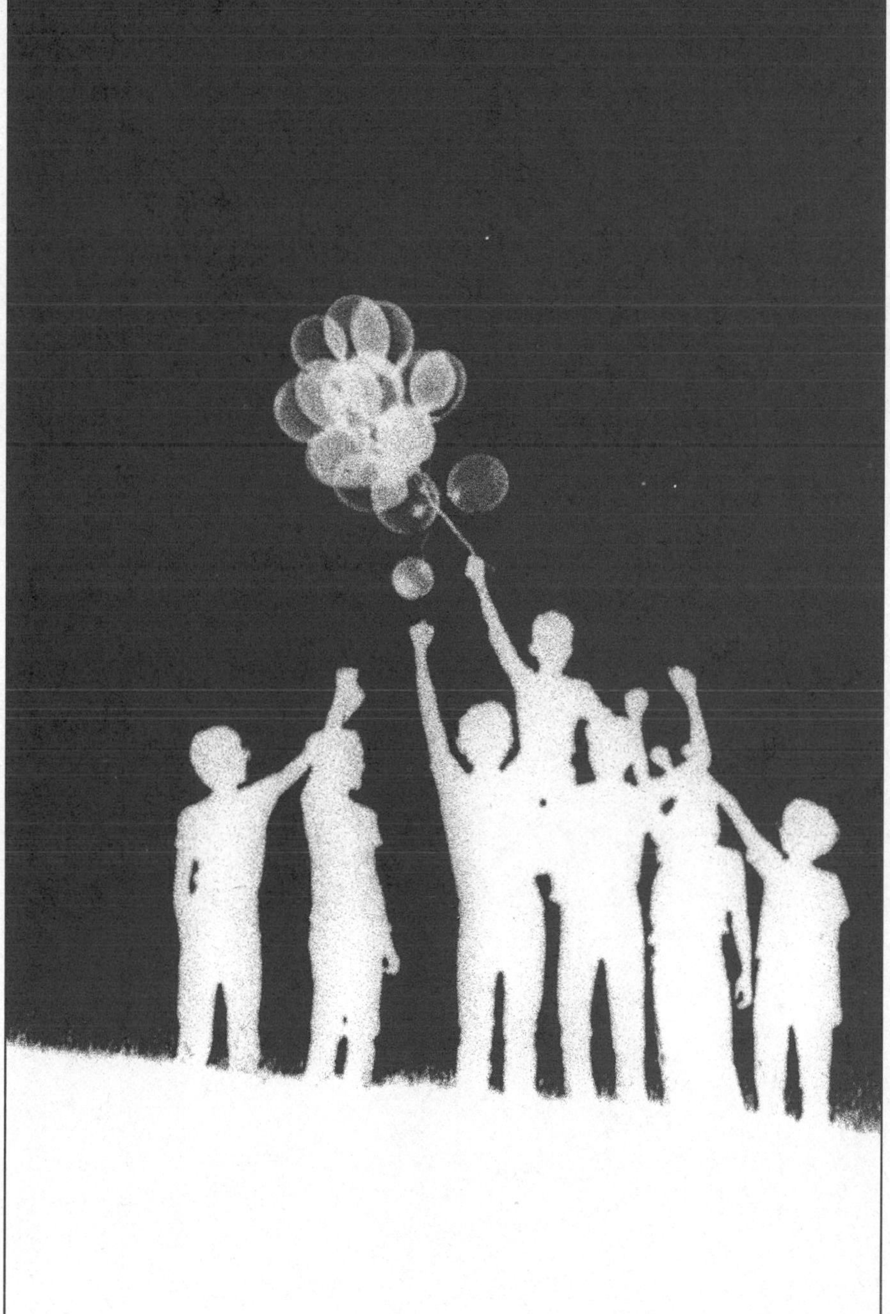

Perspectives on the Nursing Care of Children and Adolescents

Chapter 1

Roxie L. Foster

The celebrations and rituals that mark the birth and development of a child in every culture testify to the mystery and wonder that are associated with the first two decades of life. Nurses who choose to work with children and adolescents seem drawn to that mystery—perhaps not so much to unravel it as just to experience it. They are warmed more than most by a child's smile; they are touched more than most by a child's cry. They recognize the "personhood" of even their youngest client. They are genuinely interested in a child's opinion of what the moon is made of and in an adolescent's explanation for purple-striped hair. They are highly skilled—there is little room for error. They are gentle and kind—the spirit of a child is fragile. Pediatric nurses care not only *for* children and families, they care *about* children and families.

Related Topics
Nontraditional family styles, Chapter 2
Cultural assessment, Chapter 2
Assessment of religious influences, Chapter 2
Effects of culture and lifestyle on development, Chapter 3
Family assessment, Chapter 12
Safety, Chapter 17
Legal aspects of consent, Chapter 27
Injuries, Chapter 52

This chapter sets the stage for the study of pediatric nursing by examining factors that affect the health care of children and adolescents. It begins with a statement of the goal for pediatric nursing, profiles the pediatric population by common illnesses and causes of death (morbidity and mortality), examines the effects of poverty on today's youth, and describes the role of the pediatric nurse. The chapter continues with factors that influence the health care of children, including past and present social attitudes, nursing research, techniques for intercultural communication, ethical issues, and the nursing process as it relates to children and adolescents.

The Goal for Nursing Care of Children and Adolescents

The goal for nursing care of children and adolescents is best understood as it relates to the practice of nursing as a whole. Nursing has been defined by the American Nurses' Association (1980, p. 9) as "the diagnosis and treatment of human responses to actual or potential health problems." More specifically, nursing is a discipline whose focus is the well-being of persons and whose practice involves the contracting (either formally or by inference) with individual clients and/or families and communities to prevent, assess, and intervene in disease processes and to promote wellness in life and dignity in death by use of the caring and curing processes deemed morally and legally appropriate. Within the framework of that definition *the goal of pediatric nursing is to promote the healthy maturation of the child/adolescent as a physical, intellectual, and emotional-social being within the context of the family and the community.* This goal incorporates prevention and assessment of and intervention for threats to physical, intellectual, and emotional-social well-being.

Implications for Nursing Practice

The key word within the stated goal is *maturation.* It emphasizes the *uniqueness* of nursing care for children and adolescents in terms of their response to illness and their need for advocacy. The child* has developing, and, therefore, often immature physical characteristics and immature physiologic and cognitive processes. Self-concept, coping patterns, and social behaviors are also less well developed than in the adult. Because of this immaturity, the physical, cognitive, and emotional responses of the child to illness will vary with chronologic age and with achievement of developmental tasks. Also because of this immaturity, the developing child or adolescent requires adult advocacy for the maintenance and restoration of health. The overwhelming influence of the family upon all aspects of the child's health and development makes the family integral to all nursing assessment, analysis, planning, intervention, and evaluation. Generally, the term "client" in this text refers to child and family.

One of the fundamental goals of nursing is to provide family-centered nursing care. This is in part based on the premise that, since the family is a system, no one individual member can be effectively cared for if that care does not consider the other members who both affect and are affected by the member seeking nursing care. Practitioners who care for the children in families must acknowledge this relationship because it is the family that is largely responsible for that child, that most significantly enhances or hinders that child's development, and to which that child must ultimately be accountable.

Where family once referred primarily to the traditional nuclear group of two parents and one or more children, family structure is changing so that the nuclear family is no longer the standard. Nursing must consider that modern families are often headed by single parents, may be transcultural, biracial, blended, adoptive, communal, gay, or one of several other alternative or nontraditional family styles. Each family must be approached as a unique group of individuals with particular strengths and limitations. Family assessment is detailed in Chapter 12. Several of the most common types of nontraditional family styles are discussed in Chapter 2.

Desired Outcomes

The overall goal for pediatric nursing is realized when the nurse (1) recognizes developmental immaturity and distinguishes these normal characteristics from disease processes, (2) identifies threats to well-being related to physical, intellectual and emotional-social developmental processes, (3) directs nursing strate-

The assistance of Nancy Case, RN, PhD candidate, in reviewing the section on nursing ethics is gratefully acknowledged.

* The word "child" will be used in this chapter as a generic term to connote the developmental stages of infancy through adolescence.

gies to support the unique response of *this* child to issues of health and illness, and (4) supports parental advocacy and initiates professional advocacy for the child within the health care system and within the community.

A Perspective on the Pediatric Population

Three major areas are discussed in this section for the purpose of gaining a perspective on the child population and nursing activities within it. Morbidity and mortality are addressed because they speak to numbers and causes of diseases and death among children and adolescents. The effect of poverty on the pediatric population is included to detail a social issue that increasingly holds implications for the type of clients we see today and will see in the future. Finally, the role of the nurse is discussed as it pertains to care for children and adolescents.

Morbidity and Mortality

Morbidity refers to "sickness" or disease condition.

Mortality refers to the death rate.

The word morbid means diseased, unhealthy, unwholesome. Morbidity is the term used to denote the disease conditions seen within a population. The *morbidity rate* for a specific disease is the number of cases of that disease in a specified period of time (usually a year) within a specified unit (stated number, e.g., 10,000, 100,000) of the population.

The word mortal means human or subject to death. Mortality refers to the number of deaths within a stated population. The *mortality rate* for a given disease is the ratio of the number of deaths from that disease divided by the total number of reported cases of that disease. Together, morbidity and mortality provide a thumbnail sketch of the illness problems that bring children to the health care system and an indication of which diseases carry the highest risk of mortality within a given age group.

Morbidity by Diagnosis in Physicians' Offices. Nurses working in physicians' offices are most likely to attend children for well child care or who have an illness involving the respiratory tract. Although statistics vary between countries (e.g., the United States and Canada) and among regions within the United States, the following morbidity statistics are an indication of illnesses commonly encountered in American children. The University of Southern California, Los Angeles, and the US Division of Research and Medical Education, Washington, DC, found that well child care and diseases of the respiratory tract accounted for 84.5 per cent of the diagnoses made by pediatricians (Hoekelman et al, 1983). Nadler and Evans (1987) stated, "Most of the time pediatricians take care of the non-life-threatening health problems of children who arc under 10 years old and repeatedly see the same dozen or so diagnoses." Table 1-1 summarizes the five most frequent diagnoses made by pediatricians in a study by Hoekelman et al (1983) of 429 pediatricians from across the United States. Well child care and illnesses of the respiratory, gastrointestinal, dermatologic, and musculoskeletal systems accounted for 66 to 87 per cent of patient diagnosis (depending upon age group).

Table 1-1. Five Most Frequent Diagnoses by Age

	Age, Year, Per Cent of Visits*				
Primary Problem Focus	<1 (4,799)	1–4 (7,784)	5–9 (5,179)	10–14 (2,841)	15–19 (1,181)
Well patient	54.6	24.8	14.7	18.3	22.2
Upper respiratory tract†	11.3	19.0	15.2	12.2	10.0
Ears	9.4	16.7	13.1	—	—
Gastrointestinal	6.7	—	—	—	—
Skin	4.4	—	—	10.5	9.8
Mouth/throat	—	10.9	17.1	15.2	16.1
Lower respiratory tract	—	8.8	10.8	7.6	—
Musculoskeletal	—	—	—	—	7.9
Total for 5 Most Frequent Foci	**86.4**	**80.2**	**70.9**	**63.8**	**66.0**

* Number of visits of sample to pediatricians studied indicated in parentheses.
† Not localized to ears, nose, mouth, or throat.
(From Am J Dis Child *1983; 137:1059. Copyright 1983, American Medical Association.)*

Table 1-2. Distribution of Diagnoses Made by Pediatricians

	Age (Years), Per Cent of Visits*					
Primary Problem Focus	All Ages (21,784)	<1 (4,799)	1–4 (7,784)	5–9 (5,179)	10–14 (2,841)	15–19 (1,181)
Well patient	28.0	54.6	24.8	14.7	18.3	22.2
Upper respiratory tract†	15.0	11.3	19.0	15.2	12.2	10.0
Ears	12.2	9.4	16.7	13.1	6.3	3.4
Mouth/throat	10.6	3.4	10.9	17.1	7.6	16.1
Lower respiratory tract	8.5	3.9	8.8	10.8	15.2	7.4
Skin	5.5	4.4	5.4	8.2	10.5	9.8
Gastrointestinal	5.1	6.7	4.9	4.4	5.1	3.7
Nose	1.9	1.3	1.9	2.4	1.8	1.7
Skeletal	1.7	0.2	0.7	1.8	5.1	5.2
Head/neck	1.2	0.9	1.1	1.5	1.7	1.8
Emotional/behavioral	1.0	0.3	0.2	1.9	2.1	3.3
Eyes	1.0	0.9	0.9	1.3	1.2	0.7
Neurologic	0.7	0.4	0.5	0.9	1.7	0.8
Muscular	0.7	0.2	0.2	0.6	2.2	2.7
Blood/lymphatics	0.6	0.3	0.5	0.8	0.7	1.2
Renal	0.6	0.0	0.1	0.9	0.5	0.0
Circulatory (heart)	0.3	0.3	0.2	0.3	0.3	0.6
Genital (M)	0.2	0.1	0.2	0.3	0.3	0.7
Gynecologic	0.2	0.0	0.1	0.2	0.4	2.0
Endocrine	0.2	0.0	0.0	0.3	0.8	0.8
Liver/gallbladder	0.1	0.3	0.0	0.1	0.1	0.2
Breasts	0.1	0.1	0.0	0.0	0.3	0.2
Circulatory (other)	0.1	0.0	0.1	0.1	0.2	0.1
Arthritis/rheumatism	0.1	0.0	0.1	0.2	0.2	0.3
Other and multisystem	2.0	1.4	1.5	1.5	4.3	4.1

* Number of visits of sample to pediatricians studied indicated in parentheses.
† Not localized to ears, nose, mouth, or throat.
(From Am J Dis Child *1983; 137:1060. Copyright 1983, American Medical Association.)*

Table 1-2 gives the distribution of all diagnoses made by pediatricians in this study.

Morbidity by Hospital Admission. Pediatric nurses who work in acute care settings see children who have a different mix of disease conditions, depending upon whether the facility is a children's hospital or a general hospital. Children are more likely to be admitted to a *general hospital* with respiratory and gastrointestinal illnesses, surgery for tonsillectomy and adenoidectomy, and for injury-related causes. Children are more likely to be admitted to a *children's hospital* for specialized treatment for diseases such as congenital anomalies, malignancies, gastrointestinal disease, and central nervous system anomalies (Nadler and Evans, 1987). Box 1-1 details the 21 most common diagnoses of children admitted to children's hospitals. Of course, hospital admittance depends upon hospital access. If access to a local or regional children's hospital is limited by geographic or financial factors, the closest general hospital must adapt to more specialized pediatric needs. Box 1-2 is a partial listing of children's hospitals and other institutions caring for children within the United States and Canada.

Injury as a Cause of Morbidity. The importance of considering injury under the category of morbidity is emphasized by the fact that for every death attributed to injury (accident), at least 1000 other injuries occur that, although nonfatal, are serious enough to require treatment (Guyer and Gallagher, 1985). Table 1-3 illustrates the results of a Massachusetts study of medical care for injuries. These statistics will of course vary by state and location, but they imply that nurses in emergency care facilities can expect to see a large number of pediatric clients with injuries, probably fewer than 25 per cent of whom will be admitted for hospital treatment.

Table 1-3. Results of a Massachusetts Study: Distribution of Cases by Level of Medical Care for All Childhood Injuries

Level of Care	Number	Per Cent of Total
Emergency room:		
Treated and released	18,800	96.5
Admitted	668	3.4
Death	15	0.1
TOTAL	19,483	100.0

Source: Gallagher et al: Am J Pub Health *1984; Dec.*

Box 1-1
Top 21 Admission Diagnoses in Children's Hospitals

Noninfectious gastroenteritis
Asthma without status asthmaticus
Convulsions
Asthma with status asthmaticus
Hypertrophied tonsils and adenoids
Organism; pneumonia
Otitis media
Chronic tonsillitis
Bilateral inguinal hernia
Croup
Preterm infant
Maintenance chemotherapy
Acute bronchiolitis
Viral infection
Chronic serous otitis media
Viral enteritis
Lack of normal physiologic development
Extrinsic asthma with status asthmaticus
Unilateral inguinal hernia
Viral meningitis
Chronic nonsuppurative otitis media

From Nadler and Evans, The American Journal of Diseases of Children, *Jan. 1987, 141:23. Copyright 1987, American Medical Association.*

Mortality. The majority of deaths that occur in the first year of life are attributed to the neonatal period, the first 28 days of life. As illustrated in Figure 1-1, neonatal deaths significantly outrank those for the postneonatal period (after the first month of life) for both black and white infants. About 40 per cent of all deaths in the first year occur within the first 24 hours (Behrman and Vaughan, 1987). The major causes of neonatal deaths are congenital anomalies and prematurity.

Although the United States has experienced a decline in infant mortality, the rate of 11.2 deaths per 1000 live births in 1983 was still higher than for 17 other nations. Mortality rates for black infants in the United States remain significantly higher than for white infants. Note in Figure 1-1 that deaths for white neonates are actually similar to deaths for black infants older than 1 month and that the survival rates are poorest for black infants in the first 28 days of life and best for white infants in their second month of life. Figure 1-1 shows that the mortality rate for black infants in the postneonatal period (28 days to 1 year) did not dip below the level for white neonates (birth to 28 days) until 1983. Analysis of the National Infant Mortality Surveillance project revealed three factors contributing to the higher mortality rate for black infants: (1) a higher percentage of low birth weight in black infants, (2) a higher neonate mortality rate for black infants more than 2500 grams at birth compared with white infants of comparable weight, and (3) a higher postneonatal death rate for black infants in all birth weight categories (Infant mortality . . . , 1987).

Text continues on page 11

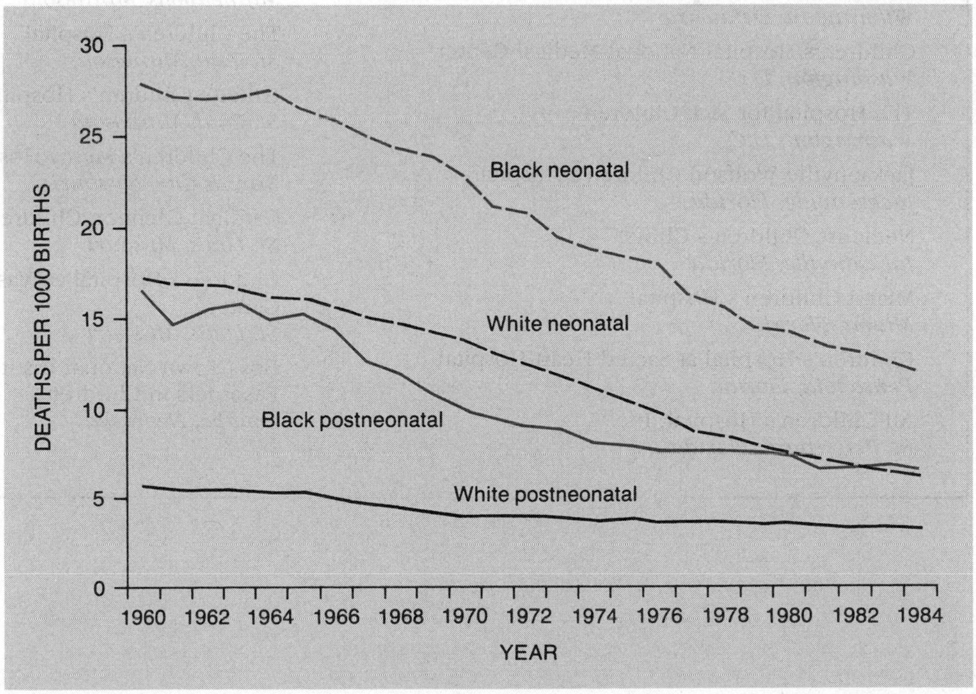

Figure 1-1. Neonatal and postneonatal mortality rates among single-delivery infants, by race and year—United States, 1960–1984. (From Infant mortality among black Americans. *Morbid Mortal Weekly Report* 1987; 36(1):2.)

Box 1-2
Children's Hospitals and Treatment Centers, United States and Canada

UNITED STATES

The Children's Hospital of Alabama
Birmingham, Alabama

Children's Health Center
St. Joseph's Hospital
Phoenix, Arizona

Phoenix Children's Hospital
Phoenix, Arizona

Arkansas Children's Hospital
Little Rock, Arkansas

Valley Children's Hospital
Fresno, California

Miller Children's Hospital
Memorial Medical Center of Long Beach
Long Beach, California

Children's Hospital of Los Angeles
Los Angeles, California

Children's Hospital Medical Center of Northern California
Oakland, California

Children's Hospital of Orange County
Orange, California

Children's Hospital at Stanford
Palo Alto, California

Children's Hospital and Health Center
San Diego, California

The Children's Hospital
Denver, Colorado

Newington Children's Hospital
Newington, Connecticut

Alfred I. duPont Institute
Wilmington, Delaware

Children's Hospital National Medical Center
Washington, D.C.

The Hospital for Sick Children
Washington, D.C.

Jacksonville Wolfson Children's Hospital
Jacksonville, Florida

Nemours Children's Clinic
Jacksonville, Florida

Miami Children's Hospital
Miami, Florida

Children's Hospital at Sacred Heart Hospital
Pensacola, Florida

All Children's Hospital, Inc.
St. Petersburg, Florida

The Henrietta Egleston Hospital for Children
Atlanta, Georgia

Scottish Rite Children's Hospital
Atlanta, Georgia

The Children's Memorial Hospital
Chicago, Illinois

LaRabida Children's Hospital and Research Center
Chicago, Illinois

James Whitcomb Riley Hospital for Children
Indianapolis, Indiana

Kosair Children's Hospital of NKC Hospitals, Inc.
Louisville, Kentucky

Children's Hospital
New Orleans, Louisiana

The Kennedy Institute for Handicapped Children
Baltimore, Maryland

Mt. Washington Pediatric Hospital, Inc.
Baltimore, Maryland

The Children's Hospital
Boston, Massachusetts

Floating Hospital for Infants and Children
New England Medical Center
Boston, Massachusetts

Joseph P. Kennedy Jr. Memorial Hospital for Children
Brighton, Massachusetts

C.S. Mott Children's Hospital
University of Michigan Hospitals
Ann Arbor, Michigan

Children's Hospital of Michigan
Detroit, Michigan

Minneapolis Children's Medical Center
Minneapolis, Minnesota

The Children's Hospital
St. Paul, Minnesota

Gillette Children's Hospital
St. Paul, Minnesota

The Children's Mercy Hospital
Kansas City, Missouri

Cardinal Glennon Children's Hospital
St. Louis, Missouri

Children's Hospital at Washington University Medical Center
St. Louis, Missouri

Boys Town National Institute for Communication Disorders in Children
Omaha, Nebraska

Children's Memorial Hospital
Omaha, Nebraska

Children's Seashore House
Atlantic City, New Jersey

Children's Specialized Hospital
Mountainside, New Jersey

Children's Hospital of New Jersey
United Hospitals Medical Center
Newark, New Jersey

Carrie Tingley Hospital for Crippled Children
Albuquerque, New Mexico

St. Mary's Hospital for Children, Inc.
Bayside, New York

The Children's Hospital of Buffalo
Buffalo, New York

Schneider Children's Hospital
New Hyde Park, New York

Blythedale Children's Hospital
Valhalla, New York

The Children's Medical and Surgical Center of Duke University Hospital
Durham, North Carolina

St. Luke's Children's Hospital
Fargo, North Dakota

Children's Hospital Medical Center of Akron
Akron, Ohio

Children's Hospital Medical Center
Cincinnati, Ohio

Health Hill Hospital for Children
Cleveland, Ohio

Children's Hospital
Columbus, Ohio

The Children's Medical Center
Dayton, Ohio

Oklahoma Children's Memorial Hospital
Oklahoma City, Oklahoma

Children's Medical Center
Tulsa, Oklahoma

Geisinger Children's Hospital Center
Danville, Pennsylvania

Children's Rehabilitation Hospital
Philadelphia, Pennsylvania

The Children's Hospital of Philadelphia
Philadelphia, Pennsylvania

St. Christopher's Hospital for Children
Philadelphia, Pennsylvania

Children's Hospital of Pittsburgh
Pittsburgh, Pennsylvania

The Rehabilitation Institute of Pittsburgh
Pittsburgh, Pennsylvania

Department of Pediatrics, Rhode Island Hospital
Providence, Rhode Island

Children's Hospital
Charleston, South Carolina

East Tennessee Children's Hospital
Knoxville, Tennessee

Le Bonheur Children's Medical Center, Inc.
Memphis, Tennessee

Children's Hospital of Vanderbilt University
Nashville, Tennessee

Children's Medical Center of Dallas
Dallas, Texas

Texas Scottish Rite Hospital for Crippled Children
Dallas, Texas

Cook-Fort Worth Children's Medical Center
Fort Worth, Texas

Children's Hospital of the King's Daughters, Inc.
Norfolk, Virginia

Children's Hospital
Richmond, Virginia

Children's Medical Center
Richmond, Virginia

Children's Hospital and Medical Center
Seattle, Washington

Mary Bridge Children's Hospital and Health Center of Multicare Medicare Center
Tacoma, Washington

Children's Hospital of West Virginia
Morgantown, West Virginia

Children's Hospital of Wisconsin
Milwaukee, Wisconsin

CANADA

Chedoke-McMaster Hospitals
Hamilton, Ontario

Children's Hospital of Eastern Ontario
Ottawa, Ontario

The Hospital for Sick Children
Toronto, Ontario

The Hugh MacMillan Medical Centre
Toronto, Ontario

(Used with permission of National Association of Children's Hospitals and Related Institutions.)

Table 1-4. Leading Causes of Death by Age Group

Rank Order in 1978	Cause of Death* and Age	Rate
	Under 1 Year—All Causes	1378.4
1	Congenital anomalies	252.1
2	Immaturity, unqualified	110.3
3	Respiratory distress syndrome	99.7
4	Asphyxia of newborn, unspecified	88.7
5	Hyaline membrane disease	80.0
6	Birth injury without mention of cause	55.5
7	Influenza and pneumonia	46.0
8	Accidents	37.9
9	Septicemia	32.8
10	Conditions of placenta	23.0
—	All other causes	552.3
	1 to 4 Years—All Causes	69.2
1	Accidents	28.8
—	Motor vehicle accidents	10.6
—	All other accidents	18.2
2	Congenital anomalies	8.4
3	Malignant neoplasms, including neoplasms of lymphatic and hematopoietic tissues	4.9
4	Influenza and pneumonia	2.9
5	Homicide	2.6
6	Diseases of heart	2.3
7	Meningitis	1.8
8	Meningococcal infections	0.9
9	Cerebrovascular diseases	0.8
10	Anemias	0.6
—	All other causes	15.1
	5 to 14 Years—All Causes	33.9
1	Accidents	17.2
—	Motor vehicle accidents	8.8
—	All other accidents	8.4
2	Malignant neoplasms, including neoplasms of lymphatic and hematopoietic tissues	4.2
3	Congenital anomalies	1.8
4	Homicide	1.3
5	Diseases of heart	1.0
6	Influenza and pneumonia	0.9
7	Cerebrovascular diseases	0.6
8	Suicide	0.4
9	Anemias	0.2
10	Benign neoplasms and neoplasms of unspecified nature	0.2
—	All other causes	6.0
	15 to 24 Years—All Causes	117.5
1	Accidents	64.5
—	Motor vehicle accidents	46.4
—	All other accidents	18.1
2	Homicide	13.2
3	Suicide	12.4
4	Malignant neoplasms, including neoplasms of lymphatic and hematopoietic tissues	6.3
5	Diseases of heart	2.7
6	Congenital anomalies	1.6
7	Influenza and pneumonia	1.3
8	Cerebrovascular diseases	1.1
9	Diabetes mellitus	0.3
10	Benign neoplasms and neoplasms of unspecified nature	0.3
—	All other causes	13.8

* Eighth Revision, *International Classification of Diseases,* Adapted, 1965.

Statistics for United States, 1978 (refers only to resident deaths occurring within the United States; rates per 100,000 population).

(Adapted from Monthly Vital Statistics Report *1980; 28(13):23, 25.)*

Table 1-5. Injury Deaths Among Children and Adolescents in the United States, 1980

Injury Type	Less Than 1 Year Old	1–4 Yr	5–14 Yr	15–19 Yr	TOTAL
Motor vehicle					
Occupant	218	493	1122	7246	79079
Pedestrian	13	435	1005	757	2210
Motorcycle	1	8	120	788	917
Pedal cycle	0	16	387	159	562
Other	20	264	285	480	1049
TOTAL	252	1216	2919	9430	13817
Bicycle	0	4	25	10	39
Burn	177	735	535	348	1795
Drowning	91	693	795	1012	2591
Choking/Suffocation	439	214	205	131	989
Foreign Body	1	4	2	2	9
Poison	22	83	52	293	450
Falls	44	111	89	209	453
Other	140	253	602	824	1819
TOTAL	1166	3313	5224	12,259	21,962

Source: National Center for Health Statistics.

Major Causes of Death. Table 1-4 lists causes of death by age group. Two of these leading causes of death, injuries and suicides, deserve additional discussion.

Injuries/Accidents. Table 1-5 details the leading causes of death attributed to injury in 1980. Guyer and Gallagher (1985) argued for use of the word "injury" to replace "accident." They stated, "Gradually the unscientific term accident, with its connotations of chance, fate, and unexpectedness, is being replaced by the description of injuries and the physical and chemical agents that cause them." The importance of this difference in perception is that injury prevention may then seem a more feasible goal. Chapter 17 deals with issues of safety for children and adolescents, and Chapter 52 covers the injured child.

Suicide. Between 1970 and 1980, the suicide rate among American teenagers and young adults (15 to 24 years) increased 40 per cent (Youth suicide, 1987). The increase is due in large part to an escalation in the rate of suicide among young white men (Fig. 1-2). The method of suicide also changed significantly in this 10-year reporting period. The proportion of suicides attributed to firearms increased sharply for both young

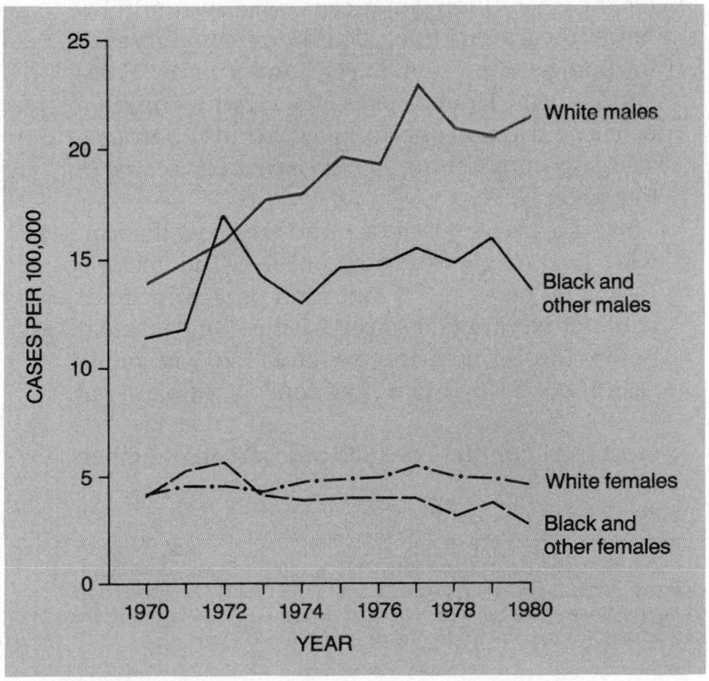

Figure 1-2. Suicide rates for persons 15 to 24 years of age—United States, 1970–1980. (From Youth suicide—United States, 1970–1980. *Morbid Mortal Weekly Report* 1987; 36(6):87.)

men and women while intentional poisoning decreased.

The Children of Today and Tomorrow: Effects of Poverty

As we enter the last decade of the 20th century we are faced with a major social problem that directly affects the young people of our nation: poverty. Despite our marvels of modern technology, despite the growing national movement toward "holism" and "caring," despite decades of antipoverty programs, and despite the emphasis placed on the American family during the 8 years of the Reagan administration, *the children of the United States are currently the poorest age group in the population.* According to the US Census Bureau, one of every five American children lives in poverty—more than 16 per cent of white children, nearly 40 per cent of Hispanic children, and half of all black youngsters. Senator Moynihan (1987) wrote, "It is fair to assume that the United States has become the first society in history in which a person is more likely to be poor if young rather than old." Moynihan reported that the poverty rates for children in the United States exceed those for children in Canada, Germany, Norway, Sweden, and the United Kingdom.* Social scientists disagree on the causes for these figures, but Moynihan suggested that major factors include the increase in teenage pregnancy, the increase in female-headed single families, unemployment, and decreasing tax exemptions for dependent family members. Moynihan and others chronicled the following facts:

- Of the 34 million Americans who currently live below the poverty line, 20 million are hungry and 2 million have no homes (O'Connor et al, 1986). Suddenly the United States is faced with a problem usually attributed only to Third World countries—a large group of children who have been reared on the street.
- The poor are not just those who are on welfare and who live in ghetto communities. The majority (about 60 per cent) of American poor who are capable of working do so but have incomes that fall below the poverty line, set at $11,203 in annual cash income for a family of four (Whitman et al, 1988).
- Most poor families in which one or more members work are white, two-parent families. The "working poor" are quite evenly divided among central cities, suburbs, and rural areas (Whitman et al, 1988).
- Pregnancy among American teenagers (15 to 19 years) reached a rate of 96 per 1000 in 1985, compared with 44 per 1000 in Canada and 14 per 1000 in the Netherlands. (To make that statistic somewhat more concrete, in 1983 one in every five births in the U.S. was to an unwed mother!)
- The number of female-headed single families in America is increasing at an alarming rate. It is estimated that during the period 1980–2000 the number of female-headed families will increase at more than five times the rate of husband-wife families.
- "Children don't vote, lobby, or make campaign contributions" (Edelman, cited in O'Connor et al, 1986, p 21). Children must rely on parents to exert political influence on their behalf. One-parent families have only half as many votes as two-parent families.
- Adults without children tend to vote for programs that will protect them in their old age and to leave the problems of childhood to "someone else."
- Between 1970 and 1984 the average elderly person receiving aid from Old-Age and Survivors Insurance saw a 54 per cent increase in cash benefits. During that same period the mother receiving aid from AFDC (Aid to Families with Dependent Children) saw dollar benefits *decline* by 34 per cent.
- Since 1985 the U.S. government has abolished the Job Corps and slashed budgets for education, nutrition, and health programs by $36.5 billion (Moynihan, 1987; O'Connor et al, 1986).
- For a medium-status four-person family, the average cost (i.e., not need, but actual expenditure) to raise a child from birth to 18 years is in excess of $82,000. That figure increases if the mother is also employed outside the home.
- In 1948, fully 75 per cent of median family income was exempt from taxation, providing in part for the cost of raising a family. By 1983, less than 33 per cent of median family income was tax exempt, thus eroding protection for the rearing of American families.
- Of the 35 million persons in the United States who lack any form of health insurance, 11 million are children (Oberg, 1987).

Implications for Nursing Practice. What do these statistics mean to the pediatric nurse? They mean that there is likely to be a significant change in the

* Although the poverty rate among children in Canada and Norway exceeds the poverty rates among the elderly in those countries, the Norwegian rates are very low, and the 9.5 per cent poverty rate among Canadian children is only half the US rate.

population of children and adolescents who present themselves for treatment in the coming years. The pediatric population in America at the turn of the 21st century may well be

- increasingly ethnically mixed (the birth rate has declined faster for white families in the United States than for people of color, and as American birth rates decline in general, the nation will be pressed to increase immigration);
- more sickly because prenatal care and well child care are luxuries in a poverty-level environment;
- more susceptible to delays in growth due to improper nutrition and improperly treated illnesses;
- more prone to drug and alcohol abuse, depression, and suicide related to unstable and non-nurturing environments.

The Challenge for Pediatric Nursing. *The challenge to the nurse who cares for children,* therefore, is to provide care of such *quality* that it can offset the potential decline in *quantity* of interactions with a child and family. Further, there is a challenge to *make a difference.* Never has there been more need for nurses to make an impact on community knowledge and attitudes about health care; to provide effective liaisons with other health care professionals; to use every aspect of their scientific knowledge and every strategy of their art in client interactions; and to base nursing practice upon nursing research. *Never has there been a greater opportunity for nurses to fulfill the societal expectations that are linked to nursing's claim to professional status.*

On some fronts, of course, the pediatric nurse will have increasing resources to help meet this challenge. Morbidity and mortality are likely to be decreased through additional organ transplants and innovations in immunotherapy and pharmacotherapy. Computerization of hospital and agency files will eventually decrease time spent in paperwork. Employment opportunities for nurse practitioners are also expected to increase as third party payment (direct payment to nurses from insurance companies) becomes more common and as health care costs force alternatives to care solely by private physicians. Nursing research will provide nursing with an increasing base for practice that is goal oriented rather than task oriented; that is, it will help eliminate mundane and repetitive tasks, freeing the nurse for additional creative and therapeutic endeavors.

The effective nurse of the coming generation will base his or her practice on sound knowledge of the nursing process and the professional role. The nurse will need to understand not only where pediatric nursing is going but the social and historical influences that have dictated practice as we know it today. Increasingly, the nurse will need to be skilled in intercultural communication and ethical decision making. The remainder of this chapter details these influences upon attainment of the goal of pediatric nursing—healthy maturation of children and adolescents.

The Role of the Pediatric Nurse

The Commitment to Excellence

Inherent in the role of every professional nurse is a commitment to society. "Entering a profession involves one in societal institutions whose goal is to serve the welfare of persons. Choosing how and where to serve involves one in surveying the environment and its social institutions in order to see how to convert this choice into action" (Quinn and Smith, 1987). Implicit in the role of the pediatric nurse is the special commitment to safeguard society's most precious resource—its youth. Though unwritten and unspoken, this commitment is communicated to the nurse through the expectations of parents and others who expect a particular dedication and excellence in the nursing care provided to children.

In fulfilling this expectation for excellence, the pediatric nurse will rely upon a formal knowledge base or *science* of nursing. In addition, the nurse will use personal attributes—physical, cognitive, and spiritual—to accomplish professional goals. This is the *art* of nursing, or therapeutic use of self. The unique qualities of the nurse-artist will dictate creativity in problem solving and skill with interpersonal relations. Those unique qualities that enhance the pediatric nurse's effective use of self are truly to be recognized and nurtured within the profession.

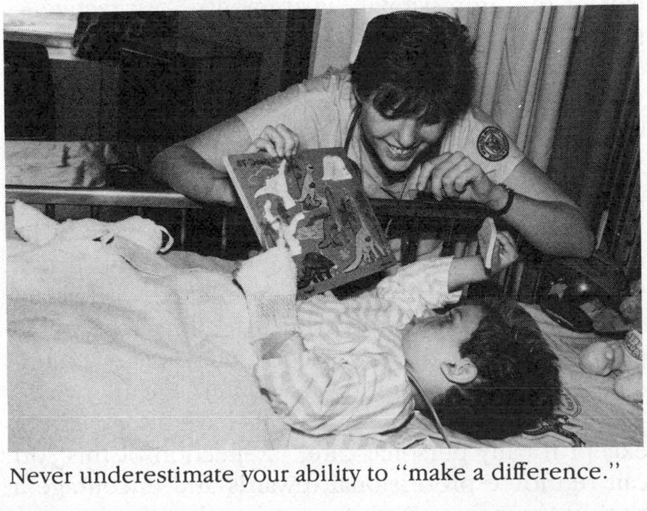

Never underestimate your ability to "make a difference."

Universal Principles of Pediatric Nursing Practice

Four "universals" of practice will serve all pediatric nurses well:

- NEVER underestimate the skills, concern, or intuition of the parent.
- NEVER betray a child's trust.
- NEVER neglect your own mental, spiritual, and physical health.
- NEVER underestimate your ability to "make a difference."

The nurse who possesses adequate self-esteem will not need to bolster a sagging ego by falsely inflating the professional role. Instead, this nurse will be able to truly *listen* to a parent's concerns and suggestions and will be able to take advantage of the parent's skill with the child. The nurse's educational preparation and professional experience qualify him or her for the role of expert *consultant* on specific aspects of wellness and illness. The parents' history with the child and sense of responsibility and love for the child qualifies them as the *expert* on their child's responses.

The nurse who recognizes the precious and fragile bond of trust offered by a child will be reluctant to betray it. Once destroyed, it is unlikely the bond can be sufficiently rebuilt within the time frame of most nurse-patient encounters. Earning and safeguarding trust is accomplished through consistent honesty, through accurate assessment of needs and responses, and through communication that tells children they are accepted and valued for their unique personhood.

The role of the pediatric nurse is as demanding as it is exciting and rewarding. Excellence in pediatric practice demands that the nurse be able to offer his or her best during the hours of professional practice. This can only be done if the nurse nurtures the most important of the professional "instruments" of practice—the self.

Most of us enter the nursing profession with a desire to make a difference. What happens to those wishes? What is it that so often makes us feel impotent? Is it the bureaucracy of the health care system, or the pervasive nature of disease, or some kind of emotional "anesthetization" that occurs over time? Whatever the reason, feelings of impotence represent a mindset that is incompatible with nursing excellence. Instead of succumbing to these occasional feelings, the nurse might ask, "How did my practice today make a difference?" "For *whom* did I make a difference and why?" "What, exactly, would my patients have done without except for my personal care?" Reflection of this sort can reinforce professional rewards and encourage a positive mindset. Each nurse has the opportunity, every day, to "make a difference" but it doesn't happen by accident. It is accomplished by the nurse who implements "making a difference" as a practice goal.

Unique Aspects of the Pediatric Nursing Role

Certain aspects of the pediatric nursing role are unique because of the vulnerability and developmental immaturity of children and adolescents. These aspects include the issues of advocacy and health teaching.

The Pediatric Nurse as Advocate. The advocacy role in pediatric nursing includes the responsibility to work with the family to substitute judgment for that of the child who is too young to make self-care decisions and to be a spokesperson for the child who is too young, too inexperienced, or too frightened to make care needs known. An advocate is someone who pleads in behalf of another. An effective advocate is knowledgeable of the values and beliefs of the child and family so that the "plea" truly represents the client's needs from the client's point of view. (See the section on intercultural communication.) The pediatric nurse will at times be the primary advocate for a child or for an entire family, but more often will join forces with the family and other health care professionals in obtaining optimum services.

An important aspect of advocacy was brought to light by Romero (1986). Her research with school-age children revealed that many of them experienced an overwhelming lack of control in the hospital situation. Several children drew pictures of themselves as "captives" in their hospital beds. The children indicated that they not only *needed* the nurse to act as an advocate in helping them gain a sense of control within the hospital environment, but also *expected* this behavior.

The Nurse as Teacher. The pediatric nurse must structure health teaching to incorporate the family's values and health beliefs. A nurse colleague tells of her experience as a nurse practitioner in an Alaskan village. She became increasingly frustrated because in the clinic mothers seemed to comprehend her instructions to use tepid water to reduce a child's fever but then repeatedly returned with febrile children and admitted they had not tried the water bath. After "time in residence" at the clinic, she learned that a family's water had to be hauled several miles across frozen tundra and that most families did not have enough "extra" water to use it for fever reduction. She recalls, with a smile, "I would have been better off to suggest they buy a can of soda pop at the local store and use it to sponge the child. Soda pop was much less costly to a family than water."

Health teaching must include both those aspects

of care the child can perform alone and more complex instructions for the adult caregiver. Encouraging the parent to allow appropriate self-care will increase the child's sense of self-esteem and will increase the probability that the child will comply with the prescribed therapy. Sometimes health teaching is best carried out through role modeling. The nurse's role modeling of appropriate child care can be especially effective when parents do not understand how to care for the child and do not have the advantage of advice from extended family.

An important component of all health teaching activities is a nonjudgmental attitude on the part of the nurse. Children and families who feel intimidated by the "knowledgeable" nurse may indicate understanding just to remove themselves from an uncomfortable teaching situation. One tactic that can set the tone for teaching encounters is, "Many children (families) tell me that this is difficult to understand. May I go over it with you?" Statements like this communicate that the client cannot be expected to know about that aspect of care and that therefore there is no disgrace in admitting the need for help.

Much health teaching will take place during nurse-client encounters for well child care. These visits afford excellent teaching opportunities because they are a time of less anxiety for the child and family and because this teaching generally concerns positive issues of the child's development. Aspects of well child care are also important topics for hospital discharge teaching. Teaching that focuses upon changes related to the child's growth and development requires a firm knowledge of developmental norms because implications for wellness promotion in the child vary with each developmental stage. The chapters in Unit II contain detailed information for anticipatory guidance of families with children at each developmental stage.

Diversity of Practice in Pediatric Nursing

Technologic advances in health care and the emphasis on wellness have dramatically increased the opportunities for varied positions within pediatric nursing. Pediatric nurses are found in clinics and doctors' offices; in schools, rehabilitation centers, summer camps, and day care centers; on cruise ships; in administrative positions related to quality assurance and control of infectious diseases; in the client's home; in acute care, intensive care, and emergency care facilities; on board flight-for-life helicopters and emergency transport craft; and virtually everywhere else there are children.

Positions vary in their requirements for educational preparation and experience. Expanded roles for nurses with master's degrees and doctorates in nursing include positions for nurse practitioners, clinical specialists, nurse administrators, nurse educators, and nurse researchers. Nursing research is a growing field with implications for nurses at all levels of practice. The current and potential influence of nursing research upon nursing care of children and adolescents is covered later in this chapter.

Legal Aspects of the Pediatric Nursing Role

Clarification of legal aspects requires that the nurse be aware that legal and ethical aspects are not synonymous. In fact, an action that is legal may not always be ethical and an act that is ethical may not always be legal. Herein lies the potential for professional conflicts.

The legality of nursing practice is determined in part by the practice acts of each state and in part by the courts that pass judgment upon cases involving nurses. Every nurse must be aware of the legal boundaries governing practice in the state in which she or he is licensed.

Legal aspects unique to the role of the pediatric nurse include state laws governing consent for treatment of a minor, laws pertaining to automobile restraints for children, and laws regarding child abuse. Each pediatric nurse is accountable for knowing the laws and institutional policies relating to individual practice. Chapter 27, Principles and Skills of Pediatric Nursing, deals with legal aspects of consent and abuse. Chaper 17 addresses laws pertaining to automobile safety.

Factors Influencing the Health Care of Children

A Historical Perspective on Societal Values

It has been suggested that in the future pediatrics will become synonymous with the science of growth and development (Nadler and Evans, 1987). In many respects, that may already be the case. Viewing pediatric practice (whether medical or nursing) as a science of growth and development emphasizes a change in focus from a time when medical practices for children consisted of adult remedies administered to smaller bodies. For example, in the early 1900s bloodletting, purging, and opiates were the mainstays of medical treatment regardless of the patient's age (Brodie, 1986). For the purpose of developing a perspective on pediatric nursing, it is pertinent to understand the historical factors that have led to changing attitudes about children in the health care community and in the whole of society.

The Relative Value of a Child: Society's Indifference to Its Young

Vaughan (1987) wrote, "The caring qualities of any society may best be measured by the concerns it manifests for its aged, its disadvantaged . . . and its young" (p 1). Historically, the young have often been among the most disadvantaged. Few historical accounts of the experience of childhood or of society's attitudes toward children exist before modern times. We can only speculate, therefore, about the reasons for what Brodie (1982) has referred to as "society's indifference to protecting and providing for its young" (p 219). Among these reasons are a shorter life span and ignorance of developmental processes.

Shorter Life Span as a Reason to Disvalue Children

The significantly shorter life span in earlier centuries (for people in general and children in particular) might have contributed to this attitude. In the 15th century it is estimated that almost 65 per cent of children died before age 5 years (Forsyth, cited in Brodie, 1986). The mortality rate had not improved by the 18th century, and it is said that even Queen Anne, who can be presumed to have had the best available care for her children, lost 18 babies in early infancy (Dolan et al, 1983). In 1900, the mortality rate in the United States remained at 23 per cent for children under 5 years of age. Today that rate has diminished to 1.3 per cent (UNICEF, 1986).

Ignorance of Developmental Processes

Another probable cause for the historical indifference to children is that *childhood,* as we know that concept today, was not born before the 16th century and not commonly recognized before the 18th century. Not until the 18th century did children come to be viewed as minors by the legal system and given sentences that differed from those handed down to adults (Brodie, 1986). Aries (cited in Levine et al, 1983) wrote:

> In medieval society the ideal of childhood did not exist; this is not to suggest that children were neglected, forsaken, or despised. The idea of childhood is not to be confused with affection for children: it corresponds to an awareness of the particular nature of childhood, that particular nature which distinguishes the child from the adult, even the young adult. In medieval society this awareness was lacking. That is why, as soon as the child could live without the constant solicitude of his mother, his nanny, or his cradle-rocker, he belonged to adult society . . .

Although it seems strange that people of any era could have failed to recognize childhood, the idea becomes more believable when one considers that the physiologic and cognitive processes of maturation had not yet been delineated. Without an understanding of the developmental differences between children and adults, there were few conclusions one could draw other than that children were miniature adults who behaved rather badly.

A Belief in the Inherent Evil of Children: Spare the Rod and Spoil the Child

Perhaps it was the difference in the social behavior of the young that led to what Brodie (1982) terms the belief in the inherent evil of children. It was the task of parents to ensure that good prevailed over this inherent evil through "swift, constant, and strong punishment" (Brodie, 1982, p 220). Brodie cited advice from an early English handbook on childrearing that admonished parents to "take a smart rod and beat them in a row till they cry mercy and their guilt well know."

Punishment as a Parental Duty. This attitude toward the evil in children bore two major implications that have an impact on our current thinking. One was that harsh punishment was a parent's *duty* as well as a parent's right. That attitude, which was as prevalent in colonial America as in Europe, is an important part of our heritage. Understanding the origin of that attitude and its prevalence throughout several hundred years lends perspective to the problems faced today in the fight against child abuse.

Albeit somewhat more subtle in the last century, the belief in the leaning of children toward evil has survived. It can be traced through such literary works as Charles Dickens' accounts of Oliver Twist's treatment in a London workhouse, Mark Twain's characterization of the attempts of religious and educational institutions to "reform" Huck Finn, and even in the strong moral fiber of Laura Ingalls Wilder's *Little House on the Prairie.* Particularly expressive of turn-of-the century attitudes toward the *guidance* of young people is a book written in 1905 by a female physician, *What Every Young Woman Ought to Know.* It underscored both a conviction of personal worth and a concern that, left to her own devices, a young woman would probably go astray:

> Life will be safer for the girl who understands her own nature and reverences her womanhood, who realizes her responsibility towards the human race and conducts herself in accordance with that realization. Life will be nobler and

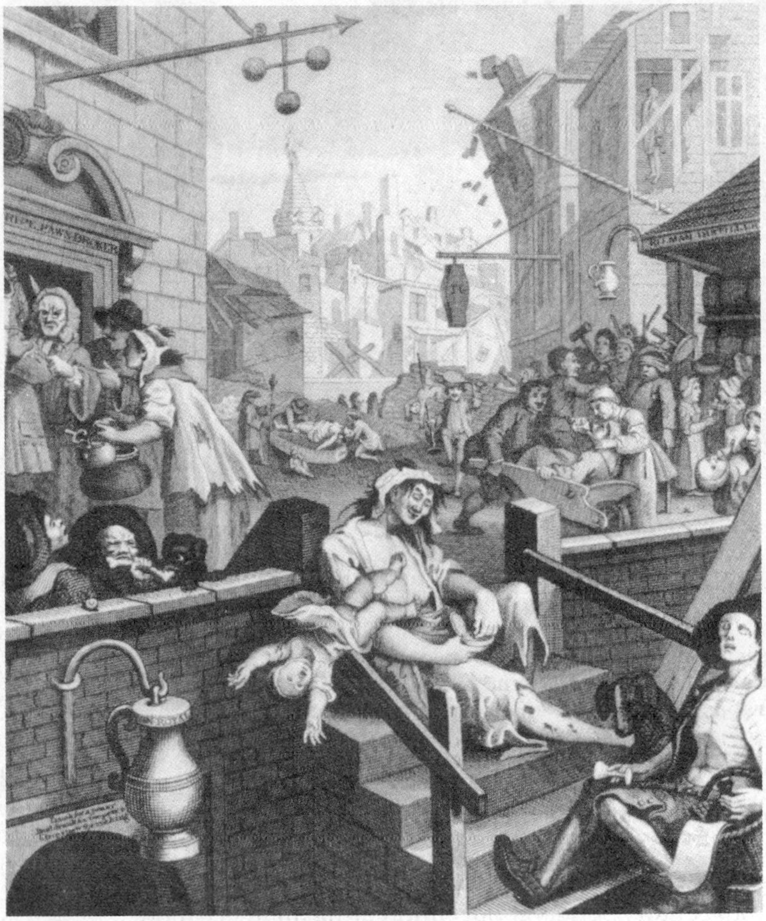

"Gin Lane," a famous picture by Hogarth, depicts the disvaluing of human life in the pleasure-craving society of the 1700s.

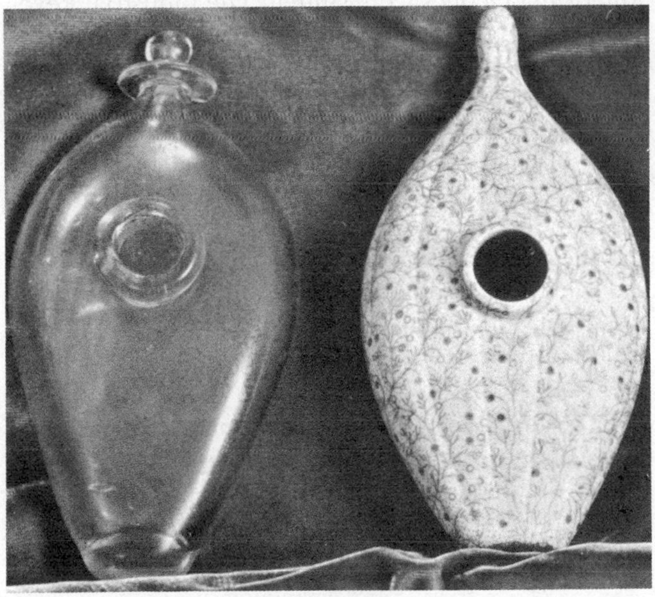

These glass and porcelain nursing bottles are examples of those used in the late 1700s and early 1800s. (From Dolan JA, et al: Nursing in Society: A Historical Perspective. 15th ed. Philadelphia, WB Saunders, 1983.)

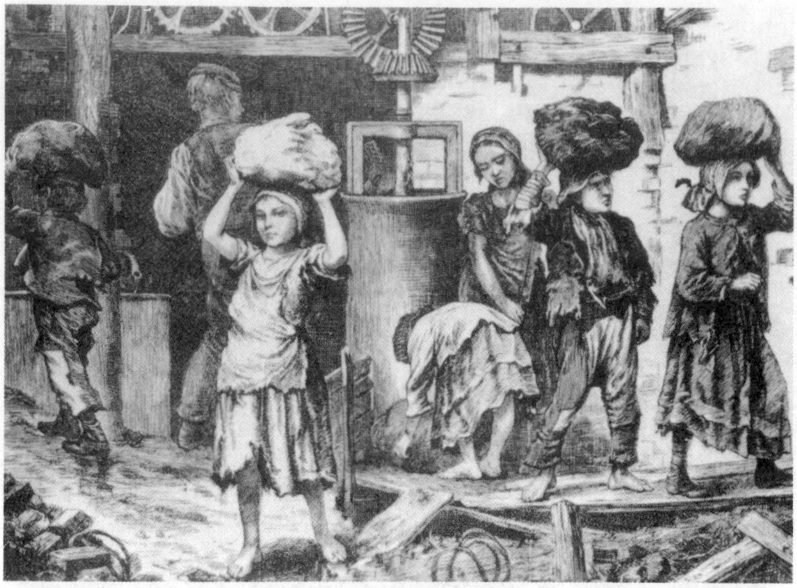

The "brick-yard children" of England included those as young as 5 years, who were forced to work 15- to 16-hour days. (From Dolan JA, et al: Nursing in Society: A Historical Perspective. 15th ed. Philadelphia, WB Saunders, 1983.)

purer in its possession and its transmission if, from childhood onward to old age, the thought has been held that "Life is a gift of God and is divine," and its physical is no less sacred than its mental or moral manifestation; if it has been understood that the foundations of character are laid in the habits formed in youth, and that a noble girlhood assures a grand maturity (Wood-Allen, 1905, pp 16–17).

Fear of Spoiling the Child. The fear of "spoiling" a child with too much affection and attention can be traced to earlier admonitions to parents to provide firm guidance for the "inherently wayward" child. Why do 16th century beliefs about childrearing influence modern practices? Modern parents, who must find that fine line between being too strict and too lenient, have "inherited" societal attitudes in the form of cultural values passed from one family generation to another. Another major influence on parenting behavior is advice given by the health care community. When not a catalyst for changing societal values, the health care community is a mirror of the current social structure. (Consider that health care professionals, when not directed by specific professional knowledge and values, can advise only from personal experience and beliefs.) With regard to attitudes toward spoiling infants, the infant bonding studies of Drs. Klaus and Kennell in the 1970s were a catalyst for change. Contrast the current emphasis upon physical closeness for appropriate parent-infant bonding with the following excerpt from instructions given to my mother in 1945:

> It is well not to pick up the youngster and hold it too much as it will soon develop into a spoiled youngster and will demand to be held at any time. If you would like to pick up the youngster and hold it, it is well to choose some certain time of the day and do it at the same time every day, inasmuch as the youngster will learn when it is to be held and will not likely demand to be picked up at any other time.

The Need to Subvert Idleness. Closely linked with "spare the rod and spoil the child" attitudes has been the belief that poverty and idleness (the latter often viewed as the effect of the former) led to "badness." This concern contributed to putting children to work prematurely. In the early 1600s, children were apprenticed to English craftsmen. Young English "vagrants" were sent in 1619 to the new American colonies to provide cheap labor (Brodie, 1982). Child labor practices were no more lenient in the 1800s. The "brick-yard children" of England were forced to work 15- to 16-hour days in exchange for a small wage and substandard food and lodging (Dolan et al, 1983). American practices were similar. The Industrial Revolution in the 19th century led to labor demands for machine operators, and children in the United States could be found working 12- to 14-hour days in factories and mills (Brodie, 1986). Although the first Child Labor Bill in the United States was signed by President Wilson in 1916, it was soon overturned by the Supreme Court in reaction to societal pressures. Not until 1941 did the Supreme Court finally uphold the legality of the Fair Labor Standards that ensured children protection from work practices that interfered with their education or their health.

The Influence of Developmental Theory on Attitudes Toward Children

Despite the beginning realization that children were distinct from adults and differed among themselves according to age, it was not until the acceptance of theories of development that the concept of *childhood* was fully realized. The delineation of physical/behavioral, psychosexual, cognitive, and psychosocial development painted an entirely new picture of childhood and irrevocably changed societal attitudes toward children and childrearing practices. The work of developmental theorists in the early 20th century remains unparalleled although it is now common to combine several of these works to form a more integrated approach to development.

The Contribution of 19th Century Authors. Although theories of child development were not conceived until the early 1900s, certain authors of the mid-19th century helped prepare the American public for a change in thinking about childrearing. Lydia Sigourney's classic, *Letters to Mothers,* published in 1838, suggested that less severe tactics might better serve the parent and the child. As cited in Levine et al (1983), she saw the primary problem of child nurture as one of "how the harp might be so tuned as not to injure its tender and intricate harmony." Catherine Beecher, a popular author of childrearing materials during the same era, echoed Sigourney's themes of valuing the child and accepting the "sacred" responsibility to guide its development to adulthood. In 1871, Jacob Abbott published *Gentle Measures in the Management and Training of the Young.* He emphasized the need to keep in mind physiologic and neurologic readiness in the moral guidance of children. This was a novel approach both in the attention to a process of development during childhood and in the assertion that "bad habits of action" were not due to inherent evil but to improper guidance of the child (Levine et al, 1983).

Gesell. With the dawn of the 20th century began an earnest interest in child development as we know it today. Arnold Gesell, in the early 1900s, was the first to use the words *child development* in describing the process of maturation. His study of age-related behaviors resulted in the first "developmental norms" for physical and behavioral maturation. He established the Clinic for Child Development at Yale University in 1911, which was the first organized effort toward the scientific study of child development. Contemporaries of Gesell included, among others, Sigmund Freud, Erik Erikson, Jean Piaget, and Charles Darwin, all of whom were instrumental in changing societal views about the purpose and experience of *childhood.*

Freud. Sigmund Freud, an Austrian physician and neuroscientist, developed a psychoanalytic theory of development. His theory postulates that psychic energy (libido) changes its focus within the body during development according to an invariant, maturational pattern. This resulted in his assertion that the psychosexual foci of development proceeded through the oral, anal, phallic, latent, and genital stages. It is interesting to note that this enduring theory was developed from the recollections of adult patients, *not* from the study of children (Lerner, 1976).

Piaget. Jean Piaget is known for his theory of cognitive development—the acquisition and utilization of knowledge. He emphasized developing cognition as an adaptation of the organism to its environment and introduced the processes of assimilation, accommodation, and equilibration. His age-related cognitive stages have since provided one of the major frameworks for childhood education and for measuring cognitive maturation in children.

Erikson. Where Freud's theory dealt with the effects of biologic factors upon the developing psyche, Erikson expanded and broadened this perspective to include the context of the child's environment, or society. Erikson's epigenetic principle presented a holistic view that has become a mainstay of our current understanding of development. As defined by Erikson (cited in Lerner, 1976), ". . . this principle states that anything that grows has a ground plan, and that out of this ground plan the parts arise, each having its time of special ascendancy, until all parts have arisen to form a functioning whole" (p 200).

Darwin. Charles Darwin's book *On the Origin of Species* (1859) and his subsequent book, *The Expression of the Emotions in Man and Animals* (1872), not only influenced societal attitudes about the evolution of the human being but also complemented and enhanced the work of developmental theorists in providing a scientific rationale for the study of development. As noted by Levine et al (1983), "His theory of the evolutionary thrust of development within life forms and across time, combined with new views of scientific study, contributed to clearer formulations of the nature and scope of human development" (p 10).

Health Care for Children in the 20th Century: The Effects of Increased Understanding and Advancing Technology

Advances in Nursing and Medical Care of Children. At the turn of the 20th century, the major health issues for children involved infection control and sanitation. Robert McCombs, a physician who wrote a book for nurses about the diseases of children, detailed the most frequent illnesses of infancy and childhood in the early 1900s:

> Diseases of the gastro-intestinal tract and bronchopneumonia are seen more often than any other diseases before the second year. The other common conditions met with during this period are affections of lymph glands, tubercular meningitis, pertussis, and measles.
>
> After the second year the following diseases are most frequently seen: Disorders of nutrition, such as rickets and scurvy; bone and joint diseases, these being usually tubercular and more rarely syphilitic; diseases of the blood; organic diseases of the heart; pneumonia, typhoid fever, the acute contagious diseases, such as measles, mumps, pertussis, varicella, scarlet fever, and diphtheria (1907, p 19).

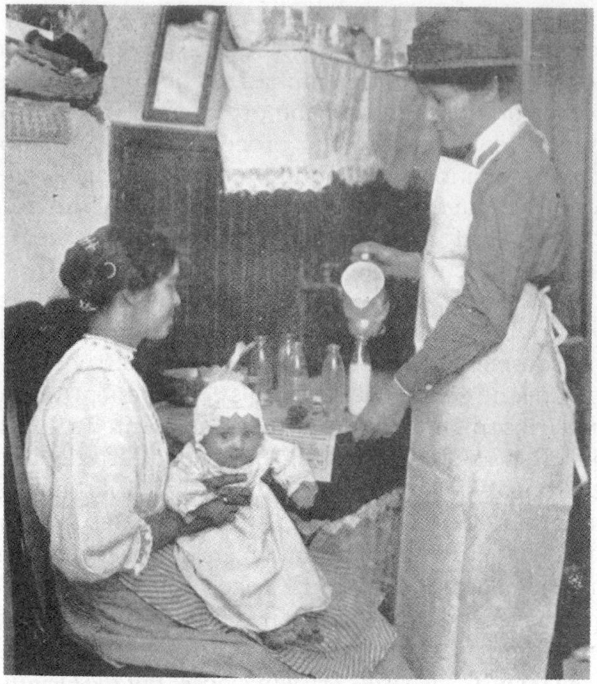

The baby welfare nurse. (From Brainard AM: The Evolution of Public Health Nursing. Philadelphia, WB Saunders, 1922.)

The contamination of the milk supply presented a major health hazard. Milk was not pasteurized and often came from cows that were diseased with tuberculosis and housed in filthy sheds. These animals were fed on distillery wastes, further reducing the quality of the milk produced. Pitchers of milk were purchased from open barrels and then stored in homes without refrigeration (Brodie, 1986). In 1889, a milk distribution center opened in New York for the purpose of providing uncontaminated milk to sick infants. While this effort was certainly a step in the right direction, it was ineffective because once the sick infant recovered contaminated milk was fed again (Dolan et al, 1983).

Nursing at this time was primarily oriented toward meeting the basic physical needs of sick children since immunization and antibiotics were not yet available and there was not yet a significant emphasis upon the preventative aspects of care. Much of the care of sick children took place in isolation units within hospitals. Family visitation was discouraged because of the concern for "containing" the infectious diseases.

Training for pediatric nurses in the late 1800s and early 1900s was just that—on-the-job training in hospitals for children rather than education about children and their health. Linda Richards, who has been called America's first trained nurse, was educated at such an institution, The New England Hospital for Women and Children. Influenced by Florence Nightingale, whom she met, she distinguished herself by advocating better training of nurses. Mary Eliza Mahoney, America's first black nurse to graduate from a school of nursing, was also a graduate of The New England Hospital for Women and Children (Dolan et al, 1983).

The work of Lillian Wald, who has been credited with founding community health nursing, was important to the health care of children. Henry Street Settlement, which she established in 1893, was the first American institution conceived and administered by a trained nurse (Silverstein, 1985). The house on Henry Street not only provided holistic nursing care and the support of social workers for the sick (and often immigrant) poor of New York City, but also established the importance of teaching health-promoting behaviors. The Henry Street Settlement still exists as a social settlement although the nursing component separated in 1944 to become the Visiting Nurse Service of New York (Silverstein, 1985). Wald encouraged the use of nurses in the schools of New York and initiated school lunch programs (Dolan et al, 1983). She was also largely responsible for establishment of the US Children's Bureau, which helped states create divisions of Maternal and Child Health.

Nursing care for children became more sophisticated as advances in medicine led to increasing knowledge about the physiology of childhood and increasing options for treatment. The establishment of the American Academy of Pediatrics in 1929 reflected the discoveries about the unique nature of health and illness in children. The 1940s and 1950s saw the introduction of penicillin and corticosteroids and immunization for diphtheria, tetanus, and pertussis. In addition, anticonvulsants and antihistamines were introduced. Classic research by Spitz and Robertson and others revealed the detrimental effects of maternal deprivation on institutionalized children. This led to the movement to allow increased family visitation and parental involvement in the care of hospitalized children. The play therapy (child life) programs, play rooms, and preparation visits for hospitalization, common today, were initiated as a result of this research.

Physicians increasingly began to devote time to well child care instead of just to the treatment of disease. Well child clinics provided another health maintenance/disease prevention role for nurses in the community. Testing for phenylketonuria (PKU) began in the 1950s, and in the next decade legislation made mandatory the reporting of child abuse. Immunology and clinical genetics developed as clinical specialties within medicine in the 1960s. Increasing knowledge of the physiology of the immune system and the role of genetics in predisposition to health and disease has influenced nursing assessment, analysis, planning, intervention, and evaluation of children.

In 1965 the University of Colorado introduced a nurse practitioner option within its master's program in nursing. The role of the nurse practitioner was developed in response to what was at that time a shortage of physicians, especially in rural areas. Nurse practitioners have advanced skills in physical assessment and health promotion. Today pediatric nurse practitioners work in clinics, in home care, in day care centers, and many other areas in the community where nurses must function with greater than usual autonomy.

Major technologic advances of the 1970s included fetal monitoring, echocardiography, and computed axial tomography. Technologic advances led to increased survival of those with several previously fatal diseases, resulting in an increase in the number of children treated for chronic illnesses. Increasing emphasis was placed upon the psychologic effects of illness and hospitalization during childhood. In a review of the literature on pediatric hospitalization since 1965, Thompson (1986) reported 306 research studies related to responses of children to hospitalization. Factors considered in relation to these responses were separation and rooming-in, parental anxiety, the unfamiliarity of the hospital setting (including specific activities of children during hospitalization, interactions with others, and sleep patterns when in the hospital), the effects of play during hospitalization, and the effects of preparation for hospitalization and for health care procedures.

Nursing care for children today recognizes the holistic nature of the child, and pediatric nurses are educated to base their practice upon physical, intellectual, and emotional-social responses to childhood illness and to consider all three of these competencies as pertinent to health promotion and health maintenance. It has become increasingly evident that the child must be viewed in the context of the family and that the "client" in pediatric nursing is often the family group. The modern nurse who cares for children must be sensitive to the changing family structure, to the increasing number of children who live in poverty, and to the changing health care milieu wherein children are generally hospitalized only for severe and involved conditions and obtain the remainder of their care in outpatient departments, in offices of physicians and nurse practitioners, and in the home.

Social Policies to Protect Children. It was not coincidental that at the time developmental theorists were defining the concept of childhood, President Theodore Roosevelt initiated the First White House Conference on Children and Youth in 1909. In 1912 the Children's Bureau was formed, an agency that served as a national repository and resource for childhood development data, which became the current Department of Health and Human Services. In 1916 a federal law was enacted to protect children from harsh labor practices. Within a year, however, this law was repealed and not re-enacted until 1940.

Under the Social Security Act of 1935, financial aid to poor families became available through Aid to Families with Dependent Children (AFDC). Despite criticism from those who would abolish welfare programs, Moynihan (1987) has called AFDC the single most important program affecting the lives of children apart from the public schools. As cited in the previous section on poverty, recent federal cuts in AFDC are directly linked to the growing ranks of children in the United States who live below the poverty level.

The decades of the 1960s and 1970s saw the reinstatement of day care under the Economic Opportunities Act and the establishment of the National Institute of Child Health and Human Development. Project Head Start began in 1965, and the Child Nutrition Act was enacted in 1966. These and other acts under Title XX of the Social Security Act (1975) reflected an era of increased social concern for children (Takanishi, 1978; Wallace, 1983).

The 1980s: The Effect of Shrinking Funds. In the 1980s, escalating health costs without resultant decreases in morbidity and mortality resulted in reduced concern for equal access to health care and increased pressure to ensure that the health care delivered was both necessary and cost effective. In 1983 the federal government instituted prospective payment for health care in the form of Diagnosis-Related Groups (DRGs). This federal mandate has had a tremendous impact upon health care delivery, resulting in earlier hospital discharge and a rapidly expanding home care market. Another economic indicator for the health care industry has been the establishment of health maintenance organizations (HMOs).

Concerns for modern health care for children were summarized in this 1981 report of the federal Select Panel for Promotion of Child Health:

- Although disease prevention and health promotion services are demonstrably effective, they are not widely available or adequately used.
- Although the overall health status of children has improved over the past 2 decades, all groups of children have not shared equally in this process.
- Although child health needs have changed considerably over the past 2 decades, the health care structure has not.
- Although the family should remain the primary source of health care and nurturing, the current system does not adequately recognize or support this system (cited in Noyes, 1985, p 136).

Today, despite our technologic advances, our clinical expertise, and our professional commitment, the health of America's children is in jeopardy. As reflected in this 1981 Select Panel Report and in the statistics cited in the previous section on childhood poverty, our role as professional advocates demands intervention at the political/social level as well as within our clinical practices.

> Many are willing to fight over children, but precious few are willing to fight for them. This fight is not always easy or popular, but even the smallest victories can touch the lives and brighten the futures of hundreds of thousands of children. As advocates, we must make it uncomfortable for the administration or Congress to destroy children's hopes (Noyes, 1985, p 139).

Research to Advance Nursing Practice

Critical to the advancement of nursing practice is nursing's ability to answer its own practice questions through research. That level of research expertise has only recently become a reality. As noted by Fawcett, "Significant progress has been made in the past several years in establishing nursing as a discipline with a corps of scholars leading its advancement. This scholarly influence is perhaps the most critical factor involved in the elimination of obstacles to nursing research . . ." (1984, p 6).

The education of a *corps of nursing scholars* has historical significance. Until the 1950s, nursing "borrowed" much of its scientific knowledge from medicine and the basic sciences. Although this provided a large, eclectic base for nursing practice, it required "modification" of research findings and theoretic explanations of phenomena to fit the unique practice of nursing. Nursing, at this time, was also limited in its ability to answer questions generated by practice. Clearly, professional advancement required that nursing define its unique subject matter (generate theories of nursing) and conduct its own research of these phenomena. The coming of age of nursing research, then, has required the education of nurses prepared in theory construction and in research methodology appropriate to nursing phenomena.

Nursing education began as training of nurses in hospitals by physicians for the purpose of providing cheap labor. It soon progressed in both the United States and Canada to in-hospital education by early nursing leaders, such as Isabel Hampton Robb and Mary Agnes Snively, and was patterned after the Nightengale system to focus upon education rather than upon hospital service. Isabel Hampton Robb was instrumental in establishing university education for nurses in the United States. Her efforts resulted in the establishment of a course in hospital economics for graduate nurses at Teacher's College, Columbia University, in 1907. Adelaide Nutting became the world's first professor of nursing at Columbia University (Dolan et al, 1983). Columbia Teacher's College has continued to be a significant force within the profession, educating many of the nursing leaders (Peplau, Henderson, Hall, Abdellah, King, Wiedenbach, and Rogers) whose theories have helped define the practice of nursing.

College education for nurses was furthered by the 1965 position paper of the American Nurses' Association, which called for preparation of nurses at the baccalaureate level. Another significant development at this time was the initiation of the federally funded "nurse scientist" program that provided support to nurses wishing to obtain doctoral degrees in the basic sciences. Although research in nursing was not new at this time (it had been advocated and conducted since the time of Florence Nightingale, and the journal *Nursing Research* had been circulating since the early 1950s), the nurse scientist program was notable for providing the first significant influx of doctorally prepared nurses who were interested in, committed to, and prepared to conduct research. Many of the nursing leaders responsible for the establishment, in the 1970s, of graduate programs in nursing were educated in the nurse scientist program. The emphasis within masters's degree programs is primarily advancement of the practice field through the preparation of clinical specialists and nurse practitioners. Nursing theory is studied rather than generated, and the research emphasis is often more upon analysis and utilization than upon conduct. The conducting of nursing research and developing of theory receive major emphasis within nursing doctoral programs, and graduates of these programs are expected to provide the leadership required to advance future "scientific inquiry."

As outlined by the American Nurses' Association Commission on Research in 1981, responsibility for research within nursing is not limited to nurses with graduate degrees. Graduates of Associate Degree Nursing Programs are expected to demonstrate an awareness of the value of nursing research and to assist in problem identification and data collection. Graduates of Baccalaureate Nursing Programs are expected to read, interpret, and evaluate research for its relevance to practice, identify researchable problems in clinical practice, gather research data, apply established research findings to practice, and share research findings with colleagues (ANA, 1981).

Nursing has prepared its corps of scholars, but this alone will not ensure professional advancement. That advancement will be realized as nurses at *all levels of professional preparation work cooperatively* to reach for excellence, to think at the level of "what if," to incorporate into practice the systematic, scientific questioning and answering that is research.

Cooperative research efforts within work settings require the guidance of nurse researchers who are prepared at the graduate (both master's and doctoral) level. These researchers serve as consultants to staff nurses to teach the research process, assist with analysis of published research, promote research utilization, assist with conduct of research studies, and model the value of nursing research through conduct and application of their own studies. The vignette in Box 1-3 is an account by a master's-prepared nurse of her role as a nurse researcher at a children's hospital.

Cooperative research efforts also require the final bridging of the gap between nursing education and nursing practice. One such attempt is NURSELINK,* a computer network that links the Center for Nursing Research at the University of Colorado Health Sciences Center with area clinical agencies. It is designed to (1) provide access to and consultation with individuals who have expertise in specific clinical areas, research methodologies, statistics, or research instruments for the purpose of facilitating clinical research and problem-solving, (2) provide a means of communication between the clinical agencies and the Center for Nursing Research, and (3) develop a readily accessible research data base. NURSELINK is the one of the first projects in the United States to link nursing practice, education, and research through computers.

Cooperative research involves sharing results (both successes and failures) through formal and informal "networking" processes such as research conferences and journal articles. Researchers have a responsibility to communicate clearly to their audience — if the researcher is unable to articulate implications for clinical nursing, it is unlikely that the staff nurse will be able to use these results in practice.

The body of nursing research has grown rapidly in recent years as nurses have begun to realize the value of generating and answering their own practice questions and as they have had increasing access to graduate-prepared nursing research consultants. Nursing re-

Box 1-3

Making Research Work at the Level of Practice: Notes from a Nurse Researcher

In my role as nurse researcher at The Children's Hospital of Denver it is exciting for me to see nurses questioning the time-honored way of carrying out a particular task or performing a procedure. Staff nurses are questioning "the way it's always been done" and they use me as a sounding board for their ideas. My relationships with staff nurses are collegial because they recognize my knowledge and skills as a clinical nurse as well as a research nurse.

In conjunction with other nurse researchers on staff, I teach a workshop on the research process to encourage staff nurses to answer their own research questions. Nurses interested in research can then receive one-on-one consultation through all phases of the re search process — from formulation of a researchable question, through selection or development of research tools (e.g., questionnaires), data collection, data analysis, and interpretation of results. We also encourage the nurses to share research results through hospital-sponsored communication sessions and at research conferences, through a research newsletter which I edit, and through publication of articles in nursing journals.

Nursing research can have a positive effect on the public's perception of the nursing role. In my own research activities I have found that children and their families are very interested in nursing research. They are quite supportive of the nurse at the bedside looking at, "researching," a new and better way to care for children. I have found that parents are very eager to have the research findings shared with them. I keep track of these families and send them research results at the completion of the study.

Nurses in our hospital are involved in a wide variety of research. We have categorized the studies according to their focus: (1) those that study children (Human Care studies), (2) those that involve families as well as children (Family Care studies), and (3) those that study nurses (Health Care Delivery System studies). Examples of research recently completed or currently in progress include:

- a study of the effectiveness of transcutaneous electrical nerve stimulation (TENS) in reducing the pain of radial artery puncture in neonates
- a comparison of regular Pedialyte and "Pedipops" for oral rehydration. ("Pedipops" was coined by the nurses who developed a Pedialyte and Koolaid solution of controlled molecular weight which is then frozen on a stick.)
- a study of the effect of increased parental involvement on the metabolic control of a child with diabetes
- an exploration of the impact of emergency transport on the child's family
- a study of nurses' attitudes about breast feeding versus bottle feeding
- development of a technique for restructuring group meetings for effectiveness

If nursing is to grow and develop with a scientific knowledge base to guide practice, we must continually evaluate what we do and how we do it. We need to be accountable for our actions, and we need to validate when those actions make a difference in the lives of our clients. Those of us in expanded roles must foster and maintain a spirit of inquiry within the profession. Providing high-quality care and support to families should be the constant challenge for all nurses. Questioning and evaluating how we practice will help us meet that challenge.

–Anne Marie Kotzer, RN, MS

* A project funded by US West Information Systems, Marilyn Stember, RN, PhD, Principal Investigator.

search is, however, still in its infancy. Application of research findings requires first that something of a "critical mass" of research accumulate to help ensure the success of implemented findings. In other words, research is much like a jigsaw puzzle; it is hard to predict the total picture from one piece. This is especially true of nursing research because of the complexity of many of the phenomena pertinent to nursing, such as pain, parent-infant attachment behaviors, health concepts of children, clinical decision making of nurses, and so on. When several pieces of research begin to fit together, one can have increased confidence in results that are congruous with those of other nurse researchers working with that same subject matter. That nursing is now achieving that critical mass of research, in at least some subject areas, is evidenced by the advent of nursing research conferences that are designed to share research ready for immediate clinical application. The ability to critique and utilize such results will become increasingly important for every professional nurse in the next decade.

A Perspective on Intercultural Communication

To promote the healthy maturation of children and adolescents, the nurse must (1) anticipate possible and probable needs of the client, (2) assess actual needs, (3) respond to communicated needs, and (4) evaluate the effectiveness of the interventions. Each of these steps involves *communication.* Communication, in turn, is inextricably linked with culture. It is important, therefore, to understand (1) how culture affects communication, and (2) techniques to enhance communication between persons of different cultures. As defined here, *culture* includes socioeconomic, ethnic, and religious factors and other characteristics that qualify an individual for membership in various identity groups. This section will define culture, delineate various cultural identity groups, detail the links between culture and communication, and discuss specific ways to enhance intercultural communication.

Understanding Culture as the Context for Communication

Formally defined, culture is "the deposit of knowledge, experiences, beliefs, values, attitudes, meanings, hierarchies, religion, timing, roles, spatial relations, concepts of the universe, and material objects and possessions acquired by a large group of people in the course of generations through individual and group striving" (Porter and Samovar, 1985, p 19). Stated more simply, culture provides the pattern for living; it has to do with the ways in which a given people organize their perceptions and their behaviors in order to make sense of the world. It gives meaning to life. *Culture is the context for communication.*

The Culture of the United States. One geographic area frequently contains more than one major cultural group. The United States is no exception. It is a young nation, settled just over 200 years ago primarily by European immigrants who failed to merge peacefully with the native Indians. Northern and southern perimeter states bear the influences of French-Canadian and Spanish explorers and of current relations with neighboring Canada, Mexico, and Cuba. Although Anglo-Americans still predominate within the United States, the early European immigrants have been joined by many others from Africa, Central America, Mexico, Asia, and other countries around the world. Despite the concept of the American "melting pot," "the many diverse groups that make up the country have proven to be surprisingly persistent in maintaining their separate identities" (Hall, 1969, p 10). The persistence of strong ethnic boundaries within the United States is a clear indication of people's need for "roots," of the sense of pride and security that is gained from ethnic heritage. It is a message, as well, of the need to have that ethnicity acknowledged.

Identity Groups Within the Larger Culture. Superimposed upon an already diverse society are innumerable identity groups that further define alliances of individuals. These groups are sometimes referred to as cultures themselves (e.g., middle-class culture or the culture of poverty), or as subgroups or subcultures, but the umbrella term *identity group* may be technically more correct. As used here, an identity group refers to "a number of people who perceive some aspects of the external world more or less similarly, and recognize (communicate) that they share that similarity of perception" (Singer, 1985, p 63). In some cases identity groups overlap with roles.

An example of identity groups for a young woman might be Spanish-Americans, Catholics, persons of the middle class, wives, mothers, kindergarten teachers, executive board members of the American Association of University Women (AAUW), and members of the teachers' union. A child's identity groups might include Caucasians of German heritage, Lutherans, 5th graders at Largent Elementary School, members of the Little League Softball, students of the same piano teacher, members of the 5th grade Sunday School class, and members of the Tuesday night Dungeons and Dragons Club. Our identification with such groups communicates something about who we believe ourselves to be.

Childhood as an Identity Group. Goodman (1976), among others, has proposed that childhood is a culture (for our purposes, an identity group) in itself.* It is pertinent for pediatric nurses to consider the characteristics and implicatons of such a group.

Perhaps more than any other subgroup within our culture, childhood contains an identity unto itself. By virtue of their stature, behavior, and youthful appearance, children and adolescents are easily identified as children or "nonadults." Their language differs from that of the adult population, first in the attempts at "baby talk," then in the school-age struggle with mastery of grammar, and later in the adolescent "stylization" of language that renders it unintelligible to many adults.

Behavior also identifies the members of the childhood group. Whether it be the clumsy curiosity of the toddler, the exuberance of mid-childhood, or the yo-yo-like behavior of the adolescent who is balancing tenuously between childhood and adulthood, the actions are different from those of an adult.

Perceptions vary between children and adults as well. Who among us fails to remember the "monsters" in our childhood closets, the "bigness" of our fathers, the unlimited "power" of the doctor and nurse to do anything they pleased to us, the "length" of one childhood hour, or the sheer delight that was a chocolate milkshake? Socially, the child is characterized by immature blunders and occasionally by endearing attempts to make amends for them. Even the adolescent struggles with social graces and with the transitions in behavior that must continually be made between the social world of peers and the social world of parents. These are but a few of the many disparities between the perceptions of children and adults. It is important to recognize the identity group of childhood because the differences in perceptions can lead to distortion in nurse-child communications. The resulting challenge is one that pediatric nurses can ill afford to ignore.

Culture as Both a Conscious and Subconscious Phenomenon

Culture is pervasive, complex, and abstract. It operates at both conscious and subconscious levels. While we can communicate quite easily about "*how* things are done where we live," it may be more difficult to explain *why* we do these things or why we hold certain values and beliefs. Culture that is so basic to our way of organizing the world as to be largely subconscious is what Hall (1984) refers to as *primary level culture.* It is "that variety of culture in which the rules are known to all, obeyed by all, but seldom if ever stated. Its rules are implicit, taken for granted, almost impossible for the average person to state as a system, and generally out of awareness" (p 230). *World view* is an example of belief operating at the primary level of culture. One's world view dictates such things as the purpose and meaning of life and the nature of truth.

To realize that world views differ significantly among cultures is to be aware that the meaning of concepts like health, illness, and parenting will vary among persons of different geographic and ethnic backgrounds. Recognizing these differences in "views of the world" is one thing; accepting them as valid in relation to one's own beliefs may be more difficult. Grosso and colleagues (1981) recounted a situation in which a young Vietnamese-American mother refused to be hospitalized for repair of a rectovaginal fistula following childbirth unless her mother and her newborn infant stayed with her during the hospitalization. The nurses were puzzled by the woman's reluctance to leave her infant during the short period of hospitalization required and also questioned why this new mother had not mentioned symptoms of the fistula while she was hospitalized for delivery. Upon further inquiry they learned that Vietnamese people believe a mother and newborn baby should be together constantly (hence the reluctance to leave the infant) and that the new mother should have help with infant care (therefore the request to have the infant's grandmother present). They also learned that Vietnamese people are uncomfortable discussing private health matters and believe that care of the sick belongs to the family. This helped explain why the Vietnamese woman had not told anyone about symptoms that would have led to earlier diagnosis of the fistula.

It must be emphasized that the nurses considered not only widely held Vietnamese beliefs but also the meaning of those beliefs to *this family.* Upon exploring the reason for the woman's request, the nurses and surgeon chose to modify hospital policy to accommodate her cultural values. Their ability to recognize and accept cultural values different from their own allowed the woman to obtain prompt treatment. Unfortunately, professionals are not always this successful at overcoming the feeling that everyone else should believe as they do, a way of thinking termed *ethnocentrism.*

Ethnocentrism: A Caveat* for the Nurse. Ethnocentrism is the mindset that causes us to judge the beliefs and behavior of others according to our own cultural rules. Ethnocentrism is not a manifestation solely of Anglo-Americans. It pervades every cultural

* The rationale for interchanging the words "culture" and "identity group" is Singer's (1985) explanation that "a pattern of perceptions and behavior which is accepted and expected by an identity group is called a culture. Since by definition each identity group has its own pattern of behavioral norms, each group may be said to have its own culture" (p 63).

* Caveat is a Latin word meaning to beware or to heed.

group. Ethnocentrism can be dangerous if we are unaware of its effect upon perceptions.

Ethnocentrism leads to cultural *stereotyping* when the majority group within a culture sets itself up as the standard by which everyone else is judged. Stereotyping emphasizes differences between the majority group and other identity groups. Values of good and bad, right and wrong are assigned according to the similarity of the subgroup's beliefs and values to those of the majority group. Ethnocentrism and stereotyping have had disastrous effects upon intercultural relations throughout the world. In the individual sense, presuming needs and preferences based upon a few manifest or easily discerned characteristics of a person negates nursing's claim to recognize and value the holistic and individualistic qualities of personhood. Lee (1976) asserted that "to view in terms of category . . . is a meager and a lazy substitute for knowing." Although it is tempting to look for easy solutions and simple guidelines in interacting with persons of different cultures, stereotyping leads to false premises. There are charts and handbooks, for example, that detail such information as "characteristic food choices" of blacks and other ethnic groups. However, knowing whether a black person is an impoverished rural resident of Alabama, a recent immigrant from Ethiopia, an upper class urban gourmet, or a college student experimenting with vegetarianism is far more relevant to his or her food preferences than is skin color. A truly therapeutic relationship is based upon knowledge of the person as an individual with unique values and needs.

Communication: A Product of Culture

"When someone observes our behavior or its residue and gives meaning to it, communication has taken place regardless of whether our behavior was conscious or unconscious, intentional or unintentional" (Porter and Samovar, 1985, p 28). That is to say, whenever behavior (e.g., spoken words or nonverbal gestures) or the product of behavior (e.g., a written note) is encountered by someone else the behavior communicates something. Further, communication is formed and patterned indelibly by culture. This paragraph communicates to the reader through my cultural language; English words are chosen for their ability to symbolize my thoughts. Even those thoughts are conceived largely according to culture. Culture dictates that certain stimuli will be attended and certain others will be ignored. To communicate effectively with persons of different cultures, one must understand the interdependence between culture and communication.

Communication, as defined by Porter and Samovar (1985), involves eight separate components: a source, an encoding process, a message, a channel for the message, a receiver, a decoding process, receiver response, and feedback. Although this is a necessarily simplified view of a dynamic and complex process, it effectively demonstrates the essential elements of communication (Fig. 1-3).

Source. The source of communication is a person with whom the communication originates. Usually, this person has a desire to share perceptions and feelings with another human being, although, as has been pointed out, communication can occur even unintentionally.

Encoding. Encoding is a process of choosing verbal and/or nonverbal symbols to represent the thoughts one wishes to communicate. The symbols are selected and arranged to form a *message* that is intended to communicate the thoughts and feelings of the source person.

Channel. The message passes between the source and the receiver by means of a channel. The channel is usually something that can be interpreted by the senses, such as the spoken voice, an object or image that can be seen, a tactile stimulus, or a particular smell. The words on this page are a visual channel for this "message" about communication. In addition to sensory channels, an intuitive channel exists. Intuition is a way of knowing that does not require sensory data. It has been described as an overall impression, a "shortcut in the reasoning process" (Rew, 1987, p 44). Others have explained it as "something experienced, not thought out, something felt rather than actively pursued or constructed" (Belenky et al, 1986, p 69). As Western views change to include more emphasis upon Eastern philosophies, intuition is becoming acknowledged as another legitimate way of knowing.

Receiver. The receiver is the human being who apprehends the message. The receiver may or may not be the person for whom the message was intended.

Decoding. Decoding is "converting external energies into a meaningful experience" (Porter and Samovar, 1985, p 18). That is, the receiver incorporates the message via the channel used and processes the information to determine the need for a response and the type of response necessary.

Receiver Response. The receiver decides what to do about the message on a continuum from ignoring the message to taking immediate action. For example, a mother in the supermarket might choose to "tune out" a message from her preschooler who wants another bag of cookies, but she would respond quickly to the child's cries of terror if he started a cookie avalanche by pulling out the bottom package on the shelf.

Feedback. Feedback is information that tells the speaker (source) whether the message sent was the message received. It is related to receiver response in that the receiver's response is a common way for the

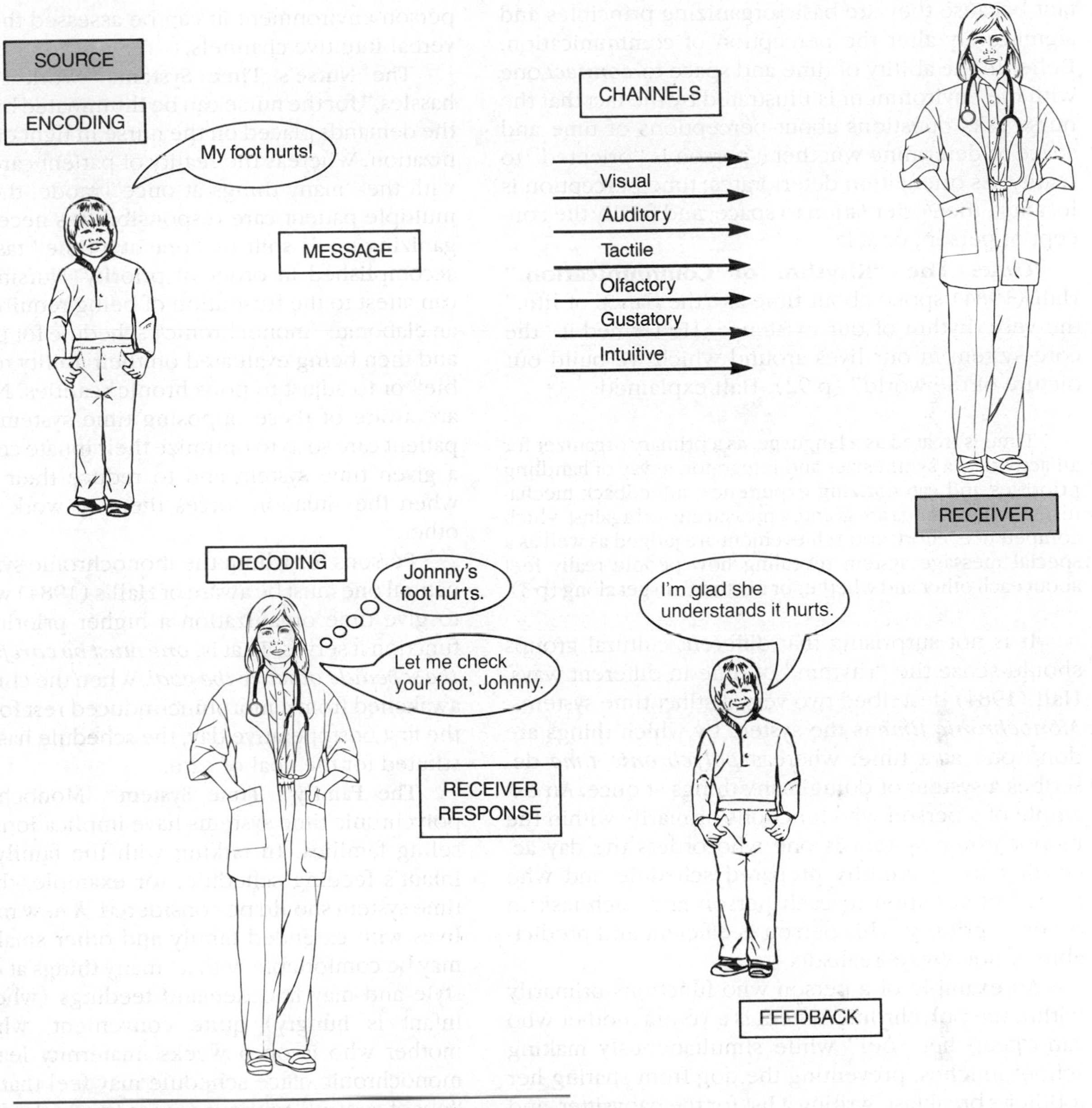

***Figure* 1-3.** Components of the communication process.

speaker to ascertain whether he or she has been understood.

Culture Determines Appropriateness of the Message. Culture is linked with each of the communication components presented. The ideas and feelings of the source person are influenced by culture because "people learn to think, feel, believe, and strive for what their culture considers proper" (Porter and Samovar, 1985, p 19). The message is encoded according to culturally determined symbols in the form of words and gestures and is sent along channels considered culturally appropriate. The message may be a hug, a symbol that encodes affection and is delivered through the tactile channel. A hug may be more appropriate among members of some identity groups than among others. One woman tells of growing up in a family (and community) where one rarely saw a public expression of affection. Visiting in another state as a young teenager, she observed her married aunt greet a brother-in-law with an affectionate hug. She recalls, "My mouth dropped open and I thought, wait till my mother hears about THIS!"

Two other important aspects of the cultural link with communication are the concepts of time and space. Perceptions of time and space vary among persons of different cultures and define the environment within which communication takes place.

Communication: The Influence of Time and Space. All communication takes place within the contexts of time and space. These concepts are important because they are basic organizing principles and significantly alter the perception of communication. Belief in the ability of time and space to *connect* one with the environment is illustrated by the fact that the nurse asks questions about perceptions of time and space to determine whether a person is "oriented" to reality. As orientation deteriorates, time perception is lost first, then orientation to space, and finally the concept of person, or self.

Time: The "Rhythm of Communication." Hall (1984) spoke about time as "the dance of life," the very rhythm of our existence. He termed it "the core system in our lives around which we build our picture of the world" (p 92). Hall explained:

> Time is treated as a language, as a primary organizer for all activities, a synthesizer and integrator, a way of handling priorities and categorizing experience, a feedback mechanism for how things are going, a measuring rod against which competence, effort, and achievement are judged as well as a special message system revealing how people really feel about each other and whether or not they can get along (p 3).

It is not surprising that different cultural groups should sense the "rhythm" of time in different ways. Hall (1984) described two very distinct time systems. *Monochronic time* is the system by which things are done one at a time, whereas *polychronic time* describes a system of doing many things at once. An example of a person who functions primarily within the monochronic system is one who orders the day according to a carefully prepared schedule and who gives full attention to each person and each task in order of priority. This person is efficient and predictable, if not always realistic.

An example of a person who functions primarily within the polychronic system is a young mother who can "keep her cool" while simultaneously making school lunches, preventing the dog from sharing her toddler's breakfast, writing a list for the babysitter, and taking a business call. A polychronic time system allows for the realities of multiple, simultaneous demands but is less predictable with regard to appointments and deadlines.

It is important to understand that each system has its pros and cons but neither is right or wrong; time systems are essentially value-free. Each person has a preference for one system or another, a preference that is influenced by cultural heritage. Situations that force one into the opposite system can be quite stressful. Time systems certainly vary within cultural groups, however, and sometimes vary even among family members. *Time systems are important to communication insofar as they enhance or disrupt the person-environment relationship.* (Remember that communication is more than verbal messages; person-environment fit can be assessed through nonverbal intuitive channels.)

The Nurse's Time System. Work stress, "job hassles," for the nurse can be illuminated by looking at the demands placed on the nurse in light of time organization. Whereas the reality of patient care fits better with the "many things at once" mode, the reality of multiple patient care responsibilities necessitates organizing one's shift by "one at a time" tasks that are accomplished in order of priority. Nursing students can attest to the frustration of being required to make an elaborate "monochronic" schedule for patient care and then being evaluated on their ability to "be flexible" or to adjust to polychronic realities. Nurses who are aware of these opposing time systems can plan patient care so as to optimize their innate comfort with a given time system and to reduce their frustration when the situation forces them to work within the other.

Persons for whom the monochronic system is the natural one must be aware of Hall's (1984) warning not to give time organization a higher priority than the function it serves. That is, *one must be careful not to let the schedule obscure the goal.* When the child must be awakened from a morphine-induced rest for a bath on the first postoperative day, the schedule has been substituted for the goal of care.

The Family's Time System. Monochronic and polychronic time systems have implications for counseling families. In talking with the family about an infant's feeding schedule, for example, the family's time system should be considered. A new mother who lives with extended family and other small children may be comfortable with a "many things at once" lifestyle and may find demand feedings (whenever the infant is hungry) quite convenient, whereas the mother who is on 6 weeks' maternity leave from a monochronic office schedule may feel that her life is "out of control" without a more fixed schedule for her infant's meals.

Time as a Context for Language. Time places words in context. When said at home, "It's time for lunch" can mean "Bring your playmates in for sandwiches and milk." Those same words in the hospital can mean "Here's a tray of salty beef broth, rubbery gelatin, and lukewarm tea. Please finish it so I can take this needle out of your arm." Similarly, the word "cut" may be nonthreatening to the preschooler playing with a scissors but can take on an entirely new dimension when heard during preparation for surgery. The nurse who is aware of the time context of communications will be more sensitive to the meaning of words for a child.

Time as a Reflection of Status. Hall (1984) made the point that *time spent waiting is a reflection of our* *status.* He noted, "The message comes through that hospital staff is in charge; they are important, the patient isn't (he's lucky to be there)" (p 75). Considering that children are afforded little status in modern society in the first place, the plight of the hospitalized child is potentially grave indeed. Added to this are the facts that (1) a child perceives time to be longer in duration than does an adult, (2) "time 'drags' when the body clock and the clock on the wall are out of sync" (Hall, 1984, p 131), and (3) fear and anxiety can significantly lengthen perceived time. To enhance the child's sense of mastery and self-esteem, the nurse must attempt to reduce unnecessary frustration and anxiety associated with periods of waiting.

Time spent in bed almost always seems interminable to a hospitalized child. Although the presence of a parent or family member is one of the best ways to counteract anxiety and boredom, other strategies should be considered as well. A common source of frustration is the difference between the client's perception of lapsed time and that of the nurse. For example, the nurse may feel she or he has moved heaven and earth to return in 10 minutes with a requested pain medication, only to be met by an icy stare or verbal query of "Why did it take so long?" Using a common "time keeper" can be helpful. If the nurse establishes that she or he will return in 10 minutes, or "when the big hand gets to here," and then returns on time, frustration can be diminished for all involved. It is necessary, however, that the child have access to an actual clock; "10 minutes" does not have a universal meaning in the culture of childhood.

Another strategy for reducing periods of waiting is to involve the child in an activity that requires focused concentration. Concentration of any sort tends to make time pass quickly. It is unrealistic to expect that a child can be this fully entertained for more than short periods of time; therefore special activities can be saved for waiting periods that promise to be the most problematic, e.g., the time until a parent can return or the time period immediately preceding an anticipated and unpleasant procedure. For this reason, thoughtful coordination with a recreational therapist may significantly alter the child's perception of the hospital experience.

Space: An Influence upon Communication. The effect of spatial context upon communication becomes apparent when one considers the changes in communication styles and in messages sent in the following scenarios. (The scenes should be considered individually, not as progressive actions.)

- A 10-year-old girl and a nurse happen to enter a hospital elevator together. The nurse acknowledges the child with a smile, the child returns a shy smile, and both persons assume the "elevator posture"—gazing at the illuminated numbers.
- A nurse and a child find themselves at the same table in the hospital cafeteria. The nurse initiates a social conversation with the child.
- The child is lying in a hospital bed, the nurse is standing at the bedside with a medicine cup containing an orange liquid. The nurse explains that the contents must be swallowed. The child stiffens and turns her head away.

Although all three scenarios take place within a hospital, the spatial context dictates a social situation in the first two instances but not in the third. Cultural practices make polite conversation unnecessary in the first case, but quite mandatory in the second. In both the social situations the two people have assumed similar postures; this fact equalizes their status somewhat even though the adult is presumably in charge. In the third instance, the context is nonsocial. The child is subjugated not only by the status of youth but by physical posture (below the nurse), and by the nurse's implied authority. Space, in each instance, defined the context for communication.

Not only is every action made within the context of space, but space changes the expectations for action. Space denotes status (e.g., size of room), determines appropriate means for communication (e.g., whether a message can be whispered or must be shouted), and invites ownership (e.g., "my room," "my bed"). Sensitivity to the spatial needs of a child and family will enhance nurse-client communications to the extent that it reduces client frustration.

The Interaction of Time and Space. Perception of space is linked to both time perception and other cultural patterning. Persons who operate principally within a polychronic time system often need less "private" space and may be less affected by crowding (as in a hospital room). Persons of monochronic tendencies, however, often protect their private space vigorously and may be quite uncomfortable with crowding and forced intimacy.

Realistically, a child's and family's space preferences are rarely considered beyond asking whether they prefer a private, semiprivate, or ward-type room. Recognizing the influence of spatial elements on behavior can be helpful, however, in planning daily care. A child who is used to sleeping in a room apart from other family members may have trouble adjusting to the noise of a roommate. This is the child for whom special rest times can be planned, with drawn curtains and a "Johnny is sleeping now" sign on the door. On the other hand, a child who usually sleeps in a room with one or more siblings may be unable to rest in the hospital because of the perceived "emptiness" of the room. This child may rest better in a room near the nurse's station, with the door open to the sound of voices, telephones, and rolling carts, and with a radio or television playing.

Space limitations in hospital rooms seem to be a universal problem. Whereas most children and families adjust to side-stepping around equipment and furniture during short hospital stays, longer periods of hospitalization may be an occasion for modifications within the hospital room. Making adjustments in the child's designated hospital "space" can communicate the priority of the child's and family's needs over the needs of the staff for spatial "uniformity."

This discussion of communication and culture has demonstrated that cultural patterning affects each aspect of the communication process and determines the context for communication. In the words of Porter and Samovar (1985):

> . . . communication is an intricate matrix of interacting social acts that occur in a complex social environment. This social environment reflects the way people live, how they come to interact with and get along in their world. This social environment is culture, and if we truly are to understand communication, we also must understand culture (p 19).

The remainder of this section deals with techniques to enhance communication among persons of different cultures and identity groups.

Social Communication: Searching for Similarities, Delighting in Differences

Getting to know someone in a social setting is often a process of searching for similarities and delighting in differences. It is perhaps unfortunate for nursing that in an attempt to be "professional" we have made such a sharp demarcation between social and professional communication. Social skills, after all, are the result of a long cultural evolution toward the most effective interpersonal techniques. Social skills can be adapted quite effectively to meet professional goals.

In a social setting, it is common for new acquaintances to search for similarities in everyday living (e.g., occupation, marital and parenting status) that can form the basis for conversation. As a conversation develops, the parties often find themselves interested in the differences among their perceptions and experiences and encourage further explanation. They may leave the encounter enriched by new ideas and enthusiastic about implementing new remedies for old problems. Persons who fail to find interest in anyone's view but their own are termed boors and are unwelcome guests.

The following section proposes a model for professional communication that draws upon this familiar social model. It delineates the elements of (1) preparing for the initial encounter with the child and family, (2) searching for similarities in identity groups, (3) appreciating differences in nurse-client experiences and perceptions, and (4) validating perceptions.

A Social Model for Intercultural Communication

Intercultural communication occurs whenever a message encoded by someone in culture A is received and decoded by someone in culture B. It involves the *probability for distortion* of the message. The term "culture," as used here, can be taken quite liberally. Porter and Samovar (1985) explained that "intercultural communication takes place in a wide variety of situations that range from interactions between people in whom cultural differences are extreme to interactions between people who are members of the same dominant culture and whose differences are reflected by membership in different subcultures or subgroups" [i.e., identity groups] (p 22). Given the diversity between the identity group of "adult" and the identity group of "childhood," it is safe to say that *the majority of interactions in pediatric nursing involve intercultural communication,* whether or not there are differences in ethnicity or nationality.

Preparing for the Initial Encounter with a Child and Family. Preparation for the initial encounter with a child and family is an activity that is often overlooked. It takes only a few moments of the nurse's time but can dramatically affect the tone of the encounter.

The purpose of preparing to meet the child and family is to clear the mind of distractions and prejudicial thoughts that could limit the nurse's ability to begin to know this child and this family for the unique individuals that they are. This preparation is necessitated because of distractions by other job-related details, and because of the human tendency to categorize this child with others of that race, age, disease process, and so on.

Values clarification is a critical part of the preparation process that begins long before the nurse considers a particular encounter. In actuality, values clarification starts with the decision to become a nurse and involves the meaning of nursing for each individual personally. It continues with values clarification exercises and discussions during nursing education and is ongoing throughout the nursing career. Values clarification means raising one's consciousness about one's own values in order to predict one's behavior in a given situation. Personal values must be identified as they relate to the meaning of life; to illness, pain, and death in children; and to various cultural characteristics. (See

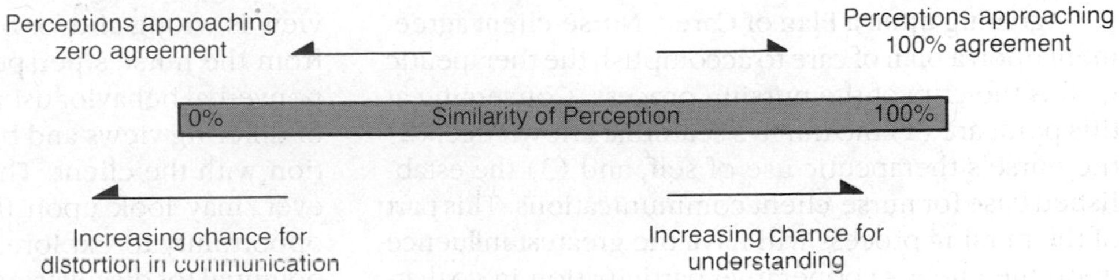

Figure 1-4. Continuum for similarity of perception.

the discussion on values clarification in the following section on ethnics.)

Values clarification is also necessary because it is very difficult to value that of which one is only vaguely aware. By identifying personal values, the nurse becomes more aware of self and thus better able to value the self. The person who is able to value the self (in full awareness of limitations as well as virtues) is prepared to learn about and to value the other. *Values clarification assists in learning about the child and family insofar as it reduces the risk that preconceived notions will take the place of meaningful communication.*

Preparation at the time of the initial encounter may take only a few moments. It involves only the nurse's brief inventory of mindset and a conscious effort toward openness and genuineness. This moment of preparation before entering the room, however, is often vividly communicated in the nurse's nonverbal behavior and can set the tone for all future encounters with this client.

Searching for Similarities in Identity Groups. Searching for similarities constitutes a major strategy for meeting two separate but interrelated nurse-client goals. The goals are (1) to establish a base for communication and (2) to agree upon a plan of care.

Establishing a Base for Communication. Just as one searches for similarities upon which to base a social conversation, it is important to identify commonalities upon which to base the nurse-client relationship. In Singer's (1985) words: "Communication tends to be easiest among individuals who identify most closely with each other, and most difficult among individuals who perceive more or less dissimilarly . . ." (p 64).

Singer proposed a continuum of similarity of perception among individuals (Fig. 1-4). On the one end, perception (and, therefore, communication) approaches, but never reaches, zero, and on the other end, it approaches, though never reaches, 100 per cent. By virtue of the fact that we are human beings and share in the experience of a communication process, our perceptions will never be zero. Even among close family members, however, perceptions are never identical because of variations in physiologic sensory processes and in past experiences. It is the nurse's goal to assess the degree of similarity (and therefore of dissimilarity) in nurse-client perceptions to establish a base of mutual acceptance and trust upon which to build a therapeutic relationship.

Nursing assessment for cultural similarities is most effective when conducted in an informal manner. Although the strategies are almost identical to those used in a social situation, the nurse is constantly aware of the goal of this encounter. Although it is often desirable in a social context to share as much about oneself as the other shares with you, in a professional situation the nurse's goal is simply to establish the existence of similarities without elaborating upon them. For example, during the course of the admission interview, the nurse might share with a rural family that she or he lived on a farm as a child, or might share with the child an understanding of what it is like to be an only child. The nurse then continues the interview, focusing upon the client. If the client asks additional details about the nurse's experiences, answers are, of course, appropriate. Rarely, however, does the *client* confuse the goal of the conversation. Rarely, too, does the client fail to recognize the identified similarities as a basis for trust and support. Often the child or parent will seize the opportunity "to talk with someone who must understand how I feel."

The more identity groups two people share in common, the more similar will be their perceptions in a given situation. It follows that the more dissimilar they are, the greater the probability for misunderstandings. Dissimilarities such as race, religion, or geographic origin can often be offset by similarities in other areas, e.g., age, occupation, marital and parenting status, and so on. But what if dissimilarities between the nurse and client remain significant? We are reminded again that culture is important *to the extent* that it affects communication. If progress toward the goal is unimpeded by cultural differences, those differences are unimportant. If, however, communication suffers to the extent that it affects progress toward the therapeutic goal, it is the professional responsibility of the nurse to recognize this fact and to cooperatively adjust nursing assignments to effect a better nurse-client "match."

Agreeing upon a Plan of Care. Nurse-client agreement upon a plan of care to accomplish the therapeutic goal is the crux of the nursing process. Converging at this point are (1) the nurse's scientific knowledge, (2) the nurse's therapeutic use of self, and (3) the established base for nurse-client communications. This part of the nursing process will have the greatest influence upon the client's cooperative participation in goal attainment and upon the client's overall perception of the nurse's importance and expertise.

As explained in the section on nursing process, agreement upon a plan of care should be obtained as soon as possible after the client is encountered in the care setting. *The purpose of the meeting is to obtain the client's agreement that the problems perceived by the nurse and physician are shared by the client, and that the strategies proposed to meet the therapeutic goals are in keeping with the beliefs and values of the client.*

Through this process any cultural values and beliefs and other attitudes of the client pertaining to health care can be explored. It is therefore important that the nurse emphasize the importance of the client's input into both the goals and strategies for care.

Discussing the plan of care will address all pertinent cultural aspects of nursing care, such as dietary practices, religious practices, health beliefs, and so on. At the same time, this approach guards the client's privacy in areas that do not relate to current care. *The only cultural values and cultural practices that are pertinent for nursing consideration are those that have a direct bearing on either the plan of care or on nurse-client communication.*

Appreciating Differences in Nurse-Client Experiences and Perceptions. Differences in nurse-client experiences and perceptions can be the impetus for innovations in the nursing process and for individualization of care. To appreciate these differences, however, the nurse first must possess enough self-esteem to view differences as nonthreatening. The nurse who values the self is prepared to value the other.

Differences are *appreciated* when they are identified and met with openness and genuineness. Appreciating differences, therefore, requires (1) a genuine attempt to discern the client's perspective of the situation, (2) identification of ways in which that perspective is similar and dissimilar to the nurse's perspective, and (3) exploration of the reasons for differences in attitudes and perceptions. When these differences are the result of misunderstanding on the part of the nurse or client, further discussion can alleviate potential problems. When these differences result from dissimilar experiences and differing world views, the nurse can base further nursing interactions on one of two premises: The nurse may conclude that the client's view is wrong and/or old-fashioned because it differs from the nurse's perspective. In this case the nurse's nonverbal behavior usually communicates intolerance of differing views and blocks therapeutic communication with the client. The more informed nurse, however, may look upon the identified difference as an opportunity to explore another viewpoint and as the potential for discovering other viable ways to approach a problem. The nurse who approaches a difference in experience or perceptions in this way communicates that the client is a valued member of the "treatment team." The client then feels more free to express preferences and ideas about health care practices and to ask questions about other aspects of treatment. This is the basis of therapeutic communication. *Appreciating differences means recognizing the potential of every interpersonal encounter to expand and enrich existing knowledge.*

Validating Perceptions. Validating perceptions is, of course, integral to the three preceding elements of this model for intercultural communication. Its importance to the success of this model, however, warrants its inclusion as a separate topic. It involves determining whether the message sent was the message received and incorporates the communication elements of receiver response and feedback.

Nonverbal response is often more important to validation than is verbal response. This is especially true when a language barrier exists, such as between a child and a nurse or between an English-speaking nurse and a non-English-speaking client. The importance of nonverbal communication within our culture in general is emphasized by Hall's (1984) estimate that only 10 per cent of communication is accomplished verbally. This cultural propensity for nonverbal communication is a benefit to the pediatric nurse because it means one enters the profession with a certain amount of expertise in reading nonverbal signals. The pediatric nurse who refines these observations will greatly enhance professional communication skills.

Perceptions must be validated almost continuously when there are great disparities between the cultural "identities" of persons involved. When, for example, a language barrier exists, validation by nonverbal gestures and the help of an interpreter may be necessary. Ironically, because of aggressive efforts, often we are better at validation of perceptions in these extreme circumstances. We must be careful, as well, to validate perceptions with the client who seems "more like" us. We have but to reflect upon missed communications within our own families to remember that perceptions can never be taken for granted.

Culture molds values and beliefs, influences perceptions of space and time, and patterns communications. Culture has a complex and pervasive influence upon every individual. The nurse and client come together as products of culture to attempt understanding through communication, which is also culturally patterned. This means that nurse-client interactions often involve intercultural communication. This section has proposed a model for intercultural communication, one which

- prepares the nurse to meet the client nonjudgmentally, with openness and genuineness,
- establishes similarities for the purposes of building a trusting relationship and assessing whether the client's values and beliefs are in keeping with the goals and strategies of care,
- encourages exploration of value differences to enrich the nurse's awareness and appreciation of other ideas, and
- evaluates the effectiveness of communication through continual validation of perceptions.

This overview of intercultural communication has established the importance of recognizing the interdependence of culture and communication as they influence the practice of pediatric nursing. Detailed nursing strategies related to culture and communication are also included in this text. Chapter 2 provides a framework for cultural assessment and details those aspects of culture that may influence health behaviors. Specific nursing strategies for communicating with children and parents can be found in Chapter 11.

A Perspective on Ethical Influences

Achieving the goal of pediatric nursing will involve decisions about appropriate assessments and the meaning of the assessment data; choices of strategies within a therapeutic plan and various means of delivering the care; and judgments about the effectiveness of the interventions. When determining what should or ought to be done for a client, nurses are often faced with ethical decisions. *Ethics deals with "practical problems that arise from human conduct when an individual is faced with a choice between alternative values"* (Sigman, 1986, p 26).

Ethical Practice in the Nursing of Children and Adolescents

Values and Beliefs. Culture and ethics both relate to values and beliefs (Fig. 1-5). Culture is the way in which values are transmitted to an individual through various identity groups that either are part of the individual's heritage (that is, race, gender, religion), or are groups with which the individual decides to align (e.g., education, occupation, marital status). Ethics determines how those values and beliefs are used to make choices.

Ethics can be thought of as standards of moral behavior shared by a community. Viewed in the broadest sense (the community of mankind), ethics is a branch of philosophy. Under the umbrella of ethics in this

Figure 1-5. The effects of culture and ethics upon individual values and beliefs.

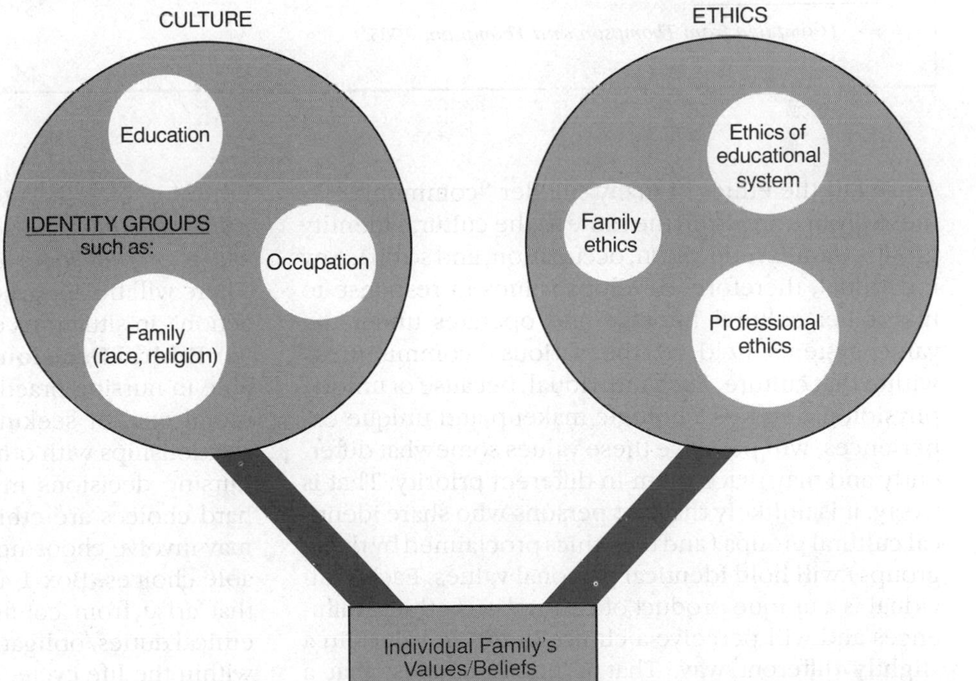

Box 1-4
Ethical Issues

ISSUES OF PRINCIPLE

Autonomy, self-determination of patients and professionals
Do good, do no harm (beneficence, nonmaleficence)
Justice, fairness (allocation of resources)
Truth telling (veracity)
Informed consent
Quality of life/sanctity of life
The Golden Rule

ISSUES OF ETHICAL RIGHTS

Right to privacy (confidentiality)
Right to decide what happens to oneself/one's body (self-determination)
Right to health care (currently debatable; some say equal access only, others say not a right at all)
Right to information (informed consent, access to records)
Right to choose whom you care for (frequently limited to physicians in nonemergency situations)
Right to live, right to die
Rights of children

ISSUES OF ETHICAL DUTIES/OBLIGATIONS

Respect persons
Be accountable for decisions/actions
Maintain competence (professionals)
Exercise informed judgment in professional practice
Implement and improve standards of profession
Participate in activities contributing to profession's knowledge base
Safeguard clients from incompetent, unethical, or illegal practice of any person
Promote efforts to meet health needs of public
Participate in the formulation of public policy

ISSUES OF ETHICAL LOYALTY

Professional-patient relationship (covenant fidelity, contract, seller of services)
Accountability to whom as employee
Professional-professional relationships
Professional-patient family relationships
Who decides?

ISSUES OF CONCERN IN LIFE CYCLE

Contraception and sterilization
Genetic engineering and embryo transfer
Abortion (When does life begin?)
Infanticide
Adolescent sexuality
Allocation of scarce resources
Lifestyle
Euthanasia

(Compiled from Thompson and Thompson, 1985.)

sense fall the ethics of many smaller "communities"; these groups are often the same as the cultural identity groups (family, education, occupation, and so on). Any individual, therefore, develops values in response to his or her cultural heritage and operates under the value systems held by the various "communities" within that culture. Each individual, because of unique physiologic and psychologic makeup and unique experiences, will perceive these values somewhat differently and may place them in different priority. That is to say, it is unlikely that two persons who share identical cultural groups (and the ethics proclaimed by those groups) will hold identical personal values. Each individual is a unique product of cultural and ethical influences and will perceive a choice between values in a slightly different way. That is not to suggest that a group of individuals cannot arrive at consensus in an ethical choice; it is to say that *the complexity of our cultural/ethical personhood makes it almost impossible to avoid some conflicts among value systems.* There will be disagreements about "the best course of action" in situations of health care.

Ethical Decisions. Ethical decisions are inescapable in nursing practice because nursing involves the moral goal of seeking good for others and involves relationships with other persons (Curtin, 1986). Many nursing decisions involve hard choices, but not all hard choices are ethical decisions. Ethical decisions may involve choosing between two equally unacceptable choices. Box 1-4 lists examples of ethical issues that arise from conflicts of principle, ethical rights, ethical duties/obligations, ethical loyalty, and concern within the life cycle. Although the grouping of issues in Box 1-4 shows extensive overlapping, the value of this classification is in listing examples of common ethical issues.

Sometimes an ethical decision is of such consequence to society as to make media headlines, such as the sensitive process for allocating scarce donor organs for transplant. Though the nurse may at some point be involved in a headline case, the types of ethical decisions that follow are more reflective of day-to-day practice. It is important that these common decisions be identified as ethical issues so that the nurse will know to employ the correct approach in their solution.

- The nurse is exhausted and is concerned about the ability to stay alert during the shift, but the unit is already short-staffed; if this nurse leaves, the patients may receive even less care.
- A 16-year-old victim of an auto accident confides in the nurse that she is sexually active and wants counseling about birth control. She says that her parents would not understand because of their religious convictions.
- An 8-year-old boy with leukemia refuses to undergo another round of chemotherapy. The parents ask the nurse whether they should respect his wishes or go ahead with the therapy.
- The foster mother leaves instructions that the young child's biologic mother is not to visit because she upsets the child. The biologic mother arrives on the unit and looks through the window at her son who begins crying "Mommy" and holding his arms out to her.
- The father of an adolescent boy with an inoperable tumor requests that his son not be told the truth about his diagnosis.

The Nurse's Unique Perspective. "Nursing ethics is different from biomedical ethics, not in process but in substance" (Sigman, 1986, p 33). Nurses have a unique perspective on the values of the client because they spend more time with the client and because clients are often less intimidated by nurses than by physicians and tend to confide in them. The nurse is also in a position of liaison between the client and other health care professional and often can understand the rationale for differing values among all the parties involved.

The Issue of Autonomy in Pediatric Nursing. Pediatric nursing is unique in the number of ethical decisions involving autonomy. Since infants and small children do not possess the knowledge to make decisions for themselves and since children under age 18, under normal circumstances, cannot sign consent forms, the judgment of adults often must be substituted for that of the child. Issues of substituted judgment involve decisions made for the child by either the nurse or the parent(s). Sometimes these decisions must be carried out against the will of the child, such as when the nurse must administer an oral medication to a resisting toddler or give a preoperative injection to a resisting 10-year-old. Although this is not a pleasant part of the nursing role, the choice to administer the medications seems clear-cut in these two examples. What about the child in the earlier example who refused chemotherapy, however? Does the child have some rights in a decision that has such a profound bodily effect? At what age can a child make a personal decision? Should the wishes of a chronically ill or terminally ill child be given more consideration than those of an acutely ill child? There are no general answers. The ambiguity of the autonomy issue is a concern for every pediatric nurse.

Resources for Ethical Decision Making

Surely there must be rules and guidelines for making such decisions. Yes and no. Yes, there are guidelines in the form of ethical theories, codes of ethics, and various linear problem-solving procedures. No, these guidelines, do not always lead to clear-cut answers. In gathering the facts about an ethical dilemma, one must consider not only the broad theoretic principles offered by various guidelines but also the facts as they relate to the unique situation. This approach is necessary because aspects of the issue that emphasize only universal principles tend to be insensitive to the unique aspects of the case, and aspects that emphasize only the unique characteristics are easily clouded by emotion.

In addition to the failure of broad principles to consider the uniqueness in a situation, there is no way to assure that the principles upon which ethical theories are based are true. "The ethical principles that we develop from our philosophy are no more certain than the philosophy on which they are based, and these principles raise additional uncertainties about how to apply them to specific situations" (Quinn and Smith, 1987, p 52). That is one reason why there is no universal ethical theory upon which everyone agrees. Persons tend to favor one theory or another because the tenets of the theory are more in keeping with their own value system. The best chance for making a good decision in an ethical conflict is to have an education that includes a base in the arts and humanities, an awareness of guidelines from ethical theories, an awareness of professional and personal ethics, an openness to the values and perspectives of others, and knowledge of one's professional resources.

Ethical Theories. While it is beyond the scope of this chapter to present all of the ethical theories in

Box 1-5

United Nations Declaration of the Rights of the Child

Preamble

Whereas the peoples of the United Nations have, in the Charter, reaffirmed their faith in fundamental human rights, and in the dignity and worth of the human person, and have determined to promote social progress and better standards of life in larger freedom,

Whereas the United Nations has, in the Universal Declaration of Human Rights, proclaimed that everyone is entitled to all the rights and freedoms set forth therein, without distinction of any kind, such as race, color, sex, language, religion, political or other opinion, national or social origin, property, birth or other status,

Whereas the child, by reason of his physical and mental immaturity, needs special safeguards and care, including appropriate legal protection, before as well as after birth,

Whereas the need for such special safeguards has been stated in the Geneva Declaration of the Rights of the Child of 1924, and recognized in the Universal Declaration of Human Rights and in the statutes of specialized agencies and international organizations concerned with welfare of children,

Whereas mankind owes to the child the best it has to give

Now therefore the General Assembly proclaims

This Declaration of the Rights of the Child to the end that he may have a happy childhood and enjoy for his own good and for the good of society the rights and freedoms herein set forth, and calls upon parents, upon men and women as individuals and upon voluntary organizations, local authorities and national governments to recognize these rights and strive for their observance by legislative and other measures progressively taken in accordance with the following principles:

PRINCIPLE 1

The child shall enjoy all the rights set forth in this Declaration. All children, without any exception whatsoever, shall be entitled to these rights, without distinction or discrimination on account of race, color, sex, language, religion, political or other opinion, national or social origin, property, birth or other status, whether of himself or of his family.

PRINCIPLE 2

The child shall enjoy special protection, and shall be given opportunities and facilities, by law and by other means, to enable him to develop physically, mentally, morally, spiritually and socially in a healthy and normal manner and in conditions of freedom and dignity. In the enactment of laws for this purpose the best interests of the child shall be the paramount consideration.

PRINCIPLE 3

The child shall be entitled from his birth to a name and a nationality.

PRINCIPLE 4

The child shall enjoy the benefits of social security. He shall be entitled to grow and develop in health; to this end special care and protection shall be provided both to him and to his mother, including adequate pre-natal and post-natal care. The child shall have the right to adequate nutrition, housing, recreation and medical services.

PRINCIPLE 5

The child who is physically, mentally or socially handicapped shall be given the special treatment, education and care required by his particular condition.

PRINCIPLE 6

The child, for the full and harmonious development of his personality, needs love and understanding. He shall, wherever possible, grow up in the care and under the responsibility of his parents, and in any case in an atmosphere of affection and of moral and maternal security; a child of tender years shall not, save in exceptional circumstances, be separated from his mother. Society and the public authorities shall have the duty to extend particular care to children without a family and to those without adequate means of support. Payment of state and other assistance toward the maintenance of children of large families is desirable.

PRINCIPLE 7

The child is entitled to receive education, which shall be free and compulsory, at least in the elementary stages. He shall be given an education which will promote his general culture, and enable him on a basis of equal opportunity to develop his abilities, his individual judgment, and his sense of moral and social responsibility, and to become a useful member of society.

The best interests of the child shall be the building principle of those responsible for his education and guidance; that responsibility lies in the first place with his parents.

The child shall have full opportunity for play and recreation, which shall be directed to the same purposes as education; society and the public authorities shall endeavor to promote the enjoyment of this right.

PRINCIPLE 8

The child shall in all circumstances be among the first to receive protection and relief.

PRINCIPLE 9

The child shall be protected against all forms of neglect, cruelty and exploitation. He shall not be the subject of traffic, in any form.

The child shall not be admitted to employment before an appropriate minimum age; he shall in no case be caused or permitted to engage in any occupation or employment which would prejudice his health or education, or interfere with his physical, mental or moral development.

PRINCIPLE 10

The child shall be protected from practices which may foster racial, religious and any other form of discrimination. He shall be brought up in a spirit of understanding, tolerance, friendship among peoples, peace and universal brotherhood and in full consciousness that his energy and talents should be devoted to the service of his fellow men.

depth, two prevalent theories, utilitarianism and deontology, will be briefly outlined as examples of what theory can lend to an ethical decision. The reader is encouraged to use the references and bibliography at the end of this chapter for recommendations of current textbooks that deal in more depth with these and other ethical theories. The more familiar one is with ethical theories, the easier it will be to understand other perspectives in an ethical issue. Also, the more one knows about an ethical theory and its strengths and limitations, the more confident one can be in either applying it or discarding it in a specific situation.

Utilitarianism. "Utilitarianism holds that an action is morally correct if its consequences produce the greatest amount of happiness for the greatest number of people, including the actor" (Fromer, 1986, p 82). This is the theory often characterized as "the greatest good for the greatest number." Utilitarianism is known as a *consequentialist* theory because of its emphasis upon the results of actions. Under this theory, no action is inherently good or bad in itself but is judged only in the results it brings (Quinn and Smith, 1987). Triage is an example of a nursing action that follows the utilitarian theory. The goal is to save as many persons as possible when not everyone can be saved. Another example of utilitarianism is that it is justifiable to deceive a patient about a diagnosis (e.g., terminal cancer) if, in so doing, the patient is spared some anxiety. Whether or not to "spare" the child the anxiety of a serious diagnosis is a common issue in pediatric nursing. (See Chapter 26 on the dying child.)

Deontology. Deontology holds that "we have an ethical *duty* or obligation to do or to avoid doing some things regardless of the consequences" (Quinn and Smith, 1987, p 19). The deontologic focus upon duties leads to the related aspects of rights. "The belief that people have a right is the belief that they are legitimately entitled to something, that it is owed to them" (Quinn and Smith, 1987, p 23). If the nurse has a duty to a patient, the patient has the right to that action from the nurse. (See Box 1-5, The United Nations Declaration of the Rights of the Child.)

The four principles most common to deontology are those of autonomy, nonmaleficence, beneficence, and justice. Deontologists believe that several principles can be effectively applied to one problem. Of course, this necessitates assigning priority to the principles involved, depending upon the views of the problem solver, in order to arrive at a decision based upon principle (Fromer, 1986). The reader is cautioned that deontologic principles are very complex and have no universal meanings. The principles

Box 1-6
Code for Nurses

1. The nurse provides services with respect for human dignity and the uniqueness of the client unrestricted by considerations of social or economic status, personal attributes, or the nature of health problems.
2. The nurse safeguards the client's right to privacy by judiciously protecting information of a confidential nature.
3. The nurse acts to safeguard the client and the public when health care and safety are affected by the incompetent, unethical, or illegal practice of any person.
4. The nurse assumes responsibility and accountability for individual nursing judgments and actions.
5. The nurse maintains competence in nursing.
6. The nurse exercises informed judgment and uses individual competence and qualifications as criteria in seeking consultation, accepting responsibilities, and delegating nursing activities to others.
7. The nurse participates in activities that contribute to the ongoing development of the profession's body of knowledge.
8. The nurse participates in the profession's efforts to implement and improve standards of nursing.
9. The nurse participates in the profession's efforts to establish and maintain conditions of employment conducive to high-quality nursing care.
10. The nurse participates in the profession's effort to protect the public from misinformation and misrepresentation and to maintain the integrity of nursing.
11. The nurse collaborates with members of the health professions and other citizens in promoting community and national efforts to meet the health needs of the public.

(From Code for Nurses with Interpretive Statements, *American Nurses' Association, 2420 Pershing Road, Kansas City, MO, 1985.)*

sketched here briefly, however, will acquaint the reader with some of the more obvious applications of these principles to pediatric issues.

Autonomy can be seen as a client right; it is "personal liberty of action and implies independence, self-reliance, freedom of choice, and the ability to make decisions" (Fromer, 1986, p 83). Autonomy was discussed previously in regard to the need for substituted judgments in pediatric nursing. It is employed in issues such as "At what age and under what conditions should pediatric patients be granted autonomy?"

Nonmaleficence is the duty to "first do no harm." It involves examination of the risks of action or nonaction. Nonmaleficence comes into play when nurses are asked to perform procedures with which they are not familiar. If the nurse attempts the procedure, she or he may inadvertently harm the patient.

Beneficence is the duty to do good. It involves the benefits of an action. It also involves balancing risk/benefit ratios and determining whether the potential for good outweighs the risk of harm. Does one take the risk of performing a new procedure without help if no help is available? Does one participate in a therapeutic abortion if the mother is a 13-year-old rape victim?

Justice is the principle that concerns fairness of practice. It involves rights of individuals, groups, and societies. "It is thought that justice is served when an individual receives his or her 'just desserts,' or what is owed him or her by another individual or by society" (Fromer, 1986, p 84). A common application of justice is in the allocation of scarce resources, such as the nurse's time. How does one allocate time among three infants who all want to be fed at once? Decisions of time allocation are common and are very difficult. Fromer stated that justice is the most complex and the most difficult principle to apply to nursing. ***It is important to remember that ALL ethical choices should be made from the basis of the professional ethic and based upon the available facts, and not upon personal preference or emotional involvement.***

Distinguishing Between Personal and Professional Ethics. Upon becoming a professional, one implicitly agrees to abide by the stated ethics of that profession. It behooves the nurse, therefore, to be well versed in the implications of the American Nurses' Association Code and in the ANA Standards of Maternal–Child Health Practice. (See Boxes 1-6 and 1-7.)

Ethical decision making will be enhanced by the nurse's ability to differentiate between personal and professional values. Box 1-8 lists questions that may be helpful in this type of values clarification. Once values have been explored, the nurse is in a better position to act autonomously because the values that drive behavior will be known entities instead of subconscious motivators.

Occasionally the nurse may be caught in a conflict between personal and professional values. Perhaps the most common example is the nurse who holds strong personal values against abortion but recognizes the professional value of allowing the client to make her own decision. In such an instance it is not just permissible but advisable for the nurse to remove herself or himself from the situation if another nurse is available and willing to help. The nurse has the right not to compromise strong personal values, and the client has the right to nursing care that is nonjudgmental.

Box 1-7
American Nurses' Association Standards of Maternal–Child Health Nursing Practice

STANDARD I

The nurse helps children and parents attain and maintain optimum health.

STANDARD II

The nurse assists families to achieve and maintain a balance between the personal growth needs of individual family members and optimum family functioning.

STANDARD III

The nurse intervenes with vulnerable clients and families at risk to prevent potential developmental and health problems.

STANDARD IV

The nurse promotes an environment free of hazards to reproduction, growth and development, wellness, and recovery from illness.

STANDARD V

The nurse detects changes in health status and deviations from optimum development.

STANDARD VI

The nurse carries out appropriate interventions and treatment to facilitate survival and recovery from illness.

STANDARD VII

The nurse assists clients and families to understand and cope with developmental and traumatic situations during illness, childbearing, childrearing, and childhood.

STANDARD VIII

The nurse actively pursues strategies to enhance access to and utilization of adequate health care services.

STANDARD IX

The nurse improves maternal and child health nursing practice through evaluation of practice, education, and research.

(*From* Standards of Maternal-Child Health Nursing Practice, *American Nurses' Association, 2420 Pershing Road, Kansas City, MO, 1983.)*

Openness to the Values of Others. The nurse who has explored personal and professional values is better prepared to be open and accepting of the values of others. Conversely, the nurse who operates only from subconscious, gut-level feelings (values) of right and wrong is less likely to be aware that right and wrong are relative concepts and is likely to disagree with anyone who holds a different view. The nurse must be sincerely open to other values in order to adequately explore the perspectives of each person involved in an ethical issue. Without such exploration, the actual problem (specific value conflicts) may never be identified.

Professional Resources. The nurse has several professional resources to help with decision making: knowledge of the arts and humanities, knowledge of ethical theories, professional codes, client bills of rights, senior staff members who have had more experience with ethical decisions (e.g., shift supervisor, head nurse, assistant head nurse), and, where available, the hospital or agency ethics committee (i.e., through either a formal presentation to the committee

Box 1-8
Clarifying Personal and Professional Values

1. Choose an ethical issue from Box 1-5. Then ask yourself the following questions.
2. "What do I believe about this issue?" If applicable, break the issue into component parts and think about values in relation to each part. It may help to think about what your "first impulse" would be if you were in this situation.
3. "What would my parents say about this issue?"
4. "How did I feel about this issue when I was in high school?" If your values have changed, ask why?
5. "To what extent has my nursing education influenced my thinking on this issue?"
6. "What explicit and implicit guidelines are contained in the ANA Code and the ANA Standards of Practice that can clarify the professional position on this issue?"
7. "Do my personal values agree or disagree with my professional values on this issue?"
8. "What course of action will I take if faced with a decision involving a similar issue?"

(Based upon Thompson and Thompson, 1985.)

or a consultation with a nursing representative on the committee). In addition, several models exist for ethical decision making. Some of these models are more appropriate for groups like an ethics committee, but others, such as the one proposed by Thompson and Thompson (1985), are equally applicable to individual decision making. (See Box 1-9.)

Ethics and Excellence

"The willingness to enter with a patient that predicament which he cannot face alone is an expression of moral responsibility; the quality of the moral commitment is a measure of the nurse's excellence" (Levine, 1977, p 845). More recently Levine's sentiments were echoed by Bishop and Scudder (1987): "Since nursing practice aims at the well-being of the patient, the first moral responsibility of any nurse is excellence of practice" (p 36).

What constitutes excellence of practice? Benner (1984) described the expert nurse as one who "with an enormous background of experience now has an intuitive grasp of each situation and zeroes in on the accurate region of the problem without wasteful consideration of a large range of unfruitful, alternative diagnoses and solutions" (p 32). In light of this definition of excellence, perhaps one might amend Bishop and Scudder's statement to include the notion that the first moral responsibility of any nurse is to first *develop* excellence in practice. The novice nurse is not expected to be an expert in ethical decision making. He or she is expected, however, to be prepared to develop that expertise.

Summary

Because nursing depends upon human relationships in every aspect of practice, and because each individual holds a unique value system, the nurse cannot escape making decisions among conflicting values in the course of providing patient care. The development of excellence in practice is contingent upon the nurse's ability to identify ethical issues as such and to base decisions upon facts and upon professional values. The nurse's ability to discover pertinent facts and to clarify professional values is enhanced by knowledge of the arts and humanities, by knowledge of ethical theories and professional codes of conduct, and by clarification of personal and professional values.

The Nursing Process as It Relates to Children and Adolescents

The nursing process is a method of problem solving that incorporates five steps:

- assessment
- analysis

Box 1-9
Ethical Decision Making: The MORAL Process

M Massage the dilemma
Identify and define the real issue

O Outline the options
Include opposing viewpoints

R Resolve the issue
Review driving and restraining forces

A Act
Base act on what you can control, influence, and anticipate

L Look back
Evaluate all aspects of the processes

(Based on Stockton, cited in Halloran, 1982.)

Box 1-10
Assessment Guide for Children and Adolescents

I. PHYSICAL FUNCTION
- A. Sleep-rest
  1. Client patterns
  2. Family patterns
- B. Nutrition-metabolism
  1. Skin integrity
  2. Nutrition
  3. Fluid balance/electrolytes
  4. Teeth
  5. Height, weight, status on growth chart
  6. Temperature
  7. Client and family eating patterns
- C. Elimination
  1. Urinary, toilet training
  2. Bowel, toilet training
  3. Client patterns
- D. Activity-exercise
  1. Pulse, respirations, blood pressure
  2. Client and family patterns
  3. Self-care/family/care deficit
  4. Airway/gas exchange/breathing
  5. Diversional/play activities
  6. Tissue perfusion/cardiac output
  7. Neuromuscular integrity
  8. Developmental level

II. EMOTIONAL-SOCIAL FUNCTION
- A. Self-perception/self-concept
  1. Self-concept
     a. body image
     b. self esteem
     c. role performance
     d. identity
  2. Parenting patterns
     a. child safety
     b. family beliefs/values
     c. social behaviors and roles
     d. self-regulation and independence of child
- B. Sexuality
  1. Appropriate to developmental stage
  2. Related family values and beliefs
- C. Coping-stress-tolerance patterns
  1. Client patterns
  2. Family patterns
  3. Fear/anxiety
  4. Coping strategies appropriate to developmental stage
  5. Resources
- D. Spiritual health
  1. Sense of purpose
  2. Sense of hope
  3. Sense of wholeness
  4. Sense of peace

III. INTELLECTUAL-PERCEPTUAL FUNCTION
- A. Health perception/management
  1. Child's perception of illness
  2. Parent's perception of illness
  3. Health beliefs/cultural values
- B. Knowledge of illness/health management
  1. Anticipatory guidance and discharge planning related to
     a. disease process
     b. home management
     c. well child care
     d. prevention of physical injury, poisoning, trauma, suffocation
- C. Pain
- D. Sensory perceptual alterations

(Adapted from Gordon, 1987.)

- planning
- implementing
- evaluating

The nursing process as it relates to children and adolescents takes into account the central role of the family.

Assessment

The first phase of nursing assessment answers the question, "What do I need to find out about this client in order to provide the best care?" Data gathering in this regard requires a framework or guideline designed to remind the nurse of all the aspects of care that must be considered for any client.

A Framework for Assessment

The framework used in this textbook has been adapted from Gordon's (1987) functional health patterns (Box 1-10). The three major assessment areas correspond to the three major aspects of personhood: physical, emotional-social, and intellectual-perceptual. It is by no means necessary to use this framework to utilize the nursing process plans and other nursing guidelines within this text. The point is that without a framework of some sort, the nurse must rely upon memory and may well neglect an important area of assessment.

It is emphasized that an assessment framework is a *guideline*. It would not be practical to include each point in the guideline in every client assessment. Instead, a framework helps assure that the nurse will cover all the aspects of assessment (both subjective and objective) *pertinent to this client*.

Subjective Assessment. Subjective information includes all information supplied by the client. It is information unavailable to the nurse unless communicated by the child or parent. Figure 1-6 is an excerpt from Table 31-2: Nursing Process Plan for the Hospitalized Child (page 972). This excerpt shows pertinent subjective and objective information related to physiologic function for the child being admitted to the hospital.

Subjective information for the pediatric patient often will be supplied by a combination of answers from the child and the parent. The child should be allowed to answer questions whenever possible, because the parent's and child's perceptions may differ on a given issue. Often the parent may not even be aware of this difference of opinion. Because the child is the focus of the assessment, his or her perceptions are vital to the entire nursing process. Acknowledgment of the child's knowledge and opinions at this point in the nursing process also allows the child a feeling of control that is so important to a sense of security, coping, and mastery.

Objective Assessment. Objective information is obtained directly by the nurse examiner (Fig. 1-6). It includes all observable responses of the child, results of physical examination, and results of diagnostic tests.

Analysis: Nursing Diagnosis

Nursing diagnoses answer the question, "What do the assessment data mean?" Nursing diagnoses describe actual or potential health problems that nurses by virtue of their education and experience are capable and licensed to treat (Gordon, 1987). The nursing diagnoses used in this text are those approved by the Eighth Conference of the North American Nursing Diagnosis Association (NANDA) in 1988. Appendix One contains the complete listing of these diagnoses and their definitions.

Components of the Nursing Diagnosis. A nursing diagnosis has three major components: the problem statement (contained in the NANDA-approved diagnoses), the etiology, and the list of defining signs and symptoms. In this text the Nursing Process Plans list all three of these components. The nursing diagnosis sections accompanying specific diseases formally list the first two components and incorporate the signs and symptoms under the heading, "Clinical Manifestations."

The *problem statement* is the result of thoughtful analysis of the meaning of *these* data for *this* particular client. It is chosen on the basis of the lowest common denominator of meaning. That is, one should strive to select the diagnosis that is most meaningful and the most concrete for nursing practice. It is obtained by repeatedly asking oneself, "What does this mean for the child?" For example, the nurse legitimately could choose any of the following nursing diagnoses for a child with the medical diagnosis of anemia:

- Impaired gas exchange
- Altered tissue perfusion
- Activity intolerance

Impairment of the oxygen-carrying components of the blood in anemia leads logically to either of the first two diagnoses, but the question "What does this mean?" will further reduce the diagnosis to activity intolerance because it, in turn, is the result of impaired gas exchange and altered tissue perfusion. It is, therefore, the most concrete level to which the nursing diagnosis can be reduced. By reducing the diagnosis to the most concrete level of meaning for the client, the nurse can more accurately delineate therapeutic nursing actions to achieve the goal associated with the diagnosis.

Sometimes qualifying information must be added to a NANDA nursing diagnosis to make it more meaningful. When this occurs, the qualifying data are attached to the NANDA stem with a colon, as the following example:

Diversional activity deficit: *altered play behavior*

The diagnosis is more meaningful if one knows the *type* of diversional activity that is being addressed.

When choosing a nursing diagnosis from the NANDA list, it is important to make sure the definition of that diagnosis matches the child's condition. For example, the diagnoses *Altered Family Processes* and *Ineffective Family Coping* might seem quite interchangeable if one failed to consider their definitions. *Altered Family Processes* describes a family that normally functions effectively but is challenged by a stressor that has altered or may alter the family's function. This diagnosis differs from *Ineffective Family Coping*, which describes a family that has a pattern of ineffective responses (Appendix One).

A problem statement may be *qualified* by the words *potential* or *possible* (Carpenito, 1984). A potential problem is one that may develop in the absence of certain nursing strategies. A possible problem is one that may actually exist but that requires additional as-

1 SUBJECTIVE ASSESSMENT
Information supplied by the client (child, parent, or guardian)

2 OBJECTIVE ASSESSMENT
Information obtained directly through observation, physical examination, and interpretation of diagnostic test results

3 ANALYSIS: NURSING DIAGNOSIS
Problem statement and etiology

4 DEFINING CHARACTERISTICS
Signs and symptoms that support the nursing diagnosis

5 CLIENT GOAL
The desired change in client condition or behavior, agreed upon by the client and nurse

6 EVALUATION CRITERIA
The observable and/or measurable indications that the client's condition or behavior has changed

7 NURSING GOALS/STRATEGIES
The plan and actions the nurse undertakes

8 (SELECTED RATIONALE)
Explanations or further clarification of nursing goals and strategies

Table 31-2.
Nursing Process Plan: The Hospitalized Child

By Roxie Foster

I. Assessment of Physical Function

Sleep/Rest
Nutrition/Metabolism
Elimination
Activity/Exercise

Subjective Assessment	***Objective Assessment***
Upon admission: Report from child and/or parent(s) regarding usual patterns of sleep/rest, eating, bowel and bladder elimination, activity/exercise patterns, self-care, play/diversion; current developmental level *During hospitalization:* Self-report or parental report of changes in baseline behaviors established upon admission	*Upon admission:* General appearance (whether well-nourished), specific gravity of urine, number of teeth, height and weight, percentiles on growth chart, vital signs, assessment of respiratory, cardiovascular, neuromuscular, integumentary, and genitourinary systems; developmental status *During hospitalization:* Observable changes in baseline data established upon admission
1	2

Analysis: Nursing Diagnosis 1

Sleep pattern disturbance (child), related to anxiety associated with
- *unfamiliar environment*
- *separation from parents/family*
- *discomfort of illness*
- *medications*

3

Defining Characteristics

Subjective: Self-report or parental report of sleeplessness, restlessness, marked irritability	***Objective:*** Pale to grayish skin tones, dark circles under eyes, lethargy, frequent dozing but no prolonged periods of sleep

4

Client Goal/Evaluation Criteria	***Nursing Goals/Strategies (Selected Rationale)***
1.1. The client† will obtain sufficient sleep to meet needs, as evidenced by:	
5 a. agreeing to sleep and rest at the times client usually does so at home b. rested appearance c. decreased irritability d. increased energy for and interest in play 6	*Determine usual sleep patterns,* including naptime and bedtime routines and rituals 7 (the younger the child, the more important these familiar activities are to promote sleep). 8
	7 *Provide for continuity of care.* When parents cannot be present to prepare the child for sleep, the primary nurse can assume this responsibility. *Establish a record of sleep.* • If the hospital uses a flow sheet, label one column for sleep; cumulatively total hours of sleep over the 24-hour period. • Compare the child's usual sleep patterns with this guide from Chapter 20 and determine appropriate adjustments to meet the body's increased need for sleep and rest during illness.

Neonate	20–22 hr/24 hr
6 weeks	14–16 hr/24 hr
6 mo–1 year	12–16 hr/24 hr
1–3 years	10–14 hr/24 hr
3–5 years	12–14 hr/24 hr
6–9 years	11–12 hr/24 hr
10–12 years	9–10 hr/24 hr
Adolescent	8–10 hr/24 hr

Enforce naptimes by posting a sign such as, "Jeremy is asleep; please come back at 3:30." Usually other health care professionals will observe the request.
Decrease the child's anxiety related to hospitalization. (See Section II, diagnoses 8 and 10 of this nursing process plan.)
Plan the administration of analgesic medications so that discomfort does not interfere with sleep.
Assess whether sleeplessness may be a side effect of medications given, e.g., theophylline. Alert the physician as appropriate.

Figure 1-6. Elements of the nursing process plan.

sessment data for validation. The absence of these qualifying words implies that the nurse has sufficient assessment data to validate the diagnosis.

The *etiology* component of the nursing diagnosis gives precise information about the cause of the problem and is separated from the problem statement by the words "related to" (Carpenito, 1983). When the diagnosis relates to physical illness, the etiology often includes pathophysiologic mechanisms of disease. It is important that the etiology be as complete and as descriptive as possible. It is appropriate to list more than one cause. For example, the following diagnosis from Table 31-2 lists four specific causes for the altered play behavior:

> Diversional activity deficit: altered play behavior, related to

- separation from usual playmates/friends
- lack of interesting toys/diversional materials
- isolation associated with communicable disease
- immobility or discomfort associated with disease process or its treatment

The nursing diagnoses in this text frequently list multiple causes because these diagnoses serve as guidelines and need to be as inclusive as possible. In actual care planning the nurse would identify and list only those causes applicable to a *particular* client.

Sometimes the etiology will be so complex as to require more information than can be communicated in the "related to" clause. In this case the etiology statement can be extended by using the words *associated with.* The information in the "associated with" clause further explains the "related to" statement as in the following example:

> Ineffective individual coping related to crisis of hospitalization associated with multiple stressors of

- separation from parents and significant others
- unfamiliar environment
- harm, injury, and pain
- unclear limits and expectations
- loss of control

Clearly, the information added to this nursing diagnosis after "crisis of hospitalization" is important to direct the nurse's plan and execution of care.

Defining characteristics justify the assignment of the diagnosis. They communicate why the nurse has identified this particular problem. They usually include a combination of subjective and objective assessment data as in the following example from Table 31-2:

> Sleep pattern disturbance, related to anxiety associated with

- unfamiliar environment
- separation from parents/family
- discomfort of illness
- medications

> Definining Characteristics
> **Subjective:** Self-report or parental report of sleeplessness, restless, marked irritability
> **Objective:** Pale to grayish skin tones, dark circles under eyes, lethargy, frequent dozing but no prolonged periods of sleep

Developing a Plan of Care

In the planning phase, the nurse identifies client goals and outcome measures and the nursing goals and strategies that will accomplish them. Figure 1-6 provides an example of a plan that leads quite logically from the preceding diagnosis, *sleep pattern disturbance.*

As demonstrated in Figure 1-6, the client goal is actually the desired outcome of the nursing strategies. (Students who conceptualize client goals in this way may find them less troublesome to formulate.) The client goal is usually complex enough to require a specific list of evaluation criteria by which the nurse will know whether the goal has been met. The evaluation criteria usually refer back to, and attempt to reverse, the defining characteristics. (Compare the defining characteristics (④) with the evaluation criteria (⑥) in Figure 1-6.)

The nursing strategies section should be as specific as possible since the plan is designed to provide guidance for nurses who care for a child in the absence of the nurse who formulated the plan. *Nursing goals* for the strategies in Figure 1-6 are italicized. When nursing strategies are complex, the care plan will benefit from the assignment of nursing goals for each strategy grouping.

Within this text the word *strategies* often will be used to refer to nursing *interventions.* The term *strategies* is used deliberately to reflect the complex reasoning process used by the nurse in developing an action that is designed to accomplish a goal. We believe the word *strategy* connotes a more professional level of performance than the word *intervention.*

Nursing Process Plan Versus Individualized Care Plans. An important distinction exists between a nursing process plan and a care plan: a Nursing Process Plan provides general guidelines for *any* child with a similar condition; a care plan is individualized for a *specific* client. Nursing Process Plans, such as those found throughout this text, provide standards of

Table 1-6. Individualizing the Plan of Care from a Nursing Process Plan

Nursing Process Plan	Individualized Plan of Care
Determine usual sleep patterns, including naptime and bedtime routines and rituals	Johnny's usual sleep patterns: • Naps from 1–3 PM • Sleeps from 8 PM to 6 AM • Goes to sleep with pacifier and teddy bear. Pull drapes in PM to darken the room

excellence to guide the nurse in formulating a care plan specific to the needs of an individual child. They ensure that the major diagnoses commonly associated with a given condition will be considered in designing an individual plan of care and help maintain continuity and excellence in care among unit staff. *A Nursing Process Plan is never intended to be used without modification for individual needs.* When possible and where applicable, strategies in the individualized care plan should detail *what* will be done *when, where,* and *how.* Table 1-6 provides an example of individual modifications that might be made for the plan presented in Figure 1-6.

Implementing the Plan

Implementing the plan of care is a two-step process. Before actually implementing the strategies, they must be discussed with the client.

Discussing the Plan of Care with the Client.* The first phase of implementation is to discuss the plan with the child and at least one family member. *Failure to apprise the child and family of goals for care and proposed strategies to meet those goals communicates that their input and cooperation are unnecessary and that they have little or no control and few if any rights in the situation.* As detailed in the preceding section on intercultural communication, this discussion also affords the nurse the opportunity to ensure that goals and strategies are in accord with the family's values and beliefs. Goals and strategies that are attempted in ignorance of value conflicts (or in spite of them) have little chance for success.

Ideally, the plan of care should be presented to the family within a few hours of the child's admission. It need not be written in final form at this time because information gained during the interaction often results in additions or modifications. It usually takes only a few minutes to discuss the plan of care and to obtain input from the child and family. The information gained in this exchange of ideas will save the nurse a great deal of time in implementation and usually results in a more cooperative and less frightened parent and youngster.

Implementing the Plan. The implementation of a well-conceived plan is one of the joys of the nursing of children. At this point the nurse may realize some of the greatest rewards of the nursing role: the quieting of a fussy infant who cuddles into the nurse's arms, the smile on the face of a previously distraught child as pain is relieved, the relief in a parent's face when the treatment process is explained, the satisfaction of achieving a successful venipuncture. Quite frankly, isn't this the part of the nursing process that you envisioned as the whole of nursing when you first began your education? It is the "doing" phase. Every nurse must remember, however, that *doing* without adequate *planning* results, at best, in mediocrity.

Evaluating the Success of Nursing Strategies

Evaluation is often accomplished simultaneously with implementation. At this point the linear, point-by-point discussion of the nursing process breaks down. Evaluation is the least "linear" of any of the components. Rather, it is the impetus for recycling—for going back for more assessment and analysis, further planning, additional modifications, and new strategies. Evaluation is so natural to the experienced nurse as to be an integrated and essential part of each of the other components. Evaluation answers the question, "Did it work?" "Is this child making progress toward the goal, and if not, why not?" "Did I obtain the necessary data?" "Can I rely upon my findings and upon my interpretation?" "Is this an appropriate goal for this client?" "Are there more appropriate or more descriptive evaluation criteria for the goal?" "Did the strategies accomplish what I intended them to?" "Are there other strategies that might work better or faster?" "Is there a way to accomplish this with less stress to the child?"

Evaluation will be most effective when client input (subjective information) is elicited and used to make modifications in the plan. When working with children evaluation is often hindered by their lack of socialization into adult patterns of illness behavior. This factor makes it necessary to validate evaluation criteria with the child and parent. For example, a nurse who administered a pain medication 30 minutes ago and now finds the child lying quietly, watching television, might assume the medication was effective in reducing the pain. Upon questioning the child, however, the

**Client* is used to convey the child/family unit or any part of that unit. Since pediatric nursing so often involves at least one family member, the word *client* provides a concise way to connote consideration of the family.

Table 1-7. Nursing Process Plans

Chapter 27: Principles and Skills Adapted to the Care of Children	Nursing Process Plan: Perioperative Care
Chapter 29: Nursing Management of Pain in Children	Nursing Process Plan: The Child in Pain
Chapter 31: Nursing Care During Hospitalization	Nursing Process Plan: The Hospitalized Child
Chapter 32: Principles and Strategies of Home Care	Nursing Process Plan: Home Care
Chapter 35: Nursing Strategies: Emotional-Social Disturbances	Nursing Process Plan: The Child with Failure to Thrive
Chapter 38: Nursing Strategies: Altered Respiratory Function	(1) Nursing Process Plan: The Child with Respiratory Tract Dysfunction (2) Nursing Process Plan: The Child with an Acute Asthma Attack
Chapter 39: Nursing Strategies: Altered Cardiovascular Function	Nursing Process Plan: The Child with Congestive Heart Failure
Chapter 40: Nursing Strategies: Altered Hematologic Function	Nursing Process Plan: The Child with Anemia
Chapter 41: Nursing Strategies: Altered Digestive Function	Nursing Process Plan: The Child Following Abdominal Surgery
Chapter 42: Nursing Strategies: Altered Genitourinary Function	Nursing Process Plan: The Child Undergoing Dialysis Secondary to Chronic Renal Failure
Chapter 43: Nursing Strategies: Problems of the Immune System	(1) Nursing Process Plan: The Child on Corticosteroid Therapy (2) Nursing Process Plan: The Child with Atopic Dermatitis
Chapter 46: Nursing Strategies: Altered Neurologic Function	Nursing Process Plan: The Child with Increased Intracranial Pressure
Chapter 47: Nursing Strategies: Altered Musculoskeletal Function	Nursing Process Plan: The Child at Risk for Neurovascular Impairment Associated with Trauma, Traction or Casting
Chapter 48: Nursing Strategies: Aberrant Cell Growth	Nursing Process Plan: The Child Undergoing Chemotherapy
Chapter 49: Nursing Strategies: Altered Endocrine Function	Nursing Process Plan: The Child with Diabetic Ketoacidosis
Chapter 50: Nursing Strategies: Altered Metabolic Function	Nursing Process Plan: The Family in Need of Genetic Counseling
Chapter 51: Nursing Strategies: Sensory and Communication Alterations	Nursing Process Plan: The Child with an Identified Sensory Impairment
Chapter 52: Nursing Strategies: The Injured Child	Nursing Process Plan: The Child with Severe Burns

nurse might learn that "The hurt is still there, but it helps if I lie real still and try not to think about it." The action taken by the nurse in the latter instance would differ significantly from an action based upon the former evaluation.

The nursing process embodies the role of the professional nurse. This text provides information about illnesses in a nursing process format and includes nursing process plans designed to be applicable across a broad span of disease conditions. (Table 1-7 lists the Nursing Process Plans.) Nursing diagnoses are incorporated throughout the text to familiarize the reader with the use of NANDA-approved diagnoses. Unit III contains boxes detailing nursing diagnoses applicable to health promotion and related nursing goals and strategies.

References

American Nurses' Association: *Standards of Maternal–Child Health Nursing Practice.* Kansas City, MO, American Nurses'Association, 1973.

American Nurses' Association Commission on Nursing Research: *Guidelines for the Investigative Function of Nurses.* Kansas City, MO, ANA, 1981.
Austin G: A new age for pediatrics: change, challenge, and cost. *Pediatrics* 1982; 70(4):643–645.
Behrman RE, Vaughan VC: *Nelson's Textbook of Pediatrics.* Philadelphia, WB Saunders, 1987.
Belenky MF, Clinchy BM, Goldberger NR, et al: *Women's Ways of Knowing.* New York, Basic Books, 1986.
Benner P: *From Novice to Expert.* Menlo Park, CA, Addison-Wesley, 1984.
Bishop AH, Scudder JR: Nursing ethics in an age of controversy. *Adv Nurs Sci* 1987; 9(3):34–43.
Brodie B: Children: a glance at the past. *MCN* 1982; 7(4):219–20.
Brodie B: Yesterday, today and tomorrow's pediatric world. *CHC* 1986, Winter; 14(3):168–173.
Carpenito LJ: *Handbook of Nursing Diagnosis.* Philadelphia, JB Lippincott, 1983.
Carpenito LJ: *Nursing Diagnosis.* Philadelphia, JB Lippincott, 1984.
Cherry BS, Carty RM: Changing concepts of childhood in society. *Pediatr Nurs* 1986; 112(6):421–424.
Curtin LL: The nurse as advocate: a philosophical foundation for nursing. *In* Chinn PL (ed): *Ethical Issues in Nursing.* Rockville, MD, Aspen Systems Corporation, 1986, 11–20.
Dolan JA, Fitzpatrick ML, Herrmann EK: *Nursing in Society: A Historical Perspective,* 15th ed. Philadelphia, WB Saunders, 1983.
Fawcett J: Hallmarks of success in nursing research. *Adv Nurs Sci* 1984 Oct; 7(1):1–11.
Foster RL: A prism model for nursing within the new paradigm. Unpublished manuscript, University of Colorado Health Services Center, 1986.
Fromer MJ: Solving ethical dilemmas in nursing practice. *In* Chinn PL (ed): *Ethical Issues in Nursing.* Rockville, MD, Aspen Systems Corporation, 1986, 81–87.
Goodman MA: The culture of childhood. New York, Teacher's College Press, Columbia University, 1970.
Gordon M: *Nursing Diagnosis; Process and Application.* New York, McGraw-Hill, 1987.
Green M, Hoekelman RA: Trends in the education of pediatricians. *Pediatrics* 1982; 29:325–350.
Grosso C, Barden M, Henry C, et al: The Vietnamese American family . . . and grandma makes three. *MCN* 1981, May/Jun; 6:177–180.
Guyer B, Gallagher SS: An approach to the epidemiology of childhood injuries. *Pediatr Clin North Am* 1985; 32(1):5–15.
Hall ET: *The Hidden Dimension.* New York, Anchor Books, 1969.
Hall ET: *The Dance of Life.* New York, Anchor Books, 1984.
Halloran MC: Rational ethical judgments utilizing a decision-making tool. *Heart Lung* 1982; 11(6):566–570.
Hoekelman RA, Starfield B, McCormick M, et al: A profile of pediatric practice in the United States. *Am J Dis Child* 1983; 137:1057–1060.
Infant mortality among black Americans. *Morbid Mortal Weekly Report* 1987; 36(1):1–4, 9–10.
Lee DD: *Valuing the Self: What We Can Learn from Other Cultures.* Englewood Cliffs, NJ, Prentice-Hall, 1976.
Lerner RM: *Concepts and Theories of Human Development.* Menlo Park, CA, Addison-Wesley, 1976.
Levine ME: Nursing ethics and the ethical nurse. *Am J Nurs* 1977; 77(5):845.
Levine MD, Carey WB, Crocker AC, et al: *Developmental-Behavioral Pediatrics.* Philadelphia, WB Saunders, 1983.
McCombs RS: *Diseases of Children for Nurses.* Philadelphia, WB Saunders, 1907.
Magrab PR: Services for children: challenge for the 1980s. *J Pediatr Psychol* 1982; 7(2):105–110.
Meleis AI: *Theoretical Nursing: Development and Progress.* Philadelphia, JB Lippincott, 1985.
Moynihan DP: *Family and Nation.* San Diego, Harcourt, Brace, Jovanovich, 1987.
Nadler HL, Evans WJ: The future of pediatrics. *Am J Dis Child* 1987; 141(1):21–27.
Noyes EJ: Children: a priority? *Nurs Econ* 1985; 3(3):136–139.
Oberg CN: Pediatrics and poverty. *Pediatrics* 1987; 79(4):567–568.
O'Conner C, Murr A, Wingert P: Affluent America's forgotten children. *Newsweek,* 1986 Jun 2:20–21.
Patient Mix by Diagnostic Categories 1983. National Association of Children's Hospitals and Related Institutions, 1985.
Pedersen AB, Pedersen PB: The cultural grid: a personal cultural orientation. *In* Samovar LA, Porter RE (eds): *Intercultural Communication: A Reader.* 4th ed. Belmont, CA, Wadsworth Publishing Company, 1985, 50–61.
Porter RE, Samovar LA: Approaching intercultural communication. *In* Samovar LA, Porter RE (eds): *Intercultural Communication: A Reader.* 4th ed. Belmont, CA, Wadsworth Publishing Company, 1985, 15 39.
Quinn CA, Smith MD: *The Professional Commitment: Issues and Ethics in Nursing.* Philadelphia, WB Saunders, 1987.
Rew L: Nursing intuition. Too powerful—and too valuable—to ignore. *Nurs 87* 1987; 17(7):43–45.
Romero R: Autobiographical scrapbooks: a coping tool for hospitalized school children. *Issues Compr Pediatr Nurs* 1986; 9(4):247–258.
Sigman P: Ethical choice in nursing. *In* Chinn PL (ed): *Ethical Issues in Nursing.* Rockville, MD, Aspen Systems Corporation, 1986, 21–36.
Silverstein NG: Lillian Wald at Henry Street, 1893–1895. *Adv Nurs Sci* 1985, Jan; 7(2):1–12.
Singer MR: Culture: a perceptual approach. *In* Samovar LA, Porter RE (eds): *Intercultural Communication: A Reader.* 4th ed. Belmont, CA, Wadsworth Publishing Company, 1985.
Takanishi R: Childhood as a social issue: historical roots of contemporary child advocacy. *J Social Issues* 1978;23(2):8–28
Thompson RH: Where we stand: twenty years of research on pediatric hospitalization and health care. Child Health Care 1986 Spring; 14(4):200–210.
Thompson JE, Thompson HO: *Bioethical Decision Making*

for Nurses. Norwalk, CT, Appleton-Century-Crofts, 1985.

UNICEF: *The State of the World's Children.* Oxfordshire, UK, Oxford University Press, 1986.

Vaughan VC: The field of pediatrics. *In* Behrman RE, Vaughan VC (eds): *Nelson Textbook of Pediatrics.* 13th ed. Philadelphia, WB Saunders, 1987, 1-5.

Wallace H: Policies regarding health and social welfare of mothers and children in the United States. *Clin Pediatr* 1983; 22(1):14-21.

Wegman ME: Annual summary of vital statistics—1984. *Pediatrics* 1985; 76(6):861-871.

Whitman D, Thornton J, Shapiro JP, et al: America's hidden poor. US News World Report 1988 Jan 11; 104(1):18-24.

Wood-Allen M: *What a Young Woman Ought to Know.* London, Vir Publishing Company, 1905.

Youth suicide—United States, 1970-1980. *Morbid Mortal Weekly Report* 1987; 36(6):87-88.

Bibliography

Bailey CF: Withholding or withdrawing treatment on handicapped newborns. *Pediatr Nurs* 1986 12(6):413-416.

Baretich DM, Anderson LB: Should we diagnose strengths? No: stick to the problems. *Am J Nurs* 1987 Sept; 87(9):1211-1212.

Bishop AH, Scudder JR (eds): *Caring, Curing, Coping: Nurse, Physician, Patient Relationships.* Birmingham, University of Alabama, 1985.

Bushweller E: Why pediatric office nursing? *MCN* 1985; 10(6):408-410.

DeMaio D: Self-determination, the right of a profession. *J NY State Nurs Assoc* 1982 Dec; 13(4):8-17.

Feldman HR: Practice may make perfect but research makes a difference. Nurs 87 1987 Mar; 17(3):34-35.

Fleming JW: Maternal-child nursing in the decade ahead. *MCN* 1985; 10(6):369-376.

Frick S: Pediatric psychosocial research: a concern of all children's health care professionals. *Child Health Care* 1986 Spring; 14(4):196-197.

Heineken J, Roberts FB: Confirming, not disconfirming: communicating in a more positive manner. *MCN* 1983; 8(1):78-80.

Hoskins LM, McFarlane EA, Rubenfeld MG, et al: Nursing diagnosis in the chronically ill: methodology for clinical validation. *Adv Nurs Sci* 1986 Apr; 8(3):80-89.

Jackson PL, Runyon N: Caring for children from divorced families. *MCN* 1983; 8(2):126-130.

Landis D, Brislin RW: *Handbook of intercultural training.* Vol II. New York, Pergamon Press, 1983.

Leacock EB: *The Culture of Poverty.* New York, Simon & Schuster, 1971.

Leff EW: Ethics and patient teaching. *MCN* 1986; 11:375-378.

McClowry SG: Research and treatment: ethical distinction related to the care of children. *J Pediatr Nurs* 1987; 2(1):23-29.

Miller CA, Fine A, Adams-Taylor S, et al: *Monitoring Children's Health: Key Indicators.* Washington DC, American Public Health Association, 1986.

Mitchell C, Rutherford PA: Dilemmas in practice: the fragile survivor. *AJN* 1987; 87(5):603-606.

Popkess-Vawter S, Pinnell N: Should we diagnose strengths? Yes: accentuate the positive. *Am J Nurs* 1987 Sept; 87(9):1211,1216.

Rae WA, Fournier CJ: Ethical issues in pediatric research: preserving psychosocial care in scientific inquiry. *Child Health Care* 1986; 14(4):242-248.

Sandelowski M: The politics of parenthood. *MCN* 1986; 11(4):235-238.

Switzer KH, Kelly JT: The nurse: a member of the school team. *MCN* 1981; 6(3):189-192.

Van Steenkiste S: Adoptive parents need special reassurance. *MCN* 1981; 6(2):122.

Veatch RM, Fry ST: *Case Studies in Nursing Ethics.* Philadelphia, JB Lippincott, 1987.

Walker LO: Identifying parents in need: an approach to adoptive parenting. *MCN* 1981; 6(2):118-123.

Withrow C, Fleming JW: Pediatric social illness: a challenge to nurses. *Issues Compr Pediatr Nurs* 1983; Jul-Aug; 6(4):261-275.

Yura H, Walsh MB: *The Nursing Process.* 4th ed. Norwalk, CT, Appleton-Century-Crofts, 1983.

The Developing Family

Chapter 2

Anna Frances Z. Wenger
Jo Joyce Anderson

The quality of family life and the health of its members form a symbiotic relationship. No other aspect of a child's life has a more lasting impact on the child's development — physically, socially, culturally — than the family experience.

This chapter introduces the facets of healthy family life — its structure, functions, and roles — in its many constructs. The chapter also familiarizes the reader with the cultural and lifestyle factors that serve as a milieu for the family unit's growth and development. This knowledge is valuable to the pediatric nurse in any setting since the family system is the critical variable in the success or failure of each child to achieve optimal health.

Related Topics
The effects of poverty on child health, Chapter 1
Intercultural communication, Chapter 1
The effect of culture and lifestyle on development, Chapter 3
Communicating with children and families, Chapter 11
Assessing and promoting family health, Chapter 12
Promoting healthy parenting, Chapter 13

A child is a transient who comes into the lives of parents for a brief period. He stays only a few years before he must be on his way to his own fulfillment. Mothers and fathers should live with each child so that they are happy to greet that child when he comes to them and happy to see him go when the time comes for going.

—*Margaret and Willard Beecher*

Defining Family

In a world that places ever-increasing and changing demands on the family, a very fluid definition is required: *The family unit is a living, open system of reacting and interacting persons who group themselves together with a central purpose to create and maintain a common culture that aims to promote progressive and holistic development of each of its members.*

Regardless of how the members of the family units group themselves together or whether they reside in the same household, their effect upon each other is significant and generically similar. In each family unit there are (1) *relationships* that are distinctly *purposeful and highly intimate,* (2) *shared values and goals,* and (3) *extensive communication systems* to which each member makes a contribution.

This concept of the family as an interacting whole in an open system with an intimate environment encourages the nurse to work with the client in the context of the family (i.e., family-centered nursing). Comprehensive planning will yield more effective interventions of longer-lasting impact. Because families are highly individualistic in structure, lifestyle, and interactions viewing them in a developmental sequence helps the nurse make some predictions about a family's behaviors, needs, and potential conflicts.

Family: A Historical Perspective

Looking at how the family has evolved historically helps one better understand the realities of contemporary family life. *Nurses must learn not to inappropriately diagnose as unhealthy or aberrant those family forms with which they are unfamiliar.* When one recognizes the changing forms of "family" through history, one can be objective about the many options in family composition that are possible today. A historical perspective also reinforces the premise of anthropologists that, while the form or composition of "family" varies greatly, certain *functions* or *tasks* continue constant for families through history and regardless of the form chosen.

Historically the family has taken the form of *extension* (an extended family pattern in which parents, children, and other related kin sustain themselves either under the same roof or on attached or nearby homesteads, with shared daily activities) and *contraction* (a nuclear family pattern in which a couple and their children exist separate from other relatives and maintain their separate routine of daily activities). The rhythm of these modes follows modification of the political order and economic conditions. Throughout time, people have continually shown imagination in the construction of various styles of family living and different ways of relating the family to the larger community, each experiment again reaffirming the family as the basic unit of human living, of social stability, and of health. A growth process is continually in evidence, moving the family, in its hundred variations, toward a more symmetric form of living. We have progressed from a preindustrial (agricultural) family, housed rurally, to an industrial (traditional) family in urban residence, and, further, to a postindustrial (modern) family with a suburban or small town abode. Table 2-1 illustrates some of the differences in each stage of this historical growth process.

These stages are presented here as a frame of reference for the nurse because, even though we are today in a postindustrial social era, the socioeconomic status of an individual family often will influence what particular stage a given family is in, with the accompanying characteristics of that stage. For example, a family of lower socioeconomic status in this postindustrial era still may closely resemble an early industrial (Stage II) family with some Stage I (preindustrial) elements; a "blue-collar" middle class family in this post-industrial era still often resembles the Stage II (industrial) family; the "white-collar" middle and upper classes are most likely to reflect the Stage III (postindustrial) family in their lifestyle. Familiarity with the characteristics that accompany these stages of family living will help the nurse identify the lifestyle patterns and attitudes that the family with whom she is interacting is likely to show. The nurse can then relate to them in a way that accommodates their living patterns and considers their family attitudes.

Regardless of its lifestyle, the family provides for some satisfactions that are hard to come by and sustain anywhere but in a family setting. The healthy family unit provides "roots" for its members, offering them love, intimacy, and companionship that is ongoing and noncontingent. A link between the past and future, one's family offers a foundation for the present and for one's continuity and stability through time. The family continues to be the most economic and efficient agent for the raising of children, although child care responsibilities change, owing to factors such as decreased family size, increased leisure hours, increased num-

Our thanks to Dee Gerken, who contributed to the section on alternative family lifestyles.

Table 2-1. A Historical Perspective on the Stages of Symmetric Growth in Family Living

Purpose	Goal	Motivation	Structure/Roles	Orientation	Societal Expectations
I Preindustrial (agricultural)					
Economic unit of production	Self-sufficiency	Survival	Closed system; patriarchal structure; dictatorial governance; rigidly defined roles; childrearing = 54% of married life	Children were economic necessities, assets, viewed as possessions. Treated as miniature adults with early indoctrination into adult responsibilities and strong lines between right and wrong	Economic security; protection; religious training; recreation; education; reproduction; health care
II Industrial (traditional)					
Consumptive unit; work-oriented	Success, domesticity	Quantity of living; accumulation of goods; power	Emerging open system; less patriarchal, but husband still head of household and final authority. Autocratic governance; clearly defined roles but not rigid	Children seen as an economic liability after enactment of child labor laws. Early assumption of adult role—contribute to the family income by age 16 or 18	Reproduction; religious training; class and status-conferring; privacy; identity-conferring
III Postindustrial (modern)					
Consumptive unit; leisure-oriented	Self-actualization of members and independence; enhancing potentials of members	Quality of living; harmony	Open symmetric system; shared equalitarian structure. Democratic governance; de-differentiation of roles—flexible and negotiable, depending on who is available and the situation; childrearing = 18% of married life	Children seen as an economic liability borne by choice, viewed as persons in their own right. Late assumption of adult role, average at age 21–22 years. Obligation to family is to develop own potentials	Provision of physical needs; fulfillment of emotional and love needs. Nurturing—preparing child's personality for modern world; companionship

bers of mothers in the work force, and increases in single-parent family structures.

Establishing a Family System: Family Coping

A family system may take various forms and is established through legal (marriage) or extralegal (living together) means. Its members demonstrate a commitment to the family unit, with the intent of some degree of permanence. The commitment is usually based on emotional attachments among the family members, and the unit's permanance primarily depends on a continuation of those attachments. Every healthy family system contains some tensions, produced as a result of the attachments between various family members. A family unit that displays excessive tension (enmeshed) or no tension (disengaged) is usually dysfunctional. (See Chapter 12 for a discussion of dysfunctional families.) Family goals, structure, and functioning are all adaptive in an attempt to achieve and maintain equilibrium within the family system.

Coping Through Family Goals and Values

Family goals and values must be considered on three levels: (1) goals and values of the total family unit; (2) goals and values of the marital dyad or parental members; and (3) goals and values of each individual family member. The goals of a family satisfy the affiliation

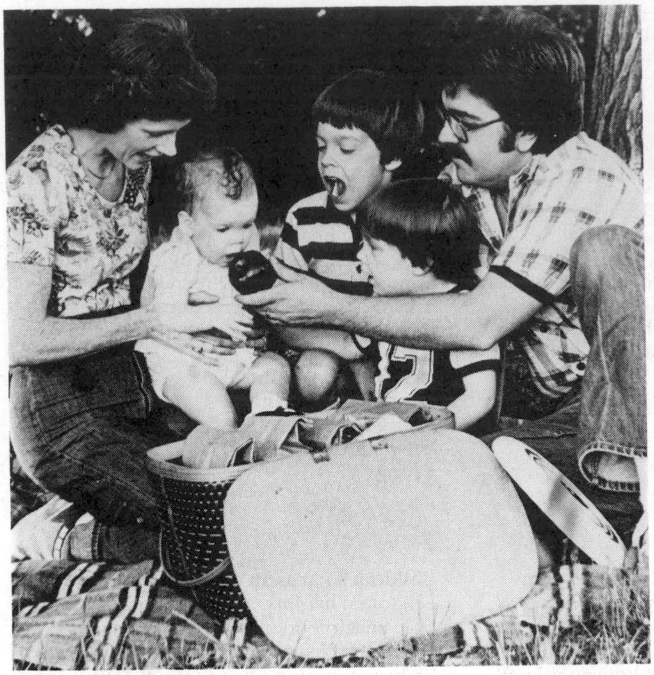

Families structure time for their members. Strong families plan frequent joint activities.

needs of each member and maintain family cohesiveness. They determine the way a family accomplishes its activities of daily living (lifestyle) and the degree to which a family relies on other institutions for its socialization (e.g., family-created recreation as opposed to recreation obtained at the "Y" or the park recreation program). Their goals reflect the family members' social status, their value systems, and how they feel about their reason for being. The nurse who knows a family's goals knows the family's priorities. For example, is present gratification most important, or has the family a future orientation? Are children valued as important members of the family, or are they seen primarily as expensive liabilities produced and tolerated out of social expectation? Are healthy life habits a purposeful part of family behavior or merely present by accident or circumstance?

Family goals also profoundly influence developmental tasks at every phase in the family life cycle. In the emerging family, the way two individuals go about adjusting to living as a married couple (a developmental task) greatly depends on the family goals they have formed. An expanding* family can be expected to care for and nurture its children to the extent that such activities are consistent with family goals and values. A contracting† family will release its young adults from the family unit in a manner that does not compromise family goals.

All families are obligated to meet certain societally defined goals in order to assist their members to develop socially acceptable relationships. These goals validate the necessity for and existence of families. They can be categorized into four major areas of responsibility:

- Security and survival
- Emotional and social development and maintenance
- Sexual differentiation and teaching
- Growth of individual members

Security and Survival. The family unit is responsible for its own physical and biologic maintenance. This involves providing for food, clothing, and shelter; managing reproductive considerations of planning and controlling family size; recruiting and releasing family members; obtaining health care for members; apportioning both tangible (goods, facilities, income) and intangible (space, affection, authority) resources; and maintaining reasonable divisions of labor (assigning responsibility for income, household tasks, child care, and so forth). Because this responsibility is a societal expectation in North America, social institutions have developed to assist families who do not or cannot meet it on their own.

Emotional and Social Development and Maintenance. Responsibilities of this goal include support to family members during periods of stress (morale maintenance), enforcement of a system of social controls that involves rewards and punishment (motivation maintenance), support and acknowledgement of efforts to achieve (ego maintenance), channeling of sexual and affectional drives and establishing effective patterns of communication (maintenance of order), enculturation, and preparing members for a place in society by protecting them from undesirable outside influences and by establishing each member's ties and status within the family, the community, and its institutions. Although American society sets some primarily legal minimums on this family responsibility, there is great latitude in what families assume.

Sexual Differentiation and Teaching. This goal involves the family's responsibility for nurturing its members, especially child care and rearing, teaching members their roles and responsibilities, fostering the development of conscience, and supporting the learning of hobbies and skills that will produce healthy, capable adults. American society fluctuates culturally and geographically in the degree to which social institutions (mostly schools) help families fulfill this responsibility.

Growth of Individual Members. Responsibility here is to guide the internalization of increasingly

* Expanding means that the number of family members is increasing through birth, adoption, etc.

† Contracting means family members within the household are decreasing through going off to college, marriage, death, etc.

mature and acceptable patterns of physical, intellectual, and emotional-social behavior in each member (socialization, personality development) by fostering gradually expanding independence, encouraging problem solving, and supporting each member's efforts to adjust to her or his changing body. Schools have a steadily increasing involvement with families in achieving this goal, especially as more children are introduced to school or day care at younger ages.

The manner in which these four goals are performed and the degree to which they are accomplished varies with the family's socioeconomic status, cultural orientation, and place within its life cycle; but these responsibilities do confront all families regardless of the integrative or destructive factors involved.

Division of family goals into these four categories facilitates the nurse's assessment of where the family is in its development of responsibility for itself and its members. Using this assessment to implement the nursing process is discussed in Chapter 12.

Coping Through Family Structure

Family structure refers to the pattern of inter-relatedness within the family unit. A unique feature of family structure is intimacy.

Today's rapidly changing expectations and demands make this characteristic of families highly appealing. In an era when little remains constant and most relationships outside the family are temporary and founded on numerous contingencies, which lends them a fragile nature, the source of security is ideally the noncontingent, love-based, enduring, and close relationships at home. In a healthy, intimate climate, family members learn to live in harmony despite their differences, children become social beings, and the foundation for happiness and health is derived. In such a home, members can be themselves, experience and express a diversity of feelings, and know that they are still accepted. No other institution in modern society allows this degree of intimacy or unconditional caring. However, it is unrealistic to believe that all homes actually create this desirable environment. The nurse needs to assess the extent to which this characteristic exists in a family and intervene, with the help of the health care team, when deficiencies are apparent (see Chapter 12).

The family structure is a complexity of interaction (subsystems) and communication patterns that are controlled by boundaries. Through these interaction-communication patterns a family relates to life outside and one member's actions are stimulated by the behaviors of other members. In simplest terms, family interaction is the sum total of all the roles performed within a given family. The roles (goal-directed patterns of behaving that an individual carries out in interactions with a given role partner) of family members are defined by the boundaries within the family and those established by society.

Boundaries are like rules. They define the degree of input one subsystem will accept from other subsystems and specify who may participate in a particular subsystem. These boundaries, or norms, also define the extent that one can interact with members of other subsystems. A boundary may be healthy or unhealthy, and its permeability varies. A particular norm may be so rigid that little or no input is tolerated from other subsystems or that a member of a particular subsystem is virtually isolated from one or more other subsystems. Conversely, a boundary may be so diffuse that a subsystem's membership is ambiguous, or the communication permitted is unclear or inconsistent.

Each family member participates in various subsystems or interactions and has different functions, influence, and power within each. One's position in a given situation or subsystem is the basis for the role(s) assumed, and thus both position and role may fluctuate, depending on who the role partner is in an interaction. For example, a man might enact roles as follows with the accompanying role partners:

Position Role	*Position Partner*
Husband	Wife
Father	Child
Son	Father
Brother	Sibling
Employee	Employer

A broader discussion of role prescriptions within a family unit will be presented later in this chapter.

The roles acquired (e.g., oldest child, female) or achieved or adopted (e.g., breadwinner,* parent, spouse) by family members largely determine the nature of family communication and with whom it occurs. As a society takes over more of the functions of a family or its members through agencies outside the family unit, fewer roles are required of each member. As the number of roles a family member has decreases, the remaining roles become increasingly significant and are performed more ardently. This societally imposed decrease in roles tends to produce within the family more intense relationships. Simultaneously, having fewer roles with their entailed responsibility allows for more freedom and time to experiment with the remaining roles (role flexibility) and for role fluidity (exchanges in role tasks among members as the family situation dictates).

Minuchin's (1974) classic investigation of family structure disclosed three extremely significant subsystems within the family: (1) spousal, (2) parental, and (3) sibling.

---

* A role open to either or both spouses in many homes today.

Spousal Subsystem. In a healthy *spousal subsystem* each spouse supports the other, being mutually interdependent while yielding some separateness. If the boundaries of this subsystem are too rigid the spouses become isolated, whereas diffuse boundaries leave the spousal subsystem vulnerable to intrusion and disruption by other subsystems. This theory of spousal harmony was reinforced by Schlesinger (1983), whose research investigated the factors that make the spousal subsystem durable and permanent. He found ten consistent factors, listed here in order of importance: (1) respect for each other; (2) trust in each other; (3) loyalty; (4) love for each other; (5) being able to rely on each other; (6) consideration by each for the other's needs; (7) providing emotional support to each other; (8) commitment by both to making the marriage last; (9) fidelity; and (10) give-and-take in communication and in tasks of daily living. Scott and Scott (1983) investigated the spousal relationship and found that in the spousal subsystem in healthy families, a "love style" was demonstrated by each spouse and each observed boundaries providing both private and mutual territory in work, play, and decision making.

Parental Subsystem. The power and authority established by the *parental subsystem* is also important to family harmony. Children, says Minuchin (1974), need access to the parental subsystem but not to the spousal subsystem. The parental subsystem forms when the spousal subsystem differentiates to care for children. The most critical aspect of the parental coalition is decision making and task allocation. The spousal subsystem serves as a mutual support system to the parental subsystem.

In single-parent families, the spousal and parental subsystems are either absent or are created in a surrogate fashion. A child (often the oldest) may be singled out to help the single parent accomplish parenting responsibilities. Or a live-in adult partner of the single parent may assume a surrogate spousal subsystem, parental subsystem, or both. In blended families the spousal and parental subsystems are potentially compromised by numerous stressors unique to the stepparent situation. (See Chapter 13 for further discussion of these family structures in relation to parenting.)

Sibling Subsystem. Siblings tend to identify with each other and to make comparisons of their skills. This identification leads either to competition in trying to outdo each other or to the intentional development of very different behaviors and skills to gain each other's respect and parental recognition. Birth order significantly affects the boundaries within sibling subsystems (Toman, 1976). Oldest siblings tend to have the advantage of more personal attention from their parents but have higher expectations placed upon them. Successive children experience fewer expectations and have more leeway for individualism; however, they also tend to receive less of their parents' time and attention. In the process of learning how to cope effectively with each other, siblings learn how to relate to peers. Though the sibling subsystem may appear within the home environment to be wracked with rivalry, it tends to be cohesive and supportive when a sibling faces adversity from outside the subsystem. It is not unusual to see siblings who are seemingly continual irritants to each other stand shoulder to shoulder in support of each other when confronted by the "neighborhood bully." The children in sibling subsystems need relative autonomy without undue parental interference.

Coping through Family Functioning

The matrix for family functioning, i.e., the process by which a family operates to accomplish its goals, is communication. All transactions within the family, its subsystems, and its supra systems (school, church) depend upon the clarity and congruence of that communication.

Communication is a complex process through which families relate feelings (affective communication) and information (instrumental communication). Through feedback a family provides output to its suprasystems and receives from these systems input that helps determine how well they are functioning. Some families require the assistance of health professionals to interpret feedback and make changes.

Some families have difficulty functioning satisfactorily because they have *deficits in resources* with which to achieve their goals. Poverty, an increasing problem in America affecting one of every five children, usually means a deficit in most, if not all, of the resources needed to function at a level consistent with societal expectations. One in six Caucasian children, about 40 per cent of Hispanics, and half of black children come from such resource-scarce, impoverished homes (US Census Bureau, 1984). Depleted resources may include problem-solving skills, information, money, health, friends, and so on.

A great deal of energy is discernible in interactions among family members. Energy may be dispersed as spontaneity, as tension, or as conflict. Spontaneous energy is conveyed through attentiveness, directness, and eye contact between members. Such communication contains more humor, touch, and laughing. Tension is inherent in all family systems, though the degree varies. The tension may be generated from inside or outside the system and is more prevalent when autonomy is threatened. The normal changes produced by individual and family development generate much psychic tension. Tension is sometimes released through family arguments. The health professional should not confuse such stress-releasing behaviors with disagreement. Arguments can be helpful to family members in clarifying issues or negotiating differences. The energy released in conflict is usually the result of a building up of tensions that produces a disturbance in the positive feelings or bonds experienced by members. The effect is family disequilibrium. Occasional family conflict that results in negotiations and problem resolution within the family is a normal process in a closely aligned group (Murphy, 1983). For example, a young working couple with an ill child may find themselves in conflict over which of them is going to cancel business appointments to stay home until their son is over the flu and can return to the day care center. They will need to bargain and negotiate to arrive at an arrangement that both find fair. Nursing intervention is not needed in this type of episodic conflict. Intervention is in order, however, if conflict becomes the usual mode of interaction among family members, leading to constant disequilibrium and perhaps even to family violence. At this point the nurse should encourage the family to see a psychologist or professional family counselor to help them break the unhealthy cycle. For in depth discussion of family dysfunction, see Chapter 12.

What holds families together in light of the many elements that can cause tension, conflict, or family dissolution? Family bonds are the emotional ties that initially draw a family together and, if nurtured, hold the family together. The strength of these bonds greatly affects the quality of family living. When bonding is flexible and adaptive, shared values and family consensus can be maintained much of the time. If these bonds erode without suitable replacement in the form of new attachments, the family's ability to resolve conflict is diminished, children become uneasy and display stressful behaviors, and the likelihood increases that one or both spouses will look outside the family unit for alternative bonds.

Four characteristic forms of bonding may be observed in the family unit (Miller and Janosik, 1980). *Membership gratification bonds* give the individual a sense of esteem and validation through association with the family group or subsystems within the family. These bonds may not be strong enough or compelling enough to endure over time, especially if family position is not particularly prestigious or if membership involves conflict. *Task bonds* develop when goals to be achieved cannot be achieved alone. These bonds are usually ongoing and cumulative even though specific goals may change. *Person bonds* may result from a desire to associate with or emulate a family member(s) seen as highly desirable or who has valued traits. These bonds may also develop as a response to another family member's admiration, e.g., big brother–little sister bonds. Such bonds are usually strong and increase over time, especially if reciprocal. The strongest, most enduring and unwavering bonds are *crescive bonds.* These bonds emerge from time shared or invested together, blended with memories and shared experiences. They usually involve a substantial interdependence and sense of responsibility toward each other. Such bonds are built on communication at varying levels and are supported by one's sense that the other person's well being is closely related to one's own actions.

Family Life Cycle and Developmental Tasks: Potential for Stress

Families, like children, are born, develop, mature, and age. At each stage families, like children, are faced with new developmental tasks requiring a reorganization of roles, communication patterns, and goals. Families, like children, are affected by situational crises (illness, change or loss of income, change in family composition), maturational crises of individual members, or altered social and environmental conditions (inflation, war, move to a new locale).

Duvall's (1977) eight stages in the family life cycle are presented in Table 2-2. Remember that clear-cut stages can be described only for families with one child. Stages in family developmental tasks overlap in multiple-child families. Still, the family life cycle approach emphasizes the dynamics of family interaction as shifting and changing from one period to another in a family's life span. This approach also helps illustrate how family developmental tasks parallel those of individual family members, sometimes complementing each other. For example, in beginning families a developmental task of the unit is the establishment of satisfactory sexual relations, a task that complements or facilitates each spouses' developmental task of achieving intimacy. At other times tasks are in conflict: for example, in a childrearing family a family developmental task is to provide sufficient income to meet the increasing costs of family living, which usually requires that the parent(s) be away from home a great deal, yet the individual task of the parent now is to become an effective parent (generativity), which requires time investments within the home. The nurse's role is to act as facilitator or change agent to promote acceptance and successful accomplishment of tasks by the family (refer to Table 2-2).

At whatever stage in the life cycle a family is when a nurse interacts with it, the family's developing relationships should be assessed and supported. Interventions should be planned so that the family members can be kept together as much as possible, and action should promote progressive mastery of individual member and family group tasks by the family unit. Ongoing anticipatory guidance at each stage facilitates

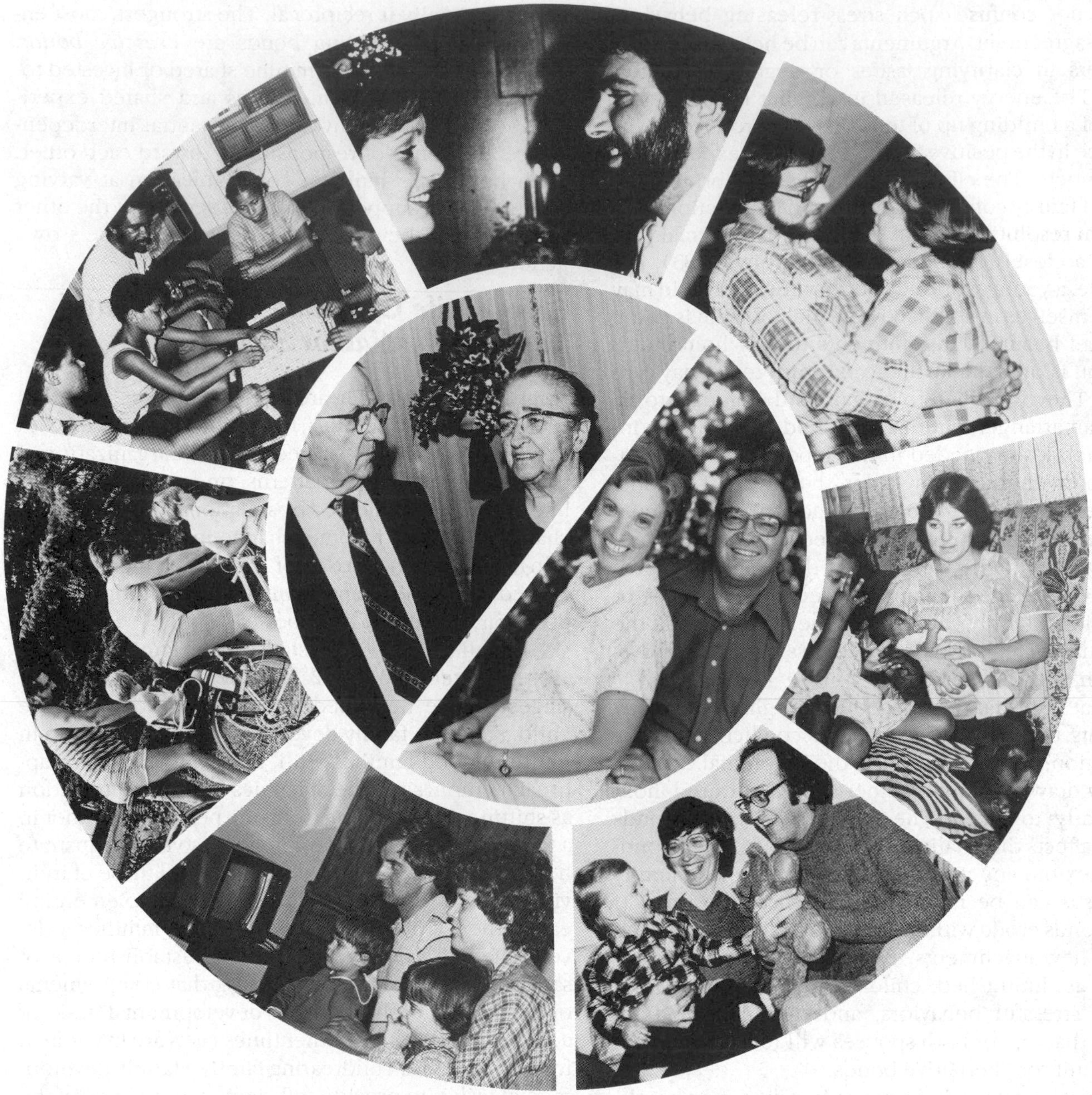

The cycle of family growth: Families, like children, are born, develop, mature, and age.

the nurse's aim of helping the family members help themselves and accept assistance confidently when it is needed.

Family Coping and Role Prescriptions

Although each stage has unique developmental tasks for the family, the nurse can use some tasks common to all stages as an assessment guide as to how the family is generally coping with their development. These common tasks are summarized on page 62.

Traditional roles, that is, roles clearly defined on the basis of sex and family position, are not functional in most families today. Clearly defined roles do not allow for individual uniqueness or particular family needs, both of which are major concerns in modern families. Rigidly fixed roles can suppress valuable aspects of the role-bearer's personality and foster guilt when the individual's feeling and desires do not agree with rigid role expectations. Contrary to earlier beliefs, clearly differentiated roles do not seem necessary for

Text continues on page 61

Table 2-2. The Family Life Cycle and Associated Developmental Tasks

Stage	Individual/Positional Developmental Tasks	Family Group Developmental Tasks
The Emerging Family		
Stage 1 (approx. 2 years) **Beginning Family** (Married couple without children)		
Establishment phase (Wedding day to confirmation of first pregnancy)	Individual adults: intimacy Spouses: adjustment to life as a couple without loss of individual identity	Establish the marriage Sexual adjustment • Relinquish childhood inhibitions, prohibitions • Achieve reciprocal gratification • Family planning Reshape family and social relationships • Establish own home unit • Develop workable philosophy of life as a couple • Accept separation from parents • Establish mutual friends compatible with the marriage Accept new roles as husband and wife and as potential parents • Mutually satisfying, realistic economic arrangement (income and budget) • System of open communication • Ways of expressing and accommodating differences creatively • Satisfactory division of labor, responsibility
Expectant phase (Confirmation of pregnancy to birth of baby)	Individual adults: continuing intimacy and emerging generativity Spouses: maintaining a basic relationship as a married couple while beginning integration of a perception of selves as parents	Adjustment to pregnancy Re-evaluate division of labor and responsibility Adapt sexual relations to pregnant state Adapt relationship with relatives and friends to realities of pregnancy Maintain family members' morales Preparation for the parent role Develop new economic arrangements to accommodate changes in income/expenses as needed Expand communication system to consider present heightened emotional needs and addition of new child Acquire knowledge about and plan for specifics of pregnancy, childbirth, parenthood Arrange for the physical care of the expected baby Adjust family goals to incorporate new roles
The Expanding Family		
Stage 2 (approx. 2.5 years) **Childbearing Family** (From birth of first child until 30 months old)		
Exaltation phase (From birth until parents take baby home)	Individual adults: accept parenthood (generativity) Spouses: accept each other as parents and companions Parents: learn basic infant care	Realizing the child really exists Accept new or added responsibility (Re)orient to parent role Begin bonding with child

continued

Table 2-2. *(continued)*

Stage	Individual/Positional Developmental Tasks	Family Group Developmental Tasks
	Infant: trust; develop physiological skills of survival (sleep, suck, swallow, primitive coordination)	Adjusting family life to incorporate new baby
Homecoming phase (From time child is taken home to third month)	Spouses: regain intimacy and develop marital relationship Parents: develop confidence and competence in parenting role and child care; learn baby's cues Infant: settling into a routine Siblings: trust → autonomy; begin separation from mother; make room for new baby in relationships with parents	Support during members' mood swings (postpartum blues, baby settling in, sibling jealousy) Realignment of division of labor and responsibility to compensate for member fatigue and 24-hour care Father accept provider role at least temporarily (or some external resource if single parent family, e.g., mother's parents, government supplement program such as ADC)
Stabilization phase (3rd through 30th month of baby's life)	Parents: learning to accept growth and development of child(ren), to accept displays of selfhood, to recognize "teachable moments" in child's development Child(ren): learn to handle self and own will	Establishing a stable family unit; making a home for all members Adapt resources to accommodate child(ren) • Provide adequate housing—space for parental privacy • Childproof home environment • Adjust budget • Reshape division of labor and responsibility to include care of children without taxing any one member and provide opportunities for child to contribute as able • Plan for future children Re-establishing relationships to include children but retain parental privacy • Maintain working relationships with relatives that allow exposure to child(ren) • Revitalize mutually satisfying sexual relations • Allocate time and funds for spouses to get away occasionally and participate in social, community activities Rework family philosophy to: • See satisfaction in parenthood • Value persons above things • Establish healthy independence among members • Resolve conflicts in developmental tasks of members and unit in constructive ways • Accept help in a spirit of appreciation and growth
Stage 3 (approx. 3.5 years) **Family with Preschooler** (Oldest child 2.5 to 5 years; usually one or two other children)		
	Individual adults; expanding generativity (concern for children generally in the community, not just one's own) Spouses: marital maintenance Parents: nurturing children; learning to separate from children Preschooler: initiative Younger children: trust → autonomy Siblings; adjustment to shared relationship with parents and to ordinal position roles	Supplying adequate space, facilities, equipment for a larger and progressively more active family Meeting predictable and unexpected costs of family life • more illness and health maintenance costs • home ownership costs Maintaining satisfactory sexual relations, setting controls on family affectional behaviors (oedipal period), and planning for future children

Table 2-2. *(continued)*

Stage	Individual/Positional Developmental Tasks	Family Group Developmental Tasks
		Creating and maintaining effective communication that allows for the increasing expressive skills of the children and yet allows for individual privacy Cultivating fuller relationships with relatives as resources to help impart cultural and familial values and enrichment between generations Realistically apportioning responsibilities and home duties among members, including children but not overburdening any one member Enjoying contacts outside home • Time away from each other • Time for developing individual friendships, interests
Stage 4 (approx. 7 years) **Family with School Child** (Oldest child between 5 or 6 and 12; may have younger children in all developmental stages)		
	Individual adults: fostering a home atmosphere of love; continuing own development of skills; enlarging generativity to concern for all children in nation Spouses: continue to satisfy each other as married persons Parents: socialization and education of children; learning to accept rejection by school child without deserting him or her School child: industry Younger children: trust → industry depending on age Siblings: continued adjustment to shared relationships with parents and sibs and to occasional changes in ordinal position roles	Reorganizing to adapt family living to expanding world of school-age child • Provide for children's activities and parent(s)' privacy • "Let go" of school child so she or he can grow socially • Cooperation by all members to get things done • Participation in parent-child affairs/activities • Feeling close to relatives • Tying in with life outside the family (PTO, athletic groups, clubs) Keeping financially solvent • Mother may go to work • Father may hold two jobs • Single parent may supplement basic employment with babysitting or a second job Effectively utilizing family communication • Time for each child to get individual attention • More verbal discussion of member differences • Try to see life through child's eyes • Increased effort for spouse (or spouse surrogate) companionship
The Maturing Family		
Stage 5 (approx. 7 years) **Family with Teenagers** (Oldest child 13 years until time he leaves home; may have children in all developmental stages)		
	Individual adults: keeping "up to date" while adjusting to realities of impending middle age; generativity evolved to concern for children throughout world Spouses: remaining compatible allies in the midst of developmental conflicts among family members Parents: balancing teen's freedom and responsibility; building a new life that allows release of young adults	Loosening family ties to allow readiness for releasing young adults in-the-making Provision of facilities for widely differing needs of members Assignment of greater responsibility and freedom to children in the division of labor and responsibility Keep communication systems open • allow nonjudgmental exchange of ideas among members

continued

Table 2-2. *(continued)*

Stage	Individual/Positional Developmental Tasks	Family Group Developmental Tasks
	Teenager: identity; beginning emancipation from parents; establishing self with peers of both sexes Other children: trust → identity, depending on ages Siblings: adjusting to sharing of resources with sibs who have increased demands for them	• members keep themselves available to each other to listen and support • alter affectional guidelines among family members and with friends and dates • allow each member space for private thoughts • maintain contact with extended family as a valuable support system Work out money conflicts during this period of escalated school and personal expenses • part-time jobs for children • reasonable allowances • democratically determined family budgeting Put marriage relationship into focus • spouses manage time alone and to get away together • get reaquainted, re-establishing common interests • reorganize social relations with peers
The Contracting Family		
Stage 6 (approx. 6.5 years) **Family as Launching Center and Recruiter** (Oldest child leaves home until last child leaves home)		
	Individual adults: adjust to middle age; develop postparental interests Spouses: rediscover each other as a couple and as friends Young adults: identity → intimacy Other children: trust → identity, depending on ages Siblings: adjusting to absence of other sibs from home and to changing availability of resources in the home	Reorganize family to maintain unity while releasing matured and maturing children into lives of their own Rearranging physical facilities and resources in accordance with decreased need or use Managing income to meet costs during this peak expenditure period • determine how costs of college/marriage will be covered • plan for retirement expenses Reallocate responsibilities and household tasks among grown and growing children Widen family circle by recruiting new members through marriage of children Come to terms with selves as husband and wife • accept reality of gradual alterations in body appearance and function • adapt to menopausal changes • adjust to decreased vigor and health Maintain open communication within family and the family members recruited • keep a secure home where children and their families are welcome • accept comfortably the way of life children choose • reconcile conflicting values and loyalties among members
Stage 7 (approx. 15 years) **Family in the Middle Years** (Empty nest until retirement)		
	Individual adults: maintain activity that promotes self-fulfillment and moves one toward ego integrity Spouses: reignite conjugal relations; re-establish marital dyad	Re-emergence of the marital dyad. Single parent often seeks marriage or housemate now that children do not consume time Maintain a pleasant, comfortable home • share household responsibilities and decrease their number

Table 2-2. *(continued)*

Stage	Individual/Positional Developmental Tasks	Family Group Developmental Tasks
	Parents: accept separation and individuation of children as they establish their own families and colleagueships Grandparents: contribute to enrichment of grandchildren's concepts of life and to their historical roots	• reaffirm those values and routines that have meaning Assure security for later years while income is at its peak • provide for care of aging parent(s) • arrange for steady income after retirement • arrange for coverage of health costs that are predictable as aging occurs • Keep a system of open communication within and outside of family unit • maintain links with older and younger generations • invest energy in new interests and peer relationships • participate in community life • keep in touch with siblings and aged parents • maintain periodic contact with grown children and their families • draw closer together as a couple
The Declining Family		
Stage 8 (approx. 16 years) **Family in Later Years** (Retirement until death of one or both spouses)		
	Individual adults: ego integrity; learning ways to deal constructively with aging, loneliness, death Spouses: helping each other find life meaningful after retirement Grandparents/great grandparents: develop a feeling of kinship in warm, meaningful interactions that transmit the familial history and orientation	Adjust to and accept retirement • Adjust to retirement income • Establish comfortable household routines • Find a satisfactory home for later years Face aging, loneliness, death, and manage grief constructively • Cope with final independence from own parents as they die • Cope with final independence from spouse when he/she dies • Accept own impending infirmity and death Maintain communication within and outside of family • Nurture each other as spouses • Maintain contact with children and their families • Involve self with people and activities outside family (senior citizens groups, religious groups)

(From Duvall, 1977; Hymovich and Barnard, 1979.)

development of a secure sexual identity. What is important is how fully one incorporates the notion of one's sex, how acceptable that gender is to one, and how comfortable one is being that sex. These factors depend primarily on how the family originally accepted the infant's sex and whether the family allowed the child to develop at his or her own rate, not on how precisely roles were defined in the family unit.

The husband and wife roles that prevailed (and still do in homes that reflect a preindustrial or industrial character) before the 1970s described the wife's role as being expressive and integrative. She fulfilled that role if she kept the home in order and did most of the childrearing, healed the emotional wounds of family members, and offered unconditional love. A husband's role was instrumental or task oriented. He complied with the description of his role if he maintained a position of final authority at home, resided as breadwinner and taskmaster, and offered his love to members on a conditional basis that demanded respect for his contribution and authority in the family.

Postindustrial society added a role to the position

Table 2-3. Assessing Family Developmental Task Mastery

Tasks Common to All Developmental Stages	Assessment Factors (also refer to Table 2-2)	Nursing Strategies to Facilitate Coping
Maintenance of family internal system	Communication and interaction reflect family goals/values Respect for members' and family's needs by each member Decision making/problem solving adequate to manage crises and adapt to necessary developmental changes Mutual age-appropriate attempts by members to gratify needs and maintain family harmony Consideration given to situational variables such as fatigue, being busy, illness, and to constant variables of personality, age and experience, resources available	Be a role model of effective communication patterns Demonstrate respect for members Provide anticipatory guidance regarding age-related and situation-related needs Help members interpret feedback from members and problem solve to make changes Provide or refer for counseling if dysfunction persists
Meeting physical needs	Basic necessities (food, clothing, shelter, health care) provided Resources recognized and used appropriately	Reinforce attempts and successes in providing basic needs Help family identify and obtain access to helpful resources
Family member and group integration into external environment	Amount and type of involvement by each member and by family unit is church, school, work force, health care facilities, community activities Any isolated member(s) Family leisure activity patterns Extended family relationships Friendships outside family membership	Help family problem solve in identification of barriers to positive interaction with the external world Help family identify resources to aid in making opportunities for socialization outside the family and as a family within the community Reinforce attempts at external socialization
Helping members meet individual developmental tasks	How family adjusts when member moves from one developmental stage to another Degree of consistent nurturing for each member. Any member not receiving/not offering nurturance. Protective behavior displaced proportionate to member's abilities or need for autonomy Toddlerhood and adolescence seem most difficult for many families; both stages require a careful balancing between nurturance and allowing autonomy Family identify impact of developmental needs on family values, priorities, goals, relationships	Provide anticipatory guidance regarding developmental stages/tasks/needs. Have family describe necessary changes to family priorities, relationships, goals Reinforce nurturing behaviors Demonstrate nurturing behaviors Help family identify support systems and resources to assist them in coping with changes required as children's developmental needs change and/or when complicatons in task accomplishment arise. Provide or refer for counseling if dysfunctional behaviors persist

of wife, primarily out of economic necessity, to allow her to hold at least a part-time job outside the home, but this role addition did not shift any of her other clearly defined tasks to the husband; it simply added one more task to those she already performed. The stress created by this situation for the working mother is similar to that experienced by the *single parent,* who must essentially fulfill both spousal roles in the nurturance of children.

The shared-role ideology that emerged to accommodate the looser-knit "equalitarian" marriage of the eighties involves both spouses sharing economic, household, and childrearing tasks and responsibilities. Although the loosely defined roles of this ideology produce tension (some strain exists in all roles, regardless of how well prescribed they are), they allow for much greater flexibility, creativity, and general happiness among family members. Although couples are permitting greater role flexibility in their relationships, the true equalitarian marriage is still rare among American families. Fathers spend more time with their children, but their influence is more often through play than through actual caretaking activities. These tasks are still largely left to the mother whether or not she works out of the home (Beail, 1983; Winborn, 1983).

There are many possible causes of role strain; knowing the source of the conflict can aid the individual (with the nurse's help, if involved) in abating the conflict. Common sources of role strain include:

1. The role is acquired too quickly for the necessary modification in self-concept to occur for role acceptance. Many rituals have developed such as bridal and baby showers and graduation ceremonies, to help persons adapt to their self-concept more rapidly.
2. The role demanded by a position is in conflict with a characteristic of the individual's personality, as when a man of mild temperament is placed in a position requiring assertiveness.
3. Conflicting pressures of the "middleman role" that make role fulfillment difficult (woman as arbitrator between her child's needs and her husband's demands).
4. Two antagonistic roles, making it difficult for adequate performance in either role (a woman who is both housewife and jobholder).
5. The role is incongruent with the person's emotional needs (an ill child who tries to continue carrying out the role of a well child in the family).

How well a person resolves role conflicts or adjusts to a new role is largely determined by the quality and con sistency of responses the role evokes, especially from one's "significant others"; how well each partner's roles complement each other; the extent to which the role either satiates emotional needs or stimulates creative tendencies; and how much energy one invests in learning the role.

The following family role prescriptions are discussed here: spouse, mother, father, child, sibling and grandparent. See Chapter 13 for a discussion of roles created as a result of alternative family structures.

Being a Spouse. The condition of a marriage lays the foundation for the successes or failures in a family's development. Therefore, how well a man and a woman perform the role prescription of spouse is crucial to the family's well-being. Goldstine and colleagues (1977) have identified the features most likely to produce happy, healthy interactions: each spouse is able to accept affection from and express affection for each other, has confidence about the mate's fidelity, and is committed to personal fidelity. Each spouse displays a democratic or equalitarian attitude toward the other, performs sexually in a manner that satisfies both, and exerts energy to maintain harmony with the spouse and to develop shared interests. The spouse's actions are judged with charity, an attempt is made to remain attractive to the spouse through the years, and each is committed to the permanence of the marriage. Communication is open and honest, offering outlet for both intellectual and emotional expression.

As most married couples will attest, achieving this role prescription requires hard work, with many ups and downs of daily living—obviously a task requiring maturity.

Being a Mother. The mother role is performed best when the mother integrates attitudes learned from observation of and interaction with her own mother, the development of motherliness (a feeling of emotional bond with the child), and the acquisition of child care skills and some knowledge of child development. Enacting the mother role prescription effectively requires resolution of some basic conflicts inherent in being both a person and a mother. Some of these basic conflicts include (1) the idealized mother projected by the mass media onto the woman's own fantasies about motherhood against her feelings of inadequacy as a mother; (2) vacillation between her own need to be dependent and the need to be independent and responsible; (3) love for versus resentment of the child; (4) demands made by the child for her love and energy versus those made by her husband or spousal surrogate; and (5) self-actualization versus successful motherhood.

From the arbitration of these conflicts, the modern mother attempts to carry out a role prescription characterized by either providing or obtaining child care that satisfies the child's growing needs and enhances development. She also allocates time with her children that emphasizes quality rather than quantity. Her role involves allowing her children enough freedom to develop autonomy, initiative, and independence; supporting them when they succeed and when they fail; permitting them to experience life and the continuum of feelings associated with living fully; and providing a role model of acceptable adult behaviors. Obviously the role prescript just described is an ideal toward which mothers aspire. But this achievement is not always possible and largely depends upon a mother's own understanding of her mothering goals, her individual capacities to fulfill the prescription, and the available resources or support systems to accomplish the role. Family lifestyle does not seem to be as critical a factor in fulfilling the mother role as are the mother's personal characteristics and her knowledge of a child's growth and development needs. Cultural norms also have a strong impact on how the mother role is carried out. In some cultures certain aspects of the mother role are delegated to other family members or to an extended family member such as the grandmother. Chapter 13 further describes the mother role prescription relative to parenting.

Being a Father. To be more human, more responsive, and more fully functional is a freedom being offered men by equality of the sexes that will surely gratify and complement the role of father. The new

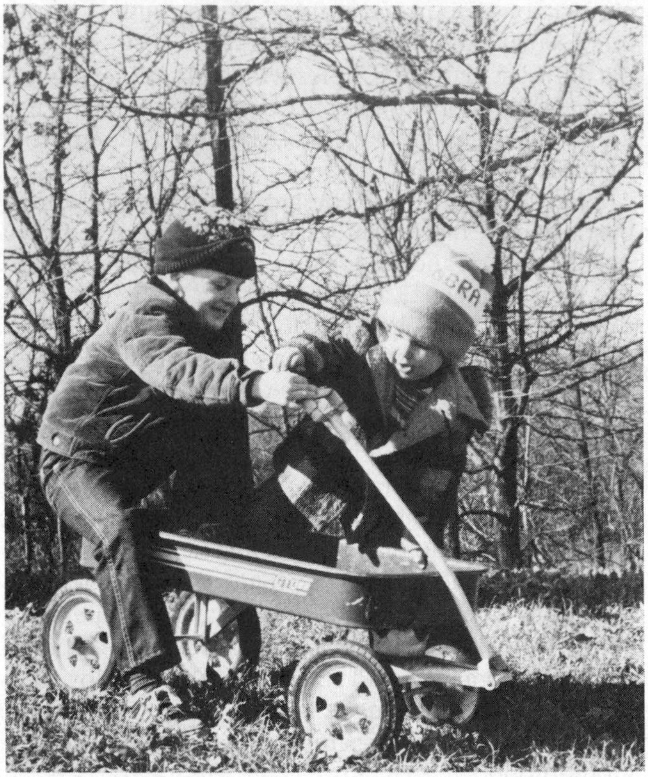

A feature all siblings have in common is that they must learn to share.

measures of a man's masculinity are no longer based on sexual exploits or stoic unemotionalism but on how he manages his life, whether his conduct with other people recognizes his and their humanness, his ability to make decisions, and how perceptive he is as to the consequences of those decisions. Measuring up to this yardstick of manliness supports rather than compromises his effectiveness as a father.

A man's role prescription as a father can, by today's emerging standards, reflect his manliness. The role involves being a beloved friend and teacher to his child and a stimulating source for awakening the emotional potential in his child. He is to be a model of mature social and vocational behavior; an ego ideal for masculine love, ethics, and morality; and a protector and counselor as his child develops. The father's role, like the mother's, is best performed when it blends the attitudes he learned from observing and interacting with his own father, the development of fatherliness (a feeling of emotional bond with his child, more easily achieved when he has been actively involved at all stages of the pregnancy and birth), and the acquisition of child care skills and some knowledge of growth and development.

As with the mother role prescription, that of the father described here is an ambitious goal toward which to strive. The father who is a single parent is left with fewer choices and is more likely to blend the mother-father roles. Likewise, the father who is absent from his children much of the time because of occupation or divorce is less able to fulfill his parenting role expectations. His own personal characteristics, his cultural membership, and his insights into a child's developmental needs also have an impact on how his father role is carried out.

Sharing roles allows the two people involved in parenting to exchange components of the role prescriptions, without fear of personal or social reprisal, as family need or circumstance demands and on either a temporary or permanent basis. Since no society has yet devised a foolproof system within which all men and women become equally felicitous and satisfactory parents for all their children, this ideology is a contemporary solution in the individual's and family's best interests. Because of this trend toward blending of the mother and father roles, a *parenting* role prescription is probably most appropriate for the nurse to focus on in assessment and nursing strategies. Chapter 13 addresses the parenting role in greater detail.

Being a Child. Although a child's role in the family is not static, some aspects of the role prescription remain constant. The child role requires behaviors that will result in acquisition of (1) a psychic structure that produces a secure identity and constructive self-esteem (see Chapter 16), (2) skills for independent functioning, (3) an education, and (4) experience in peer relationships. Other components of the child role prescription fluctuate depending on the child's age and the techniques of parenting with which she or he must cope. The age-related role prescriptions of being a child are discussed in those chapters that correspond to each age (Chapters 5 through 9).

Being a Sibling. Every child in a family learns different lessons about self and life depending on ordinal position (eldest, middle, youngest child), sex, the age span between siblings, whether or not the child was planned or wanted, and the socioeconomic state of the family at the birth. But beyond all the prescription features unique to the sibling role, every sibling has a feature in common with brothers and sisters: learning to share. Siblings have to learn to share parents, toys, space, and what seems to them to be their entire world. The younger the sibling, the more conflict this sharing involves. Felson (1983), in his research on aggression and violence between siblings, found that siblings have less conflict when parents stay uninvolved in their interactions. He also discovered that both sexes are equally aggressive and that aggressive behavior is more often verbal than physical. The wider the age span between siblings, the less threat the sib prescription to share creates for them.

Being a Grandparent. Although the majority of families do not house the grandparents, the parents do, at intervals, either visit or bring to their home these

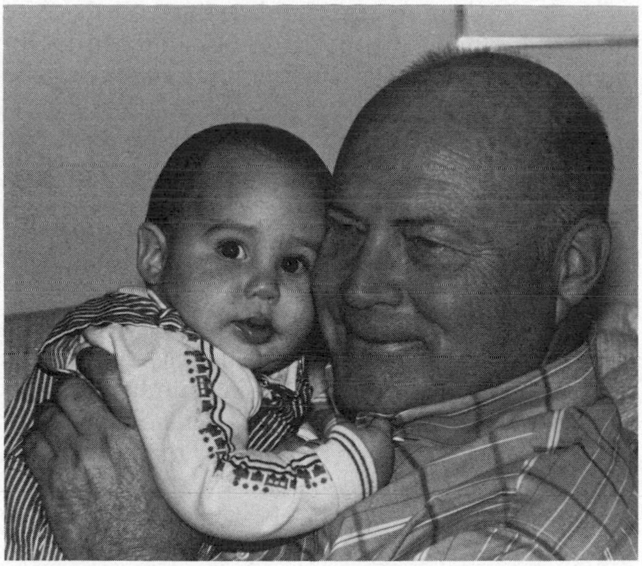

The patience and wisdom of a grandparent can be a wonderful resource for young families.

special people in a child's life. By the time parents become grandparents they have usually learned how to cope with life's unknowns in a relatively effective manner. Exposure of children to grandparents provides them with role models who have learned the lesson of living each day fully and to live a day at a time. Grandparents can offer a generational and cultural richness to children's understanding through the stories they tell, the rituals they practice, and the general experience they avail of communicating with and loving older people.

Grandparents should be encouraged by parents and by health care providers to be good listeners, to ask questions, and to add to their grandchildren's knowledge through storytelling so that they can fulfill their guidance role as grandparents (Strom and Strom, 1983).

Grandparenting tends to be characterized by two styles of interaction (Hymovich and Barnard, 1979). One is the indulgent grandparent who seeks pleasure and enjoyment from grandchildren; the other is grandparents who remain aloof, preferring infrequent contact, usually during holidays or ritual occasions. Whichever the style, the grandparents should keep in mind the parents' primary position with their children and be aware of those rules of childrearing that parents do not want breached under any circumstances. Grandparents also may assist at intervals when the parents seek further education or experience illness. The role may be more enduring in divorce or if the grandparents are providing child care for dual-career spouses' children. As grandparents convey respect for their grandchildren, they will be delighted at the love and respect they receive in return.

Family Living: An Adaptive Process

Family living is an adaptive process that involves establishing an equilibrium between the family's integrative features (strengths) and its disruptive aspects (limitations). When family members' strengths predominate in their daily living, they evidence capacity and motivation to successfully master their individual and family group developmental tasks. When the family's strengths waver because of disruptive events (role conflict, loss of a support system, maturational changes, accidental interruptions such as illness), its members experience a period of crisis during which the help of external support systems (extended family, community agencies, health professionals) may be needed.

The nurse who understands the goals, structure, roles, functions, and tasks of families and the changes inherent in periods of transition from one life stage to another can be useful to families in times of crisis. During periods of equilibrium, the nurse with this knowledge base can anticipate the needs of families and their members, can help them identify ways to satisfactorily perform their roles and adapt to role changes with minimal stress, can help them recognize their present and potential strengths, and can support their developmental efforts as a growing, healthy family unit.

During times of crisis the nurse can apply this same knowledge base to help the family surmount its problems. By assessing how well the family is meeting its own and society's goals for it and how well the family is achieving its developmental tasks, the nurse can identify those strengths in the family that can be organized to combat the problem. These strengths should be drawn on when planning interventions. Family members and their support systems should be included in the planning process, and ways to involve other potential resources should be devised. The nurse's intervention should include support to family members as they apply their strengths and resources to the problem, and positive reinforcement for attempts to develop latent strengths should be offered. The evaluative process is an opportunity for the nurse to help the family accept the fact that sometimes help is needed and that seeking help at those times is itself a strength. It also affords the nurse the opportunity to help family members determine how this crisis has prepared them to handle future crises by sharpening or adding to their store of strengths. The nursing diagnosis, *Family coping: potential for growth,* highlights the possible benefit of a family crisis.

Family life at its best fulfills a human need not fully met by any other arrangement or institution. The family, despite all its limitations, remains the most powerful influence in most of our lives.

Milieu for Family Growth and Development: Culture and Life Style

In a discussion about the structure and function of the family within the cultural context and social system, Malinowski, a well-known anthropologist, states that family is one of the universal institutions of mankind (Leininger, 1984). Although the concept of family may be universal, the structure, role, function, status, and developmental process of the family are culture-bound variables that depend on the social system for meaning. Beliefs and values of a particular cultural group are important to nursing because they determine the perceptions of health and illness and the health care practices of individuals and families.

The Concept of Culture

Theorists have debated and refined the concept of culture for many years. Cultural explanations are determined by the way in which culture is conceptualized (Harris, 1968; Aamodt, 1978). In this discussion, *culture refers to the shared values, beliefs, and practices of a particular group, all of which guide their thoughts, decisions, and actions in patterned and recurrent ways through time* (Leininger, 1978, 1984). These cultural lifeways are passed from one generation to the next and are known by the cultural group members. The existence and continuity of cultural values do not depend upon particular persons, even though parents do impart cultural values and beliefs to their children (Rambo, 1984). Grandparents, relatives, and other caregivers in the cultural group influence children to share the group's world view or perspective on life.

Some differentiate readily observable cultural products (e.g., dress, religion, childrearing practices) from those that are covert or not as obvious (e.g., ideals and values). However, culture can be viewed as the pervasive, dynamic aspect of social interaction which forms the material and nonmaterial matrix of life for the individual and the family.

It is important to bear in mind that the production of culture is a human enterprise. In a very real sense, *people create their culture and are created by it.* Culture is invented and transmitted by humans who are themselves shaped by the culture in which they participate. Culture is probably the most important part of the human environment, because it defines the way of life for a group of people (Leininger, 1978).

When viewed over a short span of time, cultures seem stable, so that one might mistakenly conclude that they are static or unchanging. On the contrary, cultures are dynamic, although some seem to change more slowly than others. The direction and shape of future alterations grow out of present cultural forms. In other words, the seeds of a given cultural epoch can be identified in earlier periods of the group's history. Since culture is not a completely harmonious system, change can result from internal conflict, strains, or maladjustments. In the words of Benedict, "It is, so far as we can see, an ultimate fact of human nature that man builds up his culture out of disparate elements, combining and recombining" (Benedict, 1959).

Culture should not be equated with ethnicity. Culture is determined by more than ethnicity. Ethnicity is but one identity group with which an individual may align because of common origins and some form of distinctiveness. Common origins may refer to cultural heritage, (e.g., a rural community in South Dakota) but the ethnic affiliation could relate to nationality or genetic ancestry (e.g., Norwegian-American). (Additional discussion of identity groups is found in Chapter 1.)

Ethnicity is determined subjectively and objectively. Ethnic affiliation is partially a notion of self-identification. That is, persons can choose to identify with an ethnic group, if they share some aspects of the ethnic criteria. However, ethnicity is also objective in that language, genetic ancestry, and other demographic conditions set the boundaries between ethnic groups. Ethnic affiliation is often attributed to subcultures by persons in the dominant culture. The term "ethnic minorities" is used for persons whose race, language, or cultural lifeways differ from the dominant or majority culture. Most Anglo-Americans would not view themselves as belonging to an ethnic group, whereas Japanese-Americans or Native Americans would. Increasingly in the United States, persons belonging to ethnic minorities are proud of their ethnicity and choose to emphasize their cultural or racial differences.

For nurses to provide culture-congruent nursing care, they need to learn about cultural similarities and differences related to health. For instance, Suzuki (1980) states that Asian-American mothers tend to be more permissive with young infants than their Anglo-American counterparts. Asian-American children are weaned at a later age, toilet-trained more gradually, and often are allowed to sleep with the parents. These approaches to childrearing may seem like indulgences to Anglo-American parents who focus on encouraging independence and autonomy in the developmental process. For the Asian-American, priority is given to developing close affective ties within the family and the child's sense of belonging to the family (Leininger, 1979; Chinn, 1980; Rambo, 1984). Horn (1978) found in her study of childrearing among Muckleshoot Indians that children were taught not to ask questions. As a result, children were sometimes perceived by outsiders to be dull because of their quiet and reticent attitude; instead, the Indian children were practicing a cultural value they had been carefully taught. *Nurses cannot know all the specific cultural differences and similarities of their patients but rather need to choose a conceptual framework for cultural assessments.*

Framework for Transcultural Nursing

Leininger, a nurse-anthropologist, has proposed a transcultural nursing conceptual model, postulating that care is the essence of nursing and that nursing, as a practice profession and as a scientific discipline, should consider cultural diversity. A major premise of the theory is that "care and health differ with cultural cognitions, values, and practices among cultures with some identifiable universal features" (Leininger, 1984, p 135). Cultural care diversity is influenced by social structure factors, language contexts, and folk and professional health care systems. Social structure factors, such as technology, religion, kinship, cultural values, economics, politics, and education, influence the health, illness, and care patterns of cultural groups as they choose and utilize folk and/or professional health care services.

The goal for nurses using this model is to do an ethnonursing assessment, which results in one or a combination of three types of ethnonursing care: (1) cultural care accommodation, (2) cultural care preservation, or (3) cultural care repatterning (Leininger, 1985).

- *Ethnonursing* refers to nursing care that is based on culturally derived ethnographic data on health and health care.
- Cultural care *accommodation* refers to those culturally based assistive, facilitative, or enabling acts that reflect ways to adapt or adjust services to fit client needs.
- Cultural care *preservation* refers to those culturally based assistive, facilitative, or enabling acts that preserve cultural lifeways in the caregiving services.
- Cultural care *repatterning* refers to those altered ways of assisting others that are substantially different from original cultural lifeways or patterns.

In ethnonursing, the nurse relates to the client in a manner that is acceptable in that culture. Box 2-1 lists selected references that can help the nurse learn more about a particular cultural group. For instance, the Native American mother may avoid eye contact when speaking because that is considered to be impolite. This action may make uncomfortable the nurse who is used to using eye contact for cues in a therapeutic relationship. The nurse may stand or sit alongside rather than directly in front of the mother so as to encourage her to speak without facing the nurse directly. In so doing, the nurse uses accommodation, which recognizes a cultural value, while at the same time maintaining a therapeutic relationship in which the mother can discuss her childrearing concerns with the nurse.

Cultural care accommodation is more difficult in acute care settings where policies and procedures are used to standardize nursing care. However, an increasing number of agencies encourage the nurse to interact with clients in ways that encourage cultural accommodation if the nurse uses cultural assessment in the nursing process to propose accommodative actions. Sevcovic (1979) reported a study of maternity care of the Navajo people in which hospital policies and procedures were completely revised to accommodate Navajo cultural lifeways. Nurse-midwives assist during labor, flexible rooming-in policies allow family members to have contact with the new member of the family, and babies sometimes sleep in their mother's bed in the hospital. At the family's request, the infant's cord is saved by the nurses and given to the family. These and other accommodations in providing culture-congruent care required many in-service meetings of hospital personnel but resulted in more satisfied clients and a decrease in client-initiated premature discharges from the hospital.

Sometimes cultural care patterns should be preserved even when they may not be the nursing intervention of choice or when folk health care is used that diminishes the need for professional nursing care. Cultural patterns are interrelated and complex. Interventions, viewed as helpful and positive by the nurse, may disturb other interdependent care patterns. For example, in Amish families grandparents usually live on the family farm in a separate small house or in an addition added to the farmhouse for the express purpose of providing a place for the grandparents. Grandparents assist with child care and relate to their married children and grandchildren, often being asked for their guidance and wisdom. In a study of ethnic elderly, Tripp-Reimer and Schrock (1982) reported that 75 per cent of the Amish elderly preferred to live with relatives. Children learn caring responsibilities by assisting their grandparents as they become physically less able to care for themselves. Preserving the caregiving and -receiving network within the Amish extended family is seen as more important than the potential gain of professional nursing care in a nursing home. Amish are known for their persistence in preserving their cultural caring patterns and selective use of professional health care services.

At times the action of choice is cultural care repatterning. This is more difficult than the other two types

Box 2-1
Annotated List of Readings about Culture

Choi ES, Hamilton RK: The effects of culture on mother-infant interaction. JOGNN 1986 May/Jun; 15(3):256.

Reports nursing research using the Brazelton Neonatal Behavioral Assessment Scale to study infants of Korean and American mothers. The conclusions and literature review point out what is and is not known about cultural differences in infant behavior.

Clark AL: *Culture, Childbearing, Health Professionals.* Philadelphia, FA Davis, 1978.

Provides health professionals with a detailed look at the childbearing experiences of a number of cultures in America. Each chapter focuses on the ways a particular culture values children, uses conception control, regards marriage and pregnancy as well as the care of children.

Henderson G, Primeaux M: *Transcultural Health Care.* Menlo Park, CA, Addison-Wesley, 1981.

Focuses primarily on Third World cultures but includes American Indian and other American subcultures. It is divided into three parts: sociocultural dimensions of health care, folk medicine, and patient care. A chapter on biologic variations is included.

Jordan B: *Birth in Four Cultures: A Crosscultural Investigation of Childbirth in Yucatan, Holland, Sweden and the United States.* Montreal, Eden Press, 1980.

In the United States, birth generally falls into the medical domain. This small book gives an enlightening view of the sociocultural as well as biologic aspects of the process of childbirth.

Leininger M: *Transcultural Nursing: Concepts, Theories and Practices.* New York, John Wiley and Sons, 1978.

Leininger began her pioneering efforts to consider nursing care within the cultural context as early as 1955. This book contains several original transcultural nursing studies within the United States and four from foreign countries, including several on childbearing. Chapter 5 on cultural assessment domains in nursing practice is especially helpful for the clinical nurse.

Leininger M: *Reference Sources for Transcultural Health and Nursing.* Thorofare, NJ, Slack, Inc., 1984.

Nursing students and professional nurses will find this resource invaluable. It provides complete references to films, articles, books, and chapters on cultures and subcultures in the United States and several other countries. Special topics such as transcultural pain phenomena, folk health care practices, poverty, and rural, urban, and migrant subcultures are included.

Leininger M: Transcultural care diversity and universality: a theory of nursing. *Nursing and Health Care* 1985; 6(4):209-212.

Leininger's theory is briefly described. Included are general theory statements, definitions, and assumptions. The Sunrise Model is visually presented and discussed. This model can help nurses to discover what care means to people of various cultures.

Rambo BJ: Adaption and cultural diversity. *In* Rambo BJ: *Adaptation Nursing: Assessment and Intervention.* Philadelphia, WB Saunders, 1984, pp 346-361.

This chapter presents the nature and assessment of culture. The dominant cultural values in the United States are compared with those of the Black American, Mexican-American, and American Indian cultures. Application to clinical practice is included.

Rosenberg JA: Health care for Cambodian children: integrating treatment plans. *Pediatric Nursing* Mar/Apr 1986; 12(2).

Focuses on childrearing practices of a recent immigrant group, Cambodians. The discussion of how some practices have been misinterpreted by American health professionals provides insight into the need for understanding the cultural base of families and children.

Tripp-Reimer T, Brink PJ: Culture brokerage. *In* Bulecheck G, McCloskey J: *Nursing Interventions: Treatments for Nursing Diagnosis.* Philadelphia, WB Saunders, 1985, pp 352-364.

This pragmatic and stimulating chapter provides nurses with a self-view that incorporates cultural concepts in nursing interactions. As a nursing intervention, cultural brokerage involves nurses acting as a mediator between clients and members of the health care professions. The article provides succinct strategies and case studies.

Tripp-Reimer T, Brink PJ, Saunders JM: Cultural assessment: Content and process. *Nursing Outlook* 1978; 32(2):78-82.

Nurses need to be prepared to work with clients from various cultures. A variety of assessment tools and guides help in this process. This article presents the process of cultural assessment in two phases: data collection and data organization. A list of questions the nurse may use in collecting cultural information is included.

(By Anna Frances Z. Wenger.)

of nursing actions since it involves cultural change. Repatterning is only possible if the clients understand and accept the needed changes. Many Asian immigrants need to incorporate cultural care changes as they adapt to life in the United States. Some of the disciplining patterns for children have been interpreted by the dominant Anglo-American culture as child abuse. These immigrant families need assistance in repatterning some of their parent-child relationships as they become acculturated. Cultural care changes should occur slowly so that the adaptation has integrity with the other cultural patterns.

Cultural Assessment

Cultural assessment should always involve a shared negotiation between the nurse and the client. It does not involve data on all aspects of the culture. *Assessments should focus on those values, beliefs, and practices that influence the particular setting or health care concern.* Tripp-Reimer et al (1984) suggest a two-phase process in cultural assessment that involves data collection and data organization. They state the purpose of cultural assessments quite succinctly:

> A thorough cultural assessment differs from assessments of systems that have generally accepted standards. The purpose of assessing biological and psychological domains is to determine where deviations occur from normal and then bring the client into alignment with the "standards." For cultural assessments, the purpose is different. Here, the assessment is done to identify deviations in cultural parameters with the goal of modifying the client's system or modifying the health care professional's system in order to increase congruence between them (p. 81).

In the data collection phase of cultural assessment, the nurse collects subjective data from the client using the client's own words as much as possible, since language provides clues for understanding cultural meaning. Objective and subjective data are collected without drawing conclusions or making generalizations. The collected data must then be placed in a context. In nursing practice, the context includes three interrelated cultures each with its own set of standards related to the specific health care concern: (1) the client's identified culture, (2) the nurse's professional culture, and (3) the professional health care system or, more specifically, the health care facility in which the interaction takes place. When areas of incongruence are identified, the nurse and client negotiate until agreement is reached and a nursing care plan evolves that is based on the principles of cultural care accommodation, preservation, or repatterning.

Leininger's conceptual model can serve as a framework for the cultural assessment process. The social structure factors constitute an array for eliciting cultural information. To provide some examples of culturally relevant data, each of the categories of factors are discussed next, citing content that nurses might consider when making cultural assessments of individuals, families, or specific cultural groups.

Technologic Factors. People in the United States, Canada, Japan, and Western Europe are reminded every day of the vast array of technical and electronic equipment that influences and sometimes governs their lives. Some cultures are more likely to be overwhelmed by mechanical systems than other cultures. Americans are generally able to adjust rather quickly to new advances in technology. Nevertheless, even in the United States, there are cultural groups who have less access to technology because of poverty or geographic location. Also, some cultural groups choose to limit their use of technology for such reasons as religion or a cultural belief that technology detracts from human interactions.

Religious/Philosophic Factors. Clients' religious or philosophic beliefs greatly influence their values related to health and their health care practices. The impact of religion on family life in general and on behavior related to health and sickness in particular is readily evident. Often religious preference is also intermeshed with the ethnic or cultural background of families, making it an even more salient aspect of the lifestyle. Among the family patterns affected by a family's religion are sanctioned relationships among its members, family power configurations, responsibilities of parents and children, diet, use of leisure time and finances, attitudes toward family planning and divorce, beliefs regarding health and illness, and use of health care resources.

In general, religion is seen as supportive of family strength by its tenets that place value on respect for others, mutual helping, commitment, and other such interpersonal behaviors. Religion also provides activities in which all family members may participate, thus increasing the time that families can spend together. In some faiths divorce or extramarital sexual activity is strongly prohibited.

A number of religious groups emphasize the approved roles and power relationships within the family. For instance, some of the fundamentalist groups advocate the father as family leader and primary decision maker and tend to emphasize the mother/homemaker roles as most desirable for women. Various groups provide rules regarding the use of family planning methods or stress values related to optimal family size. The duty of adult children to care for aging parents is enjoined on some religiously conscientious families in the light of the biblical fifth commandment.

Groups such as the Church of Jesus Christ of Latter-Day Saints (Mormons) or the Seventh-Day Adventists advocate healthy dietary habits and abstinence from stimulants and depressants. These practices, along with other lifestyle factors, seem to have had the effect of prolonging the life expectancy of the adherents of these faiths beyond national averages.

A number of religions affect family health care behavior through precepts determining which, if any, medical or health-related procedures are appropriate for their followers. This has often led to conflict between families and health care providers, especially when certain interventions were refused on behalf of dependent children. Such situations have sometimes been resolved by having the child temporarily declared a ward of the court.

In assessing the religious aspects of family, the nurse must maintain an open and nonjudgmental attitude. Often the family may value adherence to their religious convictions much more highly than a conflicting health goal that is valued by the nurse. It is also important to avoid the pitfall of religious stereotyping of the family: that is, failing to assess accurately the extent to which each individual family adheres to the tenets of their religious preference and the extent to which they may have made alternative decisions. The nurse should be alert to cues that the family or its individual members are experiencing guilt or conflict in relation to religious concerns. In these instances as well as others involving interpersonal or intrapersonal distress (designated by the nursing diagnosis *spiritual distress*), the nurse should keep in mind the possibility of collaboration with or referral to a clergyman or other family-designated religious advisor in a team approach to family care implementation.

Kinship and Social Factors. Health care roles in families and social groups are related to kin and social alignments (Leininger, 1978). For example, in some cultures the grandmother is included in health care decision making. In many Hispanic families, the husband is consulted and often chooses to be present when a physician or nurse examines his wife or child. In most cultures health care knowledge is considered to be the responsibility of the women and is passed on from mother to daughter. In some cultures, there is differentiation between care activities, which are women's work, and cure activities, which may be the domain of men (Leininger, 1978). Social status and kin relationships may determine the order in which health care is made available within the cultural group. For instance, male children may receive more health care attention than females because of their status within the cultural group. These role expectations may not be congruent with the nurse's value system of equality in health care services. Nevertheless, the nurse should attempt to understand the cultural views of the clients and identify areas of potential conflict and/or need for accommodation or repatterning.

Cultural Factors. Among the cultural factors that influence health and illness beliefs and practices are the concepts of *care, space,* and *time.* The cultural concept of *care,* naturally, is of great importance in nursing. Cultures vary in how they express care. In some cultures touch is used to express care among adults and children quite frequently and openly, whereas in other cultures touch is not as important and even inappropriate in contexts other than intimate family settings. Among Mexican-Americans, respect is a primary expression of care. In general, the elderly are accorded more respect than the young. Respect for age is carefully taught throughout childhood in many cultures including Hispanic, American Indian, and Asian-American.

Cultures vary in their use of folk health care. Belief patterns may undergird the specific practices. Many of the American Indian folk health practices are based on the need to live in harmony with nature. Illness is a sign that a person is not in harmony with nature. A similar belief, the need for balance of human energy with the universe, is the basis for Asian folk health care. For example, an improper diet or anxiety may be caused by an imbalance in energy. In many Latin American cultures as well as Haitian and Jamaican cultures, good health is related to the balance of hot and cold "humors" derived from beliefs in humoral pathology. Foods, herbs, beverages, medicines, and other treatments are classified as hot or cold. The cause and the treatment must be balanced according to their hot or cold properties. Nurses may not be familiar with these inter- and intracultural variations but should respect and be willing to learn about their client's folk health care beliefs and practices. Persons in all cultures are influenced to some degree by cultural health care beliefs.

Health professionals should realize that traditional practitioners such as shamans, herbalists, and medicine men are often sought in preference to physicians and nurses. In the past the typical reaction has been to discourage and ridicule the use of the traditional practitioner. As more is learned about the relationship between belief and healing, progressive health professionals are learning to work cooperatively with traditional practitioners for the benefit of the client. Even if families are willing to accept Western health care providers, they often wish to use folk remedies or have treatment applied in ways that do not violate cultural beliefs. For example, the Southern black woman may come to the hospital for delivery but continue to hold the belief that a knife placed under the bed will "cut the pain." When family values have been explored, the nurse is able to add an important dimension to care planning by incorporating the family's cultural health beliefs.

Personal space is another relevant factor in cultural assessment. Personal space needs determine the amount of physical distance the person must maintain in interaction with others. Territorial dominance needs relate to the space over which a person desires to maintain control, such as a bedroom or an office. Since a family is made up of interacting individuals with differing spatial requirements, these concerns may be potential sources of conflict. Many adolescents, especially in Western cultures, for instance, pass through a developmental period when the need for privacy and control of their own bedroom is greatly valued and fiercely defended, a situation that may lead to clashes with siblings or parents.

Anglo-Americans are especially sensitive to the perceived need for space that allows family members to have their "own" rooms. Personal ownership of toys and, later on, furniture or other equipment is emphasized at an early age. These extensions of the individual person require space and respect for that ownership of space by all members of the family. Cultures that emphasize group relationships, communal ownerships, and extended family housing arrangements tend to want less individual space. This does not mean that privacy is not valued, but rather that the expression of privacy needs may be more covert than overt.

Consideration of family space characteristics may be included in the nursing assessment, plan, and intervention. The following questions may be relevant:

- What are the perceived spatial needs of individual family members and to what extent are these being met?
- What is the relationship of the amount of living space to the size of the family group?
- Does the family perceive this space as being adequate?
- If there is a lack of space, does this represent a problem to the functioning of the family or its members?
- Is space organized and used to promote or inhibit family interaction?
- Is the allocation of space a source of conflict for the family?
- Are there areas in the home for both privacy and family togetherness?
- Do members tend to congregate in certain areas for common or individual pursuits?
- What is the family's perception of and level of satisfaction with its home area and neighborhood?

Time is another example of a cultural factor related to health. The dominant American culture is very time conscious. Time is viewed as a continuum divided into past, present, and future. Time is objectified so we can do many things like manage time, control time, spend time, save time, or waste time. Time is very different for people like the Hopi whose language has no past, present, and future tense in verbs (Hall, 1983). Their verbs indicate the relationship between the speaker and the experience but do not indicate time as we know it. Some cultures are more present oriented whereas others focus on the future. Waiting time and "being on time" have varying acceptable limits. For Americans who are future oriented and time conscious, "being on time" for an appointment means being punctual or 5 minutes early, whereas for some Latin American cultures "being on time" may allow one to arrive 30 minutes past the appointed time.

A number of important time-related assessments can be made in the nurse's work with a family. The nurse may want to obtain a comprehensive view of how family time is structured:

- In what types of activities is the family together and how much time is used for them?
- Are meals, recreation, or religious occasions a time for family interaction?
- Are there periods during the day for quiet or private communication between husband and wife, parent and child, or for individual solitude?
- What value do the family members seem to place on time and how are they oriented to its use?
- Are they extremely relaxed or very compulsive in their modes of responding to time commitments?
- How much freedom is accorded individual family members to schedule their personal activities?
- Is there satisfaction or dissatisfaction in the family concerning its overall use of time?

The answers to these questions will aid the nurse in assessing the effect of time on family function.

Political/Legal Factors. The political system is reflected in the power and influential strategies that individuals and groups have on each other. The political system is a powerful determinant of available health care programs and often influences whether an outside health professional may enter a culture to provide health services (Leininger, 1978). The Old Order Amish have refused to participate in some health care programs, not because they were opposed to the health care services, but because the health care services were linked to governmental controls with which they did not choose to be associated.

Many governmental policies influence trends in health care, as well as availability of health care services. One facet of the advocate role of the nurse is to assist the family in coping with governmental policies that might tend to impair its integrity or functioning. A related professional responsibility involves providing knowledgeable and active input, either individually or through organizations that aid in the development of public policies and programs sensitive to and supportive of family well-being.

Economic Factors. It has been said that, no matter what their income, people think they would be financially secure if their income were increased by 25 per cent. As incomes rise for United States families, their perceived needs also rise and, with increased affluence, spending and indebtedness increase rapidly. Thus higher-income families tend to be more in debt than do middle- or lower-income families. Much of this debt results from attempts to meet the family's demands for more and better goods and services. The general affluence of society, the ready supply of luxury items and services, and constant advertising pressure that creates artificial needs combine to generate an almost irresistible urge to acquire. A lack of skill in financial management may be present in many families. It has been estimated that during the husband's lifetime approximately half a million dollars will pass through the hands of the typical United States middle-class family, and yet most of the time the family will be experiencing financial problems.

Poverty is sometimes viewed as a culture. Economics and other sociocultural factors contribute to continuation of poverty lifeways which are passed on from one generation to the next. As nurses plan to provide services to poor families, they should be aware of the special health problems that may be implied. They must know the relationship between lack of adequate income and the family's inability to provide itself with resources to maintain and restore health.

Educational Factors. Nursing has increasingly given attention to educational principles in health promotion and health care. Formal educational levels, reading ability and developmental stages are assessed. But these assessments are usually made in reference to Anglo-American public education norms. In this multicultural society, differences exist in educational interests and in the manner in which information is learned and assimilated into the culture.

Nurses need to learn about the educational patterns within the cultures they encounter. Do the people use gestures or elaborate examples in passing on information? Are books and other written resources available in their homes? Is television a major resource for information? Are proverbs or folk tales used to instruct and inculcate values? Are there persons, such as the grandmother, to whom the family members look for health care knowledge? Data from questions like these will assist the nurse to use educational modes that are culturally appropriate.

These sociocultural factors (technical, religious/philosophical, kinship/social, cultural, political/legal, economic, and educational) provide a useful framework for the nurse to make culture-specific observations and to ask appropriate questions.

Cultural assessment questions are best stated in a manner that allows clients to choose their style of disclosing cultural information. Suggested examples are: "Who do you call family?" "When you need help, to whom do you go in your family?" "Tell me how the children are cared for when they are ill." "When something important like a birth or a death or an illness happens, who in your family helps?" "How do they help?" Questions like these allow the nurse to learn cultural factors from the client's point of view. In ethnonursing, it is essential that the nurse assume the role of *learner,* always listening and observing for cues that will provide cultural information. The data collected about religion, ethnic group affiliation, education, kinship, technology, cultural values, economic factors, patterns of decision making, language, styles of communication, norms of etiquette, and folk health care practices are used by the nurse and client to design mutually beneficial nursing interventions.

• *The nurse should always include children in the cultural assessment.* Health care professionals often fail to perceive the extent of children's perceptions and their ability to understand relationships. Children at all stages in the developmental process are active participants in enculturation. Any culture has customs about the nature, capacities, and behavior of children. Nurses should consider the culture of childhood as well as the larger societal culture (Tiedeman, 1981).

Alternative Family Lifestyles

When one is confronted with unfamiliar family lifestyles and childrearing practices, it is difficult to remain objective. One's own values influence how one perceives and reacts to situations. Nurses must attempt to understand their own values about the single-parent's ability to parent, the decisions of parents to divorce, the mobility of migrant families, foster parents' attachment to the children, adoptive parents' ability to love their children unconditionally, communal sharing of childrearing responsibilities, and gay and lesbian parents. To examine one's values does not mean one agrees with the choices others have made regarding lifestyles. It does mean that one attempts to understand the grid through which one views another's lifestyle. In doing so, the nurse will be able to focus on the assessment of the family system and the ways in which it responds to the basic needs of the children for nurturing, caretaking, education, and development of family values.

In this section, common alternative family lifestyles in contemporary Western society are defined, with particular attention to childrearing practices and child-adult relationships. Some of the unique aspects of the variant styles will be compared with the traditional nuclear family, which was discussed earlier. The goal of these descriptions is to provide a basis for nurse interaction with many differing family systems. Therefore, whenever applicable, suggestions for nurse interaction patterns are included. Most of the suggestions are general and could be used by any health care provider. However, the educational preparation of the professional nurse and the unique contribution of nursing practice to health care have been considered in formulating the specific suggestions. In Chapter 3, alternative family lifestyles as a factor in the development of children are discussed.

Single-Parent Families

The single-parent family consists of one parent who is caring for his or her children, in his or her home, and who is a single parent due to widowhood, divorce, or separation or who is unmarried. The current concern about the increasing incidence of single-parent families ignores the fact that there have always been single parents in this country. High death rates and mobility of the breadwinner who sought an improved livelihood by westward migration meant that children in early America had fewer parental surrogates than today (Sussman, 1978). Single parenting because of death is not increasing, but as society embraces more values for individual fulfillment, the incidence of divorce and remaining single by choice has increased. Most single-parent families are headed by women, but the number of male single-parent families is increasing (Nieto, 1982; Moynihan, 1987).

Male Single-Parent Families

The general assumption that children should live with mothers is challenged daily in families working through the process of separation. The feminist movement has given impetus for women and men to discard traditional roles. New laws on custody provide indication that single male parenting will likely increase.

A research study on male single-parent families showed that the most important factor in the health of the family was whether the situation was chosen by the father or was accidental (Mendes, 1979). The father's initial reaction to the child is based on that factor. The assenters (acceded but did not seek the role) needed assistance most but were least likely to seek out supportive services. These fathers wanted to prove their abilities as single parents. The seekers (chose the role) more readily expressed their needs and concerns about parenting, such as concern about normal childhood, adolescent behavior, disciplinary problems, and daughters' sexual development (Mendes, 1979).

In other research studies of motherless families, it was shown that the fathers take on homemaking, child guidance, and nurturing responsibilities as well as the more traditional father role of financial support and house maintenance (Klein, 1973; Mendes, 1979; Chang and Deinard, 1982). The most difficult area of responsibility for single male parents is the nurturing of the children. Many expressed insecurity in responding to their children's feelings. The men usually report that they feel closer to their children as a result of increased nurturing responsibilities.

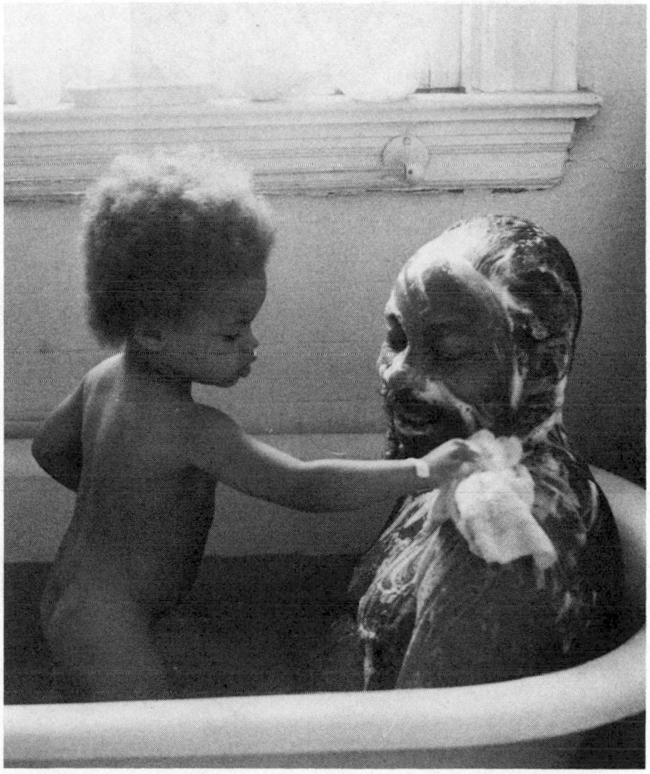

Today more single fathers are taking on homemaking, child guidance, and nurturing responsibilities. (Anna Kaufman Moon/Stock, Boston, Inc.)

Male single parents also rely on grandmothers, sisters, and other female relatives to supplement nurturing.

Because men earn more than women, financial problems are not the predominant stress for fathers as they are for female-headed families. Table 2-4 identifies the common problems of the male single-parent family and nursing roles that can facilitate resolution of those concerns.

The roles of father and husband have usually been viewed as inseparable and compatible. Some fathers are finding it necessary to challenge this assumption. Some are successfully demonstrating that they can and want to care for and nurture their children without the support of a wife (Scanzoni, 1981). As society comes to regard emotional responsiveness as a male trait as well as a female trait, single male parents will be better

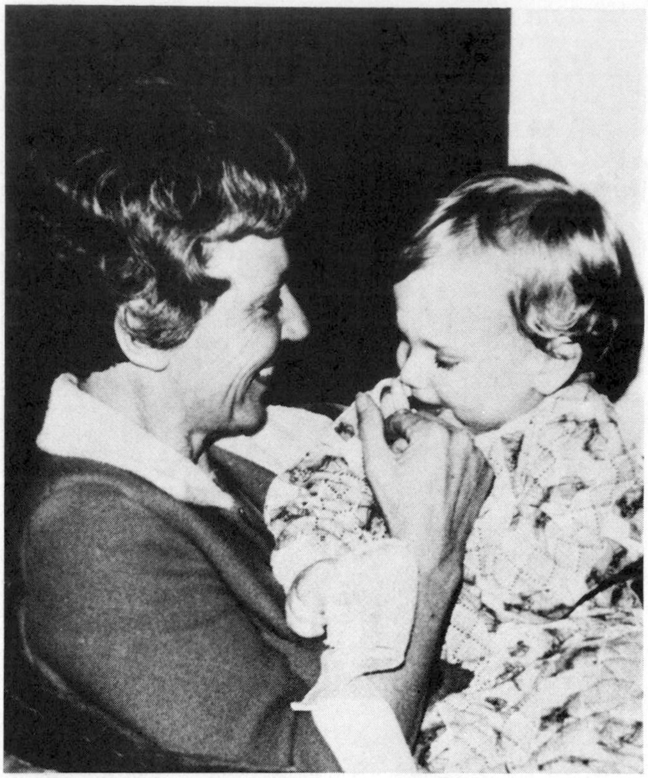

Grandparents are special people in a child's life.

prepared for the nurturing responsibilities and privileges of parenthood.

Female Single-Parent Families

Since homemaking, child care, and nurturing traditionally have been female family responsibilities, mothers who have become heads of household by accident or by choice continue to assume these important family functions. In addition, they are confronted with the burden of economic provision and other traditional male family tasks (automotive repair, house maintenance, and some child discipline). Two of three single mothers work outside the home (Norton and Glick, 1986). In divorce situations, courts generally have granted custody of children to mothers rather than to fathers. This practice is changing, but the majority of single-parent families are still headed by women.

Mothers who become single parents not by choice sometimes work outside the home for the first time. Home and child care tasks that formerly consumed all their time now are relegated to marginal time, often when they are tired. The children's view of the change in their mother's priorities can be interpreted as rejection, making the emotional climate even more unstable. Nurses relating to these families can be helpful in encouraging the mothers and the children to verbalize their views of the home responsibilities and relationships. The mothers and children may need assistance in setting priorities and in securing help from friends and relatives or community resources.

The purported negative impact on male children in female-headed families has been a focus of research and discussion (Klein, 1973). Black female-headed families are often perceived to be female dominated when, in reality, several male relatives and friends may be influential in the setting (Hall and King, 1982). A high degree of normal psychosocial development was found in the female single-parent families that had the support of other family members and relatives. In fact, such families functioned better than many two-parent families. The key seems to be support from relatives and friends, who serve to strengthen the mother's parental role and who serve as male and female role models.

Research into the sexual attitudes of one-parent children concludes that "inappropriate" attitudes result less from having been raised by only one parent than from the attitudes of that parent (Klein, 1973; Eiduson, 1980). Children may experience a variety of problems that relate to poor sexual identification if single parents have conflicting feelings toward the opposite sex. This conflict may focus on one member of the opposite sex, such as the absent father. A mother may react to her son negatively because of her unresolved feelings toward her absent spouse. Some mothers react with overprotection of the son, whereas others may reject the son. The nurse's responsibility is to assess the family interaction patterns, to assist the family members in finding professional counseling,

Table 2-4. Nursing Strategies to Maximize the Male Single-Parent Family Experience

Situational Factors	Nursing Strategies
Father's need for support in child nurturing	Identify community support groups
Support groups need masculine role models	Influence community agencies to include men in organizing and conducting groups for single-parent fathers
Assistance needed in learning physical care of children and home-making tasks	Assess family needs for child care. Teach physical care of children and/or mobilize community resources
Children's need for mother role models	Assist in identifying surrogate mothers and adult women role models within father's support group of relatives, friends, schools

Table 2-5. Nursing Strategies to Maximize the Female-Single-Parent Family Experience

Situational Factors	Nursing Strategies
Mothers may need assistance with financial matters and home repair	Assess need areas. Identify resources such as financial counseling, home repair courses, or community groups that assist in home repair
Children's need for father role models	Assist in identifying surrogate fathers and adult male role models within the mother's group of relatives, friends, schools

and to encourage widening the circle of their relationships. (The foregoing discussion on sexual identification and attitudes pertains to both sexes but is presented in this section because of the popular concerns about single-parent mother-son relationships.)

Table 2-5 identifies the major concerns in the female single-parent family and appropriate nursing strategies to help such problems.

Single-Parent Families Through Divorce

It is estimated that 100,000 Canadian children and 1,000,000 American children are in families experiencing marital breakdown (Shamsie, 1985). Only 50 years ago, divorce was scandalous. Now it is common to find in every classroom some children whose parents are separated or divorced. In fact, these children are a distinct category, "children of divorce," in professional literature (Jenkins, 1978; Wallerstein, 1983).

The attitudinal and economic barriers against divorce have weakened in the last two decades partly because of the women's rights movement. Women and men are increasingly concerned about self fulfillment; it is also an obligation to realize one's potential for growth. For some persons who are struggling with disenchantment with their marriage, professional marriage counseling and support from friends and family do not seem to be enough to stabilize the marriage. For some, economic factors, too-early marriage commitments, the demands of parenting, and the lack of support systems seem to make dissolution of the marriage the only viable option.

Children of these families are caught in the matrix of the parents' frustration and changing lifestyles. The responses of the children depend on several variables, such as the developmental stages of the children, the elapsed time since the event of separation, predivorce family interaction, and postdivorce family structures. The adjustment of children of divorced parents tends to be measured against the norm of children from intact, presumably well-functioning families rather than against children in homes in which there is considerable parental dissension, the predivorce norm (Jenkins, 1978). In addition, there has been little follow-up study of children after the initial crisis.

A longitudinal study following 131 children from 60 divorced families over many years has been done in California by Wallerstein and Kelly (Wallerstein and Kelly, 1980; Wallerstein, 1983). This study is age related and involves children's responses in four developmental periods: preschool, early latency, later latency, and adolescence. The sample is composed of 92 per cent white families, 3 per cent black, and 5 per cent interracial, including Oriental and Hispanic parents. Although replication in samples with a broader class and ethnic base is needed, some salient factors can be noted from this significant research.

The latency period was divided into two distinct groups because of the evidence from the interviews. The latency period is usually viewed as one developmental stage, but the children's responses to divorce were significantly different in the early latency (7 to 8 years) and later latency (9 to 10 years) periods. The children and their parents were seen by an interdisciplinary team during four to six individual clinical sessions conducted over a 6-week span of time. Indepen-

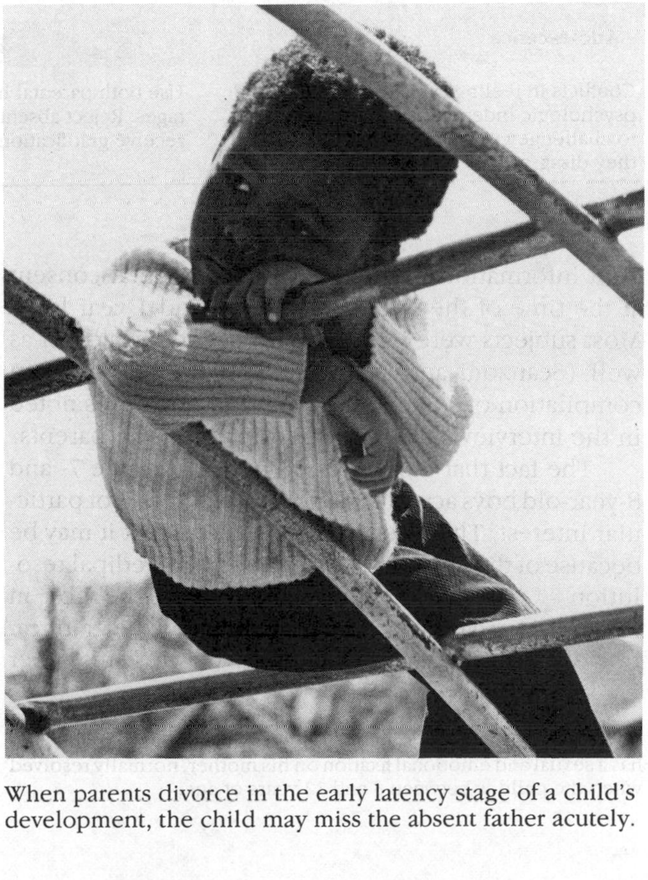

When parents divorce in the early latency stage of a child's development, the child may miss the absent father acutely.

Table 2-6. Children's Responses to Divorce at the Time of Initial Counseling and 1 Year Later

Initial Responses	One Year Later
Preschool	
Use of denial through fantasy. Assumed responsibility for precipitating the divorce. Rise in aggression and irritability	5- to 6-year-olds cling to hope of reconciliation
Early Latency (7- to 8-year-olds)	
Pervasive sadness. Awareness of their own suffering with difficulty gaining relief. Family dissolution perceived as threat to their whole life; fantasies of deprivation. Absent father missed acutely, especially by young boys. Anger toward custodial mother (most lived with mother). Fear of antagonizing mother. Conflicts with loyalty, need to hold on to both parents	Modified responses. Sad, resigned attitude. Reluctantly accept finality of divorce. View life as more difficult; less gratification. Cling to absent fathers, even when fathers are disinterested
Later Latency (9- to 10-year-olds)	
Initial poise, presence, and courage. Age-available coping noted; denial, courage, bravado keeping in motion, conscious avoidance, seeking support. Layering of psychologic functioning, use of coping mechanisms, and simultaneously succumbing to anguish or pain. Conscious, intense anger; organized and object-directed moral stance in judgment against parents. Feelings of vulnerability and lack of security. Variety of somatic complaints	Muted responses; accepting situation. Align with custodial parent. Precocious thrust into adolescent preoccupation with sexuality and assertiveness. Reject absent fathers if they do not receive gratification from them
Adolescence	
Conflicts in feelings toward parents. Some psychologic independence. More freedom to challenge custodial parent's position, if they disagree	Use both parental homes to their advantages. Reject absent fathers if they do not receive gratification

dent information was obtained with parental consent at the time of the initial counseling and 1 year later. Most subjects were interviewed a second year later as well (Scanzoni and Scanzoni, 1981). Table 2-6 is a compilation of some of the common responses noted in the interviews with the children and their parents.

The fact that more than 50 per cent of the 7- and 8-year-old boys acutely missed their fathers is of particular interest. The researchers, postulate that it may be because of the closeness in time of their "oedipal resolution."* Developmentally considered, the boy in early latency has only recently renounced the gratification of his mother, but in divorce he may lose his father as well. It may also threaten to disrupt the process of identification with his father that has been evolving since birth.

As noted, these responses of a middle class, largely white sample cannot be used as generalizations for other social classes and ethnic or racial groups. However, they do serve as a model for raising questions about other groups of families enmeshed in the complexities of divorce. Professional nurses can be cognizant of the probable differences between the early and later latency responses and the resulting needs of the children. In this study no consistent parallels between behavior at home and in school could be noted. The effect of divorce on school performance showed wide variation. Sometimes there was increased success in school and in other cases a decline in school achievement was noted. This is important because too fre-

* The psychologic stage in a boy's development in which he has a sexual and emotional fixation on his mother, normally resolved when the child is between 8 and 12 years of age.

quently expectations for children's behavior in school are formed according to what is known about their home situation.

The nurse's role in the dilemma of divorce will depend on the period of time elapsed since the parental separation, the child care arrangements, and the ages and sexes of the children. When nurses are the primary care providers, they may be the key people who can help the family members obtain professional counseling. In the community they may be instrumental in the development of support groups for divorced parents or children of divorce or both. They often may serve as the liaison between the home and the school when the reasons for a child's behavior are being sought. The effects of divorce on the well-being of the client should always be a concern for nurses. Box 2-2 contains an annotated list of books that may be helpful to children and parents in divorce.

Divorce remains a topic for continued concern and careful research. Predictions are that marital separation will continue to increase. The parents and the children affected need various levels of support not only during the initial crisis but also until some measure of equilibrium is found in which all family members feel a sense of identity, security, and encouragement for growth.

Single-Parent Families Through Death

The possibility of losing a parent by death is seldom discussed in families, and yet it is a reality for many children. The reactions and adjustments of children to the death of a parent depend on their development stages, the openness with which their dual-parent family discussed death, and the support that they have to discuss their feelings after the death of the parent.

In the last two decades professional literature and popular magazines have contained many articles encouraging people to deal openly with fears of death and to consider death as a part of life. Probably the researcher who has had the greatest impact, especially among professionals, is Elisabeth Kübler-Ross (Kübler-Ross, 1975), who conducted a series of research projects in which she has learned about the experience of imminent death from children and adults who are dying. She and her fellow researchers recorded and analyzed the responses of dying persons and their families. She says that we routinely shelter children from death and dying, thinking we are protecting them from harm. But it is clear that we do them a disservice by depriving them of the experience. By making dying a taboo subject and keeping children away from people who are dying, we create unnecessary fear.

Grieving is necessary for all children who are separated from a parent by death. Preschool children faced with the death of a parent cannot comprehend the finality of death. For them, death is reversible. If encouraged, these young children will verbalize and, in their play, act out their fantasies of the parent's return. Children in the latency period who understand the finality of death may react with sadness, withdrawal, regression, and anger. They may be very reluctant to verbalize their feelings but often become adept at drawing pictures depicting their emotions. Adolescents are more sophisticated in their range of coping mechanisms and may feel the need to mask their intense feelings of loss. They respond according to what they think is an appropriate adult response (that is, denial of death). They too need supportive persons around them who will listen but not insist on verbalization.

The remaining parent may be so involved in his or her own grief that it is difficult to respond to the developmental level of the children's needs. Nurses involved in the situation should assess this burden for the remaining spouse and help each family member find resource persons who can be available to them.

The children's later responses to living in a single-parent family will depend largely on their ability to work through the grief process. The finality of death, even though painful and difficult, needs to be psychologically dealt with by children of all ages. It is essential that the children receive sustained and open support as they incorporate this painful experience into their lives (Jewett, 1982).

Never-Married Single-Parent Families

In considering persons who are parents but have never been married, the factor of choice and nonchoice is relevant. Although questions have often been raised about the covert psychologic need of the unwed mother to bear a child, the fact remains that if she chooses to bear the child, she must either have the child adopted, or become a single parent. In the past, the majority of unwed mothers did not consciously choose that role, and society at large did not accord single unwed mothers respect. In fact, historically children born out of wedlock have been referred to as illegitimate children or bastards, a stigma that affected their lives adversely. The social stigma of illegitimacy has stemmed, in part, from the expectation that children without a father would not be provided for properly. As women establish themselves socially and in the work place, the single woman who chooses to have children is better able to provide them with access to the social world and the resources once considered solely a father's contribution. Although the term *illegit-*

Box 2-2

Selected Books for Parents and Children about Divorce. Stepparenting, and Alternative Families

BOOKS FOR YOUNG CHILDREN

Baum L: *One More Time*. New York, William Morrow and Company, 1986. ($10.25) *A young boy's "visitation" time with his father is treated with gentle humor. The point is made that although the "goodbye" is hard at the end of the day, it is made easier by knowing there will be another day together soon.*

Boegehold B: *Daddy Doesn't Live Here Any More*. New York, A Golden Book, 1985. ($3.50) *A story detailing a little girl's feelings about her parents' divorce. Contains foreword with suggestions for parents about talking with young children.*

Boyd L: *The Not-So-Wicked Stepmother*. New York, Viking Kestrel, 1987. *A story about a young child's fears and anxieties in meeting the new stepmother. Details how the little girl works through her confused feelings when the stepmother she is determined to hate turns out to be nice.*

Brown LK, Brown M: *Dinosaurs Divorce: A Guide for Changing Families*. Boston, Little, Brown and Company, 1986. ($13.95) *A story of a dinosaur family going through divorce and remarriage, living with stepbrothers and stepsisters. Allows the child to view a sensitive subject from a safe distance. Contains a list of definitions of "divorce" words, including lawyer, visiting rights, judge, half brother or half sister.*

Lindsay JW: *Do I Have a Daddy? A Story about a Single-Parent Child*. Buena Park, CA, Morning Glory Press, 1982. ($3.95) *In this story the young child's question about his father is triggered by questions from his peers. Offers suggestions about answering peer questions and looks at the possibility that his mother may someday remarry. Appendix addressed to parents, including those single through divorce and those never married.*

Magid K, Schreibman W: *Divorce Is . . . A Kids' Coloring Book*. Gretna, LA, Pelican Publishing Company, 1980. ($5.95) *Pictures to color are based upon "the 25 top problem questions" children ask about divorce and are paired with answers to the questions. For example, a picture of a child being physically pulled between parents has the caption, "Sometimes I feel I have to choose between Mom and Dad." It is followed by two "answer" pages. The first shows the child and father at the zoo: "Even though Mom and Dad don't live together anymore I can still have fun with Dad . . ." The second shows the child with Mom at an amusement park: ". . . or do something special with Mom."*

BOOKS FOR SCHOOL-AGE CHILDREN

Dragonwagon C: *Dianna, Maybe*. New York, Macmillan Publishing Company, 1987. ($11.95) *A whimsical story of a school-age girl who dreams of someday meeting her half-sister, her father's child from a previous marriage. Explores feelings of "belonging" and the parent's sadness at the failed first relationship.*

Fassler D, Lash M, Ives SB: Changing Families: A Guide for Kids and Grown-Ups. Burlington, VT, Waterfront Books, 1988. ($14.95) *A book of children's drawings about the changes associated with separation, divorce, and remarriage. Some pages encourage the child to draw his or her own picture. Designed to be used by parents or professionals to help a child talk about and work through feelings.*

Gardner RA: *The Boys and Girls Book about Divorce*. New York, Bantam Books, 1970. ($3.50) *Now in its 15th printing, this book provides answers to questions children frequently ask about divorce. Based upon the author's psychiatric practice with children of divorce and their families.*

Gardner RA: *The Boys and Girls Book about Step-Families*. Cresskill, NJ, Creative Therapeutics, 1982. ($3.50) *Provides answers to questions frequently asked about living with a stepfamily. Includes parent living with an unmarried partner, adoption by a stepparent, and when and where to seek counseling. Reading level is for age 10 years or older.*

Jong E: *Megan's Book of Divorce*. New York, New American Library, 1984. ($10.50) *The story of divorce through the eyes of a 4-year-old girl. Treated with humor and irony and details her antics in trying to make trouble between each parent and their new love interest. For example: "I tell him: 'Don't hug Mommy.' He says: 'Somebody has to hug your Mommy.' I say: 'I will do it! Or let Doug.' He says to Mommy: 'Who the heck is Doug?'" Although advertised as "a kid's book for adults", seems more appropriate for school-age children or even adolescents who could identify with the feelings but feel enough "removed" from the preschool age to find some emotional release in the humor.*

Krementz J: *How It Feels When Parents Divorce*. New York, Alfred A. Knopf, 1984. ($12.95) *Children from 7 to 16 years of age were interviewed and photographed, and the children's own words are used in the stories. The point is made that they agreed to share these feelings so other children would know they're not alone.*

Nystrom C: *Mike's Lonely Summer. A Child's Guide to Divorce*. Belleville, MI, Lion Publishing Company, 1986. ($6.95) *Story details a 10-year-old boy's feelings about divorce and, in the end, helps him find meaning through his religious faith.*

BOOKS FOR ADOLESCENTS

Brogan JP, Maiden U: *The Kids' Guide to Divorce*. New York: Ballantine, 1986. ($2.95) *Includes a loss inventory scale that the reader completes to calculate the impact of divorce on his or her lifestyle.*

Dolmetsch P, Shih A (eds): *The Kids' Book about Single-Parent Families*. New York, Doubleday, 1985. ($7.95) *Children ages 11 to 15 years talk about their lives after divorce, death of a parent, or in never-*

married, single-parent families. Designed to recognize the richness of life that is possible in single parent families.

Getzoff A, McClenahan C: *Step Kids. A Survival Guide for Teenagers in Stepfamilies.* New York, Walker and Company, 1984. ($8.95) *Includes discussion of a parent in a homosexual relationship. Sections throughout contain advice on "how to cope," "how to say it," and "how not to say it."*

Willis I, Richards A: *How to Get It Together When Your Parents Are Coming Apart.* Summit, NJ, Willard Press, 1976. ($9.95) *A psychologist and high school teacher team up to discuss the process of family quarrels, divorce, and the aftermath. Includes causes for divorce such as a homosexual or alcoholic parent. Each section begins with a short vignette of a teen in a particular situation and then goes on to discuss the feelings involved and to give the reader suggestions for action.*

BOOKS FOR PARENTS

Berman C: *Making It as a Stepparent.* New York, Harper and Row, 1986. ($6.95) *Based on interviews with hundreds of blended families. Includes discussion of money matters, visitation rights, use of family names, discipline, and "the instant parent syndrome."*

Burns C: *Stepmotherhood. How to Survive Without Feeling Frustrated, Left Out, or Wicked.* New York, Harper and Row, 1985. ($6.95) *Looks at the range of stepparenting experiences with humor, "avoiding glib reassurance and false cheer." Suggests many stepparents either underestimate the demands or expect too much from the role.*

Goldstein S, Solnit AJ: *Divorce and Your Child: Practical Suggestions for Parents.* New Haven, CT, Yale University Press, 1984. ($5.95) *A lawyer and child psychiatrist discuss implications of divorce for children and give practical suggestions for handling both legal and emotional problems.*

Rogers F, O'Brien C: *Mister Rogers Talks with Families about Divorce.* New York, Berkley Publishing Company, 1987. ($6.95) *A book to help parents deal with children of divorce from toddlers to teens. Describes experiences of other families. Includes a read-aloud story for younger children.*

Roosevelt R, Lofas J: *Living in step. A Remarriage Manual for Parents and Children.* New York, McGraw-Hill Book Company, 1977. ($5.95) *Identifies roots of resentment in stepfamilies and shows how some families have handled "merging" of families. Designed to help stepfamilies achieve harmony. Includes the parent with and without custody and "the myth of instant love."*

(Compiled by Roxie Foster.)

imate is still used in the courts and in federal statistics, the social stigma is decreasing.

Second only to divorced persons, the most rapidly growing category of single parents, especially since 1970, has been the never-married mother (Bronfenbrenner, 1977). In part, this has been due to the changing values in American society, such as increasing acceptance of extramarital intercourse, single mothers keeping their babies in lieu of adoption or abortion, and single-parent adoption of children. (Single-parent adoptions are discussed later in this chapter in the section on adoption.)

The most important factor in discussing parenthood outside of marriage is the preparation and desire of the parent to provide for and nurture children. When parenthood is voluntarily chosen by a single person who is equipped to provide the child with the necessary resources, the experience can be beneficial and satisfying to both parent and child (Scanzoni and Scanzoni, 1981). These mothers consider parenting a role that will give them satisfaction and believe that they have a contribution to make to their children.

Eiduson (1978) reports three distinct categories of single mothers: nest builders — women who consciously chose and planned to have a baby and start a new household; post-hoc adaptors — women who had not planned to become pregnant but adjusted happily to this circumstance; and a small group of unwed mothers — more like the unwed mothers of yesteryear in attitudes and circumstances. The levels of education and of professional development, income status, and general lifestyle were distinctive for each group, with the nest builders being the most self-sufficient women, whose goals were most closely tied to those of the women's movement. Roles and responsibilities toward the child also differed among the groups, depending on the availability of economic, psychologic, and social support.

Stepfamilies

An increasing number of children in the United States live in stepfamilies. In 1985, over 15 million children in the United States were living in stepfamilies (Reutter and Strang, 1986.) Families reconstitute for many reasons; also, there are many possible relationships among family members, depending on the number of previous marriages and children involved. An 8-year-old child was overheard exclaiming to her friend, "You have so many different mothers and grandmothers and brothers and fathers, how can you keep them all straight!" Her friend replied nonchalantly, "Well, it is no problem for me." Although there may be special problems in stepfamilies with their varied relationships, they are not insurmountable.

The terms used to describe stepfamilies are also varied. The term *step* is derived from an Old English word meaning *to bereave* (Scanzoni and Scanzoni, 1981). When a stepfamily is formed because of the death of a spouse, the term is appropriate. However, in remarriage after divorce the child has both biologic parents as well as a stepparent, which is an additional parent rather than a replacement. Stepfamilies are now frequently referred to as *blended families* or *merged families.* Just as there are inadequate kinship terms, there are also inadequate guidelines for responding to the needs of these new relationships.

Children in stepfamilies face adjustments that may be overwhelming, especially in the early stages. Disequilibrium should be expected, because the children have been developing values that now may be in conflict with those of the stepparent. Stern (1982) states that family cultural beliefs that shape children's value patterns may differ sharply among the members of the new family constellation. Beliefs about proper behavior, especially regarding childrearing and discipline, are internalized and become part of each person's cultural perspective. If there is dramatic disparity between the birth parent's and stepparent's cultural rules and cultural norms for enforcing rules, conflict will arise about whose rules should be enforced.

The process of assimilation should be a major concern for families in which various combinations of birth parent and stepparent relationships with children exist. Two one-parent families may be brought together into a single household, or a single parent may marry a spouse without children. The family system becomes even more involved if birth parents with whom the children continue a viable relationship live elsewhere. Some children live with a birth parent and a stepparent and spend weekends with the other birth parent and a different stepparent.

When a parent dies and the remaining parent remarries, the stepparent may have to deal with the overidealization of the dead parent by some children (Krementz, 1981). Some children make comparisons between the idealized parent and the stepparent as a way to hold onto the memory of the dead parent. The best way to cope with the situation is to discuss the good points of the deceased parent and yet not agree to the comparison.

The responses and needs of the children depend to a great extent on the relationships established in the previous family system. If there was unresolved hostility and anger, with little parental support for the children, they may respond with eagerness to a new avenue of love. Or they may have difficulty trusting the stepparent, afraid to invest in another failure. Some of the child's anger at the absent birth parent may be displaced onto the stepparent, since the child may feel safer in doing this. The nurse should encourage the stepparent not to take this anger personally, because he or she obviously is not responsible for it. To react angrily in retaliation may only verify the child's feelings that she or he was correct in the first place, and this may interfere with full acceptance of good feelings about the stepparent. See Box 2-2, an annotated list of books that may be helpful to parents and children in stepfamilies.

The ages of the children also determine their responses to the stepparent (Longfellow, 1979; Wallerstein and Kelly, 1980). Developmental tasks may be interrupted by the change in family relationships. At some ages the bonding between parent and child seems to be more crucial. For instance, the 10-month-old infant who has been cared for primarily by the mother and enters a relationship with a stepfather may be able to adjust rather quickly because of the sustained relationship with the birth mother. However, the 5-year-old son who is sorting through oedipal relationships and begins a new relationship with a stepfather may have more difficulties in the assimilation process. Adolescents who are in the process of self-identity and are fluctuating between the need for parental guidance and self-reliance sometimes find the relationship with the stepparent most difficult (Wald, 1981).

The individual members in the new family system have ongoing developmental tasks now placed within the complex context of a family that is forming a new identity in which marital roles and parental roles must be assumed simultaneously (Wald, 1981). Privacy, time, and energy available to new couples without children are not readily accessible in newly constituted stepfamilies. The ambivalent feelings expressed in a stepfamily about new family relationships need to be viewed as a developmental task of establishing the family roles and rules of behavior.

Sometimes single parent units, such as the mother and her children and the father and his children, resist the tasks of stabilization of the new family unit by maintaining prior single-parent family patterns (Wald, 1981). In these situations, schisms develop whereby the children do not accept parenting by the stepparent. Ideally, all family members need to work at establishing a balance between the old and the new bonds so that the rights and needs of all are recognized.

Even though the incidence of stepfamily relationships is increasing in the United States, there is still little research on stepfamily development, behavior, and outcomes. Most research focuses on stepfather families (Wallerstein and Kelly, 1980; Biller, 1981; Hetherington et al, 1982; Santrock et al, 1982; Stern, 1982). Until recently, mothers most often were given custody of the children in divorce settlements. Hence, when these mothers remarried, it was the stepfather who joined the mother-child/children family unit. The longitudinal studies of divorced and remarried families reported by Wallerstein and Kelly (1980) emphasize that although conflicts may arise between the children and the stepfather, a relationship with an interested stepfather appeared to have positive effects.

As a result of their research, Hetherington et al (1982) stress the importance of a child's continuing relationship with the divorced parent as well as the parents in the stepfamily. In their study, children benefited when the continuing relationship with the divorced parent was associated with positive attitudes toward childrearing expressed by the stepfather.

Stepfamily relationships can be very complex. Nurses and other health care professionals should focus on intervention processes that "facilitate the building of empathetic bridges among all family members and move the family from a small group of strangers to one that has identified realistic goals in the service of achieving a workable family balance" (Wald, 1981).

Many families benefit from support groups. Local communities may have a stepparents' support group sponsored by a church or other social agency. Contact can also be made with the Stepfamily Association of America, Inc.*

Recognition of the problems and potentials in the steprelationship is necessary for the parents as well as the children. Sussman (1978) summarizes the strengths and limitations in Box 2-3.

> Box 2-3
> *Strengths and Weaknesses in Stepparenting*
>
> **STRENGTHS**
>
> Previous marital experiences may result in an increased number (actual incidence unknown) of stable marriages.
>
> Parenting, which may formerly have been the function of a single adult, may be shared with the new partner and his or her older children.
>
> For some, there is improved economic status as a consequence of shared income.
>
> **WEAKNESSES**
>
> The difficulties in blending two formerly independent households into one functioning unit may result in extreme emotional stress for some members.
>
> Formations consisting of two large families may require substantial economic help, counseling, and other supports to survive.
>
> Economic and social commitments to individuals of previous marriages may restrict the development of adequate, stable relationships in the new marriage.

Foster Parents

Foster care of children refers to parenting by persons who are not the biologic or adoptive parents of the children involved. The foster child is not an orphan; one or both birth parents are living (Guerney, 1982). For various reasons the care of the child by the birth parents or parent has been interrupted temporarily or permanently. This has necessitated placement of the child in another family.

Placement in families can be a formal or informal process. If a social agency assumes jurisdiction for the child's welfare, the placement process is a carefully detailed procedure whereby the foster parents must meet criteria before becoming approved. Payment, usually minimal, is involved. Some persons or families assume foster parenting responsibilities through friendship or familial ties with the birth parent who is unable to care for the child. This arrangement is more often temporary; for instance, the child stays with the foster family until the birth parent again gets a job or remarries or recovers from some other family crisis.

Permanence is increasingly becoming a major issue in foster care (Fanshel and Shinn, 1978). In the recent past and even today, many foster children are moved from foster home to foster home, sometimes with intermittent periods of time with their birth parent. Anyone with even limited knowledge of the developmental tasks and needs for nurturing of children can speculate about the problems of these children. There is an important difference between protecting children from the extremes of neglect or abuse and providing care that ensures permanency in living arrangements and continuity of relationships.

Fanshel and Shinn (1978) report in their longitudinal study of children in foster care that:

> It is no longer considered sufficient that a child be afforded a placement situation in which his basic needs are being cared for in terms of shelter, food and clothing, and a benign environment in which positive emotional growth can be enhanced. A newly emphasized criterion is being used to assess the adequacy of an agency's performance, namely whether a child can be assured permanency in his living

* Stepfamily Association of America, Inc., 28 Allegheny Avenue, Suite 307, Baltimore, MD 21204.

arrangements and continuity of relationship. It is not enough that he might be placed in a foster family home that offers him family-like care. If he cannot regard the people he is living with as his family, on a permanent basis, his situation is increasingly regarded as reflecting something less than an adequate resolution to his life situation.

Permanency planning must begin early in foster care. This means intensive work with the birth parents to achieve a decision on their child's future. Care must be given to balancing the rights and wishes of the parents and the rights and needs of the children, especially when the need for continuity is added to the child's rights.

The pediatric nurse who cares for foster children should be aware of the physical and psychologic impact of foster care. Large segments of the past may not be known or may be incomplete. The child may be beset with chronic feelings of inadequacy, unworthiness, and low self-esteem. He or she may have difficulty relating emotionally, often developing shallow relationships, afraid to get attached to any person because of fear of loss or separation.

The nurse tries to ensure a nonthreatening environment for the child. The foster parents need support in understanding that the anger the child may display toward them is rarely a direct attack against them as caretakers. These children often have been hurt, disappointed, and deserted. They need an environment where they can express themselves and receive loving care and guidance. The nurse and foster parents need to watch for clues of past trauma. The present situation may awaken emotional reactions of the past. The child needs safe and acceptable avenues to express feelings from the past without being rejected. This attitude requires investment of time and effort. In many nonverbal and verbal ways the child forces the issue, asking, "You really care above me, don't you?" The foster parents' and the nurse's gratification comes from the glimmer of hope in the child's eyes with each new invitation to trust others in his or her world.

Migrant Children

Children of migrant laborers know transience as a way of life, since the family moves with the job. Farm labor is seasonal; families may move to another state or from one section of a state to another, as do the fruit harvesters in Florida, or they may travel from Mexico to the northern midwestern states. In this case the change means contact with a different culture and language.

These children are sometimes referred to as "children who follow the sun" or "children of the road" (Park, 1976). They are born into one of the grimmest poverty situations in the country. The living accommodations are often make-shift, minimal, and crowded. Illnesses such as rickets, scurvy, pinworms, anemia, and malnutrition abound. At an early age the children join their parents in the fields, and many spend the rest of their lives working in similar situations. Their school life is interrupted frequently — in fact, every few weeks at the peak harvest season. School records seldom move with the children, increasing the problems of continuity. Lack of health records poses the same problem, sometimes necessitating repeated immunizations; at other times tests and immunizations are missed.

Since 1966 the federal government has taken special interest in the welfare of migrant children. Title I of the Elementary Education Act was amended to give the US Office of Education authority and funds to improve educational programs and to offer supplemental services for these children (Park, 1976). Continuity of instruction, health care, nutrition, and psychologic services have high priority.

In 1974, Public Law 93-380 authorized the use of the Migrant Student Record Transfer System, a computer data bank located in Little Rock, Arkansas, which can trace the whereabouts of each migrating child (Park, 1976). This service makes student placement easier, indicates where special help is needed, and eliminates repetition of tests and physical examinations. In one instance it was used to find more than 200 children who were potential victims or carriers of typhoid fever.

There has been improvement in educational, health, and social services for migrant children; however, the greatest barrier remaining is the manner in which these services are delivered. Ida Brownlee Bragdon, herself once a migrant child and now an oral language specialist working with migrants, identifies the masks of nonverbal behavior, periodic tuning-out, blank stares, ignorance, and hostility that these children wear and suggests ways to lift the masks (Bragdon, 1976). Environmental, economic, and social factors as well as lack of communication between the migrant children and providers of education and health services help produce these defense mechanisms. The most effective way to reach these children is to recognize their strengths (Table 2-7) (Bragdon, 1976). Health care strategies should be built on the positive attributes of these families.

Adoption

Adoption refers to the process of surrogate parents assuming legal custody of children who were not born to them. Various types are dual parents, single parents, transracial adoptions, transcultural adoptions, intercountry adoptions, and stepchild adoptions. The adoption process is also varied, involving adoptions through public and private adoption agencies, those arranged through physicians and lawyers, and some

Table 2-7. Potential Strengths of Migrant Children

Strength	Rationale
Eager to please	Families emphasize respect for authority
Responsible	Care for younger children, contribute to family income
Loved	Families welcome children with enthusiasm
Adaptable	Move frequently, adjust quickly
Perceptive and sensitive	Language barriers increase need to read visual cues
Express themselves vividly with family	Little contact outside migrant group
Want education	Encouraged to continue to enroll in school
Curious	Have had many and diverse living situations
Possess a culture	Beliefs, values, and behavior based on survival in life they know

These strengths may not apply to all migrant children. Other positive attributes will then need to be identified to serve as a basis for health care strategies.

arranged by other intermediaries functioning between the birth parents and the adoptive parents. State laws govern adoption and, although generally similar, they vary in specific details that should be known to all involved in the adoption process. Intercountry adoptions sometimes involve a prolonged process during which each country's adoption laws are being satisfied.

The overt and covert reasons for the formation of adoptive families are also many and varied. Some persons adopt children for social conscience motives: population control, assisting handicapped children, or breaking race barriers and poverty cycles. Others adopt because of needs for personal fulfillment through parenting when bearing children is not possible or feasible: infertility problems, personal choice to circumvent pregnancy and labor, single parenthood. Still others respond to extended family or godparent commitments when children are separated from birth parents by death or desertion.

Each adoptive family is the result of a unique combination of factors, all of which have a bearing on the relationships. Nurses may not know these factors, but they should be sensitive to the complex and unique qualities of each adoptive situation, which cannot be discussed here in detail. Some aspects of adoption that can help the nurse interact positively with families will be discussed.

Development of Entitlement. The purpose of adoption is the creation of a continuing relationship not formed by birth. This relationship must be viewed as being as real as the biologic one. The length of time it takes for entitlement (the right of adopted children and adults to fully belong) to develop varies according to the age of the child at the time of adoption and the psychologic reaction of the parents to the adoption. If the parents feel that conception and pregnancy are necessary for complete parent-child bonding, they may never view the adopted child as really "theirs." The child will always be "their adopted child," rather than simply "their child." If the sense of belongingness is not developed, the adults can never be successful parents. If it is partially developed, the adults can parent some of the time but may have problems with discipline, with allowing the child to separate from them, or with telling the child about the adoption (Depp, 1982).

Persons outside the family sometimes verbalize their awe or disbelief that the parents and siblings do not differentiate their feelings of belonging between children born into the family and those adopted. Families with only adopted children do not know how they might feel with children born to them, but families with children both born to them and adopted by them can attest to their bonding with each child in the family. All children in the family need to be included in the development of entitlement.

It is best for the family members to openly acknowledge their feelings of belongingness with each other. This may be difficult for some, but if adoption is an acceptable topic of discussion and related to the developmental age of the children, it can be a rewarding process, a growth experience for all members of the family. All persons need to acknowledge their self-identity at various stages in life. The family with adopted members is forced by circumstances to deal with this issue and can be healthier for it. Some may need assistance in discussing their relationships and feelings about adoption. Nurses can encourage and guide this process or help the family find professional counseling services in the community.

Adoption does not have a negative effect on self-concept. Studies have shown no significant difference in self-concept of adolescent adoptees and nonadoptees (Norvell and Guy, 1977). The initial motive of the parents to adopt is the most important factor in successful adjustment. Therefore, nurses should carefully assess the parents' views of bonding with their adopted children and assist parents in developing realistic and healthy attitudes in their parenting roles.

Telling or not telling children about their adoption has been an ongoing topic of discussion among professionals and lay persons (Dukette, 1984). In most communities stories still circulate with variations on the theme of tragic results when persons learned of their adoptive state at inopportune times in their lives. Some families and communities have not fully dealt with entitlement.

At the same time, many heartening changes are taking place in sociocultural values and agency policies. Attention is being given to the value of adoptive ties that weave adoptees and their families into a complete life experience, with a beginning as well as a future (Dukette, 1984; Pannor and Barron, 1984).

Open Adoption. Open adoption is a recent trend in adoption. It refers to the policy in which the birth mother and father, if he is available, participate in the choice of the adoptive family and, in some instances, maintain contact with the child throughout his or her life (Haithman, 1984; Pannor and Barron, 1984). Open adoptions have occurred informally for years, but the development of adoption agency policies that encourage and assist the birth parents and the adoptive parents in relating to the child in an open, supportive manner is relatively recent.

A number of societal trends have encouraged open adoption. The increasing divorce rate has meant that many children and adults have needed to relate to both birth parents and stepparents, often involving adoption. Research has indicated that it is desirable for children to maintain relationships with these sets of parents in many situations (Wallerstein and Kelly, 1980). Adoption laws changed in 1975 to allow adult adoptees to obtain information about birth parents if birth parents did not forbid it. Therefore, many persons argue that it is reasonable to share the information at the outset (Hall and King, 1982). Sociocultural sanctions regarding out-of-wedlock pregnancies have changed in recent years. Many birth mothers who have relinquished their children for adoption have been resentful about the abruptness with which the separation took place. Proponents of open adoption believe that a more humane process in adoption will encourage mothers, especially teenage mothers, to consider it. The birth mother who chooses open adoption can have a major role in determining the adoptive couple and deciding on the appropriateness of a continuing relationship with her child.

It is important to understand that agencies that espouse open adoption insist that arrangements cannot be finalized until after the baby is born. The birth parent is supported in the decision-making process during the prenatal period, but after the birth she or they must have the opportunity to reconsider. This is difficult for the potential adoptive couple, and they will need much support during that period.

In open adoption the adoptive parents become the legal guardians of the child in the same manner as in traditional adoptions. In other words, the adoption laws have not changed. Rather, it is a bureaucratic and a social change, not a legal one. Any agreement to share relationships with the child following adoption is strictly voluntary on the part of the adoptive parents and the birth parents.

In some instances the adoptive parents attend the birth, some even providing coaching during labor. The birth parents quite commonly choose adoptive families that resemble their own, and the relationship is thus more likely to be compatible. However, there are many variations in the process and frequency of continuing the relationship. For some, the contact between the birth parent, adoptive family, and child continues to be made through the agency. The visits may be negotiated, such as only two per year between the child and the birth parent. In contrast, the birth mother may be used as a babysitter for the child.

As more reports on open adoption are circulated in the media and more agencies consider the advantages and disadvantages of open adoption, this option is likely to increase. Research is needed on the longitudinal effects on all parties. In the meantime, nurses relating to adoptive families and birth parents should be knowledgeable about this option and should increase their skills in offering support and counsel to families who choose open adoption. One adoptive family summed it up this way (Wallace, 1984):

> For the birth mother, open adoption affords continuing reassurance through letters and photographs that her baby is loved and prospering. For us there is a link to our son's past, an inalienable part of him. For our son, there is evidence that he was loved from the moment of his birth and before.

Transracial Adoption. Some families adopt children of a different race. These families cannot easily choose when to tell their child about adoption because the child's skin color or physical features are unlike those of the parents. Strangers often assume that they are not a family.

One family tells of an incident in which their 4-year-old child (he was mulatto and they were white) wandered about a restaurant until the waiter brought the family's food, whereupon he again joined his parents to eat. The proprietor came to the table and said, "Friendly little fellow, just comes and eats with you." "But he is our son," the mother replied. "No, he is not," the proprietor insisted, "he belongs to that other family." There was also a Mexican-American family in the restaurant. It took further discussion to convince the proprietor that the child and parents indeed belonged together.

In transracial adoption, parents and children must establish their relationship in their own way when others question their identity as a family unit. One child, becoming aware of his appearance with the family, would look at himself often in the mirror, sometimes calling himself derogatory names. His mother once asked, "If you could have anything in the world you wanted, what would it be?" He laid his brown arm alongside her pale one and said, "To look like you, Mommy." With love and with constancy, yet not with-

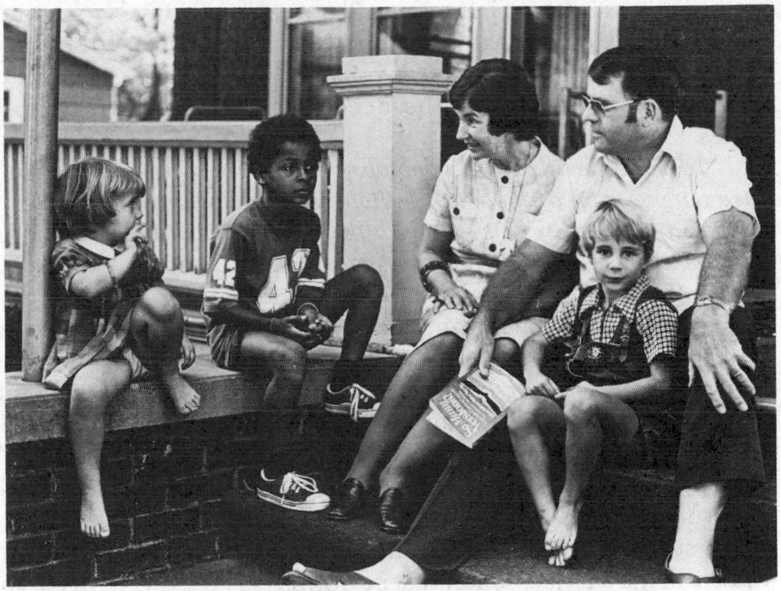

In adoptive families, parents and children in their own ways must establish their identity as a family unit. Parents are able to bond with each of their children, whether the child is born to them or adopted, of the same race or different. (Photograph by Alice Roth.)

out sadness and hurts, this family supported each other in recognizing the child's identity as he continued to work through who he was. When he was 12 years old, in class, the teacher asked which skin color is the best. "The color you *are*," he volunteered.

Some professionals, as well as some racial groups, are very critical of transracial adoptions. There is little question that it is preferable for children to be adopted into families who are as similar to the child as possible, if these families are capable of providing loving support and encouragement. If such parents are not available, the child's present need for food, shelter, and a home is considered by some to be more important than future psychologic and pyschosocial needs (McRoy et al, 1982). When the parents are comfortable in the parenting role and recognize the problems in transracial adoption, they can support the child as he or she develops an identity in the transracial setting. In fact, the home can become a microcosm of what the world community is really like. Multiracial appreciation is not only discussed but also acted upon.

Single-Parent Adoption. What makes single women or single men choose a role that many divorcees and widowed persons find stressful? Dougherty (1978) sought the answer to this question and reports on the increasing incidence of single-parent adoptions. The majority of mothers studied were willing to accept responsibility for the child, and all were highly educated. Other single parents, friends, and family provided the needed support. Moral support was a recognized need, but few wanted institutional help. Adjustments focused on scheduling, new financial arrangements, and change in friends. Some of these persons experienced a broadening of their circle of friends to include couples with children, but they also lost some of their previous friends who did not care to adjust to the needs of children in the single-parent's home.

Surrogate Pregnancies and in Vitro Fertilization

In recent years some new options have been made available for couples in which the prospective mother is unable to conceive or maintain a pregnancy. *In vitro fertilization* and *surrogate pregnancy* are two such options. Both options are controversial, raising ethical and legal questions.

In surrogate pregnancies, the infertile couple contracts with a woman who is artificially inseminated with the husband's semen (Reame, 1984). After the baby is born, the surrogate mother relinquishes all parental rights to the biologic father and his wife, usually at the time of delivery. The couple pays a fee, which has raised the ethical issue of whether surrogate mothering is "baby selling."

The surrogate mother and the couple whose child she is bearing need support and guidance as they separately or together deal with the complexities in the situation. The surrogate mother must handle her family's and friends' reactions to her pregnancy, her own feelings about maternal-infant bonding, any obstetric complications that may develop, relationships with the adoptive couple, and eventual relinquishing of the infant after birth (Reame, 1984; Reame and Parker, 1984). The biologic father and his wife, while pleased with the possibility of a child entering their family, may be concerned about the possibility of a miscarriage, their relationship to the surrogate mother, and the possibility of her changing her mind and not relinquishing the child. The emotional, legal, and ethical problems in surrogate mothering are numerous, and state or federal legislation is likely to be needed to clarify the issues.

"In vitro fertilization involves recovering a mature oocyte from an ovarian follicle through laparoscopy and fertilizing this egg with the man's sperm in a Petri dish filled with culture medium" (Garner, 1983). If fertilization occurs, the embryo is transferred into the uterus of the woman. In vitro fertilization (IVF) and embryo transfer (ET) may be indicated for approximately 40 per cent of infertile couples and therefore offers hope for an estimated four million couples (Garner, 1983).

The nurse's role with the couple who is attempting in vitro fertilization and embryo transfer is that of educator, support person, and counselor. For the nurse who is on the staff at a center that performs IVF/ET, the nursing functions include providing factual information and emotional support for the couple, pre- and postoperative teaching, and assisting with the technical procedures in estradiol monitoring and embryo transfer.

When couples do not achieve pregnancy with the embryo transfer, the nurse is involved with grief counseling, since the grief reaction may be similar to that following miscarriage. The nurse's role is especially strategic because usually very few of the couple's friends know of their participation in the IVF program (Garner, 1983.)

In contrast, when pregnancies result, the nurse's role includes the opportunity for early prenatal teaching. From a medical standpoint, they become a "normal pregnant couple." Nevertheless, the couple need continuing support as they deal with their own feelings and the general public's reactions to this comparatively new phenomenon creating family life with "test-tube babies," as the media have chosen to dub this approach to infertility.

Communal Families

Communes are intentional communities that are formed of biologically unrelated people who live together in order to build a kind of large chosen family (Scanzoni and Scanzoni, 1981). Commune members are interdependent and expect a commitment from one another. Communal living is not a new phenomenon; the practice stretches far back into history, even to biblical times (Acts 2:44–45). The best known modern communal society is the kibbutz movement in Israel.

Communes are organized for a variety of reasons. Many have been organized to avoid, challenge, or replace the highly competitive materialistic atmosphere spawned in the urban-industrial society. Others have sought family systems that foster individual growth. Whatever the goals, communes tend to be formed by groups of people who are actively searching for a better way of life. Their motivation may be religious, political, economic, psychosocial, or a combination of these.

Communal childrearing is a convenient way of caring for children since the responsibility is shared by the group (Scanzoni and Scanzoni, 1981). It is often the means by which the commune's ideals are taught. This is exemplified by the Oneida Community,* in which a basic tenet was for all people to love each other equally. A special relationship between parent and child was considered out of keeping with universal love. This view is different from that of the kibbutz, in which childrearing is shared but parents can visit young children in the Children's House at any time and have special times when the children can join them in their private quarters (Spiro, 1967).

Spiro contends that the kibbutz is a child-oriented society par excellence (Spiro, 1967). Children are prized above all else, and no sacrifice is too great to make for them. Collective education may be strict and formal but the amount of energy, money, and services provided for the children is noteworthy. The functions of the parent and the "nurse" (nurse in the sense of caretaker for children) can be divided into four categories: caretaking, nurturing, training, and values. The "nurse" is responsible for nurturing and caretaking only. After the child is 2 years old, the sole responsibility of kibbutz parents is "to love" their child.

Development of the child is a result of continity in the kibbutz educational-childbearing process and the ideals upon which the kibbutz is founded. There is consistency between the child's world and the community which makes easier the transition from childhood to adulthood. Adolescents are involved in the social and work ideals of the community. By contrast, many Western adolescents are isolated in their own world of peers during adolescence. Kibbutz children learn by doing — how to work, think, relate to others, and take responsibility. Kibbutz youth criticize the adult society, but their criticism is thoughtful and specific, usually including their views on solutions to problems (Rabin, 1982).

Children's age makes an important difference in communal child care. In Berger's (1972) research

*The Oneida Community was a mid-nineteenth century commune located in New York State along the Oneida Creek. It survived for more than a generation, disbanding in 1879 because of lack of an adequate leader and increasing external pressures. Some of the features of the community included group marriage, scientific breeding, and sexual equality.

study, American infants and early toddlers were almost universally in the charge of their mothers. Children from 2 to 4 years of age belonged to the commune to a greater extent, although they received a good deal of fathering. Strong traditions required fathers to be involved in child-nurturing. After age 4 or 5 years, the child was the responsibility of any adult in the group. All children were viewed as intrinsically worthy of love and respect, but not necessarily of attention. The role of parents in such communes is to facilitate child development, which is essentially exemplary rather than paternalistic or didactic. Every attempt is made to allow children to grow naturally, to be as autonomous as possible.

An important comparison is made by Berger and his co-workers in their studies of parent-child relationships in communal families and traditional nuclear families. The most important belief governing the relation between children and adults in communes is that the experiences of children are their own and do not reflect upon parenting practices. This is in contrast to both preindustrial and middle class views in which the behavior of children reflects upon their parents who are in some sense responsible for it (Berger, 1972).

Commune members generally say communes are good for children. They may provide important continuity between generations. Most studies of contemporary communes, except for the kibbutzim, have involved only preadolescent children. Longitudinal studies may provide data for distinctive child development practices. Professional nurses who have contact with communal families should make every effort to understand the basic values of the specific commune as they respond to the families' health care needs.

Homosexual Parents

It is estimated that in the United States the number of children who have lesbian or gay parents may be between 6 and 10 million (Bozett, 1987b, p 4). Although homosexuality is discussed more openly today than in previous decades, many surveys show that the majority of Americans continue to disapprove of it.

The concerns researchers have about the sexual preference of the parents are generally in two areas: its influence on the child's development of a sexual identity and the possibility that the child might be stigmatized and have difficulty developing normal peer relationships. A number of comparative studies have found no major differences in adjustment between children of lesbians and heterosexual single mothers (Nungesser, 1980; Pagelow, 1980; Hoeffer, 1981; Kirkpatrick et al, 1981; Hotvedt and Mandel 1982). To date, there are no known studies on the development of sexual identity of children of gay fathers (Bozett, 1987a, p. 47).

Regarding the fear that children might be stigmatized and have conflict with their peer groups, it is known that children of interracial marriages have overcome similar problems. Further, it is believed that the degree of stress experienced will be related to the amount of support given by the parent. The use of parental discretion can minimize negative reactions (Fishel, 1983). A study by Hotvedt and Mandel (1982) found no differences in sons of lesbian mothers and heterosexual single mothers with regard to self-ratings of popularity with other boys and girls. In that study, daughters of lesbian mothers rated themselves more popular with girls and boys than did daughters of heterosexual mothers.

Bozett finds that children of gays can "respond to society's reaction to their father, to society's reaction to themselves as the child of a gay father, or to both on the basis of their imputed or 'virtual social identity,' that is, the negative identity society attributes to gays, rather than to their 'actual social identity' (Goffman, 1963, p 2)" (Bozett, in press). It is the child's self-concept, tempered perhaps by the openness and relaxation of a parent regarding his or her sexual orientation, realism, and understanding of the child that influences the degree to which the child feels stigmatized (Pennington, 1987).

For various reasons, not the least of which is the fear of losing custody of the child(ren), some lesbian and gay parents choose not to disclose their affectional ties even when living with a partner. However, one researcher found communication and other psychologic problems to result when lesbian orientation was not disclosed (Pennington, 1987). Other parents openly discuss their situation with their children. Parents have to consider the risk of the children learning of their emotional attachment/sexual attraction (Switzer and Switzer, 1980) from others. When and how parents discuss the situation with children depends on the parents' comfort with their own sexual preference and their own ability to respond to the demands of children, partners, and society.

When first learning of their parents' lifestyle, the response of children of lesbian or gay parents is varied. In his sample, Bozett found that the overriding concern was the "fear that others would think that they, too, were gay" (1987a, p 40). In her study, Pennington found that "children around 7 years of age and younger were more concerned with the parents' separation or divorce rather than with their mother being a lesbian. They expressed concern that they might be deprived of parental attention" (1987, p 62). Older children often realize that same-sex relationships are not generally accepted and fear that ostracism and isolation could result from other children finding out about their mother's lesbianism (Pennington, 1987).

Although gay marriages do not have legal status, many lesbians and gays do form unions that provide permanence, faithfulness, and a shared life (Berger, 1984). Lesbian mothers now win 15 per cent of child custody battles, versus 1 per cent in 1970 (McCandlish, 1987), whereas fewer gay men are custodial parents (Bozett, 1987a). Families with lesbian or gay parents can have any configuration. Some are single-parent families, some are in heterosexual marriages, some have adopted children or foster children. Some live with a partner who may serve as stepparent (Baptiste, 1987). Some lesbians choose to be artificially inseminated.

While there has been an increase in alternative family life styles in the recent past, there also has been a change in parent-child, and care-giver and care-receiver relationships. Maier (1982) states that there has been a change from child rearing and parenting as activities directed toward children to a focus on caring as a process of reciprocal, continuous interaction between parent and child. Whatever the family lifestyle, children need an environment and relationships where they are assured a pattern of reliable dependence and where they repeatedly find freedom to grow. The challenge is to offer children all the love, warmth, and security they need while nudging them toward independence and the ability to be self-reliant, contributing members of society.

References

Aamodt AM: Culture. *In* Clark AL: *Culture, Childbearing, Health Professionals.* Philadelphia, FA Davis, 1978, 3-19.

Baptiste DA Jr: Gay and lesbian stepparent family. *In* Bozett FW (ed): *Gay and Lesbian Parents.* New York, Praeger, 1987, 112-137.

Beail N: The psychology of fatherhood. *Bull Br Psychol Soc* 1983 Sep; 312-314.

Benedict RF: *An Anthropologist at Work: Writings on Ruth Benedict* (edited by Margaret Mead). Philadelphia, JB Lippincott, 1959.

Berger B, et al: The communal family. *Fam Coordinator,* 1972 19 Oct; 419.

Berger R: Realities of gay and lesbian aging. *Social Work* 1984 Jan/Feb; 57.

Billar HB: Father absence, divorce, and personality development. *In* Lamb M: *The Role of the Father in Child Development.* New York, John Wiley and Sons, 1981.

Bozett FW: Identity management: social control of identity by children of gay fathers when they know their father is a homosexual. *West Nurs Res,* in press.

Bozett FW: Children of gay fathers. *In* Bozett FW (ed): *Gay and Lesbian Parents.* New York, Praeger, 1987a, 39-57.

Bozett FW: Gay fathers. *In* Bozett FW (ed); *Gay and Lesbian Parents.* New York, Praeger, 1987b, 3-22.

Bragdon I: How to help migrant children. *Today's Educ* 1976 Jan/Feb.

Bronfenbrenner U: The changing American family. *In* Hetherington M, Parke R: *Contemporary Readings in Child Psychology.* New York, McGraw-Hill, 1977, 317.

Chang PN, Deinard AS: Single father caretakers: demographic characteristics and adjustment processes. *Am J Orthopsychiatr* 1982 Apr; 52(2):236-243.

Char EL: The Chinese American. *In* Clark AL: *Culture and Childrearing.* Philadelphia, FA Davis, 1980, 141-164.

Chinn P: *Child Health Maintenance: Concepts in Family-Centered Care.* 2nd ed. St. Louis, CV Mosby, 1980.

Coser R: *The Family: Its Structures and Functions.* New York, St. Martin's Press, 1974.

Depp CH: After reunion: perceptions of adult adoptees, adoptive parents and birth parents. *Child Welfare* 1982 Feb; 115.

Dougherty SA: Single adoptive mothers and their children. *Social Work* 1978 Jul; 311.

Dukette R: Values issues in present day adoptions. *Child Welfare* 1984 May/Jun; 234.

Duvall E: *Marriage and Family Development.* Philadelphia, JB Lippincott, 1977.

Eiduson B: Child development in emergent family styles. *Child Today* 1978 Mar/Apr; 24.

Eiduson B: Changing sex roles in alternative family styles: implications for young children. *In* Anthony E, Chiland C: *The Child and His Family: Changing Roles of Children and Parents.* New York, Wiley Interscience, 1980.

Fanshel D, Shinn E: *Children in Foster Care: A Longitudinal Investigation.* New York, Columbia University Press, 1978.

Felson R: Aggression and violence between siblings. *Social Psychol Q* 1983 Dec; 271-285.

Fishel AH: Gay parents. *Issues Health Care Women* 1983; 4:139-164.

Garner CH: In vitro fertilization and embryo transfer. *J Obstet Gynecol Nurs* 1983 Mar/Apr; 75.

Gerken DA: *Social Competence and Behavioral Problems in Children of Lesbians.* Unpublished master's thesis, Azusa Pacific University, Azusa, CA, 1988.

Goldstine D et al: The three stages of marriage. *Family Circle* 1977 3 May; 10.

Gottschalk E Jr: Exploding the myths about the American family. *Family Circle,* 1977 13 Dec; 72.

Guerney L: The effectiveness of foster care as supplemental parenting. *In* Kostelnik M, et al: *Child Nurturance: Patterns of Supplementary Parenting.* Vol 2. New York, Plenum Press, 1982.

Haithman D: And baby makes five: pros and cons of the new open adoption. *Chicago Tribune,* 1984 30 Jul; 1.

Hall EH, King GC: Working with the strength of black families. *Child Welfare* 1982 Nov/Dec; 536.

Hall ET: *Beyond Culture.* New York, Anchor Press/Doubleday, 1976.

Hall ET: *The Dance of Life: The Other Dimension of Time.* New York, Anchor Press/Doubleday, 1983.

Harris M: *The Rise of Anthropological Theory.* New York, Thomas Y. Crowell, 1968.

Henderson G, Primeaux M: *Transcultural Health Care.* Reading, MA, Addison-Wesley Publishing Company, 1981.

Hetherington E, Cox M, Cox R: Effects of divorce on parents and children. *In* Lamb M: *Nontraditional Families: Parenting and Child Development.* Hillsdale, NJ, Lawrence Erlbaum Associates, 1982.

Hicks GL, Leis PE: *Ethnic Encounters: Identities and Contexts.* North Scituate, MA, Duxbury Press, 1977.

Hoeffer B: (1981). Children's acquisition of sex-role behavior in lesbian mother families. *Am J Orthopsychiatr* 1981; 51:536-544.

Horn BM: Transcultural nursing and childrearing of the Muckleshoot people. *In* Leininger MM: *Transcultural Nursing: Concepts, Theories and Practices.* New York, John Wiley and Sons, 1978, 223-266.

Hotvedt M, Mandel J: Children of lesbian mothers. *In* Paul W, et al (eds): *Homosexuality: Social, Psychological, and Biological Issues.* Beverly Hills, CA, Sage Publishers, 1982, 275-285.

Howe L (ed): *The Future of the Family.* New York, Simon & Schuster, 1972.

Hymnovich D, Barnard M: *Family Health Care: Developmental and Situational Crises.* Vol 2. New York, McGraw-Hill, 1979.

Jenkins S: Children of divorce. *Child Today* 1978 Mar/Apr; 16.

Jewett C: *Helping Children Cope with Separation and Loss.* Cambridge, MA, The Harvard Common Press, 1982.

Keniston K, Carnegie Council on Children: *All Our Children: The American Family Under Pressure.* New York, Harcourt Brace Jovanovich, 1977.

Kirkpatrick M, Smith C, Ray R: Lesbian mothers and their children: a comparative survey. *Orthopsychiatr* 1981; 51:545-551.

Klein C: *The Single Parent Experience.* New York, Walker and Company, 1973.

Krementz J: *How It Feels When a Parent Dies.* New York, Alfred A. Knopf Publishers, 1981.

Kübler-Ross, E: *Death: The Final Stage of Growth.* Englewood Cliffs, NJ, Prentice-Hall, 1975.

Leininger M: *Transcultural Nursing: Concepts, Theories, and Practices.* New York, John Wiley and Sons, 1978.

Leininger M: *Transcultural Nursing — 79.* New York, Masson Publishing USA, 1979.

Leininger M: *Care: The Essence of Nursing and Health.* Thorofare, NJ, Slack Inc, 1984.

Leininger M: Transcultural care diversity and universality: a theory of nursing. *Nurs Health Care* 1985; June: 209–212.

Leininger M: *Transcultural Care Theory.* Thorofare, NJ, Slack Inc, in press.

Lindsey D: Achievements for children in foster care. *Social Work* 1982; 27(6): 491-496.

Longfellow C: Divorce in context: its impact on children. *In* Levinger G, Moles O: *Divorce and Separation: Context, Causes and Consequences.* New York, Basic Books, 1979.

Maier HW: To be attached and free: the challenge of child development in the eighties. *Child Welfare* 1982 Feb; 67.

Malinowski B: The group and the individual in functional analysis. *Am J Sociol* 1939; 938-964.

Martin D, Lyon P: *Lesbian Woman.* New York, Bantam Books, 1972.

McCandlish BM: Against all odds: lesbian mother family dynamics. *In* Bozett FW (ed): *Gay and Lesbian Parents.* New York, Praeger, 1987, 23-36.

McRoy R, et al: Self-esteem and social identity in transracial and inracial adoptees. *Social Work,* 1982 Nov; 522.

Mendes H: Single-parent families: a typology of life styles. *Social Work* 1979 May; 193.

Meyer C: Who is for the American family? *Social Work,* 1982 Nov; 471.

Miller J, Janosik E: *Family Focused Care.* New York, McGraw-Hill, 1980.

Minuchin S: *Families and Family Therapy.* Cambridge, MA, Harvard University Press, 1974.

Moynihan DP: *Family and Nation.* San Diego, Harcourt, Brace, Jovanovich, 1987.

Murphy JF: Conflict theory. *In* Clements IW, Robert FB (eds): *Family Health: A Theoretical Approach to Nursing Care.* New York, John Wiley & Sons, 1983.

Nieto D: Aiding the single father. *Social Work* 27(6) 1982; 473-478.

Norton AJ, Glick PC: One parent families: a social and economic profile. *Fam Relations* 1986; 35:9-17.

Norvell M, Guy RF: Comparison of self-concept in adopted and nonadopted adolescents. *Adolescence* 1977 Fall; 443.

Nungesser LG: Theoretical bases for research on the acquisition of social sex-roles by children of lesbian mothers. *Homosexual* 1980; 5:177-187.

Nurse service for surrogate mothers. *Clin Aspects High Risk Pregn* 1983 Dec; 1.

Pagelow MD: Heterosexual and lesbian single mothers: a comparison of problems, coping and solutions. *Homosexual* 1980; 5:189-204.

Pannor R, Baron A: Open adoption as standard practice. *Child Welfare* 1984 May/June; 245.

Park J: Children who follow the sun. *Today's Educ* 1976 Jan/Feb; 53.

Pennington SB: Children of lesbian mothers. *In* Bozett FW (ed): *Gay and Lesbian Parents.* New York, Praeger, 1987, 58-74.

Rabin A: Supplementary parenting in the kibbutz childrearing system. *In* Kostelnik M, et al: *Child Nurturance: Patterns of Supplementary Parenting.* Vol 2. New York, Plenum Press, 1982.

Rambo BJ: *Adaptation Nursing: Assessment and Intervention.* Philadelphia; WB Saunders, 1984.

Reame N: The development of a perinatal nursing service for the surrogate mother. *Obstet Gynecol Nurs* 1984 Jan/Feb; 59.

Reame N, Parker P: Effects of surrogate pregnancy on obstetrical performance. *Fertil Steril* 1984 Feb; 97.

Reinhardt A, Quinn M: *Family-Centered Community Nursing: A Sociocultural Framework.* St. Louis, CV Mosby, 1973.

Ruetter L, Strang V: Yours, mine and ours: stepparents and their children. *MCN* 11:264-266, 1986.

Rosenblatt PC, Cunningham MR: Television watching and family tensions. *J Marriage Fam* 1976 Feb; 105.

Rosenthal K, Keshet H: *Fathers Without Partners.* Totowa, NJ, Rowman and Littlefield, 1981.

Safilios-Rothschild C: Trends in the family: a cross-cultural perspective. *Child Today* 1978 Mar/Apr; 38.

Santrock J, Warshek R, Elliott G: Social development and parent-child interaction in father-custody and stepmother families. *In* Lamb M: *Nontraditional Families: Parenting and Child Development.* Hillsdale, NJ, Lawrence Erlbaum Associates, 1982.

Scanzoni L, Scanzoni J: *Men, Women and Change: A Sociology of Marriage and Family.* New York, McGraw-Hill, 1981.

Schlesinger B: Lasting marriages in the 1980's. *Can J Commun Mental Health* 1983 Sep; 45-56.

Schulz D: *The Changing Family: Its Functions and Future.* Englewood Cliffs, NJ, Prentice-Hall, 1976.

Scott E, Scott K: Healthy families. *Int Offender Ther Comp Criminol* 1983; 27(1):71-78.

Sevcovic L: Traditions of pregnancy which influence maternity care of the Navajo people. *In* Leininger M: *Transcultural Nursing-79.* New York, Masson Publishing USA, 1979.

Shamsie J: Family breakdown and its effects on emotional disorders in children. *Can J Psychiatr* 1985; 30:281-287.

Smith D, Sherwen L: *Mothers and Their Adopted Children: The Bonding Process.* New York, Tiresias Press, 1983.

Smith J, Miroff F: *You're Our Child: A Social/Psychological Approach to Adoption.* Lanham, MD, University Press of America, 1981.

Sobol E. Robischon P: *Family Nursing: A Study Guide* St. Louis, CV Mosby, 1975.

Spiro M. *Children of the Kibbutz.* New York, Schocken Books, 1967.

Stern P: Conflicting family culture: an impediment to integration in stepfather families. *Psychiatr Nurs Mental Health Nurs* 1982 Oct; 27.

Strom R, Strom S: Redefining the grandparent role. *Cambridge Educ* 1983; 13(1):71-78.

Suppe F: The Bell and Weinberg study: future priorities for research on homosexuality. *J Homosexual* 1981 Summer; 69.

Sussman M: The family today. *Child Today* 1978 Mar/Apr; 32.

Suzuki BH: The Asian-American family. *In* Fantini MD, Cardenas R (eds): *Parenting in a Multicultural Society.* New York, Longman Inc., 1980.

Switzer DK, Switzer S: *Parents of the Homosexual.* Philadelphia, Westminster Press, 1980.

Tapia J: The nursing process in family health. *Nurs Outlook* 1972 Apr.

Tiedeman ME: *Children's Perceptions of Health and Illness: A Comparison of Two Cultures.* Unpublished paper. Detroit, Wayne State University College of Nursing, 1981.

Toman W: *Family Constellations.* New York, Springer Publishers, 1976.

Tripp-Reimer T, Brink PJ, Saunders JM: Cultural assessment: content and process. *Nurs Outlook* 1984 Mar/Apr; 78-82.

Tripp-Reimer T, Schrock M: Residential patterns and preferences of ethnic aged: implications for transcultural nursing. *In* Uhl CN, Uhl J (eds): *Transcultural Nursing Conference Proceedings.* Transcultural Nursing Society, 1982, 144-157.

US Bureau of the Census: *Money Income and Poverty Status.* 1984, pp 21, 22.

Visher E, Visher J: *Stepfamilies: A Guide to Working with Stepparents and Stepchildren.* New York, Brunner/Mazel Publishing, 1979.

Wald E: *The Remarried Family: Challenge and Promise.* Milwaukee, WI, Family Service Association of America, 1981.

Wallace R. Jr: Double blessing of adoption. *The Goshen News,* Goshen, IN, 1984 14 Dec; 10.

Wallerstein J: Children of divorce: stress and developmental tasks. *In* Garmezy N, Rutter M: *Stress, Coping and Development in Children.* New York, McGraw-Hill, 1983.

Wallerstein J, Kelly J: California's children of divorce. *Psychol Today* 1980; 67.

Wallerstein J, Kelly J: *Surviving the Breakup: How Children and Parents Cope with Divorce.* New York, Basic Books, 1980.

Weiss R: Growing up a little faster: children in single-parent households. *Child Today* 1981 May/Jun; 22.

Wenger AFZ: *Health and Care Phenomena Among Soviet Jewish Immigrants in the Acculturation Process: A Mini Ethnonursing Study.* Unpublished field study. Detroit, Wayne State University College of Nursing, 1983.

Winborn R: Adapting to parenthood: negotiating new roles. *Social Casework* 1983 Dec; 618-624.

Bibliography

Crane D, Griffin W: Personal space: an objective measure of marital quality. *J Marital Fam Ther* 1983 Jul; 325-327.

Eshleman JR: *The Family.* 3rd ed. New York, Allyn/Bacon, 1981.

Fawcett J: The family as a living open system: an emerging conceptual framework for nursing. *Int Nurs Rev* 1975 Oct; 113.

Gecas V: The socialization and child care roles. *In* Nye I (ed): *Role Structure and Analysis of the Family.* Beverly Hills, CA, Sage Publishing Company, 1976.

Goody E: *Contexts of Kinship: An Essay in the Family Sociology of the Gonja of Northern Ghana.* New York, Cambridge University Press, 1973.

Hawkins J, Weisberg C, Roy D: Marital communication style and social class. *J Marriage Fam* 1977; 39(3):479-490.

Hymovich D, Barnard M: *Family Health Care: General Perspectives.* Vol 1. New York, McGraw-Hill, 1979.

Keesing RM: Theories of culture. *In* Seigel BJ, Beals AR, Tyler SA (eds): *Annual Review of Anthropology.* Palo Alto, CA, Annual Reviews, Inc., 1974, 73-97.

Kogan K, Wimberger H: Interaction patterns in disadvantaged families. *J Clin Psychol* 1969; 25(4):347-352.

Kornhaber A: The vital connection — 1983; grandparents are coming of age in America. *Child Today* 1983 Jul/Aug; 31-33.

Leininger M: *Caring: An Essential Human Need.* Thorofare, NJ, Slack Inc., 1981.

Spradley JP: *Participant Observation.* New York, Holt, Rinehart and Winston, 1980.

Spradley JP: *The Ethnographic Interview.* New York, Holt, Rinehart and Winston, 1979.

Swanson A, et al: Family systems: values and value conflicts. *J Psychosoc Nurs Mental Health Serv* 1983 Jul; 24-30.

Toffler A: *Future Shock.* New York, Random House, 1970.

Walsh F: Normal family ideologies: myths and realities. *Family Therapy Collections* 1983; 1-14.

Recommended Reading

Bonkowski S, Bequette S, Boomhower S: A group design to help children adjust to parental divorce. *Social Casework* 1984 Mar; 131.

Curry H, Clifford D: *A Legal Guide for Lesbian and Gay Couples.* Reading, MA, Addison-Wesley, 1980.

Fantini MD, Cardenas R (eds): *Parenting in a Multicultural Society.* New York, Longman, Inc., 1980.

Flynne L, Hamm W: Team: parent-agency partnership in adoption. *Child Today* 1983 Mar/Apr.

Henderson G, Premeaux M: *Transcultural Health Care.* Reading, MA, Addison-Wesley Publishing Company, 1981.

Krementz J: *How It Feels to Be Adopted.* New York, Alfred A. Knopf, 1983.

Lonetto R: *Children's Conceptions of Death.* New York, Springer Publishing Co., 1980.

Ladner J: Adopting the cross-cultural child. *Psychiatr Ann* 1982 Sep; 849.

Orgue MS, Bloch B, Monrroy LSA: *Ethnic Nursing Care.* St. Louis, CV Mosby, 1983.

Rowe P: Bridging the gap: from foster care to independent living. *Child Today* 1983 Sep/Oct; 28.

Smardo FA, Schmidt V: Developing multicultural awareness. *Child Today* 1983 May/Jun; 23-25.

Tamez EG: Familism, machismo and child rearing practices among Mexican Americans. *J Psychosoc Nurs Mental Health Serv* 1981 Sep; 21-25.

Zepeda M: Selected maternal-infant care practices of Spanish-speaking women. *J Obstet Gynecol Nurs* 1982 Nov/Dec; 371-374.

Developing Children

Chapter 3

Jo Joyce Anderson

Growth and development are the words that succinctly describe the process of maturation from childhood to adulthood. Chapter 1 described the goal of pediatric nursing: promoting healthy maturation of the child/adolescent as a physical, intellectual, and emotional-social being within the context of the family and the community. To accomplish that goal, nurses must be knowledgeable about developmental theories and about the ways in which heredity and environment interact to affect maturation.

This chapter builds the foundation for all the specific growth and development chapters in the next unit. Theories are introduced to help explain and predict physical, intellectual, and emotional-social development. Growth, development, and maturation are defined and specific principles examined. Development is considered as a process of maturation, learning, conflict resolution, cognitive change, and cultural adaptation. Various factors within the child's environment are explored for their influence upon growth and development: culture and family lifestyle, school, socioeconomic status, neighborhood, mass media, and certain physical aspects varying from intrauterine environment to climate. Genetic influences are discussed in Chapter 4.

Related Topics

Expanded discussion of the influences of poverty, Chapter 1
Expanded discussion of culture, family lifestyles, Chapter 2
Religious influences, Chapter 2
Genetic influences on development, Chapter 4
Development of health concepts, Chapter 10
Development of self-esteem, Chapter 16
Nutritional influences on growth, Chapter 18
Development of dentition, Chapter 19
Play and exercise, Chapter 21
Sexual development, Chapter 22
Concepts of stress and coping in childhood, Chapter 23

Why Study Growth and Development? Nursing Implications

Anyone who has watched a sleeping infant, studied closely the determined way toddlers force their whole body into mobility, listened to the imaginative conversation of two preschoolers at play, tolerated the teasing of an active school-age child, or cried over the tense struggle of an identity-seeking adolescent cannot deny the miraculous fascination of the young human being. Researchers and professionals in the helping arts attest to the intricacies and complexities that interplay to create a whole being who is totally unique and yet shares a core of commonalities with all others of the species.

By studying these commonalities in our existence, we can better understand how we grow, develop, and mature into unique individuals who seek to achieve our full potential. But the reward of knowledge alone is not adequate reason for the extensive and intense study of human development that is a part of studying the nursing of children. Nurses who work with children use their knowledge of the commonalities of development as a basis for recognition of potential and actual deviations from or alterations in growth and development. Also, as health professionals, nurses must sometimes intervene in this growth and development relationship in order to deal with disease, abnormality, or other factors threatening health, and we ought to know with what we are interfering. Nurses and other health professionals are expected not only to understand human developmental processes but also capably to treat and prevent those conditions that might adversely affect these processes. Therefore, studying human development helps the nurse to know what to expect of individuals at any given stage of development. Such knowledge is needed for the nurse to develop and deliver a plan of care that is developmentally appropriate and relevant to the needs of the client. Understanding human developmental processes also helps us see the reasons why many conditions or illnesses occur more frequently or are more threatening in certain age groups. Nurses working with childbearing and childrearing families require developmental knowledge to provide anticipatory guidance to parents, so that parents can contribute positively to their children's attainment of optimal growth and development.

The primary concern of the nurse working with children and their families involves the individual needs of that child-family unit in the development of life competencies (i.e., successful achievement of individual and family group tasks which forestall the occurrence of alterations in family processes). Any factors enhancing or altering development of those competencies become essential aspects of the nursing assessment and contribute to the nursing diagnosis and plan of care.

Altered growth and development is a key nursing diagnosis for the nurse who works with children. A clear problem statement will usually require that this diagnosis be further explained by one or more of the three competency categories of growth and development: physical, intellectual, or emotional-social. For example, a diagnosis might read, *altered growth and development: physical related to inadequate oxygen transport associated with a congenital heart defect.*

When assessing the impact of a disorder or situation upon the child's growth and development, the nurse must consider (1) that "growth" and "development" are not synonymous terms (see page 113) and (2) that the family's development may also be altered by the child's illness. Altered family development can be defined through diagnoses such as *altered in family process, ineffective family coping: compromised,* and *ineffective family coping: disabling.*

Using Chronologic and Competency Approaches to Study Growth and Development

As the previous discussion implies, a child's development is a complicated, intertwined process. To facilitate learning, the chapters on growth and development are divided according to widely recognized chronologic divisions. Although any chronologic division is somewhat arbitrary, the list of stages that follows is based upon the performance or competency criteria that signal change or that progress from one developmental stage to another. It must be remembered that these chronologic divisions and associated developmental stages are not such obvious divisions in the real child's life. *The nurse in practice would do well to assign developmental norms to an individual child based on behaviors of the child, rather than on the chronologic age of the child.*

The terms used to describe the chronology of development are:

- *Prenatal life*—period of life from conception to birth
- *Newborn or neonatal life*—period extending from birth through the first month of life

We appreciate the critical review of this chapter by Sandra Frick, RN, Ph D, and her contributions to it.

- *Infancy*—period beginning at the end of the first month of life and ending at 1 year of age
- *Toddlerhood*—period extending from age 1 year through the 36th month of life
- *Preschool years*—period extending from the beginning of the third year to the end of the fifth year of life
- *School-age years* or *middle childhood*—period from the start of the sixth to the end of the 11th year
- *Adolescence and young adulthood*—period from the beginning of the 12th to the end of the 21st year of life

Furthermore, since the whole person is more easily understood if described in terms of broad categories, this book describes the child's development as three facets of the self called *competencies: physical, intellectual,* and *emotional-social.* Again, the division is arbitrary and often not clear-cut, since change in each developmental competency affects development in the other spheres as well.

The three competency areas described in this book are defined as follows:

- *Physical competency* involves the child's ability to apply various motor, neurologic, and biologic capacities to steadily achieve more mature self-care abilities requiring mobility and manipulative skills. Aspects of this competency include physical health, body build and configuration, size, strength, rate of motor, neurologic and biologic maturation, and motor skill performance.
- *Intellectual competency* involves development of language and reasoning to the point of mature abstract thought and the development of perceptions and communication skills. Some aspects of intellectual competency are perceptual level, memory, problem solving and reasoning ability, language skills, academic achievement, and IQ.
- *Emotional-social competency* concerns development of an inner sense of security that is supported by self-awareness and acceptance and evidenced by the capacity to form productive interpersonal relationships with individuals and groups. Temperament, interpersonal relations skills, emotional adjustment, and development of sexuality and morality are measures of this competency.

Developmental Theories

"It is the child's growing capacity to take in his world, rework experiences and give it out again in speech or song, craft or art, in all the activities in which men engage, that is the source of individuality."

—Margaret Mead, from *Family* by M. Mead and K. Heyman, Macmillan, 1965.

Description of the whole person and his or her competencies—physical, intellectual, and emotional-social—is often facilitated when facts or data about the person are organized according to a conceptual framework. Theories of human growth and development provide conceptual frameworks that allow child health care professionals to describe typical behaviors of different-age children, explain the significance of these behaviors, predict behaviors that might occur in a given situation, or control behavioral manifestations. Since human growth and development is highly complex and multifaceted, many developmental theories deal only with one aspect or domain of development.

Understanding of development can be enhanced by the study of several theories. This text emphasizes two major theories, Piaget's theory of intellectual (cognitive) development and Erikson's theory of emotional-social (psychosocial) development, and incorporates other theories as they are applicable.

Since different theories can explain the same behavioral phenomena differently, an individual's use of a particular theoretical framework will influence the approach to nursing assessment and intervention. It is useful to analyze different theories of growth and development to determine their utility in guiding nursing practice. Table 3-1 provides a comparison of nine theories of human growth and development.

Physical Competency

Intellectual and emotional-social competencies are both deeply rooted in and influenced by the capacities and needs of one's physical competency. Underlying each developmental advance is a physical maturational or functional change. Likewise, a child's feelings and behavior are directly affected by both physical state and current physical needs. An example of this is the peak period of misbehavior typical just prior to a child's usual mealtimes, when there is a physical need for food.

Because physical development is mostly quantitative, it is easily measured. Physical development also displays some conspicuous age uniformities, so it is a useful means of evaluating the relative health status of a child (see Chapter 15, Physical Assessment, for examples of methods to evaluate physical competency). The level of physical competency achieved by a given child is compared with established norms or averages. These norms are defined from the mathematical average obtained by measuring many children of similar age on a given trait. The norm is more truly representative when the children measured are drawn from vary-

Text continues on page 98

Table 3-1. Comparison of Theories of Human Growth and Development

Underlying Theoretical Motivation for Behavior	Theoretical Assumptions	Use	Nursing Strategies
Theorist: GESELL. Description of typical physical and mental characteristics of infants, children, and adolescents. Focus: Motor skills and hygiene, language skills, and personal-social skills, including play and past-times, school, emotional expression, fears, dreams, self and sex, ethical sense, and philosophical outlook			
Development is genetically programmed. Cycles of behavioral stages influenced by genetic inheritance alternate between equilibrium (in which the child is in harmony with the environment) and disequilibrium (or periods of disharmony). Environment has little effect on development. Individual differences are explained in relation to genetically determined body types (somatotype).	Behavioral cycles tend to occur at specified chronologic ages in all children. Prior practice or training does not influence age at which behaviors occur. Readiness for developmental progression of behaviors is genetically preprogrammed.	Primarily descriptive. Explains prior behaviors. Predicts future development.	Allows for comparisons of individual child with average behaviors for age to assess developmental level. Can be used in parent teaching and anticipatory guidance of parents to help them understand their child in relation to other children of same age. Does not allow for control of future development.
Theorist: HAVIGHURST. Description of physical, cognitive, affective, and social developmental tasks			
Heredity and environment interact to produce biologic, psychologic, and cultural tasks that the child strives to accomplish. Accomplishment leads to happiness and future success. Failure to accomplish leads to unhappiness, lack of future success, and lack of approval from society.	Critical periods are assumed for some tasks, whereas other tasks tend to recur in successive stages. Theory implies optimal age range for teaching to facilitate achievement of critical period tasks.	Primarily descriptive, does not explain. Describes how child is and was, does not explain why. Can be used to predict future development.	Allows for comparison of individual child with average behaviors for age to assess developmental level. Can be used in parent teaching and anticipatory guidance of parents to suggest ways environment can be structured to facilitate task achievement. Also assists parents in ability to predict readiness for future tasks.
Theorist: FREUD. Psychosexual; emphasis on development of personality			
Developing child is essentially a passive recipient of two internal, biologic forces or instinctual urges: the urge to survive and procreate (libido) and a death urge that governs aggressive or destructive acts. Libido or life force is predominant. Satisfaction of urges results in tension reduction or pleasure; frustration of urges results in increased tension or pain. Motivation for behavior, simply stated, is to achieve pleasure and avoid pain.	Invariable sequence of four stages (oral, anal, phallic, latency) is assumed in which pleasure is invested in a different erogenous zone or modality. Sensual pleasure is derived from use of this zone. Three personality components (id, ego, superego) develop sequentially during birth, toddlerhood, and preschool years, respectively. Id is raw libido seeking pleasure. Ego is reality component which mediates conflicts occurring when id urges are frustrated by environmental realities. Defense mechanisms are ego creations which allow for tension reduction when urges are frustrated. Superego (conscience) arises from the ego and puts good or bad labels on behavior. According to Freud, psychosexual development is essentially complete at approximately 6 years of age.	Allows for explanation of past and present behaviors. Not useful in predicting specific future behaviors. Limited control of behavior is implied in pleasure motive.	Can be used in parent teaching and anticipatory guidance of parents to explain basis for past and present behaviors, guide parenting behaviors to facilitate healthy development. Care of the infant focuses on provision of pleasurable sensory experiences and protection from unnecessary frustration of pleasure motive. As child enters toddlerhood, care will include careful guidance for learning of environmental realities and appropriate problem-solving to attain pleasurable goals. Care in preschool years includes setting reasonable standards of right and wrong and appropriate limits to enforce these standards. Awareness of sensory zone or modality for age and stage allows nurses to avoid painful or intrusive procedures involving that modality if possible (e.g., axillary rather than rectal temperatures when anal zone is predominant)
Theorist: ERIKSON. Psychosocial development			
Forces within the individual interact with societal and cultural forces to produce a series of eight tasks, conflicts, or crises which the individual strives to successfully resolve. Each stage's task is represented by opposite extremes between a positive and a negative aspect. The individual strives and is	Stages are invariant with each stage being built upon and dependent upon the preceding stages (epigenesis). Critical periods exist during which resolution of the central crisis must occur in order for optimal future development to occur. Each new stage requires that important aspects of the previous	Little attention to individual differences decreases ability to use in describing development in relation to other children. Explains past and present	Provides a useful framework for helping parents understand behaviors and development of their child. Useful in anticipatory guidance of parents in helping them to structure the environment and to use parenting skills that will facilitate healthy development. Highly useful as a theoretical

continued

Table 3-1. (continued)

Underlying Theoretical Motivation for Behavior	Theoretical Assumptions	Use	Nursing Strategies
impelled by social and cultural forces to establish equilibrium between these opposite aspects, ideally with a predominance of the qualities of the positive aspect. Successful resolution of the conflict or task of one stage produces in the individual the attributes which are necessary for meeting the task of the next stage.	stage must be relinquished, at least in part. For example, in order to achieve a sense of autonomy, the dependence of trust must be relinquished. Prior practice and teaching do not facilitate passage through stages. Psychologic and social readiness must be present for this to occur.	development. Predicts what might occur in future development.	framework for nursing interaction with and provision of nursing care to children. Awareness of the current developmental characteristics allows for interventions that would promote achievement at the positive extreme for the crisis of that stage and avoid imposition of negative aspects of that stage. Especially useful in the structuring of dramatic play sessions to assist the child in working through his or her feelings. Can be used to provide nursing care in a way that will ensure maximum compliance.
Theorist: PIAGET. Cognitive development			
Heredity, or innate biological structure, and environment (physical and social) interact. Individuals are seen as active organisms who initiate acts which result in development. All individuals have a tendency to organize their mental activities in order to be able to deal with their environment (adaptation). Adaptation involves the attempt to maintain a balance (equilibration) between the taking in of new information that fits existing mental structures (assimilation) and the changing of mental structures to allow contrary information to fit these structures (accommodation).	Cognitive development proceeds in an invariant sequence of four stages for all children. Each stage has substages. Prior practice or teaching has little effect on development of new cognitive skills and progression to the next stage until suitable cognitive maturity or readiness for that stage has occurred.	Little attention to individual differences decreases ability to use in describing development in relation to other children. Explains past and present; predicts patterns of future cognitive development.	Useful in parent teaching and anticipatory guidance of parents to help explain to them the nature of their child's understanding of the environment at different stages. Of high practical utility in structuring of patient teaching. Implies definite guidelines for the kinds and amount of information which the child will require. Allows nurses to know types of misperceptions that can occur as a result of the level of mental operations that occur at different stages and to assess and intervene in relation to these perceptions.
Theorist: KOHLBERG. Moral development			
Extension of Piaget's theory and theorizes same or similar behavioral motivation. Standards of the social environment and social rewards play a major role in motivation for movement to higher levels of moral reasoning. Urges within the child beginning with premoral urge to satisfy own needs also interact with societal standards. Modeling is also recognized as influential in development of moral standards.	Moral development proceeds in an invariant sequence of six stages. Heavily tied to Piagetian cognitive stages; acquisition of higher levels of moral reasoning cannot occur until appropriate cognitive development has occurred.	Little attention to individual differences decreases ability to use in describing development in relation to other children. Explains past and present. Predicts what can occur within appropriate societal context in future.	Main utility is in parental guidance and in counseling of adolescents. Higher levels of moral reasoning can be facilitated by setting realistic standards of right and wrong; teaching the child ways to avoid misbehavior; emphasizing the rights and need of others; and providing multiple opportunities to explore the elements of moral problems and their possible solutions.
Theorist: SKINNER, WATSON (Learning Theory; Behaviorism). Focus is entirely on behavior. Internal processes such as thoughts, feelings while sometimes acknowledged are not dealt with			
Behavior is determined (conditioned) by environmental events or experiences or consequences. Behaviors that are rewarded (reinforced) are repeated. Behaviors that are not rewarded or are punished are not repeated.	A previously neutral stimulus can be paired with a response that elicits a behavior so that the behavior is elicited by the neutral stimulus (classic conditioning). Making a reward contingent upon the emission of a certain behavior increases the strength of that behavior's occurrence (operant or instrumental conditioning). Development does not occur in stages but is recurrent throughout the lifespan.	Allows for prediction and control of behavior.	High practical utility. Childrearing and nursing care can be focused on ways to encourage desired behaviors. Extremely useful in discipline issues and in compliance issues related to medical and nursing treatment regimens. Not suited to in-depth explanations of internal processes such as thinking, feeling, and so on.

Table 3-1. *(continued)*

Underlying Theoretical Motivation for Behavior	Theoretical Assumptions	Use	Nursing Strategies
Theorist: BANDURA, BANDURA, AND WALTERS (Social Learning or Observational Learning Theories). Focuses on how behaviors that are appropriate to age, sex, and social class are learned			
Motivation is primarily environmental. Child will imitate or model behaviors that he or she observes, especially if those behaviors are perceived as being rewarded. These imitated behaviors are then reinforced when performed by the child. If the individual modeling a behavior is a significant individual in the life of the child, the behavior may be imitated even if no reward is perceived (vicarious reinforcement).	Theory is heavily dependent on operant conditioning model. Accepts internal mental processes as an aspect of behavior. Memory is acknowledged in that behaviors may not be emitted until long after they are observed. Idea of free choice is incorporated in that individuals are seen as being able to deliberate on the consequences of observed behaviors. Modeling as a motivator of behavior and behavioral change is seen as recurrent throughout the lifespan.	Explains past development. Does not predict future. Allows for control of behaviors instrumental in development.	Great practical utility, especially in guidance of parents regarding childrearing. Parents can be taught to model as well as preach those behaviors that they desire in their children and to encourage association with positive models. This would involve the "do as I do" approach to parenting. Includes useful nursing implications in that exposure of children to others who successfully and appropriately cope with procedures and treatment regimens would provide a model for their coping behaviors.
Theorist: SEARS. Social learning theory applied to socialization. Focus on overt behaviors			
As in observational learning, child imitates observed or modeled behaviors which are rewarded or which are emitted by significant others. A secondary source of reward is intrinsic to the act of imitation itself, in that the child experiences a pleasurable sense of closeness to the significant other whose behavior is emitted. Internal and external motivational sources interact in that reduction of anxiety and psychic tension is seen as significant in reward system for imitated behaviors.	Modeling as a motivator of behavior and behavioral change is recurrent throughout the lifespan. New behaviors that are then rewarded can become the basis for learning even newer behaviors.	Explains past development. Does not predict future. Allows for control of behaviors instrumental in development.	Great practical utility, especially in guidance of parents regarding childrearing. Parents can be taught to model as well as preach those behaviors which they desire in their children and to encourage association with positive models. Specific implications for child discipline are included. Physical punishment is viewed as modeling of aggressive behavior. This would involve "do as I do" approach to parenting. Includes useful nursing implications in that exposure of children to others who successfully and appropriately cope with procedures and treatment regimens would provide a model for their coping behaviors.
Theorist: MASLOW (Humanistic Theory). Focuses on attributes or characteristics that contribute to healthy personality development and are not traditionally dealt with in other theories, e.g., love, creativity, self			
Humans are motivated by two need systems. Basic or deficiency needs such as food, water, and shelter are imposed and rewarded by the environment. Growth needs or metaneeds such as the needs for beauty and self-fulfillment are internally motivated and reinforced. These need systems are hierarchically arranged with lower level needs assuming dominance or prepotency over higher level needs. When one need level is satisfied, the next becomes prepotent.	Does not address developmental stages or shaping of human behaviors. Concerned with the uniqueness and the potential of individuals.	Not intended for use in describing individuals or groups of individuals. Explains behavior only in reference to need systems. Cannot be used to predict or control development except as this is related to ability to meet individual needs.	Primary utility lies in awareness of needs hierarchy. Parenting and nursing care practices that meet basic needs will assist the individual in reaching the next need state.

(By Sandra Frick, RN, PhD.)

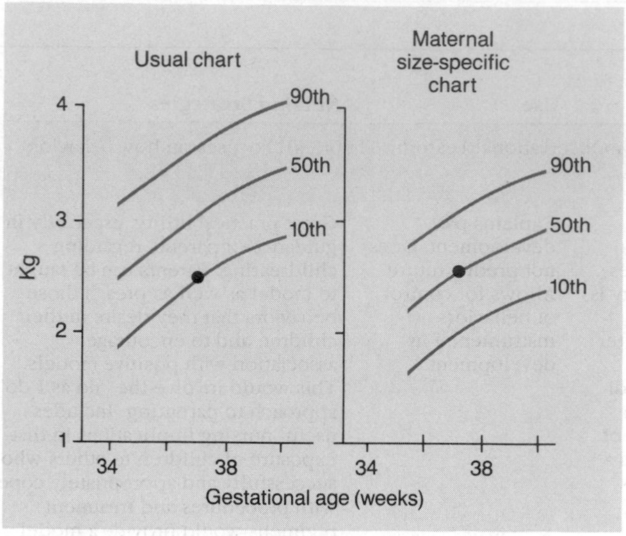

Figure 3-1. The weight of a 5-pound newborn baby, born of a 4-foot, 11-inch, 88-pound mother, plotted on a usual growth grid *(left)* and on one that is specific for the maternal size *(right)*. (Redrawn from Winick M: Biological correlations. *Am J Dis Child* 1970; 120:416 (left) and Thomson AM, et al: The assessment of fetal growth. *J Obstet Gynecol Br Comm* 1968; 75:903 (right).)

ing social and cultural groups. However, if a group of children digress significantly from the norm for a given trait, many of them should be measured for that trait to establish an appropriate average.

Growth charts for height and weight represent an example of norms established to determine physical competency. These grids are especially helpful when a pattern is obtained over a period of time for the child and compared for consistency in height and weight gains. Growth charts are now available that allow for consideration of parental size when evaluating a child's growth. The influence of parental size on these evaluations is shown in Figure 3-1.

Body weight has proved to be a useful index of nutritional status and correlates positively with height increases. For example, a child at 4 to 6 months is considered to have adequate caloric intake if the weight has doubled from what it was at birth. Beyond that age weight increases usually correspond closely to height increases.

Head circumference also is used to monitor physical development. Growth charts for head circumference are available for evaluating a child in relation to established norms. Head circumference is usually a part of the physical appraisal until about age 4 or 5. This is because a composite of these measurements provides an estimate of the rate of brain growth. The normal range is narrow for each age group. Brain and nerve cell growth specialization are most rapid from birth to approximately 4 years of age, at which point there should be a significant slowing. Thus, this age span is considered a ***critical period*** for protein and caloric intake and for intellectual development. A critical period in growth or development, or both, is one in which optimal growth must occur. If it is delayed, growth will not occur or will be delayed significantly. There are critical periods in all domains of development. If growth does not occur during a critical period, catch-up growth can be facilitated in some instances. Figure 3-2 shows some organ tissues for which critical growth periods exist. Brain growth is almost complete by 2 years of age, when 80 per cent of the adult head size has been attained. These first 2 years, then, represent the most critical period for brain growth. Factors that interfere significantly with brain growth during the first 2 years of life can mean lifelong problems. The most readily available method of assessing brain growth is by measuring head circumference. See Chapter 15 for further explanation of this measurement.

Another measurement of physical development is skeletal growth or bone age. Skeletal growth is most rapid during infancy and adolescence. Norms have also been established for dental development and vital signs (temperature, pulse, respirations, and blood pressure) for children at various ages, which are also measures of physical competency. Likewise, laboratory determinations important to routine health appraisal have established normative values for children at different ages. Normative ranges for vision and hearing performance at different ages also exist.

Nutritional patterns and intake needs at different ages also have been determined through averages. An estimation of the child's nutritional adequacy is an important aspect of the evaluation of physical competency.

Physical activity patterns associated with sleep, rest, exercise, and elimination are also significant fea-

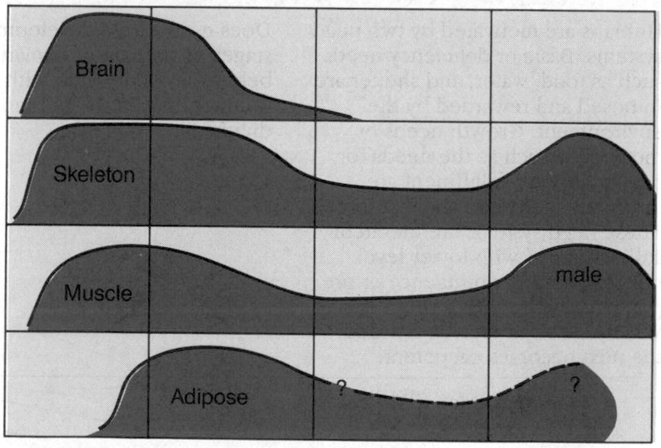

Figure 3-2. Critical periods of increasing cell number for several organ tissues. (Redrawn from Smith DW, Bierman EL: *The Biologic Ages of Man.* Philadelphia, WB Saunders, 1973.)

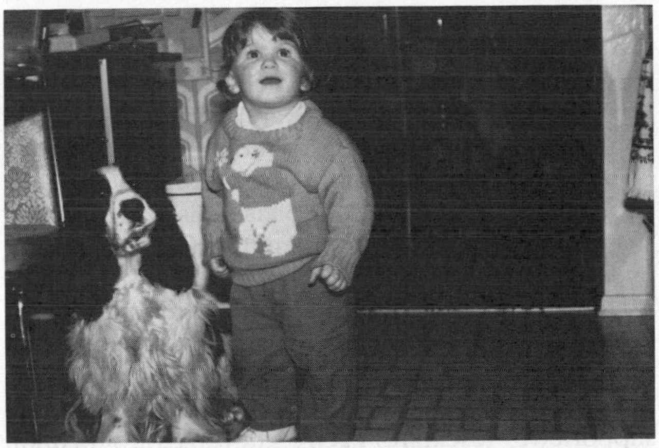

Figure 3-3. The child's growing capacity to take in the world is the source of individuality.

tures of physical competency for which normative ranges exist. However, these must be evaluated in context with the typical patterns of the family unit also.

In evaluating physical competency in those areas for which norms are not measurable, such as motor skills, screening tools are useful. The Denver Developmental Screening Test (DDST), which evaluates fine and gross motor development, is an example of such tools.

Specific norms of physical competency are presented in Chapter 15, in the age-related chapters on growth and development, and in the appendices.

Keen observation is required by the nurse assessing a child's physical development and physical needs. Children, especially those under 5 or 6,* have difficulty identifying and describing their physical discomforts or needs in ways adults can understand. Also, physical changes in children often occur quite suddenly and without any accompanying warning signs.

Obtaining accurate physical measurements from a crying, squirming infant or from actively protesting toddlers and preschoolers can be quite a challenge to even the most skilled nurse. However, knowledge of age-effective approaches to children, coupled with keen observational skills, usually yields successful evaluations.

The nurse caring for children should always keep in mind that the physical care offered is not only supportive to the child's physical needs and development but is also a means of communicating support for emotional-social and intellectual needs. The nurse's understanding of physical development and recognition of the alterations to physical development caused by stress—whether accidental (illness) or maturational (change in structure or function) or environmental (inadequate diet related to poor socioeconomic status of family unit)—will give direction for nursing strategies to prevent, minimize or remedy those stresses and for strategies to enhance the child's environment in ways that support healthy physical development.

Intellectual Competency

Intellect is a composite of skills, behaviors, and adaptive abilities that makes it possible for an individual to adjust to new situations, to think abstractly, and to profit from his or her experiences. Although only ambiguous measures of intellect exist, it is demonstrable in the way a person solves problems and in how appropriate his or her response is in any given situation. By 1 year of age children show increasingly overt evidence of their developing mind. They can make some of their own decisions and can accept the decisions of others with whom they feel secure. They have achieved the ability to wait because they can intellectually recognize the cues and sounds in their environment that assure them their needs will momentarily be met. Their intellectual advances by 1 year have also taught them that they can anticipate certain routines from their environment. Evidence of a young infant's developing mind is seen when he or she registers the sounds of bottle preparation. Children learn that these sounds mean they will soon be fed, so they await the bottle in alertness rather than expressing their need by crying. They evidence here the rudimentary notion of cause and effect.

Intelligence, once believed to be genetically fixed, has been found, in longitudinal studies, to be fluctuating (Pulaski, 1971). These findings illustrate the effect of environment on intellectual development and function. Neither can the maturational factor be ignored. Intellectual development cannot advance until the structures for thought exist to assimilate the experience. However, a variety of sensory and motor stimuli are needed before learning will occur. Learning cannot be accomplished for children. They must do their own learning from their experiences with movement, touch, sounds, visual images, and taste. It is from these manipulations that thoughts arise that are necessary for the formation of mental images. A child cannot intellectually categorize the mental image of a cow simply by being offered a verbal description of one. The image will not occur until the child has at least seen a picture of a cow, or felt one or watched one in real life.

These findings on the effect of environment on intellect have resulted in a rising concern for the provision of primary or early learning opportunities. Evidence of this concern has been exemplified in the

*Language and intellectual development has not progressed enough before this age to allow clarity in verbalization of mental processes.

movements for development of Head Start or Get Set programs, preschool or kindergarten education, nursery schools, play programs for children during confinement, and similar social structures whose aim is to counteract any sensory deprivations that a child might experience because of any sociocultural or physical limitations in the child's early life. Other programs that have arisen out of a recognition of the importance of motor and sensory stimulation early on are the stimulation programs for immature babies and infant-stimulation programs for any infant with signs of developmental lag.

Knowledge of intellectual development and intellectual needs of children at various ages is extremely valuable to the nurse who interacts with children. *Understanding the child's level of intellectual thought and function helps the nurse to decipher more meaningfully a child's communications, to more accurately interpret the behaviors and the processes that motivate them, and to realize more emphatically the meaning various experiences have for the child.* This understanding should be demonstrated in the nursing strategies planned, the approach with which those interventions are offered, and the age-appropriateness of nurse-child communication. Because the nurse often deals with children under circumstances that have placed limits on them and their environmental exposure, it is of utmost importance that the necessity for stimulating and interactional experiences be recognized and provided for as an essential aspect of nursing care.

Although most tests available for measuring predictive intellectual capacity or estimating level of intellectual function are done by personnel in other health-related professions, the nurse should be familiar with existing tests and the caution with which they must be interpreted. The nurse should also be aware of the variability of test results in young children and of the limited correlation that exists between results of these early tests and of tests conducted later in the child's life, although more consistency usually exists after age 5.

The construct of the test will vary, depending upon the age of the child being evaluated. Performance-type tests are usually used with infants and toddlers; the DDST is an example. Pre-school and early school-age children who have not yet mastered reading cannot respond to the written tests offered literate school-age children. Young adults are usually given verbal tests. Any of these tests, however, are more fair measures of predictive capacity when interpreted in conjunction with achievement and school readiness tests.

The one individual who has perhaps contributed most toward our understanding of intellectual or cognitive development is the Swiss psychologist Jean Piaget. He and his Geneva colleagues, through a variety of ingenious studies, derived the stage theory about children's intellectual activity and how it undergoes qualitative changes over the span of childhood.

According to Piaget, there are four major stages of cognitive development: sensorimotor, preoperational, concrete operational, and formal operational. Each stage has its own substages or phases. Each of the major stages of cognitive development represents a qualitative change in the way the individual thinks or behaves. All individuals progress through the stages of cognitive development in the same order and no stage of development is skipped. (This idea of invariance of occurrence of stages of cognitive development has been supported by research.) Each of the stages is built upon what occurred in the previous stage and each stage provides the basis for the next stage. In the following overview of Piaget's theory, the terminology of the theory, summarized in Box 3-1, is used.

Piaget believed that during early infancy, primitive reflexes determine behavior. Later, experience modifies reflexes into purposeful activities. He believed that the cognitive development of individuals is governed by two major organizing principles. *Organization* is the tendency of all species to integrate all cognitive processes into one overall system. *Adaptation* is the tendency for all species to deal with their environment. Piaget further asserted that adaptation involves continuous twin processes, *assimilation* and *accommodation.* Assimilation allows the individual to deal with or adapt to his or her environment through the use of already existing behaviors. Accommodation requires the development of new behaviors in order for adaptation to occur.

Through the process of cognitive development, adaptation allows the individual to deal with an ever wider and more complex environment. At each stage of development, the individual has mental representations or cognitive structures of his or her world called *schemata.* Each schema becomes more complex, more realistic, more abstract as development progresses. Each schema involves a mental representation of some facet of the world and an observable behavior. What we learn about an individual's cognitive development, we learn from the behaviors we observe. Schemata become more highly developed through the processes of assimilation and accommodation.

Assimilation is the process of incorporating new information into one's current activity or way of thinking (making the unfamiliar seem familiar). New information is assimilated via all of the senses. Therefore, one's schema for an object or event can consist of multiple types of sensory information. For example, a child will form a schema for dog by assimilating visual information (two ears, a tail, four legs), auditory information (bark), and tactile information (texture of fur, the feel of a wet tongue). As different dogs are encoun-

Box 3-1
Definition of Piagetian Terms

Schema (Plural, schemata)

Mental representation or cognitive structure representing objects, events, ideas; known by its observable behavior.

Assimilation

Mental process that involves the taking in of new sensory information that fits or matches with existing schemata.

Accommodation

Mental process that involves the changing of schemata in order to include new information that does not fit the existing schemata.

Adaptation

Tendency for all species to adapt to (or deal with) their environment; an equilibrium between assimilation and accommodation.

Organization

Tendency of all species to integrate all cognitive processes into one overall system; the proper inter-relationship among schemata.

Equilibrium

Cognitive balance between assimilation and accommodation.

Equilibration

Process involved in equilibrium.

Operations

Mental activities that develop from manipulation of objects.

(By Sandra Frick, RN, PhD.)

tered they can be assimilated into the existing dog schema so long as no change in mental representation must occur.

Accommodation is a process involving the changing of mental representations in order to include new information that does not fit the existing schema. Accommodation therefore involves an ability to adjust a schema to fit new information or new circumstances. Since schemata (and changes in schemata) are known by behaviors of the individual, the process of accommodation can be described by looking at a series of behaviors. Early in life a baby obtains food by crying and subsequently sucking on the nipple that is offered. The baby's schema for obtaining food changes when solids are offered from a spoon. The baby must accommodate his or her schema for obtaining food by changing the way in which it is ingested and the sensory qualities of what is ingested. Later the baby will again accommodate when self-feeding begins.

Assimilation allows for the addition of new perceptions to a schema with existing capabilities; accomodation requires that existing schema be changed to fit more complex circumstances. Assimilation and accommodation function together to bring about a cognitive balance called *equilibrium.* The process of *equilibrium* allows the individual to form a mental representation of the world which is suitable to existing capabilities and which allows for growth and change. As the individual grows and capabilities increase, the balance or equilibrium between assimilation and accommodation is threatened. The individual is thereby motivated to maintain equilibrium by altering old ways of thinking to solve new problems. Figure 3-4 illustrates the flow of the intellectual processes for adaptation.

The following is an outline of the sequence theorized by Piaget as the development of intellect.

Sensorimotor Period—First 2 Years of Life

The child moves from neonatal birth reflexes to the construct of symbolic images during this period. The task involved is mastery of coordinating simple sensorimotor activity. During this stage children are dependent upon their bodies for self-expression and communication. They work to create an organized world that links their desires for physical satisfaction to their sensory experiences.

There are six substages in the sensorimotor period.

Substage 1—use of reflexes (birth to 1 month). This stage is characterized by automatic innate or reflex responses to external stimuli. Body movements are random. The infant is completely self-centered and does not perceive the accomplishments of reflexive behaviors. Genuine intelligent behavior is absent; however, the continual practice of reflexes leads to their maturation and a sense of order for the neonate.

Substage 2—primary circular reactions (1–4 months). Circular reactions stimulate their own repetition or continuation. Primary circular reactions involve an active effort to reproduce a behavior that was first achieved by chance through some random activity. The infant's repetitive use of the primitive reflexes, coupled with neurologic and physical maturation,

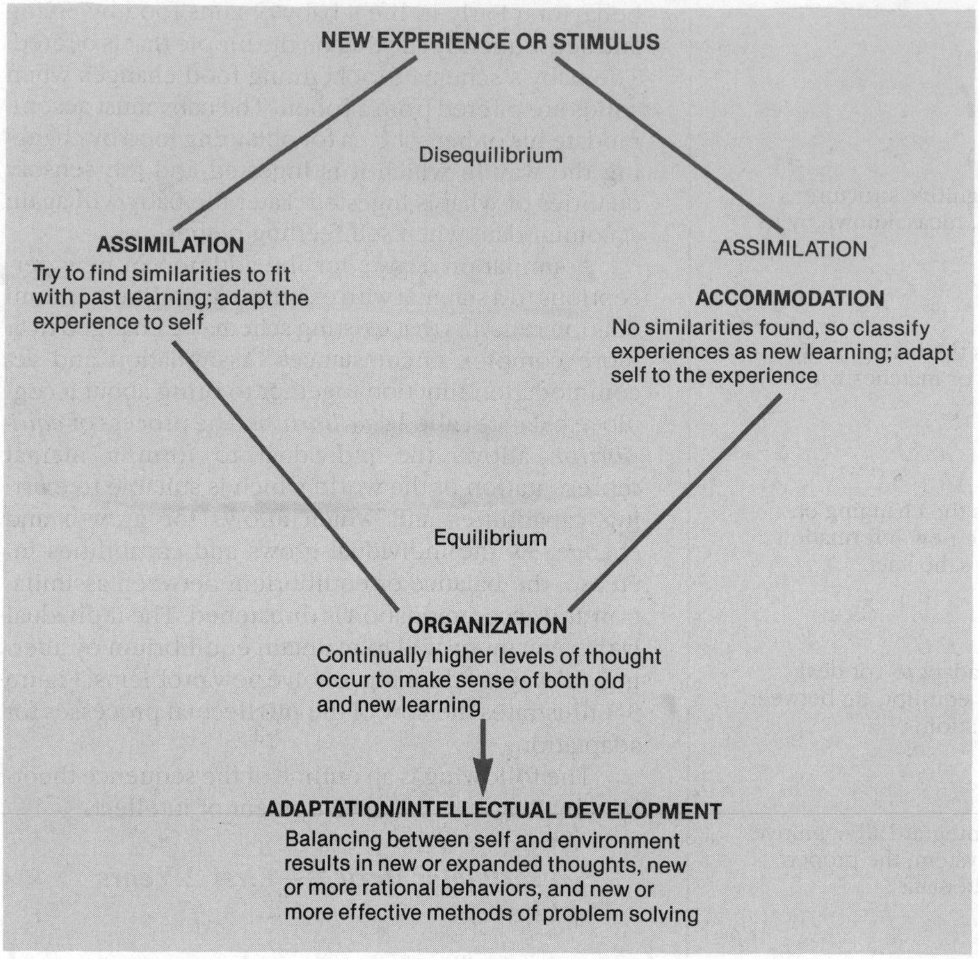

***Figure* 3-4.** Intellectual process in adaptation (a diagrammatic presentation of Piaget's theory of intellectual development as an adaptive process).

tends to produce habits. These new behaviors, or habits, are repeated purely for the pleasure they produce.* For example, random arm movement places the fist at the infant's mouth at a moment he or she happens to be making sucking movements. The baby repeats this movement combination because of the discovery that sucking the fist is satisfying; thus, the accidentally acquired behavior becomes a new sensorimotor habit.

Substage 3—secondary circular reactions (4–8 months). Behaviors during this substage involve concern with the external (or secondary) environment rather than with one's own body. The baby continues to repeat primary circular reactions, but now a greater awareness of the surrounding world produces an increasing interest in the results of the actions. New behavior is repeated as a means of reproducing an interesting alteration in the environment that was initially discovered by accident. An example of this is when a rattle is placed in the infant's fist and random arm movement makes it rattle. The infant will repeat the arm movement over and over to re-create the noise that occurs—having discovered that the action produces a given result. This is the basis for play.

At this point the infant is beginning to associate events that occur close together. The position of cradling at the breast is associated with time to eat and the infant roots and makes sucking movements. In fact, the first notion of causality derives from recognizing that certain actions have certain results. The infant also gains a dim awareness of *before* and *after* in the sequence of events (i.e., a rudimentary notion of time); recognizing the breast as a part of the sequence is evidence of a dawning recognition of symbols. Eye-hand coordination is achieved during this stage. Also during this stage the concept of object permanence begins to develop. Infants will search for an object if part of the object is visible but will not do so if the object is completely hidden—even if they saw it being hidden.

Substage 4—coordination of secondary circular reactions (8–12 months). Secondary circular reactions are coordinated to form new, more complex, behaviors that are unquestionably intentional. The baby in this substage can solve simple problems using

*This initially reflexive behavior gradually becomes behavior that is consciously motivated, by about 2 months of age.

behaviors that have already been mastered. Infants will push aside obstacles or use sources close at hand to get what they want. For example, pulling on the mother's hand that has a bottle in it can bring the bottle into reach. Infants in this substage also exhibit anticipatory behavior. Previously they have mastered the ability to let go of objects; now they will anticipate the landing of a toy dropped over the side of the crib.

The concept of object permanence is more highly developed. Infants will now search for a totally hidden object if they saw it being hidden; however, if the object is moved while the baby watches, he or she will continue to search in the first hiding place.

Substage 5—tertiary circular reactions (12–18 months). In this substage rudimentary trial-and-error behavior occurs through active experimentation to discover different ways of getting results or solving simple problems. By varying their actions, babies look for the most effective way of attaining a goal. For example, they discover that pulling at a blanket corner brings a toy into reach. These activities are evidence of beginning reasoning. Serious interest in the construction of objects fosters various manipulations of them—the baby pulls at a toy and pokes, pats, and bites it. The concept of object permanence is evident in the fact that children now seek an object in the place they saw it moved to, not in its original location. The fact that they continue to seek the nonvisible object indicates memory and retention.

Substage 6—invention of new means through deduction (18–24 months). Children in this substage have a well-developed understanding of the nature of objects. A basic concept of causality has been formed. Their ability to use symbols mentally allows these children to "figure out" solutions to problems. They can also remember, plan, imagine, and imitate someone else's previous actions. These children begin to see themselves as separate from others in their environment, motivating emotional attitudes of competition and rivalry. Object permanence is now well developed. The child understands visible and unseen displacement of objects; so he or she can see a series of object displacements and search for an object in its last hiding place. The child will search for an object even if he or she did not see it hidden.

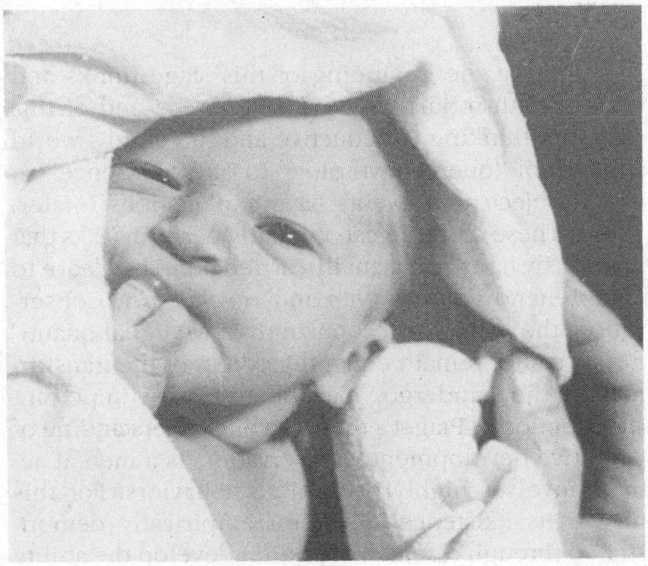

Primitive reflexes, accidentally produced (stage 1), are repeated for pleasure (stage 2) during the sensorimotor period.

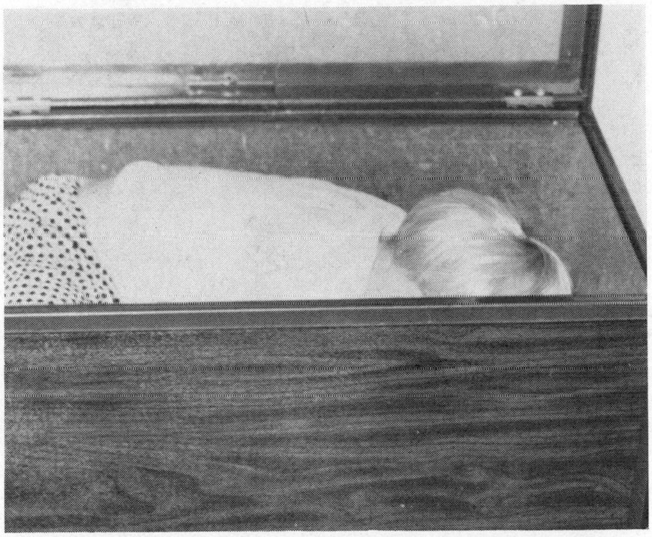

During the preoperational stage children see things only from their own point of view. This child of age 2½ thinks that because he cannot see anyone he cannot be seen.

Preoperational Period—2 to 7 Years

The major qualitative change in cognitive function from the sensorimotor to the preoperational period involves the ability to use symbols. This period continues to be characterized by egocentric* thought that is expressed in animism,† artificialism,‡ realism,§ and magic omnipotence.** The child at this state continues to seem illogical to adults. The child's task is to use language and memory to begin to understand the past, present, and immediate future. These children display progressively more socialized behavior in this period as they move steadily away from egocentric thought. The irreversibility of this stage evolves into a

* The child sees things only from his or her own point of view.

† The child attributes lifelike qualities to inanimate objects.

‡ The child perceives that all things are designed by human beings.

§ Everything is considered real by a child in this stage—even dreams.

** The child believes that things can be made to happen just by thinking them and that the world exists for the child alone.

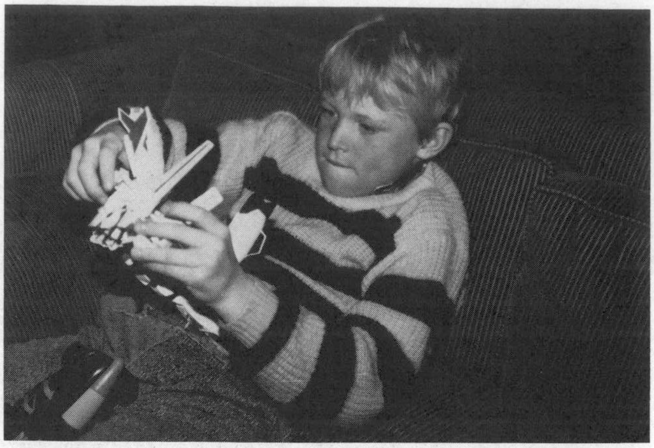

Children in the stage of concrete operations develop increasing capacity for problem solving.

conception of reversibility in the concrete state. If a preschooler is asked whether he has a brother, he will say "yes." If asked whether his brother has a brother, he will say "no."

Stage 1 (preconceptual stage)—2 to 4 years. Children now form mental images to stand for things they cannot see (symbolic thought), including their various properties. These concepts are reinforced through drawings, language, dreams, and "make believe" and "imitative" play. Play involving language, action, and symbolic imitation is this child's primary tool for adaptation and consumes most of his or her waking hours. A child uses symbolic thought in play which focuses on deferred imitation of previously viewed activities such as Mommy washing dishes or daddy fixing the car. Symbolic thought is also evident in play in which one object is made to stand for something else. For the preoperational child a packing carton has endless possibilities as a car, a spaceship, a house, a swimming pool, and so on. Most play at this stage is parallel. Because of children's egocentrism, they are engrossed in their own thoughts, feelings, and experiences, so are not able to give attention to what someone else is doing or may want. This egocentrism is also operational in their perception of objects and events. For example, these children cannot visualize the other side of a box or the other side of a profile of a face. They wonder if ocean waves stop at night when they are asleep (i.e., all else in the world sleeps when they sleep). Children comprehend "doing what they are told" and relate it causally to pleasing their parents. They take their instructions literally, therefore needing specific instruction in behaviors to be carried out; "be good" is not specific enough for children in this stage to enact.

Stage 2 (perceptual or intuitive stage)—4 to 7 years. Prelogical reasoning appears, based on perceptions that do not acknowledge intrinsic aspects. Experiences and objects are judged by outside appearances and results. For example, given an equal number each of toothpicks and pencils, a child may insist there are more pencils because they are bigger or they take up more space. Nor can the child accept that two 4 ounce glasses both contain the same amount of water because one is short and wide and the other tall and narrow. Selective attention is also present in that the child can concentrate only upon one characteristic of an object at a time. For example, red balls cannot at the same time be rubber balls, even though the child's image of the object attributes to it multiple properties. This focus on only one aspect of a situation at a time is called *centration*. Not until the next period of cognitive development will the child be capable of decentration. Children at this stage begin to use words to express their thoughts, but during the first couple of years in this stage some thoughts are still acted out. During the first half of this stage the child still perceives anything that moves or is active as being alive. Play becomes gradually more social, demanding collective rules, organized games, and fantasy enactments of the rules and values of the child's elders. An additional limitation of preoperational thought is *transductive reasoning*. There are two kinds of logical reasoning: deductive reasoning goes from general to particular; inductive reasoning goes from particular to general. The preoperational child goes from particular to particular without considering the general situation. This type of illogical thinking can result in the child's assuming the existence of a cause-and-effect relationship between two unrelated events: "I was a bad boy, so I got sick."

Concrete Operational Period—7 to 11 Years

The child at the beginning of this stage thinks and reasons with inductive logic, but by the end of this stage the thinking is deductive and the child's world shifts from "one of mythology to one of science" in which objects and events have explanations (Maier, 1969). These children can mentally perform tasks that previously had to be actually carried out. They learn to comprehend *conservation* and *reversibility*. Conservation, the ability to recognize that two equal quantities of matter remain equal regardless of the transformation they undergo, may be the most important contribution of Piaget's theory to our understanding of cognitive development. Conservation as a mental activity involves highly observable behaviors. For this reason its existence has been empirically demonstrated through research. Children develop the ability to conserve for different qualities of matter at different times. The abilities to conserve for length and number occur early in the period, while the abilities to conserve for space and volume do not occur until the end of the period. Examples of the different types of conservation and the tasks through which they are demonstrated are shown in Table 3-2. Learning about one kind of conservation cannot be transferred to another kind of conservation. Each kind is learned separately through manipulation of the different qualities of matter. (This is an example of just how concrete mental operations are during this period.) In addition to providing the correct response to problems, children must demonstrate by their justification of their response that they truly understand the conservation principle. Acceptance justifications include those that justify according to reversibility (if you poured it back in the other glass, rolled it back into a ball, moved them back to the corners, it/they would be the same); identity (it is the same water, same clay, same horses); or compensation (one glass is shorter but it's fatter; the snake is skinnier but it's longer). The tasks involved in conservation assist one in the understanding of concrete operations.

> "The term *concrete* does not mean that the child must see or touch the actual objects as he works through a problem. Rather . . . that the problems involve identifiable objects that are either directly perceived or imagined."
>
> Thomas, 1979, p. 313

The concrete operational child is capable of *decentration,* the ability to focus on multiple aspects of an object, event, or situation at the same time. These children understand that most actions can be reversed. They also understand the value of rules, and base judgments on reason. The future and the abstract are still beyond comprehension. Concrete operational children invest much energy into efforts to order and classify the objects and experiences in their lives, as evidenced by their endless collections and scrapbooks.* By the end of this stage children can comprehend that they belong to a family, a city, and a country simultaneously. Play and conversation now serve to establish progressive mutuality and equality in their relationships. Notions of animism and artificialism continue during this period but gradually decrease.

Formal Operational Period—From 11 Years On

This stage is characterized by logical reasoning and the ability to think about the hypothetical and abstract. It is no longer necessary for mental problems to deal with concrete objects. Children in this period can systematically analyze abstract problems and arrive at their possible solutions. Relative realism exists, by which they can separate what is thought from what is of the real world. Thought patterns incorporate the past, present, and future.

Piaget's theories can help nurses better understand children's concepts about their bodies and their world and about health care experiences. Not all of Piaget's concepts are universally accepted. Research evidence is accumulating that suggests the need to reject or revise some of Piaget's concepts. A large body of research has been carried out (and continues), however, that provides empirical validation of many of Piaget's concepts (Halford et al, 1986; Kruger and Tomasello, 1986; Madden, 1986; Miller, 1986).

Developmental assessment of a child should always include a focus on cognitive development. In addition to gaining data that might contribute to a nursing diagnosis of altered growth and development, information about the child's level of cognitive development will help the nurse to know how to structure the provision of information to the child. For example, research has been carried out that explains children's understanding of the CAT scan procedure, using Piaget's concepts as a framework (Hellier, Ptak, and Cerreto, 1986).

Behavioral Learning Theory

Another developmental focus that should be included in the nurse's consideration of a child's intellectual development (as well as other domains of development) is the behavioral learning theory focus. Piaget's theory of cognitive development is a stage theory. Learning theories, in contrast to stage theories, see development as not necessarily sequential or fixed. Stage theories focus on different processes (e.g., centration, irreversibility) that occur at various stages of development. Learning theories focus on the same processes (e.g., conditioning, social imitation) throughout the life cycle. Stage theorists stress changes in internal structures that impel development, while learning theorists stress the influence of environmental forces on behavior.

Learning, defined as a change in behavior, is seen as occurring through the process of classic conditioning, operant conditioning, and imitation of social models.

Classic conditioning, a method of using environmental stimuli to bring about a change in behavior, was demonstrated by the Russian psychologist Ivan Pavlov. Classic conditioning involves a process of stimulus substitution in which a new, previously neutral stimulus is substituted for the stimulus that originally elicited the response. In classic conditioning the stimulus elicits the response. Pavlov rang a bell whenever food

*These children are able to sort objects into categories according to characteristics such as color or shape, an act also referred to as *seriation.*

Table 3-2. Conservation Abilities and Tasks Used to Detect Their Existence

Conservation Ability	Conservation Task	Conserving Response
Number		
The ability to recognize that number is not changed if arrangement or physical properties of items changes	Arrange five pennies in a row close together and another five pennies in a row but spaced at a distance from one another. Ask the child which row has more pennies	Both have the same number of pennies
	Show the child four blue marbles and two red marbles. Ask whether there are more red marbles or more blue marbles	There are more marbles
Length		
The ability to recognize that length is not changed if configuration changes	Show a child two straight strings of identical length. Curve one string into an S curve. Ask the child which string is longer	Both strings are the same
Liquid Amount		
The ability to recognize that the amount of liquid is not changed by the shape of the container into which it is poured	Show a child a short, wide container filled to the brim with colored water. Pour the colored water into a tall narrow container that holds the same amount of liquid as the first container. Ask the child which glass holds the most water	They both hold the same amount of water
Solid Amount (Substance)		
The ability to recognize that the amount of a solid substance is not changed by altering the shape of the substance	Show a child two identical balls of clay. Roll one ball into a "snake." Ask the child which ball has more clay	They both have the same amount of clay
	Show the child two identical bags of potato chips. Smash one bag so that the chips are broken into crumbs. Ask the child which bag has more potato chips	They both have the same amount of potato chips
Space (Area)		
The ability to recognize that the amount of area on a surface is not changed by rearrangement of the objects on it	Show a child two identical green square "farmyards" with a farm building placed on each corner of each square. Move all four buildings to the center of one square. Ask the child which farmyard has more green grassy space	They both have the same amount of grassy space
Weight		
The ability to recognize that the weight of a substance or object is not changed by altering the shape of the substance	Show a child two identical balls of clay evenly balanced on a scale. Remove them from the scale. Flatten one ball. Ask the child which ball will now weigh the most	They both still weigh the same
Volume		
The ability to recognize that displacement of liquids results from the volume of an object and will not be changed by altering the shape of the object	Show a child two containers of water. Drop identical balls of clay into the water and tell the child to watch how high the water rises. Remove one ball of clay from its container and alter its shape by flattening or elongating it or dividing into several separate balls of clay. Ask the child which water will be higher when the clay is again dropped into the water	The water level will be the same in both containers.

(By Sandra Frick, RN, PhD.)

was presented to a dog; soon the stimulus of ringing the bell was all that was needed to elicit the response of salivation.

Benjamin F. Skinner extended the concept of classical conditioning to *operant conditioning,* a type of conditioning in which a behavior or response is altered by the stimuli or consequences that follow the response. There are two types of consequences, *reinforcers* and *punishers.* A punisher is a consequence that follows a response that has the effect of decreasing the frequency of the response it follows. A reinforcer is a consequence that follows a response that has the effect of increasing the frequency of the response it follows. *Behavior modification* involves the use of reinforcement and punishment to alter behavior.

Social learning theory, also called observational learning theory and modeling theory, builds upon the principles of classic and operant conditioning. Social learning theory posits that one does not have to have the opportunity of actually making a particular new response in order to learn the new response. Social learning theory says that new responses can be learned by watching the behavior of socially competent people (models).

Learning theories are useful to nurses in their interactions with children and families. Nurses can use behavior modification techniques to help shape desired behaviors in children and can teach parents these strategies. Nurses often learn novel parenting strategies from some parents that can be shared with other families. For example, one young couple taught their infant son to look straight ahead and open his mouth for the spoonful of solid food by only putting the food in his mouth in response to that behavior. Anyone who has ever "chased" a little mouth in an effort to feed an infant solid food can appreciate the logic in the strategies used by these parents.

Role modeling is another important teaching strategy for showing parents how to care for their well or ill children and for demonstrating to children appropriate self-care. These learning theory strategies are detailed for specific situations throughout this text.

Development of Language

Language is an important aspect of intellectual development that has only recently gained much attention by researcher and health professionals. Language development involves an increasingly complex expansion of receptive (comprehension of language) and expressive (speaking of language) skills over time. Language efforts that are rewarded with approval from parents and other adults in the child's environment (socially reinforced) seem to result in more effective language skills. Nurses should apply this knowledge in

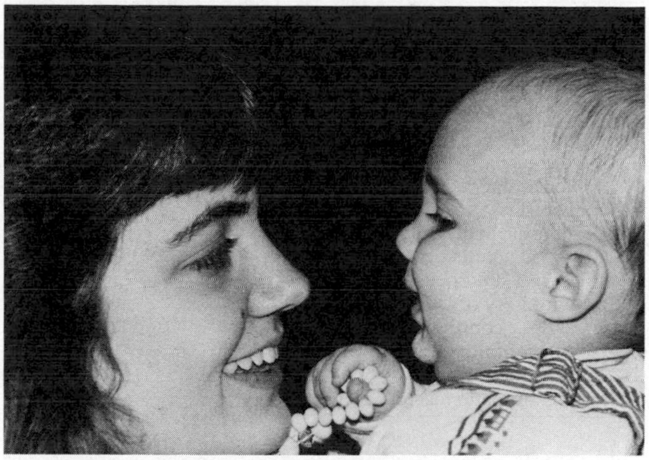

Children's interactions with adults stimulate their language development.

their own verbal interactions with children and in their child guidance instruction to parents.

It is also known that receptive language skills are achieved earlier than expressive language skills, as is evidenced in the early toddler's ability to follow an instruction before he or she has learned the vocabulary skills to acknowledge that instruction. Nurses can apply this fact in their nursing care, too. ***Even infants have a less stressful response to nursing procedures if they are spoken to before, during, and for a brief interval after the procedure.***

As with all other realms of development, language development is influenced by both nurturing and natural forces.

Children's interaction with adults stimulates their language development, so when that interaction is diminished, language skills take longer to develop. Females evidence earlier language acquisition than males. It has been speculated that parents' interactions with their daughters may be more verbal, whereas their interactions with their sons may more often be physical in nature.

Twins usually are slower in language achievement than are children born singly. This may be because there is less conversation between each of them and their mother, most likely due to the fact that they are so close with each other that the mother often addresses them as one.

Socioeconomic influences on language also exist, with language mastery occurring earlier in children from middle and upper class homes. Children from bilingual backgrounds may have difficulty with mastery of one or both languages. When children are expected to learn two languages at once with differing rules and letter pronunciation, they become confused. Learning a second language is usually easier once one language has been mastered well enough for the child

Table 3-3. Age Ranges of Language Developmental Stages

Cooing stage	0–2 months
Babbling stage	2–6 months
First word, usually imitated	12–18 months
Rapid vocabulary acquisition	18 months–3 years
Open and pivot words	
Telegraphic sentences	
Steady word acquisition	3–5 years
Multiword sentences	
Basic mastery of language by end	
Progressively complex sentences	6–11+ years
Use of pronouns, proper nouns, prepositions	
Basic grammatic mastery by end	

to be comfortable with it. However, the single most influential factor in learning a second language is whether the child is being reprimanded for trying to use one of the languages (Hurlock, 1978). Dialects (language variations) are structured by professional association (incorporation by professional jargon-terminology into language), age (adolescent slang is usually unique to that generation alone), geographic location (usually different inflections or pronunciations of the same words, called colloquialisms, from one locale to another), and socioeconomic class (more complex word forms are used in upper classes).

Theories of Language Development

Three theories of language development seem equally viable to our current knowledge of language development (Evans and McCandless, 1978; Helms and Turner, 1978). Noam Chomsky's research supports an *innate theory* in which he depicts language development as genetically determined. Through this innate capacity of brain cells to act upon linguistic input, triggered by a system known as a *language acquisition device* (LAD), native language learning occurs. LAD enables the child to select and fit together properties of language and concrete experiences, eventually synthesizing them into language competency.

B.F. Skinner has applied *reinforcement theory,* also called behavior modification theory and stimulus-response theory, to language development. He supports the concept that language, as with all behavior, is acquired or learned as a result of one's environmental interactions through which behaviors that produce language are reinforced.

Social learning theory describes the development of language as a modeling process, resulting from the child's imitation of adult remarks and from caretakers' expansion of his or her utterances.

All three theories are most likely functioning in language development, each being a description of one facet of yet another complex component of human development.

Moreover, all three theories are in accord as to the approximate age range during which various stages of language acquisition occur. The progression of language development is seen in Table 3-3.

Emotional-Social Competency

A child's personality is the integration of feelings, attitudes, and relationships as expressed by behavior patterns. The adult measure of a healthy personality (i.e., the goal of emotional-social development) is one's capacity to love, to achieve, and to become interdependent in function. Yet emotional-social development is not something that has been mastered by adulthood. It is, rather, a process that unfolds throughout the individual's lifetime, with each stage of life having its own tasks to be mastered and the leftover tasks of other life stages to be re-resolved.

Erikson's theory on the psychosocial development of human beings illustrates this lifelong struggle for emotional-social equilibrium. Erikson's theory is unique in that it describes psychosocial development throughout the entire life span. Psychoanalyst Erik Homburger Erikson extended Sigmund Freud's theory of psychosexual development. Freud emphasized the id and biosexual connotations of human behavior. Erikson's theory emphasizes the ego and social connotations of human behavior.

According to Erikson, individual development occurs within the context of the social and cultural environment. Social and cultural factors influence or impinge on development at all stages, and only when these factors are taken into account can psychosocial (or emotional-social) development be understood. External social and cultural factors do not operate alone. Each individual possesses within him- or herself an internal or innate capacity to interact with the environment.

In Erikson's theory there are eight stages of psychosocial development (Erikson's eight ages of man). During each stage of development, the individual is presented with a basic developmental task (also referred to as dominant central problem or crisis). This task, problem, or crisis requires the individual to resolve a conflict between two opposing forces (one positive and one negative). The individual cannot progress to the next stage until the conflict of the previous stage is resolved. Ideal resolution results in a greater predominance of the positive psychologic attribute (ego qualities) for the stage. Many individuals misinterpret the meaning of crisis resolution. Erikson was adamant that healthy psychologic development does

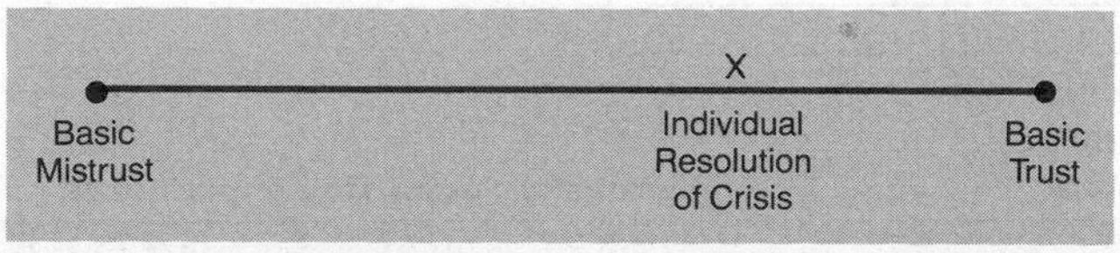

Figure 3-5. Example of positive resolution of Erikson's first developmental crisis.

not mean that the individual develops all characteristics of the positive psychologic attributes (e.g., trust, autonomy, initiative) and no characteristics of the negative psychologic attributes (e.g., mistrust, shame and doubt, guilt). Rather, development of these attributes should be viewed as occurring on a continuum. Ideal development would involve more positive than negative attributes, but some of the negative should be present. For example, an individual who develops all trust and no mistrust would be at risk for danger and discomfort. Similar statements can be made about the negative attributes of later stages. The individual who develops all autonomy and no shame and doubt, all initiative and no guilt will have difficulty coping in society. Optimal resolution of the first developmental crisis is diagrammed in Figure 3-5. As soon as the central task or crisis of one stage is resolved, a new set of societal and cultural factors come to bear on the individual. At the same time new skills and qualities have developed within the individual as a result of dealing with the crisis of the previous stage. These skills and qualities enable the individual to master the new task set by society and culture. Each succeeding task therefore is built upon what occurred in the previous stage of development. Table 3-4 illustrates Erikson's eight stages, the approximate age at which each task or crisis is experienced, the negative counterpart of unsuccessful task mastery, and the significant interpersonal relationships and experiences in the environment of the person needed to support him or her in task accomplishment. To show the relationship between Erikson's theory and that of Freud, Freud's stages are shown in parentheses after the appropriate Erikson's stage.

Erikson stresses that the negative counterparts to each stage's task are never completely conquered but must be retackled at various times throughout life; however, it is healthy if favorable mastery exists most of the time and if healthy compensations are used when mastery totters.

Illness or accident can compound the problems confronting a child who is already at the peak of a psychologic crisis. The nurse who is a part of the child's environment can support development if he or she knows the task being faced. Regression to a previous task level, or reversion in the direction of the negative counterpart of a task level currently confronting the child, is common in children (and parents) during extreme or continued stress. The nurse should respect the individual's need to regress, help the child and his parents to accept that fact and the accompanying increased dependency, support them as they rework those tasks and provide an environment that fosters a return to their age-appropriate tasks.

As Erikson's model illustrates, parents too are in the process of developing and may require assistance from nurses in (1) building constructive relationships with each other and with their children, (2) feeling satisfaction and confidence in parenting skills, (3) learning to cope with the stresses confronting their children and in knowing their responsibility in helping the child manage those stresses.

Another component of a child's emotional-social development is his or her sexuality development. Although sex is determined genetically at conception, a child's total sexuality is influenced by his or her development progress in all three competency areas (physical, intellectual, emotional-social). Sexuality also affects development of those competencies.

A third component of emotional-social development is moral development. Morality is composed of developmental tasks in two areas. Children must achieve a realistic acceptance of their social responsibility. They must also integrate personal principles of justice and reciprocity that are based on empathy, mutual respect, and regard for the integrity and rights of others.

One of the leading theorists in the area of moral development is Lawrence Kohlberg.* He states that moral development is prefaced by the child's ability to reason, thus moral development follows a sequence that corresponds with the development of intellect. Kohlberg's model describes three phases of moral development. In the first phase, *preconventional* or *premoral morality* (4 to 7 years), children perceive rules as absolute and unalterable. This perception is congruent with the intellectual egocentrism and realism of children this age. A punishment and obedience orientation prompts acceptable moral behavior at this phase. This "do what's right or be punished" attitude, coupled with a naive instrumental hedonism (doing right earns one favor or rewards), makes the child in this phase fairly compliant to adult-set rules.

The *conventional morality* phase (7 to 11 years) is based on the child's perception of rules as existing for the good of all, to preserve order and to protect people. Children in this phase comply with rules because of their desire to please or help others and to maintain approval as a "good" child, which helps them to avoid

*Because Kohlberg and Piaget have very similar theories about moral development, only one is discussed.

Table 3-4. An Expansion Chart of the Eight Stages in the Human Life Cycle

Task and Subtasks	Task's Negative Counterpart	Significant Persons	Significant Supporting Experiences
Infancy (Oral)* (0 to 1 Year)			
Sense of trust: realization of hope. Getting; tolerating frustration in small doses; recognizing mother as distinct from others and self	Mistrust	Primary caregiver	Consistency and quality in the care received
Toddler (Anal) (1 to 3 Years)			
Sense of autonomy: realization of will. Child will try out new powers of speech; beginning acceptance of reality vs. pleasure principle	Shame and doubt	Parent(s)	Opportunity to attain some self-control based on a feeling of self-esteem rather than fear
Preschool (Oedipal) (3 to 6 Years)			
Sense of initiative: realization of purpose. Questioning; exploring own body and environment; differentiation of sexes	Guilt	Basic family	Opportunity to do for self with a balance between imaginative exploration and set limits
School Age (Latent) (6 to 12 Years)			
Sense of industry: realization of competence. Learning to win recognition by producing things; exploring, collecting; learning to relate to own sex	Inferiority	Neighborhood; school; same-sex peers; adult, nonparent idols	Opportunity to achieve success and recognition by engaging in manageable tasks in the child's social world so he or she can learn responsibility, social and work skills, cooperation and fair play
Adolescence (Mature) (12 to ? Years)			
Sense of identity: realization of fidelity. Moving toward heterosexuality; selecting vocation; beginning separation from family; integrating personality (e.g., altruism)	Identity diffusion	Peer groups and out groups; models of leadership	Opportunity to establish who the child is and what her or his purpose in society is to be through both private and social experiences that build self-esteem, foster increased need for independence, and cushion periods of feeling of not belonging
Late Adolescence and Young Adult			
Sense of intimacy and solidarity: realization of love. Becoming capable of establishing a lasting relationship with a member of the opposite sex; learning to be creative and productive	Isolation	Partner in friendship, sex, competition, cooperation	Opportunity to experience close, shared relationships with individuals of own and opposite sex in which the child's identity is verified and accepted and he or she accepts the identity of others.
Adulthood			
Sense of generativity: realization of care. Learning effective skills in communicating with and managing children; developing active interest in the next generation	Self-absorption and stagnation	Spouse; children; friends and work associates	Opportunity for involvement in activities that arouse concern for and advocacy for the next generation
Late Adulthood			
Sense of integrity: realization of wisdom. Reconciling life accomplishments; learning to accept death; putting life in order; accepting retirement without quitting life	Despair	Spouse: children and grandchildren; friends	Opportunity to be acknowledged for life accomplishments by self, children, peers in a manner that looks at what was achieved rather than what was not so that end of life can be dealt with gracefully and peaceably

* The corresponding stage in Freud's theory of development is listed in parenthesis.
(Based on Erikson, 1963; Maier, 1969.)

the feelings of guilt they experience by not "being good."

Principled morality (12 years on), the last phase in Kohlberg's schema, is the period when individuals accept rules on the basis of their own judgments of what is universally ethical and on the basis of their personal conscience. Their moral conduct is prompted by (1) a sense of obligation to social contract and democratic law and (2) a desire to avoid loss of respect among peers and in the wider community.

Temperament

Temperament is yet another facet of emotional-social development that needs to be discussed. A behavioral style that makes unique one's approach to people and situations, temperament is bound in those genetic or constitutional traits that cause individuality. The characteristics of one's temperament are evidenced from birth and are predictive of one's adult personality. Although the traits that make up one's temperament may become less prominent over time, the chances of actually averting them is slim, and the fact that they continue to exist will be evident as they reappear during new or stressful situations. (Thomas et al, 1968). Whether the behaviors typical of a given temperamental characteristic will present in acceptable or aberrant ways depends largely on how the significant others in one's life respond to those characteristics. Additionally, any situation* or demand that strongly conflicts with one's temperament produces severe stress, during which time signs and symptoms of behavior problems may arise.

Although temperament has been found to have a genetic origin,† it has been shown that one's environment can heighten, diminish, or otherwise modify temperamental characteristics but not abolish them. In fact, some research even suggests that these apparent changes are in actuality only fronts enacted to gain social acceptance (Thomas et al, 1968). This tendency of temperament to remain basically unchanged despite environmental pressures is called *persistence in personality and self-concept.* If any modifications are possible in these genetically transmitted traits and the associated self-concept, they are more likely to occur in early childhood than at any other time in one's life—thus the importance of an environment that fosters these traits as assets and that positively reinforces self-concept from the beginning of life.

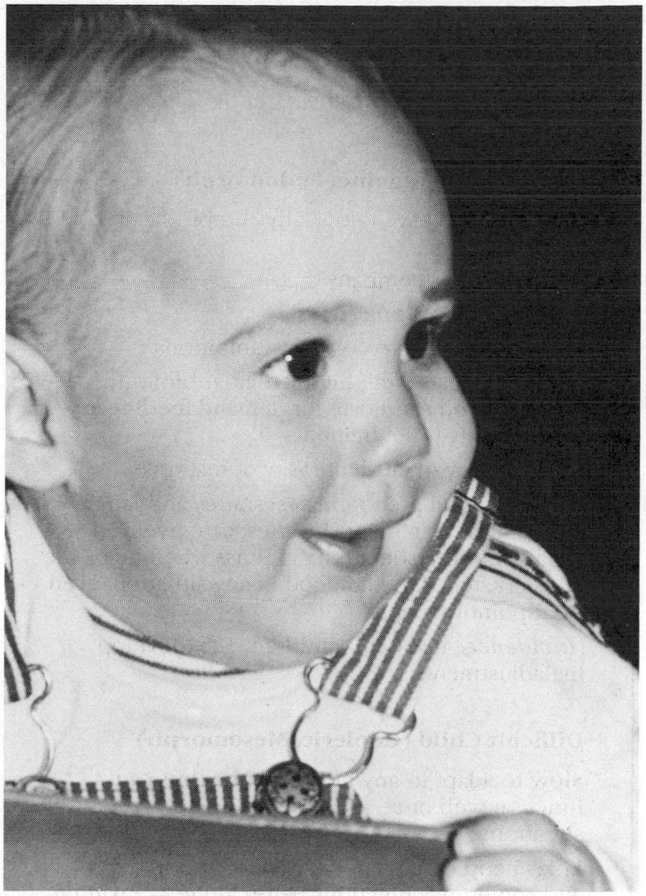

The characteristics of temperament are evidenced from birth and are predictive of the child's adult personality.

Extensive research conducted by Thomas and coworkers (1968) indicated nine clearly recognizable characteristics, or traits, of temperament. They are categorized according to reactivity.

1. Motor activity—the intensity and frequency of activity or motility
2. Rhythmicity—regularity of repetitive biological functions such as sleep and wakefulness, eating patterns, bowel and bladder patterns
3. Approach to the new—withdrawal from or acceptance of it—the child's initial reaction to a new stimulus
4. Adaptability—the ease or difficulty with which initial responses to new stimuli can be modified
5. Intensity of response—degree or amount of energy invested in reactions to stimuli
6. Threshold of responsiveness—level of external stimulation necessary to evoke an overt response
7. Quality of mood—general cheerfulness or unhappiness, amount of pleasant and friendly behavior as

* Such situations might include inconsistent care, inappropriate performance expectations, a series of traumatic events, imitations of aberrant behavior in other member(s) at home.

† Similar research studies carried out in Norway by Ann Torgurson and in America by Thomas and others resulted in remarkably similar findings. The same distribution of temperament types was found, despite marked differences in culture, parenting style, socioeconomic status and racial factors.

Box 3-2
Incidence and Characteristics of the Three Personality Types

Easy Child (Sanguine, Endomorph)

Well adjusted psychologically and physically; adapts rapidly

Friendly, likes company

Seeks people during stress

May need urging to complete ambitions

Sleeps and eats well; highly regular biologic rhythm, good candidate for demand feeding as infant; easily toilet trained

Displays low to mild intensity of response

Positive mood predominates; smiles and laughs much more than he or she cries; caregiver can usually be sure something is amiss when he or she does cry; tends to find good in any situation, even disappointing ones.

Incidence: 40% of all children; 18% develop maladjustments

Difficult Child (Choleric, Mesomorph)

Slow to adapt to any new situation, but can function well once she or he "learns the rules" of situation

Likes people but is not dependent upon them and sometimes functions better alone—a natural leader

Seeks activity during stress; needs acceptable outlets for her or his vigor and aggressive motor drive; competitive

Seems to be constantly moving and highly destructive; intense in reactions; needs unbreakable, well-constructed toys and clothing

Displays mostly negative withdrawal responses to new situations; frustration expressed in tantrums or destruction; pleasure expressed loudly and boisterously, but these outbursts do not necessarily reflect the value of the situation to child—his or her responses simply have an "all or nothing" quality

Has irregular biologic functioning; sleeps poorly and lightly and requires less sleep; erratic in appetite and frequency of hunger; not a good candidate for demand feeding as an infant and much patience and time is required for toilet training, with more frequent accidents

Negative mood predominates; seems to fuss or cry constantly; finds reasons to be unhappy; tends to be an "I can't" person; seldom a good scholar

Incidence: 10% of all children;* 70% develop maladjustments

Slow-to-Warm-up Child (Phlegmatic, Ectomorph)

Slow adaptive capacity; usually quietly withdraws but is watchful and contemplative all the while

Primarily a loner; usually prefers only one or two close friends; socially shy

Seeks to be alone during stress; avid reader

Often matures late; oversensitive and immature compared with most peers

Poor relaxer; frequently experiences disturbed sleep and eating patterns

Displays low intensity of reaction

Fairly high frequency of negative mood, although it sometimes is not immediately noticeable because of low intensity with which it is expressed

Incidence: 15% of all children; 40% develop maladjustments

---

*Research by Someroff and Zax at the University of Rochester showed that women who were highly anxious or who had a psychological disorder during the prenatal period have a higher incidence of difficult children.

(Compiled from Thomas et al, 1968; Gesell, 1974; Segal and Yahroes, 1978.)

opposed to unpleasant and unfriendly behavior

8. Distractibility—effectiveness of extraneous environmental stimuli in altering the direction of ongoing behavior

9. Attention span and persistence—length of time an activity is pursued, whether self-initiated or planned or structured, and the amount of frustration tolerated in activity despite obstacles (Thomas et al, 1968).

These traits tend to combine to form three clearly different personality structures.* Box 3-2 describes the incidence and traits of these three personalities.

The nurse who is able to recognize these three personality structures or temperaments is able to make a more reasoned judgment about the child's behavior and about the approach to him that will be most effective. Knowledge of temperament is especially helpful

---

*Approximately one third of the population does not fit neatly into these three categories but are instead blends not clearly separable.

to parents. Knowing that some aspects of their child's behavior are due to his or her nature helps to relieve many parents of guilt feelings and of undue pressure caused by their belief that their parenting methods are creating the behavior. Understanding the parenting methods most effective with the various personality types can aid parents in adopting the method most appropriate for each of their children. (See Chapter 13 for further discussion of temperament and parenting style.)

A child's feelings may appear irrational at times; nonetheless they are very real. The most loving thing adults can do is to let a child experience the full range of all these feelings—sadness as well as happiness. This deepens children's sense of self and helps them to discover that feelings change. Acknowledging and respecting the feelings children are experiencing allows them to do the same. This acknowledgment and respect also comforts children because they then know they are not alone in this experience. In the long run this freedom to express feelings allows children to use their own inner resources to manage the challenge at hand; they feel less burdened by the feelings themselves and can focus more of their energy on dealing with the problem.

Because children's feelings are an expression of who they are, they are an important description of their emotional-social health status. Nurses and parents who are attuned to the children's feelings are given insight into where they are developmentally, which tasks are presently confronting them, and in which areas they need support. The feelings and behaviors that children use to express themselves are their cues to their significant others of where they are headed next. With knowledge of human development, the nurse who heeds those cues can recognize signs of the child's readiness for new experiences that the nurse or the parents can help to provide. The nurse's awareness of the child's cues, along with the understanding of every child's need for satisfying achievements and relationships, and the recognition of the importance of maintaining and protecting the child's relationships with the family, will bring the nurse a long way toward the construction of a holistic plan of care, effectively delivered.

Defining Growth, Development, and Maturation

Growth and development are not synonymous terms, but in the healthy child these two processes do parallel each other and are interdependent in function. The ways the whole child changes over time are both *quantitative* and *qualitative* in nature.

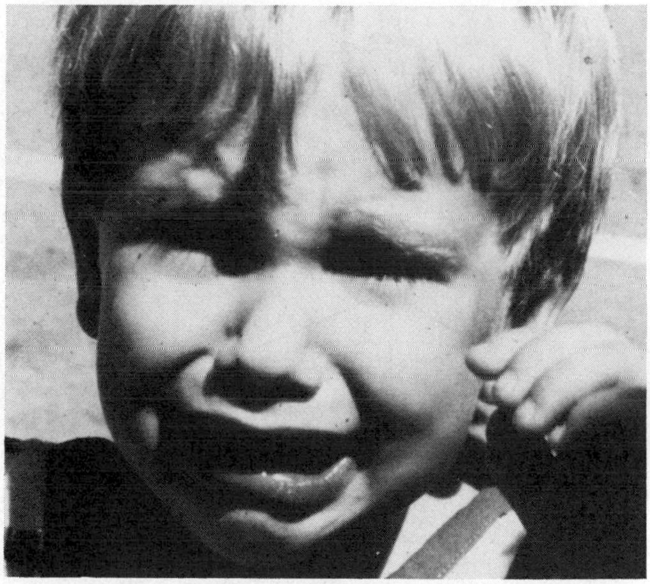

Children need to experience the full range of emotions—the sad as well as the happy.

Growth comprises *quantitative* change, involving an increase in size of the whole child or in size and number of any body parts. The change is measurable—usually either in centimeters or inches (height), kilograms or pounds (increased organ mass, weight), or by an increase in numbers present (increased vocabulary, increased number of relationships with others, increased number of physical skills able to perform)—and is easily observed or studied.

Qualitative changes are the "leaps" (increased skill or capacity) in function that result from mastering a series of smaller steps.* The qualitative component, called *development,* is more complex and less easily measured or studied.

The timing of these quantitative and qualitative changes is to some extent controlled by a maturational process that involves the child's biologic (genetic) ability and environmental opportunity to relinquish previous functions and learning or to integrate new functions and learning into his or her existing structure for more mature performance, or to perform both these actions. For example, the child relinquishes the palmar grasp in favor of the more manipulative pincer grasp that will allow better investigation of the environment, but not until he or she has developed the biologic structures—increased muscle cells and nerve cell specialization—necessary to perform this action.

* Piaget's steps of progressive intelligence, Erikson's stages of progressive sociability, Kohlberg's steps to adult morality, Freud's steps of sexuality formation illustrate qualitative change.

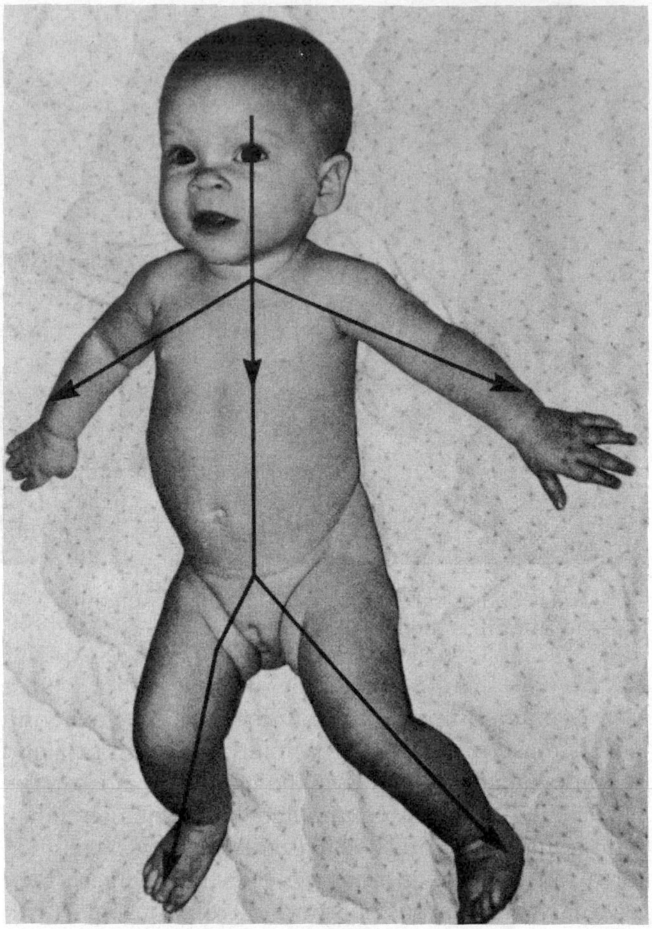

Figure 3-6. The development of muscular control proceeds from head to tail (cephalocaudal), and from the center of the body to its periphery.

Principles Evident in Growth and Development

Primary to a discussion of the principles or commonalities in human development is the concept of the child as an open system who receives from and gives to the environment and who has adaptive potential (ability for both qualitative and quantitative changes) within the limits of his or her inheritance. A second relevant concept is that an interactive heredity and environment shape that open system into a unique human being. Another important concept is that self-realization or self-actualization (i.e., achieving one's potential) is the ultimate goal of human development.

Derived from these concepts are some commonalities of development, typically referred to as *principles of growth and development.*

Development Is *Complex*

Human development is a continuous, irreversible, and complex process that is lifelong. Inherent in this developmental process is aging, which, interestingly enough, is most rapid during the fetal stage, and is also lifelong.

Development Has *Direction*

Human development is progressive and orderly (i.e., follows a sequence). It proceeds:

1. From simple to complex.

This is exemplified in the child's ability to make basic "cooing" sounds before learning to refine those sounds into speech.

2. From general to specific.

Illustrative of this principle is the infant's acquisition of palmar grasp before learning the finer control of pincer grasp.

3. From head to toe (cephalocaudally).

An example is the fact that an infant gains neck and head control before being able to control the movements of trunk and limbs (Fig. 3-6).

4. From inner to outer (proximodistally).

This principle is similar to the cephalocaudal principle in that the child learns control of the near structures before the structures farther away from the body center. The ability to coordinate the arms to reach for an object occurs before learning the hand and finger coordination necessary to grasp it (Fig. 3-6).

Development Is Predictable

The orderly sequence of development is invariable and although the precise age for the sequential steps to occur varies for each child, there is a general chronology that involves wide norm ranges to allow for these individual differences. For example, the age range for learning to walk is usually given as 9 to 15 months, with the average age being 12 months. Walking can occur as late as 28 months and still be considered normal.

A child will usually follow a consistent pattern with respect to either an early or late rate of development. Therefore, *deviation from the child's own pattern may be more indicative of a problem than lack of conformance to the norm.*

However, the characteristics of growth and behavior at each age, and the maturational changes that occur with increasing age, bear obvious resemblances among children. The child cannot walk until creeping is mastered, regardless of whether the pattern for achieving these characteristic behaviors or changes is early or late.

Children Develop Uniquely

Each child has his or her own genetic potential for growth and development that cannot be exceeded but may be deterred or modified at any stage in the sequence. For example, although intellect is primarily set by genetic inheritance, a child's experiences during the critical periods will either stimulate or discourage intellectual achievement. If affected by poor nutrition, confined to the crib or playpen, and offered few interactions with the people in the environment, the child may not achieve intellectually, regardless of genetic potential. Conversely, offered opportunities to experience the world from a number of positions (crib, playpen, floor, shoulder, tabletop), sustained on a nutritionally balanced diet and provided with regular opportunities to interact (be spoken to, played with, cuddled) with the important people and objects in the environment, the child is on the way to achieving intellectual potential.

Knowledge of growth and development principles is as important to the nurse as knowledge of discrete norms for growth and development skills and behaviors and knowledge of theoretical assumptions that assist in the description, explanation, prediction, and control of behaviors. The nurse can use these principles as a kind of basic yardstick in assessment for possible alterations in growth and development. They are also invaluable in anticipatory guidance of parents (see Table 3-1). Parents should know that the norms for developmental attainments exist in a wide range, and any comparisons with other children should be in the context of these ranges.

Theoretical Perspectives on Development

Developmental research has led to several points of view or theoretical conceptualizations of how children reach adulthood (see Table 3-1). Each is an attempt to describe systematically the phenomenon of human growth and development. A collective view that incorporates all these perspectives probably gives the most holistic view of how children proceed to adulthood.

Development as Maturation: Critical Periods

This perspective holds that the development of human behavior and physiologic growth occurs in predictable patterns as the child ages, i.e., reaches a new level of maturity. The child's increasing age results in the behavioral and physiologic changes. Human variations in the maturational process are the result of genetic and temperament differences. Thus, development as maturation means that a child develops at an individual but predictable pace, according to an inherited biologic schedule for maturation. Within this maturational process are critical periods. A critical period is a specific timeframe during which certain environmental events or stimuli have their greatest impact on a child's development. The timeframe involved is either that point when maximum capacity for a particular aspect of development is first present or that point when the structures to be developed are undergoing their most rapid growth.

During these critical periods some form of minimal sensory stimulation is necessary for normal progression in development. If the stimuli are not introduced during this critical period, the task in question cannot be mastered, at least not without much difficulty (Evans and McCandless, 1978). After this critical period the child can be either totally unaffected by certain stimuli or resistant to them. For example, a fetus is not affected by maternally contracted rubella virus after the critical first 3 months of fetal development. Deficits of appropriate sensory stimulation during the critical periods are cumulative and can progressively interfere with future development of other

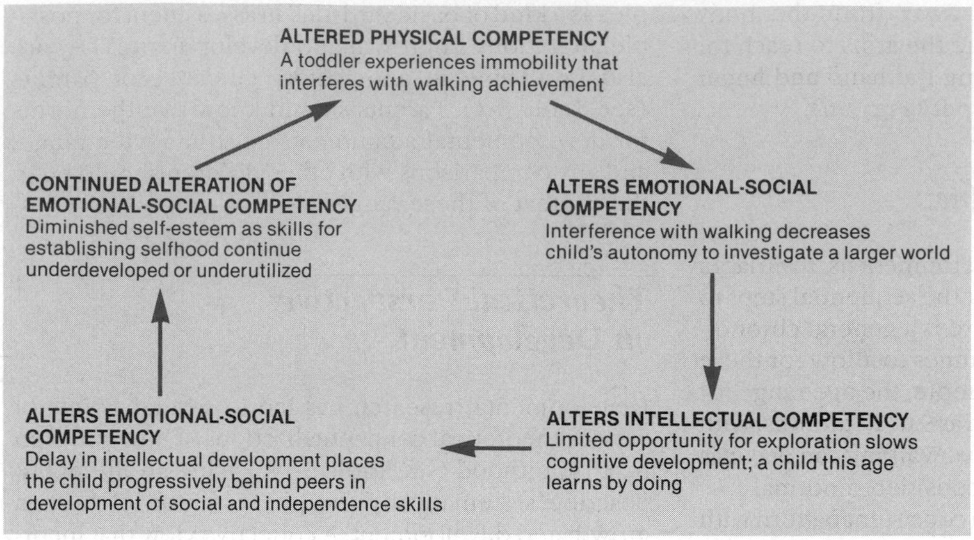

ALTERED PHYSICAL COMPETENCY
A toddler experiences immobility that interferes with walking achievement
ALTERS EMOTIONAL-SOCIAL COMPETENCY
Interference with walking decreases child's autonomy to investigate a larger world
ALTERS INTELLECTUAL COMPETENCY
Limited opportunity for exploration slows cognitive development; a child this age learns by doing
ALTERS EMOTIONAL-SOCIAL COMPETENCY
Delay in intellectual development places the child progressively behind peers in development of social and independence skills
CONTINUED ALTERATION OF EMOTIONAL-SOCIAL COMPETENCY
Diminished self-esteem as skills for establishing selfhood continue underdeveloped or underutilized

Figure 3-7. Alteration of one competency interferes with development of other competencies.

competencies besides the one competency involved during the critical period (Erikson, 1963). Figure 3-7 illustrates this relationship.

Conversely, sensory stimuli necessary to development of a particular skill or task that are exerted upon a child before the critical period will have negligible, if any, effect (Evans and McCandless, 1978). For example, infants cannot learn to read regardless of how often they are exposed to the media that would produce reading skills, whereas children at the right age and stage in their development have a "readiness" to read; that is, during their critical period they acquire reading skills fairly rapidly.

Related to this theoretical perspective, Gesell, Brazleton, and many others have formulated scales and tests to measure whether an individual child's maturity is on course and how far the child departs from the norm of the species. The pediatric nurse can use these to reassure parents that their child's growth and behavior are consistent with the predicted pattern for development. These scales and tests can also be used as guidelines for parents and health care providers on what nurturance to provide the child so that his or her biologic clock (critical periods) will receive appropriate stimuli to produce steadily progressive maturity.

Development as Learning: Reinforcements

Researchers holding this perspective attempt to understand development by studying the child's personal history and environmental and social interactions. This view perceives the child as being shaped by the environment while reacting to the events in that environment. The child will choose various ways of behaving, depending on the consequences (rewards or punishment). A given behavior or practice is repeated because some factor in the external environment prompts or reinforces that action, or does both. Pavlov, Watson, Skinner, and Bandura's writings reflect this theoretical position. This conceptualization is also the premise upon which behavior modification programs are based. The success of these programs lends credibility to this theoretical view. However, if one accepts this viewpoint to the exclusion of all others, when a child's development is difficult, the burden of guilt may be seen to rest with the child's caregivers since the child's development is often directly the result of the reinforcements provided by caregivers.

Development as Resolution of Conflict: Adapting to Challenges

This theoretical construct incorporates and expands upon the maturational theory described earlier. This model sees the child as being continually torn between activity and passivity and between natural instincts (physiologic impulses) and social constraints as he or she moves from one maturational stage to another.

Social expectations for each developmental or maturation stage exist; these are called developmental tasks. The task of each stage is to overcome the problem or challenge that confronts a child because of his or her age. Delay or failure in task achievement makes further development more difficult. Examples of developmental tasks follow: (1) Erikson defines the infant's emotional-social task as resolving inner and environmental conflicts so as to develop more trust than mistrust; (2) Piaget defines the school-age child's intellectual task as learning to use symbols and the concepts they represent; (3) a physical task of the toddler is learning to walk without aid.

Each stage in the developmental sequence has intervals of equilibrium, or balance, and disequilibrium. For example, at age 2 years life runs smoothly. These toddlers have a calm willingness to do what they can but do not try too hard to do things they cannot manage; but at 2 ½ their lives pose marked disequilibrium. They become rigid and inflexible, demanding rituals and routines that must not be altered. They shuttle endlessly between any two extremes of a situation.

Conflict arises out of children's motivation to master their environment and their lack of competency needed for that mastery. Equilibrium exists before the new environmental or maturational stimulus occurs that demands adaptation by the child, and after the child has developed the necessary competence to adapt to the stimulus. Disequilibrium exists in the interval from recognition of and desire to master (adapt to) the new stimulus until mastery is accomplished. Growing children repeatedly evidence their strength and competence to adapt and achieve if their environment gives them at least some support.

Development as Cognitive Change: Practice and Energy Investment

This theoretical viewpoint, described most fully in the research by Piaget and Kohlberg, presents development as a series of maturational changes in the comprehension of self, the world, and how one deals with this knowledge. Through a process of assimilation and accommodation children adapt to the changes in themselves and in the world, both inanimate and social, around them.

Developmental energy flow is invested most heavily in certain competency areas at any given time, depending on the child's current level of comprehension, so that different aspects of development progress at different rates. Earlier achievements in one competency area may even regress temporarily while some other aspect of that competency area or another competency area is being stimulated, because a strong preoccupation exists to practice and perfect the skill required for mastery of the newly confronted stimulus. For example, during infancy the central focus of energy is on sensorimotor and physical growth. The toddler's energy concentration is invested in his or her developing selfhood and body control, while the preschooler's investment is in language development. Intellectual development and sociability require the bulk of the school-age child's energy, and the teenager exerts massive energy into development of sexual and social identity and capacity for intimacy.

Development as Cultural Adaptation

Research into the cultural variations in development is relatively recent. Only in the past 30 years have ethnic variations and social class variations been considered in accounting for the nonuniform and unusual. Although there is now increased sensitivity to the child's assimilation of his or her culture, the research is incomplete on the actual impact on development. What is clear is that mastery of developmental tasks occurs within the context of the cultural and ethnic group characteristics of the child's primary care provider(s). This influence is second only to gender socialization in shaping the child's developing attitudes and behaviors (Levine et al, 1983). This understanding is useful to the pediatric nurse when evaluating a child's development. It is important to remember that cultural variations only indicate *differences* in development, not *deficiencies.*

In summary, human development, although complex, is continuous, follows an orderly sequence and general chronologic pattern that may vary slightly among different cultures, involves task mastery, and requires concentrations of energy upon the task confronting the child at that particular time. However, task achievement in one competency area is not accomplished in isolation but interacts upon skills in other competency areas simultaneously to result in characteristic ways of behaving.

Factors Influencing Child Development

Anyone who has in some way been involved with the study of children has had exposure to the nature versus nurture (heredity versus environment) controversy that has been a key developmental issue of the 19th and 20th centuries. No one really knows the total effect of each of these forces upon developmental process. One thing studies have revealed is that these forces are *interactive* with the individual organism to influence development.

It is generally accepted that nature sets the limits on potential development, while nurturing forces present the realm of opportunities or possibilities for attaining that potential. Research has demonstrated that physical development is primarily influenced by natural forces and that long-term deprivation in nurturing is required to interfere with physical development. However, research to date also has shown that intellectual and emotional-social development, although controlled by nature with regard to ultimate capacity for development, is much more influenced by nurturing forces (i.e., environmental stimuli), allowing individuals either to maximize their genetic (natu-

> **Box 3-3**
> *Issues and Situations in Which Consideration of Temperament May Be Significant for the Clinician*
>
> Reassurance of parents that child's deviation from culturally desirable norm does not mean pathology in child or bad parenting. Especially true with difficult or slow-to-warm-up child
>
> Child-care advice specified in terms of child's temperament, such as approach to weaning, toilet-training, and the like
>
> Evaluation of severity of acute physical illness by estimating deviation of child's behavior from usual temperament. Also, temperament may affect reaction to illness
>
> Evaluation and management of specific symptoms such as colic, night-awakening, or "hyperactivity" as partially influenced by temperament
>
> Child's adaptation to beginning nursery school or day-care center as influenced by reactions to new situation and speed of adaptation
>
> Ease or difficulty of child's establishment of peer relations
>
> School functioning—optimal style of classwork and homework schedule in relation to degree of persistence and distractibility
>
> In behavior disorders, identification of influence of temperament and the specific pattern of "poorness of fit"
>
> Special influences of temperament in the physically handicapped and the mentally retarded
>
> *(From Levine et al, 1983.)*

ral) potential or to allow it to depreciate. These are examples of the usefulness of an interactional model of heredity and environment.

The interactional model, popular since the 1970s, has several implications for parenting, anticipatory guidance, and health assessment and intervention. One implication is that early development, while important, is not irreversible or irreparable. Development does not stop at age 5 or at adolescence, but continues through all ages till death. When there is goodness of fit (i.e., when properties of the environment and its expectations and demands are in accord with the individual's own capabilities, motivations, and temperament or behavior style), then consonance exists, which permits optimal development in a progressive, positive direction. In poorness of fit (i.e., when there is a discrepancy between the individual and the environment), dissonance is produced. The excessive stress created by dissonance usually results in distorted and maladaptive functioning. Poorness or goodness of fit is rarely constant. At any age, for any individual, certain environmental demands are consonant with individual capabilities and coping mechanisms, while others are dissonant. What environmental demands create consonance or dissonance may shift at different ages (Levine et al, 1983).

A second implication of this model is the flexibility of development, which requires one to acknowledge that developmental sequence and standards for measurement of growth and development are not fixed. Rather, *there are many pathways to task mastery and to effective social functioning* (the goals of development), depending on the characteristics of the child and the nature of the environment. The sensitivity to ethnic variations in recent years has done much to further this concept.

A third implication of the interactional model is that the expression of one's temperament (the way one behaves) is influenced by environmental factors. (A discussion of temperament constellations is found on page 552.) What must be emphasized to health care providers and to parents is that the different temperamental constellations represent the wide range of behavioral styles exhibited by people and are all variations within normal limits. Box 3-3 lists some of the situations when temperament should be considered by the health clinician in planning intervention. It is also valuable for the practitioner and parents to keep in mind that most minor behavior problems are often related to dissonance between the child's temperament and the environment.

The premise of the interactional model for development is that there is a constant reciprocal interaction between the child's biologic make-up and the environment. The interaction produces stress, which is a developmental motivator, and, unless the demands are excessively stressful, the developmental effects are positive. Maturation is sequential and progressive, allowing for positive interactions with the environment that are increasingly complex.

Social Milieu and Physical Environment as Forces in Development

Culture and Lifestyle as Milieu

A child's developmental task mastery, though dependent on biologic potential and maturation, occurs "within the context of the cultural and ethnic group characteristics of the child's primary care providers" (Eiduson, 1983). Cultural input* is second only to gender socialization, which is itself culturally affected,

*Cultural input refers to ethnicity, demographic setting, socioeconomic class, parental occupation, and family structure.

in its impact on a child's development. That input may contribute either constructively or deleteriously to development. See Chapters 1 (section on intercultural communication) and 2 for a more detailed discussion of cultural and ethnic factors affecting individual and family development.

Family lifestyle is also a part of the milieu that shapes a child's development. During the late 1970s and early 1980s there was a growing recognition of the existence of family structures other than the two parent nuclear family. Hanson and Sporakowski (1986) listed the possible types of families as traditional (two parents, father working, mother at home); dual earner; step-parent; single parent; househusband; communal; and gay. An additional family type—the black extended family—was described by Wilson (1986).

Much of the attention on alternate family structures has been focused on single-parent families, also called one parent, lone parent, and solo parent families (Hanson and Sporakowski, 1986). By 1984 25.7 per cent of all family groups were headed by one parent, twice as many as had been single-parent families in 1978; during the same time period the number of two-parent families decreased by 13 per cent (Hanson and Sporakowski, 1986). The majority (88 per cent) of single-parent families were mother-child families, and more single-parent families were black than white (Hanson and Sporakowski, 1986; Norton and Glick, 1986). Of these mother-child families, 38.8 per cent were headed by divorced mothers, 24.4 per cent by never-married mothers, and 18.5 per cent by separated mothers (Hanson and Sporakowski, 1986).

Fathers maintaining single-parent families were better educated than mothers of mother-child families. This factor contributed to the greater economic well-being of father-child households than of mother-child households (60 per cent of mother-child families had incomes below the poverty level). Education seems to be an important variable in relation to both father- and mother-maintained single parent families. The fewer years of school completed by a parent, the more likely they are to be maintaining a single-parent family. Single parents are more likely to have a high school education, while married parents are more likely to be college graduates (Norton and Glick, 1986).

The primary cause of the increase in single-parent families is divorce (Norton and Glick, 1986). One estimate stated that 100,000 Canadian children and 1,000,000 United States children were in families undergoing marital breakdown (Shamsie, 1985). An increasing number of custody disputes in divorce actions involves preschool children (Fine, 1987; Wallerstein, 1985). The effects of divorce on children have been extensively studied. Much of this research indicates that divorce can have deleterious effects on children (Hetherington et al, 1979; Kalter et al, 1984). Zill (1984) found that children in divorcing families were more likely to develop emotional disorders than children in intact families. Hetherington and colleagues (1985) found that divorce had more negative, long-term effects on boys than it did on girls; however, girls whose parents were separated were more likely to engage in problem behaviors such as promiscuity, substance abuse, and running away than girls in intact families (Kalter et al, 1985). Santrock and Warshak (1979) believe that the sex of the custodial parent is related to outcomes in the child; children living with the same-sex parent seem to have fewer problems than those living with an opposite-sex parent.

It is possible that children's problems relating to divorce are inter-related with problems experienced by their parents. One study described single parents as significantly less satisfied and well-adjusted and as having more problems with their children than married parents (Fine et al, 1986). Dealing with the absent parent is seen by divorced parents as one of their greatest problems (Melli, 1986). Divorced parents who are able to resolve their differences do better than those who cannot. A study of 51 families showed that those who "did well" were individuals who showed respect for each other, were able to empathize with their children and with the other parent, had high self-esteem, were flexible, and were open to help (Steinman et al, 1985).

Nurses who work with families in which divorce has occurred can use their knowledge of factors that promote parental well-being to facilitate effective family coping. A counseling program focusing on social support and skills in childrearing and household maintenance for single parents can result in positive outcomes (Bloom et al, 1985). Similar counseling programs for children that focus on stressors they experience are also beneficial (Kaltar, 1984). Sometimes just the provision of information is helpful. Nelson (1986) described the use of a newsletter to provide information and support to single-parent families, and reported increased knowledge and positive behavioral outcomes in subscribers.

Descriptive information about single-parent families helps the nurse plan interventions that will correct problematic family coping and alteration in family processes. For example, since two out of three single mothers of children under age 18 work outside the home (Norton and Glick, 1986), the nurse will need to work with the mother to provide for reliable child care while she is at work. (See Chapter 7 for a discussion of child care.) Employed single mothers are also at risk for *ineffective individual coping.* Because of their multiple responsibilities in and out of the home, employed single mothers have less time for personal care, recreation, and household tasks than their married counterparts (Sanik and Mauldin, 1986). The nurse can assist the employed single mother in setting realistic priorities for use of her limited free time.

One descriptive study of single-parent families provided information that is highly useful to the nurse in planning wellness promotion and illness prevention strategies. Hanson (1986) found relationships between physical and mental health of single parents and positive parent-child communication and social support. Similar relationships were found between physical and mental health of children of single parents and parent-child communication, social support, and religiousness. Nursing interventions that focus on the development and improvement of these areas have a high probability of bringing about effective individual and family coping.

Less information is available about father-child single-parent families. It is known, as was previously stated, that single fathers are better educated and have higher incomes than single mothers. One study of the parenting of single fathers described them as perceiving themselves as competent parents who demonstrate concern for making their homes child-centered, report spending considerable time with their children, are concerned regarding the health care of their children, and feel emotionally close and affectionate toward their children (Risman, 1986).

A family type that frequently occurs as a result of divorce is the stepfamily, also called the remarried, blended, or reconstituted family (Reutter and Strang, 1986). Stepfamilies consist of two adults married to each other, at least one of whom has a child from a previous family. In 1985, more than 15 million children in the United States were living with remarried parents (Romanczuk, 1987). Some authorities believe that stepfamilies may eventually become the most common form of family life in contemporary society. Reutter and Strang (1986) listed the following differences between stepfamilies and nuclear families:

- In stepfamilies, at least one spouse and one child have suffered the ending of a relationship
- When a couple with children divorce, a "double single-parent stage" commences, in which children become members of two single-parent families. The parent-child bond that is formed may be resistant to the integration of a step-parent.
- Members of stepfamilies are characterized by dual family membership, lack of common history, instant multiple relationships, and lack of norms and societal support.

Problem areas for stepchildren and step-parents include loss through death or divorce, conflicts of loyalty, questions regarding belonging, and the need to adjust to two sets of rules in two separate households (Visher and Visher, 1982).

Given these factors it is not surprising that members of stepfamilies and the families as a group are at risk for ineffective or maladaptive coping. Reutter and Strang (1986) summarized the ways in which nurses can assist the family and its members to cope as follows:

> Nurses can acknowledge and help stepfamilies appreciate the complex issues involved in stepfamily development. We can empathize with them and help them to anticipate and deal with feelings related to loss. We can work to dispel myths and to foster positive social attitudes about them. Finally we can encourage stepfamilies to tolerate ambiguity as, over time, they work out mutually satisfying relationships.

Nurses who work with families in which remarriage will result in the creation of a stepfamily can provide anticipatory guidance to the members. The Stepfamily Association of America recommends professional counseling for couples in those families (Romanczuk, 1987).

The black extended family was described by Wilson (1986). The nuclear family expands by marriage. In the black extended family expansion occurs through childbirth to an adolescent mother and through absorption of a divorced member or other dependent adult or child. Elderly family members are continually involved in the family. This family pattern, which is being adopted by an increasing number of white families, provides advantages in that it makes resources available to one-parent families. Some researchers have also described negative attributes of such a family structure. Jarrett (1982) believes that parenting practices of adolescent mothers in these families are not always optimal. The nurse who works with children born to adolescent members of black extended families should include adult extended family members in interventions designed to improve the parenting practice of the adolescent.

In 1974 researchers at the University of California, Los Angeles, initiated a longitudinal study to investigate the effects of non-traditional family lifestyles on child development (Eiduson, 1978). Included in the nontraditional family lifestyles were single mothers, unmarried social contract groups, and people living in communal groups. No major differences have been found in physical or mental development of the children or in childrearing practices of the parents (Weisner and Eiduson, 1986). Growth rates are comparable, as are health practices generally. Diets are comparable, although mothers who breastfeed in alternative families generally do so slightly longer. There are no differences in use of vitamins, in immunizations, or in medical care sought. Neither group was more or less prone to illness. Intellectual development, including language, showed no significant differences. Children in alternative families showed earlier motor mastery during the first months of life, but the difference disappeared after the first year of life. Nor were there any differences in attachment or separation behaviors among the children.

This study indicated that children from alternative families seem to develop early an ability to adapt to change, perhaps because alternative families tend to seek solutions to stress and conflict through change (whether in location, job, mate, or time away from family unit) more than do traditional families. Despite these changes, nontraditional families' children were no less stable or withdrawn than children of traditional families. Children from single-parent and extended family units were slightly more cooperative and more independent at all ages and showed strong social sensitivity. They were more creative in problem solving and more apt to participate in group decision making, while their traditional family counterparts tended to show stronger motivation from academic achievement.

The UCLA studies reflect thus far that each family style offers trade-offs. No one type of lifestyle consistently is associated with a particular problem or dysfunction in the child's development. As with all elements of living, each family style has some very competent and some less committed parents as well.

Demographers estimate that today more than 50 per cent of all children under age 18 will spend part of their childhood in other than their two-parent original birth family. Assessment of family structure and composition should be a routine part of history taking in all settings.(See Chapter 2 for further discussion of alternate family lifestyles.)

Family Environment as Milieu

Family interaction, especially parenting (see Chapter 13 for a detailed discussion of parenting), is a source of influence on particular facets of child development. There is a definite reciprocal dependency between family development and the individual child's development (Lerner and Spanier, 1978). Other family relationships affect and are affected by the dyadic (parent-child) relationship. Likewise, the dyadic relationship changes over time, primarily as a function of the child's developmental changes. Most parents are not equally adept at parenting at all the different developmental stages, thus the quality of parenting is also likely to change as the child develops, fostering either positive or negative consequences in the child's developmental progress.

Birth order and family size are aspects of family interaction that also have demonstrated their effect on a child's development. The middle child's exposure to older siblings fosters earlier and easier learning, particularly of motor, social, and language skills. Only children usually have earlier intellectual development because of their constant exposure to adults but slower motor development because adults are doing things for them and they have no sibling to encourage their motor performance through active play. Youngest children are often slower in some areas of development (language, motor skills) because they have had less encouragement or opportunity to express themselves. Oldest children display more neurotic behavior, while later born children display more antisocial behavior and are greater risk takers, which makes them also more accident prone. Children spaced more than 5 years apart tend to develop as though they were all first borns.

School as Milieu

As children grow older their siblings, and later their peers, have an increasingly greater impact. The school milieu contributes to their development in the form of skill training, cultural transmission, and self-actualization. Again, the relationship between school progression and the child's development is reciprocal. As the child develops and matures, the curriculum and how it is offered also changes, presumably to reflect different developmental needs. Table 3-5 describes the five major transitions within the school milieu, which are intended to foster progressive intellectual and social development and problem areas likely to arise when there is a mismatch of developmental tasks at each transition. Whether or not each transition affects development positively depends upon the particular school system and its approach to facilitating the child's adaptation to each transition and upon the particular child. If the child's individual maturation is not consistent with the norm, a misfit may occur between the child's developmental readiness and the school-critical developmental tasks the transition requires of the student.

Likewise, if the child's temperament is one that adapts to changes slowly or with difficulty, each new transition is likely to pose some developmental conflict. Wesley and Wesley (1977), among others, have documented that boys generally lag behind girls about 12 months in neurologic development during the early school years, which helps explain why more boys experience reading failure in those early school years.

Although these mismatches between child and school expectations do occur, more often the problem is one in which parents' expectations of their child's school performance are unrealistic for that child, either developmentally or relative to that child's personality. Rutter's (1979, 1980) extensive studies of school outcomes for children reflected that those facets of the school milieu that most obviously influence school

Table 3-5. Developmental Transitions of the School Milieu

School-Critical Developmental Tasks	Potential Conflicts
School Entry (Age 3–5 Years*)	
Peer interaction–sharing, taking turns	Demands do not match motor or mental capabilities
Social development–basic self-care skills	No previous exposure to other children
Following directions	No previous experience with separation from parent(s)
Developing language skills	
Academic Reading Instruction (Age 5–7 Years)	
Learning fundamentals of reading	Neurologic or cognitive unreadiness; success interferences such as moving, family upsets, poor self-concept
Reading To Learn (2nd–3rd Grade)	
Content of reading becomes important	Poor mastery of reading fundamentals results in poor reading skills with resultant behavior or attendance problems Learning deficits associated with neurologic immaturity or experiential naivety
Start Middle School (Junior High)	
Subject-oriented emphasis Change to multiteacher and multiclass experience Often change in school building and administrative personnel.	Output failure is greatest potential problem due to: (1) difficulty for child in having a relationship with a single caring adult (2) risk of losing sight of child's specific or special needs (3) troublesome nature of organizational structure for child with more rigid personality
Start High School (9th or 10th Grade)	
Change building and administrative personnel Student selection of courses to coincide with career goals Student responsible for balancing academic and social obligations	Removes familiar supportive adults and records/information about child's specific/special needs Student may not have identified any career goals yet Diminished special education focus and of special education resources Vocational education now available but too late for failure prone child whose academic problems began at junior high level or earlier Serious mismatch of developmental rate and school expectations has greatest likelihood in this transition

* Earlier if handicapped.

problems are (1) increased expectations that do not fit with the child's developmental/emotional status, (2) changes in important personnel such as teachers or principal, (3) repeated incidences of intimidation by peers or a teacher, and (4) a coercive, unstable teacher.

Socioeconomic Status as Milieu

Poverty can be an obvious deterrent to healthy development. The Census Bureau has specified the poverty line so that family income should be sufficient to provide an adequate diet. The line is defined in relationship to the number of family members and is adjusted each year to the cost-of-living index. More than 16 per cent of white children in the United States live below the poverty line and nearly 40 per cent of Hispanic children and 50 per cent of black children (Moynihan, 1987). Poverty among Canadian children is half the United States rate. These poor families tend to be characterized by lack of education, high unemployment rates, larger families headed by women, residential crowding, and lack of adequate bathroom facilities. The poor are five times more likely than the nonpoor to perceive their health status as only fair or poor. Poverty and minority status are inversely related to life expectancy. Those residents in poverty areas show higher crude death rates for tuberculosis and homicide than residents in nonpoverty areas. Infant mortality rates among blacks remain significantly higher than the rates for whites despite an overall decrease in infant mortality rates in past years. (MMWR, 1987).

Learning disabilities, language delays, and mental retardation (50 to 80 per cent of all cases are from low income homes) are disproportionately present in the poverty level population (Levine et al, 1983). Behavior problems are much more common than in the general population, probably associated with the greater exposure to antisocial behaviors in adults. There is also a higher incidence of accidents, mostly related to structural deficiencies in the environment.

Significant national policy changes are necessary that go beyond the health care system and its professionals to reverse the deleterious effects of poverty on children's development. Some measures can be taken, however, to help offset these deficits, such as the availability of preventive health services in areas accessible to these families and the mobilization of community support groups to impact local and regional services.

As nurses plan to provide services to poor families, they should be aware of the special health problems that may be implied. They must know the relationship between lack of adequate income and the family's inability to provide itself with resources to maintain and restore health. When subsistence is a problem, health is not a primary family goal. When the family is struggling to pay the rent and provide food, clothing, and

Box 3-4
Home Call: Mother and Child

There's so little
here: one table, not
laden, one curtain, ripped,
one blind shut. One bulb
hung straight down. One woman,

not well (a cigarette,
and that look—someone who won't
talk, because they've been beaten
so the bruises
don't show), and one

boy, dancing over, no
diaper, eager for the coin
or cheap candy you lay in his
hand. How he aches

upward, a tendril attaching,
reaching out of the dark, leaning into
your yellow dress, unfurling his last

leaf for you. She watches
you, the one who has
everything—a house she imagines half
glass, where light
pours in, and everything
is already paid for, your
yellow dress, the shine of health
you wear with such casualness, the look
of wealth and the power to make the right

phonecalls, calls to people like you,
who, when you call,
will do what you say, pay
what you tell them, when and to

whom. You,
who have at least two
of everything, you lift her son
to your yellow breast, that well-lighted
place, where the air
is clean and there's meat
(lean) on the plate, the colors
are bright,

and you don't
hate yourself, waiting in line
to pay for a sack of
potatoes. Take me, her son
begs, take me with you.

She waits to see
what you will do. You who
have things, you who can
do things, you
who can do what you
choose to, you
who can do something for them,
if you choose to,
a little something

or nothing.

—Marilyn Krysl

Reprinted with permission of the author and the Center for Human Caring, University of Colorado Health Services Center, Denver, CO.

other basic necessities, the parents may not be able to keep the children's immunizations up to date, especially when this involves long waits, paternalistic and condescending attitudes displayed by health care providers, and transportation problems that a public clinic visit often entails. Since the majority of professional nurses are white, middle class women, differences between their values and those of the poor families they serve may result in labeling and blaming if the family's behavior is evaluated in light of the nurse's own value system. The poem in Box 3-4 provides a poignant view of such a clash in lifestyles. Commissioned by the Center for Human Caring at the University of Colorado Health Sciences Center to study and "capture" the phenomenon of "caring" in nursing, Marilyn Krysl described this poem as "the nurse's very complex and intelligent reactions to the complicated situation of her client" (Krysl and Watson, 1988).

Another facet of nursing care for poor families is advocacy. The nurse who assumes the advocate role represents the family's interest as it seeks to cope with the health and welfare systems. In this role the nurse perceives herself as primarily accountable to the family rather than to an institution or agency. Intervention by the nurse-advocate is often vital to the effective functioning of the poor family. Faced with a bewildering array of health and social welfare agencies, the family is often at a loss as to how to proceed. A nurse with the ability to coordinate the family's interaction with the health department, Big Brothers or Big Sisters, and the many offices of governmental social service departments such as Protective Services and Aid for Families with Dependent Children (AFDC) performs an invaluable service.

In a larger sense the nurse may act as advocate for poor families by participation in the political process. Individually and collectively, nurses may actively support legislation to ameliorate the social and economic stresses affecting poor families while concomitantly affirming the dignity of each family and maintaining family integrity. Political action is necessary at local, state, and federal levels by nurses who have knowledge of the legislative process and skill in the application of pressure to gain political ends.

Affluence, too, can adversely affect children's development. Often parent-child relationships are lacking as a result of long or frequent absences by the parents or general inattentiveness to their children's needs as they get caught up in social and business pressures. As a result substitute care takers often replace parents, further disrupting parent-child bonds. Parents may also fail to set sufficient standards or goals for their children beyond material success, resulting in extraordinary pressure on their children to measure up to a relatively narrow definition of success. These children also experience little opportunity to learn how to delay gratification of their wants, to do without, or to learn to make choices. Drug abuse and accidents, particularly from automobiles, is higher among affluent children because of the easier access (Burquest, 1981; Grinker, 1978; Wixen, 1979).

Neighborhood as Milieu

A child's neighborhood is the child's first and most impressionable exposure to the world outside the home. To foster healthy development, that environment should be protective, friendly, and familiar. The neighborhood ideally offers the child an opportunity to experience the world outside home as accepting, supportive of a child's physical and psychosocial needs, and reinforcing of the child's self-confidence and safety. The availability of such neighborhood experiences today, however, is rapidly diminishing. Zill (1982) found, when he surveyed children from communities of various sizes and socio-economic levels of affluence, that an overwhelming majority of children, regardless of the neighborhood they resided in, perceived that neighborhood as dangerous and unsupportive of children. Some of the fear is admittedly stimulated from media exposure to the vandalism, violence, and abuse occurring within the community rather than from directly experiencing these things. However, the effect is the same in that most children perceive the world outside home negatively, and this breeds fear; inhibits learning, socialization, and recreational activities; and disturbs children's development of trust and confidence.

Health professionals can exert civic and political influence in an effort to reduce and control crime in their neighborhoods and to encourage supportive informal neighborhood networks to ensure a safe environment for children. Safety precautions—being always in groups and not alone, accepting no rides, avoiding fights, and so on—should be taught on a community-wide scale.

Mass Media as Milieu

A powerful modern influence is television. The power of this medium is felt in both individual and family life. Despite the many studies that have been done to investigate the manner and extent of television's influence, we continue to have a very poor understanding of its effect. Such questions as what the relationship is between the sex and violence portrayed on television and violent crime in society, what effect child-oriented advertising has on the children's minds, and how involvement with visual imagery affects desire and ability to relate to the written word are among the many queries to which we have no answers.

The vast financial investment in this medium and the powerful interests involved in its control create tremendous pressure that may, unfortunately, contaminate the objectivity of some investigations. The tension between the Federal Communications Commission (FCC), a regulatory body of the federal government charged with guarding the public interest, and the huge monied corporations and advertising interests concerned with amassing wealth and control often leads to conflict. In addition, various public interest organizations have entered the arena, seeking to promote or safeguard certain ideas or groups. For instance, the American Academy of Pediatrics is currently asking for a ban on television advertising directly to children, and this is being strongly opposed by those industries that are dependent on advertising appeals to the young, such as cereal and toy manufacturers.

Action for Children's Television (ACT) and other groups are also pressuring the Federal Trade Commission to regulate television advertising aimed at children, beginning with control of ads for heavily sugared candy and cereal. In response, some manufacturers have produced research findings which they say prove that sugar is not harmful to the general health of children and does not predispose to dental caries. Some religious groups are attempting to apply moral censorship in the areas of sexuality, violence, and profanity. A basic dilemma revolves around the issue of safeguarding the public interest while maintaining First Amendment guarantees of free speech and free press.

Television is said to be the most pervasive force in United States society. It is the primary source for socializing children and their major source of information about the world. There is at least one television set in 98 per cent of homes, and many homes have several sets. By the time of high school graduation, the average child in the United States will have spent more time in front of the television set (15,000 hours) than in school (11,000 hours) (Rothenberg, 1985). A child from a home where television is not available will often watch at the home of a friend. Television is described as the dominant diversional activity of hospitalized children (Bordeaux, 1986). The financial importance of children's television is demonstrated by the fact that advertisers spend $600 million a year on children's shows. Broadcasters realize 25 per cent of their overall profits from the 7 per cent of their programming aimed specifically at children (Kittrell, 1978).

The effect of television watching on family life is of concern. Many parents and children argue over what to watch, and there is speculation that mass communication may be replacing interpersonal communication. Rosenblatt and Cunningham (1976) see television contributing to troubled family relationships in two ways. The operation of a television set creates frustrations rising from the noise and distraction it produces as well as the tension caused by differing preferences for programs or sound volume. It may be difficult to carry on other activities in proximity to the television set, such as reading, conversing, telephoning, or sleeping. If living quarters are cramped, this problem is intensified, since alternative space for other activities may not be available. The second problem that television creates for the family lies in its use as a coping mechanism that allows escape from family problems. The family may use television watching to avoid tension-laden interactions and to provide an outlet for anger and aggression.

Rosenblatt and Cunningham (1976) found a strong positive correlation between the amount of time television sets were on in the home and scores on a scale measuring family tension. Families with few members in relation to amount of available space tended to operate the set less than families with relatively high population density. We wish to note that this is consistent with the hypothesis that, despite the frustration that may stem from television set operation, watching television is used to head off tense interaction. Rosenblatt and Cunningham conclude that in families with a great deal of space in the dwelling enabling them to get away from each other, television set operation is frustrating, but in families with little space, operation of the set is an acceptable avoidance mechanism to escape unpleasant interaction.

There is an average of six times more violence during 1 hour of children's television than there is in 1 hour of adult television. By high school graduation, the average child will have witnessed approximately 18,000 murders, most of them bloodless and painless (Fosarelli, 1986) and numerous episodes of violence such as beating, robbery, and arson (Rothenberg, 1985). The "catharsis hypothesis," a well-known psychologic theory on aggression reduction, suggests that people can make unconscious impulses less harmful by bringing them to the surface. According to this theory, children will become less likely to act out aggressive impulses if they view violence and aggression on television. In reviewing the literature in this area, Heaps (1977) found only one study that supports this hypothesis. By contrast, the majority of studies on the subject have shown that aggressive tendencies are stimulated rather than reduced by viewing television violence (Rubenstein, 1983). In fact, it has been found that children actually learn aggressive behavior from "film-mediated models" (Heaps, 1977). Rothenberg (1985) reviewed research literature and concluded that: "(a) children are likely to learn and remember new forms of aggressive behavior by watching the kind of violence presented in the mass media; (b) repetition of violence in the mass media results in a decreased emotional sensitivity to media violence and an increased probability for decreased emotional sensitivity to actual aggressive behavior in real-life situations; (c) watching the kind of aggression shown in the media does not result in aggression catharsis . . . but in the opposite; and (d) aggression can be inhibited by the reminder that the aggression was morally wrong in terms of the viewer's own ethical principles and by an awareness of the bloody, painful aftermath of aggression." (p. 148). Two processes are involved in the child's response to the observation of television violence (Heaps, 1977). The first relates to the child's learning of new aggressive modes of behavior that were previously not part of the child's repertoire. The child becomes an imitator of novel types of violence that are observed on the screen. The second process involves the release of inhibitions revolving around violent and aggressive patterns of behavior already in the child's repertoire. In other words, the child not only may learn new patterns of aggressive behavior but also is stimulated to act out those patterns that are already known.

Another consideration raised by viewing many of the cartoons that children watch is the unrealistic protrayal of the physical and moral consequences of violence and aggression. Cartoon characters are virtually indestructible. Humans and animals are beaten, shot, bombed, knifed, thrown from windows, pushed over cliffs, smashed with jackhammers, squashed by falling boulders, and subjected to any number of other traumas, and yet—after a brief period of looking frazzled and a bit foolish—they are always completely restored to their former condition. The character perpetrating this mayhem is often the hero of the episode. What does this teach the child about the result of violent behavior? It certainly does not show that it is harmful in an immediate or long-range sense. Nor does it teach the child that there is anything morally wrong with the infliction of pain and harm on others. The child is stimulated to perform actions without accurate information as to the results.

Kittrell (1978) compares television watching to drug taking. Both of these activities tend to withdraw

Box 3-5
Effects of Heavy Television Watching

Increased aggressive behavior and acceptance of violence

Difficulty in distinguishing between fantasy and reality

Distorted perceptions of reality in relation to importance of consumption of products and services; extent of violence and role of minorities

Trivialization of sex and sexuality

Increased passivity and disengagement

Negative effects on cognitive learning

Potential to inform, teach, and promote "prosocial" behavior not fully realized

(From Levine et al, 1983.)

the child from the environment and to obliterate the real world, and both may be used as a means of escape. Both are basically passive states that require little thought or preparation. The desired effect is achieved with no exertion or commitment. Television, like a drug, can act as a stimulant or a sedative, depending on the child and the program watched. A parent may prescribe a dose of television to relax a child. Most parents are aware of the various effects of television on their children but do not know how to deal with them. Kittrell (1978) views this "narcotic" effect of television on children, not violence or advertising, as the fundamental issue. He contends that television violence and advertising can be handled through laws and regulations, but "dealing with the effects of television, on the other hand, will require creative, individual responses from parents and children."

Rothenberg (1985) also expresses concern about the promotion of materialistic values and "consumerism" in children as a result of television commercials. His research review revealed that children under age 8 cannot distinguish between program content and commercial content. This could lead them to believe that television character role models are endorsing products advertised in commercials. Rothenberg also points out documented cases of injuries to children trying to imitate stunts performed on television.

Kittrell (1978) and Rothenberg (1985) raise several questions regarding the effects of television viewing on children. What role does television play in the development of role models and value systems? Does the enforced passivity brought about by television decrease the child's opportunities to observe and imitate the behavior of meaningful adults in order to learn appropriate patterns of social and emotional interaction? Does television viewing result in a decrease in the normal physical activity that is one of the hallmarks of childhood? Does television produce a passive attitude to life, blunt the imagination, or inhibit the child's ability to engage in creative play? Do "flashy" educational programs such as "Sesame Street" or "3-2-1 Contact" cause lack of interest in the more mundane, regimented, and difficult world of classroom learning? Does television, by occupying the child's leisure time, discourage personal emotional discoveries that the child could be making? These are questions to which we have no answers at present, but certainly parents should be made aware of these issues as they make decisions about television for their children. The facts do exist that while a child is watching television he or she is not playing, sleeping, conversing, reading, or participating in outdoor or social recreational activities, and that whatever the child may be learning is happening vicariously (and not necessarily with information reflective of the real world) rather than through direct experience. Box 3-5 lists some effects of heavy television watching that have been derived from studies conducted by the National Institute of Mental Health (1982) and from studies by Comstock and coworkers (1978, 1980) and Rubenstein (1978).

O'Bryant and Corder-Bolz (1978) report research findings that indicate that the most effective control of television's influence on children can be exerted from the home rather than from outside organizations. A research project revealed that only about one third of parents studied tried to control the amount of television their children watched. The study showed that children are most likely to adopt the television habits of their parents. Adolescents were the only group who did not display this behavior, probably as part of the rebellion against parents characterizing this developmental stage.

Parents were found to use television as reward and punishment. This practice was viewed as detrimental in several ways. A general rule of discipline is that reward and punishment should be specifically related to the behavior to which the parent is responding. Granting television viewing privileges as a reward may become a crutch to parents too lazy or unimaginative to think of other means of showing approval. Denial of viewing privileges as punishment may mean that the child misses a documentary or a show that has been assigned in school. A major consideration is that use of television viewing as reward and punishment places too much emphasis and value on television viewing.

O'Bryant and Corder-Bolz (1978) suggest that parents interrupt during television programs and interpret what is seen by children to help them understand and organize their visual perceptions, as well as to separate the real and the unreal. By becoming an active participant the parent can influence what the child learns and retains, and the attitudes that he develops.

Indirect mediation is recommended as a technique that parents can use to intervene in the television watching of teenagers. This is accomplished by a parent making a comment to the spouse or another family member in the teenager's hearing. The comment should express approval or disapproval of things seen on television in relation to family values. This gives the teenager the opportunity to compare what is watched with values the parent hopes to impart. The parent's silence when television presents material that conflicts with family values and attitudes is misleading to the adolescent, who is likely to interpret this silence as consent or agreement. Parents should view television purposefully, selecting and planning what is to be watched; critically evaluate what is seen and verbally express their criticism; and use television to lead to the discussion of topics that might otherwise be postponed or neglected, such as drugs, rape, teenage pregnancy and other controversial or sensitive issues.

What are the nursing implications related to the effects of television on the child? If comprehensive family care is a nursing goal, the nurse must critically evaluate the often contradictory findings of research in the area and present accurate information to families. Here are a few recommendations that may help guide the nurse during counseling:

1. Parents should be in control of the use of television. They have the responsibility to guide their children in wise choices.
2. Parents need to spend time with their children, both when they are watching television and when engaged in other activities.
3. Television watching must not be allowed to occupy completely the time individuals and families need for exercise, reading, talking together, and pursuing other activities.
4. Television should not be used as reward or punishment.
5. Television should not be used as a babysitter.
6. Parents should be able to inculcate their own values and attitudes; if television interferes with this process, they must re-evaluate its use.
7. As they develop children should be learning progressively to appreciate the difference between reality and unreality. Parents must be careful that use of television does not impede this process.

Nurses can ask about the type and amount of television watching as a part of the history-taking phase of child assessment. An obvious way that nurses can become familiar enough with children's programming to make evaluative judgments about it is to watch the programs children watch (Fosarelli, 1986). This is especially important in families with communication problems or in those in which children have behavioral problems. Parents can be asked if any problematic behaviors, such as fears or heightened aggression, customarily follow their child's television viewing (Fosarelli, 1986). Nurses can teach parents to use television selectively and creatively.

Physical Environment as Milieu

Research is increasingly supporting the idea that the physical environment has a very significant effect on one's overall development. In the fetal stage of development certain intrauterine conditions may jeopardize development. A few obvious examples are nutritional deficits; malposition; maternal metabolic or endocrine imbalances; the impact of teratogenic agents such as maternal exposure to radiation, smoking, or drug use during pregnancy; and Rh incompatibility.

Climate and season also affect development. Climatic influences are secondarily related to sanitary problems posed by warm or temperate climates. Growth spurts are seasonally correlated; for example, height gains correlate positively with the coming of spring.

One's state of general health also has an impact upon developmental progression. Illness or injury with associated disability, nutritional impairment, immobility, and energy diversion for recovery rather than learning all hamper progress in some facets of development.

In summary, there is substantial evidence to support the interactional theory that both biologic environment and social milieu and physical environment affect any individual child's developmental progress. The implication for assessing and impacting that environment by health professionals is of obvious importance to promoting and maintaining the healthy development of human beings at all ages.

References

Bandura A: The role of modeling processes in personality development. *In* Hartup WW, Smothergill NL (eds): *The Young Child Review of Research, 42–58.* Washington, DC; National Association for the Education of Young Children, 1967.

Bandura A: *A Social Learning Theory.* Englewood Cliffs, NJ, Prentice-Hall, 1977.

Bandura A, Walters R: *Social Learning and Personality Development.* New York, Holt, Rinehart and Winston, 1963.

Bloom BL, Hodges WF, Kern MB, McFaddin SC: A preventive intervention program for the newly separated—Final evaluation. *Am J Orthopsychiatr* 1985; 55:9–26.

Bordeaux BR: Television viewing patterns of hospitalized school-aged children and adolescents. *Child Health Care* 1986; 15:70–75.

Burquest B: The search for structure. *American Society for Adolescent Psychiatry:* A Paper, 1981.

Comstock G: *Television in America.* Beverly Hills, CA, Sage Publications, 1980.

Comstock G, et al: *Television and Human Behavior.* New York, Columbia University Press, 1978.

Cox RD, Cox MJ: Children in contemporary American families: divorce and remarriage. *In* Walraich M, Routh D (eds): *Advances in Developmental and Behavioral Pediatrics.* Greenwich, CT, Jai Press, 1984, pp 1–31.

Eiduson B: Culture and ethnicity. *In* Levine M, et al: *Developmental-Behavioral Pediatrics.* Philadelphia, WB Saunders, 1983.

Eiduson B: Emerging families of the 1970's: values, practices, and impact on children. *In* Reiss D, Hoffman H (eds): *The Family: Dying or Developing.* New York, Plenum Press, 1978.

Erikson EH: *Childhood and Society.* 2nd ed. New York, Norton, 1963.

Erikson EH: *The Challenge of Youth.* New York, Doubleday Anchor, 1965.

Erikson EH: *Identity, Youth and Crisis.* New York, Norton, 1968.

Fine MA, Donnelly BW, Voydanoff P: Adjustment and satisfaction of parents *J Fam Issues* 1986; 7:391–404.

Fine S: Children in divorce, custody and access situations: an update. *J Child Psychol Psychiatr* 1987; 3:361–364.

Fosarelli P: In my opinion . . . advocacy for children's appropriate viewing of television: What can we do? *Child Health Care* 1986; 15:79–81.

Freud S: Beyond the pleasure principle. *In* Strachey J (ed): *The Standard Edition of the Complete Psychological Works of Sigmund Freud.* Vol 18. London, Hogarth, 1957.

Freud S: Some psychological consequences of the anatomical distinction between the sexes. *In* Collected Papers. Vol. 5, London, Hogarth, 1950.

Gesell A, Ilg F, Bates Ames L: *Infant and Child in the Culture of Today.* New York, Harper & Row, 1974.

Gordon M: *Manual of Nursing Diagnosis.* New York, McGraw-Hill, 1987.

Grinker R Jr: The poor rich: the children of the super rich. *Am J Psychiatr* 1978; 135:913.

Halford GS, Brown CA, Thompson RMcL: Children's concept of volume and flotation. *Dev Psychol* 1986; 22:218–222.

Hanson SMH: Healthy single parent families. *Fam Relations* 1986; 35:125–132.

Hanson SMH, Sporakowski MJ: Single parent families. *Fam Relations* 1986; 35:3–8.

Havighurst RJ: *Developmental Tasks and Education.* 3rd ed. New York, David McKay, 1972.

Health of the Disadvantaged. Chartbook. USDHEW (HRA) 77–728, 1977.

Heaps L: Effect of exposure to television violence on aggressive behavior. *Fam Perspect* 1977 Winter; 35.

Hellier A, Ptak H, Cerreto M: CATS inside my brain: children's understanding of the cerebral computed tomography scan procedure. *Child Health Care* 1986; 14:211–217.

Hetherington EM, Cox M, Cox R: Family intervention and social and emotional and cognitive development of children following divorce. *In* Vaughn L, Brazelton TB (eds): *The Family Setting Priorities.* New York, Science and Medical, 1979, 89–128.

Hetherington EM, Cox M, Cox R: Long-term effects of divorce and remarriage on the adjustment of children. *J Am Acad Child Psychiatr* 1985; 24:518–530.

Hurlock EB: *Child Growth and Development.* 5th ed. New York, McGraw-Hill, 1978.

Jarrett GE: Childrearing patterns of young mothers: expectations, knowledge, and practices. *MCN* 1982; 7:119–124.

Kalter N, Pickar J, Lesowitz M: School-based developmental facilitation groups for children of divorce: a preventive intervention. *Am J Orthopsychiatr* 1984; 54:613–623.

Kalter N, Riemes B, Brickman A, Chen JW: Implications of parental divorce for female development. *J Am Acad Child Psychiatr* 1985; 24:538–544.

Kittrell E: Children and television: the electronic fix. *Child Today* 1978 May/Jun; 20.

Koch H: *Twins and Their Relations.* Chicago, University of Chicago Press, 1966.

Kohlberg L: Moral development and identification. *In* Stevenson HW (ed): *Child Psychology.* Sixty-second Yearbook of the National Society for the Study of Education, Part 1. Chicago, University of Chicago Press, 1963.

Kohlberg L: The cognitive-developmental approach to moral education. *Phi Delta Kappan* 1975; 46:670–677.

Kruger AC, Tomasello M: Transactive discussions with peers and adults. *Dev Psychol* 1986; 22:681–685.

Krysl M, Watson J: Existential moments of caring: facets of nursing and social support. *Adv Nurs Sci* 1988 Jan; 10(2):12–17.

Lerner R, Spanier G (eds): *Child Influences on Marital and Family Interaction.* New York, Academic Press, 1978.

Levine M, et al: *Developmental-Behavioral Pediatrics.* Philadelphia, WB Saunders, 1983.

Madden J: The effects of schemes on children's drawings and the results of transformations. *Child Dev* 1986; 57:924–933.

Maslow AH: *Motivation and Personality.* New York, Harper & Row, 1970.

Maslow AH: *The Farther Reaches of Human Nature.* New York, Viking Press, 1971.

Melli MS: The changing legal status of the single parent. *Fam Relations* 1986; 35:31–35.

Miller SA: Certainty and necessity in the understanding of Piagetian concepts. *Dev Psychol* 1986; 22:3–18.

Morbidity Mortality Weekly Report 1987; 36(1).

Moynihan DP: *Family and Nation* San Diego: Harcourt Brace Jovanovich, 1987.

Murray JP: *Television and youth—25 years of research and controversy.* Boys Town, NE, Boys Town Center for the Study of Youth Development, 1984.

National Institute of Mental Health: *Television and Behavior.* Rockville, MD, NIMH, 1982.

Nelson, PT: Newsletters: an effective delivery mode for providing educational information and emotional support to single parent families? *Fam Relations* 1986; 35:183–188.

Norton AJ, Glick PC: One parent families: a social and economic profile. *Fam Relations* 1986; 35:9–17.

O'Bryant S, Corder-Bolz C: Tackling "the tube" with family teamwork. *Child Today* 1978 May/Jun; 21.

Piaget J: *The Origins of Intelligence in Children.* New York, International Universities Press, 1952.

Piaget J: Piaget's theory. *In* Mussen PH (ed): *Carmichael's Manual of Child Psychology.* Vol 1. New York, John Wiley, 1970.

Piaget J, Inhelder B: *The Psychology of the Child.* New York, Basic Books, 1969.

Reuter L, Strang V: Yours, mine and ours: stepparents and their children. *MCN* 1986; 11:264–266.

Risman BJ: Can men "mother"? Life as a single father. *Fam Relations* 1986; 35:95–102.

Romanczuk AN: Helping the stepparent parent. *MCN* 1987; 12:106–110.

Rosenblatt P, Cunningham M: Television watching and family tensions. *J Marriage Fam* 1976 Feb; 105.

Rothenberg MB: In my opinion . . . role of television in shaping the attitudes of children. *Child Health Care* 1985; 13:148–149.

Rubenstein EA: Television and behavior. *Am Psychol* 1983; 38:820–825.

Rubenstein E: Television and the young viewer. *Am Sci* 1978 Jun; 685.

Rutter M: *Fifteen Thousand Hours.* Cambridge, MA, Harvard University Press, 1979.

Rutter M: *Scientific Foundations of Developmental Psychiatry.* London, Heinemann Medical, 1980.

Sanik MM, Mauldin T: Single versus two parent families: a comparison of mother's time. *Fam Relations* 1986; 35:53–56.

Santrock WJ, Warshak RA: Father custody and social development in boys and girls. *J Soc Issues* 1979; 35:112–125.

Sears RR: Identification as a form of behavioral development. *In* Harris DB (ed): *The Concept of Development.* Minneapolis, University of Minnesota Press, 1957.

Sears RR: Personality development in the family. *In* Seedman JM (ed): *The Child: Handbook of Readings.* New York, Holt, Rinehart & Winston, 1958.

Segal J, Yahroes H: *A Child's Journey: Forces That Shape the Lives of Our Young.* New York, McGraw-Hill, 1978.

Shamsie J: Family breakdown and its effects on emotional disorders in children. *Can J Psychiatr* 1985; 30:281–287.

Skinner BF: *The Behavior of Organisms.* New York, Appleton, 1938.

Steinman SB, Zemmelman SE, Knoblauch TM: A study of parents who sought joint custody following divorces: who reaches agreement and sustains joint custody and who returns to court. *J Am Acad Child Psychiatr* 1985; 24:554–562.

Thomas A, Chess S, Birch H: *Temperament and Behavior Disorders in Children.* New York, New York University Press, 1968.

Thomas RM: *Comparing Theories of Child Development.* Belmont, CA, Wadsworth, 1979.

Visher EB, Visher JS: Children in stepfamilies. *Psychiatr Ann* 1982; 12:832–841.

Wallerstein J: Children of divorce—emerging trends. *Psychiatr Clin North Am* 1985; 8:837–855.

Watson JB: *Behavior: An Introduction to Comparative Psychology.* New York, Holt, 1914.

Weisner TS, Eiduson BT: The children of the 60's as parents. *Psychol Today* 1986; 20:60–66.

Wesley F, Wesley C: *Sex-Role Psychology.* New York, Human Sciences Press, 1977.

Wilson MN: The Black extended family: an analytical consideration. *Dev Psychol* 1986; 22:246–258.

Wixen B: Children of the rich. *In* Noshpitz J (ed): *Basic Handbook of Child Psychiatry.* New York, Basic Books, 1979.

Zill N: *American Children: Happy, Healthy and Insecure.* New York, Doubleday, 1982.

Zill N: *Happy, Healthy, and Secure.* New York, Doubleday, 1984.

Bibliography

Aldous J: *Family Careers: Developmental Change in Families.* New York, John Wiley and Sons, 1978.

Bloom B, White S, Asher S: Mental disruption as a stressful life event. *In* Levinger G, Moles O (eds): *Divorce and Separation.* New York, Basic Books, 1979.

Borolby J: *Attachment and Loss: Loss.* Vol III. New York, Basic Books, 1980.

Cohen J, Eiduson B: Changing patterns of childrearing in alternative life styles: Implications for development. *In* Davids A (ed): *Child Personality and Psychopathology: Current Topics.* New York, John Wiley and Sons, 1975.

Coles R: *Privileged Ones, The Well-Off and the Rich in America.* Vol V, *Children in Crisis.* Boston, Atlantic-Little, Brown Books, 1977.

Dail PW, Way WL: What do parents observe about parenting from prime time television? *Fam Rel* 1985; 34:491–499.

Donaldson M: *Children's Minds.* New York, WW Norton, 1978.

Eldred C, et al: Some aspects of adoption in selected samples of adult adoptees. *Am J Orthopsychiatr* 1976; 46:279.

Erikson E: *Childhood and Society.* New York, WW Norton, 1963.

Evans E, McCandless B: *Children and Youth: Psychosocial Development.* New York, Holt, Rinehart and Winston, 1978.

Furman E: *A Child's Parent Dies.* New Haven, CT, Yale University Press, 1974.

Glick P: Remarriage: Some recent changes and variations. *J Fam Issues* 1980 Jan; 455.

Harrington C: Culture as a manifestation of human diversity. *In* Gordon E (ed): *Human Diversity and Pedagogy.* Westport, CT, Mediax, Inc., 1982.

Helms D, Turner J: *Exploring Child Behavior: Basic Principles.* Philadelphia, WB Saunders, 1978.

Hinde R: *Toward Understanding Relationships.* London, Academic Press, 1979.

Kadushin A: *Adopting Older Children.* New York, Columbia University Press, 1970.

Kayes L: *Developing Your Child's Temperament.* New York, Dell Books, 1979.

Kelly J, Wallerstein J: Part-time parents, part-time child: Visiting after divorce. *J Clin Child Psychol* 1977 Jun; 51.

Macoby E: *Social Development: Psychological Growth and the Parent Child Relationships.* New York, Harcourt Brace Jovanovich, 1980.

Macoby E, Jacklin C: *The Psychology of Sex Difference.* Stanford, CA, Stanford University Press, 1974.

Maier H: *Three Theories of Child Development.* New York, Harper and Row, 1969.

McCall RB: Nature-nurture and the two realms of development: a proposed integration with respect to mental development. *Child Dev* 1981; 52:1.

Moody K: *Growing Up on Television.* New York, Time Books, 1980.

Mullen PD: Promoting child health: channels of socialization. *Fam Commun Health* 1983; 6(1):52–68.

Murray J, Lonnborg B: *Children and Television: A Primer for Parents.* Boys Town, NE, The Boys Town Center, 1981.

Papilla D, Olds S: *Human Development.* New York, McGraw Hill, 1978.

Pearl D, Bouthilet L, Lazar J (eds): *Television and Behavior: Ten Years of Scientific Progress and Implications for the Eighties.* Vols 1 and 2. Rockville, MD, National Institute of Mental Health, 1982.

Persson-Blennow I, McNeil TF: Temperament characteristics of children in relation to gender, birth order, and social class. *Am J Orthopsychiatr* 1977; 51(4):107–113.

Pulaski MS: *Understanding Piaget: An Introduction to Children's Cognitive Development.* New York, Harper and Row, 1971.

Roche A: Secular trends in human growth, maturation and development. *Monogr Soc Res Child Dev.* 1979; 44(3).

Rothbart MK: Measurement of temperament in infancy. *Child Dev* 1981; 52:569–578.

Sahin S: The multifaceted role of the nurse as genetic counselor. *J MCN* 1976 Jul/Aug; 211.

Singer D, Singer J, Zuckerman D: *Teaching Television: How to Use Television to Your Child's Advantage.* New York, Dial Press, 1981.

Sutterly D, Donnelly G: *Perspectives in Human Development: Nursing Throughout the Life Cycle.* Philadelphia, JB Lippincott, 1978.

Thomas A, Chess S: *Temperament and Development.* New York, Brunner/Mazel, 1977.

Thomas A, Chess S, Brick H: *Temperament and Behavior Disorders in Children.* New York, New York University Press, 1968.

Visher J, Visher E: Stepfamilies and stepchildren. In Berlin I, Stone E (eds): *Basic Handbook of Child Psychiatry.* New York, Basic Books, 1979.

Wallerstein J: Children of divorce stress and developmental tasks. *In* Garmezy N, Rutter M (eds): *Stress, Coping and Development.* New York, McGraw-Hill, 1983.

Weingarten J: Remarriage and well-being: national survey evidence of social and psychological effects. *J Fam Issues* 1980 Jan; 583.

Wilson E: *On Human Nature.* Cambridge, MA, Harvard University Press, 1978.

Wittig W, Peterson A: *Sex Related Differences in Cognitive Functioning.* New York, Academic Press, 1979.

Zuckerman DM, Zuckerman BS: Television's impact on children. *Pediatrics* 1985; 75:233–240.

Principles of Genetic Inheritance

Chapter 4

Maureen H. Clark
Roxie L. Foster

Nurses who care for children have a unique responsibility to "developing families." During the childbearing years a family is most in need of counseling concerning the likelihood their offspring will be affected by inherited tendencies or genetic alterations. This chapter begins with an overview of the basic principles of inheritance, identifies the major causes of genetic disorders, provides information to help the nurse identify families in need of genetic counseling, specifies the goals of genetic counseling, and, finally, applies these facts to nursing strategies for support of families who are experiencing a genetic disorder. Specific genetic disorders are discussed throughout the text in relation to the involved body systems. Table 4-1 provides a broad overview of known genetic disorders. Chapter 43 includes a Nursing Process Plan for the family in need of genetic counseling. Box 4-1 provides a glossary of terms specific to the study of genetic disorders.

Related Topics
Nursing Process Plan for the Family in Need of Genetic Counseling, Table 50-3
Specific hereditary diseases in related body systems chapters
Further discussion of Down syndrome, mental retardation, Chapter 34

Table 4-1. Selected Single Gene Disorders

Genetic Disease	Pathophysiology and Clinical Manifestations	Therapeutic Management
Autosomal Recessive		
Congenital adrenal hyperplasia (Chapter 49)	Deficiency of enzyme(s) (usually 21-hydroxylase) required for normal synthesis of cortisol. May affect aldosterone production as well. Excess testosterone is produced, leading to virilization and development of secondary sex characteristics	Corticosteroid replacement therapy
Albinism	The absence of the enzyme tyrosine leads to a defect in formation of melanin, the pigment normally found in the hair, skin, and eyes. The child has extremely fair skin and fine, white hair. Irises appear gray or blue in color; refractive errors, strabismus, nystagmus, and photophobia are common, along with a persistent loss of visual acuity	Supportive; assess for neoplasms
Alpha$_1$-antitrypsin deficiency (AAT)	AAT is a plasma protein synthesized in the liver, which protects the body from the effects of trypsin and other proteolytic enzymes that are released with cell injury. Liver and lungs are organs most often affected by AAT deficiency, with resultant hepatitis, cirrhosis, or emphysema	Supportive; liver transplantation; avoid inhaling industrial fumes, cigarette smoke
Cystic fibrosis (Chapter 38)	A generalized dysfunction of the exocrine (mucus-producing) glands leads to fibrosis of the pancreas (with failure to secrete proteolytic enzymes needed for digestion), chronic lung obstruction, and other problems	Proteolytic enzyme replacement; supportive pulmonary treatment
Familial dysautonomia (Riley-Day syndrome)	Deficiency of the enzyme dopamine-beta-hydroxylase results in failure to convert dopamine to norepinephrine. This leads to disturbances in the autonomic nervous system, including altered sensation (including lack of pain sensation), neuromuscular disturbances, and absence of tear formation. Prognosis is poor, with death usually occurring before adulthood	Supportive: control of respiratory infections, prevention of corneal ulceration
Galactosemia (Chapter 50)	Absence of the enzyme galactose-1-phosphate uridyltransferase results in inability to convert galactose to glucose. Cellular accumulation of galactose and its abnormal metabolites leads to cirrhosis and mental retardation if diagnosis is not made at birth	Elimination of galactose from the diet
Homocystinuria (homocystinemia)	Deficiency of cystathionine synthetase results in accumulation of homocysteine, which is produced in the degradation of methionine (an essential amino acid). Progressive mental retardation and eye problems are common as well as skeletal abnormalities	High doses of vitamin B and dietary restriction of methionine
Hurler syndrome (Chapter 50)	Deficiency of the enzyme alpha-1-iduronidase leads to accumulation of unmetabolized mucopolysaccharides resulting in mental retardation, coarse facies, skeletal and joint deformities, deafness, dwarfism and corneal clouding. This progressive disease usually leads to death by age 10 years	Supportive
Maple syrup urine disease (Chapter 50)	Absence of the enzymes needed for normal metabolism of leucine, isoleucine, and valine (essential amino acids) results in disrupted protein synthesis for neurologic development. Even with early, vigorous treatment, few children achieve normal physical and mental development	Dietary control of leucine, isoleucine, and valine
Metachromatic leukodystrophy	Deficiency of arylsulfatase A leads to demyelinization of the white matter of the brain with resultant loss of neuromuscular function. Children typically live only a few years after diagnosis	Supportive
Phenylketonuria (PKU) (Chapter 50)	Absence or deficiency of the enzymes phenylethylamine and dihydropteridine reductase results in failure to convert excess phenylalanine (an essential amino acid) to tyrosine. Increased serum levels of phenylalanine and its abnormal metabolites lead to mental retardation	Dietary regulation of phenylalanine
Sanfilippo syndrome	Deficiency of heparan N-sulfatase leads to tissue accumulation of heparan sulfate with resulting damage to neurons and profound mental retardation. Gait disturbances and hyperactivity are characteristic. Death usually occurs during adolescence	Supportive

Table 4-1. *(continued)*

Genetic Disease	Pathophysiology and Clinical Manifestations	Therapeutic Management
Sickle cell disease (Chapter 40)	Sickle hemoglobin is produced instead of normal hemoglobin, resulting in hematologic crises triggered by infection, dehydration, hypoxia, fever, high environmental temperature, high altitude, vigorous exercise, or emotional stress	Supportive: avoidance of predisposing conditions
Tay-Sachs disease	Deficiency of hexosaminidase leads to ineffective degradation of lipids found in cell membranes of the nervous system. The resulting accumulation results in neuromuscular deterioration, head enlargement, mental retardation, and blindness, with death typically occurring before age 4 years. Occurs primarily in Ashkenazi Jews	Supportive
Thalassemia major (Cooley anemia) (Chapter 40)	A defect in hemoglobin synthesis results in a severe, progressive hemolytic anemia	Blood transfusion
Vitamin D–dependent rickets (Chapter 50)	Defective production of calcitriol or ineffectiveness of vitamin D at the receptor level leads to poor calcium absorption. This leads to bowing of the legs and resultant short stature.	Large daily doses of vitamin D
Werdnig-Hoffmann disease (infantile spinal muscular atrophy)	Atrophy of anterior horn cells in the spinal cord and of motor nuclei in the brain result in weakness and lax muscle tone, with a characteristic frog-leg position in infants. Intelligence is normal. Death usually occurs before adulthood and is often related to respiratory failure	Supportive
Wilson disease (Chapter 50)	A defect in the synthesis of ceruloplasmin, a protein needed for copper transport, results in copper accumulation in the liver, brain, and cornea leading to cirrhosis, neurologic abnormalities, and Kayser-Fleischer rings of the cornea. Renal damage may also occur	Chelating agents to remove serum copper
Autosomal Dominant		
Achondroplasia (Chapter 49)	Abnormal skeletal growth results in short stature, short limbs, and a large head. This disease is associated with increased paternal age. The life span is usually normal	Supportive for psychosocial effects of short stature
Epidermolysis bullosa (EB)	EB is the general term for a group of diseases, some inherited through autosomal dominant genes, others as an autosomal recessive trait. The diseases are characterized by blisters brought on by mechanical trauma and high environmental temperature. They vary in severity from mild (epidermolytic EB) to life-threatening (junctional EB).	Supportive; nonirritating clothes, no hot baths or tape on skin; drainage of large blisters
Familial hypercholesterolemia (Chapter 39)	Lipoprotein metabolism is altered such that there is a marked increase in low density lipoproteins (LDL) from birth. Premature atherosclerosis, the most important manifestation, usually does not develop until middle age. Affected children usually have total cholesterol level >250 mg/dl.	Diet low in cholesterol and oral cholestyramine
Huntington disease	Progressive degeneration of basal ganglia leads to dementia, choreiform movements, and an irregular, dancing gait. Onset is more common in middle age than in childhood	Supportive
Marfan syndrome (Chapter 4)	A disease of connective tissue, Marfan syndrome results in a tall, thin stature; long, slender fingers and hands; refractive errors in vision; and cardiac defects.	Ongoing evaluation for heart disease
Neurofibromatosis (von Recklinghausen disease) (Chapter 46)	May be related to defective nerve growth factor, a neurohormone needed to differentiate neurologic cells. The classic signs include >6 café-au-lait spots and multiple cutaneous and subcutaneous neurofibromas (tumors of peripheral nerves). The tumors may become malignant and this disease has the potential for becoming a prototype for the association between cancer and certain dominant genes. Symptoms worsen with puberty and pregnancy	Excision of tumors that cause pain or impair function; ongoing evaluation for malignancy
Noonan syndrome	Probably associated with autosomal dominant inheritance, this syndrome characterizes children who have certain anomalies in common with females with Turner syndrome. Common abnormalities include short stature, webbed neck, chest malformation, congenital heart disease, eye and ear abnormalities, and micrognathia (small chin.)	Supportive

continued

Table 4-1. (continued)

Genetic Disease	Pathophysiology and Clinical Manifestations	Therapeutic Management
Osteogenesis imperfecta (OI) (Chapter 47)	The name for a group of hereditary diseases, some of which are transmitted by autosomal dominant traits and some by autosomal recessive inheritance. OI is characterized by bone fragility, blue sclera, presenile deafness, and a fragile appearance of skin. Cataracts are common, and teeth may be deformed.	Prevention and treatment of fractures and deformity
Progeria (Hutchinson-Gilford syndrome)	Noted for the characteristic appearance of premature aging, syndrome may be associated with autosomal dominant inheritance. Advanced paternal age seems to be an inheritance factor. Although motor and mental development are normal, profound growth failure occurs in the first year. Other common signs are characteristic facies, alopecia, loss of subcutaneous fat, abnormal posture, stiffness of joints, atherosclerosis, and "aging" skin. The median life span is about 13 years, with death from cardiac or cerebral vascular disease.	Supportive
Retinoblastoma (Chapter 48)	A malignant tumor of the retina characterized by the cat's eye reflex (white reflex of the pupil instead of the normal red reflex), loss of vision, redness of the eye, and pain. Glaucoma may be present. Heterochromia (eyes of different colors or different colors within one iris) is sometimes associated	Radiation therapy, cobalt plaque applicators, cryotherapy, photo coagulation, enucleation
Treacher Collins syndrome	Characterized by deformities of facial bones, pinnas, and palate and by malocclusion of the teeth. Deafness is common	Supportive
Tuberous sclerosis (Bourneville disease) (Chapter 46)	Sclerotic cerebral lesions (tubers) occur throughout the cortical gray matter. The lesions, present at birth, gradually enlarge and calcify and cause mental retardation and intractable seizures. Benign tumors develop in organs such as the kidneys, heart, liver, spleen, and lungs. Prognosis varies with the degree of involvement	Treatment of seizures, excision of large tumors
von Willebrand disease (Chapter 40)	Deficiency or absence of factor VIII (necessary for platelet aggregation) leads to prolonged bleeding time, bleeding from mucous membranes, heavy and prolonged menses	Infusion of DDAVP
Waardenburg syndrome	Characterized by congenital deafness, abnormal pigmentation of the hair and eyes (a white forelock of hair and eyes which are either different colors or very pale in color). Skin also may be very light in color	Supportive for deafness
X-Linked		
Color blindness	Carrier females pass this trait to their male children. It results in the inability to distinguish among certain colors: a) red, blue, and green, b) yellow and blue, c) green and purple	None
Duchenne muscular dystrophy (pseudohypertrophic MD) (Chapter 47)	Primarily affecting males, this type of MD results in progressive muscular weakness, atrophy, and contractures. Death usually results from involvement of respiratory muscles	Supportive; keep active and ambulatory as long as possible
Glucose-6-phosphate dehydrogenase (G6PD) deficiency	Deficiency of this enzyme leads to episodes of hemolytic anemia associated with infections or certain drugs and to a chronic type of hemolytic anemia. Most common in males of Greek, southern Italian, Sephardic Jew, Filipino, southern Chinese, black, or Thai descent	Males of ethnic risk should be tested for G6PD before oxidant drugs are administered
Hemophilia A (factor VIII deficiency, classic hemophilia) (Chapter 40)	Deficiency of Factor VIII leads to a coagulation disorder in which hemarthrosis (bleeding into a joint) is common as is bleeding into tissues following minor trauma. Severity depends upon the amount of functioning factor VIII	Intravenous factor VIII replacement
Hemophilia B (factor IX deficiency, Christmas disease) (Chapter 40)	Deficiency of blood factor IX leads to a coagulation disorder as in hemophilia A	Intravenous factor IX replacement
Hunter syndrome	This mucopolysaccharide disease is similar to, but milder than, Hurler syndrome. Unmetabolized mucopolysaccharides are stored in tissues, leading to coarse facial features, short stature, joint stiffness, mental retardation, hepatosplenomegaly, and hernias.	Supportive

Table 4-1. (continued)

Genetic Disease	Pathophysiology and Clinical Manifestations	Therapeutic Management
Menkes disease (Chapter 50)	The inability to absorb copper from the gastrointestinal tract leads to failure to thrive, hypothermia, kinky hair, and progressive neurologic deterioration. Much of the damage occurs in fetal life and is irreversible, leading to death, often within the first year of life	Parenteral administration of copper
Retinitis pigmentosa	A progressive degeneration of the retina leads to vision loss with impairment of night vision as an early symptom. This disorder may also be passed by autosomal dominant or recessive traits	Supportive
Wiskott-Aldrich syndrome	Characterized by thrombocytopenia, decreased immune competence, draining ears, and eczema	Splenectomy, bone marrow transplant

Human genetics, the science of human variations, explains the similarities and accounts for the differences among human beings. People have recognized these differences and illustrated them in their paintings and sculpture in many cultures for centuries (Kunze and Nippert, 1986). From a combination of specific inherited characteristics and environmental exposure, each infant emerges a unique person. Yet a spectrum of differences arises among individuals and among cultures.

Science is only beginning to unlock the secrets of the genetic codes that determine our gender; height; weight distribution; the color of our skin, eyes, and hair; the shape and size of our facial features and other body parts; the uniqueness of intricate physiologic processes; our intellectual capacity; and perhaps even our personalities. Genetics appears to be basic and pervasive not only to physical appearance and the ability to sustain life, but to the *experience* of life.

Researchers in many scientific disciplines have long asked: If the complete genetic code were known, could it alone describe, predict, and control every aspect of the human being? This is the essence of what has been called the "nature versus nurture" controversy. Psychologists have conducted studies on identical twins who were raised, since birth, in different environments in an attempt to sort out the effects of heredity versus those of environment. Sociologists have studied humans raised in the wild by animals and anthropologists have studied people of vastly differing cultures in an attempt to differentiate between culturally acquired and genetically programmed behavior. The results of the studies, taken individually, are inconclusive. Their cumulative answer, however, is one of compromise: it is now commonly agreed that neither heredity nor environment can, in itself, explain the human, but that we are the products of unique combinations of those elements. The interrelatedness of heredity and environment is an important concept for nursing because it underscores the fact that individuals have choices, that lives are not predetermined on the basis of heredity. A young life is shaped by a nurturing family; optimal growth and development can be reached in the proper environment; health behaviors can offset the predisposition for disease.

As researchers study the sequences of chemical subunits (bases) that make up the genes, they are searching for new answers to many health questions: Given the same exposure to a virus, why does one person contract the illness and another person remain well? Why do some people manufacture more endorphins (natural opiates) than others? Why does the same dose of a drug act differently in different people? What part does heredity play in heart disease, cancer, autoimmune disease, and other illnesses? If the complete genetic code were known would all disease be preventable or curable? Although the answers to these questions still elude modern science, genetic research promises to have a major influence on health care in the next decade and beyond.

The practice of pediatric nursing is uniquely affected by principles of genetic inheritance. While there is ample room for genetic variation within a range that science has defined as *normal*, some genetic variations cause disease or affect normal growth and development. The nurse who works with children must be adept at distinguishing normal variations from those that indicate the need for further evaluation.

Genetic disorders are not limited, however, to those discovered in infancy or early childhood. Every nurse, regardless of specialty area, will encounter clients affected by a genetic disorder. Genetic alterations can become apparent later in life and affect persons at all phases of the life cycle (Table 4-2). Genetic alterations span all areas of nursing practice, including the workplace, school, hospital, clinic, office, mental health facility, and community health agency (Cohen, 1984). It is important, therefore, that nurses (1) have a basic knowledge of genetic inheritance, (2) know the goals of genetic counseling in order to identify those needs not met in the counseling process, and (3) be prepared to plan, execute, and evaluate strategies to support the family prior to genetic counseling, during the decision-making period that follows the formal counseling sessions, and during the months or years of follow-up care for the affected child.

For the nurse who is interested in a more in-depth discussion of human genetics than this chapter provides, it would be helpful to take a course in human genetics or consult a textbook on basic human genetics (e.g., Cohen, 1984; Thompson and Thompson, 1986).

Basic Principles of Inheritance

Since Hippocrates' time in the 5th century, the contributions of both the mother and the father have been recognized as important to the genetic characteristics of the child. The blueprints for these traits are carried in the nucleus of each gamete. Genetic characteristics are irrevocably established at the moment of the union of the sperm and the egg. The genetic information carried in the fertilized ovum, when combined with environmental influences, determines the physical

Box 4-1
Glossary of Genetic Terms

ALLELE

One of two or more alternative forms of a gene at the same site in a chromosome, which determines alternative characters in inheritance.

AUTOSOME

Somatic chromosomes; any chromosomes other than the X and Y sex chromosomes.

CARRIER

An individual who has, and therefore can transmit, a particular gene or chromosomal abnormality but who does not show the trait.

CHROMOSOMES

Microscopic units located within the nucleus of every cell, which contain the basic hereditary factors in the form of genes. There are 46 chromosomes in every cell except the reproductive cells (egg and sperm cells), which each contain 23.

CONGENITAL

Relating to a characteristic present at or dating from birth, either of genetic or environmental origin.

CONSANGUINITY

The state of being "related by blood," that is, of being descended from at least one common ancestor.

DIZYGOSITY

Unidentical, or fraternal, twins resulting from the fertilization of two eggs by two sperm cells. They can be of the same or opposite sex.

DNA

Deoxyribonucleic acid; the nucleic acid of the chromosomes, which carries the genetic code.

DOMINANT

A gene that produces the same characteristic when it is present in a single dose, along with a specified allele (heterozygous), as it does in a double dose (homozygous).

FAMILIAL

A condition more often present in two or more members of a family group than would be expected in the population as a whole.

GAMETE

The haploid cell which is the product of meiosis and which, by combination with a gamete from the opposite sex, produces a zygote.

GENE

A segment of a DNA molecule.

GENETIC COUNSELING

Provision of information bearing upon the problems related to the occurrence, or risk of occurrence, of a genetic disorder in a family. The process is concerned with the risk and burden of the disorder and the options available for dealing with it.

GENETIC SCREENING

Testing on a population basis to identify individuals at risk of having a specific genetic disorder or of having a child with a specific genetic disorder.

GENOTYPE

The genetic makeup of the individual.

HAPLOID

Having half the number of chromosomes characteristically found in the somatic (diploid) cells.

HETEROZYGOTE

An individual who has two different alleles, one of which is the normal allele, at a given locus on a pair of homologous chromosomes (e.g., notation: Aa).

HOMOLOGOUS CHROMOSOMES

A "matched pair" of chromosomes, one from each parent, having the same gene loci in the same order.

HOMOZYGOTE

An individual possessing a pair of identical alleles at a given locus on a pair of homologous chromosomes (e.g., notation: aa).

INBORN ERROR

A genetically determined biochemical disorder in which a specific enzyme is missing or is present in insufficient quantities.

KARYOTYPE

The chromosomal constitution of the cell nucleus; by extension, the photomicrograph of chromosomes arranged in numerical order.

LOCUS

The position of a gene on a chromosome.

MEIOSIS

The special type of cell division occurring in the germ cells by which gametes containing the haploid chromosome number are produced from diploid cells. Two meiotic divisions occur: the first and the second (meiosis I and meiosis II). Reduction in number takes place during meiosis I. To be distinguished from mitosis.

MITOSIS

The ordinary process of cell division which results in the formation of two daughter cells and by which the body replaces dead cells. The two daughter cells receive identical diploid complements of chromosomes (46) which are characteristic of somatic cells.

MONOZYGOTIC TWINS

Twins derived from a single fertilized ovum. Identical twins.

MOSAIC

An individual or tissue with at least two cell lines differing in genotype or karyotype; derived from a single zygote.

MULTIFACTORIAL

Arising as the result of the interaction of several genes or of genetic and nongenetic factors, each with only a minor effect by itself. (Synonym: polygenic.)

MUTATION

A permanent heritable change in the genetic material.

NONDISJUNCTION

The failure of two members of the same pair of chromosomes to separate into the newly formed daughter cells, resulting in one cell with one chromosome less than the normal amount and one cell with an extra chromosome.

PEDIGREE

A diagrammatic representation of a family history, indicating the affected individuals and their relationship to the person who is the basis for the genetic study.

PHENOTYPE

The entire physical, biochemical, and physiologic nature of an individual, as determined by the genotype and the environment in which the person develops.

POLYDACTYLY

Extra fingers and/or toes.

POLYGENIC

Determined by many genes at different loci.

RECESSIVE

A gene that will only produce its character when present in homozygous combination (i.e., must be present in both parents).

SEX LINKAGE

Location of a gene on a sex chromosome: X-linkage on the X chromosome and Y-linkage on the Y chromosome.

TERATOGEN

Any substance that is potentially harmful to an individual or to an unborn fetus.

TRANSLOCATION

The transfer of a segment of one chromosome to a nonhomologous chromosome.

TRISOMY

The state of having three of a given chromosome instead of the usual pair, as in trisomy 21 (Down syndrome).

X CHROMOSOME

A sex chromosome found paired in the normal female and singly in the male.

Y CHROMOSOME

The sex chromosome that occurs singly in the normal male and is absent in the normal female.

ZYGOTE

A fertilized egg.

Table 4-2. Usual Stage of Manifestation of Selected Genetic Disorders

Age of Onset	Disorder
0–6 months	Cystic fibrosis
0–12 months	Tay-Sachs disease
6 months–3 years	Sickle cell anemia
2–6 years	Duchenne muscular dystrophy
0–puberty	Turner syndrome
12–16 years	Marfan syndrome
8–20 years	Wilson disease
20+ years	Glaucoma, Huntington disease

and intellectual characteristics and capabilities of the developing child.

Characteristics of Heredity

The *gene* is the basic unit of inheritance. It is the physical basis for the transmission of traits from parents to children. Genes, made of DNA (deoxyribonucleic acid), are located within the cell nucleus and are arranged in a linear order in each chromosome. The DNA has the now-famous double helix structure (Fig. 4-1) made up of series of different combinations of four nitrogenous bases. The sequence of these bases in a stretch of DNA strand makes up a gene. These genes code for specific proteins.

Chromosomes occur in pairs, one of each pair being supplied by the mother and the other by the father. Every organism has a definite number of chromosomes, but each species maintains a consistent size, number, and shape of its own. There are 23 pairs of human chromosomes, 22 autosomes (chromosomes common to both sexes), and one pair of sex chromosomes (XX in females and XY in males).

Cytogeneticists (scientists who work with chromosomes) visualize human chromosomes by using a blood sample (leukocytes) or tissue sample such as skin or bone marrow. The samples are cultured and with the use of sophisticated laboratory methods the cells are stimulated to divide (mitosis) since it is only during the division phase of the cell cycle that chromosomes are condensed enough to be visible by light microscopy. The chromosomes are processed,

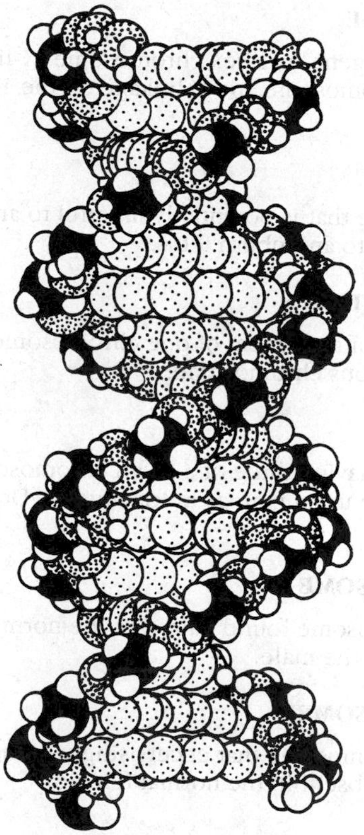

Figure 4-1. Double helix structure of DNA. (Courtesy of Genetics Screening and Counseling Service, Texas Department of Mental Health and Mental Retardation.)

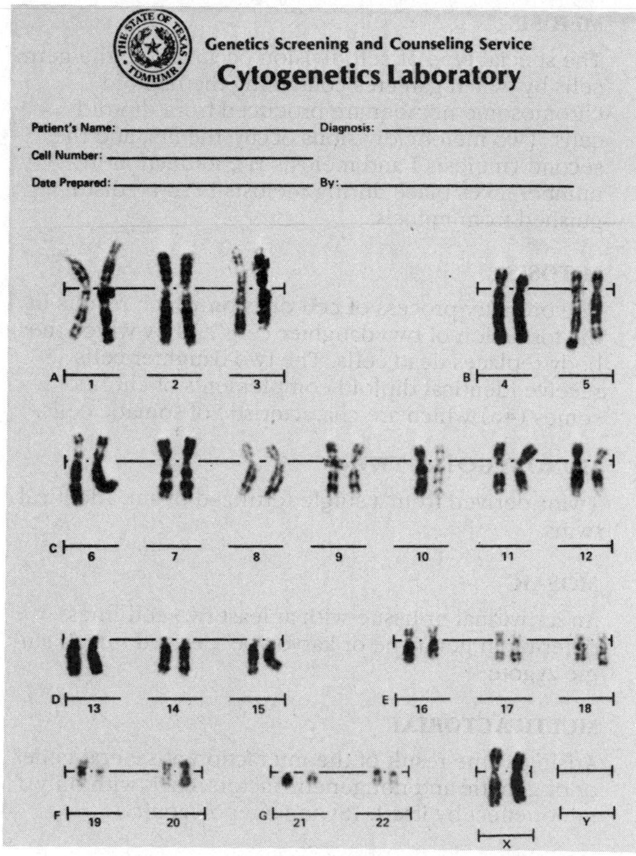

Figure 4-2. Normal female karyotype. (Courtesy of Genetics Screening and Counseling Service, Texas Department of Mental Health and Mental Retardation.)

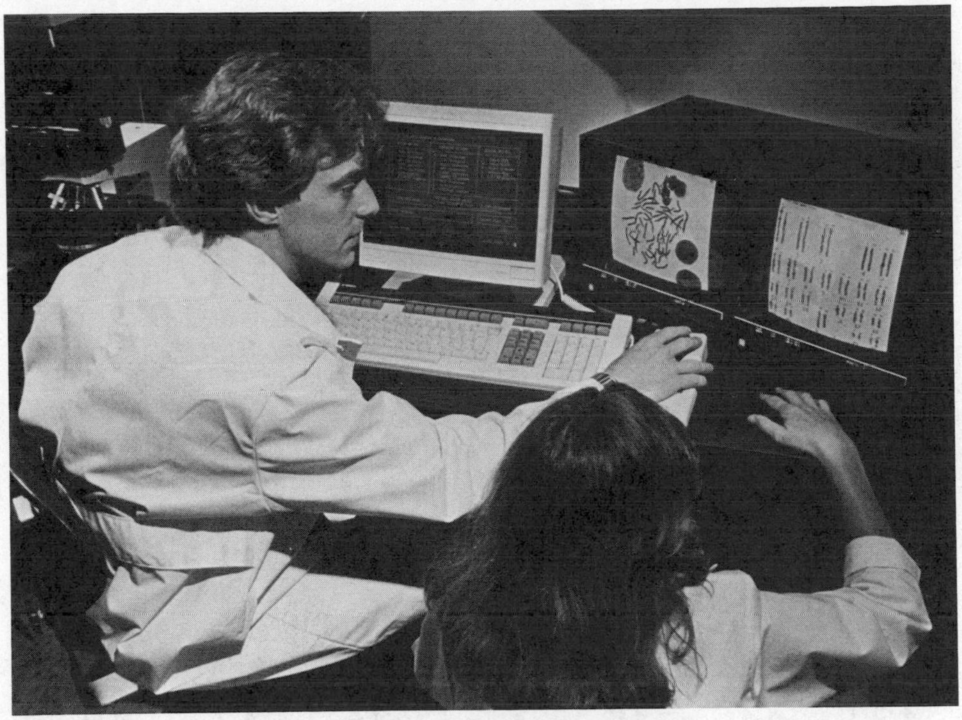

***Figure* 4-3.** Use of computer enhancement to produce karyotypes. (Courtesy of Genetics Screening and Counseling Service, Texas Department of Mental Health and Mental Retardation.)

stained, and photographed by a camera attached to a high-resolution microscope. Individual chromosomes are cut out from the photographs and arranged according to a standard classification system used throughout the world. The graph-like pattern is a karyotype (Fig. 4-2). The chromosomes are assigned places on the karyograph sheets according to their size, shape, and configuration. The paired chromosomes are arranged in decreasing length and are assigned a number (1 to 22) for reference. The sex chromosomes, X and Y, are paired separately.

Prior to modern banding techniques (until the 1960s), chromosomes were placed in seven major groups, A to G. You may still see references to conditions using these letters when the specific chromosome has not been identified. Banding (staining) of chromosomes permits identification of each chromosome individually due to the pattern of light and dark areas that will distinguish various regions within each chromosome.

This complex procedure of preparing a banded karyotype is used in the majority of laboratories. Today, however, in a handful of centers across the United States, this can now be done by digitalized images generated by a computer that is highly efficient. It was developed by image enhancement computer experts at the National Aeronautic and Space Administration using the latest in digital technology and shortens the amount of time laboratory technicians need to prepare karyotypes (Figs. 4-3 and 4-4).

Chromosome disorders occur as an alteration in either chromosome structure or number. *Meiosis* is the two-step process of cell division through which sperms and eggs (gametes) are formed (Fig. 4-5). These cells contain one half the number of chromosomes present in other body tissues. When, at fertilization, the male and female gametes (each with 23 single chromosomes) are united, the resulting zygote contains 46 chromosomes (23 pairs).

Occasionally, during meiosis, an error occurs in which the sperm or egg will have an extra chromosome resulting in the zygote having more than the normal 46 chromosomes. The most common errors in alteration of number of chromosomes occur as a trisomy, a condition in which there is one extra chromosome in each cell. The most common autosomal trisomies are 21 (Down syndrome), 18 (Patau syndrome) and 13 (Edwards syndrome). The most common sex chromosome abnormalities include one or more extra X chromosomes in a male (Klinefelter syndrome) and a missing X chromosome in a female (Turner syndrome).

Mitosis is the ordinary process in which new cells are made in the developing fetus, during childhood growth, and in the replacement of dead cells in the adult (Fig. 4-6). Normally chromosomes in the new cells have the exact number and structure of the original. An error can occur in mitosis during early embryonic development in which division is unequal, resulting in a cell with an extra (duplication), lost

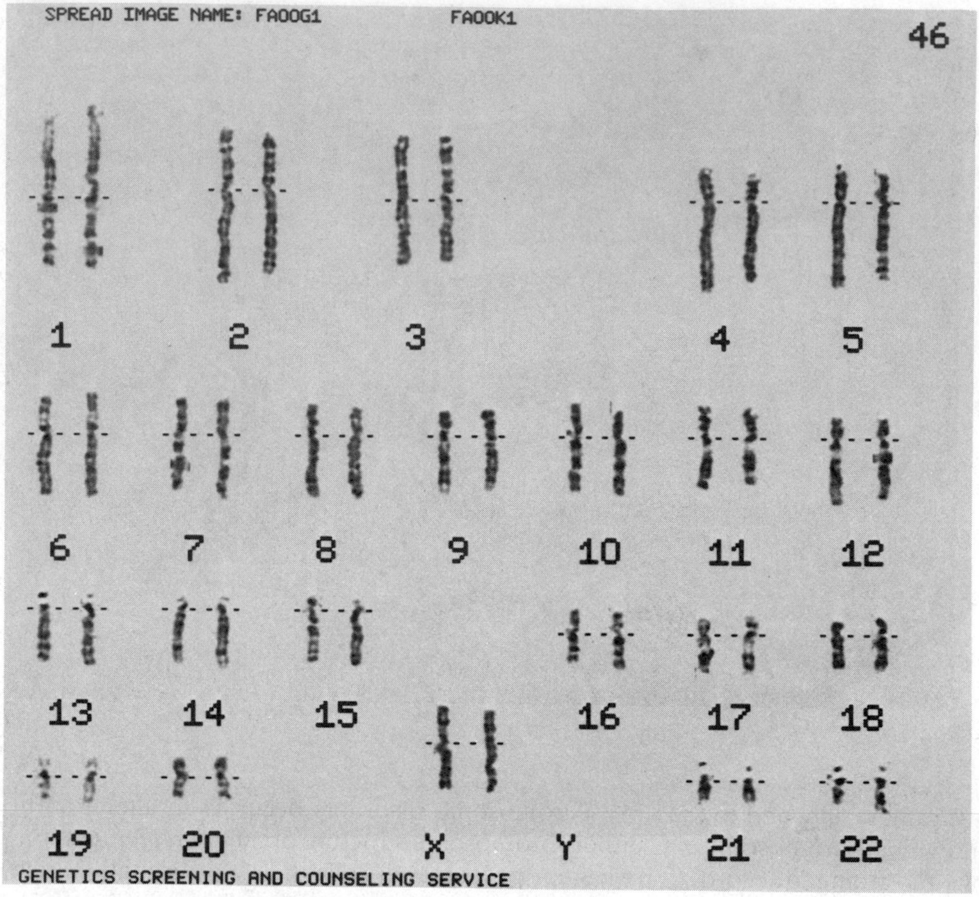

***Figure* 4-4.** Karyotype produced by computer enhancement. Note that all the chromosomes have been straightened. (Courtesy of Genetics and Counseling Service, Texas Department of Mental Health and Mental Retardation.)

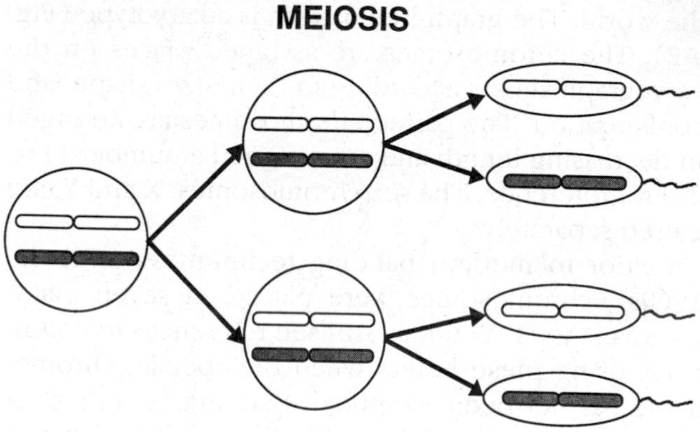

***Figure* 4-5.** A simplified illustration of meiosis, showing the end product (sperm) with half the number of chromosomes the original had. In oogenesis, the original cell develops into three cells with half the number of chromosomes: an ovum and two polar bodies. (Courtesy of Genetics and Counseling Service, Texas Department of Mental Health and Mental Retardation.)

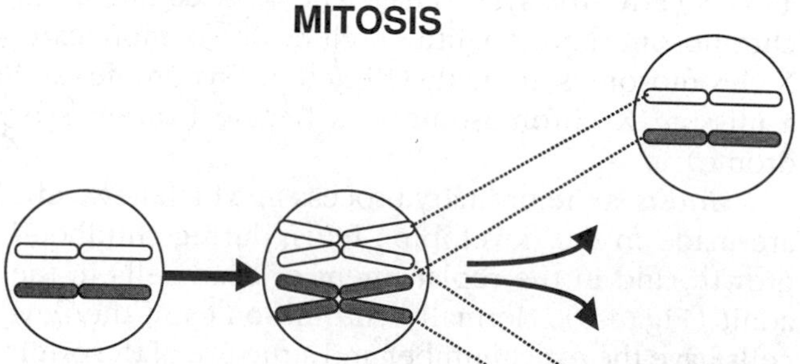

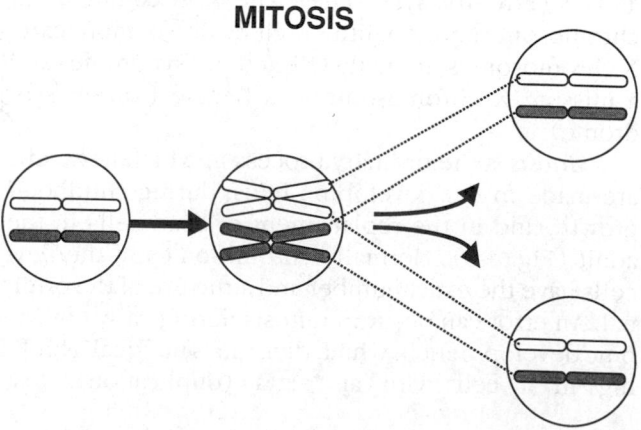

***Figure* 4-6.** Mitosis. (Courtesy of Genetics/Screening and Counseling Service, Texas Department of Mental Health and Mental Retardation.)

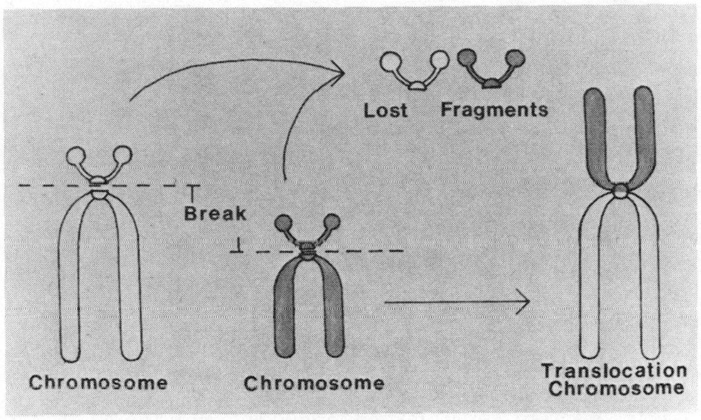

Figure 4-7. Translocation. (Courtesy of Genetics Screening and Counseling Service, Texas Department of Mental Health and Mental Retardation.)

(deletion), or broken and rearranged chromosome (either autosome or sex chromosome). The individual's body can then carry two types of cell lines with different chromosomal makeup, a condition called *mosaicism*. The significance of the mosaic etiology is that the individual develops in a unique pattern according to the proportion of abnormal cells.

In either meiosis or mitosis, chromosomes can be broken and reattached (*translocated*) to other chromosomes (Fig. 4-7). Occasionally, an entire chromosome or piece of a chromosome will attach itself to another. An individual who has no *extra or missing* chromosomal material is termed a balanced translocation carrier and is normal physically and mentally. However, these translocated chromosomes are very difficult to copy (that is, to divide exactly in half) for the formation of a sperm or an egg. Therefore, a translocation carrier has a significant risk of having children with extra and/or missing portions of chromosomes, the effect of which is extremely variable. Even a very tiny portion of missing or extra material can cause mental and physical handicaps. Rarely, both ends of a chromosome can be broken off and the ends attached to each other, resulting in a "ring" chromosome (Fig. 4-8). Chromosome deletions or duplications are known to occur from many causes, including exposure to radiation and chemical mutagens, some of which occur naturally in the environment.

Major Causes of Genetic Disorders

Faulty transmission of genetic information is responsible for three major types of genetic disorders:

- Chromosome disorders (disorders of autosomes and of sex chromosomes)
- Single gene disorders
- Multifactorial disorders (Thompson and Thompson, 1986)

This chapter presents only the principles underlying nursing care for families in need of genetic counseling. In-depth coverage of the major disorders resulting from genetic alterations is reserved for chapters relating to the body systems most affected by the disorder (Table 4-1).

Disorders of Autosomes

Trisomy 21 (Down Syndrome)

This syndrome, widely known in the medical community since the 1930s, was the first chromosome abnormality to be identified, in 1959. It occurs in all races, in both sexes, in about 1 in 1,000 live births. Individuals with Down syndrome have characteristic facial features: upslanting palpebral fissures, a small nasal bridge, Brushfield spots in the irises, a small nose and a large tongue. (See protocol for genetic assessment, Box 4-4; see also Fig. 4-9.)

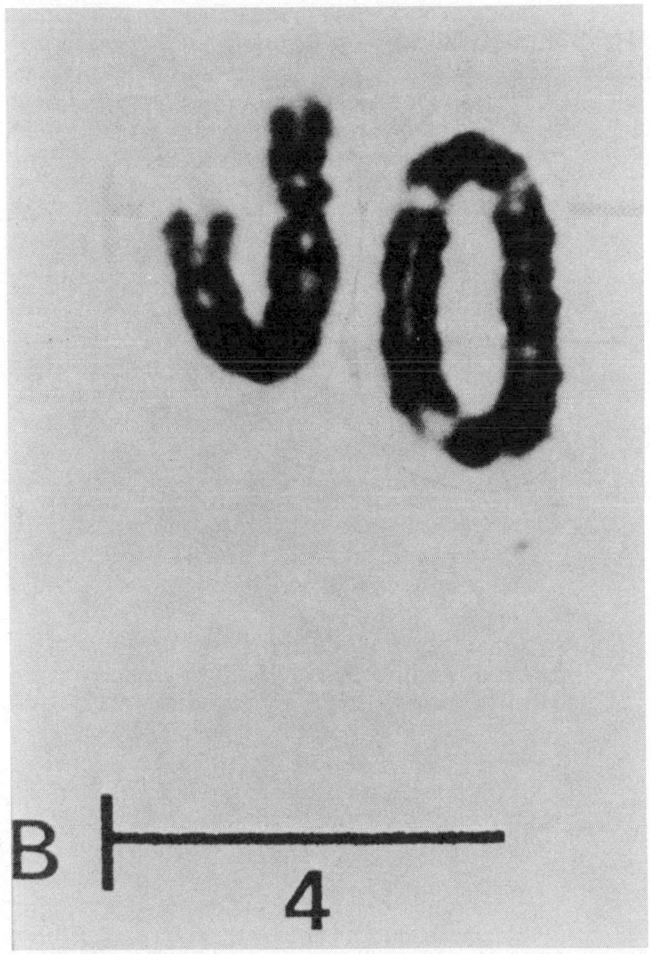

Figure 4-8. Fractured chromosomes. (Courtesy of Genetics Screening and Counseling Service, Texas Department of Mental Health and Mental Retardation.)

They often have brachycephaly, small ears, clinodactyly (incurved finger) of the fifth finger, simian crease (single palmar line), and short stature. The most striking feature a newborn nursery nurse will identify is hypotonia (lax muscle tone). Some individuals with Down syndrome have congenital heart defects. Approximately 40 per cent have ventricular septal defect (VSD). Mental retardation is present, with most in the moderate-to-severe range.

The majority of Down syndrome cases (approximately 95 per cent) are the result of an extra number 21 chromosome present in the sperm or egg, resulting in the zygote having three number 21 chromosomes. (This is called nondisjunction because the number 21 chromosomes did not "disjoin," or separate, in meiosis) (Figs. 4-9, 4-10, and 4-11). Parents of an infant with the nondisjunction form of trisomy 21 have a 1 to 2 per cent risk of having another child with trisomy 21. The number of individuals born with this type of Down syndrome increases with advanced maternal age (Table 4-3). Translocation of chromosomes is responsible for about 4 per cent of cases. If the mother is the translocation carrier, there is a 10 to 15 per cent chance that the child will have Down syndrome. If the father is the carrier, the risk is reduced to 5 to 8 per cent. The translocation type of Down syndrome is not influenced by age. Mosaicism is the cause of Down syndrome in about 1 per cent of the cases (Hirschhorn, 1987).

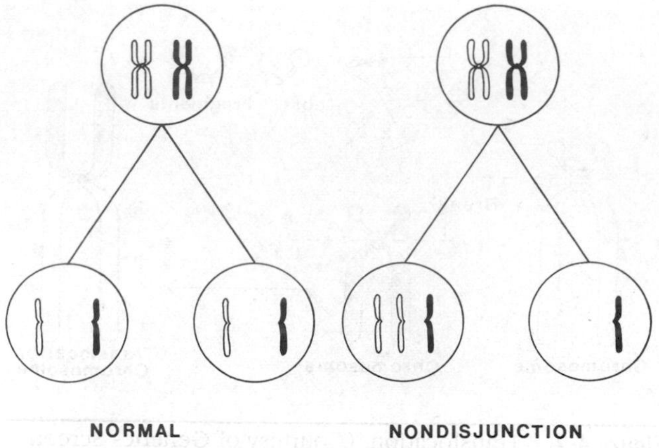

***Figure* 4-10.** Nondisjunction. (Courtesy of Genetics Screening and Counseling Service, Texas Department of Mental Health and Mental Retardation.)

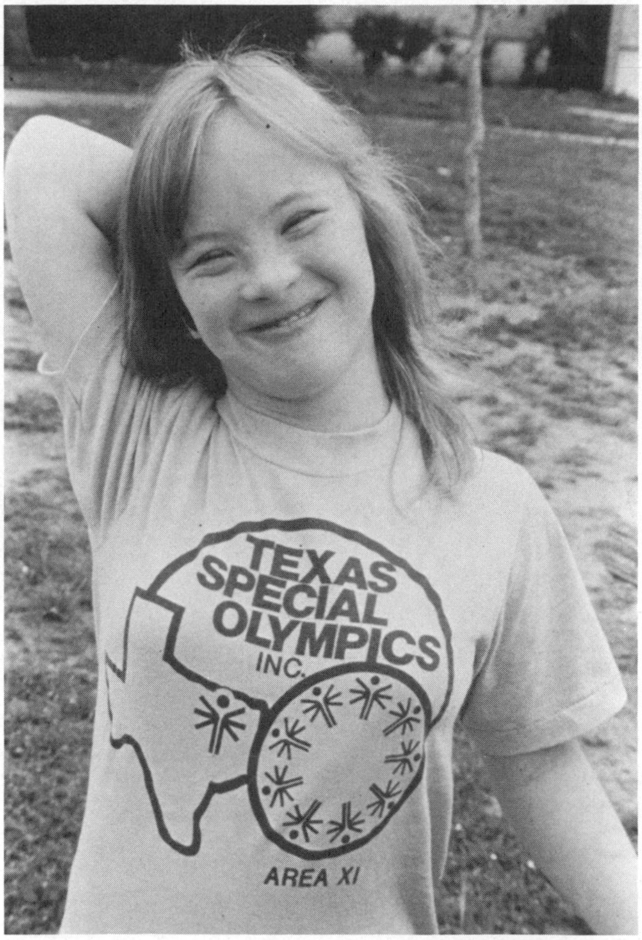

***Figure* 4-9.** Child with Down syndrome. (Courtesy of Genetics Screening and Counseling Service, Texas Department of Mental Health and Mental Retardation.)

Trisomy 18 (Edwards Syndrome)

Trisomy 18 occurs much less frequently than trisomy 21 and affects the individual much more severely (Table 4-4). The female-to-male ratio is 2:1, and it occurs in all races. More than 95 per cent of persons with trisomy 18 have heart defects. Common features include small stature, head, eyes, nose, and mouth; and malformed and low-set ears. A baby with trisomy 18 often fails to thrive. Many have a characteristic way of clenching their hands with their smallest finger overlapping the ring finger and the pointer finger overlapping the middle one. Some individuals have very prominent heels and/or rocker bottom feet (Box 4-4, page 155). Most of the infants born with trisomy 18 do not survive one year and those who do survive are profoundly mentally retarded. As with trisomy 21, advanced maternal age is associated with increased incidence.

Trisomy 13 (Patau Syndrome)

This is the least frequent of the three major autosomal trisomies; its incidence increases with maternal age (Hirschhorn, 1987). The anomalies are more severe than those seen in trisomy 21 and 18. Almost 80 per cent have irreversible heart defects. Many have abnormalities of the formation of the midbrain, abnormali-

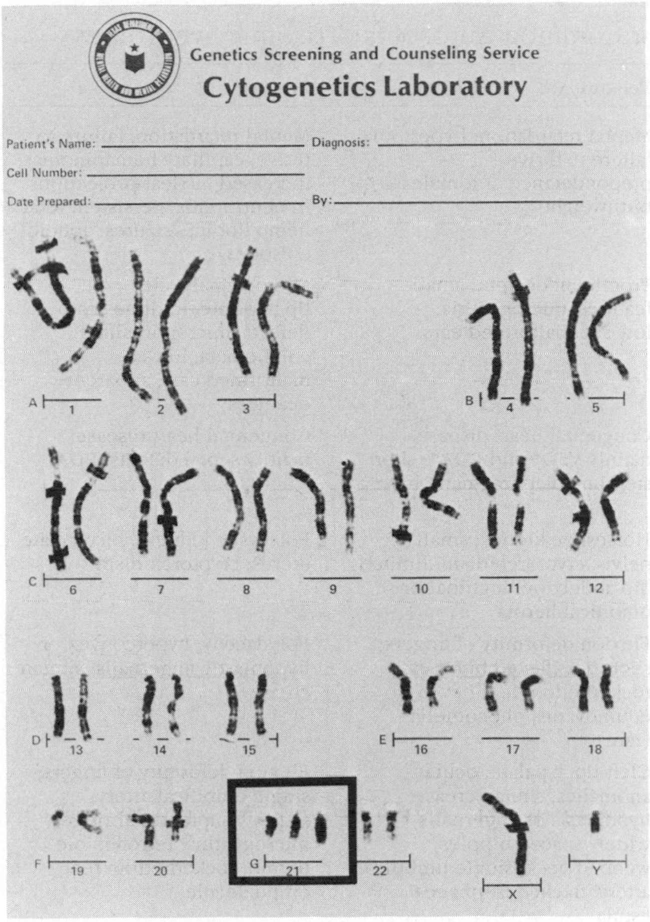

***Figure* 4-11.** Trisomy 21 karyotype. (Courtesy of Genetics Screening and Counseling Service, Texas Department of Mental Health and Mental Retardation.)

ties of midfacial structures that include cleft lip and palate, and severe eye defects. Urogenital anomalies are also common. Fewer than 20 per cent of infants live beyond the first year of life (Cohen, 1984).

***Table* 4-3.** Risk of Down Syndrome in Live Births

Maternal Age*	Frequency of Down Syndrome Live Births
-19	1/1550
20-24	1/1550
25-29	1/1050
30-34	1/700
35	1/350
36	1/300
37	1/225
38	1/175
39	1/150
40	1/100
41	1/85
42	1/65
43	1/50
44	1/40
45+	1/25

* Approximate (rounded) estimates chiefly from data of Hook EB: Rates of chromosome abnormalities at different maternal ages. *Obstet Gynecol* 1981; 58:282-285.
(Modified from Thompson and Thompson, 1986, p 121.)

Disorders of Sex Chromosomes

Compared with autosomal disorders, alterations in the sex chromosomes are more common and affect the individual less severely. Unless detected by neonatal screening, a sex chromosome defect may not be diagnosed until early adolescence when secondary sexual characteristics may be slow or fail to develop, or until fertility problems arise (Cohen, 1984). A chromosome analysis is performed as a basis for genetic counseling and treatment.

Klinefelter Syndrome

Klinefelter syndrome is the most common of the sex chromosome disorders, with a chromosomal constitution (genotype) of 47,XXY. The child born with this syndrome is considered a male because of the presence of the Y chromosome (in the absence of the Y chromosome, the child would develop as a female). It is important to note that the presence of the extra X chromosome does *not* imply any tendency toward homosexuality (Cohen, 1984).

Most affected men can lead normal lives and may not be diagnosed until they seek treatment for infertility (Hirschhorn, 1987). Not all men with Klinefelter syndrome are sterile, however, and some can produce normal offspring. Affected males do share certain physical characteristics, notably, tall stature, sparse facial and pubic hair, enlarged breasts (gynecomastia), and small testes. The potential for and severity of mental retardation increases with the number of additional X chromosomes present.

Turner Syndrome

The majority of females with Turner syndrome have a single X chromosome (instead of the normal XX), resulting in a genotype of 45,X (or 45,XO, with O representing the missing chromosome). It is estimated that the number of girls born with Turner syndrome represents only 5 per cent or fewer of those conceived (Hirschhorn, 1987). The other 95 per cent of pregnancies of this chromosomal constitution (genotype) end in spontaneous abortion.

The missing X chromosome has significant implications for normal sexual development. Occasionally called "the syndrome of sexual infantilism," Turner syndrome is characterized by short stature, failure to develop secondary sexual characteristics, incomplete development of ovaries, and infertility (Thompson and Thompson, 1986). Intelligence is usually normal although there may be associated specific learning disabilities. The newborn infant may have a low hair line, a webbed neck, a heart defect, and puffiness (lymph-

Table 4-4. Major Clinical Features of the Three Most Common Autosomal Trisomic Syndromes

Characteristic Features	Trisomy 21	Trisomy 18	Trisomy 13
General	Mental retardation; hypotonia	Mental retardation; hypertonia; failure to thrive; preponderance of females; low birthweight	Mental retardation; failure to thrive; capillary hemangiomas; increased nuclear projections in neutrophils; persistent fetal hemoglobin; seizures; apneic episodes
Craniofacies	Flat occiput; oblique palpebral fissures; epicanthic folds; speckled irides (Brushfield spots); protruding tongue; prominent, malformed ears; flat nasal bridge	Prominent occiput; small features; micrognathia; low-set, malformed ears	Microcephaly; cleft lip ± palate; midline scalp defects; microphthalmia; colobomata; low-set malformed ears; apparent deafness
Thorax	Congenital heart disease, mainly septal defects, especially of the endocardial cushion	Congenital heart disease, mainly VSD* and PDA*; short sternum; diaphragmatic hernia	Congenital heart disease, mainly septal defects, PDA
Abdomen and pelvis	Decreased acetabular and iliac angles; small penis; cryptorchidism	Horseshoe kidney; small pelvis; cryptorchidism; limited hip abduction; inguinal or umbilical hernia	Polycystic kidneys, bicornuate uterus; cryptorchidism
Hands and feet	Simian crease; short, broad hands; hypoplasia of middle phalanx of 5th finger; gap between 1st and 2nd toes	Flexion deformity of fingers; short dorsiflexed big toes; rockerbottom feet or equinovarus; phocomelia (rare)	Polydactyly; hyperconvex or hypoplastic fingernails; simian crease
Other features observed with significant frequency	High-arched palate; strabismus; broad, short neck; small teeth; furrowed tongue; intestinal atresia; imperforate anus; Hirschsprung disease	Cleft lip ± palate; ocular anomalies; simian crease; hypoplasia of fingernails; widely spaced nipples; webbed neck; single umbilical artery; tracheoesophageal fistula	Flexion deformity of fingers; single umbilical artery; shallow supraorbital ridges; micrognathia; retroflexible thumb; rockerbottom feet; omphalocele

* VSD = ventricular defect; PDA = patent ductus arteriosus.
(From Hirschhorn, 1987.)

edema) of the hands and feet. The nurse can be instrumental in obtaining cytogenetic studies that will confirm the diagnosis. Estrogen therapy may be instituted in the early teen years to produce some breast enlargement, increased pubic hair growth, and initiation of menstruation. However, infertility remains. Growth hormone is being used experimentally to increase the predicted adult height of about 5 feet. The parents will need genetic counseling concerning the risk of recurrence.

Fragile X Syndrome

Fragile X syndrome falls into a category of heritable diseases in which the X chromosome has a fragile site at the tip of the long arm. The fragile site appears very thin and extended compared with the rest of the chromosome. It results in a syndrome characterized by nonspecific mental retardation (in about 80 per cent of males), large testes, large protuberant ears, a prominent chin, and a jocular (joking) speech defect (Thompson and Thompson, 1986). Fragile X syndrome accounts for up to 30 per cent of X-linked mental retardation in males and up to 10 per cent of all mild mental retardation in females. In frequency it is second only to Down syndrome in males (Hirschhorn, 1987). Carrier females are either of normal intelligence or are less severely retarded than males because they have one normal X chromosome as well as the defective X.

Single Gene Disorders

Principles of Mendelian Inheritance

Since our chromosomes come in pairs (one from our father, one from our mother), our genes, which make up the chromosomes, come in pairs. Within a pair of genes for the same trait only one gene is normally expressed. The gene that is manifested is referred to as *dominant.* The other gene, which is present but not expressed, is termed *recessive* (expressed only when no dominant gene is present on either chromosome) (Thompson and Thompson, 1986). For illustrative purposes, let's assume eye color is determined by one pair of genes and brown is dominant over blue. If the

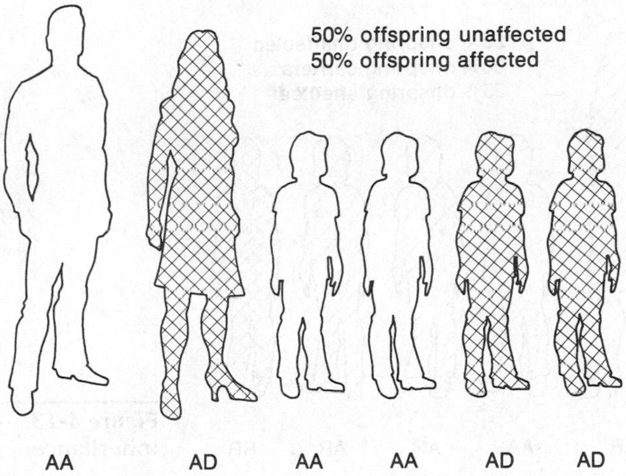

Figure 4-12. Pattern of dominant inheritance.

gene pair (genotype) for eye color contains one gene for blue and one for brown, the child will have brown eyes. For a recessive trait such as blue eyes to be expressed, both genes of the gene pair must be identical or *homozygous*: for example, two genes for blue eyes. When dissimilar genes appear in the genotype (e.g., one gene for blue eyes and one for brown) the individual is said to be *heterozygous* for that trait.

Replication of DNA

At conception, the *zygote* (fertilized ovum) is a single cell. Miraculously, this one cell contains all the genetic information necessary to form a new human life. For the fetus to develop normally, however, exact replication of DNA is required. If an error in DNA replication occurs in development of the sperm or the ovum (meiosis) or during the multiplication of cells of the zygote (mitosis), genetic alterations may be evident in the child.

In some cases mutations are beneficial because they enhance adaptation to a unique environment. It has been found that persons who carry one abnormal gene that codes for sickle cell (i.e., a carrier for the disease) have increased resistance to malaria. Most genetic mutations, however, result in disease or death.

Dominant Disorders

One abnormal, dominant gene can cause a genetic syndrome. A mutation, or change, in one gene in meiosis (formation of the gamete) or in mitosis of the first few divisions of the zygote can cause abnormalities to occur. New mutations occur with increasing frequency with advanced paternal age. Individuals who have a disease caused by one abnormal dominant gene have a 50 per cent risk of passing it to their children (Fig. 4-12). Diseases caused by dominant genes are seen in both males and females. Dominant genes have a great variability (are expressed in various ways) in different individuals even within the same family. For example, in neurofibromatosis one person may have only 6 or 7 café-au-lait (the color of coffee and cream) spots on the skin, while the child or parent of that person could be mentally retarded, have a seizure disorder and deafness, and many skin lesions. Examples of dominant disorders include achondroplastic dwarfism, tuberous sclerosis, polydactyly, Huntington disease, and Marfan syndrome (see Table 4-1).

Marfan syndrome, a genetic disease of connective tissue, is an example of a syndrome that produces a variety of seemingly unrelated signs and symptoms. The nurse should be alert for the possibility of Marfan syndrome in the young adolescent who stands taller than family and peers, is abnormally thin, has long slender fingers and hands, wears corrective lenses, and has associated cardiac defects. This syndrome is a single gene, autosomal dominant disorder. Therefore, there is a 50 per cent chance that an affected parent will pass the disease to offspring. Abraham Lincoln is thought by many geneticists to have had Marfan syndrome.

Recessive Disorders

In recessive disorders both parents may appear normal but still carry the recessive gene. The parent's normal gene on the matching chromosome does the necessary work. If the child receives an abnormal recessive gene from each parent, the child has no normal gene to do the work. If both parents carry the *same* abnormal recessive gene, they have a 25 per cent risk of having a child with the disease, a 50 per cent chance of having a child who is a carrier, and a 25 per cent chance of having a child who does not have the disease and is not a carrier (Fig. 4-13).* It is necessary for both parents to carry the *same* abnormal recessive gene to have a child with a recessive disorder. It is more likely that a couple

* This risk is the same for *each* pregnancy.

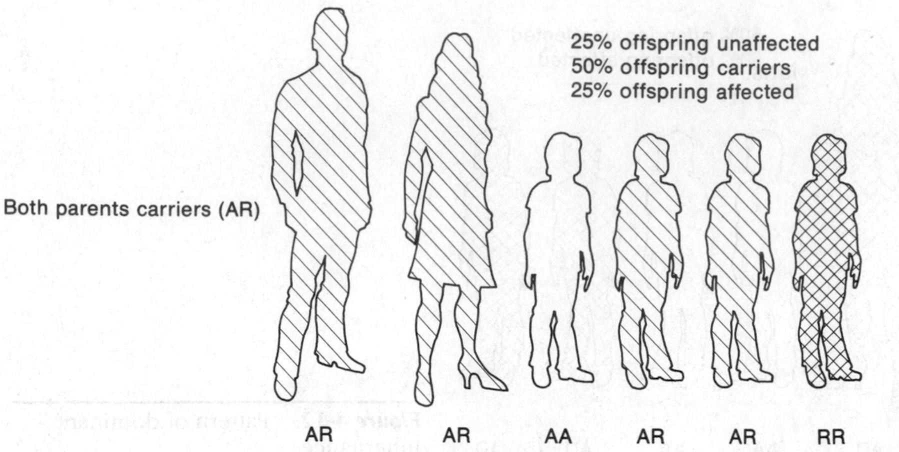

***Figure* 4-13.** Pattern of recessive inheritance.

will carry the *same* abnormal gene if they are related. Therefore, a union between related (consanguineous) people is more likely to produce children with recessive disorders than is a union of nonrelated people. Both males and females have disorders caused by recessive genes and some diseases are seen in higher frequencies in specific populations. Examples of recessive disorders include cystic fibrosis (Caucasian), sickle cell anemia (black), phenylketonuria (Australian), and galactosemia and albinism (all populations) (see Table 4-1).

Cystic fibrosis is one of the most common diseases caused by recessive genes, occuring in about 1 in 2000 births. Individuals with cystic fibrosis have abnormally thick mucous secretions in the pancreas and bronchial tree. They require extensive home care to prevent pneumonia due to the thick bronchial mucus and require dietary supplementation and medical management related to the abnormal pancreatic function.

Sex-Linked Recessive Disorders

Some disorders are caused by a recessive gene on the X chromosome (Fig. 4-14). A female can have one abnormal gene and not show any evidence of disease since she has another X chromosome with a normal gene to do the work. However, if she gives her son the X with the abnormal gene, he will be affected with the disorder since his other sex chromosome is a Y from the father, and that leaves him with no normal gene to do the work. If a woman carries an abnormal gene on her X chromosome, she has a 50 per cent chance to pass it on to her son, who will be affected, and a 50 per cent chance to pass it to her daughter, who will be a carrier. In X-linked disorders, females are carriers and males are usually affected. (Rare exceptions occur.) Examples of X-linked disorders include hemophilia, color blindness, and Duchenne muscular dystrophy (see Table 4-1).

Gene Mutation Leading to Enzyme Deficiency

Many inherited disorders, while classified as dominant, recessive, or sex-linked, are understood to be the result of specific mutant genes. Each gene controls the formation of a specific single protein and its metabolic reaction. This "one gene/one enzyme" principle means that every metabolic process is regulated by an enzyme (or enzyme substrate) and controlled by a specific gene. An absence or deficiency of the enzyme can produce specific defects in the individual.

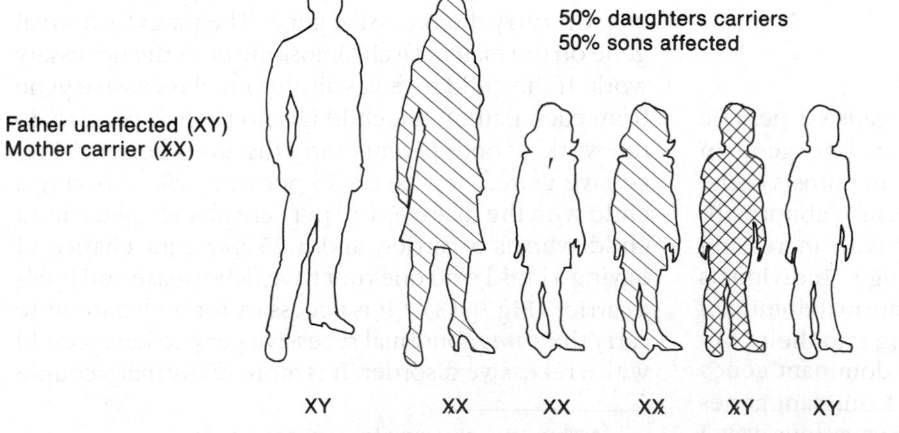

***Figure* 4-14.** Pattern of X-linked inheritance.

The most common and best known of these disorders is *PKU* (phenylketonuria), a recessive disorder affecting one in every 10,000 to 20,000 Caucasians. The genetic defect in this disorder is an absence or deficiency of the enzyme phenylalanine hydroxylase, which is needed to metabolize the essential amino acid phenylalanine. In this disorder excessive amounts of phenylpyruvic acid accumulate in the blood, tissues, and urine, which can lead to severe mental retardation if left untreated. Although a diet low in phenylalanine cannot reverse existing brain damage, it can limit further progression. If an infant is placed on the diet soon after birth, intelligence can be normal. (See Chapter 50 for a complete discussion of PKU.)

Whether the odds or estimates of risk for passing on a disorder are made from knowledge that a certain syndrome or birth defect is dominant, recessive, or sex-linked or are the conclusion from analysis of a family tree (pedigree), the risks hold true for *each* pregnancy. When an affected child is born, the parents cannot assume either that no other children will have the disorder or that all successive children will be affected.

Multifactorial Disorders

A large number of birth defects and genetic disorders cannot be classified in strict mendelian patterns of inheritance or by chromosomal aberrations. Many disorders are caused by the *combined influence* of each child's specific genetic makeup and a variety of environmental factors, such as the mother's pregnancy, the health status and ages of the parents, exposure to infectious disease, and environmental hazards like radiation and pollutants. This combined influence of genetic and environmental factors is termed *multifactorial*, or *polygenic*.

It is not known how many of the genetic disorders are a result of multifactorial inheritance, but some of the more common anomalies attributed to this category include neural tube defects (spina bifida and anencephaly) (Ch. 46), clubfoot and congenital hip dislocation (Ch. 47), pyloric stenosis and cleft lip/palate (Ch. 41), and many congenital heart defects (Ch. 39). These and other multifactorial disorders tend to recur in families. ***It is important to recognize that the risk for recurrence of a multifactorial genetic disorder is higher when more than one family member is affected.*** This is in contrast to single gene disorders in which the risk for affected children remains the same for every pregnancy regardless of the number of family members who display that genotype. For example, the risk for cystic fibrosis, with two carrier parents, remains at 25 per cent for each pregnancy, but for the family who has a child with spina bifida the risk for another affected child increases from 1/2000 (for the general population) to 1/40 (March of Dimes, 1985). A second child born with spina bifida will double the parents' risk that a third will be born with a neural tube disorder (defect of the spine and/or brain).

Determining the Need for Genetic Counseling

The Family History

The family history can indicate two major categories of information pertinent to genetic assessment: (1) genetic disorders that have occurred within that family in recent generations, and (2) evidence of environmental hazards that could lead to or contribute to alterations in genetic makeup. Box 4-2 contains examples of questions that may be used to elicit information about hereditary and environmental factors. Important information includes any family member with learning difficulties or physical abnormalities. Histories of stillbirths, miscarriages, or infertility can give important clues. Many first-trimester spontaneous abortions are due to chromosomal imbalances. Infertility may be caused by a sex chromosome disorder. In other cases, a person may have a translocation that causes severe chromosome imbalances in the embryo, leading to miscarriage within days after conception. Diseases known to recur in families, such as high blood pressure, diabetes, and cancer, should be ascertained in a complete family history.

The Family Pedigree

History-taking and pedigree-taking skills can promote an understanding of how genetic information relates to a comprehensive family health assessment. The pedigree includes medical, health, social, and ethnic background information about the patient and the family (Box 4-3). First-degree relatives (i.e., parents, siblings and children) and second-degree relatives such as grandparents, aunts, uncles, nephews, and nieces are usually included. The family may have an informal historian, perhaps a grandparent, who can supplement information provided by the parent and child. When combined with the objective data from physical assessment of the child, the subjective information gained in the family genetic history and the resulting pedigree chart will provide the basis for decisions regarding the family's need for genetic counseling.

Physical Examination of the Child

Box 4-4 details a protocol for genetic assessment during physical examination of the child. The nurse

Text continued on page 156

Box 4-2
Examples of Questions to Be Included in the Genetic Family History

Questions Pertaining to Familial Hereditary Factors

"Are all the members of your immediate family—grandparents, parents, aunts, uncles, brothers, sisters, and cousins—living and well?"

"Do you know of anyone in your family who has (or had) a birth defect of any kind?"

"Was anyone in your family born with a heart defect?"

"Is there anyone in your family who is considered very different from the other family members in appearance or in health status?"

"What is your ethnic origin?"

Questions Pertaining to Environmental Factors

"Are you often exposed to radiation, temperature extremes, chemicals, pesticides, animal wastes, microorganisms, or air pollutants?"

"How often do you take over-the-counter medications such as vitamins, minerals, diet or sleep aids, cold and cough formulas, and pain relievers?"

"Do you take any prescription medications?"

"Have you ever used street drugs?"

"Do you smoke tobacco or drink beer, wine, or mixed alcoholic drinks? If so, how much/how often?"

"Are you (or is anyone in your family) allergic to any foods?"

Box 4-3
Protocol for Genetic Assessment: The Health History and Family Pedigree

THE HEALTH HISTORY

Information specific to genetic assessment can be collected during any health history. Genetic assessment requires, however, that the nurse obtain specific information about disease conditions. For instance, if the family reports a history of heart disease, a number of specific questions are to be asked, such as, "When was the problem diagnosed?" "Was surgery required?" "What is the current health status of the affected person?" These questions can help the clinician distinguish between a birth defect, such as congenital heart disease, and an acquired health problem, such as coronary artery disease.

Often during the interview, the family will volunteer much more information than appears to be useful for construction of the pedigree. Some of the more common diseases they disclose can be selectively chosen for inclusion in the pedigree. The remaining problems and concerns can be noted in a summary statement accompanying the completed pedigree. Finally, the nurse should keep in mind that the family may feel that their information is considered important only when the nurse is writing or recording it. Therefore, notekeeping should be consistent throughout the interview process. Ideally, each family member should be given the chance to present personal information in private. Personal information such as the history of an elective termination of a pregnancy or paternity may arise, and while nurses can explore whether or not other family members know this information, they must respect the individual's right to confidentiality.

When there is little time for information gathering, such as after the birth of a child with multiple congenital problems or a syndrome requiring immediate surgery, history taking can be accomplished in stages. The questions can be tailored to focus on the immediate problem, while other areas of inquiry can be postponed. This initial interview process can serve to establish rapport and trust, while at the same time helping the family focus on the particular problem at hand. Once the immediate crisis has been attended to, the nurse can complete the assessment process.

PEDIGREE CONSTRUCTION

After the data have been gathered from the interview and organized, construction of an actual pedigree can begin in collaboration with the genetics specialist. The symbols used in the pedigree may vary slightly, but basically they are uniform in the United States. The figure on the next page lists the most commonly used symbols. The pedigree represents a diagrammatic drawing of the family health history at a glance. Patterns of inherited disorders and affected and at-risk relatives can be noted. The nurse can begin to construct a pedigree from information available in the medical record.

Basic guidelines to be used in the construction of a pedigree:

- Identify one person to be studied as the index case (proband).
- The consultand (indicated by C) is the individual who seeks counseling. The proband (indicated by an arrow) is the most immediate family member affected. An affected child is usually the proband.
- Locate the male partner on the left of the mating line whenever possible.

- Designate birth dates (not current ages) for the proband and for each person designated on the pedigree.
- Previous generations and ancestors are listed at the top of the pedigree. It is seldom necessary or reliable to collect information farther back than three generations (Cohen, 1984; Thompson and Thompson, 1986).
- In general, marriages are represented by a double line between husband and wife (A=O). Maiden names are written in parentheses after first names. They should be noted for the proband or spouse, mother of proband, each affected family member, and at-risk married women. Married names should be noted for each married woman who is affected, is a carrier, or is at risk.
- Siblings (designated by Arabic numerals), stillbirths, and abortions should be arranged in chronologic order, with the oldest on the left.
- Causes of death and/or health problems should be noted for the various family members above or below their respective symbols.

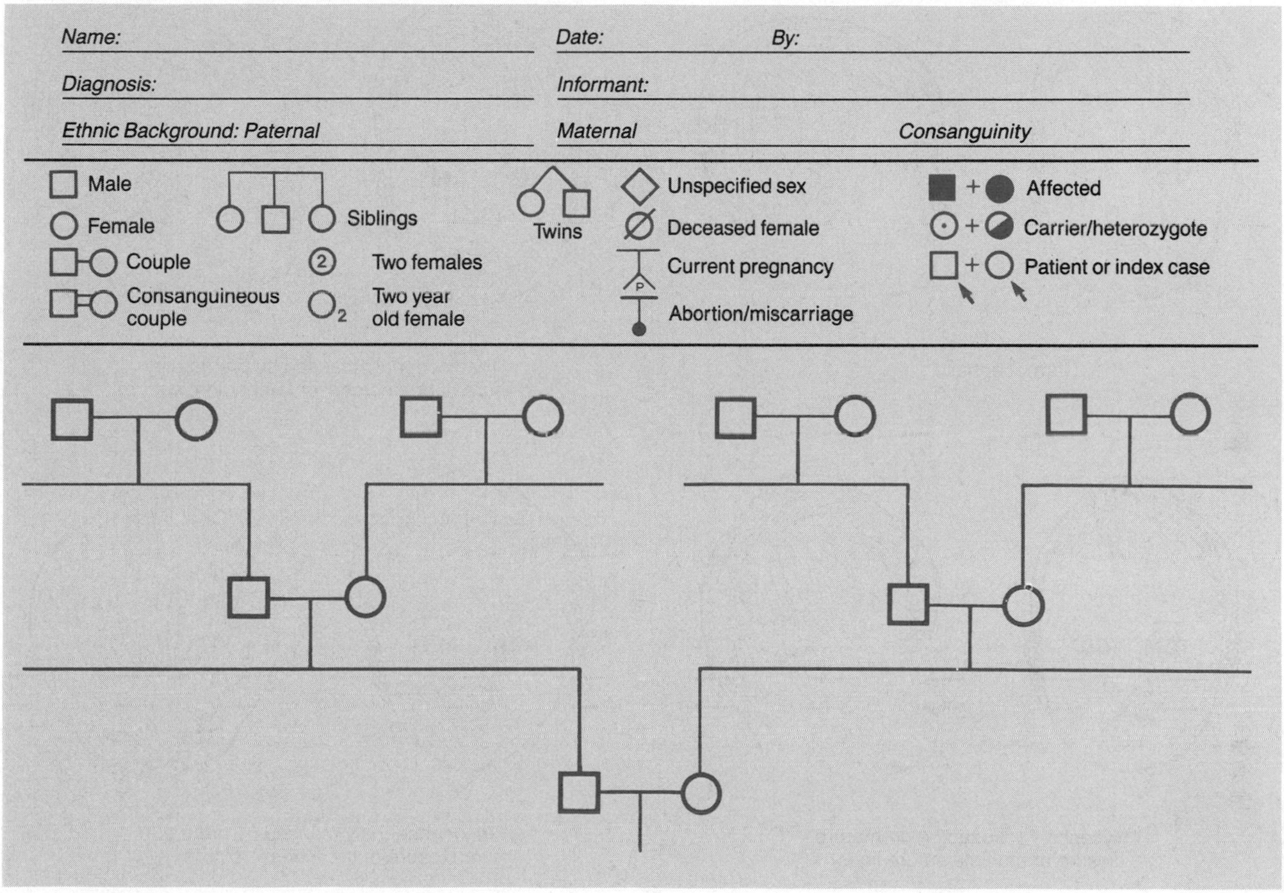

COMMON CONCERNS IN CONSTRUCTING A PEDIGREE

Often during the construction of a personal pedigree, concerns arise as to why the collected data do not explain the presence of what is thought to be a genetic problem or syndrome. A negative family history can result from a new genetic mutation, nonpaternity, adoption, or a trait so rare or minimally expressed that it may be missed in that examination.

Finally, the clinician should remember that family health records, radiographs, and autopsy reports can provide additional information. Even church, school, employment, and military records may yield useful information. No source of possible information is too trivial to pursue. Final interpretation of the pedigree should be done by a clinical geneticist, trained genetic counselor, or genetics nursing specialist. However, the staff or office nurse can use the information-gathering process of pedigree construction as a time to establish rapport and trust with the family. This, in turn, provides a foundation upon which quality nursing care can be built and continued for generations to come.

(Based on Clark et al, J Pediatr Nurs, *in press.)*

Box 4-4

Protocol for Genetic Assessment: Physical Examination of the Child

GENERAL ASSESSMENT

Begin the physical assessment by noting the child's general appearance and any distinctive or unusual odor. If there is anything unusual about the child's general appearance, it is helpful to take body measurements for comparison with established standards. Observe the parent(s) for the same unusual feature or minor anomaly noticed in the child. Although the appearance of the same anomaly in the parent may lessen concerns, it can also be a clue of a dominant inherited trait.

HEAD

The *size* of the head is extremely important because the first two years of the child's life are vital for brain growth. The normal size of a child's head is 34.5 cm at birth to 49 cm by 2 years of age for boys and 34 cm at birth to 48 cm

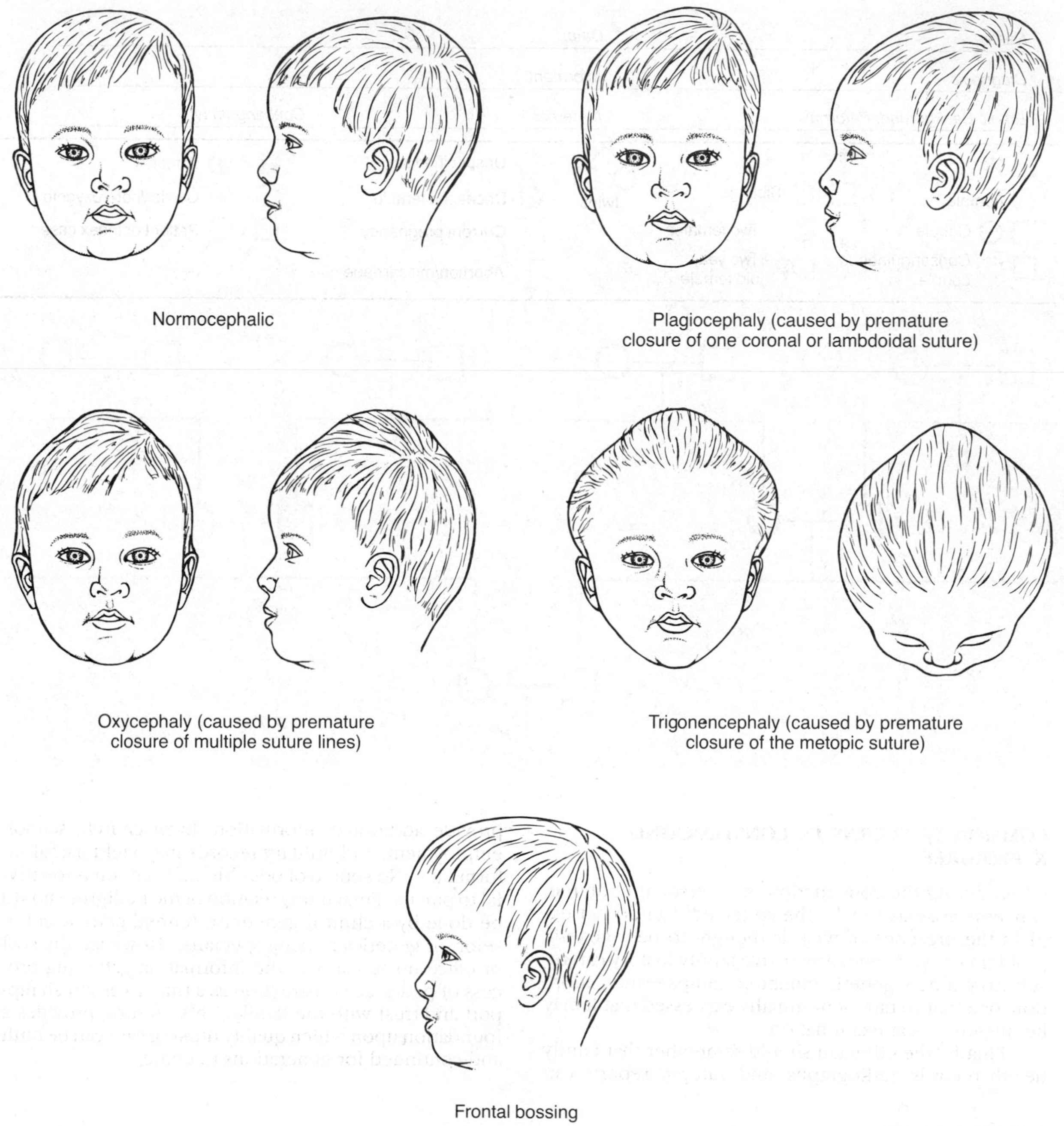

***Figure* 4-15.** Head shapes.

at 2 years of age for girls. A series of measurements is the most useful. Measurements should be taken at the widest circumference of the head.

Among abnormal findings is *microcephaly*, which is the result of limited brain size causing the head to be 2 or more standard deviations below normal parameters. This may be caused by infection, brain trauma, or genetic abnormalities. Brain tissue may be abnormal in some cases. *Macrocephaly* is an increased head size. *Hydrocephaly* is an increase in the amount of cerebrospinal fluid. Macrocephaly with or without hydrocephaly is seen in some genetic syndromes along with other anomalies.

The *shape* of the child's head should be *normocephalic* (Fig. 4-15). Normal closure of fontanels is usually completed between 9 and 19 months. Late closure could indicate cretinism, Down syndrome, rickets, osteogenesis imperfecta, hydrocephalus, or syphilis. An anterior fontanel diameter that measures either two standard deviations above or below 2.1 cm (0.6 and 3.6 cm, respectively) is important. Posterior fontanels rarely exceed measurements of 0.5 cm. *Premature closing of suture lines* is termed craniosynostosis; this disorder is detailed in Chapter 46. A prominent forehead, or *bossing* (Fig. 4-15), is found in several genetic conditions such as Hurler syndrome and fragile X syndrome.

EARS

By drawing an imaginary line from the outside corner of the eye straight back, one can determine whether the ears are set in a normal *position* (Fig. 4-16). The upper part of the *pinna* should meet this line. If it is below the line the ears can be described as low set. The rotation of the ear can be determined by drawing a vertical line from the lobe of the ear straight up crossing the horizontal line. When the angle of the slope of the ear exceeds 10 degrees from the horizontal line, then a definite rotation exists. Abnormally shaped and positioned ears are found in various disorders and should be reported. Check to see whether both ears are at the same level. Do they appear to be protruding? Are they bigger or smaller than normal (Fig. 4-17)? Check the size and complete-

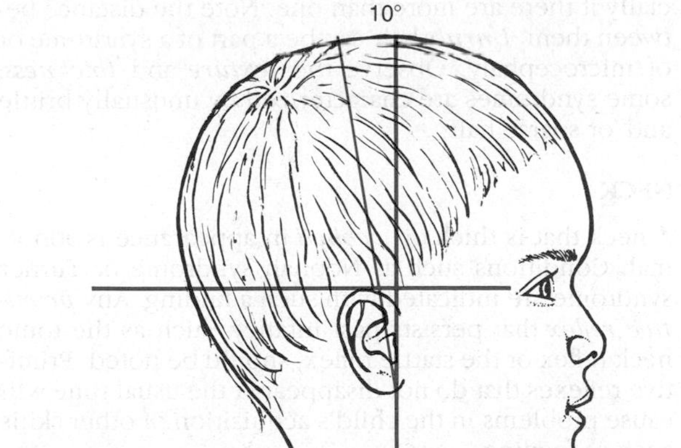

Figure 4-16. Normal placement of the ear.

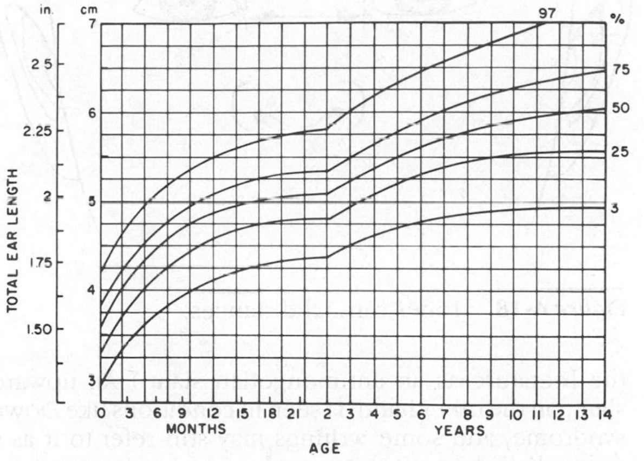

Figure 4-17. Maximum ear length. (From Feingold M, Bossert WH: Normal values for selected physical parameters. *Birth Defects* 1974: 10(13):1-16.)

ness of ear *lobes.* Check for sinuses or tags of skin on the ears. Children with fragile X syndrome have ears longer in length than normal and they are often posteriorly rotated. Hypoplasia of *cartilage* causes ears to be soft and flexible. Practice looking at ears of your colleagues closely so that you can recognize minor anomalies of structure and placement.

FACE

Observe for *spacing* of features, *symmetry*, and signs of *weakness* or *paralysis.* The normal *width* of a newborn infant's face is approximately 8 cm. Children with fragile X syndrome have long, thin, narrow facies and midface hypoplasia (flattening of cheekbones). Many genetic syndromes are associated with asymmetry of the face. Some are due to structure, as in hemifacial microsomia, and some are due to unbalanced movements of musculature, as in Moebius syndrome (maldevelopment of cranial nerves).

Eyes

Normally, eyes are the same *level* and are within standardized measurements for *space* between the eyes (Fig. 4-18). *Hypertelorism* of the eyes refers to wide-spaced orbits and is often associated with some syndromes of mental retardation. The mean distance between inner canthi for term infants is 2 cm. A distance of 3 cm is associated with hypertelorism. *Hypotelorism* is defined as abnormally close-set eyes. This may be associated with the lack of a nasal bridge, or trigonocephaly. *Microphthalmia* (moderate-to-severe reduction in eye size) may indicate encephalo-ophthalmic dysplasia, toxoplasmosis, or retrolental fibroplasia. A *protruding supraorbital ridge* is found in conditions such as mucopolysaccharidosis and Marfan disease. *Ptosis of the lids* (incomplete opening of the eyelids) may indicate some neurologic problems such as myasthenia gravis, but may also be an inherited trait. *Slant of the eyes,* such as a downward slant, may indicate conditions such as Treacher Collins syndrome. (This is often referred to in

Continued

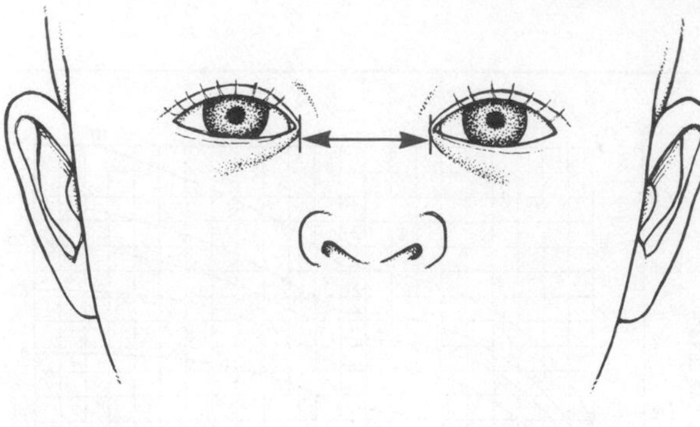

Figure 4-18. Inner canthal distances.

the literature as an antimongolian slant.) An upward slant, on the other hand, is seen in conditions like Down syndrome, and some writings may still refer to it as a mongolian slant.

Epicanthal folds (a vertical fold of skin over the angle of the inner canthus of the eye) may be present as a result of Down syndrome, glycogen storage disease, renal agenesis, or hypercalcemia. The condition may be present in some normal children but most often will disappear by age 10 years. *Synophrys,* which is a midline meeting of the eyebrows, is found in de Lange syndrome and others. Bushy or thick curly *eyelashes* may be found in such disorders as Hurler syndrome. If absent on the inner two thirds of the lid, it may indicate Treacher Collins syndrome.

The color of the *iris* is established by the age of 1 year. Pinkish coloration may indicate albinism. Light or white speckling (Brushfield spots) are found in 80 per cent of children with Down syndrome and 20 per cent of the general population. *Sclerae* with a blue cast are normal in the neonate, but persistence of this characteristic may indicate osteogenesis imperfecta, Russell-Silver syndrome, or other genetic problems. A *lens* with an absent red reflex may indicate cataracts. This condition can also be due to several conditions leading to mental retardation, such as toxoplasmosis. A dislocated lens may be the result of Marfan syndrome or homocystinuria.

Nose

A normally placed nose is found in the middle and upper portion of the face. The *shape* of the nose is important because in many syndromes one sees a great deal of variation. Notice whether the nose is broad and flat, small and up-turned, or sharply pointed. Note whether the nose is straight and whether the *nares* are symmetric. Palpate to examine the *bone* and *cartilage.* Check the *septum* with a penlight to determine whether a perforation exists by shining the light into one naris and observing to see whether the light escapes into the other naris. Occasionally the tip of the nose will have a tiny vertical indentation. Nose shape is usually unremarkable by itself, but an asymmetric nose or a nose not symmetrically placed may be important in combination with other abnormalities.

Mouth

The mouth should be symmetric. Note the *lips* to see whether they are turned down, sag to one side, or are the same size on both sides. Look for tiny dimples or pits. Are there clefts in the lip or *palate*? Drooling starts at about 3 months of age and continues until the child learns to swallow saliva at about 9 to 12 months. Examine the palate for a gentle slope. Report a high arched palate or one that is notched at the junction of the soft and hard palates. Note *micrognathia* (an excessively small lower jaw) or *macrognathia* (a large jaw), which may indicate genetic problems that should be further evaluated. For instance, a prominent jaw is found in many children with fragile X syndrome. *Teeth* that have a delayed eruption past 1 year of age may result from cretinism. *Gums* that are discolored with a dark line along the margin may indicate a high concentration of lead in the child's system. (Do not confuse this with the normal dark pigmentation seen on the gums of black children).

Note the size of the *tongue.* A tongue that appears large for the mouth is found in conditions such as Down syndrome, cretinism, or Hurler syndrome. Tongue protrusion is a common finding in children who are mentally retarded. Note the normal milestones in feeding patterns. It is important to note *reflexes,* such as the rooting, sucking-swallowing, gag, chewing, and bite reflexes. Rooting disappears by 2 months; the sucking-swallowing reflex disappears at approximately 6 months; the gag reflex diminishes after the chewing reflex begins at approximately 7 months; and the bite reflex ceases at about 5 months. *Lip closure* begins at about 6 to 8 months. Facial features are described as coarse if they are broad and fleshy. Always check previous pictures of the individual to see if the features are becoming more coarse, a common sign of metabolic diseases.

HAIR

Some syndromes are noted by hair *distribution* far down on the neck (Fig. 4-19) (Noonan or Turner syndrome) or low down on the forehead (Hurler syndrome). Hair on other parts of the body, such as patches low on the spine, should be reported. *Color* is important because white hair in young people may indicate albinism; a white patch may indicate Waardenburg syndrome. Diets deficient in protein cause reddish or gray color changes in hair. The majority of hair *whorls* are normally located on the left side of the crown in a clockwide rotation (Fig. 4-19). The location of the whorl should be noted, especially if there are more than one. Note the distance between them. *Unruly* hair can be a part of a syndrome or of microcephaly. Observe the *texture* and *thickness*; some syndromes are characterized by unusually brittle and/or sparse hair.

NECK

A neck that is thick or *webbed* in appearance is abnormal. Conditions such as Noonan syndrome or Turner syndrome are indicated with such a finding. Any *primitive reflex* that persists past infancy, such as the tonic neck reflex or the startle reflex, should be noted. Primitive reflexes that do not disappear at the usual time will cause problems in the child's acquisition of other skills such as feeding.

CHEST

The *shape* of the chest should be noted for any irregularities. A protruding *sternum* or a funnel-shaped sternum

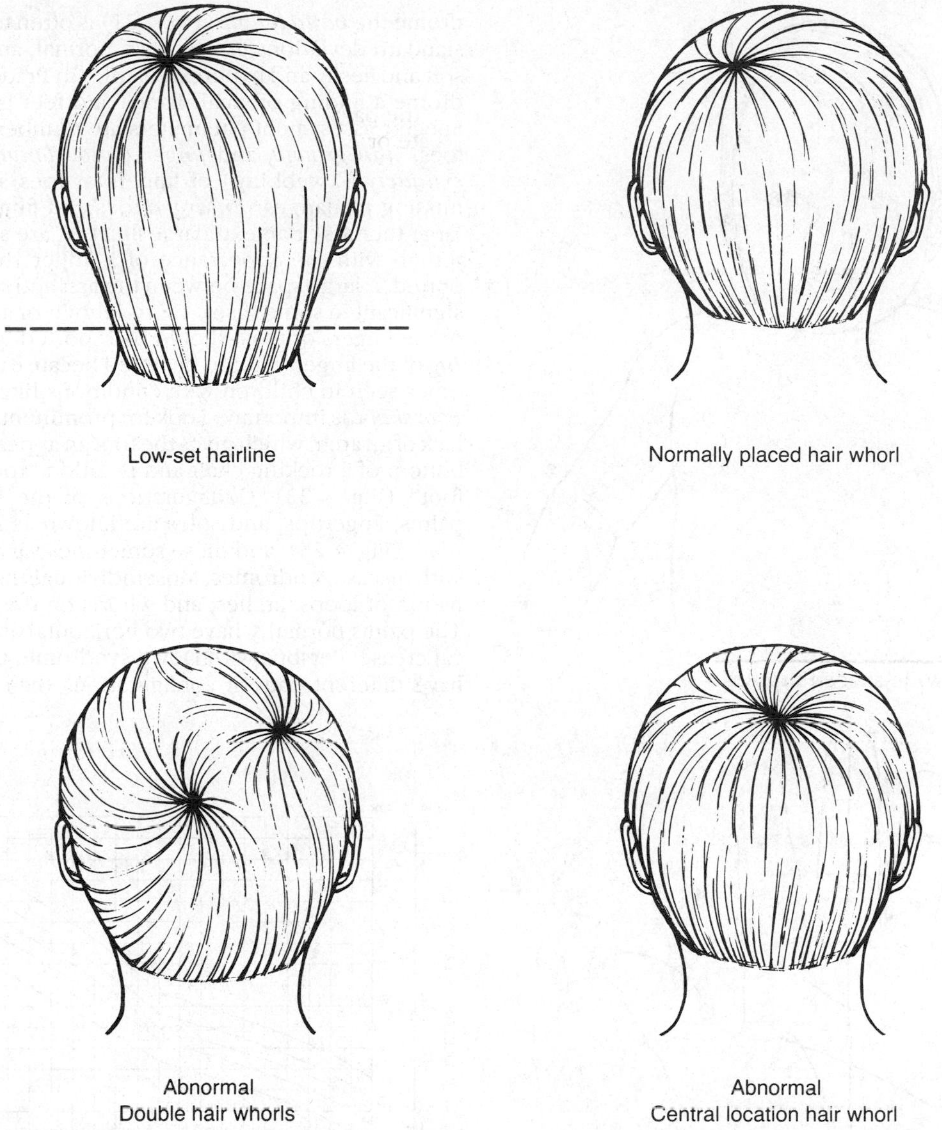

Figure 4-19. Whorls and hairline.

is often seen in Marfan syndrome or Marquio disease. An indentation of the chest is termed pectus excavatum and a protrusion is pectus carinatum. Does the chest seem to "match" the body in proportion? Look at the *nipples* and record whether they are wide set (Fig 4-20) or hypoplastic. Wide-set nipples are determined in infants by using the formula:

$$\frac{\text{Intermamillary distance } (\text{cm} \times 100)}{\text{Circumference}} = \text{Wide set if} > 28 \text{ cm}$$

ABDOMEN AND BACK

In the newborn infant it is important to note the usual presence of two arteries and one vein in the *umbilicus*. An *omphalocele* is a herniation of abdominal viscera into the base of the umbilical cord. It is important to remember that up to one half of children with omphalocele have other defects. Many of these associated defects are related to genetic and developmental factors. Palpate for a large liver and spleen, which may indicate a metabolic disease. A dimpling in the *spine* can be associated with *spina bifida*. The spinal column and *hips* should be evaluated radiologically for defects if dimpling is found.

HEART

Listen for adventitious heart *sounds* or sounds that are irregular, slow, or excessively fast. Many syndromes are accompanied by heart anomalies.

ARMS, LEGS, HANDS, AND FEET

Children with genetic problems often are found to have defects of the extremities. For instance, in fragile X syn-

Continued

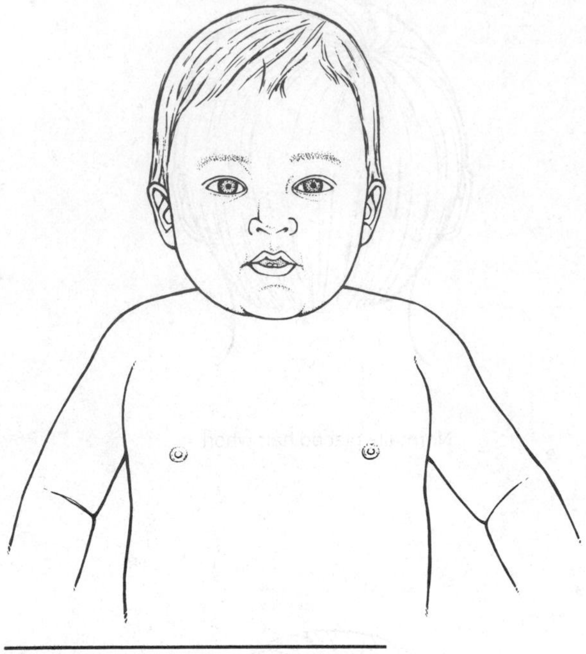

Figure 4-20. Wide-spaced nipples.

drome the *hand length* (Fig. 4-21) is often found to be 2 standard deviations greater than normal, and hands are soft and fleshy and hyperextensible. In Prader-Willi syndrome a finding of small hands and feet is significant. Specific assessment parameters are numbers of fingers, toes, *nail growth*, and *finger or toe length*. Note any *syndactyly* (webbing) of fingers or toes and short or missing phalanges. *Enlarged* toes and fingers, such as large thumbs or an extralarge first toe, are significant. A thumb with the appearance of a finger should be reported. A large space between the first and second toe is significant in some cases. *Clinodactyly,* or an in-curving or the fingers or toes, should be reported. Any *overriding* of the fingers should be noted because this is sometimes seen in children with conditions like trisomy 18. *Foot shape* is important. Look for prominent heels or the lack of an arch, which gives the foot an appearance of the bottom of a rocking chair and is called "rocker bottom foot" (Fig. 4-22). Configurations of the lines in the palms, fingertips, and soles are known as *dermatoglyphics* (Fig. 4-23), and these sometimes vary in children with disease syndromes. Most individuals have a combination of loops, arches, and whorls on their fingertips. The palms normally have two horizontal and one vertical crease. Persons with Down syndrome, in particular, have different pattern configurations than the normal

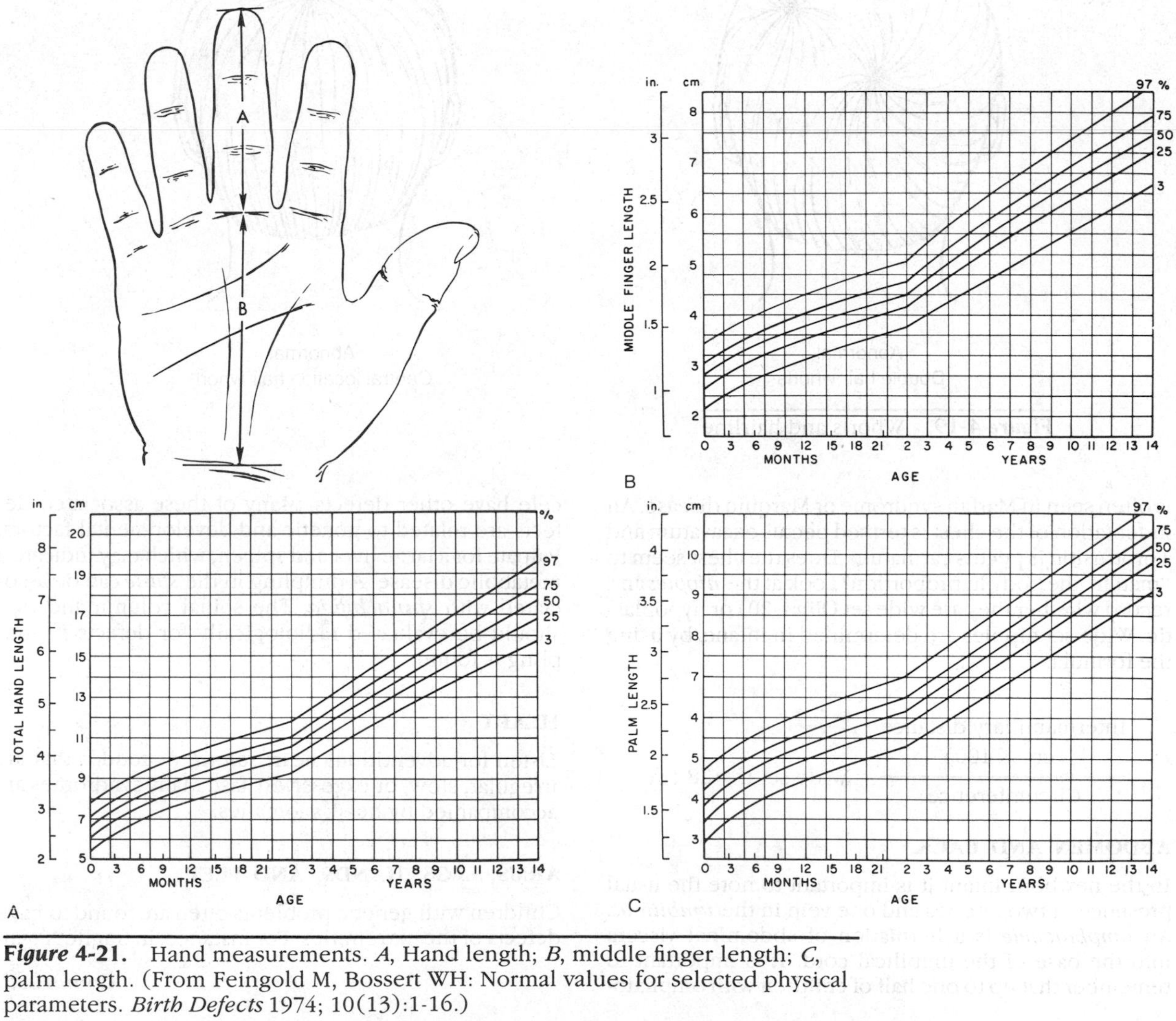

Figure 4-21. Hand measurements. *A*, Hand length; *B*, middle finger length; *C*, palm length. (From Feingold M, Bossert WH: Normal values for selected physical parameters. *Birth Defects* 1974; 10(13):1-16.)

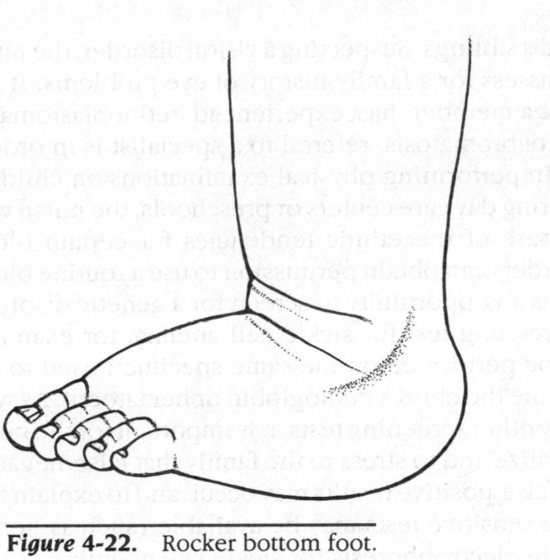

Figure 4-22. Rocker bottom foot.

population. An increased *carrying angle* of the *elbows* (Fig. 4-24) should alert the nurse to the possibility of conditions such as Klinefelter syndrome in males or other genetic conditions that are found in females as well.

GENITALIA

Observe for *hypospadias* (an abnormal placement of the urethral opening), *position*, and *size* of the *penis*. A small penis is a minor anomaly seen in many syndromes. Check to see whether the *testes* are descended and that the *scrotum* is placed normally and is of normal size. (Several companies sell models that can help estimate testicular volume.)

In girls, observe for hypoplastic *labia* or an enlarged *clitoris*. In some syndromes the genitalia are ambiguous and it is necessary to perform an emergency chromosome study to determine gender. Assess for signs of *puberty*. It is important to note any deviations in the development of genitalia when associated with normal milestones. Growth occurring too *early* may indicate endocrine problems. *Missing* secondary sexual characteristics may be the result of genetic defects such as Klinefelter or Turner syndrome. In young boys, abnormal genital *enlargement* often may be the result of neurogenic or idiopathic sexual precocity. After puberty, significantly enlarged testes in males may be the result of fragile X syndrome.

SKIN

Lack of *pigment* or increased pigmentation can indicate disease syndromes, and unusual colors like yellow or blue can indicate illness. Observe skin for color consistent with genetic heritage. Observe for symmetry of color. Look for spots on the skin (white, light brown, and red) and record the location, size, regularity of

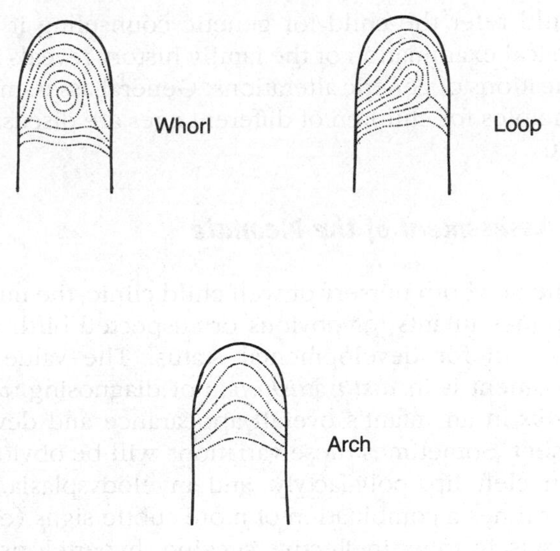

Figure 4-23. Fingertip dermatoglyphics.

border, texture, and whether or not they are raised. Determine by observation or history whether the person's *perspiration* is normal. Too much or too little sweating is characteristic of some genetic syndromes. Abnormal *odor* of the sweat can indicate a metabolic syndrome. A reported salty *taste* to the perspiration is characteristic of cystic fibrosis.

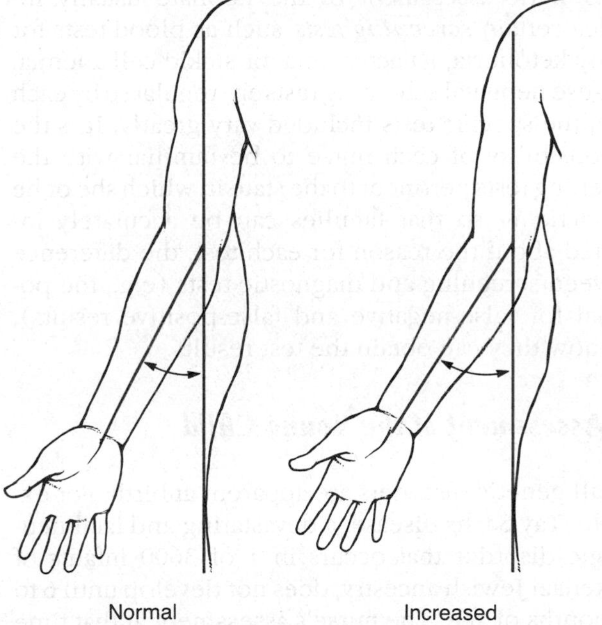

Figure 4-24. Carrying angle of the elbows.

By Peggy Drapo, RN, PhD, and Becky Althaus, RN, MS.

We thank the Genetics Screening and Counseling Service, Texas Department of Mental Health and Mental Retardation, Denton, for all illustrations used in this box, except Figures 4-19 and 4-23.

should refer the child for genetic counseling if the physical examination or the family history reveals any indications of genetic alterations. General assessment principles for children of different ages are discussed next.

Assessment of the Neonate

In the newborn nursery or well child clinic, the nurse examines infants for obvious or suspected birth defects and for developmental status. The value of assessment is in *distinguishing*, not diagnosing, *variations* in an infant's overall appearance and development. Sometimes these variations will be obvious, as in cleft lip, polydactyly, and myelodysplasia. At other times a combination of more subtle signs (e.g., lax muscle tone, ineffective sucking, hypertelorism) leads the nurse to request further genetic evaluation. Whereas one minor birth defect will be found in about 13 per cent of otherwise normal infants, fewer than 1 per cent will have two anomalies (Cohen, 1984). *Therefore, the presence of two or more anomalies, however minor, should alert the nurse to the potential for more serious genetic alterations and to the possible need for genetic counseling.* The opportunity for early detection of genetic disorders can sometimes reduce the severity by providing timely treatment.

Genetic assessment of the neonate usually includes certain *screening tests*, such as blood tests for phenylketonuria, galactosemia, or sickle cell anemia. Because neonatal screening tests are regulated by each state, the specific tests included vary greatly. It is the responsibility of each nurse to be familiar with the screening tests pertinent to the state in which she or he is practicing so that families can be accurately informed about the reason for each test, the difference between screening and diagnostic tests (e.g., the potential for false-negative and false-positive results), and how they can obtain the test results.

Assessment of the Young Child

Not all genetic disorders are apparent at birth. For example, Tay-Sachs disease, a devastating and fatal neurologic disorder that occurs in 1 of 3600 infants of Ashkenazi Jewish ancestry, does not develop until 6 to 12 months of age. The nurse's assessment at that time may reveal a discrepancy with the growth chart standards for height and weight and delay in meeting developmental tasks.

Community health nurses and office nurses routinely screen preschool and young elementary school children for hearing and vision disorders. Knowing that about 50 per cent of all hearing disorders are hereditary, the nurse can initiate screening for an affected child's siblings. Suspecting a vision disorder, the nurse can assess for a family history of eye problems. If any family member has experienced retinoblastoma or neurofibromatosis, referral to a specialist is in order.

In performing physical examinations on children entering day care centers or preschools, the nurse who is aware of the ethnic tendencies for certain blood disorders can obtain permission to use a routine blood test as an opportunity to screen for a genetic disorder. A screening test for sickle cell anemia, for example, can be performed on the same specimen used to determine the child's hemoglobin or hematocrit. As with many other screening tests, it is important for the nurse to realize and to stress to the family that false-negative and false-positive results may occur, and to explain that more sensitive tests may be available (such as hemoglobin electrophoresis for sickle cell anemia).

When the nurse assesses a child's growth and development, both developmental achievements and delays are noted. Although only about 5 per cent of mental retardation and developmental disabilities have a genetic origin, those genetic disorders have profound effects upon the child's future physical and cognitive development. Disorders such as PKU, galactosemia, hypothyroidism, and homocystinuria can result in severe mental retardation unless detected and treated soon after birth. Others, such as trisomy 18, trisomy 21 and fragile X syndrome result in varying degrees of mental retardation and developmental delay.

Assessment of School-Age Children and Adolescents

Two of the more common genetic disorders that may become manifest in the young school-age child are *cystic fibrosis* (although this may be diagnosed in the neonate) and *Duchenne muscular dystrophy*. Clinical manifestations of these disorders and the impact of these chronic diseases upon children and their families are discussed in Chapters 38 and 47, respectively.

Insulin-dependent diabetes mellitus (IDDM) usually has its onset in persons under 20 years of age. Although the inherited tendency for diabetes to occur in families seems unquestioned, the mode of inheritance and a specific gene have not been identified. Health professionals aware of one family member with diabetes need to offer screening and information to siblings and first-degree relatives who are also at risk. (See Chapter 49 for further information about IDDM.)

As discussed previously, Klinefelter syndrome and Turner syndrome may not become evident until early adolescence. These and other *sex chromosome disorders* may show problems of menstrual irregularity, lack of secondary sexual characteristics, and impotence.

Box 4-5
Indications for Genetic Referral

Family history of genetic disease
Any abnormality affecting more than one family member
Major congenital anomalies or the occurrence of two or more minor anomalies in the same child
Unexplained delays in growth or disproportionate growth
Unexplained delays in physical, cognitive, or sexual development
Blindness or deafness
Familial occurrence of neoplasms
Consideration of marriage to a blood relative
Women exposed to radiation, infectious diseases, toxic agents, or potent drugs immediately before or during pregnancy
Men who are planning fatherhood and have been exposed to radiation, toxic agents, or potent drugs
Members of ethnic groups in which certain genetic disorders are frequent and where appropriate screening or prenatal diagnosis exists for the disorder
Unexpected reactions to drugs or anesthesia

(Compiled from Cohen, 1984.)

Making the Referral

Indications for genetic referral are summarized in Box 4-5. If in doubt about the appropriateness of a referral, the nurse can contact the genetic counselor or genetic nursing specialist to discuss concerns. It is important to note that genetic referral need not be made by the physician; *nurses can and should refer clients for genetic counseling* when there is reason to suspect genetic alterations. Qualified genetic counselors can be located through the local chapter of the March of Dimes, the American Board of Medical Genetics (which certifies genetic counselors), the National Society of Genetic Counselors, the schools of nursing or medicine at a local university, health professionals at specialty clinics, or the state public health department.

The Process of Genetic Counseling

Genetic counseling is a new specialty that has arisen in the last 20 years; it provides an interpretation of medical information about the risk of occurrence and recurrence of suspected or known genetic disorders within a family. The nurse prepared as a genetic counselor practices prevention, counseling, and education, as well as intervention.

The genetic counseling process hopes to fulfill the following objectives:

- **Provide medical data.** Most genetic disorders occur in frequencies less than 1 in 5000. The genetics personnel must provide the family with information concerning the health maintenance and prognosis of an individual diagnosed with a genetic disease.
- **Provide recurrence risk.** The parents' chances of having another child with the same disorder are described and illustrated. The risks of the parents' siblings, the affected child's siblings, and the affected child having children with similar problems are also included.
- **Discuss options.** These include prenatal diagnosis, adoption, taking their chances, artificial insemination by donor, having no more children, and carrier detection. Of course, these vary according to the methods of inheritance that apply to a particular family.
- **Provide support and referral to community resources.**

Genetic counseling is usually intended to be nondirective; that is, facts and options are presented in order that the persons involved can make an informed decision. In nondirective counseling the counselor's personal values should not influence the decision in any way.

The Role of the Nurse Generalist in Support of Families Experiencing Genetic Alterations

Although some nurses may seek additional education and training to become genetic counselors, the great majority of nurses who interact with families experiencing genetic alterations will be nurse generalists.

Families experiencing any health-related crisis with a child need three types of support from nurses: *help in dealing with the feelings evoked by the diagnosis, information, and help in interpreting that information* for its meaning in their daily lives. Families reacting to the possibility of or actual diagnosis of a genetic disorder in a child in particular will need information and emotional support during all three phases: (1) the initial diagnostic phase of the disorder prior to genetic counseling, (2) the process of decision making with regard to future pregnancies, and (3) follow-up care for affected children.

Supporting the Family During the Diagnostic Phase

Whether the diagnosis of a genetic defect occurs at birth or during childhood or adolescence, it can carry with it some particularly harsh realties for the child, the parents, and, often, for siblings and other close relatives. The family must face the fact that this is something that will not ever "go away," something that may involve time-consuming and costly treatments, something that may claim the child's life, something that may affect future children. They deal with feelings of guilt (*whether or not justified*) about having "passed on" a defective gene or about activities during pregnancy that they perceive could have harmed the developing baby. They must tell friends and relatives about the child's diagnosis and deal with the resultant well-meaning, but often unfounded, advice and speculations of cause. They may experience fear, disbelief, guilt, frustration, loneliness, and anger. They may feel "that the joy of becoming parents [or brothers or sisters] is slipping away" (March of Dimes, 1982, p 7).

The skilled and caring nurse can make a difference in the family's ability to work through these initial feelings and to begin to focus upon their role in helping the child develop to full potential. *The nurse's ability to be an effective source of support depends upon previous values clarification with respect to genetic disorders and upon the realization that support at this time is primarily a function of listening and reflecting the family's feelings.*

The Importance of Values Clarification

Values clarification allows nurses to come to terms with personal feelings about genetic disorders and to clarify the attitudes they wish to project to families in their care.* When overwhelmed with technical information and overcome with emotion pertaining to the diagnosis, families tend to take cues from health care professionals as to what the diagnosis "really means." Have no doubt—the personal attitudes of health care professionals in regard to the genetic disorder will be projected, whether verbally or nonverbally. Professionals must consider whether their personal attitudes are appropriate professional attitudes and must take care that personal "discomfort" with a disorder does not become a barrier to their ability to offer therapeutic support. Consider the different attitudes displayed in the following two accounts related by the mothers of children with genetic anomalies:

My husband had gone out briefly to make phone calls when the doctor came in. He started talking before he quite got to my bed and he wouldn't meet my eyes. He just sort of paced around and his voice was real gruff. He said, "Your baby appears to have several birth defects." I don't think I heard the next few sentences but I remember him saying something like, "His brain didn't develop right and he will probably be severely retarded." Then he said we should consider putting him in an institution because we'd never be able to care for him at home. My mind was whirling, I couldn't even comprehend what he was saying; I just kept thinking it must be a mistake—I had seen my son in the delivery room and he looked fine. When I looked up to ask how this could be true, the doctor was gone. I called for my nurse and demanded to see my baby. She said she couldn't bring him in right then because he needed special attention in the nursery. I asked her what was wrong, but she just said I'd have to talk with the doctor about that and she left. The nurses didn't come in much after that, only when they had to and they didn't stay long. I wondered if they were afraid of me—like if they would catch something that would make *their* babies sick.

Dr. J. came in to talk with John and me right after the delivery. He pulled up a chair and asked John to sit down too. He reached out and put his hand on mine and then he said, "Mary and John, the baby has Down syndrome. Let's talk about what that means." I don't remember much of that first discussion but we felt Dr. J's concern for us and we knew he was there for us. The nurses were great too. I had one special nurse—I think they call it a primary nurse—she was there every day. She brought Judy in to us the first time that we saw her after delivery. She asked if one of us would like to hold Judy and I took her. Then she said, "Let's talk first about why they suspected Judy has Down syndrome" and she showed us Judy's eyes and her little short fingers and talked about—you know—the ways in which Judy is a little different. I thought, "Well, this isn't so bad—Judy looked so cute and cuddly and all." I'm glad she talked about those things first because John and I were so scared that's all we could think about. Then, when she did a physical exam on Judy and showed us all the ways she was a normal, healthy baby, we could start to get some perspective on what it meant—the Down syndrome. Of course, it took a lot longer than that for it all to sink in and for us to understand what it would mean for our lives, but we felt so much better after that first time. The nurses were always there to answer questions and sometimes Sara, that was my primary nurse, would just come and bring me a glass of juice and sit with me for awhile. She didn't make me talk if I didn't want to and she didn't talk a lot either—she was just there for me.

There is little question that the physician and nurses in the second situation were more effective in supporting the parents during the initial diagnostic phase. It seems a safe assumption that those professionals had worked through personal feelings about genetic disorders so that they were able to focus their interactions therapeutically to deal with the parents' feelings instead of with their own.

The Art of Listening

A prime reason for nurses' discomfort when dealing with children and families during periods of diagnosis

*See also the section on values clarification in Chapter 1.

or at other stressful times is the mistaken notion that it is necessary to offer solutions to the problems raised. After all, *intervention* follows assessment and diagnosis in the nursing process. It is often a relief for nurses to realize that they cannot be expected to solve all the problems of their clients. The following excerpts help illustrate that point. They are taken from a poem entitled "Listen," in Bauer and Hill (1986, p 101); the author is unknown.

When I ask you to listen to me
and you start giving advice,
you have not done what I asked.

When I ask you to listen to me
and you begin to tell me why I shouldn't feel that way,
you are trampling on my feelings.

When I ask you to listen to me
and you feel you have to do something to solve my problem,
you have failed me, strange as that may seem.

Listen! All I asked, was that you listen,
not talk or do—just hear me.
Advice is cheap: 25 cents will get you both Dear Abby and Billy Graham in the same newspaper.
And I can do for myself: I'm not helpless;
Maybe discouraged and faltering, but not helpless.

When you do something for me that I can and need to do
for myself, you contribute to my fear and weakness.

But, when you accept as a simple fact that I do feel what I feel,
no matter how irrational, then I can quit trying to convince
you and can get about the business of understanding what's behind this irrational feeling.
And when that's clear, the answers are obvious and I don't need advice.

Irrational feelings make sense when we understand what's behind them . . .

The process described in these verses might be called active listening (Gordon, 1970) or reflective listening. In this type of listening the nurse tries to interpret what the client is communicating (that means noticing nonverbal as well as verbal cues), and then reflects that interpretation back to the client for clarification. It is a process in which the client is encouraged to explore his or her feelings for the purpose of working through the emotional reaction to the situation and surveying appropriate actions. "The goal of the provider in active listening is to always keep the door open" (Bauer and Hill, 1986, p 99).

Listening to Children

It is important to make the point that this process works equally well to help children (both the ill child and the siblings) clarify their feelings and begin adaptive problem solving. Too often we adults "close the door" on communications with children, perhaps because we feel they either cannot, will not, or should not be thinking or communicating about the issue (such as the diagnosis of a genetic disorder) or that they are developmentally incapable of coping with it. Numerous investigators and researchers describing coping in children, however (Murphy, 1974; Pless and Pinkerton, 1975; Bluebond-Langer, 1978; Garmezy and Rutter, 1983; Rose & Thomas, 1987; and others) have shown that children are quite capable of accepting and coping with major changes in lifestyle and with serious diagnoses, even at young ages. Jampolsky and Taylor, in a foreword to a book of drawings by children with cancer, conveyed a sense of respect and even awe for the coping abilities of their young patients. They wrote, "We have found that love is the fuel that allows for the joining of minds, and that age is not a factor in telling us who our teachers are" (There is a rainbow, 1978, p 3).

Siblings are affected in several ways by a family member with a genetic disorder. They may feel slighted because of the amount of time parents spend in caring for the affected child. They may have to assume extra family responsibilities as family roles shift to accommodate the increased work load. They may resent the different structure that is necessitated within their family by the affected child, such as the need for constant supervision and the strain this puts on family activities and outings. They usually suffer to some extent from what Goffman has termed a "courtesy stigma," or stigma by association. This means that because their sibling has a genetic disorder they are stigmatized by the fear and suspicion of uninformed people who believe they must be affected also. Nursing interventions that facilitate family communication about these issues can help resolve them. In addition, siblings often can benefit from support groups of others their age who are experiencing similar lifestyles.

Nurses can support both adult and child family members during the diagnostic period by encouraging them to express and explore their feelings, by correcting misinformation, and by reinforcing adaptive problem solving. Unit IV, Impact of Stress and Illness on Children and Families, deals in depth with these therapeutic interactions.

Exploring Other Sources of Support

It is important that nurse-client interactions include reflective listening, and it is also important not to underestimate the potential for the nurse to be a therapeutic agent. It is unrealistic, however, to think that any one nurse can "be all things" to any one family.

Therefore, the nurse must assess the family's resources for emotional support among family and friends and determine the need for referral to other sources of counseling and physical support. Support groups can be particularly effective because they put the family in touch with other families who have experienced the same or similar disorders and can offer both emotional support and valuable advice about such things as equipment rental, respite care, and financial aid. Genetics clinics and the March of Dimes are good resources.

Supporting the Family During the Period of Decision Making

The role of the nurse generalist in support of the family during the period of decision making is to assist, as needed, with clarification of information gained during genetic counseling sessions and, through active listening, to help the family recognize and deal with the feelings evoked by this new information. The nurse generalist's role arises from two facts related to the genetic counseling process: (1) the primary goal of genetic counseling is to provide the parents with information about the results of diagnostic tests and the risk of occurrence or recurrence of a heritable condition, and (2) the genetic counselor's contact with the family is usually limited to formally scheduled appointments. The nurse who works with the family either in the acute care setting, in the clinic, or in the home often has the opportunity to help the parents and children clarify both technical information and help them cope with their reactions to it. If additional information or more extensive emotional counseling is needed, the nurse can either make or instigate (depending upon institutional policies and state licensing laws) the proper referrals.

The Value of Time in Gaining Perspective. The nurse can be helpful in recognizing and supporting the family's need for time to come to a comfortable decision. The following excerpt from an interview reported by Kelly (1977, p 130) illustrates that point. The couple in this scenario had originally decided to accept amniocentesis as a method of detecting a sex-linked genetic disorder, but when the wife became pregnant again they decide to complete the pregnancy without amniocentesis. The husband elaborated upon their decision:

> I think what happened with us—and you may find this happening with other patients—is that when patients are exposed to an idea such as amniocentesis for the first time, in a framework of a disease that we have, it's something that sounds like an alternative that was never present before, and just because it is a fresh approach it's good. It's an alternative that seems positive at the time, and one's tendency is to go with the new suggestion. And I think to some extent that happened with us. Like, "Hey, here's something else we can do! We don't have to make these other decisions. There are other alternatives." And suddenly because it's there, it becomes at the time what seems the right way to go. But you need six months—you need a year! You need two years maybe to really sift all this out, let it fall into perspective with the other alternatives that you have before you can start to really make a choice and be intelligent about it, before you can really know your own feelings about that choice.

Supporting the Family During Follow-Up Care for Children with Genetic Disorders

Nurses who care for children in any setting will encounter families who are dealing with the day-to-day realities of a genetic disorder. Specific assessments and interventions for the major genetic disorders are covered in Unit VII, Nursing Strategies in Physiologic Alterations. This section will highlight those aspects of the nurse generalist's role that are common to all genetic disorders.

The role of the nurse generalist in supporting families affected by a genetic disorder is to

- promote the child's optimal growth and development,
- help the family and other health care professionals control the effects of the genetic disorder,
- promote adaptive family coping.

Promoting Optimal Growth and Development

The process of helping the child develop to full potential begins at diagnosis. The nurse can be instrumental in identifying those aspects of the child's physical, cognitive, and spiritual makeup that reflect normal needs in relation to growth and development and those that will require special attention. Parents thus can be made aware of ways in which their child's needs for nutrition, sleep, stimulation, safety, maintenance of physiologic function, communication, social activity, and attainment of developmental tasks are like those of other children and ways in which these needs are modified by the disorder.

Promoting optimal growth and development calls for frequent assessment of those parameters and for realistic interpretation of the findings. Some middle ground must be found between depriving the family of realistic hope for this child's future achievements and inflating the child's potential to make everyone (including the nurse) feel better about the situation. It is particularly easy to become overly optimistic when the child is diagnosed in infancy because the child may seem to be meeting early developmental milestones quite normally. It must be realized that attainment of developmental tasks will probably become more noticeably delayed as the tasks become more complex.

We are reminded of a particular blond and cuddly baby boy with cerebral palsy who at age 3 months was nearly on line with developmental norms for infants his age. It became easy to deny the medical diagnosis and to hope that *this* child would prove the exception. But by 6 months of age he had not progressed through the developmental tasks for infants of 4 months, and the expectations of nurses and parents alike had to be realigned.

Controlling the Effects of the Genetic Disorder

The nurse will be responsible for providing information and helping the family learn techniques to manage the day-to-day care of the child. At times the alterations in daily living will be minimal and time-limited, (e.g., caring for an infant who has been casted to correct club foot), and in other instances the impact upon the family's lifestyle will be significant (e.g., caring for the child with cystic fibrosis, including the administration of enzyme supplements, and provision of respiratory therapy treatments).

The family will expect the nurse to possess a basic understanding of the genetic disorder, including the principles of inheritance, and the impact of the disorder upon the child's physical, mental, emotional, and social development. The nurse can make a significant contribution by establishing communication with the child's school to open the way for cooperation between school support services (e.g., the special education team) and the primary health care provider.

Promoting Adaptive Family Coping

As elaborated in Chapter 2, family goals, structure, and functioning are ways in which a family adapts to internal and external strains and attempts to maintain a cohesive family unit. Guidelines for family assessment are detailed in Chapter 12 and include investigation of roles, relationships, and functions. Chapter 25, Impact of Chronic Illness, provides additional background for understanding the emotional and social toll of chronic illness on family life.

Family assessment can highlight both strengths and limitations of the family unit in regard to ongoing care of the child with a genetic disorder. The nurse will be effective to the extent she or he is able to support and reinforce family strengths and to help the family find sources of support for limitations. As noted in Chapter 12, family limitations that are unchangeable help provide realistic boundaries for goal setting.

Cohen (1984, p 342) lists the following signs of successful family adjustment to a genetic disorder: an intact family unit, the resumption of sexual relationships between partners, appropriate plans for future reproduction in light of genetic counseling and family goals, ability to help other parents, realistic plans for management of the affected child, retention of the family health care practitioner, and ability to relate to others.

Promoting Adaptation in Infancy. The developmental stages of infancy, childhood, and adolescence will color the meaning of a genetic disorder for the affected child. Development of self-image begins in infancy. The infant who is loved and accepted by parents and siblings has the basis for a positive view of self. Nursing interventions may be needed at this time to increase the family's "comfort" with the infant. Parents and siblings can be helped to put the genetic disorder in perspective by recognizing the ways in which the infant is like all other infants, the ways in which he or she responds to their affection, and the ways in which their interactions can be modified, if necessary, to produce the desired response. For example, see Chapter 51 for suggested interactions with the infant who is visually or hearing impaired.

Promoting Adaptation in Childhood. The affected toddler or preschooler may experience a crisis in the development of autonomy. Parents and siblings who have had good reason to focus upon the affected child's increased needs for safety may need extra support in allowing the child an appropriate measure of independence. When they understand the importance of autonomy to the child's development, this allowance is often made more easily. Also at this age, the young child's self-image will be affected by the comments and behaviors of peers and other persons in the widening social environment; unkind remarks and behavior are likely to have a negative effect. The nurse can teach family members to deal with these situations by educating extended family, friends, teachers, and others in the children's social environment to the facts of the disorder. Facts can help dispel the fear that prompts discourtesies. The nursing process plan in Chapter 51 provides additional details of interventions to reduce social stigma.

In later childhood affected children must find something at which they can excel. In minor disorders impediments to the child's attainment of this developmental task may be few. In more severe disorders, however, the family may benefit from the support and suggestions of the nurse. Other families who have gone through this stage of childhood with their youngster can also be good resources.

Promoting Adaptation During Adolescence. The impact of a genetic disorder can be quite a problem during adolescence. When other adolescents are gaining increasing independence by learning to drive and earning their own spending money, the affected adolescent may feel terribly constrained. In addition, the tasks of establishing satisfactory relationships with members of the opposite sex and planning for further education, marriage and a career will be affected by the heritability of the disorder and by the physical and cognitive limitations it manifests. Adolescents tend to turn increasingly outside their families for emotional support. The nurse, therefore, can be a valuable resource to the adolescent in helping clarify risks of occurrence, explaining how to obtain genetic counseling with a potential mate, and assisting the young person to focus upon strengths instead of upon limitations in the struggle to find a place in the world.

Effective coping in both the ill child and the siblings will be reflected in their ability to develop and maintain a positive self-image and meet attainable developmental tasks (that is, tasks dealing with physical, cognitive, emotional, and social development). Children who reflect these adaptive traits almost always reflect, in turn, a healthy family, and a healthy family is often one that in time of need has found information and emotional support within the health care system.

References

Bauer BB, Hill SS: *Essentials of Mental Health Care: Planning and Interventions.* Philadelphia, WB Saunders, 1986.

Bluebond-Langer N: *The Private Worlds of Dying Children.* Princeton, NJ, Princeton University Press, 1978.

Cohen FL: *Clinical Genetics in Nursing Practice.* Philadelphia, JB Lippincott, 1984.

Emery AEH, Pullen I: *Psychological Aspects of Genetic Counseling.* Orlando, FL, Academic Press, 1984.

Garmezy N, Rutter M: *Stress, Coping, and Development in Children.* New York, McGraw-Hill, 1983.

Gordon T: *P.E.T.: Parent Effectiveness Training.* New York, Peter H. Wyden, 1970.

Hirschhorn K: Chromosomes and their abnormalities. *In* Behrman RE, Vaughan VC (eds): *Nelson Textbook of Pediatrics.* 13th ed. Philadelphia, WB Saunders, 1987, 247–267.

Kelly PT: *Dealing with Dilemma: A Manual for Genetic Counselors.* New York, Springer-Verlag, 1977.

Kunze J, Nippert I: *Genetics and Malformations in Art.* Berlin, Grosse-Verlag, 1986.

March of Dimes: Your special child. Pamphlet White Plains, NY, March of Dimes Birth Defects Foundation, 1982.

March of Dimes: Spina bifida. Pamphlet White Plains, NY, March of Dimes Birth Defects Foundation, 1985.

Murphy LB: Coping, vulnerability, and resilience in children. *In* Coelho CV, Hamburg DA, Adams JE (eds): *Coping and Adaptation.* New York, Basic Books, 1974.

Pless IB, Pinkerton P: *Chronic Childhood Disorder: Promoting Patterns of Adjustment.* Chicago, Year Book Medical Publishers, 1975.

Rose MH, Thomas RB: *Children with Chronic Conditions: Nursing in a Family and Community Context.* Orlando, FL, Grune & Stratton, 1987.

There is a rainbow behind every dark cloud. Millbrae, CA, Celestial Arts, 1978.

Thompson JS, Thompson MW: *Genetics in Medicine.* 4th ed. Philadelphia, WB Saunders, 1986.

Bibliography

Bergsma D: *Malformation Syndromes.* Baltimore, Johns Hopkins Press, 1975.

Concise Book of Genetics. Scarborough, Canada: Prentice-Hall, 1982.

Emery A, Pullen I, (eds): *Psychological Aspects of Genetic Counseling.* London, Academic Press, 1984.

Feingold M, Pashayan H: *Genetics and Birth Defects in Clinical Practice.* Boston, Little, Brown, 1983.

Fuhrmann W, Vogel F: *Genetic Counseling.* New York, Springer-Verlag, 1983.

Hsia Y, Hirschhorn K: *Counseling in Genetics.* New York, Alan Liss, 1979.

Kaback M (ed): *Tay-Sachs Disease: Screening and Prevention.* New York, Alan Liss, 1977.

Otto J, Towie A: *Modern Biology.* New York, Holt, Rinehart and Winston, 1982.

Pueschel S (ed): *Down Syndrome.* Kansas City: Sheed Andrews, 1978.

Schwarz R, Yaffe S: *Drug and Chemical Risks to the Fetus and Newborn.* New York, Alan Liss, 1980.

Shepard T: *Catalog of Teratogenic Agents.* Baltimore, Johns Hopkins Press, 1980.

Smith D: *Recognizable Patterns of Human Malformation.* Philadelphia, WB Saunders, 1982.

Strategies in genetic counseling. *Birth Defects* 1984; 20(6).

Tinley ST: Nurses' and geneticists' role expectations for the nurse clinician. *J Pediatr Nurs* 1987; 2(4):259-264.

Growth and Development of Children within Families

Unit Two

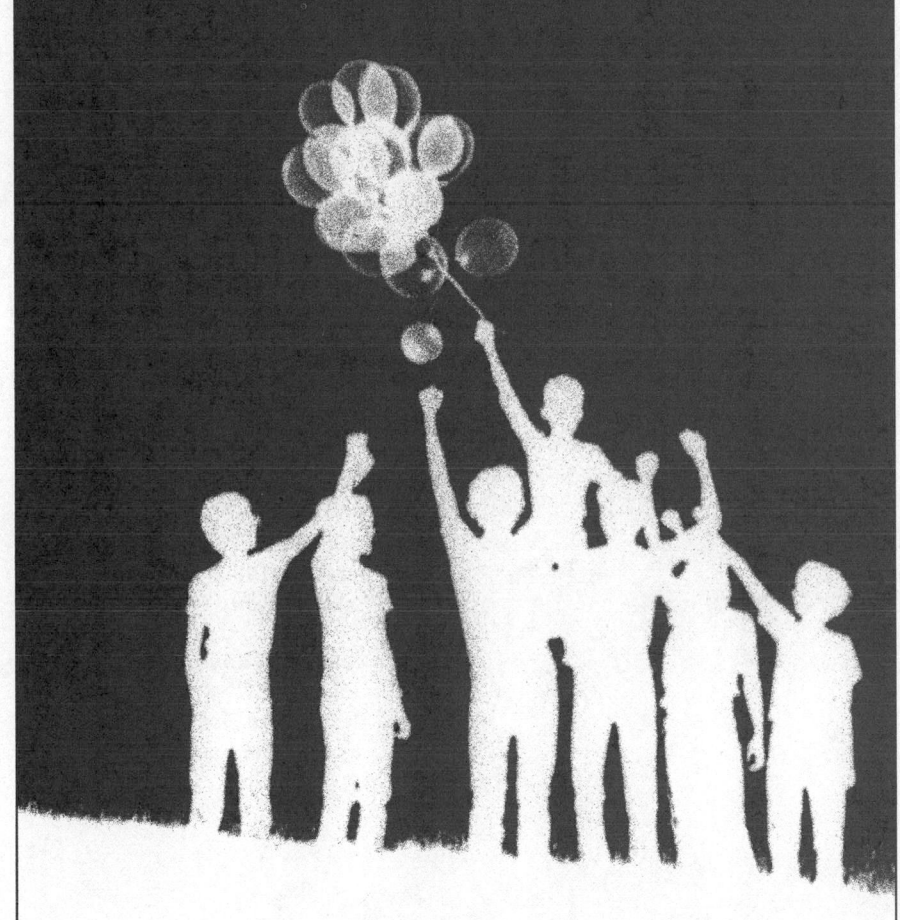

Families with Infants — Chapter 5

Related Topics
Developmental theories, Chapter 3
Promoting healthy parenting, Chapter 13
Child health assessment, Chapter 15
Infant nutrition, Chapter 18
Infant sleep, Chapter 20
Gavage feedings, Chapter 27
Bronchopulmonary dysplasia, Chapter 38
Oxygen administration, Chapter 38
Neonatal sepsis, Chapter 40
Retinopathy of prematurity, Chapter 51

The birth of an infant is an event filled with wonder and joy for most families. Adjustments in personal and family roles are required, however, to incorporate the new family member. The first section of this chapter discusses the developmental and adaptational processes associated with assuming the parent role. Nursing strategies to promote healthy parenting are detailed.

The remaining sections of this chapter involve health concerns and strategies for health promotion in the first year of life. Physical assessment of the newborn infant is discussed in detail, because the nursing role in identifying potential neonatal problems is an important one. Infants with problems at birth frequently are those born early or late or whose weight differs from the norm. These infants and their families have special problems and care needs, which are detailed in later chapters. Here an overview is given of their needs, so that the nurse may see how the future development of child and family might be affected.

The final section of the chapter presents the exciting story of the infant's first year of development.

Development and Adaptation of the Family with an Infant

Jo Joyce Anderson

Family life cycle transitions are important because all families experience them and because they frequently are associated with family crises. The birth of a first baby initiates a life cycle transition for the family. This life cycle transition to beginning parenthood is generally looked forward to by prospective parents as a period of joy and emotional enhancement rather than as a period of family crisis. Therefore, new parents frequently are unprepared for experiencing the variety of stresses that may accompany the arrival of their infant. They soon discover that they are sensitive and vulnerable at this time. Reality does not measure up to anticipated expectations generated during the childbearing period.

The major task of a family with an infant is *the healthy incorporation of a new person into the existing family.* This process requires the family to (1) internalize the infant's existence, (2) make necessary adjustments, (3) maintain morale, and (4) adapt available resources. Each of these facets of incorporation has potential stressors that are commonly experienced. The pediatric nurse working with the new family can do much to foster healthy adaptation by being personally aware of these potential stressors and, when indicated, by educating family members as to what to expect, offering reassurance regarding the "normality" of these stressors, and helping them problem solve preventively to minimize the number and intensity of stressors actually experienced. Many of the stressors that are encountered by new parents are also the defining characteristics or risk factors for the nursing diagnosis: *altered parenting: potential.* The nurse should include these defining characteristics in the assessment of all prospective parents to identify families that may need special help with parenting.

Internalizing the Infant's Existence

Prenatal Attachment

Health professionals have begun to realize the valuable experiences families can have prenatally to facilitate bonding to the yet unborn child. These experi-

We appreciate the critical review of this chapter by Sandra Frick, RN, PhD, and her contributions to it.

ences can help the family to be more receptive to the infant from birth. Scientific advances such as the Doppler device that permits early audibility of the fetus' heartbeat, ultrasound that permits visualization of the fetus and sometimes even identification of its sex, as well as greater awareness of the effects of external environment on fetal movement, have all intensified parents' and siblings' awareness of the baby's realness and existence even before birth. Preliminary research has been carried out that suggests that nursing interventions to promote prenatal maternal-infant bonding increase the frequency of maternal attachment behaviors (Carter-Jessup, 1981). Such interaction with the fetus facilitates the family's internalization of the infant's existence by the time it is born (Grace, 1984).

Carter-Jessup's (1981) findings that postnatal bonding is facilitated by intrauterine attachment interventions are suspect, however, because of the small sample size (N = 10) and because the questionnaire used to assess postpartum attachment had no established reliability (Davis and Akridge, 1987). A test that has no proven reliability can be likened to a ruler made of elastic; one cannot be sure if the results of the study are due to actual differences in the subjects or to inaccuracies in the measuring device. The questions arising from Carter-Jessup's work have prompted other research, some that support Carter-Jessup's findings (such as the study by Anisfeld and Lopper, 1983) and others that find no difference in postnatal attachment between women who received interventions to direct their attention toward their fetuses and those who received no such interventions (such as the study by Davis and Akridge, 1987, which attempted to replicate the Carter-Jessup work).

Despite the inconclusiveness of research in prenatal attachment, it seems likely that parents can be helped to prepare for their infant's birth by nursing strategies designed to help them perceive the baby as a real, growing person. The nurse can ask questions such as, "Do you ever think about what your baby looks like?" "Do you have a pet name for the baby?" "What do you think your baby's personality will be like, judging from the way he or she moves inside you?"

Parents who seem the least attached to their unborn fetus will require the most intense and innovative nursing care to help them prepare for the reality of their child. While it has been speculated that a high-risk pregnancy (i.e., one involving significant danger to the fetus or the mother) might affect prenatal attachment to the fetus, a study by Kemp and Page (1987) found no difference between the prenatal attachment scores of women in the normal and high-risk groups. In addition, they found no significant relationships between the attachment scores and any of the following demographic variables: educational level, age, race, whether the pregnancy was planned, whether the women had a sonogram, or the ordinal position of the infant in the family.

Identification: Attachment After Birth

The identification and claiming process is an important first step in the family's incorporation of the "real" baby into their family. According to Mercer (1977), after the baby's birth, the mother establishes a realistic image of her infant and absorbs the infant into her self and her social systems through an acquaintance-attachment process. Rubin (1961) has described the typical manner in which a mother identifies and claims her infant. She examines the baby's soft and tiny features first by touching them with her fingertips and then with her palms and finally she enfolds the baby in her arms and looks directly into the baby's eyes – an en face position. Klaus and Kennell (1976) define *en face* as the position in which the mother's face is rotated so that her eyes and those of the infant meet fully in the same vertical plane of rotation.

Whether a mother touches her newborn infant along this orderly pattern, however, should not be used as a single measure of the quality of the beginning relationship. Trevathon (1981), in a study of 66 mothers during the first postpartum hour, found no evidence of a pattern of touch but noted that the pattern of tactile exploration varied with gender of the infant, parity (the number of infants the woman has delivered), and socioeconomic or sociocultural background of the mother. The tactile identification process that most mothers demonstrate in a variety of forms confirms to them the existence of a separate person and an object to which attachment can be made (Luddington-Hoe, 1977).

Reaching is another indication of identification work. At first, the mother may receive her baby passively, but over the next few days most mothers progress toward active reaching for the baby. Active reaching indicates a desire to take the infant into the mother's personal body space and to get closer (Luddington-Hoe, 1977).

The father of a newborn infant also must identify the infant as a real person joining his family. Opportunities to be with his infant will increase his involvement with the baby and the mother; he becomes part of the family unit. The nurse must recognize the importance of the father and include him in the assessment and plan of care.

The process of the family in identifying and claiming the infant can be facilitated by nurses who recognize the significance of this initial step. The nurse present at the birth and afterward can provide opportunities for all family members to relate to the neonate. Nursing intervention in this early stage can assist in the prevention of actual alterations in parenting.

Traditional hospital practices often interfere with the process of identification and claiming by isolating the baby from some family members. Fortunately, these practices have changed in many places. Within the confines of the setting, the nurse minimizes or prevents interruption of contact between the infant and family members.

The nurse also can model methods of interacting with the baby by pointing out characteristics of the baby that resemble family traits, by encouraging the unwrapping and examination of the whole baby, and by talking to the baby and responding to his or her behavior. The nurse thus gives permission and endorsement to the family to proceed with their developmental task of identifying and claiming this baby as theirs.

Forming a Bond

The term *bonding,* introduced by Kennell and Klaus (1976), and the term *attachment* are sometimes used interchangeably, but have different meanings. Bonding generally refers to a parent's tie to a child and is thought of as a fairly rapid process that occurs immediately after birth (Campbell and Taylor, 1980). Bonding is unidirectional from parent to child. Attachment is somewhat different, referring to an affectional tie between parents and infants that is a two-way process. Attachment develops gradually during the first year of an infant's life.

Theories of bonding and attachment have their roots in studies of animal behavior. Highly predictable behavior can be elicited in a certain species by specific stimuli at a time when the organism is in a state of readiness (Campbell and Taylor, 1980).

Brief experimental separation of certain animals (rats, goats, monkeys) from their mothers has resulted in disturbed maternal caretaking following the separation. Such animal experiments gave rise to the speculation that for humans also an especially sensitive period, known as a "critical period," may exist, during which time optimal mother-infant bonding could take place. Based on these findings from animal studies, Klaus and Kennell (1976) suggested that a sensitive period exists immediately after birth during which the maternal-infant bond was most likely to be established.

Klaus and Kennell published articles in the early 1970's reporting on studies in which early and extended contact was provided between mother and infant dyads. These infants were followed to study the effect of such early contact on later parent-infant relationships and child development.

These early studies reported some positive outcomes in their experimental groups, such as mothers being more attentive, exhibiting more soothing and fondling behavior, and more *en face* positioning (Klaus et al, 1972). Research studies proliferated which further examined whether a sensitive period exists and, if it does, whether maternal-infant contact during that time would have a lasting effect on subsequent parent-child relationships and child development. The chart on page 169 summarizes the findings of some of the major research studies.

Reviews and critiques of the bonding/attachment literature are also listed in this chart. Most reviewers conclude that there is insufficient evidence to support the idea that a human sensitive period exists during which time optimal parent-infant bonding takes place. Some of the studies have shown that early mother-infant contact may have a positive effect on maternal-infant bonding, but long-term effects have been difficult to demonstrate. In addition, confusion exists about a valid measure of maternal-infant bonding and populations used in the studies have varied widely in racial and cultural backgrounds; in general, the results from bonding studies have not been clearly positive.

Although there is consensus that early contact between mother and infant has been over-rated, few would disagree that the studies of Kennell and Klaus have influenced modern maternal-infant care in a positive way and have humanized hospital procedures. The trend today is to encourage early mother-infant contact, which sets into motion the ongoing process of developing an affectional tie. At the same time, many parents miss the early moments of being with their infant, and it is important for health care professionals to recognize that parents can form strong emotional bonds to their infants despite this. Mothers may require anesthesia for obstetric reasons, or the infant may be whisked away to an intensive care unit. Mothers who are fatigued and prefer to rest rather than spend extra time with their infants should not be made to feel less worthwhile. Adoptive parents and fathers who missed their infant's birth also form emotional bonds with their infants and should not be made to feel that they have missed the crucial moment of beginning a relationship.

Mother-Infant Bond

A healthy mother-child relationship does not spontaneously occur at the birth of a child but has to develop as the mother and child learn to respond to each other. A mother may not always feel the enormous happiness that she expected to feel at the birth of her baby. Instead, she often feels disoriented and tired.

A Summary of Major Research on Bonding

Author and Date of Study	Brief Description	Findings
Klaus et al, 1972	A group of mothers and infants experienced early contact and were compared with a control group who received routine care	Mothers with early contact exhibited more attentive, soothing, and fondling behaviors at 1 month postexperiment
Kennell et al, 1974	Same group of mothers (as above) were examined at 1 year postexperiment	Mothers with early contact reported missing baby when they returned to work to a greater extent than routine care group
Hales et al, 1977 (First study to look at *timing* of extra contact)	Twenty mothers had 45 minutes of early contact, compared with twenty who had a 45-minute contact at 12 hours	Early contact group engaged in more kissing, smiling, talking, and *en face*. No differences in proximity or caregiving
de Chateau and Wiberg, 1977	Fifteen minutes of skin-to-skin contact immediately after delivery; mother, father, and infant together 2 hours in delivery. Compared with routine care: contact 1 of every 4 hours for first 2 days then daytime rooming-in. Evaluated at 36 hours, 3 months, and 1 year	Contact group at 30 hours showed more *en face*, kissing, baby smiles. By 3 months, contact group reported more breastfeeding problems. By 1 year of age, contact group breastfed for 175 days versus 108 days for controls
Craig et al, 1982 (Controls in this study had more early contact [≤10 min] than most controls in other studies)	Twenty-six mothers given 1 hour of skin-to-skin contact after delivery were compared with ≤10-minute contact (baby wrapped)	At 1 month of age no difference was noted between groups on any measures
Svejda et al, 1980	Contact given for 15–25 minutes after birth + 45 minutes in own room and an extra hour at each feed. Control group given 5 minutes at delivery and 30 minutes every 4 hours	No differences in any discrete behaviors or in categories of behaviors

(Some critiques and reviews of the bonding literature can be found in Campbell and Taylor, 1980; Chess and Thomas, 1982; Goldberg, 1983; Klaus and Kennell, 1982; Lamb and Hwang, 1982; Mitchell and Mills, 1983; Svejda et al, 1982.)

Brazelton (1973) has researched mother-infant interactions by studying videotape recordings. He found that infants exhibit a cycle that is characterized by eight stages of interaction.

- Initiation: The infant's attention is attracted by the mother and the infant looks back at her.
- Orientation: The infant orients body to face the mother.
- State of Attention: The infant alternately sends and receives cues.
- Acceleration: There are fewer oscillations of attention and inattention.
- Vocalizing: Cooing.
- Peak of Excitement: The infant whirls arms and kicks legs, exhibits jerky activity.
- Deceleration: Activity, eye contact, and vocalization gradually decrease.
- Withdrawal: The infant withdraws from looking and interacting.

The infant's overtures must be perceived and reciprocated by the mother for their interrelationship. It is clear that both mother and baby are active participants in the attachment process.

The term *maternicity* has been used to mean the characteristic quality of a woman's personality that supplies her with the emotional energy for feeling that her infant occupies an essential part of her life as determined by bonds of affection. These bonds include feelings of warmth, devotion, and protectiveness toward the infant, concern for the infant's well-being, and pleasant anticipation of continuing contact. Maternicity develops as the mother and infant are in close contact and indicates a high probability for the successful development of a healthy mother-child relationship.

In assessing the development of maternicity in the mother of an infant, the nurse should remember that observation of eye-to-eye contact (en face position) between mother and infant is of primary importance.

The mother's style of feeding and bathing her infant is also an indicator of maternal behavior. Luddington-Hoe (1977) suggests parameters to observe in mothers for the development of maternicity:

- Initial identifying behaviors prior to and after delivery,
- Active and passive reaching behavior,
- Touch progression: Fingertip to palm or to hand; hand to arm embrace,
- Positioning of the infant to the left of mother's sternum, *en face* positioning (in right-handed mothers),
- Eye-to-eye contact,
- Verbal identifying behaviors: Association and pronoun identification,
- Developmental phases: Taking-in phase of dependency; taking-hold phase of task execution; letting go of predelivery expectations,
- Rhythm-reciprocity patterns,* and
- Cooing behaviors.

Absence of these behaviors suggests further evaluation of the mother-infant attachment.

Assessment of deviations and early therapeutic intervention when maladaptive maternal behaviors exist may prevent child abuse, mental illness, and many psychosomatic and learning disorders. This type of assessment may be compromised by the current trend toward early discharge of mothers and babies. The nurse should be alert to the need for home follow-up to prevent future problems.

Father-Infant Bond

Although mothers require a period of time to separate from the image they have developed of the baby as an integral part of them, the father's image of his baby is one of separateness. Before the early 1970s, very little was known about father-infant attachment. Bowen and Miller (1980) found that bonding may be stronger in fathers present at the delivery of their infant. Greenberg and Morris (1974) found indications that the first 3 days after birth are an important time for father-infant bonding to occur. In a sample of 30 first-time fathers from three British maternity hospitals, all manifested "engrossment" in their newborn infants—a sense of bonding, absorption, and preoccupation with their child. The researchers interpreted this as an innate potential "released" in fathers by exposure to the infant.

Weiser and Castiglia (1984), in reviewing research-based characteristics of father-infant bonding, identify the following as key elements of assessing father-infant attachment:

Inspection: Does the father look at the infant, assume an *en face* position, smile at the infant, express awareness of distinct characteristics of the infant, or turn away from the infant?

Verbalization: Does the father vocalize to the infant, does he call the baby by name, does he use affectionate terms for the infant?

Tactile contact: Does the father touch the baby with fingertips and whole hand? Does he rock, kiss, or hold the infant? Does he refuse to hold the infant?

Caretaking: Does the father feed the infant? Does he burp, clean, or diaper the infant? Does he respond to the infant's cues and demands for attention?

The infant's state of activity during interactions with the father may also indicate father-infant attachment. Is the infant active and alert or inactive and passive? Has the father been with the infant only during periods of sleeping or crying? What is the behavior of the father when he is alone with the infant? When the mother, infant, and father are together?

One reason early father-infant bonding is important today is because the extended family is seldom available for new parents as it was in the past; thus, fathers need to contribute to the early emotional and physical care of new infants in the nuclear family.

Sibling-Infant Bond

The attachment between infant and siblings has been explored and documented far less than has parent-infant attachment. When older children are prepared to expect a new baby in the family, they will be able to handle their jealous feelings at displacement with less stress. Furman (1978) says, "To the children, and to young children in particular, this baby was not looked forward to as a cherished newcomer—it was a potential rival without whom they could have easily gotten along happily in life." Even though a young child cannot verbalize these feelings, it is logical that he or she might be thinking, "Where have I failed? Mommy and Daddy wanted to have another baby. They must not have been satisfied with me." A child's excitement at meeting a new brother or sister is often tempered by these negative feelings.

With these factors in mind, some hospitals are providing prenatal classes for siblings and allowing siblings in the delivery room to view the birth of their brother or sister. The older child's attachment to a new sibling seems to be facilitated when parents help the child understand what is happening, explain that this is the child's baby as well as theirs, and reassure him or her of their continuing love by verbal expression and

---

*That is, the rhythm and reciprocity of the behaviors and responses between mother and infant, resulting in a cyclic exchange indicating mutual satisfaction.

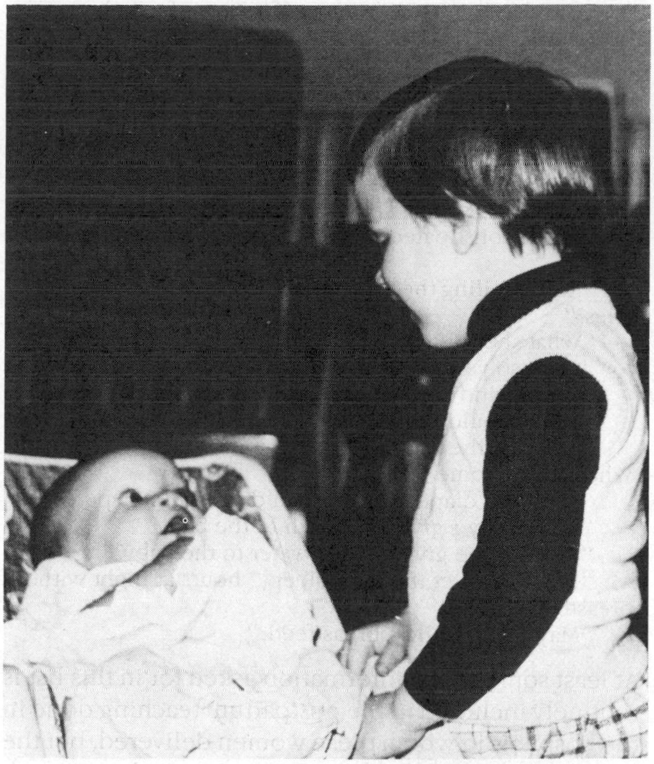

The attachment of older children to a new infant seems to be enhanced by understanding that the new infant belongs to them as well as to the parents. (Photograph by Jim Tackett.)

by demonstration. The infant's responses to the older sibling will also be influential in establishing a bond between them. As children have an opportunity to examine, touch, and interact with their new sibling, their negative feelings can be altered and finally replaced by feelings of protectiveness and love.

Nursing Strategies

Supporting and reinforcing parents and siblings during the early infant acquaintance process is an important nursing function. For this, the nurse observes the quality and progress of interactions between parents and children and offers reinforcement when they observe their infant, talk to the baby, and comment about his or her behaviors. The nurse can also teach family members to interpret their infant's behaviors appropriately.

Nurses can do much to provide extensive opportunities for parent-infant interaction. One group of nurses planned, carried out, and evaluated a highly structured intervention session designed to facilitate the bonding process (Dean, Morgan, and Towle, 1982). Each neonate was individually assessed by a nurse before the intervention session. During the session, the baby's identifying characteristics were explained to the mother; the individuality and uniqueness of the infant were emphasized. Any variations from expected newborn characteristics were thoroughly discussed. The infant's hearing, sight, and reflexes were demonstrated and explained. The atmosphere was deliberately kept warm, gentle, and interactive. At the end of the session, each mother received a written record of material covered to reinforce what had been learned. Mothers who participated had lower anxiety scores than mothers who did not. In every contact nurses can reinforce parents' strengths and capacity to cope, thereby improving parents' self-images and increasing the self-confidence they pass on to their babies.

However, the nurse should realize that attachment is a multifactorial process and should intervene at all periods of development to strengthen parent-child relationships (Mitchell and Mills, 1983). Any practices that humanize or enrich the childbearing and child-rearing experiences for the family should be encouraged as a means of enhancing parental satisfaction and self-esteem, which correlate directly with healthy parent-child attachments and contribute to healthy parenting.

The nurse can also offer reassurances to parents who, for whatever reason, are not afforded the early contact with their infant. These parents need reassurance that this does not automatically mean there will be deficits in their relationships with that child. The bonding process, in most instances, has already begun prenatally. Nursing actions that help foster parental satisfaction and self-esteem despite limited opportunity for direct contact with the infant will facilitate the maintenance and building of the bonding process when direct contact does become possible.

Accepting Responsibility for the Infant

Another task that is a part of internalizing the infant's existence is the acceptance of new or added responsibilities associated with the infant. For some people, having a baby may satisfy a need for purpose and responsibility. For others, the responsibility for another's survival is overwhelming. A nurse who suspects that the family is experiencing feelings of being overwhelmed should consider a possible diagnosis of *ineffective family coping*. The feeling of being overwhelmed by the new responsibilities is emphasized when parents first realize that the parent role is irrevocable.

One of the most crucial needs often felt by an infant's parents is based on their sense of insufficient knowledge. Nurses who work with such parents should include in their care plan an ongoing assessment of parental knowledge of basic infant care. This assessment will allow them to recognize when a diagnosis of *knowledge deficit* is appropriate, as well as ensuring that the specific area in which knowledge is lacking is noted. If the criteria for making a nursing diagnosis are followed, the nurse will include in the diagnostic process the etiologic factors related to the problem of knowledge deficit. Interventions can then be directed toward these etiologic factors and, if the etiology is a matter of lack of exposure to information, nursing interventions will focus upon client-appropriate teaching of the necessary information.

Basic infant care is taught before and after the baby is born, prenatally in classes and postnatally in the hospital or home. However, two factors make this teaching less effective than it might be at a different time. The baby care found in a prenatal class is taught before the baby is born, and parents tend to forget this information because they cannot relate it to their baby until they can see and hold him or her. The teaching done in the hospital following the birth comes at a time when the mother feels very dependent and is not yet ready to think in terms of caring for her baby. She has a need for care herself. Much of what a mother is taught in the first days after the birth of her baby is not retained after discharge. In the couples studied by Williams (1977), 74 per cent said they would like to have included in postnatal classes information on the physical care of infants, such as bathing and feeding. These topics had been taught in the postpartum units of each hospital in which these women delivered.

The effectiveness of in-hospital teaching cannot be discounted, however. In a study of 140 postpartum mothers, Rutledge and Pridham (1987) found that in-hospital teaching significantly increased perceptions of competence for infant feeding and care.

Other etiologies for the nursing diagnosis of *knowledge deficit* include anxiety, lack of interest or motivation, and cultural-language differences that interfere with the use of learning resources. Teaching infant care skills would be an inappropriate intervention for these etiologic factors. Therefore, subjective and objective assessment of parents and accurate use of the diagnosis *knowledge deficit* are important.

A group of 14 baccalaureate nursing students at Goshen College in Goshen, Indiana, visited 28 families in their homes in the early days and weeks after their babies were born. This was designed to be a learning activity in a nursing elective course on the "fourth trimester" (the 3 months following the birth of a child). One goal of the students in visiting the families was to identify the knowledge needs expressed by the parents or observed by themselves. The knowledge needs they identified were in the areas of baby care and feeding; mother's self-care; infant characteristics, growth, and development; family planning; and sibling adjustments and discipline. Some representative questions raised by the parents in relation to baby care were:

"How can I tell if the baby is dressed warmly enough?"
"He sleeps such a short time. Why is he so fussy?"
"Is she constipated if she has no bowel movement one day?"
"Am I spoiling the baby by picking him up every time he cries?"
"What should I do for diaper rash?"
"She's so yellow. Should I take her to the doctor?"
"Is one kind of pacifier better than another?"
"What should I do about hiccoughs?"
"May I lay the baby on his abdomen if the cord is not off? When will it come off?"
"Are cloth diapers better than disposable diapers?"
"When may I give a tub bath to the baby?"
"Should I be giving sugar water to the baby?"
"Is it OK to let the baby sleep 7 hours at night without breastfeeding?"
"May I diet while I breastfeed?"

At least some of the information asked for in this list is routinely included in the postpartum teaching done in the hospitals in which these women delivered, but the questions remain when the parents have sole responsibility for the baby at home.

Nursing Strategies

The need for parenting education has become ever more acute with early discharge of mothers and babies from maternity units (within 24 to 72 hours after birth for most healthy babies). Just as nurses have led in the development of childbirth education classes for expectant families, community parenting support offers many professional opportunities for the nurse.

Some instructional activities nurses can undertake include:

- Making parenting literature and bibliographies available in doctor's offices, clinics, and at discharge from maternity units
- Teaching prenatal classes and postnatal parenting classes through hospitals, community organizations, or independent practice
- Structuring and scheduling teaching opportunities in hospitals before discharge, in pediatrician's offices, and in well-baby clinics
- Organizing parent coffee get-togethers or discussion groups and functioning as a resource person in groups
- Implementing fourth trimester (the 3 months following birth of a child) follow-up by telephone or home visiting after early discharge
- Becoming involved in community education programs

- Establishing education programs for adolescent mothers through school systems

Knowledge deficit as an etiologic factor for the nursing diagnoses of *ineffective individual coping: parent; fear; disturbance in self-concept: self-esteem; powerlessness;* and *disturbance in self-concept: role performance* has been traditionally recognized; well-developed interventions to remedy knowledge deficit are available. Nurses must be aware that the problem area may not be knowledge deficit and be prepared to include interventions that are appropriate to other problems in their plan of care.

When the parental stresses of insecurity, fear, and low self-esteem exist, the nurse's major intervention is one of reassurance and of identification of the parents' strengths. The parental need for reassurance is poignant even in those families in which the knowledge base is strong; they frequently ask, "What am I doing wrong?" "Do other mothers feel this way?" "Do bottle-fed babies cry this much?"

Parents' security and self-esteem as parents will be enhanced when they are given opportunities to define their concerns, to state what they believe to be effective solutions to their problems, to describe actions they have tried, and to express what they want to do next. Erikson (1978) states: "Mothers and fathers are creative and resourceful. More importantly, by including them we encourage them to feel more personally responsible for their child's care." *The nurse can help parents become problem-solvers rather than merely help-seekers and thereby facilitate effective coping.*

Adjusting Family Life to Incorporate a New Baby

Perhaps no single event in human growth and development requires the number of adjustments the birth of a baby requires in the life of a family. Adjustments in relation to role changes and maintaining family morale will be discussed here.

Assuming New Roles

The new responsibilities associated with the infant require that all members in the infant's family assume some new roles. The addition of parental or sibling roles creates critical role transition periods while each family member works out an accommodation among new and old roles. Making a transition from husband-wife to father-mother requires development of several new inter-related roles. What these new roles are perceived to be and how they are internalized varies according to the individual's own experiences, feelings, and needs. A parent who has been an only child or the youngest child in a family has had fewer opportunities for exposure to infant and child-care responsibilities and may be unprepared for what to expect of infant behaviors.

Any situation that involves a change in roles or in which new roles are perceived as conflicting with existing roles has the potential for a resulting *disturbance in self-concept: role performance.* Nursing assessment must include consideration of the defining characteristics of this nursing diagnosis. Awareness of the facets of the roles of mother, father, and sibling contributes to the nursing assessment.

Mother Role

The mother in the family of an infant usually experiences the greatest change in her position. Her maternal roles usually require at least temporary interruption of her occupational role and often most of her other extrafamilial responsibilities.

Nursing interventions incorporate recognizing mother's dependency needs. During this time the new mother is overloaded. It is an especially hard time for the educated career woman who is used to being in control. Support groups for new mothers in this category can be particularly helpful for dealing with feelings of frustration and anxiety that can arise when the employed woman perceives herself less competent in the mothering role than in her professional role.

The nurse's reassurance of the mother will help build her self-confidence. At no time should a nurse's behavior communicate that she or he is better able to care for the baby than the mother; instead the nurse must use every opportunity to foster feelings of adequacy in the mother.

Father Role

Not only are fathers able to be involved with their infants, many also want to have this involvement as a parent. Their involvement makes a difference to the baby's well-being. Nurses in contact with the families of infants can promote opportunities for fathers to be with their infants in the hospital and to encourage their family involvement at home. The changes in attitudes regarding a father's involvement are evident in the changing policies within hospitals. In the 1970s barely one fourth of hospitals allowed fathers in the delivery room. Now nearly all do, even during cesarean births; many hospitals accommodate the presence of siblings as well.

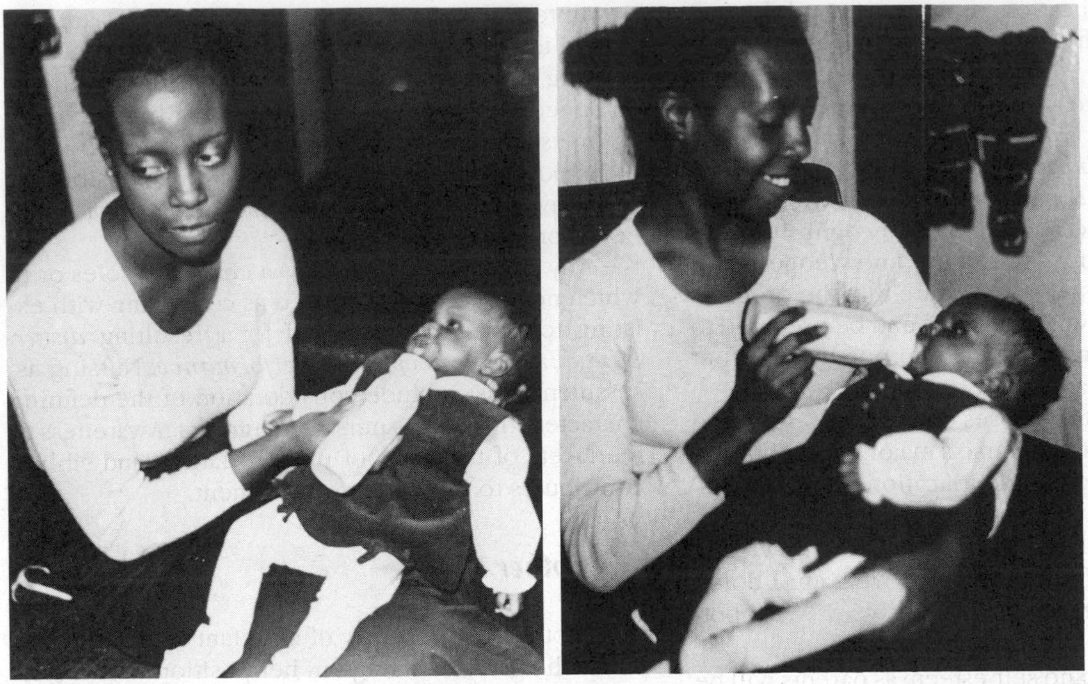

Subtle messages convey the conflict (left) or health (right) of parent-infant interaction (posed photos). (Photographs by Jim Tackett.)

The father's involvement in the home may call for the development of sociocultural support systems such as paternity leaves from employment after the birth of a baby. This type of social change may be hastened by nurses who recognize the importance of the father-infant involvement to the baby, the father, and the total family. Such nurses can seek opportunities to increase community awareness of this and make contacts with persons in positions of power to help bring about changes in policies.

The foregoing discussion about the assumption of parental roles may lead one to think that the responses of parents to each child as it is born are similar. This is not so. The baby actually molds or triggers adult behavior. It is the individual characteristics of the child that set up specific parental responses and influence their feelings and nurturing. The mother's and father's orientation to their parental roles surely will be influenced by this particular baby as they learn to communicate and to stimulate the baby's further development.

Sibling Role

Just as parents must assume new roles in relation to the neonate, older children in the family have the sibling role thrust upon them by the baby's arrival. The need to assume this developmental task comes at a time when support structures are not as available and predictable as usual. If the birth occurs at a hospital, the older children likely will be separated from their mother for one or more days and nights. As the father tries to establish an early relationship with his infant, he too may be separated from the older child for extended periods of time. Some hospital maternity units are attempting to reduce the older child's stress at being separated from the mother by promoting sibling visitation at the hospital.

Some changes have been observed in the nature of the relationship between the mother and the older child when a new baby arrives. A new baby's arrival seems to stimulate higher expectations by the mother for her older children, as she pressures them to master additional developmental tasks without as much maternal encouragement. The children may resent the family newcomer whose presence seems to have prompted these changes in their mother's behaviors.

Older children will be able to assume the sibling role in a healthier way if they can express to an understanding person—preferably the parents—their honest feelings about the changes they are experiencing and also can have their personal needs for affection and security met.

A complete discussion of factors involved in preparing a child for the birth of a new sibling is presented in Chapter 6.

Potential Stresses: Realignment of Member Tasks

Each couple needs to determine the appropriate division of labor for itself. The decisions will not be appropriate, however, until they are satisfactory to both members of the couple. These decisions frequently are not discussed openly, so one spouse's feelings of unfair distribution of duties may not be known by the other (Broom, 1984). The older children in the family who may assume some responsibility for certain household tasks should not be required to sacrifice all of their personal time for this purpose, because such demands may foster the development of resentment toward the baby and their parents.

One of the nurse's greatest contributions to relieving stress related to the family's division of labor is the promotion of open communication. If the family members are not able to discuss their feelings on this topic, the nurse can help by asking questions, interpreting feelings, and facilitating decision making.

Nurse researchers working with married couples during the period of adjustment to parenthood suggest that health care providers need to place more emphasis upon enhancing communication between the husband and wife, both prenatally and postnatally (Broom, 1984; Tomlinson, 1987). Broom (1984) compiled a list of the concerns most often expressed by parents (Box 5-1), which could be effectively used to stimulate conversation in couples preparing for childbirth. As Broom noted, "with increased understanding

Box 5-1
Potential Concerns of New Parents

PRACTICAL

A. Family income

Baby clothing and equipment expenses.

Fewer shared decisions on economic issues

Less money available to spend on "couple" activities

Loss of income due to spouse's leave from work

Economic responsibility imposed by arrival of baby

Child-care expenses

B. Household tasks

Conflict over amount of sharing in household tasks

Conflict over amount of sharing in child-care tasks

Balancing demands of spouse, housework/job, and child

Feeling too busy, having too much to do

Amount of time and energy required to care for baby

PERSONAL

A. Physical affection

Having sexual play

Concern that sexual intercourse will never be the same due to physical changes resulting from the birth process

Reduced spontaneity of sexual relationships

Reduced leisureliness of sexual relations

Beginning sexual intercourse again

Return of my/my wife's figure

Discomfort from stitches (episiotomy) will interfere with sexual pleasure

Methods of birth control

Breast soreness will interfere with sexual pleasure

B. Empathy

Spouse will not understand my moodiness, depression, tension

Emotional tension

Feeling tied down

Husband will feel excluded from family life due to breastfeeding

Husband will feel excluded from family life due to work schedule

Feeling "blue," "depressed," "down"

Conflict (about baby) with in-laws will cause conflict with spouse

C. Companionship

Less time for shared leisure activity with spouse

Level of social activity (as a couple) will change

Less communication with spouse

Less time to be alone with spouse

Activities will have to be worked around baby's schedule

Communication with spouse will be centered on baby

Little time/energy to devote to giving special attention to spouse

Spouse will be less stimulating intellectually

(From Broom, 1984.)

of the other's views, couples can more efficiently define problems and offer each other needed support."

Potential Stresses: Family Relationships and Communication

Friedemann and Emrich (1978) developed a formula for the number of interpersonal relationships within a family, in which x equals the number of interpersonal relationships and y the number of persons:

$$x = \frac{y^2 - y}{2}$$

Therefore, in a two-parent family of four persons, six interpersonal relationships exist: husband-wife, mother-child, mother-infant, father-child, father-infant, and child-infant (Fig. 5-1). The potential for the development of stress when new relationships are established with the arrival of the infant is understandable.

The nurse can be helpful to couples who identify problems and seek help with their marital relationship, by interpreting the dynamics of how the spouses may be feeling and promoting open communication between them. Serious disturbances in the relationship may require referral to a marriage or family counselor if the nurse is not educated in counseling methods. In a study of 96 couples recruited from childbirth education classes, Tomlinson (1987) found that the greatest determinant of postbirth marital satisfaction was the couple's marital satisfaction before birth of the new infant.

Nontraditional families experience role stress as well. A single mother who lives with her family of origin must determine how much of the parenting role she will assume and how much she will relinquish to *her* parents. In some families cultural traditions will be influential in these role determinations. The nurse can enhance problem solving by encouraging the expectant mother to discuss these role issues before the infant's birth with the significant others with whom she lives.

Stresses on nontraditional families are often different from those for the nuclear family. The single mother who does not live with extended family or in a communal arrangement may be the only person available to meet the demands of the new infant as well as those of older siblings. This fatiguing role can be compounded by early hospital discharge. If this is the mother's first child, she may not realize how much time is required to care for a newborn (Broom, 1984) or just how much her sleep will be disrupted. The nurse can be instrumental in helping this single parent realize the need to call upon extended family or friends for help in the first days and weeks. If the woman does not have such resources, follow-up home visits are advisable.

Maintaining Morale

The effect of the physical and psychologic upheaval experienced by families in the transition to parenthood often takes the form of mood swings and low morale. It is important to note that new coping mechanisms are needed to maintain the family's morale.

Duvall (1977) lists five attitudes or behaviors that help families in the childbearing stage to cope and maintain good morale:

1. Seeing beyond the drudgeries to the fundamental satisfactions of parenthood
2. Valuing persons above things
3. Resolving the conflicts inherent in the contradictory developmental tasks of parents and young children, and of fathers and mothers
4. Establishing healthy independence as a married couple
5. Accepting help in a spirit of appreciation and growth

These attitudes and behaviors help to keep priorities in proper perspective for the family.

Edwards (1974) has identified some questions that the new mother might explore, ideally with her husband, in the attempt to promote good morale in the family during this period of transition:

Am I doing important things as a mother?

What is my fantasy mother (concept of what a mother ought to be and ought to do) asking me to do?

Is it possible and helpful to me and my family to do them?

If I'm important, then how can I get some sleep and eat better?

Did my fantasy mother have fun?

Do I want to be like her?

What can I do for fun everyday? Can I dance alone, listen to music, sing while I nurse?

What did I decide to give up for "fourth trimester": ironing, working on a business at home, cleaning rooms that are seldom used?

What did I decide I wouldn't give up for "fourth trimester": employment, playing the piano, reading to my 2-year-old?

How can I feel better now with my dirty house and demanding baby?

For the employed mother who returns to work outside the home 6 to 8 weeks after the birth of the child, these questions must be modified and some additional ones asked. This mother's tasks include devis-

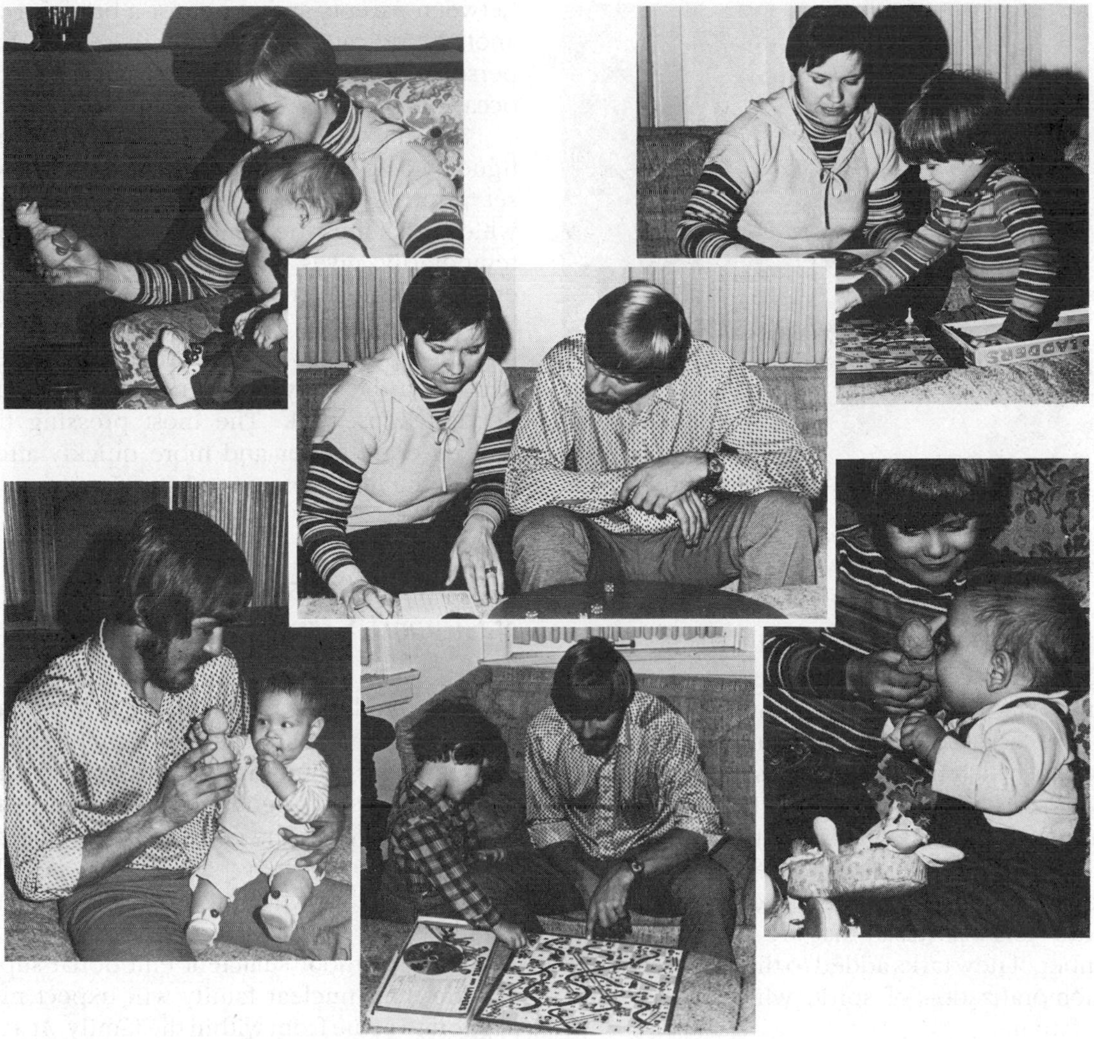

Figure 5-1. In a family of two persons, one relationship exists; in a family of three, three relationships. Adding one more family member increases the number of relationships to six. (Photographs by Jim Tackett.)

ing viable ways to meet her role responsibilities as wife and mother while attending to responsibilities in the workplace. If she has already established a workable childcare arrangement for her older children, this task may be relatively simple. However, the employed mother will have to add to her list of questions those that focus on her feelings about leaving the new baby in the care of others. Again, the nurse can provide a real service to the mother by providing information and by helping her identify unrealistic demands she may be placing on herself. Some of the mother's self-imposed demands may be the results of guilt that she is feeling about leaving her baby in someone else's care. Some research has shown that babies of employed mothers are at greater risk for emotional-social problems (Barglow, Vaughn, and Molitor, 1987). However, a growing body of evidence indicates that the mother's feelings about employment and her relationship with her baby are more important influences than is the fact that she is working outside the home. In mothers who preferred outside work to staying home, anxiety about separation from their first-born infants decreased sooner and to a greater extent than in mothers who preferred staying home (DeMeis, McBride, and Hock, 1986). More importantly, mothers who had warm, accepting relationships toward and with their infant sons demonstrated secure attachment with their babies, and neither the form nor the stability of the childcare arrangements were associated with the quality of that attachment (Benn, 1986).

Potential Stresses: Parental Fatigue

People are not at their best when tired, and the parents of infants have many reasons for their chronic fatigue.

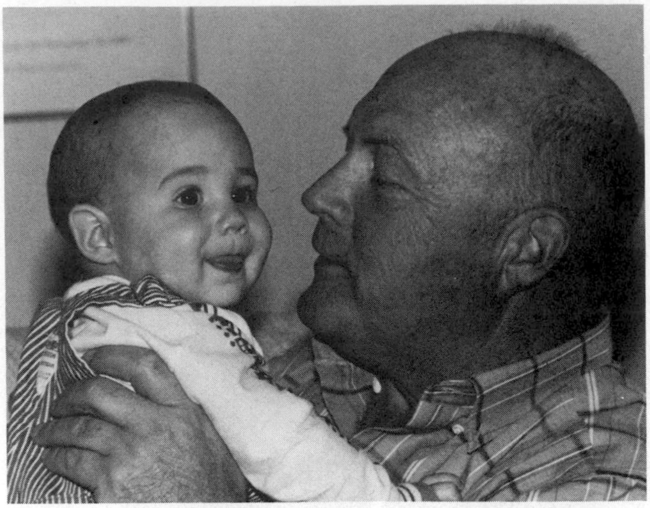

Grandparents can sometimes relieve the parent from the intensity of infant care.

The mother recently has had a dramatic change in her physiologic and psychologic status as a result of the baby's birth. The unpredictable nature of the baby's needs in the early weeks of life causes an irregular "schedule" to which the parents must adjust. This irregularity in schedule is responsible for parental loss of sleep as well as a sense of disorientation. The pressures inherent in the transition to new roles cause a certain degree of physical and emotional exhaustion. The inability to finish tasks that are begun plus the sheer number of new tasks added to the daily schedule cause a demoralization of spirit, which adds to the feeling of fatigue.

It is not difficult to understand why postpartum depression and a general disenchantment with the parenting role might afflict the parents of an infant, particularly during the early weeks after the birth. As the infant develops, he or she usually sleeps longer between feedings and establishes a more predictable and regular schedule that allows the parents to get more rest.

For the mother, chronic fatigue lessens her enjoyment of the maternal role, her self-confidence, her feeling of attractiveness to her husband, and her patience with the infant's siblings.

The father may resent the fatigue he feels from needing to earn the living and then assuming heavy family responsibilities upon his return home, plus having his sleep interrupted by the baby's crying. Tensions are likely to build between the parents in such an atmosphere.

Infants can sense tensions in parents by the way they are held and spoken to. When they sense tension, they often respond by crying or being fussy and irritable, which in turn causes more tension in the parents. This cycle must be broken by putting some distance between parents and infant for a brief period. This is another indication of the family's need for support persons to relieve them of child care responsibility occasionally.

The nurse can help parents prevent extreme fatigue by helping them to think through how they will set priorities. The nurse, by helping to determine which tasks must be done and which can be ignored temporarily, gives professional reassurance that parents should not try to do everything they did before the baby came plus the many new tasks associated with the baby. A top priority for the fatigued mother may be to nap when the baby sleeps rather than to do a lot of needed housework. The most pressing housework will be done better and more quickly after she has rested; the less pressing tasks can wait.

Potential Stresses: Parents' Lack of Support Structures

In the United States, availability of jobs has been at least partially responsible for young couples moving away from the communities in which their parents live. Society views independence as desirable for young couples. However, the geographic distances between the couples and their parents removes the family support structure when an infant is born to the young couple.

Those without sufficient emotional support from outside their nuclear family will expect most of the support to come from within the family. At a time when transition to new roles is occurring among nuclear family members, this support for one another may be limited. Research has demonstrated that mothers of infants are more satisfied with their lives when they perceive that they are receiving support from their husbands (Levitt, Weber, and Clark, 1986). A couple with self-esteem is able to trust one another. When a couple lacks trust based on self-esteem, husband and wife each feels there is barely enough to sustain his or her own life, let alone help the other. The mother and father in such a family lack emotional support at a time when it is sorely needed, and this lack of support brings a sense of social isolation as well. Lack of adult companionship and stimulation from outside relationships produces stress.

The mother and father who feel alone with their new responsibilities may develop resentment toward the infant, whom they see as having brought about this situation, or they may become so totally involved with the infant and his or her needs that their own personal development and self-confidence suffer. This decreasing confidence actually may cause them to withdraw from opportunities for social interaction.

When friends or relatives are available, they can alleviate some of the stress felt by the parent. Crnic and colleagues (1983) found evidence that mothers with greater stress had less positive attitudes and behaviors toward their baby, and mothers with greater support had more positive attitudes and behaviors toward their baby. Additionally, support from friends and relatives can be helpful by giving older children in the family special personal attention. This eases the child's jealousy of the attention devoted to the baby. If this special attention is given to the older child when away from home, he or she will have unique experiences to share with the family upon returning. The time away from home also temporarily gives the child's parent some lessened responsibility. When these opportunities do not exist, some potential richness is lacking from the older children's lives. As individuals within the family find support outside the family, the whole family benefits because of greater personal fulfillment of its members.

Nurses in contact with families with an infant may find themselves in a good position to fulfill a strong nurturing, supportive role. The beginning goal should be to establish a helping relationship with the mother and concentrate on her needs. Identifying observed family strengths rather than focusing on problems will contribute to the support the family members feel. Parents' strengths are the qualities that can be relied on as they cope and for which they do not need the professional's help. What the professional health care worker can offer is support and encouragement for their strengths.

Some hospitals, birthing centers, and community health agencies offer telephone follow-up or home visits to provide support during the transition to parenthood.

When nurses make the initial follow-up phonecall, they have the maternal and infant Kardex care plans, plus the postpartum follow-up care plan, in front of them. They assess the mother's psychosocial adjustment; knowledge of health concepts including nutrition, hygiene, sexual matters, rest, and activity; understanding of basic infant care, feeding, hygiene, safety, growth, and nurturing; maternal attachment; paternal engrossment (process of father identifying and claiming the infant as his, focusing attention and investing emotionally in the baby); and the nature of parental expectations for this baby.

During the home visit the nurse typically performs physical examinations of the mother and infant, weighs and measures the infant, draws blood samples and obtains laboratory specimens if indicated, assesses parenting skill, and encourages questions about infant care and the mother's self-care. Nurses also discuss family role adjustments associated with the birth of the new infant. During follow-up the nurse is committed to promoting confidence, competence, and independence among families. This is done by nurturing their growth and strengths. This type of program provides much support and professional help to new parents.

Nurses should be aware of professional and community sources of support to which they can refer clients. An informed referral should be based on an assessment of needs and an evaluation of the service offered (Gosha and Brucker, 1986). Nurses can systematically obtain data from clients regarding the value of services received and keep those data on file to use in future referrals.

Adapting Resources

The addition of an infant to a family unit can strain family resources. This kind of strain on family resources can result in *impaired home maintenance management*. This nursing diagnosis should be considered especially when several of the following defining characteristics of the diagnosis are detected in the nursing assessment (Gordon, 1987):

- Household members express difficulty in maintaining their home in a comfortable fashion. Basic needs such as heat in winter or running water may not be met, if finances are a problem
- Household members describe outstanding debts or financial crisis
- Unwashed or unavailable cooking equipment, clothes, or linen
- Overtaxed family members (e.g., exhausted, anxious parents)
- Household members request assistance with home maintenance
- Accumulation of dirt, food wastes, or hygienic wastes
- Offensive odors
- Lack of necessary equipment or aids

Nursing Strategies

The adaptation of resources to accommodate the infant cannot be prescribed generally because the resources available to families vary extensively. However, some basic considerations in the decision making include individuals' needs for privacy, personal attention, and finances, as well as the need for family planning.

Providing Space for Individual and Couple Privacy. Providing space for privacy may be difficult in some settings. During the early days at home with an infant, parents often find it convenient to keep the infant's bed near their own because of the baby's need for care at night. However, when the baby begins to sleep through the night, it is advisable for parents to get some distance from the infant. Physically, distance means that parents are not disturbed by normal baby noises and movement and the baby is not disturbed by parental voices and movements. Psychologically, the distance provided by moving the baby's bed outside the parents' room gives the parents a sense of privacy for intimacy and for a respite from the demands of the family. When separate rooms are not possible, portable screens or dividers may be useful.

Each family member should be allowed to have some space that is his or her own to arrange, keep "treasures" in, and go to for time alone. Although this may not necessarily be an entire room, even some section of a room can be useful.

For the mother who regularly is at home caring for the infant and possibly other children, the greatest sense of privacy may come when she is relieved of all household and child care responsibilities for a period of time to go outside the home and do what she pleases. Time away from home may also be the best arrangement for the couple to have some privacy if someone can provide child care. Recognizing the need for time alone and a place for each individual to call his or her own can stimulate creative planning and be one factor in establishing a stable family unit.

Providing for Individual Attention. Finding a time and place for each family member's privacy may be difficult, but equally difficult is finding time to give attention to each family member. The importance of maintenance of existing family relationships has been discussed previously. Ways parents can maintain loving relationships with their children, and wives or husbands with their mates, have also been presented.

Adapting Financial Resources. Another significant adjustment that many families face upon the birth of an infant is in the financial realm. Few young families can escape the burden of needing to plan very carefully for adequate funds for their needs. The many expenses that accompany the birth experience and the needs of the infant can often strain the family budget.

Financial management is always a challenge that requires self-discipline and some maturity to handle successfully. The family that experienced financial problems before the birth (e.g., poverty; unemployment; mismanagement due to gambling, or alcohol or substance abuse) may be at special risk. *Although nurses cannot provide financial security for any family, they should be aware of and sensitive to the importance of financial resources as a family or single mother adapts to a new infant.* If the neonate has been born with problems that require hospitalization or other medical care at home, the cost of care is another stress on the family.

Nursing Strategies

A significant contribution can be made by a well-prepared, perceptive, and supportive professional nurse. However, the nurse's role in working with these families will depend upon his or her opportunities to have contact with them.

Typical points of nurse-family contact today are in the hospital after birth, in physicians' offices and clinics, in parenting classes, in community health department channels, and in informal neighborhood contacts.

It is rarely mother alone, father alone, schools alone, friends alone—or any one factor alone—that shapes the destiny of the child. Children from birth onward are affected by a mosaic of forces. However, *the most significant influences on a child's life are parental relationships and family experience.* This is why nurses who are prepared to assess the needs of families and to plan and intervene to meet these needs can play a significant role in identifying stress within families of infants and can initiate care to alleviate or reduce this stress.

The Normal Neonate

Carolyn G. Pedigo

The newborn period is defined as from birth to 1 month of age. The adjectival form of neonate, *neonatal,* will be used interchangeably with *newborn* in this chapter.

This section focuses on the appraisal and care of the normal full-term neonate. "Normal" refers to the absence of problematic physiologic, pathologic, or neuromuscular conditions, or all three. Minor deviations are common and considered normal; therefore, they are included in this section. "Full-term" refers to gestational age. The full-term neonate is one born following 38 to 42 weeks of gestation in utero.

Nursing assessment and care are best learned first with the normal full-term neonate. Working from a normal base, the nurse can begin to recognize deviations from normal as minor or major, formulate appropriate nursing diagnoses, and carry out appropriate nursing interventions.

"It's a girl!" "It's a boy!" A baby has been born. The whole gamut of emotional responses might be compressed into this exclamation. After 9 months of waiting, the momentous event has occurred. Parental adaptation to the birth may be influenced by many factors: whether or not the pregnancy was planned, whether or not the pregnancy was normal, the length of time and degree of difficulty in labor and delivery; the medications administered during labor and delivery; and the sex and appearance of the newborn infant. Nursing interventions are geared toward identifying those factors—parental or neonatal, or both—that might interfere with a positive adaptation.

The birth transition from intrauterine to extrauterine existence may enhance or interfere with neonatal adaptation. In the neonate born at term, all systems are considered mature enough to adapt and support life outside the uterus. Following a 9-month existence in an environment that is totally protected and nurturing, the fetus is suddenly and sometimes painfully propelled through a narrow, constricted passage into the bright, cold, and noisy environment of the delivery room. To facilitate extrauterine adaptation, the neonate's nose and mouth are suctioned with a bulb syringe to remove mucus, which may obstruct respiratory passages. Once the umbilical cord is clamped and cut, the child is forced to establish independent life-sustaining functions. At no other time in an individual's life are greater physiologic adjustments required than during the first hour after birth.

Initial Assessment of the Neonate

Assessment of the neonate includes the initial Apgar scoring and comprehensive physical assessment, including gestational age and size (weight and length), and assessment of behavioral characteristics. Assessment is done to determine how satisfactorily the neonate is adapting to extrauterine life and to rule out any risk factors that might compromise growth or life or both.

Apgar Score

Dr. Virginia Apgar (1953) developed this tool for evaluating the infant's condition at birth. Assessment is done at 1 minute and again at 5 minutes, using five standardized observations (heart rate, respiratory effort, reflex irritability, muscle tone and color). The 1-minute assessment is valuable because it provides a rapid method of determining the infant's ability to adapt to extrauterine life. With the 1-minute Apgar score, one can identify specifically the resuscitative measures that should be taken. The purpose of the 5-minute score is to re-evaluate the newborn's condition, particularly the response to resuscitative measures.

As soon as delivery is complete a timer is started, so that the neonate can be assessed at exactly 1 minute. The *heart rate* is the first and most important observation made, providing the most useful diagnostic and prognostic information. It should be counted for a full minute either through auscultation of the precordium or palpation of the umbilical cord pulse located at the junction of the umbilical cord and the abdominal wall.

The second most important observation is *respiratory effort.* Only the neonate's unassisted respiratory rate is counted. Respiratory rate should be assessed by counting the number of inspirations within 1 full minute in order to note any delays in inspiratory effort. The rate may be determined by auscultation of the chest or observation of chest wall excursions.

Reflex irritability is assessed by stimulating the newborn infant in order to evoke a response. Suctioning the nares, gently rubbing the back, or lightly flicking the sole of the foot are examples of stimuli used. The more alert the neonate, the more easily one can evoke a response.

Muscle tone is assessed by observing the infant's spontaneous return to a state of flexion; that is, when limbs are extended, they should return rapidly to their original position when released. The examiner should attempt to extend the extremities, noting the presence or absence of resistance and the rapidness of return to flexion. The infant's appearance in flexion is discussed later under the heading "General Appearance."

Color is the last observation, and according to Dr. Apgar, of least significance. All babies are cyanotic at birth. With the onset of respirations the skin becomes pink, except for the extremities, which may remain slightly cyanotic *(acrocyanosis)* for the first few hours of life. Acrocyanosis is due to insufficient circulation to the extremities, a condition that becomes reversed with adaptation to extrauterine life.

The Apgar Scoring Chart is found in Table 5-1. Each of the five observation areas should receive a score of 0, 1, or 2 according to the descriptions found in the score chart. When each of the five areas is scored, the sum total equals the Apgar score. A score of 10 is the highest possible, 0 the lowest. An infant who has a score of 7 to 10 is in good condition and will only need suction of the nose and mouth and routine care and observation. A score of 3 to 6 indicates a moderately depressed infant who will need some form of resuscitation along with close observation during the first 24 hours of life. An infant who receives a score of 0, 1, or 2 is considered severely depressed and will need ventilatory assistance and intensive care as part of resuscitative measures.

Table 5-1. Apgar Score Chart

Observation	Score: 0	1	2
Heart rate	Absent	Slow (below 100)	Over 100
Respiratory effort	Absent (apneic)	Slow, irregular, shallow	Good, sustained cry; regular respirations
Reflex irritability	No response	Grimace, frown	Sneeze, cough, cry
Muscle tone	Limp, completely flaccid	Some flexion of extremities; some resistance to extension of extremities	Active motion, good muscle tone, spontaneous flexion
Color	Cyanotic, pale	Body pink, extremities pale	Completely pink

(From Apgar, 1953.)

Table 5-2. Score Sheet for External Physical Characteristics

External Sign	Points: 0	1	2	3	4	Score
Edema	Obvious edema of hands and feet; pitting over tibia	No obvious edema of hands and feet; pitting over tibia	No edema			
Skin texture	Very thin, gelatinous	Thin and smooth	Smooth; medium thickness. Rash or superficial peeling	Slight thickening and peeling especially of hands and feet	Thick and parchment-like; superficial or deep cracking	
Skin color	Dark red	Uniformly pink	Pale pink; variable over body	Pale; only pink over ears, lips, palms, or soles		
Skin opacity (trunk)	Numerous veins and venules clearly seen, especially over abdomen	Veins and tributaries seen	A few large vessels clearly seen over abdomen	A few large vessels seen indistinctly over abdomen	No blood vessels seen	
Lanugo (over back)	No lanugo	Abundant; long and thick over whole back	Hair thinning especially over lower back	Small amount of lanugo and bald areas	At least 1/2 of back devoid of lanugo	
Plantar creases	No skin creases	Faint red marks over anterior half of sole	Definite red marks over > anterior 1/2; indentations over < 1/3	Indentations over > anterior 1/3	Definite deep indentations over > anterior 1/3	
Nipple formation	Nipple barely visible, no areola	Nipple well defined; areola smooth and flat, diameter <0.75 cm	Areola stippled, edge not raised, diameter <0.75 cm	Areola stippled, edge raised, diameter >0.75 cm		
Breast size	No breast tissue palpable	Breast tissue on one or both sides, <0.5 cm. diameter	Breast tissue both sides; one or both 0.5–1.0 cm	Breast tissue both sides; one or both >1 cm		
Ear form	Pinna flat and shapeless, little or no incurving of edge	Incurving of part of edge of pinna	Partial incurving whole of upper pinna	Well-defined incurving whole of upper pinna		
Ear firmness	Pinna soft, easily folded, no recoil	Pinna soft, easily folded, slow recoil	Cartilage to edge of pinna, but soft in places, ready recoil	Pinna firm, cartilage to edge; instant recoil		
Genitals						
Male	Neither testis in scrotum	At least one testis high in scrotum	At least one testis right down			
Female (with hips 1/2 abducted)	Labia majora widely separated, labia minora protruding	Labia majora almost cover labia minora	Labia majora completely cover labia minora			
					EXTERNAL TOTAL:	

(From Dubowitz et al, 1970.)

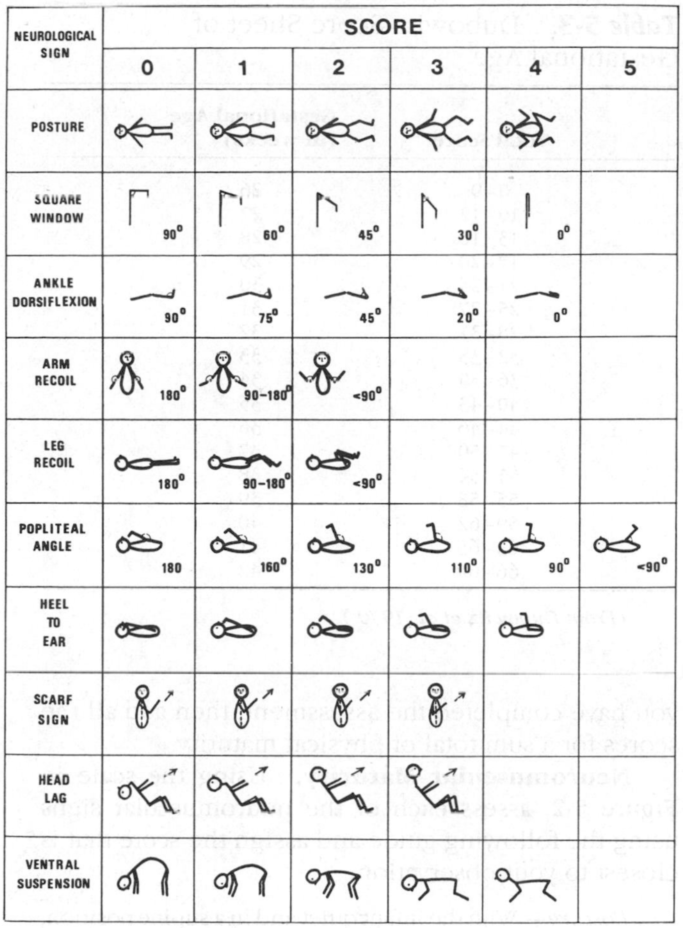
NEUROLOGICAL SIGN
SCORE
0
1
2
3
4
5
POSTURE
SQUARE WINDOW
90°
60°
45°
30°
0°
ANKLE DORSIFLEXION
90°
75°
45°
20°
0°
ARM RECOIL
180°
90-180°
<90°
LEG RECOIL
180°
90-180°
<90°
POPLITEAL ANGLE
180
160°
130°
110°
90°
<90°
HEEL TO EAR
SCARF SIGN
HEAD LAG
VENTRAL SUSPENSION

Figure 5-2. Score sheet for neurologic characteristics. (From Dubowitz L, et al: Clinical assessment of gestational age in the newborn infant. *J Pediatr* 1970 July; 1.)

Gross physical assessment is performed immediately after delivery to identify risk factors that could potentially interfere with life or growth. Within the first 24 hours of life a thorough physical examination, including assessment of physical, neurologic, and behavioral characteristics, should be performed to provide a normal data base for comparison as the newborn baby progresses through life.

Dubowitz Assessment for Estimation of Gestational Age

A standard set of criteria should be used for estimation of gestational age (GA) as an indicator of maturity. GA is defined as the number of weeks spent in utero to the time of birth. Dr. Lillian Dubowitz and her colleagues (1970) developed a standardized tool, using 11 external signs and 10 neurologic signs for estimating the gestational age of the neonate.

External physical characteristics should be assessed as soon as possible after birth. These physical characteristics are external signs of progressive tissue development. They provide data for evaluating the degree of physical maturity of the neonate.

The neurologic signs provide data for evaluating neurologic development and maturity through passive and active muscle tone. The infant should be alert and quiet during the neurologic testing to obtain valid results. Any signs that deviate from normal should be reassessed within 24 hours. The gestational age of the neonate is estimated by combining the score from the physical maturity chart (Table 5-2) and the score from the neurologic maturity chart (Fig. 5-2). The final score is then compared with the maturity rating scale (Table 5-3) to determine estimated gestational age. The full-term infant is 38 to 42 weeks of gestation.

The sections following are designed to provide experience in actual evaluation of an infant.

Physical Maturity. With the neonate on an examining surface and using the scale in Table 5-2, assess each of the following physical characteristics: edema, skin texture, skin color, skin opacity, lanugo, plantar creases, nipple formation, breast size, ear formation, ear firmness, and genitalia. The descriptions for each area range from 0 to 4 beginning with less mature development and progressing to mature tissue. After assessing the presence or absence of edema, find the description in the scale that best describes your observation and give the neonate the appropriate score. Proceed in the same manner with each characteristic until

Table 5-3. Dubowitz Score Sheet of Gestational Age

Total Score	Gestational Age (in weeks)
0–9	26
10–12	27
13–16	28
17–20	29
21–24	30
25–27	31
28–31	32
32–35	33
36–39	34
40–43	35
44–46	36
47–50	37
51–54	38
55–58	39
59–62	40
63–65	41
66–69	42

(From Dubowitz et al, 1970.)

you have completed the assessment, then add all the scores for a sum total of physical maturity.

Neuromuscular Maturity. Using the scale in Figure 5-2, assess each of the neuromuscular signs using the following guide and assign the score that is closest to your observation.

Posture—With the infant quiet and in a supine position, observe the degree of flexion in the arms and legs. Muscle tone and degree of flexion increase with maturity. Full flexion of the arms and the legs = 4.

Square window—Without rotating the wrist, flex the hand with enough pressure to get as great a degree of flexion as possible. Measure the angle between the base of the thumb and the anterior aspect of the forearm. Full flexion = 4.

Ankle dorsiflexion—At the ankle, flex the foot onto the shin with sufficient pressure to provide maximum flexion ability. Measure the angle between the dorsum of the foot and the anterior aspect of the leg. A 20 degree angle = 3.

Arm recoil—With the baby in a supine position, fully flex both arms, hold for 5 seconds, fully extend and rapidly release arms. Recoil to a state of flexion should occur instantly. A brisk return to full flexion = 2.

Leg recoil—With the baby in a supine position, fully flex both legs without lifting the hips up from the surface. Hold flexed for 5 seconds, fully extend, and rapidly release. Recoil to a state of flexion should occur instantaneously. A brisk return to full flexion (less than 90 degrees at knees and hips) = 2.

Popliteal angle—With the neonate in a supine position, flex one thigh on the abdomen. Be certain to keep body alignment straight and hips flat on the surface. While maintaining flexion of the thigh, attempt to straighten the leg toward the head until resistance is met. Measure the popliteal angle and score. Less than 90 degrees = 5.

Heel to ear—With the neonate supine, pelvis flat on examining surface, attempt to pull the feet toward the head. When resistance is met, determine the distance between the heels and the ears and score according to distance.

Scarf sign—With the neonate in a supine position, place the arm across the chest so that the hand touches the opposite shoulder. The elbow may be lifted across the body (Fig. 5-3). The score is determined by the location of the elbow. If the elbow does not reach the midline of the thorax, the score = 3.

Head lag—With the neonate supine, grasp both arms and slowly pull the infant up to a sitting position. Observe the relationship of the head to the trunk during the procedure. If the neonate has sufficient muscle tone to hold the head slightly forward of the body, the score = 3.

Ventral suspension—With the newborn infant prone, place the palm of your hand supporting the chest. Raise the infant off the examining surface and observe the infant's independent postural change. Straightening of the back with slight hyperextension of the head = 4.

The sum total of these observations will yield the score for neuromuscular maturity. Find the sum total of the physical maturity scale and the neuromuscular maturity scale. Using Table 5-3, compare the score with the maturity rating scale to determine the neonate's estimated gestational age. This score is accurate within 2 weeks of the neonate's actual gestational age. After 5 days of life, the scoring becomes less accurate due to neurologic and tissue maturation.

Appropriateness of Size for Gestational Age

Once the gestational age (GA) has been determined, the examiner can assess the neonate's size in relation to the estimated gestational age (EGA). In their research, Dr. Lula Lubchenco and co-workers (1963; 1966) developed standardized tools for assessing weight, length and head circumference related to GA in order to determine whether the neonate is appropriate for gestational age (AGA), small for gestational age (SGA), or large for gestational age (LGA). According to Figure 5-4, the AGA newborn has an average gestation

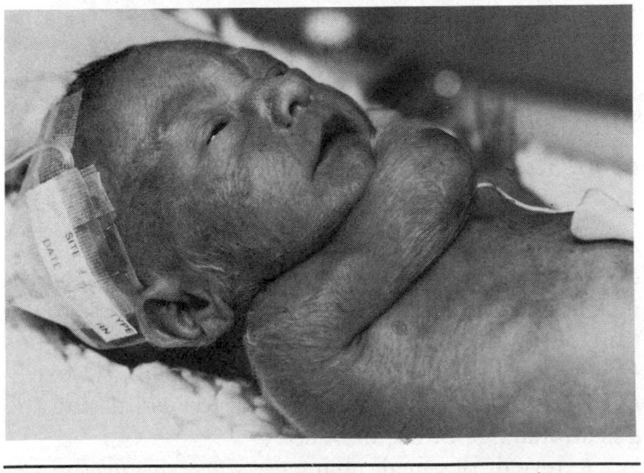

Figure 5-3. Scarf sign. A neonate born at 28 weeks' gestation. On assessment, elbow can be brought to midline without resistance. As the infant matures, this movement is resisted.

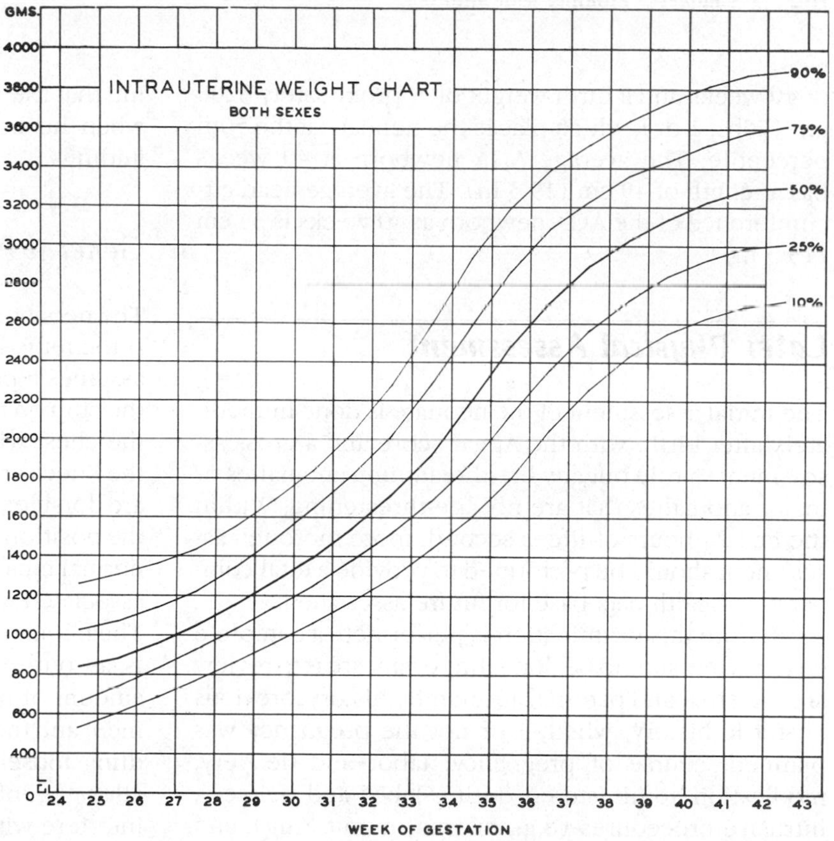

Figure 5-4. Intrauterine length, weight, and head circumference charts. (From Lubchenco L, et al: Intrauterine growth as estimated from liveborn birthweight data at 24 to 42 weeks of gestation. *Pediatrics* 1963 Oct; 793.)

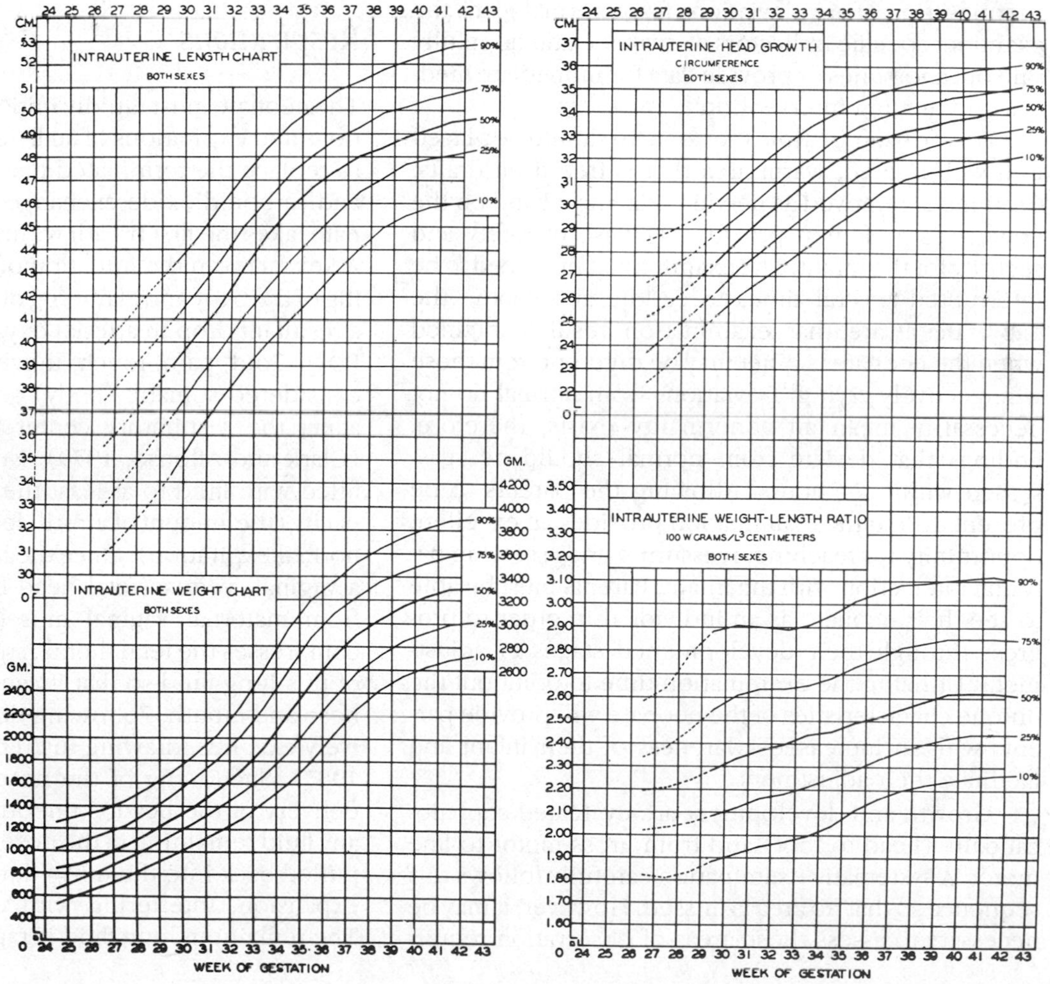

of 40 weeks and a birth weight of approximately 3200 gm (7 lbs, 1 oz), which places the neonate at the 50th percentile. The average AGA newborn at 40 weeks has a length of 49 cm (19.3 in). The average head circumference of the AGA newborn at 40 weeks is 34 cm (13.5 in).

Later Physical Assessment

The initial assessment of the neonate is done immediately after birth, with the Apgar score and a gross assessment to rule out any life-threatening anomalies or major anomalies that are not life-threatening. Within the first 24 hours of life, a second, more thorough assessment should be performed to provide a total comparative health data base for future assessment.

Before this examination is performed, a complete chart review should be done. Important areas to review are maternal and paternal age, family history, previous obstetric history, whether or not the pregnancy was planned, course of pregnancy, labor and delivery, medication administered during labor and delivery, intrusive procedures (e.g., internal monitoring), and Apgar scores with appropriate resuscitative measures. Identification of any deviations from normal gives the examiner specific indicators to evaluate and hopefully rule out anomalies or provide data for immediate medical and nursing intervention.

For the examination, the neonate should be placed in a well-lighted, warm area that is free from drafts. Clothing is removed as needed. Placing a hand on the newborn's abdomen provides a sense of safety and security for the infant. The examination may need to be interrupted several times to cuddle and soothe the baby. Be aware that examination results obtained when the neonate is quiet may be different from those when actively crying. Deviations from normal do not necessarily mean an abnormality exists; therefore, findings that deviate from normal should be reassessed within 24 hours. Allowing the parents to be present during the examination provides an excellent opportunity for teaching, reassuring and assessing parental interaction with the infant. Parents must be able to see their neonate as an individual in order to progress through their developmental stages of adjustment. Utilizing the examination time to point out the unique characteristics of the neonate will provide parents with an increased awareness of their infant and facilitate their adjustment.

Growth and development are evaluated cephalocaudally (head to foot) and from gross motor to fine motor. A systematic examination carefully follows this sequence so that no area is missed. However, it may be necessary to assess those areas of observation requiring that the infant be in a quiet state first, or at a point when he or she becomes quiet, to ensure accurate findings.

General Appearance

The neonate assumes a posture similar to that in utero. If the fetus was in a vertex position, the infant readily assumes a posture of flexion. The head is flexed with the chin on the chest, arms are flexed and held close to the chest with hands fisted, the back is slightly bent, the knees are flexed with thighs on abdomen and feet are dorsiflexed on the anterior aspect of the leg. This is the position of comfort for the baby and is indicative of normal muscle tone. A decrease in muscle tone may be associated with trauma, sedation, or preterm gestation. The neonate's size appropriateness for gestational age is as outlined in Table 5-3. Flexion decreases the amount of body surface area exposed to the environment and thereby decreases the rate of heat loss. Swaddling loosely or covering lightly with a blanket will allow the infant to assume a position of flexion, yet not interfere with freedom of movement.

Respirations

The neonate must rapidly initiate and maintain inspirations and expirations of sufficient depth and regularity to replace the terminated placental source of oxygen and carbon dioxide exchange. The normal term neonate takes the first breath within 30 seconds after birth. A key factor in the initiation of respiration is the cooling of the baby and clamping of the umbilical cord with a resultant drop in arterial oxygen or hypoxemia (low PO_2). Cold, pain, touch, movement, and light are all considered somatic (body) sensory stimuli that also affect the respiratory center to stimulate breathing (Clark and Affonso, 1979). Normally, fetal lungs are filled with fluid to at least the functional residual capacity (the amount of air still left in the lungs following normal expiration). Once the head is delivered during a vaginal, vertex (fetal head first) delivery, pressure from maternal vaginal muscles and tissue actually compresses the fetal thorax, squeezing out almost half of this lung fluid so that it can be suctioned from the nose and mouth. Following delivery, the chest reflexively expands, drawing in 20 to 40 ml of air (Reeder, 1987). Suctioning of the nose and mouth following delivery of the head is important, because without it any fluid remaining in the nose and trachea will also be pulled back into the lungs during reflexive chest wall expansion, interfering with efficient gas exchange. The remaining lung fluid is rapidly absorbed within 6 to 24 hours. It moves from the lungs into the pulmonary capillaries and lymphatic system, then into the main circulation for excretion through the kidneys (Reeder, 1987).

The baby delivered by cesarean section does not have the benefit of vaginal compression of the thorax; therefore, considerable lung fluid remains and must be cleared for maximum gas exchange to occur.

Respirations may be irregular and should be assessed by counting the number of inspirations for a full minute. The normal respiratory rate following successful adaptation to extrauterine life is 40 to 60 breaths per minute. After the first 24 hours, the rate drops to 30 to 50 breaths per minute (Sharping, 1983).

Circulatory Changes

Fetal circulation and the changes that occur after birth are shown in detail in Chapter 39.

The peripheral circulation may be somewhat sluggish, accounting for transient cyanosis of the hands and feet *(acrocyanosis)* and around the mouth *(circumoral cyanosis)*.

At the time of birth, if the cord is allowed to cease pulsating before being clamped and cut, the baby will receive an additional 50 to 100 ml of blood from the placenta. The appropriate time to cut the cord is debatable. Some authorities think that the neonate can benefit from the additional volume of iron-rich oxygenated blood. Others believe that the additional volume is an overload for the infant's system.

Assessment of the heart is done by auscultating the apical pulse. The first and second heart sounds should be clearly distinct. The rate may be rapid but should be regular, between 120 and 150 beats per minute during the quiet, alert state. During crying periods the heart rate may increase to 190 beats per minute, and, during sleep, may decrease to 70 to 90 beats per minute (Sharping, 1983). Since activity influences the heart rate, the baby should be quiet for an accurate assessment.

Skin Assessment

The skin of the neonate provides an index of growth. Well-nourished neonates have well-defined layers of subcutaneous fat over their bodies, which provide thermoregulation and a barrier against infection. Lack of subcutaneous fat may indicate prematurity or malnutrition. The skin should be observed closely for breaks as this may be a portal of entry for bacteria.

Skin Color. Immediately after birth the term neonate's skin is erythematous (beefy red), then fades to its normal color within a few hours. Acrocyanosis is a normal transient phenomenon caused by vasomotor instability, capillary stasis, and high hemoglobin. Persistent generalized cyanosis indicates underlying distress.

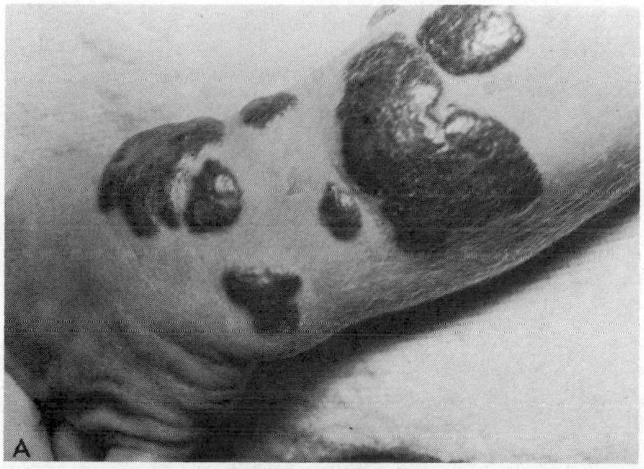

Figure 5-5. Strawberry hemangioma. (Courtesy of Mary Lou Moore.)

Cyanosis is assessed in the white neonate by looking at the skin and by inspection of the mucous membranes of the mouth, eyes, and nailbeds of the hands and feet. In assessment of the infant with darker skin color, the mucous membranes and nailbeds are the most reliable indicators of cyanosis.

Harlequin Color Change. When the neonate is placed in a side-lying position, the side next to the mattress will turn pink while the upper side remains pale. This is known as harlequin color change and has no known significance. However, color distribution should remain even, in supine or prone position.

Telangiectatic Nevi (Stork Bites). These are common on the upper eyelids, back of the neck, and occiput. They are flat, localized, reddened areas created by capillary dilation and should disappear during the first year of life.

Strawberry Hemangiomas. These may be present at birth or appear up to 2 weeks following birth. They resemble strawberry clusters and consist of dilated capillaries in the dermal and subdermal layers (Fig. 5-5). They are elevated and may continue to grow up to 1 year of age. Absorption and shrinkage takes place slowly and usually requires 7 to 10 years for completion. Although hemangiomas are unsightly and may be disturbing to parents, they are best left untreated. However, large or multiple hemangiomas may signal the presence of internal involvement. These children should be referred for evaluation of this possibility.

Mongolian Spots. Bluish-gray or purple patches of pigmentation are sometimes seen across the sacrum or buttocks (Fig. 5-6). Known as mongolian spots, the pigmentation begins at birth in the basal layer of the epidermis and is prevalent among children of Asian,

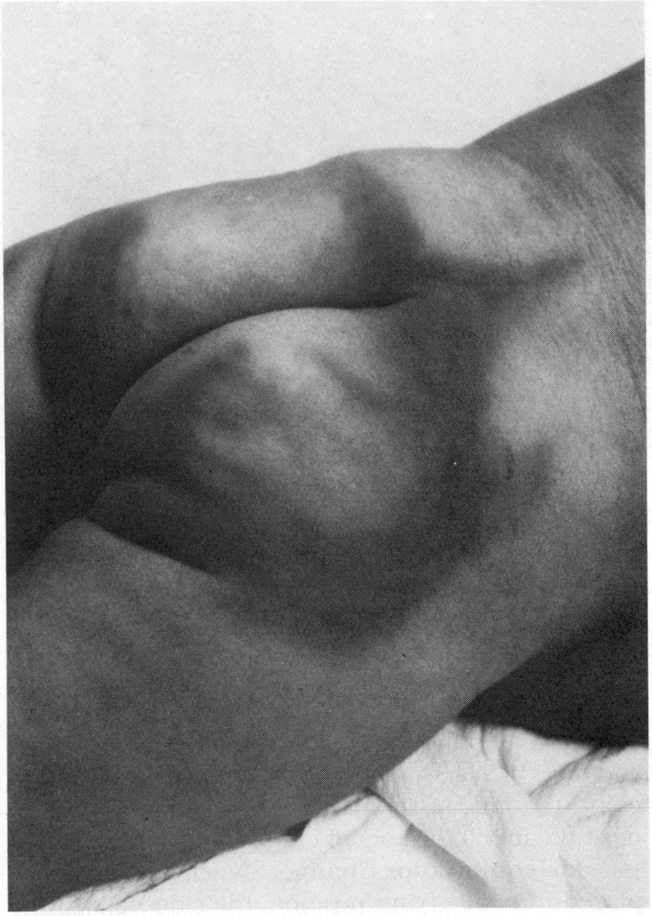

Figure 5-6. Mongolian spots. (Courtesy of Mead Johnson & Company, Nutritional Division.)

southern European, and African descent. These spots disappear by school-age without treatment.

Port Wine Stain. This is reddish discoloration of the skin of the face or neck. This vascular birthmark usually involves serious deformity because of the large skin area that is typically involved.

Lanugo. These are fine, downy hairs that cover the neonate's body. They are often concentrated over the shoulders and back. These hairs disappear without treatment.

Milia. The small, shiny, whitish nodules beneath the skin, found on the nose and chin, are called milia. They are caused by retention of sebaceous gland secretions. They disappear spontaneously.

Skin Turgor. Turgor is related to tissue hydration and is present in the normal neonate. Transient edema may also be present around the eyes and dorsal aspects of the extremities due to birth trauma. Lack of skin turgor may indicate malnutrition in utero or metabolic disorders. To assess turgor, grasp the skin with thumb and forefinger and gently turn. The skin should feel elastic and return to a smooth surface when released.

Head and Neck Assessment

The head of the neonate is proportionately large (approximately one fourth the total length of the newborn). The forehead is prominent and the chin recedes.

Head circumference is measured by placing the tape above the eyebrows and around the most prominent aspect of the occiput. Measurement may need to be repeated several times for accuracy. Accurate assessment of circumference provides a baseline for future assessment of cephalic development.

Molding. With a vaginal, vertex delivery, the neonate's head molds to fit the birth canal more easily by gradual overlapping of the calvarium bones and narrowing or over-riding of the sutures. Molding is usually not present following a cesarean birth. Parents may be anxious about the presence of molding; they need reassurance that it will disappear in a few days.

Fontanels and Suture Lines. The fontanels are soft membranous spaces where the skull bones join (Fig. 5-7). The anterior fontanel (soft spot) is diamond shaped and lies between the sagittal and coronal sutures. It is approximately 2 to 3 cm wide and 3 to 4 cm long. It closes at 12 to 18 months of age. The posterior fontanel is triangular and lies between the sagittal and lambdoidal sutures. It is approximately 1 cm long and closes at about 2 months. The nurse should feel and measure the fontanels. Bulging fontanels are indicative of increased intracranial pressure and depressed or sunken fontanels of dehydration. Parents are sometimes afraid to touch the "soft spot" for fear of causing brain damage. Actually it is as tough as canvas and needs the same amount of stimulation as the rest of the scalp. The suture lines denote the separation of the cranial bones and are either closely approximated or over-riding. They should never appear or feel separated; this is indicative of increased intracranial pressure.

Caput Succedaneum. This is the result of diffuse edema (margins of swelling are indistinct) of the soft tissues of the scalp which may extend across suture lines (Fig. 5-8). It is caused by continuous pressure on the scalp during labor and is most pronounced following prolonged labor. It is gradually absorbed and disappears within a few days. Ecchymotic coloration (black and blue bruises) may be present; this may cause feelings of guilt and anxiety in parents. Nursing intervention should be directed toward helping parents resolve these feelings.

Cephalhematoma. In this condition, a collection of blood from ruptured blood vessels forms between the skull bone and the periosteum because of trauma to the head during the birth process (Fig. 5-9). It does not cross suture lines, because it is confined to

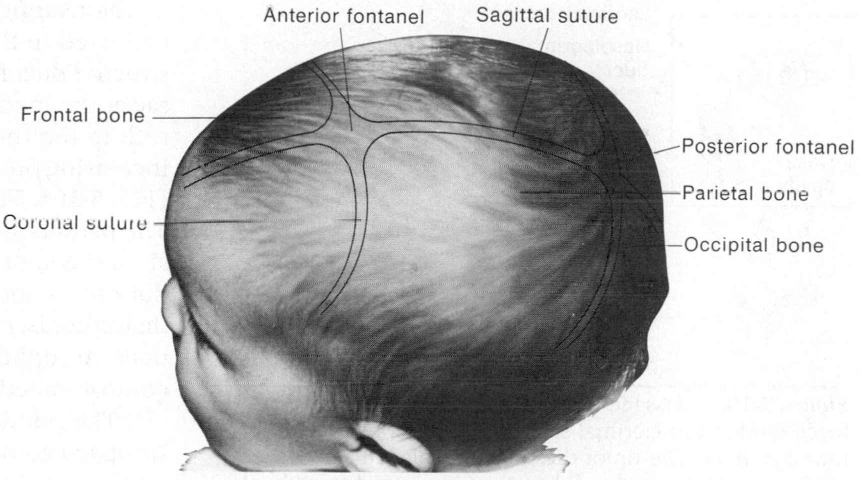

Figure 5-7. Location of the anterior and posterior fontanels.

one bone. Obvious swelling develops within 24 to 48 hours after birth. The area may be ecchymotic due to the presence of coagulated blood. Absorption of a cephalhematoma may take 2 to 3 weeks or longer. As with caput succedaneum, parents may experience guilt. The nurse should help absolve them of this feeling.

Scalp. The nurse should palpate and inspect the scalp for lesions, bleeding or coarse, brittle hair. If an internal monitor was used during labor, the neonate will have a small puncture wound in the occipital area of the scalp. This area should be kept clean and dry and inspected for signs of infection.

Face. The face should be inspected for symmetry of parts and symmetry between the left and right sides. Some asymmetry may be due to position—that is, resuming a position that was maintained in utero. This will disappear within a few weeks or months. Facial asymmetry may indicate facial nerve palsy due to birth trauma.

Eyes. The eyes should appear clear without redness or purulent discharge. Occasionally, the eyelids are puffy with a purulent discharge during the first 24 hours. This is a transient chemical conjunctivitis due to silver nitrate ($AgNO_3$) drops administered to prevent ophthalmia neonatorum (gonorrheal conjunctivitis). In 1980, the American Academy of Pediatrics recommended the use of 1 per cent tetracycline or 0.5 per cent erythromycin in place of silver nitrate. Silver nitrate is effective in preventing gonococcal ophthalmia but is not thought to prevent chlamydial ophthalmia caused by *Chlamydia trachomatis.* The incidence of chlamydial ophthalmia has surpassed that of gonococcal ophthalmia in the United States (Bryant, 1984). Erythromycin seems to be the drug of choice in pre-

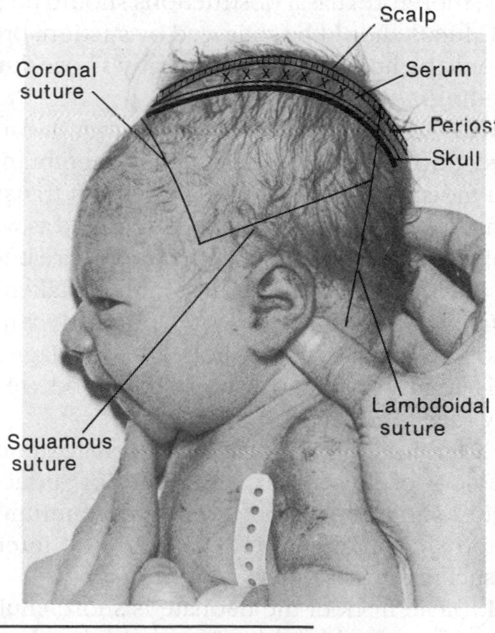

Figure 5-8. Caput succedaneum.

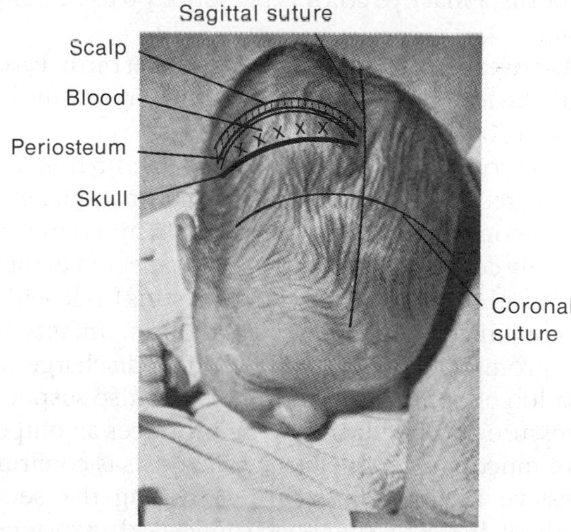

Figure 5-9. Cephalhematoma.

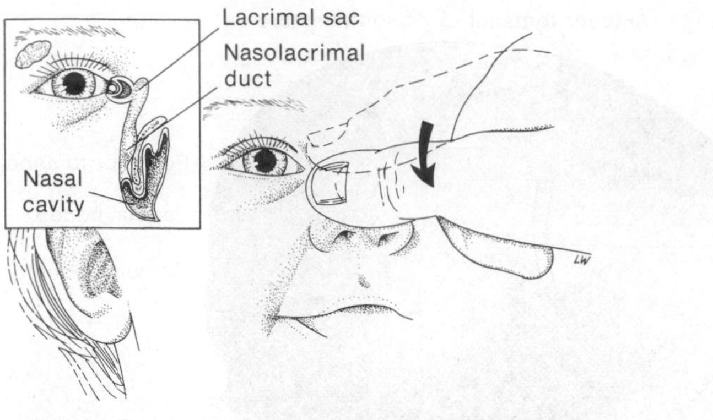

***Figure* 5-10.** Massage of the lacrimal drainage tract to force fluid in the lacrimal sac through the obstructed drainage tract. The tip of the thumb is placed above the sac at the medial angle of the eye. Slowly and steadily, the thumb is rolled downward.

vention of both chlamydial ophthalmia and gonococcal ophthalmia with no evidence of chemical conjunctivitis (Bryant, 1984).

The eyelids of the neonate are closed most of the time. Attempts to force the eyelids open will meet with resistance. Holding the infant in an upright position and gently rocking the head back and forth will usually stimulate opening of the eyelids. Bright lights, loud noises, and touching the eyelashes will cause the neonate to promptly close the eyes.

The sclera has a slightly bluish tint. When jaundice is present, the sclera becomes yellowish; this may be the first indication of jaundice because the ruddy skin color may mask it elsewhere. Occasionally, small conjunctival vessels rupture during the pressure of labor and delivery, causing a bright-red streak near the iris. This is a subconjunctival hemorrhage and will disappear spontaneously within 2 to 3 weeks.

The iris is usually dark or grayish-blue in most newborns. Final eye color is present by 6 to 12 months of age.

Lacrimal gland ducts are immature at birth. Parents should be told not to expect tears with crying until 1 to 3 months of age.

Dacryostenosis is a congenital lacrimal stenosis that creates an obstruction of the lacrimal duct and is often accompanied by dacryocystitis. This condition is relatively common in infancy. It is suspected in infants with purulent discharge (dacryocystitis) but without any conjunctival injection or irritation. Infants who have prompt recurrence of purulent discharge after cessation of ophthalmic antibiotics are also suspected. If pressure over the lacrimal sac produces an outpouring of mucopurulent material, diagnosis is confirmed. Excessive lacrimation (tearing) during the second month of life is a sign that suggests dacryostenosis which may be readily noticed by the nurse during infant examinations.

Nonsurgical correction involves forcing the fluid collected in the affected lacrimal sac through the obstructed duct by placing the tip of one thumb over the sac at the medial angle of the eye and slowly, steadily rolling the thumb toward the duct opening, thereby increasing pressure on the stenosis to gradually open it (Fig. 5-10). This is done four times daily for a month. The parents should be instructed in the procedure and should demonstrate its use satisfactorily. If this procedure does not open the duct within a month, an ophthalmologist can open the duct by probing the lacrimal tract. An ophthalmic antibiotic may be prescribed to control infection until the obstruction is cleared.

The pupils should be observed for any whiteness or opacities that indicate congenital cataracts. This is particularly important if the mother had rubella during pregnancy.

Incoordinate eye movements, "setting sun" eyes, and the doll's eye phenomenon are transient reflections of neuromuscular immaturity. They usually disappear after 10 days. However, setting sun eyes may also be indicative of hydrocephaly.

Ears. Cartilage formation is present in the ears, although not complete. This allows the pinna to bend easily, but it should rebound. It is important to assess the position of the ears. The top of the external ear should be slightly above the level of the eyes. Low-set ears are seen in infants with chromosomal abnormalities; these abnormalities include other physical defects and mental retardation. Low-set ears may also be associated with renal disorders.

Nose. The neonate's nose may appear large or slightly flattened. This discrepancy will disappear as the face grows. Remember that neonates are nose breathers; therefore, nasal obstructions should be prevented. (Mucus should be removed by suction; breast tissue should be held away from the baby's nose during breastfeeding.)

Mouth. The inside of the infant's mouth can be visualized during crying. The mucous membrane is pink and moist. Thrush, a candida infection transmitted during the birth process, may be identified as white or gray patches on the tongue, gums, and entire buccal mucosa. Occasionally, milk curds are mistaken for thrush. Irrigating with sterile water or gently wiping with a tongue blade should help in the diagnosis. Thrush is highly contagious and should be treated promptly (see also page 1661).

The frenulum linguae (mucous fold extending from the floor of the mouth to the interior surface of the tongue) should be inspected. If the frenulum linguae is too short (tongue-tie) there will be interference in sucking and speech.

Neck. The neck of the neonate is short, chubby, and creased with skinfolds. It should be flexible enough to rotate from side to side and from flexion to extension. The nurse should closely examine the folds by raising the shoulders and hyperextending the neck. Excessive folds (webbing) may be associated with pathologic conditions.

Although the neck is not strong enough to support the head, some degree of head control should be evident. Hyperextension (opisthotonus) may be associated with neurologic disease. Decreased muscle tone (hypotonia) is manifested by inability to lift the head. This may be indicative of prematurity, pathology, or hypoxia.

Torso and Extremities

Chest. The overall appearance of the chest should be symmetric. Breast engorgement may occur in both boys and girls owing to circulating maternal hormones. Occasionally, a thin, watery fluid may be secreted from the nipples. Engorgement and fluid will disappear within 2 weeks. Fluid should not be expressed from the breasts.

Abdomen. The abdomen of the neonate is slightly protuberant. The nurse should observe for signs of distention such as tight skin that makes subcutaneous vessels visible.

The umbilical stump is bluish, moist, and shiny. It should contain two arteries and one vein. An umbilical cord containing only one artery may be associated with congenital anomalies. The cord stump begins to dry, darken, and slough off by the sixth to tenth day.

The cord stump should be inspected for bleeding and signs of infection. Swabbing the cord stump with alcohol facilitates the drying process. Bellybands should not be used, since they interfere with drying and provide a dark, warm, moist environment conducive to bacterial growth.

Anogenital Area. The anus should be inspected for patency. An imperforate (closed) anus interferes with the passage of stools. The first stool should be passed within 24 hours. This condition may also be diagnosed when it is impossible to insert a rectal thermometer.

The female genitals consist of the *labia majora,* the *labia minora,* the *clitoris,* and the *vaginal opening.* The labia majora covers the labia minora. The hymenal tag is a fleshy pink tag protruding from the base of the vagina. It is present in nearly all female newborns, but gradually atrophies and disappears by the end of the fourth week. The labia may be engorged due to the influence of circulating maternal hormones. Hormones are also responsible for a milky vaginal discharge tinged with mucus or blood or both. Both the edema and the discharge should disappear as soon as the hormones have cleared from the neonate's system. The urinary meatus is difficult to visualize; therefore, the number of voidings should be observed and recorded.

In male neonates, the scrotum is edematous and covered with rugae. Both testes can be palpated in the sac. Occasionally, one or both testicles may recede temporarily into the body cavity through the inguinal ring when the baby is exposed to cold. *Cryptorchidism* is a condition in which one or both testes have not descended. This condition requires referral to determine the cause and treatment.

The *glans penis* (head of the penis) is covered by the *prepuce* (foreskin). The foreskin is not retractable and cannot be displaced until 4 to 6 months of age. The foreskin should never be forcefully retracted, not even for cleansing purposes. The prepuce should be examined to rule out stenosis. The external *urinary meatus* (a small slit) is located near the tip of the glans penis and should be easily visualized. Occasionally, the meatal opening is located on the ventral portion of the glans penis *(hypospadias)* or dorsal portion *(epispadias).*

Circumcision (surgical removal of the prepuce) is a common practice today. For Jews circumcision is a religious practice and takes place in a ceremony on the male infant's eighth day of life. The American Academy of Pediatrics (1975) has stated that medical indications for routine circumcision are nonexistent. Only rarely is it required to correct a defect, as when the foreskin is so constricted that it interferes with voiding or circulation (phimosis). Circumcision is contraindicated in the presence of hypospadias because the foreskin will be used during surgical reconstruction of the meatal opening at a later time.

Extremities. The arms and legs of the neonate appear short. They should be symmetric in shape and movement. The nurse should observe the position (flexion) assumed at rest and inspect fingers and toes for extra digits, clubbing of fingers, fusion, or webbing. The hands are examined for palmar creases. A simian crease (single line crease across the palm) is associated with Down syndrome. The feet are inspected for sole creases and clubbing.

Hip dislocation is determined by placing the neonate in a supine position and testing for Ortolani's sign. Both legs are flexed and abducted (away from the body) to nearly touch the examining surface. A click may be felt or heard if a dislocation is present. With the infant in a prone position, the nurse should note the creases of the buttocks and thighs. They should be symmetric and the legs should be the same length. Movement should be noted, as fine tremors of the extremities may indicate hypoglycemia.

Back. The back is examined and palpated for spinal defects and curvature. Tufts of hair may indicate *spina bifida.* The coccygeal area (base of the spine) should be examined for pilonidal dimples, or cysts.

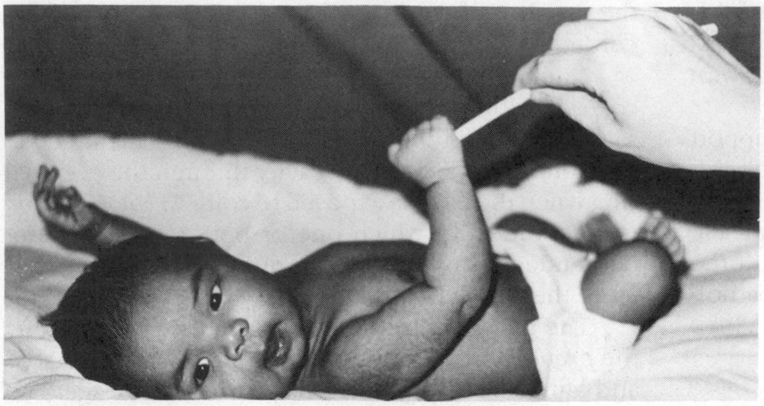

***Figure* 5-11.** Palmar grasp reflex.

Neurologic and Sensory Examination

Reflexes

Reflex responses provide important data on the status of neurologic functioning. Abnormal signs that are present in the first days or weeks of life may disappear and be followed by abnormal findings months or years later. Therefore, every physical examination should include assessment of reflexes. Since this may be a tedious, tiring experience for the neonate, the total examination may have to be performed in stages. Also remember that neonatal central nervous system function may be decreased by narcotics administered to the mother during labor.

Rooting Reflex. Lightly stroking the cheek at the side of the mouth will stimulate the newborn infant to turn the head in that direction in order to find food. The rooting reflex disappears at 9 to 12 weeks, when it is no longer needed. If the mother grasps both cheeks in an effort to turn the neonate's head in the direction of breast or bottle, she creates confusion with this double stimulus. Absence, weakness, or asymmetry of responses may indicate CNS depression or dysfunction.

Sucking Reflex. The sucking reflex is stimulated by touching the baby's lips or placing an object in the mouth. Sucking should be rhythmic and strong enough to obtain nourishment from breast or bottle. If the sucking reflex is unstimulated it will disappear rapidly.

Swallowing Reflex. The swallowing reflex is stimulated by food on the posterior portion of the tongue. Swallowing is spontaneous, but the neonate may need a little time to coordinate sucking and swallowing effectively. Gag, cough, and sneeze reflexes are protective methods of maintaining a clear airway. These are particularly evident during early feedings when the baby has to handle mucus in addition to nursing.

Grasp Reflexes: Palmar and Plantar. Exerting pressure on the palmar surface of the hand will stimulate curling or grasping of the fingers (Fig. 5-11). The grasp is so strong that the neonate can be raised momentarily by the examiner's finger. This reflex disappears at 6 weeks to 3 months of age.

Placing an object on the plantar surface (sole) of the foot will stimulate curling or grasping of the toes (Fig. 5-12). This reflex disappears at about 8 to 9 months of age.

Traction Response. This response is elicited by placing the neonate in a supine position and slowly pulling him or her to a sitting position by holding the wrists. Response should be extension of the arms with some degree of head control.

Moro Reflex (Startle Response). *The Moro reflex is the single most significant response denoting CNS status.* This response can be elicited by startling the baby with a loud noise or by bumping the crib. The nurse can place the neonate in a supine position, grasp both arms, allow the head to remain on the examination surface, and raise the shoulders by gentle traction on the arms; then release arms, allowing shoulders to drop to the surface, and observe the response. A normal response includes two phases: (1) Quick flexion at elbows is followed by abduction (away from the body) of the upper limbs at the shoulders, extension of the forearms at the elbows and extension of the fingers and legs; (2) subsequent adduction (toward the body) of the arms at the shoulders and the legs against the abdomen (Fig. 5-13). Observe the completeness and symmetry of the response and the degree of difficulty in eliciting it.

The Moro reflex is strong during the first 8 weeks of life and fades by the end of the second or third month.

Yawn, Stretch, and Hiccough Reflexes. These reflexes are demonstrated spontaneously by the neonate and have been related to increasing oxygen intake and elimination of gas. Parents generally express concern and want to know how to intervene when the baby develops hiccoughs. The nurse can reassure them that this hiccoughing is normal. However, increased yawn-

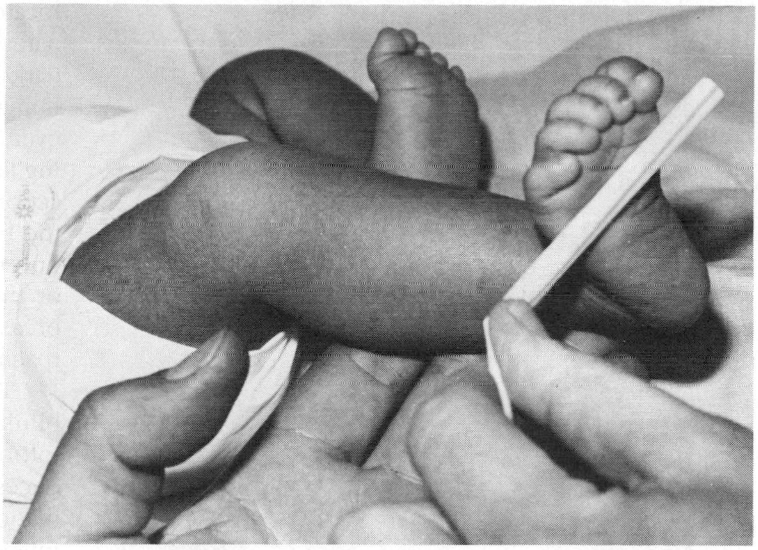

***Figure* 5-12.** Plantar grasp reflex.

ing, sneezing, and hiccoughing are frequently observed in infants of heroin-addicted mothers as they experience withdrawal syndrome.

Trunk Incurvation Reflex. With the neonate in a prone position, touching along one side of the vertebral column will elicit curvature of the spine toward the stimulated side. This is a good test of spinal cord integrity.

Placing and Stepping Reflexes. Holding the infant in an upright position and allowing the dorsal part of the foot to lightly touch one edge of the examining surface will result in spontaneous lifting of the foot by flexion of the knees and hips. The neonate looks as though he or she is *placing* each foot alternately on the examining surface. This reflex disappears after 4 to 6 weeks.

The stepping reflex is stimulated with the neonate in an upright position. When the soles of the feet touch a hard surface, the infant will take a few quick alternating steps (Fig. 5-14). The stepping reflex disappears by 3 months.

Tonic Neck Reflex (TNR). TNR is known as the "fencing position" because it simulates the position assumed by someone preparing to fence. Place the baby in a supine position and turn the head to one side. Observe extension of the arm and leg on the side to which the head is turned and flexion of the opposite arm and leg (Fig. 5-15). This reflex disappears at about 6 months of age.

Babinski Reflex. The reflex is stimulated by stroking the sole of the foot from heel to toe. The response is dorsiflexion of the big toe and fanning or spreading of the other toes (Fig. 5-16). The Babinski reflex is present until 3 months of age but may persist until the child walks, at which time an adult response of flexion is elicited.

***Figure* 5-13.** Moro reflex (startle response).

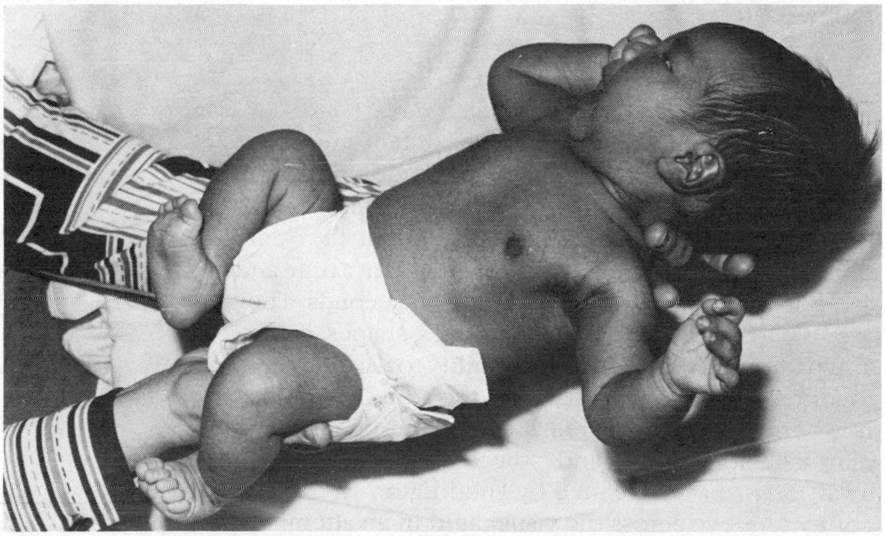

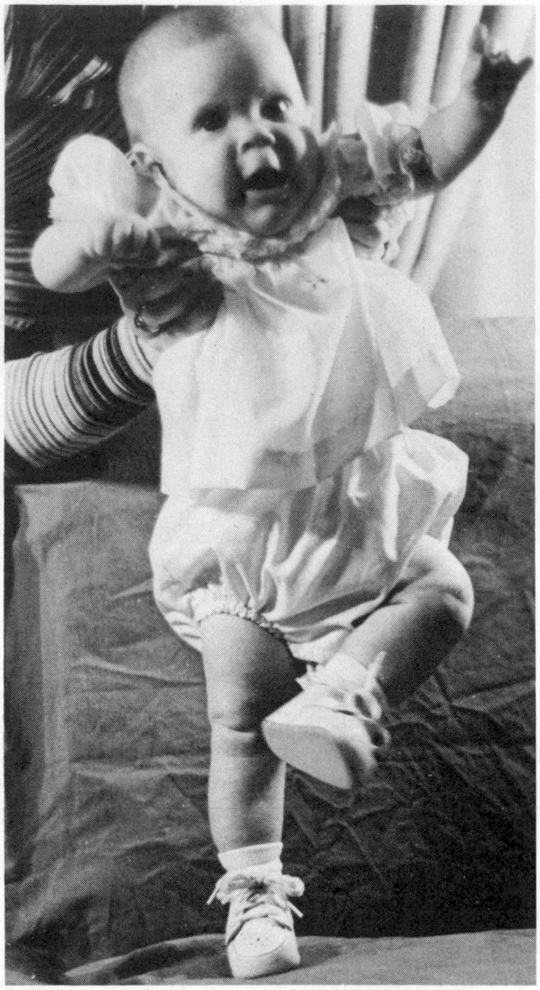

Figure 5-14. Stepping reflex (dancing).

There are many other reflexes to include in a thorough neurologic examination; however, the ones discussed here are of greatest importance in performing a nursing assessment of the central nervous system of the neonate.

Senses

Vision. Visual abilities of the infant are better developed than once thought. Luddington-Hoe (1983) reported the following characteristics of newborn vision: neonates can *fixate* (look at the same point with both eyes) for up to 10 seconds at a time and can refixate at intervals of every 1 to 1.5 seconds. They are able to *discriminate* between sizes, shapes, colors, and patterns. *Conjugation* (the ability to use both eyes together) is nearly on a par with the adult except that newborn infants must refixate more frequently and may take longer to "find" the object after looking away. *Scanning* is defined by Luddington-Hoe as the ability to move across the visual field in an attempt to locate the most satisfying object. She reports that neonates have the ability to scan and prefer areas of sharp dark-light contrast; they also show a preference for the human face over inanimate objects. Neonates, however, are unable to *accommodate* to distance (requiring flattening or thickening of the lens in response to action of the ciliary muscle). This means that during the first month of life objects are in perfect focus at only one point in space; this distance is about 8 inches, or the distance between the mother's face and her breast when she is feeding the infant. Accommodation reaches the adult level by 4 months of age.

The eyes are sensitive to light, and the neonate will blink or squint in response to light. Parents need to be informed of the baby's visual capabilities and preferences so that they can provide appropriate visual stimulation such as appropriate mobiles and changes in the infant's environment.

Hearing. Hearing is present at birth, although temporarily hindered by amniotic fluid in the middle ear. Within a few hours after birth, the fluid is absorbed and replaced by air. Behavioral manifestations of hearing include *alerting* (seems to stop and listen), eye movements, startle reaction, and crying. The neonate's ability to determine the cause and direction of sound does not develop until weeks later.

The infant will respond to various sounds in a reflexive manner (Moro, blink). An actively crying infant will respond to a soothing voice by abruptly ceasing all activity as though alerting to the sound. From 3 to 14 weeks of age, eye response to noise includes opening the eyes or squinting. Some head movement may also occur.

Taste. The neonate can differentiate between

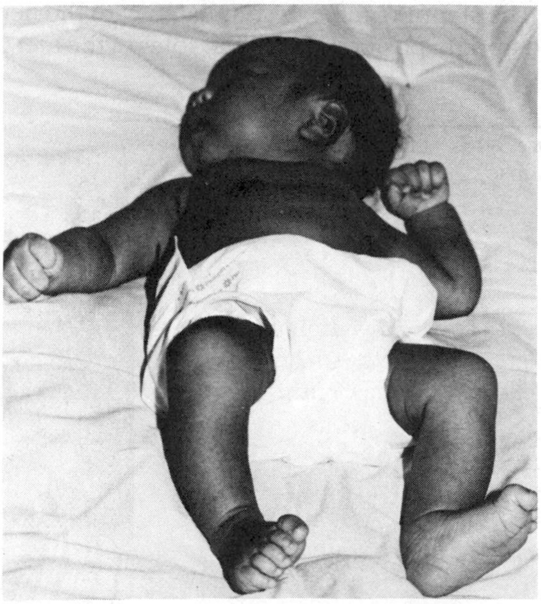

Figure 5-15. Tonic neck response (fencing position).

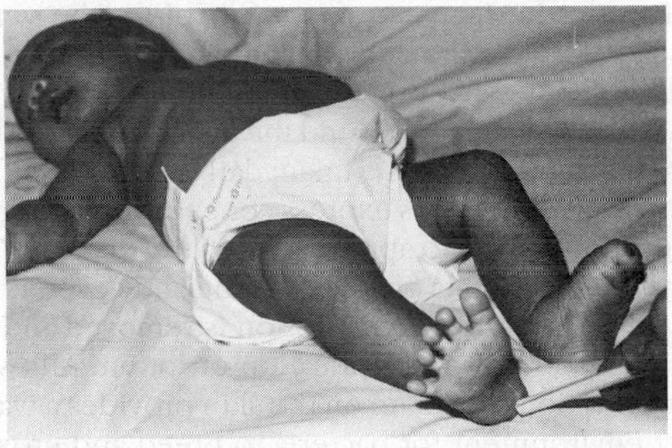

Figure 5-16. Babinski reflex.

bitter and sweet tastes. Pleasurable flavors will elicit active sucking, whereas bitter or unpleasant flavors will cause tongue protrusion and active turning away.

Smell. The sense of smell is present as soon as the nose is clear of amniotic fluid and mucus, although the degree of development is unclear. Some researchers speculate that the neonate learns to differentiate his or her mother by recognizing her own particular body scent.

Touch. Tactile sensation is well developed at birth, particularly in the facial area (rooting, sucking). Sensitivity to pain and extreme temperatures seems to be present, but not distinct, at first. By the tenth day, a definite reaction to painful stimuli is observed.

Care of the Neonate

Thermoregulation

Thermal balance is maintained by regulation of heat loss and heat production. The environment plays a major role in heat loss; therefore, maintenance of an optimal thermal environment is one of the most important aspects of neonatal care. Heat exchange (loss) between the body and the environment occurs by evaporation, conduction, convection, and radiation.

Heat Loss

Evaporation. Immediately after delivery the neonate is covered with amniotic fluid (liquid), which is converted to a vapor utilizing thermal energy. Evaporation with heat loss is increased when the environmental humidity is low. Drying the neonate thoroughly with warm towels will interfere with heat loss through evaporation. Bathing the neonate may also contribute to evaporative heat loss. Therefore, bathing should not be performed until the body temperature is normal and stable. In many institutions vital signs (especially temperature) are taken before a bath is given. This is a good way to determine the appropriateness of the planned bath.

Conduction. Loss of body heat through conduction occurs when the skin is in direct contact with a cooler surface. Body heat rapidly moves to the cooler surface to equalize the different temperatures. The naked neonate should always be placed on a padded, warm surface to prevent conductive heat loss. This is important to remember when bathing and examining.

Convection. Loss of body heat via convection occurs when the surrounding air is cool. Heat moves from the body surface to the cooler surrounding air. Temperature, air movement, and humidity all contribute to the rate of convection. Convective heat loss can be reduced by maintaining an ideal environmental temperature and humidity (72 to 76°F; 40 to 60 per cent humidity); however, air temperature will have no significant effect on heat loss by radiation or evaporation.

Radiation. Radiant heat loss occurs by transfer of body heat to a cooler solid object that is not in direct contact with the neonate. If the warmer or incubator has a warm padded surface, the environmental temperature is warm, and the infant is dry, then heat loss may still occur if the newborn unit is placed in close proximity to a cold window or wall or other sources of coldness. The amount of heat loss through radiation is directly related to the distance from a cold surface. The implications are obvious for placement of the neonate in the delivery room, neonatal nursery, and home nursery.

Heat Production

Discussion of the four modalities of exchange of heat between the body and the environment has focused on heat loss for the neonate. However, body heat gains may occur in the same manner from external sources. Precautions should be taken to prevent excess heat loss or heat gain when caring for the neonate.

The neonate who is exposed to a heat-loss environment will compensate by increasing heat production through increased metabolic activity. The full-term infant who is exposed to cold can increase the thermogenic rate 2½ times over the resting state to a level that almost equals that of the adult (Korones et al., 1981).

The neonate exposed to cold stress increases heat production through a mechanism called *nonshivering thermogenesis.* This refers to heat that is produced by an increased metabolic rate in a cold environment. This in turn requires increased oxygen consumption. The type of body fat known as brown fat seems to be the major source of heat that is produced by nonshivering thermogenesis. Brown fat composes 2 to 6 per cent of the neonate's body weight. It usually disappears some weeks after birth when it is no longer needed.

Exposure to cold will deplete stores of brown fat. If the depletion is severe, as with prolonged cold stress, it is hypothesized that effective thermogenic capacity is eliminated (Korones et al., 1981). The cold-stressed neonate is also at risk for developing hypoxemia, metabolic acidosis, rapid depletion of glycogen stores, and reduction of blood glucose levels *(hypoglycemia)*.

Thermal Management

All neonates lose some body heat immediately after delivery. Physiologically, cold stimuli are probably essential to the initiation of extrauterine respirations; however, too much is hazardous. The temperature of the infant's skin signals the presence of a metabolic response to heat loss. A drop in skin temperature indicates a heat loss environment that requires warming. The metabolic responses to cold stress will be triggered before core (deep tissue) temperature changes occur. Rectal temperature may be normal in the cold-stressed newborn infant in the beginning. Axillary temperatures may be falsely high owing to the presence of brown fat padding. During the first few hours after birth, when the neonate has difficulty regulating and maintaining body temperature, a heat-sensitive probe taped to the abdomen is the most accurate method of continually assessing body temperature status. The probe should remain uncovered to assure accuracy of skin temperature recordings. Once the infant's temperature has stabilized, rectal temperature readings are sufficiently accurate.

Parents should be taught how to use a rectal thermometer on their baby: lubricate the tip with petroleum jelly and gently insert the tip (about ¼ inch) into the rectum. The thermometer can be held in place with one hand while the infant's legs are grasped at the ankles with the other hand. This prevents kicking, which may cause the thermometer to be inserted deeper. If using a glass thermometer, hold it in place for 3 minutes before reading.

Bathing

The purpose of bathing is to provide skin stimulation and maintain cleanliness while allowing inspection. Because neonates do not perspire, they do not need to be bathed daily. The face, chin, and neck should be cleansed after each feeding, and the entire diaper area cleansed with each diaper change. The condition of the skin and the environmental temperature are good guidelines in assessing the need for a bath. During the summer when it is hot and humid a daily bath may be refreshing, whereas during the winter, bathing the infant three to four times per week is sufficient.

During the first few days after birth, the vernix gradually disappears and the skin becomes dry and scaling. There may even be slight bleeding where the skin becomes cracked around the hands and feet. This is normal, but to bathe the infant daily can increase this drying process. Parents express concern about dryness and generally wish to apply lotion to the dry skin. The use of lotion benefits only the parents; however, it will cause no harm if the excess lotion is removed and the area washed before reapplication of lotion. Allowing layers of lotion to remain on the skin provides a warm, moist environment for bacteria to breed and grow. A neonate should not be immersed in a tub of water until the umbilical cord has dropped off and the stump has healed (approximately 10 days maximum). During that time, sponge bathing is appropriate.

Bath time should be planned some time before a meal and when the baby is not fussy. Bathing right after a feeding may cause the newborn infant to spit up. Bath time should be fun for the parents and the baby. Infant-bathing instruction that occurs during the hospital stay is an important part of discharge preparation.

The neonate can be bathed in a baby bathtub or while placed on the kitchen table or a bed. The bath area should be warm, draft-free, and at a comfortable height to prevent the parent from becoming overly tired (stretching and bending). The area should also be big enough to work comfortably. Some parents enjoy using the kitchen sink. If the sink is used, a few safety factors must be kept in mind:

- Clean the sink thoroughly.
- Place a folded towel in the bottom of the sink for padding.
- Prepare the water and then turn the faucet away from the baby before placing the baby in the water. Accidental burns could occur if the temperature should change while water is allowed to flow directly over the newborn.
- If the sink has a window over it, the window should be closed to prevent drafts.

The bath water should be comfortably warm. Feeling the water with the inner aspect of the forearm is a good way to test the water. The elbow is not sufficiently sensitive to temperature to detect water that would be too hot for the infant. Other articles needed are a clean towel and washcloth, a bar of mild soap, a comb or soft brush, and clean diaper and clothing. The use of lotions, creams, or powders is unnecessary. Baby powder has a tendency to "pill" where skin surfaces rub together and can thus result in skin irritation. It can also be aspirated by the infant. Everything should be arranged in the bathing area before beginning.

Once the procedure is begun, the neonate must not be left unattended for any reason. *One hand should be kept on the baby at all times.* This is an important safety rule to be applied in all areas of infant care.

Place the neonate on a padded surface and wash the eyes and face gently with clear water. Use a different portion of the washcloth for each eye and clean by wiping from the edge of the nose outward (inner canthus to outer canthus). Two cotton balls wrung out in clear water will also cleanse the eyes rapidly and safely. Some babies do not like to have their faces covered. Gentle, soothing touch and speaking or singing quietly will help the neonate learn to enjoy the experience. The ears and nose should be cleaned with a wisp of cotton or the tip of a washcloth. A Q-tip should never be inserted into these areas; damage to the delicate tissues may result.

The head should be lathered lightly and the fontanel area (soft spot) should be washed as well. There is no need for parents to be afraid to touch this area.

Cradle cap, a desquamation that may occur on the scalp (particularly over the fontanel area), can be prevented by daily washing and rinsing. If scales do occur, they can be softened with baby oil and removed with a fine-tooth comb or brush after washing. The infant should be picked up and the soap rinsed off the head. The "football carry" is a comfortable and safe way to hold the neonate. This also gives good face-to-face contact during the procedure.

Further instructions for the mother bathing the baby include placing the infant back on the padded surface and drying the head. Proceed to undress the infant and gently lather the baby's front; turn him or her on the abdomen and lather the back. It feels nice to lather the infant's head and skin with the hands; the skin-to-skin contact can be very satisfying to parents and baby. After lathering, remember that the baby is very slippery. Pick the neonate up gently, supporting head and back, and gradually lower into the water. Supporting the baby's head out of the water with one hand, use the other hand to gently swirl the water over the body. As the baby learns to enjoy the water, he or she will enjoy kicking and splashing. Allow enough time for this form of play.

Cord Care

The cord should be kept dry until it falls off and the stump has healed. The process generally requires 5 to 10 days. There should be no active bleeding at the site. A few drops of blood are not uncommon when the cord begins to separate. The parents should inspect the area for signs of infection (redness, edema, drainage).

A drying agent may be used. Some physicians recommend applying triple dye once a day or swabbing the cord and base with alcohol at each diaper change. The use of bellybands is contraindicated: they do not prevent umbilical hernias and may cause infection by delaying or preventing the drying process. Diapers and rubber pants should be folded down to keep the cord area dry.

Circumcision Care

Circumcision is the surgical removal of the foreskin. Care following a circumcision is based on general principles of postoperative care: keep the wound clean and dry, and observe for signs of bleeding or infection or both.

Following the circumcision, a sterile dressing with petroleum jelly is applied to the area. This should be changed with each voiding unless the physician wishes it to remain securely in place to serve as a pressure dressing for 24 hours. Keep the neonate off the abdomen for the first 12 hours to eliminate discomfort, pressure, or friction rubbing. The penis should be observed for bleeding at least every hour during the first 6 hours postoperatively.

The neonate may be fussy. Crying is due to the restrained position during the procedure and to the pain caused by the procedure. Taking the baby out to the mother as soon as possible for nursing, comforting, and cuddling is reassuring and helpful for both.

Clothing

Parents tend to overdress the neonate. They mistakenly conclude that cool, slightly bluish hands and feet mean that the baby is cold. The infant who is overheated must activate heat-loss physiologic mechanisms. Conversely, room temperatures that are comfortable for the adult may cause the neonate to initiate heat production. The nurse should explain to parents the importance of sufficient, but not excessive, clothing. Generally, the neonate will be comfortable when dressed in the same amount of clothing as the adult, plus one additional layer. The extremities will feel slightly cool, while the trunk is warm to touch.

Feeding

Feeding is one of the first tasks the new parents must accomplish in learning to care for their baby. The method of feeding (breast or bottle) is a choice that must be made with guidance and without undue pressure. Information should be provided as needed and the decision supported rather than judged. Parents not

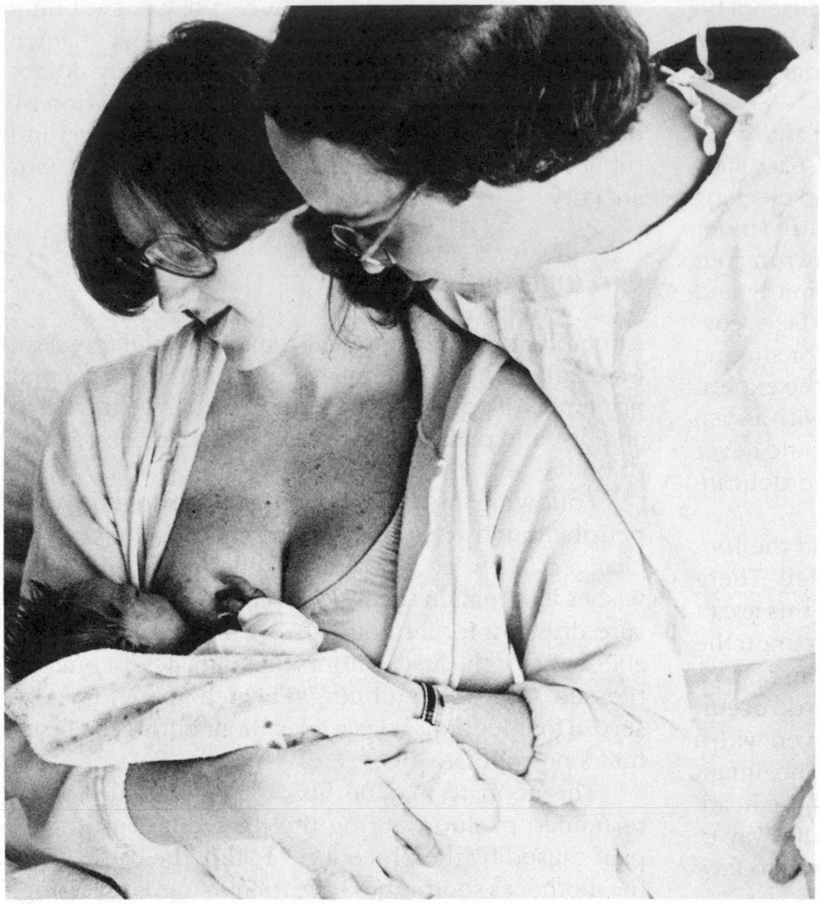

Parents and baby derive pleasure and form bonds of attachment during feeding.

only must learn to successfully feed their infant, they must also learn to assess his or her hunger. Readiness for feeding can be determined by observing the infant's behavior. Rooting and sucking, hand-to-mouth activity, crying, and alertness are clues that the baby is hungry. These behaviors should be explained and demonstrated to both parents. The nurse can ensure a happy, satisfying feeding time for baby and parent by showing the parent how to hold, feed, and burp the infant successfully and by providing positive feedback to strengthen healthy interaction and feeding activity.

Parents should be urged to hold their baby for feedings and to spend a few minutes talking with and stroking the infant before feeding to facilitate both their own and the baby's relaxation. Prefeeding relaxation reduces the incidence of vomiting and colic and encourages attachment.

Nutritional Needs

Unless the mother or infant develops health problems, breastfeeding is often begun immediately after birth, during the first period of reactivity. This can be a very meaningful experience, since the neonate is alert and interested in sucking at this time. Breastfeeding after delivery is not done to supply nutritional intake but to promote closeness and attachment. This is also an opportunity for mother and baby to practice the proper "latch-on" and positioning for breastfeeding (Box 5-2).

For bottlefed infants, the first milk intake usually occurs about 4 hours after delivery. Neonates require 100 to 120 calories per kilogram of body weight every 24 hours. Approximately 3 to 4 minutes sucking time at the breast, or 30 to 50 ml of formula per feeding, will meet this requirement for the first 3 to 4 days of life. As the baby gains weight, formula amounts will increase. The nurse can calculate the child's 24-hour caloric intake to ensure that caloric requirements are met. (Most commercially prepared infant formulas contain 20 calories per ounce.) The neonate averages six to eight feedings per day.

Parents should be informed of the importance of placing their baby in a position that reduces the likelihood of regurgitation or aspiration of food after feeding. Placement in an infant seat or laying the infant on the side or on the abdomen are all acceptable positions for 30 minutes to an hour after each feeding.

Box 5-2
Proper Latch-On and Positioning for Breastfeeding

SIGNS OF CORRECT LATCH-ON

- Mother states "It feels right"
- No nipple pain is experienced
- Noisy swallowing is heard once let-down occurs
- Deep jaw movements are seen and the ears may wiggle. The whole head will also move

SIGNS OF INCORRECT LATCH-ON

- Baby's cheeks are sucked in when feeding
- The nipple may appear flattened when removed from baby's mouth
- Painful, cracked, bleeding or blistered nipples
- Baby may fuss at breast, pulling on and off
- A loud clicking sound may be heard

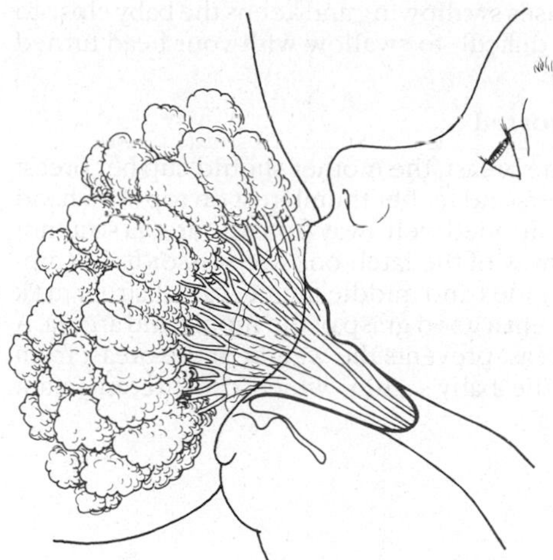

Proper position of head, lips, mouth, and tongue during breastfeeding.

Wide Mouth

Before pulling baby onto the breast, the mouth must be *open wide.* The mother can facilitate this by tickling baby's lips with the nipple. For stubborn babies, put gentle downward pressure on baby's lower jaw; this will encourage baby to open the mouth wide. Now the teat should be well back in the baby's mouth. This prevents nipple chewing, which causes pain, blisters, and cracked and bleeding nipples.

Lips Curved Back

When properly latched on, the lips should be curved back almost as though they were turned inside out, rather than the pursed lips of a bottlefed baby. The lower lip should be aimed to cover more of the lower portion of the areola. The tongue will now be in place *below* the nipple. The mother may not be able to see this looking down at her baby. If the position of the mouth is not correct, the mother should break the suction by inserting her finger gently into the corner of the mouth and reposition again.

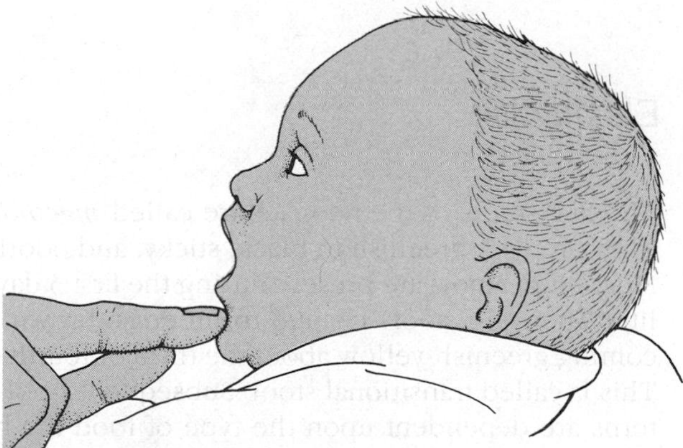

Baby can be encouraged to open mouth wide by putting gentle pressure on the lower jaw.

Head Slightly Extended

The baby's head should be extended slightly. The chin is thus pressed into the mother's breast and the nostrils are free from occlusion. Swallowing is easier in this position. The lower jaw will "milk" the breast more effectively.

Baby Close to Breast

The baby must be held as close to the mother's breast as possible. Unwrap the baby and have arms hugging the mother with one of baby's arms under the mother's arm and one arm resting on top of the breast. This helps prevent the baby from flexing the head. The nipple will not slip out of the mouth as easily, and the baby will not have to exert excess suction to keep the nipple in its mouth, thus causing nipple damage and pain.

Body Aligned

In any hold, the baby's stomach should be against the mother's body, with the mouth at the level of nipple.

Continued

Pillows can be helpful here. The body should be well supported so the head and body are in straight alignment. This eases swallowing and keeps the baby close to mother. It is difficult to swallow with your head turned to the side.

Breast Supported

To support the breast, the mother should cup her breast with her fingers and let her thumb rest on top. The hand should be positioned well away from the areola so as not to get in the way of the latch-on. The scissor hold (nipple between index and middle finger) can obstruct milk flow and prevent a good grasp of the nipple and areola. A supported breast prevents the weight of the breast from pushing on the baby's chin, which can tire an infant when nursing.

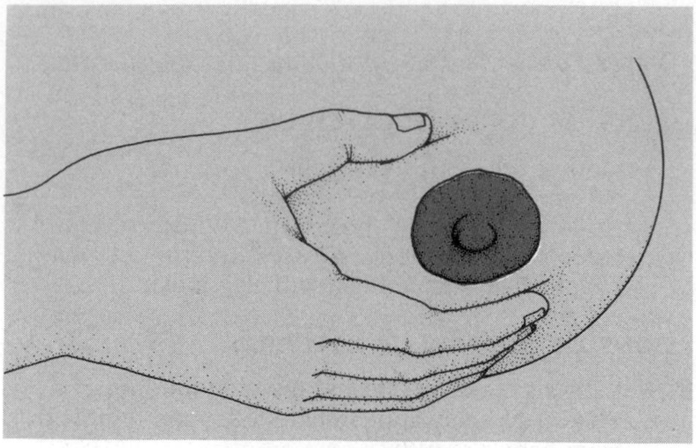

Hand is positioned well away from the areola.

(Text prepared by Ruta Valaitis, BScN, BA, MHSc, Clinical Nursing Consultant, and Lecturer, McMaster University School of Nursing, Hamilton, Ontario.)

Body Composition

Seventy-five per cent of body weight in the newborn infant is composed of water. The normal weight loss of up to 10 per cent of body weight after birth represents fluid loss. Parents can be assured that this weight loss is not harmful to the infant.

Fat constitutes about 12 per cent of the body weight, giving the neonate a somewhat thin appearance. The total protein is similar to that of other ages. The neonate has a high hematocrit and hemoglobin concentration, plus large stores of iron in the liver. This provides an iron concentration that is approximately double that of the adult. Calcium and phosphorus are present in low concentrations. The infant's bones are relatively flexible and poorly mineralized; this facilitates the birth process. Both fat-soluble and water-soluble vitamins are present in adequate amounts.

The supply of vitamin K (fat-soluble) is commonly less than adequate. Vitamin K deficiency may cause uncontrollable bleeding; therefore, an injection of vitamin K (Aquamephyton) is routinely given shortly after birth. Bacterial synthesis in the intestinal tract leads to the production of vitamin K. However, at birth, the intestinal tract of the newborn is sterile. Breastfed babies experience more vitamin K deficiency because human milk has only one fourth as much vitamin K as cow's milk does.

The digestive tract is somewhat immature, with a scant production of saliva. "Spitting up" is common until the digestive system matures. This needs to be differentiated from vomiting, which indicates that pyloric stenosis (stricture of the pyloric sphincter between the esophagus and the stomach), or other illness may be present.

Owing to immaturity of the kidneys, production of concentrated urine is limited. Therefore, in order to excrete solutes (urea, uric acid, creatinine, minerals), a large volume of water must be excreted. Improper formula preparation, excess sweating, diarrhea or insufficient fluid intake may cause dehydration.

Elimination

The first stools of the neonate are called *meconium.* They are dark greenish to black, sticky, and odorless. Meconium stools are present during the first 3 days of life. Then the stools change to greenish-brown, becoming greenish-yellow about the third or fourth day. This is called transitional stool. Subsequent stool patterns are dependent upon the type of food the baby receives.

Breastfed babies have bright, golden-yellow stools that are soft (mushy) and unformed but not watery. They are sometimes a light greenish color. Their odor is sweet smelling. Initially, a breastfed baby will have one to two stools per day, increasing to more than four per day by the second week.

Formula-fed babies have pale yellow or yellow-white stools that are firmer and more formed. The odor is foul smelling. Initially, a bottle-fed baby has more stools per day than a breastfed baby, but these decrease to about three per day by the second week.

Green, watery stools indicate diarrhea, and a physician should be notified. Stools should be observed for blood indicative of intestinal bleeding.

Most newborn infants void during the first 12 hours of life. The number of voidings should be assessed. Occasionally, urate crystals are passed with the urine. These appear as pink (brick dust) staining on the diaper. Urate is not significant but should be differentiated from blood. Urates dissolve and disappear when the diaper is placed in water; blood does not.

Keeping the neonate clean and dry will prevent diaper rash. If the baby's skin is so sensitive that rash does occur in spite of diligent efforts, short periods of exposure to air during the day can be beneficial. Petroleum jelly applied to the clean skin can serve as a protective barrier against skin breakdown from urine and stool.

Icterus Neonatorum

Jaundice (yellowish color of the skin and sclera) is a normal physiologic occurrence between the second and third days of life, appearing in about 50 per cent of all neonates. In icterus neonatorum the jaundice is a result of the breakdown and incomplete excretion of fetal red blood cells. The normal breakdown of hemoglobin in red blood cells produces bilirubin, which must be conjugated by the liver before it can bind with albumin for excretion from the body. Icterus neonatorum occurs when the neonate's liver cannot conjugate the bilirubin produced in the first days of life. This is a normal finding *unless* (1) jaundice occurs in the first 24 hours or persists beyond the first week of life; (2) serum bilirubin rises at a rate greater than 4 mg per dl per 24 hours; (3) serum bilirubin is greater than 12 mg per dl in full-term or 14 mg per dl in preterm infants; or (4) direct-reacting bilirubin is greater than 1 mg per dl at any time (Behrman and Vaughan, 1987). If any of these conditions occur, *hyperbilirubinemia* may be present.

Kernicterus is the most dangerous complication of hyperbilirubinemia. It occurs when unconjugated bilirubin crosses the blood-brain barrier and damages brain cells. Kernicterus can be fatal or cause various short- and long-term sequelae, i.e, irritability, seizures, cerebral palsy, mental retardation, hearing loss, hypotonia, or hypertonia. The serum bilirubin level at which kernicterus occurs is uncertain. The level most commonly accepted is 20 mg per dl (340 μmol/L). However, lower levels may be toxic when associated with certain factors, e.g., prematurity, low serum protein levels, acidosis, elevated levels of fatty acids, and certain drugs.

Phototherapy treatment may be instituted if the indirect bilirubin level rises significantly. Guidelines for the initiation of phototherapy vary somewhat from institution to institution. Generally, the indications depend upon the infant's gestational age, birth weight, related illnesses, and rate of rise of serum bilirubin concentration. When the bilirubin in the skin surface is exposed to the special phototherapy lights, it is transformed or isomerized into water-soluble molecules. These molecules can then be excreted in the bile. The ideal light source appears to be special blue fluorescent bulbs with wavelengths ranging from 400 to 500 nm. These blue lights are used in conjunction with white lights so as not to obscure signs of cyanosis. An acrylic plastic shield is also required to block out infrared and ultraviolet light. Knowledge of the following complications should be incorporated into the nursing care of all infants receiving phototherapy:

- phototherapy lights can increase the infant's temperature so that special attention is given to thermoregulation;
- insensible water loss increases due to the increased temperature, so the infant should be monitored for signs of dehydration;
- diarrhea and lactose intolerance have been found to be complications of the gastrointestinal tract;
- retinal damage in animals has been caused by phototherapy, so the use of opaque eye patches is an essential part of care;
- rashes and burns have been known to occur as a result of phototherapy, therefore careful attention is given to skin care.

The goal of *exchange transfusions* is to prevent the toxic effects of the bilirubin by removing it from the circulation. Specific guidelines for the use of this treatment also have not been well established. It is indicated when phototherapy is not effective or when the bilirubin levels rise to dangerous levels too quickly. The use of phototherapy has decreased the need for exchange transfusions.

Home Phototherapy. Phototherapy can now be administered in the home. For the family willing to accept the responsibility of monitoring the infant's condition under the bilirubin lights, this home therapy can decrease the length of hospital stay for the infant or prevent readmission. Parents will need to be instructed about set-up and maintenance of the bilirubin lights. The nurse will explain that the blue lightbulbs are the ones that actually reduce the bilirubin levels and that the white lightbulbs are present to give the baby a more natural color for purposes of assessment. Under only blue light, the baby would appear blue.

Parents are asked to keep detailed records of the infant's axillary temperature, fluid intake, wet diapers, stools, and position. The records help the nurse making the follow-up visit verify that the infant can maintain normal body temperature despite being nude under the lights, and that intake and output are adequate to facilitate excretion of bilirubin wastes in the urine and prevent dehydration. Frequent turning of the neonate allows all skin surfaces to be exposed to the light to maximize the detoxification of bilirubin in the skin.

Once phototherapy is instituted, serum bilirubin levels will be monitored daily (or more often if levels are rising rapidly). The home care nurse will draw these blood samples for the infant on home phototherapy. Phototherapy is usually necessary for only 2 to 3 days.

Safety

Everyone caring for a newborn should wash their hands before and after handling the baby.

Safe handling techniques should be demonstrated, taught, and practiced by all who handle the baby. These include firmly supporting all body parts, especially the head; keeping a controlling hand on the infant during weighing or giving care on any surface without protective straps; placing a hand between the baby's skin and the diaper if pins are used; placing the infant on the side or abdomen for at least 30 minutes after feeding to prevent aspiration of regurgitated fluids; and carrying the infant in a protected, secure manner.

The nurse should discuss with parents the use of infant car seats before the neonate leaves the hospital. If an infant car seat has not been purchased, the nurse should encourage the family to do so. In many states the use of a car seat for children is mandated by law. If the family feels that a car seat costs too much, the nurse can suggest options such as borrowing or renting or purchasing a used seat. Many hospitals now operate their own rental programs, offering car seats for the neonate and exchanging them for larger ones as the child grows. All health care personnel should recognize their responsibility to encourage the use of proper infant and child car restraints, because automobile accidents are a prime cause of death and injury in children. Chapter 17 discusses in detail the reasons parents do or do not use car seats and nursing strategies to promote proper use.

Variations in Development Related to Gestational Age and Weight

Mary Lou Moore and Janet Pinelli

This section focuses on neonates who differ from the norm at birth because of an alteration in gestational age (the length of time from conception to birth). The general term used to describe such neonates is *dysmature.* The Dubowitz assessment of gestational age and the relationship between the infant's gestational age and weight were discussed earlier in this chapter.

A *term* infant is born between 38 to 42 weeks. Those infants who vary from the norm owing to gestation are called *preterm* (babies born at less than 38 weeks' gestation) or *post-term* (babies born at more than 42 weeks' gestation). A newborn infant of average weight for age is called *appropriate for gestational age* (AGA). An infant whose weight is not appropriate for age is called *small for gestational age* (SGA) or *large for gestational age* (LGA). Dysmature neonates are at high risk for morbidity and mortality; therefore, early identification and initiation of medical and nursing management are important. Nurses who have a good understanding of the characteristics and assessment of the normal neonate can appreciate how deviations from the norm affect the neonate's ability to survive and thrive. Most of the complications due to dysmaturity result from chemical disturbances or the inadequate functioning of organs and systems. Most disorders are described in depth in Unit Seven, which covers the body systems. When mentioned here, they are cross-referenced to those chapters.

The special needs of babies who are other than healthy term infants frequently require a period of hospitalization. Sometimes this requires transfer from a community hospital to a specialized neonatal intensive care unit (NICU) away from home. Frequently the infant and family are separated within the first minutes, hours, or days of life. Therefore, families as well as the infants need nursing intervention and support.

Descriptions of the term infant and the complete physical examination are provided earlier in this chapter. A similar approach is used to examine the dysmature infant; the initial appraisal begins at the moment of birth, with particular attention paid to the first several breaths and the ease of respiration. After respiration is well established, a careful examination of the newborn baby is completed. This examination is important to rule out the presence of major abnormalities and to determine whether or not birth injuries and minor anomalies exist.

The Preterm Infant

In the majority of cases, the specific cause for the birth of a preterm infant is unknown. Related factors that have been identified include

- concurrent maternal disease, such as renal or heart disease
- intrauterine infection
- uterine malformation
- incompetent cervix
- toxemia
- premature rupture of membranes
- spontaneous onset of labor
- fetal distress
- fetal anomalies
- multiple birth
- placenta previa or abruptio
- low socioeconomic status
- maternal age under 16 years or over 40 years
- poor maternal nutrition
- prepregnancy weight of less than 50 kilograms
- previous premature labor

The preterm infant is vulnerable because of physiologic immaturity. Physiologic homeostasis is difficult to achieve without assistance. With rapidly advancing technologic assistance, smaller and sicker babies are surviving. The outcome of these infants varies widely but all of them must be assessed with the recognition that they were born too soon. *During infancy and early childhood, growth and development of an infant born prematurely is assessed on the basis of "corrected age," i.e., the age of the child is calculated from the expected date of delivery (due date) rather than the date of actual delivery.* For example, an infant born 2 months prematurely who is assessed 4 months after birth is evaluated as an infant 2 months of age.

A wide range of time is required for these infants to catch up; some remain developmentally disabled. With technologic advances, the mortality statistics for preterm infants continue to improve. However, the increasing survival rates have resulted in such complex and long-term problems that the emphasis should be on general prevention of preterm deliveries.

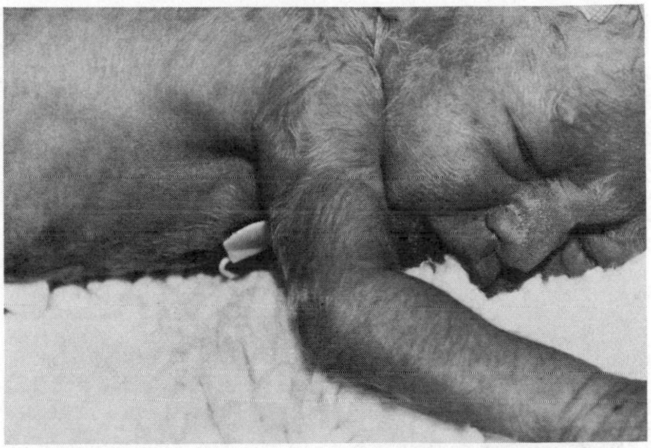

Figure 5-17. Lanugo, a downy distribution of fine hair over the body. It is most evident on the shoulders, back, extremities, forehead, and temples. It begins to appear on the fetus by about the 16th week of gestation and begins to disappear after the 32nd week. This infant is 24 hours old and was born at 28 weeks' gestation; lanugo is therefore abundant.

Age-Related Differences in the Premature Infant

Preterm infants differ from term infants in a number of ways. It is important to remember that preterm infants also differ markedly from one another. The physical characteristics, the behavior, and the needs of infants of 28 weeks (who weigh 1000 grams or less) are obviously different from those of infants of 32 weeks (who average 1500 grams) or of 36 weeks (whose weight is usually between 2000 and 2500 grams).

General Appearance of Preterm Compared with Term Infants. Differences in the general appearance of term and preterm infants are evaluated through the use of the Dubowitz assessment (see Neonatal Assessment). The external criteria used in the assessment describe some of the most obvious physical differences. Because of the cephalocaudal progression of development, the younger the gestational age of the baby, the larger its head will be in proportion to its body. Because testes do not descend until the 8th month of gestation, genitalia will be less well developed in preterm infant boys. In girls, the labia majora do not cover the labia minora until their age approaches that of a term baby. Lanugo is abundant on the body of an immature infant (Fig. 5-17), except in extreme prematurity in which case it is absent. The preterm infant's head hair is in fine, woolly bunches, whereas the term baby's hair is silky and flat, with individual strands.

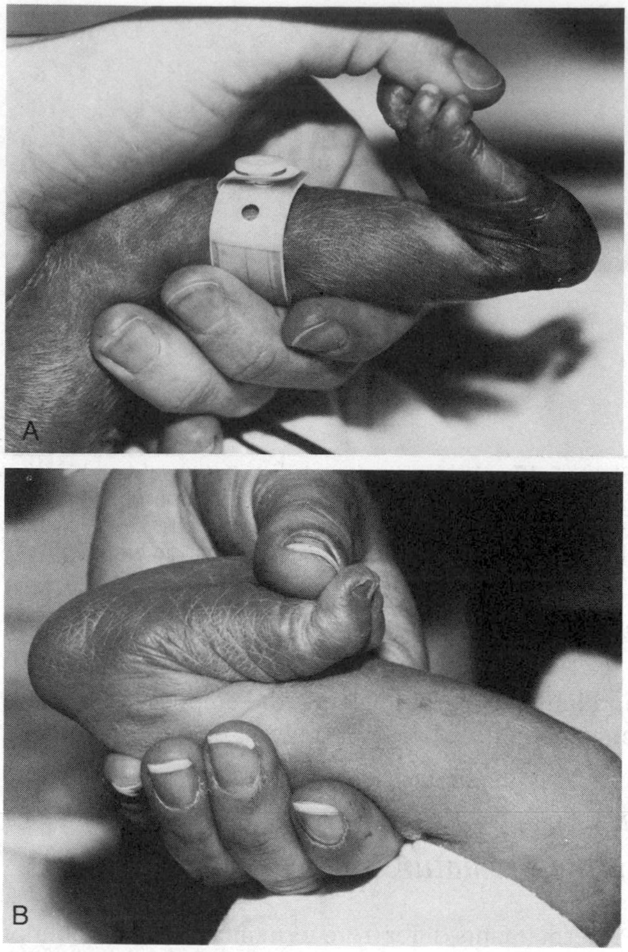

Figure 5-18. Ankle dorsiflexion. Increasing flexor responses reflect maturation. A decreasing angle between the dorsum of the foot and the anterior aspect of the leg occurs with maturation. *A*, Premature infant at 28 weeks' gestation. *B*, Full-term infant.

The skin of a preterm infant is thin, with numerous veins and tributaries visible. Even infants as old as 34 weeks' gestational age have relatively little subcutaneous fat; that layer is deposited chiefly in the 4 weeks prior to term.

Neurologic Development and Function. The nervous system of both preterm and term neonates is quite immature structurally. It is also functionally different from that of adults. In particular, neurons are immature in function, and there is limited myelination of the conduction pathways. In the premature neonate, neurologic function is largely directed by the brain stem and spinal cord rather than the cortex.

There are some distinct differences in the neurologic function of infants at various gestational ages. Some functions are present in neonates at 28 weeks and at term, but they vary in the consistency and quality of neurologic response to stimuli. These functions include vision, pupillary response, hearing, pain response, level of alertness, and limb movement. Other responses, such as primitive reflexes, are not present until a specific gestational age.

The appearance of these reflexes, or a change in their quality, forms the basis of the neurologic criteria used in the Dubowitz assessment. Generally, the development and suppression of primitive reflexes follows a specific sequence that can be used to determine gestational age. Increasing flexor responses reflect this development as the infant reaches 40 weeks' gestation (Fig. 5-18). This is followed by decreasing flexion and increasing extensor responses as the infant reaches 2 to 3 months post-term. The overall posture of the baby also reflects increasing flexion. The posture of a preterm baby is one of general extension, whereas in the term baby the posture is one of general flexion (Fig. 5-19).

The majority of acute neurologic problems in premature infants have occurred secondary to circulatory, metabolic, infectious, environmental, or physical conditions that impair function temporarily or permanently (Klaus and Fanaroff, 1986, p. 356). It is, therefore, critical that these systemic disorders be diagnosed and treated promptly. The common pathologic conditions associated with premature infants will be discussed in the Special Needs section.

Respiratory Development and Function. Of all the differences between preterm and term infants, none is more significant than the development of the respiratory tract. *Respiratory development is the crucial difference between viability and nonviability.* Before 26 to 28 weeks' gestational age there is limited development of the alveoli (the tiny air sacs at the terminal end of the respiratory system through which oxygen and carbon dioxide are exchanged) and of the alveolar capillaries. There are two types of cells within the alveoli: Type I cells give structure to the alveolus, and Type II cells produce several compounds collectively termed surfactant. The most abundant of the surfactant compounds is lecithin, accounting for 50 to 70 per cent of surfactant. The function of lecithin and other surfactant compounds is to prevent the collapse of the alveoli on expiration. Surfactant production may be inadequate because of the immaturity, impairment, or death of the surfactant-producing cells that line the alveoli. Neonatal stress diminishes the production of surfactant whereas stress to the fetus in utero increases production. When surfactant production is inadequate, respiratory distress syndrome (RDS or hyaline membrane disease) results.

Preterm infants also differ from term infants in the characteristics of their breathing; respirations are more irregular, with periodic apnea. Both the relative weakness of respiratory muscles and the decreased rigidity of the thoracic cage lead to hypoventilation, which in

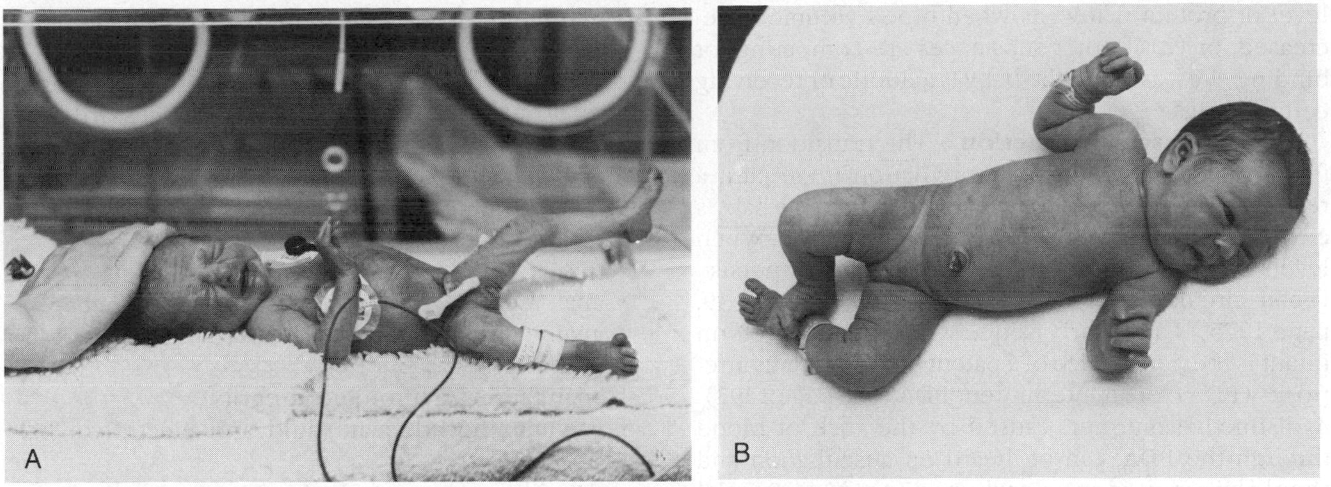

***Figure* 5-19.** Muscle tone and degree of flexion increases with maturity. *A*, The posture of a premature infant is one of general extension. *B*, The posture of a term baby is one of general flexion.

turn results in the retention of carbon dioxide and subsequent acidosis. Respiratory complications may occur because of the weak cough and gag reflexes of preterm babies, which increase the possibility of aspiration. The goal of treatment of respiratory distress in preterm infants is to correct these problems (see Special Needs of Preterm Infants discussed later in this section).

Gastrointestinal Development and Function. The gastrointestinal tract in preterm infants differs from that in the term infant in several ways. Gastrointestinal motility is decreased; stools may be infrequent, with abdominal distention. A glycerin suppository usually will stimulate defecation.

Before 34 weeks' gestation, the sucking and swallowing reflexes of the preterm baby may not be sufficiently coordinated to allow direct feeding from breast or bottle, so that alternate feeding methods may be necessary (gavage, intravenous feedings).

The immature digestive system of the preterm baby makes certain dietary adjustments necessary. Not only must the type of carbohydrate, fat, and protein be adapted to the special needs of the preterm baby, but factors such as renal solute load also must be considered.

Lactose is the carbohydrate of human and cow's milk and of many commercially prepared formulas. The enzyme lactase is necessary for lactose digestion. Since lactase enzymes do not attain maximal activity until 9 months' gestation, preterm infants may have impaired lactose tolerance.

Fats, even those digested rather easily by term infants, are not believed to be well assimilated by preterm babies. Triglycerides, however, are readily absorbed into the blood.

Preterm infants with respiratory distress syndrome have higher caloric needs because of an increased respiratory rate and thus an increased metabolic rate. When glucose alone is supplied to meet caloric needs, negative nitrogen balance results. Thus, protein breakdown is very high at a time when the body needs protein for brain development.

Provision of minerals is also a major problem. Lack of calcium can lead to undermineralization of the skeleton; however, it is not clear whether calcium supplementation is of any value. Since iron is stored by the fetus during the last trimester of pregnancy, preterm infants have minimal iron stores.

Liver Function. The liver of a preterm infant is less mature than that of a term infant. A less mature liver increases the likelihood of hyperbilirubinemia and toxicity from drugs that must be excreted through the liver.

Bilirubin is a product of red blood cell destruction. Indirect bilirubin is fat soluble and cannot be excreted in the bile or via the kidneys. Through the glucuronyl transferase enzyme system in the liver, conjugation of indirect bilirubin occurs. This converted or direct bilirubin is water soluble and thus can be excreted in the bile or via the kidneys. It is the unconjugated, or indirect, bilirubin that may cause kernicterus, a form of serious and nonreversible brain damage in neonates.

When the liver is immature, the ability to conjugate bilirubin (convert indirect bilirubin to direct bilirubin) is decreased; this is one of the factors causing hyperbilirubinemia of preterm infants. Another factor that may be as significant, or even more important, is the decreased number of Y and Z carrier proteins in the liver cells to which bilirubin must bind in the conjugation process. There is a danger of kernicterus (1) if the level of protein is low, as when blood volume is decreased, or (2) if other substances are competing for binding sites, as when the baby is acidotic or receiving certain drugs.

Cardiovascular Function. The transition from fetal circulation to neonatal circulation is, in part, a response to the increased level of oxygen in the baby's circulatory system following initial respiration. When levels of oxygen are low, fetal circulation may persist. (Fetal circulation is shown in detail in Chapter 39, page 1275.) Particularly frequent in the small preterm infant is the persistence of a patent (open) ductus arteriosus (PDA), or an intermittent PDA (see page 1292). A distinctive murmur, caused by the rush of blood through the PDA, can be heard on auscultation and should be reported and closely monitored (see Special Needs).

Renal Function. Because of a reduced glomerular filtration rate, preterm infants are more likely to retain fluid and to excrete drugs poorly. Moreover, when blood pressure is low, kidney perfusion, and therefore urinary output, will be diminished. When body water is diminished, however, the kidneys are not able to concentrate urine in order to conserve water; consequently, the baby may become easily dehydrated.

Within the renal tubules, both reduced tubular absorption and reduced tubular secretion may occur. Reduced absorption of glucose and amino acids may result in glucose and protein being spilled into the urine at lower serum levels than in more mature infants or older children. Metabolic acidosis is more likely because of the decreased ability to retain bicarbonate. Reduced secretion in the tubules, like the reduced glomerular filtration rate, limits drug clearance. The doses of medication given to preterm infants are very small but nevertheless they may accumulate in the body.

Immunologic Competence. Immunologic competence refers to the ability of an organism to resist infection. Immunologic competence involves cellular and humoral immune factors such as white blood cells, factors that enhance the ability of white blood cells to destroy bacteria, and immunoglobulins such as IgG, IgM, and IgA. For a variety of reasons, white blood cells are less effective in their action in these babies. The immunoglobulin IgG crosses the placenta and provides the neonate with immunity to certain infections to which the infant's mother is immune (e.g., diphtheria, measles, tetanus). The preterm infant has a deficit of IgG because transplacental passage of IgG occurs primarily in the third trimester. IgA, the primary immunoglobulin of colostrum, is not available to the baby who does not receive breast milk, and many preterm babies do not.

Special Needs of Preterm Infants

Though basic needs of preterm infants are similar to those of any neonate, nursing care necessarily becomes highly specialized in view of these infants' unique characteristics.

The main nursing considerations and common complications are related to

- maintaining a neutral thermal environment
- maintaining adequate gas exchange and tissue perfusion
- maintaining neurologic integrity
- maintaining adequate fluid and electrolyte balance
- providing adequate nutrition
- preventing infection
- maintaining skin integrity
- maintaining a sensory environment appropriate to gestational age and health status

Special needs of the family will be addressed later in this section.

Maintaining a Neutral Thermal Environment. The basic need of all neonates for warmth has been described earlier in this chapter. Thermoregulation for a preterm infant, especially an infant weighing less than 1500 grams, requires special consideration.

"Neutral thermal environment" refers to the narrow range of temperatures in which the neonate can maintain normal body temperature with the least amount of oxygen consumption and lowest metabolic rate. The goal is to maintain a core or rectal temperature in the range of 35.5 to 37.5°C (96 to 99.5°F) or an abdominal skin temperature of 36.5°C (97.7°F).

Except for very low birthweight infants (less than 1000 grams), heat production is not the problem in thermoregulation; the problem is heat loss. This excessive heat loss is due to the relative increase in overall body surface of the premature infant proportionate to weight, the limited development of subcutaneous fat, and the extension of limbs that increases the body surface exposed to the environment. As described on page 195, infants lose heat through four modalities: convection, radiation, evaporation, and conduction. *Convection* refers to the ambient temperature and the rate of air flow around the infant. An example of loss by this modality is the loss of heat through inappropriate incubator air temperature. *Radiation* refers to the loss of heat to cooler solid surfaces that are close to the infant. An example of this is radiant loss to an Isolette wall. *Evaporation* refers to the loss of heat through conversion of liquid to a vapor. An infant in an environment of very low humidity will increase its insensible water loss, which results in a decreased core tempera-

PULMONARY DISORDERS

Common

- Respiratory distress syndrome
- Transient tachypnea
- Meconium aspiration
- Pneumonia
- Pneumothorax

Less Common

- Pulmonary hypoplasia
- Upper airway obstruction
- Rib cage abnormalities
- Space-occupying lesions
- Pulmonary hemorrhage

EXTRAPULMONARY DISORDERS

Vascular

- Persistent fetal circulation
- Congenital heart disease
- Hypovolemia, anemia
- Polycythemia

Metabolic

- Acidosis
- Hypoglycemia
- Hypothermia

Neuromuscular

- Cerebral edema
- Cerebral hemorrhage
- Drugs
- Muscle disorders
- Spinal cord problems
- Phrenic nerve damage

***Figure* 5-20.** Differential diagnosis of neonatal respiratory disorders. (From Klaus MH, Fanaroff AA: *Care of the High Risk Neonate.* 3rd ed. Philadelphia, WB Saunders, 1986, 179.)

ture. The last modality is *conduction;* this refers to the loss of heat through direct contact with a cooler solid surface, e.g., a blanket (not prewarmed) from a bedside table placed under a nude infant in an Isolette.

When exposed to cold, the neonate will conserve heat by two mechanisms. The first mechanism is constriction of peripheral blood vessels. This will decrease blood flow nearest the skin, which will minimize heat loss through conduction. The second mechanism is nonshivering thermogenesis, through which heat production occurs from an increase in metabolism. The major energy source in nonshivering thermogenesis is brown fat. An infant of fewer than 30 weeks' gestation has almost no brown fat stores. Accordingly, an increase in metabolism, which results in increased oxygen demands, leads to anaerobic metabolism and metabolic acidosis. Continued cold stress will quickly deplete the brown fat and glycogen stores of a premature infant and will result in the same consequences, namely metabolic acidosis, hypoxemia, and hypoglycemia.

There is no doubt that cold stress will increase the risk of morbidity and mortality in premature infants. The prevention of hypothermia, therefore, is a crucial aspect of nursing care.

Infants of less than 1800 grams, or infants who cannot maintain a temperature of 36.4°C (97.6°F) in room air, should be cared for in an Isolette or radiant warmer. The baby's temperature is maintained at a constant level by a heat-sensitive probe that is taped to the abdomen or back. The unit heater is activated automatically when the baby's temperature falls below the desired level of thermoneutrality. The baby's axillary temperature also should be monitored at frequent intervals as a check of the accuracy of the probe. Other important nursing care strategies that will facilitate thermoregulation in the premature infant include judicious bathing, minimizing drafts into and around the Isolette/warmer, prewarming all surfaces that will contact the baby, using a radiant heat source for procedures that necessitate removal of the infant from the Isolette, use of a heat shield for very low birth weight infants, and use of knitted caps and booties.

Maintaining Adequate Gas Exchange and Tissue Perfusion. Respiratory problems are the most frequent cause of neonatal mortality and morbidity. Although most are a result of underlying lung disease, respiratory disorders may be caused by other problems, summarized in Figure 5-20. While many of these disorders have multisystem involvement, this section will deal with problems related to *ventilation.* Despite the differences in the underlying cause of the various disorders, much of the nursing care is similar. The main thrust of care is directed toward maintaining adequate gas exchange and tissue perfusion. Alterations common to the premature infant that affect oxygenation status are discussed next.

Respiratory Distress Syndrome (RDS). Respiratory distress syndrome (RDS), also known as hyaline membrane disease (HMD), is an acute respiratory disorder that occurs primarily in premature infants. Its occurrence increases as birth weight decreases. Recent reduction in the incidence and severity of respiratory distress syndrome have occurred chiefly as a result of prenatal therapies that inhibit premature labor, i.e., bed rest, tocolytic drugs, and the use of steroids given to the mother prior to delivery to stimulate lung maturation in the fetus. The use of surfactant replacement therapy, although less well established, likely will also reduce the rate of occurrence.

In effect, RDS occurs in infants born before completion of their lung maturation. Due to surfactant deficiency and structural immaturity, these infants are unable to establish effective respirations and, therefore, are unable to maintain adequate gas exchange. The presence of adequate surfactant allows alveoli to remain stable and not collapse following each breath. In the absence of surfactant, progressive collapse of the alveolar sacs occurs (atelectasis), leading to pulmonary hypoperfusion. These factors impair gas exchange and produce hypoxia and hypercapnia. Prolonged hypoxia results in metabolic acidosis; retention of carbon dioxide causes respiratory acidosis. Typical clinical symptoms include nasal flaring, expiratory grunting, use of accessory chest wall muscles in breathing (sternal and intercostal retractions), tachypnea, diminished air entry by auscultation, cyanosis, and apnea. The classic chest radiograph shows congested lung fields with a ground-glass appearance.

Treatment in the acute phase of the disease, i.e., the first 3 to 5 days, includes the use of supplemental oxygen; providing a neutral thermal environment; intravenous therapy; and frequent monitoring of color, activity, respiratory rate and effort, heart rate, body temperature, blood pH, arterial oxygen tension (PaO_2), arterial carbon dioxide tension ($PaCO_2$), and bicarbonate (HCO_3). Approximately 10 to 30 per cent of infants with RDS also require assisted mechanical ventilation to maintain adequate gas exchange and tissue perfusion (Klaus and Fanaroff, 1986). The two major nodes of mechanical ventilation are continuous positive airway pressure (CPAP), alone or alternatively, in conjunction with intermittent mandatory ventilation (IMV). CPAP provides positive pressure at end-expiration for infants who can breathe spontaneously but who are experiencing alveolar collapse. Intermittent mandatory ventilation delivers a combination of end-expiratory pressure and inspiratory pressure at a specific respiratory rate and pattern. Both of these forms of assisted ventilation involve the use of an endotracheal or nasopharyngeal tube and, frequently, supplemental oxygen. High-frequency jet ventilation and high-frequency oscillation are two new modes of mechanical ventilation under research. It is hoped that they may decrease the long-term effects of the trauma to the lungs from current modes. (See Chapter 38 for further discussion of respiratory therapy.)

Because of the risks involved in the use of too much or too little oxygen in premature infants, discussed later in this section, continuous monitoring of the oxygen levels in the blood is a crucial part of care. This monitoring includes frequent measure of the ambient oxygen concentration and of the level of oxygen in the blood. The latter is accomplished directly by blood sampling or indirectly through the use of transcutaneous oxygen monitors and oxygen saturation monitors (refer to Chapter 38 for discussion of monitoring of oxygen levels).

Patent Ductus Arteriosus. The ductus arteriosus remains patent in about 20 per cent of preterm infants weighing less than 1750 grams, but increases to 75 to 80 per cent of infants of less than 30 weeks' gestation with hyaline membrane disease (Cotton, 1987). As pulmonary vascular pressure decreases to a normal level, it falls below aortic pressure. This leads to a pressure gradient causing blood to flow from left to right through the ductus (refer to Chapter 39, page 1273 for review of fetal circulation). Hyperperfusion of the lungs and pulmonary edema result, which can cause congestive heart failure if prolonged. Patent ductus arteriosus is characterized by recurrent apnea or ventilatory failure, increased inspired oxygen concentration, a characteristic heart murmur, visual and palpable cardiac impulse over the precordium, bounding brachial and femoral pulses, crepitant rales in the lungs, and decreased peripheral perfusion. None or all of these symptoms may be present. The echocardiogram and Doppler assessment are considered the most reliable diagnostic modality. Treatment of PDA will depend on the severity of the symptoms caused. Symptomatic PDA refers to a compromise in pulmonary or cardiovascular function. Serious morbidity and mortality can occur if a symptomatic PDA is left to progress untreated. Supportive treatment measures include fluid restriction and maintaining adequate systemic perfusion through the administration of packed cells, providing a neutral thermal environment, and minimizing handling. Definitive treatment is closure of the ductus by indomethacin and, as a last resort, by surgical ligation.

Persistent Pulmonary Hypertension. A patent ductus arteriosus is also involved in another, more serious disorder: persistent pulmonary hypertension of the neonate (PPHN). This disease results from pulmonary arteriolar constriction, which may be brought about by a number of causes. Basically, pulmonary vasoconstriction causes pulmonary artery pressure to rise above aortic pressure and results in a right to left shunt across the ductus arteriosus. Pressure in the right atrium of the heart may be greater than in the left atrium, causing further shunting through the foramen ovale. Vasoconstriction also results in pulmonary hypoperfusion and decreased blood return to the left atrium, which causes severe hypoxemia. Persistent pulmonary hypertension of the neonate can occur with hyaline membrane disease, pneumonia (especially Group B streptococcal), meconium aspiration, diaphragmatic hernia, cold stress, rapid changes in inspired oxygen concentration, and perinatal asphyxia. The treatment of this disorder is very difficult and complex and includes oxygen therapy, assisted mechanical ventilation, vasodilators and vasopressors, and treatment of metabolic imbalances. (See Chapter 39 for the hemodynamics of PDA.)

Meconium Aspiration. Distress of the fetus in utero can result in release of meconium into the amniotic fluid, which may then be aspirated at the time of delivery. The ensuing cardiorespiratory problems result from a combination of airway obstruction and chemical inflammation. The initial fetal distress, if prolonged, can result in acidosis and hypoxemia, pulmonary vasoconstriction, and, finally, persistent pulmonary hypertension.

In addition to the effects from the intrauterine hypoxemic insult, the airway obstruction can lead to various air leak disorders of the lungs, which will be discussed later in this section. The most important treatment for this disorder is to minimize the aspiration of meconium at the time of delivery. This includes suctioning of the nasopharynx following delivery of the head, prior to delivery of the shoulders and before the infant takes the first breath. In the presence of significant meconium a laryngoscopy should be performed to allow direct suctioning of the trachea. The need for mechanical ventilation, supplemental oxygen, and further respiratory support can then be assessed.

Transient Tachypnea of the Neonate. Like meconium aspiration, this affects infants at, or close to, term. There is no underlying lung pathology in this syndrome, and it appears to result from slow absorption of fetal lung fluid. This syndrome is frequently referred to as "wet lung." Respiratory symptoms are similar to but usually less severe than in HMD. The chest radiograph usually can distinguish it from HMD and meconium aspiration, but it may be indistinguishable from Group B streptococcal pneumonia. These infants require frequent monitoring and may need supplemental oxygen. They rarely require mechanical ventilation or drug therapy.

Apnea. "Apnea is probably the most common respiratory event occurring in the high-risk neonate" (Marchal et al, 1987). Two major clinical circumstances involve apnea: (1) apnea in full-term or preterm neonates as part of respiratory distress, cardiovascular compromise, sepsis, and intrauterine hypoxic insult, or (2) apnea and bradycardia in premature neonates without other symptoms.

Severe or recurrent apneic episodes result in inadequate gas exchange, causing hypoxemia and bradycardia. This can lead to decreased cardiac output, decreased blood pressure, and decreased cerebral blood flow.

Apnea also may result from hyper- or hypothermia, metabolic imbalances, abdominal distention, vagal stimulation, and certain drugs. Apnea not related to any other cause is thought to result in premature infants, from weak upper airway musculature, decreased brain stem respiratory control, and response to hypoxemia by hypoventilating.

Immediate treatment includes cutaneous stimulation; if no response is obtained, then bag and mask ventilation is applied. Recurrent apneas may be treated with low CPAP, supplemental oxygen, a pulsating waterbed, and methylxanthine or doxapram drug therapy. Nursing care includes a prompt response to stimulate the apneic infant, a neutral thermal environment, proper suctioning technique, efficient gavage tube insertion, feeding infant on the right side or in a prone position with neutral neck flexion, and monitoring for toxic drug symptoms.

Complications of Respiratory Management. The treatment for most of the preceding respiratory disorders includes supplemental oxygen therapy or assisted mechanical ventilation or both. Note that these treatments are not without complications. Three major complications have been associated with one or both of these common therapies: air leak syndromes, chronic lung changes, and retinopathy of prematurity.

Air leak syndromes are the most frequent life-threatening complications of assisted mechanical ventilation. They can also occur spontaneously or in association with obstructive disorders, such as meconium aspiration. Pulmonary interstitial emphysema, pneumothorax, and pneumomediastinum are the most common types of air leak syndromes.

Pulmonary interstitial emphysema (PIE) is characterized by air leaks that travel along the outside of the blood vessels in the lung tissue. This air causes pressure on the vessels, which compresses them, resulting in circulatory impairment. Air may also travel along the vessels toward the hilum of the lungs and invade the mediastinum (pneumomediastinum). Air bubbles can accumulate at the hilum to such an extent that the area ruptures, releasing air into the pleural space (pneumothorax). This final type of air leak may require immediate medical intervention. Pulmonary interstitial emphysema can be diagnosed only by radiologic examination and will resolve only when mechanical ventilation is discontinued as the underlying lung disease resolves. Pneumothorax and pneumomediastinum vary in the extent of their clinical manifestations. No outward clinical symptoms may be evident, and radiologic examination may be required for a diagnosis. Symptoms vary with the extent and severity of the air leak but can include tachypnea, muffled heart sounds, diminished breath sounds, and cyanosis.

Chronic lung changes can occur following oxygen therapy or mechanical ventilation. These changes, which include thickening and necrosis of alveolar walls, atelectasis, and fibrosis, have been identified as bronchopulmonary dysplasia (BPD). The majority of these infants will survive and develop normal cardiorespiratory function by 5 to 6 years of age. The disease is characterized by long-term supplemental oxygen dependency, poor weight gain, recurrent acute infections, and cardiac changes. Nursing care implications include the need to ensure adequate oxygen to avoid hypoxemia, the need to monitor the infant for signs of respiratory distress and cardiac failure, protecting from infection, and minimizing unnecessary oxygen consumption for feeding and handling. Bronchopulmonary dysplasia is covered further in Chapter 38, page 1250.

Retinopathy of prematurity (ROP) is also known as retrolental fibroplasia. Etiology is discussed in Chapter 51. The incidence of ROP appears to be greatest in infants of very low birth weight. Time spent in oxygen has also been identified as an associated factor. Retinopathy of prematurity is a progressive disease of the retinal vasculature. It is characterized by the development of abnormal blood vessels on the retinal surface, following capillary constricture.

The progression of the disease involves leakage of fluid or hemorrhage from these abnormal vessels into the vitreous body. Scar tissue, which may then form, may result in detachment of the retina. Retinopathy of prematurity has a wide spectrum of severity, ranging from minimal vascular changes with no visual impairment to severe fibrovascular proliferation and retinal detachment leading to blindness. A classification system has been developed to define the extent of the disease (Shapiro, 1986). Nursing implications include cautious and judicious use of supplemental oxygen, and continuous assessment and monitoring of respiratory status, cardiac status, and activity. As the infant improves, oxygen requirements will decrease; the nurse is in a key position to recommend a decrease in therapy promptly.

Maintaining Neurologic Integrity

One of the greatest fears of parents of premature infants is that their child will be neurologically impaired. The maintenance of neurologic integrity, therefore, is of prime importance. Congenital and chromosomal abnormalities cause neurologic malfunction in neonates. However, this section will address only neurologic sequelae of (consequences occurring secondary to) oxygen deprivation prior to or during the birth process, hyperbilirubinemia, mechanical trauma, and metabolic imbalances. Neurologic malfunction related to infections in infants is addressed in Chapter 46.

Hypoxic-Ischemic Insult. Neurologic insult can occur as a result of inadequate oxygenation of brain tissue, either from decreased perfusion or decreased oxygen in the blood or both. This hypoxic-ischemic insult can be chronic and can occur prenatally from a variety of maternal conditions: toxemia, placental insufficiency, diabetes, drugs. It can also be acute, occurring at the time of birth. Common causes of hypoxic ischemia during labor and delivery include abruptio placentae, cord compression, meconium aspiration, placenta previa, and subdural and subarachnoid hemorrhage.

Clinical manifestations of hypoxic-ischemic insult at the time of birth vary from severe to subtle signs and may include hypo- or hypertonia, respiratory and cardiac depression, and decreased perfusion. Seizures are not usually visible before 6 hours of age.

Brain damage related to inadequate oxygenation can be temporary or permanent, with a wide gradation of functional impact. Cell damage and functional impairment of varying degree can also occur in organs other than the brain. These complications can be summarized by organ systems, as seen in Box 5-3.

The long-term sequelae of hypoxic-ischemic encephalopathy can include seizures, hydrocephalus, motor deficits, and mental retardation. In general, the more prolonged and extensive the hypoxic-ischemic insult, the higher the risk for severe long-term effects.

The significant damage resulting from hypoxia and decreased tissue perfusion has been discussed in relation to prenatal and intrapartum events. Note, however, that similar complications can occur in the postnatal stage. *Infants are at risk for neurologic damage whenever their systems are deprived of oxygen or adequate perfusion.* This may occur during apneic/bradycardic episodes, during cardiac arrests, from respiratory equipment malfunction, from cold stress, or from seizures.

Periventricular-Intraventricular Hemorrhage. Periventricular-intraventricular hemorrhage is of particular significance to preterm infants. One half of all preterm infants will have a periventricular-intraventricular hemorrhage, and this will be the major determinant of their neurologic morbidity (Avery, 1987). Preterm infants are susceptible to this particular type of intracerebral hemorrhage because of several factors related to their developmental immaturity. The site of hemorrhage is usually found in the subependymal germinal matrix at the head of the caudate nucleus. This matrix is composed of highly proliferative cells that are the precursors of neuronal or glial cells. The matrix is perfused by abundant but very fragile capillaries that are weakly supported by gelatinous tissue. Preterm infants also have an immature vascular autoregulatory system and increased fibrinolytic activity in the periventricular region.

The situation in which the preterm infant often finds itself contributes to these factors and can result in a hemorrhage of varying degree. Abrupt increases in

Box 5-3
Complications in Main Organ Systems Effected by Perinatal Hypoxic-Ischemic Insult

RESPIRATORY

respiratory distress
pneumonia
pulmonary hemorrhage
hypercapnia

CARDIOVASCULAR

dysrhythmias
cardiogenic shock
persistent fetal circulation
disseminated intravascular coagulation
hypotension

GASTROINTESTINAL

necrotizing enterocolitis
release of meconium into amniotic fluid

URINARY

acute tubular necrosis
renal failure

NEUROLOGIC

cerebral edema
cerebral necrosis
intraventricular-periventricular hemorrhage
intracerebral/cerebellar hemorrhage
subdural/subarachnoid hemorrhage
seizures
hypoxic-ischemic encephalopathy
periventricular leukomalacia

ENDOCRINE/METABOLIC

syndrome of inappropriate antidiuretic hormone secretion (SIADH)
hypoglycemia
acidosis

arterial blood pressure, such as those secondary to resuscitation efforts or infusion of hyperosmolar solutions, can rupture the sensitive capillaries in the germinal matrix. The increased fibrinolytic activity may then allow the hemorrhage to spread throughout the subependyma or into the ventricles themselves. Abrupt changes in cerebral blood flow, such as those caused by hypoxia and rapid reperfusion, can also rupture blood vessels. Lastly, increased venous pressure, resulting from mechanical ventilation or pneumothorax, which impede venous return, may contribute to capillary rupture.

Many hemorrhages of this type will occur on the first day of life. The smaller and younger the infant, the higher the risk of hemorrhage. The clinical features may be rapid, severe deterioration or can be much more subtle in nature. Since many intraventricular hemorrhages may be missed, most NICUs do routine real-time ultrasonography on all infants at risk, those under 1500 to 1800 grams, or those with a history of trauma or hypoxia, during the first few days of life.

It is very difficult to give parents a definite prognosis when a periventricular-intraventricular hemorrhage has occurred. There is still much that is not known about the process, and many of these infants have had other insults that complicate the prognosis. Follow-up studies will continue to provide data in this area.

Generally speaking, the more severe the hemorrhage, the poorer the outcome. The severity of the hemorrhage is determined by the extent of the bleeding and the structures involved. Hemorrhages confined to the subependymal region are more likely to have a better outcome than those that extend into the ventricles or into the cerebral parenchyma. Many of the moderate and most of the severe hemorrhages will result in the development of some degree of hydrocephalus. This is the reason that all hemorrhages initially detected by ultrasonography are then monitored by serial testing and computed tomography (Faerber, 1986).

Ventricular dilatation usually begins within 2 weeks of the onset of the hemorrhage. Hydrocephalus may occur days or weeks following the dilatation. There may be no dilatation, however, and the hemorrhage will resolve over time. (Hydrocephalus is discussed in Chapter 46, page 1742).

Hyperbilirubinemia. Neurotoxicity can also result from severe hyperbilirubinemia. Because of the immaturity of a premature infant's liver, the potential for kernicterus to develop is increased compared to a full-term newborn. (See page 201 for discussion of icterus neonatorum in the full-term neonate.) Because of the higher level of unconjugated bilirubin free to enter brain cells in a premature infant, this danger of kernicterus exists even when total bilirubin levels may not be excessively high. An increased susceptibility to bruising in preterm infants leads to increased red blood cell destruction, increasing the risk of hyperbilirubinemia. Delayed feeding, which may allow reabsorption of bilirubin from the bowel, also increases the likelihood that hyperbilirubinemia will develop. For all these reasons, serum bilirubin is monitored very closely in preterm infants.

Prior to initiation of treatment, the underlying cause of the hyperbilirubinemia must be determined.

This is usually done through various laboratory examinations.

Causes of indirect hyperbilirubinemia include:

- hemolytic diseases
- infections
- excessive breakdown of blood products from polycythemia, bruising, cephalhematoma
- metabolic disorders
- increased enterohepatic circulation from bowel obstruction, pyloric stenosis
- poor fluid/caloric intake (Osborn, 1986).

The two major treatments for moderate-to-severe hyperbilirubinemia are phototherapy and exchange transfusion. (See page 201 for discussion of these two forms of treatment.)

Therapeutic Management and Nursing Strategies to Maintain Neurologic Integrity. Treatments for pathologic conditions of the neurologic system are to correct the underlying problems or to support the infant as much as possible. Adequate oxygenation and ventilation are primary to maintaining neurologic integrity. In many circumstances, this can be achieved only through the use of mechanical respirators and supplemental oxygen, as previously discussed. Tissue perfusion, including the brain cells, also may be facilitated through the use of blood volume expanders, vasodilators, or inotropic drugs. On the contrary, in the case of hypoxic-ischemic encephalopathy, blood volume expansion is not desirable because of the associated cerebral edema that is largely responsible for decreased cerebral blood flow. The goal of treatment, under these circumstances, is to minimize interstitial fluid volume through fluid restriction.

Nursing interventions in relation to neurologic integrity include prevention of hypothermia and maintaining adequate gas exchange and tissue perfusion. Additionally, the nurse focuses on maintaining adequate fluid and electrolyte balance, providing adequate nutrition, preventing infection, and providing an appropriate sensory environment. A major component of care is the identification and management of seizures.

Because neonatal seizures are the most common neurologic problem leading to investigation, it is crucial that nurses become skilled at detecting them. Seizures of any type and of any etiology require prompt medical attention. Increasing evidence indicates that seizures may cause severe damage.

"The neonate's seizure is a disorganized event, often insidious in onset and progression" (Torrence, 1985). The premature infant's seizure is even more subtle. In neonates, jitteriness is often confused with seizure activity. Jitteriness must be distinguished from seizures. Seizures are not stimulus dependent and will not cease, as will jitteriness, when the limb is gently restrained. Seizures are caused by a wide variety of disorders. The main causes include hypoxia, intracranial hemorrhage, infection, hypoglycemia, hypocalcemia, hyperbilirubinemia, and maternal drug use (Torrence, 1985).

Behaviors associated with subtle seizures may include blinking or fluttering eyelids, sucking or mouthing movements, tonic posturing of a single limb, bicycling movements of the legs, rowing movements of the arms, and apnea. These may or may not be associated with any change in color, respiratory rate, or cardiac rate. Nursing care of an infant with seizures is discussed in Chapter 46, page 1719.

Maintaining Adequate Fluid and Electrolyte Balance

The body composition of a premature infant is 90 per cent water, compared with 75 per cent water in the term infant and 50 to 60 per cent water in the adult. There is, therefore, a difference in the composition of electrolytes in premature infants compared with adults or children. In the first 5 to 7 days of life, a term neonate normally will lose up to 10 per cent of its birth weight. A premature neonate will lose up to 15 per cent.

Neonates require water to replace fluid losses and to support growth. Water is lost from the body in four ways: through insensible loss, from skin and respiratory tract; through urine; through fecal water; and through sweat. Premature infants have increased insensible water loss due to the immaturity of their skin; increased permeability of the skin epidermis to water; increased skin blood flow relative to the metabolic rate; a larger body surface in proportion to weight; and lack of subcutaneous fat.

Electrolyte concentration affects fluid distribution maintaining the proper fluid balance in the major compartments, namely, *extracellular* and *intracellular*. Therefore, an imbalance in one will be reflected in a change in the other. (See Chapter 30 for further discussion of fluid and electrolyte balance.)

Fluid disturbances in neonates can be caused by a variety of disease states, but may also be caused by phototherapy, radiant warmers, increased ambient heat, increased loss by conduction or convection, increased insensible water loss (by mechanical ventilation, increased motor activity, crying, suctioning), and blood loss. Electrolyte disturbances occur primarily as a result of fluid imbalance, malfunction of regulatory organs (i.e., kidneys, skin, respiratory tract, gastrointestinal tract) or increased demands by the body.

Table 5-4. Problems and Interventions in Maintaining the Preterm Infant's Nutrition

Problems	Interventions
Small energy stores Relatively higher energy needs	Early provision of adequate calories
Glucose intolerance Hypoglycemia Hyperglycemia	Careful monitoring of blood glucose and glucose intake
Immature gastrointestinal system Impaired lactose tolerance Relative inability to digest fats Increased nitrogen catabolism with respiratory distress syndrome	Feedings adjusted to the special needs of the preterm baby
Immature sucking and swallowing reflexes	Alternate routes of feeding, including gavage, intravenous feedings
Treatment for respiratory distress may interfere with oral or gavage feeding	Intravenous feeding

These disturbances are usually imbalances in glucose, calcium, sodium chloride, and phosphates or acid-base imbalances.

Premature infants and ill or at-risk term infants require frequent adjustment of their fluid and electrolyte intakes, based on careful monitoring of their status. This monitoring includes daily calculation of intake of fluids and electrolytes, measuring urine output, daily or twice-daily checking of weight, and identifying excessive loss of fluid through gastrointestinal or respiratory tracts. Further, certain blood or urine tests are indicators of fluid and electrolyte balance, that is, serum sodium, potassium, phosphorus, calcium, chloride, glucose, hemoglobin, hematocrit, urea, and creatinine. Urine is checked for specific gravity, osmolality, sodium, and potassium. The most important nursing monitoring that is done, however, takes place through the clinical assessment of physical signs and symptoms. Physical signs of dehydration in a neonate may include decreased fontanel tension, skin turgor, blood pressure, peripheral perfusion, weight, and urine output and dry mucous membranes. Physical signs of overhydration may include increased weight, tachypnea, tachycardia, a patent ductus arteriosus murmur, and edema.

Providing Adequate Nutrition

Providing adequate nutrition in the premature, low birthweight infant is often the most challenging aspect of care (see Table 5-4). Because of the increasing complexity involved in this issue and because of the surge of research being conducted, the role of the nutritionist likely will assume increasing prominence on neonatal health care teams.

Two significant issues are involved in the provision of adequate nutrition in low birthweight infants: (1) determination of the types of nutrients that are required to achieve a specific goal, and (2) the method of delivery of these nutrients. Although there are no definitive answers to many of the questions involving neonatal nutrition, several generally accepted practices may be recommended.

The "gold standard" for growth of premature infants is controversial; a growth assessment can be performed by using either intrauterine or extrauterine standards. Frequent measurements are taken of the premature infant and include weight, length, and head circumference. These measurements can then be compared to a standard of similar populations to determine the adequacy of the nutritional regimen. For example, a desired weight gain for most premature infants who are appropriate for gestational age is 15 to 20 grams per kilogram per day. Acceptable head circumference growth is approximately 0.5 to 1 centimeter per week (3/8 inch).

A number of studies have attempted to determine the amount of specific nutrients that are required to achieve the desired rate of growth. These studies have resulted in recommendations for the intake of protein, fat, carbohydrate, vitamins, and minerals. Generally, daily energy intakes of 114 to 181 Kcal per kg per day is suitable for most infants. The standard used most frequently for the amount of nutrients adequate for growth is human milk. However, the nutritional adequacy of human milk is not as well established for preterm infants as it is for full-term infants. The composition of milk supplied by mothers of preterm infants is different from that of term mothers. Because of this difference, it is regarded by many as suitable for premature infants. The special properties of preterm milk provide the basis for the recommendation against the use of banked human milk (which is term milk) for the growing preterm infant. Required trace elements (Ca, P, Na, Fe, Cu, and Zn) are thought not to be adequate in banked human milk. Vitamin supplementation for premature infants is also controversial, whether infants are receiving human milk or a special formula. Although in theory both human milk and special formula contain the required vitamins, proponents of supplementation argue that premature infants are born with low body stores, experience rapid growth, and have reduced gastrointestinal absorption, reduced daily intake of formula, and frequent illness states that increase requirements. As a result, practices of vitamin and mineral supplementation vary and will continue to change only as significant research data become available. (See Chapter 18 for further discussion of vitamin and mineral supplementation.)

In addition to the controversies involved in the type and amount of nutrients required for preterm infants, each method for the ideal delivery of nutrients has its proponent. Nutrients can be delivered by an enteral method, i.e., through a gastrointestinal route; or by a parenteral method, i.e., through an intravenous route.

For infants who have not yet developed the ability to suck and swallow in a coordinated fashion, or whose ability is impaired by disease, tube feedings are the method of choice. The three methods commonly used are: *gavage* (intermittent gastric), *continuous transpyloric,* and *continuous gastric feedings.* An oral or nasal tube is inserted into the stomach or into the distal duodenum or jejunum (transpyloric), depending on the method chosen, and breast milk or formula is delivered by bolus at frequent intervals (1 to 4 hours) or continuously. (Gavage feedings are further discussed on page 1387.) Determination of the tolerance to enteral feeding is made by noting the amount and frequency of vomiting/regurgitation, abdominal distention, and stools. In the case of intermittent feeds, the amount of residual (formula still present in the stomach just prior to the next feeding) can be determined by aspirating stomach contents with a syringe attached to the feeding tube. A large amount of residual may indicate the need to decrease the amount given at each feeding or, with an older premature, to extend the length of time between feedings (usually from 2 to 3 per hour). Intolerance to feeding also may be an indication of developing sepsis or other disease processes and should be reported and investigated.

Although intermittent gastric feeding is used most commonly, there may be indications for continuous feeding: short bowel syndrome, severe gastroesophageal reflux, delayed gastric emptying time, and so on. More clinical studies are needed to determine the effectiveness of the various feeding techniques.

Feeding implications are vitally important to nurses. Safe and effective delivery of feeding by tube includes skill in tube insertion and removal, proper positioning of the infant, instillation of milk at a controlled rate, and careful observation for signs of intolerance or distress during or following feeds.

Nutrients are delivered via the parenteral route when the premature or term infant is unable to receive any or enough of them enterally, as in congenital gastrointestinal anomalies, necrotizing enterocolitis, severe respiratory distress syndrome, and other conditions. Total parenteral nutrition (TPN) may be administered by either central or peripheral veins. Complete nutrient requirements can be met by total parenteral nutrition through a combination of specific components: protein is supplied in the form of amino acids, dextrose is the primary energy source, fats are supplied as lipid emulsions, and vitamins and minerals are added. The amount and type of TPN components used in practice vary, but are usually similar to those listed (Ohio Neonatal Nutritionists, 1985).

Complications of the administration of total parenteral nutrition include infection, hyperglycemia, cholestasis, lipemia, and rickets. Frequent laboratory assessments are essential, and growth is monitored as for infants receiving enteral nutrition.

The key aspects of nursing care during total parenteral nutrition are maintenance of the venous line through aseptic techniques and judicious handling and restraint of the infant so that the line does not become dislodged. (See Chapter 30, page 922, for further discussion of TPN.)

Preventing Infection

Premature infants suffer decreased transplacental transfer of immunoglobins from the mother. Immunoglobins provide the infant with passive immunity to a myriad of infectious agents. Not receiving such immunity, the premature infant is at risk for infection (sepsis). In addition, the premature's immature immunologic system is capable of only a minimal anti-inflammatory response when exposure to infectious agents occurs.

The two major sources of infection in infants are intrauterine-acquired and hospital-acquired (nosocomial). Nosocomial infections can develop endogenously from the invasion of bacteria from the skin, respiratory tract, or gastrointestinal tract. They can also develop from exogenously acquired bacteria or viruses, such as respiratory syncytial virus (RSV), influenza A, shigella, or salmonella. A specific infection commonly seen in premature infants is necrotizing enterocolitis (NEC). (See Chapter 41, page 1433, for further discussion of NEC.)

In view of the premature infant's minimal ability to resist infection, health professionals must assume major responsibility for prevention of infection. Several simple measures can be taken to diminish the likelihood of exposure to infectious agents. The most important measure, and yet the one most frequently ignored, is thorough handwashing with a bactericidal solution. Hands must be washed both before and after contact with each infant and his or her equipment. Gowning practices vary from institution to institution. Generally, gowns are worn when in direct contact with an infant and are changed between patients.

No one who is ill should be in contact with patients in a neonatal intensive care unit (NICU). As well, strict procedures for the routine cleaning of all equipment should be followed. For infants with specific infections, further isolation precautions may be initiated. Certain treatment modalities have been associated with an increased risk of infection, such as umbilical catheters, indwelling peripheral or central venous catheters, peripheral arterial catheters, and respiratory therapy equipment. Scrupulous aseptic technique must be followed by all personnel involved in these procedures.

The prognosis for premature infants with sepsis depends on prompt recognition and treatment of the disease. Clinical symptoms are usually very subtle in onset. They include apnea, decreased peripheral perfusion, temperature instability, hyperbilirubinemia, feeding intolerance, acidosis, hypoglycemia, tachypnea, and tachycardia. Changes in the blood count, especially leukocytes, platelets, and neutrophils, or pathogenic organism growth from a cultured specimen lead to a definitive diagnosis. Infants who are suspected of having an infection are started on antibiotics before test results are known, however. It is common, therefore, to find a high proportion of sick neonates in an NICU receiving antibiotics.

Antibiotics given most frequently to preterm infants include ampicillin (50 to 100 mg per kg per day) and gentamicin (5 mg per kg per day). Because drugs are excreted more slowly by the immature kidneys of neonates, blood levels of antibiotics remain high for a longer period of time than in older children or adults. For this reason the 24-hour dose is divided in two and given at 12-hour intervals.

The widespread and intense use of antibiotics in neonatal intensive care units has encouraged the emergence of resistant strains of various organisms. As a result, new drugs are constantly being developed. The rapid changes related to premature and term neonates in the pharmacology field have led to the addition of a pharmacist to the health care team in many neonatal intensive care units.

Maintaining Skin Integrity

As stated, the immaturity of infants' skin is a source of difficulty in maintaining body temperature. The increased permeability also results in greater opportunity for pathogenic organisms to invade the tissues. In addition, there is a risk for toxicity from absorption of chemicals through the skin.

The preterm infant is at greater risk than older infants for skin damage from the removal of tapes, electrodes, or collection bags. This is due to the diminished cohesion between the dermis and epidermis and to the immaturity of the stratum corneum.

Part of the protective function of the skin results from the acid mantle that it produces. This acidic quality provides a barrier to the growth of normal flora on the skin. Frequent bathing with alkaline soaps and moisturizers can raise the skin pH. This may, in turn, cause bacteria to increase in number.

The nursing implications in maintaining skin integrity are

- avoid use of caustic solutions to clean the skin
- minimize use of tapes
- minimize friction to skin
- avoid the use of alkaline-based soaps
- use mild solvent to remove adhesive tape

Maintaining a Sensory Environment Appropriate to Gestational Age and Health Status

Though our understanding of the sensory needs of preterm infants remains limited, research indicates that appropriate sensory stimulation may be significant in the baby's development. The long-term effects of stimulation programs for preterm infants have not been well documented, however. Numerous methodologic problems have been associated with many of the studies that have been conducted.

General agreement exists, however, that stimulation of premature infants, especially those ill and those extremely premature, must be approached with caution. The very immature or sick infant's general homeostatic mechanisms are fragile and may be easily overwhelmed by almost any extra stimuli. The NICU environment contributes to pleasant stimuli and sensory deprivation of excessive stimulation from noxious stimuli. Therefore, it is important to protect these infants from the noxious stimuli in order to promote stabilization of their basic biologic processes.

The differences in the behavior of preterm infants and full-term infants may be related to the differences in neurologic development and to any illnesses that are superimposed on the situation. Infants born prematurely must cope with performing all the vital functions that were previously assumed by their mothers. Premature infants are also deprived of the regulatory influences of their mothers' biorhythms and of the entirety of the intrauterine sensory experience. Finally, they are exposed to the highly technologic environment of an intensive care unit that includes excessive painful and intrusive stimuli.

Many of the current stimulation programs incorporate these principles:

- (1) the approach should be modified according to each infant's stage of development and temperament;
- (2) the timing and type of intervention used should be determined and modified based upon observation of the infant's behavior and responses;
- (3) parents should be involved as much as possible;
- (4) prior to initiation of any program, the existing environmental conditions should be assessed.

Various forms of tactile, vestibular, and oral stimulation have been advocated, as well as proper positioning and range-of-motion exercises.

The goals for care, which are congruent with these principles, should include withdrawing stimuli when the infant demonstrates avoidance behaviors, supporting approach behaviors, and observing and recording responses to interventions. Gorski (1985) found that distress signs following caregiver tasks often did not occur until 5 minutes later. He also found that social interaction could produce as much stress in weak infants as did painful stimuli. Oehler (1985) studied well, moderately ill, and very ill premature infants. She found that sicker babies differed in their response to stimuli and could tolerate only minimal stimulation in a single modality.

Adverse or avoidance behaviors of premature infants that have been associated with overstimulation include gaze aversion, arching of trunk, finger splaying, crying, and yawning. Responses may also be more severe, such as mottled or cyanotic skin, apnea, bradycardia, blood pressure instability, and hypoxemia.

Regardless of the approach to infant stimulation that is advocated in any institution, nurses involved in the caretaking of premature and ill neonates can incorporate certain basic measures into their plan of care. In general, an effort is made to avoid or minimize noxious stimuli. Nursing care should be organized so as to disturb the premature infant as little as possible, especially during the night. It is important to observe carefully and document the infant's positive and negative responses to various stimuli. Consistency in caregivers should be promoted. Observations of the infant's responses in various situations should be shared with the parents. Any unnecessary equipment noise in the neonatal intensive care unit should be eliminated or minimized. An example of this is keeping respiratory tubing free of excess water, which creates additional noise. The preterm infant should be handled and moved in a smooth, slow manner. Sufficient support to the spine, head, and extremities is required to avoid rapid extension and startling.

The manner in which the preterm neonate is handled may influence progress in growth and development and overall health. Special attention must be paid to these infants to ensure that their need for a balance between stimulation and rest is not overlooked.

Significance of Prematurity for Long-Term Development

What does being born prematurely mean for infants as they become toddlers, older children, and, ultimately, adolescents? As technology has enabled us to sustain life at an earlier gestational age, concern has grown about the quality of life of these tiny babies who survive. Early studies of babies born in the 1950s found that a large percentage of preterm infants had major neurologic damage (Lubchenco, 1972). Numerous recent studies, however, have concluded that most of the individual children do well (Kopp and Parmelee, 1979; Cohen, 1986). In groups of survivors weighing less than 1500 grams at birth, 80 per cent were quite normal (Stewart et al, 1981; Hack et al, 1983). Other studies that included infants weighing 500 to 800 grams at birth found approximately 35 per cent to be profoundly handicapped (Bennett et al, 1983; Kitchen et al, 1983; Buckwald et al, 1984).

Follow-up of preterm infants through the school-age years is ongoing. Such studies will help predict specific infants at risk to determine the effects of biologic and social factors and to determine the causes of some of the major handicaps thought to be associated with prematurity.

Post-Term Infants

Up to 12 per cent of neonates have a gestational age of more than 42 weeks and therefore are considered postmature. Some of these infants have a characteristic appearance that includes absence of vernix caseosa;

dry, cracking skin; long nails; decreased subcutaneous fat; oligohydramnios; and meconium staining of the skin and nails. The body appears long and thin. The mortality rate is increased compared with full-term infants, especially in those born to primiparous women and women over 35 years of age. There is also an increased incidence of cephalopelvic disproportion, cesarean section, and birth injuries in post-term infants, due to their increased size.

Specific clinical complications have been associated with post-term infants. These include fetal distress with subsequent hypoxic-ischemic insult and/or meconium aspiration, inadequate nutrition, thermal instability, small for gestational age, hypoglycemia, and polycythemia-hyperviscosity syndrome.

The Infant Who Is Small for Gestational Age

At any gestational age, an infant's weight may fall below the 10th percentile, according to standard growth charts. This infant will be termed *small for gestational age* (SGA). Approximately one third of all babies weighing less than 2500 grams at birth are SGA rather than preterm. These infants may also be said to have *intrauterine growth retardation* (IUGR). The clinical picture of retarded intrauterine growth is related to the duration, severity, and time of initial onset.

One type of IUGR is *asymmetric* or *hypotrophic* growth retardation, in which the neonate's length and head circumference fall within normal limits on the growth curves. Only the weight is abnormal. At birth, these infants appear thin and wasted. There is little subcutaneous tissue so that the skin appears loose; it is often peeling and meconium-stained. This type of growth failure occurs late in pregnancy; its causes include toxemia, hypertension, Class C diabetes, and cardiac and renal disease. These infants are often distressed at birth and rapidly become hypoxemic and acidotic; therefore, they require resuscitation. They may also have aspirated meconium, thereby exacerbating the distress. Following birth, infants with asymmetric growth retardation do not lose weight but rather soon experience a period of rapid weight gain. In the absence of severe hypoxic-ischemic insult or other problems, these infants usually do well.

The second type of intrauterine growth retardation is *symmetric* or *hypoplastic*. In this type, all the aforementioned growth parameters are below normal. The infant does not appear wasted since growth in body weight stopped weeks before birth, prior to the development of adipose tissue. This chronic growth failure occurs as a result of intrauterine infections (such as congenital rubella and cytomegalovirus); congenital and chromosomal abnormalities (such as dwarfism, cri-du-chat syndrome), and maternal malnutrition. These infants are also distressed at birth, but their distress is often due to hyaline membrane disease.

Because SGA infants have small reserves of both glycogen and fat, hypoglycemia can be a significant problem. If glucose is not supplied from the time of birth, central nervous system damage can result.

Polycythemia (an excess of red blood cells) is frequent and is probably an intrauterine response to chronic fetal hypoxia. When the hematocrit is greater than 65 per cent, the blood becomes sufficiently viscous to reduce its flow.

Because the incidence of congenital malformation is increased in these infants, especially meticulous physical assessment is indicated.

If congenital infection is suspected, blood from both mother and baby is examined for the presence of antibodies to the TORCH groups of infections (toxoplasmosis, others [e.g., syphilis and infectious hepatitis], rubella, cytomegalovirus, and herpes simplex.)

Other factors are associated with SGA infants. Multiple births may be a problem, especially with twin-to-twin transfusion. Twin-to-twin transfusion refers to an artery-to-vein anastomosis in the placenta. Blood is chronically shunted away from one twin, resulting in growth retardation. Maternal factors include high altitudes, smoking, low socioeconomic status, narcotic abuse, anticonvulsant therapy, antimetabolite therapy, and chronic alcoholism. There is also a 23 per cent incidence of mental deficiency in fetal alcohol syndrome. These infants commonly have dysmorphic features and cardiocirculatory abnormalities. (See Chapter 52 for further discussion of fetal alcohol syndrome.)

The Infant Who Is Large for Gestational Age

When an infant's birth weight exceeds the 90th percentile for gestational age, that infant is considered *large for gestational age* (LGA). A birth weight of over 4000 grams often reflects a genetic predisposition; infants of diabetic mothers are the exception.

LGA babies weigh more and have proportionally larger heads and length. Infants of diabetic mothers (IDM) are disproportionately heavier. This excessive weight is related to the deposition of fat from elevated maternal blood sugars. This occurs because the infant is not capable of excreting sufficient insulin to handle the elevated blood sugar.

Hypoglycemia is a major concern in infants of diabetic mothers because of the following sequence: increased maternal blood glucose results in a higher level of glucose crossing the placenta; fetal insulin production increases to metabolize the glucose that is stored as glycogen; at birth, maternal glucose is no longer available, but insulin production remains increased, leading rapidly to hypoglycemia. Respiratory distress, hypocalcemia, and hyperbilirubinemia are also common in infants of diabetic mothers.

Typical clinical complications associated with LGA infants include: hypoxic-ischemic insult, spontaneous air leaks, transposition of the great vessels, and birth trauma, all of which increase the mortality rate for large for gestational age babies.

Family of the Infant with Problems Due to Gestational Age or Illness

The families of infants who require intensive care at birth are confronted with many stressors. Parents are separated from their neonates because the infant is transferred either to a special unit within the hospital of birth or to a referral center some distance away. They often face the uncertainty of the initial diagnosis as well as the long-term outcome. Mothers of high-risk newborns may be ill themselves and therefore have additional physical stressors. All mothers also experience the normal physiologic changes that occur following delivery. Families may lack financial, social, and internal supports, all of which will exacerbate the stress caused by the birth of their baby.

When a baby needs specialized care because of prematurity or illness, the reactions and needs of the family are similar to those of families of an infant born with a congenital defect (see discussion in Chapter 25). Parents must grieve for the lost baby of their dreams so that they can then accept their baby as he or she really is. When the infant is critically ill, this grief may be compounded by an anticipatory grief through which parents try to prepare themselves for their infant's death. Sadness, denial, guilt, diminished self-esteem, and anger are some of the emotions parents express before reaching a stage at which adaptation to the reality of their situation begins.

Just as parents of babies with anomalies look within themselves for possible reasons for the defect, parents of preterm infants and infants who are ill at birth search for reasons. The diabetic mother of a large for gestational age infant may feel particularly guilty if her infant has more than transient problems, because she sees a direct link between her own condition and the baby's problems.

As with all parents and new babies, it is essential that a relationship of love and caring be established in the early stages of development. When the attachment process does not occur, child abuse or long-term psychologic difficulties for the child and family may result. An important goal of nursing care, therefore, is to facilitate the attachment process. This goal is applicable to all parents of high-risk newborns, even when the infant may not survive.

Research indicates that the grieving process is facilitated when parents have tangible, specific memories and events relating to their deceased baby. Resolution of grief may not occur, or may be delayed for months or years, in parents who have never seen or touched their newborn babies. Understandably, parents are often reluctant to allow themselves to become attached to a baby who may die.

It is just as important to individualize care for the parents and families of ill or premature neonates as for the infants themselves. The meaning of this crisis event and its impact may be very different for the mother than for the father; it may vary considerably from family to family. Each person may have a unique way of coping with the situation.

To plan appropriate interventions, therefore, an assessment should be made of each parent and of the family unit as a whole. This assessment should include the parent's perception of the event, what things the parent finds stressful or helpful, how she or he is coping with the situation, and what resources are available and useful to the individual or family. With this information, an initial plan of care can then be devised and discussed with the parents. It is imperative that the plan of care be revised regularly, since parents' perceptions often change over time. A critically ill or very premature infant may remain in the hospital for many weeks, during which time the health status will change frequently. This "roller coaster" situation necessitates ongoing assessment of parental responses. In some units, the primary nurse is responsible for the family plan of care. In other units, the care of the family may be coordinated by a clinical nurse specialist or social worker.

Providing around-the-clock opportunities for visiting and telephoning, careful explanation of day-to-day changes in the baby's condition and treatments, and opportunities for participation by parents in care contribute to parental adaptation. (See Figure 5-21.)

The opportunity for parents to discuss their feelings, particularly their negative feelings, is significant as well. Many intensive care nurseries sponsor group discussions in which parents can share feelings with one another as well as with staff members. Before their first visit to the NICU, parents should be prepared for their infant's appearance, the equipment involved in treatment, how treatment is contributing to the recovery, and what they may expect to do to help with the baby's care. The nurse should be nearby during the parents' visits but should allow them some degree of privacy. Most parents require some direction regarding the level of interaction appropriate for their baby's age and state of health. The nurse can take each opportunity available to point out the infant's positive features and progress. As the parents indicate readiness and the infant's condition warrants, they may be taught how to perform their infant's basic care. This may include changing the baby's diaper, holding the syringe during a gavage feeding, stimulating the baby orally during feeding, talking to or stroking the baby, and bringing in personal items for the baby. (Refer to previous section on Environment for more details.) Another important and unique contribution to the baby's care can be made by the mother, namely, the provision of breast milk for her infant. Mothers who wish to take on this task require additional support, encouragement, and teaching.

In caring for parents and their infant with gestational age or health problems, it is easy to overlook the siblings of that infant. Parents, too, are frequently so involved with their own feelings that they are unable to adequately provide for the needs of their other children. Preschool children, with their limited understanding of cause and effect, and a focus that is primarily self-centered, are especially likely to feel responsible for the baby's illness. Nursing assessment includes checking with parents about what siblings have said or what the parents may have observed in sibling behavior. One could say: "Brothers and sisters often have worries about their baby brother (sister). Has (name) asked about the baby?" Many intensive care nurseries provide opportunities for children to visit briefly with new siblings.

The parents' division of time between children who need them at home and their own need to be with their baby in the hospital can be discussed in groups as well as individually. There is no one satisfactory answer, but helping parents recognize the issue is a beginning.

Planning for Transfer or Discharge

Planning for transfer or discharge begins at birth, with activities that enhance the developing relationship between parents and infants, and continues throughout hospitalization. Parents frequently approach the day of transfer or discharge with mixed feelings of anxiety and joy. Their anxiety results from concern regarding their own ability or the ability of the receiving unit to care for a baby who is still small or who has required highly specialized care. A smooth transition will occur only if there has been adequate planning, preparation, and support of the family and communication with the receiving unit.

Ongoing assessment is required for effective planning. A multidisciplinary approach is used in most units. Team members may include staff nurses, physicians, community health nurse, follow-up or home care coordinator, physical or occupational therapists, social worker, and clinical nurse specialist. The needs of the family and of the child dictate the type of referrals and follow-up that will be required.

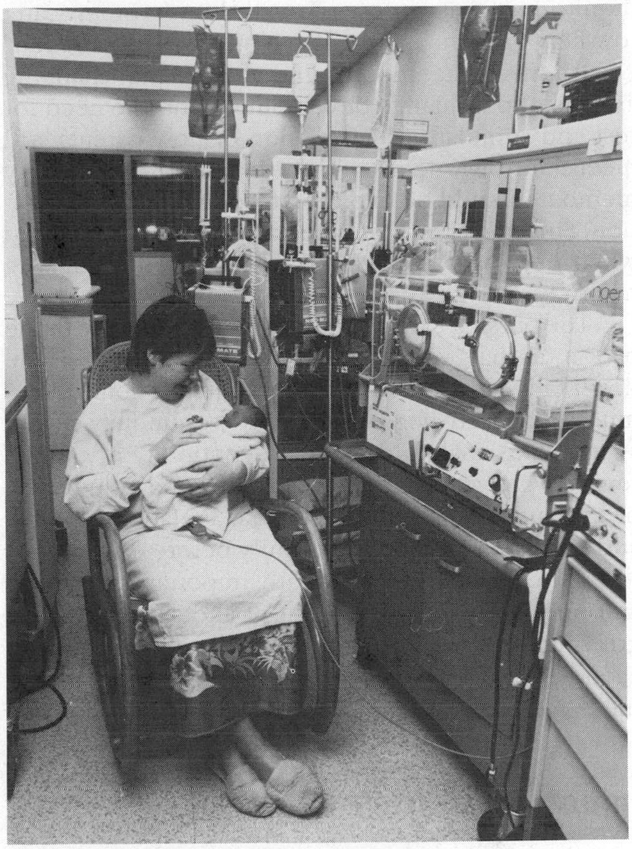

Figure 5-21. If given the support and opportunity, parents of critically ill infants can develop a relationship of love and caring even though their baby is in the midst of an overwhelming technical environment.

Criteria for transfer or discharge may include the following: resolution of acute illnesses or stability of chronic illnesses, adequate weight gain, adequate enteral fluid and caloric intake, apnea controlled or resolved, medication levels at therapeutic range with documented side effects, and a specific plan for any special needs. Frequent discharge medications include methylxanthines, anticonvulsants, digoxin, diuretics, and vitamin and mineral supplements (Colangelo et al, 1987).

Parents will need certain knowledge and skills to provide care for their infants at home. They must be comfortable with basic infant care tasks such as safety, feeding, diapering, and bathing. Second, parents need to understand fully the special health needs of their infant, which may include infection and environmental control; signs and symptoms of recurrent illness; administration and side effects of medications; home monitoring; ventriculoperitoneal shunts; ostomy care; low flow oxygen; and cardiopulmonary resuscitation.

Parents also should understand the changing aspects of the infant's development and the need for rest and stimulation. Discussion of how parents will meet their own needs and the needs of other family members should be explored throughout hospitalization. Finally, parents need to know how to obtain help when necessary and what the plans are for ongoing health care follow-up.

The nursing care of families does not end with the baby's discharge from the hospital or even with the death of a baby. When the infant returns home, communication between hospital and community health agency nurses should facilitate continuity of care. If referrals are made before discharge, the community health nurse can begin to establish a relationship with and provide support to the family before discharge.

If the baby dies, it is equally important to provide an opportunity for assessment of and support during grieving. This may be done through community health agencies or return visits to the medical center where the baby received care.

Infants in Multiple Gestations

Approximately 1 in 87 births in the United States and in Canada is a twin birth. Triplets are far less frequent, occurring approximately once in 7569 births. Twins may be *monozygotic* or *dizygotic*. Monozygotic twins develop from a single fertilized ovum that divides to form two embryos within the first 14 days following fertilization; this occurs approximately once in every 200 pregnancies. Dizygotic, or fraternal, twins result from double ovulation. Rates of dizygotic twins are influenced by race (higher in black and lower in Oriental women), by maternal age (increased incidence as maternal age increases), and by family history of dizygotic twins.

Placentas in twin pregnancies may be *monochorionic* (i.e., with one chorion and either one or two amnions) or *dichorionic* (with two chorions and two amnions). When the placenta is monochorionic, a vascular connection usually exists between the twins; when this connection is artery-to-vein, there is a fetal-to-fetal transfusion (fetal transfusion syndrome). Such transfusion occurs in approximately 15 per cent of twins with monochorionic placentas.

Intrauterine development of twins is much like that of a single fetus during the first 29 to 32 weeks or to the time when the combined weight of the fetuses is approximately 3000 grams. After that time, the placenta may no longer be able to meet rapidly increasing growth needs and intrauterine growth retardation can occur. Intervention that enhances uterine blood flow, such as rest in the left lateral position, may enhance fetal growth.

Meeting the Immediate Physiologic Needs of Infants in Multiple Births

When a multiple birth is expected, adequate nursing and medical personnel must be present at the delivery to assure that each infant receives sufficient care immediately following delivery. Twin births are considered "high risk" and include a higher risk of prematurity and being small for gestational age.

The possibility of fetal transfusion syndrome may be suspected when maternal hydramnios occurs in a twin pregnancy. Ultrasound may reveal a major disparity in twin size; birth weights may differ by as much as 1000 grams (2.2 pounds).

Each twin will have specific problems that require immediate attention. The twin at the arterial side of the transfusion will be small, malnourished, pale, anemic, and hypovolemic. Frequently the baby is in shock. Immediate care, as in any anemic, hypovolemic neonate, involves careful assessment of infant status and transfusion to replace volume and red blood cells. The baby is critically ill and requires all the support and intensive nursing care of a very sick neonate.

The recipient twin, in contrast, is well nourished, plethoric, polycythemic, and hypervolemic. The heart is enlarged, and the baby may have heart failure. Secondary to polycythemia, jaundice or thrombosis may occur. If the central hematocrit is greater than 65 to 70 per cent, a partial exchange transfusion may be in order to replace the more viscous blood with normal blood. At slightly lower levels, intravenous fluids may alleviate hyperviscosity if there are no symptoms of problems.

Attachment in Twin and Multiple Births

The first sight of their newborn infant and the moments of "togetherness" that follow are among the important steps in the attachment process. In multiple births, of course, the arrival of the first baby may result in a very different physical sensation for the mother; she may feel the other fetus or fetuses moving inside her. Between the delivery of the first baby and subsequent babies, both parents' attention is necessarily divided between the activities of the second stage of labor and the baby already born.

When twins are premature or ill, the period immediately following birth will be like that of any other neonate with similar problems, and nursing actions to support attachment will be similar. If the babies are term and healthy, both (all) may be with the mother during the fourth stage of labor, and breast feeding, if desired, may be initiated.

During the first days after birth, both during hospitalization and at home, parents need extra help to integrate the babies into their lives. Not surprisingly, parents may also require additional guidance in relation to organization of time and energy. With twice the workload, fatigue is a major source of stress for parents of twins. Finances also may be a problem due to the increased need for clothing and equipment.

Mothers-of-Twins Club, a national organization, provides emotional support and very practical advice for new parents. Ideally, contact will be made with a local group prior to the time of birth. If not, nurses who care for the mother following delivery should provide her with information. A local La Leche group may have a member experienced in the care of twins who may be particularly helpful to the breastfeeding mother. In smaller communities where no formal support structure may be available, nurses can help parents identify sources of support among their own family and friends and in the community.

The Feeding of Twins (and Infants in Multiple Births)

Twins can be fed, just as any other infant, in a manner appropriate to gestational age, any special needs of the baby, and the desires of the mother. Though some mothers overlook the possibility of breast feeding when multiple neonates are expected, breast feeding offers several advantages. Because more bottles and formula will be required, breast feeding is economical of both money and preparation time. Mother will need a well-balanced diet high in calories and protein, a high fluid intake, and opportunity for rest at intervals during the day as well as night. If these conditions are met, milk supply is usually adequate, because the stimulus of two nursing babies enhances milk supply.

Mothers of twins may want to feed each twin individually at first, but work toward nursing both babies at the same time, allowing more time for rest and other activities between feeding time. Several positions for joint feeding are possible. The babies may be held longitudinally facing the mother (not comfortable in the first days following cesarean delivery), or in a "football" hold with feet toward the mother's sides. Other alternatives are positioning the babies in parallel, both facing the same way, or holding one baby in each arm with their bodies crossed. At first, mothers of twins, like all mothers, will need help in experimenting with positions that are most comfortable for them and their babies.

When twins are bottle fed or alternately breast and bottle fed, the mother may have help at feeding time, from father or others. Parents need factual information about costs and time for various feeding methods.

Growth and Development of the Infant

Linda Upton

The nurse must incorporate many inter-related aspects of growth and development, while promoting the health of the infant within the family. The nurse provides information to parents and reinforces their self-confidence in caring for their infant. Table 5-5 contains a summary of infant growth and development.

Physical Competency

The development of physical competency in the infant covers many aspects of his or her life. It is this competency that many people use to judge the infant's health and, indirectly, the competence of the family as caregivers. Although competency is not the only measure of health, it is useful to explore this competency in some depth, since it does significantly affect the infant's total functioning.

Height and Weight

From birth through the first year of the infant's life, one of the first questions asked is "How much does the baby weigh?" The rate of growth of the infant is usually more important than the actual height and weight (see height and weight charts, Appendices Two and Three). Birth weight is generally doubled by 4 to 6 months and tripled by 1 year of age. Height increases about 50 per cent in the first year of life. No accurate predictions can be made about the infant's ultimate height and weight from the absolute or percentile height and weight figures of infancy.

Anticipatory Guidance: Height and Weight

Height and weight charts are most valuable when used at each periodic health assessment. The nurse should

Table 5-5. Summary of Infant Growth and Development

Physical Competency	Emotional-Social Competency	Intellectual Competency
1 to 2 Months		
Holds head in alignment when prone; Moro reflex to loud sound; follows objects; smiles	Gratification through sucking and basic needs being promptly met; smiles at people	Reflex activity; vowel sounds produced
2 to 4 Months		
Turns back to side; raises head and chest 45–90° off bed and supports weight on arms; reaches for objects; follows object through midline; drools; begins to localize sounds; prefers configuration of face	Social responsiveness; awareness of those who are not primary caregiver; smiles in response to familiar face	Reproduces behavior initially achieved by random activity; imitates behavior previously done. Visually studies objects; locates sounds; makes cooing sounds; does not look for objects removed from presence
4 to 6 Months		
Birth weight doubled; teeth eruption may begin; sits with stable head and back control; rolls from abdomen to back; picks up object with palmar grasp	Prefers primary caregiver; sucking needs decrease; laughs in pleasure	Some intentional actions; some sense of object permanence, looks on same path for vanished object; recognizes partially hidden objects; more systematic in imitative behavior; babbles
6 to 8 Months		
Turns back to stomach; sits alone; crawls; transfers objects hand to hand; turns to sound behind	Differentiated response to nonprimary caretakers; evidence of "stranger" or "separation" anxiety	Continued development as in 4–6 months
8 to 10 Months		
Creeps; pulls to stand; pincer grasp	Attachment process complete	Actions more goal directed; able to solve simple problems by using previously mastered responses. Actively searches for an object that disappears
10 to 12 Months		
Birth weight tripled; cruises; stands by self; may use spoon	Begins to explore and separate briefly from parent	Begins to imitate behavior done before but not seen self do. Understands words being said; may say 1–4 words. Intentionality is present.

share infant growth charts with the parents, taking into account the multiple factors such as parental size that can affect an infant's height and weight, while assisting the family in evaluating the appropriateness of their infant's growth. Sharing this information with the family can be a useful teaching tool in pointing out some of the factors affecting growth. The nurse can clearly identify the infant's pattern of growth as well as the actual height and weight. Reassurance that the infant is growing at an appropriate rate, if such is the case, is an important nursing intervention. Further assessment is indicated if there has been significant change in the usual weight percentile or a slower consistent change upward or downward. An infant who is consistently above the 97th percentile in weight or below the 3rd percentile needs to be assessed more fully.

Body Proportions

The body proportions of the infant are also changing. The head is most developed at birth. The trunk and legs are not as fully developed as the head but begin to slowly catch up with head growth during the first year. By 6 months of age the thorax circumference may be larger than the head circumference, although there is great variability in this ratio.

Table 5-5 *(continued)*

Nutrition	Play	Safety
1 to 2 Months		
Breastfed or fortified formula	Variety of positions. Caretaker should hold and talk to infant; large; brightly colored objects	Car carrier; proper use of infant seat
2 to 4 Months		
As for 1–2 months	Talk to and hold. Musical toys; rattle, mobile. Variety of objects of different color, size and texture; mirror, crib toys, variety of settings	Do not leave unattended on couch, bed, etc. Remove any small objects that infant could choke on
4 to 6 Months		
Introduction of solids; initial store of iron depleted	Talk to and hold. Provide open space to move and objects to grasp	Keep environment free of safety hazards; check toys for sharp edges and small pieces that might break
6 to 8 Months		
	Provide place to explore. Stack toys, blocks; nursery rhymes	Check infant's expanding environment for hazards
8 to 10 Months		
As for 6–8 months	Games: hide and seek, peek-a-boo, pat-a-cake, looking at pictures in a book	Keep: electrical outlets plugged, cords out of reach, stairs blocked, coffee and end tables cleared of hazards. Do not leave alone in bathtub Keep poisons out of reach and locked Continue use of safety seat in car
10 to 12 Months		
More solids than liquids; increasing use of cup; begin to wean	Increase space; read to infant. Name and point to body parts.Water; sand play; ball	As for 8–10 months

Head Circumference

The brain grows faster than do other tissues and organs during infancy. Rapid brain growth results from an increase in both cell number and cell size. Because the cranial bones have not completely fused, fontanels and cranial sutures are still open. This allows for growth of the skull as the brain expands. In fact, the growth rate of the skull is mainly determined by the growth rate of the brain. Growth of the skull, as determined by increasing head circumference, is a much more accurate index of brain growth than is the presence or size of fontanels (Silver et al, 1983). The anterior fontanel normally closes by 12 to 18 months and the posterior fontanel by 2 months. The size and shape of the fontanel may be affected by conditions other than the rate of brain growth, such as hydration and intracranial pressure.

The head circumference is an important measurement in the physical assessment of the infant. The circumference of the head increases from an average of 35 cm at birth to 47 cm at 1 year (Silver et al, 1983). The use of head circumference charts is valuable in determining the absolute growth as well as the rate of growth of the skull. Deviations from the normal pattern need to be assessed in detail by a physician.

Anticipatory Guidance: Head Circumference

While measuring the head circumference the nurse has an opportunity to point out to the family why this measurement is being taken. This is also a good time to reiterate the information that the fontanel, which may be referred to as the "soft spot," is covered by a very strong membrane, so there is no substance to the common belief that the brain can be damaged by touching the area. Since the young infant's skull is pliable, the skull may be flattened if the infant spends a great deal of time in the same position. This flattening does not cause brain damage and usually is gradually corrected as the skull continues to grow and the infant spends more and more time with the head erect. If the infant's head has become flattened and the hair rubbed off in one spot, the nurse should explore in more detail the infant's daily routine: these signs may be a clue that the infant is spending a majority of the day in the same position. This, in turn, *might* suggest a lack of parental attention to the infant. The nurse should offer suggestions about positioning the infant on the abdomen, on the side, and in a sitting position. Placement of colorful stimuli in a variety of locations can stimulate infants to turn themselves at the age of 5 to 6 months.

Mouth

Mature sucking, which occurs at about 16 weeks of age, is an acquired function of the orofacial muscles with the tongue moving back and forth. The oral cavity is growing larger so that the tongue no longer fills the mouth. The tongue is growing differentially at the tip. These two features allow the tongue more mobility. The longer tongue can be protruded to receive and pass food between the gum pads and erupting teeth, allowing mastication (Pipes, 1985). Around 24 to 28 weeks the up-and-down movement of the jaw occurs.

Teeth

Another landmark that nurses and families readily observe as an index of physical competency is the eruption of teeth. The eruption of the first tooth often occurs about 4 to 6 months of age but may not occur until the end of the first year. For the usual pattern of tooth eruption see Chapter 19, where fluoride needs of the infant are also discussed.

Anticipatory Guidance: Teeth. Parents have many questions about teething. The nurse should discuss the general pattern of tooth eruption with the family when the infant is about 3 months old. Drooling occurs at about this time. Saliva is now being produced, but the infant has not yet learned to swallow it. This drooling at 3 months is not directly associated with teething. There are many myths about the supposed responses of the body to eruption of the teeth (e.g., fever, diarrhea, vomiting). However, a cause-and-effect relationship between teething and these symptoms has not been established. Since teething usually extends over quite a long period and infants have frequent minor illnesses, teething has perhaps been unjustly blamed for at least some of these. Parents need to be encouraged to consult with health care providers about any signs and symptoms that would cause concern if the infant were not teething. "The greatest danger of inaccurately ascribing the cause of such signs and symptoms to teething is that parents will delay medical treatment for a serious illness" (Bradshaw, 1981).

Teething does cause discomfort to many infants. They often are irritable, rub at their gums, and display a desire to bite. Their gums are often red and swollen. Chewing on hard, clean objects such as teething rings, hard rubber toys, or Zwieback toast may bring some relief. Preparations containing alcohol should be avoided. Nurses and parents need to be aware that some teething lotions contain a high percentage of alcohol. Alcohol-containing products are potentially toxic to infants and could have systemic effects (American Academy of Pediatrics, 1984).

Bradshaw (1981) provided the following guidelines for nurses who are working with parents of teething infants:

- Do not belittle the parents for their beliefs and concerns about teething. Attacking firm ethnic, cultural, or socioeconomic group beliefs about teething runs the risk of alienating the family.
- Do not discourage home remedies for teething unless they are definitely harmful.
- Acetaminophen (10 to 15 mg/kg every 3 to 4 hours) can help relieve teething pain that does not respond to nonpharmacologic comfort measures.
- The practice of placing an aspirin tablet against the painful area should be avoided. An aspirin tablet can erode gingival tissues and can be easily aspirated.

Nurses can also provide guidance to prevent a tragic and needlessly occurring dental condition, *"milk bottle syndrome."* Milk bottle syndrome occurs in older infants and toddlers who fall asleep with a bottle of milk or other sweetened fluids in their mouth. Treatment consists of prevention. Children older than 10 to 12 months of age should not be permitted to sleep with a bottle in their mouth. Anticipatory guidance given to parents to avoid this practice when the infant is young is a nursing responsibility. If the older infant is accustomed to going to sleep with a bottle, plain water may be substituted for the milk or sugar-containing liquids. Eventually, if untreated, the rampant decay of milk bottle syndrome may cause alterations in the permanent teeth as well as great discomfort to the infant. It should be noted that allowing a child to fall asleep with a bottle in the mouth, if the infant is unattended (as in the practice of bottle propping), could result in aspiration of formula and resultant pneumonia or even asphyxia. See Chapter 19 for further discussion of this syndrome. Additional guidance of parents will focus on care of their baby's teeth. Following each bottle or meal with water will help to prevent prolonged contact of food sugars with teeth. The baby's teeth can also be lightly rubbed with a gauze-wrapped finger.

Motor Development

The rapid development of neuromuscular control is an extremely important aspect of physical competency. The maturation of the central nervous system provides progressively better control and integration of muscular movements throughout the first year of life.

The coordination of nerves and muscle which results in body movements is referred to as motor development. Much of the physical development in infancy centers around motor development. The infant's motor development is inextricably inter-related with cognitive and emotional-social competencies. The infant learns about and interacts with the world through increasing motor abilities. The two major motor tasks that the infant must learn are upright postural control or locomotion, and fine motor manipulation, including prehension or grasping. Even though the age when each motor skill is attained may differ among babies, all will follow the same sequence.

Upright Postural Control or Locomotion

The sequence of motor skills involved in the achievement of upright postural control or locomotion is a visible example of the principle that states that growth and development proceed in a cephalocaudal direction. (See Figure 3-6, page 114.)

Head Control. One of the major motor tasks of early infancy is head control, which is necessary for the infant to sit and eventually to walk. Head control develops in the following order:

Birth	Turns head when prone
↓	Holds head up momentarily while prone
	Holds head 45 to 95 degrees while prone
	Holds head in fairly good control in a variety of positions
	No head lag when pulled to sit
4 months	Sits with stable head and back control

Sitting. Another important skill is sitting alone. Infants must achieve head control before they can sit

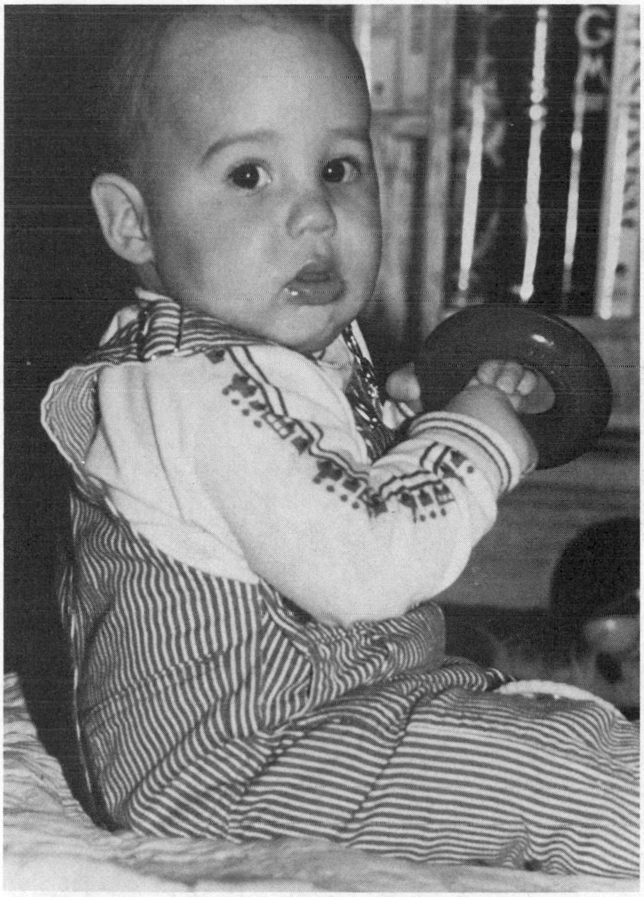

At 7 to 8 months, the infant can sit alone without support. To do so, the infant must be able to sit with the back straight.

alone. The ability to sit alone develops gradually from 4 to 8 months:

4 months	Sits with support
6 months	Sits alone momentarily with own hand for support
7 months	Sits alone briefly
8 months	Sits without support

Locomotion. During this same period infants are learning a variety of locomotion skills that will prepare them for walking. The ability to roll over develops from approximately 2 to 6 or 7 months:

2 months	Rolls from side to back
4 months	Rolls from back to side
5 to 6 months	Rolls from abdomen to side
6 to 7 months	Rolls from back to stomach

Many infants use this rolling ability to get from one place to another, and may be able to move about much farther than the parent or nurse expects.

Another means of locomotion is hitching or scooting (moving along while sitting up), which appears at about 6 months. Crawling (wriggling on abdomen,

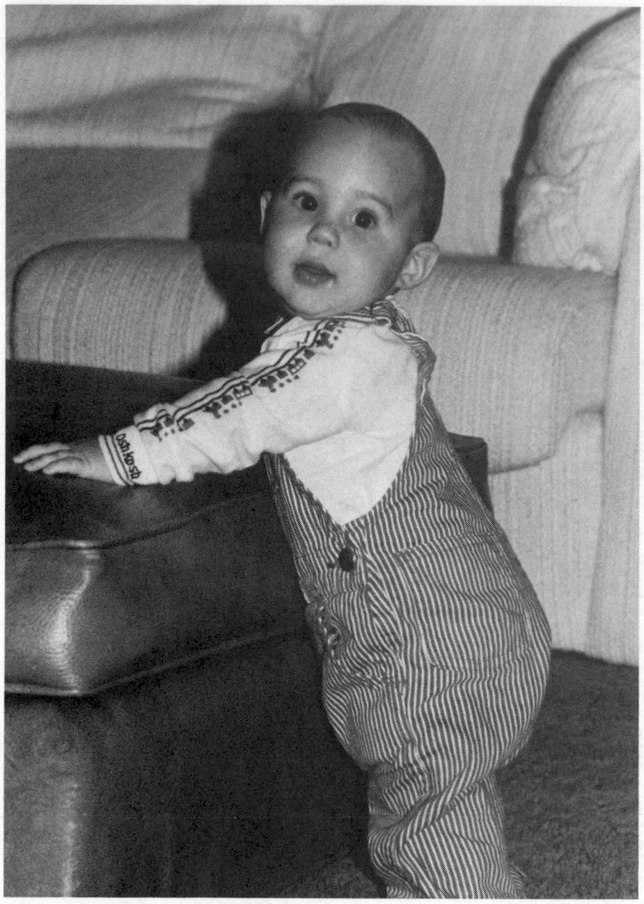

The infant of 7 to 8 months can stand for short periods with support.

pulling with arms) usually appears by 8 months. Creeping (on hands, knees, with trunk off floor) usually appears by 9 months. Some infants may use hitching or crawling as a substitute for creeping and progress to walking without creeping. At about 10 months of age infants begin to pull themselves to a standing position and soon stand with assistance. They then begin to cruise around furniture (walking sideways while holding onto supporting object).

Once the infant is able to stand alone it is usually not long (about 1 month) before he or she attempts to walk unassisted. The average infant can walk alone well by 15 months. Throughout the first year of life the infant has mastered many incremental steps in learning to walk.

Fine Motor Manipulation

The infant is also rapidly developing fine motor skills that greatly assist in manipulating his or her environment. Fine motor development is complex and involves eye-to-hand coordination. Fine motor skills, as with other aspects of physical competency, seem to occur in an orderly sequence.

Prehension or Grasping. One of the fine motor skills to be developed is that of grasping an object. The sequence of skills involved in the development of the ability to grasp provides an example of the general to specific and proximal to distal principles of growth and development.

The neonate has a grasp reflex that gradually gives way to an intentional grasp. Before this skill has developed it may appear to the parents that the infant actually has lost a skill he or she once had. Alerting parents to the normal sequence of this developmental task can be reassuring to them.

The sequence of events in development of the infant's ability to grasp is as follows:

3 months	Object placed in hands retained briefly
4 months	Reaches for objects and picks them up with raking action of fingers
6 months	Picks up objects deftly with palmar grasp
6 to 7 months	Transfers objects from hand to hand Bangs objects together
8 to 9 months	Pincer grasp developed

The infant develops the visual skill to follow objects past midline by 2 or 3 months of age. He or she is usually able to follow objects through 180 degrees by the age of 3 to 4 months. This skill, in combination with the neonate's increasing skill of grasping objects, gives the infant ever-increasing ability to manipulate the environment.

Anticipatory Guidance: Motor Development

From the preceding discussion it can be seen that much information about motor development can be shared with parents. They need to know the sequence of development and the fact that the exact time of appearance of each skill depends on the individual. Nurses can help parents explore ways to promote the motor development of their infant.

Specific suggestions can be made as to how to promote head control. The infant can be periodically placed in a prone position; he or she will be able to lift the head more easily in this position. This assists development of the necessary muscles for head control.

Parents should be alerted early to the developmental benefits of laying the infant on the abdomen. An infant who has few opportunities to be prone will often prefer the supine position and will cry when put on the abdomen. The infant also needs to have an opportunity to be placed in a sitting position and to practice holding the head erect. Once the head is fairly steady in the sitting position, pulling the infant to a

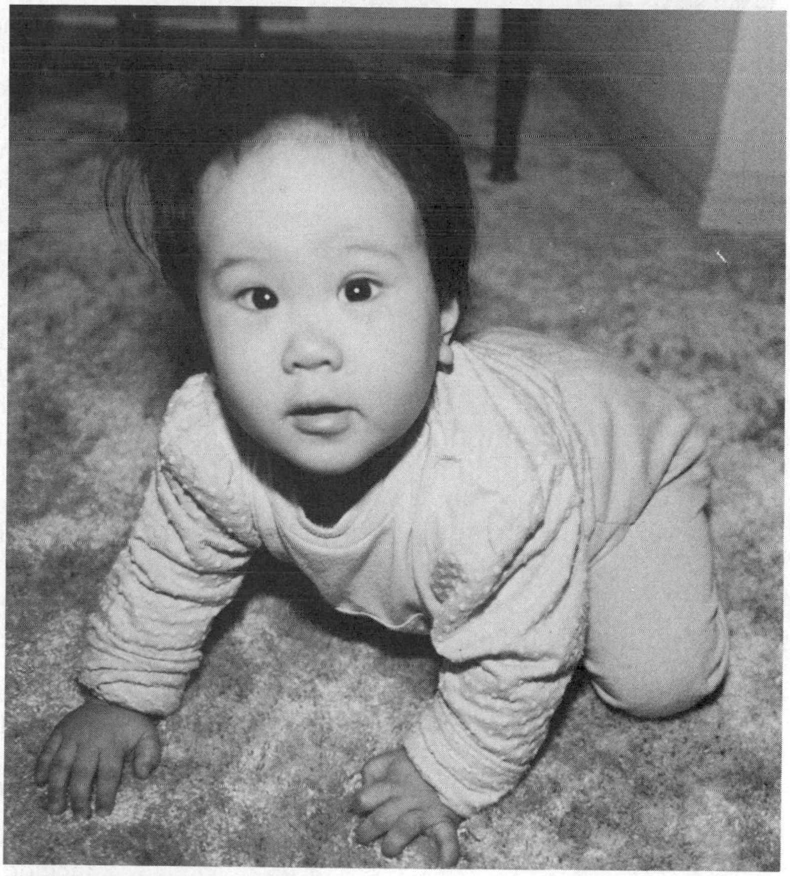

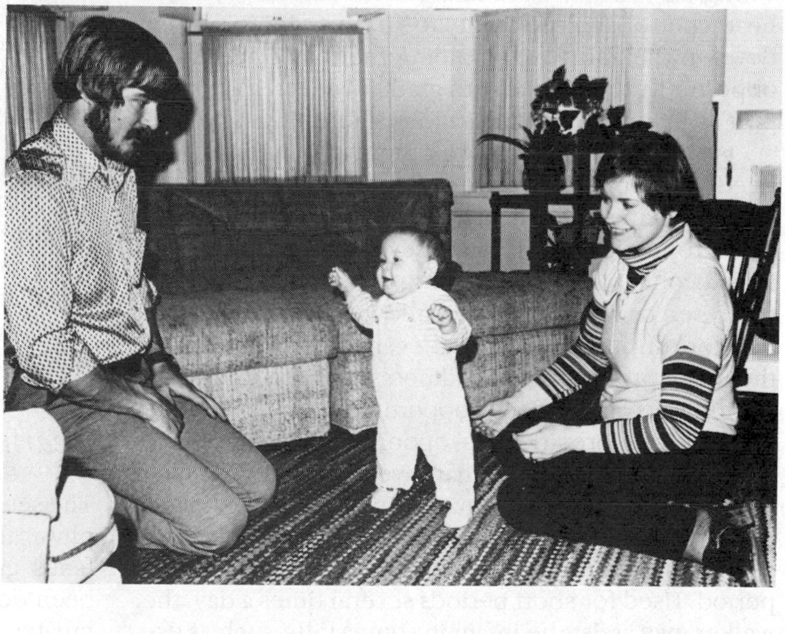

Creeping is one of the incremental steps that the infant masters in learning to walk. Infant and parents alike delight in those first steps taken alone.

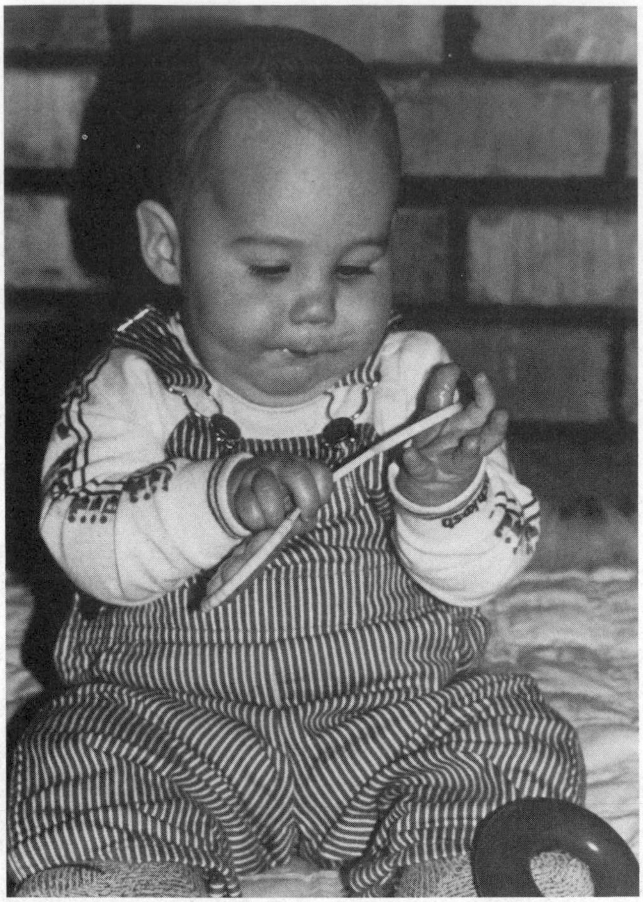

The infant of 6 to 7 months can transfer objects between hands.

sitting position will promote further development of head control and the ability to sit. In order to further develop the ability to sit alone, the infant needs the opportunity to practice with gradually decreasing support as he or she becomes more stable.

As locomotion is developing, the infant again needs the opportunity to try out and practice these skills. Placing the infant on the floor and allowing space to move will promote development of the various locomotion skills. Keeping the infant confined to a playpen or walker does not allow sufficient opportunity for turning, rolling, and eventually creeping. As the infant progresses in readiness to pull to a standing position he or she needs opportunities to do so. The playpen can provide this opportunity, as can safe, sturdy pieces of furniture that have no sharp edges. The infant needs the opportunity to practice the skills of cruising around items and eventually walking. There is some controversy over the use of "walkers" in this period. Used for short periods several times a day, the walker may assist the infant in some skills, such as use of leg muscles and balance. However, walkers can limit the developing locomotion and exploratory skills of infants if used in place of opportunities for crawling, cruising, and walking on their own. In addition, the use of walkers is accompanied by hazards such as tipping over, rolling down stairs, and so forth.

There are a variety of ways that parents can promote their infant's fine motor development. In order to develop the infant's grasp, attractive objects can be presented within reach by 3 to 4 months. Chapter 21 describes age-appropriate objects for infant stimulation. These objects also encourage the infant to develop the skill of banging objects together and transferring them from hand to hand. To encourage the pincer grasp as the infant approaches 9 months, smaller objects need to be provided, but with supervision to prevent aspiration. Giving the infant dry cereals for self-feeding can be one mechanism to promote the pincer grasp.

At the same time, the infant can be given activities to stimulate development of the ability to follow objects and further increase eye-hand coordination. The placement of mobiles and brightly colored objects within the infant's range of vision is useful. Many of the same objects that promote grasp also can be used to promote hand-eye coordination. Placing the infant in a variety of settings and positions stimulates him or her to look at and reach for new objects. Expensive toys are not necessary; items commonly found in the home can be used, such as colorful plastic cups.

Nursing Implications: Motor Development

Nurses who work with children in health care settings include consideration of all aspects of development in their plan of care. Safety factors in relation to the child's motor development will influence decisions regarding positioning and the use of restraints. The nurse who is aware of the importance of motor development will be more likely to provide for supervised removal of restraints whenever possible and allow for motor movement of extremities. If locomotion will be restricted for extended periods due to treatment devices such as casts and braces, the nurse can encourage exploration of the environment by placing the child in a wagon or cart and by moving the crib to other areas such as the playroom.

Hearing and Vision

The senses of hearing and vision are another aspect of physical competency that significantly affect the infant's growth and development. Much research has been done recently that shows that the newborn has greater development in these areas than was once thought (Klaus and Kennell, 1982; Luddington-Hoe, 1983). The neonate's auditory system is functioning and is developed well enough to detect differences in sound. If both visual and auditory cues are presented, there are no age-related differences in localization of sound. If only auditory cues are presented, the ability to localize sound develops gradually over the first 1½ years of life (Morrongiello and Rocca, 1987). Chapters 15 and 51 discuss assessment of vision and hearing in the infant.

Anticipatory Guidance: Vision and Hearing

The nurse can point out to parents the infant's visual and auditory capabilities and fascination with human faces. The infant needs to be exposed to a variety of visual and auditory stimuli. The importance of a variety of colors and shapes in the neonate's environment can be stressed. The young infant responds well to black-white contrast (Luddington-Hoe, 1983).

The human voice is an important and readily available sound stimulus. Neonates prefer the sound of their mother's voice over that of other individuals (Roberts, 1987). The infant also responds well to musical toys and toys that make different sounds. Stimulation needs of individual infants will vary. Infants do need periods of rest during which they are not bombarded by visual and auditory stimuli.

Sleep

Sleep as an aspect of the infant's developing physical competency is of special interest to parents. The developmental changes in sleep in the first year involve length and timing of the sleep periods, as well as the type of sleep. Individual differences in sleep patterns for infants are significant. All too often a long sleep pattern becomes equated with "a good infant." Chapter 20 describes the normal variations and maturational changes in sleep patterns during infancy.

Anticipatory Guidance: Sleep

Parents can be assisted to understand sleep patterns and the individual needs of their infant. The nurse can point out that sleep patterns (longer periods of sleep and diurnal cycles) are signs of maturation in the infant. Parents need not be left with only the general impression that infants sleep a lot.

Sleeping arrangements for the infant vary from family to family. The nurse should ascertain common cultural practices in order to assist parents realistically. In some Asian cultures, for example, children typically sleep with parents.

Elimination

Another area of physical competency that becomes somewhat regular in the first year is the timing of elimination. Both breast-fed and bottle-fed infants progress to a pattern of fewer number of stools per day after the first month or two. Stools of breast-fed infants remain less formed than those of bottle-fed infants. Stool color varies, especially with the introduction of solid food. The timing and number of stools per day tends to be stable by 6 months of age, although a large number of infants remain unpredictable. The kidneys are continuing to mature. Rectal and urethral sphincters are not mature enough for control in most infants until after a year of age.

Anticipatory Guidance: Elimination

Parents often need help to understand that even though the infant's voiding and stooling patterns have become more regular, he or she is not developmentally ready to achieve self-control. The infant must be cognitively aware of elimination before true readiness exists. Also, the young infant often strains during a bowel movement, and some parents assume that this straining means the infant is constipated. This straining may be due to the immaturity of muscle coordination rather than to constipation. If the bowel movement pattern is regular for that infant (may range from several per day to one every 4 to 5 days) and the stool is not hard, no intervention is necessary.

Nutritional Requirements

There have been many opinions expressed about the nutritional needs of the infant. As research in this area continues, recommendations and opinions will change; however, some basic facts about nutritional requirements remain fairly consistent. Infant nutritional requirements are based on what is considered necessary to support life, to provide for growth, and to maintain health. Components to meet the nutritional needs of the infant include water, nutrients (protein, fat, carbohydrates), vitamins, and minerals. Since the first year of life is a period of rapid change, the nutritional requirements of this period also change.

Water

The percentage of body weight provided by water is greater in the newborn infant than after a year of age, going from 75 per cent at birth to 60 per cent at 1 year (Pipes, 1985). Infants have a relatively greater need for

Table 5-6. Summary of Infant's Nutritional Requirements

	Daily Requirements	
Component	1–6 Months	6–12 Months
Water	100 mg/kg for the first 10 kg; 50 mg/kg for the next 10 kg; then 20 mg/kg thereafter	
Calories	100–120 Kcal/kg	100–120 Kcal/kg
Protein	2.2 gm/kg	2 gm/kg
Fat	30–50% of total calories	30–50% of total calories
Carbohydrate	50–100 gm	50–100 gm
Vitamins		
A	1400 IU	2000 IU
D	400IU	400IU
E	4 IU	5 IU
C	35 mg	35 mg
Thiamine	0.5 mg/1000 Kcal	0.5 mg/1000 Kcal
Riboflavin	0.6 mg/1000 Kcal	0.6 mg/1000 Kcal
Niacin	8 mg/1000 Kcal	8 mg/1000 Kcal
Pyridoxine	0.3 mg	0.3 mg
Folate	50 μg	50 μg
Minerals		
Calcium	360 mg	540 mg
Phosphorus	240 mg	400 mg
Magnesium	60 mg	70 mg
Iron	10 mg (1.5 mg/kg)	15 mg
Iodine	35 mcg	45 mcg
Zinc	3 mg	5 mg
Fluoride	0.25 mg	0.25 mg

water than do children and adults, and they are therefore more vulnerable to water imbalance. Water lost by evaporation in infancy is 60 per cent of that needed to maintain homeostasis compared with 40 to 50 per cent in the adult (Pipes, 1985). The young infant has functionally immature kidneys. The faster rate of the infant's metabolism is a factor in the need for relatively more fluid than is needed by the adult. Also, young infants are unable to let adults know when they are thirsty. The usual diets of most infants meet this basic water requirement.

The sources of water are fluids (mostly milk) and food. Most strained foods are 75 to 85 per cent water. Difficulties may occur in meeting the water requirements if formulas are improperly prepared, if infants ingest a limited amount of milk (especially with illness), if fever exists during hot weather, or if diarrhea and vomiting are present. Dehydration results much more rapidly from these difficulties in the infant because of the factors previously outlined.

Nutrients

Infants must take in adequate nutrients to promote growth as well as to provide fuel. The infant's body size and composition, physical activity and rate of growth all affect the amount of energy expended to maintain life. The energy requirement for infants is much greater per unit of body weight than for adults. There is a gradual decrease in energy requirements per unit of body weight throughout the first year of life from 120 kcal/kg/day at birth to 100 kcal/kg/day at 1 year. There are several reasons for these changes in energy requirements of infants. The higher basal metabolic demand in early infancy is thought to be due to a larger loss of heat because of relatively greater body surface and a larger proportion of metabolic tissue (Pipes, 1985). Decreasing rate of growth throughout the first year results in decreasing energy requirements per unit of body weight.

For the infant, milk (human or fortified formula) meets most of or all of the nutritional needs of the infant through most of the first year of life if consumed in appropriate quantities (Table 5-6). Especially in the first 6 months of life there have been no data to support the theory that solid foods are needed in order to meet the nutritional needs of the infant. Breast milk provides necessary nutrients, except possibly for vitamin D, iron, and fluoride, although there is no consensus on this point. Formula-fed infants may need no supplements, depending on the formula used. Labels on formula need to be checked carefully for information on its nutritional adequacy. The American Academy of Pediatrics (AAP, Committee on Nutrition, 1983) does not recommend vitamin D supplements for breast-fed infants, unless the mother's vitamin D nutrition is inadequate. A water-soluble form of vitamin D has been found in human milk.

Normal infants of well-nourished mothers are born with adequate stores of iron to meet their needs for 4 to 6 months. Small and preterm infants' neonatal iron stores meet their needs for 2 months. In the past, iron supplements have been recommended for the breast-fed infant and are still recommended by some professionals (Foman, 1977). It has been discovered that the trace quantities of iron found in breast milk are extremely absorbable, so that iron supplementation is not believed to be needed by term infants until their weight triples (Chow et al, 1984). Iron-fortified formulas are recommended for the bottle-fed infant in the first year of life.

Intellectual Competency

Intelligence

Another major competency area that undergoes rapid change in the infancy period is intellectual development. There are a number of factors in intellectual development that are essential for the nurse to be aware of while assessing the growth, development, and total health status of the infant.

The Swiss psychologist Piaget has made significant contributions to what is known about the intellectual development of the infant. His theory is discussed in Chapter 3. The infant is in the sensorimotor stage as described by Piaget. The infant progresses from responding primarily through reflex activity to beginning to organize sensorimotor activities in relation to the environment.

The concept of the permanent object is an important achievement of the sensorimotor period. The permanent object has a reality of its own and continues to exist even though the infant cannot see, hear, feel, taste, or smell it. Within the sensorimotor stage Piaget outlines six substages in the development of the concept of object permanency. Four of these substages are usually developed in the first year of life. The first substage (0 to 1 month) is a period basically consisting of reflex activity that allows the infant to adapt and survive. Learning occurs in this substage but is confined to the sphere of reflexes. The section of this chapter on The Normal Neonate contains further information about neonatal reflex activity. The second substage (1 to 4 months) is characterized as that of primary circular reactions. At this time the infant makes an active effort to reproduce a behavior that is initially achieved by random activity. The behavior must have some value to the baby, such as the pleasure produced by placing his or her thumb in the mouth. Another example is when the infant accidentally shakes a toy, producing an interesting sound; the infant can then be observed actively trying to reproduce both of these behaviors. Infants study objects, including faces, during this period. They begin to develop hand-eye coordination. As activities of looking and grasping begin to extend infants' environment, they are attracted to objects that are moderately novel. Piaget believes the curiosity of infants at this stage is stimulated by objects that are not too familiar to them. However, an object that is completely foreign to infants does not seem to attract them as readily, perhaps because they cannot relate it to anything with which they are familiar, and therefore it has little meaning to them. Piaget called this phenomenon the principle of moderate novelty. Infants (1 to 4 months) have not developed a true concept of object permanence. When an object is removed from their presence they do not look for it; it is as if the object no longer exists. This can be seen clearly when the infant is being held and is attracted to the eyeglasses of the adult. If the adult removes the glasses and places them behind a book on the table the infant does not look for the glasses but moves on to some other activity.

The third substage (4 to 8 months) is described as that of secondary circular reactions. Infants are now beginning to show evidence of intentional action. Their horizons are expanding and their reactions involve events in the external environment. Infants are becoming interested in the results of their actions. They have perceived an interesting external result from an accidental movement and, connecting the results to their actions, they want to repeat the result. One can note this particular sequence as the infant accidentally knocks over a tower of blocks, expresses pleasure, and repeats the action over and over. Given the opportunity, infants learn to prolong an interesting activity. They have become interested in their external environment and are beginning to have an impact on it. They are gradually differentiating between means and ends. Secondary circular reactions do have limitations in that they are not fully intentional; with them, infants do not attempt to invent new behaviors. For instance, in the block episode the infant does not build the tower initially for the purpose of knocking it over.

During this substage (4 to 8 months) the infant makes progress in the formation of the concept of object permanence, but it is far from the mature concept. Infants indicate by various behaviors that they have some sense of object permanence. They begin to look for objects that have disappeared, but only under special conditions. The searching behavior must lead to early discovery of the lost object, or it ceases. Infants do not pause and renew the search for the object. This behavior seems to relate to the infant's own actions rather than to the independent individual existence of the object. Another indication of some progress in the concept of object permanence is the infant's ability to recognize and seek objects that are partially hidden. A favorite toy partially covered by a blanket will now attract the infant's attention.

Substage four (8 to 12 months) is that of coordination of secondary circular reactions and their application to new situations. Infants' actions now are becoming increasingly goal directed. They can solve simple problems by using responses they have previously mastered. If an obstacle arises that prevents the infant from attaining his or her goals, new means for removing the obstacle must be developed in order to achieve the desired end. The new means developed by the infant have limitations. The infant can generalize patterns of previously learned behavior, modify them slightly, and coordinate two secondary behaviors to achieve the desired ends by removing the obstacle. An example of this kind of activity is seen when an older sibling grabs a toy away from the infant. The infant may initially just try to grab randomly for the object. Soon, however, he or she will first push aside the sibling's hand and then grab the toy. The infant has not invented new means (behaviors) but has coordinated two previously learned behaviors: those of pushing aside a hand and grasping a toy. The infant has removed an obstacle (the hand) to achieve the end (holding the toy).

Infants also make great strides in their developing concept of object permanence. Their improved manipulatory skills contribute significantly because they can more readily explore the objects. As they explore and move the object, infants become aware that it remains the same even though their visual perception of it changes. They thus begin to recognize the permanence and substance of the object. At this point infants will actively search for an object that vanishes. Hiding the eyeglasses behind a book on the table no longer works. There are some limitations to infants' concept of object permanence at this stage. If the movement of the object becomes too complicated (number or complexity of movements), the object again takes on subjective qualities and becomes related to the infants' past actions. They thus search for the object in the place where they succeeded in discovering the object previously, rather than looking for it where they last saw it. This concept can be illustrated by hiding a cracker in the presence of the infant who is at this stage of development. If a cracker is hidden under a napkin while he or she watches, the infant will search for the cracker, push aside the napkin, and retrieve the cracker. Then, while the infant still watches, the cracker is placed under the napkin, taken out and shown to the infant, and then placed under a bowl. The infant will look for the cracker under the napkin.

A number of types of learning are a part of the infant's developing intellectual competency. Imitative learning seems to be one of the most important types during infancy. A number of investigators, including Piaget and Uzgiris, have explored the steps in the development of imitative behavior and have arrived at similar sequences. By about 3 months old infants imitate certain behaviors, but only those that they have previously spontaneously performed themselves (such as cooing). Around 4 to 8 months infants become more systematic in their imitative behavior. They are more interested in the action of others. As they develop more behaviors of their own they are capable of imitating more behaviors. Infants still imitate only those acts they have previously been able to watch themselves do (such as clapping their hands). At times it appears as if they will imitate only enough of the behavior to get the other person to repeat the behavior.

By 10 to 12 months infants have made progress in their use of imitation. They begin to imitate actions that they have done before but never watched themselves do (such as forming facial expressions). They can make a connection between what they see and the corresponding movement of their own body parts. They may begin to imitate new actions. There are limitations in the accuracy of the infants' imitations and their ability to imitate new actions.

During the last 20 years, there has been a proliferation of research evidence regarding the intellectual competencies of infants. Whereas little was known previously, infant development, including cognitive development, is now a field that supports several specialty journals, textbooks, whole college courses, and other courses of study. For example, very young babies are capable of discriminating between tastes and smells as well as between visual sensory stimuli (Lewis, 1979; Meltzoff, 1985). Babies are able to recognize facial expressions signifying emotions (Nelson, 1987), tend to prefer complex visual stimuli over simple ones, can differentiate between shapes and colors, prefer female voices to male, and have a beginning ability to categorize (Friedrich, 1983). Many of the sensory and cognitive capabilities of the infant have been demonstrated to exist in the fetus (Bernhardt, 1987).

Anticipatory Guidance: Intelligence

Many of the activities that stimulate development of the infant's physical competency also promote the intellectual competency, since this is the sensorimotor period. The infant of 1 to 4 months needs a variety of objects to study. Studies have shown that a positive relationship exists between measures of cognitive

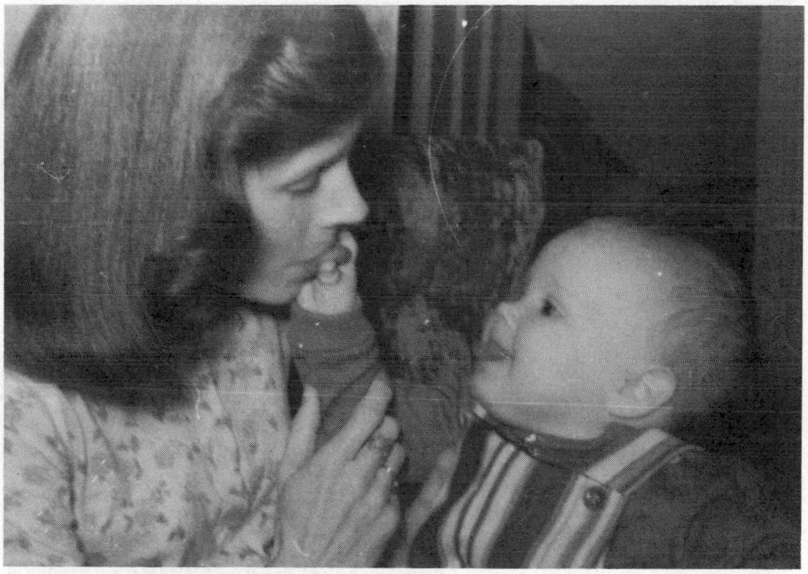

By 10 months, the infant can imitate facial expressions. (Photograph by David Trainor.)

competence and the availability of objects for exploration in the home (Parke, 1978; Power and Chapieski, 1986; Wachs and Gruen, 1982). Parents need to know that they should introduce new objects into the environment to stimulate this curiosity. Infants need objects to manipulate in order to associate their random activities with specific results. Infants need the opportunity to explore objects fully. These activities will promote development of their sense of object permanence. Infants also need the opportunity to explore and get to know their environment.

Between 4 and 8 months of age, parents can initiate games with infants to help them develop the concept of object permanence. Hiding and recovering objects, dropping and recovering objects, and hide-and-seek with people are all appropriate activities.

As infants progress to the next stage at 8 to 12 months, their actions become more goal-directed. Stacking, nesting, and ring games are interesting and challenging to infants. This allows them to perceive connections between events, such as placing a certain block on top of another and building a tower. Toys or household items that can be placed in containers and taken out easily also contribute to infants' goal-directed abilities and development of the concept of object permanence. By this time, because infants do imitate new actions, demonstration by the parents may assist them to learn activities. Infants enjoy imitating facial expressions and body movements. Throughout discussion with parents the nurse should include the rationale for the suggested activities.

In recent years a controversy has arisen regarding programs to develop infant intellectual competencies early. Programs and centers have been developed to teach reading, math skills, music appreciation, and other topics to babies and very young children. Many parents see these programs as a desirable way to produce an exceptional child. Opponents of these programs argue that overstimulation occurring too early might have an adverse effect on long-term developmental abilities. Parents need guidance to help them to see the drawbacks as well as the benefits of any program. They need to consider whether the program under consideration allows the baby time and opportunity to experience and explore the environment spontaneously, as well as rest periods from intense stimulation. Additionally, even though many skills may be gained through reinforcement, the baby is not truly aware of the meaning of what has been acquired. Early infant training programs have not been in existence long enough to establish through research whether the long-term outcomes are beneficial or detrimental.

Questions are often raised about the feasibility of measuring infant intelligence. Intelligence is a difficult concept to define and measure, especially for infants. Since infants do not have command of language, they cannot be tested for thinking or reasoning. Their range of behaviors is limited. In addition, their motivation cannot be controlled. There is almost no predictability between an infant's score on various infant intelligence tests and scores on intelligence tests given later. This may be because tests for infants measure behavior and tests for older children can measure additional cognitive processes. Tests such as the Bayley Scale of Infant Development (1965) are useful in finding deviations from normal development.

Language

Language development is an important aspect of intellectual competency. It has been repeatedly noted that children throughout the world go through the same

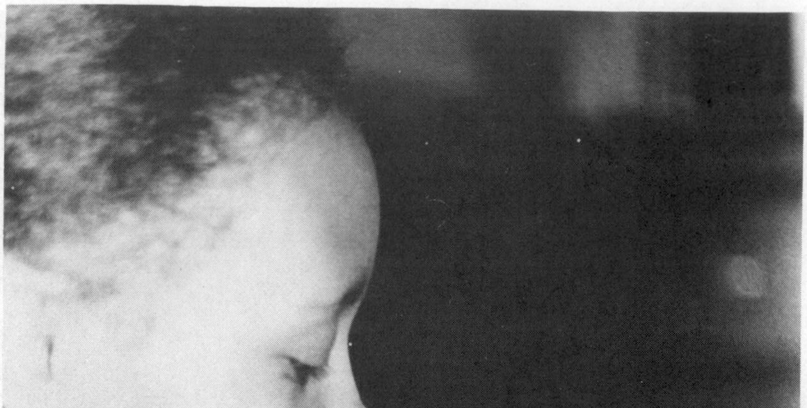

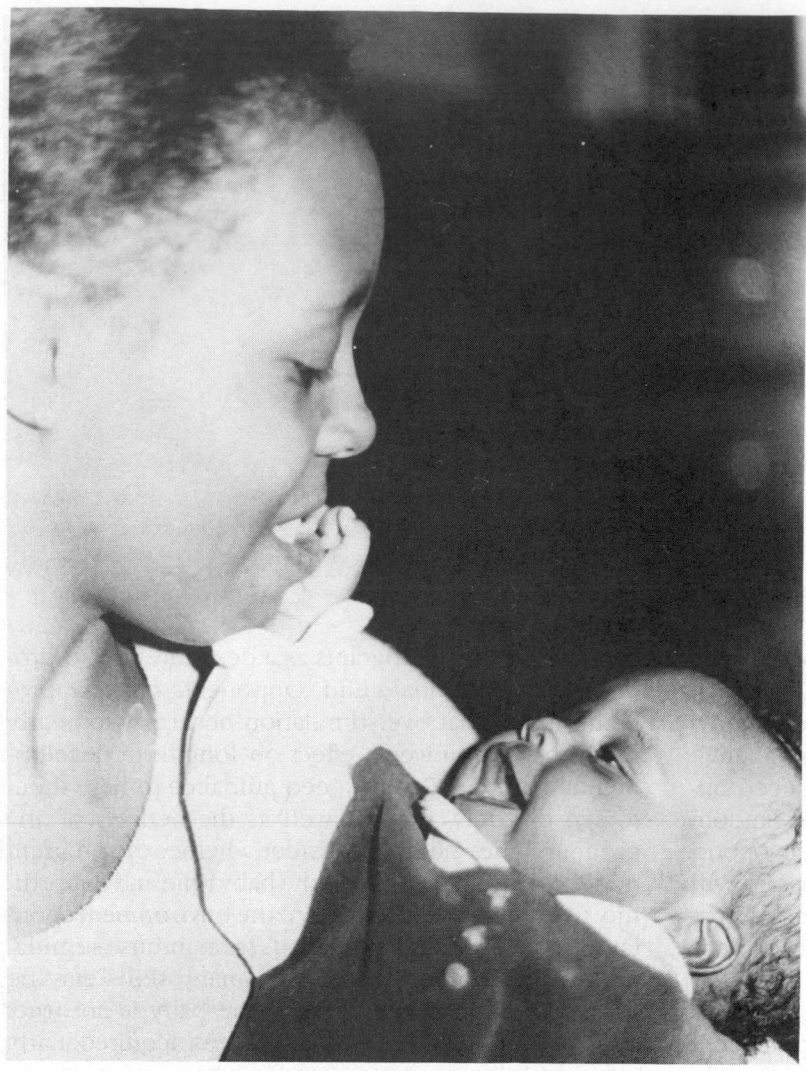

Talking to the infant encourages vocalizations that lead to the first words.

basic stages of language acquisition. Language development is affected by intellectual development, maturation of the central nervous system, development of the organs of speech, and exposure to human language. Receptive language (what a person understands) and expressive language (what a person says) are both important to consider. The infant appears to be especially attuned to the types of sound needed for language development. It can be observed that by about 10 months of age infants understand some of the words being said to them, such as "bye-bye" and "peek-a-boo."

Vocalization in infancy follows a definite sequence. During the first 2 months most of the sounds produced are vowels and are made mostly in the front part of the mouth (Smart and Smart, 1978). Crying is a means of communication during this period. Cooing sounds are noted at about 2 to 3 months; they consist of a variety of simple vowel-like sounds. These sounds are usually produced when the infant is happy and is responding to an adult's social smiling and vocalizing. Around 4 to 6 months babbling appears, which consists of sounds of vowels and consonants resembling syllables. The most common sounds are "ma," "mu," "da," "di." By 9 to 10 months these sounds are repeated as two syllables. The infant is attempting to imitate sounds at this point. Sounds are mixed with play such as bubble-blowing or gurgling. By 12 months words such as "mama" and "dada" are emerging. All normal children learn their native language and show similarities in this learning.

Anticipatory Guidance: Language

The nurse, in order to assist the parent most effectively, needs to make sure they understand the process of language development in their infant. A number of activities are appropriate to promote language development in the infant. Keeping in mind the receptive abilities of even the very young infant, parents can be encouraged to talk to infants while holding or handling them. They can be encouraged to observe the response of the infant to adult vocalization. Incorporating smiling and eye-to-eye contact while talking with the infant can make this type of interaction positive for adult and infant. As the infant starts making sounds, the parents can imitate the sounds and vocalize in response to the infant. Infants seem to enjoy vocalization during activities such as eating, bathing, and dressing. Toys and household items that produce sounds also elicit responses from the infant. As the infant approaches 9 to 10 months it is helpful to accompany simple verbal directions with gestures, to repeat the directions, and to have the infant participate in the activity. Repeating the names of familiar objects to the infant is also helpful. Continued vocalizing with the infant during activities remains important. Parents can make sounds such as tongue-clicking or lip-smacking that the infant can imitate.

Infants at 1 year of age have made enormous strides in their intellectual competency which is consistently influencing and being influenced by the development of competence in other areas.

Emotional-Social Competency

The emotional-social competency is another essential and rapidly changing area during infancy. A number of theories have been devised to explain this phase of infant development. No one theory adequately explains all that is happening in the emotional-social areas.

Freud's theory postulated the development of three facets of personality—the id, ego, and superego. The newborn infant was seen as being governed by id impulses. The id was the driving force of personality, operating to obtain pleasure and avoid pain. A frequent explanation of id motivation is worded, "I want what I want when I want it." Pleasure (gratification of id impulses or tension reduction) is centered in different body areas or zones. In the infant this body area is the mouth. Through sucking the infant derives pleasure. Freud's theory focuses mainly on forces (or tensions) within the individual as motivators of development.

As stated in Chapter 3, Erik Erikson's theory takes into account cultural and societal influences on development. The central task, conflict, or crisis for the infant is that of basic trust versus basic mistrust. Infants have innate capacities that facilitate their interaction with the environment as they strive to develop more trust than mistrust. Infants must learn to trust individuals in their environment in order to be able to achieve a sense of trust in themselves. Erikson sees the feeding situation as central to resolution of the trust-mistrust conflict. The very young infant cannot tolerate much frustration when hungry. The quality of the mother's/caretaker's interaction when providing the breast or bottle is crucial to the development of trust. Eventually, infants begin to develop self-trust as feelings of hunger are consistently rewarded. They can rely on their own behaviors to obtain food and are therefore able to tolerate some delay. Other interactions between the infant and mother/caretaker are also seen as contributing to the development of a sense of trust. Trust results from being held, talked to, cuddled, warmed, changed, rocked, and so on. Erikson sees "sense of" as having three components: a conscious experience that is felt within oneself, a way of behaving that is observable by others, and an inner state that can only be verified by psychoanalytic interpretation. A sense of trust therefore would involve, for infants, feelings within themselves of comfort and security. Trusting infants could also be recognized by their behaviors. Erikson stated that a trusting baby is one who eats well, sleeps deeply, and enjoys bowel relaxation. This view exemplifies one criticism of Erikson's theory—that it does not take into account individual differences. It is possible that babies with different temperaments may demonstrate trust in different ways. There are also differences in caretakers, and behaviors differ at different times. A tired baby is less likely to fit Erikson's picture of trust than is a rested baby.

Erikson believes, however, that the actual skill used in handling and caring for the infant is of little importance when compared with the underlying motivation of the caretaker. Infants must learn that those who care for them can be relied upon to satisfy their basic needs for survival and comfort. The trust-mistrust crisis provides a useful conceptual basis for describing, explaining, and predicting infant emotional-social behaviors.

Attachment

Bonding of parents to their infant and beginning attachment of infants to their parents was discussed earlier in this chapter. These processes continue to be an important component of the developing emotional-social competency of the infant. Keep in mind that infant-to-parent attachment and parent-to-infant bonding are two different processes. Often, the terms attachment and bonding are used interchangeably, which can lead to confusion. Whatever the terms used, the process is a two-way one—parent-to-infant and infant-to-parent.

It has not been very long since the prevailing view of the infant's social responses held that infants responded to all humans with little or no discrimination for the first 3 to 4 months of life. It is now known that newborns prefer the sound of their mother's voice over those of other females (Roberts, 1987). Infants also display social responsiveness earlier than was once thought. Babies as young as 12 days will imitate adult facial expressions (Meltzoff, 1985). Social responses of infants are important to the process involved in the infant becoming attached to parents. By the time their infant is 6 to 8 weeks of age most parents have identified and are responding to at least two social responses of their baby. They notice that the baby follows them (and other objects) visually when they are within the direct line of vision and that the baby smiles in response to social stimuli. By 2 to 4 months of age the baby will smile spontaneously at a human face.

Ainsworth (1973) characterized the initial phase of infant attachment to the parents as nondiscriminating because the babies did not appear to discriminate between their parents and other humans in these social responses. In the second phase infants progress to discrimination in their social responsiveness. By 6 months their responses clearly indicate that the primary caregiver is preferred. By the third phase at 9 to 10 months of age most authorities believe infants are truly attached. They actively initiate proximity-seeking, contact-seeking behaviors and maintain contact with their parent(s) or other primary caregivers. They may relate easily to others, but with discrimination. The attachment behaviors of smiling, gazing, vocalization, and motor approach are of a different quality and intensity toward people to whom infants are attached. They do not seek the same kind of contact with people to whom they are not attached.

A new set of behaviors that occurs around 8 to 9 months of age can be seen as evidence of the infants' attachment to their parents. The 9-month-old baby will tend to respond to strangers with a serious, sometimes wary expression. "Stranger anxiety" occurs by this age and is manifested in overt distress when the stranger attempts to approach the baby. This can be devastating to grandparents who were welcomed with smiles and coos when they last visited. This stranger anxiety can be seen as evidence of the baby's strong attachment to the familiar parents. (The baby can also be said to be demonstrating a strong sense of trust in the familiar—the parents—and a healthy sense of mistrust in the unfamiliar.) Several studies have clearly indicated that formation of a secure attachment to at least one parent (or caregiving person) is necessary before 9- to 12-month-old infants will explore and start to separate from their parents, as they begin the process of developing autonomy (Ainsworth, 1973). A strong attachment serves as a secure base from which to explore. Infants do form attachments to more than one person, although not to large numbers. Once the infant is attached to a parent, attachment behaviors, rather than autonomy behaviors, are likely to increase following separation.

Anticipatory Guidance: Oral, Trust, and Attachment Needs

The nurse can assist parents to understand the developing emotional-social competency of their infant and their role in promoting his or her sense of trust and attachment. The nurse can give support to the parents as they respond to the needs of their infant and can discuss the reciprocity between bonding of the parents to their infant and the infant's attachment to them. Parents generally bond earlier and more quickly to their infant; later the infant attaches to the parents. In addition, the nurse can point out the specific attachment behaviors of the infant to the parents and stress the importance of promptly responding to these behaviors. The parents should be given reinforcement for responding to attachment behaviors of their infant. The nurse can encourage parents to provide periods of close contact with their infant. The infant needs to be held, cuddled, and carried. The use of infant carriers that allow the infant contact with the parents could be encouraged.

Discussion about meeting the basic needs of the infant for survival and comfort is appropriate. The prompt meeting of the infant's basic needs in a consistent manner helps to give the infant a secure and trusting view of the environment. The technical skill of the parents is not the key factor in meeting these needs. It is the manner (warm, consistent, caring) in which these needs are met that is the key factor. The infant is not concerned with how neatly the diaper is secured or how few wasted motions the parents use in giving the bath. What is important in these interactions is the fact that the parents responded to the infant's need to be clean and dry, in a social, caring manner. *Parents need to feel confident about their ability to meet the needs of their infant.*

The importance of the oral sense to the infant should be discussed with parents. Sucking is an important way for the infant to meet nutritional needs. The mouth is also used as an organ for touch. In addition, sucking in itself seems to be an important need for the infant. Some infants have greater sucking needs than other infants. Parents may need assistance in determining if their infant is hungry or has a non-nutritive sucking need. Overfeeding can result if sucking needs are interpreted as hunger needs. Non-nutritive sucking need is greatest in the first 4 to 6 months of life. Satisfying the need for sucking provides comfort to the infant and does not lead to dependency on sucking.

Many parents, professionals, family members, and friends have strong positive or negative feelings about the use of a pacifier. The nurse can provide information about its appropriate use and can help parents determine if their infant requires this mechanism to meet sucking needs. If the pacifier is given, infants can be held and cuddled while they use it. It should not be used constantly or to substitute for holding and other ways of meeting the infant's needs. Pacifier use should be eliminated when the infant evidences a diminishing need to suck (usually at about 4 to 5 months of age). When used in this manner pacifiers do not become habit-forming. However, use of pacifiers beyond infancy or as a substitute for caretaking may lead to a habit that is difficult to overcome. Some infants may substitute a thumb for the pacifier. The type of pacifier used (size, shape) does not justify its prolonged use. Parents may choose the shape of pacifier that corresponds to the type of nipple used during feeding.

Parents may want to discuss coping with the changing needs of the infant as he or she progresses in the stages of attachment. In the first few months of life the infant needs opportunity to interact with the parents; some parents express the idea that it does not seem to matter to the infant who takes care of him or her. Infants seem to respond in the same way to all caretakers. These parents need assistance in understanding that discrimination in response and ultimate attachment is a process that is enhanced by these early opportunities for interaction.

Parents often ask how much time is actually necessary to allow attachment to occur, or what effect there is on the infant if both parents work outside the home. The nurse must realize that there are no specific answers. In light of what is known about attachment, the nurse can assist parents to arrive at a satisfactory plan to promote attachment of their infant as well as meet the family's needs. It is certainly clear that there is flexibility in the amount of time needed for interaction between parents and infant and that quality of interaction is more important than quantity.

Parents need assistance in anticipating that as infants become attached to one or both parents, they will respond differently to other family members and friends and caretakers. Parents can then help others (such as grandparents) not to feel rejected. It may help to suggest a little distance in these persons' interaction with infants until they give clues they are ready for more interaction with them.

Parents need opportunities to discuss their feelings as the infant begins to demonstrate exploratory and independent behaviors. All of a sudden their infant seems not to want them as much or to be as close to them. In reality, of course, the infant needs them as much as ever, but in a slightly different way. As infants explore, they need parents as a secure, consistent base to come back to for support. In this period, if infants have been separated from their parents for even a few hours they may demonstrate more contact-seeking attachment behaviors, such as clinging and wishing to be held. Parents need to understand that this is not regressive or spoiled behavior. Infants still need close contact with their parents and are not capable of functioning independently. They use attachment behaviors to maintain the support from their parents and to build on their developing sense of trust. This period can be confusing to parents as they try to meet the attachment needs of their infant as well as his or her beginning needs for independence.

Temperament

As in all areas of infant development, infant temperament has been studied in a variety of ways since the early 1980s. Previous research had sometimes looked at infant temperament without taking into account its inter-relationship with other variables. It is now generally accepted that temperament is inter-related with many other variables and that negative effects of temperament can be mediated by other psychosocial variables. Current thinking also holds that it is more likely that infant temperament affects the mode of expression of security or insecurity than whether or not these feelings actually develop (Belsky and Rovine, 1987). A promising measure of infant temperament, the Infant Behavior Questionnaire, or IBQ (Rothbart, 1986), can be used by the nurse while working with parents to promote optimal well-being of the infant. The tool is useful in a general discussion of the differences in infant temperament. It can assist the nurse and family to better understand and meet individual infant needs.

Anticipatory Guidance: Temperament

The nurse has to take into account the effect the infant's temperament has on the family, friends, and health care providers. In order to understand an infant's behavior more fully the parents and nurse need to be aware of the specific characteristics of the infant. If the family and nurse are aware that some infants have intense reactions and slow adaptation to change in their environment, they will approach the issue of changing the sleeping location in a different way for such infants than they would for infants who have low-intensity reactions and who readily adapt. This does not mean the parents cannot change the infant's place of sleep; rather, the best or least disturbing approach can be sought. Families need assistance in recognizing that infants, even within the same family, may have very different temperaments. The infant's temperament characteristics will affect how family members and others respond to him or her. The characteristics and responses do not indicate that either the infant or parent is good or bad. The nurse can help the family

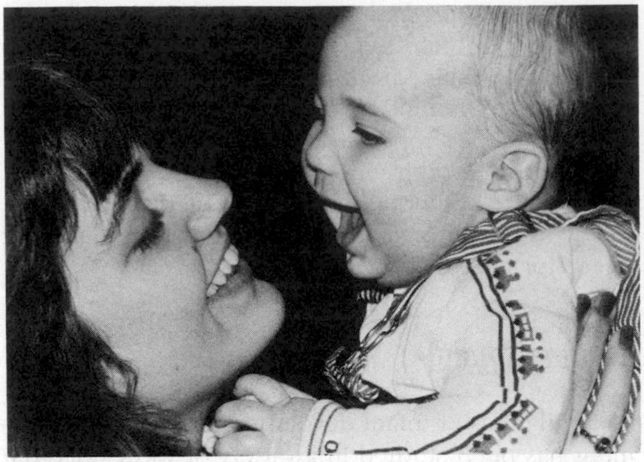

Optimal emotional development in the infant depends on satisfying interactions with significant others.

look at approaches to childrearing, taking into account the temperament of this infant and their response to his or her temperament.

Emotions

There has been much controversy over when emotions appear in the infant. Infants do not seem to have a range of emotions from an early age. However, they do not express emotions as adults do, nor are infant emotions likely to be exactly like those of adults. The smiles and cries of infants seem to give evidence of differentiation at an early age and are definite means of communication. Parents and professionals must be cautious about interpreting these clues (cries and smiles) the same as they would adult cries and smiles.

The smile of the infant is considered an important developmental milestone. Many emotional connotations are placed in the powerful smile of the infant. It certainly plays an important role in promoting contact between the infant and adults. Initially the smile of the infant is spontaneous, but by 1 month of age the infant directs the smile toward people. By 2 to 3 months the smile is in response to the face of a familiar person. The smile often occurs in conjunction with the gratification and comfort associated with these interaction experiences. These experiences help the infant to develop the association between pleasure and smiling.

Optimal emotional development in infants depends on interaction with individuals around them, particularly the mother. There is evidence that the young infant can recognize facial expressions of emotion, although this recognition develops slowly and is still rudimentary at the end of the first 2 years of life (Nelson, 1987). This ability to recognize facial expressions influences emotional-social development during infancy. When faced with an unfamiliar situation, the infant will look to the mother's facial expression and behave in a way that demonstrates that the baby was influenced by that facial expression (Hornick et al, 1987; Klinnert et al, 1986).

Another evidence of the developing differentiation of emotions is the temperament characteristics of the infant, previously discussed. The overall regularity in patterns of functioning of the infant also influences how adults view the baby's emotions. For example, an infant with a slow-to-warm temperament might be viewed as displaying the emotion of fear. Physiologically the infant may not have progressed to regularity in sleep, elimination, and so forth, and this unpredictability might be interpreted as emotions of anger or unhappiness.

Wolff (1969) has identified a variety of infant cries: (1) basic rhythmic cry, (2) mad or angry cry, (3) pain cry, and (4) cry of frustration. Infants do develop certain individual crying patterns. Parents need assistance in understanding crying as one of the methods of communication available to the infant. Although there are no scientific bases for saying that certain amounts of crying are "good" for the infant, families may have strong opinions on this subject. At times, crying does seem to allow the infant to release some tension.

Anticipatory Guidance: Emotions

Nurses need to assist parents to understand behaviors of infants and our limited ability to assess adequately the emotional state of the infant. Infants do show different behaviors that indicate a range of emotions, but we do not know if the emotions differ in degree or substance or both from adult emotional responses. Parents need opportunities to discuss their particular infant and his or her behaviors that have emotional connotations.

It is helpful for parents to know that their baby's responses are influenced by the parents' facial expressions and emotions. This information can assist them to modulate their own expression if they believe this is appropriate in a situation. It is important to respond promptly to an infant's behavior (smiling or crying). The nurse can help parents try to understand their infant and their responses to him or her.

Guiding Parents to Promote Their Infant's Development

As was indicated throughout discussion of the growth and development of the infant, parents' perceptions, characteristics, needs, and developmental level greatly influence the development of the infant, and vice versa. In addition to their perceptions of their infant, parents are influenced by the special concerns of being parents of an infant. They are becoming acquainted with and bonded to a new member of the family who has unique needs. The interaction patterns within the family have been increased. The parents are just beginning to sort out their roles as parents with this particular infant and to deal with childrearing issues and their expectations of the infant. They are dealing with an individual who is dependent on them and limited in his or her ability to express needs. In addition, the infant is changing so rapidly that it is difficult for parents to establish a pattern of anticipating and meeting the infant's needs. The addition of this new member to the family calls for adjustments in the life of all family members.

The nurse who works with the parents of an infant must be aware that all of these factors can contribute to a nursing diagnosis of *altered parenting: actual or potential.* The nursing assessment should include this diagnosis as a focus so that positive parenting can be reinforced, potential alterations prevented, and actual alterations treated.

Parents need a great deal of support for the difficult but rewarding task of raising an infant. They may have been given little information about development expectations for the infant. Parents need an opportunity to discuss their concerns with a knowledgeable nonjudgmental person. The nurse must acknowledge the parents as people with their own needs and concerns. The nurse will find it useful to get some sense of how parents view the health of the infant, including growth and development, in order to begin to recognize how the parents view health and development (e.g., do they believe they can affect their infant's health?). Also, the nurse can assess how competent parents seem to feel. Counseling can be geared to the unique needs of this particular family. The parents may need assistance in recognizing they still have needs of their own. The nurse can help them look at their pattern of communication with each other, now that an infant is part of the family, and at the impact of an infant on their total situation.

The parents will be the people providing most of the health care for the infant. The nurse should assist parents as they care for their infant to promote his or her optimum growth and development without neglecting their own developmental needs. Throughout this chapter growth and development knowledge and issues have been discussed that are pertinent to nurses as they provide assistance to parents through education, discussion of concerns, guidance, and counseling on the needs of their developing infants. If the parents know what to expect in the process of healthy growth and development of their infant, they will be better prepared to meet these needs and feel more capable as parents. In addition to providing anticipatory guidance on the developing competencies of the infant, the nurse can help parents see their infant's needs in the areas of nutrition, play, safety, and immunizations. Included should be an emphasis on the individual differences between infants. Nurses can use their knowledge of theories of growth and development as a basis for describing and explaining the baby's behaviors and for predicting outcomes of interactions between the baby and parents.

Nutrition

Alterations in nutrition can occur in infants if parents do not follow sound feeding practices. The defining characteristics for the nursing diagnosis, *altered nutrition: less than body requirements,* would be essentially the same for infants as those found in most nursing diagnosis references. An additional defining characteristic, weight below the fifth percentile, should be added. Similarly, a defining characteristic that addresses excessive growth percentiles for weight should be included in the defining characteristics of the nursing diagnosis, *altered nutrition: more than body requirements.* If either of these diagnoses is suspected, the etiology must be closely examined. If the etiology is underfeeding or overfeeding by the parents, then the reason must be explored. Only when the underlying cause is treated can this problem of nutritional deficit or obesity be alleviated.

Introduction of Solids

Introduction of solid foods to the infant's diet is an issue of interest to parents and health professionals. Current information supports the view that the infant does not need solid foods for adequate nutrition until at least 6 months of age. Previous recommendations had been for early introduction of solids, from 2 to 6 weeks of age. Solids were introduced at this early age because of developmental expectations and several beliefs: that the infants needed the solids to grow, that they were hungry, that they needed to practice feeding skills, and that solids would help them sleep through the night. None of these beliefs has been supported by sound research data. However, some parents and professionals have used this pattern of early introduction of foods satisfactorily, and see no need to change.

Those persons advocating later introduction of foods do so primarily on that basis of three assumptions: (1) young infants do not require solids for adequate nutrition; (2) in allergy-prone infants food allergies are more likely to occur early because of the incomplete digestion of food; and (3) the tendency to give too many calories, producing an overweight infant. All these assumptions have some research data to support them.

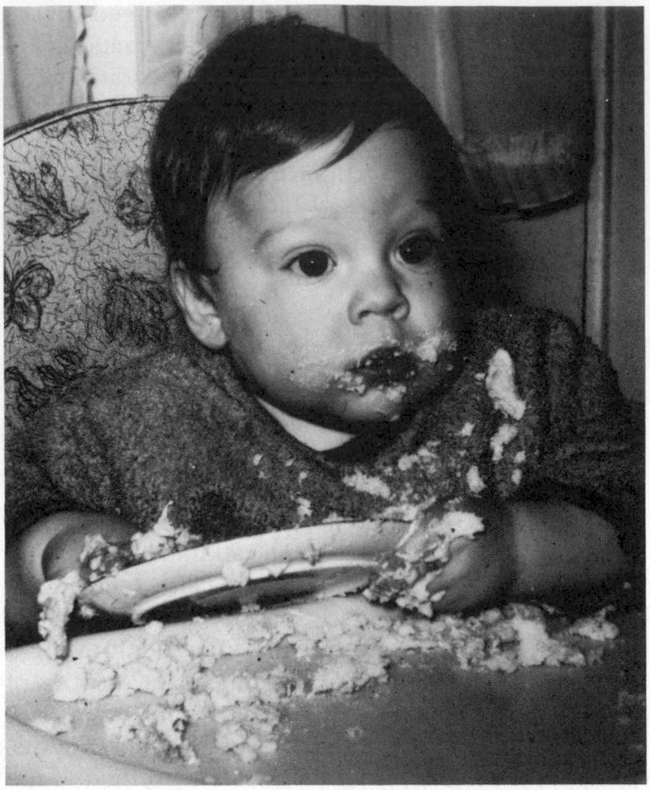

Feeding time can become messy as the infant's drive to explore includes food. (Photograph by David Trainor.)

Developmental skills give some guidance for the introduction of solids. Maturation of the central nervous system controls motor skills that influence the infant's ability to eat and drink. Illingsworth and Listen (cited in Pipes, 1985) point out that an infant learns to chew at about 6 to 7 months of age and therefore is ready developmentally to consume food. The sucking pattern of the infant changes in the first year as maturation alters both the form of the oral structure and the way the infant takes liquid from a nipple (Pipes, 1981). By 4 to 6 months the oral cavity has grown, mature sucking and jaw motion have developed and these indicate the readiness of the infant to start solid foods. At the same time the infant has achieved other developmental skills that affect feeding: ability to grasp, hand-to-mouth movements, and ability to sit. The infant is truly ready to handle solid foods, including finger foods. At this age the tongue is still better able to handle spoon-feeding than drinking from a cup.

The nurse can assist parents by relaying information about the nutritional requirements of infants and developmental skills that aid feeding, and the rationale for current recommendations about introduction of solids. Parents often have many questions about the sequence and methods of introducing solids. No one sequence is consistently recommended. However, some concepts that will aid the nurse in helping parents establish the pattern they will use in introduction of solids can be identified. The addition of food to the diet should be individualized to the infant and should never be forced. The infant will need some practice as he or she learns the new skill of eating solids, changing gradually from a sucking to a chewing motion. One new food should be introduced at a time, and a number of days (two to seven) should intervene before another new food is introduced, so that an allergic response could be more easily identified.

It has been generally recommended that the first food offered to the infant be rice cereal, as it is considered to be the least allergenic of the cereal grains and because most cereals are fortified with iron. Parents should give only cereals that are fortified with iron. Labels on the numerous cereal products available need to be read carefully. These products vary significantly in their nutritional value. Fruits are often the next solid introduced. It is thought that infants find fruits better tasting than some other foods; this may be an adult bias. Vegetables are introduced next, followed by meats and eggs.

Frequently parents ask about the merits of using commercially prepared strained food as opposed to making their own strained foods. Either method can safely meet the nutritional needs of the infant. Some parents prefer to use a combination of these methods. If using commercially prepared foods, the parents should be encouraged to read the labels carefully. An item to look for is the amount of sugar and salt contained in the product; foods containing less of these are preferred. A number of companies in the last few years have altered or removed the additives in their baby food products. The nurse should also point out that the mixed dinner labels should be examined with care. There is usually substantially less meat in the dinner labeled "vegetable and meat" than in the "meat and vegetable" dinners. Even the latter type of dinner may not contain an adequate amount of meat relative to cost. Many of the commercial dessert items have a high content of starch filler and add little to the diet other than calories. If parents are preparing the strained food themselves, they must be sure to prepare a well-balanced diet. If baby foods are prepared at home, parents should remove the baby's portion before salt, sugar, or other spices or condiments are added. They may prepare just enough food to be fed immediately. If they prepare extra food, it can be mixed with a little water or milk, frozen in ice cube trays, placed in storage bags and kept frozen until immediately before use.

At about the same time or soon after strained foods are introduced, table (finger) foods also may be given. Chewing can be done with the gums, so teeth are not necessary. Infants can feed themselves such items as melba toast, crackers, and Zwieback. As the infant gains skill in chewing, other bite-sized finger foods may be gradually added, including cereals, chicken, vegetables, cheese, and canned fruits. Finger foods should be cut to a size that is easily handled in the infant's mouth to prevent choking. Foods that are small and hard and easily aspirated, such as nuts, popcorn, kernels of corn, and chunks of meat should not be given to infants.

Parents need to be aware that feeding time can become quite messy. However, this is normal as the infant explores food as well as everything else. Near the end of the first year infants are beginning to exert independence, self-control, and mastery of skills that include self-feeding. Coordination of skills needed to finger-feed themselves eventually becomes transferred to skill in using utensils. By the end of the first year infants have begun to feed themselves and in the next year will perfect the skills.

Use of Cup

Along with learning the skills associated with feeding himself, the infant is also developing the ability to drink from a cup. As indicated by the earlier discussion related to developmental skills achieved because of neuromuscular maturation, the infant can begin to drink from the cup by 6 months of age. Most infants can drink from a cup by 12 months.

Weaning occurs as infants move from a primarily liquid diet to a more solid diet. As they increase their solid intake and begin to drink from a cup, they will need less from the bottle or breast. The issue of when to wean a particular infant fully often arises when the baby is 6 to 12 months of age. There is no one right time or way to wean an infant. The nurse must assist parents in their individual approach to weaning their infant. Factors to be considered as this process is discussed with the parents include developmental readiness of the infant, the baby's sucking needs, parents' beliefs and feelings, environmental pressures (family, job), finances, nutritional requirements, and past experiences of family.

Play

The needs of the infant for play are implicit throughout the discussion of promotion of infant growth and development. Play provides opportunities for the infant to learn and develop many skills. The importance of a variety of play opportunities can be pointed out to parents. Play is not just an extra activity that serves no purpose (see Chapter 21), but rather the way infants learn about themselves and their environment. As the reader reflects on the discussion of the activities that promote development of physical and intellectual competencies, it becomes clear that many of these activities are usually classified as play activities. Expensive toys are not necessary for play; articles commonly found in the home are perfectly adequate. The nurse can assist the family to creatively use the resources available to them. Play activities promote cognitive and emotional-social development of infants as they separate themselves from their environment. Many such activities foster interaction of the infant with other people. Play can stimulate the attachment of the infant to parents and the eventual ability of the infant to separate. It can provide many pleasurable experiences for infants as they learn to trust and adapt to their world.

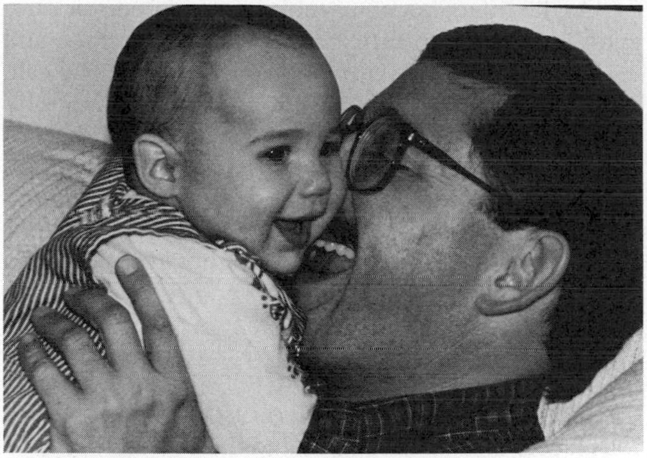

Social interactions with parents are a significant part of "play" for the infant.

Safety

Safety is another key issue implicit in the discussion of infant growth and development. While discussing the developing competencies of the infant, the nurse can help parents look at the environment in terms of the hazards these developing skills may introduce. The nurse can use the nursing diagnoses of *potential for injury: falls, potential for injury: poisoning,* and *potential for injury: suffocation/aspiration* as a framework for discussing hazards to the safety of the infant.

Parents need to recognize that even very young infants soon will be turning and rolling over. Thus, it is not safe to leave infants unrestrained on any object they might roll off of, such as a bed or changing table. As the infant becomes able to reach items and grasp and bring them to the mouth, parents must be even more alert to what is within reach. Small objects such as coins, buttons, and pins must be removed from the baby's territory. Nothing should be tied around the infant's neck, including pacifiers on strings.

As the infant becomes mobile, the parents or caretaker must learn to anticipate this ability to creep and crawl farther and faster than they think he or she can. An infant's ability to explore the environment increases every day. The parents must anticipate that the baby will soon be able to pull up to a standing position and begin to walk around objects. Safety hazards are covered in more detail in Chapter 17. The infant must be protected from the risks of his or her ever-widening environment.

Immunizations

Chapter 14 provides a detailed discussion of the various facets of immunizations and the currently recommended immunization schedule. The following schedule is currently recommended during infancy:

2 months:	DPT, OPV
4 months:	DPT, OPV
6 months:	DPT, OPV

Immunizations are an important component of anticipatory guidance. Parents need to be informed about the benefits of immunization procedures and the rationale for the procedure. Parents must be informed of the risks as well as the benefits of immunizations. The Committee on Infectious Disease of the American Academy of Pediatrics recommends immunization schedules. These are revised periodically as new information arises. The nurse should consult current resources such as latest editions of AAP's *Report of the Committee on Infectious Disease (Red Book)* for detailed information about immunizations. The nurse also needs to help prepare parents for possible reaction of the infant to certain immunizations and related interventions.

References

Ainsworth M: The development of the infant-mother attachment. *In* Caldwell BM, Ricuiti HN (eds): *Review of Child Development Research.* Vol 3. Chicago, University of Chicago Press, 1973.

American Academy of Pediatrics, Committee on Fetus and Newborn: Report of the Ad Hoc Task Force on Circumcision. *Pediatrics* 1975 Oct; 610.

American Academy of Pediatrics, Committee on Fetus and Newborn, Committee on Infectious Diseases: Prophylaxis and treatment of neonatal gonococcal infections. *Pediatrics* 1980 May; 1047.

American Academy of Pediatrics, Committee on Nutrition: Toward a prudent diet for children. *Pediatrics* Vol 71, Jan 1983.

Anisfeld E, Lopper E: Early contact, social support, and mother-infant bonding. *Pediatrics* 1983; 72:79–83.

Apgar V: A proposal for a new method of evaluating the newborn infant. *Curr Res Anesth Analg* 1953 Jul/Aug; 260.

Babson S, et al: *Management of High Risk Pregnancy and Intensive Care of the Neonate.* St. Louis, CV Mosby, 1975.

Banagale P, Donn S: Asphyxia neonatorum. *J Fam Pract* 1986; 22:539–546.

Barglow P, Vaughn BE, Molitor N: Effects of maternal absence due to employment on the quality of infant-mother attachment in a low-risk sample. *Child Dev* 1987; 58:945–954.

Bayley N: Comparisons of mental and motor test scores for 1–15 months by sex, birth order, race, geographical location and education of parents. *Child Dev* 1965 Jun; 379.

Behrman RE, Vaughan VC III (eds): *Nelson's Textbook of Pediatrics.* 13th ed. Philadelphia, WB Saunders, 1987.

Bell EF, Oh W: Fluid and electrolyte management. *In:* Avery G (ed): *Neonatology: Pathophysiology and Management of the Newborn.* 3rd ed. Toronto and Philadelphia, JB Lippincott, 1987.

Belsky J, Rovine M: Temperament and attachment security in the strange situation: an empirical rapprochement. *Child Dev* 1987; 58:787–795.

Benn RK: Factors promoting secure attachment relationships between employed mothers and their sons. *Child Dev* 1986; 57:1224–1231.

Bennett FC, Robinson NM, Sells CJ: Growth and development of infants weighing less than 900 grams at birth. *Pediatrics* 1983; 71:319–323.

Bernhardt J: Sensory capabilities of the fetus. *MCN* 1987; 12:44–46.

Bocchese J, Merker A: Seizure disorders in the neonate. *Crit Care Nurse* 1983; 3:42–51.

Bowen SM, Miller BC: Paternal attachment behavior as related to presence at delivery and preparenthood classes: a pilot study. *Nurs Res* 1980; 29:307–311.

Bowlby J: *Attachment and Loss.* Vol 1. New York, Basic Books, 1969.

Bradshaw TW: Teething. *Pediatr Nurs* 1981 May/Jun; 41–42.

Brazelton T: *The Neonatal Behavioral Assessment Scale.* Philadelphia, JB Lippincott, 1973.

Brazelton T: The remarkable talents of the newborn. *Birth Fam J* 1978 Winter; 187.

Britton C: Early mother-infant contact and infant temperature stabilization. *JOGNN* 1980 Mar/Apr; 84.

Broom BL: Consensus about the marital relationship during transition to parenthood. *Nurs Res* 1984 Jul/Aug; 33 (4):223–228.

Brune K, Lacey L: Common hematologic problems of the immediate newborn period. *JOGNN* 1983; 12:195–265.

Bryant BG: Unit dose erythromycin ophthalmic ointment for neonatal ocular prophylaxis. *JOGNN* 1984 Mar/Apr; 83.

Buckwald S, Zorn WA, Eagan EA: Mortality and follow-up data for neonates weighing 500–800 grams at birth. *Am J Dis Child* 1984; 138:779.

Campbell S, Taylor PM: Bonding and attachment: theoretical issues. *Semin Perinatol* 1980; 3:3–14.

Canadian Paediatric Society, Fetus and Newborn Committee: *Use of Phototherapy for Neonatal Hyperbilirubinemia.* 1986; 134:1237–1245.

Carter-Jessop L: Promoting maternal attachment through prenatal intervention. *MCN* 1981 Mar/Apr; 6(2):107–112.

Censullo M: Home care of the high risk newborn. *JOGNN* 1986, 15:146–153.

Chess S, Thomas A: Infant bonding: mystique and reality. *Am J Orthopsychiatr,* 1982 Apr; 213–222.

Chow M, et al: *Handbook of Pediatric Primary Care.* 2nd ed. New York, Wiley Medical, 1984.

Clark A, Affonso D: *Childbearing: a Nursing Perspective.* Philadelphia, FA Davis, 1979.

Cohen S: Longitudinal studies of preterm infants. *In* Taeusch HW, Yogman M (eds): *Follow-up Management of the High-Risk Infant.* Toronto and Boston, Little, Brown, 1987.

Cohen SE: The low-birthweight infant and learning disabilities. *In* Lewis M (ed): *Prenatal and Perinatal Factors Relevant to Learning Disabilities.* Champaign, IL, University of Illinois Press, 1986.

Colangelo A, Vento T, Taeusch HW: Discharge planning. *In* Taeusch HW, Yogman M (eds): *Follow-up Management of the High Risk Infant.* Toronto and Boston, Little, Brown, 1987.

Cole J: Infant stimulation reexamined: an environmental and behavioral based approach. *Neonatal Network* 1985; 3:24–31.

Cotton R: The relationship of symptomatic patent ductus arteriosus to respiratory distress in premature newborn infants. *Clin Perinatol* 1987; 14:621–633.

Craig S, et al: The effect of early contact on maternal perception of infant behavior. *Early Hum Dev* 1982; 6:197–204.

Crnic KA, Greenberg MT, Ragozin AS, et al: Effects of stress and social support on mothers and premature full-term infants. *Child Dev* 1983; 54:209–217.

Crouse D, Philips J: Persistent pulmonary hypertension of the newborn. *Perinatology-Neonatology* 1987; 11:10–20.

Davis MS, Akridge K: The effect of promoting intrauterine attachment in primiparas on postdelivery attachment. *JOGNN* 1987 Nov/Dec; 430–437.

Dean PG, Morgan P, Towle JM: Making baby's acquaintance: a unique attachment strategy. *MCN* 1982 Jan/Feb; 7:37–41.

de Chateau P, Wiberg J: Long-term effect on mother-infant behavior of extra contact during the first hour postpartum. I: First observations at 36 hours. II. A follow-up at three months. *Acta Paediatr Scand* 1977; 66:137–151.

DeMeis DK, McBride SL, Hock E: The balance of employment and motherhood: longitudinal study of mothers' feelings about separation from their first-born infants. *Dev Psychol* 1986; 22:627–632.

Dubowitz L, et al: Clinical assessment of gestational age in the newborn infant. *J Pediatr* 1970 Jul; 1.

Erickson M: Trends in assessing the newborn with his parents. *MCN* 1978 Mar/Apr; 99.

Faerber E: *Cranial Computed Tomography in Infants and Children.* Oxford, England, Blackwell Scientific Publications, 1986.

Foley K: Caring for the parents of newborn twins. *MCN* 1979; 4:221–226.

Fomon S: *Nutritional Disorders of Children.* Washington, DC, USDHEW Publication No. (HSA) 77–5105, 1977.

Friedemann M, Emrich K: Emergence of infant sleep-wake patterns in the first three months after birth. *Int J Nurs Stud* 1978; 15:5–16.

Friedrich O: What do babies know? *Time* 1983 Aug 15; 52–59.

Furman E: The death of a newborn: care of the parents. *Birth Fam J* 1978 Winter; 214.

Goldberg S: Parent-infant bonding: another look. *Child Dev* 1983; 54:1355–1382.

Gorski P: Behavioral and environmental care: new frontiers in neonatal nursing. *Neonatal Network* 1985; 3:8–11.

Gosha J, Brucker MC: A self-help group for new mothers. An evaluation. *MCN* 1986; 11:20–23.

Gottfried A, Hodgman J, Brown K: How intensive is newborn intensive care? An environmental analysis. *Pediatrics* 1984; 74:292–294.

Grace J: Does a mother's knowledge of fetal gender affect attachment? *MCN* 1984 Jan/Feb; 42–45.

Greenberg M, Morris N: Engrossment: the newborn's impact upon the father. *Am J Pathol* 1974; 44:520–531.

Gromada K: Maternal-infants attachment: the first step toward individualizing twins. *MCN* 1981; 6:129–134.

Hack M, Caron B, Rivers A, et al: The very low birth weight infant: the broader spectrum of morbidity during infancy and early childhood. *J Dev Behav Pediatr* 1983; 4:243.

Hales DJ, et al: Defining the limits of the maternal sensitive period. *Dev Med Child Neurol* 1977; 19:454–461.

Harlow H: The nature of love. *Am Psychol* 1958; 673.

Harned H Jr: Respiration and the respiratory system. *In* Stave U (ed): *Perinatal Physiology.* New York, Plenum, 1978, 53.

Hill S, Shronk L: The effect of early parent-infant contact on newborn body temperature. *JOGNN* 1979 Sep/Oct; 287.

Hornick R, Risenhover N, Gunnar M: The effects of maternal positive, neutral, and negative affective communications on infant responses to new toys. *Child Dev* 1987; 58:937–944.

Inwood S, Finley GA, Fitzhardinge PM: High-frequency oscillation: a new mode of ventilation for the neonate. *Neonate Network* 1986; 4:53–58.

Karp T, Solon J, Olson D, et al: High frequency jet ventilation: a neonatal nursing perspective. *Neonatal Network* 1986; 4:42–50.

Kemp VH, Page CK: Maternal prenatal attachment in normal and high-risk pregnancies. *JOGNN* 1987 May/Jun; 179–184.

Kennell JH, et al: Maternal behavior one year after early and extended postpartum contact. *Dev Med Child Neuro* 1974; 16:172–179.

Kitchen WH, Yu V, Orgill A, et al: Collaborative study of very-low-birthweight infants. *Am J Dis Child* 1983; 137:555.

Klaus M, Fanaroff A: *Care of the High-Risk Neonate.* 3rd ed. Toronto and Philadelphia, WB Saunders, 1986, 184.

Klaus M, Kennell J: *Maternal-Infant Bonding.* St Louis, CV Mosby, 1976.

Klaus M, Kennell J: *Parent-Infant Bonding.* 2nd ed. St Louis, CV Mosby, 1982.

Klaus MH, et al: Maternal attachment: importance of the first postpartum days. *N Engl J Med* 1972; 286:460–463.

Kling P: Respiratory distress syndrome in the tiny baby. *Neonatal Network* 1986; 4:7–13.

Klinner MD, Emde RN, Butterfield P, et al: Social referencing: the infant's use of emotional signals from a friendly adult with mother present. *Dev Psychol* 1986; 22:427–432.

Kopp CB, Parmelee AH: Prenatal and perinatal influences on infant behavior. *In* Osofsky J (ed): *Handbook for Infant Development.* New York, John Wiley and Son, 1979.

Korner A: Intervention with preterm infants: rationale, aims and means. *In* Smeriglio VL (ed): *Newborns and Parents.* Edited by Hillsdale, NJ, Lawrence Erlbaum Associates, 1981.

Korones S: *High-Risk Newborn Infants.* 4th ed. Toronto and St. Louis, CV Mosby, 1986.

Kuller JM: Skin development and function—Part I. *Neonatal Network* 1984; 3:18–23.

Lamb M: Second thoughts on first touch. *Psychol Today* 1982 Apr; 9–11.

Lamb ME, Hwang CP: Maternal attachment and mother-neonatal bonding: a critical review. *In* Lamb ME, Brown AL (eds): *Advances in Developmental Psychology.* Hillsdale, NJ, Erlbaum, 1982.

Lawson M: Persistent pulmonary hypertension of the newborn: current trends in classification and diagnosis. *Neonatal Network* 1987; 6:27–35.

Lemons P, Stuart M, Lemons J: Breast-feeding the premature infant. *Clin Perinatol* 1986; 13:111–122.

Levitt MJ, Weber RA, Clark MC: Social network relationships as sources of maternal support and well being. *Dev Psychol* 1986; 22:310–316.

Lewis M, Brooks-Gunn J: *Social Cognition and the Acquisition of Self.* New York, Plenum Books, 1979.

Linn P, Horowitz F, Fox H: Stimulation in the NICU: is more necessarily better? *Clin Perinatol* 1985; 12:407–422.

Lubchenco L, et al: Intrauterine growth in length and head circumference as estimated from live births at gestational ages from 26–42 weeks. *Pediatrics* 1966 Mar; 403.

Lubchenco L, et al: Intrauterine growth as estimated from liveborn birth-weight data at 24 to 42 weeks of gestation. *Pediatrics* 1963 Oct; 793.

Lubchenco L, et al: Long-term follow-up studies of prematurely born infants. II. Influence of birth weight and gestational age on sequelae. *J Pediatr* 1972 Mar; 509.

Luddington-Hoe S: What can newborns really see? *AJN* 1983 Sep; 1286–1289.

Maltz H: Imprinting: empirical basis and theoretical significance. *Psychol Bull* 1960; 57:291–314.

Manning FA, et al: Fetal breathing. *In* McNall L, Galeener J (eds): *Current Practice in Obstetric and Gynecologic Nursing.* Vol 2, St. Louis, CV Mosby, 1977, 108.

Marchal F, Bairam A, Vert P: Neonatal apnea and apneic syndromes. *Clin Perinatol* 1987; 14:509–523.

Meltzoff AN: Immediate and deferred imitation in 14 and 24 month old infants. *Child Dev* 1985; 56:62–72.

Mercer R: Postpartum illness and acquaintance-attachment process. *Am J Nurs* 1977 Jul; 1174.

Miller D, Baird S: Helping parents to be parents—a special center. *MCN* 1978 Mar/Apr; 117.

Mitchell K, Mills N: Is the sensitive period in parent-infant bonding over-rated? *Pediatr Nurs* 1983 Mar/Apr; 91–94.

Monin P, Vert P: The management of bronchopulmonary dysplasia. *Clin Perinatol* 1987; 14:531–545.

Moore M: Total parenteral nutrition for infants. *Neonatal Network* 1987; 6:33–40.

Morrongiello BA, Rocca PT: Infant's localization of sounds in the horizontal plane: effects of auditory and visual cues. *Child Dev* 1987; 58:918–927.

Nelson CA: The recognition of facial expressions in the first two years of life. *Child Dev* 1987; 58:889–909.

Nelson NM: Respiration and circulation after birth. *In* Smith CA, Nelson NM (eds): *The Physiology of the Newborn Infant,* Springfield, IL, Charles C Thomas, 1976, 117.

Nugent J: Extracorporeal membrane oxygenation in the neonate. *Neonatal Network* 1986; 4:27–38.

O'Connor S, et al: The effect of extended postpartum contact on problems with parenting: a controlled study of 301 families. *Birth Fam J* 1978 May; 231–234.

Oehler J: Examining the issue of tactile stimulation for preterm infants. *Neonatal Network* 1985; 4:25–33.

Ohio Neonatal Nutritionists: Fluid needs and management. *In: Nutritional Care for High Risk Newborns.* Philadelphia, George F. Stickley Company, 1985.

Osborn L: Management of neonatal jaundice. *Nurse Pract* 1986; 11:41–52.

Parke RD: Children's home environments: social and cognitive effects. *In* Altman I, Wohwill JF (eds): *Children and the Environment.* Vol 3. New York, Plenum Press, 1978, 33–81.

Parmelee A: Sensory stimulation in the nursery: how much and when? *Dev Behav Pediatr* 1985; 6:242–243.

Pipes P: *Nutrition in Infancy and Childhood.* 2nd ed. St. Louis, CV Mosby, 1985.

Power TG, Chapieski ML: Childrearing and impulse control in toddlers: a naturalistic investigation. *Dev Psychol* 1986; 22:271–275.

Rapoport R, et al: *Fathers, Mothers and Society.* New York, Basic Books, 1977.

Reeder S, et al: *Maternity Nursing.* Philadelphia, JB Lippincott, 1987.

Roberts M: Class before birth. *Psychol Today* 1987 May; 41.

Rothbart MK: Longitudinal observation of infant temperament. *Dev Psychol* 1986; 22:356–365.

Rushton C: Promoting normal growth and development in the hospital environment. *Neonatal Network* 1986; 4:21–30.

Rutledge DL, Pridham KF: Postpartum mothers' perceptions of competence for infant care. *JOGNN* 1987 May/Jun; 185–194.

Scherf R: Total patient care of the newborn infant who develops bronchopulmonary dysplasia. *Neonatal Network* 1985; 3:28–37.

Shapiro C: Retrolental fibroplasia: what we know and what we don't know. *Neonatal Network* 1986; 4:33–44.

Sharping EM: Physiological measurements of the neonate. *MCN* 1983 Jan/Feb; 70.

Siegal E: A critical examination of studies of parent-infant bonding. *In* Klaus M, Robertson M (eds): *Birth, Interaction and Attachment.* Edison, NJ, Johnson and Johnson, 1982, 51–61.

Silver H, Kempe C, Bruyn H: *Handbook of Pediatrics.* East Norwalk, CT, Lange Medical Publications, 1983.

Stark A: Twins. *In* Cloherty J, Stark A (eds): *Manual of Neonatal Care.* Boston, Little, Brown, 1980.

Steichen J, Krug-Wispe S, Tsang R: Breastfeeding the low birth weight preterm infant. *Clin Perinatol* 1987; 14:131–171.

Stewart AL, Reynolds EOR, Lipscomb AP: Outcome for infants of very low birth weight. Survey of world literature. *Lancet* 1981; 2:1038.

Svejda MJ, et al: Mother-infant bonding: failure to generalize. *Child Dev* 1980; 51:775–779.

Svejda MJ, et al: Parent-to-infant attachment: a critique of the early "bonding" model. *In* Emde RN, Harmon RJ (eds): *Attachment and Affiliative Systems.* New York, Plenum Press, 1982.

Thibeault D: Pulmonary barotrauma: interstitial emphysema, pneumomediastinum and pneumothorax. *In* Thibeault D, Gregory G (eds): *Neonatal Pulmonary Care.* 2nd ed. Norwalk, CT, Appleton-Century-Crofts, 1986, 499–517.

Tobin C: Dispelling common myths—Part II. *Neonatal Network.* 1984; 3:24–27.

Tomlinson PS: Spousal differences in marital satisfaction during transition to parenthood. *Nurs Res* 1987 Jul/Aug; 36 (4):239–243.

Torrence C: Neonatal seizures: Part I and Part II. *Neonatal Network* 1985; 4:9–15, 21–26.

Trevathon WR: Maternal touch at first contact with the newborn infant. *Dev Psychobiol* 1981 Dec; 14:549–558.

Wachs TD, Gruen GE: *Early Experience and Human Development.* New York, Plenum Press, 1982.

Weiser MA, Castiglia PT: Assessing early father-infant attachment. *MCN* 1984; 9:104–105.

Wolff P: The natural history of crying and other vocalizations in early infancy *In* Foss F (ed): *Determinants of Infant Behaviors.* New York, Methuen and Company, Ltd, 1969.

Wood A: Sequelae of perinatal asphyxia. *Neonatal Network* 1987; 5:21–23.

Bibliography

American Academy of Pediatrics, Committee on Drugs: Ethanolin liquid preparations intended for children. *Pediatrics* 1981 Mar; 73(3).

American Academy of Pediatrics, Committee on Nutrition: Vitamin and mineral supplemental needs in normal children. *Pediatrics* 1980 Dec; Vol 66.

Anderson E: Enhancing reciprocity between mother and neonate. *Nurs Res* 1987 Mar/Apr; 89–93.

Bell SM, Ainsworth M: Infant crying and maternal responsiveness. *Child Dev* 1972 Sep; 1171.

Biller H, Meredith D: *Father Power.* New York, Anchor Press–Doubleday, 1975.

Bower TGR: *Development in Infancy.* 2nd ed. New York, WH Freeman and Company, 1982.

Brazelton T: *Infants and Mothers: Differences in Development.* New York, Delacorte Press, 1969.

Brazelton T: Future care of the infant. *Birth Fam J* 1978 Winter; 242.

Brenner A: The blues: how postpartum depression affects both mother and child. *Am Baby* 1979 Mar; 50.

Brodish M: Relationship of early bonding to initial infant feeding patterns in bottle-fed newborns. *JOGNN* 1982 Jul/Aug; 248–252.

Brody S: The concepts of attachment and bonding. *J Am Psychol Assoc* 1981 Apr; 815–829.

Buckner E: Use of Brazelton Neonatal Behavioral Assessment in planning care for parents and newborns. *JOGNN* 1983 Jan/Feb; 26.

Carey W: Clinical application of infant temperament measurements. *J Pediatr* 1972 Oct; 823.

Chess S, Thomas A, Birch H: *Your Child Is a Person: A Psychological Approach to Parenthood Without Guilt.* New York, Viking Press, 1972.

Colombo J: The critical period concept: research, methodology and theoretical issues. *Psychol Bull* 1982 Feb; 260–275.

DeAngelis C: *Pediatric Primary Care.* 3rd ed. Boston, Little, Brown, 1984.

Donaldson N: Fourth trimester follow-up. *AJN* 1977 Jul; 1176.

Erickson M: *Assessment and Management of Developmental Changes in Children.* St. Louis, CV Mosby, 1976.

Erikson E: *Childhood and Society.* New York, Norton, 1950.

Foman S: *Infant Nutrition.* Philadelphia, WB Saunders, 1974.

Food and Nutrition Board, National Research Council: *Recommended Daily Dietary Allowances.* Washington, DC, National Academy of Sciences, 1980.

Funke J, Irby M: An instrument to assess the quality of maternal behavior. *JOGNN* 1978 Oct; 19.

Gesell A, Amatruda C: *Developmental Diagnosis: Normal and Abnormal Child Development.* 2nd ed. New York, (Haeber) Harper, 1949.

Ginsberg H, Opper S: *Piaget's Theory of Intellectual Development.* Englewood Cliffs, NJ, Prentice-Hall, 1969.

Hangsleben K: Transition to fatherhood: an explanatory study. *JOGNN* 1983 Jul/Aug; 265.

Harris J: When babies cry. *Can Nurse* 1979 Feb; 32.

Harrison M: The experience of home-start. *Health Visitor* 1984 June.

Hersh S, Levin K: How love begins between parent and child. *Child Today* 1978 Mar/Apr; 2.

Honig JC: Preparing preschool-aged children to be siblings. *MCN* 1986; 11:37–43.

Hymovich D, Chamberlin R: *Child and Family Development—Implications for Primary Health Care.* New York, McGraw-Hill, 1980.

Illingsworth R: *The Development of the Infant and Young Child.* 8th ed. New York, Churchill Livingstone, 1983.

Klaus M: The biology of parent-to-infant attachment. *Birth Fam J* 1978 Winter; 200.

Klaus M: Future care of the parents. *Birth Fam J* 1978 Winter; 246.

Klaus MH, Fanaroff AA: *Care of the High Risk Neonate.* Philadelphia, WB Saunders, 1986.

Klaus M, Kennell J: Bonding—another view. *Perinatol-Neonatol* 1984 Mar/Apr; 72–73.

Kohn C, et al: Gravidas' responses to realtime ultrasound fetal image. *JOGNN* 1980 Mar/Apr; 77–80.

Korsch BM: More on parent-infant bonding. *J Pediatr* 1983 Feb; 249.

Maier H: *Three Theories of Child Development.* New York, Harper & Row, 1969.

Maisels MJ, et al: Circumcision: the effect of information on parental decision making. *Pediatrics* 1983 Mar; 453.

Milne L, Rich O: Cognitive and affective aspects of the responses of pregnant women and sonography. *Matern Child Nurs J* 1981 Spring; 15–39.

Murphy L, Moriarty A: *Vulnerability, Coping and Growth from Infancy to Adolescence.* New Haven, CT, Yale University Press, 1976.

Newton L: Helping parents cope with infant crying. *JOGNN* 1983 May/Jun; 179.

O'Connor S, et al: Reduced incidence of parenting inadequacy following rooming in. *Pediatrics* 1980; 66:176–180.

Porter R, Cernoch J, Perry S: The importance of odors in mother-infant interactions. *Matern Child Nurs J* 1983 Fall; 147–154.

Righi FC, Krozy RE: The child in the car: what every nurse should know about safety. *Am J Nurs* 1983 Oct; 1421.

Snow C: The development of conversation between mothers and babies. *J Child Language* 1976 May; 1.

Sullivan R, et al: Determining a newborn's gestational age. *MCN* 1979 Jan/Feb; 38.

Wranesch BL: The effect of sibling visitation on bacterial colonization rate in neonates. *JOGNN* 1982 Jul/Aug; 211.

Families with Toddlers

Chapter 6

Jo Joyce Anderson
Mabel Hunsberger

Related Topics
Developmental theories, Chapter 3
Child health assessment, Chapter 15
Promoting safety, childproofing the home, Chapter 17
Promoting dental health, Chapter 19
Promoting healthy play for toddlers, Chapter 21

The parents in the childbearing stage of the life cycle who now have a toddler rambling through their home, perhaps along with older children, find themselves faced with a revised set of family developmental tasks. The overall task of the family with a toddler is the establishment and maintenance of a stable home that values each member's contributions and responds to the changing needs of each. To accomplish this task the family must (1) successfully adapt its resources to accommodate an active child or children, (2) reorganize relationships within and outside the home to include the child without disrupting intimate marital bonds, and (3) continue to derive satisfaction from parenthood. This section looks at those tasks and their impact on each member, as well as each member's responsibility in accomplishing those tasks. The nurse's role in assisting families to adapt in healthy ways to these task demands is described, with consideration given to common stressors of the family with a toddler. The following section details toddler growth and development, including anticipatory guidance for the parent(s).

Development and Adaptation of the Family with a Toddler

The most commonly encountered stresses in families with toddlers are those related to parenting and either the threat of, or actual, breakdown in family relationships (husband and wife, parent and child, child and sibling). The family with a toddler is "ripe" for stress or crisis because of several developmentally associated factors. Toddlers, in their unique developmental crises or transitional states, are in disequilibrium much of the time between dependence and striving for independence; this puts extra stress on their relationships with family members. The parents are at a decisive point in the establishment of their childrearing goals and methods as their infants become mobile and aware of themselves as individuals, an area in which they may discover that conflicting values exist. Siblings must now learn the lessons of sharing not only their mother and father but also toys, play space, and perhaps even their bedrooms or beds as a sibling moves into toddlerhood. Or if toddlers are presented with a new baby brother or sister, they will find the demands on their immature coping skills quite draining. And so goes the hotbed of potentially stressful situations and relationships in the home with a toddler.

Knowing about the potential stresses to families with toddlers is extremely valuable to nurses who will interact frequently, and perhaps regularly, with this family. They can be involved in helping the toddler and his or her family manage stress in ways that will continue to foster healthy development both of the family as a unit and of the individuals in it.

Adapting Resources to Accommodate a Toddler

Managing this task involves adjusting family philosophy to incorporate a higher valuation of people than of possessions, reallocation of space and facilities within the home, reappraising the environment to ensure the safety of a now mobile child, and reprioritizing the family budget to handle new expenses.

Valuing Persons Above Things

The family that values people over possessions and individual accomplishment over obedience will find satisfaction and stimulation in their years with a toddler. The family seeking, instead, to gather in material success and to demand authority will find adapting to a toddler a stifling and frustrating experience. This issue of values is a prime concern in the family with a toddler.

A stable family life is built with people as the central value. Person-centered homes nourish toddlers' evolving, unique personalities and make it possible for them to incorporate a respect for themselves and the people important to them. Parents who have developed a family philosophy that places prime value on the persons in it will respond to the unique personality of each child rather than treating the child and siblings alike.

Reallocation of Space and Facilities

Once a baby has taken the first steps that propel him or her into toddlerhood, the family quickly becomes aware of how much space this mobility requires. The baby who was satisfied to be contained in a crib or playpen where a small repertoire of toys could also be confined refuses to accept such limitations in space as a toddler. Furthermore, at this stage, children's selection of toys is expanding and they want their play things to accompany them wherever they happen to meander.

It is often at this point that families decide it is time to add another bedroom, to invest in a larger home, or perhaps to buy their first home to escape the small quarters. Other families decide to adapt to their limitations in space and to improvise as necessary to ensure private retreats for each family member. Whichever decision is made, the American norm is to provide children with some space of their own, separate from that of their parents, by the time the children approach toddlerhood. If the family's socioeconomic situation and values about privacy make it feasible, this means that each child has his or her own bedroom or at least one that is shared with a same-sex sibling. If budget or values do not support such an arrangement, the toddler's private retreat may be a large closet renovated into play and sleep areas or a section of a room that can be closed off with folding doors or pull-around drapes. Privacy, not the size of the area, is the important consideration.

Aside from a need for a space of their own, toddlers' demands for space to play and discover must also be reckoned with by the family unit. Again, depending on their attitudes about children and values about people and possessions, each family manages this situation differently. The more traditional family in terms of attitudes and values is motivated to manage this concern in a manner that keeps the child or children out of the the adults' way but still considers the child's comfort. The modern family with a developmental orientation that places greater value on persons is motivated to provide whatever space is needed to help the child grow and develop at his or her best. Either approach can allow the toddler opportunities to move about, explore, and manipulate; but the modern family approach tends to grant the toddler the range of the home. The traditional approach usually means confinement of toys and explorative activities to certain rooms or certain areas in rooms within the home.

Whichever approach is used, a consideration for the needs and safety of all family members should be included.

Another change that families with expressive toddlers must make is with emotional space. Toddlers' caregivers will foster their development of self-control by allowing them space for making choices and for emotional expression. For example, toddlers might choose the toys they will take to bed with them or which pajamas to wear. As long as the choices and emotional expressions are healthy, are conducive to their development, and will cause no one harm, as much choice as their ages warrant should be given. When their choices or emotional expressions breach these considerations, limits must be be imposed. Usually this is to the child's relief, because he or she is aware of the loss of control and finds it frightening.

The parents' responsibility with regard to space and facilities is to make such allocations and, if limits exist in relation to the space provided, to make those limits realistic and clearly understood by the toddler.* Consistent enforcement of these limits is important so toddlers know where the boundaries are and need not worry about whether they are inside or outside their limits "this time."

Toddlers' responsibilities in achieving the family task of allocation of space and facilities are to learn to enjoy and discover their world within whatever space their parents can grant them, to incorporate a respect for whatever limits are imposed, and attempt to comply with them. Children's motivation to comply arises from a desire to please their parents; therefore, they are more likely to continue compliance if their cooperation is acknowledged and praised occasionally.

Childproofing

Each new move to independence in a child's life is an intrusion into his parents' life, and parents become especially conscious of this intrusion when their baby begins toddling after them at their every step and toward every precious possession in their home. Their message—that this is the baby's home, too—comes through loud and clear once the child has achieved even amateur mobility (crawling and pulling himself up). This is the time for parents to make a careful study of the home for environmental hazards and possible relocation of precious possessions. They need to become aware that special vigilance and firm discipline can prevent accidental injury to their child.

Although some families choose to leave the home unaltered and teach their toddler what he or she may handle and what must be left alone, most families opt

*Toddlers live in the present, having not yet developed the ability to recall the past or anticipate the future conceptually. They need frequent reminders in simple terms, not a one-time discussion.

for at least minimal childproofing. Ideally, every home with a toddler is childproofed at least to the extent that medicines and poisonous or corrosive items are not available to the child. The less childproofing there is, the more continuous watchful surveillance is necessary to ensure the toddler's safety.

The need to include vigilance for defining characteristics of the nursing diagnoses *potential for injury: falls; potential for injury: poisoning;* and *potential for injury: suffocation/aspiration* as the child grows and develops was introduced in the previous chapter. This need becomes critical in the toddler group. In this age group more deaths occur from accidents than from any other cause. Nurses can use their assessment data to assist the parent in childproofing the home.

Parents must see that childproofing plans are carried out and periodically re-evaluated in light of their toddlers' progressive motor skills (eventually they will climb, unscrew caps, open latches, and unlock doors). Whatever limits are to exist must be communicated to all family members and to any of the toddler's caregivers during parental absences. Enforcement of limits should be consistently enacted, especially because the child's safety may be at stake.

Anticipatory Guidance: Resources

Because the behaviors and developmental skills of the toddler are so drastically different from those of the infant, family members may need guidance in understanding their toddlers. As in all nurse-family interactions nurses should include in their ongoing assessment awareness of cues suggesting a diagnosis of *knowledge deficit.* If the nurse determines that a knowledge deficit exists, he or she must establish the cause of the knowledge deficit before planning strategies. As in all situations in which knowledge is lacking, interventions must be directed toward the cause. If the cause is a simple lack of familiarity with necessary information, the nursing intervention will focus on education. The approach the nurse uses to accomplish this educational process is dependent to a large extent on the value emphasis (persons or material possessions) of the family. Therefore, a significantly important initial task of the nurse is to make observations and ask questions to assess the family's philosophy. This assessment not only will help the nurse identify what teaching approach will be most appropriate for the family, but also will provide guidance about the likely

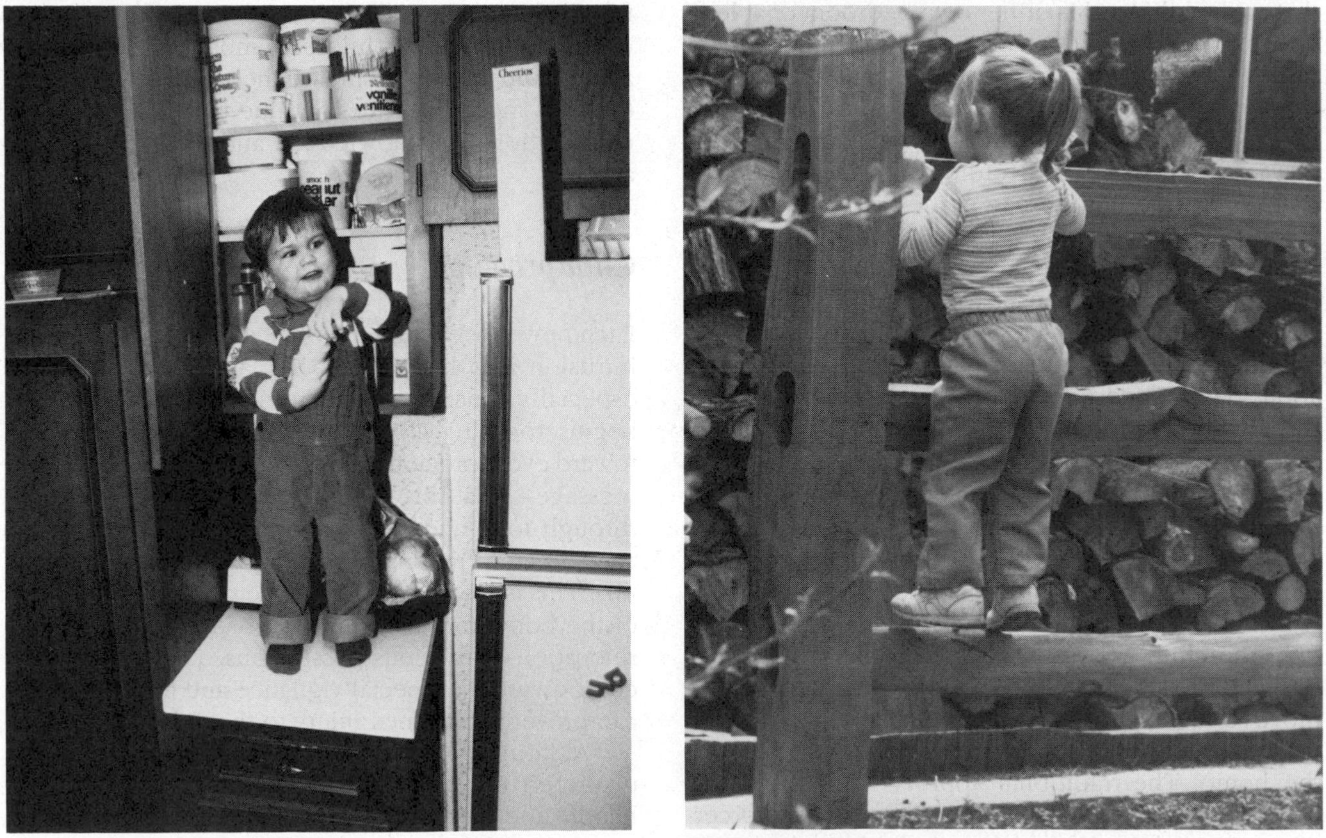

A B

(A) Toddlers' ability to climb places a new emphasis on childproofing the home.
(B) Climbing ability extends to objects outdoors as well and calls for caregiver vigilance.

potential areas of conflict. For example, the family that values material goods is going to experience more stress relative to childproofing and the toddler's innate manipulative curiosity than a family that values personal development. The philosophy held will also influence how the family accepts and nurtures the toddler's attempts at self hood.

One of the most critical aspects of teaching with the family of a toddler is related to providing information regarding the toddler's rapid (almost daily) developmental advances. Because development is still occurring at such a rapid pace, parent education will involve anticipatory guidance in relation to the multiple issues with which they will be presented. Safety risks associated with that rapid development, especially motor development, must be emphasized. The nurse may also be a useful resource to families in helping them assess their space needs (physical, emotional, and social) and in facilitating innovative problem solving that is realistic for the family budget. Acquainting the family with community resources to assist them in adapting their own resources to the needs of their toddler and family life is often needed.

Reorganizing Relationships to Encompass a Toddler

Family relationships are particularly in need of attention during the toddler years. Keeping up with a busy toddler requires distribution of labor resources to avoid energy depletion in one or more members. The increasing assertiveness and vocal participation of the toddler in family interactions places stress on parents, requiring attention to maintaining the parents' relationship or securing social support for the single parent. As the toddler's mobility increases, his or her world expands. Additional resources become essential to the toddler's safety and development. All these factors cause attention to be focused on the out-of-home environment and relative relationships.

Division of Labor to Avoid Energy Depletion

The family with a toddler is at particular risk for energy depletion in one or more of its members. (The mother or primary caregiver is by far the most frequent victim.) Any combination of the following dynamics is usually in play to cause energy depletion:

1. Toddlers work hard to get what they want; they are into everything. Exploring is their work, and the more stimulated they get, the more they like it. They will pursue such stimulation to the point of exhausting their caregivers and themselves, if not directed periodically into quiet activities.

2. When their routine is changed (friends visit and the usual nap is delayed), ritualistic toddlers find it difficult to handle this breach in their security. Family members around them can feel emotionally drained and exhausted just trying to satiate a frustrated child.

3. Because of the toddler's need to "check in" frequently, the parent has little opportunity for privacy or solitude, let alone the opportunity to pursue favorite activities. Even being alone in the bathroom becomes a challenge.

4. If the parent is employed outside the home, he or she is carrying a double load. Meeting the needs of a hungry, cranky toddler picked up from day care just as the employed person would like to relax and unwind from his or her own day can set up an explosive or dangerous situation. Toddlers (in a nuclear family) are still likely to make most of their demands upon the mother when she is around, especially during early childhood when they have not completely separated their identity from that of their mother.

5. If the division of labor is not equalized among spouse and older siblings, the mother's household responsibilities, along with the care of a busy toddler, may be quite heavy.

6. If family income is low, either or both parents may be undernourished or have other health problems because they cannot afford adequate food or medical attention for themselves.

7. The mother may be pregnant again or caring for a completely dependent infant as well as the toddler.

8. If the toddler and an older sibling or siblings share a room or even the same bed, the sleep patterns of one may interrupt or disturb the sleep of the others.* A nursing diagnosis of *sleep-pattern disturbance* is a real possibility for any member of a family with a toddler.

If the family has not developed coping mechanisms that allow healthy adaptation to any one or more of these circumstances, some member(s) of the family will eventually become chronically fatigued. When physical or emotional energy is depleted, family relationships will inevitably suffer, with potentially serious long-term results.

All these factors that contribute to energy depletion are also factors that can lead to ineffective coping. If one family member is unable to cope because of excessive demands resulting from this family developmental crisis, the result can be *ineffective family coping: compromised or disabling.* The nurse who is vigi-

*Toddlers sometimes display sleep problems in the form of waking and crying out at night or experiencing frightening dreams. They may require a night light to sleep. All these factors can interrupt the sleep of older siblings in close proximity.

lant for defining characteristics of these diagnoses can plan interventions that will result instead in the positive nursing diagnosis of *family coping: potential for growth.*

Special effort should be made to allow each family member opportunity for individual interests and stimuli. Morale and energy maintenance are two areas in which families often need assistance. The nurse is a valuable resource to the family in helping them to see where the imbalances lie and in helping them identify resources to resolve those imbalances. *A child's assessment is complete only if it includes an appraisal of the physical and emotional status of the people he or she relies on for care.*

Certainly the toddler is the most vulnerable family member and should be given first priority in terms of nursing assessment and intervention. But next in priority should be the caregiver (usually the mother), who is at greatest risk of energy depletion.

Physical energy status can be evaluated by investigating for any potentially debilitating conditions.* The caregiver's developmental status in relation to age should be investigated to determine if energy is being drained to handle more than one developmental level at once, such as a teenage mother handling simultaneous tasks of identity, intimacy, and generativity. Sleep patterns should be checked to see if any sleep extremes (under four hours a night, over 10 hours a night) exist on a regular basis. Weight should be evaluated in relation to height and eating patterns assessed to identify any distortions (inadequate intake, unbalanced diet) which interfere with physical well-being and deplete energy. An obvious, but frequently overlooked, assessment of the caregiver's general appearance should be made with particular attention to the eyes, posture, and gaze.

Emotional energy status should include an evaluation of the caregiver's experience with his or her parents as a child. The question most likely to get a useful response is, "How were you punished as a child?" The caregiver needs to be evaluated for signs of postpartum or clinical depression,† such as listlessness, tense affect, body language suggesting anxiety or withdrawal, and negative body image. Just listening to the full meaning of the caregiver's comments gives the nurse a perspective on whether his or her attitude is primarily positive or negative. The nurse should be alert, over time, to any deterioration in the caregiver's apparent level of understanding and comprehension. A nurse who visits a caregiver's home should be alert to an environment there that is either chaotic or relentlessly clean, as both are danger signals of emotional energy depletion.

All parents should be helped to realize that there will surely be bad days, even in the most smooth-running household, when there is a busy toddler around. And they should be helped to see that they have a number of options available to them when the bad days occur from which they can select without guilt. For instance, when the mother is at her wits' end, she could opt for any one of these solutions that best suit her situation and resources. She can get a sitter and leave for a time; forget about any tasks she planned to accomplish that day and indulge herself and her toddler in some unwinding, just-for-fun activities; take a walk with her toddler. Even in the rain this activity is refreshing to the spirit of most of us, especially with the delightfully curious toddler at our side to help us see the world from a fresh perspective. Or she can call a friend to come support her and share her day or select from any other options that will relieve boredom, change the scene, or put embattled relationships into a different perspective.

Nurses whose focus is on the child and his or her family will see the significance of identifying families at risk for energy depletion of one or more members. They are motivated to help members of that family build their confidence and coping capacity by praising them in their healthy efforts and backing them in the options they choose. These nurses will initiate a plan of care that has as its goal helping the family learn to problem-solve by focusing on their actual or potential stress, to recognize that options exist to resolve or minimize that stress, to select that option with which they are most comfortable and to carry it through.

Division of Labor to Include the Toddler

Many parents are hesitant about assigning responsibilities to their toddlers. Some put off making such demands out of fear they will be accused by friends and relatives of passing their own duties along to the children. Others delay because they feel unable to find the time or patience that instruction for responsibility requires. But children are not born responsible; they have to learn responsibility.

There are some times at which it is easier to teach responsibility than at other times. The opportune time for teaching toddlers responsibility is when they first show signs of willingness and readiness to do things for themselves. Whether youngsters are 1 or 2 or 3 years old, they should be given responsibilities as they convey their readiness for dressing and caring for themselves, for looking after their own possessions, for doing small tasks around the house. This is how they learn a healthy attitude toward doing their part.

---

*Elevated blood pressure; hemoglobulin under 12 grams; pain of any intensity or duration; bleeding of any type; acute or chronic infections; any generalized medical problem such as diabetes, asthma, or a cardiac condition.

†Depression is clinical if the caregiver forgets to perform child care, essentially being so drained emotionally that he or she forgets that the baby or toddler exists.

The work toddlers do is not as important as the sense of responsibility they acquire. And learning this early helps them establish proper relationships with society as they mature. Toddlers, like all of us, need to feel the tasks they are performing are necessary and helpful and not merely busy-work routines. To toddlers work is another form of play. Therefore, responsibility introduced in the toddler years helps them recognize early that work can be pleasant.

Many toddlers display an early interest in wanting to work with Mommy and Daddy. Parents should respond to this readiness for responsibility in home chores. Toddlers are not too young to learn to put away toys, empty trashbaskets, run simple errands inside the home, or put away papers and magazines. With assistance they can do a satisfactory job of dusting, watering houseplants, setting the table, or drying unbreakable dishes. They find the opportunity to help bake or fill the shopping cart a delightful experience. At this early age, of course, youngsters seldom do a perfect job; and they also tend to lose interest quickly. But parents who exercise tolerance with these early endeavors will find teaching much easier as the child grows older.

Toddlers need specific instructions when asked to do a task. "Clean up your room" means little to them, so they will be unlikely to act. If they are asked to put their toys on the shelf and put the clothes they took off in the laundry basket, toddlers usually cooperate enthusiastically.

The toddler feels amply rewarded for his or her efforts if given a hug or a big smile and told "Thank you for helping me" or "You did a good job." Just as important as praise, at this stage of developing autonomy, is recognition of the toddler's independent accomplishment. Statements such as "You did that" or "You did it all by yourself" provide reinforcement that is appropriate to the developmental tasks of the toddler stage. Permitting children to take on responsibility at home makes them feel useful in an environment that accepts them for who they are, supports what they are becoming, and helps them cope with what they cannot be.

Relationships and Involvement Outside the Home

Parents of an infant tend to temporarily withdraw from activities involving social interactions away from home. But by the time these parents have a toddler, they are rediscovering the need to maintain relationships and involvements beyond their child and family. However, retaining some satisfying contacts with friends and personal interests away from home can be a rather complicated matter when there are small children. External activities, once spontaneously followed, now must be planned ahead and arrangements made for a babysitter. The trouble associated with getting the child cared for and paying for this service is so difficult for many parents that they tend to give up and stay home.

Some innovative parents have found numerous options available to them, with a little cooperation from others in the same circumstance as they. One option is to develop social relationships with other parents who have young children and take turns entertaining in each other's homes. These same parents might arrange a reciprocal child care agreement, whereby one parent watches the other's child or children so that parent can do something special and then the favor is exchanged at another time. Mothers (or fathers) who are full-time caregivers may arrange to "take turns" watching each other's child or children so that each can get away regularly to pursue personal interests or just enjoy a quiet morning at home alone. Such breaks in child care are refreshing, renewing energy for continued child care and for other significant relationships.

Some churches and synagogues provide nurseries for small children during services and social events. In those that do not, many parents have gotten together and agreed to take turns managing a children's nursery for these times, so that the other parents can participate without the interruptions of their infant or toddler.

Times away from home as a whole family can be an exhilarating break from routine, too. A trip to the zoo or beach, a family picnic, an outing to a movie or musical production can be a refreshing and uniting experience. Neighborhood get-togethers that include the whole family, church or synagogue events, and other community activities suitable to the family's life stage are all feasible options to home confinement.

Accepting Help with Appreciation and Maturity

The tasks of the family with a toddler are not easily achieved and, owing to the rapidity with which the toddler develops, most families find themselves in an atmosphere of urgency, during which time they feel a need for increased support and guidance, whether from relatives and neighbors (grandparents become important resources again), from health and child care professionals, or from all these sources. The nursing diagnosis *altered family process* is defined as "inability of family system (household members) to meet needs of members, carry out family functions, or maintain communications for mutual growth and maturation" (Gordon, 1987). The family with a toddler is in a developmental phase with a high potential for the occurrence of altered family process. Often this problem can be resolved by assisting family members to explore and accept outside help in dealing with their situation.* Most parents are willing to make use of any outside help that will enrich what they have to offer their child or the family group, but only if they are allowed to retain their parenting responsibilities throughout the helping situation. The acceptance of help is made easier if a family's philosophy recognizes the basic interdependence of all people.

The first step in accepting help is to acknowledge those areas of family life in which limitations exist. Then the family can draw on those outside resources that enhance existing strengths and those that will help strengthen weak spots (lack of knowledge, communication breakdown, chronic illness). Utilizing outside support systems such as relatives, helping professionals, self-help support groups, or government aid programs can help build and maintain internal support systems (members themselves, their skills, their caring), making life as a family with a toddler a happy, growth-producing experience.

Anticipatory Guidance: Relationships

Many parents at this stage need help anticipating their child's new skills, identifying his or her readiness for new experiences or responsibility, and learning how they can cope with the child's developing personality. These parents will be primarily interested in the teaching and anticipatory guidance a nurse can offer them in those areas. Nurses who are effective with children and their families will have learned that a parent so enlightened is more cooperative and will evidence that learning by affording parents every possible opportunity to question and to be taught. Nurses may also be involved in helping the family recognize their strengths and limitations in the management of the tasks of this stage. They can assist the family to find ways to successfully accomplish the tasks that cause difficulty by offering them useful information that will help them move forward, by referring them to resources or support systems that can help them correct limitations to task achievement, and by reinforcing the efforts they are making to grow and develop as a family unit through praise, encouragement, and advocacy of their needs and rights.

In some situations the nurse's relationship with the toddler will be as a parent surrogate. At such times, he or she should reinforce those routines, parenting methods, affectional demonstrations, and self-care expectations that the child is accustomed to from the parents. Knowledge of these factors should be learned from the nurse's assessment and integrated into the plan of care.

*Inability to accept and receive help is a defining characteristic of *alteration in family process.*

Rework Family Philosophy to Incorporate Parenthood and Children

Managing this task involves continuing to find satisfaction in parenthood as the baby becomes a toddler, resolving the developmental task conflicts of parents and toddler, providing for healthy independence among family members, and planning for future children.

Deriving Satisfaction from Parenthood

Many parents today take parenthood seriously—they plan, they read, they keep their family size small so they can do a good job. They feel a stronger sense of obligation to do the parenting themselves. After a year they have begun to feel like parents and find that people perceive them that way. They have learned how to care for an infant and find some predictability in living with him or her. They have come to know their partner as a parent. And they have seen how society really treats families. Their parenthood is still fragile, a "work in progress," but it is more than they had before.

But now they have a toddler who changes faster than at any other time outside the womb. This series of developmental changes can provide a constant feast of fun for both parents and toddler—new words, new movements, new games, new self-care skills are an almost daily experience. The parents' satisfaction or frustration during this period depends largely on their confidence and the love, care, and attention they can give the child. Children can be a ticket back to fantasy and wonder if their parents pause and enjoy their children's new exploits. The child can now offer parents a reciprocal relationship of shared love and pleasure, bringing satisfaction in being together.

But the parental task of realistically balancing the needs and demands of this active child with the expectations of a spouse or significant other and commitments to their own personhood can leave the best intentioned parent with some bouts of ambivalence toward parenthood. Some of the ambivalent feelings experienced by parents stem not from the fact that they sometimes do not like their child or children so much, but from not knowing how to cope with either the child or the whole juggling act just described. One study demonstrated that mothers who had been rejected as children and who received little support from the father after the birth of a child were more likely to parent their toddlers in angry, punitive ways (Crockenberg, 1987). Unfortunately, this kind of parenting seems more likely to be associated with angry, noncompliant behavior in the child. During this exciting but critical period of development, parents need all the help, reinforcement, and information available so that their relationship with their toddler will be mutually satisfying and rewarding.

Toddlers' tasks in supporting their parents' satisfaction with parenthood are instinctual. They will respond to the satisfaction they feel in their parents' care with unconditional love and a physical freedom timed to revive the mother and father from even their deepest doubts. Children's shows of affection and enthusiasm for their parents is a mirrored reflection of what they sense they are receiving from their parents—and most parents find no better reward for their efforts.

This kind of reciprocal satisfaction between parents and toddlers is facilitated by cooperation between them. Part of the family's task is to learn how to cooperate with each other. Each side must be prepared to give and take appropriately. Although the parents make allowances for the demands of their toddlers, toddlers must learn that their demands will not always be in the best interests of the family.

Discipline

Parents play a major role in fostering a sense of family cooperation in their toddlers. A major portion of this task involves the ability to provide direct, purposeful discipline. Parents may be hesitant about this task, unconsciously fearing that discipline will prove traumatic to the child. The important thing they need to realize is that discipline is necessary to healthy growth and development. They may be dismayed when they realize that discipline contributes to a change in the child's image of them. Images of exclusively loving parents are gradually replaced by images of parents who make demands and punish as well as reward. It is helpful to remind parents that the ambivalence that this change in image creates in the child is a necessary step in the independence and separation process confronting him or her.

Discipline should be differentiated from punishment. Punishment involves the application of unpleasant or painful consequences as a response to wrongdoing. Discipline involves training for the purpose of enforcing the rules of conduct. Parents provide discipline so that their children may learn how to conduct themselves appropriately in their environment.

Toddlers are actively involved in testing their ability to function independently. They are single-mindedly preoccupied with asserting this independence; however, they have not learned their own limits or those of their environment. Discipline for toddlers involves setting limits for them to preserve their safety and to ensure the rights of others. This kind of discipline is based on love.

An important prerequisite for discipline based on love is that children have learned to trust. Their ability to follow parental rules of conduct is motivated by their desire to please based on the love, warmth, and trust they experience in their relationships with their parents, and their tendency to imitate. The more positive the parent-child relationship, the less likely toddlers are to thwart their parents' disciplinary efforts. Parents who have a positive relationship with their children do not need to resort to external rewards for good behavior.

The young child needs and wants only simple rewards—attention, approval, a smile, and some kind words. The toddler does not yet recognize the value the world places on material things and does not want or find meaning in material rewards.

Parents also need to share with the child their feelings about the child's behavior. Even when children are too young to understand the meaning of the words, they still understand a lot from the tone of voice and facial expressions that accompany the spoken words. Disapproval can be communicated to the young child without being physical. Research has indicated that physical punishment of toddlers is probably not effective in teaching compliance to rules and impulse control (Hammer and Drabman, 1981; Power and Chapieski, 1986). As one mother said, ". . . handling my own anger by screaming myself hoarse and slapping the smallest person in reach does not teach my child self-control or discipline. All it teaches is fear, submission, and the idea that if you eat all your greens, you'll grow up to be big enough to slug your own kid someday" (Hyde, 1980). Talking does take more time than physical punishment, but it requires thinking. As a result, the parents think through acceptable behavior and sensible limits while they are calm and reasonable instead of at a time when they are angry or tired. It is as important to express approval when rules are followed as it is to express disapproval when they are not.

The main reason for discipline during toddlerhood is to protect the child from accident or harm. Therein lies an important reason for parents to remain calm about discipline. The less often they have to express anger, the more impression it will make when they do. It is at moments of danger that the parent wants to be heard and obeyed promptly; angry behavior is best reserved for such moments.

Parents should approach discipline with a firm, consistent approach. Toddlers will test limits to see if they are firm. Consistency on the part of the parents will allow the toddler to know what to expect in a situation. Toddlers cannot be expected to know that rules can change when parents are busy, overworked, or tired. Thus, if rules are going to be changed on a given day, it is best to say so. Even young children can adjust to such changes as long as they do not occur too often. They will feel good about trying to be especially well behaved to help their parents out.

Children learn at a young age that getting in trouble gets them attention. As a result children will act out to get attention if they feel they are being neglected or otherwise ignored. Parents need to consciously offer attention when their children are behaving, so that less time needs to be spent responding to misbehavior. Toddlerhood is not too young to also begin learning that parents have needs and rights too. Parents should help their child learn this by explaining their needs (e.g., privacy, quiet) and then asserting these rights when needed. Box 6-1 summarizes guidelines for disciplining the toddler. See pages 272 to 284 of this chapter for a discussion of emotional-social development and related discipline.

Resolving Developmental Task Conflicts

Spouses in the family unit with a toddler are immersed in the task of maintaining intimacy while expanding their parental capacity to accept the growth and development of their child or children, acknowledge the child's emerging self-hood and recognize his or her teachable moments. Toddlers are working through the transition from babyhood to childhood by developing the autonomy necessary to control their bodies and their will.

This stage in the family life cycle seems full of paradoxes. Having just become settled in and comfortable as parents, the spouses find new and more difficult roles now emerge—those of limit setter, guide, and teacher. These new parental roles involve much patience; the parent must accept the child's individual pace, let him or her make mistakes and learn from them, and accept a role as assistant to rather than director of the child's activities. Some of the decisions to be made now are clear-cut, but most are not. When there are two parents, they must agree on a form of discipline that is logical, consistent, and comfortable without causing damage to the child's physical, intellectual, or emotional-social development.

The ways in which the parents resolve their conflicts and the ways they interact with each other are imitated by toddlers, who use these observations in a hundred ways to cope with their personal processes of self-development. Parents best handle the conflicts of this stage when they

- remember that their child's rebellion, expressed by contrariness, is temporary and normal and that what often appears to be destructive behavior is simply the child's curiosity in action;
- agree on democratic, shared parenting;
- support each other in their role shifts;
- work out realistic ways for each to fulfill some personal or career interests;
- learn to approach each other and their child or children positively, encouraging desirable actions through compliments and rewards for well-intentioned efforts.

Daily family rituals are also invaluable means of providing a workable daily routine that eases conflict while giving family members a sense of order, security, and satisfaction in living together.

> Box 6-1
> *Guidelines for Effective Discipline*
>
> Focus on only one or two rules of conduct at a time.
>
> Express disapproval of misconduct verbally and through tone of voice.
>
> Express approval when rules of conduct are followed.
>
> Save expressions of anger for situations which pose a threat of accident or harm to the child.
>
> Be firmly consistent in enforcing rules.
>
> If the rules must change, tell the child.

Healthy Independence Among Members

Living together with enough harmony to allow expression of a variety of feelings, enough cooperation to permit each individual self-fulfillment in his or her developmental tasks, and enough open communication to condone each member's assertion of independence and self-hood or uniqueness requires a family to be in a continuous adaptive state. Having established itself as a unit that can incorporate children and having accepted the entailed responsibilities, the family group with a toddler is now faced with the task of finding parenting patterns that meet the needs of both parents and active, mobile children and of establishing enough freedom for each member so that age-appropriate independence is possible.

This freedom for independent development in a family finds its origin in the parental relationship. Spouses who are mature enough to allow each other independent social and recreational or hobby pursuits are much more likely to recognize and permit the individual endeavors of their children. Trust in the family member's motives is at the heart of such freedom. This trust provides the security necessary to "let go" of the family member and allow him or her to develop uniqueness. In his research, Kirkpatrick (1963) found evidence that children are more independent in their activities when they can rely on (trust) parental affections. The same factor undoubtedly holds true in husband-wife independence. A spouse who knows he or she can count on a partner's affection is more likely to grant freedom in the relationship for pursuit of personal happiness.

No parents at their first child's birth would ever dream that within one brief year that child would already be beginning to insist on "being on his way to his own fulfillment." But such is the case as the infant of about a year takes those first steps that bring him or her to the doorstep of toddlerhood. In conveying their respect for toddlers' self-hood or fulfillment activities, parents certainly want to let them be as grown up as they can be without pushing them too quickly out of babyhood. Parental respect for the developing toddler's individual efforts must be focused on three aspects of this activity: (1) the child's need to explore; (2) the child's need to learn self-control of body functions and emotional expression; and (3) the child's need to develop an identity that will accommodate childhood rather than infancy. Refer to pages 272 to 275 of this chapter for further discussion of the balances between dependence and independence and the impact of separation of the toddler and family unit.

Planning Future Children

The family with a toddler has already made the decision for parenthood; the question before them now is how much parenthood. The best reason for having another child, in fact the only valid reason, is because it is truly wanted. However, the financial implications of another child are a crucial consideration. Other factors parents weigh against their desire for another child are the amount of emotional and physical energy they have to offer another child; their career goals; their ages, particularly the mother's; whether their lifestyle would accommodate another child; their feelings about family size; and, if the toddler was their first, the pros and cons of raising an only child.

If after evaluation of these factors a family decides to have another child, the next important consideration is spacing between children. It is best, from the standpoint of developmental needs of both the children and the parents, not to have children less than three years apart. This three-year spacing makes a dramatic difference in the lives of the toddler and his or her sibling. Older toddlers will have more maturity to cope constructively with their resentment of the tiny intruder, they will be developing more out-of-home interests (nursery school, peer play) with much less focus on their caregiver, which means displacement at home costs considerably less than if the toddlers were younger. Studies have shown that significantly more rivalry exists when there is less than three years between sibs; that the closer the spacing is, the more excessive is the stress to the marital relationship; and that there is a much greater emotional drain on all family members with closer spacing. (Duvall, 1977; White, 1975; Yarrow, 1979). An age gap of at least three years between children allows more enjoyable experiences for all involved. And a parent whose children are happy is also happier and vice versa.

Most professionals involved with children believe that each child should be wanted before it is born, and this is most readily ensured if parents are helped to plan their families without prohibition of marital sexual relations. The nurse is frequently the source first sought for information and guidance in this matter and, if parents do not initiate requests for assistance, the nurse has many opportunities to determine their need and offer aid. This assessment is merited from the standpoint of its significant effect on the toddler, unborn children, and the family as a whole. Whether the pediatric nurse offers assistance directly or through resource referral, the nurse's main concern is that the family understand the benefits of spacing and that the method of family planning chosen is congruent with the family's philosophy, attitudes, and values.

If by decision or accident another child is expected in the home with a toddler, certain additional tasks are demanded of family members. Parents must consider how to realistically involve their toddler in preparation and planning for the new family member. Preparation, especially for the very young toddler, should not begin too far in advance. One to two months before the new baby's due date is usually an optimal time to begin preparing the toddler. Because toddlers are so ritualistic, the manner in which they are prepared should stress how things will remain the same, to include the fact that "Mommy and Daddy will love you just the same as always." Toddlers should be told very simply what babies are like. If they know that "babies cry a lot and need to be fed and have their pants changed," the attention given to the baby to meet these needs will not seem as much like an invasion of their territory.

If the toddler will be giving up his or her crib for the new baby, the move to a new bed should be made well in advance of the birth of the new baby. An early move to a new bed can be a very positive "graduation" experience in which the child takes pride, rather than a negative experience in which the older child might feel displaced in favor of the new arrival. If the toddler is not toilet trained, instituting training close to the time that a new baby is introduced into the household is not advisable. It is not unusual for toddlers to regress to soiling themselves after the new baby has arrived.

Toddlers can participate in simple ways in the physical preparations, perhaps a month or so before the baby comes. The infant crib, the blankets, the baby clothes, and doll play help to initiate them into the upcoming event. The toddler will probably cleave to the mother as her due date draws near. Children at this age should have opportunity to become accustomed to their substitute caregivers before time of the hospitalization. Toddlers do best if kept at home during this separation and may be comforted if given some physical token of their mother. They are also comforted by frequent confirmation of where their mothers are and by the daily homecomings of their father.

Toddlers and young preschool-age children have increased problem behaviors after a new sibling is born. Problem areas include toileting, demands for bottles, clinginess, and displays of anxiety and aggression (Dunn and Kendrick, 1980; Field and Reite, 1984; Stewart et al, 1987). These behaviors tend to decrease over time, but parents will need to know that their children need assistance in adjusting to the new baby once it is brought home.

The nurse in contact with the family before the baby arrives is in a good position to help parents anticipate the adjustments that the infant's siblings will need to make when the baby is born. Some hospitals have created sibling-to-be programs in which the preschooler can learn what life will be like with the new baby (Honig, 1986). Whether or not a formal program for prospective siblings is in place, the nurse can help the parents to understand the importance of their attitudes and responses to the older children and can offer concrete suggestions for easing the child's transition into a sibling role.

Examples of such suggestions follow:

- Do not assume that the siblings will be overjoyed upon meeting the infant. Their more immediate concern is the well-being of the mother.
- It is helpful to have the father or another person carry the new baby into the house when mother and baby return home from the hospital. This allows the mother to give her undivided attention to the older children from whom she has been separated.
- Expect some negative reactions or jealous responses from the infant's siblings and express understanding about how they are feeling.
- Expect from the older children some regressive behavior more typical of an earlier stage of development when no baby was around to interfere with their relationships with their parents.
- Express interest in the older child's activities and ideas and try to spend time with each child away from the baby.
- Allow the siblings to enter into baby care and interaction as much as they care to, but set clearly understood limits as to what is safe behavior with an infant.
- Recognize that negative feelings about the baby may be expressed months after the baby's arrival.
- Avoid instituting new and possibly stressful developmental learning experiences, such as toilet training, in the period after bringing a new baby into the home.

The toddler's adjustment to the new baby does not depend so much on advance information as on a thoughtfully planned protection of his or her sense of status and prestige by the parents. The child's status does change, however, and the toddler's task is to find ways to cope with the status of being a sibling that reinforce rather than harm the child's fragile identity. Owing to the child's immature emotional state, he or she will need the parents' guidance and love to be successful.

When the siblings are of school age and older, the responses of their peers to the baby's birth are significant to them and affect their own responses to the sibling role. If the newborn is more than 10 years younger than the sibling, some embarrassment about the sexual connotations of birth may be a part of the sibling's response. Frequently, older siblings prove to be delighted to have a baby in the home. Parents should be alerted, however, not to expect parental behavior of older siblings; parents should protect the privacy of the older siblings and the safety of their possessions from the infant's explorations when the time comes.

The nurse can do much to promote effective family coping when a new baby is born. Guidelines for preparing a child for the new sibling are presented in Box 6-2. In addition to those interventions already discussed, the nurse should be aware of the many fine books that are available to facilitate coping in children when a new sibling is brought into the home. Gates (1980) and Honig (1986) provided excellent summaries of representative books (Box 6-3).

Anticipatory Guidance: Satisfaction with Parenthood

The nurse and other health professionals working with parents of toddlers can significantly influence the satisfaction parents get from parenting. Awareness of stressors that can interfere with the ability to parent effectively will assist the nurse in promoting *family coping: potential for growth* while avoiding *alterations in parenting* and subsequent *ineffective family coping* and *alteration in family process.* Nurses must

> Box 6-2
> *Preparing the Toddler for a New Baby*
>
> Prepare about 1 to 2 months ahead of time.
> Maintain the child's rituals.
> Stress how things will remain the same.
> Tell the toddler what babies are like.
> Introduce the child to a new bed early.
> Do not toilet train late in the pregnancy.
> Allow the toddler to help prepare the baby's things.
> Introduce the child to the substitute caregiver early.

Box 6-3
Selected References for Helping the Child Adjust to a New Baby

Nobody Asked Me If I Wanted a Baby Sister. (M. Alexander) New York, Dial Books for Young Readers, 1977.
Oliver, who is jealous of his baby sister Bonnie, tries to give her away. When he finds someone who will take her, she cries and cries. Oliver is the only person who can console her. He decides that she is smarter than he thought, and he happily takes her home.

When the New Baby Comes, I'm Moving Out. (M. Alexander.) New York, Dial Books for Young Readers, 1981.
In this companion book for *Nobody Asked Me If I Wanted a Baby Sister,* Oliver sees many of his old things such as his crib are being given to his new sibling. He is upset because he was not asked, and he feels displaced. After trying to throw his mother away, he decides to run away. When his mother tells him how special it is to be a "big brother," Oliver decides to stay home.

Billy and Our New Baby. (H. Arnstein.) New York, Human Sciences Press, 1973.
This book demonstrates how parents can cope with a child's verbal and physical responses to the arrival of a new baby. Billy shows off for his mother, but she does not seem to notice. Therefore, he assumes she loves the baby more than she loves him. He suggests she take the baby back to the hospital. Mother recognizes his feelings for what they are and explains that other boys and girls feel as he does when a new baby comes into the family. Later when Billy tries to push the baby away, his mother tells him she will not allow that behavior because she would not let anyone hurt Billy either.

Billy regresses somewhat; he begins crawling, creeping, and wanting a bottle. His mother copes with Billy's reactions by reminding him that being a big boy is more fun. Eventually Billy realizes that it is more fun to be big and starts helping his mother do things that an infant cannot. "But Billy still got mad at the new baby at times. Sometimes he got mad for good reasons and sometimes just because the baby made him angry."

The New Baby. (S. Berenstain and J. Berenstain.) New York, Random House, 1974.
This simple story shows that one very important advantage of having a new baby is being a big sibling. The child bear is just getting ready to move into his new bed when the baby bear arrives.

Go and Hush the Baby. (B.C. Byars.) New York, Penguin, 1982.
A young boy imaginatively attempts to quiet his crying baby brother by singing songs and performing music—all to no avail. Finally, he tells a tale about a prince and princess, and this impressive story puts his brother to sleep.

The Wonderful Story of How You Were Born. (S.H. Gruenberg.) Garden City, NY, Doubleday, 1970.
This story discusses fertilization, pregnancy, and birth. The text is simple and the pictures are soft and appealing. The real facts are presented clearly to create a healthy attitude toward sexuality and birth. For 3- to 4-year-olds, the pictures may encourage questions; for older children, the story can be read aloud or to themselves.

A Baby Sister for Frances. (R. Hoban.) New York, Harper & Row, 1976.
Frances, who is jealous of her new sister Gloria, "runs away" by hiding under the dining room table. Her mother and father miss her and talk about the specialness of being a "big sister." Frances returns to her family a happier sibling.

We Are Having a Baby. (V. Holland.) New York, Charles Scribner's Sons, 1972.
This story is a true narration by a 4-year-old about pregnancy, birth, and the new baby. Through a series of actual photographs, the child's feeling and eventually her acceptance of the new baby are portrayed. When the new baby comes home, Dana has a sad feeling in her stomach, but after she helps feed her brother, she begins to feel better.

Peter's Chair. (E.J. Keats.) New York, Harper & Row Publishers. 1983.
Peter believes that all of his possessions are being taken away and given to his baby sister. He takes his baby chair and runs away. Surprised to find out that he is too big for his chair, he begins to accept his new role as big brother by helping his father paint the chair bright pink for his sister.

Too Big (H. Keller.) New York, Greenwillow Books, 1983.
When he attempts to be like his baby brother, Henry repeatedly is told he is too big. The story depicts the difficult task the older child faces when becoming a big sibling. It is told touchingly and with humor, and young children will identify with Henry.

Mom and Dad and I Are Having A Baby! (M. Malecki.) Seattle, The Pennypress, 1979.
This book prepares children to attend the birth of a sibling. It is written honestly and openly and can be enjoyed by children of all ages.

My Mom's Having a Baby. (E. Rushnell.) New York, The Putnam Publishing Group, 1978.
Based on a television special, this book is written for the older child (preferably reading age). Both photographs and cartoons accompany the lengthy text.

That New Baby. (S.B. Stein.) New York, Walker, 1974.
This unique book is designed with separate texts for the child and the adult. The adult text serves as a resource for answering questions that may arise spontaneously as the child's text is read aloud. It presents many of the common sentiments of the older child, including jealousy, anger, distrust, disappointment, separation, and confusion.

Betsy's Baby Brother. (G. Wolde.) New York, Random House, 1982.
This short story is simply written with very colorful and uncomplicated pictures. The book describes Betsy's reaction to her baby brother, including anger, jealousy, and fantasies about being a baby. She begins to realize that she can do many things that her baby brother cannot. The story ends on a happy note.

Other good children's books about sibling rivalry are *She Come Bringing Me That Little Baby Girl.* (E. Greenfield.) Philadelphia, JB Lippincott, 1974, and *The Knee Baby.* (M. Jarrell.) New York. Farrar, Straus, and Giroux, 1973.

(Compiled from Gates, 1980; and Honig, 1986.)

continue to be vigilant in their assessment for the defining characteristics of these nursing diagnoses. If the assessment reveals strengths in parenting, family coping, and family process the nurse will be able to reinforce those strengths and potentiate a positive situation. When problems are revealed, the nurse must search for the etiologic or related factors so that interventions may be directed toward these factors. On many occasions the etiologic factors involve parent lack of satisfaction with their changing roles. Inherent in finding satisfaction is a sense of confidence in the role and a comforming of that role with the other roles of the parents. The nurse is a primary source of information and support to parents as the family adapts to having a toddler. Most parents, if they know what to expect of their toddler developmentally and if they understand the tasks facing the family unit at that developmental stage, can problem solve and plan in the toddler's and the family's best interests. The anticipatory guidance offered enthusiastically as the parents began parenting with their infant should not dwindle or be ignored as that infant emerges into toddlerhood.

This section has described the overall task of the family with a toddler, that of establishing a stable home. Components of this task are summarized in Box 6-4.

Box 6-4
Components of the Task of Establishing a Stable Home

I. Adapt resources to accommodate children
  A. Align values to place people above possessions
    1. Confirm persons in family as central focus of life
    2. Respect unique personality of each member
    3. Depend on each other as family members for fun, learning, and stimulation.
  B. Reallocate home space and facilities
    1. Provide private space for each family member
      a. Add more space
      b. Adapt existing space
    2. Manage play space
      a. Confinement to certain rooms or areas
      b. Freedom to range of house
    3. Emotional space allowed
      a. Allow choices by members
      b. Permit emotional expressions
  C. Decide about childproofing
    1. Determine extent environmental hazards will be eliminated and precious possessions removed
    2. Provide watchful surveillance for child's safety
    3. Provide firm discipline and limits for safety
II. Reorganize relationships to include children
  A. Rearrange division of labor
    1. Share tasks so no one is over taxed
    2. Assign realistic responsibilities to toddler
    3. Allow all members the right and respect to make decisions as capable
  B. Provide out-of-home involvement
    1. Social relationships with other couples in each other's homes
    2. Reciprocal child care among friends
    3. Neighborhood "take turns" arrangements
    4. Church or synagogue nursery during services
    5. Child-care cooperatives
    6. Whole-family trips and outings
  C. Accept help in a mature manner
    1. Acknowledge needs that exist
    2. Use outside help that enriches what family offers
    3. Respect basic interdependence of human beings
III. Rework family philosophy to incorporate parenthood and children
  A. Seek satisfaction in parenthood
    1. Revel in the child's naiveté, fantasies, and growth
    2. Maintain a positive parent-child relationship that supports cooperation
    3. Enact discipline needed for safety, order, and harmony in family
  B. Resolve developmental task conflicts
    1. Accept members' adjustments to new roles with patience
    2. Spouses arrive at agreement on parenting plan
    3. Accept that conflict is inevitable, is temporary, and can be managed democratically
    4. Use a positive approach to get members' cooperation
    5. Establish daily family routine and rituals
  C. Provide healthy independence among members
    1. Establish realistic limits that allow freedom for growth but protect
    2. Allow each member time to pursue personal and social interests or hobbies
    3. Trust members' motives for the private times
    4. Convey affection for members
    5. Respect toddler's needs to explore, learn self-control, and secure his or her own identity
  D. Plan future children
    1. Decide how many children are wanted and affordable
    2. Determine spacing desired between children, if more than one is wanted
    3. Institute planning options that do not prohibit marital sexual relations
    4. If another child is expected, prepare all members according to age

Growth and Development of the Toddler

The developmental changes that occur in a child from 12 to 36 months engage the entire family in a life full of drama. Within the first year of life infants have developed attachments that serve as a secure base from which as toddlers they can wander to learn and explore. As their motor abilities give them access to new territory, their rapidly expanding intellectual and language abilities enable them to attach meaning to their discoveries. Because they have had only limited experience with people and objects, toddlers are dependent on their families to rescue them from conflicts and protect them from danger. The imbalance between toddlers' motor skills and their mental capacity puts parents into the difficult position of protecting them from physical harm while nurturing their inexhaustible energy and curiosity toward the development of creative human beings.

The variations of toddlers test the family's ability to rapidly shift from scenes involving stressful conflict to those characterized by their irresistible charm. Their physical, intellectual, and emotional-social development requires mutually adaptive behaviors between toddlers and their families. Nurses use themselves, their knowledge, and their skills to promote healthy family functioning that allows each member to realize his or her full potential as the toddler grows and develops.

Physical Competency

To provide for the safety of a toddler without hindering development requires constant attention and ingenuity by the entire family. Assisting parents to identify expected physical development can contribute to their confidence and ability to cope with changes as they occur. In this chapter assessment parameters that reflect physical growth and development during the toddler years are discussed, with emphasis on the nurse's role with parents in promoting physical competency of their toddler. Table 6-1 summarizes growth and development of toddlers.

Height and Weight

The growth rate slows in late infancy and continues to decelerate until 24 months of age. From 2 years of age through the preschool years growth remains relatively stable. A toddler gains about 2.5 kg (5.5 lb) a year and usually quadruples his or her birth weight by 2 to 2½ years of age. At 2 years a toddler's height represents approximately 50 per cent of his or her eventual adult height. During the 2 years of toddlerhood a child grows approximately 20.3 cm (8 inches) compared with 25.4 cm (10 inches) during the first 12 months of life.

Anticipatory Guidance: Height and Weight

Parents continue to have a keen interest in the physical growth of their child during the toddler years. They can best understand the characteristic slowed growth rate if the height and weight of their child is plotted on a graph to show them consistency in the percentile range. Parents need assurance that the decelerated growth rate is normal for this stage of development.

Head and Chest Circumference

Head circumference reflects the growth of the brain and is an important parameter to be assessed until at least 2 years of age. At 2 years of age the brain attains approximately 90 per cent of adult size. The posterior fontanel usually closes by 2 months of age and the anterior fontanel by 18 months, but there is a wide range of normalcy. In some normal children the anterior fontanel remains slightly open past 18 months of age. Head circumference increases approximately 3.5 cm (1.8 in) during the toddler years compared with a growth of 12 cm (4.7 in) during the first year of life.

In addition to measuring head circumference and palpating fontanels, growth can be evaluated by comparing head with chest circumference. At birth the head circumference exceeds the chest circumference, but during the second year of life the head and chest circumference usually become equal. The chest circumference continues to gradually increase and during childhood exceeds head circumference.

Anticipatory Guidance: Head and Chest

The nurse should explain the expected progression of fontanel closure. It is important to explain the variability of fontanel closure that exists from one child to another because a parent may be comparing the child with a friend's child or with an older sibling.

General Appearance and Skeletal Growth

The general appearance of the toddler changes markedly between 12 and 36 months of age. When toddlers first begin to walk, the trunk is long, the legs and arms are short, and the head is proportionately large, giving them a top-heavy appearance. They walk with their feet

Table 6-1. Summary of Toddler Growth and Development and Health Maintenance

Physical Competency	Intellectual Competency	Emotional-Social Competency
General: From 1 to 3 Years		
Gains 5 kg (11 lb). Grows 20.3 cm (8 in). 12 teeth erupt. Nutritional requirements: Energy 100 Kcal/kg/day Fluid 115–125 ml/kg/day Protein 1.8 gm/kg/day See Chapter 18 for vitamins and minerals.	Learns by exploring and experimenting. Learns by imitating. Progresses from a vocabulary of three to four words at 12 months to about 900 words at 36 months.	Central crisis: to gain a sense of autonomy vs doubt and shame. Demonstrates independent behaviors. Exhibits attachment behavior strongly and regularly until third birthday. Fears persist of strange people, objects, and places and of aloneness and being abandoned. Egocentric in play (parallel play). Imitation of parents in household tasks and activities of daily living.
15 Months		
Legs appear bowed. Walks alone, climbs, slides down stairs backwards. Stacks two blocks. Scribbles spontaneously. Grasps spoon but rotates it, holds cup with both hands. Takes off socks and shoes.	Trial and error method of learning. Experiments to see what will happen. Says at least three words. Uses expressive jargon.	Shows independence by trying to feed self and helps in undressing.
18 Months		
Runs but still falls. Walks upstairs with help. Slides down stairs backwards. Stacks three to four blocks. Clumsily throws a ball. Unzips a large zipper. Takes off simple garments.	Begins to retain a mental image of an absent object. Concept of object permanence fully develops. Has vocabulary of 10 or more words. Holophrastic speech (one word used to communicate whole ideas)	Fears the water. Temper tantrums may begin. Negativism and dawdling predominate. Bedtime rituals begin. Awareness of gender identity begins. Helps with undressing.
24 Months		
Runs quickly and with fewer falls. Pulls toys and walks sideways. Walks downstairs hanging on a rail (does not alternate feet). Stacks six blocks. Turns pages of a book. Imitates vertical and circular strokes. Uses spoon with little spilling. Can feed self. Puts on simple garments. Can turn door knobs.	Enters into preconceptual phase of preoperational period: Symbolic thinking and symbolic play. Egocentric thinking, imagination and pretending are common. Has vocabulary of about 300 words. Uses two-word sentences (telegraphic speech). Engages in monologue.	Fears the dark and animals. Temper tantrums may continue. Negativism and dawdling continue. Bedtime rituals continue. Sleep resisted overtly. Usually shows readiness to begin bowel and bladder control. Explores genitalia. Brushes teeth with help. Helps with dressing and undressing.
36 Months		
Has set of deciduous teeth at about 30 months. Walks downstairs alternating feet. Rides tricycle. Walks with balance and runs well. Stacks eight to ten blocks. Can pour from a pitcher. Feeds self completely. Dresses self almost completely (does not know front from back). Cannot tie shoes.	Preconceptual phase of preoperational period as for 24 months. Uses around 900 words. Constructs complete sentences and uses all parts of speech.	Temper tantrums subside. Negativism and dawdling subside. Bedtime rituals subside. Self-care in feeding, elimination and dressing enhances self-esteem.

spread apart to create a broad base, which helps to compensate for their weight distribution and immature musculoskeletal system. They also have a normal anteroposterior curvature of the spine (lordosis) and a characteristic pot-bellied appearance until the musculoskeletal system matures. Bowed legs *(genu varum)* and flat feet are common when a toddler begins to walk. The feet appear flat because of a plantar fat pad that gradually disappears by the age of 2 years. When toddlers first begin walking they tend to walk on the medial portion of the foot, and there is a slight external rotation that straightens with ambulation around 2 years of age. These combined features account for the characteristic toddling gait of the beginning walker.

During the toddler years muscle tissue begins to replace the high proportion of adipose tissue characteristic of an infant, and bone ossification takes place. With increased ambulation and maturation a toddler's legs and arms lengthen, the body straightens, and the pot-bellied appearance disappears. The lordosis resolves as ambulation increases and muscle and bone develop. The legs retain a slightly bowed appearance

Table 6-1. *(continued)*

Nutrition	Play	Safety
General: From 1 to 3 Years		
Milk 16–24 oz. Appetite decreases. Wants to feed self. Has food jags. Never force food; give nutritious snacks. Give iron and vitamin supplementation only if poor intake.	Books at all ages. Needs physical and quiet activities, does not need expensive toys.	Never leave alone in tub. Keep poisons, including detergents and cleaning products out of reach. Use car seat. Have ipecac in house.
15 Months		
Vulnerable to iron deficiency anemia. Give table foods except for tough meat and hard vegetables. Wants to feed self.	Stuffed animals, dolls, music toys. Peek-a-boo, hide and seek. Water and sand play. Stacking toys. Roll ball on floor. Push toys on floor. Read to toddler.	Keep small items off floor (pins, buttons, clips). Child may choke on hard food. Cords and table cloths are a danger. Keep electrical outlets plugged and poisons locked away. Risk of kitchen accidents with toddler under foot.
18 Months		
Negativism may interfere with eating. Encourage self-feeding. Is easily distracted while eating. May play with food. High activity level interferes with eating.	Rocking horse. Nesting toys. Shape-sorting cube. Pencil or crayon. Pull toys. Four wheeled toy to ride. Throw ball. Running and chasing games. Rough-housing. Puzzles. Blocks. Hammer and peg board.	Falls: from riding toy in bathtub from running too fast Climbs up to get dangerous objects. Keep dangerous things out of wastebasket.
24 Months		
Requests certain foods, therefore snacks should be controlled. Imitates eating habits of others. May still play with food and especially with utensils and dish (pouring, stacking).	Clay and Play-Doh. Finger paint. Brush paint. Record player with record and story book and songs to sing along. Toys to take apart. Toy tea sets. Puppets. Puzzles.	May fall from outdoor large play equipment. Can reach farther than expected (knives, razors, and matches must be kept out of reach).
36 Months		
Sits in booster seat rather than high chair. Verbal about likes and dislikes.	Likes playing with other children, building toys, drawing and painting, doing puzzles. Imitation household objects for doll play. Nurse and doctor kits. Carpenter kits.	Protect from: turning on hot water falling from tricycle striking matches.

until around 18 months of age. After the legs have shown a resolution of the genu varum, a physiologic *genu valgum* (knock-knee) normally follows, lasting through the preschool years. This genu valgum is usually accompanied by a protective toeing in of the feet (Fig. 6-1).

Anticipatory Guidance: General Appearance and Ambulation

The nurse should prepare parents for the normal changes that will occur in physical appearance. It is especially important for the nurse to inform parents regarding the normal changes that occur as the feet and legs mature. Nurses can often intervene to discourage parents from buying corrective shoes when it is unnecessary. If the genu varum and genu valgum are not within normal growth expectations, the nurse should refer the child for further evaluation and treatment.

Parents often ask what kind of shoe should be worn by a toddler. The function of shoes is to protect the feet from trauma and temperature changes. They should be comfortable and fit properly. Support to the foot and ankle is not a function of shoes unless an abnormality is

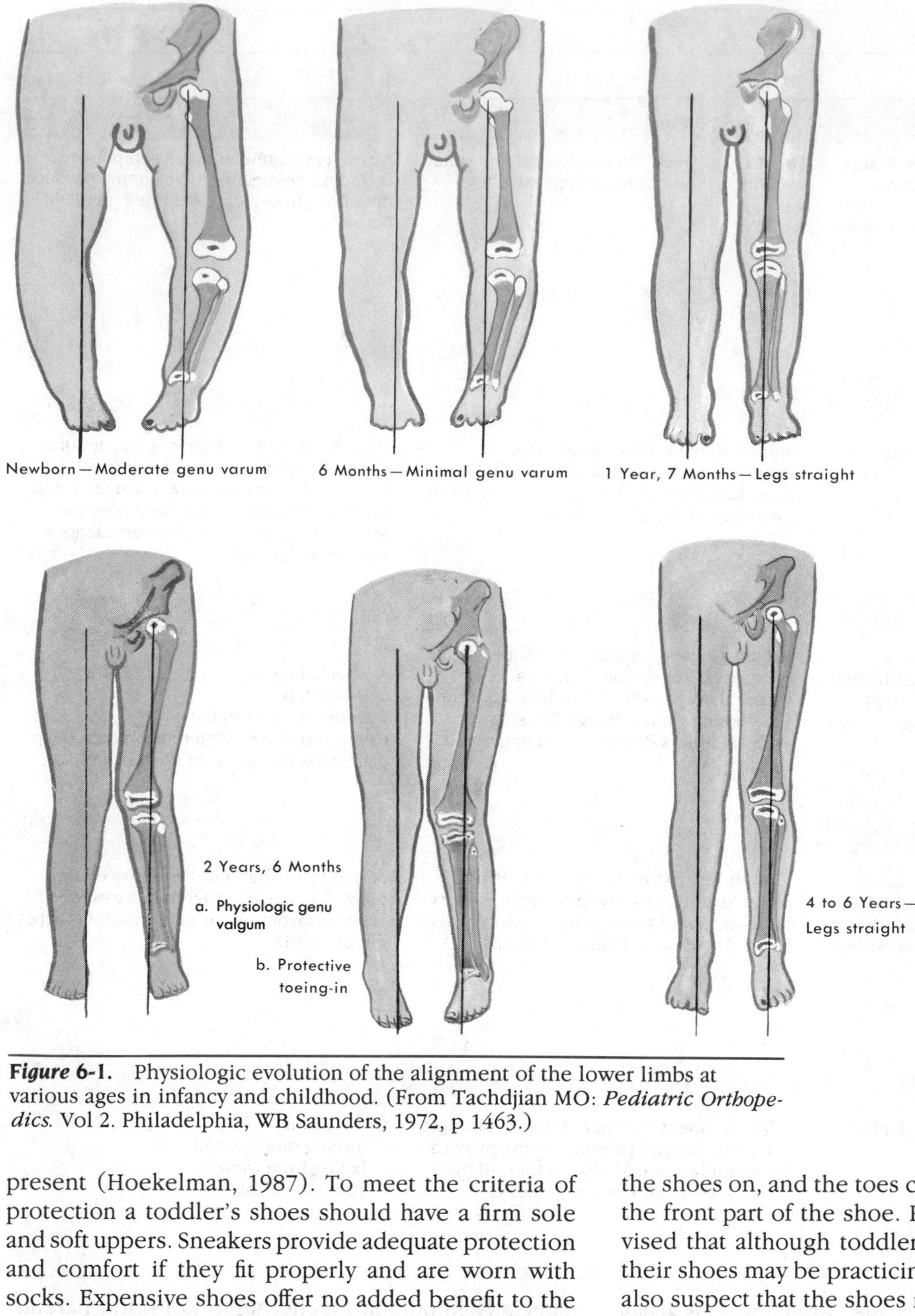

Figure 6-1. Physiologic evolution of the alignment of the lower limbs at various ages in infancy and childhood. (From Tachdjian MO: *Pediatric Orthopedics.* Vol 2. Philadelphia, WB Saunders, 1972, p 1463.)

present (Hoekelman, 1987). To meet the criteria of protection a toddler's shoes should have a firm sole and soft uppers. Sneakers provide adequate protection and comfort if they fit properly and are worn with socks. Expensive shoes offer no added benefit to the proper development of a toddler's feet.

Because a child's foot grows rapidly, it is not uncommon for children to wear shoes that fit too snugly. Parents should be taught how to examine for proper fit of their toddler's shoes. When the toddler is in a standing position there should be $\frac{3}{4}$ inch between the tip of the great toe and the front of the shoe and $\frac{1}{4}$ inch between the edge of the fifth toe and the lateral edge of the shoe when the foot is pushed medially within the shoe. Parents can identify shoes that have been outgrown because it becomes increasingly difficult to get the shoes on, and the toes can be felt pressing against the front part of the shoe. Parents should also be advised that although toddlers who constantly take off their shoes may be practicing a new skill, they should also suspect that the shoes may be too small and may hurt. Finally, parents should be told that going barefoot when it is safe to do so is actually good for the child's feet.

Dentition

The usual order of appearance and anticipatory guidance regarding toddler dentition are discussed in Chapter 19.

Many parents are not aware that care of the deciduous teeth is important for the development of healthy permanent teeth, as is evidenced by the fact that over 50 per cent of children under age 2 experience dental decay (Forrester, 1978). This presents a serious challenge to nurses to explain to parents that ossification and formation of permanent teeth take place during the toddler years even though the teeth are not visible and to provide the information and follow-up needed to help parents provide early preventive dental care. One practice against which parents should be cautioned is allowing the child to go to sleep with a nighttime bottle. Prolonged contact of milk with the child's teeth will predispose to caries.

Lymphatic System

During early childhood the lymphatic tissue increases in size, accounting for the presence of peripheral nodes, enlargement of tonsils and adenoids, and a spleen tip that is more likely to be palpable (Smith, 1977). Hyperplasia of lymphoid tissues is a phenomenon of normal physiologic growth and is thought to occur as a response to the numerous infections of childhood. The excessive swelling and hyperplasia of lymphoid tissue in a normal child may persist long after the primary infection has resolved. Lymphatic tissue shows progressive growth during the toddler years and attains maximum size by 10 to 11 years of age.

Anticipatory Guidance: Lymphatic System

The decline in surgical treatment of hypertrophied tonsils and adenoids is not always understood by parents. The nurse can gain the cooperation of parents to comply with the tedious task of repeated antibiotic treatment of upper respiratory infections if time is taken to explain the normal growth curve of lymphatic tissue. Parents are better able to cope with the stress of repeated visits to the practitioner's office if they understand that the hypertrophied tonsils and adenoids are thought to be a protective response to infection and a phenomenon of normal growth. Parents should also know that lymphatic tissue serves a protective response in the body throughout life.

Motor Development

The significant advances in motor development during the toddler years affect the child's physical, mental, and emotional-social development. Toddlers employ new skills of locomotion and manipulation to satisfy their curiosity and experience new sensations. Physical maturation coupled with opportunities for practice fosters mastery of increasingly complex skills. They rapidly develop the motor skills that enable them to comply with socially accepted standards in their daily living.

Locomotion

Important gross motor skills that are perfected during the toddler years are the ability to walk and run. The age at which these skills are perfected varies from one child to another and particularly from one culture to another. The advanced motor development that has been found to be present in black babies is thought to decrease and possibly level out during the second year of life (Smart and Smart, 1977). Ethnic differences in locomotion observed during the first year are thus generally not as observable during the toddler years.

Most children are able to walk alone by the age of 15 months, although some normal children walk as late as 21 months and others as early as 10 months. At 15 months a toddler becomes an avid climber, climbing onto chairs, sofas, and low tables, and may climb out of a crib, high chair, or stroller. At this age a toddler can quickly disappear by climbing up a staircase on hands and knees. He or she can get down stairs by going backward and sliding from one step to the next, but an occasional accident may still occur as the child slips down the stairs too quickly.

At 18 months of age toddlers walk well. If they fall, it is usually because they try to run too quickly. They now push chairs to cupboards and tables so they can climb to higher, more intriguing destinations. They can walk up stairs one step at a time if someone holds onto one hand, but they still slide down the stairs backward. They like to push and pull things while they walk

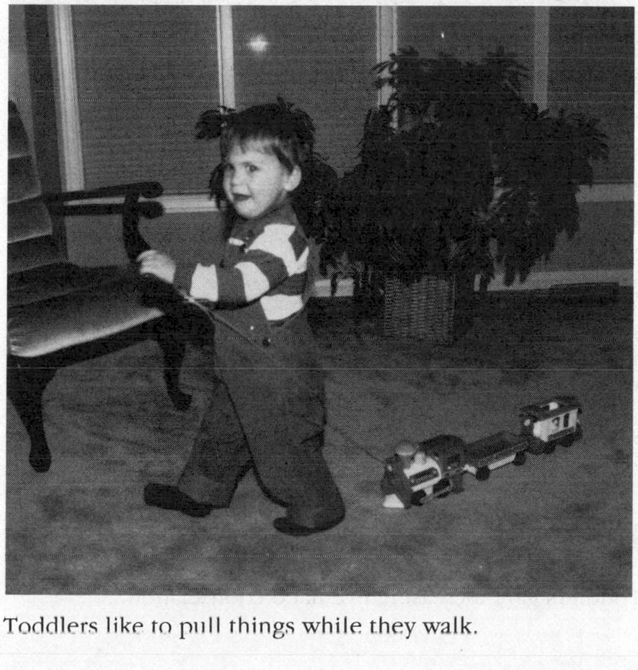

Toddlers like to pull things while they walk.

and can even walk sideways while pulling a toy, making this an ideal age for pull toys.

At 2 years of age toddlers have acquired a more steady gait and generally run well with fewer falls but are not able to stop quickly. The speed with which they are able to move is a threat to life if they venture outdoors unattended. They can now go up and down stairs alone by holding onto a handrail but do so by putting both feet on each step rather than the more advanced method of alternating feet.

From the second to third birthday toddlers become increasingly adept at all of their skills of locomotion. By 3 years of age they can walk downstairs alternating feet, can run and walk skillfully, and can ride a tricycle. Their skills of locomotion have progressed from the characteristic toddling gait to one of balance and control that qualify them for the status of preschooler.

Motor Skills Affecting Play

Toddlers' play activities are affected by all aspects of development but are restricted to boundaries as prescribed by their motor abilities. At 15 months they are still highly engaged in gross motor activities, but they also enjoy the challenge of fine motor control.

At this age toddlers stack two blocks, put objects into a container and pour them out, and scribble spontaneously if they are ingenious enough to get possession of a pencil.

At 18 months of age toddlers can build a tower of three to four blocks, which gives evidence of improving hand-eye coordination. They can also manipulate a pounding bench, although rather crudely. They will try to assist with turning the pages of a book but do so by turning two or three at a time. Although they cannot effectively kick a ball, they are able to clumsily catch and throw one without falling.

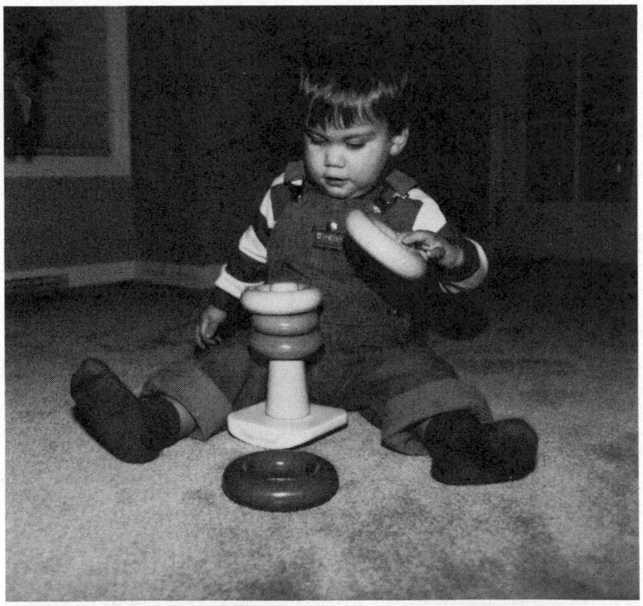

Toddlers gain increasing eye-hand coordination.

By 24 months toddlers can build a tower of six blocks and can line them horizontally to make a train. They now can turn the pages of a book one at a time and imitate vertical and circular strokes, but they still hold the crayon or pencil with a fist. By 30 months they can use their fingers to hold a pencil or a crayon and by age 3 their hands are steady enough to build a bridge, an 8- to 10-block tower, and a structure that resembles a house. See Chapter 21 for further discussion of play.

Motor Skills Affecting Eating

Toddlers make it known that they want access to eating utensils long before they can manipulate them efficiently. At 15 months of age the spoon is grasped, but because toddlers rotate the spoon, they frequently lose its contents on the way to the mouth. At this age they spend a great deal of time practicing the skill of stirring their food during mealtime. They enjoy and are able to pick up pieces of food with their fingers. They can also hold a cup by grasping it rather clumsily with both hands, and as with the spoon, they spill the contents frequently because they tilt the cup before it reaches their mouth.

From 15 months to 2 years of age toddlers demonstrate remarkable advances in their eating skills. At 18 months of age they can use a spoon and drink from a cup or glass. They are able to partially feed themselves but need adult supervision because they easily get engrossed in playing with their food. By 2 years of age they can feed themselves, hold a cup with one hand, and set it down after drinking without spilling. By 2 they have mastered the use of the spoon and spill little.

By 3 years of age toddlers can pour from a pitcher and prepare their own dishes of milk and cold cereal. They feed themselves completely and have only occasional accidents of spilling.

Motor Skills Affecting Self-Care Activities

At 15 months of age toddlers are dependent on their caregivers for most of their physical care. Toddlers at this age have the fine motor skills to take off their socks and shoes and do so as a playful, experimental activity. By 18 months they assist in undressing more than dressing and may not necessarily be undressing when it is time for bed. They can unzip a large zipper and take off simple garments. They will also try to brush teeth at this age but have not acquired sufficient fine motor skill to perform this task. By 2 years of age they are able to assist in self-care by putting on simple garments but do not differentiate front from back. They are now able to zip and unzip zippers. They can put on their shoes but are not able to buckle or tie them. They wash and dry their hands, brush teeth crudely, and, if helped to reach the sink, can turn on a water faucet. They can also turn doorknobs and open doors without assistance. By 3 toddlers dress themselves almost completely but still do not know front from back and cannot tie their shoes.

A toddler's physical development provides boundaries within which he or she performs increasingly complex activities of daily living. Although development of fine and gross motor skills determines when a child can perform a particular task, the emotional and social development of a child has tremendous impact on the accomplishment of these activities; thus, activities of daily living are further addressed in the discussion on the emotional-social development of the toddler.

Anticipatory Guidance: Motor Skills

The toddler years are a time when parents need special assistance from the nurse to provide adequate opportunity for the development of this child's motor skills. Parents need suggestions in how they can provide a safe environment without detracting from the toddler's opportunity to practice his or her motor skills. A toddler can be given the opportunity to practice stair climbing under supervision and to practice running outdoors on the grass, where a fall is less dangerous. A popular and safe toy at this age is a three-step sliding board. The nurse should also encourage parents to allow their toddler to practice fine motor skills by permitting self-feeding, assistance in dressing, and participation in other self-care activities.

Parents should be assisted in choosing play activities that promote fine and gross motor skills appropriate for the various stages of toddlerhood. If parents can regard the practice of motor skills as an essential component of their toddler's developing self-esteem as well as physical development, the frustrations that eager toddlers pose to parents may be more tolerable. Encouraging parents to provide opportunities for the development of motor skills without undue emphasis on premature perfection builds an environment within which the toddler thrives.

Vision and Hearing

During toddlerhood the normal development of vision and hearing should be evaluated on each health care visit. Impaired hearing is difficult to detect if there is a unilateral or minimal hearing loss. However, it is crucial that hearing loss be detected because a toddler who cannot hear will not progress through the normal sequence of language development. A strong indication that the toddler's hearing is impaired is the case of an infant who babbles at 6 months and who does not progress to increased sound production but rather shows a marked decrease in vocalization and eventually does not produce any sounds. See Chapter 15 and 51 for further discussion on hearing testing.

Evaluation of visual acuity continues to be difficult during the toddler years. It is not until about the age of 3 that a child can cooperate sufficiently for use of the Snellen illiterate E chart. (See Table 15-4 for a list of vision tests.) Before the age of 3, vision can be assessed by observing the child's eye-hand coordination and his or her response to bright lights and objects. The Denver Eye Examination Screening Test is an effective way to screen vision in the toddler. Despite hyperopia (farsightedness), which is normal during the toddler years, distance fixation is not well developed, so that an object must be within a six-foot range for clear vision.

The parent's description of a child's behavior can give important clues to visual problems. Usually toddlers are attentive to stimuli in their environment and will respond to new stimuli by attempts to manipulate them. The preference a child shows to sit close to a television set is not indicative of a visual problem. Many children with normal vision enjoy the stimulation of large images and sit close to a TV. Parents should always be asked for their evaluation of their toddler's vision.

Anticipatory Guidance: Vision and Hearing

The nurse should explain the relationship between hearing and language development. Parents should be taught the normal progression of language development as a preventive measure to detect hearing impairment. Parents should be encouraged to assess hearing and vision by observing their toddler's responsiveness to stimuli. The reports of parents can give the first clue to vision and hearing problems.

Nutritional Requirements

The amount of energy expended is determined by body size and composition, physical activity, and rate of growth.

A toddler needs a greater number of total calories (1000 to 1500 Kcal/day) than during infancy owing to an increase in body size, but the requirements *per unit of body weight* decrease. Two major factors affect energy requirements during the toddler years: slowed growth rate reduces energy requirements and increased activity increases energy requirements. The sum effect of these changes is only a slight decrease in requirements from 108 Kcal/kg/day in infants to 100 Kcal/kg/day in toddlers.

Although physical growth rate slows during the toddler years, protein requirements remain relatively high because of the rapid growth of muscle tissue. In spite of a decrease in appetite, under normal circumstances the toddler's protein requirements are met if a balanced diet is consumed.

By about 2 years of age the percentage of total body water is similar to that of an adult, i.e., approximately 60 per cent of total body weight. The adult 40 : 60 ratio of extracellular to intracellular water is reached by about 1 year of age. Metabolic rate remains relatively high; therefore, a toddler's fluid requirement is 115 to 125 ml/kg/day.

A balanced diet including 16 to 24 ounces of milk supplies vitamin D, calcium, and phosphorus in recommended amounts. Excessive amounts of milk may reduce a child's desire for intake of solid foods rich in iron, resulting in iron deficiency anemia. See Chapter 18 for recommended daily allowances of various nutrients during toddler years.

Intellectual Competency

A study of the intellectual development of a toddler offers some explanation of the increasing complexity with which toddlers relate to their environment. Their fascination with practicing newly learned motor skills, their experimentation by poking, tasting, and pushing, and their dramatic limitations are not explained simply. What are the mental processes accompanying this incessant activity? The question "What are they thinking?" becomes less of a mystery after toddlers reach the age of 2, when their remarkable advances in language development enable them to express their thoughts and make verbal requests. Stages of cognitive development identified by Piaget provide a theory base that the nurse can use to assess cognitive growth and development.

Stages of Cognitive Development

By 12 months of age infants have progressed through four substages of development that have resulted in numerous important accomplishments. They now search for an object that has vanished (object permanence); their actions show deliberate intention, and they have a rudimentary concept of cause and effect.

Infants enter toddlerhood with a beginning understanding of spoken words and engage in prelinguistic formation of sounds. The imitative behaviors that were begun at about 3 months of age now become particularly noticeable as they imitate new actions daily. Things learned in the first four substages continue to be practiced, and new learning emerges during the next 12 to 36 months. Cognitive developmental attainments according to Piaget are summarized in Chapter 3.

Substage five (12 to 18 months) is characterized by what Piaget has called tertiary circular reactions. This is a third type of circular reaction that differs from the other two (primary and secondary) circular reactions. In this stage children knock down a tower of blocks, help to rebuild it, and knock it down again not for the sake of repetition (primary circular) and not only to observe the results (secondary circular). Now they are searching for new ways to bring about the same results or experimenting to see if they can produce new results, or both. They may therefore push the blocks over gently one time, and the next time stand up and swing their arms to see if something new will happen. It is this "experimenting to see" that brings about new behaviors and results in trial-and-error as a predominant method of learning. Deliberate manipulation to find out what will happen fills the day of a busy toddler during this phase of development.

Substage six (18 to 24 months) marks the transition from predominantly trial-and-error behavior to thinking about solutions and consequences before carrying them out. This stage is characterized by a beginning ability to use mental images and words when referring to absent objects. Toddlers can also anticipate what will happen to the object as a result of a certain action and therefore they solve problems by thinking about the results rather than always having to carry them out by trial and error. For example, during this stage children are less fascinated with throwing a variety of objects from the high chair than they were earlier. They remember that an object falls and makes a noise without doing it every day. They also can anticipate that if they throw a fork instead of a spoon, it will also make a noise; therefore, it is not necessary to throw the fork on the floor. The breakthrough of being able to mentally try out alternate ways of accomplishing a goal has been described by Piaget as the stage of inventing new means through mental combinations.

The ability to retain an image of an object or action beyond immediate sensory experience is demonstrated when a toddler imitates a past event in the absence of the original stimuli. For example, when a child pretends he is shaving in front of the mirror hours after his father has gone to work, he is engaging in what has been described by Piaget as deferred imitation. During this stage children imitate a model in their environment that has significance and meaning to them. The process of identification takes place as they take on the behavior and values of those in their environment.

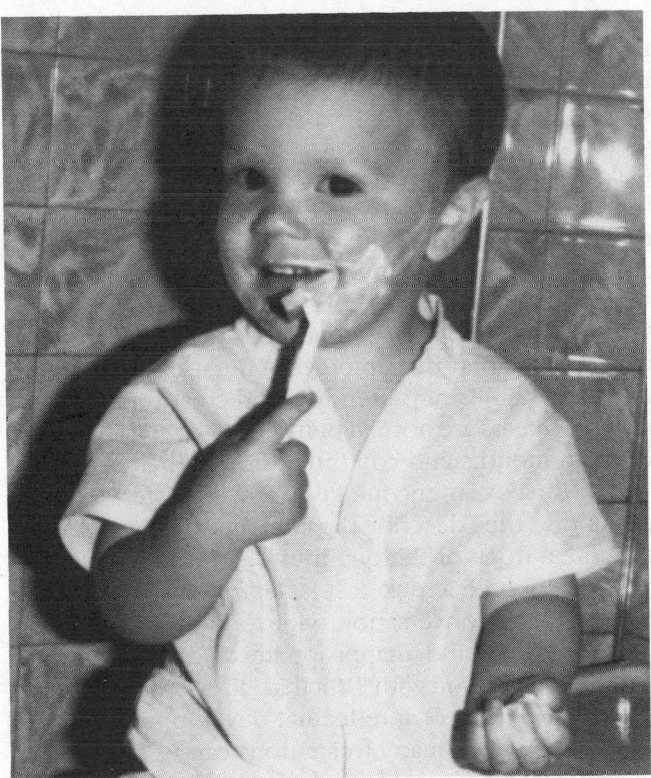

The toddler portrays deferred imitation when he pretends to be shaving with a toy razor after father has gone off to work. (Photograph by David Trainor.)

The concept of object permanence is now fully developed. If a ball rolls under the sofa, toddlers have a concept of the ball continuing to move even though they cannot see the movement. If they cannot find the ball under the sofa they will conclude that the ball has moved through to the other side and they will go around the sofa to look for the ball. It is the child's ability to retain a mental image of the ball and to think about the property of the ball that brings about this level of behavior.

Entrance into the preoperational period (2 to 7) is characterized by an increased internal representation of objects and the ability to engage in symbolic thought.* Piaget is not consistent in the use of the term "symbol," so that the difference in symbolism between the last phase of the sensorimotor period and the first stage of the preoperational period is not precise (Phillips, 1969). The preoperational child has greater ability to differentiate signifiers (blanket, teddy bear) from significates (going to bed). For example, before 2 years of age the blanket and bear might be signs that symbolize going to bed (blanket-bear-bedtime are perceived as a single unit), whereas a preoperational child can differentiate the blanket and bear from the experience of going to bed (Phillips, 1969).

The preoperational period begins with a period described as *preconceptual.* The increased use of symbols permits children to internalize what they see and experience, but these concepts are not as complete and logical as those of an adult, thus the term preconceptual. For example, all dogs will be called by the name of the child's dog. He or she is not able to comprehend that all objects within a class are not one and the same object; therefore, the child's attempts at generalization result in cognitive errors.

Although pretending and imagination show their beginnings during the latter part of the sensorimotor period, symbolic play is at its peak in children from 2 to 4 years of age. Symbolization is greatly enhanced by rapidly developing language ability during this period. Egocentric thought also facilitates symbolic play. For imagination and pretending to ensue, assimilation must outweigh accommodation so that a distortion of reality takes place (Pulaski, 1971).* Children distort reality by taking into account only the characteristics of objects that meet their immediate needs. The greater the egocentrism, the greater the distortion of reality. At times there is almost no resemblance between the object and the symbol that it is representing in the child's mind (between the stick the child is using for a carrot and an actual carrot).

Over a two-year period toddlers' cognition progresses from a predominantly trial-and-error method of object manipulation to a beginning retention of mental images which allows them to think about alternate solutions, and finally, by the age of 3, internal representation of objects enables them to make a dish or a box become a hat or a shell a cup. Reality is first copied (imitation) and later (2 to 4 years) reality is distorted (symbolic play). Symbolism and imitation eventually disappear, but during the toddler period they represent his or her efforts to adapt to reality. Pulaski suggests that during this period children's lives are polarized around their attempts to adapt to reality by pleasing their parents (imitative accommodation) and their need to escape from parental demands and satisfy their own egos (assimilative symbolic play) (Pulaski, 1971).

Anticipatory Guidance: Intellectual Development

The nurse can be in a position to evaluate how attuned the family is to their toddler's intellectual needs. Toddlers need a variety of experiences that allow them

*Symbolic thought is the ability to make something—a mental image, a word or an object—stand for something that is not present.

* See Chapter 3 for further discussion of assimilation and accommodation.

to make discoveries. Parents should be helped to understand that a toddler's intense examination and incessant manipulation of anything new is the way he or she learns. Toys and games that allow practice of cognitive skills should be encouraged. Besides being fun, playing "peek-a-boo" helps the toddler to gain the concept of object permanence. A jack-in-the-box serves a similar purpose as well as teaching cause (turn the crank) and effect (jack pops up). Toddlers are growing intellectually when they insist on examining the contents of cupboards, drawers, boxes, and anything they can reach. If a nurse will take the time to explain the meaning of such toddler behavior, a family is more likely to feel a sense of pride and even intrigue in their toddler's fascination with and scrutiny of everything and everybody he or she encounters.

The limit-setting and constant surveillance that are required by a family with a toddler are exhausting and often stressful. It is important for a nurse to explore with the family ways that encourage the development of their toddler without exhausting and immobilizing the rest of family life.

During the trial-and-error stage toddlers need parents who can patiently stand by and watch their countless attempts to complete a task without reaching in and making the final move just as they are about to accomplish it on their own. Parents must maintain a delicate balance as they support the curiosity of their children (allowing them to make their own discoveries) while having the sensitivity to know when help is needed in order to avoid undue frustration.

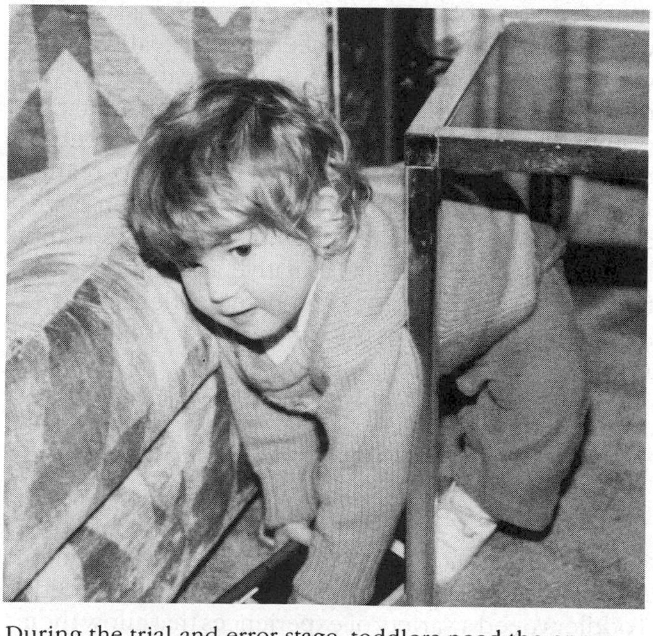

During the trial-and-error stage, toddlers need the opportunity to solve problems on their own. This toddler is trying to get both herself and her storybook out of a tight place.

It is important for the nurse to explain to families that their toddler's learning by experimentation is not restricted to planned play opportunities, but that dresser drawers, kitchen cupboards, and bathroom closets provide a source of even greater fascination. Making a special cupboard available with some kitchen utensils will please toddlers and may keep them out of the rest of the kitchen cupboards. In other areas of the house a similar approach can be taken.

As a child enters the preoperational period (around 2 years of age) parents need to be prepared for the symbolic play that emerges. A nurse can explain to them that games of pretending and creation of imaginary playmates are normal behaviors for a toddler from 24 to 36 months and continue through the preschool years. Nurses can encourage parents to listen to their toddlers as they describe the contents of a box that has become a truck or the qualities of a plastic container that has become a rocket. It is appropriate for parents to carry on a conversation with toddlers about their imagined play and inappropriate to discourage the child's imagination with "But that is a box, not a truck."

In all phases of intellectual development during the toddler years many frustrations can be avoided if the nurse helps parents to be consistent in what is allowed and to avoid setting a child up for punishment. For example, knowingly leaving new and intriguing things within reach and then punishing a child for destroying them is unreasonable. By observing the parent-child interaction and discussing activity of a normal day, the nurse can gather important clues regarding the family's encouragement of intellectual development of their toddler.

Just as nurses encourage understanding of the toddler's cognitive development by the parents, they must keep it in mind when working with the hospitalized toddler. Cognitive development can be encouraged through carefully planned play programs in hospitals. The nurse can work with the child life specialist to assure that the child is prepared for procedures in developmentally appropriate ways.

Language Development

It is the nurse's role to assess the appropriateness of the toddler's language ability and help families to provide an environment conducive to language development. Nurses must therefore be knowledgeable about (1) stages of language acquisition, (2) characteristics of toddler language, and (3) factors that contribute to language development.

Stages of Language Acquisition

By the first birthday the infant's language development has been influenced by the amount of reinforcement the child has received. It has been noted that babies babble more when people talk to them. Also, when babies have been stimulated to practice babbling, they are likely to abandon babbling in favor of speech earlier than if no reinforcement was received (Hurlock, 1978). The babbling stage (beginning at 4 to 6 months) is followed by single-word utterances at about 1 year of age. A vocabulary of three words is common for a 1-year-old, typically including ma-ma, da-da, and bye-bye.

From 15 to 18 months of age an *expressive jargon* emerges that has rhythmic intonations, but no real words can be recognized. Expressive jargon is thought to be an expression of feelings or ideas, and it is a way to make contact with another human being (Smart and Smart, 1977). Although expressive jargon does not seem to contain real words, toddlers use it in conjunction with pointing and movement toward the object or person they are "talking" about, thereby communicating their wants.

Between 18 and 24 months of age one-word utterances are commonly used to communicate increasingly complex ideas. When one-word sentences are used to express whole ideas, the accompanying gestures give clues to the meaning. For example, saying bye-bye while standing at the door and hitting on it after playing indoors for several hours may mean "I want to go bye-bye," whereas standing at the door quietly as father is leaving for work and saying "Bye-bye" probably means "Da-da is going bye-bye." If, however, hitting of the door again accompanies the utterance "Bye-bye" as Daddy leaves, it now clearly means "I want to go bye-bye with Da-da." These one-word utterances that carry whole ideas are referred to as *holophrastic speech*. Giving careful attention to the situation surrounding one-word utterances and the accompanying gestures becomes an integral part of successful communication with a toddler.

By 18 to 24 months of age most toddlers have mastered locomotion reasonably well and can put more effort into expression through language. From 18 months to 3 years of age vocabulary growth and complexity of sentence structure progress rapidly and constantly. Although there is a wide variation in the number of words a toddler is able to say, a typical vocabulary at 18 months of age is 10 or more words; by 2 years of age the child may easily progress to a phenomenal 300-word vocabulary, and by 3 he or she uses around 900 words. At about 2 years of age two-word utterances become increasingly common, by $2\frac{1}{2}$ years of age an average sentence contains three words and by 3, complete sentences are constructed using all parts of speech.

Characteristics of Toddler Speech

Around 2 years of age a characteristic pattern of speech emerges. There are a few words that seem to be used repeatedly and other less frequently used words are attached to them. The frequently used words have been described as *pivot* words and the less frequently used words as *open*. For example, "down" may emerge as a pivot word in "sit down," "put down" "go down." Sit, put, and go (open words) are less frequently used than "down." Another characteristic is that when two words are combined it is usually a noun and verb. For example, "me do" is a grammatically incorrect sentence containing only the words that carry meaning. Articles, prepositions, and adjectives are generally lacking as is typical in a telegram, which accounts for the use of the term *telegraphic sentences* to describe these phrases.

The egocentric thought that dominates in the preconceptual phase of the preoperational period (beginning at 24 months of age) is expressed in the content of a toddler's language. Toddlers in this stage engage in a monologue with little regard for a response of another child or adult who happens to be present. The function of this *egocentric speech* is that it meets the toddler's need to practice speech. This type of speech often accompanies the symbolic play which characterizes this period. As toddlers mature and are able to consider another's view, their speech becomes more socialized and they engage in increasingly more conversation with others and less monologue.

Anticipatory Guidance: Language Development

The knowledge nurses have regarding the stages and characteristics of language development facilitates their own communication with children and serves as a guide in counseling of parents. When parents have a concern that their toddler's language is not developing as rapidly as that of a sibling or other playmates, the nurse can help parents to understand the wide range of normal language acquisition and can explain the impact of other areas of their child's development. For example, pointing out that a toddler's language development is often delayed by his or her absorption in learning motor skills during the second year of life is reassuring to parents.

The nurse can also offer some practical suggestions on how parents can facilitate language development. Research has demonstrated that the mother's goals when talking to her 2-year-old and the structural characteristics of her speech do influence the child's language development (Hoff-Ginsberg, 1986). The most frequently misunderstood element of relating to a toddler has to do with "baby talk." To shape the learning of speech a child should be given the opportunity to hear correct speech. A nurse can encourage parents to respond to their toddler's speech by using correct communication and by expanding and rephrasing what he or she says in a grammatically correct statement. They should not, however, correct the child's language by saying "No, it's not wa-wa, it's water." If the parents avoid responding with "baby-talk," correct language is learned. Young children are actually more responsive to adult forms of speech such as "throw me the ball" than they are to two-word commands like "throw ball."

A nurse should also counsel parents to guard against giving toddlers what they want in response to crying and gestures. The incentive to learn to speak is dramatically hampered if a toddler's requests are granted in the absence of verbalization. Toddlers understand much more than they can say, so they will understand "tell mama" or "tell daddy what you want." Most of the time it is quicker and easier to grant the request without asking the toddler to verbalize, but this practice establishes a pattern that discourages language development.

As a toddler progresses through the various stages of language development (holophrastic sentences, jargon, telegraphic speech) with its common characteristics (egocentrism, pivot and open words), parents need to be encouraged to be attentive to the situation as well as the actual words that are spoken. Parents may need help in understanding that the repetition of favorite words is a toddler's way of practicing language and is not necessarily a request or true expression of his or her desires. At all stages of language development toddlers need a family whose members talk to them and respond to their language efforts. It is important for the nurse to stress that toddlers understand a great deal of what they hear. They certainly sense the tone and feeling of verbal language and are sensitive to the relationships that exist between family members. A toddler's language development thrives when he or she feels secure and loved and when warm, intimate relationships prevail within the family.

Emotional-Social Competency

The emotional-social development of a toddler is a dramatic unfolding of a person who has a sense of self, expresses feelings verbally and bodily, and is struggling to become increasingly more independent without giving up the security and comfort that dependency affords. Toddlers are now able to differentiate the responses of those around them. They try to curb those behaviors that result in disapproval and repeat performances that are given attention and approval. As they become increasingly aware of themselves and the world around them, they experiment with a variety of ways to gain control over what happens to them without losing the approval of their parents and significant others.

According to Freud's theory, the body area or zone in which pleasurable feelings or tension reduction is centered in the toddler is the bowels. Freud stated that pleasurable sensations are derived from moving the bowels and therefore called this the anal stage of development. Freud further believed that a conflict occurred in toddlers between the desire for the physical satisfaction of involuntarily relaxing the bowel sphincter and the emotional gratification of receiving their mother's loving approval when they did not. The process of toilet training was seen by Freud as a way of resolving this conflict and improper toilet training as a way of producing lifelong psychologic trauma.

The Eriksonian task, conflict, or crisis for the toddler is autonomy versus shame and doubt. To be autonomous is to see oneself as a separate being with a will of one's own. Once infants have learned to trust their own body, their mothers, and the world they begin to discover that they can exert a predictable effect on others. They learn that they can control. To control is synonymous with autonomy and autonomy is synonymous with independence and self-governance. Therefore, autonomy requires children to relinquish some of their dependence on or trust in others. This produces conflict in a number of ways. Some of the child's physical venturing out into his or her environment inevitably results in falls and physical hurts. These physical hurts provide toddlers with a realization of their own limits and a resulting possibility of doubt in their ability to be autonomous. Children learn that expressing autonomy by insisting on having their own way can result in punishment and shame, whereas dependent, submissive behavior is rewarded. Three major struggles during this stage—toilet training, limit setting and discipline, and sibling rivalry—all involve the conflict between autonomy and shame and doubt. Toddlers are in conflict because they wish to exercise their own will but fear situations that extend their coping capacity.

This crisis of autonomy versus doubt and shame is largely affected by how the family responds to the child's assertive behavior. If toddlers feel secure in their families, they are likely to venture farther in their exploration and take on unfamiliar tasks and territory. The family can further assist the development of healthy autonomy and avoid shame and doubt by encouraging activities that are age appropriate. Parents should know that one danger of providing toys that are too advanced is development of shame and doubt when the child fails to master them. If a family encourages and rewards age-appropriate expressions of expanding cognitive and motor development, the child gains a sense of mastery and positive self-esteem. If a toddler's explorative behaviors are discouraged and repeatedly punished, the strivings for autonomy are thwarted. However, in the life of every toddler some punishment and interruption of intent must take place to ensure his or her physical safety, to maintain the integrity of personal belongings, and to set limits that help the child gain self-control and feel secure. Healthy autonomy must be accompanied by the kind of healthy shame and doubt which protects toddlers and others around them from harm that could result if they were allowed total autonomy without limits on their behavior. See Chapter 35 for further discussion of unhealthy dependence/independence.

The emotions expressed by a toddler become socially more obvious than during infancy. Young babies show discomfort and displeasure by crying or screaming, whereas toddlers add throwing, biting, hitting, stamping their feet, and pushing or pulling to their repertoire. Their pleasant emotions are also now expressed overtly. If they feel a need to be close to their parents they have the physical ability to pull on them and to hug them, and the verbal ability to say "love ma-ma" or "love da-da." Expressions of both pleasant and unpleasant emotions elicit various responses from those in their environment. That which children experience tends to encourage or discourage certain behaviors and in this way they begin to adapt to the social demands of their families and society. If toddlers can feel loved and accepted, with some sense of control over their own destiny, they are likely to develop a sense of worth and high self-esteem. As toddlers strive to master developmental tasks, their experiences within the family to a large degree shape their emotional and social development. Each family interprets the confines of acceptable behavior and has its own ideals and expectations for its developing toddler.

There is much variation in how a family chooses to socialize its toddler. The decisions and choices that a family makes are largely a consequence of their own cultural values. Nurses must learn to relate to families from various cultures and seek to understand the ethnic differences in defining acceptable, socialized behavior for a toddler. The nurse's own cultural orientation and family experiences will influence his or her definition of acceptable behavior. Areas of development in which cultural variations are particularly evident during the toddler years are (1) time to begin toilet training, (2) handling of anger and aggressive behavior (temper tantrums), (3) use of corporal punishment, (4) tolerance for crying, (5) importance given to provision for play, (6) degree of independence encouraged, and (7) age of weaning.

Nurses who are to work effectively with families from various cultures must recognize that unique cultural patterns persist, and these differences affect socialization of a toddler. The tasks of the toddler are achieved in a way that is consistent with culturally defined family values. Expectations of the nurse may be inconsistent with those of the family, and it is important for nurses to examine the impact that their own cultural values and beliefs will have on the guidance and counseling offered to families.

Temperament

By the time a baby reaches 1 year of age a pattern of interaction within the family has been established. The temperament* of the baby and of other family members is an influential determinant in the evolving pattern of communication. If relationships are tense and stressful, the toddler's behavioral style can be adversely affected. Toddlers have so much learning and controlling of emotions to master during these years that their families may have difficulty adapting to the varied and new manifestations of the child's temperament. A toddler's emerging sense of self, the wish to control, and the insistence on having his or her own way are stressful to a family.

The temperament apparent during infancy tends to persist through toddlerhood and throughout later years, but, according to Thomas and Chess (1977), it is not immutable. This view has particular meaning for the toddler years because of the numerous demands for socialization that are encountered. The way the developmental tasks are handled by parents may indeed bring about adaptations in the basic behavioral style. The environmental influences that children experience within their families may accentuate, modify, or alter traits of temperament (Thomas and Chess, 1977).

Regardless of the temperament of the child and the expectations of parents, there is likely to be some stress and conflict between parent and toddler. The interactive process of temperament and environment has been described as being consonant or dissonant. Thomas and Chess (1977) have identified numerous areas of consonance and dissonance. These are (1) establishment of regular sleep and feeding patterns; (2) mastery of self-care (feeding, dressing, toilet training); (3) compliance to family expectations; (4) response to masturbatory experiences; and (5) the emergence and growth of interpersonal relationships within the family. The degree of consonance or dissonance between the toddler's temperament and capabilities and the demands and expectations of parents has a profound impact on the child's development.

Anticipatory Guidance: Temperament

The nurse must first help family members to express their own frustrations and concern about the tempera-

*Temperament is the way a person behaves and can be equated with a *behavioral style* (Thomas and Chess, 1977).

ment of the toddler. Especially when there are older siblings, parents may feel baffled by the dramatic differences in behavior of their children. Using disciplinary approaches that they had found successful for an older child when he or she was a toddler may not be effective this time. For example, a highly adaptable toddler may comply if told to stop turning the TV knob, an easily distractible toddler may be readily diverted, but one who is persistent may have to be picked up and carried away from the TV. Parents need assistance to understand that these temperamental variations do not constitute bad or good behavior but that toddlers of certain temperaments need responses from their families that are suited to their particular temperaments.

The way a child expresses normal toddler characteristics is consistent with his or her particular temperament. Parents of toddlers frequently compare their child's behavior with that of a friend's or relative's child in search of an answer to handling their toddler's behaviors. The nurse can be of assistance by encouraging parents to identify those behaviors that are most stressful and then helping them develop approaches that are congruent with their own temperament as well as their toddler's. (See Chapter 13 for a discussion of parenting that considers temperament.)

Attachment and Separation

The interactions between infant and caregiver from birth gradually develop into an emotional tie described by Bowlby (1969) as an effective bond. During the toddler years, attachment behavior (seeking and maintaining proximity) is neither less intense nor less frequent than at the end of the first year. According to Bowlby (1969), most children exhibit attachment behavior strongly and regularly until around their third birthday. Typical toddler attachment behaviors are watching, smiling, following, calling, and listening. Beginning in the latter half of the first year of life, children express distress when separated from their mothers or other individuals who are emotionally significant to them. This phenomenon is referred to as *separation anxiety*. As with stranger anxiety, separation anxiety demonstrates a cognitive developmental ability. Separation anxiety also has emotional-social significance. The child's distress at being separated from his or her mother demonstrates the strength of the mother-infant bond. It is a behavioral indication that a sense of basic trust has been developed. Viewing separation anxiety in this way helps to point up the normalcy of the behaviors involved. Indeed, this normalcy has been demonstrated in research which showed that 13-month-old children displayed negative emotions when separated from their mothers, with the most frequently observed emotion being anger (Shiller et al, 1986). Crying and protesting at separation from the caregivers persists during the toddler years, but Bowlby (1969, 1973) reports a change in a toddler's ability to separate at about 2 years and 9 months.

By 3 years of age children are able to engage in play with other children in their caregiver's temporary absence. Although children before 2 years and 9 months may cry for only a short time when their caregivers leave, they are likely to remain quiet and less involved in play, and constantly demand attention of the substitute caregiver (Bowlby, 1973).

The need for toddlers to visualize their caregivers is frequently demonstrated when they momentarily wander too far from the caregiver and frantically return for contact, sometimes in tears, as though it were the caregiver who separated from them. As toddlers develop attachments and feel more secure, they are able to explore and play in their caregiver's presence with only occasional "checking back" for reassurance. Toddlers who constantly seek proximity with their caregivers cannot be assumed to be more attached, because the ability to separate is an outgrowth of a healthy attachment. It should be expected, however, that when toddlers are in a novel environment they will make contact with attachment figures more frequently than when in a familiar environment.

The quality of attachment in infancy has been studied to identify its relationship to competence and adaptation during the second year of life. Matas et al (1978) studied quality of attachment in infancy and quality of play and problem-solving behavior at 2 years of age. Infants who were assessed as securely attached at 18 months were, at 2 years of age, more enthusiastic, persistent, and cooperative than insecurely attached infants. The competent 2-year-old boy in this study did not automatically comply with his mother's request, but demonstrated gradual cooperation (for example, on helping to clean up toys.) These findings are in agreement with other studies that show securely attached infants to be more socially and cognitively competent.

Anticipatory Guidance: Attachment and Separation

The nurse needs to be aware of the particular lifestyle within a family, which will affect the toddler's ongoing development of attachment. If both parents work, the nurse should help the parents to feel comfortable with their child care arrangements. Parents need reassurance when their toddlers momentarily seem more interested in continuing play than in returning home with their parents. If parents can be encouraged to take an interest in what has happened during the day—what their toddler has said, how he or she played, what he or she ate, and what discipline was required—they can feel more integrally a part of the child's development and experience an ongoing attachment. The nurse might suggest that frequent conversations be held with the substitute caregiver so that parents will feel more in control.

The nurse should also provide some guidance in helping parents understand how a toddler perceives and responds to separation. Toddlers learn from experience that parents reappear after a brief separation and that even though they are absent for short periods, the parents continue to exist. Learning to tolerate brief separations is a developmental task of a toddler that may cause some difficulty to parents. If parents understand the kinds of behavior that brief separations cause, their coping ability is enhanced. For example, a toddler, after being left with a babysitter, may become more clingy and show an increase in attachment behaviors. Conversely, he or she may ignore the parents and demonstrate an ostentatious interest in the substitute caregiver. Parents need to respond to such behaviors by providing extra attention and affection and need to guard against demanding the level of independence that their toddler exhibited before the babysitting experience. It is also helpful for parents to know that there is evidence that the quality of the mother's interactions with her toddler during play time may have an effect on the child's sense of security regarding the mother's availability and support (Slade, 1987).

These kinds of understandings must also be facilitated in parents of the hospitalized toddler. One mother, who had been hospitalized after an automobile accident, when finally reunited with her toddler, who had also been hospitalized, was devastated when the child turned her back on her. This mother was assisted by the nurse in understanding and responding to the child's behavior as expected and normal.

Fears

Each age seems to bring with it typical or characteristic *fears.* An increasing perception of their environment makes toddlers more alert to auditory, spatial, and visual changes. The types of fears that result are fear of noise, sudden movement, an approaching object and unusual sensations (height, water). Fear of the water develops most frequently around 18 to 24 months of age in relationship to being bathed. Children typically suddenly refuse to take baths and scream each time someone attempts to wash their face. Fear of strange people and strange objects and places and of aloneness persists from the latter part of the first year until the third year, then tends to diminish (Bowlby, 1973). Fear of the dark and of animals runs somewhat parallel and is not common before the age of 2 years.

The fears of children under the age of 3 are usually not a problem. If parents can be sensitive to the normal fears of their toddlers and provide the security they need, children are likely to progress through this period experiencing only the normal fears. Chapter 36 discusses the development of extreme fears in childhood and the effective management of normal and excessive fears.

Anger, Aggression, and Temper Tantrums

During the toddler years *anger* is commonly expressed through physical means. When a person's goal is blocked by an obstacle, frustration results, and aggressive behavior is a normal toddler reaction. For a toddler the obstacles encountered within a day are more frequent than many adults realize. Not only do adults interfere with a toddler's goals but the child's own ineptness leads to one predicament after another. Toys get stuck, ice cream cones fall, and balloons break, resulting in disappointment and frustration. Sometimes toddlers can be helped to accomplish their goals, but often they must learn to cope with their situations with little realization of the cause. Even though they caused their own dilemmas, they feel frustrated and angry. Expressions of anger are typically generalized and unproductive.

As toddlers develop in language and cognitive abilities, they have other options for dealing with their feelings. However, for most of the toddler years, their modes of expression of anger include varied degrees of screaming, kicking, throwing things, and even hurting themselves by banging their head or biting them selves. Sometimes toddlers will hold their breath when overcome with intense anger. When display of anger reaches an uncontrollable level it is typically referred to as a *temper tantrum.* One can hardly witness such an outburst without being impressed with its tone of desperation. It is as if the intensity of the child's feeling causes such internal distress that his or her only recourse is to release it all at once. The most common age for temper tantrums is 18 months to 3 years—the age of negativism and resistive behavior. This developmental stage makes toddlers particularly vulnerable to physical demonstrations of anger. Their struggle for independence is strong. Interference or thwarting of their self-determined course brings angry resistance, but their limited language and reasoning ability leave them little alternative but to have a tantrum.

Anticipatory Guidance: Anger, Aggression, and Temper Tantrums

Mismanagement of normal expressions of anger by a toddler can cause serious consequences to the child

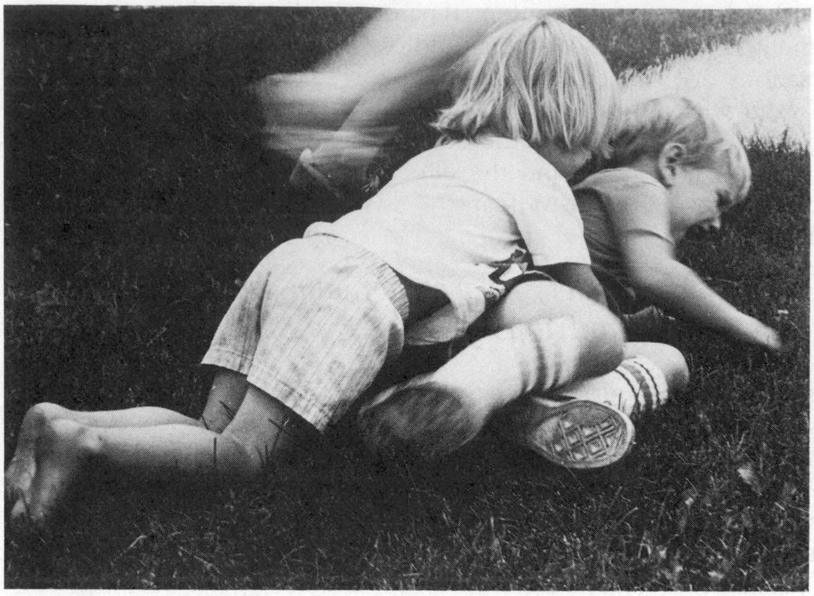

Toddlers express emotions physically through biting, hitting, or pulling. (Photo by Jim Tackett.)

and his or her family. The nurse must be sensitive to clues that suggest developing conflict. Even before a pattern of temper tantrums develops the nurse can help parents cope with small annoyances caused by resistive behavior.

Nursing management begins by encouraging parents to express the distress and embarrassment they feel when their child has a temper tantrum. This period of "telling the story" is filled with clues for management. While hearing out a parent, the nurse should seek to answer the following questions: (1) How do the parents feel about how they handle temper tantrums? (2) Are they asking for help to change their behavior? (3) In the nurse's judgment, is there a potential for child abuse? (4) Are the parents making an attempt to control situational factors such as tiredness, hunger, excessive demands, and insecurity? (5) Do the parents understand the developmental needs of a normal toddler? The goal of the nurse is to assist the family to cope with the normal developmental tasks that their toddler is mastering without making undue demands on individual family members.

When counseling parents, the nurse must also consider the varied cultural approaches to expressions of anger. There is a broad range of acceptable aggressive behaviors among cultures. That which is unacceptable behavior to the nurse may be encouraged by parents, or vice versa. The nurse's concern then is to assist the family to handle the daily expressions of anger in a way that is consistent with their own pattern of behavior.

The goal for management of their toddler's normal expression of anger is that "tantrums must achieve nothing, and the cause of the tantrum—insecurity, faulty management, or fatigue—should be looked for" (Ilingsworth, 1975). Although it is the nurse's role to help parents understand that temper tantrums are normal for this age, he or she should also assist the family to make every attempt to alter those circumstances that predictably result in a tantrum. The frequency, duration, and intensity of tantrums can be reduced if situational factors are controlled. Situational factors affecting the toddler to be examined can be pinpointed with the following questions: (1) Is the child tired and hungry? (2) Have excessive demands been made that are beyond his or her developmental capability? (3) Has the child's security been threatened? (4) Has he or she been excessively stimulated? (5) Is the child suffering from boredom? (6) Has there been physical exercise?

During the toddler years the most effective method of handling temper tantrums is to ignore the behavior. If a tantrum is to achieve nothing, parents are obliged to give nothing in response to it. If the temper tantrum is accompanied by breath holding, the parents need to know that ignoring this behavior will not result in harm. The child will resume breathing as a reflex when he or she needs to.

Two forms of ineffective responding are common, and in each case the tantrum has achieved something for the toddler. One response is to give in to such children and give them what they want. This stops the tantrum at hand but breeds repetition of the behavior because it has been rewarded. Another response by the parents is to have a tantrum of their own. Striking out at a child with violent verbal and physical aggression is just another form of reinforcing the child's aggressive behavior. A review of learning theories of development (Chapter 3) reminds us that behaviors that are rewarded are repeated. Any form of attention to a behavior can be perceived by the toddler as a reward. Any form of attention in response to a tantrum should be avoided if the parent hopes to break the inevitable cycle of repetition.

Nurses must realize that there is no foolproof method to handle temper tantrums. The counsel they give must be given with an attitude of suggestions and options rather than solutions. Whenever temper tantrums become the pattern of behavior, the nurse should assist parents to carefully evaluate the circumstances surrounding the tantrums and correct any that predictably bring on a tantrum.

Independence, Negativism, and Dawdling

Toddlers have attained numerous abilities that foster independence. Their motor, language, and cognitive skills combined with their developing sense of self have an additive effect toward independent behavior. Independence, however, does not exclude a toddler's need to be dependent. Much of a toddler's behavior is characterized by ambivalence. Although toddlers are in constant battle to strive for their independence, they continue to seek attention, approval, and physical closeness from their caregivers. When these goals are in conflict, toddlers need the understanding of parents who are able to promote their independence and to respond flexibly to their periodic pleas to be dependent.

Negativism and dawdling are manifestations of the noncompliant spirit that pervades the personality of a toddler. *Negativism* is the resistance a toddler displays around 18 months that lasts to about 3 years of age. This stage is characterized by a seeming delight in doing the opposite of what he or she is asked to do. *Dawdling* is a form of controlling others by responding to demands in a self-determined way. If children sense they are being hurried to perform or are asked to do something specifically, they may do it but prolong the activity unmercifully. Dawdling then controls to what degree they can be manipulated by others, whereas negativism is a decided resistance to being controlled by others.

The "no, no" toddlers proclaim tells more about their ego development than it does about their desired course of action. Most of the time the firm assertion "no!" is little more than an affirmation of their power to decide their own course. The telltale feature of toddlers' "no" that means "yes" is that while repeating "no, no, no" they simultaneously carry out the very thing they are resisting, as if their words had no relationship to their actions.

Dawdling is an expression of feelings similar to those reflected in the use of "no, no"; that is, toddlers have the need to assert their power to control. There is no better way for toddlers to be in control than by showing others that they decide when and at what speed they will cooperate.

When the unfolding toddler's sense of self and emanating drive to exercise his or her will are considered, negativism and dawdling can be understood as constructive behaviors toward developing autonomy and self-esteem. The nurse who works with a family of a toddler will probably, however, find that it is not so impressed with the constructive nature of these behaviors but rather finds the situation exasperating and frustrating. The assertion of the child's will to master self-control is difficult for the family.

Anticipatory Guidance: Independence, Negativism, and Dawdling

In an environment that fosters the attainment of a sense of autonomy and positive self-esteem, the family provides a graded independence with consistent application of limits. The nurse can help a family accomplish this goal by encouraging them to air their frustrations and describe those situations that cause difficulty. It is sometimes difficult for families to adjust to toddlers who want to do everything for themselves and to be held and cuddled at their own convenience. Parents need to be assured that the strivings for independence are not a rejection of their love but are actually an index of the quality of their ongoing love and affection.

Family members can learn to cope with negativism and dawdling if the nurse informs them about the developmental significance of these behaviors, gives them an opportunity to express their own frustrations, and gives suggestions to manage the behaviors. There are a number of consolations for parents with toddlers; these behaviors are normal, it is a stage that will eventually resolve, and other parents feel similar frustrations.

The following suggestions may be helpful if parents find their toddler's negativism and dawdling particularly stressful:

- avoid questions that can be answered by no,
- don't phrase a request as a choice if no choice is really available to the child,
- avoid requesting completion of tasks when the toddler is tired or hungry,
- help the child finish when he or she dawdles (at the toddler's own pace),
- pay special attention to the child when there is excessive stimulation caused by the presence of many people,
- avoid drawing attention to negativistic and dawdling behaviors.

Forewarning a family of the activities that are potential battlegrounds is a preventive nursing function.

Typical situations when toddlers are likely to exert their own will relate to eating, sleeping, elimination, and dressing.

Becoming Social

The family influence the socialization of its toddler. The drive for autonomy needs to be molded for positive social development. Toddlers who insist on their own way without modifying their behavior for the benefit of others clearly are not moving toward a socialized level of development. Social experiences of a toddler can be described as those "designed to shape behavior in accordance with goals held by his family and society" (Smart and Smart, 1977).

During the toddler years many newly acquired skills affect the process of socialization. Increased perception, mobility, manual dexterity, language acquisition, and mastery in self-care increase the child's self-esteem. With experience toddlers begin to realize that to feel accepted they must sometimes defer to the wishes of others rather than always have their own way. This conflict between the need for acceptance and the will to do as they please has been described as *growth ambivalence.* Manifestations of growth ambivalence are prevalent; eating, sleeping, toilet training, playing, and self-care activities are all affected by a need to be dependent yet independent.

Becoming Social in Eating Behavior

Toddlers move from a stage of relative dependence to one of almost complete independence in eating behavior. With practice they learn to use eating utensils and show a beginning respect for the table manners adopted by their families. Socialized eating behavior is thus a standard determined within cultures and more specifically within families. A toddler within a traditional Chinese family may be fed longer than a child in Western culture because chop-sticks are difficult to manipulate. Within some cultures utensils are not used, and eating with hands is the social norm for adults. However, in Western culture a toddler is taught to use fingers primarily for those foods prepared to be picked up.

Becoming social in eating behavior implies more than getting food into one's mouth. Toddlers also learn to control their behavior in the way they make their likes and dislikes known. Impulsive throwing of food, demanding by screaming or pounding, or refusing to sit down to eat or to eat at all are typical toddler behaviors that must eventually be altered to a more acceptable level of behavior. A toddler's perpetual motion, fascination with the varied textures of food, and clever experimentation of dumping, mixing, and stacking are typical mealtime behaviors that eventually are given up for more acceptable table manners.

The developmental characteristics of toddlers affect the gradual attainment of socialized eating behavior. At 15 months they may insist on trying to feed themselves even though they lack the physical skills to do so. From 18 to 24 months toddlers' physical skills have improved but now they become engrossed in playing with their food. They resist any interruption of their "game" and protest any infringements of their territory. By the age of 3 toddlers feed themselves with only occasional spills and less fascination with food manipulation. Their imitative behaviors, increased motor skills, and wish to be independent, coupled with their need for parental approval, bring about rapid social development in eating behavior during the toddler years. Reaching this level of independence gives them a sense of mastery and fosters their self-esteem. See Health Maintenance section for anticipatory guidance.

Developing Sleep Regularity and Routines

A toddler requires approximately 10 to 14 hours of sleep. Most toddlers take an afternoon nap, and before 2 years of age some may need a morning and an afternoon nap. Keeping toddlers on a relatively consistent sleeping schedule reduces the frequency of irritable and cranky periods. They cannot tolerate losing sleep without showing changes in their behavior.

Developmental characteristics that are displayed in sleep behaviors of toddlers are ritualism, separation anxiety, and autonomy (they resist sleep). Beginning at 18 to 21 months and continuing until 3 years, they prepare for bed by performing several activities in a precise order (washing, brushing teeth, turning a light switch, putting shoes into a certain place, and a variety of other time-consuming tasks). These rituals give toddlers a sense of security that they need when they are learning to separate themselves from their attachment figures. The child's autonomous nature is expressed in these rituals in that they provide a sense of control. Rituals can be viewed as a form of dawdling in which toddlers go to bed after they have done what they want to and when they are ready to do so. At this stage it is also common to have a favorite toy or blanket (transitional object), which is taken to bed for security.

Sleep is also resisted by more obvious behaviors, especially as toddlers approach their second birthday. Toddlers may resist so violently that they have temper tantrums or they may stand in the crib and cry for their parents. Such behaviors are eventually given up as toddlers overcome separation anxiety and as their intense need to control lessens. See Chapter 20 for further discussion of rest and sleep.

Anticipatory Guidance: Sleep Behaviors

Parents may need the counsel of a nurse as they try alternate methods of coping with normal bedtime behaviors of their toddler. Many bedtime crises can be avoided by planning approaches that take into consideration the developmental characteristics of a toddler. The incessant activity and curiosity so typical of this age leave a toddler irritable, overtired, and highly stimulated if some effort is not made to provide a quiet period before bedtime. Toddlers' engrossment in play and their need to have some control over their actions make it necessary to give them some warning before it is time for bed. To abruptly inform them that it is time for bed and that they must put their toys away is certain to bring resistance and perhaps a tantrum, especially if they are tired. Forewarning and then helping the child to put the toys away followed by reading a favorite book will more likely bring the desired result.

Helping parents cope with the bedtime rituals is another area for the nurse to consider. Parents should be advised to keep bedtime activities as simple as possible. Once a routine has been established a toddler will insist on following it; therefore it is easier to avoid adding additional rituals than it is to omit them after they have been started. It does not work to tell a toddler, "Just tonight you may turn the light switch off and on."

Bedtime can be a pleasant time if parents allow extra time for the rituals rather than altering them against the toddler's wishes. Once the usual rituals have been carried out, it is most effective if the parent says "good night" and does not return to the room. If a toddler can manipulate a parent to repeatedly return for minor requests, the behavior is likely to be repeated. If the child has a legitimate request it is only reasonable to grant it, but repeated requests are the toddler's way of postponing separation, and this is a form of sleep resistance. If a child stands in the crib and cries after the usual routines have been completed, it is better to leave and usually the child goes to sleep. He or she may cry until falling asleep, but eventually the child learns that the parents are in control of the sleep routine. It is not uncommon for toddlers to have particular difficulty separating from their mother at bedtime, in which case the fathers may have more success in getting them to bed.

A toddler's resistance to sleep can be exasperating to parents. It is helpful to point out that many of a toddler's fears are encountered at bedtime. Children's fears of separation, of the dark and of noises such as flushing the toilet and water rushing out of the tub all happen in relation to going to bed. Although fear of the dark is more common after 3 years of age, some toddlers show signs of such fear earlier. It is important for the nurse to help parents recognize that the child's fear is real and should not be ridiculed and that most bedtime fears can be dispelled with help and patience from parents. Although sleeping practices vary in cultures, it is generally recommended that children not sleep in their parents' bed.

Toilet Training

All areas of development are involved in the successful attainment of bowel and bladder control. Physical, intellectual, and emotional-social aspects of development occur simultaneously and are interdependent with the completion of this task. "Because the acquisition of mature toileting behavior is a universal developmental milestone, every major developmental theory must provide an explanation for it" (Martin et al, 1984). Neuromuscular maturation, awareness of imminent elimination, and the desire to please parents by staying clean and dry are necessary before toilet training can be achieved. In other words, successful toilet training requires physical, cognitive, and psychologic readiness.

Physical maturation of the sphincter muscles and myelination of the spinal cord are biologic requirements for the control of elimination. By the time toddlers sit and walk well (12 to 18 months), their nerve pathways have developed to the extent that they can physically control their bowel and bladder sphincters. The regularity of bowel movements is usually better established by 18 months than it was in infancy. Bowel movements are often associated with meals, with one after breakfast or one after supper or at both times. However, there is a wide variation in when toddlers develop regularity and the pattern of regularity.

In addition to the physical ability of sphincter control, the child must have cognitive awareness of elimination and the ability to communicate this awareness to the mother or caregiver. The awareness level that must accompany neuromuscular development comes later. The stages of awareness that most children go through are (1) an awareness that elimination has just occurred; (2) an awareness of the process of eliminating while doing it; and (3) an awareness that elimination is imminent. It is generally agreed that by 18 months of age toddlers have some awareness that a bowel movement is occurring and that some children even indicate by gestures that they know it is coming; however, it is usually not until closer to 2 years of age that they can give enough advance warning to be helped to the toilet. Children must also possess psychologic readiness, a desire to please their parent by holding on and letting go at appropriate times. Waiting until closer to 2 years or 30 months of age to begin toilet training increases the success rate considerably.

Some children attain bowel control before bladder control. Brazelton (1962) found that 80 per cent of

1163 children studied had achieved both by age 33.3 months, daytime control was attained earlier than nighttime control, and girls tended to attain control 2.4 months earlier than boys. Even if training is not achieved by age 5 or even later, it usually is not indicative of any pathology but rather of the individual variation that exists.

Anticipatory Guidance: Toilet Training

Toilet training is often an early source of parenting conflict, involving many emotional factors and psychologic consequences. It is therefore important to look at the effects that misdirected training attempts can have. There are three categories of unhealthy toilet training patterns: attempting to toilet train too early, placing undue emphasis on the product and cleanliness rather than on the process of toilet training, and being coercive and punitive during toilet training (Dodson, 1970; Shulz, 1976).

Attempting Training Too Early

The earlier toilet training is attempted, the longer it will take to accomplish and the greater the impact on the child's development and character (Bernstein, 1979). When children are started in training before 18 months to 2 years, they lack enough muscular control to master voluntary "letting go," and they develop a sense of failure. Because they cannot intellectually connect the toileting sequence and involuntary sphincter relaxation with the product, they cannot understand what is being requested of them; instead they develop a fear of anger or loss of affection (sensed as abandonment) from the trainer and they fear a loss of self-control, since they perceive the product as having appeared magically or by some power in the trainer. A "battle of the pot" contest is likely to ensue because children's physical mobility is restricted, the objects of their curiosity are removed, and for no apparent reason that they can perceive. There are indications that early training leads to some exaggerated character traits, including fearfulness, aggression, compulsiveness, obstinacy, and difficulty experiencing pleasure (Herbert, 1975).

Overemphasis on Product

The major problem with focusing on the product rather than the process of toilet training is that if there is no product (which can often be the case, especially if the parent rather than the child is prompting the visits to the bathroom), the parent's response shows annoyance, hostility, or even rejection, at least from the toddler's perspective. According to Freudian theorists, the child who attempts to meet these cleanliness (toileting) demands often over-responds to the point of becoming obsessed with an exaggerated need for cleanliness, orderliness, and punctuality, being scrupulous about very insignificant matters and confusing body functions and sexuality with dirtiness. It is believed that such a person has a preoccupation with bowel movements throughout life.

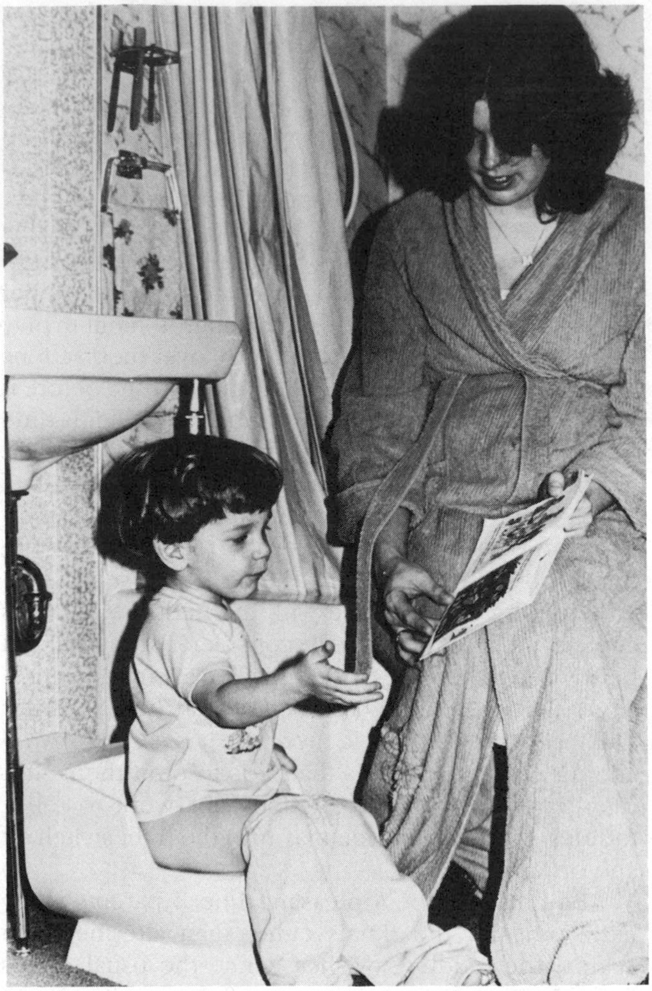

In a positive, reinforcing environment, toddlers actually train themselves. (Photo by Jim Tackett.)

Strict, Coercive Training

This type of training leads to many emotional upsets in both toddlers and trainers. Children have more accidents* and experience more punitive measures, especially physical. These toddlers learn to hate themselves and their trainers. They are in a double bind, for if they comply with their parent's demands they lose autonomy and if they do not comply they experience punishment and still do not feel autonomous because they cannot control this body function. Such children become defeated, full of frustration and undermined self-confidence. Their frustration is often expressed in

*Perhaps a subconscious form of rebellion despite the child's fear of punishment. See discussion of encopresis in older child, page 1117.

behaviors such as extreme shyness, night terrors, eating problems, or outright rebellion during any interactions with their trainers. A research finding worth noting is that the parent who is coercive in toilet training almost always restricts other "messy" activities, such as sand or water play, use of clay or finger paints, or play with food during meals (Ambron, 1977).

By introducing the subject of toilet training early a nurse can prevent the conflict of inappropriate training. Soon after their baby is 1 year of age parents may be receiving toilet training advice from friends and relatives. The nurse should therefore discuss toilet training by the time the child is 12 to 15 months old so that parents have an understanding of the developmental factors affecting successful toilet training. If they have accurate information, they will feel less compelled to begin toilet training too early. Information regarding the age at which most children complete toilet training can influence the age at which such training is begun. Martin and colleagues (1984) found support for the hypothesis that maternal pressure is strongly related to the age of onset of toilet training but not to the age at which toilet training is completed. Knowledge of this tendency might deter some parents from pressuring their children to begin toilet training before it is appropriate.

The readiness of the child and family are equally important when determining the best time to begin toilet training. The nurse should alert the family to the importance of a stable, nonstressed environment for successful toilet training. If certain stressful events can be predicted, it is better to wait until after the event has occurred and an equilibrium has been re-established. Events that cause a change in routine or environment interfere with the toddler's progress in accomplishing a new task. For example, birth of a sibling, parental change of jobs, an older sibling leaving for college, a family vacation, or geographic relocation would be felt as stresses by the toddler and the stress of toilet training should not be superimposed. If such events cannot be avoided during toilet training, the nurse has a responsibility to help the family understand and cope with the regression that such stresses cause.

The nurse should explain that there are no precise rules or schedules that can be applied to guarantee successful toilet training. From the beginning, parents need to feel relaxed and confident that their toddler will achieve the task of toilet training without undue pressure and control from them. Some useful suggestions that the nurse can offer are: (1) do not punish noncompliance, (2) do not force a toddler to sit on the toilet, (3) use praise as a reinforcer for positive results, (4) capitalize on a toddler's imitative behavior by allowing observance of adult elimination, (5) avoid creating a tense environment, (6) wait for readiness of the child, and (7) do not begin when the family is experiencing undue stress (Box 6-5).

Parents must be willing to wait for their children's readiness for toilet training and then accept their successes and relapses as they learn. In a positive, reinforcing environment toddlers actually "train" themselves. Toddlers demonstrate readiness in many ways. They develop a distaste for wet or soiled diapers, recognize when they have urinated or defecated, and tell their caregiver. They signify a need to eliminate verbally or with gestures. Willingness to release their grasp of a favorite toy on command is often a sign of readiness to "let go" in toilet training. Children who remain dry for several hours, who urinate large amounts at one time rather than frequent dribbling, and who can remove their own pants are also demonstrating signs of readiness.

Nurses who identify actual or potential stress in the area of toilet training should immediately institute interventions to relieve the stress. Their teaching should emphasize that, given time, toddlers will themselves indicate their readiness for training; it should also indicate there is no room in this matter for force or punishment, but rather the use of tactful suggestions and quiet flattery will gain the toddler's cooperation in the toileting sequence. They should teach that it is wise to wait until the child is at least 24 months of age so that training can be completed faster and easier by a toddler mature enough to perform the whole sequence alone. If a parent is patient enough (diapers do become a monotonous, bothersome feature of child care) to wait for the toddler's readiness, all he or she will have to invest in the training is an initial explanation of the toileting sequence in terms the child can understand. Then the parent can praise the successes and ignore the failures as the child masters for himself or herself the task of toileting self-control.

Box 6-5
Factors That Encourage Successful Toilet Training

Observe the time of day that child has bowel movement and place him or her on the potty prior to that time.

The potty should be comfortable and secure-feeling to the child.

Use acceptable and simple, easy to understand words and gestures to indicate to the child what is expected of him or her.

Encouraging the child to play with toys may distract from the purpose of toilet training; use distraction judiciously if at all.

10 to 15 minutes is long enough for the child to sit on the potty.

Reinforce success with verbal praise and physical affection.

Do not punish lack of success or noncompliance.

Becoming Social by Participating in Self-Care

The increasing development of motor skills enables toddlers to participate in their own care. They participate in such activities in the spirit of play, but this is how they develop the necessary skills for independence. Toddlers are generally intent on doing things for themselves before they have the necessary gross and fine motor skills to complete tasks efficiently. They gradually become adept at self-care and from 1 to 3 years of age progress from almost total dependence to a remarkably high level of independence. Participation in self-care activities helps toddlers to feel positive about their own abilities, and the praise of their parents makes them feel loved and accepted, all of which contribute to their developing self-esteem.

Becoming Social Through Play

Toddlers' play is affected by all aspects of development, and play influences their physical, intellectual, and emotional-social development. Toddlers have specific needs that can be met through play. They need to be physically active and to explore and learn about objects, people, and unfamiliar territory, to experience a variety of sensations (movement, tactile), to practice small muscle skills, to identify with significant others by imitation, to develop language skills, and to begin to relate to others through play. To facilitate a toddler's development it is important to provide a variety of play opportunities.

The characteristics of toddlers' play are determined by their developmental level. They remain primarily egocentric in play activities, showing little regard for the feelings of others. Egocentrism in play is characterized by a predominance of behaviors that prove children's own power and central position. This is how they build their self-image, which contributes to their rapidly developing awareness of themselves as persons. The type of play coming out of these needs is *parallel play,* in which children engage in similar activities while playing beside each other but not together.

During this period children learn a great deal by imitating their caregivers. They particularly enjoy helping with household tasks. They will happily squeeze water out of a sponge, carry silverware to the table, and fold clothes after a fashion. They also enjoy playing with real items that they see their parents use. The classic example is the toddler's fascination with emptying a cupboard of pots and pans. To a toddler, manipulation of pots and pans is a form of helping by imitation. Although the help toddlers give usually creates work for their parents, these imitative behaviors are an important step in development.

Another characteristic of a toddler's play is the love of active play and manipulation of objects. Exercise of both large and small muscles is necessary for toddlers to develop a sense of control over their bodies and their environments. Toddlers' needs to explore are facilitated by their gross and fine motor abilities that give them access to almost anything that intrigues them. Toddlers enjoy activities of motion such as a ride on a tricycle, stroller, wagon, or swing.

Toddlers also learn about their environment through their sensory experiences. Anyone who observes toddlers at play will note that much of what they

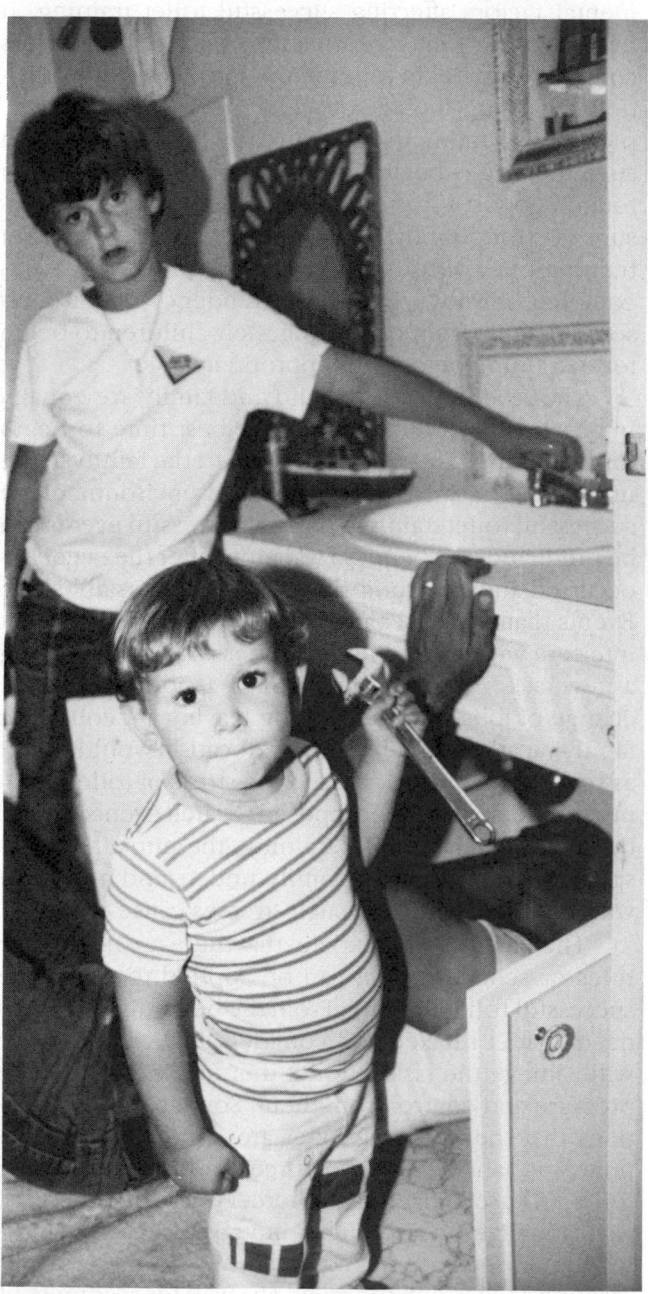

Toddlers enjoy playing with real items used by parents.

do provides sensory benefits. Toddlers touch objects to see how they feel, run their fingers over them, and still explore with their lips and tongue, although mouthing objects is now less frequent than during infancy. They are also fascinated by the various sounds they can make and experiment using voice, tongue, and lips to create new sounds or to imitate the sounds they hear.

Some quiet, sedentary activities are also appropriate for the toddler and are especially useful before bedtime. Much of a toddler's encounter with books during the period from 12 to 24 months involves identification of objects, turning pages and imitating familiar sounds of animals and objects such as trains, cars and trucks. Toddlers also enjoy having parents read to them and repeat nursery rhymes. From 2 to 3 years of age, as their attention spans increase, they become increasingly interested in listening to and imitating nursery rhymes and hearing short stories illustrated by pictures.

Children develop language through their play. Their play experiences increase their encounters with the world, requiring them to attach labels to what they do and sense. For example, toddlers who want the straddle toy that another child is using will pull on it and say "ride." They will likewise learn to say "bike-ride" if they want their parents to take them for a ride. The raw material for thinking, imagination, and language is experienced through the senses, and the more they can experience, the more they have to express.

The frustrations that toddlers experience because of their struggles with developing autonomy can be directed into suitable play activities. Simple activities of running, throwing a ball, and hammering on a peg board are ways to dissipate excess energy safely. Many sensory experiences have the added benefit of providing a means for expression of aggressive behavior. Pounding, splashing, and hitting are harmless when directed at sand, water, or soap bubbles. These energy-dissipating activities allow toddlers to express how they feel within the confines of social acceptance while gaining approval and increasing self-esteem and self-control. See Health Maintenance section for anticipatory guidance.

Gender Identity, Sex-Role Identification, and Sexuality

Gender identity is one's subjectively felt sense of being male or female. *Sex role* (or gender role) refers to the behaviors that show appropriate male or female orientation. Awareness of gender identity begins around 18 months and is fully established by 5 years of age (Armstrong, 1978). Although 2-year-olds are not aware of anatomic differences, they can distinguish between males and females by general appearance. Most toddlers know whether they are boys or girls by 3 years of age and have some notion of sex-appropriate behaviors.

During the toddler years gender identity and sex-role identification are primarily influenced by experiences within the family. When a toddler is consistently treated as being of a particular sex, the child internalizes that gender identity. For example, repeated expressions to him as a "big boy" or to her as a "sweet girl" help a child learn this identity. Rewards for proper self-identification as male or female also help the child develop normal gender identity.

Sex-role identification during the toddler years is learned through imitation and involves differences in the way parents interact with boys and girls. A toddler imitates both parents but particularly the same-sex parent, adopting appropriate roles, attitudes, and values. From the child's birth, parents generally behave differently toward boys and girls, resulting in early socialization into male and female roles. Some of the differences are that mothers talk and respond more to infant girls than to boys, boys may be handled more roughly in play, and more aggressive behavior is tolerated in boys than in girls.

A toddler learns which behaviors are appropriate for his or her sex by the responses received from parents. Such behaviors are referred to as *sex-typed behaviors.* Parents give different rewards for a certain behavior depending on whether the behavior is displayed by a boy or girl. Parents make such responses out of their own ideas of sex-appropriate behavior, resulting in a wide variety of responses from one parent to another and particularly from one culture to another. However, within most families and most cultures boys and girls behave differently.

Anticipatory Guidance: Gender Identity, Sex-Role Identification, and Sexuality

A family may feel confused about what kind of behaviors to encourage regarding sex-role identification. The question of choice of toys may be brought to the nurse because parents disagee or because parents have read about the advantages of teaching all children the sex-role behaviors of both sexes. The nurse can be most helpful by encouraging parents to make traditionally sex-typed toys equally available to male and female children if this approach is consistent with their own philosophy. Nurses' own biases will certainly influence their stance, but it is essential that their counsel not pressure parents into feeling that they must strive either to enforce or discourage sex-typed behaviors. The nurse's role is to provide information so parents can make their own decisions according to their personal and cultural orientation.

The nurse can facilitate normal development of gender identity by encouraging parents to develop a close relationship with their toddler. Parents should be assisted to plan their responsibilities so that both can spend time with the child. If only one parent is present, the nurse should explore with the parent ways in which a substitute mother or father figure can be established. Often a relationship with a relative, friend, or neighbor can play a significant role in a toddler's life and warrants the extra time and effort that a parent puts into providing such an opportunity.

It is during the toddler years that parents become aware of more deliberate genital self-exploration in their child. Also, parents begin to have concerns about their own nudity in the presence of a toddler of the opposite sex. The nurse should encourage parents to deal with these issues in a way that is comfortable for them, but they should not shame or punish a toddler for exploring his or her genitals. The way parents respond to these early sexual behaviors and interests forms the beginnings of the child's own sexuality. See Chapter 22 for further discussion of sexuality.

Health Maintenance

Throughout this chapter counseling and guidance of parents has been emphasized as an important role of the nurse. Understanding and being prepared for developmental changes before they occur gives parents a feeling of security and eases the stress that the toddler years can bring. Counseling needs vary from one family to another. Concerns that a family might bring to a nurse are discussed throughout this chapter. However, during the toddler years there are four areas of health maintenance that a nurse should discuss with each family: nutrition, play, safety and immunizations.

Nutrition and Development

Changes in each aspect of development affect nutritional intake during the toddler years. The nurse's counseling is based on a thorough assessment of (1) usual intake within a 24-hour period, (2) level of motor ability achieved in self-feeding skills, (3) effect of normal toddler development on eating behavior, and (4) concerns that parents have about their toddler's food and nutrient intake.

The nurse's role is to prepare parents by reviewing developmental changes that influence the way their toddler eats. By 1 year of age many children have been weaned from the bottle, with the exception of a nighttime bottle. The eruption of additional teeth during the second year makes it possible for toddlers to eat most adult foods. Their slowed growth decreases their requirement for food and is reflected in a decreased appetite. Their increased motor abilities enhance their eating skills, and their emotional-social development markedly influences the eating behavior. Parents who know of and are prepared for these changes can more effectively prevent or cope with the stress involving eating during these years.

Parents should be told that a decrease in appetite is common, and that they can expect a pattern of fluctuation in the amount and type of food their toddlers eat. It is difficult for parents to cope with toddlers who one day eat their meals eagerly and the next refuse to eat anything. Toddlers may insist on certain foods (food jags), which can make it difficult for parents to ensure that they have a balanced diet. These food jags cannot be easily altered but often last for only a few days. During such time toddlers may refuse to eat anything if they are not given at least a small portion of the preferred food. Other foods can be offered in small portions and within a few days they will likely request a different food as the favorite. If the nurse can adequately inform a family and offer suggestions to handle normal developmental behaviors, mealtime and eating can be associated with pleasure and satisfaction in these early impressionable years (Table 6-2).

The nurse should also discuss nutritional concerns involving dentition, iron deficiency anemia, and obesity. The major points to discuss with parents regarding nutrition and dentition are that sweets be avoided as between-meal snacks, that 16 to 24 ounces of milk be consumed daily, and that a bedtime bottle, if offered, not contain juice or milk. Iron deficiency anemia is prevented if adequate iron-rich foods are consumed and milk is limited to 24 ounces daily. This is recommended because toddlers may drink too much milk. This causes satiation that, in turn, decreases intake of solid foods rich in iron (liver, dark green vegetables, iron-enriched cereals, egg yolk). Obesity can be prevented by using skim or low-fat milk and by offering limited sweets (especially candy and sodas). Snacks should consist of small amounts of nutritious foods. Obesity in toddlerhood is also prevented by providing opportunities for physical exercise. The nurse should pay particular attention to how food is used by the parents. The practice of using food as a reward or to pacify may establish patterns that lead to obesity later.

A quantitative 24-hour dietary recall gives nurses information to help them assess the need for additional nutritional counseling or referral for further evaluation and treatment. A toddler eats approximately half as much food as an adult and should be served foods from the basic four food groups. Vitamin and iron supplementation is unnecessary unless a well-balanced diet is not consumed. Parents should be encouraged to make a serious effort to provide a balanced diet to establish healthful practices of eating rather than relying on vitamins and iron preparations. See Chapter 18 for further discussion of nutrition.

Table 6-2. Guidelines to Promote Socialized Eating Behavior

Principles	Suggestions
To develop skill in manipulating utensils, toddlers need the opportunity to practice but may need some assistance. They will often refuse assistance even though they need it.	At 15 months: help by feeding with a second spoon, provide finger foods. At 18–24 months: be supportive by helping the child get food onto spoon to mouth. Continue finger foods.
At mealtime a toddler should learn to associate mastery, pleasure, and acceptance with the experience of eating.	Avoid forcing of food. Allow self-feeding but assist on toddler's terms; avoid punishment for spills and messiness. Praise attempts at self-feeding even though many spills occur.
A toddler needs total concentration to accomplish the skills of self-feeding.	Provide a quiet place with minimal distraction; no loud music or television. Once the meal has begun, getting up from the table and returning by parents and siblings distract a toddler.
Food intake is likely to decrease if toddlers have been involved in vigorous physical activity immediately prior to a meal, or if they have had to wait a significant time past regular mealtime. They also take less interest in food if they are overtired (lacking sleep) or overfatigued (too much physical activity.)	A time of quiet before meals and regularity in mealtimes is conducive to a toddler's appetite. Keeping children on a balanced schedule of rest and activity improves their dispositions and general eating behavior.
A toddler imitates eating behaviors of his or her family.	Parents need to provide appropriate role modeling and to discipline siblings in table manners.
A toddler finds security in following certain routines and rituals.	Use the same plate, cup, and utensils, and consistency in the order of preparing the toddler for eating (washing hands, sitting in chair, serving food).
Toddlers' appetites fluctuate, as do their moods. Variation from dependence to independence is prevalent in toddlers' eating behaviors, as is a strong need to have their own way. A toddler cannot be forced to eat.	Do not try to force a child to eat. When toddlers refuse to eat and insist they want to get out of the high chair or down from the table, let them miss a meal. Avoid snacks and they will probably eat the next scheduled meal. Over a period of a week intake is usually adequate.

Play and Development

The nurse can increase a family's awareness and understanding of how play enhances the toddler's development. The motor skills that affect play (see chapter discussion on skills affecting play) can be discussed with parents, as well as the characteristics of a toddler's play, his or her developmental needs for play, and appropriate activities to meet these needs. Sharing this information helps parents to have realistic expectations regarding a toddler's interactions during play and prepares them to knowledgeably guide the child's development through play.

The nurse should encourage parents to play with their toddler. Toddlers will play alone or beside another toddler for short periods, but they also enjoy the attention and interaction that play with adults affords. Special times set aside for play with a toddler are rewarding to both the child and the adult. When siblings are present, parents especially need to provide time for play for each child separately. Household tasks and work responsibilities can be arranged in such a way that each parent is free for at least a short time each day to provide opportunities for play.

There are certain circumstances that require special effort on the part of parents to provide adequate play opportunities. When a toddler is an only child, some provision should be made for play with another child or children about the same age. When there are siblings close in age parents also have problems, such as arguments and fighting during play. Each family develops its own pattern of handling conflicts between children, but a basic rule is to let children solve their own problems as much as possible. When a babysitter cares for their toddler it is advisable that parents plan special activities such as drawing, water play, or outdoor activities to guard against excessive use of television. Instructions can be given to the babysitter regarding play as the parent would for meal preparation.

Toddlers are especially prone to injury because the excitement of play engrosses their entire being. They do not anticipate danger and are particularly vulnerable because of their insatiable curiosity and limited precision in gross and fine motor skills. The nurse should encourage parents to remove dangerous household objects and carefully evaluate the safety of toys before purchase.

The nurse should stress that a toddler needs a variety of play opportunities; however, it is unnecessary to buy expensive toys. Play with various-sized cardboard boxes, plastic containers and jar lids, access to pots and pans, permission to enjoy the sensations that nature offers, and encouragement to be the parents' helper give a toddler many of the experiences that foster development.

Suggestions for appropriate toys and play activities should be offered by the nurse for the age of the toddler (see Chapter 21). Children may play with the same toy throughout the toddler years, playing with it differently as they grow older. Therefore many of the same toys are appropriate throughout toddlerhood.

Safety and Development

Accident prevention is one of the greatest challenges that face health professionals who care for children. The stages of childhood development can be used to predict the type of accidents most likely to occur. By 1 year of age toddlers are very mobile, and as they pull themselves to standing position they pull at whatever is within reach. Hanging table cloths, dangling cords, and unstable furniture are hazards. From 1 to 2 years it is the child's curiosity without a sense of danger that makes him or her vulnerable to accidents. By the time children are 2 their speed of mobility adds still another danger to which parents must be alerted. Types of accidents that parents should guard against as common hazards to toddlers are: (1) accidents while riding in a car, (2) being hit by a moving vehicle, (3) drowning, (4) ingesting harmful substances, (5) burns, (6) aspiration of a foreign body, (7) suffocation, (8) falls, and (9) toy accidents.

A familiarity with what toddlers are likely to do is a parent's best defense. Safety should be discussed at each health care visit to keep the parents abreast of the rapid development that takes place during the toddler years. Parents need frequent reminders that toddlers are compelled by a constant drive to see "what would happen if . . ." but do not comprehend the danger involved. It is the preventive measures of their parents that keep toddlers safe, and it is the nurse's responsibility to provide the motivation and guidance required to help parents meet that obligation.

Immunization

Measles, mumps, and rubella (MMR) will be given in a combined vaccine during the toddler years. DPT and polio vaccines, as well as the *Haemophilus influenzae* B (HiB) vaccine may also be given. Refer to Chapter 14 for further information about immunizations.

References

Ambron S: *Child Development.* New York, Holt, Rinehart & Winston, 1977.

Armstrong J: Development of sexual identity. *In* Hoekelman RA, et al (eds): *Principles of Pediatrics.* New York, McGraw-Hill, 1978.

Banks M: A family's overconcern about a child in the first two years of life. *Matern Child Nurs J* 1977 Fall; 187.

Bernstein A: Toilet training without fears. *Parents* 1979 Jan; 187.

Bowlby J: *Attachment.* New York, Basic Books, 1969.

Bowlby J: *Attachment and Loss* Series: *Separation: Anxiety and Anger.* Vol. III. New York, Basic Books, 1973.

Brazelton TB: A child oriented approach to toilet training. *Pediatrics* 1962; 29:121–128.

Crockenberg S: Predictors and correlates of anger toward and punitive control of toddlers by adolescent mothers. *Child Dev* 1987; 58:964–975.

Denver Eye Examination Screening Test. Denver, CO, University of Colorado Medical Center, 1973.

Dodson F: *How to Parent.* New York, Signet Books, 1970.

Dunn T, Kendrick C: The arrival of a sibling: changes in patterns of interaction between mother and first-born child. *J Child Psychol Psychiatr* 1980; 21:119–132.

Duvall E: *Marriage and Family Development.* Philadelphia, JB Lippincott, 1977.

Field T, Reite M: Children's responses to separation from mother during the birth of another child. *Child Dev* 1984; 55:1308–1316.

Gates S: Children's literature: it can help children cope with sibling rivalry. *MCN* 1980; 5:351–353.

Gordon M: *Manual of Nursing Diagnosis.* New York, McGraw-Hill, 1987.

Hammer D, Drabman RS: Child discipline: what we know and what we can recommend. *Pediatr Nurs* 1981 May-Jun; 31–35.

Herbert M: *Problems of Childhood.* London, Pan Books Ltd, 1975.

Hoekelman RA, et al: *Primary Pediatric Care.* New York, McGraw-Hill, 1987.

Hoff-Ginsberg E: Function and structure in maternal speech: their relation to the child's development of syntax. *Dev Psychol* 1986; 22(2):155–163.

Honig JC: Preparing preschool-aged children to be siblings. *MCN* 1986; 11:37–43.

Hurlock E: *Child Development.* New York, McGraw-Hill, 1978.

Hyde C: Confessions of a nonspanker. *Parents* 1980 Oct; 86–87.

Illingworth RS: *The Normal Child.* New York, Churchill Livingstone, 1975.

Kirkpatrick E: *The Family as Process and Institution.* New York, Ronald Press, 1963.

Martin JA, King DR, Maccoby EE, et al: Secular trends and individual differences in toilet-training progress. *J Pediatr Psychol* 1984; 9:457–467.

Matas L, et al: Continuity of adaptation in the second year: the relationship between quality attachment and later competence. *Child Dev* 1978 Sep; 547.

Phillips JL: *Origins of Intellect: Piaget's Theory.* New York, WH Freeman, 1969.

Power TG, Chapieski ML: Childrearing and impulse control in toddlers: a naturalistic investigation. *Dev Psychol* 1986; 22(2):271–275.

Pulaski MA: *Understanding Piaget.* New York, Harper & Row, 1971.

Ross Laboratories: *Children are Different: Developmental Physiology.* Cleveland, Ross Laboratories, 1978.

Shiller VM, Izard CE, Hembree EA: Patterns of emotion expression during separation in the strange-situation procedure. *Dev Psychol* 1986; 22(3):378–382.

Shulz D: *The Changing Family: Its Function and Future.* Englewood Cliffs, NJ, Prentice-Hall, 1976.

Slade A: A longitudinal study of maternal involvement and symbolic play during the toddler period. *Child Dev* 1987; 58:367–375.

Smart MS, Smart RC: *Children: Development and Relationships.* 3rd ed. New York, Macmillan, 1977.

Smith DW: *Introduction to Clinical Pediatrics.* Philadelphia, WB Saunders, 1977.

Stewart RB, Mobley LA, VanTuyl SS, et al: The firstborn's adjustment to the birth of a sibling: a longitudinal assessment. *Child Dev* 1987; 58.

Thomas A, Chess S: *Temperament and Development.* New York, Brunner/Mazel, 1977.

White B: *The First Three Years of Life.* Englewood Cliffs, NJ, Prentice-Hall, 1975.

Yarrow L: Right and wrong reasons for having another baby. *Parents* 1979 Jan; 45.

Bibliography

Brazelton TB: *Toddlers and Parents.* New York, Dell Publishing, 1976.

Caplan F, Caplan T: *The Second Twelve Months.* New York, Grosset and Dunlap, 1977.

Christophersen ER: Incorporating behavioral pediatrics into primary care. *Ped Clin N Am* 1982; 29(2): 261–296.

Ditzion J, Wolf D: Beginning parenthood. *In The Woman's Health Book Collective: Ourselves, Our Children: A Book by and for Parents.* New York, Random House, 1978.

Erikson EH: *Childhood and Society.* New York, WW Norton, 1950.

Foster C: Developing responsibility in children. *Science Research Associates* 1977; No. 5-939.

Fraiberg S: *The Magic Years.* New York, Scribner, 1959.

Gulick EE: The effects of breastfeeding on toddler's health. *Pediatr Nurs* 1986 Jan–Feb; 12(1): 51–54.

Horner M, McClellan M: Toilet training: ready or not? *Pediatr Nurs* 1981 Jul; 12–18.

Hymovich D, Barnard M: *Family Health Care: Developmental Situational Crises.* Vol II. New York, McGraw-Hill, 1979.

Piaget J: *The Language and Thought of the Child.* Gabain M, Gabain R (transl). Latimer Trend, 1959.

Piaget J, Inhelder B: *The Psychology of the Child.* New York, Basic Books, 1969.

Prugh D: *The Psycho-Social Aspects of Pediatrics.* Philadelphia, Lea & Febiger, 1985.

Sande DR: Language development in infants and toddlers. *Nurse Pract* 1985 Sep; 10(9): 39–41.

Schleicher I: Teaching parents to cope with behavior problems. *Am J Nurs* 1978 May; 838.

Schulz D: *The Changing Family: Its Function and Future.* Englewood Cliffs, NJ, Prentice-Hall, 1976.

Skolnick A: *The Intimate Environment: Exploring Marriage and the Family.* Boston, Little, Brown, 1973.

Families with Preschoolers — Chapter 7

Jo Joyce Anderson

The world of the preschool child is rapidly expanding both within and beyond the confines of the family unit. All family members are changing cognitively, physically, emotionally, and socially, and those changes affect every family member's functioning. New relationships are forming within the family structure as parents and siblings relate to a preschool child. The nurse needs an awareness of these family interrelationships to effectively give guidance to families with a preschooler.

The family with a preschooler is confronted with the tasks of (1) allocating resources to meet the needs of a more active family; (2) maintaining satisfying communication that recognizes the preschooler's contribution; (3) establishing realistic expectations and responsibilities of family members, including the preschooler; and (4) cultivating relationships with relatives and the world beyond the nuclear family. These tasks are interrelated and accomplished simultaneously within the family unit. They are achieved by building upon previously established patterns of family living.

Related Topics
Theories of moral development, Chapter 3
Development of self-esteem, Chapter 16
Gifted children, Chapter 34
Alterations in development of speech and language, Chapter 51
Vision and hearing assessments, Chapter 15
Family assessment, Chapter 12
Promoting Healthy Parenting, Chapter 13
Coping with stress, Chapter 23

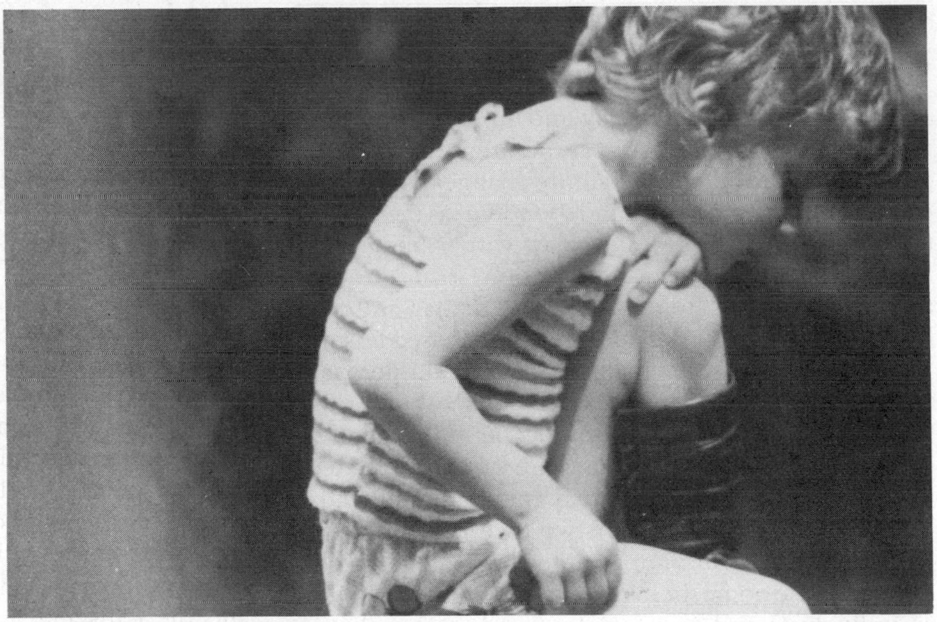

Preschoolers begin to ponder their expanding environment.

Development and Adaptation of the Family with a Preschooler

Resource Allocation

Preschool children, through their initiative, are becoming active members of their existing world. New developmental attainments and expanding interests put new demands on available family resources. A rapidly expanding interest in drawing, coloring, painting, cutting, and pasting necessitates more supplies and space. For the financially secure, employed parent, toys and equipment can be enjoyable to supply, but for the poor family, the suddenly unemployed family, or the family whose income is strained through medical expenses or other family crises, supplying the preschooler's play needs may have a low priority.

The need for larger play equipment to enhance large muscle development and the need for added space to house toys, crafts, and projects of the preschooler are a concern to parents. The child needs a larger bed; additional bedrooms and a larger dining table may be needed as the preschooler grows and matures. For families on a strict budget, these requirements demand reallocation of funds as well as innovative methods of using household materials to make play equipment (making paste and modeling dough; saving partially used paper for the preschooler to draw or paint on; saving safe, empty containers to utilize as building blocks or imaginative play items).

Preschool years are active years in which accidents are not uncommon, thereby increasing financial demands on the already strained family budget. Nursing priorities are (1) continuing to assess for the defining characteristics of the nursing diagnosis *potential for injury* and (2) stressing the importance of safety measures to minimize the probability of accidents. Teaching families how to determine when medical care is needed and teaching basic first aid measures to eliminate frequent emergency room visits may significantly decrease the medical costs of many families.

The preschooler comes into contact with many individuals beyond the nuclear family, which increases the exposure to upper respiratory infections and communicable diseases. The applicable nursing diagnosis is *potential for infection.* Health maintenance costs for families with a preschooler may be increased because of these frequent illnesses. When the preschooler contracts a communicable illness, other family members may become ill as well. Some of the expenses incurred (throat cultures, medication) may be included in insurance plans for the family. A nurse can increase the family's awareness of insurance coverage to which they are entitled or assist them in locating other sources of assistance for the costs of health maintenance, including dental care and immunizations.

We appreciate the critical review of this chapter by Sandra Frick, RN, PhD, and her contributions to it.

Maintenance of Family Communication

Parents of a preschooler may find a need to recharge their relationship after the years of intensely parenting an infant and toddler. The family changes as the children become increasingly independent, as they entertain themselves more, and play with siblings and friends. With an increased attention span, the preschooler will watch television, enjoy a sitter, and read books. All this allows many parents increased leisure, which can be used to maintain or rebuild personal interests, as well as for family activities.

Adult family members should be encouraged to have private conversations that are not child related, and that stimulate and satisfy mutual intellectual needs, interests, and goals. In two-parent families, regularly scheduled and impromptu times alone, inside or outside the home, help parents maintain themselves as individuals and as a couple, in addition to being parents.

The preschool child's questioning can disrupt family unity and test parental patience. When a child first begins the "why" questions, parents view it as a challenge to respond appropriately. However, as the "why" questions increase in frequency, often with no logical progression, parents can become frustrated with this behavior, even though the majority of parents realize the child is learning about the world through the torrent of questions. Because of the cognition level, the child may be unable to assimilate an answer given by the parent and may require repeated explanations for the same question. This cycle of events frustrates busy, tired, over-worked parents!

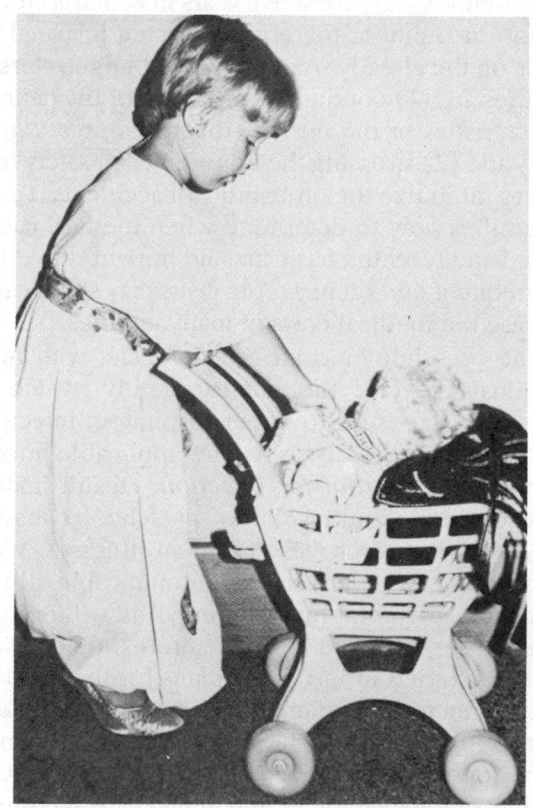

The preschooler loves to pretend.

The preschooler's curiosity is far-reaching and includes questions about sex ("Where did I come from?), death ("Where is heaven?" "What happens to people when they die?"), and about common, everyday events. Often the questions about sex cause parents discomfort. Communication and attitudinal patterns within each family dictate how parents respond to these questions. The responses range from openness to refusal to discuss sex, or to the giving of erroneous answers to a child's probing questions.

By addressing the topic of sex-related questions and the constant "whys" with parents during well-child visits, the nurse can encourage parents to think about their responses to the inevitable questions before they occur. The nurse should encourage parents to use honest and clear communication with their child, using correct terminology for body parts, to meet the child's immediate need. Information given should be directed specifically to the question asked. The preschooler is seldom ready for more than a simple explanation. Many books are available to assist parents in formulating age-appropriate answers.

Siblings will relate differently to the pre-schooler than they did to the toddler, and parents need to accept this relationship change as a natural, developmentally healthy event. Older siblings may now see the child who has become a preschooler as a nuisance—no longer a plaything but an individual with his or her own desires and needs. Verbal battles and physical aggression between siblings are common as the preschooler is increasingly capable of self-preservation. Parents need to be alert to problems of physical abuse and dominance by the older sibling so that the fragile self-concept of the preschooler is not damaged. At the same time, they must avoid overprotection of the younger child.

Jealousy between siblings may cause behavioral acting out by the preschooler or sibling. Each child needs time alone with each parent to enhance individual identity and security as well as to decrease the feelings of jealousy toward siblings or parents. There is perhaps no remedy more effective for behavioral acting out than increased quality time with the parents. Family unit play, special times for each child to discuss pertinent matters with parents or all family members, and quiet times for children to pursue individual interests may also help the family respect each member.

The preschooler may begin to imitate the sex roles

personified within the family structure. Developmentally, the child is coping with feelings of intense affection toward the parent of the opposite sex and rivalry with the parent of the same sex. This oedipal phase (Oedipus or Electra complex) (see discussion on page 307) may cause feelings of rejection and frustration for the unsuspecting same-sex parent. Nurses can help parents understand the developmental struggle with which the child is coping, relieving undue parental stress caused by the competitive preschooler. It is helpful for the parents of the preschooler to know that they do not have to give in to every affectional demand made by the preschooler. Setting limits on these demands, coupled with the preschooler's observations of displays of affection between the parents, aid in resolving the feelings of the oedipal phase.

Realistic Expectations and Responsibilities of Family Members

As preschoolers develop, increased capabilities change their behavior as well as the expectations for their behavior held by parents, peers, siblings, and relatives. Preschoolers may enjoy "helping" with household activities like sweeping, dusting, and outside chores. Nurses should encourage parents to allow and plan for preschoolers to participate and become the active family member they desire or are able to be.

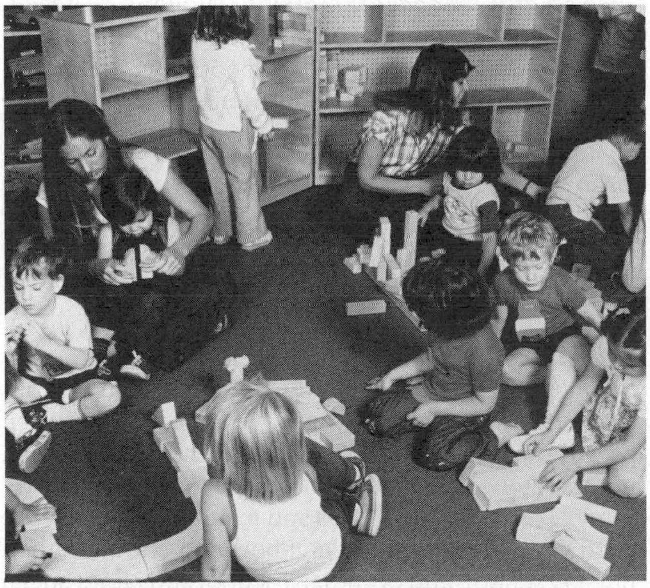

Under the supervision of skilled, competent caregivers, the preschooler has opportunities for socialization and self-expression. Note how blocks are used to develop motor skills (manipulating the blocks), social skills (working together to construct towers), and intellectual skills (identifying and matching shapes). Thus three important skills areas are practiced in what seems at first glance only to be play. (Photograph by Brian Leatart.)

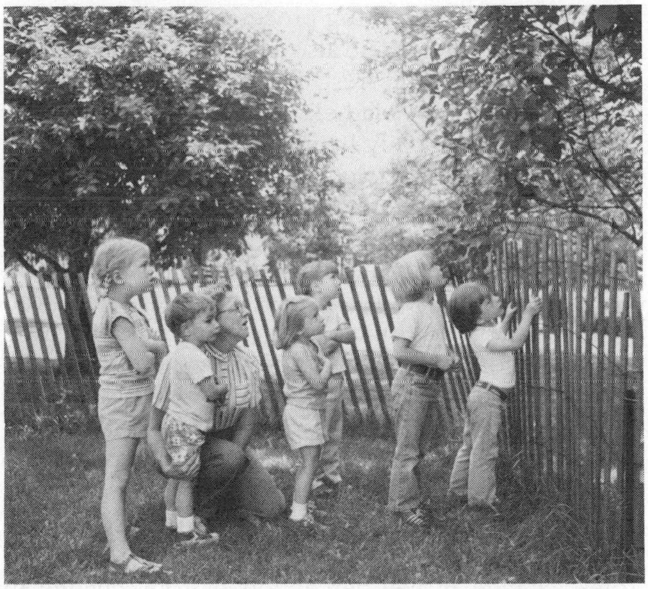

The day care center program has planned activities that are structured to stimulate the child cognitively as well as caring for physical and emotional needs. Day care homes are a popular choice of formal day care for preschools. These children learn about nature in the back yard.

This activity will help them see themselves as useful family members.

Parents need an awareness of age-appropriate expectations for the child. For example, realistically the 5-year-old child could be responsible for dressing and tidying the room, whereas the 3-year-old may not be able to perform these tasks in their entirety. Role prescriptions may change from month to month, and setbacks in behaviors are not uncommon. The use of rewards (stars pasted on a clearly designed daily worksheet or additional privileges) may be suggested to parents who have difficulty maintaining the preschooler as a contributing family member with increasing responsibilities.

Parents are also changing their role prescriptions to encompass the duties and responsibilities that correlate with expanding family needs as related to active play, crafts, reading time, formal learning activities, quiet individual times, and family group activities. The constant supervision of children's activities is mentally and physically exhausting to parents. In single parent families, the parent is especially vulnerable to physical and mental exhaustion without a network of social support. Grandparents, sisters or brothers of the parent, other single parents, or formal support groups can provide shared care-giving and respite for the single parent. The nurse can help by "giving permission" to the single parent to ask for assistance and by offering realistic suggestions to prevent social isolation.

In two-parent families, both parents can be active in planning and supervising their child(ren)'s routine tasks. This joint parenting process allows children to see parents as a team and also frees one parent to complete household tasks, rest, or pursue individual interests while the other is helping the preschooler perform activities of daily living and diversional or craft projects. Tension between spouses may accompany role changes within the family if these changes have not been anticipated or clearly delineated. Tension may be evidenced by frequent verbal or physical abuse or emotional isolation between spouses. Nurses can help parents by anticipating these possible role changes and helping parents identify their unique response to these changes.

Most of the defining characteristics of the nursing diagnosis, *disturbance in self-concept: role performance,* represent risk factors of which the nurse should be aware when working with parents of preschoolers. If a majority of these factors—denial of role, conflict in roles, change in self-perception of role, change in others' perception of role, lack of knowledge of role, or change in usual patterns of responsibilities (Gordon, 1987)—are seen, the nurse must determine the etiologic factors so that appropriate interventions may be developed.

Parents may find themselves in a continual dilemma as their preschool child develops initiative and self-confidence. Parents do not want to stifle the initiative that both they and their preschooler enjoy, yet specific limits need to be applied to the aggressive tendencies of the preschooler. Even though the preschooler's cognition remains preoperational (lack of ability to make appropriate generalizations or to reason deductively), cause-and-effect reasoning is advancing so that parents can utilize natural consequences of inappropriate actions as a disciplinary approach with their preschooler. The parenting approach can also consider the preschooler's developing ability to put off immediate need gratification to more fully enjoy a future event. For example, the preschooler who demands to finger paint immediately will agree to do this later when mother explains that the child's friend is arriving later that day with paints and then there will be a better selection of equipment.

There is a change in the kind of questions preschoolers ask and in the type of information and support they need. The nurse should be familiar with available books, magazines, and community-based parenting classes, as well as with techniques and theories of parenting to responsibly answer parents' questions. When working with parents a nurse needs sensitivity to possible individual parenting problems and to assess for alterations in parenting (Chapter 12), as well as to have the ability to give anticipatory guidance of developmental disciplinary needs. It is important that the nurse stress the individuality of each child and that proposed book methods of handling problems with the preschooler be tailored to fit the individual needs of the child.

The child's use of television is an increased responsibility for parents as, on the average, the preschooler of the Western world views 4 hours of television per day. Preschool children are impressionable and, with an increasing attention span, are enthralled with television. Violence (physical and emotional), the sedentary nature of viewing television, noncommunication between parents and children during viewing, and the potential behavioral modeling of television characters are all factors parents should consider as the preschooler views television. The nurse can encourage parents to use television as a learning tool and only minimally as a "babysitter." Television can aid preschoolers in developing social behavior by providing competent models who relate to persons with kindness and respect. Programs of this nature *(Mister Rogers' Neighborhood,* for example, and *Sesame Street)* are available in most areas.

In the modern world, in many families television has replaced valuable family group events. Unfortunately, television preempts family times of playing simple word games or card games, group games, table games, or working side by side. Such family interaction is enjoyable for the preschooler and helps advance cognitive and social skills as well as cement family relationships.

Encouraging parents to utilize as teaching tools the many educational children's magazines *(Ranger Rick's Nature Magazine, Humpty Dumpty, or World)* can greatly expand the preschooler's learning about the world, as well as provide an opportunity for intense interaction, learning, and enjoyment among all family members through reading and discussion.

Family Relationship to the World Beyond the Family

In a nuclear family, the child's world starts with only the mother and the self, and gradually expands to include the father and siblings. The nuclear family can provide security and companionship as well as a safe, nonthreatening environment for the testing of the preschooler's inquisitive ideas and mannerisms. After the third year, relatives and neighborhood children, then nursery school, and eventually school and larger social circles become part of the preschooler's world. Relatives of the preschool child fulfill various roles for the child, depending upon the physical distance between family and relatives. Grandparents, cousins, and other relatives represent roles such as censor, educator (they show the preschooler different viewpoints on subjects), authority figure, babysitter, and playmate to the child and the family (Hurlock, 1978). By cultivating fuller relationships with relatives, the parents and the child can utilize them as resource persons to enhance their understanding of the family heritage and values. Also, parenting skills can improve by learning through the experience of relatives. With this expanding social circle the preschooler learns to share people, starting with mother and father. The preschooler who belongs to an extended family has many opportunities to share with and learn from a large variety of family members (Wilson, 1986).

Cooperative play by the preschooler and peers allows the preschooler to develop friendships and playmates beyond family members.

When children first expand their social circle beyond their parents, it usually is a relationship with one other child to the exclusion of all others. Each positive friendship experience encourages the child to expand this circle to larger and larger groups. The child becomes eager to make friends, quickly learning that sharing brings approval of adults and more playmates. The ability to cooperate with others is not learned overnight but takes much time and assistance from adults, parents, and preschool teachers. When children feel secure in the love of an adult, they find it much easier to share with others.

The preschool child has increased cognitive and coping capacities as well as more communication skill, initiative, and independence, as compared with a younger child, and responds less violently to separations. Much of this response is based on previous experience and developmental readiness. The child must have developed sufficient ego strength and the emotional freedom necessary to transfer dependence from the parent to other responsible adults.

Community activities—group play, gymnastics, crafts, religous activities—add greater dimensions to the preschooler's world. Parents may notice new behaviors as a result of their preschooler's exposure to influences outside the home. The entire family can also attend events together (zoo, children's theater, and sports events).

Socialization with other families is changing. The preschooler can now play alone or play with peers for longer periods of time without direct supervision, thereby allowing parents' socializing to be more relaxed and enjoyable. In addition, parents may be more relaxed in visiting friends because the home being visited need not be as childproof as during toddlerhood. Nurses should encourage families to interact with relatives and friends, as these interactions may renew and positively influence learning for both the preschooler and parents.

Day Care

Many parents do not have the luxury of making a choice between staying home or placing their child in day care. More mothers are working outside the home, more women are delaying childbearing until their careers are established, and the number of single

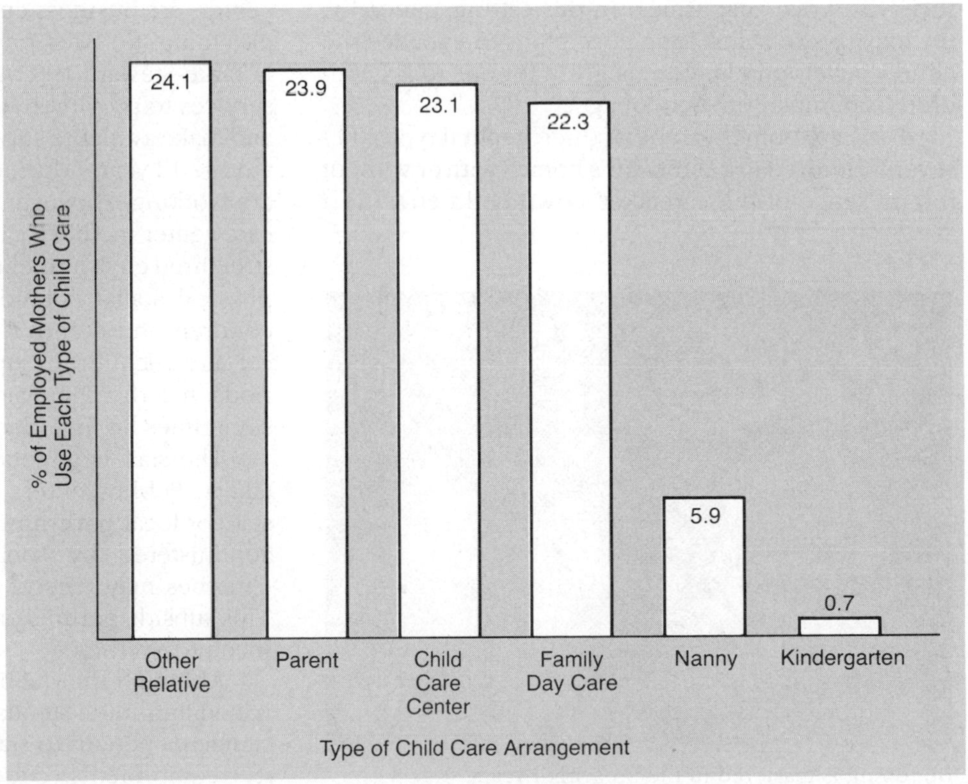

Figure 7-1. Per cent of employed mothers who use various child care arrangements for children under age 5 years. (From Dateline child care, *Child Care Inform Exch,* 1987 Jul; 56:9.)

mothers who must work to support their children is increasing (Dateline child care, 1987, 10). These three factors all contribute to the increased number of children who are cared for outside their home. It is now believed that day care alone cannot be viewed by itself as a single factor affecting a child's development. What is probably more important is to consider variables that make day care centers different from each other (Hambrick-Dixon, 1986). Different types of day care and the percentage of employed mothers who use each type are shown in Figure 7-1.

When a day care or preschool program is chosen, parents should explain what the preschool program is and why it is necessary that the child spend some time there each day. Appropriate preparation will help the preschooler avoid feeling abandoned or rejected. School should be discussed at home, and a visit made to the preschool to see what it looks like and to meet the teacher. Friends or siblings already attending school can offer positive input to the preschool child. Parents should have confidence in the preschool and convey that feeling to their child. If possible, a parent should transport the child each day and assure the child of his or her return at the end of the day, rather than entrusting this to someone whom the child does not know well.

Day Care Homes

In the family day care home the child's immediate needs are attended to satisfactorily (nutrition, safety, supervised play, nap time). In this setting, generally, no activities relate to long-term plans to enhance the child's development. Care is given for one to six children from infancy to school age.

Day care homes can be of three general types: (1) several children in a caretaker's home (with or without the presence of the caretaker's own children), (2) a nonfamily member caretaker in the family's residence, and (3) a care situation in which the children (sometimes including the caretaker's own children) are cared for by more than one caregiver. Day care homes are a popular choice of formal day care for preschoolers in the United States and worldwide. These homes are usually located relatively close to the family's residence or to the place of employment of one parent.

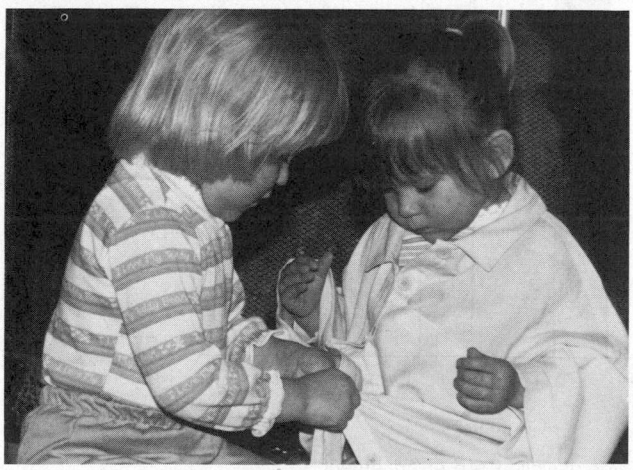

Buttoning is mastered in the preschool years.

Day care homes are not required to be licensed in many states. Some states do offer licensing standards for day care homes to assure safe, appropriate care. Licensing implies some of the following: proper adherence to the health code for the day care residence (plumbing, heating); sufficient living space for the number of children cared for; and physical and mental stability of the caretaker. Limits are also set on the number of children a home may care for at one time. Home day care provides the opportunity for children to be in a home setting for the hours in a day they are not with their parent(s). While caregivers in a day care home are less likely to have special preparation or education, this arrangement does tend to provide a stable, warm, and stimulating environment, especially for the younger preschooler (Clarke-Stewart, 1982).

Day Care Center

Day care center programs are generally located in their own facility and provide daily care for children from 2 or 3 to 6 years of age. Over 50 percent of day care centers are business enterprises, run for profit, mostly providing for the physical needs of the children (Clarke-Stewart, 1982). Many also now have extended services to provide transportation to and from school and make available supervision of school-age children (to age 12 years) during nonschool hours that parents are working. However, the long-term goal of the day care center includes careful attention to planning and structured environments for learning to provide for the physical, social, cognitive, and emotional needs of the children who attend. The day care plan includes physical care of children, supervised play activities, rest periods, health supervision, and crafts. The parent may sometimes be included in center activities.

The staff is generally composed of trained caretakers. Public centers administered by a unit of the state or local government and some voluntary centers administered by social agencies, settlements, or churches may receive federal monies for operation. This subsidy permits parents to pay according to their income level.

Although the quality varies, each state has established minimum standards for day care centers. These standards pertain to staff qualifications, physical facility requirements, code requirements, standards for child health, records and reports, nutrition, and insurance and special provisions for handicapped children. (US Department of Health and Human Services, 1971, 1984). Each state has its own definition of what constitutes a day care center.

Nursery School

The nursery school operates two to five days a week for either two or two and a half hours a day as morning or afternoon sessions. Groups can be composed of children of the same age or different ages (as 3- to 5-year-olds). Various types of nursery schools exist: guided observation schools (laboratory to study growth and development, often associated with colleges and universities); cooperative nursery schools (parents are utilized as teacher-helpers, thereby decreasing tuition costs as well as including parents in their preschooler's learning world); schools with full-time teachers and no daily solicitation of parent help (private schools such as Montessori schools); child development centers (governmental Head Start program for disadvantaged children); and schools for exceptional children (US Department of Health and Human Services, 1984). Nursery schools can be nonprofit or profit enterprises, but all exist to enrich the world of the preschooler.

The nursery school will afford the preschooler socialization opportunities as well as enhance learning about the physical environment. Free self-expression through various means allows the preschooler to develop a positive self-concept and encourages cognitive growth. A good nursery school should afford parents the opportunity to participate in some aspect(s) of the program.

Child-directed as well as teacher-directed activities are a part of the nursery school plan. Opportunities to expand language and visual acuity, develop fine and large motor coordination, and participate in school readiness activities (familiarization with numbers and letters and identification of like objects) may be a part of the curriculum. Educational models and learning objectives vary, depending upon the population served and teachers' orientation.

Play Schools

Local play schools or neighborhood play sessions are child-care alternatives that many parents find helpful for occasional use. Voluntary organizations (churches or groups of neighborhood mothers) may provide play sessions. These are short-term, with no planned curriculum other than babysitting, as the population served varies daily. These alternatives are used most often by the family that has a parent in the home full-time.

Other Day Care Alternatives

An innovative concept of day care that has the added benefit of exposing children and the elderly to each other is the provision of child day care services within nursing homes. Vujovich (1984) describes one such project, called GrandKids. The children and nursing home residents share numerous activities during the day, such as exercise time, crafts, story and music hours, play time, field trips, and pet times. This concept has increased the alertness and orientation of residents while enhancing the children's conceptions of and respect for the elderly. The arrangement provides the child with a home-like atmosphere and a richness of cultural and historical exposure not available in other day care settings (Sugarman and Brown, 1983).

Some employers are also establishing day care facilities at the work place. The City of San Francisco has passed an ordinance that requires proposed public buildings to include space for employee day care before a building permit will be awarded. This placement of day care facilities in the work place permits parents and children to interact during workbreaks and mealtimes and gives both parties more security because of

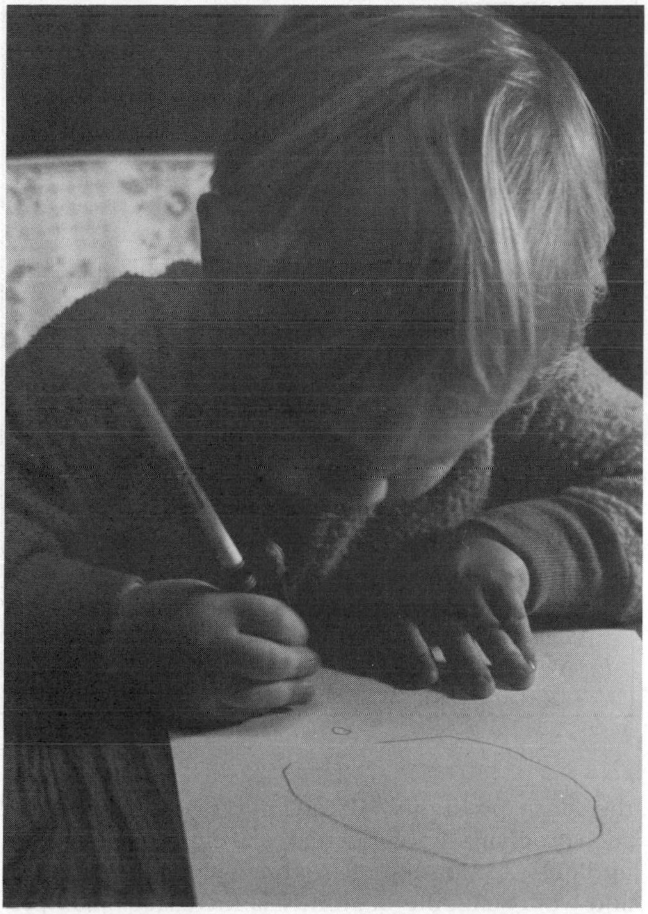
Mastery of fine motor skills requires eye-hand coordination. The 3-year-old can copy a circle.

Box 7-1
Guidelines for Parents Selecting a Day Care Facility for Their Preschooler

PURPOSE(S) OF THE PROGRAM

Is the focus to foster development of the child?

PROGRAM STRUCTURE

Can children pursue their individual interests? Are there organized, continuous experiences suited to the children attending? What are the cultural expectations? Are these expectations realistic in relation to and supportive of the preschooler's developmental tasks?

PERSONNEL

Is the ratio of children to caretaker-teacher realistic for the ages and needs of the children attending? Are the teachers professionally competent? Are the personnel and the facility certified? Do aides supplement the child-to-teacher ratio? What training and qualifications do they have? What is the general emotional climate? How do staff discipline children? How do staff spend most of their time?

FACILITIES

Is the facility easily accessible to home or employment? Is the space (indoors and outdoors) adequate for the needs of active preschoolers? Are appropriate materials and equipment provided? Are the fees and manner of payment manageable?

HEALTH AND SAFETY

Are nutritious meals and snacks provided and in sufficient quantity? Are health records kept on employees and children? What are the entry requirements regarding health status? Does the facility have an established plan for ill children? Is the health status of children identified daily? Is adequate provision made for first aid and emergency care? Is there adherence to public health codes? Do staff practice good handwashing?

SPECIAL SERVICES

Are special services provided for parents? For children with special needs? Are there financial adjustments to fees? What does the facility expect from the parents?

the close proximity. Companies that have initiated such programs report decreases in employee turnover, tardiness, and absenteeism while productivity, morale, and work schedule flexibility is increased. Such programs also improve company image and facilitate employee recruitment (Burud et al, 1983).

Another relatively new day care alternative is the day care center for sick children. These centers are designed to provide safe, competent day care to children with minor illnesses. They are staffed with nurses as well as other day care workers. Some of these centers are free-standing and some are run by hospitals. Guidelines are available for the care of ill children in traditional day care centers (Aronson, 1987).

Day Care Evaluation

Box 7-1 lists factors that nurses should encourage parents to review when contemplating any type of day care for their preschooler (Leeper, 1974; US Department of Health and Human Services, 1984). For the child about to enter day care, nurses should encourage hearing and vision screening, a complete physical and developmental assessment, and updated immunizations. Most centers for child care require health forms, immunizations, and physical examinations prior to acceptance of the child.

Families may use a combination of day care types. Parents need encouragement to evaluate child care arrangements regularly and select alternatives if one arrangement is detrimental to the child or family. The quality of any child care arrangement is not dependent upon the facility, equipment, or curriculum as much as on the caretakers and teachers (Box 7-2). The nurse should urge parents to trust their own feelings and impressions regarding the best arrangement and the best setting for their child. Nurses can help parents realize the value of preparing the child in advance for day care, help the parent and child adjust to school (separating from each other), and help parents provide continuity between the experiences of day care and life at home.

Research studies have investigated the social, emotional, and intellectual effects of day care on children's development (Webb, 1977; Gold and Andres, 1978; Etaugh, 1980; Collins and Deloria, 1983; Anderson, 1984; Smith, 1984). Later research contradicts many earlier hypotheses. Numerous researchers have found that day care does not disrupt parent-child attachment, regardless of the child's age when day care is initiated. Carefully chosen day care can have many beneficial effects on the child's development (Scarr, 1984). Parents with children in day care tend to devote more uninterrupted time to their children in talk and play than parents at home each day with their children (Belsky and Steinberg, 1978; Winett et al, 1977). Day care staff also tend to spend more time directly interacting with a child than do at-home parents. Day care has been found to enhance the cognitive development of disadvantaged children (Haskins, 1985). Although all children are not affected cognitively, most children who have experienced day care adjust more quickly to

> Box 7-2
> *Steps to Good Day Care*
>
> **STABLE CARETAKERS**
>
> Low turnover rates
> Educational and experiential background
> Assignment to specific children or specific groups of children
>
> **SMALL GROUPS**
>
> | *Centers* | *Homes* |
> |---|---|
> | 1:3 infants* | 1:5 children 2 years and under |
> | 1:4 children under 3 years | 1:6 children 3 to 6 years |
> | 1:8 children 3 to 6 years | |
>
> **RIGHT KIND OF ATTENTION**
>
> Under 3 years—frequent direct contact with a few adults; informal learning experiences
> Over 3 years—adult supervision and periodic direct contact; some formal instruction
>
> **RIGHT ACTIVITIES**
>
> More emphasis on learning about themselves, their neighborhood, and the world than on academics (math, reading, etc.)
>
> **PARENTAL INVOLVEMENT**
>
> Parental involvement welcomed, invited, and planned
> Child development and other educational workshops for children
>
> * That is, one caretaker for every three infants.
>
> *(From Scarr, 1984.)*

the school experience later (Collins and Deloria, 1983; Smith, 1984). No evidence exists that day care increases children's insecurity. On the contrary, day care children tend to adjust better to groups and to unfamiliar situations, learn social skills earlier, and are cooperative (Webb, 1977; Gold and Andres, 1978; Scarr, 1984). Some evidence exists that disadvantaged children who attend preschool programs may be more aggressive and more intelligent than children who do not attend such programs (Haskins, 1985).

Some argue that day care increases the incidence of illnesses. Over a 5-year period, Glezen and colleagues (1971) found a slightly higher respiratory illness rate (8.9/child/year) in day care children than in children cared for at home (8.3/child/year). The greater concern is regarding the "day care diseases"—shigellosis, giardiosis, and hepatitis—that have been causing problems for children in day care and their adult caretakers and parents (Ogden, 1984). These diseases can all be prevented with sound hygienic practices and sanitation. Experiments utilizing health department nursing services for health screening and assessments, health education, and counsel to teachers and parents have shown significantly decreased incidences of illness in participating day care populations (Mennie and Klinger, 1984).

The Alliance for Better Child Care (ABC) is a group working to influence legislation that will provide quality child care arrangements for all individuals (Dateline child care, 1987). This group believes that legislation is necessary that would express the following principles:

- improve access to quality child care for all families
- provide help for low and moderate income parents in paying for care
- provide sliding fee scales to promote a socioeconomic mix
- strengthen child care standards and improve their implementation
- strengthen family day care as well as center-based care
- support parental involvement in child care
- support the development of staff training programs
- encourage coordination among child care agencies
- improve the level of compensation for child care workers

School Readiness

It is a general belief in the United States that children should begin their formal education sometime between age 4½ and 6 years. However, children differ in their readiness for school just as they differ in other areas. There are no specific rules, but parents generally can identify when their child has the maturity for school. The nurse can offer parents guidance as they evaluate their child's readiness and help them recognize that school can be more complicated and threatening to children than adults realize. Reassure parents that they need not push their child into school at the earliest age the community allows. On the average, girls are more mature and thus more ready for school than boys at the same age (Granger, 1979). Table 7-1 lists the areas of maturity needed by a child in readiness for the school experience.

Kindergarten

Kindergarten is a structured learning environment available to most preschool children through local public school systems. It is generally a half-day experience, 5 days a week, utilized to provide a gradual transition from home to school. Kindergarten affords an

Table 7-1. Check List for School Readiness

Characteristic	Preparatory Experiences
Physically healthy and strong enough to enjoy the challenge of going to school and to handle the increased stresses involved	Balanced diet Adequate rest and sleep Opportunities for exercise; exposure to activities and play equipment suitable to child's age Positive reinforcement for skill mastery
Capable of separating from parent(s) and spending several hours each day in an unfamiliar place with adults and children who are largely unknown at first	Experiences with substitute caregivers in caregiver's home Day care or nursery school a few hours a day or a couple of days a week Social activities away from home such as Sunday school, play at a friend's home, supervised play with unfamiliar children at park
Long enough attention span to be able to sit fairly long and to concentrate on one thing at a time, gradually learning to enjoy the practicing and problem-solving activity involved	Listening to rather long stories Experiences working through activities that take awhile, such as large puzzles, weaving mats Sitting through a full length TV program, movie, circus show, etc.
Able to tolerate frustration of not getting immediate attention from teacher or others and to wait for and take turns	Parent should not always respond to requests immediately. Help child learn to wait till the activity of parent is finished or at a good stopping point If siblings, enforce rules about taking turns Experiences with small groups of children and a single caregiver
Has some basic hand-eye skills necessary to learning of reading and writing	Practice with child and provide toys that stimulate recognizing shapes and colors Books where child has to turn pages Experiences using a pencil and crayons Craft experiences; cutting with blunt-end scissors, pasting, painting, molding clay Exposure to simple computer games, to TV shows that enforce learning word sounds, alphabet letters, shapes and colors

opportunity for children to develop positive attitudes toward school and to complete learning of the alphabet, numbers, and application of letter sounds and combinations to form words, as well as to develop abilities to think, discover, reason, and concentrate on one activity for a period of time. A professional is responsible for teaching the classes. Emphasis is placed upon total growth and development of the individual child as well as group experiences, thus making entrance into formal learning activities of lower elementary grades an easier transition for the child.

Anticipatory Guidance: School Readiness

Parents should see themselves as educators and should share activities with their children that provide learning opportunities to prepare them for school. Nature walks, with discussions of what is seen, and visits to community buildings, post offices, city halls, or fire stations all help the children expand their knowledge. If available, art galleries and museums are good places to explore, as are zoos and parks. The city child gains insights from a visit to the farm, while the farm child needs exposure to the city. A ride on a train, a bus, and a taxi are all valuable learning experiences, and ones that parents can share. Parents can also participate in their child's learning by playing simple games, putting puzzles together, making cookies or pudding, and

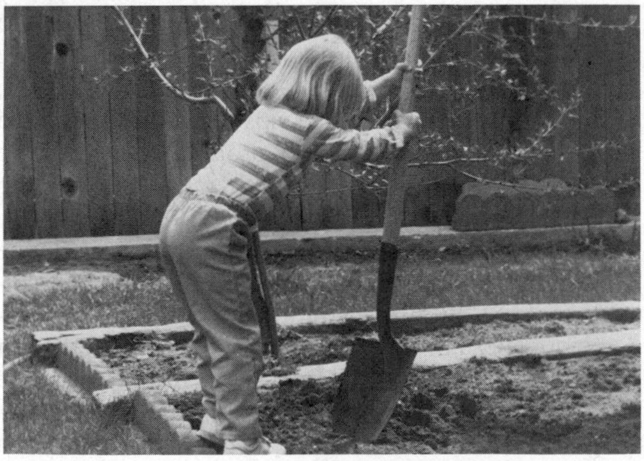

Increased coordination and strength of large muscle groups allow preschoolers to attempt increasingly difficult tasks. This preschooler is helping plant a garden.

sharing other simple forms of cooking. Providing paper, finger paints, paste, crayons, and blunt scissors allows the preschooler to be imaginative and create art work. Reading to the preschooler is probably one of the most valuable experiences. This activity should begin in infancy. Music and musical games are other opportunities for learning that the preschooler and parents can mutually enjoy.

Children should know their name, parent(s)' name, address, and age and should be able to play cooperatively, dress themselves, complete their own elimination, and follow safety principles (can cross street safely on own). For children who have not attended nursery school or day care centers, nurses should encourage parents to have their child spend a day away from home occasionally to initiate the separation process imminent with school.

Attending Sunday school and summer vacation bible school provide opportunities for children to learn to play and work with peers, particularly for the preschooler who is not in a nursery school program. In the nursery school, preschool and Sunday school setting, the child is provided with planned activities that prepare for the school experience. These same activities can be planned in the home, but valuable interaction with peers may be missing. The day care center provides interaction with peers but usually without planned school readiness activities. Parents should be aware of the differences in preschool and day care services and plan for their child's needs accordingly.

Growth and Development of the Preschooler

The child from 3 to 5 years is very active, progressing rapidly in motor abilities, cognitive function, and language development. The constant practice of these abilities and skills brings amazing changes in personality development. An individual appears. Some preschoolers are boisterous, outgoing, active, curious, and exploring constantly, whereas others are quiet, shy, passive, and withdrawing. One child is aggressive; another appears totally nonaggressive. Each child develops a "self"; some become leaders and others are content to be followers.

Physical Competency

Preschoolers become increasingly more aware of their physical competence during the years from 3 through 5. They are conscious of the skills of their peers and those of the older children they are exposed to and become frustrated when they are unable to accomplish the same tasks as other children. A refinement of gross motor skills and a progressive mastery of fine motor abilities evolve during this period. Having discovered themselves as a separate person by the end of their toddler years, their performance now directly affects their developing self-esteem.

Assessment guidelines that characterize the preschooler's physical development are presented in Table 7-2. The nurse's role is to help parents stimulate their preschoolers' physical competency. Nurses should provide information on the achievement of developmental tasks when undertaking anticipatory guidance to parents of preschoolers. The nurse should spend time playing with and talking with the child to gain the child's cooperation and trust, especially before attempting any procedures. A preschooler is usually more cooperative than a toddler during health care. When the parent is allowed to remain close, separation anxiety is minimal.

Height and Weight

The preschooler's growth continues to be slow and steady as in the toddler years. On the average the preschooler grows about 2 to 3 inches (5 to 7.5 cm) a year and gains 4 to 5 pounds (1.8 to 2.3 kg) a year. The child's weight at 1 year of age is doubled by the end of the preschool period.

Anticipatory Guidance: Height and Weight. Once the height and weight have been taken and plotted on a graph, it is important to discuss the significance of these findings with the parent. It is easy to point out graphically to parents where their child stands, and problem areas are obvious. Many times parents do not recognize obesity unless they can see evidence of it on paper. It is important to discuss diet and activity, as well as expected weight gains in the coming year. This record will help parents to see if they are overfeeding or underfeeding their child; however, it is not always the quantity of food a child eats that affects growth but also the quality of food intake. Parents should be reassured that wide variance exists in size and stature among preschoolers. As in all age groups, the size of the parents can affect the child's placement on the graph.

Table 7-2. Growth, Development, and Health Promotion for Preschoolers

Physical Competency	Intellectual Competency	Emotional-Social Competency
General Summary, 3 to 5 Years		
Gains 4.5 kg (10 lb) Grows 15 cm (6 in) 20 teeth present Nutritional requirements: Energy: 1250–1600 cal/day (or 90–100 Kcal/kg/day) Fluid: 100–125 ml/kg/day Protein: 30 gm/day (or 3 gm/kg/day) Iron: 10 mg/day	Becomes increasingly aware of self and others Vocabulary increases from 900 to 2100 words Piaget's preoperational/intuitive period	Freud's phallic stage Oedipus complex–boy Electra complex–girl Erikson's stage of Initiative vs. Guilt
3 Years		
Runs, stops suddenly Walks backward Climbs steps Jumps Pedals tricycle Undresses self Unbuttons front buttons Feeds self well	Knows own sex Desires to please Sense of humor Language—900 words Follows simple direction Uses plurals Names figure in picture Uses adjectives/adverbs	Shifts between reality and imagination Bedtime rituals Negativism decreases Animism and realism: anything that moves is alive
4 Years		
Runs well, skips clumsily Hops on one foot Heel-toe walks Up and down steps without holding rail Jumps well Dresses and undresses Buttons well, needs help with zippers, bows Brushes teeth Bathes self Draws with some form and meaning	More aware of others Uses alibis to excuse behavior Bossy Language—1500 words Talks in sentences Knows nursery rhymes Counts to 5 Highly imaginative Name calling	Focuses on present Egocentrism/unable to see the viewpoint of others, unable to understand another's inability to see own viewpoint Does not comprehend anticipatory explanation Sexual curiosity Oedipus complex Electra complex
5 Years		
Runs skillfully Jumps 3–4 steps Jumps rope, hops, skips Begins dance Roller skates Dresses without assistance Tie shoelaces Hits nail on head with hammer Draws person—6 parts Prints first name	Aware of cultural differences Knows name and address More independent More sensible/less imaginative Copies triangle, draws rectangle Knows four or more colors Language—2100 words, meaningful sentences Understands kinship Counts to 10	Continues in egocentrism Fantasy and daydreams Resolution of Oedipus/Electra complex, girls identify with mother, boys with father Body image and body boundary especially important in illness Shows tension in nail-biting, nose-picking, whining, snuffling

General Appearance and Skeletal Growth

In general, the preschooler is tall and thin as compared to the toddler, looking sturdy yet graceful and agile. The baby fat of infancy becomes muscle tissue so that the posture is erect.

At age 3 years, the head circumference for boys ranges from 47.9 to 52.7 cm with the 50th percentile at 50.4 cm, whereas the range for girls is 46.8 to 52.0 cm with the 50th percentile at 49.3 cm. Head circumference is not usually measured after 3 years of age.

When observing the child standing, the distance between the medial malleoli of the tibias should be noted, and if the distance is more than 2 cm with the knees touching, the condition of genu valgum (knock-knee) is present. This is a normal condition in the child from 3 to 5 years of age. Also, while the child is standing, the foot should be examined for arches. Many 3-year-olds will have the appearance of flat feet because of the fat pad that is normally present under the medial arch until the child has walked for a couple of years. Flat feet in even the 4- and 5-year-old child is not a problem unless it is causing some specific symptoms.

One of the best methods of evaluating the struc-

Nutrition	Play	Safety
General Summary, 3 to 5 Years		
Carbohydrate intake approximately 40–50% of calories Good food sources of essential vitamins and minerals Regular tooth brushing Parents are seen as examples; if parent won't eat it, child won't	Reading books is important at all ages Balance highly physical activities with quiet times Quiet rest period takes the place of nap time Provide sturdy play materials	Never leave alone in bath or swimming pool Keep poisons in locked cupboard; learn what household things are poisonous Use car seats and seatbelts Never leave child alone in car Remove doors from abandoned freezers and refrigerators
3 Years		
1250 cal/day Due to increased sex identity and imitation, copies parents at table and will eat what they eat Different colors and shapes of foods can increase interest	Participates in simple games Cooperates, takes turns Plays with group Uses scissors, paper Likes crayons, coloring books Enjoys being read to and "reading" Plays "dress-up" and "house" Likes fire engines	Teach safety habits early Let water out of bathtub; don't stand in tub Caution against climbing in unsafe areas, onto or under cars, unsafe buildings, drainage pipes Insist on seatbelts worn at all times in cars
4 Years		
Good nutrition 1400 cal/day Nutritious between-meal snacks essential Emphasis on quality not quantity of food eaten Mealtime should be enjoyable, not for criticism As dexterity improves, neatness increases	Longer attention span with group activities "Dress up" with more dramatic play Draws, pounds, paints Likes to make paper chains, sewing cards Scrapbooks Likes being read to, records, and rhythmic play "Helps" adults	Teach to stay out of streets, alleys Continually teach safety; child understands Teach how to handle scissors Teach what are poisons and why to avoid Never allow child to stand in moving car
5 Years		
Good nutrition 1600 cal/day Encourage regular tooth brushing Encourage quiet time before meals Can learn to cut own meat Frequent illnesses from increased exposure increases nutritional needs	Plays with trucks, cars, soldiers, dolls Likes simple games with letters or numbers Much gross motor activity: water, mud, snow, leaves, rocks Matching picture games	Teach child how to cross streets safely Teach child not to speak to strangers or get into cars of strangers Insist on seatbelts Teach child to swim

ture and function of the foot is to look at the child's shoe. Lateral wear on the heel and sole of the shoe indicates a well-functioning foot. Fair function is seen with even wearing of the heel and sole, and poor functioning is evident when the sole has become worn on the medial aspects (Trainex Corporation, 1980).

Anticipatory Guidance: General Appearance and Skeletal Growth. Parents should be informed of the normal changes that will occur in their preschooler's appearance. Information and reassurance that the knock-kneed, flat-footed characteristics of their child are normal at this age can save parents the needless expense of corrective shoes. If extreme variations in these normal preschool skeletal features exist, the nurse should refer the child for further evaluation.

Parents should also be cautioned against lifting preschoolers off the ground by one hand or wrist or yanking on the upper extremities, usually done in an effort to hurry them or lift them over an obstacle. Such movements can cause a disorder referred to as "uncles' elbow," or "nursemaids' elbow." In this disorder the child may complain of pain in the elbow or wrist or, when the shoulder is involved, may refuse to use the arm.

Motor Development

By the time a child reaches 3 years of age, gross motor skills have reached considerable maturation because of increased nerve myelinization (development of an insulating myelin sheath around the nerve fibers) and the separating of nerve fibers as the central nervous system matures. Additionally, the brain has increased in size. This allows the child greater coordination and enables such things as running, going up and down stairs easily, jumping up and down, jumping over objects and throwing a ball with some accuracy. Preschoolers are able to pedal a tricycle and balance on one foot for brief periods of time. They can undress themselves and, with some assistance, dress themselves. They can do some simple buttoning on the front of clothing.

By the age of 4 years, they can run easily, hop on one foot and sometimes skip clumsily. They can balance on one foot for up to 10 seconds, heel-toe walk forward, and climb steps without holding on to a rail; their movements are more graceful and rhythmic. They sit well balanced even while reaching forward and twisting and they are able to touch the nose with a finger when asked. They generally can dress without supervision, button well, and can tell the front from the back of clothing.

By the age of 5 years, the preschooler has developed the skill to run with speed and agility, to play games with others. Coordination increases. They can balance on their toes and begin to dance with rhythm, roller skate, hop and skip well, jump rope, and climb on a jungle gym. They can dress without supervision and tie their own shoelaces, if they have had practice with shoes that have laces instead of Velcro.

In developing finer movements involving the use of the hands and fingers, the preschooler acquires increasingly more complicated skills. Mastery of these fine motor skills requires perceptual maturation, as evidenced by progression in the development of eye-hand coordination. The 3-year-old is able to put large beads on a string, to copy a circle, to stack eight blocks on top of each other, to draw a vertical line beside another vertical line, and to cut with scissors.

By the age of 4 years, children are able to cut out pictures. They can copy a cross and imitate a square if it is demonstrated. They can draw a person with three parts and can build a bridge with blocks.

By 5 years of age, children can draw a square without assistance, draw a six-part person and other recognizable objects, and hit a nail with a hammer. Again, preschoolers will not learn these skills if they have no opportunity to practice and receive no encouragement. The development of skills is not necessarily a function of chronologic age but a progressive refinement of previously learned skills.

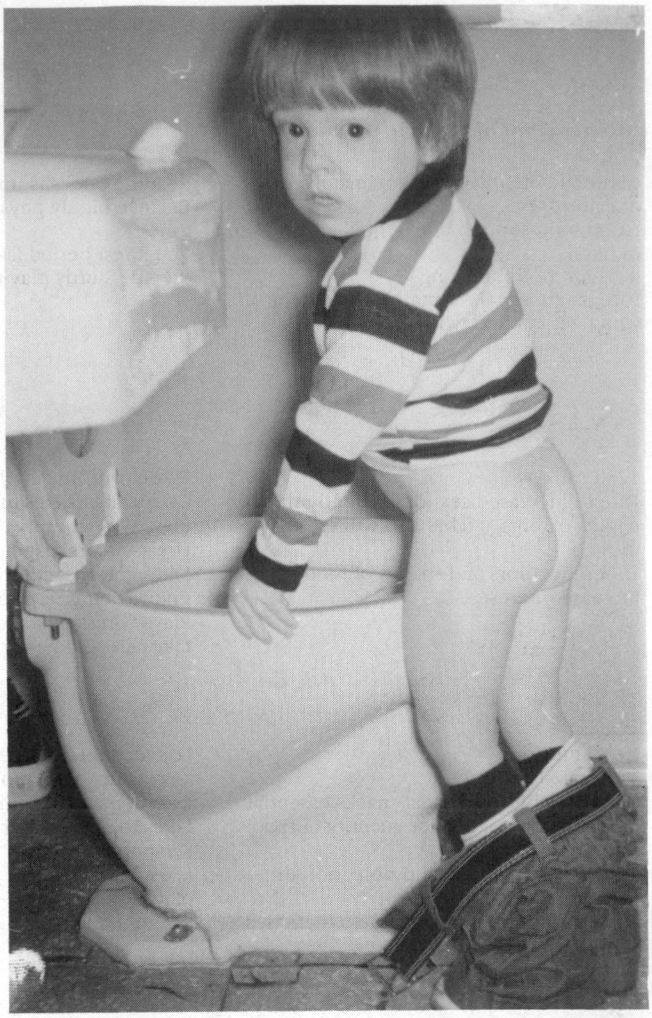

By 4 years of age, the preschooler may be independent in using the toilet. (Photograph by David Trainor.)

Anticipatory Guidance: Motor Development. Preschoolers will learn to do all these tasks provided they have been given the opportunity. Nurses can explore with parents the need for children to have some freedom and independence as they learn from their curiosity and exploration. However, safety is of utmost importance, since accidents constitute the most common cause of death in preschoolers. Nursing assessment must continue to focus on the defining characteristics of the *potential for injury* nursing diagnosis. Safety rules must be clear-cut, consistent, and simply explained to preschoolers. Children should be given praise as a reinforcement for safe behavior. Frequent punishment and constant threats eventually will be ignored, and children become resentful and rebellious.

Children must have access to paper, pencils, and crayons and be encouraged to use them. They must have clothes that need buttoning and shoes that need tying to learn those skills. The parent who does everything for a child does not help her or him learn and mature.

Dentition

Preschoolers have all their primary teeth. Permanent teeth do not begin erupting till early school age for most children. Tooth brushing should be a regular activity. Maintenance of the primary teeth is the major emphasis of anticipatory guidance during the preschool years, including the first dental visit at age 3 years. Thumbsucking, begun in infancy, sometimes persists during preschool years. Dentists usually do not express concern about thumbsucking until the permanent teeth begin erupting. The older preschooler usually can be reasoned with to attempt abandoning this habit if it has persisted to this time. See Chapter 19 for further discussion of dental development and maintenance.

Vision and Hearing

Sensory function is highly developed by the time a child becomes a preschooler. Since a child at this age who has a visual problem is unaware of it and because amblyopia (lazy eye) becomes an irreversible condition usually by the age of 6 years, preschool vision screening is essential.

Vision screening is done for the preschool child with the use of the E chart, which is similar to the standard Snellen chart with the exception that the letter E replaces the alphabet, or with the Denver Eye Screening Test (DEST, 1973). Visual acuity may reach 20/20 as early as 6 months of age.

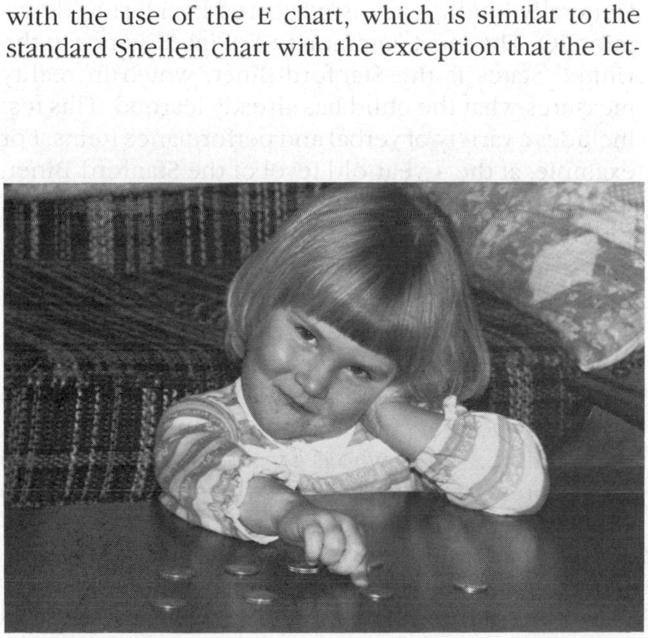

Preschoolers have not yet mastered the principle of conservation. A preschooler will indicate that there are more coins in the row which is longer.

Preschool hearing testing should be done at the same time that preschool vision testing is done. See Chapter 15 for a discussion of hearing and vision testing. Because the development of speech depends on the child's ability to hear, the nonhearing child is generally diagnosed before the preschool period. Occasionally a child of this age who has been treated for retardation will be found to have severe hearing loss.

Two types of hearing loss are seen in children. One is *conduction loss,* in which there is an interference with the transmission of sound. The most common cause of conduction loss is frequent or untreated ear infections (otitis media), which can damage the tympanic membrane. Temporary conduction loss occurs with upper respiratory infections. The other type of hearing loss is *perceptive loss,* in which there is damage to the eighth cranial nerve. This is sometimes called nerve deafness. It is seen in children who have had serious illnesses such as meningitis; in previous years it occurred with the more commonly seen contagious diseases such as measles and mumps. Some drugs, called ototoxic drugs, are capable of causing perceptive deafness. It has been suggested that the noises from incubators and intensive neonatal nurseries may contribute to perceptive deafness.

An otoscopic examination is an important part of each health appraisal during the preschool years. Preschoolers are particularly prone to upper respiratory infections and secondary ear infections. After a few ear infections the tympanic membrane may become stretched or perforated so that the child no longer expresses discomfort when infections do occur; therefore the condition of the internal ear should be monitored regularly.

Anticipatory Guidance: Vision and Hearing. Although the Snellen E test or the DEST (1973) for visual acuity can identify many visual problems while they are still treatable, parents should be informed that these tests in no way replace an ophthalmologic examination. This examination should be conducted at each health appraisal or whenever the parents notice any behaviors in their preschooler that suggest visual problems (frequent eye rubbing, squinting, attention span deficit).

Parents should be encouraged to take advantage of organized preschool vision screening programs. These programs, however, do not reach anywhere near all the children in this age group who need to be screened. Nurses can help make these programs available in areas where they do not exist, and make parents aware of those that do exist. Home test kits are also available to parents, especially those who live in areas where this screening does not exist. These kits can be obtained from the National Society for the Prevention of Blindness.*

It is important that eye safety be taught to preschoolers and their parents. Most eye injuries are preventable, and they can cause blindness. Usually they are caused when children throw small objects at their siblings or friends. Children should be taught to use silverware for eating, not as weapons, and preschoolers should never play with knives, darts, or sticks. At this age they should be well supervised during play activities. Toys should be inspected: those with small removable parts and those that can become dangerous weapons should not be allowed.

Parents should be instructed to promptly report any behaviors suggestive of hearing loss in their preschooler, such as playing alone despite the availability of peers for cooperative play, delays in speech development, or lack of response to repeated requests made in normal voice tones.

Bowel and Bladder Control

The preschooler will have bowel control and daytime bladder control, as these skills are usually learned during the toddler period. Some young preschoolers may have accidents if they become absorbed in play, so they need to be reminded to take time to go to the bathroom. Nighttime bladder control is usually accomplished between 3 and 4 years of age. By 4 years of age children can usually manage their own clothing at elimination, and by 5 years are completely responsible for the entire process.

The average urinary output in a 24-hour period for the preschooler is 500 to 780 ml. The 5-year-old voids about 4 to 6 times a day while awake, and generally sleeps through the night without getting up to void.

Anticipatory Guidance: Bowel and Bladder Control. The nurse should help parents understand that occasional bowel or bladder accidents or both are to be expected during the preschool years and that punishment will not alter this fact. Children are old enough to take responsibility for cleaning themselves and changing clothing at such times with only minimal parental assistance. Preschoolers should be reassured that their parent understands it was an accident.

Preschoolers' ability to manage their own toilet activities should be permitted and reinforced by the parent(s). If the child requests privacy during these activities, the request should be granted. However, the parent(s) should be nearby so that, if the child needs assistance, the parent is immediately aware of it and can help. Periodic reminders and checks on the child's use of hygienic measures during elimination, especially girls' use of front-to-back wiping, is appropriate during the preschool period.

Nutritional Requirements

Nutrition for the preschool child includes the same basic four groups of food needed by adults. The child's growth remains stable through the preschool years. Children's curiosity about what is going on around them persists, so they may have little interest in eating.

Calories from proteins and carbohydrates are essential for muscle growth in the preschooler. The child in the 3- to 5-year-old range requires from 90 to 100 Kcal/kg of body weight per day. Water, an essential element for life, comprises approximately 60 percent of the child's body weight. The principal source of water in the diet is fluids, although many fruits and vegetables that children eat contain up to 90 percent water. The average daily requirement of water for the child of 3 to 5 years is 100 to 125 ml per kg (1.5 to 2 oz per pound) of body weight. Protein requirements for the preschool age child are 2 to 3 gm per kg (0.9 to 1.35 gm per pound) of body weight. See Chapter 18 for vitamin, mineral, and other dietary requirements during the preschool years.

Intellectual Competency

Intelligence

Generally intelligence is measured by a test to determine IQ. The most common test of intelligence in the United States is the Stanford-Binet, which in reality measures what the child has already learned. This test includes a variety of verbal and performance items. For example, at the 4-year-old level of the Stanford-Binet, the child is asked to name pictures that illustrate a variety of common objects, to name objects from memory, to discriminate between such forms as circles, squares, and triangles, and to define such words as bat and ball. In addition, the test on this level includes repeating a ten-word sentence and counting four objects. The list is scored in terms of mental age, as a ratio of mental age over chronologic age multiplied by 100. For example, a child who is 4 years and no months old who scores a mental age of 4 years and no months would have an IQ of 100.

Another common intelligence test used with preschool-age children is the Wechsler Preschool-Primary Scale of Intelligence (WPPSI), which has a verbal scale and a performance scale. There are subtests within each scale and each subtest is scored in terms of the mean for the age group. The IQ is derived from the

*National Society for the Prevention of Blindness, Inc., 16 East 40th Street, New York, NY 10000.

total scores on all subtests. There is a high correlation between IQs derived from the Stanford-Binet and from the WPPSI, even though there are differences in the test items given and the methods of computation. The Revised Peabody Picture Vocabulary Test (PPVT-R) is a screening test for intellectual functioning in preschool children. This test should be used cautiously because of a tendency to underestimate IQ as measured by the Stanford-Binet (Altpeter, 1985).

Generally, the 3-year-old child has an attention span of 10 to 15 minutes and has a beginning comprehension of the past and the future but is primarily concerned with today. (Although children at this age are frequently characterized as having a short attention span, it is probably more correct to describe them as easily distractible.) They know their own age and can understand simple directions. They are imaginative, can organize their thoughts, and can be bargained with.

By the age of 4 years, the attention span has increased to 20 minutes, and they have developed a concept of time. They know what day of the week it is, how old they are, when the next birthday will come, and that birthdays and holidays are particular time units and are related to parties. They can count to five and understand the concepts of one, two, etc.

Children at age 5 have become less imaginative than at age 4, and are interested in detail and the definition of words. They can be reasoned with logically, become more practical and sensible, and have some understanding of money. They are beginning to understand the meaning of being related to another person. The attention span is now 30 minutes, memory is good, and they have a good sense of time, including months, years, and weeks. In addition, they should be able to solve some problems without assistance, to start and complete activities of interest, and to play without continuous supervision.

Anticipatory Guidance: Intelligence. Developing the skills that are evidence of intelligence is essential to children's enjoyment and learning in the school environment. Parents should be encouraged to help their children achieve these skills by exposing them to the concepts of time, money, and memory tasks (see Table 7-2). Much of that exposure can be achieved merely by encouraging and assisting preschoolers to become independent. They should be allowed to participate in their own care, and they should have some items of their own.

Language Development

"Where does the sun go at night? Why can't I go outdoors? Where did baby Susie come from? Why is it wrong? Why can't I see Grandma? Why? What? Where? When? How?" This is the language of the preschooler. This is the way to learn, to get information and gain attention, and for social experience and understanding. Response from others to these questions is essential for the child to relate to others and to problem solve. Without response, the preschooler will attempt to find refuge in a fantasy world and neglect the verbal communication that is necessary for the period of growth from infancy to school age.

At 3 years of age preschoolers have a vocabulary of about 900 words and are using plurals. They use language more fluently than previously, and sing simple songs. They can make up a phrase and repeat it, not seeming to care whether anyone is listening. They talk to themselves or to imaginary playmates.

By 4 years the vocabulary has increased to 1500 words, and preschoolers understand prepositions. They use "I," talk in sentences, ask many questions, and want detailed explanations. They exaggerate, tattle, and tell family problems outside the home. They are starting to know one or more colors if they have been exposed to them.

By age 5 years preschoolers have a vocabulary of 2100 words and use language correctly with meaningful sentences. They talk constantly, ask questions (about the meaning of words and how things work), and can tell a story accurately, sometimes adding a little fantasy to make it "better." They can sing fairly well, count to 10, and know some colors, again depending on exposure.

During the preschool years children gradually master vowel and consonant sounds. Box 7-3 shows ages at which the various sounds are usually mastered. Nonfluency typifies the preschoolers' language. Probably because of their incomplete mastery of sounds, their speech lacks the smoothness and rhythm of fluent speech. Egocentric speech typical of the toddler and early preschooler yields more to social speech by the end of the preschool stage as the child learns how to both listen and initiate conversation, is able to both ask and answer questions, and to offer as well as understand commands, requests, or threats.

Box 7-3
Approximate Ages for the Mastery of Vowels and Consonants

Age 3 to 4 years:	Most vowel sounds and p, b, m, h, w.
Age 4 to 5 years:	K, g, f, d, m, (ng) as in sing, (ya) as in yellow.
Age 5 to 6 years:	F, v, sh, l, th, s, z, r, ch, (jah) as in jar.

Anticipatory Guidance: Language Development. The nurse is often approached by parents about the speech of their preschooler. Parents get particularly concerned when their child mispronounces sounds or hesitates in speech. Parents should be encouraged not to expect or demand perfection in their preschooler's speech. The child should not be criticized or forced to repeat correctly mispronounced sounds or words, as such measures only serve to create speech disturbances such as stuttering. What parents can do to help their preschooler master correct pronunciation is to model the proper pronunciation of sounds in their own speech, giving special clarity to the particular sounds that the preschooler is learning at the time (see Box 7-3). Bringing to children's attention the sounds that are present in the environment (engines running, wind blowing) and talking with them about what makes the sounds helps them learn to listen to sound and to understand what they hear.

Self-talk (talking about what you are doing) and parallel talk (talking about what the child is doing) gives the child words to think with and to describe all sorts of activities and feelings. *Sesame Street* is an example of a television program that uses the technique of self-talk. Encouraging parents to watch such programs with their children may help them expand their communication skills with their preschoolers.

The nurse, parents, and others who interact with preschoolers should listen to their contributions to conversation even if they cannot be understood. This makes them feel that what is said and how it is said is important, thereby encouraging language development.

Obscure or curse words should be ignored. The more attention given to this type of language, the more it is reinforced. Omission of these words from the parent's language is usually the fastest way to eliminate them from the child's repertoire.

In addition to adults' responding to the child's attempts at communication, language is developed from their reading to the child and making reading materials available. Stories should be simple at first and colorfully illustrated to interest the child. Content should fit into the child's world of fantasy and reality, such as animals that talk as well as inanimate objects that act like humans.

Cognitive Development

Preschoolers fall into Piaget's stage of preoperational thought. During this stage, they will treat objects as symbolic of things other than what they are. For example, a block of wood becomes a car, and the children will move it around like a car, making a noise as it travels. In addition, these children cannot take into account another's point of view; they cannot imagine that the way they see something might not be the way another might see it. Piaget calls this *egocentrism.* Preschoolers seem to feel that their experiences are universal, and the world revolves around them. This becomes obvious in their speech, in which everything is centered on self.

Egocentrism is one of the constructs in Piaget's theory that has been challenged by research evidence (Donaldson, 1978). When children are given "egocentrism tasks" and questions are phrased differently than they were by Piaget, they are able to see other points of view. Therefore it is possible that egocentrism is more a facet of emotional-social development than of cognitive development.

Preschoolers have not yet learned the principle of conservation, i.e., that a certain quantity remains constant in spite of transformation of shape. If you give these children two sets of five identical coins and count for or with them the number of coins in each set, so that they know there are five in each, then lay them out in two rows, spreading one row out farther so that it is longer, preschoolers will tell you that there are more coins in the longer row than in the shorter row (see photograph, page 303). The same thing will be observed when pouring a specific amount of water from a short fat glass into a tall thin glass; the children will tell you that there is more water in the tall thin glass because it appears higher. These cognitive abilities: conservation of number and conservation of liquid amount, are described in Table 3-2 (page 106).

Another aspect of the preoperational stage is the inability of the child to classify or sort objects in any order. For example, if the child is given a group of small toys consisting of people, animals, and houses and is asked to give you all the toys that are like the horse, she or he might give you all the animals, a person, and a house. Preschoolers seem not to understand the difference.

Piaget described another characteristic of preoperational thought, called *centration.* Because of this characteristic the child is able to focus or center attention on only one aspect or characteristic of a situation at a time. Nurses who keep this characteristic in mind will realize that verbal explanations of procedures focusing on benefit in terms of wellness will probably be blocked by the child's more immediate centration on aspects such as fear of the otoscope.

Animism is another characteristic of preoperational thought described by Piaget. Animism involves endowing inanimate objects with human powers and abilities. Piaget saw animism as an example of cognitive immaturity. Recent research has demonstrated that this may not be the case. One study revealed that children personified inanimate objects selectively, indicating that animism may just be a comfortable way for the child to describe the environment (Inagaki and Hatano, 1987). Whether or not animism indicates cognitive immaturity, it is frequently used by preschoolers in verbalizations about the environment. The nurse should be aware of this and the possibility that these verbalizations represent the child's perceptions of reality. Large pieces of equipment used in the hospital, such as the x-ray machine, ECG machine, or oxygen or mist tents may be viewed as frightening or capable of attack. (One can only imagine what animism would mean in the child's perceptions of the CAT scanner!) Health care personnel, especially the nurse and the child life worker, can help a preschooler deal with and master fears through the use of dramatic play. (See Chapter 21 for a complete discussion of the uses of play.) Many hospitals have tours for children who are scheduled for hospital admission to acquaint them with the hospital and some of its equipment. (The practice of providing hospital tours for kindergarten groups and other preschoolers not scheduled for hospitalization may produce unnecessary fears in those children and is therefore not recommended.)

An additional characteristic of preoperational thought is *transductive reasoning* (see Chapter 3). Transductive reasoning proceeds from particular to particular without taking the general situation into account. This can cause the child to assume cause and effect where none exists ("I wished Mommy were dead; now she's sick; it's my fault.")

Anticipatory Guidance: Cognitive Development. Much of preschoolers' mastery of cognitive tasks arises from their discoveries during play investigation. Parents can help their child learn to classify objects through verbalization of object groups that are present in the child's activities of daily living. For example, while selecting the shirt the preschooler is going to wear, the parent might say, "These are all shirts. Which do you want to wear: the blue shirt that buttons, the red shirt that zips, the green shirt that goes over your head, or the brown shirt that snaps?"

Parents may need assistance to associate the fears and misconceptions of their preschooler as a natural developmental phenomenon created by the characteristics of the cognitive processes at this time. When parents can anticipate that objects or experiences may create fear in their preschooler because of these cognitive processes, they can prepare their child about the object or experience through appropriate books, by gradually exposing the child to the situation through pretend play opportunities, and by being present and supportive during the experience.

Reassurances should be based on knowledge of the characteristics of preoperational thought. Taking egocentrism into mind, the parent (or nurse) would begin with, "Nothing *you* did (or said, or thought) caused. . . ." Similarly, explanations of cause would deny the products of transductive reasoning. Recognition that the child's fears are real and finding ways to help the child master those fears is probably more helpful than insisting that the child is imagining things. Stephen King's book *Cujo* (1981) provides a wonderful example of how parents help their child deal with a monster in the closet by writing out words that keep the monster away.

Emotional-Social Competency

As preschoolers' environment broadens and their interests expand, they become more of a social being. At 3 years of age they are friendly but still self-centered; by 4 years they are not as pleasant and have become noisy; at 5, they are becoming more sociable (see Table 7-2). They become a companion rather than someone to care for and can be a pleasure to be around. Their imaginations assist them in learning about others. They learn to get along with both children and adults and behave in a more grown-up manner. In their play they imitate adults, mimic their conversations and manner of speaking, and love to pretend by "dressing up" in their old clothes.

The Developing Person

Psychosexual Development

According to Freud's theory of psychosexual development, in the preschooler the phallic zone is the body zone in which pleasurable sensations or tension reduction is centered. This designation indicates that Freud was more definitive in his description of psychosexual development of little boys than of little girls. According to Freud, little boys develop sexual strivings (or id impulses) toward their mothers whom they wish to have all to themselves. They perceive their fathers as rivals and wish to replace them. These wishes bring about conflict as the little boys fear retribution from the father in the form of castration. This conflict is referred to as the oedipal conflict. The little boy resolves the oedipal conflict by suppressing his sexual feelings toward his mother and developing feelings of identification with his father. Freud described a phenomenon in little girls called the Electra complex in which they note the absence of a penis and presume the mother is responsible for its loss. Penis envy in little girls was attributed by Freud as arising from the Electra complex.

The Oedipus and Electra complexes currently are not seen as valid explanations of preschool age children's behaviors or motivations for behaviors by most child development experts. In evaluating Freud's theory, it is often helpful to examine it in a historical context. Children *do* evidence castration anxiety and penis envy. Their motivation is probably quite different from that which Freud hypothesized during the Victorian age. The nurse will do well to take into account possible castration fears when preparing the preschool-age boy for diagnostic tests and other procedures (Chapter 27). Freud believed that the superego, or conscience, developed as a result of the Oedipus and Electra complexes. According to Freudian theory, the alliance with the same sex parent that occurs at this age results in role modeling not only daily tasks and behaviors, but also the parent's standards, ethics, and morals. (See the discussion of conscience development later in this chapter.)

Initiative and Self-Esteem

The preschooler is in the stage of initiative versus guilt, which is the third Eriksonian stage of development. The central task, crisis, or problem of this stage is for the child to develop a sense of initiative that outweighs any sense of guilt. Initiative may be defined as actively beginning a task, leading, readiness to begin, or enterprise. The word *enterprise,* which means a great or bold undertaking or the willingness to undertake great and bold projects, probably is closest to Erikson's intended meaning for initiative. Because they have mastered motor skills and self-care skills to the point where these can be carried out unconsciously, preschoolers are now ready to try new activities and experiences. Their curiosity and inventiveness are part of their innate capacities for developing a sense of initiative. At the same time, the environment presents them with opportunities to develop initiative, perhaps formalized, as in beginning to attend a preschool, or simply new areas for play and self-care in the home.

Erikson saw the development of a sense of initiative as being characterized by intrusiveness; and preschoolers do intrude. They physically intrude into space via their locomotion abilities as they pedal their tricycles or Big Wheels furiously into the midst of things. The danger to preschoolers is that punishment of unacceptable physical expressions of initiative can result in guilt. Preschoolers intrude into the unknown with their consuming curiosity, evidenced in their questions and play. Much imaginative play or make believe is seen during this stage of development. Excursions into fantasy may serve an important purpose in the development of a sense of initiative. Children may find it easier to tolerate the frustrations and prohibitions of the real world if they periodically can retreat into a fantasy world where those frustrations and prohibitions are mastered. However, their fantasies also can result in a sense of guilt if preschoolers know they would be unacceptable to parents ("Daddy's mean; I wish he was dead").

Guilt is a possibility because much of what preschoolers would like to do is either forbidden or they are physically or mentally unable to do it. Guilt also occurs when those they wish to please are not pleased, or when they themselves are not happy with what they have done. Because preschoolers have a rigid conscience, they frequently have unwarranted guilt feelings over obvious or secret wrongs. As in the previous developmental stages, some guilt is desirable. The individual who develops no sense of guilt is amoral (typically referred to as sociopathic). Preschoolers must learn what actions are inappropriate or wrong and should feel guilty when they commit them. At the same time, they must learn to feel a sense of initiative for developmentally appropriate acts and thoughts.

Other evidences of the initiative stage include some exaggerating and making up of stories, and tattling. An imaginary friend may be used to take the blame for undesirable actions. By the age of 5 years, preschoolers are more responsible and less rebellious. They are more truthful and cooperative and are making progress toward Erikson's fourth stage of development.

Preschoolers' developing sense of self gives a sense of belonging, which provides security and a sense of competence. A sense of competence, in turn, motivates them to perform those tasks that develop initiative. From a very early age, parents must provide safety and security in meeting the needs of their infants to start this foundation. Parents must provide both verbal and physical love that tell children they are worthwhile, thereby contributing to their sense of worth and self-esteem. During the preschool years, children judge self-worth on the basis of this competence with things, competence with parents and other adults, and competence with peers. If they have not developed a sense of belonging and self-worth, they will be hindered in the ability to move out into the bigger world of school and community (see Chapter 16).

Anticipatory Guidance: Developing Initiative. Adults, especially parents, should use praise and affection, rather than scolding and threatening in their relationships with preschoolers. Guidelines for discipline described in relation to the toddler (Chapter 6) continue to apply to the preschooler. Punishment of unacceptable behaviors by physical means, verbal threatening, attacks on the child as a person, or threats of consequences to the child (especially loss of parental approval) all can produce a child who is anxious and fearful about loss of parental love and in whom guilt predominates over initiative. When the child misbehaves, discipline should focus on the behavior, not the child. Examples of strategies that should be *avoided* when disciplining the preschooler include:

Nice boys/girls don't do that . . .

You're a bad/terrible person . . .

If you do that, Mommy won't like you . . .

Mommy/Daddy doesn't like boys/girls who . . .

Parents should refrain from comparing their preschooler with siblings or other preschoolers. Children develop at different rates, and comparing makes it difficult for the preschooler to develop a sense of competence and self-worth. Parents who are warm and accepting of their preschoolers although not necessarily always of their behavior, will help them develop a high level of initiative.

Nurses should be observant of the interactions of the family. A home visit is especially helpful to observe the family in its normal surroundings and usual activities. By becoming more observant and listening carefully to what is not being said as well as what is being said, the nurse can see what warmth, affection, and control a parent provides, and frequently what problems a child may have and why.

Developing Sex-Role Identification

Preschoolers' sense of self is given additional definition by developing sexual curiosity and an awareness of how they differ from others. They are learning about their body, what it looks like and what it can do, and all of this helps them form a sense of sex-role identification. Sex-role identification in the child includes the ability to correctly apply a gender label—male or female—to himself or herself; the acquisition of culturally prescribed gender-appropriate standards of behavior; developing a preference for one's own gender; and identification with parents of the same gender. The development of sex-role identity is explained differently by different theories of development. Freud's psychosexual theory sees sex-role identification as the resolution of the Oedipus complex. Cognitive developmental theory sees it as a function of cognitive development. Children hear and learn the labels "boy" or "girl" as symbols that stand for gender classifications. Social learning theory says that children observe that certain (sex-appropriate) behaviors are rewarded and other (inappropriate) behaviors are not rewarded.

Sex-role identity begins at birth. Fathers distribute cigars announcing the new baby's sex. Baby clothes and other items (sheets, blankets, furniture) are color coded by sex—pink for girls and blue for boys. Even hospital identification bands and bassinet labels may display such color coding. The name given usually conveys a baby's sex. Infant girls and boys are also treated differently. Fathers tend to be more physical with male infants than with female infants. Such attitudes convey subtle messages regarding sex-role identity. From infancy onward, the types of toys given to a child tend to be sex-typed. A male infant is more likely to receive a rattle shaped like a boxing glove than is a female infant.

Toddlers and preschoolers are influenced by our culture, which tends to sex-type them. Many parents have definite ideas of how boys should behave, such as "fighting back" and not crying when unhappy, whereas girls are punished for "fighting back," but tears are acceptable. Parents may also buy toys that help endorse those cultural sex-type expectations (war games for boys and dolls for girls). Boys are pressured to develop characteristics of their fathers, and girls model themselves after their mothers. By the late preschool age, the child identifies self and others by the correct sex.

Children learn and acquire behaviors that are culturally accepted as sex-appropriate through imitation of behaviors that they see rewarded. Television plays a primary role in the modeling of sex-appropriate behaviors. Television—including commercials—tells the child what to eat, what toys to desire, and how to dress and act. (See Chapter 22 for further discussion of sexuality development.)

Changing family lifestyles and numerous families in which both parents work have tended to decrease sex-role stereotyping. Children are more likely to be exposed to multiple examples of appropriate sex-role behavior. To decrease the amount of sex-typing in the family, it is important for children to observe parents doing things together, such as housework and yardwork. Parents can provide a variety of toys and encourage preschoolers to play with any toy that interests them, regardless of the sex-typing connotations traditional culture attaches to it.

The child in a single-parent family needs substitute experiences with a relative or family friend of the opposite sex to provide the relationship of a missing parent. In some two-parent families, one parent is too busy, not interested, or out of town a great deal; the same need is present and can be filled by an interested relative, neighbor, or family friend.

Anticipatory Guidance: Sex-Role Identification. Sexual exploration, masturbation, or sex play in preschool children is fairly common. Preschoolers learn by exploration; they should not be punished for attempting to satisfy their curiosity. Obviously sex play is not encouraged, and limits may be enforced regarding when or where sex organ manipulation may occur, but children should not be made to feel guilty about this very natural response to their inquisitiveness and developing sexual identity. The nurse should be aware, however, that some religious groups condemn masturbation. Sensitivity to family values is an essential characteristic for the nurse who counsels families about child behavior. It is often a good idea to preface advice with further assessment of parental values, e.g., "Some parents have religious or cultural beliefs about masturbation being wrong or harmful. Do you have concerns such as these?"

The way in which some parents verbally respond to their preschooler's masturbation can create guilt in the child. Commands like "Don't put your hand *down there,*" "Don't touch *it,*" "Stop doing *that*" may suggest to the child that the activity is so *bad* that it can't even be named. These kinds of commands are usually caused by parental discomfort. Parents who understand that masturbation is not unusual in this age range will be more comfortable in addressing the behavior openly. It is often helpful for parents to compare setting limits on masturbation to setting limits on elimination. Most parents do not have difficulty communicating to their child limits on where and when urination and defecation are appropriate. Limits on sexual expression could be expressed in statements such as, "Touching your penis* is a private thing like going pee pee," or, "Just like you don't have a bowel movement in front of people, you don't touch your vulva* in front of people." Additional guidance for the parents is advice to ignore the behavior whenever possible. Focusing attention on the behavior may be reinforcing to the child. Often the child can be distracted to another pleasurable but more socially acceptable activity. Most preschoolers gradually decrease the frequency of genital manipulation (see Chapter 22).

Developing a Conscience (Superego)

Conscience, or superego, development is the acquisition of moral beliefs. Conscience begins developing during the preschool years as children learn what behavior is acceptable to parents. When children's behavior is not acceptable, they feel guilty. The moral behavior they develop is adopted from that of the parents, as they are the judges. Preschoolers, during the process of identification, strive to become similar to the parents, especially the parent of the same sex. They therefore closely imitate all behaviors of that parent that they observe. During these preschool years, rules are absolute, passed by parents who are "perfect," and things are totally right or totally wrong, with the parent always right. Parents and nurses should realize the preschooler often believes that sickness, accidents, and hospitalization are punishment for some real or imagined transgression.

*The ability of parents to address sexual exploration or sex play openly is important for another reason. Children who know correct anatomic labels and who are comfortable in their use are more likely to be able to describe improper instances of genital manipulation and other forms of sexual abuse perpetrated on them by adults.

In addition to learning right from wrong by imitating the parents, preschoolers also become indoctrinated into the behaviors or practices evidenced by parents related to their religious and ethnic affiliation. Although preschoolers cannot yet discern the reasons for behaviors such as prayer or attendance at religious services, they eagerly participate in these practices as a part of their identification with the parents.

Likewise, preschoolers cannot comprehend the rationale that makes some behaviors acceptable and others unacceptable. Nevertheless, to facilitate cognitive development they need opportunities to question or disagree, even if they do not comprehend.

Anticipatory Guidance: Developing a Conscience. Many parents do not recognize the significant impact they have on their preschooler's developing moral, religious and ethical attitudes. Parents need to be aware of the role model they provide for their child. The attitude of parents and their relationships with each other as well as with their children all affect the conscience development of the preschool child. The nurse can help parents identify what values and attitudes they want to instill in their child and then help them to recognize their behaviors or practices that either foster or hinder their preschooler's acquisition of those values and attitudes. The nurse may encourage parents to participate actively and regularly in religious or ethnic activities that will provide their preschooler with the role models needed, if they identify these as important in their child's development.

Parents also may require assistance to understand that their child is not ready to adopt acceptable behaviors or avoid inappropriate behaviors only from discussions or explanations of why these behaviors are correct or not correct.

Becoming Social

Rest and Sleep Routines

The preschooler seems to have an endless supply of energy and may be on the go continually. Parents need to be aware of this and initiate rest periods or periods of quiet activity, such as reading. The 3-year-olds need from 10 to 14 hours of sleep daily. They may still nap during the day or at least rest quietly for 1 to 2 hours. By 5 years of age, the sleep requirement is down to 9 to 13 hours and the child seldom naps. Ritualistic bedtime routines continue during the preschool years and can be used as a means to postpone bedtime.

Many preschoolers fear the dark, and this fear is exaggerated when they are exposed to ghost stories, scary television programs, or very active play before bedtime. In addition, the child this age has a vivid imagination, and at night when it is dark, stuffed animals, designs on wallpaper, rustling leaves and blowing branches become frightening objects. Many preschoolers have dreams and nightmares that waken them during the night. (See Chapter 20 for further discussion of rest and sleep.)

Anticipatory Guidance: Rest and Sleep Routines. Parents may need guidance in the management of sleep behaviors common to preschoolers. The preschooler's wish to postpone bedtime can be dealt with in various ways. Usually a consistent, regular routine, such as taking a favorite toy or blanket to bed, with a story and prayers of a specified time limit, encourages a readiness for bed. The endless "drink of water" and "go to the bathroom" tactics can be minimized by incorporating these two activities into the bedtime routine. Solutions to bedtime fears include monitoring TV, keeping play quiet before bedtime, removing objects that can appear scary at night, and leaving a night light on.

When terrifying nightmares awaken preschoolers, they need reassurance that they are safe, and that the dream only seemed like it was real. The technique of an understanding parent sitting with the child and placing a light for her or him to see that it is safe is much preferable to that of taking the child into the parent's bed, which can easily become a habit very difficult to break. When these measures do not effectively manage the sleep disturbances or fears, additional evaluation and counselling are appropriate. (See Chapter 36 for further discussion.)

Health Maintenance

Nutrition

Mealtime for the preschooler should be a happy time within a warm atmosphere. This should be regular and planned to include all family members present at the time. A planned quiet period for the preschooler and siblings may be necessary before the mealtime. Conversation should include the preschooler.

This is a time for the child to learn socialization skills, mealtime behavior, language skills, and family rituals. Table manners at this age are best learned from observation and should not be stressed. Parents should not expect better table manners from the child than they use. Mealtime spills should be accepted, cleaned up, and forgotten.

Because preschoolers grow at a slower rate, they have a small appetite. Serving small portions with seconds allowed, or allowing children to serve themselves, is preferable to serving more food than the child can eat. It is normal for the child to want more food on some days than on others (this occurs in adults), but some parents tend to think that children should always eat a specific amount of food a day.

All preschoolers still enjoy finger foods; these should be offered in some form at mealtime.

By the age of 4 years, most children can use a fork and can spread with a knife. Many 5-year-olds are able to cut their meat with a knife. All food should be served in small amounts so children can handle it easily. As they learn colors, they become more aware of food colors, and may prefer brightly colored foods to dull ones. Chapter 18 discusses the average portions and number of servings for preschoolers per day.

Assisting in food preparation also makes eating interesting, and preschoolers can do many helpful things in the kitchen. They can help plan a menu and assist during grocery shopping, set the table, and help wash the dishes. Some parents feel that it is too time-consuming to allow them to help or to teach them about food preparation, but if parents will take the extra time, they will be rewarded by their preschooler's new interest in food. Helping the child plant vegetable seeds in a garden in the spring and watch the vegetables mature and then pick them, may increase interest in eating vegetables.

Attitudes about foods and eating habits formed during early childhood will last throughout life. It is important to introduce children to new and different foods so they can learn more about the world around them. A variety of foods increases the child's ability to select and accept those foods that contribute to a well-balanced diet. New foods should be introduced gradually and include a variety of tastes, colors, and consistencies. It is very important that foods introduced to the preschooler be accepted by adults in the home and eaten by them at mealtimes. Most preschoolers will try new foods owing to their initiative but will refuse them if other family members make disparaging remarks.

Between-meal snacks should be planned at appropriate intervals and should consist of juice, fresh fruits or raw vegetables, cheese, peanut butter on crackers, and other similar foods. Sweet foods should be offered infrequently, as they tend to contribute to dental caries, malnutrition, and obesity. Snack time should be supervised. Snacks should not be given just before mealtimes.

If the child is growing in accordance with height and weight charts for age and is happy and healthy, plays well, and has healthy teeth, parents should be advised that "not eating a thing" is probably the normal decrease in diet for the age. It is important for the nurse to go over proper diet with the parent(s) and explain the role of junk food in decreasing appetite. If the diet seems adequate, it usually is not necessary for the child to be taking supplemental vitamins.

Play

Imaginary play is a predominant form of preschool play activity. Preschoolers play house using what they observe at home and, if there are older siblings in the home, they play school. As a toddler they played alone, even if side by side with another toddler (parallel play). This play time was spent learning to use fingers and manipulate objects. The preschooler is more coordinated and is experienced in manipulation, so these activities take up much less time.

Young preschoolers start to play with at least one other preschooler *(cooperative play)*. They still remain somewhat selfish but are more interested in what is going on around them. By the age of 4 years they have a longer attention span and play with groups of children. Much of this play is noisy, aggressive, and dramatic. When children reach 5 years they can play simple games with other children and can share. All preschoolers like quiet times involving such activities as coloring, pasting, cutting, and being read to. They also like noisy, boisterous activities, active games, riding tricycles, playing with cars and trucks, and playing with water, mud, snow, leaves, and other outdoor activities. Preschoolers enjoy getting wet and getting dirty and frequently are.

Parents should provide sturdy and simple play materials. Many household articles make good play materials, and they need not be expensive. Play should provide physical activity through the use of balls, blocks, wagons, tricycles, swings, and safe climbing materials. Creative play should be encouraged with sheets of paper, crayons, finger paints, clay, scissors, boxes, cloth, and yarn scraps. Dramatic play can be stimulated by providing dolls, cars, and dress-up clothes. Quiet play can be encouraged with books, records, and puzzles. Parents should provide opportunity, equipment, space, and safety during play but should avoid attempting to structure the child's play. (See Chapter 21 for further discussion of play.)

Safety

The preschooler is old enough to start learning about safety. The desire to imitate and the sense of initiative assist in the ability to learn safety measures. Parents should take advantage of this readiness and teach the rationale for safety rules. For example, preschoolers can comprehend why it is dangerous to cross the street. They are old enough to learn to look both ways before crossing streets, and to cross busy streets only with a green light if available, or with an adult.

Car accidents are still a leading cause of injury to preschoolers, and parents need to explain the rationale for use of car seats and seat belts. If children observe the parents using seat belts, consistently, they will be more likely to comply. When the child is too short to see out of the car window, use of a car seat brings less resistance than restraint by a seat belt.

The nurse should counsel parents *to never leave a child in a car alone, even for a few minutes,* awake or asleep. A preschooler can very quickly set a car into motion while imitating the parent driving. The child could also climb out of the car and be injured by other cars, or get lost. Although it takes longer to unbuckle a child and take him or her into the store for a moment, the safety of the child is ensured. The preschooler is not mature enough to be left alone at home, responsible for self or siblings.

An area in which preschoolers sometimes get into trouble is while playing outside and hiding from others. Poor judgment and lack of experience may lead the preschooler into dangerous hiding places, such as under cars or in abandoned refrigerators and freezers. Abandoned buildings are also favorite playing places but are unsafe, and children should be cautioned about entering these. They should be taught to refuse to talk to strangers, to refuse rides, and to refuse gifts. The preschooler should learn ways to discourage inappropriate sexual advances (see Chapter 35). The preschooler should also know name, address, and phone number, and how to approach a police officer for help.

Preschoolers' drive to imitate adult roles can lead them into dangerous play if they are not supervised and taught the safe limits of experimentation with materials usually used by adults. Because of their curiosity and quick movement, it is wisest to keep them away from areas in which power tools or equipment are being used, such as lawnmowers and saws. They should be taught to use sharp objects, such as a paring knife, with extreme caution and never without supervision by an adult. Power tools should be stored out of their reach. If a gun is kept in the house, it should be stored unloaded with the bullets stored in a separate area, both preferably locked.

Preschoolers are intrigued by matches and fire, and they soon develop the dexterity to ignite them. Matches are best kept stored in a tight container out of reach. The older preschooler may be allowed to accompany a parent to the incinerator and permitted to help burn trash. This measure often helps reduce the child's interest in matches. In addition, it offers an opportunity for the parent to teach the child about fire and the safety precautions needed around fire.

During the preschool years a child's play and daily activities are less supervised than in earlier years. *Potential for injury: poisoning and suffocation* continues to be a nursing diagnosis for which the nurse should assess carefully. Parents need to be cautioned to provide adequate supervision of a preschooler to prevent falls and serious accidents during play and activities of daily living. For example, a preschooler's engrossment in play, especially imaginative play, interferes with a perception of danger. Upstairs windows should have sturdy screens or guards to prevent a serious fall by a preschooler, who may be engaged in "flying superman" play. A preschooler also must be closely supervised when playing around water to avoid drowning. Although many preschoolers are afraid of water, they may slip and fall into the water accidentally. A preschooler's independence in daily activities should be supported by providing special safety devices (adhesive strips in the tub).

Immunizations

Basic immunizations should be complete by the preschool age. Tuberculin skin testing, however, may be done before school entry, and DPT and polio boosters will be given at that time. See Chapter 14 for further discussion of immunizations.

References

Altpeter T: Use of the PPVT-R for intellectual screening with a pre-school pediatric sample. *J Pediatr Psychol* 1985; 10(2):195–198.

Anderson R, Anderson K: Day care—social, emotional and intellectual effect. *Occup Health Nurs* 1984 June; 301–306.

Aronson SS: Care of ill children in child care programs. *Child Care Inform Exch* 1987; 56:34–38.

Belsky J, Steinberg L: The effects of day care: a critical review. *Child Dev* 1978 Sep; 929–949.

Burud S, Collin R, Divine-Hawkins P: Employee support child care: everyone benefits. *Child Today* 1983 May-Jun.

Clarke-Stewart A: *Day Care.* Cambridge, MA, Harvard University Press, 1982.

Collins R, Deloria S: Headstart research: a new chapter. *Child Today* 1983 Jul/Aug.

Dateline child care. *Child Care Inform Exch* 1987; 56:9–10.

DEST. Denver, CO, University of Colorado Medical Center, 1973.

Donaldson M: *Children's Minds.* New York, WW Norton, 1978.

Etaugh C: Effect of nonmaternal care on children. *Am Psych* 1980 May; 309–319.

Glezen W, et al: Epidemiologic patterns of acute lower respiratory infections of children in a pediatric group practice. *J Pediatr* 1971 Aug; 397–406.

Gold D, Andres D: Developmental comparisons between ten year old children with employed and unemployed mothers. *Child Dev* 1978 Sep; 75–84.

Granger R: *Your Child from One to Six.* Washington, DC, US Department of HEW. Publication No. 79-30026, 1979 Aug.

Hambrick-Dixon PJ: Effects of experimentally imposed noise on task performance of Black children attending day care centers. *Dev Psychol* 1986; 22(2):271–275.

Haskins R: Public school aggression among children with varying day care experience. *Child Dev* 1985; 56:689–703.

Hurlock E: *Child Growth and Development.* New York, McGraw-Hill, 1978.

Inagaki K, Hatano G: Young children's spontaneous personification as analogy. *Child Dev* 1987; 58:1013–1020.

King S: *Cujo.* New York, Viking Press; 1981.

Leeper S, et al: *Good Schools for Young Children.* New York, Macmillan, 1974.

Mennie J, Klinger M: Health department services for preschools and day care centers. *J School Health* 1984 Apr; 160–161.

O'Bryant S, Corder-Bolz C: Tackling "the tube" with family network. *Child Today* 1978 May/Jun; 21.

Ogden L: Day care diseases. *Home Healthcare Nurse* 1984 Jan/Feb; 48–49.

Rothenberg MB: Role of television in shaping the attitudes of children. *Child Health Care* 1985; 13:148–149.

Rubenstein E, Comstock G, Murray J (eds): *Television and Social Behavior.* Report to the Surgeon General's Scientific Advisory Committee on Television and Social Behavior. US Department of Health, Education, and Welfare, 1972.

Scarr S: *Mother Care/Other Care.* New York, Basic Books, 1984.

Smith D: Myths about day care: fact or fantasy. *Pediatr Nurs* 1984 Jul/Aug; 278–280.

Sugarman J, Brown P: Child care centers in long-term care facilities. *Nurs Homes,* 1983 Nov/Dec; 4–7.

Trainex Corporation: *Physical Examination of the School Age Child: The Musculoskeletal System.* Filmstrip made by Undergraduate Dietetic Program and the Department of Nursing, California State University at Los Angeles, 1980.

US Department of Health, Education and Welfare, Office of Child Development: *Abstracts of State Day Care and Licensing Requirements Part 2: Day Care Centers.* Washington, DC, US Government Printing Office, 1971.

US Department of Health and Human Services: *A Parent's Guide to Day Care.* Washington, DC, US Government Printing Office, 1984.

Vujovich J: Child day care livens a nursing home. *Geriatr Nurs* 1984 Jan/Feb.

Webb R: *Social Development in Childhood: Day Care Programs and Research.* Baltimore, The Johns Hopkins University Press, 1977.

Werner E: *Child Care: Kith, Kin and Hired Hands.* Baltimore, University Park Press, 1983.

Wilson MN: The black extended family: an analytical consideration. *Dev Psychol* 1986; 22(2):246–258.

Winett R, et al: Children and their families in different child care environments: some data and conclusions. *J Commun Psychol* 1977 May; 149–159.

Bibliography

Advocacy Organization. Child Care Action Campaign, P.O. Box 313, New York, NY 10185. Many single-page information sheets available on various aspects of child care; including research.

Biro P, Thompson M: 1984 Screening young children for communication disorders. *MCN* 1984 Nov/Dec; 9(6): 410–413.

Butler J: A walk-in unit for pre-school children and their mothers. *Health Visitor* 1983 Nov; 411–412.

Castillo N: Framework skills for nursing day care and early childhood education managership. *Pediatr J Nurs* 1982 Jul/Dec; 29–30.

Children's Defense Fund: *The Child Care Handbook: Needs, Programs and Responsibilities.* Washington, DC, 1982.

Duvall E: *Marriage and Family Development.* Philadelphia, JB Lippincott, 1977.

Fish LJ: Identifying gifted preschoolers. *Pediatr Nurs* 1985 Mar/Apr; 11(2):125–127.

Gibson J: *Growing Up: A Study in Children.* Menlo Park, CA, Addison-Wesley, 1978.

Honig JC: Preparing preschool-aged children to be siblings. *MCN* 1986 Jan/Feb; 11(1):37–45.

Katsura H, Miller G: The difficult child in day care—a nursing challenge. *MCN* 1978 May/Jun; 166.

Kittrell E: Children and television: the electronic fix. *Child Today* 1978 May/Jun; 20.

Linley JF: Mothers' attitudes regarding health care for their children. *MCN* 1984 Jan/Feb; 9(1):37–41.

Maheady DC: Health concepts of preschool children. *Pediatr Nurs* 1986 May/Jun; 12(3):195–197.

Malinowski J: Answering a child's questions about sex and a new baby. *Am J Nurs* 1979 Nov; 1965.

Ragozin A: Attachment behavior of day care children: naturalistic and laboratory observations. *Child Dev* 1980 Jan; 409–415.

Rapoport R, Rapoport R: *Working Couples.* New York, Harper & Row, 1978.

Smith DP: Common day-care diseases: patterns and prevention. *Pediatr Nurs* 1986 May/Jun; 12(3):175–180.

Sommers KM: The generation mix: child care in the nursing home. *Nurs Homes* 1985 Jul/Aug; 34(4):27–30.

Sussman M: The family today. *Child Today* 1978 Mar/Apr; 32.

Washing out day-care infection. *Emergency Med* 1983 15 Oct; 220–222.

Werner E: Alternate caregivers for children: a perspective. *Child Today* 1983 Sep/Oct; 22–27.

Families with School-Age Children

Chapter 8

Jo Joyce Anderson

Second only to the family, the school is the major socializing agency available for transmitting values as well as knowledge to children. This chapter describes common needs of families with school-age children, presents the developmental tasks of families with children in the age group from 6 to 12 years, and considers methods of adapting to life changes encountered. Available support systems are discussed. Interventions aimed at promoting the well-being of the child and family are described.

Related Topics
Theories of cognitive and moral development, Chapter 3
Children's health perceptions and health behaviors, Chapter 10
Family assessment, Chapter 12
Promoting healthy parenting, Chapter 13
Fostering self-esteem, Chapter 16
Promoting healthy nutrition, Chapter 18
Promoting dental health, Chapter 19
Promoting healthy sexuality, Chapter 22
Substance use and abuse, Chapter 36
Common childhood infectious diseases, Chapter 45
Common childhood injuries, Chapter 52

We appreciate the critical review of this chapter by Sandra Frick, RN, PhD, and her contributions to it.

Development and Adaptation of the Family with School-Age Children

As individual family members move from one life stage to the next, family life is marked by changing relationships, with family functions at one stage superseded by responsibilities of the next. The willingness of parents to meet changes in their growing children and progress in their own relationship determines the degree and quality of the family unit's functioning.

The family with school-age children is confronted with three major areas of change that constitute the family's developmental tasks. These are (1) adapting to the child's expanding world as he or she moves into school and the world of teachers and peers, (2) expanding family communications and activities to recognize the school-ager's readiness for independent thinking and greater responsibility both within and outside the family unit, and (3) maintaining financial solvency as family costs escalate to meet the needs of school and extracurricular activities.

Table 8-1. Tasks of Children, Parents, Teachers and Nurses in Facilitating School Adjustment

Child's Tasks	Parents' and Teacher's Role In Facilitating Task Achievement	Nurse's Role in Assisting Parents, Teachers, Child
Diffusion into Larger World (5 or 6–8 yr)		
1. Must adapt to differences in teacher's and parents' disciplinary approach and behavioral expectations	1. Parents and teacher should communicate their respective expectations to identify extreme differences and to work out compromises that permit the child to meet expectations of each so that parents and teachers can mutually reinforce their expectations	1. School nurse can help organize parent-teacher interaction (e.g., preschool roundups; parent-teacher-nurse conferences) or mediate in conflicts a. During preschool roundup or school physical, learn what child's and parents' expectations for school are
2. Must compete with peers for teacher's attention and approval as teacher replaces parent for large portion of day	2. Teachers should avoid obvious favoritism in classroom, give individual attention and praise to each child, avoid comparisons of achievement	2. School nurse can offer guidance to teacher and intervene in unhealthy child-teacher relationships a. During preschool registration or school physical, evaluate parent-child relationship for problems as these often carry over to teacher-child relationships
3. Must learn to handle blatant, hurtful honesty and downright rudeness of peers without damage to self-concept	3. Peer activities and behaviors need close adult supervision	3. Nurse in well-child facilities or schools can provide this guidance to parents and teachers
4. Needs to test out new ideas and behaviors in security of home environment	4. Parents need to recognize developmental function of "trying on" ideas and behaviors incongruent with family's but set reasonable limits on how much and what type of "trying on" is to be allowed	4. Nurse in well-child facilities or schools may offer this anticipatory guidance
Disorganization Created by Disparities Between Home and School or Peers (8–10 yr)		
1. Must learn to concentrate on cognitive achievements in school life	1. Parents and teachers need open communication about cognitive tasks that are being focused on at any one time and skills the child finds difficult so that both parties can support the mastery of those skills	1. School nurse observations in classroom will help identify children having difficulty with this task. Investigation of state of health, sensory organ function, and neurologic, physical and emotional function should follow to determine source of problem in achieving task
2. Must learn to integrate peer values in a manner that does not deny family values and to transfer family values into larger world in socially acceptable ways	2. Parents and teachers must understand that just as children fall as they learn to walk so will they fall as they learn to think. These falls during school age are typically boasting, teasing, fighting, lying, cheating, sassing, and whining	2. School nurses should regularly monitor playground and classroom activities to identify extricated children and then set the task force (parents, teachers, nurses, other pertinent school or health personnel) in motion to uncover source of problem and offer help

Adapting to the Expanding World of School

One changing characteristic of all school-age children and their families is the need to adjust to a world no longer totally controlled by parents and the home environment. The school environment takes over many social functions and provides new models for children to imitate. They are faced with the need to master basic skills in reading, writing, and arithmetic. By second grade educational experiences expand beyond these basic skills to the natural sciences. The timing is congruent with the developing cognitive ability which leads children to be curious about the natural sciences.

Beginning school is an event that creates anxiety in some children; this situation can be mitigated by anticipating potential sources of difficulty. Here is an example of a successful adaptation to first grade:

Carrie Hearn began first grade last Monday. Carrie was fortunate in having had the experience of attending nursery school in her neighborhood. There she developed some friendships that could be continued since her preschool playmates also entered elementary school. In addition, Carrie's mother had accompanied her to school and had ensured that she arrived at the appropriate room, was introduced to her teacher, and became involved with another little girl who lived in the same block. Three factors helped Carrie meet the new challenge of beginning first grade: having past experiences in a school setting, encountering a new situation with the support of her mother, and locating an old friend.

As children begin school the family must deal with the new parameters presented by school and peers (Table 8-1). Children may, for the first time, experience being labeled (e.g., "Fatso," "Skinny," "the kid from Becker Street") and prejudice. With exposure to differing moral attitudes and beliefs, both children and parents must now contend with the incongruities between family beliefs and expectations and those of school peers. In addition, children now beginning to handle sibling rivalry are faced with the new situation

Table 8-1. *(continued)*

Child's Tasks	Parents' and Teacher's Role In Facilitating Task Achievement	Nurse's Role in Assisting Parents, Teachers, Child
	Teachers and parents need to develop the art of overlooking minor falls and feel comfortable seeking help for more serious or persistent falls. Children left alone with their peer group often overcome problems with peer assistance rather than adult intervention	Well-child facility and school nurse should evaluate child's behavior patterns and self-concept at each contact to pick up clues that all is not well in child's emotional and social relationships. Nurse in clinic or school should offer parental/teacher anticipatory guidance regarding handling of behavior problems
Disposition of Compromise Between Home and Larger World (10–12 yr)		
1. Must take increasing responsibility for initiating and carrying out own learning activities at school and home; find internal satisfaction in performance	1. Family and teacher must acknowledge child's ability to manage responsibility and allocate responsibilities in which child can take pride and feel success	1. Nurse in any setting in contact with parents and teachers may offer this anticipatory guidance. Nurse may role model such interactions in dealing with child
2. Must take interest in organized school and peer activities to be accepted as a group member	2. Parents need to see developmental advantage of child's involvement in organized activities and plan with child how to get to these, financially handle the expenses involved and still manage home and school responsibilities. Teachers should understand the need for such involvement and assign homework reasonably	2. Same as 1 above. Nurse may help family learn about community activities available to children this age and of financial assistance available through schools, community clubs, churches
3. Must become capable of maintaining appropriate personal conduct (control impulses, resist temptation) with little or no adult supervision	3. Child should be given increasing opportunity to go to school, religious and peer functions unattended by parents and be praised for reports of good conduct. Digression from appropriate conduct should be dealt with in accordance with the seriousness of digression. Parents need to communicate faith in child's ability to handle himself or herself adequately	3. Same as 1 above

of peer rivalry as they compete with other children for the teacher's attention and approval.

As children begin absorbing the values of the peer group and school, conflict often arises. Home becomes a testing ground for new ideas and behaviors—parents are sometimes non-judiciously compared with teachers and cooperative preschool darlings can become relentlessly sassy school-age teases. The inevitable consequence of this, even in the best-adjusted families, is some degree of conflict, particularly between parent and child; between home and school; or between home and peer groups, especially with the older school-age child. Some parents perceive the decrease in control over their child's life as threatening; they sense a progressive impotence as parents. They may respond with alarm or anger directed toward the child or the school (usually the teacher). Sometimes parents over-react as their child expresses new ideas or imitates peer behaviors, trying them on for size. Parents may impose overly strict rules or punishment in response to the experimentation. Other parents give up, refusing to set any limits at all on these experimental ideas and behaviors. Many parents, however, find comfort from sharing concerns and frustrations (not to mention the humor created by some of their children's experimental antics) with parents in similar situations. These parents, although they sometimes feel like packing their bags and running away or hiding out for a day, usually set realistic limits on their children's experimental activities.

The rapidity and extent to which adaptation by the child and family occurs primarily depend on the degree of congruence that exists among home, peer, and school values.

Teachers

As children approach and settle into school, teachers become especially significant and can represent valuable support systems to school adjustment. Caplan (1974) describes support for the child as occurring when:

> Other people are interested in him in a personalized way. They speak his language. They tell him what is expected of him and guide him in what to do. They watch what he does and judge his performance. They let him know how well he has done. They reward him for success and punish or support and comfort him if he fails. Above all, they are sensitive to his personal needs, which they deem worthy of respect and satisfaction.

Such support may be of an enduring or short-term nature. Characteristic functions of support systems are helping to mobilize psychological resources, sharing tasks, and providing extra supplies of materials, tools, skills, and cognitive guidance to improve handling of the situation.

The extent to which teachers possess the attributes of support systems allows them to function as facilitators in the child's attempt to adapt successfully to school. By making expectations clear, guiding efforts, judging products, and rewarding success or comforting failure, a teacher can influence a child's sense of industry. According to Erikson (1968), good teachers "know how to alternate play and work, games and study. They know how to recognize special efforts, how to encourage special gifts."

As the child strives to achieve and master new knowledge or skills or develop talents, the teacher can be a vital supporter.

According to Jerome Kagan (1971), the motive for mastery has as its foundation three goals: "the desire to match behavior to a standard, the desire to predict the environment, and the wish to define the self."

The first goal becomes realized as the child acquires new ideas about the world. Children try to simulate many phenomena by putting into practice some of the ideas they have learned, such as taking apart a miniature motor—similar to repairs of real cars performed by a parent. Teachers can guide children in efforts to meet standards by helping define certain strategies and persuading them that they possess intellectual talents that, if used, can lead to success. Teachers can also assist the child to recognize what standards are realistic. Many children do not realize that some goals are best met by gradually increasing the level for standards against which performance is measured. In their attempt to predict outcomes, the second goal, children strive to master unknown situations. School-agers try to predict what will happen in school, how well they will do on a test, or how many hits they will get in the afternoon baseball game. The need of school-age children to be able to predict the environment has been validated through nursing research. Frick (1985) described problems with prediction as boredom (excessive predictability) and confusion (diminished predictability). Children diagnosed as confused also scored low on a standardized achievement test and received lower grades in subject areas. In the learning environment the teacher can promote optimal predictability by structuring situations in such a way that children can confirm their predictions at least part of the time.

In terms of children's attempts to define themselves, the third goal, the teacher can play an important role in making each child aware of his or her special areas of competence. The teacher can construct work groups in which each child has one area of relatively superior skill, whether it be in music, art, physical coordination, reading, writing, or arithmetic. This process also helps build an expectancy (or prediction) of success and permits children to define themselves as people with certain skills.

In a similar fashion, the teacher can play an important part in preventing the development of feelings of inferiority in the child. Besides structuring the learning situation so a child can experience relative success, the teacher can contribute toward the maturing of positive feelings toward self and others. School-age children still greatly depend on the opinion and attitudes of significant adults as an aspect of their own self-esteem. The implications of this for teachers go beyond merely providing a warm and accepting climate. Teachers must have knowledge of childhood developmental processes in psychodynamic terms. *Maturity in children must not be equated wholly with reasonableness—there must be an appreciation for the creative potential inherent in fantasy; actions should be based on the expectation that growth will be gradual, wavering, regressive, and uneven.* The teacher who understands that conflicts occur naturally in development will be able to convey to children that doubts, fears, problems, and backslidings are acceptable parts of being a person.

Erikson (1968) indicated that "the development of a sense of inferiority, the feeling that one will never be 'any good,' is a danger which can be minimized by teachers who know how to emphasize what a child can do and who recognize a psychiatric problem when they see one." By being sensitive to a child's personal needs and deeming them worthy of respect and satisfaction, the teacher can be a source of emotional support merely by listening to and understanding problems, even if they are outside the scope of solution within the school. Thus by guiding the child's attempts to achieve and providing the cognitive skills to master situations, the teacher can enhance the attainment of a sense of industry. Likewise, by treating the child as an individual and recognizing variations in the growth process, a teacher can be instrumental in preventing feelings of inferiority. Both of these qualities are important attributes of people in support systems.

Peers

Peers can also become important members of the child's support system. From their peers children learn how to cooperate and compete and learn the meaning and importance of following rules. They are also forced to consider situations from perspectives other than their own. An extra feature of these "supporters" is that there is a greater likelihood for enduring relationships in light of the fact that children normally progress through their school years with the same peers, in contrast to the yearly exposure to different teachers. In terms of the need to develop a sense of industry, to feel good about his or her products, and to compete with others for recognition, the peer group watches and judges each child's performance, and lets the individual know how well he or she has done. Typically, this latter process is conveyed through inclusion or exclusion from group activities. Essentially, children look to their peers to measure their own skills and worth. According to Maier (1969), "A sense of accomplishment for having done well, being the strongest, best, wittiest, or fastest are the successes toward which he strives. The child wards off failure at almost any price." Thus, children look to others for approval of themselves as worthwhile people.

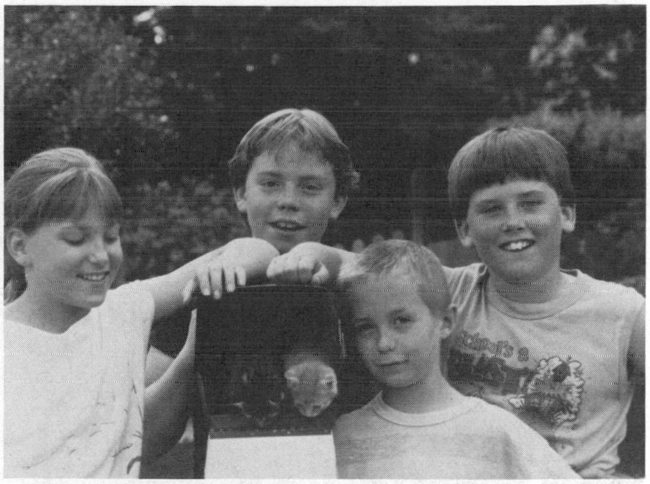

Peer groups are important to children's feelings of acceptance and self-esteem. Often, children will have one group of friends at school and another group of friends who live nearby and are available for play after school and on weekends. Neighborhood groups more often involve members of the opposite sex.

The structure of childhood social groups progresses roughly through three stages—from a global or undifferentiated group of children to a highly differentiated group with an exaggerated structure to an articulated functional unit.

Prior to age 8 or 9 years, children of both sexes socialize informally. The group composition more or less depends on who is available and is interested in the same activity. Activities are organized around playful games. There is little formality or organization; groups collect by chance and consist of whomever shows up on the sidewalk or street corner at a particular time. The children may have little other association with each other, yet there is a mutual participation in fun activities.

At about 8 or 9 years, a marked change appears in the social groupings, with a cleavage occurring between sexes, and a pattern of strong affiliation and loyalty evolving for a particular group or gang of the

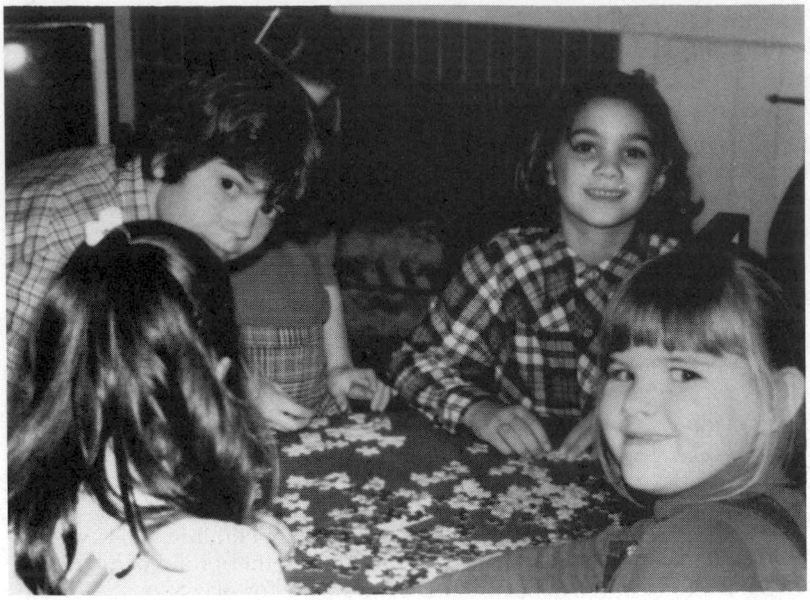

At about 8 or 9 years of age, strong affiliation for a particular group or gang of the same sex emerges. (Photograph by Dan R. Bruggeman.)

same sex. Cross-sex peer interactions are seen as taboo in children of this age group (Buhrmester and Furman, 1987). The group or gang provides the support system for children to declare independence from adult rules. Secret languages or codes and odd mannerisms of behavior and dress are developed to further this independence. The group almost takes on the form of a secret society with formal rites.

Toward the end of the school-age period, the lore of belonging to a secret society abates, and groups and gangs are more likely to be organized around particular kinds of activities and functions. There may be nature clubs, fan clubs, or secret societies with special rules, and plans may be made in advance, such as going to the movies, building a fort, or having a picnic.

At this time, too, the child's activities are focused around a best friend of the same sex with whom all areas of life can be discussed. Together they may belong to more than one group, depending on their interests. These interest groups do not require the fierce loyalty and solidarity of the previous group structure. Some chumships may be brief, but subsequent intense and exclusive relationships between one child and another usually develop within a short time.

As children progress through these social stages, they are socialized into the peer culture. At the next developmental stage, adolescence, socialization is to the social culture of the community at large.

Culture

A major change in a child's life occurs with the onset of the school-age years—the child is introduced into society and the extrafamilial culture. This is a fundamental social change resulting in greater and greater demands being placed. At the same time, the child is treated in a less personal way than previously. Individuality is lost in the large group structure of which the child becomes a part.

During the school-age years, the basic values of the culture are inculcated. In every society, even the most primitive, these are the years when the knowledge, laws, and customs of the civilization are passed on. They are crucial years both for society and for children. Basically, children bring to this stage the culture of the family and the ever-expanding cognitive skills, thirst for knowledge, and urgent sense of industry or need to

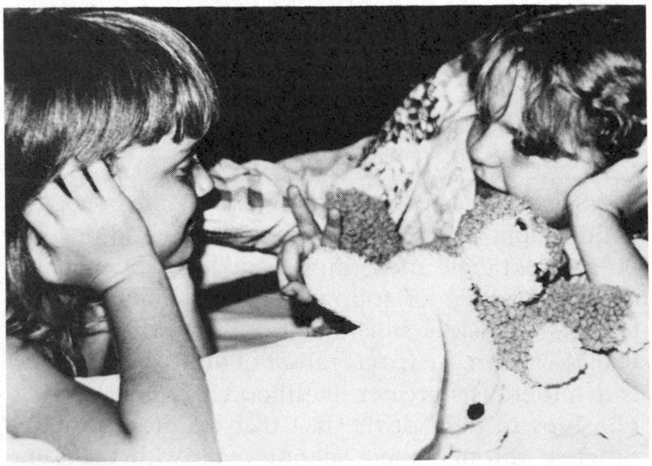

Spending the night at a best friend's home is typical of the school-age period.

master the world. The child is ripe for absorbing cultural values.

Although children are ready for it, this inculcation of culture may be somewhat traumatic, especially if the cultural values of the family differ from those of society at large or from the school or peer group. They must learn to reconcile the differing values in a way that makes sense to them and that they can live with.

Fortunately, this process of inculcation of culture and reconciliation of differing values is not thrust on the child all at once. The process is slow and gradual. It proceeds primarily through the peer group, which becomes a major force in the life of the school-age child at about age 8 or 9 years.

The cultural values inculcated through the peer group are a mixture of the family cultural values of each of the group members and the values promulgated by the schools and religious groups to which the children belong and the mass media to which the children are exposed. The children actively "try on" differing approaches, insofar as cognitive processes allow.

Conflicts may arise between the family's cultural values and those that the child is exposed to in the peer group. A family may be very prejudiced against a particular racial or ethnic group, and the peer group may not be, or vice versa. The peer group might think that experimenting with smoking or drugs is the thing to do, while the family is opposed to such activity. In such situations, the child must resolve the conflict by choosing one viewpoint or the other.

The new cultural values that are adopted, for varying periods of time, by school-age children make them somewhat of an immigrant whose new host culture is the subculture of middle childhood and whose parents live in a hopelessly old-fashioned foreign culture. Overtly, children are ostentatious in their allegiance to the peer group's rules of conduct and behavior. Covertly, however, children are still dependent on the parents for guidance, and they tend to maintain the essence of their value system. Buhrmester and Furman (1987) found that children in the middle school-age years see both parents and peers as important companions.

Our society has created one group of children who may be more susceptible to peer influences and less susceptible to parental influences than other children in their age group. "Latchkey children" is a term given to that group of children who return to their own or someone else's home after school, when no adults are present in the home. The children have their own key with which to gain access to the home, thus the term "latchkey."

One typical viewpoint about these children has been that lack of adult supervision coupled with inappropriate peer influence makes them more likely to develop problem behaviors than children who are supervised in the home or in a day care setting after school. At least one research study has demonstrated that problem behaviors relating to peer pressures may be due more to variations in supervision and setting than to the mere fact of the child being a latchkey child. Steinberg (1986), in a study of fifth, sixth, eighth, and ninth graders found that children home alone were less susceptible to peer pressures to engage in antisocial activities than children who were at a friend's house unsupervised. Those children whose parents knew where they were and who were more authoritative in parenting style were also less likely to be influenced in an antisocial way by peers. (See Chapter 13 for a complete discussion of the latchkey child.)

Prejudice

Once children reach school age, parents can no longer cushion or protect them from the prejudice of others that may exist because of the child's size, beliefs, color, ethnic background, family social status, or neighborhood of family residence. Parents can take measures, however, to help their child build self-confidence and the ability to relate tolerantly to those who are prejudiced against him or her. With these qualities the child can deal with this byproduct of life in a diverse society without severe loss of self-esteem or detriment to emotional or social development. Children also need direct, honest answers when they question why they or someone else is different. They need regular reassurance that because they are different does not mean they are "bad" or less worthy than their peers.

In dealing with a situation in which there is prejudice, parents can make use of available literature and music and provide for participation in ethnic, religious, or social events to help answer questions and to provide the child with a sense of belonging and reassurance about any differences.

When children are confronted with others' prejudice against themselves, they will react in a fashion similar to the way their parents have responded in the past. Therefore, parents should develop skill in handling prejudice in a positive way. There is no one best way to confront prejudice against oneself, but using a calm, forceful approach is probably most effective.

Children sense their parents' prejudices and imitate those same prejudices in their peer group. By school age, the best approach of a person trying to help children overcome their prejudices toward others is to discuss frankly these prejudices, encouraging children to formulate their own ideas and opinions rather than bearing the burden of a parent's preconceived ideas. Ideally, of course, the parent also works to overcome that prejudice.

Parents can expose children positively to all kinds of people. Family friendships and social interactions with families of diverse backgrounds help develop an early appreciation for the richness that people's differences can lend to living. Such a child will not adopt prejudiced ideas that arise from knowing nothing about other cultures or lifestyles.

Children need to learn that no one need tolerate discrimination and that legal assistance in dealing with and protection against discrimination do exist in the United States.

Parents may need help to realize that prejudice is learned and that parents are the primary teachers. If parents provide opportunity for exposure to the diverse cultures of America and keep communication lines open on this subject, they will be helping their child to grow up with a clearer view of the world and a self-confidence that allows tolerance of others' ignorance.

Role of the Nurse in Facilitating Adjustment

The possible implications are numerous for the nurse in the school setting to facilitate the child's adjustment within the framework of the support system afforded by teachers, peers, and family. School-age children and their families face new potential stresses that can affect coping abilities. The nurse in the school setting must continually assess children and their families in relation to coping abilities. If defining characteristics are identified which point to a nursing diagnosis of *family coping: potential for growth,* the nurse will be able to support and maintain the behaviors and characteristics which have resulted in this positive wellness state. If the defining characteristics of one of the problematic diagnoses *(ineffective individual coping, or ineffective family coping: compromised, or disabling)* are seen or if conditions exist which increase the potential likelihood for one of these diagnoses, the nurse can plan interventions for the problem. The nurse's holistic assessment is enhanced by an awareness of the factors which influence perceived stress for an individual or family.

Potential stresses of families with school-age children depend on many factors, including the behavioral style or temperament of the children, parental perception of the youth and expectations for their behavior, the marital relationship, effectiveness of family support systems, and circumstantial factors such as financial pressures, illnesses, and myriad events affecting the family. These factors influence how the family deals with "stress" and must be considered when evaluating a child's response to school, since the effects of family discord are often acted out by the youth in the school setting.

Frequently, the school nurse is a member of the interdisciplinary team that develops a treatment plan for the school-age child who is having problems; assessment of family interaction is often the nurse's task. Observations gained from family interactions provide the nurse with information about strong and weak character traits of members, the problems they face, and their methods of coping with issues. This assessment is the basis for a nursing diagnosis of *ineffective family coping: compromised or disabled.*

A family interview, preferably in the home, is essential to the nurse in gaining an understanding of problems of school-age children and in planning with families how to manage these problems. In addition to specific verbal information collected during the interview, equally important is observation of the family members' behavior during the interview itself. For example, the nurse can observe and note the father's sitting back and leaving it to the mother to tell the story and to discipline the child, the child's willingness to stay put during the recitation of problems, and the increasing restlessness and distracting activity as the nurse draws the mother's attention away from the child and to more neutral ground. From such observations can be developed a working hypothesis that the child's apparent "problem" behavior at least works in that through it the child keeps the mother's attention. An appropriate intervention might be to applaud the mother's obvious extra effort in trying to deal with the child and to engage the father in helping the mother to back off and become less involved in the child's behavior.

No behavior occurs in isolation, and no intervention is aimed at one family member alone. The nurse's energies are directed toward observing the family system in action and abstracting from that observation the repetitive patterns of interactions among family members that support the problem behavior. With this information the interdisciplinary team can establish strategies to help the family members manage their stress in a way that does not precipitate problem behavior in their school-age child.

The school nurse may be in a more advantageous position than the teacher to deal with crisis situations arising from school performance, since school performance is associated with teachers' evaluations. In any family the child's learning problems may impinge on the goals and aspirations of the parents. A child may be perceived as a psychological extension of the parents, the bearer of their genetic traits, and the product of their childrearing efforts. If the child fails in school, the parents may see themselves as failures. Feelings of guilt, doubt, and anxiety may turn into anger, which is projected onto the school. Principals, teachers, learning disabilities specialists and remedial instructors may not be able to obtain the trust and confidence of the parents because these educators are often the conveyers of bad news regarding the child's achievements. In situations such as these, the school nurse may be more successful in engaging the family in counseling and may be more effective in any therapy efforts. Thus, such actions may relieve some of the tension between school personnel and individual children.

In summary, factors that seem to foster school adjustment are a positive regard for a child's individuality by parents, teachers, and peers; a willingness among these support groups to respond appropriately to signals of need; an atmosphere within the family and school that is conducive to growth; and the availability of effective support systems. By assessing the family unit and classroom routinely for psychosocial dysfunctions, the school nurse can identify "stressors" and develop appropriate methods of intervention.

Table 8-1 summarizes the major challenges of the school-age child, parents, and teachers to achieve adequate school adjustment. Nursing actions to facilitate the child's and family's adjustment are also listed.

Expanding Family Communication and Activities

Expanding communication and activities during the school-age years involves two interwoven processes: the process of letting go by parents and the process of taking on progressively more independence and responsibility by the school child. These two processes are accomplished in the milieu of family group activities or projects as well as activities the child participates in away from home and without parental supervision.

Letting Go

Letting children go is one of the hardest tasks parents must undertake. It begins during the school-age years as the child leaves home for school and culminates in late adolescence or early adulthood when the child leaves to make a home.

All parents experience some degree of stress upon "letting go" of their youngster to the school system, which requires day-long separations. Likewise, the broader social exposure that school creates forces families to cope with attitudes of prejudice and potential threats to the child's safety during hours away from home.

Letting go requires that parents free their children to make increasingly more of their own decisions, learn from their own choices and experiences, and take progressively more responsibility for themselves and their actions. Letting go also involves allowing children to experience hurt and humiliation when choices were unwise, to feel the exuberance of having done something "all alone," and to know the satisfaction that comes from working with others because of personal choice. Parents grant this freedom by keeping their mouths closed and hands at their sides when they are tempted to give instructions, assist in tasks, or baby the child. Giving in to these temptations often alienates the child and impairs the development of independence and responsibility.

Along with this spirit of allowing freedom, parents need to communicate faith in the child's competence and resilience. Children who know that their parents believe in them and are proud of them have fewer failures and bounce back quicker when they do fail. Children who experience belittling of ideas and efforts and whose parents communicate doubt in their abilities usually comply with these expectations for failure.

Keeping an open door requires giving the child room to make mistakes and offering support or comfort during recuperation from the lapses in self-confidence and self-esteem that mistakes or failures create. The nurse can help parents understand the need for and benefits of increased autonomy to the developing child. Putting parents in touch with other parents who are now or have in the recent past gone through this stage with their children is often supportive, especially for parents who are afraid that they will be perceived as irresponsible if they allow their child this kind of independence.

Parents also need to understand the "angel at school, hellion at home" syndrome of childhood. If they recognize that the family unit is the resource to the school-age child for security and stability as the child attempts to integrate and adapt to a new world of people, ideas, and experiences, the dichotomous behavior is met with better understanding. In order to meet the social expectations outside the home, the school-ager needs to be able to come home and express all the fears, disappointments, and self-doubts imposed by the new world. These feelings are generally expressed through misbehaving, whining, or demanding behaviors. Within this dichotomy the child goes through a process of self-evaluation to achieve self-acceptance within a new framework of multiple roles and values.

The nurse who assists the family to recognize the phenomenon of development fosters healthy relationships despite the stress that is a consequence of increased independence for the child. Urging parents to consistently enforce a wide set of rules, to continue to set limits, and to provide positive feedback as their child struggles to adapt is important because such actions foster the child's developing sense of reality and self-confidence in decision making.

Ensuring that the child is being assimilated into groups that conform to family and community expectations can be comforting to parents as they cope with the gradual loss of their child's attention. This can be augmented by encouraging the establishment of contacts with other families who possess similar values and by reinforcing socialization experiences that help the child make the emotional shift from family to peers to the larger society. Parental participation in the child's activities should continue but will take different forms than it did earlier. For example, instead of playing baseball with Johnny, who now prefers to be with his peers, the father may provide transportation for the team, be a volunteer at the neighborhood recreation center where Johnny and his friends defend their title, or be a proud spectator.

Parents may need to be encouraged to invite school-age children to participate in family projects and outings that are appropriate to their interests, talents, and developmental level. The freedom to become involved in or help organize family activities and the parents' respect for that contribution to the cooperative endeavor can reinforce the school child's self-worth and convey feelings of belonging that could provide a positive frame of reference for addressing group activities outside the family. The nurse should encourage parents to speak of the unique contributions made by their children. In this manner individual differences that contribute to identity formation will be encouraged. It is important to recognize that in addition to involvement in family activities, children need separate time with parents. The nurse involved in counseling parents can bring this to their attention.

Disruptions or distortions in the normal process of parent-child separation or ''letting go'' during school-age years often are symptoms of earlier problems in these relationships (overdependency, overprotection, unreasonable developmental expectations, psychosexual conflicts) that have persisted or increased because of the child's required attendance and participation in school or the child's developmental maturation. Other stress factors may have occurred within the family that adversely affect separation, such as divorce, illness, or death of a parent, the main caretaker's working outside the home, or a geographical move with the subsequent loss of friends and change of school. Such factors, whether their effects are long-term or temporary, may upset the family balance and produce dysfunctional behavior among its members.

For example, Brody and colleagues (1986) found that an inter-relationship exists between the quality of the marital relationship and parenting practices. Parents with poorer quality relationships tend to give less positive feedback to the child and intrude more into the child's tasks. Often the conflict within the family is projected onto one member, who becomes a ''scapegoat'' or who produces symptoms indicative of emotional disturbance. If the family conflicts are displaced to the school-age child, school difficulties, peer problems, and maladaptive affectional relationships frequently are found.

Progression in Independence and Responsibility

The school-age child is ready for increased independence and responsibility both at home and away. Even early school-age children are capable of caring for their room, making their bed and helping with household tasks such as meal preparation and clean-up, vacuuming and dusting, and garden work. By age 8 most school-agers are responsible enough to run short-distance errands alone, take full charge of pet care, help wash the car and entertain younger siblings, and do other moderately demanding jobs.

By 10 years, the child is usually interested in a paper route, lawn tasks, or other after-school and summer jobs to supplement an allowance. He or she can also help with household repairs and prepare simple meals alone. By this age the child also wants to go some places alone with peers such as the movies, a ball

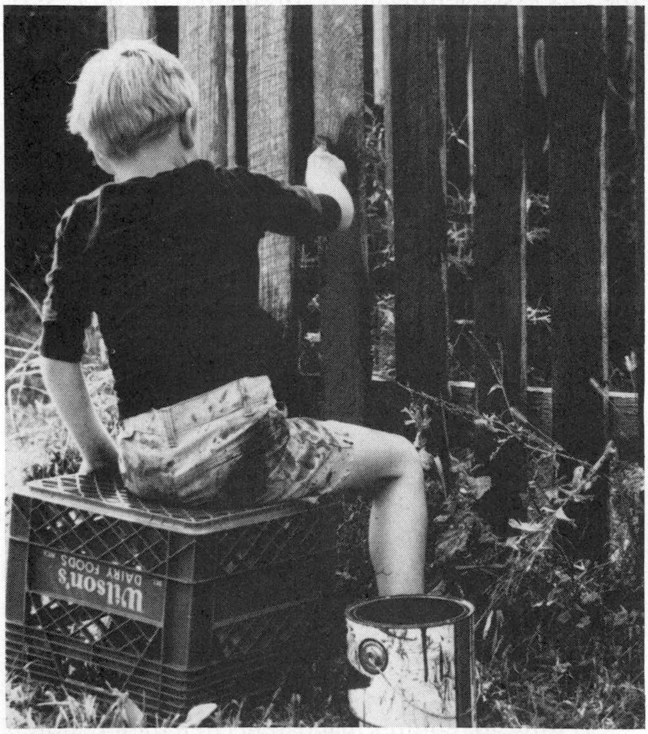

The school-age child is industrious.

game, school activities. Most grade schoolers can handle themselves adequately in public (often manifesting better behavior than they display at home) and the opportunity to go alone to public activities with peers builds their self-confidence to meet new situations.

School-age children need privacy for personal activities separate from those of other family members. The sanctity of places to keep diaries and special mementoes should be respected. Rules that safeguard the person's right to privacy need to be developed and clearly communicated to family members. Parents should use consistency in dealing with violations of these rules. As children approach adolescence, the need for more privacy must be anticipated.

The nurse's role in fostering progressive independence and responsibility in the school-age child lies primarily in the provision of information, support, and guidance to parents as they attempt to lessen their control over the child. Suggestions to parents for yielding independence and greater responsibility to their children as provided by Foster (1976) can be useful for the nurse's anticipatory guidance. Foster's recommendations are:

- Praise the child's independent efforts at responsibility; do not criticize or condemn poor results.
- Do not label tasks as being male or female responsibilities; instead, rotate all household jobs to lessen the monotony of some tasks and to diminish the likelihood of slackening quality in the job done.
- In addition to providing a variety of jobs, allow choices in duties; this permits the child to make maximum use of abilities and to explore different interests.
- If carelessness creeps into work heretofore done well, either rotate tasks or increase the challenge of the existing task.
- When children shirk their tasks, letting them suffer the natural outcome is usually the most effective management. However, flexibility in demands is needed. If they have other demands on their time such as homework, either pitch in and help with the task or temporarily take it over.
- Check work performance while the child is still around; do not tolerate slipshod work or redo it as long as it is a task within the child's capabilities to do well.

Such anticipatory guidance from the nurse may serve to prevent unnecessary family conflict. To provide opportunities for children to master competencies expected for their developmental stage yet to reasonably restrict them from situations that are beyond their coping ability requires a balance not easily obtained. To allow children to make mistakes and to learn from them is often difficult for parents. Group discussions with other parents who have successfully coped with similar situations may be useful.

Family Relations

During this stage of family development, emotional nurturance is needed by all members; there is a higher incidence of divorce during this stage (Miller and Janosick, 1980). A task of spouses who have school-agers

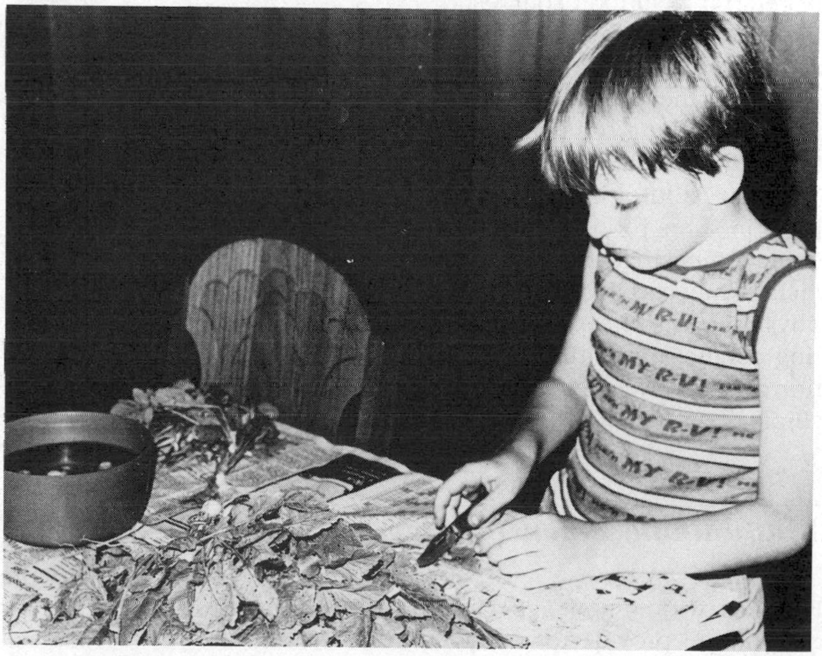

By 9 years, the child can assume responsibility for assisting with meal preparation and clean-up.

is to share the nurturing and disciplining of this child and be mutually supportive of each other. The single parent without outside support systems, e.g., Big Brothers and Big Sisters Programs or Parents Without Partners, may need help to sort out the demands and stresses of raising a school-age child.

In two-parent families a frequent source of spousal breakdown is related to the developmental crisis of each member of the couple. The mother who has a self-image invested totally in the mothering role is faced with a sense of a crumbling self as the school-ager demands less of her time and wants less input or help from her. The father and/or mother who has maintained a profession is usually at the height of the occupational role, spending many hours and energy to that end, leaving less time and energy for family demands. Parents need, during this stage, to be caring with each other and to allow refueling through personal as well as "couple" projects. If not, parents may each become self-absorbed and neglectful of the needs of their child and their mate.

Added to the stress created by the spouses' individual developmental crises and crises presented as a family unit with a school-ager, the family is frequently also faced with changes in composition either with the addition of a new sibling, the moving in of an elderly grandparent, death of a parent, career changes which often involve geographic moves, a parent who goes to work or loses a job, or the separation or divorce of parents who have not been able to cope with all the stresses.

Because of the increased risk of family stress during school-age years, the nurse should take some time at each opportunity to evaluate parents' needs and to assist them as necessary through counseling, teaching, or referral to support sources.

During this stage in family development, siblings are typically at seemingly continual odds at home and yet each other's best defender away from home. The nature of sibling conflict varies, depending largely on the number of children and the years of age difference. Younger children tend to identify with the older siblings in some form of competition. Parents need encouragement to let the children resolve their own conflicts as much as possible as long as there is no risk of physical harm. The experience of working through sibling conflicts gives the school-age child the preparation and experience needed to manage peer relationships.

Maintaining Financial Solvency

Families with school-age children are expected to continue to provide for the physical safety and economic needs of their members and to obtain enough goods, services, and resources to survive. Because of heightened financial and social pressures as children enter school and participate in extracurricular activities, and the increased time available as they attend school for longer periods of time, mothers who did not work outside the home previously may begin employment. In addition, both fathers and mothers may "moonlight," work overtime, or seek promotion to positions of greater responsibility and stress. The demands of employment will require some shifting of roles and responsibilities of some or all family members.

There are three major concerns for which the nurse can assess and offer guidance. For this age group, the school nurse may be in a position to offer the most assistance.

- Does the family have the financial resources to provide adequate food, clothing (including cold weather clothes), transportation to and from school, and needed school materials so that the child is both healthy, safe, and able to participate fully in school activities? Generally, schools have guidelines for referral for assistance to outside agencies for these basic needs. The national school lunch program has special provisions for low-income children.

- Does the child have medical, dental, hearing, or vision problems that have not been corrected because the family cannot afford care? Most schools have established programs of screening for such problems; however, it does no good to notify parents that their child needs dental work or glasses if the family cannot afford such assistance. The nurse should also be aware that family members may not be able to read or may not read English and thus may not be able to understand referrals for medical attention. Any system of health screening in schools should have a strong follow-up program and take into consideration the financial inability of some families to provide care.

- Are there conditions in the home that place undue responsibilities on the child so that he or she is not able to pursue play, outside activities, or schoolwork? Are the parents employed so many hours that the child is responsible for most or all of the care for younger children? Is the child employed so many hours in a family business or enterprise that health or welfare suffer? Has the parent or parents recently become unemployed, placing financial or emotional stress on the family? Often, family unemployment and long hours of work by children (for example, by farm workers) are community-wide problems.

The school nurse, community health nurse, or clinic nurse frequently sees the effects of financial problems in the health and behavior of children. Health promotion for children is not adequate unless it includes participation in the political process as an advocate for children.

Growth and Development of the School-Age Child

The school-age period, 6 to 12 years, is characterized by slow but steady physical growth, refinement of neuromuscular skills, and rapid expansion of cognitive and social skills. It is a time for "doing" and mastering the ever-expanding world of things and people. During this period the foundations are laid for future adult roles in the world of work, recreation, and social interaction.

Statistically, the school-age child has the lowest rates of mortality and serious morbidity of any age group. In a health interview survey conducted in the United States, 95 per cent of this age group was reported to be in good or excellent physical health (Health US., 1984).

The primary goal for the nurse in working with this age group is to promote optimal competencies within the child and to assist the child and parents to appreciate the importance of and the interrelationship between physical, intellectual, emotional, and social competencies.

Promotion of competency in health behaviors must take into account the meaning of health for each child. A study by Hester (1987) revealed that the 225, primarily Caucasian, middle-class children interviewed perceived health as a holistic, multidimensional construct. In response to the question, "Tell me what you think a healthy (unhealthy) child is like," these children responded with statements about activity-exercise, personal grooming, physical health, nutrition, behavior, emotional health, dental health, sleep, friends, family, and substance use. The results of this nursing research suggest that at least some school-age children are sophisticated enough to view health as more than the absence of physical illness. The nurse interacting with a school-age child can ask questions such as the ones used in this study to assess individual perceptions of health. When a child's response indicates a holistic understanding, the nurse can build upon this concept of health by reinforcing the child's perception and offering suggestions for age-appropriate health behaviors involving physical, emotional, and spiritual health. When the response indicates a narrower view of health, the nurse can use that opportunity to begin expanding understanding by exploring with the child how other aspects of life affect the way one feels and what responsibility a child of that age can have for various health activities. The nurse who can "plant the seed" of responsibility for self-care at this early age can contribute immeasurably to the child's future health behaviors.

Physical Development

To assess the physical competency of a school-age child, the nurse must be aware that each child has a unique growth pattern. Although the most obvious measures of physical growth are increases in height and weight, other indicators of normal development, such as neuromuscular ability, sensory organ development, tooth eruption and other measures, are included in a complete assessment of physical competency (see Table 8-2, page 346).

Body Proportions: General Appearance

Height and Weight

During the early school-age period the child's progress in height and weight is relatively slow and steady at approximately 5.5 cm (2 inches) per year for height and 2.5 kg (5.5 pounds) per year for weight.

Boys are an average of an inch taller and two pounds heavier than girls in the early school-age period. (The average weight in early school-age years is 40 to 50 pounds, and the average height is 44 to 48 inches.) The yearly increment in height and weight is comparable for boys and girls through age 9, when it begins increasing more rapidly for girls than for boys. By age 12 girls are an inch taller than boys and two pounds heavier. This preadolescent growth spurt for girls, beginning between 10 and 12 years, is an initial sign of pubertal maturation. Boys typically have to wait another two years for the acceleration in growth; that is, between 12 and 14 years.

Although a slow and steady growth pattern applies to school-age children as a population group, a given child may not follow it precisely. Growth charts (Appendices Two and Three) provide for individualization of the assessment in that increases in height and weight are plotted sequentially from year to year. Growth is not constant. Periods of acceleration occur at different times in any group of children, with the overall pattern evening out over time. Often children experience an acceleration in height during the spring and an acceleration in weight during the fall of the year.

Anticipatory Guidance: Height and Weight

Because school-age children may not receive annual health assessments, the school physical examination for the first grade is an opportune time for the nurse to discuss expectations about increases in height and weight with children and parents. With the advent of regular school attendance the child is faced, usually for the first time, with large numbers of children the same age. Comparisons of self to others are inevitable. Children and parents should be helped to understand that genetic endowment, nutrition, and exercise are major determinants of increases in height and weight in the healthy child.

Boys who are significantly shorter than their peers (of the same age) do seem to be at risk for some emotional difficulty displayed by withdrawing (Holmes et al, 1982). Family members and the nurse can assist these boys by teaching ways to assertively manage peer teasing.

The height and weight chart should be reviewed with the child and parents. Parents can be taught how to weigh and measure the child accurately so that together they can plot the child's growth between health assessment visits. The child's birthday is an opportune time for plotting height and weight. With this activity, the child can attain a sense of accomplishment through knowing the exact growth over time and learn a valuable lesson about the usefulness of self-comparison as a yardstick for progress. The natural tendency is to compare self to others, and the child this age needs to learn the value of comparison of individual progress over time.

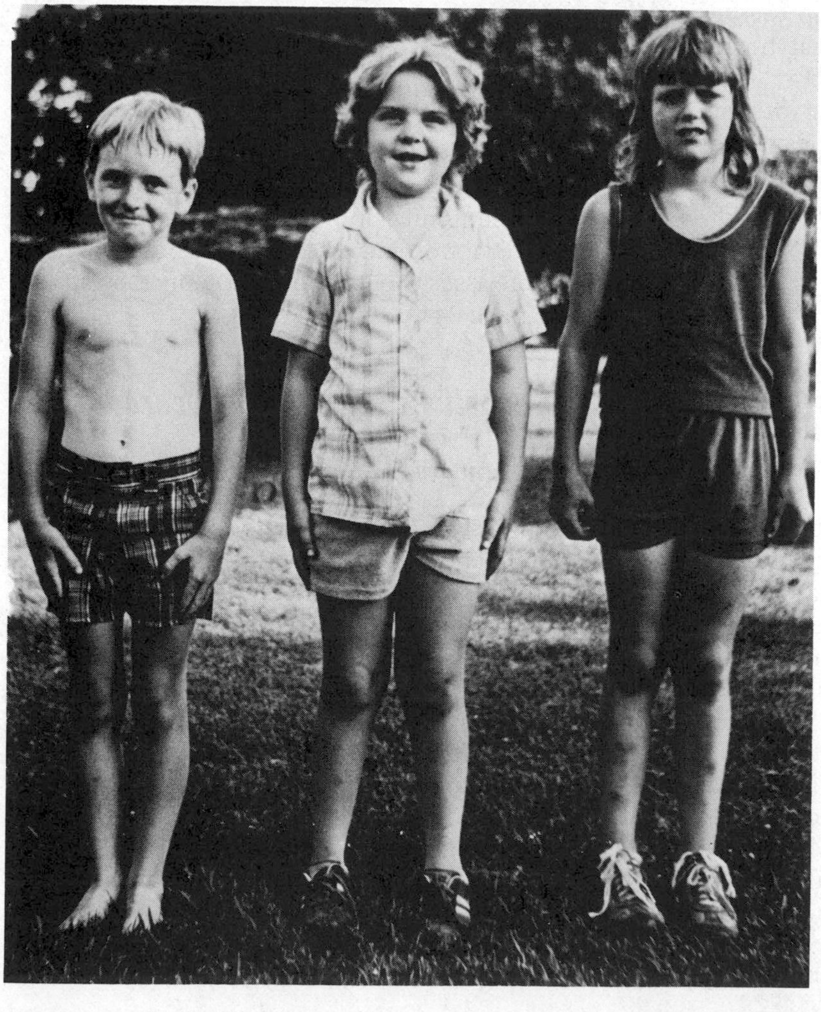

These three 9-year-olds exemplify the typical variations in size during the school years of children the same age.

Body Composition

Body composition, as measured by the percentage of body weight attributed to organ weight, muscle mass, body fat, and extracellular fluid, changes little during the school-age period. Body fat remains at approximately 15 per cent of total body weight in the school-age child. Muscle mass and extracellular fluid increase by 1 to 2 per cent at this age, while organ weight decreases by 1 to 2 per cent. Until the adolescent growth spurt, body composition for boys and girls is comparable.

The lymphatic tissues such as tonsils and adenoids grow rapidly during the school-age period, with growth reaching a peak toward the end of the period. Thereafter, involution of lymphatic tissue occurs.

Skeletal Growth

The rate of growth of the trunk and extremities continues to exceed that of the head during the school-age period. Although head circumference increases little, remodeling of facial bones occurs. The frontal sinuses, present in rudimentary form from birth, become visible by x-ray during the early school years, and the other sinuses enlarge. Because of facial bone remodeling, the eustachian tube gradually assumes a more downward, forward and inward direction than previously. This structural change is associated with a decrease in the frequency of ear infections as the child grows older.

By age 10 or 11 years, the distance from the crown of the head to the symphysis pubis is approximately equal to the distance from the symphysis to the sole of the foot, and remains so thereafter. Because of these variations in the rate of growth between the head, trunk, and extremities, the center of gravity of the body with erect posture moves from a point just below the umbilicus at age 5 to below the crest of the ilium by 13 years. Improved balance of the older school-age child is attributed to this lower center of gravity.

The overall bodily appearance of school-age children also changes—they tend to look thinner than preschool children and adolescents. As skeletal growth progresses, the "rounded" shoulders, slight lordosis, and prominent abdomen of the early school years gradually give way by the end of the period to a more erect posture.

Anticipatory Guidance: Body Composition and Skeletal Growth

Knowledge about body composition and skeletal growth can provide the nurse with a base for guiding parents and children in dealing with selected health problems that might occur during this age period. If enlarged tonsils and adenoids or susceptibility to ear infections are of concern, simple explanations about the growth patterns of lymphoid tissue and the direction in which the eustachian tube lies are helpful. Understanding that normal growth can alleviate selected health problems can be especially helpful to the child. The awareness that no relative increase in body fat is expected until the adolescent growth spurt can alert parent and child to a potential problem with obesity if the child starts to "fill out."

Adults (parents or teachers) may become unduly concerned about the posture of an early school-age child, when, in actuality, normal growth will alleviate the "rounded" shoulders, lordosis, and prominent abdomen of that age group. Posture should be considered satisfactory if a straight line can be visualized to pass from the front of the ear through the shoulder and the greater trochanter to the anterior part of the longi-

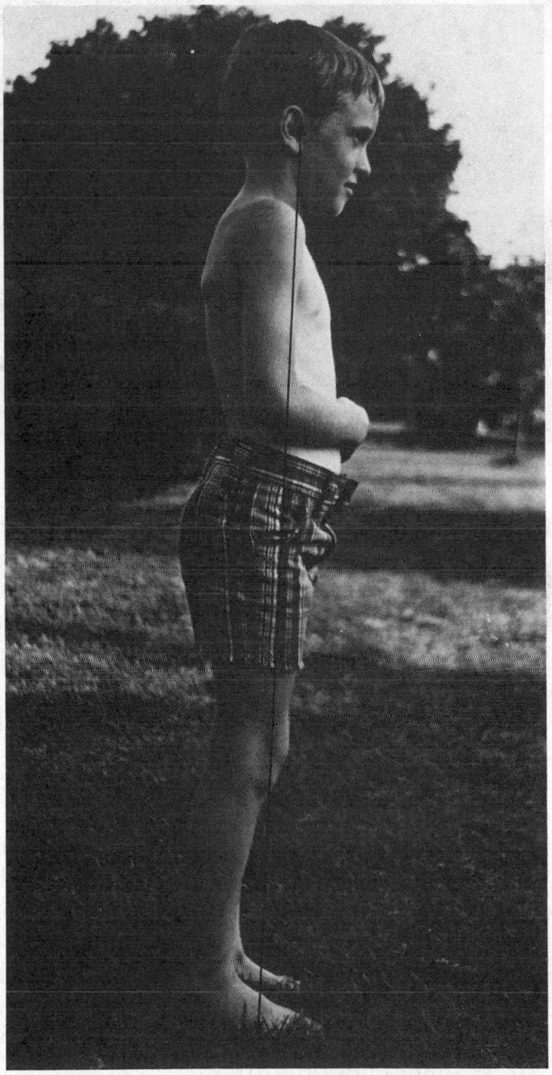

Figure 8-1. A straight line that passes from the front of the ear through the shoulder and the greater trochanter to the anterior part of the longitudinal arch of the foot indicates satisfactory posture during the school-age period. (Photograph by Jim Tackett.)

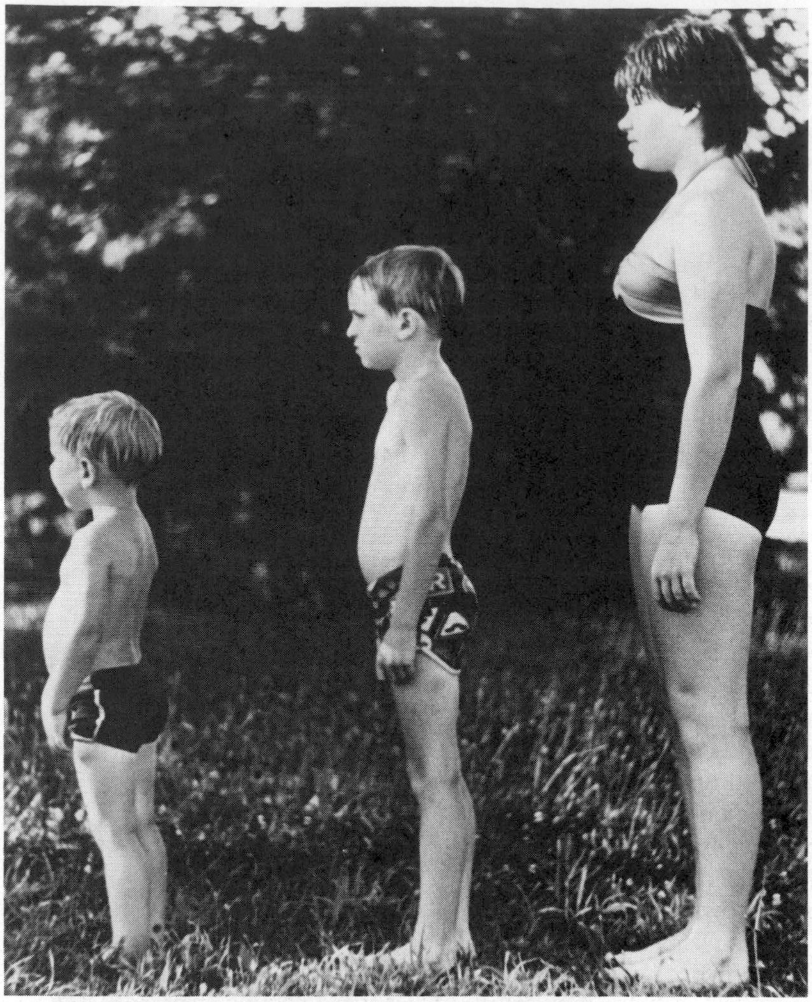

Note the changes in posture from preschool to school age and to adolescence.

tudinal arch of the foot (Fig. 8-1). Seeing that the child has regular physical activity and regular changes in position when sedentary is more effective in promoting good posture than exhortations to stand straight. A healthy, rested child typically assumes a balanced, comfortable posture.

Excessive exercise to develop a specific skill that places undue strain on a bone or joint should be avoided. Because the bones are still ossifying, they cannot tolerate pressure and muscle pull as well as mature bones can. In addition, growth of bone, muscle, tendon, and support tissues may not be synchronous, especially during the preadolescent growth spurt. For these reasons, children are more prone to injury from excessive exercise than adults. Caution also needs to be exercised in carrying heavy loads. Heavy loads, such as books or a pack of newspapers, should be shifted periodically.

Motor Development

The word that best describes the neuromuscular development of the school-age period is *refinement.* The basic mechanisms involved in neuromuscular skills already have been acquired; however, they are rudimentary. The school-age period is the time for refinement and expansion of those skills.

Gross Motor Skills

Physical activity seems to be a natural and strong impulse for the school-age child. The child seems driven to "be doing" something with his hands, feet, and body. During the early school years before refinement of motor control, physical activity seems somewhat aimless as can be observed in the restlessness of the first grader. By the time the child is ready to embark into adolescence, this physical activity is more controlled and directed toward specific goals such as those found in sports.

The six basic gross motor skills that are refined during this age period are running, jumping, sequencing foot movements, balancing, throwing, and catching. Steady improvement in all six basic motor skills is seen in school-age children, if they are given the opportunity to practice them.

Most children practice these skills during play and delight in the experience as well as in their accomplishments in skill development. The games of childhood, which seem to pass from generation to generation, provide experience in the basic gross motor skills. Examples include running in tag, hide-and-seek and red rover; jumping, sequencing foot movements and balancing in skipping, jump rope, hopscotch, bicycling, skating, skate boarding, scrimmaging, and tug of war, and throwing and catching in many games. In most games of school-age children coordination of the basic skills is required and complex movements evolve.

Even in physical activities other than play, school-age children seem intent on testing out what can be accomplished with their bodies. While engaged in a motor activity such as walking down the street, a puddle is to walk in, to see how big a splash or how small a ripple can be made. An ice-covered sidewalk is to see how far one can slide on two feet without falling. *School-age children explore the world with and through their bodies.*

Play of a child changes over time in keeping with the development of motor skills. The 6-year-old has boundless energy and rudimentary skills. Consequently, play is active, somewhat disorganized and requires rather simple skills such as running, jumping, throwing, and skipping. The 7-year-old seems more cautious, quiet, and intent on acquiring skills such as sequencing foot movements, balancing on a bicycle, throwing, and catching. The 8-year-old has greater smoothness in movements and becomes more involved in group activities than previously. The 9-year-old works intently on and takes great pride in demonstrating motor skills and strength. Competitive team sports are of interest, and disparity between the skills of individuals becomes more apparent than previously. During the tenth through twelfth year muscular control and skills in all gross motor areas are established. Just as the school-age period was ushered in on a child who experienced a great need for physical activity, it ends on the same note. The 11- to 12-year-old is energetic, although sporadically, and very active physically. Because of the preadolescent growth spurt this increased physical activity may appear more clumsy than a year or so earlier. (See Chapter 21 for further discussion of play and exercise.)

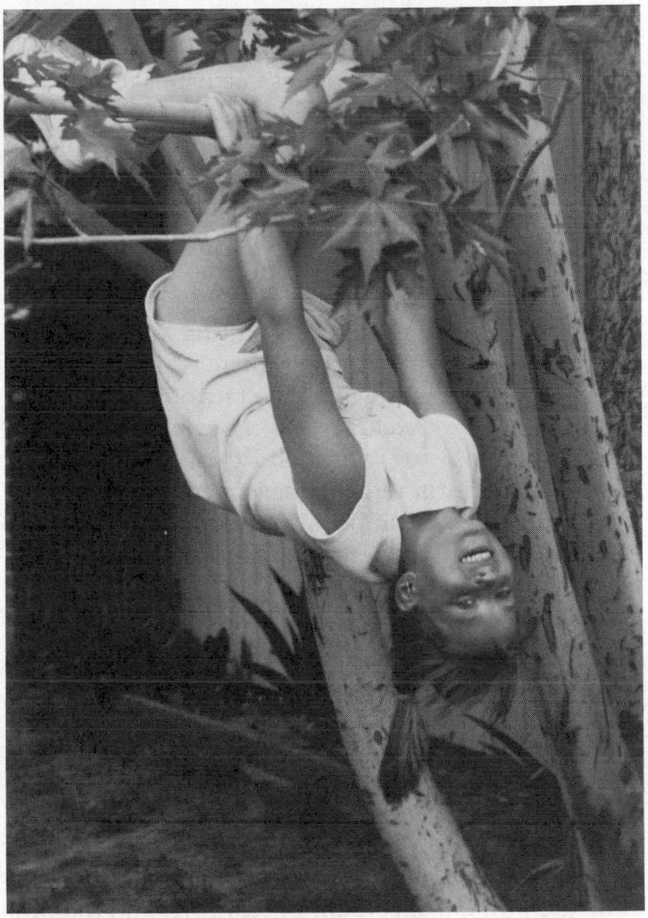

Gymnastic activities demonstrate the increased coordination of large muscle groups in school-age children. A tree becomes a jungle gym for this 11-year-old.

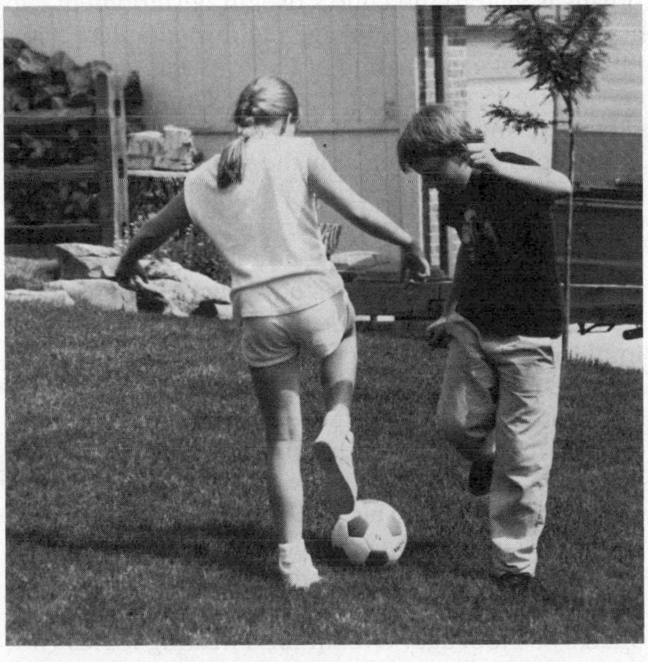

A game of soccer demonstrates the gross motor skills of running, sequencing foot movements, and balancing.

Fine Motor Skills

Although the fine motor skills lag behind gross motor skills, they progress approximately at the same rate. Six-year-olds can cut with scissors and can paste, can button and zipper their clothes, and can copy a triangle, draw a man with 12 details and use a pencil for printing. However, skill in these activities tends to be uneven in development, and they may be performed clumsily. The 7-year-old ties shoes, copies a diamond, and draws a man with 16 details. At 8 years old, cursive writing begins, and at 9 years eye-hand coordination is well developed, and the child can manipulate objects skillfully enough to benefit from hand crafts.

The reaction time or speed in performing fine motor skills, such as tapping, turning small objects, and removing and placing pegs increases rapidly from 6 to 9 or 10 years, after which the rate of improvement gradually slows. Accuracy of movement improves markedly from 5 to 9 years and then less rapidly to adolescence. Girls tend to have better dexterity of hands and fingers than boys and tend to perform fine motor skills at a greater speed and more accurately than boys (Smart and Smart, 1978).

Anticipatory Guidance: Gross and Fine Motor Skills

The healthy school-age child will pursue gross and fine motor activities if provided with the opportunity. Parents should be encouraged to provide these opportunities for a variety of reasons. The benefits of physical activity are numerous, including the promotion of bone growth, enhancement of learning, and the promotion of fitness and a physically active lifestyle.

Although the genes determine the basic growth and shape of long bones, environmental factors are influential also. The complex development of cartilage into mature adult bones entails growth in length and width, changes in bone density, and maintenance of shape and integrity. Although the exact mechanisms are not clear, intermittent energetic compression of the entire cartilage, aided by gravity, weight-bearing, and muscle contractions, is indispensable in keeping children's bones growing at the required rate (Bailey et al, 1978). Bone density also is influenced by physical activity, with inactivity resulting in deossification. Activity has even more influence on bone density than nutrition does. Only extreme deficiency of calcium and vitamin D will cause deossification, while it is often found on x-ray after only a few weeks of inactivity.

Periods of physical activity also enhance academic learning. Schools have long recognized this phenomenon and have provided recess periods for gross motor activity. Research also has demonstrated the positive influence of such motor activity on learning. One of the largest and most notable studies showed that in a school in which classroom time was decreased by one-third and that time was devoted to physical education, children performed better academically than their counterparts whose school maintained the regular schedule. Even though the time of instruction was decreased by a third, the children did as well or better on scholastic tests than their counterparts (Bailey, 1978).

Physical fitness is almost synonymous with physical activity. A physically fit child who finds pleasure in gross motor activity usually carries this fitness and pleasure into adulthood. Childhood provides a unique opportunity for promoting healthful exercise habits, because of the child's propensity for delighting in gross motor activity.

The opportunities parents provide for gross and fine motor activities need not be elaborate nor expensive. A great deal of gross physical activity can take place in a relatively small space. Walking or jogging can be a family affair. Advantage can be taken of community programs and parks.

For fine motor activities, paper, pencils, crayons, water colors, scissors, string, beads, empty food cartons, and so forth can be implements for creative activities. See Chapter 21 for further discussion.

The child should be encouraged to pursue physical activities. Limits may need to be set on television viewing if it interferes with more positive pursuits. Increased competency in skills should be rewarded by praise that is deserved but not exaggerated.

Sensory Organ Development

A major thrust of the school-age period is exploration of the world. Normal development of the senses, especially those of sight and hearing, are crucial to this exploration. Therefore, the competency of the sense organs is vital to the child's overall development. No assessment of the school-age child is complete without a careful examination of the eyes and ears.

Nearly 75 percent of ocular development is completed during the first three years of life. The final growth phase, affecting only the posterior segment of the eye, proceeds at a very slight and steady pace until approximately 15 years. The crystalline lens is the only component of the eye that continues to grow throughout life. Its growth, associated with alterations in its shape, pliability, and refractive index, has important implications for visual acuity.

The normal hyperopia of the young child gradually diminishes during the early school-age period owing to the growth of the posterior segment of the eye globe. If the eye axis grows to be longer than average, myopia results. This refractive error, which tends to manifest itself between 8 and 10 years of age, usually increases until ocular and body growth are completed.

The ear and the sense of hearing are well developed by school age. Overall mild hearing losses (not exceeding 25 decibels) usually do not produce communication problems for the school-age child. (Chapter 51 discusses hearing losses and visual losses in detail.)

Anticipatory Guidance: Sensory Organs

Parents need to be aware of the symptoms of visual problems and should be encouraged to follow through to have them corrected. If corrective lenses are prescribed, every effort should be made to help the child look upon them in positive terms and to wear them as directed.

Eyestrain should be avoided for the general well-being of the child. Causes of eyestrain include using poor lighting (either too little or glare) and poor posture while reading, reading too-small print, reading in a moving vehicle, doing close work, or watching television, films, or a computer screen for prolonged periods without rest or change of focus. The child should be taught how to rest the eyes by simply changing the gaze from near to distant vision (and vice versa) for a few minutes.

To prevent hearing problems, parents need to be aware that middle ear infections require prompt treatment and that consistent follow-up and hearing tests are indicated for recurrent otitis media. Immunizations also should be encouraged as primary prevention for complications of the communicable diseases that may cause nerve (perceptive) hearing losses. The parents and child should be informed that trying to remove wax from the ear canal with a hairpin or similar implement probably will only impact the wax more firmly against the tympanic membrane and may even damage the membrane.

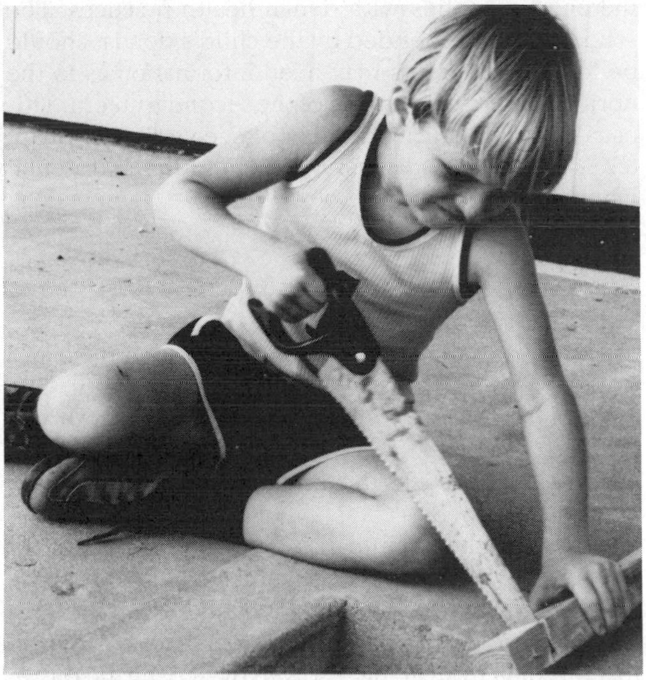

The 9-year-old has coordination of eye and hand that allows him to manipulate objects and benefit from a variety of projects and crafts.

Eye-Hand Coordination

The development of eye-hand coordination is related to development of gross and fine motor skills. By the age of 9 years, the child works well with both hands concurrently on large and small motor tasks but shows preference for either the right or left hand.

Lateral preference for using the left or right hand and foot is established during the late preschool or early school-age period. Preference is determined by asking the child to perform a task such as throwing a ball, writing, or kicking a ball. Eye dominance is typically established by 2 years of age. The child with a dominant right eye will tend to be right-handed (Behrman and Vaughan, 1987).

Ability to discriminate left from right on their own bodies is achieved after hand preference is established. Almost all children can make this discrimination on their own body by age 7. Discrimination of left and right on others follows self-discrimination. Children with visual-spatial perception problems often have delays in left-right discrimination (Behrman and Vaughan, 1987). The perceptual ability to imitate the movements of another person standing facing the child, however, presents a more difficult task, and the skill may not be acquired until adolescence.

Anticipatory Guidance: Eye-Hand Coordination

The child should be encouraged to participate in activities that promote eye-hand coordination. The lateralization for hand, foot, and eye preference is a natural process that gradually evolves over time. Parents and teachers should not pressure a child to use either right or left hand, foot, or eye. The physical activities that promote the development and refinement of gross and fine motor skills are the same activities that promote eye-hand coordination and lateralization.

Teeth

The major emphasis of dental health during school-age years is dental hygiene which helps to preserve the primary teeth until they are all lost and protects the secondary teeth as they erupt. Frequency of dental checkups will vary depending upon the general state of health of the child's mouth and teeth and how well the child complies with dental health practices. The schedule recommended by the child's dentist should be followed. Parents may need information as to the normal pattern of eruption of the secondary teeth. This usually occurs during the school-age years. See Chapter 19 for further discussion of dentition and dental maintenance.

Sleep and Rest

At the beginning of the school-age period the child usually averages 11 to 12 hours sleep per night. The amount of sleep per night gradually diminishes to an average of 9 to 10 hours per night at age 12. A healthy child ordinarily seeks the amount of sleep required to meet health needs.

If a preschool child has developed the habit of retiring for sleep at a late hour and sleeping late in the morning, difficulties can be anticipated with the start of regular school attendance. Parents can be advised that this difficulty can be resolved by making the retirement hour earlier and earlier over a period of several months before the start of school.

To promote sleep, a period of quiet activity just prior to bedtime is advised. An exciting or stimulating television program is not included in the category of quiet activity. Overstimulation, either physical, mental, or emotional, can have an adverse effect on the restful sleep that is the norm for the school-age child.

If children who usually sleep well experience sleep problems without apparent reason, they may be upset or worried about some aspect of school or home life. This cue should be followed up with the child and efforts made to alleviate the problem. See Chapter 20 for further discussion of sleep.

Elimination Skills

Most healthy school-age children experience no difficulties with elimination. Bowel and bladder control are usually well established. However, when a child is under undue stress temporary lapses are not unusual. For discussion of problems with bowel (encopresis) and bladder (enuresis) control, see Chapters 36 and 42.

Nutrition

As has been noted previously, the school-age years are characterized as a period of relatively slow and steady growth. The exception is the preadolescent growth spurt at about 10 to 12 years for girls and 12 to 14 years for boys.

Until the adolescent growth spurt, the nutritional needs of the child are relatively stable, with the need slightly increased for quantity (to accommodate the increases in height and weight) rather than quality.

Proportionately, however, in calculating the daily needs for calories, protein, and water per kilogram of body weight, a slight and steady decrease in requirements is seen. See Chapter 18 for a discussion of nutrient and caloric needs specific to age.

Just as the school-age period is noted for being probably the healthiest of any age period, it also is one with relatively few nutritional problems. The results of the biochemical tests included in the federally sponsored nutrition survey in 1971–72 indicated that fewer school-age children had nutritional deficiencies than those in age groups that precede or succeed this age. The survey would seem to indicate that as a population group the school-age child seems relatively well nourished, with the possible exception of iron and total calories.

Information about eating habits as well as kind and amount of food eaten is essential to the total evaluation of nutritional status. Snacks are common for school-age children and often consist of empty-calorie foods that can interfere with proper nutrition.

Various forms of interviews are used to assess nutritional status (see Chapters 15 and 18). From the interviews, an assessment can be made of a child's diet. The results should be compared to the recommended food intake and average size of servings for a child of that age (see Chapter 18 for recommendations). This comparison should disclose possible deficiencies that should be included in anticipatory guidance.

The concern of the federal government for the nutritional status of its youth has long been evident. The first legislation of significance to the school-age group was the National School Lunch Act of 1946, which supported and promoted nutritious school lunches at reasonable cost or free to those who cannot afford it. In 1966 a similar program to support and promote school breakfasts was initiated. By 1975, 80 per cent of the public and nonprofit private schools in the nation participated in the school lunch program.

Anticipatory Guidance: Nutrition

As a child enters school and moves from the confines of the home and its immediate environment, other influences become increasingly important to the child's health practices. These influences can be both positive and negative. Ideally, the teacher, the school nurse, and perhaps peers will have a positive influence on health practices, including eating habits.

Health education is an important and integral part of a school curriculum. The American Academy of Pediatrics has repeatedly reaffirmed its support for health education in the schools. Although school nurses can contribute directly to the health education program by teaching selected content, a more effective role is to serve as a consultant and resource person for teachers. Health education, to be truly effective, must be a consistent and integral part of daily classroom instruction—something no school nurse could possibly accomplish or schedule alone.

Education in nutrition and in dental health overlaps and therefore instruction is combined for these. An example is the fact that nutritious snacks also promote dental health. Suggestions about anticipatory guidance for dental health discussed previously apply equally to nutrition education.

In health education about nutrition, cultural factors play a greater role than in most other topics of health education. Children need to learn that a great variety of foods, taken in proper quantities, will meet their daily requirements in nutrition. Respect for their own cultural heritage and for that of others can be an indirect benefit of well-planned nutrition education.

Because school-age children do not have control over meal preparation at home, nutrition education should extend into the community to include the parents. School-age children do have control, however, over intake at meals and need to have sufficient knowledge to select appropriate types and quantities of available foods. Breakfasts and snacks need special emphasis, because they are often deficient in quantity or quality.

Obesity may be a problem in the school-age population as well as other populations. As school-age children become absorbed in school or play activities, meals may be forgotten or ignored. When children become hungry, they are often likely to fill up with nutritionally poor, calorie-laden junk foods. These foods are made desirable in the television commercials to which the child is exposed daily. The pace of life in our society has resulted in a generation of individuals who do not eat at home. Much of this eating is done in fast-food restaurants where calorie levels and fat content are quite high. In addition to eating excessively, obese children often do not exercise as much as children of average weight. A vicious cycle may ensue; the more obese the child, the more difficult it is to keep up with the other children in physical activity, and eating becomes a consolation.

The nurse should be alert to the defining characteristics of this nursing diagnosis for several reasons. For children, obesity is both an emotional social risk factor and a physiologic problem. In one study, obese children reported lower self-concept, were more depressed, and were rejected more and liked less by their nonobese peers (Strauss, Smith, Frame, and Frehand, 1985). These findings suggest that the obese school-age child may also be at risk for the development of other diagnoses such as *disturbance in self concept: self-esteem and/or body image* and *social isolation.* See Chapter 36 for a detailed discussion of obesity.

Intellectual and Language Development

Although physical development during the school-age period is characterized as slow and steady, cognitive development is characterized as rapid and expanding. It is as though physical development in general is held somewhat in abeyance so that all the child's energies can be directed toward cognitive development. That is not to say that physical development ceases; it continues unabated and contributes much to cognitive development. Neurologic development, including refinement of the corpus callosum of the brain at age 7 or 8, promotes the expansion of cognitive competency.

Intelligence

Intelligence is generally considered to be the ability to learn or acquire and retain knowledge. Included in this definition is the ability to learn from experience and to apply previously learned knowledge to a new situation. Intelligence is assessed by various tests. The Stanford-Binet test is widely used and is established as one of the most reliable intelligence tests. The Wechsler Intelligence Scale for Children is used widely also.

Results of intelligence tests must be interpreted with caution, especially the results of group testing—the usual testing method. These tests are encumbered by the problem common to any paper or pencil test—their results depend on the motivation to do well on the test and the well-being of the child at the time the test is given. Reading skill, practice on specific skills involved in the test, as well as luck in guessing correct answers, affect results; the tests may not be truly reflective of mental ability.

Since the late 1960s, intelligence tests have been the subject of controversy, primarily because of misuse of test results to "label" and track children educationally. Blacks, Hispanics and other children not exposed to white mainstream middle class experiences are at a disadvantage in taking the tests. Much effort has been devoted to development of tests that are valid and reliable across the ranges of culture and experience.

Anticipatory Guidance: Intelligence

Intelligence tests should be considered only as *screening tools* to be used to help the child reach full potential. IQ can and does change. If used appropriately, the tests can help the parent and the child recognize the child's strengths and weaknesses and set realistic goals and expectations.

The sense of competency in one's own ability is important to school-age children. Whatever the mental ability, children need to be appreciated for what they can do competently. Comparison of the child's own accomplishments and competency over time helps him or her to see individual progress and to acquire self-esteem.

Parents can promote intellectual competency by stimulating the child's desire for achievement and by offering a variety of experiences that foster mental development. The values the family holds about intellectual pursuits profoundly affect a child's achievement orientation, as well as the experiences to which he is exposed. Certainly a child who is exposed to books and magazines in the home and sees parents reading with interest will have an orientation to achievement and intellectual pursuits different from that of a child who is exposed to neither situation.

Cognitive Development

During the school-age period, the child's thought processes undergo dramatic shifts. According to Piaget (1966), at the beginning of the school-age period these thought processes are characterized as intuitive thought; they move into concrete operations at about 7 or 8 years of age and from there into formal operations at about 11 or 12 years.

The Intuitive Stage

With intuitive thought (6 to 7 years), thinking is based on immediate, unanalyzed relations between any particular environmental phenomenon and the child's own viewpoint. For example, to this child anything that moves is alive (animism). Conversations tend to be monologues because children think others think as they do (egocentrism) and can even read their minds.

Children may recognize two or more characteristics of something in the environment but focus their attention or thought on only one characteristic at a time (centration). They cannot consider wholes and parts at the same time; attention is focused either on the whole or on a part but not on both simultaneously.

These characteristics of intuitive thought lead the child to make gross misinterpretations of phenomena. They do not provide the cognitive tools for organizing the world of people, places, and things into systems. Those cognitive tools are provided through "operations"—first, concrete operations for dealing with people, places, and things that can be experienced through the senses and then formal operations for dealing with abstracts and for playing with ideas.

The Concrete Operations Stage

During the stage of *concrete operations* (approximately 7 to 11 years), children step outside their own thought processes and realize that their way of thinking is not the only way. Real conversation and sharing of information become possible. Gradually, the egocentric and fluctuating rules for games and behavior give way to democratically derived rules for games and reasonable expectations for behavior.

The children can now decenter or take into consideration more than one characteristic or attribute of an object or environmental phenomenon at the same time. They can consider the various parts of a whole while maintaining the concept of the whole. Other important characteristics of the thought processes are retracing the steps taken mentally to arrive at a conclusion. Children also realize that there may be more than one way of arriving at the same conclusion.

When children enter the stage of concrete operations, all characteristics of the stage are not necessarily available in all situations. For example, children discover the conservation of substance at 7 or 8 years by realizing that changes in shape do not change the quantity of such substances as clay. However, they do not discover the conservation of weight until they are about 9 or 10 years old and do not discover the conservation of volume until about 11 or 12 (measured by displacement of water whan an object is immersed). Conservation abilities during the concrete operational stage are detailed in Table 3-2 on page 106.

Concrete operations not only have a powerful influence on the acquisition of knowledge for school-age children but also profoundly affect the emotional and social life. Illustrative of the changes seen in the emotional and social life of children during this coordination of concrete operations are their concepts about causality and chance, moral feelings and judgments, use of rules for games, and perceptions of reality. Much of what is known about the concepts is derived from the work of Piaget and Kohlberg.

Prior to age 8 or 9 years, the concept of chance is lacking. Everything has a reason—often based on immediate, unanalyzed relations between environmental events. For example, falling down and skinning a knee may be attributed to disobeying Mother an hour or so earlier. Not only does everything have a reason, but because of the young child's egocentric thought patterns, the reason often centers on self. For example, the child may think a parent has become ill because the child angrily wished it so. With the realization at age 8 or 9 years of the concept of chance, life becomes much more benevolent than previously.

In a similar manner, the changes in moral feelings and judgment make life more benevolent during the period of concrete operations than during the intuitive stage. For the 6- or 7-year-old, the many rules of behavior are immutable. Rules are based on what adults direct and are taken literally. Children are likely to judge an act in a unidirectional way as absolutely right or absolutely wrong. They are likely to consider that an act is bad if it elicits punishment, and tend to be very harsh in the punishment they would prescribe for another child who has broken a rule.

As concrete operations become available to the child, the absolutes become tempered by the realization that the same act may be viewed in many different ways by different individuals. The intentions that prompted an act now are taken into consideration. Through interaction and cooperative endeavors with peers, the child develops respect for them and for self and realizes that rules evolve through mutual consent and the democratic process of consensus. Rules are no longer absolute and immutable but can be changed by either mutual consent or extenuating circumstances. Punishment the child would recommend now becomes less harsh, more specific for the infraction, and is no longer considered absolutely necessary. Moral judgments are increasingly more independent of adults as the solidarity between peer groups of children grows and a morality based on cooperation develops. The importance of peers in the development of moral reasoning was demonstrated in the research findings of Kruger and Tomasello (1986). They found that moral discussions between school-age peers were characterized by more spontaneous use of reasoning than were similar discussions between school-age children and adults.

Rules used for playing games also undergo the same type of change as do moral feelings. As children move away from egocentric thinking and appreciate the viewpoints of others, they become increasingly capable of cooperative play and team play involving rules. This play is in contrast to that of early school-age children, who like to play games with rules but exhibit only a partial understanding of them and think another child with whom they are playing understands the rules in the same way they do. In actuality, the age-mate may have a completely different understanding of the rules. Young children play the game as they understand it, without real concern for what others are doing. In the game nobody loses and everybody wins because the purpose of the game is to have fun in a group activity.

After age 7 or 8 years, games are characterized by increasing structure, with common observance of rules and mutual surveillance to make sure all players observe the rules. The spirit of the game is honest competition, with some players winning and others losing according to the rules. True communication, cooperative play, and mutual respect are now possible. After age 10 or 11 years, handicaps are even added to games when appropriate, for to win over a less-skilled opponent is not to win at all.

From ages 8 or 9, the behavior of children also evidences an increased perceptive ability, with attendant self-criticism of activities such as drawing. Drawings consequently seem less creative and imaginative as the child tries to replicate reality. In everyday life, the age of 9 years is known as the age of erasures, in which children demonstrate increased dissatisfaction with their efforts if the drawing does not appear realistic.

During the stage of concrete operations (8 to 10 years), children work hard to discover how the world of people, places, and things—which they can experience through their senses—functions. The concrete operational child is not yet able to work with abstractions, hypotheses, and propositions removed from the concrete and present observation—that is, to play with ideas. That ability will begin to develop at age 11 or 12 years as the child moves into adolescence and the stage of formal operations. (Additional discussion of concrete operations is included in Chapter 3.)

Anticipatory Guidance: Cognitive Development

Piaget's theory of cognitive development is particularly useful for understanding behaviors and perceptions of school-age children. Much of the research which provides empirical validation for Piaget's theory focuses on aspects of cognitive development during concrete operations, particularly conservation. For example, Piaget said that in order for children to have fully developed concrete operations, they must be certain that conservation is "true." Miller's (1986) research validated that concept. Halford and Boyle (1985) found that 3- to 4-year-old children do not understand conservation of number while 6- to 7-year-old children do.

The nurse who has a thorough knowledge of Piaget's theory will be better able to recognize the defining characteristics of *potential or actual altered growth and development.* If either of these nursing diagnoses is made, interventions will often involve guidance for the parents.

During the intuitive stage parents and teachers may utilize a variety of "think games" to nurture the development of concrete operations. (For example, several cups of different colors and progressive sizes may be used to help learn ranking and arrangement of objects by common characteristics; a variety of objects or pictures may be used to help learn to compare, contrast, and classify items that are alike and different in some way.) Similarly, games can be used with older children to help them master temporal and numerical concepts.

Parents should be encouraged to have patience and allow school-age children to do some of their own problem-solving. Parents may need to be reminded that trial and error is a valuable part of learning problem-solving. Parents should not expect the school-age child to handle more than one big problem at a time, and they should be cautioned to expect some fluctuation in the school-ager's skill at problem mastery.

Play continues to be a necessary main activity if the school-age child is to progress cognitively. Through play, group games and peer interaction the child learns the cognitive concepts necessary to cooperation, compromise, persuasion, and productivity. Parents may need help from the nurse to understand this valuable function.

Language Development

As might be expected from the profound changes in cognitive development, language development progresses rapidly during the school-age period.

An assessment of the progress in language development includes examination of the three interactive components of language itself: *phonics,* or speech sound, *syntax,* or grammar, and *semantics,* or meaning in language forms such as words and sentences. The assessment is not complete, however, without looking at the personal and social uses of language for the child.

Speech usually is fluent and the voice well-modulated in the 6-year-old. Also, *articulation,* or phonically correct speech, is usually good, with the possible exceptions of thr, shr, sk, sh, ch, s, j, and z sounds. By 7 or 8 years, however, these sounds should be pronounced correctly (Smart and Smart, 1978). Articulation difficulties may result from physical problems such as cleft palate, hearing losses, or true cultural factors. Apparent speech defects may be a consequence of the child imitating the speech patterns of the home or neighborhood environment.

Syntax, or grammar, is usually correct by 6 years of age and the child can form five- or six-word sentences. Semantically, the 6-year-old has a vocabulary of 2,500 to 3,000 words, can carry out commands involving three to four actions, and comprehends "if," "because," and "why" (Lowrey, 1978).

Research indicates that a basic qualitative change in both syntactic and semantic development takes place at around 7 years of age when concrete operations begin to be established (Lowrey, 1978). Complex and compound sentences are used increasingly after that age. Nuances of word meaning, whether standing alone or included in a sentence, are comprehended increasingly. In addition to increasing the vocabulary, the child learns new meaning and more subtle connotations for old words. Whereas younger school-age children typically define words by offering descriptions of the thing signified or examples of its functions, the older school-age child tends to employ explanations or synonyms. At the end of the school-age period, word meanings increasingly approximate those of adults.

Illustrative of the expansion in mental processes involved in language are the typical questions the child asks during the school-age period. As children advance in age, their questions become less global (Why?) and more specific (What? Who? Where? Which?), and, finally, more definitive (How?).

The language of school-age children has a distinctive quality, with unique personal and social functions. This language is a part of the culture of childhood—a culture that is learned, shared, and transmitted among children but which is shaped by the adult world around them (Goodman, 1970). Children teach other children the rhymes, chants, and rituals of childhood. Language enables school-age children to meet their abiding need to master and control their expanding world and to acquire a social identity with peers.

The function of chants, rituals, and superstition to the culture of school-age children is an example of how the many aspects of development are inextricably interrelated. While they are expressed in language and thus are important in language development, chants, rituals, and superstitions are also important aspects of emotional-social development. The countless chants and magic-making words of school-age children provide a sense of control in a sometimes frightening and bewildering world. Chants accompany many ancient games such as London bridge, ring-around-a-rosy, jump rope, and ball bouncing. Some are saved for special occasions: "Ladybug, ladybug, fly away home," "It's raining, it's pouring, the old man is snoring." Some have special powers to grant wishes or protect from unseen harm: "Star light, star bright, first star I see tonight," "Cross my heart and hope to die," "Knock on wood." Some may be verbalized or just acted out. "Hold your breath crossing a bridge." "Lift your feet crossing a railroad track." "Cross your fingers." These words tend to have a magical quality for school-age children, as well as being fun to say.

Humor is also expressed through language. Verbal humor can function just for the sheer joy of demonstrating mastery over language. This delight in language mastery is seen in "knock knock" jokes, puns, tongue-twisters, and riddles. The verbal humor of early school-age children is often expressed in riddles. Riddles can provide children with a sense of authority or power. So much of what adults say is incomprehensible or difficult to understand; a riddle can create a situation in which children are the authority with the answer. Likewise, jokes, which become more common around ages 8 or 9, often tend to disparage adults and, thus, release tensions the child may experience about his inadequacy in knowledge and power in relation to adults. Jokes can serve as a way of releasing anger, aggression, or frustration in a socially acceptable manner—for example hostility toward a sibling:

Boy, is my little sister spoiled.
She is not!
Oh yeah, you should see what the steamroller did to her!

"Cruelty" jokes are another form of verbal release of feelings:

Momma, Momma, why do I keep going in circles?
Shut up or I'll nail your other foot to the floor.

Jokes can also serve to express the very real and natural curiosity of the school-age child about sex:

Wanna hear a dirty joke?
Yes.
A boy fell in the mud. Wanna hear another one?
Yes.
A girl fell in the mud. Wanna hear another one?
Yes.
Three people came out of the mud.

Jokes can also serve as a way of releasing tension related to fears and doubts of the school-ager. These kinds of fears and doubts are seen in jokes about death, such as the "dead baby" jokes, and in little moron jokes that can express doubts about the child's competence.

Social identity with peers is promoted also through the use of chants, rituals, and humor. But social solidarity with peers to the exclusion of adults and other groups of children is attained primarily through the secret language so prevalent with peer groups after the ages of 8 or 9 years. Secret language provides the child with a sense of belonging to a particular group and a sense of power that comes with knowing something adults and other peer groups do not know. If the code of the language is broken by adults or others, the secret language is merely changed to provide another exclusive language. Nicknames are another manifestation of group solidarity. To be given a nickname by the "in" group means one really belongs. Even to be given an offensive nickname means recognition.

Language during the school-age period is the vehicle for expanding knowledge as well as personal and social growth of children.

Anticipatory Guidance: Language Development

As with other aspects of development, children need to be provided with opportunities to exercise and expand their language skills. Exposure to pronunciation and usage of society's mainstream language and to reading should be provided.

Currently, some controversy exists about encouraging use in the classroom of minority ethnic languages such as "Black English," which supposedly helps the minority child develop a positive identity. The arguments for and against such a policy are too numerous to recount here. Awareness of the controversy, however, is pertinent to the anticipatory guidance given to parents and children. The ultimate decision about language usage in the home is theirs.

Parents can facilitate language development in the expression of feelings and thoughts by encouraging discussion of their child's ideas, plans, and reactions regularly. Likewise, parents can be urged to express their own feelings, observations, and ideas to their children so that they learn the appropriate words to describe feelings and thoughts. Such discussion opportunities not only help develop vocabulary and learn correct grammar (provided proper grammar is used by the parents), but such activity helps keep communication lines open as the child approaches adolescence.

Anticipatory guidance about the personal and social uses of childhood language helps parents conjure up at least hazy memories of the chants, rituals, and secret languages they used as children, facilitating their acceptance of these language forms as a part of growing up.

Emotional and Social Development

The major thrust of emotional and social development in the school-age period is the introduction of the child into society, primarily the society of peers, and the child's evolvement as a competent doer and member of that society. This emotional and social development is related to and runs parallel with physical and intellectual development and language development. Separating them is somewhat artificial but provides for a more coherent picture of development than considering all three facets together. Included in the discussion of emotional and social development are temperament, emotions, culture, and the developing person.

Temperament

Because of their awareness of the individual differences between children that could not be accounted for by developmental theories, health professionals who deal with children have welcomed the work of Thomas and Chess (1977) on temperamental styles. Although innate characteristics of temperament seem to be relatively stable, their expressions may vary over time, being influenced by environmental and intrinsic developmental factors. Therefore, an understanding of the nine major categories of temperament provides a means of seeing how the individual child approaches learning tasks and interacts with peers and adults. The factors involved in temperament are activity level, approachability, adaptability, intensity of reaction, threshold for stimulus, mood, distractibility, attention span, and persistence.

A child's innate *activity level* is not likely to present problems in the adjustment to school if it is of an average or low level. However, a high activity level may make it difficult for the child to settle down to sedentary activities in the classroom. Opportunities for regular motor activity are important, especially for the child with a high activity level, as is patience on the part of the teacher and parent.

The child who has a personality characterized by high *approachability* responds well to new situations, people, places, and learning demands and usually is a joy for a teacher. On the other hand, the child who initially withdraws from new situations and is "slow to warm" may be misjudged by teachers and adults as being slow mentally or noncooperative. This child needs extra time or repeated exposures to new materials to function optimally and to maintain a sense of dignity and self-worth.

The quality of high *adaptability* helps to counteract the effects of high withdrawal in new situations. With extra time or repeated exposures, the child with high withdrawal and high adaptability will function well in new learning situations. However, if the child has high withdrawal and low adaptability, new learning situations will create great difficulty for both the child and the teacher. Much patience and individualized attention is needed to prevent failure in academic achievement for this type of child. Early successes in overcoming difficulties with new learning situations will help to motivate the child to persist despite high withdrawal and low adaptability in subsequent new situations.

With many children, one can judge their interest, moods, likes, and dislikes with great accuracy merely by observing their reactions to situations or people. These are children with moderate to high *intensity of reaction*. However, for those with a mild intensity of reaction, simple observations of their responses will not give an accurate evaluation. For these children, the teacher or other adult must be alert for more subtle cues to accurately assess their reactions and to respond to them appropriately.

Children vary greatly in their ability to discern visual, auditory, or tactile stimuli. The hypersensitive child with a low *threshold for stimuli* may be distracted easily in a classroom situation, while the child with a high threshold may be oblivious to the small stimuli. The child with a low threshold is likely to pick up small nuances in voice and behavior that go unnoticed by the child with a high threshold. Consequently, the child with a high threshold may need more detailed instructions to carry out a task than the child with a low threshold.

The quality of *mood* also varies among children. The good-natured child with a typically positive mood is likely to be treated more positively than the ill-natured child with a negative mood. Responses to both types of children are likely to reinforce their prevailing quality of mood. The child with negative mood may feel "picked on" and find confirmation for the feeling that a negative response is appropriate for the predominantly negative world in which he or she lives.

A child who is highly *distractible* may be aware of extraneous visual and auditory stimuli in the environment, while the child with low distractibility will be able to concentrate on the task at hand with only peripheral awareness of the extraneous stimuli. The latter child usually has the advantage in the classroom situation. However, in the social situation the child who is highly distractible often has capacities for social sensitivity, empathy, and constructive behavior that are lost to the child with low distractibility.

Attention span and *persistence* are the last two of the nine temperament characteristics. In the classroom situation long attention span and marked persistence are assets, while short attention span and low persistence are usually liabilities. However, unusually long attention span and marked persistence can lead to stubborn insistence on completing a task even if another activity is called for.

These temperamental qualities tend to occur in clusters, to form what Thomas and Chess (1968) call "easy," "slow-to-warm," and "difficult" children, each having special vulnerabilities that can be offset. The concept that temperament is a factor that can significantly influence school success has been validated in research by Schor (1985).

Anticipatory Guidance: Temperament

Awareness of the temperamental styles of a given child helps the teacher, parent, and nurse to adapt their responses to best meet the child's needs. What works with one child will not work with another of a different temperament. A "canned" preoperative teaching program may be ideal for one child but may alienate another who has a different temperament style.

The reactions of children to illness, injury, and hospitalization will vary according to temperament characteristics. The nurse must assess the temperament characteristics of the child if nursing care is to be optimal.

Easy children tend to be a joy to all and usually

adapt well to the demands for socialization and school life and in health care situations. The key to optimal response for slow-to-warm children is that they be given time to adapt at their own pace. Patience is required in working with these children. If pressured, their reactions tend to be exaggerated. Difficult children are most vulnerable to the demands of socialization, that is, the demands for altering spontaneous responses and patterns to conform to the social rules of living with family, schoolmates, and peers. However, once these children do learn the rules, they function easily, consistently, and energetically. The greatest risk period for them is the long adaptation period, and much patience and encouragement is called for in helping them adapt. The transition from home to school is a crucial period in their school life. See Chapter 3 for further discussion of temperament and management of temperament types.

Emotions

Emotions contribute to total personality patterns and enrich life if properly used. By age 6, the major emotions of anger and aggression, fear and worry, jealousy, and love and affection are fairly well established. During the school-age period, emotional expression becomes more organized and controlled. The major movement is from primarily ***physical*** expression to *verbal* expression of emotion (Williams and Stith, 1974). The intensity of emotional expression, of course, depends on the temperamental characteristics of the child.

The major task for the maturing child is to control and express emotions in a manner acceptable to the society in which the child lives. An acceptable expression, however, varies with the subcultural groups within that society. Some subcultural groups are more demonstrative in emotional expression than others. What may be acceptable at home may not be acceptable at school or with a peer group. Consequently, the child must learn not only to control the expression of emotion but also to learn acceptable ways for expression in different environments. Usually, if the home is a safe haven in which the child can count on abiding love, emotions can be expressed more openly there than in other environments.

Recent research has shown that children's knowledge of how and when to control emotional displays improves between the first and fifth grades and then levels off (Gnepp and Hess, 1986). That research demonstrated that children can understand and regulate spoken expressions of emotion better than their facial expressions. This may be because adults hold children more responsible for words than for nonverbal communications.

A major mental health goal in the school-age period is for children to accept their emotions and to learn to express them in socially acceptable ways. Anticipatory guidance for the parents and children is directed toward this goal. The discussion of the major emotions that follows includes essential considerations to include in anticipatory guidance.

Anger is a common emotion of childhood. The usual cause for anger is that children find themselves in situations in which they are not able to do what they want. The situation may be one in which the child is restrained or inhibited by adults or peers who enforce limits on behavior, by circumstances such as stormy weather, by objects such as a defective tool, or by the child's own lack of skill. Any of these situations may precipitate an outburst of anger. Physical states such as hunger or fatigue may cause an otherwise benign situation to be anger provoking. Also, if expressions of anger are rewarded by giving the child his or her own way, or if parents are overly concerned about expressions of anger, the child may use it inordinately (Williams and Stith, 1974).

Two periods during childhood are especially anger provoking for school-age children. One of these periods is during the transition from home to school, when skills are rudimentary and when many new situations are experienced that thwart the child's desires. The other period is at about 8 or 9, when children tend to tease and criticize each other excessively. During both these periods, parents need to be patient and understanding and help the child work out his or her concerns.

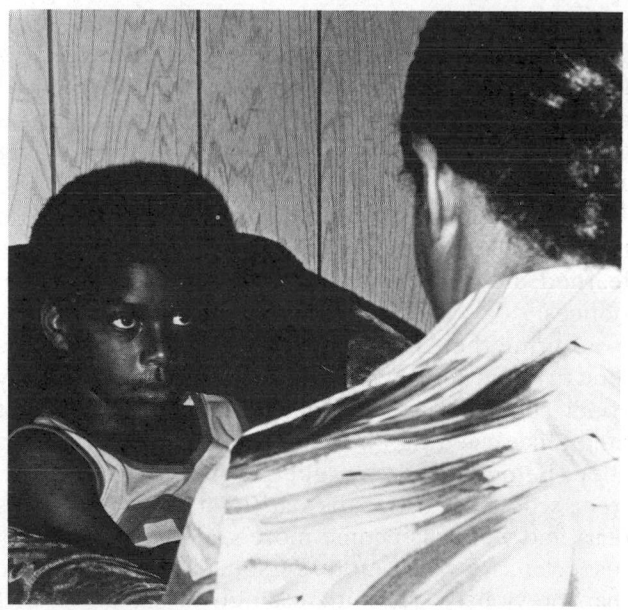

The school-age child needs help learning to verbalize anger and examine the circumstances that triggered the anger so he can learn to use the anger constructively.

As children become better able to control motor skills, to use words more glibly, and to understand rules for behavior, life becomes more reasonable and children are able to bring anger under control. Verbal rather than physical expressions of anger increase with age. The self-centered anger of the school-age years gives way increasingly to anger triggered by injustices to others or social conditions. However, such anger is more typical of the adolescent than of the school-age child. Such anger can be and is used constructively as the energizing force for social action.

As verbal expressions of anger become more available to the child, so do more covert or devious methods of expression, such as sassing, sulkiness, sneering, belittling, plotting, arguing, or scapegoating.

Probably the best way to help children learn to use anger as a constructive force is to help them verbalize the anger, to examine honestly the circumstances that triggered the anger, and to figure out how those circumstances can be changed, or what can be done about them. Providing models of acceptable expressions of anger is also important. As with adults, physical activity can take the edge off the anger. Also, role playing, either through puppetry or doll play, can help a child work through angry and aggressive feelings.

Aggressive behavior usually is a result of anger but is different from simple expressions of anger. It often involves intentional injury to an animal or human or destruction of an inanimate object. Behavior such as hitting another person is fairly common in the young school-age child. However, from age 10 years on, when aggressive tendencies are better controlled, it occurs rarely. In the younger school-age group, boys are involved in interpersonal conflicts more than girls; boys tend to use threats and physical force more than girls when in these conflicts (Miller, Danaher, & Forbes, 1986). Aggression tends to be better tolerated by society in boys than it is in girls. The same methods for helping a child control anger apply to controlling aggression.

As the world of school-age children expands, so do their worries and fears. Although fears and worries are learned, they are not necessarily related to actual experiences.

During the early school years, *fears and worries* tend to be related to family and school. Children worry about such things as parental illness or death, not being liked, getting into trouble and getting hurt, and about being harmed by supernatural beings or monsters, wild animals, or the dark. With age, children's fears and worries become more generalized in many respects, as well as more personalized and realistic than previously. They increasingly worry about self and possible failures and about scoldings or embarrassment related to specific situations. Mass media opens the door to more generalized fears such as those involving cancer, air pollution, cigarette smoke, and war. Fear of such supernatural beings as monsters is abandoned around age 10. Consequently, horror stories and films may be fun or therapeutic for the child 10 or older, while they are very frightening for the younger child.

Less overt, but demonstrable, signs of anxiety in the school-age children are nail-biting and hair-pulling or twisting. These behaviors are often seen in the school-ager who is less vocal or who has a more sensitive self-concept. Parents concerned with this behavior should be urged to encourage their child to verbalize fearful or anxious feelings and to role model such expressions of feelings themselves. Hounding the child to stop the behavior serves only to increase anxiety and, most likely, to increase the frequency of the behavior. Socially acceptable alternative behaviors such as doodling or pounding a punching bag may be suggested until the child develops the ability to verbalize feelings of anxiety.

Fear or worry can be of value if not excessive. It warns children of danger and can motivate learning or healthful behavior. Excessive fear, however, can narrow a child's field of experience and damage self-concept. *A positive self-concept is a powerful deterrent to excessive fears and worries.* Frank discussion of fears and worries, successful experiences in overcoming specific fears, and role models who display mastery over fears can help children to master their own fears and worries.

Episodes of *jealousy* are virtually unavoidable in childhood. An older sibling is often jealous of a younger one because of special privileges and the attention of parents, while the younger sibling is jealous of the older for similar reasons. The perspectives are different, but the supposed reasons are the same. Jealousy stems from insecurity in a relationship and is often accompanied by feelings of anger or inferiority. Its frequency of occurrence decreases with age. As the child matures in cognitive development and moral judgments and his concepts of rules become more mature, he is better able to ward off feelings of jealousy. A positive self-concept and time spent by parents with each child also deter feelings of jealousy.

The need for *love and affection* seems to be an innate, basic human need. The fulfillment of this need is essential for normal development. Just as a child needs to be loved, he needs to love himself and others.

Average school-age children will be able to accept and to give love, but the expressions of love and affection are less overt than with younger children. The young school-age child is usually reluctant to kiss and hug a parent in public, while the child 10 years and older will avoid such a display with vehemence. This does not mean the school-age child loves the parent less, only that love and affection are expressed in more covert ways, such as just being near parents or trying to please them. Likewise, the parent expresses love and affection by showing genuine interest in what the child is doing. With peers, expressions of affection are shown by the desire to be with them and to share experiences with them.

Joy, or happiness, is allied closely to love. Joy can be experienced by sharing an experience with a loved one. Joy is experienced also in circumstances that promote self-love or self-esteem, such as completing a difficult task. In this age period when the triumph of the sense of industry over the sense of inferiority is a major developmental achievement, joy is found in accomplishments and the sense of competency.

As in most things during this stage, peers play a major role in the emotional well-being of school-age children. Some children are more popular with their peers than others; because status with peers is so important to the child's emotional-social well-being, it has been studied intensively. Children who are popular and well liked by their peers tend to be physically attractive, self-confident, energetic, and considerate. The popularity may also be associated with behavior of the child's mother. Mothers of children who are well liked by their peers tend to be more positive and focused on feelings and less disagreeable and demanding than mothers of less popular children (Putallaz, 1987). Research such as this points out the need for nursing interventions to focus on both the child and the mother.

Children develop their basic emotional patterns and character formation during the school-age period. Character traits are stabilized as are the fundamental ways for dealing with people and things. With proper guidance and models to emulate, the pattern will be healthy and carry the child through successful adolescence and adulthood.

Nursing assessment of the school-ager must focus on the defining characteristics of nursing diagnoses which describe the child's perceptions of self and pattern of role engagements and relationships. The following diagnoses should be considered if problems are suspected: *fear; anxiety, disturbance in self concept: self esteem; social isolation; altered growth and development.* If properly channeled, even negative emotions can lead to positive outcomes. Anger that is just can lead to social concern and reform. Fear and worry can be motivators for positive action and cautions for avoiding negative action. Jealousy can promote empathy and identity. The positive emotions of affection and joy give meaning to life.

The Developing Person

The major thrust in psychosocial development in the school-age period is the establishment of the ego quality of *industry versus inferiority*—Erikson's fourth stage. As Erikson (1967) stated:

> One might say that personality at the first stage crystallizes around the conviction "I am what I am given," and that of the second, "I am what I will." The third can be characterized by "I am what I can imagine I will be." We must now approach the fourth: "I am what I learn." The child now wants to be shown how to get busy with something and how to be busy with others.

Erikson (1967) described what he meant by the term *sense of industry:*

> Children become dissatisfied and disgruntled without a sense of being useful, without a sense of being able to make things and make them well and even perfectly: this is what I call the sense of industry.

The child becomes involved in production of things, work completion, division of labor, equality of opportunity, and positive identification with those who *know* things and know how to *do* things.

As is clear from Erikson's words, the ego quality of industry versus inferiority has both personal and social implications. On the personal level, the focus is on the competency of the individual, especially in physical

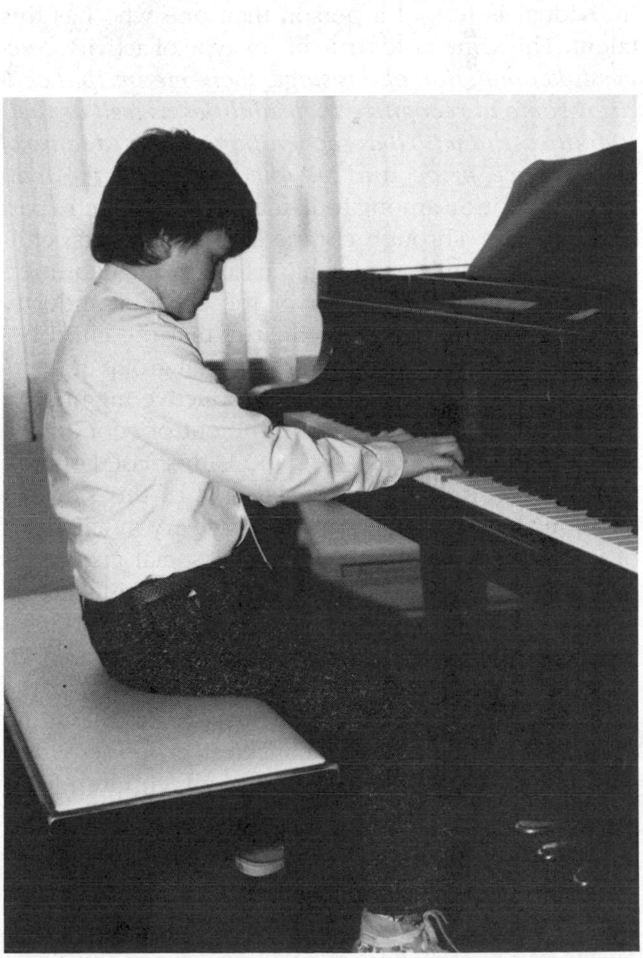

School-age children need to develop one relatively superior skill that they can be proud of.

and cognitive skills. Previous discussion of these skills demonstrates the progress the normal child makes in these areas. The child's psychic energies are directed toward the acquisition and perfection of these skills. "Industrious" is an apt description of school-age children.

The danger of this stage is that children will find their physical and cognitive skills wanting and will develop a sense of inadequacy and inferiority rather than industry and competence. Most children, however, are capable of developing competence in some area of activity. Likewise, few will be capable of developing competence in all areas of activity.

A sense of inferiority in some areas of activity is inevitable for the vast majority of children. As Erikson points out, the "versus" in the stage designations does not mean that the negative component is not present; it means only that for successful completion of the stage, the positive component must outweigh the negative component in the equation. School-age children, therefore, need to recognize their limitations and to accept them without a diminution of self-esteem. Not everyone has artistic talent, but just because an individual does not have artistic talent does not mean the individual is less of a person than one who has this talent. The same holds true of any type of activity. *Successful completion of this stage, then, means that children come to recognize their abilities as well as their liabilities and with that recognition develop a sense of competence, pride, and self-esteem for what they can do.* Competition among individuals is very much a part of this stage. Through competition with peers, children gain recognition of personal assets and liabilities.

The social implication of the stage of industry versus inferiority means primarily that the child becomes a productive member of a social group of peers in preparation for becoming a productive member of society as an adult. The development of cooperative and collaborative working relationships based on mutual respect is the major social goal of this stage of development. Again, competition is very much a part of this process, but with respect to social goals, it is group or team competition rather than individual competition. Children learn to respect the abilities of others and to take pride in the accomplishment attained through group activities. They learn that the strengths and weaknesses of individuals, including their own, can be counterbalanced in group activities. And, perhaps the hardest lesson of all, children learn that the accomplishments of others do not diminish theirs.

This major achievement of a personal and social identity as an industrious and competent individual and group member occurs rather slowly over the entire span of the school-age period. The characteristic behaviors of the child at each age from 6 to 12 years illustrate this gradual progression.

The 6-year-old is noted for almost constant activity; the whole body seems to be involved in almost anything and everything being done. Throwing a ball involves the entire body; telling a story involves gesturing with the arms and face. Much spontaneous dramatization is evident during this sixth year. The child tends to be restless and indecisive and needs activities that require use of the large muscles. Group activities are entered with enthusiasm, but children are not yet ready for cooperative play, often leaving a game if they do not get their way or if they are distracted by something else. Behavior is often explosive, with temper tantrums reaching a peak at this age. Rudeness is common, especially at home and at play. The conscious or moral judgment is strict, literal, and unreliable. Cheating is frequent but against the child's conscience. The child may behave very differently at home and at school. This is not an easy age for either child or parent. Probably the most endearing characteristics are the child's eagerness to learn and to "help" adults by performing tasks for them. Adults, parents and teacher, are very important to the child, and direct imitation of their mannerisms is frequent. Parental affection, patience, and praise are extremely important to the child throughout this difficult year.

Seven-year-olds are full of vitality and energy but are more cautious in exercising it in play than 6-year-olds. At this age children are also cautious, self-critical, and anxious to do things correctly in activities undertaken. They are talkative and start to use words to express anger rather than physical means. They enjoy songs, rhythms, fairy tales, myths, nature stories, comics, television, and movies. A rudimentary understanding of time and money values is evident. Seven-year-olds assume responsibility better than 6-year-olds and are very concerned about what is right and wrong even though they may take things that do not belong to them. They are sensitive to the feelings and attitudes of both peers and adults and want to be liked by them. A spontaneous awareness of and sensitivity about sex makes 7-year-olds modest and concerned about self-exposure. Children at this age become concerned about fairness but have difficulty accepting criticism or blame. They are especially dependent on the approval of adults and need a warm, encouraging, friendly relationship with them.

Eight-year-olds are eager to do things and do them with more smoothness and poise than previously. Group activity takes on increasing importance and the child seeks it out actively, disliking to be alone. Segregation by sexes is obvious, and the child chooses a best friend of the same sex. However, these friendships tend to be unstable, and the child may have several best friends in sequence during the year. Play outdoors may be vigorous but quiet activities are important, and dramatic play is very popular. Collections of miscellaneous objects are common and are treasured. The child is eager to learn and usually enjoys school. Areas of interest expand beyond the immediate environment. Time concepts are expanding, and the child tries to relate to the past and present. The difference between real or historic characters and fictitious ones in movies or on television can be recognized. Eight-year-olds are beginning to understand and accept other people more than previously, recognizing individual differences. They begin to see themselves in relation to others and have a beginning capacity for self-evaluation. Conscience is less rigid than previously, and they begin to resent parental authority, looking more to the group for support. Behavior is likely to be better away from home. Although children at the age of 8 move increasingly to the peer group for support, they continue to need much praise and encouragement from adults.

The 9-year-old is fairly responsible, reasonable, and dependable. Individual differences in abilities and skills between children become more distinct and clear both to adults and to the children themselves. The same-sex groups or gangs of childhood are all important. Conformity within the group is accentuated and the group may leave out a child who is different in any way. New forms of independence from adults are attained through the peer group. The parents are reappraised to a more realistic level. The former image of the parent as all powerful and all knowing is devalued down to a more human level, and new authorities are set up against parents. Hero worship becomes prominent. The child has an increased attention span and the capacity to plan and complete a fairly complex project with little or no help from adults. Interests expand rapidly. There is less interest in fairy tales and fantasy and more in the community and country and in other countries and people. The scope of interest includes babies, and both sexes enjoy interacting with babies and small children. As part of their interest in learning about the world around them, 9-year-olds are interested in learning about the origin of babies and how they grow. The 9-year-old is self-sufficient, self-critical, and somewhat of a perfectionist. A strong sense of fairness, right, and wrong plus being mature enough to accept blame for wrongdoing comes into play at this age. However, they do not like to be talked down to. The support of parents and adults is needed in the child's efforts to become more self-sufficient personally and to become a productive member of the peer group.

The most obvious change at 10 years is the differences between the sexes. Girls often start sexual maturation and are more poised and socially mature than boys, who start puberty approximately two years later. The solidarity of the sexes, however, is still very evident. Team sports and cooperative activities are prominent, and the child readily submits to the rules of the game. A stable and lasting friendship with someone of the same sex is formed, and a separation through a move to a distant new home by either child may be very traumatic for both. Collections are no longer miscellaneous but very distinct and organized and may lead to a lifelong hobby. Hero worship continues. Interests in the world of people, places, and things continue to expand and a strong moral sense of good and bad is expressed about many of them. Children continue to reappraise parents and become self-conscious of them and about them. Some children develop a "foundling" fantasy in which these ordinary people could not possibly be their parents, while fantasizing that the parents are some glamorous figures. However, they are still very dependent on the love of parents and implicitly accept certain standards of the family.

Differences between the sexes are even more apparent in 11- and 12-year-olds, because of differences in timing of onset of puberty. However, many behaviors are characteristic of both sexes. The sex cleavage is often intensified, and frequent expressions of resentment and disgust toward the opposite sex are common. Girls are the first to break down the cleavage by becoming "boy crazy." Sexual concerns are often discussed secretly with a best friend or a cohesive peer group. An increase in curiosity and physical and intellectual activity in both sexes is seen. Tension outlets of nail biting and foot twirling may appear, as may compulsive behavior, fears, and aches and pains of unknown and benign origin. The relationship with the family may be ambivalent and oscillating, with the child wanting to be independent, especially of the mother. The child is secretive and demands and needs privacy. Increased unruliness, sloppiness, and dirtiness are often evident. Parents are often astonished to hear how well these same children behave in other settings. Memberships in groups and clubs that are organized around a specific function are of increasing importance. Team games and sports are very popular. As with the other ages of the school-age period, 11- and 12-year-olds need parents' support in this difficult transitional period. Their need for privacy needs to be respected, as does their need for peer activities.

This overview of the behavioral characteristics of children as they progress through the school-age period illustrates the tremendous progress children make in personal and social competency. These are not easy years for either the child or parents. The parents' understanding of the typical behavior of the child, however, will help to provide the support the

Table 8-2. Competency Development of the School-Age Child

Physical Competency	Intellectual Competency	Emotional-Social Competency
General: 6–12 Years		
Gains an average of 2.5–3.2 kg/year (5½–7 lbs/year. Overall height gains of 5.5 cm (2 inches) per year; growth occurs in spurts and is mainly in trunk and extremities. Loses deciduous teeth; most of permanent teeth erupt. Progressively more coordinated in both gross and fine motor skills. Caloric needs increase with growth spurts.	Masters concrete operations. Moves from egocentrism; learns he or she is not always right. Learns grammar and expression of emotions and thoughts. Vocabulary increases to 3000 words or more; handles complex sentences.	Central crisis; industry vs. inferiority; wants to do and make things. Progressive sex education needed. Wants to be like friends; competition important. Fears body mutilation, alterations in body image; earlier phobias may recur, nightmares; fears death. Nervous habits common.
6 To 7 Years		
Gross motor skill exceeds fine motor coordination. Balance and rhythm are good —runs, skips, jumps, climbs, gallops. Throws and catches ball. Dresses self with little or no help.	Vocabulary of 2500 words. Learning to read and print; beginning concrete concepts of numbers, general classification of items. Knows concepts of right and left; morning, afternoon and evening; coinage. Intuitive thought process. Verbally aggressive, bossy, opinionated, argumentative. Likes simple games with basic rules.	Boisterous, outgoing, and a know-it-all, whiney; parents should sidestep power struggles, offer choices. Becomes quiet and reflective during seventh year; very sensitive. Can use telephone. Likes to make things: starts many, finishes few. Give some responsibility for household duties.
8 To 10 Years		
Myopia may appear. Secondary sex characteristics begin in girls. Hand-eye coordination and fine motor skills well established. Movements are graceful, coordinated. Cares for own physical needs completely. Constantly on move; plays and works hard; enforce balance in rest and activity.	Learning correct grammar and to express feelings in words. Likes books he or she can read alone; will read funny papers, scan newspaper. Enjoys making detailed drawings. Mastering classification, seriation, spatial and temporal, numerical concepts. Uses language as a tool; likes riddles, jokes, chants, word games. Rules guiding force in life now. Very interested in how things work, what and how weather, seasons, etc., are made.	Strong preference for same-sex peers; antagonizes opposite-sex peers. Self-assured and pragmatic at home; questions parental values and ideas. Has a strong sense of humor. Enjoys clubs, group projects, outings, large groups, camp. Modesty about own body increases over time; sex conscious. Works diligently to perfect skills he or she does best. Happy, cooperative, relaxed and casual in relationships. Increasingly courteous and well-mannered with adults. Gang stage at a peak; secret codes and rituals prevail. Responds better to suggestion than dictatorial approach.
11 To 12 Years		
Vital signs approximate adult norms. Growth spurt for girls; inequalities between sexes are increasingly noticeable; boys greater physical strength. Eruption of permanent teeth complete except for third molars. Secondary sex characteristics begin in boys. Menstruation may begin.	Able to think about social problems and prejudices; sees others' points of view. Enjoys reading mysteries, love stories. Begins playing with abstract ideas. Interested in whys of health measures and understands human reproduction. Very moralistic; religious commitment often made during this time.	Intense team loyalty; boys begin teasing girls and girls flirt with boys for attention; best friend period. Wants unreasonable independence. Rebellious about routines; wide mood swings; needs some times daily for privacy. Very critical of own work. Hero worship prevails. "Facts of life" chats with friends prevail; masturbation increases. Appears under constant tension.

Table 8-2 *(continued)*

Nutrition	Play	Safety
General: 6–12 Years		
Fluctuations in appetite due to uneven growth pattern and tendency to get involved in activities. Tendency to neglect breakfast due to rush of getting to school. Though school lunch is provided in most schools, child does not always eat it.	Plays in groups, mostly of same sex; "gang" activities predominate. Books for all ages. Bicycles important. Sports equipment. Cards, board and table games. Most of play is active games requiring little or no equipment.	Enforce continued use of safety belts during car travel. Bicycle safety must be taught and enforced. Teach safety related to hobbies, handicrafts, mechanical equipment.
6 To 7 Years		
Preschool food dislikes persist. Tendency for deficiencies in iron, vitamin A and riboflavin. 100 ml/kg of water per day. 3 gm/kg protein daily.	Still enjoys dolls, cars and trucks. Plays well alone but enjoys small groups of both sexes; begins to prefer same sex peer during 7th year. Ready to learn how to ride a bicycle. Prefers imaginary, dramatic play with real costumes. Begins collecting for quantity, not quality. Enjoys active games such as hide-and-seek, tag, jumprope, roller skating, kickball. Ready for lessons in dancing, gymnastics, music. Restrict TV time to 1–2 hours/day.	Teach and reinforce traffic safety. Still needs adult supervision of play. Teach to avoid strangers, never take anything from strangers. Teach illness prevention and reinforce continued practice of other health habits. Restrict bicycle use to home ground; no traffic areas; teach bicycle safety. Teach and set examples re harmful use of drugs, alcohol, smoking.
8 To 10 Years		
Needs about 2100 calories/day; nutritious snacks. Tends to be too busy to bother to eat. Tendency for deficiencies in calcium, iron and thiamine. Problem of obesity may begin now. Good table manners. Able to help with food preparation.	Likes hiking, sports. Enjoys cooking, woodworking, crafts. Enjoys cards and table games. Likes radio and records. Begins qualitative collecting now. Continue restriction on TV time.	Stress safety with firearms, Keep them out of reach and allow use only with adult supervision. Know who the child's friends are; parents should still have some control over friend selection. Teach water safety; swimming should be supervised by an adult.
11 To 12 Years		
Male needs 2500 calories per day; female needs 2250 (70 cal/kg/day). 75 ml/kg of water per day. 2 gm/kg protein daily.	Enjoys projects and working with hands. Likes to do errands and jobs to earn money. Very involved in sports, dancing, talking on phone. Enjoys all aspects of acting and drama.	Continue monitoring friends; Stress bicycle safety on streets and in traffic.

child needs to progress in the long struggle for a sense of industry and competency as opposed to inferiority and inadequacy.

Health Maintenance

The school-age period is a relatively healthy one for children. Morbidity and mortality are lower than at any other time during childhood.

Acute illnesses, especially respiratory illnesses, are fairly common with this age group. Over half the acute illnesses reported are due to respiratory conditions. The average number of days of restricted activity for illness per child in the 6 through 16 age group is approximately 10, with approximately 5 school days lost due to illness (Health U.S., 1984). Although acute illnesses are to be expected as a normal part of life, this information about the incidence of acute conditions indicates that prevention of respiratory conditions should be included in health promotion efforts for this age group.

The following concerns need to be included in a health promotion program: nutrition, play, safety, immunizations, sex education, and value clarification.

Nutrition

Proper nutrition, discussed previously and in Chapter 18, is essential for the health and well-being of children. A properly nourished child is less susceptible to acute illnesses and is better able to develop the physical, intellectual, emotional, and social competencies so important to this age group.

One problem area in nutrition for this age group is that children may become too busy and involved to eat properly. Children like structure and rituals, and adults can use this to the advantage of both themselves and their children. Regularity of meal and snack times gives children the structure they need around which to plan activities.

Mealtimes also should be pleasant occasions to look forward to and to provide opportunities for social interaction with the family. The 6- or 7-year-old may find it difficult to sit through a meal and may need to be excused early. By 9 years, the child's table manners are good and responsibilities for assisting with meal preparation and clean-up can be assumed. The younger child can help, too, but may be somewhat erratic in the ability to carry through on assigned tasks. Tasks for the younger child need to be simple, such as putting the napkins on the table or clearing away dishes. The child can acquire a sense of competence and pride in contributing to family welfare if undue pressure on skilled performance is not applied.

Play

It has often been said that play is the work of children. When consideration is given to what play does for the development of physical, cognitive, and social competence, this might even be considered an understatement (see Chapter 21).

Play is of vital importance to the acquisition of the ego quality of industry versus inferiority. Children acquire physical competence and skills through play involving gross and fine motor activity. Active involvement in play promotes cognitive development, and through playful experiments on the environment, the child discovers much new knowledge and many new cognitive skills. Some parents may require assistance in the continued need of this age child for ample playtime. Socialization to the peer group is acquired primarily through the play of children. Peer group and team activities are important to the school-age child's developing peer identity, not just during the school year but also during summer months. Parents may need information about community facilities, programs, and camps that provide opportunities for play experiences. A childhood without ample opportunities for play is no childhood at all. The value of play cannot be overestimated in the promotion of a healthy childhood.

Safety

Safety education is of primary importance in health maintenance efforts for the school-age group. Accidents are by far the leading cause of death. Because motor vehicle accidents account for nearly half of those deaths automobile safety should be stressed (Health U.S., 1984). Children like rituals, and one ritual that should be automatic is buckling up the seat belt. Children can learn the rules of the road also and included in the rules is proper behavior in the automobile so that the driver is not distracted from the primary task of driving the car.

Although motor vehicle accidents are a major cause of death, the other half of the accidents of this age group occur inside the house or on adjacent property (Health U.S., 1984). Home safety measures therefore also assume major importance and *potential for injury* continues to be a diagnosis of importance to the nurse. Boys are twice as likely to have accidents as girls. According to one study, the most common commercial products involved in these accidents were bicycles, glass, swings, skateboards, and nails.

Caution in play and other activities needs to be stressed. However, caution should not be overly stressed because excessive caution or fear can inhibit normal development. A certain number of skinned knees and bruises seems inevitable in the normally developing child.

Common Concerns

Sex education and drug education are two major concerns pertaining to the child that need to be faced by parents during the school-age period. The older school-age child must acquire factual knowledge and values about sex and drugs. The younger school-age child needs to have questions answered in terms appropriate to cognitive development, but the older child needs more specific information and clarification of values.

The older school-age child can assimilate factual knowledge about menstruation, nocturnal emissions, and reproduction if he or she has information about the anatomy and physiology of the human body. If sex education is given in isolation, learning is harder. If given in isolation it also gives undue emphasis to sexual function as the only bodily function of importance. If presented in context with a study of the wonders of the human body, it becomes a natural process to be respected as are all other natural processes of the body. If given in this context, certainly the 11-year old can assimilate the information, and the 9-year-old can handle introductory information (Bernstein and Cowan, 1978).

Sex education is a value-laden topic, and many adults are uncomfortable talking about it. Ideally, a child should receive information about sex and sexuality from parents. But many parents avoid discussing sexual issues with their child and rely on other sources to provide this information. More and more, sex education is provided in the school setting. Nurses who have experience teaching human sexuality can be valuable resources to school faculty responsible for teaching sex education. Seybold and Klisch (1982) described a half-day workshop held by nurses for faculty of a private grade school. They found that a primary need of workshop participants was to decrease their own discomfort in relation to sexual topics and terminology.

Whether sex education occurs in the home, in school, or both, concerned adults should be available to respond to children's questions appropriately and provide value clarification. Otherwise, questions will be answered and values clarified with the peer group only and this situation is often one of "the blind leading the blind." (See Chapter 22 for further discussion.)

With the increasing availability of drugs to younger children, children need to be made aware of the harmful effects of drugs. Rather than scare tactics, emphasis is more effectively placed on how drugs hinder the ability to accomplish all the feats so important to the age group (see Chapter 36).

References

Bailey D: The growing child and the need for physical activity. *In* Smart M, Smart R: *School-Age Children, Development and Relationships.* New York, Macmillan, 1978

Bailey D, et al: The influence of exercise, physical activity and athletic performance on the dynamics of human growth. *In* Falkner F, Tanner J (eds): *Human Growth. Vol 2: Postnatal Growth.* New York, Plenum Publications, 1978.

Bernstein A, Cowan P: Children's concepts of how people get babies. *In* Smart M, Smart R: *School-Age Children, Development and Relationships.* New York, Macmillan, 1978.

Brody GH, Pillegrin AD, Siegel IE: Marital quality and mother-child and father-child interactions with school-aged children. *Dev Psychol* 1986; 22:291–296.

Bronfenbrenner U: Response to pressure from peers versus adults among Soviet and American school children. *Int J Psychol* 1967 Feb; 199–207.

Buhrmester D, Furman W: The development of companionship and intimacy. *Child Dev* 1987; 58:1101–1113.

Caplan G: *Support Systems and Community Mental Health.* Englewood Cliffs, NJ, Behavioral Publications, 1974.

Committee on School Health of American Academy of Pediatrics. Statement on health education. *Pediatrics* 1978 1 Jul; 117.

Dess M: Lessons in letting go. *Home Life* 1976 Dec; 36.

Erikson E: Identity and the life cycle: Selected papers. *Psychol Issues Monogr* 1967 Jan.

Erikson E: *Identity, Youth and Crisis.* New York, WW Norton and Company, 1968.

Foster C: *Developing Responsibility in Children.* Ontario, Canada, Science Research Associates, 1976.

Frick SB: Diagnosing boredom, confusion, and adaptation in school children. *J School Health* 1985; 55:254–257.

Goodman NE: *The Culture of Childhood.* New York, Columbia University Teacher's College Press, 1976.

Gnepp J, Hess DLR: Children's understanding of verbal and facial display rules. *Dev Psychol* 1986; 22:103–108.

Halford GS, Boyle FM: Do young children understand conservation of number? *Child Dev* 1985; 56:165–176.

Health United States–1984. Washington, DC, US Department of Health and Human Services, Publication No. (PHS) 84-1232, 1984.

Hester NO: Health perceptions of school-age children. *Issues Compr Pediatr Nurs* 1987; 10(3):137–147.

Holmes CS, Hayford JT, Thompson RG: Personality and behavior differences in groups of boys with short stature. *Child Health Care* 1982; 11:61–63.

Kagan J: *Understanding Children—Behavior, Motives and Thought.* New York, Harcourt Brace Jovanovich, 1971.

Kruger AC, Tomasello M: Transactive discussions with peers and adults. *Dev Psychol* 1986; 22:681–685.

Lowery G: *Growth and Development of Children.* Chicago, Year Book Medical Publishers, 1978.

Maier H: *Three Theories of Child Development.* New York, Harper & Row, 1969.

Miller J, Janosik E: *Family Focused Care.* New York, McGraw-Hill, 1980.

Miller PM, Danaher DL, Forbes D: Sex-related strategies for

coping with interpersonal conflict in children aged five and seven. *Dev Psychol* 1986; 22:543–548.
Miller SA: Certainty and necessity in the understanding of Piagetian concepts. *Dev Psychol* 1986; 22:3–18.
Piaget J: *The Psychology of Intelligence.* Totowa, NJ, Littlefield, Adams & Company, 1966.
Putallaz M: Maternal behavior and children's sociometric status. *Child Dev* 1987; 58:324–340.
Schor DP: Temperament and the initial school experience. *Child Health Care* 1985; 13:129–134.
Seybold SA, Klisch ML: Preparing grade school faculty to teach family life education. *MCN* 1982; 7:50–54.
Smart M, Smart R: *School-Age Children — Development and Relationships.* New York, Macmillan, 1978.
Steinberg L: Latchkey children and susceptibility to peer pressure. *Dev Psychol* 1986; 22:433–439.
Strauss CC, Smith K, Frame C, et al: Personal and interpersonal characteristics associated with childhood obesity. *J Pediatr Psychol* 1985; 10:337–343.
Thomas A, Chess S: *Temperament and Development.* New York, Brunner/Mazel, 1977.
Williams J, Stith M: *Middle Childhood — Behavior and Development.* New York, Macmillan, 1974.

Bibliography

Allensworth DD, Kolbe LJ: The comprehensive school health program: exploring an expanded concept. *J School Health* 1987 Dec; 57(10):409–412.
Anderson AR, Clore ER: Asbestos in schools: reducing pediatric risk factors. *Pediatr Nurs* 1986 Jul/Aug; 12(4):296–297, 321.
Bausell RB: A national survey assessing pediatric preventive behaviors. *Pediatr Nurs* 1985 Nov/Dec; 11(6):438–442.
Broome ME, Hellier AP: School-age children's fears of medical experiences. *Issues Compr Pediatr Nurs* 1987 10(2):77–86.
Brosnan CA: Long-term results of an elementary sexuality program. *Pediatr Nurs* 1987 Mar-Apr; 13(2), 130–131.
Denyes MJ: Nursing research related to schoolage children and adolescents. *Annu Rev Nurs Res* 1983; 1:27–53.
Galli N, Greenberg JS, Tobin F: Health education and sensitivity to cultural, religious and ethnic beliefs. *J School Health* 1987 May; 57(5):177–180.
Hitchens-Serota JA: Assessing parent's knowledge of pediatric dental disease. *Pediatr Nurs* Nov/Dec 1986; 12(6):435–438.
Johnston PK: Getting enough to grow on . . . a vegetarian diet. *Am J Nurs* 1984 Mar; 84(3):336–339.
Jose NL: The silent gift: a project for spiritual health. *J School Health* 1987 Feb; 47(2):72–73.
Kotchabhakdi P: School-age children's conceptions of the heart and its function: methodology and findings (part 2). *Matern Child Nurs J* 1985 Winter; 14(4):203–263.
Kronmiller JE, Nirschl RF: 1985. Preventive dentistry for children. *Pediatr Nurs* 1985 Nov/Dec; 11(6):446–452.
Kuhnen KK, Chewning B, Day T, et al: Barny: a computer for teaching sex education. *MCN* 1983 Sep/Oct; 8(5):350–353.
Lamarine RJ: Self-esteem, health locus of control, and health attitudes among Native American children. *J School Health* 1987 Nov; 57(9), 371–374.
Law CM: Growth and development in childhood: 1985. *Nursing* (Oxford), 1985 Jul; 2(39):1143, 1145–1147.
Lyons JF, Hester NO: Research-generated nursing diagnoses for healthy school-age children. *Issues Compr Pediatr Nurs* 1987; 10(3): 149–159.
McClellan MA: On their own: latchkey children. *Pediatr Nurs* 1984 May-Jun; 10(3):198–202.
Millar TP: How do you give a child self-esteem? *Child Today* 1983 Sep-Oct; 12(5):2–3.
Price JH, Desmond SM, Ruppert ES, et al: School nurses' perceptions of childhood obesity. *J School Health* 1987 Oct; 57(8):332–336.
Ruddy-Wallace M: Temperament: assessing individual differences in hospitalized children. *J Pediatr Nurs* 1987 Feb; 2(1):30–36.
Ryan NM: Recurrent abdominal pain among school-aged children. *MCN* 1986 Mar/Apr; 11(2):102–107.
Shupe SD, Sandoval WM: Nutrition education: from the lunchroom to the classroom. *J School Health* 1987 Mar; 57(3):122–123.
Strother DB: Latchkey children: the fastest-growing special interest group in the schools. *J School Health* 1986 Jan; 56(1):13–16.
Thompson CE, Stroud SD: The motorized tricycle: an accident waiting to happen. *J Pediatr Nurs* 1987 Apr; 2(2):120–125.
van Reek J, Drop MJ, Joosten J: The influence of peers and parents on the smoking behavior of schoolchildren. *J School Health* 1987 Jan; 57(1):30.
Weinstein LB, Abrams RA, Ayers CS: A school program to reduce dental caries. *J School Health* 1988 Jan; 58(1):32–33

Families with Adolescents — Chapter 9

Patricia Neel Scott

The adolescent period is defined as beginning with the appearance of secondary sex characteristics at approximately 12 years of age, and ending with the completion of somatic growth at about age 19. However, adolescence must also be considered within the context of psychosocial and cognitive development, rather than just as a chronologic or physical event.

As the adolescent develops, the family develops as well, and adolescent development and family development have a reciprocal relationship. Changes during adolescence influence the family and relationships within. Normal adolescent developmental events may

Related Topics
Developmental theories, Chapter 3
Adolescents' concepts of health, Chapter 10
Health assessment, Chapter 15
Fostering self-esteem, Chapter 16
Promoting safety, Chapter 17
Promoting healthy nutrition, Chapter 18
Promoting healthy sexuality, Chapter 22
Anorexia nervosa, bulimia, Chapter 36
Substance abuse, Chapter 36
Adolescent pregnancy, Chapter 49

We appreciate the critical review of this chapter by Saundra Frick, RN, PhD, and her contributions to it.

potentially stress the family. The nurse can play a pivotal role in working with adolescents and their families, not only by aiding them during stressful times but also by helping them to maintain health. This chapter will cover growth and development of families with adolescents, potential stresses of families with adolescents, adolescent growth and development, and health care of adolescents.

Development and Adaptation of Families with Adolescents

The adolescent stage of family development begins when the oldest child is 12 years of age and ends when that child is independent. The period may be brief, as for a family whose adolescent joins the military at age 18, or may last longer, as for a family whose adolescent remains at home throughout graduate school.

Duvall (1967, 1977) lists basic tasks common to all North American families with adolescents. Successful achievement of the tasks leads to present satisfaction within the family, and eventual emancipation of an adolescent who is competent to be independent and whose family is able to let go. The overall family goal is to prepare for impending separation by promoting adolescent responsibility and by gradually loosening ties.

Family Growth and Development

Providing Facilities for Widely Different Needs

Needs of family members vary during the adolescent years. Parents need to understand their adolescent's desire to spend time away from the family and to be involved in outside activities. The relationship between parent and teen is best when the parent derives pleasure from the teen's activities. Parents should be encouraged to support activities in which the teen is interested, within their financial and time limitations. Some parents may need to be reminded not to push a teen into an activity in order to meet their own spoken or unspoken needs.

Adolescents need privacy to think and dream. It is often difficult for younger siblings to understand their older brother's or sister's need to be alone. Parents should allow the teen time or space to be without siblings or parents. Not every adolescent can have a private room, but they should be able to take a walk, sit in the yard, or go to the park occasionally without the company of brothers and sisters.

Although parents may not be able actually to increase the space available to their adolescent, they may rearrange home furnishings to include special interest areas more acceptable to the teen. They should allow the youth the opportunity to organize and decorate his or her own room to satisfy adolescent tastes.

The designation of specified places for having a conversation, listening to records and tapes, watching television, and playing musical instruments, while not eliminating the sounds of the adolescent in the home, may reduce angry feelings on the part of other family members.

Parents' needs also vary during the adolescent stage. They are usually not as bound to the home as they were earlier. They often develop or redevelop outside interests and have more time for career growth. Parents should be encouraged to pursue their interests in order to enhance personal growth.

Sharing the Tasks and Responsibilities of Family Living

The adolescent can assume greater household responsibilities than the younger child. There are a number of reasons for involving the adolescent in a greater share of these responsibilities. Adolescents are forming their sense of identity. Encouraging their participation in household responsibilities helps them to incorporate into their identity a sense of being a useful and participating member of a family unit. Adolescents should be given creative as well as routine tasks. Responsibilities should be increased as the adolescent matures. It is important for parents to recognize and commend teenagers' efforts.

Another reason adolescents may be given a greater share of household responsibilities is because their help is needed when the mother decides her children are old enough for her to return to work. This decision can create disequilibrium in the family and may place the family at risk for *ineffective family coping: compromised.* In addition to assessing for the defining characteristics of that nursing diagnosis, the nurse can assist the family in adapting to this change in the family unit. The nurse may help the family to understand that tasks the mother has performed for years may now be done in less detail or shared by other family members, with different outcomes than when done by the mother. Because the outcomes are different does not necessarily mean they are unsatisfactory. The family must agree on what is expected of each member and work together to continue to function adaptively.

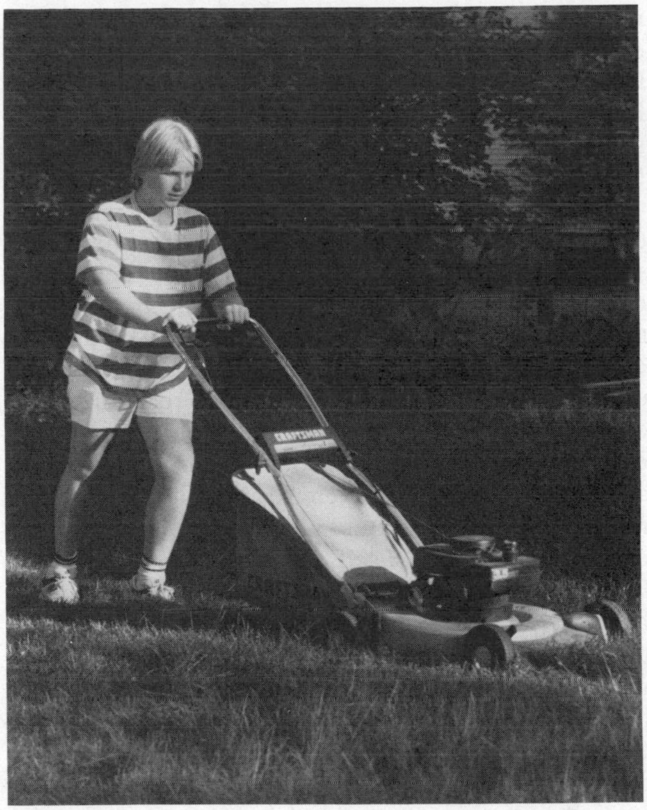

Sharing the tasks and responsibilities of family living. (Photo by Ken Kasper.)

Putting the Spousal Relationship into Focus

In families with both partners living at home, the adolescent period provides more time for the couple to be alone. This is true for traditional as well as the nontraditional couple, with the possible exception of large communal or extended families. Parenting is as demanding (and sometimes more so) as it was earlier, but absolute time spent with a teen is decreased. The couple may enjoy activities they used to do earlier or re-establish old friendships. They often begin to consider their own future together with an "empty nest." Couples may rediscover one another and the characteristics that brought them together. Physical and emotional intimacy may be rekindled. On the other hand, more time together may mean facing problems in their relationship. A loving relationship between partners provides a good model for a teen's future relationships.

Keeping Communication Systems Open

Open communication is a necessary aspect of living with an adolescent who may be loquatious, argumentive, or moody. It requires attentiveness as well as acceptance of the youth as an individual. Many parents find it trying to listen to adolescents as they talk at length about personal discoveries that they consider of universal significance or as they discuss matters that may seem trivial to adults. Listening attentively lets teenagers know that they have something worthwhile to say. Teens also need to listen to themselves and to get feedback from adults to aid in establishing opinions and values. Talking also helps develop communication and social skills.

Parents often feel threatened when teens disagree with them. Negativism is typical of young adolescents especially, as they attempt to express autonomy. Disagreements are natural in all families and should not be suppressed but rather expressed as rationally and respectfully as possible. Cognitive growth enables many teens to engage in more logical discussion than before, and adults can then appeal to reason. Parents should insist that opposing views be expressed respectfully and should express their own views respect-

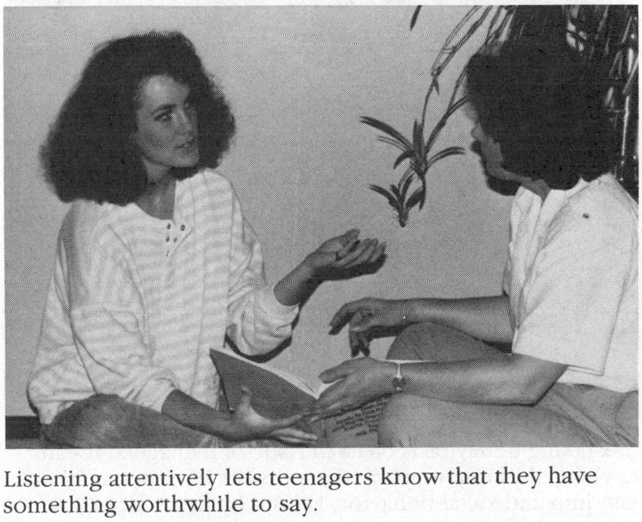

Listening attentively lets teenagers know that they have something worthwhile to say.

fully as well. Consciously humiliating an adolescent does nothing to improve the reasoning skills and can be detrimental to his or her self-esteem. Humor may help in arguments but adolescents like to be taken seriously, so the humor should be directed at the situation and not the youth.

One of the more difficult aspects of communication with the adolescent is the fluctuating emotional state. Parents may need assistance in recognizing their child's behavior as a form of communication. Sometimes parents' attempts to keep the lines of communication open are perceived by adolescents as "picking" on them. Parents should be helped to recognize that constructive criticism is necessary to help their adolescent grow, but it should be offered with compassion and should not be an exercise in fault-finding. The most destructive effect of fault-finding on the adolescent is the lowering of self-concept. This reduces confidence in the youth's ability to solve problems and in his or her interpersonal relationships. In dealing with this moodiness during adolescence, parents may be most helpful by making themselves available to comfort, advise, or listen during a low mood; understand during a quiet mood; and share the fun during a happy mood.

Maintaining Contact with the Extended Family

Families need extended family members to provide company and support and to help maintain cultural identity. Adolescents may learn religion, customs, and language from older family members. By maintaining closeness, parents of adolescents can aid one another in dealing with their teenagers. Teenagers can learn to use family support systems during times of stress.

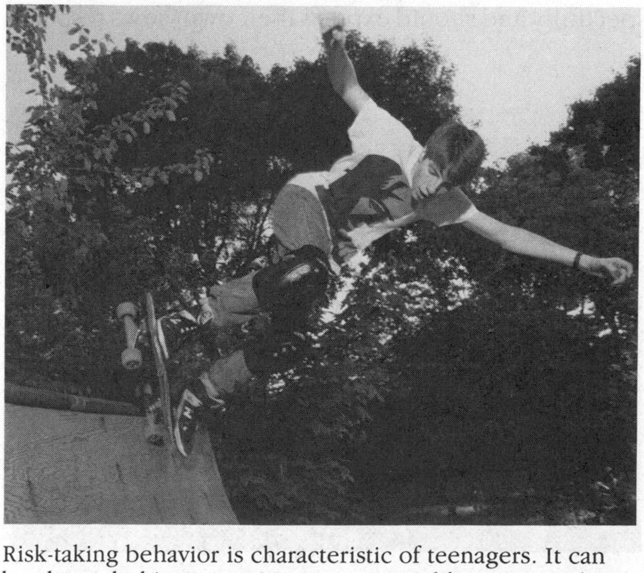

Risk-taking behavior is characteristic of teenagers. It can be channeled into constructive pursuits like sports rather than into antisocial behavior. (Photo by Ken Kasper.)

Potential Family Stresses

Potential Stress Related to Cognitive Change

Early in the formal operational period, the adolescent experiences egocentric thought characterized by feelings of indestructability and immunity to accidents (Elkind, 1970). Subsequently, teens may behave recklessly, causing stress within the family. Parents frequently and legitimately worry about their teens. Consequences of recklessness such as disability, pregnancy, or death are obvious sources of stress. Nurses can aid parents in teaching their adolescents to behave responsibly. Parents can give facts and reasons but must remember that, although teens may be able to reason to a degree, they do not necessarily use mature judgment. Adolescents therefore need, and often want, limits. For example, parents may know their child has been thoroughly instructed in driving safety, but they must still provide specific rules regarding drinking and driving and when to return the car.

Potential Stress Related to Psychosocial Change

Issues of independence and rebellion are probably the primary sources of family stress during adolescence. Impending independence is often met with ambivalence by both parents and teens. Parents look forward to the freedom, but dread letting go. Adolescents want to be treated like adults, yet expect complete financial support.

To begin the process of separation, adolescents create psychologic and physical distance between themselves and their parents. They prefer to spend time with their peers and no longer idealize parents (Buhrmester and Furman, 1987). Not all adolescents can create the necessary distance and still demonstrate love and respect. Not all parents understand the separation process; even if they can intellectualize the process, they still often feel rejected by their teens. Parents who are lonely and dependent upon their teens often feel more rejection than parents who have an adult source of support, such as a spouse. Conflicts heighten with the anger and guilt that may result. The nurse can help by listening to the parents, explaining the adolescent's behavior, and assuring them that their teen still needs them very much.

Rebellion is a natural part of seeking independence and identity (Erikson, 1959). It generally involves defiance of limits and argumentiveness. Rebellion is not usually intended to hurt the family, but many families see it as such. Parents may feel that the teen is selfish and unappreciative. Siblings may resent the attention the teen receives by "being bad." After defining with the family the extent of the rebellion, the nurse can help the family to deal with it. If the rebellion is causing harm to the teen or to others, as in vandalism or drug abuse, for example, the family will require more intensive counseling. For milder forms of rebellion, such as staying out past curfew, parents can be assured that this is not unusual and that it does not usually indicate rejection or lack of appreciation. Parents should be advised to set reasonable and specific limits and to explain the reasons for the limits (Friedman and Sarles, 1980). Both parents should be consistent in expectations and in discipline. Limits are necessary, for ignoring rebellious behavior can cause an adolescent to feel ignored and rejected, and may possibly cause more extreme rebelliousness in order to receive parental attention and demonstration of concern (Sedgwick and Hildebrand, 1980). Limits as well as privileges will need to be revised as the teen matures.

Adolescence is a time when a person seeks friends to fulfill the needs to be liked, to be accepted, and to belong to a group. The adolescent moves away from the family, and friends become the bearers of his or her ideals and standards. Making friends is an important developmental task. As adolescents become more and more resistive to parental admonitions about behavior acceptable for them, they double their efforts to act like and dress like their selected friends of the moment.

Many times the adolescent's selection of friends and allegiance to them produces a stressful situation for the family. Parents may need help to understand that this exaggerated conformity to peer groups is a manifestation of the adolescent's process of achieving identity and independence from the parents. Adolescents desperately need approval, and since they are moving away from dependence on their parents, they need the support that approval from friends provides. Once parents recognize the adolescent's desire and need to make friends, their attention becomes focused on the "desirability" of the friends selected. The nurse may assist the family to understand that the adolescent needs to test a wide variety of friendships that may include those adolescents from differing cultural, social, and economic backgrounds, and those whose values are quite different. Research focusing on peer influences on adolescent behaviors indicates that this can be a problem area. Boys tend to be more susceptible than girls to peer influences to engage in antisocial acts and misconduct (Clasen and Eicher, 1986). In one study, girls were more susceptible than boys to peer influences to abuse substances (Huba and Bentler, 1980). As one would expect, adolescents who are left without adult supervision are more susceptible to peer pressures to engage in antisocial activities than are adolescents who are supervised (Steinberg, 1986). While problem behaviors do result when peer influences are brought into play, peer pressure is seen by adolescents as more effective in relation to issues of socialization than in relation to the commission of antisocial acts. Parents are often distraught when their child engages with peers in behaviors that are unacceptable to them. It is helpful for these parents to know that continuing parental support can make a difference in the adolescent's behaviors. One finding of a study investigating the influences on adolescents to smoke was that adolescents with higher levels of parental support were less likely to smoke (Chassin et al, 1986). The choice of lasting friends can be influenced by parents making themselves available to discuss family value systems, to participate in activities of interest to the child and his or her group, and to foster strong kinship and generational ties.

Adolescent sexuality may potentially stress family relations. Parents may worry that their teen will become promiscuous, become pregnant (or cause a pregnancy), or contract a sexually transmitted disease. Conflicts may ensue if parents place unnecessarily strict restraints on the adolescent's activities or if they express lack of trust in the teen.

Parents often have difficulty conceptualizing their adolescent as a sexual being. They may, therefore, ignore the issue of sexuality at a time when adolescents need their input. Parents may also avoid discussing sex because they themselves are poorly informed (Fox, 1979) or because they believe that discussing it will promote sexual activity.

Avoidance of these conflicts is best accomplished by encouraging all parents to begin discussing sexuality with their children well before puberty. Nurses can provide anticipatory guidance to parents regarding their feelings about their child's sexuality and can teach them how to teach their children. Parents and adolescents should discuss values and morals associated with sexual behavior instead of merely focusing on the biology of reproduction and the risk of sexually transmitted diseases.

For the teen to hold positive attitudes about sex, it is essential for him or her to observe interactions of emotionally mature adults, to have a positive relationship with the parent of the opposite sex, and to see discipline used to foster growth and not to control family members. The adolescent who learns that sexual contact is most fulfilling when it involves caring, commitment, and sensitivity to the best interest of others does not generally resort to indiscriminate sexual experimentation.

The idea that sexual urges cannot be controlled is not true. The best guard against the adolescent engaging in promiscuous sexual experimentation at a time when the sex drive is high and peer pressure is excessive is for the family to promote their adolescent's self-esteem. When adolescents believe in and like themselves, they are able to take a stand on moral issues. In this context adolescents can be guided to think about the consequences of sexual activity to themselves and to others. Parents may help their children to think through some difficult situations in advance and consider the consequences of their actions. Such anticipatory guidance may help the adolescent handle difficult situations and not become caught up in the situation or the intensity of emotion. Kastner (1984) found that contraceptive use was increased among teens who had positive communication with parents about sexuality. Adolescents who may be most at risk for unplanned pregnancy are those affected by an inadequate education, poverty, social isolation, and a perceived lack of control over life situations (Burke, 1987).

The stresses that have been discussed can all represent risk factors for the occurrence of *ineffective family coping: compromised.* Since developmental crises, family role changes, and temporary family disorganization are all etiologic factors for this nursing diagnosis (Gordon, 1987), the nurse should be alert to the possibility that it exists.

Potential Stress Related to the Single-Parent Family

The preceding section has described stresses that occur in the two-parent family with an adolescent. The proportion of single-parent families continues to rise dramatically. In 1984, 25 per cent of all family groups were headed by one parent and most of those were headed by a divorced mother (Hanson and Sporakowski, 1986). The effects of divorce and its byproducts on family and child development have been studied extensively. Much of that research has revealed that children of divorced parents are more likely to engage in problem behaviors and to develop emotional disorders (Kalter et al, 1984; Zill, 1984; Hetherington et al, 1985; Steinberg, 1987) than are children from intact two-parent families. The potential for problem behaviors in the adolescent is greater in single-parent families headed by the mother (Dornbusch et al, 1985), and mother-son conflicts are more likely than mother-daughter conflicts (Gjerde, 1986).

The nurse should always obtain information regarding the family structure of the clients. Awareness of the presence of such risk factors as imminent or recent divorce or the presence of a divorced female head of family will allow the nurse to assess in greater depth for the existence of problems. A number of guides to interventions have been reported in the literature, and the nurse with education and experience in individual and family counseling should be aware of those interventions. Divorced parents who have high self-esteem, who show respect for each other, who are able to empathize with their child and the other parent, and who are flexible and open to receiving help have families with fewer difficulties (Steinman et al, 1985). School-based counseling groups have assisted children of divorced families to adjust to the new stresses confronting them (Kaltar et al, 1984). One study found that the provision of information via newsletter assisted single parents in coping with stress (Nelson, 1986). Of particular interest is a study by Hanson (1986) that demonstrated that social support and good parent-child communication predict physical and mental health of single parents, while social support, good communication, and religiousness predict physical and mental health of their children. This focus on wellness allows for the identification of specific defining characteristics of positive individual coping and *family coping: potential for growth.* The nurse can intervene in a wellness-oriented way to identify and improve those attributes that contribute to healthy family functioning.

Development and Adaptation of the Adolescent

Adolescence is characterized by physical, intellectual, and emotional-social developmental changes. The changes interact and are all dimensions of a whole process. Linked to the developmental changes are goals of adolescent development. The goals are to accept one's body, to achieve the ability for formal operational thought, to form a sense of identity, to become independent, to attain a workable value system, and to establish mutually giving relationships with others. This section will cover the physical, intellectual, and emotional-social changes of adolescents with these developmental goals in mind. Also presented are general principles relating to communicating with adolescents, confidentiality when working with teens, and adolescent health care, including implications for nursing.

Physical Growth and Development

Puberty entails the sequence of physiologic and anatomic changes resulting in physical maturity and the capability of reproduction. Once puberty begins, the events occur in the same sequence but not at the same rate for all. Adolescents begin and complete puberty at various ages.

The Growth Spurt

Adolescence is the only time after birth that the velocity of growth significantly increases. During puberty, both males and females attain the final 20 per cent of their mature height. Most of this growth occurs during a "growth spurt" that lasts 2 to 3 years. This spurt usually occurs 2 years earlier for females than for males. The beginning age is variable, from 9.5 to 14.5 years of age for girls and 10.5 to 16 years for boys.

During their growth spurt, boys average an 8-inch height gain, with 4 inches attained during the peak year (around age 14). During the growth spurt a girl's average gain is over 3 inches per year. At age 18, more than 99 per cent of growth has occurred and only about 1 inch in height remains to be gained.

Growth follows a pattern, with almost every part of the body being affected. The legs usually lengthen first, causing the youth to appear lanky and awkward, then the thighs become wider. Next the shoulders broaden, followed by trunk growth. Facial bones change, particularly the mandible and maxilla. The maxilla grows forward and the ramus of the mandible lengthens. Coordination is often affected during this time of uneven growth, and the adolescent may go through periods of clumsiness.

Body Composition

Skeletal changes are dramatic during adolescence. Skeletal mass doubles, contributing significantly to weight gain in puberty.

Muscle or lean body mass and nonlean body mass (principally fat) double during puberty. In males muscles increase both in number of individual cells and in size, while in females muscles increase only in size. This probably accounts for greater male strength, but the cause is unclear. At the time of physical maturation females average twice as much body fat as males. Total body fat in males actually decreases during puberty.

The heart, lungs, liver, spleen, kidneys, pancreas, thyroid, adrenals, gonads, phallus, and uterus double in size during puberty. It is also thought that the digestive tract enlarges. In contrast, the tissues of the lymphatic system (thymus, tonsils, adenoids, and portions of the spleen) decrease in size. Reasons for this decrease and its relationship to antibody production remain to be investigated.

Adult visual levels were attained in early childhood. Adolescents have normal adult hearing, although they are sometimes accused of "selective deafness," or hearing only what they want to hear. Pulse, respirations, and blood pressure values reach adult norms by 15 to 16 years of age. (See Chapter 15 for vital sign values during adolescence.)

Sexual Maturation

Sexual maturation involves the development of primary and secondary sexual characteristics. The total process is not considered complete until about 20 to 21 years of age. Primary sex characteristics involve the physical and hormonal changes necessary for reproduction. Secondary sex characteristics, while not necessary to reproduction, are the characteristics that externally differentiate male from female.

Regulation of this onset of puberty is a complicated and not fully understood process. Trophic hormones are produced in the pituitary gland but are thought to be the result of a "feedback" mechanism. The hypothalamus becomes less sensitive to negative feedback with increasing age and begins to produce

Table 9-1. Classification of Sex Maturity Stages in Boys

Stage	Pubic Hair	Penis	Testes
1	None	Preadolescent	Preadolescent
2	Scanty, long, slightly pigmented	Slight enlargement	Enlarged scrotum, pink texture altered
3	Darker, starts to curl, small amount	Longer	Larger
4	Resembles adult type, but less in quantity; coarse, curly	Larger; glans and breadth increase in size	Larger, scrotum dark
5	Adult distribution, spread to medial surface of thighs	Adult	Adult

(From Behrman and Vaughan, 1987.)

releasing factors. These gonadotropic-releasing hormones then signal the pituitary to secrete gonadotropic hormones such as FSH (follicle-stimulating hormone). FSH in turn stimulates both the growth of ova in the female ovary and the growth of sperm-producing cells in the male testes. Cells in the ovary and testicle produce female and male sex hormones, respectively. Estrogen (female hormone) is produced by the ovary, and testosterone (male hormone) is produced by the testes. These hormones are responsible for development of the secondary sex characteristics. Sex hormones are also produced by the adrenal gland so that both sexes have some of both male and female hormones.

Many practitioners and investigators have observed the more or less orderly (although widely variable) progression of sexual development in both sexes. The description and labeling of these stages by Tanner (1962) are generally accepted as guidelines to normal development (Tables 9-1 and 9-2). These tables enable an examiner to determine the stage of development, to detect abnormalities, and to guide the adolescent as to changes to expect next.

Female secondary sexual development during puberty involves increase in size of the ovaries, uterus, vagina, labia, and breasts. Body hair appears in the pubic area and under the arms; menarche occurs. The first visible signs of sexual maturity are pubic hair, breast buds, or both. These developments occur in orderly fashion but do not necessarily occur together. Each aspect of development (growth, pubic hair, breast appearance) must be evaluated to determine if the young woman is developing normally. For example, it is rare for a girl to reach pubic hair stage 3 or 4 without breast development. In this case, the girl should be evaluated for the presence of hypothalamic, pituitary, or gonadal dysfunction. The vast majority of girls will achieve adult breast size by age 19.

Menarche (the appearance of menstruation) has occurred earlier each generation; present-day adolescent females begin menstruating at an average age of 12 years and 3 months compared with age 17 a century ago. Reasons for these changes are unclear, but effects of environment, nutrition, and better health care are most likely responsible. Menarche occurs at about the time the growth spurt slows. About 99 per cent of girls will reach menarche within 5 years after beginning breast development. If no evidence of puberty can be seen by age 13, a medical assessment should be done. Menarche usually occurs at stage 4.

Male secondary sexual development consists of genital growth and the appearance of pubic and body hair. The first event is usually enlargement of the testes. During puberty the testes, epididymides, and prostate will increase their prepuberty size seven times. As the testes enlarge, so does the scrotum; the scrotum develops rugae and becomes darker in color. The next sign is growth of the penis and a few tufts of long, straight, and slightly pigmented pubic hair. The genitals progress to near-adult size before more pubic hair appears. The final stage of hair growth is to adult type, with hair extending to the medial thigh areas.

Ejaculation has usually occurred in boys by stage 3 and probably earlier. Spermatozoa are almost always present. Stage 4 must be reached before the full adult number of sperm are present.

Table 9-2. Classification of Sex Maturity Stages in Girls

Stage	Pubic Hair	Breasts
1	Preadolescent	Preadolescent
2	Sparse, lightly pigmented, straight, medial border of labia	Breast and papilla elevated as small mound; areolar diameter increased
3	Darker, beginning to curl, increased amount	Breast and areola enlarged, no contour separation
4	Coarse, curly, abundant but amount less than in adult	Areola and papilla form secondary mound
5	Adult feminine triangle, spread to medial surface of thighs	Mature; nipple projects, areola part of general breast contour

(From Behrman and Vaughan, 1987.)

Table 9-3. Characteristics of Adolescents

Early Adolescence (12–14 yr)	Middle Adolescence (15–16 yr)	Late Adolescence (17–21 yr)
Becomes comfortable with own body; egocentric	"Tries out" adult-like behavior	Aware of own strengths and limitations; establishes own value system
Difficulty solving problems; thinks in present; cannot use past experience to control behavior; sense of invulnerability—society's rules don't apply to him or her	Begins to solve problems, analyze, and abstract	Able to verbalize conceptually: deals with abstract moral concepts; makes decisions re future
Struggle between dependent and independent behavior; begins forming peer alliance	Established peer group alliance with associated risk-taking behavior	Peer group diminishes in importance; may develop first intimate relationship
Parent-child conflict begins; teen argues but without logic	Peak turmoil in child-family relations; able to debate issues and use some logic but not continuously	Turbulence subsides. May move away from home. More adult-like friendship with parents

The male growth spurt occurs at about the same time as penile growth and about a year after the increase in testicular size. If growth has not begun by sexual development stage 4, the boy should be evaluated for thyroid dysfunction, growth hormone adequacy, or chronic disease. Generally, a boy who is short at stage 4 will continue to grow but will be shorter than average as an adult.

Males normally experience an increase in size of breast areola. About 30 per cent or more will also experience some bilateral, nontender increase in size of the breasts. Transient breast tenderness is also common. Facial and axillary hair appear at about stage 5. Breaking and deepening of the voice also occur at this stage.

Anticipatory Guidance: Physical Development

Dramatic physical changes require adolescents to adjust to their new appearance and to develop a feeling of comfort inside their maturing physical body. Furthermore, the adolescent must cope with the emotional and social pressures that accompany these physical changes. These changes may overwhelm the adolescent or they can be used as the foundation for learning adaptation mechanisms useful later in life. The understanding of young people by parents and other adults is crucial to smooth progression through adolescence.

Both boys and girls observe their peers, see variations in development, and compare themselves with those around them. These variations produce anxiety in those who develop slightly earlier or later than their peers.

The physical assessment provides a good time to discuss physical development. Changes may be pointed out and discussed in a casual, matter-of-fact manner. Adolescents should be assured that their growth and development are normal. Because most adolescents do not ask questions they may have about their body changes or lack thereof, adults around them must anticipate questions. Characteristics of adolescent growth and development are summarized in Table 9-3.

Females

Menarche is a rather late occurrence in female sexual development. Therefore, when a girl who has not begun the growth spurt nor developed breast buds is anxious about not menstruating, the nurse can inform her of the order in which this development occurs and reassure her that sexual characteristics have a wide range of rate of development. Statistically, the adolescent girl should begin menstruation by age 13½ (or 5 years after breast development begins) and, if she has not, medical evaluation is indicated.

It is also normal for a young woman to experience irregularity in the amount of menstrual flow and in the spacing of periods. She can be reassured that for the first year or more her periods will be unpredictable. What is more, emotional changes affect the menstrual cycle; the teenage girl may find that her period is delayed during times of stress such as final examinations.

The school-age or prepubertal adolescent girl should be prepared for the onset of menstruation. Parents should be advised to obtain menstrual supplies for the girl long before she will need them. Their use should be explained and the girl allowed to become familiar with them. Myths that baths and physical exercise should be avoided during menstruation should be dispelled. Menstruation is a normal physiologic process that requires additional attention to hygiene but generally does not interrupt normal activities of the adolescent girl. If menstrual discomfort does occur, it usually does not happen until several months after menarche (after periods become ovulatory).

Another aspect of anticipatory guidance for a girl is breast self-examination. While breast cancer is rare in teenage girls, the habit of self-examination is best learned while the girl is keenly aware of and concerned about her body. See Chapter 15 for a discussion of breast examination.

Males

One of the major concerns of boys is their height; most want to be tall. If a boy's growth spurt has not occurred by the time his genitals are at stage 4, he should be medically evaluated. After an examination is done, and if no abnormalities are found, the nurse should provide an opportunity for the boy to express his feelings about being short. In 85 per cent of males who are shorter than average, the cause is familial. Health professionals should concentrate on helping the boy who will not be tall to feel good about himself.

Size of penis is also a major concern for adolescent boys and adult men. If this concern exists, the boy should be reassured that penile size is not the determining factor in being able to satisfy one's sexual partner.

Erections and nocturnal emissions (wet dreams) are signs of sexual development; however, these are often sources of great embarrassment for the young man. He should be reassured that they are normal and that the frequency of the unwanted erections will gradually decrease.

Uncircumcised boys need to be taught to retract the foreskin and carefully cleanse the glans, if they have not already learned to do so. Infections can result if this is not done. Also, the foreskin should be returned to its normal position over the glans to avoid constriction and edema of the glans.

Boys should be educated to seek medical help if they experience testicular pain. There are several conditions, some serious, that can occur in males, including injury, torsion of the testicle, and epididymitis. In addition, young men should be taught self-examination of the testicles. The best time to examine the testes is right after a hot bath. The fingers are placed under each testis and the testicle is gently rolled between the thumb and fingers. The testes are oval, measuring about 4×3 cm. The epididymis on the back of the testicle should not be confused with an abnormal lump. Lumps should be examined immediately by a doctor, as testicular cancers detected early have an excellent prognosis.

Intellectual Development

The requisites for progression to the formal operations stage are normal neurologic development, social stimulation, experience with things, a child's own cognitive reorganization occurring as a result of his or her own need to change, and the child's desire to solve a problem when concrete operations are not effective (Ginsberg and Opper, 1979). Piaget (1976) sees formal operations as a kind of reconstruction of concrete operations to a new level. Concrete operations provide the substance and pave the way for formal operations.

A concrete operational child can work well with tangible things but is limited to dealing with observable phenomena. When confronted with a problem, a school-age child can deal only with the action at hand, the here and now, and does not consider possibilities before tackling the problem (Piaget, 1976). A formal operational youth can imagine possibilities and make suppositions before acting. When solving a problem, these children can form a hypothesis, draw deductions from the hypothesis, formulate a plan to test the hypothesis, test it systematically, then interpret the results. Unexpected results are not as confusing to an adolescent as to a school-age child, because the teen has considered several possibilities (Ginsberg and Opper, 1979). Adolescents are able mentally to reverse a sequence of events so that they can better understand why something occurred (Maier, 1978). Because of the ability to form hypotheses and to reason deductively, Piaget refers to adolescent thought as *hypotheticodeductive.* Also, thought processes become more flexible and previous learning can be applied to new problems (Piaget, 1976).

Formal operational youths can understand symbolism. Metaphors or double entendres take on new meanings (Elkind, 1970). A school-age child might enjoy a metaphoric poem for the rhyme and the story it tells, but an adolescent will recognize the symbolism in the verse and realize that the image conjured is a representation of something more intangible.

Adolescents become able to understand abstract and theoretical concepts such as existentialism. They can also attach emotion to abstractions (Ginsberg and Opper, 1979). For example, a school-age child can love a puppy and hate spiders, but a teen can love peace and hate bigotry.

Future becomes a possibility. The notion of future plus the ability to make suppositions enables adolescents to construct ideals. They can think of how things "could be." In exercising this new-found ability, teens often become intolerant of people, conventional establishments, and the status quo (Elkind, 1970).

Adolescents are able to think about thinking. They think about their own thoughts and become introspective. Physical changes and introspection stimulate the self-preoccupation so typical of adolescents. They can also think about the thoughts of others. Young teens often cannot differentiate others' concerns from their own. Therefore, they erroneously believe that others are equally as interested in their behaviors, weaknesses, assets, and appearances. This is known as *adolescent egocentrism* and accounts for the characteristic self-consciousness of adolescents over things younger children and adults find insignificant. They are reacting to an *imaginary audience.* Thus, the hours attending to every detail of appearance are spent in anticipation of the audience's reaction (Elkind, 1970).

Adolescent egocentrism engenders feelings of uniqueness. Teens cannot imagine that anyone has ever been through what they have, loved as much, or suffered as much. They believe that their life events are of universal significance and that no one will ever understand them or their complex thoughts. Elkind refers to this as the *personal fable.* The feelings of uniqueness may lead to the idea that "it can never happen to me." The personal fable thus helps to explain some of the risk-taking during adolescence. By late adolescence, egocentrism diminishes. Young people begin to behave for themselves rather than for others, and discover that even though they are individuals, others have experienced similar feelings and events as they.

Progression to formal operations is not universal. Some people may never attain that level of thinking; or an individual may use formal operations in a task that has personal relevance but not in another task (Ginsberg and Opper, 1979). For example, an adolescent may use formal operations in understanding the symbolism in a play but not in solving an algebra problem.

Anticipatory Guidance: Intellectual Development

How can the foregoing knowledge help the nurse help adolescents and their parents? Sachs (1987) stresses the need to assess the cognitive developmental level of adolescent clients. Before the entry into formal operational thinking, adolescents may discuss problems with parents, but often the adolescents' arguments are critical of the parents and related to what could be or might have been. Parents' viewpoints are not easily understood or tolerated. These handicaps combined with the adolescent's limited ability to discern the emotions of other people make it important to explain one's point of view and feelings to the young adolescent patiently instead of assuming that he or she has an adult's ability to "pick up vibes" (Jersild et al, 1978).

Being unable to perceive abstractly a situation or pattern that is not immediately evident causes many young adolescents to be criticized. If an adolescent member of a family seems repeatedly to attempt a task and is unable to complete it in a mature manner, parents need to realize that the reason may be the youth's developmental stage rather than laziness or disobedience.

Upon entering the formal operational stage young people are for the first time able to think about their values and reasoning processes. Often this new ability leads adolescents to idealism. They are able to question their own and their family's religious affiliations. It may become a major time of unrest for teenagers if they find that they disagree with the basic religious values they have always considered unquestionable. Some young people feel so alienated that they become part of a counterculture, a "true believer" movement, or some "radical religion." Parents and adults should openly discuss religion and values with adolescents. They should not force their point of view but offer a point of reference.

Poor school performance is a problem experienced by some adolescents and is often a problem of cognitive development that is troublesome to parents. The process of learning is complex; after a complete history and physical examination, the school is usually the best source of advice and referral for such problems. Learning disabilities can and do lead to emotional problems and often result in the child's dropping out of school and other behavioral problems. Parents need to show interest in school work, assist with homework, and keep in close contact with teachers to be able to spot correctable problems.

Piaget's beliefs about formal operational thinking can be supplemented with the inclusion of other concepts. Some researchers see Piaget's formulations as descriptions of competencies that were never meant to allow for understanding of how particular adolescents respond to real problems in real-life situations. They believe that the effect of stress on cognitive perceptions must be taken into account. Adolescents may be able to repeat information that was provided to them but still may not be able to assimilate it and act upon it because they cannot cope with the stress it imposes. It is probably more important to focus on the content of the adolescent's thoughts than the form of those thoughts and to keep in mind the effects of individual perceptions on emotional responses to this content.

Emotional and Social Development

Identity

Formal operations enable adolescents to have an internal representation of themselves: a self-concept, or *identity.* Identity may even be a kind of cognition about the self (Ellis and Davis, 1982). Identity is displayed by one's personality. Erikson (1963) refers to the central task, crisis, or problem of the adolescent period as *identity versus role confusion.* An adolescent either develops a stable identity or remains confused, complicating adulthood with old struggles or settling on a negative identity, such as "dummy" (Maier, 1978).

Erikson (1963) believes that confusion during adolescence has several sources: The body is changing rapidly and the adolescent must come to terms with skeletal growth, development of secondary sex char-

Box 9-1
Teenage Crisis

As a teen you reach an overlook point
Where your fondest memories
And your worst fears of the past
Are put before you,
As if to test your strength.

For the past must be conquered
Before you are ready to move on.

And as you reach back through your childhood
You are forced to realize
All that you've left behind
Is now beyond your grasp.

Learning to cope with the loss
Of the you that you used to be
Is the "mid-life crisis" of a teenager.

–Andrea Foster, 1988
Age 16

acteristics, and libidinal urges. The future and the responsibilities of adulthood become real. Therefore, the sense of familiarity felt during childhood is intensely disturbed. Coming to terms with the perceived successes and failures of childhood and with the loss of the security of earlier years is a process that requires a great deal of time and emotional energy for the adolescent. The poem in Box 9-1 represents one teenager's feelings about this period. Adolescents have various means of alleviating identity confusion and of discovering their identities, including learning about their bodies and accepting the changes, experimenting with roles, seeking independence from families, identifying with a peer group, rebelling and arguing, and becoming idealistic.

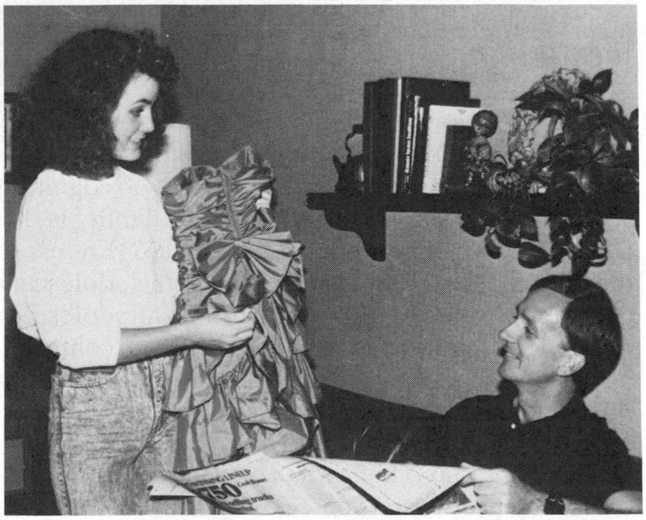
"Do you like it, Dad?" Parental support and approval can help promote development of a healthy body image.

Learning About One's Body and Accepting Its Changes

Body image is an intricate aspect of identity. It is "the picture of our own body which we form in our mind, that is to say, the way in which our body appears to ourselves" (Schilder, 1935, p. 104). Body changes and adolescent egocentrism evoke preoccupation with the body. Adolescents are acutely aware of every change. They scrutinize their bodies and compare their bodies with those of others. Preoccupation may aid in understanding and becoming familiar with one's body, and thus in gaining a clear body image (Dempsey, 1972).

Role Experimentation

An adolescent's search for identity involves experimenting with a variety of roles. A youth's earlier identifications and the roles and skills that have been learned must now be integrated (Erikson, 1963). The adolescent faces countless alternatives and combinations of choices. Adolescents' choices of roles with which to experiment are influenced by many factors such as family expectations, societal norms, and past roles that have proven effective. Teens cannot simply play multiple choice and pick the wisest alternative. They must try a role and verify its effectiveness and its consequences (Maier, 1978). This explains the changes often seen in young adolescents, such as changes in dress, academic achievement, manner of speaking, and groups of friends. Older adolescents continue some role experimentation through work or volunteer activities. For some young men and women, education and apprenticeships are still a part of role experimentation. For instance, college freshmen may change majors several times before finding a major that "fits."

Independence

Adult responsibilities and careers become tangible to adolescents. They are able to make plans for becoming independent and can suppose how independence will be. Independence from parents contributes to an adolescent's sense of individuality, and thus to his or her sense of self. The transformation from dependence to independence is a process beginning in early childhood and completed in late adolescence or early adulthood. For example, toddlers behave defiantly, school-age children walk to school without parents, young teens spend nights with friends, and older teens plan training and occupations.

Early adolescents usually use parents for role models and accept their authority. As adolescence progresses the teenager continually tests the parents and more and more freedom is demanded. By midadolescence a typical complaint is that parents give too little freedom and do not trust the adolescent. This is in conflict with parents' views: parents feel that both the freedom and trust they do offer is abused.

Parents have less and less influence in decision making as their adolescent progresses. Teens often find another adult in whom to confide. Late adolescents find their parents easier to consult. They have found ways to satisfy their need for affection and intimacy outside the home, to take responsibility for the behavioral choices they make, and to construct their values out of a sense of self rather than from rebellion so that they no longer perceive their parents as threats to their autonomy but as comrades in an adult world. During the interlude of adolescence parents must learn to be comfortable in addressing their children in an adult relationship. For many parents this task is not fully accomplished until their children become parents.

Rebellion

The process of identity formation often results in rebellious behavior. Rebellion is a way of saying, "I am different from the adults around me. I am special." Rebellion as an act of defiance, and rebellion by defending one's rights to independent thoughts and values, may engender immediate relief from parental control; therefore, feelings of self-control emerge (Friedman and Sarles, 1980). Rebellion against parental authority may be a means of affirming maturity, or an adolescent's perception of maturity. For example, a teen may think, "Children are non-drinkers. Adults are drinkers. If I drink, I can be more grown-up" (Jessor, 1982). Rebellion is harmful when it interferes with school, interpersonal relationships, physical or emotional health, or is harmful to others (vandalism or truancy, for example) (Friedman and Sarles, 1980).

Once adolescents are more confident with their own identities, they are less threatened by parental controls, philosophies, and perceived interferences (Friedman and Sarles, 1980). Although they may not conform to be like their parents, the nonconformity will be due to personal convictions, not rebellion.

Peer Group Identification

School and the peer group divisions that the school environment affords become the teen's social "miniworld." Banned from participation in adult society and insulted by the society of childhood, teenagers are forced to shape their own subculture or group identity to preserve their sense of belonging.

Belonging to a peer group helps an adolescent avoid role confusion (Erikson, 1963). Membership in a particular group provides an adolescent with a focus of identity through the clique's attitudes, behaviors, dress, and interests. Teens begin to rely on peers rather than solely on parents for sources of ideals, values, and behavior. The peer group is a kind of "social laboratory" where teens can experiment with roles and behavior (Nicholson, 1980).

As adolescents mature, they rely less on their peer group to clarify normal and accepted behavior. A clear identity enables teens to be what they want even if peers are different.

Idealism

To alleviate uncertainty, adolescents search for something enduring. The ability to imagine how things "could be" enables them to develop ideals. Ideals such as sincerity and genuineness become important, as they seem solid in a time of confusion. Teens become intolerant of things they see as being phony or hypocritical. They may not be able to understand when others do not share their ideals and often become disillusioned with people or establishments. It is very common for adolescents to devote themselves to causes such as fund-raising for the needy, ecology, or antinuclear movements (Logan, 1980). Idealism not only helps adolescents feel as if there are some enduring things in the world, but also paves the way for development of adult values and convictions (Erikson, 1963).

Anticipatory Guidance: Emotional and Social Development

"The tension between freedom and attachment and attempts to achieve the impossible union of the two" may be, as Bloom (1987) stated, "the permanent condition of man" (p. 113). Certainly, however, this tension is prevalent in the adolescent. Struggling to become a functional, stable entity independent of one's family while still maintaining needed bonds of love and support, risking one's self-esteem in forming heterosexual attachments, enduring the pain of broken relationships—such is the turbulence of this period. Add to this adolescent dilemma the fact that young people making the transition from childhood to adulthood today find themselves in a flux of societal values and traditions in which right and wrong have become relative, "situational" conditions. The struggle for identity within such ambiguous boundaries may contribute to the escalating rates of pregnancy, substance abuse, and suicide among teens. (Suicide is discussed on page 1136.)

Parents play a critical role in increasing and maintaining their adolescent's self-esteem. First, the success and self-esteem of the parents is influential in establishing self-esteem in the adolescent. Parents should pay attention to their own needs and growth. Second, parents should accept an adolescent for just *being* and express often that he or she is liked. Third, parents and teachers can emphasize positive aspects of the adolescent and not magnify negative aspects or failures. Assistance in developing strengths builds self-confidence.

The search for identity leaves the adolescent open to many influences, which can be either constructive or detrimental both to the person and to society. Adolescents often identify intensely with charismatic figures, from political personages, religious leaders, film or music stars, or professional athletes to local gang leaders. The adolescent who desperately wants "to be somebody" may, without guidance and support, settle for something which is ultimately self-destructive.

One help to developing a secure identity is investigation of vocational opportunities and the making of career plans. Parents should discuss future plans with their son or daughter. Parents cannot choose an identity for their child, however. Who or what he or she becomes must be the young person's personal choice; but parents can offer advice from their own experience when it is solicited. Open communication lines help the young person seek advice and bounce ideas off the adult without fearing ridicule or criticism.

Teenagers are old enough to get part-time, after-school, and summer jobs and should be encouraged to do so. Youth employment gives the teen a chance to explore career options and has the added advantage of helping smooth the transition from school to work. Greenberger and associates (1983) studied working youth to discover the consequences of part-time employment while still in school. They found that young people who were employed displayed a greater understanding of economic matters, demonstrated more willingness to stick to tasks, and expressed greater feelings of responsibility and self-reliance. No significant negatives appeared unless the teenager worked more than half-time, in which case these youths displayed poorer health states, demonstrated poorer academic performance, and exhibited more disturbances in family interactions. Shore (1984) describes youth employment benefits as including the following:

1. Job success builds self-esteem.
2. Money earned permits the youth greater independence from parents.
3. Because of youths' tendency to make job changes to explore various roles, there is greater exposure to different types of work before a career choice must be made.
4. The opportunity to deal with and identify with more adults exists.
5. Working provides a channel for the excess energy of youth into constructive avenues.
6. Work helps the youth test new skills against reality.

Teens should also be able to manage their own checking and savings accounts and to assist in family budgeting. Every opportunity should be used to help adolescents feel good about themselves. Recognition should be given to the teenager by providing positive verbal feedback and displaying affection and approval. Teenagers need opportunities to contribute to others. Volunteer work, running errands for an elderly neighbor, taking food to a sick friend, or any other unpaid good deed will help the teenager develop a positive self-image. Organizations such as Boy and Girl Scouts and 4-H help adolescents learn and develop a sense of pride and accomplishment.

Moral Development

Young children before the age of 9 or 10 years make moral judgments based on absolute standards of right and wrong. Preadolescents and young adolescents reach what Kohlberg (1969) calls the *conventional level of morality.* The child's judgments are based on norms and expectations of the group. The group is first the child's family, and children realize that they must live up to rules in order to win praise from parents. Later, the group is the larger society and the child's orientation is toward maintaining law and order. Older adolescents and young adults begin to realize the arbitrariness of social and legal conventions. Eventually an individual conscience and defined set of moral values are developed. Moral judgments are then founded on conscience and principles of universal understanding. Kohlberg (1969) refers to this last stage of moral development as the *postconventional* level. Preteens and young teens would approach a situation requiring moral judgment differently than would older adolescents and young adults. As an example, if presented with a story about a poor woman who must steal food in order to feed her starving children, a child in the conventional level would likely say "Stealing is bad, but the mother's duty is to provide food for her children. She should eventually pay for the food or be punished in some way." Youths at the postconventional level would discuss the story in terms of the higher principle of saving hungry children. They may conclude that the mother is morally right to steal. As with formal operations, the ability to make postconventional moral judgments is not universally attained, nor are postconventional moral judgments used exclusively.

Sex Role and Sexuality

Adolescent Sexual Development

By the time children enter first grade they have clear ideas of their own sex and of stereotypical female and male role characteristics. They have normally adopted behaviors and attitudes consistent with their gender. A child's sense of masculinity or femininity is influenced by cognitive processes and by external socialization such as family, friends, and media. During adolescence, youths integrate their present sex roles, their upsurge of sexual interest, their search for identity, and their self-esteem. Sex roles become clearer and refined and youths learn to express themselves sexually. Sexuality is thus a dimension of one's personality (Katchadourian, 1980; Graydanus, 1982).

The sexual urges felt by adolescents have generally been attributed to the same neuroendocrine process that causes puberty; however, that theory is not well founded and it is likely that psychosocial factors are equally as important as hormonal factors in "awakening" libido (Katchadourian, 1980).

As well as being a major component of identity, sexuality during adolescence may be a part of the search for identity (Erikson, 1963). Adolescents experiment with roles that make them feel more (or less) manly or womanly. They establish romantic or sexual relationships, or both, in hope of self-discovery through one another. Sexual experimentation helps adolescents to feel recognition as sexual beings and helps to answer questions regarding their normalcy (Katchadourian, 1980; Tauer, 1983).

Sexuality contributes to an individual's self-esteem. An individual's concept of having an appealing personality and body is greatly influenced by the ability to evoke desire in another (Katchadourian, 1980).

Behavioral Consequences of Adolescent Sexual Development and Implications for Nursing

Typical consequences of early adolescent sexual interest are masturbation, fantasies, attachments to same-sex friends, and crushes. Fantasies and masturbation are very natural components of sexual development. They aid a young teen to prepare mentally and physically for sexual activities (Odiorne and Tenerowicz, 1980). Teens will not generally discuss fantasies or masturbation with the health care provider, and there is usually no reason for them to; however, if teens seem anxious, the nurse can mention, during an interview or psychosocial history, that masturbation and fantasizing are very normal activities for people, especially while they are growing up.

Early teens often develop crushes on adults or

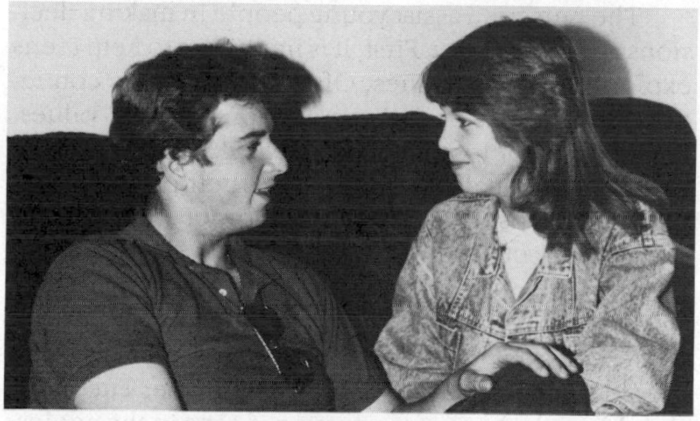

Being found attractive by a member of the opposite sex is important to an adolescent's self-esteem.

older teens of the same or opposite sex. Crushes help the adolescent choose appealing characteristics to be imitated or looked for in another. Crushes are usually short-lived and harmless unless the individual takes advantage of the adolescent's affection (Odiorne and Tenerowicz, 1980). If the parents feel concerned, they may wish to discuss the matter with the nurse, who can assure them that infatuations are normal and temporary. Naturally, the situation is different if the focus of the crush is sexually abusing the teen: then reporting the abuse, referral to the appropriate agencies, and more intensive counseling, become necessary. (See Chapter 35 for a discussion of sexual abuse.)

Attachments to same-sex friends or some experimental sexual exploration with same-sex friends is very typical of young teens. This may include spending time alone together sharing intimate secrets, practicing kissing, or comparing body parts. This kind of behavior is usually not predictive of homosexuality, but is a natural occurrence in heterosexual development. Teens and parents should be assured of the normality of experimentation and closeness of two young friends. Referral for psychotherapeutic support should be offered if the adolescent desires to be homosexual and is having psychologic stress, or if the adolescent would like to have heterosexual relationships but is having difficulty pursuing them after homosexual encounters (Committee on Adolescence, AAP, 1983).

During middle adolescence, most teens begin spending time with members of the opposite sex at school and social events and on group dates. An adolescent will eventually feel confident enough to be alone with a boy or girl and will pair off at parties or go out on single dates. By late adolescence many teens develop close relationships. Young romance teaches about loving and giving, and young people learn about qualities to look for in a future mate. The couple must decide how to deal with physical intimacy and the degree of intimacy with which they both are comfortable.

The nurse can assist young people in making decisions about sexuality. First, it is important to help teens explore their own values. Often teens' values contradict peers' values or their perception of peers' values. It sometimes helps to remind adolescents that they are unique individuals who can make their own choices. In other words, it is fine if they do not want to have sexual intercourse.

Nurses can also help the adolescent with problem solving. Formal operational thinking will enable many adolescents to think through their alternatives and consider the consequences of intercourse. The nurse should teach about reproduction if gaps in the adolescent's knowledge are discerned. Misconceptions must be dispelled. As knowledgable as adolescents may be about some aspects of sex, they often believe such myths as, "You can't get pregnant the first time." Because of a lack of experience in decision making, the nurse may need to assist by applying an everyday process of decision making. For example, in deciding which elective course to take, it may be helpful for the teen to write down alternatives and possible consequences. This makes the process seem more concrete to younger or immature adolescents. Small group discussions in the school or clinic may be helpful in sharing concerns, experiences, and practical decision making. Role-playing can also be helpful (Tauer, 1983).

Many schools now incorporate family living classes as curriculum requisites. Formal curriculum packages for use in schools, as courses in church youth programs or social agencies for youth (e.g., YM/YWCAs, ROTC, youth camps), or as college electives have also been developed, many from government grants. One such program, which has been extensively tested, refined, and evaluated across the country is a life skills education program entitled "Bridging the Gap Between Youth and Community Services" (Hofman and Cole, 1983). The premise of the 12 unit program* is that youth will make good decisions about their lives if given the information and support needed to do so. The thrust of this program is to increase youths' understanding of themselves, their feelings, and their bodies; to better understand relationships with peers, parents, and other caregivers; and to develop knowledge of community resources and how to use them. This program has received nationwide acclaim.

Nurses should always encourage parents to be involved in educating their children about sex well before adolescence as well as during adolescence. Nurses may conduct classes or provide information and instruction materials for parents. Parental discussions with children before the age of 12½ years have been shown to be very important in delaying sexual activity and its consequences (Fox, 1980).

* The program is available upon request from Peter Hofman or Elma Cole, Social Services Department, Salvation Army–Eastern Territory, New York City, New York.

General Principles of Communicating with Adolescents

Usually, young teens will come to the clinic or hospital accompanied by a parent, middle teens may come with or without a parent, and older teens may come alone. There are several ways to approach an interview with an adolescent when parents have also come. The teen may be seen first, followed by an interview and/or summary with the parent; the parent may be seen initially; or the family may be seen together for all or part of the visit. Most health care providers have an approach that is comfortable for them, or may alternate approaches depending upon the individual case. At some point, adolescents need to be seen alone so that they will feel free to discuss topics such as family problems or sexuality and so that they begin to take responsibility for their own health care (Adams, 1983).

Adolescents are frequently frightened of visiting a clinic or hospital. Younger teens especially may not be very articulate and may fear sitting and talking with an unfamiliar adult. They are also often afraid of being examined and of uncomfortable procedures that might occur. It is, therefore, important to put adolescents at ease from the beginning of the interview or visit. The nurse should discuss the events that will take place over the course of the visit and answer any questions. It may also be helpful to discuss briefly a topic of interest such as the teen's extracurricular activities (Adams, 1983).

Health care professionals often try to establish rapport with teens by behaving like teens. Adolescents seeking health care or counseling are not looking for peer support. They need health care providers to provide professional guidance, to act as adult role models, and to behave in a way that lets adolescents feel they are in competent hands. Teens view adults who try to speak and dress like teenagers as being phony. When interacting with an adolescent one can be friendly, warm, and display a good sense of humor, while still maintaining a professional manner (Felice and Friedman, 1982).

Noncommunicative or hostile behavior is usually an indication of fear. Silence may be confronted with a statement such as "I'll bet there are a lot of places you'd rather be, but I'd like to spend our time together by figuring out how I can help you." The nurse may approach an angry adolescent by a comment such as

"You seem to be pretty mad. I'm wondering if it is because you had to come here today." Sincerity and openness will often allow a teen to feel less fearful and more able to approach the subject of the interview (Adams, 1983).

Confidentiality

Confidentiality is important in good nurse-client communication. Professionals working with adolescents will often ensure confidentiality from the outset, explaining that no information shared by the teen will be discussed with the parents without the teen's permission. The adolescents should be told that the exception occurs if there is a situation that is harmful to them or others. In that instance, the nurse is responsible for talking with the parents and taking measures to remedy the situation (Adams, 1983). Adolescents will trust the nurse more, knowing he or she has been honest.

Rights of minors to give consent to treatment without parental knowledge are governed by state laws. Most states consider minors to be anyone under 18 years of age. Some states allow minors to seek and obtain health care without parental consent for sexually transmitted diseases, contraception, drug use, and abortions. Some states have *emancipated minor* provisions whereby minors may give consent for health care if they are considered by the state to be financially independent of the family. Two examples of such emancipated minors are young persons in the military and those who are married. Many courts have adopted a *mature minor rule*. The practitioner may give treatment if the minor is judged by the practitioner to be capable of understanding the nature and consequences of the treatment, and if the treatment is for the benefit of the adolescent (Dunn, 1980; Hoffman, 1980; Litt, 1983). Because of differences among state laws and the occasional alterations of laws, it is wise for nurses to be well informed of the statutes of their own state.

Health Care Services for Adolescents

The health care needs of today's youth are staggering. Of the 30 million teenagers who populate the United States, one of every two adolescents (age 15 to 19 years) is sexually active; one of every four adolescents (11 and older) drops out of school; one of every 10 adolescent girls (15 to 19) becomes pregnant each year; one of every 30 adolescents will run away from home; and one of every 600 youths (10 to 24) will die—35 per cent from motor vehicle and other accidents and 15 per cent from homicide and suicide (Alexander, 1980).

Health care is becoming specialized for adolescents. For years, it was informally considered part of both pediatrics and adult health care. Certainly the needs of adolescents are similar to those of both children and adults. However, adolescents also have unique needs based more on their stage of development than on physical differences. Teenagers have often felt out of place in both pediatric and adult health care settings. Craft (1987), studying the health care preferences of adolescents, found that adolescents tend to prefer the physician's office as a setting for health care except "when anonymity was desired for problems of substance abuse and birth control." In most instances, parents were identified as the companion of choice to accompany the adolescent. Factors such as this should be kept in mind when planning health care services for adolescents.

In the 1950s the special health needs of teenagers were recognized. Dr. Roswell Gallagher, a Boston internist, was a leader in this movement. Several outpatient clinics were opened that centered on diseases prevalent in adolescents, such as rheumatic heart disease and diabetes. These clinics were highly successful and were followed by adolescent hospital inpatient units and an increasing number of outpatient units specifically for adolescents. The federal government has begun to establish adolescent health care clinics. Some of these focus on specific needs such as birth control, while others are comprehensive in their approach and still others are research-oriented. Other services available to adolescents include school health programs and college health services. Several cities have responded to the emergency health needs of adolescents (particularly runaways) by establishing free clinics. Crisis hot lines have been set up in various cities and serve as effective entries for adolescents into the health care system. Other approaches include multiservice centers where medical and counseling services are available. Services for teenage parents are also becoming more common.

Adolescent Health Care

Adolescents should be seen by a physician or other primary care provider at least every 2 years, even if no problems arise. During routine health visits the health professional should provide guidance and counseling based on the individual needs of the adolescent. Anticipatory guidance is basic to adolescent health maintenance, as it is at any age. The health care provider working with adolescents requires knowledge in such areas as personal care, dental care, nutrition, sexually transmitted diseases, birth control, substance abuse, and accidents.

Personal Care

Adolescents may be known both for sleeping "all the time" and for chronically "burning the candle at both ends." The actual amount of sleep required by an adolescent covers a wide range. Rather than state a specific number of hours, it is wiser to advise parents to be cognizant of their adolescent's sleep patterns and symptoms of fatigue. Many other effects can result from a lack of adequate sleep, such as crankiness, accidents and frustration. If the sleep pattern changes suddenly, a call or visit to a primary care provider is in order.

Headaches are a common complaint of adolescents, and tension headaches are the most common recurrent form (Debrun, 1981). The school nurse is usually the health care provider to whom complaints of headaches are taken. Debrun (1981) stated that nursing management of the adolescent with a headache should include a complete assessment including history and measures to decrease the effects of stressors that may precipitate the headache.

A sufficient amount of exercise, sunshine, and fresh air is important to young people's emotional as well as physical health. Fresh air and change of scene can reduce tensions built up by the relative immobilization of the classroom.

Depending on when initial childhood immunizations were completed, Td boosters as well as periodic tuberculin testing will be necessary sometime during the adolescent years. (See well-child maintenance schedule in Chapter 14.)

Dental Care

A full set of permanent teeth is expected by age 13 with the exception of the wisdom teeth, which erupt by 22 to 23 years of age. Adequate dental maintenance includes proper brushing at least twice a day, daily flossing, and regular dental visits as recommended. An adequate supply of fluoride is needed to help prevent cavities and can be obtained from treated drinking water (1 part per million), from topical application in the dentist's office, or from oral fluoride tablets if the drinking supply has no fluoride. (See Chapter 19 for a full discussion.)

Nutrition

Total nutritional needs are greater during adolescence than at any other time (Marino and King, 1980). (See Chapter 18 for RDAs.) Caloric and protein requirements increase for boys from age 11 to 18. Girls at this age have a slightly increased protein need, but caloric needs decrease. The iron needed by the adolescent is almost double that needed by the adult male or the postmenopausal woman. Iodine is necessary for proper thyroid function and the need rises sharply during the growth spurt. Calcium required for skeletal and dental growth also increases during the growth spurt. Niacin and thiamine needs increase during adolescence in males. Most of these nutrient needs drop after adolescence. Chapter 18 describes nutritional assessment and the servings of each food group needed by adolescents.

Nutritional counseling should focus on the four basic food groups, and should be done with the adolescent's likes and dislikes and cultural influences in mind. Relating nutrition and appearance is an effective way to obtain a teenager's interest in nutrition. Adolescents like snacking, which is a part of most social events. The nurse can teach teens about healthy snacking and about avoidance of high-fat, high-carbohydrate "fast foods." Fad diets and overzealous dieting should be highly discouraged. (See Chapter 36 for a discussion of anorexia and obesity in adolescents.)

Nurses are often asked to advise athletes on nutrition needs. No special formulas or supplements are necessary, with the exception of the young female athlete, for whom it is recommended to take 30 to 60 mg of iron per day. The best diet for athletes is to eat from the four basic food groups as outlined in Chapter 18. The number of servings from each group will depend upon the energy requirement of the individual and the sport. Cold water is the best hydrating beverage (Marino and King, 1980; Committee on Sports Medicine, AAP, 1983).

Sexually Transmitted Diseases (STDs)

The incidence of sexually transmitted disease (STDs) is very high among adolescents in the United States. Approximately one million cases of gonorrhea are reported annually, and nearly 25 per cent of those cases involve adolescents. It is therefore imperative that sexually active adolescents be screened for STDs, even when they are asymptomatic.

Recommended tests for sexually active adolescents include:

Females: Annual (or semiannual in high risk groups) Pap smear, cervical gonorrhea culture, cervical *Chlamydia* culture, syphilis serology, and vaginal wet mount.

Males: Annual syphilis serology and in high-risk groups annual urethral cultures for gonorrhea and *Chlamydia.* Homosexual males will also need rectal and pharyngeal cultures for gonorrhea.

Adolescents at risk for AIDS and those who have had partners who were at risk for AIDS should be tested for the AIDS virus. Pretest and post-test counseling by a skilled professional is an important part of AIDS screening. See Chapter 43 for further information about AIDS.

As a part of their annual physical examinations, sexually active adolescents require careful examination of the genitalia. Too often this part of the examination is omitted to spare the patient embarrassment. Unfortunately, this results in missed cases of condylomata acuminata (genital warts), herpes, *Phthirus pubis* (crab lice), primary syphilitic chancre, and other STDs.

Education is the only way to prevent the continued rampant spread of STDs. It is the nurse's responsibility to counsel *all* adolescents about STDs, whether or not the young person is sexually active. Further discussion of STDs is found in Chapter 45.

Birth Control

The prevalence of sexual intercourse in American adolescents is high, and studies have confirmed that the rate is increasing (Zelnik and Kantner, 1980). Most adolescents are sexually active 6 to 12 months prior to seeking birth control (Zelnik and Kantner, 1980; Kalmuss, 1986). The risks are significant. Over one million teens become pregnant annually (Burke, 1987). The costs of teenage pregnancy are significant for teens, their families, and for society. As noted by Edelman (1987),*

1. Only 50 per cent of the teens who become parents graduate from high school.
2. Teen mothers are twice as likely as older mothers to be poor.
3. Infants born to teen mothers are at a significantly greater risk for low birthweight and other health problems because pregnant adolescents frequently fail to obtain adequate prenatal care.
4. Special hospital care for low birthweight babies averages $1000 per day.
5. Medicaid pays for 30 per cent of hospital deliveries for adolescents at an annual cost of about $200 million.
6. The public cost for babies born to teenage girls in 1985 was $1.4 billion.

For teens who choose to be sexually active, the nurse has a primary role in making birth control accessible and in helping teens to make informed decisions about birth control methods.

Withdrawal is a method of birth control used by some teens. It is free, involves no devices, and is always available. The couple have intercourse until just before ejaculation. Then the penis is removed from the vagina and the sperm is deposited at a distance from the vagina. The biggest problem with this method is its low rate of effectiveness. The reasons for this are that some sperm escape even before ejaculation, and timing of withdrawal before the moment of ejaculation is very difficult to control. Therefore, withdrawal is not recommended as a form of birth control.

The *condom,* or rubber, is another common birth control device used by teens. Condoms are relatively cheap, available without the need to visit a health care professional, and allow a male to control his fertility. Many clinics provide condoms at no charge. They prevent pregnancy by providing a barrier between the penis and the cervix. When used properly, the condom is very effective. When used with contraceptive foam, the effectiveness rate approaches that of oral contraceptives. *All* sexually active adolescents should be encouraged to use condoms every time they have intercourse, even if using another form of birth control. Some precautions for the young client using condoms are:

1. Use only latex condoms.
2. Keep condoms away from heat (such as body heat from keeping them in a wallet).
3. Be sure to put the condom on before the penis gets anywhere near the vagina.
4. Leave a half-inch space at the end of the condom.
5. Be sure to hold on to the condom when the penis is withdrawn from the vagina.
6. If the rubber breaks or tears, insert contraceptive foam into the vagina immediately.

Condoms are very effective in preventing the spread of venereal disease and AIDS. See page 1590 for a discussion of AIDS.

Contraceptive foam may also be used alone. The foam is placed in the vagina before intercourse by means of an applicator. The foam then blocks entry across or through the cervix and immobilizes or kills the sperm. Use with condoms greatly increases effectiveness of the foam, which also serves as a lubricant. The user must remember to:

1. Shake the can well before dispensing.
2. Fill the applicator completely full.
3. Insert the foam just before intercourse.
4. Insert more foam if she has intercourse again.
5. Insert as far as comfortably possible so the foam will cover the cervix.
6. Avoid douching for at least eight hours after intercourse.
7. Wash the applicator with soap and warm water.

Foam may also help prevent some STDs and AIDS.

* See Chapter 37 for in-depth discussion of the consequences of adolescent pregnancies.

Allergies to foam can sometimes be prevented by switching brands.

The *rhythm method,* also known as the *calendar method,* is also used by some adolescents. Unfortunately, many are grossly misinformed about this method. Its use requires knowledge, skill, and motivation to be successful; however, even when used properly, it is not very effective. The *calendar method* is based on the fact that ovulation usually occurs 14 days before the onset of menstruation in a regular 28-day cycle. Sperm live for 2 to 3 days, and the ovum survives about 24 hours. The woman must chart her cycles for at least 8 months, then subtract 18 days from her shortest cycle and 11 days from her longest cycle; the period of time between those days is her fertile time. For example, if her longest cycle (space between first days of two periods) was 30 days and her shortest was 25 days, she should abstain from sexual intercourse between days 7 and 19 of each cycle. A central problem with this method is that adolescent girls have irregular menstrual cycles. It is also not a preferred method of adolescents because it requires abstinence for a period of time each month and time calculations are complicated.

The *intrauterine device (IUD)* is one contraceptive method for which the young woman must seek medical advice. The IUD is a small plastic appliance, sometimes containing copper or progesterone, that is inserted by the practitioner into the uterus. The IUD's precise mechanism of action is unknown, but it somehow prevents implantation of the embryo on the uterine wall. Some conditions contraindicating use of an IUD include active pelvic infection, pregnancy, abnormal Pap smear, abnormal uterine bleeding, and allergy to copper (if the device contains copper). Some doctors will not insert IUDs into young women who have never been pregnant, because of their greater incidence of pelvic infection when using an IUD (Faulkner and Ory, 1976). It is not known, however, whether the IUD itself is responsible for the increased incidence of pelvic inflammatory disease, or whether girls who use IUDs are simply more sexually active and thus more prone to developing pelvic inflammatory disease (Klein, 1980).

IUDs are relatively effective in controlling pregnancy. It is somewhat easier to insert an IUD during menses, and if the device is placed at this time, a pregnancy is unlikely to exist already. Insertion is likely to cause some cramping or nausea, so it is a good idea to have someone else drive the girl home after insertion of the IUD. Precautions to warn the user about are: (1) The string should be checked monthly after each menses; (2) there is a chance that the IUD may perforate the uterus; (3) there is an increased chance of developing pelvic inflammatory disease. IUD users should call their doctor immediately if a period is missed or if symptoms of vaginal infection occur. Because of their association with pelvic inflammatory disease, IUDs are not generally recommended for adolescents. Also, many IUDs have been taken off the market because of lawsuits against the manufacturers.

The *diaphragm* is a dome-shaped latex cup with a flexible rim that is inserted into the vagina. It must be fitted by a health professional, for both size and type. The diaphragm is always used with a spermicidal cream, foam, or jelly and serves to hold the spermicidal agent against the cervical os. Effectiveness is directly correlated with proper use of the diaphragm. The diaphragm is inserted no more than 2 hours before intercourse by folding and inserting it, jelly side up, into the vagina, or by use of an applicator. It *must* be checked by inserting a finger into the vagina to feel for the cervix inside the dome's rim. Subsequent intercourse must be preceded by an application of more spermicide. To remove the diaphragm, a finger is hooked on the rim and it is pulled down and out.

The wearer must be sure to leave the diaphragm in place at least 6 hours after the last intercourse, and should not douche. The diaphragm should be washed and dried carefully, dusted with cornstarch, and kept in its case. A return visit is necessary to have the fit checked after 1 to 2 weeks of use and after a pregnancy, pelvic surgery, weight gain or loss of 10 to 20 pounds, or if any discomfort is experienced. One diaphragm should last about 2 years but should be checked regularly near a light for holes or tears.

Oral contraceptives, or birth control pills, are used by 10 to 15 million women in the United States. The oral contraceptives containing a combination of estrogen and progestogen suppress ovulation by inhibiting the secretion of hypothalamic gonadotropin-releasing hormone, and may also act directly on the pituitary to inhibit release of gonadotropins. The combination pill also causes development of "hostile cervical mucus," which decreases the chance of sperm penetration. Contraindications to using the pill include cardiovascular disorders, migraine headaches, liver problems, malignancy, and pregnancy.* Pills containing 50 mg of estrogen or less are preferred for adolescents (Klein, 1980).

The pills are taken once a day for 21 days, followed by a 7-day "off" period before another 21-day cycle is resumed. The 28-day cycle of pills (containing 7 days' worth of inert pills) is recommended for the adolescent because with it she simply takes a pill every morning instead of having to interrupt and resume the sequence.

To be given a prescription for oral contraceptives, a girl must have a complete physical examination, including a Pap smear, hematocrit, blood pressure, and

---

* For a full discussion of the various types of oral contraceptives, and their benefits and risks when used by adolescents, see *Contraceptive Technology,* published annually.

tests for sexually transmitted diseases. The worst (life-threatening) side effects of oral contraceptives are blood clots in the legs, pelvis, lungs, or brain; liver tumors; and hypertension.

The nurse can be helpful in counseling the young woman in the importance of taking her pill every day. If a pill is missed, two should be taken the next day. If two or more are missed, the girl should avoid intercourse until menses occurs or use another contraceptive method in addition to completing the rest of the pill cycle. Any side effects such as spotting, nausea, or weight gain should be reported to a doctor or nurse practitioner. Questions should be encouraged. The girl's nutritional requirements for vitamins C, B_6, and B_{12} and folic acid are increased by taking oral contraceptives. The nurse should assess the teen's diet and recommend foods that are high in B complex vitamins and vitamin C (Hatcher et al, 1978).

Adolescents are known to be poor contraceptors even after securing a birth control method (Litt et al, 1980). There is no way to ensure compliance but it may be helpful to assure confidentiality, to explain the birth control method simply and completely, to discuss the risks of pregnancy versus the risks of contraception, and to schedule frequent follow-up visits. (See Chapter 37 for an in-depth discussion of teen pregnancy and parenting.)

Substance Abuse

Abuse of psychoactive substances is a growing concern to individuals providing health care services to adolescents. Adolescents may turn to drugs and alcohol for many reasons. For some teens these substances provide "false courage" in threatening social situations or "make the world seem more bearable" when social anxiety causes withdrawal from peer interactions. Substance abuse may be subconsciously encouraged by parents, or the adolescent may use substance abuse to divert parental attention from marital problems. Some teenagers use alcohol or drugs because they believe this makes them seem grown up (Rice and Kibbee, 1983). (See page 1128 for a complete discussion of substance abuse.)

Accidents

Accidents are the leading cause of adolescent mortality. Motor vehicle accidents are the leading cause of death and are often intoxicant-related, with adolescents being passengers or drivers. Following motor vehicle accidents, the primary accidents causing death in teenagers are those caused by drowning, firearms, and poisoning (National Center for Health Statistics, 1982; United States Morbidity and Mortality Weekly Report, 1982).

Peer pressure, high energy, intoxication, and feelings of being indestructable cause recklessness in adolescents. Nurses play an instrumental role in accident prevention. They should work toward strict drinking and driving laws and support organizations that promote responsible behavior, such as MADD in the United States and PRIDE in Canada. In states where the drinking age was raised, there was a 29 per cent decrease in motor vehicle accidents (Wagnaar, 1981). If a teen has made the choice to drink alcohol or smoke marijuana, the nurse should present alternatives to driving while intoxicated. Such options include taking public transportation or calling friends or family for a ride home. Many parents would rather pick their teen up after a party than allow drunken driving.

Nurses must advise their adolescent patients to take swimming and water safety classes, and never to swim while intoxicated. Nonswimmers can take swimming classes during the winter so that they can join friends in summer swimming without taking risks.

Stricter gun control laws would very likely decrease the incidence of accidental shootings. Nurses should encourage gun control regulations. If parents insist on having guns at home, for hunting, for example, the guns must never be kept loaded at home and parents must teach their teens gun safety and proper handling.

Accidental poisonings in adolescents are most often by psychoactive substances, usually barbiturates (Leitman, 1983). Excess ingestion occurs in a teen who is already intoxicated, or in one who thinks that more is better; or fatal accidental overdose may be caused by addiction.

References

Adams BN: Adolescent health care: needs, priorities, and services. *Nurs Clin North Am* 1983; 18:237–247.

Alexander A: Adolescent health: Challenge of the 80's. *J School Health* 1980 Jan; 471.

Behrman RE, Vaughan VC (eds): *Nelson Textbook of Pediatrics.* 13th ed. Philadelphia, WB Saunders, 1987.

Bloom A: *The Closing of the American Mind: How Higher Education Has Failed Democracy and Impoverished the Souls of Today's Students.* New York, Simon and Schuster, 1987.

Buhrmester S, Furman W: The development of companionship and intimacy. *Child Dev* 1987; 58:1101–1113.

Burke PJ: Adolescents' motivation for sexual activity and pregnancy prevention. *Issues Compr Pediatr Nurs* 1987; 10:161–171.

Chassin L, et al: Changes in peer and parent influence during adolescence: longitudinal versus cross-sectional perspectives on smoking initiation. *Dev Psychol* 1986; 22:327–334.

Clasen DR, Eicher SA: Perceptions of peer pressure, peer conformity dispositions, and self-reported behavior among adolescents. *Dev Psychol* 1986; 22:521–530.

Committee on Adolescence, American Academy of Pediatrics: Homosexuality and adolescence. *Pediatrics* 1983; 72:249–250.

Committee on Sports Medicine, American Academy of Pediatrics: Nutrition and athletic performance. *In* Smith NJ (ed): *Sports Medicine: Health Care for Young Athletes.* Evanston, IL, AAP, 1983, 161–175.

Craft MJ: Health care preferences of rural adolescents: types of services and companion choices. *J Pediatr Nurs* 1987; 2:3–12.

Debrun SR: Headaches in adolescents. *MCN* 1981; 6:407–411.

Dempsey M: Development of body image in the adolescent. *Nurs Clin North Am* 1972; 7:609, 615.

Dornbusch SM, et al: Single parents, extended households, and the control of adolescents. *Child Dev* 1985; 56:326–341.

Dunn LJ: Legal aspects of communication with and about the pediatric patient. *Issues Compr Pediatr Nurs* 1980; 4:13–18.

Duvall EM: *Family Development.* 3rd ed. New York, JB Lippincott, 1967.

Duvall EM: *Marriage and Family Development.* New York, JB Lippincott, 1977.

Edelman MW: Teenage pregnancy: an epidemic takes its toll. *In* Cohn AR, Leach LA (eds): *Generations.* New York, Pantheon Books, 1987.

Elkind D: *Children and Adolescents, Interpretive Essays on Jean Piaget.* New York, Oxford University Press, 1970.

Ellis DW, Davis LT: The development of self-concept boundaries across the adolescent years. *Adolescence* 1982; 17:695–710.

Erikson EH: *Childhood and Society.* 2nd ed. New York, WW Norton, 1963.

Erikson EH: *Identity and the Life Cycle: Selected Papers, Psychological Issues* (monogr). Vol 1, No 1. New York, International Press, 1959.

Faulkner WL, Ory HW: Intra-uterine devices and acute pelvic inflammatory disease. *JAMA* 1976; 253:1851–1853.

Felice ME, Friedman SB: Behavioral considerations in the health care of adolescents. *Pediatr Clin North Am* 1982; 29:399–413.

Fox GL: *Mothers and Their Teenaged Daughters.* Detroit, The Merrill-Palmer Institute, 1979.

Fox GL: *Mother-Daughter Communication Patterns re Sexuality.* Final report. Grant No. HD11224 (NINHC), September 1, 1977, to February 3, 1980.

Friedman SV, Sarles RM: "Out of control" behavior in adolescents. *Pediatr Clin North Am* 1980; 27:99–107.

Ginsberg H, Opper S: *Piaget's Theory of Intellectual Development.* 2nd ed. Englewood Cliffs, NJ, Prentice-Hall, 1979.

Gjerde PF: The interpersonal structure of family interaction settings: parent-adolescent relations in dyads and triads. *Dev Psychol* 1986; 22:297–304.

Gordon M: *Manual of Nursing Diagnosis.* New York, McGraw-Hill, 1987.

Greenberger E, Steinberg L: Statement on proposed changes in Child Labor Regulations. *Am Psychol* 1983 Jan; 38(1):105–109.

Greydanus DE: Adolescent sexuality: an overview and perspective for the 1980s. *Pediatr Ann* 1982; 11:714–726.

Hanson SMH: Healthy single-parent families. *Fam Rel* 1986; 35:125–132.

Hanson SMH, Sporakowski MJ: Single parent families. *Fam Rel* 1986; 35:3–8.

Hatcher RA, et al: *Contraceptive Technology 1978–1979.* New York, Irvington Publishers, 1978.

Hetherington EM, Cox M, Cox R: Long-term effects of divorce and remarriage on the adjustment of children. *J Am Acad Child Psychiatr* 1985; 24:518–530.

Hoffman AD: A rational policy toward consent and confidentiality in adolescent health care. *J Adolesc Health Care* 1980; 1:9–17.

Hofman P, Cole E: Bridging the gap between youth and community services: a life skills education program. *Child Today* 1983 May/Jun; 17–22.

Huba GJ, Bentler PM: The role of peer and adult models for drug taking at different stages in adolescence. *J Youth Adolesc* 1980; 9:449–465.

Jersild AT, et al: *The Psychology of Adolescence.* New York, Macmillan, 1978.

Jessor R: Problem behavior and developmental transition in adolescence. *J Sch Health* 1982; 52:295–300.

Kalmuss D: Contraceptive use: a comparison between ever- and never-pregnant adolescents. *J Adolesc Health Care* 1986; 7:3332–3337.

Kaltar N, Pickar J, Lesowitz M: School-based development facilitation groups for children of divorce: a preventive intervention. *Am J Orthopsychiatr* 1984; 54:613–623.

Kastner LS: Ecological factors predicting adolescent contraceptive use: implications for intervention. *J Adolesc Health Care* 1984 Apr; 5(2):79–86.

Katchadourian H: Adolescent sexuality. *Pediatr Clin North Am* 1980; 27:17–28.

Klein JR: Update: adolescent gynecology. *Pediatr Clin North Am* 1980; 27:141–152.

Kohlberg L: *Stages in the Development of Moral Thought and Action.* New York, Holt, Rinehart, and Winston, 1969.

Kuhnen KK, et al: A computer for teaching sex education. *MCN* 1983; 8:350–353.

Leitman PS: Chemical and drug poisoning. *In* Behrman RE, Vaughan VC (eds): *Nelson Textbook of Pediatrics.* 12th ed. Philadelphia, WB Saunders, 1983, pp 1786–1797.

Litt IF: Legal issues in adolescent care. *In* Behrman RE, Vaughan VC, (eds): *Nelson Textbook of Pediatrics.* 12th ed. Philadelphia, WB Saunders, 1983, p 1529.

Litt IF, Cuskey WR, Rudd ST: Identifying the adolescent at risk for contraceptive non-compliance. *J Pediatr* 1980; 96:742–745.

Logan RD: Identity, purity, and ecology. *Adolescence* 1980; 15:409–413.

Maier HW: *Three Theories of Child Development.* 3rd ed. New York, Harper and Row, 1978.

Marino DD, King JC: Nutritional concerns during adolescence. *Pediatr Clin North Am* 1980; 27:125–139.

Miller H: *Approaches to Adolescent Health Care in the 1970's.* Washington, DC, DHEW Pub (HSA) 76-5014, 1975.

National Center for Health Statistics: *Vital Statistics of the United States, 1978.* Hyattsville, MD, 1982.

Nelms BC: What is a normal adolescent? *MCN* 1981; 6:402–406.

Nelson PT: Newsletters: an effective delivery mode for providing educational information and emotional support to single-parent families? *Fam Rel* 1986; 35:183–188.

Nicholson SW: Growth and development. *In* Howe J (ed): *Nursing Care of Adolescents.* New York, McGraw-Hill, 1980, pp 1–31.

Odiorne J, Tenerowicz C: Adolescent sexuality. *In* Howe J (ed): *Nursing Care of Adolescents.* New York, McGraw-Hill, 1980, pp 246–280.

Piaget J, Inhelder B: *The Growth of Logical Thinking from Childhood to Adolescence* (trans Parson A, Seagrin S). New York, Basic Books, 1958.

Piaget J: *The Psychology of Intelligence.* Towota, NJ, Littlefield, Adams and Co, 1976.

Rice MA, Kibbee PE: Review: identifying the adolescent substance abuser. *MCN* 1983 Mar–Apr; 8(2): 139–142.

Sachs B: Cognitive screening for adolescent health education. *J Pediatr Nurs* 1987; 2:113–119.

Schilder P: *The Image and Appearance of the Human Body.* London, Kegan Paul, 1935.

Sedgwick R, Hildebrand S: The adolescent at risk: crisis, the delicate balance. *In* Howe J (ed): *Nursing Care of Adolescents.* New York, McGraw-Hill, 1980, pp 281–304.

Shore M: Youth employment: curse or blessing? *Child Today* 1984 Jan/Feb; 6–8.

Steinberg L: Latchkey children and susceptibility to peer pressure: an ecological analysis. *Dev Psychol* 1986; 22:433–439.

Steinberg L: Single parents, stepparents, and the susceptibility of adolescents to antisocial peer pressure. *Child Dev* 1987; 58:269–275.

Steinman SB, Zemmelman SE, Knoblauch TM: A study of parents who sought joint custody following divorce: who reaches agreement and sustains joint custody and who returns to court. *J Am Acad Child Psychiatr* 1985; 24:554–562.

Tanner JM: *Growth at Adolescence.* Oxford, Blackwell Scientific Publications, 1962.

Tauer KM: Promoting effective decision-making in sexually active adolescents. *Nurs Clin North Am* 1983; 18:275–292.

United States Morbidity and Mortality Weekly Report: Alcohol-related highway fatalities among young drivers. *MMWR* 1982; 31:641–644.

Wagnaar A: The raising of the legal drinking age in Michigan and Maine. Rockville, MD, National Institute on Alcohol and Alcoholism, 1981.

Zelnik M, Kantner J: Sexual activity, contraceptive use, and pregnancy among metropolitan-area teenagers: 1971–1979. *Fam Plann Perspect* 1980 Sep-Oct; 12(5):230–237.

Zill N: *Happy, Healthy, and Insecure.* New York, Doubleday, 1984.

Bibliography

Babington MA: Adolescent use of oral contraception. *MCN* 1984; 10:111–114.

Bearinger L: Priorities for adolescent health: recommendations of a national conference. *MCN* 1987 May-Jun; 12(3):161–162, 164.

Catrone C, Sadler LS: A developmental model for teen-age parent education. *J School Health* 1984; 54:63–67.

Chard M: An approach to examining the adolescent male. *MCN* 1976 Jan/Feb; 1:41.

Church JL: Examination of the adolescent: a practical guide. *J Pediatr Health Care* 1987 Feb; 2(1):3–12; Mar-Apr; 1(2):65–72.

Craft JM: Health care preferences of rural adolescents: types of service and companion choices. *J Pediatr Nurs* 1987 Feb; 2(1):3–12.

Daniel W: *Adolescents for Health and Disease.* St Louis, CV Mosby, 1977.

Daniel W, Brown R: Adolescent physical maturation. *J Curr Adolesc Med* 1979 Jun.

Elkind D: Teenagers and sex. *Parents* 1987 Jan; 62(1):127.

Fam Plann Perspect 1980; 12:320–337.

Finklestein JW: The endocrinology of adolescence. *Pediatr Clin North Am* 1980; 27:53–69.

Gibbs JT: Black adolescents and youth: an endangered species. *Am J Orthopsychiatr* 1984; 54:6–21.

Harlan W, et al: Secondary sex characteristics of boys 12 to 17 years of age: the U.S. Health Examination Survey. *J Pediatr* 1979 June; 293.

Harlan W, et al: Secondary sex characteristics of girls 12 to 17 years of age: the U.S. Health Examination Survey. *J Pediatr* 1980 June; 6.

Kosidek J: Improving health care for troubled youth. *Am J Nurs* 1976 Jan.

Magilvy JK: The health of teenagers: a focused ethnographic study. *Public Health Nurs* 1987 Mar; 4(1):35–42.

McBride AB: The secret of a good life with your teenager: thriving in the second decade of parenthood. New York, Times Books, 1987.

Mercer RT: *Perspectives on Adolescent Health Care.* Philadelphia, JB Lippincott, 1979.

Nelms BC: Adolescent health care—the need is great. *J Pediatr Health Care* 1987 Mar-Apr; 1(2):59.

Piaget J: Intellectual evolution from adolescence to adulthood. *Hum Dev* 1972; 15:1–12.

Pramik M: Too short/too tall. *Transitions* 1979; 2(2).

Wells G: Reducing the threat of a first pelvic exam. *MCN* 1977 Sep/Oct; 2:304.

Proctor SE: A developmental approach to pregnancy prevention with early adolescent females. *J School Health* 1986 Oct; 56(8):313–316.

Reichert K: *Primary Care of Young Adults.* New Hyde Park, NY, Medical Examination Publishing, 1976.

Smart M, Smart R: *Adolescents: Development and Relationships.* New York, Macmillan, 1978.

Smith J, Felice ME: Interviewing the adolescent patient. *Pediatr Ann* 1980; 9:38–44.

Stephens G: The creative contraries: a theory of sexuality. *Am J Nurs* 1978 Jan.

Thornburg HD: Adolescent sources of information on sex. *J School Health* 1981; 51:274–277.

Ticky A, Malasanos L: The physiological role of hormones in puberty. *MCN* 1976 Sep/Oct; 384.

Unit Three

Health Promotion

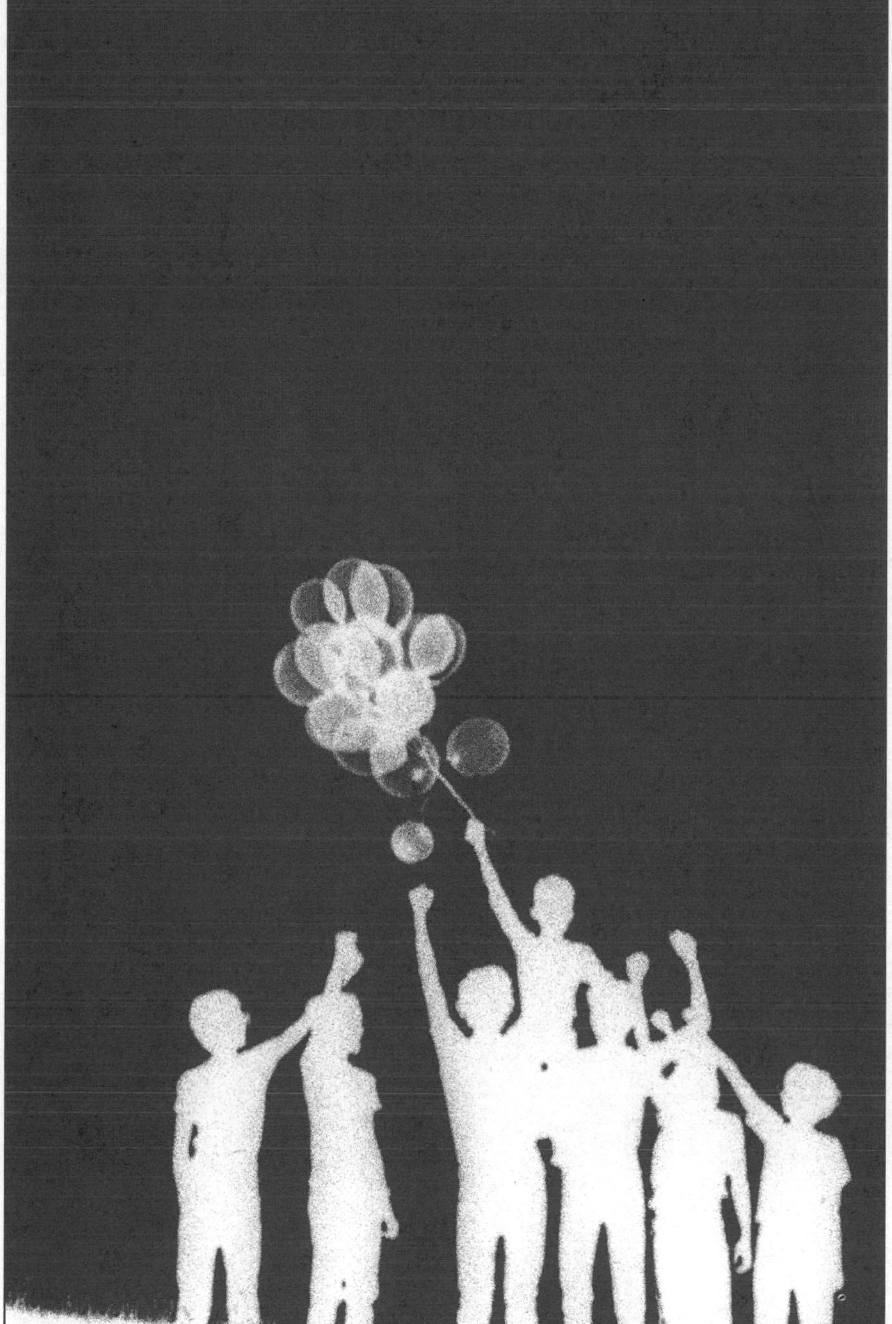

Health Concepts: Children's Perceptions and Behaviors

Chapter 10

Mabel Hunsberger

To a large extent, children's adoption of healthy behaviors is influenced by role models and environmental factors. Children's beliefs about how people stay healthy and how they get sick also influence their health practices. This chapter reviews children's concepts of health at the different developmental stages and how they affect healthy behaviors, as well as nursing strategies that promote those behaviors.

Promoting healthy behaviors in children is an exciting challenge to nurses in all health care settings. Because children model the behavior of others, health promotion of children necessarily focuses on the entire family. Self-responsibility of each family member for maintaining and improving health is the nurse's ultimate goal.

Self-care behavior involves the steps of (1) identifying personal health needs, (2) developing problem-solving skills, and (3) taking responsibility for self-care. To facilitate this process, the nurse uses many techniques and skills: (1) establishing a working relationship, (2) being supportive, (3) building parental self-esteem, (4) providing information to increase parenting success, and (5) reinforcing parental credibility. The nurse teaches, counsels, and initiates referrals.

Related Topics
Assessing and promoting family health, Chapter 12
Promoting Well Child Care, Chapter 14
Concepts of stress, coping, and illness, Chapter 23
Teaching approaches, Chapter 31

Health Concepts: Maintenance, Promotion, and Disease Prevention

Nursing Diagnoses	Nursing Goals/Strategies
Potential health maintenance alteration • *related to child's limited understanding of health associated with developmental level*	Encourage health-promoting behaviors appropriate for developmental level • Show health-promoting behaviors by example (role model) • Reward enactment of positive behaviors • Encourage child to express personal health goals and plan of action • Correct misconceptions about cause and effect relationships • Use teaching methods, materials, and approaches appropriate for developmental level (see Table 10-1)
• *related to lack of opportunity for child to participate in managing own health needs*	Promote self-care management appropriate for child's developmental level • Determine child's perception of health needs • Assist child to identify and evaluate various options available to achieve a health goal • Provide additional knowledge required to make health care decisions • Give progressively more opportunities to child for health care decisions • Teach parents to involve child in personal health care
• *related to ineffective role modeling of health-promoting behaviors*	Promote health practices in individuals and families • Involve parents in identifying the factors that influence their child's health-promoting behaviors • Raise parents' awareness about the impact of their own role modeling • Help the family members change their own behaviors through giving information and making referrals
• *related to inadequate support of caregivers in the health care of children*	Promote parenting behaviors that support child in health-promoting behaviors • Build parents' self-esteem • Provide information needed by parents to promote the child's health • Reinforce parents' credibility by complimenting them and conveying confidence in their decisions • Provide anticipatory guidance to parents, especially in areas that potentially cause conflict (see Box 10-4)

Most health care professionals agree that health promotion should be a major goal of health care. The public, too, is concerned about health hazards and is aware of the effects of lifestyle on health. Although both the professional literature and popular media reflect the importance of health promotion, whether health care focuses on *health* is debatable. More than 95 percent of health resources are directed toward treatment of illness; less than 5 percent are used for prevention of disease, health maintenance, and health promotion (Bedworth and Bedworth, 1982).

Nurses have great opportunities to promote children's health. Anticipatory guidance (counseling and teaching parents about children's health and growth and development) helps families provide a growth environment that fosters health, which must be supported by the lifestyle of the entire family. Thus, a pediatric nurse facilitates the attainment of growth and developmental milestones and promotes healthful living patterns and health habits, to the maximum satisfaction of the child and family.

Dilemmas arise in translating the goals of health promotion into practical nursing strategies because of the diversity of beliefs about two key questions: What is health? and What motivates healthy behavior? These questions are the subject of much debate and research. When applied to children, the questions are even more perplexing because (1) children's views of health are poorly defined; (2) children's views of health change over time because they are a function of cognitive development; and (3) the mechanisms that prompt children and families to carry out health behaviors are not well understood.

This chapter examines various definitions of health, identifies health subconcepts that are important to pediatric nursing, and reviews available literature concerning the development of children's health attitudes and behaviors. Practice strategies and nursing roles appropriate for the care of children and families are identified based on current knowledge concerning children's health beliefs and behaviors.

A Definition of Health

In 1974 the World Health Organization defined health as "a state of complete physical, mental, and social well-being, not merely the absence of disease or infirmity." The traditional view of health was the absence of any overt disease. The WHO definition has one shortcoming: it does not allow for the various *degrees* of health states individuals can attain. However, three characteristics of the WHO definition that are essential to a positive conceptualization of health are

- the individual is viewed as a total person rather than the sum of his or her parts;
- health is presented in the context of internal and external environments; and
- health is equated with predictive and creative living (Pender, 1987).

Although health is not a universally agreed upon concept, the WHO definition, despite criticism, has endured.

Can health and illness be viewed as a continuum, with health and illness at opposite poles? This view is criticized because it suggests that in the absence of illness a person automatically achieves health and that health cannot be achieved by someone with an illness or disability. In contrast, current nursing theories view health "as a *dynamic* state or process that changes with time and varies according to circumstances" (Chinn, 1983). The presence of a pathologic condition does not preclude achievement of health when health is viewed as a dynamic process.

The process of achieving health is viewed in a variety of ways, as seen in the numerous definitions of health. Some health definitions are based on the premise that the achievement of health is interdependent with circumstances of the environment; some view the health process as something that can be achieved largely because of the nature of the individual (Chinn, 1983). Box 10-1 presents some common definitions of health.

Subconcepts of Health

To understand the concept of health more fully, it is helpful to understand the major themes, or subconcepts, that are reflected in many of the health definitions. The major subconcepts reflected in the definitions of health in Box 10-1 — *adaptation and stability, actualization, effectiveness,* and *responsibility for one's own health*— are discussed next.

Adaptation and Stability

The subconcepts of adaptation and stability arise from the view that health exists when the organism engages in effective interaction with its physical and social environment. This model developed from the writings of Dubos (1959, 1965), who views the state of health to depend on one's ability to adjust to the various internal and external environmental tensions. In this view, disease occurs when the organism fails to adapt to and cope with changes in the environment. Adaptation and stability are common themes in current nursing models (Levine, 1971; King, 1971; Roy, 1976). From this perspective, nursing care aims to restore adaptive behavior or reduce the impact of the environment when unusual stressors or weakened coping mechanisms result in ineffectiveness. This concept has particular relevance to the care of children and families as the developing child, as well as the developing family, experiences a sequence of developmental crises that must be mastered. As children or families cope with the stresses of development, internal and external stimuli evoke either an adaptive or a maladaptive response. The nurse promotes adaptation by providing information, by counseling, and by giving emotional support. The nurse's actions, according to Roy (1976), aim to gain equilibrium and prevent difficulties. King (1971) adds the concept of achieving the maximal potential for daily living as an outcome of adaptation or adjustment. From a framework of adaptation, the nurse caring for children and families is concerned with the developmental crises of the child and the family. If achievement of optimal potential is a goal, then one must go beyond survival of the crises and foster growth and development to the optimal level.

Self-Actualization and Wellness

The wellness process is different from good health. Good health is viewed as a state of being at one point along the health continuum, whereas wellness is a process of reaching a higher level of being in which the individual actively participates to achieve self-actualization (Bruhn and Cordova, 1977). Wellness, according to Dunn (1961), is related to learning and develop-

Box 10-1
Definitions and Descriptions of Health

"High-level wellness for the individual is defined as an integrated method of functioning which is oriented toward maximizing the potential of which the individual is capable. It requires that the individual maintain a continuum of balance and purposeful direction within the environment where he is functioning."

—Dunn, 1961

"A person is well if he is able to carry on his usual daily activities. To the extent that he cannot, he is in a state of dysfunction, or deviation from well-being."

—Fanshel, 1972

Wellness is "a status in which an individual of a given state of growth and development is capable of meeting the minimum physiological, psychological, and social requirements for appropriate function in the given sex category and at the given growth and development level."

—Hadley, 1974

"A dynamic in the life cycle of an organism which implies continuous adaptation to stresses in the internal and external environment through optimum use of one's resources to achieve maximum potential for daily living."

—King, 1971

Health and disease are viewed as patterns of adaptive change with wholeness of the individual as a central theme.

—Levine, 1971

A person's health is a state of wellness or illness which is determined by four variables: physiologic, psychologic, socio-cultural, and developmental. Health is relative and in a dynamic state of flux.

—Neuman, 1982

Health is part of the life process, is a fusion of disease and non-disease that is a basic pattern unique to the person as he/she evolves toward expanded consciousness.

—Newman, 1979

A state of wholeness or integrity of the individual, his/her parts, and modes of functioning.

—Orem, 1980

Health is a value word broadly defined by cultures and individuals to denote behaviors that are of high value and low value.

—Rogers, 1970

The health-illness continuum is a continuous line representing states of degrees of health or illness that a person might experience at a given time. Health-illness is an inevitable dimension of the person's life.

—Roy, 1976

"The existence of the person is absolutely central to life and its meaning and the meaning of life is inextricably tied not only to love, creativity, and self-fulfillment but also to the liberation from material and physical values on the one hand and freedom from fear of death and dying, disease and suffering on the other."

—Schlosser, 1977

(Data from Keller, 1981; Fitzpatrick and Whall, 1983.)

ment with cumulative results, in contrast to a state of homeostasis in which there is freedom from illness. Dunn (1961) believes there is not one level of optimal wellness but that each person has the potential to reach an individualized level of wellness.

The premise that health is a process of reaching one's potential is based on the belief that optimal health for each individual is different because it is determined by past experiences, genetic potential, and environmental circumstances (Bedworth and Bedworth, 1982). In other words, optimal health criteria are different for each individual, based on environmental and physiologic constraints. An individual with a chronic illness or disability may in fact function at maximal capacity (wellness); and contrariwise a person without an illness may function at a level below his or her potential (illness). This concept has particular relevance to the care of children and families. The variations between developing children and the interacting forces within growing families are infinite. Recognition of the individual nature of what constitutes wellness is the foundation of pediatric nursing practice.

Effectiveness

According to Bedworth and Bedworth (1982), health can be thought of in terms of effectiveness. They define health as "the quality of our physical, psychological, and sociological functioning that enables us to deal adequately with self and others in a variety of situations." A similar theme is reflected by Bruhn and Cordova (1977), who include the idea of competence in their definition of wellness, describing it as "the social ability to master one's self and one's situation in life" (active coping). The ideas of effectiveness and competence are also inherent in the role-performance model (Smith, 1981), which views health as effective performance of one's roles.

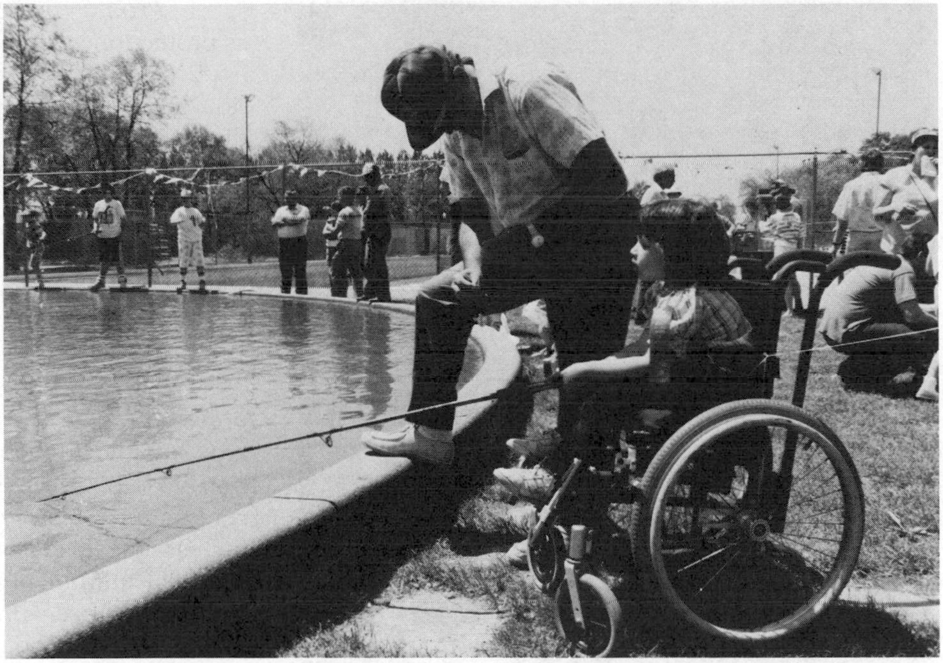

Being confined to a wheel chair is not a measure of health: functioning at one's potential capacity differentiates wellness from illness. This 10-year-old girl with spina bifida is enjoying a day at the park where she had a picnic lunch, participated in games, and went fishing.

To promote competence and effectiveness in the developing child, the scope of nursing care must broaden to include strategies that foster a child's self-esteem and support the development of a good self-concept. (See Chapter 16 for discussion of self-esteem.)

Self-Responsibility

That a healthy person has the capacity for self-responsibility in health care is a subconcept reflected in the holistic view of health. The idea of holism originates from Gestalt theory, which implies a "state of feeling complete and balanced" (Payne, 1983). It is based on the concept that each individual is an integrated whole with constant interaction of the biologic, psychologic, and sociologic dimensions.

Orem's view of health (1980) contains the idea of "wholeness, living within one's physical, biologic, and social environments to achieve some measure of one's potential." Self-care is a predominant theme in this model and is viewed as a learned behavior relative to beliefs, habits, and practices within the cultural group of an individual. It is defined as a deliberate activity, and is one's personal, ongoing contribution to one's own health and well-being.

Self-responsibility for one's own health is an important concept to incorporate into nursing practice with children and families. Children are taught to take responsibility for their health during child health visits and in special educational programs. Also, parents must be encouraged in self-responsibility so that their health behaviors are positive models. Children adopt many of their parents' health-related habits and practices; therefore, nursing strategies necessarily include the parents.

Health Behavior

Health behavior, for both parents and children, is manifested when the child or parent (1) identifies and accepts reality, (2) actively adjusts when the internal or external environment changes, (3) holds a wholesome outlook or attitude toward self and life in general, (4) effectively deals with self and others, and (5) takes on developmentally appropriate responsibility for managing her or his own health. These health behaviors should be promoted by nurses in all settings, with the recognition that an appropriate nursing goal is to extend practice beyond the cure of illness.

Health Promotion as a Nursing Goal

All persons should be supported and challenged to attain their maximal potential, a process that is not limited by the boundaries established by an illness. This emphasizes health promotion. In a review of the nursing literature, Brubaker (1983) makes the following points regarding health promotion: (1) the term is seldom defined; (2) it is sometimes used interchangeably with disease prevention and health maintenance; and (3) writers imply that health promotion and disease prevention are not synonymous even though a clear differ-

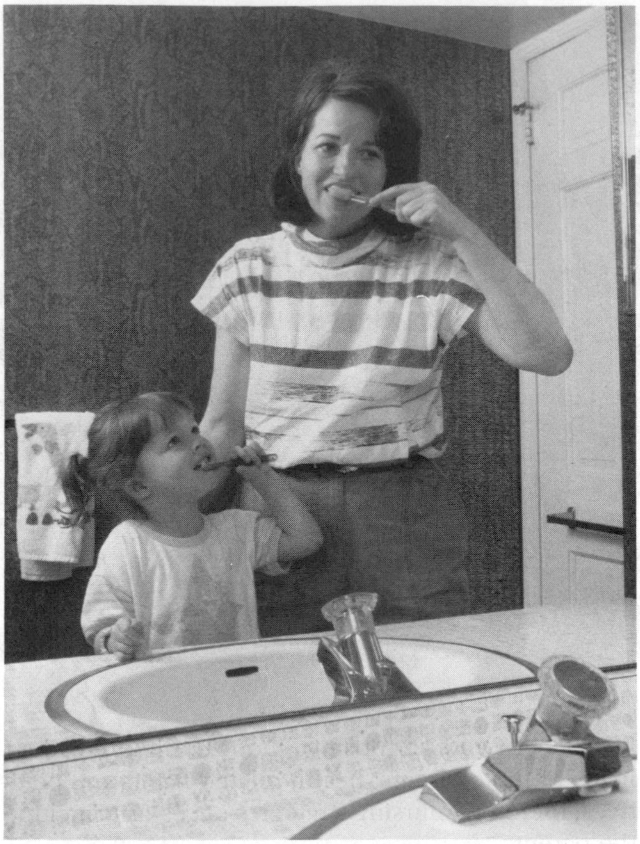

"Example is not the main thing in influencing others, it is the only thing."—Albert Schweitzer

entiation is not usually made. The terms most commonly used inconsistently are prevention (prevent the development or spread of disease), health maintenance (preserve the present state of health), and health promotion (maximize the optimal level of functioning). Health care must include all three practices (prevention, maintenance, and promotion) as well as curative and rehabilitative interventions.

The difficulty in separating these terms lies in the fact that a single activity may be carried out for numerous reasons. For example, an exercise program may be carried out to cure a health problem, to prevent a problem from developing, to maintain one's current health status, or to promote one's sense of well-being. The discussions in the literature regarding the meanings of prevention and promotion (Shamansky and Clausen, 1980; Brubaker, 1983; and Moore and Williamson, 1984) demonstrate that there is indeed significant overlap in the use of these terms.

Prevention traditionally has been described to exist at three levels: primary, secondary, and tertiary (Shamansky and Clausen, 1980), which are defined as follows:

1. *Primary prevention* is health promotion as well as protection against disease.
2. *Secondary prevention* is the early identification of disease and prompt intervention to treat the disease, resulting in shortened duration and reduced severity, with a return to normal function at the earliest possible time.
3. *Tertiary prevention* is the process of rehabilitation once the effect of a disease is fixed or irreversible. It is the process of restoring an individual to an optimal level of function within the constraints of the disability.

Primary prevention encompasses the ideas of prevention of illness, as well as maintenance and promotion of health. Pender (1987) proposes two definitions to replace the single definition of primary prevention: *health promotion* activities aim to "sustain or increase the level of well-being, self-actualization, and personal fulfillment of a given individual or group" and *primary prevention* activities aim to "decrease the probability of encountering illness, including active protection of the body against unnecessary stresses." Thus, health promotion is "maintaining the current health status or moving to a more desirable level of health," whereas prevention is "a defensive posture or set of actions taken to ward off specific illnesses or their sequelae that may threaten the quality of life or longevity."

Several factors justify and, in fact, necessitate a health promotion orientation in the nursing care of children. Children are the future of our world, and its positive progress requires not just their survival but their development as persons who are healthy physically, mentally, and socially. This means that we must attend to the environment within which they grow, develop, and are likely to adopt health values. Health promotion means that health hazards are reduced, access to health care is increased, and families within which children grow adopt healthful lifestyles, and that people take an active part in improving their own health (Bedworth and Bedworth, 1982). The quality of health of the next generation is believed to depend on the health behavior of this generation (Bedworth and Bedworth, 1982).

Children's Health Beliefs and Behaviors

The development of a child's beliefs about health and the adoption of health behavior is an expanding area of study. Despite such study, considerable gaps in our understanding remain. We simply do not know why some children engage in healthy behaviors while others do not. The child's developmental and psychologic characteristics and the environmental factors (family, school, peers, television) to which a child is exposed are influential variables. The differences in children's health may indeed be related to these factors, but the mechanisms by which they operate to influence behavior are not clearly defined.

Children's Health Concepts

Two important theoretic models used to study children's concepts of health are (1) the cognitive-developmental view (based on piagetian theory), and (2) the expectancy model (based on social psychology or social learning theory).

Cognitive-Developmental Model. It is believed that children's concepts of health change qualitatively, reflecting the progression of cognitive development, advancing from preoperational through concrete and formal operations (Kalnins and Love, 1982). A concept of health as it progresses according to cognitive development is summarized in Table 10-1. Natapoff (1978) found that younger children (termed *preoperational*) have difficulty in defining health. They tend to group events into a loose form (syncretism) and are unable to attend to more than one event at a time. They can list specific health acts, but children cannot understand the principles underlying these separate events until they are able to abstract (formal thinking). As children move from concrete to formal abstract thinking, concrete examples of health, such as proper food and actions (external cues), give way to more abstract feeling states (internal cues).

An important practical implication of how cognition affects health behavior is the child's limitation in understanding causality. Causality is not well understood until formal thought processes are acquired (after age 11 years). The notion of prevention, therefore, is not grasped until this time because it requires an understanding that a certain current action or lack of action can bring about a changed state in the future.

Expectancy Theory. Expectancy theory, drawn from the social psychology of Lewin (1935), is a central concept in social learning theory (Rotter, 1954). In expectancy theory, a behavior is performed if one expects that the behavior will bring about a desired outcome. This theory is reflected in the *health belief model* (HBM), which is a scheme to explain how health behavior decisions are made. According to the HBM, the likelihood of taking preventive actions is determined by *perceived benefits of preventive action* minus *perceived barriers to preventive action* (Pender, 1987).

The perceived benefits of preventive action are modified by the person's perceived susceptibility and threat of the disease. The greater the sense of vulnerability and the more serious the threat, the more likely a preventive action will be taken. If it is expected that the behavior can effect a positive outcome, the likelihood of action is even greater.

In regard to children's health, this means that a child's view of health and illness and understanding of cause and effect will influence the practice of healthy behaviors. If a child expects that a desired health goal will be reached by a certain behavior, then the child will be more likely to carry out that behavior. Perceived susceptibility and perceived threat of illness according to the HBM have been studied mainly by using adult populations (Mikhail, 1981).

Gochman (1971, 1977) and Gochman and Saucier (1982) have investigated children's senses of vulnerability or feelings of susceptibility to illness. These investigations focused on (1) the degree to which children perceive themselves vulnerable to a certain illness; and (2) the relationship of perceived vulnerability* to potential health behavior.† Children have been found not to be highly motivated by health and not to perceive themselves as particularly vulnerable to health problems. Although increased perceived vulnerability has been found to influence adult health behaviors positively, the same relationships have not been observed in children. On the contrary, negative correlations were observed between perceived vulnerability and various health behaviors, such as good nutritional habits, participation in sports, and patterns of sleep duration (Gochman and Saucier, 1982), meaning that as a sense of vulnerability increased, healthy behaviors decreased.

Of particular note is that perceived vulnerability in children was observed to be negatively correlated with self-concept and positively correlated with anxiety. These correlations suggest that perceived vulnerability is an anxiety-like state that makes an individual feel incapable of coping and see oneself in a basically negative way. Gochman and Saucier (1982) conclude that perceived vulnerability is a personality characteristic and part of a child's cognitive makeup. Their finding that children's reported vulnerability was generally consistent across health problems and over time further substantiates this belief. Children's receptivity to educational programs thus may be affected by different levels of perceived vulnerability or anxiety-like states.

Children's beliefs about how people stay healthy and how they get sick have been studied by Green and Bird (1986). Causes of health and illness in 82 children from grades 1 through 8 were analyzed. They found

---

*The term *vulnerability* refers to a likelihood of encountering a variety of health problems, in contrast to *susceptibility,* which is concerned with a certain isolated problem (Gochman and Saucier, 1982).

†Potential health behaviors are naturally occurring beliefs that reflect one's awareness of preventive and adaptive behaviors beneficial to health.

Table 10-1. Health Concepts, Cognitive Skills, and Self-Responsibility by Age, with Teaching Approaches to Them

Cognitive Level	Health Concept	Responsibility for Self-Initiated Care	Age-Related Teaching Approach
0–2 Years			
Sensorimotor	No concept, learns to value needs on basis of how well and how consistently they are met	Child moves from total dependence on caregiver to performance of simple tasks	Basic needs are generally met by caregiver
2–4 Years			
Preoperational (preconceptual)	No concept, merely imitates behavior of role models that are satisfying and/or earn reward	Some capacity to carry out tasks to promote own health if taught skills and allowed opportunity to take responsibility; likes to practice wellness behaviors	Continue meeting basic needs but steadily demand that child master skills of daily living; role model wellness behaviors; reward imitation. Play with child to learn the child's perceptions since they are not verbalized adequately
4–7 Years			
Preoperational (perceptual or intuitive) Egocentric, cannot consider whole and part simultaneously. Cannot conserve, i.e., cannot keep the original in mind and simultaneously consider a change	Health involves a series of health practices (eat right, brush teeth, stay clean), and health is apparent when one is able to perform usual activities. Does not consider cause and effect, cannot be part healthy and part not healthy at the same time. Sickness is unrelated to health status at another time.	Can carry out many tasks to promote own health, seeks responsibility; practice important. Can take independent action to identify many health needs and can identify some realistic solutions	Encourage any account of what the health need is, what caused it, what the child might do to resolve that need. Correct misperceptions. Use teaching techniques that provide tactile, visual, auditory, and motor experience.
7–11 Years			
Concrete operational Cause and effect are considered. Gradual increase in causal reasoning. Decentralization but still favors concrete reality. Able to conserve (consider original and changed state). Can classify objects and concrete ideas	Concept of health as sense of physical well-being, evidenced by "feeling good or being in shape." Believes can be part healthy and part not healthy	Can plan for and take initiative to carry out most health needs if has learned trust and autonomy. Can actively participate in managing own health needs. Acute interest in health education. Can consider possible risks and benefits of health behaviors if allowed to participate in problem solving	Share assessment and/or findings, to allow child to perceive changes in health status. Allow time for child to validate perceptions of needs and what actions should be taken; respect views and opinions. Give simple rationale for health practices/procedures. Make the invisible processes of health real with diagrams, models. Teach the skill/procedure (tangible, concrete) then give the rationale (abstract) in simple terms
Above 11 Years			
Formal operational Realizes realm of possible and hypothetical as well as the real. Develops theories. Craves details for egocentric purposes primarily. Can consider abstractions; deductive reason develops	Concept of health as long-term physical, emotional, social stability though superimposed brief illness may cause temporary instability. Evidenced by feeling good, being in control of self, being able to participate in desired activities. Future health is considered	Can assume full responsibility to identify health needs, determine possible resolutions, and carry them out. Can experientially apply wellness to life choices.	Significant other role models of wellness behavior crucial to overcoming peer pressures. Inform of realities of health problems and the possible outcomes; honesty imperative to child's cooperation. Present all details, relate them to child personally. Especially likes theoretic explanations and discussions. Discuss the effects of health problems and health behaviors on the future. Let child determine the possible resolutions to health needs and collaborate to determine management. Begin by presenting rationale for a skill/procedure, then give details of performing it

(Data from Bruhn and Cordova, 1977; Pidgeon, 1977; Natapoff, 1978; and Natapoff, 1982.)

that health practices over which the child had some control were mentioned most frequently as causes of health and illness. The most commonly cited cause of staying healthy was "the foods I eat." Older children ranked germs and bad weather as the most important causes of illness, whereas younger children ranked germs and weather equally with self-initiated care as causes of illness. Green and Bird think this finding may suggest that as children get older they develop a self-protective bias by learning to take personal responsibility for health but accepting less personal blame for illness.

Locus of Control

An additional psychologic variable found by Gochman (1971) to mediate health behavior in children is locus of control. An individual may believe that a reward (reinforcement for behavior) was received because of an actual behavior or as a result of forces beyond one's personal control (locus of control). Persons who perceive a reward as the result of fate, chance, or the power of others are said to be externally controlled. Persons who perceive the reward as an event that was determined by their own behavior are said to be internally controlled. It seems reasonable that an individual who expects that events are related to one's own behaviors would take more steps to change life conditions. In adult health behaviors, although research results are not altogether convincing, findings are consistent that imply that internal individuals, when faced with problems, engage in more adaptive behaviors than do external individuals. Gochman (1971) has been able to show that the degree of perceived internal control is an important factor influencing perceived vulnerability to health problems and potential health behavior. The way locus of control affects a child's beliefs about vulnerability is complex and is affected by the degree to which health is of importance or a value held by the child (salient). More internally controlled children were found to feel less vulnerable to health problems than externally controlled children (inverse relationship), but if health was not salient the relationship did not exist.

Neuhauser (1978) found that both cognitive development and locus of control are important factors in children's conceptualization of healing. Locus of control was found to influence the accessibility of knowledge about the insides of their bodies with the more internal children having greater access to internal cues. This difference was found only when the assigned task required use of the child's highest, more abstract cognitive ability. If the task was too easy or beyond their cognitive abilities, locus of control did not make a difference in their conceptualization. These findings emphasize the individual nature of each child and the differences that exist between adults and children.

Locus of control as a factor in affecting health beliefs and health behavior in children has been found to be related to other variables: internality is greater with increased age, with socioeconomic status, and in females (Perrin and Shapiro, 1985). This area of study requires further research if it is to yield nursing strategies to promote health.

Environmental Factors

Children's ideas about health are affected by their developmental level and psychologic characteristics, such as the aforementioned perceived vulnerability (an anxiety-like state) and locus of control. In addition, influential variables for each child arise from the particular situation in life to which a child is exposed. Children learn behavior from those they relate to and from the things they hear and see. Although each child is unique in ways of responding to the environment, all children learn from their family, peers, school, and media.

The family is an interactive system through which all members influence one another's behaviors: parent-child, child-parent, and sibling-sibling. The relationship of child and parental health behaviors and beliefs has been studied by Dielman et al (1982). The daily *behaviors* of parents are what influence their children whereas parental *beliefs* concerning health are seldom communicated verbally and have little direct influence (Dielman, 1982).

The extent to which the family influences a child's behavior varies with the age of the child. The greatest influence is exerted during early childhood. By early adolescence, peers become the dominant influence (Mullen, 1983). Figure 10-1 summarizes influences that affect children's health behaviors at the various stages of development. In today's society, the potential

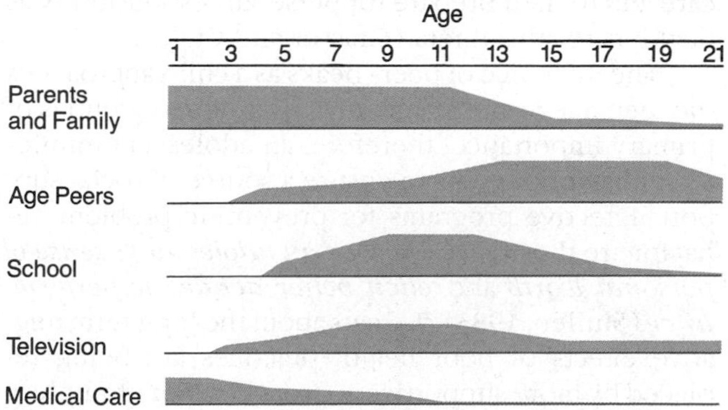

***Figure* 10-1.** Relative influences on children at various stages of development. (From Mullen PD: Promoting child health; channels of specialization. *Fam Community Health* 1983 Feb; 5(4):52–68. Reprinted with permission of Aspen Publishers, Inc.)

influence of parents even on the young child may be decreasing as the child-rearing patterns in families change. As young children spend more time in day care, preschools, and afterschool care facilities and in front of television sets, the relative influence of parents on young children may be altered. Under these circumstances it becomes even more important that the family's influence is a positive one.

Some dimensions of family functioning that are thought to affect a child's adoption of health behaviors are (1) the kind of behaviors that are modeled; (2) interaction patterns within a family; (3) the way reinforcement is used to encourage certain behaviors; (4) the opportunities provided to learn and practice health behaviors; and (5) the constraints that are put on certain behaviors (Bruhn and Parcel, 1982). These dimensions involve both the physical and mental health of children. Children not only learn principles about hygiene, diet, and sleep but also are exposed to patterns of coping and attitudes toward others.

Gaps in our knowledge about families and children's health are (1) what are the long-term effects of family influences? (2) what are the internal communication patterns of families that influence health behaviors? and (3) what are the desirable patterns for family interactions that promote children's health behavior? (Bruhn and Parcel, 1982).

As the child matures, school and peers increasingly impact on health behaviors. Schools exert their influence through formal classroom instruction, a climate of support and appropriate discipline, physical education activities, and school health services. The role of schools in health education has been to provide health information to children and to carry out early detection and preventive programs. Some schools also use humanistic education and values clarification as preventive activities to deal with mental health and improve children's self-concepts (Black and Newton, 1981). Some programs are designed to increase elementary school-age children's participation in health care and to then prepare for personal responsibility as health care consumers (Grasser and Craft, 1984).

The influence of peers peaks as a child approaches the teen-age years. Acceptance by a valued group is of primary importance; therefore, an adolescent mimics the behavior of peers to ensure a source of social support. Effective programs for preventing problem behavior are those that *improve an adolescent's sense of personal worth* and *elicit better academic performance* (Mullen, 1983). Threats about the long-term negative effects of poor health practices are being replaced by more supportive approaches. For example, a significant impact on cigarette smoking has been made by anticipating peer pressure and helping at that time with personal decision making (McAlister et al, 1980; Perry, 1980).

The impact of television on children's health attitudes and behaviors is discussed in Chapter 3. Extensive television watching can place a child into social isolation, with reduced physical activity and relating to real people. Even when peers watch a program together, social skills are not being developed. The passive nature of television watching lessens the child's opportunity to gain a sense of accomplishment from completing a project. Television watching thus has the potential to interfere with the overall healthy development of the child. On the other hand, within the boundaries of careful selection and monitoring of the number of hours, television can bring educational and creative experiences to children.

The specific content of television relating to children's health includes the messages of commercials and the health attitudes of role models depicted on the screen. Children learn from television as they do from real life: how to behave, what behaviors help them accomplish their goals, and what kinds of behaviors are likely to result in punishment (Comstock, 1981).

Specific health behaviors are learned through the portrayals of certain foods and drinks and the use of consumer products like toys and over-the-counter drugs. The average child in a single year sees approximately 20,000 commercials, the equivalent of 3 hours per week of continuous viewing of advertising (Comstock, 1981). Commercial television's effect on children is an ethical question. Is it ethical to manipulate children into desiring certain products (sugar-coated cereals and extravagant toys) through a medium such as television when they are too young to understand that the interest is sales, and not the good of the child?

Television has the potential to influence the attitudes and behaviors pertaining to many aspects of life, including health. If used selectively, it has the potential to provide a positive influence for health promotion with increased educational and health-oriented programming. It is a medium that children have incorporated into their lifestyles, but the challenge remains to use it appropriately.

Facilitating Self-Care Behavior

The societal and cultural influences that have an impact upon health differ for each family and child. The individual nature of health must be recognized as a nurse provides guidance and counsel to her clients as they engage in problem solving and decision making about health issues to reach their optimal level of functioning.

Identifying Personal Health Needs (Decision to Act)

Identifying what one considers healthy and what one needs or is required to do to preserve health is determined by subjective reality. What children or their caretakers believe to be good or right for them influences whether or not they will engage in health-promoting activities. The health needs recognized by the child or the family vary with their age, sex, education level, cultural orientation, and the parents' financial status and occupations. The more susceptible the child is believed to be to a health problem and the more serious the perceived consequence if health promotion behavior is not performed, the more likely are parents to assist their child to adopt the behavior. Children, however, do not seem to be motivated in the same way. The nurse's role with the parents and child, therefore, may differ. With the parents, the nurse's task is to help them recognize the child's susceptibility and potential consequences if health behaviors are not adopted. For the child, the nurse attempts to understand the child's cognitive ability regarding health and provide explanations appropriate to the developmental level.

Eliciting a child's understanding of the problem at hand and previous experiences related to the problem is important. A child's understanding of causality must be considered before attempting to describe consequences.

Deciding whether a problem exists that merits their attention is ultimately the family's responsibility. The nurse must work within the framework of their values and beliefs to help them see health as being vital, or necessary. The nurse's efforts will be more successful if the action required to maintain health is feasible in relation to the family's lifestyle and economic status.

Developing Problem-Solving Skills (Direction Action Will Take)

Recognizing a health need does not guarantee that the child or parents will take any action to meet that need. A prerequisite to action is knowing the possible action(s) to be taken to resolve the need. The process necessary to arrive at action alternatives is called problem solving. The family derives its problem-solving options from a variety of sources, each of which the nurse must consider in order to understand and support the decision made by the child or family. Common sources include:

1. *Family or cultural tradition.* The option a family has used in the past to deal with a health need remains as long as it seems to work. The family is most familiar with and best able to employ this option. Repetition of that option is encouraged by the endorsement received from the extended family or cultural group.
2. *Social or peer incentives.* The group with which the child or family identifies presents a recommended option. The more a child or parent feels the need for that group's approval, the more likely this option is to be selected. The role the individual holds within that group also influences to what extent he or she is expected to adopt the recommended option.
3. *Information from mass media, including health media, to the extent that the child or family is exposed to it.* The degree to which mass media information influences the option chosen depends upon how much personal meaning the message has to the child or parent. Studies have shown that mass media messages that stress personal and social consequences are more effective in influencing behavior than those stressing bodily damage (Wu, 1973). For example, an advertisement that discourages smoking because it decreases the person's ability to maintain endurance during active sports or because it causes bad breath will have more impact than an ad that discourages smoking because it leads to cancer or heart disease. The exception to this is when an individual knows someone who has experienced the bodily damage or for whom the recommended healthy behavior has worked.
4. *Information from a source who children or parents respect as knowledgeable* and who they believe cares sincerely about them as individuals. The primary caretakers of infants and young children are that source. To the extent that children's basic needs are met consistently and adequately, they are informed that those needs and the practices employed to meet them are important (valued, given priority). Figure 10-2 shows the relationship of these early experiences to the development of behavior promoting or not promoting health.

The task of the nurse becomes one of helping the family or child evaluate the various options in terms of the probable consequences of each and then to nonjudgmentally support efforts to carry out the option. The nurse can help the child and the family evaluate consequences by asking them to list the things they enjoy that they can expect to do or can continue to do if the option is carried out. They are then asked to identify the things they enjoy that they could not expect to do or could no longer do if that option is not carried out. This approach, rather than to focus on potential pathology to which they cannot relate because they have not experienced it, allows a personal identification with each option evaluated, since the child and family can relate the option to experiences with which they are familiar (things they enjoy).

Nurses must be ready to handle their feelings

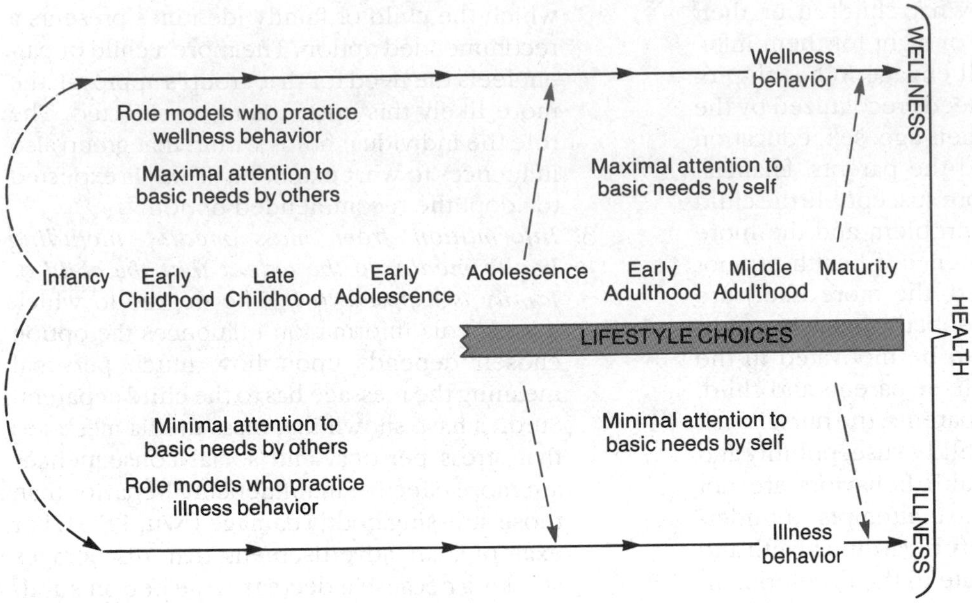

***Figure* 10-2.** Development of wellness- or illness-seeking behavior. (From Bruhn J, Cordova F: A developmental approach to learning wellness behavior. Part 1: Infancy to early adolescence. *Health Values* 1977 Nov/Dec; 246–254.)

when the option the child or family chooses is not the one they consider most desirable. Recognition that there is no one right way to maintain or promote health, that many possible actions may achieve that goal, is essential. Nurses also must realize that their preferred options are often not the most *feasible* option for a family or child. Nurses who help the child and family carry out the option they choose, even when inconsistent with their values pertaining to health, have helped them move toward the client's health goal. Success in that choice readies them to try a higher-level option. When optimal courses of action are not chosen, nurses can discuss why they chose their course and offer additional information to clarify misconceptions and augment more informed decision making. Reasonable choices should be reinforced.

The extent to which the nurse actively participates in the child's and the family's problem solving decreases as their skill in that process increases. Temporary dependence on the health professional can sometimes be healthy and necessary; we should permit parents and children to be dependent in some situations, especially during crises, whereas in other situations they are expected to be independent and self-reliant. Allowing some dependence on health care personnel while the child and the family are learning greater skill in problem solving or decision making is important to their health care and health education.

Responsibility for Self-Care (Taking Action)

Once behaviors have been identified that promote health, action must be taken to carry out those behaviors. To carry out a behavior requires knowledge of how it is performed and the ability to resolve any barriers that interfere with enacting it. Table 10-2 summarizes major factors (potential barriers) influencing behavior enactment.

In the early months of life, children are totally dependent on caretakers to carry out the behaviors that will ensure their health, but as they develop and acquire skills of daily living they are increasingly able to assume more responsibility in this. Thus, by young adulthood, children are capable of being fully responsible for their own health maintenance.

Achieving this level of responsibility requires that caregivers and health personnel allow growing children progressively more opportunity to (1) be involved in their own health care (identify their own health needs, determine how to meet those needs, and acquire knowledge, skills and attitudes essential to meet those needs), (2) assume responsibility for their own healthy and unhealthy habits and their consequences, and (3) assume responsibility for contacting and relating effectively to health care providers.

Nursing Strategies in Health Promotion

Promoting children's and families' personal responsibility for health may occur in the clinic, hospital, home, doctor's office, school, or any other setting where the nurse interacts with people.

The strategies used to promote health are the same regardless of the setting. They include establishing rapport and providing support, teaching, counseling, and therapeutic referral.

Table 10-2. Factors Influencing Preventive Health Action

Personal Readiness	Social Factors (Influence of the Environment)	Situation Factors (Attributes of the Action)
1. Recognize consequences of not adopting behavior and consider them personally important	1. Family/cultural pressure to carry out behavior	1. How likely the behavior is to maintain health
2. Accept personal vulnerability to unhealthy state	2. Social or peer group pressure to carry out behavior	2. Pleasure gained in performing the behavior
3. Adopt positive attitude about doing something to decrease that vulnerability	3. Health actions are congruent with perceived role expectations	3. Effort required to perform it
4. Believe that behaviors do exist that can decrease vulnerability or satisfy health need	4. Health actions are not in conflict with personal values and beliefs, lifestyle	4. Environmental conditions (middle column) make carrying out the behavior possible (feasibility)
5. Prove to be intellectually, emotionally and physically able to carry out behavior	5. Economic resources to carry out behavior exist	5. How appealing the behavior is to the individual
6. Know behavior(s) that will satisfy health need or decrease personal vulnerability		6. How promptly behavior can be carried out once the decision has been made to act; how often behavior must occur

(Adapted from Wu, 1973.)

Establishing a Working Relationship

The essentials for a working (cooperative) relationship are trust, empathy, and genuineness, shared by each person involved in the interaction. Participants come with their own values, needs, and perceptions of what the relationship will accomplish. *Trust* is most quickly established when the nurse responds in a consistent, nonjudgmental manner that conveys acceptance of and alliance with the child and parent. *Empathy* is communicated to the child or parent when the nurse takes seriously the concerns expressed, whether verbal or nonverbal. Questions, asked to help nurses discover the child's and parent's perceptions of their needs, show that they care, that they consider them worthwhile, and that they want to understand how they are feeling. *Being genuine* is extremely important when dealing with children, who are particularly alert to insincerity. The nurse should be honest with the child and the parent at all times and make no promises that cannot be carried out. If possible, the nurse should take a position at the child's level during any interaction and avoid artificial barriers such as desks or counters.

A working relationship is seldom established immediately, and the child will frequently test the nurse to be assured that the relationship is still stable. Often, the best approach to the child is through the medium of shared play. Parents respond more quickly when the nurse's approach considers their needs first (even small ones such as making sure they are comfortable or that they have a cup of coffee).

When the nurse models the behaviors necessary to a good working relationship, the client, whether child or adult, is given guidelines for his or her behavior in the relationship. Once the client becomes comfortable in this behavior, cooperative interaction is possible.

Supportive Nursing Actions

The modern family frequently may feel isolated from the resources that might help them make decisions regarding health, especially from the wisdom of the older generation in an extended family. The health profession has recognized this fact and accepted greater responsibility for providing information and support services that were formerly readily available within the family itself (Hansen and Aradine, 1974). Parents now expect the health professional to understand and reinforce their own strategies of parenthood and childrearing. Becoming well acquainted with the characteristics of the family that so strongly influence a child's health is economical of both the nurse's time and resources. Unless caretakers have their dependent needs met, we cannot expect that they will do well in meeting their children's developmental needs.

The support that parents or caretakers request from the nurse involves building up their confidence and self-esteem as persons and parents, providing information on meeting their child's needs successfully and encouraging the child to steadily assume responsibility for health, and giving reinforcement of their own credibility as parents.

Building Parental Self-Esteem

Very simple actions by the nurse, if genuinely employed, will build parents' self-esteem. These actions can be carried out during even brief contacts with them. The most gratifying experience for any of us is to be addressed by our name. When nurses address the parent (or child) by name, they acknowledge the parent to be recognizable and unique rather than "just another parent." A casual statement by the nurse, such as "Mrs. Jones, you are feeding Bobby properly. He is gaining just the amount in weight and height that he should be for his age," reassures the caretaker that positive changes are occurring in the child because of the care given. It takes 5 seconds to say, but it adds immeasurably to the caregiver's confidence. Equally supportive are comments that help the family see their child's positive responses to them; for example, "See how Tommy follows you with his eyes? You are important to him. He seeks you out," or "Beth talks to you frequently and pretends she is you, when she plays at the day care center. You are obviously very special to her." Not only do such statements support the caretaker's confidence as a parent, they also stimulate positive feelings in the parent toward the child.

An approach that acknowledges the feelings, needs, and well-being of the family and not just the child is also a supportive action. A statement such as "How are the rest of the family reacting to Susie's temper tantrums?" or "How are you managing your need for rest while David is ill?" communicates the nurse's understanding that the child's needs and behaviors affect all family members.

Phone calls or home visits initiated by the nurse also build parents' self-esteem. These convey personal interest in the family and their child and willingness to take their needs seriously. An additional benefit is that the nurse's assessment and diagnostic capacities are increased by this exposure to the family.

Information to Increase Parenting Success

The specific kinds of information parents (and children) need to promote the child's health are discussed later in this chapter. In addition to the specific skills the nurse can teach parents, supportive actions can be taken to enhance the parent-child relationship within which successful parenting occurs.

The nurse should use every possible opportunity to develop parents' awareness of their child's assets as well as deficits. Establishing assets (physical, mental, or social) helps to personify the child to the parents in a positive manner. Stressing the developmental normality of their child's behaviors as well as those behaviors that convey the individual's personality reassures parents that their child is progressing and that any developmentally associated negative behavior is only temporary and not caused by faulty parenting techniques.

Allowing parents (especially first-time parents) telephone access to a health professional on a 24-hour basis during stressful times is also a supportive action. Such action is seldom abused by parents; each call a parent makes to a health professional resource is a cry for support at some level.

Reinforcing Parental Credibility

The nurse has an obligation to support families within the context of their cultural beliefs, parenting practices, and selected lifestyle. Associated with that support is a responsibility to gently and tactfully introduce those scientific practices and facts essential to health in such a way that they do not conflict with the family's beliefs and values. This task admittedly challenges the nurse's most creative abilities, but it is essential to meet the goal of self-initiated healthy living. The nurse can begin by accepting the caregiver's (or child's) intentions as well as abilities. For example, during an examination of an infant with an umbilical hernia, the nurse may note that the mother has taped a coin over the hernia (a culturally motivated behavior). The nurse compliments the mother on her good intention by saying, "I see you're taking measures to attempt to correct your baby's hernia. You are right to be concerned." The nurse then introduces scientific facts that complement rather than conflict with the mother's belief that measures must be taken to reduce the hernia. "It has been discovered that placing Tommy on his tummy frequently will help reduce the hernia by strengthening his tummy muscles. Babies like to be on their tummies anyway. You can do this often, and the baby is comfortable since there's no itching or pulling from tape or a binder. This position also helps him learn the head control he needs before he can sit." Thus the nurse has praised the mother's intention to care for her baby, has given her an easier way to do so, and has done this without being in conflict with the cultural attitude that measures should be taken to reduce umbilical hernias.

Another example of complimenting intent: A mother brings her child to the clinic with an ear infection. When the nurse enters to obtain a history and examine the child, the mother states that she was going to bring the child in 2 days ago but she could not get transportation until today. An appropriate statement from the nurse might be "It was good that you tried to bring her in two days ago. The earlier we begin treating infections, the quicker they are brought under control and the less likely the child is to have serious consequences." This statement compliments the mother on her intentions and gives her factual information to utilize the next time she must make a similar decision regarding her child's health. The statement also avoids judgment or blaming by the nurse.

The nurse should make use of every opportunity to convey confidence in the parents' ability to make health judgments and to trust their own feelings and their ability to act to promote the child's health. The feeling of success the nurse helps to engender in the

The child selects the alternative(s) she will carry out. This is written down and becomes a contract between the child, the nurse, and others involved as to what must be done by each.

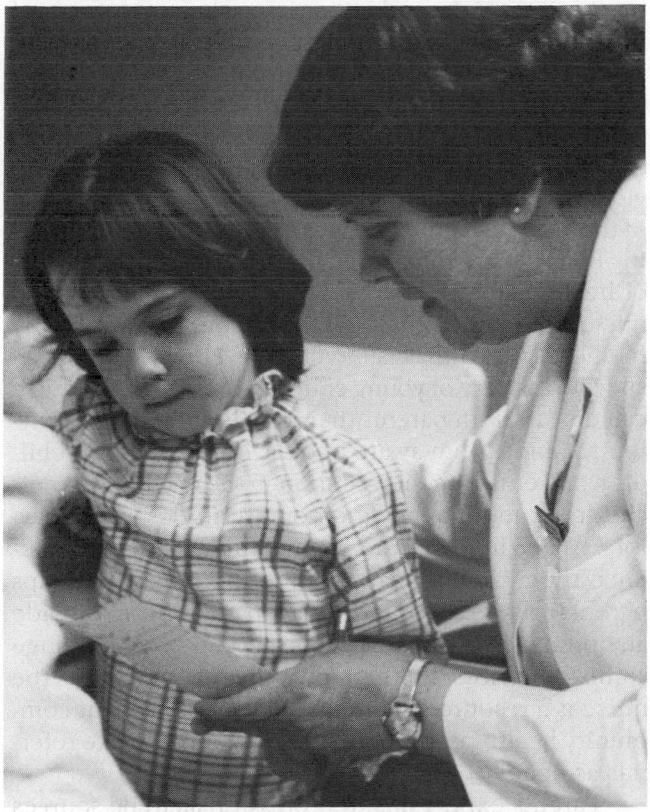

child's caregivers in one situation encourages them to act successfully in others.

The supportive actions identified here to promote healthy parenting are equally functional in supporting children as they attempt to assume self-initiated care.

The Nurse's Teaching Role

A large amount of nursing care in any setting is teaching. Through teaching the nurse fosters an atmosphere of personalized caring and attempts to help families gain information to competently initiate their own problem solving and overcome the barriers to healthy change in their lives. There is a wealth of information that parents and children can use to their advantage, and the nurse is pressed to communicate it all in the brief contacts with family members. Because of the brevity of contact, the nurse should recognize that all moments while a parent waits are precious teaching opportunities, and each procedure or treatment offered lends itself to simultaneous teaching.

Teaching may be done formally in a planned situation, such as a parent education or school health class. More often teaching is informal or incidental, occurring at any opportune moment and prompted by immediately identified need. The three most prominent forms of incidental learning are *imitation of role models, task repetition,* and *positive environmental feedback.* In any situation, active teaching is usually more effective. Active teaching utilizes actions more than words to convey the necessary information.

A technique the nurse may use in active teaching is role modeling. At any age, individuals learn more from the teacher's actions than from words. This is especially true of children and those adults who feel insecure in the parent role, since they tend to capitalize on imitation to learn skills. A second technique is demonstration to clarify verbal instruction. A third is role playing, puppet play, games using role reversal, and psychodrama. These take more time but are extremely effective in increasing the learner's sensitivity to others' feelings or circumstances. A fourth technique is learner participation in tasks, reinforced by visible or tangible rewards for effort as well as accomplishment. One learns best when performing or practicing under supervision those skills one must eventually manage on one's own. Rewards can be used to motivate repetition to master the task. As a general rule of thumb, the more educated the learner, the more likely learning can take place through verbal or written instruction and logical explanation, with or without the use of active teaching techniques.

Teaching Caregivers

The extent to which parents practice healthy behaviors greatly influences their child's development of healthy attitudes and behavior. This explains the importance of teaching parents and other caretakers the facts of healthy living to reach the goal of self-initiated responsibility for health in their children.

The nurse's role in teaching must necessarily be family focused. If children do not have the opportunity to observe health-promoting behaviors in those individuals who are influential in their lives, the likelihood of their adopting such behaviors is diminished. Changing behavior in adults is the focus of a large component of health care. It is beyond the scope of the pediatric nurse's practice to deal with each behavior of family members that they wish to change. However, with respect to the care of young children in a home, the nurse can discuss with parents their role in modeling behaviors. Making them aware of their impact on their children and enlisting their support in the teaching of their children can influence their own attitudes and behaviors. Analyzing with the parents the factors that influence their child's health-promoting behaviors helps parents understand their own responsibility to provide an optimal environment. When parents seek to change some behaviors in their own health practices, the nurse is a resource to provide information about community health promotion programs and to make referrals as needed.

Parents expect health professionals to be sources of information and education. The teaching that the nurse does concerning future events and circumstances has been called anticipatory guidance. With respect to childrearing, this means that the nurse provides information about health and developmental issues so that parents know what to expect and how to manage situations when they happen. The particular content of such teaching is somewhat predictable according to the ages and stages of development. More than 30 years ago, the Public Health Association defined anticipatory guidance as "teaching the mother what to expect before she begins to worry or make mistakes" (Committee on Child Health of the American Public Health Association, 1955). The underlying belief is that giving information assures the parents of the normality of the developmental changes and provides them with information sufficient to keep their children safe and healthy and to promote optimal growth and development. This approach has the potential to become routine and primarily oriented to "giving information" rather than creating an atmosphere for an exchange of information. A problem-solving approach has been recommended in which the knowledge and skills of both the client and the professional are used collaboratively to define the problem, goals, and solutions (Pridham et al, 1977).

The technique of anticipatory guidance, with its increased emphasis on teaching to foster healthy emotional and psychologic adjustment of the child and family, makes additional time demands on professionals. In an effort to provide a forum within which information is disseminated but professional time is minimized, the well-child visit can be carried out in groups. The group discussions with parents provide a time for mutual sharing of experiences, and the nurse is used as a resource for information (Osborn, 1982).

Hansen and Aradine (1974) have identified several critical areas in which parents expect assistance. They want information about:

1. Child development and the parents' role in fostering positive development;
2. Childrearing issues and the rationale for approaches that the health profession recommends;
3. Child behavior, including school, social, and learning behavior and how to manage it;
4. The steps to take when caring for an ill child at home and the rationale for this management;
5. Family issues and balancing the needs, care, and problems of all family members;
6. How best to utilize and relate to health professionals and other community resources;
7. Identifying and managing problems and needs that parents themselves experience;
8. Family relationships related to issues such as personal and interpersonal crises, illness, divorce or separation, single parenting, and extended family issues.

These issues are addressed throughout this book, including nursing actions to help meet the family's informational needs.

Underlying these many expectations brought to the health professional is the parents' desire to succeed in the care of their child and to receive encouragement from the professional that their parenting strategies can succeed. Health-related topics are abundant in consumer media. The nurse should stay abreast of these sources, since parents are likely to read and use that information. The nurse should answer questions that parents have about such information, validate accurate sources, and supply facts when the family has been misled. The nurse can also utilize a variety of techniques in helping parents gain knowledge and skills in parenting, applying teaching-learning theory to the approach. But the teaching done as a role model, demonstrating to parents how to respond to their child through cuddling, talking, listening, touching, and praise, is probably the most pertinent knowledge the nurse can impart.

Teaching Children

Too often health teaching about children is directed mostly toward their parents. As Pidgeon (1977) notes, "Like sponges they (children) silently absorb and ruminate over what they hear. . . . health teachings should be aimed at children as well as their parents."

The child's thoughts should be explored and concerns, questions, and opinions elicited.

If we expect children to assume more responsibility for their own health as they grow, we need to teach them how to manage stress. They must learn ways to reduce stress in their environment, acquire effective coping skills, and develop attitudes that are oriented toward health rather than illness. Children need information about what to expect (what they will hear, feel, smell, and see) during health care experiences. And, if they are to initiate their own health care, they must learn how to approach health care providers and be assertive with them.

In an elementary school program, children were given the right to seek health care based on their own decisions. This program demonstrated that such an approach helps children develop a sense of self-control and self-responsibility (Lewis and Lewis, 1982).

Acquisition of healthy behavior by children involves four processes. They must develop an *awareness* of health from their role models. They must be exposed to developmentally appropriate *information* about wellness and health practices. If they are to learn responsibility, they must be included as *active participants* (as early in life as possible) in making health choices so that they can master the problem solving required to make healthy decisions about life. And, finally, they must be *reinforced* for their attempts and their successes in practicing wellness behaviors.

Health teaching aimed at children takes into account the child's thinking ability at various ages, the concept of health that is characteristic of the age, and the degree of independent action that a child is realistically capable of at each stage of development. Box 10-2 describes such characteristics for children in the various age groups and their relevance in selecting an appropriate teaching approach.

Whatever and wherever the teaching opportunity with a child is, the nurse can take the same basic steps to help the child develop problem-solving and coping abilities in health promotion. The only alteration required is in the teaching approach taken, which must be adjusted to the child's age and cognitive capabilities. Steps according to Lewis (1974) include:

1. Ask Robert what he thinks his problem or need is (he learns problem identification) and whether the problem is important to him (he learns to make health a priority). This information gives the nurse an understanding of the child's perception of his situation and the priority that health currently is given in his family. This tells the nurse how much health information the child needs before he is likely to cooperate.
2. The nurse then gets an additional history, preferably from the child and then augmented by his caregiver, and does whatever assessment is indicated. Teaching occurs throughout this process as the nurse gives truthful explanations of what the child will see, hear, feel, smell, or taste during assessment procedures. Age-appropriate rationale is also given for each procedure. Because young children acquaint themselves with the world through their physical senses, teaching should focus on this aspect of procedures. These children also require visual examples (for example, a procedure done on a doll) to comprehend what to expect. Older school-age children can usually comprehend from verbal explanations alone. Adolescents, although

---

Box 10-2

Examples of Realistic Health Behaviors Children Have Identified at Various Ages

Early Childhood

I will brush my teeth after breakfast and at bedtime.
I will cover my coughs and sneezes with my hand or a tissue.
I will drink a glass of milk at breakfast, lunch, and supper.

Middle Childhood

I will try to remember to wash my hands after using the toilet and before eating.
Whenever possible I will change wet shoes and socks or stockings for dry ones.
I know what a good breakfast is, and I will try to eat one every day.
I will go to bed willingly when I am told to do so.

Late Childhood and Preadolescence

I will try to learn to eat some foods that are new to me or that have been prepared in a new way.
I will listen to the morning weather report and dress accordingly.
I will try to cooperate with my parents and other adults who help to keep me well.
I will keep my hands clean and will also keep them away from my face, especially from my eyes, nose, and mouth, and away from any sores.

Adolescence and Young Adulthood

I will study my own posture and try to do the things that will improve it.
I know about the four food groups (meats, vegetables, fruits, and dairy products) and I will try to eat foods from each every day.
I will take frequent baths and wash my hair at least once each week.
I will listen to my parents' point of view in areas in which we disagree and seriously evaluate their points.

they want to know what to expect, are much more interested in the rationale and consequences of each procedure.

3. The child is presented with the important findings uncovered in the nursing assessment. This is a good opportunity to teach names of body organs or explain body processes or both, and what it means when they are altered. How simple and concrete or complex and abstract this teaching must be will depend on the child's age.
4. The nurse interprets the findings to the child in terms of probable cause. For the young child who still perceives people as the cause of all events, the explanation should be prefaced by reassurance that the cause was not himself, his wishes, or the wishes of others upon him. The child in late childhood or preadolescence has usually mastered causal relationships enough to grasp a simply presented scientific explanation. The adolescent or young adult will want a detailed scientific explanation. The provision of health information is critical at this time because it now has maximal relevance to the child personally.
5. The nurse elicits the child's opinions of what he thinks ought to be done. Usually the best approach is to have the child list the alternatives he can think of and why he thinks each would help (he learns problem solving). This task should be the child's responsibility, with the nurse assisting only if the child cannot think of any alternatives on his own. Box 10-2 gives examples of some alternatives children have selected that reflect age-appropriate understanding of their problem or need. Health education is then offered to correct any misconceptions, to increase the child's knowledge of the situation so he can identify more realistic or additional alternatives, or to reinforce accurate perception of what will work and why.
6. The child selects the alternative(s) he will carry out alone or with assistance (he learns decision making). Before he makes his selection, he should be informed whether any of his alternatives are unacceptable because of rules of the setting in which they must be carried out. The child's selection should be written down for him (and/or for those who will assist him to carry it out) and documented in the nurse's records. This becomes a contract between the child, nurse, and others involved as to what must be done by each. (See Box 10-3 for a discussion of contracts.)
7. The child is asked to identify the resources (personal or in his external environment) that he will need to utilize to carry out his alternative(s). Health teaching that helps the child to become knowledgeable about available personal, family, or community resources and how to use them is appropriate.
8. The nurse asks the child what he will do if the same problem or need recurs (reinforces child's ability to be responsible for initiating his own health care).

When the child selects optimal alternatives, this should be reinforced. Inappropriate decisions are not reinforced, and the nurse provides additional information to further clarify the problem and its cause and to help the child see the inappropriateness of the decision.

This approach involves the child actively in identifying his health needs, finding viable solutions and carrying them out. The nurse applies learning, reinforcement, and decision-making theories to help the child become responsible for his own wellness behaviors.

Counseling Role

A counseling relationship, whether with child or parent, is a two-way interaction involving both verbal and nonverbal communication. Its purposes are (1) to realistically define or resolve a problem, (2) to increase the client's awareness of self and needs, and (3) to get a broader understanding of a situation causing conflict for the client. Many times counseling is the intervention initiated during developmental or situational crises. Common developmental crises in families for which the nurse is most often consulted are listed in Box 10-4. Situational crises requiring counseling include

Birth of a sibling
Death in the family
Adoption
Divorce or separation
Rape, incest, promiscuity
Child with handicaps
Entry into school and school readiness
Preparation for hospitalization

The nurse counselor, to be successful, must develop skills of astute observation, tactful questioning, objective listening, and, foremost, allowing the client to choose alternatives and solutions. (Refer to Chapters 11 and 21 for a review of communication and play theory, both of which are useful in counseling.) In determining the family members who should be included in counseling, a general rule is that all who will be affected by the situation or its resolution should participate in the decision making. This mutual participation is most successful because it allows each in-

Box 10-3
Using a Contract to Motivate Healthy Behavior

A contract is a partnership between two parties (nurse and child, parent and child, teacher and child, nurse and family) that specifies mutually agreed upon goals or behaviors and each person's role in fulfilling the contract. The contract may be informal and verbal *(mutual agreement)* or formal, written and signed by both parties *(contract)*.* If positive or negative reinforcers are included in the contract, it is called a *contingency contract.* The intent of the contingency contract is to sustain the child's motivation to specific self-care or self-control activities by providing planned consequences for attaining or not attaining the desired goal or behavior.

The contents of the contract depend upon whether it is a mutual agreement, contract, or contingency contract. A mutual agreement usually includes a statement of the goal to be reached, the date by which it is to be reached, and each person's responsibilities in achieving the goal. A contract has these same features with the addition of each person's signature to the written document. A contingency contract has all the features of the contract but specifies in addition what the child will gain (reward) for fulfilling her or his part of the contract and what he will forfeit if he does not fulfill his obligation. The second party to the contract (nurse, parent, teacher) dispenses the rewards or forfeitures as designated in the contract.

Stuart (1971) and Homme and coworkers (1970), through their research on the effectiveness of behavioral contracts, formulated several rules that increase the likelihood of successful behavior change in contingency contracting. These rules can guide the nurse in making contracts with children and their families.

* A nursing care plan is a *mutual agreement* if jointly developed with the client and a *contract* if it is jointly developed, written, and signed by the nurse and client.

Rule 1. The reward should be immediate.
Rule 2. Initial contracts for a behavior should reward small approximations of the behavior.
Rule 3. The contracts should be devised so that rewards are frequent and in small amounts.
Rule 4. Performance should be rewarded after it occurs. The reinforcing party has a tendency to become lenient or ease up on contract specifics. This usually dooms any success in changing behaviors.
Rule 5. The contract should be mutually devised and genuinely agreed on by both parties. Neither should comply out of fear.
Rule 6. Each party must clearly understand what is expected and what can be expected in return.
Rule 7. The contract must be followed consistently, otherwise the child interprets forgotten or missed reinforcements as condoning undesirable behavior. (Neglect of contract reinforces and perpetuates the undesired behavior).
Rule 8. The goal or behavior contracted for, as well as the reinforcers, must be realistic and achievable.

The contract approach to obtain healthy behaviors in children has several benefits. It clearly identifies the necessary requirements to achieve the goal or solve the problem. Clarification of responsibility minimizes confusion, contributes to a trust relationship, and provides a vehicle to help the child make a transition from behavorial management by others to self-regulation (Gelfand and Hartmann, 1975; Sheridan and Smith, 1975). The contingency contract is especially successful because human beings, like other animals, tend to behave in ways that pay off for them.

volved family member to gain perspective on the problem and his or her particular role in its management. An indirect effect is that this approach motivates a cooperative partnership among all members of the counseling relationship, including the nurse counselor.

The environment can be a valuable adjunct in promoting the counseling relationship and the desired problem solving. The decor, furniture arrangement, and opportunity provided for the client to initiate contact with the nurse all have significant impact (Johnston, 1979). Colors, style and texture of furniture and play equipment, and lighting help convey that the client is welcome, that comfort and privacy (not isolation) are the nurse's concern, and that the client's needs as well as those of the staff have been considered. The decor should emphasize living and health rather than illness and morbidity. Decor and furnishings can also be effective in reminding staff of the needs of the children and families they serve. Any room arrangements or approaches to clients should encourage eye-to-eye contact and conversation; an "assembly line" approach must be avoided. When choices are feasible (which nurse to confer with, which room to have the meeting in), they should be offered, since choices permit the client some sense of control.

The nurse's responsibility as a counselor is to help the family attain the counseling goals by evoking their sense of security and self-confidence in handling problems, by offering health information that will help them solve problems, and by guiding them in the decision-making process. However, the nurse is not to be a decision maker for them.

Box 10-4
Potential Developmental Areas of Child-Parent Conflict

Newborn and Young Infant
- Feeding
- Crying
- Sleeping
- Bathing and dressing
- Schedules

Older Infant
- Feeding
- Weaning
- Separation
- Toilet needs
- Sleeping
- Crying
- Safety measures

Toddler
- Self-feeding
- Decreasing appetite
- Toilet training
- Separation
- Tantrums
- Negativism
- Breath-holding
- Aggressive behavior
- Discipline
- Childproofing

Preschooler
- Speech
- Independence
- Sibling rivalry
- Sexual curiosity
- Bad dreams
- Phobias
- Discipline
- Safety rules

School-age
- School adjustment
- Conduct disturbances
  - Lying
  - Cheating
  - Stealing
  - Bad language
- Aggressive behavior
- School achievement
- Discipline

Adolescent
- Independence (adolescent rebellion)
- Sexual activity
- Drug experimentation
- Peer group choices
- Delinquent behaviors
  - Truancy
  - Shoplifting
- Nutrition

(Adapted from Browder, 1970.)

Box 10-5
*Some Common Resources Available to Families**

Parenting Education
- College and school academic and nonacademic courses
- Hospital and clinic classes
- Red Cross classes
- Mental health center classes
- Planned Parenthood
- Cooperative Extension Services
- State and local health departments

Parent Support
- Voluntary self-help organizations
- Parents Without Partners
- Psychologists, social workers, physicians, nurses in private or group practice
- Health department nursing services

Children's Self-Initiated Care
- School health programs
- Children's clinics
- Teen-age clinics
- Walk-in clinics
- Al-Anon and Alateen
- Youth Services Bureau
- Project Grow
- Head Start, Get Set

Crisis Assistance
- Hot lines
- Crisis centers
- Family and children's services
- Clergy
- Mental health centers
- Project Now
- Social services departments of hospitals, government
- Runaway and youth counseling services
- Legal Aid Society

Financial Assistance/Reduced Fee Health Care
- City or county health department
  - WIC Program
  - Well-Child Clinics
  - Immunization clinics
  - Communicable disease clinics
- Crippled Children's Services (government program usually located in health department or family and children's services)
- Health collectives
- Local civic clubs

* To find what is available in a specific area, begin with the yellow pages of a phone book (social services organizations, psychologists, city or county listings, Health Services headings).

The Nurse's Role in Referrals

Health promotion is a multiposition, interdisciplinary responsibility that requires a sharing of skills and cooperative division of labor. The nurse alone cannot possibly manage the complexity of needs that can exist in a family. When it becomes necessary or advantageous to solicit assistance beyond what is directly available to the nurse, the appropriate action is to refer family members to resources that can help them.

This does not absolve the nurse of responsibility for the family but rather adds to the helping role. To refer appropriately, the nurse must become acquainted with the many potential health team members on a local, regional, and state-wide basis. Nurses must know what each resource offers, what its capabilities are (its record of success in handling the problems it professes to be able to manage), and how the family can obtain those services. When a family is to be referred to the resource, the nurse is responsible for informing the family. To attain or maintain the needed services, the nurse may be called upon to act as an advocate for the client or as a liaison (negotiator, mediator) between the client and the resource provider.

If several resources are needed by the family, the nurse is often the team member selected to coordinate the various services in a manner that does not overwhelm the family. (Box 10-5 lists several types of resources.) Collaboration with those in other disciplines is not always easy; it demands that the nurse apply diplomacy and creativity if the family is to obtain the help it needs.

References

Allen M: The health dimension in nursing practice: notes on nursing in primary health care. *J Adv Nurs* 1981; 16:153–154.

American Nurses' Association: *Nursing: A Social Policy Statement,* Kansas City, MO, 1980.

Bedworth AE, Bedworth DA: *Health for Human Effectiveness.* Englewood Cliffs, NJ, Prentice-Hall, 1982

Black JL, Newton J: Should health behavior change be an objective of school health personnel? *J Sch Health* 1981 Mar; 51(3):189–190.

Browder J: Needs and techniques for counseling parents of young children. *Clin Pediatr* 1970 Oct; 599.

Brubaker BH: Health promotion: a linguistic analysis. *Adv Nurs Sci* 1983 Apr; 5(3): 1–14.

Bruhn J, Cordova F: A developmental approach to learning wellness behavior. Part 1: Infancy to early adolescence. *Health Values* 1977 Nov/Dec; 246–254.

Bruhn JG, Parcel GS: Current knowledge about the health behavior of young children: a conference summary. *Health Educ* 1982 Summer/Fall; 9(2 and 3): 142/238–165/261.

Chinn PL, Jacobs MK: *Theory and Nursing: A Systematic Approach.* St. Louis, CV Mosby, 1983.

Committee on Child Health of the American Public Health Association: *Health Supervision of Young Children.* New York, American Public Health Association, 1955.

Comstock G: Influences of mass media on child health behavior. *Health Educ Q* 1981; 8(1): 32–38.

Dielman TE, et al: Parental and child health beliefs and behavior. *Health Educ Q* 1982 Summer/Fall; 9(2 & 3):60/156.

Dubos R: *Mirage of Health.* Garden City, NY, Doubleday, 1959.

Dubos R: *Man Adapting.* New Haven, Yale University Press, 1965.

Dunn HL: *High Level Wellness,* Arlington, VA, RW Beatty Company, 1961.

Fanshel S: A meaningful measure for health for epidemiology. *In J Epidemiol* 1972 Winter; 4:319–337.

Fitzpatrick J, Whall A: *Conceptual Models of Nursing: Analysis and Application.* Bowie, MD, Robert J. Brady, 1983.

Gelfand D, Hartmann D: *Child Behavior.* New York, Pergamon Press, 1975.

Gochman DS: Some correlates of children's health beliefs and potential health behavior. *J Health Soc Behav* 1971 June; 148–154.

Gochman DS: Perceived vulnerability and its psychosocial context. *Soc Sci Med* 1977; 11:115–120.

Gochman DS, Saucier JF: Perceived vulnerability in children and adolescents. *Health Educ Q* 1982 Summer/Fall; 9(2 and 3): 46/142–58/154.

Grasser SC, Craft BJ: The patient's approach to wellness. *Nurs Clin North Am* 1984 June; 207–218.

Green KE, Bird E: The structure of children's beliefs about health and illness. *J Sch Health* 1986 Oct; 56(8):325–328.

Hadley BJ: Current concepts of wellness and illness: their relevance for nursing. *Image* 1974; 6(2):21–27.

Hansen M, Aradine C: The changing face of primary pediatrics. *Pediatr Clin North Am* 1974 Feb; 245.

Homme L, et al: *How to Use Contingency Contracting in the Classroom.* Champaign, IL Research Press, 1970.

Johnston M: Toward a culture of caring: children, their environment, and change. *MCN* 1979 Jul/Aug; 210.

Kalnins I, Love R: Children's concepts of health and illness and implications for health education. An overview. *Health Educ Q* 1982 Summer/Fall; 9(2 and 3):8/104–19/115.

Keller MJ: Toward a definition of health. *Adv Nurs Sci* 1981 Oct; 43–64.

King IM: *Toward a Theory for Nursing— General Concepts of Human Behavior.* New York, John Wiley and Sons, 1971.

Levine ME: Holistic nursing. *Nurs Clin North Am* 1971; 6:253–264.

Lewin K: *A Dynamic Theory of Personality.* New York, McGraw-Hill, 1935.

Lewis CE, Lewis MA: Children's health-related decision making. *Health Educ Q* 1982 Summer/Fall; 9(2 and 3):129/225–141/237.

Lewis M: Child-initiated care. *Am J Nurs* 1974 Apr; 652.

McAlister A, et al: Pilot study of smoking, alcohol and drug abuse prevention. *Am J Public Health* 70:, 1980; 70:719–721.

Mikhail B: The health belief model: a review and critical

evaluation of the model, research and practice. *Adv Nurs Sc* 1981 Oct; 65–80.

Moore PV, Williamson GC: Health promotion: evolution of a concept. *Nurs Clin North Am* 1984 Jun; 195–206.

Mullen PD: Promoting child health: channels of specialization. *Fam Community Health* 1983 Feb; 5(4):52–68.

Natapoff J: Children's views of health: a developmental study. *Am J Public Health* 1978 Oct; 995–999.

Natapoff J: A developmental analysis of children's ideas of health. *Health Educ Q* 1982 Summer/Fall; 130–140.

Neuhauser C, et al: Children's concepts of healing. Cognitive development and locus of control factors. *Am J Orthopsychiatr* 1978 Apr; 335–341.

Neuman B (ed): *The Neuman Systems Model.* New York, Appleton-Century-Crofts, 1982.

Newman M: *Theory Development in Nursing.* Philadelphia, FA Davis Company, 1979.

Orem DE: *Nursing: Concepts of Practice.* 2nd ed. New York, McGraw-Hill, 1980.

Osborn L: Group well-child care: an option for today's children. *Pediatr Nurs* 1982 Sept/Oct 306–308.

Payne L: Health: a basic concept in nursing theory. *J Adv Nurs* 1983; 8:393–395.

Pender NJ: *Health Promotion in Nursing Practice.* East Norwalk, CT, Appleton-Century-Crofts, 1987.

Perrin EC, Shapiro E: Health locus of control beliefs of healthy children, children with a chronic physical illness, and their mothers. *J Pediatr* 1985 Oct; 107(4):627–633.

Perry C, et al: Modifying smoking behavior of teenagers; a school-based intervention. *Am J Public Health* 1980; 70:722–725.

Pidgeon V: Characteristics of children's thinking and implications for health teaching. *Matern Child Nurs J* 1977 Spring; 1.

Pridham F, et al: Anticipatory care as problem solving in family medicine and nursing. *J Fam Pract* 1977; 4(6):1077–1081.

Rogers ME: *Introduction to the Theoretical Basis of Nursing.* Philadelphia, FA Davis Company, 1970.

Rotter JB: *Social Learning and Clinical Psychology.* Englewood Cliffs, NJ, Prentice-Hall, 1954.

Roy C: *Introduction to Nursing: An Adaptation Model.* Englewood Cliffs, NJ, Prentice-Hall, 1976.

Schlosser C: Health in a new key. *Health Values* 1977 Nov/Dec; 258–261.

Shamansky SL, Clausen CL: Levels of prevention: examination of the concept. *Nurs Outlook* 1980 Feb; 104–108.

Sheridan A, Smith R: Student-family contracts. *Nurs Outlook* 1975 Feb; 114.

Smith JA: The idea of health: a philosophical inquiry. *Adv Nurs Sci* 1981; 3(3):43–50.

Stuart R: Behavioral contracting within the families of delinquents. *J Behav Ther Exp Psychiatr* 1971 Feb; 1.

World Health Organization: *Constitution.* Geneva, 1947.

Wu R: *Behavior and Illness.* Englewood Cliffs, NJ, Prentice-Hall, 1973.

Wylie WE: Cost-benefit analysis of a school health education program: one method. *J Sch Health* 1983 Aug; 53(6):371–373.

Bibliography

Balog JE: The concepts of health and disease: a relativistic perspective. *Health Values* 1982 Sept/Oct; 6(5):7–13.

Birchfield M: Headstart health: a process for health education. *Am J Matern Child Nurs* 1977 Sept/Oct; 307.

Brazelton TB: Anticipatory guidance. *Pediatr Clin North Amer* 1975 Aug; 533–544.

Damberg CL: Strategies for promoting the health of minorities: the school-age population. *Health Values* 1986 May/Jun; 10(3):29–33.

Dane JK, et al: Determinants of wellness in children: an exploratory study. *Health Values* 1987 Jan/Feb; 11(1):p.13–18.

Eberst R: Defining health: a multidimensional model. *J Sch Health* 1985; 54(3):99–104.

Eiser C: Changes in understanding of illness as the child grows. *Arch Dis Child* 1985 May; 60(5):489–492.

Flaherty M: Preschool children's conceptions of health and health behaviors. *Matern Child Nurs J* 1986 Winter; 15(4):205–265.

Graham P: Psychology and the health of children. *J Child Psychol Psychiatr* 1985 May; 26(3):333–347.

Greenberg JS: Health and wellness: a conceptual differentiation. *J Sch Health* 1985 Dec; 55(10):403–406.

Kirscht JP: Preventive health behavior: a review of research and issues. *Health Psychol* 1983 Summer; 2(3):277–301.

Kitzman H: The nature of well child care. *Am J Nurs* 1975 Oct; 1705.

Lau RR, Hartman KA, Ware JE: Health as a value: methodological and theoretical considerations. *Health Psychol* 1986; 5(1):25–43.

Maheady DC: Health concepts of preschool children. *Pediatr Nurs* 1986 May-Jun; 12(3):195–197.

Mauksch H: A socio-scientific basis for conceptualizing family health. *Soc Sci Med* 1974 Aug; 521.

Mickalide AD: Children's understanding of health and illness: implications for health promotion. *Health Values* 1986; May/Jun; 10(3):5–21.

O'Connell JK, Price JH: Ethical theories for promoting health through behavioral change. *J Sch Health* 1983 Oct; 53(8):476–479.

Petosa R: Emerging trends in adolescent health promotion. *Health Values* 1986 May/Jun; 10(3):23–28.

Pringle SM, Ramsey BE: *Promoting the Health of Children.* St. Louis, CV Mosby, 1982.

Reichenback MB: A framework for the nature and development of health beliefs in children. *Matern Child Nurs J* 1986 Fall; 15(3):119–128.

Reisinger MD, et al: Anticipatory guidance in pediatric practice. *Pediatrics* 1980; 66:889.

Schmeiderman LJ: *The Practice of Preventive Health Care.* Reading, MA, Addison-Wesley, 1981.

Skinner R: Lifetime health monitoring, preventive care: age one through adolescence. *Patient Care* 1979 April 30.

Snegroff S: Health education and mass communications. *Health Educ* 1983 May/Jun; 8–11.

Steele S: *Child Health and the Family: Nursing Concepts and Management.* New York, Masson, 1981.

Zangari M, Duffy P: Contracting with patients in day-to-day practice. *Am J Nurs* 1980 Mar; 451.

Communicating with Children and Families

Chapter 11

Mabel Hunsberger

We are always communicating something, whether we are aware of it or not. Thoughts, feelings, and opinions are exchanged, consciously or unconsciously, through verbal and nonverbal means. Relationships are formed through a continuous process of learning about what others think and feel. From infancy, an individual becomes oriented to the physical and social world through a continuous exchange of behaviors and responses with caretakers. It is the quality of the interaction that affects the unfolding relationship between infant and caretaker.

Talking to a child differs from talking to another adult. Children's language has characteristics that adults must learn to understand in order to communicate effectively. Children may not necessarily understand when they appear to have comprehended, and the questions they ask are often less complex than adults interpret them to be. Also, children cannot express their feelings in adult-type conversations, so a variety of alternate techniques can be used to help children express what they think and feel.

The nurse who cares for children can help parents understand the process of communication and the effect this process has throughout the development of their child. Interpersonal communication is not just one of many dimensions of human life, it is "the defining dimension, the dimension through which we become human" (Stewart and D'Angelo, 1975). The health of children is promoted through the nurse's own communication with parents and children and through interventions to support quality relationships between parents and children in the home. This chapter discusses principles of communicating with children and families, with emphasis on developmental differences that affect how children think and respond.

Related Topics
Intercultural communications, Chapter 1
Interviewing children and families, Chapter 15
Promoting healthy play and exercise, Chapter 21
Children's art, Chapter 21
Therapeutic play, Chapter 27
Preparation of children for procedures, Chapter 27
Teaching children, Chapter 27

Communicating with Children and Families

Nursing Diagnoses	Nursing Goals/Strategies
Potential for impaired verbal communication, related to • *psychologic barrier associated with nurse's lack of respect for the individuality of the client/family*	Communicate in a way that makes the child and family feel respected, feel empathy, and feel culturally accepted • Show recognition by using individual's name • Assess cultural/family factors that determine communication patterns • Elicit client/family values concerning family member roles in communication (especially role of child) • Accept behaviors that are in conflict with those of the professional • Elicit client's/family's goals concerning various health issues
• *psychologic barrier associated with nurse's ineffective portrayal of empathy*	• Listen to client's/family's point of view • Refrain from giving advice concerning a point of view unless requested • Guide the client/family in problem solving with their input having dominant influence • Provide positive comments to support client/parent in performance of roles as child/parent
• *psychologic barrier associated with cultural differences (language and lifestyle) between nurse and client/family*	• Identify specific cultural norms for communication patterns • Differentiate lack of understanding associated with language barrier vs. cultural differences • Use an interpreter as required • Adapt plan of care to comply with cultural beliefs and values • Speak slowly and softly and use gestures • Use written forms of communication to supplement the usual verbal methods • Use bilingual dictionaries
• *the child's limitation in receptive and expressive language associated with developmental level*	Promote child's communication at a level consistent with age • Observe for nonverbal cues as expressions of feelings and thoughts • Respond to nonverbal communication with comforting measures, responsive gestures, and verbal expressions as appropriate • Facilitate expression of ideas using strategies of orienting, enabling, informing, sustaining, and concluding* • Use language appropriate for age determined by individual child's ability • Encourage use of alternate means of expression, e.g., play, art, storytelling, storywriting, sentence completion • Differentiate between a comfortable and a fearful silence
Potential for altered family processes, related to inappropriate use of communication techniques with child	Promote communication within the family. Teach family to: • Speak to child at physical level • Include child in decision making • Be honest in explanation even if news is unpleasant • Keep promises that are made and explain if they cannot be kept • Set limits, giving child a sense of security • Use touch to communicate love and acceptance • Avoid indiscriminate touch • Avoid interrupting child's activity • Provide privacy for a child • Give a child adequate time to warm up in a relationship

* See Box 11-1.

Nursing Diagnoses	Nursing Goals/Strategies
Potential knowledge deficit, related to communication (cognitive and language) limitations associated with developmental level	Facilitate child's understanding of information provided • Check child's understanding of communication by asking for explanations in own words • Use techniques appropriate for age to explain information (simple language, play techniques, illustrating) • Explain what will happen even if child does not fully understand • Encourage parents to re-explain information • Stay with child for comfort when understanding is lacking • Differentiate between a silence of comfort and of not understanding

The Process of Communication

The process of communication with children and parents is affected by the relationships that exist between family members as well as the relationship that the nurse has with each member. The nurse's self-understanding and awareness of the effect of personal communication are keys to the relationship with children and their parents. The way messages are formed (coded) and interpreted (decoded) is subject to the acceptance one feels in the presence of another. The nurse's goal is to facilitate communication by creating an atmosphere of acceptance.

In the communication process, a stimulus causes an individual to form a message that is transmitted to another person, the receiver. If a parent sends a message to the nurse in the presence of children, the nurse must decode that message with the realization that parents may not feel free to speak openly in front of their children. For example, the question "Do you have problems in the area of discipline?" may not bring an accurate description if the child is present. Also, when children talk in the presence of their parents, the nurse must recognize that communication is influenced not only by the nurse-child relationship but also by the acceptance the child senses from the parents. Thus the context within which the message is sent has an essential bearing on the way the message is decoded. Communication has not been accomplished until the message is received in the context within which it is sent. The receiving of a message involves decoding both the verbal and the nonverbal content of the communication. Aside from the relationship that exists between communicants, each person's biases and life experiences always affect communication. In the case of children and parents, the family within which they live largely influences their communication with each other and with those outside the family unit. (See Figure 1-3, page 27, for further descriptions of the communication process.)

The Parent-Child-Nurse Relationship

Because communication is the heart of human relationships, it is the most important skill a nurse uses when dealing with children and their families. Much of what a nurse can accomplish depends on the ability to make parents and children feel accepted and comfortable in the relationship. Parents are unlikely to reveal true feelings about their children if there is even a slight possibility that they will feel judged as incompetent parents. Children also are sensitive to lack of recognition from adults. It is important to focus on the child, giving opportunity for the child's expression of fears and concerns. Some children may look to parents to speak for them whereas others like to speak for themselves. The nurse's sensitivity to these differences is central to developing a relationship and making all members of the family feel accepted.

Respect for the individuality of each person within the relationship has particular relevance when dealing with parents and children. The way an individual thinks and feels, and therefore responds to a message, is a reflection of that person's total life experiences, including values of family, friends, community, and society. Communicating respect involves recognizing that the views that parents hold regarding childrearing, health promotion and children's roles may be in opposition to those of the nurse. To respect parents as individuals is to recognize that long-standing family and cultural patterns are an integral part of their way of life and affect their view of parenting.

Children also need to be respected as individuals.

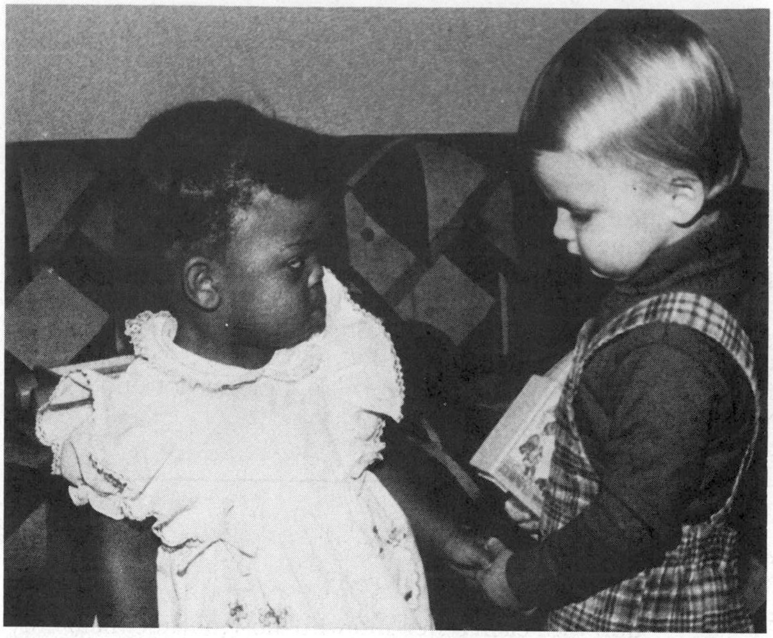

Relationships are formed as thoughts and feelings are communicated.

Although various developmental stages show characteristic behaviors, not all children of the same age act alike. Each child is exposed to a unique set of experiences that affects talking and feeling and interpreting what is communicated. When nurses can respond to the individuality of needs of each family member, that communication contributes to an effective parent-child-nurse relationship.

Implicit in respect is the idea of acceptance of the total person. To convey acceptance of a person when a behavior is not condoned can be difficult. For example, to be accepting of a parent a nurse must understand that a child's temper tantrums produce intolerable frustration in and may lead to corporal punishment by the parent. The nurse does not have to agree with corporal punishment as a means of discipline to be accepting of the parent. The nurse accepts the need that motivates the behavior and does not condemn the parent for the behavior. The nurse can show acceptance by encouraging expression of feelings and discussion of stresses that are impinging on the family. Through these discussions the nurse can help a parent identify alternate ways of expression. Communicating with children involves a similar approach. The behavior of the child does not have to be condoned even though the need of the child is accepted. When the nurse communicates acceptance of the individual, parents and children feel secure in the relationship and are likely to describe feelings and events more accurately.

Empathy is an essential element of the parent-child-nurse relationship. Nurses are empathic when they can make parents and children feel that the meanings of their life experiences are being understood. The important feature of empathy is that the recipient feels it. When dealing with children, empathy means that one has to be able to see the world through children's eyes. Children express how they feel when they are quiet, when they talk, and especially when they play. To grasp how a child feels, attention must be given to all aspects of his behavior, not only speech. Empathy requires spending enough time with the child to see, hear, and understand how the child feels. Sensitivity to a child's nonverbal communication gives the nurse the most accurate sense of the child's true feelings, because children are often unable to verbalize how they feel. If a nurse is able to "tune in" and "be with" a child as private thoughts and feelings are explored, loneliness and alienation are less likely (Dimick and Huff, 1970). Providing this comfort is one of the most important things a nurse can do for a child.

Parents also are relieved from loneliness if they feel understood. When dealing with parents empathically a nurse does not offer advice or try to change a parent's way of thinking. Attempting to alter another person's thinking in accordance with one's own biases and beliefs is evaluative, not empathic. To establish a relationship in which communication can take place, a nurse does not wish to make the parent into what the nurse feels is a good parent but hopes to create a secure environment within which parents can realize their own potential and chart their own courses. However, some individuals will seek advice. In these instances the nurse strives to engage the client in problem solving to enhance self-care abilities. Through empathic understanding, people can be helped to become less dependent on the opinions of others and able to clarify their own thinking and course of action (Dimick and Huff, 1970; Kalisch, 1973).

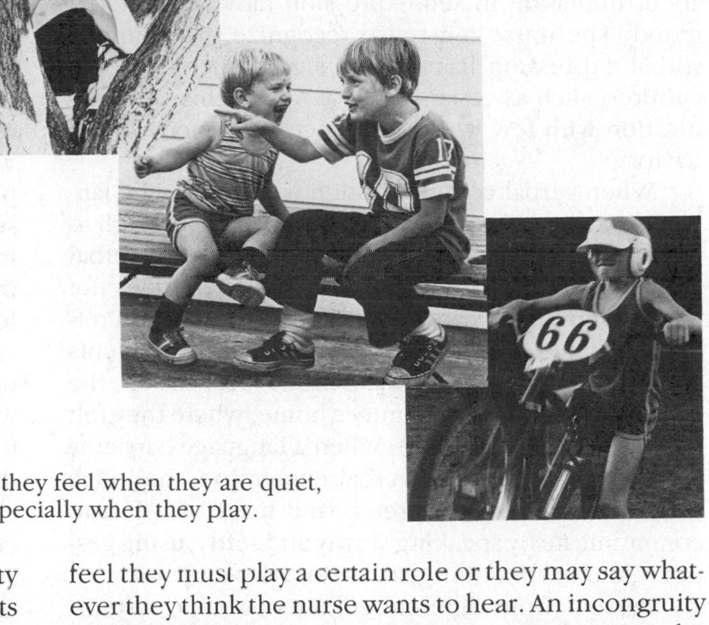

Children express how they feel when they are quiet, when they talk, and especially when they play.

The nurse's self-understanding and individuality determine the respect and acceptance given parents and children empathically. The parent-child-nurse relationship is shaped by the nurse's ability to use personal attributes in combination with skills of communication.

Types of Communication

Nonverbal

For nurses to communicate effectively, they must learn how to use and be responsive to verbal and nonverbal communication. Invariably gestures, facial expressions, and tone of voice add important dimensions to what is said. Nonverbal communication is less easily governed by conscious control than is verbal communication and is therefore more reliable. Children particularly show by their actions how they feel even before they have the language to express such feelings. Nonverbal communication is a child's natural mode of expression. Crying, staying close to a caregiver, and becoming very quiet or overactive are ways that young children express their needs. The innumerable ways that children seek attention through behavioral changes rather than verbal efforts are clues which the nurse learns to recognize.

Adults exercise more control over their nonverbal messages than do children, but tone of voice, facial expressions, and body language are hard to control even for an adult. Thus, even though parents do not necessarily verbalize their true feelings, their nonverbal communication remains an important dimension. Parents may conceal their true feelings because they feel they must play a certain role or they may say whatever they think the nurse wants to hear. An incongruity between verbal and nonverbal communication may be the nurse's only indication that parents hold feelings they hesitate to verbalize.

Verbal

The spoken word is the most obvious expression of thoughts and feelings, but it is not necessarily the most

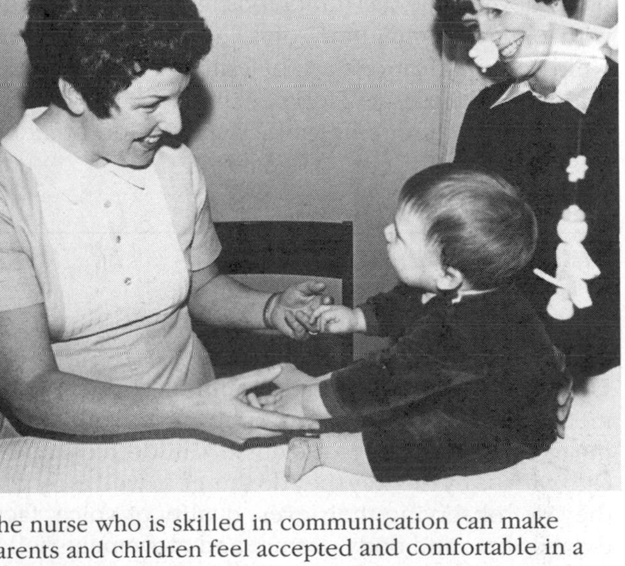

The nurse who is skilled in communication can make parents and children feel accepted and comfortable in a relationship.

accurate. Individuals vary in their ability to use language as a way to communicate: the person who is reluctant to talk may be telling the listener something about limitation in self-expression rather than about mood. The nurse must also recognize that minimal verbal expression has cultural significance. In some cultures, such as certain parts of Appalachia, communication with few words is the accepted mode of behavior.

When verbal communication is hampered by language barriers, the nurse must be sensitive enough to recognize when a nod of the head and lack of verbal communication really means that the client does not understand. When caregivers communicated with refugees from Southeast Asia, it was found that patients comprehended health instructions best when the nurse gave them in the family's home, where they felt comfortable (Leyn, 1978). When a language barrier is the reason for reduced verbal expression, the nurse should search for interpreters and make an effort to communicate by speaking slowly and softly, using gestures, and having bilingual dictionaries available.

Persons from different cultures or value systems may use the same words to communicate, but the meaning of the words varies. The parent, the child, and the nurse each have life experiences and values that affect the use and meaning of words. To communicate effectively therefore, it is important for nurses to recognize when they have not been understood and to clarify the intent when others have used language in a way unclear to them.

The use of words to communicate, even with adults, is subject to misunderstandings. Children may pose additional barriers to effective communication. Although children may be honest and straightforward, sometimes embarrassingly so, their abilities to understand what is spoken and to express their ideas have some developmental limitations. Nurses' interactions with children and their roles in supporting parent-child communications can be enhanced by an understanding of these developmental characteristics (see discussion on communicating with children later in this chapter).

Skills of Communication

Observation

Observation of nonverbal communication provides meaningful clues to what children and parents are saying to each other and to the nurse. Children communicate with us by the way they do things as well as by what they do: observing their eyes, quality of voice, facial expressions, and body posture and movements tell us how they feel about situations and people. Does a child say "I feel disappointed," or does he show us this by his sad eyes, quiet mood, or sobbing cry?

The interaction between parents and children is an integral part of communication at all times and should be the focal point of the nurse's observations. The nurse should observe how the parents respond to their child's requests for attention. Does the child receive rewards for good behavior or is attention granted only when unacceptable behavior ensues? The way a parent physically handles a child, the way questions are answered or whether they are answered at all, and the manner in which the parent elicits cooperation from the child are clues to an understanding of how parents feel about their children.

The nurse should also observe how the parents react to her or him; for instance, how they respond when the nurse demonstrates affection and care for their child. Is there a response of pride and joy, or is there some indication that the nurse's attention to their child is causing some conflict because they do not feel equally affectionate to the child? Does a parent resent attention given by the nurse because it is viewed as competition? Sensitivity to the parents' nonverbal expression of how they feel when the nurse shows affection and attachment to their children is an often-neglected link to effective communication. Observation of the multidirectional flow of nonverbal clues provides the nurse with important information needing a response in the nurse's communication with children and their parents.

Listening

To listen carefully, attention must be given to the words, the tone of voice, and the predominant theme of a conversation. Listening to communication between parents and children makes it apparent whether the child is encouraged to speak out or whether the parent completes sentences, corrects the child, and shows little regard for the ideas of the child. Children should be supported in their attempt to engage in the conversation, especially when the conversation concerns them. Addressing children by name and responding to their concerns is an important dimension of listening to children.

Listening to concerns of parents and children requires special skills of openness and acceptance by the nurse, because parent-child relationships are often highly charged with emotion, and frequently parents have difficulty acknowledging problems. The concerns that parents verbalize about themselves, their children, and each other may therefore be distorted because they do not wish to be regarded as incompetent parents, nor do they want to reveal personal difficulties in a marriage. By sensitive assessment of what is heard and seen, the nurse can develop a true perspective of how parents feel. The messages from parents should be received with the realization that they may be under a great deal of stress trying to conform to the abstract model of "good parenting."

When listening to children, an understanding of their level of language development and cognition is fundamental. Listening to the cry of an infant and trying to interpret it are the beginnings of sensitive communication with children. When children begin to talk, it is important to take the time to listen to what they say to adults and other children.

Perhaps the greatest problem for adults is not so much when children cannot use language, but rather when they *can* speak. Children speak early in life, and it is easy to assume that the thinking underlying the speech is the same as that of an adult. Children's thinking changes as they develop, and it is important to respond to children on the basis of their thinking level and not how adults think. For example, a child may ask for a drink of water or ask to see the stethoscope or to listen to the nurse's watch. What the child is asking may involve more than the obvious request. The child may be thirsty or curious; on the other hand, the child may be trying to delay the nurse because of fear of what is coming next, or may be asking for company because of fear or loneliness.

The greatest disservice we can do to a child is not to listen at all. Ignoring a request without any explanation not only cuts off communication but interferes with the basic trust relationship. If one does not have time to listen, it is important to say why and tell the child when there will be time. Rules and limits can be set to regulate when it is appropriate to talk, but they should be clear to both parties. Just as a child can accept that others have the right to speak, adults must accept a child's right to be heard.

Silence

Silence is a common medium of communication when dealing with parents and children. Children may be quiet because they are afraid, angry, or shy or because they are busy. Therefore silence cannot be understood without taking into account the individuality of the child and the surrounding stimuli. The age of the child, the usual behavior of the child, and the nature of the situation are important elements of the meaning of silence. Perhaps the parent or the child does not wish to speak about a certain topic in front of the other, or maybe the topic is a point of conflict within the family. When silence is used to block communication, it is important for the nurse to be sensitive to the unreadiness of the child or the parent to discuss the problem. The role is to resume conversation at a level that is more comfortable, thereby allowing the regaining of composure (Collins, 1983).

Silence can be used positively by the nurse to encourage communication. Silence is needed for the processing of thoughts and feelings; during silence people seek to understand the content of what has been said. An inability to understand the meaning of what has been said results in a puzzled silence. For a child, thoughtful silence may be primarily filled with fear of the unknown and the inability to express that fear. Often words do not dispel fear in a child, but the nurse's presence brings comfort. The nurse's silent presence can be one of the most effective ways to share the difficulties and fears of another's thoughtful silence. The nurse's use of silence allows the child or the parent to feel accepted in the presence of a caring person. To use silence most effectively, the nurse must evaluate its meaning with regard to the age of the child, the relationships between family members, and the nature of the situation at hand.

Communicating with Children

A basic component of communicating with children is watching and listening carefully to understand their thoughts and feelings. The impact of their families is taken into account and principles of communication are adapted to the needs of children and their families.

Impact of Family

Each child reacts to a unique set of stimuli, which combine to form his personality. What has happened to a child within the family creates the most important force in development, and within the family a child develops a style of communication. According to Satir (1975), all communication is learned. From family, a child develops ideas about self (self-concept), has experiences of interacting with others, and learns how to deal with the world. Families develop patterns of communication that have a great impact on how children relate; therefore, for a nurse to have a realistic expectation of a child's style of communication it is important to begin with an assessment of the family.

The attitude of parents toward their children within the home is the fabric from which patterns of communication evolve. Children who have been deprived of attention and affection at home may be overwilling to please and to comply with the wishes of others. When dealing with a child who interacts in this way, the nurse should respond to the need that the behavior indicates.

Communication patterns are further affected by the relationships between siblings. When sibling rivalry persists, the internal family relationships deteriorate. Friction develops between husband and wife as well as between parent and child as blame is attributed to various family members. A child who comes from a family in which relationships are strained often has difficulty developing relationships outside the home (Hurlock, 1978).

The child who is encouraged to participate in decision-making in the home is likely to take an active role in decisions outside the home. A more dependent role is to be expected when the child comes from an adult-centered home in which children are expected to be submissive and are allowed little opportunity for input into family matters.

Principles of Communicating with Children

Communication with a child is affected by the fact that the child is an individual who comes from a certain family and is at a particular developmental level.

The basic principle of communication is that *adults need to take time to listen to and talk with children.* It is most distressing for a child to be with adults and shown no recognition. Being talked about as if they were not in the room particularly upsets older children and adolescents. Children are people, have ideas, and need to feel important. Young (1965) asserts that children's resentment is not because adults "disagree and deny" but because they "disregard and ignore." Children should be involved when decisions are being made that affect them. Children should be made to feel that their ideas and thoughts are important enough to be heard and considered. Not all wishes can or need to be granted to give a sense of well-being; the important element is being given the opportunity to talk and to be heard.

A child's view about health needs to be heard and considered when health care is being planned. Natapoff (1978) found that children as young as 6 years of age have ideas about health and can talk about health matters.

For nurses to develop relationships with children in which they are trusted, they must *be honest.* Generally, adults do not consciously think they are being dishonest with a child; rather, they tend not to tell children the truth or tell half truths because they wish to protect them from hurt. A fair approach to a child's question is an honest, straightforward answer. For example, if a child asks whether an injection will hurt, the honest answer is "Yes," but this is coupled with a reassuring statement such as "Yes, a shot hurts, but it is over quickly and I am going to be right here with you." The touch, the facial expression, and the few words of simple explanation and encouragement can make that "yes" tolerable. A child can accept the truth even if it means discomfort as long as the nurse communicates a sense of caring and stays with the child.

An adult must *be reliable* in a relationship with a child so that an environment of trust is created in which the child feels secure. Promises that cannot be kept are a great disappointment to children and make them feel deceived. If you tell a child you will be back to play a game it does not matter so much when, but you must return to fulfill the promise. Should it be absolutely impossible to do so, a broken promise must be explained. Another potential deception is offering a choice when there is no choice. Small choices can be offered to a child for providing a sense of importance and some control. For example, asking whether a child wishes to take the pink medicine or the orange medicine first is significant and should not be overlooked by the nurse.

To *set limits* is to demonstrate respect and care to a child, whereas setting no limits produces feelings of insecurity. A child feels isolated and out of communication when those responsible for care are unaware of the child's activities. The "testing" of adults by children should be recognized as a normal part of how children receive feedback. Trying to crawl up on a forbidden table one more time and being prevented from doing so may be a test of whether or not that child can feel confidence in adults. Consistency and fairness in limit-setting provide security in child-adult relationships and are beneficial to the child.

Communication by touch is a sensitive dimension. Treating children as objects to be indiscriminately patted, kissed, and picked up without giving them a choice can communicate disrespect for them as persons. Adults are often unaware of the inappropriateness of their well-intended actions. A child may be engaged in planning an important course of action just when an adult comes by and abruptly picks him or her up. When adults meet their own needs by holding and cuddling with little regard for where the child was going or was about to do, touch has been used indiscriminately. A sensitive adult will observe what a child is doing and use touch in response to the child's needs and as a way to communicate affection. This approach shows respect for the child and simulateously teaches a child self-respect and self-esteem.

While recognizing that a child needs stimulation and communication from adults, the *right of privacy* must also be preserved. Even at a young age a child's private thoughts should not be interrupted. According to Young (1965), children need a private world for many reasons. They need safe retreats in which to fantasize, or quiet times to sort out stormy emotions. When the big world outside gets too confusing, they may need a psychologic refuge. To the question "What were you talking to your sister about?" a child may

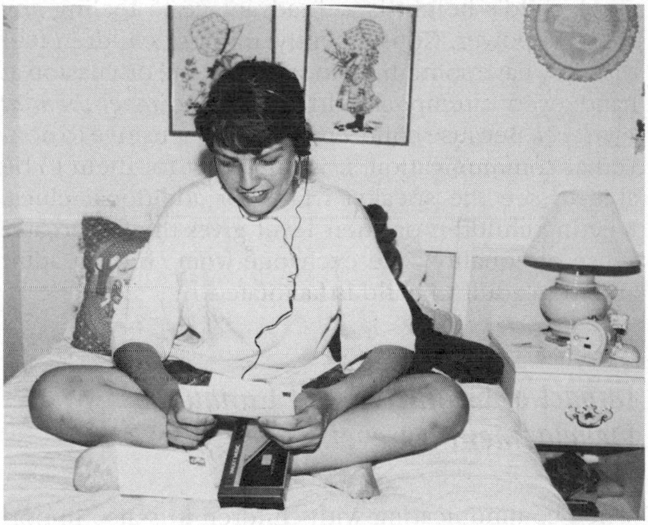

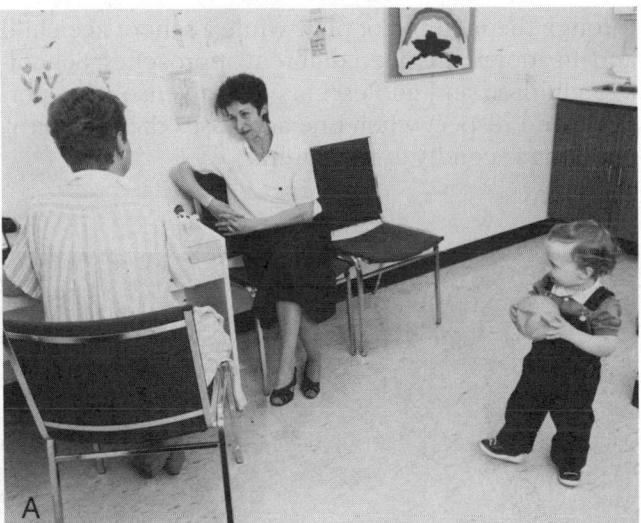

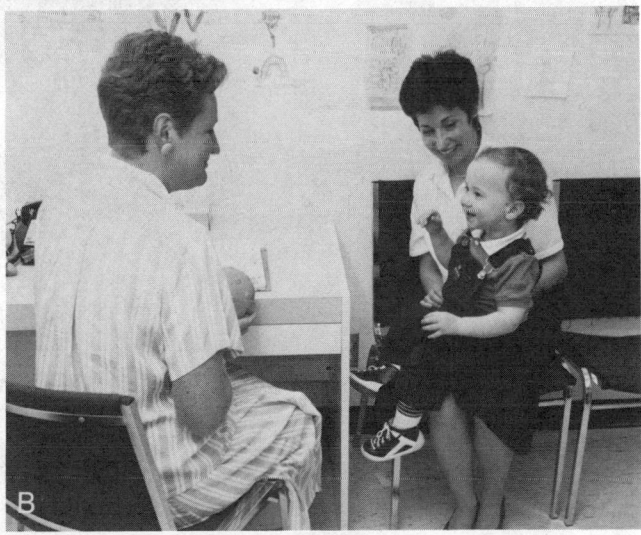

To have privacy is a child's right. Respect and confidence cannot be forced — they are won.

express the need for privacy with a retort such as "Oh, we were just talking." To have privacy is a child's right; a right to open or close a door. To communicate sensitively with children is to realize that the door cannot be commanded to be opened. The respect and confidence that children develop in their relationships with adults cannot be forced — it must be won (Young, 1965).

In relating to children effectively it is important to *respect their emotions.* Children gradually become socialized and learn to control their emotions and translate their feelings into actions as well as words. To communicate with children it is important to realize that emotions change rapidly, with hate existing one moment and love the next. Respecting emotions means that a child is allowed to cry when hurt and to become angry when thwarted. It does not mean that the child is allowed to be destructive or cause injury. If aggressive acting out becomes a pattern of behavior, action is taken to channel the aggression into constructive play and exercise or positive verbal communication and problem-solving. The goal is to learn to control emotions rather than have the emotions control the child (Davis, 1984).

The fears of a child make it imperative to *avoid rushing a child into a relationship.* Children need time to become acquainted with and check out a new environment. An infant or a toddler may be frightened if approached and spoken to directly. When a child fears strangers, it is more effective to first speak to the parent in the presence of the child and gradually to become acquainted with the child through the parent. The approach can be made by first glancing at the child while speaking to the parent and gradually moving closer to the child while making reference to him or her. It is important not to block the view of the parent so that the child will not fear the parent has disappeared.

A preschool child can often be approached

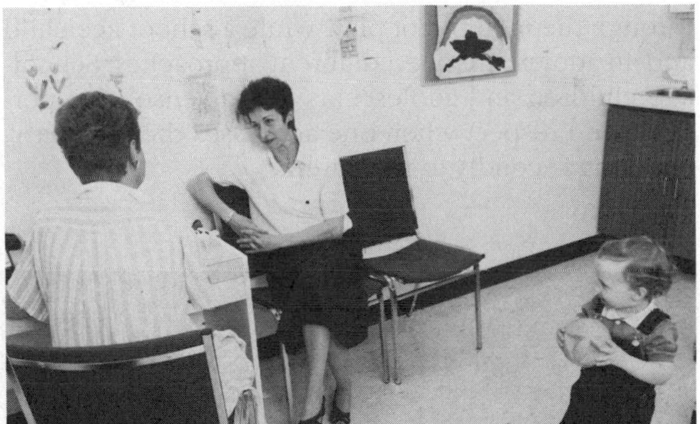

(A) Approaching a fearful child by first speaking to the parent gives a child time to accept a stranger. A child looks to a parent for the cue that "it's OK."

(B) A parent's lap is a good place from which to begin a relationship.

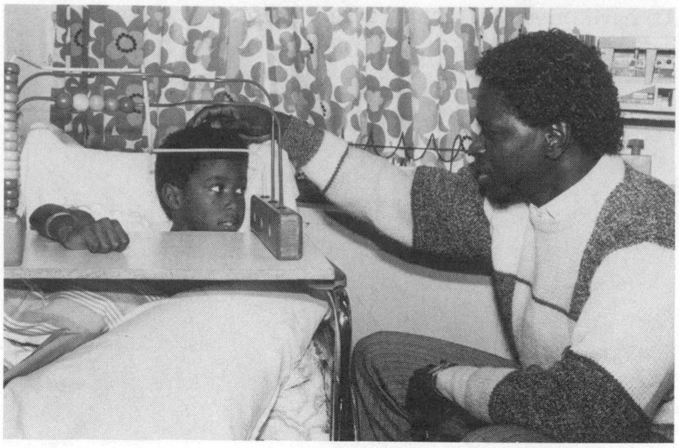

Meeting children at their eye level gives them a greater sense of equality.

through the medium of play, while a school-age child and an adolescent need different approaches. School-age children and adolescents feel a sense of importance and respect when one addresses them directly, speaking secondly to the parent.

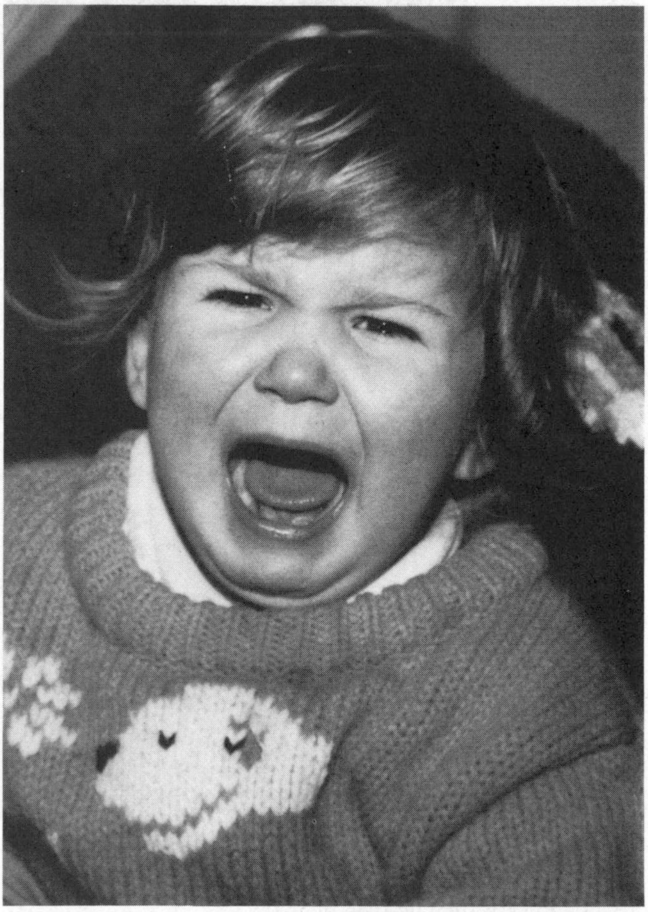

Crying is a forceful way to communicate a need. The pitch of the cry, the facial expression, and the tenseness of the child's body communicate the power of the message.

A child's height is a disadvantage to feeling any sense of power. Consequently, to make children feel that they have something to say about the discussion at hand, every attempt should be made to *meet them at eye level.* Because children are highly sensitive to nonverbal communication, it is important for them to be able to see the speaker's face for additional clues. Meeting children on their level gives them a greater sense of equality. The exchange from child to adult and from adult to child is facilitated.

Impact of Cognitive and Language Developmental Level

When communicating with children it is also important to *consider their cognitive and language abilities.*

Infant. Adults speak to infants long before they expect their words to be understood because it is a means of communicating love and attention. Although they may have no comprehension of words spoken to them, infants attend to the human voice and face, synchronizing their movements with the adult's pauses and segments of speech. Pleasure and displeasure are associated with certain voice tones because of simultaneous experiences. For example, speaking in a soft voice while rocking and feeding the baby is how an infant learns to experience pleasure in response to a soft-spoken voice. The reciprocal system between parent and child develops a sense of competence in the infant and is rewarding for the parent.

By 6 months of age vocalizations become a major form of response to their caretakers by infants. Different pitches of sound are used in response to the tone of their caretaker's voice. Crying is another forceful way in which an infant communicates various needs; different qualities of cries represent hunger, anger, tiredness, or pain. An infant's arm-waving and leg-kicking behavior is also a stimulus that elicits caring, therefore it is a way of communicating. When a parent soothes and settles a thrashing infant, the responsiveness of the infant in turn communicates that the parent is needed (Emde, 1980). Rhythmic sounds or motion is comforting and soothing to the infant and provides further sensations of love.

Toddler and Preschool. As children begin to understand and use words, it is important to know the thought processes that affect their communication. According to Piaget (1967), from 2 until 7 years of age (preoperational thought), children see things from their own points of view. It is difficult for them to understand why they cannot have a drink of water before a diagnostic test. They also make causal errors by thinking that events that happen in proximity to each other are related. To give an injection immediately after a child has been reprimanded for some unacceptable behavior causes the child to think that the behavior resulted in the shot. Verbal explanations of the relationship between treatments and a child's state of health are not understood completely, but brief, simple explanations should be given.

To increase a child's sense of well-being and security, it is paramount that acceptance and affection are communicated both verbally and non-verbally before, during and after any hurtful event. Although a child does not understand the full implication of the words, understanding (receptive language) is greater than speech (expressive language).

During the preoperational stage a child engages in pretending; this is a form of communication often difficult for adults to understand. Children's natural tendency to act out their feelings and experiences helps them cope with the real world and can provide information to others. Allowing children to act out that which is about to happen to them is frequently more beneficial than verbal explanation. If they can see and imagine the events that will occur by reproducing them with dolls or puppets or conversations, they have an acceptable and bearable perception and are able to diffuse some of the emotions pertaining to the event.

Imaginary play is frequently accompanied by talk in the form of a monologue. During this stage play is sustained by talking. In other words, children have to say what they are doing in order to do it. During this phase of language learning, children do not necessarily expect or seek responses to their utterances. More importantly, they need a "sense of a listener" (Martin, 1976). Especially when involved in imaginative play, children do not want the interruption of a real conversation.

One of the most challenging aspects of communication with children at this stage of development is that of answering the "why" question. Answering why questions is difficult because of the difference between the ways children and adults interpret the meaning of why.

According to Piaget (1967), an adult perceives "why" to have two distinct meanings: the goal ("Why are you going?") and the cause ("Why is the car moving?"). A child's "why" implies both meanings at the same time but does not appear to differentiate between the goal and cause (Piaget, 1967). Children often ask questions pertaining to phenomena even when there is no "because." They are also thought to use why questions to learn the meaning of "why." Concrete objects are easily labeled with words but children of this age have difficulty understanding the abstract concept of such words as why and how (Smart and Smart, 1977).

When answering why and how questions, it is important not to read too much into the questions and to avoid explanations that require abstract thinking. For example, "Why is that truck stopping?" is most simply answered with "Because there is a stop sign." A child of this age often responds with "But why?" Additional information such as "Because the truck will hit the car on the other road" may be sufficient to satisfy the child, but sometimes the answers stimulate further questions. Providing simple, concrete answers helps the child understand relationships and satisfies curiosity. To answer the question is of greatest importance. It must not be ignored.

Children may ask questions to satisfy curiosity, to gain information, or for other reasons. Children sometimes practice language and make social contacts by asking questions without expecting an answer. For example, a young child who sees his mother returning from the grocery store with obvious purchases of food may ask "Why did you go to the store?" This may be an effort to make his presence known rather than to discuss the activity of shopping. On some occasions it is apparent that children ask questions to gain attention or as a request for help with a problem. Persistent questioning also may be an indication of fear, insecurity, or unresolved concern. Through attempting to answer a child's questions, we gain insight into what is motivating the question. It is important to answer a child's questions since one who is not offered explanations will not learn to seek answers concerning events (Tough, 1979).

Explanations need to be given in concrete terms, with reference to familiar happenings in the child's life experience. For example, time is understood when it is explained in relation to "after you wake up, have your breakfast, and brush your teeth." Explanations like "There will be bright lights, the room will be cool, and they will take your picture with a large camera" give the child concrete facts to think about and do not leave thoughts to an imagination capable of visualizing an event as far more injurious than it really is. It is also important to avoid words such as cut or bleed when giving explanations. Because of a child's difficulty in separating fact from fantasy, it is important to explain a painful procedure just prior to its occurrence and to follow it with physical comfort. See Chapter 27 for further discussion on preparing young children for procedures.

School-Age. During the stage of concrete operations (7 to 11 years), important cognitive advancements that affect communication are made. At around age 7 years children are better able to cooperate because they begin to comprehend viewpoints other than their own. They are now able to engage in discussions about events because they are able to focus on more than one aspect of an experience. They can comprehend explanations that describe an event though still are bound to concrete thought. For example, they

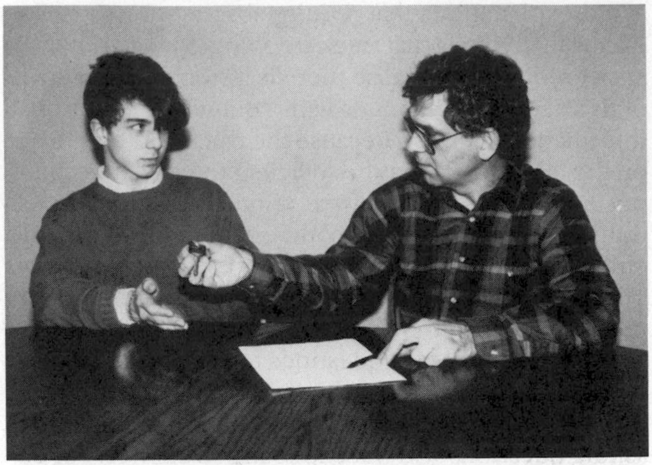

Communication between parents and adolescents involves fair negotiation in which the teenager's views are respected. Here an agreement is made between father and son about use of the family car.

can understand that it is not painful to have a chest radiograph but cannot comprehend how repeated x-ray films may be harmful to the body.

Their cognitive ability enables them to explore and consider many alternatives to a problem. School-age children need to be given the opportunity to question and explore what is being said and what will happen to them. An increased understanding of their body and environment requires that details be painstakingly explained when describing an event that pertains to the body. It is especially important to encourage expression of fears when their body integrity is threatened by invasive procedures. Their increased use of word symbols makes it possible for them to use language to express their concerns and understand more complex explanations. All such communication, however, must be confined to concrete phenomena, because they cannot solve problems or understand ideas that involve abstract thinking.

Children use language at this age as a form of gaining control. Control is experienced simply by playing with words (Martin, 1976). As children become experienced socially they discover that others seek to control them by talking and that they can control the behavior of others by their increased facility with words. At this stage parents begin to see themselves reflected in the way children use communication patterns to cope with and solve problems.

Preadolescent and Adolescent. The period of formal operations (11 to 15 years) is when abstract thinking begins so that hypothetic situations can be created. It is important to remember that during this stage there is an increased need to express feelings verbally. Adolescents, no longer bound to concrete phenomena, wish to discuss their values and ideals. They now can hypothesize about how things should be done and especially do so when it involves their own destinies. They do not wish to be told what to do but will be much more cooperative if they are included in the decisions made regarding them. For example, decisions about responsibilities in the home can be discussed and negotiated, then committed to writing. Clarity of the task and involvement of an adolescent in the decision making about what is expected can thwart daily hassles.

A major difficulty during adolescence is the confusion between ideals of how things should be and how they actually are. This preoccupation with what "could be" characterizes the thinking during the stage of formal operation and sometimes produces conflict with other people. Adolescents need to have the opportunity to express their thoughts of how things should be to help them evaluate their own ideas. Putting their ideas into words is how they formulate what they actually are and eventually resolves the confusion between the real and ideal.

Adolescent thinking is again characterized by egocentricity, as it was early in life. They often imagine other people to have thoughts and feelings they do not have but which are in reality their own (Hurlock, 1978). They have the need to engage in egocentric thinking and need the privacy to do so. A special respect for their private thoughts should be communicated by avoidance of prying into personal matters. Because of their egocentricity they often misinterpret the meaning of someone else's communication by not differentiating their own thinking from the thoughts of others. They are highly sensitive to nonverbal communication and need an environment of acceptance within which they will feel the freedom to express personal views if they so desire.

Talking to a Child

Developmental level, experiences, and personality account for the notable variations in how children communicate. Some children readily engage in conversation while others remain reticent. The process of engaging a child in conversation involves helping a child remember, sustain a line of thought, and put ideas into words. No one technique can be used successfully to engage a child in conversation, but an awareness of some of the characteristics of children's conversations and effective adult responses can promote conversation between adults and children.

Linguistic Characteristics

Maintaining a conversation within the linguistic and cognitive boundaries of the developmental level is necessary to retain children's attention. If their part in a conversation requires speech and thinking ability beyond their level, they will soon become disinterested and frustrated. Children maintain conversations with adults by using some identifiable techniques when they do not understand adult conversation.

Ambiguous Answers to Questions. Pickert and Furth (1980) identified some specific linguistic responses used by children aged 5 to 11 years. These children used ambiguous terms to answer questions they did not understand. For example, in answer to the question "How does a doctor know how to mend your bone?" a 6-year-old child answered, "Because he's special." Further clarification is needed to bring a child to an understanding of the question. "How does a doctor get to know?" leads the child to answer "By learning, like a nurse." Ambiguity in a child's answer may indicate that the question requires further clarification. Additionally, the use of qualifiers in an answer, such as "partly," "sort of," "sometimes," is another technique that children use to maintain a conversation even though they do not fully understand the question. These qualified responses permit children to maintain the topic of conversation without committing themselves to a definite answer (Pickert and Furth, 1980).

Responses to Vague Messages. One cannot be sure that young children understand the content of communication because they respond differently to vague messages than do adults. Flavell et al (1981) noted that young children may show behavioral signs of uncertainty briefly but do not request clarification for a vague message they have received. On the contrary, they resolve uncertainties by making guesses at the speaker's intended meaning. Very young children are thought to have such trust in the person sending the communication that they would be unaware that such a trusted individual could make a vague or ambiguous statement. It has also been noted that kindergarten children seem to persist on relying on nonverbal cues to determine a speaker's intent. When children rely on the physical context and the speaker's gesture to determine intent, misinterpretation can easily occur. This is especially true because young children are known to trust the speaker to correct their arbitrary interpretation of the message if it is not correct (Speer, 1984). Eventually children learn to seek clarification. Recognition of these factors points out the need for adults to explain carefully what will happen to a child and, more importantly, determine a young child's understanding *after* the explanation.

Use of Questions in Child-Adult Conversation. Too frequently in an adult-child encounter the child is bombarded with a string of questions. These questions, unfortunately, are often the same questions that everyone else asks the child. For example, "How old are you?," "What grade are you in?," and "Do you like school?" is the extent of conversation that many adults hold with a school-age child. If given the opportunity, children are capable of more than answers to these mundane and predictable questions; however, many adults lack the skill or do not take the time to engage a child in a more productive conversation.

Questions can be useful and are often necessary to help gather information. Even in an interview situation, however, it should be recognized that successive questions make demands on the child. Questions are a form of power through which the child's thoughts, attention, memories, and ideas are directed and controlled (Wood, 1982). Continued questioning can result in the suppression of a child's spontaneous volunteering of information.

The type of question used to initiate conversation with a child is important. A closed question, one which has only one answer (often a one-word answer) does little other than supply a label for an object or action. An open question, one that invites a range of possible answers, stimulates a child to think and express ideas and thoughts. For example, "What do you think will happen next?" offers the opportunity for a child to share ideas because there is no one right answer. It must be recognized that an "I don't know" answer or shrug of the shoulders means that a child may lack confidence to answer, may not understand the question, or may not have had experience considering alternative answers (Tough, 1979).

Dialogue Techniques

Conversations with children can occur at a variety of levels of communication. The following conversation was heard between a parent and a 9-year-old child concerning a school trip to an Indian museum:

Parent: "How was your trip today?"
Child: "Oh, fine."
Parent: "Did you have fun?"
Child: "Yup."
Parent: "What did you do?"
Child: "Oh, walked around and looked at things."
Parent: "What kind of things?"
Child: "Oh, you know, old things."

This questioning results in a dull conversation that

leaves both parties disinterested. However, strategies to extend this exchange into a more challenging dialogue can be used to enhance the child's social and cognitive skills and overall development. Five strategies to encourage conversation have been identified by Tough (1979) and are summarized in Box 11-1. They are labeled according to the function they have in conversation: orienting, enabling, informing, sustaining, and concluding. They are effective whether a conversation is at a simple reporting level, such as the trip to the museum, or in a more advanced problem-solving situation. Four examples of conversational processes identified by Tough (1979) are summarized in Boxes 11-2, 11-3, 11-4, and 11-5, including reporting, logical reasoning, predicting, and projecting, respectively. Each box gives examples of questions reflecting the five strategies of orienting, enabling, informing, sustaining, and concluding.

Simple *reporting on a present or past experience* (see Box 11-2) is a common form of language use. To encourage dialogue under these circumstances, the steps to include, according to Tough (1979), are

- label the components of the scene
- refer to detail (size, color, and so on)
- refer to incidents and the sequence of events
- make comparisons and identify related aspects
- make an analysis
- identify the central meaning
- reflect on the meaning of the experience (include feelings)

More complex ways of thinking are employed when language is used to engage a child in reasoning processes (see Box 11-3). Adults can foster movement toward logical reasoning by encouraging a child to

- explain a process
- identify causal and dependent relationships
- recognize problems and their solutions
- justify decisions and actions
- reflect on events and draw conclusions
- recognize principles

Even though a child's thinking is prelogical, a reasoning mode is used by some young children and can be fostered in conversation.

Encouraging the use of language to *predict or describe anticipated events* is another way to foster communication with children (see Box 11-4). To encourage a child in this type of conversation, Tough (1979) suggests the following:

- anticipate and forecast events
- anticipate the detail and sequence of events
- anticipate problems and possible solutions
- anticipate and recognize alternative courses of action
- predict the consequence of actions and events

This process is particularly useful to the child who is anticipating a painful procedure. These strategies can be employed by engaging the child in conversation or through the use of play. As the child communicates

Box 11-1
Dialogue Strategies to Promote Conversation with Children

1. **Orienting Strategies**
Comments and questions that direct the child's thinking toward a particular topic and to think in a particular way (i.e., predicting, reasoning).
2. **Enabling Strategies**
Utterances that enable a child to move toward an extended interpretation (extend meaning that a situation has for a child as far as is possible).
    a. *Follow-through strategies:*
    Statements that help child give further detail, explanations, and justifications. They follow-up the child's response and help extend a description or interpretation.
    b. *Focusing strategies:*
    A deliberate focusing of child's attention on essential features to promote a fuller interpretation of a picture, event, or experience.
    c. *Checking strategies:*
    To help the child reconsider the statements giving an opportunity to provide omitted information. For example, "Did you really mean. . . ?"
3. **Informing Strategies**
Providing information when a child seems ready to receive it or when additional information is needed to complete an idea or solve a problem.
4. **Sustaining Strategies**
Supportive comments encourage the child to say more and indicate that she or he has the attention of the listener. These strategies may be verbal, e.g., "Really?" "Good!" "What else?" or nonverbal (gestures and facial expressions). Comments also may be repetitions of what the child has said, using intonation and a pause that encourages the child to go on.
5. **Concluding Strategies**
Comments that indicate intention to bring a particular topic of discussion to a close. It is important to leave the child with a sense of satisfaction because efforts have been recognized or difficulties understood.

(Adapted from Tough J: Talking and Learning. *London, Ward Lock Educational, 1977, © School Curriculum Development Committee.)*

Box 11-2
Reporting on Present and Past Experience

TALKING ABOUT A CHILD'S DRAWING OF HIS PARTY AND RECALLING THE PARTY

Goals

1. Label the components of the scene
2. Refer to detail (size, color, etc.)
3. Refer to incidents and the sequence of events
4. Make comparisons and identify related aspects
5. Make an analysis
6. Identify central meaning
7. Reflect on the meaning of the experience (include feelings)

1. **Orienting**
Will you tell me about your picture?
That's a lovely picture of your party. I'd like you to tell me about it.
Tell me about your party yesterday.
I believe you had a party yesterday. I'd like to hear about it.
What happened at your party yesterday?
2. **Enabling**
 a. *Follow-through*
 Oh, why is he doing that?
 How do you play . . .?
 What did you do then?
 Why did Jane cry?
 And what was special about your cake?
 b. *Focusing*
 And what is this?
 Did you have good things to eat?
 Did you play games?
 Did you get some presents?
 c. *Checking*
 Did you say you didn't have a birthday cake?
 Ten o'clock—was it really so late?
 I don't think it would have ten candles, would it?
3. **Informing**
A good way to make pink is to mix red and white together.
When you play Blind Man's Bluff, you have a scarf over your eyes so you can't see and you have to catch one of the others and then guess who it is. Sometimes people play that game at parties.
4. **Sustaining**
Go on, I'd like to hear more about that.
That sounds like fun.
You did have a good time, didn't you? I wish I'd been there.
5. **Concluding**
That's a lovely picture. Would you like to put it there to dry?
I enjoyed hearing about that. You had a lovely time.
Are you going to finish your picture now?

(Reprinted with permission from Tough J: Talking and Learning. *London, Ward Lock Educational, 1977, © School Curriculum Development Committee.)*

Box 11-3
Toward Logical Reasoning

TALKING ABOUT A BIRD'S NEST

Goals

1. Explain a process
2. Identify causal and dependent relationships
3. Recognize problems and their solutions
4. Justify decisions and actions
5. Reflect on events and draw conclusions
6. Recognize principles

1. **Orienting**
Why do you think the bird needs a nest?
Why do you think the nest is in the tree?
And how do you think the bird made it?
2. **Enabling**
 a. *Follow-through*
 How does it keep safe?
 Why do you say that?
 Why doesn't it like people near?
 Why would an animal want to catch a bird?
 What would happen if an animal could get to the nest?
 b. *Focusing*
 Are there any animals that might come after the bird?
 Can you see what it's made of?
 What do you think this is?
 Do birds always build their nests in trees?
 Have you seen a nest under the roof of a house?
 c. *Checking*
 Lions and tigers! Are there any lions and tigers in the school yard?
 It looks like string, but is it really?
 Feel this, does it feel like stones?
 Would a car really be a good place for a nest?
3. **Informing**
There are lots of cats about. Cats sometimes catch birds.
They watch the bird and keep very still and then they pounce.
The bird would have to fly up with bits of dry grass in its beak. Then it would use its beak to weave the grass into the nest.
Some birds build their nests on the ground.
Here's a picture of a skylark's nest. It's in the long grass so it's not very easy to see, is it?
4. **Sustaining**
That's a good idea.
Anything else?
Did it really!
5. **Concluding**
You do know a lot about birds. Have you seen the bird book in the book corner?
Shall we put it back on the table now for the other children to look at?

(Reprinted with permission from Tough J: Talking and Learning. *London, Ward Lock Educational, 1977, © School Curriculum Development Committee.)*

Box 11-4
Predicting

TALKING ABOUT A FORT TWO CHILDREN ARE GOING TO MAKE

Goals

1. Anticipate and forecast events
2. Anticipate the detail and sequence of events
3. Anticipate problems and possible solutions
4. Anticipate and recognize alternative courses of action
5. Predict the consequences of actions and events

1. **Orienting**
   How are you going to make your fort?
   What is your fort going to be like?
   What will you do with your fort when you've made it?
2. **Enabling**
   a. *Follow-through*
      What are you going to need for it?
      Why does a fort need high walls?
      What would the soldiers do to defend their fort?
      If a real fort was made of wood, what might happen?
      What are you going to do next?
   b. *Focusing*
      Look at this picture of a fort. Can you see the gate?
      Will the walls need to be thick?
      Would it be protected if it was at the bottom of a hill?
      Will the soldiers stand on top of the wall?
   c. *Checking*
      Does a fort really have a chimney?
      There are slits? I can't see them.
      Did you mean they shoot arrows or cannon-balls?
      Is it going to be a castle or a fort?
      I'm not sure what you mean.
3. **Informing**
   I think they might have had cannons on the walls to shoot at the enemy.
   I think that there might be a moat to prevent attackers getting near the wall of the fort.
   They would have a big gate that could be shut quickly if there was an attack.
   Wood burns easily, doesn't it, and if they shoot flaming arrows onto the buildings they might catch fire.
4. **Sustaining**
   I like your idea of that.
   That should be good when you've finished.
   Yes, you could do that.
5. **Concluding**
   That sounds great. I'll come back and see it when you've finished.

(Reprinted with permission from Tough J: Talking and Learning. *London, Ward Lock Educational, 1977, © School Curriculum Development Committee.)*

Box 11-5
Projecting

PROJECTING INTO AN IMAGINED SCENE ARISING FROM PLAY WITH LARGE FLOOR BRICKS AND PLANKS

Goals

1. Project into the experiences, feelings, and reactions of others
2. Project into situations never experienced

1. **Orienting**
   I think there's a storm coming, what will happen next?
   What's happening to you in your boat?
   What will happen to all the men in your boat if a storm comes?
2. **Enabling**
   a. *Follow-through*
      The wave's coming—what will it do to the boat?
      What will all the men have to do?
      Why will you have a life jacket—what will that do?
      Why will they be frightened?
      What could they do?
      Why do you think that?
      And what will he say?
   b. *Focusing*
      Do you remember what the Air Force pilot had to save him when he fell into the sea?
      Do you know what a wireless transmitter is?
      Will you need a life jacket?
      Could the boat capsize?
   c. *Checking*
      Do you really think a fish can give you a ride on its back?
      Do you mean a television or a radio?
      Does the lifeboat sink or can it float in stormy weather if the waves have sunk the ship?
      The captain won't jump off first, will he?
3. **Informing**
   Well, boats usually have a special sort of radio so they can send out messages to other boats. So I think they could send for help.
   The captain really is in charge and the crew take orders from him. He usually stays on a boat when it's ship-wrecked until the very last.
4. **Sustaining**
   The boat's sunk—I see (remodeling the child's "The boat's sinked").
   Oh, dear—the boat's sunk.
5. **Concluding**
   That was an adventure, wasn't it? Could you begin to clear up now?
   Good—I'll come back later when you've rescued everybody.

(Reprinted with permission from Tough J: Talking and Learning. *London, Ward Lock Educational, 1977, © School Curriculum Development Committee.)*

understanding of the anticipated event, misconceptions can be clarified.

The use of language to *project into the feelings of others* is not easily done by the young child. However, Tough (1979) suggests that to teach children to appreciate another's point of view they can be encouraged to

- project into the experiences, feelings, and reactions of others
- project into situations never experienced

These various processes of reasoning, predicting, and projecting can be employed when talking to children. Encouragement of the use of language in this way encourages children to engage in more complex thinking than the mere labeling of events and experiences.

Whether one is engaging a child in conversation related to reporting, reasoning, predicting, or projecting (as just described), the five dialogue strategies in Box 11-1 facilitate achievement of the goals in each of these processes.

Indirect Communication Techniques

Nurses are frequently required to communicate with children at a time when they are encountering unusual and frightening circumstances. Children tell about their thoughts and feelings indirectly through their usual patterns of self-expression (stories, drawing, play) more readily than through a formal interview. An interview depends on the use of language for communication, and it may be misinterpreted by a young child. Furthermore, it is often too direct and confronting for children. Although nurses, unless especially prepared, are not expected to use psychotherapy, numerous indirect approaches of a nurse can promote self-expression. These techniques assess children to determine the need for additional therapy.

Useful conversation techniques are the *third-person technique* and *sentence completion.* In the third-person technique, feelings are explored through a statement like "Lots of times kids feel afraid or lonely in the hospital." Children are not directly asked how they feel but rather are allowed to accept, reject, or ignore the interpretations (Mesibov and Johnson, 1982). A discussion about how "other children" feel may eventually encourage the child's own expression of feelings. The sentence completion technique is particularly useful with school-age children and can be introduced as a game. Non-threatening topics are described by incomplete sentences, such as "The thing I like best about summer is . . ." Gradually personal statements can appear, such as "The thing I like least about being in the hospital is . . ." This approach can be expanded into having the child list as many "good things" and as many "bad things" she or he can think of about a certain event or topic.

Engaging the child in *story-telling,* whether verbally or in conjunction with drawing and writing, provides a natural medium through which children express themselves. A child can simply be asked to tell a story about being in the hospital or about a specific event the child has experienced. The technique of writing a story or drawing a picture and telling a story to accompany it is a common method of teaching in the elementary schools and is familiar to school-age children. Feelings also can be explored by showing a child predrawn pictures or a comic strip. The child is then asked either to tell or write a story to go with the pictures.

Although drawing, writing, and telling stories about ideas is a commonly used technique, some children may find it difficult to express themselves in a drawing and others have difficulty with writing or telling. One must search for the medium that best suits the abilities of each child.

Another important way to use stories is to have *books on the topics and events* that are similar to what a child is experiencing or is about to experience (bibliotherapy). Life events such as moving, starting school, birth of a sibling, adoption, divorce, illness, hospitalization, and other new or stressful experiences can be introduced through books. A child can learn about the nature of an event and is given the opportunity to express feelings and concerns about a personal situation. This technique can be combined with *story-telling, drawing, and writing stories* by using a book as a way of introducing a topic and then encouraging a child to relate personal ideas in response to the book.

A specialized technique that has been introduced by Gardner (1971) is the mutual *story-telling technique.* This is a psychotherapeutic approach designed to elicit the child's thinking but it also introduces new ways of thinking. In this technique a child is asked to tell a story for a make-believe television program. The child is instructed to tell the moral of the story. The therapist then tells a story using the same characters, but with healthier adaptations and ways of thinking. Anxiety-provoking confrontations are avoided in this method. Gardner suggests that this is not an easy technique and that proficiency in its use may require months or even years of practice.

Play as an avenue for communication, and its developmental characteristics, are discussed in Chapter 21. Play is believed to be an important activity through which children and adolescents can maximize their coping skills when encountering the stress of hospitalization and illness. Children placed into stressful circumstances are less likely to play spontaneously (Bolig, 1984). Play and its use in the hospital is discussed in Chapter 21. It should be recognized that even in less threatening places, such as clinics and offices, elementary schools, and the home, play should be introduced as a way of facilitating communication. For example, taking an interest in the child's normal play activity, use of puppets and miniature versions of office equipment, handling of unfamiliar equipment, and use of stories and drawings in these less threatening environments are important supportive nursing measures.

Art is another frequently used technique to help children express how they feel. Children can be encouraged to draw a picture and then talk about the picture. Although drawings express children's feelings and can open a door to communication, a full interpretation of drawings should not be attempted without specialized preparation (see Chapter 21 for further discussion of children's art).

Communicating with Parents

The nurse who hopes to relate to parents in a beneficial way must begin from the premise that parents are individuals. How a parent thinks and feels about the parental role differs with each one. This role is a manifestation of each person's total life experiences, including cultural, moral, and ethical dimensions. This accounts for phenomena that nurses may find troublesome: as individuals, parents may disagree with each other on parenting issues. The nurse should acknowledge the uniqueness of each parent by encouraging individual expression and giving equal recognition. The nurse's acceptance of and respect for the opinions of each can teach parents also to respect each other's individuality.

In communication with parents, the nurse must recognize that the way parents perceive their role will affect the communication process. Parents may think that they are expected to have certain feelings and respond in prescribed ways because they are parents. The nurse can dispel some of these erroneous ideas by acknowledging that their frustrations with parenting are normal reactions.

Positive feedback from the nurse that acknowledges effective parenting gives the parents needed assurance. Most parents need to hear that their children are growing and developing normally, but it is equally important for the nurse to attribute the health of children to the care and nurturing of parents. Small recognitions of positive parent-child relationships provide a significant source of encouragement to parents.

Frequently nurses do not make such assurances because they fail to realize the regard that parents have for the professional opinion of a nurse. Comments such as "You handle your baby very confidently," "You seem very calm when Mark insists on his own way," and "I notice you are careful to pay attention to your children's questions," are incidental observations that give parents added confidence in their parenting skills. This kind of feedback provides a feeling of basic acceptance that can encourage parents to express the less admirable feelings they hold regarding their children.

The nurse whose goal is to establish an atmosphere that encourages communication will be careful to avoid "talking to" but rather will use an approach that facilitates "talking with" parents. The nurse uses the skills of silence, listening, and observation in conjunction with personal characteristics of acceptance of others, respect for them, and empathy with them. A nondirective approach (using open-ended questions) often creates an environment within which a parent feels accepted and is able to think through a problem and consider new ways of approaching it. The nurse's role then is to reflect the parent's thinking so that the issues can be more easily clarified and decision making by the parent can be facilitated. The goals parents set for themselves are more likely to be reached and to bring beneficial results to the family than are those the nurse can establish for the parents.

References

Bolig R: Play in hospital settings. *In* Yawkey TD, Pellegrini AD: *Child's Play: Developmental and Applied,* Hillsdale NY, Lawrence Erlbaum Associates, 1984.

Collins M: *Communication in Health Care.* St. Louis, CV Mosby, 1983.

Davis A: *Listening and Responding.* St. Louis, CV Mosby, 1984.

Dimick KM, Huff VE: *Child Counseling.* Dubuque, IA, William C. Brown Company, Publishers, 1970.

Emde RV: Emotional availability: a reciprocal reward system for infants and parents with implications for prevention of psychosocial disorders. *In* Taylor PM: *Parent-Infant Relationships.* New York, Grune & Stratton, 1980.

Flavell JH, et al: The development of comprehension, monitoring and knowledge about communication. *Monographs Soc Res Child Dev* 1981; Serial No. 192; 46(5).

Gardner RA: *Therapeutic Communication with Children: The Mutual Storytelling Technique.* New York, Science House, 1971.

Hurlock EB: *Child Development.* New York, McGraw-Hill, 1978.

Kalisch BJ: What is empathy? *Am J Nurs* 1973 Sep; 1548.

Leyn RB: The challenge of caring for child refugees from Southeast Asia. *MCN* 1978 May/June; 178.

Martin N, et al: *Understanding Children Talking.* New York, Penguin Books, 1976.

Mesibov GB, Johnson MR: Intervention techniques in pediatric psychology. In Tuma JB: *Handbook for the Practice of Pediatric Psychology.* New York, John Wiley & Sons, 1982.

Piaget J: *Six Psychological Studies.* Translated by Tenzer; edited by Elkin. New York, Random House, 1967.

Pickert SM, Furth G: How children maintain a conversation with adults. *Hum Dev* 1980; 23:162–176.

Satir V: *Peoplemaking.* Palo Alto, CA, Science and Behavior Books, 1975.

Smart MS, Smart RG: *Children: Development and Relationships.* New York, Macmillan, 1977.

Speer JR: Two practical strategies young children use to interpret vague instructions. *Child Dev* 1984; 55:1811–1819.

Stewart J, D'Angelo G: *Together: Communicating Interpersonally.* Reading, MA, Addison-Wesley, 1975.

Tough J: *Talking and Learning.* London, Ward Lock Educational, 1979, pp 26–29.

Wood DJ: Talking to young children. *Dev Med Child Neurol* 1982 Dec; 24(6):856–859.

Young LR: *Life Among the Giants.* New York, McGraw-Hill, 1965.

Bibliography

Allen RR, Brown KL: Developing communication competence in children: ten years later. Paper presented at Annual Meeting of Central States Speech Association, Cincinnati, April 1986.

Beal CR: Repairing the message: children's monitoring and revision skills. *Child Dev* 1987; 58:401–408.

Beal CR, Flavell JM: Development of the ability to distinguish communicative intention and literal message meaning. *Child Dev* 1984; 55:920–928.

Blondis MN, Jackson BE: *Nonverbal Communication with Patients: Back to the Human Touch.* New York, John Wiley & Sons, 1977.

Brunner J: *Child's Talk: Learning to Use Language.* New York, Norton, 1983.

Chopoorian T: Communication beyond the assessment process. *In* Brandt PA (ed): *Current Practice in Pediatric Nursing.* St. Louis, CV Mosby, 1978.

Costello DE: Communication patterns in family systems. *Nurs Clin North Am* 1969 Dec; 721.

Duldt BW, et al: *Interpersonal Communication in Nursing.* Philadelphia, FA Davis, 1984.

Elmassian BJ: A practical approach to communicating with children through play. *MCN* 1979 Jul/Aug; 238–240.

Faber A, Mazlish E: *How to Talk so Kids Will Listen and Listen so Kids Will Talk.* New York, Avon Books, 1980.

Feagans L, et al: *The Origins and Growth of Communication.* Norwood, NJ, Ablex Publishing Corporation, 1984.

Flavell JH: *The Development of Role-Taking and Communication Skills in Children.* Huntington, NY, Robert E. Greiger Company, 1975.

Garvey C: *Children's Talk.* Cambridge, MA, Harvard University Press, 1984.

Green M: Interviewing children and adolescents. *Patient Care* 1986 Sep 30; 20(15):76–78.

Greenspan SI: *The Clinical Interview of the Child.* New York, McGraw-Hill, 1981.

Guralnick M, Paul-Brown D: Communicative adjustments during behavior-request episodes among children at different developmental levels. *Child Dev* 1984; 55:911–919.

Keane SP, Conger JC: The implications of communication development for social skills training. *J Pediatr Psychol* 1981; 6(4):369–381.

Kenny TJ, Clemmens RL: *Behavioral Pediatrics and Child Development.* Baltimore, Williams & Wilkins, 1975.

Klinzing DR, Klinzing DG: *The Hospitalized Child: Communication Techniques for Health Personnel.* Englewood Cliffs, NJ, Prentice-Hall, 1977.

Levin H, et al: Nurturant talk to children. *Language Speech* 1984 Apr-June; 147–162.

Lloyd P, Beveridge M: *Information and Meaning in Child Communication.* London, Academic Press, 1981.

Lyman MJ, et al: Adolescent communication: understanding its dynamics and fostering its development. *Nurs Pap* 1986 Spring; 18(1):67–77.

Milosky LM, et al: School-age children's understanding of explanation adequacy. *J Educ Psychol* 1986 Oct; 78(5):334–346.

Mitchell AC: Barriers to therapeutic communication with black clients. *Nurs Outlook* 1978 Feb; 109.

Penner SG: Parental responses to grammatical and ungrammatical child utterances. *Child Dev* 1987; 58:376–384.

Pothier PC: *Mental Health Counseling with Children: A Guide for Beginning Counselors.* Boston, Little, Brown, 1976.

Rice M: *Child Language and Cognition: Contemporary Issues.* Baltimore, University Park Press, 1984.

Rich J: *Interviewing Children and Adolescents.* New York, Macmillan, 1968.

Smith LF: Communicating with young children: an experiment with play therapy, Part 3. *Am J Nurs* December 1977 Dec; 1963.

Strodtbeck F, Perez RC: Poetry play: a method of communication with pediatric clients. *Issues Compr Pediatr Nurs* 1981 May/Jun; 5(3):129–137.

Thompson CL, Rudolph LB: *Counselling Children.* Belmont, CA, Wadsworth, 1983.

Tough J: *Focus on Meaning: Talking to Some Purpose with Young Children.* London, George Allen & Unwin, 1976.

Tough J: *Listening to Children Talking.* London, Ward Lock Educational for The Schools Council, 1976.

White JD: *Talking with a Child.* New York, Macmillan, 1976.

Wiedenbach E, Falls CE: *Communication: Key to Effective Nursing.* New York, Tiresias Press, 1978

Wood BS: *Children and Communication: Verbal and Nonverbal Language Development.* 2nd ed. Englewood Cliffs, NJ, Prentice-Hall, 1981.

Assessing and Promoting Family Health

Chapter 12

Jo Joyce Anderson
Judith Maserang

Family assessment is essential to family-centered nursing care. This chapter introduces a range of theories that can be used to assess families. An attempt is made to emphasize the nurse's role as advocate for the family, recognizing cultural variances in the structure and function of the family unit. Intervention is addressed, focusing on the benefits of an interdisciplinary approach in assisting families to stay well or cope with problems. The major goal of the chapter is to expand the nurse's understanding of how and when to assess families for actual or potential dysfunction.

Related Topics
Values clarification, Chapter 1
Alternative lifestyles, Chapter 2
The Developing Family, Chapter 2
Health Concepts: Children's Perceptions and Behaviors, Chapter 10
Communicating with Children and Families, Chapter 11
Promoting Healthy Parenting, Chapter 13
Fostering Self-Esteem, Chapter 16

Nurses who work with children know that families have a direct impact on the health potential of the child, influencing the child's health beliefs and attitudes as well as the likelihood that prescribed interventions will be carried out. With some specific legal exceptions, *the family has the initial and final say about what health care a child needs, when it should be sought, and what kind of care will be employed.*

Thus health goals set for children must involve the entire family unit if they are to be met. Successful child health care rests on identification of family attitudes, resources, and needs. This element is even more important as more children are cared for at home. To work with families to promote children's health, the nurse must know something about those families. The pediatric nurse cares for families for the child's benefit, realizing that family survival is critical to a child's well-being and that the interdependence of family, child, and health care system must be considered in all aspects of the nursing process.

Family and Society Interface

Just as the child is viewed in the context of the family, rather than as a person in isolation, the family itself is viewed in the context of the environment in which it is functioning. The family can be conceptualized as a behavioral system with unique properties. A close interrelationship exists between the psychosocial functioning of the family as a group and the emotional adaptation of its individual members.

The family can be viewed comprehensively in terms of the relationships, association, and connections that occur in a dynamic, interacting whole. A family system includes not only the family members but their relationships, their communication with one another, and their interactions with the environment.

Although families differ from one another, the family is the basic group in human societies. It provides newborn members with their initial experience of other human beings and with their earliest definitions of themselves and the world in which they are destined to live. Even though a rapidly changing society has produced a variety of family forms and lifestyles, as discussed in Chapter 2, the family is still the institution that provides new recruits for society; it is the unit charged with the overall responsibility of preparing those new recruits for assuming functional social roles as adults.

According to Delaney (1982, page 54):

> The family serves as a buffering zone or neutralizing agent between the individual and society. It provides psychosocial protection for its members and is the major vehicle for the transmission of culture. The health of the individual is interwoven with the relationships, beliefs, values, and duties in the family system. The family is a necessary and natural unit of service for the nurse.

The family and society mutually interface, resulting in alteration of norms by both family and society to meet the needs and goals of each.

The family is America's most precious resource and most important institution. The strength of our families is the key determinant of the health and well-being of our nation, of our communities, and of our lives as individuals.

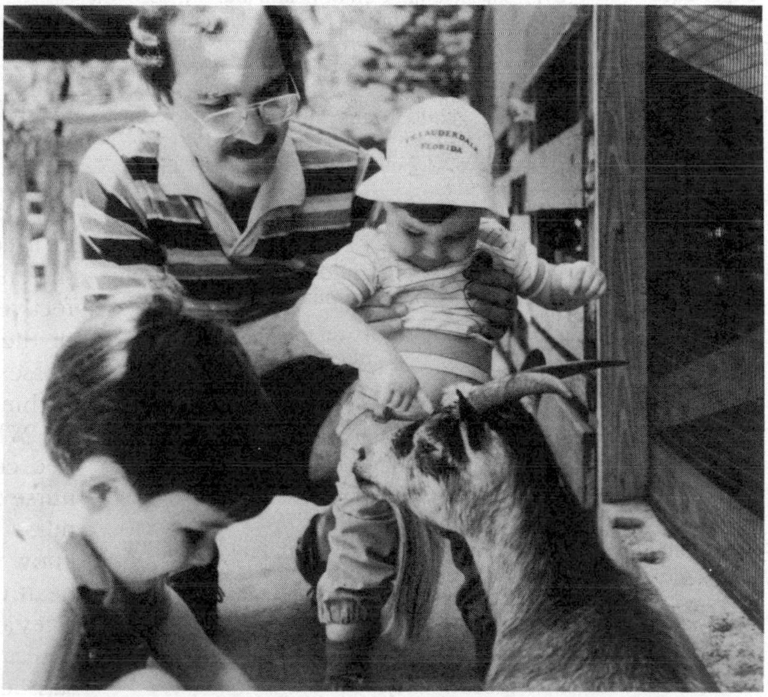

Family-Centered Nursing Roles and Child Health

Ideally, all areas of nursing practice are family centered. However, the reality is that the extent to which care is family centered is greatly influenced by the philosophy of the institution where the nurse works and the amount of contact with the family that the setting allows. Most influential is the nurse's own understanding of the significance of the family to individual members' health and the nurse's own experience in working with families. Table 12-1 describes the interrelationship between the child's health status and the family's involvement.

One frequent nursing role in pediatric practice is that of the *health educator*. The aim is to teach children responsibility for self-care and provide parents with the anticipatory guidance that will help them transcend the maturational crises of raising their children. Teaching a child about health-promoting behaviors (self-responsibility; regular balanced meals that include breakfast; age-appropriate amounts of rest and exercise; stress management; safe environment) is not effective unless the family shares the knowledge and supports these behaviors.

Table 12-1. Family Involvement According to Child's Health Status

Child's Health Status	Family Involvement
Health Promotion and Illness Prevention	Wellness strategies of the child require involvement of family system as a whole: • Improvement in entire family lifestyle may be necessary. • Wellness strategy may induce conflict due to impact on family as unit. • Child's self-view and body image as either healthy and active or sickly and frail is learned in family context.
Symptom Experience Stage	Family assesses child's health behavior and provides basic definition of health and illness: • Interprets symptoms by conveying to child the seriousness of symptoms, possible causes, significance, and degree of concern or attention to be given to symptoms. • Protects child from health hazards to extent family unit is aware of such hazards. • Family disorganization may be cause of symptoms.
Care-Seeking Stage	Family decides when ailing child is really sick and needs help. Family decides where child's illness should be treated (home, clinic, hospital).
Medical Contact Stage	Family serves as primary referral agent, deciding what type of intervention should be sought.
Dependent Patient Stage	Family defines the patient role (to what degree advice will be followed) and patient role behaviors (how soon patient is expected to recover), ranging from making no demands on patient to forcing a prompt recovery.
Rehabilitation Stage	Family determines degree of support for child's convalescence or rehabilitation. When the person's condition is serious or the person is a pivotal or crucial family member, the impact on family is more pronounced.

(Based on Friedman, 1986.)

The pediatric nurse spends a lot of time in the role of *delivering, coordinating,* and *supervising* the child's physical *care.* The aim in this role is to teach the child and family self-care and self-responsibility for health practices. This is particularly important in preparation for early discharge to home and in the home, where the nurse assesses:

- their readiness to assume part or all of that responsibility,
- the family's potential and actual expertise for delivering the care needed.

Helping the family adapt through improvisation within the home environment also requires knowledge of the family's lifestyle and home situation. The home care or community nurse visits the home to determine what adaptations to existing resources (e.g., space, equipment) can be made to minimize costs and disruptions to lifestyle for the family and still adequately provide for the child's needs.

The nurse's role as *consultant* and *counselor* has come into the forefront as emphasis shifts from physical to emotional-social and behavioral health problems. To provide consultation on behalf of a child to teachers, physicians, legislators, and probation officers, the nurse requires information about the child's family. The specific goal of counseling is to facilitate the child's and family's problem solving. This goal can be accomplished only with a realistic understanding of the environment within which they must function. Effective counseling of the child mandates a knowledge of the strengths and problem-solving skills already possessed, communication patterns, and coping styles within the family system.

When dealing with minor children who have limited control over many elements of their lives, the nurse's *advocate* role is particularly important. The nurse must ensure that children and their parents know what to expect from the health care system and health personnel, and the recommended treatment. They also need information about their rights as clients and as human beings. The degree to which the family satisfies its own dependency needs and the family's previously demonstrated ability to be their own advocate or a co-advocate on their child's behalf are important nursing assessments.

Family-Centered Nursing Process

In family-centered nursing process, the nurse uses the same steps as when nursing process is applied to the individual (see Chapter 1). The difference is that the focus of the process is the individual child and the family system at the same time. The duality makes the process more extensive and complex (Fig. 12-1). The critical point for the nurse is that family functioning cannot be determined from only one member. Nor can a child be fully understood unless viewed within the context of the whole family.

Assessment. Data come from several sources. As many family members as possible (including youngest and oldest members) should be interviewed as age-appropriate. The nurse should realize that subjective appraisal is invaluable. Different members convey different information and at varying depths. Whenever possible, objective observation of the family's interaction in the home environment should incorporate both the *action* and the *feeling* level. Additional information also may be available from records, other team members, and referral sources.

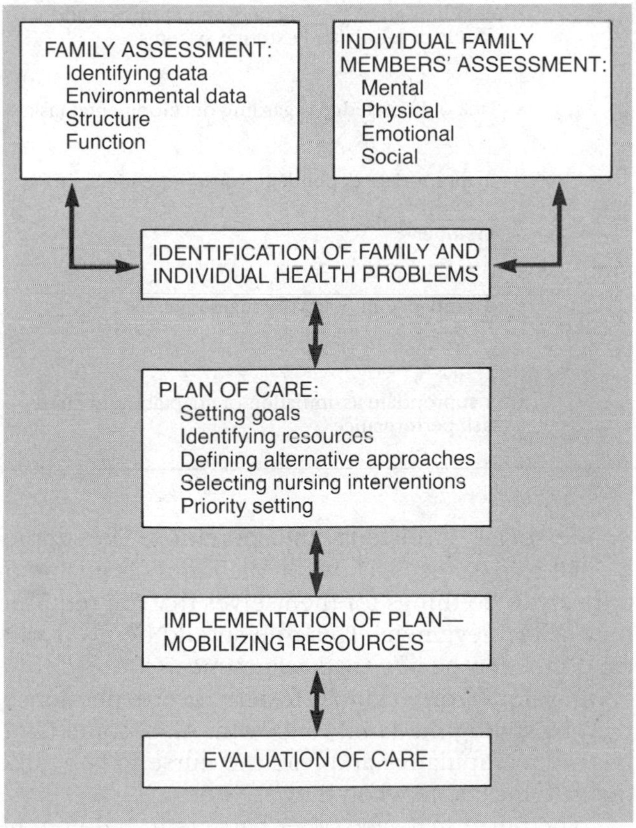

***Figure* 12-1.** Steps in the family-centered nursing process. (From Friedman M: Family Nursing—Theory and Assessment. 2nd ed. Norwalk, CT, Appleton-Century-Crofts, 1986.)

Analysis. This step in the process is ideally done together with the family. Their involvement provides a useful learning opportunity for them to see themselves in an organized, objective fashion. Analysis should include identification of both individual member and family unit health states, family and member strengths and assets, and family and member deficits and limitations (Friedman, 1986). At a family level, nursing diagnoses can be derived from any of the many frameworks or approaches available (Table 12-2).

Problems that involve at least two members (a subset) or the entire family are *family* health problems. Identified real and potential problems should be assigned priorities from the family's perspective to achieve maximal effectiveness from interventions. The most common problems are in family process, generated by ineffective family coping with actual or potential health or environmental problems. Of low priority are any needs that are impossible to fulfill, because of either client or resource restraints. Referral to appropriate community resources should be made for any problems beyond the level of expertise of the nurse.

Planning. For change to be successfully implemented, mutual goal setting, based on diagnosis priorities, should take place. The nurse's responsibility is to see that goals are clearly stated in writing and accepted by the family. Further, the nurse helps the family identify and mobilize its own resources (strengths and potentials of members, family group, and external support systems). The nurse also facilitates problem solving, by asking questions and making suggestions to help the family derive a workable approach to resolve problems.

Friedman (1986) has identified key questions the nurse should consider in assisting the family's planning or problem solving:

- Will the proposed approach(es) foster increased dependence or increased independence by the family?
- Is the proposed action(s) within the information and skill level of family members or their own resources?
- Will the proposed action(s) strengthen or weaken the family's coping abilities?
- Does sufficient commitment and motivation exist on the part of the family and its members to adhere to the plan?
- Are sufficient resources available to carry out the plan?

Table 12-2. Nursing Diagnoses for Families*

		Dysfunctional Family	
	Functional Family (Requires no intervention or health promotional intervention)	**Potential** (Requires preventive or health promotional nursing action)	**Actual** (Requires resolutional, rehabilitative nursing actions)
	Family Coping: Potential for Growth, related to:	**Altered Family Process (Actual/Potential), related to:**	
Systems Framework Analyzes communication and ability to adapt within family relationships and between family and external world	• intact subsystem: spousal, parental, parent-child, sibling • equilibrium with suprasystem: balance in community/relational exchange	• lack of intact subsystem: spousal, parental, parent-child, sibling • disequilibrium with suprasystem: community/relational over-investment; community relational underinvestment or isolation	
Structure/Function Analyzes the family's structure or organization in relation to achieving family functions	• structural organization that allows achievement of family functions	• structural disturbance • functional failure	
Interactional Framework Analyzes how family members relate to each other, focusing on roles and communication	• adaptive role transition • role congruity or adaptive resolution of role incongruity • open communication among members	• role transition • role incongruity • communication disturbances	
Developmental Framework Analyzes family group adjustment at various life stages	• congruent goal setting between members and family or family and external systems • adequate knowledge regarding developmental tasks • dependency-independence balance appropriate for family/member stage • boundary maintenance that balances input exchange with external environment • appropriate assimilation or adaptation to family task performance	• conflicting goal setting between members and family or family and external systems • lack of knowledge regarding developmental tasks • inappropriate dependency or independence for family/member stage • disturbance in boundary maintenance • inappropriate assimilation or adaptation to family task performance	

* Utilizing NANDA categories.

Once resources are identified and an approach selected, responsibilities are delineated so all involved know the nurse's responsibility, the responsibilities of the family group or its members, and what rests with other resources. Sometimes the nurse will have to accept family decisions that run counter to the advice given, but the family should not be rejected or support withdrawn because of the decision.

Intervention. The nurse's role during intervention is developmental, facilitative, or supplemental in nature (Friedman, 1986). Developmental roles involve teaching the family and supporting their own self-care and self-responsibility activities. The facilitative role is necessary when the family needs assistance in removing barriers to care. These are generally economic, social, or related to transportation. The supplemental role is necessary when the family is unable or unready to do things for themselves that are required for goal achievement. This role should be used with caution since nurses tend sometimes to overdo the "doing for" role, which fosters overdependence, thereby stifling the family's growth. Also, some families are manipulative and lead the nurse to conclude they are incapable when they are not.

The nurse may face other barriers in helping the family achieve goals. One is *apathy.* What is labeled apathy is often really a difference between the nurse's and family's cultural values or priorities. Genuine apathy can sometimes be countered by teaching the family and encouraging support groups to be involved.

Indecision is another common barrier, usually resulting from fear or powerlessness, coupled with a poor perception of the consequences of action alternatives. The outcomes of the proposed change are simply not perceived to be better than leaving things status quo. In this case, the nurse needs to engage the family in more problem solving so that pros and cons and related feelings are thoroughly understood. The other possibility is that a *de facto* (i.e., just let things happen) family pattern is characteristic. The nursing action is still the same: engage the family in more problem solving regarding consequences (Wilde et al, 1985).

Evaluation. The nursing care plan, which was the intervention blueprint, is also the evaluation framework. The written client goals become the evaluative criteria used to determine if the nurse and family are satisfied with what was achieved. Cost effectiveness (time, money, and other resources) should be considered as well as an analysis of whether the problem has been satisfactorily resolved and for what reasons success was or was not forthcoming. Evaluation is also done on a regular basis during the intervention process, to determine whether revision or more planning is needed.

Approaches to Family Analysis

The family may be assessed using several different frameworks, depending on the nurse's education and experience. In this chapter, a family developmental framework, systems framework, structural-functional, and interactional frameworks are introduced.

A Family Developmental Framework

When using a developmental framework, the family is analyzed as a small group progressing and changing through its life cycle. This framework does have a mid-

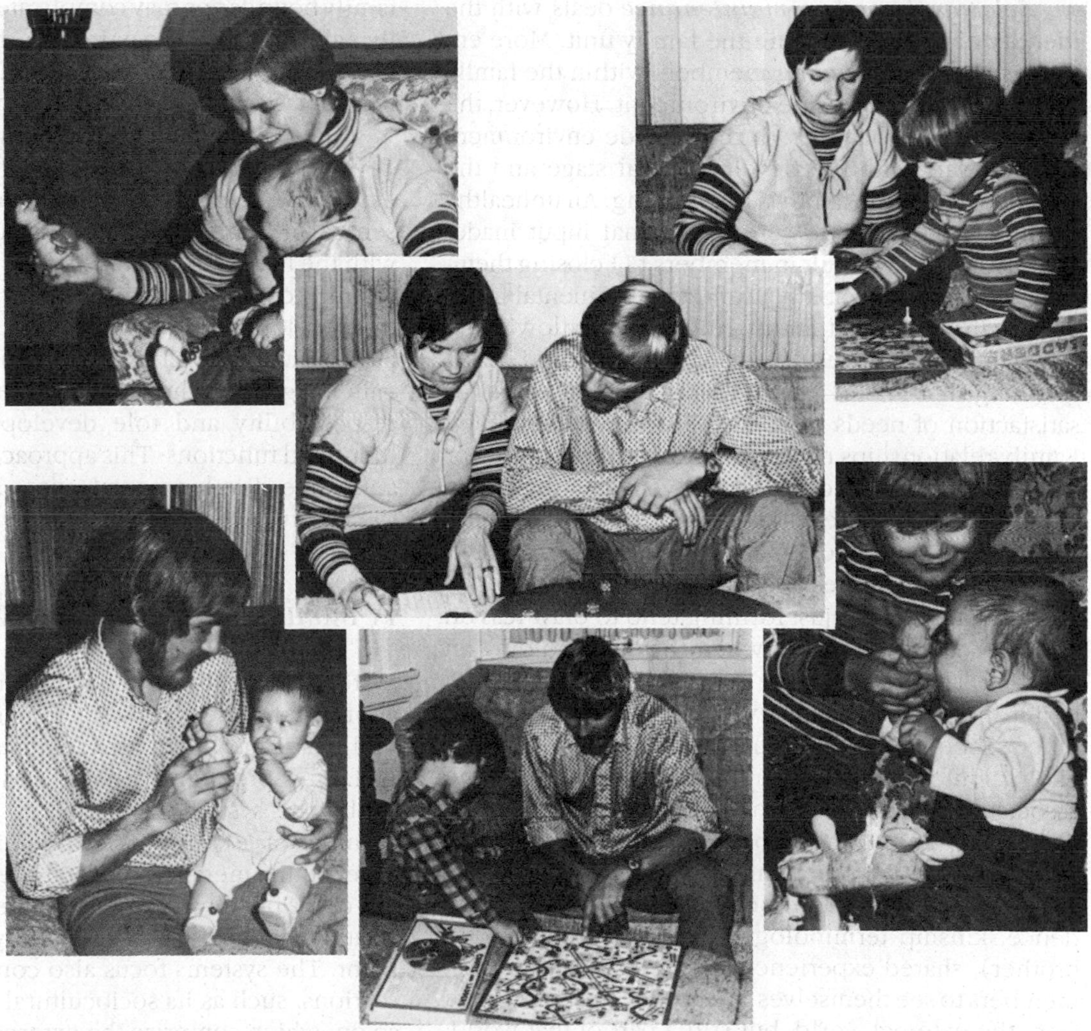

Most family assessment frameworks focus on the family as a group or on the subgroups of the family system.

dle class, nuclear family bias, but it guides the nurse to analyze the family system at different periods in its development as well as to anticipate changes in the family group over time. Aldous and D'Antonio (1983) discuss four systematic characteristics that change as the family moves through its developmental stages: (1) family interdependency, (2) selective boundary maintenance, (3) adaptability to and initiation of change, and (4) family task performance. Analyzing these aspects of family development helps the nurse identify actual or potential problem areas in adjustment as the family moves from one stage to another.

The degree of *family interdependency* will vary according to the individual's and family's stage in the life cycle. For example, a child's dependency is greatest during the younger years and lessens as the child prepares to launch from the family group. Conversely, parents' dependency on children increases during later years when their own functioning ability diminishes. Power exerted by members in family decisions may indicate the dependence of certain family members on each other, as well as the stage of family life.

Selective boundary maintenance deals with the identity of members within the family unit. More energy is exchanged among members within the family unit than with the outside environment. However, the degree of interchange with the outside environment tends to vary with the developmental stage and the effectiveness of the family's functioning. An unhealthy family system tends to screen external input inadequately. This may result in members (1) closing themselves off from potentially useful environmental information through strict family rules or (2) allowing so much input that the result is disorganization and chaos, resulting in a loss of family identity and a search for satisfaction of needs from the external environment. Family relationships may be shallow and frustrating or rigid and overcharged with stress. The healthy family displays a balanced exchange with the environment, inviting new ideas and opportunities that are then tempered by family values and goals.

Families that are just forming tend to draw less on the external environment when they are molding an identity. The same is true when new members are being incorporated. However, as children grow and enter school, the healthy unit tends to rely on more external information and support to accommodate the associated changing demands of the family unit.

Aldous and D'Antonio (1983) describe several characteristics of the family that contribute to its boundary maintenance. For example, a separate residence, kinship terminology (e.g., Dad, mother, kid brother), shared experiences, shared rituals all assist members to see themselves as a unique group separate from the external world, but still a part of that world. Family boundaries may be impinged upon by external agencies; however, external interactions can contribute resources to the family unit that assist it to retain its identity.

Adaptability to change refers to the interdependencies of family members and the boundary-setting characteristics of the family unit. The family must set goals for itself that do not conflict with goals of individual members and the expectations of external agents. In a conflict between any of these, the family may utilize feedback processes to adapt to or initiate change. Such events as the birth of a baby, marriage of a child, or a mother taking a job outside the home will require the family unit to change such things as communication patterns or decision-making processes.

Family task performance refers to the tasks or functions the family system must perform to meet family goals (see Chapter 3). Family tasks or functions vary in difficulty and importance throughout the family life cycle. For example, physical maintenance is a major task in early infancy and childhood and in retirement, whereas social control is important in early childhood and later in adolescence. Also, external influences on family boundaries may complicate or facilitate the family's ability to adapt to or initiate change when meeting its tasks. The family life cycle and associated developmental tasks are described in Table 2-2 of Chapter 2.

The family is evaluated by determining whether developmental tasks are being achieved, as well as the extent and *quality* of the performance. The tasks presented in Table 2-2 do not include tasks associated with the break-up and re-forming of blended families. If family composition differs from the nuclear makeup, the developmental tasks must be adapted. It is important to examine the functions within each family and to gain insight into the members' understanding of their responsibility and role development in respect to identified functions. This approach can also be used to anticipate developmental crises and to identify how the family copes with them.

A Family Systems Framework

Systems theory is used in many disciplines. A systems approach focuses on interactional process rather than on linear causality in the identification and resolution of family problems. Becvar and Becvar (1982) describe the systems approach as more holistic; each member of a family should be viewed in relation to other family members, as each affects and is affected by the other persons. These subsystems or sets of family relationships comprise the family's internal environment. The systems focus also considers family suprasections, such as its sociocultural group, schools, and so on, which comprise the external environment with which the family interacts. Interactions in both the internal and external environments, of course, are bidirectional.

This theory focuses on communications among family subsystems (e.g., between spouses, between siblings, between each spouse and each child) called the *family microsystem*; among the family and the immediate external environment (e.g., extended family, neighbors, and friends) called the *mesosystem*; and among the family and other social institutions (e.g., schools, health agencies, church, town, or residence) called the *macrosystem*.

The other aspect of this theory to be considered is the capacity for change, or adaptability. This refers to the ability of the family unit and its members to modify behavior toward each other and the outer world as a situation demands. The family may accept, reject, or modify input or feedback to meet its needs. Balanced adequately, this is called family *homeostasis*, which allows continual change and growth. This is demonstrated by flexibility rather than rigidity or disorganization, spontaneity rather than stagnation or inertia, and confident receptiveness to new situations rather than resistance or distress and defensive behaviors. Predictable communication patterns are characteristic of a family in a homeostatic, steady state.

Assessment, then, involves looking at the boundaries within the sets of relationships of family members and the extent to which boundaries with the external suprasystems are open and flexible. Subsystems are assessed to determine who the nurse should work with to facilitate change. Assessment of the degree of openness with suprasystems gives substantial clues about the family's capacity for change.

Structural-Functional Framework

The structural component of this framework relates to how the family is organized, such as family type (nuclear, extended), power structure (matriarchal, patriarchal), marital patterns, and family style (based on values, communication, and roles).

The functional component has been succinctly defined by Tapia (1972):

- socialization of members into productive members of society;
- reproduction;
- provision of physical necessities to members;
- coping strategies to maintain stability between external and internal environments;
- provision and allocation of sufficient economic resources; and
- affection necessary to personality development and maintenance of members.

This framework allows an autonomous assessment of the family unit and then a study of its links with outside institutions. How well the family is meeting its functional obligations is a useful assessment for the nurse in determining appropriate nurse-client relations and interventions.

Interactional Framework

This approach to viewing a family focuses strictly on internal dynamics, i.e., how family members relate to each other. Roles members assume internally and the nature of communication processes within the family are analyzed. The advantage of this framework is that it allows the nurse to do a microanalysis of family communications and role expectations, which is particularly useful when problems exist or are suspected in family roles or communication. (See "Family Role Structure" heading in Table 12-6, page 445.) A problem with this framework is that it does not take into account influences of the external environment on the family. See Chapter 2 for a discussion of family roles.

Family Health Assessment

Just as several frameworks exist from which family assessment can be approached, a multitude of tools are available as guides to achieving that assessment. The nurse should become familiar with several and select one or more according to the nurse's and employer's philosophies, the purpose for which the assessment is being conducted, the depth of family knowledge needed, and the availability of the family. The tools presented in this chapter represent only a few of the many available. Speer et al (1985) review nine family assessment tools and evaluate them on ease of administration and scoring, clinical relevance, and type of family situation in which they are appropriate.

Assessment Process

The family assessment process becomes itself an intervention if the entire family is included as team members. As the family focuses upon itself, awareness of the family's situation is enhanced. Members see their problems in a broader perspective as they identify strengths and limitations in meeting needs and coping with crisis. As roles, relationships, and functions are investigated, the family is more likely to recognize the value of interdependent responses and cooperation in problem solving. The assessment process also teaches problem-solving behaviors that increase the family's capacity to cope independent of nursing assistance in future problem situations.

Assessment information may be gained through interview and questioning, through observation of parent-child interactions, and by careful listening to family members' comments, as well as attention to what is not said. A clear picture of some aspects will require a visit to the home if this is feasible in the nurse-family relationship (community health nurse, family nurse practitioner, school nurse, hospital nurse visiting a patient before admission to or discharge from the hospital), or through feedback from other professionals who have visited the home (social worker, mental health worker). If direct family contact is impossible or impractical, assessment may need to be achieved with a questionnaire. However, the validity of information is substantially compromised. This fact should be carefully considered when using the data to establish interventions.

Family interviewing is a necessary skill in assessing and intervening with families. Ideally, a family assessment includes all members within the family group, including the younger children. At a minimum, the assessment should include the child and primary caregivers. The fullest assessment is completed entirely within the child's home environment. There the nurse can note such things as environment, sociocultural variables, and interaction patterns of family members. These observations must be documented and assessed, as must all other components in the data base. Obviously, a home visit is not possible or desirable in every circumstance. For most short-term hospital stays by a child, family assessment can be included in history taking at admission, during observations of child and family throughout the hospital visit, and as part of the discharge planning procedure.

Assessment Tools

Assessment of the family system, as with individuals, is ongoing and reliant upon the nurse's and other health team members' keenness of observation and skill in asking relevant questions.

Tables 12-3 and 12-4 and Figures 12-2 through 12-7 (discussed later) provide the reader with examples of various tools to use as guidelines in assessing a family. Whatever tool is used, the assessment data are categorized as to areas of family strengths, both actual and potential, and areas of family weakness or limitation, i.e., family needs.

Family relationships among its subsystems are presented in Figure 12-2. If family members are each asked to draw such a diagram, one gets additional information about the consistency with which different members perceive family relationships. Further, members can be asked to describe their feelings as they drew the diagram, which allows the nurse to glimpse conflicts that exist in the relationship. This assessment tool is particularly useful when a child has emotional

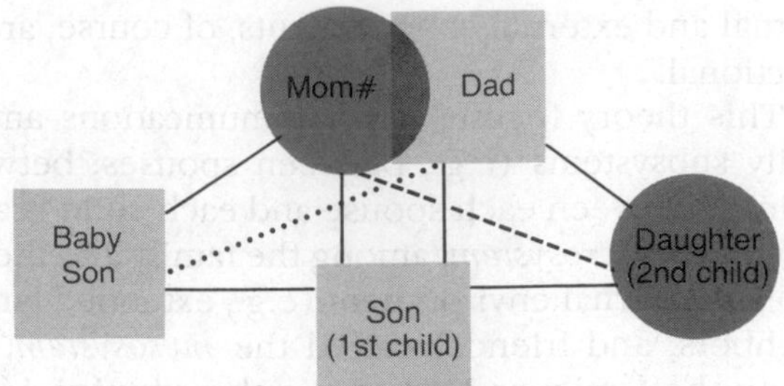

Figure 12-2. Family relationship diagram example. *Key: Circle* = female. *Square* = male. *Solid line* identifies strong bond or relationship. *Broken line* identifies some conflict in relationship. *Dotted line* identifies serious conflict in relationship. # after name is the member drawing the diagram and from whose interpretation the relationships are being described.

Interpretation (from Mom's perspective):

1. Mom and Dad have a close spousal relationship.
2. Baby son and mother have a close relationship, whereas father and baby son display serious conflict in their relationship.
3. Oldest son has a similar relationship with both mother and father. He also has a similar relationship with both siblings.
4. Daughter has a close relationship with her father, a similar relationship between her siblings, and displays some conflict in her relationship with her mother.

or behavioral problems or when psychosomatic complaints are suggested from the child's health assessment. The data can be used to identify counseling needs and to facilitate identification of etiologic factors and intervention strategies to improve dysfunctional relationships. The tool does not take long to administer. With preschool and early school-age children the nurse may have to draw the diagram by questioning; that skill is often beyond their cognitive and fine motor abilities. The tool cannot be used effectively with infants and toddlers.

Family genograms are presented in Figures 12-3 and 12-4. The genogram provides an orderly way of organizing the family and the family's history so that the family and nurse can look at it together and identify key associations—for example, the transfer of a specific disease or characteristic within the family. Figure 12-3 also denotes how to illustrate the relationships in reconstituted or blended families. This tool can also provide the nurse with information about the health and disease patterns within a family. It may be used to identify risk factors to the child's health or provide epidemiologic information of a communicable or genetic trait. The tool takes little time to administer, is usually diagrammed by the nurse while questioning family members, but is limited to the extent of the family's knowledge and recall of disease historically. It can be used to assess both physical and emotional illness patterns.

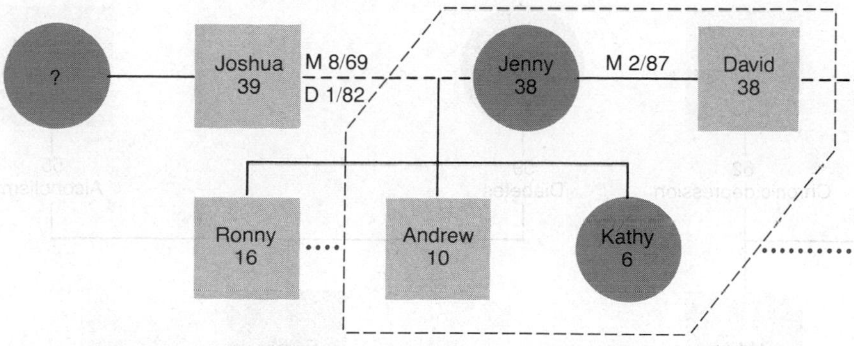

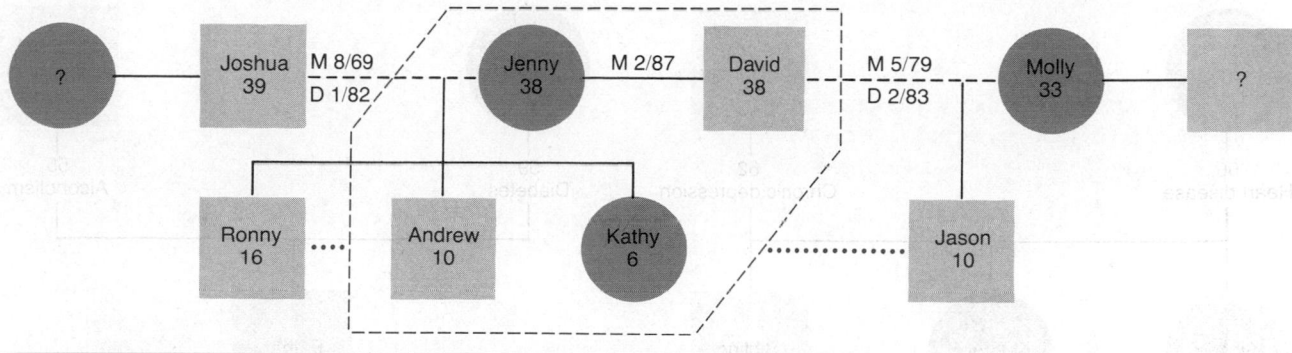

Figure 12-3. Example of a blended family genogram.
Key:
Vertical line indicates offspring
Circle indicates female
Square indicates male
Triangle indicates sex unknown
Circle and square connected by solid line horizontally is a marital pair
Circle and square connected by broken line horizontally is a divorced pair
M and date indicates date of marriage
D and date indicates date of divorce
Broken line encompassing several circles/squares indicates members who comprise household
Dotted line indicates persons who are occasional members in household
The following are types of data that can be included inside circles and squares, providing information about the individual the symbol represents:

Name
Age or birthdate
Death date (indicated by d. and followed by date of death)
Place of birth
Occupation
Health problem or cause of death (* placed after disease or accident when cause of death)
Any other data relevant to the assessment

A family ecomap of external relationships is illustrated in Figure 12-5. This tool reveals the relationship of a family unit to its external environment. This assessment is made by interview, observation, and collaboration with other agencies involved with the family. It is particularly valuable in ascertaining whether a family is primarily open or closed as a system and what, if any, resources the family already has to draw upon during crisis or distress. It can also reflect whether or not those resources are supportive or disruptive to the family. This information is particularly valuable if a child is diagnosed to have a chronic health problem or terminal illness, or when home care is being considered.

A *Comprehensive Guide to Assess Family Function* is presented in Table 12-6. (Because this table is lengthy, it has been placed at the end of this chapter on page 442.) The numbers of areas assessed, and to what depth, will be guided by the circumstances and purpose of the assessment. The nurse uses assessments of other health professionals or agencies who have already seen the family, as a part of the total database.

Smilkstein's Family APGAR (1984) is reproduced in Figure 12-6. This is a tool that can quickly measure a family's satisfaction with their general state of functioning, referred to in the tool as the family's APGAR. The questionnaire can be used to measure the APGAR of subsystem relationship functioning (i.e., husband-wife, parent(s)-child, sibling-sibling), as well as satisfaction with total family functioning. The questionnaire may be filled out by each family member or completed by the family collectively through the process of consensus, under the nurse's direction. The tool, of course, is not useful for obtaining very young children's input. It presents a quick picture of the family's overall functioning from which the nurse can then identify areas needing more thorough assessment, or it can offer clues about risk when abuse, emotional or behavioral illness, or psychosomatic disorders are suspected. Its relevance when home care is being considered is also obvious. If a family is already demonstrating coping problems, home care is probably not desirable for management of a child's health state. The nurse must remember, though, that one APGAR should not be used to determine family functioning or intervention decisions over a long period. All families experience dysfunction at one time or another; therefore, periodic reassessments are indicated.

Otto's Family Assessment Criteria Checklist, pre-

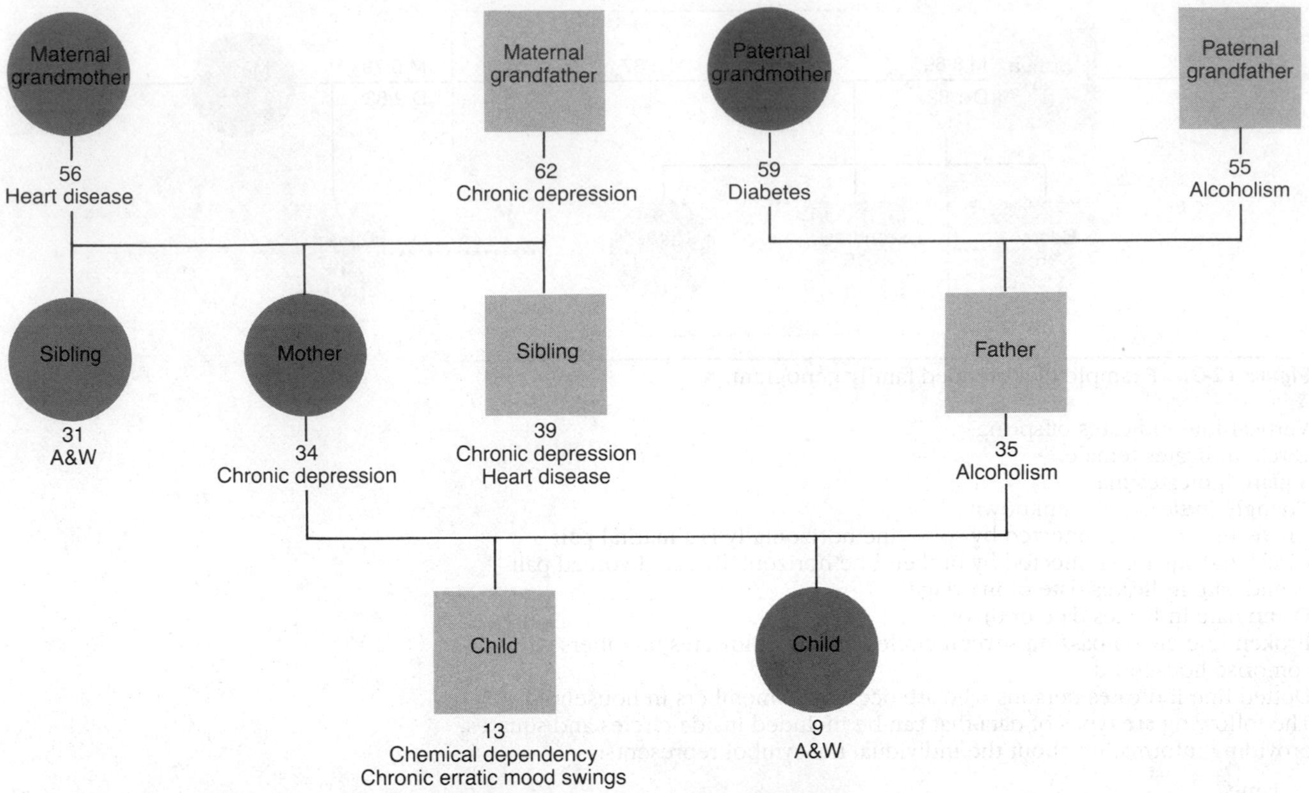

Figure 12-4. Family genogram of disease patterns. See Figure 12-3 for definition of symbols. A&W indicates alive and well, good health. An arrow indicates a specific client if the nurse is doing the assessment with regard to a particular family member. Twins are indicated by a line joining the boxes or circles.

sented in Table 12-3, has 13 assessment criteria that contribute to family unity and the development of family potential. The concept of this check list is similar to Smilkstein's (1980) Family APGAR questionnaire in that it gives the nurse a basis for determining areas of family dysfunction needing intervention. The nurse marks the check list on the basis of an assessment of each of the criteria.

The *Family Assessment Device* (FAD) is a self-report measure of family functioning (Epstein et al, 1983). This tool is based on the McMaster Model of Family Functioning (Epstein, 1978), which views the family as an interactional system. This model incorporates six dimensions of activity that are essential for family functioning:

- problem solving,
- communication,
- roles,
- affective responsiveness,
- affective involvement,
- behavior.

The FAD consists of 60 items to which respondents indicate they agree or disagree (on a 4-point scale).

From assessment data, the nurse and health care team can apply principles of change to increase, support, and reinforce family strengths or to eliminate or correct family limitations. A combination of these may be needed to produce necessary changes in knowledge, attitudes, or practices that will result in problem prevention or resolution, to foster healthier adaptation of the family unit and its individual members. Recognition of family strengths is imperative to identify family resources in order to prevent or resolve problems, as well as to plan realistic interventions. Likewise, acknowledging family limitations guides nursing diagnoses by identifying both real and potential problems. Family limitations can be seen in illness-producing, adaptation-disrupting behaviors. Family limitations that are unchangeable help provide realistic boundaries for goal setting.

Nurses need to recognize that their own values, derived from their families, influence encounters with any group. And the family is no exception. Nurses must be aware that their values will be communicated verbally and nonverbally to the family and will become embedded in the relationship. It is therefore important to recognize those values and clarify them, as nurses will always encounter families whose beliefs, values, and attitudes are different from their own.

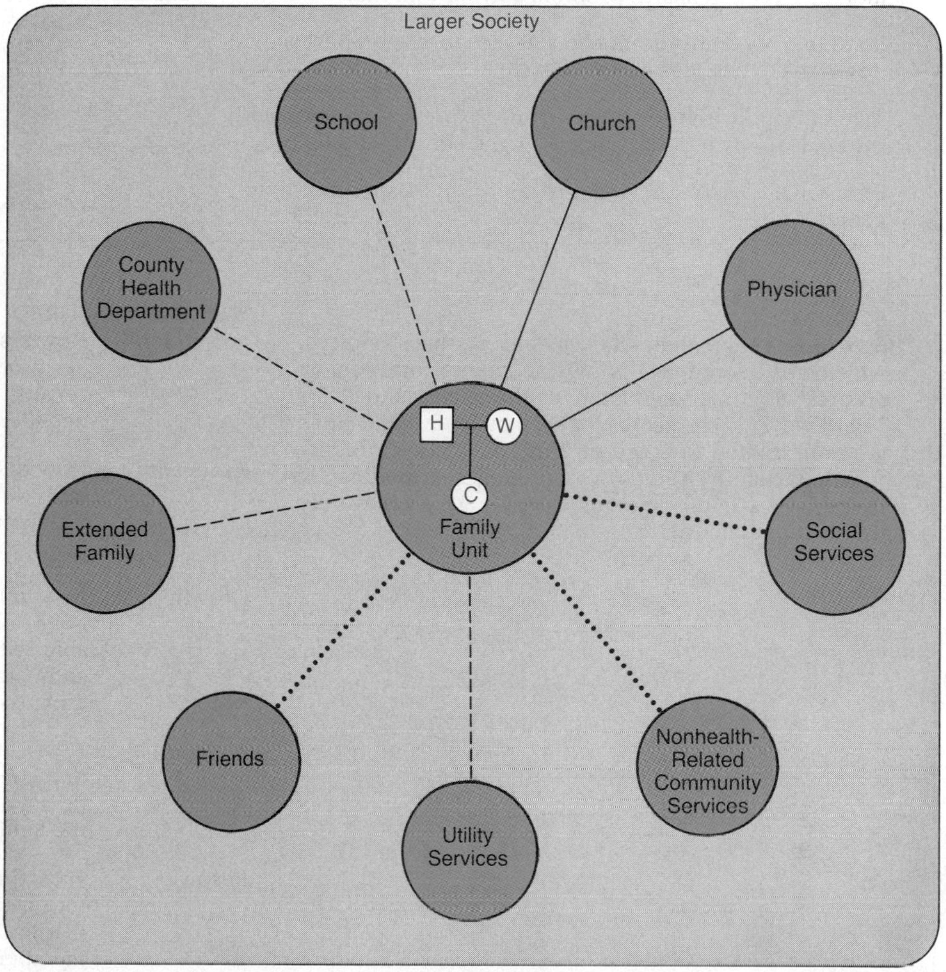

Figure 12-5. Family ecomap of external relationships. Pictured here are but a few of the many that could be considered.

Key: ______________ Strong, supportive, positive relationship.

-------------- Erratic, conflicted relationship, sometimes supportive and sometimes disruptive

. . . . Negative, disruptive, or nonexistent relationship.

The Family APGAR Questionnaire

	Almost always	Some of the time	Hardly ever
I am satisfied with the help that I receive from my family* when something is troubling me.	______	______	______
I am satisfied with the way my family discusses items of common interest and shares problem solving with me.	______	______	______
I find that my family accepts my wishes to take on new activities or make changes in my lifestyle.	______	______	______
I am satisfied with the way my family expresses affection and responds to my feelings such as anger, sorrow, and love.	______	______	______
I am satisfied with the way my family and I spend time together.	______	______	______

SCORING

Scoring: The patient checks one of three choices, which are scored as follows: 2 points for "Almost always," 1 point for "Some of the time," and 0 for "Hardly ever." The scores for each of the five questions are then totaled. A score of 7 to 10 suggests a highly functional family. A score of 4 to 6 suggests a moderately dysfunctional family. A score of 0 to 3 suggests a severely dysfunctional family.

* According to which member of the family is being interviewed, the nurse may substitute for the word "family" either spouse, significant other, parents, or children.

(Adapted from Smilkstein, 1984.)

WHAT IS MEASURED

Adaptation	How resources are shared, or the member's satisfaction with the assistance received when family resources are needed.
Partnership	How decisions are shared, or the member's satisfaction with mutuality in family communication and problem solving.
Growth	How nurturing is shared, or the member's satisfaction with the freedom available within the family to change roles and attain physical and emotional growth or maturation.
Affection	How emotional experiences are shared, or the member's satisfaction with the intimacy and emotional interaction within the family.
Resolve	How time* is shared, or the member's satisfaction with the time commitment that has been made to the family by its members.

* Besides sharing time, family members usually have a commitment to share space and money. Because of its primacy, time was the only item included in the Family APGAR; however, the nurse who is concerned with family function will enlarge understanding of the family's resolve by requiring about family member's satisfaction with shared space and money.

***Figure* 12-6.** The Family APGAR Questionnaire.

Table 12-3. Otto's Family Assessment Criteria Check List*

Assessment Criteria for Behaviors	Degree of Family Strength, Behavior Demonstrated as Family Strength: Most of the Time	Occasionally	Rarely
1. Able to meet members' physical, emotional and spiritual needs.			
2. Parents have joint responsibility and are comfortable in childrearing.			
3. Effective communication among members.			
4. Able to provide support, security, and encouragement to members.			
5. Able to initiate and maintain growth-producing relationships within and outside the family.			
6. Demonstrates responsible community relationships.			
7. Home used as matrix for growth of adult and child members.			
8. Able to help themselves and to accept help when needed.			
9. Flexible in performing functions and roles.			
10. Demonstrates mutual respect for individuality of each member.			
11. Uses crisis as a means of growth.			
12. Concern for family unity, loyalty, cooperation by members.			
13. Flexible in initiating and using family strengths.			

* Ethnic and cultural variance must be considered.
(From Otto, 1968.)

The Dysfunctional Family

When the health or development of a family member is threatened, whether parent or child, the entire family system is placed in a position of jeopardy for abnormal development or dysfunction. Knowing this, the nurse should be alert in the assessment to cues that signal a troubled family or a potential one, so that dysfunction or disintegration of the family can be averted by prompt intervention.

Assessing Dysfunction

Defining dysfunction precisely is not always possible, because family interactions are complex and the contact with families is relatively brief. All families have phases when they function well and other periods when they function poorly, even to the extent of disintegration. So nurses need to distinguish whether a dysfunctional pattern is temporary, situational, or chronic and try to foresee whether the outcome of a particular family's interaction is likely to have reversible or irreversible effects on its members.

Dysfunctional family units are not carrying out the universally accepted tasks of families and their members—that is, they are not able to provide physically or emotionally for the needs of their members. Such families display behaviors that place their children in jeopardy, physically, emotionally, socially, and intellectually. Parents in these families are unable or unwilling to assume responsibility for their own actions and life outcomes that is expected in our social structure today.

Relationship Disturbances

The assessment and intervention focus must be on the interactional patterns in such families, because disturbed relationship is the common denominator of altered health states of families in dysfunction. (See Affective Function and Socialization Function sections of Table 12-6 at the end of this chapter for assessment factors. Also see Chapter 13 on Parenting.) Common disturbances in relationships frequently found in family dysfunction are (1) inflexibility in parenting style, (2) parental misperception regarding the child, (3) inappropriate expectations of parents, and (4) parent-child mismatch.

Inflexibility in Parenting Style

An inflexibility in parenting style invites dysfunctional interaction within a family. The nurse may see parenting practices that are functional for one of the children and quite dysfunctional for another child. One basis for these differences lies in the children's temperaments, or their basic individual approaches to life. Inconsistency is apparent—one child is singled out as the scapegoat to receive the blame for all family problems. Inconsistency is also demonstrated when parental mood results in very different responses to the same behavior.

Parental Misconceptions About Children

Disturbed functioning may be stimulated by parental misconception regarding the child. We know that parents are affected by their child's unique responses to them and by their perceptions of the child. Their perception may be related to a projected attribution, not objectively to the child's looks or behavior. "He looks like Uncle John. I don't like him!" or, "She's so cute! She acts just like I did at this age" are types of parental responses. The parents begin to prescribe injunctions (prohibitions) and permissions that the child either accepts or rejects to develop her or his own life plan, or script.*

The Gouldings (1982) have described recognizable life injunctions that influence people's behavior:

> Don't be (exist or live); Don't be you (the sex you are); Don't be a child (be a parent instead, take care of me); Don't grow (stay little); Don't make it (out in the world); Don't (fearful); Don't be important; Don't be close (to others, or be sexually responsive); Don't belong (here or anywhere); Don't be well (or sane); Don't think (don't think about "X" —forbidden subject—don't think what you think, think what I think); and Don't feel (don't feel "X"—mad, sad, glad—don't feel what you feel, feel what I feel).

The positive opposites of these injunctions are permissions for living, for uniqueness, and for thinking, feeling, and doing. The injunctions and permissions are either verbalized by the parents so the child hears them as messages, or the child infers them from sensory cues and behavior. The child then makes decisions and develops a changeable script. This script dictates how the child will think, feel, and act.

*A script is a life plan people develop out of their responses to injunctions and permissions.

Inappropriate Parental Expectations

Dysfunction can result when parents relate to their children in a manner that reflects inappropriate expectations in relation to age or capabilities. Often they lack the knowledge that is required to anticipate what their child can be expected to do or comprehend. During periods of stress, even informed parents sometimes relate inappropriately to their child.

Parent-Child Mismatches

A mismatch in family members' personalities may prompt conflict. One particular child may not "fit" the parents, but this child could be loved and nurtured by another set of parents for the very qualities that produce stressful interactions within the present family (Thomas and Chess, 1977).

Cultural and ethnic differences cannot be overlooked in defining family dysfunction. A well-functioning family may be unable to adapt successfully when it is transplanted into another cultural setting. Subcultures exist in every society, and members of them may suffer deprivation and loss as a result of subtle and systematic discrimination against their efforts to "make it" in the mainstream society (Taylor, 1979).

Characteristics of Families with Dysfunctional Life Patterns

A comparison of a functional versus dysfunctional family is presented in Table 12-4. Following is a discussion of the major characteristics of dysfunctional families.

Crisis and Stress Response

A striking feature of families in dysfunction is crisis: either a series of crises or multiple concurrent crises.

Table 12-4. Comparison of Functional Versus Dysfunctional Family

Functional Family Characteristics	Dysfunctional Family Characteristics
Communication	
Two-way	One-way
Positive and negative behaviors addressed, with emphasis on positive. Open, empathetic, positive. Talk often, without fear, on any subject	Only negative behaviors addressed by parent(s). Closed, restricted to social chit-chat, self-centered, negative or sarcastic. Anxiety-laden
Clear, congruent. Self-disclosing, specifics	Vague, incongruent. Incomplete, generalized, apathetic
Elicits feedback. LISTENS. Open-ended questions, direct questions, validation	Refuses, rejects feedback. Resentment
Consistent rule enforcement	Sporadic rule enforcement
Congruency between topic and responses	Responses inconsistent with topic
Affective messages exchanged, spontaneity, introspective	Controlled, predictable affective exchanges to no affective interchanges; no introspection

Table 12-4 (continued)

Functional Family Characteristics	Dysfunctional Family Characteristics
Power and decision making based on developmental readiness and member abilities; cooperative in nature	Coercive in nature, resentment expressed in silence or anger; no mutual respect
Conflict dealt with openly to problem solve—resolve through consensus	Conflict denied or, if confronted, *total* agreement is critical; unable to stay focused on issue
Power Structure	
Flexible (egalitarian) power structure in which decisions are made together or shared and made independently. Parental coalition provides shared leadership	Chaotic or leaderless family power structure, often exists with no member making effective decisions; or a markedly dominant structure in which there is absolute control and no negotiation by the power figure, usually one spouse
Children permitted to negotiate or offer options, but with clearness of where the negotiation boundaries are and of the ultimate power hierarchy. In some family forms(e.g., single parent), some parental power may be given to older children. This usually works if parent remains clearly the primary source of decision making, control, and guidance	
Role Function	
Adults assume adult and parenting roles while children are encouraged in age- and ability-appropriate child roles	Role reversal: Adults fail to assume many or most adult and parenting roles. Children prematurely assume adult and/or parenting roles
Role consistency	Role confusion, inconsistency
	Role denial, refusal
Adaptation During Crisis	
Problem-solving behaviors demonstrated	Despairing, nonproblem-solving attitudes or anger response. Chaotic responses
Minimal or temporary disruption to family functioning during crisis. Support systems identified and utilized	No support systems recognized or tapped. Voluntary support systems often increase disruption
Family works as unit to resolve conflict	Blaming, lashing out behaviors—no cooperative effort
Support System Building	
Internal and external support network maintained	Overinvestment in a single support system; destructive support system
Take time to do things together; plan together	No family unit collaboration
Friendships and community affiliations beyond home	Isolated. No external affiliations
Accepted by community	Alienated by community
Family Life Style	
Organized, flexible	Disorganized, rigid
Scheduled routine of meals, sleep, recreation	No schedule of ADL or family activities—each member vies for self; members function as unrelated units
Orientation to time, space, social obligation	Disorientation to time, space, social obligation
Relatively stable in residence; plans any moves	Frequent moves without forwarding address or phone number; no planning
Basic trust in humanity	Suspicious of all outsiders
Parents model problem solving, caring	Parents in own world; model acting out behavior, apathy
Sense of well-being felt, as demonstrated by loyalty, integrity, honesty, sense of usefulness, and self-esteem	Uneasiness about life, as demonstrated in borderline or antisocial behaviors, low self-esteem, mistrust
Members value each other, express and receive affection, talk positively *about* and *to* each other	Members show little concern or caring for each other; talk negatively *about* and *to* each other
Commitment to each other and to family unit; encourage individual pursuits, but forego any that threaten existence as marital couple or as a family unit	No sense of commitment to anyone. Marital couple do not regard each other's individuality as important

(Based on Stinnett and De Frain, 1986, and Weitzman, 1985.)*

* This research involved over 3000 families from several countries. The sample included families from all economic levels, differing educational backgrounds and social strata, varying age groups, races and cultures; yet the findings were consistently similar.

(See Family Coping Function section of Table 12-6 for assessment factors.) In dysfunctional families, members' coping mechanisms are inadequate to meet the challenges posed by their environment in ways that foster life and health. In fact, stress response in the form of either altered health states or psychosomatic disease may be one indicator of dysfunction (Woolfolk and Richardson, 1978). When confronted with what they perceive to be painful and stressful events, family members may respond with panic, anger, or apathy. They may say, "This is just the way life is!" They may see no other way to look at their situation or may feel that they have no other choice of action. The recurring or unrelenting pressure of their problems eventually leaves them with a sense of powerlessness. Apathy is then adapted to dull the perpetual pain of not being able to cope. This strife frequently is accompanied by or creates marital discord. All energy being used up, the marriage typically stagnates, adding to the negative effects of family life on the children. Frequently one or both spouses entered the marriage seeking to be dependent, a need which the spouse fails to fulfill, particularly during crisis. They often operate in rigid, prescribed patterns learned in their family of origin. Their learned patterns limit the person's ability to think, solve problems, or leave the scene of action. It must be recognized, however, that some parents survive multiple stressors and remain effective parents, yet other parents have parenting problems even when faced with minor or temporary stress because of their limited resources and coping abilities.

Some families seek out the stimulation of stressful activities for excitement. However, they may overextend their energy resources and become fatigued so that their children are neglected. The nurse may be able to help them plan alternate periods of rest and recreation with stressful activities so that they experience pleasure. Their children, in turn, will experience more pleasant responses from their parents.

At times, dysfunctional families present a dizzying merry-go-round of activity to health professionals, making it difficult to see where intervention is possible. The sheer destructive energy and momentum of dysfunctional family systems, like centrifugal force, repel the best efforts of helping professionals to exert a counterforce.

Nurses involved with dysfunctional family systems may experience the contagion of stress, discovering in themselves symptoms of the stress response. Pulses may race with anger at the mother of twins who are failing to thrive. Nurses feel the urge to lash out with angry words, to blame the mother for getting herself into a helpless position with an alcoholic husband who does not care for her or provide for their babies. However, nurses can use the energy generated by their anger constructively to help the mother plan better care for the twins and get help through community agencies. A person who succeeds in coping with a crisis builds up self-esteem and adds options in responding to different situations. Nurses can teach families how to draw upon resources within their environment of which they were previously unaware.

Disturbed Communication Patterns

Families in dysfunction experience both verbal and nonverbal miscommunication. People who have not learned to say what they think, believe, see, hear, and feel seem to have difficulty exchanging valid information with others. The nurse may experience a surge of frustration when talking with them. A clear picture of what they are describing does not emerge and confusion may result. Incomplete sentences, distorted ideas, or grandiose or degrading epithets may be heard as the nurse or anyone else talks with family members. The nurse may check with several members to get information and may consult with other health professionals in order to get a realistic view of the family to plan its care.

Members of families with disturbed communication patterns tend to respond inappropriately to others and to situations. One woman laughed and giggled as she talked about the loss of her first baby and the severe illness of her newborn son. As a child, she had not been allowed to express her feelings or needs, especially sadness. Her parents expected her to cope on her own and not bother adults. Laughter at inappropriate moments often covers fear. Anger also may be used to cover fear or sadness, and vice versa.

Some parents respond to their children with irritation and anger much of the time, an inappropriate mode that tends to destroy creativity and problem solving. Other families have hidden "rules" that inhibit expression of feelings. Relationships between children and their parents in these families tend to be apathetic, revealing little affection or feelings. Children from such environments often seek inappropriate affectional exchanges (usually in excess) from casual acquaintances or strangers and do not portray the "stranger anxiety" that usually is characteristic of the child's developmental age. (See section on Communication Patterns in Table 12-6 at end of chapter for assessment factors.)

Role Disturbances

Dysfunctional families frequently display role confusion or role reversals among members. Family life is often parent centered, with the expectation that children "care for" their parent(s)' needs, negating their own needs. Children become the parents to their immature parent(s) or the sibling, or best friend surrogate for the isolated parent. Parents may display an inability to assume adult roles that would permit them to provide for their children's emotional and economic needs. The consequence is to rob the child of childhood; the child's need to feel protected and cared for goes unfulfilled. Parents' unmet needs cause them to push the child into a pseudoindependence before he or she is developmentally ready.

In a family with two adult members (spouses, parent–live-in partner, parent-girl/boy friend), one adult member may be competing with the child for the other adult's attention and love, resulting in unhealthy relationships. The competing adult may vent anger and rage on the child or on the other adult if she or he feels deprived. Siblings may have to provide the authority, guidance, and decision making for other siblings if parents do not assume that responsibility. The child forced prematurely into these adult roles may compete with or resent the parent and may likewise be resented by the parent. (See Family Role Structure section of Table 12-6 at end of chapter for assessment factors.)

Perpetuation of Dysfunction to Next Generation

Characteristically, families with dysfunction perpetuate their disruptive and destructive parenting practices to the next generation. Thomas Gordon (1978), the originator of Parent Effectiveness Training, says:

> Most parents, confronted with a situation where a child is experiencing a problem, respond the same way their own parents did. And because they have not had a chance to learn a better way, parents keep making the same mistakes *their* parents made.

(See Developmental History of Family section in Table 12-6 for assessment factors.)

Although the extended family can be supportive when a young family undertakes its parenting tasks, sometimes the family members are locked into dysfunctional interaction patterns. For example, well-meaning grandparents may take over care of a newborn baby and not allow the parents to establish bonding and attachment with their own child or re-establish their marital relationship in a new way following the birth of the baby. Relatives and friends are often unaware of how they may be compounding distress in the family by their efforts to be helpful.

Unhealthful parenting practices may be the parents' own unsuccessful solution to a developmental hurdle. The young parents may have gone through a difficult period at a particular age. When their own child comes to that age or stage, the parents have a difficult time nurturing the child. Instead, they react more as a sibling to their offspring. Unwed teenage mothers are often caught in this situation with their own mothers.

A woman who had a turbulent adolescence may discover that her parents had a similar upset at the same age. One mother expressed terror as her children approached their teen years, not because she herself had a hard time but because her sister did. Her sister acted out and caused much disruption in the family. This mother had been extra "good" as a teenager in order to compensate for her sister's "badness." Reliving her compensatory behavior recreated pain for herself as her children began adolescence.

Parental guilt may lead to perpetuation of dysfunctional behaviors in the next generation. When parents feel guilty, they may overnurture their children, also a disruptive parenting practice. Parents, especially in the middle class, work hard to give their children advantages they themselves may have missed. They are overinvested in their child's achievements. The children in these families may feel overwhelmed by expectations, or "swallowed up."

Behaviors characteristic of parents in dysfunctional family units are described in Box 12-1. Nurses should watch for signs of these behaviors in their own interactions with parents as well as in their observation of parent-child exchanges. Often referring agencies make note of experiencing these behaviors in their exchanges with the child or parent.

> Box 12-1
> *Parental Behaviors That Warrant a Family Assessment for Dysfunction*
>
> Minimal awareness of child's needs, activities, friends, whereabouts.
>
> No interest or participation in child's school functions, progress in school.
>
> Dissatisfaction with parenting role—history of inadequate parenting. Poor self-esteem.
>
> Intense need to be cared for; unable to demonstrate affection; immature.
>
> Limited problem-solving and communication skills—uses denial and projection as coping strategies.
>
> Cannot comprehend conceptual information or apply generalizations to own situation.
>
> No planning or organization in daily activities; unaware of personal or external resources.
>
> Passive-aggressive; little eye contact in interactions, unless a cultural characteristic.
>
> Seeks health care only during crisis.
>
> *(Data from Clark, 1986; Leatherland, 1986; Mackey, 1986.)*

Lack of a Beneficial Support Group—Isolation

Another characteristic of families in dysfunction is lack of a constructive support group, or enmeshment in a group having destructive effects on the family or its members. Relatives or friends may cling like a leech to a family that is already barely holding together. Two apparent opposites—isolation and overinvolvement in destructive relationships—are common. One woman in Parents Anonymous* belonged to a roller skating group of about 30 people. Social workers, noting that these friends were constantly in and out of the woman's house, at first thought she was not isolated. But as the caseworker got to know the woman's situation better, she discovered that this group was playing into the mother's system of neglect and abuse of her children by reinforcing it. If she could not find a baby sitter when it was time to go roller skating (she had four children under 7 years of age), her friends would urge her to go anyway and leave the children at home. Members of the group yelled at, spanked, and generally "scapegoated" her children. As the caseworker discovered later, the mother was angry because she felt the children tied her down. The group responded to the anger the mother felt, and, by supporting her behavior in this way, joined her abuse system. (See Social Support Systems section in Table 12-6 at end of chapter for assessment factors.)

Disorganization of Family Living Pattern

Families in dysfunction and crisis experience disorganized daily living patterns. (See Health Care Function section of Table 12-6 for assessment factors.) Often food is not provided for family members, meals are not prepared, and sleeping arrangements are erratic or crowded, or the children's sleep needs are disregarded in favor of adult social desires. Noise may disturb rest and sleep schedules of parents and children alike. General environmental disorder is visible. Children may have disturbed behavior such as nightmares, somnambulism, compulsive solitary rocking or head-banging, and despairing crying, whining, or wailing. These children may be ignored and their needs discounted by the parents.

These families are often disoriented as to time, space, and sequence or social obligation, evident to the nurse by their missed appointments or their coming on the wrong day, at the wrong time, or both. They move frequently; they may give relatives' addresses and phone numbers and cannot be located or reached by telephone. They are often trying to avoid creditors and bill collectors; they may view health professionals with suspicion.

Children in Jeopardy

The most extreme characteristic we see in dysfunctional families is children in jeopardy. The underlying cause of jeopardy varies. Often dysfunctional families neglect or cannot manage the fulfillment of basic human needs for food, shelter, body protection from the elements; for security and protection from harm; for rest and for stimulation; and for recognition and self-identity. (See Health Care Function section of Table 12-6 at end of chapter for assessment factors.) Nurses may be the crucial persons in the health care field who advocate understanding of children. They can help break the chains of miscommunication that

*A group that, like Alcoholics Anonymous, reinforces healthy behavior patterns through mutual support. Its members seek to channel impulses to abuse their children into constructive action.

Box 12-2
Behaviors of Children That Warrant a Family Assessment for Dysfunction

- Inattentiveness
- Frequently tired, chronic fatigue
- Poorly nourished (below 3rd percentile on growth chart)
- Inappropriate attire for weather conditions
- No interest in sharing experiences, accomplishments with parent or other appropriate adults such as teachers or coaches
- Few friendships, watches TV most of time, shallow relationships
- Unsupervised large blocks of time or left in care of strangers
- School difficulties/truancy
- Excessive behaviors: shyness, fears, aggressiveness, etc.
- Difficulty recognizing or expressing own or others' feelings; marginal communication skills
- Sadness or depression prevalent, solemn
- Affection sought from unfamiliar or inappropriate sources
- Timid or evasive toward adults, as if fearful of being struck or yelled at
- Excessive sibling rivalry
- Despairing cry or whining
- Compulsive, repetitive behaviors, such as solitary rocking or head banging
- Preoccupied (fear of loss, hunger, abandonment, harm)
- Developmental delays
- Poor physical health, frequent infections
- Arrives early and stays late at school
- Precocious sexual behavior
- Behaviors indicative of drug or alcohol abuse
- Aggressive destructive behaviors
- Cruelty toward animals
- Physical or behavioral signs of sexual abuse
- Age-inappropriate behaviors or concerns
- Persistent, excessive behaviors such as enuresis, encopresis, fire-setting

(Data from Arent, 1980; Friedman, 1986; Leatherland, 1986.)

Box 12-3
Indicators of Families at Risk for Dysfunction

Family Structure

Single parent family with inadequate supports
Blended family with inadequate supports
Adoptive family with inadequate supports
Teenage family
Young family with several children close in age
Single parent with changing live-in partner
Family with peripheral spouse—viewed by spouse as unreliable, incompetent, tyrannical
Parental separation

Family Environment

Impoverished family
Multiproblem family
Immature parents
Member(s) with handicapping, chronic, or fatal disease
Migrant or highly mobile family
Employment instability of key family members
Violence-prone family
Chemically dependent family member(s)
Chronic marital discord

(Data from Clark, 1986; Friedman, 1986; Leatherland, 1986.)

bind generations together with missed signals, anguish, and despair. Behaviors the nurse may discover during child appraisal or from school referral, which indicate that a family appraisal for dysfunction is imperative, are listed in Box 12-2.

Identifying Families at Risk for Dysfunction

A family can be considered at risk through consideration of a number of complex factors. The nurse must recognize that families may exhibit risk factors without being dysfunctional. Being at risk indicates a greater potential for dysfunctional family function; however, many families in risk categories cope very effectively and are able to meet the needs of members adequately. Obviously the more risk factors a family accumulates, or the more severe or chronic a risk factor is, the greater is the likelihood of dysfunction. Structural and environmental stressors that have a high correlation with dysfunction are identified in Box 12-3.

Intervening with Dysfunctional Families

One of the principles of change is to involve all who will be affected by that change. Therefore, intervention with dysfunctional families necessarily at some point must involve all members, including the children. Likewise, because the problems of dysfunctional families are usually multifaceted, a multidisciplinary approach is essential to any significant change.

A Multidisciplinary Team Approach

The multidisciplinary approach has numerous advantages. First, families receive several resource alternatives from which to choose. This also prevents any one resource from becoming depleted in efforts to help the family with all its needs. Professional burn-out with dysfunctional families is high because progress is slow or sometimes nonexistent. A multidisciplinary team allows professionals a collegial support group to help offset burn-out risk. A group approach also adds creative alternatives that one professional alone might not consider. Community resources frequently needed to intervene in dysfunctional families are listed in Box 12-4.

The multidisciplinary approach has potential disadvantages if the team is not organized and a coordinator is not identified. Without a coordinator the family can be pushed into further dysfunction through the intrusion, competition, and possible contradictory guidance of multiple agencies, each taking its own actions without consideration for what other agencies might be doing, resulting in *fragmentation of services.* The family ends up being overwhelmed, or manipulative behavior is fostered within the already dysfunctional unit. The coordinator role is frequently assigned to the nurse because of the more frequent contact with the family. Nurses need not be coordinators but should see that an effective one is appointed by the team.

In establishing the team members, the initial intervener should first identify with the family their needs. Next, resources currently used by the family and the degree of family involvement and satisfaction should be listed. Team members may be individually contacted by the coordinator, or team planning and evaluation meetings may be scheduled. The family should not be overlooked as team members, for success is extremely unlikely without them. The schools of the children should be considered key resources in interventions with dysfunctional families. Teachers should be educated and encouraged to identify children whose behaviors indicate family problems and families who do not demonstrate nurturance. School resources are welcomed because of their daily contact with the children whose lives and development are being affected by family dysfunction.

Obviously, the critical element in successful intervention is casefinding at the primary and secondary levels. If nurses, teachers, and other professionals who

Box 12-4

*Community Resources Commonly Needed for Interventions with Dysfunctional Families**

COUNSELING/LEGAL SERVICES

Legal Assistance services
Juvenile Authority
Tough Love Group and Hot Line
Family and/or marital counseling
Mental health centers

FINANCIAL

Housing authorities
Fuel assistance agencies
Free or sliding scale medical and dental care
ADC (Aid to Dependent Children)
Medicaid or other health financial assistance
Food stamps
Welfare
Public housing
Budget and financial incentives counseling
Emergency shelters

HEALTH CARE SERVICES

Home Health services
School health programs
Occupational health settings
Ambulatory care settings
Visiting Nurse Association
Family Planning services
Homemaker services

SUPPORT GROUPS/SELF-HELP

Religious-affiliated groups
Singles clubs
Friendly Visitor program
Parents Anonymous
Alcoholics Anonymous, Al-Anon, Ala-Teen, Ala-Tot, Narcotics Anonymous

DEVELOPMENT/REHABILITATION

Vocational rehabilitation, employment services
WIC program
Child development clinics
Child guidance centers

PARENTING ASSISTANCE

Single Parent clubs
Foster Grandparent program
Big Brothers/Big Sisters program
Surrogate Parent program
Subsidized or sliding scale child care
DCYS (Division of Child and Youth Services)
Foster care
Parent aide programs (nurturance to parents)

* The system of resources varies from state to state and community to community. Many communities develop reference books of community resources that describe services rendered, eligibility requirements, how to gain access to services, fee basis, and so on, which are available in public libraries, county health departments, or Chambers of Commerce. The yellow pages in phone books list local agencies and resources by title.

have regular contact with children and families are alert to the subtle indicators (risk factors, family characteristics, early behavioral signs) that a family is becoming dysfunctional, interventions can be initiated before the family becomes embedded in a dysfunctional life pattern and before problems become multiple and complex. The costs to family and community of dysfunction certainly attest to the fiscal soundness of preventive and early intervention programs.

As part of the intervention team, the nurse should be familiar with the rules of approach in interacting with families to combat dysfunction. A slow, warm approach is fundamental. The families usually are mistrustful, have low esteem levels, and are not socially skilled. An aggressive approach will result in family rejection of team efforts. Services or resources need to be presented positively. For example, the nurse would describe a program as designed to foster and support parenting rather than to prevent child abuse. Agencies should keep this concept in mind when they establish their organizational titles and in the way they describe their services on printed and advertising media. This positive presentation fosters cooperation rather than causing families to be defensive and diminishing further their already weak self-esteem and motivation. The family should be informed that the aim of the team is to help them look at alternatives to the weak elements of their lifestyle that jeopardize their health and happiness, so they can make choices about how to improve their current situation. This approach communicates hope to the family, conveys to them that they are not "all bad," and reminds them that they can take control of their life situations and participate in making their life better. The family should help establish intervention priorities. Family priorities take precedence, unless member safety is at stake.

Because many dysfunctional families think concretely, the team will have to effect education and change by demonstration and example, rather than by imparting concepts. For this reason, frequent home visits will be necessary to role model mature and social behavior and practice desired changes with family members. For this reason, programs in which parent aides, homemaker aides, and surrogate grandparents are used demonstrate success in helping dysfunctional families change.

Table 12-5 describes the major intervention issues in dysfunctional families and the appropriate goals and intervention strategies to manage those issues. The intervention team evaluates progress and behavior on an ongoing basis. Learned responses of family members used to please must be differentiated from real changes in behavior. Ability for this is developed primarily through experience with such families. For this reason it is good to have some "seasoned" members on the team. Frequent evaluation helps bring the little successes into focus, bolstering family esteem and motivation and offsetting professional member burnout. Likewise, frequent evaluation helps identify problem areas in family progress so these can be dealt with before they go on too long. It cannot be overemphasized that both assessments and interventions must be considered within the cultural context of each family unit. The intervention strategy should involve the family in establishing short-term goals with realistic deadlines and specific tasks, because of their concrete thought processes and present-moment orientation.

Primary Nursing Roles in Working with Families in Dysfunction

The nursing profession has a unique advantage in helping families in dysfunction. Nurses can be eclectic and select interventions from other disciplines that will be helpful to clients. Nurses can continually enlarge their repertoire of interventions by drawing from various psychotherapeutic theories and methods.

Casefinder. The nurse is often the first professional helper with whom the family shares its dysfunction. Their request for help often is not direct; their report of some symptom may lead a nurse to suspect dysfunction. The nurse, therefore, must be observant of family interactions and alert in history-taking for those patterns that characterize the dysfunctional family. The Family Coping Index shown in Figure 12-7 can be helpful. The nurse's own skills can be employed to intervene, or the family can be referred to resources that can help them.

Role Model. The first interventions are the nurses themselves—their humanity, wholeness or incompleteness, experiences in their own family of origin, and their particular stage of personal development. All these are resources the nurse can use to intervene by modeling how to relate to others in an autonomous and caring manner. The nurse can teach people how to look at things, hear things, feel, touch, and respond in ways that bring them pleasure instead of the pain of dysfunction. The nurse can model how to interact with others by encouraging family members to express what they really think, feel, need, and want in a given situation.

Teacher and Counselor. The nurse's functions as teacher or counselor require intervention to help reverse the family's dysfunction. Information can be provided to help parents correct knowledge deficits or misconceptions regarding parenting options or developmental expectations. (See Chapter 13 on parenting.) Teaching problem-solving skills is a critical need in dysfunctional families. Counseling efforts can reinforce the fact that each child is unique. To these families, their child's uniquenesses can be emphasized. Parents should be assured that temperaments do clash, but ways to cope with their own can be learned. Parents may also need guidance to develop realistic ways of interacting with their child during periods of stress.

Parenting the Parent. Nurses can lend themselves to families as parent-surrogates for a time. When nurses intervene to assist a mother or father with parenting tasks, they nurture them in the present and also may be caring for parts of their personalities that suffered deprivations and unresolved hurts in childhood. Specifically, the nurse's interventions are aimed at giving parents permission to enjoy their children and instruction in how to relate to them. Together, nurse and parents can plan how to initiate actions whereby parents can meet their own needs so they can, in turn, give to their children. These experiences can stimulate the parent to take charge of his or her own life and decide how to behave.

Team Member. Family dysfunction may require lengthy treatment because of persisting patterns of interaction; multiple interventions may be required to effect change. The nurse's therapeutic effectiveness can be increased by participating in an interdisciplinary team. The team offers the advantage of combating the multiple problems of the dysfunctional family with the energies and expertise of those in several disciplines. The involvement of representatives of several disciplines also brings to bear on the family the implied pressure of society to achieve relief of their stress and to get on with being human in a humane setting. The team offers each individual professional the emotional reinforcement needed to withstand the exacerbations that typify this family unit. The nurse's specific role within the team and interaction with the family depend on several factors, including the team's composition and the nurse's particular expertise.

Child Advocate. The nurse keeps in mind the needs of the vulnerable child and acts in her or his behalf. The nurse responsible for a child's care should act in the child's behalf during parental absence or whenever the child's development or survival is jeopardized, but within a context that attempts to preserve the family. A nurse may respond humanly and emotionally to a family situation in which it seems that the interests of the child are not best served by keeping her

Text continued on page 442

Table 12-5. Nursing Diagnoses in Dysfunctional Families, with Goals and Strategies

Nursing Diagnoses	Client Goals/Evaluation	Nursing Strategies
Altered family process, • related to communication skill deficits Defining Characteristics: No acknowledgement or expression of feelings or needs Marital discord Disengagement of members within family unit	Describes feelings toward self, spouse, children Describes personal needs Discusses an issue with other family members without disintegration of interaction (walk out, violence) Identifies needs, activities, interests of other family members	Role model appropriate feelings, needs, ideas with various family members Encourage honest discussion of feelings through open-ended questions Role play verbalization of needs, ideas, feelings among family members Refer to appropriate community resources (e.g., family or marital counseling) Praise efforts to increase communication
• related to inability to provide basic family necessities Defining Characteristics Lack of food shelter clothing safety rest and recreation	Earns income above poverty level or receives and manages public assistance optimally Manages budget to acquire low cost but adequate basic necessities Provides housing that is safe and meets at least minimal standards of heat, electricity, refrigeration, facilities, and some room furnishings	Obtain or assist family to obtain services needed to satisfy basic necessities Involve family members in obtaining/providing for these necessities Praise family group and individual efforts to meet basic needs Role model reasonable use of resources available
Ineffective family coping, • related to lack of support network Defining Characteristics: Social isolation Psychologic abandonment of family members Live in own world Negative support systems (e.g., extended family takes over, friends support neglect)	Stays in same residence Identifies persons/agencies who can/do offer positive support Establishes regular times for social interaction outside family and with family	Provide/assign family to obtain information about church, school, other family activities Encourage increased spousal activities (time away from children)—suggest child care alternatives so this is possible without leaving children unattended Introduce family to other families in area with similar interests Identify community groups where social relationships can be established (e.g., singles club, Friendly Visitor program) Praise efforts to increase social interaction
• related to problem-solving deficits Defining Characteristics: Present-oriented, need/crisis-oriented No introspection Acting-out behaviors/impulsive Concrete thought patterns	Identifies problems and contributing factors Identifies alternative coping strategies and likely consequences of alternatives Recognizes persons/agencies to contact during crisis and how to do so Identifies how family, friends can be useful in resolving needs Identifies how health care system can be helpful in resolving health-related needs	Educate family as to resources available to help them with coping (e.g., counseling service, employment service, support groups) and how to gain access to these (best to give a person's name to contact). Refer appropriately with family input Role model the problem-solving process Discuss parents' childhood and help them reflect on how that affects their present functioning Teach stress management skills in concrete manner (see Chapter 23) Praise problem-solving efforts; point out success Involve family members in assessment, intervention, and evaluation process Identify main decision maker and the distribution of power. Interest the decision maker in making changes first
Altered in parenting, related to • lack of knowledge of growth and development • lack of role model • lack of support from significant other • unmet social/emotional maturation needs of parents • presence of stress Defining Characteristics: Inconsistency in discipline Lack of parental attachment Verbalization of disappointment in infant/child	Provides safe, adequate caregiving environment Demonstrates consistency Demonstrates realistic and age-appropriate expectations Identifies disciplinary method alternatives Interacts positively more than negatively with children	(See Chapter 13 on parenting) Foster a parent/child attachment by pointing out the child's positives and by pointing out positive parenting responses Role model age-appropriate parenting, nurturance, interaction Document parenting strengths and weaknesses with parent, and help parent establish concrete way of overcoming weaknesses

Table 12-5 *(continued)*

Nursing Diagnoses	Client Goals/Evaluation	Nursing Strategies
inattention to infant/child growth and development lag in child		Listen actively to identify "cries for help" from parents. Identify behavior that places their child at risk Praise positive parenting/nurturing Help family obtain needed resources (e.g., Parents Anonymous, parent aide, surrogate parents, child guidance services, etc.) Teach growth and development and anticipatory guidance in concrete manner Establish contract for changes in parenting Teach parenting alternatives in concrete manner

(Based on Weitzman, 1985; Friedman, 1986.)

FAMILY COPING INDEX SCORING PROFILE SHEET

FAMILY NAME

COPING ESTIMATE: INITIAL PERIODIC DISCHARGE

DATE

COPING AREA	RATING X-STATUS O-EST. CHANGE	JUSTIFICATION
Physical independence	1 2 3 4 5 Not applicable ☐	
Therapeutic independence	1 2 3 4 5 Not applicable ☐	
Knowledge of condition	1 2 3 4 5 Not applicable ☐	
Application of principles of general hygiene	1 2 3 4 5 Not applicable ☐	
Attitudes toward health care	1 2 3 4 5 Not applicable ☐	
Emotional competence	1 2 3 4 5 Not applicable ☐	
Family living patterns	1 2 3 4 5 Not applicable ☐	
Physical environment	1 2 3 4 5 Not applicable ☐	
Use of community resources	1 2 3 4 5 Not applicable ☐	

Figure 12-7. The nine assessment areas of the Family Coping Index are based on nursing diagnoses established from the family's coping ability and adaptation to meet their needs. The sliding scale from 1 (no competence) to 3 (moderate competence) to 5 (complete competence) scores present functioning. The same scale is used to score anticipated functioning after multidisciplinary or nursing intervention, providing direction and guidelines for periodic evaluation. (From Freeman R, et al: *The Family Coping Index.* Johns Hopkins School of Public Health and Richmond, VA, City Health Department, Nursing Service, Cooperative Nursing Study, 1964.)

or him in a family that is dysfunctional. The legal and cultural basis of our society, however, supports the primacy of the family. The nurse is legally obligated to report abuse and neglect, but the decision to remove a child from the family is made by the social service and legal systems. (See Chapter 35 for discussion of child abuse.)

People who are taught dysfunctional life patterns fail to achieve developmental tasks within their complex family network. The outcome of their failures is often psychic pain and physical symptomatology, ranging from psychosomatic disease to physical trauma. By the time children in dysfunctional relationships receive medical or legal intervention, much damage may have been done to their bodies and their minds. Thus interdisciplinary and community effort should be focused on preventive and early intervention efforts.

The nurse is a primary resource in interventions with children and families; therefore, the nurse is in a position to offer several nursing roles for an impact on this growing social and health problem in American society. The nurse is a vital link in the lifeline of recovery for dysfunctional families.

Table 12-6. A Comprehensive Guide to Assess Family Function

Elements of Assessment	When to Assess/Reasons or Uses	Special Considerations
Identifying Data		
Family Composition Names, birth order, occupation, education, phone number and address	Get to know family, communicate interest in whole family	
Type of Family • nuclear • extended • single • blended • experimental variant	Capsule view of family in relation to contemporary organizational structures	The importance here is whether the family lifestyle permits health promotion and developmental nurturance of children
Cultural/Ethnic or Religious Orientation • Identity • Degree involved in identification, acculturation (replication in dominant culture of one's beliefs, values, practices) • Behavioral clues: Family friends of same ethnic group; ethnically homogeneous neighborhood; act within cultural group in relationships, social activities, recreation; traditional dietary habits and dress; home décor reflects culture; traditional family roles enacted; native language spoken exclusively or frequently; socialize within cultural community; family uses folk medicine or traditional healers	To understand family behavior, value system, perceived functions, and the priority of those functions	Must evaluate each family member, as acculturation may differ Important assessment in relation to potential family dysfunction, especially when a family has been transplanted into another cultural setting. (See section of chapter on Assessing Dysfunction)
Social Class Status Head of household's occupational status, income level/expenditures, educational level, inheritance	Strongest influence on life style, structure/function, characteristics, and association with external environment	Variations result from different conditions of and demands placed on family by society at large
Adequacy of financial resources: *Adequate:* solely personal resources used *Marginal:* unemployment and general relief aid *Inadequate:* solely from general relief, welfare, or self but so low can't supply basics	Gain insight into resources available, values stressed, level of teaching appropriate, what are perceived as problems and priority placed on them	Greatest overall influence on family life; influences: • early socialization • role expectations • values stressed • behavior considered positive or negative • world experiences members have
Allocation Adequacy: *Adequate:* realistic budget and spending *Marginal:* conflict over management of resources, unrealistic budget/expenditures *Poor:* impulsive spending, excessive debts resulting in family's basic needs unmet	Insight regarding function of providing necessary physical and economical resources	Poor money management alone doesn't mean child's basic welfare is endangered

Table 12-6 *(continued)*

Elements of Assessment	When to Assess/Reasons or Uses	Special Considerations
Social Class Mobility Movement up or down in social class strata. (Example: a woman who was a doctor's wife with an affluent and social lifestyle becomes divorced and is now a single parent living on a secretary's wages and in a working professional's lifestyle)	Information on potential stressors, rejection, social isolation More important assessment when drastic changes in lifestyle, upward or downward, have occurred (e.g., as a result of marriage, divorce, inheritance, move to another region or country). Such experiences may result in family dysfunction	Changes in position, status, prestige (positive or negative) are stress producing; alter interpersonal relationships in and outside family
Developmental History of Family Common and unique: Each spouse's past experiences—how accomplished or perceived Own family of origin—present and past relationship with them Begin with how met, marriage and family of origin's responses, marriage without children, life in original family and ordinal position, any other live ins, relations with in-laws, plans when first child coming, impact/plan each child, how family spends time, daily family routines	Picture of historical coping, amount of anticipatory guidance needed, idea of how adapt to change Better appreciation of parents during parents' formative years: insights into their parenting behaviors, potential risks Family dysfunction tends to be generationally perpetuated; assessment of this element is pertinent whenever family dysfunction is suspected or demonstrated. (See section in this chapter on Assessing Dysfunction)	Make sure that family is open to exploring the past and that nurse's purpose is meaningful
Family Recreational Activities Activities done together How family relaxes: diversion, self-development, social participation Subsystem activities: spouses, parent-child, sibling-sibling	Information regarding family cohesiveness and stability, resources, involvement of parents with children Information regarding relationships	There is a high positive relationship between number of leisure time factors and marital satisfaction There is positive correlation between outdoor recreation and family solidarity
Environmental Data		
Housing Adequacy of space, setting State of repair, adequacy, and facilities available for sanitation, sleep, privacy Family's subjective feelings regarding home Vermin present Safety	Insights into stressors caused by risks associated with home environment; insight into possible social isolation, access to community resources; information regarding environmental modifications needed in relation to home care Insight into territoriality, motivation, lifestyle, interests Insights regarding teaching needed	Home visit best approach. Address may give clues to adequacy Family behaves most naturally at home Home has psychologic effects; influences self-perception and life satisfaction; illness-related stressors and motivation; territoriality
Neighborhood and Community Association and Interaction: Length of residence—degree of geographic mobility Condition of structures: house, streets, sanitation, security/safety Demographic characteristics: social/ethnic characteristics, occupancy, density Resources available for basic physical/social needs: who uses what, how often, knowledge of resources Family attitudes/satisfaction regarding community	Insight into family exchange with outer environment; degree of homogeneity with neighbors; level of awareness family has of community resources; degree they seek out; degree of isolation/security	Homogeneity more influential than proximity in family friendships *Urban* more impersonal; *rural* more personal
Social Support Systems Family, friends, helping person ready to assist family Liabilities/relations with above; are interactions task-oriented or emotionally supportive Whom does family interact with, and satisfaction with interaction	Degree of isolation Resources to help family or share during crisis, coping, celebration When family dysfunction is suspected or demonstrated	Numerous research studies have identified an association between isolation and violent/abusive behaviors, among other signs of family dysfunction Lack of a support group is a common characteristic of dysfunctional families (see discussion in this chapter under Assessing Dysfunction)

continued

Table 12-6 *(continued)*

Elements of Assessment	When to Assess/Reasons or Uses	Special Considerations
Friendships established, frequency of contact		
What external resources does family have? Use? Know about? • Community based? • Formal professional services?		
Assessment questions: 1. Who has helped you when ________? 2. Whom would you get help from if ________?		
Communication Patterns		
Overt Openness and Clarity, Honesty Can discuss personal and social issues Lack of total agreement not a catastrophe Each listens Can stay focused on one issue	Evidence of acceptance of differences; permit autonomy; fostering authenticity and self-growth; ability to empathize This section is particularly important to assessment of families with suspected or demonstrated dysfunction (see section under Assessing Dysfunction in this chapter)	Functional family uses communication to create and maintain mutually beneficial relationships Cultural norms influence openness of communication in relation to modesty, privacy, sexual roles
Affective Communication (Physical and Verbal) Express caring, spontaneity, positiveness Focus on various members' needs	Evidence of fulfillment of family members' affectional needs and satisfying of affectional responsibility of family unit; degree of self-centeredness of members	Methods of appropriate expression are culturally defined Degree of verbal behavior also culturally defined
Power Hierarchy and Family Rules Is distribution of power based on family members' developmental needs and ability, resources of members? Use of cooperative vs. coercive statements Tone used in conversation	Insight into degree of relative cooperation vs. coercion; where decisions made; who to consult for planning interventions	Power relationships culturally influenced Table 12-4 provides a comparison of communication patterns in functional and dysfunctional families
Conflict Resolution Open discussion with problem-solving strategies evolved from group discussion employed Appropriate use of authority to make decisions as necessary	Insight into family's ability to reach consensus and ability to problem solve, deal with conflict	
Family Power Structure Who makes what kinds of decisions regarding • finances • social plans • major decisions, e.g., job changes, residence change • childrearing?	Insight into family's underlying value system To understand family interpersonal relations, family relations with health professionals and outside agencies. Knowledge and appreciation critical to provide effective care, especially in areas of health regimen compliance and motivation to seek/use health services—know who is health authority in family to consult and acknowledge if want family cooperation with health care or in other diagnosis-related issues	Contemporary family changes have steadily improved sharing of decision making (a measure of family power and individual power) Best way to assess is combined observation of marital, parent/child, sibling and family subgroup interactions, coupled with self-reporting by all members if possible
What is the approach to decision-making: consensus; accommodation, (bargaining, compromising, coercion); *de facto,* i.e., no decision making?	Insight into how family makes decisions	
Who makes decisions and how? *Legitimate power:* power based on shared beliefs of family members that one member has a right to control another by virtue of role or position, such as parent over child *Expert power:* power derived from having many resources desirable to family, such as the person who controls the coming in and going out of monies	Insight into how authority and power of individuals in family are derived	Power and authority not always reflected in same individual. A person can have power but not receive the recognized authority to employ it. Conversely, a person in authority may not employ the associated power

Table 12-6 *(continued)*

Elements of Assessment	When to Assess/Reasons or Uses	Special Considerations
Referent power: the influence one has over another because of the member's positive identity with them, such as a big brother by baby sister *Reward power:* power received because person being influenced expects a reward from the other person in exchange for compliance *Coercive power:* power achieved because person influenced expects punishment from the other if there is noncompliance *Information power:* power achieved because one is able to persuade or to give a persuasive message *Affective power:* power derived through manipulation of member by withdrawing or bestowing affection *Helpless power:* unconscious control of family based on helplessness or frailty		Helpless power can be very effective in families, potentially interfering with other family members' needs
Are there any intermediaries (go-betweens) in the family communication network?		Cultural differences will exist relative to how power is derived
Who enforces/implements decisions once made?	Important information for nurse relative to whom to work with once decision is made to accept interventions prescribed	Power and authority in family are frequently role assigned
Where does the family rest on the family power continuum? If dominance—who is the dominant person? To find this out, a good question is "Who usually has the last say about important family issues?" or "Who runs the family?" or "Who wins if there is disagreement?"		
Are members satisfied with the present power structure: "Are you satisfied with how decisions are made and with who makes them?"	Insight into conflicts or confusion children may experience in home, causing mental stress and physical illness	
Family Role Structure Are formal positions and roles fulfilled? (Refer to Chapter 2 for discussion of roles.) Who fills each?	To determine family strengths and resources necessary to plan interventions To determine whether role changes or problems exist, as these can create substantial disequilibrium and tension within family, compromising family and individual members' level of wellness. To understand roles/relationships of child within family and responsibility assumed by each parent in child care Important component of assessment when family dysfunction is suspected or demonstrated (see discussion under Assessing Dysfunction in this chapter)	Important for teaching and therapy purposes. Use as information/demonstration of role to family in therapy or teaching; to determine support, help or counseling needed; to assist members in adapting to new roles Gives evidence of any role strain, conflict, or confusion Cannot assume certain roles accompany certain positions as this is very individual in families, especially in contemporary society Applicable to assessment of interactional framework described earlier in this chapter
Are family members satisfied with who holds each role and with the way they carry out the role?		
Is there flexibility in roles where needed?	Provides insight into adaptive quality of family relationships and ability of members to collaborate and adjust during crisis (e.g., during illness of a member)—especially important to nurse when dealing with situations that add stress to roles and relationships, such as terminal illness of a child	A strong social class and cultural impact on roles exists. The nurse needs to be acquainted with social class and culture of family to determine whether role behaviors and role assignments are appropriate; critical issue, however, is member satisfaction with roles and role performance
Is the marital relationship strong? Have children interfered with the strength of this dyad?	Conveys basic strength and stability of family and maturity of spouses	Vital component of healthy family unit when both parents are present

continued

Table 12-6 *(continued)*

Elements of Assessment	When to Assess/Reasons or Uses	Special Considerations
Nature of the marital relationship? Three types characterize healthy marital dyads: • Complementary. Mates exhibit contrasting behaviors of dominance and submission. They accept and enjoy these differences, with strong dependency displayed between mates. The potential problem is that the growth of one or both may be stifled if roles are too rigid • Symmetric. Equality of mates exists, with each having the right to initiate action, have decision-making voice, and confront the other's behavior. Allows mutual respect, independence, spontaneity, trust, and individual growth. Potential risk is that competitiveness will be overemphasized, with diminished cooperative behavior • *Parallel, or mixed.* Considered most stable as encourages interdependence. It combines the characteristics of the complementary and symmetric types, depending on the situation and each mate's competence in that situation. Interchange and flexibility in roles enhance growth of each with minimal stress		Cultural variations must be considered
What informal or covert roles exist in the family, who plays them, and how frequently?	Gives insight into adequacy and character of subsystem dyad relationships	Need to determine whether the informal role, if it exists, is permanently assigned one member or it's transferred. If continually assumed by one individual, implies dysfunction, promoting estrangement between other family members
Are these covert roles consistent with the formal roles family members hold? Appropriate to the age, competency, and personality of individual members? What purpose does each covert role serve? Are any members labeled, thereby encouraging self-fulfilling prophecy behavior?	Gives insight into emotional climate/needs of family and its members as these roles are played out to meet those emotional needs	If informal role assumed as a result of labeling (i.e., self-fulfilling prophecy), must ascertain if having negative effect and thus interfering with that and/or other members' healthy emotional development Informal roles are necessary to fulfill the integrative and adaptive requirements of a family group. These informal roles include: • *encourager:* draws out family members so they feel important • *harmonizer:* mediator during conflict • *intermediary:* censors and transmits information between two persons with blocked communication; confidant • *initiator:* creative, encourages problem-solving ideas • *compromiser:* yields in conflict to resolve it • *blocker:* negative, illogical • *follower:* passive cooperation, serves as audience in family interaction • *dominator:* tries to assert authority by manipulating and flaunting of member with power • *recognition seeker:* strives to be center of attention • *martyr:* sacrifices for family's sake continually

Table 12-6 (continued)

Elements of Assessment	When to Assess/Reasons or Uses	Special Considerations
		• *stone face:* lectures continually on "right" way to do things • *pal:* playmate to family • *self-indulging:* stays peripheral to family interaction, doing own thing These informal roles are learned through role models, the emotional responses the behavior receives, imitation of adults (usually selects ones comfortable to age and personality to imitate) Member may accept role to fill a vacuum not being filled by members in the formal roles
In parents' early lives, who were role models of parenting and of marital relationship?	Information useful to help family members see how past models influence their present expectations and behavior Important assessment when role problems exist	
Family Values		
Compare family values with those of the dominant American culture (or of the specific ethnic culture if assessor is knowledgeable of these)	Degree of conformity or divergence is important in understanding family and family members' responses to health care delivery system and to establishing acceptable interventions	Values and norms can't be observed directly but are inferred from observation and assessment of family roles, power structure, communication, as these are strongly influenced by underlying family values
American Values Productivity Work ethic Materialism Individualism Education Consumption ethic Progress and mastery over environment Orderliness and practicality Future time orientation Rationality Cleanliness Democracy, equality, freedom, voluntarism, "doing" orientation Health		
Family Values Evaluate with family: • How important are these values to family? • Are these values consciously or unconsciously held? • Value conflicts evident in family? • How do family values affect health status or family?		
Ascertain from Comparison Extent family acculturated to American ways Extent family receives reward from society/ethnic reference group: lack apparent if marked diversity between those values and family values Health issues created by value conflicts		
Affective Function		
Family Need–Response Patterns Awareness of each family member of needs	Understand degree of mutual nurturance and identity; where teaching, support,	Fulfillment of this function is critical to healthy growth and development of family

continued

Table 12-6 *(continued)*

Elements of Assessment	When to Assess/Reasons or Uses	Special Considerations
(physical, emotional, mental) of other individuals in family	counseling are needed for one or more members	members and central base for formation and continuation of family unit
Are each member's needs, differences, interests respected by other family members? Are rights of parents and children recognized and valued? Are recognized needs of family members met by family? To what extent?	Important area to assess when family dysfunction is suspected or demonstrated. (See discussion of Relationship Disturbances under Assessing Dysfunction in this chapter)	
Mutual Nurturance, Closeness, and Understanding How much do family members support each other? How well do family members get along with each other? Expressions of affection evident? Who are resources for nurturance available to individual members during illness, rehabilitation? Are mutual understanding and bonding apparent as evidenced by empathetic statements, concern for other members' feelings and problems, interest in other members' experiences?	Useful for case finding regarding intimacy/bonding problems in relationships	
Separateness and Connectedness How does family help members who want to be together and be cohesive?	Helps to understand impact of separation/loss on family unit and members	Family connectedness essential to development of sense of belonging
Opportunity for developing separateness encouraged appropriately? Are behaviors indicative of enmeshment (subsystem boundaries are continually violated) present? In enmeshment members are too engrossed in each other. Family members speak for other members, not allowing them to speak for themselves, and there is supersensitivity when a member sends out messages for help Are behaviors indicating disengagement present, as demonstrated by • insensitivity toward other family members • underinvestment of members in each other • rigid or closed boundaries between subsystems • little or no interest or concern for member's messages for assistance?	Insight into inappropriate opportunity for mastery and freedom, over/underdependency	Age and development affect the degree of connectedness and separateness members need or feel. For example, the infant is very connected to the main caregiver and only gradually experiences separateness. Conversely, the adolescent expends much energy developing separateness and focuses on connectedness mostly during particularly stressful times or during family rituals
Socialization Function		
(See Chapter 13 regarding childrearing, which is major focus of socialization function) What are family's childrearing practices in these areas: • discipline • rewards/punishment • autonomy and independence • giving and receiving love • age appropriateness of behavior expected and training offered?	Casefinding in unhealthy parenting styles Useful to understanding anticipatory guidance needed and approach to be taken in teaching and other socialization-related interventions Important assessment when family dysfunction is suspected or demonstrated. (See Assessing Dysfunction discussion in this chapter)	Nurse must be aware of own attitudes/biases and not interject them into the assessment or analysis process. Must also evaluate reasonableness of own expectations for parents and children. Good balancing question for assessment is "How functional is this family's approach to socialization for them in their own situation?" Be aware of compliance expectations in regard to teaching—was teaching realistic or ideal?
Are family's childrearing practices realistic and adaptive for their situation?	Helps nurse temper the "idealistic with the realistic" in planning interventions	

Table 12-6 (continued)

Elements of Assessment	When to Assess/Reasons or Uses	Special Considerations
Who assumes responsibility for child care and socialization? If shared, how is that managed—is the message to children consistent?	Useful in knowing who to address about anticipatory guidance and teaching regarding parenting	
How are children regarded in family—what cultural beliefs are apparent in childrearing approach?	Essential knowledge for planning realistic interventions in relation to the child to enhance compliance	
Health Care Function		
How does family decide who's sick? Clues used? Who decides? Family's general level of knowledge regarding health, disease, hazards to health? Can family observe and report significant symptoms and changes? To what health problems does family perceive they are vulnerable or susceptible and what do they think they can do to reduce that risk? Do they carry these actions out? Adequacy of family practices (age-appropriate) in health promotion: • *Diet:* The function of mealtime for the family; adequacy of diet; shopping practices; adequacy of storage/refrigeration; way food is prepared; who is responsible for planning, shopping, preparing meals • *Sleep:* Age-appropriateness of habits; who decides when children go to bed; where they sleep; who naps; who decides how members relax • *Exercise/recreation:* Family attitudes regarding regular exercise/recreation; daily work activities permit exercise?; how manage stress release? • *Family drug habits:* Use of alcohol, tobacco, caffeine, stimulants; by whom; how much; is use perceived as problem; does use interfere with ADL performance; use of over-the-counter and prescription drugs; how long keep/reuse; properly labeled and stored safely?	Critical information in determining when discharge from hospital is appropriate and in determining whether home care is an option (also how much teaching and supervision will be necessary). Guideline for teaching Casefinding regarding health problems; actual/potential; epidemiologic information regarding contributing health practice deficits Insight into receptivity to teaching/counseling of health promoters and of how realistically family identifies needs To establish reasonableness of health service prescribed/needed, information on resources available/used by family, especially in relation to acute/chronic care Important to assess when family dysfunction is suspected or demonstrated. (See Children in Jeopardy and Disorganized Family Living Patterns under Assessing Dysfunction in this chapter)	Four primary components to health care function are: *Lifestyle practices:* diet, sleep, exercise, self-care, drug habits, stress management *Environmental practices:* cleanliness, safety *Medical-based preventive practices:* physical examinations, eye/hearing examinations, immunizations, record-keeping *Dental health* (Refer to chapters in text that discuss these in detail)
Family Health Maintenance Measures Who are health leaders for family? Health decision makers? Amount of self-care assumed by members?		
Adequacy of environmental practices; exposure to pollutants (air, noise, water, etc)		
Attention to hygiene and cleanliness		
Medically based preventive measures: age/sex/health state–appropriate actions; physical health surveillance and dental checkups; family attitudes regarding examination and immunization status;		

continued

Table 12-6 *(continued)*

Elements of Assessment	When to Assess/Reasons or Uses	Special Considerations
family medical history (genogram); attitudes toward health services; satisfaction regarding care and relationships with health care personnel (ecomap)		
What is the health care provider coverage for an emergency? If none, does family know nearest ER services available? Know how to call an ambulance service?		
What arrangements exist for paying for health services?		
Private or group plan, Medicare? An amount family must pay? Receive any free services? Does cost affect use of health care services? Knowledge of what services are covered by payment sources?		
Distance of health care services from home? Transportation to get to them? If public transportation, what problems, i.e., travel time or hourly service?		
Family Coping Function		
What stressors are impinging (long- and short-term) on family? What strengths does family perceive it has to counterbalance these? Is family able to make realistic, objective appraisal of situation and from there make decisions? Problem-solving abilities of each member?	Need this insight to know what resources family has to deal with health issues, what can be enhanced and supported, what stressors can be decreased, how weaknesses can be diminished or reverted to strengths. Knowledge of how well family does at helping itself achieve/maintain wellness Important assessment when family dysfunction is suspected or demonstrated. (See Crisis and Stress Response section of Assessing Dysfunction in this chapter)	All families have strengths *and* weaknesses Constantly faced with need (from within and outside) to modify perceptions and lives, forcing families to cope or adapt
Typical family reaction to stress situation?		
Functional Strategies? Family group relies on each other more when under stress by providing greater organization and structure until the stressor is resolved, closing family boundaries temporarily? Use of sense of humor? Sharing of feelings, thoughts, actions? Strong subsystem support? Control management of problems? Draw on external resources for support?		
Dysfunctional Strategies? These behaviors, if demonstrated in a family, should be a cue that the family is not adaptive, i.e., is not coping with some or all of life experiences in a healthy, functional manner: spousal violence, child abuse/neglect, scapegoating—one member is selected as the focus for all difficulties, considered deviant		

Table 12-6 (continued)

Elements of Assessment	When to Assess/Reasons or Uses	Special Considerations
Use of threats, e.g., suicide, divorce, separation, denying individual needs if don't stick together?		
Triangling: constant use of intermediary in dyad relationship?		
Authoritarianism: submission at emotional expense to member(s)?		
Pseudomutuality: family homeostasis at cost of affective function?		
Family myths: hold to false, distorted ideas regarding self or family?		

(Drawn from Watzlawick, 1966; Leahy et al, 1982; Olson et al, 1982; Roberts and Feetham, 1982; Wright and Leahey, 1984; Speer et al, 1985; Friedman, 1986.)

References

Aldous J, D'Antonio W: *Families and Religions.* Beverly Hills, CA, Sage Publishers, 1983.

Arent R: *The Child in Stress: Strategies for Support.* Arent and Associates, PO Box 2501, Littleton, CO 80161, 1980.

Becvar RJ, Becvar DS: *Systems Theory and Family Therapy: A Primer.* Washington, DC, University Press of America, 1982.

Clark J: Supporting the family: heading off a breakdown. *Nurs Times* 1986 Aug 6–12; 33–34.

Delaney J: Nursing assessment. *In* Griffith J, Christensen F (eds): *Nursing Process: Application of Theories, Frameworks, and Models.* St. Louis, CV Mosby, 1982.

Duvall EM, Miller B: *Marriage and Family Development.* Philadelphia, JB Lippincott, 1984.

Epstein NB, et al: The McMaster model of family functioning. *J Marr Fam Counsel* 1978; 4:19–31.

Epstein NB, et al: The McMaster Family Assessment Device. *J Marital Fam Ther* 1983; 9:171–180.

Freeman R, et al: *The Family Coping Index.* Johns Hopkins School of Public Health and Richmond, VA, City Health Department Nursing Service, Cooperative Nursing Study, 1964.

Friedman M: *Family Nursing: Theory and Assessment.* Norwalk, CT, Appleton-Century-Crofts, 1986.

Gordon T, Sands J: *P.E.T. in Action.* New York, Bantam Books, 1978.

Goulding M, Goulding R: *Changing Lives Through Redecision Therapy.* New York, Brunner/Mazel, 1982.

Johnson S: *High-Risk Parenting: Nursing Assessment and Strategies for the Family at Risk.* Philadelphia, JB Lippincott, 1986.

Leahy KM, Cobb MM, Jones MC: *Community Health Nursing.* New York, McGraw-Hill, 1982.

Leatherland J: Do you know child abuse when you see it? *R.N.* 1986 Nov; 28–36.

Mackey RT: Transactional Analysis applied to family living. *Health Educ* 1986 Aug-Sep; August-17(4):37.

Olson D, et al: *Family Inventories—Inventories in a National Survey of Families Across the Family Life Cycle.* St. Paul, University of Minnesota Press, 1982.

Otto H: Criteria for assessing family strength. *Fam Proc* 1968 Sep; 329.

Roberts C, Feetham S: Assessing family functioning across three areas of relationships. *Nurs Res* 1982 Apr; 231–235.

Smilkstein G: Assessment of family function. *In* Rosen IG, et al (eds): *Behavioral Science in Family Practice.* Norwalk, CT, Appleton-Century-Crofts, 1980.

Smilkstein G: The physician and family function assessment. *Fam Systems Med* 1984 Fall; 263–279.

Speer J, et al: Selecting the appropriate family assessment tool. *Pediatr Nurs* 1985 Sep-Oct; 349–355.

Stinnett N, DeFrain J: *Secrets of Strong Families.* Boston, Little, Brown, 1986.

Tapia J: A model for family nursing. *Nurs Outlook* 1972 Apr.

Taylor C: Cultural barriers: an anthropological perspective. *In* Hymovich D, Barnard M (eds): *Family Health Care.* New York, McGraw-Hill, 1979.

Thomas A, Chess S: *Temperament and Development.* New York, Brunner/Mazel, 1977.

Watzlawick P: A structured family interview. *Fam Proc* 1966 June; 256–271.

Weitzman J: Engaging the severely dysfunctional family in treatment: basic considerations. *Fam Proc* 1985 Dec; 473–485.

Wilde J, et al: All in the family . . . practical skills in problem-solving for the family group. *Nurs Times* 1985 May 1–7; 30–31.

Woolfolk R, Richardson R: *Stress, Sanity and Survival.* New York, Monarch (Simon and Schuster), 1978.

Wright LM, Leahey M: *Nurses and Families: A Guide to Family Assessment and Intervention.* Philadelphia, FA Davis, 1984.

Bibliography

Allen W, Stukes S: Black family life styles and the mental health of Black Americans. *In* Munoz F, Ends R: *Perspectives on Minority Group Mental Health.* Washington, DC, University Press of America, 1982.

Belsky J, et al: *The Child in the Family.* Reading, MA, Addison-Wesley, 1984.

Boss P, et al: Family boundary ambiguity: a new variable in family stress theory. *Fam Proc* 1986 Dec; 535–546.

Brown M, Hurlock J: Mothering the mother. *Am J Nurs* 1977 Mar; 439–441.

Campbell J: *Theories of Violence: Nursing Care of Victims of Family Violence.* New York, Reston Press, 1984.

Clements I, Roberts F: *Family Health. A Theoretical Approach to Nursing Care.* New York, John Wiley & Sons, 1983.

Doherty W: Family interventions in health care. *Fam Relations* 1985, Jan; 129–137.

Duffy M: Primary prevention behaviors: the female-headed one-parent family. *Res Nurs Health* 1986 June 9; 115–122.

Fraley Y: The family support center: early intervention for high-risk parents and children. *Child Today* 1983 Dec; 13–17.

Friedman R: Making family therapy easier for the therapist: burn out prevention. *Fam Proc* 1985 Dec; 549–553.

Greenspan S: Developmental morbidity in infants in multi-risk-factor families: clinical perspectives. *Public Health Reports* 1982 Jan; 16–23.

Hall M, et al: Working with neglected families. *Child Today* 1982 Feb; 6–36.

Heindl M: Who is the victim? *Nurs Clin North Am* 1981 Mar; 117–125.

Hendrix M: Home is where the hell is. *Fam Commun Health* 1981 Feb; 54–63.

Hoffman L: *Foundations of Family Therapy.* New York, Basic Books, 1981.

Hollen P, et al: The pediatric home liaison in a private practice. *Pediatr Nurs* 1980 May/Jun; 25–27.

Humenick S (ed): *Analysis of Current Assessment Strategies in the Health Care of Young Children and Childbearing Families.* New York, Appleton-Century-Crofts, 1982.

Kirley H, et al: The experience of unemployment and its effects on family life. *Health Visitor* 1986, Oct; 312–314.

Klein D: Family problem-solving and family stress. *Marriage Fam Rev* 1983 Jan/Feb; 85–112.

MacPhail D: Mental health; skills in family therapy. *Nurs Times* 1986 Jun 25–Jul 1; 49–51.

McAdoo H: Stress absorbing systems in Black families. *Fam Relations* 1982 Jan; 479–488.

McAdoo H: Societal stress and the Black family. *In* McCubbin H, Figley C (eds): *Stress and the Family.* Vol I. New York, Brunner/Mazel, 1983.

McCreery A: Scapegoating. A survival phenomenon. *In* Getty C, Humphreys W (eds): *Understanding the Family.* East Norwalk, CT, Appleton-Century-Crofts, 1981.

McCubbin H, Patterson J (eds): *Systematic Assessment of Family Stress, Resources and Coping.* St. Paul, University of Minnesota Press, 1981.

McCubbin H, et al (eds): Social stress and the family. *Marriage Fam Rev* 1983 Jan/Feb; 85–112.

McGoldrich M, et al (eds): *Ethnicity and Family Therapy.* New York, Guilford Press, 1982.

Melito R: Adaptation in family systems: a developmental perspective. *Fam Proc* 1985 Mar; 89–100.

Minuchin S: *Family Kaleidoscope.* Cambridge, MA, Harvard University Press, 1986.

Minuchin S, Fishman H: *Family Therapy Techniques.* Cambridge, Harvard University Press, 1981.

Nix H: Why Parents Anonymous? *J Psychiatr Nurs* 1980 Oct; 22–28.

Norwood R: *Women Who Love Too Much.* New York, Pocket Books, 1986.

Nover R, et al: Preventive intervention with infants in multi-risk-factor foster families. *Child Today* 1981 Oct; 27–31.

Nye I, Berardo FM: *Emerging Conceptual Frameworks in Family Analysis.* New York, Macmillan, 1981.

Olson D, et al: *Families: What Makes Them Work.* Beverly Hills, CA, Sage Publishing Company, 1983.

Peters M: "Making it" Black family style: building on the strengths of Black families. *In* Stinnett N, et al (eds): *Family Strengths: Three Roots of Well-Being.* Lincoln, NB, University of Nebraska Press, 1981.

Rhyme M: Understanding and supporting families in the process of divorce. *Nurse Pract* 1986 Dec; 31–38.

Rogers J, Durkin M: The semi-structural genogram interview. *Fam Systems Med* 1984 Summer; 176–187.

Rosen IG, et al: *Behavioral Science in Family Practice.* Norwalk, CT, Appleton-Century-Crofts, 1980.

Ruger J, Wooten R: A developmental approach to helping families at risk. *Social Casework* 1982 Mar; 3–14.

Schwartzman J: Family ethnography: a tool for clinicians. *In* Hansen J, Falicov C (eds): *Cultural Perspectives in Family Therapy.* Rockville, MD, Aspen Systems, 1983.

Sheriven L: Alternative parenting patterns: clinical implications. *Topics Clin Nurs* 1984 Oct.

Skaggs M, Barber V: *The Mother Person.* New York, Bobbs-Merrill, 1977.

Tapia J: Fractionalization of the family. *In* Schuster C: *The Process of Human Development: A Holistic Approach.* Boston, Little, Brown, 1980.

Temple H: Using research in practice: the practice of family assessment by nurses who work with children. Implications for nursing. *West J Nurs Res* 1983 Feb; 194–196.

Tomlinson P: Applying family stress theory to nursing practice. *Nurse Pract* 1986 Oct; 78, 80–81.

Vega W, et al: Family life patterns of Mexican Americans. *In* Powell J (ed): *The Psychological Development of Minority Children.* New York, Brunner/Mazel, 1983.

Weeks G, Jackson J: The power of powerlessness. *Am J Fam Ther* 1982; 44–47.

Whall A: In search of holistic family assessment: an investigation of a clinical instrument - Watzlawick's structured family interview. *Issues Mental Health Nurs* 1984; 6:105–115.

White House Conference on Families, 1978. Joint hearings before the Subcommittee on Child and Human Development of the Committee of Human Resources, US Senate, and the Subcommittee on Select Education of the Committee on Education and Labor, House of Representatives, Ninety-fifth Congress. Washington, DC, Government Printing Office, 1978.

Ybarra L: When wives work: the impact on the Chicano family. *J Marriage Fam* 1982 Feb; 169–180.

Yoak M, et al: Alternative professional roles in health care delivery: leadership patterns in self-help groups. *J Appl Behav Sci* 1985 Apr; 427–444.

Other Sources of Family Assessment Tools

Bloomquist M, Harris W: Measuring family functioning with the MMPI. *J Clin Psychol* 1984 Sep; 40(5):1209–1214.

Combrink-Graham L: A developmental model for family systems. *Fam Proc* 1985 Jun; 139–150.

Epstein N, et al: The McMaster family assessment device. *J Marital Fam Ther* 1983 Sep; 171–180.

Feetham S, Roberts C: Assessing family functioning across three areas of relationships. *Nurs Res* 1982 Apr; 231–235.

Filsinger E: *Marriage and Family Assessment.* Beverly Hills, CA, Sage Publications, 1983.

Forman B, Hogan B: Measures for evaluating total family functioning. *Fam Ther* 1984 Jan; 1–36.

Hymovich D: The chronicity impact and coping instrument. *Nurs Res* 1983 Feb; 275–281.

Massie H, Campbell B: *The Massie-Campbell scale of mother-infant attachment indicators during stress.* Children's Hospital and Medical Center of San Francisco, PO Box 3805, San Francisco, CA 94119.

Olson D, et al: *Family Inventories.* St. Paul, MN, University of Minnesota, 1982.

Pino C, et al: The children's family environment scale (CFES). *Fam Ther* 1984 Jan; 85–86.

Watzlawick P: A structured family interview. *Fam Proc* 1966 Jun; 256–271.

Promoting Healthy Parenting

Jo Joyce Anderson

Chapter 13

Parenting as a consideration for the nurse working with children is as critical as a knowledge of growth and development processes. The relationship between parent and child is unique and reciprocal; the development of one has a dynamic impact on the development of the other. The intent of this chapter is to acquaint the nurse with principles of parenting and describe the function of the nurse in assessing parental roles, values, and behavior. Emphasis is placed on nursing interventions through teaching and anticipatory guidance, counseling, and referral to guide an individual's transition in the role of parent.

Related Topics
Alternative family lifestyles, Chapter 2
Theory of developing children and families, Chapters 2 and 3
Age-appropriate parenting interventions, Unit II
The relationships between parenting style and development of self-esteem, Chapter 16
Parenting in behavioral problems, Chapter 33
Adolescent parenting, Chapter 37

The Commitment to Parent

To become a parent is probably the biggest commitment in any adult's life. Raising children is one of the most complicated, intricate, and challenging tasks to be performed by family and society and compares with no other in terms of consequence. The task encompasses a gradual shaping of the neonate into a person capable of living in our society and the generational perpetuation of the values, skills, knowledge, beliefs, and activities deemed useful for happy, healthy living.

Socialization of a baby begins in a family, is sustained by that family, but ultimately moves outside the family as the life cycle propels the child beyond family care. Children's unique temperamental traits, coupled with family and social climate, determine in large measure how much they will be influenced by previous generations and what they ultimately will pass on to the generation they create. Thus the unfolding social nature of human beings rests upon the character and quality of parenting.

In the past, society exerted great pressure on couples to become parents — often before they were ready to take on the responsibility. Many people did not think about what parenting involved until a child was on the way. Today, alternate lifestyles and scientific advances make options available to young people. They may choose to delay becoming parents until they feel ready, then have only as many children as they feel they can skillfully socialize, or choose not to become parents at all.

Many couples now talk about having a child before they make the decision to become parents. A realization of the awesomeness of the parenting responsibility has surfaced, which is motivating more couples to seek self-knowledge and some understanding of the parenting task (minimally, knowledge of human growth and development) to make them more capable of successfully meeting the demands of parenthood. The option of choice and the acquisition of preparatory skills promise to make life better for children and more rewarding for parents.

The stresses of modern living and children's earlier exposure to the conflicts of our world make the demanding work of childrearing more difficult. However, society's emerging awareness of parents' needs for assistance is resulting in many supportive actions. Education for parenting is increasing in high schools (kindergarten through grade 12 curricula exist in some regions) and is being offered by organizations devoted to the preservation and health of the family in this changing society. Professional workers in the health, psychology, and sociology fields are helping people become better parents by providing anticipatory guidance education, seminars, and literature. The women's liberation movement and the changing attitudes it has created are freeing fathers to become more active parents and mothers to be happier persons and, consequently, more effective parents. Business leaders are becoming more aware of the lifestyle changes that will make it necessary for them to do their part to support family life and healthy parenting. A few large corporations are already providing quality day care centers and accommodating part-time and split-shift schedules, especially for parents of young children. Supportive changes such as these should in time make being a good parent less difficult and more rewarding.

Whatever the support society gives, however, the quality of parenting still depends largely upon individuals. Nurses have a responsibility to assist individuals to be successful parents and to reinforce those attitudes and behaviors in parents and children that will promote healthy socialization within the context of a happy family.

Setting the Example

I'd rather see a sermon than hear one — any day.
I'd rather you would walk with me, than merely show the way.
The eye's a better pupil and more willing than the ear,
Fine counsel is confusing, but example is always clear.
The best of all the teachers are parents who live their creeds,
For, to see good in action is what every child needs.
I can say, I'll learn how to do it if you'll let me see it done;
I can watch your hand in action though your tongue too fast may run.
Although the lectures you deliver may be very wise and true,
I'd rather learn my lesson by observing what you do;
For I may misunderstand you and the fine advice you give,
But there's no misunderstanding how you act and how you live.

–Author Unknown

How Should Children Behave?

An important question for the nurse offering anticipatory guidance about parenting or assessing a child's behavior is "How *should* a child behave?" There is no single or universal answer to this question. How a child should behave will depend on the developmental stage, physical and cognitive capacities, the culture and society of the child, and the values and beliefs of home and school environments. One society's virtues regarding healthy behavior may be insignificant in another and considered vices in a third. The same is true regarding the behaviors family units consider desirable or important.

The relevant concept is that children *learn* how to behave. Most of a child's learning is motivated by a built-in desire to grow up. From this perspective, discipline stops being something parents and other adults impose but rather becomes a form of "homework" or "practice." Discipline, then, is something which children do for themselves, with adult help. The goal of parenting is to foster the child's developing self-control. Initially, during infancy and early childhood, parents provide controls for the child (referred to as external locus of control). Eventually and steadily the child, properly guided and simultaneously released by the adult caretakers, takes responsibility for that control (internal locus of control). Therefore, children do not know how to behave until they can tell themselves, no matter how successful they are at "doing as they are told" (Leach, 1984).

If all caretakers give consistent messages, children are able to pick up from these role models the basic or general principles of behavior they must learn. The daily do's and don't's simply help exemplify or reinforce those principles. Through this process the child

Promoting Healthy Parenting

Nursing Diagnoses	Nursing Goals/Strategies
Family coping: potential for growth, related to:	
• effective use of rules	Foster healthy child and family development by providing predictable environment. Teach parents to: • agree upon rules to be adopted by all family members. • consistently enforce rules and limits. • use consistent parenting methods to enforce rules.
• effective use of positive reinforcement	Motivate a repeat performance of desired behavior. Teach parents to: • reward child spontaneously during or after desired behavior. • use rewards only when merited. • wean from external rewards gradually.
• effective use of consequences to shape behavior	Curtail a repeat performance of undesirable behavior. Teach parents to: • respond fairly and immediately to correct misbehavior. • use a strategy developmentally appropriate for age of child. • give explanation (i.e., purpose of punishment and consequence of misconduct). • curtail display of strong negative emotion when enforcing restrictions.
• effective role modeling of parents and significant others	Provide effective role models for children in the home. • stress to parents the impact that parental role modeling has on children. • teach parents to monitor behavior of other caretakers (i.e., smoking, drinking, foul language).
• adaptation of parenting style to meet needs of child and parent	Promote healthy family functioning. Assist parents to: • make adaptations consistent with child's temperament to foster positive functioning. • adapt parenting as child grows and matures to foster child's self-regulatory behavior. • identify sociocultural values that affect parenting. • maintain an attitude of accepting each other's rights (between parent and child).
Potential for altered parenting, related to:	
• role conflicts associated with parenting and job/career demands in dual earner families	Prevent role conflicts in dual career families. Encourage parents to: • discuss role expectations together. • plan child care arrangements together. • maintain family social activities. • plan reasonable assistance and responsibilities for child(ren) in the home. • maintain open communication between parents and with child(ren). • use community resources as needed.

• stress associated with childrearing and lack of support from significant others	Reduce stress of childrearing: • help parents cope with children's emotional needs. • encourage parents to join single parents' group as appropriate. • help parents seek out other adult supports. • discuss co-parenting and related feelings with parents.
Potential ineffective family coping: compromised, related to:	
• temporary family disorganization and role changes associated with stages of child's development.	Promote parent's ability to cope with children in the various developmental stages. • Teach parents: normal behavior to be expected at the various ages. to achieve a balance between meeting child's needs and own needs. how to manage difficult behavior. • give parents reassurance and support. • help family identify and use personal and community resources. • make referral to parent support group. • give parents positive reinforcement for appropriate parenting. • prepare parents for difficult behavior associated with selected developmental stages. (See Table 13-3 for nursing strategies at each stage of the child's development.)

learns the culturally and societally approved behaviors that caretakers emanate. Thus the responsibility of parents, teachers, and other caretakers is to assess their own behavior and consistently demonstrate appropriate behaviors for the environment in which they and their children must live. Children can and will learn whatever behaviors are expected of them, assuming those behaviors are developmentally realistic and if those behaviors are demonstrated and reinforced in daily living (Leach, 1984).

How Children Learn to Behave: Socialization and Parental Roles

Bitter are the tears of a child: Sweeten them.
Deep are the thoughts of a child: Quiet them.
Sharp is the grief of a child: Take it from him.
Soft is the heart of a child: Do not harden it.

From "A Child"
–Lady Pamela Wyndham Glenconner

Goals and Functions of Parenting

The goals most directly motivating parenting activities are (1) to keep the child safe, (2) to instill familial beliefs and standards (includes those social and cultural aspects the family has internalized), (3) to teach social behaviors and roles, and (4) to help the child become self-regulating and independent.

Which of these goals is the strongest motivator varies with the child's age, the parents' intellectual and

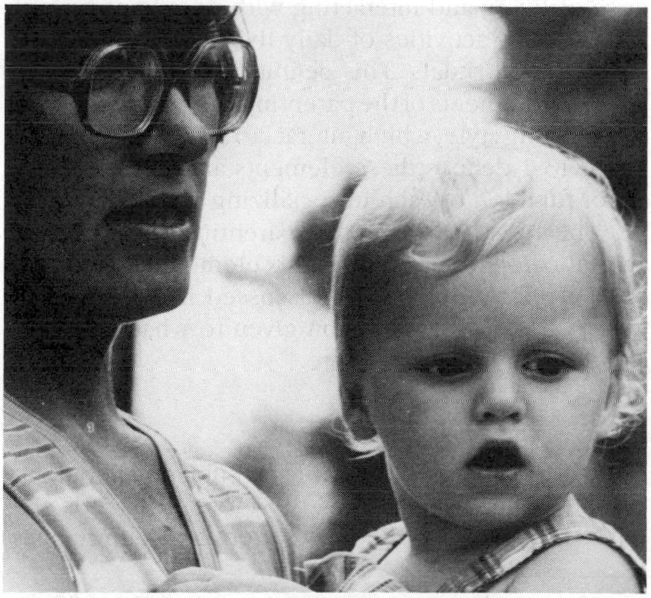

"Deep are the thoughts of a child."

social levels, the parents' interests and individual personalities, the child's temperament, and familial attitudes about parenting. These same factors determine which parenting methods are selected and influence how effective those methods are (see discussion of methods later in this chapter).

Discipline organizes the child's world. Rules consistently established and enforced make the world predictable and give the child boundaries within which to grow and develop. The predictability and boundaries increase the child's security and reinforce the developing trust of others and self. The feelings of security and trust that result from repetition of these experiences (outer controls with parent as police officer) help the child learn to cope and solve problems independently out of a sense of self-control (inner controls with parent as counselor) and self-confidence. As children progressively master the rules and roles of living, they experience a sense of accomplishment and acceptance that builds self-esteem. Positive self-esteem encourages children to make their own decisions on the basis of their own good judgment and inner convictions rather than peer suggestion or impulse, readying them for healthy adult independence. (See Chapter 16 for further discussion of self-esteem.)

A *Working Definition of Parenting**

Parenting "includes the broadest ideas on training . . . and educating the child during his early, formative years. It is (the consistent daily) love and affection which develop one's own self-esteem and self-image. It includes the pangs of guilt and punishment and the heady feelings of praise and success" (Murphy, 1976). Parenting is shaped out of the experience of living and interacting with people of various ages in play, activities of daily living, and family and sociocultural rituals. This definition implicates some essential elements of the parenting process, regardless of parenting style, which interact to socialize children. Table 13-1 defines these elements and describes the major function of each in socializing the child.

The nurse's assessment of parenting skills requires an evaluation of each of these six elements. Therefore, each of these elements is discussed in some detail, with pointers as to direction given to what the nurse should look for and evaluate.

Rules

Rules are essential to the child's mental development. Similarity in use of rules—the more frequently the same rule can be applied in a variety of circumstances—makes them easier for the child to integrate into her or his general moral code (Hurlock, 1978). When the number of rules or the character of a rule differs from one situation to another, it is harder for the child to conceptualize and incorporate the principle into the developing moral code. For example, "Be kind to others" is a rule that can be applied in the majority of situations and is therefore internalized at a fairly early age—a toddler can learn to share, not to bite or hit, to offer a friendly smile. However, "Tell the truth" varies in character depending on the situation, and the child requires many years to gain the intuition to know which degree of truth is appropriate for any given situation. As children mature, they learn when to use the absolute truth and when to avoid and modify absolute truth. One does not tell the lady at the grocery store that she is fat.

Learning rules advances the child toward greater freedom and more mastery of the environment. Although frustration is created in the process of learning rules, it is unavoidable and is not a harmful side effect. The rules the child masters will ultimately make it easier to get along in the world, because each rule mastered allows more responsibility for one's own behavior, readying one for greater independence from external (parents and other adults) guidance and control.

Clearly established rules (i.e., limit setting) give children guidelines as to what is acceptable and not acceptable. They learn that some actions are never acceptable because they are endangering, illegal, unethical, or antisocial. Conversely, they learn that some behaviors are always acceptable. They also gradually learn that a gray area exists in which some behaviors are acceptable at certain ages or in some circumstances and are unacceptable at other times.

Rules can be conveyed in a number of ways. The method most frequently used with infants and young toddlers is environmental control. Confinements in space, restrictions on play materials, and childproofing are measures taken to convey rules by environmental control. Direct verbal communication is used increasingly as a child masters language. Even though this is the most common method of teaching rules, it is the least effective. Younger children respond to a tone of voice when reprimands and explanations are given; however, direct verbal methods do not carry much weight until children reach an age (usually school age) when they can comprehend simple explanations that accompany verbal commands.

The nurse's assessment of parents' childrearing skills should include observation and discussion of the rules being communicated by the parents. The nurse can use the following guidelines:

1. Are the parents aware of the rules they are cur-

*Parenting has many synonymous terms, including childrearing, discipline, socialization.

***Table* 13-1.** Essential Elements of Parenting and Their Function in Socialization

Element	Definition	Functions in Socialization
Rules	Guidelines for behavior; may differ depending on setting and situation; establish what is and is not permitted	Educate child by identifying behaviors acceptable to cultural and social milieu. Restrain misbehavior by placing limits or boundaries on behavior. Develop moral conscience
Consistency • in rules • in required compliance • between parents in parenting methods	Maintaining uniformity or persisting in expectations for child; enforcing rules; retaining authority by using parenting methods congruent with rules, child's unique character, and situation	Speeds learning process by regular reinforcement and repetition. Provides security since child knows what is expected and what to expect from person in authority. Fosters respect for rules and authority (essential to social survival)
Punishment	Negative consequences, natural or artificial, of breaking rule (misbehavior)	Educates by emphasizing which behaviors are not acceptable and that consequence follows misbehavior. Restricts repetition of unacceptable behavior, at least temporarily. Motivates appropriate behavior following misconduct, at least temporarily
Reward	Reinforcement of behavior by physical, emotional, social, or material means that the child finds pleasurable or satisfying	Powerful motivator for acceptable behavior; stimulates repetition of desirable behavior after such behavior has occurred
Role modeling (observation)	Imitation of actions, attitudes, emotional expression of persons child perceives as competent and as possessing behaviors the child desires	Extremely effective way to educate child about acceptable behaviors and probable consequences of behaviors, especially if model provides cues to child to imitate and behavior is frequently demonstrated. Reward for imitation stimulates repetition of the behavior
Using child's imagination	Try out or rehearse behaviors through role play, free play, talking to self, stories, and children's television shows that demonstrate problem solving and behavior/consequences.	Speeds learning process through experimentation and practice. Educates about problem-solving and self-control behaviors while building self-confidence and without risk of negative consequence

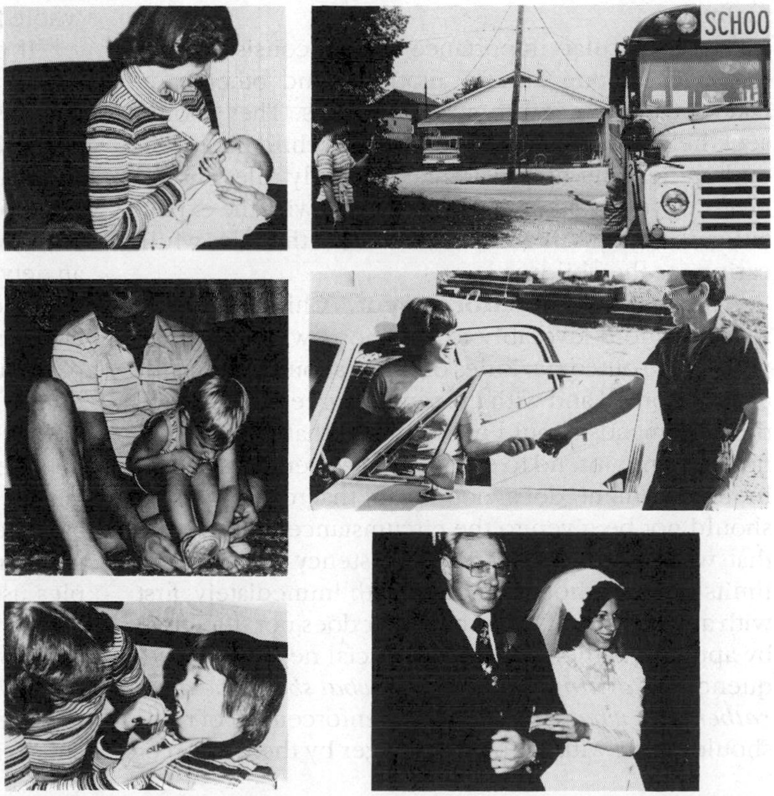

Socialization begins in and is sustained by the family but ultimately propels the child beyond the family. This series portrays the changing parent-child relationship in that socialization life cycle.

rently teaching their child? Are they able to establish rules? To say "no" when appropriate?
2. Are the rules they verbalize consistent with their own behaviors?
3. Are the number and type of rules they are currently working on realistic in terms of the child's age, temperament, and mental capacity?
4. Are the parents using age-appropriate methods to communicate the rules? Are rules being clearly communicated?
5. Are the rules logical and enforceable?
6. Is the child showing evidence of rule mastery? If so, is he or she being given the opportunity for self-regulation in that area of living?

Parents should be given positive reinforcement for those aspects of the guidelines in which they evidence parenting skill (a "yes" answer). In those areas in which their skills are lacking (a "no" answer), the nurse should institute interventions to help them develop skills.

Consistency

Consistency in Rules. Rules are learned much faster when they are consistently upheld by and applicable to all family members. Some breaches of limits may be tolerated by parents when rules are first being learned or in certain circumstances, and relapses can be anticipated during illness or fatigue. It is easier to be consistent when there are not too many rules to be maintained.

Of particular importance is the consistency of messages among fathers, mothers, and other caretakers. Parents need to agree on rules. They should seek help if they cannot agree, or the child likely will end up needing help. Parental or family rules should be conveyed to other caretakers along with the expectation that they will enforce and model the rules while caring for the children.

Consistency in Enforcement. Children usually respond more favorably to situations when they can predict the outcome. Rules or limits should be consistently enforced and with the same degree of force each time. Demands should not be made that parents cannot or do not intend to enforce. However, consistency in enforcement does not mean that consideration should not be given to the circumstances involved—that would be rigidity, not consistency. Breaches of limits or rules should be dealt with immediately, first with a warning and, if the behavior does not stop, then by applying either natural or artificial negative consequences. *Warnings ideally state what should be done rather than what should not.* The enforcement of rules should occur without obvious anger by the reinforcer and with a minimum of words. Explanations of "why" should follow the consequence, provided the child is old enough to understand. Even then, explanations should be simple and brief. Through consistently employed enforcement of rules, the child slowly learns to connect the act with the consequence and changes behavior to avoid discomfort.

Consistency in Parenting Methods. The methods used to enforce rules should be consistent with the seriousness or value placed on the rules. Fair parenting methods foster respect in the child for rules and for authority. Methods also should recognize children's individual temperaments, since some temperaments thrive better on more firmness and consistency whereas other temperaments are relatively adaptable and less dependent on consistency of method. One of the requirements of consistency is that parents agree upon and collaboratively enforce a plan of parenting.

When a couple becomes parents, ideally they develop a comprehensive parenting "master plan" that takes into account the mutual rights, privileges, and responsibilities of every family member, arrived at out of consensus. This master plan would cover the rewards and punishments allowable in that family, establish protective limits, and identify whether the parenting will be primarily the responsibility of one member or, better, a shared affair. Agreement about these issues may not be easy to achieve, especially if the parents have difficulty in communicating with each other. A nurse's assistance in developing such a parenting plan can be a true contribution to the well-being of the whole family.

If parents do not present a united front in their parenting, everyone loses. Since parenting is a daily responsibility, couples who do not stand together will become emotionally estranged owing to the constant friction their disagreement presents. The child will learn very quickly how to play one parent against the other, and all members will experience a high level of anxiety. In this circumstance the parents have progressively less control over their child's socialization. The child ends up in the middle of a parental struggle that places more pressure on him than he can bear, causing him to lose respect for the parents and even to resent one or both of them. Children need consistent limits, enforced with love, mutually endorsed by all caretakers.

The nurse's assessment in this area of potential stress in families is especially important because couples usually will not seek professional help on their own unless their disagreement is pathologically intense or until their differences have existed for some time. When nurses identify a family unit that is either at high risk for or currently displays conflicts related to childrearing attitudes, they need to help this couple talk out their childrearing differences honestly, calmly, and privately. (In extreme cases the nurse or a professional counselor may need to be present as an arbitrator in the early phases of these discussions.) The couple should be encouraged to try to understand each other's views and to work toward a satisfactory compromise in areas of opposition. Talking seldom hurts as much as silence and is essential to problem resolution in this situation. Nurses also should attempt to expand the parents' understanding of their children's differences (developmental, temperamental) so that they can select a comfortable parenting schema for their situation. Nurses may make appropriate reading materials available, teach individually, or involve the parents in parent groups, or use any other appropriate means that are available within the community.

The following checklist is helpful in assessing parents' ability to be consistent.

1. Do parents display a code of conduct that is congruent with what they are enforcing for their children?
2. Are rules realistically enforced with consideration for age, newness of rule, circumstances?
3. Do parents follow through by enforcing rules?
4. Have parents communicated rules to other caretakers?
5. Do parents agree on the rules to be enforced and share their enforcement?
6. Is enforcement promptly enacted?
7. Is rationale shared with the child age-appropriate? Simple? Concise?
8. Are enforcement methods congruent with the rules involved? The child's temperament?
9. Does the child display evidence of developing respect for rules? Authority?

Negative Reinforcement

The ground rules of negative reinforcement, if it is to be effective in encouraging desirable behavior, are that the child be informed of the consequence if misconduct occurs and that if punished, the child know why.

Punishment, or negative reinforcement, is the "fine," or price, for deviating from established rules. It may be disapproval, withdrawal of privileges, isolation, substitution, or physical punishment. *Disapproval* may be verbal or nonverbal. Often tone of voice alone conveys that the parent "means business." Numerous facial expressions and gestures can be used; their meanings are learned quickly even by young children.

Older children are more likely to respond to *privilege withdrawal.* Something they would like to do or have is withheld. The privilege withheld should be reasonable, not something critical like a birthday party or long-anticipated special event such as a prom, and the negative reinforcer should occur fairly soon after the misdeed. When possible, the withheld privilege should be something associated with the misconduct.

Isolation works with some children. As a general rule isolation periods of longer than an hour breed contempt for the parent rather than redirecting the offender's behavior. This method is not usually easily carried out before preschool age.

Substitution is a form of environmental control generally used with infants and young toddlers. The parent bodily removes the child from the situation prompting inappropriate behavior or makes a diversion with another activity or toy. It is often coupled with a disapproval action.

Although many parents use *physical punishment* with their children at some time or another, there is no evidence that it is an effective disciplinary measure. On the other hand, for parents with poor impulse control, use of physical punishment sets up a situation in which serious injury of children is a potential outcome. Some believe spanking cancels the crime, freeing the child to repeat the act.

Natural consequence may also be used as a negative reinforcer and is probably most effective in helping the child see self-regulation as a personal responsibility. For example, if a child refuses to eat at mealtime, he or she gets extremely hungry before the next meal when he can again have food. This approach does require restraint on the parents' part to not intervene but allow the natural consequence to occur. This approach is usually most successful with preschool and early school-age children.

Having the child use *positive practices* (apologizing, repairing the results of the misdeed, correcting inappropriate behavior, practicing correct behavior several times) as a negative reinforcer is often realistic and has the double advantage of also reinforcing desirable behavior (Norton, 1977).

When possible, negative reinforcement should be presented unemotionally. However, parents are only human and circumstances sometimes make unemotional intervention extremely difficult to achieve. Fairness (i.e., punishment that fits the crime) is an important factor in determining how severe the negative reinforcer should be. This does not mean all children in a family need the same form or degree of negative reinforcement; what is right for one child is not necessarily right for another.

A misdeed should be acted upon promptly, then the act should be forgotten. Children do not need reminders of their wrongdoings on a long-term basis.

The following checklist can assist the nurse's assessment of parents' use of negative reinforcement in the parenting process.

1. What forms of negative reinforcement are usually employed?
2. Is the reinforcer used age- and developmentally appropriate?
3. Is the parents' goal to educate or motivate desirable behavior or to impart revenge?
4. Is the reason for negative reinforcement explained to the child?
5. Are the parents usually able to apply punishment without emotional display?
6. Is the negative reinforcer realistic to the misdeed?
7. Are misdeeds immediately followed by negative reinforcement measures?
8. Do the parents attempt to employ positive practices as negative reinforcers whenever possible?
9. Does the child express through words or behaviors an understanding of the consequence if a rule is broken?

Positive Reinforcement

Rewarding is really another means of enforcing rules or setting limits. All of us, but especially children, need praise, encouragement, and rewards for behaving properly. Rewards should be differentiated from *bribes.* Children are bribed when they are either told beforehand that they will be rewarded or actually are rewarded in advance for a promise to avoid misbehavior. Children are rewarded when they have conducted themselves properly. The positive reinforcement is given spontaneously during or after the act (Murphy, 1976).

The use of positive reinforcement increases the likelihood that a child will repeat desired behavior. It also communicates to the child what the desired behavior is without a lot of confusing verbal exchange.

Positive reinforcers fall into five general categories. Table 13-2 describes the advantages and disadvantages of each type.

To be effective, a positive reinforcer must meet certain criteria: (1) it must be something the child finds satisfying and desirable, (2) it must be readily available, and (3) it must be accessible to the child only when the desired behavior occurs (Norton, 1977). When and how frequently the reinforcer is offered also determine its effectiveness. Whatever its form, the reinforcer or reward should be given while the child is still engaged in the desired action or immediately after it ends. Initially the behavior must be reinforced regularly, preferably each time it occurs. Gradually the reward can be given only occasionally (intermittent reinforcement). Eventually the desired behavior will become a habit, requiring no external reward. (See Chapter 33 for further discussion of behavior modification.)

Accentuating the positive aspects of behavior (i.e., catching the child in the act of being good) can eliminate a lot of parent-child conflicts. A child who perceives the parent as a supporter of the growing self is more apt to imitate that parent's values and beliefs. However, the psychology laboratory has produced evidence that both rewards (positive reinforcement) and punishment (negative reinforcement) have strong motivational effects on socializing behavior (Fisher and Fisher, 1986). Unfortunately, scientific investigation has revealed no simple formula for when to use each—that is still left to parents' intuition and judgment.

The following checklist may help assess parents' use of positive reinforcement in their parenting:

1. Do parents offer rewards or bribes? Do they know the difference?
2. What type of positive reinforcers do the parents employ? Are they appropriate to the child's developmental level?
3. Does the child communicate verbally or through behaviors that the rewards are perceived as worthwhile?
4. Are the rewards realistic and given only when merited?
5. Do the parents know how and when to wean the child from external rewards?

Learning by Observation: Role Modeling

Children naturally imitate as a way of learning. Through imitation they learn to perform specific actions; they learn attitudes and they learn emotional expression. This fact illustrates the importance of parents, older siblings, and other caregivers in providing cues that influence children's behavior. Psychologists stress that most of what we learn about our world occurs because of our observing other people. A child who is inexperienced or unsure how to behave in a situation is likely to observe and imitate someone thought to know how to behave appropriately (Norton, 1977).

This statement brings to light some factors that influence observational learning. First, children imitate people they perceive are competent and hold status—"someone thought to know how to behave appropriately." Significant others, parents, and caregivers, in particular, meet those specifications for the child, at least until adolescence, when peers begin to replace parents as role models. Second, children imitate someone who possesses behaviors the child de-

Table 13-2. Advantages and Disadvantages of Rewards

Reward Category	Advantages	Disadvantages
Objects (food, toys, trinkets, clothing)	Since object is visible, reinforcement continues each time object seen or used. Stimulates several sense modalities	Can be costly. If food is used, calories involved. Cannot always be given immediately after the desired behavior
Activities (TV, theater, roller skating, whatever activity the child finds rewarding and parents approve)	Usually inexpensive. Perceived as desirable by most children. May be contingent upon earning so many tokens or points	What appeals can change rapidly; avoid problem somewhat by giving child choices or by letting child suggest activities
Social (hugs, kisses, pats, smiles, praise)	Can use lavishly without any cost.	Must be sure to give only when earned. Needs to be combined with tangible rewards occasionally to retain effectiveness
Personal (self-satisfaction, feeling good)	Most desirable; fosters self-regulation	Must be learned, cannot be given by another. Seldom effective in child with poor self-concept
Token (stars, check marks, points)	Good for all ages, can be promptly given	Reward finally earned by accumulated tokens can be expensive

Parents are their children's first teachers.

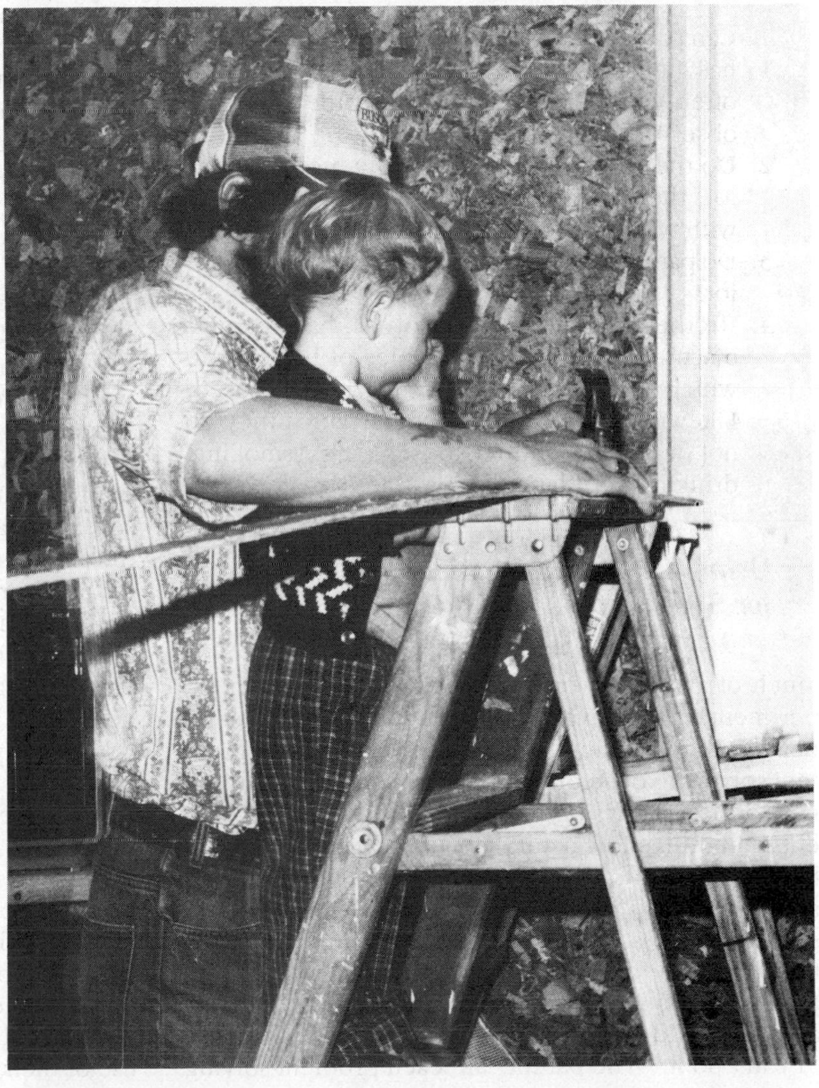

sires at the time—"when the child is unsure how to behave." Parents or caregivers are most often the resources available to the child in confronting unknown situations. Children will repeatedly imitate those who they have previously been rewarded for imitating. The child who hears, "You're a big girl— you did that just like your mother," is more likely to imitate mother again.

Children vary in how much they rely on role models to learn behavior, however. Those who have gained some skill in appropriately behaving in similar situations are more likely to handle new situations on their own than to imitate. Likewise, children who have experienced frequent successes are less likely to rely on someone else to guide their behavior. This does not mean that only inadequate children imitate—all children imitate. Parents usually can encourage imitation regardless of how children perceive their parents' competencies or their own capabilities by making sure rewards are provided for imitative behavior.

The following checklist may help assess parents' conscious use of role modeling in their parenting:

1. Can parents identify instances when their child has imitated them? Of these instances, how often was the parent aware that the child was observing?
2. Do the parents consciously role model behaviors they specifically want the child to learn or with which the child is having difficulty?
3. Do parents reward the child for imitated behavior?
4. If other caregivers are involved, have parents discussed with them examples of behavior to which they wish to have the child exposed? Likewise, specific behaviors to which they do not want the child exposed, e.g., smoking, drinking, foul language?

Using the Child's Imagination for Socialization

Much of a child's world is imaginative. Children experiment imaginatively, trying out new behaviors, rehearsing and refining behaviors, and practicing problem solving to overcome problems or fears—learning new or better ways of interacting with the world. Parents can utilize this natural activity to teach desirable behavior. Parents also can use children's tendency to talk to themselves to help them master the problem solving process. (Children talk to themselves more than adults do because they are less capable of the private communication adults call thinking.) For example, a child expresses frustration over a task, saying "I can't do it." The parent can teach problem-solving thinking by saying "Watch me. I'll show you." As mother demonstrates, she can talk aloud to herself, enumerating what must be done first and why, what second, and so on till the task is completed. Then she evaluates aloud, saying, "Now, how did I do? Yes, that's fine." By describing each of the necessary steps of the task, and why, occasionally questioning whether it is correct, and evaluating and praising the results aloud, the child learns not only the motor action required and how to deal with any complications but also how to "think through" a problem (see Box 13-1).

Many well-designed children's television programs (e.g., Sesame Street, Afternoon Youth Specials) and teaching stories can be useful in teaching children appropriate behavior. These stories and televised programs are structured to capture the child's attention, center on a particular problem faced by children, and provide a convenient way of solving the problem, with rewards to the successful problem-solver hero or heroine. Parents can fabricate their own stories to fit a particular problem or behavior facing their child, following these same guidelines and being careful not to focus so intently on the moral that the entertaining aspect of the story is lost. Or they can draw upon the child's creativity to help evolve a story. All these approaches to learning behavior are enhanced if followed by discussion between the parent and child about the intended theme and how the child might apply the information learned to a life situation.

An enjoyable teaching method for some that is similar to story participation is for a parent and child to role play. This is especially useful with older children and can be followed by a discussion of how each felt in the new role, reinforcing for the child the fact that people do not all think or feel alike in a given situation. Discussion also reveals the reasons behind each person's behavior. Role playing also can aid children in improving their behavior when they role play themselves in various problem behavior situations. Once the parent sees what is provoking the problem behavior and the responses it is receiving, the parent or nurse observer can help the child practice more desirable alternative behaviors through modeling another role. Practicing the behavior increases the child's confidence and the likelihood that it will be carried out. Additionally, the child can receive immediate feedback.

Whether teaching behavior through talking to themselves, story telling, or role playing, children are shown ways of reacting to situations, which will ultimately teach them to control their own behavior. An extra benefit is that parent and child are given an opportunity for positive interaction, which in itself fosters sociable behavior.

The following checklist can help assess parents' use of their child's imagination to teach behaviors:

1. Do the parents talk their child through the steps of tasks to aid problem solving?
2. Are parents conscious of the behaviors of their child that illustrate learning through imagination?
3. Can parents identify television programs or storybooks that help their child learn desirable behaviors? Do they expose their child to these? Do they discuss them with the child?
4. Are parents acquainted with the technique of role playing? Have they used this technique with their child? Do they seem comfortable doing a sample role play with the nurse?

> Box 13-1
> *Helping a Child Problem Solve to Elicit Appropriate Behavior*
>
> **UNSOLVABLE PROBLEMS**
> 1. Accept the child's problem as real.
> 2. Express empathy.
> 3. Try to help the child understand the situation, why it cannot be resolved.
>
> **SOLVABLE PROBLEMS**
> 1. Have the child describe the situation from his or her own perspective; get perspectives of others involved if helpful.
> 2. Help the child identify options.
> 3. Help the child determine the likely consequences of each option.
> 4. Use simulation—parent and child role play ways the child may respond to the problem if it occurs again. This helps the child realize that options exist in resolving problems and that each has its own consequences. The child can then select the most comfortable option the next time the problem arises.
> 5. Sometimes talking and simulation are not enough guidance for the child and the parent needs to structure a program of change to help the child improve responses to the problem.

Parental Roles

Children are unique individuals with their own special potential; that factor makes parenthood an exciting endeavor for those who make the commitment to parent. However, successful parents keep in mind that they are persons first and parents second.

The skills of parenting are not sex-specified. Male and female parents should combine their individual capabilities, each contributing those parenting behaviors with which they feel most comfortable and competent.

Providing a home and food is only the beginning of being a parent. The most important role of parenting is the *nurturing* of personality and development in a climate of *love* and *security* that starts a child on the road to healthy adulthood. The paradox of parenting is that we live with our children so we can teach them to live without us. This nurturing begins before the child's birth as the parent(s) prepares emotionally and intellectually for the parenting role.

We are all products of our own childhood. For parents raised in a loving home, repeating that atmosphere with their own children is usually easier. If one has experienced an unloving or insecure childhood, successful parenting may be more difficult, but it is not an impossibility. None of us chose our backgrounds, but by understanding the importance of giving love in a way children can perceive and becoming educated for parenthood, one can compensate for one's own childhood deprivations.

Parents are their children's first teachers. They teach the most important lesson of living: how to interact with other humans. Most also teach children to be happy and loving by providing them with happiness and love. Expressions of love can be woven into all the things parents do for or with their child.

An effective parent cannot be passive but must participate in the child's learning process. How a parent participates (parental role) in the learning process will change as the child grows and develops. Table 13-3 describes the primary parental roles at each developmental stage of childhood. Encouragement, approval, and positive interactions are needed from their parents by children at all ages.

Parental roles have traditionally been differentiated into mothering roles and fathering roles. In modern society this is steadily changing so that the relative impact of each parent on a child's development is also undergoing change. However, this modern concept of parenting has not existed long enough for adequate researched documentation of the changes it produces. Many families, particularly at lower middle and lower class levels, are still functioning with traditional parenting standards, discussed next. Single parenting is an increasingly common experience for children, at least during part of their childhood. It is discussed later in this chapter.

Principles of Parenting

Any set of principles to help parents select parenting techniques can only be a guide and not a blueprint. Nor

Table 13-3. Development-Related Parental Tasks and Nursing Considerations

Parental Task/Role	Nursing Diagnosis of Actual/Potential Problem	Nursing Strategies
Infancy		
Learning infant's cues and interpreting infant's needs Physical caregiver—affirm love and acceptance. Stimulator of motor development. Builder of trust by being predictable and consistent	Altered parenting related to lack of knowledge *Defining characteristics:* • diminished or inappropriate visual, tactile, or auditory stimulation of infant • verbalization of perceived or actual inadequacy (e.g., nervous, overwhelmed by demand to meet infant's needs)	Provide parenting and child care education Empathize with parent's sense of immense responsibility and offer reassurance and support that parent can learn to know child's needs Provide positive reinforcement for appropriate behavior
	Altered parenting related to change in family unit: new child *Defining characteristics:* • inappropriate parenting behaviors • lack of parental attachment behaviors • verbalization of frustration of role	Teach parents the importance of balance between infant's needs and needs of other members, including themselves—self-sacrificing not healthy Help family identify and utilize personal and community resources Provide positive reinforcement for appropriate behaviors
Early Childhood (Toddler)		
Learning to accept child's growth and development and accompanying acceptance of some loss of control while simultaneously maintaining reasonable limits Physical helper—affirm developing selfhood. Stimulator of self-regulatory body functioning. Facilitator of exploration within set limits	Altered parenting related to rebellious child *Defining characteristics:* • frequent verbalization of disappointment or dissatisfaction with child • evidence of abuse of child • verbalization of misinterpretation of child's refusals and negativism as disrespect (threatening to parent insecure in own authority and autonomy)	Teach parents about normality of child's behavior for developmental stage Reassure parents that child still loves them and needs them despite negative outbursts or refusals of parental assistance Provide information that children develop individual personalities by asserting themselves with people they trust Help family identify and obtain assistance from personal and community resources
	Altered parenting related to unmet psychosocial needs of child by parent *Defining characteristics:* • inappropriate parenting behaviors • behaviors demonstrating child is anxious because parents do not maintain limits and/or keep the child's world orderly	Provide positive reinforcement for appropriate parenting behaviors and attempts at same Teach parents how to relax and enjoy their child(ren) Teach parents how to manage rebellious behaviors
Middle Childhood (Preschooler and Early School-Age)		
Learning to become separate from child, allowing independent development, while demonstrating appropriate standards through role modeling Become comfortable with endless questions of child Provide opportunities for child to initiate activities with a sense of purpose Physical—psychologic helper—affirm creative efforts. Facilitator of emotional self-control, moral and sexual development. Stimulator of self-care skills with limits	Altered parenting related to lack of knowledge *Defining characteristics:* • evidence of abuse/neglect of child • inappropriate parenting behaviors (e.g., unable to allow child increased independence, unable to model acceptable standards *or* incongruency in verbal instructions and what is role modeled re standards, threatened and frustrated by child's natural abundance of questions)	Teach parents about normal development and associated behaviors of child this age Provide parenting education Provide positive reinforcement for appropriate parenting behaviors and attempts at same Provide reassurance that child still loves them and that they are not being disrespectful just because they question everything Help family identify and utilize personal and community resources

Table 13-3 *(continued)*

Parental Task/Role	Nursing Diagnosis of Actual/Potential Problem	Nursing Strategies
Late Childhood (School-Age and Early Adolescence)		
Learning to accept rejection without abandoning the child Psychologic helper—affirm capacity to be productive. Stimulator of mental, social, ongoing moral development. Facilitator to acceptance of changing skills and body image. Progressive freedom-giving with reasoned limit setting.	Altered parenting related to lack of knowledge *or* Altered parenting related to parents' unrealistic expectations of child *Defining characteristics:* • Overinvested parental attachment behavior (e.g., prohibit child from social participation, prevent child from assuming greater self-sufficiency, pressure child in industrious pursuits to fulfill those dreams they themselves did not accomplish) • inappropriate parenting behavior (e.g., abandonment of any roles *or* restriction to family unit, excluding any outside involvement or interests) • verbalization of perceived or actual inadequacy (e.g., full-time caregiver who has difficulty adjusting to the diminished caregiver role)	Provide parenting and child development education Make referral to parent support groups Provide reassurance the child still needs them but is shifting from a need for physical support to a need for psychologic support Encourage setting of special time each day with child, but allowing child to pursue own interests and friendships as well Help full-time caregiver to assess skills/interests and develop them as caregiver role decreases
Later Adolescence and Early Adulthood		
Learning to build a new life by adjusting to altered family roles and relationships during teen's identity crisis Provide security and reliability through clear, reasonable limits and communication of expectations for acceptable behavior Psychologic supporter—affirm developing adult image. Facilitator of open communication. Freedom-giver. Reinforcer of moral limits	Altered parenting related to history of ineffective relationship with own parent(s) *or* Altered parenting related to lack of knowledge *or* Altered parenting related to separation from nuclear family *Defining characteristics:* • frequent verbalization of disappointment/dissatisfaction with teen • verbalization of frustration with role (e.g., anxiety, over-reaction to teen's identity crisis, discomfort with social and sexual issues)	Provide parenting and child development education—relate to parents' developmental stage Reassure parents it is OK to admit when they make bad decisions; that their critical teen still loves and needs them. Prepare parents that upheavals are a normal part of this stage and stress the importance of being objective and communicating. Provide positive reinforcement for appropriate parenting and attempts at same Refer to community resources

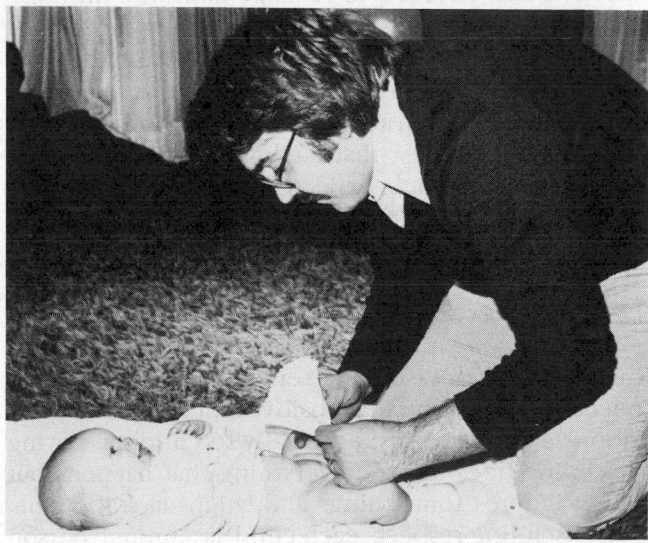

Many fathers, even in traditional homes, enjoy the closeness that helping care for their children allows them.

can the most timely childrearing manual be adopted for all children or in all homes. Any effort to do so will soon find parents filled with resentment, guilt, lowered confidence, or all three, because most manuals offer guidelines too vague to be useful or that do not take into account differences in parents or the uniqueness of a child.

Basic Guidelines

Some guidelines have been offered to parents that come from children themselves and that have applicability regardless of the child involved or the parenting methods preferred by parents.

1. *"Don't blow your class,"* or, keep the dignity of your parenthood. The first rule to maintain parental dignity is for parents to present a united front regarding rules and the disciplinary measures taken to enforce them. Although differences are likely to exist in a couple's attitudes and parenting methods, they should be resolved by compromise outside the child's hearing and, ideally, before the baby is even born.

A second rule to retain parental dignity is to avoid arguing with the child. Confrontations force someone into submission, which is deflating to self-esteem. If a parent firmly believes in the stance taken on an issue, it should simply be enforced. If the issue cannot be enforced, it should be dropped and forgotten. And if the parent has no definite stance on the issue, the child's opinion should be heard to arrive at a joint decision.

Parents also should avoid threats, promises, bribes, and sarcasm. Threats only invite misbehavior. The use of promises invalidates the parent-child relationship. Bribes communicate doubt to the child of ability to behave on his or her own initiative and insure only short-term cooperation. Sarcasm blocks communication and encourages revenge fantasies. All these diminish parenting as a teaching-learning process.

A final rule for maintenance of parental authority is to talk less and listen more. Authority calls for brevity in the administration and enforcement of rules. Brevity requires conciseness that facilitates the child's comprehension of what is expected or why the reinforcement occurred. When words are used to socialize children, the emphasis should be on what must be done. Words should be kept to a minimum and accompanied by action; they should be descriptive, not general.

2. *"Bug me a little,"* or, use firm, but fair, loving discipline. Such discipline remembers that everyone needs successes and that positive attitudes and expectations are contagious, especially to children. Loving discipline does not see everything that happens but rather ignores some things and laughs at still others. Fair discipline respects each child as a unique person and allows room within which to learn the rules of happy living. Firm, fair discipline allows the experience of feelings but sets limits on the actions taken to express them, channeling expression into acceptable forms (symbolic release, talking it out, or play). Fair discipline also respects the child's ability to absorb only a few rules at a time. Four or five rules are manageable by the average child, although those children with mental or intellectual handicaps may be able to handle only one to three rules at a time and may require a longer period for mastery. Above all else, fair and loving discipline does not involve comparisons between children.

3. *"Call my bluff,"* or, let the child see that you mean what you say. Children need limits set on their behavior until they have learned to be self-regulatory; they expect to bear the consequences of misbehavior despite the temporary anger, frustration, or disappointment it causes them. Once a rule is established and conveyed to the child, it should be promptly and consistently enforced. Rules that cannot be enforced should not be made. Parents should also allow children to solve their own problems to the extent that they are ready and able.

4. *"Light me a candle,"* or, show the child the way to maturity and faith. The majority of a child's learning occurs as a result of imitation of significant others. Thus, if parents wish to effectively socialize their children, they need to model behaviors consistent with what they are attempting to teach. Children also behave in a manner consistent with the injunctions and permissions their parents project upon them, usually unconsciously. These injunctions and permissions are conveyed to children indirectly through conversations they overhear about themselves that the parent is addressing to someone else, as well as from disciplinary feedback.

Research findings and observations of children's instinctual behavior support the validity of two other principles of parenting (Homan, 1977; Fisher and Fisher, 1986). First, parents need not waste time teaching those things that children will teach themselves when they are developmentally ready (toilet training, weaning). Instead, parents should consider the attributes society will judge once the child is an adult (dependability, honesty, creativity, ambition) and teach those. Second, parents are wise to avoid extremes—overpermissiveness or strict authoritarianism, bribery or revenge, pampering or being overly strict—as these invariably produce unhealthy responses in children.

Parenting Styles

No one method for instructing in the rules of living and conveying right or wrong has proved more effective than another, as long as the method used was not carried to extremes. No method will work until a child respects the parents and the authority a parent represents.

Three parenting themes can be derived out of the parenting behaviors within families. Any one of them, if extreme, can result in incomplete or unhealthy socialization of children. Conversely, any of them, if conducted in an atmosphere of love that positively reinforces desired behavior, can effect the healthy socialization of children. Table 13-4 summarizes these three styles.

Factors Influencing Selection of Parenting Style

Children are very different and have their own unique responses to all life's experiences and challenges, including the parenting with which they must cope on a daily basis. Parents also differ with regard to the parenting styles they can effectively and comfortably employ and in how they respond to each child. Thus there can be no one right or wrong parenting style, nor can a given parenting style be used with all children.

A child's temperament and developmental stage as well as parental interests and sociocultural values are factors that influence the effectiveness of the various parenting styles. The discussion that follows is intended to offer some guidelines that the nurse can utilize in offering guidance and counsel to parents in their efforts to socialize their children. To use the guidelines appropriately, the nurse must assess the child and parents in terms of each of these factors. (See Chapters 2 and 12 for guidance in assessment.)

Temperament or Basic Personality

Parenting methods have impact on whether children's traits develop into assets or problems. Box 13-2 de-

Table 13-4. Three Parenting Styles

Main Theme	Predominant Approach to Teach Socialization	Primary Teaching Methods	Comments
Autocratic or Authoritarian			
Obedience; respect	Favors punitive measures to curb self-will when child does not comply with code of conduct	State rules. Declare expectations. Assert parental values. Apply negative reinforcement for noncompliance, usually physically. Occasionally grant privileges or increased responsibility for compliance	Behavior evaluated in accord with a set standard of conduct, often theologically based. Tends to employ primarily negative reinforcement
Democratic or Authoritative			
Autonomous problem solving based on self-regulation and disciplined conformity. Rational, issue-related approach	Shares rationale for desired behavior with child; affirms child's efforts to comply but sets limits or boundaries for acceptable behavior. Flexibility in rules	Describe problem or explain rules. Help child find own solutions to problem or way to comply with rule based on uniqueness. Reinforce positively for compliance, negatively for noncompliance: verbally (declare pleasure or indignation), physically (actions that communicate satisfaction or dissatisfaction with behavior), in writing (notes of praise or recommended change in behavior)	Least likely to be carried to extremes. Encourages development of child's own inner controls over behavior, self-reliance. More verbal exchanges; employs both positive and negative reinforcement. Respect for child's opinion and right to disagree; however, parent retains ultimate control
Permissive			
Absence of restraints; child free of parental input	Uses reason; punitive measures seldom (if ever) used to teach socialization	Suggest rules, giving reasons for them. Give child choice of complying or not complying. Sometimes positively reinforce compliance, usually ignore or tolerate noncompliance	Does not foster development of inner controls. Few demands made for responsibility unless child chooses to have it. Tends to leave child on own, reinforcing neither positively or negatively

Box 13-2
Temperament or Basic Personality as a Factor in Parenting

EASY CHILD

1. Adapts to almost any parenting approach and is easy to manage as long as expectations are clearly defined and consistently endorsed; this avoids confusion for the child.
2. Learns rules quickly unless intellectually impaired.
3. Realistic parenting that will not be incongruent with what child finds in the world outside the home is an important consideration. These children seldom develop behavior problems, but when they do it is most often due to a conflict between home-taught values and those of the outside world.
4. Because this child adapts so readily, it is important not to initiate any practice or ritual that is undesirable to continue over time, as the child will quickly incorporate that practice into his or her living pattern.

SLOW-TO-WARM CHILD

1. A patient, relaxed, persevering approach is most effective. New situations or rules should be presented gradually, but repeatedly, without much pressure. (One reassuring feature of these children is that they gradually adapt and their noncooperation or nonparticipation until they do is usually nonbelligerent and silent.) Because of some common elements in the traits of difficult and slow-to-warm personality types, some management guidelines apply to both. Nos. 2–8 in this section apply to both.
2. Refuse to compete with the child or to force adherence to every rule of the home to its more rigid interpretation. Such action only increases a negative display of behavior.
3. Try not to explode at the child, as such fury only exaggerates the inappropriate behavior.
4. Clearly identify on a regular basis what behaviors will be accepted and what behaviors are unacceptable. (A picture chart or check list posted in rooms the child spends much time in are creative ways to regularly reinforce expectations.) These children also need help identifying what behaviors are contingent on the situation at hand; do this clarifying at times when they are not misbehaving so that they are not so tense that they cannot hear the rules. Then carry through consistently in enforcing established limits. (A democratic approach is least overwhelming to this child. However, an autocratic approach also suits the difficult child as long as it is not extreme.)
5. Since this child learns slowly, much repetition is needed.
6. Build in daily success experiences for this child.
7. Maintain established routines while child is mastering a rule or behavioral expectation.
8. Key words to management:
   - Firmness
   - Repeated exposure
   - Consistent reinforcement
   - Patience

DIFFICULT CHILD

1. A firm, consistent approach that emphasizes the positive works best. Those aspects of a child's temperament that may have undesirable consequences if allowed unrestricted expression should be controlled and limited in a calm but firm and consistent manner.
2. Patience is essential. (This child is two times more likely to receive parental criticism.) Active effort is necessary to avert negative parent-child relationships from arising out of the child's constant stressful behaviors. (Nurturing a child of this temperament places special demands on parents, and interactions are usually perceived as stressful.)
3. Parents of this "testy" child do best if they take turns coping with the child's behavior and give each other a daily chance to get away.
4. In those activities that predictably cause negative behavior, parents are wise to take turns handling the child; it is important to persist in introducing the child to this situation or expectation, however, so that he or she can eventually learn control.
5. These children need gradual and repeated reinforcement (positive and negative) of expected behaviors before they can internalize them. (Problems in behavior usually arise from conflict between the children and almost any aspect of their environment, whether it be parents, new situations, or the world outside.)
6. This child can manage only a minimum number of rules at a time (one to three). The rules need to be straightforward and unencumbered by explanations or choices.
7. Provide constructive avenues for excess emotions and energy.

MIXED-TEMPERAMENT CHILD

Respond to whichever of the other three personality types seems to predominate in this child.

(Data from Thomas and Chess, 1977.)

scribes management of the three temperaments to derive the most positive functioning of the child. The following temperament-related considerations are also useful to parents as they construct a parenting plan for each child:

1. Make demands and expectations consistent with the child's temperament, i.e., realistic for that youngster.
2. Encourage children to function at their potential; do not foster complacency or underachievement.
3. Accept that some temperaments are more demanding of tolerance than others; some are more at risk for behavior problems; it is all right to seek professional help; it is important to identify and correct problems as soon as they appear.
4. Try to accept the nature of each child and to channel negative features in a desirable direction. Occasional frustration is normal, but seek help if it is prolonged or chronic.

Age and Developmental Stage

Parents will need to adapt their basic parenting plan for each child as the child grows and matures. The need for external (parent-initiated) reinforcements diminishes as a child gets older, and the external reinforcements that are provided can become gradually less action-oriented and more reason-oriented as the child develops intellectually. Keeping a child's developmental tasks in mind at each age helps parents determine what adaptations to the basic parenting approach are needed. Table 13-5 clarifies realistic parental expectations at each age and stage of development.

Table 13-5. Age and Developmental Stage as a Factor in Parenting

Parenting Goals	**Infant (0–1 yr)**	**Toddler (1–3 yr)**	**Preschooler (3–5 yr)**	**School-Age Child (6–12 yr)**	**Adolescent/Young Adult (13–21 yr)**
Safety	Protect from falls, injuries, etc., as motor skills increase	Place limits on investigations and mobility; childproof home	Assist in protecting self. Teach safety rules	Allow unassisted activities but with safe levels of limits, as riding bike on road but not on heavily traveled streets	Self-responsibility for safety
Family beliefs and values	Child can adapt to routine ADL	Child can begin integrating religious and cultural values through practice and participation in rituals	Child can conform to home routines, take responsibility for helping with some. Able to learn manners, feel guilt. Increased participation in family practices and rituals	Ready to comprehend reasons, explanations behind values, beliefs, practices. Ready for involvement in group activities and practices	Ready to decide or choose for self what beliefs and values to accept—time to let go and allow that choice. Enforce morality rules of family until they learn to trust their own moral judgment
Social behavior and role	Enforce cooperation in ADL and care procedures. Child can learn some patience	Expect obedience most of the time. Child is able to learn respect for other's belongings, and to accept substitute caretakers	Able to cooperate, learning to share. Can increasingly control anger and aggression. Tries many roles during play. Needs sexual questions answered; will investigate	Can have regular responsibility for some home chores. Needs some limits set on friend selections. Expect acceptable school behaviors, peer tolerance	Needs limits on sexual expressions; don't expect mature judgments. Avoid overreacting to typical teen crises. Expect acceptable social behavior
Self-regulation and independence	Dependent on others to meet needs; no self-control	Can take increasing responsibility for regulation of body functions; needs to learn proper language for body and its functions. Learns to accept, respect limits. "Do it myself" really means "Let me do what I can, then help me"	Can accomplish most self-care in ADL. Will need help in more complex tasks	Able to increasingly accomplish ADL without aid; anticipate occasional regression. Increasingly socialized (internal enforcement) in behaviors, but still heavily guided by imitating significant others	Has internalized most rules of living. Able to maintain own ADL and many of home chores if given opportunity. Needs faith in abilities reinforced and support during failures; otherwise, independent, self-regulating

(Data from Norton, 1977; Erikson, 1986.)

Sociocultural Values and Interest of Parents

Values and roles become less rigidly defined with increasing socioeconomic status and when parents perform at higher intellectual levels. This seems particularly evident in the areas of parenting related to parenting style, developmental competency emphasis, and parental protectiveness.

Parenting Style. Lower class parents tend to use more power-oriented reinforcements, especially with their sons (Brown, 1977). Although a good mix in preferred parenting styles exists within the middle class, the tendency is to use a democratic approach, especially with daughters (Brown, 1977). The middle class parent uses more body contact in nurturing activities. Upper class parents show a preference for the permissive parenting style, although they are also strictest about sexual training.

Developmental Competency Emphasis. Lower class parents tend to value early self-control (physical competency), whereas middle and upper class families value earlier mastery of problem-solving skills (emotional, intellectual competence) by their children.

Parental Protectiveness. Lower class parents tend to underprotect their male children and overprotect their female children. Middle class parents are the ones most frequently involved in motivating social agencies to promote a safe environment for children. Upper class families have been reported to overprotect their children (Koller, 1974).

Specific cultural practices influencing parenting depend on the family's cultural background. Whether cultural or societal values are given precedence in parenting depends on how strong the family's bond is with their cultural heritage. A parent's personality structure influences parenting preferences. The more rigid a parent's personality (difficult or slow-to-warm temperament), the more likely that person is to employ strict or autocratic parenting methods.

Whether a parent's interests are primarily child-centered or self-centered also affects parenting style. Figure 13-1 illustrates the relationship that usually exists between parental interest level and parenting style.

Issues Related to Parenting

The number of families within the traditional family structure is steadily declining. In over 50 per cent of two-parent families in America today, both parents work; the projection is 75 per cent by 1990 (Siegel-Gorelick, 1983). Single-parent families comprise about 40 per cent of American homes at any given time. In families who suffer a parental loss through death or divorce, 80 per cent will be a blended family an average of 2 to 3 years later. A blended family results from a marriage in which one or both spouses had offspring prior to the marriage who become family unit members after the marriage. These alternative structures face added concerns about parenting that ultimately affect the socialization of the children involved.

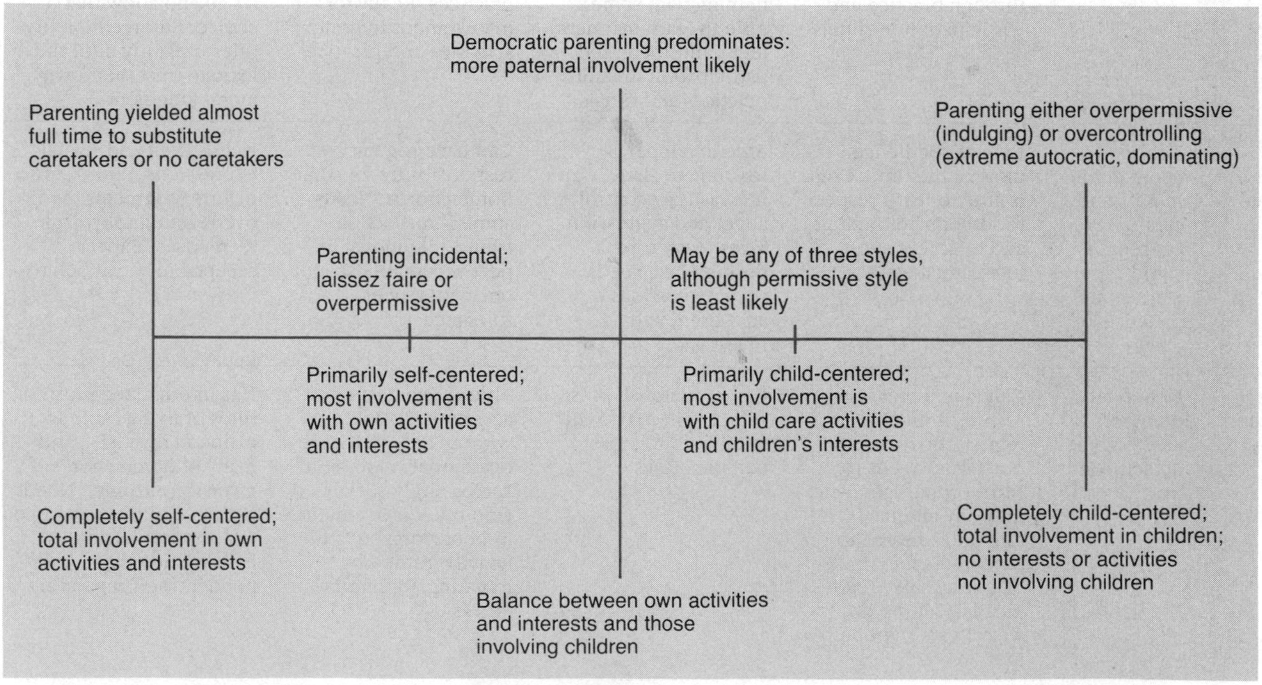

Figure 13-1. Relationship between parental interest level and parenting style.

Parenting and Dual-Earner Families*

A number of factors affect the decision for both parents to work. The most significant motive in today's society most often is financial necessity—money is needed to maintain or upgrade the family's standard of living. Meeting unanticipated medical expenses, inflationary costs of housing and food, and extra expenses of raising children, as well as family desires (music lessons, attendance at entertainment and sports events) necessitates larger incomes for families. Personal fulfillment of goals, career opportunities, or a sincere enjoyment of the challenge of the work world may influence the decision for outside employment. Part-time work by one spouse to supplement full-time employment of the other spouse, full-time work by both spouses, and part-time work by both spouses are options available to dual-earner families.

Unlike most other industrialized countries, in the United States the freedom to work is accompanied by the challenge that each family must arrange its own child care and home maintenance, usually without any economic or social support from either the employer or the government. The extent to which child care and home maintenance needs can be adequately satisfied influences parents' ability to fulfill work responsibilities successfully. Although the availability of early and extended day care and after school programs—some even employer arranged—is increasing, these are unaffordable to many parents. In addition, many programs do not accommodate parents whose work schedules do not fall within normal business hours or are not in close proximity to either home or work. When childhood illness prevents attendance at child care or school, the parent is provided with little help in the community or at work. A few sick care programs are beginning to appear; these provide care to ill children either in the home or in a special area of child care facilities for working parents, but they are still scarce and unaffordable to many parents.

In many families the mother finds she remains the primary child caretaker and housekeeper in addition to being employed outside the home (Richardson, 1983). Thus, the mother must cope with the stresses of inequitable division of household tasks, less time to attend to family needs, her own and her child's separation anxiety, and physical and mental exhaustion from her job. It is interesting that some mothers find it difficult to accept help for housework from their spouse or children (even though they may want and need the help) because of a need to maintain their own standards for household and child care (Richardson, 1983). A mother with these feelings may either attempt to complete all household tasks to maintain her standards or become frustrated with having to settle for tasks being completed by other family members and not necessarily exactly as she prefers. Adaptation to these sources of stress (expressed or implicit) may create family tensions. Many parents struggle with images of "superparent" as they try to complete home, work, and personal tasks. Parents need to learn to request and to accept help from others, including their children.

The initial separation process for young children and their working parents can be traumatic for both. If the parents are confident that the decision for both to work is a good one, if the child is cared for in a quality day care environment, and if the parents can avoid long absences from the child at times other than employment hours, the child will probably not develop undesirable long-term behaviors as a result of having dual-career parents (Howell, 1973; Nye and Hoffman, 1976; Bane, 1978; Norris and Miller, 1984). If the separation process is handled in a positive, reassuring knowledgeable manner, taking into consideration the growth and developmental level of the child, the young child learns that the parents will return. Nurses can help parents by teaching them the need for a gradual separation process. They can warn parents to expect acting-out behaviors when they pick up the child at the end of the day and remind them to reassure and express love to the child during this separation process.

The presence of young children in the family seems to contribute to lower job satisfaction for both spouses, with the mother being the most dissatisfied (Troll, 1984; Voydanoff and Kelly, 1984). This dissatisfaction may occur from societal pressures for a parent to be at home, inequality in family task prescriptions, or logistic problems in establishing child care.

If parents portray a sense of pride and fulfillment in employment and discuss this fulfillment, along with any career and home anxieties, the child and family seem able to be positive and accepting of each parent's needs. Through increased self-esteem, assertiveness learning, and positive reinforcement from their support systems (spouse, family, relatives, nurse), both parents can see themselves as complete persons in the dual roles of parent and employee.

The nurse working with dual-earner parents should explore whether specific role expectations have been discussed to avoid implicit assumptions by one or both spouses. The nurse should bring to the

---

* Dual-earner family is defined here to mean that both heads of household pursue employment and at the same time maintain a family life together. The literature uses many terms. Dual careers usually imply that the employment is a professional career that both partners hold by choice and both careers are taken seriously. Some refer to an arrangement wherein both partners work but one partner's "job" is dispensable or secondary to the other partner's as a two-job family. Dual earner encompasses both these possibilities (Cherpas, 1985).

family's attention the following special problems raised by parenting and working (Howell, 1973; Kutzner and Toussic-Weingarten, 1984):

- What are each parent's reasons for working? Are they congruent with the other parent's reasons?
- If conflicts exist, how can they be resolved? Do the jobs demand more than the parents are willing or able to give?
- What are the benefits? What problems are expected at work and at home?
- How will responsibilities be assigned or shared concerning child care, household routines, and other day-to-day decision making? Who will transport children?
- How will family integrity be maintained in the mornings as parents prepare themselves and their children for departure?
- Can child care and other community resources be found that are compatible with parental values and philosophies?
- Does each parent feel comfortable with the child care arrangements?
- Who have the parents identified as back-up child care providers for unexpected situations? What will be done if a child is ill? Who will handle any emergencies?
- Have work schedules been planned so that there is time for family activities together? Is their conscious planning for open communication channels for all family members?

The child who is a member of a dual-earner family can be encouraged to help the parents in tasks that are part of daily living activities for the family. This helps the child develop skills and feelings of self-worth. It also helps distribute family tasks. Most children develop pride in their parents' accomplishments and benefit from the increased exposure to multiple role models (Scott, 1984). An equalitarian parental role model for children is a possibility in the dual-earner family, providing the child with enriching experiences with both mother and father.

Parenting and Single-Parent Families

The single-parent family structure was discussed in Chapter 2. Divorce may affect the immediate parenting capabilities of both parents.

There is a tendency for parents after divorce to neglect or even exploit their children's emotional needs during the first weeks or even months of loss. These parents usually love their children, but they are emotionally, and sometimes physically, drained by the stresses of their marital battles and, finally, the loss of a partner. Children sometimes temporarily take on roles as miniparents toward the parent, or older children may so serve younger siblings. Fortunate children have other significant persons (grandparents, teachers, neighbors) who can help them deal with their own despair until their parent regains control and resumes appropriate parenting. Other children are left without assistance beyond their own inner resources and whatever sibling support is available until their parent "comes around." If parental recovery takes too long, the child will usually demonstrate negative behavior that will get the need for help recognized.

Eventually the wounds begin healing and the family unit stabilizes again. The unit will not ever be the same, but it can again be healthy and happy. At this time the parent has a renewal of interest in the parenting role and begins coping with the total day-to-day task of parenting.

Financial necessity forces most divorced parents to retain, regain, or obtain employment. Unless co-parenting is arranged, the parent with custody bears major responsibility for childrearing. The visiting parent becomes primarily a "playtime" parent, experiencing only brief or periodic intervals with the children. The feelings that can be engendered by both parents and by the children—guilt, jealousy, anger, sense of being overwhelmed—become obvious in such situations.

Because the single parent usually must be employed, she or he is confronted with the same parenting dilemmas as the dual-earner family. The major difference is that instead of spousal support, the single parent must seek out other adult support systems (e.g., friends, relatives, Parents Without Partners groups). If co-parenting is decided upon, the family contends not with its death, but rather its reorganization. The limited research available on joint custody and co-parenting supports it as the preferred arrangement for most children, provided the divorced couple can work together in childrearing without hostility. The "how-to-do-it" of co-parenting will vary from family to family. Decisions have to be made regarding time scheduling (do children or parents change homes and how frequently?), financial arrangements, clothes and toys (some at each place or transported back and forth), and other family-specific issues.

Latchkey Children

Millions of children in the United States are "latchkey kids." About 10 million children between the ages of 5 and 12 years and another 5 to 10 million between ages 12 and 16 years are left alone by adults to care for themselves, stay at home, play in the street, or become part of a gang. The term also refers to those children who, although there is a caretaker at home, have such loose care arrangements that they are ineffective (Long and Long, 1982; Galambos and Barbarino, 1983; McClellan, 1984).

Several factors have contributed to the development of this phenomenon. The proportion of single-parent families has steadily increased. Most are headed by women who must work but who cannot afford the luxury of child care, particularly for school-age children. In two-parent families, steadily increasing numbers of units are dual-earner and parents' work hours often overlap, leaving children without supervision for at least short intervals each day. Increased geographic mobility and the nature of modern urban living leave families in social isolation—they do not have extended family nearby and are not acquainted with their neighbors. Present-day tendencies for age-segregated housing, coupled with increasing numbers of dual-earner families, leave few alternative caretakers available within the neighborhood. These facts indicate that in many families adults are away from home for several hours a day on a regular basis; this results in less supervision and more household responsibility for millions of children.

Studies of latchkey children have not provided consistent information regarding the effects on these children. What has been discovered is that there seem to be no clear-cut negative or positive consequences that apply to all children. Three significant factors seem to be family social status, sex of the child, and type of community or neighborhood where the child resides. An increased risk of accidents or injuries and delinquent behavior seems to be associated with a lower social class and more densely populated communities. Lower class girls seem to be the only group who showed diminished academic achievement. This group was also more likely to have to come home after school, clean the house, do laundry, care for younger children, and possibly even prepare dinner. The children frequently are not permitted to "waste time" in activities considered by the parents to be unimportant. Consequently, they may not participate in school activities; they may not have friends or appear to enjoy life. The excessive demands made on them by their parents frequently result in a passive attitude toward life (McClellan, 1984).

Girls more than boys seem to benefit from having mothers who work outside the home. They appear to admire their mothers more, to be more independent, and to hold a more positive perception of being female than do their peers (McClellan, 1984). All children display more responsibility, adeptness at problem solving, and skill in self-care and household activities (Long and Long, 1984). Studies also suggest that latchkey children feel more isolated, lonely, bored, and fearful than their peers cared for by adults (Long and Long, 1984). The Longs' study revealed that children cope with their anxiety when alone by hiding, turning up the volume on television sets, and soliciting comfort from a pet. Anxiety seems to be inversely related to the closeness of the parent-child relationship.

Children should not be left alone without first establishing that they are ready for it. They should be able to manage all daily self-care activities, know how to use the telephone, especially for emergencies, and be able to anticipate possible problem situations and describe how to manage them, preferably with some trial runs. All children left alone on a regular basis need lots of adult support. A parent or back-up person should be available by phone (important phone numbers should be in plain sight near the phone). A neighbor, nearby storekeeper, or adult friend who is usually available should be established as a resource for emergencies. Parents should be urged to utilize an afterschool program as an alternative if one is available. Many schools are now providing such services, and some day care facilities are providing extended-school day care.

Parents who decide their child can cope should review and discuss several points with their child and have an opportunity for some brief trial runs. Box 13-3 identifies concerns that both the parent and child need to consider before the child is left alone.

Nurses need to be aware of latchkey children's problems and assist these children and their families. Nurses can take an active role in helping develop quality afterschool child care programs in the community if a variety of options do not exist and can counsel parents regarding selection among options if they do exist. The nurse is also a logical resource to present classes or speeches about the problems and needs of latchkey children and their families, as well as either teaching or helping develop local "survival skills" programs for children. Hotlines for latchkey children have been well utilized in communities where they exist (Guerney and Moore, 1983). The nurse might serve as a hotline counselor or help develop such a resource within the community. The nurse with research skills can contribute to the research needed on latchkey children and the effectiveness of various intervention programs. Table 13-6 identifies resources the nurse might utilize to help organize services for latchkey children in the community or to share with interested parent or community groups.

Parenting and the Blended Family*

Statistics show that the majority of people remarry two to three years after a spouse's death or departure. That

*Other names are reconstituted family, stepfamily, combined family, and remarriage.

Box 13-3
Problems and Needs of Latchkey Children

SAFETY

1. Teach children not to display keys and always to lock doors. Keep a spare key at a neighbor's house.

*2. Tell children not to go into the house after school if the door is ajar, a window is open, or if anything looks unusual. Teach child not to open the door to anyone unless the person has been approved by the parent.

*3. Walk through the after-school routine with the child. Some children have keys but cannot reach the locks. Teach child not to get in cars with strangers.

*4. Consult with fire and police officials about burglar-proofing and fire-proofing the home. Teach child what to do if a burglary attempt occurs.

5. Teach children first-aid procedures.

*6. Prepare a safety kit.

7. Teach safety rules to children who are expected to cook. Microwave ovens are the safest.

8. Emphasize such fire safety rules as:
   a. Leave the house and do not return to it if a fire starts.
   b. Practice fire drills and evacuation at home, including a safe place to meet outside the home.

9. Prevent traffic accidents.
   a. Instruct parents that children are often not ready to cross streets alone until age 7 years.
   b. Tell children not to ride bicycles in the street without adult supervision.

10. Instruct parents about the dangers of garage door openers. Children have been fatally injured when they have activated the doors and the doors closed on them.

11. Teach children about weather-related safety.
   a. Stay in the house in an electrical storm. Do not take a bath in an electrical storm.
   b. Stay in the storm cellar or in the safest part of the house during a tornado warning. Practice tornado drills with children.
   c. Keep a flashlight handy to child in case of power failures.

12. Prevent drowning.
   a. Instruct children that they should never swim without adult supervision.
   b. Teach older children caring for infants and toddlers about safe bathing methods.
   c. Keep toilet lid down. Older infants and toddlers have drowned by falling headfirst into toilets.

13. Use locked storage for firearms. Instruct children that firearms are to be handled by adults only.

TELEPHONE USE

1. Teach children to tell callers that their parents are "busy," rather than saying "They're not here."

*2. Keep police, fire department, and other important telephone numbers by the phone. Be sure child knows how to report emergencies.

*3. Investigate the neighborhood for families who will be at home and available for help with emergencies.

4. Ask police and fire officials to offer classes about when and how to call them.

5. If a "telephone hotline" for latchkey children exists, teach children how to use it.

6. Be sure children know their own telephone numbers, addresses, and parents' names.

AFTERSCHOOL ACTIVITIES

*1. Arrange for the child to spend some afternoons with friends.

*2. Provide structured activities, such as art projects.

*3. Have the child go to a public library–sponsored activity rather than watching television at home.

4. Establish clear rules with child as to what may/may not be done until parent gets home.

*5. Offer children a choice of activities.

6. Discuss with all children in a class what they do after school. Recommend specific activities other than television.

7. Teach children that independence and resourcefulness are virtues, but don't demand too much.

8. Help children feel successful in taking care of themselves.

*9. Counsel parents regarding the potential problems of having older children care for younger ones when not developmentally ready.

LONELINESS

1. Talk to children about their experiences of being alone after school.

*2. Consider getting a pet to help comfort the child.

*3. Be punctual. Children's anxiety escalates when parents don't return home as promised.

*4. Call the child when parents will be late.

*5. Leave a tape-recorded message for children to play when they arrive home.

*6. Form a group of parents with flex-time so that their children can be cared for by one of the group after school.

NETWORKING

*1. Parents, teachers, and nurses can help develop a supportive network of working parents.

2. Families may find church memberships helpful.

*Items specifically for parents.
(Adapted from McClellan, 1984. Additional reference from McKnight and Shelsby, 1984; Dennis, 1986.)

Table 13-6. Selected Resources for Assisting Latchkey Children

Program or Service	Source	Address	Functions
The School-Age Child Care Project	Wellesley College Center for Research on Women	Wellesley, MA 02181 617/431-1453	Offers technical assistance about the design and implementation of school-age child care programs
	Day Care Council of America, Inc.	711 14th Street NW Suite 507 Washington, DC 20005 202/638-2316	Provides technical information about day care for children of various ages
	The National Commission on Resources for Youth, Inc.	605 Commonwealth Avenue Boston, MA 02215 617/353-3309	Promotes programs that give children ages 10 to 18 years opportunities to contribute to their communities
Child Care Information Service	National Employer Supported Child Care Project	363 East Villa Street Pasadena, CA 91101 213/796-4341	Has written a manual for employers about initiating child care programs. Has information about employer-supported child care programs in this country
"Chatters"	Neighborhood Centers Day Care Association	5005 Fannin Houston, TX 77004 713/529-3931	Provides a telephone check-in and reassurance program for children 8 years old and older for an annual fee
"I Can Do It"	Council of Campfire	200 Statler Building Buffalo, NY 14202 716/853-6550	Provides a program for self-help skills for 2nd through 4th grade children. Held in eight afterschool sessions at low cost ($12.00)
"Prepared for Today"	National Office of Boy Scouts of America	1325 Walnut Hill Lane Irving, TX 75062 214/659-2000	Provides a program for children aged 6 to 12 years to help them deal with being at home alone, including effective communication with parents
Kids Check-In Club	Fairfax County (VA) Office for Children Betsy Shelsby, Program Director	Family Day Care Check-In Project 10396 Democracy Lane Fairfax, VA 22030	Provides package with step-by-step procedures for starting up, administering, supervising, and evaluating a neighborhood-based day care provider for upper elementary, junior high, and high school students

(Adapted from McClellan, 1984. Additional reference from McKnight and Shelsby, 1984.)

Table 13-7. Characteristics Differentiating the Blended Family from the Nuclear Family

Nuclear Family	Blended Family
Single family membership	Dual family membership
Husband-wife the central core	Custodial parent (usually mother) and children are the central core
History of family experiences, values, rituals that lend emotional cohesiveness	Lack of a common history of family experiences, values, rituals, which can lead to emotional conflict
Dyad relationship that gradually expands to include other members	Instant multiple relationships within and outside household
Norms and social support for nuclear unit	No norms or social support for blending unit; further compounded by unrealistic expectations that stepparent will instantly love children of spouse and that children will demonstrate instant obedience to stepparent
Commitment is to the nuclear unit	Commitments exist to blended unit as well as to previous family unit (emotional, monetary, visiting privileges); boundaries *must be* flexible

(Data from Stern, 1984; and Reutter et al, 1986.)

means there are over 40 million blended or stepparent family units in existence (Einstein, 1983). By 1990, blended and single-parent families will comprise more than 50 per cent of American families (Christian Science Monitor, Dec. 27, 1982). Research on children who have lost a parent to death or divorce shows that these children fare no worse than those who are raised entirely in nuclear family units (Stern, 1984). However, these children do retain the mind set that they have only one mother and one father, no matter how undesirable the lost parent may have been and no matter whether the lost parent ever makes contact with the child again. A second characteristic is that these children fantasize that someday Mom and Dad will somehow get back together. With these facts in mind, a stepparent, no matter how loving and kind, is going to be perceived as an intruder.

The blended family can assume many different,

Table 13-8. Common Barriers to Blended Family Integration and Nursing Strategies

Barriers to Family Integration	Nursing Strategies
Role Confusion	
Custodial parent after death or divorce (usually mother) has ambivalence about what role they want the stepparent to take with regard to their children and with family decision making. Stepparent shares the same ambivalence and uncertainty about options and responsibility toward the spouse's children. Feelings of jealousy, confusion, resentment, and inadequacy experienced by some or all members of new family unit.	Empathize with each member's feelings and help them anticipate and deal with the complex issues involved in blended family development through anticipatory guidance and counseling. Provide reassurance of the normality of the feelings members are experiencing and that growth and time will support healthy family and member development. Be an advocate for the blended family in the community and state. Assist spouses to recognize their ambivalence and to openly discuss it and arrive at a comfortable role description, stressing that they should not attempt to emulate either primary family but rather formulate their own role definitions that suit the needs and strengths of members. Encourage creativity in roles and emphasize that the stepparent role may differ with each child depending on the child's age, willingness to bond, and nature of the relationship with the custodial parent (i.e., allow natural relationships to develop). Foster marital bonding by helping family look at ways spouses can have time alone together and develop their own romance and friendship. Refer family to self-help support groups for stepfamilies within the community.
Conflicting Family Cultures	
At the individual family cultural level, rules are established as to where silverware goes, the things children may or may not do during meals or when adults are present, and general rules about how mothers, fathers, and children should act. When blended family develops, individual family cultural rules are brought to the union from two primary families, which produces power struggles and conflict (culture shock) during early cohabitation. Compromise gradually occurs in some areas, usually taking 2–7 years for the infinite differences to be negotiated and resolved, resulting in development of a new individual family culture. New conflicts will emerge at various developmental stages.	Facilitate open communication between family members (fear of confrontation is common because of a previous marriage failure). Refer to community self-help support group for stepfamilies or, if conflicts are serious, to family group therapy. Provide education on crisis management, culture shock, and communication skills. Support and reinforce members as they take steps toward conflict resolution.
Discipline of Children	
Discipline involves a series of lessons designed to develop behaviors that can be tolerated by adults and move children toward healthy adulthood. Obviously rules will be in conflict from the differences each primary family brings to the blended unit. Research repeatedly shows the discipline of children as a major stumbling block to integration of the blended unit. Dangers to watch for are (1) the custodial parent feels a need to monitor the stepparent's interactions with children, tends to interpret stepparent's behavior to children and vice versa, preventing stepparent and children from establishing their own relationships; or (2) stepparent insists on early assumption of co-management	Refer family to community self-help support group for stepfamilies or to family group therapy if serious conflict exists. Educate and assist stepparent to carry out "befriending/affiliating" behaviors, i.e., make friends with each stepchild before making new rules and enforcing them (single most important action to achieve success in stepparenting). Strategies: 1. Spend time with each stepchild, being sensitive to the timing of interactions; 2. Spend some money on stepchildren—will not buy love, but does earn stepparent favorable attention from children;

complex forms, depending on whether one or both parents were previously married and/or have had children, whether the children are living with them, and whether there are children from their own union. Couples who consider making a blended family must prepare themselves for some troubled times before the family unit finally adapts to peaceable relations. Table 13-7 lists the characteristics of blended families which make them different from nuclear families and which are associated with conflicts that must be overcome to achieve family integration. Table 13-8 identifies the most common barriers to blended family integration and suggests measures to help the family organize its own cultural unit in time.

A prospective stepparent should not be introduced to children until the couple has dated each other exclusively for some time, or until they have decided to marry. If children are introduced to their parents' dates

***Table* 13-8** *(continued)*

Barriers to Family Integration	Nursing Strategies
privileges and spouse agrees, but children respond with shock, resentment, and resistance or even display behavior problems because they have not had time to adjust to and learn to trust the new stepparent first.	3. Role model being a kind, friendly person; 4. Come through for the child in times of trouble; 5. Use clear communication, i.e., leveling, encouraging children to respond in kind; 6. Accept each child for who and what she or he is; 7. Have tolerance for children's inconsistent responses—remember that trust takes time to develop. Reinforce positive efforts of the stepparent and encourage open communication between spouses.
Semipermeable Boundaries (Dual-Family Membership)	
A multitude of persons are attached to former relationships, which continually surface in the blended family's life, particularly the children's other parent and children of one or both blended family spouses who do not live in the blended unit. Potential problems to watch for: 1. A tendency for any conflicts between ex-spouses and/or new spouses to be fought through the children, instead of through direct confrontation between the adults; 2. A spouse who has not been around children is likely not to have realistic expectations about the behavior of children; 3. A frequent conflict is that children who do not live with a parent are favored or given exceptions to family rules during their visits to the blended family unit. The nearer the remarriage is to the time the original family unit lost its intactness, the more resistant the single parent unit is to blending.	Educate the family about stress management, the importance of open communication, and the potential problems of relationships beyond the blended unit. Refer the family to a community self-help support group for stepfamilies or to family group therapy if serious problems exist in the family's ability to be creative and flexible. Provide parenting and growth and development education if one parent has not had experience with children. Support family through periods of crisis.
Unresolved Grief	
Unresolved grief over past failed relationships may be repressed and acted out in disguised ways by members of family. Children often have unresolved grief because of their unrelenting hope that their parents will get back together some day, and often the grief is compounded by their egocentric belief that they are responsible for the family break-up. They may extend this egocentric "power," thinking they can also break up the new marriage, if they are not offered assistance to handle their grief. Unresolved grief is a more common problem when a blended family unit is formed within a short time frame after the primary family break-up (sources vary in the time required to resolve that grief, usually 1 to 3 years). The grief related to divorce is somewhat different from other grief in that it results from a change in the nature of relationships, not a separation or loss. Feelings of vulnerability to loss, since one marriage failed, may inhibit the open dialogue necessary to resolve conflicts and to bond the blended family together. Remarriage shatters the child's hopes of a reunion of the original family unit. Children may also feel stepparents are dislodging them from the close relationship with the custodial parent developed during the single-parent stage.	Refer for individual or family group counseling. Foster open family communication through education, role modeling, positive reinforcement or communication efforts. Apply usual interventions to facilitate resolution of grief (refer to any one of the many excellent references available on this subject). Educate the family about the grief process and how members or other family resources can assist and support the grieving member(s).

(Data from Stern, 1984; Reutter et al, 1986.)

repeatedly, they develop a pattern of keeping distant so as not to have to experience grief and loss each time Mom or Dad changes "friends." Once a decision to marry is made, the couple ideally should take their time before the ceremony. Each prospective mate needs time to change gears and think in terms of several people's needs, not only about two people. Both need ample opportunity to see how they feel about sharing this parenting responsibility. If one of them has never been a parent, major emotional and physical adjustments are required. Both have to learn to deal with their resentment and jealousy when the children's demands take time from being together, and with the children's resentment toward the intruder for taking time from them and their parent. A sense of humor is critical to adaptation—all behaviors of the children cannot be taken as serious or as directed toward the prospective stepparent personally. Nonetheless, effort must be made to apply some reasoning and to empathize with the child's feelings. It is also helpful if the couple can recognize and discuss their own feelings and work through them, supporting each other. Another important fact for prospective stepparents is the importance of just being themselves—efforts to "win" the children by forcing "fun" on them or trying to be the "perfect stepparent" are perceived by the children as phoniness. Stepparents who expect jealousy, resentment, and rejection will not be surprised or destroyed by its appearance; it must be remembered that children make friends slowly with strange adults.

Another problem area is discipline. The couple should discuss privately the limits and controls and roles of each parent in disciplining so that a united front is presented to the children. If a prospective mate will not permit a sharing of discipline with the stepparent, the pattern only accelerates if they marry, ultimately damaging everyone. An argument for the stepparent's involvement is the fact that schoolteachers and police officers are not "real" parents, but they and many other authority figures tell children how to behave in a given day. A stepparent should be no different. All adults are potential instructors for children.

It is especially important to a blended marriage, because of the additional problems that will be encountered, that the couple not only be in love but also be very close friends. The ease and psychologic freedom experienced with a friend takes time, mutual life events, and open conversations about each other. If time is allowed for friendship to develop, the children also gain an opportunity to learn to know, like, and trust their second parent before the marriage. Another argument in favor of a long courtship before remarriage is the fact that the couple do not have the luxury of being alone to adjust to each other and work out living patterns—the children's needs also are to be met from the beginning. In remarriage, special effort will be needed to maintain romantic feelings while struggling to be a happy family unit; keeping romance in the relationship can help tremendously. All children can learn that parents need privacy and that parents, like children, need a daily supply of affection. Little affectionate gestures and saying "I love you" is healthy medicine for all members of the family unit.

The couple entering a remarriage will do well to learn (or review) the developmental stage characteristics of childhood. Knowing the usual struggles and behavioral characteristics helps keep children's actions in perspective and avoids blaming every misbehavior on the blended family situation. Stepparenting teenagers is noted in study after study as being by far the most difficult. Stepparents need to remember that all teens are rough on parents, even natural parents. Self-confidence is essential when rearing teens.

Instant families can survive and adapt if problems are acknowledged as they occur and faced head on. Flexibility is important. Generally, the younger the children, the more easily they accept the new parent. In time, the stepparent's presence is accepted as routine, and members start receiving emotional benefits. As the blended family adapts, the spouses can take pride in the fact that no matter how disparate life becomes within the unit, there will have been a healing of *some* wounds from the original family unit. Even if a stepchild never shows gratitude (remember, by nature children are self-absorbed and do not know adults can experience rejection), some part of him or her will be thankful for the gifts of love and care the blended unit provided.

The nurse plays an important role in assisting the blended family toward adaptation. The nurse should assess regularly the parents' knowledge of developmental behavior and the family's awareness of problems in adapting. Education, counseling, or referral should be offered as indicated. Support of each member is continuously needed. The nurse can use role playing to determine whether the couple is developing or maintaining open communication and cooperating in parenting responsibilities. Information regarding community support groups for blended families can be provided. The nurse can be an objective confidante for children to express fears, hostility, or anxiety that they do not feel ready to express at home. Younger children can be helped in self-expression by encouraging them to tell a story about someone named (*their name*). Each member needs to have positive efforts recognized and reinforced.

The key elements the nurse should assist the family to keep in perspective are that the integration into a new family cultural unit takes *time* and *tolerance* for the ambiguities in roles and of the reactions of members. Reassurance that their feelings are normal and that the stressors are surmountable is important feedback for the blended family.

Assessing Parenting Capabilities

Raising a family should not be approached as an exercise in perfection. Parenting will be affected not only by parents' strengths and flaws but also by their children's strengths and weaknesses. No family is perfect, and yet the great majority of parents do a more-than-adequate job of raising their children to be successful adults—sometimes against tremendous odds. Health professionals have a responsibility (1) to help parents free themselves from unjustified guilt when their child does not always measure up; (2) to help parents develop self-confidence and trust in their parenting instincts, enhanced by accurate information and professional guidance; and (3) to help parents find a compromise between what they expect of themselves and their children and what is realistic.

Reassurances That Parents Need

Research and surveys of parents indicate that parents need support from professionals in order to relax and enjoy realistic, guilt-free parenting enacted with self-confidence (LeShan, 1965; Fletcher, 1972; Chess, 1977; Peck, 1978; Yarrow, 1979; Fisher and Fisher, 1986). Health professionals can help parents accept three reassurances:

1. It's OK not to be perfect.
2. It's OK to exert authority.
3. It's OK not to be rich.

It's OK Not to Be Perfect

Parents need reassurance that it is all right to be themselves with their children. No one is perfect; all parents make mistakes with their children. If parents are able to admit to their human failings and imperfections, they are modeling genuineness—a useful adult concept that children will imitate and incorporate into their own moral codes. Being genuine frees a parent to admit that a situation was handled badly, from brooding or guilt, and to apologize to the child. (Such action builds rather than diminishes a child's respect.)

Genuine parents can continue being "husband and wife" as well as "mother and father" without feeling guilty that they may be inadequate parents by doing so. After all, parenting has built-in time limits; marriage does not. The modeling of a healthy male-female relationship that this action provides to children is also a valuable learning experience, preparing them for successful adulthood.

Real parents need real children. Parents who accept self-imperfections are more able to accept the imperfections of their child and the stimulation their "real" child provides in inventiveness, unpredictability, and mischievousness. Knowledge of child growth and development facilitates parents' adaptation to their real child's changing self, allowing them to relax their anxieties about those behaviors they know are a part of their child's stage of growth and guiding them in the establishment of realistic rules and limits. Parents should also realize that this knowledge of development, although it makes them more self-confident, flexible, resilient, and resourceful, cannot produce the perfect child. Setting aside in a personal "memory bank" or "emotional savings account" the wonderful things their child does gives parents a reservoir to draw from to retain their optimism on the days when their child is not so wonderful (Murphy, 1976).

Parents who are able to accept that neither they nor their children are perfect can feel comfortable accepting that their parenting actions will not always be perfect either, and that this is all right. Although there are certain minimal elements parents must provide for satisfactory parenting—rules, consistency, positive and negative reinforcements, all based on love—there is no single recipe for providing those ingredients. Parents should periodically evaluate the impact their approach is having on their child, to see whether unpleasant feelings, increased misconduct, or an atmosphere of family tension is building up. If they are prepared to modify their approach if it seems to be damaging, regardless of what manuals, relatives, or psychologists say, they can trust that their own recipe is a good one. That trust will help their children grow to trust themselves.

When parents are genuine enough to teach their child all they honestly know and believe, they have no need to feel guilty when the child chooses a different path from their own.

It's OK to Exert Authority

To raise children takes lots of energy and ingenuity and is rarely a peaceful endeavor, but parents who feel comfortable setting limits for themselves and their children make the tasks of learning and growing easier. (A sense of humor kept handy is also helpful. A smile or laugh can lighten serious moments, ease tension, reduce anger, restore perspective.) To successfully raise their children, parents sometimes need to exert authority. Relationships that are loving and caring readily withstand acts of authority, with the end result being respect and cooperation: two desirable characteristics to be developed as children grow into adults. An important aspect of parental authority is the recognition by parents and children that parents can use different reactions and parenting styles with each child and still be loving. Effective parenting does not require equal or identical parenting behaviors for each child in a family.

Expert advice from professionals can be helpful and even lifesaving, but children are not all alike and the expert does not know a child as the parents do. Parents should not be condemned if their approach does not match the recommendations in the latest manual or the beliefs of the professional. The professional's obligation is to ascertain objectively that the parental approach is not having a negative impact on the child or family. If it is not, the parents' approach should be reinforced. If a negative effect exists, parents need to be provided insight into the conflict, to be offered information that will give them broader parenting options to choose from, and to be supported in their efforts to change.

It's OK Not to Be Rich

The conflict between children's desires and the realities of the budget is a common frustration to most families today. It is important for parents to recognize the influence of finances on their parenting decisions. Parents need to realize and be reassured that children do not need everything they desire; in fact, they are often better off without the majority of things the glamorous ads make them believe they need. Every family's budget has a limit. Parents who recognize that fact are able to set priorities, ignore the cajoling media, and retain some genuine experiences rather than substituting artificial or inanimate ones for them. These positive actions establish values that will be important to the children's ability to handle money as adults.

Parents should not protect their children from the budget; it is an important skill to be learned along with the other skills of successful adult living.

Parenting Problems

As with any aspect of living, problems in parenting can and do arise. Statistics of basic research and criminal justice allow classification of parenting problems that produce disturbances in socialization into four general categories. Box 13-4 lists those categories and describes the kinds of parenting activities that are symptomatic of these problems. Nurses and other professionals who work with children and families should be watchful for any of these symptomatic behaviors each time they observe and interact with their clients.

The child's overt behavior can also be a direct barometer of the state of health of parenting. Through their knowledge of normal development and temperament, nurses can learn to distinguish temporary deviant behavior that indicates problems. Nurses should offer guidance or help parents and child obtain guidance from appropriate sources whenever they observe or receive parental reports of the following persisting behaviors:

1. A child who continually behaves outside the stereotyped norms for children of same age and temperament. Even if the behavior is later established to be normal, parents are usually grateful for guidance in how to accept and constructively interact with their perceived "atypical" child.
2. Bizarre behavior or speech that persists or receives frequent negative social response.
3. Unexpected, atypical reactions to situations for age and temperament.
4. Prolonged adverse reactions to common situations or experiences (ADL* disturbances).
5. An accumulation of several related or unrelated troubling behaviors—unhappy, confused, rebellious, "ornery" without regard for others' responses, stubborn beyond reason, lazy, oversensitive, aggressive, delinquent—that seem to be lingering, worsening, or steadily involving more of the child's time.

Seeking professional help should be a first-aid measure rather than a last resort; this often requires alertness and initiative on the professional's part to help the family acknowledge that the problem potentially exists or is developing. See Chapter 33 for a full discussion of children with behavior problems.

Another preventive measure is for the nurse to be alert to family situations that place the parents at high risk for ineffective parenting. Situational crises in the family overlying the parenting responsibility always require concern and preventive intervention by the nurse. Box 13-5 describes some of the major liabilities preventing effective parenting. See Chapter 12 on

*Activities of daily living.

Box 13-4
Parenting Problems and Symptomatic Parental Behavior

UNREALISTIC EXPECTATIONS

Parent requires more self-control from child than age, development, or circumstances make reasonable

Parent expects immediate obedience

Parent enforces too many rules at once or provides no rules (children need rules for behavior and will seek them elsewhere, often in gangs)

Parents request social skills of the child that they do not model owing to lack of knowledge or experiences

INCONSISTENCY

Family disharmony

Parents lack a united front in goals, values, parenting philosophy, or moral stance about right and wrong

Parents model behaviors and values incongruent with what they teach verbally and in rules established

Enforcement is not consistently carried out

Distortions in communication—too vague, too long, contradictory, or void

EXTREMES IN STYLE, METHODS

No limits established or no guidance and reinforcements to help child comply with limits; overpermissive

Lack of firmness; parent not respected as authority

Limits too rigid; power replaces authority and fear or anger replaces respect

Reinforcements (positive or negative) do not match deed; too excessive, too long, teach wrong lesson

Primary disciplinary methods employed are bribes, promises, threats, sarcasm

DISTURBED RELATIONSHIPS

Parent is too close to child to permit growth—intrusive control, dominance—exemplified by parent who always (1) wants to change child, (2) demands to know child's activities and conversation, (3) interferes in child's problem-solving or decision making, (4) reminds child of misdeeds

Basically unfriendly or ambivalent interaction

Interaction inappropriate for child's age, stage, or temperament

Parent is too distant for child to develop respect: (1) parent preoccupied with self and own activities or wishes, (2) child feels isolated or unwanted

Family Assessment for further guidelines in identifying problems.

Intervening in Parenting

Parenting is not a topic to be evaluated and discussed at the third yearly visit, or when negative reinforcement is not working or after deviant behavior is observable. The nurse should approach the topic with the parent(s) early in the parenting relationship. Ideally, parents would have sought and been offered information before deciding to have children. However, very few parents discuss such things before their infant arrives. The parenting process begins when the infant is born, so parents need information by this time, at least, and additional information can be added as the nurse and parents together anticipate the child's changing needs throughout the developing years.

As nurses counsel parents through their child's developing years, they should bear in mind that, within a loving, secure home (ensured through adequate bonding and attachment) with routines, parents can try any style of parenting with which they feel confident and comfortable, and most children will respond favorably as long as extremes are avoided. Occasional "mistakes" do not destroy a child for life.

In early counseling, the nurse should listen sensitively, observe the parent-child relationship and the individual temperaments involved, and then help the parents find the style they can live with and feel comfortable with on a daily basis. Ongoing assessment of the parenting process and its impact on the child should occur at each contact, with particular attention given to symptoms in the four areas mentioned earlier in which problems frequently occur.

If symptoms are suggested either by the nurse's own observations, parental report, or the child's deviant behavior, the nurse should intervene early to reverse unhealthy parenting patterns. Intervention may involve helping the family see the problem area and

Box 13-5
Liabilities Contributing to High-Risk Parenting

PHYSICAL LIABILITIES OF PARENT

Abused or neglected as child; abusive of own children; abused by partner

Drug user

Adolescent

Poor physical condition of parent, spouse, or another child

Pregnancy unwanted, complicated, or resulted in defective birth

EMOTIONAL OR DEVELOPMENTAL LIABILITIES OF PARENT

Children conceived for poorly thought out reasons; not desired by both partners; partner jealous of children

Low self-esteem—feelings of worthlessness, being unloved, ineptness

Unable to empathize with other people/children having problems

Unrealistic expectations from parents as a child; experienced mostly negative parental feedback

History of mental illness, low tolerance to disruption of own plans/goals

Marital discord exists; nonaccepting of each other as they are

Pregnancy was result of rape or incest; pregnancy denied or found distasteful or considered as a punishment

Unrealistic expectations of what child(ren) can offer emotionally; no knowledge of parenting

Mentally "deficient" or "absent" in everyday living

Adolescent parent

Shows no loyalty to family unity, members; lacks cooperation

SOCIOCULTURAL/ECONOMIC LIABILITIES OF PARENT

One or both parents will be absent frequently from home on 24-hour basis (e.g., military spouse, imprisonment)

Isolated; no friends, relatives, neighbor acquaintances to ask for help or periodically offer relief; superficial or absent social relationships

Money availability a constant problem; no insurance; history of job instability/unemployment; no job skills

Single parent

Poor communication between partners/significant others

Substandard housing/living conditions

History of coming from broken home and home with continual high distress levels

Major loss occurs during pregnancy—home, family member, job

(Based on Youngkin, 1983.)

referring its members to a competent resource for assistance. Problems that are minor, that are identified early, or that the nurse is competent to intervene in directly should be promptly managed. First, a general physical assessment of the child should be done, with special attention to the hematocrit determination and height and weight progression. A developmental assessment, such as the Denver Developmental Screening Test (DDST, see Chapter 15 and Appendix Four), also should be done. The physical and emotional status of the parents should be assessed.

The support systems available to the parents—moral, direct, personal, and professional—and whether these are having a positive or negative effect on the parenting efforts should be ascertained. If support systems exist that appear detrimental, the parents should be aided to reshape or get rid of them. If support systems appear inadequate, resources available to the family should be evaluated to strengthen those already existing or create additional ones.

When teaching or correcting parenting skills, the nurse should always work with and emphasize the strengths of the parents and child. In addition, the nurse is responsible for locating appropriate resources capable of offsetting their deficiencies. It is impossible to predict or teach all the skills germane to parenting. But if nurses can help parents develop an ability to sort out problems, look at options, and negotiate suitable interventions, they have progressed a long way toward effective preparation for the challenge. Box 13-6 highlights the main issues or guidelines which the nurse and parents can use as a base for developing successful parenting behaviors. It is important for the nurse to remember that as children grow, so should their parents, for all life experiences, positive and negative, can be growth experiences.

Box 13-6
Guidelines For Effective Parenting

FOSTER OPEN PARENT-CHILD COMMUNICATION (See also Chapter 11)

1. Listen actively
   - Accept that your child has something worthwhile to communicate and identify with the child's feelings, perceptions, and thoughts, recognizing that they are real.
   - Try not to ask questions or interrupt while the child is speaking.
   - Avoid presenting an opinion about what the child is saying; instead, share your feelings when the child is finished.
   - Do not interpret the child's speech or try to restate what you think the child was REALLY trying to say; such behavior suggests to children that their opinions are inferior.
   - Do not recommend solutions or changes in view; rather, redirect the child to identify possible resolutions and the associated likely consequences.
   - Let the child continue to the end, then seek an evaluation of the situation, rather than interrupting to interject your own evaluation or judgment.
2. Express thoughts and feelings clearly and honestly
   - Use "I messages" rather than "you messages" (see example), subjectively stating your own needs or feelings (gets a cooperative response) rather than placing judgment on the child's behavior (gets a defensive response of hostility or a power struggle). I messages also avoid overgeneralizations or character criticisms. Adding feelings to the I message allows the child to participate in relieving the situation and to be aware of your feelings too.

You Message:	"You are too noisy! Stop turning the TV louder!"
I Message:	"I need to have quiet right now so I can get this reading done. Please turn down the TV."
I Message (feelings described):	"I feel angry because I have so little time to read and no quiet in which to do it. I have a right to some quiet just as you do. I need some quiet time right now."

   - Express basic positive feelings about the child in association with requests for behavior change. (For example, "I feel you really tried harder last evening to help me have quiet, but I am still frustrated that I cannot have a quiet time every evening. I will feel more like talking or watching TV with you if I have some quiet for a half-hour after dinner each evening.") Messages that express the parent's needs by describing the behavior that needs to be changed without character criticisms allows the child to correct the behavior or offer alternative solutions without diminished self-esteem.
   - Empathize with the child while expressing your feelings or expectations. This shows the child that you understand the reason for the undesirable behavior, but that it must stop. (For example, "You must want to go play with your friends right now, but you will have to wait till you have finished clearing the table.")

MINIMIZE UNACCEPTABLE BEHAVIORS

1. Modify the environment to encourage age-appropriate independence and opportunities for learning and recreation.
   - Age-appropriate toys/resources available to child at home.
   - Specified areas reserved as each child's private place for own pursuits.
   - Quiet, sedate activities available for when child needs to "wind down," such as before meals or bedtime.
   - Opportunities in home or related to home functioning that allow self-care responsibility and contribution to family living.
   - Childproof home surroundings and set limits to extent that safety is ensured and all members can relax. Must be based on development and temperament of members.
2. Set limits
   - Firm, consistent limits foster competence and reduce anxiety in children.
   - Strive for agreement and support among adult members regarding major expectations of child. These expectations will/should change as members grow and develop.
   - Provide issue-related reasons for the limits and explain consequences for violations of limits. Child may participate in establishing limits and consequences.
   - Separate disapproval of behavior from acceptance of child by conveying love but explaining unacceptable behavior. DISAPPROVE OF THE BEHAVIOR, NOT THE CHILD. "I messages" help accomplish this.
3. Avoid win-lose conflicts
   - Accept that conflicts are likely to be frequent and are a part of "growing" for all members.
   - Allowing child as much self-care responsibility as possible eliminates the source of many parent-child power struggles.

Continued

- Strive for a "no lose" mind set that involves mutual discussion and compromise (once child has mastered basic language skills). Parent and child identify problem and discuss possible solutions. Seeking cooperation eliminates power struggles.

4. Spend time together as a family and with each child
   - Establish some time each day that is exclusively with children. Does not have to be scheduled or a certain time span but appropriate to family situation. If time occurs regularly, children can take the occasional exception in stride. Children will also have less need to compete by acting out to get time with parent(s).
   - Make time together enjoyable for all involved.
   - Communicate to child you are available as a "consultant" to talk or share concerns whenever the child feels a need and you are able.

5. Utilize a disciplinary approach that "fits" the parent and child
   - Never hesitate to seek assistance in evaluating management approaches and their appropriateness to your situation and values. (Nurses should convey that they are available to help parents with parenting concerns. Assistance includes helping them clarify key issues about their child and delineate specific target behaviors needing intervention.)
   - Recognize that good parenting can be accomplished in different ways.
   - If, or when, corporal punishment (i.e., nonbrutal physical punishment) is used in response to a child's unacceptable behavior, it should occur as promptly as possible after the behavior and be accompanied by the parent's reason and a statement of what the desired behavior is. (Try to assess whether this approach is best with the child or if it really is a stress release for the parent. If a stress release, help the parent identify other means for stress release when the urge for corporal punishment occurs.)
   - Recognize each child's need for privacy as well as one's own privacy needs and provide for this.
   - Utilize the child's creativity for discipline through expressive play activities, fantasy play activities, parallel story telling (tell a story that depicts the child's situation and reveal how the story child felt and responded; follow story with problem-solving questions to child).
   - Allow children to learn discipline through the experiencing of natural results of their misbehavior as long as their safety is not threatened by doing so and no moral judgment is involved. This involves allowing the child to choose between acceptable/unacceptable behavior. The parent provides guidance but allows the child accountability for choice and action.
   - Utilize behavior modification to reduce repetitious unacceptable behaviors and/or to increase repetition of desirable behaviors (see discussion in Chapter 33).
   - Use "time out" for stopping behaviors that cannot be allowed to simply decrease over time. Key is an environment that is unstimulating and unpleasant for a reasonably brief period (see discussion in Chapter 33).
   - Interject lots of humor into both pleasurable and stressful interactions with your child(ren).

Summary: Give your child all the courtesies you would offer any adult or nonfamily member and you will get a positive return for your effort.

(Based on Gordon, 1975; Guerney, 1979; Humenick, 1987.)

References

Brown J: Childrearing in cross-cultural perspective. *Health Values* 1977 Mar/Apr; 77.

Cherpas C: Dual-career families: terminology, typologies and work and family issues. *J Counsel Dev* 1985 June; 616–620.

Dennis L: A comparison of family characteristics and attitudes toward afterschool care for latchkey children. *Pediatr Nurs* 1986 Jul-Aug; 215–225.

Einstein E: Stepfamilies—dealing with anger and disappointment. *US News World Rep*, Jan 17, 1983; 67–68.

Erikson E: *Childhood and Society*. New York, WW Norton, 1986.

Fisher S, Fisher R: *What We Really Know about Childrearing*. New York, Aronson Publishers, 1986.

Galambos N, Barbarino J: Identifying missing links in the study of latchkey children. *Children Today* 1983 Jul/Aug; 2.

Gordon T: *Parent-Effectiveness Training*. New York, New American Library, 1975.

Guerney B: Fortifying family ties. In *Families Today*. DHEW Publ. No. 79–815. Washington, DC, US Department of Health, Education, and Welfare, 1979.

Guerney L, Moore L: Phonefriend: a prevention-oriented service for latchkey children. *Child Today* 1983 Jul/Aug; 4–5.

Howell M: Employed mothers and their families; I. *Pediatrics* 1973 Aug; 252.

Howell M: Effects of maternal employment on the child; II. *Pediatrics* 1973 Sep; 327.

Humenick S, et al.: Parenting roles: expectations versus reality. *MCN* 1987 Jan–Feb; 36–39.

Kutzner S, Toussic-Weingarten C: Working parents: the dilemma of child rearing and career. *Top Clin Nurs* 1984 Oct; 30–37.

Leach P: *The Childcare Encyclopedia.* New York, A Knopf, Publisher, 1984.

LeShan E: *How to Survive Parenthood.* New York, Random House, 1965.

Long L, Long T: *Handbook for Latchkey Children and Their Working Parents.* New York, Arbor House, 1984.

Long T, Long L: *Latchkey Children: The Child's View of Self Care.* Washington, DC, US Educational Resources Information Center. ERIC Document ED 214 666, 1982.

McClellan M: On their own: latchkey children. *Pediatr Nurs* 1984 May/Jun; 198–202.

McKnight J, Shelsby B: Checking in: an alternative for latchkey kids. *Child Today* 1984 May/Jun; 23+.

Murphy M: When parents ask about discipline. *Pediatr Nurs* 1976 Dec; 28.

Norris G, Miller J: *Working Mother's Complete Handbook.* New York, New American Library, 1984.

Reutter L, et al: Yours, mine and ours: stepparents and their children. *MCN* 1986 Jul-Aug; 264–266.

Richardson A: *Working Couples.* New York, TAB Books, 1983.

Salk L: *What Every Child Would Like His Parents to Know.* New York, Warner Paperback Library, 1984.

Scott P: What is happening to the dual career family? *Nurs Economics* 1984 Sep/Oct; 351–355.

Siegel-Gorelick B: *The Working Parent's Guide to Child Care.* Boston, Little, Brown, 1983.

Stern P: Stepfather family dynamics: an overview for therapists. *Issues Ment Health Nurs* 1984; 89–103.

Thomas A, Chess S: *Temperament and Development.* New York, Brunner/Mazel Inc, 1977.

Troll L: *Early and Middle Adulthood.* Monterey, CA, Brooks-Cole Publishing Company, 1984.

Voydanoff P, Kelly R: Determinants of work-related family problems among employed parents. *J Marriage Fam* 1984 Nov; 881–892.

When you can't be home: teach your child what to do. *Changing Times* 1984 Aug; 35–36.

Youngkin E: High-risk parenting: portfolio for success or failure. *VA Nurse* 1983 Fall; 162–165.

Bibliography

Asmundsson R: Blended families: one plus one equals more than two. *In* Getty C, Humphreys W (eds): *Understanding the Family: Stress and Change in American Family Life.* New York, Appleton-Century-Crofts, 1981.

Bach G, Wyden P: *The Intimate Enemy.* New York, Avon Books, 1981.

Chinn P: The game of parenthood. *J NY State Nurses Assoc* 1982 Dec; 30–45.

Clarke B: Improving adolescent parenting through participant modeling and self evaluation. *Nurs Clin North Am* 1983 Jun; 303–311.

Crouter A: The children of working parents. *Child Today* 1982 Jul/Aug; 25–28.

Duffy M: Primary prevention behaviors: the female headed, one-parent family. *Res Nurs Health* 1986 June 9; 115–122.

Elkind D: David Elkind discusses parental pressures. *Pediatr Nurs* 1986 Nov-Dec; 417–418.

Giraldo Z: *Public Policy and the Family: Wives and Mothers in the Labor Forces.* Lexington, MA, DC Heath and Company, 1980.

Hall D, Hall F: Stress and the two career couple. *In* Cooper C, Payne R (eds): *Current Concerns in Occupational Stress.* New York, John Wiley, 1980.

Levine K: Mother vs. mother. *Parents* 1985 Jun; 63–67.

Long L, Long T: The unspoken fears of latchkey kids. *Working Mother* 1982 May; 76+.

McGoldrick M, et al: Ethnic intermarriage: implications for therapy. *Fam Process* 1984 Sep; 347–364.

Mulvihill D: Between parent and child . . . technique called rebonding. *Can Nurse* 1987 Feb; 12+.

Papernow P: The stepfamily cycle: an experimental model of stepfamily development. *Fam Relationships* 1984 Jul; 355–363.

Pepitone-Rockwell A: *Dual-Career Couples.* London, Sage Publications, 1980.

Rhyme M: Understanding and supporting families in the process of divorce. *Nurse Pract* 1986 Dec; 37–38+.

Rowland B, et al: A survey of parents' perceptions regarding latchkey children. *Pediatr Nurs* 1986 Jul-Aug; 278–283.

Scherer M: The loneliness of the latchkey child. *Instructor* 1982 May; 38–41.

Spock B: Discipline: how much is enough? How much is too tough? *Redbook Magazine* 1983 June; 12, 16–18.

Stern P: Affiliating in stepfather families: teachable strategies leading to stepfather child friendship. *West J Nurs Res* 1982 Winter; 75–89.

Stewart M: Supporting group action for women: a self help strategy—single parents. *Can Ment Health* 1983 Sep; 11–13.

Sund K, et al: Dual earner families: stress levels and personal and lifestyle related variables . . . in the preschool stage of family development. *Nurs Res* 1985 Nov-Dec; 357–361.

Thomas A, Chess S: Temperamental differences: a critical concept in child health care. *Pediatr Nurs* 1985 May/Jun; 167–171.

Trimberger R, Maclean M: Maternal employment: the child's perspective. *J Marriage Fam* 1982 May; 469–475.

Weinberg T: Single fatherhood: how is it different? *Pediatr Nurs* 1985 May/Jun; 173–176.

Wong D: Helping parents select day care centers. *Pediatr Nurs* 1986 May-Jun; 181–187.

Promoting Well Child Care Chapter 14

Mabel Hunsberger
Jo Joyce Anderson

Well child care takes place in all settings of health care. Children have similar basic needs whether they are free of illness or are learning to cope with a long-term illness. In other words, an ill child is a well child with a particular illness. The chapters that follow in this unit provide a basis for health promotion of *all* children.

This chapter discusses the nurse's participation in promoting health of children through the specific health care strategies of (1) regular child health visits and (2) the immunization of children.

Related Topics
Health Concepts: children's perceptions and behavior, Chapter 10
History and physical assessment, Chapter 15
Promoting healthy parenting, Chapter 13
Principles of administering medications, Chapter 28
Childhood infectious diseases, Chapter 45

Child Health Visits

Although schedules for health supervision and the content of each health visit vary from one provider to another and from one region to another, all have common general goals:

- To promote general health through counseling or anticipatory guidance
- To prevent illness with immunizations and teaching healthy self-care habits
- To detect illness early through history, physical assessment, and screening
- To provide prompt treatment for asymptomatic and symptomatic illness
- To prevent complications and unnecessary disability with effective management of chronic disease.

Promoting Well Child Care

Nursing Diagnoses	Nursing Goals/Strategies
Potential for altered health maintenance: failure to comply with child health visit schedule, related to: • *lack of social support* • *lack of transportation* • *conflict of schedules* • *patient belief system in conflict with that of health care professional* • *inadequate knowledge*	Promote child health through regular child health visits according to accepted standards. • Make telephone contact (if possible) to assess parents' perception of need for child visits • Accommodate the family's time constraints to the degree possible • Assess need for financial support and make necessary referrals • Assist family to assess available social supports • Assess parents' knowledge level concerning need for health supervision • Provide new information and correct misinformation concerning health promotion and screening routines • Identify conflicts between patient's belief system and expectations of health care provider
Potential for altered health maintenance: failure to comply with routine immunization schedule, related to: • *fear of serious side effects* • *conflict of religious beliefs* (All related factors and interventions listed in preceding diagnosis also apply to this diagnosis.)	Protect all children against communicable disease with known safe vaccines. • Ask parent to explain source of fear • Acknowledge that immunizations carry a level of risk • Provide known data concerning risks associated with the actual illness compared to the immunization • Explain expected side effects of immunization when administered • Provide instructions in how to manage side effects • Encourage patient to express how religious beliefs conflict with immunization • Seek assistance from state and specific church officials to help patient resolve conflict • Retain a stance of being a child advocate in resolving conflict

Guidelines for Health Supervision

The appropriate use of periodic health visits has been studied collaboratively by the United States Preventive Services Task Force and the Canadian Task Force.

Box 14-1 describes the guidelines for health supervision set forth by the Committee on Practice and Ambulatory Medicine and the American Academy of Pediatrics (AAP) (1985). These guidelines reflect the philosophy that children are not merely small adults but at different ages have unique anatomic, physical, behavioral, and pathologic characteristics. This factor, coupled with technologic and scientific advances, environmental conditions, and changing societal norms, determines what the care provider's assessment and counseling focus with the child and family will need to be at any given time.

The content of supervision can be categorized into five general areas. The *history and physical examination* (see Chapter 15) provide the data needed to identify asymptomatic or symptomatic illness and to monitor the control of chronic illness. Any marked increase or decrease in growth is usually indicative of illness of a chronic nature. This aspect of health supervision also provides an opportunity to talk to the child and parent to pick up clues about insidious or overt psychologic problems. A *developmental and behavioral assessment* provides data about brain development as well as specific areas such as self-esteem (see Chapter 16). This assessment may be accomplished through observation, structured testing (e.g., Denver Developmental Screening Test), and/or asking questions relative to sleep and eating patterns, parental satisfaction with the child's progress, and the child's relationships.

As major organic illness in children has been

Box 14-1

Guidelines for Health Supervision

Each child and family is unique; therefore, these **Guidelines for Health Supervision of Children and Youth**[1] are designed for the care of children who are receiving competent parenting, have no manifestations of any important health problems, and are growing and developing in satisfactory fashion. **Additional visits may become necessary** if circumstances suggest variations from normal. These guidelines represent a consensus by the Committee on Practice and Ambulatory Medicine, in consultation with the membership of the American Academy of Pediatrics through the Chapter Chairmen.

The Committee emphasizes the great importance of **continuity of care** in comprehensive health supervision[2] and the need to avoid **fragmentation of care.**[3]

A **prenatal visit** by the parents for anticipatory guidance and pertinent medical history is strongly recommended.

Health supervision should begin with medical care of the neonate in the hospital.

	INFANCY						EARLY CHILDHOOD					LATE CHILDHOOD				ADOLESCENCE				
AGE[4]	**By 1 mo**	**2 mos**	**4 mos**	**6 mos**	**9 mos**	**12 mos**	**15 mos**	**18 mos**	**24 mos**	**3 yrs**	**4 yrs**	**5 yrs**	**6 yrs**	**8 yrs**	**10 yrs**	**12 yrs**	**14 yrs**	**16 yrs**	**18 yrs**	**20+ yrs**
HISTORY																				
Initial/Interval	●	●	●	●	●	●	●	●	●	●	●	●	●	●	●	●	●	●	●	●
MEASUREMENTS																				
Height and Weight	●	●	●	●	●	●	●	●	●	●	●	●	●	●	●	●	●	●	●	●
Head Circumference	●	●	●	●	●	●														
Blood Pressure										●	●	●	●	●	●	●	●	●	●	●
SENSORY SCREENING																				
Vision	S	S	S	S	S	S	S	S	S	O	O	O	O	O	S	O	O	S	O	O
Hearing	S	S	S	S	S	S	S	S	S	S	O	O	S[5]	S[5]	S[5]	O	S	S	O	S
DEVEL/BEHAV ASSESSMENT[6]	●	●	●	●	●	●	●	●	●	●	●	●	●	●	●	●	●	●	●	●
PHYSICAL EXAMINATION[7]	●	●	●	●	●	●	●	●	●	●	●	●	●	●	●	●	●	●	●	●
PROCEDURES[8]																				
Hered./Metabolic Screening[9]	●																			
Immunization[10]		●	●	●			●	●				●					●			
Tuberculin Test						●	←		●[11]	→		←		●[11]	→		←		●[11]	→
Hematocrit or Hemoglobin[12]	←				●	→	←		●	→		←		●	→		←		●	→
Urinalysis[13]	←			●		→	←		●	→		←		●	→		←		●	→
ANTICIPATORY GUIDANCE[14]	●	●	●	●	●	●	●	●	●	●	●	●	●	●	●	●	●	●	●	●
INITIAL DENTAL REFERRAL[15]										●										

1. Committee on Practice and Ambulatory Medicine, 1981.
2. Statement on Continuity of Pediatric Care, Committee on Standards of Child Health Care, 1978.
3. Statement on Fragmentation of Pediatric Care, Committee on Standards of Child Health Care, 1978.
4. If child comes under care for first time at any point on the schedule, or if any items are not accomplished at the suggested age, schedule should be brought up to date at the earliest possible time.
5. At these points, history may suffice; if problem suggested, standard testing method should be employed.
6. By history and appropriate physical examination; if suspicious, by specific objective developmental testing.
7. At each visit, complete physical examination is essential, with infant totally unclothed, older child undressed and suitably draped.
8. These may be modified, depending upon entry point into schedule and individual need.

9. PKU and thyroid testing should be done at about 2 wk. Infants initially screened before 24 hr old should be rescreened.
10. Schedule(s) per Report of Committee on Infectious Disease, ed. 18, 1982.
11. The Committee on Infectious Diseases recommends tuberculin testing at 12 mo of age and every 1–2 yr thereafter. In some areas, tuberculosis is of exceedingly low occurrence and the physician may elect not to retest routinely or to use longer intervals.
12. Present medical evidence suggests the need for reevaluation of the frequency and timing of hemoglobin or hematocrit tests. One determination is therefore suggested during each time period. Performance of additional tests is left to the individual practice experience.
13. Present medical evidence suggests the need for re-evaluation of the frequency and timing of urinalyses. One determination is therefore suggested during each time period. Performance of additional tests is left to the individual practice experience.
14. Appropriate discussion and counseling should be an integral part of each visit for care.
15. Subsequent examinations as prescribed by dentist.

N.B.: **Special chemical, immunologic, and endocrine testing** is usually carried out upon specific indications. Testing other than newborn (e.g., inborn errors of metabolism, sickle disease, lead) is discretionary with the physician.

Key: ● = to be performed; S = subjective, by history; O = objective, by a standard testing method.
(From: American Academy of Pediatrics, 1985.)

contained by medical advances, a "new morbidity" has received epidemiologic attention. This new morbidity—acting out behaviors and behavior problems, failure to thrive, alcohol and drug abuse, school failure, accidents, delinquency, and other manifestations of adjustment difficulties—needs the serious attention of health professionals. Astute behavioral assessments and appropriate counseling can help prevent or diminish these childhood disabilities that are of acute concern to parents (Breslau, 1982).

Screening tests, both clinical (e.g., vision testing) and laboratory (e.g., hemoglobin testing), provide data to complement the physical and behavioral assessments in identifying altered health states. *Immunizations* are administered, to prevent specific infectious diseases that have the potential to cause serious illness. Education about their significance is important to gain cooperation of parents in following through with the entire series. *Counseling* and *anticipatory guidance* constitute an integral part of every health visit. Information provided is adapted to the child's age and prepares parents for anticipated developmental events. Some parents only require the nurse's reassurance that they are taking care of their children properly and that their expectations for their child and themselves are realistic and appropriate. Other parents will initially need repeated reinforcement of information offered and may require assistance applying information to their own child and home circumstances. Subject areas that are generally included for anticipatory guidance during health visits are safety, nutrition, sleep, play and exercise, development, discipline, and parenting. Age-specific discussions of these subjects can be found in Unit 2; Growth and Development of Children Within Families (Chapters 5 through 9).

Support of the Parenting Role

The primary goal of counseling and anticipatory guidance is to facilitate parents' capabilities to promote their children's well-being. The effectiveness of child health maintenance services is largely dependent upon the assistance parents receive in increasing their competence and confidence to meet their children's needs. Therefore, it is exceedingly important that the pediatric nurse knows how to be effective with parents. To work with parents the nurse must: (1) understand and respect parents as individuals; (2) appreciate the tasks inherent in parenting; and (3) recognize the growth promoting (and anxiety producing) potential of parenthood.

Health professionals tend to perceive parents solely in terms of the parent role and to judge them as persons in terms of parental adequacy, communicating attitudes based on that judgment. It is important to remember that parents have many roles, relationships, and responsibilities in daily living, besides parenting, and that they will have the energy to meet their children's needs satisfactorily only if their own needs are being met (de Castro et al, 1976). It is imperative that the nurse understands and accepts each parent as an individual and demonstrates respect as well as a genuine willingness to help them be successful at parenting.

The responsibility of parenting is demanding and frequently in conflict with other roles, relationships, and aspirations. The resolution of these conflicts is another inherent, continuous task. The nurse needs to remember that conflict evokes guilt and anxiety, resulting in defensive behaviors that may interfere with the parents' ability to accept or utilize help. When such defensive behavior is evident, the nurse will need to assist parents to acknowledge the conflict and direct them, either personally or through referral, in problem solving to diminish the conflict.

Because the process of parenting is taxing, parents lacking adequate support are vulnerable to failure. The nurse has a responsibility and opportunity to identify those parents with support deficiencies early so that consistent, supportive care can be made available.

As children grow, parental tasks change. Anticipatory guidance helps parents to plan in advance for these developmental changes and the associated alterations in their own parenting role. The nurse attempts to promote a mutual love, respect, and relaxation within the parent-child relationship throughout the various phases of development occurring in the child and within the family as a whole.

Psychosocial growth is realized as the tasks of parenthood are accomplished. As parents experience success in one task, their capacity to accomplish future tasks is increased. The nurse's assistance with early parental tasks can enhance the number of successes that parents experience from the beginning. It is critical for the nurse to share professional knowledge and skills in a manner that enhances parental self-esteem (see Chapter 13 for further discussion on parenting).

Role of Nurses in Promoting Child Health

Emphasis over the last decade has been placed on developing more effective ways to deliver pediatric ambulatory and counseling services. Pediatric nurse practitioners, school nurse practitioners, and clinical nurse specialists can provide such services, strengthening the nursing role in many health care settings. The specific roles of the nurse are hard to define because of many variables unique to each setting in which they practice. Nurses increasingly are assuming responsibility for the assessment and primary care management of selected children and their families in a collaborative—not subordinate—relationship with the physician.

The nurse functions as a primary source of health promotion, as well as preventive and curative care. Nurse practitioners have been innovative in developing parent groups, newsletters, telephone information tapes, and other modes for educating and supporting parents and children. These creative approaches to provide health services have been undergoing investigation and are found to be endorsed by parents. Ryberg and Merrifield (1984) did a study to find out what parents want to know and in what manner. Parents preferred services that could be used at their convenience and discretion in contrast to services (such as parent groups) that require attendance within given timeframes. The most preferred method for gaining information regarding child health issues was telephone resources that parents could access. Nurse practitioners are most often the resources on the other end of the telephone. Additionally, many hospital pediatric and newborn nursery units have created "call for help" lines that provide parents with resources for information. Alternative methods for providing support and information to parents and alternative resources for ambulatory pediatric care and counseling through various nursing roles has helped health care professionals and parents develop a team effort to achieve the goal of optimal well-being for every child.

Promoting Health Through Immunizations

The majority of immunizations are administered during child health care visits by the primary care nurse or physician or through a local public health department. However, nurses should assess the status of immunizations in any setting. Children not protected from disease because of irregular attendance at a clinic or their physician's office can be identified by thorough history taking and specific data collection during an episode of acute illness. Thus, a pediatric nurse in *any* setting should have a good understanding of immunizations so that unimmunized children can be identified and immunized or referred for later immunization when the child is well.

Immunity and Types of Agents Used for Immunization

Immunity is a state in which the host is resistant to a specific disease. *General immunity (or natural immunity)* occurs through the host's ongoing exposure to organisms of low virulence that do not overwhelm the host. Natural immunity affords the host the ability to live in an environment that is teeming with organisms (i.e., water, soil, food, air) without becoming ill. On the contrary, highly virulent organisms possess specific characteristics that result in disease. The purpose of immunizations is to protect the host against a specific group of known microbes that have the potential to cause serious illness.

Protection against specific illness can be acquired by contracting the actual illness (i.e., one episode of chicken pox protects the child against that particular disease). This is a *natural active immunity.* Immunity is also achieved by electively inducing immunity through immunization. This type is sometimes called *artificial active immunity.* Active immunity through the artificial means of vaccination is accomplished by using vaccines or toxoids (see summary of types of agents used in immunization in Box 14-2).

Another way of acquiring immunity is through *passive immunity* in which ready-made host-defense factors are transferred to the host. These factors are not produced by the host; therefore, the resultant immunity is called passive (produced by an exogenous

Box 14-2
Types of Agents Used in Immunization

LIVE VACCINES

The objective is to induce protective immunity without producing the actual full-blown clinical illness. To accomplish this, the organisms are *attenuated*, which means the virulence has been diminished to a level where immunity is achieved but the clinical illness is avoided. Measles, mumps, rubella, varicella, and polio (Sabin) vaccines are examples of live attenuated viruses. BCG vaccine is an example of live attenuated bacteria.

KILLED VACCINES

Immunity is stimulated by the host's reaction to the killed microbe. Polio (Salk) and influenza vaccines are examples of killed viruses. Pertussis vaccine is an example of a killed bacteria.

TOXOIDS

A toxoid is a bacterial toxin that has been treated by heat or by chemicals to destroy its toxic properties but retain its antigenic quality (i.e., ability to stimulate antibody production). Tetanus toxoid and diphtheria toxoid are examples of a treated toxin.

ADSORBED AGENTS AND FLUID AGENTS

Adsorbed Agents (vaccines and toxoids) have substances added to the immunizing agent to enhance its antigenic effect. Antigens are therefore released more slowly, enhancing the response by prolonged contact. Adsorbed agents must be given intramuscularly.

Fluid agents are more rapidly absorbed and produce a more rapid secondary response. Fluid tetanus toxoid is used at the time of an injury if the victim has had the initial series of tetanus immunization.

source) and is usually temporary. Placental transfer of antibodies to the fetus is an example of *natural passive immunity. Artificial passive immunity* is produced by injecting the host with the plasma proteins (antibody) that have been produced by another human or an animal that has been actively immunized against the specific antigen. Such antibodies are of various types including human immune serum globulin or animal antiserum (antitoxin).

Human Immune Serum Globulin

Human immune serum globulin may be prepared from pooled plasma and is used to reduce the severity of diseases or to prevent diseases such as measles, viral hepatitis A, and viral hepatitis B (if specific hepatitis B immune globulin is not available). Specific human immune serum globulin is also available. This is prepared from the plasma of patients recuperating from specific illnesses such as tetanus, pertussis, hepatitis B, mumps, and varicella zoster. Plasma of a recuperating patient contains the antibody for that specific illness.

Animal Antiserum (Antitoxin)

This antibody is prepared from animal serum (horses, cows) in which the antibody has been actively produced. Because reactions to the foreign serum may occur, the individual is first pretested to determine hypersensitivity. Examples of this method of passive immunity are tetanus antitoxin and diphtheria antitoxin.

The Practice of Immunization

Routine immunization of children has dramatically reduced the incidence and prevalence of infectious diseases in the past 40 years. It is universally agreed that appropriate immunization is crucial to the promotion and maintenance of health in children.

The timing of immunizations and which ones are critical is, however, widely debated and is somewhat influenced by the geographic and socioeconomic region in which the child lives. The most often debated vaccine is pertussis because of its potential serious consequences. Within the United States, the Committee on Infectious Diseases of the American Academy of Pediatrics (AAP) and the Advisory Committee on Immunization Practices (ACIP) of the United States Public Health Services recommend immunization policies and procedures. The schedules are revised periodically as new information is discovered. The pediatric nurse should consult current resources such as the latest editions of AAP's Report of the Committee on Infectious Diseases (Red Book) and the Nurses' Drug Alert to keep abreast of changes and to acquire detailed information. The nurse should be prepared to provide children and parents with explanations of the risks, benefits, and rationale for the various immunizations.

Current Recommendations

Current recommendations of the AAP for immunization of infants and children are summarized in Table 14-1, and recommendations of the National Advisory Committee on Immunizations (Ottawa, Canada) in Box 14-3. The nurse should reinforce and praise the child and parent(s) who have initiated and kept immunizations current.

***Table* 14-1.** Recommended Schedule for Active Immunization of Normal Infants and Children (United States)*

Recommended Age	Immunization(s)	Comments
2 mo	DTP,[1] OPV[2]	Can be initiated as early as 2 wk of age in areas of high endemicity or during epidemics
4 mo	DTP, OPV	2 mo interval desired for OPV to avoid interference from previous dose
6 mo	DTP (OPV)	OPV is optional (may be given in areas with increased risk of poliovirus exposure)
15 mo	Measles, mumps, rubella (MMR)[3]	MMR preferred to individual vaccines; tuberculin testing may be done
18 mo	DTP,[4,5] OPV[5]	
24 mo	HBPV[6]	
4–6 yr[7]	DTP, OPV	At or before school entry
14–16 yr	Td[8]	Repeat every 10 yr throughout life

1. DTP—Diptheria and tetanus toxoids with pertussis vaccine.
2. OPV—Oral, poliovirus vaccine contains attenuated poliovirus types 1, 2, and 3.
3. MMR—Live measles, mumps, and rubella viruses in a combined vaccine (see text for discussion of single vaccines versus combination).
4. Should be given 6 to 12 months after the third dose.
5. May be given simultaneously with MMR at 15 months of age.
6. *Haemophilus* b polysaccharide vaccine.
7. Up to the seventh birthday.
8. Td—Adult tetanus toxoid (full dose) and diphtheria toxoid (reduced dose) in combination.

For all products used, consult manufacturer's package insert for instructions for storage, handling, and administration. Biologics prepared by different manufacturers may vary, and those of the same manufacturer may change from time to time. Therefore, the physician should be aware of the contents of the package insert.

(From Committee on Infectious Disease, AAP, 1986.)

* At the time of this writing, revised recommendations are being prepared by the Committee.

Interrupted Schedule

Interruption of the recommended schedule does not require starting over in the schedule (National Advisory Committee, 1984; American Academy of Pediatrics, 1986). The immunization is continued as if the usual time interval had elapsed.

Unimmunized Children

Children not immunized in the first year of life may be started on a schedule of primary immunization any time before the age of 7 years, according to Table 14-2 or 14-3. The goal is to provide protection as efficiently as possible. In the United States the mumps, measles, and rubella (MMR) vaccine is not given until the child is 15 months of age (in Canada it may be given as early as 12 months of age).

Children who start or continue immunization after 7 years of age should use the adult form of tetanus-

Box 14-3

Recommended Immunization Schedules for Infants and Children (Canada)

Few measures in preventive medicine are of such proven value and as easy to implement as routine immunization against infectious diseases. Immunization carried out as recommended in the following schedules will provide good basic protection for most children against the diseases shown.

With respect to tetanus and diphtheria, the schedules pertain to use of either fluid or adsorbed toxoids, but in view of their superior antigenic properties, the use of adsorbed products is recommended.

Both live and inactivated polio vaccines have been used in Canada with equal success in preventing the occurrence of paralytic poliomyelitis, and either may be used in the following schedules.

Modifications of the recommended schedule may be necessary because of missed appointments or intercurrent illness. Interruption of a recommended series does not require starting the series over again, regardless of the interval elapsed.

Routine Immunization Schedule for Infants and Children

Age	Immunization against			
2 months	Diphtheria	Pertussis	Tetanus	Poliomyelitis
4 months	Diphtheria	Pertussis	Tetanus	Poliomyelitis
6 months	Diphtheria	Pertussis	Tetanus	Poliomyelitis[1]
12 months	Measles	Mumps	Rubella[2]	
18 months	Diphtheria	Pertussis	Tetanus	Poliomyelitis
4–6 years	Diphtheria	Pertussis	Tetanus	Poliomyelitis
14–16 years	Diphtheria[3]		Tetanus[3]	Poliomyelitis[1]

1. This dose may be omitted if live (oral) polio vaccine is being used.
2. Rubella vaccine is also indicated for all girls and women of childbearing age who lack proof of immunity. At all medical visits the opportunity should be taken to check whether girls and women have received rubella vaccine.
3. Diphtheria and tetanus toxoid (Td), a combined adsorbed "adult type" preparation for use in persons ≥7 yr old, contains less diphtheria toxoid than preparations given to younger children and is less likely to cause reactions in older persons.

(From National Advisory Committee on Immunizations, 1984.)

Table 14-2. Recommended Immunization Schedules for Children Not Immunized in First Year of Life (United States)*

Recommended Time	Immunization(s)	Comments
Less Than 7 Years Old		
First visit	DTP, OPV, MMR	MMR if child ≥15 mo old; tuberculin testing may be done
Interval after first visit		
1 mo	HBPV†	For children 24–60 mo
2 mo	DTP, OPV	
4 mo	DTP (OPV)	OPV is optional (may be given in areas with increased risk of poliovirus exposure)
10–16 mo	DTP, OPV	OPV is not given if third dose was given earlier
Age 4–6 yr (at or before school entry)	DTP, OPV	DTP is not necessary if the fourth dose was given after the fourth birthday; OPV is not necessary if recommended OPV dose at 10–16 mo following first visit was given after the fourth birthday
Age 14–16 yr	Td	Repeat every 10 yr throughout life
7 Years Old and Older		
First visit	Td, OPV, MMR	
Interval after first visit		
2 mo	Td, OPV	
8–14 mo	Td, OPV	
Age 14–16 yr	Td	Repeat every 10 yr throughout life

* At the time of this writing, revised recommendations are being prepared by the Committee.

† *Haemophilus* b polysaccharide vaccine can be given, if necessary, simultaneously with DTP (at separate sites). The initial three doses of DTP can be given at 1- to 2-mo intervals; so, for the child in whom immunization is initiated at 24 mo old or older, one visit could be eliminated by giving DTP, OPV, MMR at the first visit; DTP and HBPV at the second visit (1 mo later); and DTP and OPV at the third visit (2 mo after the first visit). Subsequent DTP and OPV 10 to 16 mo after the first visit are still indicated.

(From Committee on Infectious Disease, AAP, 1986.)

diphtheria (Td) vaccine. The schedule to follow for unimmunized children 7 years of age or older is also presented in Tables 14-2 and 14-3. When immunizations are not obtained as prescribed, further assessment is required to identify those factors that are interfering with the family's response to this aspect of health care. Strategies to facilitate the achievement of adequate immunization status are instituted by the health care team.

Table 14-3. Immunization Schedules for Children Not Immunized in Early Infancy (Canada)

Timing	Immunization Against			
For Children 1 through 6 Years of Age				
First visit[4]	Diphtheria	Pertussis	Tetanus	Poliomyelitis
Interval after 1st visit				
1 month	Measles	Mumps	Rubella[2]	
2 months	Diphtheria	Pertussis	Tetanus	Poliomyelitis
4 months	Diphtheria	Pertussis	Tetanus	Poliomyelitis[1]
16 months	Diphtheria	Pertussis	Tetanus	Poliomyelitis
Pre-school[5]				
At age 14–16 years	Diphtheria[3]		Tetanus[3]	Poliomyelitis[1]
For Children 7 Years of Age and Over				
First visit[4]	Diphtheria[3]		Tetanus[3]	Poliomyelitis
Interval after 1st visit				
1 month	Measles	Mumps	Rubella[2]	Poliomyelitis[1]
2 months	Diphtheria		Tetanus	Poliomyelitis
14 months	Diphtheria		Tetanus	Poliomyelitis
10 years	Diphtheria		Tetanus	Poliomyelitis[1]

1. This dose may be omitted if live (oral) polio vaccine is being used.
2. Rubella vaccine is also indicated for all girls and women of child-bearing age who lack proof of immunity. At all medical visits the opportunity should be taken to check whether girls and women have received rubella vaccine.
3. Diphtheria and tetanus toxoid (Td), a combined adsorbed "adult type" preparation for use in persons 7 years of age or more, contains less diphtheria toxoid than preparations given to younger children and is less likely to cause reactions in older persons.
4. Measles, mumps, and rubella vaccines may also be given at the first visit if it is considered likely that a child will not return for further immunization. It has not been shown, however, that full response to all antigens will occur.
5. When the last of the aforementioned doses is given before the fourth birthday, consideration should be given to administration of an additional dose at school entry.

(From National Advisory Committee on Immunizations, 1984.)

Multiple Vaccine Administration

Protective responses and side effects of vaccines administered simultaneously have been found to be similar to those that are administered separately (American Academy of Pediatrics, 1986). It is sometimes advisable to administer vaccines simultaneously especially if it is unlikely that a child will be brought back for additional immunizations. For example, children who are 15 months old and older (but under age 7) can be given MMR, OPV, and DTP at one visit.*

* The abbreviation DPT is interchangeable with DTP.

Illness and Vaccination

It is not uncommon for a child to present with a febrile or acute illness at the time he or she is scheduled for an immunization. Minor, nonfebrile illnesses (e.g., mild upper respiratory tract infections, allergic rhinitis, or a mild episode of diarrhea) should not preclude routine vaccination. Deferring the immunization of children with minor illnesses too frequently results in children remaining unimmunized for too long, thereby subjecting them to the danger of contracting a preventable disease. However, children with *febrile* illness should not be immunized, because the fever may be symptomatic of a more serious condition. Parents are asked to bring their child for immunization as soon as the febrile illness has subsided.

Immunization of Immunocompromised Children

Children may be immunocompromised because of an underlying disease or as the result of therapy that suppresses the immune response. Generally, live virus vaccines are contraindicated in children with congenital disorders of immune function.

Other modes of management include use of inactivated vaccines and monthly administration of immune globulin. Oral poliovirus vaccine should not be given to family members of an immunocompromised child, because the virus can be transmitted through shedding.

After immunosuppressive therapy has been discontinued, the normal immunologic response does not resume until 3 months to 1 year later. Live virus vaccines can be given to patients with leukemia in remission if chemotherapy has been terminated for 3 months (American Academy of Pediatrics, 1986).

The use of a varicella vaccine in children with cancer receiving immunosuppressive therapy is being investigated because for these children the risks associated with natural varicella outweigh those involved in receiving the attenuated virus as a vaccine (American Academy of Pediatrics, 1986).

Immunization of Premature Infants

It is recommended that premature infants receive routine immunizations according to their chronologic age, and that vaccine doses are not reduced (American Academy of Pediatrics, 1986). If an infant is still in the hospital at the age of 2 months when the first immunization is received, the oral polio vaccine (OPV) is postponed until discharge. This is done to prevent cross-infection of poliovirus to the other infants in the nursery. Also, preterm infants should receive hepatitis B immune globulin if exposed to a mother who is hepatitis B surface antigen (HBsAg) positive.

Site and Route of Administration of Immunizing Agents

The preferred site for intramuscular injection is the anterolateral aspect of the thigh (vastus lateralis muscle). In older children (late school age), the deltoid muscle has usually attained sufficient size for intramuscular injection and is often preferred by the child. The gluteus muscle should not be used for immunizations, especially in infants and young children, because of the danger of damaging the sciatic nerve. (See Chapter 28 for further discussion of injection sites.)

Needles used for intramuscular injection should be of sufficient length to actually reach the muscle. The amount of fat present rather than the age of the child determines the length of needle required.

Adsorbed vaccines must be injected deep into the muscle mass to reduce the risk of local reactions. Types of agents and route of administration are summarized in Table 14-4.

Immunizing Agents

Many of the vaccines are administered in combination to reduce the number of injections required. The two major examples are DPT (diphtheria, pertussis, and tetanus) and MMR (measles, mumps, and rubella). A combination of tetanus and diphtheria (Td), instead of DPT, is used at 7 years of age and thereafter. These combinations along with polio make up the commonly used immunizations. *Haemophilus influenzae* type b is increasingly being used but remains optional.

DPT (Diphtheria Toxoid, Pertussis Vaccine, and Tetanus Toxoid)

DPT is given by intramuscular injection in a series of three doses 2 months apart, followed by a booster 1 year later (at 15 to 18 months of age), and another booster upon entry into school. A preparation DT is given to children under 7 years of age in whom pertussis vaccine is contraindicated. Children 7 years of age and older are routinely given Td. The small "d" indicates a reduced diphtheria dose containing only 20 per cent of that in DPT. It is recommended that the adult form (Td) is given at 10-year intervals. Diphtheria toxoid is a safe vaccine with a low incidence of fever

Table 14-4. Type of Immunization Agent, Side Effects, and Route of Administration

Route and Side Effects	Comments*
Diphtheria Toxoid	
Administration: Intramuscularly (if *fluid vaccine* rather than an *adsorbed vaccine* is used then it is given subcutaneously) Low incidence of fever and local soreness, redness, and swelling at injection site	Usually given in combination with tetanus and pertussis (DPT) or just DT (for the child <7 yr old who has reacted to pertussis). Td is an adult vaccine (used for children ≥7 yr). It contains the standard amount of tetanus toxoid but only 20% of the diphtheria toxoid supplied by DTP or DT
Tetanus Toxoid	
Administration: Intramuscularly (if *fluid vaccine* rather than an *adsorbed vaccine* is used then it is given subcutaneously) Low incidence of fever and mild local tenderness, redness, and swelling at injection site. Antipyretics are used for fever postinjection. Prophylactic use of antipyretics is often recommended if fever occurred following previous immunizations	Usually administered in combination with diphtheria and pertussis (DPT) to children <7 yr old and Td to children ≥7 yr and to adults
Pertussis Vaccine	
Administration: Intramuscularly (if *fluid vaccine* rather than an *adsorbed vaccine* is used then it is given subcutaneously) Over 50% have temporary local tenderness. A swelling or lump may remain at injection site for a few weeks or even months but gradually disappears. Approximately 50% of the children have fever, irritability, or lethargy. More serious reactions can occur on rare occasions. Antipyretics used for fever. Warm soaks on involved area for comfort (or warm bath)	Usually given in combination with tetanus and diphtheria toxoids (DPT). Parents need clear explanations about risks and benefits of the vaccine (see discussion in this chapter). Nurse should ask about reactions to previous pertussis vaccine before administering vaccine
Polio (trivalent oral poliovaccine, TOPV)	
Administration: Orally Virtually no side effects. A few cases of vaccine-associated paralytic disease have been reported in the primary vaccinee: 1 : 10 million. In the primary vaccinee (person vaccinated) plus close contacts: 1 : 4 million incidents of paralysis have been reported	Not administered to family members of immune deficient child. Although antibodies in breast milk can neutralize the vaccine, it does not interfere with development of immunity. Not given to premature infants until discharged from hospital, because of dissemination to other prematures (because OPV produces secretory antibodies within the intestinal tract, infection of close contact may occur). Such indirect immunization can also be beneficial to contacts
Polio (trivalent inactivated polio vaccine, TIPV)	
Administration: Subcutaneously (if fluid); intramuscularly (if adsorbed) No common reactions	Given in combination with OPT (generally not used in US but is used in some parts of Canada). Little or no locally protective antibody in pharyngeal and intestinal secretions develops
Measles	
Administration: Subcutaneously Approximately 5% of vaccinees develop fever between 6–10 days after vaccination, lasting up to 5 days. Transient rashes reported in 3–5%. Antipyretics used for fever; warm soaks or warm bath and antihistamine for rash if pruritic	Given in combination with mumps and rubella vaccines
Mumps	
Administration: Subcutaneously Rarely fever and rash	Given in combination with measles and rubella vaccines
Rubella	
Administration: Subcutaneously Approximately 30% of vaccinees have transient rash, lymphadenopathy, or arthralgia. Approximately 1% have self-limited arthritis (occurs about 2 wk after the immunization). More common in women than in children. Mild analgesic may be used for pain	Given in combination with measles and mumps vaccine

continued

Table 14-4. (continued)

Route and Side Effects	Comments*
Haemophilus influenzae **Type B, A Polysaccharide**	
Administration: Intramuscularly or subcutaneously Approximately 50% of children have fever and mild local reactions at vaccination site. Significant fever occurs in only 1% of children. Antipyretics used for fever	When this vaccine is given simultaneously with DPT, the incidence of reactions is not increased more than if DPT is given alone
Hepatitis B (Plasma-Derived) and Hepatitis B (Recombinant DNA) Vaccines	
Administration: Intramuscularly Approximately 15% of vaccinees have mild local tenderness at injection site	Indications for use of plasma-derived and recombinant DNA are similar, except plasma-derived vaccine is used for hemodialysis patients and the immunosuppressed. When an infant is born to a mother who is hepatitis B surface antigen (HBsAg) – positive, first dose should be administered within 7 days after birth. Hepatitis B immune globulin (HBIG) is given within first few hours after birth. If given at same time, a separate injection site is used
Pneumococcal Vaccine	
Administration: Intramuscularly or subcutaneously Local redness and mild soreness occurs in 50% of cases	Children under 2 yrs old do not respond to the vaccine with protective antibody titers. The safety of second doses in children has not been determined. Adults have more severe local reactions from a booster dose
Influenza Vaccine	
Administration: Intramuscularly preferred (also subcutaneously) Approximately ⅓ of vaccinees develop mild local redness and swelling at injection site. Systemic reactions of fever and malaise are infrequent. In 1976, a temporal association was noted between administration of the "swine flu" vaccine and Guillain-Barré syndrome in adults	Individuals with egg allergies should not receive the vaccine, because it is made from egg-grown viruses. November is generally accepted as the optimal time for organized vaccination campaigns

* All vaccines must be stored according to manufacturer's recommendations.

(From American Academy of Pediatrics, 1986; National Advisory Committee on Immunization, 1984; Dossett, 1987; Centers for Disease Control, 1987c; Centers for Disease Control, 1987d.)

and only minor local pain at the site of injection. The primary series of DPT is greater than 90 per cent effective in the prevention of serious cases of diphtheria.

A high level of appropriate immunization exists (96 per cent of children entering school) in the United States today. Cases of these diseases that do occur are found in unimmunized or inadequately immunized individuals (Centers for Disease Control, 1985). The Schick test may be used to determine whether older children still carry acquired immunity to diphtheria. If immunity titers do not exist, a red patch will develop at the skin test site and persist for 4 to 5 days. Because many adults have been found not to be protected against diphtheria, more emphasis should be placed on adult immunization programs (Centers for Disease Control, 1985).

Tetanus toxoid is the form of tetanus that is administered in routine immunizations. Other forms of tetanus vaccine include tetanus immune globulin (TIG) and tetanus antitoxin (usually horse serum).

Tetanus toxoid is administered routinely in the form of DPT to children under 7 years of age. In older children, the Td preparation is used because of the reaction that DPT induces in children older than age 7. Even in young children, administration of pertussis vaccine is associated with a higher incidence of reactions and complications than many of the other vaccines. One particular area of study is the possibility of an association between DPT and sudden infant death syndrome (SIDS) (Walker, 1987).

In addition to the routine immunizations, a form of tetanus immunization is sometimes required in the event of injury. A child with a minor clean wound who has received the primary immunization and a booster within 10 years prior to the injury does not require a booster of tetanus toxoid. In the event of a more serious wound to a previously appropriately immunized child, a booster is given if tetanus toxoid has not been received in the preceding 5 years (Centers for Disease Control, 1985). If the three primary injections have not been received, then a child under 7 years of age receives DPT and a child over 7 receives Td (even in the event of a minor wound). Serious wounds are treated with tetanus immune globulin to provide passive protection if the three primary injections were not received. In this event, Td is also administered. When both TIG and Td are administered, separate syringes and sites are used (American Academy of Pediatrics, 1986).

Because so many persons are hypersensitive to the tetanus antitoxin horse serum, the use of tetanus antitoxin has been largely replaced by hospital treatment of susceptible wounds in nonimmunized individuals (Leach, 1984).

Reactions to DPT vaccinations are largely due to the pertussis portion of the vaccine. Reactions are of three types: (1) local swelling and tenderness at site of injection, a slight fever, and irritability; (2) excessive tiredness, inconsolable crying that lasts 4 hours or longer, and a shock-like syndrome also lasting for several hours; and (3) neurologic reactions including occasional convulsions and in rare occasions encephalopathy with brain damage or even death (Mortimer, 1987). Reactions that are contraindications to further vaccination with pertussis vaccine include a fever greater than 105°F (40.5°C), a shock-like syndrome, allergic hypersensitivity, and neurologic reactions including convulsions and encephalopathy. Continuation of diphtheria and tetanus immunization can be provided by administering DT in a child under 7 years of age.

Although pertussis vaccine has risks, the risk of death from pertussis in the unimmunized child is estimated to be 10 times greater than in the immunized child (Dosset, 1987). Serious neurologic illness requiring hospitalization attributable to pertussis vaccine is rare; the risk is reported to be 1 : 140,000 administered doses. Concern about serious side effects has led some professionals to reduce the dose of DPT to less than 0.5 ml per dose (Centers for Disease Control, 1987a). This practice is not approved by the ACIP and AAP, and current recommendations are to give the full dose (Centers for Disease Control, 1985).

Polio Vaccine

Polio vaccine is a trivalent vaccine that produces immune titers against the three main strains of poliovirus. Two types of vaccines are available:

- oral polio vaccine (OPV), a live, attenuated trivalent polio vaccine (Sabin)
- inactivated polio vaccine (IPV), a killed trivalent polio vaccine given subcutaneously (Salk)

OPV is the recommended drug for routine immunization in the United Sates. In Canada, IPV is the commonly used preparation. Either vaccine can effectively control wild poliovirus disease* (Salk, 1988). An intended effect of live poliovirus is that it will immunize contacts by virus spread; however, there is no consistent evidence to indicate that the spread of virus significantly increases the immune status of a population (Salk, 1988). A properly timed combination of OPV and IPV is an alternative that has been used in some countries and is thought to have some advantages (Melnick, 1988).

Trivalent oral polio vaccine (TOPV) and IPV are started at the 2-month visit with a second dose at 4 months. A third dose is given at 6 months (optional when using OPV). Booster doses are recommended at 18 months of age and at school entry. IPV is the preferred vaccine for children with an immune deficiency disease. Family members of an immunosuppressed child should not receive OPV either, because of the potential for transmission of poliovirus.

MMR (*Measles, Mumps, and Rubella*) Vaccine

MMR is given as a triple vaccine in one dose that affords lifelong immunity. It is administered subcutaneously at 15 months of age in the United States and at 12 or 15 months of age in Canada. Some children who are immunized for measles before 12 months of age have contracted measles in spite of having received the vaccine. It is felt that persistent maternal antibodies can interfere with antibody production and inhibit immunity, although findings have not been consistent documenting a greater risk of outbreaks if vaccination occurs from 12 to 14 months of age compared with vaccination at or after 15 months of age (Centers for Disease Control, 1987b). In the event of a measles epidemic, measles vaccine should be given to children as young as 6 months of age. In these cases, it is recommended that the immunization be repeated after 15 months of age (Centers for Disease Control, 1987b).

Measles vaccine may be contraindicated if a child has had recent central nervous system infection (e.g., meningitis), is prone to febrile convulsions, is immunocompromised, or is allergic to eggs (the vaccine is a live attenuated virus in an egg medium). This vaccine does cause a mild version of the disease in about 30 per cent of children (Leach, 1984).

Mumps vaccine has been reported on rare occasions to cause fever and a temporary rash.

Rubella vaccine has prevented large epidemics, but small epidemics still occur regularly in high

* Poliomyelitis that is contracted by exposure to the virus that exists because of *actual* cases of poliomyelitis (poliomyelitis also can be contracted through the spread of the virus after receiving OPV).

schools, colleges, and places of employment where large numbers of young people work.

All women in prenatal clinics should be screened for rubella immunity and, if not immune, should be immunized immediately after delivery.

The primary concern associated with rubella vaccine is that young women in their first trimester of pregnancy should not receive the vaccine. Although vaccination of pregnant women is to be avoided, in cases where it has inadvertently occurred, deleterious effects to the fetus have not been reported (Dosset, 1987; Mortimer, 1987).

Hib (Haemophilus Influenzae Type B) Vaccine

Hib vaccine (*Haemophilus influenzae* type b) has been licensed for administration since 1985. The organism *Haemophilus influenzae* type b in unimmunized children causes many serious, invasive infections (e.g., bacterial meningitis, pneumonia, epiglottitis, septic arthritis). Studies to date show immunity to be most satisfactorily achieved if the vaccine is given at 18 months of age, although it may be given anytime before the fifth birthday. Immunization is not recommended before 18 months of age. Children beyond 5 years of age with a chronic illness that is known to be associated with increased risk for Hib infections should be given a single dose of vaccine. Children with Hodgkin disease should be immunized 10 to 14 days before initiation of chemotherapy or 3 months after cessation of chemotherapy.

The need for more than a single dose of vaccine for lifelong immunity has not been established. Because of the greater incidence of Hib infection in day care settings, special efforts should be made to immunize children attending day care centers (Committee on Infectious Diseases, 1985).

Yellow Fever, Cholera, Typhoid Fever, and Rabies Vaccines

Yellow fever, cholera, typhoid fever, and rabies vaccines are not recommended as a part of the routine immunization schedule in the United States. However, they are given routinely in some parts of the world and to western world children traveling to those countries. All of these vaccines have side effects, and for some individuals receiving the vaccine is inadvisable. In such cases, travel to countries where these diseases are epidemic is discouraged.

BCG (Bacillus Calmette-Guérin) Vaccine

BCG vaccine is a preparation of an attenuated strain of mycobacterium tuberculosis (bacillus Calmette-Guérin). BCG vaccine is not given routinely against tuberculosis in the United States; rather, those individuals who have been exposed, who are at high risk, or who are especially susceptible are given regular skin testing and treated prophylactically if the skin test results are positive.

Tuberculosis (TB) Testing

TB testing, while not an immunization, is part of the immunization schedule recommended by the American Academy of Pediatrics. The initial skin test is recommended at 1 year of age. It is recommended that skin tests be repeated before school entry, at age 8 years, and during adolescence (14 to 16 years of age). More frequent testing may be done in the event or likelihood of exposure.

The common tuberculosis screening tests are described in Box 14-4. Two preparations of tuberculin,

Box 14-4
Common Tuberculosis Screening Tests

MANTOUX:

PPD 5 tuberculin units (5TU) in 0.1 ml solution injected intradermally at the forearm inner (volar) surface using #27 needle tuberculin syringe, after site is cleansed and has dried. Wheal produced if injection is intracutaneous

Read in: 48–72 hr

Negative Reaction: 5 mm induration

Doubtful Reaction: 5–9 mm induration

Absolute Positive Reaction: 10-mm induration

TINE (OT):

4-prong multiple puncture button containing OT is pressed into inner (volar) surface of mid-forearm after site is cleansed and has dried

Read in: 48–72 hr

Negative Reaction: 0–2 mm induration

Doubtful Reaction: Papule 2 mm

Positive Reaction (retest with Mantoux): One or more papules 2–5 mm or larger in diameter

Absolute Positive Reaction: Vesiculation

old tuberculin (OT) and purified protein derivative (PPD), are available. PPD has largely replaced OT because it is less expensive. The tine test contains OT, whereas the Mantoux test contains PPD. The tine test is the most widely used multiple-puncture skin test. Other multiple-puncture tests used include Aplitest, Heaf, Mono-Vac, Sterneedle, and Selavo Test.

If the child has been exposed to TB, upon testing a skin reaction will develop, forming an area of induration (hard raised spots) at the site of injection. Sometimes this is accompanied by erythema. Since the nurse is responsible for administering and interpreting these skin tests, he or she must measure, or teach the parent to measure, the width of the palpated elevated area. The presence or absence of redness should be disregarded. Reactivity to a skin test may be suppressed if the child is malnourished, under severe stress, or receiving steroids or immunosuppressive drugs. Children with doubtful readings on multiple puncture tests should be retested using the Mantoux test.

Skin testing is not reliable if done within 4 weeks following a case of measles or following vaccination with live virus. Live vaccine is thought to alter the immune mechanism and may depress tuberculin sensitivity, producing a false negative TB test. Because administration of live vaccine can cause an exacerbation of tuberculosis, it is recommended that tuberculin testing be done prior to or concurrently with the administration of live vaccine when tuberculosis is endemic or suspected in an individual.

Hepatitis B (HB) Vaccine

Plasma-derived HB vaccine became available in 1982. The three major groups at risk for contracting hepatitis B are (1) persons who work in health care professions and have exposure to blood; (2) staff and clients of institutions for the developmentally disabled; and (3) staff and patients in hemodialysis units (Centers for Disease Control, 1987c). Additionally, in the pediatric population, hepatitis B vaccine is recommended for several high-risk groups, one of which is infants born to mothers who are hepatitis B surface antigen (HBsAg)–positive. Babies born to HBsAg–positive mothers should receive hepatitis B immune globulin (HBIG) at birth, with additional doses of hepatitis B vaccine at birth or within 7 days of birth, at 1 month and 6 months of age (Bureau of Communicable Disease Epidemiology, 1987; Centers for Disease Control, 1987c). Children who reside in households where chronic hepatitis B virus carriers live are at greater risk to develop the disease. It is recommended that these children receive the vaccine only.

In July 1986, a new genetically engineered vaccine called the recombinant DNA hepatitis B vaccine was licensed. The recommended dose is similar to plasma-derived vaccine (5 μg for children less than 10 years old and 10 μg for adults). Two additional doses, at 1 and 6 months after the first dose, are required. The recombinant vaccine has been demonstrated to be safe and to produce effective immunity (Centers for Disease Control, 1987c).

Pneumococcal Polysaccharide Vaccine

The pneumococcal vaccine contains the polysaccharides of 23 common pneumococcal strains. Children who should be vaccinated include those who are 2 years of age or older and those who are at risk because of asplenia, sickle cell disease, nephrotic syndrome, or other immunodeficiency syndromes. Children with Hodgkin disease should be immunized before beginning therapy (American Academy of Pediatrics, 1986).

Meningococcal Polysaccharide Vaccine

Meningococcal vaccine is available in three preparations: monovalent group A, monovalent group C, and a divalent vaccine that contains both group A and group C polysaccharides. Meningococcal vaccine is currently recommended for use only under the circumstance of epidemic outbreaks of group A or group C disease. Serogroup A vaccine is highly effective for all ages of children, whereas group C vaccine does not protect very young children (i.e., under age 2).

Varicella Vaccine

A live, attenuated varicella vaccine, developed and tested in Japan, has been found to be safe and immunogenic in children. Significant antibody titers have persisted for 5 years following immunization (Arbeter et al, 1986). However, questions remain about the duration of immunity and the effect of vaccination on varicella epidemiology. In 1985, the vaccine was licensed in five European countries (Plotkin, 1986), for use on persons with leukemia. Specific recommendations regarding the use of this vaccine have not yet been developed in the United States, but selected immunosuppressed children are likely to benefit. This vaccine has not been used widely because varicella is generally a mild disease.

Rationale for Immunizations

Parents sometimes question or do not understand the purpose of immunizations or how the immunization works to protect the body from the particular disease. Parents need explanations to help them understand that the body's immune system does not provide perfect protection from all diseases and that immunity does not occur unless the individual either experiences the disease (natural immunity) or receives an agent (by injection or orally) to stimulate the body into producing antibodies (acquired immunity). The immunizing agent is a strain of the infection-causing virus or bacteria, in either a dead or attenuated state that is incapable of causing the full blown disease. These dead or attenuated strains serve as antigens to the body, resulting in the production of antibodies making the individual resistant to the disease when exposed to the specific live virus or bacteria. (See Chapter 43 for further discussion of the immune response in relation to disease.)

It must be stressed to family members that although immunizations begin during infancy, they require boosters in later life. For some infections, boosters are necessary periodically throughout life to keep antibody titers effectively high. It is helpful and important to keep an immunization record for each family member to aid in keeping immunizations current.

The most obvious rationale for immunizing all children is to prevent unnecessary discomfort, disability, and potential mortality that can result when children get communicable diseases. It seems unreasonable to place a child's health at the risk of sterility, as a consequence of mumps, or of paralysis, as a result of poliomyelitis.

Another rationale is the threat that the presence of such diseases causes to others in society. Risks include (1) congenital malformations of the fetus if an unimmunized pregnant woman is exposed to a child with rubella; (2) more severe side effects to unimmunized adults who might contract these infectious diseases from children; (3) infants coming in contact with the disease who are too young to be immunized but too old to still have neonatal immunity; (4) the potentially fatal consequence for those children with diseases that do not permit them the privilege of receiving immunizations; and (5) the hazardous effects to elderly persons with already compromised health states.

Another rationale relates to cost factors. Today more than 60 per cent of married women work, and more than 40 per cent of families are managed by a single parent who works. Because unimmunized children who contract these diseases must be isolated, it means loss of work time for a parent or extra cost to hire home care while the child is excluded from day care or school. There is also the cost of medical care to supervise the child's illness and medication to relieve symptoms. There are also costs to the child who must be absent from school and who falls behind the class in academic and social activities. An even greater cost is incurred by the child if complications occur, which can extend the illness and discomfort and potentially result in permanent disabilities.

These are significant reasons for achieving the immunization of all children. Health care providers, particularly those caring for children, must recognize the importance of assessing the immunization status of all individuals and their responsibility in educating parents and children regarding the rationale for immunizations and providing information about how to obtain immunizations within the local community.

Legislative and Societal Actions

Governmental involvement in the issue of mass immunization has existed in varying degrees since the first vaccine was discovered. The Federal Food and Drug Administration approves and regulates the vaccines available for use on human beings. The government budget continues to include financial support for research into the development, refinement, and effectiveness of various vaccines. The World Health Organization continually studies the issue of immunizable diseases around the world, developing and recommending policies for countries to adopt and enforce. Governments, religious and health based organizations, and social cause groups have organized and funded mass public immunization programs. Within the United States, the Department of Health, Education and Welfare (now the Department of Health and Human Services) in 1977 instituted a national campaign to improve and maintain the immunization levels of children in America (Paskert, 1983). By late 1983, a 90 per cent overall immunization level had been achieved in the school-age population through legislative regulation of immunization requirements for school attendance. The current need is to focus on the preschool and infant populations in which immunization levels are substantially lower. Some measures are now being taken in which pediatric nurses can be actively involved: (1) increasing the number of health care provider–based immunization programs (independent nursing practices, pediatrician practices, health maintenance organizations, walk-in mediclinics, and so on) rather than continual dependence on government-organized programs; (2) increasing hospital, prenatal, and well baby clinic-based education programs for parents of newborns and infants; and (3) acquiring cooperation of day care, nursery school, and preschool programs to enforce proof of immunization as a prerequisite for attendance, similar to the school system.

One of the problems in achieving full immunization of children relates to the highly mobile society in which we live. A concept being considered, which has been used successfully in some European countries, is a computer-assisted, centralized immunization registry (Loeser et al, 1983). With this system, a child's name would be entered at birth. The health care provider would then input into the system each time a child receives an immunization (this is, of course, one of the potential downfalls of the system's success, as it depends on the health care provider's commitment in updating information). If a child does not receive a particular immunization or a dose in a series within 3 months after the desirable time, a printout reminder is provided to the health care provider. The cost of operating such a system is relatively inexpensive—approximately 65 cents per child per year. Once the child becomes of school age, the proof of immunization required in the school system takes over as a monitoring method.

While society as a whole supports immunization of all children, each individual family is still responsible for ensuring that immunizations are obtained by its members. Noncompliance tends most often to be associated with ignorance or misunderstandings regarding the rationale for immunizations and the potentially serious consequences of not taking such preventive actions. Many families are unaware of what immunizations are needed, when they should be received, or where they may be obtained. With so many dual-career and single working parent family units, the problem is sometimes a lack of accessibility during evening or week-end hours when parents are not at work. This is especially true in smaller communities and rural communities that do not have access to the multiplicity of medical services or to the 24-hour availability of services that exists in large cities.

Families cannot be held totally accountable for the underimmunization of infant and preschool children, however. All health care providers have not taken seriously their part of the responsibility of promoting preventive immunizations among their patients. Assessment and education regarding immunizations needs to become an automatic part of every contact with a pediatric patient, regardless of the reason for that particular contact.

Managing Immunization Reactions

The pediatric nurse should assess certain factors before administering an immunization. First, is the child acutely ill? If so, immunization should be deferred. Has the child experienced any reaction to a previous dose of the immunization? If so, subsequent doses should be given with caution or, in some cases, not given at all. Rubella vaccine is contraindicated during pregnancy. Live virus vaccines should not be given to patients with malignancies, who are pregnant, or who are immunologically compromised.

Some children do experience reactions to particular immunization vaccines. These reactions may be relatively immediate and short-term or, rarely, long-term in the form of residual effects (usually related to central nervous system function). The reaction may be localized at the injection site or systemic. It must be emphasized that rarely are reactions serious in nature. If this were the case, the vaccine would not have FDA approval and would not be advocated for mass usage.

Typically reactions can be prevented or promptly ameliorated by simple measures. The nurse should discuss both the possible reactions and interventions with the child and parents just prior to or immediately

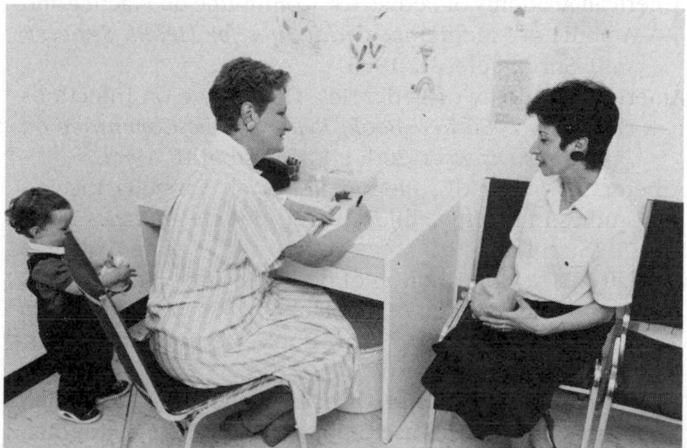

The upset that an injection causes to a child and parent may interfere with recall. Written information about what to expect and how to care for a child after an immunization can relieve a parent's anxiety at home.

after the immunization is given so they are reassured that the reaction, if one occurs, is not uncommon and is not cause for alarm. Table 14-4 identifies the common local/systemic reactions to childhood immunizations and appropriate preventive/alleviative measures. Reactions are more common in infants than in preschoolers, and more common in preschoolers than in older children (Christenson et al, 1983).

Increased publicity about adverse effects of routine childhood immunizations and concern about litigation have prompted the use of written information and consents prior to immunization. One survey of pediatricians reported that 62 per cent of pediatricians who give immunizations require a parent's signature as evidence of having received information and as consent for the immunization (Holt, 1987).

In summary, immunizations are one of the miracles of this century that can prevent a tremendous amount of discomfort and grief. An immunization program that is right for one population is not necessarily the most preferred for another at all times. For each immunization available, the cost and the benefits must be considered. Those responsible for establishing recommended schedules consider carefully (1) whether the costs involved in immunizing can be repaid monetarily or in social terms, or both; (2) how seriously and with what frequency the disease occurs in unimmunized populations; (3) what protection the immunization offers and for how long; and (4) what the risks of the vaccine itself are. All these factors are balanced against the benefits of eliminating the specific infection from the world population. The nurse has a role in all facets of these decisions, from the collection of epidemiologic data to the education of the public and the administration of immunizations to patients.

References

American Academy of Pediatrics, Committee on Infectious Diseases: Hemophilus type B polysaccharide vaccine. Unpublished paper, 1985.

American Academy of Pediatrics, Committee on Practice and Ambulatory Medicine: *Guidelines for Health Supervision.* Springfield, IL, 1985.

American Academy of Pediatrics, Committee on Infectious Diseases: *1986 Red Book; Report of the Committee on Infectious Diseases.* 20th ed. Evanston, IL, 1986.

Arbeter, AM, Starr SE, Plotkin SA, et al: Varicella vaccine studies in healthy children and adults. *Pediatrics* 1986; 78 (Suppl).

Breslau N: The contribution of pediatric nurse practitioners to child health care. *In* Breslau N: *Nurse Practitioners in Pediatrics.* Chicago, Year Book Medical Publishers, 1982.

Bureau of Communicable Disease Epidemiology, Laboratory Center for Disease Control: Statement on immunizing agents for the prevention of hepatitis. *CMAJ* 1987 Aug 15; 137:303–307.

Centers for Disease Control, Immunization Practices Advisory Committee (ACIP): Diphtheria, tetanus and pertussis: guidelines for vaccine prophylaxis and other preventive measures. *Morbid Mortal Weekly Report* 1985 Jun 12; 34:405–428.

Centers for Disease Control: Pertussis surveillance — United States, 1984 and 1985. *Morbid Mortal Weekly Report* 1987a Mar 27; 36:168–171.

Centers for Disease Control: Measles prevention. *Morbid Mortal Weekly Report* 1987b Jul 10; 36:409–425.

Centers for Disease Control: Update on hepatitis B prevention. *Morbid Mortal Weekly Report* 1987c Jun 19; 36:353–360.

Centers for Disease Control: Prevention of influenza. *Morbid Mortal Weekly Report* 1987d; 36:373–380.

Dosset JH: Immunizations. *In* Hoekelman RA, et al: *Primary Pediatric Care.* St. Louis, CV Mosby, 1987.

Holt VL, et al: Pediatricians' immunization consent practice in Washington state. *Am J Dis Child* 1987; 141:734–735.

Leach P: *The Childcare Encyclopedia.* New York, Alfred Knopf, 1984.

Loeser H, et al: The organization and evaluation of a computer-assisted, centralized immunization registry. *Am J Public Health* 1983 Nov; 1298–1301.

Melnick JL: Vaccination against poliomyelitis: present possibilities and future prospects. *Am J Public Health* 1988 Mar; 78(3):304–305.

Mortimer EA: Preventive pediatrics and epidemiology. *In* Behrman RE, Vaughan VC: *Nelson Textbook of Pediatrics.* Philadelphia, WB Saunders, 1987.

National Advisory Committee on Immunizations: *A Guide to Immunizations for Canadians.* 2nd ed. Ottawa, Health Protection Branch Laboratory, Center for Disease Control, 1984.

Paskert C: Progress and focus on the national childhood immunization program. *J School Health* 1983 Aug; 357–359.

Plotkin SA: Varicella vaccine: a point of discussion. *Pediatrics* 1986; 78(4):705–707.

Ryberg J, Merrifield E: What parents want to know. *Nurse Pract* 1984 Jun; 24–33.

Salk D: Polio immunization policy in the United States: a new challenge for a new generation. *Am J Public Health* 1988 Mar; 78(3):296–300.

Walker AM, Hershel PH, Perera DR, et al: Diphtheria-tetanus-pertussis immunization and sudden infant death syndrome. *Am J Public Health* 1987 Aug; 77(8):945–951.

Bibliography

American Academy of Pediatrics, Committee on Infectious Diseases: Pertussis vaccine. *Pediatrics* 1984 Aug; 303–305.

Barkin R, et al: DTP reactions and serologic responses with a reduced dose schedule. *J Pediatr* 1984 Aug; 189–194.

Bernbaum JC, Daft A, Anolik R, et al: Response of preterm infants to diphtheria-tetanus-pertussis immunizations. *J Pediatr* 1985; 107(2):184–188.

Chamberlain R, et al: An evaluation of efforts to educate mother about child development in pediatric office practices. *Am J Public Health* 1979 Sep; 875–886.

Christenson B, et al: Mass vaccination programmes aimed at eradicating measles, mumps and rubella in Sweden: first experience. *Br Med J* 1983 Aug 6; 389–391.

De Canis A, Golin A: *The Interdisciplinary Health Care Team.* Germantown, MD, Aspen Systems Corporation, 1979.

Ford L: Nurse practitioners: history of a new idea and predictions for the future. *In* Aiken L (ed): *Nursing in the 1980's: Crises, Opportunities and Challenges.* Philadelphia, JB Lippincott, 1982.

Frank T, et al: Pertussis immunizations? *Pediatr Nurs* 1984 Sep/Oct; 360.

Hinman A: The pertussis vaccine controversy. *Public Health Reports* 1984 May/Jun; 255–259.

Hinman AR, Koplan JP, Orenstein WA, et al: Live or inactivated poliomyelitis vaccine: an analysis of benefits and risks. *Am J Public Health* 1988 Mar; 78(3):291–295.

Linley J: Mother's attitudes regarding health care for their children. *MCN* 1984 Jan/Feb; 37–39.

Loening W, Coovadia H: Age-specific occurrence rates of measles in urban, peri-urban and rural environments: implications of time of vaccination. *Lancet* 1983 Aug 6; 324–326.

Murphy M, et al: Effect of early immunization on antibody response to immunization with measles vaccine as demonstrated by enzyme-linked immunosorbent assay. *Pediatrics* 1984 Jul; 90–93.

National Advisory Committee on Immunization (NACI). Statement on tetanus toxoid. *Can Dis Weekly Report* 1987 Aug 1; 13(6):135–138.

Osborn L: Group well-child care: an option for today's children. *Pediatr Nurs* 1982 Sep/Oct; 306–308.

Pajares K, et al: Rubella vaccination. *Pediatr Nurs* 1984 Jan/Feb; 72.

Pinchen C: Whooping cough: swings and roundabouts—pros and cons of the vaccine. *Nurs Mirror* 1982 Dec 8; 24–28.

Reisinger K, Bires J: Anticipatory guidance in pediatric practice. *Pediatrics* 1980 Jun; 889.

Rudy C: Communicating with families through a pediatric newsletter. *Pediatr Nurs* 1982 Sep/Oct; 3394.

Ryber J, Merrifield E: A questionnaire for assessment of parents' needs in a child health clinic. *Pediatr Nurs* 1982 Sep/Oct; 318–319.

Salomon ME, et al: Evaluation of the two-needle strategy for reducing reactions to DPT vaccination. *Am J Dis Child* 1987; 141:796–798.

Stetler H, et al: Severe local reactions to live measles virus vaccine following an immunization program. *Am J Public Health* 1983 Aug; 899–900.

Swarts T, et al: Comparison of inactivated polio virus vaccine and oral polio virus vaccine programs in Israel. *Rev Infect Dis* 1984 May–Jun; S556–561.

US Department of Health and Human Services: *Health Information for International Travel, 1987.* HHS Publication No. (CDC) 85-8280, Centers for Disease Control, May, 1987.

Uzark K, et al: Primary preventive health care in children with heart disease. *Pediatr Cardiol* 1983 Oct/Dec; 259–263.

Weidermann G, et al: Risks and benefits of vaccination. *Infect Control* 1984 Sep; 438–444.

Yvonnet B, et al: Immunologic effect of hepatitis B vaccine in children: comparison of two and three dose protocols. *J Med Virol* 1984 Mar/Apr; 137–139.

Assessing Child Health

Chapter 15

Janet Hadley

A vital component of the nursing process is the nursing assessment, which consists of evaluating the quality of current health status. This is done by gathering data from the interview and physical assessment and from diagnostic and developmental testing. The assessment must be multifocal to be complete and should include an evaluation of family dynamics as well as any cultural, sociologic, environmental, and religious variables that may affect the child's physical and emotional development. The goal of a comprehensive assessment is to evaluate a child's physical, intellectual, and emotional/social competence. These three categories of competence, therefore, provide the framework upon which the assessment process is structured.

Related Topics
Child development, Unit 2
Family genogram, Chapter 4
Immunization schedule, Chapter 14
Dietary history, Chapter 18
Nutritional requirements at various ages, Chapter 18
Development of visual acuity, Chapter 51

Documentation of Nursing Assessment

The information gathered by the nurse is the database. This database must be recorded in a systematic way so that other members of the health care team can use it. Each work setting has its own system for recording information, however, the following components are universally accepted as those needing to be documented:

- subjective data—history;
- objective data—physical examination, developmental assessment, screening tests, laboratory tests;
- analysis—nursing diagnosis;
- plan—nursing strategies

Taking a History

Gathering historical information will provide the nurse with the majority of the data necessary to assess overall health status. From these data the nurse will decide first what components of the physical assessment must be carried out. Then, from both the history and the physical assessment, the nurse determines what diagnostic and developmental testing needs to be done.

Historical information is gathered from two sources—the existing medical record and the interview of parent and child. A review of the medical record is done quite simply. The interview is more complex and requires attention to specific points.

Interviewing

The interview is a time for the nurse to establish a trusting relationship with both the child and parent. It should be conducted in a private, quiet, comfortable room. For younger children, all evidence of invasive, potentially painful equipment should be concealed until necessary for examination. The interview should not begin until the nurse has been introduced and explains what is about to happen.

There are several kinds of interviews, each devised to meet different needs and situations. The three types of interviews are the well-child interview, the problem interview, and the therapeutic interview.

The *well-child interview* is most frequently conducted by nurses and pediatricians working in ambulatory care settings. Initially, it includes a complete history, which is updated on subsequent visits. After completing the health history and the physical examination, the careprovider offers the child and family guidance on nutrition, safety, and growth and development.

The *problem interview*, also known as the interim health history, focuses on an immediate physical, social, or emotional problem that has been identified by the family, child, or the health care provider. Information obtained pertains primarily to a specific problem but should not be restricted to the problem. Sufficient data should be collected so that the nurse can determine the general health status of the child. The length of time of this interview varies with the particular circumstances. If the child is seen for regular well-child visits, the interview may be relatively brief. If the family generally seeks health care only when problems arise, the nurse is responsible for obtaining a total health history.

Once a problem has been identified and management begun a *therapeutic interview* may be needed. This is generally used to obtain information about how a problem—especially one that is persistent, complex, or long term—is responding to treatment.

The interview approach should be based on the developmental levels of the child and the adult. Questions should be asked in a clear and concise manner, avoiding use of jargon and medical terminology. They should also be asked in a way that is nonthreatening and nonjudgmental. For example, instead of asking the child, "Are you having any problems in school?" the nurse may ask, "What is school like for you?" This approach does not judge or threaten the child by presupposing a problem or making the child feel inferior.

The way questions are asked is very important. The type of questions may either facilitate the interview process or make it difficult and tedious. One example is the use of open as opposed to closed questions. Open questions allow the child or parent the opportunity to express views, opinions, thoughts, and feelings. The closed question does just the opposite—instead of developing rapport, it can make the interview too clinical and concise if used excessively. An example of a close-ended question would be, "Do you like school?" This allows for only a yes or no answer.

There are also direct and indirect questions. Direct questions are stated in a manner that generally require a yes or no answer or specific information, such as, "How old are you?" and "When did Amy first sit alone?"

Indirect questions do not sound like questions. They permit the client to select or elaborate on information. For example, "You must have some thoughts about discipline," or "It must be difficult to have twins" are indirect questions. They do not end in question marks but obviously invite a response. Such questions express the interviewer's interest in the child and family and offer another way to gather information.

The response to such questions gives the nurse an opportunity to learn more about a client's perception of a situation as well as information about the client's communication style.

There is another type of question that is particularly helpful to use when the nurse needs to gain the cooperation of a child for a physical examination. These are double questions. They provide the child with the opportunity to choose between two alternatives. An example would be, "Do you want me to examine your ears or nose first?" Such questions enable the child to control part of the examination, thus providing a sense of security and lessening the anxiety.

Almost every interview will contain a variety of these questions. The style of questioning will depend upon the type of information that is needed by the interviewer. Certain kinds of data lend themselves to particular techniques. For example, direct questions may be used when collecting the data in the review of body systems, whereas an open-ended question may be better when collecting data about family or social relationships. When an indirect, open-ended approach does not produce the information desired, more direct or close-ended questions may be more successful.

In addition to being able to employ a variety of questioning styles, the nurse must also be an active listener in order to conduct a successful interview. The nurse must listen carefully for what is said, what is implied, and what is omitted. Throughout the interview the nurse will need to ask for clarification of client answers. At the end of the interview the nurse should present the child and family with a summary of perceptions based upon the information gathered. This will allow the interviewee to clear up any misinterpreted statements.

Both developmental stage and age of a child are additional considerations in interviewing. The preschooler is verbal enough to tell the nurse about daily routines if questions are put in terms that can be understood. The preschooler may also be able to locate discomforts or sensations if they are being experienced during the interview or examination (e.g., stomachache); however, an accurate recall of past sensations may be vague at this age. Optimal cooperation can be more easily obtained when parents remain present throughout the interview and examination of preschoolers.

School-age children can provide the majority of current information about themselves and their family, school, and daily lives. The older school-age child can be a significant informant about health history and systems review. Encouraging an older school-age child to participate in the interview conveys to the child a sense of competence and reliability as a health care consumer. Parents can remain present during most of the interview; however, the school-age child should have some time alone with the nurse so that concerns that may not be expressed comfortably in front of a parent may be expressed to the nurse. Whether or not the parent is present during the physical examination should be decided during the child's time alone with the nurse. The child's decision should not be influenced by the parent's presence.

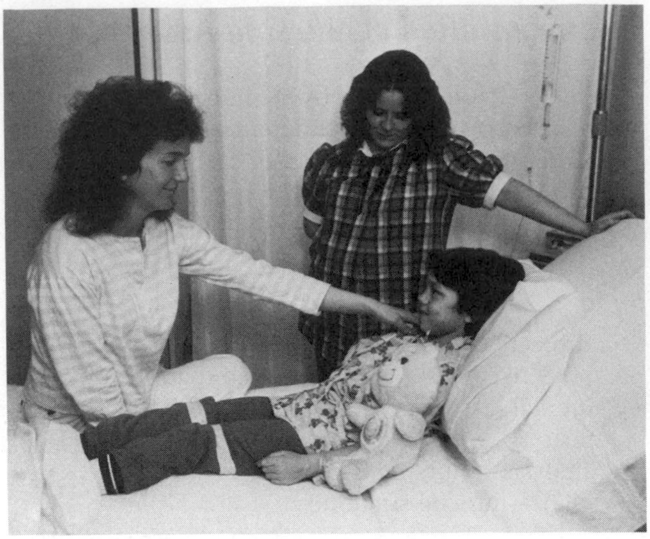

"Do you want me to examine your ears or your nose first?"

Generally, the adolescent can be independent in contributing the necessary information to the interview. Once the interview is complete and the examination done the clinical summary and planned management should be shared first with the youth and then with the youth and parent together.

Finally, the interviewer must be tuned into the nonverbal component of the interview. While actively listening to the parent and the child, the nurse should be aware of clients' body postures and facial expressions. The nurse should specifically watch to see how well the verbal message matches the nonverbal cue. An example of this may be verbal expressions of joy and contentment about a parent's relationship with a child and noticing a strained expression and rough handling of a child during an office visit.

In summary, the successful interview requires multiple skills and techniques. The interviewer must first establish appropriate environmental conditions and a rapport with the parent and child. Next, the nurse must use a sound knowledge of growth and development, a variety of direct and indirect question techniques, and appropriate verbal and nonverbal communication skills. By using all of these skills and techniques the nurse can glean from the family the information necessary to assess overall health status.

The Health History

The following discussion focuses on the type of information obtained in each category of a pediatric history. (See Box 15-1 for an example of history format.) It is one approach for gathering data in an organized manner. Titles may vary in different settings, but the con tent usually remains unchanged.

Demographic Data

This is the data that identifies the patient. Usually, it is found in the chart and need only be verified by the interviewer. Both the informant and the informant's reliability should be noted. If the child is one of the historians, note that also.

Reason for Contact (Chief Complaint)

This is the specific reason for the visit to the office, clinic, or hospital. It is a brief statement recorded in the child's or parent's own words. If there are multiple problems, the informants may have to identify the one problem that caused them to seek health care at this time.

Box 15-1
Pediatric History-Taking Outline

DEMOGRAPHIC DATA

Date of interview
Name (nickname or preferred name)
Address
Date and place of birth
Sex
Age
Race/Nationality
Religion
Primary language spoken
First names of parents
Source and reliability of informant(s)

REASON FOR CONTACT (CHIEF COMPLAINT)

1. Statement in child's or informant's own words of the reason health care is presently being sought—problem or symptom.

PRESENT ILLNESS (ANALYSIS OF CHIEF COMPLAINT)

1. Onset—events coincident with onset, sudden or gradual, previous episodes, when began.
2. Characteristics of chief complaint (analysis)
   a. Type, or *character*, of complaint (pain: dull, sharp, aching, burning, radiating, itching, tickling).
   b. *Location* (if applicable). Should be anatomically precise (ask child to point to affected area).
   c. *Severity* (annoying, uncomfortable, incapacitating) and effect on normal daily activities (eating, sleeping, elimination, playing mood).
   d. *Duration* (intermittent, persistent or continuous, interval between if intermittent).
   e. *Influencing factors* (precipitating, aggravating, relieving, ameliorating, recent illness exposure).
   f. *Past treatment* or evaluation of complaint. (When, where, and by whom, what studies were performed in the past and what were the results [blood studies, x-ray, etc.], results of past treatment, past diagnosis).
   g. *Current treatment* or evaluation of the complaint (treatment, medications, tests) and response of condition to these measures.
3. Present status of complaint (getting worse, better, unchanged).
4. Reason for seeking care now.

FAMILY PROFILE

1. Family members
2. Familial and hereditary diseases
   a. Glaucoma, cataracts, other eye disorders
   b. Tuberculosis, asthma, heart disease, hypertension
   c. Ulcers, colitis
   d. Kidney disease
   e. Arthritis, muscular dystrophy
   f. Mental disorder, epilepsy, learning disorders
   g. Allergies, diabetes, sickle cell disease, cancer, congenital anomalies
3. Family social history (see Box 15-2)
   a. Finances
   b. Resources
   c. Family relationships
   d. Residence
   e. Health attitudes and practices

PAST HEALTH HISTORY

Birth History (prenatal)

1. Mother's state of health during pregnancy
   a. Illnesses (fever, rash, vomiting, infection); month in pregnancy when occurred; treatment prescribed.
   b. Hospitalizations; month in pregnancy when hospitalized; treatment prescribed.
   c. X-rays; month in pregnancy when taken.
   d. Medications taken (over-the-counter or prescribed); month in pregnancy when taken; reason(s) taken.
   e. Diet during pregnancy; amount of weight gained.

Continued

2. Previous obstetrical history
   a. Gravida including this pregnancy
   b. Para including this pregnancy
   c. How long before this pregnancy were there any stillbirths, abortions or miscarriages and their causes, if known?
   d. Have any live-born children died? How long before this pregnancy and cause if known?
   e. Length of this pregnancy
3. Prenatal care received
   a. Mother's age with this pregnancy
   b. When was prenatal care initiated and for how much of pregnancy was it maintained?
   c. Bleeding or complications (toxemia) during this pregnancy and blood type of both parents
4. Attitude toward this pregnancy
   a. Mother describes as easy or difficult pregnancy
   b. Planned or unplanned pregnancy
   c. Child wanted by either or both parents

Birth History (Natal)

1. Circumstances of birth
   a. Where was baby born (e.g., home, birthing room, hospital)?
   b. Natural or induced labor; length of labor; any problems during labor
   c. Was fetal monitoring used? Why?
   d. Any drugs given during labor?
2. Characteristics of delivery
   a. Natural, assisted (forceps used) or C section delivery
   b. Was the father present?
   c. Mother awake during delivery?
   d. Was baby in normal position? Breech?
3. Condition of baby at birth
   a. Birth weight
   b. APGAR score
   c. Did baby cry immediately?
   d. Was mechanical suctioning or oxygen required? Was baby intubated?
   e. Was the baby put in an incubator?
   f. Any abnormalities noted at birth?

Birth History (Postnatal)

1. Weight loss or gains and amount during hospital stay
2. Any difficulties during stay in nursery (Feeding or sucking problems; cyanosis, jaundice, rashes)?
3. Length of baby's hospital stay? Nursery or rooming in? Baby and Mother went home together?
4. Feeding method
5. If male, circumcised?

Past Illnesses

Accidents
1. Age at each accident
2. Circumstances surrounding accident (cause, where occurred)
3. Facts regarding accident
   Extent of injury
   Treatment received
   Complications or residual problems
   Child's reaction
4. Any current problems associated with accident(s)?

Illnesses
1. Names of illnesses or infections
   Age when occurred
   Treatment received
   Complications or sequelae
2. Names of childhood diseases
   Age
   Severity
   Treatment
   Residual problems

Operations
1. Date and age at each operation
2. Why was surgery done?
3. Outcome of surgery
4. Child's reaction to each surgery
5. Any follow-up or complications?

Hospitalizations
1. Reason for each hospitalization
2. Dates and child's age at each
3. Length of each
4. Child's reaction to hospitalization(s)
5. Outcome
6. Complications

Allergies
1. Untoward response to medications, foods, animals, insect bites
2. Type of reaction (Hives, rash, swelling, rhinitis, nausea)
3. Do symptoms occur seasonally?
4. Do symptoms occur immediately or a few to several hours after exposure?

Immunizations

1. Type received
2. Dates received
3. Untoward reactions

DEVELOPMENTAL HISTORY

1. Motor development milestones
2. Language development milestones
3. Social development milestones
4. Current developmental status with regard to activities of daily living
   a. Diet
      How is child's's appetite?
      Bottle-fed? Breast-fed?
      If breast-fed, mother's diet and fluid intake? If bottle, what kind, how much, how formula mixed? Amount in 24 hours? Number of feedings in 24 hours, length of each feeding, how progressing? If taking solids, what kind, portion size, how often?
      What kinds of foods in diet—meats, vegetables, fruits, cereals, juices, eggs, milk, snacks? How often? What portion size? How does child eat (spoon, fork, fingers, knife)? How well does

child feed self? Is messy, neat? Does he or she use a cup?
When does child eat (alone, with family)?
Does child take vitamins (kind, how often, with or without iron)?
Food dislikes, food likes, food jags?

b. Elimination
What are child's bowel patterns? Frequency? Consistency? Discomfort?
Is child toilet trained? (At what age? Accidents? Day or night trained?) How was the child toilet trained?
Any associated stresses with elimination habits? Enuresis? (A more detailed history is found in the review of systems.)

c. Sleep
When does child go to bed? Does child sleep through night?
Nightmares, night terrors?
Difficulties with putting the child to bed?
How many hours does child sleep in 24 hours?
Naps (when, how long)? Difficulty falling asleep?
Insomnia? Where does child sleep? Does child have own bed?
How does the child awaken (alert, fussy)?
Any change in sleep patterns?

d. Development
How does child compare to siblings, peers?
What can child do now? (This should be age appropriate: 15-month-old walks, 3-year-old rides a tricycle, and so on.)
What new tasks has child accomplished since the last visit?:
What does child like to do? The developmental patterns should cover fine and gross motor activities, intellect and speech, and personal-social.
What kind of games does child like to play? How does child play with peers?

e. Personality/school performance
Unusual behaviors (thumbsucking, nail biting, masturbation)?
How does child describe herself or himself?
How does parent describe child's personality?
What are child's school interests? Grades?
School performance?
How does child interact with teachers, classmates?
How does child get along with family members?
What chores does child do?
What does child do when mad, sad, glad, scared?

f. Discipline
How is the child disciplined (verbal, physical)?
When is child disciplined? How often?

g. Sexuality
What questions is child asking?
What are parent's responses?
What is family's attitude toward masturbation, nudity?
What does child or adolescent know about secondary sexual development, sexuality, menstruation, sexual exploration?
Is child's/adolescent's information about STD and AIDS accurate?
Is adolescent sexually active? Using birth control (type, frequency of use, problems)?
Does the adolescent female know how to examine her breasts?

CHILD REVIEW OF SYSTEMS (SEE BOX 15-3)

1. General appearance
2. Skin and lymphatics
3. Eyes, ears, nose and throat
4. Cardiopulmonary system
5. Gastrointestinal system
6. Genitourinary system
7. Musculoskeletal system
8. Neurologic status

Present Illness

This portion of the history is obtained if the child presents with a specific problem. The problem may be physical, intellectual, or emotional/social. This portion of the history may be omitted if there is not a specific complaint. The present illness history consists of four components:

- a description of the onset and progression of the problem;
- identification of the characteristics of the problem;
- the present status of the problem;
- the reason for seeking health care at this time.

If more than one problem exists, they must be investigated in order of occurrence. See Box 15-1 for summary of the type of information to be gathered for these components of the present illness.

Family Profile

The primary purpose for obtaining a family health history is to discover potential hereditary or familial diseases that could affect the health of the child. The second purpose for a family health history is to identify possible stress factors that could affect the child and the family. A recent death or chronic illness of one of the family members may interfere with the normal function and developmental progress of the child. The family health history may be represented in written form or pictorially by a genogram.

Family Members

A list or diagram of family members, including their ages, sexes, and states of health, should be made. If a genogram is used, a circle represents a female and a square represents a male. Marriage is represented by a horizontal line and a vertical line indicates a descend-

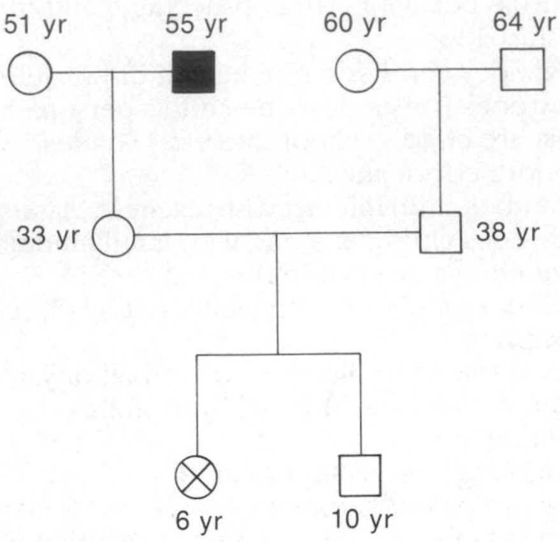

Figure 15-1. A family genogram.

ant. A blackened circle or square indicates that an individual is deceased. An "X" indicates the child or client with whom the health history is concerned. (See Figure 15-1 for an example of a basic family genogram.)

Familial or Hereditary Diseases

Information on existing or past conditions that are of a familial or hereditary nature in parents, grandparents, first aunts and uncles, and siblings should be obtained. A review of the specific problems noted in Box 15-1 will enable the nurse to identify the significant problems.

Family Social History

This portion of the history includes information on environmental, economic, personal, and social factors that influence the child's and family's overall development and health. Box 15-2 summarizes the pertinent data in this area, and the Home Observation for Measurement of the Environment (HOME) appears in Appendix Five. Much of the information requested in this section is of a sensitive and personal nature. It is important to recognize that an accurate family social history may come about only after the family has established a trusting relationship with the nurse.

Past Health History

Birth History

The birth history should include data concerning the mother's health during pregnancy, labor, and delivery, and the infant's condition immediately following birth. Box 15-1 lists questions that should be covered in a comprehensive birth history.

Past Illnesses

The past health history includes a summary of any diseases, accidents, operations, or hospitalizations that the child has experienced. Box 15-1 summarizes the questions to ask in order to document these experiences.

Box 15-2
Family Social History

FINANCES

1. Who is employed? Where? Occupation?
2. Does the family have enough money to do the things that are important to its members?
3. Are they receiving financial assistance (welfare, food stamps)?
4. Do they have health insurance?

EXTERNAL RESOURCES

1. What schools, day care or preschool facilities are being used?
2. Are there babysitters? How often used?

FAMILY RELATIONSHIPS

1. Who lives at home (parents, grandparents, significant others)?
2. What are the family interrelationships?
3. What is the marital status?
4. What is the home atmosphere like (happy, sad, cooperative, antagonistic, chaotic)?
5. Who shares in household chores?
6. Who within the family shares in caring for the children?
7. What is the level of education?
8. What are some of the family activities?
9. How were the parents disciplined as children?

RESIDENCE

1. Type of housing (house, apartment, room)?
2. Is there a yard and is it fenced?
3. Are there stairs?
4. Is a busy street nearby?
5. What is the proximity to transportation, shopping, playground, schools, health care facilities?
6. Is it a safe neighborhood?
7. Is there city or well water? Is it fluoridated?

HEALTH ATTITUDES AND PRACTICES

1. How does the family regard health services and personnel?
2. How is the family's role as health consumer perceived?
3. Who makes decisions about health issues, management of illness, when to seek health care?
4. What cultural or religious traditions exist that affect health care or childrearing practices?
5. What is the family's attitudes and participation in preventive health practices?
6. How is safety stressed in home and family living?

Immunizations

The types and dates of the child's immunizations should be noted. Pay special attention to children who have immigrated to the United States since they may have had immunizations that are not routinely administered in America. Any reactions to the immunizations and the treatment that followed should also be noted. A record of tuberculin skin testing is included with the immunizations. If a child has not been immunized for a specific reason (e.g., chronic illness, immunodeficiency, religious beliefs), it should also be noted in this section. Chapter 14 summarizes the recommended schedule of immunizations for infants and children.

Developmental History

Documentation of the age at which the child mastered developmental milestones is included in the health history. Although parental recall may be hazy, such information may give insight into a current abnormality. Milestones usually recorded include motor, language, and social development. These vary according to age and are reviewed in the growth and development chapters, 5 through 9, in Unit Two.

A review of the child's current developmental status is also summarized, particularly with regard to skills relevant to daily living (Box 15-1). Special questions asked will depend on the child's age and development.

Review of Systems

The review of systems is done for a complete database in a well child as well as for a child who presents with an illness or specific complaint. It focuses attention on any deviations from health, thus allowing the nurse a more comprehensive picture of the child's health status and potential problems. The information received in this part of the history is invaluable even when it may appear unrelated to the problem at hand. Box 15-3 is an outline of suggested areas for review of each body system. The nurse should use terms that are easily understood by the parent and child. The questions will vary depending on the age and developmental level of the child.

Box 15-3
Outline of Review of Systems

GENERAL

Overall state of health? Fatigue? Growth patterns? Recent or unexplained weight loss or weight gain? Contributing factors (illness, dieting, change in appetite)? Fevers? Chills? Exercise tolerance? General liability to perform normal daily functions?

SKIN AND LYMPH

Skin problem such as excessive dryness, pruritus, skin sensitivity? Rashes? Acne? Skin color changes? Tendency for bruising? Petechiae? Abnormalities of nail color, nail growth? Hair loss? Hair color change? Use of hair dyes, chemicals for hair straightening? Swollen lymph glands?

EYES

Known visual problems? Behaviors that may indicate visual problems: turning head to one side, sitting close to the television set,* squinting, rubbing the eyes, bumping into objects? Crossed eyes (strabismus)? Lazy eye (amblyopia)? Wears glasses or contact lenses? Eye infections? Excessive tearing or absence of tears? Burning? Edema of eyelids? Redness?

EARS

Earaches, ear infections, ear discharge? Hearing loss? Behaviors that may indicate this: turning radio or television very loud, requests to repeat in conversation, loud speech, inattentive behavior, decreased or no response to loud noises?

NOSE

Nosebleeds (episodic, recurrent, severe)? Frequent nasal congestion or runny nose? Nasal obstruction or difficulty with breathing? Frequent sneezing, sinus pain, sinus infections?

THROAT

Mouth breathing? Bleeding gums? Toothaches? Teething? Sore throats, infections, strep throats? Hoarseness? Difficulty swallowing?

CARDIORESPIRATORY

Trouble breathing, choking, turning blue? Difficulty feeding, tires easily, difficulty running or playing? Cough (where, when, position, wet, dry)? Wheezing? Keeps up with other children? Number of colds per year? Heart murmur? Anemia? Date and result of last blood count? Blood type? Blood transfusion? Rheumatic fever?

* Young children tend to sit close to TV even though no visual problem exists. In school-age or older children it may indicate a visual problem.

Continued

GASTROINTESTINAL

Bowel patterns, frequency, color, discomfort? Abdominal pain, diarrhea, constipation? Flatulence, bloody stools, bleeding, fissures, nausea, vomiting?

GENITOURINARY

Urinary stream, frequency, pain on urination, urgency, periods of dryness (as opposed to dribbling or constant wetness), bleeding, enuresis? Menstruation (when started, how often, amount, length of each menses, discomfort, problems)? Vaginal discharge, pruritus? Pain or discharge from penis? Swelling or pain of testicles? Change in testicular and penile size? Pubic hair?

MUSCULOSKELETAL

Weakness, history of fractures, strains, sprains? Painful joints, swelling, redness of joints? Clumsiness, lack of coordination, tremors, abnormal gait, restricted or painful movement?

NEUROLOGICAL

Convulsions, febrile seizures? Fainting, tremors, twitches, blackouts, dizziness, frequent headaches? Learning problems, clumsiness, coordination problems? Numbness, memory loss, speech problems, unusual habits? Taste, tactile sense? Sees, hears, smells?

Physical Assessment

Approaching the Child

There are seven key issues in approaching a child for a physical assessment:

- the atmosphere must be comfortable;
- the examination must be done quickly;
- the child's modesty must be respected;
- the examiner must take advantage of opportunities for assessment as they arise;
- the procedures need to be explained before they are done;
- the examination must be done systematically; and, lastly,
- the examiner must be skilled in the assessment techniques and have a good knowledge base in anatomy as well as child development.

Incorporating all of these components into the examination routine comes about after much practice. However, paying attention to all seven points should help minimize the child's anxiety about the examination.

Providing a comfortable environment will vary for each age group. An infant needs a warm room; a preschooler needs some toys with which to play; a school-age child may need some books to read.

Doing an examination quickly requires preparation. Before beginning the examination the nurse should develop a mental outline of the steps of the exam and prepare a list of significant findings for that system. The examination can then be conducted very quickly.

For example, if a child presents with a complaint of an earache the nurse would outline the following check list before beginning with the examination:

- Is the external ear normal in appearance?
- Is the ear canal patent?
- Is the tympanic membrane normal in appearance?
- Is the tympanic membrane mobile?

Children at any age may exhibit modesty that must be respected. Beginning in toddlerhood, all children should be offered cover gowns to wear during the examination. School-age children and adolescents will need the opportunity to dress and undress in privacy. A helpful technique with young children is to have them remove one article of clothing at a time. For example, most children will readily remove shoes and socks. The nurse can then examine the feet. Next, the child could remove pants or skirt and then be examined from the waist down. Cooperation may be extended by allowing the child to replace pants or skirt before removing shirt or blouse. Finally, children ranging in age from toddlers to adolescents usually dislike being without underwear. Often, an adequate examination of buttocks, anus, and genitalia can be done by merely pulling the undergarment to the side while inspecting the perineum.

It is helpful to take full advantage of opportunities as they arise. For example, the nurse could listen to a small child's heart and lungs when the child is lying quietly in the parent's arms because the child may begin to cry later during the examination. Other examples would be to observe the child's neurologic and growth and developmental status while the child plays with toys in the examination room. The nurse may also listen to speech and articulation as the child converses with siblings or parents.

Many children like to be involved in the health examination. This interest offers the nurse the opportunity to explain the examination to the child. The explanation given will vary with the child's ability to

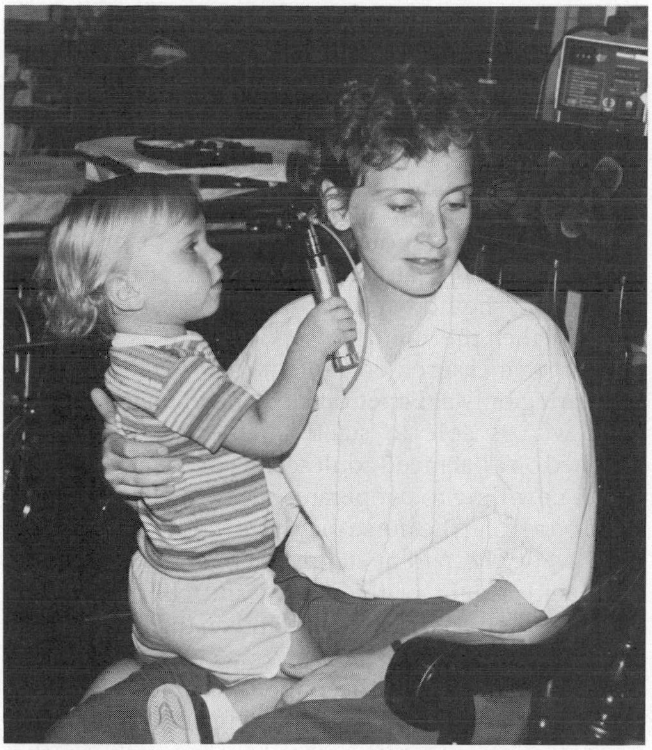

The young child may enjoy handling the equipment used for the examination and may become more confident and cooperative if allowed to examine an adult.

understand. The message needs to be simple, concise, and honest. Examples of appropriate statements may be: "I need to check your teeth to see if you are taking good care of them," or "I need to look inside your ears so I can learn about your hearing. It will not hurt, but it will feel a little funny when I give you a tiny puff of air." In addition to a verbal explanation, a child may be more cooperative if allowed to handle the equipment that will be used for the examination.

Very young children may be more cooperative if the examination is presented as a game. The toddler may enjoy playing "this little piggy went to market . . . " when the feet are examined. When palpating the abdomen, the nurse may say, "See if I can guess what you had for breakfast." If the right food is guessed, the child is delighted and generally enthralled with the process of the guessing game.

The younger school-age child may like to listen to the heart sounds. The young child may enjoy handling the equipment that will be used for the examination and may become more confident and cooperative if allowed to examine a doll or an adult. Other techniques that are sometimes helpful include the use of dolls, puppets, and stories. Sometimes pretending to examine the mother or a sibling first will also help a child to gain the necessary trust and to become cooperative.

Finally, despite multiple efforts to facilitate cooperation the child may have to be restrained or positioned for the examination to take place. The child may be held in the nurse's or a parent's lap for the abdominal and musculoskeletal examination. The parent may also need to hold the child's head against his or her shoulder for the ear examination. The ear examination can also be conducted with the child supine on the examination table while the parent restrains the knees and an assistant holds the child's arms extended straight up beside the head. The examiner then has only to control the head and otoscope. No child should be restrained without an explanation and the child should never be scolded for resisting restraint. See Figures 15-2 and 15-3 for examples of restraint.

The nurse may be able to anticipate the child's ability to cooperate by merely asking the child where the examination should take place—in the parent's lap or on the examination table. In a recent study, Moss (1983) found that children between the ages of 2 and 3 years that chose to be examined on the examination table were *always* cooperative, whereas children who chose to be examined in the parent's lap were coopera-

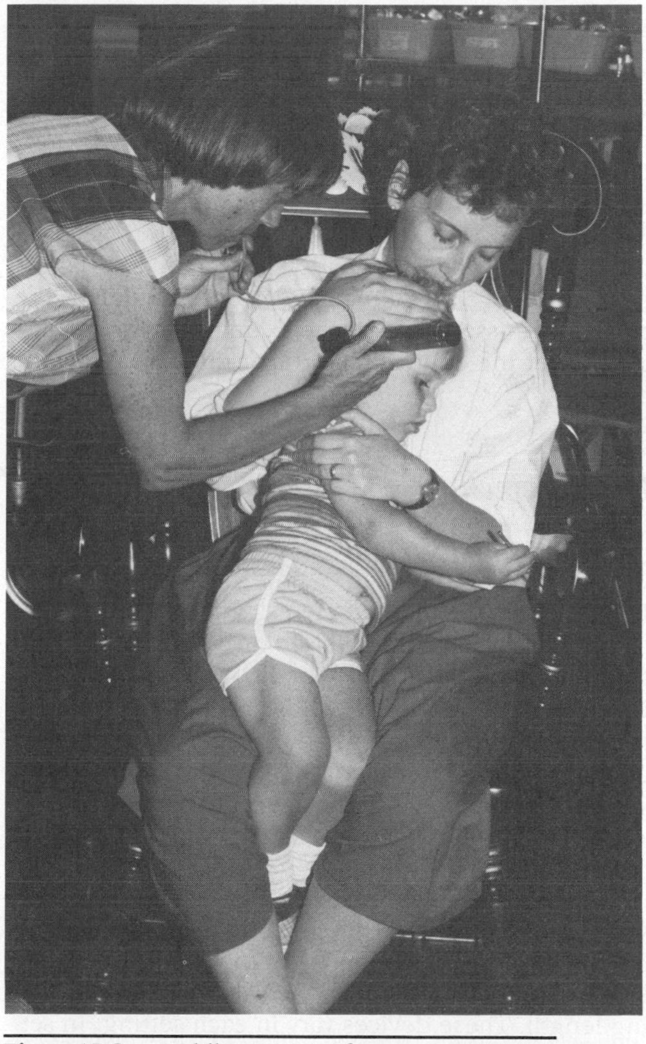

Figure 15-2. Toddler restraint for ear examination.

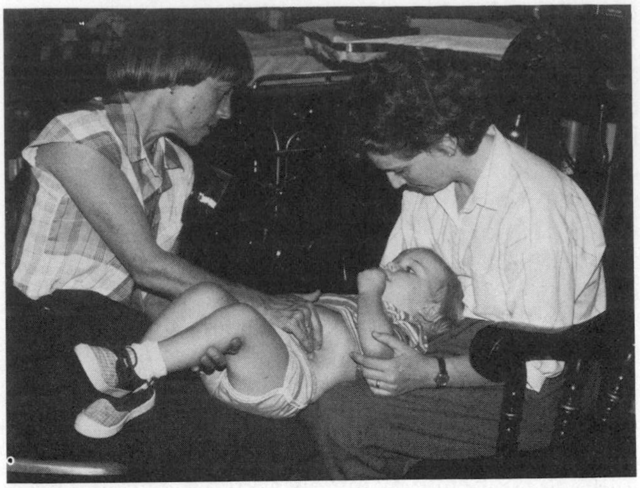

Figure 15-3. Toddler restraint for abdominal examination.

tive 50 per cent of the time. (This should not be interpreted to mean that the parent's lap is a less desirable form of restraint, since it may be that a child who chooses the table is different from one who chooses a parent's lap.)

The final key issue in physical assessment is for the nurse to develop a systematic approach to the examination. Although opportunities may present themselves for some physical evaluation (e.g., examining the child's heart and lungs while quiet in the mother's arms), the nurse should develop a routine that is adhered to for every examination. This may be a head-to-toe or toe-to-head examination or examination in another order. This systematic approach minimizes the chance of missing parts of the examination due to distraction of the child's behavior or the parent's questions.

Measurements

Height and Weight

For the child, the measurements of height and weight should be obtained and plotted on a standardized anthropometric chart at each physical examination. This is usually done at all well-child visits—approximately five times during the first year of life and once or twice a year thereafter through adolescence. Height and weight measurements reflect overall growth of the child. (See Appendices Two and Three for height and weight charts.)

The method of measuring the child's height varies with age. The preferred method for the infant or young child is to place the child in a supine position with the knees extended and to use a special device for measuring length. These devices vary in each setting. In settings where a measuring device is not available, an infant or young child can be placed in the supine position, and the nurse can mark (on the exam table paper) where the child's head and feet are and then measure the distance between the two points. The older child (after 2 years of age) can stand on a standard balanced scale with a movable rod or be measured against a wall-mounted measuring device.

Weight is also an important index of the child's growth and should be measured with every examination whether the child is well or ill. It is an easily obtainable measurement. Infants are weighed naked or wearing only a diaper on a balanced infant scale. A child who is able to stand independently may be weighed on a balanced adult scale. For the child who is afraid, unwilling to cooperate, or physically unable to stand on a scale, the nurse may have the parent hold the child while the parent stands on the scale. After the combined weight of the parent and child is noted, the nurse then has the parent stand on the scale alone. The parent's weight is then subtracted from the combined weight to give the child's weight. Whenever there are unusual conditions existing during weighing or measuring, the nurse should note such on the child's record (e.g., child weighed with shoes on).

Once measurements have been taken, they can be compared to past measurements by plotting them on a growth grid according to the child's age. Usually health care facilities use standardized percentile charts. These charts use percentiles to show the distribution of height, weight, and head circumference for a typical series of 100 children born at term. For example, the 25th percentile indicates that 75 children are taller and 25 children are shorter than the child being measured. In general, a child in the 25th percentile will continue at about this percentile throughout life. A child who suddenly has an increase to a higher or lower percentile requires further investigation. If a measurement differs greatly from previous visits, the nurse should check the technique and re-evaluate the measurement. Often the measurement has been taken incorrectly or plotted on the graft incorrectly.

Some general rules exist regarding height and weight:

- Height and weight measurements provide important information, but single measurement is of less importance than a series of measurements.
- The relationship between height and weight is significant. For example, a child who falls at a high percentile for height and at a much lower percentile for weight requires a more detailed assessment.
- Children should constantly progress in height and weight. Any persistent plateauing or weight loss needs a more detailed assessment.

Head Circumference

The brain achieves 75 per cent of its adult size by 3 years of age. One-half of total head growth occurs during the first year of life. Therefore, the head circumference should be taken at each well-child visit during the first three years.

A reliable reading of head circumference is obtained by using a metal or paper tape measure around the broadest part of the head. The tape is placed over the widest diameter of the head, the occipital protuberance and the frontal bones. If an accurate measurement is difficult to obtain, it is best to take three measurements and use the largest. Head circumference increases 4 inches (approximately 10 cm) in the first year and only 2 inches (approximately 5 cm) between the ages of 1 and 7.

The head circumference is also plotted on a growth chart (see Appendices Two and Three). As with height and weight, serial measurements provide more information than a single measurement, and marked differences should be investigated.

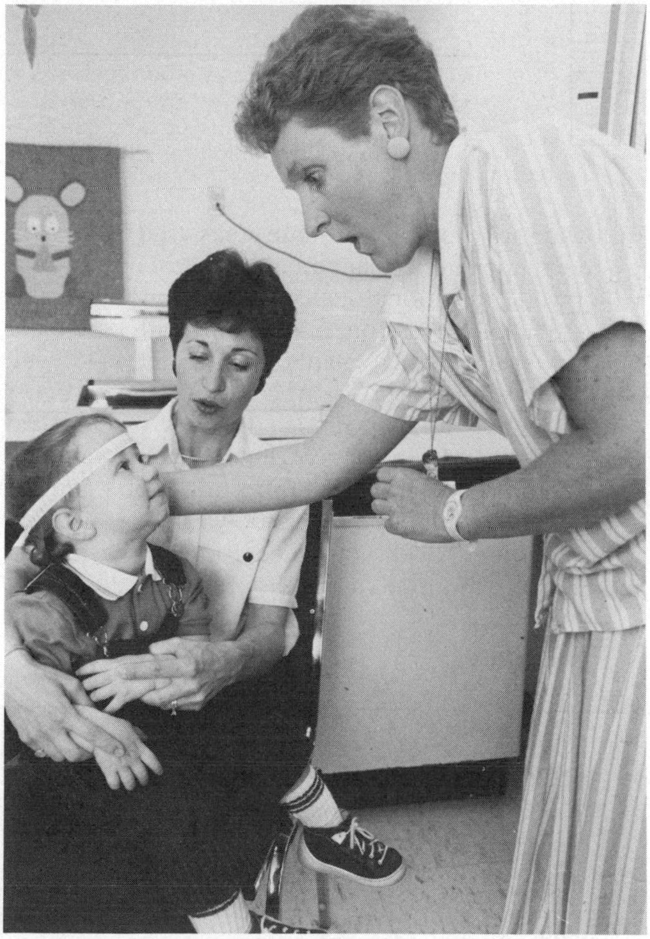

Head circumference is measured around the broadest part of the head over the occipital protuberance and the frontal bones.

Assessment of Vital Signs

As in other areas of the physical examination of children, it is important to reduce anxiety and gain cooperation when vital signs are being obtained. The same techniques to gain cooperation previously described may be employed while taking the vital signs.

The order in which vital signs are measured will depend upon the age of the child and the child's ability to understand and cooperate. A rule of thumb is to proceed from the least intrusive procedure to the most intrusive procedure. For very young children, vital signs should be taken in the following order: pulse and respirations; blood pressure; and temperature. Following this order increases cooperation and produces more accurate results, since temperature taking can produce sufficient anxiety to alter the respiratory and pulse rates.

The normal values for pulse, respiratory rate, and blood pressure will vary with the age and size of each child. Normal temperature values will depend on the route by which the temperature is measured. Generally the accepted values are between 35.5°C to 38°C (96°F to 100.4°F) for oral temperatures. There is no consensus about how much rectal and axillary temperatures differ from an oral temperature. Rectal temperatures are thought to be slightly higher than oral and axillary slightly lower than oral, but the difference is not believed to be a full degree Fahrenheit as was traditionally assumed. When temperatures are recorded, the route of measurement should be noted and the same route of measurement should be used for a particular child.

The route of temperature taking and the length of time allowed for accurate measurement depends in part on custom in various settings. With increasing frequency, careproviders recognize the anxiety produced by taking the rectal temperature of young children. Some settings use the less traumatic axillary tempera-

Table 15-1. Normal Pulse and Respiratory Rates for Specific Ages*

Age	Pulse (Beats per Minute)	Average Pulse	Respirations (Breaths per Minute)
Neonate	70–170	120	30–40
2 years	80–130	110	25–32
4 years	80–120	100	23–30
6 years	75–115	100	21–26
8 years	70–110	90	20–26
10 years	70–110	90	20–26
12 years	70–110	85	18–22
14 years	65–105	85	18–22
16 years	60–100	85	16–20
18 years	50–90	80	12–24

*These are averages and vary with the sex of the child.

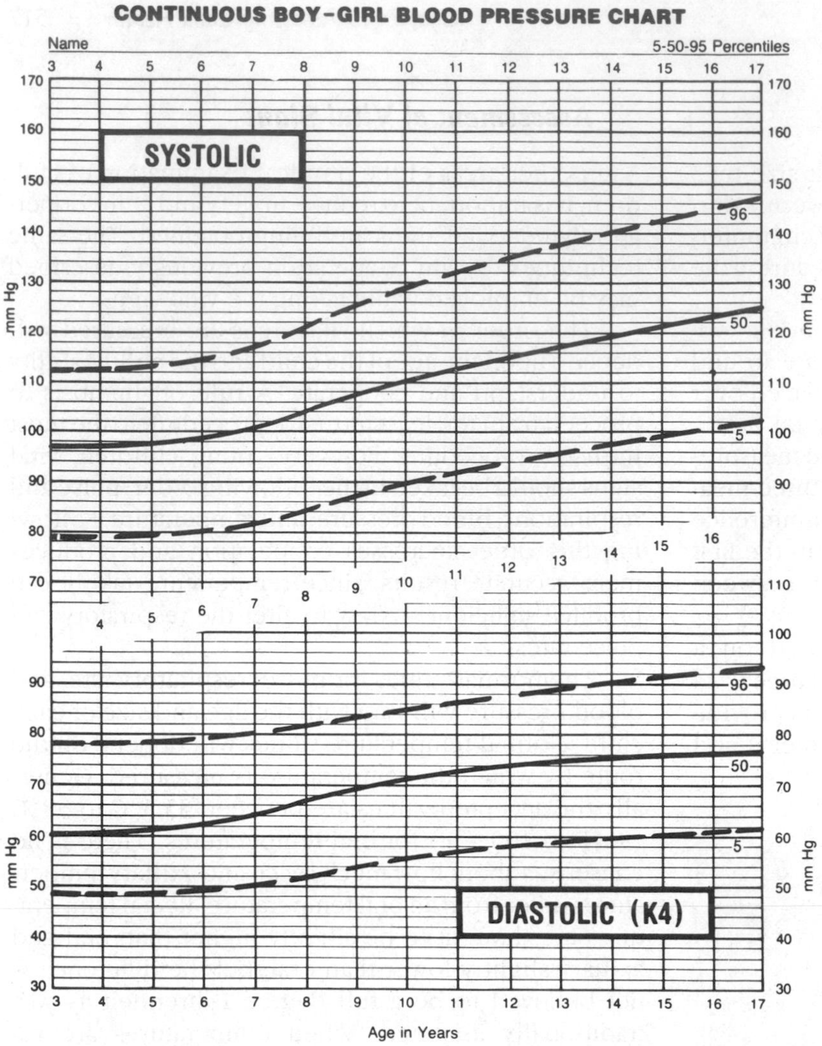

***Figure* 15-4.** Children's blood pressure chart. (From Jaworksi A: New boy-girl blood pressure chart for pediatric office use: a single sheet graph for all children. *Clin Pediatr* 1978 Sep; 699.)

tures as the routine route of measure for children who are not seriously ill. Table 15-1 describes average pulse rates and respiratory rates, and Figure 15-4 displays blood pressure readings at various ages. Chapter 27 describes in more detail some of the special techniques used in assessing vital signs in children.

The Physical Examination

Physical examination utilizes four basic assessment techniques: inspection, palpation, percussion, and auscultation. Table 15-2 describes these techniques. The examination is usually conducted from head to toe. When a body part is examined, it is usually inspected generally and then more specifically. For example, when examining the head, the general appearance is noted first, followed by the skin of the face and head. Finally, a more detailed examination of the parts of the face (e.g., nose or mouth) is carried out.

General Appearance

The examination should begin with an overall impression of the child. Observation of the child is done to formulate an impression that can be verified or disproved following a more extensive examination. The following are examples of some areas used to develop a general appearance statement: physical appearance (ill or well); nutritional status; behavior and degree of activity; facial expression; interactions with parents or nurse; developmental status; consciousness level; speech or nature of cry; gait, coordination, and posture. The general appearance focuses on physical characteristics or behaviors of the child and should be a brief summary statement. An example of a general appearance statement is as follows: Alert, smiling, well-developed, well-nourished toddler playing on mother's lap and in no acute distress.

The Skin

Techniques	**Equipment**	
Inspection	Natural lighting	
Palpation		
Examine for		
Color	Turgor	Lesions
Moisture	Edema	Hair
Texture	Temperature	Nails

Table 15-2. Techniques Utilized in Physical Assessment

Purpose	Comments
Inspection	
Evaluation of visible characteristics	Adequate exposure of area being visualized and good direct lighting necessary
Palpation	
Use of hands to touch or feel area being assessed for temperature, texture, vibration, size or position Light palpation is gentle pressure applied with the fingertips or palms Deep palpation is firm pressure applied with the fingertips to evaluate organs within the abdomen. Deeper palpation is achieved by placing the fingers of one hand over the fingers of the hand that is palpating Ballottement is application of pressure by tapping or bouncing of several fingers to note pressure within an organ (e.g., ocular pressure) or rebound tenderness (e.g., of the abdomen or a specific organ)	Temperature (e.g., of the skin) is assessed best with the dorsum of the fingers Texture, size or position (e.g., texture of the hair, size or position of an organ or mass) are best assessed with the fingertips Vibration (e.g., of air or sound moving through the lungs) is assessed best with the palms
Percussion	
A rapping motion utilized to determine the density of an area being assessed or the borders of a specific organ	Direct percussion is used most often to percuss the nasal sinuses or tendons or inflamed organs
Blunt or direct percussion is done by striking the surface being assessed with a partially flexed finger (usually the middle finger) Bimanual or indirect percussion is accomplished by placing the middle finger of one hand on the surface to be percussed. The other fingers should not rest on the surface to be percussed as this will diminish the sound created by percussion. The middle finger or index and middle fingers of the other hand strike the middle finger resting on the body surface on the upper phalange. Only the very tip of the striking finger is used	Indirect percussion may be used to percuss any area of the body. Percussion sounds include: *Tympany* (drumlike) such as is heard over the stomach or abdomen normally *Hyperresonance* (hollow sound with air interference) as is heard in pneumothorax *Resonance* (hollow sound without air interference) as is heard normally over the lung *Impaired resonance* (diminished hollow sound) as is heard when fluid has accumulated in a hollow cavity such as the lung *Dullness* is heard normally over muscle or a thick or solid tissue organ such as the liver *Flatness* is heard normally over bone
Auscultation	
Listening to the sounds arising from organs, with the aid of a stethoscope The diaphragm of the stethoscope picks up high frequency sounds and is used for auscultation of most organs The bell of the stethoscope picks up low frequency sounds such as heart murmurs	Auscultation is done over the lungs, heart and abdomen to determine the functional status of these organs. The skull, thyroid gland and carotid arteries are auscultated for bruits

The skin is examined as a whole to determine its overall condition and then more specifically as each body part is assessed.

Color

Normal skin color varies depending on race. The skin should be inspected for areas of hyperpigmentation or hypopigmentation. Hyperpigmentation is often seen in Addison's disease, hyperthyroidism, or pregnancy, or it may be the result of exposure to the ultraviolet light of the sun or a lamp. Hypopigmentation is seen in children with vitiligo (milk-white patches) or albinism.

When examining the skin, the nurse should note any signs of cyanosis or erythema. Erythema, an increased amount of oxygenated blood in the vasculature of the dermis, is found in children who are febrile, have a sunburn or a localized infection, or have been exposed to the cold. Cyanosis, a bluish tint to the skin, is caused by reduced hemoglobin in the capillaries. Usually, it is seen in children with respiratory or cardiac disease. Acrocyanosis, the bluish discoloration of the hands and feet that is frequently seen in newborns, is normal for the first few days of life. It is caused by inadequate peripheral vasculature.

Skin that is very pale demonstrates a decrease in hemoglobin content, often seen secondary to anemia or shock. In white-skinned persons pallor is noted by a loss of pink skin coloring; in black-skinned persons the skin becomes an ashen gray. Jaundice is seen as a yellow-green hue; this usually means an increased bilirubin. It occurs in children with liver disease or hemolytic blood disease. Jaundice is best discerned by blanching the skin and observing the blanched area for a yellow or yellow-green appearance. Examination of the skin for jaundice should be done in natural sunlight as opposed to fluorescent light, which gives some normal skin tones a yellow color. Areas in which jaundice is easily observed are the sclera and the hard palate and the gums, particularly in dark-skinned races. Skin that appears to be the color of yellow squash may be the result of carotenemia.

Moisture

The skin is inspected and palpated for the degree of moisture present. Sweat is produced for both excretory and heat-regulating purposes and may be due to exercise, crying, or fear. Excessive sweating may be secondary to an underlying pathology such as fever, cardiac disease, or hyperthyroidism.

Texture

Inspection and palpation of the quality and character of the skin surface is necessary for the evaluation of skin texture. Normal skin is smooth, soft, and pliable. Skin that is rough and dry often indicates an endocrine problem or is also seen in children who bathe very frequently or who are exposed to cold weather. Rough, dry skin is also seen with vitamin A deficiencies. If scaling is found, the extent and location should be described. Scaling present only between fingers and toes could be a sign of a fungal infection. Scaling of the palms and soles of the feet might be associated with scarlet fever. Eczema often causes scaling of the cheeks and behind the ears, knees, and elbows. Thick, yellow, oily scales on the scalp may indicate seborrhea, which can spread into a red maculopapular rash on the face and trunk.

Children with a velvety smooth skin may have hyperthyroidism. Palpation of the skin may also produce a crackling sensation if the child has subcutaneous emphysema caused by a lung disorder. The crackling sensation may also indicate a bone fracture of an underlying structure.

Turgor

One of the best indicators of nutrition and hydration is skin turgor. Normal skin turgor is elastic and taut. Turgor is evaluated by pinching the skin between thumb and forefinger, usually of the lower abdomen or calf, and noting the reaction of the pinched skin. If the skin returns promptly to the normal position, it is assessed as elastic. Skin that does not promptly return may indicate a loss of turgor due to dehydration or excessive exposure to ultraviolet rays. Skin that stays pinched or tented for a few seconds after the skin is released is considered flabby or decreased in turgor and may indicate chronic disease and muscle disorders.

Edema

An excess of water that is stored in the skin in the form of edema is evaluated according to whether it is pitting or nonpitting. The nurse's thumb is firmly pressed over the medial aspect of the child's malleoli for at least five seconds. After releasing the skin, any sign of indentation that lasts several seconds indicates pitting edema. Puffiness or edema that does not remain indented is nonpitting edema. Any body surface areas can be edematous and should be evaluated using the technique just described. Generalized edema, however, is often evaluated by examining the lower extremities. Edema is seen in children who have allergies, kidney or heart anomalies, and malnutrition.

Temperature

Palpation of the skin to determine its temperature is best completed by comparing body parts. Skin temperature is not an accurate reflection of the internal temperature of the body but may reflect a maladjustment in the thermoregulating mechanism of the body. Localized hyperthermia, an indication of increased blood flow, may be secondary to a burn or cellulitis. Generalized hyperthermia may be the result of generalized sunburn, fever, or hyperthyroidism. Children in shock may exhibit generalized hypothermia.

Lesions

Examination of the skin is not complete unless it has been inspected and palpated for skin lesions. Any lesions or markings on the skin should be noted and described in detail as follows: size, color, shape, location, surface characteristics, anatomic distribution, configuration, and morphology. Lesions are classified as primary, secondary, and special lesions (see Fig. 44-4).

Primary lesions are the initial lesions evident in a disease process, whereas secondary lesions are altered primary lesions that result from scratching or in response to medication or the normal healing process. Primary lesions include macules, papules, wheals, vesicles, petechiae, pustules, and bullae. Examples of secondary lesions are scales, crusts, striae, excoriation, erosion, ulcers, fissures, lichenification, and scars. Plaques may be either primary or secondary lesions. Comedones and milia are examples of special lesions.

Many skin lesions can be normal, such as capillary hemangiomas, freckles, nevi and mongolian spots. Mongolian spots are often seen in children of Black, South American, or Asian descent and usually appear on the buttocks or coccygeal area. Mongolian spots can also be differentiated from bruises in two other ways: color and appearance over time. Mongolian spots are usually slate blue overall, and they do not change in color or size from day to day as do bruises.

Other skin lesions such as cysts, port wine stains, or large, hairy moles require further evaluation and possible referral. Lesions in the form of a skin rash are seen frequently in children of all ages. Heat rash and diaper rash are common in infants and young children. Another common condition is acne. It generally begins during adolescence and can range from mild to severe. Newborns often contract a skin rash that is frequently labeled neonatal acne.

Hair

Hair is examined for color, length, distribution, cleanliness, amount, and texture. Scalp hair should be examined to determine if it is clean and shiny and if it covers the entire head. Hair texture is noted as being thick or thin, fine or coarse, soft or brittle. Nutritional and endocrine disturbances may affect hair texture. The scalp and body hair are closely inspected for alopecia, which may indicate systemic pathology or a skin infection.

Body hair is also evaluated. Hair on the eyebrows and eyelashes and any hair associated with a lesion such as a mole should be examined. Any hair on the face, axillae, pubic area, and chest should also be examined carefully at all ages. Pubic hair usually appears when the child is between 8 and 12 years of age. Axillary hair appears shortly after the onset of pubic hair. Adolescent males begin to develop facial hair approximately 6 months after the appearance of axillary hair. Hair that has appeared earlier than normal or excessive hair may be an indication of precocious puberty or could signify an endocrine problem. The spine is inspected and palpated for hair tufts of the sacral area, which are seen in children with spina bifida.

Nails

Nails are examined as part of the integumentary system. Nails are inspected and palpated for their size, shape (convex or concave), and color (pink, cyanotic, pale). Characteristics such as smoothness, pitting, ridging and clubbing are carefully noted. Clubbing is generally a sign of chronic lack of oxygen and is often seen in children with congenital heart disease or chronic pulmonary disease. It can also be a normal familial trait. Any change in color should be noted. Adolescents and children who smoke heavily may have yellow nail tips. The cuticles should be assessed for intactness, smoothness, and any splitting or hangnails.

The Lymphatic System

Techniques	**Equipment**
Inspection Palpation	None
Examine lymph nodes for	
Size Mobility Tenderness Warmth	Redness Distribution Consistency

The lymphatic system provides important information about the child's health status. A large lymph node or generalized lymphadenopathy may be the first sign of disease. Lymph nodes are inspected and palpated during the examination of the part of the body in which they are located. Palpable lymph nodes on children may be normal but should be evaluated carefully. It should be noted whether lymphadenopathy is localized or generalized. The physical examination should include evaluation of five major lymph node areas: head, neck, axillae, inguinal, and arms and legs (Fig. 15-5).

Lymph nodes are palpated by using the finger pads and gently but firmly pressing in a circular motion along the regions in which the nodes are normally present. When the nodes of the neck are palpated, the child's head should be straight with slight upward tilting without tension in the sternocleidomastoid or trapezius muscles. The examiner may find it helpful to turn the child's head 10 or 20 degrees toward the side being examined to relax the skin and muscles. The

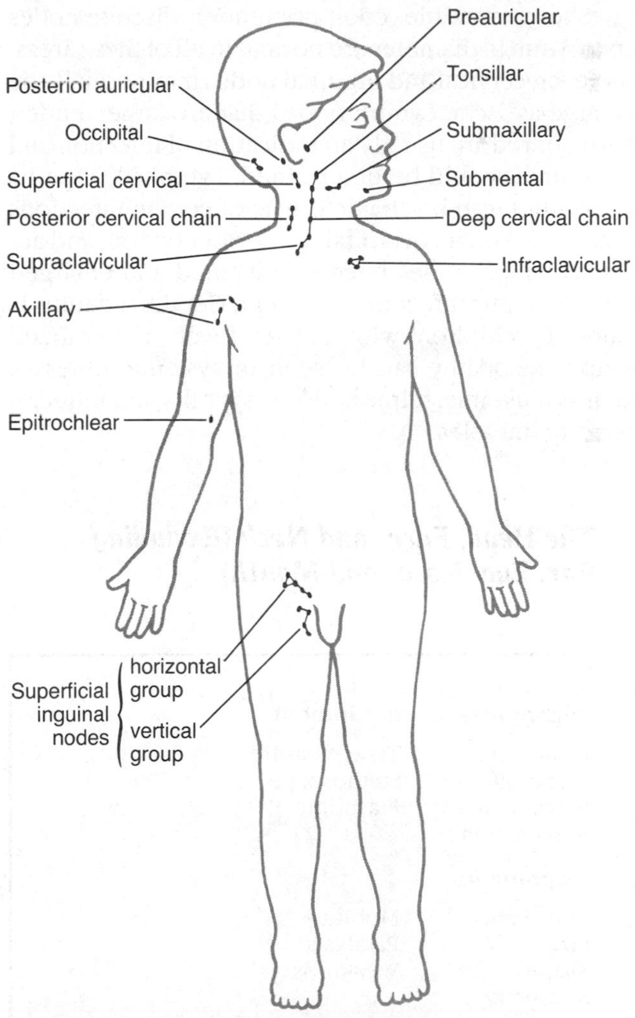

Figure 15-5. Lymph nodes of the body.

head is tilted downward slightly to allow easier palpation of the occipital chain. In order to inspect and palpate the lymph nodes located in the submental and submaxillary areas, the head may need to be tilted backward slightly.

Another examination technique used to evaluate the lymph system is to have the child shrug the shoulders slightly so the nurse may palpate the fossa when examining for supraclavicular nodes. Axillary nodes are palpated with the arms relaxed and slightly adducted, with the child's forearm resting on the examiner's forearm to eliminate pull and tension on the axillae. Often this area is very ticklish and the child may need to be distracted. Epitrochlear nodes are best examined with the arms slightly flexed. Inguinal nodes are palpated when the child is supine. Finally, the less frequently palpated popliteal nodes are located slightly medially in the popliteal fossas. These are best palpated with the knees bent at a 45-degree angle so that the muscles and tendons are relaxed. The examiner places the thumbs on the patella and reaches with the fingertips of both hands behind to the fossa, palpating deeply toward the medial aspect.

Shotty, movable, cool, nontender, discrete nodes up to 3 mm in diameter are normal in all of these areas; however, cervical and inguinal nodes may normally be as large as 1 cm. Lymph nodes that are large, tender, warm, or red are usually an indication of infection and the source should be determined. Lymphadenopathy distribution can be characteristic of certain infections (Table 15-3). The occipital, posterior cervical, and auricular lymph nodes become inflamed and enlarged when a rubella infection is present. Cervical adenitis is found in children with scarlet fever. Generalized lymphadenopathy can be seen in systemic illnesses such as leukemia, salmonellosis, syphilis, mononucleosis, and measles.

The Head, Face, and Neck (Excluding Ear, Eye, Nose, and Mouth)

Techniques	Equipment
Inspection	Tape measure
Palpation	Stethoscope
Percussion	Flashlight
Auscultation	
Examine for	
Appearance	Mobility
Size	Paralysis
Shape	Weakness
Symmetry	

Head

Inspection from all angles is necessary to determine the size, shape, and symmetry of the head. The shape of the skull is generally round but may be long or broad. Newborns frequently have asymmetrical heads due to intrauterine positioning and to molding, which may occur during the birth process. Size is best determined by obtaining a measurement of head circumference.

Suture lines and fontanels are inspected and palpated during examination of the infant's and young child's head. The head should be carefully palpated to determine if the suture lines are closed, over-riding, or separated at birth. Premature closure of suture lines can vary the shape of the head depending on which sutures are closed. The first two years of a child's life are important for brain growth; any sign of premature closure of suture should be thoroughly investigated.

There are six fontanels but generally only two, the anterior and the posterior, are of clinical significance. Fontanels are inspected and palpated for size, shape, number, and location. They are also palpated and inspected for bulging, tenseness, pulsation, or depression.

Occasionally, a third fontanel is also found. It should be evaluated in the same way as the anterior and posterior fontanels. A fontanel that is depressed may be indicative of malnutrition and dehydration. Children who have a bulging fontanel may have hydrocephaly, meningitis, lead poisoning, vitamin A poisoning, or a subdural hematoma.

Children under 6 months of age may normally have an anterior fontanel over 4 to 5 cm in diameter, but it may also be diagnostic of increased intracranial pressure, subdural hematoma, rickets, hypothyroidism, or osteogenesis imperfecta. Small, anterior fontanels should be checked closely for premature closure.

Fontanels are generally diamond shaped and should be measured in two dimensions: anterior-posterior and horizontal. The examiner uses a tape measure to measure the two dimensions.

The average anterior fontanel may be very small or absent at birth but generally enlarges to an average size of 2.5 cm by 2.5 cm. It should remain open for at least 9 to 10 months to allow for adequate head growth. Approximately 97 per cent of all anterior fontanels close between 9 and 19 months of age. Very large fontanels may not close until 2 years of age. The posterior fontanel is often not palpable at birth. If present, it averages 1 cm by 1 cm in size. It generally is not palpable after 1 to 2 months of life.

The child's scalp is inspected and palpated for scaliness, infections, and hair. Inspect the scalp closely for signs of cradle cap. This can be done by scraping the scalp lightly with a fingertip. Examine the hair as

Table 15-3. Lymphatic System

Chain	Location	Areas Drained	Clinical Significance of Enlargement
Occipital	At nape of neck (lower occipital bone)	Occipital region of scalp	Pediculosis, seborrhea, tick bites, chickenpox, rubella, external otitis, scalp lesions
Posterior auricular	Mastoid, posterior to pinna	Posterior part of temporoparietal region, pinna, posterior part of external acoustic meatus, scalp, facial skin	Rubella, skin lesions in area drained, external otitis, chickenpox, pediculosis
Preauricular	Directly in front of ear (anterior to tragus), temporal	Face, eye, lateral surface of auricula	Lesions of the eyelids (chalazions), conjunctivitis, infectious skin disorders of the face
Superficial cervical	Chain over sternocleidomastoid muscle at upper section of neck superficially	Tongue, tonsils, pinna, parotid, scalp, neck, thorax	Scalp infections, pediculosis, lesions in areas drained, scarlet fever
Deep cervical (jugular)	Begins with *tonsillar* node at the angle of jaw and continues under sternocleidomastoid muscle, ending posterior to this muscle in supraclavicular chain	Most of tongue, tonsils, pinna, parotid, oropharynx, nose, paranasal sinuses, palate, larynx, trachea, esophagus, middle ear	Tonsillitis, pharyngitis, thyroid disease, inflammatory process of areas drained, scarlet fever
Submaxillary (submandibular)	Beneath body of mandible midway between chin and ear	Medial conjunctiva, cheek, side of nose, upper lip, lateral part of lower lip, gums, submaxillary gland, anterior margin of tongue	Stomatitis, conjunctivitis
Submental	Beneath chin	Central portions of lower lip, floor of mouth, apex of tongue	Dental infections
Tonsillar	The first of the deep cervical chain at angle between ear and jaw	Mouth, pharynx, principal node for tonsil	Tonsillitis, pharyngitis
Parotid	Parotid gland; lateral wall of pharynx at junction of mandible and maxilla; occasionally in subcutaneous tissue over parotid gland	Parotid gland, tissues of face, root of nose, tympanic cavity, eyelids, frontotemporal region, external auditory canal	Parotitis, mumps, tumors
Supraclavicular	Directly over medial area of clavicle	Head, abdomen, breast, thorax, arm, lung	

discussed in the section on skin examination. Scalp hair should be examined closely for signs of alopecia, nits, and lice. Excessive hair and low-set hairlines are noted, since they may be indicative of congenital anomalies. The head should be inspected and palpated for any bulges or swellings. Cephalohematomas and caput succedaneum may be seen in the newborn period (see Chapter 5).

Control, movement, and position of the head are also observed. An infant may be observed for head lag when pulled from a supine to a sitting position. Little or no head lag should be evident after 3 months of age. The position in which the child holds his head may also indicate abnormalities. Persistent positioning at an angle may indicate torticollis or visual problems. The head should also be evaluated for full range of motion. The examiner must rotate the head of the newborn for passive range of motion, but for the older child the nurse can elicit active range of motion by having the child follow a toy or a bright light. The head should move smoothly from an extended or flexed position and from side to side. Jerky or limited movement warrants further investigation.

After the fontanel closes, a "cracked pot" sound on percussion of the skull at the junction of the frontal, temporal, and parietal bones may indicate increased intracranial pressure. Percussion is accomplished by using the direct method in which the middle finger directly percusses the child's skull.

If there is concern about head growth or shape or fontanel size, the skull may also need transillumination. To accomplish this, a flashlight is fitted with a sponge-rubber collar so that there is a tight fit when it is placed against the skull. The procedure must be done in a dark room, preferably with the child comfortably in the parent's lap. The flashlight is then placed snugly on the skull and moved across both sides and across the front and back of the skull; the halo of light extending from the rim of the flashlight is assessed. The expected halo is 1 cm in diameter in the occipital area and 2 cm in the frontoparietal area. Any increased area of light should be investigated further.

Face

The face should be inspected for shape, symmetry, paralysis, placement of features, distribution of hair, and skin color and texture. Symmetry and placement of features should be evaluated from the front and from each side. The eyes should be set at the same level and not set wide apart or close together.

The nose should be midline with symmetrical nares; the mouth should be symmetrical, and the ears set at the same level on both sides of the head. The top of the pinna (external ear) should meet or cross an imaginary line that extends from the lateral corner of the eye to the most protuberant part of the occiput. This is the eye-occiput line. Ears that do not cross this line are low set and may indicate hydrocephalus or one of many syndromes, including Potter, trisomy 13, 18, or 21, Turner, DiGeorge, Pierre Robin, and others.

Facial paralysis and asymmetry of facial movement should be closely observed. This is easily done when an infant cries or yawns. Older children can smile and wrinkle their foreheads so that the examiner can check for paralysis. Edema, twitchings, and tics should also be observed for and palpated. Facial coloring is observed, and any evidence of pallor, jaundice, cyanosis, or any unusual marking is noted.

Neck

Following examination of the head and face, the neck is inspected for control, mobility, pulsations, symmetry, size, and shape. Palpation of the neck is used to determine strength, pulsations, and position of structures such as the thyroid and the trachea. The sternocleidomastoids and trapezius muscles are palpated for tone and presence of any masses or hematomas. Strength of these muscles is evaluated by having the child move them against the resistance of the nurse's hands. Range of motion should also be determined. A child with any nuchal rigidity or opisthotonos should be referred. Enlarged veins or excessive pulsations can indicate cardiac problems.

The trachea is inspected and palpated to determine if it is midline. The examiner inspects the neck hyperextended and then palpates the trachea beginning at the suprasternal notch and moving upward. The thumb is placed on one side of the tracheal rings and the index and middle fingers on the other side to evaluate the tracheal rings and determine if the trachea is midline or deviated.

The thyroid is inspected and palpated. Inspection takes place in the hyperextended position. The examiner looks for bulges, asymmetry, or enlargement. With the neck tilted slightly forward, the examiner palpates for the hyoid bone; cricoid and thyroid cartilages; the thyroid isthmus; and finally the lobes of the thyroid gland (Fig. 15-6). The thyroid is palpated with the child in a supine or sitting position. The thumb is placed on one side of the thyroid and the index and middle finger on the opposite side. In the older child the examiner may stand behind the seated child and place the index and middle fingers of each hand on the sides of the thyroid. Having the child swallow some water moves the thyroid upward and allows for better palpation. Any nodules, enlargement, or tenderness of the thyroid gland should be considered abnormal; these signs warrant further evaluation.

Examination of the lymph nodes is done during the examination of the neck. The examiner generally begins with palpation of the occipital nodes and progresses to the posterior auricular and preauricular lymph nodes. The examiner then continues to the anterior and posterior cervical triangles. (See Figure 15-5 for locations of these nodes.)

Auscultation of the neck is done to determine the presence of bruits or murmurs. The bell of the stethoscope is placed over the carotids for this part of the examination. Finally, any hoarseness or stridor of the voice is noted. An infant's cry is evaluated for its quality. A high-pitched cry, a cat-like cry, or a low, hoarse cry are indications of abnormalities. The older child is evaluated for voice quality and speech.

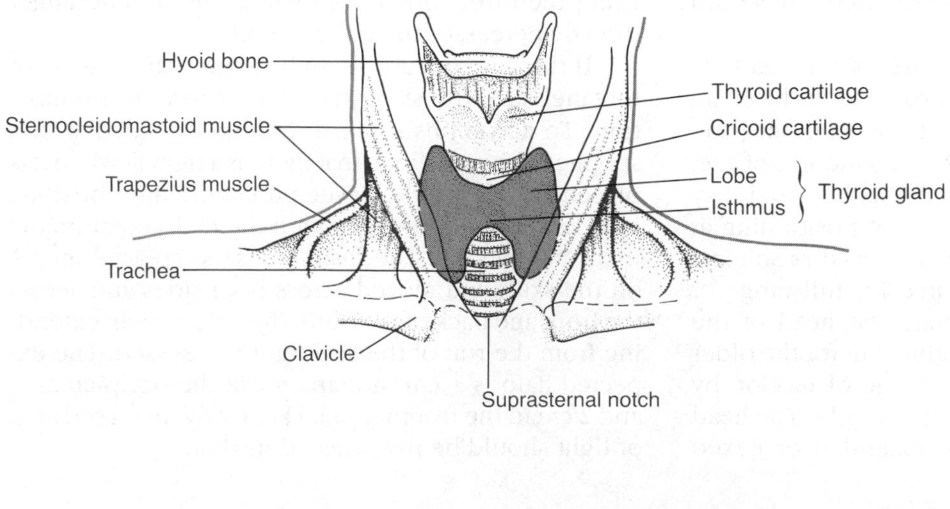

Figure 15-6. Structures of the neck.

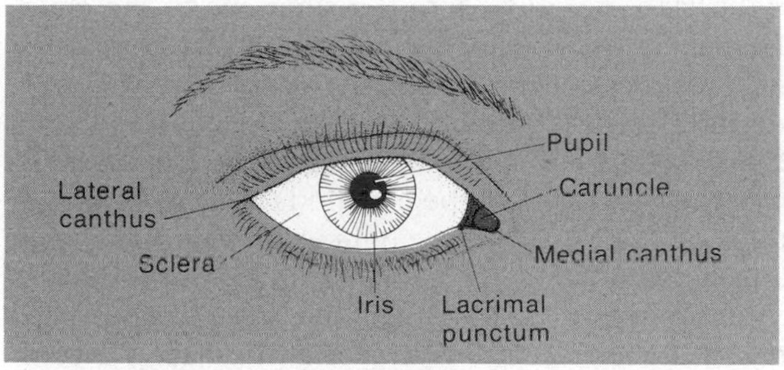

Figure 15-7. Structures of the eye.

The Eye

Techniques	**Equipment**
Inspection	Flashlight
Palpation	Tool for testing vision
Examine for	
Appearance	Color
Size	Mobility
Shape	Function

Examination of the eye (Fig. 15-7) begins with the eyelids, which are inspected for ptosis, retraction slanting, edema, redness, or epicanthal folds. They should also be inspected for styes, chalazions, boils, and blepharitis. Edema of the lids may indicate serious problems such as renal failure or may be caused by allergies, injuries, drugs, or infection.

Presence or absence of eyelashes is determined, as are their color and texture. The nasolacrimal duct should be inspected for patency, position, redness, and swelling. Eyes that tear excessively or have any discharge should be investigated further. Excessive tearing before the age of 3 months may be due to a blocked nasolacrimal duct. It may also result from infections, a foreign body, allergies or exophthalmos.

The palpebral and bulbar conjunctivae are examined next for color, moisture, and integrity. Swelling of the conjunctiva is seen with infections and allergies. The conjunctivae are also examined for pallor, inflammation, injection, growths, enlarged follicles, and drainage.

The orbit of the eye is also assessed. Children with sunken, blank eyes may be severely ill or malnourished. Small orbits usually indicate underlying pathology. Inspection of the eye orbits also determines hypotelorism, hypertelorism (abnormal width between the eyes), and prominent supraorbital ridges. The globe of the eye and the ridges are palpated for tenderness, turgor, and swelling. Exophthalmos and endophthalmos are significant findings and should be referred for evaluation.

The full range of motion of the extraocular muscles is evaluated by having the child follow an object to each of the six visual fields (Fig. 15-8). The eyes are observed closely for smooth, symmetrical tracking and any sign of nystagmus. The direction of the nystagmus should be recorded. A paralyzed extraocular muscle causes paralytic strabismus. The eye cannot follow to one or more visual fields. In concomitant strabismus the eyes do not move simultaneously but each eye can move to all quadrants during the range-of-motion exercises. Concomitant strabismus is frequently seen in the infant but should be minimal after 6 months of age.

Two screening tests are used to detect strabismus. The corneal light reflex is determined by shining a penlight at the bridge of the nose while the child looks straight ahead. Inspection of the child's eyes should then be done to determine if the reflection of light falls at the same point on each pupil. Any deviation indicates strabismus or trophia.

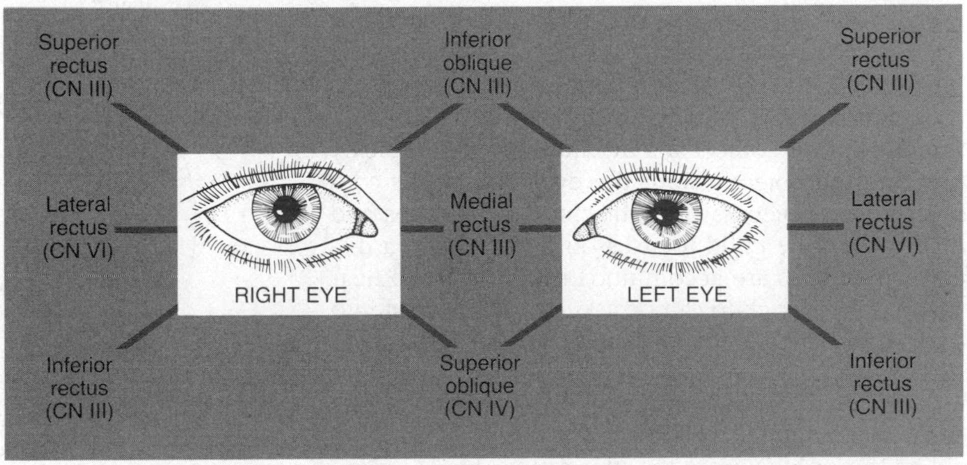

Figure 15-8. The visual fields of extraocular movement. If the child's eye is unable to move to any one of the positions, dysfunction of either that muscle or the cranial nerve (CN) is suspected. (A young child may not be able to follow instructions to move only the eyes; the nurse then should hold the child's head still.)

A cover test can also be done by holding a light 12 inches from the child's eyes and asking the child to focus on the light. The examiner occludes one of the child's eyes, making sure that both eyes remain open, and observes the uncovered eye for movement inward or outward. The occluder is then moved quickly over the other eye, and the eye that had been covered is inspected for any inward or outward deviation. The test is repeated on the opposite eye. Normally, no deviation occurs in either eye. The cover test is repeated having the child focus on a distant object. A cover test can be done on even the youngest child by having a bright, flashing object to attract attention. Older children can focus on the examiner's finger or on a picture placed on the wall. Children having a wide nasal bridge or epicanthal folds may have the appearance of having strabismus. This is referred to as pseudostrabismus. A negative cover test and an equal corneal light reflex rule out actual strabismus.

The cornea, sclera, iris, and pupil are considered to comprise the eye proper and are examined next. The cornea is inspected for clouding, enlargement, abrasions, lesions, or change in color. Abrasions or lesions are best observed by shining a light from the side across the eye. The sclera is observed for color, hemorrhage, or discoloration. The sclera of newborns is often a light blue because of its thinness, but a dark blue sclera can indicate osteogenesis imperfecta or glaucoma. A yellow sclera is often the first clinical sign of jaundice.

The iris and pupil are examined together. The size, shape, and color of the irises are noted. Any freckles, spots, or other irregularities should be noted. Pupils are examined for size, shape, equality, reaction to light, and accommodation. A difference in pupil size may be normal but can also be caused by central nervous system damage. The pupillary reaction to light can be performed by shining a light directly in the eye and noting the response—whether the pupil constricts. In addition, the nurse should shine a light in one eye and note whether or not the other pupil also constricts. Accommodation—a change in dilation and medial movements of both pupils—can be tested even in the young child by having the child focus on a brightly colored object at a distance and then quickly bringing the object toward the eye. The pupils constrict as the object is brought close to the eyes and dilate when the child focuses on the object at a distance. The eyes are accommodating from far to near vision. An older child can be asked to look far off into the distance then to focus on an object within 12 to 14 inches from the eyes.

The lens is examined by shining a light on the eyes and inspecting the lens for opacities. Finally, with the aid of the ophthalmoscope, the retina can be examined. The examiner holds the ophthalmoscope in the right hand and looks into the right eye of the child. Examination of the left eye is accomplished by reversing the process. The examination is done in a semidark room. The child should be instructed to focus on a fixed object such as a fluorescent sticker on the wall.

The ophthalmoscope is dialed to 0. The examination begins by focusing the light into the child's eyes at a distance of about 12 inches from a position that is about 15 degrees to the side of the line of vision. A red reflex is obtained at this time. An absence of a complete, circular red reflex or the appearance of an opaque density surrounded by a red reflex indicates a cataract or other pathologic condition requiring referral to a physician. In nonwhite races the red reflex is normally paler and may have a pink or salmon-colored appearance. The ophthalmoscope generally has from 15 to 20 diopters in the black (positive lens) and in the red (negative lens). (A diopter is the refractive power of the lens with a focal distance of 1 meter.) The negative lens compensates for myopia, and the positive lens compensates for hyperopia. The refractive ability of the child's eyes plus the refraction of the examiner's eyes will determine which diopters of the ophthalmoscope will be used during the examination.

Examination of the fundus (Fig. 15-9) of the eye requires a child who is cooperative and able to hold the eyes still and focused on an object for a short period of time. If the child can cooperate, the examiner approaches from the 12 inches (used to obtain a red reflex) to within 3 inches of the child. As the examiner approaches the child, each layer of the eye is inspected, beginning with the cornea, progressing to the lens, and then on to the vitreous. As the examiner moves in, the dial of the ophthalmoscope is turned to smaller numbers until red minus numbers are reached. The exact number will depend on the refractive ability of the examiner's and the child's eyes.

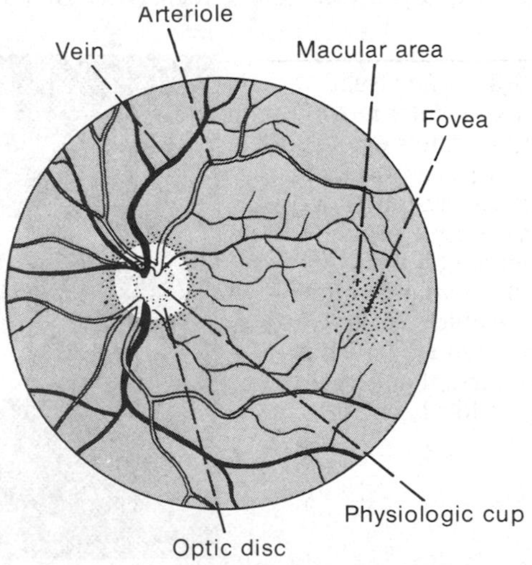

Figure 15-9. Landmarks of the ocular fundus.

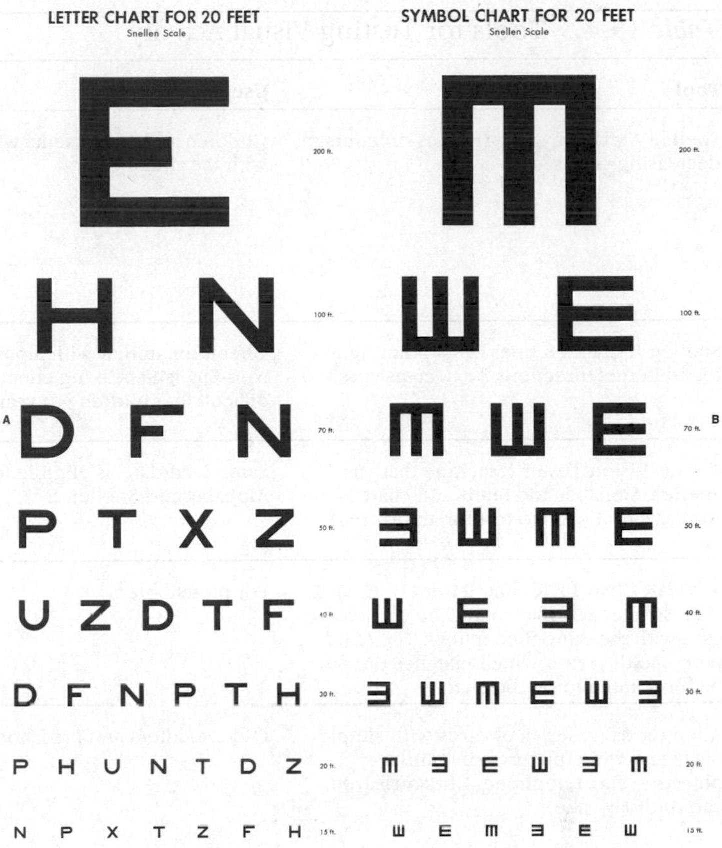

***Figure* 15-10.** Two types of visual acuity charts. The standard Snellen alphabet chart (left) can be used as early as the child's ability to name letters allows. The Snellen "E" chart can be used with younger children. The child is asked to point with hand or fingers in the direction the E points. (Courtesy of National Society to Prevent Blindness, 79 Madison Avenue, New York.)

During the internal examination of the fundus, the optic disc is located and observed for size, shape, color, margins, and physiologic depression. The disc is usually round but may, occasionally, be vertically oval. The disc is a creamy pink or pale yellow color and has a depression slightly temporal of the center that is the physiologic cup. The margins should be smooth and slightly darker than the rest of the disc.

The macula is a small circular area located 2 disc diameters temporal to the optic disc with the fovea centralis seen as a gleaming light in its center. The fundus is normally an orange-red color and should be uniform throughout. Lightness and darkness in color varies from one race to another. The fundus should be inspected for signs of hemorrhage or papilledema.

The arteries and veins should also be examined. The arteries are narrower than the veins and exhibit a light reflex from their center. Veins do not normally have a light reflex and are wider than arteries with a 3 : 2 ratio. As the vessels cross, the veins are under the arteries. Abnormalities such as tortuous vessels, hemorrhages, hypertrophied vessels, or excessive dilatation should be referred for further evaluation.

Finally, visual acuity is tested. Vision screening should begin early in life and continue at regular intervals. The infant's vision can be evaluated by watching the child's ability to focus and follow brightly colored objects or a light. The infant should be followed closely for any signs of developmental delay or an obvious lack of response to the environment, which could indicate visual problems.

Vision testing evaluates three components of vision: light perception, visual acuity, and color perception. Light perception is tested generally in the newborn by shining a light into the eyes and noting responses such as blinking, following the light, and increased alertness. A rotating black and white striped drum placed in front of the newborn's face should cause nystagmus if vision is present. The nurse should be aware of signs that may indicate visual loss, such as fixed pupils, marked strabismus, constant nystagmus, and "setting-sun" sign (this sign is characterized by the white of the eye showing between the iris and the edge of the upper eyelid).

Visual acuity is defined as the ability to see near and far objects clearly. There are a variety of tools that can be used to test visual acuity. (See Table 15-4.) Figure 15-10 gives examples of two types of visual acuity charts.

Whatever test is employed, appropriate test technique should always be used. The following items are essential for reliable testing:

- There should be adequate illumination and no glare on the eye chart;
- the chart should be at the child's eye level;

Table 15-4. Tools for Testing Visual Activity

Tool	Use	Comments
Snellen Alphabet Chart (8 lines of letters in decreasing sizes)	Children and adolescents who are familiar with the alphabet	Person being examined stands with heels 20 feet from chart. Examiner asks child, who has one eye covered, to read one line at a time. Reading the majority of letters in the line being tested constitutes a passing score. Visual acuity is noted as the line value (line 7–10 feet, line 8–15 feet) over a denominator of 20
Snellen E Chart (8 lines of Es pointing in four different directions. Es decrease in size)	Clients unfamiliar with alphabet; or Non-English-speaking clients. Often too difficult for children <6 years	Same as Snellen Alphabet chart. Sometimes helpful to refer to the E as a table and ask child to indicate which direction table legs point
Titmus Vision Tester (Machine that has Snellen Alphabet and Snellen E chart as well as a tool used to test for amblyopia)	Same candidate as eligible for Snellen Alphabet and Snellen E	Advantages of using it are a) light source is controlled, b) less distracting than testing in a room or hallway, and c) can be used in a small area
STYCAR Chart (The nine letters H, C, O, L, U, T, X, V, A are on a chart. The child has a card with the same nine letters. The child points to the letter which matches the one being pointed to on the chart)	For preschoolers	Children can easily recognize these letters
Allen Cards (A series of cards with simple black and white pictures of familiar objects—e.g., telephone, Christmas tree, car, birthday cake)	Older toddlers and preschool children	Examiner starts exam approximately 20 feet from child. If child can not identify the symbols, examiner moves to 15 feet distance and so forth. The distance in feet at which the child is able to recognize three of the pictures determines the numerator over the denominator of 30. A child who has a visual acuity difference of 5 feet between eyes should be referred
Picture Charts—e.g., Kindergarten Chart, California Clown Test, Osterberg Chart (Lines of symbols with which young child should be familiar [e.g. heart, circle, star, sailboat]. Symbols decrease in size. These charts are not as well standardized as the Snellen Charts)	Preschoolers and kindergarteners. May be used with Non-English-speaking children if someone can interpret their labels for the items	Same as Snellen Alphabet. Children may identify a symbol by an unusual name—e.g., circle may be a "tire" a "doughnut" or a "hole." Examiner need only know what the child's label is

- children should be tested individually so they do not memorize the chart while they are waiting to be examined;
- children should be pre-educated for the vision test: Have children stand a few feet away from the chart and explain what they should do; learn the names the children use for symbols if a picture chart is being used;
- occlude the nontest eye with a paper cup to prevent the child from closing that eye during the exam;
- begin the test with an easily read line and move on to a more difficult one;
- use two examiners if necessary: one to point to the chart and one to occlude the child's nontesting eye;
- expose one line of letters, Es, or symbols at a time.

Visual acuity becomes increasingly organized as the child develops. Most infants are able to see objects clearly at close range, usually 10 to 14 inches—roughly the distance between a mother's breast and face. Binocular vision is clearly established between 4 to 7 months of age and mature function of the eye muscles is generally developed by one year of age.

Children have better vision than was previously believed. See Box 51-1 for visual acuity at various ages. Any child who does not have the visual acuity expected for age should be referred. Also, any child who has a two-line difference between eyes should have further evaluation. This may indicate poorer vision in the one eye,which may be compensated for, resulting in eventual loss of vision if not corrected.

Screening for heterotropia is another important vision test. In heterotropia the child's eyes do not focus together to provide binocular vision. Heterophoria is the latent tendency for heterotropia. The corneal light reflex (Hirschberg test) is one of the most important screening tests to determine a tropia. The cover test as described previously is another screening test to help rule out a tropia or a phoria.

Finally, color vision is assessed in every child, usually at preschool age. Although color blindness is rare in females, it is important to determine the child's ability to determine colors. The child who has color blindness will need counseling for safety purposes such as interpreting traffic signals and also later regarding occupational choices. This child will also need assistance in developing the ability to coordinate colors of wearing apparel so that ridicule by peers does not become a problem. The Ishihara Plates are plates with figures composed of dots hidden in a background of similar dots. The figure is a different color so that the only way to distinguish the figure is by color. These plates are useful in children who have the skills to discriminate figure ground, letters, numbers, and geometric figures. The younger child may not be able to do this. Other tests such as matching colored yarns or putting colored tennis balls in similarly colored muffin tin compartments can be used; however, the Ishihara is the only standardized color vision test at this time.

The Ear

Techniques	**Equipment**
Inspection	Otoscope
Palpation	Cerumen spoon
Examine for	
Appearance	Placement
Shape	Mobility of the tympanic membrane
Position	

Examination of the ears begins with inspection for shape, position, and placement of the external ears. The pinna should cross the eye-occiput line and should be no more than 10 degrees posterior to a perpendicular line drawn from the eye-occiput line to the lobe (Fig. 15-11). The pinna is also inspected for color and structural anomalies. Mumps, mastoiditis, cellulitis, or congenital anomalies may cause the auricle to stand out. The pinna is palpated for cartilage formation, masses, tenderness, and cysts.

The bony prominence located immediately posterior to the ear lobe is the mastoid process. This area is inspected and palpated for erythema, swelling, and tenderness. The outer canal of the ear is then inspected for discharge. Bloody discharge is seen with a perforated tympanic membrane, foreign body in the canal, irritation or scratching of the canal, or basilar skull fracture. Purulent drainage commonly denotes a fungal or bacterial infection.

Internal structures are examined with the aid of an otoscope. The procedure is usually painless unless an infection or furuncle exists in the ear canal or the otoscope touches the bony part of the ear canal. Children may become anxious during this part of the examination, but giving adequate explanations and allowing time for the child to become familiar with the instrument often alleviates anxiety.

A child who is not able to be cooperative should be adequately restrained. The young infant can be placed on his abdomen with his head to one side. The examiner can retract the pinna with the left hand and also keep the head still while holding the otoscope in the right hand. The otoscope is held like a pencil with the right side of the hand and fifth finger resting on the child's head to cushion the otoscope if the child's head should move. The toddler or preschool child can sit on the parent's lap with the legs held firmly between the parent's legs. The parent places an arm firmly across the child's trunk and arms, and the other arm is used to hold the child's head firmly against the parent's chest. This age child can also be restrained while lying supine on an examination table with the arms extended above the head and held firmly by the parent. The examiner then leans over the child's trunk and restrains the head to one side. The examiner should be careful not to put weight on the child's chest; this could frighten the child and cause respiratory distress. Children who will sit on the examination table need only to tilt their heads to one side to allow for better visualization.

Once the child has been appropriately restrained, the ear canal may be examined. The ear canal is normally curved and must be straightened before the nurse can visualize the canal and tympanic membrane. In infants and toddlers the auricle is pulled down, and in the child over 3 years of age the auricle is pulled up and back to straighten the ear canal (Fig. 15-12). The canal is then examined internally for erythema, lesions, furuncles, or discharge. The amount and consistency of cerumen is also noted and described.

Once the canal has been inspected, the examiner proceeds to the tympanic membrane. The tympanic membrane is assessed for color, the landmarks, and mobility.

A normal tympanic membrane is a light, pearly gray color. An erythematous membrane may be seen in the child who has been crying or the child with otitis media. A dull gray or yellowish color is often seen with serous otitis and a vivid red in suppurative otitis. The

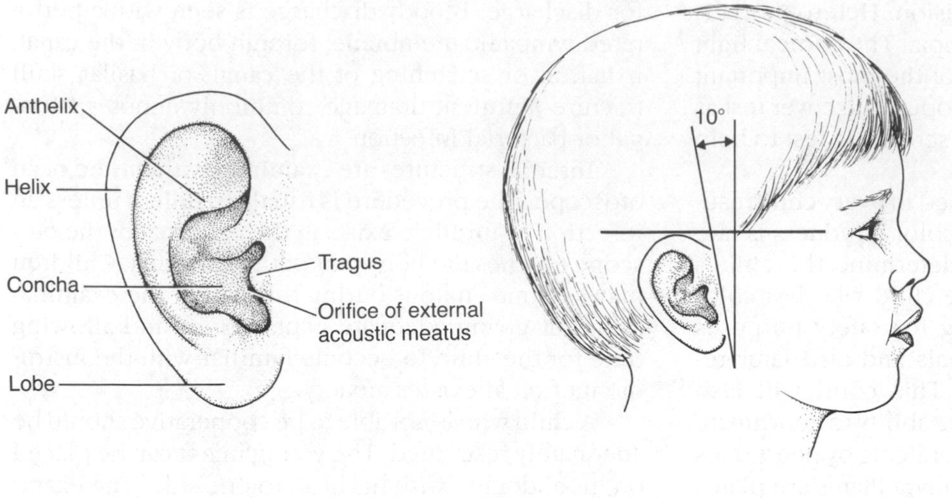

Figure 15-11. The parts of the external ear, and its normal placement on the head. The pinna should cross the eye-occiput line and be within a 10-degree angle of a perpendicular line drawn from the lobe to the eye-occiput line.

landmarks are the umbo, light reflex, long process, short process, pars flaccida, annulus, and the anterior and posterior malleolar folds (Fig. 15-13).

The light reflex is a small, triangular cone of light that is seen at the anterior inferior quadrant. It is located directly below the umbo. A diffuse, spotty, or absent cone of light may indicate infection or fluid in the middle ear. The umbo, found at the top of the cone of light, appears as a round, white fibrous area. The long process (handle of malleus) can be seen above and nasally of the umbo. The short process of the malleus looks like a sharp, white, protuberant bone through the membrane. When the membrane is retracted, the landmarks appear more pronounced; bulging makes them more obscure. A bulging or retracted tympanic membrane requires referral to a physician.

The annulus is a white fibrous ring surrounding the periphery of the eardrum. The three small bones or ossicles (malleus, incus, and stapes) lie directly behind the membrane. The incus and stapes may be seen only if the drum is very translucent or is retracted.

Evaluating the mobility of the eardrum is useful in determining the presence or absence of fluid in the middle ear. Fluid will cause the membrane to move in a restricted fashion or not at all. Mobility of the eardrum is assessed by using a pneumatic headpiece on the otoscope. This device is a piece of rubber tubing that is attached to the head of the otoscope. It must be used with a tight-fitting speculum so that the ear canal is sealed off. Air is puffed through the tubing while the examiner observes the movement of the tympanic membrane. Absent or decreased mobility indicates fluid behind the membrane.

Hearing is an essential part of the well-child examination. Since learning and language are so closely related, it is important for the nurse to be alert to clues indicating a possible hearing disorder. Children who evidence characteristics summarized in Box 15-4 should be tested for possible hearing problems. Hearing testing should be done at all ages to evaluate hearing accuracy.

For young infants and toddlers, testing is often

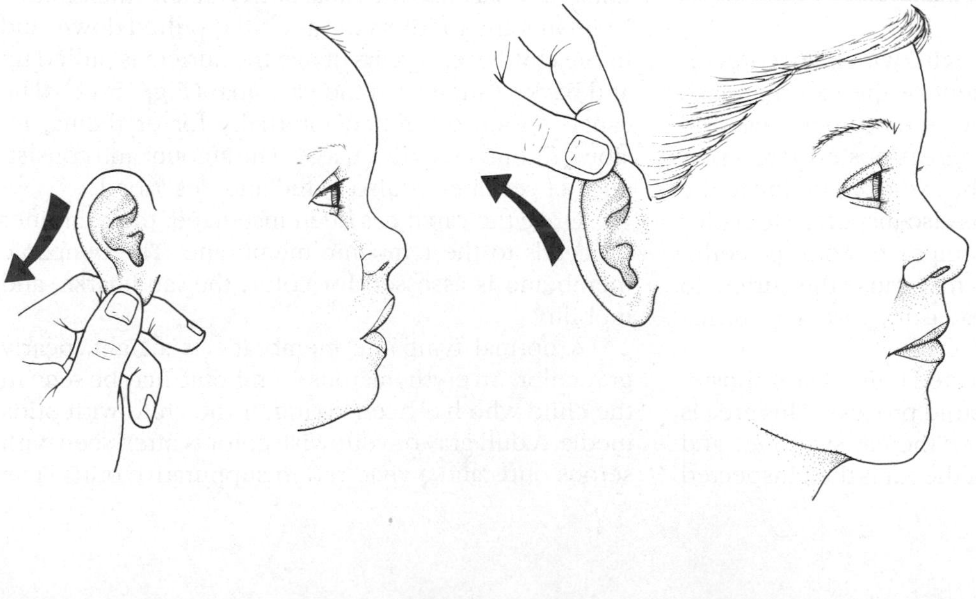

Figure 15-12. To straighten the ear canal, the auricle is pulled down in infants and children. In the child over 3 years of age, it is pulled up and back.

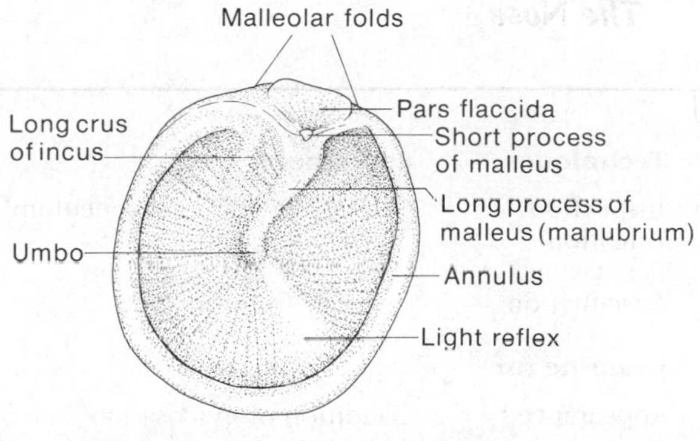

***Figure* 15-13.** Normal tympanic membrane of right ear.

Box 15-4
Characteristics of Children Who May Have Hearing or Language Deficits

RESPONSE TO AUDITORY STIMULI

(See Table 15-5 for normal development of hearing responses)
Inattentive to speech.
Does not react with a startle to loud noises during first year.
Does not react to name or commands by 6 to 9 months.
Does not turn to source of sound by 4 months.
Does not understand commands or instructions by 18 months.
Inconsistent responses to environmental sounds during first two years of life.
Turns up volume on radio or TV.

VOICE CHARACTERISTICS

Voice quality is poor.
Voice is loud or monotone.

SPEECH CHARACTERISTICS

Babbles normally until 6 months then gradually decreases sound production.
Not talking at all by age 2 years.
Speech highly unintelligible after age 3 years.
Uses mostly vowel sounds after 1 year of age.
Speech that is difficult for others to understand.
Consistently drops word endings.
Constantly misses high-pitched consonants and fricatives such as th, ch, s, sh, b, and k.
Omits initial consonants after age 3.

MEDICAL CHARACTERISTICS

History of prenatal infections, birth anomalies, prematurity, birth trauma, birth anoxia, kernicterus.
History of treatment with ototoxic drugs during infancy.
Familial history of congenital hearing impairment.
History of frequent upper respiratory or ear infections.

accomplished by using a noisemaker. The child is seated on the parent's lap and distracted visually from the front. A noisemaker is then used to one side. The child should be distracted visually by one examiner while another examiner produces the sound to one side at 18 to 24 inches from the child. The first examiner observes for the response. (Table 15-5 summarizes the characteristic responses of infants who can hear.)

The sounds produced should be of high, medium, and low frequency and should be repeated on each side. The examiner should reproduce the sound approximately 8 to 12 inches above and below the level of the ear to determine if the child can localize the sound.

Toddlers and preschoolers are difficult to examine for hearing, but it is important that adequate hearing testing is done because hearing is critical to appropriate speech development. Play audiometry is used for children over 15 months of age. The child can be tested with or without earphones; however, more specific information about each ear is gathered if the child will allow earphone testing. The child is conditioned through a play technique to respond to sound stimuli. Once the child has been conditioned to respond to the sound, by dropping the block in a box or putting a ring on a peg, the examiner can test the child with the earphones in place. Often the examiner puts several toys in front of the child, places the earphones on the child, and then requests that the child pick up a certain toy. This is done at certain frequencies and decibels. The child's responses are then recorded. By 3 to 4 years of age the child can frequently have routine audiometric pure tone testing with a minimum of preparation. Hearing and hearing loss are further discussed in Chapter 51.

Tuning forks can also be used to identify conductive or neurosensory hearing loss. This can be done only on an older child (at least 5 years of age) who can

***Table* 15-5.** Development of Hearing Responses

Age	Hearing Response
Birth	Startle reflex; blinking of eyes; attends to voice
12 weeks	Eye movement toward sound when prone
12–18 weeks	Eye movement toward sound when upright
4 months	Widening of eyes; quieting; listening posture; slight head turning; looks in same direction as sound
6 months	Turns head to source of sound; may have beginning localization; downward localization occurs before upward localization
8–12 months	Turns head 45° or more in direction of sound; localizes sound source above and below; rapid automatic response to sound by one year
12–36 months	Rapid speech development and language patterns based on hearing input

follow directions and give appropriate responses. The Weber test is performed by placing an activated tuning fork on the midline of the skull. The child should indicate if the sound can be heard equally in both ears or if it is localized to one ear. If the sound is lateralized to one ear, that ear may have a conductive hearing loss. Room noise is blocked out because of the impairment, therefore vibrations are detected better than normally. In unilateral sensorineural loss, the lateralization is to the unimpaired ear.The inner ear or nerve is affected; therefore, vibrations are not as well detected from the bone. The sound is heard better in the unaffected ear.

The Rinne test is performed by striking the tuning fork and placing the stem on the mastoid process until the child indicates it can no longer be heard. The tuning fork, still vibrating, is then placed 1 to 2 inches from the ear opening. The child is asked if the sound can still be heard. The vibrations should be heard in the air longer than the vibration on the bone because air conduction is two times longer than bone conduction. Any child who cannot hear the sound via air conduction longer than bone conduction should be referred to a physician.

Although the information received from using tuning forks is very helpful, it is not a precise assessment of the child's hearing. Audiometric hearing testing is the most reliable method to evaluate hearing. Pure-tone audiometry is done by presenting electronically generated pure tones of various frequencies and intensities to a child through earphones. Children are instructed to raise their hands as soon as they hear the sound. For children younger than 5 years of age, a play activity should be substituted for raising the hand. The child should not be able to see the audiometer controls. The usual procedure is to present the various frequencies at an intensity of 20 to 25 dB; however, a 15 to 20 dB tone is required to identify minor hearing loss caused by otitis media. Testing at 15 dB is often not done because it requires a more soundproof room. Various methods of testing are used. Downs (1981) recommends the following procedure:

1. Present a pure tone of 50 dB at 1000 Hz; this acquaints the child with the procedure. Praise the child for raising his or her hand.
2. Set the dial to 15 dB and present tones at 1000, 2000, and 4000 to one ear.
3. Switch ears; present tones in reverse sequence: 4000, 2000 and 1000 Hz.

Test results are marked on a standardized graph for each frequency. A child who fails to respond to any of the tones at 15 dB in either ear fails the test. The child should be retested later in the same day; if failure occurs again, referral is necessary.

The Nose

Techniques	**Equipment**
Inspection Palpation Percussion Auscultation	Otoscope with nasal speculum
Examine for	
Appearance Shape Patency of nares	Condition of mucosa Secretions Sinus discomfort

Determining whether the child is breathing through the nose or mouth is the first step in the examination of the nose. Patency of the nares of the newborn is assessed by placing the diaphragm of the stethoscope against one naris while blocking the other naris and listening for breath sounds. An infant who does not have patent nasal passages may experience respiratory distress. Flaring of the nares also indicates respiratory distress and can be caused by obstruction, pneumonia, fever, anoxia, and acidosis. A child who mouth breathes may have nasal polyps, allergies, enlarged adenoids, or a deviated septum.

The shape of the nose is inspected. A flat or saddle-shaped nose is seen in some races. It may also be indicative of congenital anomalies, congenital syphilis, cleft palate, and other conditions. A crease across the nose may be a result of the allergic salute in which a child frequently pushes against the tip of the nose because of rhinitis or itching. The nose is also palpated for crepitus, tenderness, and stability.

Internal examination of the nose requires a penlight or an otoscope with a nasal speculum. The otoscope provides a better visualization of the internal structures. The examiner gently pushes the tip of the nose up and places the speculum at the opening of the naris to inspect the nasal mucosa. Normal mucosa are pink and moist. Inflamed mucosa indicate irritation or infection. Pale, boggy mucosa are seen in children with allergies, and swollen gray mucosa indicate chronic rhinitis.

The examiner also determines the type and amount of nasal secretions. Thin, watery secretions are seen in children with allergies, upper respiratory infections, or foreign bodies high in the nose. Purulent discharge is commonly seen with nasal and sinus infections or foreign bodies that have been lodged for a period of time. Nasal bleeding occurs at Kesselbach's plexus, which is located at the anterior tip of the septum. Trauma, allergies, dry climate, or blood dyscra-

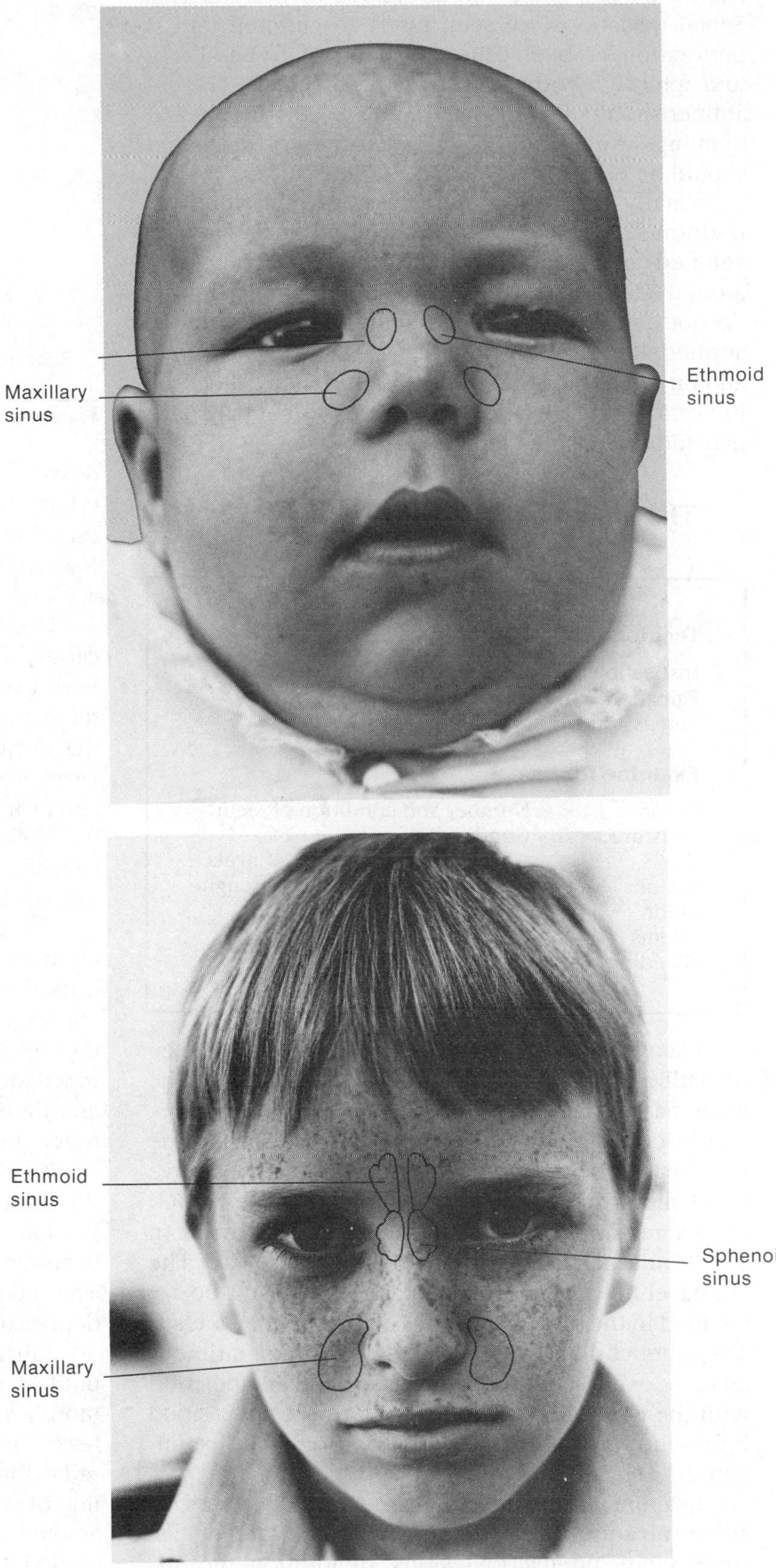

***Figure* 15-14.** Facial sinuses indicated on an infant and a child.

sias will cause epistaxis from this point. The septum should be inspected for deviations or perforations. Septal deviations are seen rarely in children unless perforation has been caused by injury of the nasal septum, a foreign body, syphilis or tuberculosis. The examiner should also inspect the turbinates and meatal openings. Any swelling, color change, or discharge should be noted.

Finally, palpation and percussion of the sinuses is performed. The maxillary and ethmoid sinuses are developed in infancy. The frontal sinuses develop around 7 to 8 years of age, while the sphenoid sinuses do not develop until after puberty. Firm pressure is applied along the supraorbital ridge, maxillary area, and on the infraorbital ridge nasally (Fig. 15-14). Any indication of tenderness with percussion or palpation may indicate a sinus infection.

The Mouth and Throat

Techniques	**Equipment**
Inspection	Otoscope or penlight
Palpation	Tongue depressor
Percussion	Disposable glove
Examine for	
Color	Number and condition of teeth
Moisture	Condition of gums
Clefts	Condition and mobility of uvula
Lesions	Condition and mobility of tongue
Odor	
Edema	
Bleeding	

Examination of the mouth (Fig. 15-15) is often difficult and traumatic for the child. This part of the examination, along with the otoscopic examination, may be done last. An attempt is always made to gain the cooperation of a child of any age. An uncooperative child should be adequately restrained to allow for a safe examination. The infant can be examined while in the supine position, arms held above the head. The young child can sit on the parent's lap and be restrained in the same way as was described for ear tests. The older child generally needs no restraint if time is taken to explain the procedure and acquaint the child with the equipment. A tongue depressor and a good light source are essential for this portion of the examination.

Examination begins with inspection of the lips for color, moisture, size, shape, asymmetry, drooping, fissures, clefts, edema, or lesions. In addition, the lips and the surrounding area are inspected for pallor or cyanosis. Cherry-red lips are seen in children with aci-

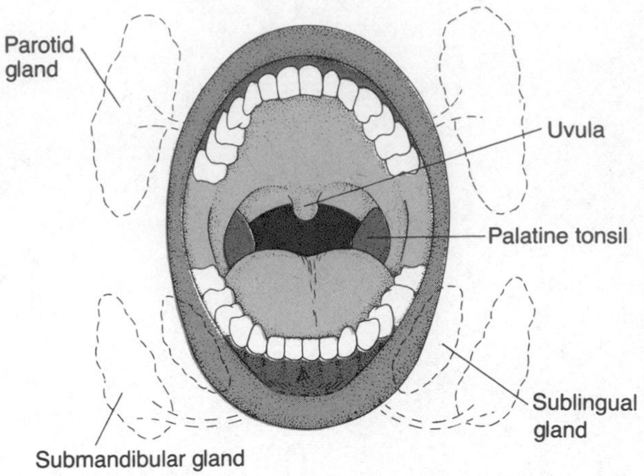

***Figure* 15-15.** Structures of the child's mouth.

dosis or carbon monoxide poisoning. Unusual mouth odors should be noted as they can be clinically significant. Unusual odors are present in children with poor oral hygiene, dental caries, sinusitis, allergies, diabetic acidosis, malnutrition, and diphtheria.

Teeth are inspected for number, type, position, caries, malocclusions, color, and hygiene. Children have two sets of teeth; the first teeth, or deciduous teeth, begin to erupt around 6 months of age. All 20 of the deciduous teeth usually are erupted by 2½ to 3 years of age. Permanent dentition begins around age 6 and progresses until all 32 permanent teeth have erupted. Delay in tooth eruption can be genetic or significant of underlying disease process. (See Chapter 19 for further discussion of teeth eruption.)

Teeth with flattened edges are usually seen in children who grind their teeth. Malocclusion is often caused by persistent thumbsucking. To determine malocclusion, the examiner inspects the alignment of the teeth. In normal occlusion the top posterior molars meet and rest snugly on the opposing bottom molars and then the upper central incisors just overlap and touch the lower incisors.

Teeth that are mottled or pitted are seen in children who have ingested excessive fluoride. Iron ingestion, antibiotic ingestion, or severe jaundice at birth can cause a green or black discoloration of teeth. The teeth should be percussed by tapping a tongue depressor on the crown and sides.

Salivation is noted. Salivary secretion is limited until 3 months of age when the salivary glands become more active. Absence of salivation may be caused by fever, dehydration, or atropine ingestion. Excessive salivation is frequently seen in children who are teething or who have caries or mouth infections. The amount, color, consistency, and odor of saliva are recorded if abnormal.

Gums should be inspected and palpated for color, moisture, inflammation, swelling, bleeding, tenderness, and ulcerations. Inflammation and swelling are secondary to infection or poor oral hygiene. A herpes virus infection or improperly fitting dental corrective appliances may cause ulcerations. Inflamed, bleeding gums may be a result of decreased vitamin C intake or pyorrhea. A black line along the margin of the gum may signify metal poisoning such as lead poisoning. Any raised or receding areas of the gums should be identified. It is important to use the tongue depressor gently to move the buccal mucosa away from the gums to allow adequate inspection of upper and lower gums.

The buccal mucosa is inspected and palpated for color, moisture, lesions, parotid ducts, and masses. The buccal mucosa is normally pink but black or brown areas may be seen in children with Addison's disease and in dark-skinned children. An enlarged, erythematous or swollen parotid duct is seen with parotitis. Koplik spots, a group of gray-white spots, are seen on the buccal mucosa opposite the molars in the prodromal stage of measles (rubeola). White patches on the oral mucosa—especially the tongue and hard palate—that cannot be scraped off indicate a yeast infection (*Candida albicans*) called thrush, or moniliasis. The floor of the mouth, the major location of oral cancer, is inspected and palpated for cysts, masses of calculi, or submaxillary glands.

Inspection of the tongue is done to determine color, moisture, size, tremors, coating, size of papillae, and the presence of lesions. The normal tongue is pink and should fit in the mouth. A large protruding tongue is seen in children with Down syndrome. Normally the tongue has conical filiform papillae; large red papillae resembling a strawberry are seen with scarlet fever. The tongue becomes tender and red with riboflavin deficiency, niacin deficiency, or severe anemia. A geographic tongue has gray, irregular borders and can be considered normal or caused by allergies, fever, or drug ingestion. The tongue should also be examined for furrows and scars. Deep furrows are seen in children with Down syndrome. Scars could be the result of trauma or previous convulsions. Gross tongue tremors when the tongue is stuck out are seen in children with cerebral palsy; fine tremors are seen with chorea or hypothyroidism. The examiner should observe the tongue closely to determine mobility. The frenulum is checked for tongue-tie and is considered abnormal if the tongue cannot extend beyond the lower alveolar ridge. The ventral surface of the tongue is inspected for distended veins. The older child is instructed to push against the tongue depressor laterally on each side to determine the tongue's strength.

The hard and soft palates are inspected and palpated for color, shape, clefts, and the presence of lesions. An abnormally high arch may be associated with congenital disorders and may result in speech problems. The palates are usually a striated pink color. Epstein's pearls are seen as firm white nodules in the midline and are of no significance. Examination of the palates is not complete until both hard and soft palates have been completely palpated for masses or nodules.

The uvula is inspected as the child is gagged or is told to say "ahh." The examiner should not attempt to gag the child until the very end of the examination. A gag reflex should also not be obtained if there is a suspicion of epiglottitis, since this may cause increased swelling and occlude the airway. The soft palate and uvula should rise when the patient gags or says "ahh." Paralysis of the soft palate or uvula, which is indicated by no movement or movement that is not midline, may signify diphtheria, poliomyelitis, or abnormality of the glossopharyngeal or vagus nerves. An exceptionally long uvula is congenital and may cause gagging or coughing.

If present, tonsils are inspected for color, size, symmetry, inflammation or exudate, and possible lesions. Tonsils are much larger during childhood and begin to shrink between the ages of 8 and 12 years. Tonsillar crypts usually indicate past infection.

The posterior pharynx is checked for color, drainage, edema, and abnormal lesions or growth. Lymphoid hyperplasia and inflammation are seen in infection. A pale, puffy mucosa usually denotes edema. Ulcers and vesicles are seen in children with viral infections. Postnasal drainage may indicate either allergy or infection of the nasopharynx or sinuses, depending on the type of discharge seen. A white membrane over the pharynx or tonsils may be a sign of diphtheria or bacterial infection.

The child is gagged by placing a tongue depressor over the root of the tongue. This allows for visualization of the epiglottis. If the child has symptoms of epiglottitis, examination is not done; the child is referred immediately. If the epiglottis is examined and found to be swollen, inflamed, or pale, the child is handled as an emergency with immediate referral to a physician.

The Chest and Lungs

Techniques	**Equipment**
Inspection Palpation Auscultation Percussion	Stethoscope
Examine for	
Location and condition of nipples Condition of breasts Condition of muscles	Condition of cartilage Condition of bones Quality of breath sounds Respiratory function

Skillful inspection, palpation, percussion and auscultation are needed to examine the thorax, breast, and lungs (Fig. 15-16). The chest is inspected for size, shape, symmetry, and movement. The shape of the chest is round in the newborn with the anterior-posterior diameter equaling the transverse diameter. With growth the chest shape becomes more oval with the transverse diameter being greater than the anterior-posterior diameter. Pigeon breast, barrel chest, funnel breast and Harrison's groove are examples of abnormal chest structure (Table 15-6). Asymmetry such as precordial bulging may indicate chronic localized chest disease, enlargement of the heart, or pneumothorax. Other causes of asymmetry include tumors, scoliosis, and congenital absence of the chest muscle. The posterior chest wall is inspected and palpated to determine equality of the scapulae, and any deformity is noted. The chest should be inspected during inspiration and expiration. Normal inspirations occur as the chest expands, the sternal angle increases, and the diaphragm descends. With expiration, the process is reversed. Paradoxical respirations (diaphragm rises on inspiration and descends on expiration) or any signs of respiratory distress should be noted. Normal respirations are abdominal in the infant and young child and become thoracic around 7 years of age, although both are normal.

Respiratory motion is also observed both during quiet respirations and during sleep respirations. It is important to note the type, rate, rhythm, and depth of respiration as well as the use of any accessory respiratory muscles.

The location and depth of retractions, if present, should be described. Retractions are usually suprasternal and severe in the presence of a high obstruction. They are usually less intense and infrasternal when there is low obstruction.

The chest is palpated to determine if any cysts,

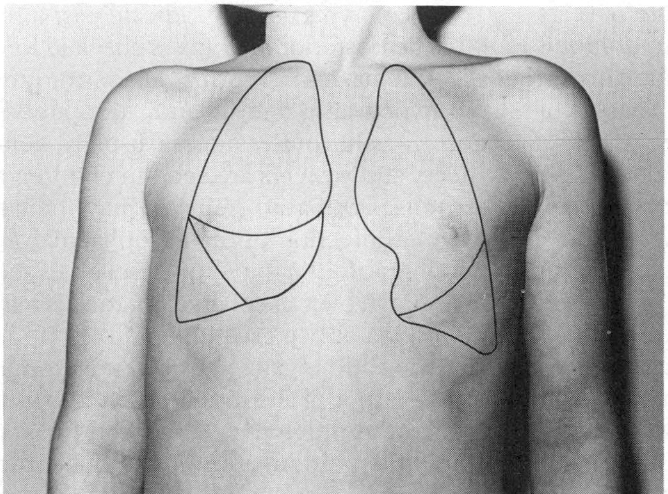

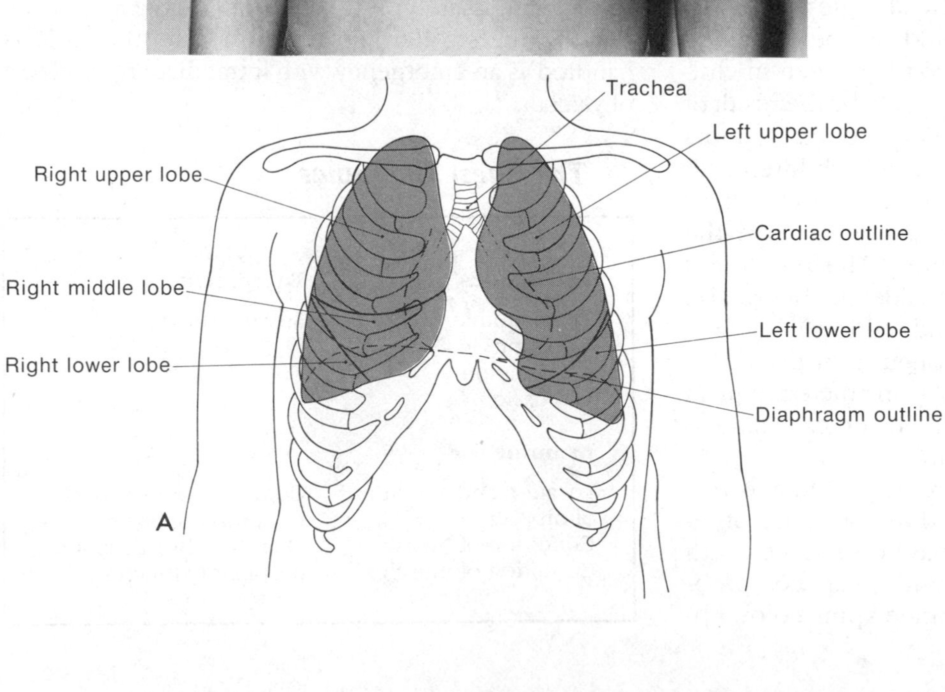

Figure 15-16. The four parts of the lung within the chest. *A*, Anterior thorax; *B*, posterior thorax; *C*, left lateral thorax; *D*, right lateral thorax.

tenderness, tumors, or abnormal growths exist. Sharp angular bumps at the costochondral junction are seen in children with vitamin D deficiency. The clavicles are palpated for crepitus and tenderness to rule out a fracture. Palpation of the ribs will indicate the number of ribs and the presence of tenderness. Lung expansion is evaluated by the examiner by placing the hands, palms down, on the child's chest, thumbs resting on the costal margin for the anterior chest or midspinally at the tenth rib for the posterior chest. The fingers are spread and placed on symmetrical areas of the chest. As the chest expands with deep inspiration, the examiner observes the thumbs to see if their movement is equal. Thumb movements should be equidistant in an upward, outward direction.

Tactile fremitus, the conduction of vocal sounds through the chest wall, is palpable by placing a hand palm down on the child's chest. Vibrations are felt best with the joints of the hands. Fremitus is felt as a tingling sensation as the child cries or when the words "99" or "blue moon" are said. The examiner's hands are placed in symmetrical bilateral positions as the chest is palpated from top to bottom both anteriorly and posteriorly. Absent or decreased tactile fremitus is seen with bronchial blockages, asthma, pleural effusion, and pneumothorax. Increased vibrations are seen with consolidation, such as pneumonia or atelectasis. The chest should also be palpated for pleural crepitus, which is felt as a coarse, crackling sensation when pressure is applied.

The indirect method is used to percuss the chest. Percussion proceeds symmetrically from side to side and downward to determine the presence, size, and density of underlying structures. Percussion should be done in the intercostal space, not on the rib, and should be just lateral to the sternum anteriorly and the spine posteriorly. Percussion starts in the supraclavicular area on the anterior chest. Dullness is percussed over the diaphragm, liver, and heart and tympany over the stomach. The liver is percussed beginning at the right fifth or sixth intercostal space in the midclavicular line. Percussion from this point downward to a point where the sound changes indicates the size of the liver. Beginning as resonant sounds, percussion sounds change to dullness over the liver then return to resonance beyond the liver border.

Posterior percussion begins at the shoulder level. The diaphragm is percussed posteriorly at the level of

Fig 15-16. *(continued)*

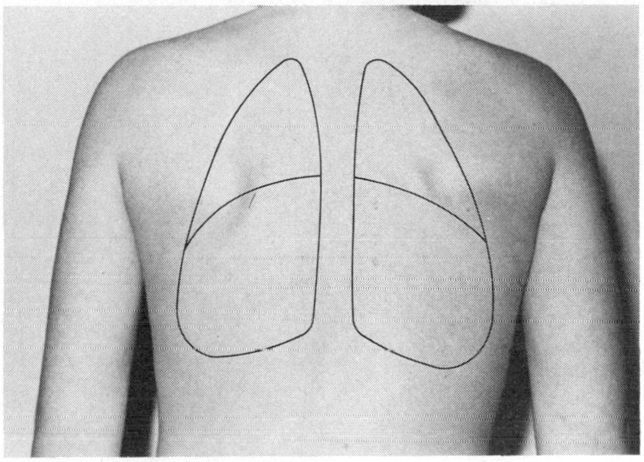

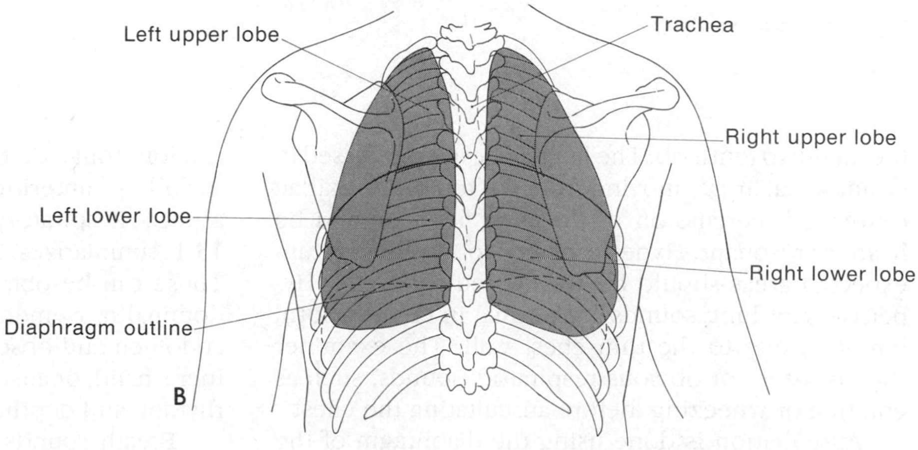

Illustration continued on following page

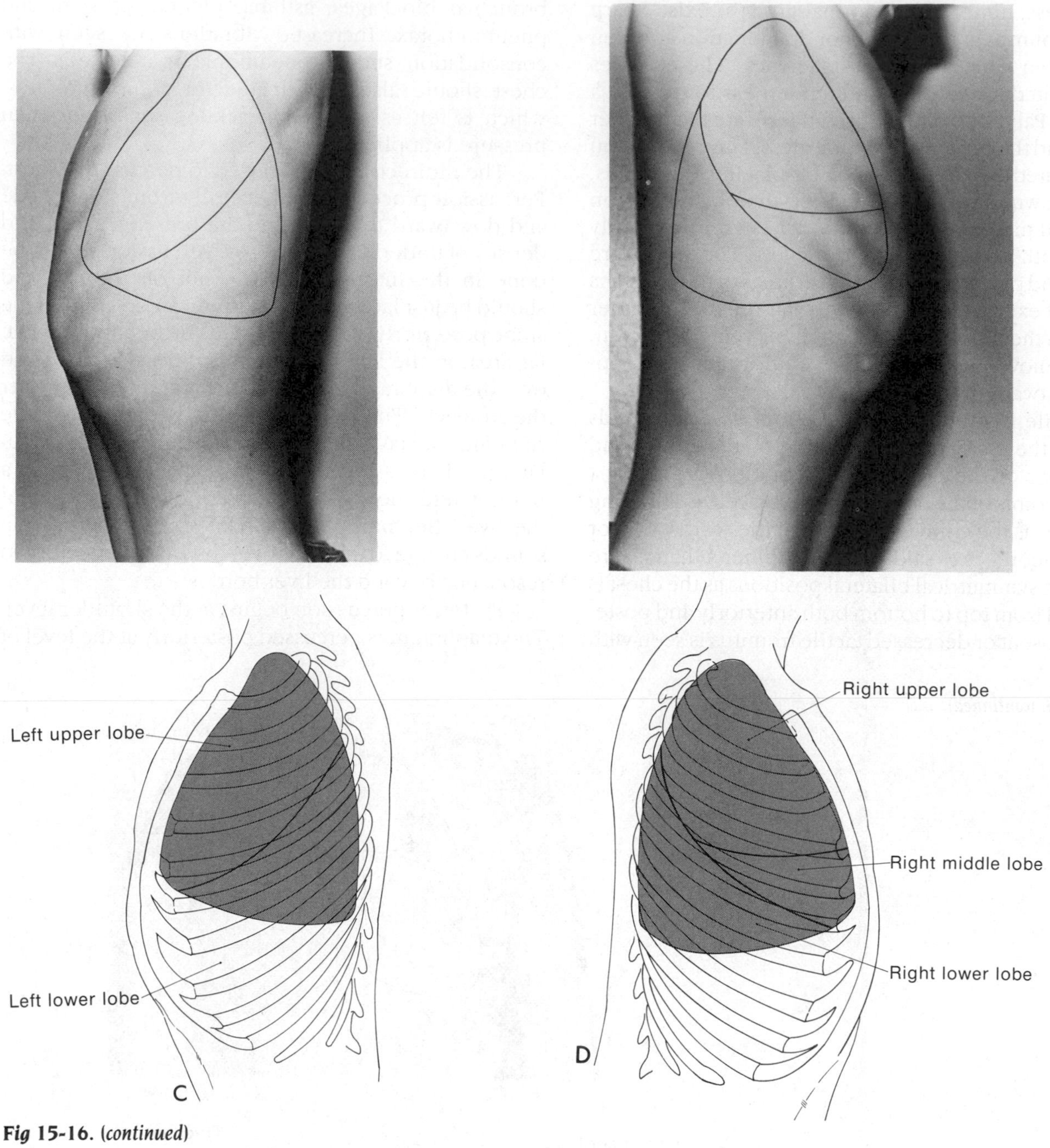

Fig 15-16. *(continued)*

the eighth to tenth rib. The lateral chest is percussed in symmetrical areas, moving from the top of the axillae downward. Percussion of the lung fields should be heard as resonant. Hyperresonance or dullness in unexpected areas should be considered abnormal. Hyperresonant lung sounds are normal in the newborn, however, due to the thin chest wall. The examiner should listen for obvious respiratory sounds, such as grunting or wheezing, before auscultating the chest.

Auscultation is done using the diaphragm of the stethoscope. The chest is auscultated in a systematic fashion from side to side moving from top to bottom, including anterior and posterior and the lateral aspects. Respiratory rate and depth are recorded. Table 15-1 summarizes average respiratory rates by age. These can be obtained by observing thoracic or abdominal movement, placing a hand on the thorax or abdomen and observing the movement of the examiner's hand, or auscultating the breath sounds for rate, rhythm, and depth.

Breath sounds are evaluated as to type, quality, pitch, duration, and intensity. Breath sounds are nor-

Table 15-6. Deformities of the Thorax

Cross-Section of Thorax | **Clinical Appearance**

Normal Infant

The chest of the normal infant is approximately round or barrel-shaped in cross-section.

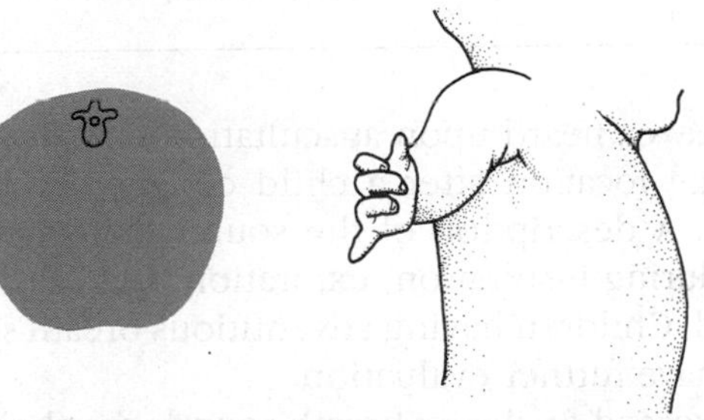

Normal Adult

As a child grows to adulthood, the transverse diameter of the thorax enlarges more than the anteroposterior diameter.

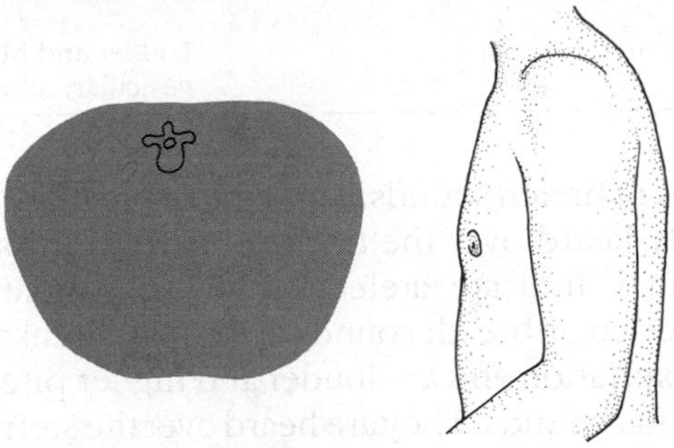

Barrel Chest

A round or barrel chest in a child after the age of 6 years suggests a chronic pulmonary disease (asthma, cystic fibrosis).

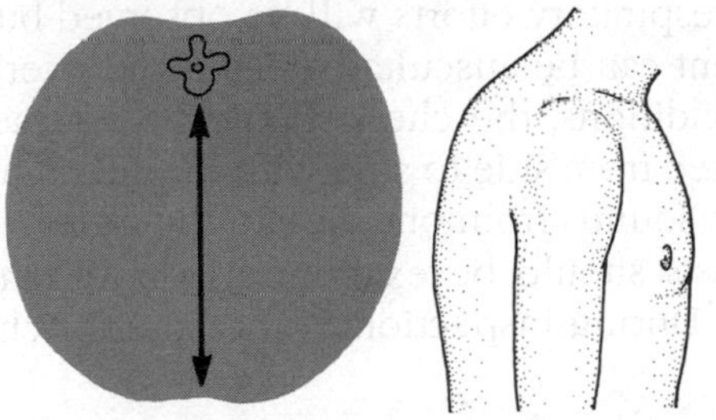

Funnel Chest (Pectus Excavatum)

A funnel chest is characterized by a depression in the lower portion of the sternum. Compression of the heart and great vessels may cause murmurs.

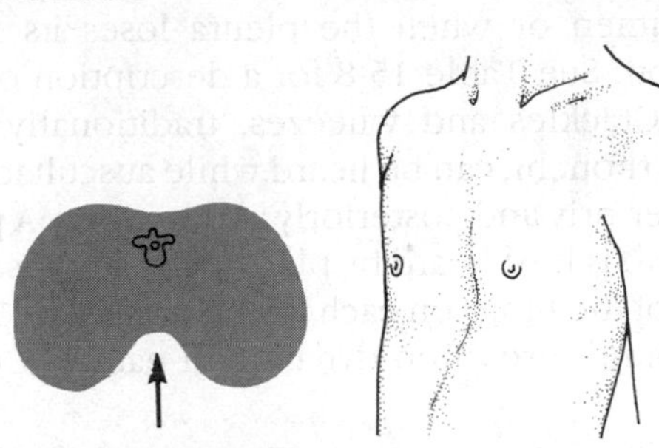

Pigeon Chest (Pectus Carinatum)

In pigeon chest, the sternum is displaced anteriorly, increasing the anteroposterior diameter. Grooves in the chest wall accentuate the deformity.

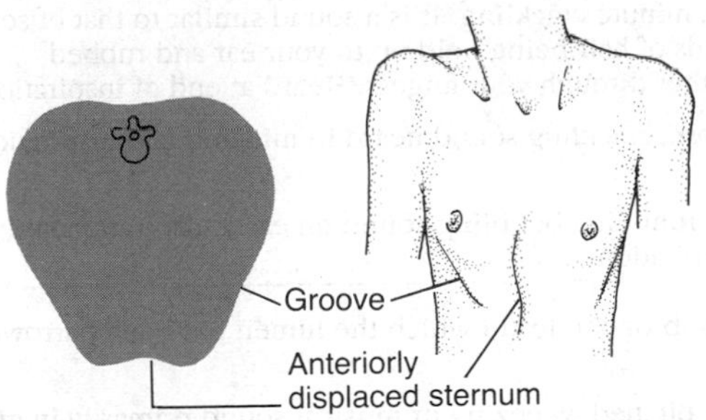

Thoracic Kyphoscoliosis

In thoracic kyphoscoliosis, the spine is curved, and the thorax shows corresponding deformities. Distortion of the underlying lungs may make interpretation of lung findings very difficult.

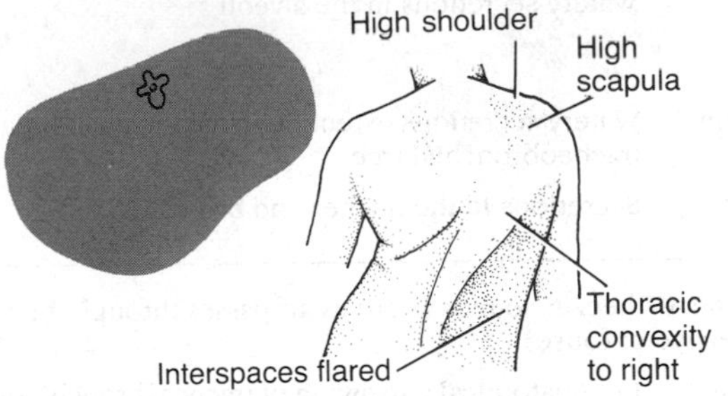

mally louder in children under 6 years of age due to the thin chest wall. There are three types of breath sounds: vesicular, bronchial, and bronchovesicular. Table 15-7 summarizes the characteristics of each. Vesicular breath sounds are louder, longer, and higher pitched in inspiration and are shorter, softer, and lower pitched in expiration. This type of breath sound is normally found all over the chest except in the areas of the sternum anteriorly and scapulae posteriorly. The ratio of the length of inspiration to the length of expirations is about 5 : 2. Vesicular sounds are exaggerated in the late stages of pneumonia, emphysema, and tuberculosis. In the early stages of pneumonia, vesicular breath sounds are diminished.

Bronchial breath sounds are shorter on inspiration than on expiration. They are usually louder than the

Table 15-7. Characteristics of Breath Sounds

Type	Length of Inspiration and Expiration	Quality and Intensity	Normal Location
Vesicular	loud soft	Softest; swishing sound	Throughout lung fields except over sternum and scapulae
Bronchial	soft loud	Loudest; blowing, hollow sound	Trachea
Bronchovesicular	same	Louder and higher pitched sound than vesicular; tubular quality	Sternum, upper intrascapular area

other types of breath sounds. This type of breath sound is normally heard over the trachea. If heard in other areas, it may indicate atelectasis or consolidation. Bronchovesicular breath sounds are equal on inspiration and expiration and are louder and higher pitched than vesicular sounds. They are heard over the sternum and upper intrascapular area.

Additional respiratory sounds not normally heard are adventitious sounds. These sounds are superimposed on normal breath sounds when air being exchanged passes through secretions or through a narrowed lumen or when the pleura loses its normal lubrication. See Table 15-8 for a description of these sounds. Crackles and wheezes, traditionally called rales and rhonchi, can be heard while auscultating the chest anteriorly and posteriorly as described. A pleural friction rub is best heard by placing the stethoscope at the base of the lungs on each lateral chest wall. Adventitious sounds are often dynamic in nature. Crackles and wheezes heard upon auscultation may disappear or change location after a child coughs or changes position. A description of the sound and whether it occurs during inspiration, expiration, or both should be noted. Children having adventitious breath sounds should have further evaluation.

Decreased or absent breath sounds are abnormal. Breath sounds are absent or decreased when the flow of air is obstructed and the sound of air exchange is not transmitted. Obstruction of air flow can be caused by a foreign object or mucus, pneumothorax, or pleural effusion. Often in children with a partially obstructed airway, respiratory efforts will be observed but no air movement can be auscultated. To avoid overlooking these conditions, the chest should be symmetrically auscultated from side to side with careful comparison of breath sounds from one side to the other.

Breasts should be examined in both males and females. During inspection of the anterior chest, the

Table 15-8. Adventitious Lung Sounds

Type	Cause	Description
*Rales** (Crackles: A crackling or bubbling sound produced by air flow through secretions)		
Fine	Watery secretions in the alveoli	Fine, minute crackling. It is a sound similar to that of several strands of hair being held up to your ear and rubbed together through your fingers. Heard at end of inspiration
Medium	Watery secretions extending from the alveoli pathway up the tracheobronchial tree	A loose, crackling sound heard in mid and late inspiration
Coarse	Secretions in the trachea and bronchi	Low, rumbling bubbling sound on early inspiration and part of expiration
*Rhonchi** (Wheeze: Sounds heard as air passes through the trachea, the bronchi, or bronchioles in which the lumen has been narrowed, irrespective of cause)		
Sibilant	(1) Anatomical narrowing of trachea, bronchi, or bronchioles or (2) bronchospasm	High-pitched wheezing or musical sound primarily in mid or late expiration but may be present throughout respiratory cycle
Sonorous	Originates in larger bronchi and the trachea. The flow of air continuously vibrates thick secretions along the airway	Loud low-pitched gurgling sound throughout the respiratory cycle that can be cleared by coughing or suctioning
Friction rub	Inflamed pleural surface with diminished lubricating fluid.	A grating sound, as if leather is being bent or rubbed together. It is heard near the end of inspiration at the lower anterolateral chest wall

* The terms *rales* and *rhonchi* are gradually being replaced by *crackles* and *wheezes,* respectively. Both sets of terms are retained here for clarity. Crackles generally include the categories of fine and coarse, whereas rales traditionally have been classified as fine, medium, and coarse.

nipples should be checked for color, spacing, placement, symmetry, fissures, inversions, secretions, scaling, and lumps. Breast bud formation usually begins around 10 to 14 years of age. One breast may begin to develop before the other and is often tender. Precocious breast development may be normal but can also indicate diethylstilbesterol ingestion or ovarian tumors. The breasts are inspected and palpated for redness, heat, tenderness, and masses. For palpation the child or adolescent lies in a supine position with the right arm extended above the head. The examiner lightly palpates the right breast with the fingertips in a rolling circular motion. Examination is begun at the center of the nipple and progresses in a counterclockwise manner in concentric rings until the entire breast and area surrounding the breast has been examined. Alternate methods of examination may be used as long as the method is systematic to ensure complete assessment of breast tissue. The axilla is also palpated for swelling, tenderness, and lymphadenopathy. The procedure is repeated on the left breast.

The breast should be examined with the child in various positions: (1) in a sitting position with hands raised above the head, (2) leaning forward, and (3) with the hands resting on the hips, pressing the elbows back and toward the midline. Inspection for dimpling, asymmetry, masses, discharge, and color takes place in each of these positions. While examining the breasts, the nurse may educate the female adolescent about self-examination techniques and the importance of routine examination.

The male breast should also be inspected and palpated for abnormalities. Any increased size should be noted, since it may be indicative of endocrine problems. The adolescent male also normally has some breast development during puberty.

The Heart

Techniques	**Equipment**
Inspection Palpation Auscultation Percussion	Stethoscope
Examine for	
Precordial abnormalities Size and shape of the heart	Quality, rate, rhythm of heart sounds Abnormal heart sounds

Inspection and palpation of the precordium is done to detect precordial bulging, thrills, lifts or heaves, precordial friction rubs, and the apical impulse. (Traditionally this has been called point of maximal impulse, PMI, but the more common terminology now used is apical impulse.) The apical impulse is palpable in the fourth or fifth intercostal space at or just medial to the midclavicular line in older children and adults. In infants, it is palpable in the fifth intercostal space (or slightly below), lateral to the midclavicular line. In thin children, the apical pulse may be visible.

A lift or heave is seen and felt when the cardiac action is abnormally forceful, actually lifting the ribs and sternum with each heartbeat. A thrill is a palpable heart murmur. It is a vibration and is often described as similar to the feel of a cat purring. Other observations related to the examination of the heart include respiratory distress, finger clubbing, edema, and cyanosis.

Percussion of the heart may be done using the direct or indirect percussion technique. Percussion of the heart outlines its size and shape. The heart normally is in the shape of an inverted triangle with the right border extending along the right side of the sternum from the second to the fifth ribs and from the right sternum at the fifth rib to the left midclavicular line at the fifth rib. The hypotenuse of the triangle is extended along the right side of the sternum at the second rib to the left midclavicular line at the fifth rib (see Fig. 15-17). The heart in an infant lies slightly more horizontally with the apex to the left of the nipple line. Percussion dullness that is located other than in the expected area could mean cardiac enlargement or heart displacement. This technique is frequently omitted during examination.

Auscultation is the most informative method of assessing cardiac function. It is used to evaluate the quality, rate, and rhythm of the heart and to detect abnormal heart sounds. There are five areas of the heart to examine when evaluating function (Fig. 15-17). (1) aortic, (2) pulmonic, (3) Erb's point, (4) apical (mitral), and (5) tricuspid (epigastric). First, the apical pulse rate, intensity, and rhythm are noted. Rapid or decreased pulse rates may be normal or may indicate pathology. The heart is auscultated with both the bell and the diaphragm of the stethoscope. The bell picks up low frequencies, and the diaphragm picks up high frequencies. The heart may be examined with the child in several positions: standing, sitting, leaning forward, supine, or left-lateral lying position. The heart should be auscultated after exercise. For routine examination the child may be examined supine or on a parent's lap.

The examiner begins by evaluating heart sounds for quality, intensity, rhythm, and unusual sounds. The first heart sound, S_1, indicates the systolic portion of the cardiac cycle; it is the "lub" of the "lub-dub." This sound is normally louder at the apex and is long and low pitched. The first heart sound is synchronous with the carotid pulse. It is caused by a closing of the mitral

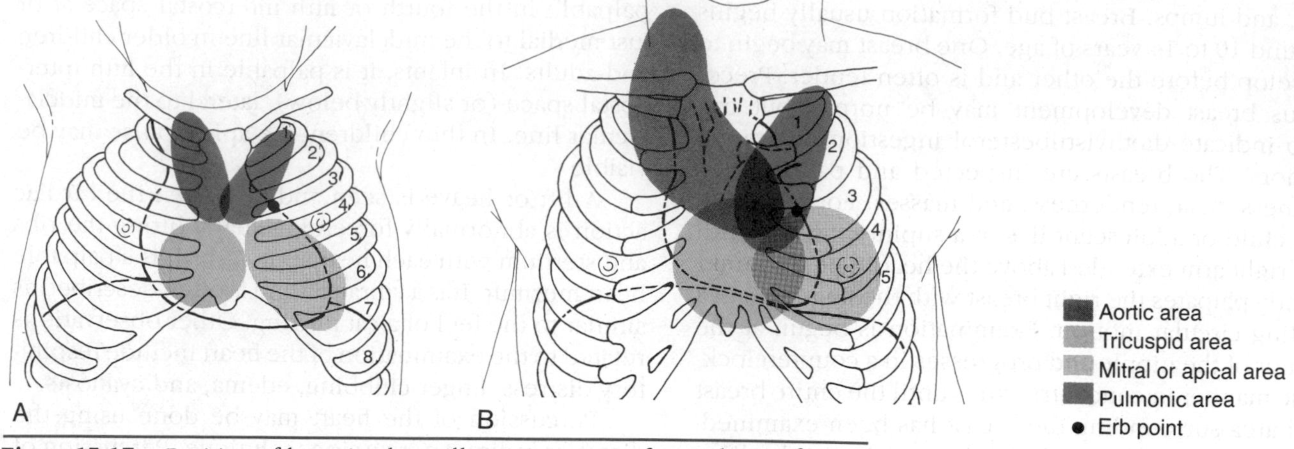

***Figure* 15-17.** Position of heart in chest, illustrating areas of auscultation for the infant (*A*) and adult (*B*). In an infant, the heart lies more horizontally in the chest because the diaphragm is higher and the rib cage is shorter than in an older child. This tends to displace the point of maximal impulse (PMI) more laterally, but it usually remains in the 5th intercostal space (or slightly below). The PMI in an infant is not higher in relation to the rib cage (i.e., it is not at the 3rd or 4th intercostal space); rather, it is the rib cage that is shorter compared with an older child. As the rib cage elongates and the diaphragm lowers with growth, the heart assumes a more vertical position; the PMI is then at the left midclavicular line in the 5th intercostal space.

The central point of each shaded area represents the most accurate area for auscultation. The perimeter of each shaded area represents the extent of radiation from each auscultation area. The location of the nipple varies considerably in both neonates and older children.

(Courtesy of Dr. R. C. Way, Director of Pediatric Cardiology, Chedoke-McMaster Hospitals, McMaster University Medical Centre Division, Hamilton, Ontario.)

and tricuspid valves. The second heart sound, S_2, is louder than S_1 at the base (aortic and pulmonic areas). This second sound reflects the diastole of the cardiac cycle and is the "dub" of the "lub-dub." It is shorter and higher in pitch than S_1 and is caused by closure of the semilunar valves (aortic and pulmonic valves). A third heart sound, S_3, is occasionally heard due to blood rushing through the mitral valve and rapidly filling the ventricle. The third heart sound is low pitched and occurs early in diastole. It is heard best at the apex. It can be normal in a child but is almost always abnormal in an adult. A fourth heart sound, S_4, may exist but is seldom normal. It is caused by an inaudible atrial contraction at the end of diastole and is heard best at the apex.

The heart sounds are evaluated for quality, intensity, and splitting. The first and second sounds should be clear and distinct. Any muffling or indistinctness may indicate pathology. Intensity refers to where each heart sound is heard best. S_1 should be heard best at the apex and S_2 heard best at the base of the heart. If this is not the case, the heart should be evaluated in more depth for a possible abnormality.

The rhythm of the heart is evaluated by listening carefully to determine if any irregularity exists. If an irregular rhythm is present, the examiner should attempt to determine a specific pattern. Sinus arrhythmia is a common irregularity in which the heart speeds up with inspiration and slows down with expiration. It should disappear when the child holds his or her breath and is considered normal in children.

One classification of unusual or abnormal heart sounds is heart murmurs. Six heart murmur classifications are presented in Chapter 39 in the section on heart anomalies. A heart murmur originates within the heart or its great vessels. The flow of blood is altered, causing an abnormal sound that is audible on auscultation. Murmurs are usually caused by (1) flow across a partial obstruction, (2) flow across an irregularity within the heart or vessel, (3) an increased amount of blood flow through a normal passageway, (4) flow from a normal passageway into a dilated area, (5) regurgitation (backward) flow through a valve or defect, and (6) flow of blood from a high pressure area through an abnormal passageway. The relationship of murmurs to other events should be noted. Murmurs may disappear or be accentuated by activity or crying or may vary with respirations. There are two types of murmurs: innocent and organic. Differentiation of the two types requires evaluation by a physician.

Finally, the cardiovascular pulses are palpated for presence or absence, regularity, and intensity. (See Table 15-1 for normal pulse rates.) The carotid, radial, femoral, popliteal, and pedal pulses are palpated and compared. The femoral and radial pulses are frequently palpated simultaneously to determine if a lag exists between the two. A femoral-radial lag or absent or diminished femoral pulses are characteristic of coarctation of the aorta. Temperature and color of the extremities should also be assessed. Cold, pale, or cyanotic extremities suggest cardiac disease or peripheral vascular disease.

A thorough examination of the heart should include blood pressure (see Figure 15-4 for normal values) and observation of the child before and after exercise or eating. Any color changes or fatigue should be noted.

The Abdomen

Techniques	**Equipment**
Inspection	Stethoscope
Auscultation	
Palpation	
Percussion	
Examine for	
Abdominal movement	Peristalsis
Abdominal shape	Muscle tone
Condition of unbilicus	Organomegaly
Herniations	Tenderness

Examination of the abdomen requires inspection, auscultation, palpation, and percussion of its four major divisions: right upper quadrant, right lower quadrant, left upper quadrant, and left lower quadrant. It is essential that the child be quiet and cooperative if the examiner is to evaluate this system thoroughly. The abdominal muscles are relaxed by flexing the child's knees slightly. Infants can be distracted or quieted by giving them a bottle in order to help relax the abdominal wall for examination. Before beginning the examination, the examiner's hands should be warm.

Inspection allows the examiner to determine shape and contour, movement and peristalsis, distention, bulges, and condition of the rectus muscle. Children normally have a pot belly that should begin to disappear by 4 or 5 years of age. The abdominal wall moves with respiration until 6 or 7 years of age; failure to do so may indicate appendicitis, peritonitis, paralytic ileus, diaphragmatic paralysis, or a large amount of air in the abdominal cavity.

Peristalsis is not generally visible in children. Visible peristaltic waves usually indicate an obstruction in the gastrointestinal tract. Pyloric stenosis is suspected if peristaltic waves occur from left to right.

Abdominal distention may be a sign of pregnancy, feces, organomegaly, ovarian cysts, ascites, or air in the abdominal cavity. The abdomen should be inspected from the front and from the sides to determine the extent of the distention; it is then palpated and percussed. Diastasis (splitting) of the rectus muscle is a protrusion in the midline from the xiphoid to the um bilicus and can be inspected and palpated. The split can be part way or the entire length between these two points. The width of the bulging can be one-half to two inches and still be considered normal. However, it may also be caused by a congenital weakness of the muscle or a chronically distended abdomen. Close follow-up with measurement of the length and width should be done.

The umbilicus is inspected closely for bulging, color, and discharge. A bluish umbilicus can be caused by intra-abdominal hemorrhage. In the newborn, the umbilical cord should be inspected for bleeding or signs of infection and for the presence of one vein and two arteries. Protrusion of the umbilicus usually indicates a hernia. Palpation of the hernia should be done to confirm a hernia after auscultation of the abdomen has been completed. Hernias are seen commonly in children up to the age of 2 or 3 years. They persist longer in black children, being seen until 7 or 8 years of age. Drainage from the umbilicus should be checked for color, odor, amount, and consistency. If infection is suspected, the fluid may be cultured. In addition to infection, a patent urachus, a remnant of fetal development, or a urachal cyst may be the cause of umbilical drainage.

Finally, the abdomen is inspected for distended veins and obvious pulsations. The skin is examined thoroughly as discussed earlier in this chapter.

Auscultation follows inspection of the abdomen so that peristaltic sounds are not disturbed by palpation or percussion. The diaphragm of the stethoscope is placed firmly over the abdomen and the examiner listens in all four quadrants for peristaltic sounds. These are metallic, short, tinkling sounds. Normally, an average of 15 to 34 bowel sounds per minute are audible. High-pitched, frequent, or hyperactive sounds are heard in children with diarrhea, gastroenteritis, and intestinal obstruction. Absence of peristaltic sounds may indicate a paralytic ileus or early peritonitis. Peristaltic sounds are very irregular and before concluding that they are absent, the examiner must listen for at least 5 or 10 minutes.

Vascular sounds may be detected by auscultation of the abdomen. A venous hum may indicate abnormality of the umbilical vein or portal obstruction. Murmurs may indicate coarctation of the aorta or a renal artery defect. Friction rubs and bruits heard in the abdomen are also abnormal and should be referred.

Percussion follows auscultation and is done with the child supine, either on his parent's lap or on the examination table. The examiner begins with the child's thorax at the left midaxillary line. The diaphragm is percussed above the spleen. Occasionally, tympany under the left diaphragm is percussed if a stomach bubble is present.

This procedure is then repeated in the right side where liver dullness is expected at the sixth interspace anteriorly and at the ninth rib posteriorly. The lower edge of the liver should be percussed at the right costal margin or occasionally 2 to 3 cm lower. With respiration the liver moves about two finger breadths. Ask the child to take a deep breath and hold it to facilitate percussion. The remainder of the abdomen is then percussed. Dullness encountered anywhere other than where it can be expected may indicate feces or a mass. Percussion should be used to outline the border and size of underlying structures. Tympany usually indicates air in the stomach and may be more pronounced in children who swallow air excessively or who have a gastrointestinal obstruction.

The final method of examination is palpation. Light palpation begins the examination and should proceed in a systematic fashion. Using the fingertips, the examiner gently and superficially palpates the quadrants in the following order: left lower, left upper, right upper, and right lower. Initially, the examiner notes if the abdomen is soft or hard, tender or distended.

After completing light palpation, the examiner proceeds in the same systematic way using deep palpation. Deep palpation is accomplished best during deep inspiration and deep expiration. The examiner may wish to place one hand on top of the other to provide firmer pressure for this examination technique. Deep palpation is useful in discovering masses, tenderness, deep vessels, and palpable organs. A pyloric tumor would be palpable at the right costal margin just to the right of the midline of the abdomen. Wilm's tumor may be palpated adjacent to the vertebral column in the kidney area.

The liver, if palpable, is felt for size, consistency, and tenderness. Any liver palpable below the costal margin should be percussed for size and evaluated for possible pathology.

The spleen can be palpated more easily if the child lies on the right side and takes a deep breath. The examiner lightly places the fingers just below the left costal margin at the midaxillary line and palpates the tip of the spleen. If more than the tip of the spleen is palpable, it is considered abnormal. In some children, the tip is not normally palpated.

To palpate the kidneys, the examiner must use very deep palpation. They are adjacent to the vertebral column and will descend slightly with inspiration. The lower pole may be felt particularly on the right, since this kidney is lower than the left. The child's flank should be firmly supported with the examiner's left hand while the right hand palpates the abdomen deeply. Normal kidneys are rarely palpable except in the newborn immediately following birth. However, palpation of the kidneys should always be attempted, since enlargement indicates significant pathology.

It is also possible to palpate the bladder in early childhood for possible distention. The intestines may also be palpable, and in intussusception, a sausage-shaped tumor may be found. Palpation is not complete until the child is checked closely for hernias. Umbilical hernias may be located and inspected with palpation. The examiner places a finger into the umbilicus and palpates for protrusion of intestines. The size of the opening through which the intestine protrudes should be noted. Hernias vary in size and should be measured at each visit to see if they are resolving. Occasionally, epigastric hernias are palpated as a small nodule protruding between the fibers of the linea alba and are often felt best when the child is standing. Examination for a femoral hernia is done by placing the right index finger on the child's femoral artery. The next finger then lies atop of the femoral vein and the ring finger is directly over the femoral canal. The standing child is then asked to strain as if having a bowel movement or to cough in order to elicit the hernia if one exists. The femoral hernia is felt or seen as a small bulge that results from a weakness in the musculature at the femoral canal. The child should be standing for this procedure (Fig. 15-18). A femoral hernia is more common in females. The technique for palpating inguinal hernias is described with assessment of male genitalia.

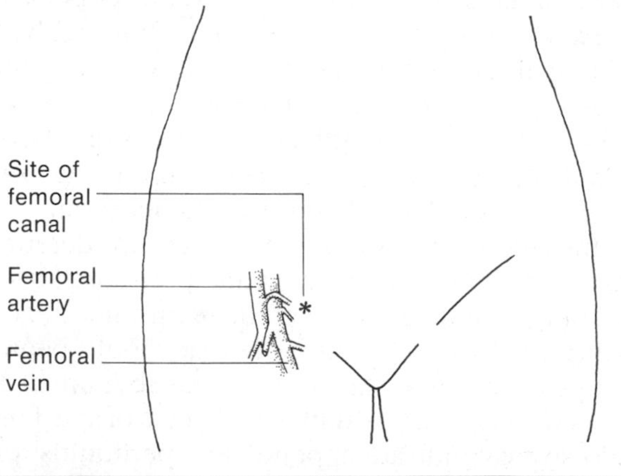

***Figure* 15-18.** The femoral area in the female. A femoral hernia, more common in females than males, is felt or seen as a small bulge at the site of the femoral canal.

The Female Genitalia

Techniques	Equipment
Inspection Palpation	Gloves
Examine for	
General appearance of anatomic structures Masses	Lesions Adhesions Size of vaginal opening

Every child should have a thorough examination of the genitalia. The examiner can complete this portion of the examination last if the child or adolescent is shy or embarrassed. This should be accomplished in a matter-of-fact manner that will put the child at ease. The female genitalia are inspected and palpated with gloved hands for presence or absence and symmetry of the external structures (Fig. 15-19). Evidence of edema, color changes, moisture, lesions, and masses should be identified and recorded. The examiner begins by inspecting the mons pubis for any masses or abnormalities. The presence or absence of pubic hair should be noted. Hair should be described according to color, quantity, texture, and distribution. It should also be inspected for lice.

The vulva is inspected for erythema, swelling, masses, and varicosities. The labia minora are normally quite large in the infant and may protrude from behind the labia majora. Swelling of the vulva could be a sign of sexual molestation, infection, a foreign body, trauma, or lymphedema.

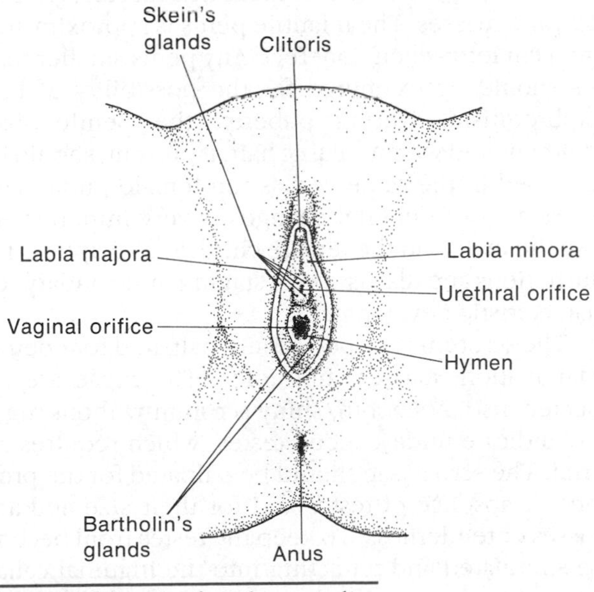

Figure 15-19. The female genitalia.

Next, inspect and palpate the Bartholin's and Skein's glands. They are not normally seen or felt. If visible or palpable, enlargement exists and is due to infection, usually gonorrhea.

The clitoris is inspected carefully to determine if its size is abnormal. It may normally be large in the newborn, while a hypertrophied clitoris in an older child may indicate labioscrotal fusion or pseudohermaphroditism. Because of its sensitivity, the clitoris should not be palpated unless there is a specific reason for doing so.

The vestibule is inspected and palpated for lesions and masses. There will be few abnormal findings here until the child is older, when the examiner may find ulcerated venereal lesions. It is also important to examine the urethral meatal opening for inflammation, erythema, and discharge. Location of the meatus should be noted for possible epispadias. Finally, the vaginal opening and hymen are checked for congenital absence of the vagina or imperforate hymen. The careprovider should note the size of the vaginal opening; an enlarged opening in a young female may be indicative of sexual abuse. Newborns may have a small amount of bloody vaginal discharge until 1 month of age as a result of absorption of the maternal hormones during fetal life. Foul-smelling discharge may be due to infection, the presence of a foreign body, or pinworms.

The Male Genitalia

Techniques	Equipment
Inspection Palpation	Good lighting Penlight Stethoscope
Examine for	
Structural anomalies Abnormal discharge	Lesions Hernias

The male genitalia (Fig. 15-20) are also examined thoroughly in a matter-of-fact efficient manner. The examiner should begin by first inspecting and palpating the penis for size and consistency. An enlarged penis may be due to precocious puberty, central nervous system lesions, or testicular tumors. It should be noted if the child has been circumcised; if not, it should be noted whether the foreskin is retractable or if adhesions are present. A controversy exists over whether or not the foreskin should be forcibly re-

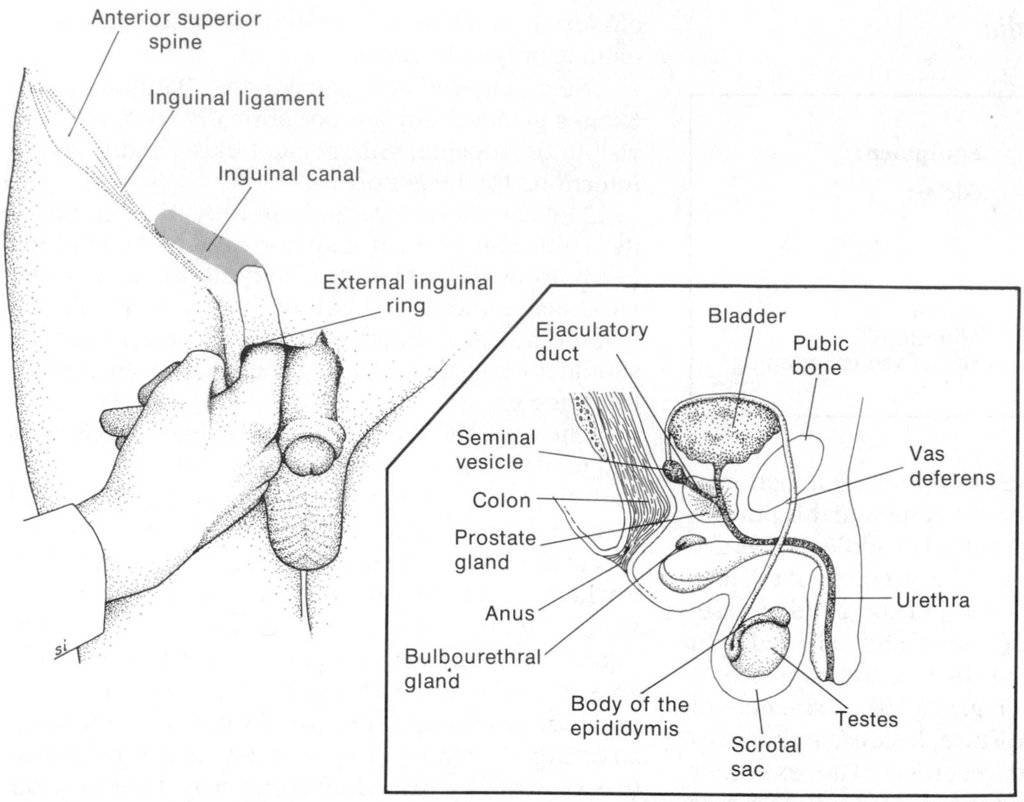

***Figure* 15-20.** The male genitalia. The inguinal canal is palpated to check for a possible hernia. In a younger child, the little (fifth) finger is used.

tracted for inspection of the glans if the child is uncircumcised. Normally, the foreskin does not retract easily for the first 2 to 3 months because of a thin membrane which connects it to the surface of the glans. At 4 months the foreskin is more easily retracted and by 4 years it is usually fully retractable. Some clinicians recommend forcible retraction beginning at birth and continued on a daily basis while others recommend retracting the foreskin only as far as possible without force. The latter clinicians feel that the trauma of forcible retraction causes scar tissue to develop when the delicate membrane has been torn, thus making retraction more difficult later. If by 4 years of age the foreskin has not gradually become retractable, the boy may be considered to have phimosis, an abnormal narrowing at the opening of the foreskin which prohibits retraction. Phimosis should be referred for physician evaluation.

The meatal opening is inspected for size, position, and any discharge. Hypospadias or epispadias is present if the opening is either on the ventral or dorsal surface of the glans penis. These conditions require medical evaluation. A pinpoint meatal opening may cause urinary obstruction. If possible, the child's urinary stream should be observed or information obtained from the child or parent during the history. A urinary stream that dribbles or is not a steady, strong stream may be seen with meatal stenosis or other anomalies. The glans is also inspected for lesions, swelling, or venereal warts.

The shaft of the penis is examined for size, varicosities, and masses. The infantile penis is approximately 2 to 3 cm long when nonerect. Any penis smaller than this should be examined for the possibility of hermaphroditism. During puberty, the penile shaft lengthens and widens. Pubic hair, if present, should be described in the same way as the female pubic hair. Assessment of pubertal changes is very important in both the male and the female child. See Chapter 9 for illustrations and discussion of staging in secondary sex characteristic development.

The scrotum is inspected and palpated for edema, inflammation, masses, and color. The rugae are inspected also. A smooth, shiny scrotum without rugae may indicate undescended testes, which requires referral. The scrotal sac should be palpated for the presence or absence of testes and for their size and any masses or tenderness. To keep the testes from becoming stimulated and retracting into the inguinal canal, the examiner occludes the inguinal canals by finger pressure. Retractile testes may not be found in the scrotal sac during examination; this disorder is referred to as pseudocryptorchidism. The spermatic cord can be palpated and followed to the testes. Any swelling, thickening, or the presence of nodules should be noted. An enlarged or pendulous scrotum should be transilluminated to determine if a hydrocele, hernia, or mass is present. This is accomplished by placing a penlight behind the scrotal sac. Illumination occurs in hydrocele but not in hernia or masses. Swelling and discoloration of the scrotum that has developed suddenly may be a sign of spermatic cord torsion, which requires immediate attention by a physician.

The inguinal canal is palpated to rule out a possible hernia (Fig. 15-20). A hernia of this type is indirect and may be congenital. It is seen in males nine times more frequently than in females and occurs more commonly on the right side. The examiner should place a finger (in a young child, the fifth [little] finger should be used) in the scrotal sac and gently approach the inguinal canal, following the spermatic cord. The finger tip should not be able to enter the canal through the external inguinal ring unless the ring is abnormally dilated. Weakness of the ring may signal a potential hernia. This weakness is tested by having the child cough or strain. The external ring is palpated for tone. The examiner also palpates the inguinal canal, noting (by pressing through the side of the abdominal wall) if any abdominal contents can be felt pressing down into the inguinal canal or if the bulge is palpable. These findings would indicate a hernia. Regional lymph nodes and the femoral canal and pulses should also be examined at this time if they were not during the abdominal survey.

The Rectum and Anus

Techniques	**Equipment**
Inspection	Glove
Palpation	Lubricant

Examine for	
Patency	Masses
Sphincter tone	Lesions
Fecal consistency	

The rectum is inspected for fissures, prolapse, hemorrhoids, polyps, inflammation, rashes, and lesions. Patency should also be determined, both with data from the history and rectal examination. Signs of scratching or irritation may be due to pinworms. Usually, a rectal examination is not done routinely in children. If history indicates the need for such an exam, it should be done. This is accomplished by inserting a gloved, lubricated finger slowly into the rectum and gently palpating the walls of the rectum as well as stool. Sphincter tone and the character, amount, and consistency of feces should be identified. Presence of masses, tenderness, or a lack of sensation should be investigated further. Fecal masses are present in children with mental deficiency, anal stenosis, psychologic difficulties, and chronic constipation. Complete absence of feces in the rectum may indicate ileus, peritonitis, or obstruction.

The Musculoskeletal System

Techniques	**Equipment**
Inspection	None
Palpation	

Examine for	
Structural anomalies	Function of extremities
Posture	Spinal deformities
Range of motion	

A general inspection of the skeletal system begins with observation as the child walks into the examination room. The child is also observed during play activities and while performing tasks such as undressing. Symmetry of movement, position, general alignment, deformities, gait, extra digits, and unusual posture are observable while the child is unaware of the examiner's scrutiny.

During the actual examination, soft tissues and muscles are inspected and palpated for symmetry, contractures, erythema, swelling, and tenderness. Muscles are inspected and palpated for symmetry, mass, tone, strength, and paralysis. The bones are palpated for shape, outline, thickening, abnormal prominence, or indentation. The examiner should determine if the temperature of one extremity seems higher than the others. All joints should be inspected and palpated for swelling, redness, or tenderness and should be actively and passively placed through full range of motion. The extremities are compared for equality of strength, length, and symmetry of movement.

With both hands simultaneously the child should squeeze the examiner's hands and fingers; this allows the examiner to evaluate strength and symmetry.

The examiner palpates the clavicles for crepitus or tenderness that would indicate a fracture. The arms are examined carefully for subluxation and for an increased carrying angle. To examine for an increased carrying angle, instruct the child to hold the arms straight out at the sides (at a right angle to the chest) with his palms facing forward. The arms should form a smooth, continuous line of approximately 180 degrees. If the lower arm is bent upward forming an angle of less than 180 degrees, the child has an increased carrying angle (see Figure 4-24, page 155). This may be normal but is also associated with gonadal dysgenesis.

The hands are checked closely for extra digits, webbing, missing digits, or abnormally short or long digits. Creases of the hands are inspected closely. Evidence of a simian crease may indicate Down syndrome but is also normal in some individuals. The knuckles should be inspected for their presence and any anomalies. Examination of the extremities should incorporate examination of the regional lymph nodes, skin, nails, hair, and pulses.

The examiner also applies pressure to the child's arms while they are held in the following positions: raised above the head, out to the sides, and straight out in front. The child should be able to maintain each of these positions while the examiner tries to force the arms in the opposite direction. The child can also stand with arms flexed across the chest while the examiner tries to straighten them, and, in reverse, the child can extend the arms while the examiner tries to flex them.

The lower extremities are observed for shape. Genu varum (bowleggedness) is present when the medial malleoli are touching and the knees are more than 1 inch apart. A child has genu valgum (knock-knees) if the knees are together and the medial malleoli are more than 1 inch apart. Genu valgum is normally seen in the child between 2½ to 3½ years of age, while genu varum is often seen in a child until walking has been established for a year. (See Figure 6-1 for diagrams of lower limb development.) The tibia should be inspected and palpated for torsion. See Chapter 47 for torsional assessment technique.

The lower extremities are checked for equality in length. The child should lie supine and with legs extended. The four malleoli should be in the same plane. The child may also be requested to stand while the examiner inspects the patellae and the crease in the popliteal fossas for symmetry. This should be done when the child is standing straight with the knees and feet together.

Strength of the legs is checked in much the same way as strength in the upper extremities. The legs are flexed, and the examiner tries to straighten them. This process is reversed by having the legs extended while the examiner exerts pressure in trying to prevent the child from flexing the legs.

Range of motion of the hips, knees, ankles, and toes should also be checked. It is particularly important to evaluate hip rotation in the infant to rule out congenital hip dislocation. See Chapter 47 for detailed assessment for a congenitally dislocated hip.

The feet are inspected for equality of size and shape and for position. If possible, the feet should be examined with the child standing. The arch is examined for unusual height or a flatness. Children have a fat pad under their medial arch until they have been walking one to two years, which gives them the appearance of having flat feet. The examiner should be able to fit at least one finger under the medial arch. An arch that allows more than one finger is high. An arch that does not allow at least one finger is considered flat. Wetting both feet and then having the child stand on a piece of paper will yield an outline of the arches.

The position of the feet should be noted. Pes valgus (toeing out) and pes varus (toeing in) refer to the entire foot turning either out or in and are caused by structural anomalies. In metatarsus varus (forefoot in) and metatarsus valgus (forefoot out), the heel is straight and midline. These conditions should be referred for further evaluation. The heels of the child's feet should be closely observed from the posterior angle. The child should stand while the examiner inspects the heel cords for deviation. Slight medial slanting before the age of 5 or 6 is normal, but after this age may be an indication of pronation. Children who have pronated feet look as if they are standing on the inner aspects of their heels and arches. The medial malleoli are frequently lower than the lateral malleoli.

Finally, children are observed for gait, balance, and stance. Children should walk, run, and skip while the examiner observes. The beginning walker (between 12 and 18 months) generally demonstrates a broad-based gait with poor balance. By 3 or 4 years of age, the gait is narrow based, and the child should be able to maintain balance on one foot for several seconds. Most children are able to skip fairly well by 5 or 6 years of age.

The child's gait and stance should be inspected from all points of view, particularly side view. The phases of the gait should be inspected for symmetry, coordination, and position of arms and legs. Any deviation should be identified in relation to the appropriate phase and stage.

Spine

At birth the spinal curve is in the shape of a C rather than the double S seen later in life. The curves present in the neonate are the thoracic and pelvic curves. Around 3 to 4 months of age the cervical curve develops. This is the time when children begin to hold their heads upright. The lumbar curve appears between 12 to 18 months when the child begins to walk. The four curves then are the cervical (a convex line), the thoracic (concave), the lumbar (ventrally convex), and, finally, the pelvic curve (concave curve directed caudally and ventrally). The cervical and lumbar curves are secondary or compensatory curves because they do not develop until after birth. It is important to remember this evolution of spinal curvatures when examining the spine in a young child.

Inspection and palpation of the spine should be done with the child standing if possible. The examiner checks for symmetry of bony landmarks, alignment and for other skin manifestations such as dimples, cysts, and tufts of hair. The spine is inspected and palpated for the presence or absence of each spinous process and for masses and tenderness. The child's posture is examined from the front, back, and side and when the child is in a flexed position. A child with an exaggerated concave curve in the thoracic region has kyphosis. On the other hand, an exaggerated convex curve in the lumbar region indicates lordosis, which may be normal in some children. Poor posture, commonly seen in adolescence, may appear as kyphosis but is usually not a permanent skeletal deformity. Scoliosis is a lateral curvature of the spine that requires medical follow-up. Positional evaluation of scoliosis is described in Chapter 47.

The Neurologic System

Techniques	**Equipment**
Observation	Reflex hammer
Interview	Familiar odors in test tubes
Examine for	Safety pin
	Tuning fork
Cerebral function	Ophthalmoscope
Cranial nerves	Small, easily recognizable objects (coin, bottlecap)
Cerebellar function	
Motor system function	Audiometer for hearing testing
Sensory capacity	
Reflex action	Developmental screening tools

A complete neurologic examination requires an in-depth knowledge of nervous system function, expertise in the performance of the examination, and an extended time period. Rarely is a complete neurologic examination performed as part of a routine physical examination. More often, the nurse uses selective tests to evaluate the baseline function of the child's nervous system. Any abnormal test results would then require further evaluation.

The neurologic examination involves testing of function within six major areas: the cerebrum, the cranial nerves, the cerebellum, the motor system, the sensory system, and reflex action.

Cerebral Function

This area is evaluated using both an interview and developmental tests. The nurse should begin by noting general behavior, level of consciousness, intellectual performance, and emotional state. In addition, the child's posture, facial expression, gestures, movement, level of activity, attention span, and speech should be noted. Observations about specific behavior should be verified with the parent.

Memory is also part of general cerebral function; immediate, recent, and remote memory should be evaluated.

Immediate recall refers to the retention of an idea or thought for a brief time; this is tested by having a child repeat numbers. A child of 4 years can usually repeat three numbers, while a child of 5 years can repeat four numbers, and a child of 6 can usually repeat five numbers correctly. Memory of an idea that lasts slightly longer is recent memory. The child can be shown an object and told to remember the object. Later, the child is asked to tell what the object was. Remote memory refers to memory for longer periods of time. Children can be asked what they ate for dinner last night or their address or birthdays.

Evaluation of specific cerebral function includes testing three functional areas:

- cortical sensory interpretation — the ability to recognize objects through the use of senses: visual, tactile, auditory, somatic;
- cortical motor integration — the ability to perform purposeful acts;
- language: expressive, receptive.

Visual sensory interpretation can be accomplished by playing the "find it" game. The examiner places several objects on a table and then instructs the child to pick up the objects as they are named. Tactile sensory integration (stereognosis) is done by placing one of several objects in the child's hands and having the object identified with the child's eyes closed. Familiar objects such as coins, bottle caps, and buttons should be used. Graphethesia is the ability to identify shapes traced in the palm or on the back of the hand. School-age children can usually identify the numbers 0, 1, 3, 7, and 8. Younger children usually identify geometric forms, parallel lines, or crossing lines. If the child cannot identify the shape, the examiner does the tracing twice and asks the child if the two are the same or different.

Evaluation of the auditory sense is done by having the child listen with closed eyes and identify different, common sounds such as a whistle or a hand clap.

Body part perception, or somatic sensory perception, can be accomplished by observing the child's response to tactile stimuli. The child's eyes are occluded. With the child's hands held out in front, the examiner touches one or two fingers and the child is asked to show which finger(s) were touched. By the age of 6 children may still occasionally confuse the third and fourth fingers, especially if two fingers were touched.

Kinesthesia, the ability to perceive direction of movement or weight, is evaluated in children over 5 by manipulating the child's finger to either an up or down position. The child's eyes should be closed for this test and the examiner should be careful to handle only the sides of the child's fingers so that the weight of the examiner's fingers does not give the child a clue to the direction. Texture discrimination can be done by having the child feel different textured items while the eyes are closed and tell whether they are smooth or rough. Visual motor integration and cortical motor integration can be tested by having the child copy various designs which are drawn or shown. A child of 3 years of age can usually draw a circle; by the age of 4 years a square can be drawn, and by 5 years the child can draw a triangle. Children 6 years of age can draw a diamond, and 7-year-olds can usually draw a British flag design.

The last specific cerebral function to be tested is the child's ability to communicate and understand both spoken and written language. Screening tests for articulation and speech may be used and are described later in this chapter. Having the child repeat numbers or nonsense syllables, testing the ability to follow directions, and testing language discrimination are other ways of evaluating language ability. An inability to repeat may indicate that the child has poor ability to perceive what is heard. Discrimination is evaluated by saying two familiar words such as fright and flight. The child is then asked if they are the same or different words.

Part of the neurologic examination of the infant is an evaluation of its cry. A high-pitched shrill cry may indicate intracranial damage, while a high-pitched screeching cry may indicate a syndrome of genetic congenital defects, especially if associated with microcephaly, low-set ears, or micrognathia.

Cranial Nerves

Evaluation of the 12 pairs of cranial nerves is easily integrated into the nurse's physical examination. Children and adolescents enjoy the active participation required for testing cranial nerve functions. Difficulty is encountered in the assessment of cranial nerves in infants and young children owing to the child's developmental level. Specific nerves and procedures for testing are indicated in Table 15-9.

Cerebellar Function

Tests for cerebellar function involve primarily assessment of balance and coordination. Developmental screening tools provide an accessible, standardized method of assessing fine and gross motor balance and coordination skills. General cerebellar examination begins with observing gait, watching the child walk heel to toe, and checking the ability to dress and undress, button, stack blocks, throw, kick, etc. Balance is specifically evaluated by observing the gait and having the child stand with the eyes both open and closed. This test of sensory equilibrium (Romberg test) is positive if the child begins to fall.

Examples of coordination tests are finger to nose, heel to shin, and various activities that involve alternating motion. For the finger-to-nose test the child stands erect with arms extended at the sides and then touches index fingers alternately to the nose. This test is repeated with the eyes closed. An abnormal response would be "past pointing," in which the child completely misses touching the nose. In the heel-to-shin test the child lies supine on the examination table and places one heel rapidly down the shin from the knee to the ankle. This is repeated using the other heel. Uncoordinated or inaccurate movements suggest a cerebellar dysfunction.

Rapid alternating motion is tested by having the child rapidly alternate pronation and supination of the hands on the knees. One hand should be tested and the other observed for mirroring movements. Slow and inaccurate movements are considered abnormal. Additional information can be obtained by having the child stand erect and balance on one foot. By the age of 4 years a child should be able to balance for about 5 seconds; by the age of 6 the child should be able to balance on one foot with arms folded across the chest. The child should balance on the right and then the left leg to evaluate symmetry. Another test would be to have the child touch each finger to the thumb of the same hand in rapid succession. This should be done with each hand to check for symmetry. The hand not performing the task should also be observed for mirroring. The cerebellar function of the infant may be grossly assessed by observing coordination in sucking, swallowing, reaching, and grasping.

Evaluating the Motor System

Examination of the motor system includes evaluation of muscle size, muscle tone, muscle strength, and abnormal muscle movements. Most of the motor system

Table 15-9. Assessment of Cranial Nerves

Cranial Nerve	Test for Function
I Olfactory (S)*	
Olfactory nerve, mucous membrane of nasal and turbinates	With eyes closed child is asked to identify familiar odors such as peanut butter, orange, peppermint. Test each nostril separately.
II Optic (S)	
Optic nerve, retinal rods and cones	Check visual acuity, peripheral vision, color vision, perception of light in infants, fundoscopic examination for normal optic disc.
III Oculomotor (M)*	
Muscles of the eye (superior rectus, inferior rectus, medial rectus, inferior oblique)	Have child follow an object or light with the eyes (EOM)* while head remains stationary. Check symmetry of corneal light reflex. Check for nystagmus (direction elicited vertical, horizontal, rotary). Check cover-uncover test.
Muscles of iris and ciliary body	Reaction of pupils to light, both direct and consensual, accommodation.
Levator palpebral muscle	Check for symmetric movement of upper eyelids. Note ptosis.
IV Trochlear (M)	
Muscles of eye (superior oblique)	Check the range of motion of the eyes downward (EOM). Check for nystagmus.
V Trigeminal (M, S)	
Muscles of mastication (M)	Have child clamp the jaws and palpate jaw muscles and temporal muscles for strength and symmetry. Ask child to move lower jaw from side to side against resistance of the examiner's hand.
Sensory innervation of face (S)	Test child for sensation using a wisp of cotton; warm and cold water in test tubes; a sharp object on the forehead, cheeks, jaw. Check corneal reflex by touching a wisp of cotton to each cornea. The normal response is blink.
VI Abducens (M)	
Muscles of eye (lateral rectus)	Have child look to each side (EOM).
VII Facial (M, S)	
Muscles for facial expression (M)	Have child make faces: look at the ceiling, frown, wrinkle forehead, blow out cheeks, smile. Check for strength, asymmetry, paralysis.
Sense of taste on anterior ⅔ of tongue. Sensation of external ear canal, lacrimal, submaxillary and sublingual glands	Have child identify salt, sugar, bitter (flavoring extract) and sour substances by placing substance on anterior sides of tongue. Keep tongue out until substance is identified. Rinse mouth between substances.
VIII Acoustic (S)	
Equilibrium (vestibular nerve)	Note equilibrium or presence of vertigo (Romberg sign).
Auditory acuity (cochlear nerve)	Test hearing. Use a tuning fork for the Weber and Rinne tests. Test by whispering and use of a watch.
IX Glossopharyngeal (M, S)	
Pharynx, tongue (M)	Check elevation of palate with "ah" or crying. Check for movement and symmetry. Stimulate posterior pharynx for gag reflex.
Sense of taste posterior third of the tongue (S)	Test sense of taste on posterior portion of tongue.
X Vagus (M, S)	
Mucous membrane of pharynx, larynx, bronchi, lungs, heart, esophagus, stomach, kidneys Posterior surface of external ear, external auditory meatus	Note same as for glossopharyngeal. Note any hoarseness, stridor. Check uvula for midline position, movement with phonation. Stimulate each side of uvula on each side with tongue depressor—should rise and deviate to stimulated side. Check gag reflex. Observe ability to swallow.
XI Accessory (M)	
Sternocleidomastoid and upper trapezius muscles	Have child shrug shoulders against mild resistance. Have child turn head to one side against resistance of examiner's hand. Repeat on the other side. Inspect and palpate muscle strength, symmetry for both maneuvers.
XII Hypoglossal (M)	
Muscles of tongue	Have child move the tongue in all directions, then stick out tongue as far as possible; check for tremors or deviations. Test strength by having child push tongue against inside cheek against resistance on outer cheek. Note strength, movement, symmetry.

* S = sensory, M = motor, EOM = extraocular movement.

Table 15-10. Evaluating the Sensory System

Sensations	Procedure
Superficial tactile sensation	Brush body part with a wisp of cotton.
Superficial pain	Evaluate ability to sense sharpness or dullness. Use both ends of a safety pin or a broken tongue depressor.
Temperature	Have child identify the temperature of test tubes filled with both warm and cold water.
Vibration	Assess the child's ability to feel a vibrating tuning fork on sternum, elbows, iliac crests, knees, and toes.
Deep pressure pain	Never evaluated unless indicated by a decreased level of consciousness. Tested by applying strong pressure on eyeballs, sternum, calf or forearm muscles, or testicles.
Motion and position	Tested as part of the evaluation of cerebellar function. (See page 550 for explanation of specific tests.)
Discriminatory sensation	With the child's eyes closed, examiner touches a body part then asks child to identify part touched.

evaluation is accomplished through the examination of the extremities and spine and developmental screening tools. Muscles should be checked for hypertrophy, atrophy, and asymmetry. Any abnormality or asymmetry should be referred.

Muscle strength is discussed in the section on examination of the extremities in this chapter. Involuntary movements are assessed by observing a child in a stationary state with hands resting on the knees or stretched out in front. Occasionally, involuntary movements can be better elicited by involving the child in a stressful conversation. If any choreic, twitching, or convulsive movements are noted, the child should be referred for further evaluation. Tremors or tics are also abnormal.

The Sensory System

Both primary and discriminatory sensation are evaluated as part of the assessment of the neurologic system. Many of the tests already discussed will give the examiner sufficient information about the sensory system for the routine examination. However, further evaluation may include an assessment of the primary, symmetrical sensation of the face, trunk, arms, and legs. See Table 15-10 for the types of sensations to be evaluated and the procedures for testing.

Reflex Action

The reflexes evaluated in the older child and adult fall into two categories: superficial and deep. Table 15-11 provides a description of the reflex and procedures employed in testing.

While superficial reflexes may not always be elicited as part of the neurologic examination, deep tendon reflexes usually are.

Deep tendon reflexes (DTR) are illustrated and described in Table 15-12. DTR responses are usually graded using the following scoring system: 0 = absent, +1 = sluggish, +2 = active, +3 = hyperactive, +4 = transient clonus, and +5 = permanent clonus. Deep reflexes are evaluated for strength and symmetry from side to side and from upper to lower extremities. The tendon should be slightly stretched and briefly tapped with a reflex hammer. The expected response is contraction of the muscle. Pathologic reflexes are particularly significant in identifying neurologic abnormality. Clonus is abnormal in the older child but can be normal in the newborn if it is mild. The child's ankle is grasped and firm pressure is exerted on the ball of the

Table 15-11. Evaluating Superficial Reflexes

Procedure for Eliciting	Normal Response	Comments
Abdominal Reflex		
Using a sharp point, the examiner strokes the four quadrants of the abdomen in a diamond or square pattern	The umbilicus moves toward the stimulus	Present after the first 2 days of life. Absence or asymmetry of response may not be significant but should be noted
Cremasteric Reflex		
Stroke the inner aspect of the thigh with a fingernail. Test both sides	Testis on the stimulated side recedes into inguinal canal	Often occurs spontaneously during exam. Abnormality could indicate pathology
Gluteal (Anal Wink)		
Examiner separates the buttocks and strokes the perianal area with a wisp of cotton	A brisk contraction of the anal sphincter	

Table 15-12. Evaluating Deep Tendon Reflexes (DTR)

Name	Procedure for Eliciting	Normal Response	Comments
Triceps 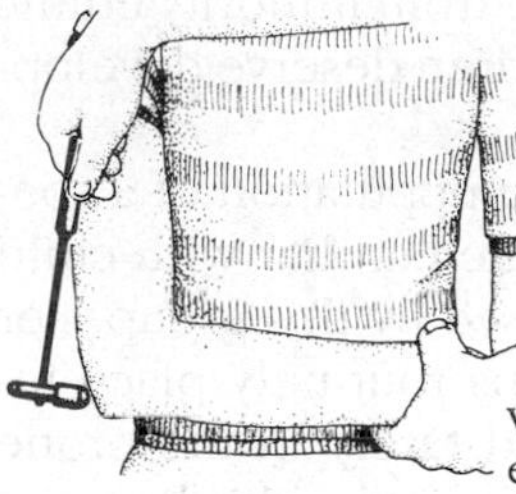	With the child's arm flexed at the elbow, the tendon is struck just above olecranon process.	Muscles of the forearm contract	Grade response, evaluate symmetry.
Biceps 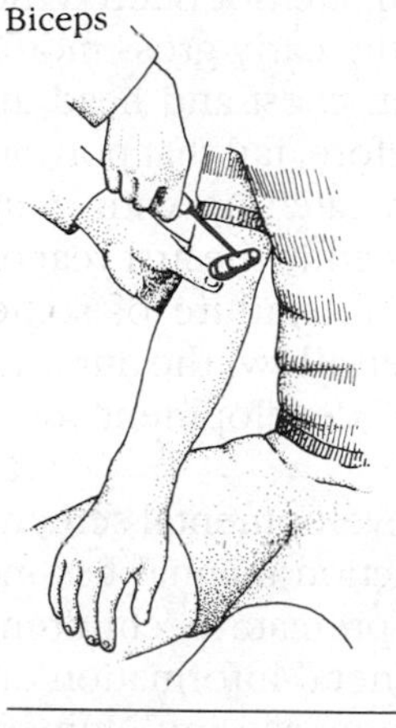	With the child's arm semiflexed at the elbow, slightly pronated, and with the elbow resting on the examiner's arm, the examiner places a thumb over the tendon and strikes the thumb.	Contraction of biceps and forearm.	Grade response, evaluate symmetry.
Brachioradialis reflex 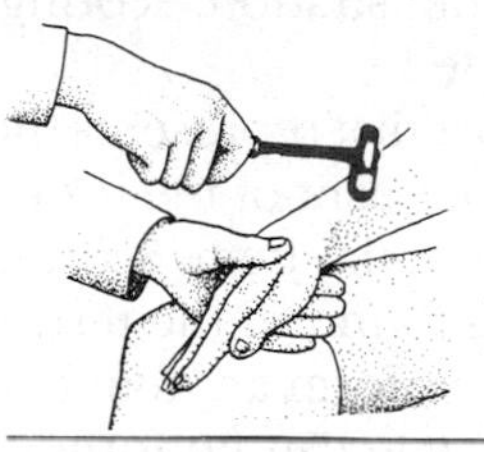	The styloid process of the radius is tapped sharply with the reflex hammer.	Elbow flexion and forearm pronation	Grade response, evaluate symmetry.
Patellar reflex 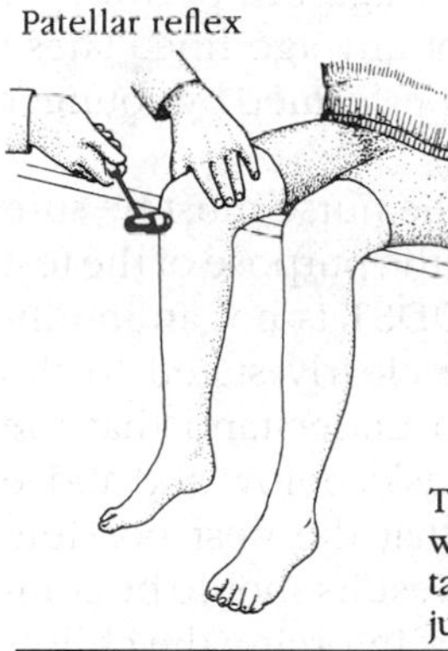	The child is in a sitting position with legs dangling freely over table edge. The patellar tendon—just below patella—is struck.	Contraction of quadriceps, and extension of lower leg.	Grade response, evaluate symmetry.
Achilles reflex 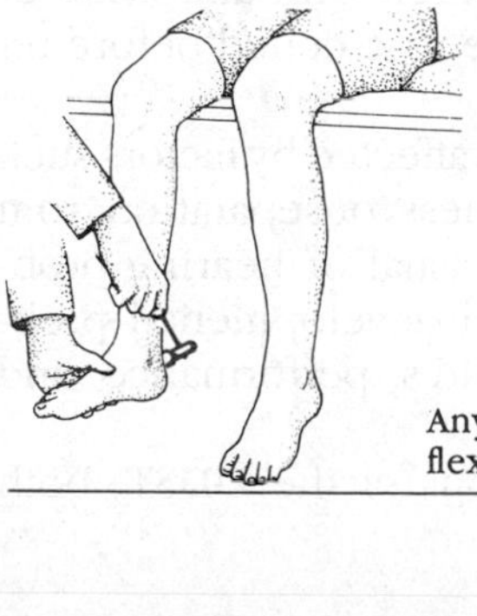	Any position where foot can be flexed to stretch tendon.	Plantar flexion of foot	Grade response, evaluate symmetry.

foot, quickly dorsiflexing the foot. Clonus is present when the foot alternately moves up and down. Sustained clonus is significantly abnormal and requires further investigation.

The Babinski reflex is one of the most significant neurologic signs. It is elicited by stimulating the lateral aspect of the sole on the foot with a blunt point or fingernail. The stimulus begins at the midpoint of the heel and moves upward on the lateral aspect of the sole and across the ball of the foot toward the great toe. A Babinski response consists of fanning of the toes and dorsiflexion of the great toe. This is accompanied by dorsiflexion of the foot at the ankle and flexion at the knee and hip. A Babinski response is normal only in the newborn and infant until approximately 18 months of age. The primary reflexes looked for in the infant are described in Chapter 5.

Soft neurologic signs are frequently discussed in pediatric neurology. There is controversy, however, regarding the existence, definition, interpretation, and significance of such signs. In general, this term is applied to subtle behaviors or signs whose significance is viewed differently. Examples of soft neurologic signs are clumsiness, hyperactivity, perceptual difficulties, short attention span, language disturbances, mirroring movement, confused laterality, articulation defects and difficulty with balance. Many clinicians believe that soft neurologic signs are very significant and as such should be given careful consideration. A child with any significant neurologic finding should be referred for appropriate medical follow-up.

Developmental Screening

Developmental screening is an absolutely vital component of child health assessment. Unfortunately, it is often omitted during routine health assessment. Without the use of formal developmental screening tools, children with developmental disabilities can remain unidentified. However, if, through screening, problems are identified early in the developmental process, treatment is more likely to be successful.

Many tools are available for developmental screening. One of the most widely used tools is the Denver Developmental Screening Test (DDST), shown in Appendix Four. This tool is used to assess the child from birth to 6 years in four skill areas: personal-social, fine motor-adaptive, language, and gross motor.

The DDST has been found to be reliable and valid. There are positive correlations with psychometric tests such as the Cattell Infant Intelligence Scale and the Revised Bayley Infant Scale. Children with questionable or abnormal scores are at risk for developing school problems despite intelligence.

One limitation of the DDST involves its value in the testing of minority ethnic groups. However, no screening tests currently available do allow for reliable, valid screening of children from minority ethnic groups. Nonetheless, these children deserve developmental screening.

Nurses working with a large population of a specific ethnic group should become familiar with child care practices that are widely used by this group. For example, Southeast Asian groups routinely place infants in the supine position and rarely in the prone position in the early months of life. These children, not often being in the prone position, are not offered the opportunity to practice some of the early gross motor skills (e.g., holding head upright, chest and head up with arm support) and may, therefore, fail that portion of the DDST. These children do catch up with their peers on these gross motor skills within the first year of life. Understanding the reasons for failure of some portions of a developmental screen allows the nurse to develop an informal standard of development for a particular ethnic group.

It is important to carry out developmental screening accurately. The DDST instruction manual has information calculating ages for premature children, scoring criteria for each item, general information on scoring, and symbols used for proper scoring. Numerous pointers on preparation, administration, scoring, and interpretation are also provided.

Each item is designated as a bar that represents the ages at which 25, 50, 70, and 90 per cent of the tested population could perform the particular item. Scoring is based on the number of delays found in the test. A delay is defined as the failure to perform an item that 90 per cent of children the same age can perform or failure in any item to the left of any age line. These items are those which could be performed by younger children.

Before beginning the test, the nurse must be sure to adequately explain to parents the purpose of the test and how it is performed. The DDST is not an intelligence test, and this should be clearly stated to the parent. The parent should also understand that the child will be asked to perform tasks below and above the expected performance so that the best possible performance is obtained. DDST results should be completely explained to the parent, reinforcing the child's satisfactory performance. Children with abnormal or questionable results should be rescreened before referral for diagnostic testing.

The child's performance is affected by factors such as fatigue, anxiety, illness, shyness, or separation from the parent. Also, undetected visual or hearing problems or neurologic or familial developmental problems may influence the child's performance and should be considered.

There are two modifications of the DDST, both

devised to do some prescreening of large groups of children. The first is the DDST Revised. It takes approximately 5 to 7 minutes to administer. The items to be assessed are those to the left of, but not touching, the age line. If any of the 12 items tested are failed or refused, a complete DDST is required.

Another modification of the DDST frequently used is the Denver Prescreening Developmental Questionnaire (PDQ). It is a questionnaire of 97 questions that can be answered rapidly. The questionnaire is divided according to the child's age and is given to the parent to fill out. Because of the wording of the questions and instructions, it is used most successfully with parents who have completed high school. The parent answers 10 questions from the appropriate category. This takes between 3 to 6 minutes to complete. The nurse then reviews the answers and provides time for the parent to express concerns or ask questions. Indications that a child has a developmental delay require follow-up with a complete DDST.

The Developmental Profile II is a developmental screening tool consisting of 168 items covering five developmental areas: physical, self-help, social, academic, and communication. It relies largely on verbal responses from the parent, teachers, older sibling, or other individuals acquainted with the child. It provides an individual profile that can be compared with data on what is normal for specific ages at which children in the standardized population perform developmental skills.

Although much attention has been focused on assessing the child's development, concern is also directed at assessing the environment, which may foster or impede the developmental processes. Using both clinical and home visit observations, Dr. Bettye Caldwell developed an assessment tool designed to identify characteristics of the environment of children from birth to 3 years and 3 to 6 years. The instrument is the Home Observation for Measurement of the Environment (HOME) (see Appendix Five for these forms). The birth to 3 years inventory measures six subscales: emotional and verbal responsiveness of the mother, avoidance of restriction and punishment, organization of physical and temporal environment, provision of appropriate play materials, maternal involvement with the child, and opportunities for variety in daily stimulation.

The inventory for 3- to 6-year-olds measures seven subscales: provision of stimulation through equipment, toys, and experiences; stimulation of mature behavior; provision of stimulating physical and language environment; avoidance of restriction and punishment; pride, affection and thoughtfulness; masculine stimulation; and independence from parental control. The purpose for both scales is to identify certain aspects of the quantity and quality of the social, emotional, and cognitive environmental supports available to the young child in his home.

This tool must be administered by a person who goes into the home and observes the child when awake during the normal daily routine. It takes approximately an hour to obtain the data. The parent should be notified of the forthcoming visit. The HOME can be used in combination with other screening tools to assist parents to solve current problems and prevent development of other problems by providing anticipatory guidance for appropriate parenting.

Obtaining a profile of the child's temperament can also be useful in planning anticipatory guidance regarding parenting. The Carey Infant Temperament Questionnaire is a clinical screening instrument used to study the temperament of the infant between 4 and 8 months of age. Carey identifies temperament as an important variable in infant development that influences the relationship between parents and infant and other caregivers. The child's patterns—feeding, sleeping, eliminating, and playing—are some of the areas identified in the questionnaire completed by the parent. The items also look at the infant's responses to different situations. There are also refinements of this questionnaire that can be used to assess temperament of the toddler, the 3 to 7 year old and the 8 to 12 year old.

The Washington Guide to Promoting Development in the Young Child is an assessment tool that can help in an evaluation of progress in the child's development. This instrument identifies expected tasks for age groups from 1 month to 52 months in functional activity areas such as sleep, feeding, motor skills, play, language, discipline, and toilet training. Corresponding to the expected performance is a suggested activity that can be recommended to the parent to help the child accomplish developmental tasks.

Speech Screening

No developmental screening would be complete without a speech evaluation. One easily administered test for children who speak English is the Denver Articulation Screening Examination (DASE) (Appendix Six), which is a word imitative procedure. The child repeats 22 different words while the examiner listens for errors in the articulation of 30 different sound elements. See Appendix Six for a copy of the examination with instructions for its use.

Intelligibility is also scored by selection of one of four categories ranging from easy to understand to cannot evaluate. The DASE is designed to pinpoint significant speech delays and normal variations in the acquisition of speech sounds. Abnormal conditions such as tongue thrust, lisp, hypernasality, and hyponasality can also be detected. Speech and language development is also evaluated by direct observation of the child's verbal skills, in addition to speech patterns and history of speech patterns and development.

Nutritional Assessment

Nutrition is a significant factor that influences and is influenced by growth and development. Physical competency is especially affected by nutritional status. Nutritional requirements are based on what is considered necessary to support life, to provide for growth, and to maintain health. Nutritional assessment is discussed in Chapter 18, with specific requirements according to age presented in Chapters 5 through 9 on growth and development.

The nurse should learn basic principles of nutritional assessment and counseling applicable at all ages. There are four major purposes for assessing food intake: (1) to identify dietary practices of the family, (2) to obtain baseline data on caloric and nutrient intake and appropriate anthropometric measurements from which progress can be measured, (3) to promote healthful dietary practices through counseling and teaching, and (4) to provide parents with the opportunity to ask questions about nutrition and feeding behaviors.

Before obtaining a nutritional history the nurse must be prepared to ask questions in a nonjudgmental way. Food and feeding practices can be extremely sensitive issues, especially for parents whose children are having problems involving body weight. Also, it is important to listen carefully to what parents are saying and what it appears they are practicing. Parents of young children can recite an appropriate diet for their child and deny the frequent use of junk food while the examiner looks at the child eating lollipops with badly decayed teeth. The nurse must also be prepared to accept some cultural food practices with which she or he may not be familiar. For example, some cultures may not give any solids for the first year of life while another may give an infant food that has first been chewed by the mother to make it an appropriate consistency.

The details of a nutritional assessment are discussed in Chapter 18, including the use of a 24-hour intake and other approaches such as a 3-day or 7-day food diary. Recommended Dietary Allowances (RDAs) are presented in Table 18-1 and physical indicators of nutritional status in Table 18-7.

The parents and child should be counseled regarding modification of the child's diet if necessary. It is important to include both the parents and the child in the plans for change. It is also important that they know the reasons why change is needed and how their beliefs, attitudes, and actions are affecting the nutrition of the child. The parents and the child may need support and help in dealing not only with their feelings and behaviors but also those of friends and relatives. See Chapter 18 for further discussion of nutritional counseling and related concerns and issues.

Laboratory Screening

Laboratory tests are used as diagnostic or screening aids; when combined with subjective and objective findings, they provide a complete database. Many of the laboratory specimens needed for diagnostic examination of children are obtained the same as they are for adults. The older child is often able to cooperate and follow directions adequately to assist in obtaining the laboratory specimens. Appendix Seven gives normal laboratory values for children.

Blood Specimens

Most blood samples are obtained by the laboratory staff or physicians. The nurse is often responsible for making certain that the parent and child understand the procedure, assisting in restraint, and making certain that the correct equipment is available. In some areas, however, such as the intensive care and outpatient clinics, the nurse is responsible for collecting specimens needed.

Most blood screening tests can be performed on either venous or capillary blood specimens.

Whatever method is used to collect the blood specimen, it is essential that the parent and child be adequately prepared for the procedure and adequate restraint be provided if the child is unable to cooperate. See Chapter 27 for discussion of specific techniques used to collect blood and the preparation of children for procedures.

As after any painful procedure, the child should be comforted by the parent. The infant should be cuddled, the toddler held and praised, the preschooler and early school-age child should be rewarded with praise and perhaps a small token, e.g., a sticker.

Hematocrit

One of the most frequently used laboratory screening tests is the hematocrit. The hematocrit is a comparison of packed red blood cell volume and the volume of whole blood. This is generally a screening test used for anemia. Using the procedure described in Chapter 27 for obtaining capillary blood, two capillary tubes of blood are filled to be centrifuged. Normal hematocrit values at sea level vary according to the age of the child. See Appendix Seven for normal ranges listed according to age.

Hemoglobin

A hemoglobin refers to the measurement of hemaglobin, a protein, within each blood cell. Since the hematocrit measures the number of red blood cells and the hemoglobin measures the hemoglobin within each cell, it is frequently important to measure both to determine if anemia is present. Depending on the type of method used to determine the hemoglobin, either capillary or venous blood is obtained. Hemoglobin values are expressed in grams per dl of blood or mmol/L of blood (The latter expression is in international units).

The hemoglobin and hematocrit are always done if there is a suggestion of possible anemia by history or physical findings. The child should be screened at 6 to 9 months of age, between 12 and 18 months, and again during adolescence. These are the ages that the child is most frequently at risk for developing iron deficiency anemia. The 6 to 9 month test may be omitted if the child is still drinking iron-fortified formula.

Sickledex

A simple screening procedure for sickle cell anemia is the Sickledex. This disease is a defect in the structure of the red blood cell, which loses its round shape and becomes sickled by stress or lack of oxygen. Approximately 10 per cent of the black American population has this condition. The test is done only on black children over 6 months of age due to the amount of fetal hemoglobin present before that age. The Sickledex is a screening test and any positive test should be referred for more specific diagnostic testing.

Phenylketonuria

Phenylketonuria (PKU), a disorder of amino acid metabolism, causes an abnormal accumulation of the amino acid phenylalanine in the blood, resulting in brain damage. Testing for PKU has become mandatory on all newborns in most states. The test is more reliable if done between the second and sixth day of life after the child has ingested any protein substance, usually milk formula, for 24 to 48 hours. However, the practice of early discharge has prompted the American Academy of Pediatrics (1982) to recommend that all neonates be tested before they leave the nursery regardless of age. Furthermore, all sick or premature neonates are to be tested by the seventh day of age, regardless of the feeding pattern.

The practice of routine screening at 2 weeks of age has been challenged on the basis of cost. The American Academy of Pediatrics (1982) recommends that infants initially screened before 24 hours of age should be rescreened before the third week of life.

The infant's heel is pricked with a lancet, and three drops of blood are pressed to a special absorbent filter paper. (Chapter 50 describes the details of this test.)

Lead

Screening for lead toxicity is done by both blood and urine testing. Blood testing requires venous blood. Screening varies according to whether a child is considered to be at risk. Blood lead concentration and erythrocyte-protoporphyrin (EP) level are the commonly used tests. (See Chapter 52 for a further discussion of screening for lead toxicity.)

Urine Specimens

One of the most painless and effective ways to evaluate the functioning of the entire body is examination of the urine. The various techniques for collecting urine specimens are described in Chapter 27. Older children and adolescents can readily provide a specimen with correct instructions but may be embarrassed by carrying specimens through hallways. If this is the case, a paper bag should be provided or the specimen may be retrieved discreetly. Adolescent females who are menstruating should delay providing a specimen or a notation should be made on the laboratory slip to explain the presence of red blood cells.

School-age children are cooperative but, like adolescents, are very curious and concerned regarding the reasons for obtaining the specimen. Explanations of the method and reasons for obtaining a urine sample will greatly expedite the procedure.

Preschoolers and toddlers are less able to cooperate. Before trying to obtain a specimen, the nurse should offer liquids and wait 20 to 30 minutes. Fluids are not given in excessively large amounts as this may distort the results of the test. The parent should be questioned as to the child's terminology for this bodily function, and these words should be used. Children who have difficulty voiding in an unfamiliar receptacle may be provided with a clean or sterilized potty chair or bed pan placed on the toilet. Toddlers in particular may have difficulty voiding in unfamiliar surroundings since they have undoubtedly been admonished for voiding in places not approved by parents during the toilet training phase. The parents may need to reassure the child it is all right to void in the bed pan.

A standard urinalysis includes an examination for

the color, pH, and specific gravity; testing for glucose, ketones, and protein; and a microscopic determination for cells, bacteria, and crystalline content. Simple qualitative screening tests can be done for pH, glucose, protein, blood, and other substances by using reagent-covered test strips that are dipped directly into the urine or pressed between two urine-saturated surfaces of a diaper. The presence of the test substance causes a color change on the strip, which is then compared to the colors identified on a chart or on the test strip bottle. The odor should also be noted, as it can indicate an abnormality. Microscopic examination of the urine is done by an experienced laboratory clinician. Further information on collection of urine specimens is presented in Chapter 27.

Urine cultures are done on children who are suspected of having a urinary tract infection and on children with routine urinalysis results indicating abnormal microscopic findings. Techniques for obtaining urine specimens for culture are described in Chapter 27.

References

American Academy of Pediatrics: *Report on the Committee on Infectious Diseases.* 20th ed. Elk Grove Village, IL, 1986.

American Academy of Pediatrics, Committee on Genetics: New issues in newborn screening for phenylketonuria and congenital hypothyroidism. *Pediatrics* 1982; 69:104–106.

Barrus DH: A comparison of rectal and axillary temperatures by electronic thermometer measurement in preschool children. *Pediatr Nurs* 1983; 9(6)424–425.

Brown MS, Murphy MA: *Ambulatory Pediatrics for Nurses.* 2nd ed. New York, McGraw-Hill, 1981.

Castiglia PT, Petrini MA: Selecting a developmental screening tool. *Pediatr Nurs* 1985; 11(1)8–17.

Downs MP: Early identification of hearing loss. *In* Lass N, et al (eds): *Speech, Language and Hearing.* Philadelphia, WB Saunders, 1981.

Fandal AW, Kemper MB, Frankenburg WK: Needed: routine developmental screening for all children. *Pediatric Basics,* Gerber Products Co. 1978.

Jaworski A: A new boy-girl blood pressure chart for pediatric office use: a single-sheet graph for all children. *Clin Pediatr* 1978 Sep; 699.

Kempe CH, Silver HK, O'Brien D: *Current Pediatric Diagnosis and Treatment.* 8th ed. Los Altos, CA, Lange Medical Publications, 1984.

Moss JR: Predicting young children's cooperation with the physical examination. *Pediatr Nurs* 1983; 9(3)188–190.

Roberts PH: Nursing assessments: screening for developmental problems. *In* Krajicek M, Tomlinson AT (eds): *Detection of Developmental Problems in Children.* 2nd ed. Baltimore, University Park Press, 1983, 9–40.

Bibliography

Barnes LSA: *Manual of Pediatric Physical Diagnosis.* 5th ed. Chicago, Year Book, 1981.

Cadman D, et al: The usefulness of the DDST to predict kindergarten problems in a general community population. *Am J Public Health* 1984; 74(10):1093–1097.

Elliman AM, et al: Denver Developmental Screening Test and preterm infants. *Arch Dis Child* 1985; 60:20–24.

Frankenburg WF, Dodds JB: Denver Developmental Screening Test. *J Pediatr* 1967;71:181–191.

Frankenburg WF, et al: Development of preschool-aged children of different social and ethnic groups: implications for developmental screening. *J Pediatr* 1975;87:125–132.

Frankenburg WF, et al: The newly abbreviated and revised Denver Developmental Screening Test. *J Pediatr* 1981; 99:995–999.

Frankenburg WF, et al: Revision of Denver Prescreening Developmental Questionnaire. *J Pediatr* 1987 Apr; 110(4):653–657.

Fung K, Lau S: Denver Developmental Screening Test: cultural variables. *J Pediatr* 1985;106(2):343.

Green M, Haggerty RJ: *Ambulatory Pediatrics III.* Philadelphia, WB Saunders, 1984.

Hall DMB, Baird G: Developmental tests and scales. *Arch Dis Child* 1986; 61:213–215.

Hoekelman RA: The physical examination of infants and children. *In* Bates B: *A Guide to Physical Examination and History Taking.* 4th ed. Philadelphia, JB Lippincott, 1987, 525–598.

Kotzer AM, McCabe ERB: Newborn screening for inherited metabolic disease: principles and practice. *Neonatal Network* 1988; 6(4):15–19.

Moss JR: Predicting children's co-operation with the physical examination. *Pediatr Nurs* 1983; 9(3):188–190.

Sciarillo WG, et al: Effectiveness of the DDST with biologically vulnerable infants. *Dev Behav Pediatr* 1986; 7(2):77–83.

Shapira Y, Harel S: Standardization of the DDST for Israeli children. *Israel J Med Sci* 1983; 19:246–251.

Sturner RA, et al: Adaptation of the DDST: a study of preschool screening. *Pediatrics* 1982; 69:346–350.

Tudor M: Developmental screening. *Issues Compr Pediatr Nurs* 1977; 2(2):1–13.

Fostering Self-Esteem

Chapter 16

Jo Joyce Anderson

Self-esteem development is perhaps one of the most crucial elements of an individual's growth process, permeating who one is, how one expresses oneself, and the position or station one takes throughout life. Health professionals, as diagnosticians, educators, researchers, and caregivers, need to know how self-esteem develops, how that development is influenced by people and experiences, and how self-esteem contributes to attaining an adaptive lifestyle. This chapter exposes the reader to the self-system and the influences on the self-system, introduces measures for building and maintaining the healthy self-system, and acquaints the nurse with some assessment tools that can be used in the practice setting.

Related Topics
Concepts of child development, Chapter 3
Development of children at different stages, Unit Two
Communication, a significant component of self-esteem development, Chapter 10
Family dynamics and development of self-esteem, Chapter 12
Impact of parenting on self-esteem, Chapter 13
Self-esteem and altered behavior patterns, Chapter 33

Fostering Self-Esteem

Nursing Diagnoses	Nursing Goals/Strategies*
Self-esteem disturbance • *related to feelings of insecurity and not belonging*	Provide an environment that facilitates child's development of a sense of security and belonging • Be honest in interactions • Set clear, reasonable limits • Maintain routines • Have child participate in self-monitoring • Encourage participation in family and social groups • Teach child the responsibility of group membership
• *related to ineffective enhancement of the self-system*	Promote behaviors in the child that enhance the self-system • Encourage legitimate self-praise by children • Teach child to accept love and praise, and to receive compliments • Help child accept occasional failure • Provide opportunity to steadily increase personal responsibility for making and maintaining decisions about own health care
Potential for disturbance in self-concept: personal identity, related to ineffective portrayal of love and acceptance	Provide a supportive environment of love and acceptance • Provide positive feedback and encourage same from teachers, Scout leaders, etc. • Make demands that are realistic and not excessive in number and type • Verbally acknowledge a task well done • Support child in the acknowledgement of limitations • Communicate love and affection through touch, active listening, and verbal expressions
Potential for disturbance in self-concept: role performance, related to lack of sense of purpose	Provide feedback and experiences that provide the child with a sense of purpose • Set reasonable expectations for child • Assist child to set reasonable expectations for self • Institute contracts to assist in the achievement of goals • Expose children to a variety of new experiences • Let child identify and pursue interests of choice

* Strategies listed are used by nurses and are taught to parents (caretakers).

Children who master healthy adaptation skills in childhood have the basis for a self-actualized adulthood. This mastery involves developing coping strategies to achieve growth and gain equilibrium as the child is confronted with the maturational and situational stressors of the world. The child instinctively strives to manage her or his world better by experimenting with and adopting behaviors that help reduce the anxiety associated with the problems and challenges of living. The behaviors learned are influenced by the child's previous experiences, the developmental stage and temperament, environmental demands, and the behaviors role-modeled by the significant people in the child's world (see Chapter 13 on parenting). If the learned behaviors are adaptive, they will serve the child successfully in later experiences. If maladaptive, the behaviors will increase the child's stress, disrupt learning potential, and result in dysfunctional behavior patterns (see Chapter 33).

A key element influencing acquisition of adaptive or maladaptive behavior is the child's self-perceptions. According to Maslow's hierarchy of needs (1968), self-esteem is an extremely important component of healthy living, preceded only by satisfaction of physiologic and safety needs and one's need to be loved. Maslow *defines the need for self-esteem as including self-respect, others' respect, self-confidence and feelings of competence, independence, success, and recognition from others.*

Defining the Self-System

The terms *self, self-concept,* and *identity* are used loosely in the literature. Whichever term is used, it is the self-system that accounts for the uniqueness of a person. *While some aspects of the self-system may change over time, the central core of this system appears to remain intact and to endure over time* (Levine et al, 1983). In fact, maintenance and enhancement of this highly stable aspect of self is the major motivational force behind all behavior. Behavioral research consistently demonstrates that maladaptive or antisocial behaviors and mental-emotional imbalance can be causally linked with an underdeveloped self-system (Crosby, 1982; Levine et al, 1983; Murray and Huelskoetter, 1983).

In this chapter the terms *self-system* and *self-concept* are used synonymously. Self-concept is a broad generic term that encompasses many smaller constructs (e.g., self-image, self-esteem, self-ideal) (Roy, 1984). Figure 16-1 defines the aspects of the self-system. Self-concept, then, is the central core of personality development that gives rise to one's uniqueness or *identity* (Sullivan, 1953). Self-concept is arrived at through self-definition and self-evaluation, which require interpersonal interactions so that the self can be seen through the reactions of others.

As children receive feedback from their interactions, they evaluate whether they are a "good person" or a "bad person." Those behaviors that generate extremely negative feedback and thus extreme anxiety are rejected as "not me" and denied. "Good person" perceptions result from consistent approval or positive feedback from significant others. "Bad person" perceptions are derived from consistent disapproval or negative feedback from significant others. Box 16-1 describes characteristics of children that reflect the level of regard they hold of themselves. Once this basic core of self-regard is established in the young child, it becomes an important factor in the adaptive strategies chosen, task mastery accomplished, and social competence achieved in later developmental stages.

Beyond early childhood, barring environmental changes of a radical nature, the "self-fulfilling prophesy" phenomenon occurs (i.e., I do not measure up to my significant others' expectations, I get negative reinforcement, I must be bad, so I behave badly—or vice versa). The child who holds a realistic regard for self feels good about self, participates eagerly in activities, and knows and feels comfortable about personal strengths and limitations. The child achieves positive resolution of developmental tasks and crises, receives adequate support from significant others, and establishes trust in self and the world.

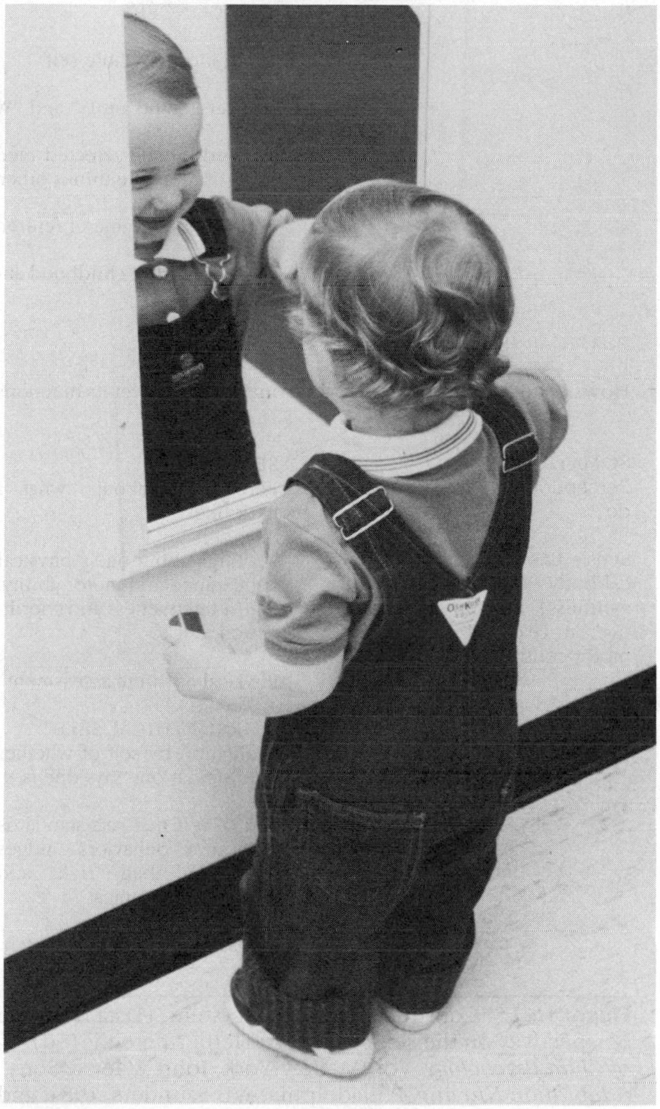

A mirror image of the physical self contributes to the child's perception about "what I look like."

Influences on Self-System Development

Children are not born with an identity, or self-concept. The self-system is developed gradually, with different constructs of the system receiving emphasis and maturing at differing times. Acquisition does not follow a smooth continuum yet is somewhat predictable, as re-

SELF-CONCEPT

Perception of whole self

Answers "Who am I?" and "What am I?"

Formed by self-selected mental images and attitudes plus reflections of how one thinks others see one

Fundamental frame of reference for all behavior

Learned during childhood and is a product of socialization

PHYSICAL SELF

How one feels about one's body and one's control over its functions

SOMATIC SELF
Perceptions about "what I can do"

Sensations about one's physical body (size, shape, state of wellness) and one's control over it (ease of movement, motor control over functions)

Skill assessment

SELF-IMAGE
Perceptions about "what I look like"

Feelings about one's physical appearance and motor ability, e.g., attractiveness and coordination

Physical attribute assessment

PERSONAL SELF

Personality part of self, e.g., self-esteem

How one feels about "who one is" in relation to "who one ought to be"

Formed by 5 years of age

Overall perception of one's worth

Inverse relationship exists between self-esteem and anxiety

MORAL-ETHICAL SELF
Evaluation by self of whether one is what one says one is

Part of self that sets standards for one's behaviors, judges good and bad, right and wrong, fair or unjust

Assessment of motive, intentions

SELF-CONSISTENCY
Expression of one's identity

Responses to everyday events and situations

Coping style

Assessment of one's temperamental or emotional character

SELF-IDEAL
Perception of "what one would like to be"

Behavioral guide to goal achievement

Assessment of how competitive one needs to be

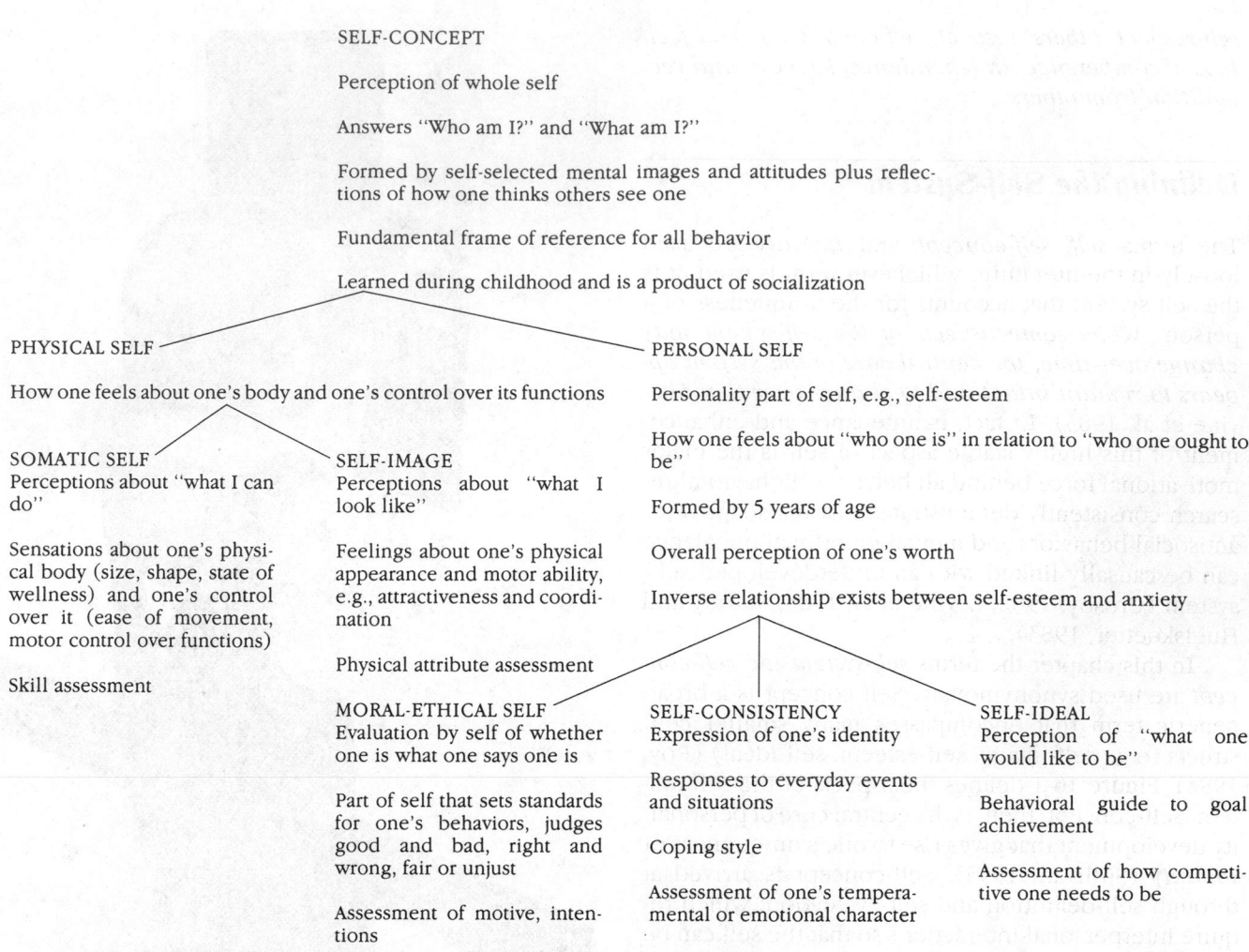

Figure 16-1. Constructs of the self-system. (Data from Harter S: Developmental perspectives on the self-system. *In* Hetherington E (ed): *Carmichael's Manual of Child Psychology.* Vol IV. New York, John Wiley & Sons, 1982; Rambo B: *Adaptation Nursing.* Philadelphia, WB Saunders, 1984; and Roy C: *Introduction to Nursing; An Adaptation Model.* Englewood Cliffs, NJ, Prentice-Hall, 1984.)

flected in personality theories. (See Kohlberg's theory of moral development, Erikson's theory of psychosocial development, and others in Chapter 3.)

Several elements of experience seem especially pertinent to development of the self-system: (1) developmental psychosocial crises, (2) significant others' expectations, (3) social role expectations and cultural factors, (4) physical health status, and (5) temperamental coping style. Development of the self-system, and of self-esteem in particular, forms the basis for trying out new skills and relationships at each new developmental stage. In response to satisfaction in skill mastery and to the information received from others, the child will try to enhance self-esteem by seeking situations and social interactions that gratify and reinforce the sense of self.

Developmental Psychosocial Crises as Factors

Early childhood is identified by many theorists as a crucial time for the healthy development of the core component of the self-system, self-concept. A sense of trust and relative success in early motor and verbal experiences seem to be essentials to the healthy progression of the self-system toward a positive self-concept and high self-esteem. These experiences, interfaced with sufficient and positive interpersonal interactions, produce an individual with a self-system sturdy enough to be self-actualized during adulthood (Fig. 16-2). Some believe the experiences that contribute to a person's eventual self-esteem may begin even before birth (Satir, 1972; Kegan, 1982). Table 16-1 de-

Box 16-1
Characteristics of Children with High and Low Self-Regard

BEHAVIORS DEMONSTRATING HIGH SELF-REGARD	BEHAVIORS DEMONSTRATING LOW SELF-REGARD
More active—seek activities and new experiences	Hesitant to participate in activities and anxiety is provoked by new experiences
Self-confidence. Inner assuredness of success and of positive responses from people	Feel inferior. Assume others will respond negatively. Pessimistic
Demonstrate leadership skills in groups, independence	Tend to follow or watch others achieve. Unable to function in groups
Recognize self as more skillful in some areas than in others and this is OK (self-coping)	Easily discouraged. Inner pressure to resort to self-defeating behaviors rather than coping directly (defensive coping), e.g., rebellious, acting-out behaviors
Handle criticism, hold realistic world view	Cannot stand losing, not being first. Self-centered and egotistic
Express feelings of being likable, worthwhile, important	Express feelings of being unlikable, unacceptable, undesirable, insignificant
Behaviors reflect self-respect, pride in self and achievements	Doubt own ability to do well or have friends. Boast to cover up fragile sense of worth
Steadily increase and willingly assume self-control (internal locus of control), effectiveness in solving problems	Hesitate or refuse to assume self-control (external locus of control). Dependent on acceptance for control
Expressive, happy, optimistic, enjoy interpersonal interaction	Depressed, timid, poor social interactions

(Data from Coopersmith, 1967; Harter, 1982; Millar, 1983.)

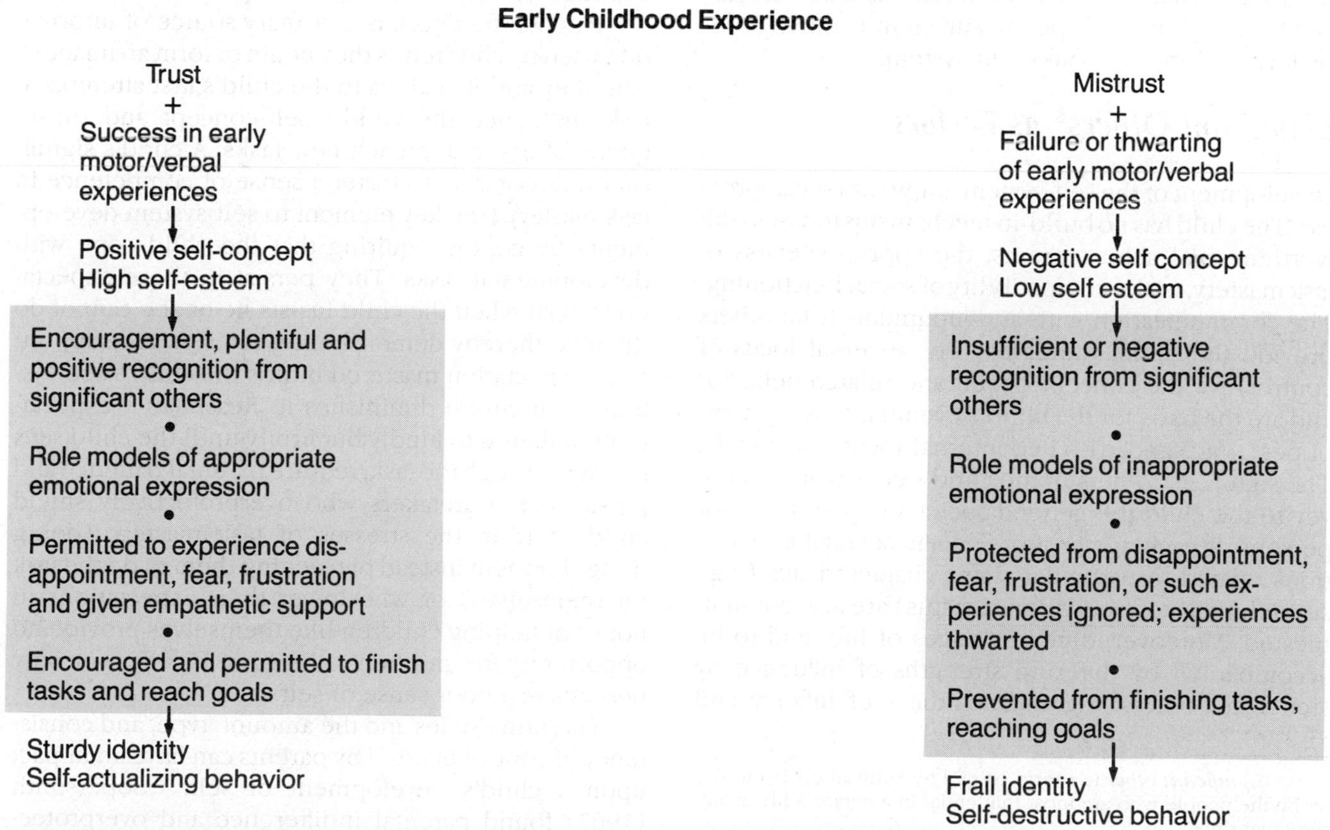

Figure 16-2. Requisites of childhood self-system development to support adult self-actualization.

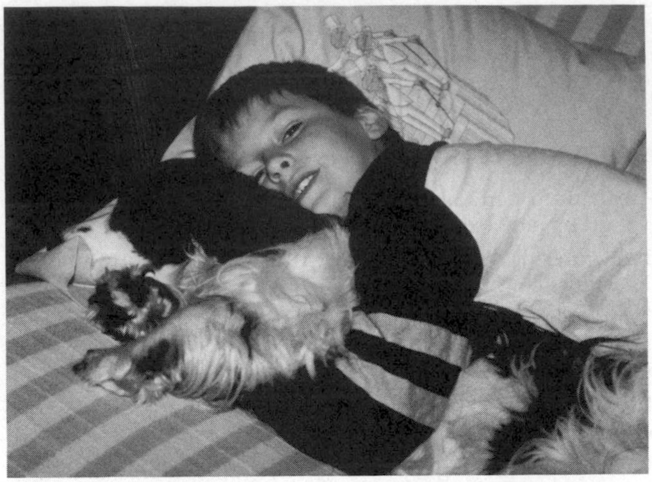

Pets give unconditional love and can be a "significant other." As a child cares for a pet, feelings of closeness and acceptance are experienced.

scribes the developmental progress of the self-system according to the child's age. Developmental theorists identify the school years as a particular threat to the self-system because of the onslaught of daily evaluation from teachers and peers in physical, social, and intellectual realms. Early adolescence, however, is realized as a potential opportunity to resolve a poor self-concept, which has developed because of insufficient caretaker feedback. As the youth establishes close, caring relationships with peers, sufficient positive feedback can reform the shaky self-system.

Significant Others* as Factors

Development of the self-system is always a social process. The child has no build-in mechanisms to assess the worthiness of achievements, the appropriateness of task mastery, or the compatibility of social functioning. The communication with and judgments from others provide the initial standards (i.e., external locus of control) for the concept of self and related behavior and are the basis for the child's eventual development of personal standards (i.e., internal locus of control). The significant others in the child's environment convey to the child the general societal expectations for persons of each age group. Specific societal expectations related to particular status characteristics (e.g., sex, ethnicity, socioeconomic status) are also communicated. Moreover, different stages of life tend to be accompanied by differing strengths of influence by significant others. Significant others of infancy and early childhood are primarily family members and other primary caretakers. When school begins, teachers and, increasingly, peers become predominant significant others. Late school years and adolescence result in stronger peer significance as well as the added influences of recreational and work alliances.

Although a child's feelings of competence regarding task mastery are the key element in development of a healthy self-system, compliance and non-compliance with societal expectations for role-specific behavior typically result in judgments of personal worth as well as more public consequences; thus, success in meeting such expectations in social interactions carries profound implications for development of the self-system (Stanwyck, 1983).

Family as Significant Others. A healthy concept of self is not a gift from parent to child. Development of self comes from within. The most that parents and other caretakers can do is provide an environment for its growth. Something besides parental valuing and approval is necessary to the construction of a healthy self-system in a child. Totally rejected children are going to have an unhealthy self-system, but so do many children whose parents care deeply and value them tremendously (Millar, 1983). Unless the child has an opportunity to cope with normal life expectations, a healthy self-system is jeopardized because through coping a healthy self-system is built.

Parental feedback is a primary source of information used by children as they begin to form an image of who they are. Reactions to the child's first attempts at tasks influence the child's self-concept and subsequent efforts to approach new tasks. A child's significant others can help foster a sense of competence in task mastery (the key element to self-system development) by gently requiring that the child cope with developmental tasks. They persist in these expectations even when the child insists he or she cannot do the task, thereby demonstrating interest and support. Each expectation mastered builds the child's self-system; each failure diminishes it. Reasonable expectations, adhered to kindly but firmly until the child sees the way through the task, require parental patience and persistence. Caretakers who overprotectively shield children from the stresses of task mastery (doing things for them instead of teaching them to do the task for themselves) or who lower their expectations in hopes of helping children like themselves provide no opportunity for children to build self-esteem or only perpetuate a poor sense of self.

Parenting styles and the amount, type, and consistency of control exerted by parents can have an impact upon a child's development of self. Coopersmith (1967) found parental indifference and overprotec-

* *Significant other* is a term coined by Sullivan (1950) to describe the people who are most influential in a person's life at any particular time.

Table 16-1. Stages of Healthy Self-System Development During the Childhood Years

Phase	Level of Self-Mastery	Critical Experiences
Infancy *Psychosocial crisis:* Trust vs. Mistrust	Learns to trust others to gratify needs (basis for confidence or hesitancy in child's approach later to tasks or self-responsibility)	Prompt, consistent responses to needs
	Sensitive to anxiety or contentment of caretakers, empathetic; struggles to feel secure and avoid anxiety	Tenderness from caretakers. Relative freedom from caretaker's anxieties
	Learns responses or consequences behavior gets from others	Realistic responses to behaviors; not *un*critical nor *over*critical
Early Childhood *Psychosocial crisis:* Autonomy vs. Shame or Doubt	Self-recognition (self-concept and -identity) and self-pride (self-esteem) evolve. "I" can produce changes in my environment. "I" can accomplish this task (mostly motor tasks)	Grant autonomous experiences and behaviors Consistent, realistic limits; not *un*critical nor *over*critical Experience delays in gratification—opportunity to accept interference with wish fulfillment
	Modifies actions to suit social role expectations (sex roles, peer roles, family member roles). Has developed personal view of world and place and value in it	Role models as guidance to appropriate emotional expression
	Uses movement and language to avoid anxiety and to build self-competence. Develops general strategy for dealing with world	Reasonable opportunities to master skills without assistance but with encouragement and affirmation. Avoid too little or too much freedom
Middle Childhood *Psychosocial crisis:* Industry or Mastery vs. Inferiority	Learns to accept subordination to authority figures outside family	Teachers who hold realistic but not underestimated expectations for child
	Develops intellectual competence, initiative, achievement	Opportunity to explore and change own world. Follow through on projects to closure
	Self-status and role stabilized. Develops consideration and concerns outside the self	Peer chumships with mutual caring and acceptance
	Comparisons made of real self and ideal self. Internal locus of control begins forming	Challenges to set goals and carry them out
Early Adolescence *Psychosocial crisis:* Identity vs. Lack of Self-Clarity	Capable of participating in genuine love relationships with others	Peer relations offer a corrective opportunity for the self-esteem of the child who previously experienced deprivation in feedback from caretakers
	Sexual self receives emphasis. Early development tends to enhance self-esteem, especially in boys	Heterosexual peer relationships, dating experiences
	Interpersonal relationships are anxiety-producing as adolescent learns to master adult level independence and satisfactory relations with the opposite sex	Realistic increases in opportunities to assume adult tasks and responsibilities Social opportunities outside family events
Late Adolescence and Early Adulthood *Psychosocial crisis:* Intimacy vs. Isolation	Establishes durable, responsible relationships Sense of self as integrated and sexual being	Opportunity for intimate relationships Diminished family unit interactions with movement toward establishment of own residence or college attendance
	Uses communication skills to protect self from conflicts with others. Behaviors based on internal locus of control; moral self established	Many social and personal relationships outside family. Job or career relations

(Data from Sullivan, 1953; Helms and Turner, 1976; Freiberg, 1983; Stanwyck, 1983.)

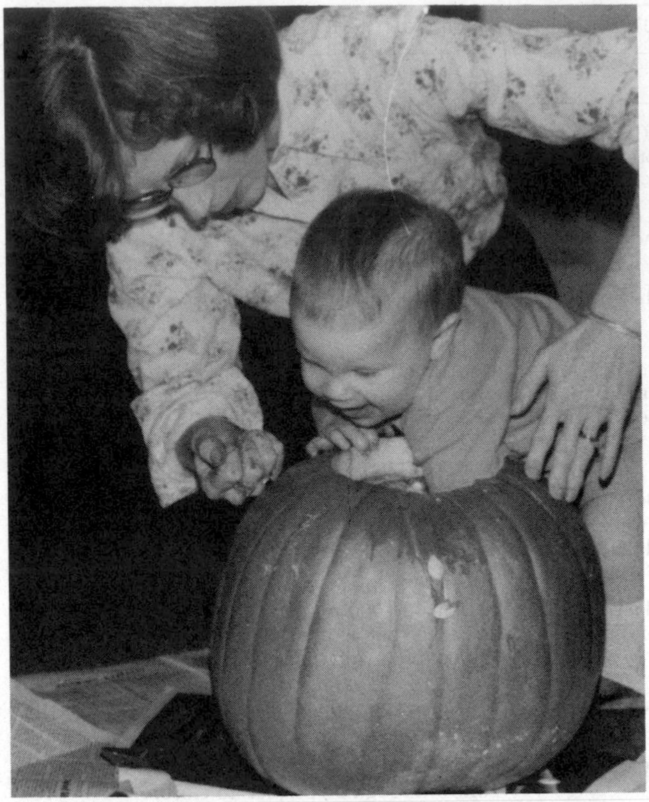

Reactions to the child's first attempts at tasks influence the child's self-concept and subsequent efforts to approach new tasks.

tiveness to be more damaging than physical punishment or rejection. Generally it has been found that when there is consistent enforcement of demands and rules combined with warmth, acceptance, respect, and open communication, children grow up to be more self-controlled and are able to approach new situations with confidence and to initiate and complete tasks (Baumrind, 1967, 1971).

A summary of the three parenting styles discussed in Chapter 3 and their impact on self-concept development is provided in Table 16-2. It should be recognized that parents from different cultures or socioeconomic backgrounds institute varying child-rearing practices. The studies summarized in Table 16-2 are based on findings in North American children, therefore are not necessarily applicable to children in all cultures.

The environment provided within the family is critical to the development of a healthy self-system. A direct correlation exists between maternal self-esteem, the perceptions and feelings a mother holds about her child, and how the child feels about self (Coopersmith, 1967; Sears, 1970; Reasoner, 1983). From his extensive work, Coopersmith (1967) identified three elements of the home environment that appear critical to development of a healthy self-system: acceptance of the child, clearly defined limits, and respectful treatment. Children assume that what adults tell them about themselves is true. Thus parental approval, love, and support based on realistic expectations validate feelings of "good me," whereas parental disapproval, distance, and indifference based on unrealistic expectations validate feelings of "bad me." Humans structure daily activities around hopes of receiving acknowledgement of their existence. If they cannot obtain positive strokes acknowledging "OKness," they will satisfy themselves with negative strokes (un-OKness) so that they are at least acknowledged for their existence.

Siblings as Significant Others. In extensive observations of family relationships and their influence on self-concept development and behavior, Toman (1966) discovered that in a family of two or more children, the children tend to turn to each other for interaction. Thus siblings may more strongly affect devel-

***Table* 16-2.** Three Parenting Styles: Impact on Self-Concept Development

Parenting Style	Main Theme	Predominant Approach	Impact on Child's Self-Concept
Democratic or authoritative (most effective)	Autonomous problem solving based on self-regulation and disciplined conformity	Shares rationale for desired behavior with child: affirms child's efforts to comply but sets limits or boundaries for acceptable behavior	High in self-esteem (Coopersmith, 1967). Competent, self-controlled, independent (Baumrind, 1967, 1971)
Autocratic or authoritarian	Obedience: respect	Favors punitive measures to curb self-will when child does not comply with code of conduct	Low in self-esteem (Coopersmith, 1967). Poor internalization of moral standards and seeks external rewards and punishment (Baldwin, 1948). Lacking in independence (Baumrind, 1971)
Permissive or low level of demands	Provide minimal direction to child's behavior	Uses reason: punitive measures seldom (if ever) used to teach socialization	High level of aggression (Sears, Maccoby and Levin, 1957). Impulses poorly controlled. Immaturity (Baumrind, 1967)

opment of a child's self-system development than do parents, particularly prior to exposure to peers in school. Altus (1966) and Koch (1957) also noted the increasing amount of influence the closer siblings are in age. Birth order–sex combination also seems to be important, with second-born boys at greatest risk for poor self-system development (McCandless, 1970; Tackett, 1972). Second-born children tend to be more dependent and "controlled" more by the older sibling. These studies suggest that second-born siblings may need extra amounts of positive reinforcement, and parents may need to monitor the sibling relationship to ensure that their second-born has experiences as a leader and opportunities to develop independence.

Teachers and Peers as Significant Others. Entering school poses a substantial challenge to autonomous behavior. Many new teacher- and peer-imposed rules are met, and virtually every behavior is subject to evaluation. These experiences pose a threat to self-concept, particularly for the child with a primarily external locus of control. If teacher and peer evaluations and the child's self-image agree, that image is confirmed; if they do not, self-esteem may be adjusted toward the majority of evaluations. The child with a high internal locus of control (does not need others' appraisals continually to feel good about self) will accept only those evaluations consistent with his or her self-esteem, rejecting or ignoring all other evaluations. Children with low self-esteem tend to set unrealistically high or low goals for their school performance so that consequent positive evaluation is either impossible or meaningless (self-fulfilling prophesy is demonstrated). Studies have shown a striking correlation between students' academic self-expectations and teacher expectations (Stanwyck, 1983; Sieman, 1978). A pattern of success or failure set in the early school years is likely to be perpetuated through the child's school and later employment careers unless significant interventions occur (Bandura, 1982; Stanwyck, 1983). Therefore, the established sense of self is further refined during school years as children compare themselves with peers, receive additional adult feedback, and are faced with many tasks to master.

Modeling Significant Others' Behavior. Developing children imitate the prominent behavioral strategies of significant others as they experiment with adapting to stressful interactions and frustrating situations. Modeled behaviors that are even temporarily functional are repeated and become patterned (Stanwyck, 1983). Modeled behaviors that encourage autonomy and independence (internal locus of control formation) enhance esteem. Conversely, modeled behaviors that encourage strict conformity and dependence (external locus of control formation) are costly and disruptive to healthy esteem development; the result is that the child is stifled from too little freedom or frightened to move because of too much freedom.

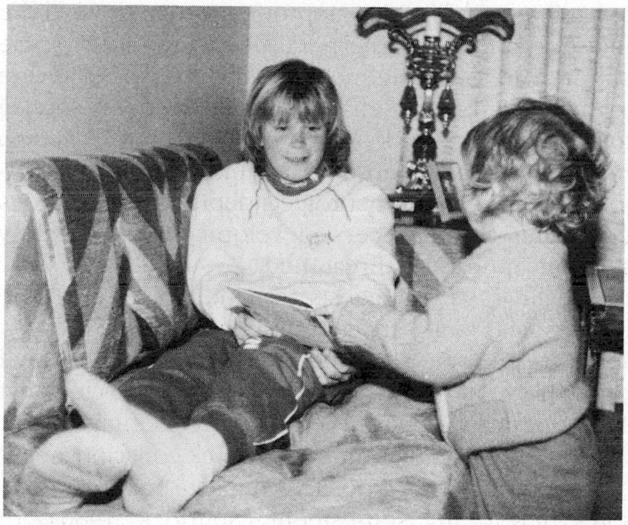
In a family of two or more, children tend to turn to each other for interaction. Siblings strongly affect the development of a child's self-system.

Social Roles and Culture as Factors

Since most socialization experiences are perceived in reference to one's gender role, culture, and ethnicity, these are three powerful forces in the definition of self and the development of personal identity (Levine et al, 1983). Whether a certain behavior is considered adaptive is strongly entwined in one's cultural and ethnic memberships. Thus, the child's emerging identity and self-definition are rooted in cultural and ethnic experiences from which family influence cannot be separated. Culture influences the developing self-system of the child from both a functional and status perspective.

Social status distinctions determine how one uses the resources and power available. A child's social class identity will influence the self-system's sense of power and control, the view of life as fatalistic or futuristic, and the perception of the world as hostile or filled with promise. Feshback's studies (1973) tied these differences to economics more than to variances in personalities among different ethnic groups.

Culture and ethnicity are functional in that they are vehicles for development of self-definition and -identity. They provide clues to the children about their affiliation with the rest of the world and serve as frames of reference as children define their worth, make judgments, and set standards for the self-system (Levine et al, 1983). Thomas and Chess (1980) studied the effects on self-concept of discriminatory experiences among children. They found that while many children are able to recognize the source of the threat to their self-system's integrity, develop appropriate anger toward the injustice, and reject the prejudiced judgments, some children are overwhelmed and suffer serious damage to their self-system. Self-attitudes develop in response to how children think others see them — i.e., *reflected appraisals* (Rosenberg and Simmons, 1971). Therefore when the majority projects depreciating attitudes upon minority members, development of a healthy self-concept can be threatened.

Lewin (1948) suggests that individuals from the lower social strata are greatly influenced by the low self-esteem projected upon them. Before the civil rights movement of the 1960s, studies reflected that Afro-American children held negative feelings about the self but since that time the "black consciousness" movement has had a positive impact on a black person's developing self-esteem (Spurlock, 1986). In contrast to the literature before the 1960s, Rosenberg and Simmons (1971) reviewed studies conducted between 1960 and 1968 and found no significant racial differences in self-esteem between blacks and Caucasians. Furthermore, Velasco-Barraza and Muller (1982) reported development of self-concept, self-esteem, and self-ideal to be similar across national groups, including Chile, Mexico, and the United States.

Although the existence of differences in self-esteem across cultures is not generally supported in recent literature, it should not be overlooked that living and working in a dissonant social situation and experiencing conflict can negatively affect self-concept (Lazarus et al, 1985). For example, a Native American boy who enters an Anglo-American school may begin to compare himself to the child of the dominant culture, and these comparisons may have a detrimental effect on his self-esteem. If, however, a Native American girl goes to school on a tribal reservation, her self-concept is not threatened because she compares herself to peers of the same culture (Lazarus et al, 1985). What affects the development of self-concept is children's perception of their living conditions and the views that they believe others hold of them.

Physical Health State as a Factor

Numerous studies have demonstrated that a child's attitude toward the body strongly influences self-concept development (Watson and Johnson, 1985; Havighurst, 1963; Zion, 1965). Illness may impose any number of coping problems that affect the physical self-concept. Diseases or injuries related to sexual identity and task performance affect the body image; the extent depends primarily on how much the physical problem impedes normal functioning, and the feedback received from significant others (Levine et al, 1983). A substantial change in weight also requires adjustments in body image. Losses of body parts or of function can be battering to the child's body image. Levine et al (1983) contend that although such persons may appear to accept and adjust to these body changes, they tend to retain an image of an intact body. The physically or mentally handicapped child experiences special stress in efforts to achieve mastery and competence, making a positive self-concept harder but not impossible to accomplish.

Antonucci and Jackson (1983) contend that although empirical studies establishing a causal relationship between self-esteem and physical or mental illness are few, there is definitely a link. They hypothesize that high self-esteem can insulate the individual from certain debilitating physical problems. They also suspect an association between low self-esteem and poor adjustment during illness and greater severity of symptoms when health problems are experienced.

Temperamental Coping Style as a Factor

Temperament* seems to influence the child's tolerance or coping level when confronted with tasks or challenges. Children of easy temperament are stimulated and respond positively, reflecting characteristics typical of the individual with high self-regard (see Box 16-1). The more characteristically difficult the temperament, the less the child seems able to display qualities indicating high self-regard. Research investigating the correlational nature of self-concept with temperament is substantially lacking. However, most parents who have children of both temperaments will insist that some correlation surely exists. Children with difficult temperaments seem to have fragile coping systems that leave them vulnerable to less adaptive perceptions about themselves and their experiences. Adults will be faced with the task of conscientiously providing the environmental conditions known to foster healthy self-system development when their child has a difficult temperament.

Nurse's Role in Fostering Self-Esteem

The nurse working with children and families has opportunities to foster the self-esteem of developing children both directly and indirectly. The nursing process can be employed to measure or evaluate the child's self-system and to establish nursing strategies for either building or maintaining it.

* Refer to Chapter 3 for a review of temperament as a characteristic of personality.

Self-Concept Assessment

The nurse may use various self-concept tools to identify children who may have problems with their self-system. Causes and symptoms of low self-concept should be explored thoroughly with the child and the family.

Because a child's self-concept cannot be observed directly, there are some difficulties in assessment. However, self-concept can be inferred from behavior (see Box 16-1). Self-concept can be measured by statements that reflect self-worth, by personal competence, and by the achievement aspirations of the child (Gilberts, 1983). Coopersmith (1967) states that self-ratings and ratings of observed behavior complement each other and the use of both is preferred over either method alone.

Self-Ratings as Measures of Self-Concept. One of the major difficulties with self-ratings is children's tendency to give information about themselves that they perceive to be socially desirable or that will gain them approval, rather than to disclose their true thoughts and feelings. Coopersmith found children below grade 4 to display significant social desirability response bias. Second, children's ability to apply the necessary symbolic thinking to represent real feelings of self-worth is not well established. Verbal self-ratings, therefore, are not recommended for children before grade 6. Observational scales and draw-a-person tests are preferred for estimating the self-concept of preschool and primary grade children to circumvent these difficulties.

Draw-a-person tests are most useful in demonstrating young children's perceived body images and self-esteem. The child is asked to draw a picture of herself or himself and of one other child on the same sheet of paper. Children with poor body image or low self-esteem portray themselves as smaller than the other child. Typically, the child's self-picture bears a sad expression, shows distortion of one or more body parts or of the entire body, and, frequently, depicts the child in some antisocial behavior.

Self-esteem inventories can be used with children in grades 4 through 12. Coopersmith's (1967) inventory, one used widely, contains groups of statements about family, school, peers, self, and general social activities. The responses reflect the degree to which children rate themselves as capable, significant, successful, and worthwhile. The statements are followed by columns in which the child checks whether the statement describes a frequent feeling as being *Like Me* or *Not Like Me.* The total score reflects the child's level of self-esteem as high, medium, or low. Box 16-2 provides some general guidelines for assessing components of the self-system.

Observational Measures of Self-Concept. The question of whether anyone can adequately infer the self-concept of another person presents philosophic dilemmas. Observational methods assume that the self-concept is demonstrated in observable behaviors and relates to some criterion such as health, social adaptability, or evidences of success. Such observation scales must carefully depict pertinent behaviors that presumably measure self-esteem. Observational methods generally are more valid if children do not know they are being observed and if they are being observed in the usual environment (Gilberts, 1983). Box 16-1 describes behaviors considered reflective of high and low self-esteem.

Building/Maintaining a Healthy Self-System

Human interaction, decision making, and growth and development—the elements of living–are all based in a healthy self-concept. The nurse's role(s) in building and maintaining a child's self-system will depend largely on the context of interactions with the child and family unit. When only occasional, short-duration interaction occurs (e.g., pediatric clinic, short-term hospitalization), the nurse's major roles are likely to be to assess the stability of the child's developing self-concept and family members' understanding of their part in guiding and fostering healthy self-system development. Further, the nurse can either teach the child and family self-concept–building behaviors or refer them to appropriate resources for this assistance.

The nurse who interacts regularly or for an extended period (e.g., home care nursing, long-term hospitalization, management of chronic disorders, school health) with a child and family unit not only can assess and teach the basic behaviors of self-concept maintenance but also can support the child and family by means of frequent positive feedback, counseling, and broadened education. The nurse's opportunities as a role model are substantially enhanced by the more frequent or lengthier contact. The strategies employed by the nurse to build and maintain the child's self-system are the same as those to be taught and reinforced in the child's significant others. Further, the nurse can teach the child self-care of the self-system, particularly by demonstrating such behaviors in the maintenance of her own healthy self-system.

Building and Maintenance Strategies (External Resources)

Researchers and psychologists generally agree on some basic attitudes apparent in persons who develop

Box 16-2
Guidelines for Self-Concept Assessment

Throughout the interview, note general mood, emotional response, affect.

I. *Physical Self* (Problem: Loss)
1. Let's pretend that I'm blind and can't see you—describe yourself to me.
2. Draw a picture of yourself for me (up to 6 years of age).
3. Are you satisfied with your physical appearance? What is it that you are not satisfied with?
4. What concerns do you have now about your body or physical function?
5. How are you feeling physically now (strong, weak, tired, sexually responsive, etc.)?
6. Think of a time in your life when you lost something or someone you valued. Describe that experience for me.
7. What concerns you now about experiencing a loss? What might you do if you experience a loss again?

II. *Personal Self*

A. *Self-Consistency* (Problem: Anxiety)
1. What kind of person are you? Tell me about yourself. (Pick up on cues to facilitate description.)
2. What makes you happy? What do you do to show it?
3. What makes you irritated? What do you do to show it? Or, when you are irritated, what do you do to show it?
4. What if your whole day is organized and something happens to alter your plans, what happens then? (May need situation for child to relate to in order to get elaboration.)
5. What are your feelings right now?
6. Note verbal and nonverbal cues related to the level of anxiety.

B. *Self-Ideal* (Problem: Powerlessness)
1. Often people dream about things or engage in wishful thinking or have hopes for the future. What are your wishes and hopes for the future?
2. What is your most important plan or goal today? In a few years from now? In many years from now?
3. When are some times you feel you have control over your life?
4. When are some times you feel you do not have control over your life?

C. *Moral-Ethical Self* (Problem: Guilt)
1. Complete the sentences: "I believe in..." "I believe that I am..." "I believe that one should..."
2. Who or what helps you know what is right or wrong? (See behavioral cues regarding guilt.)

(Freely based on Roy, 1984.)

healthy, motivated self-systems: a sense of security, a sense of identity, a sense of belonging, a sense of purpose, and a sense of personal competence (Sears, 1940; Brookover, 1965; Coopersmith, 1967; Maslow, 1968; Rosenthal and Jacobsen, 1968; Reasoner, 1982). Further, environmental conditions that foster these attitudes are crucial, generating feelings within the child of self-confidence, personal competence, and independence, which are the significant elements of a healthy self-system. Adults must provide these environmental conditions by recognizing that children need to be treated as important individuals and guided to assume steadily greater responsibility for their own lives (Reasoner, 1983).

Building a Sense of Security. Children develop security through honest interactions with significant others, so that they can learn to trust and be confident in the adults responsible for them. A firm but kind approach that defines clear, reasonable limits (i.e., the child knows what behavior is required to get approval), consistently enforced, offers the child security. Children's lives also need routine. Routine tends to reduce conflicts and assist children to meet expectations. These set patterns of living add to a sense of security built from honest interactions. Children in disrupted families also can build security and reduce anxiety if both parents enforce similar standards.

Check lists, charts (pictures can be used for young children who cannot read), and calendars or tally sheets serve as reminders and reinforcers of limits while enabling children to monitor their own adherence. Such self-monitoring builds positive images and encourages responsibility for self-care. Use of logical consequences to discourage misbehavior, predetermined with the child (removal of privileges is successful with most children), as well as realistic rewards for specified behaviors, helps children learn that actions have predictable consequences. It encourages them to take responsibility for their behavior as well as for consequences. Trustworthy adults act as role models for responsibility and dependability in their own actions.

Building a Sense of Identity. The foundation for a sense of identity is love and acceptance. Identity is built through positive feedback, providing recognition to children for their strengths and demonstrating respect for their uniqueness.

Children behave in ways that are consistent with the picture they hold of themselves. Thus a child's sense of identity is an important key to understanding behavior. Children who receive positive feedback from tasks accomplished acquire a realistic view of what they can do and cannot do. Thus feedback largely determines whether children see themselves as primarily successful or as lacking important qualities (Reasoner, 1983). Children who feel successful are more apt to make use of their opportunities to grow and learn and are less daunted by the risk of failing because they recognize their "self" as a dependable, trustworthy instrument for achieving goals and making decisions. Children, therefore, need accurate feedback from adults and an environment that avails them opportunities and experiences in creativity and productivity. Feedback should include a steady supply of appreciation of traits children possess, as well as identification of skills observed. Too often adults have a tendency to pay undue attention to shortcomings of children and to overlook their achievements.

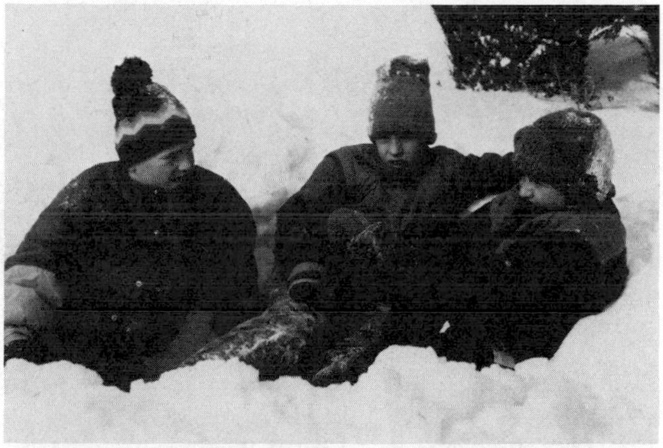

The foundation of a sense of identity for the school-age child is acceptance by peers.

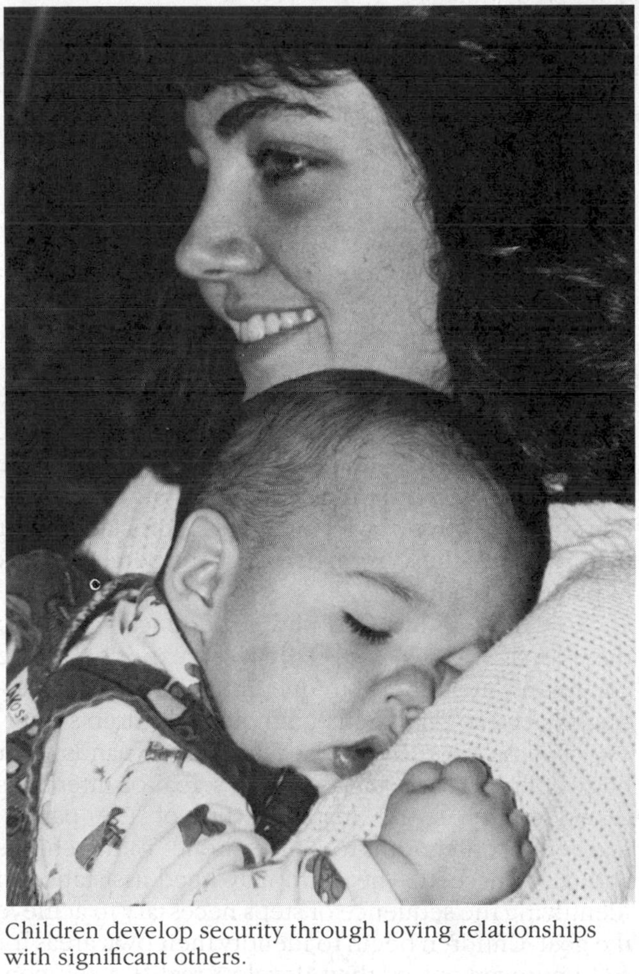

Children develop security through loving relationships with significant others.

Feedback and recognition from adults is relatively useless to children's developing self-system if these responses are not generated from a sense of love and respect for the child as a thinking, feeling individual. Touching and active listening should be combined with appropriate verbal expressions of love and affection to convey warmth and sensitivity to children. Verbal expression alone does little to provide the support children need and does not make up for a general lack of acceptance of the child.

Part of a sense of identity is self-confidence in one's own decisions and intuitions. Thus feedback from others, while extremely important, should be coupled with encouragement for the child to judge self-performance and find ways to confirm self-assessments. The educational system has many built-in opportunities for such confirmations if children have been taught to consider their own performance as part of the feedback system to their identity.

Children should also be taught that recognizing and acknowledging limitations or problems is not a sign of weakness or defect. Rather, they should be encouraged to consider appropriate sources for assistance and to accept what cannot be changed.

Building a Sense of Belonging. The need to feel accepted is important to children, peaking during adolescence. They must learn that they are simultaneously unique beings unlike anyone else and yet like everyone else. This realization is critical to the development

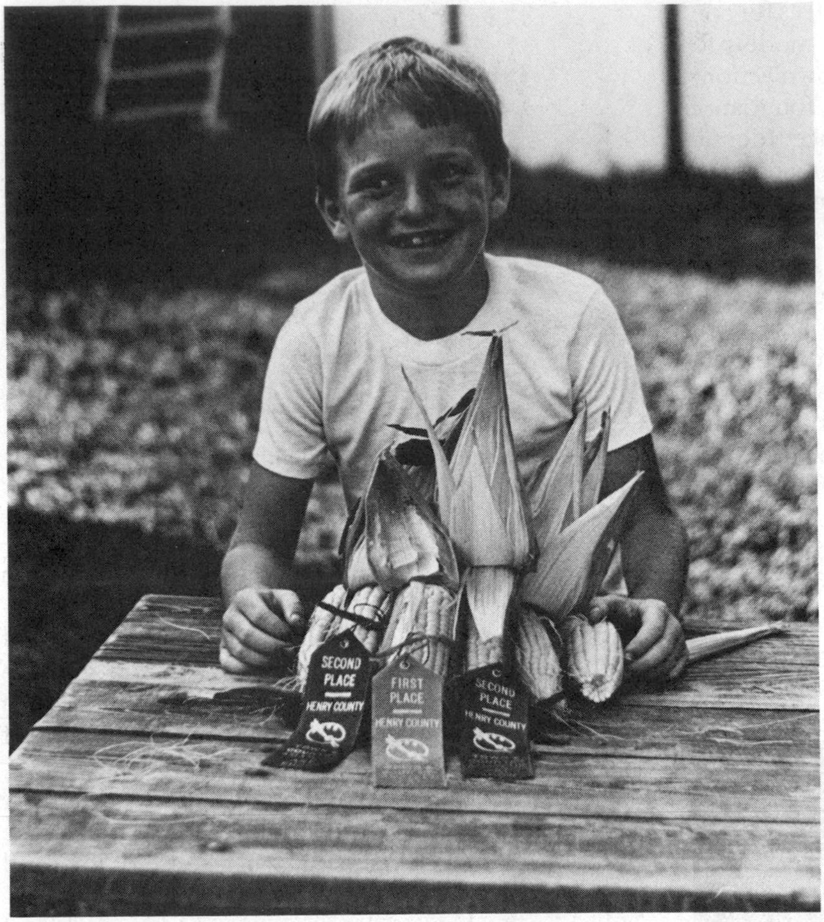

The school-age child builds self-esteem through accomplishments and evidence of competency.

of skill in differentiating when it is appropriate to be individualistic and when it is useful to function as a team or group member.

While feedback, recognition, expressed love, and acceptance help children see and develop their uniqueness, playing and working together as a family and dyadic interactions help children learn that they are also like everyone else, i.e., that they belong. Through family and group activities children realize that they cannot always be first or always have their own way, without feeling that their "self" is diminished. Through a balance of the feelings of wanting their own way and giving in, they learn the responsibility of belonging, of group membership, and the necessity of compromise. When children are encouraged to express empathy and to find ways to help others, they learn social concern and how to reduce feelings of alienation.

Building a Sense of Purpose. Purpose provides direction to life and is developed by setting realistic goals for oneself. A sense of purpose can be created by setting reasonable expectations for children, by helping them set realistic goals for themselves, and by exhibiting faith and confidence in their capability to achieve goals (Reasoner, 1983). Expectations are communicated by setting behavioral standards and limits, by identifying achievement levels as goals to work toward, and by labeling those personality characteristics that are desirable. Expectations above or below children's perceived capacity or which are too specific (e.g., an A grade in English rather than to improve writing skills) are not motivators. Challenges and contracts are effective ways to express expectations for children since these seem to reduce the perceived risk of penalty or failure.

Exposing children to new experiences can help them identify goals, especially if the experiences are congruent with their unique interests or abilities. Adults need to realize that, although children's interests may be short-lived, each interest expands their body of knowledge. Once a child's goal or interest is expressed, it is the responsibility of the parent, teacher, or other adult to convey belief in the child's ability to succeed. The child may need assistance in identifying the sequence of steps necessary to achieve the goal. Children begin to identify their own areas for self-improvement as they develop realistic self-concepts.

Building a Sense of Personal Competence. Personal competence is the feeling of being able to cope with problems or accomplish goals. A sense of competence develops from experiencing success and completing tasks. Adults can help children by providing feedback about their progress and helping them look at options when there are blocks to success or task completion. It is critical that adults not prescribe how children go about achieving their goals; telling children how to do something tends to build dependency, not confidence (Reasoner, 1983). A better approach is to discuss options with children, permitting them to make the final decision on how they will proceed. Once the child has decided on the process and resources needed, the adult's role is to monitor progress, praising both effort and accomplishment. Reward or recognition should not *always* be offered when the goal or task is accomplished, since the aim is to encourage self-motivation and self-satisfaction in success. The self-confidence that results leaves the child more receptive to new challenges, permits the child to feel less threatened by others, and provides a general sense of feeling accepted. The growth of self and success in achievements is cyclic. As one feels more self-assured, more tasks are attempted, and their successful completion, in turn, instills confidence.

Self-System Enhancement (Internal Resources)

Self-concept development, positive strokes, and success in tasks are positively correlated. However, whereas adults can and should act to increase children's self-concepts, an equally important role is to teach them to enhance their own self-concepts so that self-concept enhancement, like decision making, becomes a lifetime skill rather than a transitory state (Crosby, 1982).

Self-Praise as Enhancement. An occasional "blowing of one's own horn" can be extremely constructive to the self-system. Children will need to decipher what amount of "horn blowing" is socially tolerable before it becomes "bragging" and thus socially detrimental. The social dissonance related to self-praise can be abated in children's minds by helping them realize that the better one becomes, the more one will have to offer others. Children can also learn to offer self-praise privately. Such self-praise can have a "self-fulfilling prophecy" effect. For example, when a child, rightly or wrongly, attributes a well-done act or behavior to personal ability and effort, that child is building, and subsequently reinforcing, a healthy self-concept (Satir, 1972). Such activity helps children learn self-evaluation and also helps them acknowledge positive as well as negative behavior. An amusing exercise for teaching this concept to school-age children is to give them a "pretend" situation in which they have to justify their existences in order to be saved. They must emphasize the positive aspects of themselves and their lives, an invaluable lesson in self-concept discovery.

Adults need to give children their love, but what a given child does with that love is another matter. Children must be taught to accept love and praise, and to receive compliments in a manner that enhances rather than diminishes self. Simply teaching children by example that saying "Thank you, I'm good at that" or "Thank you, that is one of my stronger points" is a healthy response will give them another tool valuable to self-concept enhancement.

Another significant enhancement method deals with failure. Children need to learn that everyone "comes up short" sometimes but that such shortcomings are to be used as opportunities to learn from mistakes, as well as to accept occasional failure, as part of a healthy existence rather than as times to diminish self.

Self-Care as Enhancement. "In order to choose freely one must be able to believe in one's self as well as not worry about what others will think (not to be confused with considering the consequences)" (Crosby, 1982, page 435). Believing in oneself enough to be responsible for one's physical and mental health is a critical motivator, influencing personal health decisions. A strong self-concept also correlates positively with stress management ability (Girdano and Everly, 1979). Kearney and Fleischer (1979) found a highly positive or reciprocal correlation between self-care* initiative and a positive self-concept (as measured by self-confidence, achievement orientation, outgoing behaviors, and assertiveness). Thus children should be encouraged and provided opportunities to steadily increase personal responsibility for maintaining and making decisions about their own health. In so doing they further enhance their self-system.

References

Altus W: Birth order and its sequelae. *Science* 1966 Feb; 44–49.

Antonucci T, Jackson J: Physical health and self-esteem. *Fam Community Health* 1983 Aug; 1–9.

Baldwin AL: Socialization and the parent-child relationship. *Child Dev* 1948; 19:127–136.

Bandura A: Self-efficacy mechanisms in human agency. *Am Psychol* 1982; 37:122–147.

* Self-care refers to the ability of an individual to initiate and perform health activities for himself to maintain life, health, and well-being (Orem, 1978).

Baumrind D: Child care practices anteceding three patterns of preschool behavior. *Genet Psychol Monographs* 1967; 75:43–88.

Baumrind D: Current patterns of parental authority. *Dev Psychol* Monograph 1971; 4(1) Part 2.

Brookover WB, et al: *Self-Concept of Ability and School Achievement.* US Office of Education, Cooperative Research Project No. 1636. Lansing, Michigan State University, 1965.

Coopersmith S: *The Antecedents of Self Esteem.* San Francisco, WH Freeman, 1967.

Crosby R: Self-concept development. *J School Health* 1982 Sep; 432–436.

Feshback ND: Reinforcement patterns in children. *In* Pick A (ed): *Minnesota Symposium on Child Psychology.* Vol 7. Minneapolis, University of Minnesota Press, 1973.

Freiberg KL: *Human Development: A Life Span Approach.* Monterey, CA, Brooks/Cole, 1983.

Gilberts R: The evaluation of self-esteem. *Fam Community Health* 1983 Aug; 29–37.

Girdano D, Everly G: *Controlling Stress and Tension.* Englewood Cliffs, NJ, Prentice-Hall, 1979, p 106+.

Harter S: Developmental perspectives on the self-system. *In* Hetherington E (ed): *Carmichael's Manual of Child Psychology.* Vol IV. New York, John Wiley & Sons, 1982.

Havighurst R: *Human Development and Education.* New York, Longmans, 1963.

Helms D, Turner J: *Exploring Child Behavior.* Philadelphia, WB Saunders, 1976.

Kearney B, Fleischer B: Development of an instrument to measure exercise of self-care agency. *Res Nurs Health* 1979; 2:25–34.

Kegan R: *The Evolving Self.* Cambridge, MA, Harvard University Press, 1982.

Koch H: The relation in young children between characteristics of their playmates and certain attributes of their siblings. *Child Dev* 1957; 28:175–202.

Lazarus PJ, et al: Multicultural influences on the development of the young child. *In* McLoughlin CS, Guilo DF: *Young Children in Context: Impact of Self, Family and Society on Development.* Springfield, IL, Charles C Thomas, 1985, pp 183–217.

Levine M, et al: *Developmental–Behavioral Pediatrics.* Philadelphia, WB Saunders, 1983.

Lewin K: *Resolving Social Conflicts: Selected Papers on Group Dynamics.* New York, Harper and Row, 1948.

Maslow A: *Toward a Psychology of Being.* Princeton, NJ, Van Nostrand, 1968.

McCandless B: *Adolescents' Behavior and Development.* Hillsdale, IL, Dryden Press, 1970.

Millar T: How do you give a child self-esteem? *Child Today* 1983 Sep-Oct; 2–3.

Murray R, Huelskoetter M: *Psychiatric/Mental Health Nursing.* Englewood Cliffs, NJ, Prentice-Hall, 1983.

Orem D: *A General Theory of Nursing* (Tape). New York, Second Annual Nurse Educator Conference, 1978.

Rambo B: *Adaptation Nursing.* Philadelphia, WB Saunders, 1984.

Reasoner R: *Building Self-Esteem: A Comprehensive Program.* Palo Alto, CA, Consulting Psychologists Press, 1982.

Reasoner R: Enhancement of self-esteem in children and adolescents. *Fam Community Health* 1983 Aug; 51–64.

Rosenberg M, Simmons R: *Black and White Self-Esteem: The Urban Child.* Washington, DC, The American Sociological Association (published for the Arnold M. and Caroline Rose Monograph Series), 1971.

Rosenthal R, Jacobsen L: *Pygmalion in the Classroom.* New York, Holt, Rinehart and Winston, 1968.

Roy C: *Introduction to Nursing: An Adaptation Model.* Englewood Cliffs, NJ, Prentice-Hall, 1984.

Satir V: *Peoplemaking.* Palo Alto, CA, Science and Behavior Books, 1972.

Sears P: Levels of aspiration in academically successful and unsuccessful children. *J Abn Soc Psychol* 1940; 35:498–536.

Sears R: Relation of early socialization experience to self concepts and gender role in middle childhood. *Child Dev* 1970; 41:267–289.

Sears RR, Maccoby E, Levin H: *Patterns of Child Rearing.* Evanston, IL, Row Peterson, 1957.

Sieman M: Mental health in school age children. *Matern Child Nurs* 1978 Jul/Aug; 215+.

Spurlock J: Development of self-concept in Afro-American children. *Hosp Community Psychiatr* 1986 Jan; 37(1):66–70.

Stanwyck D: Self-esteem through the life span. *Fam Community Health* 1983 Aug; 11–28.

Sullivan H: *The Interpersonal Theory of Psychiatry.* New York, Norton, 1950.

Sullivan H: *Conceptions of Modern Psychiatry.* New York, Norton, 1953.

Tackett J: *Understanding Your First and Second Born.* Dissertation. Chapel Hill, NC, University of North Carolina, 1972.

Thomas A, Chess S: *Dynamics of Psychological Development.* New York, Brunner-Mazel, 1980.

Toman W: *Family Constellations: Effects on Personality and Social Behavior.* New York, Springer Company, 1966.

Velasco-Barraza CR, Muller D: Development of self-concept in children; Mexican and United States school children. *J Psychol* 1982; 110(1):21–30.

Watson E, Johnson A: The emotional significance of acquired physical disfigurement in children. *Am J Orthopsychiatr* 1985; 28:85–97.

Zion L: Body concept as it relates to self concept. *Res Q* AAHPER 1965; 36:490–495.

Bibliography

Barksdale L: *Building Self Esteem.* Los Angeles, The Barksdale Foundation, 1972.

Beier B: Enhancing positive self concept through creativity in the classroom. *Health Educ* 1981 Mar/Apr; 35.

Canfield J, Wells H: *100 Ways to Enhance Self Concept in the Classroom.* Englewood Cliffs, NJ, Prentice-Hall, 1976.

Eisenman R: Birth order, sex, self esteem and prejudice against the physically disabled. *J Psychol* 1970; 75:147–155.

Erickson E: *Identity: Youth and Crisis.* New York, Norton, 1968.

Felker D: *Building Positive Self Concepts.* Minneapolis, Burgess Press, 1974.

Hamachek D: *Encounters with the Self.* New York, Holt Rinehart and Winston, 1978.

Hester NO: Child's health self-concept scale: Its development and psychometric properties. *Adv Nurs Sci* 1984; 7:45–55.

Jaques J, Chasen K: Self esteem and low status groups: A changing scene? *Soc Q* 1977; 18:399–412.

Joseph L: Self care and the nursing process. *Nurs Clin North Am* 1980 Mar; 131–143.

Koenig F: Definitions of self and ordinal position of birth. *J Soc Psychol* 1969 Aug; 287–288.

Lynch M, et al (ed): *Self-Concept: Advances in Theory and Research.* Cambridge, MA, Ballinger, 1981.

Meisenhelder JB: Self esteem: a closer look at clinical interventions. *Int J Nurs Stud* 1985; 22(2):127–135.

Stanwyck DJ: Self-esteem through the life span. *Top Clin Nurs* 1983; 6(2):11–28.

Thomas A, Chess S: *Temperament and Development.* New York, Brunner-Mazel, 1977.

Promoting Safety

Chapter 17

Mabel Hunsberger

Safety of children is of concern to every parent, school, and community. Despite the movement toward various forms of legislation and the commitment of community organizations to promote the safety of children, accidental injury is the leading cause of death in children age 1 year to young adulthood. Accidents cause more deaths in the United States in the 1- to 14-year age group than the next six causes of death combined. The distinction of being the number one cause of death has occurred only in the past two decades because the incidence of formerly fatal diseases has been reduced through antibiotics, immunization, and chemotherapy. Accidental injury is a major threat to the life of children and adolescents, causing unnecessary pain and suffering.

One may ask, how can such a major preventable health problem persist? An accident is a phenomenon of diverse and multifactorial etiologic basis, including variation in the *host,* the *agent* (or vector), and the *environment.* The solution is not one of isolating a causative agent against which immunity can be developed, but rather involves effecting changes in human behavior through education, consumer product regulation, and legislation. This chapter addresses the epidemiology of accidents with reference to host, agent, and environmental variables and provides a review of the common types of accidents and their related nursing strategies for prevention. The care of children when an accident occurs is discussed in Chapter 52.

Related Topics
Anticipatory guidance: promoting safety, Unit 2
Toys appropriate for various developmental levels, Chapter 21
Description and use of Heimlich maneuver, Chapter 52

Promoting Safety

Nursing Diagnoses	Nursing Goals/Strategies
Potential for injury: motor vehicle accidents, related to: • *improper use of car safety devices* • *lack of knowledge regarding proper use of car safety devices* • *lack of use of car safety devices* • *lack of access to safe car safety devices*	Prevent accidental injury resulting from motor vehicle accidents. • Assess the family's and child's knowledge level about use of car seat. • Determine the existing knowledge gap from the parents' and child's perception. • Fill in knowledge gaps with information about safe use of car safety devices. • Support legislative actions to promote safety standards.
• *impaired driving and/or drug use*	Prevent accidental injury as a result of motor vehicle accidents caused by impaired driving and/or drug use. • Provide anticipatory guidance to prepare teenager for developmental changes that affect alcohol and drug use. • Emphasize appropriate use of seat belts. • Teach teenagers the dangers of driving while abilities are impaired.
Potential for injury: poisoning, related to lack of awareness of environmental hazard associated with child's developmental level	Protect child from injury by poisoning. • Teach parents to adhere to safe storage of toxic substances. • Use safety caps on toxic substances. • Supervise young children to avoid exposure to toxic substances • Keep poisonous plants out of the reach of children. • Keep poison control number at telephone. • Give specific directions to babysitters about safe monitoring of children in the vicinity of toxic substances. • Counsel parents to anticipate developmental changes that increase child's potential to access poisons (see Table 17–1). • Advise parents to keep syrup of ipecac in the home and teach parents how to use it.
Potential for injury: suffocation, related to child's lack of awareness of environmental hazard associated with child's developmental level	Prevent injury by suffocation. • Provide anticipatory guidance to prepare parents for child's developmental changes that endanger his or her life. Teach parents to: • Avoid propping an infant's bottle. • Keep plastic bags out of child's reach at all times. • Remove doors from a discarded refrigerator or freezer. • Avoid leaving child unattended in bathtubs or pools. • Avoid use of pillows in infant's crib. • Avoid hanging pacifier around infant's head. • Purchase crib that meets safety specifications.
Potential for injury: trauma, related to child's lack of awareness of environmental hazard associated with child's developmental level	Prevent accidental injury resulting from falls, burns, near drowning, and foreign body aspiration. • Provide anticipatory guidance for parents to prepare them for the expected changes that increase child's potential for injury. • Teach parents to protect children by providing a safe environment appropriate to the age of the child (see Boxes 17-3, 17-5, and 17-7 through 17-10).

Definition of Terms

The term *accident* suggests that an event happened by chance and implies that every member of the population has the same probability of being affected. Fundamental to accident prevention is the belief that accidents have causes and that these causes can be altered to prevent or modify an injury. An epidemiologic approach of identifying variables in the host, agent, and environment offers a framework that gives some predictability to accidents and therefore serves as a guide for prevention. In fact, there is some question whether an accident really is an *accident* (i.e., a random, bad luck event) (Rivara, 1982). In this chapter, the term *accident* is used, but it is not intended to convey that the event is random; the focus of this chapter is how to *prevent* accidents.

Analysis of an Accident

An understanding of the mechanism of an accident is fundamental to preventing children from suffering injury. Following is an analysis of an accident with a discussion of host characteristics, agent characteristics, and the environment.

Host Characteristics

An important variable to consider in accident prevention is the developmental level of the child. Age-related physical and cognitive skills of children and their emotional social needs are strong determinants of whether an accident is likely to happen and which type of accident is most likely to occur. Immaturity in motor skills and inexperience in how to safely discover the contents of the environment increase the chance of falls and suffocation during infancy. When curiosity is paramount and locomotion improves during late infancy, a child can no longer be protected from the environment. At this stage, the environment must be modified to protect the child. New skills and needs make older infants, toddlers, and preschoolers vulnerable to new kinds of falls and new agents, such as poisons, bodies of water, and sources of heat. During the school years, children are less supervised by their parents and they become more competitive in many of their activities. They are now trusted to new activities, such as crossing the street, playing on larger playground equipment, and riding a bicycle. As adolescence is approached, a need for independence and emancipation from childhood introduces yet more dangerous vectors, including motor vehicles. Accidents that most typically occur at the various ages are summarized in Table 17-1.

The child's sex is another variable that has been identified as a determinant in the propensity for accidental injury. In a review of the literature pertaining to childhood accidents, Rivara (1982) noted a male preponderance in pedestrian injuries, bicycle injuries, burns, home injuries, drowning, and sports injuries. The difference between male and female injury rates is not thought to be due to increased exposure but rather to behavioral differences—i.e., increased risk-taking in boys (Rivara, 1982).

A much debated issue concerning host characteristics is the idea of "accident proneness." This term refers to the notion that some individuals possess certain stable psychologic characteristics that predispose them to relatively high accident rates (Klein, 1980; Langley, 1982). Competent research has now discredited this motion, yet it lingers as a myth. It is, however, recognized that some individuals do have more accidents than others, but there has been no consistent identification of personality characteristics as direct causes of injury to explain this phenomenon (Langley, 1982). Even when traits have been identified that were thought to typify the "accident-prone" individual, the same traits were found in those without a history of repeated accidents (Rodstein, 1974). A study of infant temperament and the occurrence of accidents from infancy to age 5 does *not* clearly establish accident proneness (Nyman, 1987). Only partial support was found for the hypothesis that very difficult temperament is connected with an increased risk of accidents. The implication of "accident proneness" is that an individual who is accident prone is likely to be injured whatever the conditions of the environment, so there is little point in modifying the environment. This concept, therefore, is contradictory with the premises of accident prevention.

Accident prevention in children must take into consideration the combined physiologic and psychologic characteristics of the host that influence the likelihood and the degree of injury at the various stages. For example, children's capacity for mobility combined with their curiosity may lead them to pull hot water on themselves, and the physiologic characteristics of their skin predispose them to more severe scalding than a similar accident in an adult. Strategies for accident prevention are not static but must be altered as the child's body grows and the mind and social being develops.

Agent (Vector) Characteristics

The specific vehicle causing the injury is the agent or vector of the accident. The rate and amount of energy transferred is determined by the characteristics of the agent. For example, the design of toys, the tempera-

Table 17-1. Typical Accidents According to Developmental Age and Prevention Strategies

Prevention Strategies Requiring Repeated Monitoring Across Various Ages

Automobile:	Use of child-restraint device in automobile (check at *each* visit) Never leave child alone in car
Burns:	Reduce hot water temperature Purchase and install smoke alarm Use nonflammable clothing and toys
Poisonings:	Safe storage of drugs, corrosives, and chemicals Use child-resistant caps on drugs Syrup of ipecac in the home Poison Control Number placed at telephone
Play:	Monitor safety of toys, activities, and sports appropriate to age
Drowning:	Supervise children around water Encourage swimming lessons

Developmental Landmarks	Event and Preventive Strategies
Infant (0 to 4 Months)	
Can roll, reach, grasp, and mouth objects	Motor Vehicle Accidents Child-restraint device Falls Protect from falls during dressing, etc. Keep one hand on baby Suffocation/Aspiration Avoid use of plastic bags in and near crib and playing area Avoid bottle propping Check crib safety Do not tie pacifier around neck Keep small objects and toys with removable parts out of crib Do not use pillows or excess blankets Burns Water temperature of bath should be checked with wrist or back of hand Avoid handling hot foods or liquids near baby Drowning Nonskid bottom in tub Keep hand on baby in tub at all times
Infant (4 to 6 Months)	
Is mobile and is developing some fine motor skills Can roll over Touches, reaches, and grasps to learn about environment Begins to understand off-limit areas (e.g., stove)	Motor Vehicle Accidents Continue use of child-restraint device Falls Discourage use of walkers Use gates at stairs Highchair safety Suffocation, Aspiration, Strangulation Keep drapery cords and mobiles out of reach Avoid hard foods, such as raw vegetables, peanuts, popcorn Avoid use of toys with small parts Ingestions, Poisonings Place all harmful products out of reach (see Box 17-6) Remove poisonous plants from child's reach Burns Begin to teach meaning of "hot" and off-limit areas (see Box 17-5) Drowning Never leave child alone in tub
Infant (6 to 12 Months)	
Creeps, crawls, is inquisitive Pincer grasp has developed by 8 months Pulls self up and other things down May begin table foods around 8–9 months Holds own bottle and begins to drink from cup Teeth are developing Has the capability to chew a teething biscuit and soft cooked foods	Motor Vehicle Accidents Continue use of child-restraint device Falls (from windows, down stairs, and from outdoor play equipment) Keep crib away from window Constant supervision is required to prevent falls Suffocation, Aspiration, Strangulation Child should sit when eating to prevent aspiration Continue to avoid hard foods Cut foods into small pieces

continued

Table 17-1. *(continued)*

Developmental Landmarks	Event and Preventive Strategies
	Burns Keep vaporizer beyond child's reach Supervise constantly, especially in kitchen and bathroom (see Box 17-5) Drowning Same as for 0–6 months
Toddler (1 to 3 Years)	
Walks, runs quickly, and often darts onto the street Is more independent and developing autonomy (will stray farther from a parent) Not aware of dangers but is intent on exploration Has unsteady gait By 3 years has full set of deciduous teeth Can reach higher and open lids, can turn doorknobs May be learning to swim but continues to need supervision	Teaching of child should begin at this age Motor Vehicle Accidents (as a passenger, cyclist, and pedestrian) Reaffirm importance of car seat even if toddler resists Ride in center of back seat (restrained) Teach to stay off streets with riding toys and tricycle Cannot be trusted, therefore requires supervision Provide a fenced-in play area if possible Falls Open windows from the top Remove objects from crib that child could stand on to climb out window Suffocation, Aspiration Table foods can be given but avoid nuts and other small, hard foods Teach the danger of plastic bags and similar items Teach the child not to run with popsicle sticks or lollipops in mouth Burns Expand on teaching about hot things. Especially teach about hot water, the stove, and hot food on the stove Ingestions, Poisonings, Trauma Re-evaluate placement of poisons and medicines Keep sharp objects out of reach Use only child-resistant containers for poisons and medicines Teach child about poisons Drowning Close supervision around water Teach not to run around pools or other bodies of water Supervise in tub
Preschool (3 to 5 Years)	
Eager to learn and capable of understanding simple explanations Has the motor and coordination skills to ride a tricycle and is learning to ride a bicycle Curious and explorative, particularly outdoors Active in playground and outdoor play Motor abilities exceed cognitive skills, therefore, child engages in physical activities without foreseeing danger Is more independent and may walk or ride bike in the neighborhood with less supervision than when a toddler Engages in sex play Engages in dramatic play	All aspects of safety should be taught to child Motor Vehicle, Pedestrian, Cycle Accidents Begin to teach how to cross street safely Teach rules of the road Teach purpose of car seats and seat belts Falls, Trauma Caution against climbing into unsafe areas, marshy lands, drainage pipes, unsafe buildings Teach child how to handle scissors Suffocation, Aspiration Teach child not to run while eating Teach child not to crawl into areas where he or she could be entrapped (refrigerators, drainage pipes, excavation areas) Burns Teach fire escape rules Caution child against playing with matches Keep matches out of reach Drowning Begin organized swimming lessons Never leave alone in bath or while swimming Street Safety Teach child not to accept rides or foods without permission of parents Bodily Injury Teach child not to insert objects into body orifices Ingestion, Inhalation Expand on teaching about poisons and medicines Include teaching about cosmetics and sprays, which child may use in playing house

Table 17-1. *(continued)*

Developmental Landmarks	Event and Preventive Strategies
School-Age (6 to 12 Years)	
More coordination in motor skills Runs, skips, jumps, climbs, constantly on the move Active in sports Increasing independence and need for peer acceptance Curiosity about sexuality	All aspects of safety should be taught to child **Motor Vehicle Accidents** Pedestrian safety needs to be repeated Bicycle safety must be emphasized **Bodily Injury, Fractures** Teach how to prevent injury from cold Teach safety related to hobbies, handicrafts, sports, mechanical equipment **Drowning** Water safety Supervise water sports **Burns** Teach child appropriate use of matches and campfires **Firearms** Teach respect of firearms Avoid keeping a loaded weapon in house **Bodily Harm and Trauma** Reinforce to avoid taking things or getting into a car of anyone without parents' knowledge Teach child about harmful use of drugs, alcohol, and cigarettes Sex education to make child aware of "good touching" and "bad touching" to prevent sexual abuse
Adolescent (13 to 18 Years)	
Drive motor vehicles (cars, motorcycles) Peer pressure and their acceptance predominates Risk-taking to establish self with peers is common Activities in work and sports involve dangerous equipment Independence in all activities	All aspects of safety should be taught to adolescent **Motor Vehicle Accidents** Re-emphasize use of seat belts Emphasize the danger of alcohol and drug use (especially related to motor vehicle accidents) **Bodily Injury and Trauma** Teach proper use of equipment and maintenance of equipment **Drowning** Teach water safety Instruct in the use of emergency care equipment Teach CPR **Firearms** Close supervision regarding firearms is required No loaded weapon in house

ture of hot water in a home, or the containers in which medicines are stored influence the occurrence and nature of an accident. Intervention strategies have been directed at the agent through regulation of fireworks, packaging of drugs into child-resistant containers, and manufacturing of flame-retardant children's clothing. Regulation of speed limits and seat belt laws are examples of approaches that potentially alter the vector but still require change in human behavior. Strategies such as putting on a seat belt require repeated behaviors, and therefore, they may meet with more resistance than one-time actions, such as turning down the water temperature in a home or buying syrup of ipecac. Strategies that require passive behavior on the part of the consumer (e.g., child-resistant containers) make the greatest impact on accident reduction (Rivara, 1982). Prevention strategies that modify the agent do not necessarily prevent an accident, but the extent of injury can be modified (e.g., water temperature reduction).

Environment (Physical and Sociocultural)

Physical and sociocultural environmental factors play an important role in the initiation of injury. The influence of sociocultural factors on accidents is difficult to study, and findings are varied. High rates of injury have been correlated with single parenting, a relative lack of parental supervision, and family stress (Rivara, 1982). Matheny's (1986) findings support the notion that parental attributes and features of the home are the factors that largely affect a toddler's liability for injury. In this study, the toddler's characteristics were reported to be of less significance than social and environmental factors. Such results cannot, however, be generalized to other periods of child development. As a child reaches various developmental levels, the impact of home environment may be sharply reduced.

Klein (1980), in a review of societal influence on childhood accidents, states that reliable findings concerning the relationship between social-class level and the incidence of accidental injury do not exist. The major difficulty is that investigators use different criteria to determine social class. When income alone is used as a measure of socioeconomic status, a higher incidence of injury is demonstrated in the lower socioeconomic class (Advance Data, 1978). It is certainly recognizable that the environmental hazards that poor housing and crowding create subjects children of lower socioeconomic status to a greater risk for accidents.

The impact of television has been identified as another environmental variable in accidental injury. Imitation of television heroes during play has been identified as a mechanism that leads to accidental injury (Danen et al, 1976). Other societal influences include the value placed on autonomy, competitiveness, risk-taking, and the willingness to take on a challenge (Klein, 1980).

The creation of organizations to protect the consumer (U.S. Consumer Product Safety Commission) and legislative actions to improve safety standards (building codes, car manufacturing standards) are examples of modification of the environment. Community organizations and local governments can also act to improve safety through provision of crossing guards, development of bike paths, and placement of signs such as "Children Playing."

Prevention of Common Accidents: Nursing Strategies

The most feasible and prevalent approach to prevention of accidents in children has been education in the form of anticipatory guidance, pamphlets, posters, and counseling. However, the ability to demonstrate change in parent or child behavior through provision of information has met with some failure, resulting in a degree of pessimism (Pless and Stulginskas, 1982). For example, the widespread awareness that proper use of a child-restraint device while riding in a car reduces injuries and fatalities has *not* led to extensive use of these devices. This example points to the need for other strategies to be combined with current educational efforts. It is important that educational strategies incorporate efforts to alter the agent and environment that require only a one-time behavior rather than directing efforts primarily at host (child or parent) behavior requiring *repeated* behaviors. Modification of the agent and environment through regulation of products and legislation is another effective means that nurses should promote and support.

In 1952, the American Academy of Pediatrics (AAP) established the Committee of Accident and Poison Prevention, which has been influential in legislation concerning agents of childhood accidents, including the following:

- Federal Hazardous Substance Labeling Act
- Poison Prevention Act
- Flammable Fabrics Act
- Automotive Restraint Act
- Child Protection and Toy Safety Act
- Consumer Product Safety Act

The AAP developed The Injury Prevention Program, which is recommended to be used in anticipatory guidance for injury prevention (Krassner, 1984). It comprises three elements: (1) a parent questionnaire to identify at-risk behavior, followed by a discussion; (2) safety sheets to be handed out at the next visit to reinforce information discussed following the questionnaire; and (3) a counseling schedule. Five goals that have been highlighted in the AAP's policy statement deal with major causes of morbidity and mortality, and three of the five goals can be achieved by a single purchase or action. These goals state that parents should be advised to acquire

1. Currently approved child car seats
2. Smoke detectors in the home that would protect the child's sleeping area
3. Safe hot water temperatures at the tap
4. Window and stairway guards or gates to prevent falls
5. A 30-ml (1-oz) bottle of syrup of ipecac (Krassner, 1984).

Although these specific goals have been highlighted, the objective of this program is to make anticipatory guidance for injury prevention an integral part of all routine health supervision. Recognizing that accidents happen in a context of *host,* an *agent,* and an *environment* may help to prevent them. Following is a review of common accidents that happen during childhood and adolescence, including strategies directed at the host, agent, and environment.

Potential for Injury: Motor Vehicle Accidents

Motor vehicle accidents are the leading cause of death in children (after 1 year of age*) and adolescents. The use of properly secured child-restraint devices or seat belts has been shown to reduce the probability of death of a child by 70 to 95 per cent and for serious injury by 50 to 60 per cent. In spite of this simple recognized solution, it is reported that only 35 per cent

*Under 1 year of age, conditions associated with birth and congenital abnormalities are the leading causes of death.

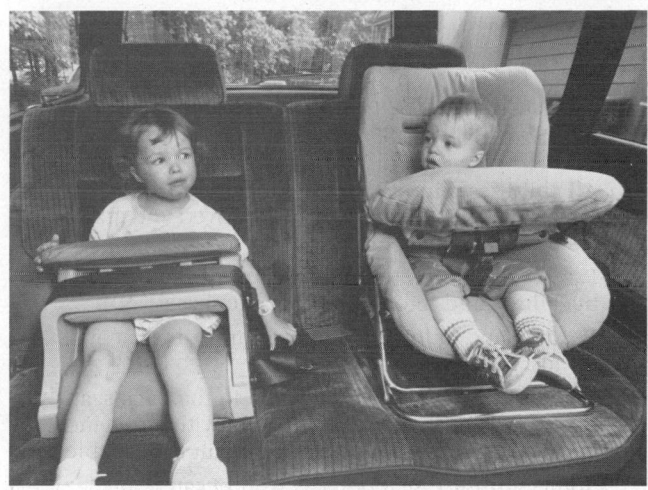

The safest place for a child to ride is in the back seat of a car, in the center. In a family with two young children, two car seats are placed in the back seat, one on each side. The car seats are (1) fastened with a tether strap through the trunk of the car and (2) properly secured with the seatbelt of the car. (3) The child is properly secured into the car seat. All three steps are essential for safety.

of children under 1 year of age and 25 per cent of children between 1 and 4 years are protected by child restraints while riding in a car (Shaw and Fluke, 1983). Despite legislation stating that infants and children must be restrained, it has been reported that two thirds of parents still do not buckle up their children even in the states with legislation requiring them to do so (Eriksen and Gielen, 1982). Additionally, car seat loaner programs and educational programs have overall not made a significant impact in this wide-scope, serious health problem.

It is also known that car seats are not used correctly (Bull and Stroup, 1985; Gunnip et al, 1987). Common car seat misuses include (1) misrouting the seat belt through the car seat frame; (2) not using the required parts, such as the top tether, internal harness, or shield; and (3) facing the seat forward rather than backward for a small infant (Gunnip et al, 1987). Specific questions can be asked by the nurse to assess the proper use of seat belts. There is a small reduction in mortality due to car accidents reported by Carraro (1982) when statistics from 1981 were compared to those in 1982. The greatest reduction (13 per cent) occurred in the 0- to 4-year-old age group and the next greatest (8 per cent) in the 15- to 19-year-old age group. This reduction was attributed to the combination of legislation concerning use of child-restraint devices, education, and more stringent drunk driving legislation.

Characteristics of the host supply important information in the study of motor vehicle accidents. The younger the child, the greater the risk of injury or fatality as a result of a collision. Infants under 6 months of age have been found to have the highest occupant death rate: 9 per 100,000 for children under 6 months of age compared with 4.8 per 100,000 for children from 6 to 12 years of age (Baker, 1979). Young children, especially infants, have a high center of gravity because of their proportionately large heads. This "topheaviness" makes a child especially prone to being propelled head first through a windshield. This difference in body weight distribution, coupled with the softness of children's skulls, makes them especially vulnerable to serious head injuries. Also, their rib cages are thinner and their internal organs are less well protected owing to the infant's prominent abdomen. These developmental characteristics explain why the most common injuries in children involve the head, chest, and abdomen. The child's spinal cord is also very vulnerable to serious injury.

Another factor thought to be related to a higher mortality rate in young infants is that adults frequently cradle an infant in their arms while riding in vehicles. This is considered the most dangerous method of holding a child, yet parents continue it because they erroneously believe this provides adequate protection. On the contrary, the impact of injury on the child is affected by the weight of the mother if she is not restrained. The forcefulness of the impact is frequently expressed by the 10-30-300 rule (see Box 17-1).

The disabled child presents a special challenge because of the need to stabilize wheelchairs and the need for support and protection of nonfunctional body parts. Although little research has been done about safety for children with disabilities, Shaw (1987) has reviewed the literature in which suggestions are made by extrapolating from information based on the nondisabled population.

Prevention Strategies

In the United States, three main approaches have been used to prevent moving vehicle accidents: consumer education, legislation, and vehicle improvements.

Consumer Education. Nurses have the opportunity to influence parents to use child-restraint devices

> Box 17-1
> **The 10-30-300 Rule**
>
> The 10-30-300 rule means that a 10 pound baby riding in an automobile going 30 miles per hour is propelled forward with a force of 300 pounds. This is analogous to falling from the third story of a building. If an adult is *not* restrained the infant risks being crushed by a force equal to the weight of the adult times the same speed factor of 30 miles per hour.

in a variety of settings. Expectant parent classes provide the best time to teach families about the importance of wearing a seat belt. Certainly the protection of their unborn child is of utmost importance, rendering seat belt use during pregnancy fairly acceptable. At this same time, parents should be taught the importance of using a child restraint device after their child is born to provide continued protection. In primary care settings, repeated assessment and encouragement is required to ensure that children and parents are properly restrained, especially as children get older. It is also advisable to include a question concerning the use of child-restraint devices on the hospital admission sheet and include appropriate teaching with discharge planning. As in the postpartum setting, the discharge note should include information concerning the use of a restraint (Nachem and Bass, 1984).

In any of these settings, nurses should be able to provide information about the different types of child restraint devices and provide some counsel about their use (see Box 17-2). A preventive program that nurses have been involved in is the AAP's "The First Ride . . . A Safe Ride" campaign introduced in 1980. The title refers to the goal of having newborn infants transported home from the hospital in an infant-restraint device. The placing of an infant into the mother's arms by a health professional for the first ride home is a practice that is now being strongly discouraged. The goals of the campaign include the following:

- Professional and in-service training for maternity and newborn ward staff and pediatricians
- Prenatal and in-hospital education of parents
- Discharge planning by hospital staff
- Legislation to make mandatory the use of child-safety restraints in each state
- Accreditation standards for hospitals and day care transportation programs
- Comprehensive public relations program (Scherz, 1982).

Many hospitals have successful "First Ride" programs. Although there seems to be some success in getting parents to buckle up their infants, as the child gets older there is a reduction in child-restraint and seat belt usage (Scherz, 1982).

It is important for the nurse to make some attempt to understand the reasons for the lack of use of child-restraint devices. Parents report a variety of reasons for not using seat belts and restraint devices, of which the most common ones include: (1) too expensive; (2) difficult and inconvenient to use; (3) fear of entrapment and increased injury; (4) forgetfulness; and (5) restrictive and uncomfortable for the child. There may be other reasons that parents express, and each of these should be addressed by the nurse.

Box 17-2

Tips on Proper Use of Child-Restraint Devices and Seat Belts

All child-restraint devices manufactured after January 1, 1981, are federally approved and crash tested at 30 miles per hour.

Parents should try the seat in their car and try buckling child into seat before purchase.

Reading and following manufacturer's instructions for installation is essential.

Whenever possible, put children in the back seat. An exception is when riding alone with an infant because easy visualization of an infant is desirable.

Adults must use seat belts as well because an unrestrained adult can be thrown into a child passenger.

Place young infants in seat with face toward rear of car.

Strategies used to increase seat belt use include both negatively and positively oriented approaches. Negative approaches include those programs that focus on vulnerability to injury or death as the result of non-use. Positive approaches used to influence parents are based on the findings that the behavior of secured children is less disruptive and judged by parents to be more appropriate than when children are not secured (Christophersen, 1977; Christophersen and Gyulay, 1981).

This information has been used to motivate parents to buckle up their children by providing a written protocol to parents describing the philosophy that children are better behaved in car seat devices. The protocol also includes guidelines for getting children to stay in their car seat. This approach has been labeled as the Behavioral Improvement Emphasis Technique (Roberts and Turner, 1984).

Some basic ideas that the nurse should share with parents to encourage the proper use of a child-restraint device are summarized in Table 17-2. Nurses should also stress the importance of not leaving a child alone in a car.

Education of children pertaining to safety and motor vehicles is another approach that must be improved. A well-designed intensive teaching program is required in the schools to teach children pedestrian safety and use of seat belts. School nurses and community health nurses can provide leadership in promoting appropriate educational programs for children beginning in preschools. The magnitude of this problem behooves all nurses in all settings to organize efforts into a highly developed plan of action with continuous evaluation and research.

Legislation. The major impact that legislation has made is in the law that requires children under a specific age to be restrained while riding in an automobile. Restraint laws are required to be passed by the states and since the first law was passed in Tennessee in 1978, restraint laws have rapidly moved toward becoming the norm. In Canada most provinces require that individuals, regardless of age, wear a seat belt or use a child-restraint device.

Legislative action has resulted in the creation of standards for child-restraint devices. Since January 1, 1981, all child-restraint devices that are manufactured are federally approved and crash tested at 30 miles per hour. Nurses can lobby for support of mandatory child-restraint legislation at the state and national levels.

Vehicle Improvements. Ongoing research to improve automobile safety is required. The potentials of air bags designed to inflate upon collision to protect the passengers continue to be studied. Also, the Department of Transportation's National Highway Traffic Safety Administration and the AAP are working toward installation of child restraint devices into all new motor vehicles (O'Shea et al, 1982). Finally, it has been suggested that manufacturers could consider designing the vehicle so that buckling of the seat belt is required to turn on the radio or even the ignition as a strategy to increase use of restraints.

Motor Vehicle Accidents and Impaired Driving

During the adolescent years (15 to 19 years of age) motor vehicle accidents cause 58.9 deaths per 100,000 in the United States. These data are similar to those of 30 countries whose mortality data were analyzed by the World Health Organization (Harvard, 1979). The explanations for such a high mortality rate among this age group includes the young people's inexperience and frequent experimentation with drugs and alcohol in association with driving a car (Litt, 1981).

Teenagers, while comprising less than 10 per cent of licensed drivers, account for 20 per cent of drinking drivers involved in fatal accidents (Fell, 1984). Findings from questionnaire-based surveys reviewed by Mayhew and colleagues (1986) suggest that driving after drinking is frequent, if not the norm, among young people. The relative risk for fatal car accidents is highest for drivers 16 to 19 years of age. The explanation for the higher number of deaths in the 16- to 19-year-olds is currently being debated and studied. Young drivers are actually no more likely than older drivers to drive while impaired by alcohol on any particular night, but owing to the greater social activity of young drivers, the opportunity for impaired driving is increased. This results in more frequent driving while impaired over time compared to older drivers. Although lack of driving exposure and experience do account for some of the increased risk for accidents, research also suggests that driver risk-taking is a major factor underlying the higher accident rate among youths (Jonah, 1986). There is considerable controversy over whether alcohol impairment actually *causes* young drivers to have accidents or whether impaired driving is rather a *correlate* of accidents in youth because of its association with the tendency for risk-taking. The greater propensity for risk-taking requires further research if its relationship to impaired driving and accidents is to be understood.

Prevention Strategies

Many programs to prevent young drivers from drinking and driving have been developed in recent years. School-based programs developed for the prevention of drinking and driving have been reviewed by Mann

Table 17-2. Educative-Counseling Issues Concerning use of Seat Belts and Child-Restraint Devices

Reason for Not Using	Educational Strategy
Prohibitive in cost	Nurse can refer client to community organizations. Many programs are available that provide a child-restraint device for a nominal fee. In most cases, a deposit is required, which is returned when the seat is returned.
Difficult and inconvenient to use	Young children accept rituals and routines and will resist less if consistently used. Some seats are more difficult to use than others, therefore before purchasing it should be tried in the car and parents should practice buckling.
Fear of entrapment and increased injury	Studies clearly show that ejection from a vehicle increases the risk of death 50 times (Physicians for Automotive Safety, 1981).
Forgetfulness	Parents should be encouraged to use their own seat belts as an example. Developing a habit of buckling up for every ride, regardless of the distance, is the best defense against forgetfulness.
Restrictive and uncomfortable (many parents do not wish to face the hassle of getting their child into a restraint and interpret resistance as discomfort)	Disruptive children have actually either directly caused or been a contributing factor in collisions. It has been found that children who are restrained exhibit less disruptive behavior (Christophersen, 1977).

Box 17-3
Swimming and Boat Safety

Never swim alone.
Do not run in pool areas.
Do not swim during electrical storms.
No false alarms (calling for help).
Pools must be fenced (4 to 6 feet in height).
Do not dive into a pool or lake that is not sufficiently deep.
Do not swim after a heavy meal, drinking, or taking medication. (See text on page 587 for discussion of children with seizures.)
Keep electrical appliances away from the water to avoid shock and electrocution hazards.
Flotation jackets should be worn by all non-swimmers and children under the age of 3 years when near water.
Nonswimmers wearing flotation devices *in* the water must be accompanied by an adult because a child can easily float into deep water.
Essential rescue devices and first-aid equipment should be easily accessible, and all swimmers should be taught how to use them.
On a boat, one adult swimmer should be present for each nonswimming child.
Do not stand in small boats.
Flotation jackets should be worn in a boat by children under 12 years of age whether they can swim or not.
Mouth-to-mouth resuscitation should be taught to all children over the age of 12 years.

(Adapted from Greensher, 1984.)

and colleagues (1986). Although it is concluded that these programs are a promising way to attack the problem of fatal car crashes associated with alcohol use, their effectiveness has not been established. Outcomes of these programs demonstrate that they are successful in bringing about short-term positive changes in knowledge and attitudes; however, these changes tend to disappear on follow-up. The traffic-safety impact of these programs has not been examined to determine whether the programs actually influence drinking-driving behavior or accident risk (Mann et al, 1986).

Another avenue for prevention is through legislation. Suggested legislation includes the need for more penalties for drunken drivers and perhaps increases in minimum driving age (O'Shea et al, 1982). Driver education has generally not been shown to decrease the number of teenagers involved in motor vehicle crashes. On the contrary, an increase in per capita crash involvement is thought to be a by-product of the increased number of licensed teenagers because of the availability of driver education (Lund et al, 1986).

Water-Related Accidents

Drowning* accidents occur at all ages in diverse environmental settings and involve different socioeconomic groups. Drowning is the second most common cause of death in children in the United States (Greensher, 1984). Death rates due to drowning are lowest for young infants, but the rate peaks at 1 year of age and again at 15 to 24 years of age. One half of all drowning victims are under 10 years old, and 75 per cent of these are boys (Pless and Stulginskas, 1982). Sixty to 70 per cent of drownings occur in fresh water, and many children drown when left unattended in a bathtub, toddlers fall into private lakes or swimming pools, school-age children drown in pools or lakes, and adolescents drown in larger bodies of water during risk-taking behavior (Quan, 1982).

Prevention Strategies

Strict supervision of children when in and near bodies of water is the single most important preventive strategy. Young children should not be left in the care of child siblings around water. For infants, even a bucket of water can present a hazard if they fall into it. Parents should be encouraged to teach children and adolescents water safety rules that are strictly enforced (see Box 17-3). Nurses should also advise parents concerning swimming lessons. Organized swimming lessons should be encouraged for children after 3 years of age. Learning how to swim properly and learning water safety provides the basic skills that all children should learn. Teaching infants to swim has also become popular. Proponents of early aquatic education stress the natural abilities of infants in water and its link to life in utero. The effect of early swimming lessons as a strategy to prevent drowning is not known (Quan, 1982), and *there is a potential for parents to feel overly secure about the abilities of their infants and toddlers who have "learned to swim."* Organized swimming instruction is not recommended for children under the age of 3 (see Chapter 21, p 676). It should be stressed that even though infants are taught to swim, they cannot be taught water safety, therefore they should be supervised as for any nonswimming child.

---

* *Drowning* is defined as suffocation by immersion in a liquid medium; *near drowning* refers to survival for more than 24 hours (with or without aspiration); *secondary drowning* means delayed death (Greensher, 1984).

Drowning is a cold weather problem also when children go on ice that is not frozen solidly and break through. The temperature must be well below freezing for several days before ice on a pond is thick enough to support a child's weight. Depending on water flow, some parts of a pond or lake may be frozen solid whereas others have only a thin layer of ice. In both rural and urban areas, children should be taught not to walk across a seemingly frozen body of water that has not been checked by an adult for safety.

Children with seizures require special attention regarding safety in water. Such children account for up to 15 per cent of the drownings and are considered to be at risk for drowning at a rate four times higher than that for other children (Quan, 1982). To prevent drowning in this high-risk group, the following counsel is recommended:

1. Encourage showering rather than bathing as many of the drownings occur during a child's bath.
2. Encourage jogging and other sports rather than swimming.
3. If water activities are done
   a. ensure that child's condition is well controlled with anti-convulsants (child should be seizure-free for 2 years)
   b. supervision is facilitated by ensuring high visibility of child (e.g., distinctive bathing caps or luminescent swimming suits have been suggested) (Quan, 1982).

The nurse's involvement in counseling about water safety should begin when the infant bath is discussed. A continued emphasis on water safety appropriate for the child's age is warranted considering the number of deaths from drowning. It is essential that parents are cautioned to know where their children are in the neighborhood and who is supervising them. One half of all home swimming pool drownings have been reported to occur in a neighbor's pool (Quan, 1982).

An awareness of neighborhood and community safety concerning water is also a responsibility of the nurse. Unsafe practices in neighborhood pools and recreational areas with water should be investigated and appropriate authorities notified. Identification and reporting of inadequate fencing or riverbank railings should be the concern of every citizen but especially of a health care professional, whose concern is the health and safety of children.

Burns and Fires

It is estimated that approximately 4000 children die of burns in the United States each year. Burn deaths rank second behind motor vehicle accidents in the 1- to 4-year-old age group and third in the 5- to 14-year age group (drowning is second). The agents involved in burn injuries include combustible materials, hot substances, electrical sources, and chemical compounds (Mofenson and Greensher, 1979). The highest incidence of burns in children occurs in 1- to 2-year-olds, and these are most frequently scalds. In children 5 years old and over, 70 per cent of burns are flame-related.

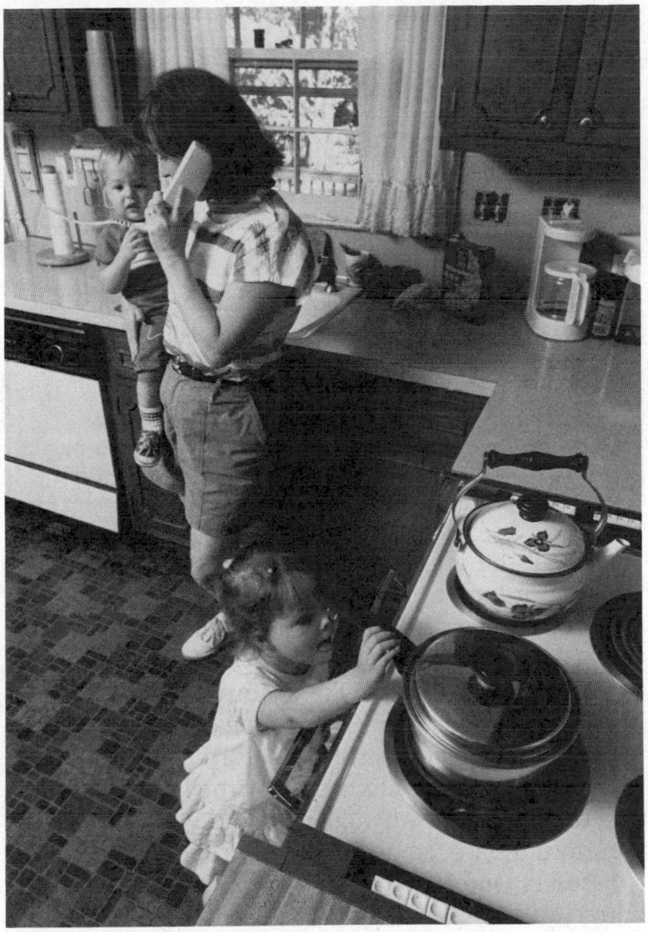

It takes only moments for the handle of a pan on the stove to be noticed by mobile, curious young children. In their attempt to see if they can reach it or see what's in it, a disastrous accident can occur.

Scalds. The type of burn accident that is likely to occur is highly related to characteristics of the child. Capabilities in locomotion and small motor skills (e.g., turning on a faucet) are involved in the events that lead to scalding. In both respects adults underestimate a child's abilities. The presence and actions of siblings must also be taken into consideration when assessing the degree of risk to which a young child is exposed. Siblings may innocently turn on a hot water faucet that injures a younger child.

> **Box 17-4**
> *Flammable Fabric Legislation*
>
> | | |
> |---|---|
> | 1972–1975 | Flammable Fabrics Act required sleepwear for children's sizes 0 to 14 to be flame resistant (flame resistance was achieved by using a chemical called Tris). |
> | 1977 | Consumer Product Safety Commission (CPSC) banned Tris in sleepwear because of its potential carcinogenic quality. |
>
> *Currently a variety of fabrics and fabric treatments are being used to attain flame retardancy.*

Of all the areas in the house, the kitchen is the most hazardous with respect to burns in young children. Boiling water, hot food, and dangling cords are the primary offenders. As new products are manufactured, new hazards arise. For example, the microwave has been reported to cause scalding of the oropharynx in relation to the heating of infant formula (Sando et al, 1984). Microwave ovens can cause the liquid temperature to be significantly higher than the bottle surface, therefore milk must be tested before feeding.

Burns Due to Flames. An important variable in injury by flames is the type of fabric used for children's clothing (agent). The mortality rate is four times as high, the surface area burned is twice as large, and the hospital stay is 50 per cent longer when clothing is ignited compared to non-clothing ignition burns (Mofenson and Greensher, 1979). See Box 17-4 about flammable fabrics.

The prevalence of flame burns in children after 5 years of age is also related to host characteristics. Children at this age are fascinated with matches and have the fine motor skills to strike a match. A relative easing off by parents in the extent of supervision provided (environment) during this stage increases the child's risk for flame burns by matches and other agents, such as campfires.

Prevention Strategies

Two preventive strategies that require the nurse's priority are to convince parents to (1) lower hot water temperatures to between 120 and 130° F; and (2) buy a smoke detector (preferably one for each level in the house).

Reducing the hazard of the agent (heat of the water) is a simple action, yet motivating parents to do so is not an easy task. The reasons for laxity have not been defined, although the concern of not having water hot enough for dishwashers has been a major drawback (Feldman, 1982).

Smoke detectors should be installed on each level of a house for the best protection. They should be placed on the ceiling (or high on the wall) where smoke and heat are most likely to accumulate first. They should be near the bedrooms so that the alarm can be heard even if the doors are closed. In case of a home fire, children should know how to proceed; therefore, an escape plan should be discussed and practiced in the home.

A major role of the nurse is to assist families in child-proofing their homes and to teach children basic fire prevention strategies. Although many of the measures to be offered seem to be common-sense suggestions, a summary of these has been provided in Box 17-5 to use as a reference when teaching caregivers burn prevention.

Poisonings

A poison is any substance that can harm one's body when exposed to it. A poisoning can occur through ingestion, inhalation, skin exposure, or eye contact, or through any other mode that causes untoward effects.

Poisoning is the fourth leading cause of death in children ages 1 to 4 years. Peak incidence occurs in 1- and 2-year-olds, a time when children become increasingly mobile, are intense explorers, and have the need to demonstrate some autonomous behavior. Although the incidence of poisonings has declined in recent years (due to childproof packaging) continued efforts and strategies are required to reduce the morbidity and mortality that results from this preventable cause.

Some epidemiologic observations concerning poisonings give some guidance for planning of prevention strategies. At least 85 per cent of all poisonings reported to poison control centers involve ingestion. Medications are responsible for approximately 50 per cent of all poisonings commonly involving aspirin, acetaminophen, vitamins, and minerals. Household products are common offenders, and many of these are extremely caustic.

Lead poisoning in children continues as a "silent epidemic" (Landrigan and Graef, 1987). Although great gains have been made in controlling childhood lead poisoning, it is now known that lead is toxic to children at levels of exposure which not long ago were considered to be safe. A syndrome of "subclinical poisoning" adversely affects the function of erythrocytes, peripheral nerves, kidneys, the immune system, bones, and the central nervous system (Landrigan and Graef, 1987).

Although there may be an absence of clinical signs and symptoms, it has been reported that daily expo-

Box 17-5
Teaching Burn Prevention to Caregivers: Effective Measures

Shelter infants from burning sun rays.

Install smoke detectors (one on each level).

Teach children 5 years old and older the proper use of matches.

Follow the recommendations of the local fire department for house checks and exit procedures, and teach these to children.

Place guards around sources of heat and fires.

Place guards over unused electrical outlets.

Teach child the meaning of "hot" early.

Insist on adult supervision of campfires and barbeques.

Adjust water heaters to a temperature between 49 and 54.4°C (120 and 130°F).

Do not store gasoline or other lighter fluids in open containers. Store these in proper, legal receptacles locked away so children cannot reach them.

Do not store matches and lighters where children can reach them. Remember that purses may have matches or lighters in them.

Do not allow candles to burn unattended.

Do not store cleaning chemicals where children can reach them.

Do not misuse extension cords or allow electrical appliances near water taps. Teach child not to chew on cords.

Do not leave children unattended while a fireplace is burning.

IN THE KITCHEN

Never leave children unattended when you are cooking. By age 7 or 8 children can use toaster and do simple cooking with supervision. Older children can use microwave oven but must be taught that foods and dishes get very hot without appearing to be.

Do not leave hot pans or food or liquids unattended on range, countertops, or tables. Do not leave handles extending over the edge of a stove or countertop.

Do not leave cords to electrical cooking appliances dangling. Children can grab them and receive severe burns from the spilled hot liquids and solids.

Do not let young children pour or serve hot food or liquids. Don't pour hot coffee or soup at the table and leave them unattended.

Do not drink coffee, tea, soup, or other hot liquids with a child on your lap. One slip or a sudden darting hand is all it takes to cause a serious scald.

IN THE BATHROOM

Check the temperature in a tub of water before you place a child in it. The skin of a 1- or 2-year-old is tender and vulnerable to scalds. Use the back of your hand to check the temperature. The water should feel warm, not hot.

Do not leave a child in the tub unattended. Many scalds occur when the child or a brother or sister turns on the hot water while playing.

Teach older children to keep hair dryers and other appliances away from water.

IN THE BEDROOM

Do not leave a hot steam vaporizer close enough to a child's crib or bed that it might be tipped or pulled over.

Do not leave hair dryers, curling irons, or other appliances plugged in with young children around.

Do not smoke in bed.

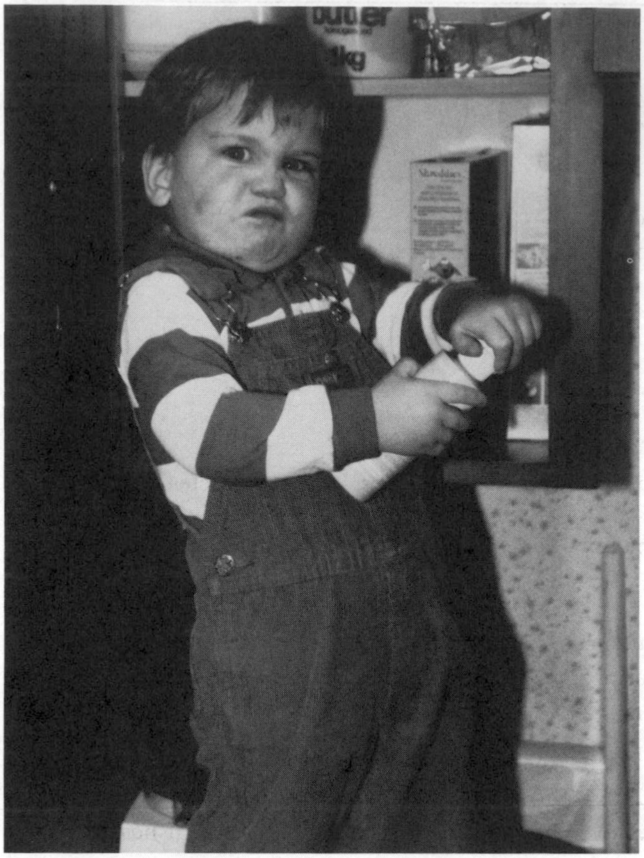

Mobility, curiosity, and manual dexterity lead a toddler to forbidden areas and dangerous substances if unsupervised. A determination to "get what I want" further endangers a toddler.

sure of children to lead in the modern urban environment can result in a neuropsychologic dysfunction affecting IQ scores (Needleman et al, 1985; Rutter, 1983). Preventive strategies have been summarized by the AAP (1980) as follows:

- Screening of preschool children for lead and for predisposing iron deficiency should be widespread;
- Screening should begin with measurement of erythrocyte protoporphyrin at 9 to 15 months of age (this coincides with hematocrit measurement);
- Vigorous abatement of all lead hazards should continue;
- Reporting of lead poisoning should be mandatory in all states.

The AAP supports the statement by the Centers for Disease Control (1987), which includes the following:

1. The definition of increased level absorption must be changed. Whole blood lead concentration of 25 μg/dl or greater (formerly 30 μg/dl or greater) is to be considered an increased lead level.

2. Lead toxicity is defined as a blood level of 25 μg/dl or greater in conjunction with an erythrocyte protoporphyrin level of 35 μg/dl or greater (formerly 50 μg/dl or greater).

Management of the child with lead poisoning is discussed in Chapter 52.

Plants are common agents that are ingested by children but fortunately a relatively small portion of plant ingestions produces severe toxic symptoms. The few plants that produce severe symptoms are extremely toxic if eaten. Highly toxic plants include rosary pea, castor bean, rhododendron, spurge laurel, tree tobacco, water hemlock, and yew. Toxic plants most frequently ingested (in order of frequency) include philodendron, dieffenbachia, jade plant, holly berries, yew, pokeweed, poinsettia, Swedish ivy, woody nightshade, black elder, and African violets (U.S. National Clearinghouse for Poison Control Centers, 1979). Other causes of poisonings include inhalation of toxic substances and exposure of the skin and eyes.

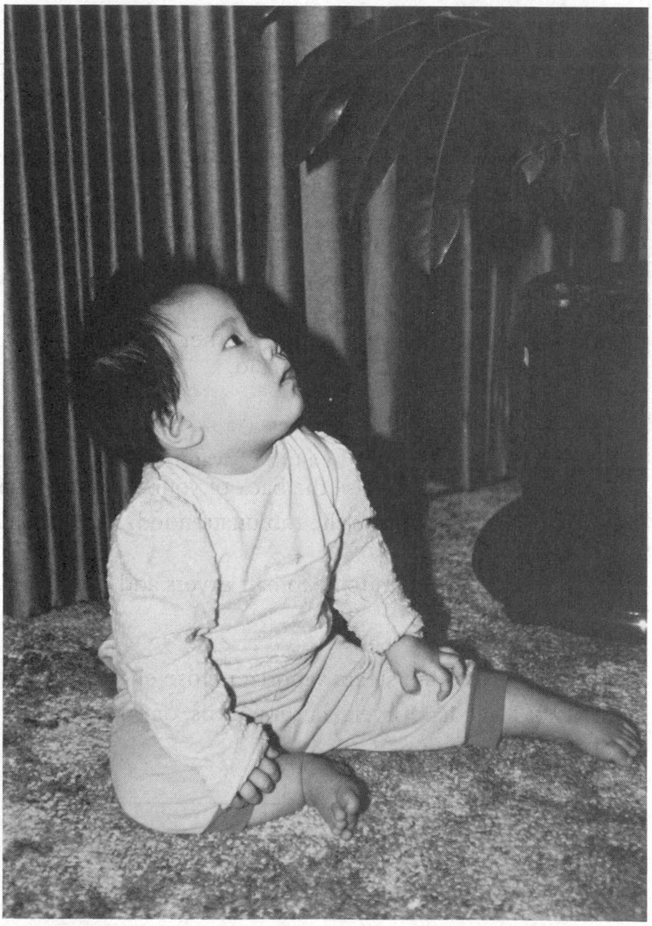

Young children are fascinated by everything they can see and reach. Plants can be a hazard if children are not properly supervised.

Numerous environmental conditions contribute to the occurrence of a poisoning. It has been noted that the late afternoon and during the dinner hours are times when calls to poison control centers occur most frequently (Temple, 1984) (purposeful overdoses are reported most frequently in the latter part of the day, with nearly half after 8 PM and into the early morning hours). Poisoning in childhood is more prevalent in circumstances of disturbed child-parent relationships, in which parents may be preoccupied with family stress. Ineffective supervision and improper child-proofing of the house for the age of the child contribute to the occurrence of poisonings.

Most childhood poisonings occur in the vicinity where common household products are stored or used (e.g., kitchen or bathroom). An important finding in poisoning episodes is that approximately 70 per cent of poisoning accidents occur while a product is being used and 50 per cent of the time a product or substance is not in its original container. Storing these substances in a familiar container (e.g., pop bottles) can lead to disaster.

Prevention Strategies

Significant prevention and management strategies that have reduced the mortality and morbidity of poisoning include the following:

1953: First poison control center established followed by a rapid spread of the movement, resulting in the existence of more than 600 centers.

1957: Bureau of Product Safety in the Food and Drug Administration established the National Clearinghouse for Poison Control Centers, which collects and standardizes product toxicology data for distribution to recognized poison control centers.

1970: Poison Prevention Packaging Act requires specified potentially hazardous household chemicals and drugs to be sold in child-resistant packaging, including aspirin or high concentrations of methylsalicylate, all prescription drugs, caustics, petroleum distillates, ethylene glycol, methanol, acetaminophen, and iron (Temple, 1984).

Although legislation has had a notable impact on poison control, nurses must continue to stress the importance of teaching families to poison-proof their homes. Basic objectives in poison prevention include the following: (1) reducing the number of poisonings, and (2) reducing the severity of the effects of the poisoning. Guidelines that can be followed to meet these objectives are summarized in Box 17-6.

An important aspect of counseling to prevent poisoning is to increase parents' awareness of potential poisoning dangers that emerge as their child develops. For example, as a child becomes more mobile and manual dexterity is increased, medicines in a mother's purse become potentially lethal to a child. The role of anticipatory guidance is to facilitate protection of the child by modifying the environment *before* the child accomplishes the next skill (e.g., crawling, climbing, opening containers). It is advised that all poison-proofing is done before the infant crawls to ensure that a new skill is not achieved when the parent least expects it.

Box 17-6
Guidelines for Poison-Proofing a Home and Poison Management

GOAL: REDUCING NUMBER OF POISONS

Keep poisonous substances in their original containers. (Never place near food, in food containers, or in pop bottles.)

Ensure that all harmful products and all medicines have child-resistant caps.

Store harmful products out of reach. (Use safety locks on cabinets.)

Teach children about poisons. Use labels such as "Mr. Yuk" to indicate which are poisons.

Know where child is and what he or she is doing at all times.

Do not refer to medicine as candy.

Discard outdated medicines by flushing down the toilet (not discarding in a waste basket).

Avoid taking medicine in front of small children.

Avoid storing medicine in a purse. (If medicine must be carried, purse must be kept out of reach at all times.)

Keep alcoholic beverages out of reach.

Use lead-free paint and do not let child chew on outdoor surfaces. Ensure that toys do not have lead-containing paint.

Teach child not to chew on plants and shrubs.

GOAL: REDUCE SEVERITY OF THE EFFECTS OF THE POISONING

Teach parents to purchase a 30-ml bottle of syrup of ipecac.

Teach parents to post the phone number of the nearest poison control center.

Teach parents first-aid do's and don'ts (see Chapter 52).

Suffocation

Suffocation is a particular threat to infants under 1 year of age because of their ability to wriggle and move but an inability to untangle or dislodge themselves from a

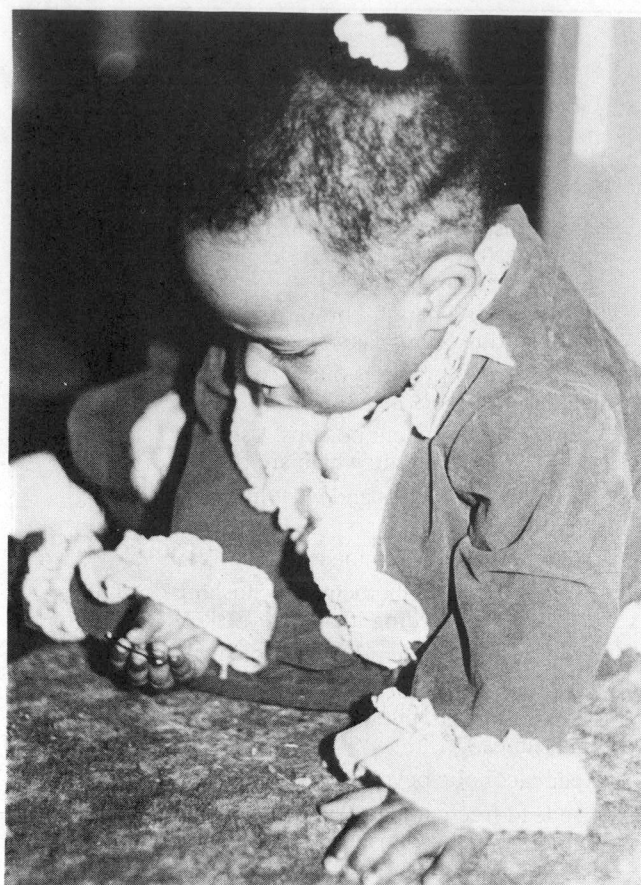

The infant's developing mobility makes child-proofing mandatory. This infant has discovered an open safety pin lying in the carpet.

constricting object. Plastic used to cover a mattress, blankets, and anything with a string (bib, pacifier on string) can strangle and suffocate an infant if it is left in the crib or near the baby's reach. Mobiles strung across cribs are not recommended once an infant begins to sit up because the child can become entangled in them. Crib and playpen slats must be no more than 2⅜ inches (6 cm) apart, and the mattress should fit the crib snugly to prevent the infant's head from getting caught between two surfaces. Decorative corner posts should not be present as the infant's head can get caught in them. As an infant becomes mobile and is able to reach, the surroundings of the crib or playpen must be carefully examined. Drapery cords are a particular hazard to an infant, who could become strangled while playing on the floor or while in the crib nearby. As a child approaches toddlerhood, abandoned refrigerators and trunks become attractive hiding places. A toddler is capable of crawling inside but does not foresee the problem of becoming entrapped. Abandoned equipment poses a danger even to the school-age child. Doors must be removed from such equipment and children of this age should be taught the dangers of playing in deserted buildings and near excavations.

Aspiration of a Foreign Body

Asphyxiation resulting from aspiration of a foreign body into the respiratory tract is the leading cause of accidental death *in the home* in children under 6 years of age. Safety pins are the most frequently aspirated object by infants from 0 to 1 year of age (Mofensen and Greensher, 1979); hard foods, especially peanuts and corn, are commonly aspirated by 2- to 4-year-olds. Infants and toddlers can find the smallest object on a thickly carpeted floor. Objects such as nails, pins, paper clips, staples, and any number of household items may be swallowed, aspirated, or stuffed into a body orifice. Coins are attractive to young children but are frequently swallowed or aspirated and should not be treated as toys. Toys need to be inspected for removable parts that could be swallowed or aspirated. Children not only put things into the mouth but also place things into the nose, ears, or any body orifice. Dangerous objects must not be put into an accessible wastebasket, as a young child will discover even the most obscure item.

The actions of parents can actually contribute to the aspiration of a foreign body. For example, propping of an infant's bottle is potentially dangerous and should be avoided. Also, during early infancy, the ingestion of baby powder can occur quite readily. Directly shaking powder onto the baby's skin can create a puff of particles that can be inhaled; therefore, it is recommended that powder should be applied to the caregiver's hands by shaking it onto the hands while holding the can away from the baby's head, then smoothing it on the infant's skin (Wagner and Hindi-Alexander, 1984). It is not uncommon to see parents permit their infant to play with the can of powder while changing a diaper. However, the top can easily come off and allow powder to spill freely into the child's mouth and face.

Aspiration of food particles while eating can be prevented by refraining from giving hard foods, such as nuts, Life Savers, small hard candies, corn, and tough meats, to infants and toddlers. Even though a 2-year-old has some molars, the ability to thoroughly chew food is not mastered until the preschool years (about 4 years of age). Prevention of aspiration is summarized in Box 17-7.

Parents should be given some basic guidance to prepare for an incident of aspiration. The following guidelines should be used when counseling parents:

Box 17-7
Prevention of Foreign Body Aspiration

FOOD

Place infant on side (usually right to facilitate digestion of food), or on stomach after feedings.

Avoid hard foods such as peanuts until chewing is well established, around 4 years of age.

Cut and break food into bite-size pieces for infants and toddlers. Encourage children to chew their food and avoid putting large pieces of food into their mouths.

Insist that children sit down to eat their food. Running and walking around the house (or on family outings) while eating predisposes to aspiration of particles.

Do not permit eating and drinking while in a lying down position.

OBJECTS

Do not permit young children to play with small objects (e.g., coins, buttons, marbles).

Balloons should be kept from infants and toddlers whether inflated or not. An uninflated balloon may be sucked into the posterior pharynx, larynx, or trachea.

Safety pins should be kept closed and not placed near the child.

Older children should not be permitted to hold objects in their mouths, such as a Lego piece, a marble, or a button.

Pacifiers should meet safety standards (mouthguard of adequate diameter—i.e., slightly under 2 inches; two ventilation holes in mouthguard; nipple portion should not separate from mouthguard; and the handle should be easily grasped). Pacifiers should not have ribbon or string attached to place around child's neck (US Consumer Product Safety Committee, 1978).

Do not permit infants and young children to play with baby powder.

1. The Heimlich maneuver has been successful in all ages and should be the first choice of emergency treatment for a life-threatening situation caused by aspiration of a foreign body. Some modification of the procedure is required for infants and children (see Chapter 52 for description of technique).
2. If a child is breathing quietly and it is known that a foreign object has been aspirated, every attempt should be made to rush the child to the nearest facility for treatment without disturbing the foreign body.
3. Do not suspend the child by the feet and pound on the back. This may dislodge a foreign body into the larynx, causing fatal obstruction.
4. Do not attempt to extract a pharyngeal or laryngeal foreign body by reaching into the mouth with one or two fingers. This is dangerous because the foreign body may be forced into the larynx more tightly, causing a partial obstruction to become a complete obstruction.

Foreign body aspiration can cause panic and incorrect treatment by parents in the home. It is the nurse's responsibility to reduce the number of fatalities and injuries from foreign body aspiration by teaching parents how to prevent its occurrence and how to correctly apply first-aid measures.

Falls

Falls account for the second highest number of accidental deaths in the general population and rank fifth in the cause of accidental death in children. Falls occur as children achieve new developmental tasks (e.g., rolling over, crawling, standing, walking) and increased supervision is not provided accordingly. Falls occur when a new skill is used to satisfy an overwhelming curiosity or simply when body movements cause something to slip or fall (e.g., a plastic infant carrier placed on a smooth counter).

The many devices that are used for children should be checked for stability and exposed parts that could cause injury. Baby walkers in particular have been reported to cause injuries, especially from falls down a flight of stairs. Prior to 1971, many walker-related injuries occurred because of exposed parts that caused fingers and toes to be caught or amputated. However, in spite of manufacturing regulations to improve their safety, walkers continue to cause injuries from falls. In one study, it was reported that 77 per cent of families used walkers. Of those children using walkers, 31 per cent experienced injuries, with a high proportion of injuries being associated with falling down stairs (Kavanaugh and Banco, 1982). The type and number of injuries from walkers warrant that health care professionals discourage their use in environments that pre-

Box 17-8
Typical Agents Causing Falls During Infancy and Childhood: Prevention Strategies

CRIB ACCIDENTS

Most falls occur while children are climbing out. Side rails should be up at all times when the infant is in the crib. Child should be moved to a bed when the height of side rail is less than 3/4 of the child's height (or when the child's height is 35 inches). If a younger child is a climber and insists on crawling out, a bed with a short side rail is recommended earlier.

HIGHCHAIRS

Child should be secured into chair and not allowed to stand in chair. Chair should be placed away from any object that can be used from which to push off. Children in highchairs should not be left unattended.

FALLS DURING INFANT CARE (DRESSING TABLES, CRIB SURFACE)

Fasten dressing table straps when the infant is on the table. Keep one hand on the child at all times when working at crib side or dressing table. If an article is required *away* from working area, pick the baby up or hold the baby with one hand and reach. *Do not turn your back on the baby without holding firmly.*

STAIRS

Place safety gate at top and bottom of any stairs to which the child has access.

INFANT SEATS

Do not place an infant on a smooth elevated surface.

WALKERS

Serious falls occur, therefore the use of walkers is not recommended.

dispose to injury. See Box 17-8 for a summary of typical falls and strategies for prevention. An injury not caused by a fall but one that is associated with mobility is injury to the arm and shoulder caused by a sudden jerk. This practice should be discouraged by nurses in their contacts with parents during health care visits.

Bicycle Accidents

Bicycle riding is a favorite activity for many children and adolescents. Unfortunately, the number of bicycle-related injuries and deaths is increasing. Injuries involving bicycles lead the U.S. Consumer Product Safety Commission's list of product-related injuries (Paulson, 1979). In 1980, 1200 deaths resulted from bike accidents; 410 deaths occurred in the 5- to 14-year age group.

Bike injuries constitute a large percentage of pediatric outpatient and hospital admissions. In 1980, the National Center for Health Statistics reported that 44 per cent of reportable injuries from bicycle accidents occurred in 5- to 14-year-olds (National Center for Health Statistics, 1980), with the greatest number occurring in boys in a ratio of 2.5 : 1.

Factors associated with bicycle accidents are multiple. Mechanical or structural defects have been reported to account for 20 per cent of children's bicycle accidents (Betz, 1983). Inappropriate frame size (too large or too small) reduces the ability to control the bike and therefore can increase the risk of injury. Young riders are reported to be at greater risk with hand brakes as compared to foot brakes (Betz, 1983).

The majority of accidents occur during daylight hours, when a child is close to home and at a time when a bicycle is used for recreational purposes rather than riding to and from school.

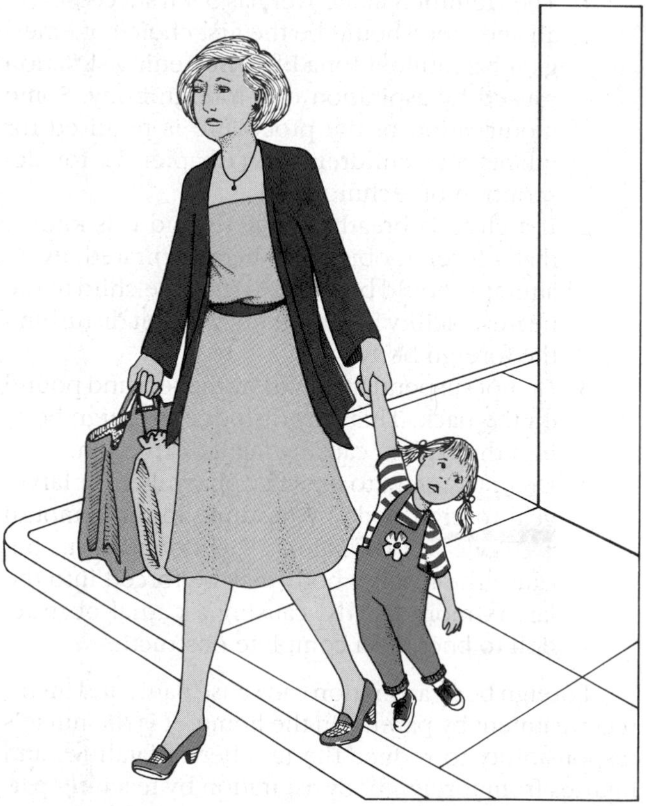

A hard upward pull or jerk on a child's arm can cause injury to tendons and muscles.

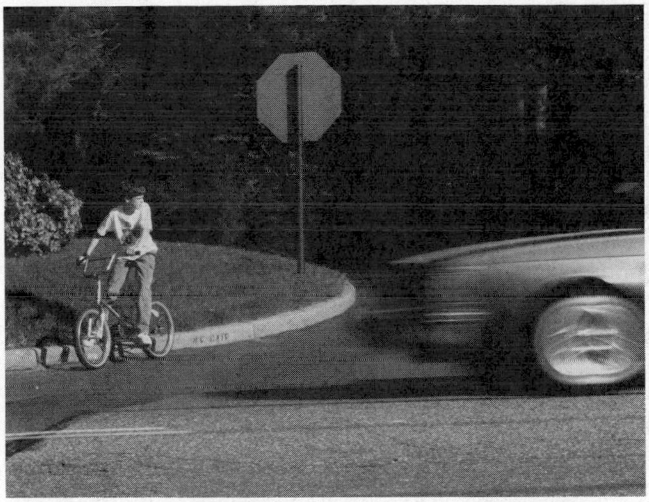

The majority of bicycle accidents occur during daylight hours close to home and involve recreational activities.

Injuries vary from mild abrasions, contusions, and lacerations requiring minimal first aid to multiple injuries of the head, trunk, and limbs. The seriousness of the injury is determined by the type of accident. Collisions with automobiles account for a high percentage of deaths from craniocerebral trauma (Paulson, 1979). Simple falls are associated with high risk for trunk injuries caused by the impact against the handle bars. Improperly worn shoulder bags can become wedged in the front wheel and cause the child to be thrown head first over the bicycle, resulting in facial injuries.

Prevention Strategies

Teaching strategies should be directed at increasing parents' and children's awareness of the simple ways that bicycle safety can be increased. The bicycle, the child, and the environment must be considered in bicycle accident prevention. Selecting a safe and appropriate bike requires the assistance of parents. The following guidelines can be used when purchasing a bicycle (Betz, 1983).

1. Child should be able to place the balls of both feet on the ground when seated on the bicycle.
2. Child should be able to straddle the center bar with both feet flat on the ground with approximately a 1-inch clearance between the crotch and the bar, or if a bike does not have a cross-bar from which to measure, the seat should be at hip level.
3. Hand brakes should be comfortably grasped, and child should be able to easily supply sufficient pressure to brake the bike. On a bicycle with foot brakes, pedal should be designed to form a good grip on the child's shoes.

The child's role in preventing a bicycle accident is primary. Children start riding bicycles during the preschool or school-age years and therefore they are old enough to learn bicycle rules. The nurse should direct teaching to the child but also impress the caregiver with the need for them to review the rules repeatedly. It is especially important to recognize that as children get older, they may take more risks, and, as they pattern their behavior after peers, rules that were respected at a younger age may gradually be dishonored. Also, as children grow older they will travel farther from home and on more dangerous roads. The wearing of a helmet is encouraged when children ride on highways and participate in racing or in any type of stunt riding. Teaching bicycle safety, therefore, must be done repeatedly and adapted to the growing independence of the child. Information on bicycle safety can be obtained from:

American Academy of Pediatrics
Educational Materials and Publications
Publication Department
1801 Hinman Avenue
Evanston, Illinois 60204

Physicians for Automotive Safety
P.O. Box 208
Rye, New York 10580

Information can also be obtained from local motor vehicle and license registration bureaus and from police departments. Some basic rules concerning bicycle safety are listed in Box 17-9.

Box 17-9
Bicycle Safety Rules

Do not ride bike with bare feet.

Inspect bike for mechanical safety regularly.

Travel in the same direction as traffic.

Ride as close as possible to the side of the road.

Walk the bike across busy intersections.

Watch for cars backing out of driveways.

Watch the road for bumps and potholes.

Stop and look all ways before entering the street from a driveway or lane.

Don't carry parcels in hands while driving.

Don't wear stereo headsets—a child needs to *hear* when a car approaches.

Don't ride two on a bicycle.

If riding at night, have appropriate lights and reflectors.

Use hand signals appropriately (arm out for left turn, up for right turn, and down for slow).

Box 17-10
What To Teach Children About Animals

Avoid strange animals, especially wild, sick, or injured ones. Parents or older child should notify health department or police of wild, sick, or injured animals.

Under parental supervision and with the permission and presence of pet's owner, have children make friends with pets in the child's immediate neighborhood.

Alert children to dangerous or nervous animals in the neighborhood. Do not let children enter yards or houses where such animals live.

Avoid riding bicycles or tricycles in areas where dogs are known to chase vehicles. Parents should notify authorities about any dog that habitually chases vehicles.

Never disturb an animal that is *eating* or *sleeping*—even an animal a child is familiar with may bite.

Teach children that pets are not toys. Pets are not to be mistreated or teased. An animal that is frightened, annoyed, teased, or mistreated may scratch, bite, or attack.

A pet should not be purchased for a child until he or she is mature enough to handle and care for the animal, around 7 or 8 years old. Parents should realize that it is *their* responsibility to teach care of the pet to the child and must not let an animal suffer because of a child's immaturity.

(Adapted from Mofensen and Greensher, 1979.)

Animal Bites

As the number of pets increases in communities so does the potential for animal-related injuries. It is estimated that the pet population in the United States includes more than 110 million cats and dogs (Greensher, 1984). More than 60,000 animal bites result in loss of sight, facial disfigurement, or other serious injury (Mofensen and Greensher, 1979). Most animal bites occur when the animal is young. Transmissible diseases also are more common among young animals (Greensher, 1984). Guidelines to use when teaching children how to interact safely with animals are summarized in Box 17-10.

Human Bites

Human bites occur in children either through roughhousing or during fights among children or as a result of child abuse. Human saliva contains a high level of bacteria; therefore, immediate treatment is required. Children should be taught not to bite and should be forewarned that if they are bitten, immediate care of the wound is required (see Chapter 52 for further discussion of care of children with a human bite).

Toys

The Consumer Product Safety Commission (CPSC) has legislative power to ban any toy that presents a risk for injury through normal use. Also, the Toy Manufacturers Association (TMA) cooperates with the government to set toy safety standards. Despite the attempts at regulation, unsafe toys appear in the marketplace, leaving the final responsibility to parents.

The safety of toys and play equipment should be brought to the attention of parents with reference to size of the toys, sharp edges, removable parts, and supervision and safety teaching in the use of chemistry sets, scissors, and electrical toys (see Chapter 21 for discussion of age-appropriate toys).

Streetproofing

As children grow and develop, the amount of protection that is afforded to them through direct surveillance decreases, and the amount of education required for self-protection correspondingly increases. Education is provided early, and its scope must encompass the dangers of places and *people.* Streetproofing is a term used to describe the process of preparing children for the potential dangers that threaten children when they embark "on the street." Streetproofing encompasses different elements according to the circumstances of the child. "The street" expands as the child grows and, according to Gossage and Gunton (1981), it is "defined by your child's travels."

The goal to protect children from the dangers of the streets should take into consideration the host (the child), the agent or vector (those who might harm the child), and the physical and emotional environment. The nurse's role begins early by encouraging parents to teach very young children about dangers associated with walking and riding on the street, play and sports activities, and being in public places. The goal is not to create a suspicion and fear that paralyzes the child but to cultivate the roots of a healthy skepticism and self-sufficiency. With appropriate teaching, a child is not restricted from play and freedom in a neighborhood but can acquire some skills to detect danger and cope with threatening situations. It is the role of all members in society to enhance the protection of children through public awareness programs and support of existing strategies in the schools and communities. The nurse has a specific obligation to address this aspect of family health through health promotion and accident prevention counseling.

Child Characteristics and Protective Behaviors

It is important for parents to know their children and their needs, their characteristics, and their vulnerabilities. Some children wander or dawdle, resulting in frequent incidents of playing alone or walking alone. Some children are more susceptible to overtures from adults that involve promise of a toy, candy, or special activity. A child who readily succumbs to peer pressure and tends to be a follower should be recognized as one who especially requires clear limits and instructions concerning the street. Although children vary considerably in the type of teaching they require, the following strategies are basic and should be brought to the attention of all children:

1. Never accept a ride from a stranger or any individual that has not been arranged and approved by a parent or caregiver (even if they say they are taking you home or to wherever your parent is).
2. Never accept candy or gifts from a stranger.
3. Do not let strangers into the house when alone.
4. If you are asked to give directions to a stranger, do not stand near the car.
5. Stay with other children or adults on the street or in public places whenever possible.

Control of the Environment: A Protective Strategy

Violence against children is a crime of situation and opportunity. The nurse can promote strategies that parents can use to control the environment of their children. Although choosing a neighborhood that is perceived as relatively safe and friendly for children is a wish of all humans, not all can afford to live in "safe" neighborhoods. Furthermore, neighborhoods cannot be guaranteed to be safe. Children must learn to protect themselves from danger and parents must, through appropriate regulation and supervision of children, reduce the risk of violence committed against their children.

A beginning strategy is to learn about the neighborhood and especially those areas which the child frequents. Taking a walk through the neighborhood with children provides the opportunity for parents to learn the characteristics of "the street" on which the child travels. The child's perception of areas and behaviors that are safe and unsafe should be elicited. Activities to be discouraged include play in abandoned buildings, vacant lots, and unlighted areas. Non-acceptable play areas should be identified and established as "off limits," and other caregivers must be informed of these. Parents should know the route their children take to school, know where they are after school, and know who their friends are. The most basic rules that a child should be asked to adhere to are the following:

- Enter only those homes which parents have approved.
- Call home as soon as they arrive at a friend's house to inform parents of their location.
- Do not stray across the agreed-upon boundaries without asking permission from parents or a designated caregiver.

Parents also need to be guided in providing a safe environment for their children. Encourage parents to gain as much information as possible about babysitters who come into the home or caregivers outside of the home. Examination of day care centers, preschools, and circumstances at school is the duty of every parent. Of most importance is that parents know where their children are. This important responsibility begins early on. Insisting that children stay with parents when in public places is essential; the child who wanders away from parents in malls, theaters, or other crowded areas can quickly become lost and abducted.

One of the most serious crimes against children in our society today is sexual abuse. Many child molesters are individuals who are known to the family. Children must be taught about inappropriate behavior of others concerning their bodies, and anyone who wants to spend excessive amounts of time with a child should be held in suspicion. When a child expresses fear of spending time alone with anyone, whether a friend, a relative, or a parent, further investigation is indicated (see Chapter 35 for further discussion of sexual abuse).

Self-Protection Strategies

Parents should be encouraged to provide specific instructions about actions to take in the event their child is approached. An individual that follows a child, starts talking to him or drives by in a car several times should be recognized as suspicious. The following basic actions should be addressed when preparing children how to deal with a suspicious encounter with an adult:

- If a child is approached or attacked, he or she should make as much noise as possible (e.g., knocking over a garbage can, screaming, or using an electronic noise-maker).
- The three basic rules are *say no, get away, and tell someone.*
- Try to remember what the person looks like, and check the license number (write it in the snow or in the dirt).
- Children must know where they can get help (e.g., block parents, police, teachers).

Barriers to Preventive Strategies: Nurse's Role

Strategies to prevent common childhood accidental injuries have been presented. To offer meaningful intervention for any of these problems, it should be recognized that despite employment of the best of methods to teach and motivate parents and children to take safety precautions, the benefits of educational strategies are inconsistent. Furthermore, efforts to increase product safety through regulation and enforcement of safety behaviors through legislation, although known to be effective, are encumbered with diversity in public opinion and various degrees of governmental bureaucracy. There is no established set of phenomena that has been isolated as underlying the inability of health professionals to bring about significant reductions in the morbidity and mortality which results from childhood accidental injury. There are, however, some basic attitudinal stances that have been proposed as forceful deterrents to successful educational programs and legislative actions.

Barriers to Safety Education and Counseling

Although it is recognized that educational strategies to increase health behaviors have not demonstrated consistent effectiveness, it is only by making an effort to understand this phenomenon that we can hope to improve the effectiveness of educational strategies. Three major attitudinal approaches that should be recognized are (1) a low level of perceived vulnerability (it won't happen to my child); (2) a fatalistic attitude (an "accident" cannot be prevented); and (3) "accidents" are to be expected during the growing-up years (children will be children).

Perceived Vulnerability

Perceived vulnerability is the degree to which people expect that a certain event will happen to them. Fortunately, most people do not have accidents; therefore, it is reasonable to believe "it won't happen to me." Furthermore, if the effort that is required to perform a safety behavior is extensive, the inconvenience is quickly perceived to outweigh the risk.

It has been suggested that the deficit in public knowledge about the extent of accidents in children "may require efforts to increase parental concern about the susceptibility of their children to serious injury and to increase the concern of the children themselves" (Fielding, 1982). This means that the nurse should repeatedly highlight the widespread injury and death that results from accidents. Although this approach should not be a punitive, judgmental one, it should be emphatic and factual. It is also reasonable to provide information that puts safety behaviors into a more attainable realm. Examples of this are suggesting an easy, effective action, such as reducing water temperature of the hot water heater or giving information that helps a parent select an easily managed child-restraint device. The overall goal is to simultaneously correct misconceptions about the prevalence of childhood accidents and reduce the perceived difficulty of performing safety behaviors.

Attitudes and Fatalism

The connotation of the word "accident" embodies the belief that people have no control over whether an accident will occur. It has been suggested that this has particular relevance to those with a low income and educational level, a situation which can contribute to a sense of relatively little control over many aspects of their lives (Klein, 1980). If the nurse is confronted with a deep-rooted attitude of fatalism, the usual methods of providing pamphlets and verbal instructions may result in colossal failures. Personalizing instructions to the family's situation, their income, and their attitudes requires an assessment of the family to determine what the family is willing and able to attempt. Strategies that require only one-time actions and that modify the agent or have the potential to reduce the severity of the injury may be more acceptable (purchase of a smoke alarm, purchase of syrup of ipecac, reduction of hot water temperature).

Children Will Be Children

The desire to permit a child the "freedom to grow" can be perceived to be in conflict with the priority of safety. In the earlier years, the freedom to explore and to attempt new skills and later to go by oneself on a bicycle are developmental needs that can increase the child's vulnerability to accidental injury. The conflict that arises emerges out of the wish to provide an environment that maximizes development but ensures safety. This conflict is best resolved through the teaching of children. Although freedom to grow is a necessity, so too is the need to learn how to keep oneself safe and to learn early on to respect the limits that are established in the home and by society. The enforcement of limits with explanations why they are important (e.g., off limits for a toddler, bicycle rules for a school-age child, and use of the family car for an adolescent) are actions that should be encouraged with all families. The attitude that children will be children with their share of accidents is too costly. Parents should be assured that "freedom to grow" is best done within limits, not only to provide safety but also to provide experiences from which a child learns some inner controls, self-preservation, and respect for rules of society.

Product Regulation and Legislation

It is recognized that strategies that do *not* require any action by the consumer (passive intervention) are more effective than those requiring repeated behaviors by the consumer (active intervention). It is also recognized that *limiting* behaviors, such as speed limit enforcement, is more easily accomplished than legislating an *action* behavior (e.g., wearing a seat belt).

The barriers concerning product regulation and government legislation of health behaviors are far-reaching—i.e., public opinion. Reluctance to support legal methods of accident prevention evolves from the deep-seated resistance to governmental interference of individual freedom and private enterprise. To even consider legislation as an option, there needs to be a high level of evidence that the intervention will work, and, as the amount of restriction on freedom increases, stronger evidence is required. Furthermore, if legislation is instituted, the costs, inconvenience, or undesirable effects that are introduced are reasons for resistance. For example, false alarms of a smoke detector, the cost of child-resistant devices, and the difficulty adults (especially the elderly*) have in opening child-resistant caps are reasons why people resist legislation.

Recognizing the barriers that exist and the magnitude of the problem of accidents in children, nurses should seek opportunities to actively support legislation that has the potential to decrease the morbidity and mortality resulting from childhood accidents. The arguments that support these actions are the following:

1. Children are different from adults in that they appreciate less the risks to which they are exposed. A proper role for government is to protect those who cannot protect themselves (the doctrine of *parens patriae*).
2. There is no substitute for safe products (e.g., observing bicycle safety rules cannot compensate for inadequate brakes).
3. Even the most vigilant parent cannot substitute for the benefits that can be derived from many of the passive interventions that are effective, e.g., fenced pools, smoke detectors, child-resistant containers (Fielding, 1982).

The nurse's understanding of the barriers that obstruct both educational and legislative efforts provides a base for accident prevention. Following are some guidelines to use in developing an approach that facilitates cooperation:

- Find out what the individual knows and wants to know.
- Assess for attitudinal barriers and correct misinformation.
- Individualize instruction according to the client's home, the particular child, and the family income.
- Recognize the degree of effort that a behavior requires and suggest options that can reduce the difficulty of performing actions.
- Promote the teaching of children by parents and in the schools, and teach children during health supervision contacts.
- Give readable (to the level of the clients) written instructions to supplement verbal ones.
- Maintain a non-punitive and non-judgmental attitude but impress clients with the scope of the problem honestly and unequivocally.

The public hardly realizes that 25,000 to 30,000 children die each year of accidental injury, and a much larger number become permanently impaired annually. It is apparent from the information presented in this chapter that nurses must become increasingly involved in designing studies to evaluate the effectiveness of current preventive strategies and to search for new, more effective approaches.

References

Adams D: Children's responses to a belt restraint program. *Pediatr Nurs* 1982 Jan/Feb; 28–30, 67.

Advance Data: U.S. Department of Health, Education and Welfare, 1978 March; 18:3–7.

*Individuals who have difficulty opening the child-resistant caps can request to have their medication placed into regular containers.

Baker SP: Motor vehicle occupant deaths in young children. *Pediatrics* 1979; 64:860–861.

Betz CL: Bicycle safety: opportunities for family education. *Pediatr Nurs* 1983 Mar/Apr; 109–111.

Bull MJ, Stroup KB: Premature infants in car seats. *Pediatrics* 1985; 75:336–339.

Carraro B: 1981 motor vehicle deaths on the down grade. *Traffic Safety* 1982 May/Jun; 20–26.

Christophersen ER: Children's behavior during automobile rides: do car seats make a difference? *Pediatrics* 1977; 60(1):69–74.

Christophersen ER, Gyulay J: Parent compliance with car seat usage: a positive approach with long-term follow-up. *J Pediatr Psychol* 1981; 6:301–312.

Daven J, O'Connor JF, Briggs R: The consequences of imitative behavior in children: The "Evel Knievel syndrome." *Pediatrics* 1976; 57(3):418–419.

Eriksen M, Gielen AC: The application of health education principles to automobile child restraint programs. *Health Educ Q* 1983 Spring; 10(1):30–40.

Feldman KW: Controlling scald burns. *In* Bergman AB: *Preventing Childhood Injuries.* Ross Roundtable on Critical Approaches to Common Pediatric Problems. Columbus, OH, Ross Laboratories, 1982; 50–54.

Fell JC: Alcohol in fatal accidents for various driver age groups. National Highway Traffic Safety Administration, *Research Notes* 1984 Apr.

Fielding JE: Public policy consideration in controlling accident behavior. Preventing Childhood Injuries. Report of the Twelfth Ross Roundtable on Critical Approaches. Columbus, OH, Ross Laboratories, 1982.

Gossage RC, Gunton MJ: *A Parent's Guide to Streetproofing Children.* Bantam Books, New York, 1981.

Greensher J: Prevention of childhood injuries. *Pediatrics* (Supplement) 1984; 74:970–975.

Gunnip A, Roberson C, Meredith J, et al: Car seats: helping parents do it right! *J Pediatr Health Care* 1987; 1:190–195.

Harvard JDJ: Mortality from motor vehicle accidents in the 15–24 year age group. *World Health Statistics Q* 1979; 32:225.

Jonah BA: Accident risk and risk-taking behavior among young drivers. *Accid Anal Prev* 1986; 18:255–271.

Kavanagh GA; Banco L: The infant walker: a previously unrecognized health hazard. *Am J Dis Child* 1982; 136:205–206.

Klein D: Societal influences on childhood accidents. *Accid Anal Prev* 1980; 12(4):275–281.

Krassner L: TIPP usage. *Pediatrics* (Supplement), 1984; 74:976–980.

Landrigan PJ, Graef JW: Pediatric lead poisoning in 1987: the silent epidemic continues. Pediatrics 1987; 79:582–583.

Langley J: The "accident-prone" child—the perpetration of a myth. *Aust Pediatr J* 1982; 18(4):243–246.

Litt IF: Compliance with automotive safety devices among adolescents. *J Pediatr* 1981; 99(3):484–485.

Lund AK, Williams AF, Zador P: High school driver education: further evaluation of the De Kalb county study. *Accid Anal Prev* 1986; 18:349–357.

Mann RE, Vingilis ER, Leigh L, et al: School-based programmes for the prevention of drinking and driving: issues and results. *Accid Anal Prev* 1986, 18:325–327.

Matheny AP: Injuries among toddlers: contributions from child, mother and family. *J Pediatr Psychol* 1986; 11:163–176.

Mayhew DR, Donelson AC, Beirness DJ, et al: Youth, alcohol and relative risk of crash involvement. *Accid Anal Prev* 1986; 18:273–287.

McKenna FP: Accident proneness; a conceptual analysis. *Accid Anal Prev* 1983; 15(1):65–71.

Mofensen HC, Greensher J, DiTomasso A, et al: Baby powder—a hazard! *Pediatrics* 1981; 68(2):265–266.

Mofensen HC, Greensher J: Childhood accidents. *In* Hoekelman RA, et al (eds): *Principles of Pediatrics.* New York, McGraw Hill, 1979, pp 1791–1823.

Nachem B, Bass RA: Children still aren't being buckled up. *MCN* 1984 Sep/Oct; 9(5):320–323.

National Center for Health Statistics: *Health: United States.* DHHS Pub. No. (PHS) 80–1232. Washington DC, US Department of Health and Human Services, 1980.

Needleman HL, Geiger SK, Frank R: Lead and IQ scores: a reanalysis. *Science* 1985; 221:701–704.

Nyman G: Infant temperament, childhood accidents and hospitalization. *Clin Pediatr* 1987; 26:398–404.

O'Shea JS, Collins EW, Butler CB: Pediatric accident prevention. *Clin Pediatr* 1982; 21(2):200–297.

Paulson J: Accidents. *In* Moss AJ (ed): *Pediatrics Update Reviews for Physicians.* New York, Elsevier, 1979.

Physicians for automotive safety: *PAS News.* 1981 Spring.

Pless IB, Stulginskas J: *Accidents and Violence as a Cause of Morbidity and Mortality in Childhood.* Chicago, Year Book Medical Publishers, 1982, pp 471–495.

Quan L: Prevention of drowning, preventing childhood accidents. Report of the Twelfth Ross Roundtable on Critical Approaches to Common Pediatric Problems. Columbus, OH, Ross Laboratories, 1982; 54–57.

Reisinger KS, Williams AF, Wells JK, et al: Effect of pediatricians' counseling on infant restraint use. *Pediatrics* 1981; 67(2):201–206.

Rivara FP: Epidemiology of childhood injuries. 1: Review of current research and presentation of conceptual framework. *Am J Dis Child* 1982; 136:399–405.

Roberts MC, Layfield DA: Promoting child passenger safety: a comparison of two positive methods. *J Pediatr Psychol* 1987; 12:257–271.

Roberts MC, Turner DS: Preventing death and injury in childhood: a synthesis of child safety efforts. *Health Educ Q* 1984; 11:181–193.

Roberts MC, Turner DS: Rewarding parents for their children's use of safety seats. *J Pediatr Psychol* 1986; 11:25–36.

Rodstein M: Accident proneness. *JAMA* 1974; 229(11):1495.

Rutter M: Low-level lead exposure: sources, effects and implications. *In* Rutter M, Russell-Jones J: Lead versus health. Chichester, England, Wiley, 1983, pp 333–370.

Sando WC, Gallagher KJ, Rodgers BM: Risk factors for microwave scald injuries in infants. *J Pediatr* 1984; 105(6):864–867.

Scherz RG: Auto safety: "the first ride . . . a safe ride" campaign. *In* Bergman AB. *Preventing Childhood Injuries.* Ross Roundtable on Critical Common Pediatric Problems. Columbus, OH, Ross Laboratories, 1982, pp 29–33.

Shaw CE, Fluke DM: A proposed campaign to increase the use of restraint systems for young children who ride in cars. *Public Health Report* 1983. Sep-Oct, 98(5):502–507.

Shaw G: Vehicular transport safety for the child with disabilities. *Am J Occup Ther* 1987; 41:1,35–42.

Temple AR: Poison prevention education. *Pediatrics* (supplement) 1984; 74:964–969.

U.S. National Clearinghouse for Poison Control Centers: *Poison Control Case Report Summaries, Toxic Case Breakdown.* Bethesda, Maryland, The Center, 1979.

U.S. Consumer Product Safety Commission: *Title 16 - Commercial Practices, Part 1511 - Requirements for Pacifiers.* February 26, 1978.

Wagner TJ, Hindi-Alexander M: Hazards of baby powder? *Pediatr Nurs* 1984; 10(2):124–125.

Bibliography

American Academy of Pediatrics, Committee on Accident and Prevention: All-terrain vehicles: two, three and four-wheeled unlicensed motorized vehicles. *Pediatrics* 1987; 79:306–308.

Amitai Y, Graef JW, Brown MJ, et al: Hazards of "deleading" homes of children with lead poisoning. *Am J Dis Child* 1987; 141:758–760.

Arena JM: The pediatrician's role in the poison control movement and poison prevention. *Am J Dis Child,* 1983; 137:870–873.

Bass JL, Mehta KA: Developmentally oriented safety surveys: reported parental and adolescent practices. *Clin Pediatr* 1980; 18(5):350–356.

Bass JL, Mehta KA, Ostrovsky M, et al: Educating parents about injury prevention. *Pediatr Clin North Am* 1985; 32(1):233–242.

Bass JL, Gallagher SS, Mehta KA: Injuries to adolescents and young adults. *Pediatr Clin North Am* 1985; 32(1):531–539.

Bergman AB: Use of education in preventing injuries. *Pediatr Clin North Am* 1982; 29(2):331–338.

Bowman JA, Sanson-Fisher RW, Webb GR: Interventions in preschools to increase the use of safety restraints by preschool children. *Pediatrics* 1987; 79:103–108.

Brown V: Providing a safe environment for children. *MCN* 1978 Jan/Feb; 3(1):53–55.

Davis RC: Prevention of childhood accidents through safety education. *Issues Compr Pediatr Nurs* 1977 May; 1(6):57–73.

Dershewitz RA, Posner MK, Paichel W: The effectiveness of health education on home use of ipecac. *Clin Pediatr* 1983 Apr 22:268–270.

Fazen LE, Felizberto PI: Baby-walker injuries. Pediatrics 1982 70(1):106–109.

Feldman KW: Prevention of childhood accidents: recent progress. *Pediatr Rev* 1980 Sep 1(3):75–82.

Friede AM, Azzara CV, Gallagher SS, et al: The epidemiology of injuries to bicycle riders. *Pediatr Clin North Am* 1985; 32(1):141–151.

Gallagher SS, Hunter P, Guger B: A home injury prevention program for children. *Pediatr Clin North Am* 1985; 32(1):95–112.

Garretson LK, Gallagher SS: Falls in children and youth. *Pediatr Clin North Am* 1985; 32(1):153–162.

Greensher J, Mofenson HC: Injuries at play. *Pediatr Clin North Am* 1985; 32(1):127–139.

Guyer B, Talbot AM, Pless IB: Pedestrian injuries to children and youth. *Pediatr Clin North Am* 1985; 32(1):163–174.

Guyer G, Gallagher SS: An approach to the epidemiology of childhood injuries. *Pediatr Clin North Am* 1985; 32(1):5–15.

Halperin SF, Bass JL, Mehta KA: Knowledge of accident prevention among parents of young children in nine Massachusetts towns. *Public Health Reports* 1983 Nov-Dec; 98(6):548–552.

Hodgson C, Woodward CA, Feldman W: A descriptive study of school injuries in a Canadian region. *Pediatr Nurs* 1984; 10(3):215–220.

Johnson N: Pacifiers: safety and security. *Pediatr Nurs* 1978; 4:58–60.

Jones JG: The child accident repeater. *Clin Pediatr* 1980; 19(4):284–288.

Langley J, McGee R, Silva P, et al: Child behavior and accidents. *J Pediatr Psychol* 1983; 8(2):181–189.

Matheney AP, Brown AM, Wilson RS: Assessment of children's behavioral characteristics: a tool in accident prevention. *Clin Pediatr* 1972; 11(8):437–439.

McLoughlin E, Crawford JD: Burns. *Pediatr Clin North Am* 1985; 32(1):61–75.

Micik SH, Alpert JJ: The pediatrician as advocate. *Pediatr Clin North Am* 1985; 32(1):243–249.

Micik SH, Miclette M: Injury prevention in the community: a systems approach. *Pediatr Clin North Am* 1985; 32(1):87–94.

Nachem B, Bass RA: Children still aren't being buckled up. *MCN* 1984; 9(5):320–323.

Reisinger KS: Preventing deaths due to fire. *In* Bergman AB (ed): Preventing childhood injuries. Ross Roundtable on Critical Approaches to Common Pediatric Problems. Columbus, OH, Ross Laboratories, 1982, pp 44–50.

Righi FC, Krozy RE: The child in the car: what every nurse should know about safety. *Am J Nurs* 1983; Oct; 1421–1434.

Robertson LS: Motor vehicles. *Pediatr Clin North Am* 1985; 32(1):251–265.

Rosser W et al: A critical look at the family. Physician's role in preventing childhood injuries. *Can Fam Physician* 1987; 33:733–740.

Schulkind ML: Preventing accidents and injuries in children. *Am Fam Practitioner* 1983 Sep; 28(3):240–245.

Wellman S, Paulson JA: Baby-walker related injuries. *Clin Pediatr* 1984 Feb; 23(2):98–99.

Zuckerman BS, Duby J: Developmental approach to injury prevention. *Pediatr Clin North Am* 1985; 32(1):17–29.

Promoting Healthy Dietary Practices

Chapter 18

Mabel Hunsberger

Health at all ages is enhanced by a diet that contains enough of the essential nutrients and avoids excessive consumption. For the young, nutrition is a primary concern because food is required not only for all maintenance and energy but also for growth. The way a child grows and develops is the result of an interplay of genetic constitution of the individual and a multitude of environmental variables. Of all the environmental factors that affect growth and development, food is one of the most influential. Both the physiologic parameters (height, weight, brain growth, and immunity) and the psychologic implications of food and feeding practices shape the growing years. It is suspected that early nutrition is associated with the development of chronic disease in adulthood (hypertension, heart disease, and some cancers), although a cause-and-effect relationship has not been established. The effectiveness of nurses in promoting a healthy diet depends on their own knowledge about nutrition and also on their understanding of the beliefs and habits, cultural variations, lifestyles, and family customs in which dietary practices are based.

This chapter begins with an overview of the scope of the problem followed by a discussion of the impact of nutrition on growth and development. A review of the nutritional requirements during childhood and adolescence is included to provide the necessary background information upon which assessments are based. The assessment process and nursing interventions are reviewed followed by a discussion of dietary issues and nutritional problems common during the developing

Related Topics
Families with Infants, Chapter 5
Families with Toddlers, Chapter 6
Families with Preschoolers, Chapter 7
Families with School-Age Children, Chapter 8
Families with Adolescents, Chapter 9
Promoting dental health—fluoride supplementation, Chapter 19
Lactose intolerance, Chapter 34
Failure to thrive, Chapter 35
Obesity, bulimia, and anorexia, Chapter 36

years. The nurse's role in the promotion of a healthful diet is addressed in this chapter; those feeding issues that arise out of specific age-related changes are discussed in the respective chapters on normal growth and development (see Chapters 5 to 9).

Nutritional Status

Lifestyle undoubtedly affects how people eat and how their children eat. In the developed countries there generally is access to adequate nutrients and nutritional messages bombard the consumer from all sides. With societal changes that have taken women into the workplace, young children to day care and babysitters, and school-age children to the afterschool activities of the season, consumers' versions of good nutrition is becoming whatever can fit into their lifestyle. In industrialized countries the trend toward malnutrition is on the side of excessive intake, intake of the wrong foods, and in some cases inadequate nutrients owing to excessive dieting. In the same society, hunger is increasingly prevalent where children live in poverty and in environments that do not provide sufficient nutrients. In these groups, children not only suffer from inadequate diets but may actually be at risk for obesity (Golden et al, 1983) because of dietary practices. A common definition of hunger is a chronic shortage of nutrients necessary for growth and good health. By that definition, 12 million children and 8 million adults, or about 9 per cent of the United States population, are hungry (Brown, 1987). Thus, whether rich or poor, nutritional problems of various types prevail.

Evaluation of nutritional status is a complex task. The Ten-State Nutrition Survey of 1968–1970, a landmark comprehensive study conducted by the U.S. Department of Health, Education, and Welfare, was the first survey of nutritional status across the ages. This study focused on populations of low income and on racial and ethnic groups most likely to be undernourished. This study evolved out of a concern during the late 1960s that Americans were suffering from hunger and malnutrition. Findings of this survey, summarized by Garn and Clark, 1975, include the following:

- Acute or severe malnutrition even in the lowest income groups was not demonstrated.
- Socioeconomic status affects size, growth, and development of children. (Children of the poor grow less well.) See Figure 18-1.

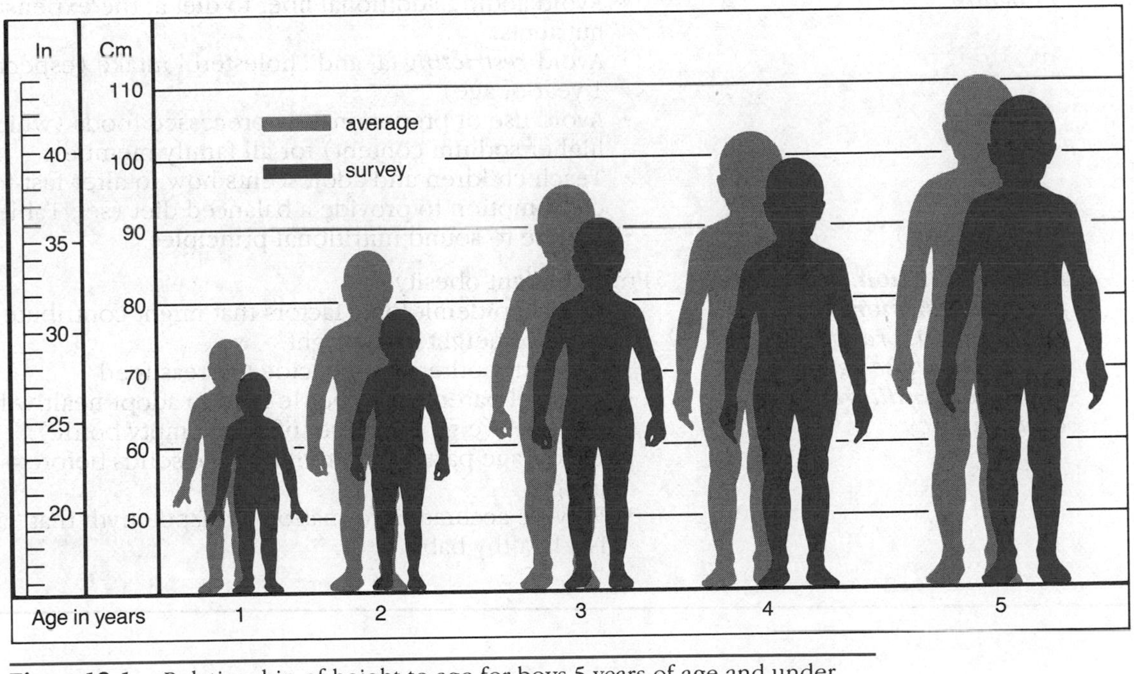

Figure 18-1. Relationship of height to age for boys 5 years of age and under, from low-income households included in the National Nutrition Survey, 1968, compared with average heights for boys.

Promoting Healthy Dietary Practices

Nursing Diagnoses	Nursing Goals/Strategies
Altered nutrition: *less than body requirements (for a child), related to* • *lack of appropriate supervision and management by adults*	Support family in the supervision and management of dietary intake appropriate for age of child. Encourage parents to: • Monitor intake of junk food. • Set limits at table regarding behavior. • Avoid snack consumption close to next meal.
• *maturational changes that diminish appetite*	Promote a balanced dietary intake consistent with child's age. Encourage parents to: • Limit milk intake to prevent child's feeling of satiety. • Avoid coercion of food intake. • Give child some control and autonomy. • Ask children to *taste* food rather than insisting on consumption of full serving. • Offer new foods at a time when the child is hungry.
• *nonconducive environment and setting*	Promote pleasant, comfortable environment at mealtime to encourage nutritionally balanced intake. Encourage parents to: • Avoid tension-producing topics. • Allow time for unhurried meals. • Provide appropriate utensils. • Seat child in an appropriate chair for comfort. • Serve food attractively.
Altered health maintenance, *related to lack of knowledge regarding impact of nutrition on health*	Provide information and correct misinformation to facilitate intake of a well-balanced diet. Encourage parents to: • Avoid adding additional fiber to diet at the expense of other nutrients. • Avoid *restricting* fat and cholesterol intake (especially before 1 year of age). • Avoid use of predominantly processed foods (which have higher sodium content) for all family members. • Teach children and adolescents how to alter fast-food consumption to provide a balanced diet (see Table 18-8). • Adhere to sound nutritional principles.
Altered nutrition: ***potential for more than body requirements,*** *related to excessive intake relative to energy expenditure during early infancy*	Prevent infant obesity. • Assess epidemiologic factors that might contribute to obesity. • Monitor height and weight. • Support mothers who decide to breastfeed. • Counsel parents who bottle-feed to adopt healthy feeding practices (e.g., not force infant to empty bottle). • Encourage parents not to introduce solids before 4–6 months of age. • Provide accurate information to dispel myth that "a fat baby is a healthy baby."

- The presently used "norms" are not appropriate for use with various races. Race-specific standards for size during growth are recommended.

The trends identified in this survey are that existing nutritional problems are related to inadequate total energy intake (quantity) rather than improper selection of nutrient intake (quality). Anemia was a common finding across all ages and was not related to income. Obesity was found to be growth-promoting (auxogenic). Those children who were obese were further developed on ossification, had larger skeletal mass, were taller, and had higher hemoglobin levels. For both sexes the poor were found to be leaner, but adolescent girls from lower income families were fatter and those from higher incomes were leaner (Garn and Clark, 1975).

Another survey, the Preschool Nutrition Survey (1968–1970) included a cross-section of children representing white, black, Hispanic, and American Indian children between the ages of 1 and 6 (Owen et al, 1974). As was found in the Ten-State survey, low economic status was correlated with smaller size. Anemia was reported at the rate of 12 per cent in black, 10 per cent in Hispanic, and 7 per cent in white children. In this survey all children seemed to have adequate protein intake (it averaged 1 to 1½ times Recommended Dietary Allowances), but 10 to 15 per cent of the children had low intake of vitamin C, a finding that correlated with socioeconomic status. As socioeconomic status improved, intake of vitamin C improved.

The Health and Nutrition Examination Survey (HANES) of 1971–1974 was the first survey carried out under the national surveillance system established by the U.S. Department of Health, Education, and Welfare. Under the direction of the National Center for Health Statistics, this survey analyzed adequacy of intake and use of nutrients. The following findings of the 1971–1974 HANES were based on a 24-hour dietary intake recall.

1. In some population groups, the mean intakes of protein, calcium, vitamin A, and ascorbic acid (vitamin C) were lower than the Recommended Daily Allowances (RDAs).
2. The mean intakes of thiamine (vitamin B_1) and riboflavin (vitamin B_2) were adequate or more than adequate in all population groups.
3. For all population subgroups (except adult white males) the mean for iron intake was below the RDA (Krause and Mahan, 1984).

The difficulties of establishing incidence and prevalence of nutritional problems are many. The impact of dietary intake on nutritional status in lower socioeconomic groups is difficult to distinguish from the impact of other factors that are associated with a low socioeconomic environment (e.g., poor housing and sanitation, and a high prevalence of illness and infections). Also, surveys that use the 24-hour recall method of evaluation have potential error because of the uncertainty that it is representative of usual dietary intake. It would be expected that inadequate intake of nutrients would show deficient biochemical values, yet the biochemical data are not shown to correlate with the level of intake indicated by some food consumption surveys (Krause and Mahan, 1984).

Malnutrition as a consequence of famine and severe food shortages is a form of nutritional inadequacy that does not exist in the industrialized world; however, nutrition-related problems prevail. Following the reduction and modification of supplemental feeding programs in the 1980s, 20 national studies have documented the extent of hunger in the United States. Among these reporting groups are the U.S. Conference of Mayors, the National Council of Churches, the U.S. Department of Agriculture, and the Physician Task Force on Hunger in America (based at the Harvard School of Public Health) (Brown, 1987). Heart disease, hypertension, obesity, anemia, dental caries, and less than optimal nutritional intake are problems that nurses encounter. The challenge is to recognize, assess, and manage problems that arise from uniquely different circumstances across families and populations. For the pediatric nurse, nutrition is particularly important because of the impact that nutrition has on the growing child. At all ages and across all populations nutrition and dietary practices affect the child's physical, intellectual, emotional, and social development.

Impact of Nutrition on Growth and Development

A child's growth and development is affected by physiologic factors such as genetic makeup, hormonal regulation (growth hormone, thyroid hormone, and insulin), and the nutrients consumed. Environmental, socioeconomic, and behavioral factors, however, determine the availability of food and the emotional climate within which food is consumed. It is the interplay of all these factors that affects the child's growth and development. Food intake and the feeding experience influence the physiologic and psychologic development of humans from birth.

Psychologic Development

The experience of eating can be viewed from various theoretical perspectives, each of which provides a unique approach to studying human development.

The psychodynamic view of Sigmund Freud views early oral experiences to be fundamental to personality development in that it is through the mouth (oral stage) that feelings (pleasurable or hostile) are expressed. Gratification of oral needs through feeding thus is viewed as an integral component of personality development. Erickson's stages of developmental crises also begin with nutrition-related activities. A sense of trust versus mistrust is developed during infancy through consistent satisfaction of hunger and sucking needs. From a behaviorist's viewpoint, feeding is seen as a stimulus-response experience. The discomfort of hunger is felt and the relief of hunger through feeding is experienced as pleasurable. According to Piaget's organic-maturation approach to development, it is through feeding that sensations of taste, smell, motion, and touch are experienced. Feeding provides an arena for mastery and learning. Increasingly complex skills are mastered so that eventually the infant can hold his or her own bottle, drink from a cup, and eat from a spoon.

According to these various theories, food and eating, especially during infancy, play a primary role in the development of the child. The experiences that are associated with feeding are a powerful component to the healthy development of children. Through feeding the process of attachment in infancy is fostered by a rhythmic giving and taking between the caregiver and the infant. Brazelton and colleagues (1974) noted that the rhythm was fostered when mothers were sensitive to their infants' capacity for attention as well as their need to withdraw. Synchrony between infant and caregiver develops when the caregiver is sensitive and attentive to the infant's cues. An example of the development of synchrony is when the caregiver responds to the infant's need to pace the feeding. Newborn infants have a natural, regular, rhythmic sucking pattern consisting of bursts of sucking followed by pauses (approximately 4 seconds in length) (Kaye, 1977). As the caregiver recognizes that stimulation of the infant (such as rigorous jiggling of the bottle or stroking of the cheek) does not cause the infant to resume sucking, a more sensitive pattern emerges. Mothers have been reported to change their response by stimulating their infant only briefly and then waiting for their infant to respond (Kaye, 1977). A lack of synchrony and lack of attachment between the infant and caregiver can result in numerous feeding problems and cause difficulties in parent-child relationships (see Chapter 35).

As the child grows and strives for independence, mealtime continues to be an experience at which positive relationships can be fostered or during which struggle and conflicts emerge as the predominant feelings. Beginning from infancy children should learn to rely on their own cues for satiety rather than being forced to finish a bottle. Mealtime is an arena in which children develop confidence and a sense of well-being in their ability to function in an increasingly social role. When maladaptive responses to feeding occur, longstanding nutritional problems such as bulimia, anorexia nervosa, and obesity can result (see Chapter 36).

Physiologic Development

The influence of nutrition on the physiologic state of the human body is a complex science. Although it is widely recognized that *severe* nutritional deficits have serious consequences, the impact of marginal nutritional imbalances is less well understood. An important phase of development that is believed to be affected by nutrition is the intrauterine period of growth. Although many questions remain concerning the impact of nutrition on fetal development, the following have been reported.

- Poor nutrition of the mother during pregnancy (especially during the last trimester) is associated with low birthweight infants.
- Poor prepregnancy nutritional status of the mother is associated with low birthweight infants.
- When nutritional status is poor at the outset of pregnancy provision of supplemental foods increases the infant's birthweight.
- Previously well-nourished women will have babies of reduced birthweight if their diets are severely limited during pregnancy (Stanfield, 1982; Creasy and Resnik, 1984).

A healthy diet during pregnancy and early childhood is of particular significance when it is recognized that the brain growth spurt begins in mid-pregnancy and continues well into the second postnatal year (Dobbing, 1984). Also, severe nutritional deficits during childhood result in reduced height and weight, a delay in puberty, and a delay in epiphyseal closure (Pipes, 1985).

The impact of nutrition during growth and later achievement remains controversial. Although many undernourished children may achieve poorly in later life, the dilemma remains whether nutrition plays a discrete role or whether the interplay of associated environmental factors determines achievement. Dobbing (1984) summarizes this issue by stating that "it may be reasonable to propose that nutrition indeed plays a role in later achievement but in the darkness of present ignorance it may well be quite a small one."

Because brain growth is linked to body growth and because there is no known method to promote brain growth, consumption of a balanced, healthful diet to promote *optimal* growth is the best solution. This raises yet another problem, that of infant obesity. Although infant obesity is a health concern, from the point of brain growth it has been suggested that a slight excess of intake is preferred to infant undernutrition (Dobbing, 1984).

A recent area of study is the effects of dietary intake on immune competence. It has long been recognized in the developing countries that malnutrition increases susceptibility to infection. It appears that malnutrition primarily affects cell-mediated immunity* rather than humoral immunity. As a consequence, children in underdeveloped countries with a profound nutritional deficiency readily become afflicted with viral disease (measles can be fatal in a malnourished child).

In the United States it has been observed through experience that malnourished children may actually be more resistant to colds than their better nourished siblings (Krieger, 1982). Data from animal experiments showing that chronic malnutrition improves cell-mediated immunity offer some explanation, although this phenomenon has not been directly studied. Thus, the degree of malnutrition may play a role in its effect on immunity. For example, in animal experiments, protein restriction of 5 per cent has been reported to enhance cell-mediated immunity, whereas further restriction had an adverse effect (Krieger, 1982). Furthermore, obesity has been associated with higher frequency of infection owing to impairment of cell-mediated immunity and neutrophil function (Chandra, 1981). Continued research is required to further define the effects of dietary deficiency on the nature and degree of impairment in the development of immunity. Identification of the effects of specific nutrient deficiencies and information on how to reverse the immunologic deficit once it has occurred is required.

The relationship of nutrition to health and disease is of high priority to many consumers of health care, but is of particular interest to parents who are concerned about the growth and development of their children. Nurses can promote children's health through nutritional assessment, education, and counseling in acute and ambulatory care, school nursing, and community nursing. Early attention given to the assessment of physical growth as well as parent-infant relationships and psychosocial environment provides the nurse with important data on which to base subsequent health promotion activities.

The components of promoting a healthful diet include knowledge concerning requirements, an awareness of the factors that affect dietary practices, and familiarity with measurement criteria used to assess nutritional status.

*T-lymphocytes (thymus-derived) function in cell-mediated immunity by becoming sensitized to the invading antigen and releasing enzymes to destroy it. B-lymphocytes (bone marrow–derived) function in humoral immunity by transforming into plasma cells, which subsequently produce antibodies.

Nutritional Requirements

The two basic nutritional guidelines that have been established are the Recommended Dietary Allowances (RDAs) (Committee on Dietary Allowances, 1980) and the basic four food groups, including (1) milk; (2) meat; (3) fruits and vegetables; and (4) breads and cereals (see Tables 18-1 and 18-2). During periods of rapid growth, such as infancy and again during the adolescent years, assessment of the level of nutrition with respect to adequacy is particularly important. During these periods of growth there is an increased risk of nutritional deficiency of all nutrients but especially vitamins and minerals. There is a wide variation in nutrient requirements according to age, sex, activity level, disease, growth rate, and genetic and environmental variables. Although optimal dietary intake is desirable, the range of food intake that provides *adequate* nutrition is not as narrow as many may think it might be (MacLean and Graham, 1982). Use of the recommended dietary allowances is universally accepted as the standard for nutritional intake (Table 18-1). It is intended that these standards are met by a *variety* of foods. It should be recognized that these standards represent a high estimate of nutrients (except for energy), to ensure that individual variations are met, reducing the risk for deficiency diseases (Box 18-1). Consequently, an individual whose diet does not fully meet the RDA is not necessarily undernourished. The RDAs are guidelines for healthy populations and do not account for special nutrient needs related to premature birth, infectious disease, or chronic illness.

Box 18-1
Recommended Dietary Allowances

Recommended Dietary Allowances (RDA) are the levels of intake of essential nutrients considered, in the judgment of the Committee on Dietary Allowances of the Food and Nutrition Board on the basis of available scientific knowledge, to be adequate to meet the known nutritional needs of practically all healthy persons.

Table 18-1. Food and Nutrition Board, National Academy of Sciences—National Research Council Recommended Daily Dietary Allowances,* Revised 1980

DESIGNED FOR THE MAINTENANCE OF GOOD NUTRITION OF PRACTICALLY ALL HEALTHY PEOPLE IN THE U.S.A.

		Weight		Height			Fat-Soluble Vitamins			Water-Soluble Vitamins							Minerals						
	Age (years)	(kg)	(lb)	(cm)	(In)	Protein (g)	Vitamin A (μg RE)†	Vitamin D (μg)‡	Vitamin E (mg α-TE)§	Vitamin C (mg)	Thiamine (mg)	Riboflavin (mg)	Niacin (mg NE)¶	Vitamin B_6 (mg)	Folacin** (μg)	Vitamin B_{12} (μg)	Calcium (mg)	Phosphorus (mg)	Magnesium (mg)	Iron (mg)	Zinc (mg)	Iodine (μg)	Energy Needs (kcal)
INFANTS	0.0–0.5	6	13	60	24	kg × 2.2	420	10	3	35	0.3	0.4	6	0.3	30	0.5††	360	240	50	10	3	40	kg × 115
	0.5–1.0	9	20	71	28	kg × 2.0	400	10	4	35	0.5	0.6	8	0.6	45	1.5	540	360	70	15	5	50	kg × 105
CHILDREN	1–3	13	29	90	35	23	400	10	5	45	0.7	0.8	9	0.9	100	2.0	800	800	150	15	10	70	1300
	4–6	20	44	112	44	30	500	10	6	45	0.9	1.0	11	1.3	200	2.5	800	800	200	10	10	90	1700
	7–10	28	62	132	52	34	700	10	7	45	1.2	1.4	16	1.6	300	3.0	800	800	250	10	10	120	2400
PREGNANT						+30	+200	+5	+2	+20	+0.4	+0.3	+2	+0.6	+400	+1.0	+400	+400	+150	‡‡	+5	+25	+300
LACTATING						+20	+400	+5	+3	+40	+0.5	+0.5	+5	+0.5	+100	+1.0	+400	+400	+150	‡‡	+10	+50	+500

* The allowances are intended to provide for individual variations among most normal persons as they live in the United States under usual environmental stresses. Diets should be based on a variety of common foods in order to provide other nutrients for which human requirements have been less well defined.

† Retinol equivalents. 1 retinol equivalent = 1 μg retinol or 6 μg β carotene = 3.3 IV vitamin A.

‡ As cholecalciferol. 10 μg cholecalciferol = 400 IU of vitamin D.

§ α-Tocopherol equivalents; 1 mg *d*-α tocopherol = 1 α-TE.

¶ 1 NE (niacin equivalent) is equal to 1 mg of niacin or 60 mg of dietary tryptophan.

** The folacin allowances refer to dietary sources as determined by *Lactobacillus casei* assay after treatment with enzymes (conjugases) to make polyglutamyl forms of the vitamin available to the test organism.

†† The recommended dietary allowance for vitamin B_{12} in infants is based on average concentration of the vitamin in human milk. The allowances after weaning are based on energy intake (as recommended by the American Academy of Pediatrics) and consideration of other factors, such as intestinal absorption.

‡‡ The increased requirement during pregnancy cannot be met by the iron content of habitual American diets nor by the existing iron stores of many women; therefore the use of 30–60 mg of supplemental iron is recommended. Iron needs during lactation are not substantially different from those of nonpregnant women, but continued supplementation of the mother for 2–3 months after parturition is advisable in order to replenish stores depleted by pregnancy.

Table 18-2. Recommended Food Intake For Good Nutrition According To Food Groups and The Average Size of Servings at Different Age Levels

Food Group	Servings Per Day	Average Size of Servings: 1 year	2–3 years	4–5 years	6–9 years	10–12 years	13–15 years
Milk and cheese (1.5 oz cheese – 1 C milk)	4	½ C*	½–¾ C	½–¾ C	½–1 C	½–1 C	½–1 C
Meat group (protein foods)	3 or more						
Egg		1	1	1	1	1	1 or more
Lean meat, fish, poultry (liver once a week)		2 Tbsp†	2 Tbsp	4 Tbsp	2–3 oz (4–6 Tbsp)	3–4 oz	4 oz or more
Peanut butter			1 Tbsp	2 Tbsp	2–3 Tbsp	3 Tbsp	3 Tbsp
Fruits and vegetables	At least 4, including:	⅓ C (citrus)	½ C	½ C	1 medium orange	1 medium orange	1 medium orange
Vitamin C source (citrus fruits, berries, tomato, cabbage, cantaloupe)	1 or more (twice as much tomato as citrus)						
Vitamin A source (green or yellow fruits and vegetables)	1 or more	2 Tbsp	3 Tbsp	4 Tbsp (¼ C)	¼ C	⅓ C	½ C
Other vegetables (potato and legumes, etc.) *or*	2	2 Tbsp	3 Tbsp	4 Tbsp (¼ C)	⅓ C	½ C	¾ C
Other fruits (apple, banana, etc.)		¼ C	⅓ C	½ C	1 medium	1 medium	1 medium
Cereals (whole-grain or enriched)	At least 4						
Bread		½ slice	1 slice	1½ slices	1–2 slices	2 slices	2 slices
Ready-to-eat cereals		½ oz	¾ oz	1 oz	1 oz	1 oz	1 oz
Cooked cereal (including macaroni, spaghetti, rice, etc.)		¼ C	⅓ C	½ C	½ C	¾ C	1 C or more
Fats and carbohydrates	To meet caloric needs						
Butter, margarine, mayonnaise, oils: 1 Tbsp = 100 calories (kcal)		1 Tbsp	1 Tbsp	1 Tbsp	2 Tbsp	2 Tbsp	2–4 Tbsp
Desserts and sweets: 100-calorie portions as follows. ½ C pudding or ice cream, 2 3″ cookies, 1 oz cake, 1⅓ oz pie, 2 tbsp jelly, jam, honey, sugar		1 portion	1½ portions	1½ portions	3 portions	3 portions	3–6 portions

*C = 1 cup or 8 oz or 240 ml.
† Tbsp = Tablespoon (1 Tbsp = ca. 15 ml = ca. ½ oz).
(Modified with M. J. Bennett, PhD, from "Four Food Groups of the Daily Food Guide," Institute of Home Economics, USDA, and Publication #30, Children's Bureau of the United States Department of Health, Education, and Welfare.)

Children should consume a healthy diet that supports and maintains cells, provides for growth, and promotes an optimal level of nutritional status. Following is a discussion of the components of a healthy diet, including energy (calories), water, and nutrients (protein, fat, carbohydrates, vitamins, and minerals).

Energy

The energy content of food is expressed in kilocalories (The large calorie) or in kilojoules (Boxes 18-2 and 18-3). Energy is required to support basal metabolism, physical activity, growth, and the specific dynamic action (SDA)* of food. Body size and composition, rate of growth, and degree of activity all affect the amount of energy expended. The energy requirements due to physical activity are as variable in infants as in other age groups. Some infants are much more active than others. Some fuel for energy is lost in stools. Thus, precise requirements are difficult to predict for a specific child. However, the recommended energy

*The process of food consumption gives a stimulus to metabolism, but not all foods have the same effect. This stimulus is called SDA and represents the energy needed to digest, absorb, and assimilate the various nutrients.

Box 18-2
Calorie and Kilocalorie

The calorie, or small calorie, is a standard unit for measuring heat; it is the amount of heat energy required to raise the temperature of 1 gram of water by 1 degree Celsius (C or centigrade).

The kilocalorie (or large Calorie) is equal to 1000 small calories, or the amount of heat energy required to raise the temperature of 1 kilogram of water by 1 degree Celsius (C or centigrade).

1 Cal = 1 kcal = 1000 cal.

amounts meet the needs of the average child and can be used as a basis for adjustments for a specific child.

The variation in expenditure of calories at various ages is shown in Figure 18-2. Compared to adults, infants have a higher basal metabolic rate (55 kcal/kg/24 hr) owing to a proportionately larger surface area and a larger proportion of metabolic tissue. Thus, energy requirements are greatest per unit of size during the first year of life (100 to 120 kcal/kg/24 hr) and decrease about 10 kcal/kg/24 hr for each succeeding 3-year period to adolescence. Consequently, as children grow they require a greater number of absolute calories, but the requirement per unit of size decreases (Table 18-3). During periods of rapid growth and development, such as at puberty, increased caloric intake is required.

The distribution of calories in an infant's diet of predominantly breast milk or formula is similar to the diet in later childhood, with approximately 15 per cent of the calories being derived from protein, 35 per cent from fat, and 50 per cent from carbohydrates.

Box 18-3
Kilocalorie and Kilojoule

The International Organization for Standardization (ISO) recommended the adoption of the joule (j) as the preferred unit of energy measurements, which was adopted by the United States National Bureau of Standards in 1964.

1. The kilocalorie is a measure of thermal energy and cannot be as precise as the joule, which is a measure of mechanical energy.

2. The conversion factor to convert kilocalories to kilojoules is 4.184, or approximately 4.2 (1 kilocalorie = 4.2 kilojoules).

3. The energy provided by the nutrients are:
4 kcal or 17 kj per gram of carbohydrates
4 kcal or 17 kj per gram of protein
9 kcal or 38 kj per gram of fat

4. Currently tables use both kcal and kj but in popular usage kcal is most often heard.

Water

Water is the most essential element in the diet. Water is part of every cell and is an important solvent. It is necessary for digestion, nutrient transport to the cells, and the removal of body wastes. The percentage of body weight provided by water is greater in the newborn infant than after 1 year of age, going from 75 to 80 per cent at birth to 65 per cent at 1 year and remaining at 55 to 60 per cent during the remainder of childhood and during the adult years. Daily consumption of fluid by an infant approximates 15 per cent of body weight, whereas it constitutes only 5 per cent in an older child and 2 to 4 per cent in the adult.

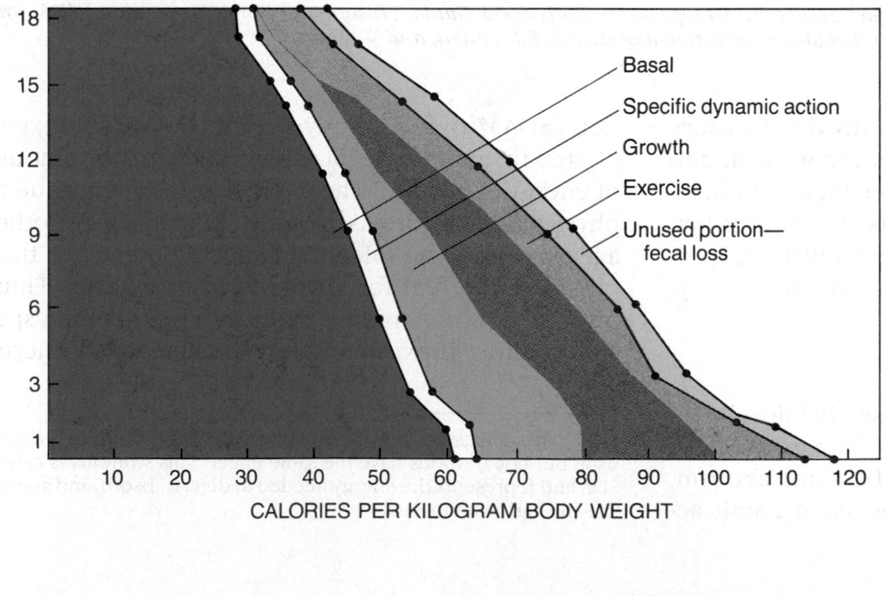

Figure 18-2. Total daily expenditure of calories with approximate distribution among individual factors in relation to age and weight. (Calorie = large calorie = 1 kcal = 1 Cal.) (From Behrman RE, Vaughan VS: *Nelson Textbook of Pediatrics.* 13th ed. Philadelphia, WB Saunders, 1987.)

Table 18-3. Mean Heights and Weights and Recommended Energy Intake

Category	Age (years)	Weight kg	Weight lb	Height cm	Height in	Energy Needs (with Range) kcal	Energy Needs (with Range) Mj*
Infants	0.0–0.5	6	13	60	24	kg × 115(95–145)	kg × 0.48
	0.5–1.0	9	20	71	28	kg × 105(80–135)	kg × 0.44
Children	1–3	13	29	90	35	1300 (900–1800)	5.5
	4–6	20	44	112	44	1700(1300–2300)	7.1
	7–10	28	62	132	52	2400(1650–3300)	10.1
Males	11–14	45	99	157	62	2700(2000–3700)	11.3
	15–18	66	145	176	69	2800(2100–3900)	11.8
	19–22	70	154	177	70	2900(2500–3300)	12.2
Females	11–14	46	101	157	62	2200(1500–3000)	9.2
	15–18	55	120	163	64	2100(1200–3000)	8.8
	19–22	55	120	163	64	2100(1700–2500)	8.8
Pregnancy						+300	
Lactation						+500	

Note: Energy allowances for children through age 18 are based on median energy intakes of children of these ages followed in longitudinal growth studies. The values in parentheses are 10th and 90th percentiles of energy intake.

* One thousand kilocalories equals 4.184 megajoules (Mj).

(From Committee on Dietary Allowances, 1980.)

The infant has a relatively greater need for water than do children and adults (Table 18-4) and is therefore more vulnerable to water imbalance. Water lost by evaporation in infancy is 60 per cent of that needed to maintain homeostasis compared to 40 to 50 per cent in the adult (Pipes, 1985). The young infant also has functionally immature kidneys and produces a more dilute urine. The faster rate of the infant's metabolism is another factor that increases the need for relatively more fluid than is needed by the adult. Also, young infants are unable to let adults know when they are thirsty. The usual diets of most infants meet this basic water requirement.

Table 18-4. Range of Average Water Requirements of Children Under Ordinary Conditions

Age	Average Body Weight (kg)	Total Water in 24 Hours (ml)	Water per kg Body Wt in 24 Hours (ml)
3 days	3.0	250–300	80–100
10 days	3.2	400–500	125–150
3 mo	5.4	750–850	140–160
6 mo	7.3	950–1100	130–155
9 mo	8.6	1100–1250	125–145
1 yr	9.5	1150–1300	120–135
2 yr	11.8	1350–1500	115–125
4 yr	16.2	1600–1800	100–110
6 yr	20.0	1800–2000	90–100
10 yr	28.7	2000–2500	70–85
14 yr	45.0	2200–2700	50–60
18 yr	54.0	2200–2700	40–50

(From Behrman and Vaughan, 1987.)

The sources of water are fluids (mostly milk for infants) and food. Most strained foods are 75 to 85 per cent water. Difficulties may occur in meeting the water requirements if formulas are improperly prepared, if infants ingest a limited amount of milk (especially with illness), if fever exists during hot weather, or if diarrhea and vomiting are present. Dehydration results much more rapidly from these difficulties in the infant because of the factors previously outlined. See Chapter 30 for additional discussion on fluid balance in infants and children.

Protein

Proteins are necessary as a source of amino acids. Large protein molecules are broken down into individual amino acids, which are required for growth and tissue repair and for the production of enzymes, antibodies, and hormones. Amino acids are classified as essential and nonessential (Box 18-4). Lack of intake of just one essential amino acid will result in negative nitrogen balance. Excess amino acids are broken down (catabolized) in the liver, and urea is formed and then eliminated by the kidney. During the first month of life excess protein may not be broken down and eliminated effectively; therefore, excessive intake may result in neurologic damage (Hughes and Griffith, 1984).

Recommended daily intakes of protein are shown in Table 18-1. During growth a proportionately higher amount of protein per unit of body weight is required. During the first 2 months of life 50 per cent of the RDA of protein is required for growth, by 2 to 3 years only 11

Box 18-4
Essential Amino Acids

Essential amino acids must be provided in the diet because the body cannot synthesize them. Absence or deficiency of one such amino acid results in negative nitrogen balance. *Nonessential amino acids* can be synthesized by the body; therefore, they are not essential in the diet.

ESSENTIAL AMINO ACIDS

Threonine	Tryptophan
Valine	Phenylalanine
Leucine	Methionine
Isoleucine	Histidine
Lysine	

In addition, low birthweight infants need
Arginine
Cystine
Taurine (perhaps)

(From Behrman and Vaughan, 1987.)

per cent is required, and after the adolescent growth spurt, 0 per cent is needed for growth.

Proteins do not all have the same nutritive value. Protein quality is a term used to describe the ability of protein to meet the body's requirements for *essential* amino acids. Requirements for essential amino acids are higher in the infant and small child than in the older child or adult (MacLean and Graham, 1982). Low birthweight infants require additional essential amino acids because enzymes are missing to synthesize them (Box 18-4). The predominant protein in cow's milk is casein, which is low in cystine and taurine. In contrast, proteins in human milk and the whey of cow's milk provide these amino acids. Consequently, now many infant formulas have been adjusted to be closer in composition to breast milk—i.e., a whey/casein ratio of 60:40 (in cow's milk the whey/casein ratio is 18:82). Animal proteins in general provide all the essential amino acids in sufficient amounts after the first year of life. In contrast, vegetable proteins are somewhat deficient in at least one of the essential amino acids, and they are substantially less digestible. Protein adequacy of vegetarian diets for the growing child therefore is important to consider (see later discussion in this chapter on vegetarianism).

Most children in developed countries consume sufficient protein; however, protein deficiency does exist in cases where milk has been withheld indiscriminantly, or in the case of poorly planned vegetarian diets. It is important to understand that sufficient calories in the form of fat and carbohydrate must also be provided in the diet, otherwise protein will be deaminated and used for energy. Excessive protein intake (except in the young infant) has not been known to cause damage. Protein intakes greater than 20 per cent of total calories increase water requirements because of the renal solute load and may result in dehydration in infants (Hughes and Griffith, 1984). The Committee on Nutrition of the American Academy of Pediatrics has set the minimum standard for infant formula at 1.8 gm of protein per 100 kcal (Committee on Nutrition, 1976).

Carbohydrates

Carbohydrates provide the greatest source of energy but are not considered a dietary essential because they can be synthesized from amino acids. There are no specific recommendations for intake, but a minimum intake of 50 to 100 gm/day has been suggested, or approximately 40 to 50 per cent of total calorie intake (Pipes, 1985).

Carbohydrates are broken down by a series of enzymatic and chemical reactions into simple sugars and are stored as glycogen in the liver and muscles. Carbohydrate that is not oxidized or stored as glycogen is converted to fat. The infant's liver is 10 per cent the size of the adult's and the muscle only 2 per cent; consequently, the infant has a smaller glycogen reserve than older children and adults and requires large carbohydrate intake for immediate energy. Ingestion of less than 5 per cent of the daily caloric needs may result in use of protein (ketosis) for growth and repair of tissue (Hughes and Griffith, 1984).

During infancy the primary source of carbohydrate is lactose (a disaccharide), found in human and cow's milk. Intestinal amylase is present in reduced amounts during the first 4 months of life, therefore the introduction of large quantities of starch (polysaccharides) may result in diarrhea. As solid foods are added (4 to 6 months of age) amylase is present and starches become the major source of carbohydrates. High carbohydrate intake, particularly of refined sugars, may be associated with atherosclerosis, although further research is required. Regardless of findings concerning such an association, high intake of refined sugars should be discouraged because they dull the appetite for other nutritious foods and are cariogenic.

Fats

In the infant diet, calories from fats provide 40 to 50 per cent of the energy requirements whereas in older children approximately 35 per cent of the energy requirements is provided by fat. Fats have a high caloric density; thus, they are protein sparing. Fat consumption is essential during growth when tissue synthesis is primary. Fats are a source of essential fatty acids in cellular structure, serve as carriers for fat soluble vitamins (A,D,E,K), and make food more palatable.

Polyunsaturated linoleic acid is an essential fatty acid for children and adults. Linoleic and arachidonic* acids may also be essential fatty acids. The American Academy of Pediatrics (AAP) suggests that 3 per cent of total energy in the diet should be derived from *essential* fatty acids (American Academy of Pediatrics, 1985). Essential fatty acids play a key role in growth, platelet function, normal skin and hair, reproduction, and synthesis of prostaglandins. The fatty acids that are essential for the human body are abundant in human milk and in commercially prepared formulas. Approximately 4 per cent of calories are derived from linoleic acid in human milk, compared with 1 per cent in cow's milk. Commercially prepared formulas, however, contain vegetable oils and provide appreciably greater amounts of linoleic acid than even human milk.

The effectiveness of substituting polyunsaturated fats for saturated fats in the diet in an effort to reduce atheromatous changes has not been established (see later discussion).

Vitamims

Vitamins are nutrients that the body requires in small amounts to catalyze cellular metabolism essential for maintenance and growth. Most vitamins cannot be synthesized by the body therefore must be supplied by dietary intake. Vitamins are classified into two groups: (1) fat-soluble (A,D,E,K) and water-soluble (the B vitamins, and ascorbic acid [vitamin C]). Any fat malabsorption illness may also result in malabsorption of vitamins A, D, or K because these three are absorbed and transported in a manner similar to lipids (Hughes and Griffith, 1984). The specific vitamins, including their function, source, and effects of excess or deficiency, are summarized in Table 18-5.

The best way to make vitamins available to the body is through the consumption of a balanced diet. Vitamin supplementation during infancy and childhood has given rise to considerable controversy. The major issues concerning vitamin supplementation are summarized in Table 18-5. Fat-soluble vitamins can be stored and cause toxicity. For example, hypervitaminoses A and D have been well documented. Vitamins that are most often lacking are vitamins A and C. Persons who are most at risk for vitamin deficiencies include

- children from deprived families;
- children who have poor eating habits or are dieting;
- pregnant teenagers; and
- children who consume a vegan diet (Pipes, 1985).

Minerals

The Food and Nutrition Board of the National Research Council has established recommended allowances for six minerals (calcium, phosphorus, magnesium, iron, zinc, and iodine). Additional minerals that are relatively abundant include sodium, chloride, potassium, and sulfur. The minerals in which diets are most likely to be lacking are calcium, iron, iodine, and possibly zinc in early infancy (Hughes and Griffith, 1984). Important minerals and their functions, sources, and effects of excess or deficiency are summarized in Table 18-6. Zinc deficiency may result from diets that are high in phytate and fiber. Any illness that causes intestinal malabsorption may result in zinc deficiency. Zinc plays an important role in cell growth; therefore its deficiency is manifested in growth failure and delayed sexual maturation (Hughes and Griffith, 1984). The major issues concerning mineral supplementation are summarized in Table 18-6.

Assessment and Counseling

There are four major purposes for doing a nutritional assessment: (1) to identify dietary practices of the family; (2) to obtain baseline data concerning calorie and nutrient intake and appropriate anthropometric measurements; (3) to promote healthful dietary practices through counseling and teaching; and (4) to provide parents with the opportunity to express concerns and to ask questions about nutrition and feeding behaviors.

Assessment of Dietary Practices

Variations in food consumption occur because of individual physical differences (stage of growth, exercise, genetic and hormonal) and because of environmental and sociocultural variations. Cultural differences, family relationships and lifestyle, peers and social influences (including television), and economic status are some of the nonphysiologic variants that predominantly affect the development of food habits.

Cultural variations, which dictate the kinds of foods that are preferred, must be respected by the nurse. It is usually desirable to maintain the basic food pattern and employ the use of *supplementation* rather than changing the staple foods. Milk and milk product use is limited in many cultures; therefore, substitutes may need to be made. The types of vegetables used may be unfamiliar to the nurse and the use of certain

*Arachidonic acid can be synthesized from linoleic acid.

Text continues on page 618

Table 18-5. Vitamins: Functions, Sources, and Supplementation

Significance in Development and Function	Deficiency Symptoms	Toxicity Symptoms	Important Sources	Supplementation
Fat-Soluble Vitamins				
		Vitamin A		
Formation of retinal pigments (rhodopsin and iodopsin) for cone (color) vision and vision in dim light Bone and tooth development Formation and maturation of epithelial tissue (skin, mucous membranes, lining of digestive tract) therefore increase resistance to infection Bile is necessary for Vit A absorption and mineral oil interferes with its absorption	Night and glare blindness Inflammation of the eye Rough, scaly skin Dry mucous membranes, causing a general lowered resistance to microbe invasion Poor tooth formation	Anorexia Fatigue Weight loss Irritability Skin lesions—dry, scaly, itching Joint and bone pains Spleen and liver enlargement Loss of hair Increased intracranial pressure and headache	Liver and liver sausage Butter, cream, whole milk Egg yolks Green and yellow vegetables Yellow fruits Ripe tomatoes Fortified margarine Fish liver oils	Prophylactic: 2000–5000 IU daily Hypervitaminosis A can occur when doses in excess of ten times the prophylactic dose are given Supplementation should be considered if there are not sufficient fruits and vegetables in the diet
		Vitamin D		
Regulates absorption and deposition of calcium and phosphorus (likely by affecting permeability of intestinal membrane) Reabsorption of phosphate and maintenance of serum calcium level (in conjunction with parathyroid hormone)	Soft bones Bowed legs Poor tooth development Lowered amount of calcium and phosphorus in the blood Poor posture, protruding abdomen	Anorexia Fatigue Weight loss Nausea and vomiting Diarrhea and polyuria Weakness Headache Renal damage Calcification in the soft tissues of the heart, blood vessels, lungs, stomach, renal tubules	Vitamin D milk Small amounts in butter, egg yolk, liver, saltwater fish Fish liver oils	Prophylactic: 400–800 I.U. Vitamin D supplementation is not usually necessary except in the following circumstances: • a breast-fed infant if mother's intake of vitamin D is inadequate and if infant does not benefit from sunlight (e.g., dark skin or little exposure) • if commercial cow's milk formula is *not* used for bottle-fed infant (e.g., goat's milk, evaporated milk, if not fortified with vitamin D)
		Vitamin E		
Mechanism of action unknown Vitamin E may protect erythrocytes from hemolysis			Vegetable oils Green leafy vegetables Margarine Egg yolk Milk fat Nuts	Premature infants requiring high concentrations of oxygen at high pressures are prone to develop retrolental fibroplasia Vitamin E is currently being used in clinical trials to reduce severity of retrolental fibroplasia (RLF) in prematurity

Table 18-5. *(continued)*

Significance in Development and Function	Deficiency Symptoms	Toxicity Symptoms	Important Sources	Supplementation
Vitamin E may protect vitamin A and polyunsaturated fats from oxidation			Wheat germ oil	Dosage varies with amount of unsaturated fats in formula
		Vitamin K		
Important in the formation of factor II (prothrombin) and other clotting factors (VII, IX, X)	Prolonged clotting time of the blood Hemorrhagic disease in newborn	Hyperbilirubinemia In infants: Jaundice Kernicterus Mild hemolytic anemia	Green leafy vegetables Liver Cauliflower Cabbage Soybean oil	A single intramuscular dose of 0.5–1 mg or an oral dose of 1.0–2.0 mg is given to all newborns
Water-Soluble Vitamins				
		Vitamin C		
Maintains intracellular substance preserving capillary walls; promotes healing of wounds and fractures and reduces potential for infection Aids in absorption of iron Essential for collagen formation (basic substance in connective tissue)	Sour mouth Stiff, aching joints Weak-walled capillaries (hemorrhages in joints, muscles, subcutaneous tissue, gums) Lassitude Impaired wound healing Improper bone and cartilage development		Fresh fruits, especially citrus, strawberries, cantaloupe Canned fruit juices Tomatoes, fresh or canned Raw vegetables, especially greens, cabbage, broccoli, peppers Potatoes	Prophylactic: 35 mg for children up to 11 years of age 60 mg/day for children after 11 years of age (½ cup of orange juice provides 60 mg of vitamin C) May be necessary in home-prepared formula
		Vitamin B_1 (Thiamine)		
Functions as part of co-carboxylase (coenzyme) during oxidation of carbohydrates. Important for growth, normal appetite, digestion, and nervous system function.	Anorexia Fatigue Constipation, atonic Depression Irritability Tenderness of the leg calf with some loss of muscular coordination Abnormal carbohydrate metabolism		Meat, especially pork Whole grain and enriched cereals Organs, especially liver Nuts and peanut butter Legumes especially soybeans Milk, dairy foods Eggs Brewer's yeast and wheat germ	No supplementation necessary in usual diet
		Vitamin B_2 (Riboflavin)		
Essential for growth Functions in tissue oxidation-reduction processes to produce energy	Burning and itching eyes Blurred and dim vision Eyes sensitive to light Inflammation of the lips and the tongue		Milk, dairy foods Organs, especially liver Meat, legumes Eggs	Supplementation not common If milk is avoided, such as in some vegetarian diets, a food equivalent can be used

continued

Table 18-5. *(continued)*

Significance in Development and Function	Deficiency Symptoms	Toxicity Symptoms	Important Sources	Supplementation
Essential for healthy eyes and skin	Lesions in the angles of the mouth Digestive disturbances Greasy, scaly skin		Enriched and whole grain cereals and breads Green leafy vegetables Brewer's yeast, liver concentrates	
		Niacin		
Acts in metabolism of carbohydrates and amino acids Involved in glycolysis fat synthesis and tissue respiration Prevents nervous depression Promotes healthy skin, nerves, and digestion	Fatigue and lassitude Dermatitis Sore mouth, especially the tongue Gastrointestinal disturbances (diarrhea and vomiting) Nervous disturbances Mental depression Weakness Anorexia		Meat, especially liver Fish Poultry Whole grain and enriched cereals Nuts Legumes, peanuts Brewer's yeast, liver concentrates	Supplementation not common

(Modified from Howe, 1981)

Table 18-6. Minerals: Functions, Sources and Supplementation

Function	Deficiency Symptoms	Sources	Supplementation
Calcium			
Development of strong bones and teeth Helps muscles contract and relax normally Utilization of iron Normal blood clotting Maintenance of body neutrality Normal action of heart muscle	Rickets Porous bones Bowed legs Stunted growth Slow clotting of blood Poor tooth formation Tetany	Milk, cheese Mustard, turnip greens Clams, oysters Broccoli, cauliflower, cabbage Molasses Small amount in egg, carrot, celery, orange, grapefruit, figs, and bread made with milk	No supplementation except for premature infants Dosage varies with type of milk feeding and growth rate
Phosphorus			
Development of bones and teeth Multiplication of cells Activation of some enzymes and vitamins Maintenance of body neutrality Participates in carbohydrate metabolism	Rickets Porous bone Bowed legs Stunted growth Poor tooth formation	Milk Cheese Meat Egg yolk Fish Nuts Whole grain cereals Legumes	No supplementation except for premature infants Dosage varies with type of milk feeding and growth rate

Table 18-6. *(continued)*

Function	Deficiency Symptoms	Sources	Supplementation
Iron			
Constituent of hemoglobin, which carries oxygen to the tissues	Nutritional anemia Pallor Weight loss Fatigue Weakness Retarded growth	Red meats, especially liver Green vegetables Yellow fruits Prunes Raisins Legumes Whole grain and enriched cereals Molasses Egg yolk Potatoes	Bottle-fed infant should receive iron-fortified formula Breast-fed infant should receive iron supplementation at 4 months (1 mg/kg/24 hr) if full term and at 2 months (2 mg/kg/24 hr) if premature After 6 months of age fortified cereals provide iron, therefore supplementation is not necessary if dietary intake is sufficient.
Iodine			
Constituent of thyroxin, which is a regulator of metabolism	Enlarged thyroid gland Low metabolic rate Stunted growth Retarded mental growth	Iodized salt Sea foods Food grown in nongoiterous regions	No supplementation
Sodium			
Constituent of extracellular fluid Maintenance of body neutrality Osmotic pressure Muscle and nerve irritability	Muscle cramps Weaknesses Headache Nausea Anorexia Vascular collapse	Sodium chloride (table salt) Sodium bicarbonate (baking powder, baking soda) Monosodium glutamate (Accent) Milk, cheese Meat, egg white	No supplementation
Fluorine			
Resistance to dental caries Deposition of bone calcium	Tendency to have dental caries	Water supply containing 1 ppm Small amount in many foods	Formula-fed infants need no supplement Supplementation is controversial If breast-fed, initiate at 2 weeks of age Dosage varies with concentration of fluoride in the local water supply (see Table 19-1).
Potassium			
Acid-base balance Carbohydrate metabolism Conduction of nerve impulses Contraction of muscle fibers	Apathy Muscular weakness Poor gastrointestinal tone Respiratory muscle failure Tachychardia Cardiac arrest	Whole grains Meat Legumes Some fruit and vegetables	No supplementation

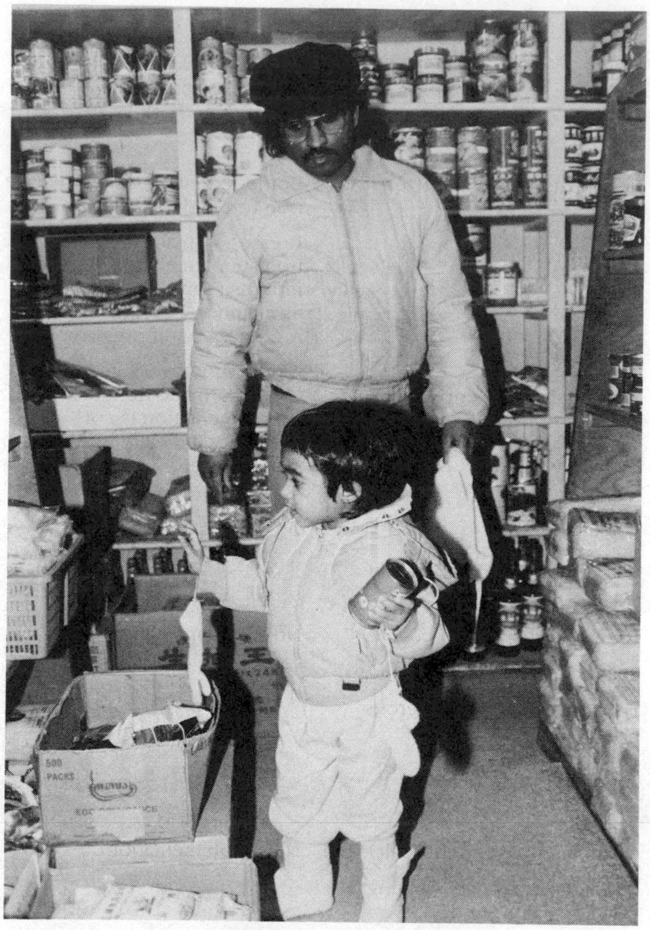

The availability of specialty foods increases the likelihood that children will be introduced to the preferences of a particular ethnic group.

staples varies from one culture to another. Beans, rice, ground corn, and soybean products are staples in many ethnic diets and are preferred over the bread products typical of the North American diet. Making generalizations about a child's or family's food preferences related to culture can be misleading. Burtis and colleagues identify cultural groups that may have characteristic food preferences, but warn that "individuals from any culture have different tastes and preferences; therefore, it is important not to stereotype cultural groups" (Burtis et al, 1987, p 332). Within the United States, regional preferences and specialties are strong in some families and not in others. School-age children who immigrate with their families may become acculturated quickly and may prefer fast-food style eating to traditional family foods. In hospital, school, or camp settings, children may dislike an unfamiliar method of preparation more than the actual food selections. Box 18-5 lists various cultural groups and some food traditions. How closely a family follows a cultural food tradition depends on several factors, including

1. whether it is an immigrant family or a first, second, or third generation family
2. how prevalent the particular group is in the community and how available specialty foods are
3. the economic status of the family

It is important, however, for the nurse to understand the nutritional adequacy of various diets and recommend only those changes that are necessary to maintain a healthy diet and to avoid making suggestions that are inconsistent with an individual's particular situation. For example, absence of the enzyme lactose in some persons makes milk digestion a problem. Thus, recommending an increased milk intake would be inappropriate. Suggesting the use of raw vegetables to someone who has been reared in a culture in which all vegetables are boiled for sanitary reasons also is unlikely to be effective.

Family relationships and lifestyle affect children's mealtime experience. Children and parents seem to be highly susceptible to conflicts and outright battles at mealtime. The underlying relationship and method of discipline largely determine the outcome of these battles. The emotional environment at mealtime should be such that children and parents feel relaxed and positive toward one another. Children whose parents show by "nagging" how concerned they are about eating soon learn how much control they can have by refusing to eat. Parents frequently need to be reassured that a healthy, hungry child *will* eat if a calm atmosphere is provided.

The family's degree of concern in insisting on a time when the family "eats together" affects the amount of experience children have in associating eating with positive socialization within the family. The hurried lifestyle of the modern family with high time demands on individual family members works against the goal of calm, unhurried mealtime experience. The negative impact that a continued pattern of hurried-up meals and tension-related eating experiences can potentially have should be considered when assessing nutritional status of children. Additionally, the tendency for families to rely on fast foods should be recognized as a pattern that can potentially lead to an imbalance of nutrients if fast foods are not varied and representative of a balanced diet.

Peers and social influences increasingly affect dietary habits as children become older, especially during the school-age years. Permission to ride a bike to a "corner store" where peers congregate enhances a child's sense of belonging and acceptance. The consumption of junk food thus becomes a socially related

Box 18-5
Some Food Traditions from Various Cultural Groups

BLACK AMERICAN

Food choices not significantly different from others in same geographic area. Southern black and white cooking tradition includes greens (collard, turnip, etc.), okra, pork products, cornbread, hominy grits.

NATIVE AMERICAN

Traditional foods vary among tribes. Corn, beans, squashes, chili peppers common. Availability and cost of fresh fruits, vegetables, and meat are major problems for those living on reservations.

MEXICAN AMERICAN

Mexican food includes influences from Spanish and Native American food. In some areas of the United States, persons of a Mexican-Hispanic background area constitute 25 per cent or more of the population, and food preferences are part of the mainstream eating patterns. Characteristic foods include tortillas (the bread of Mexican culture), tamales, tacos, enchiladas. Beans, rice, tomatoes, carrots, onions, and chili peppers are used in traditional cooking. Milk drinking is low; cheese is used.

PUERTO RICAN AND CUBAN

Spanish and Indian heritage seen in use of rice and red and white beans. In Caribbean areas, a wide range of fruits and vegetables is used—plantain, sweet potato, green bananas, cassava, breadfruit, guava, acerola, mango, avocado, okra, citrus fruits. In mainland cities, diets may suffer because these are not available or are too expensive.

CHINESE

Wide range of cooking traditions, depending on area of China family is from. Cooking style emphasizes foods being cut into very small pieces and cooked quickly. Rice is a staple in some regions, wheat flour noodles or dumplings in others. Soybean products (bean curd, also called tofu, oil, sauce) are used widely; there is a wide range of cooked vegetables including bok choy, bean sprouts, bamboo shoots, greens, mushrooms, snow peas, gourds.

JAPANESE

Fish, soybean products, rice, noodles, vegetables (seaweed, bamboo shoots, broccoli, cauliflower) use is prevalent. Traditional Japanese diets include little meat but raw fish is common; second and third generation families in United States often adopt Westernized diets. Green tea is the traditional beverage.

MIDDLE EASTERN

The countries around the eastern Mediterranean (Greece, Turkey, Lebanon, Syria, Iraq, Iran, Israel, Jordan, and Egypt) share certain food traditions. However, religious dietary differences between Moslems, Jews, and Christians are important. Lamb and goat are staple meats; beef is rare. Ground meat mixed with rice and spices and wrapped with leaves or stuffed in vegetables is a common dish. Bread, rice, beans, lentils, chick peas, olives, and eggplant are staples. Moslems and Jews avoid pork products; Moslems also avoid animal shortenings. Milk is used little in some groups; yoghurt is popular in most.

ETHIOPIAN

Ethiopian food is an example of a highly individualized cuisine brought to the United States by recent immigration. The Ethiopian staple is injera, a thick fluffy pancake-like bread. The basic meal consists of a meat or lentil stew (wat) eaten with injera. Wat is very highly spiced by a number of ground peppers and spices. In native Ethiopian meals, the amount of meat is usually small. In United States–adapted cooking, meat increases and injera becomes an accompaniment.

activity, and parents must be supported in their effort to curtail activities that grossly interfere with a balanced diet.

Television has been demonstrated to have an impact on children's eating habits. Advertisements for low nutrition foods tend to increase total calorie consumption (boys more than girls) yet pro-nutrition advertisements have not been demonstrated to be effective in promoting healthy food consumption (Jeffrey et al, 1982).

Socioeconomic factors account for a high degree of inequity between and within societies. Ability to purchase food, distribution of food, and access to health care services are common variables across populations. Consequently, when assessing nutritional adequacy, it is important to distinguish between resource issues and knowledge about nutrition as a cause of an unhealthy diet. The reasons for poor dietary intake vary according to socioeconomic variables. Malnutrition in developing countries is generally the result of marginal dietary intake and is often associated with a high frequency of illness, whereas malnutrition in industrialized countries has its roots in psychosocial causes (Pradilla, 1984).

Developmental level of the child affects the child's feeding experience and significance of food. As the

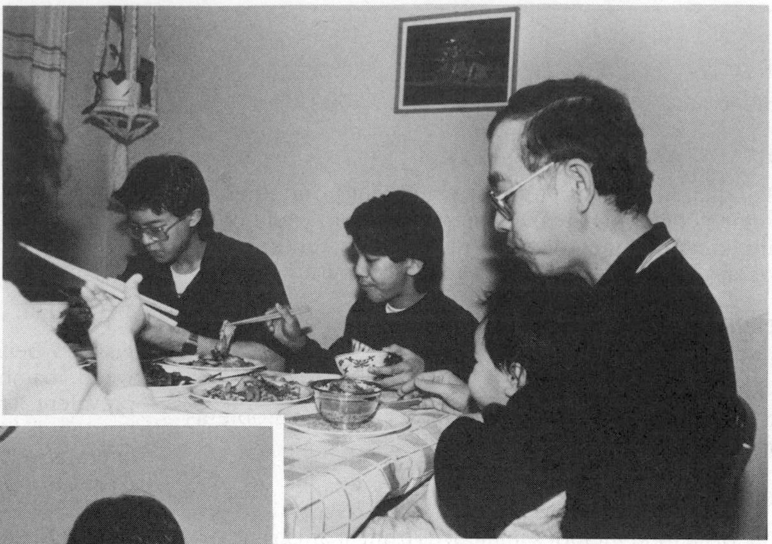

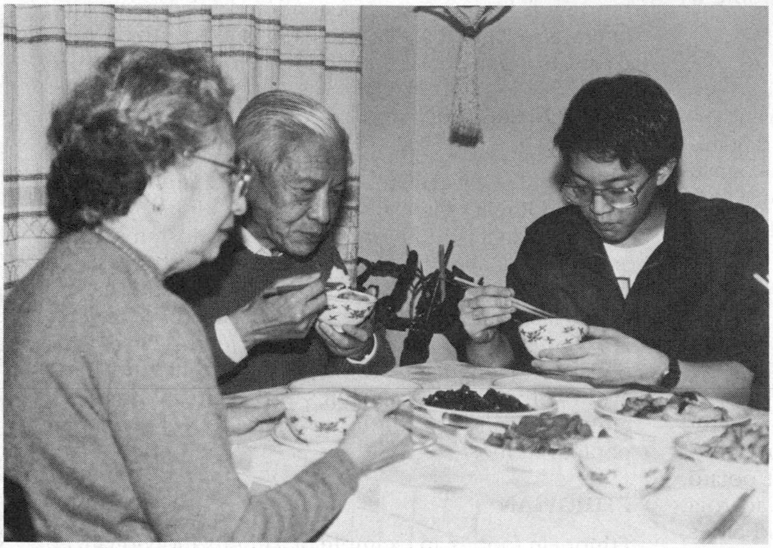

The Chinese tradition of the extended family and the custom of eating a variety of authentically prepared foods gives mealtime a place of prominence in this home, not to be exchanged for "eating fast foods on the run."

child develops cognitively his or her understanding of the meaning and importance of food changes. Developmental issues concerning food and eating that arise at the various ages are discussed in the respective normal growth and development chapters (5 through 9).

Baseline Data Gathering

A nutritional history is obtained for a 24-hour period of intake. For recall, questions about when the child got up and activities that took place at different times during the day can be asked. If more specific information is needed, a 3-day or 7-day food diary is kept. A food diary is helpful in establishing food intake and the time of day and type of food consumed. Methods of preparation and household measures (cup, teaspoon) of amounts of food consumed are recorded. Mixed dishes should have the recipe or ingredients included. Additional supplements such as vitamins or minerals should also be recorded. Although this method provides comprehensive information, it is time consuming and requires much cooperation and motivation on the part of the child and parents. It is especially helpful, however, in working with obese children to help them see exactly how much they consume. Another interview method is to ask about the frequency with which specific foods are eaten. The specific foods are grouped in the major categories and the person is asked to respond to whether they are rarely eaten (less than once a week), sometimes eaten (once a week), or eaten every day.

A total assessment of the child's nutritional status includes a record of dietary intake, clinical evaluation, including anthropometric measurements, and biochemical evaluation of nutrients within the body. Box 18-6 identifies information that a nutrition history would include. It is essential that this information be obtained in a nonjudgmental manner. It is important to remember that parents have been exposed to many ideas about nutrition and may be confused by the conflicting information available. Direct questions should be avoided if possible; open questions should be asked instead, such as, "What do you add to the cereal?" This approach avoids suggestion, criticism, or judgmental statements. The interviewer's attitude and nonverbal cues are frequently helpful in alleviating

Box 18-6
Format of a Nutritional History

I. Age
II. Concerns of parents or child about current nutrition or feeding behaviors
III. Infant history (used when client is an infant)
  A. Type of feeding method (bottle, breast)
  B. Formula feeding
    1. Type used
    2. How prepared
    3. When formula was started
    4. Other formulas used
    5. Number of bottles and ounces consumed in 24 hours
    6. Frequency of feedings and number of ounces at each feeding
    7. Amount of time required for feeding
    8. Approach to feeding (propped bottle, held in arms, etc.)
  C. Breastfeeding
    1. Number of times nursed in 24-hour period
    2. Length of time nursed at each breast, at each feeding
    3. Problems with breasts (cracked nipples, swollen breasts)
    4. Diet, medications and fluid intake history of mother
    5. Notice of milk letdown reflex by mother
    6. History of stress, fatigue in mother
  D. Additional intake
    1. Vitamins, iron, fluoride supplements
    2. Solid foods
      a. Type
      b. Frequency
      c. Amounts
      d. When started and how introduced
      e. How fed (feeds crackers, solids in bottle)
    3. Other fluids (juices, water, sugar water)
  E. Feeding behaviors/habits
    1. Satisfaction of child following feeding
    2. Use of pacifier or thumbsucking
    3. Nighttime nutrition
    4. Sleeping through night
    5. Elimination patterns
    6. Vomiting, spitting up
    7. Response to foods (spitting, colic, diarrhea, rash)
    8. Activity and personality (crying, irritable, sleeping) after feeding
  F. Family involvement with feeding
    1. Family attitudes/beliefs of food, feeding practices (how food is used)
    2. Participation in feeding (father, siblings)
    3. Response of family to feeding
      a. Breastfeeding
      b. Self-feeding by infant and inevitable mess
      c. Response of parent/child to new foods when introduced
IV. Toddler, preschooler, school-age, and adolescent history
  A. Number of meals eaten per day
  B. Where meals are eaten (school, fast-food chain, home)
  C. Method of feeding (fingers, utensils used)
  D. Amount of milk intake in 24 hours
  E. Snacking
    1. Type of foods
    2. Amounts
    3. Where snacks eaten
    4. Frequency and nearness to mealtimes
  F. Food preferences and dislikes
  G. Who plans, buys, and cooks food
  H. Finances
    1. Amount of money available for food
    2. Food programs (food stamps, Head Start Breakfast, school lunch)
  I. Dietary recall for past 24 hours
  J. Developmental behavior of eating (utensils, chewing)
  K. Habits (same as infant)
  L. Response of family to eating behavior of child
  M. Last dental visit
V. Past medical history
  A. Prenatal nutrition of mother
  B. Birthweight
  C. PKU results
  D. Developmental history
    1. Feeding behaviors (use of cup, spoon, fingerfeeding)
    2. Age of weaning
    3. Pica
  E. Allergies
  F. Chronic problems
VI. Family history
  A. Hypertension
  B. Obesity
  C. Stroke
  D. Diabetes
  E. Heart problems
  F. Allergies
  G. Hyperlipidemias
  H. Anorexia nervosa

(Adapted from Fox and Elsberry, 1980.)

Table 18-7. Physical Indications of Nutritional Status of the Child

Well-Nourished Child	Malnourished Child	Deficiency
Height and Weight		
Within growth norms—steady gain and increase from year to year	Above or below growth norms—failure to gain or excessive weight gain each year	Protein calorie, other essential nutrients
Skin		
Clear, smooth, elastic and firm	Rough, dry, scaly, xerosis	Vitamin A
Reddish-pink mucous membranes	Petechiae, ecchymoses, poor wound healing	Vitamin C
	Depigmentation of skin	Protein, calorie
	Lesions	Riboflavin
	Dermatitis, sensitivity of skin to sunlight	Niacin
	Pallor	Vitamin B_{12}, iron, folacin
Musculoskeletal		
Well-developed, erect posture	Head sags, winged scapula, bowed legs, costochondral beading, cranial bossing	Calcium, vitamin D
Shoulder blades flat		
Arms and legs straight		
Skull and jaw well developed	Epiphyseal enlargement of wrists	Vitamins D, C
Firm muscles with good tonus	Small flabby muscles, muscle weakness	Phosphorus, protein
Moderate amount of fat	Faulty epiphyseal bone formation	Vitamin A
	Pretibial edema bilateral	Protein, calorie, thiamine
Head		
Hair—smooth, good amount, lustrous	Dull, dry, depigmented, abnormal texture, easily pluckable, thin	Protein, calorie
Eyes—clear and bright	Dull with dark circles and hollows. Bitot's spots, conjunctivitis, xerosis, night blindness (nyctalopia), light sensitivity (photophobia)	Vitamin A, riboflavin
Mouth—pink, moist lips; pink, firm gums; full set of teeth	Cracking and scaling lips, cheilosis, fissuring of mouth corners	Riboflavin
	Spongy, swollen gums, bleed easily (gingiva)	Vitamin C
	Irregular or missing teeth with cavities; defective tooth enamel	Vitamin D,A
	Glossitis	Folacin, vitamin B_{12}, niacin, iron
	Tongue fissuring	Niacin
Neck		
Normal size	Enlarged thyroid	Iodine
	Enlarged parotids	Protein, calorie
Neurologic		
	Listless	Protein, calorie
	Loss of ankle- and knee-jerk reflexes, motor weakness, sensory loss	Thiamine
	Headache	Niacin, thiamine
	Polyneuritis, motor weakness	Thiamine
Abdomen		
Flat	Distended, protrudes, hepatomegaly	Protein, calorie
Cardiac		
Normal heart size and sounds	Cardiac enlargement and tachycardia	Thiamine, potassium
	Murmur	Iron

(From Pearson, 1977.)

parental anxiety. A calm, accepting attitude helps parents provide accurate data without feeling defensive.

Additional information can be obtained by observing the parent-child interaction during feeding. Observing a mother breastfeeding or bottle-feeding may provide useful information from which an assessment may be made and counseling provided. Feeding behaviors frequently reflect the child's development; delays in feeding behaviors may also indicate delays in other areas. Also, children may not be provided the opportunity to develop certain skills, such as using a cup or spoon, and the parent may need counseling in this area.

The nurse also determines nutritional status through *objective examination.* A thorough physical examination should identify areas of concern if undernourishment or overnourishment exists. Anthropometric measurements including height, weight, and head circumference provide essential information for evaluation of nutritional status. In some instances measurement of skin folds using a caliper may be beneficial. Physical indications of nutritional status are shown in Table 18-7. One or more of the signs of malnutrition indicates the need for a careful interview about food intake and eating habits. Additional helpful information about nutritional status may be obtained from hematocrit or hemoglobin tests to detect anemia; routine analysis for albumin and sugar; a 24-hour urinary creatinine excretion;* and, in children at risk, determination of cholesterol levels.

Promotion of a Healthful Diet

The goal for each child is that nutrition be of the quality to support optimal growth and development. Equal attention is given to nutrition whether a child is well or has a nutritional problem. Positive reinforcement for healthful dietary practices is encouragement that parents and children need. Identification of deficits in nutrient intake and dietary practices that interfere with health should be explored. Nutritional deficits are identified by comparing collected data with standards such as RDAs, the "basic four" food groups, height and weight charts, and normal ranges for biochemical laboratory data.

The nutrition history helps uncover long-standing nutritional problems and provides information about the family's knowledge and beliefs concerning nutrition. The 24-hour intake recall provides more precise information regarding adequacy of intake and a 3- to 7-day intake record gives the necessary data to learn about variety in a diet. The physical examination and clinical signs of nutritional problems are evaluated. Anthropometric measures must be evaluated by plotting a series of readings. Chapter 15 gives an explanation of how to use growth charts. See Appendices Two and Three for examples of growth charts.

Obvious changes or deficits in the growth pattern may require adjustments in the diet. Parents are the decision makers for the young child, but the older child has practical decision-making powers regarding nutrition. The parent and child should be counseled regarding modification of the child's diet if necessary. It is important to include both parent and child in the plans for change, so that they know the reasons why change is needed and how their beliefs, attitudes, and actions are affecting the nutrition of the child. Conditions that indicate nutritional counseling may be necessary are when the child's growth is below the 10th percentile or greater than the 90th percentile, when a child is underweight or overweight for height, when a certain nutrient is deficient in the diet (Pipes, 1985), or when the parent identifies a concern.

Common Concerns and Issues: Nursing Strategies

Nutrition is a rapidly developing science. Many cause-and-effect relationships have not been established concerning nutrition and disease. These uncertainties give rise to considerable confusion and differences of opinion concerning nutrition. Common issues and concerns that the nurse should be prepared to address are discussed in the following paragraphs.

Eating Behaviors, Limit Setting, and Socialization

Children adopt the eating behaviors of those they observe. They also learn by repeated reinforcement those behaviors that are acceptable and unacceptable. *Appropriate supervision* and *management by parents* are required to instill healthy dietary habits. Clear establishment of rules concerning food highlights important family values and attitudes. Parents should be encouraged to exercise their authority concerning behavior at the table, consumption of sweets and junk foods, and variety in their child's diet. Refusal to eat a varied diet of nutritious foods and excessive consumption of sweets and junk foods can only continue if parents purchase the food and do not monitor their child's intake. Monitoring intake of junk foods becomes increasingly difficult as the child approaches late school-age; however, parents have the responsibility

*The 24-hour urinary creatinine excretion correlates well with lean body mass if the child is on a creatine-free diet for several days before and during the test (MacLean and Graham, 1982).

to teach their children and set limits concerning food intake. The dessert crisis is not always easily resolved. Each family must develop their own rules, and these should be understood by the child. For example, a nutritionally adequate first course should be eaten before dessert is permitted. If limits are not put on desserts and snacks, excessive intake of sugar can interfere with adequate dietary intake.

The effect maturational changes have on appetite is important for parents to understand. The frustration of "getting children to eat" is a common problem experienced by parents. It should be stressed that if sweets are curtailed and excessive milk intake is not permitted, a healthy child will eat when hungry without coercion. Strategies to gain a child's cooperation at mealtime should be employed. Children can be given some control and autonomy by letting them place food on their own plates (with some supervision depending on age and maturity of child), giving some choices, and not insisting on an empty plate if the child is satiated. A child who persistently does not eat should be further evaluated. In some cases, children control their parents by not eating, in which case parents should be counseled to put less emphasis on food intake. Lack of sufficient exercise, inadequate sleep and rest, and an underlying illness should also be considered when a child persistently does not eat. The normal changes in appetite and food intake, however, should be recognized as factors that affect a child's intake (e.g., toddlers and some preschoolers are notorious for being picky eaters).

A nonconducive environment for mealtime can detract from optimal nutritional intake. Mealtime should be a pleasant, social experience. Parents are encouraged to avoid tension-producing topics and should plan for sufficient time to eat an unhurried meal. The physical aspects, such as comfortable seating, appropriate utensils, and attractive serving of food, are also amenities that children deserve. Another concern that parents frequently express is their children's resistance to trying new foods or eating certain foods, such as vegetables. It is important to recognize that children have likes and dislikes but that learning to eat new foods requires work; it does not just happen. Children learn to like food by tasting it time after time; therefore, even though a food is refused, the process of taking a small bite each time can eventually change the child's response. New foods are better accepted if they are offered when the child is hungry so that a pleasant sensation is associated with that particular food. Also, not permitting a second helping of a desired food (e.g., bread, potatoes) before the vegetables have been consumed allows consumption of the less desired food at a time when the child is not satiated. Always leaving the least desired food until last reduces the likelihood that a pleasant sensation is associated with that food.

Nutrition and Disease

Potential association between childhood nutrition and risk of development of adult disease is a relatively recent concept. Common areas of concern are the effects of intake of refined sugar, salt, and fat and cholesterol. Additionally, recent emphasis has been given to the benefits of a high fiber diet. The American Academy of Pediatrics Committee on Nutrition cautions that the safety of diets that

1. decrease caloric intake;
2. increase consumption of complex carbohydrates (fiber);
3. decrease consumption of fat and cholesterol; and
4. limit sodium intake

has *not* been established in children and pregnant women (Committee on Nutrition, 1983; 1986). Although restrictive diets are not recommended in children, it is useful for nurses to have current information concerning these issues so that they can counsel parents and children appropriately. Sugar consumption as a factor in the development of coronary heart disease, hyperactivity in children, and the increasing incidence of obesity has not been documented with scientific data (Krause and Mahan, 1984). The major offending characteristic of sugar on children's health is its cariogenic property (see Chapter 19).

In recent years, the potential protective role of fiber in the diet has been studied. A reduced fiber intake has been implicated in the development of cancer of the colon and has been identified as a factor contributing to high blood pressure (Anderson, 1983). Diets for children that contain fiber at the expense of animal protein may, however, result in deficits in vitamins and minerals. Fiber also promotes a laxative effect, which is beneficial but to be avoided in excess. With respect to fiber, a balanced diet according to the basic four groups is recommended.

A continuing area of study is the diet–heart disease relationship. The focus of recent research is the advisability of reducing the fat and cholesterol content of diets for infants and children. Atherosclerosis is a disease process that begins with the appearance of fatty streaks in the aorta during childhood. By the age of 10, virtually all children, regardless of their dietary intake and the incidence of coronary heart disease, have fatty streaks in their aortas (Roy and Galeano, 1985). Dietary recommendations have been made for adults to consume low-fat and low-cholesterol diets to reduce the risk factors for the development of atherosclerosis. However, limiting fat and cholesterol intake has been questioned with respect to children because of their needs for growth and because the effect of altering fat and cholesterol intake during the early years has not been demonstrated to reduce adult atherosclerosis. Breast milk, which contains cholesterol, is considered an ideal food for infants; it has been suggested that cholesterol may be necessary and important during the entire growing period for the formation of bile acids, hormones, and special tissues (Committee on Nutrition, 1983).

The amount of sodium in infant foods became a public concern in the middle 1960s. Since that time, there has been a gradual decrease in the sodium concentration of infant foods and, since 1977, the addition of salt to infant foods has been discontinued. The hypothesis that the sodium content of infant foods contributes to hypertension in later life has not been confirmed (Committee on Nutrition, 1981a). The important aspect to consider is that it is thought that salt preference is learned and that reduction of dietary sodium can cause taste preference to shift to lower levels of salt in food (Beauchamp et al, 1983). The overall recommendation that nurses can make for children is to eat a well-balanced diet and avoid excesses. The recommendation of the Committee on Nutrition (1983) is that "current dietary trends in the United States toward a decreased consumption of saturated fats, cholesterol and salt, and an increased intake of polyunsaturated fats should be followed with moderation. Diets that avoid extremes are safe for children."

Nutritional counseling is a major responsibility of the nurse. The relationship of nutrition and disease is an area of health care that is subject to misinformation and misinterpretation. A major source of information that can be used to guide the nurse in counseling is the *Pediatric Nutrition Handbook* published by the American Academy of Pediatrics (1985).

The nurse's role is to listen to the opinions of the clients (parent, child, or adolescent) and seek to understand any inaccuracies that might be harmful to their health. Some differences in opinion may actually not require intervention if there is no potential for actual harm. The basic principles used for management are (1) *generally discourage restrictive diets for children* and (2) *maintain a balanced diet.*

Another role of the nurse in health maintenance is identification of early signs of illness. Detection of obesity by measuring height, weight, and skin fold thickness and detection of hypertension by measuring blood pressure are nursing responsibilities. Screening of children more than 2 years of age who are at risk for hypercholesterolemia because of family history should consist of at least two serum cholesterol measurements. The high density lipoprotein cholesterol is measured when levels are consistently above the 95th percentile for age and sex (Committee on Nutrition, 1983; American Academy of Pediatrics, 1985).

Food Additives

Many consumers believe that some food additives may cause cancer and that childhood hyperactivity is associated with intake of additives. An increased use of convenience foods and the transportation and storage of food in industrialized nations makes the use of food additives necessary. The demand of the consumer for attractive foods with reduced perishability continues to promote acceptability of additives in spite of the potential disadvantages.

A food additive is a substance that is added to food for the purpose of enhancing its quality and shelf-life. The purposes of food additives vary, including (1) addition of nutritional value; (2) preservation of food; (3) aid in processing and preparation; and (4) improvement of the flavor, color, odor, and texture (Krause and Mahan, 1984).

Food additives in common use have been subjected to extensive study through large doses in animals by the Food and Drug Administration (FDA). The FDA has enforced the "Delaney Clause," which makes it necessary for any additive to be removed from the market if it has been found to induce cancer in humans or animals. The use of saccharin (a sugar substitute) has been controversial; however, it is still available as a non-prescription drug. A newer acceptable sweetener is aspartame, which was approved for use by the FDA in 1981; however, it can only be used in cold foods, and *it is not to be used by someone with phenylketonuria because it is made from the amino acid phenylalanine.*

Nitrites and nitrates used to cure meat and poultry products have also come under attack because of their potential carcinogenic qualities. Nitrate, however, is also a normal constituent of many vegetables, especially lettuce, beets, celery, and spinach (Green and Harry, 1981), and the intake through additives is considerably less than through dietary sources.

Although the claim by Feingold (1975) that chemicals added to food cause hyperactivity received wide attention, scientific research has not consistently demonstrated a relationship. A conclusion was reached by the National Institutes of Health in 1982 that (1) a few children may be helped by the Feingold (additive-

Table 18-8. Concerns Related to Fast-Food Consumption

	Nutrient Availability	Suggested Diet Alterations
High Caloric Intake	A typical fast-food meal (large hamburger, french fries and milkshake) contains approximately 1000 calories. This caloric level is too high for all individuals except perhaps a teenage male.	Choosing a smaller hamburger or low fat milk instead of a milkshake can reduce the calories significantly.
Protein	Protein is abundant in fast foods.	Protein may even be excessive. Therefore, a smaller hamburger is sufficient.
Vitamin A	Vitamin A is usually present in low quantities (pizza and tacos are an exception.)	Food from a salad bar will compensate for this deficiency.
Vitamin C	Vitamin C is generally present in low quantities, but inclusion of french fries is beneficial.	Food from a salad bar will compensate for this deficiency.
Fiber/Roughage	The fiber content is usually low. The only fiber is present in the slice of tomato and the lettuce on a sandwich.	Include a salad if available.
Sodium Content	Sodium content is generally high.	Refrain from adding salt.

free) diet, and (2) a few children respond adversely to synthetic food dyes (American Academy of Pediatrics, 1985). Lipton and Mayo (1983) provide further support for the position that some hyperactive children may benefit from the additive-free diet, but that there is no support for the breadth of Feingold's original claims (see Chapter 34 for further discussion of management of the hyperactive child). The nurse's ongoing awareness of developments in research findings concerning food additives is information required to counsel parents.

Fast Foods

The largest proportion of meals served in the United States today is through fast-food industries. The popularity of fast-food restaurants matches the fast pace of modern life. The family with young children finds avoiding meal preparation and clean-up a joy and an outing to a restaurant fun. Equally so, fast-food restaurants appeal to adolescents who congregate in groups for a meal or snack that is relatively inexpensive.

The food served in fast-food restaurants is severely criticized by some nutritionists. The generalization that these foods are junk foods, however, needs to be put into perspective. As many fast foods are consumed by teenagers, so-called junk-food intake has the potential to become the source of conflict between adolescents and parents. Because fast-food consumption has reached such high proportions, the nurse who cares for children and families requires some knowledge to distinguish between legitimate concerns and those that can be dispelled.

Some fast-food chains now make nutrition analyses available to the consumer. Nutrition data is also estimated from standard food composition tables. Independent food testing by a laboratory has been done for some industries; however, it is reasonable to believe that estimates made from the accepted standard food tables are sufficiently accurate. Concerns expressed about nutritional value of fast foods include high fat content, high in calories, protein inadequacy, vitamin A and vitamin C inadequacy, low fiber or roughage, and high sodium content. These concerns and comments about actual nutritional values with suggestions of how to alter a diet to compensate for these potential problems are summarized in Table 18-8. The overall concern that some express is that there is not a sufficient variety of foods offered. Some fast-food chains have introduced salad bars; however, adolescents often have a narrow range of preferences; therefore, availability of salads does not necessarily improve their diet (MacLean and Graham, 1982). Consuming several meals a week in a fast-food restaurant should present no nutritional problems if a few guidelines are followed in food selection and if meals consumed elsewhere consist of a balanced diet.

Vegetarianism

Throughout history people of various religions and cultures have adhered to a vegetarian diet. In North American society the past quarter century has seen an emergence of vegetarians from new religious, philosophic, or counterculture groups. Vegetarian diets can be compatible with nutritional balance if they are based on established nutritional principles.

The term *vegetarianism* is used to describe a diet that consists primarily of plant foods and excludes the consumption of meat, fowl, and fish, with or without

Box 18-7
Types of Vegetarian Diets

Lacto-ovo-vegetarians	Plant foods plus eggs and dairy products
Lacto-vegetarians	Plant foods plus dairy products (eggs excluded)
Ovo-vegetarians	Plant foods plus eggs (dairy products excluded)
Vegan	Plant foods only (dairy products and eggs excluded)

eggs and dairy foods (see Box 18-7). The main types of vegetarians are described in Box 18-8. In today's culture the term vegetarian is used in a variety of ways; some people use it loosely to indicate only that red meat is avoided. Therefore, it is important to establish from the outset what a client means by being a "vegetarian."

Understanding the reasons a person chooses to be a vegetarian is useful in establishing a working relationship (see Box 18-9). Frequently the reasons for choosing vegetarianism determine the degree of strictness with which the diet is observed. Since vegetarians may lack confidence in or be suspicious of those who hold or advocate traditional views of nutrition, it is important to communicate an attitude of support.

The American Dietetic Association has put forth a position paper on a vegetarian approach to eating which states that "well-planned vegetarian diets are consistent with good nutritional status" (American Dietetic Association, 1980). However, it is important to recognize that *poorly planned vegetarian diets* can increase the risk of diet-related nutritional disorders, especially during the growing years.

The increasing concern for health and nutrition and the benefits of predominantly vegetarian diets have led to increases in their popularity. It has been substantially documented that vegetarians have lower serum cholesterol and lower incidence of obesity, both of which are thought to be related to coronary artery disease. The possibility that vegetarian diets may reduce the risk for cancer has not been proved. There is some evidence to support the hypothesis that dietary fat and cholesterol affect the concentration and activity of bacteria in the colon. The altered bacterial activity is thought to produce tumorigenic compounds from bile acids and cholesterol metabolites (Reddy, 1976; Wynder et al, 1977). Colon cancer has also been studied in relation to fiber intake (with high fiber leading to reduced risk), although firm experimental data are lacking to support this relationship. However, because a vegetarian diet is composed of high fiber and contains reduced fat and cholesterol content, it has gained increasing acceptance as a preventive measure against cancer. The potential reduction in risk for developing disease later in life is one major reason why families make the personal choice to raise their children as vegetarians.

Nursing Strategies. Successful support of children on vegetarian diets depends on the nurse's acceptance of the clients' preference. The goal thus becomes one of working out a diet suitable to the parents and child within the family's preferred dietary prac-

Box 18-8
Types of Vegetarians

TRADITIONAL VEGETARIANS

Many vegetarians have been raised within cultural or religious groups with long-standing customs of vegetarianism (e.g., Seventh Day Adventist). Among these groups there is adherence to some degree of animal food exclusion but less emphasis on the use of unrefined or naturally occurring food sources.

NEW VEGETARIANS

Since 1960 there has been a heavy influence of Eastern thought in the Western world, resulting in various philosophic, quasi-religious, or religious groups who have adopted some form of vegetarianism. It is these groups that avoid animal food but in addition avoid other foods that are refined, are processed, or are not organic or natural. Health food stores are the primary suppliers of such foods in the market. These groups vary considerably, and include

- *Yogi Vegetarians* (lacto-ovo-vegetarian with a stress on "natural foods");
- *Hare Krishnas* (lacto-vegetarian with a stress on "natural foods"); and
- *Macrobiotics* (vegan diets with strict avoidance of animal fat sources and extensive use of "natural foods").

PERSONAL CHOICE

Individuals who for a variety of reasons choose to eat a diet primarily composed of vegetables, without affiliation with a specific religious or quasi-religious group. (See possible reasons in Box 18-9)

ECONOMIC CIRCUMSTANCES

A segment of the population within developed countries and large numbers of individuals in underdeveloped countries consume diets that exclude animal foods because of inadequate income.

Box 18-9
Reasons Why People Choose to Be Vegetarians

Ecologic

Consumption of foods that are "lower" on the food chain (i.e., those fed to livestock) is thought to be a way to reduce world hunger.

Economic

Vegetables and grains are cheaper than animal products.

Religion or philosophical beliefs

Reasons are many, combining ideas concerning violence (killing of animals) and health issues.

Health

Foods are lower in fat and lower in cholesterol, higher in complex carbohydrates, and perhaps lower in sugar.

tices. An understanding of the potential problems must be acquired to provide appropriate and relevant counsel. Although experienced vegetarian parents have a reasonable knowledge of what constitutes a healthful vegetarian diet for themselves, they may not be fully aware of the increased potential for deficiencies that exist with respect to the growing child. Potential problems and information to use in planning interventions are summarized in Table 18-9. Adolescents who choose to become vegetarians against the wishes of their parents also need basic nutritional counseling.

A vegetarian diet can be nutritionally sound if a few guidelines are followed:

- Combine legumes with grains or nuts and seeds to ensure a proper balance of dietary protein.
- Vitamin B_{12} is not contained in plant foods; therefore, if possible, supplement the diet with dairy products and eggs, or use fortified soy milk, or take a vitamin B_{12} supplement.
- Encourage breastfeeding (with attention to mother's vitamin B_{12} intake). Infants on breast milk should receive iron and vitamin D supplementation, and vitamin B_{12} (if mother's intake is not adequate).
- Consume a variety of foods.
- Provide a dietary source of vitamin C (it enhances nonheme iron absorption).
- Reduce amount of vegetables consumed that contain oxalate and phytate (they impair iron absorption).

When planning a vegetarian diet, the principles of the basic four food groups should be followed daily:

- 1 serving of nuts or seeds
- 2 servings of vitamin B_{12}-fortified vegetable protein or soy milk
- 3 servings of vegetables (include dark green leafy)
- 4 servings of fruit (at least one rich in vitamin C)
- 3 to 5 servings of grains (depending on age of child)

The goals of a complete protein at each meal and generally a wide variety of food intake should be stressed.

Nutritional Alterations

Nutritional alterations discussed in this chapter are infant obesity, severe protein-calorie malnutrition, and vitamin D deficiency rickets.

Infant Obesity

Wide variations exist in infant feeding practices. The consequences of various feeding practices are not clearly established; therefore, recommendations regarding infant nutrition are speculative and must be considered tentative (Fomon et al, 1979). Infants fed in a variety of ways may appear equally healthy either because the consequences of a poor diet are too subtle or because differences can be verified only by long-term observations (Fomon et al, 1979). Some of the questions on the long-term consequences of early eating habits that remain unanswered are the following: (1) What is the relationship of intake of cholesterol during infancy to the later development of atherosclerosis? (2) How does salt intake in infancy affect blood pressure in later life? (3) Are faulty eating habits of infancy and infant obesity an important determinant of obesity in later childhood and adulthood? (The theory that the critical period for the development of obesity is during the first year or two of life has been challenged (Taitz, 1977; Filer, 1978). It has also been suggested that onset of obesity in later childhood is more predictive of adult obesity than obesity of infantile onset. While we wait for conclusive studies regarding the effects of infant obesity, infants at risk must be identified and families need assistance to establish healthful feeding practices.

Nursing Assessment. Carrying out a thorough nutritional assessment will assist the nurse in identifying those infants at risk for obesity. Intake is evaluated in terms of the total caloric intake, amount of fluid intake, and balance of nutrients.

Epidemiologic factors associated with obesity should be recognized in an effort to identify high risk infants. Parental obesity, older or single parents, single

Table 18-9. Vegetarianism: Potential Nutritional Problems and Nursing Strategies

Explanation of the Problem	Suggested Strategies with Explanation
Protein Deficit:	Complementation of proteins compensates for this deficit
Vegetable proteins have a lower percentage of total nitrogen in the form of amino acids and all are relatively deficient in one or more of the essential amino acids (e.g., lysine is low in cereal grains and methionine is low in legumes)	Complementation of proteins is the combining of certain foods to ensure intake of quality protein (e.g., methionine-deficient legumes that have an adequate lysine content (beans, peas) should be complemented by methionine-adequate but lysine-deficient grains (rice, corn, oats) or nuts Other examples: peanut butter on whole wheat bread, bean and corn salad, corn and lima beans
Energy: It is difficult to supply adequate energy sources because: • bulkiness of the foods cause children to feel satiated. Their consumption of sufficient quantities presents a problem • some vegetables are poorly digested • vegetarian diets are lower in fat	This problem can be overcome if sufficient fats are eaten The greater the variety of food the more likely it is that energy requirements are met
Energy is more potentially a problem during the growth periods of infancy and adolescence	
Vitamins:	Vitamin B_{12} can be provided by a supplement or by fortified foods such as soybean milk or meat analogues
Vitamin B_{12}: Currently there is no known plant food that contains Vitamin B_{12}	It is also contained in yeast grown on vitamin B_{12} enriched media, seaweed, or fermented soy
This is particularly a problem for the breast-fed infant whose mother is on a strict vegetarian diet and does not take a Vitamin B_{12} supplement	If eggs and milk are included in the diet vitamin B_{12} is usually adequate
Vitamin D: Vitamin D is not found in foods of plant origin; therefore it must be supplemented in the vegan diet	Vitamin D can be supplied by exposure of skin to sunlight but this is not a reliable source
Risk of nutritional rickets in certain populations of vegetarian children persists (Dwyer et al, 1979; Hellebostad, 1985).	A supplementary source of vitamin D, such as cod-liver oil, is required if fortified soybean milk or cow's milk is excluded Egg yolks, which are also excluded in a vegan diet, are a good source of Vitamin D
Riboflavin:	Large amounts of dark green vegetables, legumes, and whole grains must be consumed to achieve riboflavin in amounts equivalent to 1 cup of milk
Riboflavin is adequate in vegetarian diets that include dairy products but marginal if such products are excluded	High intake of these plant foods is not without consequence in that they inhibit calcium and zinc absorption (see below)
Minerals	Dark green leafy vegetables, legumes, fortified soybean milk, nuts, and seeds are sources of calcium
Calcium: Milk and milk products are the most common source of calcium; therefore when these are excluded, other sources must be provided	Vegetables with high oxalic acid content (spinach, chard, beet greens) interfere with calcium absorption Oxalic acid combines with calcium oxalate (bound calcium) and therefore inhibit calcium absorption Whole grains and nuts that contain phytates can also interfere with calcium utilization The most reliable source of calcium is fortified soybean milk
Zinc: The bioavailability of zinc in plant foods is questionable The phytates in whole grains and nuts tend to form zinc-phytate complexes inhibiting zinc	Yeast fermentation of whole wheat flour (i.e, as occurs in bread-making) reduces phytates, increasing zinc availability; thus, if bread with yeast is included in the diet, the problem is reduced
Iron: Iron is absorbed form heme iron, which is animal in origin and from non-heme iron which is from plant foods	Non-heme iron absorption is enhanced by the presence of animal protein and vitamin C in the diet
Absorption of heme iron is higher than that of non-heme iron Also, non-heme iron is decreased by phytates and vegetable fiber	It should be recommended that *each meal* contain a food source of vitamin C to enhance availability of non-heme iron

(Data from American Dietetic Association, 1980; Rudy, 1984.)

children, or children in small families are epidemiologic categories that are associated with childhood obesity. Obesity in parents in particular is a risk factor. According to a 10-state nutritional survey, a child of obese parents is three times more likely to be obese than if the parents are not obese; if one child is obese, there is a 40 per cent chance that a sibling will also be obese (U.S. Department of Health, Education, and Welfare, 1972). The similarity of obesity patterns between parents and children cannot, however, be interpreted as having only a genetic base because there is considerable similarity between spouses in terms of obesity (Garn and Clark, 1975). Family eating patterns and values placed on food are important factors to assess when parents and siblings of an infant are obese.

Obesity is an "excessive ratio of fat to fat-free body mass" (Fomon and Ziegler, 1976). A general definition of obesity is (1) weight for height greater than the 95th percentile and (2) skin fold thickness greater than the 95th percentile (Fomon and Ziegler, 1976).

Height and weight measurements made at each health visit are the nurse's primary method of detecting infants at risk for obesity. Height and weight are plotted on a percentile chart to identify rapid or disproportionate weight gain. In some instances bone and muscle structure may give the erroneous clinical impression that an infant is obese. An evaluation of fat disposition also can be obtained by measuring skin fold thickness of the triceps and subscapular area. The triceps muscle, the most widely advocated site for testing, is also the easiest site to use (Rowe, 1980). (See Chapter 15 for percentile growth charts.) Use of calipers has some disadvantage in that when measurements are taken by various personnel a certain amount of error occurs owing to varying techniques and subjective readings.

Nursing Strategies: Prevention and Counseling. During infancy the goal in managing obesity is not to *reduce* the infant's weight but rather to *slow the rate* of weight gain. Prevention and management of obesity involve two approaches: (1) an increase in exercise and (2) a reduction in caloric intake. During infancy certain boundaries determine the type of interventions that are appropriate. The infant's developmental capabilities may limit the type of physical activity to only kicking, creeping, crawling, rolling, and reaching. Parents should be made aware of the importance of providing adequate space and opportunity to engage in such developmentally appropriate exercise. Also, the infant's high nutritional requirements cannot be overlooked. It is necessary to maintain a level of caloric intake that supports growth and daily energy needs.

Obesity in childhood can adversely affect a child's developing body image and self-esteem. The nurse can make an important contribution in the prevention and management of obesity by helping parents to (1) avoid feeding practices that could contribute to infant obesity and (2) recognize and correct those patterns of interaction with their baby that potentiate the tendency to become obese.

Feeding Practices That Contribute to Infant Obesity. The advantages of breastfeeding to infants are sufficiently established to warrant active encouragement of mothers to breastfeed (Cunningham, 1979, 1986). Although studies do not consistently show that bottle-fed infants tend to become more obese than breast-fed infants, it has been observed that bottle-fed infants gain weight more rapidly (Cunningham, 1979; Fomon, 1974). It has been suggested that bottle-feeding invites the problem of obesity by a caregiver's tendency to encourage an infant to suck until the bottle is empty, whereas in breast-feeding the mother no longer offers the breast when an infant stops sucking (Filer, 1978). Thus, a preventive role of the nurse is to counsel parents who bottle-feed to avoid forcing their infant to empty the bottle at each feeding. Although the protective effects of breastfeeding with respect to obesity have not been proved, breastfeeding should be supported and encouraged. It is not justified, however, to say that breastfeeding prevents obesity.

Introduction of solid foods before 4 to 6 months of age adds extra calories. However, it has not been demonstrated that early introduction of solid foods causes obesity (Committee on Nutrition, 1981b). Parents should be assured that infants before the age of 4 to 6 months do not need the additional calories that solid foods supply. They should particularly be advised against the addition of sugar and other sweets to the baby's diet. In counseling parents about solid foods for their baby, the nurse must recognize that parents start solid foods early for various reasons. Common reasons include a belief that milk does not supply adequate nutrition, social pressure exerted by family and friends, and a belief that giving solid food will cause the baby to sleep through the night (Markesbury and Wong, 1979). The nurse can help families to understand what constitutes normal infant nutrition and assist them to establish healthful feeding practices.

Parental Responses That Contribute to Infant Obesity. The stereotype that a fat baby is a healthy baby is a myth that has been transmitted from one generation to another. These beliefs are deeply rooted in some families and are not easily altered. Overfeeding babies thus can stem from a cultural or familial orientation on the part of parents to "fatten" their babies because it is believed that this is a sign of good parenting. The nurse can work with parents over a period of time, pointing out sufficient positive aspects of their parenting; eventually they can give up the need to overfeed their baby.

The use of food to quiet and satisfy the infant can lead to obesity. To always offer additional breast or bottle feedings or solid food to quiet the baby can establish a pattern whereby food is used by the child in response to anxiety rather than in response to hunger. This practice teaches an infant that internal needs can be satisfied by food and institutes a behavior pattern in which all internal tensions are interpreted as indicative of the need for food. The nurse can manage this problem by suggesting alternative methods of responding when the baby cries. Visual stimulation, cuddling, change of position, exercise, or a drink of water may quiet the baby.

Counseling Role of the Nurse. It is believed that the important variable affecting risk of persistence of obesity in infancy is the *severity* of the problem. Weight in excess of 120 per cent of ideal weight in infants who appear fat requires further investigation. This is especially true when obesity is associated with epidemiologic risk factors such as parental obesity, older or single parents, or only children (Dietz, 1984).

Severe dietary restrictions are not recommended during the first year of life, but the family may need assistance to calculate recommended dietary intake. Infants are particularly prone to become obese during the period from 6 months to 1 year of age. As solid foods are added, the nurse should teach parents to check the labels for caloric content and help them to feed according to the caloric needs of their infant. If the daily milk and food intake exceeds the required caloric amount,* water feedings can be used to replace excess caloric intake. Skim milk is not recommended in the diet of an infant under 1 year of age. It has been recommended by some nutritionists that 2 per cent fat milk may be used in the case of severe obesity in older infants (Taitz, 1977).

The question of whether frequent small feedings are better than three meals a day is not clearly answered. In adults, widely spaced large meals lead to increased serum concentrations of cholesterol and impaired glucose tolerance; the effects of feeding frequency have not been studied as they pertain to infants. The dilution of formula to increase volume intake without increasing caloric intake may not be the correct approach. Moreover, Fomon (1974) suggests that regular consumption of enormous volumes of calorically dilute food is not likely to achieve the goal of developing the habit of eating in moderation.

Although many questions regarding infant obesity remain unanswered, the nurse can play an important role in prevention by using the information that is available. Assisting families to establish healthy feeding practices for their infants is a primary role of the nurse. If a family tends to overfeed an infant, the nurse must carefully assess the parents' values and cultural orientation to food, instituting a gradual teaching program whereby parents can learn to relate to their infant in a way that fosters eating in moderation.

*Daily requirements of calories: 1 to 6 months = 117 kcal/kg; 6 to 12 months = 108 kcal/kg.

Severe Protein and Calorie Malnutrition

Marasmus and kwashiorkor are two serious forms of protein and calorie malnutrition. Both are rare in the United States and common in developing countries. However, since 1981 a reduction and modification of supplemental feeding programs has occurred, which has resulted in hunger becoming more widespread in the United States (Brown, 1987). A large proportion of children in the world do not get enough to eat, are subjected to poor hygienic conditions, and have inadequate health care; these factors produce malnourishment. The incidence of protein and calorie malnutrition is markedly increased in these areas as a result of repeated bouts of gastroenteritis. Severe protein and calorie malnutrition typically results after an infant is weaned to a grossly inadequate diet. Malnutrition can also result under other circumstances, including metabolic disturbances, chronic renal insufficiency, and maladaptive parent-child relations (nonorganic failure to thrive) (see Chapter 35). There have also been reports of malnutrition occurring as a result of a prolonged clear liquid diet in the face of infantile diarrhea (Kaplowitz and Isely, 1979). The nurse has a primary role in teaching families proper and safe administration of fluids typically prescribed for diarrhea to assist in the prevention of such an occurrence.

Marasmus is a condition of gradual wasting in the presence of grossly inadequate calories and protein. The caloric deficit is so severe that there is a marked reduction of subcutaneous fat, causing the skin to become wrinkled and loose. This results in an "old man" and "wasted" appearance. The marasmic infant is retarded in growth and development and appears restless, is fretful, and eventually becomes apathetic and listless. A starvation type of diarrhea may further complicate the dehydrated and undernourished state of the infant.

Kwashiorkor is primarily a deficiency of protein resulting in severe muscle wasting. It means "deposed child" (i.e., the child who no longer is breast-fed because a younger sibling is born). There is also a deficit in calories, but it is the protein deficit that accounts for the principal symptoms (Barness, 1987). The child is usually edematous; this varies in degree from a slight localized edema (primarily eyelids and feet) to a marked generalized edema. When edema is generalized, it may mask the muscle atrophy. Skin changes occur, beginning with erythema and progressing through a sequence of hyperpigmentation, desquamation (peeling), and finally depigmentation (loss of color). During the peeling stage, the skin readily becomes infected; the risk of infection is increased by picking off the desquamating skin (Rudolph, 1982). Another characteristic symptom is the fine, sparse, reddish-tinted hair. Alternating periods of adequate and inadequate dietary intake are mirrored in the streaked hair that results. When dietary intake is adequate, hair is pigmented, and when it is inadequate, it is depigmented. The general depleted nutritional state is frequently further compromised by infections. Most commonly acute diarrhea, measles, or parasitic infestations precede or accompany kwashiorkor in underdeveloped countries. Children suffering from kwashiorkor become irritable and apathetic and are typically sullen and withdrawn.

Therapeutic Management of Severe Protein-Calorie Malnutrition

These children are in a severe state of nutritional imbalance. The replacement of fluids, electrolytes, and nutrients requires a highly specialized therapeutic approach. Furthermore, many infections either precede the undernourished state or occur as a result of it. Treatment consists of administration of fluids and electrolytes, antibiotic therapy to treat infections, and a gradual dietary rehabilitation.

Nursing Strategies

The nurse has a responsibility to care for the infant and to become actively involved in the process of identifying those factors that led to development of the condition. The nurse must try to prevent infection or reinfection of an already debilitated child, provide meticulous skin care in the presence of edema or skin desquamation, and carefully monitor dietary and fluid intake. Although physical care of the infant is immediate, the nurse must simultaneously begin a careful collection of data and establish a relationship of sensitive interaction with the family to assist in identifying the cause of the malnutrition.

The nurse who cares for infants and families should also make every effort to identify those children with more moderate forms of malnutrition and especially evaluate the nutritional status of those children who show growth retardation and a developmental lag. Although many factors contribute to the problem of malnutrition, the one consistent finding is poverty. The nurse's efforts to educate families in adequate nutritional intake can be most effective if equal importance is given toward increasing availability of food. Studies show a clear relationship between poverty and malnutrition so that it is safe to say "malnutrition when looked for will be found in the poor of every community" (Mauer, 1975).

One of the most important roles of the nurse is to participate in the prevention of malnutrition in developed countries.

Careful management of fluid administration, avoiding prolonged clear fluids, teaching correct preparation of formula, and counseling teenagers regarding fad diets are areas in which the nurse becomes involved in various settings. Particularly, the management of infant diarrhea at home is an area that requires careful telephone advice and follow-up.

Vitamin D Deficiency Rickets

Vitamin D deficiency results in poor mineralization of the growing parts of the skeleton, leading to the disease of rickets. Vitamin D deficiency rickets is most common in children from 4 months to 2 years of age. Vitamin D is required for (1) absorption of dietary calcium and phosphorus from the intestines, (2) conservation of phosphorus by the renal tubular cells, and (3) mobilization of calcium from bone to maintain serum calcium levels when oral intake is inadequate.

The vitamin is supplied by ingestion or through ultraviolet radiation. Sunlight converts a hormone (7-dehydrocholesterol) in the skin to vitamin D_3 (cholecalciferol). Vitamin D_3, whether ingested or synthesized in the skin, must be metabolized into an active form of vitamin D. Biochemical alterations called hydroxylation first occur in the liver, then in the kidneys.

Rickets may be caused by a poor dietary intake of vitamin D or because of lack of exposure to sunlight. Black children are particularly susceptible to rickets either due to their skin pigmentation or because of inadequate penetration of sunlight (Barness, 1987). Other circumstances that may produce rickets include (1) disorders of absorption in which vitamin D, calcium, or both are not absorbed; (2) hepatic disease, which may decrease absorption of vitamin D or calcium or interfere with hydroxylation of vitamin D_3; (3) kidney disease, which interferes in the production of active vitamin D; (4) genetic factors, as in familial vitamin D resistant rickets with hypophosphatemia (discussed in Chapter 50); (5) anticonvulsant therapy (the complication of rickets is a rare occurrence); or (6) administration of glucocorticoids (Barness, 1987) (glucocorticoids appear to be antagonistic to vitamin D in calcium transport).

Premature infants are especially prone to disturbances in vitamin D metabolism, primarily due to a lack of sufficient phosphate and calcium to adequately mineralize the rapidly growing bones. This occurs because during the last trimester, significant amounts of calcium and phosphate are transferred daily from mother to fetus. Even with formula feedings, preterm infants receive much less calcium and phosphate than they would have received in utero (Koo and Tsang, 1987).

Laboratory Findings. A series of physiologic processes account for the typical laboratory findings in rickets. Whether from faulty intake, or absorption, or inadequate sunlight, the vitamin D deficiency leads to impaired absorption of calcium and phosphorus, so that these minerals are lost in increasing amounts through urine and feces. Consequently, serum phosphorus concentration is usually lowered; serum calcium level is usually normal* or slightly reduced. Children with rickets also have elevated serum alkaline phosphatase levels. Elevation of this enzyme reflects increased osteoblastic activity. These laboratory findings are apparent before any histologic bone changes are noted.

Clinical Manifestations. An early clinical manifestation of rickets in an infant under 6 months of age is craniotabes. Craniotabes results from a thinning or softening of the skull, usually in the occipitoparietal area. The thin skull bone can be indented by pressing it with a finger and, on the release of pressure, it rebounds with a crackle like that of a ping-pong ball. After the first 6 months, it is more common to see frontal bossing (prominence of frontal and parietal bones) and delayed closure of the fontanels. Rachitic rosary (enlarged costochondral junction) may be palpable in the early stages of rickets and in later stages may be seen as well as felt (Barness, 1987).

In later stages of rickets, softening of the bones causes additional skeletal changes. The chest is pigeon-shaped (the sternum protrudes) and a depression is apparent along the lower border of the chest (Harrison's groove). This groove is produced by the pull of the diaphragm on the pliable rib structure (Rudolph, 1982). Deformities of the spinal column, including scoliosis, kyphosis, and lordosis, also occur in advanced stages of rickets. In children with lordosis, deformities of the pelvis frequently occur; in the past, such deformities caused dystocia (difficult labor) in women who have had rickets in infancy (Barness, 1987). Also, epiphyseal enlargements at the wrists and ankles can be seen or palpated as a "thickening" in these areas in the early phase of rickets, and later this enlargement becomes even more apparent. The enlarged epiphyses consist of cartilage and uncalcified bone tissue; therefore, they are not visible on an x-ray (Barness, 1987). With weight-bearing, bending of the femur, tibia, and fibula results in bowlegs (genu varum) or knock knees (genu valgum) during development of the legs in infancy and early childhood, a degree of genu varum and genu valgum is normal and should not be mistaken for rickets (see Chapter 6 for further discussion on assessment of the stages of normal development of the legs).

Severe vitamin D deficiency can result in certain delays in growth and development. The appearance of the deciduous teeth may be delayed and out of normal progression. The quality of both the deciduous and permanent teeth may be affected, especially that of the enamel. Poorly developed muscles may be cause for the persisting pot belly (usually a child slims after toddler years) and delayed development in skills such as standing and walking.

Therapeutic Management. Vitamin D deficiency rickets is treated with the oral administration of vitamin D (1500 to 5000 IU daily). Healing can be demonstrated on x-rays in 2 to 4 weeks after the beginning of treatment (except in vitamin D resistant rickets) (see Chapter 50) (Barness, 1987). Another method of treatment is to give a beginning single dose of 60,000 IU or 1500 μg of vitamin D. This results in more rapid healing, and the differentiation between vitamin D deficiency rickets and vitamin D resistant rickets can be made more rapidly. If no healing occurs, the rickets is probably resistant to vitamin D (Barness, 1987). Once healing is complete, 400 IU vitamin D or 10 μg (normal daily requirement) is administered daily.

Nursing Strategies: Early Identification Strategies. The nurse has an important role in the assessment of infants and children by contributing to the prevention and early detection of vitamin D deficiency. Although vitamin D deficiency may begin to have biochemical effects in the infant in the first few months of life, visible skeletal changes may not be identified until months later. Also, a newborn infant has some reserves of vitamin D that act as a temporary protection in the event of dietary deficiency, but a history of the early diet is essential to identify those children at risk. The nurse can play a preventive role by recommending vitamin D supplementation for premature infants, artificially fed infants who do not receive vitamin D fortified formula, and infants who are breastfed. The Committee on Nutrition of the American Academy of Pediatrics (1980) has recommended that when the mother's vitamin intake is deficient and the infant's exposure to sunlight is inadequate, infants should receive vitamin D supplementation. The recommended requirement is 10 μg or 400 IU/day. The nurse should particularly assess for vitamin D defi-

*The serum calcium level may be normal because as serum calcium level is lowered, parathyroidhormone is secreted. Parathyroidhormone mobilizes calcium and phosphorus from the bone but it increases renal tubular calcium reabsorption. Thus, the serum calcium concentration may ultimately be maintained at a normal level.

ciency in black children, who are more vulnerable to development of rickets than are non-blacks. It has also been reported that Asians required longer exposure to ultraviolet radiation to produce a response in vitamin D production that is similar to that of Caucasians (Belton, 1986). Environmental conditions also need to be assessed. Those children who live in heavy smog areas and who have limited opportunity to play outdoors and those living in temperate zones are more prone to vitamin D deficiency.

Complications and Prognosis. The nurse who cares for a child being treated for rickets must be on guard for various complications. Hypocalcemic tetany is a complication of rickets that requires the nurse to make provisions for the occurrence of seizures. If the large dose (60,000 IU or 1500 μg) vitamin D therapy regimen is used, calcium balance in the body is restored more quickly than when vitamin D is given in moderate daily doses. In any event, if hypocalcemic tetany does occur, it is treated with 5 to 10 ml of 10 per cent calcium gluconate administered intravenously. The nurse involved in such therapy assists in the careful monitoring of the heart rate to prevent bradycardia and cardiac arrest, which can result from too rapid an elevation of serum calcium level. Also, children with rickets are more prone to respiratory infections such as bronchitis or bronchopneumonia, pulmonary atelectasis due to chest deformities, and chronic gastrointestinal disturbances of diarrhea or constipation (Barness, 1987). These potential complications, identified early by the nurse, are important observations that can contribute to early treatment.

Some of the osseous changes that result from rickets may take months or years to disappear. In advanced cases, some permanent alterations may persist. The nurse's role during recovery thus varies according to the severity of the disease but continues to be one of attempting to prevent those complications to which the child is vulnerable, assisting the child and family to a healthy recovery, and preventing a repetition of circumstances that make the child vulnerable to rickets.

References

American Academy of Pediatrics, Committee on Nutrition: Fluoride supplementation. *Pediatrics* 1986; 77:758–761.

American Academy of Pediatrics, Committee on Nutrition: *Pediatric Nutrition Handbook.* 2nd ed. Elk Grove Village, IL, American Academy of Pediatrics, 1985.

American Dietetic Association: Position paper on the vegetarian approach to eating. *J Am Diet Assoc* 1980 July; pp 61–68.

Anderson JW: Plant fiber and blood pressure. *Ann Intern Med* 1983; 98:842–846.

Barness LA: Nutrition and nutritional disorders. *In* Behrman RE, Vaughan VC: *Nelson Textbook of Pediatrics.* 13th ed. Philadelphia, WB Saunders, 1987.

Beauchamp GK, et al: Modification of salt and taste. *Ann Intern Med* 1983; 98:763–769.

Belton NR: Rickets—not only the "English disease." *Acta Paediatr Scand* (Suppl) 1986; 323:68–75.

Brazelton TB, et al: The origins of reciprocity. *In* Lewis M, Rosenbaum L (eds): *The Effects of the Infant on Its Caregiver.* New York, Ivan Wille and Sons, 1974.

Brown JL: Hunger in the U.S. *Sci Am* 1987 Feb; 256(2):37–41.

Burtis G, Davis J, Martin S: *Applied Nutrition and Diet Therapy.* Philadelphia, WB Saunders, 1987.

Chandra RK: Nutritional deficiency, immune function and susceptibility to infection. *In* Yeung DL: *Essays on Pediatric Nutrition.* Ottawa, Canadian Public Health Association, 1981, pp 137–153.

Committee on Dietary Allowances, Food and Nutrition Board, National Research Council: *Recommended Dietary Allowances.* 9th ed. Washington, DC, National Academy of Sciences, 1980.

Committee on Nutrition, American Academy of Pediatrics: Commentary on breastfeeding and infant formula. *Pediatrics* 1976; 57:278–285.

Committee on Nutrition, American Academy of Pediatrics: Sodium intake of infants in the United States. *Pediatrics* 1981a; 68:444–445.

Committee on Nutrition, American Academy of Pediatrics: Nutritional aspects of obesity in infancy and childhood. *Pediatrics* 1981b; 68:880–883.

Committee on Nutrition, American Academy of Pediatrics: Toward a prudent diet for children. *Pediatrics* 1983; 71:78–80.

Committee on Nutrition, American Academy of Pediatrics: Prudent lifestyle for children: dietary fat and cholesterol. *Pediatrics* 1986; 78(3):521.

Creasy RK, Resnik R: *Maternal-Fetal Medicine; Principles and Practice.* Philadelphia, WB Saunders, 1984.

Cunningham AS: Morbidity in breast-fed and artificially fed infants II. *J Pediatr* 1979; 95:685–689.

Cunningham AS: Breast-feeding and health. *J Pediatr* 1986; 110:658–659.

Dietz WH: Obesity in infancy. *In* Howard RB, Winter HS: *Nutrition and Feeding of Infants and Toddlers.* Boston, Little, Brown, 1984, pp 297–307.

Dobbing J: Infant nutrition and later achievement. *Nutr Rev* 1984; 42(1):1–7.

Feingold BF: Why Your Child Is Hyperactive. New York, Random House, 1975.

Filer LJ: Early nutrition: its long-term role. *Hosp Pract* 1978 Feb; 13(2):87–95.

Fomon SJ: *Infant Nutrition.* 2nd ed. Philadelphia, WB Saunders, 1974.

Fomon SJ, et al: Recommendations for feeding normal infants. *Pediatrics* 1979; 63:52–59.

Fomon SJ, Ziegler EE: Prevention of obesity. *In Nutritional Disorders of Children.* Washington, DC, US Department of Health, Education, and Welfare, No. (HSA) 78-5104, 1976.

Fox J, Elsberry C: *Primary Health Care of the Young.* New York, McGraw-Hill, 1980.

Garn SM, Clark DC: Nutrition, growth, development, and maturation: findings from the Ten-State Nutrition Survey of 1968–1970. *Pediatrics* 1975; 56:306–319.

Golden MP, et al: Obesity and socioeconomic class in children and their mothers. *J Dev Behav Pediatr* 1983 Jun; 4(2):113–118.

Hellebostad T, et al: Vitamin D deficiency rickets and vitamin B_{12} deficiency in vegetarian children. *Acta Paediatr Scand* 1985; 74:191–195.

Hughes JG, Griffith JF: *Synopsis of Pediatrics.* 6th ed. St. Louis, CV Mosby, 1984.

Jeffrey DB, et al: The development of children's eating habits: The role of television commercials. *Health Educ Q* 1982 Summer/Fall; 9(2,3):78, 174–193, 189.

Kaplowitz P, Isley RB: Marasmus-kwashiorkor in an 8-week-old infant with prolonged clear liquids for diarrhea. *Clin Pediatr* 1979 Sep; 18:5–75.

Kaye K: Towards the origin of dialogue. *In* Schaffer HR (ed): *Studies in Mother-Infant Interaction.* New York, Academic Press, 1977.

Koo WWK, Tsang RC: Calcium and magnesium homeostasis in the newborn. *In* Avery GB (ed): *Neonatology: Pathophysiology and Management of the Newborn.* 3rd ed. Philadelphia, JB Lippincott, 1987.

Krause MV, Mahan LK: *Food, Nutrition and Diet Therapy.* 7th ed. Philadelphia, WB Saunders, 1984.

Krieger I: *Pediatric Disorders of Feeding, Nutrition and Metabolism.* New York, John Wiley & Sons, 1982.

Lipton MA, Mayo JP: Diet and hyperkinesis—an update. *J Am Diet Assoc* 1983; 83:132.

MacLean WC, Graham G: *Pediatric Nutrition in Clinical Practice.* Reading, MA, Addison-Wesley, 1982.

Markesbery BA, Wong WM: Watching baby's diet: a professional and parental guide. *Am J MCN* 1979 May/Jun; 4(3):177–180.

Marsh AG, et al: Cortical bone density of adult lacto-ovo-vegetarian and omnivorous women. *J Am Diet Assoc* 1980 Feb; 76:148–151.

Mauer AM: Malnutrition—still a common problem for children in the United States. *Clin Pediatr* 1975; 14(1):23–24.

Owen GM, et al: A study of nutritional status of pre-school children in the United States, 1968–1970. *Pediatrics* 1974; 53:597–646.

Pipes PL: *Nutrition in Infancy and Childhood.* 3rd ed. St. Louis, CV Mosby, 1985.

Pradilla A: Nutrition: facts and hopes. *World Health.* 1984 Oct; pp 2–4.

Reddy BS: Dietary factors and cancer of the large bowel. *Semin Oncol* 1976; 3:351.

Rowe NR: Childhood obesity: growth charts vs. calipers. *Pediatr Nurs* 1980 Mar/Apr; p 24.

Roy CC, Galeano N: Childhood antecedents of adult degenerative disease. *Pediatr Clin North Am* 1985 Apr; 32:517–533.

Rudolph A: *Pediatrics.* New York, Appleton-Century-Crofts, 1982.

Rudy DA: Vegetarian diets for children. *Pediatr Nurs* 1984 Sep/Oct; 10(5):329–333.

Smith NJ: Nutrition in infancy and childhood including obesity. *In* Smith DW (ed): *Introduction to Clinical Pediatrics.* Philadelphia, WB Saunders, 1977.

Stanfield JP: The influence of malnutrition on development. *Practitioner* 1982 Nov; 226:1929–1940.

Taitz LS: Obesity in pediatric practice: infantile obesity. *Pediatr Clin North Am* 1977 Feb; 24:107–115.

US Department of Health, Education, and Welfare: Ten-State Nutrition Survey 1968–1970. Washington, DC, DHEW Publication No. (HSM) 72-8130, Centers for Disease Control, 1972.

Vander AJ, et al: *Human Physiology—The Mechanism of Body Function.* New York, McGraw-Hill, 1980.

Wynder EL, et al: Diet and cancer of the gastrointestinal tract. *Adv Intern Med* 1977; 22:397–419.

Bibliography

Bragdon DB: A basis for the nursing management of feeding the premature infant. *JOGN Nurs* (suppl) 1983 May/Jun; 12:51s–57s.

Burson JZ, Brannigan N: The use of play in the nutritional support of hospitalized children. *Issues Compr Pediatr Nurs* 1984; 7:283–289.

Burt BA, Ismail AI: Diet, nutrition, and food cariogenicity. *J Dent Res* 1986 Dec (special issue); 65:1475–1484.

Chandra RK: Nutrition and immunity: practical applications of research findings. *Can Fam Physician* 1987 Jun; 33:1417–1420.

Chase HP: Kwashiorkor in the United States. *Pediatrics* 1980; 66:972.

Contento M: Children's thinking about food and eating—a Piagetian-based study. *J Nutr Educ* (suppl) 1981; 13(1):86–90.

Cooper A: Nutritional assessment of the pediatric patient. *Am J Clin Nutr* (suppl) 1982; 35:1132–1141.

Curtis JA, et al: Nutritional rickets in vegetarian children. *Can Med Assoc J* 1983 Jan 15; 128:150–152.

Davis SS: A nutritional education program for pre-school children. *J Nutr Educ* 1983 Mar; 15(1):4–5.

D'Onofrio CN, Singer R: Unplanned nutrition education in the schools: sugar in elementary reading texts. *J School Health* 1983 Nov; 53(9):521–526.

Ellerstein NS, Ostrov BE: Growth patterns in children hospitalized because of caloric-deprivation failure to thrive. *Am J Dis Child* 1985 Feb; 139:164–166.

Forsyth BWC, et al: Mother's perception of problems of feeding and crying behaviors. *Am J Dis Child* 1985 Mar; 139:269–272.

Galler JR, et al: The influence of early malnutrition on subsequent behavioral development. IV. Soft neurologic signs. *Pediatr Res* 1984; 18:826–832.

Glueck CG, Morrison JA: Relationships of pediatric nutrients to lipids, lipoproteins, and ultimate risk of atherosclerosis. *Pediatr Ann* 1981; 10(11):45–51.

Green ML, Harry J: *Nutrition in Contemporary Nursing Practice.* New York, John Wiley & Sons, 1981.

Guthrie HA, Sheehe MP: Nutrition messages in elementary school textbooks. *J School Health* 1984 Mar; 54(3):126–127.

Hanning RM, Zlotkin SH: Unconventional eating practices and their health implications. *Pediatr Clin North Am* 1985 Apr; 32(2):429–445.

Hegsted DM: What is a healthful diet? *Primary Care* 1982 Sep; 9(3):445–473.

Helsing E: Malnutrition in an affluent society. *World Health* 1984 Oct; pp 14–15.

Hertzler AA: Children's food patterns—a review. I. Food preferences and feeding problems. II. Family and group behavior. *J Am Diet Assoc* 1983; 83(5):551–554; 555–560.

Jaycox W, et al: Theory-based health education activities for third to sixth grade children. *J School Health* 1983 Dec; 53(10):584–588.

Johnston P: Getting enough to grow on. *Am J Nurs* 1984 Mar; 84(3):336–339.

Keusch GT: Immune function in the malnourished host. *Pediatr Ann* 1982 Dec; 11(2):1004–1014.

Kramer MS: Do breast-feeding and delayed introduction of solid foods protect against subsequent obesity? *J Pediatr* 1981 Jun; 98(6):883–887.

Laing IA, Glass EJ, Hendry GMA, et al: Rickets of prematurity: calcium and phosphorus supplementation. *J Pediatr* 1985; 106:265–268.

Larson-Brown LB: Nutritional education: How to get students to eat it up. *Health Educ* 1983 Jan/Feb; 14(1):38–41.

Lowe CU, et al: Reflections of dietary studies with children in the ten-state survey of 1968–1970. *Pediatrics* 1975 Aug; 56(2):306–326.

MacLean WC, Graham GG: Vegetarianism in Children. *Am J Dis Child* 1980 May; 134(5):513–519.

Mila PJ: The weanling's gut. *Acta Paediatr Scand* (suppl) 1986; 323:5–13.

Phillips MG: Nutrition education for preschoolers: the Head Start experience. *Children Today* 1983 Jul/Aug; 12(4):20–24.

Register UD, Sonnenberg LM: The vegetarian diet. *J Am Diet Assoc* 1973 Mar; 62(3):253–260.

Rowe KS: Annotation—food additives. *Austr Pediatr J* 1974 Aug; 20(3):171–174.

Santos JI, et al: Nutrition, infection and immunity. *Pediatr Ann* 1983 Mar; 12(3):182–194.

Shamberger R: The subtle signs of chronic vitamin undernutrition: fat-soluble vitamins. *Diagn Med* 1984; 7(3):75–78, 80, 82.

Skinner JE, Woodburn MJ: Nutrition knowledge of teenagers. *J School Health* 1984 Feb; 54(2):71–74.

Sinatra F, Merritt P: Iatrogenic kwashiorkor in infants. *Am J Dis Child* 1981; 135:21–23.

Zerfas AJ, et al: Office assessment of nutritional status. *Pediatr Clin North Am* 1977 Feb; 24(1):253–271.

Promoting Dental Health — Chapter 19

Jo Joyce Anderson
Mabel Hunsberger

Tooth development begins during the prenatal period and is influenced by the mother's health status. A pediatric nurse often has the opportunity to provide health information to pregnant mothers of children they care for. Dental health care also is promoted as the nurse teaches parents how to care for their baby's teeth. This chapter reviews the sequence of eruption and shedding of teeth and describes the main components of a dental assessment and the nurse's role in teaching parents and children how to care for teeth properly.

Introduction of a child to care by a dentist is an important experience in a child's life. This chapter reviews the techniques that can be used to obtain the child's cooperation and to reduce the likelihood of establishing lifelong negative memories. The special approaches required by children with disabilities are also addressed.

Finally, the actions that can be taken to prevent *specific* dental problems are discussed, with a description of how the various dental problems occur and a review of selected forms of therapy.

Related Topics
Effects of teething, Chapter 5
Assessment of teeth, Chapter 15

Tooth Development and Eruption

Dental development during childhood involves the eruption of two sets of teeth, deciduous and permanent (Fig. 19-1). There are 20 deciduous teeth, also called primary or baby teeth. These are gradually replaced by 32 permanent teeth.

Tooth eruption varies among children. Genetic factors are the major sources of differences between individuals in tooth development and eruption. For example, siblings tend to resemble each other more in the timing of eruption than do unrelated individuals. Tooth development in females is slightly ahead of that in males, as is that of United States blacks when compared with whites.

Although variation in eruption is normal, the sequence of shedding of primary teeth and emergence of permanent teeth is important to proper occlusion; that is, the alignment of the chewing surface of the maxillary (upper) teeth to the mandibular (lower) teeth

Promoting Dental Health

Nursing Diagnoses	Nursing Goals/Strategies
Potential knowledge deficit: care of deciduous teeth, related to: • *lack of exposure to information* • *lack of recall* • *information misinterpretation* • *cognitive limitation* • *lack of motivation to learn*	Provide information about the importance of teeth of the infant and child. Teach basics of dental care to parents and child as appropriate: • Clean the teeth of infants. • Avoid putting child to bed with bottle containing sugary liquid or milk. • Limit intake of foods with high sugar content. • Supplement with fluoride as necessary (see Table 19–1). • Take child to dentist by 2 years of age. (Some recommend 1 year of age). Provide information to child as appropriate for age and setting (use teaching opportunities in school, camp, or other settings). Explain relationship of healthy deciduous teeth to later dental health. Reinforce information on each subsequent visit.
Potential self-care deficit: dental care, related to: • *lack of necessary developmental skills to perform care* • *lack of opportunity to practice skills* • *lack of knowledge* • *lack of appropriate equipment and supplies*	Promote self-care of teeth as appropriate for age. Encourage parents to: • Teach toddlers to brush teeth. • Monitor brushing by toddlers and preschoolers. • Use disclosing tablets to show children whether brushing is adequate. • Teach 8- to 9-yr-olds to floss teeth. • Role model regular dental care. • Foster child's independence in dental care, beginning in the toddler years. • Have appropriate-size brush, dental floss, and mirror available for child to use. • Give fluoride supplement as required (see Table 19-1). • If sweet snacks are permitted, offer them *with* meals rather than between meals. Provide assistance with equipment and teaching for children with physical or developmental disabilities.
Potential for fear development: dental visit, related to: • *learned response as modeled by parents or siblings* • *separation from support systems* • *knowledge deficit* • *forboding appearance of equipment* • *lack of preparation*	Allay child's fears of visiting the dentist. Encourage parents to: • Permit child to accompany parents on a dentist visit to observe. • Provide factual and sensory information about the environment and painful stimuli. • Stay with child during the dental examination.
Potential impaired skin integrity: gums and mouth, related to: • *inadequate brushing and flossing of teeth*	Maintain skin integrity of gums and mouth. Teach family to: • Teach child proper brushing techniques. • Monitor and periodically supervise child's brushing and flossing techniques. • Provide healthy diet. • Restrict child's sugar intake. • Maintain regular dentist appointments.

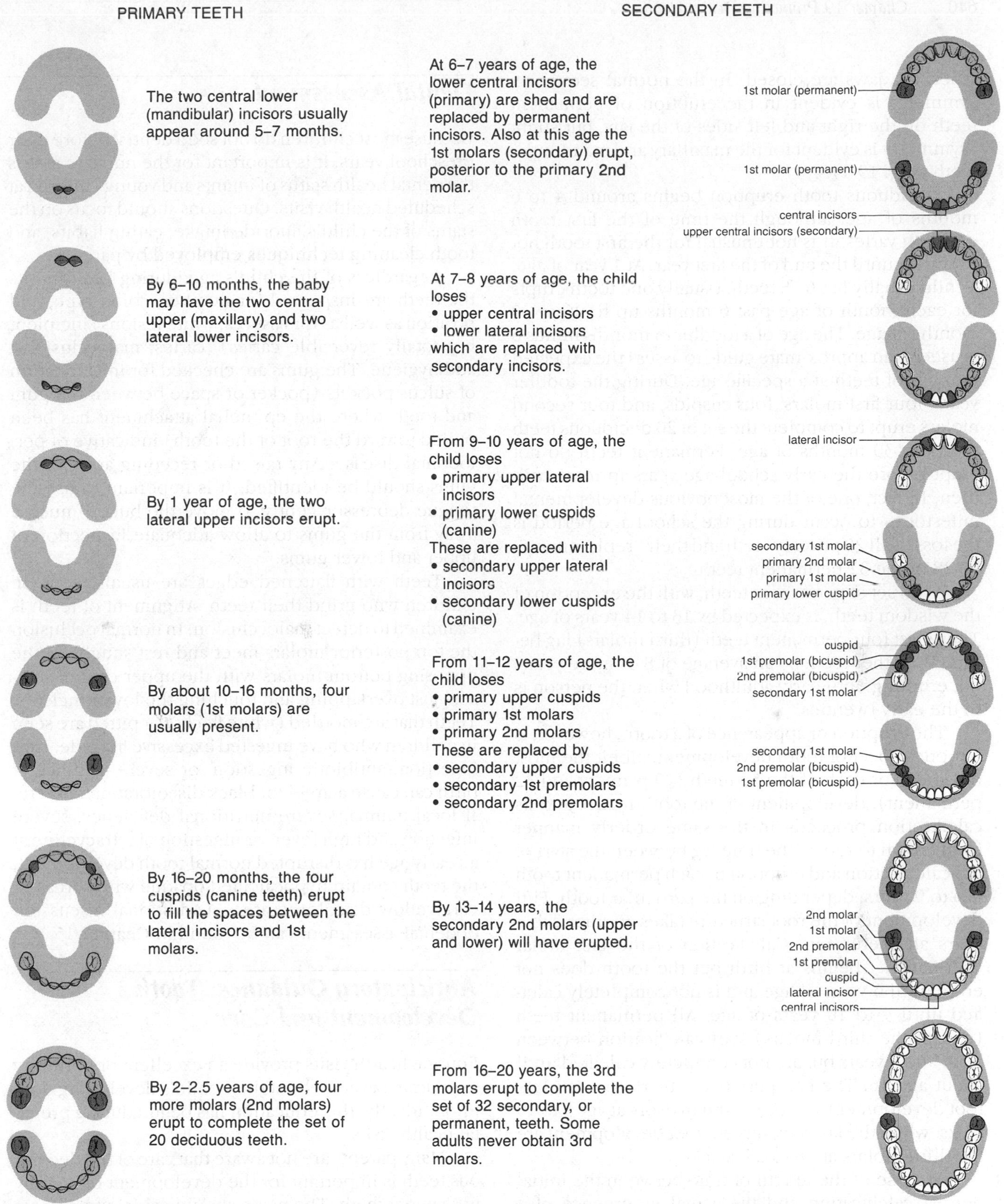
PRIMARY TEETH
SECONDARY TEETH
The two central lower (mandibular) incisors usually appear around 5–7 months.
By 6–10 months, the baby may have the two central upper (maxillary) and two lateral lower incisors.
By 1 year of age, the two lateral upper incisors erupt.
By about 10–16 months, four molars (1st molars) are usually present.
By 16–20 months, the four cuspids (canine teeth) erupt to fill the spaces between the lateral incisors and 1st molars.
By 2–2.5 years of age, four more molars (2nd molars) erupt to complete the set of 20 deciduous teeth.
At 6–7 years of age, the lower central incisors (primary) are shed and are replaced by permanent incisors. Also at this age the 1st molars (secondary) erupt, posterior to the primary 2nd molar.
At 7–8 years of age, the child loses
• upper central incisors
• lower lateral incisors
which are replaced with secondary incisors.
From 9–10 years of age, the child loses
• primary upper lateral incisors
• primary lower cuspids (canine)
These are replaced with
• secondary upper lateral incisors
• secondary lower cuspids (canine)
From 11–12 years of age, the child loses
• primary upper cuspids
• primary 1st molars
• primary 2nd molars
These are replaced by
• secondary upper cuspids
• secondary 1st premolars
• secondary 2nd premolars
By 13–14 years, the secondary 2nd molars (upper and lower) will have erupted.
From 16–20 years, the 3rd molars erupt to complete the set of 32 secondary, or permanent, teeth. Some adults never obtain 3rd molars.
1st molar (permanent)
1st molar (permanent)
central incisors
upper central incisors (secondary)
lateral incisor
secondary 1st molar
primary 2nd molar
primary 1st molar
primary lower cuspid
cuspid
1st premolar (bicuspid)
2nd premolar (bicuspid)
secondary 1st molar
secondary 1st molar
2nd premolar (bicuspid)
1st premolar (bicuspid)
2nd molar
1st molar
2nd premolar
1st premolar
cuspid
lateral incisor
central incisors
newly erupted primary teeth
previously erupted primary teeth
newly erupted (secondary) teeth
primary teeth
previously erupted (secondary) teeth

Figure 19-1. Development of teeth. A combination of primary and secondary teeth is present in the child's mouth simultaneously during the process of eruption and shedding.

when the jaws are closed. In the normal sequence, symmetry is evident in the eruption of permanent teeth on the right and left sides of the jaw, but slight asymmetry is evident for the maxillary and mandibular teeth (Fig. 19-1).

Deciduous tooth eruption begins around 4 to 6 months of age, although the time of the first tooth eruption varies. It is not unusual for the first tooth not to appear until the end of the first year. At 1 year of age, a child usually has 6–8 teeth. Usually one tooth erupts for each month of age past 6 months up to 26 to 30 months of age. The age of a toddler in months minus 6 is used as an approximate guide to assess the expected number of teeth at a specific age. During the toddler years, four first molars, four cuspids, and four second molars erupt to complete the set of 20 deciduous teeth by about 30 months of age. Permanent teeth do not erupt before the early school-age years in most children. In fact, one of the most obvious developmental milestones to occur during the school-age period is the loss of all 20 primary teeth and their "replacement" by 28 of the 32 permanent teeth.

A full set of permanent teeth, with the exception of the wisdom teeth, is expected by 13 to 14 years of age. These last four permanent teeth (third molars) lag behind the other teeth by an average of 8 or more years, not erupting until early adulthood when the person is in the early twenties.

The eruption or appearance of a tooth, however, is but one aspect of tooth development, albeit the most obvious. For each of the 52 teeth (20 primary and 32 permanent), development of the tooth matrix and its calcification proceeds in the same orderly manner from crown to roots. The time lag between the start of the calcification and eruption of each permanent tooth is 6 to 9 years, depending on the particular tooth. Full development of the root structure takes another 2 to 4 years after eruption. Calcification of the first molar (permanent) begins at birth but the tooth does not erupt until 6 years of age and is not completely calcified until 9 to 10 years of age. All permanent teeth (except the third molars) start calcification between birth and 3 years but are not completely calcified until about age 16. The first permanent teeth to complete root development are the central incisors at age 9 to 10 years, while the last to complete root development are the third molars at 18 to 25 years.

Because of the length of time between the initiation of calcification and the actual emergence of a tooth, its soundness at eruption is not as dependent on current health and nutritional status as on previous health status. Because teeth and bones are of different embryologic origins, there is little correlation between stature or onset of puberty with tooth development. Tooth development, therefore, seems relatively independent of other body systems (Demirjian, 1978).

Dental Assessment

Because most children do not see a dentist before their preschool years, it is important for the nurse to assess the dental health status of infants and young children at scheduled health visits. Questions should focus on the status of the child's fluoride intake, eating habits, and tooth cleaning techniques employed by parents.

Regardless of the child's age, during health visits the teeth are inspected for number, color, type, and position as well as for fissures, white lesions (incipient but totally reversible caries), caries, malocclusions, and hygiene. The gums are checked for inflammation of sulcus pockets (pocket or space between the gum and tooth where the epithelial attachment has been pulled toward the root of the tooth) indicative of periodontal disease. Any raised or receding areas of the gums should be identified. It is important to use the tongue depressor gently to move the buccal mucosa away from the gums to allow adequate inspection of upper and lower gums.

Teeth with flattened edges are usually seen in children who grind their teeth. Alignment of teeth is examined to detect malocclusion. In normal occlusion the top posterior molars meet and rest snugly on the opposing bottom molars with the upper central incisors just overlapping and touching the lower incisors. Teeth that are mottled (white flecks) or pitted are seen in children who have ingested excessive fluoride. Iron ingestion, antibiotic ingestion, or severe jaundice at birth can cause a green or black discoloration of teeth. If local trauma, severe nutritional deficiency, severe infection and high fever, or ingestion of tetracycline at an early age has disrupted normal tooth development, the teeth contain hypocalcified opaque white areas or dark-yellow discolored areas. (Additional discussion of dental assessment can be found in Chapter 15.)

Anticipatory Guidance: Tooth Development and Care

Routine health visits provide an excellent opportunity to educate parents about their child's developing dentition. Ideally, this education has begun during prenatal health visits.

Many parents are not aware that care of the deciduous teeth is important for the development of healthy permanent teeth. The nurse should explain to parents that ossification and formation of the permanent teeth take place all through childhood, long before and for some time after the teeth are visible. Preservation of these primary teeth is important to maintain proper spacing for the permanent teeth, to prevent decay in forming permanent tooth buds, and for chewing. In particular, the temporary 6-year molar stabilizes the dental arch and affects the ultimate shape of the jaw (Litt and Vaughn, 1987). Optimal fluoride requirements, nutritional factors, the importance of early cleaning, and the time for initial dental visits should be discussed. Information should be offered about the eruption of teeth and possible effects of teething (see Chapter 5), the effects of digital habits beyond age 6 on occlusion, development, and a description of dental disease and its effect on teeth and gums. Over 50 per cent of all children under the age of 2 have already experienced dental decay (Forrester, 1978). Twenty-five per cent of school-age children are reported to have five or more teeth that are decayed, filled, or missing (Hermann and Roberts, 1987). This presents a serious challenge to nurses to not only give information but also spend the necessary time for explanation and follow-up that will help parents to provide early preventive dental care. The tedious care of a child's teeth requires that parents believe in its value; otherwise short-cuts will likely be taken.

Guidelines for care of the teeth should be discussed with parents initially when the child is a newborn infant and readdressed during each phase of childhood. Thus, the nurse's role in dental guidance is not a one-time teaching event, but one in which dental care is stressed regularly and from various perspectives. As cognitive and motor skills develop, the child should become increasingly involved in learning about preventive practices and in assuming responsibility for his or her own dental health.

General Maintenance

Adequate dental maintenance includes proper tooth cleaning, adequate fluoride intake, regular visits to a dentist, and a balanced dietary intake that limits fermentable carbohydrates.

Tooth Cleaning

To protect the first teeth, the gums and teeth can be massaged with a soft, moist, clean cloth after each feeding. A fluoride toothpaste (an amount about the size of a small pea) is applied to the cloth and all sides of each tooth wiped.

Toothbrushing is recommended by 18 months of age, when the gingival tissue is no longer so easily damaged and a considerable number of teeth are usually present. A toddler's teeth should be brushed twice a day, and parents should continue to assist with toothbrushing after the child begins to brush his or her own teeth. Toddlers will want to brush their own teeth by the age of 2, but they need supervision.

When toddlers brush their own teeth, they need to be taught not to chew on toothpaste tubes, because they may contain lead. An unsupervised toddler may eat toothpaste, possibly consuming excessive amounts of fluoride; therefore, parents should be cautioned to use only small amounts of toothpaste and keep the toothpaste out of a toddler's reach.

The nurse should speak directly to the toddler when teaching proper brushing technique. Both the child and parents should be instructed to avoid a vigorous back-and-forth scrubbing motion, which a 2-year-old child is prone to use. Short back-and-forth or simple up-and-down brushing is easier for a child to learn than is the rotary motion (Fig. 19-2). Because toddlers and preschoolers enjoy imitating, it is good for them to observe adults brushing. Parents should monitor the child's toothbrushing and should assist the older toddler or preschooler in brushing at least once a day. Most dentists encourage the use of dental floss to clean between the teeth once the spacing between teeth that exists in the infant and young child has disappeared. Usually flossing must be completed by the parent, since a great deal of manual dexterity is required (Fig. 19-3).

Although 6- to 8-year-olds usually do not possess the required fine motor skills to be totally responsible for flossing their teeth, they should be able to do a fairly adequate job of brushing them. Children of this age lack the cognitive skills to appreciate the reasons for performing the preventive measures (i.e., increasing resistance of tooth to acid, reducing bacterial activity, and reducing the amount of fermentable carbohydrates in the mouth) and are not future-oriented enough to appreciate preventive practices. However, these children are still very dependent on adults and look to parents and teachers for guidance. Good dental health practices instituted at this age will be followed because they are the "thing to do" or the "rules." Parents should check the adequacy of the child's technique. Teachers as well can be very influential and effective during this period in promoting good dental health practices.

From the age of 9 years on, the child has sufficient fine motor and cognitive skills and is future-oriented enough not only to assume total responsibility for dental health practices but also to understand simple explanations and appreciate the rationale for preventive dental health practices. By this age, a child is also able to employ the rotary-motion brushing technique. Effectiveness of brushing at any age can be tested by use of disclosing tablets or by painting teeth with food coloring that stains the plaque. The child can then be instructed to correct the brushing technique to include the areas where plaque has formed. Children can also be encouraged by providing positive feedback to reinforce correct flossing and brushing techniques (see

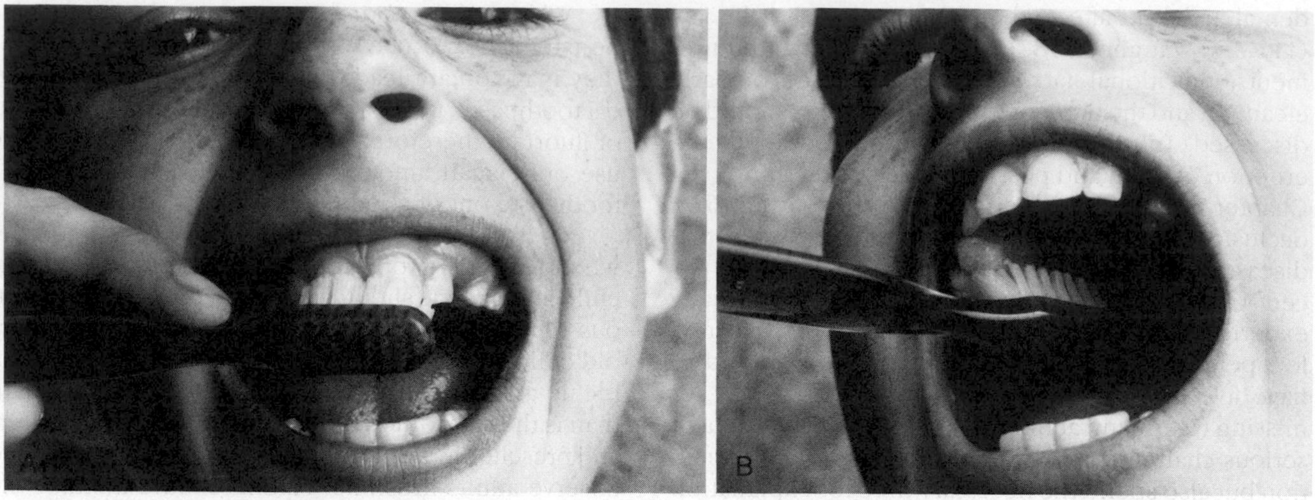

Figure 19-2. Proper brushing. Short back-and-forth or simple up-and-down brushing is easier for a child to learn than is rotary motion. (Photos by Ken Kasper.)

Fig. 19-2 for proper flossing). Dahlquist and coworkers (1985) demonstrated clinically significant plaque reduction by use of behavioral intervention including instruction and rewards.

Fluoride Ingestion

An adequate supply of fluoride is needed to help prevent cavities. Fluoride is provided in most communities through the water supply system at a concentration of 1 part per million (ppm). Some schools add fluoride to their drinking water in areas where local water lacks fluoride. In communities where water is not fluoridated, a daily supplement of sodium fluoride should be given orally for healthy development of the permanent teeth buds in the gums. Table 19-1 describes the amount of fluoride supplement desirable on the basis of age and fluoride content of the water.

Topical application of stannous fluoride is available through the dentist, in tooth dentifrices and in fluoride mouth rinse. Due to its mottling effect if taken in excessive amounts, parents should be cautioned against using more than the prescribed dose of fluoride. The nurse should be prepared to discuss up-to-date findings pertaining to use of fluoride. Recommendations are periodically provided by the American Academy of Pediatrics (1986) and the American Dental Association (1984).

Dental Visits

Dentists' views vary regarding the frequency of routine dental visits. Decisions about when a child's initial visit should occur and how often asymptomatic children need visits should be based on the child's overall health status, family dental history, and the availability of systemic fluorides. Most dentists agree, however, that the first visit to the dentist should be made by 2 years of age, preferably before any dental work needs to be done. A first visit no later than 12 months of age is recommended by some authorities (Goepferd, 1986) to initiate preventive measures and intercept potential problems. The American Academy of Pediatrics encourages dental visits to be initiated 6 months after the first primary tooth erupts, if the infant's history reflects any of the following: (1) a high risk factor in any aspect of the child's health status since birth; (2) no systemic fluoride being ingested; or (3) a family history of dental disease. Unless at high risk for dental disease, asymptomatic children may be sufficiently monitored with dental visits annually and at any time the parents notice a problem.

A cooperative dentist will let the young child look around the office, ride up and down in the dental chair, and become familiar with the instruments. The dentist's approach to the child can greatly influence future visits. Many children's books are available to prepare children for routine dental visits as well as for specific dental procedures. Books should be evaluated for accuracy before they are shared with the child (see Smardo et al, 1983, for a list of evaluated books).

Adolescent years are peak years for dental caries, and yet preventive and therapeutic treatment by dental professionals is one of the most neglected needs of teenagers. Dental care is often a low financial priority of families. Several important reasons exist for making the repair and maintenance of adolescents' teeth a priority. Adequate nutrition is nearly impossible when teeth hurt or are missing. Fresh fruit and vegetables, for example, are difficult to eat with missing, aching, or decayed teeth. Appearance is extremely important to teenagers; teens with decayed teeth usually have problems with self-esteem, while healthy white teeth help the teenager develop a positive self-concept.

Dietary Habits

A diet that is low in sweets and high in nutritious food should be stressed for sound dental health. Natural snacks should be encouraged such as fresh fruit, raw vegetables, cheese, and popcorn. When a child chews gum, it should be the sugar-free variety. A classic study showing the relationship between dietary factors and etiology of dental caries is the Swedish Vipeholm study (Wei, 1981). This study showed a higher risk of caries with increased carbohydrate intake, the risk being greatest when the carbohydrate was sticky or when it was eaten between meals rather than with meals. This finding has been confirmed in numerous other studies since the Vipeholm study.

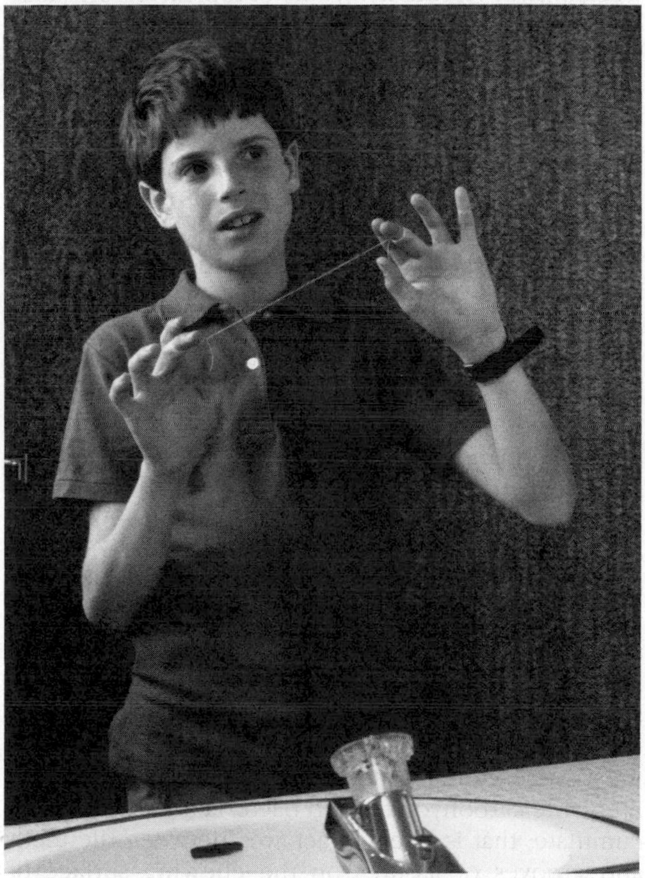

***Figure* 19-3.** Flossing of teeth. Instituting flossing during the early school years introduces a preventive practice that is required for a lifetime. (Photo by Ken Kasper.)

***Table* 19-1.** Fluoride Supplementation Schedule for Infants and Children

Age (yr)	Fluoride Concentration in Local Water Supply (ppm)		
	<0.3	0.3–0.7	>0.7
0–2	0.25*	0	0
2–3	0.50	0.25	0
3–16	1.00	0.50	0

*Values are milligrams of fluoride supplement per day. Supplementation should begin in the first 2 weeks after birth.
(From American Academy of Pediatrics, 1986.)

Dental Care for the Handicapped Child

Children with disabilities may require special care to achieve dental health. The type of diet that is required may subject their teeth to a more caries-producing environment. For example, the carbohydrates in pureed foods tend to stick to the teeth where the bacteria in plaque can then use them to produce acids that result in tooth decay. Also, a disabled child may need to drink from a bottle for an extended period of time. Sometimes small frequent meals are required, thereby exposing teeth to a more continuous environment of food. Medications can also increase the potential for tooth decay. Not only the sugar base of many medications but also the actions of drugs themselves constitute factors that potentiate decay. For example, phenytoin (Dilantin) causes gum hyperplasia and periodontal problems, and sedatives, barbiturates, or antihistamines may reduce saliva flow, thus interfering with the natural washing effect of saliva.

An interprofessional approach is required to maintain dental health for many of these children. Careful planning of the dietary intake and medication administration, in conjunction with regular dental visits, is required. Learning to care for teeth independently is a difficult task for some children, thus requiring special approaches to assist parents and children. Special adaptations can be made, such as enlarging toothbrush handles with a bicycle handle or ball, to assist the child to brush teeth independently. The dentist, public health nurse, or medical supply services may provide additional assistance.

Dental Problems

The majority of dental problems can be prevented by adherence to the dental maintenance program just discussed. The nurse plays a major role in motivating parents to be responsible for their child's teeth in the early years and in teaching children progressive responsibility for personal care of their teeth to the extent they are developmentally able.

Bottle Mouth Syndrome

While the infant is still young, the nurse should encourage parents to prepare to wean their infant from bedtime bottles once tooth eruption begins. If the child still takes a bedtime bottle, encourage the parent to feed the whole bottle before the child falls asleep. However, if the older infant is accustomed to going to sleep with a bottle, plain water should be substituted for the milk or sugar-containing liquids. Otherwise, rampant decay may eventually occur, causing alterations in permanent teeth as well as great discomfort to the infant.

Bottle mouth syndrome is a tragic and unnecessary condition that may occur in older infants and toddlers who fall asleep with a bottle of milk or of another sweetened fluid in their mouth or who are breast-fed over prolonged periods at night. These fluids pool in the oral cavity, particularly around the upper front teeth. Frequent feedings of fermentable carbohydrates, especially sucrose, have been documented as a caries-producing practice. These carbohydrates are acted upon by mouth bacteria, particularly streptococci, and metabolic acids are produced. These acids decalcify the tooth enamel and destroy its protein structures, resulting in total destruction of the tooth. Early severe dental caries of the deciduous teeth result (Fig. 19-4). The lower front teeth are less involved, probably because they are protected by the tongue and the nipple.

Treatment is primarily preventive. Once tooth eruption begins, infants should not be permitted to sleep with a bottle containing anything other than water. Parents need considerable support to avoid the practice of putting their infant to bed with a bottle of juice or milk, especially when it is common practice among their associates. Despite evidence that this practice damages the teeth, it is reported that parents frequently place fluids other than water into bedtime bottles (Hitchens-Serota, 1986).

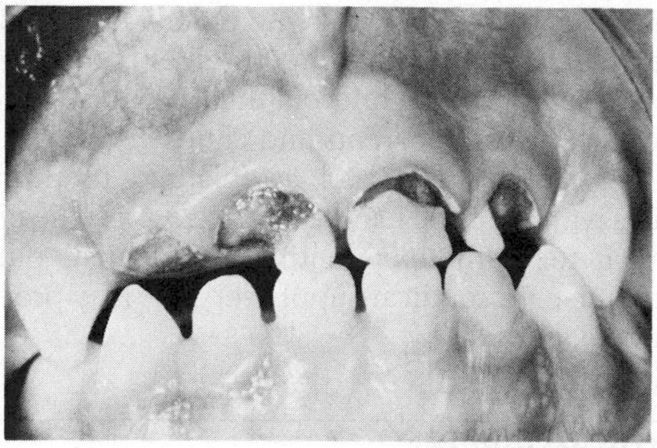

Figure 19-4. Clinical photograph of a 3-year-old suffering from "baby bottle syndrome." The four upper anterior teeth are severely decayed, while the rest of the mouth is caries free. This child always went to sleep at night with a bottle containing Kool-Aid. (From Caldwell RC, Stallard RE: *A Textbook of Preventive Dentistry.* Philadelphia, WB Saunders, 1977.)

Canker Sores

A canker sore is a small, painful, crater-like ulcer on the mucous membranes of the oral cavity, appearing singly or in groups. These ulcerations occur most often in the 10- to 20-year-old. Some people are more prone to develop the ulcers than others. Most children will call their parents' attention to a canker sore. There is no known cause of canker sores, although various etiologies are suspected, including food hypersensitivity, allergies, toxic drug reactions, endocrine factors, emotional stress, and trauma. It has also been suggested that an autoimmune reaction of the oral epithelium may cause ulcer formation. There is no specific treatment and the ulcers will heal spontaneously within a week or two. Viscous xylocaine or topical steroids may decrease the discomfort or shorten the course.

Dental Caries

By far the most important and prevalent dental problem is caries, affecting approximately 98 per cent of the population. The United States Commission of the International Year of the Child reported that 47 per cent of children under age 12 have never had any dental care (Sinkford, 1981). In addition, dental caries and malocclusions are interactive, with a major cause of tooth loss being decay from dental caries. This holds true for both premature loss of primary teeth and for loss of permanent teeth. Dental caries thus constitutes a problem of major significance.

The widely accepted explanation for the formation of dental caries is that the tooth enamel and dentin are decalcified by acidogenic (acid-forming) microorganisms, which are maintained in the mouth by fermentable carbohydrates (Fig. 19-5). The microorganisms most commonly involved are lactobacilli and aciduric streptococci, and the fermentable carbohydrates most commonly involved are sugars. The tooth surfaces most susceptible to attack are located where the fermentable carbohydrates and bacteria are prone to accumulate; that is, the contact area between the teeth and grooves or fissures on the chewing surface of teeth. This accumulation takes the form of plaque, a sticky transparent coating that becomes firmly attached to the tooth surface.

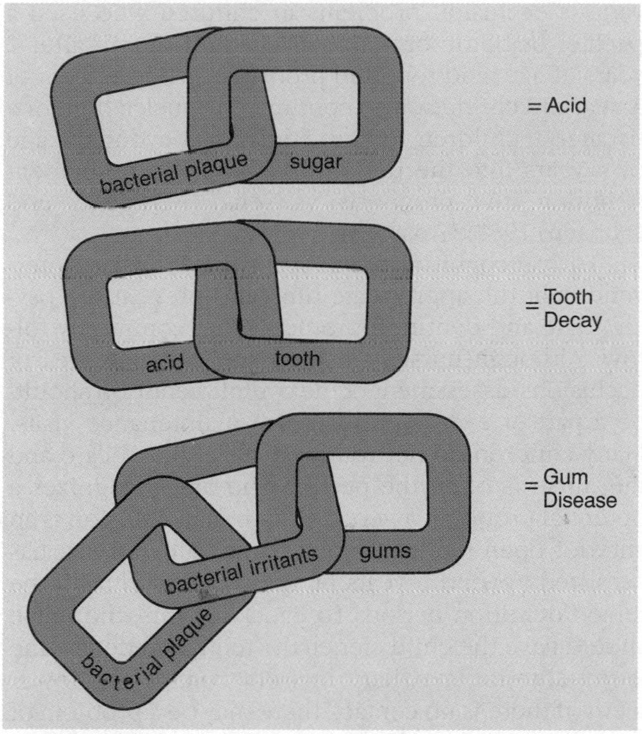

Figure 19-5. Showing the results of "poor brushing" as simple line drawings increases the child's understanding of abstract ideas.

This explanation for dental caries leads to a three-pronged approach to a prevention program: (1) increase the tooth's resistance to acids, (2) reduce the activity of microorganisms, and (3) reduce the amount of fermentable carbohydrates in the mouth. Preventive measures against dental caries and their effect are reviewed by Horowitz (1984).

The ingestion or topical application of fluoride increases the resistance of tooth enamel to acids. For maximum benefit, ingestion should be consistent throughout tooth development, which takes place throughout childhood.

Brushing and flossing remove caries-producing bacteria from the mouth and if done properly can contribute to the prevention of gum disease (Horowitz, 1984). Teeth should be brushed with a fluoride dentifrice after each meal if possible. Brushing before bedtime is especially important because the acid-producing activity of bacteria normally increases in the environment of the mouth during sleep. If brushing is not possible after eating, the mouth should be rinsed with water or an antimicrobial mouth rinse. To cleanse between the teeth where bacteria and plaque are likely to accumulate, dental floss or a water pic should be used at least once a day. A fluoride-containing mouth rinse swished through the mouth adds the advantage of getting some fluoride into the spaces between teeth.

Restoration of deep developmental grooves and fissures in the teeth and repair of cavities also reduce bacterial activity. The advent of the use of dental sealants, applied to the pits and fissures of the grindary surfaces of molars, can diminish the likelihood of tooth decay on the chewing surfaces, which is not completely prevented by fluoridation. Most studies indicate that if the sealant remains intact until the child is 6 months old, it is likely to remain for a number of years (Starr and Gravitz, 1985). The National Institute of Dental Research recommends the use of sealants to coat the teeth of most children, since decay of the chewing surfaces is the focal point of most juvenile tooth decay (Lyons, 1984).

A recent discovery of the genes responsible for the production of tooth enamel in the body is anticipated to advance greatly both the prevention and the treatment of dental caries. Altered yeast cells could be implanted in cavities, where they would grow cloned enamel crystals that would be virtually indistinguishable from normal tooth enamel. The result is a more attractive, longer-lasting tooth that is less sensitive to extremes of heat and cold (Lyons, 1984).

For children at high risk for tooth decay or in whom decay has already begun, semiannual visits to the dentist are recommended so that early repair and restoration are accomplished before extensive damage is done to the tooth.

Reducing the amount of fermentable carbohydrates in the mouth to prevent dental caries is a major nursing care goal. Minimal intake of sticky carbohydrates and elimination of snacks of fermentable carbohydrates between meals can reduce the incidence of tooth decay significantly. Such dietary restraints should be taught early since dietary habits, once established, are hard to change.

Periodontal Disease

The major cause of oral health problems and tooth loss is periodontal disease. While this is a disease of adults, children as young as 5 or 6 years of age can show beginning signs of it. Periodontal disease refers to an alteration "around the tooth." The gums, bones, and other structures that hold the teeth in place are affected.

Daily brushing and flossing are the major interventions to prevent periodontal disease. It is the collection of plaque on the teeth that causes the disease. When plaque is not removed daily, it hardens into calculus (or tartar) and collects under the gumline. A series of events then begins that eventually causes teeth to be lost. As more plaque forms on top of the calculus, brushing can no longer remove the underlying calculus. If the process continues, the plaque irritates the gums, leading to eventual gingivitis. Professional cleaning can reverse this condition, but if gingivitis continues, the final result is damage of structure that supports the teeth.

In periodontal disease, the irritated gums pull away from the teeth allowing the bacteria and pus to collect in pockets between the teeth and gums. This disease progresses slowly and can only be prevented by the establishment of rigorous dental care including brushing and flossing started during childhood. Children should be assessed for the warning signs of periodontal disease, which include

- gums that bleed during brushing
- gums that are pulled away from the teeth
- loose permanent teeth
- changes in the way teeth fit while biting
- bad breath
- pus that can be pushed out between teeth and gums when gums are pressed (American Dental Association, 1987)

The only strategy to prevent this disease is regular teeth cleaning. Because it is an insidious and initially painless disease, early detection through careful assessment is important. Habits such as nail biting or teeth grinding can make gums more susceptible to disease but the single major cause is inadequate cleaning.

Malocclusion

Dental orthodontia is a specialized area in dentistry in which malocclusions are treated. "Malocclusion" is a term used to describe the condition when the teeth of the upper and lower dental arches are not in proper alignment. If a severe malocclusion is present, the child may experience speech dysfluency, mastication problems, facial deformities, and eventual loss of teeth in adulthood. Significant psychologic problems often occur in the child with an untreated malocclusion (Klima et al, 1979). Peer or sibling rejection will perpetuate the child's poor body image.

Malocclusions are skeletal deformities of the mandible and maxilla, usually genetically caused (Klima et al, 1979). Skeletal facial development may predispose an individual to malocclusion: jaw bone size may not correspond to tooth size, the mandible may deviate posteriorly or may be hypertrophic, or the face may be asymmetrical. The child with premature loss or prolonged retention of primary teeth, or tooth loss that interferes with the normal chewing position, may also develop a bite problem. Nurses are often asked by concerned parents if their child's teeth will be damaged by thumb- or fingersucking. The likelihood of long-term effects from thumbsucking remains an area of controversy. Modier and colleagues (1982) noted various occlusion problems in children who used a pacifier or bottle or who sucked their thumb after 2 years of age, and reported problems in 30 per cent of 4-year-old children who continued to suck a digit or a pacifier. If children continue the habit beyond the age of 6 years into the period of mixed and permanent dentition, the prognosis worsens (Berkowitz and Johnson, 1987; Grossman, 1987).

Early recognition of malocclusion will allow intervention at the appropriate time and prevent the psychologic and dentition problems that commonly follow. Although nurses are not experts in the area of occlusions, assessment of the overall dentition should be a part of every child's health maintenance visits. Many children do not routinely have dental care and the nurse is often the person who first recognizes a potential problem. A very common malocclusion is an anterior open bite caused by digital sucking that has persisted beyond 6 years of age—that is, during the mixed dentition period. To check for this, the nurse should have the child clench the teeth and determine if the anterior maxillary incisors contact the lower teeth. If there is no contact, there may be a problem of occlusion. The presence of jumbled, crossed, or missing teeth should also alert the nurse to the possibility of an occlusion problem.

Convincing parents that a pedodontic or orthodontic referral is needed may be difficult, especially if the parent has not formerly recognized the problem or is not a firm believer in the necessity of dental care. An explanation of eventual long-term problems should be provided. Orthodontic treatment is expensive and many families cannot afford to receive treatment. Nurses may be able to help the family obtain financial help from community service groups or refer the child to a dental college that may provide treatment for a reduced fee.

Diagnosis should be made by a specialist in orthodontics or children's dentistry (pedodontist). Skull radiographs will be needed to establish the extent of the problem.

The child's acceptance of the need for treatment will depend on his or her prior experience with dentists and the child's present awareness of the problem. Children need a thorough explanation of the problem, including why treatment is necessary, although children who have been teased about their teeth will usually readily accept treatment.

Orthodontic treatment improves children's occlusion and thus their facial appearance. The type of treatment depends on the age of the child and the type of problem. Use of appliances, fixed or removable, is the usual treatment. Appliances are seldom used until the child reaches school age.

Removable acrylic appliances require a great deal of cooperation from the child, since it is the child who

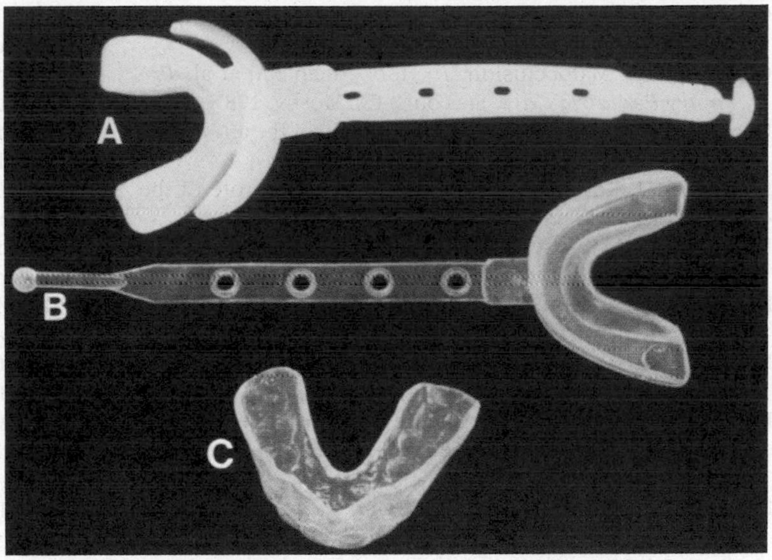

The wearing of a mouth guard while playing contact sports protects a child's teeth from unnecessary injury. *A*, stock mouth guard; *B*, mouth-formed protector; *C*, custom-fit mouth guard. (From Pinkham JR, et al: *Pediatric Dentistry: Infancy Through Adolescence.* Philadelphia, WB Saunders, 1988.)

is responsible for wearing the device and he or she may see the dentist only every 6 months. Children with fixed appliances are seen every 2 to 3 weeks. Headgear that provides cervical traction may be used to reduce the treatment time and aid in a more permanent occlusion correction (Orr, 1977).

Appliances require conscientious oral hygiene measures. Proper brushing after meals is necessary to prevent the development of caries beneath the appliance. School nurses can be helpful in encouraging the child to follow through on brushing and to reinforce intake of a nutritious diet. The child will also need verbal support that the treatment is effective. Pointing out the changes on x-ray films and taking periodic photographs are tangible means through which progress can be substantiated. Children may feel self-conscious wearing appliances around their peers and may need the encouragement of the school nurse and teacher to make the adjustment.

Dental Emergencies

Dental emergencies are rare, but they can happen. Parents should learn how their child's dentist can be reached if the unexpected happens. If a dentist is not accessible in an emergency, parents should be instructed to go to a hospital or clinic emergency room.

When a child knocks out a secondary tooth completely, the chances of implanting it are excellent *if* the child gets care within 30 minutes. Few teeth reimplanted after 2 hours survive (McTigue, 1988). The dislodged tooth should be rinsed gently, carefully avoiding any scraping of the root. The tooth should then be placed back in the socket and held in place by having the child bite on a wash cloth until emergency care is received. Such care should be sought immediately. If the tooth cannot be put back in place, it should be placed in milk and emergency care sought immediately. *Time is critical!* If a primary tooth is avulsed, it is not reimplanted because it could damage the underlying secondary tooth. A dentist is consulted because it may be necessary to provide treatment that maintains the space properly (Baker, 1987).

Dental emergencies are most often the result of sports injuries and children's rough-housing. Children who play contact sports such as football or soccer should wear mouth protectors. A catcher's mask should be worn by children who play catcher in softball or baseball. Children should be taught the consequences of pushing and shoving in general—and particularly around play equipment and at the water fountain.

References

American Academy of Pediatrics, Committee on Nutrition: Fluoride supplementation. *Pediatrics* 1986; 77:758–761.

American Dental Association: Fluoride compounds. *In Accepted Dental Therapeutics.* Chicago, American Dental Association, 1984.

Baker B: Emergency dental treatment for the family physician. *Can Fam Physician* 1987; 33:1521–1524.

Berkowitz RJ, Johnson DC: Malocclusion. *In* Behrman RE, Vaughan VC (eds): *Nelson Textbook of Pediatrics.* 13th ed. Philadelphia, WB Saunders, 1987.

Demirjian A: Dentition. *In* Falkner F, Tanner J (eds): *Human Growth.* Vol 2: *Postnatal Growth.* New York, Plenum Press, 1978.

Fluoridation and dental health. *Public Health Reports* (suppl). 1983 Sep/Oct: 94–97.

Forrester DJ: Preventive aspects of dental care. *In* Hoekelman RA, et al: *Principles of Pediatrics.* New York, McGraw-Hill, 1978.

Goepferd SJ: Infant oral health: a protocol. *J Dent Child* 1986;53(4):261–264.

Grossman LK: Malocclusion. *In* Hoekelman RA, et al: *Primary Pediatric Care.* St. Louis, CV Mosby, 1987.

Harris N. Controlling dental diseases: state of the art. *Health Values* 1984 Jan/Feb: 31–37.

Hermann HJ, Roberts MW: Preventive care: the role of the pediatrician. *Pediatrics* 1987; 80:107–110.

Hitchens-Serota J: Assessing parents' knowledge of pediatric dental disease. *Pediatr Nurs* 1986; 12:435–438, 464.

Horowitz AM: Community oriented preventive dental programs that work. *Health Values* 1984 Jan/Feb: 21–29.

Klima R, et al: Body image, self concept, and the orthodontic patient. *Am J Orthod* 1979 May; 507.

Litt IF, Vaughan VC: Growth and development. *In* Behrman RE, Vaughan VC (eds): Nelson Textbook of Pediatrics. Philadelphia, WB Saunders, 1987.

Lyons R: Look Ma, no cavities. *St. Louis Post Dispatch* 1984 March 25; 7.

McTigue DJ: Managing traumatic injuries in the young permanent dentition. *In* Pinkham JR, et al: *Pediatric Dentistry; Infancy Through Adolescence.* Philadelphia, WB Saunders, 1988.

Modier T, et al: Sucking habits and their relation to posterior crossbite in four year old children. *Scan J Dent Res* 1982; 90:323–330.

Orr F: Headgear. *In* Cohen M: *Minor Tooth Movement in the Growing Child* Philadelphia, WB Saunders, 1977.

Smardo F, et al: Looking critically at dental health books for children. *J School Health* 1983 Dec; 626–629.

Sinkford JC: Dental health needs of children and adolescents. *JADA* 1981; 103:901–905.

Starr RM, Gravitz RF: Pit and fissure sealants in the prevention of tooth decay. *Pediatr Nurs* 1985; 11:289–290.

Wei S: Nutrition, diet, fluoride and dental health. *Pediatr Basics* 1981 Aug; 30:4–7.

Bibliography

American Dental Association: Guide to dental health. *JADA* (Special Issue), 1987.

Ashton B, et al: Improving dental health education. Dental health knowledge. *Health Visitor* 1983 Oct; 362–363.

Christen AG: The development of positive dental health values. *Health Values* 1984 Jan/Feb; 5–12.

Cipes M, et al: Differences in dental experiences, practices and beliefs of inner city and suburban adolescents. *Am J Pub Health* 1983 Nov; 1305–1307.

Dahlquist LM, et al: The effects of behavioral intervention on dental flossing skills in children. *J Pediatr Psychol* 1985; 10:403–412.

Gillin M: Digital sucking and tongue thrusting in children. *Dent Clin North Am* 1979; 187.

Goepferd SJ: Infant oral health: a rationale. *J Dent Child* 1986; 53:257–260.

Ismail AI: Findings from the dental care supplement of the National Health Interview Survey, 1983. *JADA* 1987; 114:617–621.

Klein SP, et al: The cost and effectiveness of school-based preventive dental care. *Am J Pub Health* 1985; 75:382–391.

McDonald R, Avery D:*Dentistry for the Child and Adolescent.* St. Louis, CV Mosby, 1978.

Medford H, et al: Acute care of severe tooth fractures. *Ann Emerg Med* 1983 Jan; 364–366.

Misselman R: Oral facial development and oral habits. *Pediatr Basics* 1981 Aug; 30:12–14.

Nizel A: Preventing dental caries: the nutrition factors. *Pediatr Clin North Am* 1977 Feb; 141.

Nowak A: Infant dental care. *Pediatr Basics* 1981 Aug; 30:9–12.

Pinkham JR, et al: *Pediatric Dentistry; Infancy Through Adolescence.* Philadelphia, WB Saunders, 1988.

Schwaninger B, Vickers-Schwaninger N: Developing an effective oral hygiene program for the orthodontic patient: review, rationale and recommendations. *Am J Orthod* 1979 April; 447.

Weinstein P, et al: The use of nitrous oxide in the treatment of children: results of a controlled study. *JADA* 1986; 112:325–331.

Promoting Healthy Sleep Patterns

Chapter 20

Mabel Hunsberger

Sleep patterns change throughout the lifespan. The various states of sleep and arousal are now extensively studied in sleep laboratories. Electrophysiologic data are extending our understanding of the physiology and pathology of sleep states.

The sleep of neonates has received particular attention. Although pathologic sleep disorders are not widespread in children, getting a child to sleep and keeping the child asleep for the night consumes a large amount of parental energy. An improved understanding of the unique sleep patterns at the various ages helps professionals and parents have reasonable expectations.

The importance of sleep lies in its effect on the growth and development of the child, as well as the adjustment of the family.

This chapter focuses on an understanding of sleep and related developmental changes, the role of the nurse in assessment and promotion of restful sleep, and intervention options for minor sleep disturbances. Although many of the sleep problems of children do resolve over time, interventions during periods of transition when sleep disturbances may evolve can promote healthier parent-child relationships.

Related Topics
Growth and development, Chapters 5 through 9
Hospitalization, Chapter 31

The ability to sleep well, for both young and old, often provides an index of a person's general well-being. Many functions have been proposed for sleep. Sleep generally is believed to be a time for maturation and restoration of physiologic and neurochemical processes (Chuman, 1983; Busby and Pivik, 1983).

With health promotion as a goal, the nurse explores ways in which satisfying experiences related to bedtime and sleep can be achieved throughout the various developmental stages of childhood. Nurses can help parents learn the characteristic sleep behaviors that change as the child grows and develops. A family with young children is acutely aware of the disruption caused by a child who does not sleep through the night or who resists bedtime. Day-by-day living can become an exhausting and frustrating battle between parents and child. Unfortunately, many parents do not seek help until a difficult, habitual pattern

Promoting Healthy Sleep Patterns

Nursing Diagnoses	Nursing Goals/Strategies
Potential sleep pattern disturbance • *related to lack of parental understanding of their child's sleep and sleep-related behaviors*	Promote appropriate age-related rest and sleep patterns • Assess need for health information concerning sleep • Provide information to parents about normal sleep needs at various ages • Teach child/parents strategies to promote rest and sleep appropriate for age (see Table 20–3)
• *related to lack of environment conducive to sleep*	Promote rest and sleep by providing an environment that is conducive to sleep • Provide a physically comfortable and safe place to sleep • Provide an area that is free from excessive noise • Maintain a comfortable temperature in room • Provide separate sleeping or co-sleeping according to family cultural standards • Provide a night light if appropriate for age
• *related to inadequate preparation for sleep*	Promote rest and sleep by preparing child • Provide a quiet, relaxing period before bedtime • Follow a routine to the degree possible • Maintain a supportive, pleasant attitude during the "going to bed" routine • Set limits to discourage unreasonable requests

has evolved, because they expect the problem to solve itself as the child matures, or they do not realize that solutions are possible. It is important for the nurse to assess the sleep needs of children when there are no problems and to recognize difficulties early. The suffering and maladaptation that can result from escalating sleep problems warrant early attention to this area of developmental assessment.

Sleep States and Development

From birth the human organism alternates between awake and sleep states. Both these states are active physiologic and biochemical processes. A complex interaction of neural regulation (nerve cells in the brain stem and diencephalon), biochemical regulation (involving serotonin, norepinephrine, dopamine, acetylcholine, amino acids, and peptides), and the ascending reticular activating system (ARAS) results in the sleep-wake cycle. When we sleep and when we are awake is determined by our circadian rhythm (circadian rhythm is the phenomenon of rhythmic repetitions of certain processes in living organisms at about the same time during a period of approximately 24 hours each day). As the circadian rhythm of an infant matures, the sleep pattern evolves into a pattern of being awake during the day and asleep at night. This mechanism is thought to be controlled by the hypothalamus. A light impulse from the optic tract is delivered to the hypothalamus, resetting the rhythm each day (Hobson, 1982).

Wakefulness

The awake cycle depends on intact cerebral hemispheres interacting with the thalamus, hypothalamus, and brain stem. Stimulation of the ascending reticular activating system (ARAS) results in arousal, whereas destruction of the ARAS results in coma. However, decreased activity of the ARAS alone does not initiate sleep, therefore it is postulated that sleep is an active process involving the deactivation of the ARAS and the activation of sleep centers in the brain (Chuman, 1983). Furthermore, according to Jouvet (1969), catecholaminergic neuron activity is involved in arousal, wakefulness, and REM sleep whereas serotonergic mechanisms appear to be involved with sleep initiation.

The electroencephalogram (EEG) of an awake person is characterized by spontaneous, low-voltage, fast electrical activity, and the pattern is desynchron-

Table 20-1. Characteristics of REM and NREM Sleep States

Characteristics	REM Sleep State	NREM Sleep State
General State	Highly activated	Highly regulated
Eye Movements	Rapid eye movements present under closed lids	Lacks rapid eye movements
EEG Characteristics	Low voltage, asynchronous, fast, cortical activity	*Stage I:* Low voltage, fast pattern *Stage II*:* Sleep spindles with low voltage background *Stages III and IV*:* Slow, high-voltage waves called slow wave sleep (SWS)
Brain Activity	Marked. Most dreams occur during REM sleep	Resting phase
Muscle Activity	Suppression except for bursts of twitching	Muscle tone and muscle activity are diminished
Vital Signs	Pulse, respiratory rate, and blood pressure are faster and more irregular than in NREM sleep	Decrease in pulse rate, respiratory rate, blood pressure, and body temperature

*Stages II, III, and IV do not begin to appear until after the second month of life.
(Data from Anders and Guilleminault, 1976; Anders et al, 1980; Chuman, 1983.)

ized (Chuman, 1983). A high level of muscle activity is present, and the individual is alert and responsive.

Sleep States

Current understanding of sleep states dates from the observations in the 1950s by Aserinsky and Kleitman (1953), who noted rapid eye movements under the closed eyelids of sleeping infants. Before these findings, sleep was thought to be a single state of lowered central nervous system arousal. Sleep is now recognized to be an active rather than passive state and is composed of two distinct states of physiologic activity in the central nervous system. A state of sleep in which rapid eye movements (REM) occur and one in which there are no rapid eye movements (NREM) follow each other in a regular fashion to comprise the sleep cycle (see Table 20-1).

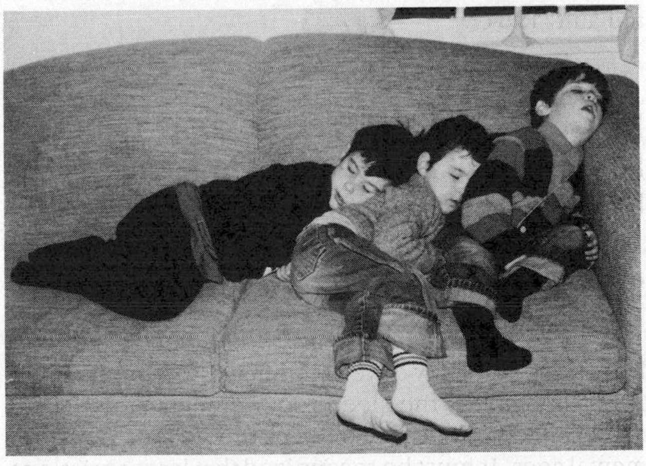

When one sleeps and is awake is determined by circadian rhythm. Children have less tolerance for disruption of regular sleep patterns and are known to fall asleep around their usual bedtime.

REM sleep is sometimes referred to as paradoxic sleep because of the presence of a fast-frequency EEG pattern (characteristic of wakefulness) co-existing with a diminished muscle tone (associated with a sleep state). The REM sleep state has two components: the *tonic or continuous* event, which refers to the overall inhibition of spinal neurons and reduced deep tendon reflexes, and the *phasic or intermittent* component, during which there are bursts of REM, muscle twitching, and variation in vital signs and oxygen consumption (Chuman, 1983). The REM sleep state has also been called the *active sleep state.*

NREM sleep is characterized by four stages of EEG activity numbered I through IV (see Table 20-1). Some notable physiologic differences are characteristic of the NREM phase. In normal states of wakefulness, carbon dioxide has a vasodilator effect. During NREM sleep, there appears to be a decreased cerebral vasomotor carbon dioxide responsiveness. Regional cerebral blood flow thus decreases, especially during short wave sleep (SWS), in spite of a slight elevation in PCO_2 (Chuman, 1983).

The speculation that sleep enhances tissue restoration is associated with the pattern of growth hormone secretion. Growth hormone is secreted during NREM sleep, with the peak occurring during SWS (shortly after the onset of nocturnal sleep) (Takahashi, 1979).

Table 20-2. Comparison of Infant and Adult Sleep Patterns

Characteristic	Infant	Adult
Proportion of REM : NREM	50 : 50 REM : NREM. By age 5 or 6 years, REM : NREM proportions are similar to those of adult. Infants spend more relative and absolute time in REM state	20 : 80 REM : NREM
Length of REM-NREM Cycles	50–60 minutes	90–100 minutes; adult pattern is achieved by adolescence
Sleep Onset	Sleep is entered through an initial REM period. During the latter half of the first year, sleep onset resembles that in adulthood	NREM sleep precedes REM sleep. REM sleep period is entered approximately 90 minutes after sleep onset
Timing (Temporal Organization) of REM-NREM States During a Night of Sleep	Length of REM period is as long in the early part of sleep as it is in the latter part. By 6 weeks of age the diurnal pattern emerges, resulting in shortened REM periods during the early part of the night; longer REM periods (such as in the adult) begin to appear during the latter part of the night	NREM (Stages III and IV) predominate in the first third of the night and the REM state predominates in the last third of the night

Growth hormone enhances amino acid transport into cells and stimulates synthesis of RNA, resulting in stimulation of protein synthesis; this explains the importance of sleep during periods of growth and recuperation from illness or injury.

Sleep behavior in infants differs from that of adults. These differences are summarized in Table 20-2. The proportion of REM sleep diminishes as the central nervous system (CNS) matures. Roffwarg and associates (1966) have proposed that the large proportion of REM sleep and its reduction with maturation occur because (1) the immature nervous system lacks inhibitory control; therefore, a reduced amount of REM sleep reflects maturation of the central nervous system, and (2) REM sleep serves to stimulate the central nervous system, thus facilitates growth and maturation. The larger quantities of REM sleep are thought to occur because of the need for more stimulation of the cortex than can be provided by sensory stimulation from external sources during the short awake periods. The REM sleep thus provides an endogenous source of stimulation that is important for development (Roffwarg et al, 1966).

Two notable changes occur with maturation: *(1) a gradual reduction in the total number of required hours of sleep, and (2) development of consolidated sleep and awake periods into a day/night cycle.* Consolidation of sleep (sleep condensed into fewer periods of longer duration) and a diurnal cycle (sleeping through the night with alternating daytime wakefulness) develop over time. The ability to prolong periods of sleep and wakefulness depends on central nervous system maturation (Jacklin et al, 1980). Although sleep has begun to consolidate and follow a diurnal pattern by 6 weeks of age, it has been reported that sleep onset time at approximately 8:00 P.M. does not become stable until age 4.5 months. By 6 months, the longest sleep period follows the longest wake period, and the time of day at which the wake-to-sleep transition occurs is relatively fixed (Coons and Guilleminault, 1984).

Nurse's Role: Assessment and Promotion of Positive Sleep-Related Experiences

Assessment

The nurse's assessment of a child's sleep-related behaviors is part of any developmental assessment. Table 20-3 summarizes the sleep requirements and characteristics that can be expected at the various developmental ages. It must be recognized that large variations in sleep patterns can be within normal limits.

An important component of a sleep assessment is to determine whether the parent(s) feel that the child

Table 20-3. Developmental Characteristics of Sleep-Related Behavior

Characteristic Sleep Behaviors	Sleep-Related Health Promotion
Neonates	
7–8 short naps. High proportion of REM (active) sleep. *20–22 hours of sleep per 24 hr*	Wrapping snuggly in a blanket promotes sleep
6 Weeks	
Diurnal pattern emerges (sleeps more of the night and is awake for longer periods during the day). *14–16 hours of sleep per 24 hr*	Release into sleep varies with infants; some are more tense than others. The safest position during infancy (before child is able to roll) is on the right side or abdomen after feeding. A light-weight cover is used to prevent chilling because metabolic rate decreases during sleep, thus production of body heat is reduced
6 Months	
Nightwaking begins in the latter half of the first year; begins to resist separation. Has 2–3 naps/day. *12–16 hours of sleep per 24 hr*	See text for management of nightwaking. An established routine facilitates getting infant to sleep
1 Year	
Usually has morning and afternoon naps. *12–14 hours of sleep per 24 hr*	Avoid putting child to bed with bottle (with milk, juice, or other sugar-containing liquid), to prevent nursing bottle mouth syndrome
Toddler (1–3 Years)	
May need morning and afternoon nap but usually by 1.5–2 years one nap is sufficient. Dawdling and delay tactics are used to resist sleep. Child resists sleep because cannot tolerate the separation. As child approaches 3 years of age, may also fear the dark. Also, may find it difficult to "unwind" because of high motor activity during the day. *10–14 hours of sleep per 24 hr*	Don't insist that child sleep during nap time, but a quiet time in the crib after lunch is encouraged. Following a routine at bedtime is essential. A few minutes' warning that bedtime is approaching, a warm bath, and a bedtime story help promote sleep. A special blanket, doll, or toy gives comfort to alleviate the pain of separation. This is usually the period when a hall-light, night light, or small table light must be left on. Usually, advance from crib to bed by the end of the toddler period
Preschool (3–5 Years)	
Some children continue to need an afternoon nap (1–2 hr) whereas others do not. Imagination and fantasies result in dreaming and increasing fears of the dark. Nightmares and night terrors are characteristic of this age. Fear of going to sleep may be related to fear of having a bad dream. *12–14 hours of sleep per 24 hr*	A rest period after lunch should be encouraged even though child does not sleep. Bedtime stories should not contain scary themes. Some form of lighting is often required
School-Age (6–12 Years)	
Child no longer takes naps or rest periods. Verbalizes many excuses to not go to bed. Bargains for special privileges to stay up. Watches the clock concerning bedtime. May try to begin a project close to bedtime. Sleepwalking and sleeptalking are common during these years (discussed in this chapter). *11–12 hours of sleep per 24 hr for 6- to 9-year-olds, 9–12 hours of sleep per 24 hr for 10- to 12-year-olds*	Continue with a bedtime routine. Avoid sending to bed as a punishment. Maintain a positive attitude about bedtime by keeping conversations pleasant. Introduce more responsibility for the child concerning getting ready for bed and performing all the related tasks without being reminded. Regular bedtime and sufficient sleep are necessary for school achievement
Adolescence	
Sleep is important because of the increased growth, strenuous physical activity (if in sports), and increased social and emotional demands. Loss of sleep typically results in late sleeping and daytime sleepiness. Symptoms of narcolepsy are often first recognized during adolescence and should be differentiated from the usual complaint of tiredness. *8–10 hours of sleep per 24 hr*	Parental encouragement to get more sleep is resisted during adolescence. The usual rules of discipline concerning curfew times need to be enforced

has a sleep problem. Asking the parents to describe their concerns about their child's sleep can yield important information. Information requested of the parent(s) and/or child assesses the effectiveness and normality of sleep-related practices. The nurse should elicit the following information:

1. History of family sleep disorders.
2. History of sleep problems in this child.
3. A description of the daily sleep duration of the infant/child/adolescent (bedtime and awakening times).
4. Number and duration of naps (if appropriate).
5. Reaction of child at bedtime and awake times.
6. Where the child sleeps (bed, crib, separate room, lighting, noise level).
7. How child is prepared for bedtime (quiet times, reading, routines that are followed).
8. Interaction of child and parent at bedtime (attitudes, limit setting, feelings).
9. School performance.
10. Presence of sleep disturbances.
11. Problems as described by parent(s) or child/adolescent.

Parents may not mention sleep problems that might be embarrassing to the child or that make the child feel odd or different if discussed in front of the child (e.g., enuresis, fears of the dark, night terrors).

Promotion of healthful sleep experiences in each age group should incorporate an understanding of (1) developmental differences, (2) environmental comfort, (3) the importance of routine and limit setting, and (4) the influence of cultural differences.

Developmental Differences

The expectations that parents have for their children related to sleep should be realistic. Recognizing some of the common variations that exist within the range of normal can provide comfort and solace to those parents having difficulty. Although not all children have similar sleep behaviors, an understanding of the various sleep needs and age-related behaviors can provide important guidelines when counseling parents (see Table 20-3).

Environmental Comfort and Cultural Differences

A child's sleeping conditions vary according to parental values and cultural differences. Common environmental conditions used to promote restful, safe sleep are a firm mattress, no pillow during infancy, a safe bed or crib, a night light as needed, a warm bath before bed, an environment free from excessive noise, and, for some parents, a separate room. These standards are commonly encouraged in an effort to provide the maximal opportunity for restful sleep. A firm mattress provides the needed support for comfort; avoiding a pillow prevents suffocation; cribs with slats no farther than 6 cm (2⅜ inches) apart are used to prevent strangulation, and a warm bath promotes rest and relaxation.

Sleeping in a room and bed separate from parents is encouraged by many to avoid later problems of adjusting to a separate bed, to promote the development of independence, and to prevent parents from being awakened by every movement of their child. However, whether or not a child sleeps in the same bed as the parents is largely influenced by personal attitudes and cultural variations. Co-sleeping (parents and children in the same bed) is a common practice in many cultures and was routine in American culture until the 20th century (Thevenin, 1976). Although pediatric health professionals commonly advise against co-sleeping, a growing number of people (including parents) are questioning this advice (Thevenin, 1976; Brazelton, 1979; Hymovich and Chamberlin, 1980) and studying the practice of co-sleeping (Lozoff et al, 1984). Advice against co-sleeping arises out of concerns about potential ill effects, summarized by Lozoff and associates (1984):

1. Interference with a child's development toward independence.
2. It may become habitual and later weaning may be difficult.
3. The likelihood is great that children will witness sexual intercourse.
4. Intimate body contact may be overstimulating to children.
5. It may reflect disturbances in family relationships (parent-child or parent-parent).
6. Sleep problems may arise.

How prevalent the practice of co-sleeping is and the extent of ill effects (if any) are unknown. In a study by Lozoff and associates (1984), co-sleeping in white families was found to be more common in high-school educated and nonprofessional parents and when family stress, maternal ambivalence, and disruptive sleep problems were present. Although the findings of this study support an association between co-sleeping and sleep problems, the explanation for the association is not obvious. Co-sleeping may *contribute* to sleep problems through reinforcement. Furthermore, delaying resolution of the underlying cause of a problem and not giving children the opportunity to regulate their own sleep patterns may contribute to sleep problems. Conversely, co-sleeping may occur primarily in response to an existing sleep disturbance, and it is conceivable that a sleep problem could be compounded by not permitting co-sleeping (Lozoff et al, 1984).

Nursing strategies to change practices that are rooted in cultural and individual values must be particularly sensitive and insightful. If co-sleeping creates a problem for parents or their children or if co-sleeping is found to be part of a more general pattern of overprotection, then intervention by the nurse may be indicated. If, on the other hand, a family chooses to experience closeness in this way and it is comforting to all family members, then the values of the health care professional cannot be the determining factor in decision making.

Brazelton (1979) reports on what parents think about their children sleeping alone (expressed in a thousand letters in response to a previous article). These parents did not agree that children should be left in their cribs alone, nor did they view nightwaking as a problem. On the contrary, separation from the child at night was cited by these parents as a possible contributor to the problem of nightwaking. The important point is that parents will make decisions regarding sleep based on their own experiences and values. A rigid approach to the issue of separate sleeping for children does not permit parents to seek helpful counsel if they do eventually find the practice to present difficulties. An attitude of acceptance and support, with a knowledge of potential difficulties, thus provides the nurse with the qualities most supportive to parents.

Preparation for Sleep: Routine and Limit Setting

Appropriate preparation of a child for bedtime is an essential component of healthful sleep behaviors. A 5- to 10-minute warning in advance of bedtime permits the child to prepare mentally. A period of quiet play or a reading time of nonscary books is an important prelude to the settling and quieting that is required to get to sleep.

Preparing a child for bed by following the same routine each night promotes more successful bedtime experiences for parents and children. Bedtime routines become particularly important during the toddler and preschool developmental ages when the struggle for autonomy and self-control influences behavior. Routines of the necessary activities of bath, brushing teeth, toileting, and undressing are established and maintained. Young children cooperate when they are not asked to adapt to new situations. Particularly at this developmental level, routines provide an element of security at a time when children resist being separated from their parents. It is also common for children to enhance their sense of security by taking their favorite stuffed animal, doll, or blanket to bed. Devotion to a "security blanket" may continue into adolescence.

Maintaining a positive attitude promotes successful bedtime experiences. Parents should be encouraged to avoid reprimand and discussion of unpleasant happenings of the day. Pleasant experiences and positive feelings should be reinforced to provide the child with a feeling of contentment and acceptance.

Bedtime could become a time of conflict and frustration. Limit setting is essential to prevent unreasonable requests and expectations from a child. Preparing a child for bedtime and following through with the stated time for bedtime is important. A child who resists bedtime should not be granted a later hour for bedtime because of the degree of insistence. This practice promotes additional resisting efforts because the behavior is reinforced. After the usual reading time, bedtime snack, and drink of water have been provided, additional requests should be handled firmly, without, however, becoming insensitively rigid and missing the special needs that children have at bedtime.

After the routine story, a hug and kiss, and a drink of water, a 6-year-old called out to his mother from his bed.

Michael: "Mom, I want to tell you something."

Mother (standing at the bottom of the steps): "You can tell me, I can hear you." (Thinking, he's just trying to get me to come back into the room.)

Michael: "No, I can't tell you from there."

Mother (still thinking he is merely putting off going to sleep): "Why, I can hear from here."

Michael: "But I just can't tell you."

Mother (with some hesitation goes to room): "Yes?"

Michael: "You know that Christmas tree decoration I told you I found? Well, I lied, I didn't find it, I stole it off the Christmas tree in Daddy's office."

Establishment of routine and firmness are principles to guide behaviors at bedtime, but they cannot override a personal sensitivity and caring for the individual child and circumstance (perhaps at the risk of being manipulated on occasion).

Sleep Disturbances

Developmental sleep variations are managed in a variety of ways by parents and by professionals. Parents' expectations of their children concerning sleep behavior arise out of a set of beliefs and attitudes that have evolved over time; therefore, that which is viewed as a problem by one individual may be acceptable to another.

Managing the sleep of a child is a component of parenting, consequently assessment and intervention strategies concerning sleep must consider the parenting style that has been adopted. The methods suggested by a professional of dealing with children's

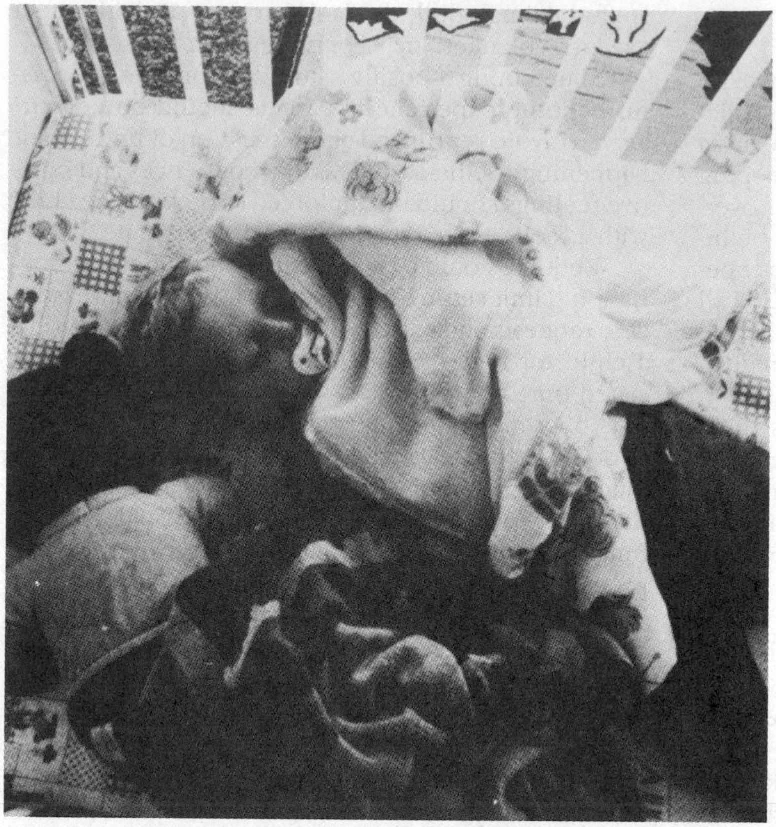

Sometimes children choose an array of transitional security symbols and want them all at one time. This child felt comfortable with a teddy-bear, a special towel, a blanket, and a pacifier.

sleep may vary considerably, depending on the parents' beliefs and attitudes and the circumstances of the situation. The professional's own set of beliefs may need to be tempered in order to relate to the parents' concerns.

Problems related to sleep are often associated with feeding, resistance to separation, and normal fears. Changes in sleep behavior are recognized as children develop, and they vary according to daytime stresses and activities. Sleep disorders can be expected to emerge at times of stress (physical or psychic) and during times of rapid maturation, particularly at ages when sleep organization (i.e., the diurnal and REM-NREM temporal pattern) is changing.

Nightwaking

Sleeping through the night, or "settling in," is a developmental milestone that parents welcome with relief. This indicates to them that their infant is maturing and that they have provided the appropriate nurturing. Moore and Ucko (1957) defined sleeping through the night as not waking from midnight to 5:00 A.M. Using this criterion, sleeping through the night was reported in 70 per cent of infants by 3 months of age, 83 per cent of infants by 6 months of age, and 90 per cent of infants by 1 year of age.

What comes as a surprise to many parents is that nightwaking resumes during the latter part of the first year and during the second year of life. It can occur as early as 1 month after sleeping through the night has been achieved. The reported frequency of nightwaking ranges from 25 per cent (Carey, 1974) to 50 per cent (Moore and Ucko, 1957).

Episodes of nightwaking occur without an identifiable cause, although temperamental, environmental, and maturational factors are thought to be relevant variables. Introducing solid foods has been found not to be associated with sleeping through the night.

Nightwaking has been reported to be associated with temperaments characterized by low sensory thresholds (determined by the Carey Infant Temperament Scale) (Carey, 1974; Weissbluth, 1981). Breastfeeding beyond 6 months of age is reported to be associated with nightwaking by some (Carey, 1975) but not others (Weissbluth et al, 1981). Osterholm and colleagues (1983) found breastfeeding, sleeping in the same room as parents, and tooth eruption to be more prevalent in infants (6 to 12 months) who did not sleep through the night. Healy (1972) reported nightwaking to be associated with sleeping in the parents' room, strained parent-child relationships, and maternal overprotection.

Several developmental factors may be associated with nightwaking. During the first several years of life, diurnal regulation and transitions between REM and NREM sleep states mature. The mechanisms responsible for the maturation of sleep states may be associated with nightwaking (Anders and Keener, 1983). In the early months, infants may awaken and console themselves and return to sleep on their own. During the latter part of the first year separation from parents begins to be resisted, therefore infants cry out when they awaken rather than getting back to sleep on their own. Furthermore, it has been suggested that infants who have rarely been placed into their crib awake expect to be rocked back to sleep if they awaken in the night. The high prevalence of nightwaking in breastfed infants may be related to a difference in comforting practices. The breastfeeding mother may be more likely to comfort her fussing baby by offering the breast; therefore, the baby learns to expect this response (Schmitt, 1981).

Management options for nightwaking depend on the way parents respond to the situation. The parents who seek alternatives to getting up at night require intervention by the nurse. If parents are satisfied with their approach to handling nightwaking, then suggested options may not be welcomed. Parents need to be highly motivated to break the cycle of night crying.

Nightwaking has been described by Schmitt (1986) as "trained night crying." Trained night crying is thought to occur because of a reinforcing response to an infant's cry. Consistently responding to awake infants by holding and rocking them at night "trains" them to expect comforting. Crying is reinforced by the secondary gain of being held. If parents are seeking to break this cycle of crying and holding each night, they will need to decrease the secondary reinforcers gradually. Younger (1982) has reported a specific behavior modification method in which going to the baby's room is prohibited. Although this may result in an excessively long period of crying on the first night, it is reported that by the fourth night the infant nearly always sleeps through.

Schmitt (1981, 1986), on the other hand, suggests that parents have great difficulty letting their baby cry. It is therefore suggested that parents wait for 5 minutes before going to their baby's room and then go for a very brief time (1 minute or less). They should try to refrain from holding and cuddling the infant but rather give pats and make a few reassuring remarks.

Similarly, Ferber (1985a) recommends that each night the parents can let their infant cry slightly longer before intervening, and the parent should stay with the infant only briefly to reassure. Asking parents to simply let a child cry for long periods until he or she falls asleep is also discouraged by Jones and Verduyn (1983) because it emphasizes the crying. What is important is that the child have practice falling asleep alone rather than while being held and rocked. Most children do not cry longer than 15 to 20 minutes unless something is wrong or unless longer crying periods have been reinforced. (Letting a baby cry for a long period of time and then holding or rocking the infant reinforces the behavior so that next time the child will cry equally long, expecting the same comfort.)

Nightwaking is usually a transient developmental phase but has the potential to result in strained parent-child relationships. Sedation is generally not recommended for nightwaking.

Sleeptalking and Sleepwalking

Sleeptalking (somniloquy) and sleepwalking (somnambulism) occur most commonly during the school-age years. Approximately 15 per cent of children between the ages of 5 and 12 years have walked in their sleep at least once. Persistent sleepwalking occurs in only 1 to 6 per cent of children.

Sleeptalking and sleepwalking are associated with neurologic immaturity and occur during the transition from Stages III and IV of NREM sleep to the first REM period (approximately 1 to 2 hours after sleep onset) (Fig. 20-1). Sleeptalkers are *not* revealing their deep secrets, and most children outgrow this problem. Sleepwalking similarly resolves spontaneously. Those adults with persistent sleepwalking have usually begun it in adolescence rather than during the school-age years. Table 20-4 summarizes characteristics and management of sleeptalking and sleepwalking.

Nightmares and Night Terrors

Night terrors must be differentiated from the more common nightmare. (See Table 20-4 for a description of each.) Sleep problems, particularly night terrors, peak during the preschool years, whereas nightmares are seen more frequently in older children (Wender, 1984). Dreams are an essential part of sleep and average five or more in number nightly (Herbert, 1975). Young children confuse waking and dreaming experiences easily, and their dreams are extremely vivid and real; thus, a dream may frighten a child whether it is pleasant or scary, simply because it looms as so real. The fright is heightened by the fact that dreams usually focus on the dreamer as the active participant or central figure rather than as a passive observer (Herbert, 1975).

A young child's dream life is influenced by life experiences and circumstances. Dreams are more likely to be negative during periods of poor health or family stress. A negative-theme dream life is also more likely in children who display exaggerated fear of the dark. Most children express some fear of the dark during the preschool years, but those exposed to signifi-

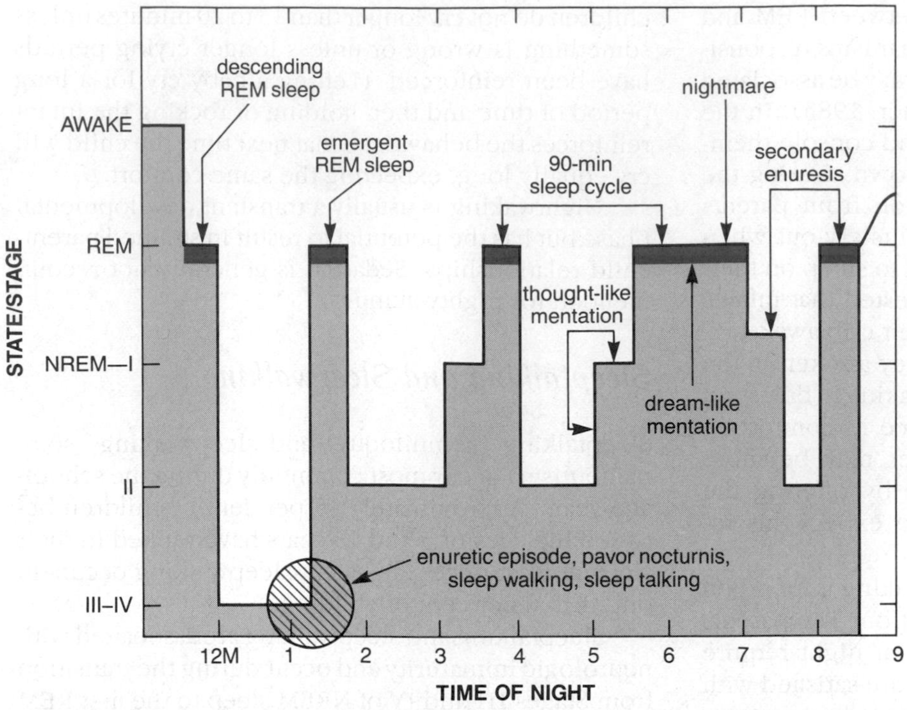

Figure 20-1. Association of parasomnias with sleep stages in an idealized sleep-wake histogram. Arousal disorders tend to occur late during the first NREM sleep period of the night. Secondary enuresis and tyical nightmares tend to occur in a later portion of sleep. (Redrawn from Anders TF, Carskadon MA, Dement WC: Sleep and sleepiness in children and adolescents. *Pediatric Clin North Am* 1980 Feb; 27(1):29–44.)

cant others (parents, siblings, peers) who show apprehension of the dark, those for whom darkness has been used as a punishment, and those for whom death has been equated with sleep are most at risk to develop phobic fears of the dark (Jones, 1969; Herbert, 1975; Winter, 1976). The fear of darkness expressed by a child is best acknowledged as real and should be combined with a program of positive reinforcement and weaning from the fear. Two weaning programs that have been successful with preschoolers are described in Box 20-1.

Disturbed Psychodynamics and Clinical Manifestations

Normal sleep disturbances in young children are basically temporary and show a variety of themes. A recurrent negative theme that exists over time is symptomatic of some underlying emotional disturbance that needs intervention. Fortunately, children express their feelings simply and clearly in their dream life, seldom with the distortion of symbolism typical of adult dreams (Herbert, 1975). Therefore the problem is usually identifiable within the child's description of the dream. Nightmares may be stimulated by disturbing or overexciting experiences or by repressed unacceptable feelings of rivalry, hostility, or sexual attraction to the parent (Prugh, 1983). Nightmares arise out of REM sleep and involve imagery over time in a story fashion (Ferber, 1985b). The child is fully awake after a nightmare and can usually recall parts of it.

Night terrors differ from nightmares in pathology. The child is not fully awake, appears to be hallucinating, and is very difficult to awaken and comfort. They occur at the moment of arousal from slow wave sleep and are associated with little or no imagery. Usually, the child has no memory of the experience. Table 20-4 describes the characteristics of these dream patterns and how each is most effectively managed.

Strategies to Eliminate Sleep Disorders

The definitive action to be taken in alleviating nightmares is to identify the underlying cause and eliminate it (Herbert, 1975). This requires an evaluation of the child's reactions to various situations, coupled with consideration of the content of the nightmares (remember that children do not dream symbolically). Parents may need assistance with this process, or they may require a psychologic expert's input.

Intervention to diminish night terrors is less easily accomplished. Since central nervous system immaturity is a primary factor, terrors cannot be completely eliminated until the central nervous system becomes more mature. Actions can be taken to eliminate environmental or psychologic stresses that may be intensifying or increasing the frequency of the night terrors. This is done as for nightmares, although professional assistance to decipher the dream may be needed, since the child often recalls only a single image.

The following practices can help a child approach bedtime positively:

Table 20-4. Characteristics and Management of Sleep Disturbances

Description	Behavior Manifested	Management During Episode
Sleepwalking (Somnambulism)		
More common in boys. Onset is usually before age 10 years and usually resolves by age 15 years. One to four episodes per week may occur	Sits upright abruptly for 15–30 seconds, climbs out of bed, and wanders around room or house, from a few min to as long as 30 min. Unconscious of environment: although eyes are open, child is not awake. Movements are rigid, repetitive, and not purposeful. Answers in monosyllables if spoken to. Speech is slurred and mumbled.	Do not attempt to wake child but protect from injury. Keep doors to basement, outdoors, and other areas of potential danger locked. Allow child's own return to bed. If guided back to bed before ready, child usually will get up again anyway Diazepam (Valium) may be considered for child with severe, intractable sleepwalking
Sleeptalking (Somniloquy)		
Occurs on occasion in the sleep of most children and adults. Is thought by some to reflect anxiety-provoking daytime experiences	Speech is usually monosyllabic and incomprehensible. Sometimes the sound of one's own voice causes individual to awaken	One should not try to awaken the child. It should not be a cause for alarm
Nightmares		
Psychologic motivation. Anxiety expressed, worked through in negative theme. Occurs during REM sleep. If child awakens, can recall all or most of dream; no recall if not awakened	Moves around restlessly in bed, may whimper or cry but not hysterically. May or may not wake. Face may show facial grimace or expression of fear	Do not overreact. If child cries, parent who wishes to respond to it should satisfy self that nothing is wrong (not caught in blankets, not fallen out of bed, no fever) then leave without waking child. If awakens, give reassurance that it was only a dream and child can safely go back to sleep. Then leave; making a fuss over the child only reinforces the behavior
Night Terrors		
Physiologic motivation: result of immature CNS function; psychologic factors determine theme. Occurs during NREM sleep. Child usually can recall only a single frightening image, if anything; usually repetitive	Sits up in bed screaming, or assumes bizarre crouching posture; pulse and respirations increase, pupils dilated. Senses doom, intensely anxious and agitated. Appears to be staring at something with eyes wide open. Disoriented. Does not recognize persons who respond to the distress but will gradually respond to a soothing voice	Although the child does not recognize the adult who responds to the shrieks, reassurance and cuddling do eventually calm the child, allowing return to sleep. One can do little to alter the course of events during the episode

(Data from Herbert, 1975; Wender, 1984; Ferber, 1985b; Anders, 1987.)

1. Use the hour before bedtime as a cooling-down period by participating with the child in some quiet, mutually enjoyable activity such as reading a mild, happy bedtime story or talking through the day's pleasant events.
2. Help the child establish some before-bed rituals that help indoctrinate her or him emotionally for bed, such as a warm bath, brushing the teeth, putting dolls or cars or teddy bear to bed, hugs from family members. Then put the child to bed.
3. Distinguish between bedtime and sleep time. Allow quiet play in bed until sleep overcomes the child.
4. Teach the child where the hands on the clock are when it is bedtime so that the clock becomes a "neutral" teller of bedtime, making a game of bedtime rather than a battle of wills.
5. Do not make the child feel isolated at bedtime. Allow comforts such as a light on, the door open, soft music, to give the child a feeling of company. Also reassure that the parent is nearby throughout the night and that the child will awaken safe and sound in the morning. Some parents even remind the child of some pleasant event to look forward to the next day.

Whatever the child's sleep problem is and regardless of its frequency, parents should be cautioned by the nurse not to overreact to the child's behavior or the child will learn to use the sleep disturbance to manipulate them. Discussion of family tensions and conflicts may be appropriate when the problem is marked or persistent. Occasionally the child and family may need referral for psychotherapy.

Narcolepsy

Narcolepsy is characterized by periods of excessive sleepiness during the day. REM attacks occur during wakefulness. These sleepy states are resisted and may last only a few minutes, but sometimes sleepiness increases so much that a REM nap takes place. Daytime sleepiness begins 3 to 4 hours after waking and may occur repeatedly throughout the day. Narcolepsy can be differentiated from similar episodes of sleepiness that can normally occur during driving or lectures. Narcoleptic attacks are often accompanied by cataplexy (loss of muscle tone precipitated by surprise or emotion, which may cause knees to weaken, resulting in a fall), sleep paralysis (an inability to move voluntary muscles when falling asleep), and hypnagogic hallucinations (vivid visual hallucinations at sleep onset). These symptoms often result in an intense fear to fall asleep. The peak onset of narcolepsy is between 15 and 25 years of age.

Daytime sleepiness may be counteracted by excessive activity in an attempt to stay awake. Learning difficulties may arise and be the first indication of a problem. Narcolepsy is thought to be a genetic disorder. The incidence in families with narcolepsy has been found to be 60 times greater than in the general population (Anders and Keener, 1983).

Treatment for narcolepsy remains inadequate. The adolescent, parents, and teacher require information about the disorder to help them understand the nature of the problem. Narcolepsy does not indicate an increased need for nocturnal sleep or daytime naps. Drug therapy may reduce attacks to some extent. Methylphenidate hydrochloride (Ritalin) may be prescribed to reduce the sleep attacks and imipramine (Tofranil) is more useful for the symptoms of sleep paralysis, cataplexy, and hypnagogic hallucinations.

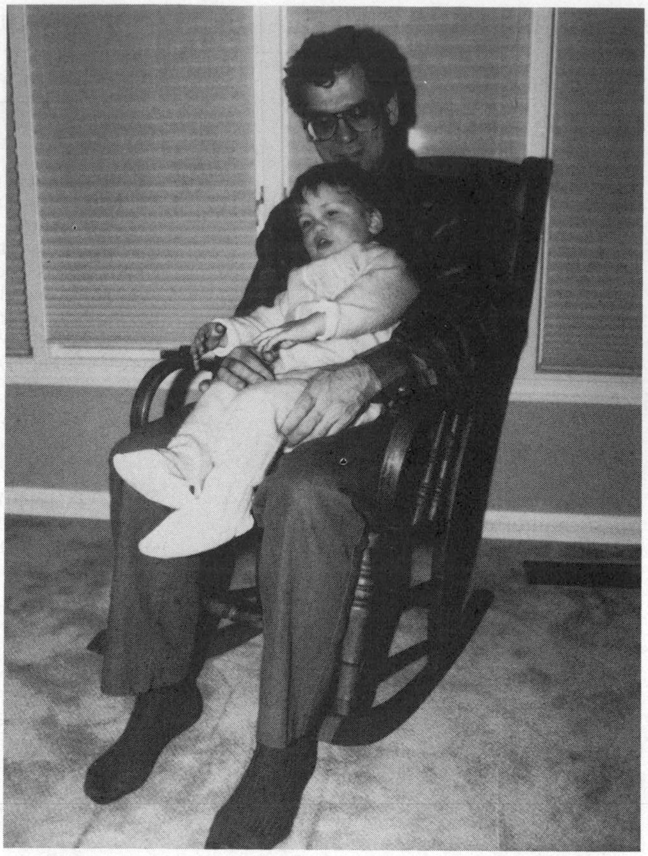

Use the hour before bedtime as a cooling down period for children who have difficulty falling asleep.

Box 20-1
Managing Phobic Fear of the Dark

PROGRAM 1

Leave a lamp on in the child's room on the floor near the bed. Move it gradually farther from the bed and eventually out of the room. How quickly this can be done will vary with the child. (The average is to move farther away every two to three nights.) If the lamp is moved and the child reacts negatively move it back to its former position a few more nights, then try again. Once the lamp is out of the room a few nights, turn it off after the child is asleep. Then, a few nights later, try not turning it on at all. The child who tolerates that for several nights has been weaned from fear, and the lamp can be removed completely. If the child regresses during illness or other upset, go to the room and give comfort but without holding her or him or turning on the light, and the child will overcome the fear.

PROGRAM 2

Place the child in bed with the room light on, but turn it off once the child is asleep, keeping the door of the room open and a hall light on. During the daytime teach the child how to turn the light on during the night. Once the child knows how to do it, the parent praises the child as a big boy or girl who can be responsible to turn it on when wanted at night, and enforces that expectation. Each time the child turns the light on, the parent turns if off again after the child is again asleep. The child will eventually tire of getting up to turn on the light and will just go back to sleep.

References

Anders TF: Nightmares and other sleep disturbances. *In* Hoekelman RH, et al: *Primary Pediatric Care.* St. Louis, CV Mosby, 1987, pp 744–748.

Anders TF, Guilleminault C: The pathophysiology of sleep disorders in pediatrics. Part I. Sleep in infancy. *Adv Pediatr* 1976; 22:137–150.

Anders TF, Keener MA: Sleep-wake state development and disorders of sleep in infants, children, and adolescents. *In* Levine MD, et al: *Developmental–Behavioral Pediatrics.* Philadelphia, WB Saunders, 1983, pp. 596–606.

Anders TF, et al: Sleep and sleepiness in children and adolescents. *Pediatr Clin North Am* 1980 Feb; 27(1):29–43.

Aserinsky E, Kleitman H: Regularly occurring periods of eye motility and concomitant phenomena during sleep. *Science* 1953 Sep 4; 118:273–274.

Brazelton TB: What parents told me about handling children's sleep problems. *Redbook* 1979 June; 51–54.

Busby K, Pivik RT: Failure of high intensity auditory stimuli to affect behavioral arousal in children during the first sleep cycle. *Pediatr Res* 1983 Oct; 17(10):802–805.

Carey W: Night waking and temperament in infancy. *J Pediatr* 1974 May; 84(5):756–758.

Carey WB: Breast feeding and night waking. *J Pediatr* 1975 Aug; 87(2):327.

Chuman M: The neurological basis of sleep. *Heart Lung* 1983 Mar; 12(2):178–181.

Coons S, Guilleminault C: Development of consolidated sleep and wakeful periods in relation to the day/night cycle in infancy. *Dev Med Child Neurol* 1984; 26:169–176.

Ferber R: *Solve Your Child's Sleep Problems.* New York, Simon and Schuster, 1985a.

Ferber R: Sleep disorders in infants and children. *In* Riley TL (ed): *Clinical Aspects of Sleep and Sleep Disturbance.* Stoneham, MA, Butterworth Publishers, 1985b.

Healy A: The sleep patterns of preschool children: general principles and current knowledge. *Clin Pediatr* 1972 Mar; 11:174–177.

Herbert M: *Problems of Childhood.* Pam Brooks, Ltd., 1975.

Hobson JA: Sleep and its disorders. *In* Wyngaarden JB, Smith LH: *Cecil Textbook of Medicine.* 16th ed. Philadelphia, WB Saunders, 1982, pp. 1930–1935.

Hymovich DP, Chamberlin RW: *Child and Family Development: Implications for Primary Health Care.* New York, McGraw-Hill, 1980, p 298.

Jacklin CN, et al: Sleep pattern development from 6 through 33 months. *J Pediatr Psychol* 1980; 5(3):295–303.

Jones DPH, Verduyn CM: Behavioral management of sleep problems. *Arch Dis Child* 1983; 58:442–444.

Jones M: A laboratory study of fear: the case of Peter. *In* Gelfand D: *Social Learning of Childhood.* Monterey, CA, Brooks/Cole Publishing, 1969.

Jouvet M: Biogenic amines and the state of sleep. *Science* 1969 Jan 3; 163:32–41.

Lozoff B, et al: Cosleeping in urban families with young children in the United States. *Pediatrics* 1984 Aug; 74(2):171–182.

Moore T, Ucko C: Night waking in early infancy: Part I. *Arch Dis Child* 1957 Aug; 32:333–342.

Osterholm P, et al: Sleep disturbance in infants aged 6 to 12 months. *Pediatr Nurs* 1983 Jul/Aug; 269–271.

Prugh DG: *The Psychosocial Aspects of Pediatrics.* Philadelphia, Lea & Febiger, 1983.

Roffwarg H, et al: Ontogenic development of human sleep-dream cycle. *Science* 1966 Apr 29; 152:604–618.

Schmitt BD: Infants who do not sleep through the night. *J Dev Behav Pediatr* 1981 Mar; 2(1):20–23.

Schmitt BD: The prevention of sleep problems and colic. *Pediatr Clin North Am* 1986 Aug; 33(4):763–744.

Takahashi Y: Growth hormone secretion related to the sleep and waking rhythm. *In* Drucker-Colin R, et al: *The Function of Sleep.* New York, Academic Press, 1979, p 113.

Thevenin T: *The Family Bed: An Age Old Concept in Childrearing.* Minneapolis, Tine Thevenin, 1976.

Weissbluth M: Sleep duration and infant temperament. *J Pediatr* 1981 Nov; 99(5):817–819.

Wender E: Common behavior problems in preschool children. *In* Shelov SP, et al (eds): *Primary Care Pediatrics: A Symptomatic Approach.* Norwalk, CT, Appleton-Century-Croft, 1984, pp 265–282.

Younger JB: The management of night waking in older infants. *Pediatr Nurs* 1982 May/Jun; 8(3):155–158.

Bibliography

Denenberg V, Thoman E: Evidence for a functional role for active (REM) sleep in infancy. *Sleep* 1981; 4(2):185–191.

Green M: Sleep disorders. *In* Green M, Haggerty RJ: *Ambulatory Pediatrics.* Philadelphia, WB Saunders, 1984, pp 249–252.

Gross PT: Evaluation of sleep disorders. *Med Clin North Am* 1986 Nov; 70(6):1349–1360.

Haslam D: *Sleepless Children: A Handbook for Parents.* New York, Simon and Schuster, 1984.

Lozoff B, et al: Sleep problems seen in pediatric practice. *Pediatrics* 1985; 75(3):477–483.

Price VA, et al: Prevalence and correlates of poor sleep among adolescents. *Am J Dis Child* 1978 Jun; 132:583–586.

Rapoff MA, et al: The management of common bedtime problems by pediatric nurse practitioners. *J Pediatr Psychol* 1982; 7(2):179–196.

Rosenfield AA, et al: Sleeping patterns in upper-middle-class families when the child awakens ill or frightened. *Arch Gen Psychiatr* 1982 Aug; 39:943–947.

Salzarulo P, Chevalier A: Sleep problems in children and their relationship with early disturbances of the waking-sleeping rhythms. *Sleep* 1983; 6(1):47–51.

Schumann MJ: A method for inducing sleep in young children. *Pediatr Nurs* 1981; 7(5):9–13.

Weissbluth M, et al: Night waking in 4 to 8 month old infants. *J Pediatr* 1984 Mar; 104(3):477–480.

White L: Sleep in chidren and adolescents: a review with implications for primary prevention. *J Preventive Psychiatr* 1987; 3(2):117–146.

Promoting Healthy Play and Exercise

Chapter 21

Mabel Hunsberger

The play of children has been examined by theorists for centuries. The most enduring interpretation is that children play to have fun. The character of play changes as a child matures, but children at all ages play. Play contributes to and is an expression of development. As children play, physical, emotional, social, and cognitive skills are developed. Children take a special interest in certain types of play, such as sports or art, that require practice and discipline to develop skill. Encouragement in the child's area of interest results in play for enjoyment. Children who develop in an environment where appropriate play is encouraged have a greater chance to achieve their maximum potential than those in homes where play opportunities are lacking.

A special benefit of play is its use during a health care encounter. Play can be used to assess a child's level of development. When children are hospitalized, play is used as recreation, as a diversion from thoughts about the hospital, and in therapeutic play to help a child cope with a stressful or painful experience.

Related Topics
Developing children, Chapters 3 and 5–9
Assessing Child Health, Chapter 15
Preparation and support of children requiring procedures, Chapter 27
Preoperative and postoperative nursing care, Chapter 27
Nursing care during hospitalization, Chapter 31

This chapter reviews theories of play as a framework for understanding the elements of play. The contributions of play to the developing child and the character of play at the various stages of development are discussed. The nurse's role in fostering the child's development through direct play with children and teaching parents how to play with their children is presented.

A child who plays is thought to be a healthy, happy child. We expect children to play but do not ask them to enumerate a series of accomplishments as we do of ourselves at the end of a day. For a child to describe the day with "Oh, I played" is sufficient. Herein lies the beauty and mystery of play. Although play is not for the *sake* of certain accomplishments, children are productive during play. Play also profoundly influences and is a form of communication with those in a child's environment.

We are beginning to understand that, through the medium of play, a child "learns what no one can teach him" (Hartley and Goldenson, 1963). One needs only to watch an inquisitive child examine the texture of each item on the dinner plate to appreciate the child's preoccupation with learning while playing. Through play children orient themselves to their expanding world of people and objects and gradually learn how to relate to them effectively. Much of this learning is accomplished by the creation of a make-believe world in which children can assume roles that offer safe expression of their fears and re-enactment of the conflicts felt in the real world. In this way a child can adapt to the expectations of those in the environment. The beauty of childhood is that the "work" of growing and developing is done in the name of play.

Watching children play is an encounter with the content of their lives. Play is a reflection of a child's developing physical, intellectual, and emotional-social competencies. Through play children are in a continuous state of telling about themselves — what they can do, how they think, and how they feel. Careful attention to the language of play gives an adult entrance into a child's world.

Adult expectations and the boundaries of permission granted to children have an impact upon the direction and scope of activities in which a child will engage. Parents' goals for their children concerning physical, social, emotional, and intellectual development translate into permission and denial of specific activities. Enrollment of young children in various sports, dance, and gymnastic programs is a reflection of how parents expect their children to play. The same parent, on the contrary, may set limits on the child's activity during free play if it is viewed as a nuisance and disruption to the parent's schedule and orderliness for that particular moment. Opportunities for free play are increasingly being placed at a premium in our society, in which day care for the young and highly organized sports programs for school-age children are the norm. Play is thus increasingly dominated and directed by adults. As parents invest more and more time in the organized play of their children, there is a danger for expectations about accomplishments and outcomes to detract from the benefits of play.

The nurse's role in the area of health care is to assess each family's situation to determine how the development of each child and the relationships within families can be maximized through play. The nurse can help parents provide an appropriate environment in which a child is permitted and encouraged to play in order to gain maximal benefit. Regardless of the nature of the health care setting, attention given to the play of a child is appropriate and feasible. The nurse's role is to draw attention to the importance of the child's play and to assist parents in their selection of play activities.

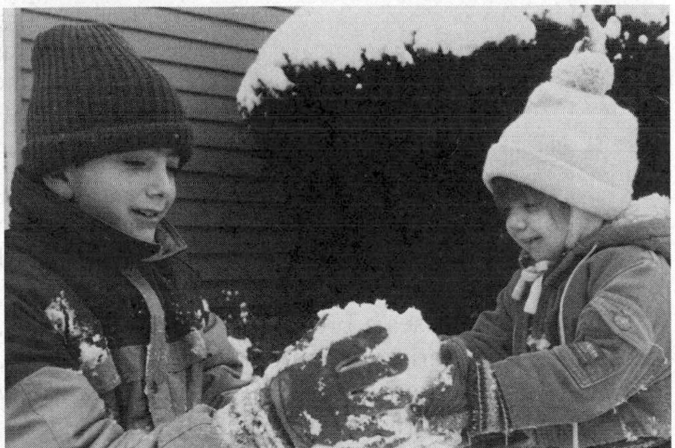

Opportunities for free play are enjoyed by most children. While having fun, these children are learning about the environment, developing social skills, increasing their manual dexterity, and having an opportunity to create whatever they choose.

Promoting Healthy Play and Exercise

Nursing Diagnoses	Nursing Goals/Strategies
Potential for altered growth and development, related to lack of appropriate play opportunities	Provide play opportunities that promote development. • Assess resources in the home (space, time, finances). • Discuss the importance of play at each health visit. • Teach parents about appropriate play at the various developmental levels (see Table 21-2). • Assist parents in choosing inexpensive toys that promote development and are safe. • Teach parents to avoid excessive numbers of stimulating toys simultaneously. • Encourage parents to provide the opportunity for children to participate in sports and exercise. • Teach parents and children how to practice safety in sports. • Role model to parents how to engage children in interactive play. • Encourage parents to play *with* their children. • Compliment parents on their interactions, choice of toys, and time given to play.
Potential for sensory-perceptual alteration: sensory deprivation/overstimulation, related to deprived/overstimulating environment	Facilitate creation of an environment with an appropriate degree of stimulation. • Assess home environment to determine appropriateness of sensory stimulation. • Assist parents to choose a variety of stimuli (shapes, colors, textures, sounds, human touch, human voice). • Role model use of touch, voice, toys during health visit. • Discuss with parents the disadvantages of overstimulation of their infant.
Potential for ineffective individual coping, related to lack of appropriate play opportunities during health care encounters	Promote maximum adjustment to stress of health care encounter. • Assess child's coping through observation of play. • Provide play opportunities to support a child's coping: diversionary, recreational, and therapeutic. • Encourage parents to provide special toys from home to give child comfort. • Use therapeutic play in combination with pharmacologic approaches to control pain, fear, and anxiety.

Parents also should be encouraged to relate to their children through play by watching them play and playing with them.

Play encompasses a broad range of experiences, beginning with early encounters with sound, color, texture, and movement. A supportive family; a safe play space; access to simple, basic materials; and the freedom to engage in play are some of the necessary characteristics of a child's environment. The nurse must approach each family with recognition of the individual circumstances that affect the child's play experiences. This chapter provides a theoretical base from which the nurse can provide counsel in the area of play.

Theories of Play

Numerous theories have been offered to explain why and how children play. An examination of them gives one an appreciation for the complexity of an activity as seemingly simple as play.

Traditional Theories

Play theories at the turn of the century were biologically based, stressing that play is instinctive and has a physiologic function. It was viewed as a phenomenon that revived the individual and thus conserved energy or expended surplus energy.

Surplus Energy Theory. Herbert Spencer, an English philosopher of the mid-19th century, hypothesized that children play because of excess energy accumulation, necessitating release through play. The exuberant activities of children were recognized to be a normal part of their development, but play was not thought to accomplish any immediate goal (Garvey, 1977). The notion of surplus energy is identifiable in the high premium that schools and families pay to provide yards and gymnasiums for the physical activity of children.

Instinctive Practice Theory. Karl Groos, a German philosopher and writer of the late 19th century, viewed play as instinctual and as a preparation for adult life (Bijou, 1976). To him the function of play was to practice skills necessary for adult life. He was particularly aware of the imaginations of children and interpreted imaginative play as "pre-exercise" for adult living. The value of Groos's theory is that he recognized the functional value of play: practicing and perfecting the skills needed in adult life. From this perspective play can be viewed as preparation for "real life" and its harshness. Sports training is therefore "training" for life.

Play as Recreation. Lazarus, another German philosopher in the late 19th century, interpreted play to be a method of recuperation from fatigue and near exhaustion. Play was viewed as "relaxation" because it replenishes one's physical energy and alleviates boredom and psychologic tension.

20th Century Theories

At the turn of the century, environment and learning were regarded as the important factors influencing human development. John Watson, the father of "behaviorism," in 1919 denounced the idea of "instinct" as a foundation from which to explain play. The three streams of thought that evolved out of the background of biologically based traditional theories were psychoanalytic, behavioral, and cognitive. These three psychologically based theories are not completely independent of each other, therefore some overlap can be seen.

Psychoanalytic Theory. Psychoanalytic theorists, particularly Freud and Erikson, stress the *cathartic* benefit children gain through play. Freud stated that "in their play children repeat everything that has made a great impression on them in real life" (Freud, 1975). To illustrate, a child who has been punished for running onto a busy street later may be seen acting out the scene in doll play, in which the child first scolds the doll, then comforts it. The repetition of the experience affords an opportunity to express hostile feelings and provide assurance that the act of running onto the street will not result in rejection. According to this theory, the playing out of such anxieties is thought to help a child gain mastery over fears, feelings, people, and things. The use of play therapy to treat emotionally disturbed children is an outgrowth of the psychoanalytic view of play.

Play as *ego mastery* was also a focus of psychoanalytic theory. It is an attempt by the child to gradually master the environment and not become overwhelmed by anxiety. According to Erikson, who extended and elaborated Freud's theory, play is a means through which a child attempts to bring into harmony the desires of the self and social processes, i.e., societal roles. The idea that a child's play is a method to gain mastery thus supposes some purpose to play.

Behaviorism. Behaviorism is a school of thought that is less introspective than the psychoanalytic view. Behaviorists emphasize learned behavior and environmental influence in the interpretation of play.

Play Through Secondary Reinforcement (A Drive-Reduction Theory). According to Hull (1943), children's play is explained by the phenomenon of secondary reinforcement theory. Satisfaction of secondary drives (i.e., drives for achievement, affiliation, and independence) occurs through play. As a drive is reduced, reinforcement of a behavior occurs.

Play as Imitative Learning. Miller and Dollard (1941) extended Hull's view by explaining play as imitative learning. Imitation occurs not only in response to rewards but also through environmental cues. For example, children who develop a specific skill in a game become aware of cues that they have leadership qualities. They then begin to imitate individuals in leadership roles. Thus play is sparked by an "acquired imitative drive."

Play as Exploration and Investigation (An Arousal-Seeking Theory). This interprets play as an avenue through which investigative and explorative needs are met. Exploratory play behavior, according to Berlyne (1960), is an attempt to reduce conflict by acquiring more information about the environment. A novel situation provides a particularly strong stimulus to investigate or explore. Therefore, play behavior is believed to be associated with arousal (Berlyne, 1960; Fiske and Maddi, 1961). Arousal-seeking theory is based on the notion that "there is an optimal arousal state that lies between the two extremes of quiescence and excitement." The theory suggests that a certain level of stimulation is comfortable for an organism. If the organism is faced with novelty or incongruity, the resultant curiosity leads to exploration and information gathering so as to reduce the uncertainty or arousal level.

Berlyne (1960) and Fiske and Maddi (1961) propose that the organism seeks tension and varied experiences and stimulation at a level suitable to one's unique biologic and sociocultural makeup. Play is regarded as the set of behaviors that maintains an optimal level of stimulation for the individual (Levy, 1978).

Play as a Need for Competence. White (1959) draws heavily on freudian theory. According to this theory play behavior is motivated by an intrinsic need to achieve competence; the drive for excellence and achievement becomes an end in itself.

Cognitive Theory. According to cognitive theorists, a child's play is the way in which reality can be explored and assimilated into the mental structure. The Swiss psychologist Piaget distinguishes between play and imitation (Piaget, 1951). The process of assimilation predominates when a child is playing. Conversely, when accommodation predominates, the result is imitation. When assimilation and accommodation are in equilibrium, intellectual adaptation occurs. (See Chapter 3 for further discussion of assimilation and accommodation.) To illustrate, intellectual adaptation occurs when a child uses mental processes to discover that raisins can be obtained from a bottle by dumping them out. Once the child has mastered this skill and repeats it for the pleasure and fun of doing it, Piaget describes that as play. If, on the other hand, a child has observed another person dumping raisins out of the bottle and then mimics the activity, that is imitation. Whether a single activity is play, imitation, or intellectual adaptation is not easily discerned on random observation.

Piaget's theory of play correlates with his theory of intellectual development (see Chapter 3). The way a child plays and the nature of imitation vary throughout the stages of development. The games that characterize certain periods of development reflect one's intellectual processes. Practice games, which predominate in the sensorimotor period of development (0 to 2 years), are repetitive actions done for the pleasure they bring. Those activities for gaining mastery or increasing understanding are not considered by authorities to be practice games (Rubin and Pepler, 1982). When mastery has been achieved, play occurs.

The period of symbolic games or make-believe play (2 to 7 years) is the stage when children are egotistic in thought and, through fantasy, transform reality to be consistent with their immediate need (assimilation). At a given time a child can pretend that an object is an animal and moments later transform that object into a person, whichever is consistent with the needs of the moment. In addition to meeting the conscious needs of a child, symbolic play functions in the realm of the unconscious. Emotional experiences are reproduced in play in an effort to diffuse the anxieties that are produced by the real world. These enactments of real-life impressions are often distorted owing to the egocentricity of thought that prevails during this stage. Gradually a child's increasing participation in the natural and social world eliminates the need for symbolic games, which are replaced by games with rules.

Games with rules (7 to 11 years) are representative of a child's increased social interaction and developing reasoning abilities. These games have sensorimotor components (races, ball games) and intellectual ones (cards, chess) and are guided by rules, within which competition and cooperation can take place. This social interactive forum facilitates the decline of egocentric thought and the development of cognitive competence (Piaget, 1951).

A variation on Piaget's cognitive theory is the enjoyment or hedonism theory. Hurlock (1978) and the Sutton-Smiths (1974) believe that play should be enjoyable and that its end result is of little consequence. According to this theory, an activity is not play unless the player is engaged merely for the enjoyment it gives. When actions are carried out with the end result as a primary goal, then the activity is more rightly called work. The differences between mastery activities and play activities are not easily identified, because one cannot be sure of the intent of the player. What this view brings to mind is that not all that children do is necessarily play. Whether a child's activity is for the purpose of mastery or play, a great deal of it does appear to provide enjoyment.

A Definition of Play

The foregoing theories provide a framework from which to formulate an understanding of play. Play is viewed from different perspectives, but each theory contributes important ideas about play. A recurring theme is that play should be pleasurable and enjoyable. If children enjoy what they do, they are likely to do it again and experiment with variations of the activity. This is how play leads to discovery and subsequent advancement in growth and development. If, on the other hand, an activity is not pleasurable, it is not likely to be continued, and the potential benefits of play are diminished. If play is not enjoyable, it follows that growth and developmental benefits will not be realized.

The idea that play is practice for adult living is a plausible interpretation because of the contributions of play to the total child. As long as the end goal of developmental advancement does not take precedence over the value of the pleasure derived from play, then the activity is play. This is not to say that play does not contribute to growth and development. The important point is that a child should be allowed to play

> Box 21-1
> *Characteristics of Play*
>
> 1. Play is a complex group of behaviors characterized by fun.
> 2. Play is sensory, neuromuscular, mental, or a combination of these characteristics with variations in the form it takes at different developmental stages.
> 3. Play involves repetition of experience, exploration, experimentation, and imitation. Risk taking and mastery are common features of play.
> 4. Play has its own time and space boundaries. The child's own interpretation of reality and fantasy provide some boundaries.
> 5. Play provides an avenue for the integration of internal and external worlds.
> 6. Play follows a sequential developmental progression (quantitative and qualitative changes occur over time).
>
> *(Adapted from Florey, 1981.)*

for enjoyment without the confines of adult standards of what has to be accomplished.

A completely satisfactory definition of play has not been established. Common elements constituting play have been summarized by Christie and Johnsen (1983) as behavior that is (1) spontaneous and arises from within (self-generated), (2) pleasurable or associated with positive emotions (not serious), (3) variable from one child to another and across situations (play is flexible), and (4) imaginary (not literal).

In a review of play theories by Florey (1981), six characteristics of play were identified as themes common to most major theories. They are listed in Box 21-1.

The question of how play contributes to what is not play (creativity, problem solving , language learning) continues to motivate research. Although the exact dynamics of how play contributes to all aspects of normal growth and development is not clear, some observations can be made. The following discussion identifies major contributions of play to the physical, intellectual, and emotional-social development of children.

Contributions of Play to the Developing Child

The varied theories of play conjure up the concept that play has something to do with every aspect of the developing child. Although a single play activity is likely to contribute to all aspects of development simultaneously, each sphere is discussed separately here to facilitate a clearer understanding of play.

Physical Development

The physical activity of play contributes to the development and coordination of the body throughout the life span. Children's play varies from one developmental stage to the next in part because of the physical maturation of their bodies. During infancy, play is dominated by sensorimotor activities such as looking, tasting, touching, and manipulating the environment. Through reaching, grasping, and mouthing objects repetitively, the *senses are developed* and *muscles are coordinated.* Hand-eye coordination is a competency that requires practice through play and maturation through growth. Through play, children develop control of their bodies as they practice creeping, crawling, and walking. The skillful movements and coordination required to take them to new territories for exploration are practiced incessantly. As children grow older they continue to increase their physical competency by engaging in activities that demand more precision, such as athletics, bicycle riding, swimming, dancing, and skating. Thus through play a person progresses from a randomly reflexive repertoire of behavior in infancy to skillfully coordinated movement in adulthood.

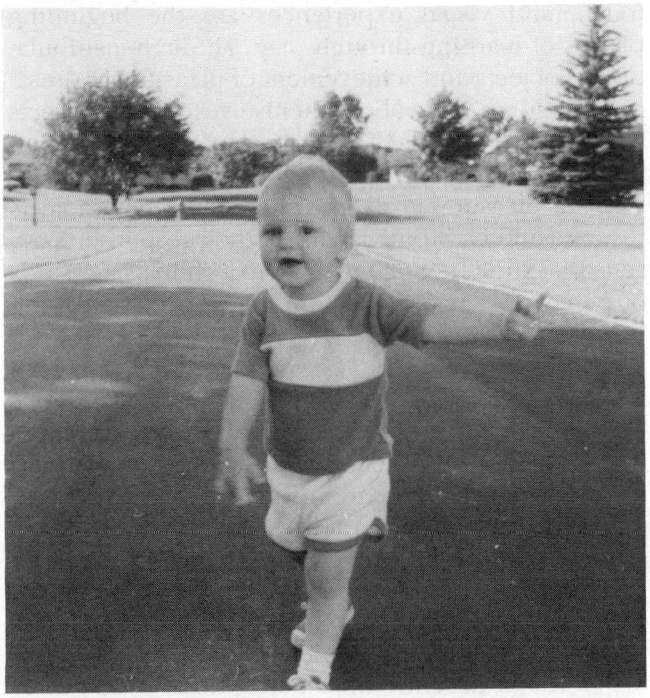

The physical activity of play contributes to the development and coordination of the body throughout life.

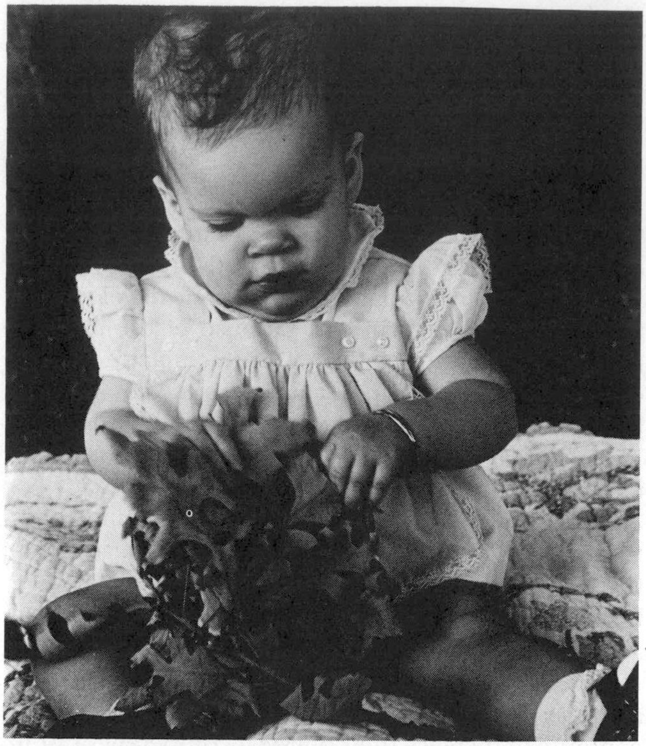

Through play the child discovers the world.

Cognitive Development

Through play children *discover the real world.* They learn about the composition of their world and relationships within that world. Earliest sound, movement, touch, and visual experiences are the beginning phases of learning through play. Through manipulation of objects and achievement of pleasurable sensations children learn about themselves and the objects in their environment. The pastime of repetitively putting objects into a receptacle and then dumping them out is a pleasurable exercise in seeing how objects respond and how one can affect their response. Early sensory experiences contribute to a child's later skills of perception and abstraction, necessary for reading (Caplan and Caplan, 1973).

Through play a child engages in extensive experimentation with sound and words to enhance *language development.* Nonsense syllables (sound play) and word substitutions are commonly observed in young children. Even before children are able to use words to describe what they see, their experiences with space, sound, color, and relationships help them form impressions about the environment. Experimentation with some objects provides an opportunity to discover their softness and smoothness before children have the words to describe their perceptions. These early experiences and the formation of multiple images help children put words into use (Caplan and Caplan, 1973). Play situations promote the use of words and phrases as children express their thoughts and wishes regarding the objects and events that comprise their play world.

As children become more social in their play, they need to increase their word usage to make their ideas known to their playmates. Language is an important tool in the expression of their innermost thoughts and feelings. Some language improvements were noted after training sessions in sociodramatic play and thematic fantasy play for groups of socioeconomically deprived children (Similansky, 1968; Freyberg, 1973; Saltz et al, 1977). Although a difference in language usage was noted following these training sessions, it is difficult to evaluate whether the findings are a result of play per se or of adult interaction and instruction (Saltz and Brodie, 1982).

Problem solving has its beginnings in play. To understand how play contributes to problem solving, it is useful to define what constitutes a problem. A problem is a situation in which a child has no ready response to deal with a presenting set of stimuli (Bijou, 1976). Play contributes to problem solving because experiences with objects, people, and ideas give the child a familiarity with how things work and to what degree one's own capacities can affect the environment. For example, if Tommy wishes to get a cookie out of a jar on a counter, he can solve the problem by drawing on previous play experiences, even though this particular problem has never been solved by him. Based on his experience he knows (1) I can move the chair, (2) I can crawl onto the chair, (3) I can open a jar. Each of these experiences has been practiced in play, but now they can be combined to solve the new problem of getting the cookie. Thus play supplies the knowledge and abilities necessary for problem solving.

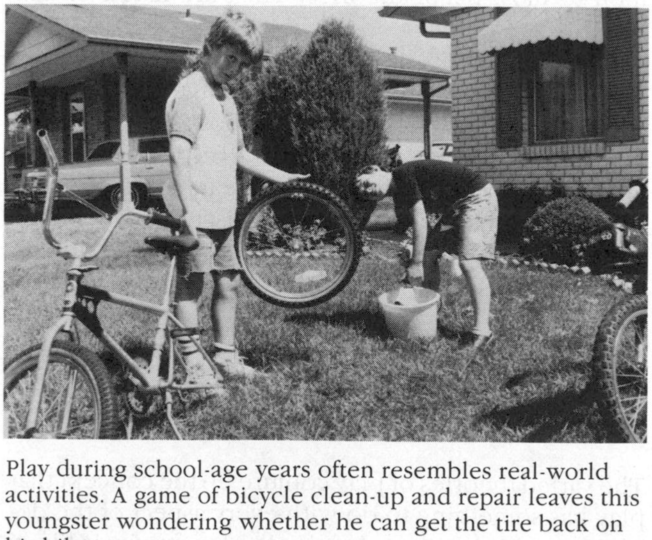

Play during school-age years often resembles real-world activities. A game of bicycle clean-up and repair leaves this youngster wondering whether he can get the tire back on his bike.

Play materials to learn problem solving are often real objects in the child's world. For example, taking things apart and putting them back together challenges a child's problem-solving skills.

Research has demonstrated that children who are given the opportunity to play with an object that is to be used in a subsequent problem-solving situation are better able to solve a particular problem than children who were not given the opportunity for prior play (Smith and Dutton, 1979; Vandenberg, 1981). It has been suggested that in these studies a play experience prior to the problem-solving situation may (1) cause children to approach the testing situation with a more playful attitude, resulting in greater flexibility, curiosity, spontaneity, and interest, (2) provide an opportunity for experimentation with objects that leads to a wide variety of ways to manipulate objects, facilitating later problem solving, or (3) facilitate abstract thinking through symbolic play (Rubin and Pepler, 1982).

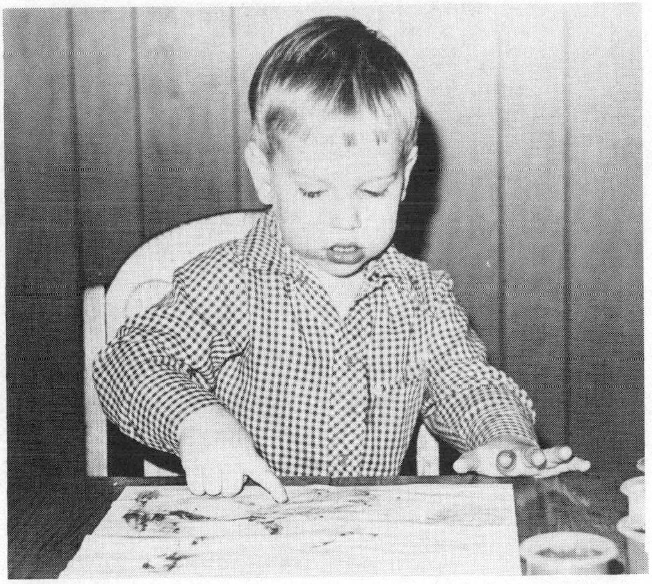

Play provides many possibilities for creativity.

Play *promotes a child's interest and concentration,* and *expands knowledge.* Children have a natural tendency to explore and learn about their environment. It is easy to capture a child's attention with novel objects and new ideas for play. Exposure to books, trips to museums, and strategy games are activities in which children happily participate. These activities increase their ability to concentrate and enlarge their mental capacity.

If a child is given the opportunity to be creative, play can be a natural avenue for *creative expression.* Creativity is so loosely defined that it is difficult to be assured of a mutual understanding without some clarification of its meaning. Creativity is the process of combining old ideas into forms that are new for the individual (Sutton-Smith, 1974). Through play children can experiment with new combinations of materials and ideas to create something they have never produced before. Children can be creative with very simple materials if left to their own imagination. Play opportunities provide many possibilities for creativity, some of which are object manipulation, dramatic play, drawing and painting, and daydreaming. Piaget (1951) suggests that adults supply appropriate materials for children's play but let them do their own experimenting: "Every time we teach a child something, we keep him from inventing it himself."

Emotional-Social Development

Play allows children to experiment with thoughts, feelings, and actions until they learn to adapt their emotions in a socially acceptable manner.

Self-awareness is developed through exploration of self and of others in relationship to self. The interpersonal experiences of smiling, crying, cooing, and touching are the beginning behaviors that lead to an awareness of the various responses a child can evoke within the environment. Through this exchange and experimentation children learn a great deal about the specific effects of their own actions and thereby develop an increasing sense of who they are relative to their environment. As children's territory widens and their relationships increase, so does their sense of self. Through play children develop an increasing sense of who they are, what they can do, and how others perceive them. These perceptions combine and contribute to the development of self-esteem.

Expression of emotions is a life-long learning process. During the developmental process, children engage in fantasy play to explore feelings, lessen fears, and work through conflicts. In games of pretending, imaginary playmates are safe recipients of aggressive impulses. Experiences that have frightened or excited a child may be re-enacted in play with imaginary participants. Through such play activities a child can express those intense feelings that may not be perceived as acceptable forms of behavior in the real world.

Independence and self-care skills are learned and practiced in a child's play. The delight children experience in seeing their own accomplishments during play gives them the confidence to begin doing things for themselves in other aspects of living. As children realize that they can stack their own blocks, they also demand that they be given control over their own bodies. In everyday activities of living such as eating, dressing, bathing, and preparation for sleep, play continues as children experiment with their own skills and become increasingly more independent.

The *moral development* of a child depends on

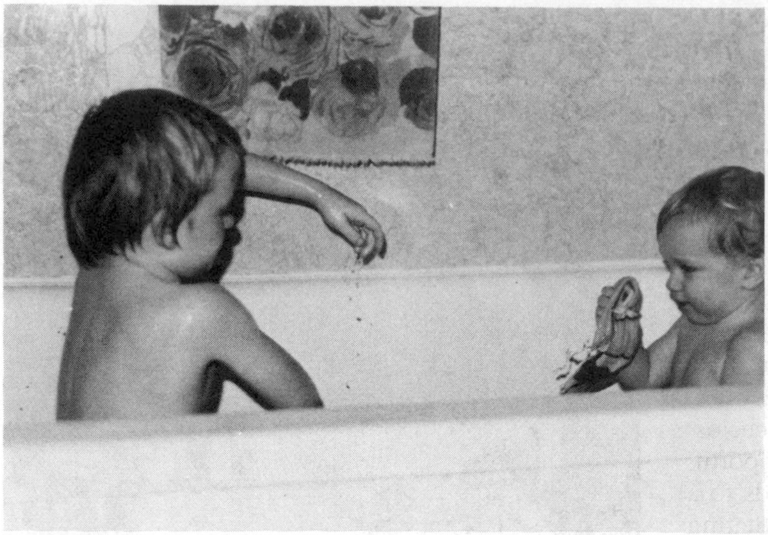

Everyday activities like bathing take on the character of play as new sensations are experienced. Through these experiences, self-care skills are learned and independence is achieved.

intellectual development and on social interactions. Children learn right from wrong in play because of the positive and negative reinforcement they receive from their family, peers, and society. Some play is rewarded and some is punished. Although learning right from wrong is an integral part of moral or ethical behavior, moral development consists of more than obeying the rules and behaving properly. The significance of play in moral development is that it helps children develop an understanding of the feelings of others and the ability to share. Ambron (1981) suggests that ethical behavior entails "understanding that the needs of others are as valid as our own." During play, rules are enforced by peers, and cheaters are ostracized. The interaction patterns developed through these play experiences contribute significantly to the moral development of children.

Cooperation is developed gradually through play as a child becomes less egocentric. As interpersonal relationships extend beyond the home to peers, children quickly learn the give and take of life during play. They learn to share playthings, agree to make a sandcastle by another's specifications, and wait until later for their turn to fly a plane. Play gives children the opportunity to show regard for the ideas of another.

Developmental Characteristics of Play

The kind of play in which children engage is largely determined by their developmental stage. Children progress through stages of play that reflect a range of thoughts and abilities. As children grow and develop, their environment changes and so do their needs. The social character and the content of play provide two developmental classifications of play to use in examining these changes.

Developmental Stages and Social Character of Play

In 1932, Parten identified different types of play in a group of 2- to 5-year-old children. The behaviors were observed in normal preschoolers and are considered typical for that age. Play behavior reflects a progression of sociability, ranging from playing alone to playing alongside another child as a toddler to cooperative play at about 5 years of age. Although Parten observed children aged 2 to 5 years, the characteristics identified are common in other age groups as well, as described next.

Unoccupied behavior describes a child who does not appear to be playing but focuses on anything that happens to be of momentary interest. When nothing exciting is taking place, the child examines his or her own body, gets on and off chairs, or just stands around or sits, looking. This type of behavior is common in toddlers and young preschoolers but occurs at all ages.

Onlooker behavior is when a child watches other children play. The child may talk to the children being watched, may ask questions or give suggestions, but does not join in the play. This type differs from unoccupied behavior in that the onlooker is observing the play of other children rather than any event in the environment. The child often takes up a position close to the group to see and hear everything that takes place. This type of play is most typical of toddlers but is seen in older children when they are in strange environments.

Solitary independent play describes the child

who plays alone with toys that are different from those used by the children in the same territory. A child may be within speaking distance of other children but make no effort to get close to them. These children pursue their own activity without reference to what others are doing. This type of play is most common in toddlers but occurs in older children if the environment is unfamiliar.

Parallel activity typically occurs during the toddler years. The child plays independently, but the activity chosen naturally brings her or him among other children. These children play with toys that are similar to those of children around them but do not try to influence or modify the activity of the children nearby. Children play *beside* rather than *with* each other. They seem to be aware of each other but make no attempt to control one another.

Associative play is more typical in the preschool and early school-age years. Children play *with* each other and talk about what they are doing. They borrow and lend play material and follow one another with similar playthings. There is no division of labor and no organization of the activity into a common group goal. Instead of subordinating individual interest to that of the group, each child acts as he or she wishes, but they play together with similar playthings or in similar activities.

Cooperative or organized supplementary play was noted by Parten (1932) in 5-year-olds, but this type of play is also typical of school-age children. Children play in a group that is organized for the purpose of attaining a group goal. They work together to make something or play in a formal game. There is a marked sense of belonging or of not belonging to the group. The control of the group situation is in the hands of one or two of the members. The children work together with a division of labor; different roles are taken by the various group members; and activity is organized so that the efforts of one child are supplemented by those of another.

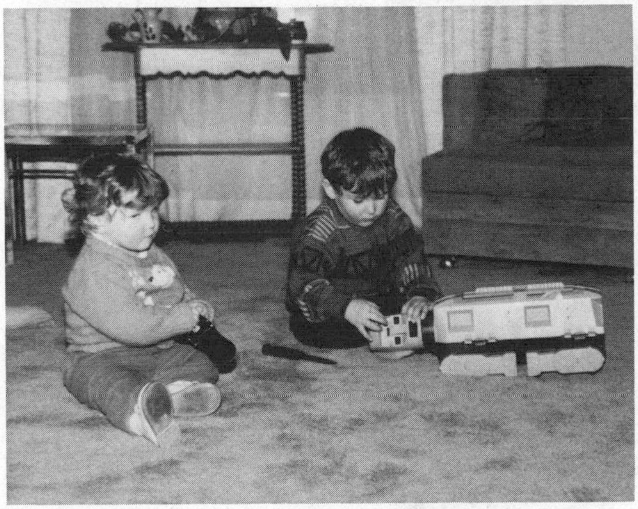

Toddlers play in close proximity in similar activities but do not try to influence or modify the activity of other children nearby.

Further discussion of play specific to each developmental level is included in the respective chapters on growth and development (Chapters 5 through 9).

Developmental Stages and Content of Play

Stone and Church (1983) have provided a useful approach to play by categorizing it according to content. The six categories of play they identified are (1) social-affective, (2) sense-pleasure, (3) skill, (4) dramatic, (5) formal, and (6) competitive.

They propose that play begins as *social-affective play*. Parents stimulate their infants by cooing, fondling, and other playful gestures. The infant's responses of pleasure are a reward to the parent, and a cyclic pattern of play develops.

Sense-pleasure play is nonsocial play that originates outside the infant. It is nonsocial in that it is stimulated by environmental variations in color, movement, sound, taste, and texture. The experience of sensing these variations is pleasurable, thus the term sense-pleasure. For infants, pleasurable experiences are expanded when they develop the manipulative and locomotor ability to experiment with the sensations derived from play with water, sand, and food. Activities of movement such as swinging, bouncing, and rocking are examples of sense-pleasure play, as is exploration of one's own body.

Skill play begins when infants have developed the ability to reach out, grasp, and manipulate. It consists of the repetitive practice of newly discovered abilities. There can be an element of sense-pleasure in skill play, depending on the type of activity, but it is the practicing and accomplishment of a task that intrigues a child rather than the pleasure derived during the activity. For example, the challenge of learning to ride a bike rather than the sensation of riding it motivates the child in skill play. Skill play is motivated by the challenge of taking on a task that one is hardly capable of accomplishing. People of all ages are subject to this fascination.

Various combinations of social-affective, sense-pleasure, and skill play continue during the toddler and preschool years. Also at this time a new motif emerges: *dramatic play*. Here a child tries out roles and identities drawn first from domestic life and later from the world at large. The imitative quality of this play is obvious when a child mimics adults by talking

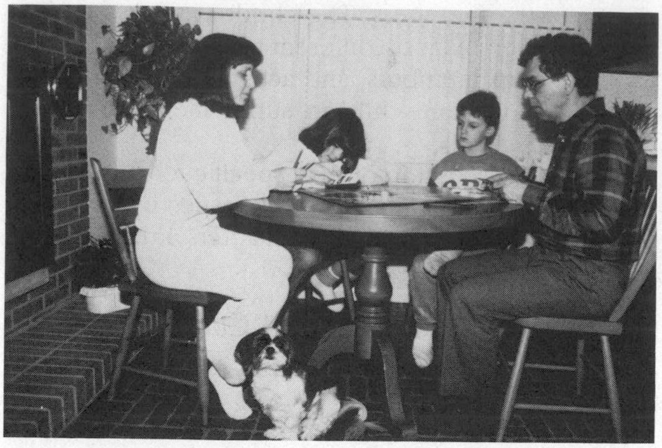

During the school-age years, table games provide opportunities for family interactions.

on the telephone, pretending to be shaving, and dressing up in adult clothing. Through imitation a child is identifying with those prominent persons in the environment.

When a child re-enacts scenes and events of everyday life, it may take the form of reproductive dramatic play or productive dramatic play. In reproductive dramatic play children try to re-create in their play a situation they have observed in real life or in the mass media. By contrast, in productive dramatic play children create characters and themes that may be taken either from real life experiences or from their imagination (Hurlock, 1978).

Formal games are simple, noncompetitive exercises such as ring-around-a-rosy and London Bridge. As children get older, their play becomes competitive and ranges from table games to sports.

The progression from social-affective play to formal games and from solitary play to cooperative play reflects the child's developing physical, intellectual, and social skills. This developmental process is influenced by the opportunities and nurturing provided by the family. Family relationships provide the basis for a child's social relationships with others and contribute to a developing sense of self-esteem. If parents play with their children, the excitement of discovery and creativity is shared, and children feel accepted and encouraged in their play. If children feel that parents are interested in what they can do, they are also stimulated to try new things in play. The characteristics of play (social character and content) are determined by the stage of development of a child but are subject to the quality of relationships within the family.

Anticipatory Guidance: Promoting Development Through Play

Nurses' understanding of what constitutes normal, healthy play is fundamental to their role in the care of children and their families. Nurses can prepare parents to expect the normal changes in the social character and content of play at various stages of development. Helping parents appreciate their child's play as an expression of development should be the goal in counseling parents about play. If parents can be helped to

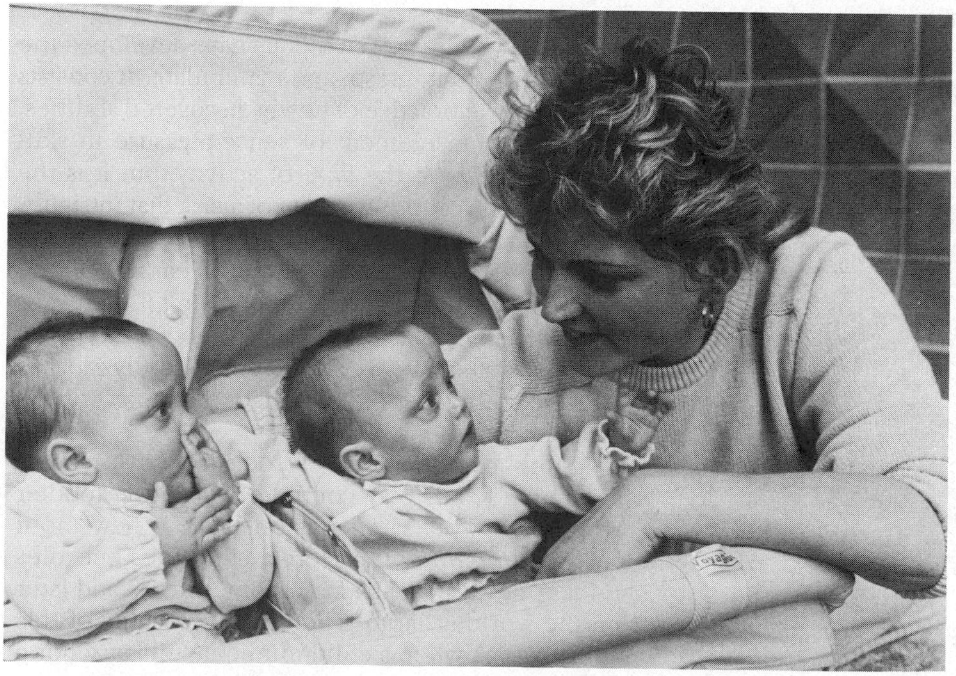

Parents and infants engaging in social exchanges of sounds, movement, and facial expressions is a form of interactive play. These 6-month-old twins readily respond to their mother's attempt to engage them in interactive play.

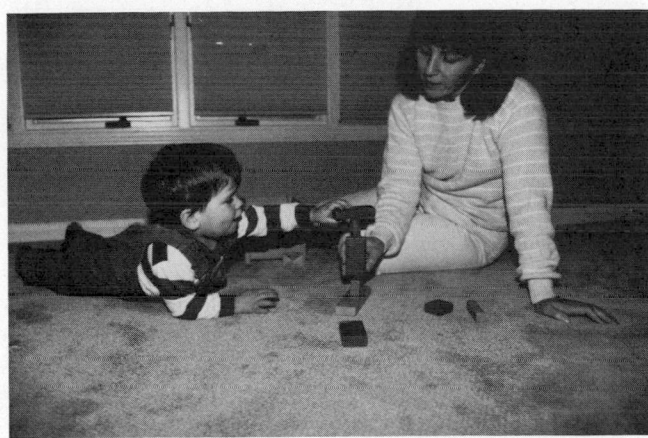

A stacking toy develops eye-hand coordination as well as a sense of accomplishment when a tower is built, and gleeful power when it is knocked down. Parents are encouraged to foster their child's development through appropriate play experience.

recognize and understand the association between their child's play and development, they can support that development more sensitively.

Parents are an excellent resource to the nurse with respect to a child's play. To counsel effectively, the nurse first gains an understanding of the home situation and the availability of resources, including space, time, and playthings. It is important to adapt what is told to parents to the parameters that are feasible for the individual family's situation. Focusing part of each health care visit on play gives it the appropriate priority. From infancy, an appreciation of play can be fostered by identifying the sensorimotor activities that the infant displays. Encouraging parents to reciprocate with sounds, movement, and facial expressions is how the beginnings of play are appreciated and encouraged. Role modeling interactive play with an infant during a health care visit is an influential aspect of promoting the beginning of healthy play behavior. As the child develops, parents need support and guidance to provide the variety of opportunities that children need. Opportunities for gross and fine motor activities, experiences in discovery and exploration, tactile and kinesthetic experiences, social interaction, and problem solving are some of the many characteristics of play opportunities that can be discussed with parents as their child develops.

Parents often do not appreciate that children's play experiences can be fostered. Because play is something that children "do naturally," parents may not recognize that their child's efforts to play can be enhanced by their support and interest. For example, a young child who wants to paint a piece of wood that is serving as a stage for a puppet performance may hear "No, I don't have time to help you — just do something else." These are the situations that can be troublesome to parents, because time and effort are required to support their child's development through play. It is not always feasible to help a child at a particular time, but nurses can help parents appreciate and understand that making time for their child's play is important in development. Parents should understand that one activity promotes development in several areas, yet the overall goal of "play is fun" should not be lost in the drive to advance the child. Examples of development promoted by certain activities or toys are summarized in Table 21-1.

Choosing safe, durable toys and encouraging activities suitable to their child's developmental level is a task in which parents may need guidance. A summary of toys and activities geared to a child's age is found in Table 21-2. We stress that it is not necessary to buy expensive toys. Excellent opportunities for a child's progress are provided by common household equipment and the sounds and textures of the outdoors.

The proper use of toys should also be addressed in counseling about play. Too many toys can be confusing and overstimulating to children. Excessive use of toys also can thwart the child's own resourcefulness in creating play situations out of natural stimuli in the environment. Self-expression and the freedom of play according to their own needs are most beneficial to children.

Parents should be encouraged to play with their children but also should be helped to realize that there may be times when they should not play, as when irritable and tired. At times, a child's greatest desire is to have a parent *watch* her or him play. Whether parents encourage the play of children by playing with them or watching them, it should be pleasurable for both generations. The nurse's role is to encourage parents to provide opportunities for play, play with their children when appropriate, and participate in the thoughts and feelings of their children by watching them play.

Promoting Development Through Special Play Activities: Nurse's Role in Anticipatory Guidance

It is important to recognize the special interests and abilities of individual children. A single child may have a broad range of interests, which may differ from those of the parents. Manipulating youngsters' activities to satisfy the parents' goals can deter a child from reaching personal goals. Parents should be encouraged to respect their child's individuality and to recognize the range of activities that provide developmental bene-

Table 21-1. Promoting Growth and Development Through Toys and Activities

Activity or Toy	Developmental Aspects Promoted
Music boxes	Auditory stimulation, awareness of environment, introduction to variety of sounds
Mobiles	Visual stimulation, awareness of environment, introduction to variety of colors and shapes
Rattles with small handles	Auditory stimulation, visual stimulation, manipulation skills, cause and effect relationships
Talking, singing to infant	Promote social responsiveness, auditory stimulation, promote attachment, facilitate language development
Pull toys	Stimulate gross motor development, sense of accomplishment in making toy do something
Books with large colorful pictures	Facilitate language development, enhance fine motor skills through page turning, teach about objects in environment through pictures; introduction to colors, shapes, and naming of objects. Foster social interaction when someone looks at books with the child
Stacking toys	Stimulate size discrimination, introduce colors, stimulate active experimentation through trial and error, muscle development through hand manipulation, eye-hand coordination, creativity through varying orders of stacking
Peek-a-boo	Encourages social interaction that is pleasurable, demonstrates permanence of objects
Clay, play dough	Promotes fine motor skills, enhance creativity and self-expression, a vehicle for expression of fantasy
Puppets	Provide outlet for handling own fears and aggressive feelings; stimulate imaginary play
Punching bags	Provide outlet for aggressive feelings and tension and direct energy into a channel that does not harm others; promote gross motor skills and coordination
Art, crafts, construction toys, drama, creative writing	Fine motor skills, stimulate creativity and self-expression, enhance eye-hand coordination, develop a sense of accomplishment
Sports (team play)	Enhance ability to adhere to rules, outlet for energy and to reduce tension, stimulate large muscle development, enhance social development, teach give and take of relationships
Tricycles, bicycles, and other riding toys	Enhance large motor skills, develop balance, promote a sense of accomplishment
Collections of stamps, rocks, coins, and other items	Teach relationships, categorization, fine discrimination of properties, responsibility, and organization
Puzzles, table games	Stimulate problem solving; rule learning and fair play promote socialization; promote concentration and mental skills of memory, discrimination, categorization; depending on game, teach fine motor skills

fits. The nurse's role is to promote the development of children by encouraging participation in a variety of activities.

Included in this section is a discussion of the role of physical activity and sports, children's art, and environmental stimulation in the development of children.

Exercise and Sports

The way children and adults play has changed appreciably in the past 20 years. We live in an era when play and recreation are organized and scheduled. The availability of exercise programs for the very young, the noon-hour physical fitness program for the executive, and the emphasis placed on sports in our society exemplify the mounting interest in physical fitness and exercise. Although young children naturally run and explore actively much of the day, our society embraces an abundance of programs and resources to teach parents how to promote exercise and direct energy into specific skill development programs for their children. Recognizing the confusion that parents may experience, it is important to address exercise and sports as part of the routine anticipatory guidance given at all ages. The nurse can use the following basic guidelines.

Assessment

An important role that a nurse often assumes is performing a history and physical assessment to screen for conditions that would jeopardize the health of a child who participates in sports. Important aspects to consider are family history of heart disease, endurance while running (twice around a quarter-mile track without stopping), a history of fainting or being knocked out, current medications being taken, a history of any illness or injury that caused missing a game or practice, admission to a hospital, or surgery (Smith, 1981). During the physical examination the nurse should check particularly for abdominal, heart, and lung abnormali-

Table 21-2. Age-Appropriate Activities for Children and Adolescents

Activities and Toys	Developmental Characteristics
Infant (0 to 6 Months)	
Solitary, sensorimotor play Crib mobile, soft squeeze toys, rattles, musical toys, stuffed animals, mirror. Place infant in various positions and take for walks, rock, use stroller, swing (for short periods). Talk, sing, and laugh with infant, splash water during bath, crinkle paper for infant to hear. Read to infant	Play at times of day that infant is content. Provide variety of textures, colors, sounds, movement. Human interaction is important; respond to sounds and cues of infant. Keep infants safe as they become more mobile
Infant (6 to 12 Months)	
Solitary, sensorimotor play Provide push-pull toys (if walking). Blocks, stack toys, nesting toys, activity box on crib. Water and sand play (supervised). Nursery rhymes, play music, read to child. Games such as peek-a-boo, pat-a-cake, and naming of body parts	Provide for larger, safe spaces in which to crawl and explore. Use household utensils as toys (check for rough edges and loose parts). Continue human interactions and variety of stimuli as for younger infant
Toddler (1 to 3 Years)	
Parallel play Push-pull toys, riding toys, throw and catch large ball, rocking horse, climbing opportunities. Sand and water play, soap bubbles, clay and play dough, blocks to build and knock down, access to certain cupboards and drawers that are safe, painting and coloring	Energetic and physically active, therefore large motor skills are being practiced. Enjoys varied textures and exploration of the environment. Aggressiveness and creativity can be expressed through manipulation of various toys and objects
Stacking toys, nesting toys, cars, trucks, dolls, large-size Legos or Loc-blocks, puzzles	Enjoys manipulative activities and miniatures of real-life objects
Dressing up, nurse and doctor kits, story telling, read to child, music to promote rhythm	Creative and educational toys and activities are to be encouraged. Imaginative play is prominent
Preschool (3 to 5 Years)	
Cooperative play Riding toys, tricycles, gym and climbing equipment, sleds. Swimming, ice skating, roller skating and skiing are common	Need provision for continued refinement of motor skills. A beginning involvement in sports activities enhances peer relationships
Sandbox and wading pool, clay and play dough, soap bubbles	Continues to enjoy varied textures and freedom to explore
Cutting, pasting, stringing beads, drawing, coloring, painting	Fine motor skills are improving and there is increased constructive use of materials
Dressing up, cooking, making things with wood	Imitation of grown-ups is predominant. Originality and creativity are demonstrated. Imaginary play
Music, records, read to child, story telling	More quiet play is enjoyed. Need to achieve a balance between active and quiet play
Continues to play with trucks, trains, cars, planes, dolls, building blocks, Legos and Loc-blocks, puzzles, Tinker Toys, and some simple card games. Television becomes a preferred activity and needs to be restricted	Now has longer attention span, therefore building projects provide long hours of play; increased sharing is evident in much of play
School-age (6 to 12 Years)	
Group play (formalized play) Continues to play with cars, trucks, and dolls, but play is more organized	Organized group play provides opportunity for sharing of common interests and encourages cooperation
Swimming, skating, gymnastics, hiking, bike riding, rough and tumble games, and many other sports	Physical activity becomes more directed into skill development and sports
Collecting, hobbies, books, movies, table and board games, music, and theater. Likes to have own music tapes and tape recorder. A pocket radio with a headset is popular at this age; this continues into adolescence	Quiet activities which require longer attention spans and concentration are now enjoyed. Aware of rules of a game
Projects using real equipment in sewing, woodworking, cooking; makes many things out of household materials. Dramatic play with real costumes and performing in plays and shows that the group has created	Many creative projects are designed. These activities require cooperation and support from parents in that rooms become cluttered and disorganized with an abundance of unfinished and finished projects that might appear useless to parents

continued

Table 21-2 *(continued)*

Activities and Toys	Developmental Characteristics
Adolescent (13 to 18 Years)	
Organized play and recreational play	
Sports interests continue, with special interest developing for certain ones. Recreation like fishing, camping, hiking, and canoeing is enjoyed	May become competitive and concentrate on maximal skill development and achievement in sports
Video arcades, home computers, and video games are challenges. The bicycle gives way to the car during adolescence and driving the car with peers (without a destination) is recreational	Much of play is determined by what is popular with peers. Activities that provide independence from parents are preferred
For the young adolescents making things, models and school projects occupy many hours. As they approach adulthood, afterschool jobs and summer jobs consume more and more of their time and energy	Many adolescents prefer less demanding and less strenuous physical activities Gradually more time is devoted to becoming economically independent

ties, dental prosthesis, hernia, and orthopedic problems. Disqualifying conditions for collision sports that have been recommended by Smith include (1) absence of any of the paired organs (lung, eye, kidney, testes), and (2) poorly controlled seizure disorders (advised not to participate in water sports). The maturation level should also be assessed, and late-maturing individuals should be advised against collision sports (see later discussion on maturation).

Counseling and Common Concerns

The nurse's counseling role is to facilitate decision making by parents and child by proffering support. Areas of concern in which a nurse can provide some information are choice of activities appropriate for age, maturational variation, male and female opportunities, and potential negative effects of sports and exercise.

Development and Appropriate Activities. During infancy, coordination, balance, and motor skill can be fostered through exercise games. Swimming has gained considerable interest as an activity for infants. The American Academy of Pediatrics Committee on Pediatric Aspects of Physical Fitness, Recreation, and Sports (1980) has recommended that organized group swimming instructions begin after 3 years of age, based on the following concerns: (1) the inability to teach young children water safety; (2) the danger of providing parents with false security that their infant can swim; and (3) incontinence of infants in pools and effectiveness of chlorination.

The use of devices like infant walkers to promote exercise and movement is generally unnecessary, and they can be hazardous (see Chapter 17 on safety). A restrictive device such as a playpen should not be used for long periods of time as both movement and variety of stimulation are hampered.

As children reach preschool age, physical activity in the form of running, sliding, swinging, climbing, and jumping comprises a considerable part of the normal day. Skill activities like tricycle riding, skating, and swimming (with an adult) provide exercise as well as a sense of accomplishment. Such activities should be fun for a preschooler. Parents should be aware that a child's lack of self-discipline and short attention span may require short, nonintensive practice periods. Other activities such as kindergym (gym for the preschooler) and dance provide the opportunity for children to socialize in a play situation and develop an appreciation for rhythm and music. The important aspect to stress is that these activities provide enjoyment to the child and thereby are rewarding to the parent.

If a child resists an activity, it should be determined whether the event can be presented to the child in a more acceptable way. If a child does not wish to participate in any planned activities, encouragement and support from parents may need to be increased. Despite this, a child may resist for a time, but as the skill is mastered, the feeling of success and enjoyment may take over. The decision whether to encourage a child to continue in a distasteful activity is an individual matter. If participation at a parent's insistence introduces ongoing conflict and stress for both parent and child, most often it is advisable to wait until the next class or season.

As the child enters school, the issue of organized sports becomes a central concern. The nurse should assess whether participation in sports and recreational activity is an enjoyable experience or whether it is putting undue pressure on the child. For example, the 6-year-old child who misses the ball in minor league baseball and turns to a parent who is watching on the sideline with "Sorry, Dad" or "Sorry, Mom" exemplifies how "play" can be abused. Our society's emphasis on competition and winning may or may not be of value to a child. When a child no longer finds pleasure in an activity, it can hardly be construed as play. Placing excessive pressure on children to perform is inappropriate.

A child's maturity should be considered in determining appropriateness of a particular sport. Recommended chronologic guidelines from Belkengren and Sapala (1982) are:

- Age 6: Noncontact sports, including swimming, gymnastics, track and field, martial arts, tennis, and skating
- Age 8: With trained supervision: basketball, volleyball, softball, soccer, and wrestling
- Age 12: Collision sports: football, rugby, and hockey.

As the child approaches adolescence, parents and adolescents face still newer problems pertaining to physical fitness and sports. Common issues that may be raised at this time pertain to maturational variations, opportunities in sports for young men and women, and adverse effects of rigorous physical training.

Maturational Variations. Individual differences in growth rates of adolescents reflect the variation in onset of sexual maturation. The Tanner staging techniques (see Chapter 9) can be used to assess maturation. In boys, sexual maturity correlates with muscle development, strength, and epiphyseal maturity (Smith, 1984). The late maturer and early maturer both may have problems, but of a different nature. The late maturer needs to be held back and advised not to participate in collision sports (football, wrestling, ice hockey). Competitive strength, endurance potential, and the skeletal maturation required are not sufficient until Tanner's Stage 5 of development is approached (Smith, 1984).

Peak height velocity usually occurs around Stage 3; this is the time of greatest vulnerability to epiphyseal injury (see Chapter 47 regarding bone growth and ossification). An early maturer may experience success in sports because of advanced biologic age. As peers reach comparable levels of physical maturity, the early maturer's performance is no longer exceptional or outstanding. The pressure that parents place on the early maturer at this time sometimes may be excessive.

The emotional stress of participation in sports is important to discuss with the child and parent. It has been observed in a group of high school students that failing in a competitive area with one's peers is one of a child's most stressful life events (Coddington, 1972).

Sports are important in the lives of adolescents, thus the entire family is affected by the rigorous schedules and interruption of family routines.

Opportunities of Boys and Girls. Prepubescent boys and girls can safely compete in sports. The strength and body proportions of both sexes are essentially the same until the beginning of adolescence. After puberty, boys become taller and stronger than girls and develop greater muscular strength and cardiovascular endurance. Separate but equal participation by girls and boys should then be available. Federal regulations require that both sexes have equal opportunity in athletics (Belkengren and Sapala, 1982).

Sports and Potential Negative Effects. Sports activities have grown at a phenomenal rate in most communities in recent decades. The physical and emotional impact of these large-scale programs has not been established with sound quantitative data. The risk of injury in prepubescent children appears to be considerably less than in postpubescent youth because of their reduced size, strength, power, and speed. The two most common types of injuries are acute lesions (sprains, strains, and, to a lesser extent, fractures) and overuse. A special problem in children is injury of the epiphyseal plate resulting in altered growth potential (Greene, 1983); the younger the child at the time of injury, the more serious the growth disturbance. (See Chapter 47 for further discussion of skeletal injuries.)

Another exercise-related injury in the young child is heat-induced illness. Children do not tolerate climatic extremes as well as adults do. Thermoregulation in children is hampered by (1) a lower sweating capacity (an unexplained mechanism increases the ability to sweat during puberty); (2) a greater metabolic heat production per mass unit; (3) a reduced ability to convey heat by blood from muscle to skin; and (4) a greater relative surface area, which results in a greater heat transfer between the environment and the body (American Academy of Pediatrics, 1983).

Precautions that can be taken to prevent heat-induced illness are that strenuous periods of activity should not exceed 30 minutes when temperature and humidity are in zone 3 (Fig. 21-1); acclimatization to a warm climate should take place by gradually increasing intensity and duration of exercise over a period of 10 to 14 days; prior to prolonged physical activity the child should be well hydrated, and dehydration during the activity should be prevented by scheduled drinking (150 ml of cold tap water each 30 minutes for a child weighing 40 kg); clothing should be lightweight (one layer), and sweat-saturated garments should be changed (American Academy of Pediatrics, 1982).

Concerns about injury to the female athlete often are based on misinformation. Concern that *serious breast injury* occurs in female sports has not been found to be true. Breast soreness has been reported; however, a sports bra can be recommended to alleviate

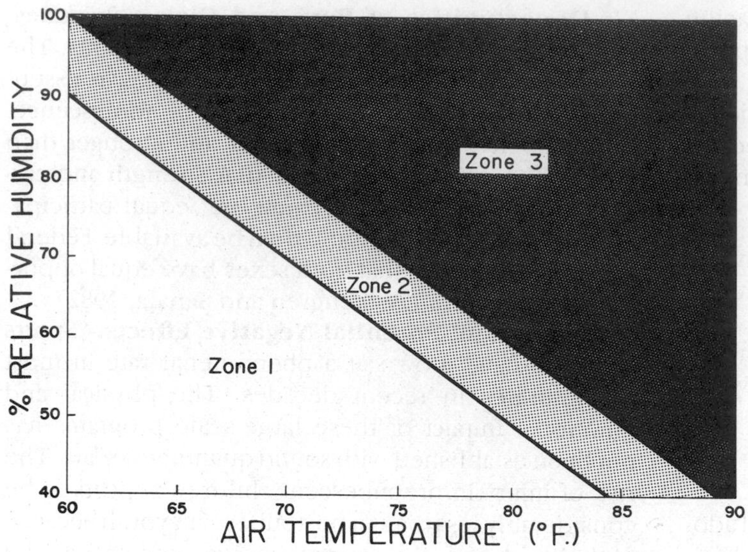

Figure 21-1. Weather guide for prevention of heat illness during prolonged strenuous exercise. (From Mathews DK, Fox EL: *The Physiological Basis of Physical Education and Athletics.* 3rd ed. New York, CBC College Publishing, Holt, Rinehart & Winston, 1981.)

this problem (Belkengren and Sapala, 1982; Gehlsen and Albohm, 1980). *Amenorrhea* can occur with intense physical training and is thought to be related to a body fat ratio of less than 10 to 12 per cent (Smith, 1981). It is important to explain to the athlete and parent that amenorrhea is not synonymous with anovulation. Usually a regular menstrual cycle can be expected after intense training has been reduced and body fat levels have been increased (Greene, 1983). However, secondary amenorrhea is not to be disregarded and should be evaluated to determine whether it is a normal variation of athletic activity, a separate problem, or a pregnancy (Belkengren and Sapala, 1982). Whether training with weights will cause muscle bulging in females may be a concern. Weight training increases strength and muscle tone, but minimal hypertrophy has been reported in girls as a result of this activity. Muscular hypertrophy is influenced by the hormone testosterone, therefore girls and women do not acquire excessive bulging of muscles (Belkengren and Sapala, 1982).

The emotional and behavioral benefits or problems that arise from sports programs have not been documented. The stress on the child that winning is essential is a potential problem in the home. The excessive demands on time to participate in practice and in games also can be stressful to a busy family. It is important for parents to assure children that their worth is not dependent on winning the game. Some positive outcomes are that children are able to enjoy the game, they learn how to win and lose, and they develop a sense of responsibility through the care of sports equipment and by being a dependable team member for practice and games. The sense of well-being derived from physical fitness, from belonging to a group, and from playing a game to their best ability is a positive outcome as long as the benefits are not offset by anxiety associated with parental pressure and expectations from an untrained coach.

Children's Art

Children's art production progresses in a developmental and universal fashion throughout childhood. From the graphic scribbles of the young toddler, later forms of art emerge. For young children, art serves as an educational and exploratory activity through which they can experiment with various colors, forms, and textures. Creation of a tangible finished product arouses feelings of accomplishment from the praise of others and simply by seeing the artwork displayed. It is a creative means through which their own thoughts, perceptions, and feelings can be communicated. Art can provide insight into the thoughts of children who may have difficulty expressing them verbally. Interpretation of art is beyond the scope of this text; however, an understanding of the developmental characteristics of art can complement other assessment tools in the care of children.

Infancy and Toddlerhood: Scribbles and Perfecting Scribbles

Scribbles are not meaningless lines on a piece of paper. Kellogg and O'Dell (1967) have identified 20 basic scribbles, which, they contend, are contained in every form of graphic art. The evolution of scribbles follows a fairly predictable pattern:

1. Shortly after 1 year of age, initial attempts at scribbling are made. The scribble is a continuous back and forth movement made of mostly

horizontal strokes, followed by circular movements. These markings result primarily from a banging action of the arm, and many markings extend off the page.
2. Around 16 to 20 months of age, a freer movement is noted; however, markings continue to extend off the page and are primarily horizontal, circular, and marks that flare in all directions.
3. Toward the end of age 2 years, the child's scribbling becomes more controlled, evidenced by the ability to keep the scribbles on the paper. The scribbles are now more circular or angular, and there is greater experimentation with amounts of pressure exerted on the pen or crayon.

Early Childhood: Preschematic Drawing

The increased ability for fine motor control in the preschooler is evidenced by the distinguishable shapes among the scribbles. By the time a child turns 3, a pencil is usually held by resting the shaft of the pencil at the juncture of the index finger and thumb, resulting in less arm movement and more finger movement. An interesting and universal shape that is frequently drawn by 3- to 5-year-olds is a figure referred to as a "mandala." A mandala is a crossed circle (may also take the form of a crossed square), a figure which has been identified on jungle stones and walls of prehistoric caves (Kellogg, 1970). From this figure a child proceeds to drawings of other objects, such as the sun, radials (spokes that spray out from a circle), and eventually human figures. A preschool and early school-age child enters the preschematic stage (4 to 7 years), when drawings represent the child's mental images (i.e., the largest objects in the drawing frequently have the greatest significance for the child). Usually one or two basic shapes are combined when drawing the human body. The progression of development represented in children's drawings is as follows:

1. Three-year-old: Shapes and forms begin to be fused together to form designs, and a crude figure is sometimes recognizable (i.e., head, eyes, mouth).
2. Four-year-old: A three-part man can be drawn. Longitudinal marks are used to represent the body, giving the human figure a tadpole shape. The eyes often dominate children's drawings at this age because of their awareness of people's eyes. Drawings of animals, trees, and flowers also are represented with similar graphics (i.e., various shapes and attached lines).
3. Five-year-old: Attains the skill to draw a six-part man (usually head, eyes, nose, mouth, body, and legs) (Fig. 21-2).

School-Age Child: Schematic Drawing

Children's drawings at this age have a highly expressive quality and reflect a boundless imagination. The magic of children's art during the school-age years, particularly around 6 and 7 years of age, is not likely to be surpassed at any other stage of development. Limitless freedom permits these young children to convey their inner feelings and express what is in their minds rather than what they necessarily see in real life. For example, realistic colors are not always used: a sun may be green or the grass may be blue, depending on what pleases a child at a certain time.

During the school-age years, children's undeveloped perceptual skills are reflected in their artwork. People and objects have highly disproportionate qualities. A flower may be as tall as a house and a head as large as or larger than the rest of the body. Children continue to exaggerate those object parts that have special significance, therefore reality is distorted. Spatial relationships, however, are better maintained by a newly acquired concept, the base line. Around the age of 6 years a child begins to use a line drawn horizontally across the page; people, flowers, and trees are drawn on this line.

A school-age child's art may appear perceptually erroneous to the casual observer. A technique called *projected animism* is common. At this age children make their subjects appear lifelike because of their belief that inanimate objects are alive. Human qualities such as smiling faces or the wearing of clothes may be associated with objects. The *x-ray technique* is another perceptual variation characteristic of this age group. Both the inside and outside of a person or object are depicted on the same drawing. Although a child does not see this in real life, it is normal in children's drawings and is not a sign of perceptual difficulties.

Some notable changes occur during the later part of the school-age years. The older school-age child (10 to 12 years) no longer exaggerates the most significant parts of an object but begins to draw important aspects with greater detail. Also, there is a greater tendency to differentiate male figures from female figures as the child's awareness of identity increases.

The developmental progression of artwork during the school-age years is

1. Six-year-old: Draws a seven- to nine-part per-

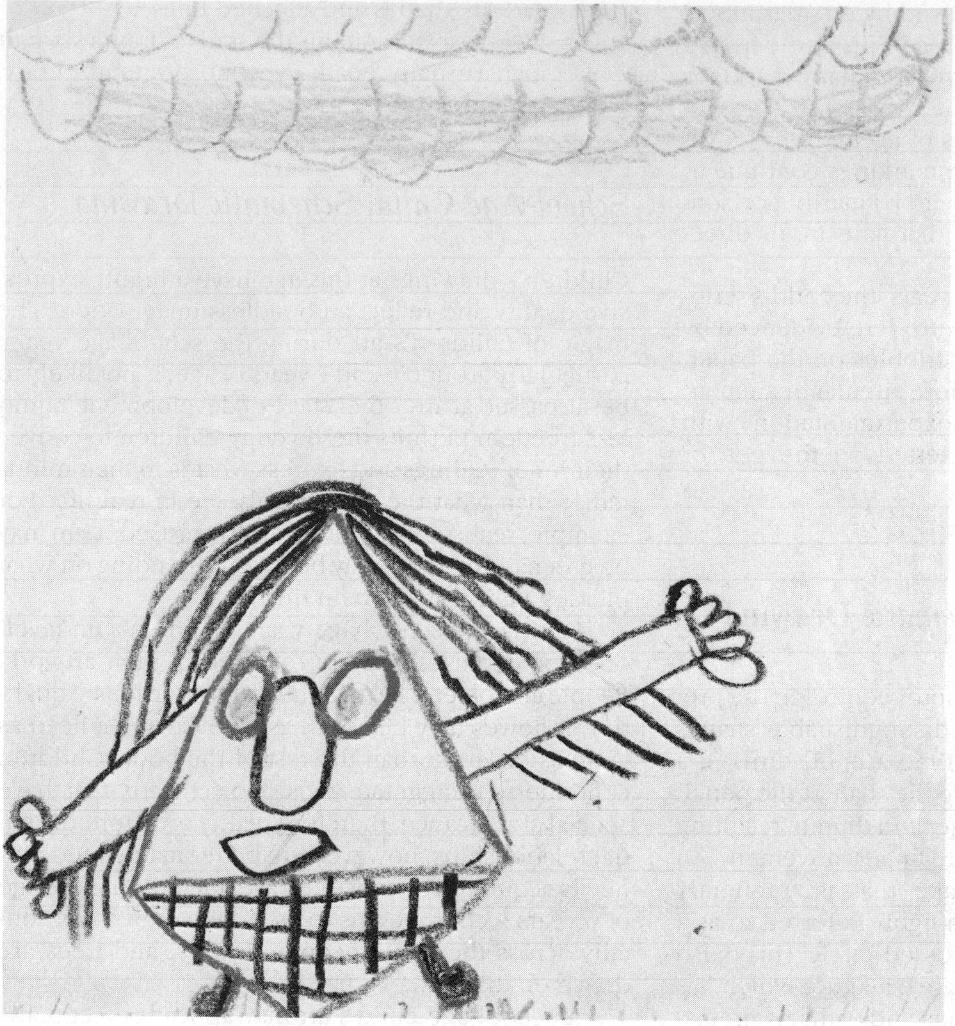

Figure 21-2. From 4 to 7 years of age, children's drawings are *preschematic.* One or two basic shapes combine to represent the human body. In this drawing by a 6-year-old child, typical features are represented: (1) disproportionate qualities (head larger than rest of body); (2) newly acquired concept of a base line (i.e., the grass); (3) 7- to 9-part person (hair, eyes, nose, mouth, arms, legs, hands, feet); (4) undeveloped perceptual skill (arms coming off head).

son. Acquires the concept of a base line. Significant parts are exaggerated; use of color is imaginative.

2. Seven- to nine-year-old: Draws a 9- to 11-part person at 7 years of age and a 10- to 12-part person at 9 years of age. Begins to draw schematically between the ages of 7 and 9 years. Has sufficient fine motor skill to produce recognizable pictures that contain some order in space. Uses x-ray technique around 7 to 9 years of age.
3. Ten- to twelve-year-old: At age 10 to 11 years, draws a 13-part person and at age 12 years, a 14-part person. Differentiates male from female figures; spatial relationships are further improved. Important objects are no longer exaggerated in size but are drawn in detail. At around 11 to 12 years of age, more attention is given to the basic features of art, such as lines, shapes, color, and space, and increased use is seen of sketching skills, such as shadows and shading.

Adolescence: Technique Development

During this period there is an increase in artistic skills. Some youngsters, of course, develop more skill than others. Artistic development during adolescence and thereafter is a matter of technique, and if no advancement in technique is developed then adults are not able to draw any better than during their early adolescence. Even though in adolescence there is an increase in artistic skill and an increased exposure to new experiences out of which artistic work could emerge, this period actually shows a decline in artistic expression and a reduced interest in art. The use of art as a form of graphic language declines because now speaking and writing skills are more efficient as a form of communication. Also, many other interests are pursued, so there is a limited amount of time available to devote to artwork. Fear of failure and ridicule pertaining to one's artwork is now common and may interfere with freedom of expression through art. The self-doubts that prevail during this phase of development can hinder artistic development (Helms and Turner, 1981).

Developmental Assessment Through Art

A difference in artistic ability from one child to another exists; however, certain characteristics of art, as just described, can be expected to emerge at the various age levels. A child's drawings can thus be assessed to ascertain whether a child is progressing normally. Any assessment based on children's art should be done with the recognition that it is a general guide to be used in conjunction with other tools and that more than one piece of art must be reviewed.

The use of art to determine psychologic pathology is beyond the scope of this discussion; considerable contradiction is seen in the way thoughts and emotions are interpreted through children's art (McLeavey, 1979).

Some general beliefs about the meaning of drawings with respect to a child's inner feelings are (1) excessively large or small drawings symbolize aggressiveness and very small ones depict insecurity; (2) exaggeration or absence of certain body parts represents a concern about that part (e.g., head for intellect, feet for security, arms for power); (3) the sun represents parental love and support; (4) excessive erasures may indicate anxiety and uncertainty; (5) shading of certain parts is related to anxiety regarding that part; (6) heavy line pressure is related to more aggressive, high-energy children and light line pressure symbolizes shyness and inhibition; and (7) stick figures are often drawn by children who are hesitant to reveal themselves. Interpretation of children's art is a process that takes place over time and is based on many pictures, includes the child's verbal explanation of the drawing, and is done by specially trained professionals.

The significance of the various colors used in drawings has also received considerable attention, but some writers caution against inferring too much from color. Marzolf and Kirchner (1973) observed that the significance of color is different for boys and girls. The significance of color discussed in the literature has been summarized by Klepsch and Logie (1982) as follows:

Red may be related to violence or excessive emotion; it has also been associated with cheerfulness; nursery-level children who emphasize it are happy, well-adjusted, and emotional in their personal reactions.

Yellow is suggestive of hostility, dependency, and infantile behavior. Yellow used with green to depict grass or a landscape is normal.

Orange often suggests a good relationship with surroundings; may suggest areas of discomfort.

Blue equates with controlled reactions and self-restraint.

Green: Blue and green are similar and represent controlled behavior. Much blue and green used together in drawings indicates that a child feels secure as long as she or he is able to maintain control.

Black: controlled reactions, intellectual, compulsive.

Brown: timidity; may be used in times of regression. Brown and black used together suggest anxiety and depression.

Excessive use of any one color may indicate that a child is constricted and is somewhat emotionally unstable, since well-adjusted children are thought to use a variety of color (Klepsch and Logie, 1982).

Encouragement and Support of Children's Art

The nurse can be instrumental in encouraging parents to provide the opportunity for their children to express themselves through art. It is one activity that can provide hours of enjoyment with minimal cost to the family. Pencils, wax crayons, washable-ink felt-tipped pens, colored pencils, watercolors, poster paints, and finger paints provide a variety of activities with different results with which a child likes to experiment. Although painting with watercolor and paints requires some supervision, some basic hints can be offered to keep the activity enjoyable for both parent and child.

1. The smaller the child, the bigger the brush.
2. The smaller the child, the thicker the paint.
3. Muffin tins or sectioned aluminum trays can be used for mixing paints.
4. Table and floor must be washable, otherwise use plastic to protect surfaces from paint.
5. Provide the child with a paint smock.
6. Teach the child how to clean up.

To promote creativity in children through art, parents should be encouraged to verbally support their children about their drawings. Many well-meaning adults frequently respond to a drawing with the question "What is it?" It is believed by some that this question limits children's spontaneity by being asked to give meaning that they never intended. Children are somewhat hesitant and frequently need to think about it when asked "What is it?" Reinforcing remarks communicating praise and approval for the artwork often will initiate conversation about the drawing, and in

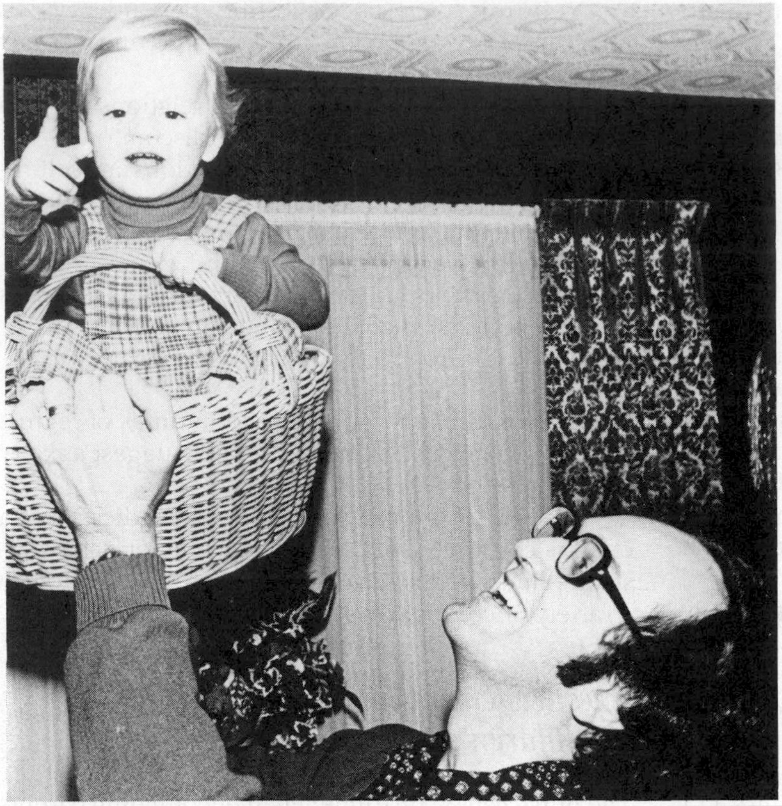

The sensation of flying is an exhilarating, happy experience when a trusted one is at the controls.

their own time children may explain. Comments such as "You have done a good job on that" or "That is something to be proud of" encourage a child to feel a sense of pride in accomplishment.

Environmental Stimulation

An important determinant of the play behavior of children is the environment in which they play. It has been recognized that an environment devoid of interesting objects, sound, and people curtails their play and development. Excessive stimulation (high intensity or prolonged exposure), on the other hand, has the potential to exhaust and tire an individual. It is important to recognize that optimal play and development are associated with a level of stimuli appropriate for a particular individual. One cannot determine an environment that is maximally suitable for all.

What is stimulation? Those features in our environment that evoke a response or activate an individual can be called stimuli. Stimuli are received internally (thoughts, memories, experiences) as well as externally (sounds, sights, touch, movement). The activation level that exists at any point in time is a function of the total stimulation impact on the individual. The salient dimensions of stimulation that are generally believed to arouse or capture one's attention are variation, novelty, meaning, some intensity, complexity, and an element of surprise or incongruity. The role of teachers, child care workers, parents, and nurses is to provide an environment that offers these dimensions in an appropriate combination for each child.

Common types of stimulation include the varied sounds and movements that are used in interactive play with an infant. The variation in shapes, colors, textures, and sounds that selected toys can provide and the human touch, face, and voice are modes of stimulation to promote play and development. Certain types of toys and activities have been found to be more beneficial than others. McCall (1979) demonstrated that toys that can be made to do something (pots and pans, mobiles, music toys) are preferred. In recent years it has been suggested that neonates see objects of varied dark and light geometric shapes and with geometric designs better than the traditionally provided brightly colored animals and objects (Ludington-Hoe, 1983).

A special area of interest that is gaining increasing attention is the effect of stimulation on premature infants. Smaller infants are now surviving, with increasing potential for neurodevelopmental deficits. Prolonged hospitalization and tremendous advances in technology have resulted in their spending the first few months of life in a highly sophisticated, technologic environment, with buzzers, incubator noises, bright lights, and the continuous hum of voices and machines. Barnard and Bee (1983) suggest that preterm infants suffer from inappropriate rather than insufficient stimulation and that the unpredictable quality of stimulation contributes to the premature baby's inability to organize reactions to external events. Infant stimulation programs continue to be studied, but the optimal type, amount, and effectiveness of stimulation are not known. Field (1980) has noted that mothers of preterm infants may tend to overstimulate their infants in their attempt to compensate for a premature baby's depressed responsiveness. For further reading, see Harrison's (1985) review of 24 studies on the effects of supplemental stimulation of prematures.

Exposure to increasingly higher levels of stimulation is evident in our society and is making it increasingly difficult to foster interest in the more aesthetic and artistic aspects of life. A quiet day in the woods or a day at an art museum is not as attractive for most children as the level of stimulation that is offered by the video arcade, a rousing television show, or the abundance of toys and electronic devices in the home. Generally, high levels of noise, the violence on television, crowded playgrounds, and constant talking are stimuli that most individuals avoid and from which children should be protected.

Additionally, it has been questioned whether the noise and crowding urban life create have the potential to alter the arousal threshold so that one is addicted to high levels of noise (Levy, 1978). Societal affluence permits more families to buy excessively and provide an abundance of motorized toys and technical gadgets in the home. The challenge today is to keep stimuli within a healthful range. The challenge of raising children in an environment that has potentially too much stimulation is as great a challenge as providing sufficient stimulation in disadvantaged environments. The nurse's support of the family who actively tries to avoid excessive stimulation for their children can be an important motivator for such a family.

On the other hand, many families do not have the resources or the information to provide a sufficiently stimulating environment and continue to need assistance from the nurse to learn of this need and how to overcome it.

The Benefits of Play During a Health Care Encounter

Entry to the health care system occurs under a variety of circumstances. There is an element of mystery, fear, and the unknown for a child who faces even minimally intrusive encounters. An x-ray machine, a blood pressure cuff, or a thermometer is a potential threat to a child. The benefits of play are reflected in the general acceptance of play programs and use of play in the home, physician's office and inpatient and outpatient settings to help a child cope with stress and understand a procedure. Play is a natural medium through which a child can express fears, sadness, comfort, or joy. With the advent of the philosophy that children should be cared for at home or through outpatient facilities, the play programs that are now well established in inpatient settings will need to be adapted for transferral to the community.

An appreciation of the various uses of play in health care, whether in the home or hospital, is an important component of nursing care for children. The discussion that follows is of the nurse's use of play as an assessment tool, as a diversion from a threat, as recreation, and as therapeutic play.

Assessment: Play as a Tool

A child who is stressed and afraid can sometimes be made to feel more comfortable if permitted to play. Typically, a young child who is directly approached by a health professional will retreat. However, if a play area is available a child will be attracted to that area and become less attentive to the new person or environment. Using play during the history and physical examination is instrumental in gaining the child's cooperation. The child's developmental level is assessed through play with developmental screening tests, such as the Bayley and Denver Developmental screening tests (see DDST form in Appendix Four).

Watching a child informally playing in any setting provides information about motor skills, cognitive abilities, social skills, and general mood and well-being. Any health care encounter may result in play behavior that is only temporary and may be a reaction to the immediate event. For example, a hospitalized child's diminished motor skills may be temporary because of a period of immobility rather than a developmental delay. Similarly, disinterest in socializing at an appropriate age level may be related to a response to hospitalization rather than poor social development. Aggressive play during hospitalization may also be a coping response rather than evidence of deep-seated hostile feelings.

The play of a child during a health care encounter, therefore, should be interpreted by conferring with parents to determine whether the child's performance is typical of usual behavior.

Diversion Through Play

Engaging a child in activities that are unrelated to the events associated with health care can distract the child and provide a means of avoiding the associated threats

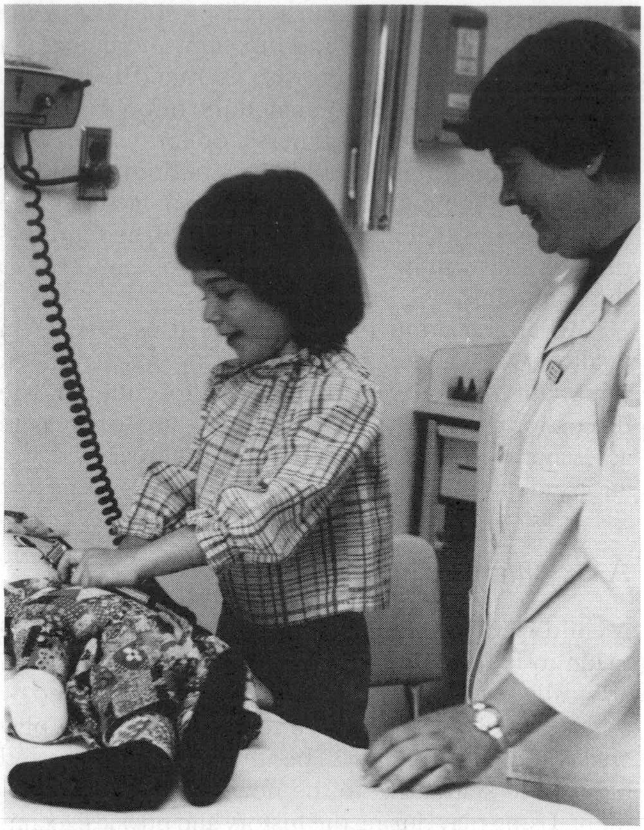

The school-age child will benefit from therapeutic play. A girl gives her doll an examination just after she herself has undergone one. (Photograph by Cynthia Stewart.)

the child may feel. This type of play is often used during hospitalization and during procedures. Simply providing toys or engaging a child in group play is diversionary because the child is focusing on something other than hospitalization or related events. A play program that consists solely of diversionary play may reduce the child's anxiety because of the distraction. The disadvantage of this approach as a single strategy is that it is not sufficiently goal-directed to encourage expression of feelings and mastery of one's environment.

Play as Recreation

Play programs on a recreation/activity model are based on three premises (Bolig, 1984):

- *Doing* is essential to maintain function and skills,
- *Doing* is relaxing because it simultaneously reduces stress,
- *Participation* must be voluntary.

The underlying belief of this approach is that in activity a sense of mastery is achieved. Planned activities focus on the "doing and participation" of a child rather than their content or meaning. Such group activities as arts and crafts, cooking, and playing cards or board games are viewed as stress reducers because of the effect of being actively involved in play.

Therapeutic Play

The therapeutic approach to play is based on psychoanalytic theories. Therapeutic play is not intended to be diversional or recreational. Its purpose is to allow children to overcome anxieties, at least to the degree that they can cope with the events in their environment. Puppets, creative play materials, dolls, and hospital and medical toys are used to familiarize the child with the health care environment and people as well as the novel equipment. Puppet play is a universal way to communicate with and gain insights about young children. Puppets are usually successful in drawing out even the slowest-to-warm-up child. Puppets may be dressed to represent health care professionals, parents and siblings, animals, or popular TV characters. The puppet seems to free the child to express ideas, feelings, and fears not shared in direct conversation.

Release is also found in creative play materials (fingerpaints, water, crayons) and "aggression toys" (bean bags, pounding boards, balls, clay). Through role playing using dolls or stuffed animals, health care objects, or miniature-sized medical toys, the child can become nurse or doctor, and the doll or animal becomes the patient.

During therapeutic play, children can subject others (a doll, stuffed animal, parent or nurse volunteer) to the very event they fear as they experiment with various ways of reacting to it. In the process they acquaint themselves with the tools (the toys in this form of play), procedures, and roles of patient and "procedure-doer" that they believe to be part of the event creating stress. During therapeutic play, the nurse has an opportunity to gain insights into the perceptions, feelings, and needs related to the event(s) the child is enacting.

The use of therapeutic play as a coping strategy for healthy children is a widely accepted practice. Despite indications that a child's play is disrupted while in the hospital, the literature also suggests that this type of play is a strategy used by children in the hospital to facilitate coping (Thompson, 1986). Therapeutic play has been a long-standing component of health care in hospitals and its use is also reported in outpatient settings (Williams and Powell, 1980; Meer, 1985). Although the benefits of this play are difficult to measure, the literature indicates that it is an effective means to reduce anxiety associated with hospitalization and related events (Clatworthy, 1981; Poster, 1982; Poster and Betz, 1983; Schwartz et al, 1983; Ellerton et al, 1985).

Play therapy differs from therapeutic play. Play therapy is a form of psychotherapy, with the goal to help children understand their own behaviors and feelings. To accomplish this goal the therapist may at times be directive and at other times nondirective. Play therapy is used by professionals with specialized skills and is used by nurses only if they have advanced preparation.

References

Ambron S: *Child Development.* 2nd ed. New York, Holt, Rinehart and Winston, 1981.

American Academy of Pediatrics Committee on Pediatric Aspects of Physical Fitness, Recreation, and Sports: Swimming instructions for infants. *Pediatrics* 1980 Apr; 847.

American Academy of Pediatrics Committee on Sports Medicine: *Health Care for Young Athletes.* Evanston, IL, 1983.

American Academy of Pediatrics Committee on Sports Medicine: Climatic heat stress and the exercising child. *Pediatrics* 1982 Jun; 808–809.

Barnard KE, Bee HL: The impact of temporally patterned stimulation on the development of preterm infants. *Child Dev* 1983; 54:1156–1167.

Belkengren RP, Sapala S: Physical fitness from infancy through adolescence. *Pediatr Nurs* 1982 Jul/Aug; 249–257.

Berlyne DE: *Conflict, Arousal, and Curiosity.* New York, McGraw-Hill, 1960.

Berlyne DE: Determinants of subjective novelty. *Percept Psychophys* 1960; 3(6):415–423.

Bijou S: *Child Development: The Basic Stage of Early Childhood.* Century Psychology Series. Englewood Cliffs, NJ, Prentice-Hall, 1976.

Bolig R: Play in hospital settings. *In* Yawkey TO, Pellegria AD: *Child's Play: Developmental and Applied.* Hillsdale, NY, Lawrence Erlbaum Associates, 1984.

Caplan F, Caplan T: *The Power of Play.* New York, Doubleday (Anchor Press), 1973.

Christie JF, Johnsen EP: The role of play in social-intellectual development. *Rev Educ Res* 1983 Spring; 53(1):83–115.

Clatworthy S: Therapeutic play: Effects on hospitalized children. Children's Health Care: Journal of the Association for the Care of Children's Health, Vol. 9, 1981, pp 108–113.

Coddington RD: The significance of life events as etiologic factors in the disease of children. II. The study of a normal population. *J Psychosom Med* 1972; 16:205.

Ellerton ML, et al: Helping young children master intrusive procedures through play. *Child Health Care* 1985 Spring; 13(4):167–173.

Field TM: Interactions of high-risk infants: quantitative and qualitative differences. *In* Sawin DB, et al: *Exceptional Infant-Psychosocial Risks in Infant-Environment Transactions.* Vol. 4. New York, Brunner/Mazel, 1980.

Fiske DW, Maddi SRA: *Functions of Varied Experience.* Homewood, IL, Dorsey Series in Psychology, 1961.

Florey LL: Studies of play: implications for growth, development, and for clinical practice. *Am J Occup Ther* 1981 Aug; 35(2):519–524.

Freud S: *Beyond the Pleasure Principle.* Strachey J (trans). New York, Norton, 1975.

Freyberg J: Increasing the imaginative play of urban disadvantaged children through systematic training. *In* Singer JL: *The Child's World of Make-Believe.* New York, Academic Press, 1973.

Garritson JS: *Child Arts: Integrating Curriculum Through the Arts.* Reading, MA, Addison-Wesley, 1979.

Garvey C: Play. *In* Brunner J, et al (eds): The Developing Child Series. Cambridge, MA, Harvard University Press, 1977.

Gehlsen G, Albohm M: Evaluation of sports bras. *Physician Sports Med* 1980; 10:89–96.

Goodnow J: *Children Drawing.* Cambridge, MA, Harvard University Press, 1977.

Greene JC: Prevention and treatment of sports injuries. *Nurse Pract* 1983 Nov/Dec; 39–44.

Hagstrom J, Morrill J: *Games Babies Play and More Games Babies Play.* New York, Pocket Books, 1981.

Harrison L: Effects of early supplemental stimulation programs for premature infants: review of the literature. *Matern Child Nurs J* 1985 Summer; 14(2):69–90.

Hartley R, Goldenson R: *A Complete Book of Play.* New York, Thomas Y. Crowell Company, 1963.

Helms DB, Turner JS: *Exploring Child Behavior.* 2nd ed. New York, Holt, Rinehart and Winston, 1981.

Hull CL: *Principles of Behavior.* New York, Appleton-Century-Croft, 1943.

Hurlock E: *Child Development.* 6th ed. New York, McGraw-Hill, 1978.

Kellogg R: Understanding children's art. *In* DeCecco JP: *Readings in Educational Psychology Today.* Del Mar, CA, CRM Books, 1970.

Kellogg R, O'Dell S: *The Psychology of Children's Art.* New York, CRM Books, Random House, 1967.

Klepsch M, Logie L: *Children Draw and Tell.* New York, Brunner/Mazel, 1982.

Levy J: *Play Behavior.* New York, John Wiley & Son, 1978.

Lowenfeld V, Brittain WL: *Creative and Mental Growth.* 6th ed. New York, Macmillan, 1975.

Ludington-Hoe SM: What can newborns really see? *Am J Nurs* 1983 Sep; 1286–1289.

Marzolf SS, Kirchner JH: Personality traits and color choices for house-tree-person drawings. *J Clin Psychol* 1973; 29:240–245.

McCall R: *Infants.* Cambridge, MA, Harvard University Press, 1979.

McLeavey KA: Children's art as an assessment tool. *Pediatr Nurs* 1979 Mar/Apr; 9–14.

Meer PA: Using play therapy in outpatient settings. *MCN* 1985 Nov/Dec; 10:378–380.

Miller NE, Dollard J: *Social Learning and Imitation.* New Haven, CT, Yale University Press, 1941.

Parten M: Social participation among preschool children. *J Abn Soc Psychol* 1932; 243.

Piaget J: *Play, Dreams and Imitation in Childhood.* (Gattegno C, Hodgson FM, trans). Boston, Routledge and Kegan Paul, 1951.

Poster EC: Stress immunization: techniques to help children cope with hospitalization. *Matern Child Nurs J* 1982; 11:119–131.

Poster EC, Betz CL: Allaying the anxiety of hospitalized children using stress immunization techniques. *Issues Compr Pediatr Nurs* 1983; 6:227–233.

Rubin KH, Pepler DJ: Children's play: Piaget's views reconsidered. *Contemp Educ Psychol* 1982; 7:289–299.

Saltz E, Brodie J: Pretend-play training in childhood: a review and critique. *Contrib Hum Dev* 1982; 6:97–113.

Saltz E, et al: Training disadvantaged preschoolers on various fantasy activities: effects on cognitive functioning and impulse control. *Child Dev* 1977; 48:367–380.

Schwartz BH, et al: Effects of psychological preparation on children hospitalized for dental operations. *J Pediatr* 1983; 102:634–638.

Similansky S: *The Effects of Sociodramatic Play on Disadvantaged Preschool Children.* New York, John Wiley & Sons, 1968.

Smith NJ: Some health care needs of young athletes. *Adv Pediatr* 1981; 28:187–228.

Smith NJ: Children and parents: growth, development and sports. *In* Strauss RH: *Sports Medicine.* Philadelphia, WB Saunders, 1984, pp 207–217.

Smith PK, Dutton S: Play and training in direct and innovative problem-solving. *Child Dev* 1979; 50:830–836.

Stone LJ, Church J: *Childhood and Adolescence.* 3rd ed. New York, Random House, 1983.

Sutton-Smith B: *Play and Learning.* New York, Gardner, 1980.

Sutton-Smith B, Sutton-Smith S: *How to Play with Your Children (and When Not to).* New York, Hawthorn Books, 1974.

Thompson RH: Where we stand; twenty years of research on pediatric hospitalization and health care. *Child Health Care* 1986 Spring; 14(4):200–210.

Vandenberg B: The role of play in the development of insightful tool-using strategies. *Merrill-Palmer Q,* 1981.

White RW: Motivation reconsidered: the concept of competence. *Psychol Rev* 1959; 66:297–333.

Williams YB, Powell M: Documenting the value of supervised play in a pediatric ambulatory care clinic. *Child Health Care* 1980 Summer; 9(1):15–20.

Bibliography

Bledsoe NP, et al: A study of reliability and validity of a preschool play scale. *Am J Occup Ther* 1982 Dec; 783–788.

Cass E: *Helping Children Grow Through Play.* New York, Schocken Books, 1973.

Duncan B, et al: A controlled trial of a physical fitness program for fifth grade students. *J School Health* 1983 Oct; 467–471.

Froelich MAR: A comparison of the effect of music therapy and medical play therapy on the verbalization behavior of pediatric patients. *J Music Ther* 1984; 21:2–15.

Garot PA: Therapeutic play: work of both child and nurse. *J Pediatr Nurs* 1986 Apr; 1(2):111–116.

Gibbons M: When parents ask about play. *Pediatr Nurs* 1977 Nov/Dec; 19.

Gordon J: *Baby Learning Through Baby Play.* New York, St. Martin's Press, 1970.

Hartley E, et al: *Understanding Children's Play.* New York, Columbia University Press, 1952.

Kuczaj SA: *Crib Speech and Language Play.* New York, Springer-Verlag, 1983.

Lee J, Fowler MD: Merely child's play? Development work and play things. *J Pediatr Nurs* 1986 Aug; 1(4):270.

Levy J: *Play Behavior.* New York, Krieger, 1983.

Mergen B: *Play and Play Things: A Reference Guide.* Westport, CT, Greenwood Press, 1982.

Millar S: *The Psychology of Play.* New York, Penguin Books, 1968.

Nadler HS: Art experiences and hospitalized children. *Child Health Care* 1983 Spring; 11(4):160–164.

Piers P: *Play and Development.* New York, WW Norton, 1972.

Pepler PJ, Rubin KH: *Play of Children: Current Theory and Research.* Basel, S. Karger, 1982.

Sparling J, Lewis I: Six learning games to play with your infant. *Parents* 1979 Oct; 35.

Tauber MA: Parental socialization techniques and sex differences in children's play. *Child Dev* 1979 Mar; 225.

Tizard B, Harvey D: *Biology of Play.* Philadelphia, JB Lippincott, 1977.

Zaichkowsky LD, et al: *Growth and Development: The Child and Physical Activity.* St. Louis, CV Mosby, 1980.

Promoting Healthy Sexuality Chapter 22

Lynn Rew

Human sexuality begins with conception and continues to develop throughout the lifespan. The term *sexuality* connotes the totality of being human, including the sex act as well as intimate feelings and meaningful relationships, whereas the term *sex* has a biologic meaning. An integration of biologic, psychologic, and sociologic aspects of sexuality takes place as a child develops a sense of self. Parents, peers, and health care professionals have an impact upon the development of attitudes, values, and sexual behavior as a child matures. Nurses have the opportunity to counsel children and their parents as the phases of sexual development are encountered. Each developmental stage brings new issues and concerns about which parents and children may require some assistance and guidance.

This chapter includes a discussion of the development of attitudes, sexual behaviors, and learning needs of children from birth to adolescence. Nursing implications relevant to each stage of sexual development are discussed.

Related Topics
Growth and development, Chapters 5–9
Use of contraceptives, Chapter 9
Prevention of AIDS, Chapter 43
Prevention of sexually transmitted diseases, Chapter 45

Promoting Healthy Sexuality

Nursing Diagnoses	Nursing Goals/Strategies
Potential altered sexual patterns • *related to development of negative attitudes about sexuality associated with early childhood experiences*	Development of healthy sexual behavior by child and family. • Help child develop self-awareness of feelings about sexuality. • Permit normal developmental expressions of sexuality. • Foster development of healthy attitudes about sexuality by open discussions with child at appropriate level of age. • Use correct anatomic terminology when referring to sex organs and sex-related topics. • Avoid reprimand for age-appropriate sexual exploration, such as masturbation and toddler or preschooler sex play. • Teach child to protect self from sexual abuse.
• *related to lack of information about sexuality*	• Assess child's and family's needs and knowledge deficit. • Encourage children and families to discuss sexuality openly at a level appropriate for age. • Provide age-appropriate information about reproduction. • Prepare school-age child for physical and emotional maturational changes during adolescence. • Provide information about contraception, pregnancy, and sexually transmitted diseases to late school-age children and adolescents. • Develop or implement teaching programs for school and community organizations.

Every human being is sexual. The sexuality of human beings refers to those characteristics associated with being male or female. One's sexuality originates before birth. Biologic, psychologic, and social factors contribute to the marvelous unfolding of each new person as one learns to live in the world as a female or male.

As the embryonic cell mass gradually differentiates into a feminine or masculine fetus, changes occur in the external world as parents plan and anticipate the process of birth. This continuous interaction of internal change with external attitudes and behaviors results in the sexuality expressed by the individual throughout life.

The interactive process that occurs at each stage of development has nursing implications. Nursing implications are derived from the development of attitude, sexual behaviors, and learning needs of the child in each stage of sexual development. See Table 22-1 for a summary.

An individual is born into a family unit, and the sexual characteristics of this child—in addition to those of siblings, parents, and extended family members—have an impact on the child's acquisition of attitudes, knowledge, and behavior.

Prenatal Development

The sexuality of every individual begins with conception. Physical differentiation, which is influenced by hormones, follows the genetic blueprint of gender determination. In addition to the physical process, a psychosocial process begins as parents and other family members prepare for the arrival of the infant. The psychosocial environment influences the attitudes and behaviors of the child as an individual sexual identity develops.

Genetic Determination and Differentiation

At the moment of conception, when a sperm carrying an X chromosome combines with an ovum (all of which carry X chromosomes), the result is a female embryo (XX configuration). When a sperm carrying a Y chromosome combines with the X chromosome from the ovum, the XY configuration yields a male embryo.

Within 2 weeks of conception the embryonic cell mass begins its transformation into a sexually identifi-

***Table* 22-1.** Summary of Stages in Sexual Development of Children

Factors Affecting Attitude Development	Behaviors	Learning Needs
Prenatal		
Parental expectations	Genetic determination Differentiation	Anticipated role change of parents and siblings
Infancy (0 to 1 Year)		
Tone of voice, touch Caregiver's acceptance	Sucking Random self-discovery Pelvic rocking Erection, lubrication	Language Trust Physical and emotional well-being
Toddler (1 to 3 Years)		
Parental reactions Freedom to explore	Names body parts Draws body parts Games such as "house" Gender roles Explores body orifices	Language (correct terminology) Social appropriateness Assertive rights Facts of reproduction
Preschooler (3 to 5 Years)		
Approaches to nudity and privacy in the home Increasing influence outside home	Masturbation, orgasm Name calling Curious manipulation of other child's genitalia Games with sex roles	Social appropriateness Respect of privacy Assertive rights Facts of reproduction repeated with more detail
School-Age (6 to 12 Years)		
Interaction with peers, school authorities Influence from mass media	Sex-linked play—role modeling Kissing, hugging, dancing with opposite sex Close friendships Voyeurism	Re-explanation about facts of reproduction and clarification of terminology heard at school Preparation for changes of adolescence Decision making about sex behaviors Basic information about consequences of sexual activity
Adolescent (13 to 18 Years)		
Audience of peers Pressure to belong by conforming	Adjustment to changing body Purposeful masturbation Experimentation with others	Express feelings Values clarification Decision making Contraception STD/AIDS

able fetus. Three primary germ layers form, and from these all tissues, organs, and systems evolve. At 6 weeks of gestation the embryonic sex glands appear. The gonad, or genital gland, originates from the epithelial cell mass. Genital ducts develop from the gonads and are the forerunners of mature structures.

The process of differentiation, by which the female is distinguished as different from the male, begins by the seventh week of gestation. Internal structures modify to become ovaries and a uterus in the female and testes in the male. In the following week the external genitalia appear similar in both sexes, arising from a site between the umbilical cord and the tail of the embryo. Each begins with a genital tubercle, followed by a groove with two folds or swellings on either side of the groove (Fig. 22-1). In the female the genital tubercle becomes the *clitoris* whereas in the male it develops into the *penis*. The groove becomes the *vagina* in the female and the *penile urethra* in the male. The two folds become the *labia majora* in the female and the *scrotum* in the male.

By 16 weeks of gestation, sex determination is possible from examination of the external genitalia. The external structures of the male develop quickly and are definitive by the tenth week. Those of the female pursue a slower course, with the gradual development of the vestibule and labia minora.

In spite of similarities in early development, the male and female embryos show distinct differences to hormonal stimulation. In the genetic male embryo (XY configuration), masculine tissues and organs develop only in the presence of the male hormone androgen. If the embryo is denied this stimulus, the primitive organs develop into those of a female. No such hormonal dependence exists in the female embryo (Diamond, 1977).

Parental and Family Attitudes and Expectations

Attitude refers to the values and feelings one has toward self and others. Parental values, hopes, and dreams color the unique setting into which each child is born. Parents of first-born children may display unrealistic expectations for themselves and for their infants. Among the expectations may be a preferred gender of the unborn child, which is followed by joy or disappointment at the time of birth. Especially when there are older children in the family, a child of a specific gender may be anticipated. The disappointment experienced by a new parent may be transmitted to the neonate, and feelings of uncertainty may be directed toward oneself as a parent. Such attitudes and behaviors of parents can influence the child's attitudes about sex and affect the development of a sexual identity. Advances in prenatal diagnostic tools are rapidly altering a family's knowledge about their unborn child. The use of ultrasonography routinely as a screening device is currently debatable, but as it gains advocates for its use the gender of the unborn child can be determined as well.

When the family prepares for the birth of another child, the older siblings need special preparation which includes acceptance of either sex unless gender has been identified prenatally. In general, parents should prepare siblings for the birth by helping children explore their feelings of what a brother or sister will mean to them. (See Chapter 6 for discussion of sibling preparation when an infant is born.)

Nursing Strategies

Nurses primarily provide anticipatory guidance in the prenatal period. Specific interventions include discussing the following with one or both parents:

1. Anticipate and assist parents to define role changes for themselves and other family members.
2. Assist other children in expressing their feelings and identifying anticipated changes in family routines.
3. Identify expectations for the gender of the unborn child.
4. Describe the sexual anatomy and physiology of the neonate, including natural behaviors such as self-exploration, pelvic rocking, and erections.
5. Prepare the mother for possible erotic feelings she may experience during childbirth and breastfeeding and assure her that these are normal.
6. Discuss parents' resuming their sexual relationship following the birth.

Infant Development (Birth to 1 Year)

The first year of life, or the infancy period, brings rapid changes in the physical and psychosocial aspects of the child. The infant's sexual attitudes, behaviors, and learning needs must be addressed.

Attitude Development

Attitudes about sexuality begin to develop in the first few hours of life. Tone of voice and touch communicate the psychosocial makeup of the delivery. Touching the skin is the basic communication from which

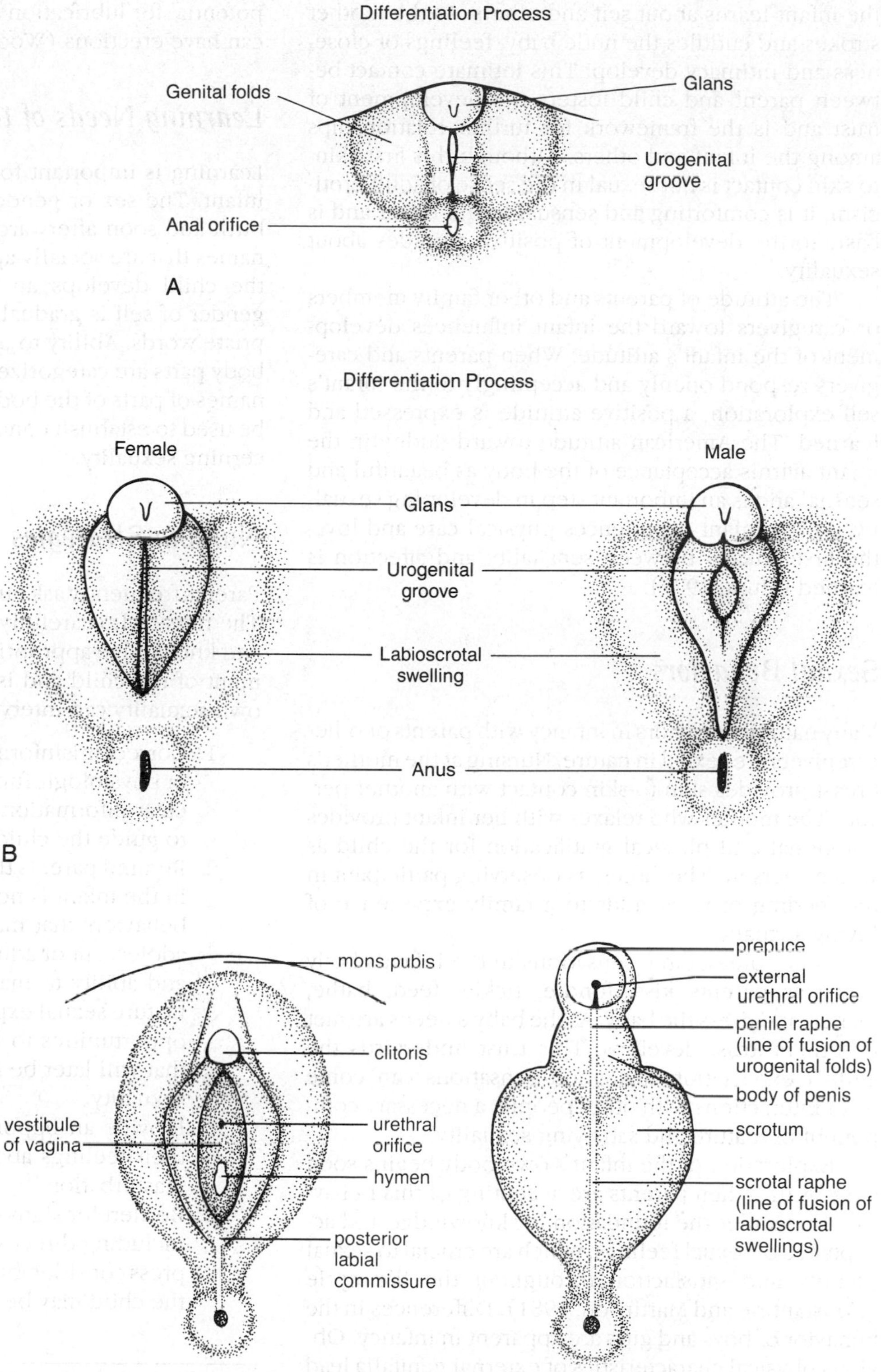

Figure 22-1. *A*, Prenatal sexual development: undifferentiated (prior to 7 weeks' gestation). *B*, Prenatal sexual development: differentiating process at 9 weeks. *C*, Prenatal sexual development: differentiated male and female fetuses.

the infant learns about self and others. As the mother strokes and cuddles the nude baby, feelings of closeness and intimacy develop. This intimate contact between parent and child fosters the development of trust and is the framework for further relationships among the infant and others. Although this first skin-to-skin contact is not sexual in the sense of adult eroticism, it is comforting and sensual to the infant and is basic to the development of positive attitudes about sexuality.

The attitude of parents and other family members or caregivers toward the infant influences development of the infant's attitude. When parents and caregivers respond openly and acceptingly to the infant's self-exploration, a positive attitude is expressed and learned. The American attitude toward nudity in the infant affirms acceptance of the body as beautiful and sensual and is an important step in developing sexuality. As the infant experiences physical care and love, the first linkage between sensuality and affection is learned (Hunt, 1977).

Sexual Behaviors

Many natural behaviors in infancy with parents or other caregivers are sexual in nature. Nursing at the mother's breast provides skin-to-skin contact with another person. The mother who relaxes with her infant provides emotional and physical gratification for the child as well as herself. The father, as observing participant in the feeding process, adds to a family experience of loving sexuality.

Other pleasurable sensations in the infant's body occur as parents kiss, fondle, tickle, feed, bathe, diaper, and dress the baby. As the baby's needs are met by others, trust develops. This trust undergirds the child's expectation that good sensations can come from interactions with other people, a necessary component of mature and satisfying sexuality.

Exploration of the infant's own body begins soon after birth. When parents are accepting of this behavior, it becomes the foundation for knowledge and acceptance of sexual feelings, which are crucial to sexual identity and satisfaction throughout the life cycle (Constantine and Martinson, 1981). Differences in the behavior of boys and girls are apparent in infancy. Obvious physical characteristics of external genitalia lead to differences in self-discovery as the little boy discovers his penis and the pleasurable sensation that accompanies touch before the little girl finds similar sensations upon discovery of her genitalia.

Masters and Johnson (1966) documented the fact that baby boys are often born with erections and baby girls with vaginal lubrication. Female infants have the potential for lubrication and orgasm, and male infants can have erections (Woods, 1984).

Learning Needs of the Infant

Learning is important for sexual development in the infant. The sex or gender of the child is assigned at birth and soon afterward the child hears sounds and names that are socially appropriate for sex-rearing. As the child develops an understanding of language, gender of self is gradually associated with the appropriate words. Ability to use the language follows, and body parts are categorized. As language develops, the names of parts of the body, including the genitals, can be used to establish comfortable communication concerning sexuality.

Nursing Strategies

Parents frequently ask questions about infant behavior. The nurse who carefully reviews attitudes, behaviors, and knowledge appropriate for each stage of development of the child and is comfortable with her or his own sexuality can intervene in these ways:

1. Correct misinformation about anatomic names or physiologic functions of the body. Direct and clear information enhances the parents' ability to guide the child.
2. Remind parents that sensual pleasure observed in the infant is not to be confused with similar behaviors that may be explicitly sexual in the adolescent or adult. An infant lacks experience and ability to make decisions associated with mature sexual expression but needs these early opportunities to learn attitudes and behaviors that will later be part of a healthy repertoire of sexuality.
3. Provide an opportunity for parents to discuss their feelings about sexual behaviors, such as masturbation.
4. Be alert for signs of possible abuse of the child, including direct sexual abuse. Parents who express considerable concern about the gender of the child may be at risk for abuse.

Toddler Development (12 to 36 Months)

The toddler between 1 and 3 years of age explores the world with new independence. Driven by curiosity, toddlers seek to learn more about the world and their unique relationship to everything and everyone in it.

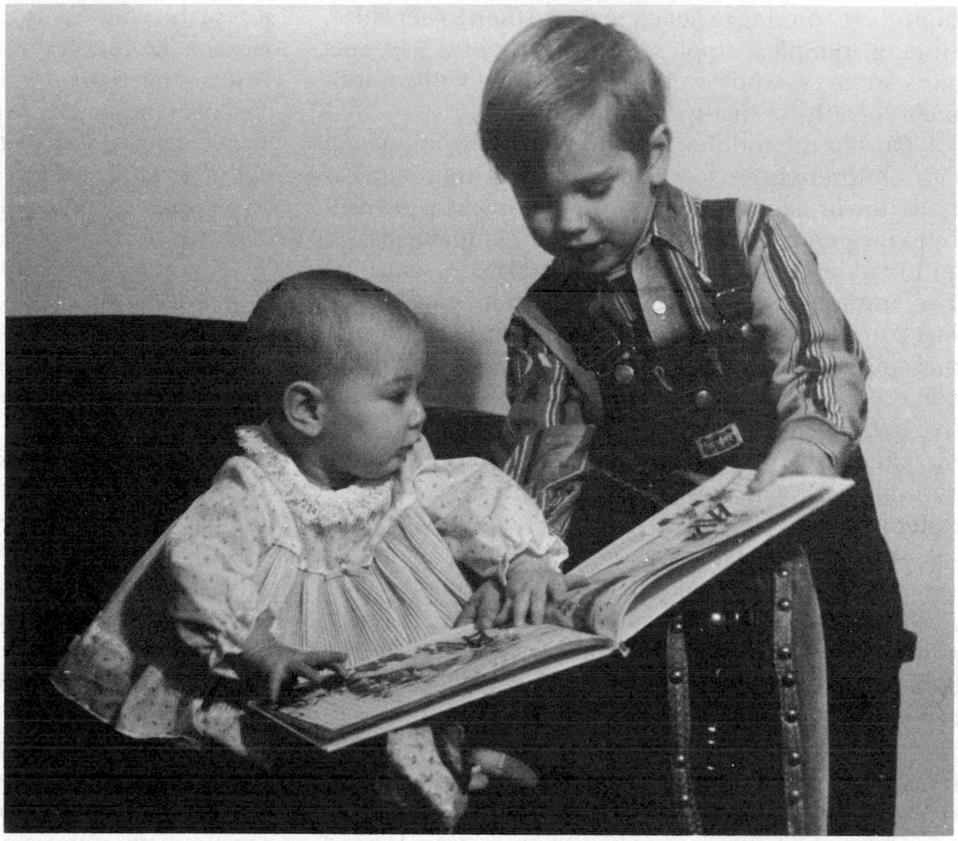

Although some parents consciously try to raise their children in ways they consider to be nonsexist, other parents sincerely believe the appropriateness of sex role differences and choose their children's clothing in accordance with their beliefs. (Photo by Jim Tackett.)

Attitude Development

The toddler as a curious and independent creature develops more awareness of self as a sexual being. Mastery of gender identity begins to some extent at this age, as evidenced by the 3-year-old child who can identify self or others as girl or boy. Through interaction with others, toddlers learn attitudes about the acceptability of their gender. Adults reinforce identity through tone of voice when encouraging specific types of play; by providing sex-linked toys, clothing, and room decor; and by linking socially approved behavior with being girl or boy.

Parental reactions to their child's play and self-exploration affect the toddler's developing attitude toward sexuality. The parent who reacts with alarm or disgust when discovering sex play among children contributes destructive negativism to attitude development. Likewise, the adult who fears that a child will be harmed by masturbation and slaps the child's hand and threatens that blindness will result conveys an attitude that sexual feelings and expressions are harmful or bad. Some parents are less obvious about their feelings. They may themselves fear that masturbation is harmful but express their feelings by avoiding *any* discussion with their child. Without explanation, a toddler is repeatedly told not to touch the genital area. Such behaviors also introduce negative feelings that the child associates with sexuality. If parents can be tolerant of sex play among toddlers, with gradual limit setting as the child matures, positive attitudes can develop. Sometimes sex play among children is unsafe and requires limit setting by parents. Providing safety and maintaining a sense of humor about the child's exploration of the world communicates a positive attitude, as illustrated in the following anecdote from a mother:

> When my husband gave Gordie a bath that night, he found that his anus was black. They had colored each other's anuses! Gordie just said, "We were coloring each other's behinds." I said we didn't think that Magic Marker was that healthy to be on his anus. We said it wasn't very healthy to do that, and please, they shouldn't do it again (Study Group of New York, 1983, p 98).

Sexual Behaviors

Sexual behavior in the toddler reflects the curiosity and independence of this developmental stage. Toddlers learn new words and find new categories for their experiences. With delight the toddler shares these with others, as did the 2-year-old sitting in her high chair pointing to her cheeks and then to her chest, singing "dimples, nipples, dimples, nipples." Parents and caregivers who accept this as natural will contribute to healthy sexuality in the young child.

During the toddler years a major developmental task children strive to achieve is toilet training. Because the urinary and anal orifices are in close proximity to the genitalia, it is important that achieving bowel and bladder control not be confused with sexuality. The attitudes of disapproval, anger, and impatience that parents so easily convey when a child is not progressing according to parental expectations may become associated with sexuality. Parents who are sensitive to the readiness of the child to learn, considering the child's interest, mastery of language, and muscle coordination, will avoid power conflicts and separate toilet training from sexual issues.

Other sexual behaviors of the toddler include a variety of types of sex play. It is not uncommon to find that toddlers place small objects into ears, nostrils, anuses, or vaginas. For example, a 3-year-old in the bath is enjoying a new plastic toy boat that has a flag on top of a pole. He discovers that the flag can be removed from the pole and is just the right size to hide in his rectum. However, in a short while the flag is gone and cannot be retrieved. The child may not tell the parent what happened. Parents and health professionals need to be aware that this type of natural behavior may happen so that they are alert to the possibility of injury or infection.

Sex play with other children is natural and a part of normal development. Many games of "doctor" and "house" have sexual overtones and at times contain overtly sexual behaviors. Describing the play of toddlers, Pitcher and Schultz (1983) found that girls frequently assumed child-care roles whereas boys exhibited this role play much less. Girls were also more likely to play both traditionally male and female roles (e.g., "mommy" or "firefighter") than were boys. This sex-linked play is part of the practice for *gender role* typical of the toddler. Gender role is learned behavior that is undifferentiated or neutral at birth. With the acquisition of language, such roles become unique to each sex as toddlers model the roles of significant others. Gender roles do not represent opposite ends of a spectrum but are identifiable along a continuum (Sears, 1974). For example, aggressive play may be seen more in boys than in girls at this age but is not limited to boys.

Learning Needs of the Toddler

The toddler spends much time learning names and categories for things and experiences, practicing new terms until they are mastered. Names that are socially acceptable and easily understood by others are necessary for the toddler to continue mastering the world. Terms are not always understood by a young toddler, but an attempt is made to use them to be acceptable. A mother explained that the proper word for "going potty" is to "urinate." The child understood this as "your nate." The toddler tried to use the appropriate term but continued to say I have to do "my nate."

Self-exploration and the innocent exploration of another toddler's body may be appropriate playful behavior among toddlers and should not be punished. However, sexual games and behavior are not appropriate when playing with older children or adults. Because young children are vulnerable, they need to learn to say "NO" to older children or adults who may try to take advantage of them. Children at this age are not particularly concerned about privacy, but they should be taught that older children and adults are not to be allowed to touch their genitals. The incidence of sexual abuse among the very young makes this kind of learning essential to the well-being of the toddler.

Frequently toddlers ask questions about reproduction and hear stories that may confuse them. Bernstein (1978) found that a group of toddlers thought babies came from a duck because the book used for their sex education showed baby ducks and then baby people. Although using animals in teaching is common and not inappropriate, this example shows that the stories read to young children must be carefully interpreted.

Nursing Strategies

The nurse working with the toddler and family should keep the following guidelines in mind:

1. Use correct terms for anatomy and physiology. Encourage parents to use correct terminology and to provide information consistent with the child's understanding.
2. Discriminate between terms known by the toddler for toileting and for genitalia. Avoid confusion of the two.
3. Avoid making stereotypical comments about gender roles.
4. Tolerate innocent sex play between toddlers, but provide limits. Provide adequate supervision and alternative activities to limit sex play.
5. Plan for safety. Avoid giving toddlers toys with small parts that may be placed in body openings.
6. Show positive attitudes toward the child and the characteristics that are gender related.
7. Accept masturbation as a natural, but private, behavior. Teach toddlers that touching private body parts is done in private.

8. Advise parents to teach hygiene with toileting, preventing urinary infections by wiping the female's vulva from front to back and keeping fingernails short and clean.

Preschooler (3 to 6 Years)

The child from 3 to 6 years of age experiences an expanded world. Independence and curiosity continue to motivate the child to master more of the world through social contact.

Attitude Development

The attitude of the young child develops as new feelings are experienced associated with life events. Issues that emerge at this stage of development include nudity and privacy. While most parents are comfortable with their own nudity and that of their infant or toddler, they express concern as the child gets older. Some parents fear that their own nudity may be provocative to children. Nudity within a healthy family actually has little impact other than validation of the similarities and differences between children and adults. Privacy is needed for the sexual expression between parents. At this stage parents are often concerned about the preschooler unexpectedly finding them during sexual intercourse. The interruption handled in a matter-of-fact way is not harmful to the child. Parents are cautioned that young children may be frightened or confused by explicit sexual acts which they may confuse with violence. Explanations should be given to the preschooler by the parents together to help the child understand that both parents agree on what is explained. If a preschooler is treated with acceptance and respect, the experience is not likely to cause any difficulty.

Sexual Behaviors

As an extension of the toddler's experience, the preschooler continues self-exploratory behavior, engaging in masturbation or sex play with siblings or peers. Reports from parents suggest that children at this age engage in purposeful behavior leading to orgasm. This play may be solitary or with other children and in most instances is part of the normal sequence of development. The Study Group of New York (1983) cited many examples, such as the following:

> Penelope described an incident in which her own daughter and the daughter of a friend were riding a Brahma bull statue at the local library. "My child said to my girlfriend's child, 'If you ride real fast it feels really good when it rubs your vagina.' They continued riding until my daughter got a very delirious expression on her face" (p 122).

Other types of play include pretending to give birth to dolls or stuffed animals, playing house with Mommy and Daddy sleeping together, or other imitations of the expanded roles in which they now see their parents. They enjoy calling each other names, sometimes using vocabulary that is associated with their genitalia and bodily functions such as "pee-nose," "pooh-head," and the like.

As experience and ability increase, the preschooler continues to engage in self-manipulation of the genitalia when bathing or curiously manipulating the genitalia of another child sharing a bath or shower. Experimentation with body parts and orifices continues as a natural behavior but requires some supervision. A 5-year-old boy was brought to the emergency room after allegedly falling out of his wagon and injuring his penis, which was red and swollen. Being unable to urinate, he had made up the story about falling rather than telling his parents that he had put his older sister's tiny rubber band (from her braces) around the glans of his penis. Fortunately a nurse discovered the band prior to a catheterization procedure and removed it.

Learning Needs of the Preschooler

The preschooler needs to learn what behaviors, including use of language, are socially acceptable and appropriate. The use of sexual terms for name calling may occur as children repeat words they overhear. The parents' decision and value system determines what language is considered acceptable. Parents can control the use of such language by not overreacting but matter-of-factly stating that these are not words their family uses.

The preschooler learns to respect the privacy of others in using the bathroom and of the need of parents to retreat to their own bedroom. Finding that others have times and places when they wish to be alone allows the child to learn to value privacy.

The sex education of the preschooler is a continuation of information given in earlier years. It is important to realize that even though a toddler was given correct terms and accurate explanations of how babies are born, this information may need to be repeated when the child is older, with more detail given as time and experience allow. Questions can be answered simply and directly.

The preschooler also needs to learn to say "NO" to adults or older children whose intention may be to exploit the child sexually. Although this should not be stressed to children to the extent that they become suspicious of all adults, sexual abuse of young children by adults whom they have trusted does occur, and children must be taught assertiveness while minimizing fear. (Recognition of sexual abuse and interventions are discussed in Chapter 35.)

Nursing Strategies

The nurse uses the following principles with preschoolers:

1. Determine the level of vocabulary used by the child to refer to body parts and functions, clarifying or providing correct terms when needed.
2. Guide parents in anticipating how they would handle an invasion of privacy by a curious preschooler.
3. When intrusive procedures are required (i.e., catheterization or pelvic examination), explain them to the child, realizing that the young child may feel embarrassed or exploited.
4. Be firm and matter-of-fact in setting limits about where and with whom the child sleeps outside of the family. Generally, brothers and sisters, children and parents in certain circumstances sleep together at this age.
5. When discovering a child masturbating in private, the nurse ignores the behavior and proceeds with the task. If repetitive masturbating is done in the nurse's presence, it is appropriate to ask the child to wait until he or she can do so in privacy. Excessive masturbation can be handled by providing additional opportunity for social interaction and play.

School Age (6 to 12 Years)

The child from 6 to 12 years of age continues to develop sexual awareness and purposeful sexual behaviors. The psychoanalytic term *latency* used to describe this stage of psychosexual development is now considered a myth (Janus and Bess, 1981).

Attitude Development

The attitude of the school-age child continues to form in response to increasing influence from outside the family. Interaction with peers, school authorities, and the mass media shape the developing attitudes.

According to the developmental psychologist Erik Erikson (1963), the 6- to-12-year-old child's task is to resolve the crisis of industry versus inferiority. The child has an intense desire for recognition as more skill and knowledge are acquired. If instead of encouragement and affirmation the child receives criticism, a perception of inferiority and inadequacy may result.

Sexual identity, although not well differentiated at age 5 years, gradually develops during the school-age years (Cramer, 1980). Girls show more consistent and rapid development of sexual identity than do boys. This parallels their more rapid physical growth and development. Many studies show that parental attitudes and values are significant in the child's formation of sexual identity (Fisher, 1973). However, peer influence is more important in this age group than previously.

Sexual Behaviors

Children in the lower grades (ages 5 and 6 years) may engage in sex play such as "house" or "doctor," each of which may include direct physical contact of a sexual nature. Play becomes more explicit at this age as girls experiment with wearing makeup, placing pillows under their skirts to mimic pregnancy, and kissing little boys. Boys play at fighting to show their prowess and feign peeking under the skirts of girls.

Children in second and third grades (ages 7 to 9 years) behave with greater sophistication. More interest is shown in sex role–related objects, such as clothing and perfume. Both sexes are interested in peeking at the bodies of members of the opposite sex, and boys begin to practice street-wise sexual vocabulary (Janus and Bess, 1981).

From grades four through junior high school, preadolescent behavior includes both same sex and opposite sex contacts. The formation of close friendships within the same sex is necessary for confirming sexual identity, while increasing physical contact with members of the opposite sex prepares the individual for mature heterosexual relationships. Sexual activity gradually progresses to hugging, kissing, and dancing with members of the opposite sex. Voyeurism continues, gradually being replaced by explicit magazines, movies, and drawings. By the end of fifth grade (age 11 years), some boys and many girls already begin to acquire mature sexual characteristics with development of breast and hip tissue and growth of pubic, underarm, and facial hair.

Masturbation and orgasm are normal in sixth graders (ages 11 and 12 years) of both sexes. Self-stimulation of the genitalia may be direct or indirect. Although some girls may give up masturbation during the school years, they continue to engage in activities like bicycle riding, sliding down ropes and bannisters, gymnastics, and horseback riding, which they report as providing pleasurable sensations in the genitalia (Clower, 1975). Both boys and girls engage in sex-related fantasies: girls enjoy those related to romance and boys enjoy those more directly concerned with specific sexual acts, such as intercourse.

The genital urgings of boys are more overt and may result in transient sexual contact with other boys throughout the school years. Such encounters are normal and may or may not culminate in adult homosexual preference. The medical literature on biologic differences influencing sexual orientation is contradictory, but most authorities agree that adult homosexual behavior is influenced by several variables and that sexual experimentation during childhood is common and normal and does not necessarily predict adult orientation (Ledwitz-Rigby, 1980).

Learning Needs of the School-Age Child

The school-age years span a time when learning needs change dramatically. In the early school-age years, more detailed explanations about the facts of reproduction are required. Children now hear interpretations at school, along with a variety of new words that require definitions. A school-age child may not necessarily bring up the subject of sexuality, therefore parents should be encouraged to give the school-ager an opportunity to have uncertainties clarified.

During the early school years (ages 8 to 10 years), children also should be prepared for the changes that will occur during adolescence. Learning needs include information for making decisions about sex behaviors and ongoing education about maturational changes. Basic information about the consequences of various sexual activities is introduced during the school-age years (i.e., pregnancy, sexually transmitted diseases, and AIDS).

Nursing Strategies

The following principles provide guidelines for the nurse to use with the school-age child and family.

1. Stress to parents the importance of maintaining a comfortable, open atmosphere at home about sexuality to encourage a school-ager to discuss questions about sex and sexuality.
2. Encourage parents to provide re-explanations about the process of reproduction. Scientific understanding is often sought at this age, but parents frequently need to take the initiative to discuss it.
3. Because of the prevalence of sex-related conversations among peers, parents are encouraged to use and explain correct terms.
4. A school-age child may wish to speak to a nurse in private.
5. The nurse provides information to the child and to the parents concerning bodily changes that occur during preadolescence and adolescence.
6. As a school-ager's television viewing expands into movies that have sexual implications, parents are encouraged to view television shows *with* their child to provide opportunities for discussion.
7. School-age children are exposed to conversation about sex preferences at school, therefore parents are encouraged to discuss a child's understanding of what is heard at school.
8. Consequences of sexual activity may be difficult for parents to discuss, but such discussions should be encouraged to make their children aware of pregnancy, sexually transmitted diseases, and AIDS. The nurse can provide parents and children with accurate information and help them find appropriate community resources as needed.

Adolescence (13 to 18 Years)

The transition from child to adult occurs gradually or suddenly between the ages of 13 to 18 years. Changes in body characteristics and functions are accompanied by shifting moods and behaviors that alternate between instability and maturity.

Attitude Development

Often before physical changes are apparent, hormonal changes occur in both boys and girls, accounting for some rapid alterations in mood and attitude. With physical changes that render the individual capable of reproduction come social responsibilities for behaviors associated with increased libido. Identity formation is a major task in an adolescent's development. During this stage an adolescent's primary influential group changes from family to peers. Developmental tasks are now achieved in the context of society in general rather than primarily one's family. In our society, strong sexual messages through films, advertising, and popular music are part of society's input. Adolescents are pushed into early intimate relationships in our society. If early sexual contact precedes formation of a sense of self, an adolescent may have difficulty resolving other developmental tasks into a firm identity (Howe, 1986).

The young adolescent is preoccupied with self, easily embarrassed, and frequently unsure. The attitude toward a body that is changing, sexual urges, and social responsibilities can be overwhelming. Encouragement and affirmation from significant others, such as family and peers, influence positive attitudes.

Sexual Behaviors

Although no longer engaged in the fantasy play of childhood, the adolescent begins to live as though responding to an imaginary audience of peers (Elkind, 1978). Consistent with development of a mature identity is the need to conform with peers in matters of dress and behavior. The need for approval drives the adolescent to experiment in a variety of ways. Equipped with a changed body capable of mature sexual behavior, the adolescent may feel peer pressure to have sexual intercourse.

Both girls and boys adopt specific behaviors related to the changes in their bodies. Girls engage in new hygienic measures and altered clothing as they adjust to menstruation and breast development, which begins between ages 8 and 18 years. Boys adjust to unpredictable erections and nocturnal emissions. Preoccupation with the size of the penis is a frequent subject of locker room comparisons. Penis size depends on stage of development; eventual mature size cannot be known at this time.

Masturbation continues in adolescence. Boys typically increase this activity as a way to relieve sexual tension whereas girls may increase it to minimize feelings of loneliness. Fantasies of boys tend to focus on performance whereas those of girls focus on romance.

Homosexual and heterosexual attraction leads to specific behaviors that may vary from minimal mutual exploration to mutual masturbation, intercourse, or oral-genital contact. Sexually transmitted diseases (STD), including acquired immune deficiency syndrome (AIDS), and pregnancy are consequences that adolescents may be aware of but not sufficiently informed about to act responsibly.

Early in adolescence, relationships are based on close friendships with members of the same sex. In mid-adolescence, direct contact is sought with members of the opposite sex in group situations. Such contacts may be sexually arousing and give the individuals opportunities to experiment with a variety of identities. The final stage of adolescence consists of explicit sexual behaviors of a transitory or permanent nature. The adolescent with homosexual orientation faces considerably more conflict about identity and may "feel different" for approximately 2 years until the term *gay* or *lesbian* is applied to the personal self (Lion, 1982). Those with homosexual preferences are few compared with those with heterosexual preferences, and a sense of belonging may not be resolved until early or middle adulthood.

Learning Needs of the Adolescent

The need to learn about sexuality increases rapidly in adolescence. Learning to express feelings and resolve conflicts is essential to formation of sexual identity. Clarification of values about sexual behavior is essential for the adolescent. Sexual values depend on one's religious, family, social, and cultural context. The development of responsibility for one's own behavior must be stressed for both boys and girls. Increased peer pressure may generate internal conflict, making values clarification counseling beneficial for adolescents.

Exploring alternatives is essential to the decisions the adolescent must make with regard to sexual behaviors. The choice of whether or not to be sexually active, with whom, for what purpose, and in what context of responsibility is a critical issue at this age.

Nursing Strategies

In addition to clarifying personal attitudes and values toward sexuality, the following interventions are appropriate for the nurse working with adolescents:

1. Review anatomy and reproductive processes, clarifying terms.
2. Provide reliable information about menstruation, physical development, pregnancy, contraception, and sexually transmitted diseases.
3. Clarify values regarding orientation and responsibility.
4. Explore alternatives in the decision-making process.
5. Reflect feelings and support during crises.
6. Encourage involvement of parents with adolescents.
7. Support community projects to educate the sexually active adolescent.

See Chapter 9 for further discussion of adolescent sexual behavior and use of contraceptives; Chapter 43 for prevention of AIDS; and Chapter 45 for prevention of sexually transmitted diseases.

References

Belotti EG: *What Are Little Girls Made of?* New York, Schocken Books, 1976.

Bernstein A: *The Flight of the Stork.* New York, Delacorte Press, 1978.

Clower VL: Significance of masturbation in female sexual development and function. *In* Marcus IM, Francis JJ (eds): *Masturbation from Infancy to Senescence.* New York, International Universities Press, 1975.

Constantine LL, Martinson FM: *Children and Sex: New Findings, New Perspectives.* Boston, Little, Brown, 1981.

Cramer P: The development of sexual identity. *J Personality Assess* 1980; 44:604–612.

Diamond M: *Human Sexuality in Four Perspectives.* Baltimore, The Johns Hopkins University Press, 1977.

Elkind D: Understanding the young adolescent. *Adolescence* 1978; 12:126–134.

Erikson EH: *Childhood and Society.* 2nd ed. New York, Norton, 1963.

Fisher S: *The Female Orgasm.* New York, Basic Books, 1973.

Goldman R, Goldman J: *Children's Sexual Thinking.* Boston, Routledge and Kegan Paul Ltd, 1982.

Howe C: Developmental theory and adolescent sexual behavior. *Nurse Pract* 1986 Feb; 65–71.

Hunt M: Changes in sexual behavior in the past generation. *In* Byrne D, Byrne LA (eds): *Exploring Human Sexuality.* New York, Thomas Y. Crowell, 1977.

Hyde JS: *Understanding Human Sexuality.* New York, McGraw-Hill, 1979.

Janus SS, Bess BE: Latency: fact or fiction? *In* Constantine LL, Martinson FM (eds): *Children and Sex: New Findings, New Perspectives.* Boston, Little, Brown, 1981.

Klaus MH, Kennell JH: *Maternal-Infant Bonding.* St. Louis, CV Mosby, 1976.

Ledwitz-Rigby F: Biochemical and neurophysiological influences on human sexual behavior. *In* Parsons JE (ed): *The Psychobiology of Sex Differences and Sex Roles.* Washington, DC, Hemisphere Publishing Corporation, 1980.

Lion EM: *Human Sexuality in Nursing Process.* New York, John Wiley & Sons, 1982.

Masters WM, Johnson VE: *Human Sexual Response.* Boston, Little, Brown, 1966.

Pitcher EG, Schultz LH: *Boys and Girls at Play—The Development of Sex Roles.* South Hadley, MA, Bergin and Garvey Publishers, 1983.

Sears RR: Development of gender role. *In* Beach FA (ed): *Sex and Behavior.* New York, Robert E. Krieger Publishing Company, 1974.

Study Group of New York: *Children and Sex: The Parents Speak.* New York, Facts on File, 1983.

Woods NF: *Human Sexuality in Health and Illness.* 3rd ed. St. Louis, CV Mosby, 1984.

Bibliography

Antonovsky HF: *Adolescent Sexuality.* Lexington, MA, Lexington Books, 1980.

Barrett JE: Family life education—parental involvement. *J School Health* 1979; 49:15–19.

DeMoya D, DeMoya A, Lewis HR: *RN's Sex Q.& A.* Oradell, NJ, Medical Economics Books, 1984.

Ellis A, Abarbanel A: *The Encyclopedia of Sexual Behavior.* New York, Jason Aronson, 1973.

Feinauer L: Rape: a family crisis. *Am J Fam Ther,* 1982 10:35–39.

Feldman SS, Nash SC: Sex differences in responsiveness to babies among mature adults. *Dev Psychol* 1979; 15:430–436.

Fisher TD: Parent-child communication about sex and young adolescents' sexual knowledge and attitudes. *Adolescence* 1986; 21(83):517–527.

Higgins LP, Hawkins JW: *Human Sexuality Across the Life Span.* Monterey, CA, Wadsworth Health Sciences Division, 1984.

Hite S: *The Hite Report.* New York, Dell Publishing Company, 1976.

Klein MM, Schulman S: Adolescent masculinity-femininity in relation to parental models of masculinity-femininity and marital adjustment. *Adolescence* 1981; 41:45-48.

Lewis M, Weinraub M: Origins of early sex-role development. *Sex Roles* 1979; 5:135–153.

Marlowe M: Boyhood sex-role development: implications for counseling and school practices—three stage model of development. *Personnel Guidance* 1981; 60:210–214.

McCary JL: *McCary's Human Sexuality.* New York, D. Van Nostrand Company, 1982.

McNab WL: Sexual attitude development in children and the parent's role. *J School Health* 1976; 66:537–542.

Parcel GS, Coreil J: Parental evaluations of a sex education course for young adolescents. *J School Health* 1985; 55:9–12.

Roesel R: The nurse's role in primary prevention in sexual health. *Imprint* 1980; 27:27–28.

Silverstein CD, Buck GM: Parental preferences regarding sex education topics for sixth graders. *Adolescence* 1986; 21(84):971–980.

Sobiesk BI: Adult interpretations of child behavior. *Sex Roles* 1978; 4:579–588.

Unit Four

Impact of Stress and Illness on Children and Families

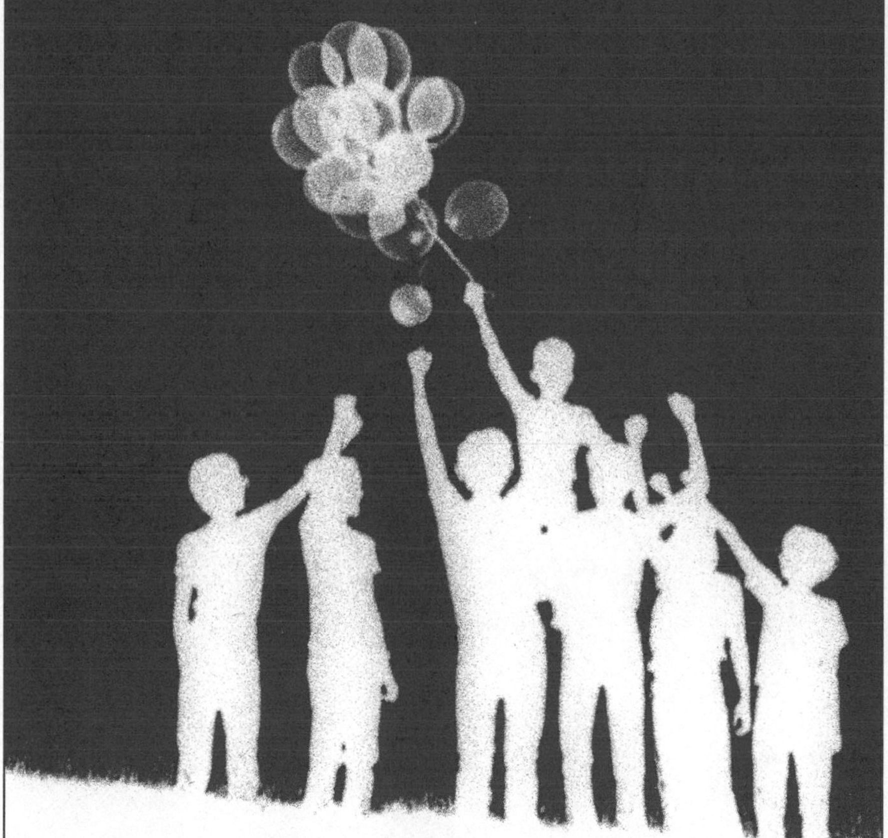

Concepts of Illness: Stress, Crisis, and Coping

Chapter 23

Carolyn Byrne
Mabel Hunsberger

A certain amount of stress is healthy, motivating, and supportive to the well-being of a child or family. It is when stress is excessive or prolonged or when it is imposed on those who are most vulnerable that negative effects result. Developing children face a series of challenges that potentially bring stress into their lives. The process of maturation itself makes demands on children, placing them into a position of vulnerability. Not only are children coping with the usual developmental crises (i.e., achieving autonomy, formulating an identity), but they encounter other situational stress to varying degrees, depending on their life circumstances. These stresses can include such events as illness, pain, hospitalization, parent separation or divorce, abuse or neglect, or their own death—all at a time when they are only beginning to develop the inner resources available to adults.

The various stresses that children face are discussed throughout this text in the chapters listed under Related Topics. This chapter presents an overview of the concepts of stress, crises, and coping and then relates these concepts to children and families who have experienced illness. Coping with specific degrees of illness (i.e., acute and chronic illness, as well as dying and death) are discussed in the chapters that follow.

Related Topics
Health Concepts: Children's Perceptions and Behaviors, Chapter 10
Assessing and Promoting Family Health, Chapter 12
Impact of Acute Illness, Chapter 24
Impact of Chronic Illness, Chapter 25
Impact of Death and Dying, Chapter 26

The Nature of Stress

Stress is a word that has no agreed-upon definition. It encompasses the idea of a *stimulus* and the person's *response* to that stimulus. The word stress is used so broadly that it carries the meaning of a form of stimulus (or stressor), a force requiring the host to change or adapt (strain), a mental state (distress), or a bodily reaction (Rutter, 1978; Garmezy, 1983).

Hans Selye, a noted stress researcher, defined stress as "the non-specific response of the body to any demand" (Selye, 1976). This nonspecific response is always the same; it is the degree of the response that changes. Selye viewed the response as a process that enabled the body to resist the stimulus (or stressor) in the best possible way, by enhancing the functioning of the organ or system best able to respond to it. Through Selye's research with animals, he identified three stages that occur in adapting to stress. This is referred to as the general adaptation syndrome (GAS).

The first stage is the *alarm reaction stage* where the body shows generalized arousal (increased adrenocorticotropic hormone [ACTH] secretion) but with no specific system being affected. The second stage, the *stage of resistance,* is characterized by a specific system dealing with the stimulus (stressor). At this stage there is a decrease in the body's ability to respond to other stimuli. The final stage is one of *exhaustion* whereby the stimulus (or stressor) is sufficiently severe and prolonged that the system dealing with it becomes exhausted and is unable to adapt to the stress (Selye, 1980).

The Body's Response to Stress

Although every system of the body is involved at some point in the stress response, the nervous and endocrine systems are central to the stress response.

Figure 23-1 illustrates how the body responds to stress. A stimulus is perceived and interpreted by the cerebral cortex (1) to be a stressor. The cortex then triggers the hypothalamus (2). The hypothalamus is one of the major areas of the brain which regulates the activities of the autonomic nervous system. It prepares the body for action by increasing the discharge of hormones. The hypothalamus' intimate relationship to the pituitary gland (3) provides the link between the nervous and endocrine systems.

The hypothalamus then triggers the two lobes of the pituitary gland—the posterior (4) and anterior (5) pituitary gland. The posterior lobe is mostly neural tissue and when stimulated it releases the hormone vasopressin (6). Contraction of the arteries and a rise in blood pressure are due to vasopressin.

The anterior pituitary gland (5) is responsible for six of the major hormones. Two of these are involved in the stress response: thyrotropin (7) and adrenocorticotropin hormone (8) (ACTH).

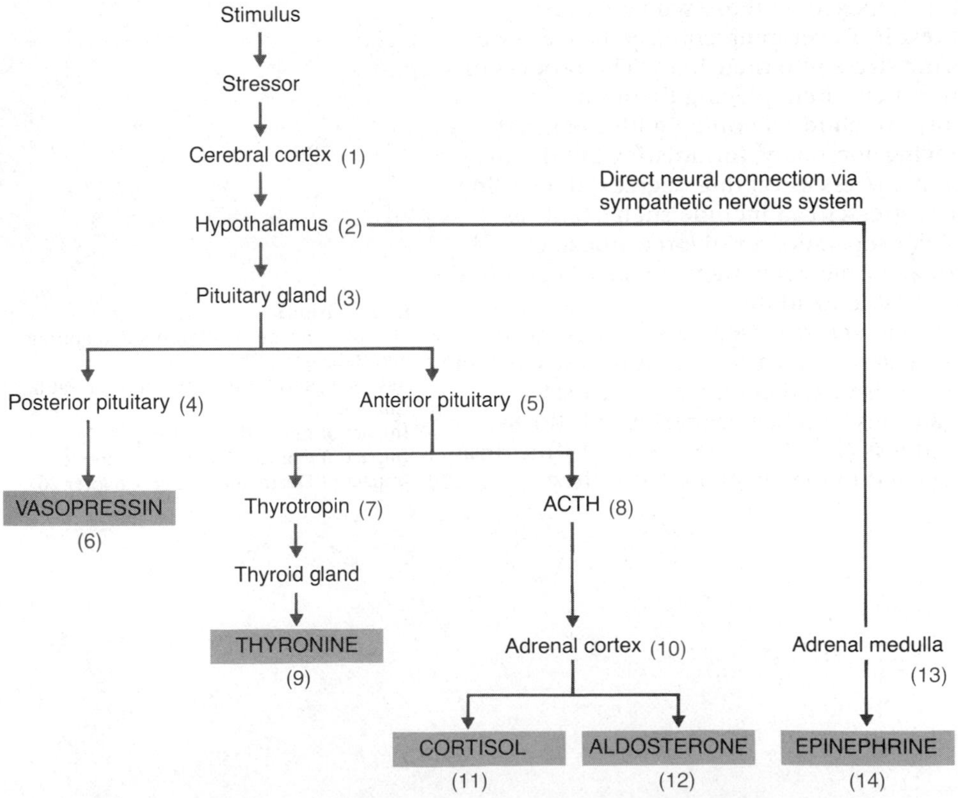

Figure 23-1. How the body reacts to stress.

Thyrotropin (7) stimulates the thyroid gland which secretes thyroxine (9). Thyroxine raises the metabolic rate to prepare the body to take action. The heart rate increases and breathing becomes deep and rapid.

ACTH (8) triggers the adrenal cortex (10) of the adrenal gland. The adrenal cortex is stimulated and, in turn, secretes hormones into the blood. The two primary secretions of the adrenal cortex are the glucocorticoids—primarily cortisol (11)—and the mineral corticoids—primarily aldosterone (12).

Cortisol (11) increases the metabolic process of the liver (gluconeogenesis) and forms glucose, the most efficient source of energy, during an accelerated period of activity. Through the process of gluconeogenesis cortisol mobilizes both fats and proteins in the blood. The mobilization of protein reduces the stores of protein in body cells. If this process is maintained because of a prolonged stress response, there may not be enough protein available for the formation of mature white blood cells and antibodies.

The increase in aldosterone (12) helps the body prepare itself for increased muscular activity and better dissipation of heat and waste products. The body retains extra sodium which results in increased water retention, blood volume, and blood pressure.

The adrenal medulla (13) is the other part of the adrenal gland that is involved with the stress response. The adrenal medulla is connected to the hypothalamus (2) by sympathetic nerves. When the hypothalamus is stimulated, the impulse is carried to the medulla, and the hormone epinephrine (14) is released. The effects of this hormone are primarily cardiovascular: increased heart rate, increased cardiac output, and increased blood pressure (Guyton, 1987).

Stress also demands psychologic adaptation and adjustment. Not only are physiologic functions affected by stress, but psychologic and behavioral responses occur. Selye's ideas have been criticized for focusing on the biology of stress and ignoring psychologic aspects and ramifications. Others believe that the psysiologic response is secondary and occurs only after the event is perceived to be threatening and the individual has responded behaviorally (Mason, 1971; Mondt and Lazarus, 1977). Regardless of which type of response occurs first, both physiologic and psychologic responses to stress do occur. Table 23-1 identifies the common signs and symptoms of stress.

Stress and Illness

Stress is a phenomenon that is universally experienced by all persons and groups of persons. There is no anticipated or common response to stress, since all persons respond in a highly individualistic manner. An individual child copes with stress in his or her own way as does a family group. What is stress for one child or family may not be for another. While it is true that all children and families experience stress from day to day, excessive stress can be damaging.

One particular type of stress that has received considerable attention in both children and adults is the number of stressful life events and their relationship to

Table 23-1. Signs and Symptoms of Stress

Physical	Emotional	Intellectual
Increased heart rate	Irritability, overreaction to some relatively minor situation	Forgetfulness, preoccupation
Elevated blood pressure	Angry outbursts, short-tempered reactions, hostility	Blocking
Tightness of chest	Lack of interest, withdrawn, apathetic, cannot get up in the morning	Increased fantasy life
Breathing difficulty	Crying tendencies	Decreased concentration, especially on complicated jobs
Headaches, migraine	Blaming others, suspicious attitude	Inattention to detail
Fatigue, exhaustion	Diminished initiative	Past-oriented rather than present-oriented
Insomnia	Reduction of personal involvement with others	Decreased creativity
Gastrointestinal problems: nausea, diarrhea, vomiting, intestinal disturbances, ulcers, colitis, stomach aches	Depression, worrying	Slower thinking, slower reactions, difficulty learning subjects
Restlessness, hyperactivity	Negative attitude, cynical	"Couldn't care less" attitude, mentally lazy, inclined to path of least resistance
Vague somatic complaints, feeling run down, minor ailments, psychosomatic complaints	General dissatisfaction	
Frequent or prolonged colds or flu		
Urinary frequency		
Weight gain or weight loss of more than 10 pounds		

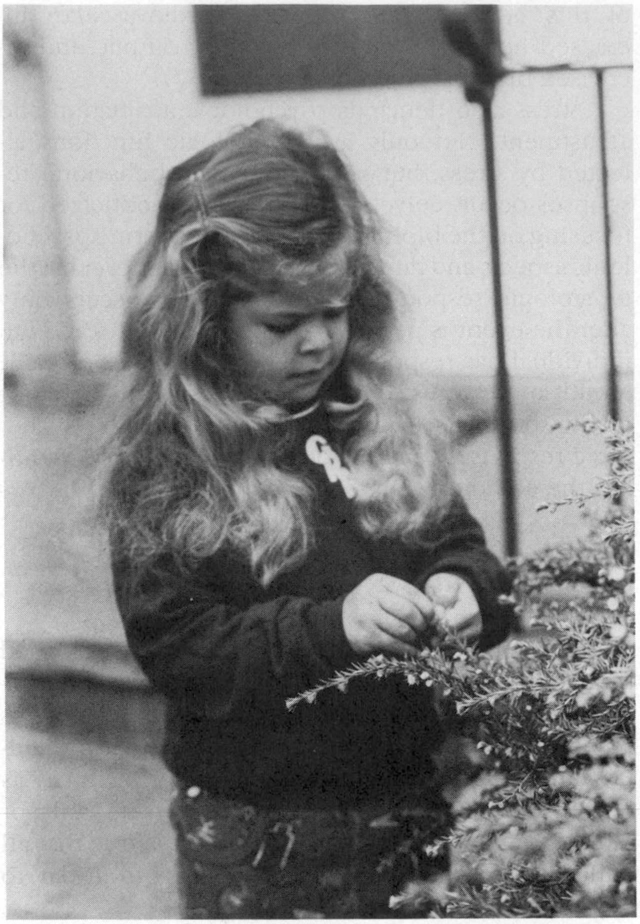

Persons respond in a highly individualistic manner to stress. Even young children may need just to be alone and think for a while.

anxiety and disease. Holmes and Rahe (1967) provided the major impetus to the scaling of life events in developing the "Social Readjustment Rating Scale." This scale, developed for adults, ranks important life events and assigns a specific value to each one on the basis of the amount of coping behavior needed by the individual to deal with the event. As the score increases, the likelihood of illness occurring is thought to increase.

Coddington (1972) developed life event scales for children based on Holmes and Rahe's work. He asked professionals working with children to judge the intensity of change required by each of the events and assigned a numerical value to each event. Examples of Coddington's life event scales for the various age groups are given in Table 23-2. Each life event has been assigned a weighting of the degree of change required to manage the event. The rationale behind these life event scales is that many changes, either positive or negative, occurring in a short space of time will disrupt the stability in an individual's life. It is felt

Table 23-2. Life Event Scales for Children

Rank	Life Event	Life Change Units
Preschool Age Group		
1	Beginning nursery school	42
2	Increase in number of arguments with parents	39
3	Change in parents' financial status	21
4	Birth of a brother or sister	50
5	Decrease in number of arguments between parents	21
6	Change of father's occupation requiring increased absence from home	39
7	Death of a grandparent	30
8	Outstanding personal achievement	23
9	Serious illness requiring hospitalization of parent	51
10	Brother or sister leaving home	39
11	Serious illness requiring hospitalization of brother or sister	37
12	Mother beginning to work	47
13	Change to a new nursery school	33
14	Change in child's acceptance by peers	38
15	Decrease in number of arguments with parents	22
16	Increase in number of arguments between parents	44
17	Serious illness requiring hospitalization of child	59
18	Loss of job by a parent	23
19	Death of a close friend	38
20	Having a visible congenital deformity	39
21	Addition of third adult to family	39
22	Marital separation of parents	74
23	Discovery of being an adopted child	33
24	Jail sentence of parent for 30 days or less	34
25	Death of a parent	89
26	Divorce of parents	78
27	Acquiring a visible deformity	52
28	Death of brother or sister	59
29	Marriage of parent to step-parent	62
30	Jail sentence of parent for 1 year or more	67
Elementary Age Group		
1	Beginning another school year	27
2	Outstanding personal achievement	39
3	Beginning school	46
4	Move to a new school district	46
5	Increase in number of arguments with parents	47
6	Change in parents' financial status	29
7	Death of a grandparent	38
8	Decrease in number of arguments between parents	25
9	Mother beginning to work	44
10	Becoming a full-fledged member of a church	25
11	Brother or sister leaving home	36
12	Serious illness requiring hospitalization of parent	55
13	Decrease in number of arguments with parents	27
14	Change in father's occupation requiring increased absence from home	45
15	Change in child's acceptance by peers	51
16	Increase in number of arguments between parents	51
17	Death of a close friend	53

Table 23-2 *(continued)*

Rank	Life Event	Life Change Units
18	Birth of a brother or sister	50
19	Pregnancy in unwed teenage sister	36
20	Serious illness requiring hospitalization of brother or sister	41
21	Loss of job by a parent	38
22	Failure of a grade in school	57
23	Divorce of parents	84
24	Suspension from school	46
25	Addition of third adult to family	41
26	Marital separation of parents	78
27	Serious illness requiring hospitalization of child	62
28	Marriage of parent to step-parent	65
29	Having a visible congenital deformity	60
30	Acquiring a visible deformity	69
31	Death of a brother or sister	68
32	Discovery of being an adopted child	52
33	Becoming involved with drugs or alcohol	61
34	Jail sentence of parent for 30 days or less	44
35	Jail sentence of parent for 1 year or more	67
Junior High Age Group		
1	Outstanding personal achievement	45
2	Breaking up with a boyfriend or girlfriend	47
3	Increase in number of arguments with parents	46
4	Beginning junior high school	45
5	Beginning to date	55
6	Brother or sister leaving home	33
7	Decrease in number of arguments between parents	29
8	Suspension from school	54
9	Not making an extracurricular activity he/she wanted to be involved in	24
10	Becoming a full-fledged member of a church	28
11	Death of a grandparent	35
12	Death of a close friend	65
13	Increase in number of arguments between parents	48
14	Becoming involved with drugs or alcohol	70
15	Mother beginning to work	36
16	Decrease in number of arguments with parents	29
17	Change in parents' financial status	40
18	Move to a new school district	52
19	Serious illness requiring hospitalization of parent	54
20	Serious illness requiring hospitalization of brother or sister	44
21	Failure of a grade in school	62
22	Change in child's acceptance by peers	68
23	Change in father's occupation requiring increased absence from home	42
24	Pregnancy in unwed teenage sister	60
25	Loss of job by a parent	48
26	Birth of a brother or sister	50
27	Divorce of parents	84
28	Addition of third adult to family	34
29	Serious illness requiring hospitalization of child	59
30	Marital separation of parents	77
31	Marriage of parent to step-parent	63
32	Death of a parent	94
33	Having a visible congenital deformity	70
34	Fathering an unwed pregnancy	76
35	Acquiring a visible deformity	83
36	Jail sentence of a parent for 30 days or less	50
37	Death of a brother or sister	71
38	Unwed pregnancy of child	95
39	Discovery of being an adopted child	70
40	Jail sentence of a parent for 1 yr or more	76
Senior High Age Group		
1	Breaking up with boy or girlfriend	53
2	Increase in number of arguments with parents	47
3	Beginning senior high school	42
4	Beginning to date	51
5	Outstanding personal achievement	46
6	Becoming involved with drugs or alcohol	76
7	Brother or sister leaving home	37
8	Not making an extracurricular activity he/she wanted to be involved in	55
9	Decrease in number of arguments with parents	26
10	Decrease in number of arguments between parents	27
11	Change in parents' financial status	45
12	Death of a close friend	63
13	Increase in number of arguments between parents	46
14	Death of a grandparent	36
15	Mother beginning to work	26
16	Suspension from school	50
17	Becoming a full fledged member of a church	31
18	Serious illness requiring hospitalization of parent	55
19	Change in child's acceptance by peers	67
20	Move to a new school district	56
21	Change in father's occupation requiring increased absence from home	38
22	Failure of a grade in school	56
23	Serious illness requiring hospitalization of brother or sister	41
24	Loss of job by a parent	46
25	Being accepted at a college of his/her choice	43
26	Pregnancy in unwed teenage sister	54
27	Birth of a brother or sister	50
28	Marital separation of parents	69
29	Serious illness requiring hospitalization of child	58
30	Divorce of parents	77
31	Fathering an unwed pregnancy	77
32	Addition of third adult to family	34
33	Marriage of parent to step-parent	63
34	Unwed pregnancy of child	92
35	Having a visible congenital deformity	62
36	Getting married	101
37	Death of parent	87
38	Discovery of being an adopted child	64
39	Death of a brother or sister	68
40	Jail sentence of a parent for 30 days or less	53
41	Acquiring a visible deformity	81
42	Jail sentence of a parent for 1 yr or more	75

(Reprinted with permission from Coddington RD: The significance of life events as etiologic factors in the diseases of children. J Psychosom Res © *1972; 16:7–18, 205–213.)*

that too many changes can cause a state of sustained arousal that can lead to exhaustion, interference with task completion, and illness.

Unfortunately, conclusions regarding the impact of life events on the health of a child are far from definite. Investigators studying life events and illness onset report that illness occurs after stressful life events more often than can be accounted for by chance (Creed, 1985; Reale, 1987). However, this research has been the subject of much criticism (Minter and Kimball, 1980; Dohrenwend and Shrout, 1985). Using only life event scales to measure stress has been met with some criticism. First, the scales often do not consider that individuals perceive events differently. What is perceived by one child to be extremely stressful may not be perceived as such by another. Second, these scales alone do not consider other factors that may influence stress, such as the type of supports available and the temperament of the child. Third, they do not measure whether the events have been anticipated. Some evidence suggests that anticipated events are less stressful than those that are not (Streiner et al, 1981). Fourth, the measurement of life events does not give an indication of "daily hassles," which may be more stressful than the major life events (Kanner et al, 1981; Oppenheimer, 1987). Finally, the life event scales for children under the age of 12 years are completed by parents and consequently parents are reporting events *they* remember, not necessarily what the *child* remembers as a life event.

More recent work on life event scales for children has led to the development of scales that latency age children can complete themselves (Lewis et al, 1984; Elwood, 1987). One such set of scales was generated by asking children for their opinions (Elwood, 1987). Box 23-1 lists events that children in grade 4 considered as daily hassles. This scale differs from the major life events scale in that it measures the daily occurrences that can affect the child's life.*

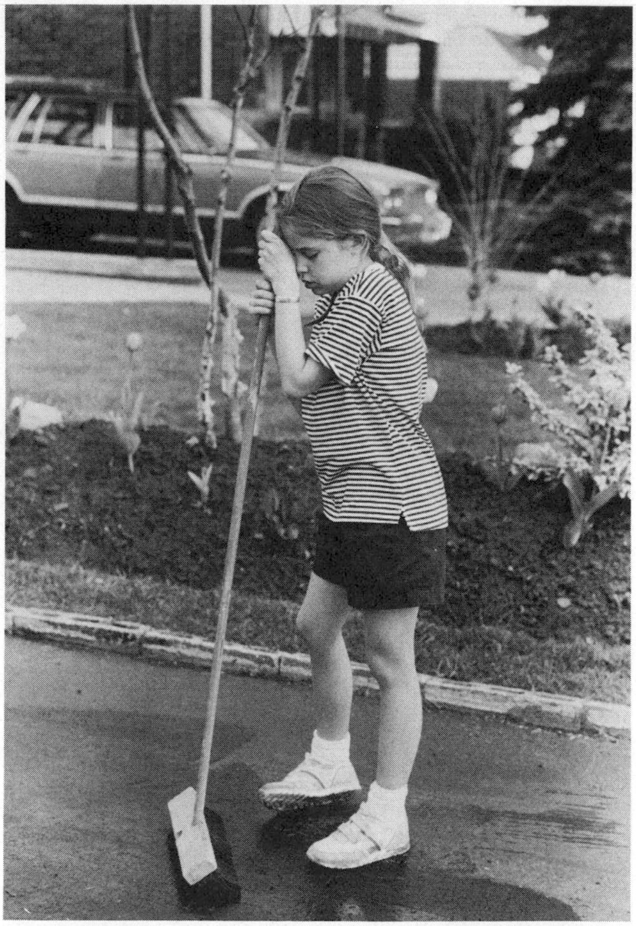

Too much stress can lead eventually to exhaustion, interference with task completion, and eventually illness.

Box 23-1
Daily Hassle Inventory (Grade 4, Age 9)

1. Something of mine was broken, lost or taken away.
2. I started to do (or planned to do somtehing) but then before I could get it done, I was told to do something else.
3. Other people teased me really badly.
4. I got into a fight or had trouble with:
   friends
   parents
   others
5. I was punished.
6. There were just too many things to do or going on at one time.
7. No one listened to me when I had something really important to tell.
8. I had to do something that was too hard for me.
9. I had to do something that I didn't like.
10. My parents or other people important to me were arguing.
11. My parents or other people important to me were upset or in a bad mood.
12. Other people were disappointed with what I said.
13. I had to make a big decision.
14. I got hurt or was very sick.
15. I didn't understand what was happening.
16. I was afraid of making a mistake.
17. I couldn't do or have something that I wanted very very much.

* In the actual tool, the child rates each item on a scale of 1 to 4 to indicate degree of hassle. (Elwood, 1987.)

Nursing Implications for Assessing Stress

Despite the controversy over life event scales, they can be used very effectively by the nurse to assess stress in children and their families. It is important to recognize the signs and symptoms of stress and then to identify the source of stress. Frequently what appears to be stressful may be compounded by many other events. Evaluating stressful changes in the child's or parent's life may assist in understanding the ways they have tried to cope. New alternatives to deal with the stress can then be developed.

The following example illustrates how understanding stressful events assists in managing stress.

Gillian, an active 8-year-old in grade 3, had been a bright and happy child who enjoyed school until this past month. Recently, every morning she would be very difficult to get out of bed and would state she did not want to go to school because she was tired. As she had not altered her bedtime, her mother checked with the school to see whether there were changes there. The teacher at school reported no change in Gillian's performance or activities but did notice she was more quiet than she had been when she joined the class 4 months ago. The teacher, however, was not concerned. The mother took Gillian to the family doctor for a check-up and found she was physically healthy. In talking with the nurse about events at home, the following became apparent.

Eight months ago Gillian's father had received a promotion at work that would keep him away from home more. To reduce his time away from home as much as possible, the family moved closer to the father's business. This move necessitated a change in school for Gillian. The family moved during the summer and in the fall Gillian settled into her new school very well. In the fall, after having settled from the move, Gillian's mother, who had been wanting to return to work for several years, found a job. She returned to work 2 months ago. With the mother's return to work, family members had to take on new responsibilities around the home. Despite a few arguments, the mother felt the family adjusted well to her return to work.

In viewing the events that had occurred in the past 8 months, it became clear that Gillian had to adjust to several changes: father away from home more, a move, change in school, mother returning to work, and increased responsibility at home. Understanding this, the mother talked with Gillian about the changes. This discussion revealed that although Gillian liked her new home and school she did not yet feel she had a good friend to talk to. Her father was busy and now so was her mother. She wanted to stay home from school with her mother so they could spend some time together.

Once this was recognized, both the mother and father began spending their own "special" time with Gillian and the difficulties in the morning disappeared.

The nurse, in assessing for stress, was able to assist the mother in identifying and understanding the stress the child was experiencing. The parents were able to find ways of reducing the stress and altering potentially problematic behavior.

Invulnerability to Stress

Nurses frequently work with individual children who seem to encounter high amounts of stress or come from disadvantaged environments yet do not appear to suffer any physical, emotional, or psychologic ill effects. These children seem invulnerable to stress and their behavior is marked by adaptation and competence. This is often noted in the self-sufficient way children handle day-to-day stresses.

A beginning understanding of invulnerability or resilience to stress has come from research investigating factors that place children at risk for poor outcomes. This research has identified that a portion of

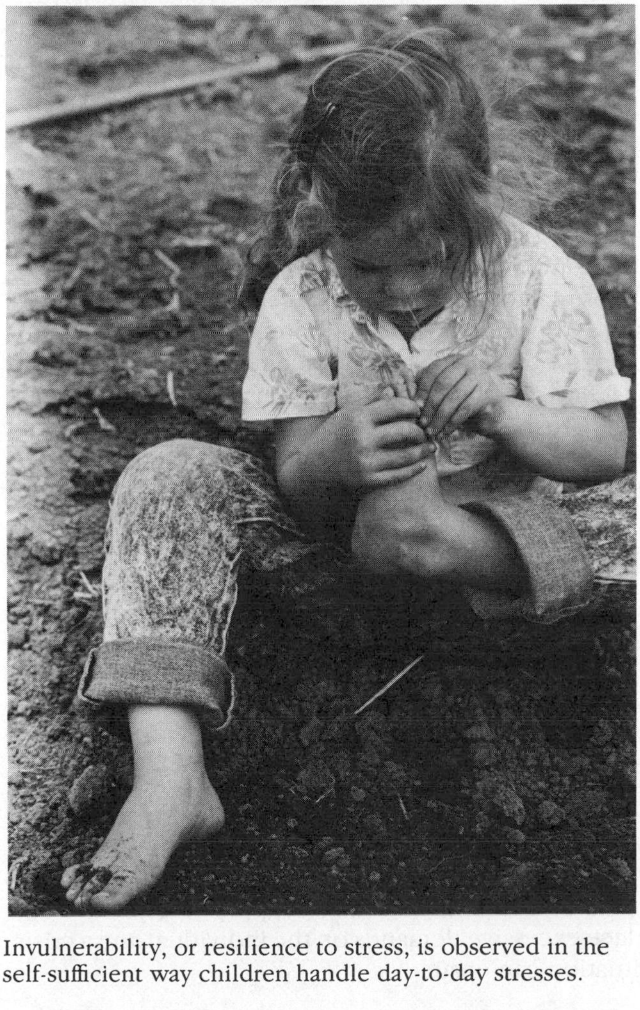

Invulnerability, or resilience to stress, is observed in the self-sufficient way children handle day-to-day stresses.

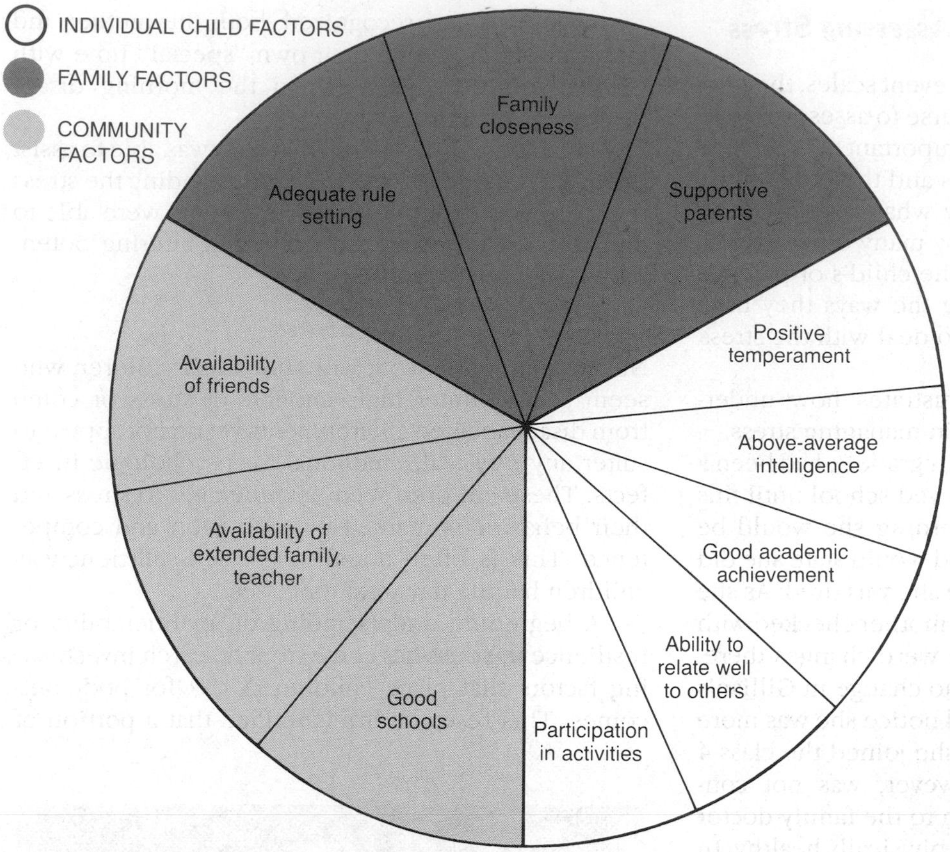

Figure 23-2. Factors found to contribute to invulnerability in children.

children thought to be at risk for problems do remarkably well (Garmezy, 1983; Burke and Wiskin, 1984; Steffman and Jung, 1986). This has led to an interest in determining the factors that protect children from responding negatively to stress.

Rutter (1985) has defined protective factors as "those factors that modify, ameliorate, or alter a person's response to some environmental hazard that predisposes to a maladaptive outcome." Protective factors that have been identified through research can be classified to be within the child, within the family, or within the community at large (Rutter, 1985; Garmezy, 1985; Rae-Grant et al, in press). They are illustrated in Figure 23-2. Although the work in this area is still in its infancy, the move toward identifying the factors that contribute to healthy functioning is a positive one. In the future these factors may well be used in preventive programs aimed at equipping children with resources to manage stress.

Crisis

Stress is necessary for survival, and certain degrees of it can assist the individual to grow in new ways. However, too much stress that is inappropriately timed can place excessive demands on the individual and a crisis situation can ensue.

Stress is present during a crisis but in itself does not constitute a crisis event. Stress produces a crisis state when the usual coping mechanisms fail. Crisis is defined as occurring "when a person faces an obstacle to important life goals that is, for a time, insurmountable through the utilization of customary methods of problem solving. A period of disorganization ensues, a

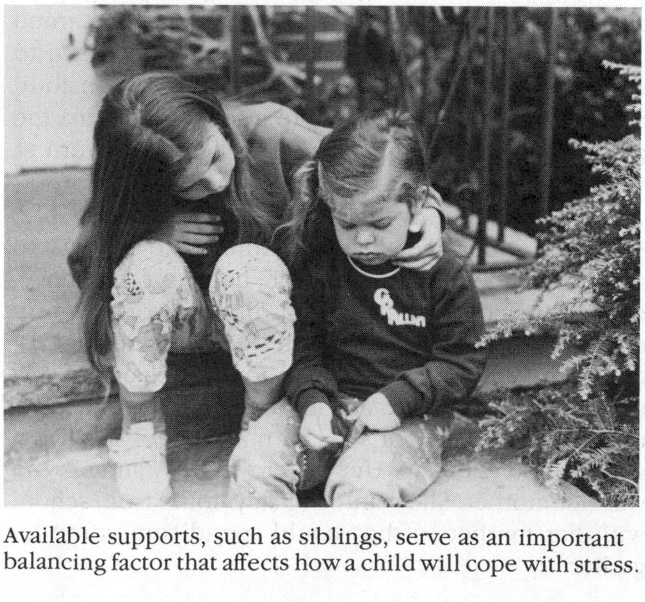

Available supports, such as siblings, serve as an important balancing factor that affects how a child will cope with stress.

period of upset, during which many abortive attempts at solution are made" (Caplan, 1961).

Phases of Crisis

Caplan (1964), the theorist most widely known in the development of crisis theory, has identified four phases of a crisis. In the *first phase* the anxiety stimulates one's usual methods of coping into action. If, however, these do not bring relief and there is no support, the individual moves into the *second phase* in which he or she becomes even more anxious as a result of the failure of the coping mechanisms. In the *third phase* the individual tries out new coping mechanisms or redefines the threat so that old ones can work; resolution can occur at this point. If resolution does not occur, the *fourth phase* brings about severe levels of anxiety. Box 23-2 illustrates the phases of a crisis and the physical, emotional, and cognitive symptoms that are associated with each stage.

Many factors influence how individuals and families react to and cope with crisis situations. Aguilera and Messick (1986) have identified balancing factors that affect the equilibrium of individuals and families. The balancing factors are the *perception of the event,* the *available situational supports,* and *coping mechanisms.* They feel that successful resolution of the crisis is more likely if the individual's perception of the events is more realistic than distorted; if there are available supports so that others can assist in dealing with the crisis; and if the individual has adequate coping mechanisms to alleviate anxiety. These balancing factors are represented in the paradigm developed by Aguilera and Messick (Fig. 23-3).

Box 23-2
Phases of Crises: Individual Responses

PHYSICAL, EMOTIONAL AND COGNITIVE SYMPTOMS

Phase One: Initial impact; crisis event; usual methods of coping fail

Somatic distress, shortness of breath, hyperventilation, weakness, fatigue
Anxiety, feeling overwhelmed, panicky
Hyperactivity or inability to carry out activities
Disorganized thinking

Phase Two: Increased anxiety

Often a denial of any physical complaints
Increased tenseness and anxiety
May try different coping strategies to resolve crisis
Withdrawal or hyperactivity
Disorganized behavior
Problem-solving abilities become increasingly more disorganized—thinking appears scattered

Phase Three: Resolution or defeat

Reoccurrence of physical complaints (tired, GI upsets)
Tension and anxiety rise
Attempts to redefine problem
Try new ways to cope
Crisis can be resolved—equilibrium restored *or* tension increases

Phase Four: Severe levels of anxiety

Many somatic complaints
Feelings of helplessness and hopelessness
Confused—problem-solving impaired
Disorganized thinking
Withdrawal
Depression

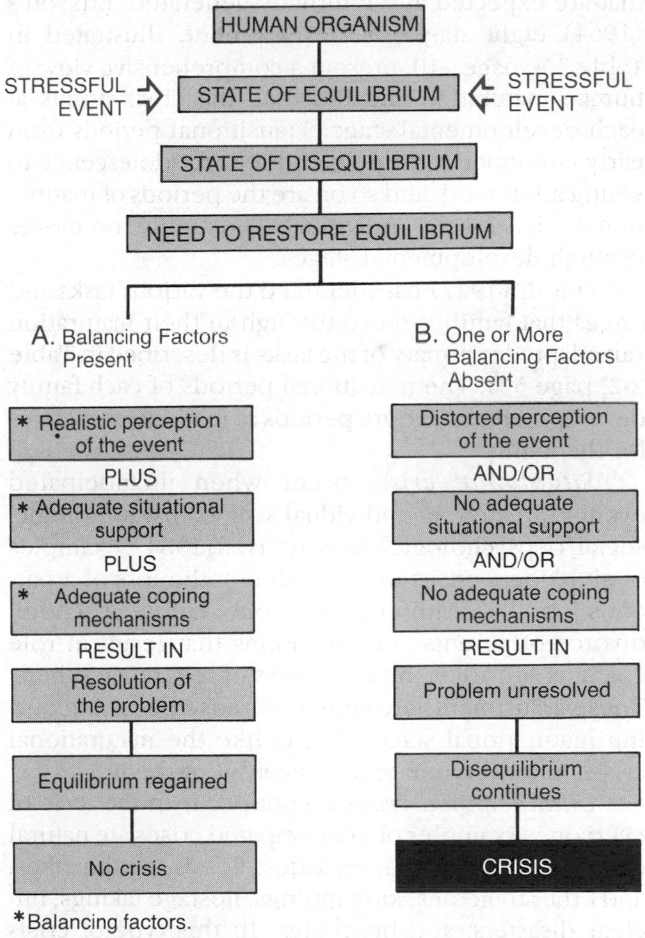

Figure 23-3. The effect of balancing factors in a stressful event. (From Aguilera DC, Messick JM: *Crisis Intervention.* 5th ed. New York, CV Mosby, 1985.)

As illustrated in Figure 23-3, the individual's or family's state of equilibrium is affected by a stressful event. This then causes disequilibrium and a need to return to the steady state. A crisis is averted if the balancing factors (*A*) are present; the problem is resolved and equilibrium is regained. However, if the balancing factors are absent (*B*), the family or individual has a distorted perception of the event, has little or no supports, and has inadequate coping mechanisms, the problem will remain unresolved, disequilibrium will continue, and a crisis will ensue.

Types of Crisis

There are three types of crisis: *maturational, situational,* and *unanticipated.* Maturational crises are also called developmental crises and require role change. Situational crises occur when an external event upsets the equilibrium of the individual or family. Unanticipated crises are accidental, out of the ordinary, and unexpected.

Maturational or developmental crises are ones that are expected and internally generated. Erikson's (1964) eight stages of development, illustrated in Table 3-4, page 110, present a comprehensive view of human maturation and illustrate the crisis points at each developmental stage. Transitional periods from early childhood to middle childhood, adolescence to young adulthood, and so on are the periods of maturational crisis for the individual. The family too moves through developmental stages.

Duvall (1977) has identified the various tasks and stages that families move through in their maturation (an adapted summary of the tasks is described in Table 2-2, page 57). The transitional periods of each family developmental stage are periods of maturational crises for the family.

Situational crises occur when unanticipated events threaten an individual's or family's biologic, social, or psychologic integrity (Hoff, 1984). Examples of situational crises include illness, the loss of a parent's job, the death of a loved one, failure at school, divorce of parents—all situations that result in role changes and adjustments in ways of relating to others. These adjustments are similar to those occurring during maturational stages, but unlike the maturational crises, not everyone experiences all of them.

Unanticipated crises do not occur in the lives of everyone. Examples of unanticipated crises are natural disasters such as fires, tornados, floods, earthquakes, and other tragedies; kidnappings, hostage takings, nuclear disasters, and hijackings. In this type of crisis disaster-precipitated emotional problems can surface weeks or months after the initial crisis period (Hargreaves, 1980; Palmer, 1980; Friedman, 1981; Frederick and Garrison, 1981; Terr, 1981).

Crisis Intervention

In reviewing the phases of crisis (Box 23-2), it becomes apparent that the individual or family experiencing a crisis is less psychologically defended and because of this is perhaps more amenable to change. In addition, the distress experienced during a crisis may serve as a motivating factor to examine new ways of dealing with the crisis. Intervention during this crisis period is to help resolve the crisis and restore the individual or family to the previous level of functioning or better (Aguilera and Messick, 1986).

There are four steps in crisis intervention: assessment, planning, intervention, and evaluation (Morley et al, 1967). These steps parallel those of the nursing process.

Assessment

This phase consists of obtaining a clear understanding of the problem. During this phase, rapport is established with the individual or family. Understanding the balancing factors outlined in Figure 23-3 is helpful in the assessment phase. Box 23-3 identifies questions to ask in assessing whether the balancing factors are present.

Determine the Precipitating Event. The individual or family may be aware of being under stress but not aware of the event that caused the stress. At times it is useful to review when the symptoms began and what events were occurring when the symptoms were first

Box 23-3
Crisis Intervention: Questions to Ask in Assessment Phase

Determine the precipitating event

- What event or events in your life have contributed to your feeling upset/anxious?
- What has happened in your life that is different?

Determine the perception of the event

- How does this event affect your life now?
- How will it affect your future?
- How does this event affect others around you?

Determine the presence or absence of situational support

- Who do you have in your life to support you?
- Who do you have to talk to about this?

Determine coping mechanisms

- Has anything like this happened before?
- How did you handle it?
- Have you had other stressful times in your life?
- What did you do to manage?

noticed. Reviewing the life events discussed earlier can assist in clarifying stressors. It is also important to determine how the event has affected the individuals or family's life. The nurse needs to assess the individual's or family's ability to meet basic needs as well as to assess how the problem is affecting life at the present.

Determine the Perception of the Event. Events can be interpreted in different ways by different people. It is important to gain an understanding of what meaning the event is given by the individual or family (Lazarus and Folkman, 1982). Does the individual or family view the event as a harm, loss, threat, or challenge? How do they feel it will impact or change their life? Since most crises involve some type of loss or a potential loss, it may be useful for the nurse to keep this in mind when exploring the perceptions of the event.

Determine the Presence or Absence of Situational Support. Information regarding the present and potential sources of support is useful in determining whether supports are adequate. When dealing with an individual: whom does the person live with? With whom is she or he close? Who understands? When dealing with a family: who supports whom in the family? What outside supports does the family have?

Determine Coping Mechanisms. The nurse needs to assess and understand the individual's or family's previous coping strategies. How did they handle previous crises? It is useful to have an understanding of the previous coping styles, as they may be strengths that could be built on in the present crisis.

Nursing Diagnosis. The final step in the assessment phase is the formulation of nursing diagnoses. This then will guide the planning and interventions. Box 23-4 identifies possible nursing diagnoses related to crisis intervention.

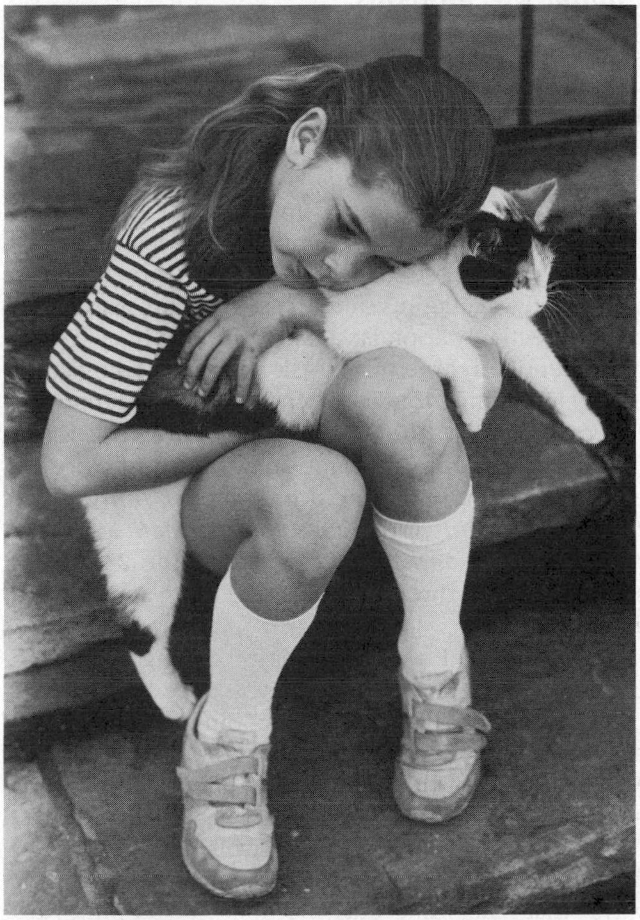

Talking about "who understands" may be important to a stressed child.

Planning

In the planning phase, the data collected in the assessment are reviewed with the individual and family to establish goals and planning action. The nature of the crisis and the individuals' and families' precrisis functioning need to be considered when planning ways to facilitate coping. Interventions should be planned that are realistic, clear, time-limited, and flexible.

Intervention

Interventions will vary depending on the individual or family and the nature of the crisis. Several guidelines can be applied to any crisis intervention:

Box 23-4
Nursing Diagnoses Related to Crisis Intervention

Altered growth and development
Altered family process
Altered health maintenance
Altered parenting
Anxiety
Decisional conflicts
Defensive coping
Disturbance in self-concept
Fear
Grieving
Impaired adjustment
Ineffective denial
Ineffective individual coping
Ineffective family coping
Knowledge deficit
Post-trauma response
Social isolation

- Help the individual and family gain an understanding of the crisis. Connections made between the meaning of the event and the crisis allow for an understanding and appreciation of why this is a crisis.
- Involve those concerned in decision making. This allows the individual or family some control and say on the approach to be taken to deal with the crisis.
- Allow time to discuss feelings. Often solutions are sought before individuals or family members have had a chance to identify normal feelings.
- Utilize the individual's or family's strengths. The use of previous successful coping strategies can give the individual or family some sense of control or mastery and assist them in having the confidence to try new ways to cope.
- Involve support systems. Using previous supports or establishing new supports can help in client assistance and gratification and establish outlets for tension. (See also page 985.)

Evaluation

Crisis resolution and anticipatory planning are the final steps in crisis intervention. The nurse and individual or family review the coping mechanisms that have been used successfully to reduce the crisis. The present management of the crisis is used to focus on ways of managing future crises.

Coping

Murphy (1974) described coping as a process that consists of a variety of behaviors used in a flexible way to deal with the challenges in the environment. Lazarus and Folkman (1984) define coping as changing those cognitive and behavioral approaches used to manage specific external and/or internal demands that are viewed as taxing and excessive of the person's resources. The individual's effort to manage and shape the stress experience involves two interacting processes, appraisal and coping (Lazarus, 1966; Lazarus and Folkman, 1982).

Appraisal of the Event

Lazarus and Folkman view the individual's perception or appraisal of a stressful event as a critical factor in the process of coping. They identify two types of appraisal, primary and secondary.

Primary appraisal is the evaluation of the significance of an event by individuals when they evaluate a stressful situation as damaging or potentially damaging. Lazarus identifies three ways that individuals perceive stress. The first is that the stress is viewed *as a harm or a loss;* the damage has already been done. Second, the stress is perceived *as a threat;* future damage is anticipated. Third, the stress is viewed *as a challenge;* the perception is that the stress will result in positive growth or mastery.

Factors thought to affect this primary appraisal of a stressful event are the priority of an individual's life commitments or purpose in life; how much control the individual feels in the situation; whether the event was anticipated or not; and if the event is ambiguous or clear (Haan, 1977; Fontana et al, 1979; Streiner, 1981).

Secondary appraisal is the individual's evaluation of personal coping resources or mechanisms to assist in dealing with the stressful event (Holroyd and Lazarus, 1982). It is thought that more effective coping results when there is a match between primary and secondary appraisal.

Additional resources that have been found helpful in assisting individuals in coping with a stressful event are economic assets, social supports, physical health and energy, problem-solving abilities, and social skills (Mechanic, 1977, 1978; Lazarus et al, 1984).

Coping Mechanisms

Coping mechanisms are a complex set of strategies that the individual uses to assist in managing stress or anxiety. Two major types of mechanisms can be used in dealing with stress or crisis: task-oriented strategies and ego-oriented strategies.

Task-oriented strategies involve the use of an individual's behavioral and cognitive abilities in an attempt to manage stress and crisis. They are aimed at realistically managing the stress situation which has been objectively appraised. Moos and Billings (1982) have identified three major task-oriented coping strategies, including *active cognitive coping, active behavioral coping, and avoidance coping.* The focus of these three coping methods may be any one or several of five techniques, including *logical analysis, information seeking, problem solving, affective regulation,* and *emotional discharge.* See Table 23-3 for a summary of the three methods of coping and the five areas of focus.

As illustrated, the methods of coping are active cognitive, active behavioral, or avoidance strategies. It could be argued that avoidance coping is a behavioral and, to some extent, a cognitive method of coping but Moos (1982) felt that it should be identified by itself since the function of avoidance coping is very different than the more active cognitive and behavioral methods. The focus of coping strategies centers on the ways that the different methods of coping are achieved. The method of coping may involve several of

Table 23-3. Task-oriented Coping Strategies

Strategy	Function	Examples
Method of Coping		
1. Active cognitive coping	Change the perceptions of a problem by identifying both positive and negative aspects	Consider several alternatives for handling the problem Tried to step back from the situation and be more objective Tried to see the positive side of the situation
2. Active behavioral coping	Seeking out others to help in solving problems Making decisions Changing to activities that are more rewarding	Talked with friend about problem Got busy with other things to keep mind off problem Made a plan of action and followed it Got away from things for awhile
3. Avoidance coping	Denying problem by trying to forget Avoidance of the problem Avoidance of people	Tried to reduce tension by drinking more Refused to believe that it happened Avoided people in general
Focus of Coping Strategies		
1. Logical analysis	Careful scrutiny of problem Attempt to identify cause of problem	Drew on past experiences Went over the situation to try and understand it
2. Information seeking	Obtaining information that will guide further actions	Tried to find out more about the situation Sought help from persons or groups with similar experiences
3. Problem solving	Outlining options Compromise	Tried not to act too hastily or follow first hunch Bargained to get something positive from the situation
4. Affective regulation	Control emotions arising from problem	Tried to reduce tension by exercising more
5. Emotional discharge	Verbal or physical activity to release tension	Took it out on other people when I felt angry or depressed Let my feelings out somehow

(Adapted from Moos and Billings, 1982.)

the strategies listed. For example, logical analyses, problem solving, and information seeking may all be used in active cognitive coping.

Ego-oriented strategies (also called defense mechanisms) are unconscious defenses to protect individuals from feelings of inadequacy and anxiety. Table 23-4 illustrates and explains the common ego defenses with examples of how they are used by children and adults.

These strategies are often viewed as negative ways of coping due to their unconscious nature. They can, however, serve as an initial protection following a stressful event (Elliott, 1980). The degree to which the defense mechanism is used to impair progress toward equilibrium or to protect the individual from being responsive to the reality of the stressful situation needs evaluation. For example, it can be adaptive for a family to deny the implications of their child's having acute myelogenous leukemia when the child is in remission and doing well. This assists in coping and managing life from day to day. It could be detrimental to the family and child to continue using this defense if the child relapses.

The overview of concepts of stress, crisis, and coping should provide a basic knowledge for examining in more depth stress, crisis, and coping in children, parents, and families during illness.

Childhood Stress, Crisis, and Coping

Children are expected to adapt to increasingly complex situations in a rapidly changing world. Children are being pressured to grow up faster, fewer adults now live with children, and child abuse in all forms is increasing (Brenner, 1984; Elkind, 1986).

Sources of Stress and Crisis for Children

The source of tension for a child can arise from the microsystem, exosystem, and macrosystem within which the child lives (Belsky, 1980; Brenner, 1984; Bronfenbrenner, 1979). The three systems can be visualized as concentric circles and are described by Brenner (1984) as follows.

The microsystem can cause stress to the child through the demands of growing and developing. The processes of maturing physically, intellectually, emotionally, and socially are stressors for a child. Increasing expectations to obey rules and to become more responsible for self and others requires continuous learning, role change, and adjustment of a child. As new family members are added to the system, stress is brought to the entire family as a whole and to individual children within the family. These types of stresses

Table 23-4. A Description of Defense Mechanisms with Examples of Their Use by Children

Description	Example
Regression	
A return to an earlier stage of development in thought, feeling, or behavior	*Child:* A 4 year old, Jillian, who has been toilet trained for over a year, begins to wet her pants when she is admitted into hospital for surgery. *Adult:* Jillian's father has a temper tantrum when he is frustrated with the admission procedure.
Denial	
A failure to acknowledge a stressful reality	*Child:* Jillian, who has been told she will be staying in the hospital for a few days, tells the child in the bed next to her she is going home with her mother. *Adult:* Jillian's mother keeps forgetting her appointment for a Pap smear.
Displacement	
Placing ideas, emotions, or feelings upon a subject other than the one to which the feelings rightly belong	*Child:* Matthew, 5 years old, is angry: he has just been punished for eating a popsicle without permission before supper. He goes up to his room and plays war with his transformers. *Adult:* Matthew's mother has had a difficult day at work. She has heard she did not get the promotion she wanted. She begins yelling at her husband, Matthew, and the other children.
Repression	
Painful experiences are barred from consciousness, awareness	*Child:* Jenny, age 18, does not remember spending 4 months in a body cast at the age of 5. *Adult:* Mrs. B. does not remember her father's death when she was 7 years old.
Projection	
Attributing one's own thoughts or impulses to another person	*Child:* John, who is envious of his sister's high academic achievements, accuses her of being envious of him. *Adult:* Wife accuses husband of infidelity when she is sexually attracted to a male co-worker.
Sublimation	
Transformation of unpleasant or blocked expressions into socially acceptable persuits	*Child:* Rick, 13 years old, would like to walk home every day with the attractive girl who sits next to him in math class. Instead, he works out in the school gym. *Adult:* Halina's husband has just left her for a younger woman. She spends much of her time reading murder mysteries.
Identification	
Process by which a person becomes like something or someone else by taking on thoughts or mannerisms	*Child:* Two 15-year-olds walking to school look exactly like the rock star on the billboard. *Adult:* The new aspiring mayor of a small town looks and acts like Ronald Reagan.
Reaction Formation	
Development of behavior that is exactly the opposite to what one would like to do	*Child:* Jean is angry at her mother for not letting her watch television. She goes into the kitchen to help with supper preparations. *Adult:* Cathy is furious with one of her co-workers who has left a considerable amount of work to be completed. She goes out of her way to be pleasant to this person.
Rationalization	
A logical, socially acceptable explanation to make something acceptable that would be otherwise unacceptable	*Child:* A 14-year-old not picked for the hockey team explains to his friends that the coach felt he should try out for a more senior team. *Adult:* A young woman fails her driving test after going through a stop sign and says that the driving instructor was biased against women drivers.

Table 23-4 *(continued)*

Description	Example
Intellectualization	
Excessive reasoning is used to allay disturbing feelings	*Child:* A 17-year-old, Jackie, is fearful of dating. She tells her friends she does not wish to date because it would interfere with her school work, and she has yet to meet anyone with enough intelligence to interest her. *Adult:* Jane becomes anxious in large crowded areas and explains her reasons for never going into shopping malls as a distaste for the crass consumerism of American society.

may be viewed as potential maturational crises for the child.

The exosystem produces stress when changes are made that affect the family's social connections (for example: when a family moves, joins or leaves religious groups, or makes changes in employment status). These types of stresses may be viewed as potential situational crises for the child.

The macrosystem brings stress to a child and family when established cultural norms are not adhered to. In addition, stressful events occurring within the community at large such as floods, tornados, or environmental disasters can bring stress to the child and family. These types of stress are unanticipated crises for the child.

The three systems interact to affect the way a child experiences individual stressors (i.e., starting school). Whenever a major stress compounds the usual stresses, a child is extremely vulnerable and may be in crisis. Illness is an example of a major stress that has the potential to cause a crisis for the child or the entire family.

Reviewing the body's stress response at the beginning of this chapter should provide a basis for understanding the physiologic response to stress in the child. Box 23-5 highlights the major physiologic indicators of both acute and chronic stress in children. As can be seen in Box 23-5, the physiologic manifestations can be quite diverse and nonspecific. Data on behavioral and cognitive coping strategies are also assessed to determine the well-being of children. An important understanding for nurses is that children view illness differently than adults do. They way illness is perceived has an impact upon how children handle the stress associated with illness (Chandler, 1982, 1985; Grey and Hayman, 1987).

Box 23-5
Physiologic Indicators of Acute and Chronic Stress in Children

Acute Stress

Vital signs increase
Blood glucose increases
Glucose may be found in urine if renal threshold exceeded
Dilated pupils
Decreased GI function
Cold perspiring skin
Tense back muscles
Increased basal metabolic rate (BMR)
Increased temperature
Alterations in hunger/satiety
Alteration in alertness/arousal

Chronic Stress

Weight may increase or decrease
Height may fail to maintain percentile rank
Developmental milestones may be delayed
Blood glucose may increase or decrease
Changes in the immune response may occur
Increase in free fatty acids and amino acids in blood

Stress and Perceptions of Illness

The way children respond to illness and cope with the discomfort and unpleasant sensations can be affected by their age. How effectively one communicates with an ill child is dependent on one's understanding of the child's fears and misunderstandings that arise out of cognitive limitations. The nurse's lack of understanding leads not only to a disregard of the child's actual experience but can cause the nurse to unknowingly increase the child's fears and fantasies by using inappropriate word choices when giving explanations (i.e., telling a young child a "dye will be used" for a test may indeed arouse the fear of dying in a preoperational child).

Children's conceptualization of the causes, preventive measures, and treatments of illness influences their ability to cooperate and participate in illness management. For example, the young child who cannot cognitively understand that medicine (especially a shot) will speed recovery is likely to kick and scream in resistance. Likewise, the older school-age child and adolescent who has the cognitive ability to understand cause and effect relationships suffers equally if explanations are *not* provided. It has been demonstrated that the conceptualization of illness advances through stages consistent with a Piagetian theoretical framework (Bibace and Walsh, 1980). This cognitive progression begins with magical/fantasy viewpoints advancing to increasingly more abstract thinking and reasoning ability. Bibace and Walsh (1980) identified stages of illness concept development, including:

- incomprehension;
- phenomenism;
- contagion;
- contamination;
- internalization;
- physiologic comprehension; and
- psychophysiologic comprehension.

Each of these illness concepts develops at corresponding developmental stages.

Infant

Bibace and Walsh (1980) used the term *incomprehension* to describe those children who were too young to explain illness. Due to the immaturity of the child's communication ability, little is known about a child's perception of illness before 2 years of age.

Toddler and Preschooler

According to Piaget (1958) prelogical thinking is typical of children from 2 to 6 years of age. A salient characteristic of the preoperational child is that cause-effect relationships are explained in terms of immediate temporal and/or spatial cues (Blos, 1978; Bibace and Walsh, 1980). Concepts of illness in this prelogical stage have been described by some as global and undifferentiated (Perrin and Gerrity, 1981; Simeonsson, et al, 1979). Two types of prelogical explanations of illness identified by Bibace and Walsh (1980) are phenomenism and contagion.

Phenomenism is the most developmentally immature explanation of illness. The cause of illness is an external phenomenon (usually sensory) that is spatially remote and inappropriate. The relationships between the phenomenon and the illness cannot be explained; the causal link is one of magic or merely that the illness and the phenomenon occur at the same time. For example, in response to a question about how someone got a certain illness, a preschooler might say "from the sun" or "from the wind." A 4-year old's explanation of illness as quoted by Bibace and Walsh (1980) follows: How do people get colds? "From the sun." How does the sun give you a cold? "It just does, that's all." How do people get measles? "From God." How does God give people measles? "God does it in the sky."

These examples reflect the preschooler's centering on a concrete, single phenomenon of his or her own experience and without any specification of the causal link.

Contagion is an explanation offered by more mature prelogical children. The child defines illness in terms of external persons, objects, or events, but the source is *near* to the ill person, or the causative event occurred *before* the illness. A child who perceives illness in this way still cannot explain the causal link; illness, if explained, is merely done so in terms of spatial or temporal proximity or magic. An example of this from the study by Bibace and Walsh (1980) follows:

> How do people get colds? "From outside." How do they get them from outside? "They just do that's all. They come when someone else gets near you." How? "I don't know—by magic I think."

The connection between the source of illness (or cure) and the actual illness is not explained; however, compared with phenomenism the identified source is closer to the person and generally more appropriate.

School-Age Child

The school-age child (7 to 10 years of age) is in the concrete logical stage of development (Piaget, 1958). The major developmental advancement that characterizes this stage is differentiation of self from nonself. This enables a child to distinguish between that which is inside and outside oneself. Multiple causes of illness are now stated including the child's actions (Brewster, 1982; Carandang et al, 1979). Rule violations are often given as the reason for illness without identifying a causal link to the illness (Perrin and Gerrity, 1981).

The concept of contamination is an explanation used by younger children in the concrete logical stage. These children do not differentiate between the mind and the body, therefore, illness in their minds can be caused by bad behavior or by contact with germs. The cause or source is still external but the bad behavior or germs are seen as being able to affect the body through surface contact. The concept of contamination is evident in the following example (Bibace and Walsh, 1980).

> How do people get a cold? "You're outside without a hat and you start sneezing. Your head would get cold, the cold would touch it, and then it would go all over your body."

The beginning of concrete operational thinking is evident in that the child begins to explain a connection between the source of the illness and the illness itself.

Older children in the concrete logical stage of development define illness in terms of an internal body part, hence the term *internalization*. The source of illness is still an external object or person (i.e., dirt, germs) or an unhealthy condition (i.e., obesity, old age), but it is seen as being able to have a direct effect on internal organs. At this stage the process of internalization (i.e., swallowing or inhaling) can be explained, but the effect that it has on the internal body is vague and undifferentiated:

> How do people get colds? "From germs in the air, you breathe them in." How does this give you a cold? "The germs, they get in your blood." And? "They give you a cold I guess."

At this stage the primary focus is not on what happens physiologically but on the process of internalization. (i.e., inhaling or swallowing). The ability to understand reversibility enables a child in this stage to understand that a person who becomes sick can become well and that illness prevention is possible through proper care.

Adolescent

According to Piaget (1958), the formal-logical stage of development occurs around 11 years of age. Children can then apply logic to abstract concepts because they are no longer bound by concrete reality. Thinking now extends into thoughts about what might be and generation of hypotheses.

The *physiologic stage* is used for younger children in the formal-logical stage of development who describe illness to be a malfunctioning of specific internal body parts or processes. Although the cause is triggered by external events, a child at this stage is more concerned with describing the internal functions. For example, explaining the effect of an infected organism in the lungs is foremost compared with how the organism was acquired. A child senses increased control over the onset and cure of illness and has a clearer perception that personal actions can contribute to outcome.

The most mature understanding of illness is when the child can describe internal physiologic processes but can also include psychologic factors as alternative causes of illness. This is the *psychophysiologic stage.* The young adolescent is now aware that a person's thoughts and feelings can cause illness; however, the cure is still viewed to be in the realm of biologic remedies such as medicine.

These stages of illness concept development, as described by Bibace and Walsh (1980), reflect a progression in the degree of control that children sense as they mature. In the very early phase (phenomenism) children perceive objects over which they have no control, such as the sun or wind, as causing illness whereas by early school age (contamination), illness is viewed as punishment; this, at least, brings illness into a more controllable perspective. Being good can thus also help one get better. By later school age (internalization), even greater control is evident, and a child is now able to understand that illness can be prevented by certain health behaviors.

A child's concept of illness is affected by other factors besides the developmental level. Studies have shown that healthy children view illness differently than do ill, hospitalized children. Although a significant number of healthy children believed they "had to be good in order to get better," they rejected the idea that illness is a punishment, whereas ill, hospitalized children do believe that illness is a punishment for wrongdoing. Children who were found to be generally anxious (but not ill) also believed that illness was a form of punishment. In families in which a sibling has been ill, Carandang et al (1979) found that the well siblings, especially those in the formal, logical stage of development, demonstrated a lower level conceptualization of illness than did children with healthy siblings. Coddington (1972) reported that sibling illness ranked among the most stressful of 42 life events for children, thus, a plausible explanation is that the stress of illness in the family is intrusive and may affect the perception of stress of healthy siblings. It has been suggested that the effect on adolescents, in particular, may be related to the fact that they, for the first time, may understand their own vulnerability to their sibling's disease. Thus, the nurse's interventions should take into account not only the child's developmental level but also individual factors such as experience with illness and general anxiety of the child.

Coping Strategies

A child's ability to cope with a stressful event or crisis is dependent on many factors. The primary and secondary appraisals suggested by Lazarus and Folkman (1982), discussed earlier in this chapter, are operative for children but are influenced by factors different from those influencing adults. Children are exposed to differing life circumstances and are born with an individual genetic makeup. Furthermore, children are developing and maturing. All of these factors affect coping.

Differing temperaments in children have been identified. The role of temperament in how a child reacts to stress events is not well studied. Rutter (1978) has reported that children with adverse temperamental characteristics were twice as likely as other children to be the target of parental criticism. Such interactions may well affect how children cope as these criticisms can affect how children perceive their own inner resources.

To a large degree young children appraise a stress through the eyes of their parents. Parents and significant others play a mediator role between the child and the larger world. They act as a filter, interpreting the stress situation and giving meaning to the situation for the child. A sensitive child quickly perceives the adult's ease or level of anxiety in a stress situation (Chandler, 1982).

Murphy (1974) feels that coping and adapting to stress in children involves four levels of behavior: an initial response with reflexes and instincts; a response with coping behaviors; mastery, which results from effectively establishing coping efforts; and competence, which results from a collection of skills accomplished through repeated mastery and achievement.

The repertoire of coping strategies used by children expands from birth to maturity. During infancy, the major coping mechanisms are through motor activity, crying, and sucking behaviors. As the infant progresses to the toddler and preschool stage, there is a beginning use of a variety of behaviors and responses to stress, which often includes active behavioral styles such as motoric expression of anger. During the school years, a larger range of defense mechanisms are used with the increase in experience and cognitive skills. The adolescent has gained experience in the use of a wide variety of coping mechanisms and has adopted those strategies that require increased cognitive abilities. Box 23-6 builds on the coping strategies identified earlier in the chapter and presents coping strategies used at the various developmental stages.

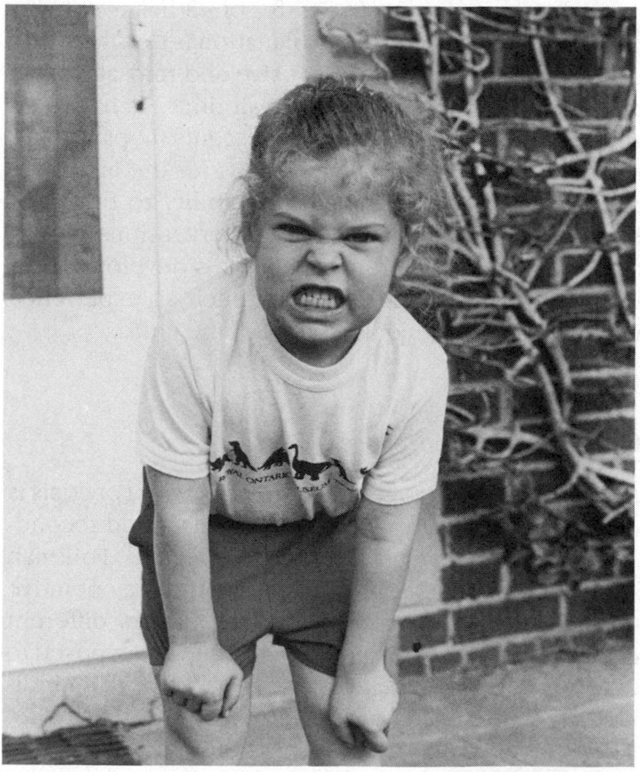

During toddler and preschool years, children use active behavioral coping styles, including motoric expression of anger.

Box 23-6
Coping Strategies Used by Various Age Groups

INFANT

movement
restlessness
rocking body
playing with toys
crying
thumb/finger sucking
sleeping

TODDLER/ PRESCHOOLER

Active Cognitive
asking questions (why)
wanting order (routine)
has favorite toy
practicing—trial and error

Active Behavioral
motor activity
play
temper tantrums
aggression
practicing—trial and error
thumb sucking

Avoidance Coping
withdrawal

Use of Ego-Oriented Mechanisms
regression
denial
repression
projection

SCHOOL-AGE CHILD

Active Cognitive
tries problem solving
communicates (talkative)
asks questions
wants to be boss/ controlling

Active Behavioral
play—acts out situations
friendships, play
aggression

Avoidance Coping
active fantasy life
withdrawal, quiet

Use of Ego-Oriented Mechanisms
regression
denial
repression
projection
sublimation
reaction information

ADOLESCENT

Active Cognitive
problem solving
reasoning through philosophical discussions
abstract ideas

Active Behavioral
conforms with peers activities
personal interests
asserts control
acting out

Avoidance Coping
use of drugs/alcohol
withdrawal

Use of Ego-Oriented Mechanisms
regression
denial
repression
projection
sublimation
reaction information
rationalization
intellectualization

Parental Stress and Coping with Childhood Illness

In this highly technological, fast-paced world, parents face a variety of different potential stressors arising from their personal, work, or family life. The functions, tasks, and responsibilities of parenting discussed in Chapter 13 highlight the complexity of the parenting role. The next several chapters in this section focus on the child who is ill. The illness of a child, whether it be acute or chronic, places the parents under stress. Sources of parental stress in the intensive care unit have been studied by Miles and Carter (1982). (These are discussed in Chapter 24 and summarized in Box 24-2, page 733.) Chesler and Yoak (1984) have categorized the types of different stresses parents undergo when their child has a chronic illness. They identify the stress as being intellectual, instrumental, interpersonal, emotional, and existential.

Intellectual stress requires the parents to understand their child's illness: what it is and the treatment implications. For the parents of a child with a minor illness, this may require information about the type of antibiotic the child is on. Parents with a child with a more serious illness may need to know more detailed information about the disease progress, symptoms, danger signals and treatment options. The process of obtaining this information can add to this stress, as often the parents are met with health professionals who vary in their degree of giving information.

Instrumental stress involves the parents' concrete ways of arranging their day-to-day functioning to manage the child's illness. In families in which both parents work, it may mean one parent staying home or finding a babysitter. If the child is hospitalized, it may

Table 23-5. Coping Strategies for Parents with an Ill Child

Type of Stress	Task-Oriented Positive Coping Strategies	Nursing Strategies to Promote Coping
Intellectual Lack of knowledge regarding illness	*Active Behavioral* Seeks out others *Active Cognitive* Requests information Interprets medical terms *Avoidance Coping* Protects against getting too much information (overload)	Be available to answer questions Provide information—through books/pamphlets, etc Teach (i.e., illness, treatment, etc) Assess for information overload by asking parents if they have been told too much, too little Be available in future to answer further questions Be aware of other resources if needed—physicians, other parents, films
Instrumental Day to day tasks	*Active Behavioral* Arranges to help at home—baby sitters/cleaners Rearranges work time, extra help Caring for sick child	Assist parents in understanding that they may need to rearrange or alter tasks and functions Assist parents in identifying resources to help them: family, friends, neighbors, colleagues at work, community resources
Interpersonal Alteration in relationships	*Active Behavioral* Seeking out others to help Maintains relationships with family Discusses and shares with others *Active Cognitive* Becoming aware of how others perceive the problem *Avoidance Coping* Avoid others who are not supportive	Assist parents in understanding the changes in their particular situation (i.e., things that all new people have to deal with) Be available to listen Assist parents in understanding how others may want to avoid problem
Emotional Personal stress	*Active Behavioral* Seek help (counseling) Care for sick child Care for self (sleep, eat, etc.) *Active Cognitive* Deal with feelings of hope, anger, fear *Avoidance Coping* Take time to be by self, away from others	Assist in identifying how the stress is manifested in individual Assess ways of coping with stress in past Clarify feelings
Existential Challenge to previous commitments	*Active Behavioral* Seek out other's ideas and opinions; reading Go to place of worship or seek other ways of support, groups *Active Cognitive* Seek meaning and explanations for illness Seek new meaning of personal life	Assist parents in understanding that child's illness has forced them into examining life

mean new role allocations, caring for the child in the hospital, caring for other family members, and maintaining household and job-related tasks.

Interpersonal stress arises as the allocation of roles changes. Additionally, the parents are having to form new relationships in relation to their child's illness (nurses, physicians, family, friends) (Hymovich, 1976). Other children in the family may need or demand more time. As the parents encounter or change their role with each person, that person becomes a potential stressor.

Emotional stress is the personal stress each parent individually experiences when their child is ill. This is a very individual experience and can depend on many factors, one of which is the severity of the child's illness.

Existential stress forces parents to question and challenge their previous commitments and life goals. It is often experienced in more serious illness when the normal order of life and death is being questioned. Often parents will question the importance of their life and try to make sense out of this experience.

The way parents experience these stressors depends on many of the factors discussed earlier in the chapter. Table 23-5 identifies the types of stress, some task-oriented coping strategies to manage the stress, and nursing strategies to enhance coping during these periods.

Family, Stress, Crisis, and Coping with Illness

The family as a system is made up of persons who are interdependent. Each member has a role to fulfill and others rely on that person to fulfill his or her role. The clarity of roles for each member is necessary and useful so that the family system can function effectively. The clarity of roles contributes to the family's maintaining a steady state as a system.

Families that are functioning effectively are able to problem solve, communicate, respond, and involve themselves together to determine roles, set rules, and care for each other. These activities contribute to the success and strength of the family unit.

When stress is introduced into the family system, significant changes and reactions occur. Within the communication network, stress affects the transfer of information. Inadequate message transmission and reception occur as stress is increased. Ineffective transmission of messages results in communication network breakdown.

Other types of stress situations that bring about dysfunction in the family system are lack of role clarity, vagueness of expectation, unresolved conflict, and conflict between the family system and other systems, such as church, school, police (Sedgewick, 1978; Tomlinson, 1986). The lack of role clarity results in family members being unable to identify their positions within the family structure. For younger family members, if there is a vagueness of what is expected from them, individual stress levels can increase and result in dysfunctional interpersonal relationships. Conflicts that are unresolved add to the dysfunctional quality of interaction. The continued elevation of stress levels in unresolved conflicts draws enormous amounts of energy from the family system that could otherwise be used in problem solving. Within the family system, when one member experiences stress all members experience stress. It must be remembered that stress does not automatically lead to crisis. It is only when the family's balancing factors are inadequate that a crisis occurs. Because a family is a system, a crisis for one member will have an indirect or "ripple" effect on all other members of that family system. A crisis directly experienced by one member of a family will unsettle the equilibrium of the family system.

It makes logical sense then that the illness of a child will have an effect on all parts of the family system. A family's response to the illness of the child will depend on the perceived severity of the illness, the supports available to the family and the individual child, and sibling and parental coping responses to the illness. The importance of working with families, approaches to understanding them, and ways of assessing families have been discussed in detail in Chapter 12. The next chapters on acute and chronic illness in children identify the effects on family life and ways families cope with illness.

References

Aguilera D, Messick J: *Crisis Intervention Theory & Methodology.* 5th ed. St. Louis, CV Mosby, 1986.

Belsky J: Child maltreatment: an ecological integration. *Am Psychol* 1980; 35:320–335.

Bibace R, Walsh ME: Development of children's concepts of illness. *Pediatrics* 1980 Dec; 66(6):912–917.

Blos P: Children think about illness: their concepts and beliefs. *In* Gellert E (ed): *Psychosocial Aspects of Pediatric Care.* New York, Grune and Stratton, 1978.

Brenner A: *Helping Children Cope with Stress.* New York, DC Heath, 1984.

Brewster AB: Chronically ill hospitalized children's concepts of their illness. *Pediatrics* 1982; 69:355–362.

Brodie B: Views of healthy children toward illness. *Am J Public Health* 1974 Dec; 64(12):1156–1159.

Bronfenbrenner U: *The Ecology of Human Development.* Cambridge, MA, Harvard University Press, 1979.

Burke SO, Wiskin N: Invulnerable handicapped children: clinician validation of characteristic amenability to change. *In* Kravitz M, Lauren J (eds): Nursing Papers;

Proceedings of National Nursing Research Conference (Suppl). 1984; 50–61.

Byrne C: The social competence of children following a burn injury. *Burn Care Rehab* 1986; 7(3):247–252.

Caplan G: Guidance for divorcing parents. *Arch Dis Child* 1987; 62:752–753.

Caplan G: *An Approach to Community Mental Health.* New York, Grune and Stratton, 1961

Caplan G: *Principles of Preventive Psychiatry.* New York, Basic Books, 1964.

Carandang ML, et al: The role of cognitive level and sibling illness in children's conceptualizations of illness. *Am J Orthopsychiatr* 1979 Jul; 49(3):474–481.

Chandler LA: *Assessing Stress in Children.* New York, Praeger, 1985.

Chandler LA: *Children Under Stress: Understanding Emotional Adjustment Reactions.* Springfield, IL, Charles C Thomas, 1982.

Chesler M, Yoak M: Self-help group for parents of children with cancer. *In* Roback HB (ed): *Helping Patients and Their Families Cope with Medical Problems.* San Francisco, Jossey-Bass Publishers, 1984.

Coddington RD: The significance of life events as etiologic factors in the diseases of children. I: A survey of professional workers. II: A study of a normal population. *J Psychosom Res* 1972; 16:7–18, 205–213.

Creed F: Life events and physical illness. *J Psychosom Res* 1985; 29:113–116.

Dohrenwend BP, Shrout PE: Hassles in the conceptualization of measurement of life stress variables. *Am Psychol* 1985; 40, 780–785.

Duvall EM: *Marriage and Family Development.* Philadelphia, JB Lippincott, 1977.

Elkind D: Parental pressures. *Pediatr Nurs* 1986; 12(6): 417–418.

Elliott S: Denial as an effective mechanism to allay anxiety following a stressful event. *J Psychiatr Nurs* 1980; 18:11–14.

Elwood SW: Stressor and coping response: inventories for children. *Psychol Rep* 1987; 60:931–947.

Erikson EH: *Childhood and Society.* New York, WW Norton, 1964.

Fontana A, et al: Subjective evaluation of life events. *J Consult Clin Psychol* 1979; 47:906–911.

Fredrick C, Garrison J: Disaster and mental health: an overview. *Behav Today* 1981; 12:32.

Friedman MJ: Post-Vietnam syndrome: recognition and management. *Psychosomatics* 1981; 22:54.

Garmezy N: Stressors of childhood. *In* Garmezy N, Rutter M (eds): *Stress, Coping, and Development in Children.* New York, McGraw-Hill, 1983, 43–84.

Garmezy N: Stress-resistant children: the search for protective factors. *In* Stevenson JE (ed): *Aspects of Current Child Psychiatry Research. J Child Psychol Psychiatr* Book Suppl No. 4. Oxford, Pergamon, 1985.

Grey M, Hayman L: Assessing stress in children: research and clinical implications. *J Pediatr Nurs* 1987; 2(5):316–327.

Guyton AC: *Human Physiology and Mechanisms of Disease.* 4th ed. Philadelphia, WB Saunders Company, 1987.

Haan N: *Coping and Defending: Processes of Self, Environment, Organization.* New York, Academic Press, 1977.

Hargreaves A: Coping with disaster. *Am J Nurs* 1980; 80(4):683.

Hoff LA: *People in Crises: Understanding and Helping.* 2nd ed. Menlo Park, CA, Addison Wesley, 1984.

Holmes TH, Rahe RH: The social readjustment rating scale. *J Psychosom Res* 1967; 11:213–218.

Holroyd KA, Lazarus RS: Stress, coping and somatic adaptation. *In* Goldberger C, Brenznitz S (eds): *Handbook of Stress: Theoretical and Clinical Aspects.* New York, The Free Press (Division of Macmillan), 1982.

Hymovich D: Parents of sick children: their needs and tasks. *Pediatr Clin North Am* 1976; 23:225–232.

Kanner AD, et al: Comparison and two modes of stress measurement: daily hassles and uplifts versus major life events. *J Behav Med* 1981; 4:1–39.

Lazarus RS: *Psychological Stress and the Coping Process.* New York, McGraw-Hill, 1966.

Lazarus RS, Folkman S: Coping and adaptation. *In* Gentry WD: *The Handbook of Behavioral Medicine.* New York, Guilford, 1982.

Lazarus RS, Folkman S: *Stress, Appraisal, and Coping.* New York, Springer, 1984.

Lewis CE, et al: Feeling bad. Exploring sources of stress among pre-adolescent children. *Am J Public Health* 1984; 74:117–122.

Mason J: A re-evaluation of the concept of non-specificity in stress theory. *J Psychiatr Res* 1971; 8:323–333.

Mechanic D: *Students Under Stress: A Study in the Social Psychology of Adaptation.* Madison, University of Wisconsin Press, 1978.

Mechanic D: Illness behaviour, social adaptation and the management of illness. *J Nerv Ment Dis* 1977; 165(2):79–83.

Miles MS, Carter MC: Sources of parental stress in pediatric intensive care units. *Child Health Care* 1982 Fall; 11:2:65–69.

Minter RE, Kimball CP: Life events, personality traits and illness. *In* Kutash IC, Schlesinger LB (eds): *Handbook on Stress and Anxiety.* New York, Jossey-Bass Publishers, 1980, 189–206.

Mondt A, Lazarus R (eds): *Stress and Coping: An Anthology.* New York, Columbia University Press, 1977.

Moos RH, Billings AG: Conceptualizing and measuring coping resources and processes. *In* Goldberger L, Brenznitz S (eds): *Handbook of Stress: Theoretical and Clinical Aspects.* New York, Free Press, 1982.

Morley WE, et al: Crisis: paradigms of intervention. *J Psychiatr Nurs* 1967; 5:537–544.

Murphy LB: Coping, vulnerability, and resilience in childhood. *In* Coelho GV, et al (eds): *Coping and Adaptation.* New York, Basic Books, 1974, 69–100.

Oppenheimer K: The impact of daily stressors on women's adjustment to marital separation. *J Fam Pract* 1987; 24(5):507–511.

Palmer E: Student reactions to disaster. *Am J Nurs* 1980; 80(4):680–682.

Perrin E, Gerrity S: There's a demand in your belly: children's understanding of illness. Pediatrics 1981; 67(6):841–849.

Piaget J: *The Growth of Logical Thinking From Childhood to Adolescence.* Parson A, Seagren S (trans). New York, Basic Books, 1958.

Rae-Grant N, et al: Risk and protective factors and the prevalence of behavioral and emotional disorders in children and adolescents. *J Am Acad Child Psychiatr*, in press.

Reale J: Life changes; can they cause disease? *Nursing* 1987; 17(7):52–55.

Rutter M: Early sources of security and competence. *In* Bruner JS, Garton A (eds): *Human Growth and Development.* London, Oxford University Press, 1978.

Rutter M: Stress, coping, and development: some issues and some questions. *In* Garmezy N, Rutter M (eds): *Stress, Coping and Development in Children.* New York, McGraw-Hill, 1978, 1–41.

Rutter M: Resilience in the face of adversity: protective factors and resistance to psychiatric disorder. *Br J Psychiatr* 1985; 147:598–611.

Sedgewick R: The family as a system: a network of relationships. *In Psychiatric/Mental Health Nursing: Contemporary Readings.* New York, D. Van Nostrand Company, 1978.

Selye H: The stress concept today. *In* Kutash IC, Schlesinger LB (eds): *Handbook on Stress and Anxiety.* New York, Jossey-Bass Publishers, 1980, 127–144.

Selye H: *The Stress of Life.* 2nd ed. New York, McGraw-Hill, 1976.

Simeonsson R, Buckley L, Manson L: Conceptions of illness causality in hospitalized children. *J Pediatr Psychol* 1979; 4:77.

Steffman AR, et al: A multivariate risk model for child behavioral problems. *Am J Orthopsychiatr* 1986; 56(2):204–211.

Streiner DL, et al: Quality of life events and their relationship to strain. *Schizo Bull* 1981; 7(1):34–42.

Terr LC: Psychic trauma in children: observations following the Chowchilla schoolbus kidnapping. *Am J Psychiatr* 1981; 138(14).

Tomlinson PS: Applying family stress theory to nursing practice. *Nurse Pract* 1986; 11(10):78–81.

Bibliography

Brown JM: Developmental changes in children's cognition to stressful and painful situations. *J Pediatr Psychol* 1986 Sep; 2(3):343–359.

Colton JA: Childhood stress: perceptions of children and professionals. *J Psychopathol Behav Assess* 1985; 7(2):155–173.

Fife PA: Development of a clinical assessment scale: evaluation of the psychosocial impact of childhood illness on the family. *Issues Compr Pediatr Nurs* 1986; 9:11.

Grey M, Hayman LL: Assessing stress in children: research and clinical implications. *J Pediatr Nurs* 1987 Oct; 2(5):316–327.

Keltikangas-Järvinen L: Psychological meaning of illness and coping with disease. *Psychother Psychosom* 1986; 45:84–90.

Impact of Acute Illness

Chapter 24

Mabel Hunsberger

The term "acute illness" transcends those conditions that require simple home remedies to ones that depend on using complex life-saving machinery. For the purpose of this chapter, acute illness will be used to describe those illnesses in which change occurs over a short period of time, reaches a peak, and then subsides. Acute illness thus includes a broad range of alterations, from common childhood upsets to circumstances of serious illness or trauma, but is differentiated from chronic illness. Whereas chronic illness requires a life-long adaptation, acute illness has peak levels which, in the case of minor illness, can leave a child achy and miserable but which, in the case of serious illness, may threaten survival.

Intrusive procedures and the need for hospitalization are circumstances that may be associated with any illness—whether acute or chronic—and are discussed in Chapters 27 and 31 respectively.

This chapter describes the child's and family's responses to the experience of an acute illness, including minor as well as serious illness, and identifies the various roles that a nurse assumes when acute illness strikes. The nurse's role ranges from telephone counseling during the peak level of a common illness treated at home to moment-by-moment monitoring of a trauma victim in an intensive care unit. The upset and stress experience when an acute illness strikes can be alleviated by nursing strategies that support the child and family in the process of coping and adaptation.

Related Topics
Parent-infant interaction, Chapter 5
Age-appropriate play activities, Chapter 21
Care of child undergoing intrusive procedures, Chapter 27
Care of the hospitalized child, Chapter 31
Childhood infectious diseases, Chapter 45
Care of the injured child, Chapter 52

The child's and family's behavioral response to acute illness in a child depends on

1. The nature of the illness (minor or serious)
2. Amount and location of discomfort
3. Extent to which activities of daily living are interrupted
4. Age of the child
5. Previous experiences with illness (personally or in others)
6. Sociocultural values and beliefs about illness
7. Child's concept of illness
8. Preconceived ideas about health care providers
9. Extent of knowledge about the illness
10. Response of significant others in their environment to the illness (Bellack, 1974; Wu, 1973)

When an illness becomes apparent over a short time period, there is minimal time for parents to learn about it and even less time to prepare a child for the experience. It is similar for the siblings—they too are ill prepared, yet they are affected by the disruption it may bring to the family in the ensuing days or weeks.

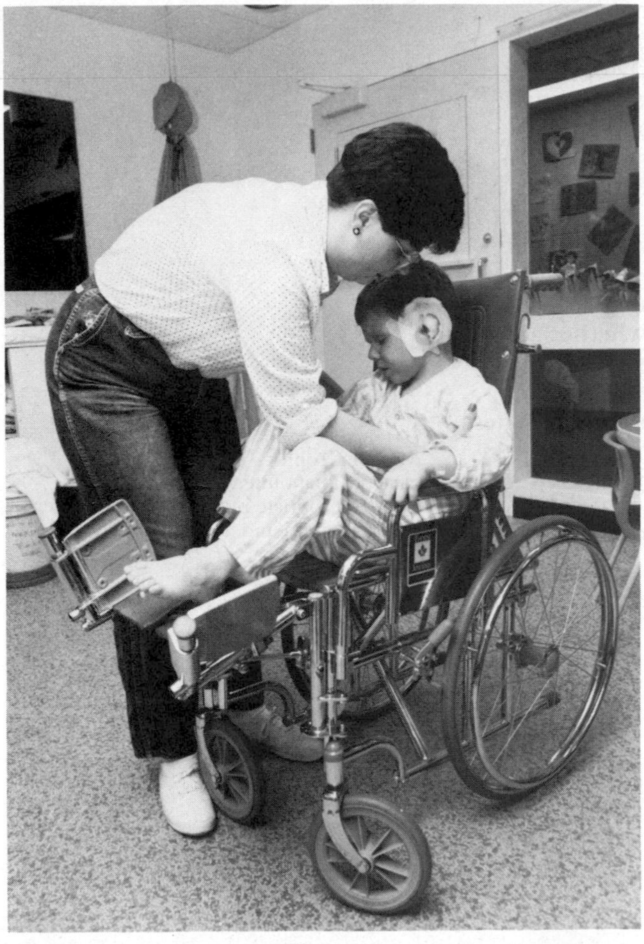

Acute illness is time-limited but causes major disruptions in a child's usual activities and routines. The discomfort that accompanies even minor surgery makes children feel sad and often irritable.

Longstanding family plans may need to be canceled for future rescheduling. Uncertainty about how long the illness will last and how quickly recovery might take place brings added stress. The severity of the illness experienced has a large impact on the nature of the stress and adaptive abilities of the child.

Minor Illness

Most minor acute illness causes a disruption in the child's usual activities and routines. Caretakers may experience interruption of sleep when called upon to soothe their irritable, uncomfortable, or sleepless child or to administer the necessary symptomatic treatments. Particularly while symptoms are most acute, parental anxiety exists about whether to seek help from a health professional, whether their judgment is adequate to determine if the child is improving or getting worse, and what measures they should take to relieve their child's discomfort.

Since care is usually administered at home, the caretaker who works away from home must either miss work or secure an adequate substitute caretaker for the sick child at home during work hours. The question of who will stay home from work may cause some antagonism between the parents. It is the rearrangements of work schedules and conflicts concerning roles that can upset the child and family even in the face of minor illness.

The impact of minor illness on children and families is not an area that has been afforded the attention of researchers to a large extent. Mattsson and Weisberg (1970) interpreted reactions by preschoolers during minor illnesses as a function of their attachment needs and their struggle for autonomy. During the acute phase of illness, all of the children studied showed some behavioral changes including reduced activity, longer periods of sleep, and a reduced appetite. Children younger than 4 years of age showed a temporary set-back in their willingness to assist in daily routines such as dressing and undressing. All children became more irritable, especially with their mothers.

Two distinct patterns emerged regarding their relationship with their mother in particular. Reaction I (primarily in 2-year-olds) was characterized by a clinging, whiny dependence with extreme irritability and intolerance of frustration. Reaction II (in those older than 3 years of age) was characterized by a diminished interest in physical and verbal contact with a withdrawal into a "self-contained, undemanding state." These children appeared at times to be "more independent than usual" and "easy to manage." The self-contained behavior may suggest a withdrawal of the child's interest in the environment and an increased focus on the body and its needs during illness (Mattsson and Weisberg, 1970).

During the convalescent phase, as the previous state of health is re-established, a change in behavior may be demonstrated. Mattsson and Weisberg noted in all children, regardless of age, an increased irritability and episodes of anger of 1 to 5 days' duration during convalescence. Thus, when young children are expected to behave as usual because they are getting better, they may actually become more irritable and difficult to handle.

Behavior responses to minor illness were examined by Haskins and colleagues (1981) in a study of 6- to 12-month-old infants in a day care center. Infants recognized as ill were noted to move less, play with toys less, and remain closer to teachers during illness. They touched teachers more and vocalized less, but cried more than when they were well. Teachers in turn gave more attention to ill infants, regarded their cries, and touched and held them more than when they were well. Haskins suggests that such social interactions related to illness may have a positive effect on responses to subsequent illness and may have a positive impact on other social interactional behavior as well.

Parmalee (1986) also suggests that minor illness experiences may contribute to the behavioral development of children in a positive way. Illness behaviors demonstrate a type of coping in which social relationships with the primary caregivers help to reduce their feelings of distress. Parmalee (1986) suggests that these recurring illnesses of short duration help children to expand experiences with "their physical selves, with associated mood changes, feeling of distress, and loss of vigour." Furthermore, minor illnesses often spread through the family, and children can observe and share in the caring of one another in a family. Such experiences can contribute to the development of the understanding of appropriate illness and wellness behavior and give a child some experience in differentiating physical from emotional causes of distressed feelings.

Nurse's Role in Identification and Management of Minor Illness

The nurse's interaction with children and families during an acute illness may take place on the phone, in a clinic, in a hospital, or at home. The interaction begins with a health assessment of the child's condition; then the problem is identified and, in collaboration with the parents and other professionals, interventions are planned and carried out. A primary role in the care of a child with minor illness is to teach the family how to assess and evaluate the condition of their child and how to care for their child at home. Follow-up care in the home or clinic for various diseases or illnesses is included throughout this text, placed at the end of the main discussion of the particular conditions.

Anticipatory guidance early in parenthood should cover some basic information that will be useful to parents when their child becomes ill. This information should include (1) when to seek nurse or physician assistance, (2) facts to gather before calling for assistance, (3) what to do during the office or clinic visit, and (4) instruction and practice in basic treatment of common symptoms (measures to reduce fever, evaluating respirations) and symptom assessment (temperature taking, throat inspection). The nurse also plays an active part in offering education and health services that can *prevent* many of the minor illnesses.

When to Seek Assistance. Parents need to know the early signs of illness if they are to make judgments about intervention. Illness is usually preceded by a change in the child's normal behavior, especially related to play and eating. A sudden or dramatic decrease in appetite and unusual irritability and lassitude are definite signs that all is not well. Fever and pain are also common precursors to illness. Although there is some variation in management of minor illness, parents are usually given guidelines about when to seek professional advice. Generally, parents are advised to call if they "think something is wrong." Parents know their children, and their observations are very important and should be taken seriously. Situations that warrant a professional's advice include:

1. A child under 6 months of age with a fever of 37.8°C (100°F) or above.
2. Any child with a persistent high fever of 39.2°C (102.5°F) or above.
3. An irritable or lethargic child.
4. A child who has received a serious blow to the head or other serious injury.
5. A child who has any signs of respiratory difficulty.
6. A child with persistent vomiting or diarrhea.
7. A child with pain.
8. When a parent recognizes a combination of changes in the child (e.g., does not eat, play, or sleep well).

Facts to Gather. Before parents seek assistance, they should look their child over for symptoms, take the temperature, and take note of the child's behavior so that the nurse's or doctor's questions can be answered. Table 24-1 outlines the observations caregivers should be taught to note and write down just prior to seeking assistance, whether by phone or during a clinic visit. From this information the health professional can decide how urgent the problem is and how it should be managed (e.g., over the phone, in the office, in the hospital, or at home).

Table 24-1. Information Parents Should Be Prepared to Provide Before Seeking Assistance

Child's Age	(Symptoms may change suddenly in children under 6 months; age may affect treatment prescribed.)*
When Child Last Well	(If symptoms are mild and recent, physician or nurse will probably follow by phone. If symptoms worsen or have lasted several days, child should be seen.)
Behavior	Is the child irritable? Lost interest in play? Decreased appetite? For how long has this been the case? (Child acting sick more than 24 hours should be seen by doctor or nurse even if symptoms are minor.)
Fever	What is child's temperature? Rectally or orally? How long has the fever existed? What has been done for it—results? (Consult physician if fever is high, longer than 3 days, if infant under 6 months, if accompanied by a stiff neck and if child is dehydrated).
Pain	Difficulty swallowing? Stiff neck? Pulling or holding ear—which one? Headache? Stomach ache—where? Pain when extremities moved? Hurt to breathe? (Consult physician immediately for acute, persistent pain; physician or nurse if child presents with no other symptoms or if minor injury is associated.)
Breathing	Slow or fast? Any noise? Coughing? Stuffy or runny nose? Unable to eat or drink? Any extra effort made to breathe? Any blueness around mouth? (See physician immediately if any distress or noise! See physician or nurse if breathing difficulty interferes with feeding, or if cough interrupts sleep.)
Skin	Cool or hot? Dry or moist? Blotchy? Any rash—flat or raised, color, location, single or several together, itchy? (See physician or nurse if child's neck is also stiff, has swollen glands, or if child looks very sick.)
Any Vomiting/Diarrhea	How many times today? How long has it been occurring? Any mucus? What does it look like? (See physician or nurse if frequent or constant, blood present, dehydration exists, possible poison or drug ingestion.)
Eyes	Dull? Tearing? Discharge—amount and color? Partly closed? (See physician or nurse if discharge present or if, coupled with other symptoms, dehydration suggested.)
Other	Any other family members ill presently or recently (past 2 weeks)? Any similar illness in neighborhood or school? Any major changes in routines? Any recent family crises? Child have any chronic conditions? (A chronically ill child should be seen by physician even if symptoms are mild.)
What Has Been Tried	Any medicines given? Have any of the things tried helped? (Gives some clue to caregiver's judgment re interventions. If questionable, child should be seen, as other observations may be inaccurate.)
What Is Caregiver Most Worried About	(If other family situations are being affected by the illness (party, trip, work) it may be important to the family for the child to be seen even if symptoms are mild.)

* The material in parentheses is a guide to the nurse in determining whether the child should be seen and by whom.

Teaching Parents Symptomatic Care. The ultimate success of the family's involvement in home treatment is largely determined by their ability and preparation to participate in it. Evaluating signs of illness, including how to take rectal and oral temperatures, is an important aspect of home care to teach parents. Additional home care management to teach parents includes fever control; dietary measures for mild vomiting or diarrhea; emergency first-aid procedures (including those for bleeding and choking, and artificial respiration and circulation); aseptic measures, including the management of contagions; and how to measure and administer medicines according to the child's age. Obviously caretakers cannot absorb all this information at one time. Therefore, information is introduced gradually and supplemented with written materials. Many school health curricula are including such information so that perhaps eventually adults will enter parenthood with some knowledge about home management measures during minor illness.

Caregivers may also need assistance in developing convalescent activities for their recuperating youngster. The key elements of successful convalescent activities is that they encourage age-appropriate motor development. Keep the child involved in an activity that is enjoyable and promotes cognitive development. Many household items lend themselves to creative play and help to pass the time. Macaroni, paper plates, paper bags, old magazines or catalogues, or fabric scraps (the possibilities are almost endless) coupled with scissors, paste, watercolor paints, and crayons can occupy many hours. Have children create stories based on a name, a character, or a situation, or perhaps write their own life story. If they are too young to write, they can dictate the story into a tape recorder or draw pictures. (See Chapter 21 for other age-appropriate play activities.)

Children are also helped through their convalescence if they are allowed to get at least partly dressed every day and occasionally to be on the living room couch, if possible. If the child cannot join the family at mealtimes, each member (except those susceptible to the disease if it is contagious) can take turns having dinner with the ill child.

Children confined to bed should still have family responsibilities if their condition permits. Activities such as sorting socks, snapping beans, sewing buttons, and licking stamps help to make children feel they are recuperating. Even very small children should be given a chance at some tasks, and if achievement expectations are not too great they will succeed. Older

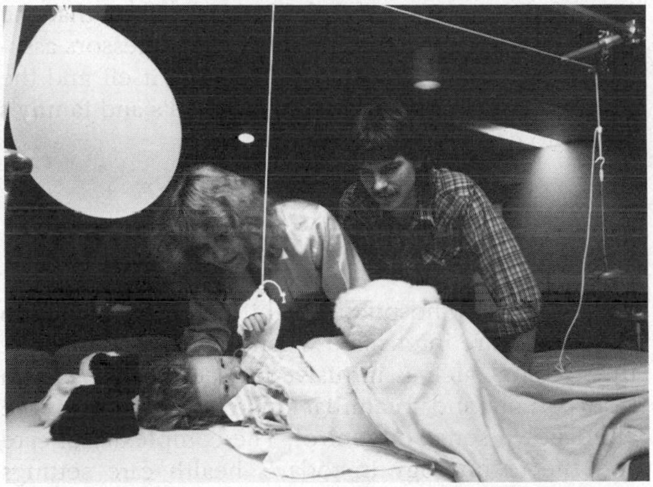

A broken bone brings considerable upset to a child. Even though this child's pain is controlled and she has supportive parents, the confinement and discomfort are stressful to a young child. Although adults know and understand that the experience is time-limited, to a 3-year-old the only reality is the misery of each day.

children can take charge of answering the phone on an extension during their waking hours and take messages or call family members to the phone with a small bell. Some time to watch favorite television shows can be allowed, but children soon tire of television as their only source of entertainment. Human contact at regular intervals is imperative to their recovery and emotional contentment. Usually parents need only a few examples of ways to occupy their child before their own imagination takes over.

Acute Illness Requiring Short-Term Hospitalization

When children require hospitalization, an additional burden is placed upon the child and family. The discomforts of "feeling sick" are now compounded with "feeling scared." Parents also have added worries. Illnesses requiring hospitalization are usually more threatening and are accompanied by more pain and discomfort than minor illnesses managed at home. (See Chapter 31 for a discussion of the stressors of hospitalization.)

The Seriously Ill Child

Serious illness threatening the life of a child brings a family into one of the most stressful circumstances they will ever experience. A child who is critically ill usually requires hospitalization for intensive therapy and management. During this phase, the experience of illness itself is a stressor, and environmental factors (unfamiliar environment, separation from family, loss of routine) account for added stress. (See Chapter 31 for a discussion of the care of a hospitalized child.)

In addition to the environmental stressors that are associated with hospitalization, one's ability to cope with any illness, whether the child is hospitalized or at home, is affected by situational and personal stressors. When illness occurs suddenly, parents have little time to make the necessary adjustments in family responsibilities that direct necessary attention toward the ill child. Uncertainty concerning the child's future is another situational stressor that places the family in a vulnerable position.

Personal stressors such as past experiences with death and illness, financial or family problems, or other life stresses are added factors that affect the family's ability to cope (Miles and Carter, 1982). Regard-

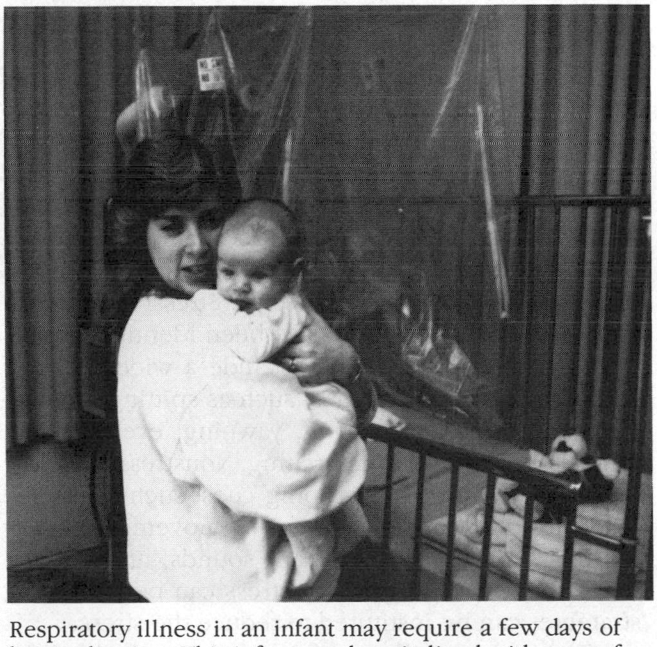

Respiratory illness in an infant may require a few days of hospitalization. This infant was hospitalized with croup for 3 days and is now ready for discharge. Although such an illness is of short duration, it causes considerable upset for the infant and family. Having to place an infant in a mist tent, the distress of seeing an infant having difficulty breathing, and daily visits to the hospital can make parents feel exhausted and irritable.

less of the setting, critical illness requires that the nurse give appropriate attention to the stressors associated with the situation of the illness itself and the individual factors that hinder the child's and family's ability to cope.

Stress of Critical Care

The stresses for hospitalized children as presented in Chapter 31 are intensified when the child is critically ill. Stressors such as intrusive procedures, separation from parents, and unfamiliar environments destroy the child's own sense of control. The complexity of care and the technology in today's health care settings makes children and parents feel dependent on others' decision making. The overwhelming environment and uncertainties about outcome present a situation that produces an intense level of stress for all concerned, including the caretaker.

Impact of Acute Illness on Child and Family

The response of neonates to the intensive care unit (ICU) environment is receiving increasing attention by caretakers and researchers. Environmental stresses such as lighting, noise level, kinesthetic factors, and tactile and visual stimuli can negatively affect the neonate's normal physiologic circadian rhythm (Updike et al, 1985). Five subsystems of the infant have been identified by Brazelton (1984) to include autonomic, motor, state, attentional-interactive, and self-regulation. In a full-term infant, these five subsystems are fairly well organized and contribute to the infant's adaptive behavior. The premature infant is less organized and signals a level of stress through greater disorganization of these subsystems. Stressful and nonstressful behavioral clues have been identified by Als (1982). Stressful behaviors include a wide range of withdrawal/avoidance cues, such as spitting up, gagging, hiccoughs, grimacing, yawning, eye aversion, finger splaying, and body arching. Nonstressful behaviors include approach/groping cues, such as tongue extension, sucking, hand-to-mouth movements, finger folding, hand clasping, infant sounds, and cooing. Once the infant's signals of stress can be identified, strategies can be instituted to reduce the stress.

The impact of illness of a neonate on the family is immense. The loss of "the perfect child" evokes feelings of disappointment and loss, and an overall sense of uncertainty. Infants may be sick at birth because of prematurity, perinatal complications, or congenital

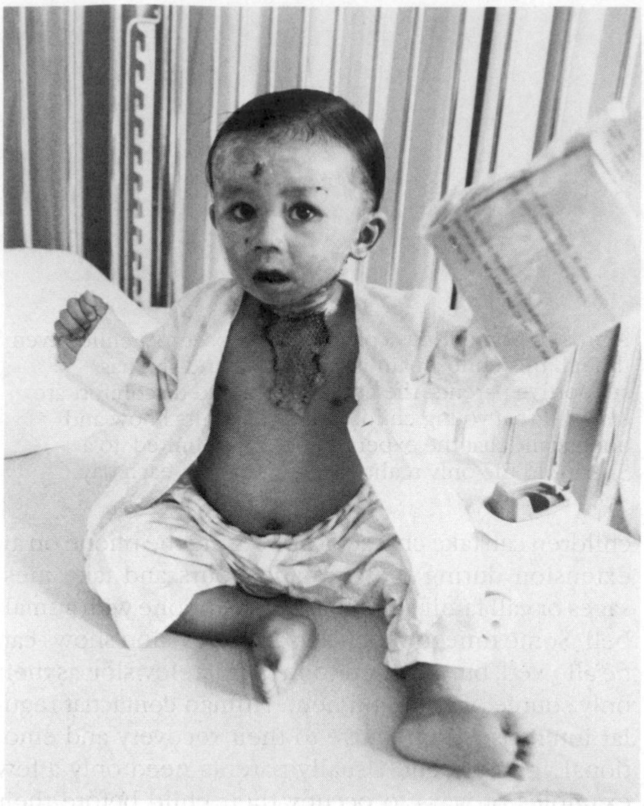

When serious illness occurs, uncertainty concerning the child's future is a stressor that places the family in a vulnerable position. This Vietnamese boy pulled the cord of a rice cooker and had serious facial and chest burns that required skin grafting. Although the final outcome is good, the family endured several weeks of uncertainty.

defects. Although there is a broad range of degree of illness, *any* illness at birth is a crisis. The seriousness of the child's condition is often unclear at birth and the outcome often is unpredictable. The uncertainty that these crises evoke places the family and professionals under extreme stress.

When the illness is a correctable anomaly, the outcome can often be more clearly stated, but it often introduces the additional stress of a surgical procedure. When prematurity compounds the situation, parents are particularly stressed because of the increased risk involved in treating premature infants.

The stresses introduced by a neonatal intensive care unit (NICU) also compound the stressful experience of parents. The intensity of care, the foreboding technical environment, and the uncertainty of prognosis leave parents distraught. The crisis of a sick newborn infant presents parents with three major issues to be resolved: (1) coping with loss, (2) overcoming barriers to bonding, and (3) getting information about the infant's current and future needs (Steele, 1987).

The more serious the infant's illness, the more

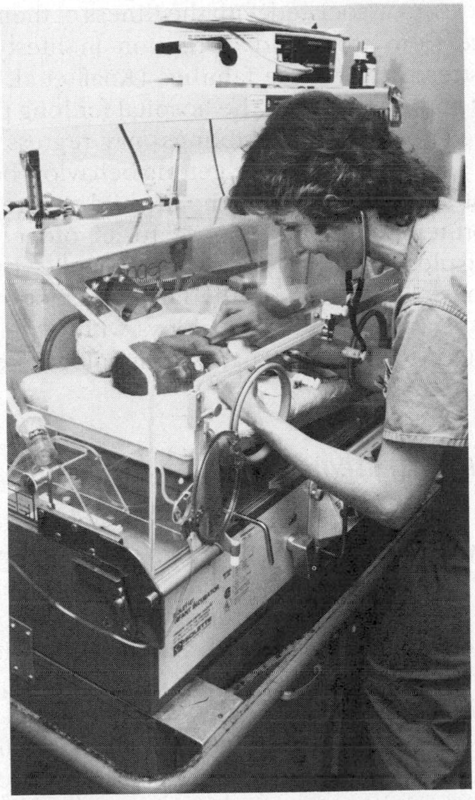

A premature infant placed into a stressful environment benefits from a nurse who uses gentle touch during procedures and attends to the infant's individual grimaces and movements.

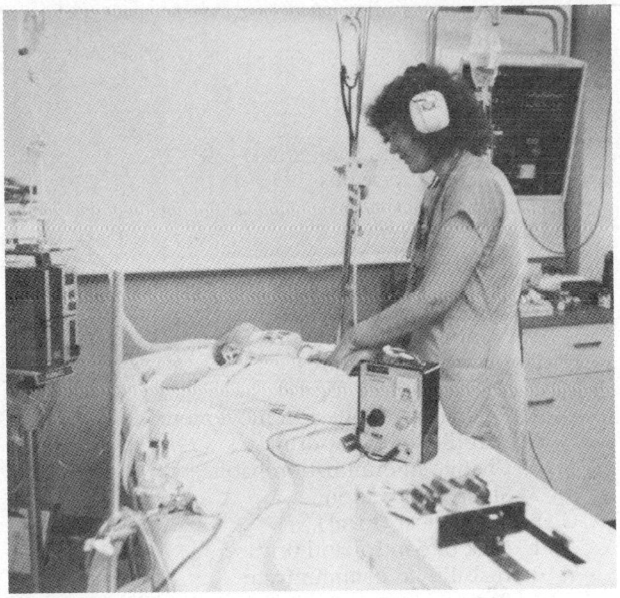

This infant is recuperating from cardiac surgery and requires close monitoring. The postoperative phase of major surgery is extremely stressful because of the threatening appearance of equipment and the uncertainty of the outcome.

likely it is that the parent-infant acquaintance is disrupted. The two-way interaction between infant and parents is how attitudes and feelings develop. When an infant is acutely ill, the caretaker may be discouraged from trying to engage the infant in exchanges of smiles, cooing, and eye contact. Instead, responses may be elicited by soothing and comforting actions such as rocking and stroking, with less active prodding for the infant's response. The sensations of discomfort and general lack of well-being can result in excessive periods of crying and a general disposition of irritability, both of which compromise the "getting acquainted" phases. (See further discussion of parents and the high-risk infant in Chapter 5.)

Although scientific investigation of the impact of being in an ICU has been done on adult patients, little attention other than anecdotal reporting has been given to the study of children's behavioral responses to confinement in a pediatric intensive care unit (PICU). Studies by Barnes (1974, 1975) are two of the most comprehensive studies available. In a study of 13 school-age children, a high sensitivity to the PICU environment was noted (especially regarding invasive procedures and treatments), and sleeplessness was reported as a problem. Other findings were that even though children were alert to hear doctors' conversations, they could not comprehend their meaning; it was also noted that the children demonstrated a high degree of concern for the welfare of other PICU patients, and sometimes misinterpreted events. In another study by Munn and Tichy (1987), 10 staff nurses were asked to identify factors in the PICU that they believed to be stressful to school-age children and adolescents. From the nurses' responses, stressors were categorized to be environmental, physical, psychologic, and social, encompassing 21 stressors (see Box 24-1). Lybarger (1979) examined children after discharge and found that children exhibited irritability and fearfulness, and needed extra sleep at home. These children had been in the PICU for 3 or 4 days.

These reports indicate that the PICU experiences have a negative effect on children, but further research is required to interpret the behaviors of critically ill children.

Behavioral reactions of parents to the ICU vary according to the circumstances of admission, severity of the child's illness, past experiences and coping styles of the parent, environmental stimuli, quality of communications, and emotional support systems (Etzler, 1984). Parents who experience an unexpected admission of their child to the ICU are reported to have significantly more anxiety than those parents who know their child is to be admitted (Eberly et al, 1985).

Reactions of parents are reported to include with-

Box 24-1
Categories of Stressors

A. Environmental (contextual)
   1. Doctors' activities
   2. Nurses' activities
   3. Other patients
   4. Equipment
   5. Design of the PICU (sights and sounds)
B. Physical (focal)
   1. Noninvasive procedures
   2. Invasive procedures
   3. Pain and discomfort
   4. Restraints on physical movement
   5. Inability to eat or drink
   6. Change in elimination habits
   7. Sleep deprivation
C. Psychological (focal)
   1. Lack of control and privacy
   2. Inability to communicate
   3. Parental behavior
   4. Lack of knowledge and understanding
   5. ICU admission and severity of illness
D. Social (Residual)
   1. Concerns with school
   2. Separation from peers
   3. Separation from family
   4. Play deprivation

(From Munn and Tichy, 1987.)

drawal, shock, helplessness, guilt, anger, and the inability to remember information that has been provided (Soupios et al, 1980; Rothstein, 1980). Active seeking of information and needing to feel hope have also been identified as characteristic of parents of critically ill children (Kirschbaum, 1983).

Stressors affecting parents have been extensively studied (Miles and Carter, 1982, 1983, 1985; Miles et al, 1985; Carter et al, 1985; Eberly et al, 1985). Seven areas of stress were identified by interviewing parents of children who had been recently discharged from a pediatric intensive care unit (Box 24-2). See Miles and Carter, 1983, for a discussion of their conceptual model. Their findings on parental stress and coping include:

1. Mothers are more stressed than fathers by the child's appearance and behavior and by the alteration required in the parental role.

2. Parents of children admitted unexpectedly are more stressed.

3. Parents of infants have more stress than parents of other age groups.

4. Uncertainty (an illness-related variable) contributed greatly to parental stress (Miles 1988).

In addition to the stress of the ICU, parents suffer other stresses associated with the illness of their child. Absence from work and disruption in lifestyle are major stressors for these families (Knafl et al, 1982). Parents may be staying at the hospital for long periods and become exhausted. Siblings may regress or engage in aggressive attention-getting behaviors because of the attention required by the ill child. A parent may be short-tempered in response to an older child's whining plea for attention, only to be rebuked by his or her spouse. The drain on the family's emotional resources is acute, and the usual joys within the family are muted by the stress that each member is experiencing.

Nursing Strategies

A variety of nursing strategies are routinely performed in many ICU settings, even though their effectiveness has not been examined. Parents are usually encouraged to touch or hold children as soon as possible and to participate in their care. Communication with parents is the intervention of importance most frequently cited in the literature (Etzler, 1984). Although physicians are noted to be the primary source of initial information, nurses build on initial explanations and assist parents to ask questions (Etzler, 1984).

An important intervention of the nurse is to assist the parents to enter the ICU to see their child. From this first moment of seeing the child, parents are thought to begin to feel a sense of role deprivation (Rennick, 1986). Because they are no longer responsible for the care of their child, they begin to sense a loss of control.

Nurses can help parents focus on the normal aspects of their child. Pointing out something normal about their child and helping them to overcome the initial shock of tubes and machinery attached to their child is an important initial strategy.

Development of a trusting relationship with the nurse is an important forerunner of a parent's ability to participate in caretaking activities. The nurse continually assesses the family for their readiness to participate in their child's care. Judgments are made about when parents are ready to proceed from simple to more complicated tasks. As parents make known their readiness to participate, the nurse shows them how they can help. As they become more involved in their child's care, they regain their sense of control and their parental role is re-established (Rennick, 1986). Aspects of the ICU experience that affect the parent-child relationship have been reported to be more stressful than the actual physical environment (Carter et al, 1985). Nursing strategies that focus on the parent-child relationship suggested by Carter and colleagues include "parental education, on-going emotional support, and enhancement of the parental role."

Box 24-2
Potential Stressors in Pediatric Intensive Care Units

Sights and sounds:
General physical environment such as:
- Steady beep and sudden alarms of monitor
- Sounds of the equipment
- Constant bright lights
- Sights of other sick children

Child's appearance:
- Tubes, restraints, and equipment
- Bruises, cuts, and incisions
- Covered eyes
- Puffiness, nakedness

Child's behavior:
- Confusion
- Rebellion
- Whining
- Demanding behavior
- Withdrawal
- Inactivity
- Uncooperativeness
- Unresponsiveness
- Pain behavior
- Loss of bowel and bladder control

Child's emotional responses:
Emotions of fear, anger, sadness, and depression
Procedures
- Suctioning
- Giving injections
- Starting and running intravenous fluids
- Drawing blood
- Oxygen administration
- Monitoring temperature and blood pressure
- Bandage changes
- Tube insertion
- Tube feedings
- Deep breathing and coughing
- Postural drainage
- Respiration therapy

Staff communications:
How the communication was done
- Explaining things too fast
- Using words not understood
- Inconsistent reports about the child's condition
- Having too many people talking to parents
- Telling parents the child's condition was the same day after day
- Talking too much about matters not related to child
- Giving too much information

Communication not done
- Not stating what was wrong with the child
- Not communicating how sick the child was
- Not telling parents about tests and treatments
- Not talking to them
- Not giving emotional support
- Not encouraging repeated questioning
- Staff not identifying themselves by name or role in care of child
- Sending parents out of the room suddenly without explanation

Staff behaviors:
- Rushing around
- Joking and laughing
- Acting as if they did not like child or did not understand child's needs or behaviors
- Looking worried about child
- Acting distant
- Acting as if they did not like having parents around
- Constantly disturbing child when resting

Parental role deprivation:
- Separation from child for long periods
- Not being able to care for and hold their child
- Not being able to see or visit the child at any time
- Not being able to minimize child's fears and protect child from pain
- Not being able to be with child while crying
- Being afraid to touch child
- Not knowing how to help child during the crisis

(Compiled from Miles and Carter, 1983.)

Impact on Siblings

Siblings of an ill child generally experience some guilt; they feel they had something to do with the sibling's becoming ill. During minor illness at home, a sibling may feel that the ill child is receiving unwarranted attention. It is beneficial if siblings can participate in the care of the ill child. Involvement in their sick sibling's illness not only helps reduce guilt, it also allows these children to have a better understanding of what their ill sibling is going through and why the sibling needs their parents' attention, thereby minimizing jealous feelings. Sibling involvement also allows the brothers and sisters to maintain a relationship and increases the helping siblings' self-esteem and the sick sibling's morale.

Siblings who have direct contact with a sick sibling in an intensive care unit should be prepared beforehand for what to expect (what they may see, hear, or do while visiting the child at the hospital) and for their sibling's physical appearance. The well sibling should then be encouraged to discuss feelings evoked by a visit to the ICU.

Parents should be cautioned by the nurse that well children express their feelings regarding the sibling's sickness and the family disruption in many nonverbal ways. Characteristic nonverbal expressions of their distress include: (1) somatic distress (sighing, weakness, fatigue, gastrointestinal complaints); (2) preoccupation with the image or memories of the sick sibling when he or she was well (especially if treatment must be conducted away from home); (3) self-blaming evidenced by irritability, impatience, social withdrawal, frequent crying; or (4) inability to maintain normal patterns of conduct and function (overactivity, restlessness, lack of initiative, regression, escalation of usual misbehaviors (Schoenberg et al, 1973).

The nurse's objective in meeting the needs of the sick child, the parents, and siblings, regardless of the duration of the illness or the setting for care, is to promote or regain family unity, or both, during the course of the child's illness. When each family member's needs are considered and met, more energy is available for each not only to adjust to the crisis but also to work together to help the sick child adapt to the stress of being ill. (See Chapter 31 for further discussion of the impact of illness on siblings.)

Maintenance of Family Relationships

The nurse can intervene by helping family members to maintain optimal relationships. Parents frequently need the nurse to help them recognize that their own resources are being exhausted and that they need the assistance of relatives, neighbors, or friends when a child is acutely ill.

The nurse should encourage parents to ease the stress for siblings by having one parent available to them most of the time. Help can be sought from support persons to prepare meals and do laundry and other household chores, but a parent should be available to provide such securities as reading to siblings at bed time and being there when they awaken. With some outside help, the couple's own relationship can also be maintained as some of the household duties are taken on by others.

References

Als H et al: *Manual for the Assessment of Preterm Infant's Behavior.* New York, Plenum Press, 1982.

Barnes C: School-age children's recall of the intensive care unit. *In ANA Clinical Sessions.* New York, Appleton-Century-Crofts, 1974, 73–91.

Barnes C: Levels of consciousness as indicated by responses of children to phenomena in the intensive care unit. *Matern Child Nurs J* 1975; 4:215–290.

Bellack J: Helping a child cope with the stress of injury. *Am J Nurs* 1974 Aug; 1491.

Brazelton TB: *The Neonatal Behavioral Assessment Scale.* 2nd ed. Philadelphia, JB Lippincott, 1984.

Carter MC, Miles MS: Parental stressor scale: pediatric intensive care. Unpublished manual available from the University of Kansas School of Nursing, Kansas City, Kansas, 1983.

Carter MC, et al: Parental environmental stress in pediatric intensive care units. *Dimen Crit Care Nurs* 1985 Jun; 4(3):180–188.

Eberly CW, et al: Parental stress after the unexpected admission of a child to the intensive care unit. *Crit Care Q* 1985 Jun; 8(1):57–65.

Etzler AC: Parents' reactions to pediatric critical care settings: a review of the literature. *Iss Compr Pediatr Nurs* 1984; 7:319–331.

Haskins R: Minor illness and social behavior of infants and caregivers. *J Appl Dev Psychol* 1981; 2:117–128.

Kirschbaum MS: *Needs of Parents of Critically Ill Children.* Unpublished thesis, University of Illinois, 1983.

Knafl KA, Deatrick JA, Kodadek S: How parents manage jobs and a child's hospitalization. *MCN* 1982; 7:125.

Lybarger P: The intensive care environment: Its effect on the child and parents. *Issues Compr Pediatr Nurs* 1979; 3(6):50–54.

Mattsson A, Weisberg I: Behavioral reactions to minor illness in preschool children. *Pediatrics* 1970 Oct; 46:604.

Miles MS: Personal communication, 1988.

Miles MS, Carter MC: Sources of parental stress in pediatric intensive care units. *Child Health Care* 1982; 11(1):65–69.

Miles MS, Carter MC: Assessing parental stress in intensive care units. *MCN* 1983; 8:354–358.

Miles MS, et al: Maternal and paternal reactions when a child is admitted to a pediatric ICU. *Issues Compr Pediatr Nurs* 1985; 7:333–342.

Munn VA, Tichy AM: Nurses' perceptions of stressors in pediatric intensive care. *J Pediatr Nurs* 1987; 2(6):405–411.

Parmalee AH: Children's illnesses: their beneficial effects on behavioral development. *Child Dev* 1986; 57:1–10.

Rennick J: Reestablishing the parental role in a pediatric intensive care unit. *J Pediatr Nurs* 1986; 1(1):40–44.

Schoenberg B, et al: *Loss and Grief: Psychological Management in Medical Practice.* New York, Columbia University Press, 1973.

Shulman J: *Coping with Tragedy: Successfully Facing the Problem of a Seriously Ill Child.* Fallet Publishing, 1976.

Soupios M, et al: Nursing aspects of pediatric intensive care in a general hospital. *Pediatr Clin North Am* 1980; 27:621.

Updike PA, et al: Physiologic circadian rhythmicity in preterm infants. *Nurs Res* 1985; 34(3):160–163.

Wu R: *Behavior and Illness.* Englewood Cliffs, NJ, Prentice-Hall, 1973.

Bibliography

Bernardo ML: A conceptual model of children's cognitive adaptation to physical disability. *J Adv Nurs* 1982 Nov; 7(6):595–601.

Bibace R, Walsh ME: Developmental concepts of illness. *Pediatrics* 1980 Dec; 66(6):912–917.

Brewster AB: Chronically ill hospitalized children's concepts of their illness. *Pediatrics* 1982 Mar; 69(3):355–362.

Fosarelli PD: The telephone in pediatric medicine. *Clin Pediatr* 1983 Apr; 22(4):293–296.

Harris J: Stressors and stress in critical care. *Crit Care Nurse* 1984; 4(1):84–97.

Hedenkamp EA: Humanizing the intensive care unit for children. *Crit Care Q* 1980; 3:63.

Lewandowski LA: Stresses and coping styles of parents of children undergoing open-heart surgery. *Crit Care Q* 1980; 3:75.

Mahan CK: Care of the family of the critically ill neonate. *Crit Care Q* 1981; 4:89.

Marten GW, Mauer AM: Interaction of health-care professionals with critically ill children and their parents. *Clin Pediatr* 1982 Sep; 21(9):540–544.

Mechanic D: Adolescent health and illness behavior: review of the literature and a new hypothesis for the study of stress. *J Hum Stress* 1983 Jun; 9(2):4–13.

Millstein SG, et al: Conceptions of illness in young adolescents. *Pediatrics* 1981 Dec; 68(6): 834–839.

Mishel MH: The measurements of uncertainty in illness. *Nurs Res* 1981 Sep/Oct; 30(5):258–263.

Pennebaker, JW: *The Psychology of Physical Symptoms.* New York, Springer-Verlag, 1982.

Perrin EC, Perrin JM: Clinicians' assessments of children's understanding of illness. *Am J Dis Child* 1983 Sep; 137(9):874–878.

Pidgeon VA: Children's concepts of illness: implications for health teaching. *Matern Child Nurs J* 1985 Spr; 14(1):23–35.

Redpath CC, Rogers CS: Healthy young children's concepts of hospitals, medical personnel, operations and illness. *J Pediatr Psychol* 1984 Mar; 9(1):29–40.

Ritchie JA, et al: Concerns of acutely ill, chronically ill, and healthy preschool children. *Res Nurs Health* 1984; 7:265–274.

Stevens K: Humanistic nursing care for critically ill children. *Nurs Clin North Am* 1981; 16:611–622.

Thayer, MB: Telephone management. *Pediatr Nurs* 1984 Mar/Apr; 10(2):121–122, 154.

Thornbury KM: Coping: implications for health practitioners. *Patient Counsel Health Educ* 1982; 4(1):3–9.

Steele KH: Caring for parents of critically ill neonates during hospitalization: strategies for health care professionals. *Matern Child Nurs J* 1987; 16(1):13–27.

Impact of Chronic Illness

Chapter 25

Bonnie Stevens

The knowledge that a child has a chronic illness may come suddenly, or it may be feared over a period of time with a gradual realization that a child requires special care. Even when the news comes suddenly, the impact of what the illness means to the child and family takes a lifetime to understand. Although remarkable advances in science and technology have made it possible to normalize the life of a child who has a chronic illness, the adjustment required by the child and the entire family is immense.

Some children adapt more easily than others, as do families. The challenge to health care professionals is to recognize the uniqueness of each child in his or her situation. Optimal adaptation can be promoted only by examining the *individual* child's personal and family strengths and vulnerabilities. This chapter examines the concept of chronic illness, with a description of the nurse's role in supporting the child and family in making a lifelong adaptation to chronic illness.

Nursing Process Plan
NPP: The Family in Need of Genetic Counseling, Table 50-3
NPP: The Child with an Identified Sensory Impairment, Table 51-10

Related Topics
Principles of genetic inheritance, Chapter 4
Children's concepts of health, Chapter 10
Children's concepts of illness, Chapter 23
Children's perceptions of death, Chapter 26
Supporting children during procedures, Chapter 27
Nursing management of the child in pain, Chapter 29
Nursing care of a child during hospitalization, Chapter 31
Home care, Chapter 32

The population of children and adults with a chronic illness is steadily increasing. Improved health care and scientific discovery have lengthened the life expectancy of children with severe and life-threatening illnesses. These scientific and technologic advancements combined with a social climate supportive of a life-oriented value system have resulted in larger numbers of individuals surviving with a chronic illness (Gruenberg, 1977; Blackburn, 1982; Ketterick, 1982; Burr et al, 1983; Hobbs et al, 1983). Although the main health burdens in developing countries are still related to acute illness, chronic illness is one of the leading health problems in the industrialized world.

Definition, Terminology, and Classification

Many definitions for chronic illness exist. An early definition evolved from the keynote address in 1956 of L. Mayo, who was then chairman of the influential National Commission on Chronic Illness. This definition of chronic illness is often still used today: "All impairments or deviations from normal which have one or more of the following characteristics: are permanent, leave residual disability, are caused by non-reversible pathological alteration, require special training of the individual for rehabilitation, and may be expected to require a long period of supervision, observation or care." Another definition of chronic illness by Mattsson (1972) is also popular: "A disorder with a protracted course which can be progressive and fatal, or associated with a relatively normal life span despite impaired physical or mental functioning."

Terms that are similar to chronic illness are often used interchangeably and include *long-term illness* and *chronic condition.* Thomas (1983) describes a chronic condition as any anatomic or physiologic impairment that interferes with the individual's ability to function fully in the environment. Chronic conditions often have stable periods that are characteristically interrupted by acute episodes requiring medical intervention. Chronic conditions are managed by individual and family efforts.

A child can be identified as being a "chronically ill child" or a "child with a chronic condition." As Thomas (1987) notes, if the child is labeled as a "chronically ill child," no aspect of the child is identified other than the illness. However, when the child is perceived as having a condition, it is easier to think of the total child with ordinary developmentally appropriate behaviors as opposed to focusing entirely on the "illness."

In addition to a variety of definitions, several terms are used to describe an illness or condition that is long-term and incurable and imposes limitations on the individual. Commonly used alternative labels in the literature include "impairment," "handicap," and "disability." Researchers who use this alternate terminology tend to focus on a particular aspect of chronic illness. For example, impairment generally refers to physiologic or anatomic abnormalities such as diabetes or asthma. Handicap describes the social consequences of the impairment resulting in an inability to attain satisfactory role fulfillment, especially the social response of others in the individual's environment. Disability has been widely defined and generally has some reference to functional limitations and the psychologic response resulting from the specific disease condition.

Although the use of some of these alternate terms is thought to be declining, they still continue to be used either consciously or unconsciously. Such labels have the potential to influence the response of the individual, family, health care provider, and society at large (Diamond and Jones, 1983). This often negative response to individuals who are not physically attractive, intact, and fully functional is also known as the process of "stigmatization" (Goffman, 1963). The individual who deviates from the social norm is devalued. The child and/or his family are in some ways held responsible or blamed for the child's differences.

Chronic illnesses can also be classified into various categories depending on their severity or visibility to others. Categories may include life-threatening illnesses (leukemia or brain tumors) or non-life-threatening illness (epilepsy, cerebral palsy) and/or illnesses visible to others (blindness, mental retardation) or invisible to others (diabetes, colitis). However, these categories are neither exhaustive nor mutually exclusive. A child with a brain tumor, for example, may have a life-threatening but invisible chronic illness. The categories of chronic illness have also been subject to change over time. The cancers were previously classified as terminal illnesses but due to medical technology and increased survival rates many childhood cancers are no longer considered life threatening.

Incidence and Prevalence

The incidence and prevalence of chronic illness in children are difficult, if not impossible, to calculate. Ireys (1981) estimated that 7.2 to 10.8 million or between 10 and 15 per cent of American children under the age of 18 have a chronic condition. This estimate is consistent with other studies which have calculated overall rates of 10 to 20 per cent (Rutter et al, 1970; Haggerty et al, 1975; Walker et al, 1981; Walker and Gortmaker, 1983). If the definition of chronic illness includes visual, hearing, and speech impairments; learning and behavior disorders; and mental retardation, estimates climb as high as 30 to 40 per cent (Mattsson, 1972). As well, according to data from the National Health Interview Survey (National Center for Health Statistics, 1981a) over 2 million American children under the age of 17 years are affected by a chronic condition that causes some limitation of activity. Respiratory diseases are the leading cause of all activity limitations in this group of children. Although the numbers of children who have an activity-limiting chronic illness are relatively small (3.8 per cent), they consume a disproportionate share of the total medical care used (Newacheck et al, 1986). In 1979, these children accounted for 9 per cent of all physician visits and 30 per cent of all inpatient visits reported for all noninstitutionalized children (National Center for Health Statistics, 1981b).

The wide variation of reported statistics for chronic illness in childhood is greatly dependent on the width of the definition, the methods used for data collection, and the source of the information. Although there has been little change in the incidence of chronic illness over the years, survival estimates of children with a variety of chronic diseases have shown considerable change over time. There has been an approximate sevenfold increase in the survival of children with cystic fibrosis (Dynesen and Flensborg, 1978) and increases in survival of two- to sevenfold for some congenital heart defects. Another group of children with chronic conditions has been created with socially sanctioned life-saving technology. Although exact numbers of these technologically dependent children are unavailable at present, this population will likely continue to increase with the widespread utilization of equipment such as respirators for long-term care. These changes in survival rate and technology have direct implications for increasing the population prevalence and the number of older children and adults surviving with a chronic illness.

Roles and Behaviors in Health/Illness

As providers of care to children with chronic illness and their families, nurses need to develop an understanding of the factors that influence an individual's responses to chronic illness. In an attempt to gain this understanding, the roles and behaviors in chronic illness are discussed including: (a) health and wellness behavior; (b) sick role; (c) illness behavior; and (d) at-risk role.

Health and Wellness Behavior

For children with chronic illness, it is especially important to view health care not as cure but as improvement of the quality of life and health promotion. Children with chronic illness are most likely unable to meet the "absence of illness" criteria of the conventional definitions of health but can achieve a level of optimal well-being. In reading about chronic illness, remember that children usually tend to define health in terms of an absence of illness.

Illness is more tangible than health for children especially in terms of its consequences. Healthy children can easily identify with sensations such as the pain of a scraped knee or a needle. Children with a chronic illness can, in addition, usually relate to painful procedures such as blood tests and lumbar punctures. Illness is more threatening to their well-being and often interrupts the activities (such as play and school) central to childhood. A hypoglycemic reaction or a seizure is an event which causes fear and disruption in children and those around them. Illness and its consequences make an impression because of their unusualness and uniqueness in a child's normally healthy world. Based on this thinking it may be reasonable to expect that children with a chronic illness may have a concept of illness but not necessarily of health.

Two major reasons may exist for children's poorly developed concept of health. First, children tend not to receive reinforcement for health behaviors (such as feeling good, energetic, or rested) whereas they do receive extra attention for illness symptoms (especially if the child is known to have a chronic illness). The child with chronic bowel disease who complains of stomach cramps will certainly receive more immediate attention than the healthy child who complains of the same symptoms. The child with Crohn disease may be rushed off to the doctor while the well child may receive little attention. The urgency of the attention may heighten the sense of being sick in this child while the lack of attention may decrease the healthy child's personal perception of being ill.

Second, children receive diffuse and often contradictory messages about health and illness from a variety of sources including the family, school, media, and peers. Children are taught either to engage in or refrain from certain behaviors to stay healthy. Most children view television commercials which promote alcohol and smoking. Yet, these same children are often taught by parents and teachers that smoking and drinking are detrimental to their health. As a result, there may be some sense of personal irresponsibility if the child experiences health problems due to the use of these products (Lewis and Lewis, 1974). Also, the child with a chronic respiratory illness such as asthma may feel a heightened sense of guilt if the illness is exacerbated by even minimal contact with products or environmental situations deemed to be detrimental to the child's health.

Children with chronic illness can function at their optimal level, which means the child is achieving wellness. Bruhn and Cordova (1977) define wellness in children as:

> "the development of behavior that increases the child's ability to actively seek changes in his or her life situation so that it is possible to function at his or her perceived capacity to achieve satisfaction."

Wellness behavior can be learned at either home or school, but the child's behavior will ultimately be influenced by the value placed on health and wellness by the parents. Parents who care for their own health needs (e.g., regular dental practices, sound nutritional practices and abstinence from smoking and consuming alcohol and drugs) stimulate children to develop the motivation to care for themselves.

Children also learn wellness behavior by increasing their knowledge, by being active participants, and by receiving reinforcement for practicing wellness behavior. For example, children suffering from chronic obesity during adolescence can increase their knowledge of nutrition and take over some of the responsibility for their own food preparation and intake. If these children can manage to adhere to their diets and receive positive reinforcement for their behavior from their parents and peers, the goal of practicing wellness behavior will have been achieved.

See Chapter 10 for further discussion of health and wellness and children's health attitudes and behaviors.

Sick Role

When a child is diagnosed with a chronic illness, subsequent behavioral changes are due in part to characteristics of illness, in part to the family and others' reactions to the illness, and in part to the maturity and coping ability of the child and family. A sequela which often accompanies the diagnosis of a child with a chronic illness is the "sick role."

In Parson's (1951) classic model of the sick role, an individual is (a) not responsible for the illness condition; (b) exempt from social role obligations; (c) obligated to get well; and (d) obligated to seek and accept professional care. Many health professionals and families with children with chronic illness function within this model. However, a basic problem with Parson's model is that it is reflective of acute and not chronic illness, in which time or length of illness is a contributing factor. In a child, exemption from normal social obligations or friends and schooling cannot be justified indefinitely. The child will need to eventually resume part or all of these responsibilities or suffer from peer isolation and poor grades if not doing so.

A second aspect of this sick role which may not fit children with chronic illness is the obligation of children or their parents to seek treatment. Parents almost always seek initial treatment for sick children. However, if the treatment involves painful procedures, unpleasant side effects from drugs, and impingement on currently acceptable lifestyle, parents balance the effectiveness of the medical help with the quality of life of the children in their decision whether or not to return for follow up visits.

Many similar considerations face parents in relation to being cooperative or compliant with the prescribed medical regimen. In chronic illness, parents or children are, in essence, the direct managers of day-to-day care. They often modify the treatment plan to fit their lifestyles and eliminate the symptoms most distressing to them rather than comply with a regimen that does not always make personal sense. If a diabetic child screams continuously when having a finger pricked for blood glucose tests, parents may abandon this component of the regimen in favor of much less distressing urine tests or no testing procedure at all.

In the case of childhood chronic illness, the care of the family and other nonprofessional supports is essential. Whole families, involving several individuals, may need to adapt to the demands of the child with chronic illness.

Fraser (1980) has expanded on Parson's (1951) model and views the sick role as one of a number of factors which handicap a child with a chronic condition. Fraser (1980) has categorized these factors into three distinct types including:

- handicapping factors A which are structural or functional deficits;
- handicapping factors B which are restrictions on the child's experiences resulting from the physical and social environment; and
- handicapping factors C that result from the attitudes toward the child's impairment in the social environment (including the social role of sickness, preconceived notions of abilities and expectation and overprotective behaviors).

Fraser (1980) considers that the sick role does free the individual from certain responsibilities and obligations. In children with chronic conditions, this may lead to exclusion from learning experiences since they may not be encouraged to develop skills and abilities normally demanded of healthy children. This exclusion also results in misunderstanding and exclusion by peers from play and social interactions. Lack of normal peer interaction, mitigated by the sick role, can compromise the child's emotional maturation and have a profound effect on personal and social development (Isaacs and McElroy, 1980; Bullard and Dohnal, 1984).

Illness Behavior

Illness behavior during chronic illness relates to the way individuals perceive, evaluate, and take action around the given symptoms of their diseases (Mechanic, 1962). In chronic illness, the goal may not be to eliminate certain symptoms but to successfully manage the existing symptoms in order to keep them from interfering with one's life's activities.

Illness behavior (or managing symptoms) depends on several factors including:

- the nature of the child's symptoms (i.e., severity, frequency);
- the meaning of the symptoms to the child and family;
- the age and level of development of the child;
- coping ability of the child and family;
- degree of interference with the child's normal activities;
- response from others; and
- nature of the child's illness (i.e., prognosis, imposed limitations).

For example, a teenage child with cystic fibrosis may suffer from repeated bouts of difficult breathing. If the child has adequate knowledge of how to manage the symptoms of these episodes and has coped well in the past, she or he is apt to manage the present situation well. A reasonable self-concept and acceptance of the illness by peers also promotes the adolescent's participation in activities and peer relationships. However, if the symptoms have been uncontrolled or required timely attention from parents and peers, a child may not cope well with ongoing symptoms. Poor coping with symptoms of a chronic condition often leads to restricted or curtailed activities and a lowered self-esteem.

At-Risk Role

Risk can be defined as the presence of potentially stressful factors in a person's environment (Anthony, 1974). Recent attention has been given to identifying factors that contribute to risk in the environment (such as noise, sanitation or pollution) and factors that protect or promote health. For the child with a chronic illness, a factor that promotes health may be the social support provided by parents, peers, or caretakers in the environment. Several authors have suggested that social support has both a direct and positive effect on the health status and physical and psychosocial level of stress in the individual (Cassel, 1976; Cobb, 1976; Kaplan et al, 1977). Based on this thinking, children who have the support of their parents and peers will benefit from attachment, social integration, feelings of worth, and opportunities for nurturance and guidance.

Vulnerability is a term that is often interchanged with risk. Although many definitions exist, there seems to be agreement that vulnerability relates to personal components and is characterized by both constitutional and acquired factors. Constitutional factors are characteristics that are inherited and are reflected in the neuroanatomy of the organism; acquired factors result from a variety of life events that enhance or inhibit subsequent disorders. Risk appears to be primarily associated with environmental factors such as pollution, bacteria, and viruses. Risk and vulnerability appear to affect one another in a dynamic way (Murphy and Moriarty, 1976; Rose and Killien, 1983).

By definition, children with a chronic illness have inherited and/or acquired characteristics which cause them to be vulnerable. Anthony (1974) describes the vulnerable child as one who is susceptible to a variety of forces in the environment. Families of children with chronic illnesses can also be considered psychologically vulnerable when affected by factors such as stigma.

When children have chronic illnesses, the major task is to maintain control of the symptoms in order to reduce risk and vulnerability. A control of symptoms may mean that a child is not presently ill but is at risk for an exacerbation of illness if a treatment plan is not followed. This at-risk role has only duties attached to it and no privileges as in the sick role.

In chronic illness, levels of risk or vulnerability are not static. To illustrate this point, consider the child born with a heart defect requiring surgical repair. At birth, the child was vulnerable due to the pathophysiology which caused physical distress. However, following the surgical repair this primary vulnerability may decrease or even disappear but secondary vulnerabilities such as emotional and social lags in development are created (Murphy and Moriarity, 1976). Secondary vulnerabilities often develop when concerned parents or health professionals create an overprotective and restrictive atmosphere rather than one that promotes the total development of the child.

Since chronic illness is often characterized by long periods of time, active management by the child and family, and the necessity to comply with an often cumbersome medical regimen, the "at-risk" role may be a more appropriate framework than is the sick role.

Health professionals need to understand these models and how to modify both risk and vulnerability factors in order to improve the state of health or to prevent deterioration in illness.

Impact of Chronic Illness on the Child and Family

Each chronic illness has its own symptoms, causes, treatments, and prognosis. However, many common features in chronic illness produce stress for children and their families. The family's central role in managing the child's illness throughout his or her lifetime is of major importance to the impact of the illness on the child.

Chronic illness can occur at all ages and stages of a child's development. The impact of the illness and the response to it will vary considerably depending on the stage of growth and development of both the child and the family. The various theories of physical, cognitive, and psychosocial development of the child are reviewed in Chapter 3. The child's perception of illness at various ages and cognitive stages is discussed in Chapter 23.

Impact of Chronic Illness on the Child

The child's response to chronic illness is often based on a number of factors which either separately or in combination are present throughout an illness. Some general characteristics of chronic illness which are of primary importance to the child include: (a) the nature of the illness; (b) separation caused by hospitalization; (c) sensory impairment, physical restriction, and social isolation; (d) dependency; (e) fear of treatments and procedures and the pain they may cause; (f) concern about death; and (g) the effect of the illness on the child's activities.

Chronic illness influences the child's physical, cognitive, social, and emotional development. The degree to which children perceive themselves as different from other children depends largely on the nature of the chronic illness (i.e., symptoms, treatment, and prognosis). For example, certain types of brain dysfunction may not limit physical functioning but may cause poor attention span, hyperactivity, and aggressive behavior thus limiting perception and learning in a normally intelligent child. Conversely, the child with spina bifida may have normal cognitive functioning but may be severely affected in mobility and self-concept due to physical limitations.

Chronic illness may cause children to experience separation from their parents due to frequent hospitalizations or the need to travel long distances for specialized treatments. Separation is particularly upsetting for children between the ages of 6 months and 4 years but may also cause problems for older children. Bowlby (1973) describes three stages of the child's reaction to separation including:

- protest—crying and resistant behavior and frequent demands for parents;
- despair—withdrawal, lack of interest in the surroundings, and loss of hope for the parents' return; and
- detachment—regaining appetite and activities but avoidance of attachment to any particular individual and avoidance of the parents when they visit.

A more in-depth discussion of the effects of separation due to hospitalization can be found in Chapter 31.

Research which has examined the effects of hospitalization indicates that children can experience temporary anxiety and distress both during and following hospitalization. Whether these effects are long term or not is unclear. The vulnerability of the child to separation effects depends largely on age, the number of previous hospitalizations, and, more importantly, the quality of previous hospital experiences. In chronic illness, less tangible factors such as the child's coping abilities and the parents' perception of the experience are also important.

Some illnesses require that the child be isolated from familiar people and environments. This isolation can also occur if the child's mobility is severely limited such as a child in traction. In addition, certain illnesses can impose sensory deficits such as blindness, deafness, or the loss of tactile perception (e.g., the burned child). All of these limitations may interfere with normal growth and development and the child's ability to cope with the illness. Toddlers need to be mobile in order to explore their environment and develop cognitive skills, while school-age children need to interact with peers to gain a sense of industry and pride in their endeavors. Children who cannot experience these freedoms often withdraw into an imaginary world riddled with fears and unrealistic expectations in regard to their illness.

Many children with chronic illnesses choose to remain dependent on their parents because it is less difficult than striving to be independent. Parents, who often feel responsible or guilty about their child's illness, unconsciously gratify these dependency behaviors in order to make the child feel more comfortable and secure. The child's dependency may also serve to make parents feel more needed and involved in the child's care. However, such actions, which unintentionally extend beyond the actual needs of the child, may hinder independence and promote poor levels of self-confidence. Nurses need to encourage parents to allow dependence during acute exacerbations of illness and then gradually revert to more independence for the child whenever possible.

Children with chronic illnesses are often fearful of procedures and treatments and of the pain that goes along with them. A child's pain may be dependent on the actual tissue damage, level of cognitive and emotional development, past pain experiences, and relationship with parents. Pain is also a subjective, abstract concept which is easily interwoven with other feeling states such as anxiety, fear, and loneliness. Therefore, the child who complains of pain may actually be experiencing distress due to anxiety or fear. These feelings are often the result of separation anxiety in the younger child, fears of mutilation in the school-age child, and loss of self-esteem and body image in the adolescent. A more detailed discussion of pain in both chronic and acute illness is found in Chapter 29.

Although scientific and technologic advances have substantially improved survival rates in several chronic illnesses, many children develop concerns about death. These concerns may be influenced by personal perceptions and those of significant others regarding the nature of the particular illness. Until recently, most childhood cancer was regarded by many as a fatal illness. Adolescents with cancer who experience extended periods of stress associated with treatment and the threat of recurrence are especially vulnerable to developing fears of death. As well, children who spend considerable amounts of time in the hospital may be exposed to other children who die. Fears of death are related to the child's cognitive and emotional development. Younger children most often view death as a sleeping period or temporary separation from their parents. After the age of 9 or 10, and as the capacity for abstract thought develops, children begin to understand the universality and permanence of death and the fragility of their own mortality. Parents and caretakers dealing with these feelings will need to be sensitive to their own fears in order to effectively reduce the child's level of anxiety. A further discussion of the child's perception of death is addressed in Chapter 26.

Another important factor that determines the impact that chronic illness has on the child is the extent to which the illness interferes with normal activities and developmental tasks. The degree of interference is largely dependent on the child's stage of growth and development at diagnosis and the ability of the family to adjust to the child's chronic condition. Since the child's activities are such an integral component of family functioning, a discussion of the effect that chronic illness imposes on normal activities and developmental tasks will be combined with the following section on the impact of chronic illness on the family.

Impact of Chronic Illness on the Family

Many authors have described the stresses imposed on the child and family when a child is diagnosed with a chronic illness (Mattson, 1972; Featherstone, 1980; Gliedman and Roth, 1980; Lavigne and Burns, 1981; McCollum, 1981; Figley and McCubbin, 1983). Understanding the impact of a child's chronic illness on the family is a difficult task. To accurately assess the effect that a child's illness has on the family system, we need to know how the family functioned prior to the diagnosis as well as after. However, we rarely have access to this valuable retrospective information.

The impact of chronic illness can affect many spheres of family life including financial, social, emotional, behavioral, and cognitive. Although specific chronic conditions vary in the stresses they impose, any chronic illness brings increased tasks, time commitments, and financial burdens to the family. Often, the child's illness strains the family's financial resources through hospitalization, treatment, and medication costs. Few insurance plans cover *all* health care services in the hospital and even fewer cover home care expenses for long-term chronic conditions. Families who live outside of metropolitan areas may spend a sizeable sum on transportation to and from health care centers. Some families even find it necessary to move to be closer to a facility that provides the necessary specialized care. It is possible that at least one parent may have to give up working or reduce his or her time in the work force, which may result in substantially less income.

A child's chronic condition may reduce the potential for healthy socialization of the child as well as the family. Children with chronic illnesses may cause fear, anxiety, confusion, and embarrassment in the social environment. These responses of society may cause more distress to the child and family than the chronic condition itself (Gliedman and Roth, 1980). Difficulty in finding caretakers for the child or problems in transporting a disabled child may lead to social isolation. Other parents and children often do not know how to interact with children with a chronic illness; they may be embarrassed or uncomfortable. The ill child and the family often feel rejected and devalued.

Social support can act as a mediator for families under such stress. Support from peers and family as well as the health care system can often decrease feelings of social isolation. However, parents still struggle in the areas of child care guidance and problem solving around the child's special needs. Extended family members provide the most consistent support (Featherstone, 1980) as the strain of chronicity tends to "burn out" nonfamily networks (Neill, 1979; Featherstone, 1980).

Emotionally, the family is faced with stresses due to the child's physical vulnerability, personal grief reactions, and feelings of guilt and blame. The grieving process is continual and is often reactivated with each new development in the child's condition (Sargent and Liebman, 1985). If mastery over grief reactions does not occur, disagreements between family members may lead to subsequent difficulties as the course of the child's illness progresses. The child may suffer from altered self-esteem and self-concept. These changes require skilled management on the part of family members and health professionals in order to ensure that children can accept their differences as well as their similarities when compared to other children. The family must continually strive to strike a balance between normal functioning and sensitivity toward their child's special needs.

Cognitively, the family needs to understand the nature of the illness, the treatment procedures, predictable and unpredictable complications, and the expected course of events. They need to be aware of the rationale behind the various aspects of treatment. They must also have an understanding of the impact the illness and its consequences have on the social and emotional well-being of the child.

The family also faces the challenge of adapting behavior patterns and activities to accommodate treatment regimens into their daily lives. The family and child's developmental needs, the age of the parents, the time the family has been established as a unit, and the family's previous coping abilities are all factors which influence the family's reaction to the illness and their ability to maintain normal functioning. The child's growth and developmental stage is a crucial factor in determining the impact of the illness on the family's behavioral, cognitive, and emotional well-being and developmental tasks. Therefore, the impact of the child's chronic condition on the child and family will be discussed according to age.

Infant

The main developmental task for the infant is to develop a sense of basic trust in self (Erikson, 1964) and the caring adults in the environment. A long-term illness or congenital defect may affect the relationship between parents and infant and impair the development of trust.

Specific limitations of the chronic illness may limit the infant's normal growth and development. The physically disabled infant's mobility is often restricted; he or she is unable to explore the environment through touching, manipulating, and mouthing objects. Lags in physical and cognitive development may result. Infants also need to experience events for themselves in order to begin to develop a frame of reference. Very young children, although able to feel pain, do not understand their discomfort because they have no other experiences to compare it to. They have no prior expectations and do not comprehend that the often painful procedures, anxious parents, or physical restrictions relate to or result from their chronic illness.

To a great extent, the most critical factor that determines how infants experience and adapt to their chronic illnesses depends on the degree to which their parents accept the condition. All pregnant couples dream of the ideal, perfect, healthy baby. When a baby is born or diagnosed with a chronic illness, the parents feel a great sense of loss and sorrow and grieve for the healthy baby that they feel they had the right to expect. To the parents, a child is an extension of themselves and, therefore, producing an unhealthy or defective child leads to a loss of self-esteem and positive self-concept.

Chronic illness during infancy can potentially disrupt the parents' attachment behaviors with the infant and the smooth transition into parenthood and family life. Parents take pride in the growth and development of their babies. However, if the child is irritable or listless and does not grow at the expected rate, parents may feel less adequate in their parenting role and less gratified for their efforts. Also, the contented infant who can be held, fed, and fondled is much more socially responsive and provides tremendous reinforcement for the family. Infants who are socially less responsive due to the constraints of their illnesses or physical deformities (such as a cleft lip or hydrocephalus) provide less social gratification.

The parents of an infant with long-term illness experience the grieving process but also have to contend with the day-to-day reality of their child's chronic condition. Such "chronic sorrow" (Olshansky, 1962) imposes stress on family functioning long after the diagnostic crisis is resolved. The family may feel that there is no escape from this situation, and it will be a lifelong stress. If the prognosis does not include a normal life span, the parents may feel even more intense sorrow, alienation, and powerlessness. The resulting disequilibrium may cause distortions in family relationships that ultimately necessitate a permanent alteration in family roles and goals. However, many families do resolve these initial grief feelings and are able to both meet the needs of their ill or handicapped infants and receive satisfaction from them.

Toddlers

The toddler's developmental task is to acquire a sense of autonomy and self-control. Erikson (1964) describes the child from 18 months to 3 years as striving to conquer the maturational crisis of autonomy. Healthy children of this age rapidly develop motor and communication skills which allow them to explore their environment more fully and tell the world about it. If children do not accomplish this task, they may feel shame and doubt because they feel they are not in control of either themselves or their world. Toddlers develop confidence in their abilities and a sense of social competence. Toddlers want to do "everything" for themselves and take great pride in controlling and manipulating their world. Thinking in imaginative and magical ways allows toddlers to be egocentric and omnipotent enough to believe that they can make things happen. They do not understand causality through logic but rather through magic.

When long-term illness is either present or diagnosed at this stage, there is potential for a major upset in this struggle for autonomy. Cognitively, if children are restricted in their activities and movements, they will have difficulty developing a sense of self and seeing themselves as separate and intact human beings. Immobilization may also seem intolerable and very frustrating to toddlers who desire to be on the move. Frequently, toddlers with a chronic condition develop increased dependency, difficulty with separation during hospitalizations, an uncertain self-image, and poor impulse control. Some studies (Sibinga and Friedman, 1971; Dowd et al, 1977) even suggest that there is potential for delay in physical, psychosocial, and language skills as a result of physical restraint during these early formative years.

As children progress beyond the dependent stage of infancy, parents need to begin to relinquish some of the supervision and total care that they assumed when the child was younger. When children have a chronic illness and may be suffering from repeated episodes of pain, immobility, loss of control, and separation, releasing parental control may be difficult. Children who are not allowed to make some choices in their lives or have some control over them may become apathetic, passive, and clinging. These behaviors tend to induce overprotectiveness and restrictiveness from the parents. Such compensating behaviors may affect the child's abilities to master autonomy and become more independent. If toddlers have decreased energy for activity, the caretakers are faced with the challenge of assisting their children to reach their maximum potential without compromising their physical health.

Parents are also confronted with attempting to deal with the ill child's behavior which may lead to conflict around discipline. In the case of toddlers, the opportunity to control their activities and lives may be sharply diminished when they are diagnosed with a chronic illness. Therefore, those situations that a toddler can control take on new and exaggerated importance. Control of feeding and elimination may, for example, be characteristic of assertiveness. Refusing to eat, playing with food, or throwing food and eating utensils in the kitchen may be behaviors typical of the toddler's negativistic nature. As well, young children may choose to control or not control their elimination or smear their stool all over their environment. Their choice to behave in certain ways is strongly influenced by the parents' response to the illness as well as by the child's natural desire to please them. In these situations, parents may also be reluctant to set appropriate limits or take disciplinary action for fear they might interfere with the child's normal development of impulse control.

During toddlerhood, children normally experience great anxiety when separated from parents even for a short period of time. With the potential for multiple hospitalizations or medical procedures in chronic illness, children are particularly vulnerable to separation anxiety. They need their family to protect them from fears of the unknown; they are often unable to cope without them. Parents will also feel guilty and see themselves, rather than the situation, as being directly responsible for this behavior.

A toddler diagnosed with chronic illness can have tremendous effects on family relationships. The family is often young, and the parents are striving to develop a marital relationship and financial stability. The diagnosis of an ill child can either cement relationships or sever them completely. In addition, an ill child will make increased demands on the parents' personal energy and finances. The parents may find it difficult to separate themselves for even brief amounts of time from the clinging and often emotional child and feel guilty when they do so. However, occasional or regular time-outs for the parents may be their only means of coping with this difficult situation.

Preschoolers

Children from 4 to 6 years old are increasingly active, are intent on mastering new skills, and have a need to be productive. Preschoolers win approval by mastering new tasks and taking responsibility for themselves, other things, and other people in their world. They need to attain desired goals and receive approval for this attainment, particularly from their parents and peers. Children who complete this stage successfully develop a sense of purpose, competence, and self-confidence in their own abilities. Unsuccessful completion of developmental tasks may result in a sense of defeat, guilt, and reluctance to attempt the accomplishment of new goals.

Cognitively, the preschooler is in Piaget's (1969) preoperational stage which is characterized by illogical and egocentric thought and the inability to generalize from isolated concrete experiences. Preschoolers are beginning to develop an awareness of the course of events, but they fail to understand the multiple complexities of causal relationships. Children of this age often describe phenomena by overt perceptual characteristics.

The diagnosis of chronic illness may limit the child's ability to achieve motor and social competence. Physical limitations may subdue his energy and enthusiasm for pursuing goal-directed efforts. Parents often limit their ill children in order to protect them. Because these preschoolers often cannot accomplish their desired goals and, therefore, receive less social approval, they may become fearful, irritable, demanding, and excessively dependent on adults.

Most preschool children can function within the limitations imposed by their disability if they can find a different route to accomplish tasks of development according to their capacity. Also, children at this stage may require assistance in identifying and accepting their limitations. The attitudes of others, especially their parents, determine how preschoolers perceive themselves and their potentials. They are particularly inquisitive about their illnesses including the inherent restrictions, procedures, and treatments. However, developmentally, preschoolers will probably interpret their illnesses as punishments for their actions or thoughts. Children in this age group need positive family and social interaction to help them obtain a realistic picture of their assets and limitations.

The reaction of the family to the chronic illness of the preschooler depends on whether the child has been diagnosed with chronic illness during the preschool years. If the child has been healthy up until age 4 to 6 years, the family has experienced the child as normal. When these parents learn of their child's diagnosis, they experience an acute sense of loss because they must alter expectations and hopes for the child's potential.

Normally, during the preschool years, children develop self-care skills that give them independence and give the parents freedom to pursue their own personal and career activities. However, preschoolers with a chronic illness may not master these self-care skills and their parents may be restricted in the pursuit of their own interests and personal and career goals. Handicapped children often make ongoing demands on the parents' time and may cause the parents to feel guilty and resentful. To compensate for these feelings, parent may reject or misplace the burden of the child's care on siblings or significant others.

The chronically ill preschooler may require early remedial education which, coupled with dependency demands, presents a separation conflict for the parents. This conflict fosters the parents' anxiety that the child cannot function without them. Overprotective parents who have not provided their preschooler with opportunities to develop self-sufficiency within the limitations of the handicap have an even greater problem separating from the child.

School-Age Child

From 6 to 12 years of age most children shift their focus to the school environment and peers. Children strive to become more independent from their parents and family and begin to desire more conformity and social approval from their peers. School-age children need to become proficient in accomplishing tasks, or in acquiring a sense of industry (Erikson, 1964). If they are unable to perform tasks or meet their own personal demands and those of peers, they begin to feel inferior rather than competent and adequate.

Cognitively, school-age children are no longer guided by superficial perceptions since they are able to generalize rules and principles from one experience to another. In fact, at this age children are often rule-bound; these new rules add stability to previously unstable concepts such as time and causality. However, since the child is still thinking in a very concrete manner, the rules are viewed in very inflexible and absolute terms.

The presence of chronic illness in this age group may interfere with the transition from parental to peer approval. The child's differences may become more visible to both the child and his peers. For example, the child with diabetes may be seen as always eating differently, and the child with juvenile arthritis may be characterized by his inability to participate in activities. Any child with a chronic illness may need to be absent from school for doctor's appointments or frequent hospitalizations. These differences may become the primary identification of the child, an observation that is immediately made by peers. Often differences in chronically ill children stimulate feelings of fear or discomfort in other children, and they react by avoiding or ostracizing the ill child. Children frequently deal with the pain of being different by developing feelings that their bodies are separate and unintegrated parts of their psychologic selves (Geist, 1979; Rodgers et al, 1981). This thinking is reinforced by health care professionals who refer to children as disease entities rather than "real" people.

The time at which a child enters school often brings renewed or additional sadness to the parents of the chronically ill child. At this time, parents too are made acutely aware of the physical and functional differences between their child and other children. The greater the perceived differences by the parent, the greater the parental sorrow is likely to be. Parents often attempt to minimize their child's differences by encouraging them not to tell peers and teachers of their illness, medications, or treatment. This approach, however, rarely is successful as the child feels overwhelmed with an extra burden of secrecy as well as all the other stresses that are being juggled. It is helpful if the parents can recognize the child's desperate need for peer acceptance and attempt to structure positive, socially reinforcing experiences. As well, since school-age children are more capable of understanding the nature of their illness, it is important for parents to answer all their questions in order for them to feel knowledgable in the eyes of their peers.

Parents of the chronically ill school-age child may also need to make decisions with regard to the type of school experience or setting that would be appropriate at this time. The child with a chronic handicap such as blindness or deafness may prosper better in a setting designed to deal with these specific handicaps. Also, an autistic child or a child with mental retardation may find less stress in a program geared to those special education needs rather than the regular school streams. These decisions may impose additional stress on the child and family as well as the need to absorb the extra costs and energy any special schooling or ancillary services may create.

The most difficult problem for families at this time, however, is relinquishing at least part of their child's care either to the child or to another responsible adult. Children need to become more responsible for themselves and to develop self-care skills in order to begin to feel a sense of control and self-esteem in the parents' absence. For children to become involved in school and its associated activities, the parents need to entrust part of the child's care to teachers, other parents, or caregivers. This "letting go" process may be more difficult for some families than others, so some

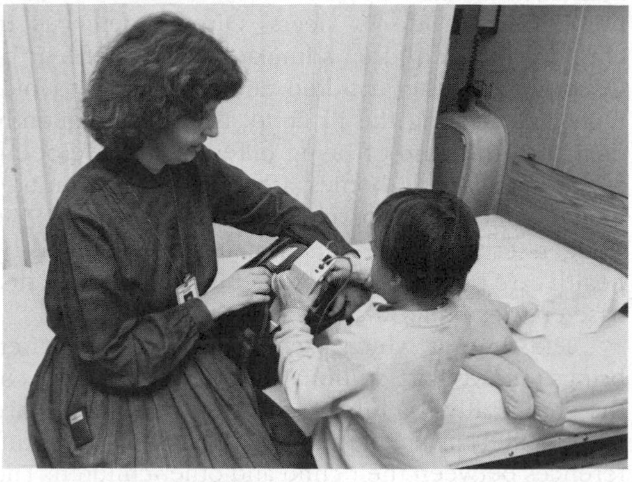

Nurses can foster independence in school-age children by letting them be responsible for their own care as they are able. Here a 10-year-old child is packing up her dialysis equipment on discharge from the hospital, as she does daily when she gets ready for school.

may benefit from the support of families who have experienced similar adjustments. Additional support from parent groups and health team members may be particularly helpful during this time of potential crisis.

Adolescent

The developmental period between 13 and 18 years of age is characterized by ambivalence, upheaval, and reevaluation. Adolescents are in a transition phase from a state of dependence (child) to independence (adult). They are also in the process of taking on a multitude of new social and emotional roles as well as coping with altered bodily functions. At this age, children are struggling for independence; in loosening the ties with the family, adolescents are constantly searching for peer approval. They want to "conform to the norm." Thus, the development of a satisfactory body image and a sense of self-esteem is crucial.

Cognitively, the adolescent phase of development coincides with Piaget's (1969) stage of formal operations when thinking becomes less concrete and more abstract. Questioning theories, generating hypotheses, and developing an awareness of values and beliefs are all part of this new intellectual mode. When adolescents have a chronic illness, all of their developmental struggles are intensified. Their illness often makes them feel dependent and lacking in autonomy at a time when they are trying to achieve independence. They are faced with a drastic blow to their self-concept and self-esteem at a time when they are trying to stabilize their identity. Adolescence is also a time when many children and their families are forced to face the limitations that a lifelong illness or handicap will place on vocational, educational, and social and sexual opportunities.

Adolescents with chronic illness stand out as different, and different, in their minds, may mean imperfect. All of these physical, psychological, and intellectual changes create a continuous atmosphere of tension and change to which they need to adapt. It is not unusual at this time for adolescents to respond to these stresses by becoming actively rebellious, noncompliant, and even guilty of sabotaging their medical regimens. At the same time, they may also become passive, overdependent, and depressed.

Adolescents with chronic illnesses are constantly struggling with independence. At the same time, their illnesses often keep them tied—physically, emotionally, and financially—to their families. The ability to successfully cope with these internal and external pressures is critically influenced by the parents' support and encouragement and by the reactions and understanding of peers.

Families need to allow the adolescent the freedom and responsibility of learning to manage the illness or handicap. Although this process may be painful for the parents to watch, it is a vital transition period and one which the adolescent must experience in order to maintain self-esteem and confidence. Young people need frequent encouragement that they are doing well at managing the illness and handling normal developmental crises. They will want to be treated as adults and have the freedom to make their own decisions as much as possible.

Many parents tend to encourage dependency in some situations and assume more of the adolescent's care than necessary in order to maintain their individual and family integrity. However, this kind of "smothering" may lead adolescents to fear independence, thinking that they may be unable to survive by themselves. Parents need to be encouraged to allow the adolescent physical and emotional freedom even if the result is temporary floundering. In most cases, both the adolescent and the illness will regain a state of equilibrium once the adjustments to independence, responsibility, and self-care have occurred.

Impact of Chronic Illness on Roles and Relationships

Chronic illness in a child has an impact on each individual family member and the total fabric of family life. Childhood chronic illness has been shown to increase stress, disrupt relationships, and interfere with family developmental tasks. As well, chronic illness in one member may be an underlying cause of a variety of symptoms in other family members. Chronic illness may disrupt communication patterns, impose financial hardships, and bring about changes in housing, careers, and sleep and recreation patterns. Disruptions in roles, resentment among siblings, and feelings of parental guilt, anxiety, helplessness, and despair can all be manifestations of the presence of a child with chronic illness in a family.

The effects on maternal and paternal roles, the parents' marital relationship, and the extended family are discussed individually.

Maternal Role

Most research on the effect that chronic illness has on families has focused on the mother and the relationship she has established with her child. Reasons for this maternal focus could include the fact that mothers are often most involved with the day-to-day care and responsibility for taking their child to the physician's office, clinic, or hospital setting. Thus, they are most visible to health care professionals as the primary caretaker and most available to participate in research studies. Generally, the literature reports wide variations in mothers' responses to their children's illness.

Mothers may feel particularly responsible since they actually give birth to the child and tend to be most influential in their child's care. Mothers experience all stages of grieving—shock, disbelief, anger, resentment, and sadness—and often become stalled at a particular stage or engage in self-blame. Mothers must be given the opportunity to mourn for the "wished-for perfect child" and accept the child which they now have. Thoughts and feelings experienced in relation to the chronically ill child may inappropriately spill over into relationships with other people establishing cause for concern. Most mothers are plagued with thoughts about what they did wrong and what they didn't do to prevent the illness.

Many researchers have described an increased prevalence of depression in mothers of chronically ill children (Walker et al, 1971; Allan et al, 1974; McCrae et al, 1973). Mercer (1974) investigated mothers' responses to infants with physical impairments for a 3-month period following the birth of the child. Findings in this study indicated that evaluation of social behaviors (particularly the mothers' evaluation of how others responded to their children) was the most frequent of all behaviors engaged in by the mothers. In a later study (1977), Mercer determined that visible impairments, particularly facial, were less socially acceptable and had the greatest influence on the parents' reactions to their children. Variation in maternal responses may be attributed to the mother's own family history, her past coping experience, her future hopes for her child, her current family and marital situation, and the presence of social support systems.

Paternal Role

There is considerably less information about the impact of chronic illness on fathers, largely because they have not been observed or studied as much as mothers. In North American society, family life is often perceived as mother centered, with fathers being involved only peripherally. This perception is often accompanied by the belief that fathers are less involved with or emotionally affected by their child's chronic illness.

These ideas have been challenged in the literature, and the importance of the father-child relationship has been explored (McKeever, 1981; Sabbeth, 1984). Some reports are that fathers did not consider themselves as secondary to mothers in the family functioning but rather as having equal responsibility for childrearing and the daily care of their ill children. Other studies suggest that differences appear to exist between fathers of children with various illnesses in

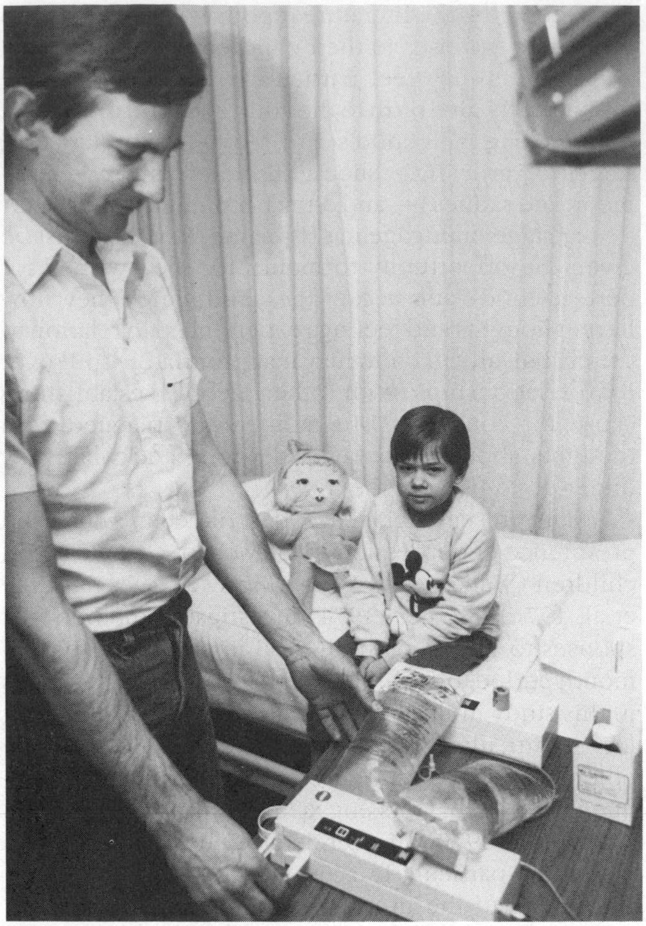

Many fathers share responsibility for their child's care. Although this 10-year-old can perform her own peritoneal dialysis, it is important for parents also to learn the procedure.

relation to the time and extent fathers participated in their child's care. For example, in one study by Barsch (1968), 89 per cent of fathers of children with Down syndrome—as compared with 38 per cent of fathers of children with organic brain disease—participated on a regular, high-quality basis in child care tasks. Many fathers share equal responsibility for their child's care with their wives while others find ways to absent themselves from the situation. An example of this absenting behavior which may be pathologic would be when the father buries himself in his work and thus spends long hours away from home and the family. Regardless of the time that fathers actually participate in their child's care, most researchers agree that a father's life is profoundly affected by his child's long-term illness (Burton, 1975).

A study by Sabbeth (1984) indicated that fathers were, for the most part, psychologically very involved with their ill children. A decrease in their own participation in child care as well as the lack of potentially helpful medical interventions available to their children left fathers feeling helpless and particularly undone by their lack of control over their child's illness. McKeever (1981) found that fathers experienced acute grief reactions at the time of diagnosis of their child's illness. However, in spite of their own feelings, they felt the need to demonstrate strength in order to support their wives during this time of crisis. Fathers also reported that their career mobility and social activities outside the family were curtailed due to the necessity of first considering the needs of the ill child and then the rest of the family. Although fathers of chronically ill children may experience these reactions and adjustments in their lives, due to frequently working conventional hours and longer absences from the home, they receive less information or support than mothers from health professionals.

Marital Relationship

Several reports in the literature suggest that a child's chronic illness has a strong and often negative impact on the marital relationship (Hughes, 1976; Bruhn, 1977; Magrab and Calcagno, 1978; Friedrich and Friedrich, 1981). However, the research to support such findings is often plagued by (a) missing or inadequate control groups; (b) lack of long-term follow-up through the course of the child's illness; (c) little consideration for differences among chronic illnesses; (d) inconsistency in methods of assessment between studies; and (e) use of instruments with unknown reliability and validity (Sabbeth and Leventhal, 1984).

Some may assume that a negative impact on parents may lead to higher divorce rates in this group. However, several sources (Burton, 1975; Darling, 1979; Friedrich and Friedrich, 1981; Sabbeth and Leventhal, 1984) have consistently suggested that divorce in families with a chronically ill child did not appear to be more frequent than in nonaffected families.

Burton (1975) found that the underlying stress and apprehension related to the child's chronic illness put severe strains on the marriage partners, allowing them less time and energy to spend together in adult activities. Parents often report feeling guilty and somehow responsible for causing the child's illness. Some decide not to have additional children. This decision is often based on either evidence of genetic transmission of the disease or the additional strain that another child would impose on a family that is already struggling to survive.

Other couples report that the stress resulting from the child's condition led to increased communication and feelings of closeness (Hewett et al, 1970; Burton, 1975; Howard, 1978; Darling, 1979). These parents also felt that they had grown in their roles and relationship and had become better people as a result of the related stresses. These findings dispell the myth that chronic illness in a child leads to the breakup of families. The outcome, rather, is determined by a combination of factors within a family.

A potential source of strain on the marital relationship is parents' coping style. Spouses often have different coping styles that tend to conflict. One partner may cope best by experiencing closeness and sharing emotions while the other partner may cope best by staying aloof and working through the stress internally. These differences are often the basis for yet another source of marital stress.

The child's illness may also cause a need for long-term changes in role expectations of one or both spouses. These changes may cause resentment or nonacceptance on the part of one or both of the marital partners. Extra care of the ill child, disruption of home routines, and extra financial burdens may all lead to increased stress and communication breakdown at a time when strengthening of relationships is needed by the marriage partners. Parents need to be encouraged to discuss their philosophies of childrearing and care and work out the most equitable solution to meet individual and family needs. If parents cannot find workable solutions to their marital problems, appropriate professional assistance should be sought.

Other Family Members

Siblings. Chronic illness in one family member is a potential source of stress for all other family members. Several reports have suggested that healthy siblings' adjustment may be disrupted by their brother's or sister's chronic condition (Power and Dell Orto, 1980; Sourkes, 1980; Kramer, 1984). Parents are also reported to struggle with the simultaneous time and energy demands of a chronically ill child and their healthy siblings (McCollum, 1981; Drotar and Crawford, 1985; Phillips et al, 1985). Sibling relationships begin at birth and often endure over an entire lifetime. As well as the length of these relationships (i.e., they may last for half a century or more), they are often characterized by their intensity of involvement. Siblings yearn for an equal relationship where they can play, share secrets, and discuss parents. For better or worse, children may spend more hours, days, and years together than any other family subsystem (Bank, 1981). Through forced interaction over the early years, children may have considerable influence on the shaping of each other's identity.

All children in the family are attempting to cope with various developmental stresses. However, siblings most vulnerable to the additional stress posed by experience of a sibling with a chronic illness are those: (a) in the midst of their own developmental transition (e.g., entry into adolescence); (b) with poorly developed coping skills (e.g., very young children); and (c) with poor parental relationships (Siemon, 1984). Some earlier research also indicates that older sisters have the most difficulty adjusting to the needs of the chronically ill sibling (Gath, 1974). Gath's research on children with Down syndrome revealed that the brunt of having a mentally handicapped brother or sister appeared to be borne by the older sisters who were exposed to more domestic responsibility than normal for their age. Gath attributed this overburdening of domestic responsibility as a possible explanation for their difficulty in adjustment.

Siblings of chronically ill children often experience feelings of anger, loss, confusion, neglect, and guilt. They often feel torn between loyalty to their brother or sister who is being teased or rejected and their own need for friends and acceptance. Siblings may feel stigmatized by their ill brother or sister to the point where their own normality is compromised. These feelings can then lead to embarassment, shame, jealousy, and resentment, even though they still love their brother or sister (Featherstone, 1980). Healthy children struggle with being loyal to their family and ill sibling and the desire to be rid of the whole situation in the hopes of becoming normal. Children in two-child families may feel an acute sense of loss when their sole sibling is ill, and there are no other similar relationships to nurture.

Siblings most commonly complain of feelings of confusion. Ambivalence exists in regard to the sibling relationship in general and the effect that chronic illness has on the family as a whole. Siblings often have questions about the cause and progress of the chronic condition, their own vulnerability to the illness, conflicting emotions, and the future. A sample of typical questions asked by siblings of children with chronic illnesses is summarized in Box 25-1.

Although parents would like to shield their healthy siblings from stress, anxiety, and hurt, it is impossible to do so.

Children who live with a chronic illness learn to live with some degree of adversity. Siblings of chronically ill children require special understanding of their particular situation. However, parents may feel burdened by the demands of the ill child and have little energy for the emotional needs of their other children. Children sense this obstacle instinctively and attempt not to burden their parents. However, this avoidance may result in isolation of individual family members, decreased sources of support and comfort, and an increased risk for the development of psychosocial problems (Tew and Laurence, 1973; Vance et al, 1980).

Parents need to experience the support and accomplishments of their healthy children in order to survive, even if understanding a sibling's distress can threaten their own ability to cope (Featherstone, 1980). The most important resources parents can offer

Box 25-1
Questions Commonly Asked by Siblings

CAUSE/PROGNOSIS

What caused ________'s illness?
Will ________ get better/worse?
Will ________ die?
Why did ________ get this illness?
Did my parents do anything to cause ________'s illness?

PERSONAL VULNERABILITY

Can I get the same illness as ________?
If so, How? When?
Do my parents love ________ more because of the illness?
Do my parents expect me to do better because of ________'s illness?
Why do I have to help care for my brother/sister?
How do I explain ________'s illness to my friends?

CONFLICTING EMOTIONS

Why did this have to happen to me? Our family?
Why do mom and dad act differently towards ________ than me?
Why do I love/hate ________?
Why do I have to protect ________ from the other kids?
Why am I embarrassed sometimes by ________?
What can I do to make life better for ________?
Does anyone know that I'm important, too?
Am I supposed to make up for ________'s inability?

THE FUTURE

What will happen to ________ when he/she grows up?
Will my parents be able to care for ________ when he/she grows up?
Will I have to care for ________ when my parents can't?
Will I be able to pursue a career/life of my own?
Will I have children like ________?

(Adapted from Klein, 1972; Featherstone, 1980; Siemon, 1984; Trahd, 1986.)

their other children are honesty, open communication, and emotional support. This can often be accomplished through frequent family conferences. Parents also need to assist healthy siblings to develop their own identities and allow them to achieve success without guilt. They also need to respect their child's reluctance to include their sibling with special needs in their activities. Siblings can also benefit from other children in similar situations who can affirm their experiences, understand their burdens, and help in explaining to others what it's like to live with a brother or sister with special needs. Sibling networks are beginning to flourish. These groups provide links with other children in similar circumstances and often provide extended support and encouragement.

Special events such as birthdays and holidays need to be celebrated in the usual family tradition. Well siblings need to continue with their usual activities and social relationships. If the children themselves have a basic understanding of their brother or sister's illness, they can often provide satisfactory explanations to their friends, thus achieving a more comfortable atmosphere for everyone.

Nurses can make a significant contribution to siblings of chronically ill children. They can help parents to anticipate the course of the illness in order to help them prepare the siblings for impending events well in advance. They can also interact directly with siblings in order to answer their many questions. Health care professionals can encourage parents to involve others who play a significant role (e.g., grandparents, babysitters) in the children's lives to be aware of the siblings' needs. During family conferences, nurses can include siblings in discussion and seek out specific information about how they are managing. They can assist parents in interpreting coping strategies to siblings and in finding realistic ways that they can participate in care. Nurses can also act as advocates for sibling hospital visitation, phone calls, participation in therapy, or anything else to promote a supportive relationship between the children. As siblings get older, they need to be encouraged in discussions about future caretaking arrangements for their sibling. With these nursing actions, there comes the awareness that the illness is not solely the child's problem but that of everyone in the family.

Grandparents. Some families are fortunate enough to include grandparents as members who are close enough either physically or emotionally to be involved in the care of chronically ill children and their families. These older relatives may have retired from active careers and have both the time and inclination to be involved in the lives of their grandchildren. Grandparents often view grandchildren as the rewards of their life's work. The joy that grandparents experience is reflected in their continuous stories about their grandchildren and the numerous pictures adorning their walls and mantles.

When a grandchild is diagnosed with a chronic illness, grandparents often feel intense dismay and sorrow. They may even feel guilt if the illness is hereditary. They often go through the grieving process, similar to parents of the child. However, their grief is difficult because they are not the parent, and they are not as intimately involved in the child's life. They may ini-

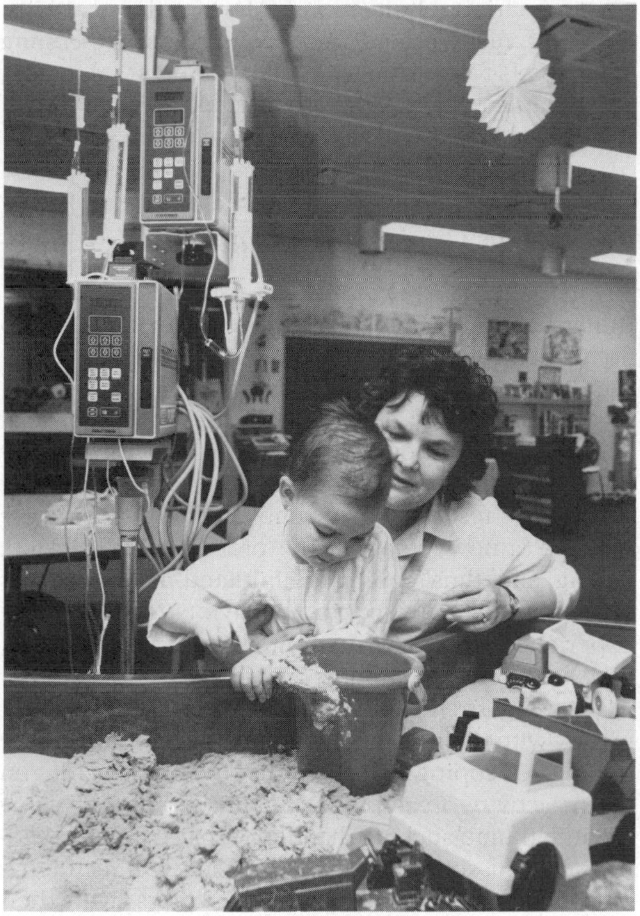

Grandparents are a stabilizing force to the child and family and help make the hospital seem more "like home."

tially not be able to offer compassion because the child's illness forces them to face their own mortality. The grandparents' reaction may be either to overindulge or avoid the ill grandchild. Also, their interaction with the grandchild may be limited due to decreased energy and a distancing that is exerted by the child's parents as a protective device for both the sake of the ill child and that of the grandparents. Thus, the grandparents may not feel included in the immediate family circle and subsequently indulge in a sense of anguish and helplessness. Parents need to be encouraged to include willing and able grandparents in the lives of the chronically ill child and the siblings as they often have much to offer. They often serve as a sounding board for the sick child's distraught parents. Grandparents may be able to assist with practical needs such as providing transportation or accompanying the child and parent during outpatient care or hospitalization. Help with nonschool routines is usually greatly appreciated. They may baby sit or give special attention to the siblings to help fill the void when their parents are occupied with the ill child. Grandparents often model the strength, patience, and faith that the family needs to learn as they adjust to living with chronic illness.

Coping with Chronic Illness

The child with chronic illness is often forced to incorporate numerous treatments and procedures, threats of exacerbations, lifestyle restrictions, lasting impairments, and, at times, a shortened life expectancy into his life experience. Other common concerns include financial constraints, restrictions on social life, sibling rivalry, alterations in routines, guilt, and uncertainty. All concerned need to develop techniques to master psychologic and physical threats in order to achieve personal and social goals and combat the daily strain of living with a chronic illness. This adjustment or mastery process has been labeled as coping by several theorists (Rose, 1972; Kaplan, 1973; Murphy, 1974; Lazarus and Folkman, 1984).

Murphy (1974) has described coping as a process of dealing with challenges from the environment. The coping process consists of strategies and flexible management of available resources to deal with problems or needs. Murphy sees the coping process as adaptive and incorporating both active efforts and defense mechanisms. Earlier in her work, Murphy identified four aspects of childhood coping resources, including

- the range of gratification available;
- the range and flexibility of the child's coping strategies;
- possession of a positive attitude toward life; and
- the ability to temporarily regress to a less demanding level of functioning.

Rose (1972) has further conceptualized the process of coping to include three levels of involvement. These include:

- inactive coping or silent and nonparticipatory behavior;
- precoping or behavior to become familiar with the environment (i.e., listening or asking questions); and
- active coping or the process of dealing with threatening, frustrating, or challenging situations either (a) by attempting to control or change the situation, (b) by resisting attempts to be controlled, or (c) by being cooperative and compliant with those who are making demands.

Lazarus and Folkman (1984) define coping as "constantly changing cognitive and behavioral efforts to manage specific external and/or internal demands that are appraised as taxing or exceeding the resources of the person" (page 141). Coping refers to a cognitive appraisal of the processes that intervene between the encounter and the reaction. Lazarus and Folkman (1984) consider that there are three kinds of cognitive appraisal which can be influenced by both personal and situational factors. These include:

- primary appraisal or judging whether an encounter is irrelevant, benign, or stressful;
- secondary appraisal or judging what might and can be done; and
- reappraisal or an altered evaluation of a situation based on new information from either the individual or the environment.

The concept of vulnerability is closely related to cognitive appraisal and coping in chronic illness (Lazarus and Folkman, 1984; Rose, 1984). Children's interactions with people and objects in their environment may produce vulnerabilities which will affect their ability to cope with the every day challenges of being a child. Murphy and Moriarty (1976) developed a list of primary and secondary vulnerabilities which affect a child's ability to cope with a situation. Primary vulnerabilities develop early in life and include such things as the child's level of growth and development, temperament, emotional lability, perceptual-cognitive abilities, and social support. All primary vulnerabilities influence the child's adaptive processes. Secondary vulnerabilities result from difficulty in integrating primary vulnerabilities.

Coping theorists generally agree that securing adequate information about a situation, maintaining autonomy, and using available intrapsychic processes are important in the coping-adaptive process. However, in chronic illness, high levels of vulnerability may interfere with the child's ability to engage in these processes.

There is little clear evidence that coping changes from one developmental level to another. We know that as young children begin to understand their world, they also become aware of more complex and emotion-laden ways of coping. Murphy (1974) and Murphy and Moriarty (1976) have suggested that although changes occur in coping behavior (from primitive reactions to more complex cognitive processes) the basis for shutting out, exploring, and aggression develops at an early age and continues to influence how an individual copes over time. The techniques one utilizes to bring about relief, reward, quiescence, or equilibrium in relation to a perceived problem are coping strategies (Weisman and Worden, 1976). Some theorists consider that similar coping strategies can be utilized by both the family (i.e., parents) and the child across a variety of situations (Moos and Tsu, 1977). However, many others found contrasts in the coping behaviors of children and their parents (Mattsson, 1972; Kaplan et al, 1973; Drotar et al, 1975). Some of these strategies are discussed below.

Childhood Coping Strategies

Bullard and Dohnal (1984) suggest that children do not work through a problem, as with a particular symptom, nor do they get over it, as with a developmental crisis. Rather, they develop patterns of psychosocial adjustment that they will utilize for the rest of their lives. This adjustment process involves both learning and reality testing. For example, when a child encounters a new situation, the processes of learning, testing, and, thus, coping are initiated. In the process of learning effective coping behaviors, children may experience anger, frustration, discovery, challenge, and, finally, gratification.

Coping strategies utilized by children will vary greatly with their age and cognitive development. The infant uses coping behaviors that center primarily on motor activity. Examples of infant coping behaviors include thumb sucking, hand-mouth activity, restlessness (i.e., fussing), crying, body rocking, and clinging to familiar people and objects. Toddlers, with their increasing communication and locomotor skills, often cope in stressful situations by regressing to earlier familiar infant coping strategies. As well, toddlers use protest (temper tantrums), withdrawal, fantasy, controlling behaviors and ritualization as coping mechanisms. Temporary use of any of these behaviors in a stressful situation is indicative of healthy childhood coping. Once children reach the age of 6 or 7 they have sufficient ability in cognitive functions such as memory, speech, language, and reality testing to have a beginning understanding of their illness and an interest in its management. The school-age child and adolescent cope successfully by finding satisfaction in a variety of compensatory activities (physical and intellectual) and identifying with other young patients afflicted with a chronic handicap. The appropriate expression of anxious, sad, impatient, and angry feelings is an essential and healthy aspect of coping.

Children with a chronic illness need to learn to cope with the difficult realities that they may face on a daily basis. Children who do not experience debilitating psychological symptoms cope by using adaptive defenses (Mattsson, 1972; Geist, 1979). Some of these defenses can be fostered in children to bring about effective coping skills. See Table 23-4, page 716, for a review of defense mechanisms used by children.

Intellectualization. The following situation characterizes the process of intellectualization.

The young nurse went into the room to prepare 12-year-old Jenny for the insertion of a central venous device to be used for parenteral feeds in the treatment of Crohn disease. When the nurse asked her how she felt about being in the hospital, Jenny replied:

"I've had Crohn's disease for about a year. I'm a bit young to have it because the most common age of diagnosis is in the teen years. I know that Crohn's is an inflammatory bowel disorder that affects part of my GI system. If I'm not careful, I may get a bowel obstruction. They have treated me with a high-protein diet, antibiotic drugs, and some steroids too. But this time I need TPN because I've lost too much weight, and my doctor doesn't want me to starve to death."

This situation illustrates that Jenny was dealing with her anxiety about her illness by providing factual information instead of discussing her feelings about hospitalization. She knew much of what was possible about the disease and its management. Other children who cope in this manner may also know death rates, surgical corrective procedures, and equipment. They acquire this information at times from their own reading but most often by questioning people (e.g., health professionals) who know the answers. Younger children who use this technique often know the medical jargon but rarely understand its meaning. For older children, intellectualization is a way of gaining control over something they feel is uncontrollable. It allows children to step outside their feelings and look at the chronic condition from a more objective vantage point. Adults can assist children in using this defense mechanism by being honest and providing them with disease-related information at an age-appropriate level.

Identification with Health Care Professionals. Strong identification with health care staff may accompany the intellectualization process or the child's preoccupation with the illness and its management. This identification is sometimes accounted for by the desire to acquire the same scientific aloofness or curative powers which the child believes the doctor or nurse possesses. Identification with health care staff is more frequently utilized as a coping mechanism in children who have the ability or desire to care for themselves rather than those who do not.

Ritualization. Children with chronic illness often develop a set of ritualistic behaviors to aid in dealing with anxiety in situations where they feel they have little or no control. For example, one youngster, during his chemotherapy, insisted that a paper bag with a picture of Dracula be placed over the red intravenous fluid because it reminded him of blood. Another child with an amputated foot demanded a particular organization of all the equipment used in his dressing change and that certain music be played while the procedure occurred. Finally, a 4-year-old child with aplastic anemia demanded a blue finger puppet each time her blood was drawn. All of these ritualistic behaviors are the child's way of exerting control over a particular situation. Even though these behaviors often appear unique and bizarre to others, they should not be disrupted unless they are self-destructive to the patient. In fact, these rituals often mutually develop between patients and their caretakers. The rituals bind them together in a shared nonpathologic way.

Erikson (1966) considered that ritualistic behavior is often based on the reciprocal needs of two individuals. It heightens a sense of both belongingness and personal distinctiveness in a playful yet formalized way. For example, when the 4-year-old with aplastic anemia was readmitted to hospital, her primary nurse sought out her favorite toys—blankets and the bag of treasured blue finger puppets—hours before her arrival. When the child arrived in her room and saw her favorite things, a broad smile crept across the faces of both the child and her nurse. The adherence to the rituals served to bond the child and her nurse in their attempts to cope with the difficult situation.

Denial and Hope. Chronically ill children often alternate between recognizing the realities of their illness and denying its existence. For example, a child demands to be left in bed because he's "sick," yet yearns to be up in the playroom because he feels well and not "sick at all." These opposing feelings often help to temporarily eliminate the painful reality of the illness and its threat to a child's well-being while allowing the courage and hope to endure pain and suffering. Denial in the service of hope needs to be differentiated from neurotic denial which interferes with the patient's ability to manage his illness on a day-to-day basis and realistically plan for the future. This adaptive form of denial allows the child to rest from the burden of the illness and for a short time be like "every other kid." Adaptive defenses allow the child to vent feelings of frustration and anxiety and gain some control over his illness and its treatment. Adult intervention is necessary only if these normal defenses become compulsive and interfere with growth and adaptation. Otherwise, they should be encouraged and fostered.

All children with chronic illnesses employ some form of coping strategies in an attempt to adjust to their illnesses. Research indicates that the nature of the illness appears to be less influential in this adjustment process than the child's developmental level, available coping techniques, the quality of the parent-child-sibling relationships and the family's acceptance of the handicapped member (Siemon, 1987). Children who cope well with their chronic illness achieve personal satisfaction from functioning effectively at home, in school, and with their peers. Any limitations in activity are imposed by the disease itself rather than by people in the child's environment. Also, well-adapted children exhibit age-appropriate dependence on their parents and do not tend to use their illness to elicit the attention or sympathy offered by the illness.

However, not all children are able to use adaptive defenses effectively to cope with their chronic condition. Exclusion from activities, learned inferiority, and nonacceptance take their toll on emotional well-being. Table 25-1 outlines common patterns of maladjustment that may be manifested in the child and family with a chronic illness. No one of these patterns will cripple a child or family's adjustment. However, it is the cumulative effect of these defenses, perceptual distortions, and behavioral responses that breed unhealthy attitudes and diminish motivation (Bullard and Dohnal, 1984). Nursing strategies used to promote adjustment are also presented in Table 25-1.

***Table* 25-1.** Patterns of Maladjustment in Chronic Illness and Nursing Strategies to Promote Adjustment

Child Characteristics	Family Characteristics	Nursing Strategies
Fear		
Frightened of everything Exaggerated normal fears Few friends Gives up easily on tasks	Make unrealistic demands Do not praise successes; resentful of child's limitations	Teach parents skills to enhance the child's confidence and independence
Pseudoadult		
Dependent on adults Companionship with adults instead of children Manipulative to attain the attention of adults Controlling and demanding behavior Deprived of normal peer relationships	Parents often narcissistic with little time to nurture child Resentful of care Wanting to spend less and less time with child	Encourage more normal peer relationships for child Teach parents skills to manage controlling, manipulative, and demanding behavior
Invisibility		
Unobtrusive in all social situations Wants to achieve obscurity and not draw attention to self Indifferent and withdrawn Speaks in a soft and quiet voice All child's attention goes into self-defense	Family often impulsive Allows other siblings to take control Family babies child and allows to be a productive member	Assist family to become less threatening to the child Establish structure and limits to create an atmosphere that enhances security and encourages the child's development
Fantasy		
Creates an imaginary world Escapes from unattractive and undesirable thoughts Real needs neglected in favor of unrealistic and unattainable daydreams Helpless and dependent deterioration Misses out on social interactions with peers	Denial by family of the child's fears and anger Allows child to be more dependent Failure to set realistic and unattainable goals Feelings of helplessness	Assist child and family to face reality Develop improved problem-solving skills
Overinvolvement in Medical Care		
Rigidly independent Aloof Adept at medical jargon regarding own illness and treatment Verbally assertive but makes no demands Always follows medical regimes, not upset by changes in plans Strives to please and make others feel better	Mistake child for coping maturely with his/her illness Ignore underlying problems of child Often nonassertive, letting child take control of the situation Compliant with child's wishes	Assist family to identify child's underlying struggle Assist child in expressing anger and depression

continued

Table 25-1 *(continued)*

Child Characteristics	Family Characteristics	Nursing Strategies
Humor		
Keeps everyone laughing Appears happy Keeps a distance from others and does not form close relationships Fears others may not like him or her Frustrated with trying to prove self Insecure and has heightened dependency Often immature for age	Enjoy the child's humor Fail to identify child's underlying anger and sadness Allow child to be dependent	Assist child to express anger and sadness Encourage parents to see beyond humor and develop ways for child to express self
Encouraging Favoritism		
Liked by family and peers Considered "special" because of disability Talked to and treated as if much younger Aims to please and strives not to hurt others Very frustrated and wants to be liked for self Feels inferior and has low self-esteem	Pitied by family members Categorized as special so there is no need to relate at appropriate level Often feels guilty and embarrassed about own feelings toward child	Encourage child to recognize worth Encourage parents to treat more appropriately to promote normal development Teach child to be more assertive
"The China Doll"		
Dressed and groomed perfectly Isolated from other children Inappropriate play skills Often disruptive behavior	Parents unable to face and accept disabilities Do not meet child's internal needs Avoid situations where they have to confront the realities of their child's illness Display child but keep away from real world	Assist parents to confront own guilt and fears Encourage less perfection on the exterior and more expression of inner thoughts
Explosive Anger		
Frequent temper tantrums and rages Clings to others Unreasonable anger and physical attacks against others Blames others for misfortune and is jealous of others Feels life is unfair Does not take responsibility for actions and projects blame on others	Unresolved mourning by all family members Permit dependence Often fearful of the child's behavior and in a dilemma as to appropriate management	Assist child to recognize underlying causes for rage and take responsibility for it Encourage parents to set reasonable expectations and guidelines and stick to them
Giving Up		
No incentive or motivation to grow, care for self or succeed Infantile helplessness Ostracized by peers Blames others for personal inadequacies Expects to be waited on	Excuse all of child's behavior Anticipate all child's needs and rescue from all problems Dependence is reinforced by doing everything for child No appropriate discipline or behavioral restrictions	Encourage parents to stop pitying, realize child's potential, and be encouraged to set realistic goals Help child to recognize helpless behavior and learn new appropriate ways of gaining attention
Overdependence		
Extreme awareness of limitations Thinks of self as unable to accomplish anything Afraid to try Fear of failing	Feel threatened by the child's chronic condition and have become very overprotective Believe in and reinforce helplessness and inability	Encourage parents to reinforce ability and give praise for trying Encourage independence and a sense of self in the child

(Adapted from Siemon, 1987.)

Family Coping Strategies

Several theorists and clinicians have examined how families cope with their child's chronic illness (Kaplan et al, 1976; Spinetta, 1980; Venters, 1981). For example, Kaplan and associates (1976) reported that only 12 per cent of all families with a leukemic child remained intact after the child's death. In Kaplan's work, initial coping responses after diagnosis were an indicator of how the family would cope later on. Kaplan categorized family coping into:

- *adaptive coping*—parents understand the nature of the child's illness and communicate about the illness to family members and each family member can grieve;
- *maladaptive coping*—the parents experience hostile reactions to sudden changes in life, and go to great lengths to protect the child from learning the diagnosis (the opposite of adaptive coping); and
- *discrepant coping*—there is a difference in coping abilities within the family (e.g., mother coping and father not coping) which often leads to a decrease in or lack of communication.

Spinetta (1980) measured the child's: (a) nondefensive personal posture; (b) closeness to parents; (c) happiness with self; and (d) freedom to express negative feelings as an indication of coping ability. Results from both Spinetta's and Kaplan's work suggest that the level of family communication is directly related to the child's ability to cope and ultimately adapt to the chronic illness.

Venters (1981) studied responses in families with children who have cystic fibrosis. In this research, Venters found that coping strategies utilized to minimize illness-related hardships were associated with the adequacy of family functioning. Two coping strategies which strengthened family functioning included *sharing the burdens of the illness* (both among family members and outside the family unit) and *assigning meaning to the illness.*

When a child is initially diagnosed with a chronic illness, parents experience feelings of fear and anxiety related to the possible fatal outcome. If the child's initial symptoms subside (as in diabetes mellitus) or if the child goes into a remission (as in acute lymphoblastic leukemia), the parents may go through a stage of disbelief of the diagnosis. During this time, it is not unnatural for the parents to seek out a second medical opinion. If the diagnosis is reconfirmed, the parents begin to feel anger, guilt, and a sense of loss. When the parents begin to recognize and verbalize their concerns and emotions, they begin to accept the reality of their child's illness and its impact on the rest of the family (Mattsson, 1972).

Any disability in a child represents a loss for both the child and family. A chronic illness represents a loss not only of bodily function but also of abilities, potential, and the wish for a healthy child. Before children and parents can adapt to this loss, they require a time to mourn (Furman, 1973; Geist, 1979). Some children and parents will move through these various stages of mourning relatively quickly while others may never reach the final acceptance phase. A crucial hurdle for parents is the ability to resolve the stage of self-blame. Those who do not conquer this stage often harbor feelings of guilt and inadequacy. These feelings may lead to altered parental responses and childrearing practices.

Maladaptive Coping

The child's adaptation can be hindered when maladaptive childrearing patterns are used. Overprotection and rejection are two mechanisms that families may need help in avoiding.

Overprotection. As parents face the reality of their child's chronic condition, they also struggle with their own feelings of guilt. In an attempt to relieve this guilt, they aim to make their child's life as easy and pain-free as possible. A pattern of overindulgence and overprotection emerges which greatly restricts the child's growth and development. Parents shield the child from all failure, anticipate their every need and pay excessive attention to the disability. The child is sheltered from all stress and fails to develop problem-solving skills necessary for successful adaptation. Despite the good intentions of parents, overprotectiveness is only functional within the family system. Peers, teachers, and extended family members will not tolerate the excessive demands of the manipulative, overprotected child. This leads to further isolation and rejection.

Rejection. Rejection is the opposite of overprotection. Both, however, represent the parents' attempts to relieve some of their own guilt and a failure to recognize the child's needs. Rejection may be overt, or it may be apparent in less obvious forms. Rejection may be portrayed as either denial of love or conditional love for the child. Parents may place unreasonable demands on the child or demand promises that are impossible for the child to keep. Failure to recognize the child's progress is also a form of rejection. For example, a parent may show no recognition for the child's accomplishments in self-care if their expectation is for the child to walk and run normally. The child's chronic condition becomes the focus of the parent-child relationship leaving the child feeling useless and unworthy of the attention of others.

Adaptive Coping

Parents who successfully cope with their chronically ill child's symptoms may use strategies including normalization, denial, rationalization, assigning meaning to the illness, and utilization of resources.

Normalization. One of the most common coping strategies used by parents of children with chronic illness is normalization. In the normalization process, the emphasis is on deconstructing the disease label and/or maximizing the child's abilities (Anderson, 1981; Siemon, 1987). The extent to which this process is successful depends on two related factors including the characteristics of the child (e.g., age, nature and severity of the chronic condition) and existence of external support (e.g., validation from outside the family, the existence of appropriate educational and treatment programs and parents' adequate knowledge of the child's chronic condition) (Roskies, 1972; Voysey, 1975; Darling, 1979).

In normalization, families acknowledge that an impairment exists and engage in behaviors that demonstrate that family life is relatively normal. Families who insist that the impairment does not exist are engaged in denial. Families who practice normalization usually define the social consequences of their situation as minimal, yet engage in lifestyle adjustments in an attempt to reorganize the family around the ill child. This reorganization may include changing the family's diet to that of the ill child or moving close to the treatment center so that the child can receive outpatient treatments. These family changes often result in at least one parent remaining at home and resisting career advancement opportunities in order to maintain family equilibrium.

Denial. Parents tend to disavow and isolate their anxious and helpless emotions from time to time in order to cope with the constant strain of the child's illness. This denial behavior may occur at crisis points (e.g., when the leukemic child is having a bone marrow aspiration to determine whether he has relapsed) and allows the parents the calmness and composure to endure the medical crisis. When the crisis subsides, many parents experience a rebound phenomenon most commonly exhibited in the form of depression and irritability. This delayed reaction allows the parents to experience their feelings of fear, anger, and guilt at a much less stressful time than during the crisis.

Rationalization. Closely related to denial is the process of rationalization. This is a process where individuals protect themselves from painful emotions by providing explanations for any occurrence related to the child's illness. These explanations may be valid or invalid. For example, the mother of a child with multiple learning disabilities explains:

> Mark's teacher has called me several times to complain about his disruptive behavior in school. She complains that he won't sit still, can't concentrate on anything and disrupts his classmates while they are trying to work. I know it takes Mark longer to learn and his concentration is poor, but he's also 6 years old and has to burn off all his energy somehow. I think that teacher is making too much of this situation.

In this situation, the parent is attempting to protect both her child and herself from addressing the realities of the child's problem. Instead, the mother is attempting to rationalize the child's behavior by emphasizing the appropriateness of this behavior for the child's developmental level and by refocusing blame on the teacher's "unreasonable expectations."

Assigning Meaning to the Illness. Many parents, like their children, use intellectual processes to compensate for the pain of their child's illness. They often attempt to learn everything they can about all aspects of the disease or handicapping process. In gathering information, parents try to decrease their anxiety through familiarization of what lies ahead. "Information reduces the ambiguity of the situation by assigning a meaning to the events that lead to the establishment of feelings of mastery and self-sufficiency by family members, page 364 (Holaday, 1984)." This process takes time, and it is not until parents experience the grieving process and begin to reorganize and reconstruct the family system that they seek medical information from both health professionals and parents of other children with the same illness. Offering disease-related information too soon after the child's diagnosis often leads to misunderstandings and difficulties with comprehension. Parents need time to mourn prior to learning new facts and skills related to the chronic illness of their child.

The particular meaning that is attached to the illness depends on the educational and cultural background of the parents. Families use religious, cultural, or scientific explanations for the illness. Any approach can be effective provided there is reduction of stress surrounding the uncertainties of their child's illness.

Effective Use of Resources. Parents who cope well tend to use personal and extrapersonal resources effectively. However, they often need assistance to meet the practical demands of the child's illness, to sustain their own personal self-worth, and to promote the morale of other family members over time (Venters, 1981). In order to balance the needs of their child, family, and self, parents must learn to utilize adaptive defenses effectively. Successfully coping parents learn to set concrete goals and expectations for all concerned in order to provide realistic opportunities for achievement. Personal control often leads to a perceived sense of control over the situation which, in turn, maintains individual and family integrity (Craig and Edwards, 1983).

Role of the Nurse in Chronic Illness

When disease of a long-term or lifelong nature compounds the normal growth and development crises of childhood, the results can be potentially devastating for both the child and the family. The nurse is usually involved in some manner in the initial diagnosis of the child's chronic illness in either the hospital, clinic, or office setting and, therefore, has the opportunity to interact and become involved with the ill child and the family from the very beginning. Skill in utilizing the various steps of the nursing process—assessment, planning, intervention, and evaluation—can ensure specific and holistic nursing care both at the time of the child's diagnosis and throughout the course of the illness.

Essential nursing goals in chronic illness focus on:

- Assisting the child and family in the psychosocial adaptation to the child's chronic illness;
- Promoting optimal potential for the child's and family's growth and development; and
- Encouraging families to make appropriate use of resources within the health care system.

Promoting Psychosocial Adaptation

When a child is diagnosed with a chronic, long-term, or life-threatening illness, the nurse experiences feelings of helplessness, discomfort, frustration, powerlessness, and, occasionally, incompetence. In order to deal effectively with these negative emotions, the nurse needs to focus on the child's and the family's responses to the chronic illness and its sequelae.

Children will develop either adaptive or maladaptive responses to their chronic illness depending on the conditions that persist in relationships with parents, peers, and society in general. Regardless of the combination of coping strategies used, underlying anxiety and stress often remain. Some common nursing strategies that promote psychosocial adaptation of children include:

- assist parents to develop realistic goals;
- facilitate mourning;
- promote self-worth;
- encourage independence;
- develop open channels of communication with their child and the health care system.

See Box 25-2 for a summary of how to promote psychosocial adaptation by using these strategies.

Adaptive families have confidence in their ability to handle whatever situations may arise. They have a sense of control yet allow each family member to maintain lifestyles that meet their own needs in a variety of roles. They are tolerant and patient and possess an ability to accept their own ambivalence at times. They have the capacity to deal with failure and hurt as well as success. Most importantly, they have a closeness and cohesiveness which allows them to laugh at themselves and start each day with a clean slate.

Parents who cope with their child's condition do not label the child negatively but, rather, attempt to set realistic goals and challenge their child to achieve them. They attempt to be hopeful in order to allow the child to develop the skills to cope with the stress of having a chronic illness.

Promoting Optimal Potential for Growth and Development

A second goal for nursing in chronic illness is to promote optimal potential for the child and family to achieve the various tasks at each stage of growth and development. The role of the nurse varies considerably and, therefore, is addressed separately for each developmental stage.

Infancy

Parents of chronically ill infants are often devastated at the diagnosis and suffer from a decrease of self-esteem. A nurse that is experienced in dealing with families during the grieving process will be most suited to deal with this situation. The nurse should arrange to get the parents and preferably the infant together as soon as possible after the delivery in order for them to be told by the health care team about the child's illness or handicap. Parents need brief, clear, basic information at first presented slowly and repeated several times. The nurse needs to be careful not to present confusing or confounding information. Also, the nurse should be aware of her or his own behavior and communication so as not to interfere with the parents' grieving process. Examples of nursing actions which may hinder this process include:

- separating the mother and the ill child from healthy mothers and babies;
- placing the ill baby at the back of the nursery; and
- stating to the parents that, "You can have another baby," "You'll be fine," or "You'll get over it."

These actions are usually not intentional and come from nurses' personal feelings of grief, frustration, and a sense of helplessness. Nurses need to recognize their own feelings and attempt to find outlets for their emotions outside of the child's family. Then, rather than engaging in meaningless or intrusive conversation

Box 25-2
Nurses' Role in Promoting Psychosocial Adaptation of the Family

DEVELOPING REALISTIC GOALS

Assist parents to gain an understanding of how their child is similar to and different from other children

Encourage parents to help their children develop realistic goals, maximizing their similarities and minimizing their differences

Encourage parents to be honest with their children about their condition by representing a realistic picture—being hopeful but not offering false promises of cures and miracles

Teach parents and children to set short-term rather than long-term goals in cases of uncertain medical courses

Facilitate evaluation of goals by the child and family on a regular basis—encourage families to let go of unrealistic goals to prevent frustration and disappointment

FACILITATING MOURNING

Encourage children and their families to express and share feelings of guilt, sadness, loss, anticipated physical deterioration, and fear of death

Facilitate discussion to allow families to ask questions about the chronic illness related to causation: "Why me?" "What have I done?" "How will we ever manage?"

Teach parents how to recognize and deal with their child's self-blame and personal guilt for the illness

Encourage parents to communicate about the present and future, not solely about the past

Teach parents the importance of letting their children take on their normal roles within the family enhancing their self-concept

Encourage parents to re-engage in own roles within family

Allow a reasonable, but not indefinite, time for mourning so that parents can acknowledge present limitations and future potentials

PROMOTION OF THE CHILD'S SELF-WORTH

Encourage child and family to stress individual and family abilities rather than disabilities

Remind parents that how children feel about themselves is influenced by what they hear their parents say about them

Teach parents the importance of letting their children take on their normal roles within the family enhancing their self-concept

Encourage parents to allow their child to have some say in what others know about them

Assist parents in gaining empathy with their child's situation from the child's perspective

Encourage parents not to be too overprotective as children require exposure to real-life situations with peers in order to learn to handle cruelty, adversity, and misunderstanding

Assist parents in understanding the need to set the same rules, have similar responsibilities, and receive the same discipline with all children in the family to avoid developing feelings of partiality or favoritism for the child with the illness

Teach parents to be able to recognize the child's need to be similar to peers in hairstyles and clothes, teach parents how to make compromises to accommodate disabilities

Encourage the child and family to put their "best foot forward"

Encourage parents to promote initiative and realistic areas of accomplishment

Discuss with parents the need for children to try new activities in order to develop creativity and problem-solving

Nurses and parents can support the efforts and provide role models

DEVELOPING AN APPROPRIATE LEVEL OF INDEPENDENCE

Assist parents in developing realistic, age-appropriate goals for independence

Encourage families to allow children to function at home, school, and play with as few limits as possible

Give children an appropriate amount of information about their condition to allow them to adapt to the necessary limits and take responsibility for their own care

Encourage family discussions to allow children and their parents to vent concerns about dependence and independence

Encourage parents to reward independence, attempts at self-care, and appropriate social interaction

OPEN COMMUNICATION WITHIN THE FAMILY UNIT

Teach parents the importance of frequent family discussions

Encourage parents to let children speak for themselves and present their own ideas

Teach parents to recognize and communicate with their children in nonverbal ways

Assist parents to be advocates for their children by insisting that others ask the children for their input and participation in discussion

with families, they can be sensitive to the parents' needs for privacy and support. Support and sensitivity can be shown by sharing silences and engaging in frequent and empathetic visits to the mother's room.

The nurse should also assess the infant's functioning and attempt to emphasize to parents those areas where the child is performing normally. In this way, parents will not maximize the defect to the point where they cannot see the child's positive as well as negative attributes.

Nurses working with infants should familiarize themselves with the most valid and reliable instruments for assessing infant functioning. Examples of instruments that assess the infant's functioning include the Bayley Scales of Infant Development (Bayley, 1969) and the Brazelton Neonatal Behavioral Assessment Scale (Brazelton, 1973). The Bayley Scales have been developed to assess the developmental status of infants from 2 to 30 months of age in the areas of mental, motor, and behavioral competency. These scales are the most well-standardized infant tests currently available. The Brazelton Neonatal Behavioral Assessment Scale is an interactive examination measuring various aspects of infant behavior. This scale measures individual progress at an earlier stage than the Bayley Scales but requires more expertise on the part of the examiner in order to administer. Other tools such as the Neonatal Perception Inventory (Broussard, 1978) and the Maternal Attachment Assessment Strategy (Avant, 1980) which focus on maternal perceptions of the newborn and maternal attachment strategies may also be useful to the nurse in her initial assessment of the infant and the maternal-child relationship.

As well as assessing the maternal-child relationship, the nurse can also promote parent-infant bonding by acting as a positive role model. She can call the baby by name, cuddle the child, make good eye contact with the baby, and emphasize the child's normal characteristics. The nurse can foster family involvement and provide positive reinforcement of the parents' efforts to participate in the child's care. Since many babies will not be able to respond to their parents' advances, the nurse will need to encourage parents not to become discouraged and continue to try since, eventually, each child responds in his or her own unique way. Once parents become attached to their child, they may experience the grieving process all over again as the realities of the illness become clarified, and they fear the potential loss.

Toddlerhood

Parents of toddlers struggle with their child's need to develop a sense of autonomy. Nursing intervention to facilitate autonomy may take many forms. First, the nurse should assess the child's developmental level using one of a number of standardized screening tools such as the Denver Developmental Screening Test (DDST) (see Appendix Four and Chapter 15, Child Health Appraisal). Parents should be made aware of the results of the assessment in order to provide added stimulation in areas of developmental lag and, more importantly, to emphasize the child's normal development and progress.

The family needs to be assisted to understand the need for independence. This can be done by allowing the toddler to participate and make small decisions in daily care such as taking medicine from a cup or a spoon. Power struggles should be avoided if possible. Yet, it is important to emphasize to parents that in spite of the chronic illness, the toddler needs consistency, appropriate limits, and a stable routine to provide a sense of order.

Parents may need to learn how to provide activities and toys that will stimulate toddlers who have chronic illnesses. Play items such as drums, punching bags, and bean bags provide children with an outlet for their frustrations. If energy needs to be conserved, parents can be encouraged to give appropriate assistance and limit play times. Body contact, a soothing voice, and distraction (e.g., a walk) may soothe the frustrations of children of this age.

During toddlerhood, children normally experience intense anxiety when separated from their parents. Children with chronic illness are often separated from their parents during hospitalization and diagnostic and treatment procedures. Nurses can be instrumental in decreasing the amount of separation or by minimizing its impact. This is accomplished by encouraging parents to room in or to be present as much as possible when stressful procedures occur.

Primary care nursing is another effective means of assisting the child to cope with separation. This mode of care provides one or a minimal number of caretakers to interact with the child; this establishes consistency and a close relationship with a substitute caretaker. The impact of separation can also be minimized by maintaining, as closely as possible, the child's home routine. This intervention gives the child a sense of security and facilitates the child's return home upon discharge. See Chapter 31 for a discussion of the hospitalized toddler and separation.

Limitations imposed by the illness may stifle the child's social, intellectual, and cognitive development. Parents need to be encouraged to maximize the child's competencies while keeping within his or her limitations. Home visits by the nurse can be useful in assisting parents to realize where safety limits should be imposed and how to make modifications in the home environment.

The diagnosis of chronic illness during the toddler years has an enormous impact on the family. Parents find little energy to devote time to themselves. Nurses can make parents aware of the means of accessing and mobilizing community resources, including suitable child care arrangements to allow parental time-out opportunities. Parents need to be encouraged to share their feelings of anger and frustration and, often, find special support groups of assistance. If parents know what to expect of their ill child, they can prepare for their future care and begin to understand the needs of other family members as well.

Preschooler

During the preschool years, children develop increasing abilities to provide self-care. Preschoolers with chronic illnesses may experience limitations in the development of these self-care skills and wonder why they are different from their peers. They may blame themselves or their parents for their limitations. The parents of preschoolers need assistance to foster the developmental potential and independence of their child and to maintain family equilibrium.

To help family members maintain or achieve a balance between their own needs and the needs of their handicapped preschooler, the nurse must begin by helping parents identify those needs unique to their own situation. Preschoolers need to develop social skills and increase their ability to separate from the family. Therefore, the nurse can support both the preschooler's and family's needs by helping to institute measures such as substitute caretaking, remedial education, or visiting friends or relatives for a day or two. This brief interlude fosters the preschooler's independence and gives parents the opportunity to pursue their own needs. The nurse can assist in finding or suggesting these resources and help to resolve any conflict that may arise when they temporarily transfer the responsibility of their child's care to another person.

As with previous stages, parents need to be aware of normal growth and developmental tasks and how their child is progressing. Preschoolers are at an age at which they are moving from dependency to becoming more independent school-age children. For parents with a handicapped child, this process is complicated by the child's additional dependency needs. Parents may gain support from other families in similar circumstances and, often, benefit from becoming involved in the child's remedial education program. In this setting, they gain insight into approaches that facilitate maximum development of potential while gaining reassurance that their own style of parenting for their child is appropriate.

School-Age Child

During the school-age years, peers and their influence become increasingly important in child development. Also, children need to develop a sense of industry and accomplishment rather than feeling inferior and ashamed. School often brings conflict for children with chronic illnesses. By virtue of periodic interruptions for treatments or hospitalization, peers begin to label the child as being different. School nurses or community health nurses usually provide much of the necessary medical intervention when the child is able to attend school. They also keep the teacher and others involved in supervising the child's academic activities aware of the disease status. The nurse also takes on the role of educator in order to provide school personnel with information and instruction regarding the disease and its management. This contact is necessary when the illness affects the child's school functioning or when treatment or medication must be administered during school hours.

A positive approach avoids needless restrictions, keeps the child at as-near-normal activity as possible, and provides substitute activities when limitations are necessary. Effort should be made to keep the child involved with healthy peers and included in their activities. Since there is a greater incidence of "school phobia" in children with chronic disease, the nurse should be alert to early signs of this behavior. Characteristic examples include frequent, unjustifiable complaints to the school nurse or frequent, unexplained (or flimsily explained) absences. The nurse, teacher, and parent should encourage and, if necessary, insist on daily school attendance. Parents may require substantial encouragement and support from the nurse while they convince their child to attend school. The school nurse is also responsible to see that a homebound teacher is arranged when needed.

To protect the child from additional disease or complications, school nurses may need to remind other parents to keep their healthy child's childhood immunizations up to date to prevent the spread of infectious diseases. They also need to inform parents of the chronically ill child of any infectious outbreaks for which their child may be at special risk. A cooperative endeavor between home and school can help eliminate or minimize the conflicts a child with chronic illness would otherwise experience at school.

School-age children should be gaining progressively more independence in their activities of daily living and in personal decision-making. School-age children with chronic illnesses may have limitations that hinder their independent development in one or more areas of living. Sometimes, the limitation is not within the children but is externally imposed by parents, teachers, peers, or other segments of society that disallow progressive independence in functioning or thinking. The nurse should regularly assess the child's social environment for evidence of unnecessary restrictions. Additional education or professional counseling may be needed to help the child or the restricting individuals to see the limitations in a more realistic manner.

The health team supervising the child's long-term care should be especially alert to conflict related to school entry and school continuation. Extra support and contact should be provided by the health care team during this time of potential crisis as a preventive measure. If the child's family, healthcare providers, and school personnel pull together as a team, they can help to make the child's school years as happy, productive, and memorable as they are for any other child.

Adolescent

Adolescents with a chronic illness are forced to consider the limitations that the illness places on independence and on vocational, educational, and sexual development. Teenagers need to be treated as adults as much as possible and given increasing responsibility for their own care as they adapt to their illness. A major emphasis for nursing of this age group is patient education. Teenagers need accurate, detailed information about their illness—what causes it, what to expect from it, what it means in terms of educational or vocational interests, how it will affect their appearance and sexual function, and how independent it will permit them to be. The "can do's" rather than the "can't do's" should be emphasized. To give the adolescent a model, someone who can provide peer support, the nurse could involve (in the teaching process) another youth who is coping with a similar illness.

Nurses have successfully used groups to provide patient or family support. For example, adolescent support groups or informal teen activity groups have been established for hospitalized patients. Community support groups or advocacy groups have been founded in many communities and provide physical and psychological support as well as current information about treatment and research. Nurses can help adolescents to think of acceptable, appealing activities that will allow peer contact without exceeding limitations set by the physician. For example, if strenuous physical activity is limited, the student could still be a part of many team sports by acting as a student manager. Within an institutional setting, it is especially important to structure acceptable ways for an adolescent to express aggressiveness, independence, and sexuality.

Teenagers should be encouraged to participate in clubs, activities, and other social interaction with peers who have similar interests not just with peers who have a similar disability. A regular school setting with modified activities is best for adjustment; however, teachers need honest information about the child's disease and capabilities. With this kind of exposure, teenagers learn to live openly with their handicaps and to answer questions gracefully. They learn that they are special and capable.

Utilization of Resources

All families with chronically ill children, although requiring the services of health professionals from time to time, struggle to regain their family equilibrium and become independent again. The nurse can have an important role in promoting an environment which stimulates self-care activities and patient/family confidence, in both the hospital and community settings.

In the hospital setting, such environmental structuring includes:

- unconditional acceptance of the patient and the family by the hospital staff;
- presenting the child's condition in a realistic manner so that the child and family can work through the grieving process appropriately;
- providing competent and continuous patient care with increasing involvement by the child and family as they are ready, both in the hospital setting and at home;
- providing opportunities for the child and family to feel valued in the hospital unit, thus, later at home and in the community;
- promotion of a familiar environment and assurance that procedures and treatments will be explained; and
- promotion of privacy for the child alone and with the family.

With the advantageous structuring of the hospital setting, patients and their families can ideally feel more comfortable and supported. However, the hospital model has historically dealt primarily with acute care and only reluctantly become involved in chronicity (Haggerty et al, 1975). Nurses who are used to functioning in well-equipped units with the support of medical technology and the availability of emergency teams also have difficulty preparing the patient and the family for community care. The issue of control over "the patient" is one that needs to be resolved. Parenting and nursing roles become blurred with parents taking on decision-making roles and attempting to be compliant with the medical management of the patient while at the same time striving to integrate the child as a functioning family member.

In the community, nurses have the potential to use their knowledge and expertise in the roles of resource person, evaluator, educator, and organizer.

As resource persons, nurses can use their knowledge of various illnesses, growth and development of children and families, and common coping strategies used by children and families. This can be done by a formal approach such as in a parent support group where the nurse can take either an active educator role or a facilitative role to encourage parent leadership and directiveness. As well, the nurse may want to interact individually with children in the school setting and their parents in the community. In this way, the nurse can monitor the child's disease process and growth and developmental achievements, as well as being a support for parents and a resource person alerting families to community facilities and services.

As an evaluator, the nurse in the community can monitor the child's physical and psychosocial adaptation to illness and the family's adaptation to the child's illness. Several tools for child assessment have been mentioned previously. The nurse should also evaluate the stressors that families with chronically ill children experience. These stressors may include strain on the marital relationship, decreased attention and time for siblings, and difficulty in managing caregiving tasks. Although extended families may provide assistance, they also struggle with uncertainty of the child's medical requirements and fear of interfering with the family functioning.

Although trained personnel are usually available to assist families in metropolitan areas, resources are not always available in rural areas. Even if resources are available in these areas, the people are not always adequately trained to manage the needs of the child and family. Out of frustration, parents are beginning to form advocacy groups to draw attention to their child's special needs. The nurse needs to carefully evaluate both the needs of the child and the competency of available health care personnel in the community. If community adaptation to chronically ill children and their families is to be successful, careful planning prior to the child's discharge from the hospital is necessary. This planning needs to address the needs of the patient, family, and community.

As an educator, the nurse in the community can follow up on the activities instituted by the hospital nurse to promote self-care. In the home, the community nurse can assess the impact that particular cultures have on the child's care. Also, the nurse can attempt to gain some measure of how the family is adapting in the presence of their ill child. Although some evaluation instruments have been developed to measure family adjustment to chronic illness (Pless and Satterwhite, 1973; Spitzer et al, 1971), the measurement remains limited within the field of child health. Qualitative approaches and open-ended interviewing (Satterwhite, 1976; Black et al, 1978) have been employed in some studies but, to date, few comprehensive measures which can quantify the impact of a child's illness on the family have been developed.

Stein and Riessman's (1980) Impact-on-Family Scale is an exception, but this instrument is in its early developmental stages and requires further refinements and reliability and validity testings. Hymovich (1983) has also developed the Chronicity Impact and Coping Instrument: Parent Questionnaire to measure parental perceptions of stressors, problematic situations, or resources. The instrument also provides a protocol for assessing the needs of chronically ill children. Although some initial validity and reliability have been established, more rigorous study is required before measurement properties are fully understood. Finally, Roberts and Feetham (1982) have developed the Feetham Family Functioning Survey to measure parents' perceptions of relationships among family members and their functioning in the outside world. This instrument needs to be used more widely and tested to determine if it is capable of detecting changes over time. Even with the lack of specific instruments, nurses can utilize their knowledge of chronic illness in children and families, growth and development, and coping strategies to generally evaluate the child and family's current functional state.

The role of the case manager is one that could be taken on by the nurse in the community. Unfortunately, there are often two case managers—one in the hospital and one in the community—which can lead to duplication of efforts, increased costs, and confusion for the child and family.

As a case manager, the community nurse can assist the family in the organization and coordination of their child's health care. It is not uncommon for children with a chronic illness to see a multiplicity of health professionals in regard to their illness and its sequalae, growth and developmental needs, educational needs, adjustment needs, and an array of other services in relation to financial, social, and psychological stresses. Often, many of these health professionals have no idea of the demands placed on the family by other caretakers. The family is literally "run ragged" going from one appointment to the other. The nurse can carefully collect information regarding all the health care agencies with which the family is involved in an attempt to assist them in managing the many conflicting demands.

Ness and Huchala (1987) have suggested the need for a community care plan. This plan is based on a multitude of factors which may be assessed to ensure successful community entry. Prior to discharge from the hospital, the issues of the availability of trained personnel, funds, equipment, and supplies need to be addressed. If training of nurses needs to take place, this should happen in collaboration with nursing specialists within the hospital system and prior to the child's discharge.

The family also needs to be aggressively involved in developing the community care plan. They need to express a willingness to care for the child at home. As well, they need to know if community supports are available, if their home can accommodate equipment and if there will be assistance for other family members during the transition period. Finally, several community issues need to be addressed. Are the community medical and nursing professionals ready to accept responsibility for the child's care? Are electrical and telephone services adequate? Are transportation, emergency, and educational resources adequate? A community care plan would assist in addressing some of these issues of the hospital, family, and community. As well, common standards of care could be developed for all health professionals practicing in both institutional and community settings.

References

Allan J, Townley R, Phelan P: Family response to cystic fibrosis. *Aust Paediatr J* 1974; 10: 136–146.

Anderson JM: The social construction of illness experience: families with a chronically ill child. *J Ad Nurs* 1981; 6:427–434.

Anthony EJ: The syndrome of the psychologically invulnerable child. *In* Anthony EJ, Koupernik C, Chiland C (eds): *The Child in His Family: Children at Psychiatric Risk.* New York, NY, John Wiley and Sons, 1974.

Avant PK: Maternal attachment and anxiety: an exploratory study. (Doctoral dissertation, Texas Women's University, 1978.) *Dissertation Abstracts International* 1980; 40:165B.

Bank S: *Sibling Bond.* New York, NY, Basic Books, 1981.

Barsch R: *The Parent of a Handicapped Child: Study of Child Rearing Practices.* Springfield, IL, Charles C Thomas, 1968.

Bayley N: *Bayley Scales of Infant Development.* New York, The Psychological Corporation, 1969.

Bibace R, Walsh ME: Development of children's concepts of illness. *Pediatrics* 1980; 66:912–917.

Black L, Hersher L, Stenschneider A: Impact of the apnea monitor on family life. Pediatrics 1978; 62:681.

Blackburn S: The neonatal ICU: a high risk environment. *Am J Nurs* 1982; 82:1708–1712.

Bowlby J: *Attachment and Loss.* New York, Basic Books, 1973.

Brazelton TB: *Neonatal Behavioral Assessment Scale.* Philadelphia, JB Lippincott, 1973.

Brewster AB: Chronically ill hospitalized children's concepts of their illness. *Pediatrics* 1982; 69:355–362.

Broussard ER: Psychosocial disorders in children: early assessment of infants at risk. *Cont Educ Fam Phys* 1978 Feb; 44, 47–48, 55–57.

Bruhn J, Cordova F: A developmental approach to learning wellness behavior. Part 1: Infancy to early adolescence. *Health Values* 1977 Nov/Dec; 246.

Bullard ID, Dohnal JT: The community deals with the child who has a handicap. *Nurs Clin North Am* 1984; 19(2):309–318.

Burr BH, Guyer B, Todres ID, Abraham B, Chiodo T: Home care for children on respirators. *N Engl J Med* 1983; 309:1319–1323.

Burton L: *The Family Life of Sick Children: A Study of Families Coping with Chronic Childhood Disease.* London, Routledge and Kegan Paul, 1975.

Cassel J: The contribution of the social environment to the host resistance. *Am J Epidemiol* 1976; 104:107–123.

Cobb S: Social support as a moderator of life stress. *Psychosom Med* 1976; 38:300–314.

Craig HM, Edwards JE: Adaptation in chronic illness: an eclectic model for nurses. *J Adv Nurs* 1983; 8:397–404.

Darling R: *Families Against Society: A Study of Reactions to Children with Birth Defects.* Beverly Hills, CA, Sage Publications, 1979.

Darling R, Darling J: *Children Who Are Different: Meeting the Challenges of Birth Defects in Society.* St. Louis, CV Mosby, 1982.

Diamond M, Jones SL: *Chronic Illness Across the Life Span.* Norwalk, CT, Appleton-Century-Crofts, 1983.

Dowd EL, et al: Releasing the hospitalized child from restraints. *MCN* 1977 Nov/Dec; 370.

Drotar D, Baskiewicz BA, Irvin N, Kennell J, Klaus M: The adaptation of parents to the birth of an infant with a congenital malformation: a hypothetical model. *Pediatrics* 1975; 56:710–717.

Drotar D, Crawford P: Psychological adaptation of siblings of chronically ill children: research and practice implications. *Dev Behav Pediatr* 1985; 6(6):355–362.

Duvall EM: *Family Development.* Philadelphia, JB Lippincott, 1971.

Dynesen AH, Flensborg EW: Prognosen for cystik fibrose 1 Danmark 1945–1974. *Videnskab Praksis* 1978; 463–470.

Erikson EH: *Childhood and Society.* 2nd ed. New York, WW Norton, 1964.

Erikson E: Ontogeny of ritualization. *In* Lowerstein R et al (eds): *Psychoanalysis—A General Psychology: Essays in Honour of Heinz Hartman.* New York, International Universities Press, 1966.

Featherstone H: *A Difference in the Family: Life with a Disabled Child.* New York, Basic Books, 1980.

Figley CR, McCubbin HI (eds): *Stress and the Family. Vol II, Coping with Catastrophe.* New York, Brunner/Mazel, 1983.

Fraser BC: The meaning of handicap in children. *Child Care, Health Dev* 1980; 6:83–91.

Freud A: *The Ego and the Mechanisms of Defense.* New York, International Universities Press, 1966.

Friedrich WN, Friedrich WL: Psychological assets of parents of handicapped and nonhandicapped children. *Am J Neonatal Defic* 1981; 85:551–553.

Furman R: A child's capacity for mourning. *In* Anthony E, Koupernik C (eds): *The Child in His Family: The Impact of Disease and Death.* New York, John Wiley and Sons, 1973.

Gath A: Sibling reactions to mental handicap: a comparison of the brothers and sisters of mongol children. *J Child Psychol Psychiatr* 1974; 15:187–198.

Geist RA: Onset of chronic illness in children and adolescents: psychotherapeutic and consultative intervention. *Am J Orthopsychiatr* 1979; 49(1):4–23.

Gliedman J, Roth W: *The Unexpected Minority: Handi-*

capped Children in America. New York, Harcourt, Brace, Jovanovich, 1980.

Gruenberg EM: The failures of success. *Milbank Mem Func Q* 1977 Winter; 3–24.

Haber M, Smith RT: Disability and deviance; normative adaptations of role behavior. *Am Sociolog Rev* 1971; 36:87–97.

Haggerty RJ: *Child Health and the Community.* New York, John Wiley and Sons, 1975.

Hewett S, Newson J, Newson E: *The Family and the Handicapped Child.* London, George Allen and Unwin, 1970.

Hobbs N et al: Public policies affecting chronically ill children and their families. Preliminary report of project: Chronically ill children in America. Nashville, TN, Vanderbilt Institute for Public Policy Studies, 1983.

Holaday B: Challenges of rearing a chronically ill child. *Nurs Clin North Am* 1984; 19:361–368.

Howard J: *Families.* New York, Berkley Books, 1978.

Hughes JG: The emotional impact of chronic disease. *Am J Disabled Child* 1976; 130:1199–1203.

Hymovich D: The chronicity impact and coping instrument: parent questionnaire. *Nurs Res* 1983; 32:275–281.

Ireys HT: Health care for chronically disabled children and their families. *In* Schorr LB: *Better Health for our Children: A National Strategy. Vol 4: Report of the Select Panel for Promotion of Child Health.* Washington, DC, DHHS (PHS) Pub. #79–55071, 1981.

Isaccs J, McElroy MR: Psychosocial aspects of chronic illness in children. *J School Health* 1980 August; 318–321.

Kaplan BH, Cassel JC, Gore S: Social support and health. *Med Care* 1977; 15(5, suppl):47–57.

Kaplan D, Grobstein R, Smith A: Predicting the impact of severe illness in families. *Health Soc Work* 1976; 1(3):71–82.

Kaplan D, et al: Family mediation of stress. *Social Work* 1973; 18:60–69.

Ketterick RG: The Pennsylvania program: Case example: The ventilator dependent child. *In* DHHS Pub. No. PHS–83–50194, Report of the Surgeon General's Workshop on Children with Handicaps and Their Families. Washington, DC, US Government Printing Office, 1982.

Klein S: Brother to sister, sister to brother: interview with siblings of disabled children, Parts I and II. *Except Parent* 1972; 2:10–15, 24–27.

Knafl KA, Deatrick JA: How families manage chronic conditions: an analysis of the concept of normalization. *Res Nurs Health* 1986; 9:215–222.

Kramer RF: Living with childhood cancer: impact on the healthy siblings. *Oncol Nurs Forum* 1984; 11:44–51.

Lavigne JV, Burns WT: *Pediatric Psychology: An Introduction for Pediatricians and Psychologists.* New York, Grune and Stratton, 1981.

Lazarus RS, Folkman S: *Stress, Appraisal and Coping.* New York, Springer Publishing Company, 1984.

Lewis CE, Lewis MA: The impact of television commercials on health-related belief and behavior of children. *Pediatrics* 1974; 53:431.

Mattsson A: Long term illness in childhood: a challenge to psychosocial adaptation. *Paediatrics* 1972; 50:801–805.

Mattsson A, Weisberg I: Behavioral reactions to minor illness in preschool children. *Pediatrics* 1970; 4:604.

McCollum AT: *The Chronically Ill Child: A Guide for Parents and Professionals.* New Haven, CT, Yale University Press, 1981.

McCrae W, Cull A, Burton L: Cystic fibrosis: parents' responses to the genetic basis of the disease. *Lancet* 1973; 2:11–143.

McKeever P: Fathering the chronically ill child. *Matern Child Nurs J* 1981; 6(2):124–128.

Mechanic D: The concept of illness behavior. *J Chron Dis* 1962; 15:189–194.

Mercer RT: When the infant has a defect. *In Nursing Care for Parents at Risk.* Thorofare, NJ, Charles B. Slack, 1977; 41–75.

Mercer RT: Mothers' responses to their infants with defects. *Nurs Res* 1974; 23:133–137.

Moos RH, Tsu VD: The crisis of physical illness: an overview. *In* Moos RH (ed): *Coping with Physical Illness.* New York, Plenum, 1977.

Murphy LB: Coping, vulnerability and resilience in childhood. *In* Coelho GV et al (eds): *Coping and Adaptation.* New York, Basic Books, 1974.

Murphy LB, Moriarty AE: *Vulnerability, Coping, and Growth.* New Haven, CT, Yale University Press, 1976.

National Center for Health Statistics: *Current Estimates from the National Health Interview Survey: United States, 1979,* Series 10, Number 136. DHHS Pub. No. (PHS) 81–1564. Hyattsville, MD, NCHS, 1981a.

National Center for Health Statistics: *Health Characteristics of Persons with Chronic Activity Limitation: United States, 1979,* Series 10, Number 137. DHHS Pub. No. (PHS) 82–1565. Hyattsville, MD, NCHS, 1981b.

Neill K: Behavioral aspects of chronic physical disease. *Nurs Clin North Am* 1979; 14:443–456.

Ness PL, Huchala B: Adaptation of the community to children with chronic conditions and their families. *In* Rose MH, Thomas RB (eds): *Children with Chronic Conditions: Nursing in a Family and Community Context.* Orlando, FL, Grune and Stratton, 1987.

Newacheck PW, Halfon N, Budetti PR: Prevalence of activity limiting chronic conditions among children based on household interviews. *J Chron Dis* 1986; 39(2):63–71.

Olshansky S: Chronic sorrow: a response to having a mentally defective child. *J Pediatr* 1962; 43, 190–193.

Parsons T: *The Social System.* New York, Free Press, 1951.

Phillips S, et al: Parent interview findings regarding the impact of cystic fibrosis on families. *Dev Behav Pediatr* 1985; 6:122–127.

Piaget J: *The Early Growth of Logic in the Child.* New York, WW Norton, 1969.

Pless IB, Satterwhite B: A measure of family functioning and its application. *Soc Sci Med* 1973; 7:613–621.

Power PW, Dell Orto AE (eds): *Role of the Family in the Rehabilitation of the Physically Disabled.* Baltimore, University Park Press, 1980.

Roberts C, Feetham S: Assessing family functioning across three areas of relationships. *Nurs Res* 1982; 31:231–235.

Rodgers BM, et al: Depression in the chronically ill or handicapped school-age child. *MCN* 1981; 6:266–273.

Rose M, Killien M: Risk and vulnerability: a case for differentiation. *Adv Nurs Sci* 1983; 5(3):60–73.

Rose MH: The concepts of coping and vulnerability as applied to children with chronic conditions. *Iss Compr Pediatr Nurs* 1984; 7:177–186.

Rose MH: The effects of hospitalization on the coping behaviors of children. Unpublished doctoral dissertation, Chicago, 1972.

Roskies E: *Abnormality and Normality: The Mothering of Thalidomide Children.* Ithaca, NY, Cornell University Press, 1972.

Rutter M, Tizard J, Whitmore K: *Education, Health and Behavior.* London, Longman, 1970.

Sabbeth B: Understanding the impact of chronic childhood illness on families. *Pediatr Clin North Am* 1984; 31(1):47–57.

Sabbeth BF, Leventhal JM: Marital adjustment to chronic childhood illness: a critique of the literature. *Pediatrics* 1984; 73(6):762–768.

Sargent J, Liebman R: Childhood chronic illness: issues for psychotherapists. *Commun Mental Health J* 1985 Winter; 21(4):294–311.

Satterwhite B: Impact of chronic illness on child and family: an overview based on five surveys with implications for management. St. Louis, Paper presented to Ambulatory Pediatric Association Annual Meeting, 1976.

Sibinga MS, Friedman DJ: Restraint and speech. *Pediatrics* 1971; 116.

Siemon M: Siblings of the chronically ill or disabled child: meeting their needs. *Nurs Clin North Am* 1984; 19(2):295–307.

Siemon M: Patterns of impairment: cognitive/emotional. *In* Rose MH, Thomas RB (eds): *Children with Chronic Conditions: Nursing in a Family and Community Context.* Orlando, FL, Grune and Stratton, 1987.

Simeonsson RJ, Buckley Z, Monson L: Conceptions of illness causability in hospitalized children. *J Pediatr Psychol* 1979; 4:77–84.

Sourkes BM: Siblings of the pediatric cancer patient. *In* Kellerman J (ed): *Psychological Aspects of Childhood Cancer.* Springfield, IL, Charles C Thomas, 1980.

Spinetta J: Disease-related communication: how to tell. *In* Kellerman J (ed): *Psychological Aspects of Childhood Cancer.* Springfield, IL, Charles C Thomas, 1980.

Spitzer RL, Gibbon M, Endicott J: Family evaluation form. New York State Department of Mental Hygiene, Biometrics Research, 1971.

Stein REK, Reissman CK: The development of an impact-on-family scale: preliminary findings. Med Care 1980; XVIII(4):465–472.

Susser MW, Watson W: *Sociology in Medicine.* 2nd ed. London, Oxford University Press, 1971.

Tew B, Laurence KM: Mothers, brothers and sisters of patients with spina bifida. *Dev Med Child Neurol* 1973; 15:69–76.

Thomas RB: Introduction and conceptual framework. *In* Rose MH, Thomas RB (eds): *Children with Chronic Conditions: Nursing in a Family and Community Context.* Orlando, FL, Grune and Stratton, 1987.

Thomas RB: Family response to the birth of a child with a chronic condition. Unpublished manuscript. Seattle, University of Washington School of Sociology, 1983.

Trahd GE: Siblings of chronically ill children: helping them cope. *Pediatr Nurs* 1986; 12(3):191–193.

Vance J, et al: Effects of nephrotic syndrome on the family: a controlled study. *Pediatrics* 1980; 65:948–956.

Venters M: Familial coping with chronic and severe childhood illness: the case of cystic fibrosis. *Social Sci Med* 1981; 289–297.

Voysey M: *A Constant Burden: The Reconstruction of Family Life.* London, Routledge and Kegan Paul, 1975.

Walker DK, Gortmaker SL: Final Report: Community Child Health Studies (Grant MC–R–250437). Springfield, VA, National Technical Information Service, 1983.

Walker DK, Gortmaker SL, Wietzman MD: Chronic Illness and Psychosocial Problems Among Children in Genessee County. Community Child Health Studies, Harvard School of Public Health, 1981.

Walker J, Thomas M, Russell I: Spina bifida—and the parents. *Dev Med Child Neurol* 1971; 13:462–476.

Weisman AD, Worden JW: The existential plight in cancer: significance of the first 100 days. *Int J Psychiatr Med* 1976; 7:1–15.

Bibliography

Bernardo M: A conceptual model of children's cognitive adaptation to physical disability. *J Adv Nurs* 1982; 7:595–601.

Ferrari M: Perceptions of social support by parents of chronically ill versus healthy children. *Child Health Care* 1986 Summer; 15(1):26–31.

Haase JE: Components of courage in chronically ill adolescents: a phenomenological study. *Adv Nurs Sci* 1987; 9(2):64–80.

Hobbs N, Perrin JM (eds): *Issues in the Care of Children with Chronic Illness: a Sourcebook on Problems, Services and Policies.* San Francisco, Jossey-Bass, 1985.

Horner MM, et al: How parents of children with chronic conditions perceive their own needs. *MCN* 1987 Jan/Feb; 12(1):40–43.

Miller JF: *Coping with Chronic Illness: Overcoming Powerlessness.* Philadelphia, FA Davis, 1983.

Muscari ME: Adolescent suicide attempts by acetaminophen ingestion. *MCN* 1987 Jan/Feb; 12(1):32–35.

Nelms BC (ed): More similar than different: children with chronic illness. *J Pediatr Health Care* 1988 Mar-Apr; 2(2):55–56.

Oremland EK: Communicating over chronic illness: dilemmas of affected school-aged children. *Child Health Care* 1986 Spring; 14(4):218–223.

Potter PC, Roberts MC: Children's perceptions of chronic illness: the roles of disease symptoms, cognitive development, and information. *J Pediatr Psychol* 1984; 9:13–27.

Strauss AL, et al: *Chronic Illness and the Quality of Life.* 2nd ed. St. Louis, CV Mosby, 1984.

Vipperman J, Rager P: Childhood coping; how nurses can help. *Pediatr Nurs* 1980 Mar/Apr; 11–18.

Zeltzer LK, LeBaron S: Fantasy in children and adolescents with chronic illness. *Dev Behav Pediatr* 1986; 7(3):195–198.

Impact of Death and Dying Chapter 26

Darlene McCown

Death signals the end of life as we know it. It touches each of us—even children. Death is usually associated with old age and is a subject people may try to avoid until they are faced with their own death or the death of their loved one. When the loved one is their child, the emotional upheaval created by the threat of loss or actual loss is immense.

Health care professionals assume an important role in events associated with death. A major role of the nurse is to assist family members through the adjustments required by the terminal illness, death, and grief response. It is important for the nurse to understand the meaning of life-threatening illness and death to the child and parents, and what the loss of the child means to the family. This chapter presents an overview of the grieving process, children's concepts of death, the child's and family's response to illness and loss, and the nurse's role in helping children and families cope with death and dying.

Related Topics
Communicating with Children and Families, Chapter 11
Concepts of Illness: Stress, Crisis, and Coping, Chapter 23
Nursing care during hospitalization, Chapter 25
Nursing Management of Pain in Children, Chapter 29

Stages of Coping with Life-Threatening Illness

Kubler-Ross pioneered the effort to study individuals' responses to terminal illness (Kubler-Ross, 1969). Her classic work focused on dying adults, but the coping strategies she identified have been observed in parents and family members facing a life-threatening illness in their child. Five stages in the response to impending death have been recognized.

Denial and Isolation

The first stage, *denial* and *isolation,* begins with the initial diagnosis of a potentially fatal disease and is reflected in the response, "No, not me." Denial lessens the impact and allows time to adjust to the dreadful news of a life-threatening illness. It is temporary and gives way to a gradual awareness of reality. Facts and information given to the family during this phase often are not heard.

If possible, the nurse should be present when the family learns the diagnosis. The nurse helps the family by demonstrating an attitude of genuine concern and caring, by answering their questions, and by restating, interpreting, and clarifying the information given to them. The nurse's role at this time is to be supportive and insure that the parents have adequate understanding of the situation in order to make decisions about treatment. Families in this phase may find it helpful to seek another opinion to confirm the diagnosis. The nurse's acceptance of the family's need to use denial without reinforcing it helps bring the child and family to a gradual awareness and psychologic adaptation to reality.

Anger

Anger occurs in the second stage, when denial can no longer be maintained. The parent demands, "Why *my* child?" This stage is associated with feelings of sadness, depression, guilt, and anger and with somatic complaints. Guilt and anger are probably the most universal or typical reactions of parents when their child is dying. Parents need to be assured and reassured by the nurse that the child's illness is not their fault. Feelings of guilt may lead to many reactions that can cause problems for their dying child, one of which is the tendency for parents to become overly permissive or overly protective.

Anger is displaced in all directions. It is often directed at health professionals and other healthy children. The family may refuse certain caregivers or particular aspects of treatment. The parents may feel they have lost control of their ability to provide the care needed by their child. The nurse helps them maintain control of as much of their child's care as possible, such as routine activities like feeding, bathing, and playing. They can be instructed in methods for special care such as managing intravenous lines, tube feedings, and dressing changes. Participation increases parental competence and provides an outlet for emotional energy. Listening to parents ventilate their angry feelings in an accepting manner helps them establish trust and confidence in those providing their child's care and gives release to their feelings of guilt and anger.

The dying child, as well as those observing the terminal illness, may express anger and guilt in various ways. This anger may be expressed through open verbal hostilities or by withdrawal, rejection, or a variety of complaints. The nurse intervenes by allowing expression of angry feelings without compounding the guilt.

Gradually the dying child and family enter a period called *bargaining.* The person engages in an agreement that is an attempt to postpone the death. The parents often set a specific time extension related to a particular event such as starting school, a birthday, or a special day like Christmas. Bargaining sets a deadline and includes a promise that one will not ask for more after the one favor. Bargains may be with God, the health team, or significant others. Dying children may bargain for a chance to go home. The nurse can help parents make arrangements to take their child home.

Depression

As the process of dying demands more and more of the child and family, there comes a deep sense of loss and *depression.* Depression has two phases: reactive depression (thinking of past losses) and preparatory depression (thinking of impending losses). In reactive depression the concern is for loss of the happiness and joy experienced before illness (physical activity, body image, future development, and general sense of well-being). The preparatory depression phase is characterized by the knowledge of impending loss and separation from loved ones. During this phase, those experiencing death become quiet and sorrowful. Attempts to cheer and brighten their day are inappropriate — it is a time to be present and quiet so that their sorrow can be felt.

Acceptance

Now there is little interest in present or future activities. Children wish only for their parents to be present, and parents want each other or a significant other. The child and family are not happy but not terribly sad. This stage is a time for tender loving care, when touch, quietness, attention to comfort, and gentle handling become the avenue of communication. The nurse must take care not to abandon the family but to remain attentive to its need for privacy, comfort, and meticulous physical care of the ill child.

Resolving Grief

Time is a great healer. But time alone is not enough to heal grief. The help and support received in the days and months following a loss facilitates recovery from and resolution of the loss. Social support systems can be both informal and formal. Friends, neighbors, and family surround the bereaved with *informal support* in the form of companionship, material assistance such as food, and aid in decision making. Their empathetic understanding allows them to support the bereaved. The concepts of *empathy* and sympathy differ. Sympathy focuses on one's own feelings and projects those feelings to others. Empathy focuses on the feelings and experiences of the bereaved person. It contains a loss of self and a concern and appreciation for the experience of the other. An empathetic person learns to vicariously experience and understand the feelings of another person. *Formal support* comes from organized groups, which preserve the societal responses to death and thereby facilitate and encourage the mourning process. Self-help and death-related support groups aid families in the grief process. (See Box 26-1.) The religious community offers answers to the questions of the ultimate meaning of life. It provides comfort and hope for the bereaved.

Signs of Recovery

Recovery from loss takes time. Each aspect of the grief process must be experienced in its intensity before grief can be resolved. Emotional energy must be released from thoughts of the deceased and invested in daily living. Facing loss can be a maturing experience, but if loss is denied or avoided, the individual may lose the opportunity to grow and may actually regress. Grief must be resolved before replacement of the loss, otherwise it will interfere with effective investment in new relationships. The course of grief depends on the ability of the bereaved to do the work needed to separate from the lost object and reinvest in new interests. Recovery from grief begins at the point when the bereaved returns to normal activities with full capacity for pleasure and life.

Box 26-1
Community Support Groups

Candlelighters
Suite 1011
2025 Eye Street, NW
Washington, DC 20006
Families of children with cancer

Compassionate Friends
P O Box 1347
Oak Brook, Illinois 60421
Parents who have lost children of all ages

SIDS Support Groups
National SIDS Institute
275 Carpenter Drive
Atlanta, Georgia 30328
Families following SIDS loss of an infant

Theories of Grief and Mourning

Various theoretical approaches have been used to explain the process of grief and mourning. Each of the following individuals have contributed to the present understanding of human response to loss.

Freud's Psychoanalytic View. The psychoanalytic view of grief emphasizes the human instinct toward life. The struggle of the neonate to breathe and to balance physiologic processes is an example of the drive for life. Psychoanalysts believe that individuals fear death and consequently develop grief as a symptom in response to the fear of death. Freud identified four major characteristics of mourning: dejection, lack of interest in the world, loss of capacity to love, and inhibition of activity. He saw grief as a departure from normal psychologic functioning and labeled it a pathologic condition.

Lindemann's Concept. Lindemann (1944) established the concept of "acute grief." His classic grief theory resulted from work with 101 bereaved persons. A pattern of grief symptoms and responses became apparent. Common responses include

- Sensations of somatic distress,
- Preoccupation with the image of the deceased,
- Feelings of guilt,
- Hostile reactions,
- Loss of usual patterns of conduct,
- Assuming behaviors of the deceased.

Lindemann viewed grief as a normal response to the cessation of a social interaction. Grief work entails emancipation from emotional bondage to the deceased, readjustment to life without the deceased, and formation of new relationships. The nurse can help the family members accomplish "grief work" by encouraging them to face the pain and allow emotional expression of it.

Engel's Phases. Engel (1964) described four distinct phases in the grief process following a death. The initial reaction is *shock* and *disbelief,* accompanied by a sense of numbness and immobility. As the reality of the death and the meaning of the loss penetrate one's consciousness, acute periods of anguish and pain are experienced.

Awareness of the loss is often coupled with physical pain, emptiness, and anger. Crying typifies this period and appears to be functional in helping the bereaved acknowledge the loss by allowing a temporary dependent state and the need of help. Engel believed that the inability to cry interferes with the normal grief process.

Restitution signifies the third stage of grief. Cultural rituals, funerals, and visits with friends and family clarify the reality of the loss as well as provide comfort, activity, and support. As the reality of the death is accepted, *resolution* of the loss occurs. This phase takes place in steps. The bereaved feels a painful emptiness and frequently a lessening of self-esteem and difficulty in forming new relationships. Physical ailments similar to those experienced by the deceased may develop as a means of suffering and maintaining a bond with the deceased. Preoccupation with thoughts of the deceased range from a focus on personal effects of the loss to physical aspects of the deceased. Gradually, a positive mental image of the deceased person develops. When the mourner's interest in new relationships and life returns, the grief process is completed. Evidence of successful healing is the ability to remember comfortably and realistically both the pleasures and disappointments of the lost relationship. The nurse will see evidence of this stage in parents who return to the hospital for a visit several months or a year after the death of their child. A few moments spent with the family at these return visits, calling them by name, and talking about their child is a very meaningful experience for them.

Definitions of Loss and Grief

The death of a loved one is followed by grief, bereavement, and mourning. Grief and mourning signify the painful, emotional, physical, and cultural reaction to death.

Bereavement (*bereave:* to deprive of, to leave desolate) represents the process of responding to the loss of a loved one. It has two primary aspects—grief and mourning (Averill, 1968).

Grief reflects the intense emotional and physical feelings aroused by a loss. It is characterized by suffering, distress, sorrow, and regret and includes feelings of despair and bewilderment. Friends and relatives respond to the suffering by offering help, companionship, and other forms of concern. Grief functions to maintain bonds and affection between people.

Mourning is the behavioral aspect of grieving, including expressions of sadness and weeping. There are also some cultural responses to loss such as a funeral, wearing of subdued clothing, and family gatherings. Participation in these societal rituals is believed to facilitate the mourning process.

Anticipatory Grief. In expectation of the death of a loved one, the family members may suffer the symptoms of grief described earlier. Anticipatory grief occurs prior to the actual loss, when the probability of the loss is realized. Unlike conventional grief, anticipatory grief has a definite ending point—the time of actual death. Conventional grief eases with time whereas anticipatory grief increases to the point of death (Aldrich, 1974). Anticipation of the loss gives family members time to prepare and may actually give the bereaved more energy to cope at the time of death.

A study of children with cancer showed that both fathers and mothers experienced anticipatory grief (Koocher and O'Malley, 1981). The difference between mothers and fathers appeared in the intensity and duration of feelings expressed. Mothers experienced stronger responses that extended over a longer time period.

The nurse may care for dying children whose parents have grieved in anticipation and have begun to detach emotionally from the child prior to death. In these circumstances family members may need assistance to understand their feelings and reactions. The nurse can help them find specific ways of parenting their child to the end. Physical presence, holding, and talking to the child will maintain a bond, relieve the parents' guilt, and provide comfort for the ill child. Anticipatory grief is therapeutic as it allows time to say good-bye, express love, and fulfill the secret wishes exchanged in meaningful moments.

Influences on the Grieving Process

Among factors influencing the grief response of children, age and developmental level are important (Bloom-Feshbach and Bloom-Feshbach, 1987).

Researchers and therapists also do not agree about the age at which the grieving process is the most difficult. Some experts feel that children under 5 years of age are most vulnerable; others believe adolescence is the significant phase. My research indicates that children in the 6- to 7-year transition are at greatest risk for developing maladaptive responses to the experience of death (McCown, 1987). Research suggests that girls may be more sensitive to death events and losses. Social support is known to influence grief behavior; when the parent dies, the child loses the primary support system. If a grandparent, sibling, or other close relative dies, the parent is also grieving and may be unable to provide adequate support for the child. Cultural and religious practices of the family always will affect a child's grieving process. As much as possible, professionals should become familiar with the family's individual practices.

Adolescent response to loss is particularly affected by the cognitive level of development. A model of adolescent grief developed by Corr and McNeil (1986), relates loss to the tasks and conflicts of normal adolescent development. They identified five core issues around which bereaved teenagers attempt to gain resolution of personal conflicts characteristic of the age group. These core issues include predictability of events, self-image, belonging, fairness/justice, and mastery/control. Although adolescents react to loss on cognitive, behavioral, and affective levels, the focus here will be primarily on the cognitive aspects of their understanding of death and grief.

On the cognitive level, the young adolescent aged 11 to 14 years recognizes that "I am different." Bereaved young teens may view the world as unsafe and feel vulnerable and recognize the unpredictability of events in life. They may be overly cautious or display risk-taking behaviors. They may believe that only peers understand them and seek peer support. These youngsters may ask "Why did my loved one die?" and exhibit self-protective or self-destructive behaviors. Finally, as an attempt to master the event, the dead person is idealized or perhaps characteristics very different from the survivor are attributed to the deceased.

The middle adolescent sees the world from the perspective of "I can do anything." Teens between ages 14 and 17 years know that the world is unsafe and that they are vulnerable. They will face the situation with a response of independent action and risk-taking behaviors. They feel that they can handle the event but fear loss of competence in the situation. These young people perceive that belonging to a group enhances their self-confidence so they seek peer recognition and approval. Many times teens have a sense of not belonging and feelings of being misunderstood. A feeling of mastery over the death is sought by believing that the teen can do anything. This is indicated by intense academic and social pursuits. These children may assume additional responsibilities in an effort to show that they are capable of self-protection.

The older adolescent, ages 17 to 21 years, operates from the cognitive principle that "I can trust." This idea is disrupted when they realize that the world is unpredictable and that they cannot protect their loved ones from death. They attempt to overcome this by investing in another person in order to gain affection and safety. The self-image of the adolescent may be threatened, and they may feel alone and isolated. They may experience a profound need for belonging in another's life. Their sense of justice may force an answer to the question, "Why"? Older adolescents may feel that they cannot risk or trust because of the threat of losing the other to death.

Development of Death Concepts

The question arises concerning when in the course of development a person develops the capacity to mourn the loss of a relationship. Some theorists speak of the "absence of grief" in children (Deutsch, 1937; Fleming & Altschul, 1963). Others advance the notion that mourning can be experienced early in childhood (Furman, 1964). Furman describes preconditions for mourning as including both a concept of death and object constancy, which are possible by age 4 years. Wolfenstein (1966) presents the view that mourning cannot occur until after the adolescent experience of separation from the parents. In other words, not until the young person has been forced to give up the parental love object and childhood past can true mourning occur.

Children learn about death through the regular course of life events and begin early to formulate a concept of death. Their understanding of death changes with developmental level, which generally corresponds with age.

Ages Birth to 5 years. A child under 2 years of age is often described as unaware of death. However, Maurer (1966) suggests that awareness of death begins at birth with the first physiologic struggles to obtain oxygen. Maurer contended that infant sleep/wake patterns and "peek-a-boo" games reflect infant awareness of states of existence and nonexistence.

For the young dying infant, the experience can be one of solitude if his or her developmental requirement for a consistently available, loving person, (intensified by the dying state) is not met. The infant under 4 months of age primarily experiences a life-threatening health state through overwhelming physical sensations (Caughill, 1976). During infancy (4 to 12 months) the baby progressively experiences dying as a fear of separation and a recognizable, hurtful sensation.

Since babies do not perceive time, the infant cannot conceive of the irreversibleness of death but rather equates it with abandonment: a sense of being left all alone. This infant's needs for a loving, consistent caregiver are paramount.

Intervention, whether by the nurse or ideally by the parents, should provide safety, trust, and comfort. Development should be kept as normal as possible through tactile, auditory, and visual stimulation without overstimulation.

The most valuable stimulation to the infant is touch. The ill infant needs the comfort offered by contact with caring persons and gentleness in feeding, holding, rocking, and cuddling. Sounds are part of the dying infant's environment. The baby should be spoken to before and during procedures. Anyone who ap-

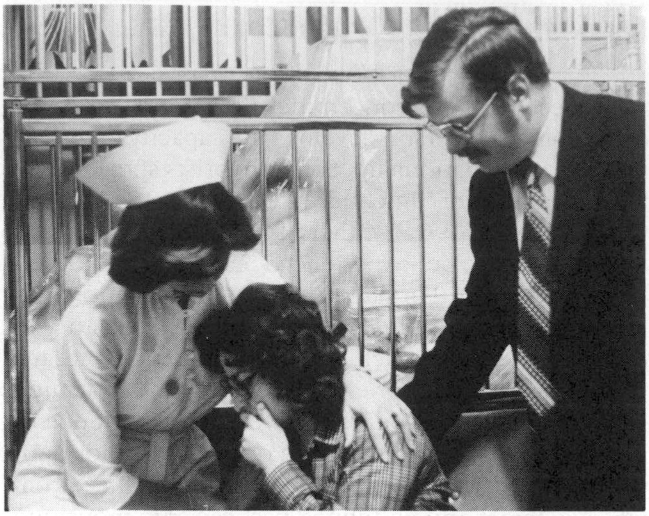

Just being near is often the most supportive nursing action for grieving parents.

proaches or provides care for the child should use soft, soothing, reassuring voice tones that will provide a sense of security. Tapes of parents' voices can have an especially calming effect during their absence or when the infant appears anxious or restless. Singing softly or playing a music box is appropriate. The visual stimulation given any other child of this age should also be available to the dying infant. *En face* positions help the infant establish relationships with caregivers, reducing the sense of being alone to die.

All these caring tasks may best be performed by the parents, who know and love the baby (or who may need to learn to know and love the infant before the death so that they can appropriately separate after the death). The nurse caring for the dying infant does not necessarily give direct care to the infant but rather helps the parents provide care. The nurse then reinforces their actions and decisions by teaching, counseling, and supporting them with verbal affirmation. Often parents are supported by the nurse's presence only.

Children between 3 and 5 years understand death as departure or sleep. They believe it is temporary and reversible (Nagy, 1948; Lonetto, 1980). Toddlers and preschoolers are egocentric, believing the world revolves around them. Because of this they are unable to differentiate self from the world or distinguish living fron nonliving. Children this age think the dead live on under new circumstances. They give life processes and thoughts to the dead. Death is associated with a lack of movement and with old age. Drawings of children aged 3 to 5 years show that they view death as male in gender (Lonetto, 1980). Preschoolers talk openly about death, indicating a lack of realization about its finality. They speak in fantasy about going to heaven on a cloud.

The course of a life-threatening illness is incongruent with all the landmarks young children are striving to achieve — autonomy, self-control, and initiative. As the illness progresses toward death, the 3- to 5-year-old exhibits discomfort, anxiety over separation, regression, and fear because of loss of control due to irregular routines and repeated traumatic experiences. The greatest need of dying toddlers and preschoolers is to be free from pain and fear of separation from their parents. It is the nurse's responsibility to relieve pain and to assure the presence of the child's parents if at all possible, or to provide for a consistent substitute if the parents are unavailable.

Ages 5 to 9 Years. Children this age think in terms of concrete perceptions. School-age children develop and reorganize their concept of death as they gain exposure to death and examine dead things. The dead fly on the windowsill, the dead plant, the squashed bug, the dead dog that was hit by a car in the road, the dead bird, the goldfish floating on its side on the top of a fish tank in the classroom all stimulate questions about death. They move gradually from understanding death as a reversible, temporary phenomenon to one of irreversibility and permanency. Schoolagers develop generalizations based on observable facts. They attribute specific characteristics to death and give it traits such as scary, dangerous, and mean. Death is associated with sadness and the old and ill. It comes in the night and snatches one away. Death is often identified with the dead object, not as a process. Children this age correctly relate biologic aspects of heart and lung activity with death. Diseases involving these organs may be particularly frightening to children and their families. They focus on concrete specifics of burial and graveyards. Death is frequently linked to external forces and violence. Comfort comes from physical closeness with familiar people and things and obeying the rules.

The nurse working with children this age may be faced with questions from the child about death — his or her own or that of others. General questions about death can be answered truthfully and directly. The nurse must recognize that unless the well-being of the child is in serious jeopardy the parents must make the decision to discuss death with a child with life-threatening illness. They are the most effective providers of support to the child. The child can be reached and helped through the parents. Often the decision clearly becomes one of what and when to tell rather than to tell or not to tell. It is quite clear, though, that "who should tell" is the parents. The nurse can assist the parents to know what and how to explain a terminal illness and death to their child. Many resources for explaining death to children are available. Pediatric

Box 26-2
Helpful Literature for Parents of Dying Children

L. Buscaglia: *Love.* Charles B. Slack Inc., 1982.

M. Colgrove, et al: *How to Survive the Loss of a Love.* Bantam Books, 1977.

W. Easson: *The Dying Child: The Management of the Child or Adolescent Who Is Dying.* Charles C Thomas, 1981.

E. Grollman: *Talking About Death: A Dialogue Between Parent and Child.* Beacon Press, 1976.

E.N. Jackson: *Telling a Child About Death.* (Hawthorn Books) Dutton, 1965.

N. Klein: *Sunshine.* Avon Books, 1982.

E. Kübler-Ross: *On Children and Death.* Macmillan, 1985.

Kübler-Ross: *Questions and Answers on Death and Dying.* MacMillan, 1974.

D. Lund: *Eric.* Dell Books, 1976.

J. Morris: *Brian Piccolo: A Short Season.* Dell Books, 1972.

D. Evans Rogers: *Angel Unaware.* Jove Publications, 1984.

E. Valens: *The Other Side of the Mountain.* Warner Publishing, 1975; Part 2, 1978.

units and clinics can maintain a supply of these materials for this purpose (Box 26-2).

The choice that most often proves harmful to the relationships within the family is maintaining the conspiracy of silence. This occurs if the family does not talk with the child at all about the reason for hospitalizations, treatments, or tests. During this process the seriously ill child easily misinterprets what is happening and why it is happening and does not have the opportunity to validate perceptions or clarify the reasons for what is happening to his or her body and physical abilities. However, if the family relationship prior to the diagnosis of a terminal illness was fraught with difficulties and stresses, it is unlikely that during this highly stressful time the family will begin to communicate clearly. In fact, the added stresses may provide the stimulus for family disintegration.

Ages 10 to 12 Years. By age 10 years, the child views death as inevitable and universal (Anthony, 1940; Nagy, 1948; Safier, 1964). It is a lawful process that happens to all living things. And, it is final. Children at this age reflect feelings of sadness, loneliness, and fear related to death (Maurer, 1966; McCown, 1970). Death becomes associated with pain as well as disease. Drawings of children between 9 and 12 years of age demonstrate progression of thought by the use of symbols, colors (black and purple), and details.

Adolescence. The teenager experiences marked physical and emotional changes; these periods of rapid change are often times of vulnerability to fears and loss. Fears of death are especially acute for teens (Alexander and Alderstein, 1958). Adolescents live in the present and future, which contributes to the impact of death as a forth-coming event. They go to extremes to challenge their fears by feats of bravado and daring. Like adults, teens understand death as a final, universal, and personal experience.

Dying adolescents fully understand what is happening to them. They struggle to find ways to accept the process. The experience of dying for teenagers is completely incongruent with all they find important —physical appearance and prowess is replaced by dysfunction and weakness. Adolescents may react to a terminal illness with extreme anger, which drives away those they need most.

The nurse needs to recognize that overt behaviors often are not a true expression of the adolescent's needs. The nurse can encourage family and friends to maintain a supportive relationship with the teen. Peer relationships among hospitalized youth can be facilitated for mutual support and understanding. The nurse needs to allow time to just sit quietly and talk with the teenager. The dying young person needs time and a trusting atmosphere that will allow facing the fact that death is happening.

The dying adolescent needs to be treated as autonomously as possible, since she or he is usually struggling to remain as independent as possible during this period of high stress. Noncompliance may be viewed as an attempt to control self-care or as an attempt to deny the seriousness of the condition. Patience and support must be provided during this time. Parents also may be feeling a great deal of ambiguity as they try to support the independence of the adolescent and also do "what is best." They may feel extreme frustration in trying to reach both these goals. Information about the disease process, treatment plans and rationale, and prognosis is essential to the adolescent at this time. The realities of the situation must be made explicit so that informed decisions about care and self-care may be made. Some parents take on the role of decision maker at this time. They become overprotective and actually set limits to the behavior that they consider acceptable. Many adolescents need the security that these parameters provide, whereas others need to be able to make their own decisions regarding the quality and length of their lives.

Adolescents may find that they sometimes need to become dependent upon their parents again, and they may be very angry, even enraged, at the injustice, asking "Why me?" and declaring "It isn't fair." The nurse

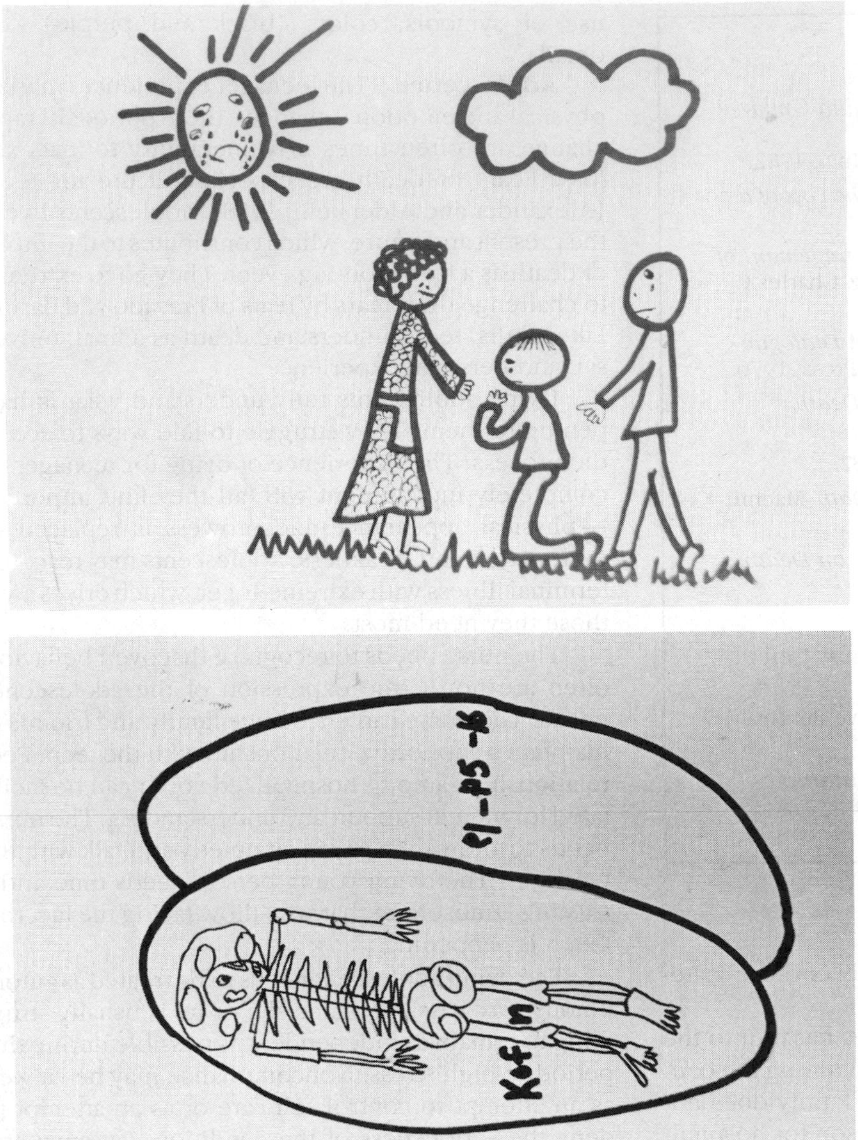

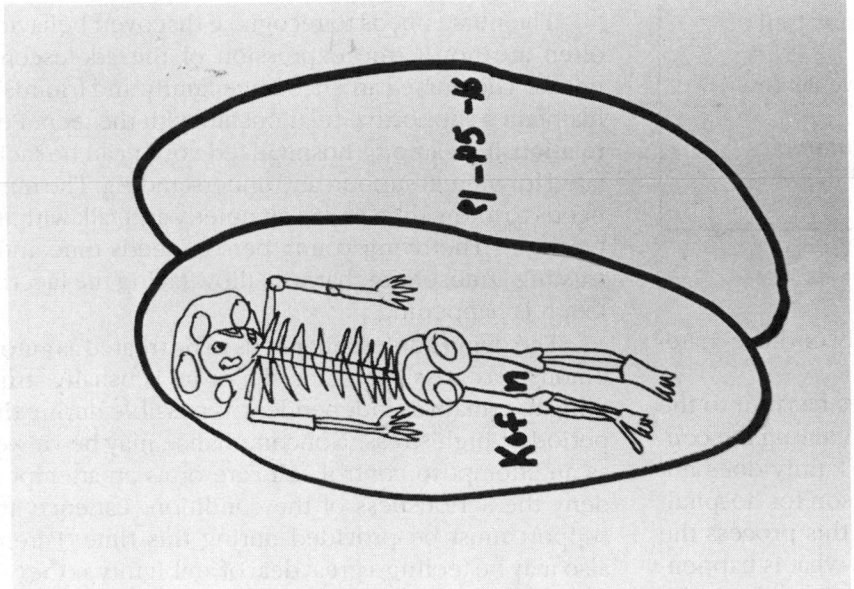

A

B

A, "A little boy dying on his front lawn—his mother and father are watching over him. They are sad. The sun is sad, too." *B*, "This is somebody dead." The school-age child is intrigued with the process of dying and with death. The two pictures illustrate a school-age child's concept of death.

can assist the adolescent and family to accept the somewhat unpredictable expressions of anger that are usually projected toward the staff and parents. By identifying the normality of the behavior under the circumstances, the nurse provides support to the family unit. The nurse can also provide opportunities for the adolescent to make decisions about self-care. The nurse can deliberately ask for the youth's opinions, suggestions, preferences, or choices, and, whenever possible, these choices and preferences should be honored, thereby assisting the dying adolescent in the quest for independence and self-respect.

With the advanced modalities available for treating young children with life-threatening illnesses, there is an increased likelihood that these children will survive to adolescence. Consequently, the nurse will sometimes need to help such adolescents cope with impending death. The death of adolescents or young adults affects all who have come in contact with them. Their zest for living and their wonderment at accomplishment are unmatched at any other stage of development. It is difficult to see such lives shortened by fatal illness, but it is sometimes awesome to see the courage with which they confront death.

Explaining Death to Children

Few guidelines are available to parents for discussing death with their dying child. The nurse has an obligation, however, to help parents become aware of the aids that do exist. Parents should be encouraged to begin by evaluating their own feelings about death. This introspection helps them know and understand

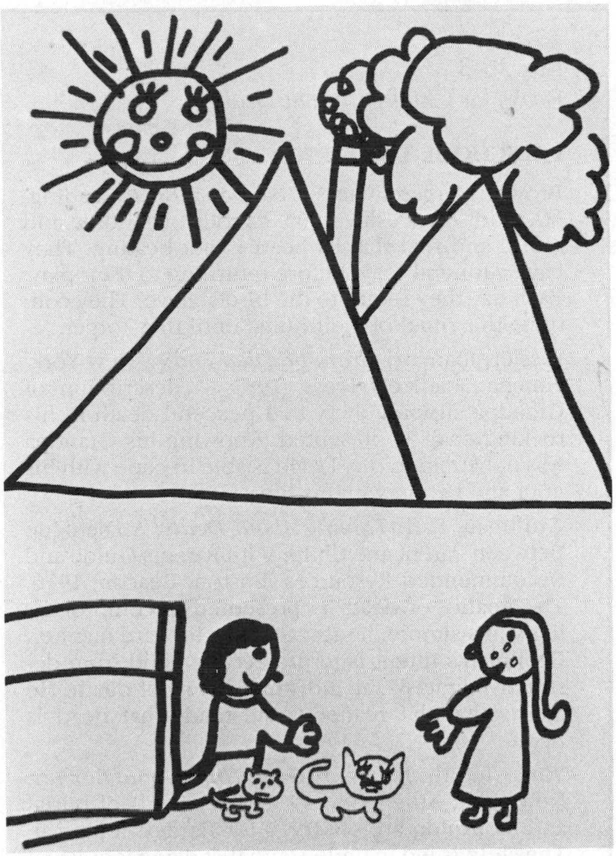

C

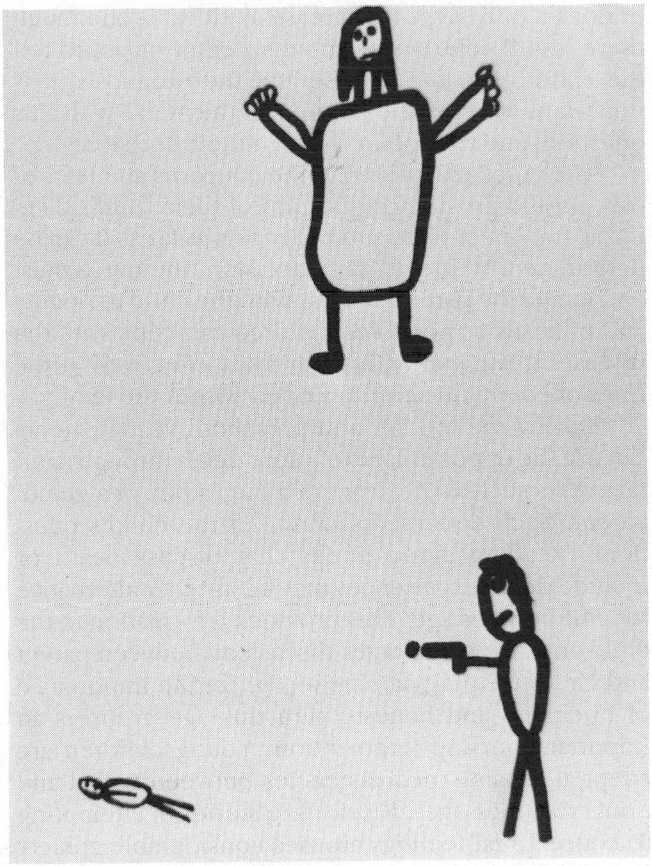

D

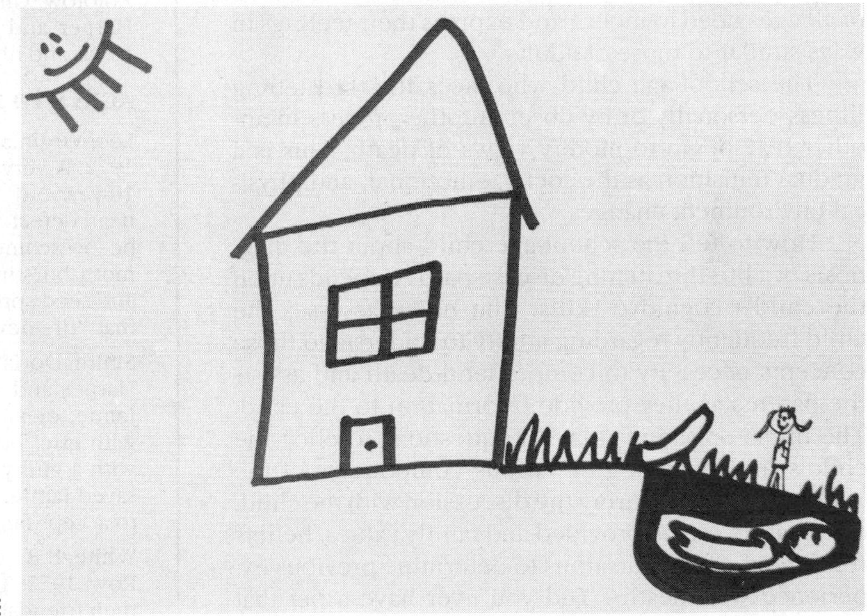

E

C, "This is when my kitten died. Mrs. Jones from next door came over to help the cat have her babies and I was sick that day. The baby kittens died because the mother cat had an infection in her tummy and if we didn't take her to the doctor she would have died." *D*, "This guy shot him and that's God up there." The school age child perceives the causes of death to include accidents, violence, illness or pain. *E*, "The little girl was digging a hole with her shovel and she buried her grandpa and she's first praying and then she's going back to her house. She's supposed to be kneeling." The school-age child concludes from experience that death comes to animals and old people.

their own feelings and fears before dealing with their child's concept and emotions. Personal beliefs, religious convictions, cultural background, and comfort with the topic will influence the parents' responses to the dying child and to questions. The ultimate decision of what to tell the child must be left up to the parents. Because adults tend to protect and shelter children from knowledge of or experiences with death, the decision concerning sharing information about the diagnosis of a life-threatening disease with a child is a major task for most parents. Authorities disagree on whether or not the knowledge of having a terminal illness in fact changes the child's concept of death—does it accelerate conceptual development, or does it only serve to increase anxiety? Even though there is still controversy about whether or not to tell the child about the disease and the prognosis, it is important to assist the parents as they deal with this question, and to support them in their decision.

The nurse must listen to the concerns and fears of parents and provide clarification of their child's diagnosis, treatment plan, and prognosis as far as it can be determined. Whatever their decision, the nurse must encourage the parents to deal with the child as openly and honestly as possible. Children can cope with the disease, treatment, and death most effectively if the lines of communication are open within the family.

During the toddler and preschool years, parents can use the opportunity to explore death through natural events such as the death of a bug, a pet, or a grandparent. Such discussions draw out the child's questions. Reading aloud books that discuss death or include death experiences may be another alternative for children this age. This provides information to the child and also encourages discussion between parent and child. Helping parents recognize the importance of openness and honesty with this age group is an important nursing intervention. Young children are adept at sensing inconsistencies between verbal and nonverbal messages. Fabricating stories or attempting to conceal real feelings arouses considerable anxiety in toddlers and threatens the child's sense of security. Parents should also be helped to realize that children of all ages need to mourn and express their feelings in ways similar to those of adults.

The school-age child who faces life-threatening illness personally or by observing the process in another may begin to modify views of death. This is a gradual transition as the social, emotional, and physical environment changes.

How to tell the school-age child about the diagnosis of a life-threatening disease partly depends upon the child's cognitive skills. The nurse assesses the child frequently regarding ability to understand those concepts necessary to comprehend death and assists the parents as they provide information to the child. The nurse or parents may use questions to elicit the child's understanding of various components of the concept of death. During the discussion with the child, clarification can be provided and family values/beliefs reinforced. Some questions to determine previous experience with death: "Did you ever have a pet that died?" "Did you ever know a person who died?"

At times, children's perceptions about a previous experience with death may differ from those of parents. Often parents assume that the child was too young to remember when a friend, family member, or pet died. Some children assume that someone is dead who has not been seen or heard from. One young school-age child, for example, was asked in a Den-

Box 26-3
Books for Children About Death

PRESCHOOL TO AGE 7 YEARS

Brown, Margaret Wise: *The Dead Bird.* Reading, MA, Addison-Wesley, 1965. A group of children find a bird and feel that its heart is not beating. They have a funeral for it before returning to their play. Each day they return to the bird's grave. They continue this ritual of mourning "until they forget."

Fassler, Joan: *My Grandpa Died Today.* New York, Human Science's Press, 1983. A description of Grandpa slipping away to a peaceful death in his rocking chair is presented. Knowing his Grandpa was not afraid to die, David is able to cope with his grief and get on with his life.

Grollman, Earl: *Talking About Death:* A Dialogue Between Parent and Child; With Parents Guide and Recommended Resources. Boston, Beacon, 1976. The finality of death is presented uncompromisingly in a simple, honest, straight-forward manner. Grollman's intent is to protect the child from destructive fantasy and a distorted view of death. He insists that the reader understands that dead is *dead.*

Viorst, Judith: *The Tenth Good Thing About Barney.* New York, Atheneum, 1971. The rituals of burial and mourning are observed for Barney, a pet cat. The child is led to understand that dying is as usual as living. Death is a part of life.

Zolotow, Charlotte: *My Grandson Lew.* New York, Harper and Row, 1974. Remembrances between Lewis and his mother, making them a little less sad.

AGES 8 TO 11 YEARS

Lee, Virginia: *The Magic Moth.* New York, Seabury, 1972. A very supportive family bravely copes with 10-year-old Maryanne's illness and death from a heart defect. The story tells the problems that had to be overcome for the family to work together. A moth bursting from its cocoon as Maryanne dies and seed sprouting just after her funeral symbolize that "life never ends—it just changes."

Smith, Doris B.: *A Taste of Blackberries.* New York, Harper and Row, 1973. A little boy's best friend, Jamie, dies of a bee sting. The boy is confronted with grief because of the loss and comes to terms with a guilty feeling that somehow he might have saved Jamie. After a period of grief, the boy comes to accept Jamie's death.

White, E.B.: *Charlotte's Web.* New York, Harper and Row, 1952. This is a story about a pig and a rat and their friendship with Charlotte, a spider. Charlotte's death and the birth of her child depict the life cycle. A classic.

AGE 12 AND OVER

Gunther, John: *Death Be Not Proud* (Memorial edition). New York, Harper, 1971. The author writes of the courage of his 17-year-old son while facing death. It is more difficult for his parents than for Johnnie to accept his death.

Hunter, Mollie: *A Sound of Chariots.* New York, Harper, 1972. Bridie McShane's happy early childhood during World War I in Scotland is interrupted by the death of her beloved father. As she matures, her life is marred by her sorrow, leading her to morbid reflections on time and death, which she finally learns to deal with through her desire to write poetry.

Zindel, B., and Zindel P.: *A Star for the Latecomer.* New York, Harper and Row, 1980. A story about a teenager whose mother has advanced bone cancer. The daughter tries to become a star in a theatrical career before her mother dies.

ver Developmental Screening Test (DDST) to complete the analogy "Mother is a woman, Dad is a ________." After a few moments of thought, the child answered "soul." The mother was very shocked since the father was not dead, but the parents had been separated for a year and a half. The perception could then be clarified. Questions to help determine the child's knowledge of death include: "What happens after something dies?" "Does it hurt to die?" "What do people do after they die?" Misconceptions about death can then be corrected depending on the child's responses.

A list of children's books by age group that present concepts of death is given in Box 26-3.

The Family Response to Impending Death of a Child

The death of a child in our society is untimely and out of step with the usual cycle of life. Most families have not experienced such an event and are unprepared to deal with it. Significant others are also at a loss to offer help and support during a child's terminal illness. The process of events usually begins abruptly, perhaps an accident or sudden recognition of signs of ill health in the child. The child is taken to the doctor, who makes a tentative diagnosis, followed by clarifying diagnostic tests and often hospitalization of the child. Frequently another doctor or specialist joins the medical team to provide consultation and a second opinion. By this time the parents have a dread awareness of a serious threat to their child's life.

To understand fully the reactions of various family members to a child's life-threatening illness and impending death, often it is necessary to explore the child's uniqueness to the family unit. The way a child is perceived and appreciated by the family may indirectly affect the attention and care he or she receives from them during the course of illness. Factors that influence a child's status within a family include the events surrounding birth and delivery, birth order, ages of other children, parents' relationship, economic situation at home, and how easy the child is to nurture and love. Insights into the dynamics of the parent-child relationship will help in understanding the meaning the child's death has for parents and siblings (Codden, 1977).

Parental Response

If the final diagnosis forecasts a poor prognosis and a threat to life, the parents may respond with shock and denial in the first stages of anticipatory grieving. The nurse helps them by providing them with a private place to recover from the impact of the terrible news and stays with them and participates as the health care team together answers their questions about the diagnosis and plan of care. Attitudes of warmth and concern and competence in providing the necessary care are important in helping families cope with the situation. Parents also may need assistance to seek out supportive friends and family who can be with them during this difficult time.

Some expression of anger, hostility, and guilt may be expected. Such feelings may be directed at the nurse but should not be taken personally. Parents may need the help of nurses and other professionals to verbalize these feelings. As parents and older children become interested in the illness, they seek information and details about it. Parents will feel saddened as the information obtained indicates a poor prognosis and the likelihood of death. The nurse needs to recognize that the strong emotions of anger, hostility, fear, guilt, and anxiety experienced by the parents may cause a change in the parenting style with both their ill and well children. Parents can be helped to understand their own behavior and be supported in their attempt to maintain their usual patterns of child care.

Guilt is a common feeling experienced by parents of dying children. One study reported that one third of their families experienced guilt feelings (Stehbens and Lascari, 1974). Parents often try to recall minor symptoms of the child that they overlooked and blame themselves for not seeking care sooner. They reflect on earlier events, even the pregnancy, searching for reasons for their child's illness. Guilt may result in blaming one's spouse or overindulging the ill child. Goldberg (1973) gives several reasons why parents may experience guilt after the child is dead: (1) an ambivalent relationship while the child was alive, marked by hostility; (2) a previous desire for the child's death; (3) feelings of anger at the deceased for dying; (4) a wish that more had been given of oneself while the child was living.

Caring for an ill child at home demands extra time, energy, and resources from the family members. Hospitalization brings the additional time and energy drain of staying or visiting with the ill child. Meanwhile the remaining family members and home must also be cared for. An increased work load added to immense anxiety, possible guilt, and depression contribute to a severe crisis for the parents. It seems reasonable to expect that these parents would have little energy left to spend on their well children or each other.

Parents may cater to or overindulge the child to maintain a role in the child's life and relieve their own guilt and sadness. Fear of separation surfaces and the parents may actually cling to their child. When a child is dying, the mother's perceptions of the child's needs may be altered. In a study of 21 children and their mothers, dying children's self-perceived needs for affection, control, and inclusion were examined (Natterson and Knudson, 1960). The researchers also studied the mothers' awareness of the children's needs. Children with life-threatening illnesses wanted additional affection but were unable to express this desire directly, and mothers of dying children tended not to perceive their child's needs accurately. At a time when children need understanding to help overcome the great losses they are experiencing, mothers may be unable to perceive accurately the needs. Nurses can point out clues the child gives and suggest ways to meet the child's needs, such as holding, gentle touching, rubbing, and talking softly to their child.

Role Adjustments

When a child is diagnosed to have a life-threatening condition, health care personnel are granted authority in the life of the child because of their knowledge and expertise. Even the ill child transfers authority to the medical staff. Parents may feel they are losing control of their child and their parental role. Relinquishment of their parental role may explain parenting behaviors frequently observed such as lack of discipline, permissiveness, and even neglect.

Fathers and mothers do not react to their child's illness and death in the same way. Parents may experience the process of mourning differently and sense a lack of support and understanding from each other. This has been labeled the "isolated wife" syndrome. The child's mother often feels she carries the whole burden of the illness. Such feelings place a stress on the marital relationship and the parents need to make a special effort to spend time together and each alone with the ill child to maintain relationships.

Caring for a terminally ill child demands tremendous energy and results in parental fatigue, which further compromises their relationship. They need assistance from supportive friends and relatives and are encouraged to plan time away from the demands of the situation. The stress placed on families requires altered patterns of living and a shift in expectations. The illness causes many changes, ranging from financial problems to changes in social status because of increased social isolation. Problems with siblings generally arise because of the time factor associated with the illness. The well sibling's perception of the mother as having limited time leads to feelings of hostility and rejection, especially when there is poor understanding of the child's illness.

Extended Family

During severe stress parents may need the help and emotional support of the grandparents. Friedman and associates (1963) found, in a 2-year study of 46 parents of children with cancer, that grandparents tended to be less accepting of the diagnosis than the parents. Reasons for grandparent difficulty with the dying child may be a fear of their own impending death; they may also feel guilty that it is not they who are facing death but the child; they may be blaming their daughter or son for the child's ill health. All these emotions can interfere with their ability to support and help the adult children cope with the crisis of a child's death.

Dying Child's Response

The dying child's reaction to the illness is influenced by the developmental stage of the child. Children's major concerns vary with age. The child prior to 5 years of age fears separation from the parent. A child 5 to 10 years old fears traumatic procedures, whereas children over 10 years of age fear death itself.

Illness and physical degeneration are a paradox for the growing, developing child. The children's limited awareness of life itself makes them vulnerable to anger and resentment toward their parents for allowing them to hurt and suffer. These feelings have been reflected in a play situation in which dying children placed distance between themselves and their families (Bluebond-Langer, 1978). The child's anger toward the parent and others or withdrawal from or clinging to the parent contributes to difficult parent-child relationships. The loss of physical function, the increased dependency, and regression of the dying child further compromises the relationship because of the tendency of parents to overprotect and indulge their child at this stage.

Research has demonstrated that dying children are aware of their fatal illnesses (Waechter, 1971; Bluebond-Langer, 1978). Indications of the child's awareness of the terminal illness include a lack of interest in the future, fears of being at home, and a desire to be in the hospital, decreased conversations about drugs, and comments about others who have died (Bluebond-Langer, 1978). Parents need help to recognize these behaviors and need support from the nurse to establish open communication with their child to allow for exchange of love and concern and expression of fears and anxieties.

Sibling Response

Siblings of dying children may exhibit behavior problems such as crying, school problems, somatic complaints, nightmares, death fears, enuresis, depression, excessive talking, and antisocial behavior. Recent research using standardized measures of behavior problems indicates that about one fourth of the siblings of deceased children have "disturbed" behavior following the death. Both boys and girls seem to be equally affected (McCown, 1987).

Qualitative research by Kramer (1987) of 11 healthy siblings of children dying of cancer revealed both negative and positive responses. The negative impact on the siblings resulted from three primary sources of stress: emotional realignment within the family, separation from family members, and disruptions caused by the ill child's therapeutic regimen. Emotional deprivation, decreased parental tolerance, and increased parental expectations contributed to emotional realignment. Lack of information, decreased family involvement, and insufficient social support resulted in feelings of separation. Watching the ill child's physical and personality changes, seeing the anxiety and pain, and adjusting to changes in family routine contributed to the negative impact of the therapeutic regimen. Positive aspects for surviving siblings included increased sensitivity and empathy for the ill child, personal maturation, and an increase in family cohesion.

Helping Siblings Cope with Life-Threatening Illness

The nurse working with dying children assesses and discusses with parents their responsibilities to their other children to promote healthy relationships for all family members to return to after the child has died. Stressing that the quality of time spent with their children is more significant than quantity may alleviate the guilt parents experience in trying to divide their attention and time equally among the children. The nurse encourages parents to be honest and open with their children, reassuring them of their love. Parents are made aware that the siblings may be fearful of having wished the child ill or dead, or of becoming sick like their sibling. Expression of these fears should be encouraged through open communication with the parents.

After the death, siblings may also need help with the ongoing hostility they feel toward the dead child who took so much time from their parents. To dissipate this hostility, siblings may need to talk to parents, the nurse, or counselors about it. They need to be reassured that this hostility and these feelings are normal and that they are not bad for feeling them.

The deceased child's toys, books, and clothing may be shared with surviving siblings. Young children (those with the concept of the reversibility of death) may be afraid that the deceased child will return to reclaim the toys. Parents may need help understanding that the sibling's concern is characteristic of a young child's way of thinking about death.

Siblings may need time to think about what has happened with the family. They may need reassurance that they will not also die of the disease that has claimed brother or sister (unless, of course, they also have a genetically caused disease). If this is the case, special follow-up help will be needed as the children prepare for their own life and death.

The interactions of parents with siblings may change after the death of one child. They may become overprotective of the surviving children. The sadness that they feel is of a different nature than the sadness of the siblings. Parents may mourn well beyond the time that siblings are actively mourning, and unconscious anger may develop toward the siblings.

The Nurse's Role in Assisting the Family to Cope with Terminal Illness

Helping the Family Cope with the Length of the Illness. The parents' grief reaction and pattern of adaptation will depend a great deal on the course of illness. If the death of their child is sudden and unexpected, a variety of shock responses can be anticipated, ranging from immobilization or hysteria to complete control of the situation. Although their reactions vary, it is clear that family members do not fully comprehend what is communicated during this shock stage. Once the shock begins to diminish they have a strong need to communicate their feelings regarding what has happened. The nurse may be the only person available to help the grievers work through their feelings and thoughts about what has occurred. Because they have not had time to prepare for the death, they are deprived of the advantages of anticipatory grief. They also may feel great remorse or guilt for not having done things differently for their child. The nurse may be able to comfort them physically and psychologically through touch, active listening, or providing a comfortable, private place for the family to grieve.

If the death is not immediate but the child lingers

days or weeks, family members may begin their anticipatory grief work, if they have accepted the diagnosis and are encouraged to mourn. On the other hand, a long-term life-threatening illness brings additional stresses, such as relapses and repeated hospitalizations. Parents not only have to live with the uncertainty of the future but also provide care for the child while they are actively mourning the expected death.

Several strategies are effective with these parents to direct their grief into constructive actions. One is to encourage parents whose children have the same medical problems or prognosis to meet in groups. Within the group, reactions, fears, and feelings are shared with others who have experienced or are experiencing them. Another is to involve parents in the care and planning of their child's treatment. Mothers may be more willing to enter into these activities, but the most benefit accrues when both parents are involved in the care. When parents are a part of the plan, their anxiety, guilt, or anger subsides; they usually become more cooperative, outgoing, and accepting of the treatment. Parents' wishes and desires regarding the care of their child should be respected; they should be allowed to take part in determining whether certain treatments should be continued if there is little hope for improvement. Parents need to be given the option to take the child home to die if they feel no cure is possible. If they do, they are informed about possible problems (pain, incontinence) or complications they may experience at home and are assured that someone will be available if help is needed.

During this time the nurse begins to prepare the family to deal with the reactions of surviving children. Childhood Death Awareness Inventory (Box 26-4)

Box 26-4
Childhood Death Awareness Inventory

Family Name__________ Date__________

Address__________

Child's Name__________

Age__________

Name of Deceased__________

Age__________

Relationship to Child__________

Date of Death__________

I. ***Child's Experience with Death***

What experiences has the child had with death?

a. Pet(s)__________ Date of death__________

Child's reaction and comments:

____

____

b. Distant relative__________ Date of death__________

Name__________

Relationship__________

Child's reaction and comments:

____

____

c. Close relative__________ Date of death__________

Name__________

Relationship__________

Child's reaction and comments:

____

____

d. Friends____________________ Date of death____________________

Name____________________

Relationship____________________

Child's reaction and comments:

____

____

e. Community (teacher, pastor, schoolmates)

Name____________________ Date of death____________________

Relationship____________________

Child's reaction and comments:

____

____

II. *Rituals of Death*

a. Has the child seen a dead person? Yes__ No__

b. Has the child seen a dead animal? Yes__ No__

c. Has the child attended a funeral or memorial service? Yes__ No__

d. Has the child visited a cemetery? Yes__ No__

III. *Beliefs about Death*

a. What beliefs about death are held by the child?

____

____

____

b. What beliefs about death are held by the family?

____

____

____

c. Is the child familiar with the church (synagogue) building? Yes__ No__

IV. *Explanation of Death*

a. What has the child been told about the (possible) death?

____

____

b. What has the child been told about the disposal of the body?

____

____

c. What has the child been told about the final services (funeral, memorial service)?

____

____

V. *Expected Reaction*

How do you expect (child) to respond to the loss?

____

____

Continued

b. What adjustments will be difficult for the child?

____

____

VI. *Supportive Measures*

a. What actions will comfort your child?

____

____

b. Who are the people who can help your child? Have you notified them of the possible death/death?

____

____

c. What literature have you read about death and grief?

____

d. What questions do you have about your child and death?

____

____

(From McCown, 1988.)

may help the parents focus on and recognize their well children's level of understanding about death and possible responses to it. Using the information gathered on the inventory, the nurse can discuss with the parents methods for explaining the situation to the well children.

Decision to Discontinue Treatment. At some point the physicians caring for a child with a life-threatening illness may suggest discontinuation of treatment based upon the lack of response to medical therapy. This decision is made in conjunction with the family. There may also come a time when the family reaches this decision before the physician mentions it. The family may request no further treatment so as to avoid further pain, frustration, or stress for their child. This decision is actually a statement that the family is giving up hope for survival—an acceptance of death as an inevitable end. It is also based on the realization that the child is not responding to treatment.

This is always a difficult decision for the family and for the health team. Respect for the quality of the child's remaining life must be the basis of the decision. Ultimately, the choice must be the family's. The nurse can be supportive to the family during this difficult decision-making time by helping them clarify their own thoughts and feel comfortable in their decision.

Decision on Alternative Environments for Terminal Care. The option of receiving supportive care and symptom management care in a hospital or in the home should be discussed with the family. Most communities have community-based programs or hospice groups to provide home care for dying children and adults. The hospice concept is that when the goal of curing cannot be realized, appropriate places other than the traditional hospitals can provide vital care during this critical time. Some cities provide hospice care to families of dying children by providing space within their hospitals; others set special places aside, such as an extended care facility. Some hospice programs are essentially home care programs. Many public health nurses are currently providing support to parents who are caring for their dying children in their own homes. Allowing a child to die in the home allows the family to design and control the environment. It allows them to parent their child when needed the most.

Criteria developed by Martinson and colleagues (1980) for the choice of home care include:

- Cure-oriented treatment has been discontinued.
- The child wants to be at home.
- The parents desire to have the child at home.
- The parents recognize their own ability to care for their ill child; the fact that they can care for the child until death is frequently not recognized until later.
- The nurse is willing to be available 24 hours a day to facilitate care.
- The child's physician is willing to be an on-call consultant.

Making the decision to care for the dying child at home is extremely difficult. During the dying process the parents may sometimes feel inept at providing the best care possible; they may wonder about their decision and may feel guilty that their child is not in the hospital. Inability to relieve pain is often a major reason why parents feel they cannot care for their child in the home, but with proper instruction and support pain management can be achieved without much difficulty. Medications for the relief of pain, either in oral, rectal, or parenteral form, can be provided to the family.

Helping Families Cope During the Final Stages of Illness. At this time some families may begin to redirect their energies away from the child, whereas others will continue to hold onto the child until the final breath. In either case, their fears of death and pain are overwhelming. Often the greatest fear is that their child is experiencing pain. Although the child may appear comfortable, it is important to understand that the parents' anxiety may also reflect their sense of inevitable loss. Providing the child maximal comfort and relief of pain during this period is critical. (See Chapter 29 for a discussion of pain management in children.)

Maintaining adequate nutrition leads to increased energy levels and improved physical appearance, which contribute to a sense of well-being in the ill child and family. Ill children who are dying should be allowed to eat whatever they desire. Special attention to diet may be needed to ensure comfort in regard to intake.

Nausea, vomiting, and *fullness,* are frequently associated with the terminal process and the treatment, especially if the child receives chemotherapy and radiation. Between one half and three fourths of cancer patients report nausea and vomiting. Outpatients report less vomiting, only about one fourth (Grant, 1982). Nausea and vomiting may result from obstruction of the digestive tract from physical defects or tumor, or from imbalances in body fluids and electrolytes. The combination of nausea and vomiting is a common side effect of the drugs used to control many chronic diseases.

Nausea and vomiting can be treated in part by diet. Dry foods such as crackers, plain cookies, or toast decrease nausea, especially in the morning. Avoid fried or greasy foods. Cold, clear liquids are easier to retain. Offer the child frequent small quantities of food. Avoid too much food in the stomach at one time by reducing liquids at mealtime and offering them an hour before or after meals. Have the child lie down or sit quietly after meals to aid the digestive process.

In addition to diet, medications are available to relieve nausea and vomiting. Antiemetics, such as one of the phenothiazines, can be useful and can be given rectally as well as orally. There is some support of the use of delta-9-tetrahydrocannabinol (THc), the antiemetic potion, or marijuana, for use in children for whom phenothiazines are ineffective. The doctor can prescribe these medications if needed.

Anorexia is loss of the desire for eating, often experienced by seriously ill persons. Decreased appetite may be related to by products (lactic acid) produced by the tumor cells (Grant, 1982). It may also be caused by alterations in smell and taste mechanisms. Food may become associated with the unpleasantness of nausea and vomiting resulting from drugs and disease. Lack of appetite may occur from decreased activity levels and general depression of mood, or an alteration in taste sensation.

Some people with cancer find protein foods bitter to the taste, but its ingestion should be encouraged for nutritional requirements. A metallic taste may be experienced by those on medications or chemotherapy. The taste of foods can be enhanced by adding seasonings like lemon, salt, sugar, spices, and herbs. Protein intake may be encouraged by serving the food cold or at room temperature. Cheese, luncheon meats, eggs, and puddings are easily served cold and are palatable to children. Marinating meats in fruit juices may also help. Providing small meals frequently, varying the type of food, serving it in "fun" ways—clown faces and animal shapes—all may increase nutritional intake for children.

High-calorie, high-protein *nutritional supplements* are available to increase the child's daily intake. Fruit flavors and chocolate are preferred by children. They taste better cold. These supplements, such as Instant Breakfast, Sustocal, or Ensure, are easy to prepare but tend to be filling. The preparations can be enhanced by the addition of eggs or yogurt. Recipes for using supplements are available from the manufacturers of the products.

Vitamins may be added to the child's diet. If the child is on methotrexate, vitamins without folic acid should be used. The physician will provide instruction regarding supplemental vitamins. The ethical implications of possibly prolonging a dying child's suffering by adding supplements to the diet need to be explored with the family and physician.

Constipation is inability to evacuate the bowel or difficulty in passing stool. Ill children are at high risk for constipation due to disease process, muscle weakness, decreased activity levels, medications, and diets low in fluids and fiber. Normal bowel patterns vary widely and range between three stools per day to three stools per week (Cimpich, 1982).

Management of constipation in the seriously ill child is best achieved by preventive interventions. Maintaining a diet sufficient in fluids and fibers and encouraging activity and regular toilet patterns assist in passing a stool. This is especially difficult in anorexic young children. Oral stool-softening agents such as dioctyl sodium sulfocuccinate may be useful to keep the consistency of the stool soft enough for defecation. Glycerin suppositories may also aid stool passage by mechanical action. Chemical laxatives and enemas should be judiciously used and confirmed with the attending physician.

Anemia is a frequent problem for dying children, especially those with cancer. It may be caused by loss of blood, destruction of red blood cells by medications, and decreased production of red blood cells by the disease or treatment processes.

A diet high in iron and proteins is one measure that can be instituted at home. Often, however, blood transfusions are needed to increase the child's hemoglobin and hematocrit to normal levels. A child who is anemic will also experience fatigue, decreased energy, lethargy, and irritability.

Terminal Phase. The parents of a dying child need information about the events leading to death so they can be prepared for the final moments. Many times exhausted parents, not realizing the immediacy of the death, have gone home to rest or out to eat when the event occurred. It is difficult for nurses and doctors to predict the exact time of death but certain signs usually precede it (Birenbaum et al, 1986). One sign of death in children is a change in normal respirations to a Cheyne-Stokes pattern. Dying children often become less alert, and periods of wakefulness decrease. They may be difficult to arouse; their eyes are glazed and may roll back. The child's skin color becomes poor, often mottled, and cool to touch. Muscle tone decreases and the child may become incontinent. Hearing is one of the last senses to fade, so the child may be comforted by hearing the parents' voices. Semicomatose dying children have been observed orienting to the mother's or father's voice in the final hours of life. If possible, parents should be encouraged to stay and comfort their child until the time of death.

Organ and Tissue Procurement. Recent years have brought dramatic improvements in the success of organ transplantation. As these changes take place, the nurse's responsibility with the family of a dying child also changes. It is important for nurses to keep abreast of the federal and state laws that affect practice and that the appropriate educational opportunities be provided to prepare nurses for these new responsibilities.

As the technology for organ transplantation advances, there is an urgent need for organs; the organs needed far outnumber those made available. The United States government has responded to the pressing need for transplantable organs by establishing a Department of Health and Human Services Task Force on Organ Transplantation. This task force placed responsibility on the entire health care team and hospital administration to be aware of the question of organ donation (Report of the Task Force on Organ Transplantation, 1986). By October, 1986, 28 states had enacted laws dealing with procurement of organs. Federal legislation in October, 1987, amended previous legislation and mandated that all hospitals have in place protocols that deal with organ transplantation and tissue procurement. State statutes vary; some *require* a request for organ donation from family members of all patients pronounced "brain dead," whereas others require that hospitals notify local organ procurement agencies of any potential organ donors.

Enactment of laws concerning organ and tissue procurement has created ethical dilemmas and imposes a difficult responsibility on nurses. As these laws go into effect, nurses will be increasingly involved in dealing with families regarding the sensitive issue of organ and tissue donation. Nurses are often the best known team member to families because they have spent the most time with them during their child's illness and hospitalization. Although it is a difficult task to approach a family about organ donation, it is known that parents who agree to donate their child's organ may have their own grief lessened by helping another child (Frauman and Miles, 1987).

As organ donation becomes more widespread, the need for organs will continue to increase. Areas in which the nurse needs educational opportunities include brain death criteria (Drake and Schneider, 1986; Volpe, 1987; American Academy of Pediatrics, 1987), the specific responsibilities of the nurse (Hazinski, 1987), statutes that regulate organ donation, and a forum in which to discuss ethical issues related to organ procurement and donation (Bouressa and O'Mara, 1987). A publication that reviews state-by-state legislation is updated annually,* and government information can be obtained from the Office of Organ Transplantation.†

After Death. After the death, the body must be cared for. The body should be cleaned, carefully positioned, and covered with a blanket for viewing and goodbyes. The parents may assist in the preparations if they wish. It is a difficult time for both the parents and the nurse. It is appropriate for the nurse to express emotion and share feelings of sorrow with the family. However, total loss of control by the nurse would add a burden on the grieving family and is inappropriate. The family should not be hurried when spending time with the body. Their behavior should be accepted without judgment as part of the grief response.

An autopsy on the child will answer questions about the cause of death. It also aids physicians in obtaining exact knowledge about the disease process. By giving permission for an autopsy, parents may feel that they are contributing to medical science, which may give meaning and value to their child's death.

---

* South-Eastern Organ Procurement Foundation (SEOPF), 3001 Hungary Spring Rd., P.O. Box 28060, Richmond, VA 23228.

† Federal Register Department of Health and Human Services, Office of Organ Transplantation, Washington, DC; (301)443-7577.

Helping Surviving Children

Telling About the Death. Children deserve a factual and accurate account of the death. This will help them develop a clear, real picture of the cycles of life. It will help give them an appreciation for life. The unpleasant details of death can be minimized but not avoided. The parent may explain how the child died, what happened to the body and plans for a funeral or memorial service. The parents can share their philosophical beliefs as well as feelings of loss and grief. Words like "God took" should be avoided, since the child may come to fear and hate a God who destroys loved ones.

Expressing Feeling. The parent should be encouraged to express sorrow and shed tears in a controlled manner when talking about the death to siblings. (Hysterical crying decreases the child's sense of security.) Many children do not cry; they should be allowed to but not forced. They should be encouraged to ask questions if desired. Opportunity for indirect expression of feelings through physical exercise and creative play should be provided and encouraged. Doll house items and paper, crayons, or painting materials as well as music, poetry, and stories allow emotional expression. The surviving children and parents need private periods of time alone with each other following a death. This allows grieving parents the chance to assure the children that they too are loved and cherished equally as much as the one that is mourned.

Funerals. Should surviving children attend the funeral? Some experts say "yes" because the funeral allows children to see firsthand the reality of the death, and they may receive comfort and support from friends. A sense of closure may be helpful (Salladay and Royal, 1981; Scholwalter, 1976). Children's fantasies regarding the funeral event may be much worse than the reality (Grollmon, 1979). On the other hand, some studies of children and funerals show that behavior problems may develop that are related to funeral attendance (McCown, 1984). Children under 7 years of age and girls are more sensitive to funeral activities. This does not mean that children should not attend funerals, but it does indicate that they should be given a choice and if they attend they need preparation. They should be told what they will see and what is expected. A close, friendly adult should stay with the child during the funeral service and provide encouragement and an explanation of the ritual. After the funeral children need an opportunity to discuss the events. If a child chooses not to attend the funeral, he or she may go to the funeral home or church to say a private goodbye to the loved one.

Guidelines. Several clear guidelines for helping surviving children with death can be summarized:

- The child should be encouraged to discuss, ask questions about, and express feelings about death.
- The child should be told about the death as soon as possible in truthful, clear, simple terms appropriate to understanding.
- A specific pattern of grief behavior should not be imposed on the child.
- Adults in the child's world should feel free to cry and to share their feelings of sadness with the child in a *controlled* manner.
- Time with the child and loved adults should be set aside in the immediate days following the death to assure the child of his or her value and importance.
- The caretaking needs of the child should continue to be met by a warm, loving person.
- The child should be given a choice regarding funeral attendance.
- Other important people (e.g., teacher, doctor, coach) in the child's life should be told of the death.
- The child should be allowed and encouraged to resume normal activities directly following the death.
- At each new cognitive developmental level, the child will need to review and reinterpret the death in light of a new understanding of death.

Death Education. Parents and close family members exert a major influence on children's understanding of and reaction to death. Preparation for understanding death begins in the first years of life. It begins with the early experiences of separation from loved objects and people. Awareness of death grows as the child experiences the deaths of plants and pets. These losses and emotional recovery should not be avoided but encouraged. Children often imitate funeral rituals of burial and graveside when a pet dies. These activities should not be denied as they provide a chance to practice grief behaviors and say goodbye to the cherished pet. These activities release energy for emotional growth and the formulation of new relationships.

Ownership and care of a pet is thought to aid development of sound personality traits in children. Loving and caring for a pet may be a step toward deeper love, care, and assuming responsibility for another. Animals are nonjudgmental companions. They can become a sounding board for thoughts and feelings unable to be expressed to human ears. Humans often develop close, affectionate relations with companion animals. The relatively short life span of animals increases the opportunity for experiences of death and loss of the pet. Children are particularly vulnerable to the loss of a pet because it may be their first experience with death of a loved object.

Immediate attempts to replace lost animals should be avoided. Immediate replacement tends to devalue

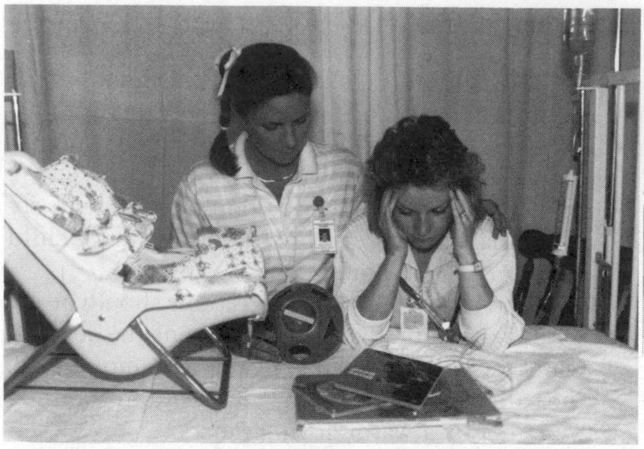

There is a strong sentiment in our culture that it is a tremendous injustice when a child suffers or dies. When given the needed support from another nurse, this nurse can acknowledge her own struggle in dealing with the death of an infant.

the sanctity of life and the uniqueness of each relationship. After resolution of grief, the child will be able to welcome a new animal and the new relationship.

Nurses' Response to Dying Children and Death

The severe stress placed upon the entire family continues to have a profound impact after the death of a child. The period after death is critical for continued support and involvement of hospital staff, if possible. Parents often complain that after their child has died they are forgotten by the staff. This period is characterized by intense grief and mourning during which the family may also renew socialization, reorganize, and make decisions. Nurses may wish to share in the funeral services or public memorial services. Phone calls, letters, or visits to the family may be appropriate and therapeutic.

Recognizing Their Own Needs. The greatest disservice that nurses can do themselves and a dying child and family is to disregard their own personal needs. Denying one's own feelings makes one less than human and takes away the child's and family's right to experience the support of a truly human relationship. All nurses have stresses and experiences in day-to-day living that shape their unique ways of relating to those in stress. It is inhuman to expect nurses to somehow be unaffected by those minor mood changes and "bad days" that we afford the rest of society the right to experience. When nurses can acknowledge that some days they feel limited or unable to cope with a dying child and family, they can then seek support from other professions to help them through the day or week. It is important to recognize that "We can give to others only from our abundance, and some days the cupboard is bare" (Kavanaugh, 1976).

Feelings of Nurses. Nurses experience a myriad of feelings in caring for a dying child. A particular child may remind nurses of their own child or a relative or close friend's child. The illness causing the suffering may remind nurses of an experience within their own family. Thus the dynamics of each parent-child-nurse relationship are unique, and when death is imminent the feelings that emerge are intense and stressful.

Nurses cope with stress in a manner similar to that of the child and family. Denial is used for protection from the reality of impending death. Real feelings are suppressed and a façade of "all is well" pervades in dealings with the child, family, and health team members.

Anger and guilt are commonly felt by nurses who care for a dying child. In our culture these are results of the sentiment that it is a tremendous injustice when a child suffers or dies. Nurses may direct anger toward a supernatural being, or they may blame parents for not seeking treatment earlier. When nurses are struggling to accept the death of a child, they may become intolerant of the many questions and demands from parents. Anger may also be directed toward the physician or to themselves for not being able to cure the child. Nurses may feel guilty because painful procedures need to be done, the child is hurting, and yet there is no hope. These feelings of anger and guilt emerge out of sensitive, caring nurses who are groping to right the wrong.

When given the needed support from other nurses and team members, nurses can feel free to acknowledge their own struggles in dealing with death. When nurses can share their feelings of anger and guilt and can break out of the shield of denial, the work of grief ensues.

Nurses' Expressions of Grief. People express grief according to their own styles of coping. Grief expression by nurses also varies according to the degree of involvement with a particular child and family, a variation that must be respected from one nurse to another. Grief is always a complex emotion but, when people have overextended themselves, behaviors of one nurse may appear inappropriate to another; each must recognize that the other needs to resolve grief in a personal way (Kavanaugh, 1976).

Grief needs an outlet such as the health care team, in which support is ready-made if "stuffy professionalism" does not thwart the process of grieving. The pretense of successful coping can seriously hamper the grieving process among professionals.

Nurses need to become increasingly aware of the toll of what Kavanaugh (1976) describes as *institutional grief*. An entire staff can become depressed and lose sight of their goals if grief remains unresolved.

Opportunities must be provided for nurses to share their feelings and anxieties about working with special families in stress. Support systems cannot be left to each individual's personal contacts such as family and friends. These are usually not prepared to hear out the feelings and expressions regarding a child who is dying. Professional support groups must be deliberately planned — institutional grief cannot be left to resolve itself. These periods of professional sharing should be ongoing, so that feelings during the process of death as well as after the death can be shared.

If nurses can ventilate their feelings in an atmosphere of openness, the child and family will gain. The sensitive exchange of feelings may bring to light that a nurse needs a period away from a particular child and family. The nurse who cares enough about the child and family is willing to take the professional risk of reaching out for help to face a new day; it may mean a temporary change of assignment to a unit away from dying children.

Nurses must take an active role in planning group sessions. Group members can be asked to privately respond to a group of statements and then provide an opportunity for the sharing of feelings (Box 26-5).

Box 26-5

A Nurse's Feeling About Caring for a Dying Child: Statements for Nurses to Respond to in a Group Session

1. I expect to feel uncomfortable when I have to talk to a dying child and to the family.
2. I feel at a loss to know what to say, especially when the child and family are aware that death is imminent.
3. I cannot imagine that anyone is ever free of the fear of dying.
4. I think I can help a child and family cope with the reality of death.
5. I am frightened at the thought of caring for a dying child.
6. I am afraid the child will ask me whether she or he is dying.
7. I feel terrible about causing tiny discomforts during a treatment when I know a child is dying anyway.
8. I feel I have to hide my own feelings of sadness so as not to make the child and family feel upset.
9. If I cry with a child or family member it disturbs me for the rest of the day.
10. I don't really have anyone to tell how I feel about (child's name) suffering.

Statements with reference to a particular situation could easily be developed by the primary nurse to facilitate sharing of personal needs and feelings about experiences with other families.

Sharing of feelings and personal difficulties in regard to care of the dying brings human experiences into focus. Nurses who respect their own humaneness recognize that they are vulnerable to the same feelings of denial, anger, fear, depression, and grief that the family experiences. If nurses can support each other during these experiences, the pain of caring for a dying child and the family can be experienced rather than repressed. When nurses feel the pain of loss, they can provide what the child and family need — the presence of a human being.

References

Aldrich C: Some dynamics of anticipatory grief. *In* Schoenberg B, et al (eds): *Anticipatory Grief.* New York, Columbia University Press, 1974.

Alexander J, Alderstein A: Affective responses to the concept of death in a population of children and early adolescents. *J Genet Psychol* 93, 1958; 93:167–177.

American Academy of Pediatrics, Task Force on Brain Death in Children: Guidelines for the determination of brain death in children. *Pediatrics* 1987 Aug; 80(2):298–300.

Anthony S: *The Child's Discovery of Death.* New York, Harcourt Press, 1940.

Averill J: Grief: its nature and significance. *Psychol Bull* 1968; 70(6): 721.

Birenbaum L, McCown D, Nunneley C: *Nurses Manual for Family Childhood Cancer Study.* Portland, OR, Oregon Health Sciences University, 1986.

Bloom-Feshbach J, Bloom-Feshbach S: *The Psychology of Separation and Loss.* San Francisco, Josey-Bass, 1987.

Bluebond-Langer M: *The Private Worlds of Dying Children.* Princeton, NJ, Princeton University Press, 1978.

Bouressa G, O'Mara M: Ethical dilemmas in organ procurement and donation. *Crit Care Nurs Q* 1987; 10(2):37–47.

Caughill R: *The Dying Patient.* Boston, Little, Brown, 1976.

Cimpich B: Symptom Management. New York, American Cancer Society Proceedings, 1982, 120.

Codden P: The meaning of death for the parent and child. Matern Child Nurs J 1977 Spring; 9.

Corr C, McNeil J: *Adolescence and Death.* New York, Springer-Verlag, 1986, 97–118.

Deutsch H: Absence of grief. *Psychoanal Q* 1937; 6:12–22.

Drake B, et al: Determination of cerebral death in the pediatric intensive care unit. *Pediatrics* 1986 July; 78(1):107–112.

Engel G: Grief and grieving. *Am J Nurs* 1964; 64:93.

Fleming J, Altschul S: Activation of mourning and growth by psychoanalysis. *Int J Psychoanal* 1963; 44:419–431.

Frauman A, Miles M: Parental willingness to donate organs. *ANNA J* 1987 Dec.

Friedman S, Chodoff P, Mason G, et al: Behavioral observations of parents anticipating the death of a child. *Pediatrics* 1963; 32:610–625.

Furman R: Death and the young child: some preliminary considerations. *Psychoanal Study Child* 1964; 19:321–333.

Goldberg S: Family tasks and reactions in the crisis of death. *Social Work* 1973; 54(7):398–405.

Grant M: Nausea and Vomiting. New York, American Cancer Society Proceedings, 1982, 111.

Grollman E (ed): *Explaining Death to Children.* Boston, Beacon Press, 1979.

Hazinski MF: Pediatric organ donation: responsibilities of the critical care nurse. *Pediatr Nurs* 1987 Sep-Oct; 13(5):354–357.

Kavanaugh R: Dealing naturally with the dying. Nursing '76 1976 Oct; 23.

Koocher G, O'Malley J: *The Damocles Syndrome.* New York, McGraw-Hill, 1981.

Kramer RF: Living with childhood cancer: impact on the healthy siblings. *In* Krulik J, Holaday B, Martinson IM: *The Child and Family Facing Life-Threatening Illness.* Philadelphia, JB Lippincott, 1987.

Kübler-Ross E: *On Death and Dying.* New York, Macmillan, 1969.

Lascari A: The dying child and the family. *J Fam Pract* 1978; *6*(6):1279–1286.

Lindemann E: Symptomatology and the management of acute grief. *Am J Psychiatr* 1944 Sep; 101:141–148.

Lonetto R: Children's conceptions of death. New York, Springer, 1980.

Martinson I (Principal Investigator): *Home Care for the Child with Cancer—Final Report.* National Cancer Institute Grant CA1 9490. Minneapolis, University of Minnesota, 1980.

Maurer A: Maturation of concepts of death. *Br J Med Psychol* 1966; 39:35–41.

McCown D: Death and Children Interviews. Unpublished audiotapes. Charlottesville, Medical College of Virginia, 1970.

McCown D: Children cremation and funerals. *J Death Ed* 1984; 8:349–363.

McCown D: Factors related to bereaved children's behavioral adjustment. *In* Barnes C (ed): *Recent Advances in Nursing Series: Caring for Sick Children.* London, Churchill-Livingstone, 1987.

McCown D: Helping children face death in the family. *J Pediatr Health Care.* 1988; 2(1):14–19.

Nagy M: The child's theories concerning death. *J Genet Psychol* 1948; 73:3–27.

Natterson JH, Knudson A: Observations concerning fear of death in fatally ill children and their mothers. *Psychosom Med* 1960; 22:456–465.

Orbach C, et al: Psychological impact of cancer and its treatment. III. The adaptation of mothers to the threatened loss of their children through leukemia. *Cancer* 1955; 8:20–38.

Report of the Task Force on Organ Transplantation: *Organ Transplantation. Issues and Recommendations.* Washington, DC, Department of Health and Human Services, Office of Organ Transplantation, April, 1986.

Safier G: A study of relationships between life and death concepts in children. *J Genet Psychol* 1964; 105:283–294.

Salladay S, Royal M: Children and death: guidelines for grief work. *Child Psychiatr Hum Dev* 1981; 11(4):203–212.

Samaniego L, Caldwell H, Witchke R, et al: Exploring the physically ill child's self-perceptions and the mother's perceptions of her child's needs; insights gained from the FIRO-BC, a behavior test for use with children. *Clin Pediatr* 1977; 16(2):154–159.

Schowalter J: How do children and funerals mix? *J Pediatr* 1976; 89:139–142.

Spinetta J, Rigler D, Karon M: Anxiety in the dying child. *Pediatrics* 1973; 52:841–845.

Stehbens J, Lasacari A: Psychological follow-ups of families with childhood leukemia. *J Clin Psychol* 1974; 30:394–397.

Volpe JJ: Brain death determination in the newborn. *Pediatrics* 1987 Aug; 80(2):293–297.

Waechter E: Children's awareness of fatal illness. *Am J Nurs* 1971 Jun; 71:1168–1172.

Wolfenstein M: How is mourning possible? *Psychoanal Study Child* 1966; 21:93–123.

Bibliography

Balk D: Effects of sibling death on teenagers. *J Public Health* 1983; 53(1):14–18.

Betz CL, Poster EC: Children's concepts of death. *Nurs Clin North Am* 1984; 19(2):341–349.

Elizur E, Kaufman M: Factors Influencing the severity of childhood bereavement reactions. *Am J Orthopsychiatr* 1982; 2:474–480.

Furman R: *Child's Parent Dies: Studies in Childhood Bereavement.* New Haven, CT, Yale University Press, 1974.

Gardner SL, Merenstein GB: Helping families deal with perinatal loss. *Neonatal Network* 1986; 5(2):17–33.

Garland KR: Grief: the transitional process. *Neonatal Network* 1986; 5(3):7–10.

Garland KR: Unresolved grief. *Neonatal Network* 1986, 5(3):29–37.

Guylay J: *The Dying Child.* New York, McGraw-Hill, 1978.

Krulik T, et al: *The Child and Family Facing Life-Threatening Illness.* Philadelphia, JB Lippincott, 1987.

Leahey M, Wright LM: *Families and Life-Threatening Illness.* Springhouse, PA, Springhouse Corporation, 1987.

Martinson IM, et al: The long-term effects of sibling death on self-concept. *J Pediatr Nurs* 1987; 2(4):227–235.

Miles M: Emotional symptoms and physical health in bereaved parents. *Nurs Res* 1985; 34(2):76–81.

Petix M: Explaining death to school-age children. *Pediatr Nurs* 1987; 13(6):394–396.

Rapheal B: *The Anatomy of Bereavement.* New York, Basic Books, 1983.

Schowalter JE: Twenty years of pediatric thanatology. *Child Health Care* 1986; 14(3):157–162.

Swoiskin-Schwartz S, et al: Parents' views about having a child after a SIDS death. *J Pediatr Nurs* 1988: 3(1):24–28.

Van Eerdwegh M, et al: The bereaved child. *Br J Psychiatr* 1982; 140:23–29.

Wass H, Corr C (eds): *Children and Death.* New York, Hemisphere, 1984.

Managing Illness

Unit Five

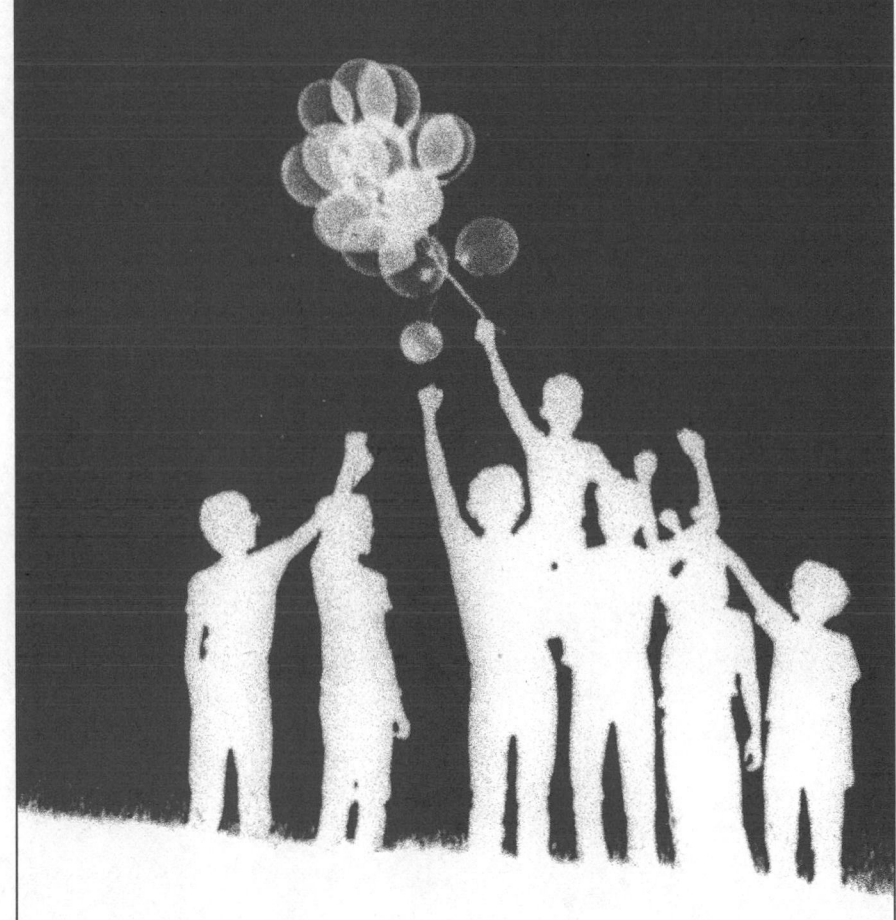

Principles and Skills Adapted to the Care of Children

Chapter 27

Mabel Hunsberger

Nursing Process Plan:
NPP: Perioperative Care, page 835

Related Topics
Communication, Chapter 11
Physical assessment and history-taking techniques, Chapter 15
Promoting safety, Chapter 17
Use of play, Chapter 21
Nursing management of pain in children, Chapter 29
Fluid and electrolyte balance, Chapter 30
Nursing care during hospitalization, Chapter 31

Children's needs differ from those of adults under most circumstances but especially during health care encounters. Everything a nurse does in health care is adapted according to the unique physical, intellectual, emotional, and social developmental levels of each child to ease the child's and family's experience and to promote their well-being.

This approach fosters trust and cooperation from a child who does not understand the goals of care. The purpose of this chapter is to discuss adaptation of nursing care in specific circumstances, including

1. Informed consent/assent
2. Education of children and families during the health care encounter
3. Performance of selected procedures
4. Care of children during illness
   a. When a child needs restraints
   b. When a child is placed in isolation
   c. When a child has a fever
   d. When a child requires surgery

Informed Consent

Informed consent involves cognitive tasks that children are not able to perform. It implies that not only has a person freely agreed to a specific intervention but that he or she also has done so with a complete understanding. Children cannot comprehend explanations of what is to be done to them or why, leaving them both *uninformed* and *unable to consent*. Fully understanding the legal and ethical implications of diagnostic and therapeutic interventions means the recipient comprehends the potential risks and benefits, consequences, and possible outcomes.

Written informed consent is required for many diagnostic procedures as well as for any surgery. The consent form signed during hospital admission represents an overall consent for treatment but does not encompass specific procedures, tests, and surgery. Any procedure with an element of risk and all major and minor operations require the signing of a special form that documents informed consent.

Although it is the physician's responsibility to inform the client, the nurse may be responsible for requesting and witnessing the signature. If the nurse has not been present to hear the physician's explanation, some have suggested that the nurse should write on the form "witnessing signature only" (Northrop, 1984). Any query about the procedure to be performed should be directed to the physician responsible for the procedure.

We appreciate the contribution of Mary Jean Yablonky, CRNA, MA, to this chapter.

Other situations requiring consent on the behalf of children include taking photographs, using medical records, performing postmortem examinations, and conducting research.

Informed Consent for Treatment

Parents or legal guardians are entrusted with the authority to give informed consent for their children who are minors. As long as the parents or legal guardians are available and the decision to be made does not involve legal and ethical dilemmas, informed consent is easily obtained. Clarification of informed consent in exceptional circumstances follows.

Mature and Emancipated Minors

States vary in their designated age of majority and definitions of emancipation. In many states, a boy or girl is considered an adult upon reaching the 18th birthday, but state laws vary and change over time. Provision exists in many states for a minor to obtain treatment without parental consent under certain circumstances; such a child is not classified as an emancipated minor but rather as a *mature minor*. The age is designated by the state and is usually set at 15 or 16 years. Treatment as a mature minor may include emergency care and areas involving private and personal issues such as contraception, drug and alcohol abuse, and care during pregnancy. Treatment with respect to abortion is affected by abortion laws, which continue to change over time and vary considerably from state to state.

An *emancipated minor* is an individual who is below the age of majority but whose life circumstances are recognized by law to set him or her free from the restrictions of childhood. Life circumstances that may qualify a minor to become emancipated include pregnancy, marriage, graduation from high school, independent living arrangements, and military service.

Particular state laws designating mature minors and emancipated minors should be familiar to the nurse in pediatric practice.

Emergency Care When Parents (or Legal Guardian) Are Unavailable

Emergency care of minors in the absence of parents or legal guardian is handled in a variety of ways. Every attempt is made to reach the parents or legal guardian to obtain consent in person or by telephone. A second nurse can listen in on another telephone to verify such verbal consent. When all efforts to reach the parents or legal guardian fail, a search is made for grandparents or other relatives to give permission for treatment. School officials, babysitters, and social workers cannot give permission for treatment without written authority from a parent or legal guardian to do so.

If the caretaker has no written permission, parents cannot be reached, and no relatives can be located, the health care team then has the legal right to proceed with treatment in the event of a life-threatening situation. When situations are not life-threatening, the search is continued for the parents or legal guardian, grandparents, or other relative to authorize treatment.

Nontreatment of Children

Parents have the right and responsibility to grant informed consent for medical procedures. This does not mean that they have freedom to withhold consent for procedures necessary for the survival of a child, even if the quality of life for the child is doubtful. In the past 20 years, surgical procedures and mechanical equipment have been developed that enable children with severe physical problems to survive. In 1982, a public debate over nontreatment resulted from a baby born with Down syndrome, who came to be known as "Baby Doe." The infant also had intestinal obstruction, but a decision was made by the family and medical team not to perform corrective surgery. The state court supported their right to do so, but the Federal Department of Health and Human Services issued a directive in 1983 aimed at ensuring that handicapped infants would receive life-saving treatment, without regard to quality of life. The directive mandated that hospital staff report any case of suspected nontreatment. This directive was strongly opposed by the medical community as interfering with the family's rights and the physician-family (patient) relationship and sparked various court test cases. The mandated reporting was ultimately overruled and the directive withdrawn.

However, the Child Abuse Prevention and Treatment Act of 1984 includes provisions for institutional review to prevent the withholding of indicated treatment from handicapped infants with life-threatening disorders. This bill sanctions institutional ethics committees, state agencies, and, if necessary, the courts to safeguard against withholding of treatment.

Informed Consent and Assent for Research

A child's parents or guardians have legal authority to give informed consent for research that involves their child. A parent's or guardian's consent does not, however, fulfill a researcher's full obligation to the child. A child's assent also should be obtained as age appropriate. *A child's assent is an expression of willingness to participate in the research after an explanation of the procedures and general purpose of the research has been provided.*

The United States Department of Health and Human Services stipulates that children must be given an explanation, in language developmentally appropriate that describes the study and what they would be expected to do or undergo, before they are asked to consent to the research. Assent is an affirmative agreement as opposed to simply not disagreeing (Lynn, 1986).

Children over the developmental age of 7 years are believed able to understand the basic purpose of the research and what is expected of them and to express a preference about their involvement (Weithorn and Campbell, 1982). However, many researchers are seeking assent from children as young as 4 years of age.

Patient Education

A primary role of the nurse in health care encounters is to prepare and teach children and parents. Patient education is an interactive process that communicates an interest and concern for the client's welfare. It is an exchange of information focusing on the client's needs and concerns. In pediatric settings, the form and content of patient education are adapted to involve parents and to facilitate participation of the child at the appropriate developmental level. Both formal and informal teaching should occur. Specific times may be scheduled during which a formal teaching session is held (e.g., teaching CPR or gavage feeding). Additionally, teaching is an informal process whereby the child and family are kept informed about the child's care and are involved in making decisions about care.

Assessment of Child and Family

The initial step in any teaching situation is to assess the factors that will affect outcomes of the educational process, including learning needs, child and family personal resources, anxiety level of the child and parent, family relationships, lifestyle and cultural patterns, coping styles, and the developmental level of the child.

Learning Needs

A simple but often overlooked task is to find out what the child and family initially know about the topic, to avoid the reteaching of previously learned information. This provides an opportunity to give praise and reinforce the client's correct information. The child and family's level of understanding can be ascertained by asking for a description in their own words. It is particularly useful to ask a child to tell you what he or she knows about the event. If the child uses technical terms, it is important to ask for clarification, as some children repeat professional language because they hear it, while having only a vague understanding of its meaning. For example, a child who states "they have to take my blood" may have no concept of how that will be done or of how it will feel. Many children fantasize that the procedure involves a much more extensive intrusion than actually occurs if no true explanation is provided. A child may think "taking blood" involves going for an operation and having an IV inserted. Watching the child's and parents' facial expressions as they explain what they know can also reveal underlying fears and uncertainties. Responding to such anxieties is important before introducing new information. Encouraging parents and children to identify what they do not understand and areas in which they require further explanation gets them involved from the beginning and develops a positive working relationship.

In many instances, it is important to speak to the parent or to the child alone. Parents often have fears that they do not wish to discuss with the child present, yet they may not seek such clarification unless a private session is suggested. It is most important that such conversations are held without the child's knowledge, so he or she does not fear that something more serious is happening. Similarly, preadolescents and adolescents appreciate being given the chance to speak to the health professional in private.

The nurse can also recognize learning needs by assessing behavior. Recognizing an incongruity between what a person says and what he or she appears to be feeling is an important clue. Children in particular cannot necessarily express their fears but demonstrate their need instead by *not* playing, *not* talking, or *not* eating.

Seeking to understand the client's learning need through verbal expressions and behavioral manifestations is an important component of the teaching process. Through this sensitivity individual needs can be met and what has been called the "patient uniformity myth" avoided (Williams and Kendall, 1985).

Child and Family Personal Resources

As parents and children increasingly engage in self-care, nurses take an active role in assessing the client's resources. Three categories of human learning are taken into consideration: (1) cognitive; (2) psychomotor; and (3) affective (attitude) (Bloom, 1956). All are relevant to patient education. The three questions to be asked are:

- Does the parent or child have the intellectual capacity to learn the relevant information?
- Does the parent or child have the physical capabilities to perform the task or procedure? (It is possible to understand how to perform an activity yet be unable to perform it.)
- Is the parent or child ready and motivated to perform the task? Is the parent or child responsible and accountable?

Assessment of these capabilities is an on-going process. If outcomes are not being achieved, the nurse's role is to reassess the client's resources and determine whether increased confidence-building is required or whether alternate approaches are needed. Once it is established that the parent or child can perform certain tasks or learn selected information, the nurse should then assess the anxiety level experienced by parents and children.

Anxiety Level of Child and Parent

The nurse's perception of the severity of an illness may be a poor indicator of the degree of parental anxiety. Individuals respond differently to similar situations. A painful procedure, even though a momentary event, may produce an enormous amount of upset for some children and parents.

It should also be recognized that the parents of an injured, sick, or upset child usually feel distressed. Extremely anxious parents and children do not hear what is explained. Readiness and motivation to learn are blocked if fears and concerns distract an individual from listening. For example, parents being taught to insert a gavage tube may be distracted by the fear that the procedure is causing pain to their child. Similarly, a child who is being taught how to inject insulin may be anxious about too much blood running out of the body. These concerns must be addressed before learning can take place. Anxiety may be expressed through avoidance, forgetting, and not paying attention. Parents and children should be given the opportunity to express verbally how they feel about the learning situation. Children may not be able to describe their anxious feelings but can be encouraged to tell a story, draw a picture, or engage in a sentence-completion activity. Also, more specific tools have been developed to measure anxiety. Because fear, anxiety, and pain are interrelated feelings, assessment tools actually measure a variety of emotions. Observation rating scales to assess distress level in children have been used by Katz and colleagues (1981), Elliot and Olson (1983), and Melamed and associates (1983). The State-Trait Anxiety Inventory (Spielberger et al, 1970; Spielberger et al, 1973) provides information regarding the individual's general disposition (trait anxiety) as well as the response to a specific situation (state anxiety). Instruments to measure anxiety are useful when assessments are being made to measure teaching effectiveness and outcomes.

Family Relationships

A healthy relationship between the parent and child is an asset to learning. Children who feel supported by their parents have the freedom to express feelings of concern and will seek explanations. Parents who can encourage their children to participate in their own care are an asset to the children's adaptation.

A trusting relationship among family members also facilitates the learning process. Children need to know what will happen, and they need to have confidence that they are being told the truth. These established patterns of communication between child and parent are assessed when planning parental involvement in the care of the children. For example, it may be necessary first to support the parents and help them cope with telling their child unpleasant information, rather than simply asking parents to tell a child unpleasant news. The nurse can role-play how to teach a child and can engage the parent in the teaching process.

Lifestyle and Cultural Patterns

The lifestyle of individuals sets the parameters within which new behaviors and responsibilities can be performed. When assessing parents and children with respect to teaching, it becomes particularly important to consider the amount of time available, economic resources, and the feasibility of the new behavior. For example, in teaching parents how to provide a balanced meal with dietary restrictions (such as for children with diabetes), fast foods may have to be included if both parents work. Similarly, guidance concerning childrearing and the discipline of children must take into account cultural beliefs and customs. It is ineffective to impart knowledge and instruct clients to adapt behaviors that are inconsistent with their lifestyle and beliefs. Breastfeeding, weaning, and toilet training are examples of issues that have cultural components.

Coping Styles

Differences in coping styles have been identified in children and adults. Individual differences in response to health care procedures must be taken into account when planning support strategies. Adults have been identified as *sensitizers* (those who expressed emotions like fear or anxiety); *avoiders* (those who denied negative feelings); and *neutrals* (those with both types of responses) (Andrew, 1970). Similar categories (copers, avoiders, and neutrals) have been identified by Delong (1971) and Shipley and co-workers (1979), who have concluded that *sensitizers* should be prepared extensively and *repressors* left alone or at least left with their defenses. Similarly, two classes of children have been identified by Burnstein and Meichenbaum (1979):

Group 1. Children who did not use defensive behaviors extensively prior to hospitalization, were relatively nonstressed during hospitalization, and were minimally anxious after surgery.

Group 2. Children who were defensive prior to hospitalization and demonstrated behaviors of avoidance and anxiety during hospitalization.

The nurse's assessment of coping styles of both parents and children guides the development of appropriate strategies for child and parent teaching (see Chapter 23 for further discussion on coping).

Developmental Level of Child

The child's level of development in the three categories of human learning (cognitive, psychomotor, and affective) determines the content, timing, and method of education used with children. The cognitive abilities that particularly affect the child's understanding include extent of language development, concept of time, understanding of cause-and-effect relationships, and reasoning and abstracting ability. Psychomotor abilities that affect the child learner in particular are gross and fine motor development, eye-hand coordination, and organizational skills. Finally, the child's feeling state (affective) largely contributes to how much can be learned. Developmental characteristics and implications for teaching are summarized in Table 27-1.

Table 27-1. Educational Strategies According to Age of Child

Developmental Characteristics of Child	Educational Strategies
Infants (0–12 Months)	
Unable to understand explanations but are sensitive to gentleness of voice, touch, and movement. Infants can anticipate what will occur by physical signs (i.e., preparation of equipment, certain sounds associated with an activity).	Main focus is to teach parents and caregiver. Tone of voice and gentle handling communicate support to infant. Prepare equipment and proceed with the activity as quickly as possible to reduce the amount of anticipated distress. Talk to and touch infant before beginning a procedure.
Familiarity is a source of comfort Stranger anxiety occurs at 6–8 mo of age	Provide infant with favorite toy as soon as preparation begins. Spend time with child before beginning a procedure or new activity. Involve parent in activity.
Toddler (1–3 Years)	
Separation from parents is primary threat Egocentric thinking. View of world is that events are related to self.	Encourage presence of parents for stressful events. Careful explanations of reasons for events should be provided. Machines and equipment should be described according to what they do and the sounds they make.
Has developed limited coping skills and ability to express emotions and feelings is limited	Use play as a method of expression. Tell child it is okay to cry.
Fantasizes about what will happen and why things are as they are	Use simple words child can understand. Encourage expression of thoughts through doll and puppet play and verbal expression (e.g., "How does your puppet feel about . . .").
Attention span short but can be increased with inclusion of sensory experiences	Teaching sessions must be short (5–10 min) and should include equipment to touch and explore or a visual aid such as a book.
Language skills limited	May interpret words literally; therefore, careful choice of simple words and short sentences is necessary.
Concept of time is limited	Explanations should be given just prior to a procedure of short duration such as an injection. If the procedure or event is more involved the child should be told 2–3 hr before it occurs.
Preschooler (3–6 Years)	
Egocentric thinking continues	Explain why things are as they are. Repeat such explanations to reduce potential for child feeling he has *caused* the situation.
Magical thinking continues	Children should be asked to "repeat back" their perception and understanding of what has been told to them. Reduce misconceptions by avoiding threatening words such as "cut." Instead say "make an opening."
Coping behaviors continue to be limited	Encourage presence of parents for stressful events.
Fears of body mutilation peak at this age	Give clear explanations about which body parts will and will not be affected (be clear about *how* it will be affected). Feelings can be expressed through doll play, with demonstration of the procedure (i.e., where is the tube, the bandage, or the opening).
Ability to understand how body works increases	Use visual aids of body models or picture outlines to enhance teaching. Use correct anatomic terms.
Attention span is increasing	Continue to provide information in short sessions (10–15 min). Involve child in the teaching sessions by doing something (i.e., handling equipment, drawing, or demonstrating on a doll).
Has increased verbal skills and questions "why." (Questioning is child's way to learn about the events and people in the environment)	Provide opportunity for child to phrase questions. Take the time to encourage further expression of questions, then provide information in a simple, clear response. Questions at this age do not require long, complicated answers.
Understands concrete explanations—only what he or she sees and touches	Actual equipment or miniature forms of equipment gives child an understanding of environment.

Table 27-1 *(continued)*

Developmental Characteristics of Child	Educational Strategies
Interprets words literally	Some words used in health care are confusing (e.g., "take your vital signs" and "take your pulse"). It is better to explain *what* you will do (e.g., "listen to your heart").
Inability to conceptualize effect of event	Explain about the sensations that will be experienced.
School-Age (6–12 Years)	
Mastery becomes important at this age. Is eager to learn and accomplish new skills and increase understanding of environment. Has also acquired more skills such as reading and verbal expression of ideas	Can use more books that teach the information through drawings, coloring books, and a variety of pencil and paper activities. Encourage child to use language ability now to verbalize fears.
Is beginning to have better understanding of causation but still cannot apply logic to abstract problems	Teaching should continue to focus on concrete aspects of the event. Clarify misconceptions about causation.
Concept of time has improved	Procedural information can be provided a day or two in advance.
Attention span	Can pay attention for 30–45 min if actively involved.
Peers are important support	Can hold educational sessions with groups of children who have similar problems.
Increased neuromuscular development	Child can now perform skills that involve manipulation of equipment.
Now more interested in self-management	Parents are still required for support but child can be given more responsibility and in many instances can be given information separate from parents. Children at this age may express some fears more freely to the health professional than to parents.
Continues to view hospitalization as punishment	Continue to reassure and give explanations that reduce child's feelings of being the cause for the situation.
Competitive behavior	Devise games that contain content to be learned.
Adolescents	
Struggling with identity versus role confusion. Trying to answer the question "Who am I?" Concerned about body image	Include a clear explanation about how the body is affected by an illness or treatment. Anticipate feelings of anger and grief in response to change in body image. Assist patient to identify ways to adapt to experienced changes.
Peers extremely important	Invite peers with a similar experience to teach an adolescent. Education sessions with a group of peers.
Independence versus dependence. Is struggling with autonomy. Wants to be autonomous but still needs some dependence	Give adolescent some control over when teaching sessions will be held, methods of learning that are preferred, and encourage collaborative decision making.
Able to think abstractly and understand complex language. Can verbalize fears	Scientific names (with explanations) can be used to describe illnesses, procedures, and techniques. Use diagrams, literature, and pamphlets. Encourage verbal expression of fears. Explain what symptoms are expected in an illness and when it is necessary to seek further advice.
Need for privacy	Explore with adolescent whether he or she wants parents involved in educational sessions. Teach parents separately if adolescent prefers.
Coping behaviors now well established	Involving the adolescent in planning can facilitate coping. Assess adolescent's coping resources and provide opportunity for expression of anxieties. Provide information honestly. Recognize that regression is common during stress; therefore, adapt teaching accordingly. Increase amount of teaching according to adolescent's readiness.

Table 27-2. Developmental Description of Children's Responses and Coping Abilities During Stressful Experiences, and Supportive Nursing Strategies

Main Fears	Verbal Response	Nonverbal Response	Ability to Cope	Nursing Actions to Facilitate Coping During Stressful Situations
Infant and Toddler (0–2 Years)				
Sudden movements Loud noises Separation from caretakers Strangers	Cries, yells, "No!" protests	Clings to caretaker Tries to return to and visually searches for caretaker if separated Tries to get away	Limited ability to cope, especially with pain Cannot hold still on own during stress	Simple explanations of what is to be done and what sensations will occur; actively involve child if old enough Keep caretaker present to calm child with touch and voice and preferably by holding child Gentle restraint introduced as "Let me help you hold still" Perform what must be done as promptly, painlessly and quickly as possible. Allow presence of special object or toy during experiences. Explain source of any loud noise and reassure while noise exists. Keep number of strangers in room minimal
Preschooler (3–5 Years)				
Dark Bodily harm Being alone Moving equipment	Cries, whimpers, screams Verbalizes pain, fear, anger Groaning, whining protests Uses postponement tactics	Seeks caretaker verbally and with eyes Holds rigidly still Turns away, shuts eyes Kicks, bites, scratches, frowns, flinches, pulls away Preoccupied with where the hurt is and nurse's actions	Believes being punished for wrongdoing Will try to cooperate if he senses care given is trustworthy Needs some assistance to hold still	Give alternative outlet for pain (cry, yell, squeeze hand) Keep caretaker present "Let me help you hold still" approach to restraint Permit special object, toy or invisible friend during experience Allow child to see and handle equipment before procedures or to see facility before going there for care Brief verbal preparation before and during stressful experience; stress what child will experience with senses; involve child actively Be honest, friendly, reassuring During stressful experience continually reassure and praise child's efforts to cooperate Avoid reprimands or after-the-fact statements that reinforce child's concept of experience as punishment Allow child to take home clean, disposable supplies for therapeutic play Tangible rewards after stressful situation at least occasionally; not based on child's being cooperative but because makes him or her feel good
School-age (6–10 Years)				
Large machines Bodily injury Loss of self-control	Verbalizes pain, anger, fear Protests and trys to postpone Whines, cries, screams	Passively seeks support and body contact from caretaker by facial expression, not verbally Sits or lies quietly, concentrating on maintaining control Holds rigidly still Turns away, closes eyes; kicks, pulls away	Will try to cooperate if knows what to expect Progressively more able to hold still on own. Tries to control anxiety	Give alternative outlet for pain (squeeze hand, count, talk about topic of interest) Describe or allow child to see equipment before procedure or the health facility before child receives treatment there Verbal explanations before a stressful situation; stress sensations to be expected and what child can do to help Keep caregiver present Encourage verbalization of fears, questions Ascertain child's perception of what will happen Correct erroneous thinking During stressful situation periodically reassure, remind child how to help, and praise cooperation efforts Allow child to take home clean disposable supplies for therapeutic play and to display before friends
Preadolescent and Adolescent (11+ Years)				
Loss of self control Disturbance to body appearance Death Drug effects	Verbalizes pain and fear in adult manner Tries to postpone until gains control Groans	Sits or lies quietly in attempt to maintain control, be brave Turns away, winces	Able to recognize and control anxiety. Tolerates pain poorly	Prepare with explanations as would an adult Encourage verbalization of questions Describe procedures and instruments, stressing effect they will have on body's appearance and for how long Tell youth how to assist (gives sense of self-control) Caregiver's presence or absence the child's choice

Nursing Diagnoses

The nurse makes individual diagnoses appropriate for each child and family encountered. The nurse's effectiveness as a teacher is influenced by an understanding of the child's knowledge deficit, the child's coping skills, and the impact of the illness on the family. Nursing diagnoses relevant to the teaching situation include:

Knowledge deficit, *related to*
- *cognitive limitations associated with child's developmental level*
- *low readiness for reception of information associated with anxiety level (parent and child), short attention span, and limited language skills*
- *denial of health care needs associated with threat to the personal self*

Ineffective individual coping, *related to*
- *separation from family and home associated with hospitalization*
- *limited coping skills associated with egocentric thinking, magical thinking, and inability to abstract*

Altered family processes, *related to*
- *disruption in family routines associated with care of ill child*
- *change in family roles associated with health care needs of ill child*
- *child's discomfort associated with child's illness*

Nursing Strategies

Children and parents can be motivated to participate in self-care through effective nursing approaches for the age of the child. Interest in health and in learning about one's health problem varies from child to child, but with individualized approaches a nurse can be a motivating force for behavior change. Strategies for teaching children at various ages are in Table 27-1; nursing strategies to facilitate coping are in Table 27-2.

Patient Safety

Potential dangers to children in the various environments of daily living are addressed in Chapter 17. When a child enters the health care system, the child is exposed to additional potential dangers because of special equipment and environmental variations. Needles, glass bottles, medications, and various types of machinery basic to any medical environment are common dangers. An identification band attached to each child at the time of admission to a hospital is a basic rule of safety. Children do not realize the consequences of pretending about their identity. One child may be in another child's bed or may even try to fool the nurse by answering to the wrong name.

Nursing Assessment

Each child and family unit is individually assessed to determine how threatening an environment is to this child. One can quickly determine how active and inquisitive a child is by watching him or her explore the environment. The parents' level of watchfulness and how long it takes them to intervene and rescue the child or the equipment are important clues to the nurse. A child who is permitted indiscriminately to explore expensive equipment and play with it as if it were a toy or who is allowed to wander away from a parent down a hall in a busy clinic can quickly become injured.

Many situations also need to be assessed for potential dangers. Placing children on carts, chairs, and wagons may put them at risk of falling if they are not appropriately restrained. Although restraints protect children, they themselves can cause harm if not properly applied. An on-going discriminating approach concerning the dangers imposed by the health care setting is an important component of a nursing assessment.

Nursing Diagnoses

The specific nursing diagnoses vary according to the age of the child, the family circumstances, and the setting. The following apply to most circumstances and health care settings:

Potential for injury, *related to environmental hazards associated with:*
- *inadequate footwear to prevent falls and punctures*
- *improper use and placement of sockets and cords*
- *inadequate supervision around stairs, elevators, and doors*
- *use of unsafe toys and recreational equipment*
- *inappropriate supervision during use of faucets and bath tubs*
- *inappropriate supervision during mealtime*
- *inappropriate use of supplies, equipment, and furniture*

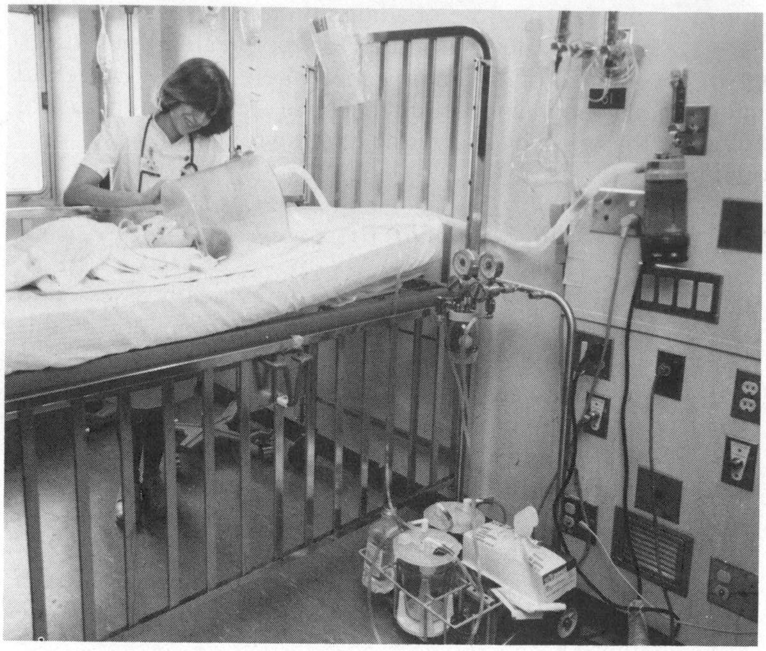

Figure 27-1. The wheels of cribs must be locked and the crib placed a sufficient distance from electrical outlets to prevent young children from poking objects into sockets. (Note: the crib side is in the down position for the photograph only.)

Potential for injury, related to transportation of child associated with:
- *inappropriate choice of vehicle for transport*
- *inappropriate or lack of use of safety belt*
- *inadequate preparation of child about where he or she is going and what will happen*

Nursing Strategies

To ensure a child's safety, the nurse identifies potential hazards in each child's immediate environment. This often involves intervening when other health professionals or parents do not adhere to safety standards. Ensuring a child's safety requires the full cooperation of all individuals involved in the child's care. The nurse also provides important input into decision-making groups who set hospital or clinic safety policies.

Environmental Safety

The environment of any health care setting is unfamiliar to the child and family compared with their home setting; thus, it is more difficult for them to predict what might happen and where dangers lie. Furthermore, when children are ill, parents and health care team members alike may assume they will be less active and not as inquisitive. Consequently, fewer precautions are taken, and accidents are more likely to happen. Regardless of the purpose of the visit or hospitalization, safety measures should be taken that are consistent with the child's development and usual level of activity (as described by the child's parents). For example, one cannot assume that an ill child will lie quietly in the crib while the nurse briefly turns away or moves a short distance away.

Special attention must be given to (1) floors, sockets, and cords; (2) stairs, elevators, and doors; (3) toys and recreational supplies; (4) faucets and bathtubs; (5) eating arrangements and utensils; and (6) furniture, especially cribs. Precautions in these areas affect safety regarding the child's mobility, play and recreational activities, and activities of daily living.

The mobility of children in hospitals is to be encouraged and should not introduce unnecessary dangers. Floors should be free of clutter; they should be clean and not slippery. A highly polished, waxed floor is inappropriate for a children's unit. Children should not be allowed to walk around in bare feet or socks. Properly fitting disposable slippers or skid-free shoes from home should be worn. Slick-soled shoes can be made safe by placing a wide strip of tape along the sole. Children should be instructed to walk, not run, in corridors, and they should never be allowed to be mobile with objects on a stick (e.g., lollipops and popsicles) in their mouths.

Numerous electrical cords and sockets are necessary in most health care settings. Cribs need to be placed so that children cannot reach sockets and appliances (Fig. 27-1). Young children out of bed must be supervised to protect them from falling over cords.

In most hospitals, children may leave the unit for

short periods to go to the gift shop or snack bar, if they are attended by a family member or hospital personnel. On the unit, children must be protected from wandering into dangerous areas such as treatment rooms, stairwells, and elevators. A lock placed at the upper corner of a door permits adults to enter but keeps children safe.

Safe toys and recreational equipment are basic to the care of all children. The potential problem in hospitals is that toys and equipment are in poor repair and cleaned improperly because no one in particular is assigned this responsibility. Thus, each nurse must take individual responsibility to ensure that play equipment is maintained and properly cleaned and that activities are safe for the age of the child (see Chapter 21 for discussion of age-appropriate toys and activities). Common sources of danger are removable parts that can be swallowed (especially the metal insert on squeak toys), rough and sharp edges, movable parts that readily pinch fingers, and toys and equipment that are too advanced for the child's age.

Daily care needs of the child in the hospital are the same as at home, but the unfamiliar environment may introduce additional dangers. A young child who knows which faucet is hot and which is cold at home may inadvertently turn on the hot water in the hospital. Older children who are relatively independent at home may need more supervision in the hospital because of differences in the height and contour of the tub and the placement of faucets.

Mealtime requires supervision to protect children from unfamiliar dangers. For example, some hospital kitchens use metal covers that are hot and must be removed before the meal is served. Also, a child may not be accustomed to the size of the fork or cup that is used in the hospital, or may inadvertently by served food that is not age-appropriate, causing him or her to choke.

One of the greatest dangers to a child anywhere involves use of hazardous supplies, equipment, or furniture. Cribs must be in good repair and should be used appropriately. For example, depending on the age and size of a child, an enclosed crib (Fig. 27-2), with or without pads around its edges, may be necessary to prevent falls and injuries. These decisions are made by the nurse and require immediate attention on admission of a child to the unit. Any crib with a broken latch must immediately be repaired properly; taping the side rail in place, regardless of how firmly, is unsafe.

Falls from cribs are an even greater threat in the hospital than at home. Hospital cribs are high, and the floors rarely have rugs or carpeting to cushion the fall. Furthermore, many people who attend to the child in the crib may not be particularly familiar with potential dangers of a crib and may inadvertently leave a siderail

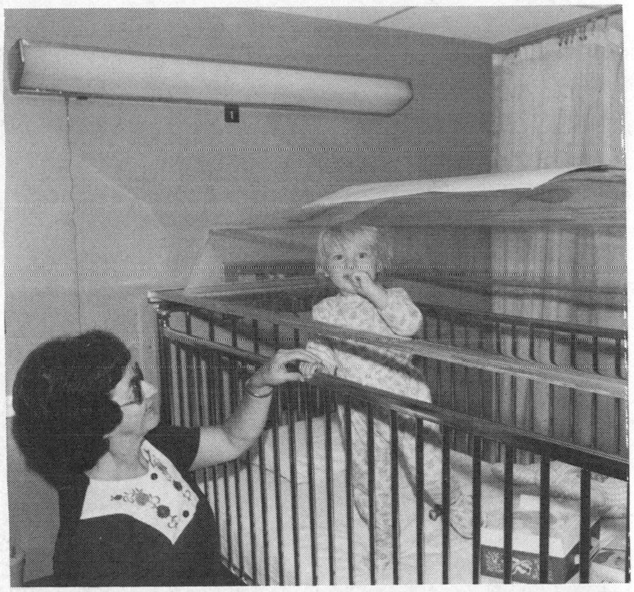

Figure 27-2. An enclosed, see-through crib keeps the toddler safe from falls but allows freedom to move. Note the large poster lying across the top of the crib to provide an interesting view for the toddler while lying in the crib.

down. Even parents, in a strange environment, may unthinkingly turn their backs on their child in the crib while the siderail is down. A siderail should never be left down — *not even momentarily*— without someone fully attending to the child. Several situations which are particularly prone to result in a fall require special caution and reminders. These include:

- infants who unexpectedly roll over
- when a mist tent is on the bed, giving the illusion that the child cannot roll out
- small infants strapped into infant chairs that could tip over
- children who are restrained but manage to free themselves from the restraint

Under these circumstances, novices might assume that a child is safe while they are obtaining something from across the room. This can also happen to experienced people because they forget that the siderail is down because of a mist tent or infant seat. ***Except while giving care, the nurse must insist that at all times siderails must remain up all the way.*** An exception may be made when an infant who cannot roll over or stand is receiving fluids intravenously. Then it is often more practical to drape the tubing across a siderail that is pulled up only halfway.

A basic principle that must be adhered to with *all* individuals who care for children in isolettes and cribs is to keep one hand *always* securely on the child. If one's back is turned to reach for something, one hand

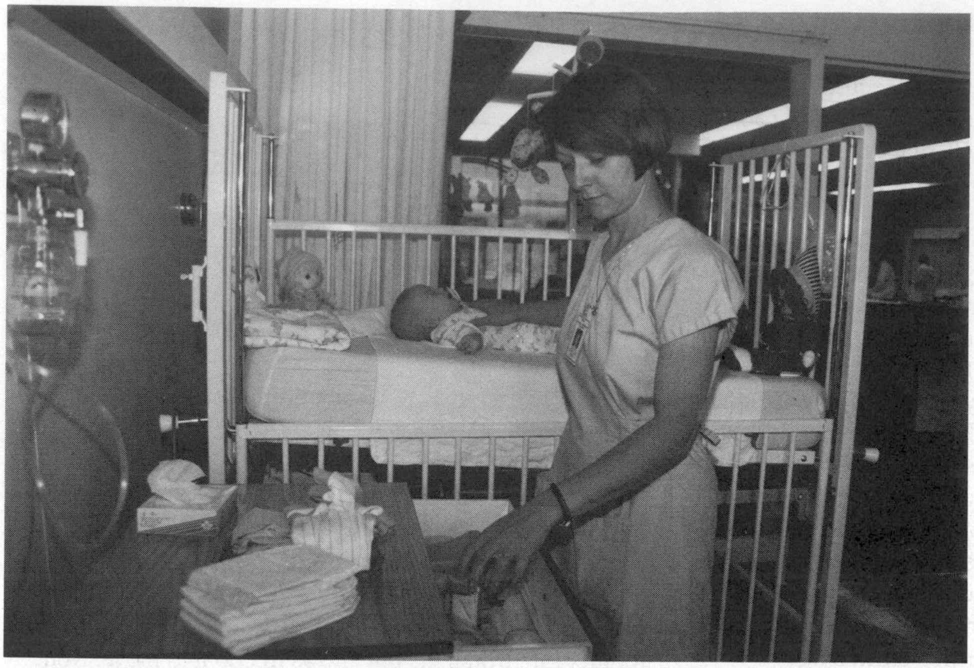

Accidents happen quickly. *Always keep one hand firmly on the child.*

must be firmly gripping the child to avoid a fall. Falls from cribs are disastrous, and the nurse must keep a watchful eye on children in cribs, especially during busy times such as at mealtimes and when rounds are being made.

Another aspect of care that requires strict safety adherence is the use of highchairs. A child in a highchair should be restrained, the wheels on a chair should be locked, and the child should not be able to reach the wall or sturdy furniture. If these precautions are not adhered to, a child can pull on or push off from a sturdy object until the chair tips and falls. A child is safe in a highchair only if not left unattended. Active toddlers can even rock themselves from side to side in a chair until it tips; restraints, regardless of how secure, are not foolproof to an ingenious toddler.

Furniture should be sturdy, and child-sized tables and chairs should be available for playing and eating. Dangerous supplies such as electrical equipment, medications, soaps and shampoos, needles, razors, and scissors must be appropriately stored. Rooms and cupboards where such articles are stored should be locked.

Transportation of Children

The hospitalized child frequently must be transported to another unit of the hospital for diagnostic or therapeutic procedures. An infant should not be carried to another part of the hospital, as the person carrying him or her could slip and fall. Appropriate ways to transport infants are by crib, baby carriage, or stroller. Older children can be transported in their bed or by stretchers, wheelchairs, wagons, or specially made carts that allow for semi-Fowler's position. In any transport, the child must be securely belted for safety.

The same safety precautions used in transporting adults apply to children. Of particular importance is ensuring that the child is adequately identified, that the IV chamber will not run dry while the child is away from the unit, and that the child will be attended while waiting in another department. *Children may even manipulate the IV flow-rate regulator out of curiosity and seriously endanger themselves.* Careful monitoring of the IV is always important, but especially during transport because of the additional hazards.

Children will be less resistive to prodecures if they are told ahead of time when and where they are going. Thus, an indirect way to maintain the child's physical safety is to prepare him or her psychologically before the actual move.

Bathing and Hygiene

The daily hygienic care children need is similar to that needed by any patient; however, the astute nurse will use this time to meet more than just hygienic needs. It is a time to observe the child's physical and developmental status, encourage appropriate self-care, and teach safety and daily health habits. For parents, the child's bath, grooming, and hygiene provide opportunities for them to participate. It is an excellent time to assist parents with concerns about their child's health. For the older child, it is a time to exercise some control over his or her own body, and for the younger child, bath time can be an enjoyable and sensual playtime.

Nursing Assessment

Decisions about how to bathe an infant or a child and whether a bath is needed are approached with various goals in mind. The child's safety, with respect to age and physical condition, largely determines whether a tub bath, shower, or bed bath is given. The nurse also assesses how to involve the parents in a way that benefits both child and family.

Nursing Diagnoses

Bathing and hygiene care of infants and children require the supervision of a caretaker because of developmental level, potential for injury, and the special care particular physical conditions require. Nursing diagnoses related to the bathing and hygiene care of infants and children include:

Self-care deficit: bathing and hygiene, *related to*
- *child's physical level of development*
- *parents' unfamiliarity with hospital routine*
- *child's knowledge deficit*
- *child's fears in unfamiliar environment*

Potential for injury: suffocation, *related to*
- *immersion in water associated with lack of safety precautions by caretaker during bathing of an infant/child*
- *lack of supervision by an adult during infant's/child's bath*

Potential for injury: trauma, *related to excessive temperature of bath water associated with:*
- *caretaker's knowledge deficit*
- *lack of supervision by an adult during infant's/child's bath*

Potential for impaired skin integrity, *related to child's physical condition associated with:*
- *restraint*
- *hyperthermia*
- *immobility*
- *excretions and secretions*
- *humidity*
- *fragility of skin*
- *immunologic immaturity*

Nursing Strategies

The child's hospital bath routine should be as similar as possible to the home bath routine. Adhering as closely as possible to the home rituals of bathing and other routines may help minimize the trauma of hospitalization. Unless the child's physical condition contraindicates, children can be bathed in an infant tub at the bedside or in a standard bathtub or shower.

Parents should be allowed to provide as much of the child's care as possible. Because parents frequently are unsure of their role in the hospital or are reluctant to participate because of the child's physical condition, they need clear instructions from the nurse about any bathing restrictions. When parents take on the responsibility of bathing and hygiene, the nurse is still responsible for the safety of these activities and must ensure that appropriate measures are taken to avoid slipping, scalding, falling, or drowning of the child in the tub. This sometimes means that a nurse must intervene when parents are not observing the necessary safety measures.

As with all procedures, the initial task is to gather all the necessary equipment before beginning, both for efficiency and to ensure that the child is not left unattended. The bath temperature should be about 37.8° to 40.6°C (100° to 105°F), although checking the water with a thermometer is usually not necessary. The water can be tested for comfort against the wrist or inner aspect of forearm, or older children can check the water themselves before getting into the tub.

Infants are usually bathed in a small infant tub at the bedside. *Soapy, wet infants are very slippery;* therefore, the bottom of the tub can be lined with a towel to avoid injury. For those infants unable to sit, the nurse should keep a secure grip on the baby throughout the bath. One hand grasps the infant's arm while the wrist and lower arm support the infant's head. The other hand is then free to bathe the infant.

The eyes should be wiped with a clean washcloth, without soap, working from the inner canthus outward. The auricle and external canal of the ears are washed with soapy water and a washcloth. Do not use cotton swabs as this may impact the cerumen and could possibly damage the tympanic membrane or canal. To clean the female genitalia, separate the labia and gently wipe from front to back. To wash the genitalia of an uncircumcised male, current practice is not to retract the foreskin. Retraction of the foreskin can cause tearing with eventual scarring and phimosis.

The amount of supervision required for an older

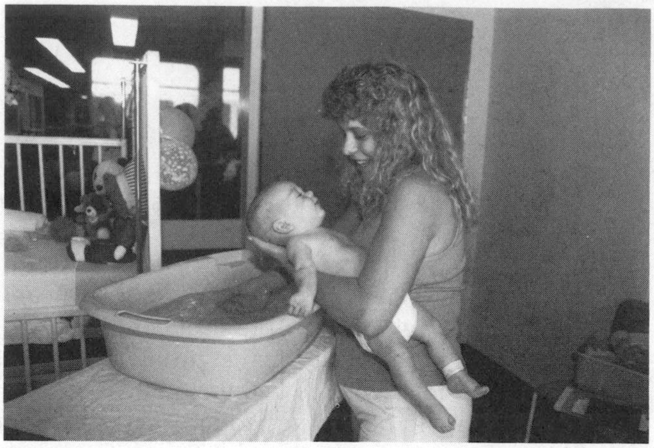

A secure hold of the baby can be accomplished by supporting the head and shoulders with one hand and firmly holding the baby against the caregiver's hip (football hold). The other hand is then free to wash the baby's hair.

child varies. Many preschool- and school-age children are baffled by taking a bath in bed and usually require some instruction and explanation. To them it is a strange request and if left to their own devices they may do a minimal job. Parents can often help supervise when the child's embarrassment makes it awkward for the nurse to check on the child's performance in bathing and hygiene.

Bubble bath products and other additives are frequently requested by children. These are contraindicated for use by children with frequent urinary tract or vaginal infections. At the first sign of skin irritation, the use of these products should be discontinued. There is routinely no need for creams or powders after a bath. Occasionally a lotion is applied to dry skin or a medicated lotion is ordered for specific dermatologic conditions.

Care of the teeth is an area of health care that is frequently neglected while children are in the hospital. If a toothbrush is not provided by the hospital, the nurse should ask the parents to bring one to the hospital for their child. Teethbrushing is an activity that some children do without reminding, but it too is an activity that requires the nurse's supervision and monitoring. It provides an excellent opportunity for nurses to teach about an important health area.

Mouth care for children involves primarily teethbrushing unless mouth ulcers develop. A soft sponge toothbrush is available in most hospitals and can be used if no toothbrush is available or when teethbrushing is contraindicated by the child's physical condition (i.e., low platelet count or mouth ulcers). Mouthwashes can be used in school-age children, but they must be clearly told not to swallow the solution. Lemon glycerin swabs are composed of an alcohol, which dries the mouth, and lemon, which may be painful if the mucosa is already irritated.

Hair care is an important comfort measure to include. An infant's head is washed as part of the daily bath. Older children may resist a hair wash; however, for any child who is hospitalized or confined to bed longer than 2 or 3 days, hair care is important. As much as possible, the technique used to wash and care for the child's hair should be similar to the one used at home. If a hair wash is impossible, then dry shampooing should be considered.

Children who have thick, coarse, or very curly hair need particular attention because this hair-type mats and tangles easily, which may cause breakage. Before matted hair is shampooed, the tangles should be removed as much as possible. To do this, use a wide-tooth comb and work in a small section at a time. Beginning at the ends of the hair, gently fluff and lift the hair. Repeat this step each time, inserting the comb farther into the hair. Pulling on the scalp is painful; *be gentle.* Application of a lubricant (Dermassage, mineral oil, or commercial hair preparations) to the hair may help disentangle it and help prevent breakage if the hair is dry. This process may have to be done in several sittings, as it is uncomfortable and difficult for a child to remain still long enough for the entire head of hair to be finished. Braiding the child's hair may prevent further tangles but care must be taken not to braid too tightly. *When special care is required, parents should be consulted and their assistance encouraged.*

Nursing Care of Children During Procedures

Nurses consider many procedures they do to be common, routine, nonthreatening events. However, for a child, having blood pressure or temperature checked may evoke anxiety and upset if the child is not prepared and supported. Procedures often involve removal of clothing, restriction of movement, and pain or discomfort. These intrusions are particularly feared by young children, who misinterpret the extent of what might occur. Thus, a child should be prepared for the event before beginning a procedure, regardless of how common and nonthreatening it may seem to the nurse.

The nurse plays a major role in allowing procedures to be performed safely and efficiently. Proper positioning and effective restraint to maintain the position avoids injury to the child and shortens the procedure. One cannot generally assume that a child will hold still without some assistance. The nurse's grip must be firm but not painful to the child. The torso and arms of the nurse can be used to block the child's movement. However, care must be taken to avoid pressure from fingertips, injury to internal organs from leaning on the child, and respiratory embarrassment from occluding the airway.

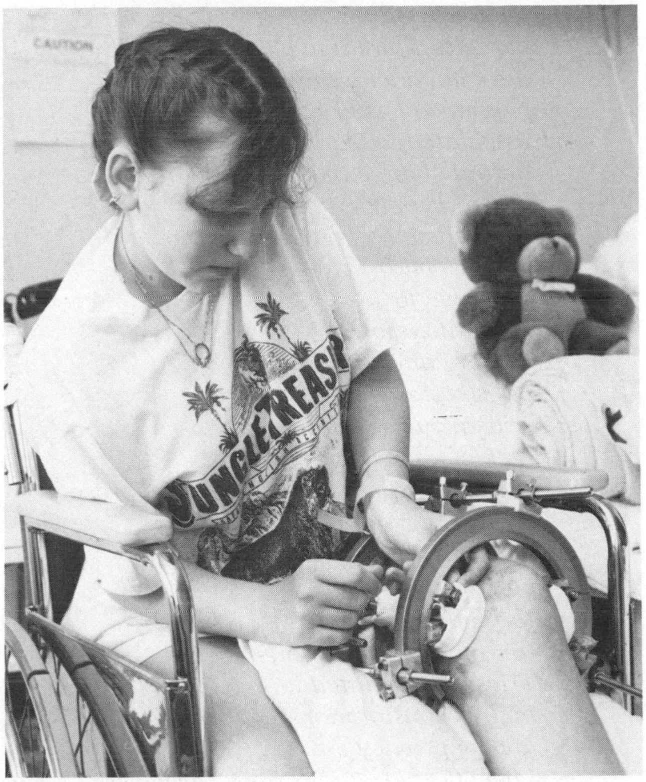

Children and adolescents should be encouraged to participate in procedures whenever possible to give them a sense of control.

Nursing Assessment and Planning

Before beginning a procedure, the nurse must prepare the child and assess the level of cooperation and potential strength of resistance. In many instances, one nurse can position and restrain a child effectively; however, for some children, additional help may be needed. Young children who do not understand an explanation but who have sufficient physical strength to resist with their whole body particularly need careful restraint. The nurse should summon additional help before beginning a procedure for these children.

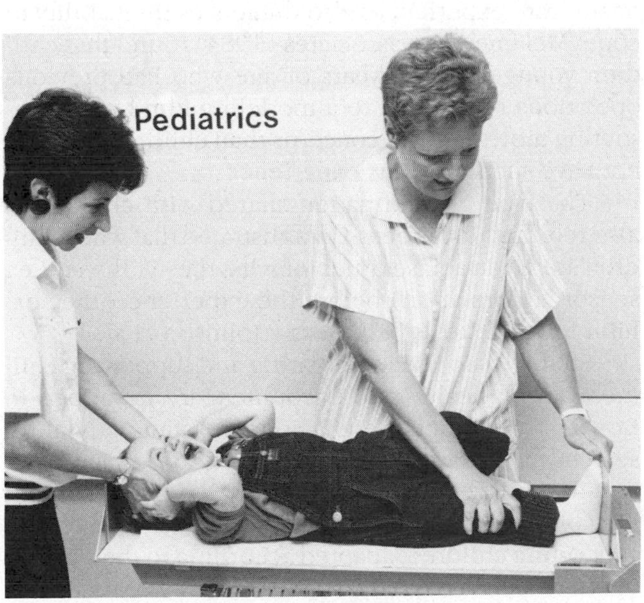

Such a seemingly simple procedure as measuring a toddler's length is resisted vigorously in spite of a prior explanation.

Before a procedure is performed, it should be explained to the child and parents. Whenever possible and appropriate, parents should be encouraged to support the child by being present. The appropriateness of a parent's presence varies with the type of procedure and the wishes of the child and the parent. In many circumstances children and adolescents can participate and should be given the option to do so.

Nursing Diagnoses

The nurse assesses a particular child undergoing a specific procedure and makes appropriate diagnoses. Most children experience some degree of anxiety, fear, powerlessness, pain, and altered coping in association with intrusive procedures, as summarized in the following diagnoses.

Anxiety, *related to*

- *perceived threat to biologic integrity associated with invasive procedures*
- *perceived loss of significant other associated with temporary separation*
- *actual change in environment associated with hospitalization*
- *transmission of parents' anxiety to infant/child*

Fear, *related to*

- *hospitalization*
- *surgery and its outcome*
- *anesthesia*
- *appearance of equipment*
- *lack of knowledge*
- *previous experience of a painful procedure*
- *potential for body mutilation*
- *potential for pain*
- *unfamiliar people*
- *unfamiliar environment*

Powerlessness, *related to*

- *lack of consultation regarding decisions*
- *lack of privacy*
- *lack of explanations from caregivers*
- *lack of parental presence*
- *limitations in cognition, communication, and physical strength due to developmental level*

Ineffective individual coping, *related to*

- *strange environment*
- *pain associated with intrusive procedure*
- *cognitive limitations*
- *separation from support system*
- *lack of opportunity for therapeutic play*
- *lack of appropriate information and preparation for procedure*

Altered comfort (pain), *related to*

- *performance of intrusive diagnostic tests*
- *excessive restraint*
- *improper positioning*
- *chemical irritants (medication)*
- *anxiety level*

Nursing Strategies

The goal of nursing intervention is to attain the maximum therapeutic benefit with the least amount of disruption to the life of the child and the family.

Procedures should be done in the treatment room whenever possible rather than at the child's bedside; thus, trauma is not observed by other children, and needles and equipment are not inadvertently left at a child's bedside. In the child's mind, the bed should be a place that is safe and comfortable. Although children cannot be taken to a treatment room for each intramuscular injection, the nurse should ensure that the more lengthy traumatic procedures are done there. Infants particularly need comfort to feel secure because they lack the cognitive skills to understand intrusive procedures.

The various approaches used to help children and parents cope with health care procedures have been reviewed by Hunsberger and colleagues (1984), Williams and Kendall (1985), and Lutz (1986). Many of the approaches are similar to those used with adults. The child's ability to express fears through play is one of the most influential resources for the nurse. Bringing an activity or event into the child's realm by using play equipment or making up a related game gains the child's attention and brings an element of familiarity to the strangeness of the environment and experience (see Chapter 21 for a discussion on the use of therapeutic play).

The use of parents to support the child is another important aspect. The nurse should recognize that parents' anxiety can directly influence the child's anxiety (Skipper and Leonard, 1978). Parents, therefore, need information and emotional support to reduce anxiety.

The timing of preparation must be adapted to the child's capabilities. Older children (above 6 or 7 years of age) may benefit from *advance preparation,* (before admission) whereas younger children have been reported to benefit from a modeling film* *at the time of admission* to the hospital (Ferguson, 1975; Melamed et al, 1976). Very young children expect events to occur immediately after being informed (Pridham, 1987). Whether children have had earlier traumatic health care experiences also influences their ability to cope. Melamed and associates (1983) found that children younger than 8 years of age who had previous operations responded to a modeling film by demonstrating more medical concerns than children who did not have such previous experiences.

The type of information shared with children is also relevant. It has been demonstrated that when children are given a description of what they will *feel* (i.e., sensory information) before the experience, they exhibit fewer distress behaviors (Johnson et al, 1975).

Strategies to use in preparing and supporting children during health care encounters are described in Box 27-1. Although there is an increasing body of research, further investigation of psychologic preparation for children is required before assuming the efficacy of the various approaches. Approaches useful in supporting children, adapted according to their developmental characteristics, are summarized in Table 27-2.

*A modeling film shows a peer in a similar situation modeling adaptive behaviour.

Box 27-1
Strategies to Help Children Cope with Procedures

INFORMATION THROUGH VERBAL EXPLANATIONS

Verbal description of the procedure explaining the steps and when and where it will take place and who will be involved is called *procedural information*. Additionally, *sensory information* should be provided, including explanation of the sensations that will be felt (Johnson et al, 1975).

STRESS-POINT NURSING

Providing a combination of strategies immediately prior to stressful events (i.e., before a blood test, an injection, or just before leaving for a procedure or the OR). The intervention includes giving procedural and sensory information, identification of the child's role in the event, and rehearsal of behaviors coupled with continued supportive care (contact with the same caregiver) (Wolfer and Visintainer, 1975).

MODELING

Exposure of a child to another peer model in a film in a similar situation. The individual in the film demonstrates coping by first exhibiting fearful behavior but is shown to gradually overcome such fear (coping model). Another model is one who demonstrates an ideal set of behaviors from the outset, not showing fear (mastery model). The coping model has been found to be more effective than the mastery model. Melamed and Siegel (1975) indicate that a modeling film may initially increase arousal (on the Palmer Sweat Index) but that it is instrumental in reducing stress later (pre- and postoperatively).

PRESENCE OF PARENTS

If parents are sufficiently supported, it is generally believed that they can in turn provide emotional support to their child. Although research to demonstrate the effectiveness of parental presence during procedures is lacking, nursing practice in many centers includes parents as a support for their child during stressful events. It should be recognized, however, that not all parents choose to accompany their child during such events and that for some procedures it may be less beneficial than others.

MOTOR ACTIVITIES

A preverbal child lacking the cognitive coping abilities of an older child needs other means to achieve coping. Motor activities that do not interfere with the actual procedure can be encouraged; i.e., allow child to (1) squeeze nerf ball or other object with hands or between knees; (2) squeeze hands of nurse or parent; (3) pound on a pillow (if procedure is on lower extremities); (4) kick against a pillow (if procedure is on upper portion of body). Movement of "procedure area" can be restricted without restricting *all* movement of the child.

PLAY

The use of play to prepare children for procedures, hospitalization, and surgery is prevalent in many hospitals and clinics today. There is considerable anecdotal literature but only a few controlled studies to support the effectiveness of play. (See Chapter 21 for discussion of therapeutic play.)

EMOTIONAL SUPPORT

Emotional support is the provision of an environment within which the parent and child feel comfortable to express feelings and ask questions. Emotional support in combination with information provision has been demonstrated as a beneficial approach (Fassler, 1980; Wolfer and Visintainer, 1975). In some instances emotional support is described as providing contact with the same nurse over a certain series of events (Wolfer and Visintainer, 1975).

PROGRESSIVE MUSCLE RELAXATION

This is a technique in which a child learns to relax his or her own body in a nonstressful situation. The technique must be practiced repeatedly until mastery is achieved and incorporated into their coping repertoire; otherwise, under stress the child reverts to his "usual" patterns of coping. If practiced, at a later time when the child is faced with a stressful situation, the previously learned relaxation techniques can be used. The technique involves learning to tense and relax certain muscle groups and performing breathing exercises. Imagery (having the child imagine a relaxing scene) is used in conjunction with the relaxation exercises. The child can gain a sense of control or mastery by using this technique during a painful procedure and it serves to refocus the child's attention from the procedure to the technique of relaxation. Progressive muscle relaxation exercises for children have been developed by Cautela and Groden (1978).

DESENSITIZATION

This technique requires considerable professional input as it is accomplished over a period of time. A threatening event is reduced to a list of events (stimuli) that lead up to the final threatening procedure. The hierarchy of events (from the least to the most frightening) is introduced one event at a time, enabling the child to cope with each event. As the child is desensitized to each stimulus he or she moves up to the next most frightening one, until the original feared stimulus no longer elicits a fearful response (Walpe and Lazarus, 1973).

SELF-TALK

Self-talk has been used as part of a coping skills package (Siegel and Peterson, 1980) in which children were taught to use relaxation, deep breathing, imagery, and calming self-talk. For example, statements such as "I will be alright soon" or "It will soon be over," are made repeatedly by the child during the procedure.

DISTRACTION

Various methods of distraction are used during painful events. For example, relaxation, imagery, and self-talk are forms of distraction. Other suggestions are counting, squeezing someone's hand, holding a favorite toy or blanket, talking to a favorite toy animal, or actually participate in the procedure (i.e., by opening packages of 4×4's or preparing tape).

Performing Specific Procedures

The unique developmental needs of children dictate precautions that must be taken and serve as a guide for determining how to approach and teach the child. Many procedures need to be altered in terms of size of equipment and approach to the patient. Numerous procedures are specific to the care of children (such as the attaching of a urinary collection bag and applying a mummy restraint).

The child's illness and therapeutic regimen largely determine the procedures the child will undergo. Specific procedures are described in the chapter in which a particular illness is discussed (Chapters 38 to 52). Procedures required by most children regardless of illness include the assessment of vital signs, collection of specimens, and administration of medications and intravenous therapy. Medication administration and intravenous therapy are discussed in Chapters 28 and 30, respectively. Following is a discussion of the nurse's responsibility in assessment of vital signs and collection of specimens.

Assessment of Vital Signs

Children are fascinated by medical equipment; cooperation can often be gained by letting a child touch and briefly use equipment on a doll or stuffed animal. It is especially important to take the time to familiarize a child with equipment when they first encounter these procedures.

Temperature. A child's temperature is usually checked orally, rectally, or by the axillary method. Activity and excessive crying can elevate a child's temperature; it is most accurate if the child is quiet and at rest. Temperature assessment is surrounded by a variety of myths, unknowns, and unfounded strong beliefs. Consequently, there is no consistency of practice among institutions. Policies evolve from a combination of individual biases and minimal research findings.

Temperature assessment in children has been made much easier, more accurate, and safer with new electronic devices. Traditionally, the use of the glass thermometer limited how quickly a temperature could be measured and excluded the oral route as an option in young children. Because circumstances exist in which glass thermometers continue to be used, both methods will be addressed.

It is now possible to obtain an accurate temperature reading from a child in a short time electronically. One commonly used device is the IVAC electronic clinical thermometer. This is a hand-held rechargeable unit that is taken to the bedside to be used. The unit has two probes (rectal has a red end and oral has a blue end) with disposable covers. Patient positioning and indication of selection of route are similar to those for the use of a glass thermometer. The major advantage is that it takes only several seconds to obtain the temperature reading, which is indicated by an audible signal. After use, it is necessary to return the device to the storage unit, where it is recharged.

An oral temperature cannot be taken with a glass thermometer in infants and young children who cannot hold the thermometer in place or who might bite the thermometer, resulting in injury from broken glass or release of mercury into a child's mouth. Some institutions have a specific age restriction (5 or 6 years of age) under which an oral temperature by glass thermometer is not permitted. A disoriented or mentally retarded child must also be protected from this danger.

A glass thermometer is placed under the tongue slightly to the right or left of the midline so that it rests in the sublingual pocket. It is left in place 3 to 5 minutes with the mouth closed. With an electronic thermometer, contact is maintained until the buzzer sounds and the read-out is stabilized.

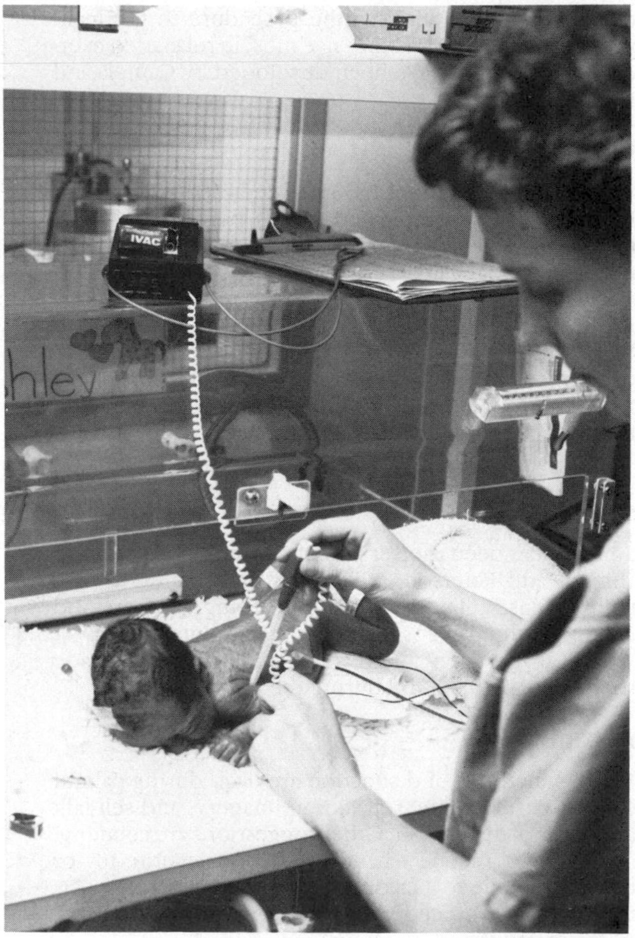

An electronic thermometer is used to obtain an axillary temperature. This equipment provides an accurate reading quickly and safely for this premature infant.

Because an oral reading may be inaccurate if taken immediately after the child drinks or eats, it is necessary to wait 15 minutes after anything is taken by mouth before measuring temperature orally. Furthermore, any condition that causes the child to mouth-breathe is a contraindication for taking a temperature orally. Oxygen therapy by tent or nasal cannula has been reported not to cause a significant change in oral temperature (Graas, 1974). Mask-administered oxygen may cause an oral reading that does not reflect the true body temperature.

Opinion varies as to the accuracy of axillary temperatures. Axillary temperatures are less intrusive than rectal temperatures and safer than oral temperatures for young children. The disadvantage is the length of time it takes to get an accurate reading. The thermometer is placed in the axilla against the skin. Care must be taken to ensure that the thermometer remains in contact with the skin during the entire procedure. A glass thermometer is left in place for 7 to 10 minutes (an electronic thermometer, usually less than 1 minute). Although some professionals believe axillary temperatures are not as accurate as rectal temperatures, there are few published studies from which to make a judgment. In neonates, a high correlation has been reported (Buntain et al, 1977; Eoff et al, 1974) between axillary and rectal temperatures measured with glass thermometers. Similarly, in a study of 50 patients (25 toddlers and 25 preschoolers) axillary and rectal temperature readings with glass thermometers were highly correlated (Eoff and Joyce, 1981). A study in which an electronic thermometer was used to compare rectal and axillary temperatures of 50 preschool children further confirms the accuracy of axillary temperatures (Barrus, 1983). The mean difference between rectal and axillary temperatures in this study was 0.42°C (0.76°F).

To take a rectal temperature, the child is positioned prone or supine with the hips flexed. The supine position is preferable as it allows the caretaker to talk to the child and maintain eye contact, but the most important consideration is that the child is held securely to prevent squirming. The thermometer is lubricated with a water-soluble jelly and is then inserted about 1/2 to 1 inch into the rectum. Safety is enhanced by holding the thermometer between two fingers while resting the hand securely over the buttocks for stabilization (i.e., preventing the thermometer from slipping further in or out). This way, if the child moves, the nurse's hand will move with the child, thus maintaining the position of the thermometer. Frequently, insertion of the thermometer stimulates the child to defecate. If the child passes stool, remove the thermometer, allow the child to complete the bowel movement and begin again. Hold a glass thermometer in place for 3 minutes (an electronic thermometer usually less than 1 minute), then gently withdraw the thermometer. Rectal temperatures are usually not recommended for children who have severe diarrhea (they may increase stooling), those who have had rectal surgery (due to trauma), and low birthweight infants. Many institutions have policies prohibiting rectal temperatures prior to 6 weeks of age because of the danger of puncturing friable rectal mucosa.

Pulse. When assessing a child's pulse, not only is the rate considered but also the rhythm and quality. The pulse should be assessed when the child is quiet, as activity or crying increases the rate. For this reason, it is best to check it before beginning any procedures to be done at the same time. Common descriptive terms for quality of the pulse are "thready," "bounding," or "faint."

The apical rather than the peripheral pulse is usually assessed in young children. To do this, palpate the apical pulse (also called point of maximal impulse) and place the diaphragm of the stethoscope on this point (palpation of apical pulse is discussed in Chapter 15). Listen closely, noting the rate, rhythm, and quality of the pulsation. If the pulse is of regular rhythm, it is acceptable to listen for 30 seconds and multiply by 2 to determine the beats per minute. An exception to this procedure is when the child has a cardiac problem, in which case auscultation for a full minute is recommended.

Respiration. Respiratory rate is assessed by noting the number of inspirations per minute. Activity or excitement may cause an increase in the respiratory rate, so this assessment should be done when the child is quiet. In addition to rate, it is important to observe for increased respiratory effort. Indicators of this are retractions (e.g., substernal, intercostal, and supraclavicular), nasal flaring, and use of abdominal muscles to breathe. Respiratory difficulty may cause grunting or wheezing and apprehension. These signs should be noted as signals of distress which may indicate the child needs prompt attention.

An accurate respiratory rate for a neonate is obtained during sleep or quiet rest, usually through auscultation (placing a stethoscope on the infant's thorax and counting respirations) or palpation (placing the hand on the abdomen to count respirations). It is also possible to obtain the abdominal respiratory rate in some infants (infants have primarily diaphragmatic respirations) by observing abdominal movement. An infant's respirations are frequently irregular and must be counted for a full minute. After infancy, the respiratory rate of a child is obtained by observing chest movement for 30 seconds and multiplying by 2 unless the child has respiratory illness; in this case auscultation for a full minute is recommended.

Blood Pressure. Blood pressure measurement is a reading often neglected in children unless the child presents with a diagnosis such as renal disease, cardiac disease, or head trauma. The American Academy of Pediatrics recommends that all children 3 years of age and older have their blood pressure measured annually as part of their routine health assessment. This is a necessary step in identifying individuals at risk for developing hypertension as adults and to prevent the long-term complications for hypertensive individuals.

The most important factor in taking an accurate blood pressure reading is the size of the cuff. The cuff should cover two thirds of the upper arm. The cuff's bladder should be one fifth longer than the circumference of the child's arm. A cuff that is too narrow or too short may result in a falsely high reading, and a too-large cuff may cause a falsely low reading.

The first step in taking a blood pressure reading in a child is to explain the procedure to the child and to allow him or her to handle the equipment. Apprehension can cause the blood pressure reading to be higher than is normal for the child; therefore, every effort should be made to help the child relax. As with adults, the child is seated with the right arm resting at heart level. The right arm is used whenever possible, as this is the arm used in the development of standardized charts. The procedure from this point on is identical to that used with adults.

Electronic equipment has simplified blood pressure measurement in children. The cuff is applied to the arm and attached to an electronic machine which pumps up the cuff and gives the systolic and diastolic pulse rates and pulse pressure within seconds. An Electronic Doppler apparatus, used in some institutions for small infants, gives more accurate systolic and diastolic readings than the conventional blood pressure apparatus.

Occasionally blood pressure cannot be auscultated and electronic equipment is not available. Blood pressure measurement by palpation is an alternative method. The steps in this method are:

1. Place the proper size of cuff on the arm.
2. Palpate the brachial pulse and keep fingertips over pulse site with sufficient pressure to feel the pulse but not obliterate it.
3. Inflate the cuff until the pulse is no longer felt.
4. Deflate the cuff until the pulse is again felt.

The point at which the pulse is again felt is the systolic pressure and is recorded 98/P, indicating the palpation method has been used.

Obtaining blood pressure measurement on an infant is a more difficult procedure and is not routinely done during well-child examinations. When it is necessary, electronic units are most accurate. If this equipment is not available and attempts to auscultate the blood pressure are not successful, a "flush" blood pressure measurement can be obtained. This method is less accurate and reveals only the mean pressure. The steps in this procedure are:

1. Place the proper size of cuff on the arm.
2. Raise the arm and snugly wrap an elastic bandage around it, starting from the fingers and proceeding up to the cuff.
3. Inflate the cuff and remove the elastic bandage. The arm should be blanched (paler than its normal coloring).
4. Slowly deflate the cuff.
5. Note when the arm flushes. This is the mean pressure.

It is possible to obtain a blood pressure reading by placing a cuff on the thigh of a child. This is done if there is no access to the arms or if a cardiac abnormality is suspected. The proper size of cuff is placed around the thigh and the femoral artery in the popliteal space is palpated. The procedure then is the same as that used to obtain a reading with the arm. In infants under 1 year old, the reading is normally the same as in the arm. After age 1 year, the systolic reading is normally higher in the thigh than in the arm. A lower thigh reading suggests coarctation of the aorta.

Collection of Specimens

Children are frequently unable to cooperate to produce the needed specimen. Young children do not have the cognitive ability to understand instructions and in many instances lack the physiologic capability to produce the specimen. Thus, specimen collection for the child is often an intrusive, frightening experience requiring some degree of body manipulation and restraint. Special adaptations are necessary to collect specimens from children in a way that is technically accurate yet produces minimal disruption and frustration in the child.

Specimens, once collected, must be clearly labeled and immediately processed. The nurse should be sure that the correct laboratory slip accompanies the specimen when it is sent to the laboratory.

Collection of Urine Specimens. Urine specimens are collected in various ways, depending on the age of the child and the purpose of the specimen. The major difficulty is the collection of specimens from children who are not toilet trained. Routine urine specimens are collected by using a clean plastic urine bag which is applied to the perineum or over the penis. Twenty-four hour urine specimens require a special collecting bag with tubing. Specimens for culture are collected by using a sterile urine bag. In some instances, either catheterization or suprapubic needle aspiration of urine from the bladder is indicated to collect a specimen for culture.

If contamination by skin does not alter the results

of the required tests (e.g., specific gravity), urine can be squeezed from a diaper or drawn out of a diaper with a syringe from which the needle has been removed. If a disposable diaper is not saturated enough, some of the wettest cotton batting can be extracted (using disposable gloves) from the diaper and squeezed to obtain the urine, or the cotton batting can be placed into the barrel of a 3 cc syringe (without a needle) and the plunger inserted to push out urine from the cotton batting. One drop of urine squeezed from a diaper is sufficient to test specific gravity with a fractometer. Reams and Deane (1988), compared laboratory values of specific gravity, blood, protein, ketones, and glucose from bagged versus diaper urine specimens and reported no significant difference.

Routine Urine Specimen. A specimen for routine urinalysis is collected from an infant or young child by using the following guidelines:

1. Wash hands well, then cleanse the perineum or penis with soap and water; rinse and dry. This should be done before collection of any urine specimen from a child who is not toilet trained.
2. The bag can be applied using various techniques. If applied from side to side, the paper backing from one side is peeled off and folded back. That side of the bag is then attached to the skin starting at the bottom and moving upward. The paper backing is then peeled off completely and the other side of the bag attached similarly. If applied from bottom to top, the paper backing from the lower half of the bag is removed and the lower portion is secured. Once the lower part is carefully secured the paper backing from the upper portion is removed and the top half of the bag secured. In either method, the single most important factor is that the bag securely adheres to the skin, especially along the lower edge where leakage and contamination are most likely to occur. For females the perineum is pulled slightly taut during application of the lower portion of the bag. In young male infants, placing the penis and scrotum inside the bag facilitates a better seal at the lower edge. For older male infants and toddlers, the bag can be applied on top of the scrotum with only the penis inside.
3. Secure a diaper over the bag to prevent loosening of the bag by pulling or kicking.
4. Place the infant or child into a semi-Fowler's position to facilitate flow of urine by gravity into the urine bag.
5. Give the usual amount of fluids. Overhydration may produce inaccurate results.
6. Check urine bag frequently (every 20 to 30 minutes) because the weight of the urine in the bag may cause it to loosen. Also, for the most accurate laboratory analysis, urine should be collected as soon as possible after the child has voided.
7. After the child voids, remove the bag gently to avoid skin irritation; then cleanse the area and rediaper the child.
8. When the specimen has been obtained, transfer it to a clean specimen container. Either refrigerate it or deliver it to the laboratory promptly. If a urine specimen cannot be delivered to the laboratory within 1 to 2 hours, it should be refrigerated. A urine specimen that is stored in the refrigerator preferably should not be stored longer than overnight.

Clean-Catch Specimen for Culture. With older children, the collection of a clean-catch or midstream urine specimen is done in a similar manner as with adults. The major differences are that more supervision is required and that the required supervision may embarrass the child.

The nurse should carefully explain why the specimen is needed and what the procedure entails, as well as forewarning the child about the coldness of the cleansing solution. Parents should be invited to accompany the child to collect the specimen if the child so desires; however, preferably the nurse should take responsibility for supervision to ensure that the urine is collected properly. Proper collection of a cleanly voided specimen may obviate the need for catheterization of a child.

Girls are asked to sit in the usual position on the toilet. The nurse wears a sterile glove to spread the labia to cleanse the meatus. The perineum is cleansed with an antiseptic solution or soap and water by wiping from front to back along each side of the meatus and directly across the meatus using a clean sponge for each wipe. The perineum is then rinsed with sterile water or saline and patted dry with a sterile gauze sponge. It is important to dry the area well because the presence of an antiseptic in the urine specimen may prevent bacterial growth, giving a false-negative report. The girl is then asked to void while the labia are spread apart. After the stream is started, a midstream sample of urine is collected in a sterile container, after which the child finishes voiding.

Boys are asked to stand in the usual position to void. The meatus and glans penis are cleaned with antiseptic solution or soap and water. If the boy is uncircumcised, the foreskin is retracted sufficiently to cleanse the meatus and glans penis. The area is then rinsed and patted dry and a midstream urine sample collected. For an uncircumcised boy, care is taken to slide the foreskin to its original position to prevent constriction of the penis.

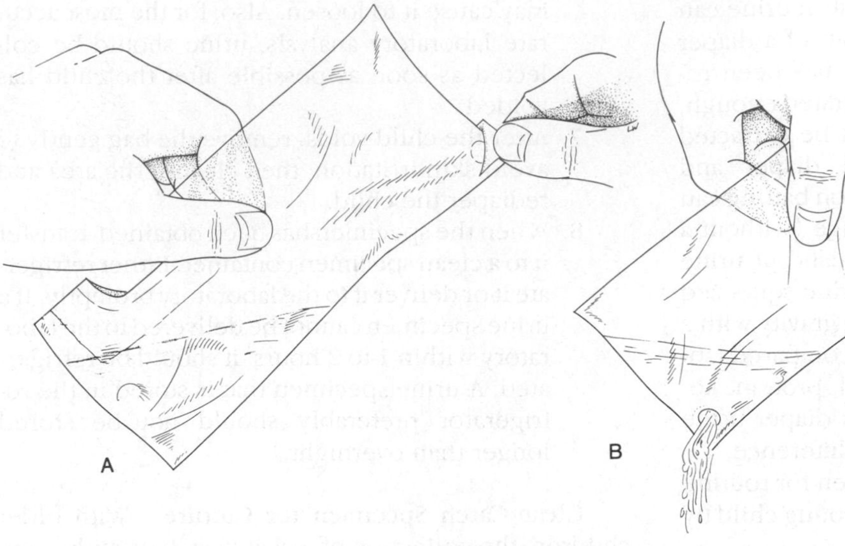

Figure 27-3. Emptying urine for culture from a sterile urine bag. *A*, To drain urine into a specimen bottle, tip the bag to one side with blue tab at upper edge. Remove blue tab. Be careful to avoid spilling or contaminating urine at large opening of bag. *B*, Turn bag with exposed small hole at lower edge and pour into sterile container. Apply lid, label, and send to laboratory.

During specimen collection for urine culture, the open edge of the container used to collect the voided specimen is not to touch the child's skin. The nurse immediately closes the container with a sterile lid and care is taken not to touch the open edge or the inside of the container. The specimen should be delivered to the laboratory as soon as possible. Urine specimens for culture must be tested promptly because of the rapidity of bacterial growth. At room temperature, bacteria double every 20 to 30 minutes.

For infants and young children, urine for culture is collected by using a sterile urine bag. The perineum or penis is cleansed in the same way as just described for a clean-catch urine specimen, using antiseptic solution or soap and water. After the area is thoroughly dry, a sterile urine bag is applied in the same manner as for a routine urine specimen. A sterile urine bag has a small hole on the lower edge to one side of the bag that is covered with a blue tab (Fig. 27-3). To empty the bag, it is held in such a way that the area with the tab is free of urine. After the tab is pulled off, the bag is then tipped into a position that permits drainage of the urine through the small hole that was under the tab. A urine culture requires at least 1 to 2 ml of urine.

Collection of a 24-Hour Urinary Output. For infants and children who do not have bladder control, a special collecting device is used to collect urinary output for a 24-hour period. The plastic urine bag is similar to those used for routine urine collection except that a long drainage tube is connected to one corner of the lower edge of the bag (Fig. 27-4). As the child voids, the urine can be drained via this tube without removing the bag.

The urine bag is applied using the same technique

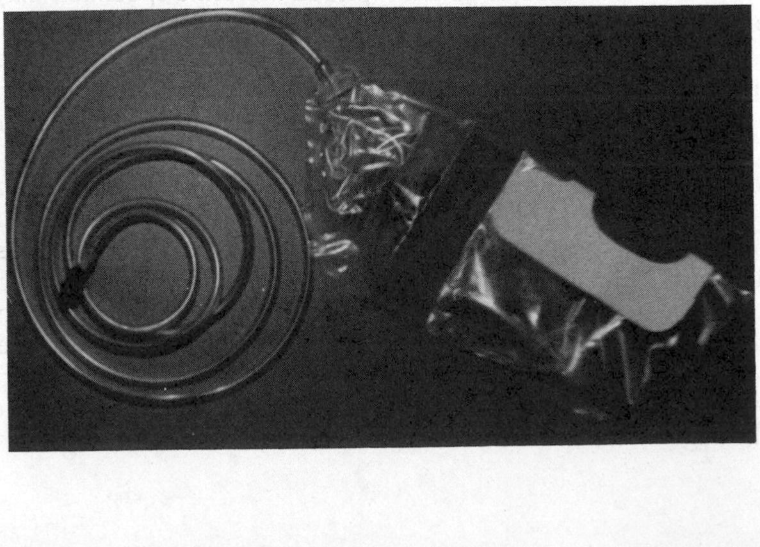

Figure 27-4. Urine collector for 24-hour specimen. The tube can remain coiled inside the child's diaper. The end of the tube has a cap that is removed frequently to empty urine. After the paper backing is removed, the designated edge must form a tight seal against the skin by use of an adhesive dressing. The lower edge of bag is applied first, using either side-to-side or bottom-to-top method.

as for routine urine collection, except for the use of an adhesive skin preparation such as tincture of benzoin to form a sticky surface before applying the bag. Tincture of benzoin (or a similar solution) is painted with a cotton-tipped applicator onto the area that will come in contact with the sealing edge of the urine bag; within a few minutes the area becomes sticky, providing an adhesive surface for attachment of the urine bag.

It is of prime importance that the bag be securely attached to prevent leakage, contamination, or loss of the entire voiding because loss of specimens interferes with the accuracy of the test. Numerous methods are used to keep the bag in position, many requiring some form of restraint. When the long tube is uncoiled and attached to a drainage bottle, restraints may be necessary to prevent the child from grasping the tube with the hands or creating a pull on it with the feet and legs.

Contamination by stool is one of the most frequently occurring problems, and necessitates restarting the 24-hour urine collection. Various forms of restraint on a sling or frame are sometimes used to avoid stool contamination. In this method, a bedpan is placed beneath the frame and the child placed on the frame without a diaper, allowing the stool to fall away from the urine bag. This method is frustrating to the child and parents and is usually unnecessary. An alternate method not involving restraint is to leave the tube coiled within the diaper. The tube has a removable cap that is opened periodically to drain the urine from the bag. With this method, the bag must be checked and emptied frequently because the weight of the urine creates a pull on the bag. Frequent checking of the urine bag also decreases the likelihood of losing the specimen owing to stool contamination. Parents can help the nurse decide how frequently the urine bag must be checked because they are generally aware of how frequently their child's diaper needs to be changed. This method is usually effective, only presenting a problem when a child has diarrhea.

The nurse is responsible for managing the collection of a 24-hour urine specimen. It is started just after the child has voided. Urine from this first voiding is discarded, but the time of the voiding is recorded as the starting time. For infants and children, it is more difficult to know the exact time of voiding. A dry diaper is checked frequently until the child voids. The bag is applied immediately after the wet diaper is noted.

During the collection period, the nurse must ensure that the urine is being stored according to specification from the laboratory. A nurse who is not certain how to store the urine should call the hospital laboratory. The bag is removed 24 hours after the time of the discarded specimen or wet diaper, and the specimen is delivered promptly to the laboratory. Improperly managing the collection of a 24-hour urine specimen may cause delay in the child's discharge; every attempt must be made to apply the bag securely, check the bag frequently, store the urine properly, and deliver it to the laboratory promptly.

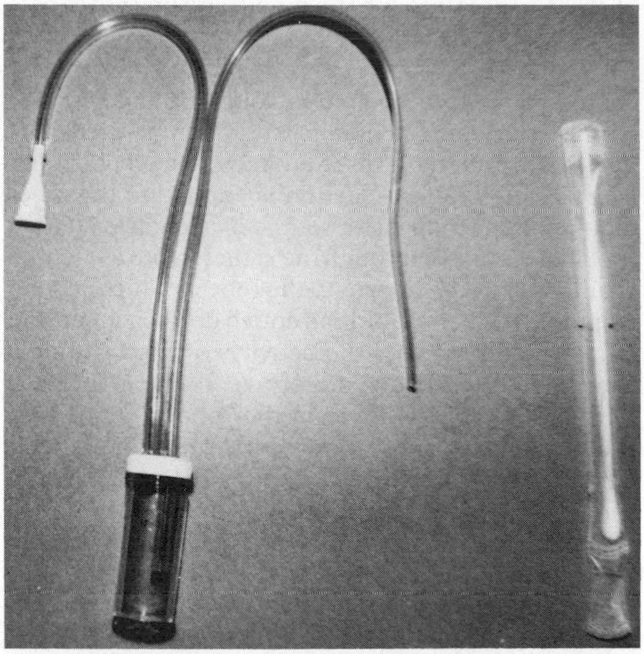

Figure 27-5. Devices used to collect throat and sputum specimens. *Left,* a mucus trap for sputum collection. Suction is applied via the tube curved to the left; the tube on the right side is the catheter tip that is inserted to the trachea. *Right,* sterile culture swab with transport media used for culture.

Throat, Nasopharyngeal, and Sputum Specimens. Specimen collection from the nose and throat is unpleasant. It should be done as efficiently and accurately as possible to avoid having to repeat the procedure. A brief explanation just before performing the procedure is appropriate for children of all ages. To obtain a throat culture, a sterile swab that contains transport medium is used (Fig. 27-5). Transport medium prevents specimens from drying before reaching the laboratory. To culture the throat, the swab should touch the most inflamed and purulent area. The swab should be passed with a rolling motion deep into the throat and across the tonsils without touching the tongue on entry or exit of the mouth. This procedure should stimulate the gag reflex if done properly. If the child cannot cooperate by opening the mouth wide, a tongue depressor should be used to hold the tongue while entering the throat with the swab. The swab is returned to the holder and pushed into the lower chamber, which holds the transport media. Various types of tubes are available whose operation is similar in principle.

To culture the nasopharynx, a swab on a flexible wire is used. Entry can be made through the nasal passages, flexing the wire downward to reach the nasopharynx or pass through the mouth and upward to pass under the uvula.

To collect a sputum specimen from children who are too young to cooperate in coughing and expectorating, a device called a mucus trap can be used (Fig. 27-5). The catheter is inserted into the trachea, stimulating a cough reflex. Suction is applied to the other tube by connecting it to a source of suction. A sputum specimen is drawn through the catheter into the mucus chamber (it is not drawn up the tube to which suction is applied). When a child can cough up a specimen, the nurse should monitor the activity to avoid getting a specimen that has been merely cleared from the back of the throat. Located within the bronchi and lungs, sputum can be removed only by a deep cough (Marchiondo, 1979). The best time to collect a sputum specimen is when the patient awakens in the morning. Specimens from the respiratory tract are collected in sterile containers. The edges and inside of the container should be kept free of contamination. The outside of the container should also be free of contamination from secretions to protect personnel handling the specimen. Collection time should be marked on the container, and it should be delivered to the laboratory immediately.

Stool Specimens. To obtain a stool sample, the tip of a tongue blade is used to transfer stool into a clean cup (a sterile container is not necessary for stool specimens). Frequently, a stool specimen must be obtained from a child with diarrhea who is not yet toilet trained; a sample of stool can be obtained by scraping a tongue blade across the diaper. If even a minute amount of stool remains on the blade, this can be broken off into the cup. When it is not possible to obtain a stool specimen, a rectal swab is done; however, only in shigellosis, gonorrhea, and a few other infections do the organisms live on the rectal walls rather than exclusively in the feces (Marchiondo, 1979). A rectal swab is done by gently inserting a swab into the rectum and slightly twisting it as it is removed. The swab is inserted approximately as far as when a rectal temperature is taken. Stool specimens and rectal swabs should be sent to the laboratory immediately. Specimens for ova and parasites need to be delivered to the laboratory immediately unless a fixating solution is used.

Blood Specimens. Collection of blood specimens is one of the most commonly performed procedures, but to a child it can be terrifying. The appearance of the equipment and the thought of having a "hole where blood can come out" can set a child off into a fit of terror. Children often begin crying fretfully at the sight of the person in white who draws blood.

Anticipation of having blood drawn causes anxiety that some children experience unnecessarily because they have not been told that a blood test is not required for them. Whenever possible, children should be protected from seeing and hearing other children go through the experience of having blood drawn. Assuring a child that he or she will not have blood drawn (when that is the case) is important to allay such fears.

Those children who do require a blood test should receive an explanation when approached. For them, the fear that is evoked can be lessened but usually not eliminated. The nurse tells the child it must be done, explains what the child can do to help, and consoles the child before and after the procedure. Giving the child a finger puppet to play with after the procedure can also help to relieve the distress. The nurse should be present whenever possible to assist laboratory personnel in restraining the child and to provide explanations and support to the child and parent(s).

Proper care of the venipuncture site after the procedure includes application of pressure to stop the bleeding and appropriate covering of the puncture site. A small Bandaid is sufficient and welcomed by most children, especially if someone takes the time to draw a happy face or animal face with whiskers on the Bandaid. Cotton balls applied with a piece of tape should be avoided because a young child may remove the cotton ball and aspirate a piece of cotton fluff.

The three sources of blood used for diagnostic purposes are venous, arterial, and capillary.

Venous Sampling. Venipunctures are done either by laboratory technicians or specially trained nurses. A site is selected, taking into consideration its accessibility, its safety, and its size. The vein must be large enough to contain the amount of blood needed for the sample. If an IV is infusing, a site in another extremity is chosen.

Veins of the antecubital fossa are usually the site of

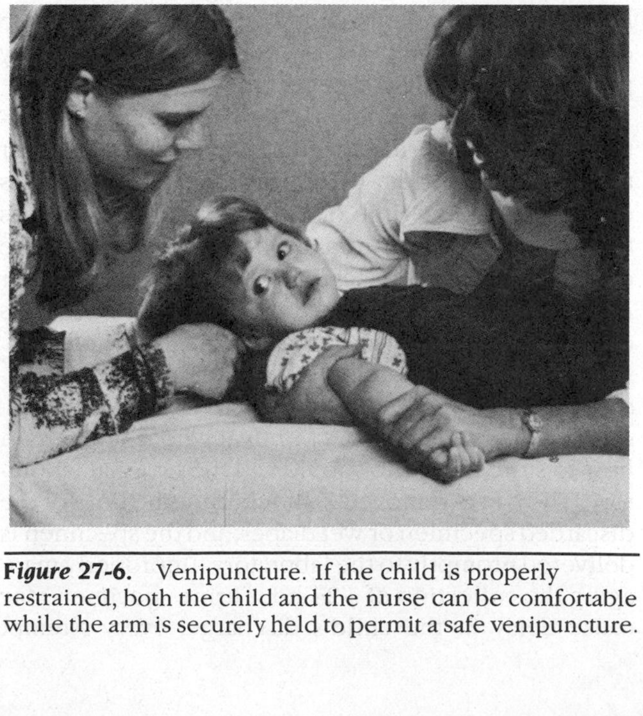

Figure 27-6. Venipuncture. If the child is properly restrained, both the child and the nurse can be comfortable while the arm is securely held to permit a safe venipuncture.

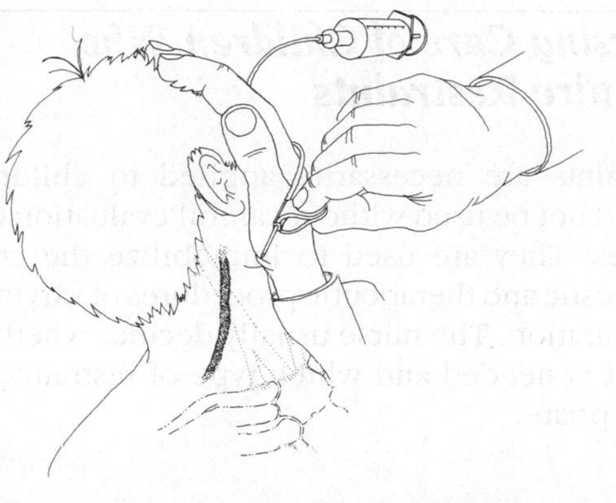

Figure 27-7. The external jugular vein. (From Hughes WT, Buescher ES: *Pediatric Procedures.* 2nd ed. Philadelphia, WB Saunders, 1980.)

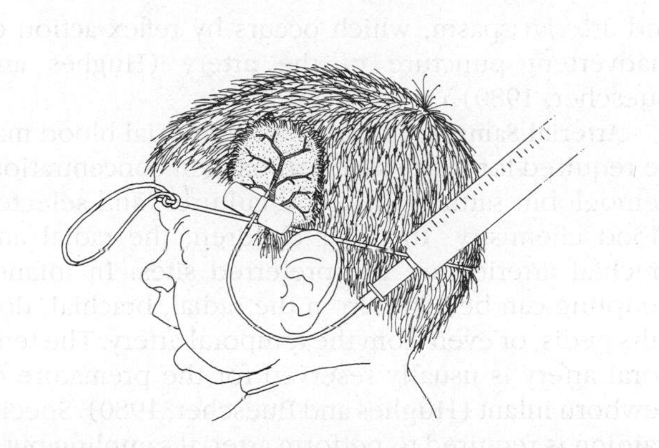

Figure 27-8. Venipuncture of the scalp veins. Site of the superficial temporal vein. (From Hughes WT, Buescher ES: *Pediatric Procedures,* 2nd ed. Philadelphia, WB Saunders, 1980.)

choice for children older than 2 years of age. Veins in this location are commonly both visible and palpable.

With the child in a supine position, the nurse can extend the child's arm, slightly hyperextending the elbow. The other hand is used to grasp the child's shoulder by placing it around the back of the child's neck (Fig. 27-6). The child's unused arm is secured behind the nurse's back. The nurse's torso can lean across the child but the weight is on the nurse's elbow, not on the child. This position is effective to restrain the child for the venipuncture and also allows talking and maintaining eye contact because the nurse's face will be in direct alignment with the child's face.

In children older than age 2, the veins of the dorsum of the hand and foot are sometimes used. If a child is on bedrest, puncture of the lower extremity is less desirable because of the risk of thrombophlebitis or embolism. In infants less than 1 year of age, the external jugular vein is used if withdrawal from other sites has been unsuccessful. The infant is placed in a mummy restraint (see Fig. 27-10) and in a supine position with the infant's head and neck supported in the nurse's hands. The infant's head is held off the edge of the table with the shoulders resting on the table. The infant's head is turned approximately 45 to 60 degrees to one side of the midline (Fig. 27-7). Key elements that enhance the success of this procedure are sufficient rotation of the head to cause stretching of the vein, stimulating the infant to cry, and ensuring that the infant's head does not move after the needle has been inserted into the vein (Hughes and Buescher, 1980). Stimulating the infant to cry during the procedure promotes filling of the vessel, which facilitates blood withdrawal. Immediately after withdrawing the needle, the infant should be brought to an upright position and pressure applied to the site to reduce bleeding from the site. In infants less than 1 year old, it is also possible to obtain a blood specimen from a superficial vein of the scalp. This method is reserved for times when other methods are unsuccessful (because the baby's hair must be shaved to select the vein). A rubberband placed around the head is often used as a tourniquet (Fig. 27-8). To be successful, traction is applied to the skin around the vein to stabilize it, and the needle is inserted against the direction of blood flow.

The femoral vein is used whenever a more superficial vein is not accessible. The child is placed in a supine position on a padded but firm table with the nurse at the child's head. The nurse assists by restraining the child; to do this, the nurse's arms must be extended along each side of the child, grasping the child's knees. The child's legs are flexed and abducted (Fig. 27-9), and the pelvis and knees are held firmly against the table while the blood is drawn. When the specimen has been collected, pressure is applied over the site with a dry sterile gauze pad as the needle is withdrawn; slight pressure over the site is maintained for at least 3 minutes after the needle is withdrawn. This method of blood sampling is undesirable because it is associated with hazards of infection, hematoma,

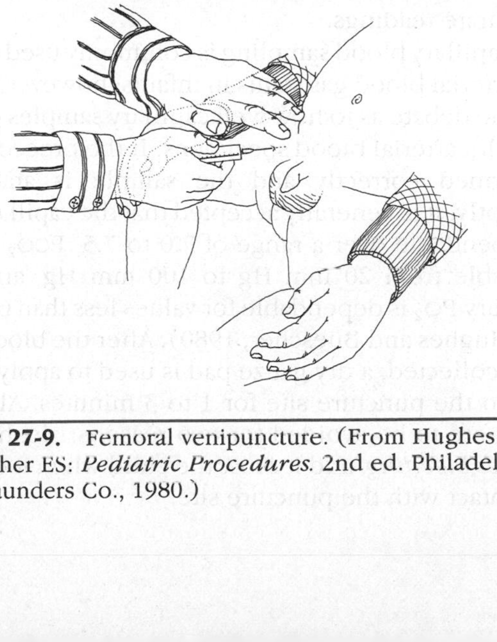

Figure 27-9. Femoral venipuncture. (From Hughes WT, Buescher ES: *Pediatric Procedures.* 2nd ed. Philadelphia, WB Saunders Co., 1980.)

and arterial spasm, which occurs by reflex action or inadvertent puncture of the artery (Hughes and Buescher, 1980).

Arterial Sampling. Samples of arterial blood may be required for studies such as oxygen concentration, hemoglobin saturation, blood cultures, and selected blood chemistry. In older children, the radial and brachial arteries are the preferred sites. In infants, sampling can be taken from the radial, brachial, dorsalis pedis, or even from the temporal artery. The temporal artery is usually reserved for the premature or newborn infant (Hughes and Buescher, 1980). Special training is required to perform arterial sampling but it has become a nursing responsibility in many intensive care settings. After the specimen is collected, a dry sterile gauze pad is used to apply firm pressure for 3 to 5 minutes with one finger centered on the site of puncture, while avoiding excessive pressure that may occlude the artery.

Capillary Blood Sampling. Capillary blood samples are also called "arterialized" samples. If the specimen is properly collected, a puncture wound of the skin can supply satisfactory specimens for micro samples for routine laboratory analysis, capillary blood gas analysis, and micro blood culture. Samples can be drawn from the heel for infants under age 2, from the finger (index, middle, or ring) or great toe in older infants and children, and from the earlobe in children if other sites are inaccessible.

The area to be sampled is warmed to accelerate blood flow through the vascular bed. Severe squeezing or "milking" causes the blood to pool in the area and interferes with blood flow (venostasis). Such manipulation also results in tissue damage, which causes the cells to lyse. Clotting factors are released and hematocrit and hemoglobin units are elevated because as the cells are damaged, hemoglobin is released into the plasma. Potassium levels are also elevated as a result of tissue damage caused by squeezing. Severe vasoconstriction, polycythemia, or local edema also result in inaccurate readings.

Capillary blood sampling is commonly used to follow arterial blood gas status in infants; however, there is some debate as to how well capillary samples correlate with arterial blood specimens. If the procedure is performed correctly and the sample is analyzed promptly, it is generally accepted that the capillary pH is dependable over a range of 7.0 to 7.5, P_{CO_2} is dependable from 20 mm Hg to 100 mm Hg, and the capillary P_{O_2} is dependable for values less than 60 mm Hg (Hughes and Buescher, 1980). After the blood has been collected, a dry gauze pad is used to apply pressure to the puncture site for 1 to 3 minutes. Alcohol swabs are to be avoided for two reasons: alcohol *increases bleeding,* and it *hurts* the child when it comes in contact with the puncture site.

Nursing Care of Children Who Require Restraints

Restraints are necessarily applied to children but should not be used without careful evaluation of alternatives. They are used to immobilize the child for diagnostic and therapeutic procedures of varying types and duration. The nurse usually decides whether a restraint is needed and which type of restraint is most appropriate.

Type of Restraint

Commonly used restraints in the care of children are (1) mummy restraints, (2) elbow restraints, (3) jacket restraints, and (4) arm and leg restraints.

A *mummy restraint* is used to immobilize an infant or small child for a short time as required for examination or treatment of the head, neck, or chest. The purpose of this technique is to secure the arms and legs within a blanket in a way that prevents the child from wriggling free. The nurse is thus free to hold the child securely to prevent movement of his or her entire body without attending to flailing arms and legs. This technique is particularly useful for jugular punctures, insertion of nasogastric tubes, scalp vein needle insertion, and detailed examination of the eye, ear, nose, and throat (Fig. 27-10).

The *modified mummy restraint* is used for procedures that require an exposed chest. Figure 27-11 details steps in securing the infant in a modified mummy restraint.

The purpose of an *elbow restraint* is to keep the child from reaching his or her face or head by preventing flexion of the elbow. This type of restraint may be needed to preserve plastic surgery of the face, a scalp vein needle, or eye patches, or to prevent scratching of the face in various skin disorders. The restraint usually covers most of the arm but it should not push into the child's axilla nor rub the wrist. A cloth (usually muslin) restraint with pockets for tongue depressors is commonly used (Fig. 27-12). A large blade made especially for these restraints or two tongue blades taped together should be placed into *each pocket.* Each blade *must* extend the entire length of the pocket to prevent the restraint from slipping to a position above or below the child's elbow. Care must also be taken to avoid using a tongue blade that is too long, which would result in pressure in the axilla. Similar types of restraints can be improvised. A padded cylinder can be made out of a cardboard or plastic container. Such restraints must be placed over the child's shirt and secured with pins, ties, or tape to keep it from slipping off (Figure 27-13 illustrates alternate elbow restraints).

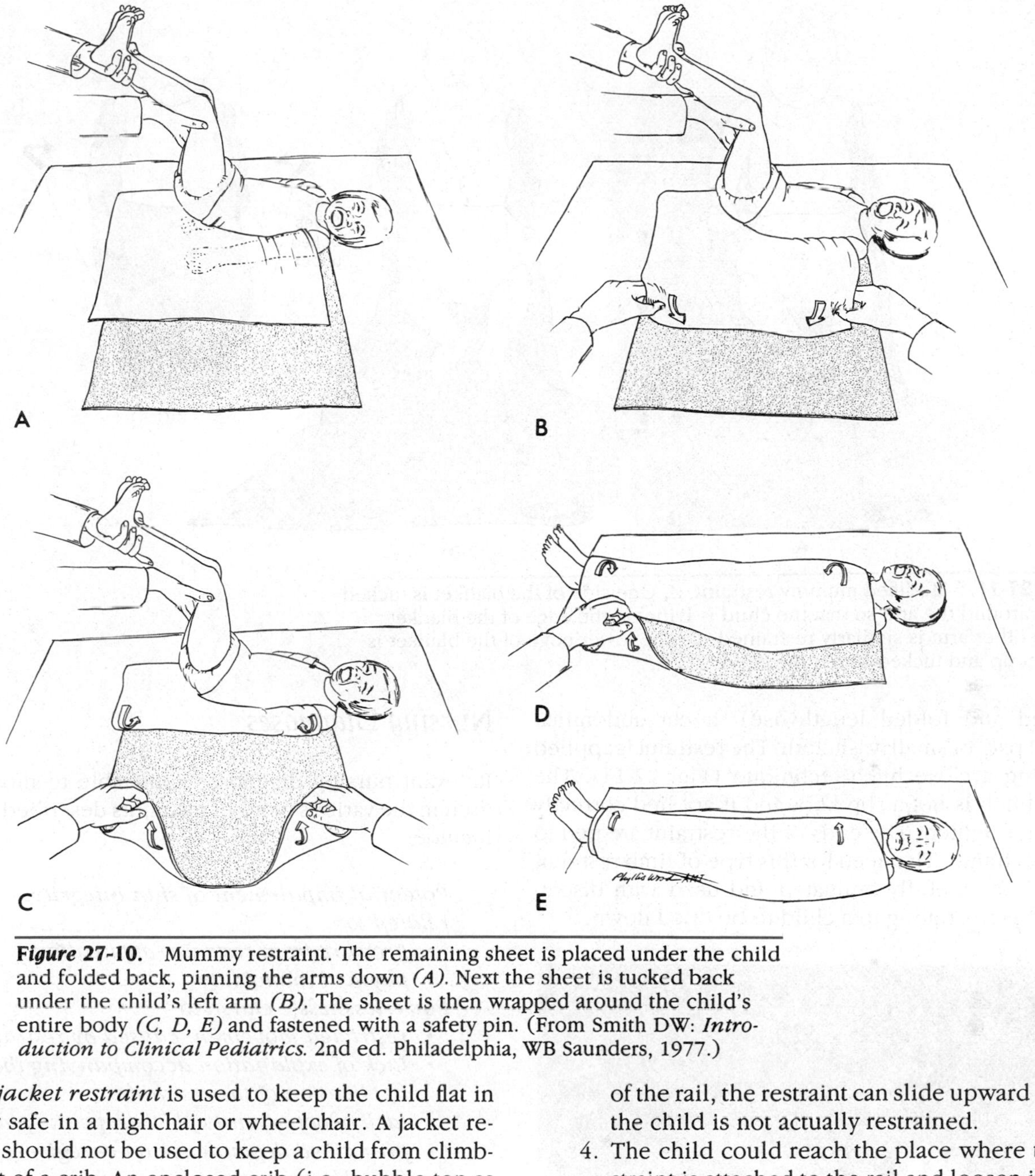

Figure 27-10. Mummy restraint. The remaining sheet is placed under the child and folded back, pinning the arms down *(A)*. Next the sheet is tucked back under the child's left arm *(B)*. The sheet is then wrapped around the child's entire body *(C, D, E)* and fastened with a safety pin. (From Smith DW: *Introduction to Clinical Pediatrics.* 2nd ed. Philadelphia, WB Saunders, 1977.)

A *jacket restraint* is used to keep the child flat in bed or safe in a highchair or wheelchair. A jacket restraint should not be used to keep a child from climbing out of a crib. An enclosed crib (i.e., bubble-top as shown in Figure 27-2) permits the child to move around and play in the crib. A jacket restraint is tied at the back to keep the child from untying it, and the long tapes on the sides of the jacket should be tied to the crib frames and not to the siderails. No restraint of any kind is to be secured to the crib railing for important reasons:

1. When the siderail is inadvertently put down, the child can be seriously injured because of the abrupt pull on the limb being restrained.
2. With this method of attachment, a siderail cannot be quickly lowered in an emergency.
3. If the restraint is secured only on a vertical bar of the rail, the restraint can slide upward so that the child is not actually restrained.
4. The child could reach the place where the restraint is attached to the rail and loosen it more easily.

A jacket restraint may be used during an intravenous infusion, to keep the child from sitting up and pulling out the IV; for cleft lip surgery, to keep the child from rolling onto the face; or whenever the supine position is necessary. With the prevalent use of various types of catheters for infusion rather than butterfly needles, the need for this type of restraint has diminished appreciably.

Arm and leg restraints are used to immobilize one or more extremities. The restraint can be a muslin strip, roller gauze, Kerlix, or similar material. First, the wrist or ankle is padded with gauze (one or two 4 by 4's

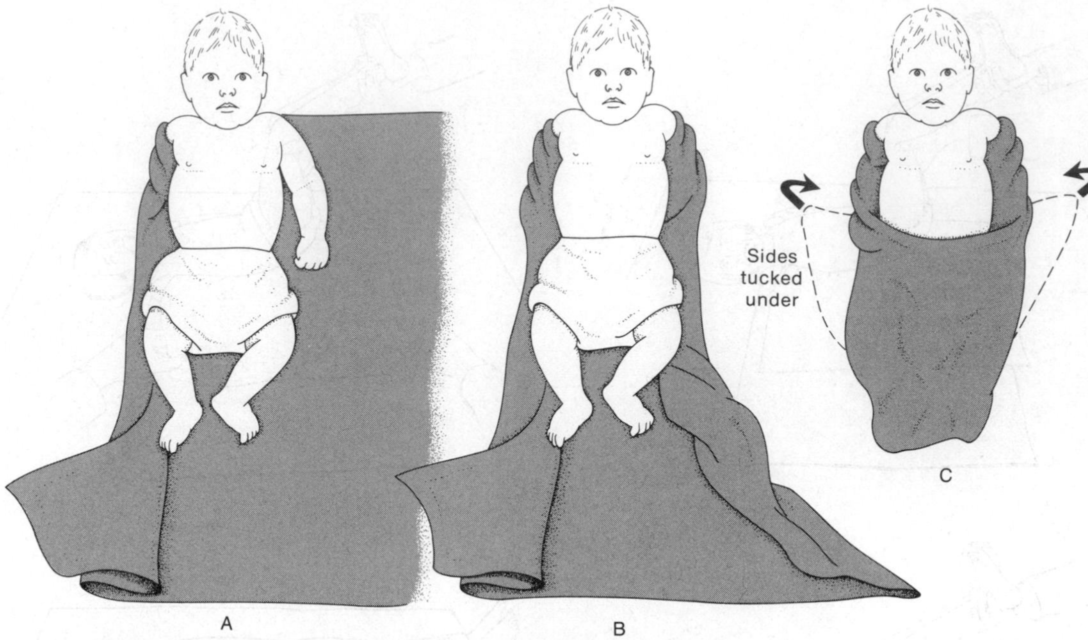

Figure 27-11. Modified mummy restraint. *A*, One side of the blanket is tucked snugly around the arm so that the child is lying on the edge of the blanket. *B*, The other arm is similarly restrained. *C*, The lower edge of the blanket is brought up and tucked *under* the child.

opened and folded lengthwise), a cut abdominal (ABD) pad, or small washcloth. The restraint is applied by using a clove hitch technique (Fig. 27-14). The clove hitch is not a slip knot and if applied correctly does not tighten. The ends of the restraint are tied to the crib frame. The need for this type of limb restraint should be carefully evaluated and used with discretion. It is frustrating to a child to be "tied down."

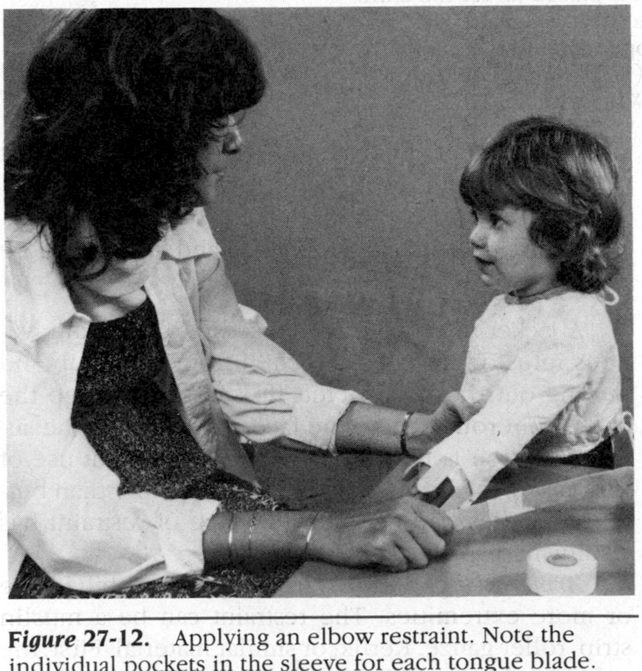

Figure 27-12. Applying an elbow restraint. Note the individual pockets in the sleeve for each tongue blade. This child requires two tongue blades taped together to provide sufficient length to keep her from bending her arm.

Nursing Diagnoses

Relevant nursing diagnoses applicable to most children in the various types of restraints described earlier include:

Potential impairment of skin integrity, related to
- *pressure from restraint application*
- *physical immobility*

Powerlessness, related to
- *restricted movement caused by restraint*
- *lack of explanation accompanying the application of the restraint*
- *lack of opportunity for therapeutic play*
- *prescribed dependence on caregivers for self-care activities*
- *interference with usual motor coping strategies*

Diversional activity deficit, related to
- *physical immobility*
- *lack of appropriate play materials*
- *ineffective use of available resources*

Nursing Strategies

The child in restraints must be continually re-evaluated to see whether restraint is still needed. The minimum amount of restraint necessary to meet the therapeutic goal should be used. The basic principle is to

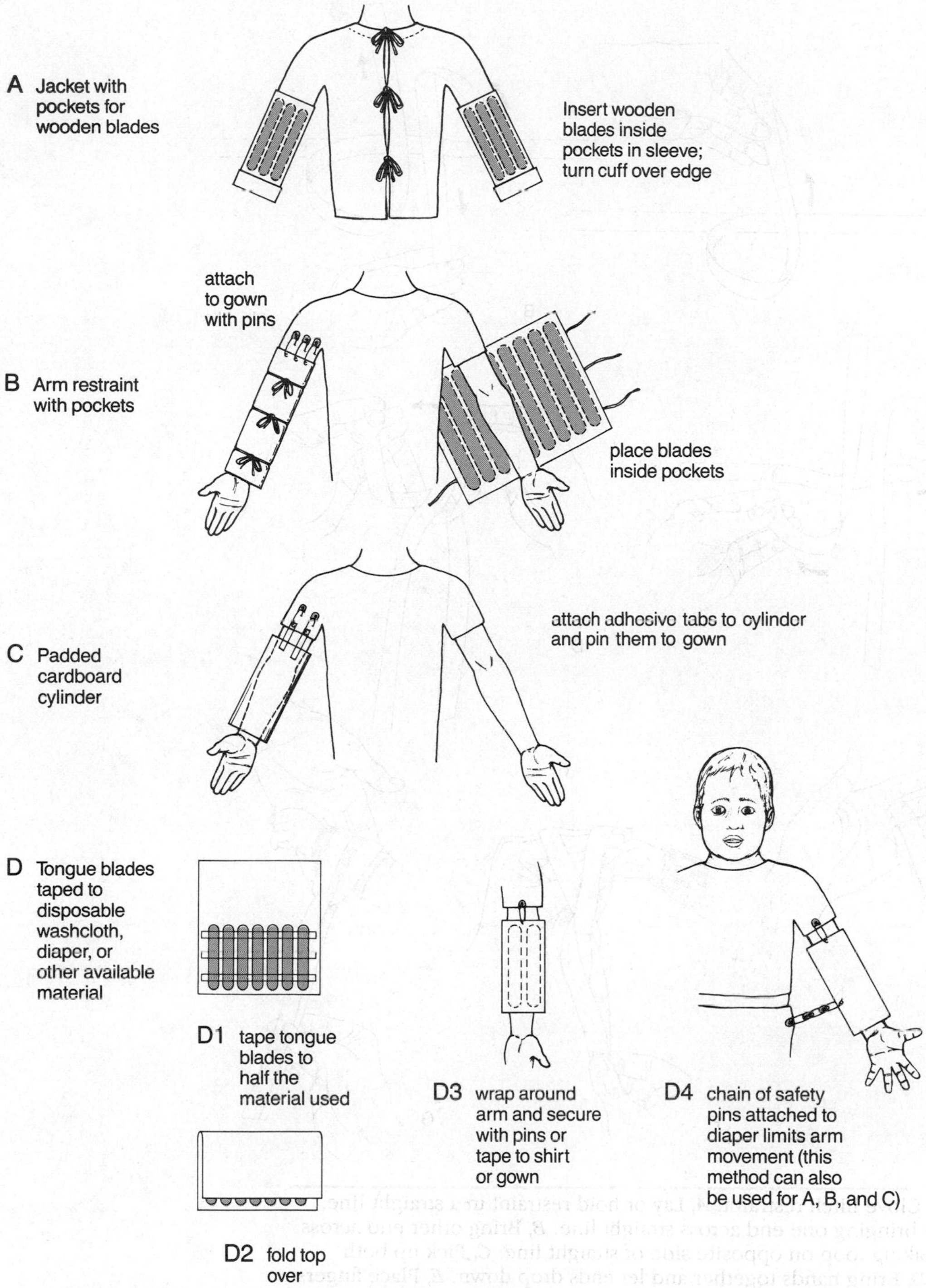
A Jacket with pockets for wooden blades
Insert wooden blades inside pockets in sleeve; turn cuff over edge
attach to gown with pins
B Arm restraint with pockets
place blades inside pockets
attach adhesive tabs to cylinder and pin them to gown
C Padded cardboard cylinder
D Tongue blades taped to disposable washcloth, diaper, or other available material
D1 tape tongue blades to half the material used
D2 fold top over
D3 wrap around arm and secure with pins or tape to shirt or gown
D4 chain of safety pins attached to diaper limits arm movement (this method can also be used for A, B, and C)

***Figure* 27-13.** Alternative methods to restrain elbows.

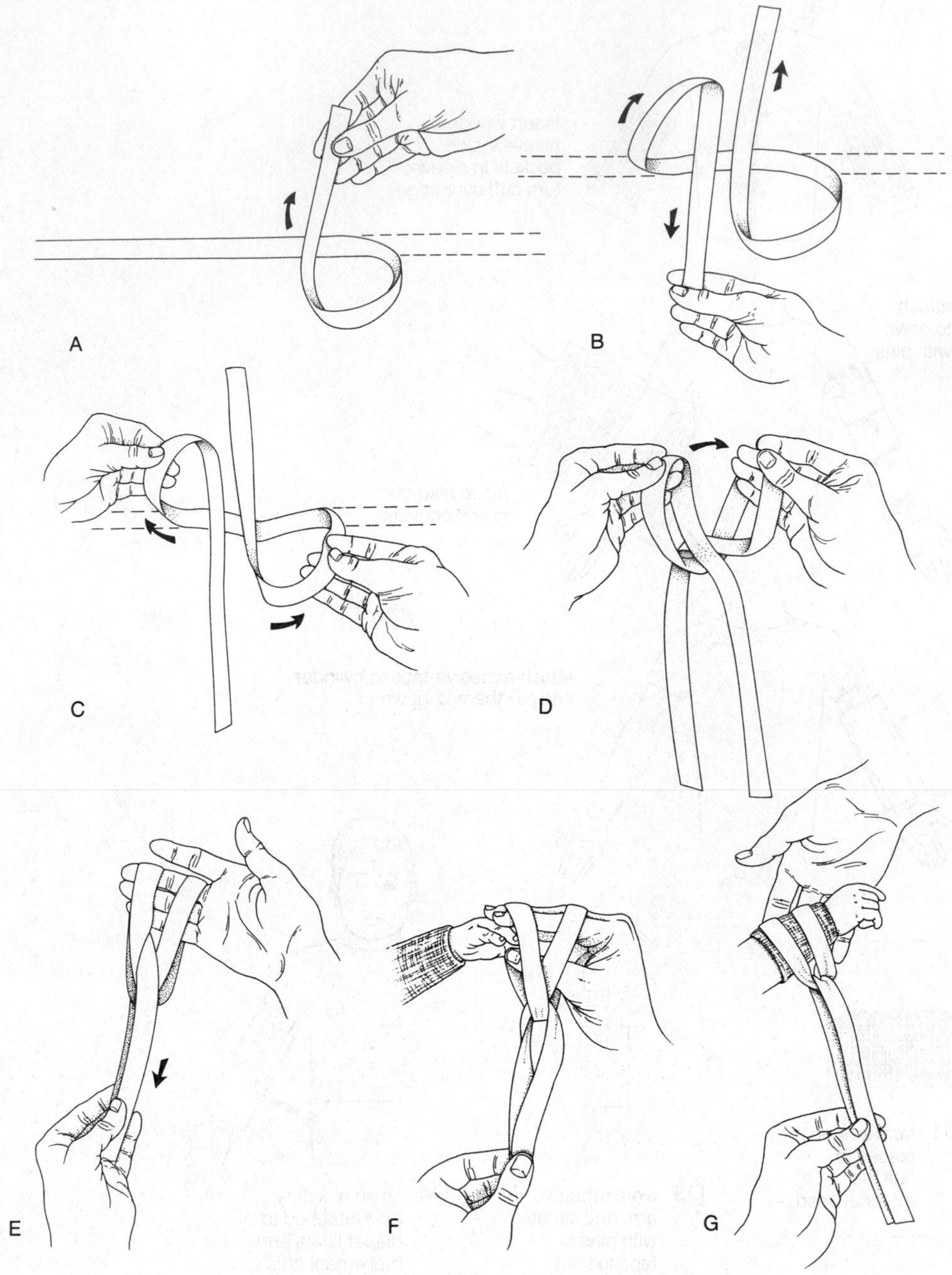

Figure 27-14. Clove hitch restraint. *A*, Lay or hold restraint in a straight line. Make a loop by bringing one end across straight line. *B*, Bring other end across straight line, making loop on opposite side of straight line. *C*, Pick up both loops at once. *D*, Bring hands together and let ends drop down. *E*, Place fingers through both loops and pull ends firmly. *F*, Slip clove hitch over padded wrist or ankle. *G*, Tighten restraint by pulling alternately on the ends of the restraint. The knot is firmly secured against the padded extremity but should not impair circulation.

allow maximum mobility while meeting the need for restraint.

The nurse should work with the family to help them understand the need for restraints. Depending on the reason for the restraint, parents can be permitted to release the child from restraints for varying lengths of time. If restraints are being used to prevent trauma to an operative site, one restraint is removed at a time.

Preventing Skin Breakdown

If restraints are applied properly, the potential for complications is minimized. If the child is not restless each extremity should be checked at least every hour, but for a restless child these should be checked more frequently. The nurse should also periodically remove restraints to exercise the involved extremity and give the child freedom of movement. It has been suggested that this should be done under supervision every 2 hours for a 10-minute period (Dowd et al, 1977). Meticulous bathing and drying of the skin is important for all children but especially when immobilized by restraints.

Increasing Child's Sense of Power and Control

Nursing strategies for a child in restraints should reduce the sense of powerlessness associated with immobility. Development of physical, intellectual, and emotional social competencies is affected by the child's inability to be mobile. When restrained, a child's major form of expression and means of coping are lost. Restrained children cannot defend themselves by running away or by physically striking out; often they cannot even suck their thumb for comfort (Dowd et al, 1977). They feel helpless, frustrated, and anxious. Immobility at a young age has also been identified as a factor in language delay and problems of articulation (Sibinga and Freedman, 1971). Limitation of activity reduces muscle strength and increases excretion of calcium, potassium, and sodium. The nurse has a responsibility to ensure that children are released for short periods, that parents are taught how to release restraints and protect their child while unrestrained, and that children are not restrained to an unnecessary degree or for excessive duration.

Although children may not fully understand the explanations, the powerlessness a child experiences can be reduced by preparing the child through explanations and playing out a similar scenario using a doll.

Providing Diversional Activities to Reduce Discomfort

Special attention is given to the child's need to engage in a form of play activity. Appropriate use of mobiles, music, and stories on records and tapes can help maintain a level of activity that engages the child's mind and attention. Although a child is restrained, he or she can be moved to the playroom with other children and be drawn into activities, if someone assists in the manipulation of materials. Caretakers must take more time with a restrained child to try to prevent the child's boredom and depression.

Nursing Care of Children Who Need to be Isolated

Confinement of a child to a separate room within the hospital is necessary in a variety of circumstances. Short-term isolation for infectious disease is a familiar precaution in pediatric settings. Also, children who receive chemotherapy for cancer in a germ-free protected environment (laminar air flow) present a special challenge to the health care team. The most extreme form of isolation is those children who are placed into a plastic "bubble" because of an immunodeficiency disease.

The length of time and strictness of isolation are important variables affecting a child's experience. A limited amount of research is available on the effects of isolation on children.

Children may have distorted perceptions of illness and hospitalization. One predominant perception is that hospitalization and illness are forms of punishment, mutilation, or rejection, and children also suffer from fears of abandonment and death (Vernon et al, 1965; Prugh, 1969). Creation of physical barriers such as masks, gloves, gowns, and closed doors can add to the confusion of a child who is feeling threatened, fearful, and alone in a hospital.

A Child's Concept of Isolation

Children and their parents often must be prepared for the need to be isolated in the midst of the crises of admission to the hospital or at the time of a new diagnosis. Too frequently the focus of preparation is limited to giving instructions about how to gown and mask, where and when to wash hands, and clarification of rules about visitors. Some explanation about the purpose of isolation is given by the physician or nurse or both. Besides explaining to parents, it is also important to explain to the child in understandable terms. Although these are important responsibilities, the nurse should try to alleviate the child's fears.

Children's perceptions of isolation have been examined by only a few researchers (Pidgeon, 1967; Broeder, 1985). Children's understanding of isolation attire has been identified as an area of misconception. The purpose of isolation attire is seen by children to be primarily associated with procedures. A child's expression about the nurse in isolation attire summarizes this misconception well: "She needs to do something to you. You don't know what, you just wait and see" (Broeder, 1985).

The child's level of language development limits comprehension about isolation. For example, the word "germ" was reported to be not well understood by young school-age children (6 to 7 years); by 9 years of age, children were more logical in explaining the concept of germs (Broeder, 1985).

Children's Responses

Few research studies have examined children's responses to isolation. In a study of six children (6 to 10 years of age) isolated for a minimum of 2 weeks for burns, Keuffner (1975) identified three stages in the hospitalization of burned children:

Stage I (agony) begins when child is hospitalized and persists until child feels condition is improving.

Stage II (hope) begins when improvement is noted and lasts until a discharge date is planned.

Stage III (reorganization) extends from the time a discharge date is planned until actual discharge from hospital.

Keuffner (1975) also found that although children often felt "aloneness" in solitary confinement, they did not always seem distressed by being alone, and sometimes even seemed to prefer it. Four children placed in a laminar air flow room during chemotherapy were studied by Hallenbeck and co-workers (1980). During the first few weeks, these children were active (talking, playing, crying). Gradually passivity became the predominant characteristic, of these children while in isolation, but when removed from isolation they again became more vocal (Hallenbeck et al, 1980). Broeder (1985), in a study of six school-age children (6 to 9 years of age) in isolation, found that they expressed feelings of deprivation (i.e., wished for food, people, and playtime).

Nursing Diagnoses

Children are isolated for a wide variety of reasons and under many circumstances. The following diagnoses are relevant to most situations for which children require isolation:

Knowledge deficit, related to
- *cognitive misconceptions about purpose of isolation*
- *misinterpretation of purpose of gowns and masks*

Sensory-perceptual alteration: input deficit, *related to*
- *physical separation from other children, family, and caretakers*
- *social isolation due to terminal or infectious disease*
- *ineffective use of resources to provide stimulation*

Potential for infection, related to
- *immature immune system*
- *invasion of a pathogenic agent*
- *medications that suppress immunologic function*
- *surgical intervention*

Nursing Strategies

Children require special care during isolation because of their cognitive, social, and biologic needs. With appropriate interventions, the negative psychologic impact of isolation can be diminished and the effectiveness of the control of organisms enhanced.

Correcting Misconceptions About Isolation

Focus on helping the child understand the purpose of isolation. Misconceptions about wrongdoing and the purpose of isolation attire should be corrected. In Broeder's study (1985), procedures were identified as the most stressful experience for children hospitalized and in isolation, and children tend to think that nurses are gowned for the purpose of performing a procedure. Sitting, talking, and playing games with children in isolation facilitates differentiation between isolation and procedures (Broeder, 1985).

Providing Sensory Stimulation and Psychologic Support

The feelings of aloneness, agony, and deprivation can be lessened by spending time with children in isolation and by encouraging parents to stay with their child when possible. Also, since children cannot see a person's face when masked, they should be allowed to see who is visiting them *before* masking to increase the

Table 27-3. Center for Disease Control Categories Used in Category-Specific Isolation System

Category of Isolation	Description of Category
Strict isolation	The most vigorous form of isolation designed to prevent transmission of pathogens that may be spread by both air and contact
Contact isolation	Designed to prevent transmission of easily transmitted or epidemiologically important infections (or colonization) that do not require strict isolation
Respiratory isolation	Designed to prevent airborne infections (droplet transmission) primarily over short distances and prevent contact with contaminated droplets and secretions
Tuberculosis isolation (AFB isolation)	This is an isolation category for TB. This category identified as acid-fast bacilli (AFB)
Enteric precautions	Designed to prevent the transmission of pathogens through direct or indirect contact with feces. Hepatitis A included in this category
Drainage/secretion precautions (includes infections formerly categorized as Wound and Skin Precautions, Discharge and Secretion Precautions)	Designed to prevent spread of organisms by direct or indirect contact with purulent material or drainage from an infected area in the body. Infectious diseases included in this category are ones that produce infective purulent material, drainage, or secretions. *Minor* skin, wound, or burn infections are included in this category, whereas *major* skin, wound, and burn infections are included in contact isolation
Blood/body fluid precautions	Designed to prevent infections that are transmitted by direct or indirect contact with infected blood or body fluids

(Adapted from Garner and Simmon, 1983.)

sense of relationship and thereby reduce feelings of aloneness and alienation.

Feelings about being in isolation also can be expressed through drawings and therapeutic play. Favorite blankets or toys should be allowed in the room to enhance the child's sense of security. Many toys can be autoclaved, washed with disinfectants, or exposed to the sun, so play can be normal.

The decision to isolate a child should always carefully consider the child's psychologic comfort. Once it has been determined that isolation is required, the procedure should be followed consistently by all professionals and visitors.

The health care team should assess regularly the child's psychologic response and physiologic status. Isolation should end at the earliest possible time the physiologic status permits.

Reducing Potential for Transmission of Organisms

Specific instructions for each type of isolation are developed by each institution. *Proper handwashing should be stressed at all times for all conditions and with all individuals entering and leaving the room.* This is the most important precaution to take when caring for children in isolation, especially because they do not necessarily adhere to some of the basic hygienic principles, such as covering the mouth when coughing and sneezing. Also, they may not routinely wash their hands yet tend to touch everything in the room, thus articles tend to be more easily contaminated.

The two major isolation precaution systems outlined in the Centers for Disease Control (CDC) Guidelines for Isolation are the disease-specific isolation system and the category-specific isolation system.

1. **Disease-specific isolation:** Precautions are outlined for *each* infectious disease or condition whereby transmission of a specific organism is interrupted.
2. **Category-specific isolation:** This system has been in use for some time. Similar infectious diseases are grouped into a category and precautions prescribed for each category.

The major categories and the purpose for each are summarized in Table 27-3. Because the isolation system and precautions vary among institutions and change over time, it is safest to become familiar with the specific procedures in the institution in which you are working.

Protective isolation (or reverse isolation) has traditionally been instituted to protect immunosuppressed patients from acquiring an infection. Traditionally, gowns, masks, and gloves were worn by the health care personnel. Research has demonstrated that strict adherence to correct handwashing provides protection equal to that of wearing gowns, masks, and gloves. Protective isolation has been removed by CDC

Table 27-4. Fever: Mechanism, Causes, and Interventions

Mechanism of Temperature Elevation	Types of Condition That Cause the Mechanism	Interventions
Set-point is raised	Infection, malignancy, allergy, CNS lesion, radiation	Antipyretics to lower set-point. Supply sufficient clothing to avoid shivering
Excessive heat production. Set-point is normal	Hyperthyroidism, ASA overdose, malignant hyperthermia	Undressing, sponging. Antipyretic administration not effective
Heat loss mechanism defective. Set-point is normal	Ectodermal dysplasia, burns, heat stroke	Undressing. Cool environment. Antipyretic administration not effective

from their new guidelines (Garner and Simmon, 1983).

Nursing Care of a Child with a Fever

Fever is an obvious indicator to parents that their child is sick. It prompts families to seek medical care for children in 30 per cent of visits (Stern, 1977). Almost every child will at some time have a fever in the range of 37.8° to 40.0°C (100° to 104°F) (Schmitt, 1984).

Pathophysiology of Fever

Body temperature is regulated by the hypothalamus, which contains sensitive neurons. The temperature of blood entering the brain is assessed by a hypothalamic "thermostat" that determines whether heat loss or heat gain is required, and the set-point is altered accordingly (similar to a thermostat in a house). This mechanism is a complex feedback system involving norepinephrine, acetylcholine, and changes in concentration of sodium, calcium, and some prostaglandins (Stern, 1977).

A fever is an abnormal elevation of the central body temperature caused by (1) a high thermostatic set-point; (2) metabolic heat production or excessive environmental heat that exceeds heat loss capacities, or (3) impairment of the body's heat loss capabilities (Table 27-4 gives examples of conditions).

Parents usually have greater fears and concerns about the hazards of fever than most temperature elevations warrant. Fever does not generally rise to harmful levels unless there is interference with the body's mechanism of dissipating heat. Fever by itself does not cause brain damage unless it reaches at least 41.7°C (107°F) (Schmitt, 1984). Fever from infection rarely poses a threat; however, heat exhaustion, thermal burns, or malignant hyperthermia are usually more serious causes of fever. Additionally, fever can be harmful to children with congestive heart failure, respiratory failure, acute neurologic disease, or endotoxic shock (Lorin, 1982).

Although normal children are usually not harmed by fever, parents fear their child will have a seizure. Only about 4 per cent of children who experience a fever are likely to have a convulsion. Some have even questioned whether fever per se causes a seizure or whether another mechanism associated with the illness is the cause. Many children have seizures at relatively low temperatures (i.e., 38.4°C or 101°F) at the onset of illness and during the illness, yet when the child's fever spikes, a seizure does not occur (Fruthaler, 1985).

Fever is triggered by many foreign substances, the most common being bacteria and viruses. Fever begins when an endogenous pyrogen is produced in response to a foreign substance. Fever is caused by complex interactions between an endogenous pyrogen and receptors near the thermosensitive neurons in the anterior hypothalamus. Mediators in this reaction are thought to include prostaglandins, monoamines, and cyclic AMP (Kleinman, 1984). Information is finally sent to the posterior hypothalamus and vasomotor centers, which act upon peripheral vessels to cause constriction. This results in a decrease in heat dissipation and a rise in the core temperature (Kleinman, 1984). When the set-point is raised, the body's sense of coldness triggers heat production through muscular contraction (shivering). Shivering is the body's defense against cold. In response to cold sensation, vasoconstriction occurs with an eventual rise in body temperature. If the rise in the set-point is rapid, severe chills may result. In children, severe shaking and chills frequently accompany pneumonia or urinary tract infections (Fruthaler, 1985).

Recently, the potential benefits of fever have been recognized. It has been hypothesized that fever may produce an environment in which endogenous pyrogen production is curtailed. Fever has also been noted to potentiate the action of antibodies (Mackowiak et al, 1982) and enhance defense mechanisms such as the inflammatory response (Schmitt, 1984).

Nursing Assessment

There is a normal diurnal variation of body temperature, with the lowest temperature occurring between 2 and 4 A.M. and the highest between 6 and 10 P.M. A similar diurnal pattern is demonstrated in most febrile illnesses.

In children, an oral temperature in excess of 38.0°C (100.4°F) or a rectal temperature in excess of 38.8°C (101.8°F) is considered by most to be a fever (Kleinman, 1984). In neonates, however, a rectal temperature of 37.5°C (99.5°F) can represent serious illness; the neonate can also have an infection without a fever and more commonly has hypothermia with sepsis.

Age is an important variable to consider when assessing fever. It is generally accepted that fever in any child under 6 months of age is more likely to be caused by serious illness than when the same degree of elevation occurs in an older child (Wright et al, 1981). It is also agreed upon by most experts that a febrile neonate should be seen promptly by a physician. Furthermore, fever in a compromised child (e.g., one who has sickle cell disease) can often indicate a more serious bacterial infection (McIntosh et al, 1980). Also, children who do *not* have associated clinical signs of infection (e.g., sore throat, runny nose) are more likely to have serious underlying disease (Younger and Brown, 1985). Fevers that persist longer than a week require diagnostic and laboratory evaluation.

The level and pattern of fever can provide important information but should be supplemented with a careful individual clinical assessment of the child. A child's spontaneous activity, play, appetite, and general behavior and disposition are significant. The child's visual movement (eyes look at observer and around room) and motor behavior (ability to move limbs, sit, stand, walk) should be noted. Any changes in behavior demonstrated at home can be identified by consulting with the parent. A history should consist of the fever pattern and an assessment of the child including age, presence of a chronic condition, length of illness, presence of associated physical signs, and a general behavioral assessment. Additional data such as complete blood count (CBC), urinalysis, urine culture, chest radiograph, and blood culture may also be obtained. The presence of serious illness, however, cannot be predicted with accuracy. Suggested parameters (Teele et al, 1979) on which to base a prediction of bacteremia when the source of infection is not identifiable are:

- age less than 2 years
- fever in excess of 38.8°C (102°F)
- white blood cell count in excess of 20.0×1000 cell/mm³ (μL)

Management

Since fever is part of the body's defense mechanism, it could be argued that fever reduction is undesirable. A child with a fever, however, often has a headache or arthralgia and may suffer from malaise. It is therefore reasonable that antipyretic medication orders are not necessarily prescribed for a specific temperature level but for discomfort.

Fever management is controversial. Fluid administration is recommended to reduce fever under most circumstances. Antipyretics, removal of clothing, and sponging are other common methods used.

Antipyretics are to be used with caution. Aspirin should not be used in children with varicella or influenza because its use is associated with subsequent development of Reye syndrome (American Academy of Pediatrics [AAP], 1982). Although the studies that demonstrated the association have methodologic weaknesses, the AAP (1982) believes that "until contradictory information is available, the present evidence is sufficient to warrant this recommendation." One advantage of using aspirin instead of acetaminophen under certain circumstances is its anti-inflammatory effect. Aspirin, however, is more likely to accumulate, resulting in an increased potential for toxicity (salicylism). Also, aspirin in normal doses can cause gastrointestinal bleeding. Acetaminophen has the disadvantage of being more costly. Currently, there is no indication for alternating acetaminophen and aspirin at 2-hour intervals (Schmitt, 1984).

There is a general overuse of antipyretics, a practice that is continually being challenged (Schmitt, 1984; Younger and Brown, 1985). Because antipyretics lower the set-point, their use is appropriate in infections, malignancy, central nervous system lesions, and allergy but not when heat production is excessive (as in malignant hyperthermia) or when the mechanism for heat loss is defective (as in burns and heat stroke). In these conditions, removal of clothing and sponging are more appropriate.

The use of tepid water to moisten the child's skin systematically is called sponging. It can be performed while the child is lying in bed or in the bath tub. Some evidence in the literature indicates that sponging does

Box 27-2
Acetaminophen (Tylenol) and Acetylsalicylic Acid (Aspirin) Preparations and Dosages

ACETAMINOPHEN PREPARATIONS (TYLENOL)

Tempra drops	80 mg/1 ml
Tempra syrup	80 mg/5 ml
Tylenol drops	80 mg/1 ml
Tylenol elixir	160 mg/5 ml
Tylenol chewable tabs	1 tab = 80 mg
Dosage	
Acetaminophen	30–40 mg/kg/24 hr in divided doses every 4–6 hr prn

ACETYLSALICYLIC ACID (ASPIRIN) PREPARATIONS

Chewable tablets (baby)	1 tab = 80 mg
Adult tablets	1 tab = 325 mg
Dosage	
Acetylsalicylic acid (ASA)	30–65 mg/kg/24 hr in divided doses every 4–6 hr prn

not have an antipyretic effect (Newman, 1985), but because it continues to be a technique that is used, it is important for health professionals to ensure that it is performed properly to avoid disastrous results. The evaporation of water from the skin surface has a cooling effect. In the past, sponge baths to reduce a fever included the use of alcohol in water. This was believed to speed cooling by more rapid evaporation. This technique is dangerous and should not be practiced because of the absorption of alcohol and too-rapid heat loss. It is important to use tepid, not cold, water (29.4° to 32.2°C), as cold water may cause shivering. If sponging is used when the set-point is raised, antipyretic drugs must be given 30 minutes before sponging. If sponging is done *before* the antipyretic drug is given, the hypothalamus attempts to offset the lowered body temperature. The child will therefore shiver (muscle contraction to produce heat), and as soon as sponging is discontinued temperature will return to the previous level (Schmitt, 1984). However, under some circumstances, such as the presence of delirium, a seizure from fever, or a fever greater than 41.1°C (106°F), Schmitt (1984) recommends immediate sponging and use of cooler water.

Sponging is noted to work more quickly than immersion. A child should be placed into a bathtub with approximately 2 inches of water, while the skin is being wet continuously. Shivering is a natural mechanism that occurs with rapid cooling and causes the body temperature to increase. Thus, if a child begins to shiver, the water temperature should be raised (Schmitt, 1984). If shivering continues, the cooling treatment should be discontinued.

Hospitalized children with persistent high fevers are frequently placed on hypothermia mattresses. These are pads with internal coils to circulate cool water. The pads should be covered with a bath blanket for comfort. It is important to watch for shivering and to discontinue the treatment if this occurs.

Parents who are treating their child's fever at home should be instructed in antipyretic therapy and told to offer fluids and not be concerned about a child's refusal to eat solids. Available antipyretic preparations and their use are summarized in Box 27-2. The nurse should review the signs of dehydration with parents and encourage them to call if the fever is not controlled.

Perioperative Nursing Care*

Parents expect the nurse to answer their questions and assist in the effective management of their child's perioperative experience. To meet these expectations satisfactorily, the nurse must be skilled in handling the unique responses of a child and family, allowing for the child's age and the particular family circumstances. The nurse must also be knowledgeable in caring for a child undergoing anesthesia and provide the specialized care required for the specific surgical procedure performed.

Specific age-related approaches to children requiring hospitalization and surgery are discussed in Chapter 31. Specialized nursing care for the various surgical problems is discussed throughout this text as applicable. The following is a general discussion on perioperative nursing care of a child undergoing surgery. See Table 27-7, page 835, for a Nursing Process Plan: Perioperative Nursing Care.

Preoperative Nursing Care

Pediatric patients are given anesthetics in conjunction with almost all surgical procedures. Anesthetics may also be administered to pediatric patients to facilitate nonsurgical procedures requiring patient immobility

*We appreciate the authorship of this section on perioperative preparation and anesthetic management of children by Mary Jean Yablonky, CRNA, MA, Chief Nurse Anesthetist, employed at Horizon Surgery Center, Livonia, Michigan.

or patient cooperation for an extended time, such as radiation therapy, radiographic procedures, cast applications, and certain types of examinations. Psychologic upsets resulting in personality changes in children have been traced to anesthesia, the hospital experience, or both (Eckenhoff, 1953; Vernon et al, 1966). Although evidence of postoperative psychologic disturbances has not been uniformly substantiated (Davenport and Werry, 1970), the induction of general anesthesia produces a stress reaction in most children (Schwartz et al, 1983). To minimize as much as possible the potentially adverse effects of the anesthesia/surgery experience, children must be prepared adequately. Since parents often represent the child's primary source of information, parental comprehension of anesthesia and surgery must be ensured (Hanna and Sherlock, 1983).

Usually, the child is admitted the day before surgery, allowing time for orientation to the unit and for preparation for the events of the following day. Parents are encouraged to stay with their child during this preparation period, their presence is comforting to the child and provides an opportunity for the nurse and family to become acquainted.

A history and nursing assessment are completed upon admission, just as for any other hospitalization (see Chapter 31). Upon admission for surgery, special attention is given to gathering information about the child's and family's understanding of the operation. In many institutions, parents may visit on a 24-hour basis and may spend the entire preoperative night in the hospital. When this is not the policy, parents are told what time the surgery will take place and are encouraged to arrive at least an hour before that time to allow time to visit with their child.

Preparation to Minimize Stress

Approaches to minimize stress for surgery and anesthesia are similar to those described for procedural preparation (see page 798) and for admission to the hospital (see Chapter 31).

Specific stresses associated with surgery identified by Wolfer and Visintainer (1975) include:

1. Admission time
2. Withdrawal of blood for blood test
3. The afternoon of the day before surgery
4. Preoperative medication injection
5. Before and during transportation to the operating room
6. Return from the recovery room

Specific interventions, based on the child's developmental level, are used to support the child at these particular times and throughout the surgical experience.

Infants and Young Children

To a young infant, the most distressing aspect of hospitalization is separation from primary caregivers. Since limited cognitive development in infancy precludes adequate psychologic preparation, reducing the length of separation from the parents and familiar surroundings is most beneficial. Out-patient surgery has had a significant impact on reducing the length of child-parent separation.

Infants and children between the ages of 6 months and 3 years appear to be the most affected by their anesthesia experience (Eckenhoff, 1953): behavioral disturbances after hospitalization are greatest in this age group. The behavioral disturbances that surface are related to fears: fear of strangers, fear of the dark, and fear of separation from parents. As with infants, separation from parents poses a significant threat to preschool children, as they are young enough to be dependent on their parents yet old enough to be aware of their separation from them. Other reasons children in this age group are most vulnerable to psychologic stress are that their defense mechanisms, which would help them cope with the stress, are limited, as is their comprehension of the need for their surgery. To allay some of the fears of separation, preschoolers should be encouraged to bring a favorite toy or blanket with them to the operating room. Parents should be encouraged to stay with their child in the immediate preanesthetic period and to be there as soon as possible after the child awakens. Some hospitals encourage parents to visit with their children in the recovery room before their physical condition warrants transfer to the nursing unit.

The preschool child between 2 and 5 years of age is prone to numerous fears, most notably that of mutilation and physical injury (Korsch, 1975). Unable to understand the rationale for specific treatments and procedures and to distinguish between reality and fantasy, preschoolers need to be reassured that their operation will "fix" their tonsils, eyes, hernia, leg, or other body part. Preschoolers should be told that they will awaken after surgery in the recovery room, that different nurses and doctors will be caring for them, and that there will be a bandage over their operative site.

School-age

School-age children seem to worry about the actual anesthetic. They are curious as to how they will go to sleep and fearful that they may awaken during the operation. "What if I'm not tired?" and "What if I wake up before the surgery is finished?" are common questions. Explaining that "anesthesia sleep" is a special kind of sleep caused by "medicines" that work even when the child is not tired and that the "anesthesia medicines" will not be turned off until the surgery is finished may help to dispel some of these fears. School-age children may welcome the opportunity to select the method of anesthesia induction if a choice is suitable to the child's medical condition.

The concept of sleep itself may be anxiety provoking to some children. Children who have been told that a dead person is "sleeping" or that a pet has been "put to sleep" may equate sleep with death. These children might view anesthesia sleep as permanent. Reassure them that anesthesia is a special type of sleep from which they will awaken at the completion of their surgical procedure. Comments from parents and the nurse about seeing the child after the operation are most reassuring.

Adolescents

Adolescents suffer intense anxiety over their self-image and identity. They are often concerned about what will happen to them while under the influence of anesthetics and may feel unsure of their ability to cope appropriately. It is important to assess their level of anxiety preoperatively. Adolescents may benefit from having a preoperative tranquilizer to reduce their anxiety. Diazepam is advantageous. Given orally, it has a significantly greater anxiolytic effect than when given intramuscularly (Assaf et al, 1975). Premedication, however, does not preclude the need for adequate preparation. Adolescents should be given information about their proposed anesthesia and surgery to reduce psychologic stress and enlist more cooperation. If their medical condition permits a choice, they should be allowed to select the manner in which anesthesia will be induced. They should be informed that monitoring is a routine aspect of anesthesia care and told which monitors will be applied before anesthesia induction. The nurse should describe the specific sensations the adolescent can anticipate as a result of the pharmacologic agents given. The adolescent should be informed that an airway tube will be inserted after the loss of consciousness to allow oxygen and additional anesthetics to be given, ensuring unconsciousness throughout the operation. Since only the surgical site will be exposed and the anesthetic will render them immobile as well as unconscious, adolescents can be assured that they need not fear doing or saying anything in the operating room that could cause them embarrassment.

All patients scheduled to receive an anesthetic should have a preanesthetic visit by the person who will be administering their anesthetic. The purpose of the visit is twofold: (1) to gather pertinent medical data critical to safe anesthetic management; and (2) to establish a rapport with the patient and parents as well as to communicate with the nurses caring for the patient. As parental anxiety is often transmitted to the child, every effort is made to gain parental confidence by explaining the anesthetic procedure and the sequence of events to them as well as to the child.

Parents should be told about the importance of the preoperative fast in preventing gastric aspiration during induction of anesthesia. It is hoped that informing them of the time after which all oral intake should cease will ensure an appropriately fasted child. The technique and agent used for induction of anesthesia should also be explained to the parents. At many institutions, the child and parents can also arrange for a tour of the recovery room to familiarize themselves with the room, to meet the nurses who will be caring for them, and to have recovery-related questions answered.

Honesty is mandatory in preparing children of all ages. The anesthetic procedure should be explained in language the patient can understand so as to dispel some of their fears and misconceptions. The nurse should be present whenever possible for at least part of the anesthetist's visit to be able to reinforce accurately the explanations.

Preoperative preparation of children can reduce anxiety and fears. Children cope more effectively, exhibit less upset behavior and more cooperation, and show fewer posthospital adjustment problems (Wolfer and Visintainer, 1975; Schwartz et al, 1983).

A check list in Box 27-3 can be adapted to the specific needs of a particular situation and institution. As each phase of preparation is completed, the check list is initialed to avoid repetition when more than one nurse is involved in the preoperative stage (Treloar, 1978).

The nurse also is responsible for physical preparation of the child. Ensure that the child has an appropriate identification bracelet on the wrist or ankle and that the bed is clearly marked. The nurse should check the chart to be sure that the routine complete blood count and urinalysis on admission have been done. Any abnormal laboratory results or unusual clinical findings

Table 27-5. Number of Hours Child Is Kept NPO Prior to an Elective Surgical Procedure

Age (mo)	Solid Foods and/or Milk	Clear Liquids
0–1	4 hr	2 hr
6–12	6 hr	4 hr
12–24	8 hr	6 hr
>24	From midnight prior to the day of surgery	8 hr

Box 27-3
Pediatric Psychologic Check List For Surgery

PATIENT'S NAME:

UNIT #:

ROOM #:

SERVICE:

DIRECTIONS:
1. The following items will be covered before surgery or procedures.
2. All explanations will include parents or some other responsible person(s).
3. All explanations will consider the child's developmental level.

1. Explain operation or procedure. Have patient verbalize understanding.
2. Explain and get return demonstration of coughing, deep breathing, and using spirometer or blow bottles. Emphasize importance and rationale.
3. Explain dietary limitations, if any.
4. Explain preoperative and postoperative use of equipment, bandages, tubes, restraints. Use pictures if necessary. Provide opportunity for therapeutic play (see Chapter 21).
5. Explain about the "stretcher person," who wears green and will take the child to the operating room on a stretcher. Explain that OR personnel also wear green suits and that someone will be with the child at all times. Allow the child to play with OR hats, masks, gloves, and so on.
6. Ensure child has security object to take to OR.
7. Let child know that parent will wait close-by for child's return.
8. Explain about the method of inducing anesthesia. Emphasize that the doctor will wake the child up only when the operation is over. For those 7 years old and younger, anesthesia is administered via face mask. Let child play with demonstration mask. For those at least 8 years old, IV medication is used.
9. Explain about the recovery room and how the child will stay there until awake. Emphasize that child will be cared for by special nurses wearing green.
10. Explain postoperative care and events:
    - an IV will be running on return from OR
    - nurse will monitor vital signs
    - medication for pain is available as needed
    - child will be requested to cough and deep breathe
11. Inform child of preoperative injections. Be honest: it will hurt. Tell child, if it is known, that he or she will *not* receive an injection. (Discussion about an injection should be introduced at the end of other teaching so that child's anxiety level about the injection does not interfere with other learning.)
12. Allow child to select gift from the Toy Chest.
13. Answer questions.

COMMENTS:

(Adapted from Treloar, 1978.)

(especially elevated temperature) should be reported to the surgeon and documented in the chart.

On the evening before surgery, the child is prepared for bed and offered a drink, as all fluids will be removed from the room during the night or early morning. All children who are to receive an anesthetic must undergo a period of fasting before surgery to eliminate the risk of aspiration upon induction of anesthesia. The length of the fasting period is determined on the basis of the child's age and should be specified in the preoperative orders (Table 27-5). The nurse should explain to the child and parents the reason for the fast and should make sure the child takes nothing by mouth, as ordered. On the morning of surgery, the child is given mouth care and again reminded that he or she is not allowed to have anything to eat or drink. Besides having the usual NPO signs at the bedside, note that children do wander around the unit and into the playroom. Placing a broad piece of tape across the front of the child's gown with "I may not eat or drink" printed on it usually ensures that an uninformed adult will not break the preoperative fast. It is helpful if, during breakfast, the parent or a nurse can engage the child in an activity in an area away from where other children are eating. If oral intake inadvertently occurs, the nurse should notify the anesthesia staff immediately as this may necessitate the cancellation or postponement of the child's surgery rather than risking aspiration.

Children should be properly prepared for the operating room before the premedicant is administered, if one is ordered. The child is bathed either at bedtime or early in the morning. Any special surgical preparations such as washes and scrubs are completed. The nurse then sees that the child is properly attired and, when applicable, that jewelry, makeup, nailpolish, and any prosthetic devices have been removed.

Children are not routinely premedicated prior to surgery. The decision to order a premedicant is determined by the anesthetist after careful consideration of the patient's physical and emotional state and the proposed operative procedure. A premedication may be given for one of the following reasons:

1. To prevent excessive airway secretions
2. To allay anxiety
3. To produce sedation and facilitate induction
4. To supplement a planned balanced anesthetic and reduce the intraoperative anesthetic requirements

If a premedication is ordered, the nurse should instruct the older child to void prior to administering the medication. This is necessary to eliminate the risk of having a sedated child attempt to get out of bed to go to the bathroom and possibly fall and get hurt. Voiding at this time also decreases the risk of bladder distention during anesthesia.

After the child has been prepared, the medication is brought to the room. If it is an injection, the child is told that it will hurt for a short time and then it will make her or him sleepy. Strategies to help the child cope with the injection are used as described earlier in this chapter. After the preoperative medication is given, the child is kept in bed with the siderails up or is quietly held in the parent's arms, whichever is most soothing to the child, to derive maximal benefit from the sedative effects of the medication.

Just before the child is taken to the operating room, the nurse should check again to be sure that the names on the chart, on the child, and on the bed coincide. The nurse must also see that the young child has a source of comfort to take along, such as a special blanket, teddy bear, or other security object.

A preoperative check list placed on the front of the child's chart is a useful strategy to ensure completion of all the nurse's responsibilities (Box 27-4). These lists vary according to hospital routines. As it is completed, the item on the list may be initialed or checked off.

If the child is asleep from the premedication, the parents should be discouraged from awakening the child to give a kiss or say goodbye. Medicated children may be disoriented and arousing them will only add to their anxiety.

Anesthetic Management of Children

Although the nurses on the unit are not required to participate in the anesthetic management of their patients, an understanding of the anesthetic period provides nurses with information to answer both patient and parental questions and to provide safe postoperative nursing care. Upon arrival in the operating suite, the child is quickly examined by the anesthetist to determine whether any changes have developed since the preanesthetic interview (for example, temperature elevation or change in sensorium). The chart is reviewed and laboratory data not available at the time of the interview are checked. If a premedicant was ordered, the time it was administered and the effect of the drug are noted. Before taking the child into the operating room, consent forms for surgery and anesthesia are checked to determine that they are properly signed.

In the operating room, anesthesia induction should proceed as quickly as possible. Unnecessary conversation and the opening of instruments should cease. Everyone's attention should focus on the child and every effort made to eliminate stress before and during the induction of anesthesia.

Induction of Anesthesia

Many methods exist for the induction of anesthesia in infants and children. No one method is effective in all situations. In general, anesthetists employ the technique they are most familiar with and one that will provide a safe and rapid onset of unconsciousness. The methods frequently used include rectally administered drugs, intramuscular agents, intravenous induction, and mask induction.

Inducing sleep with rectally administered drugs is beneficial to frightened children (Goresky and Steward, 1979) for it enables them to fall asleep in the arms of their parents. This procedure is done in a room just outside the operating room, thus eliminating separation anxiety. The procedure is relatively painless and not unlike having a rectal temperature taken. A small, short, lubricated catheter is inserted into the rectum and a calculated dose of either methohexital (25

Box 27-4
Preoperative Care Check List

1. Vital signs are taken and recorded on the chart, preferably also on the preoperative check list. Temperature, pulse, and respirations are always recorded; blood pressure is usually taken on any child over age 3 years, varying with child's condition and institution's policy. Any abnormal findings are reported to the surgeon and a note attached to the front of the chart drawing attention to such findings. The nurse should also record in the chart that the surgeon has been notified, including the time.
2. The child's height and weight are recorded on the chart and check list.
3. All preoperative laboratory tests are completed (including blood type and crossmatch, if ordered). Any abnormalities have been reported to the surgeon and the chart marked accordingly.
4. The child is assessed for allergies, and these are clearly marked on the chart.
5. All external objects such as ribbons, barrettes, glasses, contact lenses, and jewelry are removed. Long hair is kept in place by a rubberband. Nailpolish is removed.
6. The mouth is checked for braces and loose teeth. Braces are removed and given to parents. Loose teeth are brought to the attention of the anesthetist.
7. The ID band is correct and secure, and the crib or bed is marked correctly.
8. Child and parents should receive appropriate information and psychologic preparation (see Box 27-3).
9. The consent form (anesthetic and operative) is placed on the chart and correctly signed and witnessed.
10. All surgical preparation procedures are completed (e.g., skin prep, enema, NPO maintained, nasogastric tube insertion).
11. The child has voided.
12. The child is bathed and has clean gown and underpants or diaper.

mg/kg) or thiopental (20 to 30 mg/kg) is administered. The onset of sleep may take a little longer; mean time is 8.3 minutes after methohexital administration (Liu et al, 1985), but it is time well spent in avoiding a traumatic induction. In addition to eliminating separation anxiety, the method avoids the use of needles or placement of a mask on a frightened child's face. The major disadvantage is that occasionally the child may have a bowel movement after the drug is administered. If an adequate plasma concentration of the drug is not achieved, resulting in inadequate sedation (Liu et al, 1985), an additional dose may be administered.

When the child is asleep, he or she is transported to the operating room by the anesthetist. Anesthesia induction continues with one of the volatile agents.

Anesthesia can also be induced by intramuscular injection with ketamine (Wyant, 1971) or methohexital (Khazzam and Farkas, 1972). An intramuscular induction is particularly advantageous in patients who are uncooperative, who cannot be reasoned with, and in whom venous access is difficult. The advantages are the rapid onset of anesthesia and the ease of administration. The disadvantages of this technique include pain on injection, variable reabsorption if peripheral perfusion is reduced, and the occasional development of a sterile abscess if too large a volume of solution is injected at a single site. A high incidence of emergence reactions characterized by unpleasant dreams and hallucinations is also a relative disadvantage of ketamine (White et al, 1982). Once induced, intravenous access is established and additional medication is administered to maintain anesthesia.

Intravenous induction is common for adults and older children, less common in infants and small children because the anesthetist may not be able to find a suitable vein without causing significant pain. In some instances, (e.g., a hemodynamically unstable child or a child with a full stomach) intravenous induction is the method of choice.

A needle is inserted into a vein, usually on the dorsum of the hand, and anesthesia is induced with a barbiturate or ketamine. Most anesthetists use plastic cannulas rather than metal needles to start intravenous lines, since they are less likely to infiltrate. The child's attention should be diverted during the actual intravenous insertion and the extremity restrained gently but firmly. The most common intravenous induction agent is thiopental. The onset of unconsciousness is rapid, usually 30 to 60 seconds, and the cardiovascular effects minimal in an otherwise healthy patient. After the child loses consciousness, a mask is placed on the face and anesthesia proceeds with a volatile agent, narcotic, and muscle relaxant, or a combination of agents and intravenous drugs to achieve the desired result.

The most common method of inducing anesthesia in the pediatric patient population is by placing a mask over the nose and mouth and having the child breathe a potent anesthetic. This technique is generally well tol-

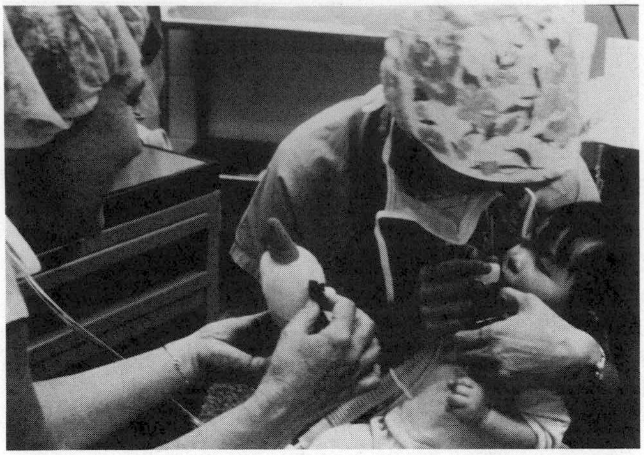

Figure 27-15. Inhalation induction of anesthesia using the anesthetist's hand and anesthesia circuit. This avoids placing a mask directly on the child's face. The child is held by the anesthetist rather than lying on the operating table. (Courtesy of University of Michigan Medical Center.)

erated by children and avoids injection. The most common agent is halothane (Warner et al, 1984). (See Box 27-5 for a summary of inhalation anesthetic agents.)

Some children prefer to hold the mask themselves during the induction. This gives them a sense of control as well as a feeling of participation in their anesthetic administration. If the child objects to the mask being placed on the face, the anesthetist can hold the anesthesia hose through the fingers and cup the hand in front of the child's face (Fig. 27-15). As the child drifts to sleep, the hand is moved closer to the face, eventually being replaced by the mask when the child loses consciousness. Throughout an inhalation induction, the anesthetist should talk to the child in a reassuring voice, diverting the child's attention away from the actual mechanics of breathing. Hypnotic suggestions that the eyes are getting heavy and that the child feels as though she or he is floating are very helpful.

Once the induction is completed, anesthesia is maintained throughout the operative procedure. This is accomplished with a variety of agents and drugs, depending on the child's condition, the type of surgical procedure, and the anesthetist's choice. The child's physiologic response to the anesthetic is assessed throughout the procedure with adjustments made in technique and agents administered based on response. In addition, intravenous fluids and, when indicated, blood products are administered.

Anesthesia Maintenance

The goal of anesthesia maintenance is to establish for the patient a reversible state of unconsciousness that is associated with amnesia, analgesia, and cardiovascular stability and to provide the surgeon with optimal operating conditions. (Box 27-5 lists the common inhalation anesthetics.)

The anesthetic agents used in children are the same agents used in adults. The major differences are that the rate of uptake of inhaled anesthetics is faster in infants than in adults and the anesthetic requirements are greater in the child than in the adult.

The minimum alveolar concentration (MAC) is the accepted measure of anesthetic potency (Eger et al, 1965). MAC is the minimum alveolar concentration of an inhaled anesthetic at 1 atmosphere that prevents movement in 50 per cent of the patients in response to skin incision. The MAC requirements for volatile anesthetics are greatest in infants between 1 and 6 months of age (Lerman et al, 1983). After age 6 months, MAC requirements decrease inversely proportional to age. Neonates, however, have lower MAC requirements than infants (Lerman et al, 1983). In general, greater than 1 MAC concentrations of inhaled anesthetics are required during surgery in healthy patients.

Induction of anesthesia with inhaled anesthetics is faster in infants and children than in adults (Salanitre and Rackow, 1969; Steward and Creighton, 1978). The rapid rise in alveolar concentrations of inhaled anesthetics is related to physiologic differences, which are most pronounced in infancy: increased cardiac output, greater alveolar ventilation, and a proportionally larger compartment of well-perfused tissues relative to body mass.

Emergence from Anesthesia

At the conclusion of the operative procedure, the anesthetic agents are discontinued. The patient's cardiac and respiratory status is assessed. The patient is extubated if blood pressure and heart rate and rhythm are within normal limits and if respiratory rate and tidal volume are adequate. The child should be positioned on the side on the transport stretcher to ensure a patent airway and reduce the likelihood of secretion aspiration. Cardiorespiratory stability should be determined before transporting to the recovery room.

Recovering from Anesthesia

The recovery room nurse's responsibility is to see that the child emerges safely from the anesthetic. All children should receive oxygen in the immediate postanesthetic period to prevent postoperative hypoxemia (Marshall and Wyche, 1972). Vital signs are monitored frequently. The nurse should alert the child's physician to any signs and symptoms of shock (decreasing blood pressure; increasing heart rate; weak, thready

Box 27-5
Inhalation Anesthetic Agents

NITROUS OXIDE (N_2O)

A weak anesthetic agent, since minimum alveolar concentration (MAC) requirements cannot be achieved at atmospheric pressure, it is used frequently in pediatric anesthesia for its analgesic properties, reducing the dose requirements of the more potent inhalation anesthetics. Induction and recovery are rapid. Myocardial and respiratory depression is minimal. It is contraindicated in patients with closed air-containing spaces (i.e., pneumothorax), as the solubility difference between nitrous oxide and nitrogen would result in expansion of the space.

HALOTHANE

Introduced in 1956, this remains the most popular of the potent inhalation agents in pediatric anesthesia because of wide patient acceptance, ease of administration, and rapid onset of action and emergence. Circulatory depression occurs due to direct myocardial depression and suppression of normal baroreceptor-mediated tachycardia, an effect that can be minimized by administering atropine. It depresses airway reflexes and is a potent bronchodilator, which makes it particularly useful in asthmatic patients. A relatively poor analgesic agent; administration is often combined with nitrous oxide or narcotics. It sensitizes the myocardium to exogenous catecholamines; it decreases cerebral metabolic requirements for oxygen ($CMRO_2$) but increases cerebral blood flow (CBF) resulting in elevation of intracranial pressure.

ENFLURANE

Introduced in 1973, induction times are generally longer with enflurane than with halothane because breath-holding is more likely to occur, causing a prolonged period of excitement. Enflurane produces a dose-dependent, reversible depression of myocardial contractility, although bradycardia does not usually occur as with halothane. Peripheral vasodilation is greater than with halothane. Arrhythmias are less common since it is less sensitizing to the myocardium in the presence of exogenous catecholamines. It is a most potent respiratory depressant; it also decreases airway resistance. Since CNS seizure activity has been noted with higher concentrations and/or hypocarbia it is generally avoided in patients with a seizure history. Skeletal muscle relaxation is greater compared with halothane and may reduce the requirement of muscle relaxants. There is evidence in adults that prolonged administration produces inorganic fluoride ion, which may cause a defect in urine-concentrating ability. This possible action may preclude its use in patients with compromised renal function.

ISOFLURANE

The most recently introduced agent (1981), its use in pediatrics is limited by its pungent aroma and irritant effect on the airway, resulting in increased secretions, coughing, and laryngospasm during inhalation induction. Cardiac output is generally maintained since the decrease in systemic vascular resistance is offset by an increase in heart rate. It does not sensitize the heart to catecholamines. It is similar to enflurane in producing skeletal muscle relaxation. A significant advantage is its use in neurosurgical patients. It produces smaller increases in CBF compared to halothane or enflurane that are more readily reversed by passive hyperventilation. It undergoes limited metabolism and hepatic and renal toxicity have not been reported to date.

pulse; cool, clammy skin). Because children are prone to laryngeal and tracheal edema, especially after endoscopic procedures and endotracheal intubation, they must be carefully observed for signs of postintubation croup. Children with stridor should be evaluated by the anesthetist.

The operative site should be checked for bleeding and any increased or continual bleeding reported to the child's physician. Some children may become delirious during emergence from anesthesia. These children need to be restrained to protect them from harm. If a muscle relaxant or narcotic was used as part of the anesthetic, the child should be observed for signs and symptoms of respiratory depression, which may be caused by narcotics or the inadequate reversal of muscle relaxants.

As children awaken from the anesthetic, their perception of pain increases (Mather and Mackie, 1983). The need for postoperative analgesia should be assessed by the recovery room nurse. Adequate medication to control pain should be ordered and administered as needed. (See Chapter 29 for pain management.)

Postanesthesia Recovery

In the postanesthesia recovery unit (PARU), the anesthetist transfers the care of the child to a nurse experienced in caring for children recovering from anesthesia. The nurse is given a report on the surgical procedure that was performed, the child's physical and psychologic preoperative status, the type of anesthetic that was administered, and response to the anesthetic agent. The recovery room nurse is always informed of all fluids and blood or blood products that were administered intraoperatively and any additional medication that was given (e.g., antibiotics), as well as the dose and time of administration.

Table 27-6. Postanesthesia Recovery Score System

	Criteria	Score
Color:	Pink	2
	Pale/dusky/mottled	1
	Cyanotic	0
Airway:	Clear	2
	Airway in place	1
	Obstruction/requires attention	0
Ventilation:	Exchanging well	2
	Diminished	1
	Unresponsive	0
Level of Consciousness:	Fully awake	2
	Arousable	1
	Unresponsive	0
Movement of Extremities:	Purposeful/appropriate for age	2
	Involuntary	1
	No movement	0
	TOTAL	

(Courtesy of C.S. Mott Children's Hospital PARU, Ann Arbor, MI.)

Discharge from the recovery unit occurs when the child's condition is stable and predetermined discharge criteria are met. Using a scoring system, such as shown in Table 27-6, children are discharged from the recovery unit to an in-patient general care unit when they have attained a score of between 8 and 10. Children with scores of less than 7 are discharged from the recovery unit if they are to be admitted to an intensive care or moderate care unit. Children whose preoperative status precludes attainment of a postanesthesia recovery (PAR) score of 8 to 10 may be discharged when they have returned to their normal preanesthetic state. If a child is fully awakened from the anesthetic but the medical condition warrants additional monitoring in a PARU, arrangements should be made to have the parents visit with the child in the recovery room to alleviate both parental and child anxiety caused by separation.

For every patient, the anesthetist should perform a postanesthesia assessment and document it on the patient's chart within 24 hours of discharge from the recovery unit. Any untoward developments related to the anesthetic should be noted and appropriate interventions initiated. If the recovery from anesthesia was uneventful and the patient's condition is stable, no further follow-up by the anesthetist is warranted.

Postoperative Nursing Care

The nurse's responsibility in caring for a child postoperatively is multifaceted. The nurse needs to know about the effect of anesthesia, the type of surgery performed, and the effect of the experience on the child and family. The nurse also must be skilled in the various nursing procedures that must be performed and in watching for postoperative complications.

Before a child returns to the room, the nurse should have received a thorough report on his or her status. This report should contain information regarding:

1. Type of operation performed and anesthesia and medication received
2. Amount of blood loss
3. Stability of vital signs
4. Presence of drains, dressings, or appliances
5. Whether the child has voided
6. The presence, rate, and site of the IV
7. Presence of cough and gag reflex
8. Level of consciousness
9. Any difficulties encountered during surgery
10. Any concerns expressed by the child or parents just before or since the operation
11. What the family has been told by the surgeon regarding the success of the operation
12. Need for any special equipment such as mist tent, oxygen tent, or suction machine.

When the child returns to the unit, the nurse should attend to the patient immediately. The person transporting the child cannot leave until the nurse is in attendance. An immediate general assessment is done, observing the IV site, the child's color and respirations, the level of consciousness, the pain status, dressings, any tubes or drains, and the tightness of any restraints. Preferably the nurse has immediate access to the postoperative orders and can review them at the bedside before beginning a more detailed assessment. Vital signs are then taken and the nurse should check that the IV has the proper solution and is being delivered at the proper rate. The patient is assessed every 15 minutes for vital signs, level of consciousness, condition and intactness of dressing, and functioning of any other tubes or appliances. The frequency of checking vital signs varies according to the surgeon's order or the policy established within the institution. A general guideline is every 15 minutes for 1 hour, then every half hour for 2 hours, then every 2 hours until bedtime. During he first postoperative night, vital signs are typically checked every 4 hours. The nurse's assessment of the child's general status is just as important as checking vital signs. For example, it is expected that in the event of hemorrhage a change in the saturation of a patient's dressing will be noted before a change in the patient's vital signs.

Text continues on page 841

Table 27-7
Nursing Process Plan: Perioperative Nursing Care

By Roxie Foster

Assessment of Physical Function*

Subjective Assessment

Upon admission: Self-report or parental report of previous operations, response to pain medications, prodromal symptoms of illness, loose teeth, last oral intake (if "same day" surgery), and developmental level. Establish legal custody or guardianship of child for purposes of surgical consent

Postoperative: Comfort level; passage of flatus

Objective Assessment

Upon admission: Physical examination by admitting nurse to establish baseline, noting carefully abnormalities such as congenital anisocoria or congenitally absent pedal pulses that will be pertinent to postoperative assessment; diagnostic tests: complete blood count, bleeding time, urinalysis

Postoperative: Adequacy of systemic ventilation/perfusion; level of consciousness; status of breath sounds; effectiveness of cough; bladder distention; bowel sounds, passage of flatus; abdominal distention; status of restraints; placement and patency of IV, drains, catheters, and other tubes inserted in surgery; status of dressings; amount of spontaneous turning/activity

Preoperative Analysis: Nursing Diagnosis 1

Potential injury: physiologic, related to the trauma of surgery superimposed upon a concurrent febrile illness or systemic infection

Defining Characteristics

Subjective: Report of aching, discomfort, e.g., sore throat, stomach pain, headache. Parental report of unusual irritability

Objective: Fever, enlarged lymph nodes, tugging at ear, vomiting, diarrhea, or other signs of infection; increased WBC, decreased hemoglobin and hematocrit, $> 5-10$ polymorphonuclear leukocytes per high power field in a cleanly voided urine specimen (Green, 1986)

Client Goal/ Evaluation Criteria	Nursing Goals/Strategies (Selected Rationale)
1. The client will be free of detectable evidence of systemic infection at the time of surgery as evidenced by: a. being afebrile b. showing no evidence of infection c. results of complete blood count and urinalysis within normal limits	*Assess for evidence of infection.* • Measure temperature every 4 hours preoperatively. Report fever to physician. • Perform a thorough physical assessment upon admission, alerting the physician and/or anesthesiologist to any evidence of infection or any report from mother or child of suspicious symptoms. (It is not uncommon for evidence of an infection [particularly viral] to develop quickly between the time of the doctor's preoperative examination and the time of surgery.)

* See Table 31-2 for a nursing process plan pertaining to Emotional/Social and Intellectual/Perceptual function of the hospitalized child.

Continued

Client Goal/ Evaluation Criteria	Nursing Goals/Strategies (Selected Rationale)
	• Alert the physician and/or anesthesiologist about increased WBC, decreased hemoglobin and hematocrit, prolonged bleeding time, increased leukocytes in urine. (Laboratory results often are not available until just prior to surgery, and the nurse may be the first to see them. If results indicate the possibility of infection, most surgeons will appreciate being alerted before the child is prepared for surgery.)

Preoperative Analysis: Nursing Diagnosis 2

Potential injury: falls, related to failure to adequately protect/supervise the child during the sedative effects of preoperative medications

Defining Characteristics: Preoperative sedation administered

Client Goal/ Evaluation Criteria	Nursing Goals/Strategies (Selected Rationale)
1. The client will not experience a fall associated with preoperative sedation	*Institute safety precautions.* • Have the child bathe and void before administering the preoperative medication. • Explain to the child and family the expected effects of the medication. Caution them about the importance of the child remaining in bed from this point on. • Keep the side rails up. Place the call bell, telephone, and urinal (or bedpan) within easy reach (to decrease the need to leave the bed.) • Encourage family to stay with the child during this time. Check back frequently.

Intraoperative Analysis: Nursing Diagnosis 3

Potential for aspiration, related to
- *dislodging of a loose tooth during placement of an oral airway or endotracheal tube*
- *vomiting during surgery*

Defining Characteristics: Signs of foreign body aspiration or vomiting during the surgical procedure

Client Goals/ Evaluation Criteria	Nursing Goals/Strategies (Selected Rationale)
3.1 The client will not lose a tooth during the surgical procedure. 3.2 The client will consume no liquids or solids during the specified preoperative fasting time.	*Implement measures to avoid aspiration.* • Assess for loose teeth. Alert the anesthesiologist if any are reported or detected. • Record the findings of teeth assessment on the pre-op check list. • Prominently post NPO signs on the door to the child's room and on the bed. • Enlist the help of family members by explaining the importance of this precaution. • Remove water and all food from bedside table.

Postoperative Analysis: Nursing Diagnosis 4

Ineffective airway clearance, related to poor cough effort, associated with
- *sedative effects of anesthesia and analgesics*
- *incisional pain*
- *inability to cooperate because of developmental level*
- *inadequate preoperative explanations and opportunity to practice cough*

Defining Characteristics: Adventitious lung sounds, tachypnea, tachycardia, pallor of skin and mucous membranes

Client Goal/ Evaluation Criteria	Nursing Goals/Strategies (Selected Rationale)
1. The client will maintain airway patency as evidenced by: a. clear lung sounds b. pulse and respirations within normal limits c. mucous membranes pink, skin color normal for race	*Monitor for evidence of ineffective airway clearance* every 2–4 hours, depending upon postoperative status. *Institute strategies to promote airway clearance.* • Preoperatively, teach techniques for splinting incision, deep breathing, coughing, and use of incentive spirometer or blow bottles. • Allow the infant or toddler to cry for a few seconds before comforting. (This will ensure deep breathing in a child too young to cooperate. If secretions are present, coughing will follow the deep breaths as a reflex action.) • Plan deep-breathing and coughing efforts to correspond with peak effects of pain medication. (Since respiratory exercises should be carried out every 2 hours, continual analgesic administration [i.e., every 3–4 hours as ordered] should be considered in the immediate postoperative period.) *Alert the physician* if evidence develops of impaired gas exchange (change in mental status, restlessness, cyanosis, dyspnea, increasing tachycardia, decrease in SO_2 [as monitored by pulse oximetry]).

Postoperative Analysis: Nursing Diagnosis 5

Altered tissue perfusion: systemic, related to
- *hypovolemia associated with postoperative hemorrhage*
- *pooling of blood in lower extremities associated with immobility*

Defining Characteristics: Restlessness, increased pulse and respirations, decreased blood pressure, decreased peripheral pulses, capillary refill > 3 seconds, decrease in urine output, skin cool and pale, possible external evidence of bleeding

Client Goal/ Evaluation Criteria	Nursing Goals/Strategies (Selected Rationale)
1. The client will maintain adequate tissue perfusion as evidenced by: a. usual mental status	*Monitor for adequacy of perfusion* every 15 minutes initially, then at least every 4 hours during the postoperative period. Check under dressings as well as on top. (Blood that fails to be "wicked" into dressing will run under child.)

Continued

Client Goal/ Evaluation Criteria	Nursing Goals/Strategies (Selected Rationale)
b. normal vital signs c. palpable peripheral pulses d. capillary refill < 3 seconds e. urine output ≥ 1 ml/kg/hr or 30–50 ml/hr for a child ≥30 kg f. skin warm and of normal color for race g. dressings dry	*Initiate strategies to improve tissue perfusion.* • Maintain IV replacement of fluids (to ensure adequate vascular volume). • Ensure frequent position changes. Infants and small children usually move spontaneously if pain is kept under control. Older children and adolescents can be encouraged to change position at least every hour and taught to alternately dorsiflex and extend the feet (to facilitate venous return.) • Discourage prolonged sitting positions, raising the knee gatch in the bed, or pillows under the knees. (These positions compromise vascular flow.) • *Alert the physician* to any sudden or significant change in perfusion.

Postoperative Analysis: Nursing Diagnosis 6

Altered fluid volume: excess, related to excessive infusion of IV fluids in the immediate postoperative period, when increased ADH and aldosterone are being produced as part of the physiologic response to stress

Defining Characteristics: Periorbital edema, tachycardia, dyspnea with grunting respirations and adventitious lung sounds

Client Goal/ Evaluation Criteria	Nursing Goals/Strategies (Selected Rationale)
1. The client will not experience hypervolemia as evidenced by: a. absence of periorbital edema b. pulse and respirations within normal limits c. clear lung sounds d. hourly IV intake of no more than prescribed amount of fluid	*Monitor for fluid volume excess* hourly in the infant and small child (whose cardiovascular systems are least well equipped to handle a sudden bolus of intravascular fluid) and at least every 2 hours in the older child. (Periorbital edema is often present before alterations in vital signs. Note especially the dependent eye if the child is lying on a side. If noted early, the IV rate can be decreased before cardiovascular function is compromised.) *Institute strategies to prevent fluid volume excess:* • Use a graduated fluid chamber for IV administration and put only 1 hour's fluid in the chamber. • Use an infusion pump whenever possible. • Monitor and record intake and output hourly on the graphic record. (Because of increased ADH and aldosterone, intake will usually exceed output during the first 24 hours postop. Output < 1 ml/kg/hr, however, may signal inadequate kidney perfusion associated with heart failure.) • If the infusion pump does not have child-proof controls, ensure safety by putting wide adhesive tape over the controls, keeping the pump out of the child's reach, or restraining the child. *Alert the physician* immediately to evidence of fluid volume excess.

Postoperative Analysis: Nursing Diagnosis 7

Altered electrolyte balance: metabolic alkalosis, related to vomiting and/or nasogastric suction

Defining Characteristics: Decreased rate and depth of respirations, latent or manifest tetany (Robson, 1983)

Client Goal/ Evaluation Criteria	Nursing Goals/Strategies (Selected Rationale)
1. The client will not experience metabolic alkalosis postoperatively as evidenced by: a. respirations within normal limits b. absence of tetany	*Monitor for evidence of metabolic alkalosis* if vomiting or significant drainage from a nasogastric tube occurs. Measure respirations hourly in this situation; compare with baseline. Note muscle tone. (This condition is more likely to occur in the infant because of the more tenuous fluid and electrolyte balance at that age.) *Alert the physician* immediately if evidence is present.

Postoperative Analysis: Nursing Diagnosis 8

Altered comfort: pain, related to
- *stimulation of sensitive nerve endings in the incisional area*
- *abdominal distention associated with anesthetic and narcotic analgesics, immobility, and manipulation of bowels during surgery*

Defining Characteristics

Subjective: Irritability, crying, reports of pain

Objective: Changes in usual behavior, obvious "guarding," increased pulse, respirations, unusual lack of movement. See Table 29-2 for other potential pain behaviors by developmental age

Client Goal/ Evaluation Criteria	Nursing Goals/Strategies (Selected Rationale)
1. The client will be free of prolonged periods of intense pain as evidenced by: a. denying discomfort within 30 minutes of analgesic administration b. comfort indicated by child pain assessment tools c. physical activities that approach normal d. vital signs within normal limits e. abdomen soft f. bowel sounds present in all four quadrants within 48–72 hours (or as expected by condition)	*Monitor for pain.* • Expect the child to experience pain similar to that of an adult in a similar situation. • Enlist the help of parents in detecting pain (although the parents' objectivity in this situation is as yet unproved). • Use the pain assessment tools and techniques detailed in Chapter 29. • Monitor abdominal distention and bowel function every 4 hours. *Institute pain-relieving strategies.* • See Table 29-4, Nursing Process Plan: The Child in Pain. • If abdominal distention develops, encourage ambulation rather than medicating. (Narcotic analgesics decrease bowel motility; ambulation increases it.) *Alert the physician* if the analgesic ordered fails to relieve the pain or if abdominal distention develops that is unrelieved by ambulation.

Continued

Postoperative Analysis: Nursing Diagnosis 9

Potential for infection, related to
- *original illness or trauma*
- *transmission of pathogenic organisms from the hands of client, visitors, or health care professionals*
- *ineffective airway clearance*
- *decreased immune response associated with the physiologic stress response*

Defining Characteristics: The potential for infection exists if the original illness or trauma involved infectious organisms (e.g., an inflamed or ruptured appendix may lead to peritonitis; a deep puncture wound may lead to osteomyelitis). The potential for nosocomial infection and respiratory infection always exists postoperatively. Actual infection is signaled by fever, lymphadenopathy, localized inflammation, and positive culture results.

Client Goal/ Evaluation Criteria	Nursing Goals/Strategies (Selected Rationale)
1. The client will remain free of infection in the postoperative period, as evidenced by: a. remaining afebrile b. incision free of purulent drainage, marked redness, or induration c. clear lung sounds d. negative cultures of wound aspirate and sputum	*Monitor for signs of infection* at least every 4 hours. *Institute and teach the client and family strategies to prevent infection.* • The importance of meticulous handwashing cannot be over emphasized. The hands of infants and toddlers should be washed for them by parents and nurses. • Encourage compliance with respiratory therapy protocol, including frequent position change. • Use sterile technique for dressing changes. • Encourage optimal rest, nutrients, and fluids (to enhance the body's immunologic defenses.)

Postoperative Assessment: Nursing Diagnosis 10

Urinary retention, related to
- *effects of anesthesia on the bladder muscle*
- *manipulation of the bladder during surgery*
- *abnormal voiding position*

Defining Characteristics: Inability to void within 6–8 hours after surgery; bladder palpable above the pubis.

Client Goal/ Evaluation Criteria	Nursing Goals/Strategies (Selected Rationale)
1. The client will void within 8 hours after surgery	*Monitor urinary status.* • Frequently ask whether the child feels the need to void. Enlist the help of the family members (especially with the child who is developing modesty). • Palpate for bladder distention. • Note fluid intake since preoperative void.

Client Goal/ Evaluation Criteria	Nursing Goals/Strategies (Selected Rationale)
	Facilitate normal voiding. • If possible, place toilet-trained children in the normal voiding position. Often they can be carried to the bathroom or allowed to use a potty chair at bedside. • If positioning alone is insufficient, try running warm water over the pubic area, letting the child hear water run into a sink, applying moderate pressure with the hand over the bladder area, or (if not contraindicated by condition), place your hand on the child's abdomen, tell the child to take a big breath and hold it, and then to push away your hand by pushing out his or her abdomen (this will apply pressure from abdominal muscles to the area of the bladder). *Alert the physician* if the child has a distended bladder and is unable to void after 8 hours.

Although specific postoperative care varies according to the child's age and type of operation, many aspects of care are similar regardless of these factors. Accurate monitoring of fluid and electrolyte balance is a primary nursing responsibility. Potassium should not be added to the IV until the child has voided (see Chapter 30 on fluid and electrolytes). Accurate intake and output records should be kept during intravenous infusion, even if there is no specific order to do so.

Assessment and management of pain in children is another important aspect of postoperative care. That children require proportionately less pain medication than adults is a myth; the difference may be that the child is less able to communicate the pain. Irritability and a lowered frustration tolerance are common in children who have pain (McCaffery, 1977). Pain may be manifested by facial grimacing, crying, muscle rigidity, clenching of fists, and twisting and turning away from the painful stimulus. A physiologic response of elevated vital signs or pallor can also occur. In some cases, pain may cause enough fatigue so that the child finally goes to sleep. The nurse should observe for such signs of pain in addition to asking a child who can communicate about the sensation of pain. (See Chapter 29 for an in-depth discussion of pain management.)

Painful procedures and activities can be done in conjunction with the administration of pain medication. Coughing and deep breathing, change of position, and early ambulation are common postoperative activities that may cause pain. Giving medication 10 to 15 minutes before carrying out these procedures may increase the child's ability to cooperate. Pain medication is not necessarily given every time a procedure is performed, but nursing care should be adapted whenever possible to allow procedures to be done at the time pain medication has become most effective.

As soon as the nurse has read the postoperative orders, he or she should explain the required care to the parents and child. Parents can help watch the child so that restraints for the IV may be unnecessary. They can also assist with coughing and deep breathing, introduction of fluids, positioning, and ambulation. Care by parents is a great asset to the child; therefore, parents should be given adequate explanations immediately postoperatively to make them feel comfortable in assisting with care.

Regardless of the type of operation, the nurse plays an important role in coordination of postoperative care. Parents frequently ask questions that must be answered by the surgeon. The nurse can reduce their anxiety by telling them how to contact the surgeon or making the telephone call for them. Questions that can be answered by the nurse should be answered promptly. Involvement of the parents throughout the postoperative course prepares them for an easier transition when it is time to take the child home.

Reactions to hospitalization and the experience of surgery vary with the age of the child. The nurse should prepare the family for some behavioral changes that may occur when the child returns home. The nurse should also give explicit instructions to the family and child (when appropriate) on follow-up care and care at home, both verbally and in writing. A system that provides for continuity of care and a method of follow-up is to use a discharge form in triplicate: one copy stays on the chart, one is given to the parents, and one is sent to the physician's office. The nurse should always clarify when the child should return to the physician's office or clinic, how to give medications and their major side effects, how to perform any procedures to be done at home, and what restrictions in activity or diet, if any, should be followed. The nurse assesses the type of care and support that is needed at home and makes a referral to agencies that may assist the family as necessary.

Same-Day Surgery

Same-day surgery reduces the stress caused by separation and staying in an unfamiliar environment. Children enter the hospital in the morning, have surgery, and return home on the same day. The introduction of this practice increases the need for excellent communication between the family's physician and the same-day surgery unit in the hospital. It is important for the nurse to be familiar with the patient's instructional needs after each type of operation because of the short time available in which to teach the family. Careful preoperative teaching is essential to ensure the patient is prepared for self-care upon discharge. In these circumstances, written information given to the patient preoperatively is particularly appropriate. Nurses in the community also need to be prepared to provide the necessary follow-up care with special skills in postoperative assessment and management.

References

American Academy of Pediatrics: Aspirin and Reye's syndrome. Special Report. *Pediatrics* 1982 June; 69(6): 810–812.

Andrew J: Recovery from surgery, with and without preparatory instruction, for three coping styles. *J Pers Soc Psychol* 1970; 15:223–226.

Assaf RAE, et al: The influence of the route of administration on the clinical action of diazepam. *Anaesthesia* 1975; 30:3152–3158.

Avery GB: The morality of drastic intervention in the ICU. *In* Avery GB: *Neonatology: Pathophysiology and Management of the Newborn.* 3rd ed. Philadelphia, JB Lippincott, 1987, 9–12.

Barrus DH: A comparison of rectal and axillary temperatures by electronic thermometer measurement in preschool children. *Pediatr Nurs* 1983 Nov/Dec; 9(6):424–425.

Bloom BS: *Taxonomy of Educational Objectives: The Classification of Education Goals, Handbook I: Cognitive Domain.* New York, David McKay Company, 1956.

Broeder J: School-age children's perceptions of isolation after hospital discharge. *Matern Child Nurs J* 1985 Fall; 14(3):153–174.

Buntain WL, et al: Axillary versus rectal temperature: a comparative study. J La State Med Soc 1977 Jan; 129(1):5–8.

Burnstein S, Meichenbaum D: The work of worrying in children undergoing surgery. *J Abnorm Child Psychol* 1979; 7:121–132.

Cautela JR, Groden J: *Relaxation: A Comprehensive Manual for Adults, Children and Children with Specific Needs.* Champaign, IL, Research Press, 1978.

Davenport HT, Werry JS: The effect of general anesthesia, surgery and hospitalization upon the behavior of children. *Am J Orthopsychiatry* 1970 Oct; 40:806–824.

Delong RD: Individual differences in patterns of anxiety arousal, stress-relevant information, and recovery from surgery. PhD dissertation, University of California, Los Angeles, 1970. *Dissert Abstr Int* 1971; 32:554B.

Dowd EL, et al: Releasing the hospitalized child from restraints. *MCN* 1977 Nov/Dec; 370.

Eckenhoff JE: Relationship of anesthesia to postoperative personality changes in children. *Am J Dis Child* 1953 Nov; 587–591.

Eger EI, et al: Minimum alveolar anesthetic concentration: a standard of anesthetic potency. *Anesthesiology* 1965 Nov-Dec; 20:156–163.

Elliot CH, Olson RA: The management of children's distress in response to painful medical treatment for burn injuries. *Behav Res Ther* 1983; 21:675–683.

Eoff MJ, et al: Temperature measurement in infants. *Nurs Res* 1974 Nov/Dec; 23:457–460.

Eoff MJ, Joyce B: Temperature measurement in children. *Am J Nurs* 1981 May; 81:1010–1011.

Fassler D: Reducing preoperative anxiety in children: information versus emotional support. *Patient Counsel Health Educ* 1980; 2:130–134.

Ferguson BF: Preparing young children for hospitalization: a comparison of two methods. *Pediatrics* 1975 Nov; 64(5):656–664.

Fruthaler GJ: Fever in children: phobia vs facts. *Hosp Pract* 1985 Nov 30; 20(11A):49–53.

Garner JS, Simmon BP: Guidelines for isolation precautions in hospitals. *Infect Control* 1983 Jul-Aug; (Suppl)4:245.

Goresky GV, Steward DJ: Rectal methohexitone for induction of anesthesia in children. *Can Anaesth Soc J* 1979 May; 26:213–215.

Graas S: Thermometer sites and oxygen. *Am J Nurs* 1974 October; 1867.

Green M: *Pediatric Diagnosis. Interpretation of Symptoms and Signs in Different Age Periods.* 4th ed. Philadelphia, WB Saunders, 1986.

Hallenbeck AR, et al: Children with serious illness: behavioral correlates of separation and isolation. *Child Psychiatry Hum Dev* 1980 Fall; 11(1):3–11.

Hanna WJ, Sherlock H: Recall and fears of anaesthesia and surgery in 50 Jamaican pediatric patients. *W Ind Med J* 1983; 32:75–82.

Hughes WT, Buescher ES: *Pediatric Procedures.* 2nd ed. Philadelphia, WB Saunders, 1980.

Hunsberger M, et al: A review of current approaches used to help children and parents cope with health care procedures. *Matern Child Nurs J* 1984 Fall; 13(3):145–165.

Johnson JE, et al: Altering children's distress behavior during orthopedic cast removal. *Nurs Res* 1975 Nov-Dec; 24(6):405–410.

Katz ER, et al: Behavioral distress in children with cancer undergoing medical procedures: developmental considerations. *J Consult Clin Psychol* 1981; 48(3):356–365.

Keuffner M: Passage through hospitalization of severely burned isolated schoolage children. *Commun Nurs Res* 1975; 7:181–197.

Khazzam A, Farkas A: Intramuscular sodium methohexital as a sole pediatric anesthetic-analgesic agent. *Anesth Analg* 1972 Nov-Dec; 51:895–898.

Kleinman MB: Fever. *In* Green M, Haggerty RJ: *Ambulatory Pediatrics.* Vol 3. Philadelphia, WB Saunders, 1984, 106–111.

Koka BV, et al: Post intubation croup in children. *Anesth Analg* 1977; 56:501–505.

Korsch BM: The child and the operating room. *Anesthesiology* 1975 Aug; 43:251–257.

Lerman J, et al: Anesthetic requirements for halothane in young children 0–1 month and 1–6 months of age. *Anesthesiology* 1983; 59:421–424.

Liu LMP, et al: Methohexital plasma concentrations in children following rectal administration. *Anesthesiology* 1985; 62:567–570.

Lorin MI: *The Febrile Child: Clinical Management of Fever and Other Types of Pyrexia.* New York, John Wiley & Sons, 1982.

Lutz W: Helping hospitalized children and their parents cope with painful procedures. *J Pediatr Nurs* 1986 Feb; 1(1):24–32.

Lynn MR: Children have rights too. *J Pediatr Nurs* 1986 Oct; 1(5):345–348.

Mackowiak PA, et al: Effects of temperature on antimicrobial susceptibility of bacteria. *J Infect Dis* 1982; 145:550–553.

Marchiondo K: The very fine art of collecting culture specimens. *Nurs 79* 1979 Apr; 9:34–42.

Marshall BE, Wyche MQ: Hypoxemia during and after anesthesia. *Anesthesiology* 1972 Aug; 37:178–209.

Mather L, Mackie J: The incidence of postoperative pain in children. *Pain* 1983; 13:271–282.

McCaffery M: Pain relief for the child: problem areas and selected nonpharmacological methods. *Pediatr Nurs* 1977 Jul-Aug; 11.

McIntosh S, et al: Fever in young children with sickle cell disease. *J Pediatrics* 1980; 96:199.

Melamed BG, et al: Necessary considerations for surgery preparation: age and previous experience. *Psychosom Med* 1983; 45:517–524.

Melamed BG, Siegel LJ: Reduction of anxiety in children facing hospitalization and surgery by use of filmed modeling. *J Consult Clin Psychol* 1975; 43:511–521.

Melamed BG, et al: The influence of time and type of preparation on children's adjustment to hospitalization. *J Pediatr Psychol* 1976; 1(4):31–37.

Newman J: Evaluation of sponging to reduce body temperature in febrile children. *Can Med Assoc J* 1985, Mar 15; 132:641–642.

Northrop C: Legal aspects of nursing. *In* Flynn JB, Heffron PB: *Nursing From Concept to Practice.* Bowie, MD, Brady Communications Company, 1984, 205–236.

Pidgeon VA: *Children's Concepts of the Rationale of Isolation Technique.* ANA Clinical Sessions, 1966, San Francisco. Norwalk, CT, Appleton-Century-Crofts, 1967, 21–27.

Pridham KF, et al: Helping children deal with procedures in a clinic setting: a developmental approach . . . competence and self-esteem. *J Pediatr Nurs* 1987 Feb; 2(1):13–22.

Prugh DG: Emotional aspects of hospitalization of children. *In* Shore MF: *Red is the Color of Hurting.* Public Health Service Publication No. 1583. Washington, DC, US Government Printing Office, 1969; 17–34.

Rae WA, Fournier CJ: Ethical issues in pediatric research: preserving psychosocial care in scientific inquiry. *Child Health Care* 1986 Spring; 14(4):242–248.

Reams PK, Deane DM: Bogged versus diaper urine specimens and laboratory values. *Neonatal Network* 1988 Jun; 6(6):17–20.

Robson AM: The pathophysiology of body fluids. *In* Behrman RE, Vaughan VC (eds): *Nelson Textbook of Pediatrics.* 13th ed. Philadelphia, WB Saunders, 1987, pp 172–207.

Salanitre E, Rackow H: The pulmonary exchange of nitrous oxide and halothane in infants and children. *Anesthesiology* 1969 April; 30:388–394.

Schmitt BD: Fever in childhood (Pt 2). *Pediatrics* 1984 Nov; 74(5):929–936.

Schwartz BH, et al: Effects of psychological preparation on children hospitalized for dental operations. *J Pediatr* 1983 Apr; 102:634–638.

Shipley RH, et al: Preparation to re-experience a stressful medical examination: effect of repetitious videotape exposure and coping style. *J Consult Clin Psychol* 1979; 47:485–492.

Sibinga MS, Freedman CJ: Restraint and speech. *Pediatrics* 1971 Jul; 116.

Siegel LJ, Peterson L: Stress reduction in young dental patients through coping skills and sensory information. *J Consult Clin Psychol* 1980; 48:785–787.

Skipper J, Leonard R: Children, stress and hospitalization. *J Health Soc Behav* 1978; 9:275.

Spielberger CD, et al: *Manual for the State-Trait Anxiety Inventory.* Palo Alto, CA, Consulting Psychologists Press, 1970.

Spielberger CD, et al: *The State-Trait Anxiety Inventory for Children.* Palo Alto, CA, Consulting Psychologists Press, 1973.

Stern RC: Pathophysiologic basis for symptomatic treatment of fever. *Pediatrics* 1977 Jan; 59(1):92–97.

Steward DJ, Creighton RE: The uptake and excretion of nitrous oxide in the newborn. *Can Anaesth Soc J* 1978 May; 25:215–217.

Teele DW, et al: Unsuspected bacteremia in young children. *Pediatr Clin North Am* 1979; 20:773.

Treloar D: Ready, set—no: something is missing from pediatric pre-op operation. *MCN* 1978 Jan/Feb; 3:50–51.

Vernon DT, et al: *Psychological Responses of Children to Hospitalization and Illness: A Review of the Literature.* Springfield, IL, CC Thomas, 1965.

Vernon DTA, et al: Changes in children's behavior after hospitalization. *Am J Dis Child* 1966 Jun; 3:581–593.

Warner LO, et al: Halothane and children: the first quarter century. *Anesth Analg* 1984; 63:838–840.

Weithorn LA, Campbell SB: The competency of children and adolescents to make informed treatment decisions. *Child Dev* 1982; 53:1589–1598.

White PF, et al: Ketamine—its pharmacology and therapeutic uses. *Anesthesiology* 1982; 56:119–136.

Williams CL, Kendall PC: Psychological aspects of patient education for stressful medical procedures. *Health Educ Q* 1985 Summer; 12(2):135–150.

Wolfer JA, Visintainer MA: Pediatric surgical patients' and parents' stress responses and adjustment as a function of psychologic preparation and stress-point nursing care. *Nurs Res* 1975; 24:244–255.

Wright PF, et al: Patterns of illness in the highly febrile child: epidemiologic, clinical and laboratory correlates. *Pediatrics* 1981; 67:694–700.

Wyant GM: Intramuscular ketalar (CI-581) in paediatric anaesthesia. *Can Anaesthet Soc J* 1971; 18:72–83.

Younger JB, Brown BS: Fever management: rational or ritual? *Pediatr Nurs* 1985 Jan/Feb; 11(1):26–29.

Bibliography

Aho AC, Erickson MT: Effects of grade, gender and hospitalization on children's medical fears. *J Dev Behav Pediatr* 1985 Jun; 6(3):146–153.

Betz CC: After the operation—postprocedural sessions to allay anxiety. *MCN* 1982; 7(4):260–263.

Broome ME: The relationship between children's fears and behavior during a painful event. *Child Health Care* 1986 Winter; 14(3):142–145.

Droske SC, Francis SA: *Pediatric Diagnostic Procedures.* New York, John Wiley & Sons, 1981.

Gregory GA: *Pediatric Anesthesia.* Vols I & II. New York, Churchill-Livingston, 1983.

Hansen BD: Preparing a child for procedures. *MCN* 1982 Nov/Dec; 392–397.

King EE, et al: *Pediatric Nursing Procedures.* Philadelphia, JB Lippincott, 1983.

LaMontagne LL: Facilitating children's coping—preoperative assessment interviews. *AORN J* 1985 Nov; 42(5):718–723.

Leifer G: *Principles and Techniques in Pediatric Nursing.* Philadelphia, WB Saunders, 1982.

McCutcheon ML: The febrile infant. *J Fam Pract* 1985 Jun; 20(6):584–588.

McGravey A, et al: Evaluation of the febrile child under 2 years of age. *J Emerg Med* 1984; 1(4):299–305.

Osborn LM, et al: Temperature and fever in the full-term newborn. *J Fam Pract* 1985 Mar; 20(3):261–264.

Parker S: *Pediatric Care: A Guide for Patient Education.* Norwalk, CT, Appleton-Century-Crofts, 1983.

Redman BK: *The Process of Patient Education.* 5th ed. St. Louis, CV Mosby, 1984.

Ryan JF, et al: *A Practice of Anesthesia for Infants and Children.* New York, Grune & Stratton, 1986.

Scharping EM: Physiological measurements of the neonate: methods for accurately measuring vital signs. *MCN* 1983 Jan-Feb; 8(1):70–73.

Strain JE: AAP periodicity guidelines: a framework for educating patients. *Pediatr Patient Educ* 1984; 74 (Suppl.): 924–927.

Trouten F: Psychological preparation of children for surgery. *Dimens Health Serv* 1981 Mar; 58:9–10.

Wilson JF: Behavioral preparation for surgery: benefit or harm. *J Behav Med* 1981 Mar; 79–102.

Woldrum KM, et al: *Patient Education: Foundations of Practice.* Rockville, MD, Aspen Systems Corp, 1985.

Pharmacologic Principles Applied to the Care of Children

Chapter 28

Mabel Hunsberger

Getting better, in most children's minds, is associated with taking medicine. At a very early age, children are introduced to medications like acetaminophen and aspirin when they have a fever and feel miserable. By 2 months of age, most children receive their first immunization, an event that many parents dread. When a more serious illness befalls a child, invasive techniques and drugs with a wide range of side effects may be required. What is most dreaded by the child is "getting a shot," and parents feel equally helpless when their child is overwhelmed with fear.

Today, the giving of injections to children is avoided whenever possible, but when an injection *must* be given, supportive techniques are used to reduce the child's fears about the experience. Simultaneously, parents are given information about the drug and are involved in supporting their child during the experience.

Nurses play a key role in supporting the child and family and in decision-making regarding the pharmacologic aspect of the plan of care. Although physicians *write* the order for drugs, the nurse is the one to *administer* them; therefore, the nurse has a legal responsibility to know that the drug is reasonable in kind, dose, and route for the condition and age of the child.

This chapter presents an overview of how drugs work in the body, the principles of safe administration of drugs, and practical suggestions about how to gain the cooperation of the child.

Related Topics
Procedural preparations, Chapter 27
Mummy restraint, Chapter 27
Pain management, Chapter 29
Fluid and electrolyte maintenance, Chapter 30

A child is completely dependent on the nurse to ensure that the right *medicine* is given in the right *dose,* to the right *patient* at the right *time* in the right way *(route).* The goal of all nurses is to meet these criteria each time a medication is administered while paying attention to the child's physiologic characteristics and psychologic needs.

Physiologic Factors

During the past decade there has been a rapid growth in the understanding of how the disposition of drugs in the body is affected by the growth process. Although there is a paucity of information regarding drug disposition in infants and children, the action of drugs in the body is known to be affected by maturation of body organs and changes in composition of tissue (Holbrook and Schaible, 1983). To understand the effect of the developing child on the action of drugs, a review of basic pharmacologic principles is helpful.

Principles of Drug Action

The action of all drugs is at the cellular level. Drugs act either on the cell surface, within the cell membrane, or by combining chemically with internal cellular components. Although the action of drugs is not fully understood, it is believed that in most cases a drug combines with an enzyme or another cellular component (Asperheim, 1985). The cellular component that interacts with the drug to produce its effect is called the *receptor,* and the locus of action is the *receptor site.* It is believed that drug receptors have a chemical or structural attraction for a specific drug. After a drug is administered (orally, intramuscularly, sublingually, or rectally), it passes from the administration site into the fluids of the body, which transport it to the receptor site. Physical, chemical, and physiologic factors determine the rate and extension of absorption, known as *bioavailability* of a drug. Intravenous administration of a drug ensures its complete availability.

After the drug reaches the plasma it becomes bound to plasma proteins or other tissue components. The amount of drug that is bound is in equilibrium with the free drug, but only the free drug can interact with the receptor to bring about a therapeutic effect. As the drug is eliminated from the body, additional drug dissociates from the plasma protein binding site to interact with the receptor. This sustains the therapeutic effect of the drug. The extent of binding with plasma proteins, however, varies from one drug to another. Therefore, *the amount and concentration of drug available to the receptor site are not directly proportional to dose.*

It is important to recognize that the response of a patient to a drug ultimately determines its therapeutic effect. The state of illness, drug interactions, age, sex, and individual differences in drug metabolism and excretion influence the concentration of drug achieved and maintained at the receptor site.

Elimination of drugs occurs primarily through the kidney, for which drugs must be fairly soluble in water, therefore, they must undergo metabolism or biotransformation. Most drug metabolism occurs in the liver. The liver contains microsomal enzymes that react with the drug to produce drug metabolites. Unchanged drugs and their metabolites are then eliminated from the body, either through the kidney, feces, respiratory tract, saliva, sweat, or breast milk. The drug or metabolite is most commonly filtered through the glomerulus into the renal tubules. In many cases drugs are partially reabsorbed back into the bloodstream through the walls of the proximal and distal tubules. A more rapid mechanism of elimination is by tubular secretion. The epithelium of the renal tubule secretes the drug into the lumen of the tubule, making it available for elimination (Reiss and Melick, 1984).

Age-Related Differences

The goal of drug therapy is to produce the desired therapeutic effect in each child and to avoid toxicity. Variation in drug disposition depends on age-related differences in body mechanisms; an infant or child cannot be treated with drugs as a miniature adult. In the neonate, especially the premature infant, the physiologic immaturity results in a reduced *rate* of drug disposition. By the age of 6 to 10 years, children utilize drugs twice as fast as adults do but from this time until death the rate of drug disposition again gradually decreases (Pippenger, 1980).

It is not fully understood at what age a child's drug disposition patterns approximate those of an adult. However, drug utilization in children changes rapidly over a period of a few months at the initial onset of puberty. It has been suggested that increasing concentrations of sex hormones at this time result in a competition between sex steroids and drugs for metabolic sites in the hepatic microsomal enyzmes (Pippenger, 1980).

Effect of Age on Absorption. Absorption is the process by which a drug passes into the body fluids, which then carry it to its receptor site (site of action). The sites at which drugs can be administered are either

We appreciate the critical review of this chapter by Shari Gray, Clinical Neonatal Pharmacist, Chedoke-Master Hospital, Hamilton, Ontario.

intravascular (intravenous or intra-arterial) or extravascular (oral, sublingual, buccal, intramuscular, subcutaneous, or rectal). In order for extravascularly administered drugs to reach the receptor sites, they must be absorbed. The absorption of a drug is by passive diffusion and is affected by the properties of the drug, the properties of the membrane it is crossing, the pH of the environment, and local blood flow (Roberts, 1984).

Absorption of orally administered drugs is often delayed in neonates and young infants. This is primarily due to differences in the pH of their gastrointestinal tract and their reduced gastric motility. For most drugs, absorption in the gastrointestinal tract occurs by passive diffusion. For a drug to pass the lipid barrier of the cell membrane, it must remain un-ionized.

Ionization of acidic drugs occurs in alkaline environments and ionization of basic drugs occurs in acidic environments. Acidic drugs remain un-ionized in an acidic environment and therefore are better absorbed. Immediately after birth, gastric pH is high. By 4 months of age gastric pH values have reached 50 per cent of the adult value, which is 1 to 3.5, and by 3 years of age they are thought to reach adult levels (Yeh, 1985). Thus the pH of gastric contents remains less acidic during infancy and early childhood. Acidic drugs, such as nalidixic acid, phenobarbital, and phenytoin, therefore are less well absorbed because they are best absorbed from an acid environment. On the contrary, the absorption of acid-labile drugs such as the penicillins may be enhanced (Morselli, 1980).

Reduced gastric motility in the neonate and young infant also affects absorption. Gastric emptying time in the neonate is 6 to 8 hours; by 6 to 8 months of age it reaches the adult time of 2 hours (Howry et al, 1981). Prolonged exposure of certain drugs to the gastric contents can increase the risk of destroying unstable drugs and delays their entry into the lower gastrointestinal tract where more absorption takes place. Reduced gastric motility and irregular peristalsis of the neonate and young infant thus delay drug absorption and attainment of peak serum concentrations.

The immaturity of intestinal transport mechanisms that carry medications to the blood stream can delay absorption of some drugs further. Such drugs must be given less frequently in the neonate. For example, it has been shown that the older infant and adult can absorb riboflavin within 3 to 4 hours whereas the neonate requires 16 hours for absorption to occur because riboflavin is absorbed by passive diffusion (Holbrook and Schaible, 1983). It is important to recognize that the total amount of drug is eventually absorbed, thus overdose can occur when passively absorbed drugs are given for extended periods of time. Examples of drugs that are orally administered and absorbed slowly by the premature baby include triple sulfonamide, chloramphenicol, and erythromycin (Kagan, 1983). The osmolarity of the vehicle conveying the drug is also important to consider. For example, the high osmolarity of elixirs may cause diarrhea and thereby reduce drug absorption.

Rectal administration of a drug is an alternative that is used for the pediatric patient. Although information concerning the bioavailability of rectally administered drugs is limited, a few drugs are known to be effectively absorbed. Sodium valproate serum concentrations after oral and rectal administrations are comparable; a rectally administered solution of sodium diazepam is more rapidly absorbed than is an intramuscularly administered dose (Magnussen, 1979).

Absorption after intramuscular or subcutaneous administration depends primarily on tissue perfusion in the area of administration. Absorption from intramuscular or subcutaneous injection sites in the neonate is often reduced because of immaturity of blood flow to the various muscles and tissues and because of reduced muscle tissue and subcutaneous fat tissue (Yeh, 1985). Drug administration to the sick neonate is predominantly by the intravenous method to circumvent these absorption uncertainties.

Effect of Age on Distribution. After a drug is absorbed, it is carried by the blood to various organs and tissues of the body. Factors that influence distribution are the fluid composition of the body and drug–protein binding.

The amount of water available in the body is an important variable determining the ultimate drug concentration achieved. In the preterm infant, total body water (TBW) comprises 80 to 85 per cent of body weight; 75 per cent in the full term infant; and 60 per cent (same as the adult) by the end of the second year of life. Thus, when administering a drug to an infant in the same dosage (according to weight) as for an adult, lower plasma concentrations of the drug result because it is diluted by the larger proportion of body water. Consequently, the loading doses required to attain the desired plasma concentration of the drug are frequently proportionately higher in infants (Holbrook and Schaible, 1983).

Drug distribution also depends on plasma protein-binding. Plasma albumin is the primary binding site for drugs. Neonatal albumin has a lower binding capacity for certain drugs (phenytoin, penicillin) compared with its binding capacity for bilirubin, although this has not been extensively studied (Udkow, 1987). (Neonatal albumin binds more bilirubin than does adult albumin.) On the contrary, some drugs have an affinity for albumin (e.g., sulfonamide, aspirin, vitamin K) and compete for available binding sites with bilirubin. The competitive drug binding in the neonate increases the potential for the infant to suffer ill effects of increased concentrations of unbound, unconjugated bilirubin (Sheridan et al, 1982).

The type and amount of albumin affect binding capacity and drug disposition. The reduced capacity for neonatal albumin to bind certain drugs results in proportionately more free or unbound drug. In addition, neonates, especially premature infants, may have low albumin concentration (Udkow, 1987). This physiologic difference is compensated for by administering albumin to neonates when indicated. The variability in albumin drug-binding capacity in infants requires further research.

Effect of Age on Metabolism (Biotransformation). Metabolism and excretion together make up the body's mechanism of eliminating drugs. Drugs undergo metabolism to convert them into compounds that are more water soluble for excretion by the kidney. Most biotransformation takes place within the liver and is performed by hepatic microsomal enzymes. Immaturity of the liver in premature infants and neonates generally reduces the biotransformation of drugs, although this varies depending on the specific drug. Immaturity of the liver can result in prolonged excessive serum concentration of drugs and lead to drug toxicity in the neonate. Microsomal enzymes that metabolize chloramphenicol are particularly immature during the first 2 weeks. Chloramphenicol toxicity (known as the gray syndrome) is known to occur when the drug is administered to premature infants in a dosage based on body weight.

The rate of metabolism through early childhood may exceed adult values. For example, clearance rates for theophylline are low in infancy but increase fivefold by 4 years of age and then slowly decline over the years (Weinberger et al, 1981). Theophylline has also been shown to be metabolized to caffeine in the neonate. Both of these drugs (theophylline and caffeine) are methylxanthines with a similar pharmacologic action and, therefore, can produce toxicity through their additive effects, whereas adults rapidly metabolize theophylline to inactive metabolites (Yeh, 1985).

Another factor affecting drug metabolism is the relative change in hepatic size. A fetal liver is 4 per cent of total body weight whereas the adult liver is 2 per cent of body weight. This helps explain why children eliminate many drugs more rapidly and have proportionately higher dosage requirements.

Effect of Age on Elimination. Urinary excretion is the major route for elimination of drugs and their metabolites. Drugs also can be excreted in bile and feces. Although the kidney of the neonate has almost as many cells as the adult kidney, it does not function as a mature kidney. Glomerular filtration rates (GFR) and renal blood flow in the neonate are only 30 to 40 per cent of those in adults. Within the first 2 weeks of life, the GFR doubles in both preterm and full-term infants (Guignard, 1982) and reaches adult values at between 2.5 and 5 months of age (Giacoia and Gorodisher, 1975).

Tubular secretion, another mechanism by which drugs are eliminated, is less efficient. In the infant, drugs such as the penicillins which are secreted mainly by tubular secretion, thus have a half-life* 300 per cent longer than that of the adult (Howry et al, 1981). Tubule secreting abilities mature over the first few months of life and reach adult values at around 7 months of age (Giacoia and Gorodisher, 1975). Excretion of drugs is also affected by tubular reabsorption (absorption from tubule lumens back into the blood stream). The pH of the urine in the newborn infant is lower (more acidic) than that of the adult, which promotes reabsorption and prolongs the half-life of weakly acidic drugs. This occurs because acidic urine promotes non-ionization of acidic drugs, leading to greater reabsorption (Howry et al, 1981). The net effect of these immaturities is the potential for a drug to accumulate in the body.

Assessment

A large component of a child's fears in the hospital are associated with the experience of receiving medications, especially when a needle is involved. Much fear can be relieved by a nurse who approaches the child appropriately and gives medications properly. An important step is to make a careful assessment of the child's and family's needs regarding support and information about the drug. An assessment of a child often needs to be done quickly to determine the best approach and technique. Parents can offer important information. Pertinent issues to address with parents before attempting to give any kind of medication include:

- Does the child have any allergies?
- How does the child usually respond to taking medication?
- How are medications administered at home or how have they been given by other nurses (i.e., equipment used, child's position, is drug mixed with something)?
- Will a parent be available to be with the child? (Leave the option open for parents not to stay if that is their wish.)
- Is the child/parent familiar with the action, purpose, and potential side effects of the drug?
- Is there anything else the nurse should know about the child that is relevant to giving medications?

* The half-life of a drug is the length of time it takes for one half of the drug to be excreted.

Simultaneously the nurse makes a quick assessment of the appropriate technique to use for the situation and developmental level of the child: the appropriate needle gauge and length for an injection, whether the child can swallow a capsule or requires liquid medication, and how and when to prepare the child for the medication. Some medications also require special assessments such as checking a pulse before giving digoxin or assessing output before giving potassium chloride.

Administering medications is a frequent activity of the nurse, under a variety of circumstances. In some cases it is an emergency; in others, the drug is routine. Sometimes it is a child's first injection; sometimes a medication with which both child and parent are familiar. In all circumstances, the nurse should prepare the child and family, involve the parents in the administration of the drug as appropriate, and respond to the individual needs of children and parents. The potential dangers involved in drug administration and the side effects of the various drugs given are information that is fundamental to the safe administration of medications.

Nursing Diagnoses

Nursing diagnoses applicable to most situations involving drug administration to children include:

***Potential for injury**, related to inappropriate administration of medication, associated with*

- *inaccurate identification of patient*
- *inaccurate drug dose, time, or route*
- *excessive restraint of child*
- *unsafe technique of administration*
- *inappropriate medication for child's condition*
- *failure to rotate sites*

***Altered comfort: pain**, related to*

- *physical trauma by needle*
- *tissue response to drug*
- *anxiety associated with an unknown experience*

***Fear**, related to*

- *previous negative experience associated with receiving medication*
- *separation from parents when receiving medication*
- *lack of relevant preparation for experience*
- *unfamiliarity of person giving medication*
- *too long a waiting period until injection is given once told about it*

***Potential impaired tissue integrity**, related to damage by a chemical irritant (medication), associated with*

- *use of too short a needle for intramuscular injection*
- *injection of too large a volume of medication at one site*
- *injection of too concentrated a medication into tissue*
- *injection of medication into an inappropriate site for age of child (i.e. gluteus maximus under age 6 years)*
- *toxicity of drug*

***Knowledge deficit (child/family)**, related to lack of familiarity with*

- *drug administration*
- *side effects of drugs*
- *purpose of drug*

***Family coping: potential for growth**, related to*

- *participation in decision making concerning child's drug regimen*
- *participation in preparing child for painful experience*
- *ability to give emotional support to child during painful experience*
- *involvement in providing child with diversional activity during a painful experience*
- *knowledge acquisition of side effects associated with child's medications*

***Powerlessness**, related to*

- *excessive restraint during medication administration*
- *lack of choice in procedure of medication administration*
- *lack of opportunity to be involved in decision making concerning medication regimen*

***Ineffective individual coping**, related to*

- *inadequate support for developmental needs*
- *knowledge deficit regarding the procedure*
- *inability to understand explanations, associated with immaturity*

Nursing Strategies

Administration of medications requires skill and sensitivity from the nurse. Achieving the task with the least amount of hurt to the child yet obtaining the desired benefit is the goal.

Reducing Fear: Preparation and Support of Child

As is true for all procedures, parents and children (as appropriate for age) require information about the procedure and the medication. An explanation of why the drug is given, what is expected of the child, and how the parent can participate and support the child is given (see discussion on procedural preparation in Chapter 27).

The child's developmental level guides how to approach and support the child. Infants need the support of a parent and the comfort of being held and rocked after a medication. Resistive toddlers and preschoolers do not necessarily understand even a simple explanation but when one makes the effort to prepare them a degree of trust is generated. Doll play with medical toys in this age group is a common approach to defuse a child's fears. School-age children require more specific information about the medication and specific instructions on how they can help. Participation, when appropriate, enhances cooperation and becomes a form of distraction from the potential hurt. Adolescents respond well to a full explanation and an opportunity to ask questions about the medication. They may wish to see the syringe or medication and want to be informed about the plan of therapy, including how often and how long the medication will be required.

Preventing Injury: Safe Technique of Administration

Until the late school-age years, children have great difficulty understanding the meaning of the events that accompany illness. To accomplish accurate and safe administration of medications with the least amount of hurt and discomfort, the nurse needs skill in the technique of administration and knowledge about a child's physiologic and developmental vulnerabilities. A child's lack of understanding results in severe physical resistance. In spite of preparation through explanations and doll play, kicking, flailing, and hitting are resistive behaviors often encountered. Parents may be able to suggest a method of administration for their child or give the medication themselves when appropriate.

Avoidance of physical injury to the child during the process is essential. Restraining a child too forcefully or leaning on a child can cause physical and psychologic harm. Furthermore, a struggling child can get jabbed, poked, or scratched with a syringe, cup, or needle. The way a child is positioned can guard against injury. The position will depend on the type of medication that is being given, but in all cases it is important to firmly stabilize the part of the body that is involved to avoid injury.

Preventing Injury: Administration of Safe Dose

A child is not a small adult, therefore drugs are not calculated according to formulas based on adult dosages. When preparing to administer a drug, the therapeutic dosage is checked by calculating according to the weight or surface area of the child.

For example, the recommended dose of a drug is 100 to 200 mg per kg daily in three to four divided doses. You have an order for 500 mg of the drug to be given every 6 hours to a child who weighs 12 kg. Calculations to check the appropriateness of the drug dose:

A. Amount of drug appropriate for patient in 24 hours:
   12 kg × 200 mg (maximum dose) = 2400 mg
   Amount of drug permitted per dose:
   2400 mg ÷ 4 doses = 600 mg
   Ordered dose of 500 mg is less than permitted dose, therefore can be administered safely

Drug dosage can also be calculated according to body surface area. The surface area is computed as a relationship between height and weight by using a nomogram (Fig. 28-1). The surface area is the point at which a straight line drawn from height to weight intersects the surface area column. Calculation to find the safe range of a drug dose:

B. Surface area of child (m^2) × dose/m^2/24 hr = dose to be administered in a 24-hour period

To use this formula: the recommended dose/m^2/24 hr of a specific drug is found in a reference source. That number is then multiplied by the surface area of the child (as determined from the nomogram) to calculate the recommended dose for a 24-hour period. After the dose for a 24-hour period is known, calculations as in *A* above are required to determine the appropriate amount to be administered per dose.

Becoming familiar with calculation of small doses requires supervised practice. Boxes 28-1; 28-2; and 28-3 summarize key facts and principles to use in calculating pediatric doses.

Maintain Tissue Integrity

It is now known that immaturity of the body systems of premature infants, neonates, and young infants can affect the disposition of a drug that is administered (see previous discussion on physiologic factors). The im-

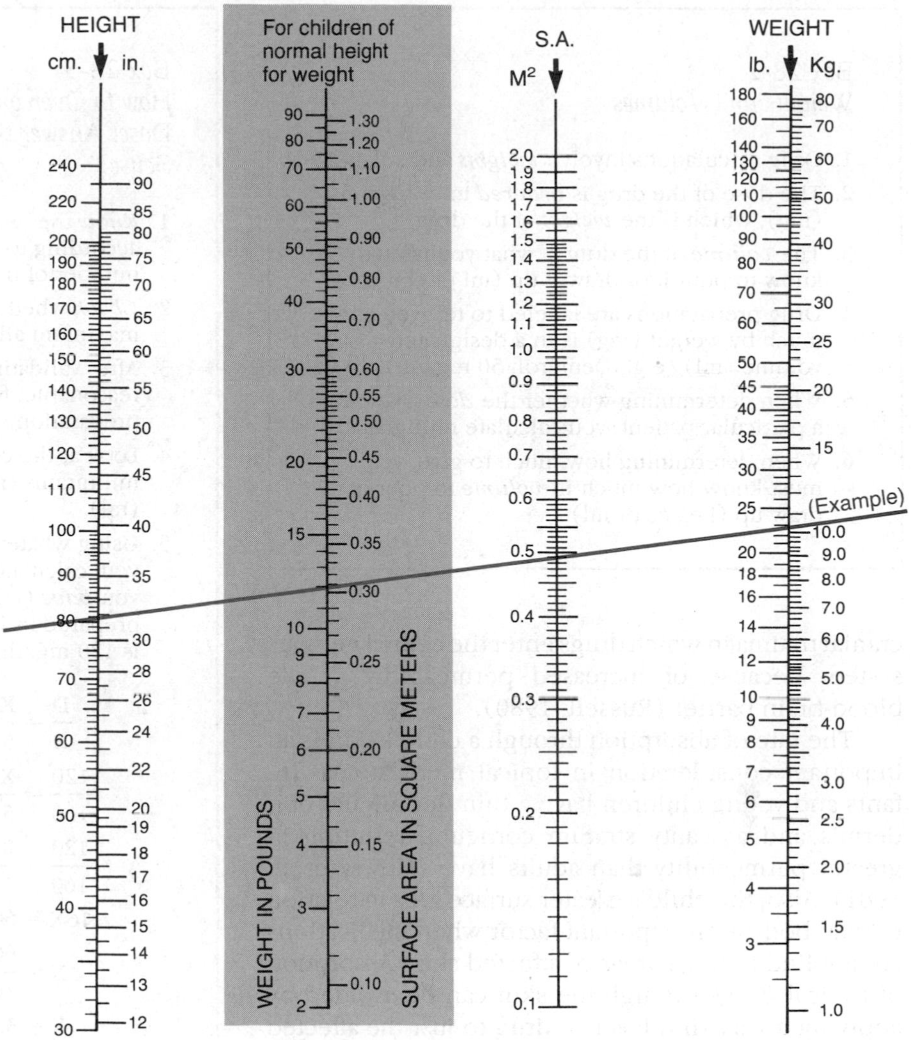

***Figure* 28-1.** Nomogram for calculating body surface area. The surface area is indicated at the intersection of a straight line connecting the height and weight column with the surface area column; if the patient is of roughly average size, it is determined by the weight alone (enclosed area). (Nomogram modified from data of E. Boyd by C. D. West.)

mature enzyme system in the liver, the reduced protein binding of drugs, and the immature renal system are factors associated with toxicity of drugs.

Drugs that disturb acid-base balance affect toxicity. For example, overdose with salicylate easily leads to metabolic acidosis in children; the same blood salicylate levels rarely lead to metabolic acidosis in adults. Careful monitoring of drug levels, urinary output, and side effects of the drug are nursing strategies to prevent drug toxicity.

Fluid and electrolyte regulation bears extremely close monitoring during certain drug therapy. Administration of diuretics to children results in depletion of sodium and potassium more readily than in adults (Kagan, 1983). The neonate has limited ability to concentrate urine, making it important to ensure adequate fluid intake for secretion of drugs and their metabolites. Intake and output should be closely monitored during drug therapy in infants as states of dehydration can increase the potential for drug toxicity.

The immature development of the blood-brain barrier is also associated with drug toxicity. Immature myelinization of the central nervous system enhances permeability of the blood-brain barrier, making it possible for drugs and bilirubin to enter the central nervous system. Myelinization to create this barrier is not mature until 2 years of age (Howry et al, 1981). The nurse is particularly careful to observe for side effects of drugs in illnesses like meningitis, brain tumors, and

Box 28-1
Most Frequently Used Equivalents in Calculation of Pediatric Doses

Volume	**Weights**
1 cc = 1 ml	1000 mg = 1 gm
1 tsp = 4–5 cc or 4–5 ml	1000 gm = 1 kg
1 oz = 30 cc or 30 ml	1 kg = 2.2 lb

Box 28-2
Weights and Volumes

1. Drug calculations involve *weights* and *volumes.*
2. The dose of the drug is *ordered* in milligrams (mg), which is the *weight* of the drug.
3. The *volume* of the drug is what you need to know to pour it or draw it up (ml or cc).
4. Drug preparations are labeled to tell you how much by weight (mg) is in a designated volume (ml) (e.g., Demerol, 50 mg/ml).
5. When determining whether the *dose* is safe for a particular patient, you calculate milligrams.
6. When determining how much to give, you must know how much in *volume* to pour or draw up (i.e., cc or ml).

Box 28-3
How to Overcome the Fear of Giving a Wrong Dose: Answer the Question, "Does It Make Sense?"

1. *Know* the recommended 24-hour dose allowed according to the weight of the child, i.e., number of mg/kg/24 hours.
2. *Check* whether the dose ordered exceeds the maximum allowed in 24 hours.
3. After validating that the ordered dose is reasonable, find the correct drug in the correct preparation.
4. Look at the container to determine how many milligrams (mg) contained in each milliliter (ml).
5. Using whatever formula or system is familiar to you, calculate what is *desired* (D) from what you *have* (H). For example, acetaminophen is prepared in 160 mg/5 ml. If the desired dose is 120 mg, the calculation may be as follows:

$$\frac{D}{H} = \frac{X}{5} \quad \text{(amount in ml to be given)}$$

$$\frac{120}{160} = \frac{X}{5}$$

$$\frac{12\emptyset}{16\emptyset} = \frac{X}{5}$$

$$16X = 60$$

$$X = \frac{60}{16}$$

$$X = 3.75 \text{ ml}$$

6. The final step is to determine mentally whether your answer *makes sense.* The mental process goes something like this:
   I had 160 mg in 5 ml.
   The amount I am asked to give is 120 mg, which is more than half of 160 mg, but is less than 160 mg.
   The amount I will give (in ml), therefore, will be more than half of 5 ml, but less than 5 ml.
   The answer is 3.75 ml, which *makes sense.*
   This process provides a check to catch any decimal point errors that might have been made in the calculation.

cranial trauma in which drugs enter the central nervous system because of increased permeability of the blood-brain barrier (Russell, 1980).

The rate of absorption through a child's skin is an important consideration in topical medications. Infants and young children have a thin dermis and epidermis and a scanty stratum corneum, resulting in greater permeability than adults have (Howry et al, 1981). Also, the child's greater surface area in relation to total body is an important factor when medications are applied to large areas of affected skin. Absorption of topical drugs through the skin can be avoided by applying a very thin layer of drug to just the affected area. Repeated topical application of steroids is avoided because of potential systemic absorption and resultant suppression of adrenal steroid production (Howry et al, 1981).

The nurse also monitors children for drug sensitivity. Sensitivity to a drug depends on the age of the child and also the developmental stage of the particular system affected by the drug. For example, inhibition of skeletal growth results when long-term therapy with adrenocortical steroids is required. Conversely, androgens such as testosterone stimulate the rate of growth but also speed up epiphyseal closure, resulting in reduced height (Kagan, 1983). The nurse's awareness of these potential side effects is an important aspect of drug administration.

Meeting Developmental Needs of the Individual Child

Medications are administered to children at all ages through different routes. The following discussion of the nurse's approach to children when giving medication by various routes of administration integrates strategies for handling children's fear, injury, powerlessness, and coping throughout the various stages of development. Table 28-1 provides guidelines for oral administration.

Oral Medication

Infant (Table 28-1). For security and comfort, the infant should be held on the nurse's or parent's lap

Table 28-1. Guidelines for Administration of Oral Medication

Nursing Actions	Rationale Based on Developmental Characteristics
1 to 3 Months	
Support head well during administration	Head control not yet developed, therefore head bobs
Keep infant's arms and palms away from face	Randomly moves arms and has a strong palmar grasp: may spill medication
Alternate methods of administration can be used:	
1. Medication can be put into a nipple. As a baby sucks and empties the nipple, more medication is added slowly	Has a strong sucking reflex which increases up to around 3 months of age. Choking or drooling, with loss of correct dosage, can occur if infant sucks medication too rapidly
2. A syringe or dropper is used by placing it to one side of the mouth along the gums toward the back of the mouth	Medication placed on the front of the tongue is easily lost because of tongue thrust normally present at this stage
3. Can be given *slowly* from a small spoon or spouted cup in small amounts	If the baby drools, the medication can be caught off the face with the spoon and re-fed
Hold the infant momentarily and lay on stomach or on the side after medication is given	Aspiration occurs more readily in the supine position
Medication is given slowly regardless of method	The strong taste of medication may cause the baby to choke if given too rapidly
Let parent give the medication as appropriate	The familiarity of the infant with parents increases cooperation
Cradle infant in arms during medication administration whenever possible	A comfortable, relaxed holding position makes infant feel secure and provides a situation similar to feeding, which encourages cooperation
3 to 12 Months	
Comfortably hold infant during medication administration	The comfort of being held makes infant feel secure and encourages cooperation
Older infants may require gentle restraint of arms (i.e., one arm held behind nurse's back and one held by nurse's hand, or use of mummy restraint, if necessary)	Infant's increasing muscle strength may be used to refuse medication more forcefully
Take special precaution to keep medication out of reach of infant who is developing rapidly	Is rapidly developing gross and fine motor muscle control, therefore can reach, grasp, and open containers
Alternative methods of medication administration can be used as appropriate developmentally (syringe, spoon, cup)	By 4 months of age an infant can take medication from a spoon more easily. As an infant approaches 12 months, the task of drinking from a cup is achieved, therefore, a small medicine cup is often used for medication. Medication that is spit out can be retrieved by using a spoon or medicine cup
Let parents give the medication as the nurse stands by	Around 7–8 months, infants develop a fear of strangers. A sense of fear makes an infant resist what strangers do
Immediately after medicine is placed into infant's mouth, encourage swallowing by gently pulling up infant's chin with thumb. Also can stroke infant's neck	Infant can forcefully spit out medicine
Respond to individual needs if expressed	As an infant approaches 12 months, specific wishes can be made known by single words or gestures, i.e., the wish to be held versus sitting in a chair
Comfort infant after medication is given by holding, stroking, and rocking	Is responsive to tactile stimuli and facial expressions at this stage
12 to 18 Months	
Keep medicine cabinets locked and keep medicine away from child's bedside	Advances from standing to independent walking and can crawl to get most things in sight
Explain what the child is to do before beginning. Involve the child in some choices regarding medication	Can indicate wants by gestures; by 18 months uses 6–20 recognizable words and understands many more. Has developed independence and resists being forced to do something
Can use cup, syringe, or spoon according to the needs of the child	May have a preference because of home routines
May need to disguise crushed tablets in small amounts of nonessential solids or liquids (i.e., pudding or soda)	Bitter-tasting medications resisted. Such medication should not be mixed into essential foods such as milk because of potential for child refusing milk thereafter

continued

Table 28-1 *(continued)*

Nursing Actions	Rationale Based on Developmental Characteristics
18 to 36 Months	
Keep medication cabinets locked and keep medication away from child's bedside	Children wander to restricted areas and explore the environment
Prepare child by doll playing and demonstration	Cooperation is important because at this age the mouth can be clamped tightly in resistance. Imaginary play is prevalent at this age
Be honest about the taste of the medication	Resistance may be transferred to all requests if nurse is dishonest
Alternative methods of medication administration can be used (syringe, spoon, cup, or chewable tablet) by about 2 years of age. Crushed tablets when not of the chewable type, may need to be disguised as aforementioned	Child is able to swallow well and chew a chewable tablet if instructions are given. Second molars erupt about 20 months of age
Use a firm, consistent approach	Reactive behavior is prominent in this age group. Limit setting makes a child feel more secure and cooperative
Let child make some choices and be as independent as able; e.g., choose between cup and syringe and holding the cup or syringe	Child does not experience a sense of loss of control if able to participate
Give simple directions such as "pick up the cup, take a drink, and now swallow"	Can follow two or three directions given at one time
Give immediate, positive tactile and verbal response for the child's participation and cooperation in taking medicine. Resistive behavior is ignored	Positive feedback encourages child to participate next time to receive again the acceptance and praise
3 to 6 Years	
Continue to keep all medications under lock and key	Although beginning to comprehend the danger of medications, will ingest dangerous amounts if unsupervised
Explain the options of medication available (i.e., liquid, chewable tablets, or capsule). Let child make some choices about how the medication is administered whenever possible	Able to comprehend explanations and has likely had some experience to know which option is preferred. Capsules may be swallowed by some children at 5 or 6 years of age, depending on the size and texture
Explain the purpose of the medication in simple terms	Though the explanation may not be completely understandable, child attaches importance to taking medication correctly if an explanation is given
Avoid prolonged reasoning and arguing, but rather set limits firmly about the need to take medication	May need assistance to achieve control and will feel better if such control is achieved and the task is accomplished
Parent or nurse can give medication; whoever can gain the child's cooperation should do it	May be more cooperative for the nurse than the parents because the child views the nurse as an authority figure and is learning to adhere to society rules (similar to what is required of the child in school)
Use therapeutic play, letting child pretend to give medicine by syringe or cup to a doll or stuffed animal to encourage cooperation	Achieves a sense of control and acts out feelings during such activities
Praise child immediately after giving medication	Future cooperation is encouraged if immediate feedback is given
6 to 12 Years	
Explain to child the purpose of the medication	As child approaches the age of 12 years, the purpose of a medication can be understood if explained simply. Cooperation can be encouraged through explanation
Give medication in the form most suitable for each particular child. Offer chewable tablets or liquids as required	Some 6–8-year-olds have had no experience swallowing capsules and may find it difficult to swallow them, especially if large
Be firm and consistent in asking child to swallow medication in presence of the nurse	Generally, school-age children are cooperative, but if the medicine is excessively bitter, a young school-age child may willfully discard the medicine, not recognizing its importance
Principles Adhered to at All Ages	
1. Medications are not compared to candy. 2. Medications are to be swallowed in the presence of the nurse.	

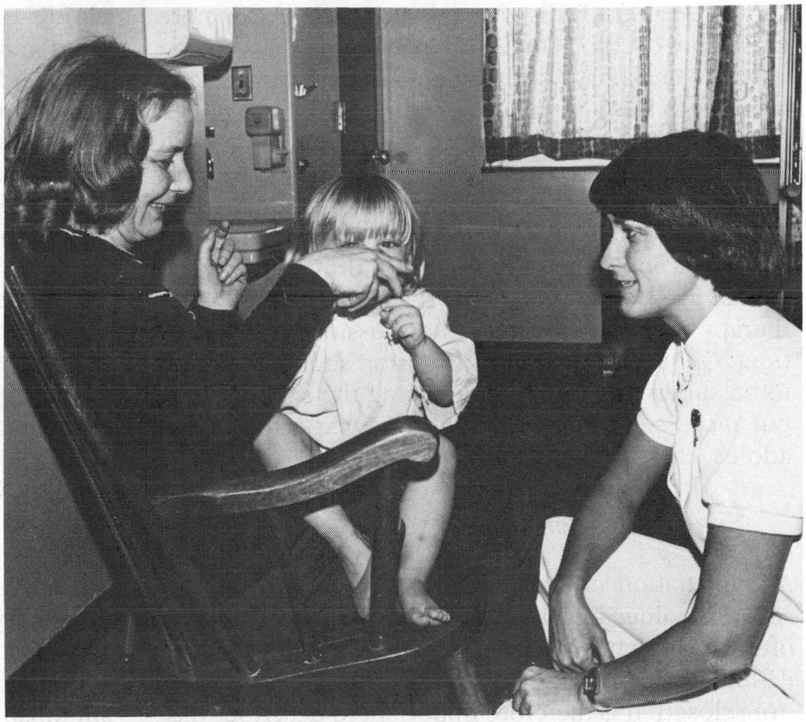

Children frequently cooperate in taking medications in a supportive environment. (Notice that the nurse gets down to the toddler's eye level.)

when oral medications are being given. If this is not possible, the infant's head usually can be lifted off the bed and cradled in the nurse's hand. Crying in an infant can lead to aspiration if medication is given too rapidly. As a general rule, tablets are crushed and mixed with a small amount of fluid unless they are chewable. Depending on the medication and individual patient restrictions, suggested fluids include water, flavored syrups, juices, or flattened soda.

Oral medications are now frequently prepared in syringes under unit dose medication systems. Medication in a syringe can be administered directly into an infant's mouth. Since the sucking reflex causes the infant to push out anything placed in the front of the mouth, the tip of the syringe should be placed in the back of the mouth and to one side and the medication given in small amounts. Medication by plastic dropper can be administered in the same manner. Small plastic medication cups bent slightly to form a spout can also be used, but since the medication is delivered at the front of the mouth, it is easily pushed out and the administration process often must be repeated. Putting the medication into a nipple is another alternative; this utilizes the infant's natural sucking responses. The nipple method is not recommended, however, in infants with sucking problems or when medication has an extremely bitter taste. Since parents often give medications with a spoon, this may be the most successful for the nurse as well. If parents are present, they are often more effective than professionals in gaining the child's cooperation to give the medication.

Toddler (Table 28-1). A spoon, a medicine cup, or a medication syringe is used to give oral liquid medication to a toddler. The usual hospital procedure is to use a medicine cup or a syringe; however, the nurse should explore whether a spoon would be more effective. When a medicine cup is used the toddler frequently wants to hold the cup or prefers that a parent hold it. The nurse should remain with the toddler until all the medication is swallowed.

When using a syringe, avoid squirting the entire contents of the syringe into the toddler's mouth at one time. The syringe should be placed to one side and toward the back of the mouth. The plunger is then pushed, injecting the portion of the medicine that the toddler is capable of swallowing at one time. (A 5-ml syringe of medication would require approximately three squirts.)

Oral medications can also be given in tablet form. Chewable tablets can usually be given to a 2-year-old. The nurse should stay with the child until the medication is chewed and swallowed. Tablets that need to be crushed can be mixed as for an infant. If the taste is extremely bitter it may be disguised in a nonessential food such as a small amount of fruit jelly. Regardless of how medications are given, the nurse must approach the child with recognition of the developmental tasks and behaviors that will affect oral administration of medications.

Preschooler (Table 28-1). Resistive behaviors to oral medications may continue to be demonstrated during the preschool years. The taste of medications cannot be as easily disguised, but resistance can more easily be counteracted with reasoning than in the younger child. Use of therapeutic play is particularly relevant to this age group.

School Age and Adolescent (Table 28-1). Swallowing of capsules or pills is usually achieved by most children by early school age. Physical resistance is not usually a problem during these years; rather, questions are raised about the purpose of the drug. During late school age and adolescence, decision making about therapy often can be made in discussion with the patient. Generally, drug administration should continue to be supervised by an adult during the school years, but more self-responsibility can be expected of the adolescent.

Eye Medication

Administration of eye medication is particularly resisted by older infants and young children. Children often resist when anyone comes near their face by flailing arms, kicking, screaming, and squeezing their eyes closed. It is therefore important to describe what will be done and to show the child the small amount of medication that will be used. Greatest success is achieved by moving quickly once the child has been told what will happen. Before administration, the medicine should be at room temperature and the eyes should be gently wiped with a moist warm cloth to remove any crusted discharge.

Administration of an eye medication may often require a second individual to restrain a resisting child. If no other person is available to assist, a mummy restraint can be used (see Chapter 27).

With the child lying supine, the shoulders and neck are raised slightly with a pillow. To administer drops, the hand holding the bottle should rest on the child's forehead. When the child's head moves, the hand moves with it. The other hand is placed on the cheekbone, and the lower conjunctival sac is exposed with the index finger (Fig. 28-2). An older child should be instructed to look up when eye drops or ointments are being being administered. The drops are placed into the conjunctival sac near the outer canthus of the eye. Ask the child to close the eye(s) and blink.

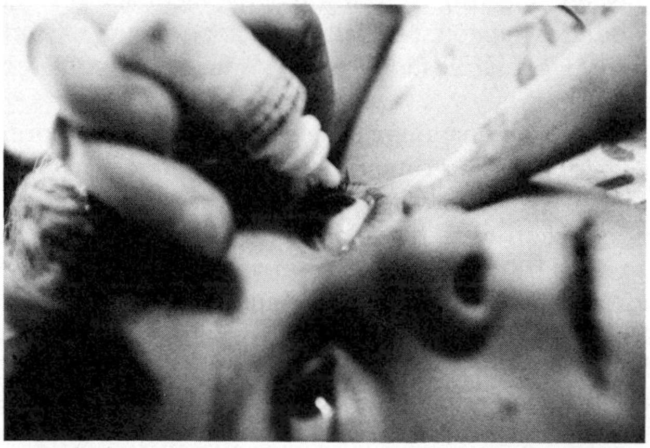

Figure 28-2. Administering eye drops. The hand holding the bottle or dropper rests on the forehead. The index finger gently pulls the skin down, exposing the lower conjunctival sac.

To administer eye ointment, the index finger is placed on the upper eyelid and the thumb of the same hand on the child's cheekbone. The thumb and index finger are then spread apart to open the eye. The ointment is applied by placing a thin streak along the child's lower conjunctival sac from the inner to outer canthus. When the child subsequently blinks the medication will spread across the eye. The excess is then gently wiped outward with a cotton ball or tissue.

If a child resists the procedure vigorously, it is extremely difficult for one person to give eye medication safely. It is advisable to stop the procedure and summon assistance from another person to ensure safe administration.

Nose Drops

Nose drops should be at room temperature. Preparation of the child includes an explanation of the position to be assumed, the number of drops to be administered, and a warning that the drops may be tasted momentarily after administration. An infant can be held supine on the parent's or nurse's lap, with the head tilted down. An older child should be placed on the back with a pillow under the shoulders to facilitate tilting the head back. The drops are instilled into each nostril without touching the nostrils or any other part of the child's face. The nostrils can be opened farther by applying gentle upward pressure to the tip of the nose. The head must be kept in its lowered position for 1 to 2 minutes after administration to allow the drops to penetrate the swollen nasal passages by gravity flow. Vigorous sniffing should be discouraged as this may suck medication into the sinuses. Watch for signs of aspiration such as coughing; the child should sit up if coughing occurs.

Ear Drops

Ear drops should be warmed to room temperature before administration to avoid pain and discomfort. The procedure is begun after an explanation has been given and questions have been answered. The external ear should be cleansed with a moistened cotton ball preceding drug administration.

Ear drops are most readily administered if an infant or young child is held on the nurse's or parent's lap. A young child often resists lying flat but can be held in a side-lying position while the nurse pulls down and back (in children under 3 years of age) or up and back (in children over 3 years of age) on the pinna. An older child should lie flat in bed with the head turned to one side, making the affected ear accessible. The medication is dropped onto the wall of the external ear canal, therefore the pinna should be held in position until the medication has progressed down the canal to the eardrum. Pressing the tragus (the area directly in front of the ear) two or three times assists the drops to move down the canal. A side-lying position should be maintained for several minutes after drops have been instilled. Placing cotton balls in the ears after administration has some disadvantages in infants and young children. A child may remove the cotton and put it into the mouth or push it into the ears farther than is recommended. If cotton is used it should be placed gently and loosely so that in the event of ear discharge secretions are not trapped in the ear.

Inhalation

Medications are also administered via inhalation to facilitate a direct therapeutic effect in the respiratory tract. Inhalation medicants are often given in conjunction with percussion and postural drainage; they should not be given immediately after a meal, therefore, because of the potential for vomiting and aspiration.

Administration of a medication via inhalation is a form of aerosol therapy, usually delivered in normal saline. The prescribed medication is mixed with the prescribed amount of normal saline and placed into the nebulizer. Either compressed air or an oxygen flow forms the particles that will reach the respiratory tract. The speed of administration is controlled by the gas flow. The usual length of time an aerosol with medication is administered is 10 to 15 minutes.

A mask is placed over the mouth and nose, and the chamber containing the medication is attached below the mask. Production of a mist indicates that the equipment is functioning properly. The mist may also be delivered via a tube on the mist chamber. The tube can be held near the nose and mouth of an infant or small child; an older child can inhale the mist through a mouthpiece on the tube.

Children often resist having a mask against their face or having the mist directed toward them and may struggle and cry. Therefore, efforts are made to provide a calm environment. Parents often hold the child during the procedure but should be given a thorough explanation so that they feel comfortable. The parent's anxiety can readily be communicated to the child, therefore the nurse should monitor the procedure and assist the parent if any anxiety is escalating. Monitoring is also required for side effects. (See Chapter 38 for further discussion of respiratory therapy.)

Rectal Administration of Medications

Children's responses to insertion of a rectal suppository vary with their experience. A young child who is not accustomed to having a temperature checked rectally may find the experience anxiety producing and threatening. Experience with toilet training also may affect how much cooperation can be achieved. A toddler who is just becoming aware of body sensations related to defecation may try to expel the suppository. At any age, privacy should be provided by drawing curtains or closing the door.

The suppository is inserted by using the index finger in older children and the little finger in infants and young children. A finger cot or glove covers the nurse's finger. If the suppository has become too soft for easy insertion, it can be placed under cold running water for a few seconds before the paper is removed.

Position the child on the left side with the right leg drawn up. The anus can be exposed easily by placing an infant or young child on the back with knees flexed. It is not necessary to lubricate the suppository, but if a lubricant is used only a small amount should be applied to avoid interaction with the medication. Moistening it with water is sufficient to permit easy insertion. The suppository must be inserted past the rectal sphincter, then the buttocks are gently pressed together for several minutes. The suppository is not likely to dissolve for 5 to 10 minutes, but a young child generally does not tolerate having pressure applied to the buttocks for that length of time. Keeping a child quiet and briefly holding the suppository in place is usually sufficient to promote absorption. If the parents are present, they are instructed to keep their child from getting up and going to the bathroom. Holding the child and walking about to distract her or him can also be effective in preventing expulsion of the suppository. The nurse can ask the parent to check the diaper carefully the next time it is changed to be sure the suppository has not been expelled.

Intramuscular Injection

Children of all ages have a degree of fear about needles; not to mention some adults! Injections continue to be a part of health care, but awareness is increasing about children's fear and anxiety. Whether an injection is the best procedure in therapy, considering the total response of the child (see Chapter 29 on Pain Management), should be evaluated carefully.

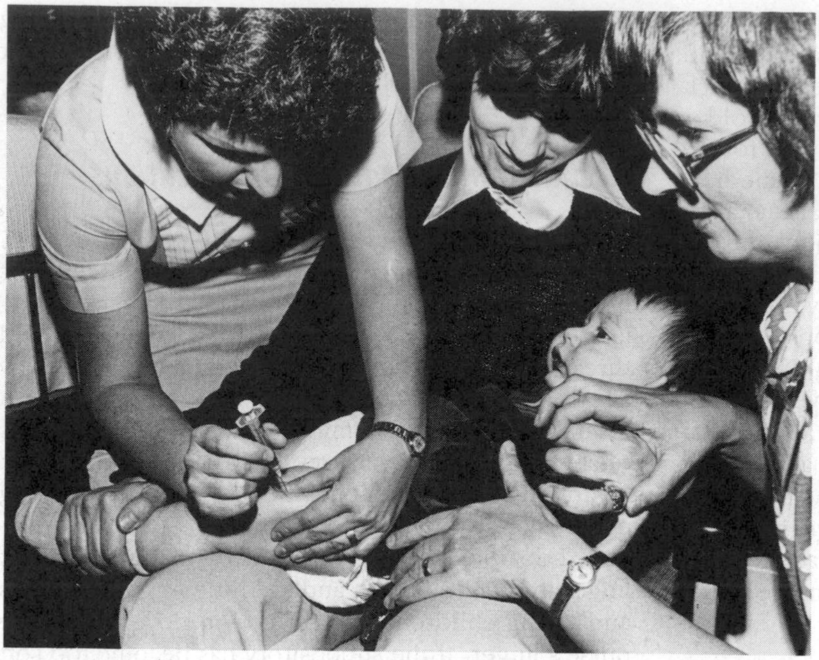

Infants tolerate procedures better in their parent's arms. Note the restraint and injection techniques.

The approach to the child and the choice of the site is determined by the child's age. In practice, how nurses prepare children and to what degree they involve parents vary greatly. There is also some variation in nursing practice concerning the technique of administration and choice of sites. Principles of practice according to the age of the child are discussed next and are listed in Table 28-2.

Infants (Table 28-2). The procedure is explained to the parents, who are asked whether or not they wish to stay with their child. If they wish to stay, the nurse explains how they can help. It is advisable to have a second individual other than the parent to assist in immobilizing the child during the procedure. It is also preferable for the nurse to spend a brief period of time with the infant before the injection is given to establish a degree of trust.

The only acceptable site to use is the vastus lateralis muscle. It is the largest muscle mass in an infant and has few major blood vessels and nerves. To locate the injection site, draw an imaginary line between the trochanter to just above the knee on the outer aspect of the thigh. The middle third of the thigh should be located by visually marking off the area from the knee to the groin into thirds; the middle third is used for the injection (Fig. 28-3).

During the procedure, the infant can be talked to or given a toy for distraction. Ensuring that the infant has a favorite toy or blanket for security is also essential. The injection is usually given with a 1-inch needle, 22 or 23 gauge, to ensure that the muscle is injected. Wipe the area with an antiseptic (wait for it to dry, particularly if alcohol is used). Pinch up the muscle tissue and insert the needle into it at a 90-degree angle. Aspirate, inject, then withdraw the needle, keeping slight pressure over the area to avoid the tissue from pulling upward as the needle is withdrawn. As with any painful procedure, infants should be held and comforted so that they do not come to associate the injection and pain with feelings of rejection.

Toddler and Preschooler (Table 28-2). The approach to a toddler and family when giving an intramuscular injection must take into account previous experience with injections, the parent-child relationship, and the child's developmental level. The parents should be told about the medication before the nurse enters the room. This explanation should be given when the child is not present, because it is likely to instill unnecessary fears. Injections are a source of fear because of the pain and intrusion of the body that is anticipated.

Toddlers and preschoolers can be prepared for injections through the use of needle play during the course of hospitalization and by a brief description of what will occur and how it will feel immediately prior to the injection (Fig. 28-4). The needle and syringe should not be flaunted or referred to in front of the toddler or preschooler nor hidden when the nurse comes to give the injection.

Once children know they are to receive an injection, it should be given promptly. Toddlers and preschoolers are usually more receptive when the injection is given by a nurse with whom they are familiar and who has spent time with them when procedures were not involved. Children of this age should also be touched, talked to, or distracted with a toy. A toddler

Table 28-2. Guidelines for Administering an Injection

Nursing Action	Rationale
Birth to 12 Months	
Spend time with the infant prior to giving an injection.	This supports the development of a sense of trust.
For the older infant, state what you are going to do and proceed with the injection.	A child this age cannot understand explanations but should not be injected without warning.
Provide something to look at or a toy to hold during the injection.	The infant is often distractible.
Provide physical comfort after the injection.	Physical comforting is more effective than verbal comforting.
Brian M., six months old, is to receive his third DPT immunization. His mother is very anxious and upset because she cannot stand to see her baby experience pain. The nurse explains the immunization procedure to Mrs. M. and asks if she'd like to leave the room. Mrs. M. decides to stay, so the nurse suggests that the mother stand close to her baby's head and talk to him so he'll be distracted from the sight of the needle and syringe. Another nurse helps restrain Brian while the injection is being administered in the right vastus lateralis *muscle. The nurse picks up Brian and immediately hands him to Mrs. M., so she can hold and cuddle him. This is an important way to help Mrs. M. deal with her feelings of helplessness as well as to comfort Brian.*	
1 to 3 Years	
State what you are going to do and proceed with the injection. Use simple words and short phrases. For example, say, "This will take only a minute and then you can play." Provide something for the child to look at, hold, or play with during the injection.	At this age the child obeys simple commands and develops a sense of time beginning at about 18 months of age. The toddler often can be distracted.
Give a simple, honest reason for the injection.	Fantasies are prominent at this age.
Use a firm, consistent approach, reward the toddler's positive behaviors, and ignore negative ones. Let the child take some part in the procedure, for example, hold the Band-Aid.	Rituals are important to toddlers, and they take pride in their accomplishments.
Provide a Band-Aid for covering the injection site.	The toddler has an incomplete sense of body boundaries and fears body contents may leak out.
Shari P., two years old, has been receiving kanamycin sulfate, 45 mg, every 6 hours intramuscularly for 48 hours. She begins to cry loudly when the nurse enters the room and tells her it is time for "the medicine in your leg." The nurse knows from the chart that Shari likes to hold the Band-Aid during the procedure. The nurse introduces Ms. Y. as "another nurse who will help you hold still." The nurse tells Shari that the alcohol "will feel cold while I wash your leg." Then she tells Shari to squeeze Ms. Y.'s hand while the medicine goes in. As soon as the needle is withdrawn, Shari lets go of Ms. Y.'s hand and the nurse asks Shari to open the Band-Aid. By the time the child accomplishes this task, she has stopped crying. The nurses and Shari's parents praise the little girl for her cooperation and remind her that it was all right to cry because it hurts. Mrs. P. picks up her daughter and cuddles her. Shari is then taken to the playroom and offered the pounding board and bean bags so she can release her aggressive feelings about the intrusive procedure.	
3 to 6 Years	
Tell the child what he or she will feel and what to do to help; for example, lying still.	A child this age remains egocentric and is a concrete thinker but also can understand simple explanations and follow directions.
Let the child see and handle equipment under supervision before the nurse gives the injection.	Seeing and handling the equipment will help the child learn, and it promotes coping.
Tell the child that injections are never used as punishment and give a simple honest explanation.	Preschoolers are developing a conscience and may view an injection as punishment for their actions, but they can understand a simple explanation.
Allow youngster a choice when possible. For example, ask in which leg to put the injection. Foster the development of coping mechanisms.	A child this age seeks to master situations and takes pride in accomplishments.
Let the child play at giving injections, including handling a needle under supervision.	Therapeutic play is an effective means of dealing with fantasies and fears, especially those associated with painful and/or intrusive procedures.

continued

Table 28-2 *(continued)*

Nursing Action	Rationale
Tracy B., 4 years old, is to have a DPT injection. She does not remember her previous immunization and is very frightened. The nurse encourages Tracy to play with the equipment before the procedure. She tells Tracy the medicine will hurt, but only for a short time. Tracy is also told she did not do anything wrong and that she can help the nurse by lying still. Tracy chooses the right leg for her injection and the nurse covers up the left leg after Tracy's jeans are removed. Tracy squeezes the nursing assistant's hands, while Mrs. B. stands near Tracy's face and comforts her. After the injection, the nurse applies a Band-Aid and gives Tracy a "hero" badge and praises her for her cooperation.	
6 to 12 Years	
Give a simple explanation of why the specific injection is needed.	A child this age has the ability to think in a logical manner and comprehend relationships.
Let the child help select the injection site, if possible, and praise the child for cooperation.	Taking part in the procedure supports the child's developmental need to master situations. This age group thrives on praise.
Provide time to sit and talk with the child.	For children of this age, talking about their fears replaces play as a method of dealing with anxiety.
Barbara H., 9 years old, had an open reduction of a fractured right humerus the previous evening. She received meperidine hydrochloride, 30 mg, intramuscularly 6 hours earlier for pain. She now is obviously in pain but denies it because she doesn't want "another shot." The nurse decides that medication should be given and tells Barbara she is going to prepare it. The nurse also explains that when Barbara is able to drink liquids, the medicine will be changed to a pill. After preparing the medication, the nurse describes to Barbara how she will feel during the injection and what she can do to help. Mrs. H. is very calm and supportive while Barbara chooses the site. The nurse suggests that Barbara hold her mother's hands and count how many seconds the injection lasts. After the medication is administered, the nurse tells Barbara how much it helped because she held so still.	
12 to 16 Years	
Provide as much information as the adolescent requests about medication, but also tell how injections will feel.	The adolescent is capable of logical, abstract thinking but may also demonstrate egocentrism, especially when under stress.
Provide privacy and permit choice of injection site whenever possible.	The adolescent experiences concern over body image and likes to feel in control of a situation.
Tony W., 15 years old, has injured his right foot on a rusty tin can while swimming in a pond. He needs a tetanus injection. The nurse explains to him why a booster injection is necessary and answers his questions. She offers him a choice of sites and Tony chooses the left deltoid. The nurse describes the steps in the procedure and tells him what he will feel. Although he is visibly anxious, Tony tries to control his fear. The nurse comments that no one likes to get a shot, and he might want to look to the other side of the room. After the injection, the nurse tells Tony that he did very well. She describes the local reaction he might have from the injection and she also tells him what he can do at home to minimize his discomfort.	

(From Evans and Hansen, 1981.)

can best be restrained if the nurse gently leans across the torso so that arms are free to move but blocked from the injection area. For many toddlers it is essential to have another nurse assist with the injection. The legs can then be restrained by one person and the other person can give the injection. Although preschoolers can often cooperate to lie still during the injection if their fears have not been given time to escalate, it is safer to have a second adult nearby to help restrain the child if necessary. Holding the child's arms in a restraining position if needed, the second adult can preserve the child's sense of self-control by simply saying "Let me help you hold still."

It is important for the nurse to remember that injections are more stressful to the preschooler (due to mutilation fears, concern about body intactness, punishment perception) than to children in any other age group.

The injection technique is the same as described for the infant. The vastus lateralis remains the only recommended site until the age of 3 years when the ventrogluteal site can be used (Fig. 28-4). The ventrogluteal site is also relatively free of major nerves and vessels. The deltoid muscle is only rarely used in children under 6 years of age and then only for very small amounts of medication. The dorsogluteal site is not utilized for any child who has not walked for at least a year, and it is strongly recommended that children under 6 years of age do not receive injections in this site. The objection is that the muscle is very small, is

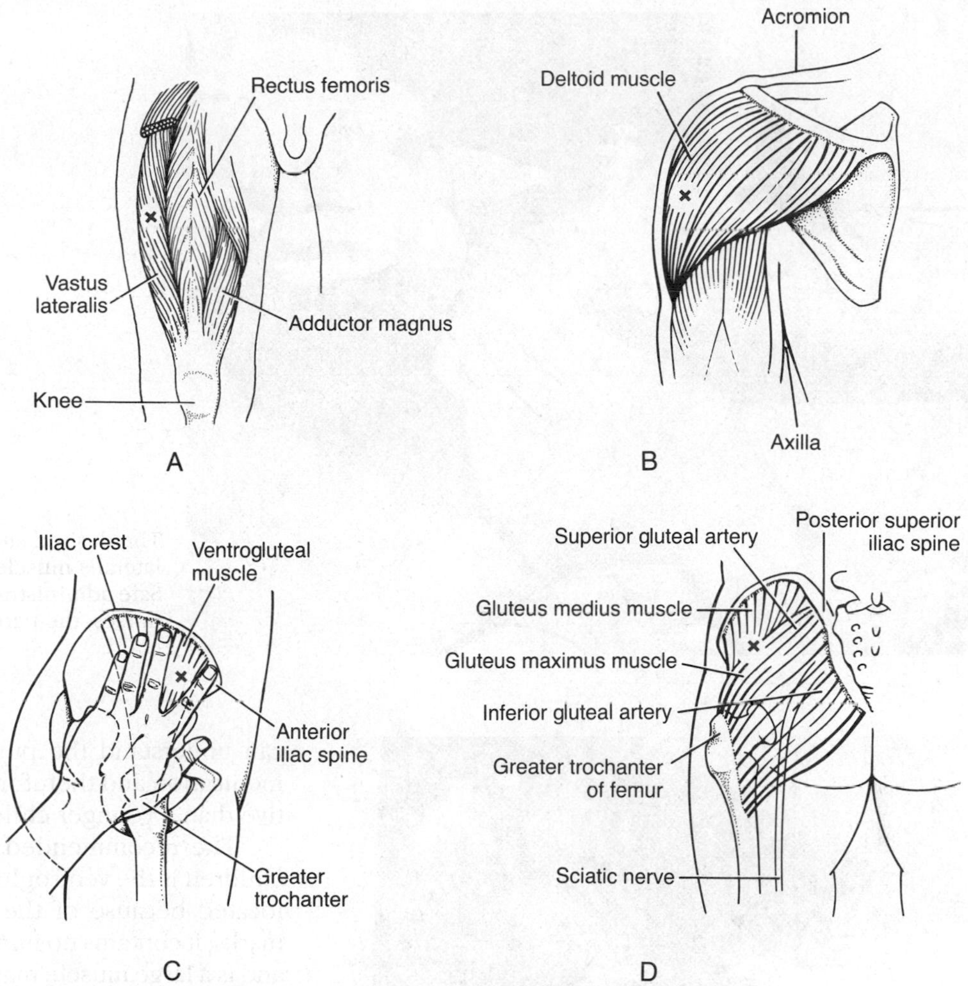

***Figure* 28-3.** Injection sites. *A*, **Vastus lateralis site,** in the midthird of the thigh. It is found by dividing the thigh into thirds from the greater trochanter to just above the knee. The area of insertion within the midthird of the thigh is found midway between imaginary lines midanteriorly and midlaterally. *B*, **Deltoid site,** in the lower part of the upper third of the deltoid. The site of insertion is midway between the acromion and the axilla on the lateral surface of the arm.

C, **Ventrogluteal site.** Place the palm on the greater trochanter and the index finger on the anterior iliac spine (this may be facilitated by the flexion of the thigh at the hip). The middle finger is extended along the iliac crest as far as possible, forming a triangle. The injection is given in the center of the triangle, or V, formed by the hand, with the needle directed slightly upward toward the iliac crest. *D*, **Gluteal region.** Injection is given into the gluteus medius. The site is found by locating the greater trochanter and posterior iliac spine. Draw an imaginary line between these two points and inject above the line into the gluteus medius.

poorly developed, and is located close to the sciatic nerve, which is comparatively large and takes up more space in young children than it does in older children.

After the injection is administered, a Band-Aid placed over the site gives comfort and helps reassure the child that his or her body is still intact (now all the blood cannot get out). The child is cuddled and praised for cooperation even if he or she had difficulty holding still.

School Age Children (Table 28-2). A school-age child still has some fears about receiving injections, but extraordinary fears are most likely to be associated with negative previous experience. Preparation of the child, therefore, includes a brief discussion about any preconceived ideas and misinformation is corrected. At this age, talking about their fears usually replaces play experiences, although the early school-age child may benefit from a play experience. A child of this age

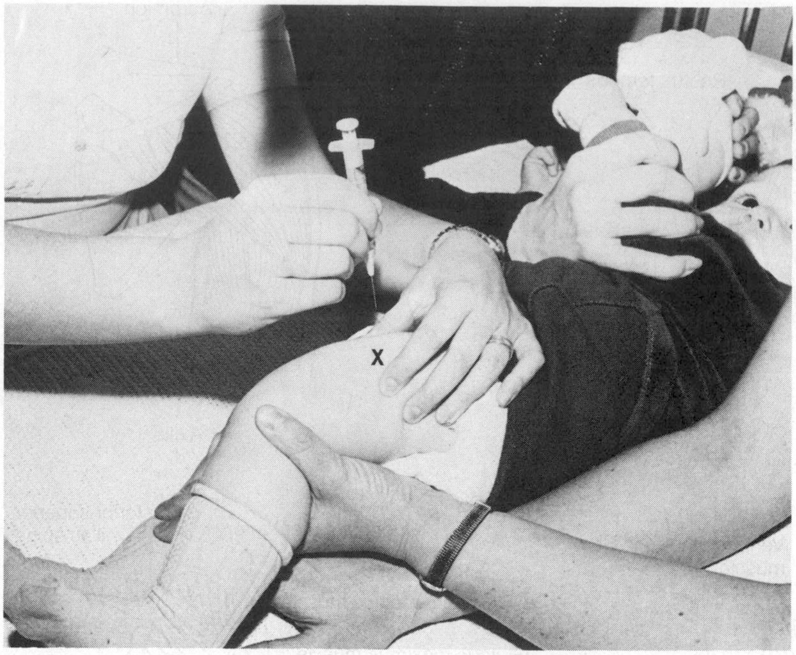

The desired site for injection is the vastus lateralis muscle (X on the photo indicates site). Safe administration is best achieved by two nurses; the parent should be free to divert the child.

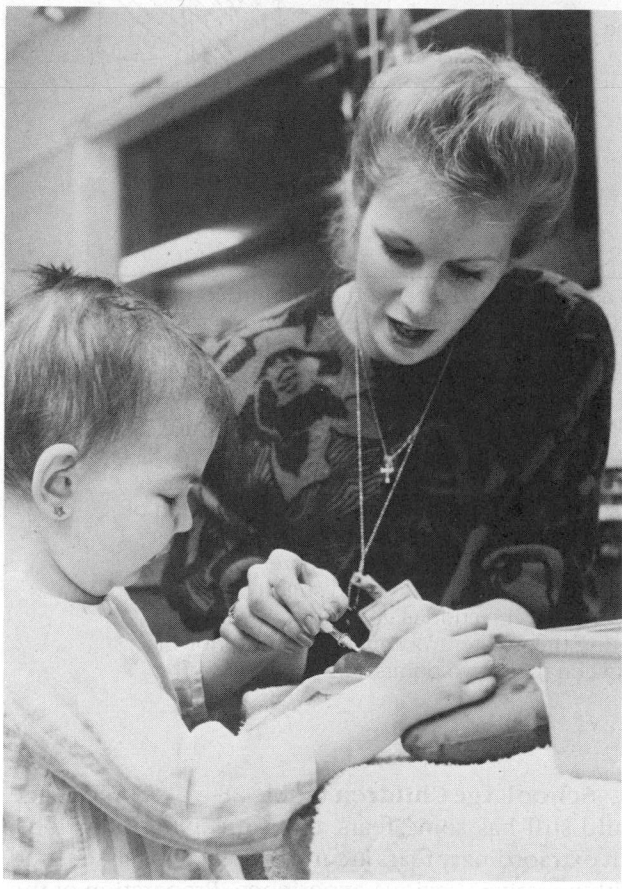

Figure 28-4. Toddlers and preschoolers eagerly participate in needle play, an activity that helps them gain a sense of mastery over their experience of receiving injections. (Courtesy of Child Life Department, Children's Hospital, Chedoke-McMaster University Medical Center, Hamilton, Ontario.)

can understand the purpose and importance of the medication and therefore can often be more cooperative than a younger child.

The recommended injection site for school-age children is the ventrogluteal muscle. This site is easily located because of the readily palpable bony landmarks; it contains no important nerves or blood vessels and is a large muscle mass with minimal subcutaneous tissue. Use of the vastus lateralis site is frequently opposed by the school-age child, but it should be used along with the ventrogluteal and dorsogluteal site when frequent injections or long-term intramuscular therapy is required. The deltoid can be used for small amounts of medication (0.5 ml), but it is not a preferred site unless rapid absorption of a drug is required. Provision of privacy during intramuscular injections is important for children of this age. Also, school-age children thrive on praise for "holding still," therefore verbal praise from the nurse is important.

Adolescent (Table 28-2). The adolescent requires a clear explanation of the purpose of the medication. The adolescent who understands the reason for the medication is more likely to participate while in the hospital and follow through at home. If choices and decisions are possible, the nurse should allow the adolescent some control. The preferred sites of administration are similar to those for an adult because the adolescent has adequate muscle tissue. However, caution must be taken to assess the amount of tissue, especially in emaciated or small adolescents. Generally the dorsogluteal, deltoid, and ventrogluteal muscles are all appropriate sites. Adolescents usually prefer the arm site if it is not contraindicated. Solutions in the deltoid should be limited to 1 ml, whereas in other sites 2 to 2.5 ml are permissible. Injections in the thigh are resisted because they seem painful, and use of the dorsogluteus is often embarrassing. The final choice can be made in collaboration with the adolescent.

Special Nursing Responsibilities

The nurse ensures that measures have been taken to provide the least discomfort and the greatest therapeutic effect possible. At all ages, intramuscular injections require special precautions. As with all medications, the five rights must be ensured, and also the following principles:

1. Proper handwashing and sterile technique when handling syringes, needles, and medications.
2. Privacy for each patient during administration.
3. Proper refrigeration of medications.
4. Accurate labeling of medications in vials for future use.
5. Safe and proper disposal of needles.
6. Rotation of sites to reduce pain and fibrosis.
7. Careful assessment of patients for the evidence of side effects.
8. Avoidance of excess amount of medication in one site.
   Guidelines:

Deltoid	6–15 years, 0.5 ml 15 years–adulthood, 1 ml
Ventrogluteal	3–6 years, 1.5 ml 6–15 years, 1.5-2.0 ml 15 years–adulthood, 2-2.5 ml
Dorsogluteal	6–15 years, 1.5-2 ml 15 years–adulthood, 2-2.5 ml
Vastus lateralis	Birth–1.5 years, 0.5 ml 1.5–3 years, 1 ml 3–6 years, 1.5 ml 6–15 years, 1.5-2 ml (Not a site preferred by older children and adults)

9. Complete and accurate documentation of drug administration.
10. Evaluation of effectiveness of drug.

References

Agunod M, et al: Correlative study of hydrochloric acid, pepsin, and intrinsic factor secretion in newborns and infants. *Am J Dig Dis* 1969; 14:400–414.

Asperheim MK: *Pharmacologic Basis of Patient Care.* 5th ed. Philadelphia, WB Saunders, 1985.

Evans ML, Hansen BD: Administering injections to different-aged children. *MCN* 1981 May/Jun; 6:194–199.

Giacoia G, Gorodisher R: Pharmacologic principles in neonatal drug therapy. *Clin Perinatol* 1975 Mar; 2(1):125–137.

Guignard JP: Renal function in the newborn infant. *Pediatr Clin North Am* 1982 Aug; 29(4):777–790.

Holbrook PR, Schaible DH: Pediatric pharmacotherapy. *In* Chernow B: *The Pharmacological Approach to the Critically Ill Patient.* Baltimore, Williams and Wilkins, 1983.

Howry LB, et al: *Pediatric Medications.* Philadelphia, JB Lippincott, 1981.

Kagan BM: Pediatric pharmacology. *In* Bevan JA, Thompson JH: *Essentials of Pharmacology.* 3rd ed. New York, Harper and Row, 1983.

Magnussen I, et al: Absorption of diazepam in man following rectal and parenteral administration. *Acta Pharmacol Toxicol* 1979; 45:87–90.

Morselli PL: Clinical pharmacokinetics in neonates. *Clin Pharmacokin* 1976; 1:81.

Morselli PL, et al: Clinical pharmacokinetics in newborns and infants: age related differences and therapeutic implications. *Clin Pharmacokin* 1980; 5:484–527.

Ormond E, Caulfield C: A practical guide to giving oral medication to young children. *MCN* 1976 Sep/Oct; 320–325.

Pippenger CE: Rationale and clinical application of therapeutic drug monitoring. *Pediatr Clin North Am* 1980 Nov; 27(4):896–925.

Reiss BS, Melick ME: *Pharmacological Aspects of Nursing Care.* Delmar Publishing, 1984.

Roberts RJ: *Drug Therapy in Infants: Pharmacologic Principles and Clinical Experience.* Philadelphia, WB Saunders, 1984.

Russell H: *Pediatric Drugs and Nursing Interventions.* New York, McGraw-Hill, 1980.

Sheridan E, et al: *Falconer's The Drug, The Nurse, The Patient.* 7th ed. Philadelphia, WB Saunders, 1982.

Udkow GP: Clinical Pharamacology. *In* Hoekelman, RA, et al: *Primary Pediatric Care.* St. Louis, CV Mosby, 1987.

Weinberger M, et al: Clinical pharmacology of drugs used in asthma. *Pediatr Clin North Am* 1981; 28:47.

Yeh TF: *Drug Therapy in the Neonate and Small Infant.* Chicago, Year Book Medical Publishers, 1985.

Bibliography

Cohen SN, et al: Drug therapy. *In* Behrman RE, Vaughan VC: *Nelson Textbook of Pediatrics.* Philadelphia, WB Saunders, 1987, 231–237.

Nursing Photobook: *Nursing Pediatric Patients.* Spring House, PA, Nursing 85 Books, 1985.

Roberts RJ: Intravenous administration of medication in pediatric patients: problems and solutions. *Pediatr Clin North Am* 1981, Feb; 28(1):23–24.

Trang JM, et al: Pharmacokinetics for pediatric nurses. *Pediatr Nurs* 1984 Jul/Aug; 267–274.

Yaffe SJ: *Pediatric Pharmacology: Therapeutic Principles in Practice.* Orlando, FL, Grune and Stratton, 1980.

Nursing Management of Pain in Children

Chapter 29

Bonnie Stevens

Pain—a concept so familiar, yet so elusive that it has been termed the most complex of human stressors (Chapman and Bonica, 1983). Pain—a common companion to illness, a common concern for nurses who seek to comfort, and yet a phenomenon that is unique to the experiencing individual. By what signs and symptoms can one recognize its existence? By what measure can one determine its intensity? By what strategies can one relieve it? These and related questions have been the subject of a burgeoning body of literature associated with pain in recent years. Although fewer data exist about the experience of pain in children than in adults, progress is being made toward building a research base for pain assessment and pain relief in pediatric nursing. This chapter presents various definitions related to pain and the pain experience, pain theories, currently available methods for pain assessment in children, and strategies for pain relief.

Nursing Process Plan
NPP: The Child in Pain, page 878

Related Topics
Communicating with children and families, Chapters 1 and 11
Concepts of stress and coping, Chapter 23
Preparing children for procedures, Chapter 27
Strategies of medication administration, Chapter 28
Pharmacologic principles, Chapter 28

Definitions of Pain and Pain Properties

The complexity of pain has made it difficult to define the concept in terms that are representative across individuals. As noted by Melzack (1973, page 45):

> Pain is not a single quality of experience . . . . The word "pain" represents a category of experiences, signifying a multitude of different, unique events having different causes, and characterized by different qualities varying along a number of sensory and affective dimensions.

Because of this complexity, pain continues to be defined in different ways by different disciplines. A neurophysiologist may think of pain in terms of patterns of action potentials in neural centers, whereas a psychologist may view pain in terms of behavioral or emotional responses. In an attempt to develop a definition of pain that could be useful to scientists and practitioners across disciplines, the International Association for the Study of Pain (IASP) proposed that pain is "an unpleasant sensory and emotional experience associated with actual or potential tissue damage, or described in terms of such damage" (Bonica, 1979, page 250). The limitation of this definition is that, although the emotional component is identified, the emphasis is upon physiologic aspects of pain.

McCaffery (1972) proposed a definition of pain from the nursing perspective: "Pain is what the patient says it is and exists when he says it does." The strength of this definition is its emphasis upon the uniqueness of the pain experience and the fact that most of the information about pain must come from *subjective* data. This definition has been widely accepted and used by nurses in recent years. As with all definitions, however, it has its limitations. How does one assess the preverbal child or the child who refuses to cooperate with pain assessment? It is also important to remember that *the child who chooses to tolerate pain rather than report it, still suffers* (Kushner, 1985). It seems that a truly universal definition of pain, particularly one that is applicable to children, is still to be found.

It is somewhat easier to define certain properties of pain than it is to define the concept of pain itself. Pain *threshold* is the point at which an individual first perceives that an unpleasant stimulus or sensation exists. Pain *tolerance* refers to the point at which the individual can no longer endure the unpleasant sensation at that magnitude or intensity (Woolf, 1983). Pain threshold is most often associated with physiologic variables whereas pain tolerance is primarily related to psychologic factors (Crook, 1985). Pain tolerance varies from person to person (Fabrega and Tyma, 1976) and from time to time within the individual. That pain tolerance is moderated by psychologic factors can be illustrated by the boy who chooses to endure moderate pain in the presence of peers rather than appear to be a "sissy," but later asks for medication for what he describes as less severe pain.

Pain *duration* is the length of time since pain onset. Duration is expressed in units of time such as minutes, hours, days, or months. For descriptive purposes, duration is usually combined with some measure of intensity; the chart may read, "Melissa has been complaining of severe pain in her leg for the past 1/2 hour." Pain duration may modify pain tolerance in that pain of long duration may fatigue the child and make the pain less bearable.

Acute Versus Chronic Pain

Pain can also be classified as acute or chronic. Acute pain is often characterized by its sudden onset and limited duration. Acute pain may originate as an emotional reaction to some unpleasant or noxious stimulus and functions as an adaptive biologic warning signal (e.g., the pain of appendicitis) or a protective mechanism against injury (limiting further tissue damage by discouraging motion) (Chapman and Bonica, 1983). As noted by Ross and Ross (1988), however, the warning function is undermined by the fact that the severity of pain does not necessarily relate to the seriousness of the injury.

Acute pain is often modified by the suddenness with which it occurs. Fear and anxiety of the precipitating event may heighten the perception of pain. This is frequently a consideration for children undergoing diagnostic or therapeutic interventions. Fear may stem either from previous experience (e.g., an injection) or from unfamiliarity with equipment that looks "scary" but inflicts no pain(e.g., an x-ray machine). Katz and associates (1981) suggest that anxiety is the basic affective state that modulates pain perception.

Chronic pain is often considered to be pain lasting longer than 6 months (Escobar, 1985). Some researchers consider the psychosocial impact of pain (interference with activities of daily living) as well as its duration in defining chronicity (McGrath and Unruh, 1987). Crue (1985) described four types of long-term pain:

- *recurrent acute*, or pain from underlying continued nociceptive input (e.g., the pain from systemic juvenile rheumatoid arthritis);
- *ongoing acute*, as the pain from malignant disease and its metastasis;
- *chronic benign pain*, or the ongoing pain that has no known nociceptive cause but permits adequate coping; and
- *chronic benign intractable pain*, which is

chronic, long-term pain with which the patient is not able to cope adequately.

Clearly, there is some overlap in the symptoms of chronic versus acute pain. However, in acute pain, the unpleasant sensation usually disappears after the pathology or noxious stimulus is resolved, whereas in chronic pain the pain may persist for much longer, even after the pathology (or other cause) has been resolved (Bonica, 1977).

Pain Theories

Theories of pain attempt to describe and explain the phenomenon called pain. Most of the early pain theories tended to focus on neurophysiologic mechanisms and did not consider psychologic, social, cultural, or developmental factors. Three pain theories that have dominated the pain literature up to 1965 include the affect theory (Marchall, 1894), the specificity theory (Mountcastle, 1975) and the pattern theory (Crue and Carregal, 1975).

Affect Theory

The affect theory dates back to the time of Aristotle and suggests that pain is an emotion rather than a physiologic sensation. According to affect theorists, this emotion had the potential to color all sensory events. Although this theory is relatively simplistic and outdated, it introduced the idea of an emotional component in the pain experience and has profoundly affected the way pain is viewed today.

Specificity Theory

Another early pain theory, the specificity theory, was originated by Descartes. The specificity theorists believed that for each sensation there was a specific energy. The specificity theorists therefore proposed that there was a specific pain modality based upon a specialized set of peripheral nerve fibers that are nociceptive (Mountcastle, 1975). In this theory, specified free nerve endings are thought to transmit the pain sensation via certain pain fibers and spinothalamic tracts to specific pain centers in the brain. In other words, the specificity theory proposed that a fixed direct-line communication system from the skin to the brain exists and that different sensations provoke different nerves. However, more recent pain experts point out that, if the specificity theory is valid, then one needs to question why two people given an identical stimulus do not consistently interpret it as pain (McCaffery, 1977).

Pattern Theory

Another pain theory, the pattern theory, evolved from the specificity theory but opposes the notion that pain has its own specialized receptors. Pain theorists who subscribe to this explanation of pain suggested that there are temporal and spatial patterns of nerve impulses. According to this theory, pain is a result of stimulus intensity (pain exceeding a certain threshold) and central summation (central interpretation of pain from receptor sites) (Crue and Carregal, 1975).

Gate Control Theory

In 1965, Melzack and Wall proposed the gate control theory of pain. This theory holds that psychologic aspects of pain are as important as physiologic aspects. As well, the gate control theory aims to account for clinical symptoms such as the spread of pain and its existence after removal of the noxious stimulus.The basic premise of the gate control theory is that pain is modulated by a gating mechanism in the spinal cord as well as by central nervous system (CNS) activity. Melzack and Wall (1965) proposed that stimulation of the skin evokes nerve impulses that are transmitted to three spinal cord systems including the substantia gelatinosa (SG) in the dorsal horn, the dorsal column fibers, and the central transmission cells (T cells) in the dorsal horn. In this theoretical explanation of pain, three mechanisms interact:

1. the SG acts as a gate control system and modulates the flow of nerve impulses from the peripheral fibers in the skin to the central nervous system;
2. the dorsal column fibers activate selective central brain processes, which in turn influence the modulating mechanism of the gate control system; and
3. the T cells activate certain neural mechanisms which are responsible for the individual's pain perception and response.

Although the exact mechanisms involved in gate control are not clear, this theory does incorporate sensory, cognitive, and emotional elements. It proposes that past experiences, distraction activities, and various emotional states such as anxiety and anticipation can act on the gate control system (higher cortical areas involved in discrimination and motivational systems) and block the individual's perception of pain.

Biochemical Theory

Another approach to pain is the biochemical theory (Lindahl, 1974). In this theory, the presence of pain is explained by a biochemical change or reaction in a nerve or in the vicinity of a nerve ending. Other biochemical research indicates that pain is suppressed

Box 29-1
Myths and Misconceptions

1. Children do not experience as much pain as adults because of the lack of development of the nervous system.
2. Children recover from pain-producing situations at a much faster rate than adults.
3. Narcotic analgesics may lead to addiction in the child.
4. Narcotic use is dangerous because of the high incidence of respiratory depression in children.
5. Children cannot describe the intensity or location of their pain.
6. Nurses who give injections are viewed negatively by patients and their families.

(From McCaffery, 1982; Hawley, 1984.)

when certain peptides (i.e., enkephalins, endorphins, dynorphin) bind with opiate receptor sites throughout the nervous system. These sites are thought to line neural pathways that transmit pain to higher pain centers.

The Child's Experience of Pain

This section will explore some common myths and misconceptions about pain in children, propose a model for conceptualizing the pain experience in children, and discuss selected research dealing with the child's experience of pain.

Myths and Misconceptions About Pain in Children

Common myths and misconceptions about pain in children, as compiled by McCaffery (1982) and Hawley (1984) are summarized in Box 29-1. There is little doubt that these myths have contributed to the undertreatment of children in pain. Research refuting many of these myths is addressed throughout this chapter.

A Framework for Studying Pain in Children

When studying complex phenomena such as pain, it can be helpful to organize the related concepts according to a conceptual framework. Figure 29-1 illustrates one such framework. This model considers three components of the child's pain: physiologic, psychologic, and experiential, all of which are modified by the child's growth and development. The physiologic component accounts for the sensation of pain that is related to actual or potential tissue damage. The psychologic component attempts to explain the individual's perception of the unpleasant sensation. The experiential component encompasses the process of assigning meaning to the pain experience.

Sheredy (1984) listed additional factors that influence the pain response of the hospitalized child.

- type of anesthesia (local or general)
- type of surgery performed (how extensive)
- nature of procedures (e.g., catheterization versus burn debridement)
- pain medication
- frequency and duration of hospitalization
- presence or absence of parents
- education (e.g., preoperative teaching)
- attitudes of parents toward particular conditions or procedures
- attitudes of nurses about pain

The Effects of Growth and Development

Physiologic Aspects of Pain

The developmental stage at which the child feels pain as a sensation and perceives this stimulus as unpleasant is a source of continuing debate. Early research upheld the concept that complete nerve myelination was required for the function of the nerve tracts (Flechsig, 1920; Angulo and Gonzales, 1929; Langworthy, 1933). Based on this thinking, the widespread assumption that infants either did not experience or perceive pain in the same way as adults (or in some

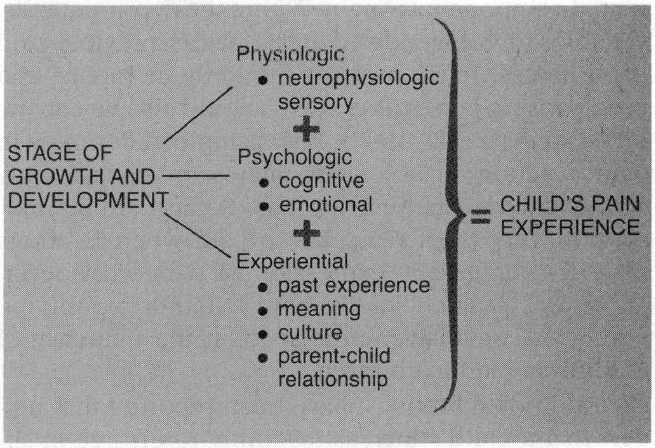

Figure 29-1. The child's pain experience. (From Stevens BJ, Hunsberger M, Browne G: Pain in children—theoretical, research, and practice dilemmas. *J Pediatr Nurs* 1987 May/Jun; 3:154–166.)

cases not at all) has persisted for many years. This thinking resulted in performance of a variety of procedures and operations on infants and young children without anesthetic.

Considerable research has now shown that pain is experienced even in young infants. The process of myelination begins in utero, and by birth myelination of the sensory roots has begun (Volpe, 1981). In clinical practice research, infants withdraw from a painful stimulus such as the heel lance (heelprick) (Wachter-Shikora, 1981) and are noted to cry within 2 to 5 seconds of the heelprick (Owens and Todd, 1984). These responses are an indication that the infant is experiencing pain and perceiving the incident as unpleasant. Grunau and Craig (1987) assessed the infant's cry and facial activity as a response to heelprick. They concluded that neonates appear to react to this noxious stimulus in a way that was interpreted as pain.

Psychologic Aspects of Pain

Behavioral responses to pain also vary with age. Children under the age of 5 years undergoing medical procedures are reported to exhibit "distress" in more intense, overt, and motoric modes than older children (Katz et al, 1980; Jay et al, 1983). A dramatic decrease in this type of expression is noted at approximately 7 years of age, which, according to Piaget, is the time at which more concrete operational thinking begins. At this stage children should theoretically have the ability to engage in more logical and realistic thinking, thus increasing their understanding of the need for medical procedures with a reduction in their anxiety (Katz et al, 1980; Jay et al, 1983).

These observations of children's pain experiences and perceptions at different ages illustrate the importance of the underlying stage of development and its influence on the physiologic, psychologic, and experiential components of pain. Within these components, variables such as gender, cultural factors, previous pain experiences, relationship with family members, and predisposing personality styles should also be considered (Stevens et al, 1987). For example, differences in pain reaction or tolerance may vary considerably across different cultural groups. Some cultures may support very overt reactions to pain whereas others may discourage any expression of pain whatsoever. However, research studies have failed to report consistent or conclusive findings about the influence of culture on pain in children.

Additional findings, have been reported that suggest that a child's increasing ability to engage in abstract thinking (thus attributing meaning to pain) can increase pain sensitivity. Beales and coworkers (1983), in studies of children with juvenile rheumatoid arthritis, indicated that older children (12 to 17 years) reported more pain than a group of younger (6 to 11 years) children. A possible explanation for this may be that older children are reminded of their potentially disabling illness when they experience pain and that they have an increased awareness of what is happening to their joints, whereas younger children do not share that understanding of arthritis. However, when the younger children actually saw a concrete surface wound (not requiring abstract thinking to comprehend the nature of the injury), their reactions to pain were like those of their older counterparts (Beales et al, 1983).

Nursing Assessment of Pain in Children

The issues that arise in attempting to assess the child's pain experience center primarily on measurement. In general, pain in children (especially in young children under the age of 5 years) is more difficult to assess than pain in adults because of

- the varying levels of comprehension and language development among children;
- the confounding influence of anxiety, fear, or loneliness upon the pain experience (Sternback, 1968; Merskey, 1978; Katz et al, 1980);
- the lack of a good understanding of the pain phenomenon; and
- the relative lack of reliable and valid instruments to accurately measure the painful experience (Beyer et al, 1983; Jeans, 1983; Beyer and Knapp, 1986).

Because of the complexity of the pain experience and the problems of measurement in children, pain assessment and analysis require a multifaceted approach. *The nurse must use every available means of assessment and consider all findings in the analysis of the child's pain.* A discussion follows of various subjective and objective assessment strategies for use with children.

Subjective Assessment

Subjective assessment of pain involves input from the child or from a family member about the presence and the quality of pain. Aspects of subjective assessment described in this section include a pain experience history and pain interview, instruments that assist the

Box 29-2
Pain Experience History

Name of child: ________ **Informant:** ________
Age: ______ **Sex:** ______ **Ethnicity:** ________

CHILD INFORMANT

Tell me what pain is.
Tell me about the hurt you have had before.
What do you do when you hurt?
Do you tell others when you hurt?
What do you want others to do for you when you hurt?
What don't you want others to do for you when you hurt?
What helps the most to take away your hurt?
Is there anything special that you want me to know about you when you hurt? (If yes, have child describe.)

PARENT INFORMANT

Describe any pain your child has had before.
How does your child usually react to pain?
Does your child tell you or others when he or she is hurting?
How do you know when your child is in pain?
What do you do for your child when he or she is hurting?
What does your child do for self when hurting?
Which of these actions work best to decrease or take away your child's pain?
Is there anything special that you would like me to know about your child and pain? (If yes, have parent[s] describe.)

(From Hester and Barcus, 1986.)

child to describe pain, and family involvement in pain assessment.

The Pain Experience History and Pain Interview

The pain experience is influenced by past experiences with pain and with its treatment. Interventions for pain are more likely to be successful when they are based upon knowledge of prior pain experiences and pain treatments. Hester and Barcus (1986) proposed obtaining a pain experience history (Box 29-2) prior to the onset of pain, such as during a well child examination or as a component of preparations before surgery or painful procedures. Information gained from the pain history can provide a base for planning intervention strategies. It also provides a base for future communication about the experience of pain.

Instruments to Assess Pain in Children

Several nurse researchers have developed instruments to assist the child in communicating about pain (Table 29-1, page 873). Although validity and reliability of many of the tools have been addressed by research, questions remain. Questions of validity concern whether the child's self-report of pain, using one of these tools, is a true measure of the pain being experienced. Questions of reliability concern whether, under identical pain circumstances, the child would again give the same response on that instrument. The fact that assessment instruments may not be totally valid and reliable, however, is no reason to discard them. They provide a concrete means for children to communicate about pain. *Nursing assessment that fails to take advantage of these communication aids risks missing valuable subjective input.* Used in conjunction with other modes of subjective and objective assessment, instruments for pain assessment can provide valuable confirmation or suggest the need to re-evaluate assumptions about the child's pain.

Color Tool. Several pediatric researchers have developed creative ways to obtain subjective reports about pain from children. Eland (1974) pioneered these projective techniques with a series of cartoon pictures designed to elicit the child's pain intensity. Included in the series of pictures (which the child was asked to rank order) was one of a dog in a similar situation to that experienced by the child. Although this particular technique was later abandoned, the popularity of this useful approach led to the more recent development of a color tool (Eland, 1981) (originally designed by Stewart, 1977). Children are prepared to use this tool prior to a painful experience by matching specific colors with their perception of various degrees of pain intensity. After the pain experience, they are asked to choose one of the previously selected colors to describe their actual pain experience (Fig. 29-2). The intensity of their pain can then be determined from the child's own prior ranking. Eland has shown through some of her research that this instrument is able to pick up both sensation and distress components of pain. A summary of the interview protocol for Eland's color tool and the accompanying diagrams for the child to indicate the location of pain are shown in Box 29-3.

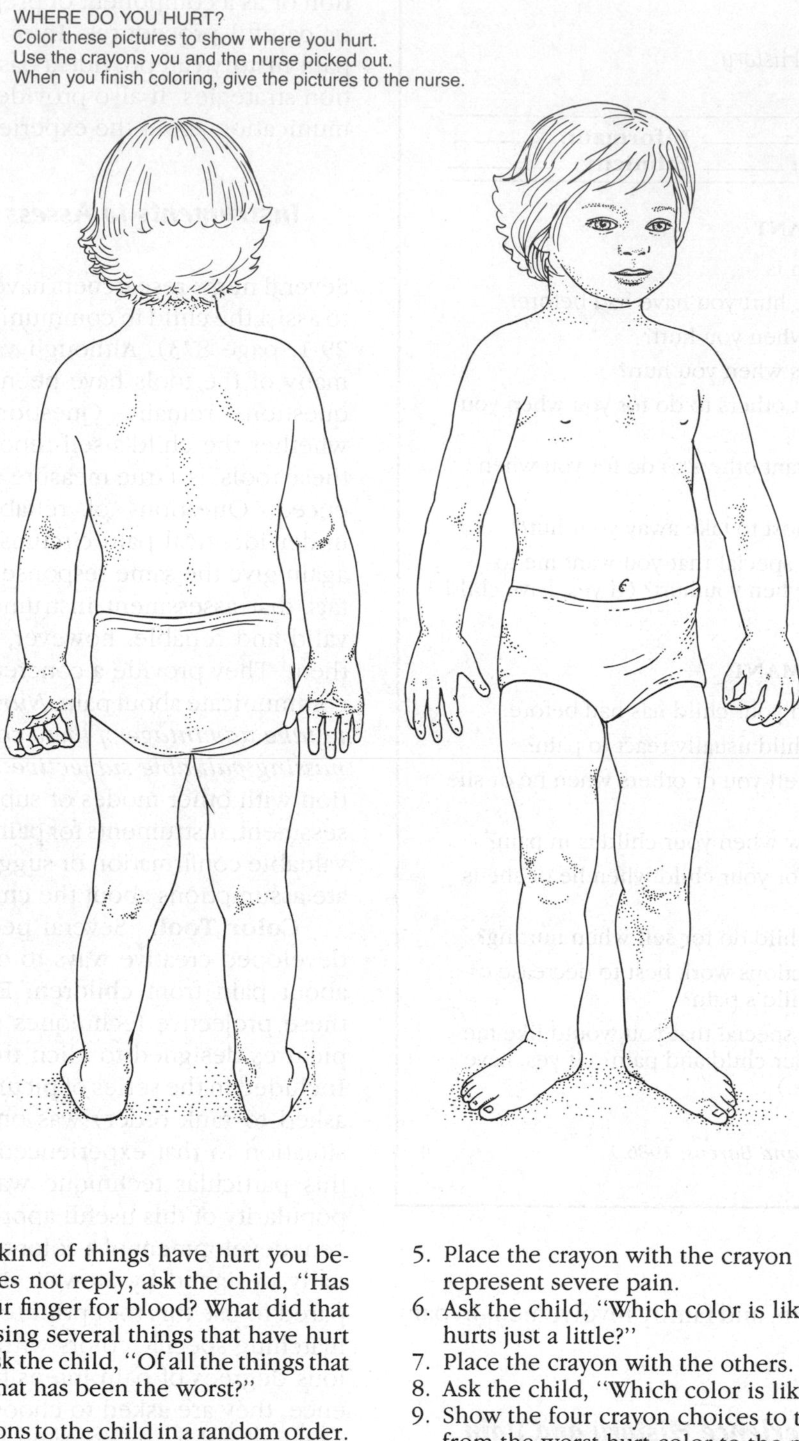
WHERE DO YOU HURT?
Color these pictures to show where you hurt.
Use the crayons you and the nurse picked out.
When you finish coloring, give the pictures to the nurse.

Eland's Color Tool.

Box 29-3
Interview Protocol

Ask the child, "What kind of things have hurt you before?" If the child does not reply, ask the child, "Has anyone ever stuck your finger for blood? What did that feel like? After discussing several things that have hurt the child in the past, ask the child, "Of all the things that have ever hurt you, what has been the worst?"

1. Present eight crayons to the child in a random order.
2. Ask the child, "Of these colors, which color is like . . ." (the event identified by the child as hurting the most).
3. Place the crayon away from the other crayons. (Represents severe pain).
4. Ask the child, "Which color is like a hurt, but not quite as much . . ."
5. Place the crayon with the crayon chosen to represent severe pain.
6. Ask the child, "Which color is like something that hurts just a little?"
7. Place the crayon with the others.
8. Ask the child, "Which color is like no hurt at all."
9. Show the four crayon choices to the child in order from the worst hurt color to the no hurt color.
10. Ask the child to show on the body outline where it hurts using the crayon for worst, middle, little or no hurt. Then ask if the hurt is "right now" or "from earlier in the day." Ask why the area hurts.
11. Document all the child's responses using his or her own words.

(From Eland, 1986.)

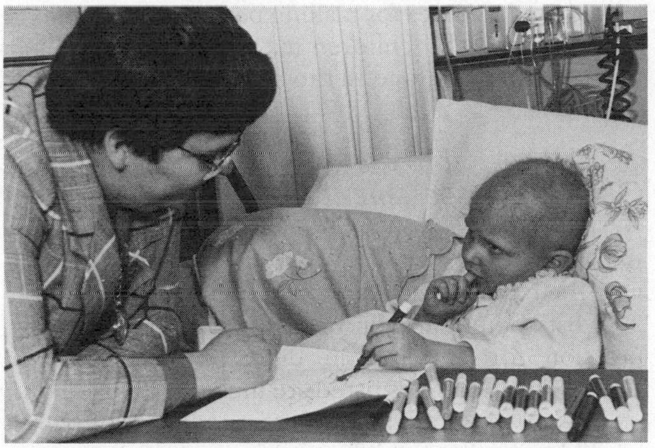

Figure 29-2. Dr. Joann Eland evaluating a child's pain by use of the color tool.

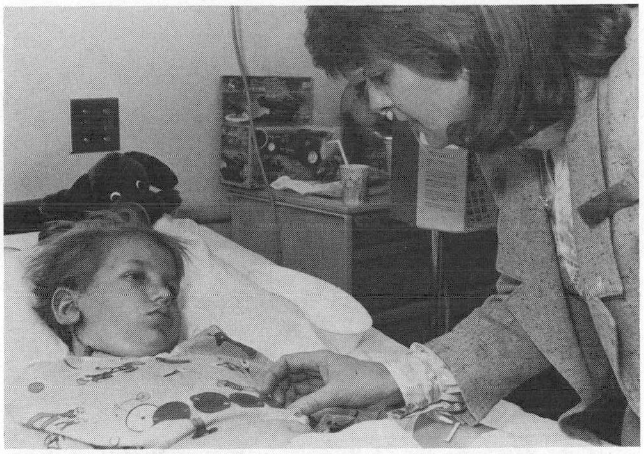

Figure 29-3. Dr. Nancy Hester explains use of the poker chip tool to a child after surgery.

Poker Chip Tool. Hester (1979) developed a pain intensity measure called the "poker chip tool." In this approach, each poker chip represents a "piece of hurt" and children are asked to describe their pain in terms of the poker chips, with one chip indicating "a little hurt" and four chips representing "as much hurt as you could ever have" (Fig. 29-3).

Visual Analogue Scale. A visual analogue scale is a visual representation of gradations of pain. This scale is commonly a 10-cm line with anchors at each end representing "no pain at all" and "as much pain as you could imagine" (represented at bottom of page). Abu-Saad and Holzemer (1981) used a 10-cm visual analogue scale in a research study with 9- to 15-year-olds to measure their postoperative pain. They were able to demonstrate a relationship between the severity of the pain and physiologic parameters such as body movements, facial expressions, and vocalizations. Several other tools have been developed as adaptations of the visual analogue scale (Huskisson, 1983).

"Hurt" Thermometer. Molsberry (1979) developed a rating scale called the "hurt thermometer." Children are asked to rate their pain by moving a red indicator from 0 to 4 degrees of pain.

Oucher. Beyer (1984; Beyer and Aradine, 1986a,b) developed a scale called the "Oucher" (Fig. 29-4). In this instrument, younger children are asked to represent their pain by choosing one of six photographs of children. The expression on the photographed child's face ranges from "no hurt" (a bottom picture) to the "biggest hurt you could ever have" (top picture). Older children are instructed to use the linear analogue scale with numerical indicators from 0 to 100 along the opposite side of the instrument. The decision as to which scale to use is based on children's abilities to count to 100. If they can, they use the numerical scale; if they cannot, they use the photographic scale. The dual measurement approach incorporated in this instrument makes it useful for pain assessment across a wide age span.

Drawings. A more open-ended self-report strategy to promote a child's description of pain has been employed using drawings. Unruh and colleagues (1983) used drawings with school-age children in an attempt to evaluate the recurrent pain associated with migraine headaches. Jeans and Gordon (1981) combined the use of drawings with an interview to study the meaning of pain in healthy 9- to 13-year-olds. Jerrett (1985) also combined drawings and an interview to assess pain in 5- to 9-year-olds receiving medical supervision for an acute health problem. Jerrett found that all the children were able to complete the drawing task and that a great deal of information regarding the child's perception, location, and intensity of the pain could be obtained. As well, there was good evidence that children could share their feelings and ideas about pain in spite of limited verbal skills. The benefit of using drawings to elicit information about the child's pain experience lies in its familiarity; children often use art to convey their feelings and express meaning in educational settings. DiLeo (1973) considers that children often communicate more clearly and openly through their art than they do verbally. A more detailed discussion of children's art can be found in Chapter 21. Variations in interpretation of children's art work raise questions about the validity and reliability of this technique. It is advisable to talk with the child, whenever possible, to discern whether the child's explanation of

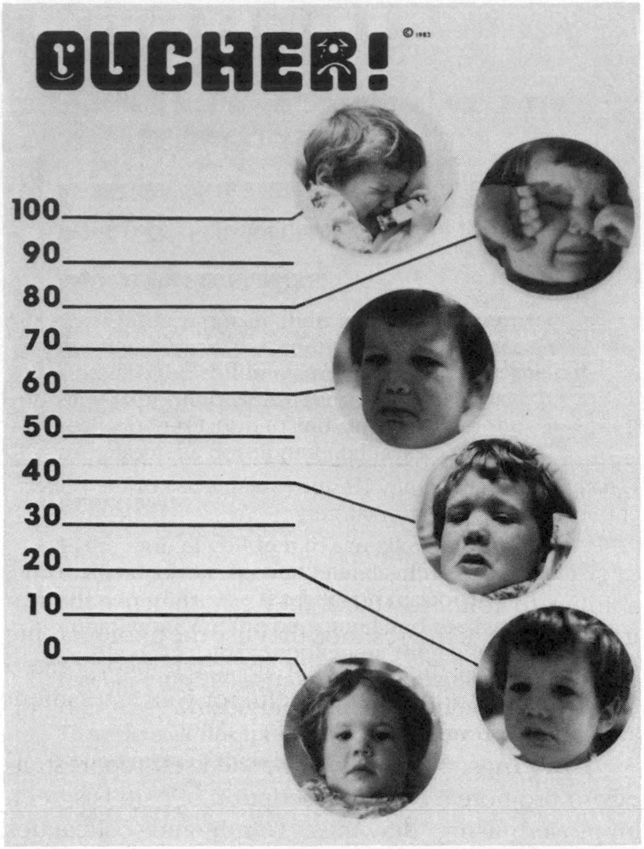

Figure 29-4. The Oucher. (From Beyer JE: *The Oucher: A User's Manual and Technical Report.* Evanston, IL, The Hospital Play Equipment Company, 1984. Copyright, The University of Virginia Alumni Patents Foundation, Charlottesville.)

the drawing is in keeping with the nurse's interpretation.

Family Involvement in Pain Assessment

Sometimes the parent who asks for pain medication for the child is labeled "overanxious." Could it be, however, that the parent's assessment of the child's pain is sometimes more accurate than the nurse's assessment? Considering the parent's extensive knowledge of the child's pain history and behavioral reactions to distress, nurses who fail to include parents in the pain assessment risk missing valuable data. A study in progress (Hester and Foster, 1988) is investigating the pain ratings given by parents (versus those given by the child and the nurse) and the cues used by both parents and nurses in making the pain assessments. Preliminary data analysis indicates that it is clear that some parents are particularly adept at identifying pain behaviors in their children and that they may use different cues than do nurses for making pain assessments. The implication is that children may benefit when nurses and parents work together to manage pain.

Objective Assessment

Behavioral observation and physiologic measures provide the basis for objective assessment of pain. Table 29-2 lists potential pain behaviors and modes of expression for children in different developmental stages. The behaviors listed are meant to be used *only as guidelines.* Often an important indicator of pain is any behavior that is "different" from normal. A parent can be helpful in defining "normal" behavior for a particular child.

Behavioral Observation

Behavioral observation involves assessment of nonverbal behavior. Pain may be expressed, either consciously or unconsciously, through any number of motor behaviors and facial expressions. Involuntary body movements (e.g., shaking, trembling) may also be evidence of pain. Behavioral observation is used most effectively in conjunction with subjective assessment (including both verbalizations and vocalizations) and physiologic parameters.

Whereas motor activity ranging from flailing of the limbs to a clenched jaw can indicate pain, the *absence* of movement can also be an important cue. Immobility is sometimes observed in infants and children following surgery. Preschoolers and older children have been known to hold the entire body rigid such that they voluntarily move only their eyes. When movement (and crying) increase pain, quiet immobility can be an attempt to control pain.

Behavioral observation should include the child's general reaction to the surroundings. Are there alterations in normal patterns of sleep, eating, play, mental concentration, and emotional expression? Does the child seem to be aware of and interested in nearby sights and sounds? Is the child able to engage in a diversional activity such as a book, game, telephone call, or television program? Does behavior become more normal as the result of medication or other comfort measures?

Behavioral observation is an important strategy for assessing pain in infants and toddlers who are unable to report pain verbally. Infants use numerous behaviors to communicate their emotional and physical states, including crying, withdrawal, irritability, and facial expression. Yet, nurses often fail to recognize that these behaviors indicate pain (Taylor, 1983). Vid-

Table 29-1. Instruments Measuring Pain in Children

Approach	Instrument	Dimension Measured	Appropriate Age
Self-report, Projective	Beyer: "Oucher" (1984) (photographic scale)	Pain intensity	3–12 years
	Eland: "Color Tool" (1981)	Pain	4–10 years
	Hester: "Poker Chip Tool" (1979)	Pain intensity	4–13 years
	Scott: "Projective Test" (1978)	Pain perception	4–10 years
	Unruh et al: "Children's Drawings" (1983)	Pain perception (categories)	5–18 years
Rating Scales and Other Assessment Techniques	Beyer: "Oucher" (1984) (numerical scale)	Pain intensity	3–12 years
	Molsberry: "Hurt Thermometer" (1979)	Pain intensity	4–8 years
	Abu-Saad and Holzemer (1981)	Perceived pain Pain intensity	9–15 years
	Hawley: "Pain Communication Tool" (1984)	Frequency, duration, type of pain	3–10 years
	Jeans and Gordon: Drawings and Interview (1981)	Quality-quantity of pain	5–13 years
	Jerrett: Drawings and Interview (1985)	Quality-quantity of pain	5–9 years
	Savedra et al (1981)	Description, causes of pain	9–12 years
	McGrath et al: "Multidimensional Pain Assessment in Children" (1985)	Pain intensity and pain affect	Over 5 years
Behavioral Observation	Katz et al: "Procedure Behavioral Rating Scale" (1980)	Behavioral distress Pain/anxiety	8 months–17 years
	Jay et al: "Observation Scale of Behavioral Distress" (1983)	Behavioral distress Pain/anxiety	2–20 years
	Lollar et al: "Pediatric Pain Inventory" (1982)	Pain perception, intensity and duration	4–19 years
	McGrath et al: "The Children's Hospital of Eastern Ontario Pain Scale (CHEOPS)" (1985)	Pain expression	1–5 years
	Dale (1986)	Pain intensity and duration	Infants, 2–4½ months

(From Stevens et al, 1987.)

eotapes and spectrographic analysis of vocalizations in infants have confirmed that the cries of distress, pain, and hunger are distinguishable from each other (Levine and Gordon, 1982; Johnston and Strada, 1986; Fuller et al, 1988). By combining behavioral observations of vocalizations, facial expressions, autonomic responses (e.g., heart rate), and body movements, Dale (1986) was able to assess the intensity and duration of infants' pain during routine immunization. This was an initial step in the development of a multidimensional tool for pain in infants. In another study, Franck (1986) used photogrammetric techniques to record the responses to heelprick at just 4 hours of age, showing that quantitative parameters of infant behavior can be obtained almost at birth with the aid of sophisticated equipment. However, many more questions have been raised than answers supplied with respect to the pain experience of infants.

Several researchers and clinicians suggest that certain behaviors and vocalizations are characteristic of pain in children (Abu-Saad and Holzemer, 1981; McCaffery, 1983; Dale, 1986). However, other researchers (Jeans, 1983; Beyer and Byers, 1985) question the usefulness of assessing behavior as a measure of the child's pain owing to strong developmental influences that may influence behavior. Clinical experi-

Table 29-2. Pain Behaviors, Expressions, Fears and Sources of Comfort – the Various Stages of Growth and Development

Developmental Stage	Potential Pain Behaviors	Potential Modes of Expression	Predominant Fears	Potential Sources of Comfort
Infant (0–12 months): Dependent on others for all needs. Forms meaningful relationship with primary caregiver. Develops trust when needs consistently and effectively met and anxiety and mistrust when they are not. "Stranger" anxiety develops at ≃8 months. Receives stimulation and gratification through mouth.	Total body movements Lack of responsiveness to feeding Changes in alertness Lack of contentment Sleep disturbances Poor responsiveness to caregivers Withdrawal, unusual stillness	Crying (quality) Whimpering Facial expression	Separation from parents Fear of strangers	Presence of primary caregiver or consistent nurses Sucking, self-comforting (soother, blanket, etc.) Holding, rocking Favorite toy, object, photograph Medication
Toddler (1–3 years): Develops autonomy through exploration. Shame and doubt if assertiveness nonacceptable or actions ineffective. Egocentric. Tolerates minimal separation from primary caregiver only. Opposes everything—"no." "Separation anxiety" 8–24 months. Gratification from control of muscles. Thought derives from sensation and movement.	Clinging to primary caregiver Rejection of all others Refusing food/toileting; regression to infant behaviors ↓ Exploration of the environment Flailing arms and legs, holding body rigid Touching hurting body part	Crying (varies from whimpering to outright scream) Refusal of everything Withdrawal Anxious facial expression or hiding face Describing pain as "hurt" or "owie" (location not specific)	Separation from parents or primary caregivers Fear of immobility and restraint	Presence of primary caregiver or consistent nurses Special toys or objects Rocking, holding Distraction activities—stories, television, music Self-comforting-sucking, holding on to special blanket Medication
Preschooler (3–5 years): Becoming more of an individual and tolerating longer separation. Mastering of play and movement, control of bowel and bladder functions, ability to initiate interactions. Magical thinking—some difficulty distinguishing fantasy and reality. Develops conscience and learns to share.	Immobility, rigidity Clinging to anyone Crying, kicking Regression to previous stages (e.g., loss of bowel and bladder control) Disinterest in normal play and tasks Anxiety	Crying (screaming) Shrieking (without tears) Withdrawal Concerned only with how pain affects him or her Able to describe pain's location and intensity "bad tummy ache" or "legs hurt" Fearful of pain-relieving interventions and incessantly questions, "What are you doing?" "Why?"	Separation from parents, siblings, home environment Fear that pain is punishment Fear of body mutilation	Presence of family, consistent staff Familiar toys, books, etc. Games and play activities (distraction techniques) Regular caregivers performing painful procedures Fantasy Increased mobility (e.g., going to the playroom) Asking child what has helped relieve pain in the past and using child's suggestions and simple participation Simple routines and explanations Medication

Table 29-2 *(continued)*

Developmental Stage	Potential Pain Behaviors	Potential Modes of Expression	Predominant Fears	Potential Sources of Comfort
School-age Child (6–12 years): Develops industry through mastery of new skills and rewards for them or inferiority if not. Enjoys structure and rules. Becomes competitive. Values peers. Bases conclusions on perceptions—beginning of logical thought.	Wide variance in behavior from hyperactivity to extreme passivity Unstable moods and temperament Demanding Overt aggression, anger Not caring for self Temper outbursts Withdrawal, extreme quietness, lying with eyes closed, "tuning out" Regression to earlier behaviors—e.g., panic attacks, bedwetting, impulsiveness Anxious facial expressions and poor eye contact	Able to more accurately describe location and intensity of pain May groan, wince, scream, but try to hold back tears and "be brave" May deny any pain in presence of peers Demand scientific explanations of how pain treatments and procedures affect body functioning May ask for pain medications providing they are *not* injections	Fear of feeling inferior Separation from peers Fear of mutilation Fear of rejection Fear of loss of self-control	Relationships with peers Ability to engage in tasks Presence of supportive, understanding adult Explanations at a level the child can understand Encourage participation in care Hypnosis and biofeedback Medication
Adolescent (13+ years): Vacillates between dependence and independence. Logical thought and deductive reasoning. Peer acceptance crucial. Self-control, body image, body changes, sexuality, and role development are very prominent concerns.	As above, there may be a wide range of behaviors and regression to previous stages Withdrawal, depression Aggressiveness, teasing Manipulation Poor eating and hygiene Refusal of care	Able to describe pain—location, intensity, and duration May verbalize desire for pain medications May refuse pain interventions in presence of peers	Fear of losing control Fear of changes in self-concept and body image Fear of loss of independence Separation from peers Concerns re: future (e.g., relationships, sexual competency, fertility, etc.)	Relationships with peers and friends Consistency of roommates Consistency of caregivers Interests; hobbies Family members—may prefer siblings to parents at times Self-hypnosis, self-relaxation Control over the situation Solitude Medication

ences suggest that preschool children may hide pain if they think they may get a "shot" or have to drink bad-tasting oral medication. At this age they may also think that their pain is a punishment for misbehavior and therefore conceal it. School-age children may fear body mutilation and adolescents may tend to hide their pain if they feel self-conscious or if their independence is threatened.

Behavioral Measurement Instruments

Several measurement tools have been developed to assess behavior changes associated with pain. CHEOPS (Children's Hospital of Eastern Ontario Pain Scale) by McGrath and co-workers (1985), Pediatric Pain Inventory by Lollar and colleagues (1982), and Observational Scale of Behavioral Distress by Jay and associates (1983) are examples of tools that categorize and enumerate behavioral manifestations of pain. These three instruments are applicable at the various developmental levels of children and have been subjected to considerable testing for reliability and validity.

Behavioral observation tools can provide information regarding the intensity of the general distress experience based on discrete behaviors rather than an observer's perception (McGrath et al, 1985). However, the range of possible behavioral reactions is large and no particular set has been shown to be consistent with particular pain experiences (Beyer and Byers, 1985; Dale, 1986). Similar to self-report techniques (especially those that are projective), behavioral observation tools are open to variation in their meaning and interpretation.

The CHEOPS (McGrath et al, 1985) is an example of a time sampling behavioral pain scale originally developed to use with postoperative patients between the ages of birth and 5 years. It includes subjective (verbal and vocal) as well as objective (nonverbal behavior) components. Categories, developed with input from experienced pediatric nurses, include behavioral observation of the child's cry, facial expression, verbal communication, torso motion, touch, and leg motion. An assessment is made by observing the child for 5 seconds, followed by 25 seconds to record the rating. A scoring method was devised to transform the descriptive data to numerical values as follows:

0 = behavior that is the antithesis of pain
1 = behavior that indicates neither pain nor the antithesis of pain
2 = behavior that indicates mild or moderate pain
3 = behavior that indicates severe pain

Using this method, possible pain scores can range from 4 to 13 representing no pain to severe pain. The behavioral definitions and scoring of the CHEOPS are presented in Table 29-3.

Physiologic Indicators

A final objective approach is the measurement of physiologic signs. Certain signs of autonomic arousal, in-

Table 29-3. Behavioral Definitions and Scoring of the CHEOPS

Behavior	Score	Definition
Cry		
No crying	1	Child is not crying.
Moaning	2	Child is moaning or quietly vocalizing, silent cry.
Crying	2	Child is crying but the cry is gentle or whimpering.
Scream	3	Child is in a full-lunged cry; sobbing; may be scored with complaint or without complaints.
Facial		
Composed	1	Neutral facial expression.
Grimacing	2	Score only if definitive negative facial expression.
Smiling	0	Score only if definite positive facial expression.
Child Verbal		
None	1	Child not talking.
Other Complaints	1	Child complains but not about pain; e.g., "I want to see Mommy" or "I am thirsty."
Pain Complaints	2	Child complains about pain.
Both Complaints	2	Child complains about pain and about things; e.g., "It hurts; I want Mommy."
Positive	0	Child makes any positive statement or talks about other things without complaint.
Torso		
Neutral	1	Body (not limbs) is at rest, torso is inactive.
Shifting	2	Body is in motion in a shifting or serpentine fashion.
Tense	2	Body is arched or rigid.
Shivering	2	Body is shuddering or shaking involuntarily.
Upright	2	Body is in a vertical or upright position.
Restrained	2	Body is restrained.
Touch		
Not Touching	1	Child is not touching or grabbing at wound.
Reaching	2	Child is reaching for but not touching wound.
Touching	2	Child is gently touching wound or wound area.
Grabbing	2	Child is grabbing vigorously at wound.
Restrained	2	Child's arms are restrained.
Legs		
Neutral	2	Legs may be in any position but are relaxed. Includes gentle swimming or serpentine-like movements.
Squirming/Kicking	2	Definitive uneasy or restless movements in the legs and/or striking out with foot or feet.
Drawn up/Tensed	2	Legs tensed and/or pulled up tightly to body and kept there.
Standing	2	Standing, crouching, or kneeling.
Restrained	2	Child's legs are being held down.

(From McGrath et al, 1985.)

cluding increased temperature, pulse, blood pressure, restlessness, and dilated pupils are associated with pain. These responses are termed "activation" (McCaffery, 1982). They have been demonstrated to occur during the first second of a painful experience and may be sustained for up to 1 hour (Cannon, 1929). During "activation" (also known as the "fight or flight" response), the sympathetic nervous system is active. Blood moves from the superficial and peripheral vessels to those organs that are essential for muscle exertion, including the lungs, heart, and central nervous system. The bronchioles dilate to increase oxygenation, and the heart rate increases to distribute the oxygenated blood. To meet the body's increased energy needs, the liver releases stored glycogen. These activities of the sympathetic nervous system are sustained by the release of epinephrine (see Fig. 23-1).

Following activation and the initial brief but intense response, the body *rebounds* and the parasympathetic nervous system takes over. During this phase, symptoms opposite to those in the activation stage are seen, with a drop in respiratory rate, heart rate, and blood pressure. The body *adapts* to these stressors within a short period of time and regains a state of homeostasis. *These physiologic indicators are short-lived, are not specific for pain, and occur inconsistently* (Johnson, 1977); therefore, they are seldom helpful in assessing the existence and intensity of pain unless combined with other assessment data. If used in combination with other pain assessment approaches during acute pain episodes, physiologic measures may provide significant information. In infants, physiologic measures have been shown to correlate with spectrographic cry analysis (Johnston and Strada, 1986).

Nursing Interventions for Pain

The undertreatment of children in pain has been documented in nursing research since the pioneering work of Eland (Eland and Anderson, 1977). Despite ongoing research related to this problem, the 1986 Consensus Development Conference on the Integrated Approach to the Management of Pain noted that even when pain is reported by the client or accurately assessed by the nurse, pain management may be inadequate.

Hester and Barcus (1986) proposed several reasons for undertreatment of pain in children. First, the myth that children do not experience pain has lingered despite research to the contrary. Second, some nurses question whether children's self-reports of pain can be believed. Third, children's pain responses are inconsistent and therefore difficult to evaluate. Fourth, nurses are sometimes fearful of adverse effects of medications, such as respiratory depression. Fifth, nurses have traditionally received little formal education related to pain assessment and pain management. Finally, there is the fact that effective pain management is time consuming, and other nursing responsibilities may take priority.

What, then, can nurses do to prevent and relieve pain in the children in their care? The following strategies are recommended:

- Recognize that ill children are *likely* to experience pain.
- *Assume responsibility* for pain management.
- Be knowledgeable about this child's unique pain history and response to pain relief measures.
- Work with the child, family, and physician to develop strategies for pain assessment and pain relief.
- Daily evaluate the effectiveness of pain management measures and alter the plan of care accordingly.

The nursing process plan (Table 29-4) provides further guidance for pain management.

Interventions to control and relieve pain involve measures to reduce fear and anxiety, strategies to enhance the child's sense of control, pharmacologic comfort measures, and nonpharmacologic measures.

Reducing Fear and Anxiety

Reducing fear and anxiety can alter the child's perception of pain and therefore enhance the child's ability to cope with the experience. Often, the first step in reducing the child's fear is reducing the parent's anxiety. Table 31-2 presents strategies to reduce the child's and family's anxiety associated with hospitalization. Many of these strategies can be adapted to other health care and home care settings. Preparation for painful procedures and for surgery can alter the cognitive perception of pain. Chapter 27 details age-appropriate preparation strategies.

The environment can have a significant influence on the child's pain experience. If children are isolated from their families, peers, and other patients they are likely to be anxious and depressed. Children can also feel isolated when information is kept from them. Johnson (1977) has shown that patients can benefit from several types of information, including what will be done to them, how long it will take, and how it feels. For example, if children who are facing a cast application can first apply a cast to a toy animal or doll in the playroom, they have the opportunity to ask questions

Table 29-4
Nursing Process Plan: The Child in Pain

By Roxie Foster

Assessment of Intellectual-Perceptual Function

Pain

Subjective Assessment: Vocalization and verbalization of level of comfort, perception of the situation, meaning attributed to the experience, score on pain assessment tool*

Objective Assessment: Changes in usual behavior, physiologic indicators of autonomic response, length of time since last analgesic

Analysis: Nursing Diagnosis 1

Altered comfort: pain, related to
- *tissue damage*
- *perception of the stressor*
- *meaning attributed to the experience*

Defining Characteristics

Subjective: Grunting, whining, crying, screaming; verbalization of the nature, location, duration and/or intensity of discomfort; verbalization of perception of painful stimulus and of the meaning attached to it; pain indicated by assessment tool

Objective: Behaviors associated with pain (see Table 29–2 for examples of behaviors by developmental stage), or significant change in usual behavior; possible increased pulse, respirations, and blood pressure; effective analgesic decreasing

Client Goals/ Evaluation Criteria	Nursing Goals/Strategies (Selected Rationale)
1.1 The client will experience reduction or elimination of pain, as evidenced by: a. vocalization indicating relief b. verbalizing increased level of comfort c. reduction/absence in physical behavior associated with pain d. vital signs and pupil response within normal limits	*Administer analgesics.* (See Tables 29-5 through 29-7.) • Administer p.r.n. analgesics prophylactically or when pain is minimal. (When pain intensity increases the ordered dose of analgesic may not be sufficient to produce relief.) • Use this opportunity to call the child's and parents' attention to signs and symptoms of pain (in order to help them better evaluate the response to the medication). • Teach the child and parent(s) about the therapeutic and side effects of the medication (to facilitate home care). • Address the common concern of addiction to narcotic analgesics by presenting facts (to correct misinformation). *Institute nonpharmacologic interventions.* • Take into account age-related coping strategies (e.g., the younger the child, the more motoric and less cognitive are coping strategies).

* Although the actual score is an objective measure, the purpose of the tool is to elicit subjective information; this type of pain assessment will therefore be categorized as subjective.

	• Provide distraction in the form of toys, play activities, visitors, etc. (Distraction interrupts the transmission of the pain sensation but works best for pain that is constant or rises slowly in intensity [Melzack and Wall, 1982]. Remember that distraction from pain does not mean absence of pain.) • Reinforce parental attempts to comfort the child through tactual, gestural, and verbal means. (For the preverbal child this may be a primary means of relaxation. For the older child it may facilitate cognitive relaxation techniques that help to control pain.) Comment, "Bobby is so much more comfortable when you hold him and sing to him." (Being able to comfort the child can give the parents a positive outlet for anxiety and can enhance the child's emotional/social environment.) • Teach and encourage parents to use massage techniques. (According to the gate control theory, stimulation of large cutaneous fibers block pain transmission.) • With the preschooler or older child teach and support cognitive techniques such as relaxation, guided imagery, and self-talk. (The gate control theory holds that cognitive techniques can also interrupt pain transmission.)
1.2 The client will experience emotional support, as evidenced by: a. verbalizing decreased fear and anxiety associated with the pain experience b. quieting and showing decreased muscular tension in response to comfort measures	*Reduce fears associated with hospitalization.* • Encourage a parent or family member to stay with children between 6 months and 5 years of age (who will be most at risk for separation anxiety). • Facilitate a trusting relationship with at least one nurse on each shift (so that the child can find comfort in a nurse's presence when family support is unavailable). • Remove the child from the room, or at least from the crib, for painful procedures (to establish a "safe" place within a frightening environment). *Provide appropriate information* in advance of potentially painful experiences (to enable the child to marshall coping abilities. This will also enhance trust and facilitate problem solving). *Provide opportunities for the child to witness adaptive coping with similar experiences.* (The principle of social modeling suggests that adaptive strategies can be learned by watching others.) • Avoid exposure of the child, whenever possible, to children with poorly managed distress. (Heightened anxiety potentiates pain and may result in perception of the stressor as unmanageable.) *Incorporate pain-relieving interventions* whenever possible. (Pain heightens anxiety.) *Encourage parental involvement.* (This may reduce their frustration and anxiety and enhance their ability to comfort the child.) • Assist parents to modify and implement any pain relief measures that are appropriate and have been effective in the past. (Parental anxiety is often lessened when their sense of powerlessness is reduced. Involving parents in interventions also allows for attention to cultural beliefs and practices.)

Continued

Client Goals/ Evaluation Criteria	Nursing Goals/Strategies (Selected Rationale)
1.3 The client will experience an increased sense of control, as evidenced by: a. verbalizing decreased fear and anxiety b. verbalizing an understanding of the cause and probable duration of the pain c. identifying strategies effective in pain management d. actively participating in pain management	*Acknowledge the pain as described.* (Identification of the problem precedes problem solving; if the child is forced to validate the pain with physical behavior, pain relief will be delayed and maladaptive behaviors may be reinforced.) *Allow the child as much control over pain relief measures as possible.* • Allow the client of school-age or older to choose an analgesic from those ordered, after explaining the expected therapeutic effects. • Assist the client to evaluate the outcome and to incorporate the experience into the next request for analgesia. (The client may actually select an injection for its pain-relieving effect, but may protest vigorously if the same injection is forced upon him or her.) • Teach nonpharmacologic measures as an alternative for or adjunct to analgesia. Allow the client to choose techniques to try. Assist in evaluation of the effectiveness of measures chosen and in modification of the measures to meet individual needs. (Nonpharmacologic methods enhance self-control because they can often be instituted by the client in the absence of the parents or nurse.) *Discuss with the child and parents the probable cause of the pain and the expected duration.* (Effective problem-solving is dependent on accurate information.) *Reinforce adaptive strategies.* (The child needs to maintain a sense of mastery over pain in order to preserve self-esteem.) • Comment on successful experiences (e.g., "You did that so well! I know it hurts to move. Pressing on your side with your hand seemed to help, didn't it?") *Involve the client and parents in evaluation of pain relief measures and discuss with them any modifications in the plan of care.* (The level of pain may be changed by the sense of control over it [Melzack and Wall, 1982].)

about the procedure as well as express their feelings through play. The importance of play as an intervention in managing a child's distress is discussed in more detail in Chapter 21.

Children's pain experiences can also be influenced by their observation of pain expressed by another child or parent. This observation may result in emotional sensitization, anxiety, and negative social modeling that leads children to act much like the person in pain that they have witnessed (Chapman and Turner, 1986). Conversely, if children can view another child coping well with a potentially painful situation, this can reduce pain expression and acting out behaviors. Melamed and Siegel (1975) have used this principle in the employment of social modeling. For example, slide tape shows and videotapes have been used successfully to prepare patients for a painful event. As well, handling of equipment and interactions with others who have undergone a similar procedure may also desensitize patients to painful episodes.

All these factors place emotional stress on the child in pain. As nurses, a major goal in providing optimal care is to either provide emotional support for the child or foster it within the child's existing support system. Nurses and parents alike need to be aware of the antecedent factors that cause emotional stress and the consequent reactions of the child. Children require the patience and understanding that only those who are significant in their lives can give. Nurses and others who are caring for the child also play a significant role in providing sensitive, caring support. Consultation and collaboration among the child, family, and health care professionals is essential.

To provide optimum emotional support for the child in pain, nurses may find the following guidelines useful:

1. Try to inform the children and parents what will be happening, how long it will take, and how they will feel. For younger children, it is also important for them to know that a painful experience is over. This can be accomplished by taking them from the area, picking them up and cuddling them, and telling them that the hurt is finished.
2. Use social modeling advantageously by providing examples of patients who have tolerated potentially painful situations well;
3. Incorporate appropriate pharmacologic and nonpharmacologic pain-relieving interventions throughout the child's care;
4. Encourage a parent or someone who is known to relate well with the child to stay with him or her as much as possible; and
5. Try to avoid exposing the child to other children who are experiencing extreme discomfort or emotional distress.

Reducing the Sense of Powerlessness/ Enhancing Control

Another method of helping children manage their pain experience is to instill in them a sense of personal control. To accomplish this, children must feel certain that they are being listened to and believed when they report their pain and that they have some role in decision-making about pain-relieving strategies and their effectiveness. To help children cope with their pain is an exhausting, demanding, and often frustrating task. The coping skills that are available for children to use are influenced by their levels of cognitive development, previous experiences, and modeling provided by parents and significant others. In a study by Jerrett (1985) 5- to 9-year-olds provided a wide range of responses to the question "When you hurt or have pain, what do you do to help yourself feel better?" Their responses indicated the use of the following coping behaviors:

1. Direct action physical activities, such as holding or rubbing, treating with something special, or applying a bandage;

2. Avoidance activities, such as those behaviors involved in detachment or distraction, including resting, reading, or thinking of other things; and

3. Help-seeking activities, such as interacting with another individual (such as a parent) and including being held or taking medications.

Although these children reported direct-action physical activities and avoidance behaviors most often, they identified behaviors that were related to the presence of a parent as the most beneficial in helping them to cope with their pain. Other studies and anecdotal clinical experience would also support that parents and significant others play a major role in the child's pain experience. A study by Hester (in press) supports and expands upon many of these findings. Hester asked children how they comforted themselves when they were in pain and what others could do to comfort them. Excerpts from the interviews are presented in Box 29-4.

Pharmacologic Interventions

Pharmacologic intervention involves the administration of analgesic medications. Although analgesia is not the only way to relieve pain, it is one of the fastest and most effective. There are three main categories of analgesics: narcotics (opioids), nonsteroidal anti-inflammatory drugs (NSAIDS), and adjuvants. The common drugs in each of the categories, their actions, and usual use are summarized in Table 29-5.

Narcotic Analgesics

The most widely used drugs for pain management are the opioids. This group of drugs, which developed from opium, now has many natural and synthetic derivatives. These drugs are thought to act primarily on the central nervous system by binding to receptor sites located in the limbic system, hypothalamus, thalamus, corpus striatum, and spinal cord. Opioids produce their analgesic effect in a selective manner which does not interfere with other sensory inputs.

Concerns may arise when a child in pain is placed on a drug regimen that includes the use of narcotics (opioids). For the parents, these concerns center primarily on the issues of addiction, dependence, and tolerance. *Addiction* is a psychologic dependence in which drug-seeking behavior is more important than pain relief. *Physical dependence* occurs after prolonged use of the drug. *Tolerance* is an increasing resistance to the physiologic effects of a drug. Parents need to understand the difference between these states and realize that psychologic dependence and subsequent abuse of narcotics is very rare in adults (Miller and Jick, 1978; Porter and Jick, 1980) and has not been documented in hospitalized children.

Box 29-4

Comfort Strategies: The Child's Perspective

The comfort strategies described by the children and adolescents who participated in this study are illustrated through interview-excerpts of Mandy, David, Cindy, Jeffrey, and Alice.

Mandy

Mandy, 5 years old (the youngest child interviewed for this study) was hospitalized for the insertion of a new stomach tube. She had had extensive experience with pain, by virtue of 35 previous hospitalizations. Mandy tried to alleviate her pain by taking medicine, telling her Mom "I'm hurting," being with her "Mom and Dad," and by holding her teddy bear or her doll. Two of these strategies were under Mandy's control; she could tell someone she hurt and she could hold her toys. However, she could not take medicine by herself nor could she determine when her parents were present. Hence, two implicit caring behaviors for Mandy were to give her medicine when she was experiencing pain and to get her parents for her or to have someone stay with her. When asked what others could do for her, Mandy replied "Hold my hand" and "Tell me to do something." *Hold my hand* was a frequent response of children of all ages in this study. *Tell me to do something* is a distraction technique. Mandy described this technique as something others could use to comfort her; older children in the study initiated various forms of distraction to alleviate the pain themselves.

David

Hospitalizations were not new to David. By 7 years of age, David had had 12 operations and approximately 30 hospitalizations. At the time of the interview David had been surgically treated for a bowel obstruction. David, an expert on pain, cried when he hurt; he also would "Call for Mom." Although he said he would tell the nurses that he hurt, he couldn't tell the doctors. The following interview-excerpt illustrates the reason:

Interviewer: Do you tell your doctor?
David: My doctor? I don't have a doctor.
Interviewer: Oh.
David: He never comes by.
Interviewer: Huh?
David: He never really comes by.

David said that when he hurt he would throw his stuffed toys or blanket. But he quickly added "Well, I can hold my blanket." This blanket was a special one from home.

In response to what nurses could do for him, David said:

"They give me some medicine."
"They give me a shot through my IV."

For David, nurses were the dispensers of medicine for his pain. It is interesting that David, like many of the informants, stressed receiving a shot through the intravenous line. A shot was acceptable only if it went through the IV line; children viewed intramuscular shots negatively and with fear. An older girl specifically described an IM shot as totally unacceptable and would consider it only if she were in really bad pain.

Like Mandy, David wanted someone to hold his hand. He did not, however, want anyone to poke him. Other children also mentioned touching or poking places that hurt as a noncaring behavior of others. Unfortunately, assessment techniques for determining the status of the child often include touching or poking painful areas.

Being involved in decisions about his situation was important to David:

David: I just want them to let me have my choice.
Interviewer: Your choice? Your choice about what?
David: Because, like they have things to make choices and (they) decide things I don't like.
Interviewer: So you want to be a part of that decision?
David: Uh-huh.

Most of the children emphasized, explicitly or implicitly, participation in the decision. Following this interview, the doctor told the interviewers that David would have surgery the next day. David had yet to be informed.

Cindy

Cindy, 10 years old, had broken her leg while skiing. This was her first hospitalization. Other than minor acute illnesses, knee scrapes, and cuts, Cindy had little experience with pain. She described her reaction to pain:

Well, sometimes I can control myself and not cry too much. But if it's really bad, I do cry and I hold really tight to somebody's hand or a bar or something and squeeze real hard and pull it and everything.

Later, she stressed the importance of holding Mom's hand.

Cindy would tell the nurse when she had pain:

Well, normally I would press the (call) button if the pain was really bad, like if I needed a pain pill or I would press the button . . . like if it's not too bad . . . but I just would tell them my toes hurt and they come in and check.

Caring behaviors for Cindy included staying with me, bringing me presents, making me feel good, talking with me, and checking me. Cindy did not want others to make a "big fuss about it."

I don't mind . . . if they check it and ask me if I need something to drink or eat. I don't like it when they stay and fuss . . . and say "Do you want more blankets and all that? Do you want this and that closer to you? Do you want the TV on?" I don't like it when people fuss about me like that . . .

But Cindy did not want to be ignored either:

> I don't like it when people ignore me when I'm in pain, like if I buzz the nurse and she says "Can I help you?" and I ask for a pain pill and (she) says "Well, I don't think we should give you one because you're a child."

Cindy felt ignored and she expressed her anger toward the nurse who was uninformed.

> But I've had them all the time . . . I can take them. It makes me mad because (she) should have been informed that I am able to take up to two pain pills at one time and I can take them up to three times a day.

In this situation a nurse thwarted Cindy's efforts to be in charge of pain. The nurse rejected Cindy's need for pain medication simply on the basis of Cindy's being a child.

Cindy was a very take-charge individual. Her family situation provides some insight as to why.

> Cindy: When I have pain it's difficult on my Mom because my Dad has MS. She has to take care of him . . . So when I get hurt, I sort of feel guilty sometimes because that puts more pressure on my Mom and she has to work a lot harder to take care of both of us.
>
> Interviewer: Do you ever talk to your Mom about feeling guilty?
>
> Cindy: Yeah, I told her that I'll be all right. I can take care of myself, just take care of my Dad and just check on me once in a while and I'll be fine.

Cindy not only took care of herself; she also tried to protect her mother from being overburdened both physically and emotionally.

Jeffrey

Thirteen-year old Jeffrey was hospitalized for an infected hip. Medically, Jeffrey had had little previous experience with pain; however, Jeffrey convincingly described extensive experience with pain as a football player. Unlike the other children in the study, Jeffrey concentrated on the noncaring behaviors of others. Jeffrey expressed a lot of anger in regard to his pain experiences and how poorly he had been treated.

> Interviewer: How do you feel when you hurt?
>
> Jeffrey: Like screaming. I get mad, I mean, I have a bad temper anyway and when I hurt, I want to get revenge . . . I want to grab my doctor's neck.

Jeffrey was particularly angry about how the health care professionals had treated him:

> They gave me Valium and Demerol to calm me down . . . but they gave me that too late.

He described a lack of sensitivity and understanding on the part of his doctor:

> A doctor has no way of knowing what it's going to feel like.

Later, he commented that the "doctor liked to inflict pain."

According to Jeffrey, others did not treat him in a very caring way. They ignored his requests for medication and they lacked sensitivity and understanding regarding his pain experiences. When asked what nurses did for him, he described:

> It depends on how nice of a nurse. They bring painkillers and stuff. Most of them try and understand but it's hard for somebody else to understand that you're in pain . . .

Alice

Alice, a 15-year old high student and the oldest individual to participate in the study, was hospitalized for pancreatitis for 45 days about a year prior to the interview. The lengthy hospital stay was related to surgical complications. Although Alice described things she did to comfort herself during pain experiences, during much of hospital stay she was very dependent on others to comfort her. As did the younger children, Alice told others when she had pain. When she was on the respirator, she wrote notes to the nurses regarding her pain. Holding a stuffed toy comforted Alice:

> I got a pink bear . . . (he) was there for me the whole time . . . he was my best friend . . . I slept on him . . . (he) was like a security blanket . . . they let me take him into the operating room until they put me under . . . and when I woke he was there again and that was so nice. So I think a security blanket is just something that you have all the time . . .

Alice wanted lots of love and comfort from others. Her mother was the primary person she wanted with her:

> Once in a while I would ask my Mom "Can I have a shot? Will you stay here while I go to sleep? Please stay here and don't leave until I've fallen asleep." I want that secure feeling that someone's there for me just in case I can't sleep or I need somebody to talk to for a while.

The interview excerpts from these five children vividly illustrate children's perceptions of how they can comfort themselves, what others should and shouldn't do to comfort them, and environmental factors that prevent their comfort. This information could be useful to the nurse in comforting the child in pain.

Success in comforting the child in pain will depend on a co-partnership among the nurses, the child, and the child's family. The nurses and the child's family must acknowledge the presence of pain and be willing to comfort the child. Often, children in pain are lonely, bewildered, and frightened. They have told us how to comfort them, and this knowledge places a demand on nurses to do so.

(From Hester, in press.)

Table 29-5. Categories of Commonly Used Analgesics

Action	Usual Use	Common Examples
Narcotics (Opioids)		
Bind with opiate receptors in CNS to alter perception of pain and emotional response to it.	For moderate to severe acute pain. Chronic pain associated with terminal illness (e.g., cancer).	Morphine sulfate Demerol (meperidine hydrochloride) Levodromoran (levorphanol) Codeine Dilaudid (hydromorphone hydrochloride) Talwin (pentazocine)
Nonsteroidal Anti-Inflammatory Drugs (Non-Narcotic Analgesics)		
Anti-inflammatory, antipyretic, and analgesic properties. Interfere with the synthesis of prostaglandins, thus decreasing the inflammatory process and sensitization of pain receptors. Work primarily at the level of the peripheral nervous system by decreasing local heat, redness, and swelling. Also believed to act centrally although mechanism unknown.	For mild to moderate acute pain (used alone). For moderate to severe pain if used in a schedule with narcotics. Especially useful for pain associated with inflammation.	Aspirin (acetylsalicylic acid) Tylenol (acetaminophen) Motrin (ibuprofen) Naproxyn (naproxen) Feldene (piroxicam)
Adjuvants		
Centrally acting and believed to potentiate the benefits of narcotics and diminish their adverse side effects.	Usually administered with narcotics in moderate to severe pain which is difficult to control.	Caffeine (stimulant) Atarax (antihistamine) Dilantin (phenytoin) (anticonvulsant) Tegretol (carbamazepine) (anticonvulsant) Valium

Parents need to know that their child will receive adequate analgesia and that frequent reassessment of their child's pain will be made. However, it should be emphasized that as the child's pain decreases, the narcotic regimen will also be adjusted accordingly and non-narcotic drugs introduced if necessary. Nurses need to encourage the parents to share their beliefs, fears, and concerns about the issue of drug use.

Potential Adverse Effects of Narcotics. For the nurse, a major issue in the administration of narcotics is the fear of respiratory depression. This fear, although sometimes exaggerated and often unfounded, is one reason why health professionals do not use narcotics to their full advantage. Nurses need to be aware of the risks that narcotic use presents for patients. Narcotics can initially depress respirations by decreasing the responsiveness of the regulatory center to carbon dioxide. Narcotics also affect the pontine and medullary centers that regulate respiratory rhythm. Because of the potential for changes in respiration, the nurse must check the respiratory rate, depth, and rhythm on a regular basis following the administration of narcotics (especially morphine sulfate.) Naloxone (Narcan), an antagonist to natural and synthetic opioids, should be available at the bedside of infants and high-risk children. If the patient's respiratory rate drops significantly, the nurse should stimulate the child to breathe deeply. If this does not re-establish a regular breathing pattern, administer Narcan as ordered, notify the physician immediately, and administer oxygen. Remain with the child to assess the need for resuscitation. Fortunately, occurrence of significant respiratory depression from narcotics is quite rare.

Nausea and vomiting may also occur in children receiving narcotic analgesia because of the stimulation of the chemoreceptor trigger zone of the medulla. A vestibular interaction is also possible because children who are lying down tend to exhibit less nausea and vomiting than those who are up and about. Nausea and vomiting are often sufficient cause for a change in medication.

Other nursing considerations when administering analgesics to children include choosing an appropriate route and dosage schedule. Many routes are available to administer analgesia to children, including oral, rectal, intramuscular, subcutaneous, and intravenous. Some of the common narcotic analgesics, their routes of administration, dosages, frequency, and nursing considerations are summarized in Table 29-6.

Non-Narcotic Analgesics

The two most common non-narcotic (nonopioid) analgesics are acetylsalicylic acid (ASA) and acetaminophen (Tylenol or Tempra). ASA is most commonly

Table 29-6. Narcotic Analgesics, Routes, Recommended Pediatric Dosages and Frequency, and Nursing Considerations

Route	Recommended Pediatric Dosage (mg/kg)	Recommended Frequency	Nursing Considerations
Meperidine (Demerol)			
PO	2–4	q 3 hr	For use with moderate to severe pain.
SC*	—		Drug of choice in acute pain situations (e.g., postoperatively); is less likely to affect smooth muscles.
IM	1.0–1.8	q 3–4 hr	More rapid onset and shorter duration than Morphine.
IV	1.0–1.8	q 3–4 hr	If given orally, dilute with water to avoid local anesthetic effect.
	Maximum single dosage: 100 mg		If using IV use of the lower end of the dosage range is recommended.
			Dilute IV dose (a maximum of 10 mg/ml) and run over a minimum 30 minutes with the patient recumbent.
			Cautions • May accumulate if renal function is impaired • Overdose may produce CNS irritability • Monitor for respiratory depression at peak action times
Morphine			
PO	0.6–1.2	q 4 hr	For use with moderate to severe pain (acute or chronic).
SC	0.1–0.2	q 4 hr	Drug of choice for chronic pain management; being used more frequently for postoperative pain control.
IM	0.1–0.2	q 4 hr	If giving orally, dilute with juice to reduce unpleasant taste.
IV	0.1–0.2	q 4 hr	If using for repeated administration, IM route is preferable.
Rectal†	Maximum single dosage: 15 mg		Dilute I.V. dose well, give over a minimum of 20–30 minutes with patient recumbent.
			Caution • Monitor for respiratory depression at peak action times
Codeine			
PO	0.75	q 4–6 hr	For use with mild-to-moderate pain
SC	0.5	q 4–6 hr	
IM	0.5	q 4–6 hr	
IV‡	—		
	Maximum single dosage: 60 mg		

*Not usually used s.c. to avoid tissue irritation.
†Available in rectal suppository form, but since absorption is unpredictable, this route is not recommended.
‡Not given intravenously due to increased risk for respiratory depression.
(Data from Shirkey, 1977; Knoben and Anderson, 1983; Graef and Cone, 1985; Gilman et al, 1985; Kastrup, 1986; McEvoy, 1986.)

used in children for its antipyretic and anti-inflammatory effects, but it can also be considered for its analgesic effect. ASA acts by inhibiting the conversion of arachidonic acid to various prostaglandins (Peterson, 1985). Prostaglandins appear to sensitize nociceptors to histamine and bradykinin. Therefore, ASA plays a part in desensitizing the nerve to chemical factors that may be responsible for producing pain (Schecter, 1985). ASA is now used cautiously because of recent links to Reye syndrome. Acetaminophen also acts by prostaglandin antagonism, but in a much narrower spectrum than ASA. Therefore, acetaminophen has less anti-inflammatory action. These two non-narcotic analgesics are summarized in Table 29-7.

Selecting the Route

Several factors should be considered when choosing the route of administration of an analgesic. The severity of the child's pain should be of primary importance. In the case of severe pain, intravenous medications generally have the fastest onset of action, giving relief within 10 to 15 minutes. However, the duration of intravenous medications is often shorter than that for

Table 29-7. Non-Narcotic Analgesics; Dosages, Actions, and Nursing Considerations

Recommended Pediatric Dosage	Nursing Considerations
Acetaminophen (Tylenol, Tempra)	
10–15 mg/kg *Maximum dose:* 60 mg/kg/24 hr *Route:* PO, q 3 to 4 hr *Onset:* 30 min *Peak action:* 60–120 min *Duration:* 3–4 hr (Rectal supplied in 120-mg suppositories, q 3 to 4 hr)*	Less anti-inflammatory action than ASA Liquid forms available in elixir (160 mg/5 ml) and drops (80 mg/0.8 ml) Fewer irritating adverse effects than ASA Fewer potential drug interactions than ASA
Acetylsalicylic Acid (ASA)	
10–15 mg/kg *Maximum dose:* 60 mg/kg/24 hr *Route:* PO, q 4 hr *Onset:* 30 min *Peak action:* 60–120 min *Duration:* 3–4 hr (Rectal supplied in 160-mg suppositories, q 3 to 4 hr)*	Assess for toxic effects, including tinnitus, nausea, and vomiting Increased risk of hypersensitivity reactions (e.g., in asthma patients) Irritating adverse effects (e.g., gastric) Implicated in many drug interactions No adequate liquid form No tolerance, physical dependence, or addiction

* Used rarely, as rectal absorption is very unpredictable.
(Data from Shirkey, 1977; Knoben and Anderson, 1983; Gilman et al, 1985; Graef and Cone, 1985, Kastrup, 1986; McEvoy, 1986; Trissel, 1986.)

other routes, resulting in the need for more frequent administration. In patients who have chronic pain, the oral route may be preferable for as long as the agents are tolerated (i.e., without gastric upset). This approach can then be followed successfully by intravenous administration. Rectal administration is also a possibility when the child cannot tolerate oral medications owing to nausea and vomiting. However, because rectal absorption is unpredictable and sometimes incomplete, the patient's response needs to be monitored carefully. Regional anesthetic blocks have also been utilized in some surgical and diagnostic procedures but are inappropriate for continuing analgesia.

For the child, the most painful and most feared route of administration is the intramuscular injection. Nurses often feel guilty for causing children additional pain and anxiety when they are already suffering. If nurses lose their objectivity and allow these feelings to interfere with their decision making (and thus avoid giving injections), the child may be undermedicated and suffer more pain than necessary. Admittedly, the intramuscular injection is difficult for both the nurse and the child. This route of administration can often be avoided by choosing an alternative route (e.g., oral or intravenous) of medication. However, if the alternatives are not appropriate, the nurse can minimize the impact of the experience for the child by the following means:

1. Explain what will happen and how it will feel (in terms the child can understand) immediately before the administration. Be honest and tell the child that the needle will hurt, but just for a short time. Also, tell the child that it will take some time for the medicine to help the pain get better.
2. Allow children to participate in the process by making simple decisions such as where (e.g., which hip) to have the injection.
3. Tell the child it is okay to cry.
4. Allow a parent to be present to hold (but not restrain) and comfort the child.
5. Use a topical anesthetic to minimize injection pain.
6. Praise the child for enduring the procedure and use rewards such as smiley-faced bandages or finger puppets.

Deciding upon the Dose

Often analgesic medications are ordered with a range of possible dosages, e.g., "morphine sulfate, 2 to 3 mg IV q 1 to 2 hours." Determination of the dosage to administer from this range is an important nursing responsibility. Decisions should be based upon an accurate understanding of the range ordered in comparison to the recommended therapeutic range for that drug (Foster and Hester, in press).

Administering analgesics to children is different from administering pain medications to adults because it is more difficult to determine the *relative dose* of medication being given. Whereas adult doses of narcotics and other analgesics usually vary only moderately among patients, doses for children are based individually upon body weight and vary with each kilogram of difference in weight. *The only way to know the relative dose of medication being given in relation to the maximum safe dose is to calculate the dosage.* See Box 29-5 for calculations.

The nurse who administers 2 mg of morphine (as in the foregoing order) should be aware that, for this child, 2 mg is only 35 per cent of the recommended therapeutic maximum. Perhaps this is exactly the dose the nurse desires; for example, it may be known that higher doses oversedate this particular child. However, if 2 mg is repeatedly administered for severe pain even though it fails to relieve the pain, the dosage decision is in error. The point is that 2 mg is not an appropriate dose simply because it falls within the range ordered. *Dosage determination requires professional decision making.*

Planning the Dosage Schedule

The nurse often has the opportunity to participate in the planning of the analgesic dosage schedule for patients. Two possible dosage schedules include receiving medication only as required (p.r.n.) or on an "around-the-clock" basis. There are advantages and disadvantages to both approaches. The p.r.n. approach allows the nurse to give the patient pain medication as required or as necessary (usually with a specified minimum time frame (e.g., every 3 hours p.r.n.). The around-the-clock regimen requires that analgesia be administered at fixed intervals over a 24-hour period.

In the p.r.n. approach, nurses are required to make decisions as to when they will administer the medication within the parameters provided (usually every 3 to 4 hours p.r.n.). Careful assessment of the child's pain is made to evaluate severity, location, and cause. It is important that children not experience severe pain before receiving their analgesia. Analgesia is most effective when it is administered either prophylactically (in anticipation of pain) or when the child's pain is minimal.

In the "around-the-clock" approach, the patient's analgesia requirements are calculated (e.g., based on prior experience or a careful 24- to 48-hour pain assessment) for a 24-hour period and then divided equally to be administered at fixed intervals. This regimen is ordered for patients known to have chronic pain (e.g., from cancer), well-defined pain (after some surgeries), or severe distress. Fordyce (1976) suggests that pain medications should be given to prevent pain and therefore should be given on a regular basis. Fordyce (1976) also suggests that p.r.n. administration reinforces pain complaints. Although a prescribed regimen gives nurses less flexibility (i.e., they must give the medications according to the schedule as ordered), their input in assessing the effectiveness is crucial information needed for the health care team to make informed decisions about dosage and medication changes.

> Box 29-5
> *Calculation of Medication Ordered in Relation to Recommended Therapeutic Dose*
>
> 1. Determine the maximum recommended therapeutic dose for the drug.
> 2. Determine the child's weight in kilograms (usually available on the nursing admission history).
> 3. Calculate the maximum therapeutic dose of the drug for this child.
>
>   Example:
>   *Drug:* Acetaminophen (Tylenol) with codeine elixir
>   *Maximum recommended therapeutic dose:** 1.0 mg/kg every 3 to 4 hours (Biller and Yeager, 1987)
>   *Child's weight:* 30 kg
>   *Maximum dose for this child:*
>   1.0 mg × 30 kg = 30 mg every 3 to 4 hours.
> 4. Determine the dosage ordered.
> 5. Divide the dosage ordered by the maximum recommended dosage to determine the relationship between the dose ordered and the maximum safe dose.
>
>   Example:
>   *Drug order:* Acetaminophen (Tylenol) with codeine elixir, 20 to 30 mg q 3 to 4 hours
>   *Maximum dose:* 30 mg
>   20 mg ordered/30 mg maximum = 66% of therapeutic maximum
>   30 mg ordered/30 mg maximum = 100% of therapeutic maximum
>
>   This calculation tells the nurse that the dosage options are between 66 and 100 per cent of the maximum safe dose.
>
> *(From Foster and Hester, in press.)*
> * Calculated for codeine

Nonpharmacologic Interventions

Various nonpharmacologic interventions can also be used to help ease a child's pain. Several approaches have been employed either intuitively by parents or in a more systematic way by health care professionals. Some of the nonpharmacologic approaches include distraction, interaction with a parent, muscle relaxation, guided imagery, massage, coping skills training, hypnosis and transcutaneous electrical nerve stimulation (TENS). These approaches can often be used independently to relieve the child's suffering, but are more likely to be used in combination with pharmacologic measures for the effective relief of pain.

Distraction

Distraction is the state in which the child's attention is focused on something other than the pain or hurt. It is often used intuitively and effectively by parents or those closely associated with a particular child. Nurses can sometimes gain insight into pain relief for an individual child by closely observing the techniques used by parents. For infants, distraction may be accomplished by singing or watching a mobile. For toddlers and preschoolers, activities such as looking at a book, listening to a story, and playing with puppets or a toy

Box 29-6
A Game to Promote Muscle Contraction and Relaxation

THE BIGGEST BALLOON ON EARTH GAME

1. Have children lie on the floor "in a heap" with all muscles relaxed, like a deflated balloon.
2. Ask them to contract various muscle groups as they "inflate themselves, like a balloon full of air." As they are doing this, they should slowly stand up and stretch their arms up as high as they can.
3. Encourage children to float around the room, with arms outstretched, muscles tense, pretending they, the biggest balloon on earth, are floating around the world.
4. Tell them, the balloon has sprung a leak and the air is slowly escaping. Ask them to relax various muscle groups and slowly float to the ground.
5. Children end up "in a heap—a deflated balloon once more."

may be utilized. For school-age children and adolescents, more complex strategies may be required. Often these strategies need to be self-generated to be effective. Distraction in this older group could take the form of a discussion with a nurse, family, or friend, reading, watching television, or engaging in a quiet game. Music therapy has also been shown to be beneficial in treating pain patients (Bailey, 1986). Music, ideally, is selected by the patient. Music therapy can promote relaxation, provoke an alteration in mood, and be a vehicle for self expression. For children, music and other forms of distraction can alleviate fear and anxiety while at the same time focusing their attention on more pleasant sensations.

There is always the danger that effective use of distraction will be misinterpreted to mean that the severity of the child's pain has decreased. Some nurses may question the existence of pain if the child is seen playing a few minutes before requesting analgesia. Remember that *distraction can interrupt the perception of pain during the distracting activity, but has no action beyond that period.* When the activity ends, pain returns.

Interactions

Interaction with parents or a significant other (e.g., babysitter, nanny, grandparent, or sibling) is another naturally occurring event for children in pain. An examination of the interaction of children and their parents during a painful event provided information about the nature of parental support (Hunsberger et al, 1987). Child and parent behaviors were identified and categorized into an interaction scoring grid. Although generalizability of the findings is limited by a small sample size, the study suggests that parents are able to increase their efforts at comforting children and helping them cope as the pain increases. Specific behaviors that parents used included:

- tactile: involving direct contact, as in touching, holding, rubbing, caressing, or rocking (as well as basic care needs, such as feeding and changing infants).
- gestural: involving all forms of nonverbal communication, e.g., smiling and staying near the child.
- verbal: communication, about the pain experience (e.g., "I know it hurts") or about other, nonrelated topics.

Parents were also able to use distraction techniques or promote self-initiated distraction on the part of the child. The mere presence of the parent or significant other cannot be underrated. In a study by Jerrett (1985), children rated the presence of a parent as "the most beneficial activity and the most helpful for coping with the pain."

Relaxation

Relaxation is a widely used nonpharmacologic approach to help ease pain. It is a popular approach because it can alter the activities of the autonomic nervous system, thus affecting the pain response. Relaxation can be promoted in young children by encouraging them to cuddle a favorite toy, holding or rocking them, singing or talking in a soothing voice, or allowing them to listen to soothing music. Deep breathing and muscle relaxation are techniques that can be used with older children. Cautela and Groden (1978) have developed relaxation techniques that are specifically tailored to children.

Rhythmic breathing is a combination of distraction and relaxation. In this approach, patients are asked to stare at a pleasing object, inhale slowly and deeply, and then exhale slowly. Patients can also be asked to concentrate on how the air feels as it goes in and out of their lungs. If children are able to incorporate a more complex approach, they can be encouraged to count, do arm or leg motions, or massage the painful area (e.g., as in effleurage during preparation for childbirth).

Progressive muscle relaxation involves systematic tensing and relaxing of muscle groups. Although this may sound too complex for children, it can be utilized effectively if approached as a game. An example of a game that can be used to promote muscle contraction and relaxation is given in Box 29-6. There are also commercially produced tapes and videotapes that outline the steps in progressive relaxation, but similar effects can be achieved if the following guidelines are followed.

1. Provide a quiet environment.
2. Children should lie on their backs, close their eyes, and totally relax. They should concentrate on how it "feels" to be relaxed.
3. Have children focus on a specific muscle group (e.g., facial muscles) and tense them for 5 seconds. Have them concentrate on how it feels when the muscles are tense. Have them relax the muscles again.
4. Focus on the differences between the relaxed and the tense states.
5. Move on to another muscle group and continue this exercise in some systematic way until all muscle groups in the body have been incorporated.

Guided Imagery

If the child finds muscle relaxation exercises too difficult or too boring, guided imagery can be introduced in combination with some form of relaxation therapy or by itself. Guided imagery is similar to distraction, but it requires patients to utilize their imaginations to create pleasant images. This technique can rarely be used in children who are not capable of at least some degree of abstract thinking. If children are reluctant to try this technique it can be explained and compared to something they are familiar with—such as fantasy or daydreaming. The only difference is that imagery is selective. Children will need some assistance in choosing an image that is right for them, but they should be encouraged to pursue something that they enjoy experiencing. For example, if they enjoy swimming at the beach, this might be a useful place to start in developing a composite image. If they can be convinced to incorporate several senses, such as how the water feels, how the air smells, how the splashing sounds, and even how they look with their hair soaking wet, the exercise will be more effective in giving them mastery over their pain. Most importantly, children need to be reminded of how much fun they would be having and how good they would be feeling in the imagined scenario. Relaxation exercises may help to prepare a child for guided imagery. Questions from either the nurse or a parent may help in children's descriptions of the various sensations. Parents may also benefit from guided imagery exercises, and their participation may provide an incentive and serve as a model for the child to follow.

Massage

Another nonpharmacologic intervention is massage. As discussed earlier in relation to the gate control theory, touch or rubbing the affected part is an automatic and instinctive response to pain. Examples of this behavior include young children who rub their ear when they have an ear infection or massage their gums by gnawing on a "soother" when teething. Massage is particularly useful for treating children with chronic pain, as it relaxes their muscles as well as provides comfort and sedation. Massage can either be superficial or deep, although the latter is rarely used for children.

Coping Skills Training

An approach that is often used with children suffering from recurrent pain (e.g., headaches, stomach aches) is coping skills training. This approach combines a number of nonpharmacologic interventions (such as muscle relaxation, rhythmic breathing, and guided imagery) with the major aim of helping children to manage their stress. First of all children need to recognize what stress is and what produces it. Then they are taught how to decrease that stress using relaxation, imagery, and breathing. They also learn to engage in "invisible talking to themselves" and thought stopping. The optimal outcome is for children to obtain both pain relief and a sense of pain control (McGrath, 1983).

Hypnosis

Hypnosis is a nonpharmacologic method of pain relief that has been researched most thoroughly in children diagnosed as having cancer. Hypnosis has been shown to reduce pain during painful procedures (Hilgard and LeBaron, 1982; Kellerman et al, 1983; McGrath and deVeber, in press). Zeltzer and LeBaron (1982) compared hypnosis with a combination of deep breathing, distraction, and preparation techniques. Results of this study indicated that hypnosis reduced pain from bone marrow aspiration by a large extent and that the other methods reduced pain by a smaller, but also significant, extent. Although hypnosis has been shown to be a promising intervention for reducing pain during procedures in patients with cancer, the availability of trained personnel to perform it is limited. Self-hypnosis requires extensive training before it can be used effectively.

Transcutaneous Electrical Nerve Stimulation (TENS)

Transcutaneous electrical nerve stimulation (TENS) has been used in the United States with adult patients since the 1950's. This technique employs a small unit attached to electrodes which deliver varying degrees of electrical stimulation to cutaneous nerves, depending upon the settings for amplitude, rate, and pulse width. Patients can operate the unit themselves to control pain. TENS has been studied more extensively in adults than in children, but Dr. Joann Eland, a nurse researcher, is currently studying the use of TENS for pain in childhood.

Eland (1988) reported successful pain relief in clinical trials of TENS units for children 4 years of age and older. TENS units were tested on children with varying types of pain, including subcutaneous chemotherapy, burning paresthesia from spinal cord compression, metastasis of cancer to the ribs, phantom limb pain, herpes zoster, and infusion of amphotericin. She concluded that TENS is a promising intervention for pain in children.

Other nonpharmacologic interventions for pain relief include biofeedback and acupuncture. Although these interventions are being used with some success in adults, they have been tested less extensively in children.

Evaluating Pain Management Strategies

Intervention for pain without evaluation is not only ineffective, it may be dangerous. Responses to pain interventions will vary with each child's age, development, unique drug metabolism, emotional status, cognitive perception, and other factors. Oversedation and undersedation are equally problematic. Effective pain management requires ongoing evaluation.

In the process of evaluating pain management, the nurse should ask:

- Is there a change in the child's self-report of pain?
- Are there changes in the child's behavior, appearance, or physiologic parameters that can be attributed to pain management strategies?
- Has the client goal for pain management been met?
- If not, what changes are needed in pain management strategies?

To monitor and evaluate the relief of the child's pain, nurses may find it beneficial to use a pain flow chart. This sheet could be used to record the nurse's assessment of the child's pain (e.g., intensity, location, duration), the pharmacologic and nonpharmacologic interventions employed, and their ultimate effect. Such a record, if placed on the patient's chart (or in another prominent place) can also be used by other health professionals who make decisions about managing the child's distress (e.g., physicians who prescribe medications).

References

Abu-Saad H, Holzemer W: Measuring children's self-assessment of their pain. *Issues Compr Pediatr Nurs* 1981; 5:337–349.

Angell M: The quality of mercy. *N Engl J Med* 1982; 306:98–99.

Angulo Y, Gonzales AW: Is myelinogeny an absolute index of behavioral capability? *J Comp Neurol* 1929; 48:459.

Apley J: *The Child with Abdominal Pains.* 2nd ed. London, Blackwell, 1975.

Bailey IM: Music therapy in pain management. *J Pain Symptom Manage* 1986; 1(1):25–28.

Barr RG: Pain tolerance and developmental change in pain perception. In Levine MD, et al (eds), *Developmental Behavioral Pediatrics.* Philadelphia, WB Saunders, 1982.

Beales JG: The assessment and management of pain in children. In Karoly P, Steffer DD, O'Grady D (eds), *Child Health Psychology: Concepts and Issues.* New York, Pergamon Press, 1982.

Beales JG, Kean JH, Lennox-Holt PJ: The child's perception of the disease and the experience of pain in juvenile chronic arthritis. *J Rheumatol* 1983; 10:61–65.

Beyer J: *The Oucher: A User's Manual and Technical Report.* Evanston, IL, The Hospital Play Equipment Company, 1984.

Beyer J, Aradine C: Content validity of an instrument to measure young children's perceptions of the intensity of their pain. *J Pediatr Nurs* 1986a; 1:386–395.

Beyer J, Aradine C: The convergent and discriminant validity of a self-report measure of pain intensity for children. Unpublished manuscript, 1986b.

Beyer JE, Byers ML: Knowledge of pediatric pain: the state of the art. *Child Health Care* 1985; 13(4):150–159.

Beyer JE, DeGood DE, Ashley LC, et al: Patterns of postoperative analgesic use with adults and children following cardiac surgery. *Pain* 1983; 17:71–81.

Beyer J, Knapp T: Methodological issues in the measurement of children's pain. *Child Health Care* 1986; 14:233–246.

Bibace R, Walsh M: Editors' notes. *In* Bibace R, Walsh M (eds): *Children's Conceptions of Health, Illness and Bodily Functions.* San Francisco, Jossey-Bass, 1981.

Biller JA, Yeager AM: *The Harriet Lane Handbook.* Chicago, Year Book Medical Publishers, 1987.

Boehncke H: Pain analysis in childhood. *In* Janzen R (ed): *Pain Analysis: A Guide to Diagnosis.* Bristol, England, John Wright and Sons, 1970.

Bonica JJ: Neurophysiologic and pathologic aspects of acute and chronic pain. *Arch Surg* 1977; 112:750–761.

Bonica JJ: The need for a taxonomy. *Pain* 1979; 6:247–252.

Cannon WB: *Bodily Changes in Pain, Hunger, Fear and Rage.* New York, Appleton-Century, 1929.

Cautela JR, Groden J: Relaxation: *A Comprehensive Manual for Adults, Children and Children with Special Needs.* Champaign, IL, Research Press, 1978.

Chapman CR, Bonica JJ: *Acute Pain.* Kalamazoo, MI, Upjohn, 1983. (Current Concepts Series.)

Chapman CR, Turner JA: Psychological control of acute pain medical settings. *J Pain Symptom Manage* 1986; 1(1):9–20.

Crook J: Concepts of pain and their relationship to measurement issues. *In* Copp LA (ed): *Perspective on Pain.* Edinburgh, Churchill Livingstone, 1985.

Crue BL: Foreword. *In* Aronoff GM (ed): *Evaluation and Treatment of Chronic Pain.* Baltimore, Urban and Schwarzenberg, 1985.

Crue BL, Carregal EJA: Pain begins in the dorsal horn—with a proposed classification of the primary senses. *In* Crue BL (ed): *Pain: Research and Treatment.* New York, Academic Press, 1975.

Dale JC: A multidimensional study of infants' responses to painful stimuli. *Pediatr Nurs* 1986; 12(1): 27–31.

DiLeo J: *Children's Drawings as Diagnostic Aids.* New York, Brunner/Mazel, 1973.

Dunn-Geier BJ, McGrath PJ, Rourke BP, et al: Adolescent chronic pain: The ability to cope. *Pain* 1986; 26:23–32.

Eland JM: *Children's Communication of Pain.* Unpublished master's thesis. Ames, University of Iowa, 1974.

Eland JM: Minimizing pain associated with prekindergarten intramuscular injections. *Issues Compr Pediatr Nurs* 1981; 361–372.

Eland JM: Children's pain: Developmentally appropriate efforts to improve identification of source, intensity, and relevant intervening variables. *In* Feldon G, Albert M (eds): *Nursing Research: A Monograph for Non-nurse Researchers.* Iowa City, University of Iowa Press, 1983.

Eland JM: The role of the nurse in children's pain. *In* Copp LA (ed): *Perspective on Pain.* Edinburgh, Churchill Livingstone, 1985.

Eland JM: The use of transcutaneous electrical nerve stimulation with children in pain. Paper presented at a national conference, Key Aspects of Comfort: Management of Pain, Fatigue, and Nausea, Chapel Hill, NC, Mar 1988.

Eland JM, Anderson JE: The experience of pain in children. *In* Jacox A (ed): *Pain: A Sourcebook for Nurses and Other Health Professionals.* Boston, Little, Brown, 1977.

Escobar PL: Management of chronic pain. *Nurse Pract* 1985 Jan: 24–32.

Fabrega H, Tyma S: Language and cultural influences in the description of pain. *Br J Med Psychol* 1976: 49:349–371.

Flechsig P: *Anatomie des Menchilchen Gehirns und Ruchenmarks* (Anatomy of the Human Brain and Spinal Cord). Leipzig, 1920.

Fordyce WE: *Behavioral Methods for Chronic Pain and Illness.* St. Louis, CV Mosby, 1976.

Foster RL, Hester NO: The relationship between assessment and pharmacologic interventions for pain in children. *In Key Aspects of Comfort: Management of Pain, Fatigue, and Nausea.* New York, Springer Publishing Company, in press.

Franck LS: A new method to quantitatively describe pain behavior in infants. *Nurs Res* 1986; 35(1):28–31.

Fuller BF, Horri Y, Conner D: Acoustic assessment of infant pain and arousal. Paper presented at a national conference, Key Aspects of Comfort: Management of Pain, Fatigue, and Nausea. Chapel Hill, NC, Mar 1988.

Gaffney A, Dunne EA: Developmental aspects of children's definition of pain. *Pain* 1986; 26(1):105–117.

Gaffney A, Dunne EA: Children's understanding of the causality of pain. *Pain* 1987; 29:91–104.

Gilman AG, Goodman LS, Rall TW, et al (eds): *Goodman and Gilman's The Pharmacological Basis of Therapeutics.* 7th ed. New York, Macmillan, 1985.

Graef JW, Cone TE (eds): *Manual of Pediatric Therapeutics.* 3rd ed. Toronto, Little, Brown, 1985.

Gross S, Gardner G: Child pain: Treatment approaches. *In* Smith W, Merskey H, Gross S (eds): *Pain: Meaning and Management.* New York, S.P. Medical and Scientific Books, 1980.

Grunau R, Craig K: Pain expression in neonates: Facial action and cry. *Pain* 1987; 28:395–410.

Hawley DD: Postoperative pain in children: Misconceptions, descriptions and interventions. *Pediatr Nurs* 1984; 10:20–23.

Hendler N: The anatomy and psychopharmacology of chronic pain. *J Clin Psychiatr* 1982; 43:15–20.

Hester NO: The preoperational child's reaction to immunizations. *Nurs Res* 1979; 28:250–254.

Hester NO: Comforting the child in pain. *In Key Aspects of Comfort: Management of Pain, Fatigue, and Nausea.* New York, Springer Publishing Company, in press.

Hester NO, Barcus CS: Assessment and management of pain in children. *Pediatr Nurs Update* 1986; 1(14):2–7.

Hester NO, Foster RL: Generalizability of procedures assessing pain in children. Unpublished data, 1988.

Hilgard JR, LeBaron S: Relief of anxiety and pain in children and adolescents with cancer: Quantitative measures and clinical observations. *Int J Clin Exp Hypnosis* 1982; 30:417–442.

Hunsberger M, Love B, Byrne C: A review of current approaches used to help children and parents cope with health care procedures. *Matern Child Nurs J* 1984; 13(3):145–165.

Hunsberger M, Stevens B, Browne G: *Children's Pain: A Stimulus for Parent-Child Interaction.* Paper presented at the 2nd International Nursing Research Symposium on Clinical Care of the Child and Family, Montreal, March 1987.

Huskisson EC: Visual analogue scales. *In* Melzack R (ed): *Pain Measurement and Assessment.* New York, Raven Press, 1983.

International Association for the Study of Pain, Subcommittee on Taxonomy: Pain terms, a list with definitions and notes on usage. *Pain* 1979; 6:249–252.

Izard CE, Buechler S: Emotion expressions and personality integration in infancy. *In* Izard CE (ed): *Emotions in Personality and Psychopathology.* New York, Plenum Press, 1979.

Jaffe JH, Martin WR: Opioid analgesics and antagonists. *In* Gilman AG, Goodman LS, Rall TW, et al (eds): *Goodman and Gilman's The Pharmacological Basis of Therapeutics.* 7th ed. New York, Macmillan, 1985.

Jay SM, Elliott C: Behavioural observation scales for measuring children's distress: The effects of increased methodological rigor. *J Consult Clin Psychol* 1984; 52:1106–1107.

Jay SM, Ozolins M, Elliott C, et al: Assessment of children's distress during painful medical procedures. *J Health Psychol* 1983; 2:133–147.

Jeans ME: The measurement of pain in children. *In* Melzack R (ed): *Pain Measurement and Assessment.* New York, Raven Press, 1983.

Jeans ME, Gordon DJ: *Developmental Characteristics of the Concept of Pain.* Paper presented at the 3rd World Congress on Pain, Edinburgh, Scotland, 1981.

Jerrett MD: Children and their pain experience. *Child Health Care* 1985; 14(2):83–89.

Johnson M: Assessment of clinical pain. *In* Jacox A (ed): *Pain: A Source Book for Nurses and Other Health Professionals.* Boston, Little, Brown, 1977.

Johnston CC, Strada ME: Acute pain response in infants: A multidimensional description. *Pain* 1986; 24:373–382.

Kastrup EK (ed): *Facts and Comparisons.* St. Louis, Facts and Comparisons, 1986.

Katz ER, Kellerman J, Siegel SE: Behavioral distress in children undergoing medical procedures: Developmental considerations. *J Consult Clin Psychol* 1980; 48(3):356–365.

Katz ER, Kellerman J, Siegel SE: Anxiety as an affective focus in the clinical study of acute behavioural distress: A reply to Shachman and Daut. *J Consult Clin Psychol* 1981; 49(3):470–471.

Kellerman J, Zeltzer L, Ellenberg L, et al: Adolescents with cancer: Hypnosis for the reduction of the acute pain and anxiety associated with medical procedures. *J Adol Health Care* 1983; 4:85–90.

Knoben JE, Anderson PO: *Handbook of Clinical Drug Data.* Hamilton, IL, Drug Intelligence Publications, 1983.

Kushner HS: When children and adults suffer. *Child Health Care* 1985; 14(2):68–75.

Lamonica EL: *The Nursing Process: A Humanistic Approach.* Menlo Park, CA, Addison-Wesley Publishing Company, 1979.

Langworthy OR: Development of behaviour patterns and myelinization of the nervous system in the human fetus and infant. *Carnegie Contrib Embryol* 1933; 24:3.

Lazarus RS: The stress and coping paradigm. *In* Bond LA, Rozen JC (eds): *Competence and Coping During Adulthood.* Hanover, NH, University Press of New England, 1980.

Levine JD, Gordon NC: Pain in prelingual children and its evaluation by pain-induced vocalization. *Pain* 1982; 14:85–93.

Lindahl O: Treatment of pain by changing the acid-base balance. *In* Bonica JJ (ed): *Advances in Neurology: International Symposium on Pain.* New York, Raven Press, 1974.

Lollar DJ, Smits SJ, Patterson DL: Assessment of pediatric pain: An empirical perspective. *J Pediatr Psychol* 1982; 7:267–277.

Marchall HR: *Pain, Pleasure, and Anesthesia.* New York, Macmillan, 1984.

Mather L, Mackie J: The incidence of post operative pain in children. *Pain* 1983; 15:271–282.

McCaffery M: *Nursing Management of the Patient with Pain.* Philadelphia, JB Lippincott, 1972.

McCaffery M: Pain relief for the child. *Pediatr Nurs* 1977; 3(4):11–16.

McCaffery M: Pain control in children. *In* Henning JS (ed): *The Rights of Children.* Springfield, IL, Charles C Thomas, 1982.

McEvoy AK (ed): *American Hospital Formulary Service Drug Information.* Bethesda, MD, American Society of Hospital Pharmacists, 1986.

McGrath P: Psychological aspects of recurrent abdominal pain. *Can Fam Physician* 1983; 29:1655–1659.

McGrath P, Cunningham S, Goodman J, et al: The clinical measurement of pain in children: A review. *Clin J Pain,* 1985.

McGrath P, Johnson G, Goodman JT, et al: The Children's Hospital of Eastern Ontario Pain Scale (CHEOPS): A behavioural scale for rating post-operative pain in children. *In* Fields HL, Dubner R, Cervera F (eds): *Advances in Pain Research and Therapy.* Vol 9. New York, Raven Press, 1985.

McGrath P, Unruh A: *Pain in Children and Adolescents.* New York, Elsevier (in press).

McGrath PA, DeVeber LL, Hearn MT: Multidimensional pain assessment in children. *In* Fields HL, Dubner R, Cervera F (eds): *Advances in Pain Research and Therapy.* Vol 9. New York, Raven Press, 1985.

McGrath PA, DeVeber LL: The management of acute pain evoked by medical procedures in children with cancer. *J Pain Symptom Manage* (in press).

McGrath PJ, Dunn-Geier J, Cunningham SJ, et al: Psychological guidelines for helping children cope with chronic benign intractable pain. *Clin J Pain* 1986; 1:229–233.

Meichenbaum D, Turk D, Burnstein S: The nature of coping with stress. *In* Sarason IG, Spielberger CD (eds): *Stress and Anxiety.* Vol. 2. New York, Wiley, 1975.

Melamed BG, Siegel LJ: Reduction of anxiety in children facing surgery by modeling. *J Consult Clin Psychol* 1975; 43:511–521.

Melzack R: *The Puzzle of Pain.* New York, Basic Books, 1973.

Melzack R: The McGill pain questionnaire: Major properties and scoring methods. *Pain* 1975; 1:277–299.

Melzack R: *Pain Measurement and Assessment.* New York, Raven Press, 1983.

Melzack R, Wall P: Pain mechanisms: A new theory. *Science* 1965; 150:971–979.

Melzack R, Wall P: *The Challenge of Pain.* New York, Basic Books, 1982.

Miller RR, Jick H: Clinical effects of meperdine in hospitalized medical patients. *J Clin Pharmacol* 1978; 18(4):180–189.

Molsberry D: *Young Children's Subjective Qualifications of Pain Following Surgery.* Unpublished master's thesis, University of Iowa, 1979.

Mountcastle VB: Pain and temperature sensibilities. *In* Mountcastle VB (ed): *Medical Physiology.* St. Louis, CV Mosby, 1975.

Owens ME: Pain in infancy: Conceptual and methodological issues. *Pain* 1984; 20:213–230.

Owens ME, Todd EH: Pain in infancy: Neonatal reaction to a heel lance. *Pain* 1984; 20:77–86.

Peiper A: *Cerebral Function in Infancy and Childhood.* New York, Consultants Bureau, 1963.

Peterson RG: Antipyretics and analgesics in children. *Dev Pharmacol Ther* 1985; 8(1):68–84.

Piaget J: *The Early Growth of Logic in the Child.* New York, WW Norton, 1969.

Porter J, Jick H: Addiction rare in patients treated with narcotics. *N Engl J Med* 1980; 303(2):123.

Ross DM, Ross SA: Childhood pain: The school-aged child's viewpoint. *Pain* 1984; 20:179–191.

Ross DM, Ross SA: *Childhood Pain. Current Issues, Research, and Management.* Baltimore, Urban and Schwarzenberg, 1988.

Savedra M, Tesler M, Ward, J, et al: Description of the pain experience: A study of school-age children. *Issues Compr Pediatr Nurs* 1981; 5:373–380.

Schecter NL: Pain and pain control in children. *Curr Probl Pediatr* 1985; 15:6–66.

Schroeder P: *A Descriptive Study of Pain Associated with Therapeutic Procedures in the Burned School-age Child.* Unpublished thesis, University of Cincinnati, 1983.

Scott R: It hurts red: A preliminary study of children's perceptions of pain. *Percept Mot Skills* 1978; 47:787–791.

Sheredy C: Factors to consider when assessing responses to pain. *MCN* 1984 Jul/Aug; 9(4):250–252.

Shirkey HC: *Pediatric Drug Handbook.* Philadelphia, WB Saunders, 1977.

Snyder SH: Opiate receptors and internal opiates. *Sci Am* 1977; 236:44–56.

Sternback RW: *Pain: A Psychophysiological Analysis.* New York, Academic Press, 1968.

Stevens BJ, Hunsberger M, Browne G: Pain in children: Theoretical, research and practice dilemmas. *J Pediatr Nurs* 1987 May/June; 3:154–166.

Stewart ML: Measurement of clinical pain. *In* Jacox A (ed): *A Source Book for Nurses and Other Health Care Professionals.* Boston, Little, Brown, 1977.

Taylor PL: Postoperative pain in toddler and pre-school age children. *Matern Child Nurs J* 1983; 12:35–50.

Trissel LA: *Handbook of Injectable Drugs.* 4th Ed. Bethesda, MD, American Society of Hospital Pharmacists, 1986.

Unruh A, McGrath P, Cunningham SJ, et al: Children's drawings of their pain. *Pain* 1983; 17:385–392.

Varni JW, Katz ER, Dash J: Behavioural and neurochemical aspects of pediatric pain. *In* Russo DC, Varni JW (eds): *Behavioural Pediatrics: Research and Practice.* New York, Plenum Press, 1982.

Volpe J: *Neurology of the Newborn.* Philadelphia, WB Saunders, 1981.

Wachter-Shikora NL: Pain theories and their relevance to the pediatric population. *Issues Compr Pediatr Nurs* 1981; 5:321–326.

Willis D, Elliott C, Jay S: Psychological effects of physical illness and its concomitants. *In* Tuma J (ed): *Handbook for the Practice of Pediatric Psychology.* New York, John Wiley and Sons, 1982.

Woolf BB: Laboratory methods of pain measurement. *In* Melzack R (ed): *Pain Measurement and Assessment.* New York, Raven Press, 1983.

Zeltzer L, LeBaron S: Hypnotic and non-hypnotic techniques for the reduction of pain and anxiety during painful procedures in children and adolescents with cancer. *J Pediatr* 1982; 101:1032–1035.

Bibliography

Ahman E: The child at home with chronic pain. *MCN* 1984 Jul/Aug; 9(4):264–266.

Beyer JE, Levin CR: Issues and advances in pain control in children. *Nurs Clin North Am* 1987 Sep; 22(3):661–676.

Bradshaw C, Zeanah PD: Pediatric nurses' assessments of pain in children. *J Pediatr Nurs* 1986 Oct; 1(5):314–322.

Burokas L: Factors affecting nurses' decisions to medicate pediatric patients after surgery. *Heart Lung* 1985 Jul; 14(4):373–376.

Cotanch PH, Harrison M, Roberts J: Hypnosis as an intervention for pain control. *Nurs Clin North Am* 1987 Sep; 22(3):699–704.

Coyle N: Analgesics and pain. Current concepts. *Nurs Clin North Am* 1987 Sep; 22(3):727–741.

Dale JC: A multidimensional study of infants' responses to painful stimuli. *Pediatr Nurs* 1986 Jan/Feb; 12(1):27–31.

D'Apolito K: The neonates response to pain. *MCN* 1984 Jul/Aug; 9(4):256–257.

Forlini J, Morin DM, Treacy S: Painless peds procedures. *Am J Nurs* 1987 Mar; 321–323.

Kleiman RL, et al: PCA vs. regular IM injections for severe postop pain. *Am J Nurs* 1987 Nov; 1491–1492.

Kline J: Recovery room care for the child in pain. *MCN* 1984 Jul/Aug; 9(4):261–264.

Lisson EL: Ethical issues related to pain control. *Nurs Clin North Am* 1987 Sep; 22(3):649–659.

McCaffery M: Giving meperidine for pain. Should it be so mechanical? *Nurs 87* 1987 Apr; 17(4):61–64.

National Institutes of Health Consensus Development Conference: Statement: The integrated approach to the management of pain. 1986; 6(3).

Olsson F, Parker G: A model approach to pain assessment. *Nurs 87* 1987 May; 52–57.

Paice JA: New delivery systems in pain management. *Nurs Clin North Am* 1987 Sep; 22(3):715–726.

Pridham KF, Adelson F, Hansen MF: Helping children deal with procedures in a clinic setting: a developmental approach. *J Pediatr Nurs* 1987 Feb; 2(1):13–22.

Scott JG, Rigney-Radford K: Factors affecting the management of pain. *MCN* 1984 Jul/Aug; 9(4)253–255.

Wright SM: The use of therapeutic touch in the management of pain. *Nurs Clin North Am* 1987 Sep; 22(3):705–714.

Zollo M: Management of pain in critically ill children. *MCN* 1984 Jul/Aug; 9(4):258–261.

Principles of Fluid and Electrolyte Maintenance

Chapter 30

Joan Meighan Rimar

Related Topics
Principles and skills, Chapter 27
Pharmacologic principles, Chapter 28
Altered digestive function, Chapter 41

Although alterations of function elicit predictable physiologic responses to compensate for deficits and excesses, in children developmental differences can alter the efficiency and magnitude of the body's compensatory mechanisms.

Specific illnesses that commonly result in fluid and electrolyte or acid-base imbalances are not discussed in this chapter but elsewhere in this text. Included here is a discussion of fluid and electrolyte balance and intravenous therapy as it applies to infants and children. Those processes that have particular significance in children and the unique characteristics of children that affect fluid and electrolyte balance will be addressed. Fluid and electrolyte balance and acid-base balance, inter-related mechanisms, are both addressed in this chapter. Relevant terms for understanding these concepts are reviewed in Box 30-1. For in-depth discussions of fluid and electrolytes, refer to basic science texts of biology, chemistry, and physiology.

Almost all illnesses in some way alter the intake, elimination, or need for water and electrolytes. The importance of this topic in children is that the status of infants and young children can change rapidly and insidiously when fluid and electrolyte imbalances occur.

Children are particularly vulnerable to such changes because

- their bodies have a higher proportionate water content (therefore more can be lost rapidly)
- a greater proportion of fluids is in the extracellular space (from which they are more easily lost)
- children have a higher metabolic turnover of water (if not replaced equally rapidly, imbalance occurs)
- homeostatic regulation is immature (renal function, buffering capacity, calcium-phosphorus regulation)

Body Water Compartments and Internal Distribution

Infants, especially premature infants, have a proportionately higher body fluid content than at any other time. Total body water (TBW) comprises 75 to 80 per cent of body weight in the full-term neonate and 90 per cent in the premature infant. This water is contained in two major compartments that are divided by the cell membrane: the cell and the extracellular space. The extracellular water includes the plasma, interstitial and lymphatic fluid, and connective tissue water.

During the first few days of life, the normal neonate loses about 5 to 10 per cent of body weight from water loss (Weil, 1982). Thereafter, the infant's rapid weight gain during the first year is primarily due to an increase in adipose tissue. Since there is an inverse relationship between total body water and total body fat, the infant's weight gain is accompanied by a proportionate reduction in fluid volume. In the 2-year-old child, both the percentage of TBW and its internal distribution approximate that of the adult. Table 30-1 compares fluid volume and its distribution at birth, at 1 year of age, and after 2 years of age.

The greater proportionate fluid volume and its internal distribution makes an infant vulnerable to substantial fluid loss. Because children under 1 year of age have a proportionately greater volume of extracellular fluid (primarily interstitial), which is lost first when loss occurs (e.g., through illness, trauma, or stressful environmental conditions), the infant is extremely susceptible to fluid and electrolyte imbalances.

Regulation of Fluids and Electrolytes

Despite wide variations in the dietary intake, volume and composition of body fluids are maintained in an extremely narrow range as excretion is adjusted to match intake (Rose, 1984). The regulatory mechanisms of the child, however, sometimes differ from those of the adult. Infants and young children are more vulnerable to rapid fluid and electrolyte imbalances than adults for various reasons, including (1) their relatively greater surface area to body mass, (2) a higher basal metabolic rate, and (3) immature kidney function.

The infant's *relative greater surface area to body mass* results in a relatively higher volume of insensible perspiration through the skin and lungs (the gastrointestinal tract is considered to be an extension of surface area). When calculating the relationship of surface area to body mass, it is found to be five times as great in premature infants and two to three times as great in a

My thanks go to Stephen Rimar, MD, for his review of this section.

Box 30-1
Fluid and Electrolyte Balance Definitions

ELECTROLYTES

Anion: An ion with a negative charge of electricity. *Example:* Chloride (Cl^-), bicarbonate (HCO_3^-).

Cation: An ion with a positive charge of electricity. *Example:* Hydrogen (H^+), sodium (Na^+), potassium (K^+), calcium (Ca^{++}) and magnesium (Mg^{++}).

Electrolyte: A substance that when placed into water dissociates into separately charged ions and conducts an electric current.

Ion: A particle carrying an electric charge, consisting of an atom or group of atoms with a positive (cation) or negative (anion) charge for each electrolyte gained or lost.

PRESSURE AND OSMOLALITY

Hydrostatic pressure: Pressure exerted by a fluid within a closed system (e.g., pressure of the blood within the capillaries).

Oncotic pressure: The osmotic pressure exerted by colloids in solution (e.g., proteins).

Osmolality: The osmotic pressure of a solution expressed in osmols or milliosmols of the dissolved substance per kilogram of solvent (water).

Osmolarity: The osmotic pressure of a solution expressed in osmols or milliosmols of the dissolved substance per liter of the solution.

Osmosis:The movement of a solvent through a semipermeable membrane to equalize the concentration of solvent on both sides.

Osmotic pressure: The pressure required to prevent the movement of solvent across a semipermeable membrane that separates two solutions of different concentrations (pressure exerted by the solutes that holds or draws back water that has escaped).

Solute: The dissolved, suspended, or solid component of a solution.

neonate compared to an older child or adult (Metheney, 1987). In infancy, evaporative loss of water through the skin and lungs consumes around 50 per cent of the water requirement (Chambers, 1987).

The *increased metabolic rate* is related to (1) their greater proportionate surface area through which heat is lost, (2) increased growth needs, and (3) a child's relatively larger viscera and brain. Since metabolic processes require water for the dissipation of heat and these processes proceed twice as quickly in children as they do in adults, the rate of water turnover in children is rapid (Weil, 1982). Without water intake, a baby would lose the water contained in the extracellular compartments in 5 days; it would take about 10 days for that to happen in an adult. Because the homeostatic mechanisms of the body are less mature in infants and small children, they are more prone to imbalances.

Gains and Losses

Any conditions that preclude normal oral intake of fluid or food (e.g., vomiting) are particularly harmful because they deplete the body's stores of water, electrolytes, acid, and base much more rapidly in infants and children than in adults (Winters, 1982). Losses accompanying fever and diarrhea also quickly deplete the child's reserves. The body surface area through which these losses occur—the skin, the lungs, and the gastrointestinal tract—is proportionately greater in children than in adults. In most situations, though, efficient regulation by other body systems, primarily the renal system, minimizes alterations in fluid and electrolyte homeostasis in children. Infants are particularly prone to imbalance because their kidneys are less mature and have limited concentrating ability. More water is therefore required to excrete a given amount of solute (Olson and Riddle, 1987).

Skin and Lung Regulation. Water is continually lost by evaporation through the interstices of the skin and by exhalation of water vapor through the lungs. The primary function of this loss is regulation of body temperature. Loss of body water by this route is called insensible water loss (IWL) because the individual does not sense its occurrence. IWL consists of pure

Table 30-1. Approximate Total Body Water and Internal Water Distribution at Birth, 1 Year, and After 2 Years of Age

	Percentage of Total Body Weight		
	At Birth	At 1 Year	After 2 Years
Extracellular (plasma and interstitial)*	40–45	30	20–25
Intracellular†	30–35	35	35
Total Body Water	75–80	65	55–60

* The plasma portion of extracellular fluid remains relatively constant. The major difference in the newborn infant is in interstitial fluid.

† Shows relatively small variation after birth and is essentially constant after 1 year of age.

(From Winters, 1973.)

water—there are no electrolytes. Abnormal conditions, such as those that cause hyperventilation (e.g., salicylate poisoning, pneumonia) may triple water loss from the lungs (Finberg et al, 1982). "Sensible" water loss may also occur via the skin in the form of sweat. Sweating also helps maintain temperature, but this is an intermittent rather than a continuous process. Sweat contains sodium, chloride, and potassium in addition to water.

Gastrointestinal Regulation. The gastrointestinal tract is of particular significance in maintaining homeostasis in children. Under normal conditions there is a larger exchange of fluid in a child's gastrointestinal tract than in the adult's: water and sodium (Na^+) are reabsorbed and potassium (K^+) is excreted. Therefore, any illness that affects intestinal absorption may seriously endanger the life of a child because of large, rapid gastrointestinal losses.

Renal Regulation. Although the infant's kidneys are less mature than the adult's kidneys and cannot regulate fluids and electrolytes quite as effectively, they are ideally suited to meet the infant's homeostatic requirements under most circumstances. The capacity of the infant's kidney to dilute urine is qualitatively the same as the adult's and ability to adapt to changes in sodium intake is considerable. Excessive intake of water and Na^+, however, is not tolerated as well as their deprivation, since the cortical area of the kidney is less developed than the medullary region. This predisposes the infant to problems associated with fluid overload and hypernatremia. The kidney of the premature infant cannot retain sodium efficiently and is prone to *hyponatremia*.

Renal regulation of fluid and electrolytes is also affected by hormones that respond to changes in plasma volume and Na^+ content. The primary regulating hormone is the antidiuretic hormone (ADH), which is manufactured in the hypothalamus but stored in and released from the posterior pituitary gland. An extreme example of alteration in vascular volume that results in increased ADH secretion is the patient who is losing large amounts of blood. In this case, volume-sensitive receptors in the body sense the decrease in vascular volume and stimulate secretion of ADH. Water is then reabsorbed by the kidney and intravascular volume increases.

Electrolyte imbalances also affect ADH secretion. When the plasma Na^+ level is high, as in hypertonic dehydration (see page 899), ADH is secreted in response to a stimulus from the hypothalamus, and the kidney conserves water to help restore electrolyte balance. On the other hand, when the plasma Na^+ levels are low, as can occur when patients are given large amounts of electrolyte-free intravenous solutions, the system is reversed: ADH secretion is inhibited and the result is diuresis. Thus ADH decreases urine volume (conserves water), and lack of ADH increases urine volume (promotes water loss). Pain and anxiety can also increase ADH secretion, as do some drugs (morphine, barbiturates, many anesthetic agents) (Finberg et al, 1982).

Additional renal regulation is accomplished through the renin-angiotensin system and aldosterone. Reduced blood flow to the kidney stimulates a specialized area in the glomerulus to secrete renin. Renin in turn generates angiotensin (angiotensin is produced from the plasma globulin angiotensinogen) within the blood vessels. Angiotensin constricts vessels and restores blood pressure and blood flow. The release of the adrenal hormone aldosterone is also stimulated by angiotensin. Aldosterone promotes increased blood pressure by enhancing Na^+ and water reabsorption from the renal tubules, thereby increasing vascular volume.

Cardiovascular Regulation. Proper functioning of the cardiovascular system depends upon adequate cardiac activity, intact vasculature, and sufficient volume, composition, and fluidity of blood. Alterations in any of these affect the entire organism, and if they are diffuse and severe, the organism dies. An intact circulatory system facilitates maintenance of water and Na^+ balance, but it requires reasonably normal levels of water and Na^+ to function adequately. A primary problem with either the system or the fluid and electrolyte balance can adversely affect the other, which in turn can make the primary problem worse. Fortunately the reverse is also true—improvement in one usually leads to improvement of the other.

Internal Transport of Fluids and Electrolytes

Water and electrolytes are continually exchanged between the different fluid compartments of the body. This is accomplished by active and passive mechanisms. Passive movement of fluid and particles develops spontaneously and does not require a supply of metabolic energy. Active transport, on the other hand, depends upon energy derived from metabolic processes. All movement of water in the body is passive, whereas solute movement occurs by both active and passive mechanisms (Rose, 1984).

Movement of Water: Hydrostatic and Osmotic/Oncotic Pressure. The movement of water between different fluid compartments is determined by hydrostatic pressure and osmotic pressure. The highest hydrostatic pressures in the body are in the vascular space, most importantly in the capillaries, and are generated by the contraction of the heart. Capillary hydrostatic pressure is a function of arterial pressure, resistance at the precapillary sphincter, and venous pressure. This mechanical force, if unopposed, pushes plasma fluid from the capillaries (the area of higher pressure) into the interstitium (the area of lower pressure). Plasma volume, however, is preserved by the opposing osmotic forces generated by plasma proteins.

Osmosis is the movement of a solvent through a membrane to equalize the concentration of solvent on both sides (Finberg et al, 1982). Osmotic pressure is generated in cellular and extracellular fluid by exchangeable solutes, notably Na^+ and K^+, and is proportional to the number of particles per unit volume of solvent. Each unit of osmotic pressure is an osmol. *Osmolality** (particle concentration per kilogram of water) is measured in milliosmols (mOsm). When osmolality in one fluid compartment is altered, the resultant concentration gradient causes water to shift; water diffuses passively from an area of lesser concentration of solutes to an area of greater concentration of solutes. Hypernatremia (increased serum Na^+), for example, results in water shift from the intracellular to the extracellular space, whereas hyponatremia (decreased serum Na^+) results in the opposite movement.

Osmolality, or tonicity, is an important characteristic of intravenous fluids. When intravenous fluid is added to blood and causes no change in the size of red blood cells (because it has approximately the same osmolality as the cell), the fluid is said to be isotonic. Hypertonic solution has a higher osmolality than the red blood cells and causes fluid to leave the cell and the cell to shrink. Hypotonic fluid causes cells to swell because water enters them. Examples of hypotonic, isotonic and hypertonic solutions are 0.45 per cent sodium chloride, 0.9 per cent sodium chloride, and 3 per cent sodium chloride, respectively.

Plasma oncotic pressure, a type of osmotic pressure, is created by plasma proteins and effectively balances capillary hydrostatic pressure (Rose, 1984). Under normal conditions hydrostatic and osmotic pressures are balanced. When capillary hydrostatic pressure increases or plasma oncotic pressure decreases, however, the result is an accumulation of fluid in the interstitial space (edema). In allergic conditions or burns, plasma oncotic pressure is decreased because capillary membrane integrity is altered and fluid follows leaking protein into the interstitial space.

Movement of Electrolytes. Electrolytes, such as Na^+, are transported across cell membranes by a variety of mechanisms. When these solutes move in the presence of a favorable concentration and/or electrical gradient (e.g., when they simply move from an area of greater solute concentration to an area of lesser solute concentration—"downhill movement"), passive mechanisms suffice. If solutes must move *against* gradients ("uphill movement"), active mechanisms are employed—energy is required.

Passive transport of solute across a membrane occurs in three ways:

1. Diffusion
   a. Simple diffusion: solutes freely move across a membrane until their concentration is equal on either side and until electroneutrality across the membrane is obtained
   b. Facilitated diffusion: solute-specific carriers exist on some cell membranes, and, when present, they facilitate more rapid diffusion of the solute than occurs during simple diffusion
2. Coupled transport: a carrier recognizes two solutes and promotes the transport of both across the membrane, and
3. Solvent drag: when water moves across a membrane because of an osmotic pressure gradient, frictional forces between the water and the solutes it contains results in membrane-permeable solutes being carried along with the water (Rose, 1984).

Active transport of solutes also occurs in three ways:

1. Primary active transport: mechanisms, such as the Na^+-K^+-ATPase pump* (or "sodium pump"), release energy to facilitate or prevent movement of solutes in one direction or the other
2. Secondary active transport: energy provided by some reactions (e.g., hydrolysis of ATP to ADP) may allow the co-transport of another solute against its concentration gradient, without the usual direct energy requirement
3. Endocytosis: a portion of a cell membrane can invaginate around a particle that is too large (e.g., insulin in the proximal tubule of the kidney) to cross the membrane directly and incorporate it into the cell; the energy for endocytosis is supplied by the hydrolysis of ATP (Rose, 1984).

Fluid and Electrolyte Imbalances

Numerous childhood illnesses cause fluid and electrolyte imbalances. However, the great majority of disturbances in hydration and electrolyte balance occur secondary to vomiting and diarrhea (Weil, 1982).

---

* The terms *osmolality* and *osmolarity* are used interchangeably in clinical practice because they are approximately equal although they are defined slightly differently. Osmolarity is expressed in terms of concentration of solute per unit of total volume of solution (rather than concentration of solute per unit of solvent).

* A system for active transport of sodium and potassium across cell membranes that is regulated by the enzyme sodium-potassium–activated adenosine triphosphate. The enzyme catalyzes hydrolysis of the high-energy compound ATP into the lower-energy compound adenosine diphosphate (ADP). The energy released by this reaction is used to transport the Na^+ and K^+ (Kaehny and Gabow, 1980).

Fluid and electrolyte imbalances occur when there is a total body deficit or excess of fluids and electrolytes or when the normal relationship between fluids and electrolytes has been altered. In many instances a disturbance exists in both the total body volume as well as fluid and electrolyte proportions. Edema and dehydration are two common fluid imbalances that occur in children and are often associated with electrolyte abnormalities.

Edema

Edema is a palpable swelling produced by an increase in interstitial fluid volume (Rose, 1984). The development of edema occurs with

- *Increased capillary hydrostatic pressure.* When hydrostatic pressure in the capillary exceeds the opposing forces in the extravascular space, fluid shifts from the vessel to the interstitial space.
  (Edema related to increased capillary hydrostatic pressure is seen in heart failure, renal failure, acute pulmonary edema and with the administration of many antihypertensive and nonsteroidal anti-inflammatory drugs.)
- *Decreased plasma oncotic pressure.* Excessive loss of protein, particularly albumin, results in a decrease in the oncotic pressure of plasma while the capillary hydrostatic pressure (that is normally balanced by the oncotic pressure) remains the same; the net effect of this alteration in the balance of oncotic and hydrostatic pressure is a shift of fluid to the interstitium.
  (Protein loss is associated with nephrotic syndrome and protein-losing enteropathy; reduced albumin synthesis occurs in liver disease and malnutrition.)
- *Increased capillary permeability.* Edema develops in the presence of increased capillary permeability, because (1) fluid can simply leak into the tissue when the integrity of the membrane has been altered, and (2) albumin also can move to the interstitium and pull fluid with it.
  (Burns, trauma, inflammation, allergic reactions, and adult respiratory distress syndrome disrupt the capillary membrane and increase capillary permeability.)
- *Increased interstitial oncotic pressure.* Small amounts of protein are usually filtered across the capillary and then returned to the circulation via the lymphatics. Under certain circumstances, however, proteins enter the interstitial space more quickly than they leave. Accumulation of proteins causes increased interstitial oncotic pressure. This promotes migration of fluid into tissue.
  (Lymphatic obstruction from tumors, hypothyroidism, and increased capillary permeability results in increased interstitial oncotic pressure.)

Dehydration and Sodium Imbalance

Dehydration occurs when body fluids are lost in excess of fluid gained. Common alterations that result in dehydration are due to disturbances in

- the gastrointestinal tract (vomiting, diarrhea, malabsorption, pyloric stenosis)
- the skin (burns)
- metabolism (fever, diabetes mellitus)
- the lungs (tachypnea, as in bronchiolitis)

Dehydration is often associated with Na^+ imbalance. Only isotonic dehydration occurs without this electrolyte imbalance. For this reason, isotonic dehydration will be discussed alone, but hypotonic and hypertonic dehydration will be considered as they relate to Na^+ imbalance. Management of specific problems that result in dehydration and associated electrolyte imbalance is also discussed with the various conditions throughout the text.

Isotonic Dehydration. This condition occurs when fluids and electrolytes are lost in approximately the same proportion as they exist in the body. In this type of dehydration there is no fluid shift because body fluid osmolality is not affected. There simply is a deficit of total body water. This is the most common type of dehydration encountered; it is seen in about 70 per cent of children with acute dehydration due to diarrhea (Dube, 1978). Signs associated with isotonic dehydration include increased heart rate, sunken eyes, dry mucosa, cool and mottled extremities, loss of elasticity of skin, lack of tears, weak cry, decreased urine output, and, in infants, sunken fontanel.

Hypertonic and Hypotonic Dehydration and Sodium Imbalance. Sodium imbalance exists when the plasma Na^+ level is either greater than 147 (hypernatremia) or less than 137 mEq/L (hyponatremia). Because the osmolality of the extracellular and the intracellular fluids is determined almost entirely by the extracellular fluid Na^+ concentration, alterations in Na^+ balance are almost always a reflection of abnormal water balance. A water decrease or extracellular sodium excess (hypernatremia) is a *hyperosmolar* disturbance. A water increase or extracellular sodium decrease (hyponatremia) is a *hypo-osmolar* disturbance.

Hypernatremia/Hypertonic Dehydration (Hypernatremic Dehydration). When there is decreased intake of water, increased intake of Na^+, or a proportionately greater loss of water than Na^+, this serious condition results. It can be produced when insensible water loss from the skin and respiratory tract is high, or by any clinical condition that depletes the body of water. The proportional excess of Na^+ increases the osmotic pressure of the blood, and so fluid shifts from the intracellular to the extracellular spaces. The normal defenses against this occurrence are the stimulation of thirst (i.e., intake of water) and the release of antidiuretic hormone (i.e., conservation of water by the kidneys). Infants, however, who likely have intact thirst mechanisms, cannot take advantage of this particular defense because they are unable to ask for water.

Approximately 10 to 20 per cent of infants hospitalized with dehydration have serum Na^+ values in excess of 150 mEq/L, and 90 per cent of this group are hypernatremic secondary to diarrhea (Paneth, 1980). If improper fluid therapy is initiated in patients with hypernatremia, seizures may occur because rapid rehydration may cause significant fluid shift and brain cells to swell. Mortality can be high. Early neurologic symptoms (marked lethargy and irritability on stimulation) may herald this serious complication.

Other conditions that may contribute to hypernatremia include the administration of hypertonic Na^+ intravenous fluids (Na^+ concentration > 0.9 per cent) or tube feedings with high Na^+ concentrations. Diabetes insipidus, which is characterized by complete or partial failure of ADH or of renal response to ADH, also results in hypernatremia if urine output is not quickly replaced. Conditions in which there may be significant insensible loss of water, such as burns, fever, and respiratory infections, may raise serum Na^+ levels. Circulatory disturbances are usually absent in hypertonic dehydration because of the relative increase in vascular volume.

Hyponatremia/Hypotonic Dehydration. When there is loss of Na^+ or retention of water, hyponatremia results. Water retention resulting in hyponatremia occurs almost exclusively when there is a defect in renal water excretion. Excretion is impaired in

1. effective circulating volume depletion (vomiting, diarrhea, tube drainage, bleeding, and intestinal obstruction),
2. renal failure,
3. diuretic therapy (thiazides, furosemide, and ethacrynic acid), and
4. presence of antidiuretic hormone (syndrome of inappropriate antidiuretic hormone secretion).

Hyponatremia occurs commonly in those who receive disproportionately large amounts of electrolyte-free solutions (often plain water) (Wink, 1983). The improper fluid can be given orally (too much plain water to a sick child or a postoperative patient), parenterally (intravenous fluid without sodium in it to the patient who is NPO), or rectally (tap water enemas, rather than isotonic saline ones). Even water inhaled by an infant or child in a mist tent or incubator can result in hyponatremia. On the other hand, children with cystic fibrosis may have normal water content in the body, but they excrete abnormally high amounts of Na^+ in their sweat. Regardless of the cause, the lack of sufficient Na^+ to keep water from entering the cells results in water shifting from the extracellular spaces to the intracellular spaces, where Na^+ concentration is higher. If a child is dehydrated as well as hyponatremic (i.e., hypotonic dehydration), blood pressure may be reduced and the child may border on circulatory collapse. Hypotonic dehydration is present in only about 10 per cent of dehydrated children (Metheney, 1987).

Another important cause of hyponatremia in the pediatric population is the syndrome of inappropriate antidiuretic hormone secretion (SIADH). In SIADH, ADH secretion is not due to the usual physiologic stimuli of hyperosmolality or hypovolemia. Instead, decreased venous return to the heart with stimulation of thoracic volume receptors results in water retention and subsequent hyponatremia. The stimulation may be secondary to severe.pneumonia; stimulation of the pituitary in disorders of the central nervous system, such as meningitis; head trauma or subarachnoid hemorrhage; or direct release of ADH by drugs (e.g., morphine, barbiturates, and vincristine). This syndrome can occur only when water is not restricted (Zucker and Chernow, 1983).

Potassium Imbalance

Potassium has two major physiologic functions: (1) it plays an important role in cell metabolism, participating in regulating protein and glycogen synthesis, and (2) the ratio of K^+ concentrations in the cell and the extracellular fluid is the major determinant of the resting potential across the cell membrane. The latter function helps produce normal neural and muscular function. When the plasma K^+ level is either excessive (hyperkalemia) or deficient (hypokalemia), a serious imbalance exists. The normal plasma K^+ level ranges from 4.0 to 5.6 mEq/L.

Absorption of dietary K^+ occurs readily from the small intestine. Ninety-five per cent of the body's potassium is found in intracellular fluid. The distribution of K^+ is maintained by movement of K^+ into the cells and urinary excretion of the net dietary intake. These processes are mediated by a variety of factors, including the Na^+-K^+-ATPase pump, catecholamines, insulin, and the plasma K^+ concentration. The plasma K^+ concentration is also influenced by pH. In acidemic states, some of the excess H^+ moves into the cell to be buffered, so K^+ moves out to maintain electroneutrality (i.e., equal electrical charges on both sides of the cell membrane). The result is an increased plasma K^+ concentration. This change is of most concern in some forms of metabolic acidosis due to an increase of mineral acid, as in renal failure or diarrhea, because plasma K^+ can increase 0.2 to 1.7 mEq/L for each 0.1 unit fall in blood pH in such situations. This shift is reversed in alkalemia but the change in the plasma K^+ level is less prominent (Rose, 1974). Immediate attention and constant surveillance are warranted whenever K^+ imbalance is suspected in infants and children.

Hyperkalemia. This excess of K^+ in the blood is due to increased intake of K^+, inadequate excretion of K^+, shift of K^+ from within the cells to the extracellular compartments, congenital adrenal hyperplasia, or a primary defect in K^+ transport. An increased intake most commonly occurs in children as a result of too-rapid administration of intravenous potassium chloride. Inadequate excretion of K^+ occurs in the event of renal failure, adrenal insufficiency, metabolic acidosis, and the use of K^+-sparing diuretics. A shift of K^+ from within the cells to extracellular fluid occurs with

- tissue damage (burns, destruction of tumor tissue, and massive crushing injuries in which potassium is released from the injured cells)
- hemolysis (due to sudden excessive water intake)
- digitalis overdose (results in relative inability of K^+ to enter the cells because of partial inhibition of the Na^+-K^+-ATPase pump by the drug)
- hyperosmolality (increased plasma osmolality pulls water out of the cells, with K^+ following because of solvent drag), and
- administration of succinylcholine (the drug reduces the magnitude of the resting membrane potential, thus favoring the movement of K^+ out of the cells) and arginine (presumably due to the movement of K^+ out of the cells as the cation arginine enters the cells) (Rose, 1984).

Hypokalemia. Hypokalemia occurs when there is inadequate intake of K^+, excessive loss of K^+ (gastrointestinal and renal), or a shift of extracellular K^+ to the intracellular space. Poor food intake over an extended period or administration of intravenous fluids without added K^+ may result in hypokalemia. Excessive losses occur with vomiting, diarrhea, nasogastric suctioning, excessive intake of licorice (which contains a steroid with mineralocorticoid activity that stimulates the reabsorption of Na^+ and the excretion of K^+ and H^+), and when K^+-losing diuretics, notably furosemide (Lasix), or corticosteroids are administered. A shift of K^+ from extracellular compartments to within the cells occurs with alkalosis and insulin administration. With alkalosis, H^+ ions are released from the cellular buffers and move into extracellular fluid to minimize the change in pH; to preserve electroneutrality, extracellular K^+ (and Na^+) moves into the cells. Insulin promotes entry of K^+ into skeletal muscle and hepatic cells.

Calcium Imbalance

Calcium is essential not only in the process of skeletal mineralization, but also in many intracellular and extracellular processes. Calcium is required for activation of numerous enzymes and for proper cardiac, neural, and muscular function. Calcium (Ca^{++}) imbalance occurs when the Ca^{++} level is either excessive (hypercalcemia) or deficient (hypocalcemia). Normal plasma Ca^{++} concentration ranges from 8.5 to 10.5 mg/dl (or 4.5 to 5.6 mEq/L) in adults and older children, and 11 to 13 mg/dl in infants (McFadden and Zaloga, 1983).

Calcium regulation is primarily under the control of the parathyroid glands, which secrete parathyroid hormone (PTH) and vitamin D. Deposition and resorption (loss) of bone serves as an exchange mechanism for maintaining serum Ca^{++} levels in the appropriate range. Serum Ca^{++} measurements are influenced by the serum protein concentration; for every increment or decrement in albumin (or total protein), there is a corresponding change of 0.8 mg/dl in the serum Ca^{++} level. (McFadden and Zaloga, 1983).

Hypercalcemia. This may result from excessive administration of vitamins A and D and some drugs, hyperparathyroidism, malignancy, and, most importantly in children, prolonged immobilization. The lack of postural changes to the skeleton disturbs the balance between bone formation and resorption, resulting in loss of bone mass and its minerals. Because children are developmentally in a state of rapid bone turnover, the kidney may be unable to excrete Ca^{++} quickly enough to maintain normal plasma levels. Hypercalcemia may also occur in the presence of acidosis because Ca^{++} leaves the bone and enters the plasma to allow H^+ to be buffered by the bone (Popovtzer and Knochel, 1980).

Hypocalcemia. This may occur in infants and children for many reasons. Conditions such as hypoparathyroidism, vitamin D deficiency, respiratory alkalosis, hyper- and hypomagnesemia, burns, infection, diarrhea, and renal failure, as well as a multitude of drugs, all predispose children to hypocalcemia (McFadden and Zaloga, 1983). A disorder called tetany of the newborn is seen early in infancy when cow's milk formulas with a high concentration of phosphate are given. This tetany associated wth hypocalcemia can occur because of the reciprocal relationship of Ca^{++} and phosphorus; when the phosphorus level in the plasma is high, the Ca^{++} level is low. Hypocalcemia may also occur when acidosis is corrected. Some of the Ca^{++} that moves out of the bone matrix during acidosis

Table 30-2. Clinical Manifestations of Imbalance of Sodium, Potassium, and Calcium

Electrolyte Imbalance	Clinical Manifestations
Sodium	
Hypernatremia: resulting from • sodium retention • water loss (in excess of sodium loss) Serum sodium >147 mEq/L	Dry, sticky mucous membranes Flushed skin Excessive thirst (older child) Nuchal and muscular rigidity Lethargy, weakness, irritability with stimulation Tremors, convulsions Peripheral and/or pulmonary edema Urine specific gravity (SG) >1.030
Hyponatremia: resulting from • loss of sodium • retention of water Serum sodium <137 mEq/L	Nausea → malaise → headache → lethargy → obtundation Twitching → convulsions Cool, clammy skin → hypotension → shock Urine SG <1.010
Potassium	
Hyperkalemia: resulting from • increased potassium intake • inadequate potassium excretion • potassium shift (from intracellular to extracellular compartment) Serum potassium >5.6 mEq/L	Nausea, malaise Muscle weakness → flaccid paralysis Hyper-reflexia Intestinal colic, diarrhea Oliguria → anuria Abnormal cardiac conduction: peaked, narrow T waves and shortened Q-T interval → widened QRS complex and decreased amplitude: widening and eventual loss of P wave → sine wave pattern (widened QRS merges with T wave) → ventricular fibrillation → asystole
Hypokalemia: resulting from: • inadequate potassium intake • excessive potassium loss • Potassium shift (from extracellular to intracellular compartment) Serum potassium <4.0 mEq/L	Apathy, drowsiness Muscle weakness/cramps → flaccid paralysis Hyporeflexia Abdominal distention and ileus Shallow breathing Impaired urinary concentration, polyuria, polydipsia Mild hyperglycemia Rhabdomyolysis (disintegration of muscle) and associated myoglobinuria Arrhythmias (premature atrial and ventricular beats, sinus bradycardia, paroxysmal atrial and junctional tachycardia, atrioventricular block, ventricular tachycardia, ventricular fibrillation) Abnormal cardiac conduction: ST segment depression, decreased amplitude or inversion of T wave, increased height of U wave, increased amplitude of P wave, prolonged PR interval, widened QRS complex
Calcium	
Hypercalcemia: resulting from • excessive administration of vitamin D or calcium • hyperparathyroidism • malignancy • prolonged immobilization Serum calcium >10.5 mg/dl in older children/adults and >13 mg/dl in infants	Nausea, vomiting Abdominal/flank pain Dryness of mouth Muscle hypotonicity Stupor → coma Cardiac arrest
Hypocalcemia: resulting from • ingestion of cow's milk with high phosphorus/calcium ratio • hypoparathyroidism • vitamin D deficiency • hyper- and hypomagnesemia • burns • infection • diarrhea • renal failure • drugs • during correction of acidosis (calcium returns to bone) Serum calcium <8.5 mg/dl in older children/adults and <11 mg/dl in infants	Tingling, numbness Muscle cramps → tetany Seizures Laryngospasm

(Sources: Reed, 1974; Sweeney, 1978; Metheney and Snively, 1979.)

is lost in the urine. As the acidosis corrects, Ca^{++} reenters the bones, resulting in a hypocalcemia. (Table 30-2 lists the clinical manifestations of electrolyte imbalances.)

Serum Electrolyte Values

During illness, disruption of regulatory mechanisms can result in *actual* depletion or excess of electrolytes in the body. Serum levels truly reflect electrolyte status at these times. Sometimes, though, disruption only *alters the distribution* of electrolytes—not the total body content. When this occurs, serum electrolyte values can be misleading. For example, a low serum K^+ is not common in patients with diabetic ketoacidosis (DKA), yet total body depletion of K^+ is common. In fact, the serum K^+ may be elevated. This apparent discrepancy occurs because K^+ moves from the intracellular to the extracellular compartment with DKA, but a rise in serum K^+ may be masked by concurrent urinary losses of the electrolyte. If treatment of DKA were to proceed based upon the "normal" K^+ level, very serious complications would quickly arise as the body's K^+ stores dwindled. Knowledge of electrolyte behavior in specific childhood illnesses, therefore, is essential for the pediatric nurse.

Acid-Base Balance

Homeostasis in body fluids is a function of acid-base balance, as well as a function of fluid and electrolyte balance. The acidity of body fluids is determined by hydrogen ion (H^+) concentration. Hydrogen ions are the products of cell metabolism and the metabolism of dietary proteins. Sources of additional hydrogen ions include strenuous exercise (lactic acid) and diabetic ketosis (acetoacetic and β-hydroxybutyric acid). Because free hydrogen ions are present in the body fluids in extremely small concentrations (40 nanoequivalents, or approximately one millionth of the milliequivalent per liter concentration of Na^+), the term *pH* is used to provide a means of expressing the value simply. The pH value is determined by taking the *negative* logarithm of the hydrogen ion concentration; therefore, the *more* hydrogen ions there are, the *lower* the pH is (Narins and Emmett, 1980). A relatively narrow range of pH is compatible with life, from 6.80 to 7.80, because minute changes in hydrogen ion concentration significantly affect enzymatic and physiologic processes in the body (Rose, 1984).

The terms *acidosis* and *alkalosis* refer to processes that cause acid and alkali to accumulate, and the pH tends to move in an abnormal direction when these processes occur (Narins and Emmett, 1980). An abnormally low pH (an excess of acid) in the arterial blood is called *acidemia;* an abnormally high pH (too much base or too little acid) in the blood is called *alkalemia.*

Three important points characterize the relationship of pH and hydrogen ion concentration:

- Normal arterial blood pH is 7.40 (range: 7.35 to 7.45), or a hydrogen ion concentration of 40 nanoequivalents.
- Hydrogen ion and pH concentration are inversely related; as the H ion concentration rises, the pH falls, and vice versa.
- When serum pH falls below 7.35 as hydrogen ion concentration rises, the patient is said to be acidemic; conversely, when the pH rises above 7.45 as the hydrogen ion concentration falls, the patient is said to be alkalemic (Narins and Emmett, 1980).

Regulation of Hydrogen Ion Concentration

Hydrogen ion concentration is maintained within its narrow limits by the kidneys, the lungs, a variety of chemical buffers, and some metabolic processes (Finberg et al, 1982; Rose, 1984).

A *buffered solution* is one that contains a weak acid and its conjugate base. Such a solution can minimize pH changes when either acid or base is added, by donating or absorbing H^+ as necessary and thereby minimizing their effect on total H^+ concentration. Body buffers that can absorb or donate H^+ in response to changes in acidity of extracellular fluids provide a defense against disastrous swings in pH. Hemoglobin, plasma proteins, and bone are effective buffers, but the most important extracellular buffer system is the bicarbonate–carbonic acid system. Buffering by this system proceeds rapidly via the following chemical reaction:

$$\text{(A)}\quad H^+ + \underset{\text{(base)}}{\overset{\text{bicarbonate}}{HCO_3^-}} \rightleftharpoons \underset{\text{(weak acid)}}{\overset{\text{carbonic acid}}{H_2CO_3}} \rightleftharpoons \overset{\text{carbon dioxide}}{CO_2} + \overset{\text{water}}{H_2O}$$

Whether carbonic acid dissociates (into hydrogen and bicarbonate or into carbon dioxide and water), or whether it is formed (from hydrogen and bicarbonate or from carbon dioxide and water) depends on which reaction(s) will restore the following important relationships:

1. the 20:1 ratio between bicarbonate and carbonic acid that is the normal ratio of base to acid in the blood (i.e., as long as the ratio is maintained, acid-base balance will exist, even if the absolute amounts of acid or base change), and

2. the equilibrium of the carbonic acid and dissolved carbon dioxide levels that is normally maintained in blood.

For example, when a strong acid is added to the blood, the hydrogen ions that it releases are buffered by bicarbonate, and carbonic acid is quickly formed. The carbonic acid then dissociates into carbon dioxide and water and the carbon dioxide is quickly excreted by the lungs:

$$\text{(B)}\quad H^+ + HCO_3^- \longrightarrow H_2CO_3 \longrightarrow CO_2 + H_2O$$

The formation of carbon dioxide and water from carbonic acid occurs so that the normal balance of bicarbonate and carbonic acid (20 : 1) is maintained. The subsequent excretion of the carbon dioxide by the lungs then restores the carbonic acid–carbon dioxide equilibrium. This system works so well because blood carbon dioxide can be increased or decreased within minutes by changes in breathing patterns. Variations in ventilation (that is, faster, slower, deeper, or shallower breaths) can adjust carbon dioxide concentration and therefore carbonic acid and H^+/bicarbonate concentrations within minutes. If ventilation increases when pH is normal, carbon dioxide excretion is augmented (reaction *B*), resulting in

1. a drop in the partial pressure of carbon dioxide (PCO_2*),
2. a drop in carbonic acid, to match the drop in carbon dioxide and maintain their equilibrium, and
3. a drop in hydrogen ion concentration (alkalemia) as they combine with bicarbonate (to restore the 20 : 1 ratio) in the blood.

A decrease in ventilation causes a rise in PCO_2 and the opposite reaction, with consequent accumulation of H^+ and a drop in pH (acidemia):

$$\text{(C)}\quad CO_2 + H_2O \longrightarrow H_2CO_3 \longrightarrow H^+ + HCO_3^-$$

Although carbon dioxide is not an acid or a base, it can indirectly increase or decrease the acidity of the blood. The lungs, therefore, through regulation of the PCO_2, can *compensate* for changes in pH related to *metabolic* processes. Diabetic ketoacidosis (DKA), for example, is a metabolic process. In DKA, when hydrogen ions (from the ketoacids) accumulate in the blood, they are first buffered by bicarbonate and form carbonic acid, which, in effect, holds the hydrogen ions and prevents the pH from decreasing significantly (reaction *B*). Then the carbonic acid dissociates into water and carbon dioxide, and the carbon dioxide is excreted by the lungs with deep breathing (Kussmaul respirations). On the other hand, when H^+ concentration is low (as can occur with vomiting or nasogastric suctioning of stomach secretions, which contain high concentrations of H^+), the partial pressure of carbon dioxide rises as ventilation responsively decreases, and the carbonic acid releases H^+, thereby preventing a rise in the pH (reaction *C*). The net effect of reactions in the bicarbonate–carbonic acid system is maintenance of a 20 : 1 ratio between bicarbonate and carbonic acid.

Whereas the lungs *compensate* for pH changes caused by metabolic disorders by controlling the carbon dioxide level in the blood, the kidneys react to pH variations resulting from *respiratory* abnormalities by regulating the other end of the reaction equation—the hydrogen ion and bicarbonate concentrations. Renal excretion or reabsorption of H^+ or bicarbonate, as compensation for changes in pH, depends on the plasma bicarbonate level and on the rate of H^+ secretion by the renal tubular cells. Bicarbonate is reabsorbed in exchange for hydrogen ions. The rate of H^+ excretion, and therefore the rate of bicarbonate reabsorption, is proportionate to the arterial PCO_2. With a respiratory disturbance, such as *hyper*ventilation, the partial pressure of carbon dioxide drops, carbonic acid dissociates into H^+ and bicarbonate, and the bicarbonate is slowly excreted to prevent the blood pH from increasing significantly. Compensation for *hypo*ventilation, during which the carbon dioxide level rises, also occurs in the kidney. In this case, however, hydrogen ions are excreted instead of bicarbonate to minimize the drop in pH.

The interdependence of pH, bicarbonate, and carbonic acid is summarized by the Henderson-Hasselbalch equation (a mathematical formulation of the earlier equation), where pK represents the dissociation constant of the acid:

$$\text{(D)}\qquad pH = pK + \frac{\log(HCO_3^-)}{(H_2CO_3)}\quad (p = -\log)$$

The equation demonstrates that H^+ concentration (pH) of a solution is the function of the ionization constant (K)* and concentration ratio of the buffer pair (bicarbonate/carbonic acid). The key clinical message conveyed is that acidity of blood is determined by the relative availability of acid and alkali, and that plasma concentrations of bicarbonate and carbonic acid (PCO_2) reflect that availability. The H^+ concentration, and therefore the pH, is defined by the ratio of the

* Since carbonic acid is in equilibrium with dissolved carbon dioxide, the measurement of partial pressure of carbon dioxide (PCO_2) can be used as a clinical estimate of carbonic acid concentration.

* The *ionization constant* is the term used to define an acid's strength. The pK is inversely proportional to the strength of the acid.

PCO_2 to bicarbonate and not by the absolute value of either one alone (Narins and Emmett, 1980). The components of the Henderson-Hasselbalch equation can be further described as follows:

- Bicarbonate (HCO_3^-): *metabolic component*
  a) primarily altered in metabolic disorders
  b) altered by buffering
  c) altered by renal compensation for respiratory disorders
- Carbonic acid [H_2CO_3 (or PCO_2)]: *respiratory component*
  a) primarily altered in respiratory disorders
  b) altered by respiratory compensation for metabolic disorders
- pH: the result of interplay between metabolic and respiratory components (Kaehny and Gabow, 1980)

In summary, the lungs control the partial pressure of carbon dioxide and, in effect, the carbonic acid concentration in the body. Carbon dioxide is eliminated by the lungs and is regulated by the rate of alveolar ventilation. Hyperventilation enhances carbon dioxide excretion; carbon dioxide is "blown off," thus lowering the partial pressure of carbon dioxide and increasing the pH (alkalosis). The plasma bicarbonate concentration is regulated by the changes in the rate of H^+ secretion from the kidney. Renal response to acid-base imbalance, however, is much slower than that of the lungs. Days, not minutes and hours, are required to restore balance.

Acid-Base Imbalance

Acid-base disturbances fall into four major categories: metabolic acidosis, metabolic alkalosis, respiratory acidosis, and respiratory alkalosis. Since the PCO_2 is regulated by respiration, primary abnormalities in the PCO_2 are called respiratory acidosis (high PCO_2) and respiratory alkalosis (low PCO_2). On the other hand, primary changes in the plasma bicarbonate concentration are referred to as metabolic acidosis (low bicarbonate) and metabolic alkalosis (high bicarbonate). In these disorders, compensatory renal or respiratory responses occur to minimize the change in H^+ concentration by minimizing the alteration in the PCO_2/bicarbonate ratio. Arterial blood gases can provide direct measurement of pH and PCO_2 and an approximation of bicarbonate concentration. If two of these three parameters are known, the other can be calculated. Direct measurement of serum bicarbonate also can be done.

Metabolic Acidosis

The most common cause of metabolic acidosis in children is diarrhea. This is the result of

- loss of HCO_3^- in the stool,
- increased ketone body* production from the metabolism of fat for energy,
- increased anaerobic metabolism secondary to dehydration and resulting in release of acids (lactic, pyruvic, and acetoacetic), free hydrogen ions, and carbon dioxide, and
- reduced blood volume causing the kidneys to function less effectively with a reduced excretion of hydrogen ions.

Additional causes of metabolic acidosis include renal failure, ketoacidosis, and lactic acidosis. The lactic acidosis is often secondary to hypoxia, which causes impairment of oxidation and subsequent increased conversion of pyruvate to lactate during glucose and amino acid metabolism.

Signs and symptoms associated with metabolic acidosis are noted in the pulmonary, cardiovascular, neurologic, and skeletal systems: increased depth of respirations, arrhythmias (potentially fatal), lethargy through coma, and impaired growth (rickets). Anorexia, nausea, weight loss, muscle weakness, and listlessness may also be noted.

Metabolic Alkalosis

Metabolic alkalosis is the result of hydrogen ion loss or bicarbonate retention. Hydrogen loss most commonly occurs via

1. Gastrointestinal tract
   H^+-rich gastric juices are lost with vomiting and nasogastric suctioning: The hydrogen ions from gastric juices are derived from the intracellular dissociation of carbonic acid (reaction *C* above); so, with H^+ loss, there is bicarbonate generation;
2. Renal system
   Mineralocorticoid excess: The mineralocorticoid aldosterone enhances Na^+ reabsorption; excessive Na^+ reabsorption results in concomitant hydrogen ion excretion; again, with H^+ loss, there is bicarbonate generation;
   Diuretics: Diuretics (e.g., furosemide) that cause Na^+ and water loss decrease extracellular fluid volume but leave the bicarbonate level essentially unchanged; as a result, the plasma bicarbonate level

* Ketone bodies include acetoacetic acid, β-hydroxybutyric acid, and acetone.

Table 30-3. Acid-Base Imbalances: Clinical Causes, Compensatory Mechanisms, and Clinical Manifestations

Classification	Clinical Causes	Compensatory Mechanism	Clinical Manifestations and Blood Gases
Respiratory acidosis: Impaired respiratory function with CO_2 retention	Disturbance of respiratory center (drugs, head trauma): disease affecting respiratory muscles; airway obstruction; pulmonary disease; cardiac failure; right-to-left cardiac shunts	Renal compensation: increased urinary excretion of hydrogen ion; makes and reabsorbs more bicarbonate	Respiratory distress, including tachypnea and use of accessory muscles. Hypoxemia often present due to underlying cause. Hypoxemia can lead to metabolic lactic acidosis* • Arterial pH low • pCO_2 elevated • Plasma bicarbonate moderately elevated
Respiratory alkalosis: alveolar hyperventilation results in blowing off CO_2 in excess of its production	Acute anxiety states; hyperactivity of respiratory center in association with infection (encephalitis, meningitis); salicylate ingestion (early stages); improper use of mechanical respirators; increased sensitivity of the respiratory center to pCO_2	Renal compensation: less hydrogen ion is excreted so that less bicarbonate is produced (each time a hydrogen ion is excreted by the kidney a bicarbonate ion is produced and reabsorbed); decreased conservation of filtered bicarbonate	Tetany due to decreased ionized calcium in the presence of alkalemia. • Arterial pH high • pCO_2 low • Plasma bicarbonate low
Metabolic acidosis • Increased production of hydrogen ions • Excessive loss of bicarbonate ions (hyperchloremia due to resulting elevated chloride level) • Decreased hydrogen ion excreted and decreased formation of new bicarbonate	Ketone acids (starvation, diabetes); lactic acids (usually secondary to tissue hypoxia); salicylate poisoning Via GI tract† (diarrhea, vomiting, suction, fistula drainage); via kidney (renal tubular acidosis) Occurs due to low glomerular filtration rate secondary to acute dehydration. Reduced tubular mass (chronic renal insufficiency) limits amount of ammonia kidney can produce. Excretion of hydrogen ion with ammonia is thus decreased	Respiratory compensation: Increased respirations to blow off CO_2 Renal Compensation • Acidosis also stimulates kidney to produce ammonia so that hydrogen ion can be excreted with it • As hydrogen ion is excreted new bicarbonate is generated	Deep, rapid respirations (Küssmaul breathing); severe acidosis can reduce peripheral vascular resistance and cause decreased function of the ventricles of the heart Hypotension, pulmonary edema, and tissue hypoxia may result. • Arterial pH low • pCO_2 low • Plasma bicarbonate low
Metabolic alkalosis • Loss of hydrogen ion resulting in the presence of comparatively too much base • Gain of bicarbonate • Reduced extracellular fluid volume with a greater NaCl loss than bicarbonate loss	1. Loss of hydrogen ion (gastric aspiration, persistent vomiting, e.g., pyloric stenosis) 2. Loading with bicarbonate as by: • Increased renal reabsorption of bicarbonate as in a potassium cellular deficit (reasons not clear) • When chlorides are lost as in vomiting the body releases more bicarbonate to keep the total number of anions equal • Administration of a diuretic	Respiratory compensation: Compensation is not effective, therefore the problem must be eliminated	Depressed respiration: Hypertonic muscles due to decreased ionized calcium in the presence of alkalemia‡ • Arterial pH high • pCO_2 elevated • Plasma bicarbonate elevated

* Hypoxemia can result in metabolic acidosis due to accumulation of lactic acid in presence of reduced oxygen supply to tissues. Exercise, trauma and infection are common causes of tissue hypoxia that can result in metabolic lactic acidosis.

† Large amounts of bicarbonate are present in gastrointestinal tract from a point distal of pylorus to anal sphincter.

‡ In acidosis there is a high ionization of calcium and in alkalosis a decreased ionization.

(Sources: Hoekelman et al, 1987; Metheney, 1987; Behrman and Vaughan, 1987.)

Table 30-4. Arterial Blood Gas Values in Uncompensated* Acid-Base Disturbances

Abnormality	pH	PCO_2	Calculated Bicarbonate	Base Excess
Respiratory Acidosis ↓ elimination by the lungs of CO_2 gas	↓	↑	N	N
Respiratory Alkalosis ↑ elimination by the lungs of CO_2 gas	↑	↓	N	N
Metabolic Acidosis a. acid is added (uses up HCO_3^-) or b. HCO_3^- is lost	↓	N	↓	↓
Metabolic Alkalosis a. acid is lost, or b. HCO_3^- is gained	↑	N	↑	↑

* This table presents arterial blood gas values as they exist before correction or compensation by the primarily unaffected system (i.e., respiratory or renal). Arrows indicate elevated or depressed values; N is normal.

rises (note: this is referred to as a "contraction alkalosis," and is *not* seen with K^+-sparing diuretics); and

3. Movement of hydrogen ions into the cells Hypokalemia. As plasma K^+ falls, K^+ moves out of the cells into the extracellular fluid; to maintain electroneutrality, H^+ move into the cells, causing a rise in pH.

Bicarbonate retention may result from

- massive blood transfusion—most bank blood is anticoagulated with acid-citrate-dextran; citrate is rapidly metabolized and produces bicarbonate,
- administration of sodium bicarbonate—excessive administration of sodium bicarbonate may lead to metabolic alkalosis, and
- milk-alkali syndrome—the chronic ingestion of milk and antacids containing calcium carbonate (which generates bicarbonate) (Rose, 1984).

Infants and children with a metabolic alkalosis may be asymptomatic or demonstrate signs of volume depletion (weakness, muscle cramps, postural dizziness) or hypokalemia (polyuria, polydipsia, muscle weakness).

Respiratory Acidosis

Acute respiratory acidosis in children is associated with events that depress *respiration* or interfere with *ventilation* (the movement of air in and out of the lungs). Respiration may be depressed because of head trauma or from the effect of opiates, anesthetics, sedatives, or alcohol on the respiratory center in the brain. Ingestion or administration of these substances results in too few or too shallow respirations or both and a subsequent rise in pCO_2 and a drop in pH. Aspiration of a foreign body or vomitus, severe asthma, or pneumonia directly interferes with ventilation. This also results in retention of carbon dioxide and the development of respiratory acidosis.

Neurologic abnormalities, such as headache, blurred vision, restlessness, anxiety, tremors, delirium, and somnolence (called CO_2 narcosis) may be exhibited with respiratory acidosis.

Respiratory Alkalosis

Respiratory alkalosis is often the result of hyperventilation from anxiety; fast, deep breaths cause excretion of carbon dioxide and eventual depletion of free hydrogen ions. It can, however, occur with hypoxemia, pulmonary disease, and salicylate ingestion.

Manifestations associated with respiratory alkalosis are related to increased irritability of the central and peripheral nervous systems. They include lightheadedness, altered consciousness, paresthesias of the extremities and circumoral area, cramps, and syncope. Arrhythmias may also occur. (Acid-base disturbances are summarized in Table 30-3 and arterial blood gas values in uncompensated acid-base disturbance in Table 30-4.)

Nursing Assessment of Fluid and Electrolyte and Acid-Base Balance

Specific clinical and laboratory data are necessary when fluid or electrolyte imbalance is suspected. The nurse must interview the parents regarding the child's current problem and any other condition or event that may affect identification or management of the current problem. Thereafter, clinical assessment is performed as warranted by the child's condition. Laboratory evaluation of renal (urine and serum electrolytes and specific gravity) and cardiopulmonary (arterial blood gases and electrocardiogram) function is pertinent to the care of the child with potential fluid and electrolyte imbalance. The nurse should review the data during care of such a child.

Nursing History

Questions in the nursing history that are pertinent when fluid or electrolyte imbalance is suspected include

- Has the child had any vomiting or diarrhea? If so, describe the circumstances.
- Describe the type, frequency, and amount of food and fluid given at home during the illness.
- Has the child been urinating as usual?
- Has the child had any appreciable weight loss or gain recently?
- Has the child had any recent change in behavior or activity level?
- If the child had a fever, what was its level and duration?
- Has the child had any recent evidence of infection?
- Is the child receiving any medication now or has she or he received any recently?

In addition, parents should be given the opportunity to describe any change that they have noted in their child. After the interview and throughout the child's illness, the nurse evaluates vital signs, body weight, intake and output, neurologic status, and the condition of the skin, mucous membranes, fontanels, and eyes.

Monitoring Vital Signs

A change in normal vital signs or a lack of change in abnormal vital signs must be noted and reported by the nurse to facilitate modification of the treatment plan.

Temperature. Elevation of body temperature can disrupt fluid balance in a child. Fever increases the metabolic rate. Since a heightened metabolic rate increases the amount of metabolic wastes, additional fluids are required for excretion of these wastes by the kidneys. Failure to provide the extra fluid can cause dehydration or worsen existing dehydration. Water and electrolytes are also lost in sweat, and additional fluid is lost through tachypnea, both of which can accompany fever. In the early phase of extracellular fluid volume depletion the body temperature is commonly elevated, whereas a subnormal body temperature may occur in the later stages of a volume deficit (Burgess, 1987).

Pulse. Pulse is evaluated for rate, quality, and rhythm. When extravascular fluid volume is reduced, the pulse is rapid (tachycardia), weak, and thready. This can occur in either total body fluid deficit (dehydration) or when plasma shifts from intravascular to interstitial spaces (edema). A bounding pulse is a sign of increased plasma fluid volume and occurs in hypertonic dehydration or when there is an excess of total body fluid volume. Cardiac arrhythmias first may be detected when an irregular pulse is noted. The arrhythmias can be the result of a variety of problems, including a K^+ level that is either too high or too low.

Respirations. The rate and quality of respirations provide information about the body's fluid and electrolyte status. Respirations may be

- fast with a normal depth (tachypnea)
- slow with a normal depth (bradypnea)
- deep with a normal rate (hyperpnea)
- irregular with a decreased rate (hypoventilation)
- deep with an increased rate (hyperventilation)
- absent (apnea), or
- normal (eupnea)

They are affected by fluid volume alterations, electrolyte imbalances, and acid-base imbalances. Metabolic acidosis, which accompanies many conditions in children, including dehydration, is compensated for by an increased respiratory rate. Hypokalemia and hyperkalemia result in shallow breathing caused by weakness or paralysis of the respiratory muscles. (See Table 30-3 for respiratory responses in acid-base imbalance.)

Blood Pressure

Although an accurate blood pressure reading may be difficult to obtain in an infant, it may add valuable information when evaluated along with other data. Most of the time a systolic value (which can be felt, as well as heard) is all that is necessary. (See Chapter 27 for a discussion of techniques used to measure blood pressure.) Increased blood pressure occurs in fluid volume excess or in the early phase of interstitial fluid-to-plasma shift. Blood pressure is decreased in a fluid volume deficit or when there is a plasma-to-interstitial fluid shift.

Weight

A child's weight provides important data about the state of hydration. The severity of dehydration and the degree of recovery from it are often reflected in a child's

Table 30-5. Correlation of Clinical Features with Degree of Isotonic Dehydration

Clinical Features	Mild Dehydration	Moderate Dehydration	Severe Dehydration
Loss of body weight	5%	10%	15%
Skin color	Pale	Gray	Mottled
Skin turgor	Decreased	Moderately decreased	Markedly decreased
Urine output	Decreased	Oliguria	Marked oliguria and azotemia
Blood pressure	Normal	Normal or slightly above or below normal	Low
Pulse	Normal or tachycardia	Tachycardia	Increased tachycardia and thready pulse

(From Dube, 1978.)

weight. For example, the severity of isotonic dehydration is classified as mild, moderate, or severe according to the weight that has been lost. (Table 30-5 presents a correlation of clinical symptoms with degree of dehydration.) To maximize the accuracy of this measurement, children should be weighed on the same scale, at the same time of day, by the same nurse. Changes in weight related to changes in intravenous lines, dressings, or other items should be accounted for by appropriately adding or subtracting their weight from the one obtained.

Weight gain during illness may indicate fluid retention and the presence of pulmonary edema or generalized edema. When a child gains weight suddenly, the nurse not only should recheck the weight but also look for signs of fluid retention, such as periorbital edema and pulmonary crackles.

Skin Assessment

The skin should be assessed for color, temperature, texture, moisture, and turgor* (tautness). It provides many clues to a child's state of hydration. Different types of dehydration, for example, result in characteristic skin conditions. In isotonic dehydration, the most common type of dehydration in children, the skin is pale and dry and its elasticity is poor. The peripheral blood flow may be decreased, making the extremities cool with poor capillary refill. The skin is often pale. In hypertonic dehydration the skin may be flushed and its turgor and elasticity may be normal because the extracellular fluid compartment is relatively better preserved than in isotonic dehydration (Haddow, 1974). The appearance of the child with hypotonic dehydration is the most dramatic; the skin is cool and clammy to the touch, and elasticity and turgor may be very poor. Color is generally pale and may become gray and mottled as circulatory failure progresses (Finberg, 1981).

When there is increased formation or decreased removal of interstitial fluid, edema develops. This occurs with a variety of conditions and may or may not result in a net weight change.

Anterior Fontanel and Eyes

The anterior fontanel and the eyes should be assessed when a child has a potential or actual fluid imbalance. The anterior fontanel, which remains open until approximately 16 to 18 months of age, should feel flat and firm. A tense and bulging fontanel indicates increased intracranial pressure or volume, and a sunken or depressed one is evidence of dehydration. Suture lines in the skull may also become prominent when the circulating volume is decreased. The eyes appear sunken when a child is severely dehydrated.

Intake and Output and Urine Specific Gravity

A nurse's accurate assessment and recording of intake and output are of prime importance in caring for children with fluid and electrolyte imbalances. The nurse who deems it necessary should keep an intake and output record even if one has not been ordered. Also, the nurse should routinely check the urine specific gravity of children who are receiving all their intake intravenously or who have identified or potential im-

* Skin turgor is assessed by pinching the skin and allowing it to fall back to its original position. When the skin remains slightly raised, or "tented," for a few seconds, this is called "poor skin turgor."

balances. However, it should be recognized that glucose, large amounts of protein, and radiographic dyes elevate the specific gravity, interfering with this parameter's ability to reflect hydration status accurately.

Infants are unable to concentrate urine as well as older children and adults, so their urine is normally dilute and will show a low specific gravity. In the immediate newborn period it ranges from 1.001 to 1.020 and thereafter from 1.001 to 1.030. A fluid excess in the body is reflected in a low specific gravity (1.010 or less) as the kidneys rid the body of water. A fluid deficit is reflected in a high specific gravity as the kidneys conserve fluid. After a period of fluid restriction, specific gravity is commonly greater than 1.025.

Oral fluid intake approximates urinary output daily. Fluid generated from metabolism roughly equals that which is lost through the skin, lungs, and stool. The normal range for 24-hour urinary output varies with age: in the neonate, 50 to 300 ml; in the infant, 350 to 550 ml; in the child, 500 to 1000 ml; and in the adolescent, 700 to 1400 ml. A markedly higher output of urine than fluid intake may be due to a shift of fluid from interstitial fluid to plasma, a high solute intake, lack of secretion of ADH (e.g., diabetes insipidus), or renal damage. Common pediatric conditions that may moderately increase urine production are fever and infection. This occurs because the higher metabolic rate results in increased wastes for the kidney to excrete; additional water is required to clear such wastes from the body.

Neurologic Status

The central nervous system displays signs and symptoms of dysfunction with many fluid and electrolyte imbalances. In dehydration, a child may become irritable and then lethargic, or simply lethargic with irritability on stimulation. Also, the child's cry may be high pitched and weak. Marked hypokalemia and hyperkalemia cause muscle weakness, tetany, and muscle paralysis, whereas hypocalcemia may be the reason for a child's twitching, irritability, and eventual convulsions. Acute hyponatremia causes headache, confusion, muscle twitching, eventual delirium, and, finally, convulsions. Severe hypernatremia may cause intracerebral bleeding, brain damage, and subsequent mental retardation, convulsions, and death (O'Brien, 1980).

Laboratory Assessment

Arterial blood gases are obtained from children with known or suspected acid-base imbalance to determine the presence of the imbalance and to provide a means of assessing the metabolic and respiratory components of the condition. Urine specific gravity and its signficance in evaluating hydration has been discussed. Imbalances in various serum electrolytes have also been reviewed. Urine electrolytes are often obtained from children with both fluid and electrolyte imbalances and are interpreted in light of the corresponding serum values. When both urine and serum samples are desired for comparison, it is best to wait to draw the blood until the urine is obtained. In this way, they represent the body's status at the same point in time.

The electrocardiogram (ECG) may provide the first clues to electrolyte imbalances in children, and the abnormal findings may precede the development of life-threatening arrhythmias. Potassium and Ca^{++} abnormalities, in particular, cause ECG changes. In hypokalemia the T wave is flattened and a U wave may appear, whereas in hyperkalemia the P wave is flattened, the QRS is widened, and the T wave is peaked. Hypocalcemia results in a prolonged QT interval, and hypercalcemia causes a shortened one (Catchpole, 1982). These ECG changes reflect abnormalities in the electrical activity of the heart secondary to the chemical abnormalities of the body's fluids.

It is important for the nurse to strive to gain an increased understanding of laboratory reports. The laboratory findings, however, must always be evaluated in conjunction with clinical findings. (Blood gas values in acid-base imbalance are summarized in Table 30-4.)

Nursing Diagnoses

Fluid volume excesses and deficits occur in a broad range of illnesses. Nursing diagnoses appropriate to the situation are formulated recognizing that imbalances can occur in vascular, cellular, or intracellular compartments of the body.

When *total* body volume loss or excess of fluid occurs, it is a *volume* deficit resulting in dehydration (isotonic) or a total volume excess resulting in edema. These imbalances occur with equal gains and losses of water and sodium. Fluid and electrolyte imbalance can also occur when there is an imbalance in the *proportion* of water and solute load, that is, hyperosmolarity or hypo-osmolarity. These imbalances can result in fluid shifts so that a certain body compartment may have an excess of fluid or solute, as discussed in the section on hypotonic and hypertonic dehydration. Nursing diagnoses that represent volume deficit/excess and hyperosmolar or hypo-osmolar imbalances are included as possible diagnoses to use in fluid and electrolyte imbalance.

Fluid volume deficits are conditions in which vascular, cellular, or intercellular dehydration occurs. A fluid volume deficit can be related to failure of regulatory mechanisms or active loss (Kim et al, 1987). Fluids are lost in association with illness or therapy.

Nursing Diagnosis 1

Fluid volume deficit, related to excess fluid loss associated with illness:

- *shock, hemorrhage*
- *heat prostration*
- *diarrhea, vomiting, diaphoresis*
- *burns, draining wounds, fistulas*
- *fever*
- *hyperventilation*

Nursing Diagnosis 2

Fluid volume deficit, related to excess fluid loss associated with therapy:

- *overuse of diuretics*
- *indwelling tubes*
- *high solute feeding*
- *frequent tap water enemas*
- *frequent irrigations with hypotonic solution*

Fluid volume deficits cause additional problems for children. Nursing diagnoses relevant to the care of children with fluid volume deficits include:

1. ***Potential impairment in urinary elimination patterns, related to decreased plasma volume resulting in decreased renal blood flow***
2. ***Alteration in cardiac output: decreased, due to inadequate blood volume***

Fluid volume excess is the abnormal retention of fluids and edema. It is always secondary to an increase in total body sodium content, which in turn leads to an increase in total body water (Metheney, 1987).

Nursing Diagnosis 3

Fluid volume excess, related to:

- *excessive sodium intake*
- *excessive fluid intake*
- *compromised regulatory mechanisms associated with renal and liver diseases, hormonal disturbance, nephrotic syndrome, lymphatic obstruction, congenital heart failure, and steroid excess*

Fluid volume excess causes additional problems for children. Nursing diagnoses relevant to the care of children with fluid volume excess include:

1. ***Impairment in skin integrity, related to edema***
2. ***Ineffective breathing pattern, related to circulatory overload (pulmonary edema)***
3. ***Anxiety due to development of pulmonary edema***

Hyperosmolar and hypo-osmolar states occur when there is an imbalance in the proportion of water and sodium. Nursing diagnoses relevant to the care of children with hyperosmolar imbalances include:

1. ***Potential injury, related to decreased level of consciousness associated with shrinking of cells in the central nervous system***
2. ***Potential alteration in urinary elimination patterns associated with reduced urinary output***
3. ***Potential impairment of skin integrity, related to dehydration***

Nursing diagnoses relevant to the care of children with hypo-osmolar imbalances include:

1. ***Potential for injury associated with mental confusion, disorientation, and convulsions, associated with cellular edema of the brain***
2. ***Alteration in thought process due to cerebral edema and dysfunction***
3. ***Alteration in comfort due to prescribed fluid restriction***

Therapeutic Management of Imbalances in Fluids, Electrolytes, and Acid-Base

Administration of intravenous fluids and electrolytes to children is a highly specialized technique. The nurse who participates in such therapy requires knowledge and a high level of clinical competence to meet this responsibility effectively. Nurses involved in the administration of intravenous (IV) fluids and electrolytes should strive to increase their theoretical knowledge base as well as their technical skill. The care of these children and families traverses all aspects of pediatric nursing. The chemical and physiologic processes are complex and the psychologic effects on the child and parents are far reaching. Starting and maintaining IV lines requires special skill and practice, and the mathematical calculations necessary to administer the prescribed fluid and electrolyte medication re-

Table 30-6. Maintenance Requirements of Fluids (in Ml) Based on Caloric Expenditure

Body Weight in Kg	Caloric Expenditure	Fluid Requirements*
3–10 kg	100 cal/kg/day	100 ml/kg/day
10–20 kg	1000 cal + 50 cal/kg for each kg of body weight above 10 kg	1000 ml + 50 ml/kg for each kg of body weight above 10 kg
Over 20 kg	1500 cal + 20 cal/kg for each kg of body weight above 20 kg	1500 ml + 20 ml/kg for each kg of body weight above 20 kg

* Water of oxidation provides a small daily source of fluid to the body. Water losses that must be replaced (insensible water loss and renal water loss) can be provided by 100 ml/100 cal/day; thus "cal" can be replaced by "ml" as shown in last column above.

(Adapted from Holliday and Segar, 1957.)

quire precision. Unsupervised novice practitioners should not have sole responsibility for such potentially life-threatening procedures. Student nurses and newly practicing graduate nurses deserve the security, and the children have the right, to have another, more experienced nurse check all calculations when electrolytes are added to an IV bag.

Fluid and electrolyte therapy is employed under a variety of circumstances. The goal of therapy is *to provide maintenance therapy to compensate for normal and abnormal losses and to replace pre-existing deficits.* The type of solution and the rate of administration vary according to the condition being corrected and the metabolic rate of the child.

Although nurses are not responsible for prescribing the required amount of fluids and electrolytes, they should have the knowledge to check the prescription by their own calculations and to decide whether it reflects a reasonable and safe dose for the particular child and condition being treated.

Calculation of Maintenance Fluid and Electrolyte Dose

The body is in a dynamic state. Fluids and electrolytes normally are gained and lost. Maintenance requirements are the fluids and electrolytes that are necessary to maintain homeostasis for the next balance period (usually 24 hours). Therapy must account for

- insensible or evaporative losses (through skin and lungs),
- urinary losses, and
- caloric needs.

Maintenance fluid requirements may be calculated on the basis of the patient's body weight, body surface area, or caloric expenditure. The method most widely used now because of its accuracy and ease of calculation is based on caloric expenditure. Holliday and Segar's formula (Table 30-6) can be commited to memory for easy use in the clinical area.

When the child is ill, ongoing abnormal losses (e.g., gastric secretions) must also be accounted for. Since this is not done in the calculation of maintenance or deficit (see below) requirements, it must be done separately and added to the maintenance therapy. This is referred to as replacement therapy. (Table 30-7 lists water losses under normal conditions.)

Electrolytes must also be maintained on a daily basis to keep the body in balance. Maintenance requirements of electrolytes are

1. sodium: 2.5 mEq per 100 cal,
2. chloride: 5.0 mEq per 100 cal, and
3. potassium: 2.5 mEq per 100 cal (O'Brien, 1980).

In addition to electrolytes, glucose must be provided at 5 gm/100 cal metabolized. A solution of 5 per cent glucose* in 0.2 per cent sodium chloride† (may be written as D5/0.2NS or D5/1/4NS) with potassium chloride (KCl) provides adequate maintenance therapy for short periods of time under normal conditions.

Potassium administration must be done with extreme caution. Incorrect placement of a decimal point can result in ten times the prescribed dose being administered; this error, for a child, is lethal. Some general guidelines to use for the administration of KCl:

- Always check the appropriateness of the dose
- Give no more than 40 mEq/L

* This solution contains 50 gm of glucose per liter.

† Full-strength normal saline has 0.9 per cent sodium chloride; therefore one half strength has 0.45, and one quarter strength has 0.22 or 0.2 per cent sodium chloride.

- *Never* give by IV push
- Give no more than 4 mEq/kg/day to correct hypokalemia
- Do not administer KCl in the presence of oliguria or anuria

Principles of Deficit Therapy. Deficit therapy is designed to evaluate and repair the losses of fluids and electrolytes that have already occurred. There are three essential components of this aspect of fluid therapy:

1. Estimate the degree or severity of dehydration.
2. Determine the types of deficits that have occurred (i.e., isotonic, hypertonic, or hypotonic).
3. Plan an approach for the repair of the deficit (Siegel and Lattanzi, 1985).

Treatment is most frequently described in three phases: an initial phase in which the goal is to restore extracellular fluid—especially plasma volume—and improve renal function; a repletion phase during which intracellular and extracellular deficits of water and electrolytes are replaced but at a slower rate; and a final phase during which re-equilibrium and stabilization occurs, usually beginning when oral fluids are begun (Robson, 1987).

Initial Therapy (Emergency Phase). This is designed to rapidly expand the extracellular fluid volume. Ringer's lactated solution of 0.9 per cent saline solution equal to 10 to 20 ml/kg can be administered within the first 2 hours. (If normal saline is used for a child with acidosis, the severity of the acidosis is used to determine the need for addition of sodium bicarbonate to the solution to correct the pH.) This usually restores normal circulation, but if it does not, a second or in some cases a third infusion may be necessary. If the child is severely dehydrated, 30 to 50 ml/kg of plasma or albumin should be given instead.

Repletion Therapy. The aim of this phase is to correct previous losses as well as to provide therapy for normal and abnormal ongoing losses. With hypotonic and isotonic dehydration, this is usually accomplished in 6 to 8 hours, but in hypertonic dehydration correction of the deficit takes up to 48 hours. Proceeding at this slower pace allows for observation of signs and symptoms that indicate that the brain is swelling and for slowing of the IV fluids. Potassium chloride is added to the IV fluid during this phase, but it must not be done until kidney function has been established. Replacement of other electrolytes is guided by serum electrolytes and varies according to the underlying problem.

Stabilization. Maintenance and ongoing losses, and any remaining deficit, are taken care of during this final phase. Oral intake may be resumed. Reintroduction of oral feedings usually begins with small amounts of clear liquids. Milk and solids are then gradually introduced while careful observation is being made for the body's tolerance of oral feedings.

Throughout deficit therapy, nurses have a very important role. They monitor the child's vital signs, state of consciousness, specific gravity, and general appearance. Since these parameters reflect the success or failure of treatment, it is encumbent upon nurses to make accurate observations and report abnormalities quickly.

***Table* 30-7.** Water Loss per 100 Calories Metabolized Under Normal Conditions

Route	Water Lost (Ml/100 Cal)
Insensible water loss	45 ml
Sweat	0–25 ml
Urine	50–75 ml
Stool	5–10 ml

Usual loss in absence of sweating is 100 ml/100 cal metabolized.

(Adapted from Winters, 1973.)

Fluid Therapy Related to Surgery

The principles of fluid therapy already discussed also apply to the child undergoing a surgical procedure. When careful attention is paid to them, parental therapy proceeds smoothly. Errors, nonetheless, do occur, and the most common error in perioperative administration of IV fluid is overadministration, particularly of dextrose in water.

Preoperative IV therapy is rarely required unless the child has a pre-existing deficit. Fluid administration during surgery varies according to the types of losses that occur during the procedure. Postoperative fluids are provided by the parenteral route until the child has completely recovered from anesthesia and is free of nausea and vomiting. After most minor operations, fluids can be resumed gradually within the first 24 hours. Intravenous fluids, however, are continued when the surgical intervention prohibits oral intake.

Common postoperative solutions used in pediatrics are D5/0.2NS and D5/0.45NS. Since surgery frequently causes an excess of tissue loss of K^+ secondary to trauma and an increased level of ADH related to stress, K^+ is not administered in the immediate postoperative period. Neither is it administered to the oliguric child because hyperkalemia results if kidney damage has occurred. Consequently, K^+ can be safely added to IV fluids only after urinary flow has been established.

Nursing Strategies: Maintaining Fluid and Electrolyte Balance

The nurse has an important role in the prevention of fluid and electrolyte imbalance and in the safe administration of IV therapy.

Preventing Imbalances

One of the nurse's responsibilities is to teach parents how to prevent imbalances and how to detect early symptoms. In times of minor illness, a few basic principles about fluid intake and output may help parents prevent their child from developing more serious problems.

Noting increases in air and body temperature and adjusting fluid intake and clothing accordingly may prevent development of serious imbalances. Overdressing for the environmental temperature causes increased perspiration, resulting in both fluid and electrolyte losses. Additional fluids should be offered to young children in hot weather, and time in the sun must be limited; the number of diapers used and their saturation can guide the need for additional fluids in infants. When a child becomes ill, parents also should be taught to check the child's temperature early in the illness. In the event of a fever, additional fluids should be offered, and clothing should only be sufficient to prevent shivering.

Parents should be taught to reduce solids and milk intake and to give clear fluids primarily when vomiting or diarrhea occurs. It is important, however, for parents to understand that giving plain water alone and in large amounts can be extremely dangerous and may result in seizures, coma, or death. Glucose-electrolyte solutions or a balanced combination of liquids must be used when fluid constitutes the child's only intake for a prolonged period of time. Undiluted skim milk should not be used because of its high solute content; large quantities of water are required for excretion of solutes, further depleting the body of water. How to gradually increase the child's food intake during and after illness in order to avoid starvation is also important information for parents to have (see Chapter 41 for discussion of diet for diarrhea and vomiting).

Treatment of conditions that predispose children to fluid and electrolyte imbalances can start promptly if parents have been taught to identify the early signs. Signs and symptoms they can identify:

1. *General appearance:* sunken or bulging fontanel and sunken eyes, no tears with crying
2. *Neurologic status:* irritability, high-pitched cry, difficult to awaken
3. *Renal status:* fewer wet diapers
4. *Integumentary status:* abnormal skin color, temperature, or moistness
5. *Respiratory status:* increased respiratory rate or difficulty in breathing
6. *Gastrointestinal status:* vomiting or many loose stools

Frequently the nurse can help parents prevent development of more serious problems by taking the time to discuss these few early parameters and encouraging them to seek professional assistance when their child is ill. Families with infants under 6 months of age, in particular, should be cautioned to seek assistance early, since the younger child may deteriorate more rapidly than the older child when imbalances occur.

Meeting Child's Developmental Needs

After a parenteral solution has been ordered by the physician, the nurse assumes the major responsibility for its proper, safe administration. After ascertaining that the dose prescribed (amount and rate of administration) is within safe limits, the nurse starts the IV infusion or assists another individual in doing so. The nurse

- prepares the child and family,
- is aware of preferred sites and equipment options (needles or catheters and pumps or controllers), and
- evaluates whether the child needs to be restrained, and if so, how it can be accomplished most easily.

Each of these interventions depend on the developmental characteristics of the child, which are summarized in Table 30-8.

Promoting Safety and Comfort

Choice of site varies according to the age and condition of the child and the condition of veins. The site selected should involve minimal risk and maximal efficiency, safety, and comfort. Intravenous lines may be placed in the veins of the scalp, hand, foot, or antecubital fossa. Scalp veins are often used in infants because they are prominent and because of the difficulty in finding peripheral veins. Since veins in the scalp do not have valves, the needle or catheter can be inserted in either direction. A rubber band with an adhesive tag

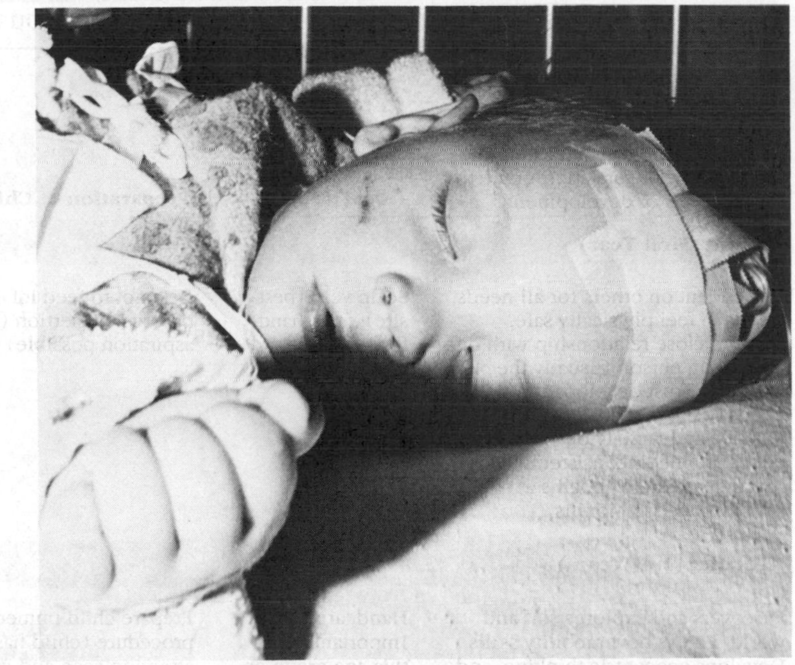

Figure 30-1. A scalp vein catheter inserted in a central position permits the child to be turned to either side.

placed around the infant's head (across the forehead) assists in distending the scalp veins. The adhesive tag facilitates quick grasping and cutting the rubber band after the catheter has been inserted. The veins of the scalp communicate with the dural sinuses, therefore, careful cleansing of head insertion sites is necessary (Metheney and Snively, 1979). Cleansing with povidone-iodine or a similar solution is more effective than using alcohol. Positioning a needle or catheter in a vein in the front center of the head rather than toward the back and side reduces the amount of hair that must be shaved and allows the baby to lie on either side and on the back (Fig. 30-1).

Peripheral veins of the hands and feet, especially those on the dorsum of the hand, are often used in children and are gaining acceptance as choice sites for intravenous therapy in infants. They allow more mobility and are less disfiguring than venipunctures of the scalp (especially if infiltration occurs). Also, the sight of an IV line in the hand (and to a lesser degree, the foot) will likely cause parents less distress than one in the head (Oelerich and Dombrowski, 1981).

Intravenous lines should not be placed in the antecubital fossa unless other sites have been exhausted. The antecubital veins overlie fleshy parts of the muscle and are difficult to enter; the brachial artery lies close to the skin in this area, making it easy to puncture. Also, IV lines inserted over any joint are likely to infiltrate most rapidly. Generally, the most distal part of the vein should always be used first since the proximal continuation of the vessel may be used for future IV therapy.

Other questions to consider: which is the infant's or child's dominant hand; how much will the child's mobility be affected (e.g., can crutches still be used); was an infiltrated IV line recently removed from that area (if yes, use another site)?

Once the preferred site has been identified, the choice of plastic catheter or stainless steel needle is made. Needles are apparently less likely to result in infection (septicemia) and phlebitis than are catheters, but they are more difficult to secure and do not bend with movement of the vein. Subsequently, they tend to last a shorter time than catheters.

Next, the appropriate catheter or needle size is chosen. The size varies according to the size of the vein. In children, 20–27 gauge catheters or needles are most commonly used. The higher the number, the smaller the diameter of the lumen. Although the smaller ones are perhaps easier to insert, the IV infusion can usually be maintained longer when the bore is large.

Regardless of the site or equipment used, the position of the catheter in the vein, the manner of taping, and the effectiveness of the restraint largely determine the duration of the IV therapy. The needle or catheter must be inserted well into the vein and the tape placed to stabilize it without covering the surrounding area needlessly. In general, catheters can be secured more easily than needles, therefore less restraint and usually none is necessary for children with catheters.

Text continues on page 918

Table 30-8. Nursing Guidelines for Pediatric IVs at Various Stages of Child's Development

Developmental Characteristics Note: Each stage builds on the earlier ones and during hospitalization many children regress to behaviors appropriate to earlier levels of development	IV Placement (Ideal Sites)	Preparation of Child	Family Involvement
Infant (First Year)			
Dependent on others for all needs. Needs to feel physically safe, through close relationship with one caretaking person (usually the mother). Trust develops through needs being met consistently. Mistrust and anxiety develop when needs are met inconsistently. "Stranger anxiety" begins at approximately 6 months	Scalp vein (best site); foot, hand, forearm	Best not to feed infant immediately before IV insertion (vomiting and aspiration possible)	Prepare family as to need for IV therapy, insertion procedure, appearance of infant with IV, and fluid needs. Encourage family to continue providing baby with tactile and verbal stimulation and TLC. Demonstrate safe ways to hold an infant with an IV. Encourage questions and clarify misconceptions
Toddler (1–3 Years)			
Discovers and explores self and world. Enjoys new mobility skills. Develops egocentric thinking, and need for parallel play. Tolerates short separations from mother. Transitional objects (security blanket, special toy) provide some comfort. Oppositional syndrome ("no" stage). Separation anxiety an important problem in hospitalized toddlers separated from mother, ages 8–24 months	Hand, arm, foot. Important: From this age group on, the less dominant extremity should be used for the IV whenever possible. Determine handedness prior to IV insertion	Prepare child immediately before procedure (child has limited attention span and is likely to become more anxious if prepared sooner). Give very simple explanation in concrete terms. Show equipment to be used. Do not offer choice. See preparation for preschool age (below) and assess ability of each child to understand	Prepare family as to need for IV therapy insertion procedure, and appearance of child with IV. Whether parents remain with the child during the procedure varies. If they stay with the child their role is to provide comfort rather than to assist with restraining. Demonstrate to parents how to safely handle child with IV
Preschool (4–6 Years)			
Magical thinking, based on what the child would like to believe. Cannot always distinguish fantasy from reality. Fears intrusive procedures. Castration fears common. Develops conscience (guilt), while asserting independence and mastering new skills. Learning to share	Hand, forearm (less dominant)	Prepare child just prior to procedure. Using small bottle, tubing, and doll or stuffed animal, explain in literal terms the need for IV, and insertion procedure. Allow child to see and touch equipment. Explain how child can help with procedure by cleaning site, opening packages, taping, etc. Allow some degree of control in the situation. Say you will help child hold still, and that it's OK to cry	As with toddlers, parents may or may not stay with the child during the procedure. If they stay, they should provide comfort and support but should not be asked to restrain the child for IV insertion. Reinforce child's need for honest, simple explanations. Reassure parents that child can still play and be active, even with IV
School Age (7–11 Years)			
Struggles between mastering new skills and failure. Enjoys school, learning skills, games with rules. Needs to succeed. Fears body mutilation. May feel need to be "brave." Can understand hospital rules. World now expanding beyond family. Peer group becomes important. Competitiveness	Hand, forearm (less dominant)	Prepare child ahead of time, but same day of insertion. Carefully explain and demonstrate equipment and reasons for IV therapy, letting patient watch you or help set up equipment. Ask child for questions about need for IV and procedure. Give child choices and let help in procedure whenever possible. Tell child crying is Ok because needles hurt, and you will help him or her hold still	Whenever possible, family and child should be prepared together, so that family can reinforce what the child has been told. Stress to family the child's need for some independence in ADL, even with an IV. Parental presence or participation in IV insertion may be appropriate, but child's preference should be considered primary

Related Nursing Actions	Protection of IV Site	**Mobility Considerations** Note: No child should be restricted to bed simply because of an IV!	Safety Needs
Infant (First Year)			
Restrain during insertion. Comfort and cuddle during and after insertion. Observe carefully during insertion for problems of vomiting, aspiration, etc. Firmly restrain extremity with IV (see next column). Use of pacifier diminishes stress, especially for NPO infants	IV may be secured with tape only or by using a paper cup with bottom cut out or a plastic medicine cup to protect insertion site. Extremity may be restrained by using a board, a sandbag, or wrist and ankle restraints	Keep restraints as loose as possible to allow for motion. Release any restrained extremities hourly for ROM. Mitten hands with cotton and stockinette to prohibit infant's grasping IV. Restraining all extremities is *rarely* necessary. Remember infant's need for sensory stimulation	Maintain strict I & O. Secure IV tubing out of range of kicking legs and flailing arms. Check restraints frequently for effectiveness and presence of adequate circulation
Toddler (1–3 Years)			
Restraining the toddler for an IV usually requires more than one person. Reassure child through verbal and tactile stimulation during procedure. Provide toys to hit or throw, for therapeutic expression of anger, after procedure and throughout hospitalization	See above (infant). A securely anchored IV is essential for the normally active toddler. Even the best site protection will not remain effective unless it is coupled with close nursing supervision, and with distracting activities for the child	Toddlers cope with the world and learn about it through action. Therefore, minimal restraints should be used, and tying the child in bed is to be avoided. Parental presence during waking hours permits the child to be constantly supervised, and makes restraints unnecessary in many cases. However, be careful to avoid setting up a situation in which the child associates parent's departure with "punishment" of restraint	Child is unaware of danger at this age and will not know that movement of IV causes pain. Constant supervision needed when out of bed. Remind frequently not to touch IV, but don't expect compliance. Distracting activities will accomplish much more than a scolding for handling the IV. Tape connections on tubing if child continues to handle tubing. Keep tubing clamps out of reach
Preschool Age (4–6 Years)			
Tell child this IV is *not* punishment. *Never* bribe or threaten with IVs (e.g., "Drink, or you'll get another IV"). Praise cooperation, or any efforts in that direction. Maintain patient privacy. Don't start an IV in view of other patients, visitors, or staff. Child needs support to cope with intrusiveness of this procedure. Show understanding	See above (infant). As with toddlers, securely anchored IVs are essential but inadequate unless coupled with food supervision and age-appropriate activities	As with infants, any restrained extremity needs hourly release for ROM. Preschoolers need maximum mobility to master surroundings. Provide a range of out-of-bed activities whenever possible	Child will be curious about IV. Is capable of understanding instructions to not touch it, but needs frequent reminders. IV clamps should be out of reach or taped over. Constant supervision needed when out of bed. Child is liable to "take off" down the hall, heedless of pole, bottle, etc. Short attention span limits duration of cooperation with instructions
School Age (7–11 Years)			
Approach child expecting cooperation (this age group likes to please adults), but expect that child will need help holding still. Allow the child to clean the site with alcohol swab, and to cut tape, prior to insertion. Praise cooperative efforts. Give child step-by-step explanation of procedure as it progresses. Child may like to take some responsibility in keeping I & O	Will need less protection than younger children owing to interest in making IV "work" correctly. May naturally protect extremity with IV. Some children will appreciate a warning sign. "Hands Off," on a piece of tape over the IV as a reminder. Utilize the child's natural curiosity and interest in learning. Tell the "rules" of safe IV handling	Show patient and family how to safely manipulate IV for out-of-bed activities (walking in hall with pole, keeping tubing out of wheelchair wheels, etc.)	Remind patient periodically about necessary caution with IV. Show patient the clamps, and caution against handling them. Teach patient signs of IV problems. Enlist child's help in the interest of good compliance, but do not entirely depend on it. Tape tubing connections. Child may forget about IV. Emphasize need for caution in some activities, especially if play includes other children

continued

Table 30-8 *(continued)*

Developmental Characteristics Note: Each stage builds on the earlier ones and during hospitalization many children regress to behaviors appropriate to earlier levels of development	IV Placement (Ideal Sites)	Preparation of Child	Family Involvement
Adolescent (12–18 Years)			
Vacillates between needs for independence and dependence. Adult cognitive abilities, deductive reasoning. Coping mechanisms: rationalization, intellectualization. Peer acceptance very important. Egocentric, rebellious at times, especially against parents and authority figures. Very concerned with body image, body changes, sexuality, and role. Searching for "who I am"	Hand, forearm (less dominant)	Prepare child several hours to a day before procedure, if possible. Needs time between preparation and insertion to absorb explanations and ask questions. For most adolescents, approach discussions on an adult level. Explain need for IV therapy and expected duration, and show equipment. May need much support for acceptance of therapy	Explain therapy needs and duration as per patient. Decision regarding parental presence during procedure should be patient's, not parents'. Stress to family the patient's need for independence and participation in decisions affecting care

(Adapted from Gublow and Kolb, 1979.)

With a scalp vein IV line, a young infant may only need positioning with a rolled blanket. Placing the tube away from the infant's body helps maintain the IV line because of random arm movements typical during this stage of development.

Starting an IV Line

To prepare IV fluids and begin administration, the following steps are suggested:

1. Prepare the IV fluid by connecting the fluid chamber to the main reservoir (small bottles of 250 or 500 ml are recommended to avoid unnecessary wasting of IV solutions).
2. Put enough fluid into the fluid chamber to fill the IV tubing (approximately 15 to 20 ml plus fluid for 1 to 2 hours).
3. "Prime" the system (i.e., run fluid through it).
4. Insert the catheter.
5. Connect the tubing to the catheter and check whether the IV runs by gravity.
6. Thread the tubing through the pump, set the desired rate, and start the pump.

Three basic methods are available for regulation of the flow of IV fluids:

- Intravenous controllers regulate fluid administration at preselected rates, but they depend on gravity for proper operation.
- Intravenous pumps automatically deliver fluid by exerting positive pressure on IV tubing (peristaltic pumps) or by pushing the fluid through a cylinder (piston and cylinder pumps) at set flow rates.
- Traditional roller clamp systems depend on gravity and are regulated by hand.

Controllers or pumps help prevent fluid overload and drug overdosage. They must be used during administration of parenteral nutrition and continuous medication infusions and when fluid restriction is necessary in small children. The IV tubing is threaded through these machines, then the dial is set for the desired rate of flow (Fig. 30-2). Intravenous pumps and controllers differ in their safety mechanisms; many have alarms that sound when the machine is not functioning properly. However, pumps often continue to infuse fluid at preset rates for a while after infiltration has occurred before alarms sound. For additional safety, a special control fluid chamber that holds a limited amount of solution and provides for accurate measurement is recommended for use in children. The pediatric minidrip set delivers 60 drops (gtts) per minute (Fig. 30-3). When roller clamp systems are used alone, adjust the flow rate when the child is quiet, if regulated when the child is crying, the rate may be too rapid when the crying stops.

Calculation of IV Rates

Calculation of the proper drip rate of fluid administered to children is simplified by the use of a system that delivers 60 gtts per minute (gtts/min). Typical fluid orders are either in number of milliliters per hour (ml/hr) or milliliters per 24 hours (ml/24 hr). The following simple calculations will convert such orders into gtts/min.

Related Nursing Actions	Protection of IV Site	Mobility Considerations Note: No child should be restricted to bed simply because of an IV!	Safety Needs
Adolescent (12–18 Years)			
Be aware of IV adding to patient's dependency status, and the need for some control. Encourage patient to keep own I & O, help in counting drip rate, etc. Privacy during insertion is very important	See above (School Age). If patient is very active, will need well-protected, well-anchored IV, as movements may be more forceful and strength greater than younger patients'	See above (School Age). Encourage mobility as much as possible as a means of independence for the adolescent	Be aware of possibility of adolescent rebellion showing itself in lack of cooperation with therapy. These patients may rebel if feeling threatened and may be very manipulative in "testing" behaviors. Consistent limits, clearly communicated to patient, parents, and staff, are needed. Instruct patient about signs of infiltration, phlebitis, etc.

When the system delivers 60 gtts/ml:

A. If the order is for ml/hr:
(Example: 40 ml/hr = 40 gtts/min*)

B. If the order is for ml/24 hr:
(Example: 960 ml/24 hr)

1. Change to ml/hr:

$$960 \div 24 \text{ hr} = 40 \text{ ml/hr}$$

2. 40 ml/hr = 40 gtts/min*

The reason that ml/hr = gtts/min is explained by the following:

Step 1:

Number of ml/hr ordered	×	number of gtts/ml delivered by system	=	number of gtts/hr
40		60		2400

Step 2:

Number of gtts/hr	÷	number of min/hr	=	number of gtts/min
2400		60		40

Because the number of seconds in a minute, the number of minutes in an hour, and the number of drops per ml are all 60, the system works out nicely. Thus, whenever the IV set is designed to deliver 60 gtts/ml, the order of 40 ml/hr can be converted immediately to 40 gtts/min without any calculations.

* Ml/hr can be equated to gtts/min only if the system delivers 60 gtts/ml.

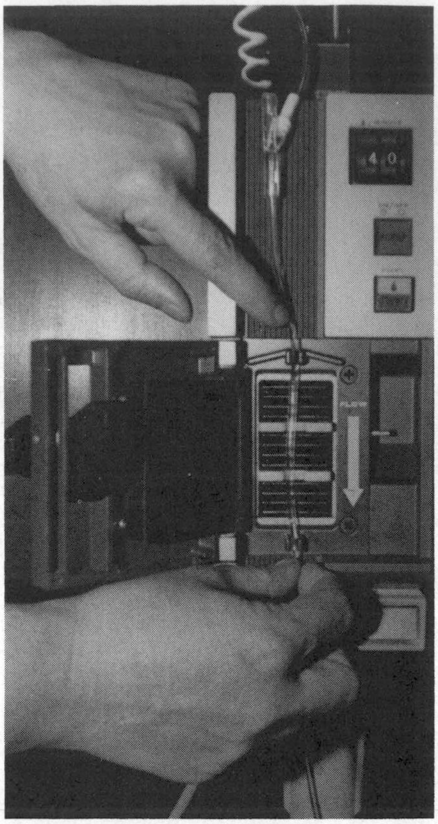

Figure 30-2. IV tubing is threaded through the pump, following the direction of the arrow on the pump. Pump designs vary; the placement of tubing through the pump may be vertical or horizontal.

Maintaining the IV Infusion

Maintaining an IV infusion entails administering fluid accurately and safely to the child. The machinery available to monitor IV therapy cannot replace nurses, but it can assist them. Pump and controller systems do not reduce work, but if used properly they increase the safety of parenteral fluid administration.

At the beginning of each shift the nurse responsible for a particular child with an IV line must make a complete check, including

1. the type of solution and electrolyte dose,
2. the date and time the bottle and tubing were hung (usually changed every 24 hours),
3. the rate; check the setting on the machine and count the actual gtts/min,
4. the tubing—check for kinks, flattening, blood, or air; check the entire length of the tubing to the insertion site,
5. the tubing for proper threading into the machine,
6. the IV site for redness, puffiness, and security of tape,
7. the security and appropriateness of restraint; check all involved extremities for warmth, color, and general appearance,
8. any medication that is running; verify that the amount is absorbed on schedule as prescribed,
9. the general status of the child, and
10. vital signs and urinary output.

The nurse should make this check in the presence of the nurse who was previously in charge of the child's care. It cannot be done without light; therefore, a flashlight must be used to make IV checks when children are asleep. A dim light from the hallway is not adequate. If there is any question regarding the site, overhead lights must be turned on even though the child or other children may awaken. Thereafter, hourly checks should include checking

1. the setting on the machine and a counting of the actual drops,
2. the entire length of tubing,
3. the site and restrained extremities,
4. the general status of the child, and
5. the amount of fluid absorbed; enter it on an IV record sheet

IV record sheets are used to monitor fluid administration. The types of forms used vary among institutions.

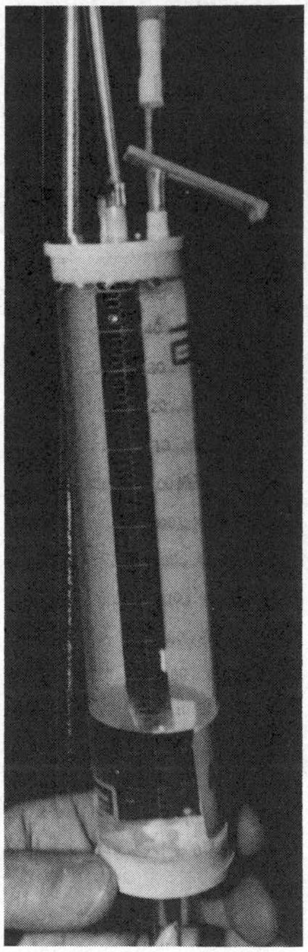

Figure 30-3. A special control chamber holds a limited amount of fluid and provides for accurate measurement of fluid administration.

Columns should be provided for the type of fluid being administered, the rate, the amount of fluid actually absorbed hourly, and a running total of fluid absorbed per shift. A column should be provided for the nurse to write her comments, and each hourly check should be documented with the nurse's initials.

The nurse is also responsible for making ongoing assessments of the child's fluid, electrolyte, and acid-base balance whenever parenteral therapy is being administered. The previous discussion on assessment of vital signs, weight, skin, anterior fontanel and eyes, intake and output and urine specific gravity, and laboratory reports describes pertinent observations that must be made during intravenous therapy.

Some environmental and clinical situations affect fluid and electrolyte balance during fluid therapy. If a child is in a hot environment, has a fever, or is tachypneic, water loss is increased. For every degree of fever above 37.8°C, 12 per cent of fluid maintenance is added. (For each degree of fever above 100°F, 8 per cent of fluid maintenance is added.) Crying may double insensible water loss in a baby. Also, a newborn infant placed under a radiant heat warmer or receiving phototherapy has increased fluid loss through evaporation. Decreases in water loss may occur in cool environments or if humidity is high (e.g., in a mist tent). If these conditions exist when a child has renal disease or has a high concentration of ADH, water intake may need to be decreased.

Preventing Complications of IV Therapy

A major responsibility of the nurse is to prevent complications of IV therapy. Complications may include

- clotting,
- infiltration,
- phlebitis,
- infection, and
- air embolism.

Clotting of IV lines occurs when the continuous flow of fluid is interrupted (e.g., the fluid chamber runs dry, the IV tubing kinks, or the IV pump is not turned on). It can occur very quickly, so measures must be taken by the nurse to prevent these problems. IV alarms should be attended to immediately.

The infiltration of IV infusions can best be prevented by use of secure restraints and proper insertion. When this common complication occurs, however, early recognition will minimize the sequelae. Signs and symptoms that the nurse must watch for include local pain, swelling, tenderness, cool skin, and blanching. IV therapy must be checked by looking at the insertion site and the surrounding area, because infiltrated fluid often collects in dependent areas. Also, if tape appears to be becoming tighter, infiltration should be suspected. When a scalp vein site infiltrates, a generalized fullness can be noted and slight asymmetry of the head may be apparent. Lack of blood return is not always proof of infiltration in children because small gauge catheters are often used and because a young child's venous pressure may not be high enough to cause backflow (Gillis, 1982). Infiltration of IV infusions, especially when medications are in the infusate, can cause enough tissue damage to require skin grafting, so prevention is of paramount importance. To guard against infiltration, take a "mental picture" of the site when the first IV check is made and carefully check its appearance hourly to compare it with its original appearance.

Phlebitis, or inflammation of the vein wall, occurs for many reasons: contaminated equipment or site, length of time the catheter is in place, difficult insertion, and chemical irritation from some drugs and solutions. It is characterized by red, hot skin, local pain, swelling, and a palpable, hardened vein. Phlebitis can be prevented by adhering to aseptic principles when inserting catheters, changing IV dressings, and handling IV solutions; changing equipment (e.g., IV tubing, solutions) frequently; and using membrane filters on all IV lines through which antibiotics or other irritating drugs are administered (Gillis, 1982).

The presence of a small amount of air in the venous system usually causes no problem. It simply travels to the lungs and is absorbed. This is not true when the amount is large (in adults, 10 ml or more) or when even a very small amount enters the circulation of a child with a right and left heart connection (e.g., ventricular or atrial septal defect). In the former, the amount may be enough to interfere with the supply of blood to a significant part of the body; in the latter, the air may cross from the venous to the arterial side of the heart and proceed to the coronary or cerebral circulation. Therefore, all IV lines in children with heart openings must have air filters on them.

It is clear from this discussion that the nurse's expertise in managing IV therapy is a skill that greatly contributes to the recovery and well being of a child.

Supporting the Child and Family During IV Therapy

Nurses are most often responsible for the preparation of the child and the family for intravenous therapy. They must also guide their participation in the process. To nurses, intravenous therapy is a common pediatric procedure. To the child and family, however, it has a

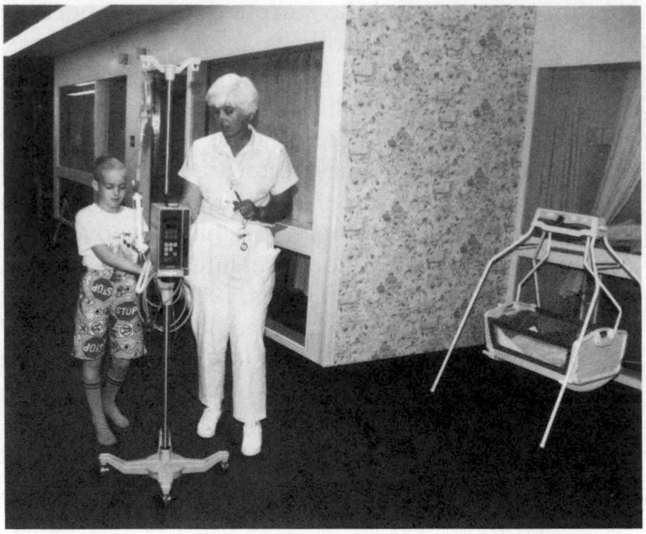

Children with intravenous lines should not be immobilized unnecessarily. Independence is fostered by allowing this 10-year-old to push his own IV pole.

variety of meanings and is the subject of numerous fears. Nurses, therefore, must approach IV therapy with the recognition that fears and questions need to be addressed. A family may interpret their child's need for IV therapy as a sign of a deteriorating condition. Responding to individual needs for reassurance and comfort is very important.

A gentle, positive approach will help gain the child's cooperation. Whether the parents should stay or leave when an IV line is started is a decision that should be made with the child, the parent and the nurse. There is no prescribed rule. Some parents wish to stay and are able to support the child. This is appropriate if the nurse's skill is not adversely affected by their presence, and it will likely be beneficial for the child to have the parents nearby. However, if the parents' fears are easily communicated to the child or if the nurse cannot work effectively with parents present, it is usually in everyone's best interest if they wait in a lounge away from the treatment room.

Children with IV lines should not be immobilized unnecessarily. Young children may require restraints when unsupervised, but parents and nurses can hold them and take them for a ride or to a play room. Older children can be up in wheelchairs, can be allowed to walk in the halls, and can go to the play area.

Age-appropriate independence to the degree the IV line permits should be fostered. Parents can be taught how to care for the child or assist the child in self-care. Too often parents fear dislodging the IV line and defer to the nurse when care is required. The physical isolation that is imposed by an IV line makes it particularly important that the nurse make every effort to assist parents to become involved to the degree that they can and want to be. The child benefits by the comfort of feeling close to the parent, and the parent derives a feeling of comfort by providing that closeness. (Guidelines for family involvement during parenteral therapy are offered in Table 30-8.)

Total Parenteral Nutrition (Hyperalimentation)

Adequate nutrition in hospitalized patients is an important factor in prompt recovery from injury or illness. When nutritional integrity cannot be maintained by oral or tube feedings, total parenteral nutrition (TPN) is indicated. This therapy provides all necessary nutrients by the intravenous route. To administer TPN safely, the nurse must be aware of the child's nutritional requirements, the composition of the solution, the indications for TPN, the implications for nursing care, and the potential complications of the therapy.

Nutritional Requirements

Under normal conditions, children ingest enough calories and protein to meet the body's needs for energy and growth. However, the spontaneous oral intake of a sick child may be inadequate to meet the body's demands, and the child may enter a catabolic state. This destructive process can be halted by the administration of carefully prescribed TPN. The TPN infusate (the solution being administered) can supply the child with protein (as crystalline amino acids), carbohydrate (as glucose), electrolytes, vitamins, and minerals. Fat, or lipid emulsions, that can be administered along with TPN supply necessary fatty acids. Fat is very important as an energy source; without it, energy requirements in the young child on peripheral TPN cannot be met. Estimation of metabolic (energy) requirements includes the calculation of basal metabolic rate (kcal/day) and the allotment of additional calories for the child's specific condition. For example, simple trauma entails a 20 per cent increment in metabolic rate, and burns may increase the rate by as much as 50 to 100 per cent, depending on the extent of thermal injury (Seashore, 1984). Other conditions that increase energy requirements include surgery, sepsis, and fever. Average energy requirements for parenterally fed infants and children are as follows (Zlotkin et al, 1985):

premature neonates		90 kcal/kg/day
infants	0–1 year	80–95 kcal/kg/day
children	2–9 years	60–70 kcal/kg/day
	10–13 years	50–60 kcal/kg/day
adolescents		40 kcal/kg/day

Amino acid requirements for the same group are (Zlotkin et al, 1985):

premature neonates		3.0 gm/kg/day
infants	0–1 year	2.5 gm/kg/day
children	2–9 yeras	1.5–2.0 gm/kg/day
	10–13 years	1.5–2.0 gm/kg/day
adolescents		1.0–1.5 gm/kg/day

Infants, children, and adults need 4, 3, and 2 gms/kg/day of fat, respectively (Seashore, 1984).

Composition of TPN Solutions

Amino acid solutions contain the eight known essential amino acids plus histidine, which is known to be essential for children. *Dextrose* (glucose) is the most important nonprotein energy source used in parenteral solutions. Trace minerals, vitamins, and electrolytes are added to base solutions. The concentration of any constituent can be changed to meet individual needs.

Total parenteral nutriton may be administered through a peripheral vein or a central vein, often the superior vena cava. The amount of dextrose to be infused is limited by the location of the intravenous catheter and the tolerance of the child and the vein to the solution. The child's tolerance is measured by serum and urine glucose levels. Hypertonic TPN is initiated slowly, and the rate and concentration of dextrose are gradually increased to allow the pancreas to respond to the increased demand for insulin (Conran, 1980). The TPN solutions with dextrose concentrations greater than 12.5 per cent must be infused centrally, where the rapid blood flow can dilute the solution and thereby decrease vein irritation. A child with a central venous catheter can receive up to 25 to 47 per cent dextrose (Conran, 1980) although these high percentages are rarely necessary if lipids can be used also. The maximal final concentration of dextrose administered through a peripheral vein is 12.5 per cent; however, adequate calories cannot be obtained with solutions of 12.5 per cent dextrose or less that are administered at conventional rates. Therefore, the calories provided by fat emulsions are especially important to those receiving peripheral TPN.

Fat or liquid emulsions are manufactured from either soybean or safflower oil, stabilized with egg phospholipid, and made isotonic with glycerol. A 10 per cent solution yields 1.1 kcal/ml, and a 20 per cent solution yields 2.0 kcal/ml (Haas-Beckert, 1987). The development of lipid emulsions makes possible adequate caloric intake in a small volume of fluid. The fat emulsion is nearly isotonic, having minimal osmotic pressure; therefore, it may be infused in either peripheral or central veins. By infusing the fat emulsion simultaneously with the dextrose and amino acid solution, the osmolality of the total infusate is decreased. Fat emulsions are also given to prevent essential fatty acid deficiency.

Electrolytes, vitamins, and trace elements are also included in the parenteral nutrition infusate. Electrolytes include potassium, sodium, chloride, calcium, phosphorus, and magnesium. Electrolyte requirements are determined by the serum levels. Daily basic electrolyte requirements must be met, along with the additional needs resulting from such factors as the particular disease process or surgery. Water- and fat-soluble vitamins are given to the child routinely. Some of these vitamins may be added to the TPN infusate. Trace element requirements for infants are still being determined; school-age children and adolescents usually receive trace elements in the solution two or more times a week. The trace elements commonly added to TPN are zinc, copper, iodide, and manganese (Conran, 1980).

The dextrose, amino acids, electrolytes, vitamins, and trace elements are mixed in one container by a pharmacist. This is done under a laminar air flow hood to decrease the risk of contamination. The fat emulsion is administered from a separate container because the addition of any other solution could disrupt the stability of the emulsion.

Indications for TPN Administration

TPN is indicated when nourishment by mouth is inadequate. A child may be malnourished, or a prolonged period without enteral feedings may be anticipated. Before TPN is chosen, the indications for each child must be weighed against the potentially life-threatening complications related to TPN infusion. The child's age, current nutritional status, and clinical status also should be considered. For example, the neonate, especially the premature neonate, has minimal nutritional reserves, so parenteral nutrition may be necessary sooner than in the older child (Conran, 1980).

Clinical conditions in the neonate and infant that may necessitate the use of parenteral nutrition include major anomalies of the gastrointestinal tract, intractable diarrhea, necrotizing enterocolitis, immune deficiency, and very low birthweight (less than 1000 gm). Indications for toddlers and older children are similar to those for adults: inflammatory bowel disease, short bowel syndrome, Crohn disease, prolonged ileus, fistulas, severe burns, major trauma, acute pancreatitis, AIDS, renal failure, and hepatic failure.

Nursing Responsibilities in TPN Administration

Nursing care to prevent complications of parenteral nutrition includes careful administration and monitoring of the TPN solution and meticulous care of the catheter.

TPN Administration

The TPN solution must be administered at a constant rate to avoid potential metabolic complications. The infusion rate is never adjusted to "catch up." An infusion pump is essential for administration, and the nurse must check the rate by counting the drops every hour. Abrupt cessation of 25 per cent glucose infusion may lead to profound hypoglycemia and seizures (Seashore, 1984). To prevent this occurrence, the nurse must assure the patency of the catheter, maintain secure connections in the line, and make sure the TPN bag never "runs dry."

The bag, IV administration tubing, and filter (if used) must be changed every 24 hours to prevent infection. Frequently the practice is to place the sterile extension tubing partly under the dressing so it is changed only with the dressing change. Prior to opening connections in the tubing system, they must be cleansed with iodophor solution to prevent yeast and bacterial growth. After reconnecting the joints, they are taped to prevent accidental separation.

Whenever a fat emulsion is being infused, it must be added aseptically below the filter because the fat particles are too large to pass through the filter. It should be added as close to the intravenous site as possible so there is minimal mixture of the two infusates. The practice of administration of fat emulsions varies. Some administer fat and TPN into the same central line whereas others administer fat emulsions into a separate peripheral line.

Some drugs are compatible with the amino acid/dextrose/mineral component of TPN, but not with the lipid emulsion (Zlotkin, 1985). The practice of administering drugs, other IV fluids, and blood products into the same intravenous site as TPN varies but is generally limited to patients in whom venous access is severely limited. Even in necessary cases, these interruptions compound the problem of inadequate nutrition (Seashore and Hoffman, 1983). Oncology patients, however, have central lines that are established for the purpose of medications and blood sampling, as well as central TPN.

Catheter Care

Central catheters for TPN are placed in the superior vena cava. In the neonate and infant, this is accomplished by inserting a silicone rubber catheter through the internal or external jugular vein to the superior vena cava. The catheter is then tunneled subcutaneously to an exit site 2 to 4 inches away from the vein insertion site. In the neonate and infant, this exit site is usually on the scalp; in the young child the site may be in the neck or chest wall (Conran, 1980). School-age and older children may have a catheter inserted into the superior vena cava via the subclavian vein. (This is also commonly used in adults.) To avoid complications resulting from infusing the hypertonic solution outside the superior vena cava, an isotonic solution must be infused until the placement of the catheter tip is confirmed by x-ray.

Proper nursing care of the catheter is vital to decrease the risk of local or systemic infection. The dressing should be changed every 48 hours and whenever it is wet or loose, using standard sterile technique. The nurse and all others in the room, including the patient, should wear masks. The nurse must also wear sterile gloves. The site should be cleaned with an acetone and alcohol solution followed by iodophor solution, cleansing from the site in an outward, circular direction. After the antibacterial and antifungal ointment is applied, the site is covered with a small sterile dressing. Then the extension tubing is changed while the child performs, or someone stimulates, the Valsalva maneuver* to prevent an air embolus. The connection between the catheter and the Luer-Lok extension tubing is then covered with part of the sterile dressing. With hypoallergenic tape, the dressing is taped occlusively, dated, and signed. Part of the extension tubing should be looped and taped on top of the secured dressing to prevent direct tension on the cath-

* The Valsalva maneuver involves forcible exhalation against the closed glottis. The child may perform this maneuver by taking a deep breath and bearing down as if having a bowel movement. This may be stimulated by applying pressure to the abdomen, if this is not contraindicated.

eter. The physician should be notified if erythema (redness), edema, drainage or any other change in the catheter placement (e.g., catheter kink or loose sutures) is noted.

Peripheral TPN in infants is commonly administered in a scalp vein; the larger arm veins are frequently used in older children. The site must be checked at least every hour for vein irritation or infiltration. If infiltration is suspected, the site must be changed immediately because of the risk of skin sloughing. Care of the IV site is the same as for any peripheral IV site.

Monitoring

The nurse must carefully monitor the child receiving parenteral nutrition. General appearance, level of activity, sense of well-being, and skin turgor are noted (Seashore, 1984). Blood pressure, pulse, respirations, and temperature must be recorded at least every 4 hours. Temperature is especially important since an increase is one of the first signs of catheter-related sepsis. An accurate daily intake and output record must be maintained to assess fluid balance. The record should indicate the type of intake and output, so that calorie and nitrogen intake and output can be determined. A diaper count may suffice for the urine output after the neonate or infant is stable on parenteral nutrition. Urine sugar/acetone fractional levels and specific gravity are checked at least every 6 to 8 hours. Glucosuria of 2^+ or greater must be corrected to prevent eventual development of hyperosmotic nonketotic coma. Dextrostix or Chemstix should be used to check the blood sugar every 4 to 8 hours upon initiation of TPN and whenever the infusion is suddenly decreased or stopped. Daily weights are obtained, and the length and head circumference of infants are measured once a week.

Laboratory assessment includes complete blood count, blood urea nitrogen (BUN), glucose, and electrolytes daily for the first 3 or 4 days, then once or twice a week. Bilirubin, SGOT, alkaline phosphatase, and ammonia levels are measured once a week (Seashore and Hoffman, 1983). Determination of serum lipid concentration should be performed frequently in children receiving fat emulsions.

Oral Hygiene

Oral hygiene is a very important but often forgotten part of nursing care. Oral hygiene must be performed at least three times a day to prevent such complications as oral lesions and parotitis and to promote comfort. Brushing teeth to prevent tooth decay is important for all children and especially for those children who are allowed to eat hard candy during TPN administration. Different-flavored mouthwashes may be offered to the child to provide some taste sensations.

Exercise

Exercise is important to maintain or regain muscle strength. Unless contraindicated, the child should be encouraged to move freely with proper protection for the IV line. Physical or occupational therapists can recommend appropriate exercises for bedridden children.

Emotional Needs

Depriving a child of food can have a significant emotional impact on the child and the family. The necessity and importance of TPN therapy must be carefully explained to everyone. The reasons for the monitoring done by the nurses and physicians and the importance of receiving nothing by mouth (NPO) and of avoiding dislodgement of the IV catheter must be explained to both the child and the family. The explanation given to the child depends on the age and level of understanding. The NPO neonate needs a pacifier so that sucking needs are met. Also, the baby should be held at regular intervals because of not being held routinely for meals. Since some children still feel hungry even when receiving adequate parenteral nutrition, they need extra attention or distraction during mealtimes and when they see food or food advertisements. Many of these children have chronic illnesses, and consequently they are hospitalized for a long time. Family members are not always able to be present, so these children need extra attention from the nursing staff.

Home Total Parenteral Nutrition (HTPN)

Since nutritional support is often required over a long period of time, home nutritional support services have been instituted. The need for long-term therapy, experience with the technique of TPN, and improvements in equipment contributed to the transition of using TPN at home.

A key factor in the institution of HTPN was the development of a Silastic catheter in the early 1970s (Broviac et al, 1974; Riella and Scribner, 1976). This catheter was very flexible and did not harden with extended use; theoretically, it could be used indefinitely (Vargas et al, 1987). A Luer-Lok at the end of the catheter made it possible to fill it with heparin and cap it when not in use. A cuff at midpoint was used to anchor the catheter to the subcutaneous tissue, preventing its dislodgement—an important feature for home use. A variety of catheters are now on the market, and they all have these key features.

A final important step contributing to sending a child home on TPN was the realization that a child's complete nutritional needs could be administered

Table 30-9. Care of Children on Home Total Parenteral Nutrition (HTPN)

Nursing Diagnoses	Nursing Goals/Strategies
Potential for infection, related to: • *contamination of PN solution* • *contamination of infusion system* • *contamination of catheter* • *contamination of catheter exit site*	*Prevent infection: instruct child and parents in* • Aseptic techniques • Catheter care • Dressing change • Capping of catheter when not in use • Handling and storage of PN solution and tubing • Preparing TPN infusion system • Attachment of infusion system to catheter • Provide an instruction manual for family
	Reduce potential for complications from an infection • Instruct parents and child about early signs and symptoms that indicate an infection (chills, diaphoresis, pyrexia of >38.5°C or 101.3°F, lethargy and weakness in the child, and redness, drainage, or odor at the catheter exit site) • Give the family a manual that contains the information taught verbally
Potential for altered nutrition: • *more than body requirements, related to excessive administration of glucose (hyperglycemia)*	*Administer the correct amount of glucose for the individual child. Instruct family:* • How to infuse the correct solution at the correct rate • To avoid rapid increases in the rate of delivery of TPN solution • Give family an instruction manual containing the correct procedure and rate required to maintain a correct balance of glucose
	Reduce potential for complications from hyperglycemia: • Instruct family about signs and symptoms of hyperglycemia (nausea, weakness, headache, increased thirst, polyuria, and increased frequency of urination) • Instruct family in a plan of action if it occurs
• *less than body requirements, related to a deficit of glucose (hypoglycemia)*	*Administer the correct amount of glucose for the individual child* • Instruct parent how to infuse the correct solution at the correct rate and to avoid rapid reduction in the rate of delivery • Give family and child an instruction manual about the correct procedure and rate required to maintain a correct balance of glucose
	Reduce potential for complications from hypoglycemia • Instruct parents and child about signs and symptoms of hypoglycemia (sweating, acute fatigue, irritability, nervousness, restlessness, seizure activity potential if prolonged) • Instruct family in a plan of action if it occurs, e.g., physician access
***Potential for ineffective family coping, (compromised)**, related to the care demands and resultant fatigue associated with HTPN*	*Promote family coping during the need for HTPN* • Acknowledge the family's experience of fatigue as an expected normal process • Suggest to the family that a relative or close friend should also learn the correct procedure of HTPN to give the family occasional relief • Encourage parents to take time for their own relationship • Help family members identify changes in relationships that are a result of need for child's TPN • Encourage family members to seek help in adjustment to change in family process that results when child requires HTPN

Nursing Diagnoses	Nursing Goals/Strategies
Potential for altered growth and development, related to the chronic illness and numerous hospitalizations that are often part of the life of a child requiring HTPN	*Foster maximal growth and development of child receiving HTPN* • Instruct parents to provide developmentally appropriate activities for child • Make a referral to occupational therapy and physiotherapy for assistance as appropriate • Provide school programs during hospitalization to maintain school performance

(Prepared by Nancy Fram, Patient Care Coordinator, Pediatric Step-Down Unit, Chedoke-McMaster Hospital (McMaster Division), Hamilton, Ontario.)

over an 8- to 12-hour infusion period if the patient was gradually introduced to such a routine (Vargas, 1987). This practice enables children to attend school and other daytime activities. The daily night-time infusion is often stressful to parents because of the daily commitment at a specific time that is required of the family.

HTPN is used either as a temporary measure or as a means of lifelong nutritional support. Vargas (1987), in a report on 102 patients, stated that the average patient received HTPN for nearly 2 years, eight received HTPN for more than 5 years, and four for a decade. The nutritional status of children on HTPN and the numerous associated complications are areas of ongoing research (Dahlstrom et al, 1985; Merritt, 1986; Vargas et al, 1987). It is speculated that bowel transplantation may be a technique to eventually obviate the need for lifelong use of HTPN (Vargas, 1987).

In some cases, parenteral nutrition is the *only* source of nutrition, that is, TPN, whereas in others, parenteral nutrition is supplemented with enteral nutrition. It is believed that enteral intake stimulates bile flow, therefore reduces the risk of cholestasis, gallstone formation, and liver disease (Postuma and Trevenen, 1979; Farrell and Balistreri, 1986).

Even small enteral feedings to interrupt the complications associated with fasting have been suggested, particularly in the care of low birthweight infants (Merritt, 1986). The nutritional value of enteral feedings, however, is affected by the amount of absorption that takes place in a particular child. The actual amount of absorption is often overestimated (Vargas, 1987). Consequently, long-term weight gain and growth have been reported to be best in children who receive 90 per cent or more of their nutrition parenterally (Dahlstrom et al, 1985).

Nursing Strategies to Support Children on HTPN

Home assessment and management of a child on TPN is a role often assumed by nurses. Nurses in acute care centers, outpatient clinics, or agencies may be called upon to provide consultation to the family with a child on HTPN. A nursing guide of potential problems and issues that families encounter is presented in Table 30-9).

References

Ackerman AD: Fluid therapy. *In* Hoekelman RA, et al: *Primary Pediatric Care.* St. Louis, CV Mosby, 1987.

Behrman RE, Vaughan VC III (eds): *Nelson Textbook of Pediatrics.* 13th ed. Philadelphia, WB Saunders, 1987.

Broviac VW, et al: A silicone rubber atrial catheter for prolonged parenteral nutrition. *Surg Gynecol Obstet* 1974; 136:602–608.

Burgess A: *The Nurse's Guide to Fluid and Electrolyte Balance.* New York, McGraw-Hill, 1987.

Catchpole M: Electrolytes, their physiological action and interaction: a review. *Assoc Nurs Anesth* 1982 Oct; 50: 476–481.

Chambers TL: Fluid therapy. *In Childhood.* Boston, Blackwell Scientific Publications, 1987.

Conran A: Nutritional support of the pediatric surgical patient. *In* Holder T, Aschcraft K (eds): *Pediatric Surgery.* Philadelphia, WB Saunders, 1980.

Dahlstrom KA, et al: Nutritional status in children receiving home parenteral nutrition. *Pediatrics* 1985; 107:219–223.

Dube SV: Metabolic emergencies. *In* Dube SK (ed): *Immediate Care of the Sick and Injured Child.* St. Louis, CV Mosby, 1978.

Farrell MK, Balistreri WF: Parenteral nutrition and hepatobiliary dysfunction. *Clin Perinatol* 1986; 13:197–212.

Finberg L: Treatment of dehydration in infancy. *Pediatr Rev* 1981 Oct; 3(4):113–120.

Finberg L, Kravath RE, Fleischman AR: *Water and Electrolytes in Pediatrics—Physiology, Pathophysiology and Treatment.* Philadelphia, WB Saunders, 1982.

Gillis A: Hazards and complications of I.V. therapy. *Dimen Health Serv* 1982 May; 60(5):9, 12–13.

Guhlow LJ, Kolb J: Pediatric IVs: special measures you should take. *RN* 1979 Mar; 40.

Haas-Beckert B: Removing the mysteries of parenteral nutrition. *Pediatr Nurs* 1987; 13:237–241.

Haddow J: Understanding and managing hypernatremic dehydration. *Pediatr Clin North Am* 1974 May; 21(2):435–441.

Hoekelman RA, et al: *Primary Pediatric Care.* New York, McGraw-Hill Book Company, 1987.

Holliday MA, Segar WE: The maintenance need for water in parenteral fluid therapy. *Pediatrics* 1957 May; 823.

Kaehny WD, Gabow PA: Pathogenesis and management of metabolic acidosis and alkalosis. *In* Schrier RW (ed): *Renal and Electrolyte Disorders.* Boston, Little, Brown, 1980.

Kim MJ, et al: *Pocket Guide to Nursing Diagnosis.* 2nd ed. St. Louis, CV Mosby, 1987.

McFadden EA, Zaloga GP: Calcium regulation. *Crit Care Q* 1983 Dec; 6(3):12–21.

Merritt RJ: Cholestasis associated with total parenteral nutrition. *J Pediatr Gastroenterol Nutr* 1986; 5:9–22.

Metheney NM: *Fluid and Electrolyte Balance.* Philadelphia, JB Lippincott, 1987.

Metheney NM, Snively WD: *Nurses' Handbook of Fluid Balance.* Philadelphia, JB Lippincott, 1979.

Narins RG, Emmett M: Simple and mixed acid-base disorders: a practical approach. *Medicine* 1980; 59(3):161–187.

O'Brien D: Fluid and electrolyte therapy. *In* Kempe CH, Silver HK, O'Brien D (eds): *Current Pediatric Diagnosis and Treatment.* Palo Alto, CA, Lange Medical Publications, 1980.

Oelerich WJ, Dombrowski JM: Mini IV patients . . . maximum precautions. *RN* 1981 Dec; 44(12):43–47.

Olson R, Riddle I: Fluid balance in infants and children. *In* Metheney NM: *Fluid and Electrolyte Balance.* Philadelphia, JB Lippincott, 1987.

Paneth N: Hypernatremic dehydration of infancy. *Am J Dis Child* 1980 Aug; 134:785–792.

Popovtzer MM, Knochel JP: Disorders of calcium, phosphorus, vitamin D and parathyroid hormone activity. *In* Schrier RW (ed): *Renal and Electrolyte Disorders.* Boston, Little, Brown, 1980.

Postuma R, Trevenen CL: Liver disease in infants receiving total parenteral nutrition. *Pediatrics* 1979; 63:110–115.

Reed GM: Confused about potassium? Here's a clear, concise guide. *Nurs 74* 1974 Mar, 20.

Riella MC, Scribner BH: Five years' experience with a right atrial catheter for prolonged parenteral nutriton at home. *Surgery* 1976; 143:295–301.

Robson AM: Parenteral fluid therapy. *In* Behrman RE, Vaughan VC III (eds): *Nelson Textbook of Pediatrics.* 13th ed. Philadelphia, WB Saunders, 1987.

Rose BD: *Clinical Physiology of Acid-Base and Electrolyte Disorders.* New York, McGraw-Hill, 1984.

Seashore JH: Nutritional support of children in the intensive care unit. *Yale J Biol Med* 1984 Mar; 57(2):111–134.

Seashore JH, Hoffman M: Use and abuse of peripheral parenteral nutrition in children. *Nutr Support Serv* 1983 Oct; 3(10):8–13.

Siegel NJ, Lattanzi WE: Fluid and electrolyte therapy in children. *In* Arieff AI, DeFronzo II (eds): *Fluid Electrolyte and Acid-Base Disorders.* New York, Churchill Livingstone, 1985.

Sweeney MJ: Fluid therapy. *In* Hoekelman RA, et al (eds): *Principles of Pediatrics.* New York, McGraw-Hill, 1978.

Vargas JH, et al: Long-term home parenteral nutrition in pediatrics: ten years of experience in 102 patients. *J Pediatr Gastroenterol Nutr* 1987; 6:24–32.

Weil WB: Fluid balance, acid-base homeostasis and gastrointestinal disease. *In* Rudolph AM, et al (eds): *Pediatrics.* 17th ed. Norwalk, CT, Appleton-Century-Crofts, 1982.

Wink DM: Fluid-induced hyponatremia in infancy: a preventable problem. *Am J Nurs* 1983 May; 83:765–767.

Winters RW (ed): *The Body Fluids in Pediatrics.* Boston, Little, Brown, 1973.

Winters RW: *Principles of Pediatric Fluid Therapy.* Boston, Little, Brown, 1982.

Zlotkin SH, Stallings VA, Pencharz PB: Total parenteral nutrition in children. *Pediatr Clin North Am* 1985 Apr; 32(2):381–400.

Zucker AR, Chernow B: Diabetes insipidus and the syndrome of inappropriate antidiuretic hormone release. *Crit Care Q* 1983 Dec; 6(3):63–74.

Bibliography

Ament ME, O'Connor MJ: Long-term cognitive development of children raised on home total parenteral nutrition. *Clin Res* 1985; 32:96A.

Costarino A, Baumgart S: Modern fluid and electrolyte management of the critically ill premature infant. *Pediatr Clin North Am* 1983; 33:153–178.

Gutcher G, Cutz E: Complications of parenteral nutrition. *Semin Perinatol* 1986; 10:196–207.

Halperin ML, et al: Acid-base, fluid and electrolyte aspects of parenteral nutrition. *In* Kokko JP, Tannen RL (eds): *Fluids and Electrolytes.* Philadelphia, WB Saunders, 1986, 817–831.

Kerner J: *Manual of Pediatric Parenteral Nutrition.* New York, John Wiley, 1983.

Lattanzi WE, Siegel NJ: A practical guide to fluid and electrolyte therapy. *Curr Prob Pediatr* 1986; 16:1.

Masiak MJ, et al: *Fluids and Electrolytes Through the Life Cycle.* Norwalk, CT, Appleton-Century-Crofts, 1985.

Smith K, Brain E: *Fluids and Electrolytes: A Conceptual Approach.* London, Churchill Livingstone, 1980.

Nursing Care During Hospitalization

Chapter 31

Mabel Hunsberger

Hospitalization is a threatening experience for everyone. For children, the stress is compounded because they do not understand why they are there or why they are hurting. New caretakers, different routines, and separation from familiar people and places are experiences counter to a young child's developmental needs. For older children and adolescents, separation from peers, the threat of the unknown, and vulnerabilities pertaining to their body image combine to make hospitalization intimidating.

Improperly managed, the experience of hospitalization can be emotionally and developmentally damaging to the child or adolescent and the family. By understanding the child's needs and how to meet them, nurses can reduce stress and promote normal development.

Nursing Process Plan
NPP: The Hospitalized Child, page 972

Related Topics
Therapeutic play, Chapter 21
Concepts of Illness: Stress, Crisis, and Coping, Chapter 23
Impact of Acute Illness, Chapter 24
Impact of Chronic Illness, Chapter 25
Preparation of children for procedures, Chapter 27
Administering medications, Chapter 28

Scope of the Problem

Hospitalization and surgery are inherently stressful for children and their families. Children between 6 months and 4 to 5 years of age exhibit the most observable responses of distress to the experience of hospitalization (Robertson, 1970). Whether this experience results in long-term sequelae has given rise to some controversy in the literature. Most early studies (Jessner et al, 1952; Prugh et al, 1953) found some indication of behavioral changes months and years after hospitalization; however, these studies have been criticized because of lack of control groups and failure to control for extraneous variables (Goslin, 1978). With improved methodology, Douglas (1975) and Quinton and Rutter (1976) found no long-term effects following *single* hospitalizations of *less* than a week. It has also been reported that some children improve behaviorally following hospitalization (Shore et al, 1965). The experience of hospitalization for children continues to be studied to further define the variables. Important variables that have been recognized so far are the child's age, type and amount of preparation, previous relevant experiences, personality and coping abilities, and the amount and nature of support received by parents and professionals. It is beyond the scope of this text to review the extensive body of literature concerning this topic. Reviews of children's hospitalization and related experiences include Vernon et al, 1965; King and Ziegler, 1981; Hodapp, 1982; Hunsberger et al, 1984; Thompson, 1985 and 1986; Bates, 1986; Byrne and Cadman, 1987. Hodapp identified five general themes:

1. The short-term effect of hospitalization depends on age. Douglas (1975) and Prugh et al (1953) found that children under 5 years of age suffered more disturbances (nervousness, crying, sleep disorders, bladder control problems) than older children, both in the hospital and in the first 1 to 2 weeks posthospitalization.
2. A single hospital experience lasting less than a week may cause a young child some short-term effects but is unlikely to result in long-term effects (Quinton and Rutter, 1976).
3. Children under 5 years of age who suffer repeated hospitalizations seem to be most seriously affected. This was found to be true even when socioeconomic and other relevant factors were controlled (Douglas, 1975; Quinton and Rutter, 1976).
4. Prehospital adjustment and personality have been identified as important factors in determining a child's adjustment to the hospital. The child's relationship with parents, especially the mother (Prugh et al, 1953), has been reported to affect the adequacy of adjustment on the ward. The child's emotional state prior to admission has been identified as a factor in later long-term disturbances (Douglas, 1975; Vernon et al., 1965).
5. The reaction of parents to a child's hospitalization affects the child's reaction. Mahaffey (1965) and Skipper and Leonard (1968) demonstrated that relief of anxiety in parents produces physiologic and psychologic changes in their hospitalized child.

Recognizing the varied responses with respect to the age, duration, and nature of the experience, the nurse assesses individual families to identify their particular needs. In all circumstances, important variables that affect the way a child and family experience hospitalization are their preparation and how the initial exposure is handled.

Preparation for Hospitalization

Communities and institutions prepare children and parents for hospitalization in a wide variety of ways and timing.

Hospital Tours for Children in the General Population

Taking groups of young children on hospital tours to expose them to the inside of a hospital is becoming an increasingly widespread practice, according to survey results (Azarnoff and Woody, 1981; Mather, 1983). It is not known whether this exposure of healthy children facilitates adjustment to hospitalization at a later time. Exposure of healthy children to the random sights and sounds of a hospital has the potential to introduce unnecessary fears and anxiety. This approach requires further study.

Preparation of well children by means of a hospital tour usually takes the following form:

1. Usually restricted to children over 4 years of age.
2. Group size ranges from 10 to 30 (1 to 3 group leaders).
3. Activities include all or various combinations of the following:

We appreciate the contribution of the section on anesthesia by Mary Jane Yablonky.

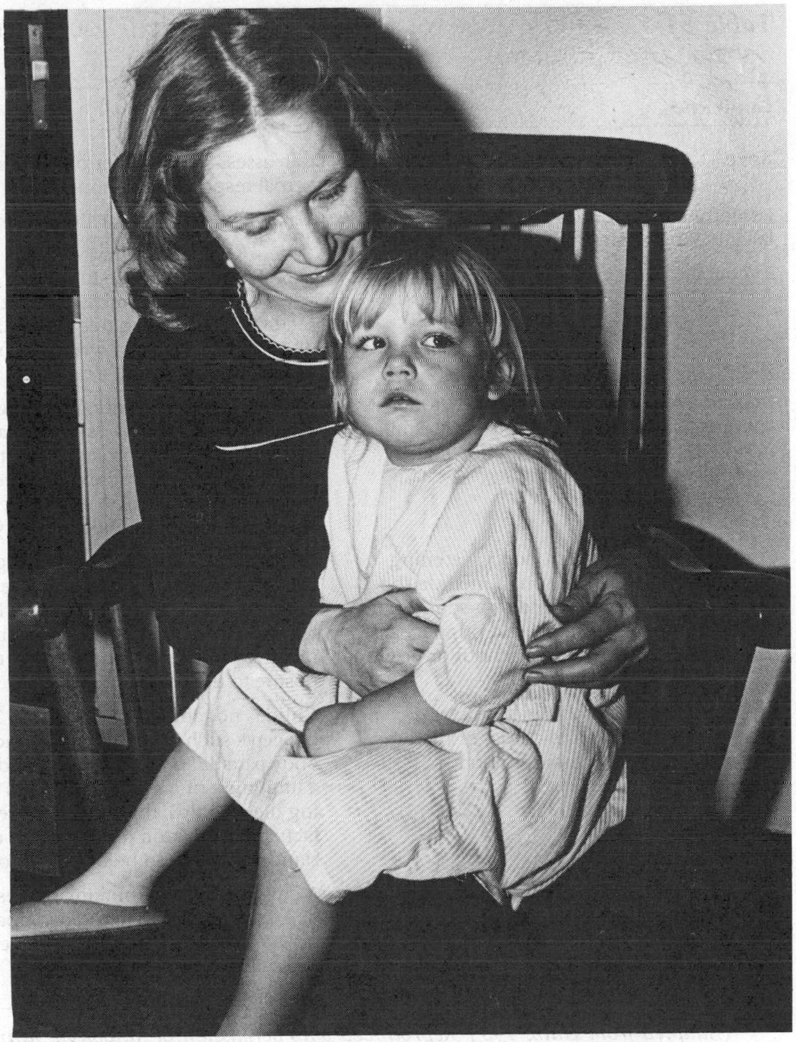

A child's stress is diminished by the presence of a parent whose anxiety has been reduced. A rocking chair is a soothing addition to a child's hospital room, both for the child and parent.

- Welcome speech
- A stop on a pediatric unit or an unused patient room
- A film or slides
- A play experience with selected medical equipment

4. Children are invited to ask questions.
5. Each child receives a coloring book about the hospital.

Guidelines for conducting hospital tours for early school-age children have been suggested by Huth (1983). Although these guidelines are not documented by research findings, rationale is provided which is based on the cognitive and psychosocial developmental stage of the child (Table 31-1).

An alternative to bringing healthy children into the hospital is for nurses to visit schools to discuss hospitalization; however, even this approach is discouraged by some and must be further researched. Robertson (1983) contends it is a fallacy to think that hospital tours and discussions at school actually prepare nonpatients for hospitalization. Because some children have difficulty differentiating between "if" and "when," they actually may be troubled with thoughts of illness, pain, and separation because they think they are really going to the hospital. Teaching about hospitalization is thought by some to be best done by parents as the occasion arises through normal life events, as when a friend, relative, or neighbor is hospitalized (Robertson, 1983; Harvey, 1983).

The child should be prepared carefully before visiting the hospital. An opportunity for further questions and discussions after the visit helps the child learn about hospitals. Should the grandparent or neighbor die in the hospital, time must be spent in dispelling the child's belief that all people who go to the hospital die there.

Preparation of healthy children for hospitalization is being studied increasingly (Roberts et al, 1982;

Table 31-1. Guidelines for Conducting Hospital Tours: Early School-Age Children

Guidelines	Rationale
Keep groups small (ten children per group)	Can assess child's reaction and promote verbal responses
Limit time length (20–30 minutes is usually long enough)	Young children have a short attention span
Encourage participation of parents	Parents can provide security and support when potentially fearful information is received. Parental anxiety also may be reduced in the event of future hospitalization of their child
Incorporate use of an indirect method (puppets, films, slides) into tour. Permit a period of play with dolls and hospital equipment	Child can express feelings through the medium of a "third person" to handle fears and anxieties. Play provides an opportunity to satisfy curiosity and express feelings toward those objects that present real or imagined threats to body integrity.
Provide information in a nonthreatening environment. In the hospital, include the playroom but avoid threatening sounds and sights. Equipment, slides, and puppets also can be taken to the child's school or home	Frightening scenes such as emergency rooms or intensive care can increase a child's anxiety. If a child will be in an intensive care unit after surgery, films or pictures may be less threatening than exposure to the actual room
Present information in concrete terms. Incorporate diagrams, models, or pictures. Avoid extensive discussions about threatening procedures	Child is not able to comprehend invisible concepts such as pain, illness, and internal body parts. Early school-age children have a multitude of fantasies and fears concerning their bodies, therefore they require factual information to help them understand but it should be brief and to the point
Allow a period for questions. Questions should be phrased to encourage the child to reveal her or his perception of the information. Areas of confusion should be dealt with thoroughly	A child's concrete thinking makes it necessary for answers to encompass an individual child's past experience so that misunderstandings are clarified

(Adapted from Huth, 1983. Reproduced with permission of Anthony J. Jannetti, Inc., publisher, Pediatric Nursing, *Nov/Dec 1983.)*

Azarnoff, 1983; Mather, 1983). Some of the data still needed have been summarized by Azarnoff (1983):

1. What types of programs are appropriate for what ages and how will the various programs be evaluated?
2. Would individual tours be more effective than group tours?
3. Would a small group tour be effective if such children were prepared for the tour (exposure to medical equipment with discussion in a nonmedical setting)?
4. Would inclusion of prepared parents on a small group tour be an effective strategy?
5. Would children prepared in a school setting respond differently with respect to stress level and information recall than a group of hospital-prepared children?

When Hospitalization Is Imminent

Children should have an opportunity to learn about and see inside the hospital before admission. Hospitals in many communities have organized programs and tours to orient children to the hospital and its environment prior to admission. During a tour children may be able to meet one of the nurses who will be caring for them. When admission to the hospital is planned for diagnostic work or surgery, the tour and parent-child teaching can be developed around that theme.

Books also provide a useful means of teaching about and preparing the child for hospitalization. Lists of age-appropriate books are available through the hospital's play or library resource person or through the local children's library (a recommended list is included at the end of this chapter). These books could be read at home before admission, during hospitalization, and again when the child and family return home. When children are old enough to read the books alone, time should be provided to discuss what they read and their reactions to it with an adult who can offer additional information and correct any misconceptions. Good film strips about the hospital experience may also be available from local libraries or the Association for the Care of Children's Health.*

Play is another common avenue used to prepare children for hospitalization. Various child-sized articles or nurse's or doctor's clothing and equipment can be made available to the children during a tour for examining and to use in dramatic play. With an opportunity to see procedures (application of a cast to a doll and its removal) and to handle equipment (IV tubing or an oxygen mask), the child can begin to work through some fears regarding illness and hospitalization. These experiences allow children to become familiar with the setting during a period when they are not under the stress of being admitted (see Chapter 21 for discussion of therapeutic play).

Some hospitals have also organized pre-readmission programs involving a home visit to help the child being rehospitalized overcome any distorted memories or fantasies left over from the first hospitalization.

Age-Related Preparation

Preparation of toddlers and preschoolers presents a special challenge. Most of the techniques that are used to prepare school-age children for hospitalization are not effective for younger children. In a review of the literature, Goslin (1978) points out that positive research findings pertinent to the preparation of children for hospitalization consistently carry qualifying statements that some children, particularly the younger ones, do not seem to benefit from preparation.

Toddlers and preschoolers must be prepared for hospitalization within the confines of their mental ability. They do not have a concept of time or causality to understand an explanation of something that is to happen in the future, nor will they understand the cause of illness or the reason for hospitalization. Stress of the younger child is most effectively reduced by the presence of a parent whose own anxiety has been reduced.

Therefore, an important role of the nurse who prepares a young child for hospitalization is preparation of the parents. To prepare parents, the nurse helps them understand the child's illness and the reason for hospitalization; she can explain the events of hospital admission and give guidelines on how to prepare their child and siblings for the hospital experience.

A common but not recommended approach used by parents when young children must be hospitalized is to protect them from the trauma of being told that they must go to the hospital. Parents are tempted to tell children that they are going to the library, to the store, to the park, or some other pleasant place. The nurse should intervene to assist parents to become comfortable with telling the truth. It is appropriate to tell toddlers about the hospitalization the morning of admission, but the explanation should be simple and truthful, with descriptions of a few of the nonthreatening events that will occur. For example, they can be told about the environment, and about the nurses, doctors, and other children they will meet. It is appropriate to tell some toddlers two or three days before admission, but the explanation should not include descriptions of threatening procedures. Toddlers also can benefit from parents reading to them about hospitalization and from playing with a nurse or doctor kit a few days before admission. Preschoolers also can be prepared a few days to a week in advance, whereas school-age children often know about the admission farther in advance because they are more involved in their own care. In all cases, discussions that are heard by the child concerning the imminent hospitalization should include the child.

Siblings should be prepared for the hospitalization of a brother or sister, including explanations of who will be at home to care for them and who will be spending time at the hospital, and how much time will be spent there. If a parent will be rooming-in, this should be explained.

Regardless of the type of preparation that a child and family have had, the nurse should recognize that hospital admission is potentially stressful under the best circumstances.

The Stress of Hospital Admission

Adams' (1965) studies revealed that most children have only vague, general, and usually distorted ideas about why they are being hospitalized and what will happen to them while they are in the hospital. In addition, Adams found that parents usually had an equally vague understanding of their child's hospitalization. This lack of knowledge was responsible for increasing

*ACCH has headquarters at 3615 Wisconsin Avenue, Washington, DC 20016.

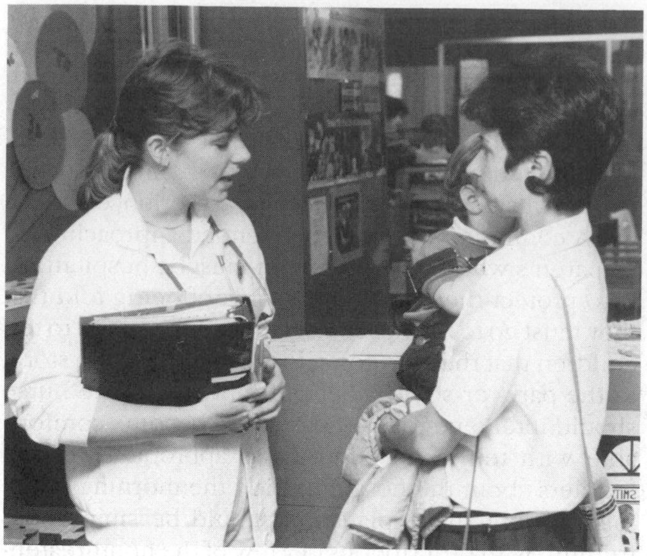

From the moment of admission, the nurse should try to understand the child's and family's fears about the experience of hospitalization.

the typical fears and anxieties associated with the child's health state and with giving over care to strangers. Parents also worry about the impending separation and effects on their other children during this crisis. A study by Rasmussen and Murphy (1977) revealed the admission experience to be confusing to the child and parents. Their suggestion to help the child adapt and maintain control during hospitalization, starting from the moment of admission, is for the nurse to look at the pediatric unit — its activities, personnel, and equipment — through the child's eyes. The nurse can then respond to children's needs, questions, and fears from their point of view.

The admission process has three aspects to which the child and caretakers will react: (1) the social environment of the admission setting, (2) the physical environment of the hospital unit to which the child is assigned, and (3) the nature of the admitting procedures to which the child is subjected. The nurse plays a critical role in influencing the child's and family's experience with each of these aspects during the admission phase, including the admission interview.

The Social Environment

When the child is admitted to the hospital, it is important that the experience be made as pleasant as possible. First impressions often linger, and a rushed, depersonalized approach is likely to have a lasting negative effect.

It is particularly important to recognize the needs of parents. They need an introduction to the people who will be caring for their child, to the facilities available for their use, and to at least one other family who has a child hospitalized on the unit. They also need information about the policies of the hospital and unit that affect them.

A warm, caring approach to parents that makes them feel welcome will considerably lessen the stress they feel. Nursing staff should convey from the beginning their recognition of the unique caretaking role of parents and provide ongoing understandable information and support that will enable the parents to utilize their strengths in supporting their child. Nursing attitudes and unit policies and facilities should provide for and encourage the presence and participation of parents and other persons most significant to the child.

During admission, children should be introduced as early as possible to their primary nurse and/or some other hospital personnel with whom they can count on regular and frequent contact during the hospital experience (director of hospital play program, volunteer grandparent, hospital teacher). They should be introduced to their roommates and to other children of

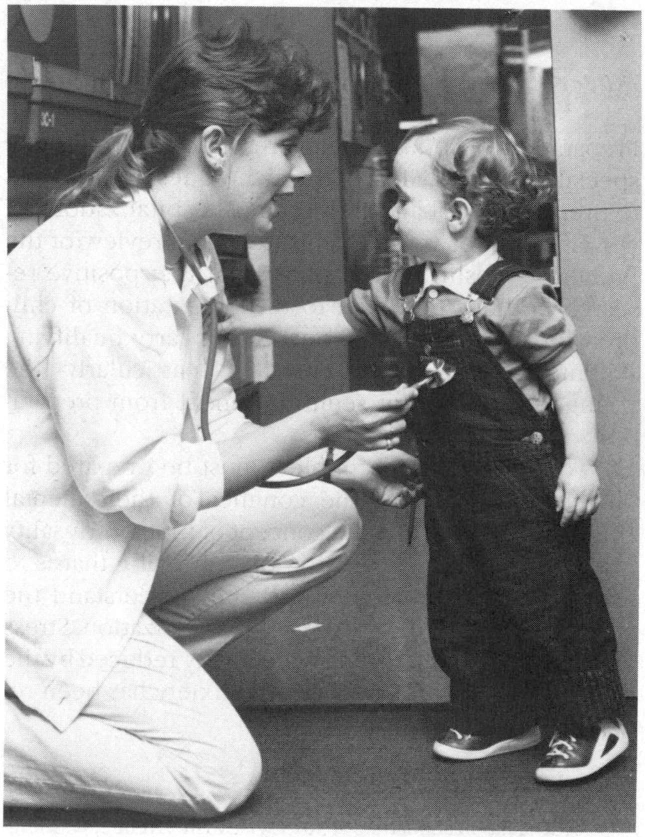

First impressions often linger. It is beneficial if they are pleasant and personalized.

similar age who are likely to be present during the hospital stay.

The Physical Environment

The actual hospital environment is another factor that may be stressful for the child and family, because of the many unfamiliar sights, sounds, and smells. In addition, children are admitted to a strange room, either alone or with children they do not know, and to an unfamiliar bed. They are removed from the objects and people they are used to at home that make them feel secure.

The nurse should encourage the parents to stay with the child at least until he or she has investigated the new environment, claimed a few of the hospital's play items as temporarily his own, and arranged his bed area to make him feel he has established his own little "place to live." Overnight accommodation for parents should be explained and parents made welcome to stay, especially when young children are concerned.

The threat of an unfamiliar environment can be reduced by giving a few suggestions to parents early. Parents should be encouraged to bring a favorite toy or blanket for younger children. School-age children may be glad to bring a favorite item such as a radio or a game. Teenagers may like having a poster of a favorite sports or movie star on a wall near their bed. These kinds of items represent the security of home and have special meaning to the child. Allowing the child to have some belongings and permitting decoration of the space helps personalize it and makes the child feel more secure.

If health permits, the child or adolescent should be given a tour of the unit and introduced to the use of the call bell, bed controls, bathroom facilities, and play area. Any rules about unit routines or restrictions should be explained to the child on admission and repeated as necessary during the hospital stay. A summary of the admitting procedure is provided in Box 31-1.

Rasmussen and Murphy (1977) suggest that, once children are situated in the room, they be asked if there are any objects in the room that they are unfamiliar with and be introduced to these objects and their function. They should be encouraged to investigate and handle these objects in the nurse's presence and should be given simple, neutral, but truthful answers to any questions the objects prompt. Children should be given opportunity to play out their admission fears with age-appropriate play materials as a part of the adaptation process. Whether they are allowed to act out their fears through active or quiet play will depend on the illness and the play facilities available (see discussion on therapeutic play in Chapter 21).

Isolation alters the physical environment, either to protect a child with an impaired immune system from contracting disease or to prevent a child with an infectious disease from spreading pathogenic organisms to other children. Nevertheless, isolation does increase stress for the child and family, particularly for the young child who has not yet developed the cognitive ability to understand its purpose. The child may wonder why mother's face is hidden behind a mask and why her familiar clothes are under a long gown. The monotony of everyone dressing alike and of being confined in the room are additional stresses to which the child must adapt. Therapeutic play becomes an extremely valuable intervention that helps to entertain the isolated child while simultaneously providing an outlet for fears and frustration. (See Chapter 27 for further discussion of caring for a child in isolation.)

Admission Procedures

Admission radiographs, drawing blood samples, and collecting urine specimens, as well as removing the child's clothing and taking blood pressure and temperature, especially rectally, are examples of procedures that may be unpleasant or frightening to the newly admitted child. If possible, admission diagnostic procedures should be done on an outpatient basis before the day of admission; if that is not possible, ideally the procedures are postponed until several hours after admission. Admission procedures should be preceded by an age-appropriate explanation to the child and completed as quickly as possible. Explanation should be given as to how the child may cooperate or participate to get procedures over quickly. The parents should also receive an explanation of the procedure and how they may assist. If it is not possible for a parent to be with the child during the procedure, a nurse to whom the child has already been introduced should offer comfort during the procedure and after it is completed. In many hospitals child life workers* are making a sizeable contribution to the support and comfort of children during procedures.

Assessment of the Hospitalized Child

A child's age and the admitting diagnosis or diagnoses provide the nurse with very basic information. As the

*Child life workers are individuals who are specifically educated to support children through a variety of approaches during hospitalization.

Box 31-1
Admitting Procedure

PRIOR TO ARRIVAL OF CHILD

Assess immediate needs of child based on history by telephone including:
- developmental age of child
- physical condition of child
- communicability of illness
- emotional status of child
- available support system

Select and prepare a room, taking into consideration the above factors

Tell roommates that a child will be coming to their room. Information about the child's condition is not shared with other children or their parents

Prepare the room with equipment required for the admission

Prepare any emergency equipment that might be required

Take toys into the room as appropriate for age

ORIENTATION TO ROOM AND UNIT

Greet the child and family as soon as they arrive

Introduce child and family to key members on the health team if they are available at the time of admission

Escort child and family to room and introduce to roommate(s) and family if present

Provide an orientation to the various areas of the children's unit, especially those that will be used by the child and family (i.e., playroom, school room, lounges, kitchen, bathrooms, linen area)

Orient the child to the room and equipment: call bell, crib/bed workings, telephone, television, supplies in bedside stand or elsewhere, special equipment such as oxygen, monitors, suction

Explain hospital policies and routines (visiting hours, mealtime, bedtime, rooming-in services)

Explain how parents may participate in the care of their child

Give child/parents a booklet about the hospital if one is available

ADMISSION PROCESS

Check identification band that name and number correctly match admitting sheet

Apply identification band if not done in admission department

Carry out any STAT orders

Perform a nursing history

Explain routine procedures to be done and use doll-play to demonstrate, then proceed with physical assessment, including temperature, pulse, respiration, blood pressure, height, weight, and head circumference (under 2 years of age or according to hospital policy)

Obtain urine specimen

Obtain other specimens specific to diagnosis

Complete admission assessment form

Give special instructions as required to child and family concerning the diagnostic and treatment plan

Make arrangements for rooming-in as desired

Write admitting nursing diagnosis and care plan

nurse gathers more specific information, the needs of the child and the family are further understood. The goal of the assessment is to obtain pertinent information for planning individual care.

Assessment of a Child's Individual Circumstances

Children respond to the same stresses in a variety of ways, reflecting their individual experiences and circumstances.

Wolff (1973) found that certain children are more vulnerable to the stress of hospitalization than others. These vulnerable children are (1) only children, (2) youngest children, (3) children living with extended families, (4) those with a history of responding poorly to strangers, (5) those who are exposed to other people only rarely, and (6) those who have experienced recent trauma, such as the death or divorce of a parent. Children with a history of poor adjustment tend to respond most adversely to hospitalization. With recognition of these factors during the admission interview, the nurse can intervene early to prevent long-term trauma associated with hospitalization.

It is also important for the nurse to carefully assess children who have been previously admitted to the hospital. Fears carried over from a previous hospital experience may linger; the nurse gives special attention to eliciting such fears and fantasies. It cannot be assumed that a second or third admission reduces a child's fears. Rutter (1981) suggests that a "first admission must in some way sensitize the child so that he is more likely to suffer the next time." A child's fears and anxiety during admission require the nurse's attention under all circumstances.

Process of Data Gathering

It is common practice to fill out an admission form to record pertinent information when a child is admitted. These forms should serve only as a guide, with careful attention being given to the individual child's and family's particular needs.

During admission an assessment is made of the child's usual level of functioning in terms of body control and self-care, the usual routines, and the rituals that are associated with activities of daily living at home. Particular attention is given to the child's eating patterns and food preferences, toilet habits and words used to describe elimination, and usual rest and exercise patterns. Whether a child is toilet trained and how parents are handling this phase are documented. The child's special fears, such as of the dark or loud noises, are identified, along with suggestions from parents about their child's usual coping strategies. The focus of the admission assessment varies according to the child's age and specific problem (see Figure 31-1 for an example of an admission form).

An appropriately handled admission interview fosters the child's and family's confidence in the ability of the staff to provide adequate care. Throughout the interview, the nurse should be sensitive to body language and convey an atmosphere of acceptance. Contact with a warm, caring person helps the child and family cope with the admission in a positive way and encourages their cooperation.

Children of preschool age and older are allowed and encouraged to participate in the interview as a beginning of participation in their treatment. Such involvement gives them a sense of control and independence that is important developmentally. The nurse should direct some questions to each parent when both are present to give equal recognition.

Time is allowed for the child and family to ask questions, to avoid making them feel rushed or pressured by the nurse's busy schedule. School-age children and adolescents should be given an opportunity to ask questions privately, without the parents' presence.

Regardless of the age or type of problem, all body systems are assessed and the findings are recorded (see Chapter 15 on child health assessment). During the assessment the entire body is inspected for the presence of rashes, scars, or injuries. Such markings must be documented at the time of admission. The child's cognitive and emotional-social functioning is also assessed (see Chapter 15 on child health assessment). It is important to recognize that the events of illness and hospitalization interfere with a child's behavior. For example, a child who is ill and afraid may not play, talk, or perform motor tasks as when in a healthy state and a familiar environment. It is important to document abnormalities or developmental lags but also to get a description of the child's usual behavior from the parents.

The child in late adolescence should be consulted about having parents present during the assessment. Certain *physical aspects* should receive special attention; a thorough reproductive assessment is indicated to determine whether puberty has occurred and to assess knowledge of reproduction. Questions about sexual activity and birth control are often more easily handled when talking about social interactions and dating. Changes in body odor occur during adolescence and create special hygiene needs, so information should be collected about the condition of skin and teeth and about cleanliness practices.

The assessment of *learning ability* is necessary to identify educational needs and plan health education. Questions about school, grades, solving problems and what is fun to learn will provide information in this area.

The *social assessment* includes learning about the adolescent's friendships with peers as well as family relationships. Information about the adolescent's hobbies, sports, and school-related activity assist the nurse to plan individualized care for the adolescent's social needs during hospitalization. Information about habits such as alcohol and drug use should be obtained. Questions as well as observations about parents' interaction with an adolescent will help in assessment of the adolescent's relationships with the parents. Finally, discussions about religion, occupational decisions, and relationships with other adults may complete the admission assessment. The understanding conveyed by the nurse during this assessment will assist in alleviating some of the adolescent's anxiety about being in the hospital. It will also provide some understanding of how the adolescent views the illness.

The end of the interview with the child and parents affords the nurse a good opportunity to talk about the purpose for hospitalization and what is likely to happen, to discuss how the child and parents will each be able to help in the plan of care, and to explain hospital policies that affect them (these policies should also be in writing). Parents should be encouraged to care for their child as they would at home and are shown how things are done and where they might find objects and facilities that they may need during the hospital stay. Explanation should be given differentiating care that parents may provide from aspects of care for which the nurse is responsible.

Assessment of the child and family's needs begins at admission and continues throughout the hospital stay. The nurse's role is to make ongoing assessments concerning the child's response to hospitalization at-

GENERAL INFORMATION

Health Care Provider	
Grade Level	Adm Date/Time
Language Spoken	Interpreter
Reason for Adm	
Brief Hx	
Medication—Prescription/Non-Prescription	

Name	Dose	Freq.	Last Dose	Comment

Way Child Takes Meds
Exposure to Contagious Illness (which, when)
Description & Time of Last Fluids & Food
Substance Use/Abuse (caffeine, alcohol, smoking, drugs)
Corrective Devices/Prosthesis/Handicaps
ALLERGIES

VITAL SIGNS/MEASUREMENTS

T	P	R	BP	Ht	Wt	OFC

ACTIVITIES OF DAILY LIVING

Breast	Bottle	Formula	
Usual Amt			
Freq			
Solids (type, amt., freq.)			
Cup	Snacks		
Feeding Skill Level/Special Utensils			
Food Likes			
Food Dislikes			
Problems/Special Diet			
Diapers	Potty Chr.	Toilet	Toilet Trained
Date Last Stool	BM Freq.		
BM Character			
Terms Child uses for Elim.			
Problems/Devices			
Bath/Hair	Dental Care	Dressing	
Menses Hx/Care			
Concerns/Problems			
Naps/Rituals/Comfort Meas./Special Needs/Habits			
Concerns/Problems			
Adm. R.N.			

A

Figure 31-1. Example of a nursing admission form used at The Children's Hospital, Denver.

tending to both the stressors and balancing factors that affect the child's experience.

Impact of Stressors and Balancing Factors on Hospitalized Child

To help the child and family in the coping process during hospitalization, it is useful to analyze the stressors and identify balancing factors that can reduce their impact.

Stressors of Hospitalization

Each child and family come to the hospital with their own vulnerabilities. Although the stressors of hospitalization vary according to the child's age and the type and seriousness of illness, Visintainer and Wolfer (1975) identified five stressors common to all hospital experiences:

1. separation from parents, peers, and trusted adults;
2. harm and injury (discomfort, pain, mutilation, and death);
3. unknown and unfamiliar events and environment;
4. unclear limits regarding expectations; and
5. loss of control and loss of competence or decision-making role.

Recognition of these stressors provides a framework to assess the hospitalized child and to devise approaches to minimize the threat.

Separation from Parents and Significant Others. The young infant (under 6 months of age) is thought to be less affected by separation from a parent because selective attachment begins during later in-

DEVELOPMENTAL INFORMATION	PSYCHOSOCIAL BACKGROUND			
Comment as appropriate on Language, Socialization, Activities/Play, Motor Levels, Sexual Behavior/Birth Control:	Health Care Experiences			
	Child's Reaction to Illness/What Child Told re: Illness/Hosp.			
		Age / Name	Usual Health Status/Comments	At Home
	Mother			
	Father			
	Guardian			
UNIT ORIENTATION	Siblings			
Bed ___ TV ___ Phone ___ BR ___ Side Rail ___ Restraints ___				
Call Light ___ Play Rm ___ Teen Lounge ___ Sib Play Ctr. ___				
Smok Pol. ___ Booklets ___ Parent Facil. ___ Isol Lev. ___	Significant Others/Pets			
Valub. ___ Prim. Nsg. ___ ID Bracelet ___ Wait for M.D. ___	Dad Working (ph#, hrs)			
Breast Pump ___ Security ___ Valet ___ Visit Rules ___	Mom Working (ph#, hrs)			
Room In ___ Visiting Plans ___				
Parent Participation in Care ___	Child Care Arrangements			
Resident/Attending notified ___	Transportation Arrangements			
	Recent Changes in Family/Situation			

DISCHARGE PLANNING	AGENCIES INVOLVED WITH FAMILY		PATIENT CARE PROVIDERS
	Name/Agency	Ph. Number	Primary R.N.
			Assoc. R.N.
			Adm. R.N.

B

fancy (6 to 8 months of age). It has been suggested that the major effect of hospitalization on the infant under 8 months of age is a disruption of routine, whereas the infant over 8 months suffers more from anxiety over separation from the mother (Blackman, 1973). Thus, for the young infant the hazard of separation is less pronounced and caretaking of the basic needs of the infant is the priority.

For the child between the ages of 6 months and 4 years, separation from parents is the most important stressor. At this stage of development, attachment to mother is "fiercely possessive, selfish, and intolerant of frustration" (Robertson, 1970). Children do not understand why they must be separated from parents, nor does their developmental level provide them with adequate coping mechanisms to withstand separation. Thus, a child at this stage is more vulnerable to psychologic upset as a result of hospitalization than at any other age. Many variables affect the way a young child experiences separation. The quality of the existing parent-child relationship, previous experiences with separation, the personality of the child, and the type of substitute caretaking are important variables that have an impact upon the young child's coping ability.

Robertson (1970) identified stages of "settling in" that an institutionalized child demonstrates when separated from the mother. These stages of protest, despair, and denial (detachment) may be recognized in hospitalized children when separated for even short periods from their parents. However, each child is unique in the response to separation, so these phases serve only as a general guide to the kinds of behavior that can be expected.

During the initial phase, *protest,* young children will cry desperately in an effort to summon the parent's usual response. They violently protest the departure of the parents by screaming and clinging as the parents try to place them in the crib. During this phase, parents experience ambivalence about visiting when they see their child pleading for them to stay. Nurses can intervene by staying with the child when the parents leave; they should realize, however, that it is not uncommon for a young child to reject the attention of the nurse during this period. It is least traumatic for the child and the parent if the parent says goodbye and then leaves. When parents return several times in desperation to comfort their child, the protests are enhanced and the parents' anxiety is increased. Parents should be truthful about their leaving even though the child protests; parents often need help from the nurse to understand the importance of not resorting to telling their child they are "just going for a cup of coffee." Recognizing the child's behavior as a normal, healthy response, the nurse explains this to parents lest they feel that their visiting is causing greater trauma than staying away would cause. The nurse clearly communicates to the parent that it is essential to their child's welfare that they not curtail their visits.

The second phase is one of *despair*, in which the child experiences a continuing conscious need of mother. Despair, or an increasing hopelessness, results when the act of protest fails to bring the parents back. The despair can be recognized by withdrawal from events and people in the environment. The child rarely resists anything that is done and seldom cries during this stage. Apathy and depression exist, but the compliant behavior is easily mistaken as a sign of adaptation to the hospital experience. During this phase the nurse must guard against misinterpreting the child's behavior when parents visit. A child is likely to cry intensely or have a temper tantrum when parents visit, as if to scold the parent for having left. The nurse who does not understand the nature of the child's anxiety concludes that she or he is "better" when the parents do not visit.

The third phase, *denial,* can result when a young child must stay for an extended period in the hospital and is cared for by a variety of nurses. In this child there is a return of interest in the environment with an appearance of having adapted; in actuality, the external appearance is the result of repression of feelings for mother. The child no longer seems upset when parents come and go and forms superficial relationships with many staff members, but avoids closeness with any one person. Typically, these children become the ward favorite because they seem to be happy and respond to everyone; what they desperately need is a trusting relationship with one individual.

For children between 6 months and 5 years of age, a variety of strategies can be considered to avoid the threat of separation. Hospitalization for elective procedures may be delayed. Day hospitals or surgeries may be used, in which the child is admitted and treated, usually in one day, and returns home at night. Parents are usually allowed and encouraged to stay with their child as much as possible in these places. Another common alternative is for the parents to stay with the child (room-in) during hospitalization (see later discussion in this chapter). A grandparent, other relative, or close neighbor could also substitute for the parent for short periods of time. When it is not possible for parents to stay near, the nurse substitutes for them to meet the child's emotional needs, to provide support to them when they can visit, and to spend extra time with the child.

Older children and teens tend to adapt more easily to separation from parents; their main fear is the possibility of bodily injury or deformity. These children have a better understanding of death, but they may fear being permanently separated from peers and family.

Harm, Injury, and Pain. Illness and hospitalization brings exposure to children of unfamiliar and uncomfortable sensations that adults label pain. These sensations are frightening and anxiety-producing for children because they usually have had little experience with pain and do not understand how one becomes ill or how recovery occurs (see Chapter 29 for discussion of pain assessment). Young children are developing an awareness about their bodies and are concerned about even the slightest injury. During the preschool and early school years, children perceive an injection as a severe threat. They fear that a large hole will be left and that blood may run out. For this reason, Band-aids are lifesavers to children of this age.

Concerns of body intactness and body integrity prevail through the preschool years, and by school age the concern encompasses fear of disability and death. By adolescence, differentiation from peers is the primary concern, therefore the degree of change in external appearance as a result of injury is of prime importance.

The nurse's ongoing assessment of children's needs concerning painful procedures is an important aspect of care. Often misconceptions exist about the purpose of the procedure and what is to be done. A child whose treatment involves daily blood sampling may fear that because so much blood is withdrawn each day, none will be left. Showing the child that 5 millimeters is only about a teaspoonful and explaining how the body replenishes its blood supply will help reduce such fears. Assuring children that pain from a needle will only last for a moment, as well as letting them play with the syringe, will help them cope with this fear. For more painful procedures such as surgery, tell children they will be given medicine to make them sleep so they will not feel the pain, and assure them that they will have special medicine to relieve discomfort after the treatment.

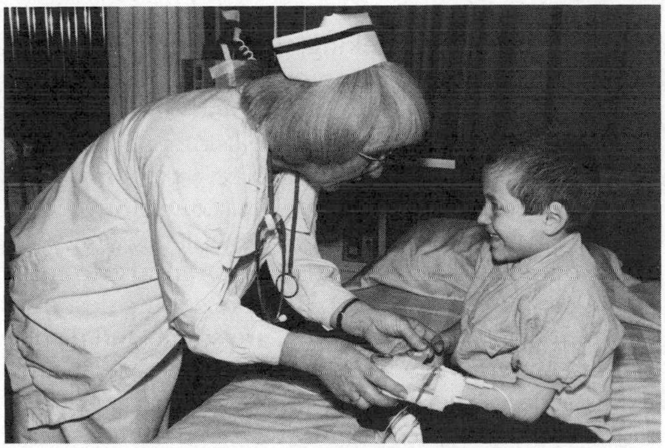

A brief explanation preceding a procedure helps a child feel secure and increases cooperation.

Other procedures, such as assessing vital signs or collecting urine or stool specimens, are fairly easily accepted by most children if they are given simple explanations. Telling a young child who needs vital signs checked frequently that the nurse has to watch him or her closely is usually sufficient explanation. Infants or very young toddlers, however, might not understand why they need to be restrained for procedures and adapt best when a parent stays to provide comfort during and after the procedure. Older children and teens will need more thorough explanations of why various procedures are done if their cooperation is to be obtained. The support of children and adolescents during procedures is discussed further in Chapter 27.

Unknown and Unfamiliar Events. Admission to the hospital not only introduces a child to a threatening environment but also to anxiety-producing unfamiliarity. Young children depend on routine and familiarity for their security. The strangeness of the sights, sounds, and smells in particular make young children feel insecure. People in the environment also are a source of stress because of their unfamiliarity and different way of relating to the child. Strategies used to reduce the stress include care by parents, preparation and education for the events of hospitalization, and therapeutic play.

Unclear Limits and Expectations. Illness and hospitalization often subject the child or adolescent to a variety of limits, including restricted movement, isolation, or altered dietary regimen. When a set of new rules is unclear, one's security is threatened. The number of people that become involved in a child's care introduces the potential for inconsistencies and communication of unclear expectations from one individual to another. When it is unclear to children and parents what is expected of them, they feel confused and threatened. Ongoing assessment of the child and family's understanding of the treatment plan and clarification of areas they do not understand can reduce the stress associated with this aspect of hospitalization.

Loss of Control. As children grow, they become more capable of accomplishing tasks and doing things for themselves. The sense of mastery that accompanies actions of self-care fosters development of self-esteem. Hospitalization potentially endangers children's developing self-esteem unless an attempt is made to permit them to participate in some way in their own care. Intrusive procedures are particularly threatening to a child's sense of control because few choices are possible and physical restraint is frequently required. The daily activities of self-care in which the child can make many personal choices are often hampered by hospital policies and rules. When daily self-care skills accomplished by a child are not identified and encouraged, a child feels a sense of frustration and loss. Assessment of the child's skills and ability to participate in care is ongoing because these may change as recovery takes place.

Balancing Factors

The stressors of hospitalization affect children differently across the ages because of their varied developmental needs. Some are more threatening at one age than another. Whether a hazard will cause a crisis for a particular individual depends on such balancing factors as (1) perceptions of the event, (2) availability of

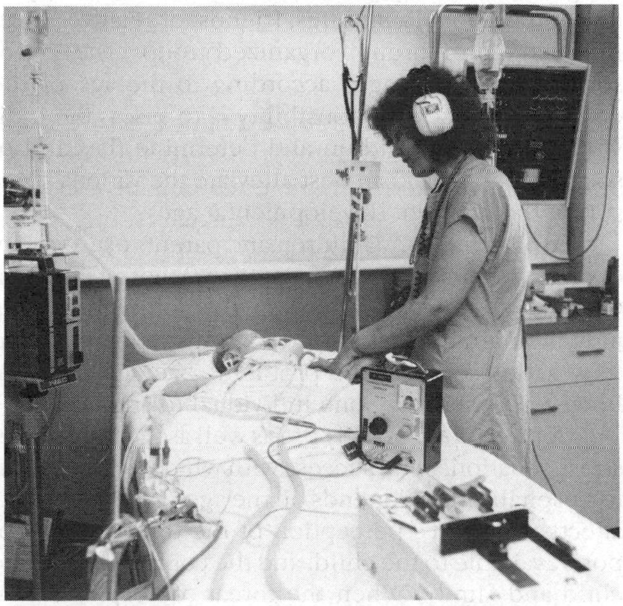

A strange environment with threatening sounds and equipment is disruptive to an infant.

social supports, and (3) the individual's coping skills (Zurlinden, 1985). The nurse's role is to assess the child and family to determine how these balancing factors can be adapted to reduce the stresses of hospitalization.

Child's Perceptions of the Event. Children's perceptions are based on their own observations, on what is told to them, and on fantasy. The cognitive limitations of children affect their own observations and the type of information that can be understood. A description of children's concepts of illness according to cognitive development is presented in Chapter 23.

The impact of the various hazards of hospitalization can be altered if the nurse recognizes that the child's perception of the event changes according to developmental stage. Careful assessment of each child's perceptions of the various stressors provides the data for planning of interventions.

Impact of Social Support. Social support has been described as a buffer or modifier of the potential deleterious effects resulting from stress (Cassel, 1976; Cobb, 1976; Kaplan et al., 1977). Social support refers to interpersonal transactions that comprise one or more of the following: affect, affirmation and aid (Kahn and Antonucci, 1980). *Affect* includes expressions of liking, respect, and love; *affirmation* refers to experiences of agreement or acknowledgement with respect to the appropriateness of verbal statements or actions; *aid* includes actions of direct help (time, money, advice). During hospitalization, children and adolescents are vulnerable because their usual sources of social support are cut off, yet they need so much more because of the stressors of hospitalization. Social support during hospitalization can be provided by parents, professionals, siblings, friends, or relatives in an informal way or through organized groups. The type of social support changes according to the age of the child. The nurse's responsibility is to assess the individual needs of children and determine the kind of social support that can best alleviate the various stressors at the different developmental ages.

Coping Skills. Children and parents use a variety of coping styles when confronted with hospitalization. Coping is generally defined as the ability to make a judgment about a situation (cognitive appraisal) and then acting to solve the problem. The action taken, however, varies from one individual to another.

Coping is part of daily life as well as the handling of stress situations. The success with which a child adapts to hospitalization depends on the age of the child (this affects the child's perception of the threat), the supports available to the child, and the coping skills of the child and family. When the threat of hospitalization overcomes the usual repertoire of behavioral responses, then coping strategies must be called upon to re-establish equilibrium.

Lazarus and Launier (1978) describe four modes of coping: information seeking, direct action, inhibition of action, and intrapsychic processes. A child responds to stress using any one of these modes. Information seeking by children may include asking questions or simply watching and exploring. Active coping deals with the threat at hand and involves controlling, cooperative, and resistive behaviors. Avoidance, ignoring, negation, and physical or verbal attack are also forms of active coping (Rose, 1972). Inactive coping describes children who are not involved, are silent, and display apathy. Intrapsychic processes use defense mechanisms such as regression, denial, repression, projection, sublimation, reaction formation, rationalization, and intellectualization. Toddlers use regression predominantly; by school age, denial is the major mechanism (Caty, 1984). Young children tend to cope by emotional expressions and by motor activity whereas school-age children and adolescents cope through greater use of their cognitive and verbal abilities. Mastery and controlling behaviors are frequent in preschool and school-age children; school-age children use controlling behaviors to cope more frequently than at any other age (Caty, 1984; Savedra and Tesler, 1981). The nurse's recognition of these behaviors and interpretation of their meaning to parents is an important nursing intervention. (See Chapter 23 for further discussion of coping with illness.)

The less ambiguous the situation, the more effective is a child's coping. The child who makes attribution (assigns causation) adapts most readily. The nurse's assessment, therefore, focuses on determining what kind of information is appropriate. Age-appropriate interventions are then planned to facilitate a child's understanding of the situation.

Impact of Hospitalization on Family

The parents of a hospitalized child also experience an increase in stress. Freiberg's (1972) research revealed that parental anxieties were increased when they lacked information about procedures and treatments their child experienced and when they lacked information about the diagnosis and its impact on the future. In addition, parents often feel guilty about their child's illness or injury, even when there is nothing they could have done to prevent it. When their child cries as they approach or leave, they feel such visits only compound their child's discomfort, thereby reinforcing their guilt feelings. Stress is further increased if the admission is an emergency rather than a planned event. The pressure to hurry and the confusion that usually accompanies emergencies add to the parent's anxiety.

Initially, parents are concerned primarily about their child's physical condition. The prolonged waiting for diagnostic procedures or the completion of surgery or for the test results adds to the parents' stress by perpetuating their sense of helplessness. Parents have a right to know about the current condition of their child, the findings from diagnostic studies, the possible and actual effects of treatments, and their child's progress. This information should be offered as soon as possible after it is available so that the parents have concrete facts with which to deal rather than the fears and fantasies that arise from not knowing. During the waiting period, a nurse should be available to the family to discuss concerns, answer questions, and clarify misconceptions.

Parents may be concerned about whether or not a particular treatment, especially if it involves much pain, is helping their child or contributing to suffering. Treatment may also involve controversial or experimental procedures, necessitate restriction of movement, or temporarily make the child's condition worse. In addition, parents may have unrealistic fears about the risk of a procedure or have unrealistic expectations with regard to its results. For example, surgery may merely reduce pain or stop progression of a deformity, whereas the parent may expect it to provide a cure. The nurse can listen, accept parents' feelings, and offer additional or clarifying information.

When a child is hospitalized, the family's routine is altered as well as that of the child. Family life tends to revolve around the needs of the hospitalized child. This can be particularly stressful for the family when the hospital is a long distance from the home and visiting requires that some members be absent from home for several days at a time.

Although the family worries about the hospitalized child and initially all work together on their extra responsibilities, they soon become weary of the extra tasks. The siblings may begin to resent the extra attention given to the hospitalized child. Parents may feel overwhelmed trying to keep up with the demands of work, home responsibilities, and being with their sick child. Siblings may begin to feel that they are being ignored. They should be kept informed of their sibling's illness and progress. Allowing siblings to visit the hospitalized brother or sister can be helpful in reducing stress. Seeing that their brother or sister is really ill helps them understand the reason for their parents' absence. They are often a source of cheer to the sick sibling as they tell the child she or he is missed and relate school, home, and neighborhood events. Older siblings may become actively involved in providing care to their sick sibling under adult supervision. Sibling visiting also provides an opportunity for the children to share in a family crisis and provides a time that parents and children can be mutually supportive.

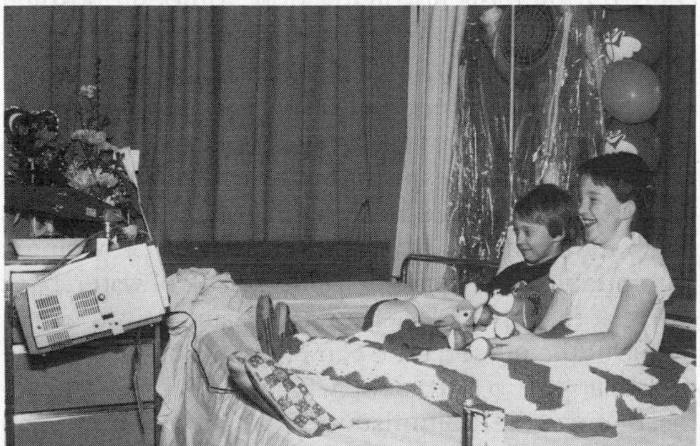
A visit from a younger brother can help to normalize a hospital environment.

Allowing hospitalized children to keep photographs of siblings at the bedside also helps keep them in their thoughts, as do photographs taken of the sick child and sent home to siblings. Notes, tape recordings, and phone calls can also help siblings and peers keep in touch with and be supportive to the hospitalized child.

Nursing Strategies

The goal of the nurse is to help the child and family adapt positively to the hospital experience and to facilitate their growth. This is done by encouraging the child and family to draw upon their strengths and healthy support systems to develop positive coping mechanisms. They can also be assisted to use the problem-solving process to convert limitations into strengths as they attempt to adapt to the new and stressful situations hospitalization poses. Reduction of the threat of hospitalization can be accomplished by designing interventions that modify the stresses of hospitalization and by strengthening the balancing factors.

Specific strategies commonly employed to facilitate the child's and family's coping include (1) maintain the usual patterns fo daily living to the degree possible, (2) meet the developmental needs of the child to facilitate coping, and (3) support and encourage the involvement of parents in the care of their child.

Maintaining Patterns of Daily Living

Hospitalization is an experience that can quickly alter the child's daily routines and patterns. Easily disrupted areas include sleep/rest, nutrition/metabolism, elimination, and activity/exercise (play) patterns.

Sleep pattern disturbance (child), related to
- *unfamiliar environment*
- *separation from parents/family*
- *discomfort of illness*
- *medications*

Refer to Table 31-2, a Nursing Process Plan, at the end of this chapter: Nursing Diagnosis Number 1.

Hospitalization for any child is a disruption of the comforts of bedtime routines and the security of being in one's own bed. The hospital environment is unfamiliar with frightening sounds and strange smells. Children are surrounded by strangers carrying unusual equipment and their own family members may be absent.

Children are vulnerable in the hospital environment because of their cognitive limitations. They misinterpret what they hear and see, harboring a myriad of scary thoughts. This feeling of insecurity and the fear of what will happen next interferes with their ability to relax and sleep. Explanations are helpful, but it should be recognized that a child is exposed to a continuous stream of sights and sounds that are not understood. Even though much of what is seen is unrelated to self, the egocentric nature of a child's thinking causes a child to have fears of which adults are unaware. These thoughts are particularly troublesome when a child tries to go to sleep at night in a strange environment.

The child's physical sense of well-being is also altered. The usual release of energy through physical activity and play is not usually possible to the same degree as when a child is at home. Furthermore, the illness introduces yet another feeling of discomfort. Pain associated with the illness and the hurts resulting from diagnostic procedures and treatments produce anxiety and physical sensations that interfere with a state of rest and sleep. The physical tiredness that children experience from a normal fun-filled day of activity is replaced with emotional distress and unpleasant physical sensations.

Nursing strategies to promote rest and sleep focus on normalizing the child's situation to the extent that is possible within the limits of hospitalization. Collaboration with the child's family, reduction of the child's anxiety, and a good communication system among health care professionals are important strategies used to promote rest and sleep.

Collaborating with the Child's Family. Upon admission, the usual sleep patterns are determined by appropriate questions in the admission history. The child's naptime, bedtime routines, and rituals are identified. The parents are asked to identify the key factors that will assist the nurses to help their child achieve adequate rest and sleep. Sometimes a child's routines interfere with another child's sleep. For example, a child may read and listen to music at home whereas in the hospital these activities may keep another child awake. Adaptations can be made, such as encouraging the child to read earlier and to listen to music through earphones. If parents and children understand the limitations within the hospital, they can be resourceful in adapting the routine without robbing the child of major forms of security. Younger children require their usual blanket or toy and bedtime feeding. Parents are encouraged to bring the child's important bedtime security object.

Reducing Anxiety of the Child. A child's anxiety during hospitalization interferes with the ability to achieve adequate rest and sleep. Major deterrents to such anxiety are the presence of supportive parents, an opportunity to play, clear expectations about procedures, and a supportive health care team. If parents can room-in with their child, many of the bedtime fears are dispelled. To have a parent read a story and provide the usual routines is the best alternative. When parents are not available, it is not usually possible for a nurse to read a bedtime story to each child, but a short story can be read to a group of children.

Opportunities to play with medical toys and clear explanations, including sensory information, are important nursing strategies that reduce a child's anxiety. Also, a child feels more secure in bed if major procedures and treatments are performed in a place other than the bed. Procedures in a children's ward that other children see and hear are distressing for all concerned. Whenever possible, these procedures should be performed in the treatment room away from other children to diminish the fearful thoughts of children that interfere with falling asleep.

A compassionate, reassuring health care team provides an atmosphere of trust for children and adolescents during their hospitalization. Although hospital rules may conflict with individual wishes (i.e., lights out at a certain time), if the child and family are treated with respect, such requests are readily honored. Every effort is made to allow individual bedtime routines to be carried out, but respect for the needs of other roommates is also required. Concern for the individual's sleep requirements is communicated by providing a comfortable environment, a story, drink of water, back rub, or other special measures of comfort. A few moments of the nurse's time can greatly contribute to the child's ability to fall asleep. If a child is experiencing discomfort, the administration of an analgesic can often be timed so that it is given at bedtime to help the child relax. Nonpharmacologic methods to relieve pain should also be used to induce sleep (see Chapter 29 on management of pain).

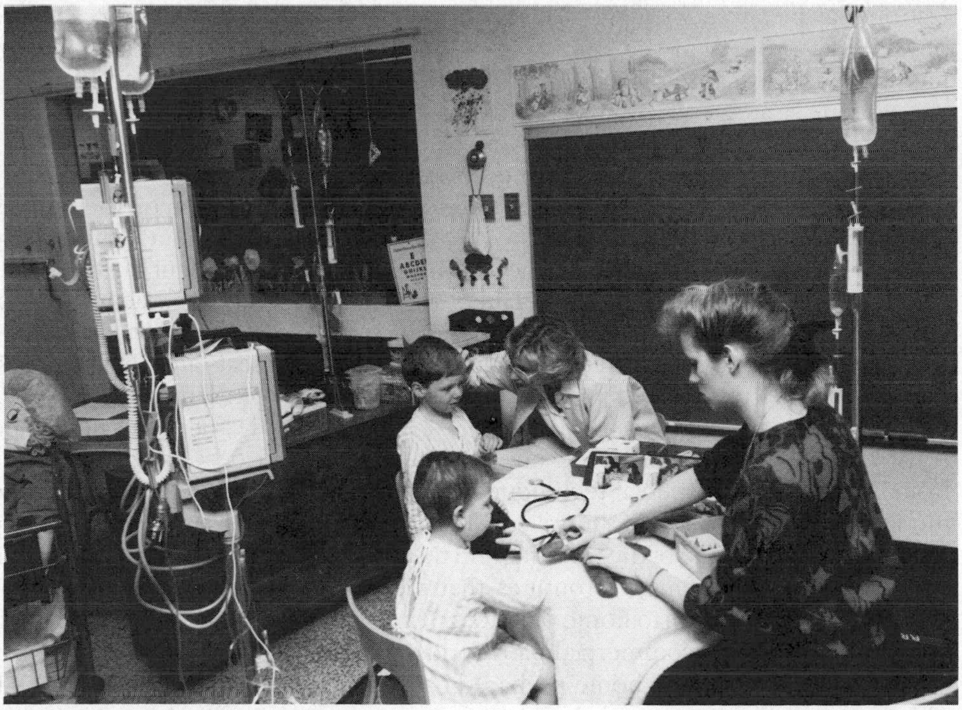

An opportunity to play with medical toys is an important strategy used in hospitals to reduce a child's anxiety. At Chedoke-McMaster Hospital, Hamilton, Ontario, a fully developed play program is provided by the Child Life Team.

The way a child's awake hours are spent should be evaluated if adequate sleep and rest are not being achieved. If a child is physically able, movement, activity, and time in the playroom or recreation lounge are encouraged. Physical activity does not need to be strenuous to provide relaxation. Even a walk to a gift shop, a snack bar, or up and down the hall should be encouraged to provide physical exercise, which in turn promotes rest and sleep. Additionally, long periods of sleep should be avoided during the day except for nap periods for younger children.

Communication Among Health Care Professionals. Hospital routines and schedules frequently do not take into account the child's need for sleep. During an illness, the child's sleep is frequently disrupted by procedures, medications, or monitoring of vital signs. When primary nursing is practiced, the nursing care can more easily be planned to avoid frequent disruptions. However, the collaboration of all team members is required to reduce the number of sequential interruptions by different professionals. The nurse is responsible for assessing the overall needs of the child and identifying with the health team ways to coordinate care to avoid frequent sleep interruptions. Alternative plans should be explored if a child is awakened frequently during the night for various medications. Accomplishment of the plan of care without interrupting sleep can often be achieved with minor alterations in scheduling. A sign posted at the bedside: "Jeremy is asleep: Please come back at 3:30" will help provide an uninterrupted period of sleep. Only the most necessary interruptions will be made if the nurse monitors the child's sleep by putting such notes at the bedside and on the nursing care plan. Including the child's need for sleep when the plan of care is discussed at team conferences is another way to alert all team members.

Altered nutrition: less than body requirements, related to

- *anxiety associated with unfamiliar surroundings*
- *variation in feeding techniques among caregivers*
- *dislike of food served associated with variations in preparation and cultural food preferences*
- *behavioral regression in eating patterns associated with anxiety of hospitalization*
- *anorexia or discomfort associated with disease process*

Refer to Table 31-2, a Nursing Process Plan, at the end of this chapter: Nursing Diagnosis Number 2.

During an illness and hospitalization, a child's appetite is often dulled. The anxiety of being in unfamiliar surroundings affects the desire to eat.

Some behavioral regression in eating patterns is noted in association with the anxiety of hospitalization. Food preparation and the type of food served are often unfamiliar to the child. Cultural preferences are not as easily accommodated in an institution, and feeding techniques of caretakers vary from those of the parents or caretaker at home. The reason for hospitalization may be another source of loss of appetite. The physiologic process of the illness or side effects of medications may cause discomfort and anorexia.

Nursing strategies to promote adequate caloric intake focus on age-appropriate feeding approaches. Specific data about eating are obtained from the parents, and any special equipment required for feeding should be brought from home.

Feeding Infants. Infants are accustomed to the smell, touch, and voice of their caretakers. Feeding is associated with the development of a sense of trust and comfort provided by the caretaker. Whenever possible, care should be planned to permit parents to feed their infant.

To provide consistency, the nurse should learn from the parents any special techniques that facilitate the suck of the infant. Use of a nipple similar to the one used at home, warming of the formula, and the order of solid and liquid feeding are routines that the nurse should follow according to home practices. If an infant is not accustomed to commercial baby foods, parents are often willing to bring home-prepared baby foods. This is generally not a good time to introduce new foods or make major changes in the infant's diet. The feeding time should be comfortable and not rushed. A comfortable place for the parents to sit to hold their infant should be provided. Breastfeeding mothers may feel more comfortable in a private area. The length of feeding time should not exceed 30 to 40 minutes, as beyond that an infant tires and expends too much energy.

Infants should enjoy the comforts of home when fed in the hospital. They should be held for their feedings; under no circumstances should bottles be propped. The practice of leaving an infant in bed with a bottle is also not condoned because it encourages dental caries (see Chapter 19 on promoting dental health). Infants are also held when being fed solids. Once they are able to sit, they are more comfortable and secure in a highchair. To ensure safety, a restraint should be fastened whenever an infant is placed in a highchair in the hospital. Independence should be encouraged by providing a plastic bottle when an infant wishes to hold the bottle, and finger foods can be held by the older infant. Infants, and toddlers, however, should not be left unattended with food and in highchairs.

Hospitalization of an infant can disrupt a mother's ability to breastfeed her infant. Usually she can continue to breastfeed if she receives the necessary support and encouragement from the health care team. If an infant can have nothing by mouth and treatments and procedures interfere with holding it, arrangements can be made to pump the mother's breasts until breastfeeding can be resumed. Even very small infants can be breastfed even though they are dependent on monitors and machines.

Burping an infant, whether breastfed or bottle fed, can be done by holding the infant upright against the nurse's shoulder or by holding the infant in a sitting position on the nurse's lap. One hand is placed under the infant's chin to support the head. In this position the infant can be readily observed for any distress. After feeding, the infant is placed on the right side to facilitate any remaining air to rise from the stomach. Infant seats and chalasia chairs are not used if the infant has a tendency for reflux (Orenstein, 1983). (See Chapter 41 for discussion of positioning of children with gastroesophageal reflux.)

Principles of Feeding Older Children. Many of the strategies used to promote an adequate intake by older hospitalized children are relevant to all ages. These include the opportunity for choice and self-regulation, companionship while eating, and appropriate presentation of food.

Opportunity for Choices, Independence, and Self-Regulation. Attainment of skills in self-feeding is an important developmental landmark. Toddlers and preschoolers should be encouraged to maintain their formerly achieved level of self-feeding during hospitalization. The nurse should be alert to notice when a child who is capable of self-feeding is too tired to eat and offer help appropriately. Children are allowed to choose desired foods from a menu with the assistance of an adult. School-age children and adolescents can be taught about their special diets.

Companionship During Meals. Young children are most comfortable if they can eat in the presence of their family members. When this is not feasible, group eating is a good alternative. Small tables and chairs are often available. Older children can help younger children as needed and can be role models for good table manners. The atmosphere of group eating encourages socialization and promotes a sense of well-being associated with eating.

Appropriate Presentation of Food. Children react to the appearance of food. Color combinations, food consistency, and the size of portions are important to consider when presenting the food tray. The way food is arranged can add to its attractiveness. For example, cutting a sandwich on the diagonal to make four small, triangular sandwiches and setting them upright can be an encouragement to eat. A small cup or specially folded napkin with a happy face can change the mood of a child. Adding preferred foods such as peanut butter from the dietary supplies kept on the children's unit may be all that is needed to interest a child in food.

The portions should be cut and some removed

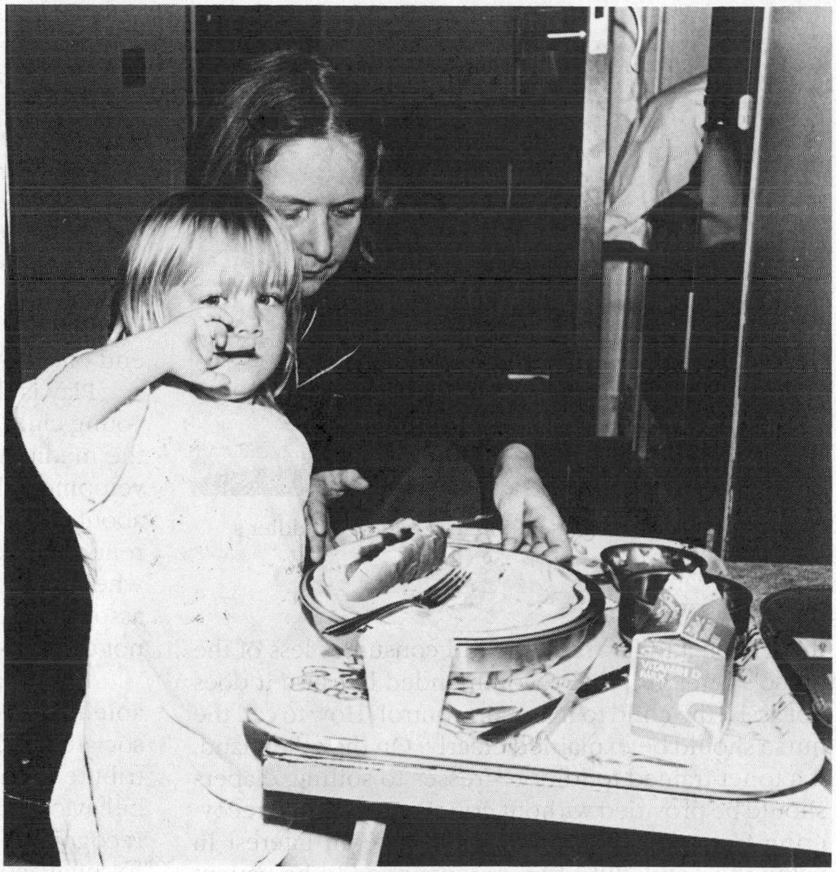

The toddler eats more willingly when served familiar foods in a parent's presence.

before serving if they are unreasonably large. Children who are not hungry are totally discouraged when approached with what they view as large mounds of food. If a child's appetite is diminished, only a small amount of liquid should be provided with the meal; a child's small stomach can soon feel a sense of fullness if a large glass of liquid starts the meal. Additional liquids can be served between meals to meet the requirements. Removal of dessert from the tray initially is sometimes necessary for a child to eat adequate portions of the main course. The way desserts are managed at home determines how a child responds in the hospital. If children have learned that they must eat a balanced meal before they may start dessert, they most likely will adhere to the same rule in the hospital.

Food should be presented attractively and a child is encouraged to eat, but food should not become a control issue between the child and the caretakers.

Children should not be forced or bribed to eat when they are not hungry. Promising to play a game if a child eats a certain amount of food is an unfair dilemma for a sick child. Further strategies for the nutrition of infants, toddlers, school-agers, and adolescents are summarized in Table 31-2.

Altered elimination: incontinence of urine and/or stool, related to regressive behavior associated with the anxiety of hospitalization

Refer to Table 31-2, a Nursing Process Plan, at the end of this chapter: Nursing Diagnosis Number 3.

The stress of hospitalization as well as the illness can alter the child's elimination pattern. Also, the changes in activity and food and certain medications can affect elimination. Parents and children (as appropriate for age) need to be kept informed of possible changes in the character of stool from certain medications.

A common problem resulting from the stress of hospitalization is regressive toileting behaviors. A toddler who has achieved bowel and bladder control just prior to hospitalization frequently becomes incontinent of stool and urine. The nurse should be supportive and not reprimand the child. Parents need reassurance that temporary loss of control while in the hospital is common. The nurse makes an attempt to help children retain bowel and bladder control by offering to assist them to the potty. Although putting

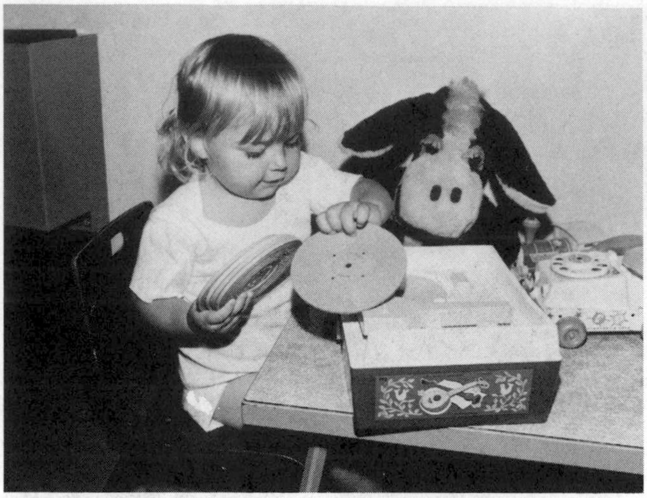

Play within the hospital is an integral part of a toddler's recovery.

diapers on a toilet-trained child consumes less of the nurse's time, it is not recommended because it does not assist the child to maintain control. How to call the nurse should be explained clearly. On the other hand, if a toilet-trained toddler regresses to soiling, diapers should be provided without criticism. The child recovering from the illness may again take an interest in using the potty, but often parents need to be patient until the child returns home. They should also be cautioned against expecting immediate mastery of the previously achieved task. Several weeks may pass before the toddler again achieves bowel and bladder control.

Older children may tend to become constipated because of inactivity or because they do not ask to go to the bathroom when they have the urge. When children are not in their home environment, they tend to put off urination and defecation because of the embarrassment they sense about elimination. Privacy is sometimes difficult to achieve, but the nurse should recognize that children from school-age on are shy to talk about toileting. Hospital gowns are generally not conducive to privacy, therefore a second gown to be worn as a robe is offered to the older child, or parents can bring a robe from home.

Children and adolescents are particularly embarrassed about using urinals and bedpans. They may not know how to use them or are afraid of spillage. If parents are available, they can help their child with the task of toileting until more comfort is achieved with the nurse. When the child is able to perform these activities, opportunities for self-care should be provided. Any assistance that the child can give should be encouraged, and a gradual return to self-care is fostered.

Diversional activity deficit: altered play behavior, *related to*
- *separation from usual playmates/friends*
- *lack of interesting toys/diversional materials*
- *isolation associated with communicable disease*
- *immobility or discomfort associated with disease process or its treatment*

Refer to Table 31-2, a Nursing Process Plan, at the end of this chapter: Nursing Diagnosis Number 4.

Play is the major activity of the waking hours of a young child. It is a natural avenue for self-expression, the medium through which children master their developmental tasks, and the major resource for learning about their world. However, at times intense stress can render a healthy child "playless." With the overwhelming stress of hospitalization and the threat of its associated hazards, many children in the hospital tend not to play spontaneously (Bolig, 1984).

The separation from usual playmates, lack of available toys, isolation, and immobility or discomfort associated with the disease process or its treatment contribute to an alteration in the hospitalized child's play behavior. Play and related activities have come to be recognized as an avenue through which the stress of hospitalization can be relieved, although scientific validation to demonstrate the effectiveness of play is lacking (Bolig, 1984). Play not only promotes development but also provides an important outlet for aggressive or hostile feelings, allowing the child to work through fears and fantasies that are multiplied during hospital experiences. It is important for nurses to integrate play into the overall plan of care and to themselves participate in this component of care. In hospitals where especially assigned individuals such as child life workers are available, both professional groups take responsibility for play to be integrated into daily caregiving. Using volunteers to supplement the nurse's role is also a common approach. In any setting, the nurse must understand clearly that play for the hospitalized child is not a "nice addition" to a plan of care but is central to meeting the holistic needs of the child.

The types of play programs vary. Some consist of little more than a play cupboard with toys, with little or no attention being given to their use in the alleviation of the stress of hospitalization. Others are based on a particular philosophy with specific goals to promote expression of feelings and mastery. It is important for the nurse to understand the various types of play and to use play effectively in nursing interventions as a balancing factor. The use of play for assessment, diversion, recreation, and reduction of anxiety common to other settings in addition to hospitals is discussed in Chapter 21. Promotion of normal growth and development through play during hospitalization is discussed next.

Play to Promote Development

In the hospital, a child's normal growth and developmental needs cannot always be met effectively through play because of limited space, impaired mobility, reduced energy, and limited toys. Also, the opportunity for socialization is thwarted because of separation from the child's family and peers. The nurse's familiarity with developmental play at different ages is an important component of nursing care. Whether or not the unit has an organized play program, the nurse can provide for the child's need to play.

Infants. To assist in preventing regression in development and a delay in the attainment of developmental milestones, an organized play period or infant stimulation program is desirable. Plank (1971) recommends that infants over 10 months of age be included in play programs. Play is intellectually stimulating for an infant and provides opportunities for continued development of motor and social skills.

When feeding, dressing, or diapering, the nurse should establish eye contact and speak to the infant. Until they have back control for sitting, infants can be propped or placed in an infant seat at intervals if their condition permits, so that they can observe the activities about them. Mobiles, mirrors, baby gyms, and music boxes provide additional auditory and visual stimulation. Every infant should have toys within reach in the crib. Some hospital auxiliaries provide small soft toys for patients if none have been brought from home.

Activities can be planned away from the crib as well. Many units have strollers, swings, and rockers. If these are not available, a mat or bath blanket can be placed on the floor to provide the older infant opportunities for crawling, rolling, and reaching.

Toddlers and Preschoolers. As the child approaches the toddler years, play becomes more active and may be severely hampered by illness and hospitalization. Toddlers and preschoolers prefer large muscle activity, but if such play is prohibited toys can be brought to the child's bed or placed on a small table in the child's room. In some hospitals, enclosed outdoor play areas permit activities to exercise large muscles. If confined to bed, it is especially important to provide for the child's needs to explore, to be independent, and to make discoveries through manipulation. Coloring, painting, and manipulating toys that stack or come apart are appropriate for young children. Large puzzles, books with cardboard pages that the child can turn, and large beads to put on a heavy string are enjoyed by young children. Toys that allow the child to dissipate energy, such as a pounding board with hammer and thick crayons that can be used to scribble vigorously, can relieve a child of some of the frustration of limited physical exercise. Creative and imaginative play activities are particularly beneficial and enjoyable.

School-Age Children. Although the school-age child preserves some of the fantasy and drama from preschool days in play, play has changed in several recognizable ways. Added are rules, ritualistic behaviors, language chants ("Step on a crack, break your mother's back"), and team activities. The person who organizes structured play activities on the school-age unit should keep these facts in mind. School-agers tend to prefer games, both active and sedentary, to unstructured group play. The school-age child also enjoys the reprieve of quiet and solitary activity (board

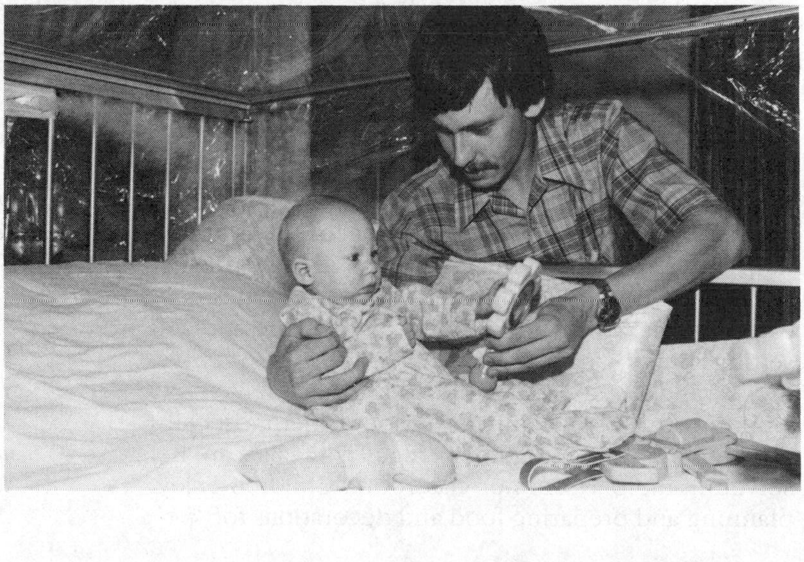

Hospitalized infants need the stimulation of play and toys to maintain their development.

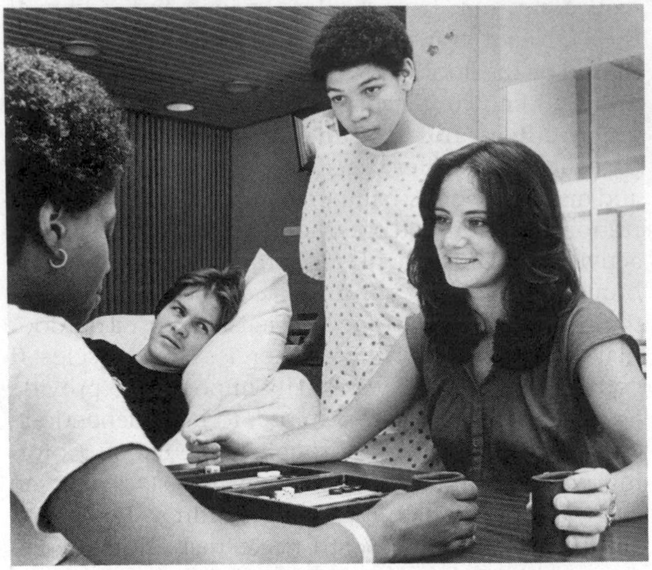

Teen activities on the hospital unit provide opportunities for establishing peer relationships and mutual support. (Courtesy of the Children's Hospital of Philadelphia.)

games, reading books, writing stories, or drawing pictures). School-age children still enjoy being read to occasionally. Therapeutic play equipment like puppets, dolls, and medical-related toys should remain available but should not be forced upon them.

Adolescents. The use of play to facilitate adjustment to hospitalization for an adolescent usually takes on a form of socialization. Group activities involving several adolescents and a place for them to gather are major recreational needs of a hospitalized adolescent. An adolescent's ability to understand explanations about the procedures and events accompanying hospitalization obviates the need for use of therapeutic play as with a younger child. Participation in recreation, games, and diversionary activities, however, is an important element in an adolescent's adjustment.

Group Activities

Group activities help reduce the stress of hospitalization for many children. The child sees how other children with problems adapt and cope, which provides ideas for adapting.

Age-appropriate group activities also offer opportunities for socialization with a number of children and help children learn to relate to those of the opposite sex. The children learn to share responsibilities and carry out tasks, and to respond to peer pressure in setting limits on behavior. Young children enjoy movies and arts and crafts; older children might enjoy working on a hospital unit newspaper. Since most children enjoy eating together, regular meals can be served in the playroom or classroom. Children enjoy planning and preparing food and decorations for special events or parties. This activity also helps children begin to utilize organizational skills. Younger children might enjoy a clown's visit or a presentation by a magician, whereas older children might enjoy a concert by a rock performer.

Group activities are especially meaningful to children who must remain hospitalized during holidays or birthdays. Whenever possible, parties should be arranged or at least allowed at these times. Perhaps more visitors can be permitted on a birthday or visiting hours extended to allow visits by family members or friends who usually are not permitted to visit.

Regardless of the type of play program that exists, a child's need to play can be integrated into the plan of care. The developmental level of the child is used as a guide when planning play and activities.

Meeting Developmental and Coping Needs During Hospitalization

Self-care deficit, *related to*
- *unfamiliar environment*
- *regressive behavior*
- *illness and treatment*

Altered growth and development:
- ***physical,*** *related to prolonged immobility associated with illness, injury, or treatment*
- ***intellectual,*** *related to decreased environmental stimulation associated with decreased mobility and decreased energy for exploration*
- ***emotional/social,*** *related to alterations in bonding, separation anxiety, or unresolved impact of hospitalization upon age-related stressors*

Disturbance in self-concept: body image and/or self-esteem, *related to effects of illness and treatment upon*
- *physical appearance*
- *physical mobility/agility*
- *intellectual function*
- *feelings of competence/mastery over the environment*
- *perceived sexuality*

Ineffective individual coping, *related to crisis of hospitalization associated with multiple stressors:*
- *separation from parents and significant others*
- *unfamiliar environment*
- *harm, injury, and pain*
- *unclear limits and expectations*
- *loss of control (Visintainer and Wolfer, 1975)*

See Table 31-2 at the end of this chapter: Nursing Diagnoses Numbers 5, 6, 7, and 8.

Hospitalized children require ongoing support from the health care team and family members to relieve the stress of hospitalization and to foster normal growth and development. The effects of hospitalization and the needs of children and parents vary according to the child's developmental level. The nurse's role in supporting the child and family to relieve the stress of hospitalization and to foster normal growth and development of children during hospitalization is discussed next.

Infant: Development and Coping. Of all the stressors of hospitalization for the infant, *separation from familiar people and routines* presents the greatest disruption. Infants as young as 10 days display a response to a change in caretakers. The young infant is likely to become subdued, whereas children over 7 months of age exhibit outward signs of stress, such as crying and clinging to parents. Therefore, rooming-in by parents is of particular importance with infants (Blackman, 1973).

An infant learns through a variety of stimuli. The usual opportunities for play, socialization, and movement should be provided for the hospitalized infant (Box 31-2). If parents cannot provide the necessary stimulation and nurturance, a primary nurse should fulfill that need.

The type of illness may influence the infant's reaction to hospitalization. The infant who is not allowed to eat or suck because of oral surgery or for any other reason may react by persistent crying or thrashing about from frustrated oral needs. The infant with a problem of the central nervous system, on the other hand, may exhibit a wide range of behavior changes. An infant's instinctive need to move freely may be affected by restraints or other means of immobilization.

The nurse should also be alert to notice the "apparently" well-adjusted infant. For example, the quiet, subdued infant in Bryant's traction may not attract the attention of the caretaker as readily as the crying, clinging child in the next bed. Although less apparent, the means of coping of the former child are equally important cues to the nurse.

Mobility is an important aspect of the development of the infant. An angry or frustrated infant frequently resorts to flailing of arms and legs. Occasionally, for safety, the infant must be restrained during procedures such as intravenous therapy and nasogastric intubation and following oral surgery. Unable to cope in the usual manner, tension is increased. Sibinga and Friedman, (1971) examined children who were restrained as infants and found a positive correlation between this restraint and later language delay and articulation problems.

Nursing strategies include (1) providing stimulation to infants while they are restrained (use of a suspended ball that could be kicked by the feet); (2) removing the restraints under supervision for 10 minutes every 2 hours to allow for random movement; and (3) changing the position while unrestrained, and at the same time, talking to, touching, and holding the infant (Dowd, 1977). Infants with orthopedic anomalies often must undergo long periods of immobility and their need for stimulation is acute.

Toddler: Development and Coping. The response of a toddler to a stress situation does not necessarily have to be one of severe anxiety and long-term adverse effects. Those aspects that are the most stress-producing can be carefully managed to minimize the threatening hospital experience. A toddler's security is particularly threatened by (1) being separated from the parents or other significant person, (2) being in an unfamiliar environment and having routines and rituals disrupted, and (3) feeling a loss of control and having autonomy threatened by procedures that are painful and necessitate restraints. The nurse and family must cooperatively plan to minimize the adverse effects of these inevitable situational crises and maximize the positive experiences that can be derived from hospitalization. This presents a unique challenge to the nurse who cares for hospitalized toddlers.

A toddler's security depends on doing things in the same way in the same environment. It is not feasible to retain every aspect of a toddler's routine, but the nurse can avoid serious disruption of the toddler's security by adapting care to coincide with established routine whenever possible. Even though parents are usually present, the nurse should be familiar with the child's most important routines.

Fear of painful procedures causes considerable stress to toddlers. Their limited cognitive ability makes them particularly likely to arrive at strange conclusions regarding painful procedures. Young children may react to threatening procedures as if they are hostile attacks and view them as punishment. The nurse's role is to prepare the toddler adequately and perform the procedures skillfully. See Chapter 27 for the supportive role of the nurse during performance of procedures.

Normal growth and development needs of the toddler can be met during hospitalization if the nurse works closely with the parents to provide individualized care. The child's physical, intellectual, and emotional and social needs must be considered when planning nursing interventions (Box 31-3). Two central themes that dominate the development of toddlers, are that they are becoming autonomous and that they develop through play.

Secure toddlers show increasingly more autonomous behaviors. Hospitalization disrupts their familiar life of people, places, and things so that they feel

Box 31-2
Developmental Needs and Nursing Strategies: Infants

PHYSICAL NEEDS

To be warm and dry

Check infant frequently and provide clean diapers and sheets as needed.

To have hunger needs met in a consistent manner

Maintain the home feeding schedule whenever possible.

Encourage the breastfeeding mother to continue. Make a breast-pump available if feeding must be curtailed for a period of time.

On admission, check with parent for type, amount, and frequency of formula (if not breastfed), and whether formula is warmed.

Encourage parents to be present for feedings whenever possible.

Ask parents about the child's usual involvement in feeding (i.e., drinking from cup, self-feeding from spoon, finger foods, holding own bottle) and foster development of such skills. (Do not prop bottle.)

Ask parents about usual position for feeding (held, highchair, infant seat, and so on).

Schedule intrusive treatments at a time other than immediately after a feeding to avoid vomiting.

To have opportunity to roll and pull self up; to reach, grasp, and mouth objects in a safe environment

Ensure that side rails are locked securely.

Provide "bubble-top" crib if child crawls up rails.

Provide crib bumper pads to avoid injury or getting caught between side rails.

Provide safe toys that can be held, transferred, and mouthed.

As condition permits, take to play area—provide mat on floor with appropriate toys (under supervision).

INTELLECTUAL NEEDS

To have opportunity to see and hear a variety of sights and sounds

Provide mobiles, music boxes, busy boxes in crib.

Take for rides in a wagon or stroller to permit varied sights and sounds.

To hear language

Speak to the infant when awake. Use appropriate language (avoid baby talk).

To learn through sensorimotor experience in a safe environment

Allow infant to learn through repetition of acts, i.e., drop and pick up toy.

Provide a variety of toys that can be manipulated so that infant can repeat performances.

Provide variety of textures to enhance experience with the environment.

Provide clean toys that can be mouthed. (Wash well after toys fall on the floor.)

EMOTIONAL-SOCIAL NEEDS

To maintain relationship with parent or primary caretaker

Encourage parent ot provide or participate in daily care (feed, bathe, hold) whenever possible.

Explain to parents whether child can be held and help parent to do so.

Suggest ways parent can participate in play and stimulation for their infant.

If parent cannot room-in, assign the same nurse whenever possible.

To develop sense of security

Handle infant gently during all care and procedures.

Cuddle infant frequently, especially after procedures.

Talk to infant during care and procedures.

Respond to infant cues by observing when infant is tired, wants to be held, or just wants to lay in crib and play.

threatened, insecure, and even punished. As they feel less secure, the spirit of "Me do it" wanes. Furthermore, hospitals are run on schedules that often do not allow for the extra time it takes to permit toddlers to do their own zipper, take off their own socks and shoes, and brush their teeth at their own pace. Toddlers dawdle to increase their sense of control, wanting to do things in their own time in their own way. When this right is taken away, development is interrupted.

The nurse who understands the importance of these behaviors will incorporate interventions into the care plan to support the toddler's developing autonomy. The tasks the toddler has accomplished should be performed whenever possible, even though it takes longer to do them. The toddler can also learn to perform new tasks while hospitalized, but major tasks such as becoming toilet trained, giving up a pacifier, or being weaned from a nighttime bottle should not be attempted during this time of stress.

The developing sense of autonomy is hampered

Box 31-3
Developmental Needs and Nursing Strategies: Toddlers

PHYSICAL NEEDS

To explore and develop muscle skill within a safe environment

Assess prehospitalization exploratory activities.

Provide small manipulative toys (boxes with lids; stack toys; nesting toys; large beads; large puzzles; equipment to color, paint, and scribble).

Provide a crib with an enclosed see-through top when a child attempts to explore by reaching for dangerous objects or crawling out of the crib.

Permit supervised activities in a playroom to explore new toys and the unfamiliar environment.

Allow exploration in child's room under supervision.

To have opportunity to engage in large muscle activity within safe limits

Assess degree of mobility attained.

Provide for supervised out-of-bed activities consistent with patterns at home as the child's condition permits.

Keep floors free of small objects.

Enforce rules about wearing of shoes or nonskid slippers when child is out of bed.

Provide toys for the large muscles (rocking horse, soft ball, indoor slide, push-and-pull toys).

To maintain physiologic function through development of self-care skills

Assess level of self-care attained (eating, elimination, dressing, hygiene, bedtime care).

Provide opportunities for participation in self-care activities.

- Eating: Provide highchair or small table and chair, bib, and usual types of food; allow child to feed self in usual manner.
- Elimination: Provide a potty chair or diapers according to usual elimination patterns. Reinforce routine as established prehospitalization.
- Dressing: Permit child to assist with those activities he or she is capable of doing.
- Hygiene: Allow child to participate in handwashing, brushing teeth, manipulating own wash cloth in tub.

INTELLECTUAL NEEDS

To have opportunity to learn via sensorimotor experience and express self through imitation and pretending

To engage in conversation with adults and children to enhance language development; to hear proper language and be encouraged to express self through language

Provide toys that encourage exploration and manipulation.

For older toddler, provide toys and equipment that can be used to reenact hospital experience.

Assess extent of child's vocabulary, especially key phrases and words pertaining to daily activities.

Allow child to complete sentences; avoid speaking for the child.

Reinforce words child has mastered and introduce new words.

Encourage group activities (play and eating) to encourage use of language among children.

To receive explanations about procedures (toddlers can understand more than they can say)

Avoid speaking about children without explanations to them as well.

Explain procedures before doing them.

EMOTIONAL-SOCIAL NEEDS

To develop sense of autonomy

Allow child to do things alone pertaining to own care.

Allow child to participate in the bedtime story, and preparation for bed according to home routines.

Give child control over some of own life: allow choices, restrain as little as possible, and praise for completed tasks.

To learn to separate from parent(s)

Encourage care by parents.

Assist family in coping with behaviors in response to hospitalization and separation.

Encourage parents to visit often even though child resists their leaving.

Provide primary nurse when parents cannot be present.

Keep image of parent in child's mind with a picture, personal belongings, or a tape recording.

To learn to adapt socially

Reinforce those socially acceptable behaviors mastered by the child before hospitalization (eating, elimination, play).

Provide play opportunities with other children.

To maintain usual routines and rituals for sense of security

Assess important rituals and routines, especially regarding bedtime (provide security objects and maintain routine; reading story, hugging, use of night light and other rituals).

Ask parents and child about preferences in foods, toys, routines regarding daily hygiene, elimination, and dressing.

Maintain as many home routines as possible.

frequently when toddlers must be firmly held during procedures or by the restraint of extremities for intravenous fluids. Although it is often necessary to restrain toddlers for a procedure, the nurse should try to gain their cooperation before resorting to the use of restraint. Toddlers who are restrained for an IV should be removed from restraints periodically. During this time they should be able to leave their room; under supervision, they may be taken to the playroom.

To accomplish the goal of forming a trusting relationship with this child, one nurse should take the responsibility for planning care so that some constancy of routine can be established. The primary nurse who plans the care should also care for the toddler when on duty. The primary nurse should attempt to have frequent interactions with the toddler throughout the day. To a toddler, several hours are an eternity; therefore, frequent contacts for shorter periods are more meaningful than only one or two contacts in an 8-hour period. The coming and going of the primary nurse during the day also gives the toddler practice in dealing with separation and increases trust that the nurse will return. Additional special methods of ongoing contact should be used. It may be feasible for a toddler to sit on the nurse's lap during charting, or sit close by in a wagon or stroller as other duties are performed.

The involvement of parents whenever a toddler must undergo a procedure is another important part of relieving stress. Parents need to learn about the procedure before it is done even if they do not plan to be present. Such a discussion should not be carried out in the presence of the toddler, who will understand some things and misinterpret others. Also, the reaction of parents to the explanation may be alarm or concern, and the toddler is particularly sensitive to the general mood of conversations even though not understanding their content.

Parents should be given the option to stay or leave when a painful procedure must be done. Some parents cannot cope with seeing their toddler being hurt, and the nurse has a responsibility to support the parent in that decision. If a parent is made to feel that he or she *must* be present, the distress of the parent is likely to be communicated to the toddler and consequently compound the anxiety. Providing the toddler with personal securities such as a blanket, teddy bear, or other special object is essential during such procedures. A young toddler who required frequent intrusive procedures used a photograph of his mother as his primary security item. When it was time for medicine or other unpleasant procedures, he would search frantically among his toys and blankets for the photo till he found it, and then calm down and cooperate with the nurse, grasping the picture throughout.

Preschoolers: Development and Coping. Even when children are prepared and development supported during the confinement, hospitalization is likely to be highly anxiety-producing for the preschooler (Galligan, 1979; Oremland et al, 1973). The experience can hinder their initiative-seeking behaviors, threaten their newly established concept of an intact body that they control, and jeopardize the progress they were making in separating from parents without conflict.

Physically, the preschooler has successfully achieved control of most body functions, allowing a fair amount of self-control in most activities of daily living. The stress of hospitalization usually leads to some degree of regression in this mastery as the preschooler attempts to cope (Tekely et al, 1978). This regression is frustrating and confusing to preschoolers. Having just mastered self-care, they find it threatening to relinquish it. Preschoolers greatly fear the loss of control over these daily routines. They need help to regain self-control so that they do not experience shame and further regression. When they are not receiving adequate assistance, preschoolers let nurses and parents know either by becoming inactive, uncooperative, and withdrawn or by becoming hyperactive and overaggressive and displaying pseudoindependence. (In pseudoindependence, preschoolers refuse comfort or assistance and act as though they do not care whether the parent is there or not) (Calkin, 1979). The withdrawal or aggression is usually expressed in relation to those activities toward which they feel a loss of control (eating, elimination, sleeping) (Tekely et al, 1978).

Intellectually, preschoolers are still egocentric. Perhaps the greatest difficulty hospitalization creates for them is feeling guilt and shame from the egocentric belief that being in the hospital is a punishment for something they did or thought (Brandt et al, 1972; Oremland et al, 1973; Azarnoff, 1974). Their thinking is intuitive and magical, out of which grows a rich fantasy life. During hospitalization, the distortion of perception that arises out of their egocentric and magical thoughts works against them. They construct unfathomable fantasies and fears stemming from the strange hospital "Land of Oz." They have usually mastered basic language skills under normal circumstances but still may have difficulty verbalizing needs and feelings during stress. With help, preschoolers can avoid or master unrealistic fears during hospitalizations and can progress in their ability to communicate their needs effectively, even under stress (Box 31-4).

Emotionally and socially preschoolers are taking initiative to gain some control over the environment and increase their independence. Upon hospitaliza-

Box 31-4
Developmental Needs and Nursing Strategies: Preschoolers

PHYSICAL NEEDS

To maintain control of body functions

Assess prehospitalization level of control and patterns for eating, elimination, and sleep. Assess words used to describe functions.

Allow normal patterns as much as possible.

Reassure when accidents in elimination occur; do not reprimand or punish.

Praise successes in self-control.

Provide age-appropriate motor stimulation.

To maintain physiologic function through increased development of self-care skills

Assess prehospitalization self-care tasks.

Allow continued self-care when possible; provide some opportunities for decisions on care, especially in aspects of care in which condition or treatment prohibits self-care.

Allow usual eating practices: provide foods child is used to, finger foods, favorite foods, and eating utensils from home; allow family members to eat with child if isolated or to feed if child must be fed; if not isolated, allow eating at child-sized table with hospitalized peers; follow child's usual rituals, such as prayer before eating.

Allow usual elimination practices: provide potty chair (from home if preferred) or regular toilet as child is accustomed to; if mobility is restricted, offer to assist child to toilet or bedpan at usual eliminating times. Keep call bell near so child may get prompt assistance at other times. (Preschoolers still have difficulty "holding off" elimination processes.) Stay with child or provide privacy as child is accustomed.

Allow usual rest and sleep practices. Allow night light if child is used to one or requests one; provide quiet, uninterrupted period during child's usual nap or rest time if nap still taken; allow usual sleep time attire to be worn; if not contraindicated, allow usual sleep position and amount of cover and pillows used at home; bring any special sleep items (blanket, pacifier, toy) from home.

Permit child to dress at least partially in own clothing during daytime.

INTELLECTUAL NEEDS

To be protected from sense of guilt, which can occur as a result of egocentric thinking

Reassure repeatedly that no one is to blame for the condition or hospitalization.

Reassure that only necessary treatments will be done, and they will not be done without telling the child first.

Provide activities (play, arts and crafts, stories) that stimulate intellectual development.

To be protected from fears created by preoperational thinking (intuitive, magical thoughts)

Explain all procedures, especially describing what child can expect to experience through the senses, before doing them.

Provide for dramatic and therapeutic play; make available safe procedural equipment and dolls during education sessions, in playroom, at bedside.

Do not talk about the child unless child is included in the conversation.

To have opportunity to use expressive language

Encourage questions and ask questions to learn fears, fantasies, and misperceptions (correct these when possible). Give opportunity for verbal expressions during stress.

Encourage child to tell stories about drawings or to tell you a "story" about hospital procedures or experiences.

Teach new words related to simple anatomy and physiology, the disease or treatment, and hospital equipment and personnel.

EMOTIONAL-SOCIAL NEEDS

To master control of the environment and develop independence

Encourage self-care in hygiene and participation in medical care and treatments. (The preschooler can cooperate if given adequate instruction and permission to participate.)

Observe safety precautions.

Promptly remove offensive smells and preserve orderliness. As a result of having mastered toilet functions, the preschooler is keenly aware of smells and disorder and is upset by them.

Permit and encourage child's own decision making regarding care and treatments when choices exist.

Praise evidence of competence in all areas of development (self-care, learning new words, helping with a treatment, cooperation during stressful procedures).

Solicit and respect child's suggestions regarding care, room environment changes, toys in room, etc.

To experience limits within environment to feel security

Enforce safety rules; give simple explanations for rules (child must be in crib or bed with rails up even if used to big bed without rails at home).

Define limits on activity due to illness (isolation from other children while disease is communicable). Since

Continued

time concept is undeveloped, give idea of how long the limitation will be by associating it with concrete things ("You can go to the playroom Saturday. That is the day that cartoons are on TV all morning" or "You can drink water and other drinks again when Nurse Smith comes to care for you this afternoon").

Learn during admission interview if parents want any home rules continued during hospitalization (only certain TV shows may be watched or TV is allowed only so many hours a day, teeth are to be brushed after each meal, limited beverages are allowed after suppertime) and enforce those not in conflict with treatment regimen.

Explain to parents reasons any cannot be enforced.

To engage in rituals to feel secure

Assess usual routines and rituals during interview. Integrate rituals into care plan as possible.

Encourage parents or other family members acquainted with the rituals to be present and help child carry out mealtime, bedtime, other significant rituals.

Ask parents to bring from home those objects related to child's rituals and other security items.

To learn to separate without conflict

Provide for a primary nurse for each shift.

Permit and encourage unlimited parental visits and participation in planning and giving care.

Allow parents to remain and comfort child, if desired during treatments or procedures parents cannot or do not wish to do. Primary nurse is present as parent surrogate to stay with and comfort child.

Let parents do as many of the "caretaking" tasks as possible.

Ask parents to bring in familiar toys, family photos, personal belongings that can be left with child as reminders of them during their absence.

During care, make up pleasant stories about home activities, including names of family members in the stories, or encourage child to tell stories about home and family activities.

Provide opportunities for child to become acquainted with other children and parents who may "fill in" as sources of comfort during parental and sibling separations.

Help parents identify ways to keep child in contact with siblings or peers who cannot visit (phone call, tape recordings, notes, pictures).

To achieve sexual identity and comfort with sexual sensations and feelings

Give thorough explanations and continued reassurance about what will happen to the child's body as a result of a treatment or procedure; it is especially important to reassure of continued presence and intactness of genitals when these body parts are involved.

Handle genitalia as little as possible and use gentleness when handling is necessary. Some children respond better if their hand is used with the nurse's in handling the genitalia.

Avoid use of intrusive procedures or treatments whenever possible (preschoolers cope with axillary or oral thermometers better than rectal).

tion, preschoolers may feel a loss of the control they had been gaining over the environment. Particularly if immobilized or isolated, they may lose the initiative to try to satisfy their curiosities. Unless nursing personnel carefully plan for preservation of the routines and rituals that they are accustomed to at home, preschoolers' sense of security is diminished. Although preschoolers now separate from parents more easily, with perhaps conflict only initially, they still will resist separation during illness and other periods of stress. They tend to perceive the separations as punishment and fear abandonment. The oedipal crisis causes them to fear body mutilation, pain, and invasion of body orifices; this is possibly the preschoolers' greatest fear during hospitalization (Oremland et al, 1973; Petrillo and Sanger, 1980). Thus, preschoolers' major task is to cope with the treatment procedures and unfamiliar individuals and equipment that are required to manage the illness. To achieve success in coping with this phase of hospitalization, the nurse and parents should (1) educate preschoolers about what to expect during the procedures and about the people and equipment involved, and (2) provide materials and opportunities for dramatic and therapeutic play so that they can work through their fears and fantasies.

School-Age Children: Development and Coping. Because of the intellectual and emotional progress made during preschool years, school-age children have fewer adjustment problems during hospitalization. They are now able to tolerate parental separation. Although not totally free of separation anxiety, they are more reality oriented. Unreasonable fantasies and fears are fewer in number and severity, and they are eager to form relationships and have experiences outside the family and home. Handled adequately, hospitalization may be perceived by school-age children as an adventure during which they can learn many new things and make new friends. Regressive behavior is less frequent in school-agers; if regression does occur, a child typically will display the type of fears characteristic of preschoolers: fears of mutilation, monsters, and separation. The predominant fears of hospitalized school-age children are of bodily injury or loss of self-control and of death. To reduce these fears, the nurse can provide procedural explanations, allow the children to participate in planning and doing their own care, and give instructions and honest answers about the illness and prognosis. Freed of excessive anxiety with the help of the nurse, school-agers are ready to make the most of their hospitalization as a growth experience.

Although school-age children adapt without too much trauma to their hospital stay, some nursing actions will facilitate the adaptation: (1) preparing them for procedures and treatments through education sessions, (2) providing opportunities for expression through play and verbal exchange, and (3) allowing and encouraging active participation in planning and carrying out the treatment regimen.

Since school-age children may be embarrassed by crying or screaming, offer alternative outlets for pain or fear, such as squeezing a parent's or nurse's hand, counting, engaging in diversional conversation, or clenching the teeth; if they do scream or cry, they should not be shamed ("Big boys don't cry") but reassured that such expression is normal and OK. (See Chapter 29 for discussion of pain management.) Most school-age children still prefer a parent's presence during procedures and passively seek contact with their eyes or through facial expressions, but they should be offered the option of having or not having a parent present. School-agers are able to hold still for a procedure and usually invest most of their energy in retaining self-control (Brandt, 1972). If they receive praise for holding still and for other evidence of cooperation or participation, the likelihood of future cooperation is increased.

School-age children's industrious drive makes them an eager candidate to participate actively in the treatment regimen. They still find security in a routine and willingly help structure what the routine will be. Their understanding of time makes them capable of "helping" the nurse stay with the planned routine. Although they will require supervision, they can perform a large variety of treatments after adequate instruction and practice. The opportunity to participate in planning and performing care bolsters school-age children's self-concept, stimulates them intellectually, and provides opportunity for refinement of motor skills. School-age children also can be invaluable in helping teach or motivate self-care in their peers.

Physically, school-age children have achieved complete control of body functions and the physical self-care required in daily living. This independence in self-care reinforces a healthy image and builds self-confidence; therefore, allowing ill children to perform their own tasks of daily living during the hospital experience, at least to the degree they can tolerate, is of obvious importance. School-age children are intent on developing their fine motor skills. They need to continue practicing fine motor tasks during hospitalization so they can keep abreast of their peers. The nurse can make use of this developmental challenge by actively involving them in education regarding their disease and treatment and by inviting them to participate in aspects of their treatment that require fine motor function (Box 35-5).

Intellectually, school-age children are testing out *concrete operations.* They base perceptions on reality progressively more often than on fantasy. Most of the fears they retain involve situations that threaten to cause loss of control or bodily injury. They accept the fact that there are various points of view beyond their own. Because they can now reason out cause-and-effect relationships, they are intrigued by the scientific process and want scientific explanations regarding their disease, the sensation they can expect during hospitalization, and the rationale underlying treatments.

Rules help school-age children think rationally. If rules are not provided, they will construct their own

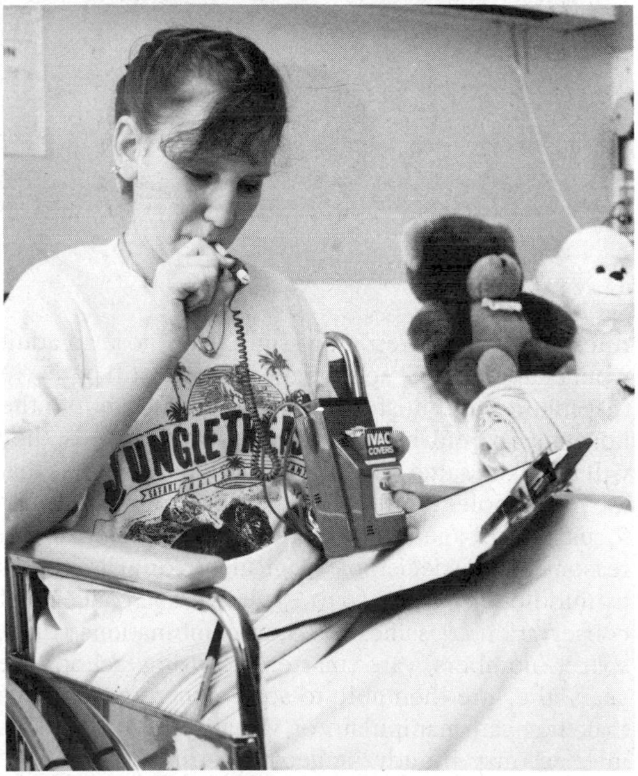

Independence and responsibility can be fostered in school-age children and adolescents by encouraging their involvement in monitoring their own vital signs.

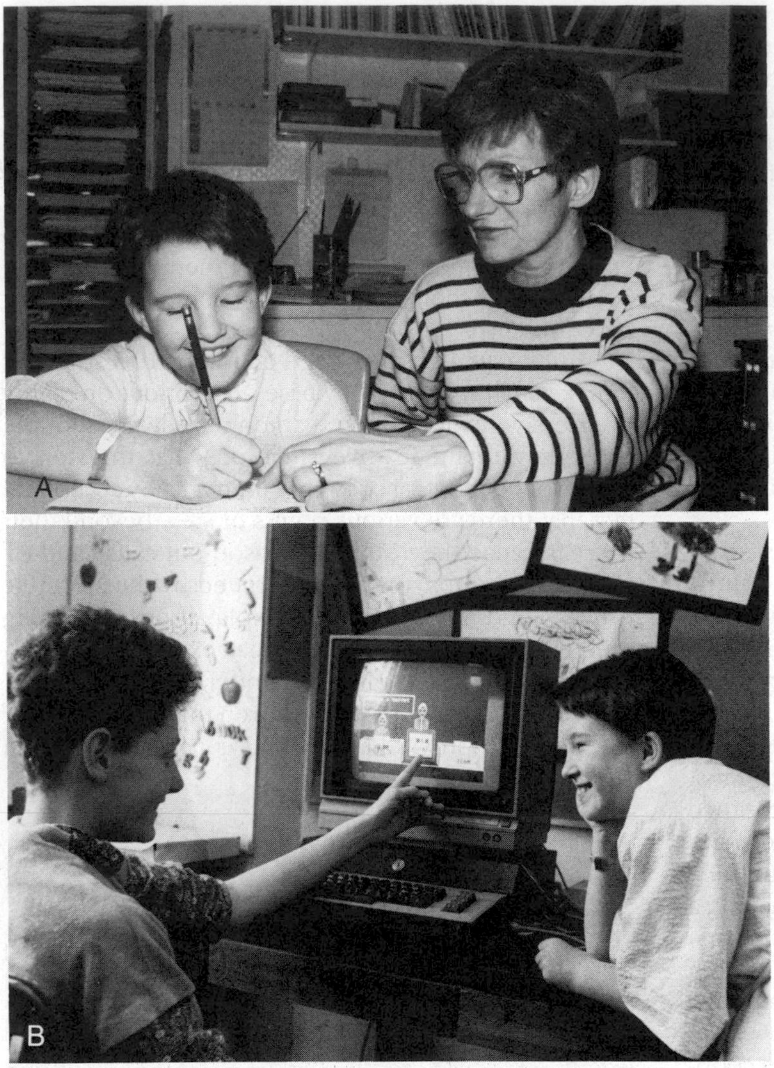

Individualized school programs are now provided to hospitalized children in some centers. Larger institutions have certified teachers and a separate classroom where equipment and supplies are available for an educational program.

rules, which are often more rigid than those an adult would supply. Early school-age children still perceive that injuries and misfortunes such as put them in the hospital are punishment for their own misdeeds; they will need the same reassurances of blamelessness that the preschooler required. As they lose their egocentric focus, school-agers rely more on past memories and reason to make decisions; magical thinking disappears by middle school-age (8 to 10 years). The concepts of conservation, classification, and combinations (time, space, numbers) are mastered during school-age years; they are then able to solve concrete problems that they can manipulate or visualize mentally. This intellect may be advantageously utilized to involve them in planning and carrying out the treatment regimen (Box 31-6).

School-age children have mastered language and are now learning to use that language to express needs and feelings during stress rather than using regressive or defiant behavior to communicate. The nurse draws out the child's unverbalized reactions, encourages communication about feelings, and teaches parents how to cope with their child's feelings and behaviors at home. If not given opportunity for verbal expression during hospitalization, school-agers will revert to the behavioral expressions characteristic of their earlier development.

Emotionally and socially, school-age children begin undertaking tasks that will lead them into healthy, productive adult relationships once the tasks are refined in adolescence. One challenge of this period (latency) is the channeling of emotional, physical, and sexual drives into socially acceptable behaviors. This period is one of general intolerance toward opposite-sex peers; same-sex peers develop gangs or clubs and engage in intimate "best friend" relation-

Box 31-5

Developmental Needs and Nursing Strategies: School-Age Children

PHYSICAL NEEDS

To complete control of body functions and self-care

Assess and maintain usual routines related to body function and self-care.

Allow independent self-care to extent feasible by treatment restrictions and child's tolerance.

Praise whatever self-care child does perform.

To develop fine motor skills

Provide materials for fine motor activities (pencils and crayons, scissors, Lego, computer games, hospital equipment safe for play that requires finger manipulation).

Encourage drawing pictures of body and body parts during discussions of disease and treatment (see Fig. 31-3). This gives nurse feedback on the accuracy of the child's interpretation of information.

Encourage child to "take notes" during patient education sessions—gives practice in fine motor dexterity for printing or writing.

Teach child to participate in treatments that give practice in fine motor skills.

INTELLLECTUAL NEEDS

To develop rational thinking, reality orientation

Provide scientific descriptions of the child's disease and body responses during educational sessions or in reply to questions.

Offer a rationale for each procedure before doing it to help the child to maintain self-control during procedures and to participate when feasible.

Provide children with rules about what they may and may not do during hospitalization, because of the disease or during a treatment. Suggest writing out a list or rules to post at bedside.

Assess whether child perceives hospitalization as a punishment; intervene as for preschooler if so.

Provide opportunities for child to make decisions about routine, treatments, and daily care whenever choices actually exist. Encourage middle school-age child to help devise a care plan.

To master concepts of conservation, constancy, and reversibility and to develop skills in classification and categorization

Allow child to participate in care by helping keep track on intake and output, writing down vital signs, counting the seconds or adding up the minutes it takes to complete a procedure.

Encourage the child who can tell time to inform the nurse when it is time for a procedure or when it is time to stop the procedure (when to take out thermometer, when to take off soaks, etc.).

Encourage scrapbook making, collection, diary keeping (according to child's interests) during hospital stay.

Utilize these concepts in teaching sessions.

Provide games that require use of these concepts (card games, board games).

Provide hospital school or tutor schoolwork.

To vocalize feelings during stress

Encourage verbalization of feelings associated with hospitalization, disease, procedures by asking questions ("How does it make you feel to have to miss school and be away from your friends?" or "Tell me what it is like to have to lie still for 30 minutes while those compresses are on").

Schedule time to talk with child, time not associated with any specific care or procedure. Let child know this is a time she or he can talk about anything or ask any questions. Encourage parents to do the same.

EMOTIONAL-SOCIAL NEEDS

To have the opportunity to channel drives into socially acceptable behaviors

Do not place girls and boys in the same room.

Provide opportunities to interact with other hospitalized school-agers.

Assess for preschool residual concerns re genitalia; manage as for preschooler.

Help maintain peer group contact via phone calls, letter writing, tape recordings, peer visitation, photo exchanges. (Teachers and parents are usually willing to help arrange these things.)

Arrange group education sessions for children with similar problems. Include discussions of how problems are similar and how they differ. Involve children in teaching each other about anatomy and physiology, disease process, treatment, under nurse supervision.

Treat any separation anxiety as for preschooler.

Encourage parents to express affection toward their hospitalized school-ager and to continue setting limits as before hospitalization.

To achieve industry and associated developing self-concept

Praise cooperation efforts, self-care accomplishments, participation in treatments, and any other achievements. Praise honestly and often.

Provide opportunities for built-in successes several times daily. (Assign tasks the child is known to be able to accomplish.)

Provide opportunities for peer cooperation (solicit roommate's help in entertaining an immobilized child).

Actively involve child in care and treatments.

Balance quiet and solitary activity with action and peer interaction as tolerated.

Box 31-6
Developmental Needs and Nursing Strategies: Adolescents

PHYSICAL NEEDS

Support of rapid skeletal growth

Provide nutritional information on diet, snacks, and weight control.

Refer to dietitian for special dietary needs.

Encourage consumption of nutritional snacks, rather than "empty calories."

To perform self-care skills associated with onset of puberty

Provide information on hygiene measures; means of independent bathing.

Answer questions and provide counseling on reproductive system and function.

Provide anticipatory guidance on preventive health maintenance, breast examinations, birth control.

Physical exercise and mobility

Assist to move out of bed and around the unit.

Recreation activities suitable to age and size.

Acknowledge need for physical expression of frustration and provide innovative means.

Encourage physical and occupational therapy to increase independence, muscle strength, and mobility.

INTELLECTUAL NEEDS

To receive scientific explanations

Thorough explanation and preparation for procedures and instructions.

Use scientific terminology to explain illness.

To participate in health care management decisions

Include client in planning guide.

Give all instructions to client as well as parent. Orient to environment, routines, and expectations.

To achieve in academics and strive toward career goals

Provide opportunity to complete schoolwork while hospitalized.

Involve school teachers in health care planning.

Reinforce realistic career goals.

EMOTIONAL-SOCIAL NEEDS

To develop healthy attitudes about body image and sexuality

Encourage verbalization of fears and concerns.

Provide privacy.

Let youth have own belongings and wear own clothes.

Assist with grooming needs (e.g., hair washing, nails).

To achieve independence

Compliment the adolescent's strengths.

Encourage self-care.

Provide flexible limits.

Provide opportunities to participate in setting goals, planning care, and choosing options.

Provide opportunities for appropriate decisions and control.

To have peer contact and approval

Provide opportunities for friends to visit and call.

Suggest recreation activities that stimulate adolescents to gather.

Arrange for unit meeting for adolescents.

Suggest passes to go home or to school or social functions.

Opportunities for appropriate calls to friends.

To receive family support

Encourage parents to visit and stay when adolescent needs or wants them.

Provide opportunities for meetings where parents can discuss issues and get support.

Encourage sibling visits.

Give support to maintain the family unit.

Encourage chaplain visits.

Encourage use of appropriate community resources.

Provide community agency referrals.

ships. From these relationships comes the learning of sex roles and the "give-and-take" prerequisite to healthy heterosexual relationships that come later in life. These factors should be considered when making room assignments and structuring activities on the hospital unit.

Hospitalized school-age children worry about whether they will retain their peer group memberships and what the group is saying and thinking about them in their absence.

To the extent that they are invested in nonfamily relationships, school-age children are able to bear parental and sibling separation (Erickson, 1967). What they need from parents during the school-age years is assurance that they are loved and that parents will provide limits to help them maintain self-control. This affection and limit setting are increasingly important during periods of crisis like hospitalization.

School-agers thrive on doing things and seeing how things work. Their industrious natures are tempered by a fear of failure. They tend to depend almost entirely on external evidence of their worth and are continually self-critical. At this most critical stage in their developing concept of self, school-agers need lots of praise, frequent built-in successes, and assistance to maintain self-control (Erickson, 1967). Although they compare themselves regularly with peers and siblings, they cannot tolerate such comparisons to be made by parents or others. Box 31-6 describes nursing actions to meet school-agers' emotional and social needs.

Adolescents: Development and Coping. Critical to an understanding of the impact of illness or hospitalization on this age group is a knowledge of the major issues or developmental tasks of the period. The nurse's role is to plan interventions that will foster the development of the adolescent.

Adolescence has been described as a period of transition, a period in which society has authorized a delay of adulthood. Time is granted for the person to integrate all the changes required to move from childhood to adulthood. Illness and hospitalization are threats to the accomplishment of this transition.

A definition of adolescence by age is somewhat arbitrary, since adolescence can begin and end at different ages for different people. The adolescent period is characterized by profound biologic and psychosocial changes. The biologic changes of rapid skeletal growth and reproductive development begin some time before the teen years (10 to 12 years old). Around the age of 12 or 13 years, the young person looks to peers and explores different adult roles in defining the personality. These movements away from home signal the beginning of psychosocial changes. Adolescence culminates at 18 to 23 years with the emergence of an independent adult. To assume the adult role, adolescents must become emancipated from parents, define their role, and answer the question "Who am I?"

The age at which illness or hospitalization occurs is significant because of the wide variances in development between 12 and 21 years of age. Young adolescents are less overwhelmed by enforced dependency and allow parents to act on their behalf. The main concern of this age group is physical appearance, function, and mobility. Illness or hospitalization is least well tolerated by the adolescent in the middle years (aged 14 to 18). The dependency and decreased control of life of hospitalization conflict with the drive for independence. Late adolescents usually use the family for support and can tolerate some dependency. A threat to the older teen is a potential blocking of career goals and lifestyle through illness.

The degree to which an adolescent's development is halted by hospitalization also depends on the nature of an illness. The adolescent has the mental capabilities to make distinctions between short-term illnesses and permanent body changes. A long-term or chronic illness, especially if disabling, may create limitations in the amount of independence achieved.

A sudden or acute illness can be devastating to the adolescent. Even though the illness and hospitalization may be short-term, they are restrictive, force dependency, and interrupt mastery and control. Stevens (1986) reported that a group of adolescents 12 to 17 years of age found four areas of stress associated with surgery: (1) anticipated and associated risks of surgery, (2) pain, (3) visible and handicapping consequences of surgery, and (4) interruption of usual lifestyles. The more time the adolescent has for preparing for and planning the absence from school and friends, the greater the degree of acceptance of the restrictions of being hospitalized. Often the season's final football game or the class dance is more important than an operation. Consequently, a planned surgical procedure is often easier to accept than injuries sustained in an accident. Automobile accidents and trauma from other accidents are frequent causes of hospitalization for the adolescent. The disfigurement, immobility, and guilt, especially if a friend has died in the accident, may lead to feelings of helplessness and despair. Adolescent accident victims require nursing interventions geared to their physical status, with a gradual increase in emphasis on the issues of returning to their family and friends. Adolescents in severe pain or acute physical distress want help immediately. They do not tolerate well the pain or the wait for relief. Prompt administration of analgesics and reduction of the adolescents' fear of losing control, or panic, are necessary nursing strategies.

Whatever the nature of the illness, the experience of being hospitalized produces anxiety for adolescents. Some of this anxiety can be attributed to internal factors, such as thoughts about the effect of illness on the body; but a large portion results from external factors. Adolescents have been removed from family and friends and now are faced with a new environment in which they have little control. Usual patterns of recreation, nutrition, sleep, and socialization are altered and controlled. Also, strange procedures and examinations invade privacy and body. Health professionals tell them what needs to be done; often they are not allowed to make independent decisions. Consequently, the hospital environment accentuates feelings of powerlessness and dependency. Maintaining contact with peers helps the adolescent cope with the strange and unfamiliar demands of hospitalization.

Anxious adolescents may cope with hospitalization by moving *toward* people, moving *against* people, or moving *away* from people (Conway, 1971). By moving *toward* people, they accept their helplessness

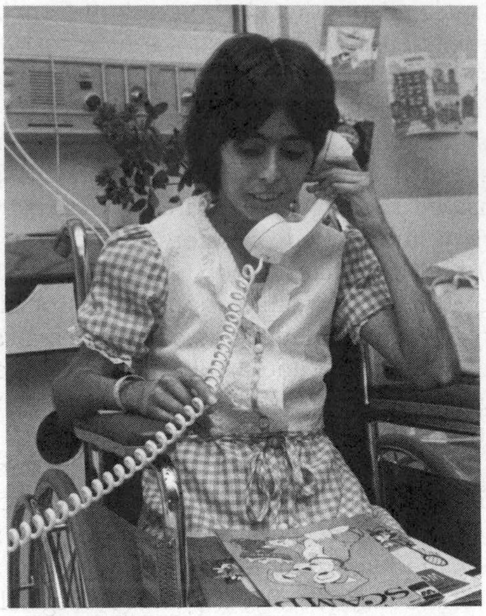

The hospitalized teen adjusts to her situation more easily if she has the means to maintain contact with her friends and family. (Courtesy of the Children's Hospital of Philadelphia.)

and, in spite of their fears, try to win the affection of others. By complying with rules and treatments, the adolescent does not feel isolated. When adolescents move *against* people, they are determined to fight and rebel. They do not trust others and strive to be strong and independent. Moving *away* from people is the way adolescents build up a world of their own. They keep apart because they believe that people do not understand them (Conway, 1971). All these coping behaviors may be exhibited by one individual, depending on the particular circumstance. Recognizing these response patterns may help the nurse understand why one day an adolescent passively goes to a test whereas the next day all assistance is opposed.

The nurse's approaches in caring for an adolescent are based on a sound knowledge of the developmental tasks being achieved at this time and also on an *individual* assessment of each situation. The physical, intellectual, and emotional-social needs of a hospitalized adolescent and related nursing strategies are summarized in Box 31-6.

The underlying anxiety about the effect of illness on their physical body, the enforced immobilization and separation from friends and family, and the conflict surrounding emotional independence from parents and other adults can be so overwhelming for adolescents that nurses perceive them as difficult or demanding. When the nurse encourages adolescents to verbalize concerns, fears, and questions, an environment is established in which they can gain information and develop trust. Ongoing interactions that emphasize strengths while promoting realistic goals help adolescents define their role and develop their identity. Arguments over nonadherence or lack of cooperation are not effective or productive. Adolescents cannot answer questions such as "Why did you do that?" They do not know why, but they can explain how difficult it is to follow a treatment plan when what they really want is freedom. Questions like "How is it living with diabetes?" will get more information and will not result in an adult-adolescent clash. Adolescents need to have some control over the environment. When health professionals allow them to make decisions and have some independence in treatment, they learn to be responsible. Rewards can be built into an adolescent treatment plan, by linking privileges to responsibilities.

In a hospital setting, some limits are necessary. Appropriate boundaries need to be established, but they need to be flexible and communicated in an understanding rather than authoritarian manner. Adolescents can be encouraged to do as much self-care as possible, but this does not decrease the nursing time they need. Thorough and scientific explanations of what is happening to them must be given. They also need to be cared for by those who are sensitive to their fears and conflicts.

Contracts often work well with adolescents because they encourage participation. A contract is an agreement between two parties that spells out expectations of each regarding a behavior or situation. A nurse and an adolescent can write out the treatment program outlining the adolescent's participation as well as the nurse's responsibilities. A contract can be as simple as an outline of things that need to be learned before going home. The adolescent agrees to learn them and the nurse and the adolescent agree upon a time when they will be taught. A contract also can be developed with specific rewards for defined accomplishments. In drawing up a contract with an adolescent, the first step is to clarify goals. Adolescents need to explain their goals and what they are willing to do to meet those goals. A sample contract is shown in Figure 31-2.

I agree to do my range-of-motion exercises at 10:00 AM, 2:00 PM, and 8:00 PM. The nurse will remind me one time.

Date: ______________________

Signatures: *Adolescent, Nurse*

***Figure* 31-2.** A sample contract.

The mechanism of contracting allows adolescents to exercise their right to choose as well as participate. This gives them control and yet allows the nurse to set limits. One important element in a contract is that the goals or behaviors are achievable by both the adolescent and the nurse. The nurse must ensure that compliance with a contract is seen as an accomplishment and not simply as obedience.

Facilitate Coping Through Teaching and Supportive Communication

Children's ability to adapt to a stressful event depends on how they perceive the event. A child's limited cognitive ability to understand the event may result in bewilderment and misinterpretations. In each developmental stage, nurses intervene in such a way that perception of the event will not interfere with adaptation. Following is a discussion of age-related teaching strategies to be used when a child is hospitalized. Also see in Table 27-1 a summary of educational strategies used for children in any health care encounter, whether at home, in a clinic, or in hospital.

Infant and Toddler. Infants and toddlers do not understand explanations about hospital events, but the nurturing caretaker who looks at them when speaking to them and explains upcoming events can communicate that they are being cared for and protected. Even though the content of an explanation is not comprehended, they can sense the feeling of caring and protection in the tone of voice, facial gestures, and physical contact. (See Chapter 27 for a discussion of helping young children cope with procedures.)

Most educational efforts for children of this age are directed at parents. Keeping parents informed about their child's condition and plan of care are useful educational strategies. Parents use problem-focused coping, such as seeking information, asking questions, talking with other parents, and being vigilant about the child's care (Miles and Carter, 1985).

Preschooler. Preschoolers need information in simple terms about their disease, including elementary anatomy and physiology, and about the procedures and treatments used to diagnose or correct it. (See Chapter 27 for a discussion of how to help preschoolers cope with procedures.) Also, any misconceptions that occur during the hospital experience should be clarified.

Preschoolers respond best when the information they need is given by the primary nurse (Galligan, 1979). After discussing with the physician the medical information he or she wants shared with the child and family,* the nurse should question the parents about their understanding of the disease or procedure and ask what they have explained to the child and how the explanation was given. The nurse can clarify any misunderstandings the parents have and provide additional information as needed. This knowledge guides the nurse's decisions about where to begin with the child. Studies show that if parents are cooperative and supportive, the preschooler benefits from their presence during teaching sessions (Oremland et al, 1973). They can be encouraged to participate in providing explanations because they usually know best the words their child is used to and the comprehension level.

Before starting a session the nurse should find out what the child already knows and understands about the topic(s) to be discussed. Questions such as "How did you know you had to come to the hospital?" or "What did your parents tell you about (topic)?" reveal the child's knowledge base, fantasies that may need correcting, the areas for reassurance, and information that should be emphasized. Denial of knowledge should not be taken at face value in preschoolers. They may think the disease will go away or the procedure will not take place if they deny its existence or knowledge about it. Preschoolers have also been known to deny having had an operation, even when shown the incision or the dressing covering it. Denial is a way of coping with an overwhelming stressor.

A story approach might be used with the denying child to obtain contributions and questions. The nurse might relate a story about a boy in the hospital who knows he is sick or that a procedure is to be done but is afraid to ask questions because he wishes it would go away or would not happen and how much better he feels when he finally asks questions. Sometimes just saying "If I were you I'd sure want to know all about (topic)" stimulates the child to talk.

The timing of the instruction is important. Children should have adequate time to work through the explanations but not enough time to let their imaginations get carried away with fantasies. If the preschooler is verbal and appears to be adapting adequately to the environment, explanations can be given the day before a procedure is to take place. The early preschooler who is not adept at verbalizing feelings and questions and any preschooler who is having trouble adjusting to hospitalization should be given an explanation shortly before the procedure. The child is given permission to object (it is OK to cry or yell) but is also given an

*Some hospitals have teaching protocols for various diseases and procedures that have been jointly approved by nursing service, medical staff, and hospital administration.

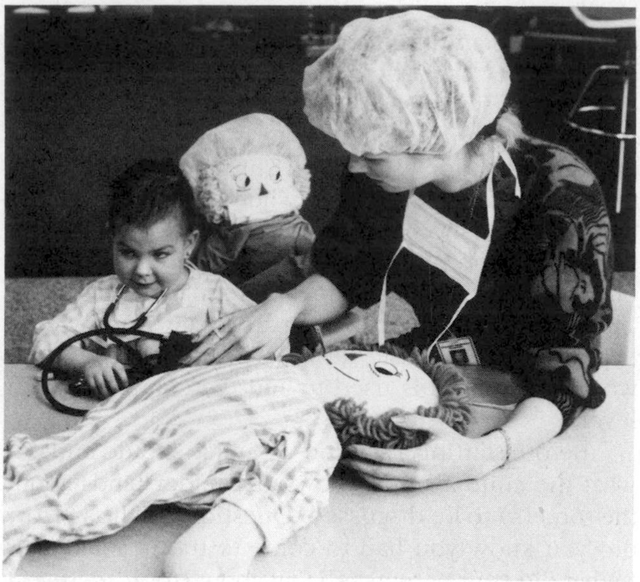

When toys or puppets accompany explanations of hospital events, preschoolers can better comprehend the event. (Courtesy of Child Life Department, Children's Hospital, Cheroke-McMaster University, Hamilton, Ontario.)

understanding that there is no choice as to whether or not the procedure will be done.

Neutral words should be used in explanations to avoid stimulating the child's imagination or producing mutilation fears. For example, in describing an operation, the nurse should say "make an opening" instead of "cut" and "the bandage may look pinkish and wet" rather than "there may be blood on the bandage." Preschoolers are very interested in what their bodies look like and the names for various parts. They are able to comprehend simple anatomy and physiology if visual aids such as body outlines, pictures, or organ models are used. Medical equipment, dolls, and puppets for play should accompany explanations. Body outlines are appealing to preschoolers because they are familiar with the concept of the flat body from storybooks and their own crude "people" drawings.

Questions should be answered honestly and briefly. The nurse must learn to pick out the actual question and answer only it; preschoolers do not want an elaborate speech. Repetition of information may be necessary before preschoolers fully understand explanations. Their lack of understanding is communicated through questions and nonverbally through uncooperativeness and defiance. The material to be taught should be covered in two or three sessions to avoid overwhelming them with information. Their attention span is usually only 10 to 15 minutes, and they lose interest in a topic if it is dealt with too many times.

School-Age Child. School-age children want explanations about the disease process and treatment plan. They need to be provided with a rationale for each procedure before it is done; this knowledge helps them to maintain control and cooperate during the procedure. (See Chapter 27 for a discussion of how to help a school-age child cope with procedures.) The teaching plan is like that for the preschooler, just discussed, but school-age children are more enthusiastic and are able to reason, so content can be more complex. Their attention span is longer, allowing them to pay attention to a topic for 30 to 45 minutes if they are actively involved in some way; they can handle slightly more content per session than can the preschooler. Questions, concerns, and feelings should be encouraged and explored. Body outlines, models, games, and puppets can be used to help them visualize verbal explanations and to solicit their active involvement (Green, 1975; Norbeta, 1976; Petrillo and Sanger, 1980). Box 31-7 summarizes what research has revealed are the typical views of the school-ager regarding the body. The nurse should determine what the school-age child's response to the use of a doll is likely to be before using one for demonstrating procedures. Sometimes acceptance is obtained by referring to the doll as a "dummy" or "model" and by using a doll that is "grown up" (Barbie and Ken dolls). Many of these children, especially those of early school age, still benefit from therapeutic play that allows handling of the equipment and doll or dummy play (Elmassian, 1979).

Procedural instruction can be provided a day or two in advance, with a quick review just before the procedure, unless the child is immature; in which case instruction should immediately precede the procedure. The nurse should be honest and specific about what parts of the body will be involved in the procedure, since the school-age child retains fear of bodily harm.

Because school-age children are preoccupied with body function and fear body injury, they need procedural instructions that cover what will happen, with an emphasis on the sensations to expect and the behaviors that are acceptable (what they may or may not do to help) (Johnson, 1976). Their developing concept of temporality makes them keenly interested in knowing the timetable of events. Allowing time for school-age children to verbalize fears and feelings permits them to grasp a better understanding of their actual fear, which increases ability to cope with the procedure and the pain involved. Shaefer (1977) found that school-age children respond positively to group education sessions and often are supportive of each other.

Adolescent. Because adolescents think about death, it is essential that they be told the nature of their illness. This explanation should be given by the physician in terms that the young person can understand. Prospects for treatment and the expected course

Box 31-7
How the School-Ager Views Her or His Body

Research conducted by Nagy (1953) and later by Gelbert (1978) revealed how children perceive their bodies in terms of content and function at various ages. Body outlines were used along with interviews to learn what children think their bodies contain, how body contents function, and where contents are located. The early school-age child (6 to 7 years) tends to maintain a preschooler view of the body that centers on what is ingested and egested (Fig. 31-3). Thus, the body is perceived to be composed of food, water, urine, and feces. In addition, the early school-ager also recognizes bones, brain, and eyes as body parts.

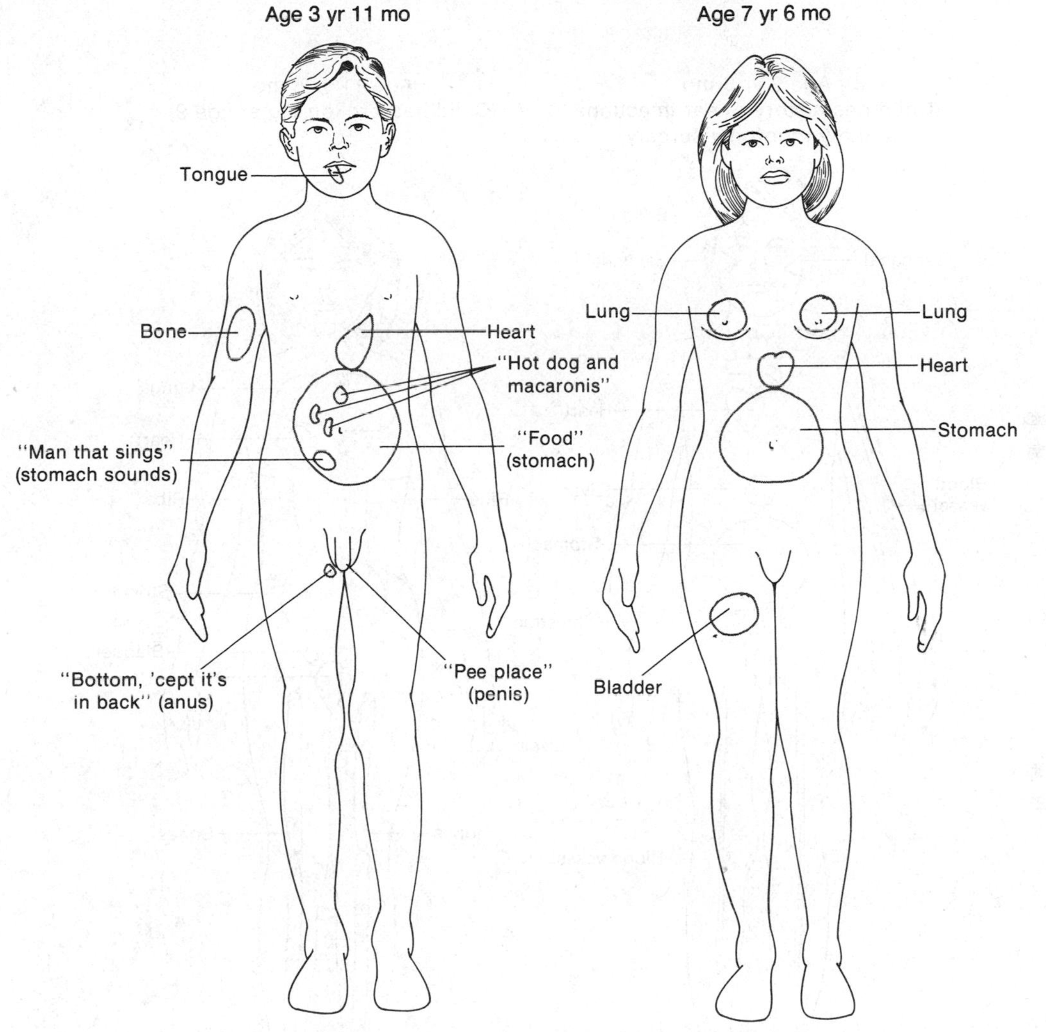

Figure 31-3. How a school-age child views the body. Examples of children's placement of body organs on a predrawn form.

Continued

Middle school-age children (8 to 10 years) concentrate more on permanent body parts, including muscles, bones, and the heart (usually drawn as a valentine shape) and blood vessels (Fig 31-3). They also identify eyes and a brain, which they believe is made of bone (probably associated with the skull). The middle school-ager usually locates the stomach low in the abdomen and overestimates its size. The liver is also included in the drawing. The heart is associated with breathing.

The older school-age child (11 to 12 years) identifies the same body parts as the middle school-ager (Fig. 31-3), although the location and size are usually more realistic with the exception of the stomach, which remains oversized and low. At this age the child begins to associate the relationship of the lungs and heart to breathing and circulation.

Individual children, regardless of age, may also identify organs with which they have had special experiences. For example, the child who has had frequent ear infections or a myringotomy includes the ear canals in the drawing. If pain or surgery has been associated with an organ, that organ often will be drawn in a distorted or oversized manner.

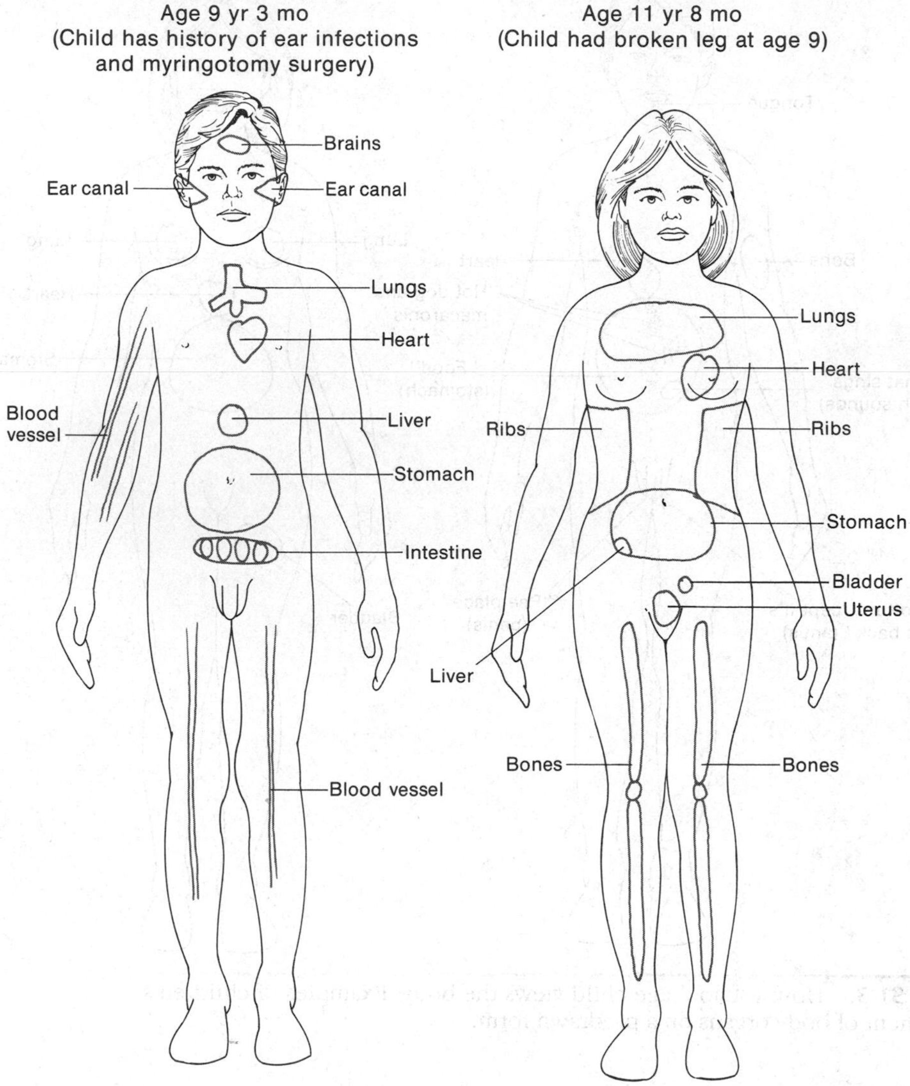

Figure 31-3 *Continued*

should also be discussed. The nurse's role is to review, support, and provide additional education as the adolescent needs it. The danger in not being honest or in not explaining to adolescents is that, if left alone, they will use their fantasy thoughts in an effort to figure out what is happening. Craft (1981) reported recurrent questions that were raised spontaneously by 40 hospitalized adolescents with an acute, chronic, or terminal illness:

1. *Illness-related:* What is the cause, how serious is it, and how long will I have the illness? What symptoms are likely to occur, and which should I report?

2. *Procedures-related:* What tests and examinations will I have and why, and how will I feel during them? What are my test and examination findings?

3. *Lifestyle changes:* How long can I expect to be in the hospital? What foods may I eat or not eat? What are the changes in exercise and athletic activities? What medications do I need and what effect do they have?

4. *Future plans:* Can I expect to make changes in school and future job plans, in friendships or dating, and in future planning for marriage and children?

Adolescents have been found to show preferences as to who should provide information: the older the adolescent, the more likely she or he is to prefer a health professional to a parent (Craft, 1981) to provide general information. On the other hand, when important topics such as cause, seriousness, symptoms, and duration of illness are discussed, adolescents seem to want the emotional support provided by the presence of their parents. It is thus important for nurses to assess the adolescents individually and discover their preferences.

Supporting the Family with a Hospitalized Child

***Altered parenting: overprotection,** related to real or perceived*
- *vulnerability of child*
- *environmental risks*

***Ineffective family coping: parents and siblings,** related to the crisis of hospitalization of the ill child*

associated with multiple stressors for the parents:
- *unfamiliar hospital environment*
- *loss of control over child's care*
- *impact of the diagnosis*
- *concern about the prognosis*
- *potential susceptibility of other family members*
- *guilt related to the etiology or the fact medical help was not sought earlier*
- *concern for the child's pain/discomfort*
- *loss of sleep of family members*
- *family and social role disruptions, including financial concerns*
- *concern about being able to manage recuperative or long-term care at home*

associated with multiple stressors for siblings:
- *guilt about the illness or injury*
- *fear of having the same illness or injury*
- *separation from parents who are with ill child*
- *loss of attention*

See Table 31-2 at the end of this chapter: Nursing Diagnoses 9 and 10.

The presence of parents in the hospital has now become the usual rather than the unusual. It has been recognized that the support provided by a child's parent cannot be equalled. The separation from familiar caretakers that hospitalization creates can be ameliorated by permitting 24-hour visiting, sleeping accommodations, involvement of parents in the care of their child, and in some instances complete care by parents. Many of the stressors of hospitalization are modified by the involvement of parents because the unfamiliar and feared is less frightening when parents are present as an advocate. From the moment of contact, the admitting nurse should communicate acceptance of the parents and tell them how important their presence is during their child's hospitalization. This is especially true for children from 6 months to approximately 4 years of age. Whether the parents room-in or visit sporadically, the nurse's priority is to maximize the quality of the parent-child relationship. The more effective the nurse is at putting parents at ease, the greater the child's security.

Parents experience stress when their child is hospitalized and their roles of primary caretakers are assumed by the hospital staff. For this reason, too, parents should be encouraged to assist with the child's care to the extent they are willing and able. They must not feel, however, that unless they provide some care their child will receive less than optimal care from the staff. The nurse should remember that parents may feel inadequate or too frightened to care for their child physically, especially if the condition is serious. In these circumstances it may be advisable to allow the parent to observe the nurse caring for the child. The nurse can use the observation time to explain the purposes of various procedures and demonstrate how they are done. As parents feel more comfortable, they may wish to increase their participation. When the parent begins to participate more actively, the nurse should assist and offer encouragement, as the parent will continue to need support and positive reinforcement. Parents also need the opportunity to ask questions and clarify information.

Parents often have useful suggestions about special approaches that may work well with their child. Some hospitals are establishing care by parent units. Nurses are available if needed, but parents provide most of the care. These can be especially helpful when the child does not require complex care or when a chronic problem requires complex care that parents have learned to provide.

When parents are able to room-in with their hospitalized child, the nurse does not leave the scene because "there is nothing to do." She continues to be responsible for the child's care, assists with daily care, and provides the specialized care pertaining to the child's illness. The more complex responsibility of the nurse, however, is that of assessing the coping level of the family and intervening to maximize the comfort of each person. At times parents feel exhausted or frustrated by the demands of caring for their sick child. The nurse should be particularly sensitive to these feelings. They need the opportunity to leave for periods of time, and they need to have contact with a nurse who makes them feel at ease to express the frustrations they are experiencing. Even infants are able to sense changes in their parents, such as anxiety or fear.

A child may respond with expressions of abandonment if the parent is feeling overwhelmed and unable to meet nurturing needs. The nurse needs considerable interaction with the child and the parents to assess whether the stress of caring for their sick child is overwhelming. When it is, the nurse can help the family identify how they can be assisted to cope with the stress of the hospital experience.

When parents can visit for only short periods and such visits are infrequent, the nurse must make a special effort to reduce the stress this produces for parents. Parents who are unable to visit when a young child is hospitalized often feel extremely guilty and need the acceptance and understanding of a sensitive nurse. It is especially important that the nurse does not compound their guilt by thoughtless, judgmental remarks. When parent-child separation is inevitable because of family circumstances, the nurse must strive to work out a plan with parents that will be most beneficial to the family as a unit. Some families may need assistance to re-evaluate their circumstances and search for alternatives that will increase their availability to their child.

Nurses should also be perceptive to the anxiety experienced by parents. Astin (1977) found that parental anxiety may subconsciously cause parents to withdraw from their child. Alexander et al (1986) reported that non-rooming-in parents were found to become more anxious the longer the child was hospitalized, especially if there were children at home. The nurse's recognition of anxiety in parents and intervention to support parents in expressing their fears and concerns are important nursing strategies to increase the parents' comfort at the bedside.

In spite of the literature that supports the positive effects of the presence of parents, many institutions still have limited visiting policies. Any nurse who works with young hospitalized children has a responsibility to work for the goal of 24-hour visitation by parents.

Support groups composed of parents of children suffering from the same or different problems can be extremely helpful in reducing stress. These groups may be planned and supervised by professionals or develop spontaneously as parents with similar needs begin to share concerns and mutually experience a relief of tension. They discuss their feelings about a treatment or test and hear how another person has coped successfully. Some of these groups continue to meet to provide information and support even after the child is discharged from the hospital.

Facilities for parents should include a lounge separate from but close to their child's room, where they can relax. Health care booklets, magazines or light reading material, television, or games provide a diversion for parents. A kitchen in which parents can make a cup of coffee, toast, or a cup of soup also may help them feel welcome. Some hospitals are able to provide a shower and dressing area for parents. In addition, some hospitals provide sleeper-lounge chairs or cots for parents, as space permits. Although comfortable facilities for parents are particularly helpful in reducing their stress, most parents respond favorably to even small attempts and gestures to make them comfortable while they stay close to their child. Referrals to appropriate resources such as the hospital's social service department can also help parents work through the day-to-day problems of transportation, lodging, finances, and home management.

Support of Parents with a Hospitalized Infant. The parent-infant relationship is threatened when an infant is hospitalized. Parents may see the activities of the nurse, in particular, as a threat to their own abilities. Their prior responsibilities of feeding, administering medications, and the like may now be taken over by persons unknown to them. From a sense of helplessness they may resort to criticism of their child's care. This means of coping on the part of parents must be understood by the nurse to be able to communicate effectively with them.

Every opportunity is provided to maintain parental

care of the infant. Encouraging parents to touch, hold, and feed their infant is the key to fostering the ongoing development of positive interactions between infant and parents. The parents are encouraged to elicit social responses from their infant, provide play opportunities, and in all ways normalize the daily activities.

The individuality of the parenting role is an important difference for nurses to respect. First-time parents of a young infant may not feel secure in their role. The hospital setting can easily compound insecure feelings; therefore, the nurse strives to strengthen the confidence of parents in their role; by verbally pointing out the infant's responses to them and identifying the normal developmental landmarks that are being achieved.

Support of Parents with a Hospitalized Toddler. The role of parents with ill toddlers is to provide the continuity of the home situation in the hospital. Toddlers desperately need their parents to feel secure. Parents are encouraged to let the toddlers do those tasks that they achieved prior to admission to maintain a sense of autonomy in this threatening environment. When a toddler is hospitalized, parents feel overwhelmed and wish to take away the hurt and anxiety they see in their child.

Parents may have difficulty setting limits in their usual way because they cannot bear to oppose their ill child's wishes. The nurse should provide an opportunity for parents to express the conflict they are experiencing and assure them that the security that the setting of limits affords toddlers is particularly important now that they are in a threatening environment. The nurse can also point out that if parents can continue to provide the limit setting in their usual manner, there will be fewer problems of readjustment for their toddler back home.

Another area of conflict is the normal resistive behaviors of toddlers. When they feel threatened with losing control over what happens to them, they may become even more resistive, with the result that parents become exhausted and frustrated. Regressive behaviors like thumbsucking and soiling (by a previously potty-trained toddler) or the whining, baby cry of a toddler may be disturbing and embarrassing to parents. Parents might even feel that they are the cause of such behaviors and begin to isolate themselves emotionally from their child, even though physically present. The nurse's responsibility then is not only to encourage parents to be there but also help them cope effectively with their child's reactions to hospitalization.

Support of Parents with a Hospitalized Preschooler. The biggest problem of hospitalized preschoolers' parents is their tendency to forget how independent their preschoolers have become. Through anticipatory guidance about the behaviors and needs of hospitalized preschoolers and through role modeling, the nurse can help parents preserve their preschoolers' independence. Involving parents in planning care communicates that they are important to their preschooler and that they know their child best (Freiberg, 1972). They can be helped to feel capable and useful by supervising their child's self-care and helping in or doing those tasks the child is unable to handle. Probably the most valuable contribution parents make to their preschooler's hospital adjustment is their participation in the child's preparation for procedures. To these children, parents are still essential interpreters and translators of the language of the outside world; therefore, their involvement in their child's education is just as important as their presence and their ability to provide comfort during hospitalization encounters.

The preschooler's stress at being hospitalized often is so great that the parents become anxious. Incorporating the parents' needs into the child's care plan results in a better adjustment to hospitalization for all.

Support of Parents with a Hospitalized School-Ager. Even though school-age children are moving away from the family toward peer influence, parents and siblings remain a major influence in their lives. They need parents now who relate as adults, not pals—someone they can turn to during stress and count on to set limits and control them when they cannot. This development becomes evident when school-agers are hospitalized. Although the continual presence of parents is not necessary, school-age children need frequent assurances that parents love them

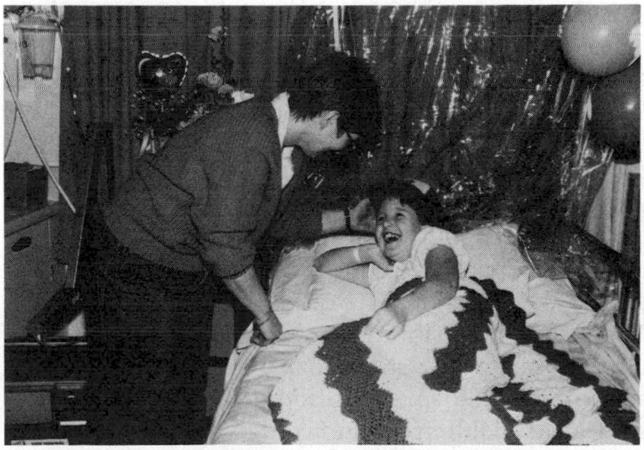

Although the continuous presence of parents is not necessary, school-age children need frequent assurances that parents love them.

and are thinking of them. They will want them present during painful procedures and when they are feeling acutely ill.

Parents may need help in respecting and permitting the child's contributions to the treatment regimen. The nurse can reassure them that the child's participation is welcomed by the staff and can encourage the parents' participation in the teaching process and in supervising their child in self-care.

Although the school-age child's family experiences the same needs, feelings, and concerns of other families when any of their children are hospitalized, they usually adapt better to the fact of hospitalization than do those with younger children. This is because the school-age child is more independent and can express feelings and needs; therefore, parents feel less pressured to be there continuously to interpret their child's needs to hospital staff.

Support of Parents with a Hospitalized Adolescent. In working with parents of the adolescent the nurse can serve as a model, showing them how to help their child during dependency states and to allow freedom and control when dependency is not desirable. Parents are often intimidated by their adolescent's anger and anxiety. The nurse can explain the relationship between developmental issues and hospitalization. Parents usually do not volunteer information about problems with the family, such as their own feelings of guilt and frustration and sibling jealousy. Parents need to talk to the nurse and be given the opportunity to receive support instead of always being expected to be pillars of strength.

Just as hospitalization is a crisis for the adolescent, it is a crisis for the parents. They have a natural concern for their son or daughter, but their ability to be supportive is influenced by their own past experiences and fears related to hospitals and illness. Parents may interpret the illness as their punishment for neglect of the adolescent and so may feel guilty. They may see themselves as failures for not preventing the illness. Parents may enjoy the nurturing role that is required when their adolescent is dependent and then may find it difficult to return to the conflicts of independence that are inevitable when the adolescent is well. The adolescent may respond better to the staff nurse's requests than to the parents' requests; this may cause the parents to resent the nurse's role as the primary caregiver. The parents and siblings may resent the time and the changes made in routines that are required to provide support to the hospitalized adolescent. The amount of support available from and contact with their parents influence the amount of anxiety experienced by adolescents. Parents are often expected to be in control and supportive without any nursing intervention or assistance. The nurse should understand the role of parents, and consider and provide support for them when their adolescent requires hospitalization.

Support of Single-Parent Families During Hospitalization of a Child. To provide the emotional support of the hospitalized child and to simultaneously maintain the family's usual level of functioning at home is often beyond what one individual can provide. The nurse's sensitivity to the special needs of single parents is an important link in effective adaptation by the child and family. Exploring alternatives with the parent and facilitating parental relief strategies can alleviate the stress experienced by both child and family.

Each family situation has its own needs and difficulties. Some alternatives to explore with a single parent are use of extended family (if available), temporary use of an adolescent in the home to take on added responsibilities, neighborhood or church group participation, or community organizations that can provide support service.

The nurse also may help by responding to the psychologic needs of a single parent. It is important for the nurse to know whether there has been a separation, divorce, or death and whether it has occurred recently. Today an increasing number of single parents raise either biologic, or adopted children, therefore it is important to clarify the circumstances early. If a recent separation, divorce, or death has occurred, or if a family is in the throes of a divorce, the nurse should know, as these determinants could result in a maladaptive response to hospitalization.

Often divorced or separated parents are present at the child's bed at the same time. The hospitalized child's condition may evoke empathic, caring responses in the parents, both for the child and for each other. To the child it may mean that the illness could be a key to the parents' reconciliation, whereas for stepparents this response between ex-spouses may arouse anger (Ahrons and Arnn, 1981). On the other hand, angry divorcing couples may use the child's hospital room as a battleground. The nurse becomes directly involved when either parent tries to control the release of information, visiting privileges, or the right to give consent for procedures. In specific cases legal consultation may be required to resolve the problems. In most circumstances, when parents are separated or divorced the parent with legal custody has the authority to consent to medical treatment without the other parent's approval; if joint custody exists, then either parent can legally sign a consent independently (Holder, 1977). Sharing of information about the child with either parent is usually appropriate (Holder, 1977).

The nurse's role in caring for a child whose parents are separated or divorced is to support the child's psychologic and emotional well-being. The nurse, therefore, cannot risk becoming involved in the parental battles. The best choice is to permit the child or either parent to express feelings but to avoid becoming involved in focusing on the "bad" qualities of either parent.

If a parent has died, the problem of loneliness, lack of support, and time and energy exists as it does for a divorced parent. The mourning family is vulnerable at the time of hospitalization, but the dead spouse generally remains as a "good" memory and the separation is complete and permanent. The nurse's role in this case is to support the family in the grieving process. If the dead parent was hospitalized before dying, the child's fears and anxieties about hospitalization and its relation to death must certainly be explored (Burns, 1984).

Support of Siblings. Traditionally, hospitals caring for children have excluded children from visiting because of the belief that children are more likely than adults to be carriers of infectious diseases. As early as 1971 the American Academy of Pediatrics stated that "experience now indicates that visiting by children and siblings is as safe as visiting by adults if those with obvious infection or known exposure to contagion are excluded" (American Academy of Pediatrics, 1971).

Proponents of sibling visits suggest that sibling rivalry can be alleviated by increasing the sibling's active involvement in the care of the hospitalized child and that a distorted perception of the ill child's situation can be corrected (Craft, 1981). In a review of the literature, Shuler and Reich (1982) found that professionals generally believe that sibling visits are helpful to both the healthy sibling and the hospitalized child; however, evidence is lacking to demonstrate the actual emotional benefits of this strategy. Scientific data are also lacking to demonstrate that sibling visits affect the prevalence of nosocomial infections (Shuler and Reich, 1982).

A general acceptance of the importance of maintaining the tie between the hospitalized child and the family is shown by the prevalence of sibling visiting. Visitation policies generally specify that the sibling should be screened for infectious disease, indicate where visiting is to take place (i.e., child's room, lounge), limit the length of the visit, and require preparation of the siblings; some include an age restriction —all without scientific data. The support that is believed to derive from these visits has led many institutions to allow completely free and open visiting. One response cited in the survey by Shuler and Reich (1982) was that restricting visiting children in any way was deemed unethical, therefore research in this area is hampered because a control group cannot ethically be provided.

The nurse can have considerable influence in supporting sibling visits and should promote this strategy of providing the necessary social support of a hospitalized child.

Preparing for Discharge

Knowledge deficit: child and parents, related to home management

See Table 31-2 at the end of this Chapter: Nursing Diagnosis Number 11.

The nurse's goal is to discharge the child or adolescent, along with the family, in optimal health. With appropriate interventions during hospitalization, the transition from hospital to home is eased.

Preparation for discharge begins when the child is admitted to the hospital. Effective discharge planning is based upon nursing knowledge of the unique meaning of *this* illness for *this* child and for *this* family and what modifications in lifestyle will be required for home management during the recuperative process. Discharge planning begins with the first explanation of the disease process and the plans for treatment.

An important component of the nurse's role in preparing a child for discharge is to encourage participation of the child in self-care. The child who is forced to comply with treatment and hospitalization without any involvement in self-care suffers a loss of control and lowered self-esteem that thwarts development and reinforces regressive behaviors. Children should be encouraged to participate in their own care according to their physical and developmental abilities. They require explanations before procedures, and their ideas should be sought when plans that concern them are developed.

Active involvement and self-care help maintain and improve coordination, muscle tone, and circulation and foster positive self-esteem and a sense of self-control. The child may have a residual chronic health problem that will require continued treatment at home. Active participation in hospital care gives the child a sense of adequacy to cope positively after hospitalization.

Text continues on page 990

Table 31-2
Nursing Process Plan: The Hospitalized Child*

By Roxie Foster

1. Assessment of Physical Function

Sleep/Rest
Nutrition/Metabolism
Elimination
Activity/Exercise

Subjective Assessment

Upon admission: Report from child and/or parent(s) regarding usual patterns of sleep/rest, eating, bowel and bladder elimination, activity/exercise patterns, self-care, play/diversion; current developmental level
During hospitalization: Self-report or parental report of changes in baseline behaviors established upon admission

Objective Assessment

Upon admission: General appearance (whether well-nourished), specific gravity of urine, number of teeth, height and weight, percentiles on growth chart, vital signs, assessment of respiratory, cardiovascular, neuromuscular, integumentary, and genitourinary systems; developmental suatus
During hospitalization: Observable changes in baseline data established upon admission

Analysis: Nursing Diagnosis 1

Sleep pattern disturbance (child), related to anxiety associated with
- *unfamiliar environment*
- *separation from parents/family*
- *discomfort of illness*
- *medications*

Defining Characteristics

Subjective: Self-report or parental report of sleeplessness, restlessness, marked irritability

Objective: Pale to grayish skin tones, dark circles under eyes, lethargy, frequent dozing but no prolonged periods of sleep

Client Goal/ Evaluation Criteria	Nursing Goals/Strategies (Selected Rationale)
1. The client† will obtain sufficient sleep to meet needs, as evidenced by:	
a. agreeing to sleep and rest at the times client usually does so at home b. rested appearance c. decreased irritability d. increased energy for and interest in play	*Determine usual sleep patterns,* including naptime and bedtime routines and rituals (the younger the child, the more important these familiar activities are to promote sleep). *Provide for continuity of care,* when parents cannot be present to prepare the child for sleep, the primary nurse can assume this responsibility. *Establish a record of sleep.* • If the hospital uses a flow sheet, label one column for sleep; cumulatively total hours of sleep over the 24-hour period.

* The interventions listed in this table are not intended to be exhaustive; see also Boxes 31-2 through 31-6 and specific interventions in Chapters 23 through 26.

† "Client" implies any hospitalized child or adolescent regardless of illness state. In addition to these general guidelines, special considerations for care of chronically and terminally ill children and adolescents are highlighted where pertinent.

- Compare the child's usual sleep patterns with this guide from Table 20-3 and determine appropriate adjustments to meet the body's increased need for sleep and rest during illness.

Neonate	20–22 hr/24 hr
6 weeks	14–16 hr/24 hr
6 mo–1 year	12–16 hr/24 hr
1–3 years	10–14 hr/24 hr
3–5 years	12–14 hr/24 hr
6–9 years	11–12 hr/24 hr
10–12 years	9–12 hr/24 hr
Adolescent	8 10 hr/24 hr

Enforce naptimes by posting a sign such as, "Jeremy is asleep; please come back at 3:30." Usually other health care professionals will observe the request.
Decrease the child's anxiety related to hospitalization. (See nursing diagnosis 9.)
Plan the administration of analgesic medications so that discomfort does not interfere with sleep.
Assess whether sleeplessness may be a side effect of medications e.g., theophylline. Alert the physician as appropriate.

Analysis: Nursing Diagnosis 2

Altered nutrition: less than body requirements, related to
- *anxiety associated with unfamiliar surroundings*
- *variation in feeding techniques among caregivers*
- *dislike of food served associated with variations in preparation and cultural food selections*
- *behavioral regression in eating patterns associated with anxiety of hospitalization*
- *anorexia and/or discomfort associated with the disease process*

Defining Characteristics

Subjective: Crying and irritability in response to food being offered. "I'm not hungry." "I don't want it." "Take it away." Expressing desire to drink from a bottle or to be fed at breast after weaning to cup

Objective: Physically trying to move away from food or to push food away, refusing nipple, spitting out food put in mouth; refusing to use eating utensils, to drink from cup, to hold finger foods, or to chew food; intake < caloric requirements; weight loss

Client Goals/ Evaluation Criteria	Nursing Goals/Strategies (Selected Rationale)
2.1 The client will meet caloric requirements, as evidenced by:	
a. nutrient intake appropriate to age, body weight, and treatment plan	*Decrease anxiety* associated with hospitalization (see nursing diagnosis 9).

Continued

Client Goals/ Evaluation Criteria	Nursing Goals/Strategies (Selected Rationale)
b. maintenance of body weight during hospitalization	*Plan for caloric requirements per 24-hr period that equal or exceed the following recommendations for the healthy child** (unless contraindicated by treatment plan): 0–6 mo—kg × 115 kcal 6–12 mo—kg × 105 kcal 1–3 yr—1300 kcal average 4–6 yr—1700 kcal average 7–10 yr—2400 kcal average 11–14 yr—2200–2700 kcal average for girls/boys 15–18 yr—2100–2800 kcal average *Adopt age-appropriate feeding strategies:* **Infant:** • Have parent feed whenever possible. • Note parent's feeding technique so that it can be copied by nurse caregivers. (This will ensure as much consistency as possible and reinforce parents' self-esteem and sense of control. Of course, teaching is indicated if inappropriate techniques are observed). • Use bottle and nipple identical to that used at home and note whether parent warms formula. • Determine whether solids or liquids are usually given first in the feeding and follow this pattern. • If the infant is not used to commercial baby food, ask the parent to bring food from home. **Toddler:** • Encourage parents and/or siblings to be present at mealtime whenever possible. • Alert parents to avoid a power struggle over food. The child should be allowed to choose the desired foods from those offered. (Given the opportunity, toddlers often use refusal of food to assert some control in a situation when they are otherwise powerless. Offered a selection of nutritious foods, usually they will choose those the body needs.) • If the toddler must eat without family, allow to eat with other youngsters whenever possible to provide a semblance of normal mealtime activity. The distraction of other children temporarily may override anxiety related to the strange environment. • Provide highchair or booster chair as close as possible to that used at home and observe usual routines, including ritualistic food preferences. • Make mealtime as pleasant as possible, avoiding administration of medication or unpleasant procedures. • Plan analgesic medication administration to decrease discomfort at mealtime. • Allow as much self-feeding as possible. (The toddler who feels partly in control will be more cooperative.)

* See also Table 18-2.

	Preschooler: • Allow child as much control over food served as possible: assist in selecting foods from printed menu, allow to help "make" toast, milkshake, etc., and to show the nurse "how Mommy makes it." (Child will feel more in control and will be less likely to demonstrate regressive behavior if newly developed language and motor skills are acknowledged.) • Encourage meals with family or other patients whenever possible. • The preschooler may like to "role model" good eating behaviors for a toddler patient. (This is in keeping with the tasks of initiative and socialization.) **School-age:** • Explain to the child which kinds of nutrients are needed for return to health, e.g., protein and vitamin C for wound healing. Allow the child to build a menu plan around favorite foods containing these nutrients. Encourage parents to supply foods from home to satisfy the choices. (Self-regulation and industry will increase the child's self-esteem and decrease anxiety; therefore, nutrient intake may also increase.) • Allow the child to record the food intake on the flow chart. (This "concrete" record makes it easier for the child to keep track of progress toward a goal.) • Allow the school-age child to "role model" eating and to entertain and help younger patients at mealtime (to increase a sense of self-worth). **Adolescent:** • Identify with the adolescent the need for proper nutrition in order to regain health. (Reasons for treatment are especially important to the young person striving to make independent decisions.) • Allow self-regulation in food selection, in eating, and in recording of intake. • Offer the adolescent a consultation with the dietitian; this may be welcomed when weight loss or muscle building is desired after hospitalization. (Information from authorities outside the family is more likely to be valued.) *Encourage family to provide food from home to meet cultural tastes.* *See individual illnesses* in Unit VII of this text for treatment of anorexia, nausea, and vomiting.
2.2. The **chronically ill** client will maintain or exceed nutrients consumed at home (unless contrary to the treatment plan.)	*Acknowledge the expertise of the parents.* (In most cases they have already established the most efficient methods of care for their child and "reinventing the wheel" by planning care without them will only lead to frustration for the parents and increased anxiety for the child.) • Encourage the parents (or child) to model feeding techniques used at home and duplicate these in nursing care whenever appropriate. (Parents and nurses can effectively share ideas for venting a gastrostomy tube, inserting a nasogastric tube, feeding the child with tongue thrust, etc.)

Continued

Client Goals/ Evaluation Criteria	Nursing Goals/Strategies (Selected Rationale)
	• Recognize that while the parents (and older child) are expert in some areas, they may have questions about others. Encourage this communication. (By recognizing their expertise, the nurse thwarts defensive behavior that might otherwise impede communication.) *Encourage the parents and child to identify any problems with nutrition that have arisen during home care and assist them with problem solving.* *Collaborate with the home care nurse.* (His or her expertise with this child can greatly facilitate delivery of care in the hospital setting.)
2.3. The **terminally ill** client will receive the nutritional intake desired (unless medically contraindicated), as evidenced by: a. Saying food tastes good b. Voicing no complaints of increased discomfort after eating	*Determine what foods the child finds most palatable* and, with the help of the family, keep a supply in the hospital. (Something that "sounds good" to the child tonight may be refused if he or she must wait for it until tomorrow.) *Identify the specific impediments to eating for this child* (e.g., stomatitis, nausea) and use all available palliative therapies. (See also Table 48-4, Nursing Process Plan: The Child Undergoing Chemotherapy.) *Allow the child as much self-regulation as possible* (since the goal of care is to increase quality of life).

Analysis: Nursing Diagnosis 3

Altered elimination: incontinence of urine and/or stool, related to regressive behavior associated with the anxiety of hospitalization

Defining Characteristics

Subjective: Failure to express need to urinate/defecate

Objective: Incontinent of urine/stool after bladder/bowel training

Client Goal/ Evaluation Criteria	Nursing Goals/Strategies (Selected Rationale)
3. The client who is toilet trained will not be repeatedly incontinent of urine or stool.	*Assess the source of anxiety and implement measures to alleviate it.* (See nursing diagnosis 9.) *Implement strategies to increase self-care.* (Allowing the child as much control as possible may help lessen frustration and anxiety.) (See nursing diagnosis 5.) *Avoid scolding or shaming the child for incontinence.* (If the incontinence is anxiety related, scolding will only compound the problem.)

Analysis: Nursing Diagnosis 4

Diversional activity deficit: altered play behavior, related to
- *separation from usual playmates/friends*
- *lack of interesting toys/diversional materials*
- *isolation associated with communicable disease*
- *immobility or discomfort associated with disease process or its treatment*

Defining Characteristics

Subjective: Crying, whining, irritability; verbal refusal to play or participate; statements of boredom

Objective: Lethargic appearance; flat facial expression; lies quietly, staring; ignores available toys and diversions; frequent dozing; watches others play but physically resists participation

Client Goals/ Evaluation Criteria	Nursing Goals/Strategies (Selected Rationale)
4.1. The client will participate in age-appropriate play or diversional activities.	*Integrate specific play times and activities into the plan of care.* *Enlist the help of parents and older siblings* by explaining that therapeutic play will help the child cope with the crisis of hospitalization. (Lay persons may not place a high priority on play activity without this explanation.) *Implement other measures to reduce the child's anxiety.* See nursing diagnosis 9. (The severely anxious child will feel too threatened to engage in play activities.) *Provide age-appropriate toys and diversional materials* (see also Table 21-2). Have a variety of toys/diversions available at the bedside, including hospital/medical toys, creative play materials, and "aggression toys." (Children often engage in anxiety-reducing play when alone with their feelings.) **Infant** (sensorimotor play) Play experienced through the senses; it elicits a motor reaction. Provide a variety of textures, colors, sounds, and movements. Human interactions are important. **Toddler** (parallel play) Active play predominant. Allow gross motor activities. Exploration of environment still important. Fine motor activities most interesting if they involve manipulation. Allow for creative, imaginative play. **Preschooler** (cooperative play) Enjoys quiet as well as active play. Imitation of grown-ups at its peak. Interested in activities that provide for refinement of motor skills. **School-age** (group play) Play more formalized, task-oriented. Likes organized group play, games with rules, activities that refine motor and cognitive skills. **Adolescent** (recreational play) "Play" activities determined by peer acceptance. Still enjoys ways to refine motor and cognitive skills toward adult levels. Needs opportunity for motor activity as well as more quiet diversions.

Continued

Client Goals/ Evaluation Criteria	Nursing Goals/Strategies (Selected Rationale)
4.2. The **terminally ill** client will use play to explore feelings about dying.	*Offer creative materials.* (Children are often able to express their perceptions of death through drawings, paintings, or clay sculptures.) • Use the play projects to engage the child and family in a conversation about fears and feelings associated with death. • Dolls or puppets can be used to portray a family dealing with grief. (This can also help work through guilt about making others unhappy.)

Analysis: Nursing Diagnosis 5

Self-care deficit, related to
- *unfamiliar environment*
- *regressive behavior*
- *illness and treatment*

Defining Characteristics

Subjective: Verbal refusal to perform usual self-care activities (e.g., dressing, brushing teeth); increased irritability when self-care is suggested

Objective: Physical refusal to perform usual self-care; inability to perform self-care because of illness, injury, or treatment

Client Goals/ Evaluation Criteria	Nursing Goals/Strategies (Selected Rationale)
5.1. The client will perform usual self-care activities as allowed by physical condition.	*Assess usual self-care activities.* *Provide opportunities for, and encourage self-care whenever possible.* (This facilitates coping by increasing self-concept and by increasing the child's sense of control.) Self-care can be enhanced by: • carefully orienting the child to the hospital environment: bed controls, release of side rails, bathroom light, use of urinal and bedpan, etc. • allowing own pajamas with familiar closures to be worn, instead of hospital gowns and hospital pants that require tying a knot or bow • encouraging parents to bring to the hospital the utensils used at home for eating, bathing, brushing teeth, etc. • providing a good mirror for bedfast clients so they can comb/curl their hair, apply makeup, etc. • arranging often-used items near enough to be easily reached • maintaining the attitude that the extra time (and perhaps extra mess) involved with self-care is well worth its benefit to the child *Teach the child modifications of care related to illness and treatment,* e.g., sitting on side of bed long enough to avoid orthostatic hypotension, using trapeze to move toward head of bed.

5.2. The **chronically ill** client will maintain or exceed usual self-care, as evidenced by:
a. performing self-care usually accomplished at home
b. performing previously learned self-care that is specific to the illness
c. learning a new self-care practice

Assess what self-care is usually performed at home rather than expecting behavior appropriate to chronologic age. (Self-care may be delayed because of repeated exacerbations of the illness, limitations in mobility, or other factors.)

Encourage self-care

- Allow the child to perform in the hospital those treatments and procedures performed at home, e.g., inserting own nasogastric tube, or self-catheterization. (This enhances coping efforts and provides an excellent opportunity to evaluate the child's technique.)
- Use this hospital experience to teach the child new self-care behaviors and more about the illness and the treatment plan.

5.3. The **terminally ill** client will achieve self-care as desired.

Allow flexibility in modes of care: the child should be supported in self-care when feeling well enough to try it but also supported with direct nursing care during periods of increased fatigue or discomfort.

Encourage the child and parents to communicate about the child's self-care needs (to avoid unnecessary feelings of guilt on either side).

Analysis: Nursing Diagnosis 6

Altered growth and development:
physical, *related to prolonged immobility associated with illness, injury, or treatment*
intellectual, *related to decreased environmental stimulation associated with decreased mobility and decreased energy for exploration*
emotional/social, *related to*

- *alterations in bonding associated with parental adjustments to the diagnosis and treatment, parent-child separations due to hospitalization*
- *separation anxiety that reaches the stage of denial*

Defining Characteristics

Subjective: Verbalizes inability to keep up with peers in motor and cognitive skills; verbalizes mistrust, shame/doubt, guilt, inferiority, role diffusion; professes to "be a loner," "not to need any one"

Objective: Inability to perform gross and fine motor tasks appropriate to age; intellectually immature for age (see developmental theories of intellectual competency, Chapter 3); inability to perform age-appropriate social tasks; failure of infant and parent to display social-affective play activity

Client Goals/Evaluation Criteria — Nursing Goals/Strategies (Selected Rationale)

6.1. Any developmental delays will be identified, as evidenced by:
a. a charted assessment of screening for physical, intellectual, and emotional/social development

Using a screening tool approved by the health care team (e.g., DDST, Chapter 15), *begin developmental assessment upon admission and complete it during the hospital stay.* (An ill child can rarely be assessed all at one time. The nurse may have to rely upon parental reports for some behaviors. Motor behavior is especially affected by the fatigue associated with illness and should be reassessed as the condition improves.)

Continued

Client Goals/ Evaluation Criteria	Nursing Goals/Strategies (Selected Rationale)
b. a referral for any abnormalities detected in screening that were previously undiagnosed	
6.2. The client will not experience developmental delays related to prolonged hospitalization, as evidenced by: a. developmental assessment at discharge showing abilities equal to or increased since admission	*Allow physical mobility within the limits of safety.* • Remove restraints every 2 hours under close supervision, to permit increased perfusion and movement. • Allow supervised play out of the crib/bed in the room and playroom. • Plan for motor play appropriate to age. • Encourage exercises for bedfast clients to maintain musculoskeletal function. *Provide a variety of sensory stimuli* appropriate to the child's age and condition, e.g., crib mobiles; music boxes; toys of various textures; music from a tape cassette; video movies; rides around the unit in a wagon; moving crib/bed out into the hall, into the playroom, or outdoors onto a sunporch. *Implement measures to reduce anxiety* (see nursing diagnosis 9). *Assess parent's knowledge of developmental tasks.* With parent, identify tasks specific to the child. Enlist parent's help, and the help of older siblings, in planning and implementing strategies to maintain or promote development during prolonged hospitalization. *Collaborate with other team members* (e.g., physical therapist) *to blend care strategies to the child's advantage.*
6.3 The **chronically ill** client will continue a prescribed therapy program to promote developmental progress.	*Identify* (through interviews with the child, parents, home care nurse, and therapists) *the protocol followed at home to promote development. Enlist the aid of these experts to plan modifications to the protocol* appropriate to the illness situation. *Implement the modified exercises* as tolerated, being as consistent as possible with home therapy. *Evaluate frequently for developmental regression* that would signal the need to further adapt the plan of care.

II. Assessment of Emotional/Social Function

A. Self-Perception/Self-Concept
B. Coping/Stress/Tolerance Patterns

Subjective Assessment

A. *Self-concept:* Self-report or parental report of feelings about self, and about self in relation to others; parenting patterns related to safety, beliefs and values, social behavior and roles, and self-regulation

Objective Assessment

A. *Self-concept:* Posture, eye contact, presence of fidgeting, attachment behavior (physical contact with parent), choice of clothing, personal hygiene

B. *Coping (child and family):* Posture, motor behavior, facial expression, eye contact, attention span, judgment, problem-solving ability, voice quality, behavior in a group, impulse control, observable role behaviors

B. *Coping (child and family):* Perception of the stressors involved with this illness and hospitalization, usual behaviors employed to deal with this kind of stress, perceptions of likelihood of resolving this crisis, availability of resources for physical and emotional support, health beliefs, religious faith, perceptions of death, perceptions of own roles and those of family members, anticipated role changes necessitated by hospitalization of child, communication patterns within the family

Analysis: Nursing Diagnosis 7

Disturbance in self-concept: body image and/or self-esteem, related to effects of illness and treatment upon

- *physical appearance*
- *physical mobility/agility*
- *intellectual function*
- *feelings of self-worth*
- *feelings of competence/mastery over the environment*
- *perceived sexuality*

Defining Characteristics

Subjective: Verbalizes feelings of inferiority, negativity, pessimism; boasts about achievements; declines opportunities for social activities, new experiences

Objective: In group situations tends to watch rather than participate; acting-out behavior; poor impulse control; poor sportsmanship; takes little pride in appearance

Client Goal/ Evaluation Criteria	Nursing Goals/Strategies (Selected Rationale)
7. The client will display an improvement in self-confidence, as evidenced by displaying one or more of the following characteristics (from Table 16-1):	
a. expressing feelings of being likable, worthwhile, important b. seeking activities, new experiences c. displaying pride in achievements d. being expressive, happy, optimistic e. enjoying interpersonal interactions	*Assess self-esteem* (see Box 16-2 for specific techniques.) *Facilitate the child's sense of security.* • Keep hospital routines for eating, bedtime, etc., as close as possible to home schedule. • Encourage a parent or family member to stay with the young child. • Limit the number of nursing personnel giving care, to enhance trusting relationships. *Facilitate the child's sense of identity.* • Encourage communication of caring through verbal and physical interactions with family.

Continued

Client Goal/ Evaluation Criteria	Nursing Goals/Strategies (Selected Rationale)
	• Comment to the child about his or her personal strengths. • Encourage the child to perform self-assessment and to think of ways the child is "special." *Facilitate the child's sense of belonging.* • Encourage visits from siblings and extended family as well as parents. • Encourage visits, phone calls, letters from friends and classmates. *Facilitate the child's sense of purpose.* • Assist the child to set realistic goals, e.g., *not* "Next time I won't cry at all," *but* "Next time I will hold my leg still, even if I cry some." *Facilitate the child's sense of personal competence.* • Allow the child to make choices from those generated through discussion. (Choosing for the child thwarts autonomy, which is basic to a positive self-concept.) • Encourage self-care (see nursing diagnosis 5).

Analysis: Nursing Diagnosis 8

Altered parenting: overprotection, related to real or perceived
- *vulnerability of the child*
- *environmental risks*

Defining Characteristics

Subjective: Child's complaints of not being allowed to do activities of peers and siblings. Parental statements, such as "Johnny has always been so sickly, he just can't do what the other children do." "No, Cindy, you can't go, you know you'll get sick if you don't have your nap"

Objective: Child delayed in self-care and in self-regulation of behavior. Parent repeatedly does things for the child that child should be doing for self

Client Goals/ Evaluation Criteria	Nursing Goals/Strategies (Selected Rationale)
8. The parent(s) will encourage at least one new self-care activity appropriate to age.	*Help the parents identify major fears pertaining to the child's illness* (see nursing diagnosis 10) *and explore any feelings of guilt they may have.* (Anxiety and guilt often lead to overprotection; this may be especially pronounced if the child is chronically or terminally ill.) *Facilitate the parents' allowance of more independence in the child.* • Using the child's behavior as an opportunity for discussion, comment that independence often makes the child feel better about self. • Act as role model for behaviors that allow the child independence. • Suggest ways for the child to attempt an age-appropriate self-care task. • Evaluate with the child and parent how the child feels about the accomplishment.

- Written materials on parenting can be helpful adjuncts and may be less personally threatening to parents. (Issues of parenting are delicate areas to approach with parents who are already stressed and who may hold cultural and social values about parenting that differ from the nurse's. Tact and sensitivity are imperative to therapeutic interactions.)
- Use an appropriate opportunity to discuss the crucial parenting roles at each stage of childhood. See Chapter 13.

Analysis: Nursing Diagnosis 9*

Ineffective individual coping, related to crisis of hospitalization associated with multiple stressors (Visintainer and Wolfer, 1975):

- *separation from parents and significant others*
- *unfamiliar environment*
- *harm, injury, and pain*
- *unclear limits and expectations*
- *loss of control*

Defining Characteristics

Subjective: Crying; irritability; verbalizing specific fears; report of nightmares; verbalizing helplessness, hopelessness, guilt, inability to "think straight"; insomnia; fatigue; anorexia or nervous overeating; diffuse somatic pains

Objective: Physical refusal to be held and comforted; wide-eyed expression; frequent visual "scanning" of environment; increased pulse and respirations; regressive and/or acting-out behavior; sleeplessness; skeletal muscle tension; shortened attention span; clinging behavior

Analysis: Nursing Diagnosis 10

Ineffective family coping: parents and siblings, related to the crisis of hospitalization of the ill child

associated with multiple stressors for the parents:

- *unfamiliar hospital environment*
- *loss of control over child's care*
- *impact of the diagnosis*
- *concern about the prognosis*
- *potential susceptibility of other family members*
- *guilt related to the etiology or the fact medical help was not sought earlier*
- *concern for the child's pain/discomfort*
- *loss of sleep*
- *family and social role disruptions, including financial concerns*

* Because the anxieties in families are so often interdependent, client and nursing goals and strategies for both individuals and families are discussed under Nursing Diagnosis 10.

Continued

Analyis: Nursing Diagnosis 10

- *concern about being able to manage recuperative or long-term care at home*

associated with multiple stressors for siblings:
- *guilt about the illness or injury*
- *fear of having the same illness or injury*
- *separation from parents who are with ill child*
- *loss of attention*

Defining Characteristics

Subjective

Parents: Verbalizing hopelessness, helplessness, guilt, frustration, "nowhere to turn," inability to "think straight," low self-esteem, insomnia, fatigue, anorexia or nervous overeating, diffuse somatic pains
Siblings: Verbalizing feelings of guilt, fear of "being punished for bad thoughts," fear of getting the hospitalized child's illness, whining and crying in presence of parents and when parents leave, complaints of diffuse somatic pains, preoccupation with thoughts of the ill child when she or he was well, irritability, impatience

Objective

Parents: Skeletal muscle tension; pacing or other restless behavior; worried facial expression; tearfulness; shortened attention span
Siblings: Social withdrawal, overactivity, restlessness, lack of initiative, regressive behavior, escalation of normal misbehaviors, clinging to parents, attention-getting behaviors

Client Goals/ Evaluation Criteria

10.1. The child/parents will experience a decrease in initial anxiety following the admission procedure, as evidenced by:
a. decreased irritability
b. increased eye contact
c. more relaxed facial expression
d. occasional smile
e. decreased skeletal muscle tension
f. increased attention span
g. verbalizing feeling "more at ease"

(For Nursing Diagnoses 9 and 10.)

Nursing Goals/Strategies (Selected Rationale)

Orient child and parents to the social environment.
- Communicate an attitude of caring and respect.
- Tell the parents, "Since you know your child best, we will rely on you to help us plan the nontechnical aspects of care in the hospital." (This immediately establishes for the parents that they are in a social climate where they are respected and are being given some control. The child's anxiety will decrease if the parents are more at ease.)
- The primary nurse should admit the client (since this is an important step in the relating process).
- Introduce the child and parents to roommates and their families.
- Provide both oral and written instructions for rules pertinent to unit and child's condition, e.g., isolation.

Orient the child and parents to the physical environment.
- Allow the child to wear own pajamas (if possible) and to have a security object. (This will decrease the threat of separation from familiar things.)
- Encourage one parent to stay with the child between 6 months and 5 years of age. Explain rooming-in policies.
- Orient the family to the facilities and items needed for self-care and parental care, e.g., bathroom, urinal, bathing facilities.
- Leave in the room a scrapbook of pictures of hospital utensils with simple explanations. (This allows clarification at a time of reduced stress and helps the child work through fears.)

	• If child's condition permits, provide a tour of the unit (playroom, etc.). • Encourage questions throughout the orientation and encourage the child to touch and manipulate unfamiliar articles. *Establish the basis for a trusting relationship.* • Convey an attitude of acceptance and respect. • Be honest, don't be afraid to say "I don't know"; the family needs a source of *reliable* information, not just an answer for every question. • Demonstrate caring and empathy. • Let the child and family know when you will be available to talk to them next, then keep the "appointment."
10.2. The child/parents will successfully adapt to the crisis of hospitalization, as evidenced by: a. identifying the source(s) of anxiety	*Provide crisis intervention as needed* (Bulecheck & McCloskey, 1985). (See also Chapter 23.) *Facilitate identification of problems* as seen by the child/parent(s). • Ask questions such as, "What is the most frightening/hardest/most frustrating thing for you about being in (or having your child in) the hospital?" "How do you feel about being here?" "How does this change your role as brother/sister/son/daughter/sibling/friend/student/mother/father/secretary/carpenter/etc.?" • Anticipate the stressors identified for nursing diagnoses 9 and 10; ask specific questions about these areas as indicated. • Accept the answers given and reinforce the right to feelings and perceptions. (The nurse's validation can facilitate the individual's acceptance; identification and acceptance of problems precedes problem solving.) • Expect identification of problems to take a period of hours to days, depending upon the meaning of the crisis to the individual.
b. discussing previously used coping strategies/solutions c. identifying external sources of support	*Facilitate identification of resources, both internal and external.* • Determine personal coping strengths and patterns. Ask, "Have you ever felt this way before?" "What did you do then?" "Did it help?" "Which of the things you did helped most?" • Determine external sources of support. Ask, "Do you have family here?" "Are there friends and neighbors who can help?" "Does your church or synagogue offer help for families of hospitalized children?" • Suggest support services of which you are aware. Refer to Social Services for others.
d. generating possible solutions to problems	*Assist with immediate needs as appropriate.* For example, Social Services may be able to provide a meal ticket or babysitting on a one-time basis. A teddy bear from the playroom may work as a replacement security object. (Beyond this initial help, allow as much self-help as possible to enhance self-esteem.) *Encourage the child and/or parent to discuss possible solutions to the identified problem(s).* • Actually listing alternatives may be helpful (this "distancing" technique can help with objectivity). • Suggest solutions detailed in this chapter, e.g., one parent staying with a young child while the other cares for siblings at home.

Continued

Client Goals/ Evaluation Criteria	Nursing Goals/Strategies (Selected Rationale)
	• Make it clear that the choice of action is theirs but that nursing support is available.
e. verbalizing "feeling in control again" f. verbalizing a decrease in symptoms of anxiety g. displaying fewer signs of anxiety	*Facilitate evaluation of the outcome.* • Ask questions such as, "How do you feel about it now?" "Are you still afraid Jennifer won't be your best friend after you leave the hospital?" "How is the babysitter working out?" • If the action was not successful, support the child/parent in retracing the problem-solving steps.
10.3. The child will display effective coping with the major stressors of hospitalization, as evidenced by:	
a. maintaining a bond with parents and significant others	*Promote relationships with family and significant others.* • Encourage a parent to remain with the child between 6 months and 5 years of age (who is at most risk for separation anxiety). • Encourage frequent family visits for the child whose parent cannot remain at the bedside. • Use pictures of family and friends, audio tapes of their voices, phone calls, and letters to help maintain the child's significant social bonds during prolonged hospitalization.
b. ability to cope with unpleasant diagnostic and treatment procedures without loss of self-esteem	*Prepare for procedures according to developmental age;* see Table 27-1. *Preserve the bed/crib as a safe place.* Remove child from the room (or if in isolation, at least from the bed or crib) to perform unpleasant procedures. *Reinforce adaptive coping* by focusing upon it and using it as an example of a coping strength, e.g., "You're holding your arm so still. It is OK to cry, but you're holding your arm so still, and that's wonderful!"
c. demonstration of understanding of most rules and expectations, with occasional questions asked about others	*Provide age-appropriate explanations and rationale for rules and policies.* • Parents can also be given these in written form. (If parents understand the rules, they can help the child interpret them.) • Provide alternative for some of the *"Nos"* and *"can'ts,"* e.g., "You may not take the tricycle to the lobby, but you may ride it to the playroom."
d. maintenance of control over some appropriate choices	*Offer actual choices as often as possible,* e.g., "Do you want your medicine in the cup or syringe?" *Do not offer choices that do not exist,* e.g., whether to take a prescribed medicine. *See also* Boxes 31-2 through 31-6 for strategies appropriate to needs at each developmental level.
10.4. The **chronically ill** or **terminally ill** client will display effective coping with the relapse of illness that prompted this hospitalization, as evidenced by: a. identifying and discussing unresolved fears from previous admissions	*Recognize that rehospitalization may be more traumatic than the first experience.* • Encourage the child to talk about previous hospitalizations. Ask, "What was the scariest part about being here before?" "What was the best part?"

b. trying at least one new method of coping with old fears	• Introduce the child to some new coping strategies (see Table 27-2 and Box 27-1). Let child choose one to practice and to try during a stressful situation. Help the child evaluate the effectiveness of this strategy and make modifications as necessary.
c. identifying and discussing the personal meaning of this change in health status	• Encourage the child to explore feelings about the relapse of the long-term illness. Ask, "Why are you in the hospital this time?" "Are you sick in the same way you were before?" "What is the scariest part about being sick?"
10.5. The parents of the **chronically ill** or **terminally ill** client will display adaptive coping with this hospitalization, as evidenced by: a. exploring the personal meaning of this relapse in the child's condition b. identifying and discussing unresolved frustration and fear associated with previous admissions c. demonstrating effective problem solving	*Recognize that each relapse/readmission may represent a greater crisis than the last* because it may signal a downward spiral in the disease process. Coping may be further impaired by physical, mental, and spiritual exhaustion from the strain of home management of the illness. • Encourage the parent to take time to consult with friends and clergy who can provide emotional and spiritual support. • Implement the steps of crisis intervention as needed (10.2). • Collaborate with the physician, home care nurse, and other involved members of the health care team in order to provide optimal information and support through a unified effort. • Provide frequent opportunities for the parents to express their feelings/concerns. One way to initiate the conversation is to state an observation, such as, "You look so sad/upset/tired." • Involve the parents in the child's care and in decision making as often as possible. (This will help thwart a sense of powerlessness.) • Reinforce effective coping and personal strengths by reminding parent of these qualities.
10.6. The **terminally ill** client and the parents will display adaptive coping with the prognosis, as evidenced by:	
a. discussing their feelings about death with each other	*Facilitate parent/child discussions about death.* • If there is initial parental reluctance to "burden" the child with the prognosis, tell parents that even small children usually know instinctively that they are going to die and may be afraid to "burden" the parent. • Discuss the benefits of open communication and mutual support to the quality of the child's and parents' lives.
b. displaying the ability to derive pleasure from loving interactions	*Encourage loving interactions.* • Allow the child to be held and cuddled by the parent as much as is desired. (Treatment protocol is secondary to quality of life at this point.) • Explain about tubes and machines to demystify them and to prevent them from forming a barrier between parent and child. • Provide privacy. • Reinforce the mutual support gained from these interactions by commenting to parents and child about how much each is helping the other.

Continued

Client Goals/ Evaluation Criteria	Nursing Goals/Strategies (Selected Rationale)
10.7. The parent(s) of the **terminally ill** client will cope effectively with a decision to discontinue life support, as evidenced by: a. verbalizing acceptance of death as inevitable b. displaying relief that the decision has been made c. verbalizing rationale for the decision	*Encourage parents to "talk through" their feelings* during the decision process. • Clarify misconceptions, offer information, listen, acknowledge their pain, but do not offer advice. (No one else can make the decision for them. The nurse can be invaluable, however, in helping them clarify their thoughts.) • Support their decision by comments like "I know this was very difficult for you." "You considered all the alternatives very carefully." "I know you love your child very much."
10.8. The siblings will display adaptive behavior in response to the ill client's hospitalization, as evidenced by maintaining usual behavior patterns: a. absence of regressive behavior b. no significant increase in attention-seeking behavior c. no unusual withdrawal or moodiness d. maintaining usual bond with ill sibling	*Alert parents to common behavioral responses of siblings.* Take care to do so in a manner nonthreatening to parenting abilities. (Anxiety increases sensitivity to guilt feelings.) *Suggest strategies to support siblings at home and maintain their bond with the ill child.* Parents can • plan time each day to spend with each child at home (if only a few minutes) when there is no competition for the parent's attention • acknowledge the normal egocentricity of childhood and adolescence and not expect the siblings to be as consumed by thoughts of the ill child as the parents are • encourage, but not force, hospital visitation, phone calls, letters, and exchange of snapshots to maintain client/sibling bonds • suggest the ill child make a picture or other simple "gift" for each sibling at home (to keep the communication of love flowing in both directions) • accept offers for child care and other help from extended family and friends (to reduce usual role stress and allow more time for family activities)
10.9. Siblings of the **chronically ill** or **terminally ill** client will display adaptive behavior to the hospitalization, as evidenced by: a. discussing new fears prompted by this change in health status	*Alert patients to fears of siblings commonly triggered by another hospitalization:* fears of their sibling's impending death, of having the same thing happen to them, of loss of security because of parents' anxiety; of further changes in family life and structure. *Discuss with parents age-appropriate ways to support siblings.* (A reminder of developmental crises and tasks can help them understand their childrens' behavior.) Parents can • encourage siblings to express their fears • discuss the child's illness and prognosis openly and honestly • give only the information asked for (which can help each sibling adjust at his or her own pace) • acknowledge that it is normal for siblings to feel angry at the ill child sometimes • encourage each sibling to develop his or her own identity/potential • keep family life and sibling responsibilities as normal as possible (Trahd, 1986)

III. Assessment of Intellectual-Perceptual Function

Knowledge of Illness
Pain (see Table 29-4, Nursing Process Plan: The Child in Pain)

Subjective Assessment

Replies to questions about knowledge of physical care: how to secure and operate equipment; necessary changes in diet, physical activity, school attendance; administration of and side effects of medications; availability of caretaker if parents both work outside the home; time and place of return appointment; signs and symptoms of relapse; whom to call for help when the clinic is closed; behavioral expectations of child after discharge

Objective Assessment

Ask parent/child to give a return demonstration of physical care, equipment operation, and medication administration as taught by nurse

Analysis: Nursing Diagnosis 11

Knowledge deficit: child and parents, related to management of the illness at home

Defining Characteristics

Subjective and/or objective evidence of the need for further instruction

Client Goal/ Evaluation Criteria	Nursing Goals/Strategies (Selected Rationale)
11. The child and/or parents will display the knowledge and skills needed for home management of the illness, as evidenced by: a. demonstrating effective physical care (e.g., dressing change) b. demonstrating effective operation of equipment and having it installed in the home prior to discharge c. identifying prescribed changes in diet, activity d. demonstrating safe medication administration and identifying major side effects e. identifying arrangements for child care as needed	*Begin discharge preparation the day of admission.* (Home management is too involved to be handled entirely on the day of discharge.) • Assess teaching needs early and list on a teaching flow sheet. • Allow the child and family to select the order for teaching from the list. • Have the child and family check off the items as they are completed. (A sense of control and responsibility will facilitate learning.) • Begin self-management and/or family management as soon as initial anxiety has decreased enough to allow it. (Repeated practice with new techniques will increase self-confidence and self-esteem and reduce anxiety.) See Table 27-1 for age-appropriate education strategies. • Whenever possible, listen to the physician's final instructions to the family (so that questions can be clarified before discharge).

Continued

Client Goals/ Evaluation Criteria	Nursing Goals/Strategies (Selected Rationale)
f. identifying signs and symptoms of relapse g. possessing written appointment notice and emergency numbers h. discussing strategies to use should the child display behavioral regression or excessive attention seeking after discharge	*Allow time for questions and clarification on the day of discharge.* • Tell the family when you can spend time with them to answer any final questions. (They can then prepare for this session.) • Provide written reminders of instructions whenever possible. • Alert parents to the possibility of behavioral reactions to hospitalization, making it clear the child may experience no behavioral change. Encourage them to give the child extra attention for a few days after discharge, increasing the attention should behavioral problems develop. *Collaborate with other members of the health care team* as appropriate to update them on the child's status after this hospitalization. Inform the parents you have called the school nurse, home care nurse, etc.

During the discharge phase, the nurse should be available to clarify any misconceptions the child or parent has about the hospital experience. The child should be encouraged to talk (a puppet is often helpful in initiating conversation) about various experiences in the hospital so that memory distortions can be identified. Photographs taken during the hospitalization will provide the child with reminders of the experience, thereby helping realistic recall and distinguishing between what was imagined and what really happened. Children also should be allowed to take safe, disposable equipment home with them so they can continue to work through their feelings in therapeutic play (Azarnoff, 1974).

The nurse should encourage parents to keep the hospitalization experience open to discussion so that their child has opportunities to reaffirm what really happened. Parents also should be informed that children need continued reassurances for weeks or months that they were not responsible for the illness or hospitalization. The child and family can be invited to return for visits to the unit after discharge. Such visits can help correct memory distortions and decrease anxiety if the child needs future hospitalization.

At home, reactions depend on the child's age and are highly individual, but older siblings may resent the loss of parental attention because of the younger child's special needs. The young patient may show regressive behaviors in developmental tasks, cling and whine, and have sleep and eating disturbances. Frequently the most recently achieved task is lost first. Parents should be informed of the possibility of these behaviors; they should be counseled to give these children additional emotional support by allowing them to be more dependent for a time and gradually weaning them back to their usual, more independent behavior. They also need to be reminded that older siblings may resent this additional attention and display attention-getting behaviors for a time.

It is equally important that nurses and parents do not have a preconceived idea that a young child will necessarily regress and become more dependent because of a hospital experience. With careful interventions to reduce stress and enhance normal growth and development, a child can mature and benefit from a hospital experience. The nurse and family must make every effort to capitalize on the unique resiliency of children.

The nurse plays a major role in the following list of the components of discharging a child and the parents from the hospital:

- Explanations of physical care
- Procuring necessary equipment to care for child's special needs
- Instructions in activities of daily living (nutrition, school attendance, physical activity)
- Behavioral counseling (i.e., posthospitalization effects)
- Counseling to prevent further illness
- Instructions concerning medications
- Assessment of capabilities of family to care for their child's additional needs
- Assessment of degree of physical and psychologic

strain that care of the child imposes on family functioning

- Assessment of appropriateness of physical environment for care of child's special needs
- Assessment of need for referrals in conjunction with an inter-disciplinary team, and make referrals as appropriate
- Coordination and consultation with community or home health nurses
- Instructions regarding date, time, place, and purpose of return appointment

Children's Books to Prepare for Hospitalization

Baznick Donna: *Becky's Story.* Washington, DC, Association for the Care of Children's Health, 1981.

Bemelmans Ludwig: *Madeline.* New York, Viking Press, 1939; New York, Penguin Books, 1977 (ages 3 to 9).

Clark Bettina: *Pop-Up Going to the Hospital.* New York, Random House, 1970 (grades K to 3).

Collier James Lincoln: *Danny Goes to the Hospital.* New York, WW Norton, 1970 (ages 5 to 8).

Hautzig D: *A Visit to the Sesame Street Hospital.* New York, Random House, 1985.

Howe J: *The Hospital Book.* New York, Crown Publishers, 1970.

Jessel C: *Paul in Hospital.* 2nd ed. New York, Methuen Children's Books, 1983.

Marsoli LA: *Things to Know About Going to the Doctor.* Lexington, MA, Silver Burdett, 1985 (ages 8 to 12).

Marsoli, LA: *Things to Know Before You Go to the Hospital.* Lexington, MA, Silver Burdett, 1985 (ages 8 to 12).

Packard Mary: *A Visit to the Dentist.* New York, Simon and Schuster, 1981.

Rey M, Rey HA: *Curious George Goes to the Hospital.* New York, Houghton Mifflin, 1966 (ages 3 to 8).

Stein Sara: *A Hospital Stay: An Open Family Book for Parents and Children Together.* New York, Workman Publishing Company, 1974 (ages 3 to 10).

Tickle Phyllis: *It's No Fun to Be Sick.* Memphis, St. Luke's Press, 1975.

Watts Marjorie Ann: *Crocodile Medicine.* New York, Frederick Warne, 1977 (ages 3 to 6).

Weber, Alfon: *Elizabeth Gets Well.* New York, Thomas Y. Crowell, 1970 (ages 5 to 9).

Ziegler, Sandra: *At the Hospital: A Surprise for Krissy.* Mankato, MN, The Child's World, affiliate of Creative Educational Society, Inc., 1976 (ages 3 to 7).

References

Adams M: The hospital through a child's eyes. *Children* 1965 Feb; 102.

Ahron C, Arnn S: When children from divorced families are hospitalized. Issues for staff. *Health Social Work* 1981; 6:21–28.

Alexander D, et al: Anxiety of non-rooming-in parents of hospitalized children. *Child Health Care* 1986 Summer; 15(1):14–20.

American Academy of Pediatrics: *Care of Children in Hospitals.* 2nd ed. Evanston, IL, 1971.

Azarnoff A: Mediating the trauma of serious illness and hospitalization in childhood. *Child Today* 1974 Jul/Aug; 12.

Azarnoff P (ed): *Preparation of Young, Healthy Children for Possible Hospitalization: The Issues.* Santa Monica, CA, Pediatric Projects, 1983. (Available from Pediatric Projects, Inc., Box 1880, Santa Monica, CA 90406.)

Azarnoff P, Woody PD: Preparation for hospitalization in acute care hospitals in the United States. *Pediatrics* 1981; 68:361.

Bates TA, Broome M: Preparation of children for hospitalization and surgery: A review of the literature. *J Pediatr Nurs* 1986 Aug; 1(4):230–239.

Blackman L: The infant in the hospital. *In* Oremland E, Oremland J (eds): *The Effects of Hospitalization on Children.* Springfield, IL, Charles C Thomas, 1973.

Blos P: Children think about illness: their concepts and beliefs. *In* Gellert E: *Psychosocial Aspects of Pediatric Care.* New York, Grune and Stratton, 1978.

Bolig P: Play in hospital settings. *In* Yawkey TD, Pellegrini AD: *Child's Play; Developmental and Applied.* Hillsdale, NJ, Lawrence Erlbaum, 1984.

Brandt P, et al: Injections in children. *Am J Nurs* 1972 Aug; 1402.

Burns C: The hospitalization experience and single-parent families. *Nurs Clin North Am* 1984 Jun; 19(2):285–293.

Byrne CM, Cadman D: Prevention of the adverse effects of hospitalization in children. *Preventive Psychiatr* 1987 Nov; 3(2):167–190.

Calkin J: Assessing small children: are hospitalized toddlers adapting to the experience as well as we think? *MCN* 1979 Jan/Feb; 18.

Cassel J: The contribution of the social environment to host resistance. *Am J Epidemiol* 1976; 104:107–123.

Caty S, et al: Coping in hospitalized children: an analysis of published case studies. *Nurs Res* 1984 Sep/Oct; 33(5):277–287.

Cobb S: Social support as a moderator of life stress. *Psychosom Med* 1976; 38:300–314.

Conway B: The effects of hospitalization on adolescence. *Adolescence* 1971 Sep; 79.

Craft M: Preferences of hospitalized adolescents for information providers. *Nurs Res* 1981 Jul-Aug; 30(4):205–211.

Douglas JWB: Early hospital admissions and later disturbances of behavior and learning. *Dev Med Child Neurol* 1975; 17:456–480.

Dowd E, et al: Releasing the hospitalized child from restraints. *MCN* 1977 Nov/Dec; 370.

Elmassian B: A practical approach to communicating with children through play. *MCN* 1979 Jul/Aug; 238.

Erickson F: Helping the sick child maintain behavioral control. *Nurs Clin North Am* 1967 Dec; 695.

Freiberg K: How parents react when their child is hospitalized. *Am J Nurs* 1972 Jul; 1270.

Galligan A: Using Roy's concept of adaptation to care for young children. *Am J Nurs* 1979 Jan/Feb; 24.

Gelbert E: What do I have inside me? How children view their bodies. *In Psychosocial Aspects of Pediatric Care.* New York, Grune and Stratton, 1978.

Gildia HH, Quirk TR: Assessing the pain experience in children. *Nurs Clin North Am* 1977 Dec; 631.

Goslin ER: Hospitalization as a life crisis for the preschool child: a critical review. *J Commun Health* 1978; 3(4):321–346.

Green C: Larry thought puppet-play "childish" but it helped him face his fears. *Nursing 75* 1975 Mar; 301.

Harvey S: Parents are the best preparers of young children. *In* Azarnoff P (ed): *Preparation of Young Healthy Children for Possible Hospitalization: The Issues.* Santa Monica, CA, Pediatric Projects, 1983.

Hennessey JA: Hospitalized toddlers' responses to mothers' tape recordings during brief separations. *Matern Child Nurs J* 1976 Summer; 69.

Hodapp RM: Effects of hospitalization on young children: implications of two theories. *Child Health Care* 1982 Winter; 10(3):83–86.

Holder A: *Legal Issues in Pediatrics and Adolescent Medicine.* New York, John Wiley, 1977.

Hunsberger M, et al: A review of current approaches used to help children and parents cope with health care procedures. *Matern Child Nurs J* 1984 Fall; 13(3):145–165.

Huth MM: Guidelines for conducting hospital tours with early school age children. *Pediatr Nurs* 1983 Nov-Dec; 9:414–415, 431.

Jackson K, et al: Behavior changes indicating emotional trauma in tonsillectomized children. *Pediatrics* 1953; 12:33.

Jessner L, et al: Emotional implications of tonsillectomy and adenoidectomy on children. *Psychoanalytic Study Child* 1952; 7:126.

Johnson J, et al: Easing children's fright during health care procedures. *MCN* 1976 Jul/Aug; 206.

Kahn RL, Antonucci TC: Convoys over the life course: attachment, roles, and social support. *In* Baltes PB, Brim OG Jr (eds): *Life Span Development and Behavior.* Vol 3. New York, Academic Press, 1980.

Kaplan BH, et al: Social support and health. *Med Care* 1977; 15(5)Suppl:47–57.

King J, Zeigler S: The effects of hospitalization on children's behavior: a review of the literature. *Child Health Care* 1981; 10(20):8.

Lazarus RS, Launier R: Stress-related transactions between person and environment. *In* Pervin LA, Lewis M (eds): *Perspectives in Interactional Psychology.* New York, Plenum Press, 1978.

Mahaffey PJ: The effects of hospitalization on children admitted for tonsillectomy and adenoidectomy. *Nurs Res* 1965; 14(1):12–19.

Mason EA: Hospital and family cooperating to reduce psychological trauma. *Commun Mental Health J* 1978; 14(2):153.

Mather PL: Current preparation research and practice in one community. *In* Azarnoff P (ed): *Preparation of Young, Healthy Children for Possible Hospitalization: The Issues.* Santa Monica, CA, Pediatric Projects, 1983.

Mather PL, Glasrud PH: Child life workers: who are they and what are they doing? *Child Health Care* 1981; 10:11.

McCaffery M: Pain relief for the child. *Pediatr Nurs* 1977 Jul/Aug; 11.

Miles MS, Carter MC: Coping strategies used by parents during their child's hospitalization in an intensive care unit. *Child Health Care* 1985 Summer; 14(1):14–21.

Nagy M: Children's concepts of some bodily functions. *J Genet Psychol* 1953 Mar; 199.

Norbeta M: Caring for children with the help of puppets. *MCN* 1976 Jan/Feb; 22.

Oremland E, et al: *The Effects of Hospitalization on Children.* Springfield, IL, Charles C Thomas, 1973.

Orenstein SR, et al: The infant seat as treatment for gastroesophageal reflux. *N Engl J Med* 1983 Sep; 309:760–763.

Petrillo M, Sanger S: *Emotional Care of Hospitalized Children.* Philadelphia, JB Lippincott, 1980.

Plank E: *Working with Children in Hospitals.* Cleveland, The Press of Case Western Reserve University, 1971.

Quinton D, Rutter M: Early hospital admissions and later disturbances of behavior: an attempted replication of Douglas' findings. *Dev Med Child Neurol* 1976; 18(4):477–479.

Rasmussen M, Murphy C: Hospital admission through a child's eyes. *Pediatr Nurs* 1977 May/Jun; 43.

Roberts MC, et al: Reduction of medical fears by use of modeling: preventive application in a general population of children. *J Pediatr Psychol* 1982; 6:293.

Robertson J: *Young Children in Hospital.* 2nd ed. London, Tavistock Publications, 1970.

Robertson J: *The Fallacy of "Preparing" Young Healthy Children for Possible Hospitalization: The Issues.* Santa Monica, CA, Pediatric Projects, 1983.

Robson AM: Parenteral fluid therapy. *In* Behrman RE, et al (eds): *Nelson Textbook of Pediatrics.* 12th ed. Philadelphia, WB Saunders, 1983, 228–249.

Rose MH: The effects of hospitalization on coping behaviors of children. Unpublished *Doctoral Dissertation.* University of Chicago, 1972.

Rutter M: *Maternal Deprivation Reassessed.* New York, Penguin Books, 1981.

Savedra M, Tesler M: Coping strategies of hospitalized school-age children. *West J Nurs Res* 1981; 3(4):371–384.

Shaefer S: Communicating with children: teaching via the play discussion group. *Am J Nurs* 1977 Dec; 1960.

Shore MF, et al: Constructive uses of a hospital experience. *Children* 1965; 12:3–8.

Shuler S, Reich C: Sibling visitation in pediatric hospitals: policies, opinions and issues. *Child Health Care* 1982 Fall; 11(2):54–60.

Sibinga M, Friedman C: Restraints and speech. *Pediatrics* 1971 Jul; 116.

Skipper JK, Leonard RC: Children, stress and hospitalization: a field experiment. *J Health Social Behav* 1968; 9:275–287.

Stevens M: Adolescents' perceptions of stressful events during hospitalization. *J Pediatr Nurs* 1986 Oct; 1(5):303–313.

Stollak G: *What Happened Today: Stories for Parents and Children.* Dubuque, IA, Kendall/Hunt Publishing Company, 1973.

Taylor SC: The effects of chronic childhood illnesses upon well siblings. *Matern Child Nurs J* 1980; 9:109–116.

Tekely K, et al: Regressive behavior in a hospitalized preschool child. *Matern Child Nurs J* 1978 Fall; 185.

Thompson, RH: *Psychosocial Research on Pediatric Hospitalization and Health Care: A Review of the Literature.* Springfield, IL, Charles C Thomas, 1985.

Thompson RH: Where we stand: twenty years of research on pediatric hospitalization and health care. *Child Health Care* 1986 Spring; 14(4):200–210.

Trahd GE: Siblings of chronically ill children: helping them cope. *Pediatr Nurs* 1986; 12(3):191–193, 244.

Vernon DTA, et al: *The Psychological Response of Children to Hospitalization.* Springfield, IL, Charles C Thomas, 1965.

Visintainer MA, Wolfer JA: Psychological preparation for surgery pediatric patients: the effects on children's and parents' stress responses and adjustment. *Pediatrics* 1975 Aug; 56:187–202.

Wolff S, *Children under Stress.* Gretna, LA, Pelican Books, 1977.

Zurlinden JK: Minimizing the impact of hospitalization for children and their families. *MCN* 1985 May/Jun; 10:178–188.

Bibliography

Ack M: Psychosocial effects of illness, hospitalization and surgery. *Child Health Care* 1983; 11:132–136.

Algren CL: Role perception of mothers who have hospitalized children. *Child Health Care* 1985 Summer; 14(1):6–9.

Altshuler A, Seidle A: Teen meetings: a way to help adolescents cope with hospitalization. *MCN* 1977 Nov/Dec; 348.

Birchfield M: Nursing care for hospitalized children based on different stages of illness. *MCN* 1981 Jan/Feb; 6:46–52.

Blos P: The child analyst looks at the young adolescent. *In Twelve to Sixteen: Early Adolescence.* New York, WW Norton, 1972.

Caldwell BS, Lockhart L: A care-by-parent unit: its planning, implementation and patient satisfaction. *Child Health Care* 1981 Summer; 10(1):4–7.

Clatworthy S: Therapeutic play: effects on hospitalized children. *Child Health Care* 1981 Spring; 9(4):108–113.

Cormier P: Identification of typologies derived from children's behaviors in the hospital as predictors of psychiatric upset. *J Psychiatr Nurs* 1979 Jun; 28.

Coucouvanis JA, Solomons HC: Handling complicated visitation problems of hospitalized children. *MCN* 1983 Mar/Apr; 8:131–134.

Denholm CJ: Hospitalization and the adolescent patient: a review and some critical questions. *Child Health Care* 1985 Winter; 13(3):109–116.

Erickson F: Play interviews of four year old hospitalized children. *Monographs Soc Res Child Dev* 1958; 33:7.

Finn K: The hospitalization of children with developmental disorders. *Child Health Care* 1982; 10:131–134.

Forest J: The contract and nursing practice. *Nurs Papers* 1975 Summer; 14.

Gellert E: What do I have inside me? How children view their bodies. *In Psychosocial Aspects of Pediatric Care.* New York, Grune and Stratton, 1978.

Guidelines for adolescent units. Developed by the Adolescent Care Study Section, Association for the Care of Children in Hospitals. Presented in Washington, DC, June, 1978.

Hardgrove CG, Dawson RB: *Parents and Children in the Hospital: The Family's Role in Pediatrics.* Boston, Little, Brown, 1972.

Honig RG: Group meetings on an adolescent medical ward. *Adolescence* 1982; 17:99–106.

Kashani JH, et al: Depression in hospitalized pediatric patients. *J Am Acad Child Psychiatr* 1981; 20:123–134.

Kellerman J, et al: Psychological effects of illness in adolescence. 1. Anxiety, self-esteem and perception of control. *J Pediatr* 1980; 97:126–131.

Knafl KA, et al: *Pediatric Hospitalization: Family and Nurse Perspectives.* Glenview, IL, Scott, Foresman and Company, 1988.

Klinzing D, Klinzing D: *Communication for Allied Health Professionals.* Dubuque, IA, William C. Brown Publishers, 1985.

Koss I, Teter M: Welcoming a family when a child is hospitalized. *MCN* 1980 Jan/Feb; 51.

Lamb JM, Rodgers DR: Assisting the hostile hospitalized child. *MCN* 1983 Sep/Oct; 8:336–339.

Liakopoulou M, et al: Developmental interventions in infancy during lengthy hospitalizations. *Dev Behav Pediatr* 1983 Sep; 4(3):213–217.

Lindsay KE: The value of music for the hospitalized infant. *Child Health Care* 1981 Spring; 9(4):104–107.

May BK, Sparks M: School-age children: Are their needs recognized and met in the hospital setting? *Child Health Care* 1983 Winter; 11(3):118–121.

McCain C: Television viewing and the hospitalized child. 1983 Jan/Feb; 33–35.

McGillicuddy M: A Study of the Relationship Between Mother's Rooming-In During Their Children's Hospitalization and Changes in Selected Areas of Children's Behavior. Doctoral dissertation, New York University Health Sciences, Nursing, 1976.

Mechanic D: Adolescent health and illness behavior: review of the literature and a new hypothesis for the study of stress. *J Human Stress* 1983; 19(2):4–13.

Melamed BG, et al: Necessary considerations for surgery preparation: age and previous experience. *Psychosom Med* 1983 Dec; 45(6):517–525.

Pass MD, Pass CM: Anticipatory guidance for parents of hospitalized children. *J Pediatr Nurs* 1987; II(4):250–258.

Porter CS: Grade school children's perceptions of their internal body parts. *Nurs Res* 1974 Sep/Oct; 23(5):384–391.

Poster EC: Stress immunization: techniques to help children cope with hospitalization. *MCN* 1983; 12:119–134.

Prugh DG: *The Psychosocial Aspects of Pediatrics.* Philadelphia, Lea and Febiger, 1983.

Rae WA: Hospitalized latency-age children: implications for psychosocial care. *Child Health Care* 1981 Winter; 9(3):59–63.

Ritchie JA, et al: Concerns of acutely ill, chronically ill, and healthy preschool children. *Res Nurs Health* 1984; 7:265–274.

Rudy-Wallace M: Temperament: assessing individual differences in hospitalized children. *J Pediatr Nurs* 1987; II(1):30–36.

Smitherman C: Parents of hospitalized children have needs, too. *Am J Nurs* 1979 Aug; 1423.

Terry G: A 5 year old boy's aggressive and compensatory behavior in response to immobilization. *Matern Child Nurs* 1979 Spring; 29.

Teyber EC, Littlehales DE: Coping with feelings: seriously ill children, their families and hospital staff. *Child Health Care* 1981; 10:58–62.

Vipperman JF, Rager PM: Childhood coping: how nurses can help. *Pediatr Nurs* 1980 Mar/Apr; 11–18.

Zeltzer L, et al: Psychologic effects of illness in adolescence. II. Impact of illness in adolescents—crucial issues and coping styles. *J Pediatr* 1980 Jul; 97(1):132–138.

Principles and Strategies of Home Care

Chapter 32

Roxie L. Foster

Home care—a term that used to apply to an illness that the parent could treat with a Bandaid or a vaporizer—has expanded in this decade to include care of very ill children in the home. This change in the location and delivery of health care services to children and families has had a profound effect on pediatric health care practices, an effect that is projected to grow rapidly in the coming years. This chapter discusses the evolution of home health care, the nursing process related to home care, and projections for the future of pediatric home care. It focuses upon the family in relation to home care; interventions are directed toward family members in general, rather than toward the ill child. Home care strategies specific for the ill child are presented for all the major illnesses in this text in sections termed *Nursing Strategies for Follow-up Care in the Home or Clinic*. (See Unit VII.)

Nursing Process Plan
NPP: Home Care, page 1009

Related Topics
Communicating with children and families, Chapters 1 and 11
Family assessment, Chapter 12
Promoting Healthy Parenting, Chapter 13
Concepts of stress and coping, Chapter 23
Impact of Acute Illness, Chapter 24
Impact of Chronic Illness, Chapter 25
Impact of Death and Dying, Chapter 26

In the nursing care of children, the term *home care* has come to represent the health care management of an ill child within the child's place of residence as implemented by one or more adult caregivers. Often the adult caregivers are parents or family members who are taught, assisted, and supervised in the child's care by nurses, physicians, and other health care professionals.

In some cases home health aides or nurses assume responsibility for intermittent or continuous care delivery to the child in the home. This may be necessary because the child requires skilled professional care at that time or because the family members themselves, for whatever reason, are unable to care for the child.

The Evolution of Home Health Care

Historic Considerations

The concept of caring for sick children at home is not new. Until the advent of modern medical technology families traditionally cared for ill members in the home. Before the 18th century the family was the source not only of health care but also work, education, religious worship, recreation, and political attitudes (Farrell and Schmitt, 1979). Family functioning and family authority were reinforced by an agrarian society. As late as 1850, the great majority of American families lived in rural areas, with health care provided by family folk remedies and by a "country doctor" who would travel among homes to tend the sick. As the industrial revolution and the lure of jobs prompted people to move to the cities, adjustments were made in family functioning. In the urban setting family members became more dependent on persons and agencies outside the family, and the family unit began to lose some of its autonomy.

At the turn of the century health care and medical technology became more sophisticated and care of the sick began to move out of the arms of the family and into clinics and hospitals. Provision was made within these facilities for patients only, and families were provided with schedules of "visiting hours." The message was clear; while care in the home was acceptable for some chronically ill elderly persons, acute illness care was primarily the domain of health care professionals within institutions.

Although the caseloads of community health nurses included some stable children with chronic illnesses, home care for children requiring more sophisticated management was given little consideration until the 1970s. At that time Ida Martinson, a professor at the University of Minnesota School of Nursing, piloted a home care program for terminally ill children. Citing enhancement of quality of life for the child and family as the rationale for the program, Martinson and her associates worked as liaisons to ensure professional support for the parents, who became the primary caregivers. In a report of their first home care program for dying children, the nurses cited a father's words of thanks (Martinson et al, 1977, page 1815):

> Seth died as we had often hoped he could—cuddled in our arms before a blazing fire, in utter quiet and peace. We have such good feelings about the peace of that moment that it has been immeasurably easier to deal with this reality. We can hardly thank you enough for permitting us the peace and dignity of that moment.

With the success of the Martinson model for home care came the question, "Why should the comfort of family support be reserved only for dying children?" Slowly health care professionals began to experiment with parental management of other illness conditions in children. Home apnea monitoring became more common, and children were sent home with central venous catheters and on continuous ambulatory peritoneal dialysis. Today, home care extends even to children who are ventilator dependent. While in 1985 children comprised only 5 to 10 per cent of the home health care market (Punch, 1985), continued growth is expected.

Social Considerations

While the Martinson home care model influenced social attitudes about the care of ill children, it is important to note that Martinson's work was the result of social trends. Societal influences have made an impact on home care since its inception in the United States in 1893, when Lillian Wald established The Visiting Nurse Service of New York City in response to public health concerns for the elderly. Home care for children has come about in response to several identifiable social factors. In particular, pediatric home care has been shaped by the need for cost containment, by increasing consumer demands for quality services, and by technologic developments.

Cost Containment

The issue of cost containment has become a reality for everyone in the health care industry. Costs for health care services have risen dramatically in recent years and insurance coverage is strained by reimbursements for costly tests and procedures and by the increasing life span of persons with chronic illnesses. It is clear that costs must be "contained"; the challenge is to cut costs without decreasing the quality of care.

Home care has been approached as one solution to cost containment. Rogatz (1985) cautioned, however, that home care must be evaluated in the light of what we are trying to achieve. If we are committed to comprehensive and effective health services as well as to cost-savings, then home care must be not only cheaper than hospital care but more cost-effective as well. Cost-effectiveness entails the provision of high quality services to the most people at the most reasonable price.

With the legislation of diagnosis-related groups (DRGs) hospitals have been given an incentive to provide care that facilitates the patient's recovery in the shortest period of time. While that might not appear to be an innovation, consider that previously hospitals could make the most money by keeping their beds full of persons whose insurance and/or Medicare plans would pay for the ongoing cost of services. DRGs dictate that, for a Medicare patient, hospitals will be paid a lump sum (or prospective fee) to treat a particular disease. That means that if the hospital can treat the illness as effectively by an alternate method of care (such as home care) a profit can be shown for that transaction.

Although DRGs at present deal only with Medicare patients, facilities that provide pediatric care are anticipating that they will be faced with similar forms of payment in the future. For this reason, and because of early reports of savings in health care dollars, pediatric institutions and private pediatricians are becoming involved in home care. Home care is cost effective if it ensures follow-up to decrease recurrent exacerbations and hospitalizations, if it minimizes the psychosocial impact of illness by maintaining a more normal environment, and if it reduces the number of salaried professionals who interact with the client.

While home care often results in substantial savings to health care institutions, it may not be cheaper for the family. Traditionally, insurance reimbursements have been more generous for hospital-based services than for those provided in the home, and families may actually be responsible for a greater percentage of the expenses if the child is cared for in the home. Another consideration is whether one parent must relinquish gainful employment to stay at home and care for the child. Even if one parent is available to provide care, the added physical and emotional burdens of continuous care for an ill child may necessitate extra expenses to relieve that parent of some of the usual household duties.

Quality of Care

Assurance of quality in the services provided entails aspects of professional and technical support and of client progress and satisfaction (see Box 32-1 and the following section on the nursing process in home care). The client's evaluation of quality care may depend, in part, upon the relative needs for technology versus quality of life. In acute or life-threatening illnesses the needs for specialized equipment and professional care are likely to be of greatest concern (and are usually best met by hospitalization), while in situations of recuperation from illness, or in chronic or terminal illness, aspects of comfort and support may be more important (and may be best addressed by home care). Figure 32-1 illustrates this changing focus of needs on a continuum from acute to terminal illness. To be most effective the method of care delivery must meet these changing needs in regard to technology and quality of life.

The issue of quality of life is particularly pertinent to home care of children. With the increasing emphasis in the professional and lay literature on the psychosocial and developmental aspects of childhood has come the realization that it is often detrimental to separate an ill child from family support. Normalization of the child's environment through home care can be effective in promoting recovery and in preventing hospital-induced psychologic trauma. Psychosocial, cultural, and economic factors that are easily overlooked in an acute care setting become much more apparent when the client is seen in the home. Solutions to illness-related problems (and resulting enhancement of the quality of life) are more likely to be effective when all aspects of the child's life are taken into consideration.

Box 32-1
Home Care Quality Assurance Components

STRUCTURAL MEASURES

Education experience of staff
Standards of care
Systems review
- What systems exist which may enhance:
  - Solving the problem
  - Identification/feedback/resolution
  - Interdisciplinary assessment, planning, intervention, evaluation
  - Interdisciplinary collaboration
  - Client's access to care
  - Staff development
  - Communication among staff, agency management and the total organization productivity

PROCESS MEASURES

Is the nursing process carried out appropriately?
Are interventions timely and accurate?
Are interventions and changing client status communicated among all involved team members?
Is the plan of care altered in conjunction with a changing client status?
Does interdisciplinary consultation occur appropriately?
Do joint visits, involving two or more disciplines, occur when needed?

OUTCOME MEASURES

Are service goals met?
Have the nursing diagnoses been resolved?
Has the client's functional level improved?
Is the client satisfied with the care?
Was the tme spent with the client effectively utilized?
Do clients within the service area have equal access to care?

(From Janz, 1985.)

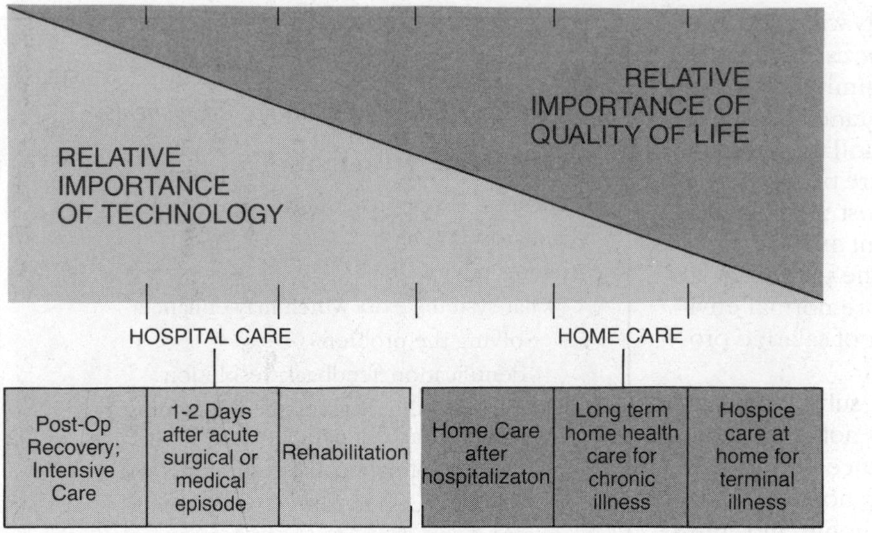

Figure 32-1. The relationship of acute and long-term illness to the importance of technology and quality of life. (From Rogatz P: Home health care: some social and economic considerations. *Home Healthcare Nurse* 1985; 3(1):41.)

Technology

The third social factor affecting pediatric home care is the technology of modern science. Recent technologic advances have resulted in the prolongation of life for infants and children who would not previously have survived. Many of these children, however, are left with chronic conditions (such as bronchopulmonary dysplasia) and need constant skilled care. Home care management by the parents, with careful teaching and follow-up by health care professionals, is often the chosen alternative for families with chronically ill children.

Another aspect of technologic advances is the equipment that has made possible home therapies that were previously only conducted in the hospital. Not only has the equipment itself become more sophisticated and reliable, but over time, health care professionals have become more comfortable with it and therefore are more willing to teach aspects of its use and maintenance to their clients. The outcome is the delivery of care in the home today that was, in some cases, considered experimental in hospitals 10 years ago.

Support services for home care equipment have also improved. Agencies that deal in home care supplies are becoming increasingly aware of the need to provide a broad range of professional services. The competition among "provider" agencies means that it is no longer enough to employ someone to deliver large green bottles of oxygen; to be competitive the agency may need to employ skilled respiratory therapists who can assist home care nurses in monitoring treatments and obtaining diagnostic data through pulse oximetry and transcutaneous monitoring.

The Nursing Process in Home Health Care

The component parts of the nursing process, as it relates to home care, become a shared responsibility between nurses (and other health care professionals) in the hospital and the nurse who will be responsible for coordination of care once the child is at home. Hospital-based nurses, in cooperation with the family and with other health care professionals, initiate the nursing process for home care by assessing whether this child and family are candidates for home care. If home care is determined to be a viable option planning continues. Being careful to clarify the perceptions of the family at each step, nursing diagnoses and clinical problems are identified and goals for treatment are set. Ideally, the home health care nurse who will be responsible for implementation and evaluation of the plan is also involved in the planning process.

Assessment

The assessment process begins in the hospital with the determination of the patient's and family's needs, strengths, and limitations in relation to home-based health care management. It results in the determination of whether this child and family are candidates for home health care. Hymovich (1976) has suggested that in order to cope with chronic illness in their child parents need (1) trust, (2) information, (3) resources, and (4) guidance and support. These criteria also apply to the child with a short-term illness and form a suitable framework for assessing family readiness for home health care.

Trust

Parents* need to trust themselves, their child, the health care professionals involved, and the treatment plan. First they must believe in their own physical and emotional ability to manage the child's care at home. Whether that care involves monitoring of equipment (such as an oxygen tank or a home apnea monitor), maintenance of indwelling tubes (such as a gastrostomy tube or central venous catheter), delivery of treatments (such as chest physical therapy or range of motion exercises), or administration of medications, parents need to feel confident in their ability to perform the tasks safely and effectively. This need for self-confidence also applies to children who are old enough to participate in self-care.

Before the parents or the child can trust themselves to deal with the treatment plan for the illness, however, they must face the illness itself. Until the reality of the illness is accepted there will be an emotional obstacle to the delivery of technical care. If they cannot come to accept the necessary dependency on the medical regimen, omission of parts of the treatment plan may result; the delivery of prescribed care will only serve as a painful reminder of the illness they might otherwise be able to deny. In order to accept the illness parents must alter the mental and emotional image of their whole and perfect child to include the reality that their child is, temporarily or permanently, dependent on a machine or tube or on certain treatments and medications. Children, in turn, must alter their self-image to incorporate the reality of the illness.

Parents and children need also to trust the ability of the treatment plan to accomplish the desired goals, which goes hand in hand with their need to trust the health care professionals involved. *The family is unlikely to comply with the treatment plan unless it addresses the problems that they have identified in a manner that is in keeping with their values.*

Certain objective assessments contribute to an understanding of trust. Competency of return demonstrations of technical tasks by the child and parents, willingness of the child and parents to participate in the technical aspects of care in the hospital setting, observable indications of parental anxiety or ease in the presence of the child, and frequency and duration of parental hospital visits are among the pertinent observable behaviors.

Trust is also indicated subjectively. The nurse must be alert for statements from the parents and child that would reveal feelings of self-confidence, feelings of acceptance of the changes necessitated by the illness, feelings of hopefulness that the desired goals can be met, feelings of some control over the situation, and feelings of being vital and valued members of the treatment team.

A family that is involved in the decision-making process is much more likely to display signs of trust in themselves and others. A prerequisite for trust is that both parties (the family and the health care professionals) accept and value each others' contributions.

If health care professionals determine that they are unable to consider the parents (and child, when appropriate) as equal participants in the treatment, they must question whether their lack of confidence is based on legitimate concerns (such as lack of mental capacity or lack of necessary manual dexterity) or whether those concerns stem only from differences in values and lifestyle. In the former case it may be appropriate to conclude that this family is not a candidate for home care or that professional help will be needed in the home. In the latter case, an unbiased re-examination of both facts and attitudes will be necessary.

Information

Assessment of information involves the determination of what discharge teaching the family and child have

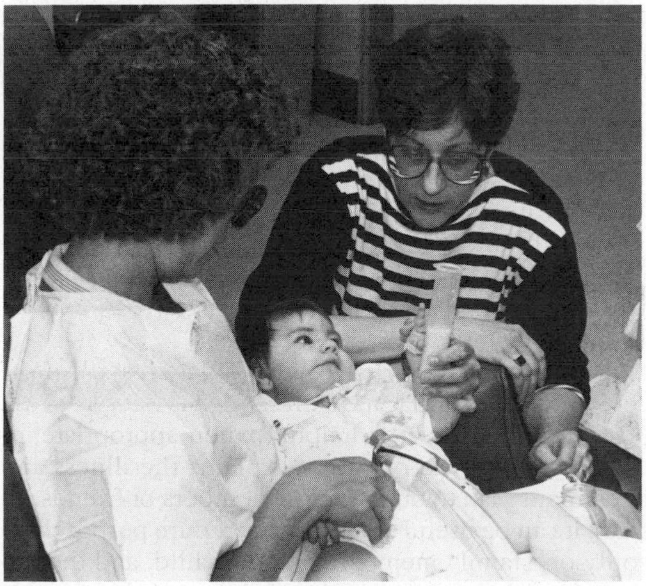

The home care nurse (seated) and the mother are both learning to care for the child in the hospital before discharge. Coordination with the child's primary nurse in the hospital ensures continuity of care. (Courtesy of Children's Home Care of The Children's Hospital, Denver.)

*Although it is acknowledged that the primary caregiver in the home may not be a parent, the term "parent(s)" will be used in this chapter to mean adult caregiver(s).

received, and whether they understand and agree with the information. If the assessment reveals a lack of understanding or agreement on the part of the child and family, the method of teaching must be evaluated.

Discharge teaching is most effective when all members of the health care team understand specifically what teaching is needed, what teaching has been done, what information needs to be covered again, and when there is agreement upon the way in which this information should be presented. Lacking such coordination, the process may be undermined by the family receiving conflicting instructions, resulting in their confusion not only about the information given but also about whom to believe.

Coordination of discharge teaching begins with a list of facts and skills to be taught.* If this list is kept at the bedside and a checklist system used for items that have been addressed, potential "teachers" among the health care professionals can be easily updated on the progress made. The form should include a column for the child and family to indicate whether, after reflecting on the information or demonstration, they have achieved a level of comfort, or whether they desire further teaching. It can be effective to allow the child and family to choose the order in which they want to cover the items on the discharge teaching list (Davis and Eyer, 1984). This provides them some control over one aspect of the hospital environment and enhances the chance for a receptive audience.

It is important to remember that anxiety decreases comprehension and to expect to discuss the same set of facts or to demonstrate the same procedure more than once. The parents and child can be "given permission" to need this additional help by statements such as, "Many children (or parents) tell me they have to do this several times before they really understand it. Would you like to do it once more?"

The issue of conflicting instructions is more likely to develop when a large number of people are interacting with and teaching the family. Control may be best achieved by designating certain "teachers" among those professionals involved and/or by frequent coordination meetings of the team responsible for discharge teaching for home care.

Assessment of whether the child and family comprehend the material and skills taught is integral to the teaching process. It is helpful, when appropriate, to listen as the child or parent explains the illness and treatment plan to other family members or friends. In fact, it can be useful to teach a procedure purposely to only one family member or to the child, and then to watch as that person teaches another of the persons who will be responsible for that part of the treatment in the home. Not only does this facilitate the nurse's evaluation of information and technical skills, but also it helps to reinforce that person's confidence by attributing to them the status and responsibility of "teacher."

There are three possible outcomes of the assessment of the scope and depth of the family's information regarding necessary aspects of the home treatment plan: (1) they may have the necessary understanding and psychomotor skills to perform the care; (2) they may show command of part of the information but require further assessment and teaching before a final determination is made regarding readiness for home care; or (3) limitations may be identified in cognitive or psychomotor abilities. These limitations may be the result of conflicts of value or other psychosocial factors that have interfered with the family's motivation to learn the needed skills. If further teaching will correct the problem, arrangements can often be made with the home care nurse for additional technical support and teaching in the first days that the child is at home. If it does not appear that further assessment and teaching will be effective, the family will not be recommended for home care.

Resources

Assessment of the family's resources includes physical, emotional, and financial considerations. *Physical resources* include individual physical characteristics, the physical environment of the home, and sources of physical support. Parents must possess the necessary physical strength and agility to perform treatments and maintain equipment, and they must be able to do so consistently. When a primary caregiver has a chronic illness, such as asthma, modificatons may be required in the plan of care. The physical strain of round-the-clock responsibility for an ill child is considerable and even the healthiest principal caregiver will need to make provisions for respite care.

The physical environment of the home must be such that the child's safety and the effectiveness of treatments are ensured. A visit to the home prior to the child's discharge is advisable when possible. During this visit the nurse or social worker can talk with the parents about such things as where the ill child will sleep and where equipment will be placed. At this time assessment can be made of the ability to heat and cool the home, of the adequacy of electrical outlets for equipment, of refrigeration to store food and medications, and of other potential safety and health hazards.

Sources of physical support include friends, extended family, and community support groups who are willing to provide such assistance as grocery shopping; help with laundry, cleaning, and meals; and babysitting for siblings of the ill child.

---

*In the illness-related chapters of this text, discharge teaching needs are itemized for many diseases under the nursing diagnosis, *knowledge deficit*.

Emotional support resources consist of those persons within the family or community who are willing to listen to the family's problems and to assist them in the problem-solving process. Families often experience numerous offers of physical and emotional support from friends and extended family at the onset of an illness. As the illness and home care situation linger on, however, few of the support persons are able to manage the weight of the family's problems in addition to their own, and the support is withdrawn. When this occurs the family begins to rely more and more upon health care professionals to meet both physical and emotional needs.

Assessment of the family's *financial* ability to meet home care costs must include the cost to implement the medical treatment plan in the home (e.g., equipment and medications); consideration for insurance coverage of prescribed treatments, home visits, and home nursing care; and the alteration of family patterns of work outside and inside the home. Will home care necessitate one parent quitting a job outside the home? Will significant expenses be incurred (e.g., additional ready-to-eat food purchases, sending shirts out to be laundered, buying ready-made clothing) because the primary caregiver does not have time to perform the usual activities within the home?

Home care of the ill child need not always be abandoned if the family's resources are inadequate to sustain this type of program. A knowledgable social worker can often help the family find sources of support for financial, emotional, and certain physical needs. It is essential, however, that the assessment process results in identification of these needs and that proper referral is made.

Guidance and Support

Guidance and support of the family by health care professionals is integral to the concept of home care. Assessment of this criterion concerns the availability of help for the family 24 hours a day, and the family's ability to reach that help. Does the family have a telephone? Can a nurse always be reached if questions arise about treatment procedures or about new signs and symptoms? If an interpreter is necessary, is there always one available? Does the family have transportation to take the child to the clinic for follow-up care? Is there ambulance service available in that area in case of an emergency? What provisions have been made, or can be made, for needed electrical equipment in case of a power outage? Is there a fire station or police station nearby that can provide oxygen and cardiopulmonary resuscitation in case of an emergency?

The needs of the child and family and the type of agency providing the home care will dictate the composition of the support team. If the home care is directed from a hospital or community health agency, it is likely that more disciplines will be involved in the care because of ease of access. If the home care is provided by a nursing registry the nurses involved often draw upon their knowledge and personal resources to provide many of the additional services themselves. In any case, the home care support team will include at least one nurse and one physician, with the involvement of educators, physical therapists, nutritionists, speech therapists, respiratory therapists, social workers, clergy, and psychologists, as necessary.

Limitations in the availability of guidance and support for the family can often be remedied by careful coordination of health care professionals and allied health care personnel. When this is not possible, it is usually because the family's insurance will not cover the costs of the necessary support services. Although insurance carriers have been slow to provide reimbursement for pediatric home care, that trend is beginning to change as the cost-effectiveness of home care becomes more evident (Kahn, 1984; Punch, 1985). According to Kaufman and Hardy-Ribakow (1988), the majority of funding for pediatric home care is provided by private insurance companies, Supplemental Security Income (Title XVI), and state crippled children's programs. They predict that more of these costs will begin to be assumed by the Title XIX Medicaid Model Waivers, designed to help individuals who currently receive or qualify for Medicaid benefits in an institutional setting.

After all of the assessment data have been gathered, the discharge planning team will determine whether the needs of the child and family can best be met by home care, by continued hospitalization, or by another care alternative such as an extended care facility. The child and family can be identified as appropriate candidates for home care if it is determined that they demonstrate adequate trust, comprehension of information, and adequate resources, and if the necessary guidance and support are available. There is one additional element, however, that must not be overlooked. Now that the family has a good understanding of the scope of their responsibilities in home care of the child, do they still consider this to be the best option? *Have they been asked that question?* The health care professionals responsible for the hospital-based assessment and planning for home care would do well to heed Elkins' (1986) caveat to home care nurses: "When working with home care patients and their families, the home health nurse must realize that she is stepping into their environment and that when she leaves they will remain in the same environment with the responsibility of care" (p. 181). Nurses and other health care professionals responsible for determining the family's readiness for home care are, at least figuratively, stepping into the lives of those persons, but they are not the ones who will carry the day-to-day burden. Care must be taken not to impose one's own values for health care on the family who will ultimately assume the responsibility for it. For home care to be successful, it is essential that the family and the professional support team have similar perceptions of the readiness for discharge and for home care.

Nursing Diagnosis

When the decision for home care has been made, nursing diagnoses form the basis for planning care. The needs of the child and family that arise from the assessment data can be stated in the form of nursing diagnoses. Family involvement in identifying these needs and problems is not only advisable but also essential. If the family is to assume the primary responsibility for care they must be actively involved in and informed about the basis of that care. The parents (and child, as development allows) should help establish each section of each nursing diagnosis (problem, etiology, and defining characteristics) and should fully participate in assigning priorities to all the problems and needs identified. *The success of the home treatment plan will depend on the family's investment in it.*

Desired Outcomes/Evaluation Criteria

The next step in the nursing process is to set realistic goals, or outcomes, that will provide direction for the treatment plan and form a basis for evaluation. The desired outcomes of home care will reflect the individualized nursing diagnoses. In some patients (e.g., children with bronchopulmonary dysplasia or cystic fibrosis) the goals may lead to the family's independence in the care of their child. In other patients (e.g., children who have terminal cancer) the desired outcomes may reflect an increased quality of life for the child, increased opportunities for caring interactions between the child and family, and the preservation of more normal family functioning. In the case of terminally ill children the involvement of the professional support team usually increases as the child's condition deteriorates.

The mutual agreement on the purpose of home care (i.e., the desired outcomes, or what is to be accomplished) is perhaps the pivot point for the rest of the home care experience. If the family is operating on one agenda and the health care professionals on another, neither party will be satisfied with the efforts of the other. The goals must be those of the child and family as well as of the health care professionals.

Agreement on the desired outcomes will be enhanced by (1) the family's involvement in determining needs and assigning priorities; (2) the family's participation in and understanding of the evaluation criteria; (3) evaluation criteria that are specific, realistic, and assigned appropriate time lines; and (4) frequent evaluation and restructuring of the desired outcomes and the methods of treatment.

Figure 32-2 illustrates part of a home care plan for 5-year-old Becky S., who has been diagnosed with cystic fibrosis and has been referred for home care. This care plan (which, in its entirety, includes nursing diagnoses, goals, and strategies for the scope of the child's illness) will be used by the parents as well as by the health care professionals who see Becky in her home. Becky's parents were involved in formulation of the care plan and agreed that Becky's lung involvement was the first priority of the treatment plan.

In the excerpt of the care plan shown in the figure, the nursing diagnosis of ineffective airway clearance is identified. This clarifies for the parents, as well as for the health care professionals, the particular lung problem and the signs and symptoms upon which the nursing diagnosis is based. The goals and strategies reflect the responses to the problem. They are written in language that Becky's parents can understand and contain specific evaluation criteria that they can use to judge their daughter's progress. The strategies (implementation) list specific instructions that reflect and reinforce the teaching the family received before Becky was discharged from the hospital. Rationale for the actions is included as a reminder of their purpose.

Although it is time consuming to construct a detailed home care plan with the family, it is cost effective. To the extent that the care plan enhances the family's sense of comfort and competence, and their trust in the treatment plan, it will increase compliance and decrease exacerbations and future hospitalizations. To the extent that it provides the parents with a basis for making decisions about minor changes in the plan and about the need for medical or nursing consultation, it reduces the number of hours of follow-up required by health care professionals. To the extent that it provides peace of mind for the family, the care plan is of immeasurable benefit in normalizing the home environment and in enhancing loving relationships among family members.

Nursing Strategies/Nursing Orders

Nursing strategies and nursing orders, or implementation of the plan of care, takes place in the home and involves the home care nurse. Before further discussion of implementation procedures, it is pertinent to explore the special qualities and preparation of the home care nurse.

Nursing Diagnosis 1

Ineffective airway clearance, related to production of thick mucus in the bronchial tree

Defining Characteristics

Recurrent wheezing, rales, and rhonchi; two episodes of *Staphylococcus aureus* pneumonia in the last 4 months; frequent cough productive of moderate-to-large amounts of thick, purulent secretions with occasional traces of bright red blood.

Client Goal/Evaluation Criteria	Parent (Nurse) Goals/Strategies (Selected/Rationale)
1. Becky will increase the clearance of mucus from her airways within 2 weeks, as evidenced by:	
a. rarely having episodes of coughing to ''get up'' mucous plugs, except when associated with respiratory treatments	Perform the respiratory therapy regimen learned in the hospital four times a day, before meals and at bedtime. (Using these times will reduce Becky's chances of vomiting. • Put the premixed solution of Alupent in the nebulizer and encourage Becky to breathe it in deeply until there are no droplets left in the nebulizer chamber. (This medicine will open Becky's airways and make it easier for the mucus to drain out.) • Clap firmly on Becky's chest for 2 minutes in each of the nine positions you were taught. Use the pictures attached to this care plan until you are more comfortable with the routine. (Percussion loosens the thick mucus in Becky's lungs and the postural drainage puts her in the best position for all of the parts of her lungs to drain.) • Encourage Becky to cough during the respiratory treatment. (Coughing is nature's way of removing mucus from the lungs.) If Becky coughs particularly hard she may still have some streaks of blood in the mucus. (This happens when small blood vessels break from the force of her coughing.) You need not be concerned about the streaks of blood unless there is considerably more bleeding than she had when she was in the hospital. If she begins coughing up a lot of blood call the home care nurse or the clinic immediately.
b. less ''noise'' and wheezing audible in her chest when parents listen to her breathe and when nurse auscultates with a stethoscope	Listen to Becky's breathing before and after the treatments. Afterwards, you should hear less wheezing and crackles and she should feel that it is easier to breathe in and out. (When the nurse visits she will take Becky's vital signs before and after a treatment, listen to her lungs, and talk with you about the effect of the treatments.)
c. *absence* of fever; chest pain; rapid, shallow breathing; a grunting sound to her breathing; and extreme tiredness	If any of these signs and symptoms of pneumonia occur, call the home care nurse or take Becky to the clinic. (If Becky develops another case of pneumonia it is important that she start on the antibiotic as soon as possible to prevent lasting effects on her lungs.)

Figure 32-2. An excerpt from a home care plan. The client is Becky S., age 5 years. Medical diagnosis is cystic fibrosis.

Preparation of Home Care Nurses

The home care nurse's preparation should include prior hospital experience with the type of patients to be seen in home care settings. It is essential that the nurse possess competence and confidence in acute care skills such as physical assessment, venipuncture, and management of indwelling tubes and equipment. In Cherryholmes' words, "The home health nurse is a higher-leveled generalist who has to be able to recognize problems and trust her own judgment and clinical skills" (1986, p. 158). She noted that knowledge of norms is necessary because there is no one in the home with whom to collaborate.

Characteristics of Home Care Nurses

Successful home care nurses tend to share certain qualities. They tend to be holistic in approach and to value flexibility and autonomy in their work settings (Mundinger, 1983; Stuart-Siddall, 1984). The home health care nurse enjoys teaching and is able to adapt teaching strategies to the full spectrum of physical and emotional climates that might be encountered. The effective nurse in the home care setting is able to communicate acceptance of a variety of lifestyles and to make judgments according to the identified outcomes for the treatment plan rather than on the basis of differences or similarities in values. In some communities it can be very helpful to be bilingual; the family will appreciate the attempt to communicate with them in their first language. Home care nurses also tend to enjoy problem solving and have the ability to help the client identify the need for change and work through the change process (Cherryholmes, 1986).

Implementation of the home care treatment plan is, in most cases, the responsibility of the family with the support of the home care nurse, the physician, and other professionals as needed. If the home care nurse was not involved in the creation of the care plan, time must be spent with the family clarifying the problems, outcomes, strategies, and evaluation criteria. A nursing process plan is presented in Table 32-1. This plan focuses upon *family* adaptation to home care. Nursing assessments, diagnoses, client goals, strategies, and evaluation criteria can be added to address the child's illness, or the child's illness can be dealt with separately in a plan meant to be used by the family as a guidline for care (Fig. 32-2).

Framework for Home Care Management

The home care nurse needs an organizational approach or personal conceptual framework for home care management (Hillman, 1986). Lenihan (1985) proposed adoption of the Wright and Leahy (1984) model for family interviewing as a conceptual framework for interactions in home care. This model offers a simple, common-sense approach to the intervention process. The steps of the model are engagement, assessment, intervention, and termination.

Engagement

Engagement is the introduction and trust-building stage of the nurse-family relationship. It is essential that this part of the process not be overlooked. Hillman (1986, p. 164) cautioned, ". . . if the home health care nurse is insensitive to the importance of the establishment of an open, ongoing relationship, she may not be able to affect a therapeutic change, regardless of the accuracy of her assessment and problem identification." The primary tool for the engagement process is an accepting attitude that communicates to the family that the nurse values their worth as human beings and their potential contributions to the treatment plan. Each family member should be acknowledged regardless of his or her involvement with the child's care (Elkins, 1986). The client in home care is the family; each member influences the environment and needs to be recognized for his or her role within the family.

Often engagement begins with a telephone call in which the nurse relates some personal qualifications and describes the services of the agency and the fees for service. At this time an appointment is made for the nurse to visit the home. The initial "engagement" visit should establish the pattern for future visits (Lenihan, 1985). The family needs to know what they can expect from the nurse and what the nurse will expect from them, such as keeping appointments and providing space for physical assessment of the child.

The nurse's communication skills, both verbal and nonverbal, will never be more challenged than during this engagement stage. A successful encounter will greatly facilitate the mutually established goals, while a less successful beginning can haunt the remainder of the relationship.

Engagement with the child must occur concurrently with the establishment of the family's trust. The young child will take cues on trust and behavior toward the nurse from the parents, and engaging their support is certainly important. The parents' acceptance of the nurse does not ensure acceptance by the child, however. Home care nurses who care for children are usually quite experienced in introducing themselves to infants and children, but it should be emphasized that the child will feel less obliged to respond politely when on home turf than when in a health care facility. Children may resent the nurse's "invasion" of the security of their home, particularly if nurses are linked with memories of painful procedures during a recent hospitalization. It is helpful to plan extra time to spend with the child on the engagement visit. The nurse should anticipate fears based on the child's developmental stage and plan ways to reassure the child about the purpose of the home visits. As always, honesty is essential. If the home visits will occasionally involve a venipuncture or other unpleasant procedure, the child needs to know this in order to best marshall coping defenses. It is best if such procedures can be avoided on the initial visit.

Assessment

Assessment begins with the first visit and continues throughout the nurse's involvement with the family. Unlike assessment in the hospital, which focuses primarily on the child's response to disease, assessment in the home is equally concerned with the *environment* in which this response takes place. The first task in assessment within the home is to clarify the perceptions of the nurse and family regarding home care.

Clarification of perceptions can be accomplished by using the same criteria that were used by the hospital-based nurse in the initial step of the nursing process: trust, information, resources, and guidance and support. As the nurse gathers data on the feelings of the child and family, these criteria will ensure discussion of the meaning of the illness, the degree of confidence in the ability to implement the plan of treatment, the degree of confidence in involved health care professionals, the adequacy of resources, and the access to guidance and support. Assessment continues throughout the home care process, to document changes in these baseline criteria as changes occur in the child's condition.

The perceptions of the child must not be equated with those of the family. Soliciting the child's impressions of the illness and of life within the family and community provides an opportunity for the nurse to correct unfounded fears and identify the child's high-priority problems. For example, Becky's mother may be most concerned about obtaining an inexpensive replacement for the broken nebulizer, while Becky's concern about her newly diagnosed cystic fibrosis is that the children in kindergarten won't play with her at recess, because they think they will catch her disease. Because of their own anxiety and concerns Becky's parents may not always realize Becky's perceptions. The nurse can facilitate family functioning by enhancing family communication.

Ongoing physical assessment of the child is the counterpart to the assessment of environmental factors. The home care nurse must be highly skilled in physical assessment in order to make judgments about the need for medical consultation or changes in the treatment plan. The nurse must be alert for untoward effects of medications, for signs and symptoms of acute secondary illnesses, and for altered growth and development. A great deal of judgment is required to distinguish between a condition that "just bears watching" and one that requires immediate referral.

Intervention

The phase of intervention combines the nurse's delivery of direct care and the supervision of the care given by the family. In both planning and implementation it is important to realize that the nurse's role in the home is different from that in an acute care facility. The major differences are

1. In the home care setting the family, not the nurse, is in charge
2. The nurse functions more often in a consultant role than in a delivery-of-care role in the home care setting
3. The home care setting changes the focus of care from illness-oriented care to wellness-oriented care
4. The "client" in home care is the entire family
5. The nurse's skills of collaboration and coordination are utilized extensively

Changes in Family Processes. Just as home care marks differences in the role of the nurse, it dictates changes in family roles and family function. Ideally, the home is a place of refuge from larger social pressures, a place where love and support is assured, a place for privacy and for being oneself. Whether or not the home fulfills such ideal functions, home care can be quite disruptive. The family living room or dining room may become the ill child's bedroom so that constant supervision is made easier. Equipment normally found only in hospitals may buzz and hiss during the day and the family may be awakened by monitor alarms at night. Mealtimes may be disrupted by the ill child's treatment schedule. Privacy is threatened by the equipment vendor who walks through the house pushing a new oxygen tank on a dolly, and by the visits from the tutor, the physical therapist, the nutritionist, and the nurse. When exhaustion of one or both parents necessitates respite care or a "night nurse" the family boundaries collapse still further. Siblings, who may at first find the changes a novelty, soon wish for their former share of the parents' attention, and behavior problems are common. It is a scenario in which the family may feel an increasing loss of control. For this reason it is important to remember that the home is the family's domain and that the family must be allowed to remain in charge. The parents must be involved in all decisions, whether those decisions involve changing the schedule for medications or only whether to move the bed across the room. Only the family can determine the emotional price they are willing to pay to keep the ill child at home.

Planning Teaching Sessions. In the role of consultant, the nurse will be evaluating the adequacy of the care given and teaching modifications of care as necessary. It is important to determine *when* the child and parents are ready to learn about additional aspects of the illness or of the treatment plan. At a time when the family is reacting to the stress of a serious or prolonged illness, their coping patterns are likely to involve both emotion-focused and problem-focused behavior (Lazarus and Folkman, 1984). Emotion-focused coping is directed at the feelings evoked by the illness, the recent hospitalization, the physical and emotional discomfort, and the frustration of an altered life style. Emotion-focused coping marks a time at which the distress is felt acutely by the individual and is dealt with by such actions as blaming self and others, by emotional outbursts, by talking about the situation, and by attempts to diminish the emotional effect through distraction or activity. When the individual is in this coping mode factual information is of limited use.

Problem-focused coping is directed at managing the problem, and since information is necessary to problem-solving, teaching will be best accepted at this time. Problem-focused coping may be distinguished from emotion-focused coping by behaviors that indicate the person is intent on the problem itself rather than on the feelings it produces. Signs of this focus in the parents and child include a less anxious demeanor, an indicated interest in learning more about the situation, close observation of the nurse's care activities, and client-initiated discussion of possible solutions to a particular aspect of the overall problem.

Treatment methods will need to be adapted to the individual home care setting, to the abilities of the caregivers, and to the family composition (e.g., small children in the home who might play with equipment settings or who might pose an increased infection risk to the ill child). Considerations specific to posthospital care of various illnesses are addressed throughout Unit Seven of this text under the sections *Nursing Strategies for Follow-Up Care in the Home or Clinic.* (Consult the index for each illness.)

Facilitating Normal Family Function. Whereas the hospital setting is illness-oriented, the home setting focuses on normalization. Meeting the needs of the child and the family will mean facilitating normal family function. This context sounds very wholesome but nurses occasionally have trouble adjusting to the change in focus. For example, normalization of family activities and inclusion of the ill child may mean hugs from a sister with dirty hands who sneezes in the ill child's face. Although the parent may have little problem with this, it will elicit a reflex shudder in many nurses. The goals of treatment, if carefully assessed, often allow such "normalization" but the key will be the ability of the nurse to be flexible and openminded and to consider the ill child's mental and spiritual health as well as the physical health.

The fact that the "client" in the home care setting is the entire family makes this one of the most demanding roles in nursing. It is one thing to give lip service to family involvement in a more traditional setting, and quite another to feel responsible for facilitating the holistic health of a family in their home during a health care crisis of one of the family members. Family assessment is essential to determine in what areas functioning is adaptive and where help is needed (see Chapter 12 for an indepth discussion of family assessment and intervention).

Coordinating Care. Because of the complexity of services involved in the home care setting someone must fill the role of care coordinator. The outcome criteria established before hospital discharge will help to determine whether the nurse is best suited for this role or whether the parents wish to assume partial or full responsibility. The nurse's collaborative skills will be important even if the parents act as care coordinators. As needs for services become apparent, the nurse is in the best position to suggest involvement of other personnel and to facilitate their smooth entry into the home care support team. If it becomes necessary for the child to be hospitalized again, the home care nurse can facilitate the hospital plan of care by sharing effective home care techniques, such as allowing the child to drink medications from a favorite red cup. *Cooperative action between home care nurses and nurses in the hospital can decrease the stress of hospitalization for the entire family.* It can also help to ensure that developmental exercises that were begun in the home are continued throughout the hospital stay so that the child does not regress unnecessarily.

Termination

Termination is that difficult, but necessary, part of the nurse-family relationship in which home visits and telephone contacts are gradually discontinued. Termination occurs when the child's condition no longer warrents professional involvement in the home, either because of death or improvement in health status, or because the family is ready to assume full responsibility for the treatment plan.

The child and family should be prepared for termination at the outset of the relationship (Lenihan, 1985). During the engagement stage the boundaries for home care involvement should be discussed in relation to the goals of treatment. This early preparation will help prevent feelings of abandonment when the support of the home care team must be terminated.

Ironically, the more successful the relationship has been, the more difficult it will be to end it. If home visits have occurred for a period of months the termination phase may find the family in a stage in which community support resources are less available. As extended family and friends become less attentive to the family's needs, reliance on the home care nurse increases. It is important, therefore, that assessment be ongoing to help the family increase and diversify its sources of support, avoiding total dependence on the home care nurse.

The child and family should be encouraged to express their feelings about the termination of services. Feelings of sadness should be acknowledged as normal and appropriate. The family should know that their feelings of insecurity are a common reaction to termination and should be reminded of their growth in skills and of their bonds with ongoing sources of care in the physician's office or clinic. If the relationship was therapeutic, the sadness that may occur with termination is offset by the growth that has been experienced by both the family and the nurse as a result of the interactions.

Evaluation

This final component is actually integral to each of the other components of the nursing process. Evaluation is made during assessment and analysis, is provided for when desired outcomes are determined, and is an essential part of intervention techniques. The danger is that certain aspects of evaluation become so natural to many nurses that other parts of evaluation can be forgotten. For effective evaluation, the progress toward desired outcomes (client goals) must be determined. If the evaluation criteria have not been met, one must ask why. Was the initial outcome, or any part of it, unrealistic or based on inaccurate assessment data? Were the strategies used to meet the goal ineffective? If the evaluation criteria were partially met, then what, if anything, needs to be done to ensure continued progress toward the desired goal? If the criteria have been fully met, which goal replaces this one in priority?

The need for effective and timely evaluation must not be underestimated. A care plan that is appropriate this week may be ineffective next week because of changes in the child's status or in the environment. The parents and nurse should discuss the adequacy of the current plan of care at each home visit, and changes should be made accordingly. For example, a child with an inoperable tumor may be discharged to home care with the understanding that pain will be controlled by oral medications and that ambulation is permitted as tolerated. A few weeks later this same child may be experiencing pain despite increased dosages of pain medications, and may now be bedridden because of weakness and vertigo. The family, at this point, could be experiencing reduced assistance from family and community support systems, might be noticing maladaptive behavior from siblings, and might be physically and emotionally unable to manage the child's care in light of the present symptoms. If the plan of care has not been revised to accommodate the changes in the child's condition, the family's position may be, "we tried it and it didn't work." The resulting frustration will undermine the family's personal sense of competence and adequacy and will complicate their future relationships with health care professionals.

Types of Home Care

The nursing process in home care will be greatly influenced by the reason for home care. The types of home care for children can be grouped into three categories: acute, chronic, and terminal.

Home Care for Acute Conditions

Care that is needed only on a short-term basis can be labeled acute home care. This type of care might be appropriate for a neonate undergoing home phototherapy for hyperbilirubinemia, or for a child requiring one or two follow-up visits after outpatient surgery.

One type of acute home care that is becoming more prevalent is perinatal home care. The perinatal home care specialist visits mothers and their neonates who have been discharged as early as 6 hours after an uncomplicated delivery. Follow-up visits occur in the home for an average of 3 days following dismissal. The mother's postpartum status is assessed and the baby is weighed and receives a physical examination. The nurse takes care to reinforce parent-infant bonding and effective parenting practices. There is an opportunity to discuss the family's adjustment to the newcomer, including infant sleep patterns and the parents' ability to get needed rest. The parents are often asked to keep a log of the infant's sleep times, feedings, and diapers. This chart is then reviewed by the nurse and discussed with the parents so that their concerns may be addressed.

Perinatal home care can be a very rewarding nursing practice. The nurse has the opportunity to affect the remainder of the parent-child relationship positively by helping the family to get off to a good start. The home setting can be optimal for teaching, and parents of newborn infants are usually anxious to learn how best to care for their baby. Learning is facilitated in this setting because parents are less anxious in their own home, and because they have had the opportunity to anticipate the visit and to prepare questions. Learning is also enhanced by the immediate "need to know." In the hospital, when there are nurses readily available to assist with the infant's care, the full weight of parental responsibility may not be as apparent. After the family is home with their baby, they are usually very receptive

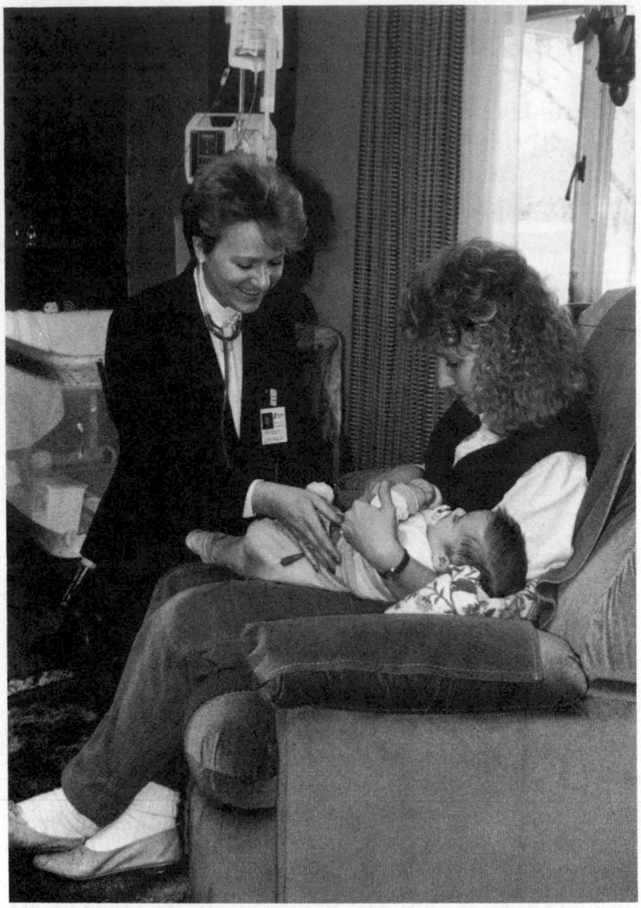

Home IV therapy can decrease the number of hospitalizations for children with either acute or chronic illness. (Courtesy of Children's Home Care of The Children's Hospital, Denver.)

to suggestions that will facilitate the necessary adjustments.

The perinatal home care specialist may also be involved in home visits to help parents work through the grief process when an infant dies at birth. Professional intervention at this time can greatly facilitate the necessary outpouring of emotion and can provide the information needed for problem solving and grief resolution.

Home Care for Chronic Conditions

This category is most accurately divided into short-term and long-term care. *Short-term care* is used to meet acute care needs in families with chronically ill children. Short-term care may also be thought of as care during the interim adjustment period between hospital-based professional management of the condition and home-based family management. A common example is the infant who is discharged from an intensive care nursery with oxygen-dependent bronchopulmonary dysplasia. Short-term home care may be instituted to ensure the family's adjustment to the baby's oxygen dependency, and will be terminated as soon as the family can manage the condition with occasional clinic visits.

Long-term care for a chronically ill child occurs when the family will need continuing support to maintain home care. Children who are multiply handicapped or who are ventilator-dependent usually require home care on a long-term basis, including some in-home direct care by a home health aide or registered nurse. The cost-effectiveness of long-term care is reflected in a report from the Children's Home Health Network of Illinois. It showed that even with home care provided by a registered nurse, the cost to manage the care of a ventilator-dependent child at home was 77 per cent less than for hospital management (Kahn, 1984).

Long-term home care for chronically ill children is often the family's only alternative to long-term institutionalization. There are obvious advantages to the child in being able to accept a role within the family and to have the opportunity for development within an optimal environment. The family itself will realize both advantages and disadvantages to long-term care. The disruption of family life and the intense physical and emotional demands experienced have been previously discussed. For many families these problems are offset by the opportunity to complete the family circle and to participate fully in the child's life.

Home Care for Terminal Conditions

The goal in home care for terminally ill children is to enhance the quality of life for the child and to give the family an opportunity to share their love and grief with the child in the privacy and comfort of the home setting. The Martinson (1977) model continues to provide a prototype for this kind of home care. The parents are supported in their efforts to provide pain control and physical comfort for the child, and open communication between the child and other family members is encouraged. Sometimes the parents will need to maintain a central venous catheter or peripheral intravenous site, but often care at this stage is devoid of the trappings of modern science. The focus instead is on the psychosocial adjustment to impending death and grief.

Termination of home care for terminally ill children occurs not at the child's death, but after the involved home care professionals have attended the funeral and provided follow-up visits to ensure that family members are either attaining a healthy adjustment or are referred for further professional support.

Text continues on page 1012

Table 32-1
Nursing Process Plan: Home Care

by Roxie Foster

Assessment of Emotional-Social Function (Family)*

Coping-Stress-Tolerance Patterns
Spiritual Health

Subjective Assessment

Roles of family members; concerns and worries related to necessary adjustments to home care; adequacy of predischarge planning; verbalizations related to adaptation/coping of family members. Ask whether family is still committed to home care of ill child

Objective Assessment

Family communication processes; organizational skills; adequacy of equipment and supplies for care of ill child; personal grooming of family members; behavior of siblings; whether caretakers appear fatigued or rested

Analysis: Nursing Diagnosis 1

Potential altered family processes, related to incomplete adjustment to the physical, intellectual, emotional, and spiritual stress of home care for an ill child

Defining Characteristics

Subjective: Verbalization of ineffective communication among family members; concerns about interactions with health care professionals, equipment vendors, community agencies, insurance companies. Verbalized feelings of being overwhelmed, fatigued, having no time for self, feeling unable to cope with "all the details" of the ill child's care in addition to other family responsibilities; feelings of guilt and inadequacy; difficulty in finding meaning and purpose in life. "Not sure we made the right decision in bringing (child) home"

Objective: Family members displaying poor eye contact with each other; tension evident in verbal exchanges. Poor organizational skills; inadequate equipment, food, clean clothing for ill child; altered decision-making skills; siblings demanding of parental attention

Client Goal/ Evaluation Criteria	Nursing Goals/Strategies (Selected Rationale)
1. The family will regain the ability to meet the physical, emotional, and spiritual needs of its members, as evidenced by: a. lessening tension in interactions between/among family members	*Determine: (1) whether disruption in family processes likely to resolve with additional time, (2) whether family resources are adequate to meet demands of adjustment period, (3) whether additional support services needed, (4) whether to recommend continuation or discontinuation of home care.* • Assess caretakers' physical, emotional ability to implement the therapeutic regimen. Evaluate whether care being performed as prescribed.

*Consult the discussions of specific illnesses for diagnoses and strategies related to physical, emotional-social, and intellectual-perceptual function of the ill child.

Continued

Client Goal/ Evaluation Criteria	Nursing Goals/Strategies (Selected Rationale)
b. effective communication with health care professionals and support services c. healthy problem solving d. caretakers receiving adequate rest e. adequate supplies on hand for ill child's care f. verbalization of increased confidence, decreased stress g. adequate organizational skills h. behavior of siblings returning to precrisis status i. verbalization of finding meaning and satisfaction in caring for ill child at home j. increasing ability to coordinate ill child's care	• Assess caretakers' perception of home care. Ask: "What is it like to care for (child) at home?" "What aspects of home care concern you most?" "What gives you the most satisfaction?" "Who can help you with that?" "Do you want to continue home care?" If no, "What do you see as alternatives?" • Assess ill child's perception of home care. Ask: "What do you like best about being at home?" "Are there things about the hospital that you miss?" "What do you wish for most?" *Support adaptive behavior.* • Recognize and praise adaptive behavior as appropriate: "(Child's) lungs sound so clear; you must be doing well with the chest physical therapy." "This medication schedule is nice, I would like to tell other families about the form you've devised." "(Child) seems so content being here with the family." "How do you manage all these tasks and still find time to read bedtime stories to the other children?" "I'm glad you took some time for yourself yesterday." "Yes, that was the right person to call. It sounds as if you have resolved the problem." *Facilitate adaptive coping.* • With the caregivers, identify specific problems and goals related to care of the ill child. • Modify the child's plan of care as the goals, strategies, and evaluation criteria change. See Figure 32–2 for an example. • Suggest time-saving ways to organize the child's care. • With the caregivers, identify problems and goals related to family processes. • Reach agreement on goals to improve family processes and discuss resources and strategies to meet the goals. • Encourage family consultation with members of the clergy or others who can help members regain peace of mind and a sense of purpose. • Make referrals to other community agencies when family resources are inadequate. Draw upon the family's resources whenever possible. (Ordinarily the overall goal is to help the family become self-reliant.) • With the family's permission contact the school nurse to obtain support for the school- age ill child and for school-age siblings. • Discuss with caregivers the need for and sources of respite care. *Encourage the family to normalize family processes as much as possible.* • Assess the family's perception of "normal" family life style. Discuss with them the aspects that are most valued and encourage them to continue those activities/relationships to the extent possible. • Discuss acceptable ways to modify the ill child's care to accommodate the usual family lifestyle. • Reinforce the importance of planning time for self, spouse, and other children. (Without this encouragement, family members may feel guilty about planning time away from the ill child.)

- Suggest that siblings be allowed to help in age-appropriate ways as family responsibilities are shifted to accommodate home care. (Helping can give siblings a feeling of worth and a sense of importance at a time when they might otherwise feel insecure.)
- Acknowledge siblings' "helper" roles when visiting the ill child (to promote their sense of self-worth and accomplishment).

Assessment of Intellectual-Perceptual Function

Health Perception/Management
Knowledge of Illness/Health Management

Subjective Assessment

Questions from caregivers/child about physical care, procedures, medications, alterations in usual activities

Objective Assessment

Ability to provide physical and emotional care related to illness and well-child care

Analysis: Nursing Diagnosis 2

Potential knowledge deficit, related to

- *procedures, medications*
- *signs and symptoms that warrant calling the nurse or physician*
- *ways to promote normal growth and development*
- *well-child care*
- *community resources*

Defining Characteristics

Subjective: Verbalizing the need for further information/instruction

Objective: Unable to perform certain aspects of care related to illness management. Concentration on illness care to the exclusion of well-child care

Client Goals/Evaluation Criteria

2.1 The child/family will display the knowledge and skills needed to perform the prescribed treatment at home, as evidenced by:
   a. effective implementation of prescribed therapy
   b. proper operation and cleaning of equipment
   c. expected progress in child's health status

Nursing Goals/Strategies (Selected Rationale)

Assess the quality of physical care.

- *Observe* therapeutic procedures instead of performing them.
- Ask to see the record of medication given and any other treatment or status records kept by the family.
- Determine caregivers' perception of progress toward the goals of therapy (to assess understanding of evaluation criteria).

Provide instructions as needed.

- Correct misconceptions and potentially harmful breaks in technique. Remain open, however, to innovations in strategies that make care easier for family members and that still accomplish the goal (i.e., evaluate whether the technique *must* be done exactly as taught in the hospital).

Continued

Client Goal/ Evaluation Criteria	Nursing Goals/Strategies (Selected Rationale)
d. identifying signs and symptoms that warrant medical intervention e. discussing appropriate emergency procedures f. demonstrating ability to perform cardiopulmonary resuscitation (CPR)	• Ensure that instruction is given tactfully and that caregivers are not admonished for being novices. Use phrases like, "This takes a great deal of practice," and "You may find it easier if you . . ." (If caregivers perceive they are being scolded for breaks in technique, they will be less likely to ask for help. Open communication is vital to a therapeutic relationship.) • Encourage questions and discussion of care. *Ensure family is prepared for an emergency.* • Ask where family keeps list of emergency numbers and when it was last updated. • Ensure that the following agencies have been notified of the family's potential need for emergency service: telephone company, electric company, fire department, emergency medical services, police department. • Periodically assist family members to update CPR skills. *Record teaching and other nursing interventions in detailed form to document the need for professional nursing care.* (Proper charting is essential to document eligibility for home care and to facilitate payment for services rendered.)
2.2 The child will receive appropriate well-child care, as evidenced by: a. keeping well-child appointments b. immunizations up to date c. expected progress in height and weight d. expected progress on developmental tasks	*Emphasize well-child needs.* • Weigh and measure the child regularly. Discuss the child's progress on growth charts. • Remind caregivers of the need to make and keep well-child appointments. (The child may be seeing a specialist for illness care and may need to have a separate appointment for routine well-child care.) • Regularly assess child's progress on developmental tasks. Alert family to pertinent tasks and discuss with them ways to help the child accomplish tasks in light of acute or chronic illness condition.

The role of the home care nurse in terminal care, or hospice care, is extremely demanding. Watters (1986) observed that "hospice is an area of work in which good will, compassion, common sense, and honesty are highly valued" (p. 222). The rewards of this type of nursing are knowing that the therapeutic relationship has met some very special needs—that it has provided a loving atmosphere for the child during the last days of life and precious memories for the family.

The Future of Home Health Care for Children

Home care for all segments of the population is expected to grow in response to the social demands for cost-effective, quality care (Coleman and Smith, 1984; Hansen, 1986). Continued growth is expected, as well, in the market for pediatric home care (Punch, 1985). The home care explosion has implications for expanded roles for nursing and for many allied health professionals. Hansen (1986) has predicted that as home health care becomes recognized as a specialty, salaries will be adjusted upward. Nursing education will soon respond with increased emphasis in undergraduate areas on adaptation of technical skills to home care settings, and masters and doctoral degrees in home health care will begin to be offered. Computerization, which is currently being piloted in many community health agencies, will simplify documentation and record keeping. Technology will spawn not only increasingly sophisticated equipment for home use but also more support services for its maintenance.

There is one part of the future of home health care that will remain the same — the basic needs of children and families involved. Whatever the technologic advances of the future may hold, the effectiveness of home care will still be dependent on the nurse who understands the effect of illness on children and families and who is prepared to support them in their adjustment.

References

Bock RH, et al: There's no place like home. *Child Health Care* 1983; 12(2):93–96.

Cherryholmes LG: The qualities of a home health care nurse. *In* Stuart-Siddall, S (ed): *Home Health Care Nursing.* Rockville, MD, Aspen Systems, 1986, pp 155–162.

Davis JH, Eyer J: Sorting out new mothers' learning priorities on home visits. *Home Healthcare Nurse* 1984; 2(5):38–42.

Elkins JL: Nursing the patient and family in their own environment. *In* Stuart-Siddal S (ed): *Home Health Care Nursing.* Rockville, MD, Aspen Systems, 1986, pp 179–188.

Farrell MP, Schmitt MH: The American family: An historical perspective. *In* Hymovich DP, Barnard MU (eds): *Family Health Care* (Vol 1). New York, McGraw-Hill, 1979, pp 57–74.

Hansen JW: Future trends in home health care. *In* Stuart-Siddall S (ed): *Home Health Care Nursing.* Rockville, MD, Aspen Systems, 1986, pp 255–270.

Hillman SM: Assessing the patient in the home environment. *In* Stuart-Siddall S (ed): *Home Health Care Nursing.* Rockville, MD, Aspen Systems, 1986, pp 163–177.

Hymovich DP: Parents of sick children: Their needs and tasks. *Pediatr Nurs* 1976, 2.9–13.

Janz KC, Burgess B: Home health care. *Stanford Nurse* 1985; 7(3):9.

Kahn L: Ventilator-dependent children heading home. *Hospitals* 1984; 58(5):54–55.

Kaufman J, Hardy-Ribakow D: Home care: a model of a comprehensive approach for technology-assisted chronically ill children. *J Pediatr Nurs* 1988 Aug; 2(4):244–249.

Lazarus RS, Folkman S: *Stress, Appraisal, and Coping.* New York, Springer, 1984.

Lenihan S: The young child and the home health care nurse: problems, challenges, and intervention strategies. *Home Healthcare Nurse* 1985; 3(6):6–9.

Martinson IM, et al: Home care for the child. *Am J Nurs* 1977; 77:1815–1817.

Mundinger MO: *Home Care Controversy.* Rockville, MD, Aspen Systems, 1983.

Pierce PM, Friedman SA: The REACH project: an innovative health delivery model for medically dependent children. *Child Health Care* 1983; 12(2):86–89.

Punch L: Pediatric home care expands as new technology is developed. *Modern Healthcare* 1985; 15(14):152, 154.

Rogatz P: Home health care: some social and economic considerations. *Home Healthcare Nurse* 1985; 3(1):38–43.

Stuart-Siddall S: What is a home health care nurse? *Home Healthcare Nurse* 1984; 2(4):1.

Watters PS: Hospice nursing. *In* Stuart-Siddall S (ed): *Home Health Care Nursing.* Rockville, MD, Aspen Systems, 1986, pp 215–223.

Wright LW, Leahy M: *Nurses and Families: A Guide to Family Assessment and Intervention.* Philadelphia, FA Davis, 1984.

Bibliography

Betz CL: The pediatric patient: strategies for improving interactions. *Home Healthcare Nurse* 1985; 3(4):11–17.

Coleman JR, Smith DS: DRGs and growth of home health care. *Nurs Economics* 1984; 2:391–395.

Edwardson SR: Using research in practice: factors associated with the adoption of a nursing innovation. *West J Nurs Res* 1984; 6(1):141–143.

Fergusson J, Hobbie W: Home visits for the child with cancer. *Nurs Clin North Am* 1985; 20(1):109–115.

Home care for children with serious handicapping conditions. Proceedings of a conference sponsored by the Association for the Care of Children's Health and the Division of Maternal and Child Health, Public Health Service, US Department of Health and Human Services, Houston, TX, May, 1984.

Ness PL, Huchala B: Adaptation of the community to children with chronic illnesses and their families. *In* Rose MH, Thomas RB: *Children with Chronic Conditions. Nursing in a Family and Community Context.* Orlando, FL, Grune & Stratton, 1987, 55–64.

No huge profit potential seen in home care. *Hospitals* 1984; 58(22):70.

Reif L: Making dollars and sense of home health policy. *Nurs Economics* 1984; 2:382–389.

Norris-Berkemeyer S, Hutchins KH: Home apnea monitoring. *Pediatr Nurs* 1986 Jul/Aug; 12(4):259–262.

Rossen S: Adapting discharge planning to prospective pricing. *Hospitals* 1984; 58(5):71–79.

Shamansky SL, Boase JC, Horn BM: Discharge planning: yesterday, today, and tomorrow. *Home Healthcare Nurse* 1984; 2(3):14–20.

Smith JB: Home care is more than Medicare regs. *Am J Nurs* 1987 Mar; 305–306.

Wildblood RA, Strezo PL: The how-to's of home IV therapy. *Pediatr Nurs* 1987 Jan/Feb; 13(1):42–46, 68.

Developmental-Behavioral Health Concerns

Unit Six

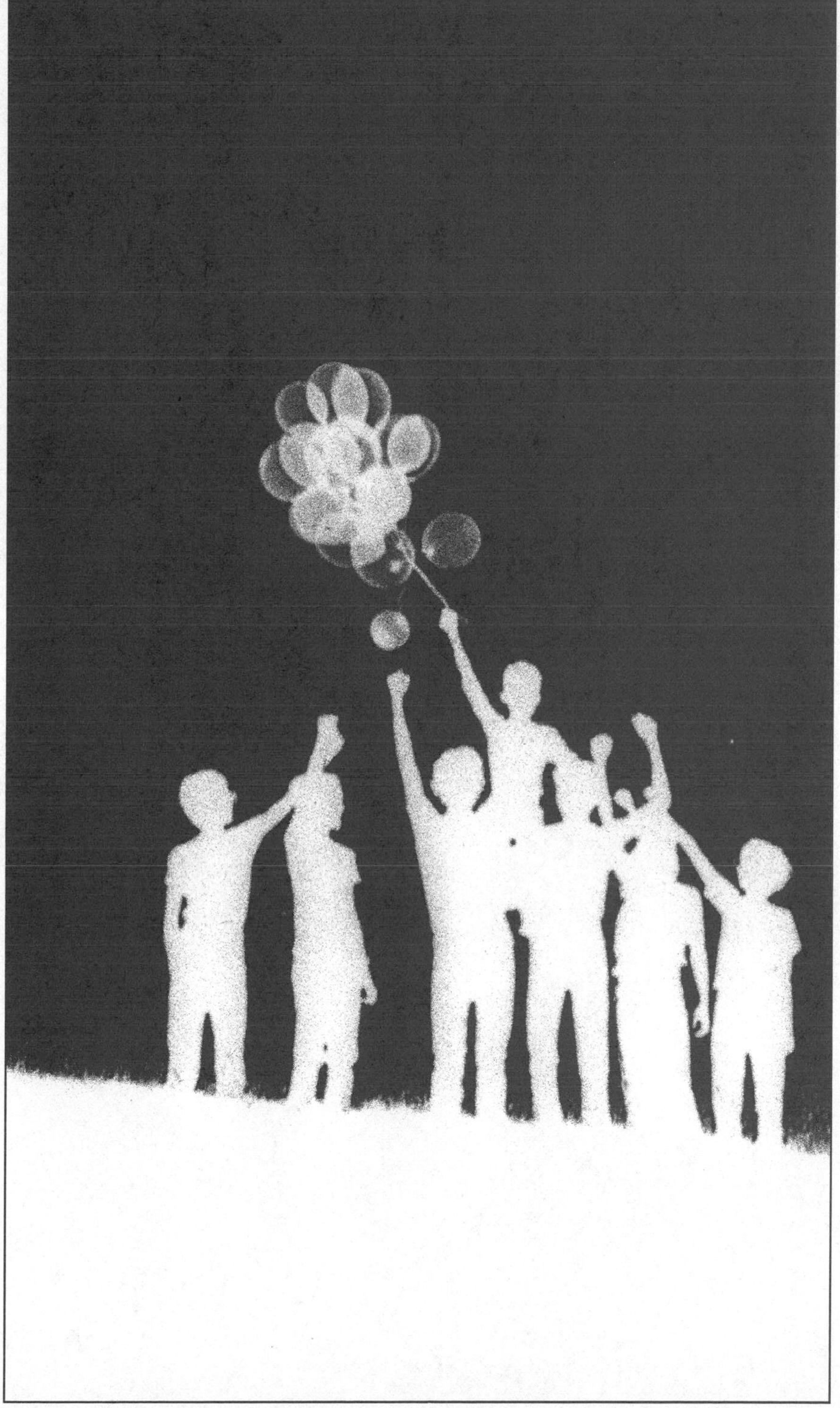

Understanding Altered Behavior

Chapter 33

Jo Joyce Anderson
Ann Wiebmer

Behavioral alteration is steadily permeating pediatric nursing practice. Behavioral assessment and management skills are a critical component of holistic pediatric practice. The intent of this chapter is to acquaint the nurse with the multifaceted dimensions of behavioral alteration etiology and present the function of the nurse in identifying and assessing behavioral alteration, participating in behavioral management, and making appropriate referral to facilitate the healthy behavioral development of children and their families. Legal, ethical, and community issues surrounding behavioral interventions are presented.

Related Topics
Development of children; inborn differences in temperament, Chapter 3
Family health appraisals and identification of high risk families, Chapter 12
Promoting healthy parenting, Chapter 13
Development of self-esteem, Chapter 16
Stress, crisis, and coping, Chapter 23
Behavioral and psychiatric disorders, Chapter 36

Assessing Behavioral Alterations

Society is concerned about and intolerant of children whose behavior is not consistent with the norms and standards adults have established for children. Thus, health care professionals have the task of identifying children with altered behavior and finding effective interventions that will redirect them toward healthier development. However, recognition of these children with problem behavior is often difficult because of the fine line that exists between "normal" and "altered" behavior.

Defining Altered Behavior

There is no rigid distinction between problem children and other children. The difference is a matter of degree. *Problematic behaviors are essentially exaggerations of, deficiencies in, or a maladaptive combination of behavior patterns common to all children.* In contrast to an emotionally disturbed child who suffers from severe and fundamental personality defects, a behaviorally disordered child shows an inability to cope with a current or ongoing situation (Taylor, 1982). The child's coping responses are considered to be behaviorally altered when the behaviors are unacceptable or inappropriate, as judged by societal standards or norms. Ten Bensel and Tobin (1975) define a behavior problem as an activity that "deviates from a discretionary social norm with a frequency or intensity that authoritative adults in the child's environment judge to be too high or too low."

Society expects that behavior is to be understandable, consistent, and controlled. The behaviorally altered child displays few or none of these characteristics. Instead, the child behaves inconsistently and unpredictably; the motivation of the behavior seems at least illogical, if not totally unintelligible. The behavior is frequently uncontrollable, regardless of the setting. It is not surprising that the child usually makes poor adjustments to societal institutions (e.g., family, school, social gatherings, camp).

Frequency, intensity, appropriateness, and predictability of behavior are not the only parameters to be used by the health professional in defining altered behavior. Age and developmental level, temperament, cultural orientation, and environmental stressors all have to be weighed.

Age and Development as Variables

An understanding of normal patterns of growth and development is needed if the health professional is to identify accurately behavioral alteration in a child. Certain behaviors that bother adults commonly occur at particular developmental stages and ages, eventually to be outgrown. While common and appropriate at one age, the behaviors may suggest behavioral disorders at another age. For example, temper tantrums are a normal demonstration of toddlers' struggles for individuality and autonomy, but a pattern of temper tantrums in a 9-year-old is not in keeping with developmental age. Likewise, behaviors such as stuttering, phobias, and nightmares, although perplexing to parents, usually arise at certain ages and gradually disappear without any consequences. The health professional who is asked for help by parents concerned about a child's behavior must know these developmental milestones to reassure parents about a normal behavior or to initiate further assessment. (Refer to Chapter 3 and Chapters 5 through 9 for a review of developmental stage characteristics.)

Temperament as a Variable

Temperament describes the way in which individuals behave or respond to their environment. (The easy, difficult, and slow-to-warm or combined temperament patterns are discussed in detail on pages 111 to 113.) An individual's temperament is relatively consistent over time and significantly influences the spontaneity with which one adapts to new situations, the intensity with which one reacts to one's environment, and the characteristic nature of one's mood tendencies. People tend to be cheerful, positive, and optimistic or to be irritable, negative, and pessimistic in response to life situations. Children with difficult temperaments are more vulnerable to behavioral problems in early and middle childhood, with 70 per cent demonstrating at least mild reactive behavioral alteration by age 10 years (Chess and Thomas, 1983). Carey's studies (1972) revealed that children with difficult temperaments who had handicaps or mental retardation were at even greater risk, and the difficult-temperament child with a mentally ill parent is at greatest risk for behavioral alteration. However, we emphasize that any child, regardless of temperament, is vulnerable to behavioral problems if the demands for change and adaptation are beyond his or her capabilities.

Various methods can be used by the health professional to determine a child's temperament pattern. Questionnaires are available (see Box 33-4 for sources) for the professional whose time permits. Temperament also can be determined through observation of and interaction with the child, through questions included in the health history (Levine et al, 1983, present a model), or by questioning the child's caretakers. This assessment is pertinent from several perspectives. The assessment process is an opportunity to discuss the child's temperament with parents and to educate them regarding temperament implications in parenting approach, health management, and child care methods. Parents of the difficult or slow-to-warm child can receive reassurance that their child's behavior is characteristic for his or her temperament and not necessarily a response to their parenting style; their child is not an antisocial misfit. This discussion also affords an opportunity for preventive counseling that might alleviate future behavioral problems stemming from parent-child conflicts because the parents did not understand their child's temperament. Box 33-1 lists situations when a child's temperament should be considered by the health professional.

The demands of socialization are particularly stressful for children with difficult and, to a lesser degree, slow-to-warm temperaments because of their slow adaptability and intense negative withdrawal reactions to new situations, places, and people. The children (and later as adults) may have difficulty sleeping through the night, may have wide swings in appetite and frequent gastrointestinal complaints, and often have diarrhea or constipation. Their delay in adapting may make them less acceptable as family members and with peers, further interfering with socialization.

Box 33-1
Issues and Situations in Which Temperament May Be Significant for the Clinician

Reassurance of parents that child's deviation from culturally desirable norm does not mean pathology in child or bad parenting. Especially true with difficult or slow-to-warm-up child.

Child care advice specified in terms of child's temperament, such as approach to weaning, toilet training, and the like.

Evaluation of severity of acute physical illness by estimating deviation of child's behavior from usual temperament. Also, temperament may affect reaction to illness.

Evaluation and management of specific symptoms such as colic, night waking, or "hyperactivity" as partially influenced by temperament.

Child's adaptation to beginning nursery school or day care center as influenced by reactions to new situation and speed of adaptation.

Ease or difficulty of child's establishment of peer relations.

School functioning—optimal style of classwork and homework schedule in relation to degree of persistence and distractability.

In behavior disorders, identification of influence of temperament and the specific pattern of "poorness of fit."

Special influences of temperament in the physically handicapped and the mentally retarded.

(From Levine et al, 1983.)

Goodness of Fit as a Variable

How a child's attributes "fit" with those of parent(s), teachers, and other caretakers influences the degree of conflict and stress the child experiences in the socialization process. The phenomenon of the "problem fit" needs to be considered by the health professional (Chess et al, 1970; Thomas and Chess, 1977, 1980; Chess and Thomas, 1983). Depending upon the temperaments of the parents and the child, with goodness of fit the child develops into one described as "just like me," or with poorness of fit becomes a "problem child." It is difficult to differentiate between the child whose behavior represents a maladaptive attempt to cope with life experiences and the child whose temperament confounds the tolerance of the caretakers. A temperamentally hard-to-please child born to temperamentally hard-to-please parents portends conflict and interactional problems, whereas a temperamentally hard-to-please child born to easy-going parents may represent a joyful challenge.

A *goodness of fit* exists when the properties of a child's environment and expectations (i.e., parental demands, lifestyle, values) are in harmony with the child's own capacities, motivations, and behavioral style. This does not mean that stress or conflict is absent, but that it is not excessive or continuous. *Poorness of fit* exists when discrepencies and dissonances exist between the child's characteristics and the environmental experiences. Distortions in development and maladaptive behaviors are then more likely. Shonkoff (1983) believes that altered behaviors in children are often "secondary symptoms and self-fulfilling prophecies" that emerge from the parent-child conflicts resulting from poorness of fit.

Some stress and conflict foster constructive growth when in keeping with a child's developmental stage, capacity, and character. The issue in behavioral disturbances is rather one of *excessive* stress created by the poorness of fit.

Excessive Demands and Stress as Variables

Research and observation of people and animals have demonstrated that the most effective coping strategy is to engage the stressor directly. If the result is a partially or completely successful outcome or resolution, self-esteem and confidence increase, preparing one for confrontation with more stressful situations. This is the story of development and healthy living.

However, problems arise when the stressor (expectation or demand) is excessive, unrelenting, or beyond the individual's capabilities to overcome. (Overprotecting the child from normal stress can be equally detrimental.) Defensive strategies are likely to ensue, such as behavioral responses of regression, denial, or avoidance, which are attempts to cope with stressors that the individual cannot or will not confront directly (Levine, 1983). (See Chapter 23 for a full discussion of stress and coping strategies.) These defensive strategies vary in frequency and their effect on development. Sometimes they may be employed temporarily as a stall in a healthy way to allow time to organize one's strengths and capacities for eventual positive resolution of the stressor. This behavior is common in children with slow-to-warm temperaments.

The nurse should investigate the cause when a child demonstrates repeated or excessive use of defense strategies. It is difficult to decide exactly when a child's behavior becomes *excessive.* Brink (1982) suggests that any behavior lasting 3 or more months be considered long-term or excessive. Stewart (1981) suggests that the behavior has reached a serious level when a consistent pattern of several deliberate behavioral alterations is seen for at least a year.

Behavioral alterations in children do indicate some degree of underlying emotional problem, but these children are not "mentally ill." The mentally ill child (also called emotionally disturbed) shows behaviors consonant with personality disorganization. The behaviorally disordered child, on the other hand, maintains an intact sense of self. These children have a lower tolerance of stressful situations, in contrast to "well-adjusted" children. Clunn and Payne (1985) view behavioral disturbances as reactive disorders, which depend less on the severity of the stimulus or stressor than upon the child's reactions and ability to cope adaptively. Problem behaviors are by-products of a child's attempt to cope with how he or she feels about stressful conditions. The child is attempting to deal with life experiences, but a "backfiring" occurs instead. The coping behaviors adopted are ineffective, inappropriate, or self-defeating, resulting in unfavorable consequences for the child and frequently for others. Consequently, behaviorally disordered children are susceptible to developing a "bad me" self-concept that further intensifies their difficulties in socialization.

Self-Concept as a Variable

Behavior is a reflection of self-perception. Self-perception is very much influenced by relationships with others. Even a well-adjusted child sometimes becomes mystified by the complexities of interrelationships. This mystification magnifies in the child whose self-concept is vulnerable. (See Chapter 16 for a discussion of self-concept development.) For example, a child who purposely breaks a toy because a sibling has just received praise from a parent is experiencing jealousy or rivalry, the reaction to which elicits a response from the parent. Even a negative parental response is a reward, for the child is getting something (attention, consideration) in return for the behavior. The child with a vulnerable self-concept learns to use problem behavior to gain notice from others. Social interactions become highly distressful, producing intense anxiety, which results in distortion of the child's judgment of appropriate versus inappropriate behaviors. A child will "shop around" to find those behaviors that get the most responses from those whose attention is sought. The child will also use problem behavior as a strategy to dominate or manipulate people and situations over which the child otherwise feels powerless. The problem behavior, and the response it earns, reinforces the "bad me" perception of the child. A self-fulfilling prophecy is seen: "I think I'm bad—I act bad—I'm told I am bad—I must be bad." Reinforced by this self-concept, the child becomes more and more socially ill at ease. Often the end result is a lonely and estranged individual.

The Etiology of Altered Behavior

Successful socialization has three major components:

- conformity to society's rules;
- pleasurable interpersonal exchanges; and
- satisfaction obtained from the realization of one's capabilities.

From the previous discussion it appears that several variables can influence whether and how successfully a child masters these components. Still the question remains as to why *certain* children embrace problem behaviors, whereas other children learn to behave with

Table 33-1. Variables Predisposing to Healthy Versus Altered Behavior

Variables Predisposing to Healthy Behavior	Variables Predisposing to Altered Behavior
Biologic Factors	
Easy temperament	Slow-to-warm or difficult temperament
Parents with healthy mental state	Genetically transferable mental illness in one or both parents
Physical health intact	Health erratic; or chronic illness, trauma
Normal brain function	Brain damage
Average or better intelligence	Extremely high or low intelligence
Environmental Factors	
Goodness of fit	Poorness of fit
Healthy bonding, attachment	Emotional/maternal deprivation
Parents provide role models for healthy social behavior	Parental deviance modeled
Marital/family harmony	Marital/family discord
Stable home	Unstable, broken home
Personal autonomy and self-care supported	Overprotection, dependency fostered
School success	School difficulties
Positive reinforcement predominates	Negative reinforcement predominates
Self-concept Factors	
Intact self-concept	Vulnerable self-concept
"Good child" cognition	"Bad child" cognition

(Compiled from Herbert, 1975; Levine, 1983.)

social or normative appropriateness. The answer is best found in an interactional perspective that recognizes the interplay of biologic factors, environmental forces, and self-concept cognition (Table 33-1). Herbert (1975) has used the "loaded gun" concept to illustrate the vulnerable child: The child perceives a crisis (precipitating event). The trigger (precipitating event) only fires the already loaded (predisposing factors) gun, releasing the bullet (manifested altered behavior). Predisposing factors may exist long before their effects are seen, but they set the stage for the trigger to snap when a crisis or stressor comes along. When the crisis occurs, the behavior promptly follows. If circumstances exist to perpetuate the behavior, it will be repeated again as a coping behavior, regardless of its effectiveness or consequence. Figure 33-1 diagrams the relationship of these elements.

The health professional must recognize this interplay of variables in the assessment and identification of altered behavior. However, keep in mind that a child's developmental progress may reinforce, modify, or change specific behavior patterns. Early life experiences, while important to development, are not indicative of later behavior, nor are early behavior patterns reliable predictors of later behavior. The health professional acknowledges that there is no single cause of altered behavior patterns. An interactional approach to assessment and, later, to intervention is necessary.

Assessment Criteria and Methods

Criteria have been developed, based on societal norms, to distinguish altered or maladaptive behavior from normal. These criteria must be considered rela-

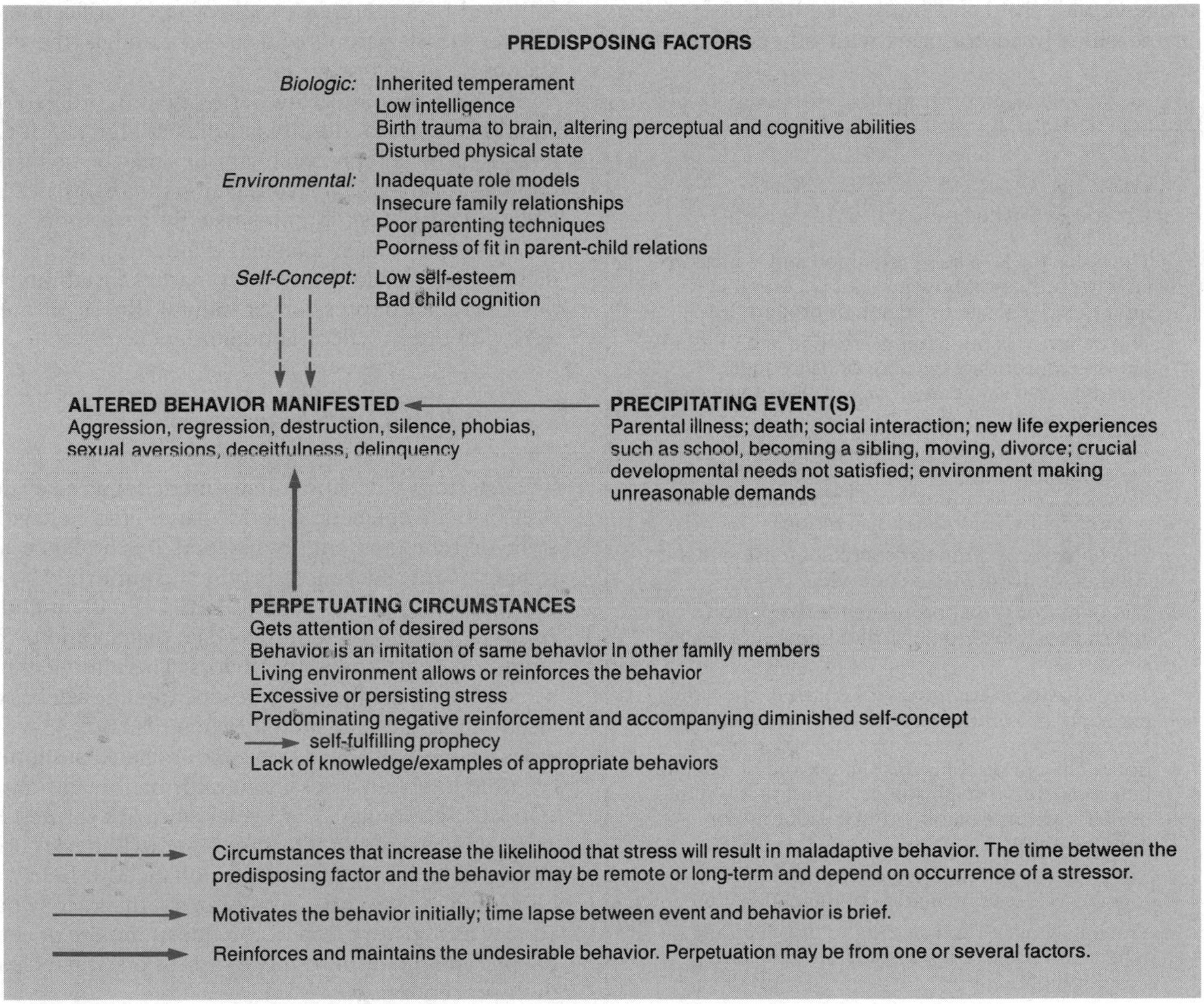
PREDISPOSING FACTORS
Biologic: Inherited temperament
Low intelligence
Birth trauma to brain, altering perceptual and cognitive abilities
Disturbed physical state
Environmental: Inadequate role models
Insecure family relationships
Poor parenting techniques
Poorness of fit in parent-child relations
Self-Concept: Low self-esteem
Bad child cognition
ALTERED BEHAVIOR MANIFESTED
Aggression, regression, destruction, silence, phobias, sexual aversions, deceitfulness, delinquency
PRECIPITATING EVENT(S)
Parental illness; death; social interaction; new life experiences such as school, becoming a sibling, moving, divorce; crucial developmental needs not satisfied; environment making unreasonable demands
PERPETUATING CIRCUMSTANCES
Gets attention of desired persons
Behavior is an imitation of same behavior in other family members
Living environment allows or reinforces the behavior
Excessive or persisting stress
Predominating negative reinforcement and accompanying diminished self-concept
self-fulfilling prophecy
Lack of knowledge/examples of appropriate behaviors
Circumstances that increase the likelihood that stress will result in maladaptive behavior. The time between the predisposing factor and the behavior may be remote or long-term and depend on occurrence of a stressor.
Motivates the behavior initially; time lapse between event and behavior is brief.
Reinforces and maintains the undesirable behavior. Perpetuation may be from one or several factors.

Figure 33-1. An interactional perspective of altered behavior etiology. (Adapted from Herbert M: *Problems of Childhood.* New York, Pan Books, Ltd., 1975; Levine M, et al: *Developmental-Behavioral Pediatrics.* Philadelphia, WB Saunders, 1983.)

tive, however, since "maladaptive" is differently defined by various cultures and socioeconomic groups, by each sex, and according to the age of the person displaying the behavior. Box 33-2 lists useful criteria for diagnosing behavioral disorder. Blackman and Silberman (1975) have defined altered behavior criteria from a slightly different perspective:

- the behavior must occur with sufficient frequency;
- the behavior pattern must be one that will be harmful to the child or the child's environment if the behavior continues over time; and
- the behavior pattern must hinder future healthy development.

Determining the meaning and etiology of a child's behavior usually requires time and use of a variety of assessment methods. Ideally, assessment includes interviews with child and family members, observations of the child in interactions with others (particularly family members), data-gathering from questionnaires or behavior checklists, and parental recordings of the child's behavior (Forehand and McMahon, 1981; Levine, 1983; Eyberg, 1985). Table 33-2 summarizes the basic components of any behavioral assessment.

Since a child's behavior may vary in different settings, the health professional obtains information from as many sources as possible (home, day care center, school, playground, peers' or grandparents' homes) to comprehend fully the dimensions of the child's problem. The nurse cannot directly observe the child's behavior in all these settings, therefore assessment relies on informant data from parents, teachers, adult significant others, siblings, peers, and other professionals who have contact with the child. When personal interviews are not possible, the telephone may be used. Also, these sources could complete a questionnaire or a behavior check list which, mailed back, could be followed by a telephone call for any clarification. At the very least, parents and, if old enough, the child should be interviewed.

During the interviews, the health professional should be alert to identify families at high risk for interactional problems. Such families may be using one child as a scapegoat to avoid facing the real issues in a situation. High-risk families usually have little or no social support, have financial difficulties, and are afflicted singly or multiply with marital instability, illness, parental depression or mental illness, or members with drug or alcohol dependencies.

Box 33-2
Criteria for Behavior Requiring Intervention

The behavior is to be condemned and is unacceptable regardless of how rarely it occurs (incest, intentional damage to person or property).

The behavior is not inappropriate in and of itself but is inappropriate because of its frequency, because it is exaggerated, or because of when or where it occurs.

The behavior is absent or deficient in that the person rarely or never displays a behavior society deems necessary and normal (never smiles, never or rarely talks, seldom pays attention).

The behavior is a regular source of tension to the child or family members or both.

The behavior is inappropriate for the person's age and stage of development, intelligence, or social situation.

The behavior is compulsively enacted, appearing to "come out of the blue" without any precipitating circumstances (obscure or bizarre motivation). The child seems unable to avoid or stop the behavior even though she or he knows it is futile or that it will inevitably bring disapproval or punishment.

The behavior is one of several others that together affect several areas of the child's life.

The behavior brings suffering to the child and others and interferes with socialization and development.

(Compiled from Herbert, 1975; Hersoo, 1977; LeBow, 1979; Levine, 1983.)

The Behavioral Assessment

A satisfactory behavioral assessment requires evaluation of both behavioral performance and behavioral style or temperament. Behavioral performance and temperament assessment is best accomplished by *observation,* after problem areas have been identified by *interview.* Box 33-3 identifies data that should be obtained on questionable behaviors. The interview may be conducted using guidelines the interviewer has devised or using established instruments (Box 33-4 provides examples). A questionnaire or checklist shortens the time to obtain assessment information and can be standardized for age. Care is taken to ask for *descriptions* of behavior, not interpretations of behavior. Reliability and validity of data are enhanced if behaviors being questioned are current or of the recent past. Having each parent complete a questionnaire or check list provides an opportunity to assess discrepancies in their perceptions.

Check lists are particularly useful in determining whether the child has multiple problems and the extent to which parental expectations are realistic (Liptak and Chamberlain, 1983). Check lists are often pre-

Table 33-2. Components of a Thorough Behavioral Assessment

Biologic Factors	Environmental Factors	Self-Concept Factors
Birth History Normal pregnancy Complications in pregnancy or delivery	**Early Bonding/Attachment Experiences** Primary caregiver first year of life Involvement of each parent in infant/child care Is child a lot "like parent" or a lot "different from parent"? Parental attitude about this Is child adopted; when; does child know?	**Peer Relationships** Does child have friends? What activities does child participate in with friends? Does child prefer single play or play with peers? Describe child's relationship with peers
Developmental History Milestone achievements Feeding difficulty, sleep irregularity Toilet training age and any difficulties Any unusual early childhood experiences	**Educational History** Schools attended Was child in any special education classes? Were any problems experienced during first year of school? Present grade Any grades skipped Average grades earned Has child ever dropped out or been expelled from school? Any school problems Subjects child likes, dislikes	**Emotional Development** Has child had any losses: deaths, separation or divorce, moving? How does child handle losses? How does the child get attention? Any phobias, fears, recurring nightmares; what age? Does child experience restless sleep, night waking, bedwetting? Any significant behavior change recently?
Medical History (See Chapter 15) Any early childhood illness, trauma, high temperatures Any seizures or convulsions Any severe blows to head Any chronic illness of medical nature Any medication taken	**Discipline/Parenting History** What behaviors warrant discipline? What discipline measures are used? Who usually administers discipline? Child's reaction to discipline Are siblings disciplined in same way for same thing? In parents' families who did the disciplining? How were parents disciplined?	**Self-Esteem Development** How does child feel about self? What are child's strengths? What are child's interests, hobbies? Describe child's relationship with parents, siblings, teachers, other adults, authority figures
Temperamental History Disposition as baby; any changes with growth Response to new situations Activity level of child	**Family History** Has either parent received treatment for an emotional problem? Has either parent a chronic illness; any siblings with chronic illness? Any significant change in child's environment, living situation, household members Child's response to changes in environment Family members in home; outside home Child living with both natural parents; if not, how long has one parent been out of the home; has that parent remarried; does child see/visit that parent? In parents' families were both parents present? Where were child's parents born? Home address; how long? Parents' occupations What activities are enjoyed as a family; how often?	
	Social History Any change in how child spends leisure time or with whom Does child have own room? What behaviors prompted seeking assistance? Does child spend more time alone or with peers?	

(Compiled from Levine, 1983; Barnard, 1985; Eyberg, 1985; Kline, 1986.)

ferred to questionnaires for completion by teachers, day care workers, or adolescent siblings or peers.

Parents can be asked to keep records of their child's disturbing behavior at home. These records should include a description of antecedents (preceding events) and consequences of the behavior and its frequency, intensity, and duration. How long records will need to be kept depends on the frequency. Disturbing behavior that occurs several times a day generally needs to be recorded for only 3 to 5 days for sufficient data. Less frequently occurring disturbing behavior will need to be recorded over 2 to 3 weeks to obtain an adequate sample.

Children may also do self-monitoring and record their own behavior. Accuracy is probably greater if the behavior children are asked to record is something they themselves are concerned about. A pleasant side effect is that often the self-monitoring results in increased positive behavior and reduced negative behavior (Kazdin, 1974; Shapiro, 1984; Eyberg, 1985).

Interviews supplement and verify paper and pencil methods of collecting information. The child's interview is uniquely suited for observation of nonverbal cues of anxiety. The interviewer should note at what points the child showed increased body movement, muscle tension, flushing, and voice tremor.

Box 33-3
Data to Be Collected for Questionable Behavior

- Frequency of occurrence of behavior
- Intensity with which behavior is displayed
- How long an episode lasts
- What circumstances immediately precede enactment of the behavior
- What circumstances immediately follow enactment of the behavior, i.e., consequences, parental response
- Situations during which behavior occurs (specific locations, persons, activities; certain times of day)
- Disciplinary style generally used by the parents with the child
- Any threat to self, others, property in enactment of behavior
- How long the behavior has been occurring (weeks, months, years); onset age
- Any unusual event near the time of onset

Any child over preschool age should be interviewed. Information from school-age children found to be reliable includes knowledge about *behavior,* such as daily activities and responses to various problem situations; *environmental factors,* such as demographic data and potential reinforcers; and *self-awareness cognitions* such as feelings about self, about the health professional, and about parents, as well as perceptions of the reasons for the behavior being questioned. The child is the best informant regarding inner feelings like fears or worries. The most difficult questions for children to answer are those concerning the reasons for their behavior (Nelson, 1977; Hodges et al, 1981; Eyberg, 1985; O'Leary and Johnson, 1986).

Interviewing should be complemented by observation. Observation in the home and school is desirable but may be impractical. Then the nurse will need to rely on observations made by family members, school personnel, or other professionals who have had observational opportunities. If behavioral observation is done in a "clinical" setting, the assessor must keep in mind that a strange environment and an observer's presence can affect the child's behavior. Of course, the assessor also must have a sound knowledge of child development.

Observation may be spontaneous or structured. To structure observation of behavior, the assessor may use role playing or staging. Webster-Stratton (1983) describes staging as ideal for the clinic setting. One-way mirrors, with or without use of videotape equipment, eliminate the observer influence on the child's behavior. Research findings support laboratory or clinic observation or staging as a valid predictor of behavior when the individuals and activity are similar to the natural situation (Kniskern et al, 1983; Eyberg, 1985). In staging, one or both parents are asked to play two games with the child, each lasting 5 minutes. The child selects the game and its rules the first time; the parents choose the second game. After the second game, the parents ask the child to put the toys away. During an office visit or home observation the observer can also utilize natural circumstances, encouraging the parent to handle any acting-out behaviors just as they would if the observer were not present. During the parent-child interaction the health professional observes parent-child exchange, noting how much the parents and child play together and how much attention they give to one another. Communication is noted for clarity, how much listening to one another occurs, whether the exchange is one-sided. The observer notes how much praise and positive acceptance parents offer contrasted with negative commands and criticism. Other observations include the amount of ordering or competition for control that exists, who leads or gives commands during interaction, whether parents or child seeks approval frequently, and how much each accepts and complies with rules. The observer is looking for pervasive trends in the interchange. DPICS (Dyadic Parent-Child Interaction Coding System) is a validated tool with instructions for observation of staging (Eyberg, 1985; Eyberg and Robinson, 1983). This method of observation is comprehensive, yet achievable within a therapy hour, requires only one observer, and can be done without special equipment.

Although children generally are not hospitalized for evaluation or treatment of a behavior problem (Box 33-6 lists exceptions), some may be hospitalized for other illness and the nurses should be aware that behavior problems may occur. An admission history should include information about how the child relates to peers and adults; how the child responds to new situations and to authority; and how the child is usually disciplined. Interactions observed during the child's hospital stay may suggest behavior problems, though the possibility that the child's illness or hospitalization is altering usual behavior and interaction should be considered. Follow-up of the child may be a relevant part of discharge planning.

Considerations in Planning Interventions: A Professional Tightrope

In a society that strives for uniformity, one can anticipate that "differentness" may create a substantial personal cost. Paradoxically, our society also espouses the

Box 33-4

Tools for Assessing Elements of the Behavioral Evaluation

TEMPERAMENT

1. Infant Temperament Questionnaires (available for birth to 4 months and 4 to 8 months)
   Address William Carey, MD
   319 W. Front St., Media, PA 19063
2. Toddler Temperament Questionnaire (1 to 3 years)
   Address William Fullard, PhD
   Dept. of Educational Psychology, Temple University
   Philadelphia, PA 19122
3. Parent Temperament Questionnaire and Teacher Temperament Questionnaire (both for ages 3 to 7 years)
   Available in Thomas and Chess: *Temperament and Development,* Brunner/Mazel, 1977
4. Behavioral Style Questionnaire (3 to 7 years)
   Address Sean McDevitt, PhD
   Deveraux Center, 6436 E. Sweetwater, Scottsdale, AZ 85254
5. Middle Childhood Temperament Questionnaire (8 to 12 years)
   Address Ms. Robin Hegvik
   307 N. Wayne Ave., Wayne, PA 19087
6. Temperament Assessment Across the Life Span: The Dimensions of Temperament Survey
   Available in Child Development (Lerner et al), 53:149, 1982

ADAPTIVE BEHAVIOR

1. Child Behavior Checklist (4 to 16 years)
   Available in Monograms of Social Research in Child Development (Achenbach and Edelbrock), 46:1-81, 1981
2. Parent Questionnaire (10 to 11 years)
   Available in British Journal of Psychiatry (Graham and Rutter), 114:581-592, 1968
3. Social Competence and Symptom Scales (preschool)
   Available in Developmental Psychology (Kohn and Rosman), 6:430-444, 1972
4. Behavior Questionnaire for Teachers (7 to 13 years)
   Available in Journal of Child Psychology (Rutter), 8:1-11, 1967
5. Brazelton Neonatal Assessment Scale (infancy)
   Available in Clinics of Developmental Medicine (Brazelton), #50, Philadelphia, JB Lippincott, 1973, and in Chapter 5
6. Personality Inventory for Children
   Address R. Wirt, Western Psychological Services, Los Angeles, 1977
7. Adolescent Life Assessment Checklist
   Available in Journal of Adolescent Health Care (Gleser et al) 1:30-36, 1980
8. Eyberg Child Behavior Inventory (2 to 17 years)
   Available in Journal of Clinical Child Psychology (Eyberg et al), 9:22-28, 1980
9. Minnesota Child Development Inventories
   a. Minnesota Child Development Inventory (1 to 6 years)
   b. Preschool Development Inventory (3 to 5.5 years)
   c. Minnesota Infant Development Inventory (birth to 15 months)
   Address Behavior Science Systems, Inc. Box 1108, Minneapolis, MN 55440

HOME ENVIRONMENT

1. Home Screening Inventory (infant to preschool)
   Available in Developmental Screening (Frankenburg, ed), Denver, University of Colorado Medical Center, 1977
2. Home Scale
   Available in Advances in Behavioral Pediatrics, (Camp, ed), Greenwich, CT, JAI Press, 1981, and in Appendix Five

INTERACTIONS WITH OTHERS

1. Mother-Infant Form (post delivery)
   Available in Seminars on Perinatology (Gray et al), 3:85-90, 1979
2. Attachment Indicators During Stress (AIDS) (birth to 18 months)
   Address H. Massie and K. Campbell
   Detroit, Wayne State University Press, 1980
3. Adolescent Interaction Scale
   Available in Journal of Adolescent Health Care (Kaplan et al), 2:101-106, 1981

CLINICAL OBSERVATIONS OF BEHAVIOR AND INTERACTION

1. Dyadic Parent-Child Interaction Coding System (approximately 2 to 12 years)
   Available in Psychological Documents (Eyberg S, Robinson E), #13, MS 2582, 1983; also from Sheila Eyberg, Department of Medical Psychology, Oregon Health Sciences University, Portland, OR 97201

INTELLIGENCE

1. Ordinal Scales of Infant Psychological Development (birth to 24 months)
   Available in Assessment in Infancy (Uzgiris and Hunt), Urbana, University of Illinois Press, 1975
2. Merrill-Palmer Scale of Mental Tests (preschool) (Check at any University Department of Psychology)
3. Wechsler Primary and Preschool Test of Intelligence (4 to 6½ years); also Wechsler Intelligence Scale for Children (6 to 17 years)
   Available from Psychological Corporation, Harcourt Brace Jovanovich, Inc., 1250 Sixth Ave., San Diego, CA 92101
4. Stanford-Binet Intelligence Scale (2 years through adulthood)
   Available from Houghton-Mifflin, #1 Beacon Street, Boston, MA 02101

"right" to be different. Thus, the health professional must consider personal attitudes and the ethical, moral, legal, and economic trends of our society in the planning of interventions and care for the "different" child.

Moral and Ethical Considerations

A "bad child" is culturally and societally defined, as is the appropriate intervention. Before the 17th century, society had no separate standards for children; they were considered miniature adults and were treated as such. The Puritan ethic of the 18th century resulted in a "bad child" concept because children's natures made them incongruent with adult expectations. The child's efforts at autonomy were perceived as disobedience, which was sinful. Play and sexual exploration were signs of idleness that were believed to lead to self-pollution and poverty. The Puritan ethic lingered in the 19th century, with idleness, illiteracy, and mischievousness characterizing the "bad child." Until the 20th century children were not permitted the behavioral liberties of what we today call childhood. Health care professionals had no role in the behavioral-emotional health of children beyond diagnosis. The belt was the treatment for minor infringements and jail or a reformatory for more serious problems (Levine, 1983).

The human rights movement has helped *children's rights* move forward over the past 30 years. The rights advanced for exceptional children (and adults) were primarily ones most people expect, such as the right to live within one's own family environment or, if that is not possible, then in a simulated family-type setting; the right to have the same educational opportunities as other children without physical/emotional/mental handicaps, within a normal school environment; and the right of confidentiality for health records (that is, they are not available to others without the parent's or guardian's written consent.) With this advancement of children's rights has come the realization that all minors must be protected from unsafe or inappropriate medical treatment, harmful environmental influences, and infringements upon their future rights of self-choice.

Labeling is another moral-ethical issue that has an impact on the health professional. Assignment of diagnostic labels to children with altered behavior has been much discussed. There is some advantage to labeling in clinical and educational settings. For example, children with similar problems, who are thus labeled, can be assigned to special subjects, teachers, or classrooms organized to address the problem area. A particular label tells the health professional that a child displays a certain category of behaviors, needing a specialized set of services or interventions. Consumer advocacy groups also can utilize this label or category to raise funds or seek resources. However, the label can be seriously detrimental to the child. There is risk of encouraging self-fulfilling prophecies or of biasing the intervention plan. Mandell and Fiscus (1981) have studied and summarized the risks of diagnostic labeling:

- Labeling may interfere with the development of appropriate *individualized* programs of treatment.
- Once bestowed, labels are difficult to remove. The label may affect how others view the child and how the child perceives self.
- Labeling fosters categorical placement which, particularly in the educational setting, may limit the opportunities for interaction with "normal" children.
- Labeling tends to diminish the significance of societal and environmental factors or to discriminately focus on the wrong primary etiology, consequently thwarting the mobilization of a much-needed multifaceted intervention program.
- Mislabeling can occur as a result of the training and disciplinary biases of the labeler. One professional might use a label of "emotional disturbance" and another relate the same observable phenomena of school problems to "minimal brain damage."
- The semantics of labeling can greatly affect how the world views and treats the child. Consider, for example, "highly independent" versus "socially maladjusted" as labels for the same behavior. One implies an eccentricity (a term rarely permitted to describe children) or behavior that will be desirable as the child grows older; the other implies undesirable or pathologic behavior with which society deals differently.

Another issue is a child's *right to "specialize."* Adults are not expected to be always cheerful and moderate in temperament; they are allowed good days and bad days, to be eccentric or " to do their own thing," and to be better at some things than at others. Yet the prevailing expectation of children is that they be constantly cooperative in interactions, always conform willingly to adult directives, and be able to accomplish well, and be interested in all tasks put before them. Children are human beings and have a right to specialize and to be "individuals." They may need the help of health professionals in resisting the over-riding drive of adults to make them good at almost everything. Specialization, a right seemingly reserved for adults, needs to be afforded to children too. History is full of examples of people who did not fit in particularly comfortably during childhood but who were destined to be more effective adults than they were children, often achieving fame. A classic example is Albert Einstein, who as a child was accused of being a day-dreamer and unmotivated.

Legal Considerations

As a health professional involved in promoting health and life adjustment of children, the nurse needs to be aware of the legal issues relating to such care. Laws pertinent to health care exist in the areas of privacy, confidentiality, and informed consent; these have only recently been applied to children, primarily as a result of court cases that established legal doctrine by precedent.* At present children are not considered to be "holders of legal privilege" due to their status as minors. Parents or legal guardians generally have been considered the legal holder of privilege for the child. But the court cases regarding children's rights in the past several years have generally upheld children's rights to confidentiality and reasonable privacy. In the area of informed consent, health providers still must seek a parent's consent or the consent of another person standing in loco parentis to treat a child. In emergencies the courts discard the need for informed consent; likewise, courts have recognized the consent of a minor for simple treatment of a non-urgent nature if the child can demonstrate an understanding of the risks and benefits of treatment.

Of particular importance to this discussion is the issue of laws regarding behavior control. Intervening in someone's life to change her or his behavior may represent deprivation of liberty sufficient to raise constitutional questions, particularly if the control procedures are unduly restrictive or harsh or abrogate personal freedom without due process (violations of the Eighth and Fourteenth Amendments). The courts tend to support the child's rights to autonomy, due process, protection against harm, least restrictive alternatives in treatment, freedom from involuntary servitude, and minimum care standards (Schwitzgebel and Schwitzgebel, 1980; Martin, 1981; Rosoff, 1981).

Two particular issues regarding a child's right to autonomy are the use of psychotropic drugs or electroconvulsive therapy to control behavior and the use of behavior modification. Court cases have established precedent that a child cannot receive psychotropic drugs or electroconvulsive therapy without consent of the parent or guardian or a court order and that it must be demonstrated that less restrictive treatment procedures have been exhausted before considering medication or electroconvulsive therapy.

The only acceptable objective for behavior modification should be to change overt behavior, not to change a person's mind or attitude (Martin, 1975). The courts have ruled in support of behavior modification that increases a child's autonomy, but not through measures that abuse the child's rights as an individual human being. States and professional organizations (e.g., The Association for the Advancement of Behavior Therapy) have established guidelines of acceptable behavior modification procedures. Many institutions which utilize this therapy regularly have established Human Rights Committees to establish policy and monitor practice to assure that legal parameters are upheld.

Protection from harm is a significant legal issue for the pediatric patient with altered behavior. A procedure to control behavior may "constitute cruel and unusual punishment if it violates minimum standards of decency, is wholly disproportionate to the alleged offense, or goes beyond what is necessary" (Schwitzgebel and Schwitzgebel, 1980, p 84). Examples of illegal practices that have been employed with children to control behavior include deprivation of basic amenities (e.g., clothing, bed); forceful drug injection as a disciplinary consequence; degrading statements or actions intended to reduce self-esteem; and unnecessary use of corporal punishment, restraint, or isolation. Case law has set forth the following as guidelines in regard to restraint and isolation for behavior control (Levine, 1983):

- A child is not to be placed alone in a locked room either as punishment or for any purpose. Legitimate time out methods may be used under close, direct professional supervision. Placement shall be in an unlocked room with staff constantly nearby to supervise the child.
- These methods will be used only when less restrictive measures do not work.
- The child should have access to bathroom facilities when needed.
- The period of segregation shall not be greater than 12 hours without renewal by a qualified professional. The restriction or isolation will require a written professional order except in emergency where it is likely the child would harm himself or others. The order must specify the terms and conditions and the rationale for the decision. Emergency use shall be for a period no greater than one hour.

Case law has established that work which serves no purpose (e.g., moving rocks from one pile to another) violates the Eighth Amendment. A child can be required to do such housekeeping tasks as would be performed at home without pay, provided nothing in the child's treatment plan contraindicates work.

* For a thorough discussion of court cases setting policy by precedent in pediatrics and a general discussion of legal policy in the areas just cited, consult Levine (1983) and textbooks whose specific subject is legal issues.

Minimum standards for child care have been addressed by the courts in the areas of physical environment, educational services, and Joint Commission for Accreditation of Health Care Organizations regulations.

Because pediatric patients are essentially powerless to prevent attempts by others to control their behavior, continuous development of legal parameters is imperative as is monitoring by professionals to ensure the child's safety both physically and psychologically.

The nurse will sometimes become involved with the legal system when a minor's behavioral alterations violate the law or otherwise necessitate involvement of law enforcement agencies. To participate effectively the nurse must be knowledgeable about local laws regarding children and the nurse's responsibilities for reporting to and working with the appropriate authorities when necessary. Rehabilitation, training, and prevention of delinquency in children are concerns health professionals and the juvenile courts share. Nurses who have interviewed or worked with children and families may be required to submit a report to the court. Such reports should be clearly written in lay language, using verbatim quotes when possible. *Facts rather than interpretations of facts* by the nurse should be presented unless interpretations are specifically requested.

Dilemma—Who Is Responsible? Who Needs the Support?

A dilemma that faces the health professional is the issue of who is responsible for the child's altered behavior. An accurate answer to this question seems critical to behavior change. Modern psychology is invaluable in helping us understand human behavior. However, a psychologic cause-and-effect assumption can lead therapists to an oversimplification that only helps destructive children avoid the consequences of real life (York et al, 1985). Such an approach that assumes a parental etiology leaves parents responsible and reduces the chances that the child will change for the better. Why should they change when the therapist has excused them and blamed their parents? The child's conclusion is "Let Mom and Dad change. It's their fault!"

It is true that parents significantly influence, particularly as role models and by their parenting practices, how a child learns to behave. But when a child fails to be acceptably socialized, is the parent at fault for providing inadequate external controls or perhaps not providing an environment that allows the child to develop adequate internal controls? Or is the child also responsible for the behavioral choices made? The truth is it really does not matter who or what is responsible for how the child came to have behavioral problems. What is needed is solutions. Not blame. Not guilt. Solutions begin by dealing with the here and now situation. The past cannot be relived, it cannot be changed. Often therapists, intrigued by grasping the underlying factors in the behavior, lose sight of the need to deal with the *now.* And *now* the child and parents all need support. The child requires support and guidance to learn better ways to get needs met, and parents require support to learn better ways to respond to their child so that behavioral change is accomplished.

In other words, the health professional should help families find a "mutual respect balance" that does not allow infringement on the rights of either parent or child but rather respects and recognizes the rights and needs of each. Parents have the right to expect their child to abide by certain rules, limits, rights, and responsibilities; the child has a right to expect that parents will make these expectations explicit, provide sufficient guidelines for their achievement, and be flexible enough to adapt expectations to the child's changing developmental needs. A middle ground between over- and under-control, overpermissiveness and rigidity, intrusiveness and neglect is needed. Imbalances can be expected temporarily during stress periods. What must be watched for is the development of a vicious cycle of imbalance that leads to a longstanding, disordered parent-child relationship. A greater risk for such imbalance exists when those variables that predispose to altered behavior (see Table 33-1) exist in the family.

Community and Family Responses to Behavioral Variation

Levine (1983) uses one word that deftly describes the response that typifies the community's, family's, and child's response to altered behavior: "bewilderment." Bewilderment is a form of fear that results from uncertainty and lack of understanding.

Communities, representing society at large, have handled this bewilderment in various ways. Sometimes the behaviorally variant individual has been socially ostracized. At other times communities have chosen to deny the problem by segregating or isolating these persons so their existence does not have to be dealt with by the mainstream populace. More recently communities have demonstrated empathy, acting to reform the social and legal conscience of society to provide resources and support for these persons. The greatest movement in this regard for children has been in the area of education. High as the costs for these resources may be, they are still less costly than the outcomes of neglecting the situation are likely to be.

The child is bewildered by the reactions and responses received. Out of synchrony with peers, this child is often robbed of positive feedback and support. The unusual child's self-image may take tremendous abuse at the hands of a world he or she never made.

Differentness has its toll on the parents and family members of behaviorally altered children. Featherstone (1981) documents the universal responses of guilt, fear, loneliness, and anger felt by parents of these children. Crocker (1981) states that similar effects exist for siblings, though the effects are usually manageable.

The degree of impact on family members depends largely on how maladaptive they perceive the behavior to be, how much the behavior disrupts family living, and how the child is received by society (school, friends, legal institutions).

Other factors, unique to a particular family, may also have an impact on the family's reactions to a child's pattern of behavior. The size of the family, the health status of individual family members, the availability of support systems, and parenting style (permissive, controlling) all contribute to the family's tolerance of a child's behavior.

Just how a family contends with a behaviorally disordered child depends upon the functional status of the family system itself. At the very least, the family is facing a serious threat to its equilibrium. A basically healthy family may become more closely unified because managing their "problem child" fosters improved communication and better understanding of each member's developmental needs. These are families that are not afraid to change ineffective patterns of communicating and relating. However, in many families, the effect of a "problem child" is the further disruption of family functioning, or even disbanding of the family unit. Satir (1982) suggests that, in dysfunctional families, one child is singled out to be the "identified patient." This is the child whose behavior is actually a reflection of dysfunction within the family system. The misbehavior of the child camouflages problems existing in the family unit, thereby creating an illusion that only the child "needs fixing." With assistance, these families can learn healthier coping patterns and develop constructive and supportive relationships with each other. The problem child may then be able to overcome or adapt to the predisposing factors that led to the maladaptive behavior.

Intervening in Altered Behavior

Table 33-3 outlines some problem behavior patterns for which parents and teachers frequently seek help; management guidelines are included. The behavioral alterations discussed in Chapter 36 may include one or more of these behavior patterns.

Often nurses have more contact with children and their families than do other health care providers. They therefore are in key positions to identify problem behavior. The nurse is also the team member who has the greatest opportunity to directly intervene with the child and the family. Optimally, intervention is aimed at two levels: one, to teach family members, especially parents, how to change their responses to the child. The second is to help the child learn healthier coping behaviors—in particular, helping her or him unlearn self-limiting assumptions about self and the world and then to relearn what was previously misunderstood. Box 33-5 identifies other principles of assessment and management the intervention team should keep in mind.

Prevention as Management

As community members and health care providers, nurses can have a significant impact on the prevention of behavioral disturbances. Nurses can initiate prenatal and parenting classes for parents in obstetric and pediatric clinics, in hospitals and physicians' offices, and in adult education departments of public schools. In these classes they can discuss not only the physical effects but also the psychologic and social effects an infant may have on family life. They can help prospective parents begin to think of their unborn child as a unique individual who will have needs, feelings, and personality quirks just like they do.

Nurses can intervene with parents in situations of high-risk pregnancy, in premature birth and cesarean section, and in instances of other early parent-child stress, such as the birth of a defective child. Postnatally, nurses can help parents learn and interpret their child's cues and gain positive self-esteem from their interactions. Nurses can praise parents when they observe healthy parent-child interactions. Well child examinations provide an excellent opportunity for the nurse to model and teach positive parenting techniques.

Education about child development, temperament, and children's perceptions or cognitions at various ages is a key element of preventive management. The nurse can use this anticipatory guidance as a basis from which to help parents watch for and manage potential problem situations common to various stages. As a primary care provider, the nurse can alert parents to clues that signify trouble may be developing. Early identification and education for prevention is the most effective management of problem behavior.

Intervention Options to Manage Altered Behavior

The focus in managing altered behavior is on developing the child's and family's abilities. Intervention is

Table 33-3. Frequent Patterns of Disturbing Behavior and Management Guidelines

Behavior Pattern and Characteristics	General Management Guidelines
Infantile Behavior Pattern	
Child functions below actual age; "babylike"	Practice firm, consistent limit setting
Prone to temper tantrums, soiling, whining, crying beyond when these are age-appropriate	Avoid bribing or arguing with child (these are negative reinforcers that perpetuate the behavior)
Poor peer relations because child always wants own way, tattles on others, runs to grown ups to solve problems	Ignore infantile behaviors and praise age-appropriate behaviors displayed
	Be supportive and kind but communicate clearly what are age-appropriate behaviors and expectations
	Spend positive time each day with child when he or she is not displaying infantile behavior
Excessively Shy Behavior Pattern	
Tends to stay outside a group; a "watcher" of activity	Approach gently
Does not ask to be included in activities and avoids participation; may participate if specifically encouraged to do so	Encourage initial involvement in noncompetitive group activity and, after successes, gradually introduce more competitive activities
Fears competition; often excels at individualized activities that are done alone	Never force group participation
Any peer friendships established are likely also to be with shy children	Praise group activity attempts
	Spend positive time with child daily using the time to reinforce his or her abilities
Hostile-Aggressive Behavior Pattern	
Becomes easily agitated and irritated	Requires absolute consistency in discipline and limit setting
Displays negative attitude toward almost everything	Role model appropriate management of frustration and anger
May physically or mentally abuse others	Absolutely do not react with anger to child's behavior (to do so mirrors child's behavior and is a reinforcer that perpetuates the behavior)
May be destructive to property	When possible, remove child from the situation before child becomes volatile
	Observe/supervise closely
	Praise attempts to handle frustrating situations and anger appropriately. Spend positive time with child daily when *not* displaying the undesirable behavior
Manipulative Behavior Pattern	
Plays one person against another	Maintain absolute consistency in limit setting
Often described as a "spoiled" child	Remain decisive and unmoving when child attempts to persuade or change your mind about something
Capitalizes on guilt feelings and fairness values of others	Avoid power struggles (these are reinforcers that perpetuate the behavior)
	Show a caring and concerned attitude toward child without "giving in"
	Praise child for appropriate behavior during interaction
	Spend positive time with child during a time each day when child is not being manipulative
Demanding Behavior Pattern	
Wants immediate satisfaction of desires	Ignore demands that compete with the needs of others
"Bossy" and insensitive to others' needs	Praise attempts of child to wait and to consider others' needs
Pouts and protests vehemently when demands are not given prompt attention	Be patient but firm in teaching the child to wait for gratification of needs

Table 33-3 *(continued)*

Behavior Pattern and Characteristics	General Management Guidelines
Demanding Behavior Pattern	
	Maintain a firm position when saying no to a demand Ask if the child needs something during those times when *not* exhibiting demanding behavior; likewise, spend time with child when he or she is not making demands

Box 33-5
Principles to Consider in Assessment and Management of Behavior Alterations

The seriousness and intensity of these behaviors vary from child to child. For example, a child who does not want to go to school on a particular day because of fear of a test cannot be considered in the same way as a child who absolutely cannot go to school at all; yet both these children have a form of school refusal, or phobia. The first child's reaction to school is mild and normal, whereas the second child and the family need some form of therapy. The importance of recognizing the degree with which each child is affected by these problems is seen when one plans management for a child and the family. Individual differences must be assessed and planned for accordingly. From this fact follows another: no one is perfect. It could be said that to a varying degree we are all behaviorally disabled.

It is important to recognize that each of the problems identified has multiple causes. Rarely is a problem only environmental or only genetic in origin. Whenever a practitioner is called upon to work with a child and family on problem behavior, the many possible causes of the condition must be carefully considered. A complete and thorough history obtained from the child, family members, teachers, peers, and other significant persons is the best tool. This multiple approach to a history gives a truer picture of the child and allows more accurate assessment of reasons for behavior. Recognizing the multiple etiology allows the nurse to use resources more skillfully during intervention.

Frequently, behavior considered a disability during childhood evolves into an advantage in later years: the child resistant to norms or who seems so distractible may become a scientist whose questioning and acute observational ability lead to important discoveries; the hyperactive child may become a highly productive employee; the egocentric child may become a strong leader; the child with erratic sleep habits may become a highly productive night person (an alternative not offered during childhood).

Every child has strengths. These should be identified during assessment and utilized as valuable resources during treatment.

Outward behavioral manifestations may be deceptive. The real cause may not be a behavior problem but rather a learning disorder, a hearing or vision problem, or a brain tumor, etc. A complete physical and neurologic evaluation, therefore, is an important component of the assessment process.

When listening to adult (parent, teacher) descriptions of the child's behavior, keep in mind that expectations for children differ greatly from those for adults. The child is expected always to display good spirits, the adult is allowed moods; children are expected to do well at everything, adults are allowed to specialize in those few things they are good at; children are expected always to conform, adults are respected for their uniqueness and individuality. Assessment helps decipher when unrealistic expectation is the real problem, not the child's behavior.

Children are developing a self-concept and as a consequence instinctively seek to avoid humiliation at all cost. Often defensive mechanisms to protect self are mistaken as a primary behavior problem.

Related to their fragile self-concept, children have minimal tolerance for failure. As a result they fall more easily into a self-perpetuating and self-destructive failure spiral. The child with a physical handicap is at specific risk.

Frequently a child's problem behavior occurs or escalates during certain moments or situations (e.g., during group activities, when singled out to perform) or in certain locations (e.g., bus stop, restroom, cafeteria, gym). Having a child recreate these "hot spots" gives the nurse a picture of events the child perceives at these times and how the child fits into the events.

It is best to avoid labels and associated dangers of self-fulfilling prophecy. This is done by identifying the problem behavior and treating the individual behavior.

Table 33-4. Intervention Options in a Multidisciplinary Management Program

Management Options*	Purpose
For The Child	
Psychotherapy • Based on premise that behavioral symptoms reflect unconscious conflicts and serve to reduce anxiety • Requires development of an emotional attachment by child with therapist *Health professional:* Psychiatrist, psychologist, social worker	Helps child understand psychologic conflicts and the symbolic meaning of the resulting behavior through use of symbolic play with children and dream and fantasy analysis with adolescents. Deals with unconscious processes and memory, not just behavior *Comment:* More useful when psychotic disorder is also present. Children with conduct disorders frequently do not benefit from psychotherapy. A long-term commitment is required for psychotherapy
Behavioral Counseling • See Table 33-5 for a differentiation of psychotherapy and counseling and Table 33-6 for a description of different types of pediatric counseling *Health professional:* Psychologist, social worker, nurse with specialized psychiatric or mental health training	Provides child and family members with individual guidance and support to achieve positive changes in behavioral responses to life experiences, that is, acquiring desirable behaviors and changing undesirable behaviors *Comment:* Age guidelines are: before age 6 years, work with parents; between ages 6 and 12, work with child and parents together; after age 12 years, work with child alone (parents may participate in part of session). Children generally cannot handle sessions of more than 20–30 minutes. Opportunity for active self-development by child through expansion of problem-solving and decision-making skills. Older children often do better with a "buddy" system of counseling in which they choose a friend, sibling, parent, or other significant adult to be with them during counseling sessions (Tauer, 1983)
Group Therapy • Counseling sessions that involve groups of children with common behavioral symptoms, or other similar problems *Health professional:* Same as for Behavioral Counseling	Adds peer perspective to support for change in behavior. Helps child see the effect on peers when displaying maladaptive and adaptive behaviors within a structured setting where feedback and support can be provided immediately.
Behavior Management • Also called behavior modification, point system, incentive system • Applies the experience derived from principles of learning and conditioning to behavior problems. • See Chapter 13 for a discussion of positive and negative reinforcement methods to achieve socialization *Health professional:* Social worker, nurse, parents, teacher	Teaches child responsibility for own behavior and effective interacting through the use of verbal and tangible incentives. Focus is on correction of behavioral deficiencies, behavioral excesses, or behavioral inappropriateness *Comment:* Basis of behavioral management is that all behavior is learned, behavior is shaped predominantly by its consequences. If a consequence is pleasant it has a greater likelihood of repetition, and conversely an unpleasant consequence has less likelihood of repetition. Temperamental differences must be considered when looking at how long reinforcers are likely to be needed before the behavior change is successful. Box 33-7 summarizes the basic components of a behavioral management system
Videotherapy • May be used alone or in conjunction with group or family therapy *Health professional:* Social worker, psychologist, nurse with mental health preparation	Provides immediate feedback to child to increase self-understanding and how one affects others
Therapeutic Recreation *Health professional:* Nurse, physical therapist, social worker	Develops cooperative and individual play skills relative to the child's developmental needs
Special Education or Occupational Therapy *Health professional:* Special education teacher, occupational therapist	Meet special educational/learning needs. Develops acceptable daily living skills, builds self-concept, expands problem-solving skills
Relaxation Training or Desensitization • Usually used in conjunction with behavioral management *Health professional:* Nurse trained in relaxation/desensitization techniques, social worker	Inhibits undesirable responses by relaxation methods. (Refer to books and training guides on this subject)
Assertiveness Training *Health professional:* Nurse trained in assertiveness training techniques, social worker	Improves interpersonal relationships and related behaviors when child is a scapegoat or when child fails to stand up for own rights or cannot express feelings or thoughts in ways that respect others' rights

Table 33-4 *(continued)*

Management Options*	Purpose
For The Child *(continued)*	
Self-Help Groups • Generally these groups use an approach similar to the 12-step concept of Alcoholics Anonymous • Tough Love is a national organization that provides assistance for the troubled child and the parents *Health Professional:* Experienced parent, social workers, nurse with mental health background	Increases child's awareness of personal responsibility for behavior choices and builds external support systems for aid during periods of stress *Comment:* Basic premise is to avoid blame, deal with the present, decentralize authority, and be action oriented
Pediatric Psychopharmacology • Used in conjunction with other therapies sparingly and for as brief a time as possible • Psychostimulants reduce hyperactivity; hypnotics and sedatives reduce agitation; tranquilizers reduce agitation and impulsiveness *Health professional:* Physician, psychiatrist, nurse, parents	Alleviates specific symptoms (high anxiety level, marked hyperactivity, marked apathy or withdrawal, when symptoms are so extreme that the child is unable to focus on behavior control) *Comment:* Criteria for use are not yet established; use raises ethical questions, poses potential dangers to physical health and development when prolonged, and gives the child a message that behavior control comes from without rather than from self-control (Popper and Famularo, 1983; Pugh-Antich and Rabinovich, 1983. Sometimes symptoms are so extreme that medication is necessary to bring the child to a functional level for application of other therapies. Medication should be available in only very small quantities to prevent suicidal misuse
For the Family—To Reinstate Child Into A Healthier Family System	
Family Therapy *Health professional:* Psychologist, social worker, nurse with specialized mental health training	Facilitates family problem solving and reintegration of child into home that supports his or her needs in a healthy fashion. Medium for reality-based interactions between child and family with professional mediation as needed
Parental Counseling • Other forms of counseling may also be indicated for individual members or the marital pair *Health professional:* Nurse, psychologist	Increases parents' role and understanding of their child's needs and behavioral management program Increases parenting skills Helps parents change their focus from organic to emotional issues. (Most parents, at least initially, want to associate a physical etiology to their child's maladaptive behavior)
Parents and Siblings Groups *Health professional:* Experienced parents or siblings with professional resources, usually nurse or social worker	Provide support and a forum for sharing opinions, common feelings, and problems; looking at possible solutions; and increasing members' awareness and understanding of behavior disorders and their management

* The treatment plan is individualized, utilizes a multidisciplinary care plan that identifies methods and outcome criteria, and incorporates the child's and family's strengths.

(Compiled from Anders and Walton, 1983; Levine et al, 1983; Gumaer, 1984; Golden, 1984; Kupchik, 1985; and Wilson et al, 1986.)

individualized to each child and family and generally requires coordination via a *multidisciplinary team.* Table 33-4 presents options for developing a characteristic multidisciplinary management program. The client may be an outpatient or inpatient. Criteria for inpatient admission are listed in Box 33-6.

Typically, several approaches to the management of behavior problems are used together to provide a comprehensive plan of intervention (see Table 33-4). Psychotherapy, behavioral counseling (Tables 33-5 and 33-6), and group therapy are used in an attempt to alter children's maladaptive behavior indirectly by changing their intrapsychic organization (the way they think or feel about themselves and, thus, perceive social situations). Psychoanalytically trained professionals manage this intervention approach. The nurse assists, particularly by teaching caretakers how to recognize and reinforce positive attitudes and behavior the child displays.

Behavior management that uses behavior modification or other point or incentive measures; self-care methodologies such as Tough Love, relaxation training, and imagery; and special education programs are based on the premise that behavior is learned and therefore can be unlearned or replaced by healthier behavior through planned changes in the child's environment. The nurse is often responsible for teaching behavioral management strategies to parents, teachers, and other significant persons in the child's environment (Box 33-7).

Box 33-6
Criteria for Inpatient Admission of a Child with Altered Behavior

Child is a danger to self, others, or property.

Child's reality testing is impaired, with inappropriate affect or disordered behavior.

Need exists for intensive and extensive medical and behavioral evaluation.

Child exhibits maladaptive behavior patterns over a prolonged period of time without response to outpatient management.

Impaired social/family/educational functioning or inadequate social/family support; child needs to be removed from an environment that cannot tolerate him or her.

Specific symptoms exist that result in dysfunctional behavior (e.g., eating disorder, learning disturbance).

Failure of outpatient or extended care management to affect behavior, or these resources are inaccessible.

Psychopharmacology is sometimes used as an adjunct to any of the other therapies. Rarely, electroconvulsive therapy may be used in a child's behavior management (generally personality disorder is associated).

Parents and teachers should be warned that the undesirable behavior often escalates with the initial treatment before it begins receding. Failure to provide this warning may cause parents to discontinue the treatment effort before adequate time has elapsed for progress to be apparent.

Perhaps the most valuable and successful intervention to emphasize when working with behaviorally disordered children is *consistency.* A predictable, congruous approach to the child's problem behavior de-

Table 33-5. Pediatric Counseling as Differentiated from Psychotherapy

Works mainly with stable children and parents
Focuses more on the present
Focuses more on behavior than on thoughts or feelings
Focuses more on normal development
Requires less extensive evaluations
Leads the interview more (provides less total listening time)
Uses more action-oriented, direct, specific approaches
Uses more empiric approaches (if an approach works, one does not need to know the theory behind it)
Uses more behavioral modification
Relies more on education, reassurance, specific advice, and environmental intervention
Provides briefer follow-up visits (20 or 30 minutes)
Provides fewer visits (two or three for most problems; six maximum)
Sets a shorter time frame (usually 3 months)

(*From Levine et al, 1983.*)

Table 33-6. Types of Pediatric Counseling

1. Releasing painful feelings with ventilation—first deal with pressing emotional issues
2. Education—supplying needed general information
3. Reassurance—specific information that counteracts fears
4. Listening and clarifying the problem—providing parents with a clearer perspective about the child's problem
5. Approval of the parents' approach—helping parents use their own resources
6. Specific advice—suggestions about altered parental handling of specific problems
7. Environmental intervention—suggestions about other changes in the child's environment
8. Extended counseling—more visits for more complicated problems

(*From Levine et al, 1983.*)

Table 33-7. Goals and Outcome Measures in Behavioral Intervention

Thorough evaluation of the problem	Evaluation is adequate to formulate an individual treatment plan and discharge plan
Increase the ability of the child, family, and significant others to manage the child's behavior	Demonstrable decrease in the severity, frequency, and duration of episodes of problem behavior
Improve specific behavioral patterns that have interfered with functioning	Improvement in daily functioning, symptom control, and learning compensation strategies. Environmental modifications are employed as indicated
Facilitate functional communication and interaction patterns within the family system	Family displays increased recognition of their own needs and those of the child. Parents are able to be firm and supportive. Family unit, including child, engages in open, honest communication exchanges.
Increase the child's and family member's personal growth, especially in the area of self-esteem	The child, and other family members as applicable, display fewer self-defeating behaviors. An increase in positive behaviors is occurring, including during periods of stress
Increased educational participation by the child	Increased attention span and improvement in the quality and amount of work produced
Child and family recognize the importance of continued work to improve conflict areas	Child and family follow through with treatment plan and periodic after-care sessions for maintenance

Box 33-7
Components of a Behavioral Management System

RULES

- Derive from parents/teachers specific statements of desired and undesired behaviors, i.e., identification of the problem behavior.*
- Post in a conspicuous place where both child and reinforcer(s) are reminded of them.
- Child is informed of the rules and why they are being posted.
- Only 2 to 3 rules should be concentrated on at any given time.

REWARDS (POSITIVE REINFORCERS)

- May be verbal, social, tangible objects, or activities.
- Examples are praise, attention, special activities with parent(s) or peers, star charts, token or point systems, candy, money (see Chapter 13).
- Purpose is to encourage child to increase a desirable behavior or acquire a behavior currently nonexistent.
- To be successful, the reward must be (1) something the child finds satisfying and desirable, (2) readily available, and (3) accessible to the child when the desired behavior occurs.

PUNISHMENT (NEGATIVE REINFORCER)

- Purpose is to cause discontinuance of undesirable behavior.
- Examples are to ignore the undesirable behavior; expressing verbal disappointment when the behavior is displayed; temporary time out or isolation (child must be quiet during this time, time does not begin till child has stopped crying or otherwise protesting, time should be brief); temporary privilege removal; physical punishment. See Chapter 13.

NOTE: If a negative relationship exists between the child and reinforcer(s), the relationship must be dealt with simultaneously or before the behavior management problem is initiated. Consistent positive reinforcement of the desired behavior and ignoring or negative reinforcement of the problem behavior is required over time to extinguish the problem behavior and/or develop the desired behavior. This system has documented success but demands energy, patience, and consistency in employment by the reinforcer.

* Priority is given to behaviors that threaten harm to the child or others, those that threaten property destruction, and those that infringe on others' rights.

(Compiled from Norton, 1977; Williams et al, 1981; and Levine et al, 1983.)

creases the child's anxiety and, as a consequence, the frequency and intensity of maladaptive behavior simultaneously decelerates. Consistency, coupled with praise and positive reinforcement, is critical to achieving and maintaining normal, appropriate behavior. Neutral emotional responses from significant others when behavior is out of line is equally significant. A neutral response is calm, matter-of-fact, and confident, removing any need in the child to be defensive or offensive in response. The most challenging aspect of intervention is always to respond primarily to the child and secondarily to the behavior.

Because of parents' sense of failure and humility, one of the most difficult tasks of nurses and other team members is motivating the family to accept outside intervention. Acknowledging how difficult their situation must be, offering a no-fault suggestion that the family deserves help, and presenting tangible intervention options is often the most effective approach. Intervention is best presented in terms of possibly resolving family suffering and should capitalize on identified strengths of the child, family members, and the family as a unit. Family and professional team members keep in mind the goals summarized in Table 33-7 as a treatment program is developed. From these program goals, healthy life adaptation of the child and family unit is promoted.

References

Anders T, Walton C: Psychotherapy with children. *In* Levine M, et al (eds): *Developmental-Behavioral Pediatrics.* Philadelphia, WB Saunders, 1983.

Barnard K: Studying patterns of behavior. *MCN* 1985; 5:358.

Brink R: How serious is the child's behavior problem? *MCN* 1982; 7:33-36.

Carey W: Clinical applications of infant temperament measurements. *Pediatr* 1972; 81:823.

Chess S, Thomas A: Individuality: dynamics of individual behavioral development. *In* Levine M, et al (eds): *Developmental-Behavioral Pediatrics.* Philadelphia, WB Saunders, 1983.

Chess S, Thomas A, Birch H: (1970). The origin of personality. *Sci Am* 1970, Aug; 102-108.

Clunn P, Payne D: *Psychiatric Mental Health Nursing.* New York, Medical Examination Publishing Company, Elsevier, 1985.

Crocker A: The involvement of siblings of children with handicaps. *In* Milunsky A (ed): *Coping with Crisis and Handicap.* New York, Plenum Publishing Corporation, 1981.

Darez-Williams P, et al: Media approach to family training in behavior management. *Issues Compr Pediatr Nurs* 1986; 2:59-77.

Eyberg S, Robinson E: *Dyadic Parent-Child Interaction Coding System: A Manual.* Psychological Documents 13, Ms 2582, 1983.

Eyberg S: Behavioral assessment: advancing methodology in pediatric psychology. *J Pediatr Psychol* 1985; 2:123-139.
Featherstone H: *A Difference in the Family: Living with a Disabled Child.* New York, Basic Books, 1981.
Forehand R, McMahon R: *Helping the Noncompliant Child: A Clinician's Guide to Parent Training.* New York, Guilford Press, 1981.
Golden L: Managing maladaptive behavior in ill children through family intervention. *J School Health* 1984; 10:389-391.
Gumaer J: *Counseling and Therapy for Children.* New York, Free Press, 1984.
Herbert M: *Problems of Childhood.* New York, Pan Books, Ltd, 1975.
Hersoo L: Emotional disorders in childhood. *Nursing Times* 1977 June 9; 864.
Hodges K, et al: The child assessment schedule: a diagnostic interview for research and clinical use. Catalog Selected Documents in Psychol 1981; 11:56.
Kazdin A: Reactive self-monitoring: the effects of response desirability, goal setting and feedback. *J Consult Clin Psychol* 1974; 42:704-716.
Kline K: Systematic data collection: key to behavioral assessment in patients with behavior problems. *Perspectives* 1986; 2:4-6.
Kniskern J, et al: Mother-child interaction in home and laboratory settings. *Child Study* 1983; 13:23-29.
Kupchik D: Prevention and management of disturbed behavior. *Can J Psychiatr Nurs* 1985; 4:9-11.
LeBow M: *Behavior Modification: A Significant Method in Nursing Practice.* Englewood Cliffs, NJ, Prentice-Hall, 1979.
Levine M, et al: *Developmental-Behavioral Pediatrics.* Philadelphia, WB Saunders, 1983.
Liptak G, Chamberlain R: Clinical assessment of behavioral performance in adjustment. *In* Levine M, et al (eds): *Developmental-Behavioral Pediatrics.* Philadelphia, WB Saunders, 1983.
Mandell C, Fiscus E: *Understanding Exceptional People.* St. Paul, West Publishing Company, 1981.
Martin R: *Legal Challenges to Behavior Modification: Trends in Schools, Corrections and Mental Health.* Champaign, IL, Research Press, 1975.
Martin R: Legal issues in preserving client rights. *In* Hannah G, et al (eds): *Presentation of Clients' Rights.* New York, Free Press, 1981.
Nelson R: Assessment and therapeutic functions of self monitoring. *In* Hersen M, et al (eds): *Progress in Behavior Modification.* New York, Academic Press, 1977.
Norton G: *Parenting.* Englewood Cliffs, NJ, Prentice-Hall, 1977.
O'Leary K, Johnson S: Psychological assessment. *In* Quay H, Werry J (eds): *Psychopathological Disorders of Childhood.* New York, John Wiley, 1986.
Popper C, Famularo R: Child and adolescent psychopharmacology. *In* Levine M, et al (eds): *Developmental-Behavioral Pediatrics.* Philadelphia, WB Saunders, 1983.
Pugh-Antich J, Rabinovich H: Major child and adolescent psychiatric disorders. *In* Levine M, et al (eds): *Developmental-Behavioral Pediatrics.* Philadelphia, WB Saunders, 1983.
Rosoff J: *Informed Consent: A Guide for Health Care Providers.* Rockville, MD, Aspen Systems Corporation, 1981.
Satir V: *Conjoint Family Therapy.* New York, Science and Behavior Books, 1982.
Schwitzgebel RL, Schwitzgebel RK: *Law and Psychological Practice.* New York, John Wiley, 1980.
Shapiro E: Self-monitoring procedures. *In* Ollendick T, Hersen M (eds): *Child Behavioral Assessment.* New York, Pergamon Press, 1984.
Shonkoff J: Preschool. *In* Levine M, et al (eds): *Developmental-Behavioral Pediatrics.* Philadelphia, WB Saunders, 1983.
Stewart M: Temper, temper: how to deal with tantrums. Parents 1981; 2:75.
Tauer K: Promoting effective decision-making in sexually active adolescents. *Nurs Clin North Am* 1983; 18:275-292.
Taylor C: *Mereness' Essentials of Psychiatric Nursing.* St. Louis, CV Mosby, 1982.
Ten Bensel R, Tobin J (eds): *Guides for Pediatric Care.* Minneapolis, Henepin County Medical Center (mimeograph), 1975, p 7.
Thomas A, Chess S: *Temperament and Development.* New York, Brunner/Mazel, 1977.
Thomas A, Chess S: *Dynamics of Psychological Development.* New York, Brunner/Mazel, 1980.
Tiernay A, Tiernay I: *Perennial Problems of Parenthood: Adopting a Behavioral Approach.* Medical Education (International) Ltd, 1983.
Webster-Stratton C: Recognizing and assessing conduct disorders in children. *Matern Child Nurs J* 1983; 5:330-335.
Williams B, et al (eds): *Pediatric-Behavioral Medicine.* New York, Praeger, 1981.
Wilson L, et al: Behavior therapy nursing: a new era. *Nurs Times* 1986; 1:48-49.
York P, et al: *Tough Love Solutions.* New York, Bantam Books, 1985.

Bibliography

Blosser C: Avoiding potential behavior problems in children. *Pediatr Nurs* 1979 May-Jun; 5.
Buckley K, Walker H: *Modifying Classroom Behavior: A Manual of Procedures for Classroom Teachers.* Champaign, IL, Research Press, 1970.
Chamberlain R: Relationships between child-rearing styles and child behavior over time. *Am J Dis Child* 1978; 155-160.
Clarizio H, McCoy G: *Behavior Disorders in Children.* Cambridge, MA, Harper and Row, 1983.
Colley K: Growing up together: the mutual respect balance. *In* Arnold L (ed): *Helping Parents Help Their Children.* New York, Brunner/Mazel, 1978.
Cone J, Hawkin R (eds): *Behavioral Assessment: New Directions in Clinical Psychology.* New York, Brunner/Mazel, 1977.
Friedman S, Sarles R: Out of control behavior in adolescents. *Pediatr Clin North Am* 1980; 27:97-107.
Gabel S (ed): *Behavioral Problems of Childhood: A Primary Care Approach.* New York, Grune and Stratton, 1981.
Green C: How to recognize hostility and what to do about it. *Am J Nurs* 1986; 11:1230-1234.

Hodges K, et al: The development of a child assessment interview for research and clinical use. *J Abn Child Psychol* 1982; 10:173-189.

Holland C: An interview guide for behavioral counseling with parents. *Behavior Therapy* 1970; 1:70-79.

Kaeppen A: Relaxation training for children. *Elem School Guid Counsel* 1974; 9:14-23.

Kelly G: Guided fantasy as a counseling technique with youth. *J Counsel Psychol* 1972; 19:355-361.

Lazarus A: *Behavior Therapy and Beyond.* New York, McGraw-Hill, 1971.

Magrab P (ed): (1984). *Psychological and Behavioral Assessment.* New York, Plenum Press, 1984.

Mahoney M: *Cognition and Behavior Modification.* Cambridge, MA, Ballinger Company, 1983.

Marholin D (ed): *Child Behavior Therapy.* New York, Gardner Press, 1978.

Martin B: Brief family intervention: effectiveness and the importance of including the father. *J Consult Clin Psychol* 1977; 45:1002-1010.

Matarazzo J: *Behavioral Health.* New York, John Wiley and Sons, 1984.

McAuley R, McAuley P: *Child Behavior Problems: An Empirical Approach to Management.* New York, Free Press, 1978.

McBrian R: Using relaxation methods with first grade boys. *Elem School Guid Counsel* 1978; 3:146-152.

Meichenbaum D: *Cognitive Behavior Modification.* New York, Plenum Press, 1977.

Nelms B: Assessing childhood depression: do parents and children agree? *Pediatr Nurs* 1986; 1:23-26.

Ollendick T, Hersen M (eds): *Child Behavioral Assessment: Principles and Procedures.* New York, Pergamon Press, 1984.

Risley T, et al: Behavioral technology for the normal middle-class family. *In* Marsh E, et al (eds): *Behavior Modification and Families.* New York, Brunner/Mazel, 1976.

Rossman H, Kahnweiler J: Relaxation training with intermediate grade students. *Elem School Guid Counsel* 1977; 4:259-266.

Schleicher I: Teaching parents to cope with behavior problems. *Am J Nurs* 1978; 78:838-839.

Stienhauer P, Rae-Grant J (eds): *Psychological Problems of the Child in the Family.* New York, Basic Books, 1983.

Thomas A, Chess S, Birch H: *Temperament and Behavior Disorders in Children.* New York, New York University Press, 1968.

Vierville E: *Behavioral Problems of Preschool Children.* Springfield, IL, Charles C Thomas, 1985.

Webster-Stratton C: Teaching mothers through videotaped modeling to change their children's behavior. *J Pediatr Psychol* 1982; 7:279-294.

Webster-Stratton C, Eyberg S: (1982). Child temperament: relationship with child behavior problems and parent-child interactions. *J Clin Psychol* 1982; 11:123-129.

Wilson D, Prentice-Dunn S: Rating scales in the assessment of child behavior. *J Clin Child Psychol* 1981; 10:112-126.

Yarrow L: Interviewing children. *In* Mussen P (ed): *Handbook of Research Methods in Child Development.* New York, John Wiley, 1960.

York M, et al: Alternative professional roles in health care delivery: leadership patterns in self-help groups. *J Appl Behav Sci,* 1985; 4:427–444.

Nursing Strategies: Alterations in Development

Chapter 34

Peggy Drapo
Charlotte Patrick

Nurses may work with developmentally disabled children and their families in a variety of settings, including the hospital, clinics, physicians' offices, schools, community agencies, and the family's home. By using the nursing process, nurses play an important role in each of these settings. Although nursing interventions will vary depending upon the nature of the child's disability, there are some commonalities in assessment and intervention with these children and their families. This chapter includes a discussion of some of these commonalities as well as some of the specifics for selected disabilities.

Related Topics
Genetic assessment, Chapter 4
Patterns of inheritance in trisomy 21, Chapter 4
The impact of chronic illness, Chapter 25
Conduct disorders, Chapter 36
Musculoskeletal aspects of cerebral palsy, Chapter 47

Developmental Alterations

The Developmental Disabilities Act of 1978 defined a developmental disability as a severe chronic state that is present before 22 years of age and is likely to continue indefinitely. The disability may be caused by either a physical or mental impairment or a combination of the two. The person who is developmentally disabled has substantial limitations in at least three of the following major life activities: self-care, receptive and expressive language, learning, mobility, self-direction, capacity for independent living, and economic self-sufficiency. The person requires individually planned and coordinated multidisciplinary care, treatment, or other services for an extended period of time or throughout his or her life.

A developmental alteration is a variation from what is classified as "normal development" for an individual. No child is 100 per cent normal; in fact, no person is 100 per cent normal. As children grow and develop, they establish and refine a set of strengths and weaknesses that is uniquely their own. Many different patterns of strengths, weaknesses, and behaviors can be classified as "normal." The term normal is in itself difficult to define because it is to some extent developmentally, culturally, and socially determined. This chapter includes information about children who have experienced the following developmental alterations: developmental delays, attention deficit disorders, learning disabilities, mental retardation, and giftedness. Considering gifted children with children who have developmental disabilities may surprise some readers. However, any alteration from the norm may bring special problems because it causes the child to depart in noticeable ways from the mainstream of society.

The medical model, for some time, has been subjected to criticism because it has centered on the condition or the variation rather than the child. Along with the medical model, Public Law 94-142 of 1975, Education for All Handicapped Children, is also responsible for describing children in terms of handicaps. For instance, the law defines children as handicapped if they are emotionally disturbed, mentally retarded, speech-language impaired, visually handicapped, hearing impaired, deaf, orthopedically impaired, physically handicapped, or learning disabled. Yet, the focus of mainstreaming, which the law seeks to legislate, is the development of whatever ability the child may have, not the disability.

Scientists and theorists have attempted to account for the development of the human being using many different approaches. Some theorists are proponents of a strong genetic explanation, whereas others have an environmental bias. Most theorists, however, generally agree that development is a combination of both genetic and environmental influences. We have learned that a person may be genetically programmed to achieve all that is deemed normal, but be subjected to social environments that can produce pathologic problems. The right social environments, on the other hand, can produce normal or near normal outcomes for those individuals with developmental disabilities. This principle of normal development applies to both handicapped and nonhandicapped individuals (Anastasiow, 1986). Although the development of children with disabilities may be slower than those without disabilities, they *will* develop. Children with such problems may only need therapies, training, or prostheses to enhance their development. The environment needed by nonhandicapped children to reach their fullest potential is also beneficial to children with disabilities.

Any developmental alteration affecting a child will influence all family members. It is, therefore, essential for the nurse to be able to work with all family members to help identify their strengths and manage the problems related to their child's disability (Hymovich, 1979). The nurse's role is to identify, prevent, and reduce the problems associated with the disabling condition. The nurse has a responsibility for recognizing babies and children who are at risk for alterations in development. Nurses are also responsible for helping parents and their children gain access to appropriate resources in the community. Nurses are beginning to use and develop tools for assessing children and families who are at risk for developmental alterations. Nurses who are caring for these children and their families will be working with different members of the health team; therefore, they need the skills required to function as effective team members. Nurses are uniquely qualified for many of the interventions needed by families of children with developmental alterations and are often the appropriate people to coordinate the family's care.

Assessment

Throughout the assessment process, the nurse's role is to establish baseline measurements, give support to the child and parents, and help the family receive the appropriate services in the community. The nurse's role includes observation of the child, administration of screening tests, recording and reporting observations and results of screening, and making appropriate referrals.

Assessment of the Child in the Hospital

Nurses in hospital settings will be working with children of all ages. Assessments are essential in order to detect infants who are at risk for developmental alterations. A series of head measurements provides one important indicator of future problems in mental and physical development. Feeding behaviors and social-behavioral parameters are also good indicators of potential risk. If possible, auditory and visual screening should be done before the infant is discharged from the nursery.

Caesar and Eggermont (1985) summarize the "alarm signs" that should alert the nurse and other professionals to infants who are at risk for neonatal neurologic problems. These signs include infants who have difficulty feeding, continuously fuss, or persistently display abnormal eye or head positions or asymmetry in posture or movements. Other risk factors are: (1) immobility, (2) apathy, (3) floppiness, (4) hyperexcitability, (5) convulsions, (6) abnormal cry sounds, and (7) abnormal head measurements. When an infant is noted to have any of these problems, all neural functions that are testable should be evaluated, using tests that are appropriate for that infant's gestational age. Although nurses may do some of the baseline neurologic screening, the physician will do further testing.

The child's physical characteristics, treatments, x-rays, and laboratory test results should all be recorded. The results of neurologic and other testing should be noted and any changes that occur should be explained carefully. These records will be invaluable to the team who will follow the child after discharge.

Although the neonatal period is a critical time for central nervous system damage, perinatal hazards are responsible for only 15 to 20 per cent of severe developmental handicaps. Because environmental, genetic, and socioeconomic factors are responsible for 80 to 85 per cent of the damage, the child is at risk for central nervous system insults up to 2 years of age while growth of the brain is still occurring (Caesar and Eggermont, 1985). Usually, major neurologic defects are identified within the first year of life. In some rural areas, where there is no ready access to medical care, children's disabilities may not be identified until after this time period. Some disorders, such as hydrocephalus, are usually diagnosed before the third month of life, whereas others, such as cerebral palsy, may not be diagnosed until toward the end of the first year (Amiel-Tison, 1985). Some neuromotor abnormalities are transient in nature, and those persons assessing the child need to be aware of this possibility, especially in the case of very low birthweight infants.

Assessment of the Child in the Community

Usually, it is a parent or relative who first notes the presence of a problem or a difference in the child. Sometimes, a routine screening by a teacher, nurse, or member of the child's health team will reveal the first indication of a problem. All young children should be screened on a yearly basis. This screening should cover general health; auditory, visual, speech, and motor development; self-help skills; behavior; and learning or thinking. Screening may be carried out by professionals in conjunction with day care providers. The medical screening may be performed by a nurse practitioner or physician. Auditory screening may be done by a nurse, audiologist, speech pathologist, or health aide (provided the aide has had special training to use an audiometer). Speech screening is usually done by a speech pathologist or therapist. Various types of screening tools can be used, such as observation checklists and commercially prepared screening instruments.

Screening Tools and Observation Checklists

Nurses need to be familiar with some of the commercially prepared screening tools. Nurses may be involved in administering these tools and helping parents understand the results of the screening. These tools are used to indicate whether more definitive testing is required. *Screening is not done to measure the child's intelligence or to make a diagnosis; it is used to define a potential problem and to indicate a child's areas of strengths and weaknesses.* Some of the more common tools are listed in Table 34-1. Other screening tools are available to measure children's intelligence (cognitive development) and adaptive behavior. Selection of screening tools depends on many factors, such as whether behavior or intelligence is being tested, the age of the child, cultural limitations, and the amount of training required for proficiency in its administration.

It is often difficult to use the more common intelligence tests for children with handicapping conditions. Some tests specifically devised for these children are the Nebraska Test of Learning Aptitude for the hearing impaired, the Perkins-Binet Intelligence Scale for the visually impaired, and the Columbia Mental Maturity Scale for those with motor and language impairments. The Merrill-Palmer Scale of Mental Tests has been adapted for children who are both speaking and hearing impaired.

Checklists can be useful tools in identifying potential problems at an early age. If you are asking a caregiver (e.g., mother, teacher) to observe behaviors and activities, provide the caregiver with a checklist and instructions for its use. Research indicates that mothers and professionals show consistent results in their assessments of a child's development if the parent has been instructed in the same strategies used by

Table 34-1. Screening Tools for Developmental Assessment

Tool	Description	Source
Brazelton Neonatal Behavioral Assessment Scale	Includes some aspects of a neurologic test but is not a neurologic examination. It is best used as a tool to assess infant interactive behavior. It can be used as a teaching tool with parents to demonstrate the baby's unique characteristics. Useful in working with high-risk infants. Requires special training for use.	JB Lippincott East Washington Square Philadelphia, PA 19105
Denver Developmental Screening Test (DDST)	Used to identify developmental lags in children from 2 weeks to 6 years. Areas observed are personal-social, fine motor-adaptive, gross motor, and fine motor skills. Reliability and validity have been demonstrated. Modifications are being made to make it more applicable to children in the lower socioeconomic group. A Spanish DDST is available.	Ladoca Project & Publishing Company East 51st Ave. and Lincoln St. Denver, CO 80216
Fathering Behavior	Designed to guide nurses in observing fathers' adaptive and maladaptive behaviors. Useful in observations of high-risk situations (e.g., divorce with the father in custody of the child, child abuse situations, or parent drug abuse situations).	Johnson SH: *Nursing Assessment and Strategies for the Family at Risk.* 2nd ed. Philadelphia, JB Lippincott, 1986.
Portage Guide to Early Development	A checklist used to measure behaviors and skills of children from birth to 6 years; cognitive development and motor skills.	Cooperative Education Services Agency 412 E. Silfer St. Portage, WI 53901
School/Home Observation and Referral System (SHORS)	A general checklist to observe a child for unusual behaviors in comparison to peers. Depending on these findings, a specific checklist is used for more detail. For children from preschool through third grade. Areas to be checked are health, motor, vision, hearing, speech, language behavior, and learning.	CTB/McGraw-Hill Del Monte Research Park Monterey, CA 93940
The Yellow Brick Road	Helps identify preschool chidren experiencing difficulty in motor, visual, auditory, and language areas. This is a game type of screening in which the child follows a path from station to station where various workers will test the child. There are 24 stations, each requiring the presence of an adult.	Christine Kallstrom Learning Concepts 2501 N. Lamar Austin, TX 78705

the professional (Beckman, 1984). There are commercially prepared observation checklists, such as the Home Observation Measurement of the Environment (HOME). This tool, developed by Caldwell and Bradley, measures the environmental support the child receives in the home. It is a checklist of responsibilities related to the mother and other items, such as the environment, discipline, and involvement with the child. Reliability and validity have been demonstrated. (See Appendix Five.)

It may be necessary to make your own checklist. If you will be observing several children, you can write the list of characteristics you want to observe (e.g., hearing, vision, specific behaviors) in a vertical column on the left side of the page, and place the children's names horizontally across the top of the page. This gives the nurse or caregiver an opportunity to see areas of deficiency, lag, or acceleration more easily when compared with other children in the same age group. Figure 34-1 is a sample checklist.

The following guidelines should be followed when you are using an observational screening tool:

1. Keep an accurate description of what the child says or does during the observational period.
2. Observe the child on several different occasions to be absolutely sure the behavior you describe is a typical one.
3. Date each observation.
4. Write down exactly what you see and hear, rather than making statements based on your opinion. Objectiveness in reporting is essential.
5. In making referrals, be specific and clear about your concerns and tell why you are making the referral.

Observer: ____________________

Date: ____________________

School: ____________________

		Children's Names			
I. Personal-Social Development	Frequent conflict with other children				
	Poor body image and self concept				
	Immature social behavior				
II. Cognitive Development	Displays lag in development				
	Discrepancy between potential and intellectual development and actual achievement				
III. Language and Speech Development	Delayed language development				
	Needs instruction repeated often				
	Inability to follow a sequence of two or more directions				
	Echoes or parrots language without understanding the meaning				
IV. Motor Development	Perseveration				
	Overactive				
	Difficulty with gross motor skills				
	Inability or difficulty in crossing midline of body				
	Distractible				
	Difficulty in fine motor skills				
	Fearful of heights				
	Inability in following directions				
V. Perceptual Motor Development	Visual perceptual problems				
	Auditory perceptual problems				
	Tactually defensive				
	Perceptual motor integration problems				

***Figure* 34-1.** A checklist for alterations in development.

Most of the observation or screening tools can be completed by teachers, health professionals, specially trained aides, or, in some cases, parents. A more definitive assessment must be done only by qualified professionals. When a child is referred to the appropriate professionals, a thorough assessment is done in an attempt to locate the problem area and to make a diagnosis. The diagnosis is made not on the basis of one test, but usually after a battery of tests are completed. This is done to ensure against labeling a child with a wrong diagnosis and a lifetime of stigma and inappropriate interventions. The tests used to further assess the child will be in the areas of intellectual, emotional, behavioral, social, physical, and language skills.

Physical Assessment

After the screening is completed, the children with alterations in development are referred to a physician for a complete examination. A complete physical examination is needed to uncover any physical problems associated with the child's developmental alteration. Of particular importance on physical examination is evidence of deviation of normal growth patterns, physical stigmata, and congenital defects. The examination will cover respiratory, cardiac, renal, neurologic, perceptual, and motor problems. In infants under 6 months of age, it is especially important to observe for asymmetric movements and the expected disappearance of primitive reflexes. Also important to note are abnormalities of gait, symmetry of muscle tone, and deep tendon reflexes as well as the presence of intact cerebellar and sensory functions (Dimond, 1984).

Children with developmental alterations may have physical problems related to genetics, such as diabetes, sickle cell anemia, hemophilia, or cystic fibrosis. Other problems may be the result of congenital malformations, such as cardiac, neurologic, and musculoskeletal conditions. Developmental alterations may also be the result of environmental problems, such as lead poisoning, and infections, such as rubella or tuberculosis.

Children with alterations in development are usually followed by a pediatrician or a physician in family practice. The physician will then establish a plan of treatment that may include referral to an agency or another professional, such as a neurologist or cardiologist. The nurse's role will include establishing baseline measurements, giving support to the child and parent, and helping the family receive the right services in the community.

Behavioral Assessment

It is important to assess children for changes in behavior and in toileting and eating behaviors. The child with developmental alterations may experience an improvement or deterioration in an existing problem. A comprehensive health assessment should include the collection of data related to the genetic and health history of the child and family members, and information about the environmental, behavioral, and social adjustment areas. It is especially helpful to have an assessment form, or series of forms, that includes all of the areas to be assessed in the evaluation. The use of such a form or forms ensures that nothing important will be omitted. Skills of daily living can also be included in a form. Analysis of these data will assist the nurse and other health professionals in taking appropriate actions for correct interventions in the client's health care.

Family Assessment

After the findings of the comprehensive evaluation are analyzed, an assessment of the child's environment is made to determine its adequacy for meeting the child's safety and special needs. The parents' perceptions of the child's condition, their expectations from treatment, and their beliefs about the child's prognosis need to be determined. This becomes an ongoing process throughout assessment and intervention. The nurse, along with other health care providers, will be involved in obtaining this information and helping the family deal with the problems they are facing.

The parent who has been dashing about with a child from one appointment to another must have a thorough explanation of all the findings and recommendations for intervention. The possible negative outcomes of the planned intervention should be discussed along with the anticipated positive outcomes.

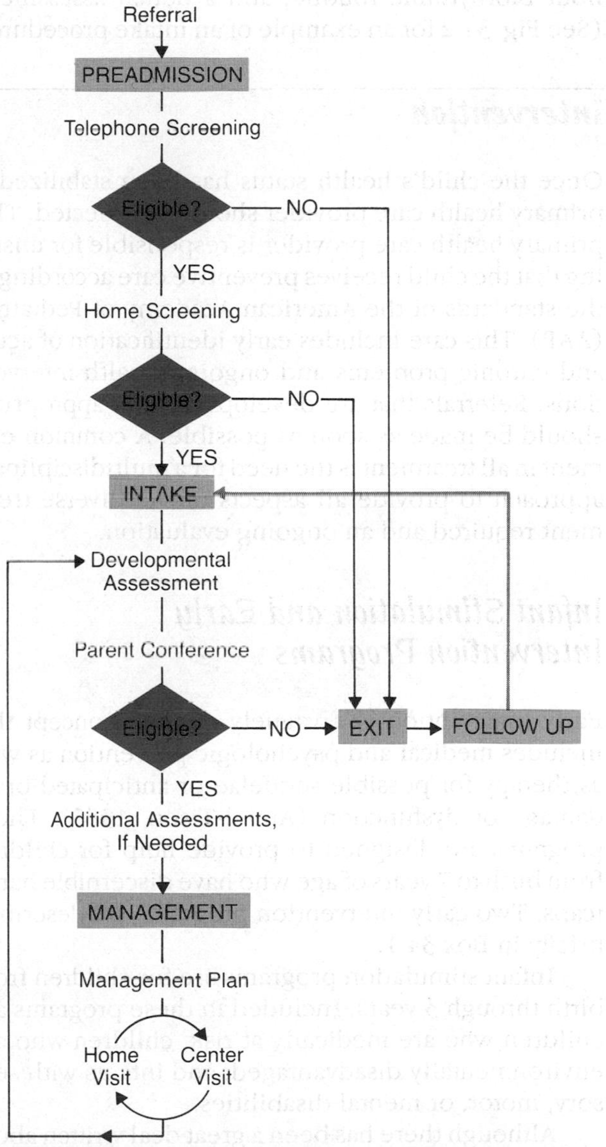

Figure 34-2. Flow chart of service delivery. (Reprinted with permission of D. Sue Schafer, Director, Child Success Through Parent Training: Final Report 1980–1983, p. 15.)

Intake Procedures

A thorough assessment of the child and family is essential before an intervention program can be instituted. The assessment by use of screening tools, discussed previously, should lead to identification of children who are likely to be developmentally delayed. The next step is a comprehensive evaluation by diagnosticians, such as physicians; audiologists; physical, speech, and occupational therapists; psychologists; community health and pediatric nurses; nutritionists; and social workers. This evaluation should include a complete physical examination with a systems review, visual and auditory screening, laboratory and genetic status, nutritional status and practices, anthropometric measurements, family history and pedigree, neurodevelopmental evaluations, normal 24-hour biorhythmic routine, and a dental assessment. (See Fig. 34-2 for an example of an intake procedure.)

Intervention

Once the child's health status has been stabilized, a primary health care provider should be selected. This primary health care provider is responsible for ensuring that the child receives preventive care according to the standards of the American Academy of Pediatrics (AAP). This care includes early identification of acute and chronic problems and ongoing health interventions. Referrals that are developmentally appropriate should be made as soon as possible. A common element in all treatment is the need for a multidisciplinary approach to provide all aspects of the diverse treatment required and an ongoing evaluation.

Infant Stimulation and Early Intervention Programs

Early intervention is a vaguely defined concept that includes medical and psychologic prevention as well as therapy for possible sequelae or anticipated brain damage or dysfunction (Amiel-Tison, 1985). These programs are designed to provide help for children from birth to 7 years of age who have discernible handicaps. Two early intervention programs are described briefly in Box 34-1.

Infant stimulation programs are for children from birth through 3 years. Included in these programs are children who are medically at risk, children who are environmentally disadvantaged, and infants with sensory, motor, or mental disabilities.

Although there has been a great deal written about the benefits of infant stimulation programs, research studies that support these views are few and far between. The exact benefits of infant stimulation programs need to be a focus of research. Barnard and Kelly (1980) state that without adequate descriptive and empirical data it is difficult to make appropriate decisions about program goals, methods of service delivery, and role descriptions for staff. They recommend that researchers begin directing their work at the effects of such programs on the child; on family adjustments; and on the change, if any, in parent-child interaction.

Amiel-Tison (1985) describes two differing viewpoints that attempt to explain how early intervention leads to improvement in the child with perinatal damage. From the brain plasticity perspective, it is suggested that an area of the brain normally intended to perform a certain skill will, in the case of brain damage, reorganize functions. For example, if a certain portion of the brain that was affected was removed before a particular age, another portion of the brain would assume these missing functions (Anastasiow, 1986). It has been suggested that motor and sensory stimulation would facilitate the mechanisms of plasticity and that the more immature the fetal brain at the time of damage, the greater the opportunity for good results.

Box 34-1
Examples of Early Intervention Programs

1. The University of California, Los Angeles (UCLA) Program for Handicapped Children affiliates with the UCLA Department of Pediatrics, Division of Child Development. This program provides year-round medical, educational, and social support services to families with developmentally disabled children. The multidisciplinary staff is made up of early childhood educators; social workers; occupational, physical, and speech therapists; a medical director; and a pediatrician. Intervention programs such as this one provide both home and center-based services (Howard and Beckwith, 1980). Broad intervention goals of the program involve working with the family to help them gain confidence and skill in raising the child, developing the child's maximum strengths, and helping the child compensate for weaknesses.
2. The Child Success Through Parent Training Program is an infant stimulation project funded by a grant written by Schafer (1984) of the School of Physical Therapy at Texas Woman's University in Denton, Texas. The goals of this program are to stimulate increased services to young handicapped children and to develop an innovative model to serve handicapped children in three counties of north Texas. The program encourages participation of parents in all activities, from the initial assessment of the child through all the interventions. The extent of parent participation is determined by the parent's interest, availability, capability, and motivation. The program capitalizes on the expertise of a team of developmental specialists.

Amiel-Tison (1985) states that she accepts the belief held by some professionals that plasticity is limited and will not yield full behavior recovery for the brain-injured child as the plasticity theorists predict. However, she is not opposed to follow-up intervention in motor function, language, fine motor skills, school adaptation, and work with the family. The second viewpoint regarding the effectiveness of infant stimulation is that there is improved function rather than reorganization. Improved function is thought to be related more to maturation than to plasticity. Some anomalies in children experiencing motor deficits at a younger age may disappear during the process of maturation. For instance, the use of physical therapy will not cure cerebral palsy, but it may improve the child's function.

Early intervention programs have a variety of philosophic and theoretical bases. Programs that are the most effective seem to have several common components: (1) intervention beginning at a very early age, (2) the inclusion of parents as full participants in their child's program, and (3) involvement of a number of disciplines in diagnosing and planning for each child. These three elements seem to be the key to providing a program that has long-range and lasting effects.

Mainstreaming

Mainstreaming means helping people who have handicaps to learn to work in settings where they will have the greatest opportunity to become as independent as possible. In the school system, mainstreaming refers to the integration of handicapped and nonhandicapped children in the same classroom. According to Kleinberg (1984), the main purpose of mainstreaming is to eliminate the dichotomy between special education classes and regular educational programs. She believes that an educational program should include a spectrum of services rather than a rigid set of choices.

There are innovative educational programs across the nation to assist children who must be absent from school frequently because of chronic health problems. These methods include the use of closed circuit television programs, flexible scheduling that allows adjustment for children with low energy levels or those on dialysis, and contracts with schools that spell out all responsibilities when children attend school with special equipment such as ventilators. These services, by necessity, are complex and require the services of many professionals with a wide range of specialized training.

Evaluation

Ongoing evaluations for preventive, maintenance, restorative, and curative activities should be carried out regularly by the health care provider. Other team members should conduct regular evaluations of the child's psychosocial development and motor, cognitive, and communicative development. Family adaptation to the child's condition should also be monitored on a regular basis.

The Impact of Developmental Alterations on the Child and the Family: The Nurse's Role

In many cases, clinical education for pediatric nursing is conducted in the hospital. When nursing instructors and students work with chidren with developmental disabilities and handicapping conditions, it is usually in the context of sick children or children who are having some surgical procedure. The nurse who sees these children only in that light develops a perception of them that is somewhat biased. Nurses, however, are not unlike the general public in this respect. Many people today still believe that children with disabilities belong in a special classroom, at home, or in an institution, or that they should not have been allowed to be born in the first place. All nurses need to take a good look at their own beliefs and values, and modify them if necessary to effectively help these children and their families.

People in the government, health care professionals, and even parents cannot agree about what is the best way to care for children with disabilities. In Texas, some recent lawsuits have brought far-reaching changes in the way in which care for children with developmental disabilities will be delivered. The Association for Retarded Citizens and the Parents' Association of Retarded in Texas have differing opinions on care and housing for these children and adults. Funding in all states is causing massive changes in services. As a result of both federal and state laws, state school institutions are being told to depopulate their facilities to more manageable levels. Public schools and communities are being required to provide for these individuals. Children who were once sent directly from the hospital nursery to institutions are now being sent home.

Nurses have many hats to wear when working with children or adults who have disabilities or problems that prevent them from achieving their full potential. The nurse's role consists of any of the following activities: case finding, direct care giving, teaching, providing guidance and support, consulting, coordinating, collaborating with other professionals, and being a child and family advocate (Hymovich, 1985). These roles may take place in a variety of settings, including the home, hospital, school, or clinic.

The Role of the Nurse as Epidemiologist

An important role for nurses in any setting is that of epidemiologist. Nurses are in an excellent position to detect children with possible developmental alterations or those who are at risk for such alterations. Knowledge of the risk factors is essential for any nurse who may come in contact with children and pregnant women.

The Role of the Nurse in Supporting the Family

The nurse has a unique opportunity to provide support to the family of a child with a developmental alteration. The response that parents exhibit when they first learn of the diagnosis is well documented. Their first reaction is often one of being overwhelmed with the knowledge that their child has a disability (Chin et al, 1979). Parents often feel guilty and begin to look for some cause of their child's disability. If they cannot find something or someone else to blame, they may turn their guilt inward. Mourning takes place for the loss of the child they had visualized in their dreams. It is quite common for parents to withdraw from friends and associates. Although such withdrawal is normal, there is a danger it may become pathologic. Parents may experience, at one time or another, feelings of rejection of their child. These feelings may lead to underexpectations for their child or to the setting of unrealistic goals (overexpectations). Trying to escape from the situation is another outcome of unresolved feelings of rejection. All of these feelings are normal, but parents often need someone to help them deal with such emotions in order to resolve them.

Nurses can be a source of support for the whole family as they deal with their feelings. The screening nurse can make referrals to others, such as community health nurses, school nurses, or home health nurses. If necessary, these nurses will be able to make additional referrals to other sources of service that will meet other needs of the family. Nurses can help parents anticipate the way in which their child's disability is likely to affect the family. The impact of developmental alterations on families is similar to the impact of chronic illness as discussed in Chapter 25.

Goldfarb and colleagues (1986) state that there are roadblocks for families in developing formal support. They describe the first block as a *bureaucratic maze* in which parents run from one agency to another seeking the services they need. As their child grows, the services they need become more complex, just as they do for nondisabled children. Nurses can direct the family to groups, such as the American Association for Retarded Citizens or the United Cerebral Palsy Association, where many services are centralized. Nurses should keep a ready resource notebook with referral sources on hand to assist parents in this tedious job.

Another roadblock for families is *cost.* The services that are available to parents in and out of the hospital are the subject of much discussion at the present time. Parents of disabled children need to know how to finance the many treatments and medications their child may need. They need to know such things as how to find information about Social Security Disability Income and Social Security Income.

There are many other roadblocks that families face, such as the *attitude of professionals* working with the family; *professional jargon* that is not explained to the family; the *stigma* that society places on the family and the person who is disabled; *time and energy* required to obtain all of the services and therapies the child requires; and finally, *lack of support* (Goldfarb et al, 1986). An advocate is needed to help families overcome these roadblocks.

Communication Skills Needed by the Nurse. Communication skills can never be taken for granted. Although they may be competent in their various fields, professionals are not necessarily adept at meeting the many needs of parents, who may be in a crisis situation. Understanding the problems faced by the parent requires certain nursing skills. Listening, gathering data, and observing the family relationships will provide the information needed to deal with the family problems brought about by the diagnosis that a family member is mentally retarded and/or developmentally delayed. (See also Chapter 11 on communication strategies.)

The Role of the Nurse as an Advocate

Perhaps the most difficult role of the nurse is the one of advocacy. Advocacy has been defined as defending and promoting the needs of a client (Monea, 1981). Collins (1983) states that advocacy is an appropriate nursing role and is used when the clients feel "alienated and unable to solve problems by their own effort."

The role of an advocate is to help the client remain independent, not to foster dependency. According to Biklen (1976), an advocate (1) helps a client remain independent and free of charity, (2) understands the handicapped as equals and realizes that they want to be treated normally, (3) does not express pity, but rather anger, for the dehumanizing conditions that exist, (4) is motivated to create change, and (5) must be willing to accept criticism from agencies and individuals who are challenged. Ways in which a person can perform the task of advocacy include writing, investigative forums, symbolic acts, boycotts, educating, negotiating, lobbying, and becoming role models (Biklen, 1976).

Advocacy, however, is not without cost. Advocates may be subjected to public criticism, political pressure, and even some subtle and not so subtle discrimination from agency officials who may feel threatened. Advocates can operate within formal systems, such as the court system, or informally by promoting the respect of client rights among the general public (Johnson, 1986a).

The Role of the Nurse in the Child's School Life

Since the passage of Public Law 94-142, the Education of All Handicapped Children, the role of those responsible for the care and education of handicapped children has been changing. The law states that all handicapped children must be afforded their right to a free and appropriate education. They must be educated with nonhandicapped students to the extent appropriate, and they are entitled to attend school at the expense of the district through the school year in which they become 21 years old or have earned a high school diploma. The law also requires that all educational agencies must locate those children who are underserved. It mandates service for those who are mentally retarded, hearing impaired, deaf, orthopedically impaired, deaf-blind, multihandicapped, speech impaired, visually handicapped, and those with specific learning disabilities. In addition, the children are to receive the following related services if they need them: transportation, speech, audiology, counseling, physical and occupational therapy, recreation, psychologic services, and medical services for evaluation and diagnostic purposes.

Handicapped youngsters are entitled to a thorough evaluation, and safeguards must be clearly established to ensure that they receive it. The evaluation of the child is to be free and must be done with the consent of the parents. Children are tested using the established guidelines and standardized tests previously discussed.

Following the evaluation, an Individualized Education Plan (IEP) is written in the public school system or an Individual Development Plan (IDP) in the day care center or home. The IEP focuses on the child's educational needs and guides special education intervention. The IDP focuses on the child's developmental needs, therapies, and related services (Child Development Program Division, 1979).

The team that works with the child in developing an IEP is made up of the school administrator, a chair person, the parent, the child (if possible), the referring teacher, the child evaluation coordinator, the child's liaison, an implementation liaison, consulting specialists, and a recorder. Goals and services and means of implementing the child's educational plan are determined and then carried out by the appropriate school personnel. The child is placed in the least restrictive environment possible for that youngster. The least restrictive environment for a child could range from a regular classroom with no assistance needed to a special class, hospital, or residential placement with a special teacher. The least restrictive environment is determined by the needs of the child that are identified at the time of evaluation and are re-evaluated on a regular basis.

Except for the requirements of Title XIX of the Social Security Act (Medicaid), the interdisciplinary team of PL 94-142 does not directly call for the inclusion of a nurse (Bureau of Community Service, 1979). However, since all children with developmental delay or disabilities have specific health problems, nurses should be included routinely on this team. The health plan should be an integral part of the total plan for each child. Unfortunately, many school and agency nurses do not see the IEP process as a function of their jobs and do not ask to be included on this team, although they could be members under the consultant classification.

Handicapped children will always be with us, and with the increasing technologic advances and the trend toward depopulating institutions, their numbers in public life are likely to increase. Therefore, it is essential that nurses become knowledgeable and skilled in working with these children and their families.

Developmental Conditions Requiring Intervention

In the previous sections of this chapter, we have presented an overall picture of the assessment tools and some intervention methods used with children experiencing developmental alterations. This section of the chapter deals with specific developmental alterations, their causes, specific problems to look for during assessment, and appropriate nursing interventions.

Developmental Delay

Delays in development can occur at any time during a child's developmental period from birth through 18 years of age. Therefore, it is important that the nurse be able to recognize the risk factors that may lead to developmental delay or handicapping conditions in infants and children. Box 34-2 contains a list of these risk factors. It is important to keep records of any risk factor

Box 34-2
Risk Factors for Developmental Delay

I. Socioeconomic Factors
  - Poverty
  - Poor housing
  - Social relationships
    - Divorce
    - Marital discord
    - Single parent
    - Teenage parent
  - Nutritional deprivation

II. Maternal Factors
  - A. Physical characteristics
    - Maternal age under 16 or over 35 years
    - Short stature (under 152 cm)
    - Weight (20 per cent below or above normal)
    - Family history of genetic problems
  - B. Problems during past pregnancies
    - Abortions
    - Infertility
    - Multiple or closely spaced pregnancies
    - Premature or prolonged labor
    - Ectopic pregnancy
    - Cesarean delivery
    - Difficult delivery (midcavity forceps)
    - Previous infant with low birthweight
    - Previous infant weighing 4 kg or more
    - Stillborn
    - Previous infant with disability
  - C. Medical Problems
    - No prenatal care
    - History of disease process or blood disorders
    - Drug addiction (including alcohol)

III. Risk Factors for the Fetus
  - Rh sensitization (also other conditions, e.g., ABO incompatibility)
  - Drugs taken during fetal developmental period of major organs
  - Viral infections during the first trimester
  - Radiation exposure (ionizing)
  - Fetal size below or above norm
  - Placental problems
  - Polyhydramnios
  - Ruptured membranes (premature or over 24 hours)

IV. Factors Associated with Labor
  - Premature or post-term
  - Prolonged labor
    - Primigravida: over 24 hours
    - Multigravida: over 12 hours (second stage over 2 hours)
  - Malposition
  - Prolapsed cord
  - Cesarean or breech delivery
  - Meconium-stained amniotic fluid

V. Risk Factors in the Newborn
  - Low birthweight: 2.5 kg and below
  - Birth weight over 4 kg
  - Apgar score 5 or below at 1 minute of life
  - Fetal distress
  - Resuscitation needed at birth
  - Respiratory distress
  - Drug-related depression
  - Depression related to other causes
  - Infection
  - Birth injury
  - Developmental malformation
  - Kernicterus
  - Intraventricular hemorrhage

noted in a child throughout the developmental period. Physicians and other health care workers may find clues to the probable cause of a child's disability by reading records that are well documented. For example, there is evidence to suggest that infants whose neurologic examinations show abnormalities or transient abnormalities are at risk for later difficulties, such as lesser cognitive function, hyperactivity, motor dysfunction, and learning disabilities (Ellison et al, 1985).

Genetic problems and congenital malformations can be responsible for delayed development. There are several thousand genetic disorders currently listed in the literature. Some are easy to discern at birth because of the obvious developmental problems they present. Others are metabolic in nature and detection results from blood tests (e.g., phenylketonuria [PKU], cretinism). There are some genetic problems that are not as easily assessed at birth and may not be recognized until the child is older and begins to show evidence of delayed development.

It is important for the nurse to recognize minor abnormalities that may be indicators of more serious problems, such as mental retardation, cerebral palsy, and heart or kidney disorders. Smith (1982) states that one minor anomaly may be found in 14 per cent of all newborn children without an appreciable increase in the incidence of major defects. In about 0.8 per cent of newborns, two minor anomalies are seen, in which case the incidence of a major defect is five times higher than those in the normal group. In 0.5 per cent of all newborn infants, there are three or more minor anomalies; in these infants, the incidence of major defects rises to 90 per cent. The findings of several minor defects is unusual, and the infant should be referred to a genetic screening and counseling center. Minor anomalies usually have no adverse medical or cosmetic consequences (Smith, 1982). Major anomalies, on the other hand, have an adverse effect on either the function or the social acceptance of the individual.

Examples of some major anomalies are hydrocephalus, anencephaly, severe microcephaly, hypertonicity, meningocele, severe micrognathia, severe hypertelorism, imperforate anus, cleft lip, or cleft palate. Minor anomalies are such things as bilateral epicanthal folds, upward or downward slanting of palpebral fissures, sparse eyebrows or thick eyebrows that grow together, a simian crease in the hand, clinodactyly, rudimentary polydactyly of the fingers or toes, and external ear anomalies, such as lack of the usual folds of the helix. All such deviations should be noted during the child's assessment. Following analysis of the findings, a decision should be made about an appropriate referral.

As the child's development progresses in the cephalocaudal direction, certain milestones are observed. Use of the observation tools and screening devices previously described will enable the child's nurse to detect areas in which the child is lagging. These tools provide a means to observe the child for basic reflexes and for neurologic, musculoskeletal, and sensory abilities.

To ensure the most normal response possible, the nurse should see that the child is warm and secure prior to testing for tone and reflexes. It is important to note when the last feeding occurred because a hungry child will suck better than one who has just eaten. A child who is crying will not do as well on testing for some reactions. Table 34-2 provides a list of infant reflexes.

One special tool not previously mentioned is the Milani Comparetti Motor Development Screening Test. It is recommended that testing of the child with this tool be done at certain key ages between 6 weeks and 24 months of age. It can be used to aid in the early detection of neuromotor delay or deficits. This is one of the tools that requires that the examiner be a physician, therapist, or nurse because of the skill level needed for its administration. The University of Nebraska Medical Center has developed a videotape and manual prepared by Trembath and associates that details the use of the Milani-Comparetti tool (Trembath, 1977).

Attention Deficit Disorder (ADD)

In the past, a wide variety of terms have been used to describe this disorder, including minimal brain dysfunction (MBD), hyperactive child syndrome, minimal brain damage, and minor cerebral dysfunction. Since 1980, the American Psychiatric Association has indicated that the name attention deficit disorder (ADD) is a more appropriate term to use because attentional difficulties are prominent and almost always present. There are three major subtypes of ADD: (1) attention deficit disorder with hyperactivity (ADDH), (2) attention deficit disorder without hyperactivity (ADDnoH), and (3) attention deficit disorder, residual type. The onset of ADD is before the age 7 years. Estimates of the presence of ADD range from 1.2 to 20 per cent of all school-age children. The syndrome occurs nine to ten times more often in boys than in girls (Botshaw and Perret, 1981; Levine and Melmed, 1982) and is more frequent in upper middle class families. The disorder has not been identified in developing countries.

Etiology

The exact cause of the syndrome is unknown. In many cases, a family history reveals a possible genetic component. Often, one of the parents may have experienced some learning difficulties or hyperactivity as a child. When there is no evidence of a genetic component, the health history may reveal possible brain damage during an early developmental period. Children who were born prematurely or who suffered apnea at birth have an increased risk for ADD (Botshaw and Perret, 1981).

Little is understood about the functions of the brain with this syndrome. Studies of the brain have identified an area called the "reticular activity system" that helps control attention (Botshaw and Perret, 1981). This reticular system allows people to block out other conversations and to pay attention. A deficit of the neurochemicals active in this system can result in malfunctioning of the reticular system. Amphetamines increase the neurochemicals that are thought to be lacking in the brain of children with ADD. This response serves as the rationale for medication therapy for these youngsters.

Assessment

The essential features of ADD (Levine and Melmed, 1982) are signs of inattention and impulsivity that are developmentally inappropriate. For children with ADDH, hyperactivity is the third essential feature. For adolescents with ADD, residual deficit, excess motor activity frequently diminishes; however, attention difficulties remain.

In school, the child does not stay at tasks; has difficulty organizing and completing work; is sloppy and impulsive; and often gives the impression of not having heard or not listening when someone speaks. Group situations are especially difficult for the child

Table 34-2. Infant Reflexes

Reason or Explanation for the Clinical Manifestation	Significance to the Nurse
Rooting-Sucking Reflex	
Hungry infant will turn head to right or left when nipple is touched to face above or below the mouth. Present in full-term babies. Lasts 3 to 4 months. May last until approximately 7 months during sleep.	Absent in small premature infants. Absence in full-term infants suggests depression of CNS. Possible causes: anesthesia (maternal), hypoxia, congenital defect Rooting reflex that persists past 7 to 8 months is abnormal. Assess child for: intact palate and lip; symmetry of facial features or abnormally shaped jaw line or chin.
Moro Reflex	
"Startle" reflexes are movements in response to stimuli. Extension and abduction of upper extremities with extension of the spine and retraction of head. Forearms are supinated and digits fan out. The arms form an arclike movement and hands are brought together over chest, then child relaxes.	Absent in some premature infants. Absence in a full-term neonate may indicate CNS disorder. If asymmetric response, assess child for fractures of humerus or clavicle or hemiplegia. Note posture and tonus, which will be pronounced if kernicterus is present. Abnormal if Moro reflex persists past 3–4 months.
Asymmetric Tonic Neck Reflex	
"Fencing" position. Present in all infants up to 12 weeks. Infant lying on back turns head to one side. The arm toward which face is pointed will extend and the other arm will flex. Lower limbs respond similarly. Becomes symmetric from 5 to 6 months.	Persistence after 7th month is abnormal: prevents the child visualizing both hands in midline. Inhibits self-feeding. Prevents standing and walking achievement. Assess child for conditions such as webbing of neck or torticollis at this time also.
Neck-Righting Reflex	
Present by 4 to 6 months of age. Passive or active rotation of head to one side is followed by rotation of shoulders, trunk, and pelvis in the direction of the face. Slight delay in turn of body with head.	Immediate turn of body with turn of head occurs in some abnormal conditions. Check infant for muscle tone that is hypotonic or hypertonic.
Landau Reflex	
When held in prone position with head, spine, and legs extended, and the head is passively flexed forward, the body flexes. Present by 3 months.	Absent in children with cerebral palsy and gross motor retardation.
Parachute Reflex	
Child is held in vertical suspension and is suddenly lowered to a flat surface. Positive response is forward extension of both arms and dorsiflexion of infant's hands. Child's visual attention is first attracted to a bright toy in front of and a little above, before he or she is suddenly lowered. Usually seen at 6–9 months. If child's vision is not distracted with a toy, the reflex may be displayed earlier, at about 3 months. May also elicit this reflex by plunging child to the side.	Abnormal if not present by 12 months. Note response that is asymmetric.

Table 34-2 *(continued)*

Reason or Explanation for the Clinical Manifestation	Significance to the Nurse
Palmar and Plantar Reflex	
Elicited by placing a finger in the child's palm or at base of toes. Fingers and toes will wrap around the finger. Found in full-term neonates	Plantar response that lasts longer than 8–9 months is significant. Palmar response weakens after 2 months. Note any asymmetry of response.
Traction	
With infant in supine position, draw the child upward by hands into sitting position. Head lags until child is upright and then falls forward over chest. Newborn infants should be able to raise head back up. Control should strengthen with age. (Care should be exercised in eliciting this response.)	Note continued head lag.
Support Reaction	
"Stepping" reaction is shown by holding infant up vertically and allowing feet to touch a firm surface. Automatic stepping observed when infant is inclined forward. Present at birth but decreases after 4–6 weeks. Able to support more weight by 10 months.	Note consistent standing on toes, scissoring of legs after 4 months.

when sustained attention is required. At home, the parents note that their child does not follow through on requests and instructions and is unable to stick to activities, including play for periods of time appropriate to age. Associated features vary with age and include obstinance, stubbornness, negativism, bossiness, bullying, increased mood lability, low frustration tolerance, temper outbursts, low self-esteem, and lack of response to discipline. Hyperactivity in the young child is evidenced by gross motor activity, such as excessive running or climbing and being constantly on the go. The older child and adolescent may be extremely restless and fidgety. The child's behavior tends to be haphazard, poorly organized, and not goal directed. Symptoms typically vary with the situation. For example, the child may be well organized and appropriate on a one-to-one basis but not in a group situation or in the classroom; or adjustment may be satisfactory at home but poor at school. It is rare for the child to display signs of disorder in all settings at all times.

In some children, nonlocalized "soft" neurologic signs, motor perceptual dysfunction (e.g., poor eye-hand coordination), and electroencephalographic (EEG) abnormalities may be present. "Soft" signs are subtle; for example, the child may have difficulty distinguishing between the left and the right hand or may have trouble standing on one foot without falling. The children are often regarded as "clumsy" by their parents. Only about 5 per cent of the children with ADD have an associated diagnosable neurologic disorder. Although the onset of ADD is typically before 3 years of age, often it is not brought to the attention of a professional until the child enters school. The peak age range for referral is 8 to 10 years.

Intervention and Nursing Care

Early diagnosis of ADD is important to avoid some of the long-lasting psychologic effects this disorder may have on a child. Treatment of the syndrome requires a team approach. A combination of medication, behavior modification, and a special education program is usually needed to treat these children. Alterations in diet (Feingold, 1975) have received popular support but little support from the scientific community.

Medication Therapy. Stimulant medications are still the treatment of choice for children with ADD. They are used to help the child respond appropriately in everyday academic and social settings. The commonly used drugs are methylphenidate (Ritalin), dextroamphetamine (Dexedrine), and amphetamine sulfate (Benzedrine). Although these drugs are often referred to on the street as "speed" or "uppers" and may be taken for their euphoric effect, they do not affect the child with ADD in the same way. They are used to enable children with ADD to control their impulses and to improve their attention spans.

It is estimated that medication-related improvements occur in 60 to 90 per cent of the children (Whalen and Henker, 1982). Studies using teacher ratings have shown an improvement in behavior and attention span of children who are taking medication. These children also performed better on visual-motor tasks, such as penmanship (Botshaw and Perret, 1981). Some studies have noted that as the dosage increased the children became quieter; however, their academic performance also declined. The child should be monitored by a physician so that the smallest effective dose can be used.

Children on medication therapy should be monitored closely for side effects. This task frequently becomes the responsibility of the school nurse. The nurse should be aware of possible side effects of loss of appetite and insomnia that are common if the medication is taken prior to meals or within 3 hours of bedtime. Some children may experience stomach cramps or irritability. Other problems with these drugs include the risk of long-term side effects, such as suppressed growth rate or altered cardiovascular functioning. The drugs may also have undesirable effects on psychosocial functioning and self-perceptions because they can undermine self-concept. Sometimes children look upon their medication as "magic pills." "The child may believe the drug controls his behavior, and that, consequently, if he forgets to take a pill, naughty behavior can be blamed on the absence of the medicine" (Botshaw and Perret, 1981, p 241). It is important that this attitude not be tolerated and that children learn to take responsibility for their behavior.

Behavior Modification. Whalen and Henker (1982) recommend treatment strategies that combine medication with non-drug interventions. They believe the most promising treatment is a combination of various forms of behavior modification and cognitive-behavioral approaches. Approaches that include contingent rewards, especially as components of token economy, or behavioral contracting programs run by highly trained parents or teachers, have proved effective. Also effective are cognitive programs that teach children self-instructional and self-reinforcement skills that they can use to guide their own behavior and systematically monitor their own progress. Some programs include metacognitive training that is designed to teach children how to analyze the components and demands of a given task, to generate appropriate problem-solving strategies, and to assess and modify their performance as necessary. Cognitive-behavioral approaches encourage children to become active agents in their own treatment programs; they teach "portable" coping strategies that the child can take from situation to situation without having to rely on external agents (parents, teachers, or pills). The initial results have been dramatic but the field is still relatively new and little is known about which techniques are best for which situations (Whalen and Henker, 1982).

Consistent management and a structured environment are vital for the child. The home and school environments should be adjusted to provide minimal external stimuli. Regular routines should be established for eating, sleeping, and doing school work. Situations that cause excitement, overstimulation, and fatigue should be avoided. When giving instructions or assigning tasks at school or at home, directions should be given one at a time, and the work should be divided into small parts.

Discipline must be consistent. Good behavior or achievement should be rewarded and inappropriate behavior ignored. Usually short contractual agreements may be used to achieve the desired goals. Achievement should be rewarded with praise rather than food. Parents will need support in managing their child with ADD, and they will need assistance in the management of their child's behavior modification program and medication therapy.

Parents of these children often harbor feelings of guilt, anger, and frustration. They will need help dealing with these normal feelings. The nurse working with the family may be able to provide the support and counseling the family needs or may need to refer the family to other health professionals for these services. Referral should be made to self-help groups such as the Association for Children with Learning Disabilities.

Learning Disabilities

The concept of learning disabilities as a specific and identifiable entity apart from mental retardation, neurologic impairment, or emotional disturbance has only come about within the past 15 or 20 years. Although learning disabilities share some common characteristics with ADD, they differ in definition and function. When Congress passed PL 94-142, The Education for All Handicapped Children Act, in 1975, it recognized learning disabilities as a handicapping condition. The Act defines a learning disability as "a disorder in one or more of the basic psychological processes involved in understanding or in using language, spoken or written, which may manifest itself as imperfect ability to listen, speak, read, write, spell, or do mathematical calculations." The definition excludes children who have learning problems attributable to mental retardation, emotional disturbance, environmental disadvantage, or visual, hearing, or motor handicaps.

Estimates of the number of children who have learning disabilities vary widely and may range from 1 to 30 per cent of the school-age population (Benton, 1976). As with attention deficit disorder, more boys than girls are affected, in a ratio of about 4 : 1. There is a higher incidence of learning disabilities among the lower socioeconomic groups. Reading problems are the most common disability (Botshaw and Perret, 1981).

There are over 100 varieties of learning disabilities. Children with learning disabilities manifest problems in language, motor skills, and behavior long before they have difficulties in school. Early identification during the preschool years is important so they can be provided with appropriate educational intervention and counseling. Usually, these children are not identified until they reach the second grade. It is hoped that with the development of early childhood screening and intervention programs, children will be identified earlier.

These children do not learn readily from past experience and may, therefore, be difficult to discipline. They also have difficulty understanding or following instructions. For example, children with visual perceptual difficulties may not understand what they see. They may be unable to trace or draw a circle or square or copy these from a blackboard. Children with auditory perceptual disabilities may not understand a series of instructions, such as the child who may not be able to carry out three consecutive directions such as "Go to your room, turn on the light, and hang up your clothes."

Although children are not hospitalized because of their learning disabilities, the symptoms can be recognized by an alert nurse. Early referral is of prime importance in assisting the child. Parents frequently recognize symptoms but may have been told their child would outgrow the condition. Many children with learning disabilities are receiving help earlier today because teachers in day care and preschool programs recognize the symptoms and initiate therapy. Parents are usually relieved to know that someone else has also recognized the problem and that help is available.

Assessment

Assessment of a child who is suspected of having a learning disability may involve a multidisciplinary approach that often includes educators, psychologists, speech pathologists, and health care personnel. It should begin with a careful history of the child's scholastic achievement and behavioral and social emotional adjustment. Physical and neurologic examinations are important, and generally the results are quite normal. School behavior ratings are made by teachers using checklists such as the Conners Teacher Questionnaire, Devereux Elementary School Behavior Rating Scale, and Pupil Rating Scale: Screening for Learning Disabilities. According to Keele (1983), learning disabilities are diagnosed by excluding mental retardation, developmental disabilities, sensory deficits, and primary psychosocial problems.

Early warning signs of learning disabilities are a child who is easily distracted, has a short attention span, needs to be told the same thing many times, and has trouble following a sequence of verbal instructions. Other early indications include delays in speech and language development, inability to repeat a sequence of numbers, frequent reversing of words in sentences, taking a long time to answer questions, and frequently asking to have instructions repeated (Easter Seal Society, 1982).

Intervention and Nursing Care

Intervention for any of the specific learning disabilities must be provided by a team. Team members should include the family, a physician, a psychologist, a teacher, a nurse, and a specialist in the discipline in which the child needs help. Various screenings must be done for auditory and visual acuity. Along with the developmental history, serologic studies, including those for lead intoxication, should be done.

Regardless of the specific diagnostic conditions, there are some general guidelines to be observed. The nurse or social worker can assist the family in implementing them:

- There must be consistency. Parents need to agree in the approach to child care. A definite time schedule for eating, sleeping, school work, and play should be planned by the family and followed consistently. Siblings and parents must evaluate their feelings, for children readily become aware of any tensions they are causing.
- Keep frustrations at a minimum. The frustration level can be increased as the child learns to function more maturely.
- Reward the child for work well done. Verbal praise is reward enough. Minimize defeats and build on strengths. Encourage positive self-concept.
- Assign simple tasks with simple directions. Show what is to be done, rather than relying on verbal commands. Give only one direction at a time.
- Special school therapy should be continued at

home. Simple motor skills can be learned through play and repetition.

One of the nurse's greatest contributions is to assist the family in using community resources. The Association for Children with Learning Disabilities (ACLD) is a parent group in which strength and support is found through exchange of concerns and ideas.

Some children need to attend special classes for learning disabilities until they are able to adapt to a more complex and confusing environment. Children, however, should be included in regular classes to the degree that they can tolerate. It is very important that they not be singled out from their peers as being different. Peers should be given a simple explanation of a learning disability so they can more readily accept the child.

The earlier an insult to the brain area is discovered, the greater the possibility of correction through remedial education. Earlier discovery in the preschool years will diminish problems in school. Many children's symptoms decrease after they reach puberty.

Children with learning disabilities require special attention, but this should not be given at the expense of siblings. Children with specific problems must be helped to learn to cope in their environments despite their handicap and should not be allowed to use this handicap as a reason for requesting special favors. Nor should they be excused from certain experiences because of lower competencies in academic skills. Nurses can encourage parents to involve the child's siblings by explaining honestly that the child has a special problem and that everyone will be required to help. This may help minimize sibling competitiveness and aid in family cooperation.

Children younger than the child with a learning disability may develop at a faster rate, and the child may be threatened and embarrassed by a normal younger sibling. All children should be praised for their accomplishments and allowed to grow at their own rate. Children should not be compared with their siblings, nor should there be a sense of competition. Children should never receive the impression that they are not loved as much as their siblings. Nurses should be supportive to parents and help them in giving each child the individual attention he or she needs. Every family member is involved in building a wholesome, nonthreatening, non-competitive, affirmative relationship.

Dyslexia

Dyslexia is the most common learning disability and is a major cause of school failure. About 15 per cent of children beginning school each year have dysfunctions in reading skills (Bruen, 1977). The term *dyslexia* is loosely used to describe children who are two or more grades below their peers in reading level. Of this group, approximately 2 to 3 per cent have either primary or developmental dyslexia (Brenton, 1976). Children with this pathologic condition should be differentiated from those with reading difficulties primarily due to lack of exposure to learning opportunities. Developmental dyslexia is more frequently found in boys than in girls. There is no known single cause of the condition.

Pathophysiology and Clinical Manifestations. It appears that *primary dyslexia* is usually familial. It may be due to weakness of one or several learning processes or immaturity of a certain part of the brain. *Developmental dyslexia* results from cerebral dysfunction and is evidenced in specific learning disorders of reading, spelling, and writing. The child can hear and understand statements but cannot read them. There seems to be a blockage or misconnection in the transmission of the written word from the eye to the higher brain centers in which the messages are integrated and relayed to the appropriate sensory area. The child with dyslexia may be unable to distinguish between similar-appearing letters, such as b and d. Letters may appear upside down or reversed. The children may read "on" for "no" or "was" for "saw." Letters are frequently seen in mirror image. Figure 34-3 helps illustrate the type of perceptual problems encountered by children with dyslexia.

Assessment. The diagnosis of dyslexia is made through a battery of tests, including appropriate psychologic evaluations. The child is usually of average or above-average intelligence. As this is not a condition that warrants hospitalization, the nurse in that setting may have limited exposure to children with dyslexia. However, as a community health person, the nurse must be aware of the symptoms and further preventive intervention. Early recognition is the key to diminishing this problem. The child needs the assistance of a reading specialist. Individualized program planning in a structured setting with limited stimuli should be provided. If therapy is initiated early, children with dyslexia can attain the same reading level as their peers within a few years. If the problem is not recognized until the child is in the third or fourth grade, the response will be less favorable.

The nurse who does vision screening using a Snellen or an E chart can aid in the detection of visual perception problems. If a problem is suspected, the family should be informed and a referral made for a differential diagnosis by an ophthalmologist.

Arriving at a definite diagnosis will relieve family tension, as family members will have been aware of a problem and may have suspected retardation or emotional disturbance. Because children with dyslexia are usually of average intelligence, they frequently act out

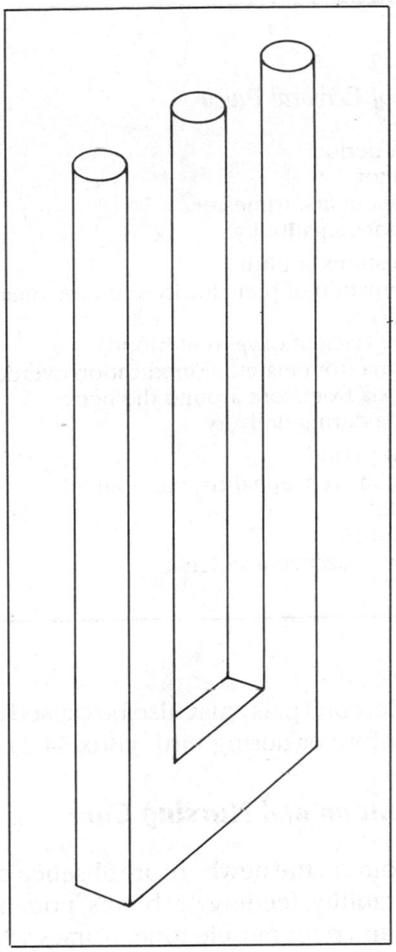

***Figure* 34-3.** This drawing causes a perceptual dysfunction similar to that encountered by the child with dyslexia in everyday activity.

their frustrations by adopting an "I don't care" attitude or by using physical strength to show competencies lacking in other areas. Very sensitive children may develop feelings of inferiority and may regress in other areas. Early detection and treatment can help prevent secondary emotional scarring.

Intervention and Nursing Care. Children should receive special help in remedial reading but should participate equally with their peers in other activities. There should be no discrimination because of lack of skill in one specific area. If their peers understand these children's specific needs, they can more readily accept the children as part of the group. The family should be encouraged not to emphasize reading excellence but to reinforce the teacher's structure and allow the child to excel in other areas until he or she gains competence in reading. The family and the school must constantly maintain open communication and help the child avoid feelings of inadequacy or of being different.

The children should be taught through repetition and reinforcement. Letters that are confusing to them can be taught by using various forms of sensory stimulation such as letting them "feel" the letter that has been cut from sandpaper, wood, soft textured material, or paper. Letters may be color-coded or traced in sand. Each letter should be mastered well before the next letter is taught. Various types of classroom learning machines to enhance reading skills are also available.

The nurse should help the family determine how it can maintain a relaxed and pleasant environment. A local parent group will be ready to share strengths and concerns. Suggestions for enhancing learning at home include those measures discussed in the section on ADD, as well as the following:

1. Provide informal learning exposure. Reading to the children will enlarge their vocabularies and create interest in the printed page. Use clocks, road maps and calendars. Teach them to recognize safety words such as "stop," "danger" and "poison." Reinforce lessons of "left" and "right" through play.
2. Improve coordination through the use of basketball hoops and playing "catch." Buy hand-eye games such as jacks or pick-up-sticks. Many games teach a child to count and involve the use of small muscles.
3. Break down complicated tasks into small steps. Be sure the children are comfortable with each step before they attempt the next. Reward with praise. Do not scold or show impatience if they do not grasp the concept right away.
4. Assure the children that they are loved and are important family members.

Cerebral Palsy

An estimated 25,000 babies are born with cerebral palsy (CP) in the United States annually. Although exact statistics are unavailable, sources estimate there are 1.5 to 5 cases per 1000 live births. Cerebral palsy involves a difficulty in controlling the voluntary muscles owing to damage to some area of the brain. It is a collective term that indicates paralysis of the pyramidal motor system, which consists of the motor cortex, cerebellum, and basal ganglia. It occurs before birth or during the early years of life. Damage is permanent and is not progressive. Children with cerebral palsy may have normal or superior intelligence, although damage to the cognitive area of the brain is frequent. Cerebral palsy is a general term that indicates a pathologic condition but does not indicate the area of damage; therefore, the term actually indicates a symptom rather than a diagnosis.

The tendency to be left- or right-brained is inherited. Constant usage establishes a pattern. Functions such as chewing, walking, and feeding become automatic with usage, but for a child with cerebral palsy they must be learned through lengthy repetition. Because one area of the brain has been damaged, the child must develop patterns through the receptors of another brain area.

Pathophysiology

A wide range of neuromuscular disability and many types of cerebral palsy exist, depending upon the brain area involved. Five major types are: (1) athetoid, (2) spastic, (3) ataxic, (4) rigidity, and (5) mixed. The child with the *athetoid* (dyskinetic) type of cerebral palsy has damage to the basal ganglia. This is recognizable by uncontrolled and involuntary movements. Because there is damage to the basal ganglia that controls involuntary movement, any stimulus causes a sudden jerking. This frequently increases in intensity during emotional stress. The incidence of accompanying hearing loss is high.

The child with *spastic* cerebral palsy has damage to the cortex. This is one of the most common types of cerebral palsy. These children are recognizable by their very tense muscles. There is total contraction to stimulus, and when the child is startled, hyperirritability of muscle tone is apparent. The child must make a conscious effort to relax. A tight heel cord causes the child to have a talipes equines (walk on toes) walk. Convulsions are more common in these children. They may have strabismus and usually have more difficulty in speech and oral musculature control.

The *ataxic* type of cerebral palsy is a less common type, and affected children have damage to the cerebellum that controls equilibrium—they appear to walk as if in a drunken stupor. Both position and touch are affected. Children with ataxia frequently have ocular problems.

The next two most common types of cerebral palsy are *rigidity* and *mixed.* The child with rigidity has resistance in both flexor and extensor muscles and is in a constant state of tension. It is not unusual for a child to have more than one type of cerebral palsy (mixed).

Many children with cerebral palsy have multiple handicaps. Over 50 per cent of the children are also mentally retarded. Other common handicaps are speech and hearing impairments, oculomotor impairment, and convulsive disorder. The most commonly associated handicaps in infancy are strabismus, nearsightedness, and hearing deficits (Taft and Matthews, 1983).

Etiology

Over half of the children with cerebral palsy received damage to the motor area of the brain during the prenatal period. Cerebral palsy may also be caused by factors occurring before or during birth (Box 34-3).

Box 34-3
Causes of Cerebral Palsy

Prenatal period
- Rh factor
- Rubella in first trimester
- ABO incompatibility

Complications at birth
- Combination of prematurity and precipitate delivery
- Anoxia (lack of oxygen in blood)
- Toxemia from maternal medication overdose
- Asphyxia from cord around the neck
- Trauma during delivery

Postnatal period
- Infections (encephalitis, meningitis)
- Trauma
- Poisonings
- Cerebral vascular accidents

Intervention and Nursing Care

Early symptoms in the newborn are absence of normal reflexes, irritability, feeding problems, poor motor development, and poor muscle tone. Nurses who recognize these symptoms should report them to the physician so that early diagnosis and treatment can be initiated. Physical or occupational therapy and infant stimulation should be begun as soon as the family has had time to consider the problem objectively. The degree of pathology will vary, but the therapeutic aim is to help the child develop skills in speech, arm coordination for feeding and self-care, and walking.

Assistance should be available through interdisciplinary teams consisting of a family member or members, a speech and hearing therapist, a pediatrician, a nurse, a social worker, an occupational or physical therapist (or both), and a neurologist. The long-term aims of management involve developing the child's abilities to the extent possible and preventing eventual deformities or complications.

Although medications such as levodopa have given relief for some athetoid children and peripheral nerve blocks have decreased symptoms in a few spastic children, the most promising specific treatment for cerebral palsy is the surgical implantation of a cerebellar pacemaker. Its exact action has not been physiologically explained, but its success in improving functioning relatively quickly has been impressive (Conway, 1977).

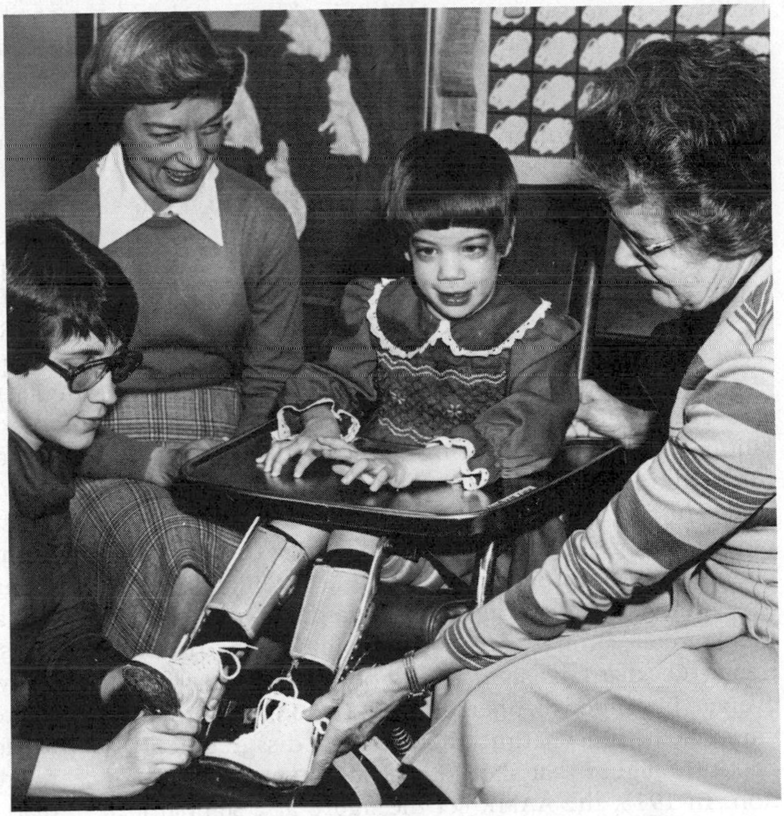

The importance of properly fitting braces is emphasized during a conference of the teacher, the school nurse, and the mother of a child with cerebral palsy. (Photograph by Howard Zehr; Joint Schools Special Education Program of Elkhart County, Indiana.)

Nursing care needs to be highly individualized for the age of the child and the degree of pathologic involvement. Most children with cerebral palsy are highly motivated toward independence. Because muscle tension increases caloric catabolism, they are given a high caloric diet. If possible, the child should be taught early to develop independent feeding skills. An adequate fluid intake is necessary. Proper positioning in a fitted chair with sturdy foot support is very important. Because many of these children wear braces, the nurse must be alert to good skin care and must be especially observant if the child is nonverbal. Drugs as relaxants or to control seizures are given, and the nurse must observe for signs of side effects. The nurse also needs to teach parents to make these observations. Early referrals for occupational and physical therapy should be made. Although these therapies will not alter the natural course of the motor dysfunction, they will help the infant achieve better functional use. Parents can also be taught to incorporate the techniques into their day-to-day management.

One of the most important aspects of quality nursing care is the emotional support given the child and the family. The interdisciplinary team must aid the family through the periods of grief and adjustment and allow them to accept the child and see him or her in perspective—as a family member who must learn to use all the abilities he or she has. The family must be aware that the pathologic condition cannot be cured but, with therapy, new patterns frequently can be established.

If children with cerebral palsy have had only minimal exposure to learning or are limited in their abilities to respond, their IQs need to be compared with their adaptive abilities. The child should be exposed to new experiences and given opportunities for learning. Through PL 94-142, educational opportunities, including transportation to classes, are now the right of the handicapped. If feasible, children with cerebral palsy should attend a regular class with peers. If needed, speech therapy or physical therapy should be provided as part of their school experiences. The children should not be singled out as being "different."

Parents and siblings should become aware of the national and community support systems available to them, such as the United Cerebral Palsy Agency. Summer camps for handicapped children or Special Olympics can help children see that they are not alone in their particular handicap, and they can gain strength from healthy relationships.

Because of heroic measures now being performed in neonatology nurseries, more children are being saved. Predictably, this has led to an increase in the number of children with handicapping conditions.

However, more research is also being done, and attempts are being made to prevent many neonatal pathologic conditions.

Communities should be aware of the needs of children with handicapping conditions. The prognosis of children with cerebral palsy depends on all factors relating to their condition and the attitude of the child, the family, and the community.

Mental Retardation

Definition

The term mental retardation (MR) describes a constellation of symptoms consisting of impaired intellectual functioning associated with impaired social adaptation. This impaired adaptive behavior must have occurred during the developmental behavior (from conception through 18 years of age). According to the American Association on Mental Retardation (AAMR), mental retardation is classified as an intelligence quotient (IQ) that falls significantly below the mean for average intelligence. Average IQ is 100 on the normal curve. At the present time, there is some disagreement about the figure that should indicate mental retardation. In 1973, the AAMR set the figure at 2 standard deviations below the mean, making it about 68 (Fig. 34-4).

According to educators, this 1973 definition of mental retardation is restrictive and excludes some students from receiving services. In a study surveying states related to their use of criteria to designate mental retardation, Frankenberger (1984) stated there was a great deal of discrepancy in the scores used to define mental retardation. Many educators continue to endorse a somewhat higher IQ cutoff of 75. The new 1983 AAMR definition continues to define mental retardation as an IQ below 70, but indicates that it may be extended up to 75 or beyond, depending upon the tests used and individual characteristics, especially in school settings (Frankenberger, 1984).

The definition of mental retardation is specifically developmental in its approach and can be differentiated from impairment following damage in adulthood. Retarded children are classified according to the developmental tasks that are appropriate for their ages. Mental retardation should not be confused with mental illness or emotional disturbance. Four levels of mental retardation are usually identified:

1. *Mild retardation.* Persons with mild retardation may be hard to identify and are often physically normal. In school, children are able to learn academic skills up to approximately sixth grade level, and as adults they often acquire vocational and social skills necessary for independent living. The majority of mentally retarded individuals are mildly retarded.
2. *Moderate retardation.* In persons with moderate retardation, intellectual functioning is of a degree that academic achievement is significantly impaired, but they can learn self-care, social, and some vocational skills.
3. *Severe retardation.* Persons with severe retardation, with special training, may be capable of a significant degree of self-care but will need supervision throughout life.
4. *Profound retardation.* Persons with profound retardation may be incapable of any self-care skills.

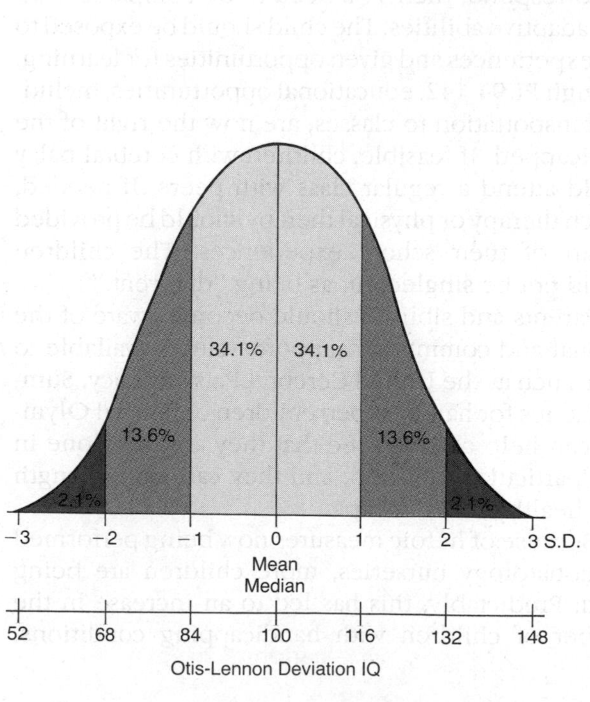

Figure 34-4. Bell-shaped curve.

Box 34-4
Factors Involved in Mental Retardation

1. Genetic Factors*
   - Phenylketonuria
   - Cerebral lipoidosis
   - Galactosemia
   - Hypoparathyroidism
   - Hypoglycemia
   - Gargoylism
   - Fragile X
2. Neonatal and Perinatal Factors
   - Inadequate prenatal care
   - Premature birth
   - Use of alcohol or drugs during pregnancy
   - Anoxia during or after delivery
   - Birth injury
   - Kernicterus (Rh factor)
   - Dehydration
   - Maternal factors
     - Rubella in first trimester
     - Malnutrition
     - Toxemia
3. Factors Operative in Infancy and Childhood
   - Infectious diseases
   - Accidents
   - Ingestion of intoxicants
   - Asphyxia
4. Social-Cultural-Familial Factors
   - Emotional rejection
   - Nutritional deficiency

* Due to an alteration of the normal genetic information stored in the DNA molecules.

Etiology

Over 250 causes of mental retardation have been identified (President's Committee, 1975). Most causes fall into four groups of etiologic factors, but some are difficult to differentiate. These etiologic classifications involve genetic, neonatal and perinatal, infancy and childhood, and social-cultural-familial factors (Box 34-4).

Incidence

There are over 6.5 million persons in the United States with a diagnosis of mental retardation. Approximately 3 per cent of the population is in the moderately to profoundly retarded range. Mild mental retardation appears to be more prevalent among the socially disadvantaged. According to the President's Commission on Mental Retardation (1975), approximately 85 to 90 per cent of cases of mild retardation that do not show identifiable organic or physical cause are associated with conditions arising from the environment.

Pathology

Causes of mental retardation can be separated into (1) true developmental malformations of the brain and (2) those occurring from acquired destructive lesions (Kepes, 1982). True developmental malformations may be those related to normal developmental steps that have not taken place or developmental steps that have occurred in an abnormal way. Acquired destructive lesions, on the other hand, cause damage to brain tissue that has already developed in a normal way. There are many areas of overlap between these two categories.

Development of the central nervous system takes place by three separate, but interrelated, means: gross organogenesis, histogenesis, and cytogenesis. *Gross organogenesis* means development of the organs. The first sign of the neural system is development of the neural plate, neural groove, and neural tube. Failure of these areas to develop normally would lead to conditions such as spina bifida. The degree of defect can be as mild as a dimple in the lumbar region of the spinal column or as severe as a meningomyelocele or meningoencephalocele. Hydrocephalus is often a secondary result of spina bifida and a further complication. Anencephaly is a closely associated problem in which the brain is not developed. When the telencephalon does not divide into two hemispheres, a condition described as telencephalon impar can occur. In a severe form of this developmental failure facial deformities may also complicate matters. (See Chapter 46 for nursing care of children with spina bifida and hydrocephalus.)

During the third and fifth fetal months, the corpus callosum is also developing. Developmental problems at this time could cause mental retardation and seizures. There are many developmental errors that can occur which affect the brain, and those mentioned are but a few of the possibilities.

Failure of cranial osseous development will expose the brain and cause severe damage. Premature closure of the sutures is responsible for preventing growth and expansion of the brain. Today surgeons have perfected procedures to open prematurely closed sutures and correct facial deformities. These surgeries allow the brain to continue its growth and in some cases prevent mental retardation. Facial surgery will not prevent mental retardation, but it may aid the individual socially and psychologically by improving appearance.(See Chapter 46 for nursing care of children with premature closure of cranial sutures, termed *craniosynostosis.*)

Histogenesis is the formation of tissues which are

groupings of specialized cells that make up organs. As the brain is developing, migrating cells eventually settle in certain areas of the brain. Neuroblasts travel to the area of the basal ganglia and others to the site of the cerebral cortex (Kepes, 1982). Much of the migration activity occurs as early as the twelfth week of gestation. Genetic and environmental problems can cause the arrest of this activity. These cells then begin to develop, abnormally, in the area of the brain where they have located at the time of insult. As they develop in wrong areas this is believed to lead to epilepsy. One severe form of mental retardation occurs as a result of agyria, in which the fissures and sulcus of the brain are undeveloped (Kepes, 1982).

Cytogenesis is the maturation of primitive neuroblasts once they have migrated to appropriate places in the brain. Depending on the role of that particular neuron, it will then enlarge and fulfill its function. Failure of development of dendrites and synapses will interfere with the progression of some neurologic impulses. This failure may result in some forms of mental retardation (Kepes, 1982).

Myelinization is not complete at birth and takes place over several years following birth. If adequate myelin is not produced to complete the process, then neurologic problems arise. Some metabolic conditions may cause this lack of production of myelin, such as maple syrup urine disease, homocystinuria, and other amino acid metabolism problems.

Genetic disorders may interfere with normal development. In some genetic conditions there is an abnormal number of chromosomes with either too few or too many chromosomes in the fertilized zygote. This results from a mishap in cell division known as *nondisjunction.* Down syndrome is an example of nondisjunction of the number 21 chromosome. Some other genetic aberrations that cause mental retardation as a result of nondisjunction of autosomes are trisomy 13 and 18. There are many others. Nondisjunction of the sex chromosomes can lead to such conditions as Turner syndrome and Klinefelter syndrome, which cause varying degrees of mental retardation.

Assessment

Diagnosis of mental retardation requires a team approach. The causes of mental retardation are many, and it may be possible to make a diagnosis immediately after birth if it accompanies gross developmental lags or deformities. On the other hand, the retardation may be mild and not picked up until the child is in school and begins to fall behind peers in academic work.

A variety of tests may be used to assess the child's intellectual and adaptive functioning. These tests are listed in Table 34-3. The Stanford-Binet Scale is among the most successful of these tests (Latham and Yando, 1982). Each of the four levels of mental retardation will vary by a point or two according to the tests used for diagnosis (Table 34-4).

The Stanford-Binet Scale (form L and M) (Latham and Yando, 1982) is designed for individuals ranging in age from 2 years through adulthood. There are six tasks that measure the IQ of children and involve manipulation and identification of objects and eye-hand coordination as well as vocabulary, sentence completion, and analogies.

The Wechsler Intelligence Scale for Children–Revised (WISC-R) is for children of ages 5 to 15 years. The Wechsler Preschool and Primary Scale of Intelligence (WPPSI) is for children of ages 4 to 7 years. It covers verbal and performance subtest areas of information, comprehension, arithmetic, similarities, digit span, and vocabulary.

Several other tests are useful to use with children who have language, sensory, or motor problems. In-

Table 34-3. Tools for Assessing Intelligence and Adaptability

Intelligence	Adaptive Behavior
Bayley Scales of Infant Development	AAMR Adaptive Behavior Scale
Catell Infant Intelligence Scale	AAMR Adaptive Behavior Scale—School Edition
Columbia Mental Maturity Scale (CMMS)	Balthazar Scales of Adaptive Behavior—Scales of Functional Independence
Gesell Schedules of Development	Minnesota Developmental Programming System—Behavioral Scales
Leiter International Performance Scale	O'Berry Developmental Tests–Behavior Maturity Checklist II
McCarthy Scales of Children's Abilities	Vineland Social Maturity Test
Peabody Picture Vocabulary Test (PPVT)	
Slosson Intelligence Test	
Stanford-Binet Scale	
Wechsler Intelligence Scale for Children—Revised (WISC-R)	
Wechsler Preschool and Primary Scale of Intelligence (WPPSI)	

Table 34-4. Levels of Mental Retardation (MR) and IQ Tests

Levels of MR	Stanford-Binet	Wechsler
Mild	68–52	69–55
Moderate	51–36	54–40
Severe	35–20	39–25
Profound	19 and below	24 and below

cluded are the Peabody Picture Vocabulary Test (PPVT), the Columbia Mental Maturity Scale (CMMS), and the Leiter International Performance Scale. The PPVT is probably the most widely used, but the most satisfactory of the three is the CMMS. The CMMS requires the child to pick out drawings on the cards. It requires perceptual discrimination of color, shape, symbols, function, missing parts, and numbers. The PPVT will produce a score slightly higher than the Wechsler and the Stanford-Binet Scale (Latham and Yando, 1982). Another test frequently used is the Vineland Social Maturity Test, which measures adaptive behavior related to specific areas of social development rather than intelligence. The tests are given under carefully controlled environmental conditions. Some measure intellectual development; some test for specific attitudes or abilities; and others test for personality related to values, problem-solving styles, interests, and attitudes.

If the child is diagnosed at a young age, the child and family may need genetic screening, medical and counseling services, and infant stimulation services. Older children will also need an educational IEP team plus a neurologist or pediatrician, or both.

The Nurse's Role

In almost every area of nursing, nurses will be involved in making referrals and working with children who are retarded. Nurses are important members of the diagnostic team. Their observational skills in noting gross and fine motor movements, visual and auditory acuity, and emotional responses are important in diagnosis. Although psychologic testing is required in the evaluation of the child's mental status, the final evaluation should be made by a team of professionals, with special attention given to adaptive behavior in the child's family environment. Intelligence testing, without considering adaptive behavior, often labels a child and limits expectations. The child's cognitive lag may be due to lack of external stimuli. In this case, with exposure to positive experiences, some degree of maturation and learning will take place.

Counseling the Family. Although it is the psychologist who will give the tests, it is imperative that nurses understand the implications of the findings. The nurse is frequently the professional sought out by parents to explain the test findings to them again after they have been presented with a diagnosis. Understanding information related to the child is, therefore, of great importance for the nurse in order to assist the family.

Parental reactions, including guilt, require the nurse to be skilled in providing interventions to help the family explore their feelings. This is done by assisting the family members to identify their feelings and giving them feedback about the appropriateness of those feelings. It is easy to imagine feelings of guilt that could occur if a retarded child is born to a mother who took drugs, either over the counter preparations or illegal drugs and alcohol during pregnancy; to a mother involved in an accident or illness; to one who has had a positive family history of genetic problems or who knowingly did anything that would prove harmful to the developing fetus. Think of the guilt a father would feel because of poverty, abuse, or even just not being supportive enough when his wife was pregnant. A sibling might suffer guilt if he or she had not wanted another brother or sister when the mother was pregnant.

To better develop communication skills among family members, the nurse helps the family develop goals for better relationships and improve family problem-solving and decision-making processes, and also promotes nurturance and growth of family members (McFarland and Wasli, 1986).

Many of the family's problems will be better solved when its members can talk to each other and help each other. We know that grieving is a normal process, but the obstructions to resolution of grief are varied. When a family member becomes stuck in a phase of grieving, it can lead to depressive states. Normally, this does not mean the family member develops a psychiatric problem. It does mean that skilled intervention is needed, though, to work through the grief process.

The family members at high risk for dysfunctional grieving are the following:

- Those family members who have had problems relating to the retarded family member.
- The family member who has shown overly cheerful, brave, or stoic behavior.
- Those who have little in the way of support systems or who perceive those systems as unsupportive.
- Those who have shown maladaptive coping mechanisms with past losses (McFarland and Wasli, 1986).

Also refer to the earlier section in this chapter on the role of the nurse as a family support for guidelines for working with families.

Mental retardation can never be an isolated diagnosis—it affects every family member. Parents and siblings need special help in understanding the pathology and their relationship with the involved child. Parents need to be especially concerned that they do not neglect other family members because of the time a retarded child demands.

Professionals should encourage parents to develop interests outside the home so that no one person is responsible for providing constant care. Guilt feelings can cause overprotection. Siblings should not be expected to forfeit their social activities and relationships for the impaired child. Although qualified babysitters are difficult to find, the family needs time away from the retarded child when internal pressures become too intense. Many communities have facilities for respite care that provide families a brief reprieve. Camps for the handicapped benefit the child and the family.

Introducing one family to another that has a child of similar ability can help both find support. Many families of retarded children become involved in local groups that provide the community with an understanding of the handicapped. The National Association of Retarded Citizens was started by a parent group. Membership in Youth NARC is open to all interested young people between the ages of 13 and 25. There are more than 600 local Youth Association for the Retarded units throughout the country.

Siblings play an important part in the child's development. When there is a healthy acceptance of the diagnosis, the child will be involved in family activities and will not be excluded from the sibling's circle of friends. The child will feel acceptance and love and will enjoy the richness of a full life. Siblings, however, need to be prepared for the onslaughts of a cruel, uninformed world that continues to tease and deride those who are disabled. Siblings have a unique role in altering public attitudes by example and education.

Nurses must remain sensitive to the daily hurts of the family and not become calloused in their attitudes. They must be aware that each family situation and child is unique and, although the family must develop its own way of adapting to changes in many life patterns, the professional team stands by supporting, caring and guiding.

The family sets the tone of acceptance for the community. If the family demonstrates care and concern for the child, the community will more likely respond with the same acceptance.

Nursing Care of the Child with Mental Retardation. Because mental retardation can accompany many other physical problems, such as cerebral palsy, hydrocephaly, spina bifida, Turner syndrome, Klinefelter syndrome, Cornelia de Lange syndrome, Down syndrome, and hundreds of other inherited or acquired disorders, the nursing care will vary. Children with mental retardation may be immobile, sensory deprived, or hearing and speech impaired. The needs of those children would be far different from those of the child who is ambulatory, aware of the environment, and able to effectively receive and express feelings and communications. Nurses are uniquely equipped to work with persons who have disabilities as a result of working with patients with other types of disease processes, such as stroke. Many of these skills can be used in working with those who have the same deficits resulting from developmental disabilities. For example, the health hazards of immobility are the same for everyone. The difference is applying this knowledge to a child.

Children who are retarded have the very same needs that all children have. Their basic needs for air, water, comfort, nutrition, love, and safety are the same. They need to learn from their environment, to explore, to manipulate, and to play. They need to learn skills of daily living. Children who are retarded have needs for attention and acceptance in order to establish a sense of self-worth (Table 34-5). Those children who cannot accomplish these things need to have a means to help facilitate these tasks. Without them the child's disability will be compounded.

Facilitating the provision of basic needs for most multihandicapped children is very difficult. Helping to facilitate independence and self-worth in a mildly retarded child is sometimes just as difficult to accomplish. Understanding some of the signs and symptoms of retardation will assist the nurse in planning interventions (Table 34-6).

The nurse may be asked to observe a child in a group who appears to be having difficulties or who is not keeping up. Observation should involve the child's language, social skills, and personal skills. Determine if the child is learning slowly or having trouble keeping up with amounts of work produced by other children. This is an important observation. The nurse should also watch the child participating in various learning areas and in different activities. An important observation is to decide if the child is lagging in many areas or whether the child is really bright but has problems in only a certain area.

Children who are retarded need to be able to believe in their own abilities. In order to do this, they must have ample opportunity to try things out and to practice. It will take them longer to master skills and learn from the environment.

Caregivers should be careful not to take over a project, but let the children have a *sense of accomplishment.* When the children are finally successful they should be rewarded. Frequently in the past we have rewarded these children with sugary treats. Dental problems and weight problems are often a result, so the rewards are best if they are of a social nature. Programs such as the Special Olympics are designed to give these children a sense of accomplishment.

Emphasis should be placed on the child's capabilities. Children should be encouraged to use all of their abilities. Parents should be asked to tell what the child does well rather than what he or she cannot do. The adage "Build on the weakness of his strength" is frequently cited. In this process, the strengths of the child

Table 34-5. Nursing Activities That Promote Self-Concept for the Child Who Is Retarded

While bathing the child	Repeat to the child, "Now I am going to wash your ears. Show me where your ears are." Do this with all body parts. With slightly older children let them show you how they wash body parts.
During bed rest periods	Have the child draw a self-portrait, trace around the hands, make fingerprints with ink pad and white paper.
	String beads.
In the hospital game room	Play "Simon Says"; move to music; trace the child's body on a long piece of butcher paper and have the child color it and label parts. Hang it in the hall by the child's door.
Before bath time	Let the child make clown faces with finger paints.
Grooming before visiting hours	Curl or braid hair and add a ribbon or flower. Let the child wear the beads that were made during rest time. Select a gown or pajamas to match.
If the child is restricted to the room	Hang up a list printed with big letters that tell the things this child likes to eat or play with, music he or she likes, favorite colors, and pets' names. Also put on the list the things the child does not like.
	Take a Polaroid picture of the child smiling and place on top of the "like" list and take a sad-face picture for the "don't like" list.
	Hang up cards from family and friends.
	Have the family bring pictures from home of family members so that the child can tell you about them.
	Have someone come to the hospital to share lunchtime with the child when possible to give the parent a break and to encourage visitors.
	Help the child call a friend on the telephone.

are reinforced, and gradually the unwholesome behavior is diminished. If the child has learned to tie shoelaces, this process might be enhanced by learning to tie other ribbons, thus developing improved finger dexterity. If retarded children have learned to feed themselves, encourage them to pour liquids from pitcher to glass or to pour sand from one bottle to another. This will improve eye-hand coordination. The process should be initiated at the point at which a child performs well. Children will want adult and peer approval, and if they receive affirmation for what they do well but no response for inappropriate behavior, they will quickly perform appropriately for approval. The inappropriate behavior will usually diminish. As the child gains competence and confidence, the negatives will lessen.

Forcing will not help the child to learn. Patience, not force, is the secret of helping a retarded child learn. Give concrete specific directions to the child and, by all means, give both physical and eye contact. Activities should be divided into small steps with one direction given at a time.

Self-help skills are very important if children are to progress in independence. They need to learn to feed themselves, bathe, brush teeth, toilet themselves, put on their clothes (appropriate to the weather), and have good hygiene. Nose picking and hair pulling will turn others away from them as they get older, although such behavior may be excusable in very small children.

These children need to learn *social skills,* which is often a very difficult project. Other children must be taught that children with handicaps are worthwhile individuals. This is one of the problems we face in mainstreaming. Built-in prejudice and wrong perceptions of the handicapped child are hard to overcome. The child frequently has no peers in the neighborhood who are similar to him or her in looks and ability. The child who is retarded does have some characteristics that are like those of all other children. When we teach others to look for our similarities they will find there are more instances of likenesses than differences. It all lies in what we dwell on, and this is one of the reasons the medical model fell into disfavor among those who are child advocates.

Nursing Care of the Adolescent. As nurses we will encounter adolescents who have not had the opportunities to learn to live in the community, and this is the direction toward which we must prepare them. As they develop into young adults they will have some very critical needs. Those needs are for

- work training
- group home living
- sex education
- safety for self and others

We can only hope that as children they have learned skills that will teach them fine motor abilities, social skills, some ability to sight read words in their environment (danger, stop, men's room, women's room, go, walk, don't walk, street signs in the neighborhood).

They now need to learn how to use the telephone, how to prepare simple meals, how to work the washing

Table 34-6. Significance of Clinical Manifestations of Mental Retardation

Clinical Manifestation and Explanation	Significance to the Nurse
Personal-Social Development	
Immature social behavior: Prefers to play with younger children Shows defective judgment by communication that does not fit situation with other children Acts out to get attention Often shows withdrawal behavior	Social skills will help a child develop self-esteem and gain acceptance from others Encourage social activities
Poor self-image: Afraid to try new tasks, withdraws from any challenge	Look for child who does not seem interested in new activities Child cries, becomes frustrated, and is anxious
Cognitive Area	
Poor problem solving: Not able to accomplish developmentally appropriate problem solving	Encourage use of games to learn colors, numbers, matching like objects Teach new words
Concrete thinking: Cannot think abstractly	Children learn best when task is concrete or functional. Learn by feeling and touching
Inability to transfer learning: Not able to apply information just learned to a new situation Poor informal learning Short attention span Short memory Difficulty with concept formation	Cannot learn by observing ideas going on around them. Need to participate Present learning in short segments Repeat lessons to reinforce words and ideas Problems learning new words and ideas Use Show and Tell sessions, role play, story telling, and dramatic play to help these children learn
Language and Speech Development	
Language delayed	
Speech problems owing to motor control and physical problems of speech area	The child with Down syndrome has small oral cavity and protruding tongue
Problems in following directions	Cannot remember the sequence of more directions than one at a time. Example: "Get your umbrella in the closet and bring it to me"
Motor Development	
Lacking in body control	Some (not all) children are clumsy or have poor balance. As a general rule, their motor control is not well developed, especially fine motor
Distractibility	The child with mental retardation would benefit from a learning center that cuts down on distraction from surroundings
Inability to follow directions	Needs simple directions given for one task at a time
Perseveration	Child may repeat some motor movement over and over again
Underactive	Tends to not become involved and to sit quietly for longer periods of time
Self-stimulating behaviors	May engage in rocking back and forth, head banging, manipulating fingers in front of their eyes, ruminating, or other distracting and disturbing activities. These activities are inappropriate but give the child some levels of feedback. Help child learn new behaviors that are appropriate Activities that will help children develop gross motor skills include rolling, jumping, hopping, crawling, tunneling, climbing, balancing, kicking, and kneeling. Reacting to music is also beneficial Fine motor skills are developed by cutting, tracing, coloring, stacking, and pasting Materials that help are finger paints, clay, beads, and watercolors

Table 34-6 *(continued)*

Clinical Manifestation and Explanation	Significance to the Nurse
Perceptual Motor Development	
Visual and auditory	Children often do not hear and see things as they really are
Problem in seeing differences	Child may have problems with a moving object. Child may be unable to see difference between two objects (pictures of apple and orange and tennis ball)
Inability to distinguish between two sounds	Child is sometimes unable to tell where sound is coming from
	Children can learn by using textured materials, such as cloth, feathers, grains, sand, foam. Materials that stimulate their sense of smell and taste are also excellent learning tools

machine and dryer, and how to prevent accidents. They will also need to know how to count money and budget their funds and to tell time. They should also learn how to use transportation, such as buses and taxis.

Personal safety is a lesson that is very difficult to instill in young people regardless of mental ability. Emotions are hard to separate from reason. Pregnancy and social disease are common to people of all walks of life. There are problems with people bent on taking advantage of others, both in our general environment and within the sheltered walls of institutions. Adolescents must learn who they can safely ask for help and who not to ask for help. It would also be important for them to have learned what people in the community can help them such as firemen, police, and medical personnel.

Body changes are occurring in the adolescent and bring special needs for understanding, hygiene, and health. Dental care, nutrition counseling, and changes in prosthetics due to growth spurts are important areas for nurses to become involved in helping the client manage. One important activity that will prove frustrating to family, client, and nurse is finding health professionals in the private sector who can and will provide health care to those persons who are retarded or handicapped.

Some health professionals have not been educated to work with clients who have disability. Owing to tight office scheduling or lack of accessibility of their facilities, these professionals are reluctant to treat individuals with special needs (Siantz, 1977).

The nurse can facilitate the visits to health professionals by attention to such details as providing the office nurse with information about the client. Some of this information includes the following:

- The client's communication skills.
- The client's physical disabilities and use of wheelchairs and other equipment. How much lifting is required?
- Financial arrangements.
- Behaviors that might be a problem and some helpful hints to deal with these behaviors.

The nurse will also need to help the family in their *preparation for the future* and for the time when the parents become elderly. For parents who have spent a lifetime "doing" for their child, this is a concept they find difficult to deal with. The thought of their child becoming independent initiates fears for the child's safety and security.

Care When the Child Is Hospitalized. *Hospitalized* children with mental retardation should be treated for the conditions for which they are admitted, but their special needs must be recognized. Their care is adapted to their specific needs, with a comprehensive and individualized plan that is geared to their developmental levels. This plan should allow for the child's self-expression, independence and progress at a slow rate.

A significant person should be permitted to stay with the hospitalized child to provide reassurance that there will be continuity of care. The care plan should have family input on the child's specific likes and dislikes, fears, favorite activities, and any other information on the child and the rituals of daily living that will make hospitalization easier. If the child does not communicate verbally, the nurse should be aware of expressions or symbols that are important.

The child with both severe mental retardation and physical handicaps presents complex problems that require a team of experts familiar with the conditions. The child with severe brain damage may have vision and hearing deficits that may not have been discovered because the child has no way of knowing that vision or hearing is impaired. The alert nurse will observe for any signs of sensory deficit.

Mentally retarded children are incapable of abstract thinking. Most can comprehend simple explanations, but concrete examples must be given. For example, instead of nurses saying that they will return after a while, they should show the children where the hand on the clock will be when they will return.

Most retarded children enjoy music. A record player and some of the child's favorite records will help ease hospital anxiety. Children should have their favorite toys with them. Toys or games that give immediate reward ("busy boxes," in which something happens when you pull a string or open a drawer) will stimulate motor activity and develop observational skills.

If the child is to have surgery, a family member, school nurse, or familiar person should stay with him or her. Procedures should be explained in simple terms. If the child is to have a tonsillectomy, a simple "The doctor is going to fix your throat so it won't hurt as much later," might be adequate. The nurse must always be honest.

Role playing and looking at pictures of doctors in their surgical attire is therapeutic. The child could be given a mask or surgical cap to play with before surgery. If the child has a fracture, a similar cast could be applied to a doll. This can be taken off to show that the cast is not permanent.

The physical needs of the mentally retarded child are basically no different from the physical needs of all people. Their body systems, for the most part, function normally, but mental and motor responses are restricted. Because all body systems are interdependent, any system might be directly or indirectly affected. It is the nurse's responsibility to observe verbal and nonverbal clues and know how to interpret them.

Medical information should be interpreted by the nurse to the family. Nurses will need to be comfortable in the role of consultant and confidante. They will frequently be asked questions produced by deep hurt and despair. Listening and observing are more important than pious words.

Because nurses are in leadership positions and have many opportunities for changing attitudes, they need to examine their own emotions of fear, discomfort, anger, or desire for escape when they are exposed to people with impairments. The child will quickly sense the attitude behind the all-important interactions with the nurse. There can be no therapeutic relationship if the child does not feel acceptance. Children are quick to recognize the emptiness of care given in a sense of duty. The nurse giving care will see a person of potential within an imprisoning shell.

Helping Parents Teach the Mentally Retarded Child. If retarded children are intellectually able to make basic decisions, they must learn to accept responsibility for their own safety. Siblings should not be held responsible or punished for actions performed by a retarded child. These children must be taught to accept responsibility for their own actions, with the same guidance their siblings received. The task and discipline should be commensurate with the child's developmental level.

One of the frustrations of the family is frequently found in the need for guidance in sexual matters. The nurse should be prepared to assist the family to establish some guidelines. The child has undoubtedly already absorbed the verbal and nonverbal cues of the family's attitude about each member's sexuality. The child's questions about sex should be answered honestly, factually, and simply. If the child has the awareness and curiosity to ask, he or she should be given an appropriate answer. Parents may need to initiate a discussion if the child does not ask. The level of comprehension (and explanation) depends upon the degree of mental impairment, but the basic approach to sex education is the same.

The school-age child is faced with physical changes, and the boy may be frightened if nocturnal emissions and penile erections are not explained. A girl should certainly have received anticipatory guidance about menstruation. Children need to know that, just as it is not socially acceptable to urinate in public, so is masturbation done in private, but parents should not make the child feel guilty. The child's sexuality is part of him or her, and an open acceptance of it frees the child to develop a better self-image. The manner in which sexual matters are discussed may be more meaningful than the verbal message.

Parents are frequently concerned with communication skills they can develop with their handicapped child. Many impaired children have speech pathologies and should be receiving speech therapy. The following suggestions will be helpful for reinforcement at home. Parents should be reminded that facial expression and voice tone are more important than words spoken. The method of communication depends upon the degree of mental impairment.

1. Let handicapped children do their own talking. Let them try to express themselves verbally as well as they can. Take time to listen.
2. Let them be an active part of family conversation, even if they are only able to contribute an occasional "yes" or "no."
3. If the child is nonverbal, teach cues for a yes or no response, such as looking down for no and smiling for yes. Ask questions that require only a yes or no answer.
4. Plan a scheduled 15 minutes each day for speech correction if necessary. This should be the only time the child's speech is corrected. Don't nag. Give praise when the child speaks properly.
5. Speak frequently to the child, using vivid explanations (the noisy, green truck; the red book; the soft, white blanket).
6. Do not accept gestures or pointing. Name the ob-

ject and encourage the child to repeat the name. If the child has the ability to speak, insist that the word be said before the object is given. For example, insist that the child say the word "milk" and do not accept pointings or gruntings. If the child makes a reasonable effort, give the milk but continue to work on quality.

7. Provide many auditory experiences by reading simple stories or playing suitable records. Allow the child to sing along or respond to rhythm.
8. Praise successful speech. Whenever the child makes an effort toward a new word, reward him or her immediately with a verbal response.
9. Use short, simple sentences and repeat words frequently.
10. Never refrain from talking to a retarded child because you do not know what to say. Speak as you would to any other child, pick cues from the child's reponse, and include him or her in group conversation.

Before children can learn to speak, they must know how to chew, suck, blow, and swallow. Speech can be reinforced at home by correlating the retarded child's self-feeding skills with the speech program. Teaching self-care skills to a retarded child requires much time, patience, and repetition, but the results are gratifying in terms of the family's satisfaction and the child's self-esteem. The child usually wants to become independent, and patterns must be established early before dependency habits become established. As children learn one skill, they develop more confidence in conquering the next.

If the child is severely retarded, developing self-feeding skills may be problematic, but in most cases the following suggestions that the nurse can make to the parent will be helpful. Have the child sit in a comfortable position with feet on a firm surface. With your hand over the child's dominant hand, provide assistance in bringing the spoon from the dish to his or her lips. There are various wrist movements involved in getting food from a dish to a spoon and then to the mouth. This procedure will need to be repeated for many sessions and may take months. Gradually move your hand from the child's hand to the wrist, and eventually you will be assisting by only a guiding touch on the elbow. Do not be concerned about spillage but encourage neatness. The same procedure can be applied to holding a cup of milk. Begin with food the child enjoys, such as applesauce. Gradually add new textures and flavors, but reward the child with a favorite food. Encourage finger foods. Be sure that food is placed in the back of the child's mouth, not just on the tip of the tongue. Peanut butter on the upper or lower gums or between the gums and cheeks encourages tongue manipulation and mandibular movement that is necessary for both speech and chewing.

Helpful hints for teaching dressing skills include:

1. If the child is learning to tie shoelaces, allow practice on an adult shoe. The child can slip his or her foot into the shoe and can play "pretend adult" games while learning.
2. Sew large buttons and enlarge the buttonholes on an adult blouse or shirt. The child can then lift the apparel and watch what he or she is doing.
3. Name tags on the neck bands of coats, slip-on sweaters and tops teach the child his or her name and identify the front and back of garments.
4. For children who have trouble getting a coat on, put the coat on the table, with the lining side up and the collar toward them. The children face the coat, put an arm in each sleeve and then raise their arms over their heads. This procedure is also used for slip-over sweaters and tee shirts. The neck label will identify the front and back.
5. To teach a child to put on socks, put the sock in position over the toes and let the child pull it over the heel and ankle.

Toilet training for a retarded child cannot be hurried. It is important that it be done at a point at which both child and mother are relaxed and ready. A routine must be established and carried out in a calm, comfortable way, with the mother explaining all actions to the child. As she takes the child to the bathroom, she says, "Here we go to the bathroom" and "Down go Jenny's pants" as she puts her hand over the the child's hands and "Up goes Jenny" as the child is placed on a comfortable stool with foot support. An adult should stay with the child so that someone is there to give immediate reward when the child performs appropriately. To be effective, the reward must be something the child particularly enjoys. If there is no result in five minutes, wipe the child and calmly remove him or her. Again, put your hands over the child's hands as you both pull the pants back into position.

Establish a pattern for bowel movements by noting on a calendar the time of elimination over a two-week span. Take the child to the bathroom a few minutes before the average time and repeat the procedure. Watch the child's face and listen for particular sounds. Dress the child in clothes that are simple to remove. If the child cries, discontinue and try a few weeks later when he or she may be more ready.

The Retarded Child in the Community. The most frequent times for recognizing mental retardation are at birth, age 3, and age 6 years. The child should receive therapy and be enrolled in a stimulating program as soon as the diagnosis is made. Because of the proliferation of preschool programs and day care centers, astute teachers are recognizing symptoms and making early referrals. Early intervention and stimulation result in greater intellectual awareness.

As retarded children progress and have adequate

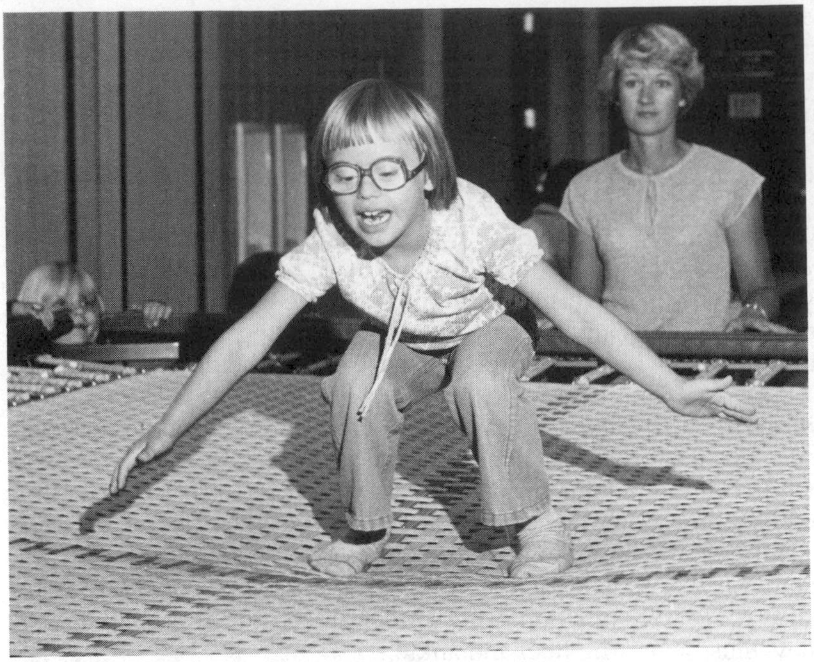

A child with Down syndrome is mainstreamed with her peers for a class in motor skills. (Photograph by Howard Zehr; Joint Schools Special Education Program of Elkhart County, Indiana.)

preparation, they should be integrated into regular classes with their peers, or "mainstreamed." This allows for normal social activities and new experiences with peers. Segregating groups of people from the mainstream of society is seen as dehumanizing. Mainstreaming gives all children an equal opportunity to participate in community and school activities. However, the teacher needs special orientation to the child and must keep open communication with the family. There is grave danger that with mainstreaming, the child will no longer receive individualized help and may regress academically. Nurses can help school personnel understand the specific needs of the retarded children they are working with.

The process of "normalization," first developed in Sweden, makes available to every retarded person opportunities and conditions of everyday life as close as possible to the norm and patterns of other people. It implies as normal a routine of life as possible. This means that children with impairments will be integrated into as many normal experiences as they are capable of participating given their condition.

Within the past few decades, great strides have been made in creating community awareness of the needs of children who are retarded. Consequently, they are more readily accepted. There will undoubtedly always be retarded children, but if today's medical and nursing personnel will focus on preventive measures, a greater percentage of children previously labeled retarded will be able to enjoy a richer and healthier physical and emotional environment.

Prevention of Mental Retardation. The nurse will note that some of the causative factors of mental retardation can be avoided. Teaching aspects of prevention cannot be overemphasized, because prevention is the most important tool in combating retardation. Nurses should always stress the need for immunization against rubella, encourage health care during pregnancy, and recommend giving human immune globulin to prevent Rh hemolytic disease. They should be sure that all infants are appropriately screened for phenylketonuria. Parents should be cautioned about the danger of fetal alcohol syndrome as a result of excessive maternal drinking. The dangers of other drugs in terms of their effects on the fetus should also be part of a prevention program. The nurse must know the community resources available and be able to follow through on referrals from the diagnostic team. If the causative factor warrants it, nurses should encourage all siblings or intellectually impaired children to have genetic counseling.

Fetal Alcohol Syndrome

Fetal alcohol syndrome (FAS) is the result of high levels of alcohol ingestion during pregnancy. Although the exact pathophysiology is not known, alcohol is thought to impair protein synthesis in the fetus (Kliegman and Behrman, 1987). Fetal exposure to alcohol may also increase the likelihood of cancer, especially neuroblastoma (Cohen, 1984). FAS occurs in an estimated 1 to 2 infants per 1000 live births (Kliegman and Behrman, 1987).

As reported by Cohen (1984), the Fetal Alcohol Study Group of the Research Society on Alcoholism has recommended that FAS be diagnosed only when the infant has signs in each of the following three categories: (1) growth retardation (prenatal or postnatal) with weight, length, or head circumference below the 10th percentile for gestational age, (2) central nervous system involvement, and (3) deformities of the head and face (e.g., microcephaly, small eyes, flattened maxilla, thin upper lip). If the syndrome is not diagnosed on appearance at birth, it may be identified later when the infant displays hirsutism (excess growth of body hair), a weak suck, irritability, and failure to thrive. Mental retardation is common, along with various behavioral problems.

There is no specific treatment for this disorder, and the prognosis for severely affected infants is poor. Intervention is best directed at teaching to prevent occurrence. Pregnant women should avoid alcohol consumption from the time of conception.

Down Syndrome

Down syndrome affects both sexes equally. It occurs approximately once in each 1000 live births. The trisomy 21 type occurs more often in children of women over the age of 35 years. As maternal age increases, the incidence of Down syndrome increases.

Normally, cells from the male and female undergo a process known as meiosis or reduction division. During the cell division, spindle fibers within the nucleus of the cell pull the paired chromosomes apart and to opposite poles of the cell. A full complement of chromosomes is 46 prior to meiosis. During meiosis, chromosome pairs separate and 23 go to one ovum and 23 chromosomes go to the second ovum. When nondisjunction of the number 21 chromosome occurs, one ovum receives two of this chromosome and increases that cell's chromosome content to 24 instead of the normal 23. The second ovum receives no number 21 chromosome and the resulting loss of genetic material is not compatible with life. If the ovum with the 24 chromosomes is then fertilized by a sperm, which has the normal complement of 23 chromosomes, the zygote will have 47 chromosomes instead of the normal 46. The odd number of chromosomes is a result of the zygote's having three number 21 chromosomes (two from the abnormal ovum and one from the sperm), or trisomy 21 (Drapo, 1986).

The developing fetus with this abnormal chromosome count will have Down syndrome (Box 34-5). Down syndrome also may occur as a result of other aberrations of the chromosomes. A second type of chromosomal disorder, known as *translocation,* occurs when a piece of a number 21 chromosome breaks off and attaches itself to another chromosome, such as the number 15 or 14 chromosome. If, during oogenesis, the chromosome with the translocated piece of number 21 and a normal 21 chromosome are grouped in the same cell and fertilized, the result is a cell with two normal 21 chromosomes (one from the father and one from the mother) and a piece of the number 21 chromosome attached to the number 15 (or 14) chromosome. This causes the same physical problems seen in trisomy 21 and accounts for 4 per cent of cases of Down syndrome.

A third condition causing Down syndrome is *mosaicism.* In this situation, some of the cells of the developing fetus are trisomy cells and some are normal cells. This occurs during early cell division following fertilization of the zygote (mitosis).

According to Steele (1982) persons with mosaicism tend to exhibit milder manifestations of mental retardation than do children with nonmosaic forms.

Signs and Symptoms. There is a striking similarity of the physical features of children with Down syndrome regardless of the manner of chromosomal aberration. Down syndrome is found in every race, culture, and creed. Characteristics are as follows:

Head: flat occiput, brachycephalic

Eyes: upslanted
iris speckled (Brushfield spots)
epicanthal folds

Nose: short with depressed nasal bridge (owing to underdevelopment of nasal bone)

Mouth: protruding tongue owing to small oral cavity; the mouth is usually open, tongue is furrowed, palate is short and narrow; dental abnormalities are common

Ears: dysplastic

Neck: short and broad

Chest: congenital heart disease is a frequent finding; lung infections are frequent

Limbs: short

Hands: hands are broad and square, and the fingers are short; clinodactyly of the fifth finger may be present; aplasia or hypoplasia of the middle phalanx also may occur

Joints: laxity of movement

Stature: short and stocky; hypotonic musculature

Dermatoglyphics: fingertips have marked increase of ulnar loops (with opening of loop on the ulnar side), usually on all 10 fingertips, associated with a decrease in whorls, arches, and radial loops

Palms: marked increase in simian creases

Feet: increase of fibular dermatoglyphic loops (opening of loop toward the fibular side) on the toes and a decrease of tibial loops on the great toe; in the area just under the great toe (the hallucal area), tibial arches are prominent; there is an increased space between the first and second toes

Dermatoglyphics in children with Down syndrome are so similar to each other and so different from the population as a whole that it is possible to

Box 34-5
Chromosome Abnormality and Nursing Significance in Down Syndrome

NONDISJUNCTION OF CHROMOSOME NUMBER 21

Accounts for 95 per cent of cases of Down syndrome in live infants.

Two thirds result from maternal meiotic error.
One third result from paternal meiotic error.

Risk increases with age in women.

Age (yr)	Risk
Under 20	1:1550 live births
30–34	1:700
Over 43	1:40

Risk for a couple who already have a child with Down syndrome for a second affected infant is about 1 per cent.

TRANSLOCATION

Accounts for 4 per cent of live births of infants with Down syndrome. Of these, 65 per cent are chromosomal accidents of that particular pregnancy (Steele, 1982).

Risk of having a second infant with this type of chromosomal accident is slightly higher than that in the general population.

Balanced Translocation (One Third of Translocation Carriers)

If this is a balanced translocation, which the parent has inherited, the risk for having a Down syndrome child at each conception is:

father: 2 per cent
mother: 10 per cent

Of the father's other children, half would tend to have normal chromosome configuration and half would have a balanced translocation like his. These latter children with balanced translocation would also produce children like their father.

Of the other children of a mother who carries a balanced translocation, half would tend to have normal chromosomes and half would be balanced translocation carriers like the mother.

A 21/21 Translocation

All children will have Down syndrome.

Mental retardation and physical stigmata are not different from those associated with trisomy 21.

MOSAIC PATTERN

About 1 per cent of children with Down syndrome have a mosaic chromosomal pattern. Recurrence is only slightly higher than for the general population.

Degree of intelligence is slightly higher in children with a mosaic configuration. Other stigmata are the same as with non-mosaic Down syndrome (Steele, 1982).

classify these persons on the basis of dermatoglyphics alone. Without looking at other features an observer can use certain index scores for dermatoglyphic patterns and score prints very accurately. In spite of such accuracy, this analysis can only be used as a supplement to a more precise means of diagnosis—the karyotype (Schaumann and Alter, 1976). (See Chapter 4 for further information on karyotypes.)

Intervention and Nursing Care. Down syndrome is readily diagnosed at birth because of some of the obvious signs. There are undoubtedly few other diagnoses that cause as much grief, confusion, and loneliness in parents as this one, ending their happy anticipation of a "normal," healthy baby. How the diagnosis is presented to the family is crucial, an event the family will always remember. This is a highly sensitive and emotional time; parents' acceptance of the child and the diagnosis cannot be rushed, for time is the only healer of the hurt. Parents have anticipated a child they do not have; they are mourning this normal child, and they feel guilty about their confused emotions. They should be assured that these are typical reactions and that no one is to blame for their child's anomaly. The nurse may be the most supportive person to stand by, listen, and help them formulate the questions they must ask.

Acceptance of the child varies with the value orientation of the family. Parents who value academic excellence may have a great deal of difficulty accepting a child with limited intellectual potential. There is a wide range of intellectual ability among children with Down syndrome. Although some are seriously affected mentally, others function at a relatively high level. Down syndrome children cannot be classified in one category, although similar signs and symptoms may be present. Most children, however, continue to function at half their chronologic age up to the age of 12. They never seem to catch up with peers.

Because of recent governmental assistance in special education, it is now mandatory that education be provided for all children with handicaps. Most communities have access to special educational facilities. The infant with Down syndrome is in some ways more fortunate than one with a hidden diagnosis, because therapy can soon be initiated. Infant stimulation increases awareness and alertness. Some children who have had early intervention are now participating in regular elementary classrooms with continued special assistance.

In years past, there was little help or support for the families and their child, and institutionalization was frequently recommended. With the academic opportunities of today, parents are encouraged to keep the child in the home setting, in which he or she can be socially and academically stimulated. One of the most important comforts the nurse can give is to assure parents that help is available. If possible, the family should establish a relationship with another family with a child who has a similar diagnosis and ability. Many communities have a parents' group in which concerns and strengths are shared. The nurse must know the community resources available.

Down syndrome children of school age usually have delayed psychomotor development. Speech is commonly delayed; the child may need speech therapy. In the classroom psychomotor activities are incorporated into the school day; children can learn much through play activity. Some children learn to read on a low level, but they cannot do abstract thinking. Although few achieve an IQ above 75, society has yet to learn what can be accomplished if the child is treated as a worthwhile member and given unlimited opportunities and exposures.

Siblings of children with Down syndrome are frequently embarrassed because of this child; older siblings have questions about heredity and wonder whether they too will produce a child with Down syndrome. They fear social ostracism because of the affected family member. Karyotyping should be done on siblings of the retarded for genetic counseling. Fetal cells obtained by amniocentesis as early as the eighth week of pregnancy may be cultured in vitro and the information made available.

The child with Down syndrome is a social person and enjoys contact with people. As the nurse helps the family members toward acceptance, they will become aware of the contribution the child can make to the family and the community. Children with Down syndrome should be among peers, as they learn much through imitation. They should be exposed to as many normal experiences as possible and should not be deprived of opportunities to learn and grow.

These individuals are commonly happy, frank, and honest people and have many lessons in values to teach us. As society learns to accept people for what they are, and not for competitive or intellectual performance, the retarded person can be valued and accepted. When children with Down syndrome are hospitalized with any medical problem, discipline and structure should be enforced, and no concessions made "because they are retarded." Children soon learn whom they can manipulate. They should be treated respectfully.

Because of modern science, these children are expected to live a normal life span. Previously they usually died of respiratory illness or cardiac pathology while fairly young. Many communities now have group homes for retarded persons where they are under adult supervision and can enjoy semi-independent living.

The Gifted Child

Children who are developmentally advanced or academically superior are called "exceptionally able" or "gifted." Gifted children represent about 3 per cent of the population. Renzulli (1978) states that giftedness is the interaction among three basic clusters of human traits: above average general ability, high levels of task commitment, and high levels of creativity. Children who are gifted and talented have, or are capable of developing, these traits and applying them to any area of human performance. These children require a wide variety of educational opportunities and services that are not usually provided through regular school programming.

In general, most gifted children move through a developmental task more rapidly than their peers. Usually, giftedness is defined on the basis of an intelligence test in which these children answer more questions correctly than their peers.

Assessment

Several parameters are relied on to determine whether a child is gifted. Early indications of giftedness in preschoolers include early achievement of developmental milestones, early language development, and boundless curiosity (Fish and Burch, 1985). Other evidence of giftedness includes the ability to understand abstract concepts, to master new skills with little repetition, to discuss experiences in unusual detail, to assemble puzzles developed for older children, and to construct interesting or unusual designs with blocks, clay, and so forth (Brink, 1982).

Test scores, teacher recommendations, grades, and IQ test scores are used to identify gifted school-age children. However, no clear relationship has been found between these measures when they are compared with one another. For example, in a study of junior high school children, Clifford (1986) found that of those students teachers identified as gifted, only 26 per cent had IQ test scores of 136 or above. In the same study, of those children who were designated as gifted on the basis of IQ test scores (136 or above), only 45 per cent had been recognized as being gifted by their teachers. Despite this lack of reliability, teacher observations remain a valuable tool in assessing ability.

Group intelligence tests and achievement test batteries are helpful as screening tools to supplement or counterbalance teacher observations. The true abilities of students with reading difficulties, emotional or motivational problems, or differing ethnic backgrounds may not necessarily be identified.

Individual intelligence (i.e., IQ) tests provide the most reliable and accurate information about a child's ability to reason. The commonly used tests are the Stanford-Binet Scale, the Wechsler Intelligence Scale for Children–Revised (WISC-R), and the Wechsler Preschool and Primary Scale of Intelligence for Children 4–6 1/2 years (WPPSI). Results of these tests do not always reflect the child's actual ability. The majority of intelligence tests are based on an educated, white, middle-class society. Minority and low income groups tend to score lower even on nonverbal portions of the tests because subcultural differences may bias a child's performance. The extremes of retardation or giftedness are more easily identified. Supposedly, the higher the IQ, the more exceptional the child's ability will be. However, intelligence tests do have serious defects when measuring exceptional ability. Tests of intelligence are basically normative and few children of exceptional ability are involved in standardization of the tests. IQ tests do not predict how well a student will perform in class or predict individual achievement (DeMaio et al, 1985; Leyden, 1985; Clifford, 1986).

Creativity is one component of intelligence that is not measured by an intelligence test. In fact, some of the most creative persons have been those who were thought unable to learn. Creativity needs to be permitted and encouraged. Opportunities must be provided to give the child a chance to think creatively. All too often, creative children are stifled owing to the lack of opportunity to express their creativity.

The truly gifted children's performance is always accelerated beyond that of their peers. Some children who in early life have received extensive stimulation in a responsive home environment are erroneously labeled "gifted." Later, as their peers gain experience, the early nontruly gifted children's intellectual development tends to level off in comparison (Anastasiow, 1986).

The local public school system is responsible for evaluating gifted children. There is still enormous controversy over what constitutes giftedness, and in some communities this may lead to confusion among professionals and parents involved with the child. The National Association for Gifted Children or the Association for the Gifted may be able to offer clarification and support if such a controversy exists.

Intervention and Nursing Care

Children who are gifted and talented are of concern to health professionals who may be called upon to help the family deal with some of the issues surrounding giftedness. Although giftedness is not a disease or illness, it is an area of significant concern to parents. The family may need help in obtaining an appropriate diagnostic evaluation of their child as well as an appropriate education. The nurse may be in a position to refer the family to the proper sources.

Levine (1983) identifies two types of gifted children who have special problems. These are the underachieving gifted and the minority gifted. Many of the underachieving gifted suffer from low self-esteem, which interferes with their ability to achieve. These students often develop inappropriate behavioral styles. The minority gifted may have been unable to achieve their potential for a variety of reasons, including economic disadvantage, bilingualism, and a lack of successful role models in the community.

Many schools have developed programs for talented and gifted children. These programs are designed to enrich and broaden the children's academic performance. The children may be placed in an enrichment program or grouped with other bright children in special classes. Although the latter program may benefit the gifted students, it deprives the other students from the stimulation these bright students provide in the classroom. Another alternative for the high achiever is to allow the student to progress or skip to a higher grade. A major drawback to this alternative is that the child's physical and emotional development may lag behind intellectual development and create problems of adjustment with the peer group. Argument over acceleration versus enrichment in the school continues to rage, but major investigators still support acceleration. This decision must be individualized depending upon the child's physical size, chronologic age, personality, family constellation, and degree of advancement.

Family life of gifted children often becomes complicated. Parents may forget natural instincts and treat the child differently. Children must often bear the burden of parental expectations, the need to excel in everything. It is necessary to keep in mind that exceptional intellectual ability may not be accompanied by the same level of physical and emotional maturity. Exceptional mental ability does not always imply equal achievement in all areas of learning (Leyden, 1985).

Difficulties in family relationships may arise. Frequently, the very bright child becomes the focus of attention within the family. As a result, the child becomes at risk for developing an unrealistic sense of importance and self-worth. This imbalance of attention may also have a negative effect on siblings. Feelings of jealousy resulting in rejection of the "favored" sibling are not uncommon. Siblings may feel inferior, especially if a younger child surpasses the older child. The uniqueness and specialness of each child should be encouraged. Siblings should have an opportunity for special time with parents. This special time and the fostering of their unique skills (e.g., athletics, music) may help the siblings feel more adequate. Parental expectations may also place an additional burden on the exceptionally bright child—e.g., to achieve success in public attention to meet their parent's own unfulfilled needs (Leyden, 1985).

Being of superior intellect does not ensure high

Date ______________

Referred by ______________

Intellect

______ Curiosity
______ Reasoning ability
______ Rapid response to new ideas
______ Learns quickly
______ Good memory
______ Extensive vocabulary
______ Imagination
______ Observation skills (good)
______ Divergent thinking
______ Other (describe)

____
____
____

Personality

______ Humor
______ High personal standards
______ Frustration
______ Impatience
______ Reacts to discrepancies in others
______ Sensitive
______ Philosophical
______ Articulate
______ Ability to make friends

Hobbies (describe)

____
____
____

Work Preference

______ Likes to work independently
______ Other (describe)

____
____
____

Leadership Skills

______ Gym class
______ Classroom
______ Clubs
______ Group play
______ Other (describe)

____
____
____

Behaviors (not extreme)*

______ Restless
______ Afraid to reveal knowledge
______ Unenthusiastic for classwork
______ Critical
______ Daydreams
______ Withdrawn
______ Other (describe)

____
____

* These behaviors are normal in many children who are gifted. However, if the behaviors become extreme, impede progress, or change in noticeable ways, the nurse should re-evaluate the student for extent of behaviors of concern.

Figure 34-5. Baseline nursing assessment for children identified as gifted.

self-esteem and emotional adjustment. On the contrary, when development does not meet "normal" expectations, whether precocious or unusually slow, the child receives a message that he or she is different. The highly intelligent child may create feelings of uneasiness among peers and adults. Intellectually gifted children may be rejected by their peer group and thus seek older children as playmates or isolate themselves. Some children will attempt to hide their abilities in the classroom and purposefully underachieve to avoid being considered different (Leyden, 1985).

Exceptional children are often handicapped by their own need to excel. These children fear failure or lack of achievement, and as a result place great stress upon themselves. For the "A student," the burden of maintaining that status increases throughout the school years. Anything less than an "A" is viewed as failure. Unrealistic expectations of self and the need to always be successful may cause some children to avoid taking risks for fear of failure.

However, not all children have difficulty adjusting to life. Terman's classic study substantiates this fact. Terman initiated a study in 1921 of 1500 middle-class school children who had Stanford-Binet IQ scores of 140 or higher. These individuals were followed until 70 to 80 years of age. They were shown to be superior in social and personal adjustments later in life as well as in productivity and longevity. Also, they were found to hold typical middle-class values of steady employment, home ownership, and family (Anastasiow, 1986; Clifford, 1986).

The nurse can support the child and family as they cope with the psychosocial problems that are often a part of being different or of living with one who is different. Parents may need support in their child-rearing practices because, either before or after finding out they have a gifted child, they often develop difficulty relating to their child. They should be told to treat the child the same way the siblings are treated. It is not wise to focus on the gifted label in front of the child or siblings. Regarding stimulation, parents should be instructed not to push their child. Materials should be child-centered and flexible so as to stimulate creativity. Access to museums, books, and other educational materials can be provided as the child expresses interest in them. The challenge faced by the nurse is to help parents learn to see their children as unique individuals with a development and personality all their own and to balance their needs with those of the family.

Counseling with Teachers

The value of nurses collaborating with other members of the school team (e.g., teachers, psychologists, social workers) cannot be overemphasized. These team members may have insights concerning the child that can be useful to the nurse, and nurses can provide additional input into the thinking of the team. There are usually discrepancies in terminology and approaches used in medicine and education, and these can be confusing to the family. The collaboration, or sharing, of everyone involved with the child can often help to eliminate some of the family's confusion. In some school districts, the school nurse is called upon to make impartial observations of the classroom behavior of students. It is important for the school nurse to work closely with teachers of children who have been identified as gifted. Figure 34-5, an assessment of gifted children, could be used by the nurse or teacher in assessing classroom behaviors. Most of the behaviors may be considered normal for gifted as well as average or below average students. However, if a behavior becomes extreme or impedes progress in a noticeable way, further evaluation is needed.

References

American Psychiatric Association: *Diagnostic and Statistical Manual of Mental Disorders.* 3rd ed. (DSM-III-R.) Washington, DC, American Psychiatric Association, 1987.

Amiel-Tison C: Neurological assessment from birth to seven years of age. *In* Harel S, Anastasiow N (eds): *The At-risk Infant: Psycho-Social-Medical Aspects.* Baltimore, Paul H. Brookes, 1985, 239–251.

Anastasiow NJ: *Development and Disability: A Psychological Analysis for Special Educators.* Baltimore, Paul H. Brookes, 1986.

Barnard KE, Erikson ML: *Teaching Children with Developmental Problems: A Family Care Approach.* 2nd ed. St. Louis, CV Mosby, 1976.

Barnard K, Kelly JF: Infant intervention: Parental considerations. In *Guidelines for Early Intervention Programs.* Salt Lake City, University of Utah, College of Nursing, 1980, 34–55. (Available from Office for Maternal-Child Health, Room 7–39, Parklawn Bldg., 5600 Fishers Lane, Rockville, MD 20857.)

Beckman P: Perceptions of young children with handicaps: A comparison of mothers and program staff. *Ment Retard* 1984; 22(4), 176–181.

Benton A: Developmental dyslexia. *J Pediatr Psychol* 1976; 1:28–31.

Biklen D: Advocacy comes of age. *Except Child* 1976; 2(6), 309.

Bleck EE: Cerebral palsy.In Bleck E (ed): *Physically Handicapped Children.* New York, Grune & Stratton, 1982, 59–127.

Botshaw ML, Perret YM: *Children with Handicaps: A Medical Primer.* Baltimore, Paul H. Brookes, 1981, 253–269.

Brenton M: Mainstreaming. *Today's Educ* 1976 Mar/Apr.

Brink RE: The gifted preschool child. *Pediatr Nurs* 1982; 8(5), 299–303.

Bruen H: The dyslexic child. *Pediatr Ann* 1977 Feb; p 129.

Bureau of Community Health Service: *Individual Service Plans in the Supplemental Security Income Disabled Children's Program.* Rockville, MD, Office of Maternal-Child Care, 1979.

Caesar P, Eggermont E: Neonatal clinical neurological assessment. *In* Harel S, Anastasiow N (eds): *The At-risk Infant.* Baltimore, Paul H. Brookes, 1985, 197–220.

Child Development Program Division: *When You Care for Handicapped Children* (TDHR Stock No. SCO943). Austin, TX, Department of Human Resources, 1979.

Chin P, Drew CJ, Logan DR: *Mental Retardation: A Life Cycle Approach.* St. Louis, CV Mosby, 1979.

Clifford T: Cognitive development of the school-ager. *In* Schuster CS, Ashburn SS (eds): *The Process of Human Development: A Holistic-Life-span Approach.* Boston, Little, Brown, 1986.

Cohen FL: *Clinical Genetics in Nursing Practice.* Philadelphia, JB Lippincott, 1984.

Collins M: *Communication in Health Care.* 2nd ed. St. Louis, CV Mosby, 1983.

Culbertson JL, Ferry PC: Learning disabilities. *Pediatr Clin North Am* 1982; 29(1), 121–136.

Curry JB, Peppe KK: *Mental Retardation: Nursing Approaches to Care.* St. Louis, CV Mosby, 1987.

Darling RB, Darling J: *Children Who Are Different.* St. Louis, CV Mosby, 1982.

DeMaio M, Shuzman E, Mott SR: *Nursing Care of Children and Families: A Holistic Approach.* Menlo Park, CA, Addison-Wesley, 1985.

Denhoff E: Current status of infant stimulation or enrichment programs for children with developmental disabilities. *Pediatrics* 1981; 67, 32–37.

Dimond DL: Delayed gross and fine motor development. *In* Shelov SP, Mezey AP, Edelmann CM, et al (eds): *Primary Care Pediatrics: A Symptomatic Approach.* Norwalk, CT, Appleton-Century-Crofts, 1984, 292–307.

Downey JA, Low NL: *The Child with Disabling Illness: Principles of Rehabilitation.* 2nd ed. New York, Raven Press, 1982.

Drapo PJ: Mental retardation. *In* Johnson BS (ed): *Psychiatric-Mental Health Nursing.* Philadelphia, JB Lippincott, 1986, 433–456.

Dubowitz L, Dubowitz V: Neurological assessment of the preterm and full term newborn infant. *In* Harel S, Anastasiow N (eds): *The At-risk Infant.* Baltimore, Paul H. Brookes, 1985, 185–196.

Easter Seal Society: *Early Warning Signs: Learning Disabilities—A Hidden Handicap.* New York, Easter Seal Society, 1982.

Ellison P, Prasse D, Siewert J, et al: The outcome of neurological abnormality in infancy. *In* Harel S, Anastasiow N (eds): *The At-risk Infant.* Baltimore, Paul H. Brookes, 1985, 253–260.

Feingold BF: Hyperkinesis and learning disabilities linked to artificial food flavors and colors. *Am J Nurs* 1975 May; 75(5):797–803.

Fish LJ, Burch KJ: Identifying gifted preschoolers. *Pediatr Nurs* 1985; 11(2), 125–127, 148.

Frankenberger W: A survey of state guidelines for identification of mental retardation. *Ment Retard* 1984; 22(1), 17–20.

Gitter MJ: Infant stimulation programs for handicapped: Rationale. *In* Hernandez-Logan C (ed): *Caregiving: A Multidisciplinary Approach.* Palo Alto, CA, R & E Research Associates, 1981, 45–49.

Goldfarb G, Brotherson MJ, Summers JA, et al: *Meeting the Challenge of Disability or Chronic Illness: A Family Guide.* Baltimore, Paul H. Brookes, 1986.

Hayes ML: Giving handicapped students the least restrictive alternative. *Educ Horizons* 1981; 59(3), 119–123.

Haynes U: *A Developmental Approach to Casefinding Among Infants and Young Children.* Rockville, MD, US Department of Health, Education, and Welfare, 1983.

Howard J, Beckwith LC: Child change in an early intervention program for the developmentally disabled. In *Guidelines for Early Intervention Programs.* Salt Lake City, University of Utah, College of Nursing, 1980, 21–32.

Hughs H, Henry D, Hughs A: The effect of frontal EMG biofeedback training on the behavior of children with activity level problems. *Biofeedback and Self-Regulation* 1980; 5, 207–219.

Hymovich DP: Assessment of the chronically ill child and family. *In* Hymovich DP, Barnard MU (eds): *Family Health Care: General Perspectives.* Vol. 2. 2nd ed. New York, McGraw-Hill, 1979, 280–293.

Hymovich DP: Nursing services. *In* Hobbs N, Perrin JM (eds): *Issues in the Care of Children with Chronic Illness.* San Francisco, Jossey-Bass, 1985, 478–497.

Johnson BS: The emotionally disturbed child. *In* Johnson B (ed): *Psychiatric-Mental Health Nursing.* Philadelphia, JB Lippincott, 1986a, 370–396.

Johnson SH: *Nursing Assessment and Strategies for the Family at Risk.* 2nd ed. Philadelphia, JB Lippincott, 1986b.

Jones EH: P.L. 94-142 and the role of school nurses in caring for handicapped children. *J School Health* 1979; 49(3), 147–156.

Kaisling PL, Kalafatich AJ: Caring for the mentally handicapped child undergoing surgery: A parent's point of view. *J Assoc Care Child Hosp* 1978; 6(3), 15–16.

Keele DK: *The Developmentally Disabled Child: A Manual for Primary Physicians.* Oradell, NJ, Medical Economics Books, 1983.

Kepes JJ: Mental retardation: Some pathological considerations. *In* Jakab I (ed): *Mental Retardation.* New York, Karger, 1982, 38–67.

Kleinberg S: Facilitating the child's entry to school and coordinating school activities during hospitalization. In *Proceedings of a Conference on Home Care for Children with Serious Handicapping Conditions.* Houston, TX, Association for the Care of Children's Health, 1984, 67–77.

Kliegman RM, Behrman RE: Metabolic disturbances. *In* Behrman RE, Vaughan VC (eds): *Nelson Textbook of Pediatrics.* 13th ed. Philadelphia, WB Saunders, 1987, 416–421.

Kosowski MM, Sopczyk DL: Feeding hospitalized children with developmental disabilities. *MCN* 1985; 10(3), 190–194.

Krajicek MJ: Developmental disability and human sexuality. *Nurs Clin North Am* 1982; 17(3), 377–378.

Krajicek MJ, Tierney W, Tomlinsin AI: *Detection of Developmental Problems in Children: Birth to Adolescence.* 2nd ed. Baltimore, University Park Press, 1983.

Latham C, Yando R: Psychological assessments of the retarded. *In* Jakab I (ed): *Mental Retardation.* New York, Karger, 1982, 120–141.

Levine MD, Melmed RD: The unhappy wanderers: Children with attention deficits. *Pediatr Clin North Am* 1982; 29(1), 105–120.

Levine MD, et al (eds): *Developmental-Behavioral Pediatrics.* Philadelphia, WB Saunders, 1983.

Leyden S: *Helping the Child of Exceptional Ability.* London, Croom Helm, 1985.

Lubar J, Shouse M: EEG and behavioral changes in a hyperkinetic child concurrent with training of the sensorimotor rhythm (SMR). *Biofeedback and Self-Regulation* 1976; 1, 293–298.

Mansheim P: Parenting children with developmental disabilities. *J Psychosoc Nurs Mental Health Serv* 1982; 20(10), 24–26.

McFarland G, Wasli E: *Nursing Diagnosis and Process in Psychiatric-Mental Health Nursing.* Philadelphia, JB Lippincott, 1986.

Monea HE: The geropsychiatric public health nurse: A model for comprehensive mental health care. *In* Ebersole P, Hess P (eds): *Toward Healthy Aging.* St. Louis, CV Mosby, 1981, 610–621.

Murphy CM: Assessment of fathering behaviors. *In* Johnson SH (ed): *Nursing Assessment and Strategies for the Family at Risk.* 2nd ed. Philadelphia, JB Lippincott, 1986, 41–60.

Olson M: Minimal cerebral dysfunction: The child referred for school-related problems. *Pediatr Ann* 1975 Aug; p 69.

Powell TH, Ogle PA: *Brothers and Sisters: A Special Part of Exceptional Families.* Baltimore, Paul H. Brookes, 1985.

President's Committee on Mental Retardation: *White House Conference on Handicapped Individuals.* Vol. 5. Washington, DC, US Government Printing Office, 1975.

Procci L, Magary JF, Tucker AS: Meeting the challenges of PL 94-142 through a continuing education program for the school nurse. *J School Health* 1981; 51(3), 154–156.

Raskin LA, Shaywitz SE, Shaywitz BA, et al: Neurochemical correlates of attention deficit disorder. *Pediatr Clin North Am* 1982; 31(2), 387–396.

Recommended guidelines for early intervention programs. In *Guidelines for Early Intervention Programs.* Salt Lake City, University of Utah, College of Nursing, 1980, 63–69.

Renzulli JS: What makes giftedness: Re-examining a definition. *Phi Kappa Deltan* 1971; 60, 180–184.

Rose TL: The Education of All Handicapped Children Act (PL 94-142): New responsibilities and opportunities for the school nurse. *J School Health* 1980; 50(1), 30–31.

Schafer SD: *Child Success Through Parent Training: A Final Report.* Denton, TX, Texas Woman's University, 1984. (Available from Sue Schafer, Texas Woman's University School of Physical Therapy, P.O. Box 22487, Denton, TX 76204.)

Schaumann B, Alter M: *Dermatoglyphics in Medical Disorders.* New York, Springer-Verlag, 1976.

Schecter NL: The gifted child. *In* Levine MD, Carey WB, Crocker AC, et al (eds): *Developmental-Behavioral Pediatrics.* Philadelphia, WB Saunders, 1983, 891–901.

Shaywitz SE, Shaywitz BA: Diagnosis and management of attention deficit disorder: A pediatric perspective. *Pediatr Clin North Am* 1982; 31(2), 429–457.

Siantz ML: *The Nurse and the Developmentally Disabled Adolescent.* Cambridge, MA, Academic Guild, 1977.

Siemon M: Siblings of the chronically ill or disabled child: Meeting their needs. *Nurs Clin North Am* 1984; 19(2), 295–308.

Simmeonson RJ, Cooper DH, Schreirier AP: A review and analysis of the effectiveness of early intervention programs. *Pediatrics* 1982; 69, 635–641.

Smith D: *Recognizable Patterns of Human Malformations.* 3rd ed. Philadelphia, WB Saunders, 1982.

Steele MW: Genetics of mental retardation. *In* Jakab I (ed): *Mental Retardation.* New York, Karger, 1982; 27–37.

Steiner P: The well child and the hospitalized disabled sibling. *J Psychosoc Nurs* 1984; 22(3), 23–26.

Strauss SS, Munton M: Common concerns of parents with disabled children. *Pediatr Nurs* 1985; 11, 371–375.

Taft LT, Matthews WS: Cerebral palsy. *In* Levine MD, Carey WB, Crocker AC, et al: *Developmental-Behavioral Pediatrics.* Philadelphia, WB Saunders, 1983; 789–800.

Tarran EC: Parents' views of medical and social-work services for families with young cerebral-palsied children. *Dev Med Child Neurol* 1981; 23, 173–182.

Trembath J: *The Milani-Comparetti Motor Development Screening Test.* Omaha, University of Nebraska Medical Center, Meyer Children's Rehabilitation Center, 1977.

Tudor M: Nursing intervention with developmentally disabled children. *MCN* 1978; 3, 25–31.

Vlasak J: Mainstreaming handicapped children: The underlying legal concept. *J School Nurs* 1980; 50(1), 30–32.

West M: The mother, developmentally disabled child and the nurse. *Topics Clin Nurs* 1984; 6(3), 19–29.

Whalen CK, Henker B: Hyperactivity and the attention deficit disorders: Expanding frontiers. *Pediatr Clin North Am* 1982; 31, 397–423.

World Health Organization: *Working Group on the Early Defects in Young Children, EURO 03332.* Copenhagen, World Health Organization Regional Office for Europe, 1966.

Zamerowski ST: Helping families cope with a handicapped child. *Topics Clin Nurs* 1982; 4, 41–56.

Bibliography

Castiglia PT, Petrini MA: Selecting a developmental screening tool. *Pediatr Nurs* 1985; 11, 8–17.

Finn K: The hospitalization of children with developmental disorders. *Child Health Care* 1982; 10(4), 131–134.

Fish LJ, Burch KJ: Identifying gifted preschoolers. *Pediatr Nurs* 1985; 11(2), 125–127, 148.

Keele DK: *The Developmentally Disabled Child: A Manual for the Primary Physician.* Oradell, NJ, Medical Economics Books, 1983.

Steele S: Young children with cerebral palsy: Practical guidelines for care. *Pediatr Nurs* 1985; 11, 259–267.

Wasch SW: Hospitalization of profoundly and severely mentally retarded children. *Child Health Care* 1981; 9(4), 126–131.

White JE: Special nursing needs of hospitalized children with learning disabilities. *MCN* 1983; 8, 209–212.

Nursing Strategies: Child Abuse and Maltreatment

Chapter 35

B. Helen Thomas

Child abuse and maltreatment are complex problems with serious immediate and long-term ramifications for children and adolescents, their families, and society. These problems transcend the health, social, and legal structures in society. Nurses may be involved in prevention, identification, and short-term and long-term treatment of abused and maltreated children and their families, whatever the setting of their employment.

The purpose of this chapter is to provide nurses with a basic understanding of these problems. This chapter presents a definition of child abuse and maltreatment, the extent of the problem, and several theoretical frameworks from which to view the problem. Potential nursing roles in the prevention, identification, and treatment of child abuse and maltreatment and the knowledge and skills required to implement the nursing roles effectively are discussed.

Nursing Process Plan
NPP: The Child with Failure-to-Thrive, page 1099

Related Topics
Maternal-infant attachment, Chapter 4
Promoting healthy parenting, Chapter 12
Assessing and Promoting Family Health, Chapter 12
Fostering Self-Esteem, Chapter 16
Understanding Altered Behavior, Chapter 33

Definition of Child Abuse and Maltreatment

One of the difficulties encountered by practitioners and researchers in the area of child abuse and maltreatment is that of definition. This difficulty exists because of deep-rooted personal values and beliefs and because of the numbers of professional disciplines and perspectives represented in the ranks of people involved in the problem.

On a philosophic level, very few would disagree with Gil's (1975) definition of child abuse and maltreatment:

> "Any act of commission or omission by which individuals, institutions, or society as a whole deprive children of equal rights and liberties and/or interfere with their optimal development constitutes, by definition, abuse or neglectful acts or conditions . . . Child abuse, neglect, and deprivation are recognized most commonly when the parent or caretaker commits an act of omission or commission which inhibits the child's development. This may be a single incident, an occasional event, or a regular pattern" (Gil, 1975).

Ultimately, the actual definition of child abuse, neglect or maltreatment is determined by the judicial system. All states in the United States and all provinces of Canada have laws defining child abuse and specifying the actions that can be taken to protect the child and punish the perpetrator. When a child's safety and health are clearly threatened, child protection agencies are empowered to separate the child from his or her family.

However, strong traditions in North American culture work against a simple definition and recognition of when child abuse is occurring. As discussed in Chapter 1 (page 16), children in the past have been considered the property of their parents. There has been a tradition that "parents know best" and that discipline is a parent's right.

Box 35-1
A Legal Definition of Child Abuse and Maltreatment

A child suffers "abuse" in any of the following circumstances:

(a) The child has suffered physical harm, either inflicted by the person having charge of the child or caused by that person's failure to adequately: (i) care and provide for that child, or (ii) supervise the child, or (iii) protect the child;

(b) The child has been sexually molested or sexually exploited by the person having charge of the child, or by another person where the person having charge of the child: (i) knows or should know of the possibility of sexual molestation or sexual exploitation, and (ii) fails to protect the child;

(c) The child requires medical treatment to cure, prevent, or alleviate physical harm or suffering and the child's parent or the person having charge of the child: (i) does not provide the treatment, or (ii) refuses to provide the treatment, or (iii) is unavailable to consent to treatment, or (iv) is unable to consent to treatment;

(d) The child has suffered emotional harm, demonstrated by: (i) severe anxiety, or (ii) severe depression, or (iii) severe withdrawal, or (iv) severe self-destructive or aggressive behavior, and the child's parent or the person having charge of the child: (1) does not provide services or treatment to remedy or alleviate the harm, (2) refuses to provide such services or treatment, (3) is unavailable to consent to such services or treatment, or (4) is unable to consent to such services or treatment;

(e) The child suffers from a mental, emotional, or developmental condition that, if not remedied, could seriously impair the child's development, and the child's parent or the person having charge of the child either (i) does not provide treatment to remedy or alleviate the condition, (ii) refuses to do so, (iii) is unavailable to consent to treatment, or (iv) is unable to consent to treatment.

MANDATORY REPORTERS OF CHILD ABUSE AND MALTREATMENT

A professional or official who, in the course of his/her duties with respect to a child, has reasonable grounds to suspect that a child: (a) is abused, or (b) may be abused, or (c) may have suffered abuse, shall report forthwith his/her suspicion and the information upon which it is based to a Children's Aid Society for investigation. The professional duty to report affects the following persons: (a) a health care professional, including a physician, nurse, dentist, pharmacist, and psychologist; (b) a teacher, or school principal; (c) a social worker or family counselor; (d) a priest, rabbi, or other member of the clergy; (e) an operator or employee of a day nursery; (f) youth and recreation workers (not a volunteer); (g) a peace officer and a coroner; (h) a solicitor; (i) a service provider and an employee of a service provider, and (j) any other person who performs professional or official duties with respect to a child.

(From Child and Family Services Act of Ontario, Canada [Government of Ontario, 1984].)

The first child abuse case ever prosecuted in the U.S. occurred in 1874, when Henry Beigh, the founder of the American Society for the Prevention of Cruelty to Animals, managed to bring a case to court by arguing that a young abused girl (Mary Ellen Wilson) deserved as much protection as animals. Up to that time no child protection statutes were in force. Over the past century, other protective laws and agencies have been created. There has been ongoing reluctance on the part of police, lawyers, physicians, and the public to interfere with the privacy of the family and rights of parents. In the United States, the Federal Child Abuse Prevention and Treatment Act of 1974 established guidelines for all states defining what constitutes abuse, neglect, and maltreatment. This act made reporting mandatory for some groups of professionals, e.g., teachers, health care workers, police, recreation leaders.

Box 35-1 spells out in detail a representative legal definition of child abuse and maltreatment and lists professionals who are required to report suspected abuse.

Reporting Child Abuse and Maltreatment

Many state laws identify two types of reporters of child abuse. *Mandatory reporters* are those required by the law to report suspected cases of child abuse: nurses should consider themselves members of this group. *Permissive reporters* are those who may, but are not required to, report suspected child abuse (Rhodes, 1987). Mandatory reporters *must* report suspected abuse; failure to do so can result in a fine or other punishment, according to individual statutes.

Two important issues related to the reporting of child abuse and maltreatment are also addressed in most statutes. First, persons reporting suspected abuse are protected from civil action unless they acted maliciously or without reasonable grounds. Second, professionals must comply with the reporting laws even if the information is deemed to be privileged or confidential. The only privileged information not subject to the reporting law is that between the solicitor and his or her client.

The main point to remember is that each professional is *independently* responsible for her or his own actions. Hospitals and agencies usually have written protocols that outline procedures to be followed when child abuse or maltreatment is suspected. These protocols should be followed. After the protocol/procedure has been carried out, if the professional who suspects possible abuse is not satisfied with the outcome, she or he can make an individual report. A person can be legally liable for not reporting suspicions, even if other people in the agency or hospital do not think abuse has occurred.

Understanding Child Abuse and Maltreatment

Although the law dictates professional practice concerning the reporting of child abuse and maltreatment, broader definitions are useful for understanding the phenomenon and working with these children and their families. One way to conceptualize abuse (of any type) is on a continuum of child and family health. This continuum is pictured in Figure 35-1. Although the health of families and children is dynamic and ever-changing, some families could be placed close to the "health" point (1 to 2) of the continuum. High-risk groups fall between point 3 (the midpoint) and point 4. Abusive families fall between point 4 and point 5. When viewed this way, it is evident that the law is concerned only with the unhealthy end of the continuum, at which continuation of the abuse could lead to severe child behavior disorder, serious physical injury or illness, or even death of a child. In contrast, health care professionals can contribute to preventing fami-

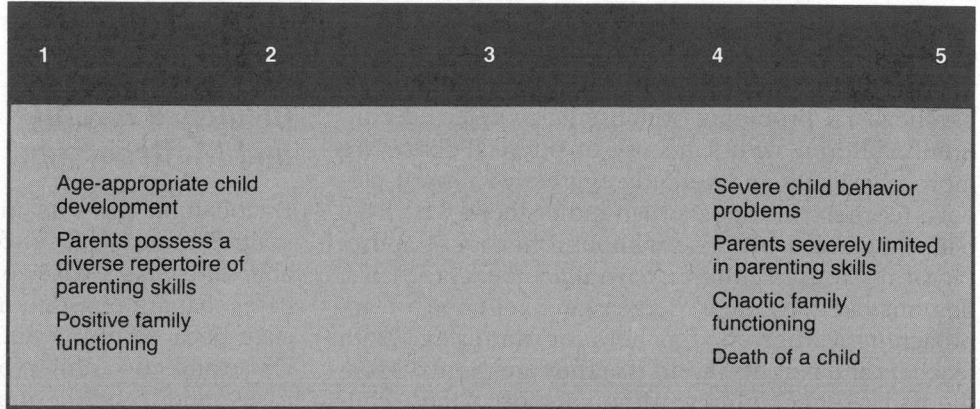

Figure 35-1. Continuum of family health related to child abuse and maltreatment.

lies from reaching high-risk status. Chapters 13 and 16 on parenting and fostering self esteem and Chapter 12 on family assessment present nursing strategies for promoting healthy families.

Another approach frequently used by professionals to understand child abuse and maltreatment is to identify subcategories of the problem. This is particularly useful in clinical practice, because there is evidence that etiology, prevention, and treatment differ, depending on the type of abuse. Abuse is commonly subcategorized as *physical abuse, physical neglect, psychologic maltreatment,* and *sexual abuse.* The perpetrators of these types of abuse, although somewhat similar, have different specific characteristics. The children who have suffered different forms of abuse demonstrate different behavior following the abuse. The long-term sequelae of various types of abuse appear to be different. Finally, the strategies for effective treatment differ, based on the type of abuse. The subcategories of abuse and maltreatment are discussed later in this chapter.

Although using categories and labels clarifies many issues for professionals, it must be remembered that for abused children there is much overlap among the categories. It is hard to imagine that a child who has been physically abused, physically neglected, or sexually abused has not also suffered psychologic maltreatment. The classic example of overlapping types of abuse is seen in children who suffer from *inorganic failure-to-thrive,* which is a combination of physical neglect and psychologic maltreatment discussed in detail later in this chapter.

Long-Term Sequelae

Regardless of how one defines child abuse and maltreatment, it is a serious problem not only because it places children at immediate risk but also because of the long-term sequelae that result if not effectively treated. The long-term problems resulting from physical abuse include functional deficits from the actual injuries as well as psychologic problems that are expressed through a variety of problem behaviors. Although the scientific evidence in this field has several consistent methodologic flaws, in a recent review of the literature Lamphear (1985) identified a number of psychosocial problems of abused or neglected children. Children with a history of physical abuse are more physically and verbally aggressive toward parents, teachers, and peers than either those who have been neglected or those without a history of abuse. Physically abused children have attachment problems, demonstrated by their decreased likelihood of approaching caregivers for help or nurturing. Both teachers and parents report that they are more disobedient than other children. Although most of these children are of normal intelligence, they do poorly at school. Their repertoire of problem-solving skills is limited. Their decreased social skills make them unpopular with peers and adults.

In a longitudinal study of children suffering various kinds of abuse, Egeland and Erickson (1987) report that physically abused children are angry, hyperactive, and noncompliant and demonstrate poor self-control and low self-esteem. Retrospective studies of convicts indicate that a high percentage have childhood histories of physical or sexual abuse or both.

Children who have been *physically neglected* or *psychologically maltreated* or both also function poorly. They are frequently emotionally withdrawn; often their physical, social, and intellectual development is delayed (Lamphear, 1985). Egeland and Erickson (1987) describe children for whom parents have been *psychologically unavailable* as very unhappy, with the least positive and most negative affect of all abused children. Their decline in intellectual functioning, attachment disturbances, and lack of social/emotional competence are enormous barriers to their subsequent development.

Sexual abuse rarely causes physical injury. McNeill and Brassard (1984) found that school-age incest victims achieve below expectations, have difficulties with peer relations, and present acting-out, hyperactive, depressive, and aggressive behaviors at home and at school. Adolescent incest victims also suffer learning difficulties. Sexual promiscuity, running away, drug abuse, and somatic complaints are common behaviors shown by adolescent incest victims (Knittle and Luana, 1980). A number of studies have revealed trends of depressive anxiety, guilt, confusion over sexual identity, and fears of sexuality among these adolescents. Adult women who experienced incest as children or adolescents report feeling isolated from others, feeling different or less worthy than their peers, and distrusting others, particularly men. They also describe problems related to their sexuality: fear of sex, promiscuity, and difficulty blending emotional intimacy with sexual contact (Brunngraber, 1986). Little is known about the long-term sequelae of sexual abuse for males.

Incidence of Child Abuse and Maltreatment

Establishing the true incidence of child abuse and maltreatment is difficult for a number of reasons. Available statistics are based on reported cases. The types of cases that are reported may be different from state to state because of the differences in the laws defining abuse and governing reporting. Because the reported cases tend to be the most severe ones, the reported

Table 35-1. Documented Child Abuse in the United States, 1983 (by Type)

Type of Abuse	Percentage of Total
Major physical injury	3.2
Other physical injury	23.7
Sexual maltreatment	8.5
Deprivation of necessities	58.4
Emotional maltreatment	10.1
Other	8.3

(From Leahey and Wright, 1987.)

incidence of child abuse and maltreatment underestimates the actual incidence. Many cases are not reported because professionals fail to recognize them, or, when abuse is identified they hesitate to report it because of ignorance of the law, fear of possible court involvement, or a critical attitude toward child protective agency intervention.

Sociologic studies suggest that at least one in three children suffer some type of abuse during their childhood. Although figures differ, depending on the source, there is consensus that the problem is common. The rate of reported child abuse and maltreatment in the United States and its territories is 23.8 of every 1000 children. Over 1.5 million American children were reported to have suffered abuse in 1983 (American Association for Protecting Children, 1985).

The proportion of these cases accounted for by the various types of abuse is displayed in Table 35-1. Deprivation of necessities appears most frequently. This is in part a reflection of poverty in our society (see Chapter 1, page 12). The high proportion of abuse from physical injury can be explained by its prevalence and also by the fact that it is the easiest type of abuse to identify.

Child abuse and maltreatment are serious common problems in our society, and nurses who care for children and their families must be able to identify them and intervene appropriately.

Theoretical Perspectives on Child Abuse and Maltreatment

An understanding of the theoretical perspectives from which child abuse and maltreatment can be viewed is essential to effective intervention. Because abuse is a complex, multifaceted problem, theoretical frameworks provide a systematic approach. Nurses need to be familiar with these frameworks to clarify their role in the plan of care, either as individuals or as part of a multidisciplinary team in the identification, treatment, and prevention of child abuse and maltreatment. Child abuse may be just one facet in a pattern of family violence (Campbell and Humphreys, 1984). Brief descriptions of six theoretical models of abusing families are given below.

Mental Illness Model. This explanation for child abuse states that parents who abuse their children are mentally ill (Spinetta and Rigler, 1972). The goal is to cure the parent, who will then stop the abuse. This model has several limitations. First, research has shown that parental psychosis accounts for very few cases of abuse: as few as 5 per cent (Justice and Justice, 1976). Second, it implies that the illness of the parent is the sole cause of the abuse and does not consider the role of the family, child, community, or society as a whole. Third, because of its narrow focus, treatment strategies from this perspective are necessarily very limited and involve only the identified perpetrator of the abuse. This model was developed very early in the identification and treatment of abuse. Subsequent models with a broader perspective are more useful.

Environmental-Stress Model. In this model, two factors interact to precipitate abuse: a violent environment and stress. The violent environment can be found either in society or the family. Sociologists and others agree that violence is tolerated to a greater degree in North American society compared with others, as evidenced by its frequent occurrence in entertainment media. Abusive parents ideologically belong to that segment of society that approves of physical violence against children in certain circumstances (Straus et al, 1980). This belief, coupled with the presence of increased acute or chronic stress, precipitates parental abuse of children to relieve the stress. According to this theory, the violence has to be a result of child behavior: abuse for no reason is unacceptable. Use of corporal punishment within schools is an example of abuse based on the environmental-stress model. Although regulations govern this practice, the underlying theory is that when a child's behavior raises the teacher's stress level beyond acceptable limits (i.e., the student breaks the rule), corporal punishment is an acceptable way to relieve the stress. Many families also subscribe to this approach.

The limitations of this model are that it fails to consider the role of family functioning or individual/family stress tolerance. For instance, using this model, it would be reasonable to expect that most poor families would be abusive because they suffer more stress than many other identifiable groups in society. Although evidence exists that the rate of abuse is higher among those of low socioeconomic status (Pelton, 1978), *abuse is not confined to this group, and many poor people do not abuse their children.* This model is used to explain intergenerational abuse: those abused as children were exposed to an environment that tolerated and even sanctioned child abuse as a method of problem solving (i.e., reducing stress).

A recent review of studies of parents abused as children concludes that *only about one third* of those who had been physically or sexually abused or psychologically maltreated perpetuated the behavior with their own children (Kaufman and Zigler, 1987). Since the rate of abuse and family stress appears to be increasing, this model does not appear sufficient to explain the behavior.

Social Learning Model. This model to explain how humans learn behavior was developed by Bandura (1973). It states that many human behaviors are learned through observation as well as through behavioral reinforcement, as proposed by Skinner. Aggression, a human behavior, can be learned in this way. Therefore, it is not necessary to experience aggression or violence but merely to observe it, to become an aggressive or violent person. Since most forms of child abuse are acts of aggression or violence, abuse can be learned through watching models. Three models that are widely available in American society are the family, the subculture, and symbolic models, especially television. This model of abuse is useful because it includes cultural and family influences.

Social-Psychologic Model. This model was proposed by Kempe and Helfer (1972), two pioneers in the field of child abuse and maltreatment research. For abuse to occur, three variables must be present: *a special parent, a special child,* and *stress.* The parent can be "special" in a number of ways, including being immature, having unrealistic expectations of the child, having poor impulse control, and failing to recognize and respect the child as a unique individual. The child can also be special or perceived by the parents to be so in several ways: "wrong" sex, physically or mentally disabled, "different" from the other children in the family, or temperamentally difficult. The stress may be acute or chronic. Helfer and Kempe state clearly that the event is perceived by the parent, not the professional, as stressful. This is important because of the frequent difference of perception of stress between the two groups and the professional's limited understanding of the parents' lifestyle and resources. This explanation of abuse is widely quoted and explains many abuse situations. Its major limitation is that it does not consider influences on abuse and maltreatment beyond the family.

Human Ecologic Model. This model to explain child abuse was developed by Garbarino (1977). It postulates that abuse is a result of interactions of the culture, the family, the parent, the child, and stress. A number of historical values in American culture lead to a predisposition to violence and to child abuse. The theoretical roots of violence in general, exploitation of children for child labor, and the belief that within families the adults are in the power position are historical cultural values. Although presently there is a sentimental belief in the great value of children to society, a comparison of the financial resources committed by government to their care and protection versus the commitment to defense or road maintenance (recognized traditional responsibilities of government), shows that children are not a public responsibility.

The inclusion of the family in this model is unique to it and useful, because then the family, not the parent or the parent–abused child dyad, is identified as the dysfunctional system, with abuse a symptom. This suggests that parents, the abused child, and other children in the family interact in such a way that abuse occurs in periods of stress. Belsky (1980) explains that since the spousal relationship is the basis for the family, dysfunction within this relationship influences parent-child dynamics. This is particularly relevant in the case of intrafamilial sexual abuse of children.

The multifactorial aspect of this model makes it useful. Much previous research supports it. Its only limitation appears to be its delineation of two types of abuse: that committed by psychotic parents and that resulting from parental role dysfunction. It seems an odd separation in view of the fact that psychosis results in role dysfunction in many areas, including parenting. In spite of this limitation, this model appears promising in providing a comprehensive approach to assessment and treatment of abusive families.

Parke (1982) has developed a social interaction model similar to the human ecologic model. A nurse researcher (Millor, 1981) has described a nursing framework for research in child abuse and neglect. This is a complicated model with components similar to those outlined in the human ecologic model. Testing of this model has not yet been reported in the literature.

Psychologic-Sociologic Model for Sexual Abuse. Although all the preceding models can be used to explain child sexual abuse as well as other forms of abuse and maltreatment, Finkelhor (1984) has presented a model specifically related to sexual abuse. It has four components, developed from an individual and a sociocultural level. First, the perpetrator must be *motivated* to sexually abuse a child. This desire is fueled by the fact that sexual contact with a child will meet an important emotional need, that the contact will be sexually gratifying, and that other sources of sexual gratification are unavailable or less satisfying. The second component necessary for sexual abuse to occur is the overcoming of internal inhibitors. For most people, child sexual abuse bears a strong cultural taboo. Use of alcohol, or a history of being sexually abused, may reduce internal inhibitors (because of the exposure and familiarity with the practice). Third, external inhibitors must be overcome. Such inhibitors include the mother's ability to protect her children, creating situations when the perpetrator and the victim are never alone. In other words, external inhibitors are any variables external to the perpetrator and victim that make the occurrence of the abuse impossible. Finally, the resistance of the child must be overcome. Although they are never to blame, children can play a role in whether they are sexually abused. Children who have a history of emotional insecurity or deprivation who lack knowledge about sexual abuse, who are in a situation of unusual trust with the perpetrator (e.g., child and father), or who find themselves in a coercive situation are most likely to be sexually abused. If the perpetrator uses force, the child's vulnerability may be irrelevant. This model incorporates societal, family, perpetrator, and child variables and is supported by much research to date.

Nursing Care of Abused and Maltreated Children and Their Families

The identification and treatment of any form of child abuse or maltreatment requires the knowledge and skills of many health, social service, and legal professionals. Nurses who work with these families must be able to identify their own role and to facilitate the smooth functioning of the team of professionals.

Attitudinal Issues for Nurses

Before nurses can learn and appropriately apply the knowledge and skills necessary to work in this field, each must clarify personal values and attitudes related to this emotionally charged issue. As well as being nurses, we are all products of our own families of origin and the broader cultural milieu within which we were raised. As a result, we have developed attitudes toward many human behaviors, including parenting and child abuse and maltreatment. For most of us the very idea of abuse raises strong negative emotions. The reality of being faced with an abused or maltreated child causes many of us to feel anger and hostility at the abusing parents or caregiver. Another common reaction is outrage at the limitations of the health and social systems that have failed to alleviate the problem. Some feel anger or disdain toward the child for being a victim: in fact, some are tempted to blame the victim. For others, an abused child revives painful childhood memories and a whole range of strong emotions toward one's own abusive or neglectful families. Those who can empathize with abusive parents may view abused and maltreated children and their families with fear: fear of their own vulnerability to the same violent behavior.

Abused children evoke a whole range of feelings among professionals who encounter them. These feelings are neither good nor bad, they just are. The first step in clarifying one's own attitude is to recognize these feelings. As human beings, we are all entitled to personal values, beliefs, and attitudes. As professionals who wish to establish a therapeutic working relationship with such families, nurses must go beyond admitting these feelings and be able to deal with them so that they are not inflicted upon the clients with whom they work. Often a greater understanding of the problem is helpful. Use of personal and professional support systems can often expand the scope of ways to view abusing families. It is necessary to view the behavior, not the perpetrator, as unacceptable.

It is important to approach families with the belief that most people care about their children. The way families demonstrate their concern for their children varies from one family to another and according to life experiences of the parents. Some questions and comments that nurses who work with abusive and maltreating families may find helpful to clarify their attitudes are listed in Box 35-2.

Box 35-2
Exploring Personal Attitudes: Some Questions

These parents are so angry I'm afraid to get involved with them. What do I know about dealing with anger?

Anyone who could treat a child like this does not have the right to have children. How can I possibly help? How can anyone help?

Why should I help Mrs. X learn how to solve her problems—all she is interested in is herself.

This is a unit for acutely ill patients, why are abused children admitted here?

Mr. Y's relationship with Susie seems very overindulgent, but she is very uncomfortable. Will they stop coming to the clinic if I ask more questions?

None of my colleagues think this case is reportable, but Mrs. M told me she is out of control and afraid she will seriously hurt Johnny. What will I do?

Mrs. A reminds me of the people in my neighborhood. She couldn't be neglecting her youngest child, could she?

How can I help the B family? I don't know anything about parenting.

I'm here to look after sick children. Teaching parents about child development and how to care for their children isn't my job.

Although hostility toward these parents is common, it impedes the therapeutic process in two important ways. First, parents are usually quite sensitive to such negative feelings. They then expend a lot of energy defending their behavior or being noncompliant with treatment rather than becoming involved with constructive plans to improve the situation for themselves and their children. Second, nurses who view families with hostility have their *rescue fantasies** reinforced. Rescue fantasies cause the nurse to respond to the child on the basis of his or her own need to rescue, rather than on what is in the best interest of the child and family (Scharer, 1978). This can have negative consequences for everyone.

Viewing the child as "very unfortunate" promotes the nurse's feelings of having to "rescue" the child from the unworthy parents. In an effort to show unconditional caring for the child, the nurse sets no parameters on the child's behavior. This leads to reinforcement of his or her socially unacceptable, sometimes provocative behavior. Opportunities for the nurse to establish a therapeutic relationship with the family are diminished, because the nurse's verbal and nonverbal behavior indicate both disdain and hostility toward the parents. Therefore, the parents do not benefit from useful learning about parenting skills. In the end, both the parents and the child may exclude the nurse. Consequently, the nurse has not successfully achieved his or her goals and the family may be discharged with no additional support, skills, or information, which can lead to another episode of child maltreatment. Awareness of personal attitudes and how they affect our professional behavior is crucial. Hostile attitudes toward parents need to be resolved before a therapeutic relationship can be established.

General Knowledge and Skills for Nurses

Although the nurse is one of many professionals who may be involved in the identification and treatment of child abuse and maltreatment, and although the precise nursing role varies according to the setting, certain knowledge and skills are required for nurses working with these children and their families, regardless of the practice setting. These are summarized in Table 35-2.

Table 35-2. General Knowledge and Skills Required to Deal with Abused and Maltreated Children and Their Families

Knowledge	Skills
Normal growth and development of children from infancy to adolescence	Assessment of physical, social, and emotional development of the identified patient/client
Normal family development	Family assessment, including structural, developmental, and functional assessment
Reactions of parents	Interviewing skills: nonjudgmental, sensitive, supportive
Nursing documentation	Objective assessment summary Concise problem identification Clear interventions Ongoing evaluation
Community resources	Communication skills: clarify options and summarize plan of action

Child Assessment

To assess a child adequately, one must have a sound knowledge base about normal physical, social, emotional, and cognitive development of children, from neonates to adolescents. The development of children through adolescence is presented in Chapters 5, 6, 7, 8, and 9 of this text. A thorough history, physical examination, and developmental assessment are performed (see Chapter 15).

Child developmental assessment tools are useful in two ways. First, they are either standardized tools or developmental guides that can assist the nurse in quickly identifying whether or not the child's behavior is within "normal" range for his or her age. Second, since several of the widely used tools (i.e., Minnesota Child Development Inventory) are paper-and-pencil questionnaires designed to be completed by parents, parental and nursing perceptions of the child's behavior can be compared. Although all these tools have limitations, appropriate selection depends upon the nurse's knowledge of the tool and skill in administering it, and a clear rationale for the use of it (i.e., different tools serve different purposes). In some institutions, such testing is performed by the psychology or psychometric department.

To provide holistic care, nurses need to understand the meaning of the scores assigned to patients on these tools. Nurses who wish to know more about tools that assess child development may refer to texts about pediatric developmental screening (e.g., Stangler et al, 1980; Lichtenstein and Ireton, 1983).

Family History and Assessment

A crucial aspect of assessment of children who are suspected of being abused or maltreated is a thorough family history and family assessment.

A number of models for family assessment are available and are reviewed in Chapter 12. The Calgary Family Assessment Model (Wright and Leahey, 1984)

* A fantasy that the child needs rescuing from a cruel family; the nurse then reaches out to the child in a way that will negate the child's bond with the family. The nurse then becomes the sole support and thereby rescues the child.

is particularly useful in this field because it assesses family structure, development, and function. It includes not only present family history but also the history of parental families of origin and the cultural milieu of current family living. Many aspects of the family development and the family function assessment sections have been adapted from the McMaster Model of Family Functioning (Epstein et al, 1981). Recently, a brief questionnaire has been demonstrated to assess these dimensions of family functioning reliably (Byles et al, 1988); it could be used for an initial assessment of family functioning.

Parental Reactions

To relate to parents who may have abused their children, the nurse should be aware of the variety of reactions parents display when confronted with the possibility of having abused or maltreated their child. Of course, the reaction depends largely upon the interviewing skills of the nurse. Nurses who recognize and are sensitive to the fact that parents in this situation have a number of emotions can minimize their denial and hostility. At this time, parents can feel any or all of the following emotions: guilty, remorseful, like a failure as a parent, inadequate as a human being, fearful that they will lose their child, and relief at the identification of the problem.

Interviews with these families should take place in a private place. The use of open-ended, clear, supportive questions facilitates parents' sharing appropriate data and allows them to state their perceptions of what happened or what has been going on. Parents are very sensitive to any signs of punitiveness from the nurse/interviewer and invariably react with defensiveness and hostility to such negative messages. Any inconsistencies or vague explanations given by parents should be identified. Parents can then be given the opportunity to clarify them.

Reactions of parents vary according to their understanding of children and their attitudes toward them. The following comments can be useful in eliciting parental knowledge and attitudes about children.

- "All parents I've ever met get angry at their kids. How do you feel when you get angry at Mary? What do you do?"
- "Being a parent is really hard work. Some of the time parents feel like they aren't doing a very good job. What do you do when you feel that way? Do you think it works?"
- "The fact that you have brought Mike here tells me you care about him. What do you think I can do to help you and him?"
- "Two-year-olds who keep saying 'no' and having temper tantrums when they don't get what they want can be very trying. Why do you think Timmy does that? What have you done to stop the annoying behavior?"
- "How were you disciplined as a child? Do you think it was useful?"

Nursing Documentation

For the nurse, the purposes of documentation are the same when dealing with abused children as with any other child. However, since more and more abuse and maltreatment cases are being dealt with in the courts, it is important to remember that if litigation ensues, the chart may be part of the evidence, and the nurse may be called to explain the documentation. The time gap between charting and court appearance can vary and is often lengthy. This makes concise, clear documentation crucial both for aiding recall and to facilitate explanations.

Initial assessment should include any physical injuries or abnormalities (e.g., bruises, scrapes, burns, unidentifiable marks). Drawings to illustrate the locations are helpful. Behavioral/developmental symptoms exhibited by the child should be recorded. These should be objectively stated (e.g., "does not make eye contact") and exclude personal interpretations of the behavior. Observations of parent-child interactions should also be objectively recorded. Actual quotes from parents should be included.

Accurate documentation of the history of the injury/complaint is essential. The initial family assessment should include data as outlined previously in this chapter. Ongoing documentation should fill in any gaps in the family history. Based on the initial assessment, short- and long-term treatment goals that are mutually negotiated with other health professionals and the family should be clearly stated. These provide direction for the development of individual patient care plans.

Ongoing nursing documentation during hospitalization includes assessment in the following areas:

- history and status of physical injuries, if any
- changes in the child's behavior
- parent-child contact—this should explain the frequency of contact, length of time the parent spends with the child, and observations of the parent-child interaction during the visit
- telephone inquiries by parents about their child
- emotional status of the parents

Community Resources

To be able to keep children and their families informed, nurses must be knowledgeable about the community resources to which these families are likely to be referred. In those situations that are by law reportable to Child Protection Services (CPS), parents should be informed about the report. This can be done in a supportive way; it is seen by many professionals as crucial in establishing a trusting, therapeutic relationship with children and families. It is important for parents to understand not only that the behavior must stop, but also that the professionals with whom the family will come in contact are primarily interested in assisting the family to function more effectively, so that abuse and maltreatment will not recur.

Because the long-term treatment of these children and their families is complex and requires the assistance of a variety of health and social service agencies, multidisciplinary community treatment teams have been developed in many areas. Representatives of agencies frequently involved with the treatment of child abuse and maltreatment form the basic core of these teams. Team participation by specific professionals is determined by the needs of each child and family. The team formulates the overall plan of management, identifies specific individual roles in implementing the plan, and, as a group, regularly evaluates and updates the plan. Professionals frequently involved in these teams include:

- Community health nurses, who provide regular one-to-one sessions with families about parenting, child development, and child safety or who may facilitate the development of parenting skills by leading parent group discussions;
- Social workers, who may provide instrumental assistance (e.g., finding better housing) or therapeutic counseling;
- Coordinators and providers of infant stimulation programs;
- Early childhood educators from day care centers;
- Mental health professionals.

For specific resources, an excellent publication is available for purchase from the American Association for Protecting Children of the American Humane Society.* Entitled "The National Directory of Children and Youth Services," this publication lists by state the social service agencies, health departments, juvenile court/youth agencies, and licensed private practitioners who serve abusive and neglectful families.

Knowledge and Skills to Deal with Specific Types of Child Abuse and Maltreatment

The specific knowledge and skills required by nurses to care for abused or maltreated children and their families depend upon the type of maltreatment and the setting in which the nurse encounters them. Each major category of child abuse will be discussed here using the human ecologic model as a framework for assessment and treatment. The nursing role in relation to the type of abuse/maltreatment will focus on the inpatient pediatric setting.

Since the treatment of child abuse and maltreatment usually takes place in both inpatient and community settings, the role of the community health nurse will be generally addressed where appropriate.

Nurses frequently deal with parents at high risk for abuse in maternity and neonatal units. The nurse's role in these settings is discussed in a later section on Prevention of Child Abuse and Maltreatment.

The indicators of potential child abuse and maltreatment (see Tables 35-3, 35-5, 35-6, and 35-7 and Box 35-3) have been developed to provide a guide for identification of these problems. The indicators are not all-inclusive, and the presence of one or two of them does not necessarily assure that abuse or maltreatment have taken place. They are meant to be used in combination with a thorough child and family history and assessment and other diagnostic tools. The presence of several of the indicators may mean that, although abuse has not occurred, the family does need some ongoing assistance as well as that dictated by the presenting problem.

Physical Abuse

Physical abuse is any nonaccidental injury to a child caused by the child's caregiver. It is most often perpetrated by parents. *These actions are rarely intentional;* rather, they result from inappropriate parental efforts to change a child's behavior. Parents with poor impulse control may vent their anger by physically lashing out at their children. Inadequate knowledge of child development or lack of parenting skills may lead to harsh, sometimes bizarre physical discipline and resulting injury to the child. Physical abuse occurs in all age groups, from young children through school-age and adolescents.

Clinical Manifestations and Diagnostic Assessment. Since children, particularly preschoolers, sustain all sorts of injuries in their normal activities, deciding which injuries are nonaccidental can sometimes be difficult. Accidental and nonaccidental sites for injury are depicted in Figure 35-2. Parental and child indicators of potential abuse are outlined in Table 35-3. The possible types of nonaccidental injuries are limited only by parental desperation or imagination. Those injuries that are not age-appropriate (e.g., fractured femur in an infant) are suspect immediately. Another major warning signal is an injury that is inconsistent with the history of the incident.

As the awareness of physical abuse has increased, so have the false allegations of child abuse and accom-

* 9725 East Hampden Avenue, Denver, CO 80231.

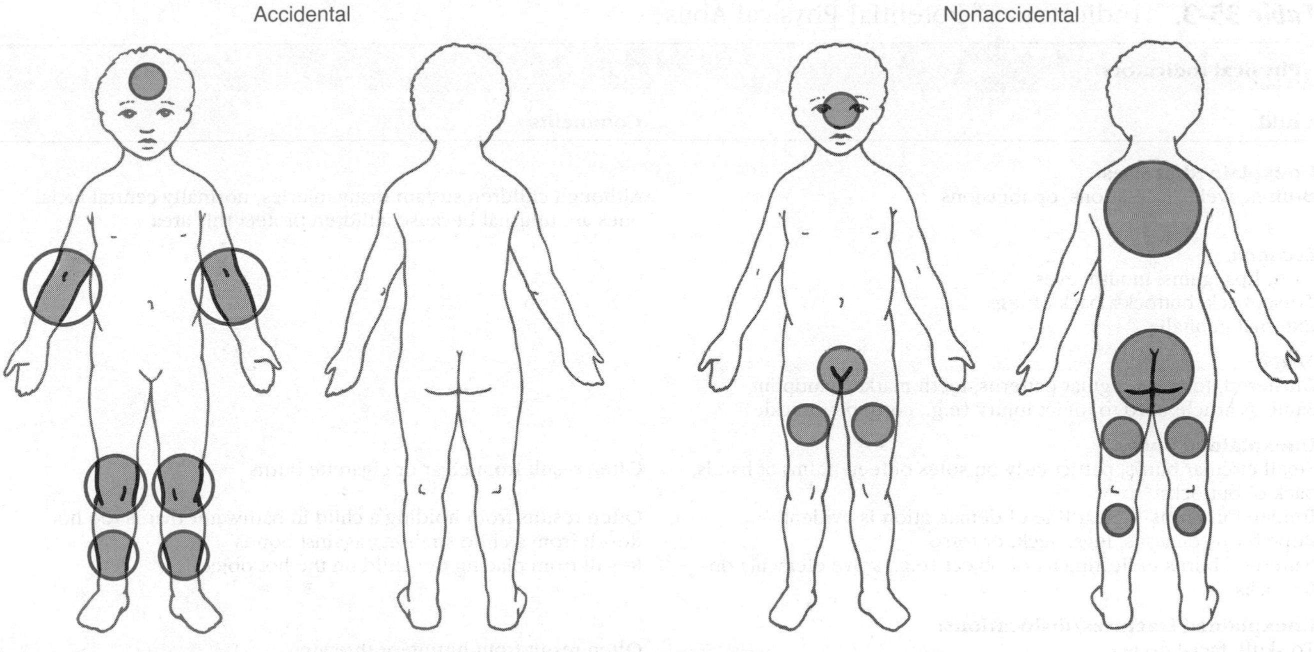

Figure 35-2. Sites of injuries to children; accidental and nonaccidental.

panying tragedies for families (Wong, 1987). Approximately 60 per cent of all child abuse allegations in 1984 were unsubstantiated by Child Protection Service agencies. The cause of this increase is unknown, but it may be related to professionals' erring on the side of caution and reporting all suspicious situations to avoid possible subsequent legal proceedings. This high rate of false allegations has led to an overburdening of CPS agencies, sometimes resulting in less-than-adequate investigations (Besharov, 1985).

Unnecessary false allegations can be minimized by an awareness of signs that may be mistakenly labeled physical abuse. Hurwoltz and Castells (1987) report two cases of osteogenesis imperfecta that were misdiagnosed as physical abuse because of an absence of a family history. Certain folk medical practices common among ethnic groups have also been mistaken as physical abuse (Levin and Levin, 1982). Although such practices may lead to physical injury and are not tolerated in our society, the treatment is very different than that for reportable physical abuse. Clinical signs of an underlying illness also may be misdiagnosed as child abuse. For example, bruises in various stages of healing are often a sign of physical abuse, but they also may occur as a result of undiagnosed bleeding disorders (O'Hare and Eden, 1984). The importance of thorough assessment is underlined by these examples of misdiagnosis.

When physical abuse is suspected, based on parent and child indicators, assessment of the level of family functioning and stress may be accomplished quickly and systematically by using the Family Stress Check List (Orkow, 1985). This check list includes a number of variables that have been empirically demonstrated to be strongly related to the presence of abuse.

The variables include:

- parental history of being abused or deprived
- parental history of being abusive/use of harsh punishment
- level of chronic and acute family stress
- low self-esteem, social isolation, or depression of parents
- poor parental impulse control
- rigid, unrealistic expectations of child behavior
- child difficult/provocative or perceived to be by parents

The presence of several of these variables strengthens the likelihood of a nonaccidental cause of injury.

Often children for whom the diagnosis of physical abuse is suspected are admitted to hospital even when treatment of the actual injury does not require inpatient care, for two reasons. First, parents are frequently overwhelmed emotionally after such an incident; hospital admission places the child in a protected environment, ensuring that immediate further abuse will not occur. It allows a cooling-off period for parents during which they are relieved of child care responsibilities. Second, having the child in hospital allows for a thorough physical, social, and emotional assessment of the child and family, for accurate diagnosis, and for initiation of treatment of the family.

Recently, an unusual form of physical abuse, termed Munchausen syndrome by proxy, has been identified (Weber, 1987). In all reported cases to date, the perpetrator is a mother who is knowledgeable

Table 35-3. Indicators of Potential Physical Abuse

Physical Indicators

Child	Comments
Unexplained bruises:	
Bruises, welts, lacerations, or abrasions	Although children sustain many injuries, normally central facial ones are unusual because children protect this area
Location:	
Face, lips, gums, mouth, eyes	
Torso, back, buttocks, back of legs	
External genitalia	
Shape:	
Clustered, forming regular patterns, teeth marks, handprint	
Same as article used to inflict injury (e.g., cord, belt buckle)	
Unexplained burns:	
Small circular burns, particularly on soles of feet, palms of hands, back of buttocks	Often result from cigar or cigarette burns
Immersion burns—clear line of demarcation is evident	Often results from holding a child in bathwater that is too hot
Rope burns on arms, legs, neck, or torso	Result from a child straining against bonds
Patterned burns indicating a hot object (e.g., stove element) on buttocks	Result from placing the child on the hot object
Unexplained fractures/dislocations:	
To skull, facial bones	Often result from hitting or throwing
Spiral fractures	Often result from pulling or twisting an arm or leg
Dislocations, particularly of shoulders or hips	
Multiple fractures in various stages of healing	On roentgenograph for the presenting complaint, other fractures in various stages of healing may be identified
Note: In children, particularly 2 years of age and under, fractures and dislocations usually result from blows, throws, or other inflicted force.	
Other forms:	
Ingestions	Result from carelessness at best, to neglect/ignorance or forced ingestion at worst
Bald patches on the scalp	Result from pulling hair out or leaving an infant in one position for extended period of time
Subdural hematomas in children under age 2	Result from severe shaking
Retinal hemorrhages	Result from severe shaking

Behavioral Indicators

Parent	Child
Explanation does not fit the injury, is inconsistent, or absent	Very wary of adults
May blame the child because he/she is bad, overactive, or defiant, and so on	Speaks in monosyllables
Parent does not support the child physically or verbally (e.g., no eye contact, touching)	Vacant stare or frozen watchfulness
Lengthy time interval between occurrence of the injury and seeking medical attention	Withstands examination and painful procedures with little movement or crying or both
Parent's reaction to the injury is inappropriate (e.g., very upset over a relatively minor injury or unconcerned over a serious one)	Does not turn to parent for support
Unaware of normal developmental stages of children	States the parent did it, although the child is to blame because he or she was bad
View the child as capable of meeting their needs	Constantly trying to please the parents and assessing parental reaction to statements
Describe their own childhood as unhappy or abusive	Role-reversal: child trying to take care of the parent
Routinely use harsh unreasonable discipline	Behavior extremes: aggressiveness or withdrawal
Express feelings of isolation, both as an individual and a parent; have no identifiable support systems	Afraid to go home
Demonstrate poor impulse control when questioned about how they handle anger	Does not participate in gym, with no apparent reason
	Inappropriately dressed (e.g., long pants and long-sleeved shirts in summer) to hide bruises
	Indiscriminately seeks affection
	Inappropriate or precocious maturity

(*From Thomas H:* Child Abuse, Neglect and Deprivation; A Handbook for Ontario Nurses, *1983.*)

about illness (e.g., a nurse). The child may be seen with actual physical symptoms of an illness. However, these symptoms have been artificially induced by the mother. An example is the addition of the mother's menstrual blood to the child's urine to simulate hematuria. In some cases, the child has a history of an illness that is fictitious (e.g., seizures) and does not respond to appropriate treatment. The reported cases are dramatic — the children have been subjected to extensive diagnostic testing, multiple operations, and lengthy periods of hospitalization. The mothers of these children rarely leave them alone during hospitalization. A warning sign of this aberration is that the symptoms disappear when the mother is absent. Another sign that Munchausen syndrome by proxy may be the underlying diagnosis is that the signs and symptoms do not make clinical sense. Clinicians may be confused by this and feel that they have never seen anything like it. If nurses and other members of the health care team are aware of the possibility of this type of physical abuse, it may be detected earlier and so minimize the trauma for children and families.

Nursing Care of Physically Abused Children and Their Families. Although hospitalization may be of short duration, the nurse has an important role. In cases of serious physical injury, appropriate nursing care of the actual injury is necessary. Other nursing strategies specific to the assessment and planning phase are summarized in Table 35-4. Generally, the nursing role is to act as a parent and child advocate. Children may be frightened and confused. The nurse should explain the reason for admission and plans for care in an age-appropriate way. Involvement of child protection services means that children and parents may be separated for an indefinite period of time. Depending on the situation, the court may rule that the child be discharged to the family with supervision or to a foster home, or may permanently terminate parental rights. The disposition, of course, is based on the perceived risk of recurrence of physical abuse.

Although children may have been severely abused, being separated from their parents is a severe loss. Many children also feel guilty because they perceive that their "bad" behavior, which led to the abuse, has resulted in the family disruption. For children who can understand, the action needs to be explained, and then they need to be given an opportunity to express their feelings. A consistent nurse is likely to be most effective in this situation because these children often have difficulty trusting others and need time to establish a relationship in which they feel safe enough to expose their true feelings.

The nursing role of parent advocate can be difficult because parents may be hostile, frightened, and confused. The nurse who can reassure the parents that bringing the child for treatment, although frightening, was a responsible act that indicates their concern for the child will often diminish parental hostility and fear.

Table 35-4. Assessment and Planning for the Physically Abused Child and Family

Nursing Role	Strategies
Child and family assessment	Use age-appropriate methods to assess development. Preverbal and young children respond to play therapy with dolls that represent family members.
	Provide age-appropriate support for the child during radiologic and other diagnostic tests
	Document physical injuries
	Document observations of child behavior that indicate psychologic and emotional status
	With other health care team members, complete the family assessment (see Chapter 12 for family assessment)
Planning and initiating care	Assess level of knowledge and skill of parent regarding child care and development
	Identify one nurse as the child's primary caregiver
	Develop a clearly defined plan of care to be followed by all nurses
	Involve older children in developing the plan for their own care
	Plan patient care to include parental participation.
Interdisciplinary participation in care	Provide positive reinforcement for family/parental strengths
	Model healthy communication and parenting behaviors
	Inform parents that child protection services are being notified, without judging or accusing parents
	Explain that the objective of involvement is to strengthen family functioning and prevent future harm to children
	Support parents during initial interviews with child protection workers
	Assist parents in identifying strategies necessary to prevent future abuse (e.g., identify other professionals as supports)

This allows parents to ask pertinent questions, to which the nurse can provide straightforward, clear answers. Through this process, parental confusion and resulting defensiveness are often reduced. Although hospitalization of physically abused children is generally of short duration, successful nursing intervention will assist in preparing parents and children to engage constructively in long-term treatment. In some cases, hospitalization is extended because there is no satisfactory placement available for the child. A legal order may be in effect keeping the child from being returned home with the parent, but no foster home or care agency may be available. Chronic shortages of quality foster care exist in some cities.

Long-term treatment of the family is to prevent recurrences of abuse. Interventions with the parents are directed toward increasing their impulse control, providing alternatives for physical abuse when they are angry, increasing their knowledge of child development, and developing age-appropriate expectations of children. Many abusive parents have such low self-esteem and so few social skills that they require one-to-one treatment until they are willing to risk entering a parent group. A number of parent group programs have reported success in changing parental attitudes and behavior. Community health nurses may provide one-to-one treatment for families and they may also lead parent groups. Self-help groups such as Parents Anonymous* provide effective support and direction for many abusive parents.

Some researchers believe that abuse results from a lack of parental empathy for the child. To empathize, parents have to recognize the emotion being demonstrated by the child and then react appropriately. Empirical evidence suggests that, compared with non-abusive mothers, abusive mothers are *unable to correctly identify child emotions,* which may explain why they respond with abuse (Kropp and Haynes, 1987). Although no programs to address this problem have been reported, the idea is an interesting one. As members of interdisciplinary child abuse teams, nurses can facilitate development and evaluation of such programs.

Recently, programs for physically abused children have been developed to help them improve their social skills, decrease their aggression, and improve their ability to relate positively to others. These programs are often implemented within day care settings for preschool children. Interest groups for older children facilitate learning of these behaviors.

Family or marital counseling or both are required by some families to improve family functioning and help families learn more constructive ways to deal with stress. Family stress sometimes can be reduced by instrumental assistance, such as budget counseling or providing parents a break from preschool children through part-time enrollment of children in nursery school/day care settings. Families and professionals may identify numerous other strategies to reduce stress in the home.

By being aware of the family dynamics and changes within the family, the community health nurse can be a valuable advocate for abused children and their families.

Physical Neglect

Physical neglect encompasses the failure of caregivers to provide the basic necessities of life: food, shelter, medical attention, clothing, safety, sleep, adequate supervision, and, in the case of the school-age child, education. It tends to be chronic in nature. It is important to distinguish between neglect and poverty. Although children suffering from physical neglect require intervention regardless of the cause, the interventions are different for physical neglect and for poverty resulting in inadequate physical care. Sometimes all children in the family are affected by neglect, but often one child is significantly more neglected than the others.

Clinical Manifestations and Diagnostic Assessment. The child's physical and behavioral indicators of physical neglect, as well as parental behavioral indicators, are contained in Table 35-5. A key diagnostic feature of physical neglect is the parental inability to influence the environment. As a result, family life is chaotic, child needs are not recognized or met, and a sense of helplessness pervades the family. In more severe situations, a particular child in the family has been neglected because she or he is or is perceived by the parents to be "different," "inferior," or "bad." These children are usually admitted to hospital because, in their neglected state, they have developed an acute illness (e.g., gastroenteritis in infants). Because of their limited resources, parents are unable to care for them at home. Accidents resulting from inadequate supervision also may result in hospitalization. For these children, physical neglect rarely occurs without being accompanied by psychologic maltreatment.

Nursing Care of Physically Neglected Children and Their Families. In hospital, children must be treated for their acute conditions. This treatment is no different than that for any other infant or child with a similar problem. However, relatively straightforward nursing goals, such as maintaining adequate nutritional intake, become difficult because these infants and children have no established eating patterns. As well, they often have not learned to eat age-appropri-

* 7120 Franklin Avenue, Los Angeles, CA 90046; telephone: 1(800)421-0353.

Table 35-5. Indicators of Potential Physical Neglect

Physical Indicators

Child	Comments
Underweight, poor growth pattern, constant hunger, wasting of subcutaneous tissue	All result from malnutrition, if other diagnoses have been ruled out. Most common cause of malnutrition is lack of food Confirmed as neglect when the child quickly gains weight when fed properly
Poor physical hygiene—severe diaper rash, skin rashes, dirty hair, dirty hands and face, persistent body odor	May result from ignorance, poverty, or neglect
Unattended physical problems or medical needs, e.g. glasses, dental work, untreated injuries	Sometimes recognized when parents have been informed of the need and have done nothing about it
Consistent lack of supervision or abandonment	
Fatigue, listlessness, lethargy	Results from inadequate rest, sometimes a result of caring for siblings, other household tasks, or lack of suitable sleeping accommodation

Behavioral Indicators

Parent	Child
Externalize blame for the situation	Infants may be dull and inactive
Describe a chaotic home life	Delay in gross motor and speech development
Lack of understanding of needs of children, e.g., food, supervision	Children may be pale, listless, thin, unkempt
Live in unsafe, dirty and/or crowded conditions	Children may beg for or steal food
May be mentally retarded or have a low I.Q.	Frequent absence from school, or arriving at school very early and leaving very late
Have little motivation or skill to effect changes in their lives	Inappropriate clothing for the weather, clothing may be dirty
Often passive, socially isolated individuals who have not experienced success	Constant squinting at the board
	Complaining of aching teeth
Unable to forego immediate gratification for long-term organization	States there is no one to look after him or her
	Assuming adult responsibilities
Describe inappropriate parenting in their childhood	Engaging in delinquent acts and/or abuse of alcohol or street drugs
Employment instability	
Lack of emotional bonds to child/children	

(From Thomas H: Child Abuse, Neglect and Deprivation; A Handbook for Ontario Nurses, *1983.)*

ate or nutritious food; feeding them requires a great deal of time, patience, and creativity.

Although these families may be followed by community health nurses and other professionals for years, during the child's hospitalization the nurse can make a valuable contribution to the ongoing care. This is an opportunity to observe parenting skills and provide much-needed modeling and reinforcement of appropriate skills. Basic adequate hygiene for infants can be reinforced by observing parents as they bathe and care for their children. As with physically abused children, a consistently assigned nurse is important to monitor changes in parental attitude and behavior toward the child and also to minimize confusion for the parents. By discharge, a thorough assessment of family strengths and ongoing needs related to child care, for use by community professionals, can be documented by this consistent nurse.

Assessment of the level of parental ability or motivation to use information and people resources to effect a positive change is essential. If Child Protection Services are involved, such assessment and evaluation often determines whether or not a court order for foster care or permanent termination of parental rights is sought. One of the factors that influences parental motivation is the teaching/learning strategies used by the nurse. Doak and associates (1985) have identified a number of issues that are useful to keep in mind when working with parents with low literacy skills. These include

- a patient's perspective tends to be limited to direct personal experience
- a patient may be insensitive to the need to give information to health care providers unless specifically asked
- a patient does not think in terms of classes of information or of categories
- a patient gives information in bits and pieces without identifiable pattern

These attributes are common among neglecting parents.

To intervene effectively, the nurse uses simple, concrete, clear questions to collect data and give simple, concrete step-by-step directions for care. To assess whether a child is obtaining enough sleep, the nurse does not ask, "How much sleep does Johnny get?" but rather leads the parent through Johnny's activities on a particular day and then deduces the amount of sleep he gets. In suggesting alterations in the daily pattern, the nurse must have information about the usual family activities, current sleeping arrangements, and other factors that impinge on Johnny's sleep. To obtain this information, a series of concrete, precise questions must be asked. Developing these communication techniques is essential for both inpatient and community nurses who wish to intervene effectively with physically neglecting families.

Since these families require long-term follow-up, liaison between inpatient and community nurses is essential for continuity of care. In the community, neglecting families often require assistance to build in some predictable daily routines for children. For many, developing adequate problem-solving skills about child care (or anything else) can be a lifelong task that requires continuous reinforcement by others. The use of lay home visitors to visit these families for several hours a day, two or three times weekly, can help overcome ignorance and chaos and develop improved parenting skills.

Since recent evidence links cognitive and emotional deficits of mentally retarded parents with neglect and since empirically tested programs (Fantuzzo et al, 1986) demonstrate that mildly retarded mothers can learn to improve their parenting skills, community nurses can be instrumental in the development of such programs.

Nursing Care of Psychologically Maltreated Children and Their Families

Psychologic Maltreatment

Psychologic maltreatment is defined as "acts of omission and commission which are judged on a combination of community standards and professional expertise to be psychologically damaging. Such acts are committed by individuals, singly or collectively, who by their characteristics are in a position of differential power that renders a child vulnerable" (Hart et al, 1983, page 2). Acts toward a child such as rejecting, degrading, terrorizing, isolating, corrupting, exploiting and denying emotional responsiveness constitute psychologic maltreatment (Brassard et al, 1987).

Although few data are available, experts generally agree that this form of abuse almost always accompanies other forms of abuse, is more prevalent than other forms of abuse, and is often more destructive in its short- and long-term impact on the lives of children (Garbarino et al, 1986). It can occur at any age.

Clinical Manifestations and Diagnostic Assessment. The parental and child behavioral indicators of potential psychologic maltreatment are summarized in Table 35-6.

Table 35-6. Indicators of Potential Psychologic Maltreatment

Parents	Child
Deny the problem or blame the child for it	**Infants**
Appear unconcerned about the child's welfare	Frozen watchfulness
Discrepancy between verbal and nonverbal communication to the child	Slow developing speech
State that they are not involved with the child in activities	Apparent cognitive or emotional developmental lag
State child is inadequate compared with others in the family	Avoids eye contact
Use predominantly negative comments to the child and about the child	Does not physically reach out to caregiver for comfort or attention
Refuse all offers of help	**Older Children and Adolescents**
	Hyperactive/disruptive behaviors
	Behavior extremes, e.g., withdrawn, aggressive and demanding
	Overly adaptive behavior, e.g., too well mannered, too clean and neat, does not cry during painful procedures
	Inhibition of play
	In play, demonstrates emotional unattachment to dolls or children
	Unusually fearful of consequences of actions, which often leads to lying
	Sleep disorders
	States no one cares about self, that he or she is no good and can't succeed
	Presents psychosomatic complaints, e.g., headache, nausea, abdominal pain
	Threatened or attempted suicide

Parental acts of omission (e.g., ignoring the child, no involvement in the child's daily activities, disinterest in the child, lack of physical intimacy with the child) or commission (e.g., yelling, criticizing, degrading, belittling) result in a lonely child with low self-esteem and decreased ability to reach out emotionally and physically to others. Although one child may be the target of psychologic maltreatment, assessment usually reveals a family in which members have difficulty sharing their feelings and emotional support for one another is minimal. These styles of relating may have evolved over a long period of time or may have been precipitated by a family crisis or stressful event.

Nurses encounter children who have been psychologically maltreated as they care for children who have been hospitalized for other reasons. Since this type of child abuse is difficult to identify, careful nursing documentation of parent-child interactions can be helpful in the process. Parents who are unable to identify a single positive attribute of the child, when asked, should alert the nurse to the possibility of psychologic maltreatment. Parents who without reason do not visit children or communicate with them by telephone are displaying signs of being uninvolved in their child's care. Now that open visiting hours for parents are encouraged in most inpatient settings and health care professionals recognize the value of parental participation in the care of hospitalized children, nurses must exercise caution in prematurely reaching conclusions about psychologic maltreatment as the reason for parental lack of involvement in child care. Many parents have obstacles to spending regular periods of time with a hospitalized child: lack of baby sitting services for other children; personal jobs outside the home; financial restrictions to public transportation; length of time to travel from home to hospital, to list a few. These obstacles may be compounded by feelings of discomfort or inadequacy about caring for the child with nursing supervision or by a belief that it is better if parents do not visit because the child gets upset when they leave. Nurses who encourage parents to visit but appreciate the difficulties involved for some families and who are able to be flexible reinforce the parent's self-esteem and decrease guilt for "abandoning" the child.

Psychologically maltreated infants and children present several nursing care challenges. The lack of responsiveness demonstrated by many of these infants can be frustrating for nurses. As with other abused and maltreated children, consistent care by one nurse is the model by which the nurse is most likely to be able to establish a therapeutic relationship.

Nurses need to be prepared to expend a lot of time and energy in relating to these children and, initially, to accept meager rewards. Once a thorough assessment of current development has been completed, nursing interactions with the infant or child focus on helping the family provide an accepting, warm, nurturing atmosphere in which subsequent developmental tasks can be achieved. Use of play therapy to stimulate development and a sense of individual control can be very helpful for infants and children.

As with others who have been abused, these children require clear plans of care, which include strategies to manage unacceptable behavior. Consistent adherence to these plans is crucial so that children who are already confused about expectations and adult reactions can learn to trust this new environment.

To effectively relate to these parents, the nurse must be supportive and empathetic to their needs. Many such parents have never known warm, supportive relationships and can initially be very suspicious. Focusing on their strengths in parent-child interactions gives parents an increased sense of self-esteem and provides positive reinforcement for the behavior.

Some parents have never learned how to enjoy their children. Through modeling games and other activities, the nurse can encourage the parent to begin to participate. Emphasizing the important and unique status of the parent in the child's life helps reassure parents that the nurse is not trying to assume this role. It also can contribute to making parents feel like worthwhile people.

When these children have been discharged from hospital, ongoing support is required to assist in the continuing improvement of family functioning. Psychologically maltreated older children can benefit from participation in adult-led activities (e.g., sports, clubs) where adults other than parents can provide positive reinforcement and the emotional support that leads to increased self-esteem. Community health nurses and others may be involved in strategies to continue to change the behavior of family members and in psychotherapy for the family and/or particular members.

Failure-to-Thrive (FTT)

There is no unanimously agreed upon definition for failure-to-thrive (FTT). The term is used to describe infants and children who fail to gain weight (or even lose weight). It results from the failure to obtain or use the necessary calories required to permit the expected velocity of growth. A parent may be offering insufficient calories because of a knowledge deficit, or the infant may be rejecting the food or not absorbing it. A weight persistently below the third percentile or 2 standard deviations below the mean on a standard growth chart characterizes the FTT child.

Failure-to-thrive is a common disorder of infancy and accounts for 2 to 3 per cent of pediatric tertiary hospital admissions. Its occurrence in the general population is not known. Failure-to-thrive is not actually a diagnosis but the term for a cluster of symptoms occurring concurrently.

Etiology. Failure-to-thrive has traditionally been classified into two categories: organic and nonorganic. A third category, mixed FTT, is now recognized as an entity caused by a combination of organic and nonorganic factors. The three categories used to describe failure-to-thrive are:

- *Organic FTT* is caused by physical factors such as congenital heart defects, gastrointestinal disorders, renal disease, central nervous system abnormalities, chronic infections, endocrine disorders, chromosomal alterations, or metabolic disorders.
- *Nonorganic FTT* is an absence of history, physical, or laboratory findings that indicate organic disease capable of causing FTT. It is rather caused by environmental factors that affect the child's intake or utilization of calories. The problem usually is due

to a complex set of interactive patterns between the infant and caregivers.

- *Mixed FTT* is caused by a combination of organic and nonorganic factors. For example, a child with a cleft lip is unable to suck adequately because of a physical deformity (organic cause). The inability to suck in turn can interfere with the mother's feelings of adequacy. She may then stimulate and caress the infant less. The interplay of positive messages and reciprocal play associated with feeding is, therefore, blocked to a degree.

Although failure-to-thrive may be due to an organic disease, it most often is the result of a disturbance in the relationship between the primary caregiver and the child. The precipitating factors underlying the disturbance are varied (Bithoney and Rathbun, 1983). Parents may lack information about infant development or nutritional requirements. They may expect responses that conflict with the child's needs, development, and abilities. For example, some young parents are disappointed to discover their baby does not "love" them, as they expected, but instead demands a lot of time and attention that they are unprepared to give. The infant may be the product of an unwanted, unplanned, or stressful pregnancy. The child's birth may have been a difficult natural one or by cesarean section. The infant's appearance or temperament may be displeasing to the parents. The baby may have been premature or have some birth-associated illness or congenital defect. The parents, especially the mother, may have been separated from the infant after delivery for a period complicated by anxiety and uncertainty about the infant's prognosis.

Historically, failure-to-thrive has been classified as a form of child neglect caused by maternal deprivation. Recently, it has been suggested that FTT is a separate pediatric illness and that the traditional view of FTT, as exclusively parentally induced, must be abandoned (Bithoney and Newberger, 1987). It is now recognized that the phenomenon of nonorganic failure-to-thrive is a complex interplay of multiple constitutional and environmental factors involving the caregivers, the infant, and their interactions. Thus, FTT could be explained within the human ecologic model of child maltreatment. Explanations that identify factors in the infant, the caregiver, and the family supersede the earlier view that FTT is caused by either medical illness or by psychologic deprivation. According to Lieberman and Birch (1984), FTT is "rooted in a specific transactional impasse between the infant and caregiver." Caregivers and the infant contribute to the impasse.

The term *maternal deprivation* has been interpreted by some professionals as unloving intentional neglect. It is now understood that a mother's inability to provide the nurture required by an infant may occur because the mother has been deprived (Gagan, 1984). Mothers may be depressed or anxious because of over concern for the child. A husband's lack of support exacerbates mother's feeling of being overwhelmed (Gagan, 1984). Furthermore, either parent may come from a background in which supportive communication patterns were undeveloped. The support of one another during the stress of child care demands is lacking within the family. A family with poor communication skills and weak social supports may be further compromised by job instability and poor living conditions. Although FTT in middle class families is well documented, it is more common in lower economic status families. Feelings of helplessness experienced by these families are often grounded in overwhelming socioeconomic conditions (Gagan, 1984).

Certain infant personalities also contribute to the impasse. They appear to fall into two extreme categories. They are described as irritable, fussy, and colicky or as passive and unresponsive. Either of these two temperaments can create negative relationships between the infant and caregiver. The dynamics between a particular dyad, (i.e., "the fit") affects the success of the relationship. The failure in the dyad is not caused by one person, rather it develops because of the characteristics of each person. For example, an irritable infant and a tense parent reinforce each other's behavior, resulting in a negative, tense relationship devoid of a positive interactive style. Similarly, a lethargic child interacting with a depressed parent results in a deficient interaction. On the other hand, an interactive infant can engage a depressed parent and an apathetic infant can be engaged by a more active parent.

Clinical Manifestations and Diagnostic Assessment. The clinical manifestations of an infant or child with failure-to-thrive can range from extreme cachexia and developmental delay to an apparently healthy-appearing infant. If weight and height are proportionately delayed, FTT may not be apparent unless a growth chart is used to evaluate the child's progress. What appears to be a healthy 9-month-old infant may be a 15-month-old child failing to thrive. Physical and behavioral indicators of potential failure-to-thrive are listed in Table 35-7.

Failure-to-thrive is a complex problem. Diagnosis is usually made by a multidisciplinary team involving a nurse, physician, social worker, nutritionist, psychologist, and occupational therapist. In the past, diagnostic assessment focused on a search for an organic cause of FTT. This approach is "diagnosis by exclusion." Another approach is to make a "diagnosis by response," in which the infant is fed and nurtured. If weight gain occurs, the cause is considered to be nonorganic (Powell, 1987). Currently, research is being done to identify specific behaviors that could distinguish nonorganic FTT from organic FTT infants. Specific behav-

Table 35-7. Indicators of Potential Failure-to-Thrive

Physical Indicators

Weight below the 3rd percentile
Sudden or rapid deceleration in the growth rate
Delay in developmental milestones
Muscular hypotonia
Decreased muscle mass
Generalized weakness
Abdominal distention

Behavioral Indicators

Avoiding eye contact
Intense watchfulness
Avoidance of physical contact with other people
Repetitive self-stimulating behaviors (e.g., rocking, head banging, head rolling, and intense sucking)
Disturbed affect (e.g., excessive irritability, apathy, or extreme compliance)
Sleep disturbances
Lack of age-appropriate stranger anxiety
Inappropriate lack of preference for parents

iors identified by Powell (1987) that differentiate organic FTT from nonorganic FTT were (1) lack of motor activity in response to stimuli, (2) lack of smile in response to stimuli, (3) general inactivity, and (4) abnormal gaze.

Nursing Care of Children with Failure-to-Thrive and Their Families. For children with possible failure-to-thrive, all the data previously outlined (General Knowledge and Skills Required for Dealing with Abused and Maltreated Children) should be collected. In addition, the prenatal history, perinatal course, and feeding history should be obtained. Since parents of FTT infants often feel inadequate, the nurse must use sensitivity and empathetic interviewing skills to elicit the assessment data. The nurse should remember that a thorough history may eliminate unnecessary laboratory testing. However, environmental failure-to-thrive should not be assumed without sufficient data. Table 35-8 describes tests commonly performed

Table 35-8. Diagnostic Approaches to Rule out Organic Disease in Failure-to-Thrive Children

Diagnostic	Purpose/Rule Out
Initial Screening	
Physical examination	R/O congenital defects; data base and measurements on admission
Denver Developmental Screening Test (DDST) (See Appendix)	Establish relation to developmental milestones
Tuberculin test	R/O tuberculosis
Bone survey radiographs of long bones, joints, skull	R/O old or recent fractures; establish bone age; check epiphyseal development
Anterior/posterior and lateral chest film	R/O pulmonary disease
Urinalysis	R/O urinary tract infection (UTI); diabetes
CBC and differential	R/O anemia, chronic or systemic infection
Sweat test	R/O cystic fibrosis
Stool testing: Reducing substance and pH Occult blood Ova and parasites	R/O mono- and disaccharide deficiency R/O milk intolerance R/O internal bleeding R/O parasitic infestation
Further Studies (When Indicated, Based on History or Failure to Gain in Hospital)	
Repeat DDST; Bayley or psychometrics	R/O mental retardation; prescribe activities for development
Detailed urinalysis: culture, 24-hour catecholamines	R/O UTI; metabolic defects
Stool testing: 72-hour fecal fat D-xylose test culture	Malabsorption Infection
PBI and T4	Hypothyroidism
Electrocardiogram; cardiac catheterization	R/O cardiac anomalies; circulatory defects
Upper and/or lower GI radiography	R/O dysphagia; anatomic abnormalities; internal injuries
Intravenous pyelogram	R/O urinary tract abnormalities; internal injuries
Biopsy: Bowel, muscle	R/O Hirschsprung disease; congenital muscular dystrophy; celiac disease

Table 35-9. Factors that Interfere with Effective Breastfeeding

Factors	Significance
The Mother	
Inadequate diet, due to dieting or inadequate intake	A marginal diet may affect the ability to nourish an infant and the quantity of milk supply
Fatigue	Most common cause of reduced milk production May inhibit let-down
Lack of confidence, stress Husband or relative disapproves of breastfeeding Stress of other life events, i.e., demands of job, family	Known to inhibit let-down reflex Lack of confidence in adequate milk supply can lead to introduction of formula and early introduction of solids
Pain, due to episiotomy, incision, sore nipples	Inhibits the let-down reflex
Difficult birth	May lead to delay in initial early feeding and limited length and frequency of feeds An exhausted mother may mean an exhausted infant and poor suck
Pain medication given in labor and delivery	May suppress infant, reducing effective sucking and early initiation to breastfeeding
Medications	
Oral contraceptives	Combined estrogen and progestin and high estrogen dose formulations appear to be associated with decreased milk production
Some diuretics	May decrease milk production
Ergot derivative (Bromocriptine)	Inhibits prolactin secretion
Pyridoxine (vitamin B_6)	Some evidence that excessive doses may have inhibiting effect on lactation
Diazepam (Valium)	Excreted into breastmilk and associated with infant weight loss, lethargy, prolonged hyperbilirubinemia
Decongestants and antihistamines	May decrease milk production
Nicotine	May interfere with let-down May inhibit production of milk by reducing prolactin levels
Alcohol	Large doses may partially inhibit the let-down reflex
Caffeine	Large doses may inhibit lactation
Breast surgery, which severs ducts or nerves in the periareolar region or 5 o'clock (left) or 7 o'clock (right breast) position	Reduces the stimulation to the hypothalamus, which reduces milk production and inhibits let-down reflex
Pregnancy	A reduced milk supply has been reported anecdotally
Hormonal deficiencies, such as hypothyroidism, antepartum estrogen deficiencies	Can result in reduced milk production
The Baby	
Poor suck, due to lethargic or medicated infant, Down syndrome, anoxia, hyper- or hypotonic infant	Leads to ineffective nipple stimulation and poor milk extraction
Illness, such as congenital heart disease, jaundice, infection, cystic fibrosis, otitis media, urinary infection, hypothyroidism	Leads to lethargy and fatigue and ineffective and less frequent sucking
Oral-facial deformities Cleft lip and palate Tongue tie (rare) Tumors of mouth	Ineffective sucking reduces nipple stimulation and ability of baby to "milk" the breast for adequate nourishment
Pacifiers	May cause nipple confusion. Delay use if possible until lactation is well established
The Dyad	
Limited length of feeding, particularly short feedings in first days postpartum	Reduces amount of nipple stimulation Reduces emptying of milk from glands required in order to reduce the pressure from milk in the glands and encourage production of more milk. Neonates need 30–40-minute feeds
Reduced frequency of feeding, such as 4-hour feeds, lack of rooming-in facilities	Reduces amount of nipple stimulation and emptying of milk
Improper positioning	Decreased *effective* nipple stimulation; decreased extraction of milk; causes pain, bleeding, cracked nipples

Table 35-9 *(continued)*

Factors	Significance
The Dyad	
Formula or water supplements, including formula samples distributed in hospital	Reduces thirst or hunger in infant, therefore reducing amount and frequency of effective nipple stimulation May cause nipple confusion in infant, leading to ineffective sucking at breast Reduces mother's confidence in her ability to supply milk Gives mixed message from health professionals regarding the importance of breastfeeding
Extended separation from mother, such as baby in NICU, baby not brought to mother at night for feedings, ill mother, etc.	Reduces length and frequency of feedings
Feeding from one breast	May be inadequate nipple stimulation

(Prepared by Ruta Valaitis, BScN, BA, MHSc, Clinical Nursing Consultant and Lecturer, School of Nursing, McMaster University, Hamilton, Ontario.)

in an effort to identify organic causes. Care should be taken not to order laboratory tests that would deprive the child of food for a period of time.

Special assessment is made of the infant's sucking technique. Failure-to-thrive may be caused by an actual deficit in nutrient intake because of ineffective sucking at the breast or bottle. (See Box 5-2, page 199, for a summary of principles related to a proper latch-on and positioning for breastfeeding.) If breast- or bottle-feeding is not successful, the mother, infant, and dyad are assessed to determine the cause (see Tables 35-9 and 35-10).

The infant should be observed interacting with his or her primary caregiver in feeding situations and in play situations, as well as observed interacting with a stranger, such as the nurse (Bithoney and Rathbun, 1983). Rosenn and associates (1980) developed a behavioral scale to quantify brief social interactions between the infant and the examiner. They found that the approach-withdrawal behaviors of infants between 6 and 16 months of age were useful in distinguishing organic and nonorganic failure-to-thrive. This scale needs further testing in the clinical area. Within 24 hours of admission, a Denver Developmental Screening Test should be done to determine the child's level of development. Ongoing documentation of the child's activity level and the infant-parent dyad is required to make a diagnosis.

The nurse's documentation of ongoing assessment is essential and should be done regularly and thoroughly. Important aspects to document about the infant-parent interaction include:

- The ways in which the child is held and fed and how eye contact is initiated by the primary caregiver(s); the facial expressions of the child and caregiver during interactions.
- What the caregiver does with the child—play, talk, hold, stroke—and the child's response.
- Whether the caregiver talks about the baby at all, and if so, how the baby is referred to. This is an indicator to others of how the caregiver perceives the child.
- The responses of the caregiver to the baby's cues. For example, what is the mother's response when the baby looks at her, cries, reaches toward her?
- The response of the infant to the caregiver's overtures, the baby's reaction to the mother's feeding rate and the way the infant is being held. What the nurse should be looking for is synchrony or disharmony, and, specifically, how this occurs.

The basic care is the same as for any child of similar age, but it may take more time, especially for feeding, with extra attention to holding the child, cuddling, eliciting eye contact, and helping parents feed their infant.

Special attention must also be given to monitoring the child's physical status. The nurse records the number, character, color, and consistency of the stools; the stools may be tested for occult blood and for reducing substances. (If the infant is malabsorbing, sugar will be present in the stool.) The pH of the stool is checked. (Less than 5.5 means that acid is present, which results when sugar breaks down into acids.) The child is weighed at the same time each day, under similar conditions. An accurate record of intake and output, including weighing the diapers, is kept. The nurse is responsible for monitoring the intake and keeping a calorie count of the food actually ingested. Calorie intake is increased above the usual recommended amounts. A referral is made to the nutritionist to plan the diet so that the child will have an optimal intake for "catch-up growth" without overfeeding.

Developmental activities appropriate for age are provided, with special attention given to motor and social deficits. The nurse may be responsible for such developmental programs or involve other team mem-

Table 35-10. Factors That Interfere with Effective Bottlefeeding

Factors	Significance
The Mother	
Anxiety related to care of infant or to other life stresses	Baby picks up anxious feelings from tensions in mother's approach, arms, and movements and becomes uncomfortable.
Fatigue	May not provide sufficient attention or time to allow for baby to receive adequate intake.
The Baby	
Poor suck related to lethargy, medication, Down syndrome, anoxia, hyper- or hypotonic infant illness	Infant gets tired and stops sucking before an adequate amount of milk has been received.
Oral-facial deformities Cleft lip and palate, tongue tie (rare)	Inefficient sucking may occur, making it impossible for baby to get sufficient calories. Lack of molding of infant's body to mother's body. A baby who does not cuddle readily makes it difficult to position the bottle to provide adequate intake.
Technique	
Characteristics of the nipple Opening too large or small, nipple too hard or soft	Hard nipples with small openings require a stronger infant suck to get the milk. The baby may become tired or frustrated and give up. Soft nipples with large openings may make the baby gag or choke because the milk is received too quickly.
Fluid level in the bottle	As the fluid level decreases, the angle of the bottle must be decreased to prevent air from being sucked into the stomach, which causes discomfort for the baby.
Temperature of formula or milk	Infants drink best if the fluid is at the same temperature at each feeding. Fluid that is too hot may burn the mouth or esophagus. Room temperature or slightly above is best (if heating, test on inside of wrist before beginning to feed).
The Dyad	
Lack of reciprocal messages of pleasure and comfort	Sounds, touch, and eye contact make the feeding experience pleasurable for both mother and infant. If these do not accompany the feeding, less pleasure is associated with eating and infants may stop because of boredom.
Tensions between the infant and caregiver	A cycle of tension is created, and if the feeding is not completed, the mother does not encourage the infant to do so.

bers, such as a child life worker and occupational therapist.

The caregiver may need "re-parenting" in those areas in which there is dysfunction. The nurse "mothers the mother" by providing emotional nurturing. This is often done most effectively through role modeling, demonstration, and positive reinforcement of the caregiver's mothering efforts by the infant's primary nurse. This re-parenting can sometimes be done even better by a foster grandmother, who may be less threatening than the nurse and nearer to the age of the mother's own mother. The parent who is not functioning well may be referred to a psychiatric social worker or psychiatrist for more intensive intervention. Social service benefits may also be required and should be explored by a social worker according to the family's needs.

In spite of all the nurse's anticipatory guidance and tact, parents may feel threatened, particularly if the child improves during hospitalization when no treatment other than feeding, nurturing, and stimulation has been provided. They need to have their insecurity alleviated and their self-esteem built up as they succeed in caring for the child. The nurse can point out their healthy behaviors specifically and the responses by the child. The parents can learn playfulness, joy, and laughter responses to their child.

The nurse can listen to the mother and help her work through her negative feelings that have disrupted healthy interactions with the child. The nurse can help allay her feeling of guilt regarding the diagnosis and reinforce healthful changes for the present and future. The mother's partner or spouse and relatives also may need guidance in relating to the child in ways that support the mother's self-esteem as an individual and as a parent. The Nursing Process Plan for the care of an infant with failure-to-thrive (Table 35-11) provides specific nursing strategies.

Table 35-11
Nursing Process Plan: The Child with Failure-to-Thrive*

By Roxie Foster

Assessment of Physical Function

Sleep-Rest
Nutrition-Metabolism
Elimination
Activity-Exercise

Assessment of Emotional-Social Function

Parenting Patterns
Coping-Stress-Tolerance Patterns
Spiritual Health

Assessment of Intellectual-Perceptual Function

Health Perception/Management

Subjective Assessment

Perinatal history; child's health history; feeding history; typical day's activities for child/caregiver; recounting of typical mealtime; reported developmental status; major family stressors/strengths; family eating patterns/health beliefs related to food; parent(s)' perceptions of child's temperament; family living conditions; family interactions

Objective Assessment

Height, weight, head circumference; patterns on growth charts; developmental status upon examination; GI, GU, cardiovascular, respiratory, and neurologic status (characteristics of stool, urine; vital signs; heart sounds; tissue perfusion; breath sounds; neuromuscular integrity); parent/child interactions during feeding/play; child's response to stranger

Analysis: Nursing Diagnosis 1

Altered growth and development: failure to thrive, related to

- *insufficient intake of calories and/or*
- *incomplete absorption of nutrients and/or*
- *other organic condition that interferes with growth and/or*
- *problematic child/caregiver interactions associated with poor "fit" between child/caregiver temperaments*
  caregiver knowledge deficit associated with development/child care needs
  family stress in excess of family strengths and available support

Defining Characteristics (some combination of these signs and symptoms)

Subjective: History of difficult or stressful pregnancy, birth, and/or inadequate incorporation of infant into family; child perceived as unattractive, irritable, not cuddly, difficult to console; report of financial difficulties which preclude purchase of food, clothing, adequate housing; marital discord, or other significant family stress; limited family resources for support; report that child does not like to eat; beliefs related to food or infant feeding that are in conflict with usual recommendations for

Objective:
Child: Height and weight below 3rd percentile or sudden, rapid deceleration in growth rate; developmental delay in several gross motor and social tasks; physical alterations—GI (e.g., chronic diarrhea, vomiting, stool positive for sugar with pH <5.5); GU (e.g., anorexia related to chronic urinary tract infection), cardiovascular (e.g., altered tissue perfusion related to congenital heart disease), respiratory (e.g., repeated pneumonia), neuromuscular (e.g.,

* Because the cause of failure-to-thrive (FTT) is often unclear initially, this plan will deal with undifferentiated FTT—i.e., not diagnosed as either organic or nonorganic.

Continued

Subjective (Continued): nutritional requirements; history of health problems; reported typical intake less than body requirements

Objective (Continued): hypotonia affecting suck and coordination of swallow); altered feeding techniques—poor suck, plays with food or nipple rather than eating, easily distracted from eating, arches back and cries in response to feeding attempts; altered social behavior—consistently looks away or physically pulls away from social advances that normally engage a child of that age, flat affect, irritable; responds to nurses' attempts to teach proper feeding techniques by steadily increasing intake and gaining weight; responds to nurses' attempts to evoke social responses such as smile, raising arms to be picked up, molding to caregiver's body when held

Child/caregiver: Altered interaction pattern—little or no eye contact; caregiver rarely talks to or smiles at child; caregiver displays flat affect and mechanical movements when caring for child; when visiting child, caregiver watches TV, reads, or talks to other visitors rather than interacting with child

Client Goals/Evaluation Criteria

1.1 The child will gain weight, as evidenced by slow, steady increase in grams each day

Nursing Goals/Strategies (Selected Rationale)

Help to identify exact cause of failure to thrive.

- Assess for physical alterations. Conduct baseline physical examination upon admission; continue to assess for additional manifestations and changes in baseline assessment.

Note especially changes in physical status related to feeding (e.g., fatigue, respiratory distress, colic-type behavior).

Note character of body secretions (vomitus, stool, urine). Conduct tests as appropriate (e.g., Hematest, Clinitest, pH).

- Assess parent/child interactions.

Note eye contact, facial expressions, whether interactions seem comfortable and pleasurable for child and parent or appear awkward and mechanical, interactions between parents, between parents and other family members or extended family.

Document behaviors, not interpretation of behaviors, e.g., "Mother read a book while feeding child," not "Mother does not seem interested in child."

Determine primary caregiver (may be extended family member, not a parent).

Encourage caregiver to talk about life with the child, major stresses, personal strengths, social support. Give permission to voice negative as well as positive feelings by such comments as, "This must be very difficult for you." "Sometimes parents feel they are being blamed for their child's failure to grow. Do you feel this way?" "Tell me what you enjoy most about your child." "Being a parent can be very stressful; what things have been most

	difficult since your child was born?" "Does parenthood feel like you thought it would?" • Assess child's feeding patterns. Note suck, food preferences, attention to eating, avoidance behaviors. *Increase caloric intake.* • Initially assess tolerance to age-appropriate food (i.e., ability to retain/absorb nutrients). • If organic cause determined, institute appropriate alterations in feeding as indicated and as ordered. Prepare discharge plan; support family in adjusting to the diagnosis and teach them appropriate care for the child at home. • If cause undetermined or nonorganic, increase intake as tolerated (diagnosis by response). Feed on demand or at least every 3 to 4 hours for infant. For toddler or older child, offer nutritious high-protein snacks between meals and small portions of a variety of foods at mealtime. • Steadily increase amount ingested per feeding (this may take several days; the child's stomach capacity may be small at first). Discourage the infant taking a few sucks or the child taking a few bites and then quitting. Gradually increase intake with each feeding. • Teach child healthy mealtime behaviors. With fingers on cheeks and under chin, gently but firmly help infant with poor suck obtain better suction on the nipple. Decrease distraction during mealtime; close door to room, turn off television, discourage interruptions by other health care professionals by posting sign outside door. Make mealtime an unhurried, pleasant experience. Provide consistent nursing care whenever possible. (Lack of consistency will confuse and frustrate the child who is trying to learn new behaviors). • Ensure that caloric intake is greater than caloric expenditure. Plan for and facilitate naps. Intervene for crying, fretfulness. Avoid tiring infant or small child with successive interventions or therapies. • Monitor intake and weight gain. Record intake and output. Record calories ingested if appropriate. Weigh at same time each day on same scale with the same clothing (e.g., nude, diaper, or underwear).
1.2 The child will demonstrate new social and motor behaviors not represented in baseline assessment of development	*Provide opportunities to practice developmental tasks.* • Provide social stimulation. Talk to child during caregiving activities, attempt to elicit smile and other age-appropriate responses. Approach children with respect for their mistrust of or lack of enthusiasm for adult interactions (allow them to view you from outside their personal space). Gradually normalize interactions as child's response permits. Document responses to social interactions. • Provide opportunities to practice motor tasks. (Interesting surroundings and the opportunity for gross motor activities are usually sufficient to elicit progress in the child who has been previously deprived). Head control and upper arm strength can be improved by placing the infant on the abdomen. If this is an unfamiliar position, the child may protest; in this case introduce the position ***Continued***

Client Goals/ Evaluation Criteria	Nursing Goals/Strategies (Selected Behavior)
	gradually with the distraction of toys or with the child closely attended. Strength of lower limbs can be enhanced by a walker and by placing a mobile at a level in the crib to encourage kicking. Provide play experiences for the toddler and preschooler to enhance developmental skills. The child life worker may be of assistance.
1.3 Interactions between the child and parent (or other caregiver) will become more caring, nurturing, and mutually pleasurable, as evidenced by a. increasing eye contact b. interactive verbalizations, vocalizations c. smiling and facial expressions of pleasure d. child molding to body of parent e. parent calling the child by given name or pet names f. parent initiating playful contact with child g. parent verbalizing pride in child	*Role model appropriate adult/child interactions.* (Role modeling is often more effective and less belittling than lecturing.) • Talk to infant or child, initiate playful interactions. Let parent see that nurse finds child attractive and enjoys the interactions. (Parent may also need to see that the nurse finds it appropriate to talk to an infant or young child and that the child can respond.) • Role model feeding behaviors and activities to promote motor development. *Provide instruction to address identified knowledge deficit.* • Include instructions with role modeling, e.g., "Babies learn to talk by listening to the people in their family. Johnnie's cooing is the first step in learning to say a word." • Explain the developmental crisis of that age child in lay terms, giving examples of the difficulties persons might have if they did not develop a greater sense of trust than mistrust, or a greater sense of autonomy than shame and doubt. Provide information about development in small segments, talking only about that pertinent for this child. (Initially, this information may seem too theoretical to apply.) Use as many different forms of materials as are available, e.g., videotapes, written brochures (to accommodate various learning styles). • It is helpful to adopt the attitude that this parent has not had the *opportunity* to learn healthy parenting behaviors, rather than to assume the parent's behavior is willful. (Nurses' attitudes will be displayed in nonverbal, if not in verbal, ways. Belittling the parent will close communications and thwart all future teaching attempts.) *Shape parental behavior by concentrating on the positive.* • Praise (appropriately and sincerely) any positive bonding or caring behaviors. (Praising the positive can illustrate for the parent the desired behavior while increasing parental self-esteem. A parent with increased self-esteem has additional strength to deal with life stress, including the tasks of parenting.) • Praise the parent in the presence of the spouse, significant other(s), and extended family members. (The primary caretaker may use the nurse's validating comment to support self-esteem or the new parenting behavior in the presence of criticism from others.) *Encourage as much parental involvement in care as is practical.* (This will enhance the caregiver's self-confidence and provide a means for evaluation.) Some units have policies that state that the primary caregiver must stay with and care for the child for a specified length of time before discharge. *Enlist the help of the physician and the social services department in ensuring follow-up home visits for this family.*

Sexual Abuse

Sexual abuse and sexual misuse are similarly defined. Brant and Tisza's (1977) definition of sexual misuse also defines sexual abuse: "exposure of the child to sexual stimulation inappropriate for the child's age, level of psychosexual development, and role in the family."

Activities that constitute sexual abuse include permitting or exposing a child to sexual acts, such as prostitution or pornography, as well as molestation, which includes exposure, fondling, masturbation, vaginal or rectal penetration, or sexual intercourse (Sgroi, 1984). About 5 to 6 per cent of all children will be victims of child sexual abuse (Finkelhor and Hotaling, 1984). Although both extrafamilial and intrafamilial sexual abuse occur, incest appears to be the most damaging to children and usually indicates severe family problems. Intrafamilial sexual abuse can involve any dyad within the family, but the most common type involves the father-daughter or the stepfather-daughter relationships. Recent evidence indicates that male victims are more common than previously acknowledged (Finkelhor, 1984; Vander Mey, 1988).

Child pornography and child prostitution represent big business in the United States and also inflict sexual abuse on increasing numbers of children. The plight of these children and the large number of runaways involved have been presented recently in the academic and popular press (Radar, 1982; Burgess, 1984).

Child sexual abuse has been identified in infants as young as 6 months. Incest usually begins with caressing and fondling and proceeds over time to sexual intercourse. It may continue on a regular or intermittent basis for years, until the child refuses to comply, leaves home, or discloses the behavior. The perpetrator of child sexual abuse is most frequently male, and in the cases of extrafamilial abuse is usually an individual the child knows. He may be a family member, friend, acquaintance, baby sitter, or, on rare occasion, a stranger.

Children who have been sexually abused are rarely admitted to hospital for the problem. They are more frequently seen in emergency rooms, outpatient clinics, schools, and private offices of physicians or nurse practitioners. Along with other health professionals, nurses in these settings may be involved in the initial interview of the child, in reporting the situation to the Child Protection Services, and in the immediate aftercare of the child (Elvik, 1986). As well, some nurses lead groups for children who have been victims of sexual abuse. Community nurses may be involved in long-term follow-up of families.

Although nurses may care for clients who have been sexually abused by any of the aforementioned perpetrators, they will most frequently encounter children who are victims of repeated intrafamilial sexual abuse. Many of the manifestations of child sexual abuse and the nursing strategies for intervention outlined in this section can be applied to all types of sexual abuse, but they are particularly relevant to incest.

Clinical Manifestations and Diagnostic Assessment. Box 35-3 summarizes the indicators of sexual abuse. It includes child physical indicators of intrafamilial or extrafamilial sexual abuse as well as behavioral indicators commonly seen in the father/stepfather, the mother, and the child when intrafamilial sexual abuse has occurred. The child behavior indicators are somewhat age dependent. For example, running away from home, drug and alcohol abuse, and promiscuity or prostitution are most commonly seen in adolescent females. Among female teens, sexual abuse is the most common reason for running away. Often the abuse has been accompanied by physical abuse as well (Felice and Friedman, 1982). Regressive behavior and age-inappropriate knowledge (advanced) about sexual activity indicate the possibility of sexual abuse in preadolescent school-age girls. Precocious sexual interest and drawings with sexual themes can reflect sexual abuse of preschool children.

It is important to recognize that seductive behavior of children/adolescents does not cause intrafamilial sexual abuse. Normal preschool females experiment with "seducing" their father or father figure. Most fathers do not use this behavior as a rationalization for beginning sexual abuse, but rather place it within the context of the father-daughter relationship. In experimenting with female roles to use outside the home, many adolescents display provocative sexual behavior at home. Again, most fathers react to this by helping the teen to evaluate it realistically. Those adults who see provocative sexual behavior of children as an opportunity to engage in incest are misinterpreting the behavior and responding inappropriately.

Since intrafamilial sexual abuse has usually gone on over a period of time, and since less than 20 per cent of the victims suffer physical trauma, identification of the problem is usually through disclosure. Disclosure can be accidental or purposeful. Accidental disclosure occurs in several ways: a third person observes the activity and reports it; during assessment of a child for an identified physical or behavioral symptom, the clinician becomes suspicious and asks the child; precocious child sexual activity arouses the suspicion of another adult who asks the child about it. Purposeful disclosure occurs when a child or adolescent reports the experience voluntarily to a teacher, health professional, or other trusted adult with whom there is contact (Sgroi, 1984). Regardless of how the disclosure occurs, it is imperative that the victim be supported in the statement. False allegations do occur, but until an initial investigative assessment has taken place, children should be believed. In the past, many profes-

Box 35-3
Indicators of Sexual Abuse

PHYSICAL INDICATORS

Child

Difficulty in walking or sitting

Pain, swelling, or itching in the genital area

Bruises, bleeding, or lacerations of the external genitalia, vaginal, or anal areas

Pregnancy, especially in early teen years

Poor sphincter tone

Dilatation of the vaginal opening

Torn, stained, or bloody clothing

Pain on urination

Recurrent urinary tract infections

Abdominal pain with no definitive cause

Vaginal/penile discharge

Sexually transmitted disease (STD) especially in preadolescents

Recurrent vaginal infections in a child under 12 years of age

Recurrent sore throat of unknown origin

BEHAVIORAL INDICATORS

Father/Stepfather

Rigid in his perception of his role within the family

Needs to dominate the family

Sees himself as a good parent

When confronted with his behaviors, often rationalizes it as being educational and pleasurable for the child

May admit guilt and be remorseful but unable to change

Describes an unsatisfactory sexual and emotional relationship with wife; may be divorced, or his wife may be dead or disabled

Lacks social and emotional contacts outside the family

Pays special attention to the child victim, usually increasing sibling rivalry

Protective and jealous of the child victim, limiting child's contacts outside the family

Mother

Often aware of the incestuous relationship

Sometimes sees it as a relief for herself, and organizes time for the two to be alone

Usually states that her relationship with her husband is poor, and may have terminated sexual relations with him

Usually a passive person who is emotionally and financially dependent on her husband

May not see herself as an integral part of the family

May want the behavior to stop, but will not risk exposing it

May blame the child for the relationship

Frequently was involved in an incestuous relationship in her family of origin

Frequently was poorly parented as a child, and has never learned how to protect herself and her children

Child/Adolescent

A. Reactions similar to those precipitated by any other severe stress, including:
- Regressive behavior in younger children (e.g., bed-wetting, thumb-sucking)
- Sudden onset of fears or phobias (e.g., of the dark, men, or particular settings, situations)
- Running away from home
- Abuse of drugs and alcohol
- Noticeable personality changes (e.g., depression, anger, hostility, aggression)
- Change in school performance
- Suicidal thoughts or attempts
- Somatic complaints (e.g., headaches, abdominal pain, eating disorders)

B. Reactions directly related to sexual abuse, including:
- Provocative drawings of a sexual nature
- Age-inappropriate sexual play
- Excessive masturbation
- Bizarre, sophisticated, or unusual sexual behavior or knowledge
- Overtly seductive behavior toward peers
- Promiscuity among adolescents
- Prostitution among adolescents
- Withdrawal from peers
- States that he or she is being sexually assaulted
- Females may state relationship with mother is poor; may be very angry because mother does not protect her
- May feel it is his or her fault

(From Thomas H: Child Abuse, Neglect and Deprivation; A Handbook for Ontario Nurses, *1983.)*

sionals regarded reports of sexual abuse as a product of childish fantasy. Recent evidence indicates that most victims, particularly preadolescent children, could not describe such incidents without personal experience.

Investigative assessment of child sexual abuse includes obtaining the history from the child through an interview (or a series of interviews), physical assessment of the child, and interviewing the alleged perpetrator. A number of researchers describe interviewing strategies for use with sexually abused children of various ages. The most salient aspects are presented here. Nurses wishing to expand their knowledge and skill in this area are encouraged to consult the original works (Sgroi, 1984; Kelley, 1985; Miller, 1985).

The initial investigative interview of the child/adolescent following disclosure of sexual abuse has several objectives:

- initial engagement of the client in a therapeutic session,
- identity of the perpetrator(s),
- history of the sexual activity (e.g., actual sexual activity, frequency, length of time from initial sexual activity to disclosure, where it occurred),
- methods used to enhance victim compliance and to keep the activity a secret (e.g., bribes, physical force, rewards, threats).
- assessment of the child's need for immediate protection,
- assessment of the extent of the child/adolescent's emotional trauma, to provide appropriate crisis intervention and begin planning for follow-up counseling services.

Because child sexual abuse is a health, social, and legal problem, information about the situation will be needed by several professionals. It is unnecessary and traumatic for the victim to have to recount the story several times. Use of a tape recorder during the initial session can minimize repeated questioning since it reproduces the facts presented. In some states and provinces, these recorded interviews are accepted in court. This means that if charges are laid, when the case is heard in court the victim does not have to recount the events. An alternative is to have the participating professionals present with an identified primary interviewer. This can be intimidating for the child but, if handled effectively, is less traumatic than having to repeat the explanation. Use of a room with a two-way mirror for professionals other than the primary interviewer can solve this problem. Parents should not be present at the interview for two reasons. First, one of them may be the perpetrator, and second, their presence may inhibit the child who feels guilty and afraid of parental disapproval or punishment.

The purpose of the interview must be clarified, in age-appropriate terms, with the child at the outset. For victims to feel comfortable enough to describe their experience, they need to be reassured that disclosure was a good thing to do, and that although what the perpetrator did was wrong, they have done nothing wrong. It is comforting for many children to know that the interviewer has talked to other children with the same problem. Because of the secrecy surrounding sexual abuse, many victims believe they are unique.

The strategies used to collect the data depend on the age of the victim. Adolescents can usually articulate answers to straightforward, clear questions. Preadolescent and younger children may have difficulty answering questions because they do not understand what is being asked, or because they are too embarrassed. A number of age-appropriate aids are available to assist these children. Anatomically correct dolls have been widely used to determine exactly what has happened. Although their usefulness is controversial and has not been empirically proved, some evidence suggests that they can be effective aids for sexually abused children between the ages of 3 and 6 years (White et al, 1986).

Two types of art work can facilitate the explanations of children (Kelley, 1984). Anatomic drawings of males and females at the different developmental stages (preschool, school-age, adolescent, adult) can be used by children to state the names they use for different body parts. Then the interviewer can ask questions using words with which the child is familiar, to help minimize confusion. Picture drawing is another useful aid for sexually abused children between 3 and 12 years of age. The children are asked to draw a picture of themselves, the perpetrator, and what happened. While they are engaged in this activity, they should be encouraged to talk about what they are drawing and how they feel about it.

Conducting investigative interviews with children who have disclosed that they have been sexually abused requires a sensitive, skilled professional who is aware of the variety of child/adolescent reasons for disclosure and of the reactions to child sexual abuse. In some settings, nurses fulfill this role; in others, nurses to whom children have disclosed sexual abuse report to the child protection services whose workers conduct the interview. In this situation, the nurse can support the child during the interview.

Physical assessment of the child follows the investigative interview, unless the disclosure occurred during the physical examination. Physical examination of the child includes assessment for physical evidence (see Box 35-3) of sexual abuse and a pediatric or adult gynecologic examination (Pascoe and Duterte, 1981).

Since child sexual abuse is a criminal offense, the initial interview with the alleged perpetrator should be conducted by the police. They are familiar with the Rules of Evidence for admission of information to court proceedings. The interviewing styles of most health and social service professionals can lead to the evidence gathered being judged inadmissible in court and thus severely weaken the prosecutor's case.

Reactions of other family members to the disclosure of intrafamilial or extrafamilial sexual abuse vary. Since intrafamilial sexual abuse has many more ramifications for the family, reactions to it are strongest. The initial reactions of the father-perpetrator to the alleged sexual abuse of his daughter include denial, anger, hostility, guilt, and remorse. Initial maternal reactions are often quite hysterical. Subsequently, mothers may express many responses, such as fear, anger, denial, hostility, and apathy. Many mothers are torn between self-blame for failing to protect their daughter and the need to protect their husband. DeJong (1988) identifies three maternal responses to the sexual abuse of their children: nonsupportive; supportive with emotional changes (e.g., sleep disturbances, mood changes, crying, somatic complaints); and supportive without emotional changes. Of these three groups, the supportive mothers with emotional changes were most likely to support legal charges against the perpetrator and to seek counseling for themselves and their children. Siblings have varied reactions as well. Those who have also been sexually abused by the perpetrator may be relieved or angry at the victim for the family disruption the disclosure has caused. Sgroi (1984) points out that all family reactions will be based on "How will this affect me?" Often, in view of the reactions of family members, victims become less motivated to maintain their position. Pressure by parents and siblings to retract the claim of sexual abuse can result in children and adolescents changing or denying their stories. This is an excellent reason for careful assessment of the victim's emotional state and demonstrates the necessity for continued support (from others outside the family) during the investigative process.

Nursing Care of Sexually Abused Children and Their Families. As members of the multidisciplinary assessment and treatment team, nurses have an important role in the care of sexually abused children and their families. Being aware of the indicators of potential sexual abuse and maintaining a high level of suspicion will alert the nurse to the possibility of child sexual abuse, regardless of the practice setting. This can result in earlier identification of the problem and facilitate treatment for the child and family. As with any other type of abuse, the nurse who suspects child sexual abuse must report it to the Child Protection Services, following the institution/agency protocol. The idea of intrafamilial sexual abuse is so horrendous for some professionals that, even in the face of overwhelming evidence, they refuse to accept it. Knowledgeable nurses can assist these professionals in dealing with their feelings and in recognizing sexual abuse when it is apparent.

An adolescent may disclose a history of sexual abuse in emergency settings, a clinic, physician's office, or the school. Nurses working in these settings must be aware of the presenting symptoms that frequently mask sexual abuse (e.g., abdominal pain, somatic complaints with no identifiable cause). They must also be able to support a patient/client after disclosure. It is tempting to begin to collect further data immediately. The nurse who understands the investigative assessment procedure will be able to judge whether it is in the best interests of the client to proceed at this time or whether to wait until the other professionals have been assembled. Regardless of the role in the assessment interview, the nurse should be present to support the child/adolescent. Nurses' suggestions about age-appropriate ways to gather data can be useful for the interviewer.

Documentation must be accurate and clear. It includes statements made by the client, physical and emotional assessment of the client, reporting procedures that have been implemented, a summary of the investigative interview, any art work done by the child, and any interaction with the parents.

In rare situations, children or adolescents who have been admitted to hospital with another problem may have been sexually abused as well. In these cases, the role of the nurse is to provide support to the patient and family and to record accurately child behavior and child-parent interactions.

As with other forms of abuse, the immediate treatment of the sexually abused child focuses on stopping the abuse. In intrafamilial sexual abuse, the initial reactions of the parents are assessed to determine whether the child can safely return home. If there appears to be a risk of further abuse, the child and perpetrator must be separated. Ideally, the perpetrator should leave the family. This is sometimes difficult to arrange and difficult to assure. In these situations, the child is removed temporarily from the family.

A number of treatment models have been developed (Giarretto, 1982; Sgroi, 1984) that provide therapy individually or in groups for the sexually abused child, the perpetrator, the marital dyad, and the family. The details are beyond the scope of this chapter. The treatment of child sexual abuse is complex and multifaceted and to be successful usually requires a substantial investment of family time and energy. Nurses working in specialty clinics or the community may be involved in the long-term treatment process. Nurses may also refer families to self-help groups for sexually abused families. Parents United and Daughters and Sons United are examples of national self-help groups with local chapters in many cities.

The objectives of treatment are

- to aid in normal psychosexual development of the child/adolescent
- to strengthen the marital bond, and
- to reintegrate the family.

In many situations, the marital relationship is beyond repair, or adolescents do not wish to remain living with either parent. In these cases, assistance in working through the trauma and stress of separation is usually necessary. A favorable prognosis for sexually abused children and families is most likely when the father can admit his guilt and remorse to his daughter, when the mother believes and does not blame her daughter, and when the victim does not feel guilty and can forgive her father.

Since child sexual abuse is also a criminal matter, perpetrators are charged and a court appearance and case disposition will take place. The abuse of the investigation and treatment of intrafamilial child sexual abuse can be as devastating as the sexual abuse itself. Incarceration for the perpetrator results in the loss of the family unit and lifestyle, including loss of family income, family need for public assistance, change of family residence, and marital separation (Tyler and Brassard, 1984). Recently, courts have been ordering perpetrators into treatment, rather than jailing them. This has at least two positive outcomes: the perpetrators are treated and the family is not so disrupted.

Nursing Roles in Prevention of Child Abuse and Maltreatment

A recent policy statement by the American Public Health Association (1987) underlines the importance of child abuse and maltreatment prevention as a national public health goal. This policy statement outlines five objectives and actions to achieve them. All have implications for nurses in practice and as concerned members of society. The nursing role in prevention of child abuse and maltreatment is addressed here using the five objectives as a framework.

I. Increase Public Awareness of the Nature and Extent of Efforts to Prevent Child Abuse

As educators, nurses can assist in achieving this goal by initiating, participating in, or expanding current community education programs. Many programs* for school-age children and adolescents have been developed to heighten their awareness of child sexual abuse and what to do if they are involved in such incidents. In evaluating these programs, it is helpful to know that important topics to be included are factual information about sexual abuse, appropriate and inappropriate touch, respective role responsibilities of parents and children, and recognition of the individuals's right to choose to engage in sexual behavior and the choice of partners. Nurses can be effective participants in school and community programs for children and adolescents, either through actual program implementation or by assisting teachers or group leaders in planning age-appropriate activities.

Nurses can participate as speakers or leaders in community programs for parents related to the prevention of sexual abuse. Parents can learn to listen to the verbal and nonverbal messages children send about their interactions with other adults and possibly prevent the occurrence of sexual abuse. This is also an opportunity to dispel myths about child sexual abuse and to highlight specific positive communication techniques for families that will enable children to discuss sexual advances of adults, if they occur.

For years, nurses have played a major role in planning and teaching prenatal classes. These classes provide an ideal setting in which to introduce the topic of parenting styles and potential problems. Providing parents with local parent support resources before they need them is another important goal that can be accomplished in these classes. Nurses can be influential in initiating parenting programs for new families in general, or for particular high-risk groups of parents (e.g., adolescent parents and single, poor mothers). The introduction of Family Life courses that move from prenatal to postnatal periods and through the ages and stages of child and family development is an idea that has received a lot of support but has not yet been implemented. Interested nurses could be involved in developing, carrying out, and evaluating such programs.

II. Increase Knowledge of Health Professionals

In the past, child abuse and maltreatment have not been emphasized in the educational curricula of health professionals. In view of its incidence, the long-term sequelae for children, and the high financial and social cost for society, it cannot be downplayed any longer. Health professionals must accept and be responsible for their role in this area of child and family care. Nurses involved in both practice and education involving the care of children and families need to provide continuing education that addresses the identification, treatment, and prevention of child abuse and maltreatment. To assure that a multidisciplinary approach is evident, consultation with other professionals involved in this field must take place.

Nursing participation in multidisciplinary community or agency child abuse prevention and treatment programs results in a more comprehensive approach to the problem. Such participation provides nurses with the opportunity to negotiate their role(s) based on their identified knowledge and skills; to increase their understanding of the issues involved in the prevention, identification, and treatment of child abuse and maltreatment; and to develop respect for the roles of other involved professionals.

* Child sexual abuse prevention resources are available from the National Committee for the Prevention of Child Abuse, Publishing Department, 332 S. Michigan Avenue, Suite 950, Chicago, IL 60604-4357; telephone: (312) 663-3520.

III. *Coordinate and Improve the Availability, Accessibility, and Quality of Health Services to Families*

There are two nursing roles related to this objective: advocacy for adequate health and social services, for all families requiring them; and early identification and treatment of families at high risk so child abuse and maltreatment can be prevented.

Advocacy for Expanded Health and Social Services for Children and Families. Nurses are in a position to know and understand the importance of meeting the health and social services needs of families in decreasing family stress and, thereby, diminishing the likelihood of child abuse and maltreatment. Nurses can participate in political lobbying at the community, state, or national level for stable funding for necessary health care for all children and families (including the working poor who are currently frequently uninsured and lack the financial resources for ongoing health care). Provision of quality day care and after-school care for children is another urgent need. Neglect is often a result of family situations in which both parents (or the sole parent) work long hours to make financial ends meet and cannot afford to pay for supervision of their children. Older children are expected to supervise younger ones, and the results are often devastating for everyone.

Nurses can help focus public concerns on issues that influence the quality of family life. These include high density living, adequate park space for inner city children, and the development of community centers where families can learn together, enjoy themselves, and meet other people. Mother-child drop-in centers are popular and decrease the social isolation of many mothers. Unfortunately, these centers do not usually have a stable funding base and are often forced to close.

Identification and Treatment of Families at High Risk for Child Abuse and Maltreatment. Families can become high risk for child abuse and maltreatment at any time. The indicators for high-risk families are outlined in Box 35-4. In an attempt to provide primary prevention programs for child abuse and maltreatment, a great deal of work has been done to identify high-risk families prenatally or during the perinatal and postnatal periods. Nurses in a clinic, physician's office, or maternity setting are in an ideal position to assess these families, because they see them over time and can develop a therapeutic trusting relationship with them. This facilitates a comprehensive family history and assessment.

Several screening instruments have been developed to assist in the identification of families at high risk:

- Child Abuse Potential Inventory (Milner and Wimberley, 1979)
- Adolescent/Adult Parenting Inventory
- Family Stress Check List (Murphy et al, 1985)
- Parenting Profile Assessment (Anderson, 1987)
- Potential Screening Scale (Avison et al, 1986)

These instruments provide a standardized, relatively quick method for assessing the level of parental risk. However, one must recognize that they have limitations. Not all of them have been adequately tested for reliability and validity. The Child Abuse Potential Inventory (Milner and Wimberley, 1979) is probably the best developed at this time. It has known psychometric properties, is designed for a grade three reading level, and asks parents to agree or disagree with 150 one-line statements. An updated version contains about 70 items, requiring less time to complete (Milner, 1988).

Selection of an instrument should be based on its purpose. For example, the Potential Screening Scale (Turner and Avison, 1985) was developed from the theory that social support is the crucial variable that differentiates abusers from nonabusers. The literature on this topic is controversial (Turner and Avison, 1985; Seagull, 1987). However, if one has a prevention program available that emphasizes the development of social support systems in preventing stress, this would be an appropriate tool to use. Other instruments are more general and based on a multifaceted approach.

Correct identification of high-risk families is the first step in prevention. The second step, engaging these families in programs to enhance their parenting and problem-solving skills continues to be a challenge for all, including nurses. There is some evidence that providing concrete assistance (e.g., loan services for car seats, toys, or cribs; respite child care; assistance with locating and moving into new homes) can enhance early participation and continued involvement (Barth et al, 1986).

Results from a Special Families Care Project indicate that intensive health care services (2 to 4 hours per week of contact for a minimum of 18 months) for high-risk parents can reduce the incidence of reported child abuse, neglect, and out-of-home placement when compared with traditional services provided at 2- or 4-week intervals (Velasquez et al, 1984). This interdisciplinary program (nurses and social workers) provided support to high-risk parents, as well as individualized plans of care based on maternal needs (e.g., developing problem-solving skills about child care, increasing knowledge about normal infant growth and development, identifying personal support systems). A unique aspect of this program was that it helped very hard-to-serve clients who do not avail themselves of group programs. Through frustration or a sense of futility, nurses often have difficulty working with these parents. This experience could be useful to nurses working with similar clients. It underlines the neces-

Box 35-4
Indicators of High-Risk Families

PRENATAL INDICATORS

Unplanned pregnancy

Children spaced less than 1½ years apart

Depression related to pregnancy

One or other parent wanted either an abortion or to relinquish the child, but they did not

Denial of pregnancy

Mothers who are extremely upset about body changes during pregnancy

Young (under 20 years of age) mothers

Single mothers

Women who do not seek prenatal care when it is available or who ignore prenatal instructions

Parents who are overconcerned with the baby's sex

Parents who have unreal expectations of the infant

Parents who voice a lot of concern about how they will cope with an infant

Parents who make no/few preparations for the infant

Parents who have few supports and are isolated (physically or emotionally) from friends and family (e.g., no phone)

PERINATAL AND POSTNATAL INDICATORS

Difficult delivery

Immediate separation of mother and infant for health reasons of either patient

Parents who avoid touching or looking at the infant after delivery

Parents who voice disappointment over sex or appearance of the infant

Parents who do not support one another

Infant with recognizable physical or mental handicaps that will require long-term treatment

Parents who do not visit the neonatal unit or inquire about the condition of the baby

Parents who do not talk to the baby

Parents who are very irritated by the infant's crying, or make little or no attempt to comfort the baby

Parents who have no understanding of infant care and appear unwilling to try, in spite of support by hospital staff

NEONATAL INDICATORS

Premature infant

Infant with a congenital abnormality

Mentally retarded infant

Parents who express unreal expectations of the infant

Parents who feel the baby is too demanding (e.g., messy eating, changing diapers, etc.)

Parents who become unduly tense and irritable when the infant cries, or who may not respond to crying

Colicky infants

Parents who express a lot of anxiety about minor or seemingly nonexistent problems (e.g., frequent calls in the middle of the night, or trips to the emergency ward). As a result, they are often labeled "anxious mothers"

Fathers jealous of the time mother spends with the infant

Parents who change health care facility frequently for vague reasons. This sometimes means *their* needs are not being met, although the infant may be treated appropriately

In interview, parents who constantly refocus on themselves vs. the infant

Parents who cannot identify any support system for themselves in times of stress

TIMES OF CRISIS

Lifestyle changes such as marital separation or moving to a new setting and a new lifestyle, resulting in loss of support systems

Sudden unemployment or other situation leading to financial difficulties for the family

Death of a spouse

Diagnosis of serious illness in one of the family members

Very ill infant or child

Birth of another child—spacing

Abuse of alcohol or drugs by either parent

(Reprinted with permission from Thomas H: Child Abuse, Neglect and Deprivation; A Handbook for Ontario Nurses, *1983.)*

sity for ingenuity, creativity, and professional support in working with hard-to-serve clients.

IV. *Develop Data Systems to Monitor the Incidence and Prevalence of All Forms of Child Abuse*

As noted, the inconsistencies of data collection systems across the country make accurate assessment of the incidence or prevalence of all forms of child abuse impossible. For nurses and others interested in planning prevention or intervention programs for these children and families, up-to-date statistics would assist in determining geographic areas where the need is greatest. Most programs are situated where they are because the people who initiated them live in that location. This is not the most effective deployment of resources, and, in these times of financial restraint for health and social services, it is insufficient criteria on which to establish programs.

Although nurses are not directly involved in this aspect of prevention, it is hoped that their appreciation of the value of a standardized method for data collection and the resulting accurate data set will inspire some to publicly advocate such a system.

V. Research

A number of issues in the field of child abuse and maltreatment need to be adequately addressed by empirical research:

- Prospective long-term longitudinal studies to document, in a systematic way, the nature, causes, consequences, long-term effects, and responses related to all forms of child abuse and maltreatment.
- Cross-cultural research in the areas of prevention and treatment program evaluation.
- Further clarification of high-risk families and effective prevention interventions.
- Further understanding of the critical differences between nonabusive and abusive families.

Nurses with the interest, knowledge, and skills may become investigators in multidisciplinary research projects designed to address any of these issues. Other nurses can become involved in ongoing projects in which their knowledge about and skill in identification and treatment of child abuse and maltreatment will be valued and used. All nurses need to develop an appreciation of the necessity for scientifically based nursing practice in this as well as other fields.

In summary, the nursing roles in the prevention of child abuse and maltreatment are several:

- educator,
- child and family advocate,
- participant in identifying parents at high risk,
- practitioner in programs designed to treat high-risk families, and
- researcher or practitioner in prevention research.

References

Altemeier WA, et al: Prospective study of antecedents for non-organic failure to thrive. *J Pediatr* 1985; 106:360–365.

American Association for Protecting Children: *Protecting Children.* Denver, American Humane Association, 1983.

American Public Health Association, 8614 (PP): Prevention of child abuse. *Am J Public Health* 1987; 77(1):111–113.

Anderson CL: Assessing parenting potential for child abuse risk. *Pediatr Nurs* 1987; 13(5):323–327.

Avison WR, et al: Screening for problem parenting: preliminary evidence on a promising instrument. *Child Abuse Neglect* 1986; 10:157–170.

Ayoub CC: Failure to thrive: parental indicators, types and outcomes. *Child Abuse Neglect* 1985; 9(4):491–499.

Bachrach S: Long-term hospitalization of non-organic failure to thrive infants. *J Dev Behav Pediatr* 1987 Jun; 8(3):188–189.

Bandura A: *Aggression: A Social Learning Analysis.* Englewood Cliffs, NJ, Prentice-Hall, 1973.

Barth RP, et al: Identifying, screening, and engaging high-risk clients in private, non-profit child abuse prevention programs. *Child Abuse Neglect* 1986; 10(1):99–110.

Belsky J: Child maltreatment: an ecological integration. *Am Psychol* 1980; 35(4):320–335.

Berowitz CD, et al: Characteristics of mother-infant interactions in non-organic failure to thrive. *J Fam Pract* 1987 Oct; 25(4):377–381.

Besharov DJ: Doing something about child abuse: the need to narrow the grounds for state intervention. *Harvard J Law Pub Pol* 1985; 8(3):539–589.

Bithoney WG: Elevated lead levels in children with non-organic failure to thrive. *Pediatrics* 1986 Nov; 78(5):891–895.

Bithoney WG, Newberger EH: Child and family attributes of failure-to-thrive. *J Dev Behav Pediatr* 1987 Feb; 8:32–36.

Bithoney WG, Rathbun JM: Failure to thrive. *In* Levine WB, et al (eds): *Developmental-Behavioral Pediatrics.* Philadelphia, WB Saunders, 1983.

Blank DM: Relating mother's anxiety and perception to infant satiety, anxiety and feeding behavior. *Nurs Res* 1986 Nov/Dec; 35:347.

Brant RST, Tisza VB: The sexually misused child. *Am J Orthopsychiatr* 1977; 4(1):80-90.

Brassard MR, et al: *Psychological Maltreatment of Children and Youth.* New York, Pergamon Press, 1987.

Brown A, Finkelhor D: Impact of child sexual abuse: a review of the literature. *Psychol Bull* 1986; 99:66–77.

Brunngraber LS: Father-daughter incest: immediate and long-term effects of sexual abuse. *Adv Nurs Sci* 1986; 8(4):15–35.

Burgess AW (eds): *Child Pornography and Sex Rings.* Lexington, MA, Lexington Books, DC Heath, 1984.

Byles J, et al: Ontario Child Health Study: reliability and validity of the general functioning subscale of the McMaster Family Assessment Device. *Fam Proc,* 1988; 27:97–104.

Call JD: Child abuse and neglect in infancy: sources of hostility within the parent-infant dyad and disorders of attachment in infancy. *Child Abuse Neglect* 1984; 8:185–202.

Campbell J, Humphreys J: *Nursing Care of Victims of Family Violence.* Reston, VA, Reston Publishing Company, 1984.

Casey PH: Failure to thrive: transitional perspective. *J Dev Behav Pediatr* 1987 Feb; 8(1):37–38.

Colton JA: Childhood stress: perceptions of children and professionals. *J Psychopathol Behav Assess* 1985; 7(2):155–173.

Daro D: *Confronting Child Abuse: Research for Effective Program Design.* New York: The Free Press (A Division of Macmillan, Inc.), 1988.

DeJong AR: Maternal responses to the sexual abuse of their children. *Pediatrics* 1988; 81(1):14–21.

Doak CC, et al: *Teaching Patients with Low Literacy Skills.* Philadelphia, JB Lippincott, 1985.

Drotar D: *New Directions in Failure to Thrive: Implications for Research and Practice.* New York, Plenum Press, 1985.

Egeland B, Erickson MF: Psychologically unavailable caregiving. *In* Brassard MR, et al: *Psychological Maltreatment of Children and Youth.* New York, Pergamon Press, 1987.

Elvik SL, et al: Child sexual abuse: the role of the N.P. *Nurse Pract* 1986; 11(1):15–22.

Epstein NB, et al: The McMaster model of family functioning: a view of the normal family. *In* Walsh F (ed): *Normal Family Processes.* New York, Guilford Press, 1981.

Fantuzzo JW, et al: Parent and social-skills training for mentally retarded mothers identified as child maltreaters. *Am J Ment Defic* 1986; 91(2):135–140.

Federation S: Sexual abuse: treatment modalities for the young child. *J Psychosoc Nurs* 1986; 24(7):21–24.

Felice ME, Friedman SB: Behavioral considerations in the health care of adolescents. *Pediatr Clin North Am* 1982; 29:399–413.

Finkelhor D: *Child Sexual Abuse: New Research and Theory.* New York, The Free Press, 1984.

Finkelhor D, Hotaling GT: Sexual abuse in the National Incidence Study of Child Abuse and Neglect. *Child Abuse Neglect* 1984; 8:23–28.

Fosson A, et al: Family interactions surrounding feedings of infants with non-organic failure to thrive. *Clin Pediatr* 1987 Oct; 26(10):518–523.

Frappier PA, et al: Nursing assessment of infant feeding problems. *J Pediatr Nurs* 1987 Feb; 2(1):37–44.

Friedman M: *Family Nursing: Theory and Assessment.* East Norwalk, CT, Appleton-Century-Crofts, 1981.

Gagan RJ: The families of children who fail to thrive: Preliminary investigations of parental deprivation among organic and non-organic cases. *Child Abuse Neglect* 1984; 8:93–103.

Garbarino J: The human ecology of child maltreatment. *J Marriage Fam* 1977; 39:721–736.

Garbarino J, et al: *The Psychologically Battered Child: Strategies for Identification, Assessment and Intervention.* San Francisco, Massey-Bass, 1986.

Giarretto H: *Integrated Treatment of Child Sexual Abuse: A Treatment and Training Manual.* Science and Behavior Books, 1982.

Gil DG: Unravelling child abuse. *Am J Orthopsychiatr* 1975; 45(4):346–356.

Goldberg S, et al: Maternal behavior and attachment in low-birth weight twins and singletons. *Child Dev* 1986 Feb; 57(1):34–46.

Goldsmith H: Roundtable: What is temperament? Four approaches. *Child Dev* 1987; 58(1):505–529.

Government of Ontario: *Child and Family Services Act,* s.o. 1984, c 55, sections 68 (i), (2), (3), (4), (7).

Hart S, et al: *Proceedings Summary of the International Conference on Psychological Abuse of Children and Youth.* Indiana University: Office for the Study of the Psychological Rights of the Child, 1983.

Hockenberry MJ, Bologna-Vaughan S: Preparation for intrusive procedures using non-invasive techniques in children with cancer: state of the art vs. new trends. *Cancer Nurs* 1985; 8:97–102.

Hurwoltz A, Castells S: Misdiagnosed child abuse and metabolic disease. *Pediatr Nurs* 1987; 13(1):33–36.

Justice B, Justice R: *The Abusing Family.* New York, Human Science Press, 1976.

Kaufman J, Zigler E: Do abused children become abusive parents? *Am J Orthopsychiatr* 1987; 57(2):186–192.

Kelley SJ: The use of art therapy with sexually abused children. *J Psychosoc Nurs Ment Health Serv* 1984; 22:12–18.

Kelley SJ: Interviewing the sexually abused child: principles and techniques. *J Emerg Nurs* 1985; 11(5):234–241.

Kempe CH, Helfer RE: *Helping the Battered Child and His Family.* Philadelphia, JB Lippincott, 1972.

Knittle BJ, Luana SJ: Group therapy as primary treatment for adolescent victims of intra-familial sexual abuse. *Clin Social Work J* 1980; 8(4):236–242.

Knutson MG, et al: Tracking infants at risk: Washington State's High Priority Infant Tracking System. *J Pediatr Health Care* 1987 Jul/Aug; 1(4):180–189.

Kristiansson B, Fallstrom S: Growth at the age of 4 years subsequent to early failure to thrive. *Child Abuse Neglect* 1987; 2:35–40.

Kropp JP, Haynes OM: Abusive and nonabusive mothers' ability to identify general and specific emotion signals of infants. *Child Dev* 1987; 58:187–190.

Lamphear US: The impact of maltreatment of children's psychosocial adjustment: a review of the research. *Child Abuse Neglect.* 1985; 9:251–263.

Leahey M, Wright LM: *Families and Psychosocial Problems.* Springhouse, PA, Springhouse Corporation, 1987, 137.

Levin NR, Levin DL: A folk medicine practice mimicking child abuse. *Hosp Pract* 1982; 17:17–20.

Lichtenstein R, Ireton H: *Preschool Screening.* New York, Grune and Stratton, 1984.

Lieberman AF, Birch M: The etiology of failure to thrive: an interactional developmental approach. *In* Drotari D: *New Directions in Failure to Thrive: Implications for Research and Practice.* New York, Plenum Press, 1984.

Lieberman C, et al: Multidisciplinary treatment of feeding disorders in the home. *Pediatr Nurs* 1987 Jul/Aug; 13:266.

MacFarlane K, et al: *Sexual Abuse of Young Children: Evaluation and Treatment.* New York, Guilford Press, 1982.

McKittrick CA: Child abuse; recognition and reporting by health professionals. *Nurs Clin North Am* 1981 Mar.

McNeill L, Brassard MR: *The Behavioral Correlates of Father-Daughter Incest with Elementary School-Aged Girls.* Paper presented at the Fifth International Congress on Child Abuse and Neglect, Montreal, 1984.

Mertin P: Maternal-infant attachment: a developmental perspective. *Aust NZ J Obstet Gynaecol* 1986 Nov; 26(4):280–283.

Miller EL: Interviewing the sexually abused child. *MCN* 1985; 10:103–105.

Millor GK: A theoretical framework for nursing research in child abuse and neglect. *Nurs Res* 1981; 30(2):78–83.

Milner JS, Wimberley RC: An inventory for the identification of child abusers. *J Clin Psychol* 1979; 35:95–100.

Milner JS: Personal communication, 1988.

Mogan J: What can nurses learn from structured observations of mother-infant interactions? *Issues Compr Pediatr Nurs* 1987; 10:67–73.

Murphy S, et al: Prenatal prediction of child abuse and neglect: a prospective study. *Child Abuse Neglect* 1985; 9:225–235.

O'Hare AE, Eden OB: Bleeding disorders and non-accidental injury. *Arch Dis Child* 1984; 59:860–864.

Orkow B: Implementation of a family stress checklist. *Child Abuse Neglect* 1985; 9:405–410.

Parke RD: Theoretical models of child abuse: their implications for prediction, prevention and modification. *In* Starr RH (ed): *Child Abuse Prediction.* Cambridge, MA, Ballinger Publishing Company, 1982.

Pascoe DJ, Duterte BO: The medical diagnosis of sexual abuse in the premenarcheal child. *Pediatr Ann* 1981; 10(5):187–190.

Pelton LH: Child abuse and neglect: the myth of classlessness. *Am J Orthopsychiatr* 1978; 48(4):608–617.

Powell GF: Behavior as a diagnostic aid in failure to thrive. *J Dev Behav Pediatr* 1987 Feb; 8(1):18–24.

Pugliese MT, et al: Parental Health beliefs as a cause of non-organic failure to thrive. *Pediatrics* 1987 Aug; 80(2):175–182.

Radar D: Child on the run: a deepening American tragedy. *Parade* 1982 Sep; 4–7.

Rhodes AM: The nurse's legal obligations for reporting child abuse. *MCN* 1987; 12:313.

Rosenn DW, et al: Differentiation of organic from non-organic failure to thrive syndrome in infancy. *Pediatrics* 1980; 66:38, 42, 689–704.

Scharer KM: Rescue fantasies: Professional impediments in working with abused families. *Am J Nurs* 1978; 78:1483–1484.

Schneider-Rosen K, et al: VII. Current perspectives in attachment theory: illustration from the study of maltreated infants. *In* Bretherton, I, Waters E (eds): *Growing Points of Attachment Theory and Research.* Chicago, University of Chicago Press, 1985, 194–210.

Seagull EAW: Social support and child maltreatment: a review of the evidence. *Child Abuse Neglect* 1987; 11:41–52.

Sgroi SM: *Handbook of Clinical Intervention in Child Sexual Abuse.* Toronto, Lexington Books, 1984, Chapter 1.

Showers J, et al: Non-organic failure to thrive: identification and intervention. *J Pediatr Nurs* 1986 Aug; 1:240.

Singer L: Long-term hospitalization of non-organic failure-to-thrive infants: patient characteristics and hospital course. *J Dev Behav Pediatr* 1987; 8(1):25–31.

Singer L: Long-term hospitalization of failure to thrive infants: developmental outcome at three years. *Child Abuse Neglect* 1986; 10(4):479–486.

Singer LT, Fagan JF: Cognitive development in the failure to thrive infant: a three year longitudinal study. *J Pediatr Psychol* 1984 Sep; 9(3):363–383.

Spinetta SS, Rigler D: The child abusing parent: a psychological review. *Psychol Bull* 1972; 77:296–304.

Stangler SR, et al: *Screening Growth and Development of Preschool Children: A Guide for Test Selection.* New York, McGraw-Hill, 1980.

Steele S: Non-organic failure to thrive: a pediatric social illness. *Issues Compr Pediatr Nurs* 1986; 9:47–58.

Straus M, et al: *Behind Closed Doors: Violence in the American Family.* New York, Anchor Press, 1980.

Thomas H: *Child Abuse, Neglect and Deprivation: A Handbook for Ontario Nurses.* Toronto, Registered Nurses Association of Ontario, 1983.

Turner RJ, Avison WR: Assessing risk factors for problem parenting: the significance of social support. *J Marr Family* 1985 Nov; 881–892.

Tyler AH, Brassard MR: Abuse in the investigation and treatment of intra-familial child sexual abuse. *Child Abuse Neglect* 1984; 8:47–53.

Vander Mey BJ: The sexual victimization of male children: a review of previous research. *Child Abuse Neglect* 1988; 12(1):61–72.

Velasquez J, et al: Intensive services help prevent child abuse. *MCN* 1984; 9:113–117.

Weber S: Munchausen syndrome by proxy. *J Pediatr Nurs* 1987; 11(1):50–54.

White S, et al: Interviewing young sexual abuse victims with anatomically correct dolls. *Child Abuse Neglect* 1986; 10:519–529.

Wong DL: False allegations of child abuse: the other side of the tragedy. *Pediatr Nurs* 1987; 13(5):329–333.

Wright LM, Leahey M: *Nurses and Families: A Guide to Family Assessment and Intervention.* Philadelphia, FA Davis, 1984.

Yoos L: Taking another look at failure to thrive. *MCN* 1984 Jan/Feb; 9:32.

Bibliography

Dale P, et al: *Dangerous Families: Assessment and Treatment of Child Abuse.* London, Tavistock, 1986.

McCormack A, et al: Runaway youths and sexual victimization: Gender differences in an adolescent runaway population. *Child Abuse Neglect* 1986; 10(3):387–396.

Miller A: *For Your Own Good: Hidden Cruelty in Child Rearing and the Roots of Violence.* New York, Farrar, Straus and Giroux, 1983.

Newberger EH, Bourne R (eds): *Unhappy Families: Clinical and Research Perspectives on Family Violence.* Littleton, MA, PSG Publishing Company, 1985.

Powers JL, Echenrode J: The maltreatment of adolescents. *Child Abuse Neglect* 1988; 12(2):189–200.

Nursing Strategies: Behavioral and Psychiatric Alterations

Chapter 36

Jo Joyce Anderson
Patricia Neel Scott
Kathleen Boggs

Related Topics
Theories of development, Chapter 3
Prevention of obesity in infants, Chapter 18
Concepts of Illness: Stress, Crisis, and Coping, Chapter 23

Many of us have heard a parent say "each of my children is so different." Individuality and uniqueness are advocated and commended in children. When individual expression of children remains within the confines of what society accepts as "normal behavior," it is met with an element of fascination and joy by family and professionals alike. However, not all children's behavior is characterized by explosions of creativity and adventure. When a child's behavior becomes maladaptive and dysfunctional, families, communities, and societies are burdened and perplexed. The complexities of how a child or adolescent becomes troubled and dysfunctional in society have created an extensive body of research and literature. General concepts related to understanding children's behavioral problems and the various methods of behavioral assessment are discussed in Chapter 33. This chapter discusses specific behavioral and psychiatric alterations that a nurse may encounter in any hospital setting, at school, or in the home. Although nurses may not be required to make independent decisions regarding the management of children with these problems, it is important to have an understanding of these alterations in order to make appropriate assessments and referrals and to work collaboratively with other disciplines in their therapy programs.

During the transition from conception to adulthood, the human being undergoes predictable and inevitable biologic changes. During this developing process a child also changes in the way the environment is perceived and understood. Relationships with people mature and take on new meaning as life experiences accumulate. As a child attempts to "find a place" and "feel important," experiences of rebuff and acceptance come and go. Over time the child develops a repertoire of behaviors and coping mechanisms that characterize the individual.

The genetic makeup and the experiences of each child shape the process of becoming a person. The interplay of biologic tendencies and the environmental milieu produces an individual score of vulnerability that is largely unmeasurable and unpredictable. Some difficulties that children encounter may be relatively short-lived and may cause minimal stress to the family, whereas others are enduring and cause lifelong worry, misery, or sadness to the child and to the family. The alterations included in this chapter span a wide range of problems; they have in common that the child's behavior varies from that deemed by individuals and society as adaptive.

Assessment

The problems discussed in this chapter have multiple causes. When assessing children's mental health, it is important to remember that a child's behavior is measured against the usual developmental responses characteristic of a certain age and a child's unique temperament and personality. Children may have difficulty in only one or two areas of function that with appropriate support will resolve.

To assess a child's mental health, an understanding of children's behavior and how children cope is required. (See Chapter 23 for a review of childhood coping and Chapter 33, Box 33-4, for various assessment tools.) Whether a specific tool is used for assessment is determined by the purpose of the assessment.

A developmental approach to observe children has been devised by Greenspan (1981), which includes assessment of patterns of relationships, mood and emotions, affect and anxiety, and thematic expressions. Observations are made of the physical aspects of the child that affect mental and psychological functioning. Special attention is given to the level of integration of the central nervous system, including gross and fine motor coordination, perceptual-motor integration, and emerging cognitive abilities (Greenspan, 1981).

Patterns of Relationships. The characteristic style and pattern of relating is observed, assessing for how one relates in a dyad (one-to-one) and one's characteristics of relating in a group.

Overall Mood or Emotional Tone. Specific emotions are assessed by direct observations of the child as well as through the topics the child discusses.

Affect and Anxiety. Consideration is given to the range of affect (rage, anger, jealousy, empathy, love), its appropriateness for the situation, and the depth of the feeling. An assessment is also made of the appropriateness of the affect for the child's age.

Anxiety is best observed in the child's verbalized fears but can also be observed indirectly through play. The nature of anxiety is noted by observing for an abrupt change of topic or activity during play or conversations (i.e., a change of topic when approaching an anxiety-producing theme).

Thematic Expressions. Observations are made about a child's ability to express organized, rich themes. This capacity is related to the child's sense of security, an inner set of controls, and the availability of a fantasy life (Greenspan, 1981).

A guide for the assessment of mental health functioning of children, compiled by Babich (1982), includes the following categories:

- general appearance and health
- self-concept
- social/relational functioning
- emotional functioning
- conscience
- cognitive/intellectual functioning
- motor functioning
- coping mechanisms

See Jellinek and colleagues (1988) for a check list to screen school-age children for psychosocial dysfunction.

Childhood Fears and Phobias

Fears are common to every child's experience. Children are afraid of different things at the various developmental stages, including the dark, imaginary creatures, certain animals, and natural events (storms, tornadoes) (Apter and Conoley, 1984). Most of these developmental fears are transient and do not interfere with the child's daily functioning. Phobias, and especially school phobia, on the contrary, can be debilitating.

A phobia is a fear to an exaggerated degree of objects or events that in reality are not dangerous and to most people do not evoke such excessive fear (Kavanaugh and Mattson, 1987). When the fear-producing stimulus is presented, a phobic child reacts with a degree of fear that is out of proportion to the stimulus (e.g., spider, thunder, elevators). When the stimulus is not present, the child's behavior is normal.

The mechanism of how a phobia develops has been explained by various theories. The traditional psychodynamic theory proposes that an internal mental conflict (most often related to sexual and aggressive feelings) is present. Negative feelings associated with the conflict are displaced onto a specific object or event. By avoiding the specified object or event, the child's anxiety can be reduced. From the viewpoint of behaviorism, phobias develop because an originally fearful situation is repeatedly avoided. The longer the situation is avoided, the more exaggerated the fear becomes.

Therapeutic techniques used to correct phobias vary. Confronting the patient with the phobic situation until tolerance is developed is rarely used in children (Kavanaugh and Mattson, 1987). Various forms of therapy are used: counter-conditioning (use of positive images or stimuli), modeling, and cognitive behavior therapy (includes coping self-statements). Children with severe specific phobias are often referred to a psychologist or psychiatrist for such therapies.

School Phobia

The child with school phobia (school refusal) presents a challenging management problem to primary caregivers and school authorities. The term *school phobia* applies to a variable set of symptoms that are "consistent with underlying anxiety in a child who is excessively absent from school" (Dale et al, 1980, page 366).

Children suffering from severe school phobia are so immobilized that they cannot attend school. Hysterical, frantic behavior will be manifested when any attempt is made to urge such a child to go to school. Different from the truant who does not want to go to school, the child with school phobia truly wishes to attend school but simply cannot force himself or herself to go when the hour arrives. The child who is truant does not stay at home when absent from school, whereas the child with school phobia does (Dworkin, 1985).

To understand school phobia more clearly, it is helpful to think of its severity as plotted on a continuum. At one end is the child with minor somatic complaints on school days when there is a test or presentation that is dreaded—a fairly normal reaction. At the other end of the continuum is the child whose anxiety is absolutely immobilizing. These are the children who become hysterical on the morning of a school day. Each child reacts to school phobia with different degrees of intensity. This is of particular significance as the management of the child is considered.

Incidence and Etiology

The prevalence of school phobia is difficult to estimate because many cases are handled by the school system or the child's primary health care provider, but it has been estimated to be 1.7 per cent per year (Dworkin, 1985). As teacher awareness of the problem increases, so do the number of referrals to mental health clinics. There are three peaks of frequency. The first is at the beginning of school life when the child is between 5 and 7 years old. The second peak is between 11 and 12 years, when the child is transferred to high school; and the third peak is around 14 years (Connell, 1985).

There are two theories about the etiology of school phobia. However, when working with school phobic children, the nurse should realize that the etiologic factors for each child may be a combination of both or part of these theories; very seldom does the phobia have a single etiology.

One theory held by some psychiatrists is that school phobia is basically a form of *separation anxiety* (Mansdorf and Lukens, 1987). The child is extremely fearful of leaving the home environment. In most studies, the mother is the parent the child feels closest to and is most fearful of leaving. The father has characteristically withdrawn from the situation, thus offering no or minimal support to the mother.

The parent (usually the mother) fosters feelings of dependency in the child. Intellectually, the mother realizes that her child must attend school; however, her dependency on this child is so great that actually having the child separate from her is extremely difficult. Phrases such as "I don't know what I'll do when you're gone" subtly reinforce the child's dependent state. It is believed that the mother has hidden hostilities toward herself for having to depend on a child and toward the child for being so dependent. In attempting to repress these unacceptable hostilities, the mother becomes overprotective of this child so that the child will not recognize these "nonmotherly" feelings. And as her overprotection increases, the child becomes more dependent on her and more reluctant to leave her to participate in normal activities such as school.

This theory might be useful in explaining why some children have dreaded school since the beginning of their school experience, but it cannot clearly explain why a child with previous good school attendance develops a school phobia.

Another theory explains why a child with normal patterns of school attendance suddenly refuses to go. Leventhal and Sills (1964) believed that children with school phobia have an unrealistic view of their abilities. They overvalue themselves—think themselves capable of feats beyond their talents. For instance, they see themselves as popular, well-liked, and competent. When their peers and teachers in school do not support this view, they feel threatened and humiliated. Their self-image is damaged, perhaps to the point that they will refuse to attend school. For these children school becomes a difficult task because they feel constantly threatened. At home they receive family input that reinforces their too-high opinion of themselves, while at school they feel insecure and uncomfortable. This theory would explain why a child with good school attendance later begins to find excuses to miss school and finally refuses to attend at all.

In both these theories, an identifiable precipitating event motivates the child's ultimate reaction to school. Events such as the birth of a sibling or unhappy experiences at school threaten the child so severely that school attendance becomes irregular or the child may cease to attend school completely.

In considering causes for a child's refusal of school, one must remember that it could be an acquired fear such as of an object, person, or situation in the school setting. A child might be bullying this child or a particular class may be too difficult. In some cases the object of fear might not be apparent to the child or family.

The theory of multicausality acknowledges that multiple factors may be involved in any given child's situation (Wright and Nader, 1983; Dworkin, 1985). A child with an unrealistically high self-image may have an overprotecting, dependent mother and additionally suffer from a particular fear.

Clinical Manifestations and Assessment

School phobia presents in the form of somatic complaints. Symptoms are varied and reflect the severity of the phobia. Abdominal pain, headaches, and general malaise are the most common symptoms; others are nausea and vomiting, anorexia, muscle aches, and occasionally a low-grade fever. The child most commonly does not complain of fear of school. As the symptomatology is so varied and nonspecific in this phobia, the primary care provider is challenged to determine the underlying issue. If a mother brings the child to the physician or nurse with the complaint of "frequent abdominal pain," an in-depth history is essential in recognizing that the primary issue is that the child does not want to go to school.

Diagnosing the child's school phobia begins with a careful, thorough history. Clarification of statements and open-ended questions are of inestimable value. A specific area on which to concentrate is the past medical history. How much illness has this child had? How frequently did illness keep the child out of school? On careful questioning, it is often evident that the school attendance of this child has been sporadic and that somatic complaints have often been the reason. Not until the parents and child start adding up these absences do they realize their frequency.

Another phenomenon that may be apparent when assessing the child's past medical history is a pattern in the timing of symptoms. Symptoms displayed by children with school phobia are rarely seen during holidays, summer vacation, or weekends. The symptoms are most prominent Sunday evenings or on a school morning and virtually disappear by afternoon. When obtaining a history from a school-age child, the nurse always should ask the child directly about school, being alert for the attitude displayed. Information from the child regarding friends and activities at school should be obtained.

Because theories support that there is a precipitating event in the life of a child with school phobia, the nurse should pay special attention to recent life events. Occurrences such as birth of a new sibling or recent death or absence of a parent or other family member could precipitate an acute episode of school phobia. Dealing with these situations may gradually eliminate the problem of school attendance.

During the initial interview and history, the nurse should pay particular attention to the nonverbal communication taking place. How do the mother and child react to one another? Is the mother dominating the conversation to the point that the child is unable to speak? If this is happening, separating the mother and child and interviewing each alone might be effective. If the father is present, an assessment should be made regarding his role in the family situation and interaction. If the father is not present, an attempt should be made to interview him at another time. Since school phobia is so intimately related to family dynamics, it is important, when obtaining the history, to have as many family members contributing as possible. When planning interventions for treatment, including all family members from the start helps ensure their commitment to participation in the management.

Because children generally present with a minor physical complaint such as a recurrent headache or stomachache, it is important for the practitioner to perform a complete physical examination, with particular attention given to the systems involved in the "chief complaint." The physical examination is done to reassure the child and the parents that the child is physically well and to rule out an organic basis for the complaint. Simple tests such as throat cultures or urinalysis are sometimes performed, depending on the reason for seeking health care. Hearing and vision screening are especially important for this child because school problems are often manifestations of difficulties in hearing and vision. The nurse also evaluates parental anxieties related to the child's blatant unhappiness, their desire to eliminate the dread of school, and their concern over how the absences will affect school work and their legal responsibility to ensure school attendance.

Therapeutic Management and Nursing Strategies

These families tend to have multiple issues facing them and long-term therapy is often the only way to manage the problems. The literature regarding school phobia generally recommends referral to a mental health provider, such as a psychiatrist or mental health nurse.

The major goal of management is to get the child back in school as rapidly as possible (Wright and Nader, 1983). Staying home from school deprives the child of the experiences needed to mature normally. The longer the child is allowed to stay out of school, the more difficult eventual return will be.

As plans are being formulated for the return to school, school authorities should be included, as their input is vital for the success of the program. The feasibility of the plan will depend on school facilities and the cooperation of teachers, counselors, and administrators. Planning for return to school must be made cooperatively with the individual child and family. If the plan does not include all these people, the chances of success are diminished. The plan could be for the child's return to school for 2 hours every day for a week in the counselor's office and then a gradual return to the classroom (desensitization technique), or an immediate return to the classroom.

Two fundamental considerations must be taken into account by the nurse in facilitating the plan: (1) school attendance is mandatory by law, and (2) the child's capability to resume a place in the community of peers.

Follow-up for guidance and support is important as the family attempts to alter long-standing patterns of behavior. The nurse is often in a position to be supportive and to help the family deal with issues that arise in school or in the family.

Prevention

As is the case in so many issues that arise in childhood, the best approach to school phobia is prevention. Early in the life of a child, the nurse can assess the separation patterns that are present. Anticipatory guidance and support to parents who have difficulty separating from their infant can prevent major separation problems from occurring later in the child's life. As the nurse works with young families, parenting skills and communication patterns can be assessed. During the preschool examination, time should be spent with the family discussing feelings the parents and child have about the child's imminent school attendance.

Encopresis

The most widely accepted definition of encopresis is dysfunction in which a child regularly passes formed or semiformed stool in inappropriate places at least once a week (Parker and Whitehead, 1982). In most cases this is associated with chronic stool retention. A few children have incontinence without clear evidence of withholding. Encopresis is further differentiated into *primary encopresis,* in which bowel control has never been achieved, and *secondary encopresis,* in which the child has been continent of stool for a period of months. Fecal soiling may occur during the day as well as at night. It frequently accompanies a time of stress in the child's life.

The incidence of encopresis is reported to be 1.5 per cent in 7- to 8-year-old children. According to Levine (1975), as many as 3 per cent of children between 4 and 10 years have encopresis. Seven per cent of children are constipated, and 7 per cent of these experience fecal soiling (Bakwin and Bakwin, 1972). Encopresis is seen more frequently in boys than in girls. It is seen in children from disrupted families more frequently than in children with intact families.

Etiology

Etiologic factors in encopresis do not seem well-defined at this time. This condition is like so many others in childhood—causes are many and components of each theory may be involved for any given child. The role of the nurse is to identify the causal factors in each child's situation so as to more effectively plan a management program. For this reason, the nurse needs to be acquainted with the various etiologic theories.

Encopresis may have a *psychologic* basis arising from a variety of possible factors. For some reason the child learns, at a very early age in some cases, to withhold stool. It could be in response to improper toilet training. Toilet training might have been started too early or coercive tactics might have been used. Having a bowel movement may be uncomfortable to the child because of a fear of the toilet or of being left alone in the bathroom. Some deep-seated emotional problem is usually present with encopresis. Two characteristics of the young child's temperament may predispose the child to constipation: intensity and irregularity (Fleisher, 1976).

Some data indicate that there may be a *genetic cause or predisposition* to encopresis. It is believed that children with encopresis absorb more water from the fecal mass as it passes through the colon, thus making the mass more difficult to expel. This theory might explain why constipation is present in these children from infancy.

Encopresis may have an *organic* basis. A neurologic problem or anatomic abnormality might cause fecal soiling and constipation. The child may have internal or external anal lesions that cause pain during the passage of stool.

Clinical Manifestations and Assessment

When a child has reached school age, bowel patterns are no longer obvious to the parents. Therefore, parents may not be aware that the child is constipated. But parents are aware when fecal soiling occurs. The initial obvious conclusion of the parent is that the child has diarrhea. This complaint of diarrhea is sometimes the reason why health care is sought by a family. Other symptoms that may or may not be present are abdominal pain, lethargy, poor appetite, and large, painful stools. Many parents approach the health professional not because of diarrhea or constipation concerns but because of the frustration and embarrassment the soiling causes and the ambivalent feelings it is creating in them and the child's peers toward the child.

The diagnosing of encopresis and constipation begins with a careful, thorough history. This history should assess the child's daily habits and the psychosocial milieu of the family. Information about family dynamics is necessary to identify causative factors and to plan successful interventions. Parenting methods should be assessed. The primary person responsible for the care of the child should be identified—the mother or father, a sibling, or a baby sitter—because of the important role the primary caregiver has in the management of this condition. While obtaining the history, the nurse should observe the child's interactions with the parents to assess the health of the parent-child relationship.

The dietary history should be explored. Junk food, whole milk, and limited fluids contribute to constipation, as do irregular eating times.

A history of toilet training should be obtained. The child's age at which bowel continence was achieved (if ever) and the approach used are important to assess. Inconsistent or coercive means to induce bowel control have been shown to contribute to the development of encopresis, as well as beginning at too young an age.

A description of elimination patterns is a necessary part of the history. Past medical history can be helpful; a long-standing problem with diarrhea or constipation might be significant. Amount and frequency of stools should be noted, with clear descriptions. The terms *diarrhea* and *constipation* should be clarified, ensuring that the nurse's and parent's use of the terms are clear to both parties. If constipation has been present, the nurse will want to determine how this constipation has been treated and with what results. The issue of fecal soiling should be discussed, giving attention to how it has been treated at home and with what results. Some practitioners believe that parents who actively intervene when their child soils are reinforcing the encopretic activity because the child finds pleasure in the attention.

A physical examination should be conducted, with special attention paid to neurologic aspects. By eliciting a normal anal "wink" (response to a pin prick to anus), one can assess the neurologic status of the anus. The abdomen may be mildly distended. Upon palpation, fecal material distending the colon may be felt. Bowel sounds may be normal or slightly diminished. Usually fecal material can be seen around the anus.

Therapeutic Management and Nursing Strategies

Once the diagnosis of encopresis has been confirmed by history and physical examination, the parents, child, and nurse can set up a management program. The goal of the program is to provide a medication, diet, and toileting ritual that encourages the child to develop normal defecation habits (Younger and Hughes, 1983).

Simple and specific explanation of the problem is the first step. Various diagrams can be drawn to explain the problem to the child and family.

The first goal of the program is to clear the impaction if it exists. The child usually has a large amount of stool distending the lower colon. Enemas are given on varying schedules until the impaction is removed. In most cases, this can be done over a 10-day to 2-week period (Levine, 1987). It may be done at home or in the hospital, depending on the family and the protocol being used. After the initial catharsis a maintenance program is instituted.

Next an oral laxative is started, and 2 tablespoons of mineral oil a day are given (refrigerated and mixed in fruit juice). A program of regular elimination patterns is also established. The child is expected to sit on the toilet for a specific amount of time at regular times during the day (usually twice a day for 10 minutes each time). There should be proper foot support for the child—the feet should be at an angle whereby pushing can be comfortably done. A diet high in residue and low in milk is started; fluids are encouraged. Exercise is promoted to increase peristalsis, which also promotes elimination of stool.

The parents and other family members will be affected by this treatment program. It may mean a diet change if they ordinarily do not eat a high-fiber diet, and an exercise program for the whole family. All members should be told to help enforce the toilet program of the child, but shame or ridicule from them will threaten a successful outcome. All family members (including siblings) should be involved in the management of encopresis.

If the child is doing well by 6 weeks, the oral laxative can be tapered off but the mineral oil is continued. In most programs, a normal bowel pattern is established by 6 months. Failures in management of encopresis are most often due to noncompliance. Giving an aura of hope to these children and involving families in the management are ways in which the nurse can motivate compliance. Follow-up every 6 weeks for the next 6 months is usually required (Levine, 1987).

Family therapy may be warranted in some cases. Knowing the family dynamics and community resources can aid the nurse in deciding whether to refer the family for counseling.

Prevention is the key to encopresis. The nurse working with families with young children should always carefully review elimination patterns with parents. Anticipatory guidance should be given regarding toilet training. (See discussion of toilet training in Chapter 6.)

Conduct Disorders

Conduct disorder is classified by the American Psychiatric Association (1987) as a subtype of attention-disordered children. Children may have an attention deficit disorder with or without a conduct disorder. (See Chapter 34 for a discussion of attention-disordered children.) Conduct disorder is described as disturbance of conduct lasting at least 6 months during which at least three of the following behaviors have been present.

1. has stolen without confrontation of a victim on more than one occasion (including forgery)
2. has run away from home overnight at least twice while living in parental or parental surrogate home (or once without returning)
3. often lies (other than to avoid physical or sexual abuse)
4. has deliberately engaged in fire-setting
5. is often truant from school (for older person, absent from work)
6. has broken into someone else's house, building, or car
7. has deliberately destroyed others' property (other than by fire-setting)
8. has been physically cruel to animals
9. has forced someone into sexual activity with him or her
10. has used a weapon in more than one fight
11. often initiates physical fights
12. has stolen with confrontation of a victim (e.g., mugging, purse-snatching, extortion, armed robbery)
13. has been physically cruel to people

Conduct disorders are more prevalent in boys than in girls in a ratio of 3 : 1 and comprise the largest group of psychiatrically disturbed children, with estimates varying from 47 to 67 per cent (Forehand and Wells, 1987). In the general population, conduct disorders have been reported to be as high as 4 per cent (Rutter et al, 1974).

The etiology of conduct disorders is unclear. It is believed that a constitutional or organic basis exists for the behavior of these children (Wells and Forehand, 1985). Certain environmental processes are also thought to be contributing factors. Patterson (1980) has suggested a "coercion hypothesis" to account for the family dynamics that contribute to conduct disorders in children. The coercive control strategies of the child, such as crying, tantrums, and screaming, are reinforced by the parent, and the parent in turn uses coercive tactics to control the child. Repeated coercive exhanges eventually result in disruption of all family members, with parents and child feeling depressed, anxious, and lacking self-esteem (Webster-Stratton, 1983).

Contrary to the adage that a child will "outgrow" behavioral problems, studies indicate that a conduct disorder at 6 years of age is a strong predictor for such a disorder at 13 or 14 years of age. Furthermore, antisocial personality in adults is strongly associated with conduct disorders in childhood (Forehand and Wells, 1987). Thus, early identification and intervention are directed at helping the family manage oppositional child behaviors effectively before coercive behavior patterns within the family become habitual. Common manifestations of conduct disorders are lying, stealing, cheating, and aggressive behaviors.

Lying

Lying is defined as a deliberate attempt to deceive others. Lying occurs at all ages. When parents, teachers, or others bring such a concern to a health professional, an attempt is made to discover whether such behavior constitutes a problem serious enough to require professional intervention. Several factors need to be considered in making this evaluation: the developmental stage and age of the child, the duration and frequency of the behavior, and whether there is actual intent to distort the truth.

Bakwin and Bakwin (1972) differentiate types of lies. The most commonly occurring lies are

1. Fantastic lies. These are the lies that come from the child's fantasy world. They are useful in helping the child learn about the real world.
2. Imitative lies. Adults are apt to embellish stories to a certain degree; the child imitates this behavior.
3. Lies of exaggeration and attention-seeking. These lies are told by the child to peers and adults for self-enhancement. These lies serve the purpose of compensating for real or imagined incompetencies or building up wavering self-esteem.
4. Lies of convention. These are the "white lies" that are told generally in order to prevent hurt to others.
5. Defensive lies. These lies are told usually to escape punishment. They may also be told in an attempt to measure up to unrealistic expectations that have been set by someone else.

Parents sometimes report that their young child tells lies, failing to understand that at this developmental age it is difficult for the child to separate reality from fantasy. Most older children tell occasional lies, especially in order to escape punishment. If the child lies frequently or deliberately lies about serious matters, an attempt is made to determine the motivation for such behavior.

When the reason for a child's lies has been determined, proper therapy can be initiated. Depending upon the experience and attitude of the nurse, the child and parents may be referred to a mental health worker. Excessive lying is often symptomatic of deeper family pathology and is appropriately referred by the nurse, who will want to follow the child's progress by communicating with the mental health counselor.

If the nurse chooses to manage this issue, a problem-solving session with parents and child might facilitate resolution. Helping the family look at communication among its members, motivation behind the child's lies, and some possible interventions may be the best approach to overcome the problem. Frequently parents will identify behaviors that might have caused the child to lie. For example, discipline measures that are too strict may force a child into lying. Supporting the parents as they begin intervening to eliminate the child's lying may be the nurse's primary role.

Prevention of a child's lying is the first defense. Parenting that promotes open communication and realistic expectations of children is encouraged by the nurse during well child visits. (See Chapter 13 for a discussion of healthy parenting.)

Stealing

A certain amount of stealing is normal in children. Young children are curious about everything around them. They love to collect things and are particularly attracted to and may "borrow" brightly colored, interesting objects. School-age children are developing a superego. Although they are learning right from wrong and "mine" from "theirs," these concepts are not fully internalized. Therefore, temptations are not always resisted—if a child sees something desirable, she or he sometimes takes it.

In the adolescent, stealing is a more serious concern. Some adolescents are challenged to swipe candy bars or other items of small value from stores, school lunchrooms, and so on, as a method of proving daring or conforming to peer norms.

When stealing occurs in older children, becomes frequent, or involves items of value, it indicates asocial behavior and is of concern. Stealing is a particularly disturbing problem to parents. The nurse may be asked for advice by parents. Bakwin and Bakwin (1972) list four causes of stealing.

1. A lack of sense of property rights. Some parents do not allow their children any privacy either in time or possessions. They do not role-model for the child any concept of ownership. Thus the child does not learn to differentiate between what does and does not belong to him or her. Certain needs of children that can be met by parents are conducive to the prevention of stealing: (1) a child needs privacy; (2) a child needs some personal possessions, especially clothes or toys; (3) a child must be taught early to respect the property of others.
2. Bribery. Children steal in order to have the means by which to obtain the favor of classmates and peers.

3. Desire to possess. One characteristic of the child in Western society is a desire to possess material goods. If not supplied with the means (allowance or pocket money) of purchasing, the child may steal items.
4. Revengeful stealing. The child may steal to "get back" at parents for some unfair disciplinary measure or too-high expectations.

To intervene effectively with children who steal, the nurse must determine the reason(s) for the stealing. The reason is not likely to be discovered until a mutually trusting relationship is established between the nurse, the child, and the parents. Family dynamics may have to be explored, depending upon the cause that is identified. This complex issue may be resolved optimally by referring the child and family to a mental health clinic. Depending upon the severity and the outcome of the stealing episodes, legal authorities may be included in the management of this problem.

The nurse may choose to work with this family regarding the issue of stealing. Suggestions from the parents about how comfortable they are in handling this problem and the intervention options that are acceptable to them should be considered first. To prevent further episodes of stealing, the parents should be encouraged to handle the situation matter-of-factly, allowing the child to see how upset they are. By clearly demonstrating to the child that stealing is unacceptable behavior and will not be tolerated, further stealing may be prevented.

Parents can also help their child stop stealing by removing tempting items. Loose change should be out of sight. Pens and pencils should be in drawers, except for the items that belong to the child. By removing "stealable" items, the parents can reduce the internal conflict experienced by a child who steals.

Cheating

Cheating is commonly seen in the early school-age years. At age 5 or 6 years, the child may not have a clear understanding of the rules of a game or activity. The child may have an extremely competitive spirit to the extent that cheating at a particular game is more tolerable than losing. The developing superego, coupled with an inability to understand rules fully, often results in cheating behavior. It is usually of a benign, innocent nature and will disappear as the child matures. If cheating should persist and influence school or social performance, the parent or school authorities may seek help for the child.

Aggression

Aggression is defined as a pattern of intentional behavior designed to produce harm to others. As a personality trait, aggressiveness is not necessarily undesirable. If channeled into socially acceptable outlets, it may serve as a positive force helping an individual become a self-assertive, competitive member of society. In the American culture, high value is placed on "rugged individualism." However, when aggression becomes disruptive to the community, the family, or the individual's lifestyle, aggressiveness may be seen as a behavior problem.

Recent child development research has identified a number of factors in aggressive behavior. Parke and Slaby (1983), in their review of current research, discuss the child's role in the development of aggressive behavior patterns; they note that at times the child elicits responses from others leading to aggressive behavior. A child's aggressive behavior is thought to have many causes, including genetically assigned instinctual survival responses, biologic factors such as hormone levels, and acquired response patterns to environmental stimuli. Aggressive behavior problems are much more common in boys than in girls. Five times as many male as female adolescents are arrested for violent crimes. Expression of aggression varies with the developmental age of the child. Physical aggression, for example, may be inhibited in favor of a verbal expression of rage in older children with a higher level of cognitive functioning.

The overly aggressive child can be disruptive to family or school, causing parents anxiety as they try to cope with outbursts of anger. The behavior may cause discord with adult caregivers and peers, eventually causing the child to become isolated from friends or involved in acts outside the legal limits of the community. Parents have several options: they may permit certain behaviors, attempt to change the aggressive behavior, tolerate certain behaviors for the time being but not actually accept them, or use anticipatory planning to avoid situations that elicit the child's aggressive behavior.

The nurse may become involved with families experiencing difficulties in handling aggressive acting-out behavior. It is important for the nurse to assess the child and behavior fully in the context in which it occurs. Observation of actual parent-child interactions can give clues to incongruent communication of parental expectations. If possible, parents can keep a diary of prosocial and antisocial child behaviors to examine precipitating factors as well as to describe the aggressive act. Specific strategies for modifying aggressive behavior naturally vary with the age of the child and the degree of aggression. Though not universally accepted by child care experts, the following are suggested as guidelines for decreasing aggressive behaviors:

- provide activities that allow for controlled release of aggression, perhaps into more socially acceptable areas such as sports,

- teach the child to modify asocial aggressive acts by substituting more acceptable responses, such as a verbal expression of anger instead of hitting,
- defuse anger-provoking experiences by exposing the child to lower levels of frustration or through use of humor or other tension relievers,
- attempt to sensitize the child to the probable consequences of aggression—pain and hurt for the victim, punishment for the child,
- decrease the child's exposure to examples of aggression, including violent television programs, toys that stimulate aggressive play, like guns, or aggressive acts by adults or peers.

Nurses can counsel parents in child management techniques, such as the need to set consistent limits, to show affection, to reward with expressions of approval for social acts, and to assist in verbalization of frustration and anger. In discussing discipline practices, the nurse can explore use of "time outs" instead of physical punishment, use of advance warning about consequences when parental tolerance limits are about to be breeched, and immediate discussion of both the child's and the parents' perceptions of what happened and what precipitated an incident. A parenting style characterized by high control and coercive actions is discouraged.

Behavioral Alterations Associated with Nutritional Conflicts

Nutritional conflicts can lead to a number of disorders, including obesity, anorexia nervosa, and bulimia. Prevention of obesity in infancy is discussed in Chapter 18. This section discusses the assessment and treatment of children and adolescents with obesity, anorexia nervosa, and bulimia and strategies for prevention at various stages of development. Obesity may occur at any stage of development; anorexia nervosa and bulimia usually begin in adolescence, occur predominantly in females, and are accompanied by mood shifts and altered thought processes.

Obesity in Children and Adolescents

Obesity is one of the most prevalent, controversial, and potentially controllable disorders affecting children's health. It is a nutritional disorder but is also seen as a body image disturbance. Besides defining obesity, this section discusses incidence and trends, etiology, associated health problems, and nursing care for obese children and their families.

Obesity is a complex disorder affecting health and body image. The etiology is controversial, but current research and epidemiology suggest that both physical and environmental factors contribute. From infancy through adolescence, assessment entails history, physical assessment, developmental-behavioral assessment, and evaluation of family interactions. The nurse's role in prevention is to teach healthy dietary practices (see Chapter 18), identify children who are at risk, participate in the treatment plan, and counsel children and families. Measures for intervention include diet, exercise, behavior modification, peer support groups, and family involvement. A combination of strategies is the most effective approach.

Definition

Obesity is defined as an excess of fat in ratio to lean body mass (Foman and Ziegler, 1976). The diagnosis is made when weight for height is greater than the 95th percentile, skinfold thickness is greater than the 95th percentile, and the individual appears obese (Brook, 1983; Dietz, 1983). Overweight is the term generally used to describe weight that is above average for height and age.

Incidence and Trends

Between 5 and 25 per cent of children and adolescents are obese (Dietz, 1983). The risk of obesity is higher for children who have obese parents than for those whose parents are lean. If one parent is obese, a child has a 40 per cent chance of becoming obese; if two parents are obese, the risk rises to 80 per cent (Wilson, 1987). The prevalence of obesity is higher among white people than black people. The prevalence generally tends to increase with socioeconomic class; however, this tendency reverses for adult females (Garn and Clark, 1976). A generalization cannot be made that fat infants become fat children, fat adolescents, and, subsequently, fat adults, as research is still inconclusive. However, obese children are at risk for remaining obese throughout their lives (Canadian Pediatric Society, 1983).

Etiology

Many theories exist about the etiology of obesity, yet there are no certain answers. Bottle-feeding and early introduction of solid foods have been implicated as causes of obesity (Taitz, 1971; Shukla et al, 1972). More recently that correlation has been challenged (Weill, 1977; Foman, 1980). See Chaper 18 for further discussion of infant obesity and infant feeding practices.

One theory is that there is a sensitive period for replication of fat cells and that obese children have an increased number and size of adipose cells (Knittle et al, 1979), which is then set for life (Brook, 1972). This theory has been challenged and there is still much to learn about its significance in the etiology and persistence of obesity. Studies of metabolic rate and regulation of energy storage do not provide irrefutable answers either. Physiologic variables may play a role in predisposition to obesity rather than causing it (Dietz, 1983).

Inactivity has been cited as a causal factor in obesity, with a cyclic pattern of inactivity, obesity, tiredness during activity, avoidance of activity, poor physical condition, and weight gain (Epstein, 1983). When activity was converted into actual energy expenditure, Waxman and Stunkard (1980) found that obese boys did not expend less energy than lean controls. It is pertinent in this study that obese boys ate much more and faster than nonobese controls, and that mothers served more food to their obese sons than to lean sons of close age.

Many variables must be considered, most notably family variables. As has been shown by large projects such as the Ten State Nutrition Survey (USDHEW, 1972) and the Tecumseh Community Health Survey (Garn et al, 1981), obesity tends to run in families, and the risk of obesity increases as the number of obese members in the family increases. This seems to indicate a genetic cause, but the tendency also exists for families with adopted children (Garn et al, 1981) and for spouses (Garn and Clark, 1976). Family correlates are strong but not explained by genetics. The epidemiology implies that conditions within the family system influence the development of obesity.

The set-point (or *appestat*) theory proposes that there is a control system in each individual that keeps body weight at a relatively stable level. The level, or set point, is maintained through metabolism; that is, when excess calories are taken in, the metabolic rate increases to burn the excess, and when calories are restricted, metabolism decreases. This theory explains why it is difficult for a thin person to gain weight and an obese person to lose weight.

A contributing factor worth mentioning is television, which perpetuates inactivity and the consumption of empty calories (Dietz and Gortmaker, 1985).

With present knowledge, it cannot be determined why some children take in more energy or expend less than others. It is prudent to consider both physiologic and environmental variables in childhood obesity.

Assessment

The major reasons for doing a nutritional assessment are (1) to identify dietary practices of the family; (2) to obtain baseline data of calorie and nutrient intake and anthropometric measurements; (3) to promote healthful dietary practices through counseling and teaching; and (4) to provide parents with the opportunity to express concerns and ask questions about nutrition and feeding behaviors. (See Chapter 18 for discussion of performing a nutritional assessment.)

When obesity is a problem, the assessment focuses on factors that might contribute to the problem. Consideration must be given to the possibility of an underlying disease. Obesity may be part of a central nervous system disorder (trauma, tumor), drugs, an endocrine disorder (hypothyroidism, Cushing syndrome), chromosomal abnormalities (Klinefelter or Turner syndrome), or a congenital syndrome such as Prader-Willi (Wilson, 1987).

The assessment also takes into consideration that physical and psychosocial problems are associated with obesity. Obesity is the primary cause of pediatric hypertension (Rames et al, 1978). Diabetes, cardiovascular disease, and orthopedic and respiratory conditions may be consequences of or aggravated by obesity (Royal College of Physicians, 1983). Children's physical fitness is compromised because of obesity (Epstein et al, 1983; Ylitalo, 1981), and it often leads to feelings of inferiority and negative self-images. During adolescence, there is a susceptibility to poor body image and feelings of being different from peers. The stress of normal changes can be compounded by obesity, especially puberty-onset obesity (Shestowsky, 1983). Whether poor self-concept is a precursor or a consequence of obesity remains unanswered.

A nutritional history should be performed (see Chapter 18), with particular attention being given to child and family interactions associated with food, including

- How is food used in the home?
- Are there rules associated with meal time and amount of food intake?
- What attempts have been made to correct obesity?
- Are there family conflicts associated with food intake?
- Are the child and family motivated to correct the problem of obesity?
- Does the child eat while watching television?

Therapeutic Management and Nursing Strategies

Obesity is managed according to the child's developmental stage. A growing infant or child has different nutritional needs than does an adolescent. The problems faced at the various ages are also quite different because of the issue of control. Who controls what the child eats becomes an important question to consider in management.

Infant and Child. *Infant* obesity is managed primarily through preventive strategies and is discussed in Chapter 18. Encouragement of breastfeeding and teaching appropriate bottle-feeding and the adding of solid foods are the major areas of intervention.

For the *child* who is obese, family involvement is also essential. When seen as a family problem, it is less likely for any one person to feel ultimately responsible for the obesity and its treatment. The child will not have the burden of guilt, thus preventing further harm to self-image. Family involvement decreases the likelihood that the child will be used as a scapegoat for other family disturbances. Counseling regarding discipline is necessary if the parents have difficulty setting limits. Implementing treatment plans will be difficult if a child is in control of the family (Dietz, 1983). Unless the family and youngster are motivated to lose weight, weight loss is unlikely to occur. Nurses need to motivate them to accomplish the loss.

Management of dietary intake is the main mode of treatment. The goal in calorie reduction is a slowing of the rate of weight gain while linear growth continues. A very low-calorie diet is contraindicated because it can result in loss of lean body mass and nutritional deficits.

For severely obese children (over 170 per cent ideal body weight) or those with complications such as hypertension, dietary restrictions will need to be more extreme (Dietz, 1983). These children require careful medical, nursing, and dietary management, and are often hospitalized. For mild-to-moderate obesity, reducing intake of fat and high-carbohydrate snacks will often result in slowing weight gain. The diet must be nutritionally adequate and individualized for a child's age, activity level, and preferences (see Box 18-1 for Recommended Dietary Allowances). Family culture and socioeconomic class need to be considered. Exchange lists, as those used for diabetic diets, are helpful in teaching and in providing variety. There is no need for separate meals or expensive dietetic foods for the child. The obese child should eat at the table with the family, not alone or in front of the television. High-calorie snacks must be removed from the house and replaced with low-calorie nutritious snacks, but an occasional treat should be allowed (Hagenbuch, 1982).

Exercise is important in improving fitness and expending energy. Toddlers and preschoolers need ample opportunity to play, jump, run, and dance. This can be encouraged if families exercise or walk together. School-age children are encouraged to participate in school, scouting, or community center activities; however, an obese child may resist these activities initially because of poor self-concept. Organized activities are especially important in summer when a child may feel bored or lonely. Unless the child is particularly eager, competitive sports are best delayed until self-confidence is improved (Hagenbuch, 1982). Biking, walking, swimming, and dancing are noncompetitive activities families can do together. It is important for all exercises to begin slowly, gradually extending effort and time.

Behavioral treatments have been shown to be highly effective in weight control (Lansky and Brownell, 1982). Based on learning theory principles, children are given positive reinforcement for desirable behaviors. Children then continue to behave in ways that are rewarded. For toddlers, praise and affection, not cookies, should be given when they remember to sit on the toilet. Preschoolers should get praise for riding a tricycle, not for emptying their plate and asking for more. A school-age child can cooperate with the family on a project of changing eating behaviors. The nurse can assist the family to agree upon behaviors to be rewarded, realistic long- and short-term goals, and appropriate rewards.

Other behavioral methods used in obesity programs are contingency contracting, self-monitoring, stimulus control, and cognitive restructuring (Brownell and Stunkard, 1978). These methods are often combined into one program. Engendering behavioral changes requires persistence. If the family is highly disorganized or inconsistent in dealing with the obese child, behavioral treatments may not be effective (Dietz, 1983). The nurse should determine whether or not a family can provide the consistency needed before helping the family implement a behavior modification program.

Evaluation is ongoing during the treatment approach. Growth variables are monitored and diet is assessed to ensure adequate nutrition. Goals and plans should be revised as appropriate to meet the final goal of designated weight loss.

Adolescent. Preventive counseling is implemented if a youth gains excess weight during puberty and is also recommended for adolescents who have obese parents. Balanced diet, not the need to lose weight, is stressed.

For the adolescent who is obese, family involvement in treatment is important. In a study by Brownell and colleagues (1983), the nature of parental involvement was found to be an important variable in weight loss in adolescents. Teens were most successful in losing weight when their mothers were involved in the program but attended separate group sessions. The best approach is to consider the adolescent's need for some degree of independence and desire to have free discussion with peers. Parents can be included in learning about such things as diet, exercise, and programs to alter eating behaviors. Group sessions can be held concurrently but separately, one for adolescents and another for parents.

The basics of nutritional treatment are the same for adolescents as for children. The diet must be balanced and based on the teen's activity level and preferences. Exchange lists are helpful. Fad diets and anorectic drugs are of no value in helping to make the long-term behavioral changes necessary in maintaining weight loss. Liquid protein diets used without competent medical supervision are not safe for adolescents. The use of drugs and surgical procedures (e.g., bypassing a portion of the intestine or occluding a large segment of the stomach) are not generally recommended for adolescents. Teens need to be warned of the hazards of overzealous dieting and encouraged to seek safe, enduring methods.

Adolescents are present-oriented and want fast results. They may give up a healthy diet when fast results are not attained. They should be told that it will take time before they see the results of their efforts. They and their families will need considerable encouragement to accomplish the goal.

Cases of morbid obesity may require severe caloric restrictions in the form of a protein-modified fast. These teens will need careful medical, nursing, and nutrition management. As adolescents are peer oriented, the group approach is very suitable. The best types of weight control programs for teens incorporate group support sessions, diet, exercise, behavior modification, and family involvement. These programs can be school-based (Nelson et al, 1983; Lansky and Brownell, 1982) or clinic-based (Brown et al, 1983; Meyer and Neumann, 1977). Both have been shown to be very effective.

Group approaches described by Cecere (1983) and Langford (1981) have sought to improve the self-images of the participants. Langford's objectives (p. 557) are

1. A peer group from which mutual support and help could be derived in dealing with a common problem
2. An atmosphere that could foster self-awareness, self-acceptance, and self-understanding
3. A place to gain confidence in social and interpersonal relationships
4. An opportunity to explore different types of physical activity in a "safe" environment
5. Encouragement to carry these newly acquired skills into everyday life

One role of nurses working with obese teens is to ensure that the total person is the focus of care. These objectives place emphasis on the adolescent and not on the fat.

As with younger children, response to treatment must be evaluated in teens. Goals will need to be reassessed and treatment plans revised.

Anorexia Nervosa

Anorexia nervosa means an abnormal or nervous lack of appetite. The term is a misnomer for a disorder that is marked by the individual's preoccupation with eating and preparing food. The appetite may, in fact, be insatiable, but the victim engages in self-starvation.

Incidence

It is estimated that this condition occurs in 1 of 100 American females between the ages of 16 and 18 years. The female-to-male ratio is 9:1. There is a bimodal distribution with one peak from 13 to 14 and another at 17 to 18 years of age. Compiled statistics from many studies indicate that only 50 per cent of anorectics who are treated recover in 2 to 5 years (Neuman and Halvorson, 1983). The other 50 per cent remain ill or follow a declining course that results in death in 15 to 21 per cent of the cases (American Psychiatric Association, 1980).

Assessment and Diagnosis

The individual who exhibits symptoms of anorexia nervosa is characteristically described by family members as an exceptional student, neat, compliant, overly sensitive, quiet, and perfectionistic. Typically, family and teachers describe the individual as a child who "never gave us any trouble." There is some indication that anorexia nervosa is a symptom of certain family characteristics. Minuchin et al (1978) identified rigidity, overprotection, enmeshment, and lack of conflict resolution as characteristics of families with an anorectic member. Selvini-Palazzoli (1985) also found denial of conflict to be a characteristic interactive pattern between the marital couple. Organic etiology such as hypothalamic-pituitary dysfunction is also considered as an explanation for this disorder.

Identification in the early stage of anorexia may be difficult because initially there are no overt signs. Complaints may be vague, such as fatigue and irritability (Crawshaw, 1985) or may include gastrointestinal disturbance, a menstrual disorder, or an athletic injury (due to compulsive exercise) (Muscari, 1987). Food rituals may be detected early in the course of the problem, including bizarre eating habits such as eating without the lips touching the utensil, weighing each bite of food, cutting food into minute pieces and pushing it around the plate, or silent chanting during the eating ritual. Other behaviors include excessive exercising and compulsive weighing of oneself; self-induced vomiting, taking diuretics, laxatives, and appetite-suppressants; and intense interest in the eating behaviors of others. Symptoms may vary as the condition becomes chronic. Initially there is weight loss, which may be reinforced by positive comments from others until it progresses to a significant and noticeable degree. As weight drops the individual may experience amenorrhea, growth of lanugo, fatigue, constipation, hypotension, dependent edema, and bradycardia. Clinical signs indicative of nutritional deficiencies are listed in Table 36-1.

Emotional symptoms of anxiety and fear are present but are usually consciously denied. With the

Table 36-1. Clinical Signs of Nutritional Deficiencies

General appearance	Lethargy, excessive or inadequate body fat, muscle wasting
Skin	Dryness, flakiness, scaling, roughness (follicular hyperkeratosis), pallor
Mouth	Angular fissures, redness at corners of mouth (cheilosis); redness, swelling or atrophic papillae on tongue; red, swollen or bleeding gums
Teeth	Severe caries
Eyes	Pale conjunctivae
Nails	Spoon-shaped, brittle or ridged
Hair	Dull, easily plucked

onset of symptoms in puberty, issues of sexuality and independence are not resolved and the behaviors may represent a regression to earlier stages of development. As the victim denies the need for food, she or he expresses an exaggerated need to control self and others. In the words of a recovered victim of the disorder, "Anorexia acts as a metaphor for all the problems of adolescence," and one solution will eradicate all the problems at once (MacLeod, 1982).

Specific criteria for the diagnosis of anorexia nervosa, provided by the American Psychiatric Association (1987) are as follows:

A. Refusal to maintain body weight over a minimal normal weight for age and height, e.g., weight loss leading to maintenance of body weight 15 per cent below that expected; or failure to make expected weight gain during period of growth, leading to body weight 15 per cent below that expected.
B. Intense fear of gaining weight or becoming fat, even though underweight.
C. Disturbance in the way in which one's body weight, size, or shape is experienced, e.g., the person claims to "feel fat" even when emaciated, believes that one area of the body is "too fat" even when obviously underweight.
D. In females, absence of at least three consecutive menstrual cycles when otherwise expected to occur (primary or secondary amenorrhea). (A woman is considered to have amenorrhea if her periods occur only following hormone, e.g., estrogen, administration.)

Therapeutic Management and Nursing Strategies

Without treatment, or when treatment is unsuccessful, the course of the disorder may be unremitting. Debilitation may then lead to death by starvation. Of those who do recover, many are left with phobias and compulsions that continue to dominate their lives.

The treatment of the individual with anorexia nervosa depends on a number of variables including age, length or chronicity of illness, physical and emotional symptoms of decompensation, family dynamics, and physical complications.

Three types of psychologic treatment have been used with some success and represent different theories of etiology and treatment. The psychodynamic approach of Hilde Bruch (1973) consists of intensive psychotherapy over long periods of time. A more aggressive approach to psychotherapy, suggested by Steven Levenkron (1982), is that of the nurturant-authoritarian. In contrast to traditional psychotherapy, the hallmark of this therapeutic approach is to help the individual accept dependence and feel safe when receiving nurturing rather than giving it. Family systems therapy has been advocated by several researchers and may be used in conjunction with other psychotherapies. Behavior modification and hospitalization may also be used to supplement family systems therapy. In this paradigm the interaction of family members is stressed and the anorexic individual is supported in communicating personal needs and anxieties within the family circle.

Behavior modification has been used extensively for those hospitalized with the disorder. With this approach a system of rewards or privileges is established to reinforce desirable behaviors conducive to weight gain and maintenance. Long-term effectiveness of this method used alone is not promising.

Hospitalization is often required when the individual has chronic symptoms. Psychoactive drugs may be needed to alter mood (particularly depression or anxiety or both), and parenteral nutrition is needed to restore electrolyte balance and nutritional deficiencies.

Nurses encounter adolescents with anorexia nervosa in a variety of professional settings. Often nurses are the first to assess behaviors, emotions, and attitudes expressed by patients or their family members that may lead to diagnosis of the disorder. Thus it is imperative that the nurse be alert to the many symptoms that may indicate a problem. More specifically, the nurse who cares for the hospitalized anorectic must be careful to monitor intake and output and observe eating patterns, family interactions, and compulsive behaviors.

Because the individuals with the disorder have such a strong need to control all variables in their life, the nurse must be cautious not to enter into a power struggle with them. Firm limits applied with kindness are more helpful than sympathetic permissiveness.

It can be very frustrating to work with victims of anorexia nervosa, because of the consistent enforcement of rules that is required. Patients require the services of a competent team in which professionals can support one another. Nurses *usually* are the profes-

> *National Organizations*
>
> American Anorexia and Bulimia Association, 133 Cedar Lane, Teaneck, NJ 07666
>
> National Association for Anorexia Nervosa and Related Disorders, Box 271, Highland Park, IL 60035
>
> National Anorexic Aid Society, The Bridge Foundation, 550 South Cleveland Ave., Suite F, Westerville, OH 43081
>
> Anorexia Nervosa and Bulimia Resource Center, 2699 South Bayshore Dr., Suite 800 F, Coconut Grove, FL 33133

sionals who monitor the individual's behavior on a daily basis during hospitalization; they particularly need the support of team members.

Organizations that provide assistance and information for anorectic patients are listed in the accompanying box.

Bulimia

Bulimia is an eating disorder characterized by episodes of binge eating alternating with purge behavior. The individual is aware that the behaviors of over-eating and then ridding the body of food are erratic. Patients often express fear that it is impossible to voluntarily control these activities.

Incidence

The precise incidence of bulimia in the United States is not known. However, the pattern of binge eating, anxiety over weight gain, and subsequent purging is on the increase. One survey of college students found that 13 per cent of the student population displayed the major symptoms of bulimia (Halmi et al, 1981). Onset of the condition is usually in adolescence, and it occurs more frequently in females than in males.

Assessment and Diagnosis

Symptoms of bulimia may not be readily apparent. Onset may be gradual and the condition becomes chronic with alternate periods of normal eating, fasting, binging, and purging. Binging consists of rapid intake of large amounts of food, usually with high caloric content and sweet taste, within a short period of time, usually less than 2 hours. Purging may consist of self-induced vomiting, excessive use of laxatives, or a combination.

Most individuals are within the normal weight range for height and age. They express undue concern about their weight and conflicts about eating and dieting. They engage in self-destructive thoughts and frequently exhibit depressed affect.

Specific diagnostic criteria are provided by the American Psychiatric Association (1987) as follows:

A. Recurrent episodes of binge eating (rapid consumption of a large amount of food in a discrete period of time).
B. A feeling of lack of control over eating behavior during the eating binges.
C. The person regularly engages in either self-induced vomiting, use of laxatives or diuretics, strict dieting or fasting, or vigorous exercise in order to prevent weight gain.
D. A minimum average of two binge eating episodes a week for at least three months.
E. Persistent overconcern with body shape and weight.

In addition to these symptoms, many individuals with the disorder experience distorted body image similar to that found in people with anorexia nervosa. They may engage in experimentation with or abuse of amphetamines, barbiturates, and alcohol. Studies have also shown that depression is common among bulimics (Killen et al, 1987; Walsh et al, 1985). Physical complications may include potassium depletion with subsequent cardiac arrest, spastic colitis, tetany, tooth discoloration and decay, hypertension, and esophageal and/or gastric perforation.

Therapeutic Management and Nursing Strategies

The treatment of individuals with bulimia consists of physiologic regulation and cognitive and behavioral therapies, in addition to psychotherapy and family counseling. Physiologic regulation of electrolyte imbalance and digestive irregularities must be provided. Antidepressive drugs may be used in conjunction with withdrawal from other abused substances.

Cognitive approaches address the self-destructive thoughts of the person. Self-affirmations and assertiveness training are used to provide cues for constructive thought processes. Behavior modification is also used to provide external rewards for appropriate eating behaviors and adaptive coping behaviors.

Psychodynamic, nurturant-authoritarian, group, and family therapies are used in treating the psychologic component. Results of these approaches are highly variable and new approaches are continuously being sought (Kelly and Liter, 1984).

The nursing process is used in assessing behaviors, thoughts, and affect of the individual with symptoms of bulimia. Following diagnosis nurses may provide inpatient physical care and/or counseling sessions with individuals, groups, or families. It is imperative that the nurse give attention to the physical, emotional, and social variables that interact within the patient. Resistance to treatment is common, and nurses must attend to their own feelings of frustration and self-doubt when working closely with these individuals. Treatment modalities aimed at physical symptoms, cognitive processes, emotional coping, and interpersonal processes are provided and evaluated. Assistance and information about eating disorders can be obtained from various organizations. (See list in the box on page 1127.)

Substance Use and Abuse

Substance use is not a new phenomenon, as it has existed throughout history. Peculiar to this decade are the specific agents used and the prevalence of substance use by adolescents. The prevalence, effects on physical and psychosocial development, and possible harmful consequences of psychoactive substances give impetus for nursing involvement.

Mood-altering substances have a substantial impact on the welfare of adolescents. Drug and alcohol abuse are associated with each of the three leading causes of death among adolescents: accidents, homicides, and suicides (Petchers et al, 1988). Some chemical substances such as caffeine, nicotine, tranquilizers, and alcohol (if used moderately) are sanctioned by society; however, these too can lead to physical and psychologic dependence.

Substance use refers to the use of drugs (including alcohol) or volatile inhalants for the purpose of altering mood, state of consciousness, or improving performance. *Substance abuse* is the use of any substance to the extent that it interferes with an individual's relationships, school, work, physical or emotional health, or is harmful to others (Williams, 1980a).

Developmental, familial, and societal factors contribute to the etiology of substance use and abuse, and the patterns of use range from experimental to dependent. All adolescents are at risk for experimental and recreational use, but those who are at risk for chronic habits are those who are unconventional in values and behavior and who come from unstable families. The nurse's role is to identify adolescent substance users and those at risk for substance abuse; to work in the prevention of intoxicant-related accidents and prevention of substance abuse; and to provide nursing care and counseling in the treatment and rehabilitation of adolescent substance abusers.

Prevalence

The drug scene is constantly changing. Cocaine has gained increasing popularity in various forms; users rose from 1.6 million in 1977 to 6 million in 1985. Use had leveled off until around 1984 when "crack" appeared on the scene, at which time the number of users again increased (Kleber, 1988). Cocaine is reported to have a dependence potential comparable to that of heroin, even when the route of administration is primarily intranasally (smoking or injecting is a more potent route) (Hasin, 1988).

The reported use of alcohol and other illicit drugs (particularly marijuana) declined from 1980 to 1984 (Johnson et al, 1986). However, 90 per cent of high school seniors report having had some experience with alcohol at least once and nearly one third of high school seniors report that all or most of their friends get drunk at least once a week (Johnson et al, 1987). Although alcohol is considered a benign drug, it is relevant that approximately 3.3 million adolescents are problem drinkers (Pallikkathayil and Tweed, 1983).

The principal psychoactive chemical in marijuana is tetrahydrocannabinol (THC). The THC concentration is much higher in marijuana sold today than it was in the 1960s. Therefore, marijuana may not be as harmless as its original users purported it to be (Silber et al, 1988). Furthermore, an increasingly serious problem related to substance abuse is the rapidly increasing occurrence of multiple substance abuse. Table 36-2 lists the main substances used by adolescents.

Etiology

Developmental Factors. Substance use may occur in school-age children. If it does, it usually denotes significant problems in the child, the family, or both, and the child and family should receive professional counseling.

Substance use is primarily a problem of adolescents and several etiologic factors are related to adolescent psychosocial development. Incentives for experimental and recreational drug use are often the same incentives as for other adolescent behavior. Developmental motives include rebelling against parental authority or the need to be independent and different from parents. Adolescents may see psychoactive substances, notably hallucinogens, as a means for self-discovery. Another motivation for substance use is the desire to be accepted into a peer group. Adolescents also learn behavior by modeling and may model substance use habits of adults whom they admire for being sophisticated, mature, or glamorous. Substance use becomes a symbol of a more mature status (Jessor, 1983). Adolescents are often simply curious and like

Table 36-2. Main Addictive Substances Used by Adolescents

Agents	Signs and Effects	Complications
Opiates		
Heroin ("H," "junk," "smack," "horse") *Route:* Inhaling ("snorting"), subcutaneous (SQ) ("skin-popping"), intravenous (IV) ("mainlining")	Drowsiness, euphoria, pain relief nausea and vomiting, miosis, needle track scars from IV use, erythema of nasal mucosa from inhaling	Constipation, menstrual disturbances, duodenal ulcer, physical and psychologic dependence, skin abscesses from IV or SQ use. From IV use: acute hepatitis, septic emboli, endocarditis *Overdose:* stupor, coma, miosis, respiratory depression, cyanosis, pulmonary edema, death *Withdrawal:* usually within 8 hours' abstinence. First yawning, then tearing, rhinorrhea, mydriasis, insomnia, "gooseflesh," cramping of voluntary muscles, vomiting, diarrhea, tachycardia, and systolic hypertension
Hallucinogens		
d-Lysergic acid diethylamide (LSD, "acid"); mescaline ("acid"); psilocybin mushrooms ("mushrooms") *Route:* by mouth (PO)	Perceptual distortions, hallucinations, mydriasis, flushing, tremors, elevations in blood pressure	Paranoia, loss of control, anxiety (bad trip), accidents, spontaneous recurrence of LSD experience (flashback), psychologic dependence *Overdose:* panic
Phencyclidine (PCP, "angel dust," "peace pills," "sheets") *Route:* PO, inhaling	Euphoria, hallucinations, perceptual distortions, emotional lability, ataxia	Accidents, anxiety, paranoia, 5–15 mg—toxic psychosis: disorientation, aggression *> 15 mg—overdose:* delirium, coma with alternating periods of wakefulness, arrhythmias, seizures, hypotension, dystonic posturing, muscular rigidity or myoclonic jerking, death
Marijuana—dried leaves and flower tops of *cannabis sativa* plant; hashish—extracted resin of plant ("grass," "joint," "reefer," "hash") *Route:* inhaled (usual), PO	Elation, relaxation, intensification of mood, acute sensory perceptions, hunger, dry oral mucosa, coughing, antiemesis, injected conjunctiva, decreased intraocular pressure	Lack of coordination, accidents, decreased concentration, short-term memory loss. Females: changes in ovulation patterns. Males: decreased testosterone levels *Large dose:* hallucinations *Chronic use:* inflammatory changes in respiratory tract, apathy, psychologic dependence *Sudden withdrawal or abstinence in chronic users:* irritability, insomnia, EEG changes
Depressants		
Alcohol *Route:* PO, beer, wine, wine coolers, whiskey	Decreased inhibitions, relaxation, diuresis, slurred speech	Impaired short-term memory, lack of coordination, impaired judgment, accidents, GI irritation, nausea and vomiting, interactions with several other drugs *Chronic abuse:* fetal alcohol syndrome in offspring of female abuser, fatty necrosis and fibrosis of liver, nutritional deficiencies. Physical and psychologic dependence (alcoholism) *Large dose:* acute gastritis, pancreatitis *Overdose:* disorientation, coma, respiratory depression, death *Withdrawal:* usually within 8 hr abstinence; anxiety, tremors, insomnia. In adolescents who have been chronic drinkers for one or more years, severe with delirium tremens and seizures
Barbiturates; usually shorter-acting: amobarbital, pentobarbital, secobarbital ("downs," "blues," "reds," "yellow jackets") *Route:* PO (usual), IV, SQ	Decreased inhibitions, sedation, slurred speech, miosis	Lack of coordination, use of amphetamines to counteract sedation, sleep deprivation due to lack of REM sleep, increased effect when used with alcohol, depression, physicial and psychologic dependence, IV or SQ complications *Overdose:* respiratory depression, coma, death *Withdrawal:* within 24 hrs. of abstinence, anxiety, headache, tremors, nausea and vomiting, cramps, tachycardia, hypotension, seizures, hallucinations
Nonbarbiturate sedatives; methaqualone (Quaalude) ("ludes") *Route:* PO	As above	Lack of coordination, use of amphetamines to counteract sedation, depression, psychologic dependence *Overdose:* respiratory depression, coma, death

continued

Table 36-2 (continued)

Agents	Signs and Effects	Complications
Stimulants		
Amphetamines (amphetamine sulfate, methamphetamine, dextroamphetamine) ("speed, uppers, bennies, dexies, black beauties") *Route:* PO, IV, SQ	Euphoria, arousal, anorexia, alertness, elevated blood pressure, mydriasis	Insomnia, use of depressants to counteract wakefulness, tachycardia, nutritional deficits, weight loss, IV and SQ complications, psychologic dependence *High dose:* anxiety, headache, tremors, impulsiveness, aggression, manic behavior, hallucinations, accidents, psychosis *Overdose:* hypertension, seizures, death *Abstinence after chronic use:* fatigue, depression
Look-alikes (contain caffeine, ephedrine, phenylpropanolamine, and mixtures of other substances); sold to look like amphetamines and advertised with the "amine" or "caine" ending *Route:* PO	Alertness, anorexia	Restlessness, weight loss, insomnia, agitation, manic behavior, hallucinations, hypertension, death
Cocaine (coke, crack, snow) *Route:* Inhaled, IV, SQ	Euphoria, increased motor activity, local anesthesia. If inhaled: injected nasal mucosa, rhinorrhea	Tachycardia, hypertension, hyperthermia, psychologic dependence, complications of IV and SQ use *Chronic use:* hallucinations, paranoid ideation, perforated nasal septum
Volatile Substances		
Substances contain toluene, hydrocarbons, or fluorocarbons: glue, gasoline, cleaning solvents, lighter fluid, typing correction fluid, thinners, lacquers, aerosol sprays *Route:* Inhaled	Giddiness, confusion, decreased inhibition, injected conjunctiva, lacrimation, rhinorrhea	Decreased coordination, hallucinations, accidents, abdominal pain, nausea and vomiting, aspiration or asphyxia from inhaling substance in plastic bag, psychologic dependence. Lead poisoning from leaded gasoline, gas encephalopathy from gasoline
Miscellaneous		
Agents used in sports; anabolic steroids *Route:* PO	No proven increase in muscle development and strength. Larger appearance sometimes due to water and sodium retention	Sodium and water retention, hypertension; alterations in liver functions, premature closure of epiphyses, short stature. Males: decreased testosterone production, testicular atrophy, decreased libido, gynecomastia if contains female hormones. Females: hirsutism, permanent deepening of voice, acne
Diuretics, stimulants *Route:* PO	Diuresis and weight loss	Dehydration, fluid and electrolyte disturbances
Tobacco *Route:* Inhaled, chewed	Perceived maturity and sophistication	Cough, staining of teeth and nails, heart disease, emphysema, lung cancer, bronchitis, smaller infants born to female smokers, physical and psychologic dependence *Withdrawal:* nervousness, fatigue, headache, tachycardia

(Data from Caddell, 1983; Cohen, 1983; Dietz, 1981; Hill et al, 1983; Horowitz et al, 1980; Iveson, 1982; Litt, 1983; McKerlie et al, 1983; Morton, 1983; Percy, 1983; Smith and Asch, 1982; Tashkin and Cohen, 1981; Williams, 1980a,b.)

excitement, especially when they can share something novel with friends.

Familial Factors. Families commonly play a role in substance use, especially when the pattern is an abusive one, not merely for experimental or recreational purposes. Adolescent substance abusers frequently come from dysfunctional families (Rice and Kibbee, 1983) and may feel the need for temporary escape from prolonged family conflicts. If the youth has become the scapegoat for family problems, substance abuse can perpetuate the problems and the scapegoating, and become a sequence in a cycle that is difficult to interrupt. Drug abuse may be a conscious or unconscious way to redirect attention from family difficulties. If an intolerable situation, such as physical abuse, exists, an adolescent may desire chemical escape (Pallikkathayil and Tweed, 1983). It is important not to conclude that all families of substance abusers have caused the problem. Sometimes family conflicts are consequences, rather than precursors, of an adolescent's habits.

Societal Factors. Societal factors contribute to the etiology of substance abuse. Enticements from the media make smoking and drinking appear glamorous. Antihistamine- and caffeine-containing diet and energy pills are openly advertised. Western culture is a drug-taking culture in which people expect quick pharmaceutical cures for all ailments. Psychoactive substances are readily available to adolescents (Parcell, 1982). In cities, dealers come to schools and parks to sell drugs. The availability of cocaine in a cheaper form (crack) has signaled a dramatic increase in its use. Drugs such as phencyclidine (PCP) are easily synthesized in school laboratories.

A lack of hope may engender substance use. If youths cannot feel optimistic about the future, it is likely for them to live for pleasures of the moment. Distraction and oblivion are appealing, particularly for adolescents who have never learned to feel competent or to feel as if anyone or anything will respond to their efforts.

Patterns of Substance Use

Experimental. The experimental use of substances is inspired by curiosity and desire to experience something new. Usually the initial experience is with an older friend or sibling. It is nonpatterned and does not interfere with daily activities. The risks of experimental use are further use and accidents.

Recreational. Recreational use mainly refers to using alcohol and marijuana at parties. It is usually controlled and nonprogressive but the risks of more intensive use and accidents exist.

Circumstantial. Circumstantial use of substances occurs when the teen feels the need for help with a problem or situation. For example, alcohol may be used to help numb the aftermath of a family argument, or amphetamines may be used to stay awake and study. Parents commonly notice changes in behavior, friends, and appearance. Circumstantial use is often the dividing line between use and abuse. The dangers are interference with relationships, school, or work, and again, further use and accidents.

Intensive. Intensive use involves daily substance abuse. The teen feels a need for the drug in order to keep performing and often uses it alone and before school. Alcohol and marijuana may be the primary drugs used; the teen may have progressed to harder drugs, such as heroin; or there may be polydrug use (use of a number of drugs). There is typically school failure and truancy. Drugs are expensive, and the adolescent may steal from parents or shops, or may sell drugs to others to get the money. Family problems surface, and intensify, and the substance abuse heightens in response to the family problems.

Dependent. *Psychologic dependence* is a "strong psychological drive to continue the use of a chemical. Though anxiety may result if the drug is discontinued, there is no associated physical symptomology" (Williams, 1980a, page 162). If *physically dependent,* the user will experience "a set of symptoms, a withdrawal syndrome, if the drug is abruptly discontinued" (Williams, 1980a, page 162). Most substances can stimulate psychologic dependence, but not all will cause physical dependence. With psychologic and physical dependence, the abuser is obsessed with the substance and with obtaining the next dose. Chemically dependent adolescents are often depressed, may be suicidal, are in poor physical condition, and may be physically ill. They may have experienced overdoses or periods of memory loss, called blackouts. They no longer attend school or work. Family members become preoccupied with the adolescent and relations within the family deteriorate (Coupey and Schonberg, 1982; Parcel, 1982; Macdonald, 1984).

Risks and Prevention

All contemporary adolescents are at risk for experimental and recreational substance use. Experience with alcohol, cocaine, and marijuana is common and may even be considered normal in the light of growing up in modern Western society. However typical substance use may be, one cannot predict which adolescents will progress to having more chronic habits. Following are risk factors for adolescents who may become substance abusers as compared with light substance users or with those who do not use drugs (Jessor, 1983):

- tend to be more rebellious
- place more emphasis on independence than academic achievement and are more distrustful of conventional establishments
- are not as certain of societal norms or of familial expectations
- have more lenient attitudes about right and wrong, are not as religious, and are not as interested in customary activities of community, school, and church
- are more likely to have other problem behaviors, such as aggression or stealing
- perceive less support and control from parents
- behavior more influenced by their peers than by their families

Unstable family situations increase the risk for substance abuse. Children of alcoholics, for example, are known to be at risk for alcoholism. It has not been determined whether this fact is explained by genetics, personality factors, or a combination thereof (US Department of Health and Human Services, 1987).

Nurse's Role in Prevention. Nurses may not be able to prevent experimental and recreational substance use, but they must help in the prevention of intoxicant-related accidents and in the prevention of more intense drug habits. Nurses can be active in preventive strategies by encouraging the raising of the drinking age and by supporting initiatives to institute strict penalties for drinking and driving.

Another role of the nurse in prevention is to participate in school-based prevention programs. Panel discussions and fear tactics have not been found to be effective approaches. Today, programs are incorporating education, peer teaching, and parental involvement. Teachers are using tactics to help teens make knowledgable and value-based choices. Programs also include teaching problem-solving skills, ways to resist social pressure, methods of improving communication with parents, and other ways of feeling good about oneself, such as creative writing or athletics. Teaching strategies can be small group discussions and role-playing (Coe et al, 1982; Pallikkathayil and Tweed 1983; Parcel, 1982).

Programs should be presented in elementary school, in junior high school, and again in high school. Pediatric nurses can help plan programs and can review teaching material to see that it is age-appropriate. Nurses can also educate teachers in how to identify pupils at risk for drug abuse and how to manage drug emergencies at school.

Summer is an especially drug-prone time for youths who are unemployed, bored, and frustrated. Nurses can encourage community leaders and businesses to support teens for camps, or for special studies or training.

When risk factors for substance abuse are identified, counseling is indicated. If the teen has a primary health care provider, he or she should be notified first. The family nurse practitioner or physician will usually know the family best and should be involved in the referral process if intensive therapy is needed. Otherwise, school nurses and counselors are excellent resources for counseling and screening for serious problems.

Assessment

Adolescents who are using substances, or who are suspected of doing so, should be interviewed alone with the assurance of confidentiality. The teen should be told that parents will not be informed of any information given in confidence unless he or she is in danger or is hurting others. If the youth, rather than parent or teacher, has initiated the visit, the chief complaint is rarely drug abuse, but instead, vague complaints of abdominal pain, headache, or fatigue (Macdonald, 1984). These physical discomforts must be evaluated first as they may be legitimate, and automatically asking, "Are you doing drugs?" will close the interview fast. After taking a routine history, the subject of substance use may be approached. The use of drugs and alcohol among friends and classmates should be discussed in a general way first. If the interviewer is nonjudgmental and conveys a caring attitude, teens will usually continue on to discuss their own substance use. They are often relieved to have a professional who can listen and help.

It is important to ascertain the specific agents used; when, where, and how often they are used; and if the teen is alone when using them. School, grades, and work should be discussed. In addition, vital questions to ask are: Do you feel lonely or depressed? How are you getting along with friends, boyfriends or girlfriends, and family? Do you believe that your substance use is interfering with school or home? Does your family see it as a problem? Have you ever done anything reckless while intoxicated? (American Academy of Pediatrics, 1983).

A complete physical assessment will need to be performed. Physical signs of substance use are not usually found unless the adolescent is intoxicated at the time or the pattern of use is intensive or dependent (see Table 36-2 for physical effects of specific drugs).

Therapeutic Management and Nursing Strategies

The pattern of substance use will be determined through the assessment. As discussed earlier, experimental or recreational use necessitates preventive measures. Circumstantial use requires counseling regarding the circumstances that are causing the substance use. Other ways of dealing with stress should be addressed. Teens who are lonely, depressed, or having school or family problems require more intensive individual or family therapy.

Patterns of abuse that are intensive or dependent clearly necessitate family or individual therapy or both. A physically dependent adolescent will need *detoxification,* "the physiologic process of reducing the toxicity of a substance" (Williams, 1980b, page 428). Whether or not an adolescent is hospitalized or placed in a detoxification unit depends on the specific agent abused and on the teen's mental and physical condition. For example, adolescents dependent on alcohol and barbiturates will need medical supervision during withdrawal. The nurse's role during withdrawal is to calm the patient, and monitor vital signs, blood pressure, fluid therapy, and intake and output. Depending on the individual situation, sedatives or seizure medicines may be ordered by the physician, and the nurse is responsible for administering the proper dose and observing the adolescent for effects of the medicine.

After detoxification, the choices for rehabilitation are either admission to residential or outpatient treatment centers or private individual, group, or family therapy. Rehabilitation is very individualized and should be based on the needs of the adolescent and recommendations of the primary health care provider and specialist in adolescent drug abuse. Nurses are often employed in drug abuse rehabilitation centers and are involved in counseling the individual and family, leading group activities, and monitoring the patient's progress.

Whether the adolescent receives residential or outpatient treatment, family involvement is essential. This may be in the form of a support group for parents or conjoint family therapy. Family communication is stressed and the focus is on the health of the family rather than the pathology.

Nurses on drug rehabilitation units should understand adolescent development and principles of communicating with adolescents. When working with troubled adolescents, it is important to treat them as individuals, not as typical adolescents. Adolescents believe that their problems are unique and resent inferences of "typical adolescent behavior." The nurse should be friendly and warm but should not behave like a peer. Teens need to feel that they are in competent hands. They need professional guidance and adult role models. Nurses who try to act like peers are often manipulated by adolescents.

Other ways nurses help in drug rehabilitation programs are by leading peer group discussions, going on group outings, and assisting with physical or creative activities. Activities are important, as teens have often become so preoccupied with the substance that they forget how good other activities can feel. Pallikkathayil and Tweed (1983) refer to "alternate high" activities as replacements for chemical highs. Examples are drama, dancing, music, art, relaxation techniques, meditation, and creative writing.

Evaluation must be a part of intervention. Throughout the treatment, the nurse will evaluate the teen's response. For example: Is the teen drug-free? Is the teen developing new skills to deal with problems? Is the family supportive but firm in their expectations? Are the adolescent and family communicating with one another? Is the adolescent making plans for school, work, or doing things with friends? Treatment may need to be revised based on evaluation of the response to the present treatment. For example, if the family can only argue when they are together, it might be better to have individual counseling sessions.

Prognosis

Prognosis depends on the extent of the problems preceding substance use, the intensity of use, and residual physical or mental effects of the substance.

Depression

Depression is generally defined as overall feelings of sadness or hopelessness. Traditionally depression was thought to occur only after about age 15; however, health professionals are increasingly recognizing the existence of depression in younger children.

Incidence

Estimates of occurrence vary considerably because of the diverse diagnostic criteria used. A few investigations of normal children suggest a prevalence as high as 2 per cent (Kazdin, 1987). Girls are more likely than boys to suffer from depression, and it is more prevalent in adolescents than in children.

Etiology

Risk factors for depression can be genetic or environmental. Depression is known to occur within families, but it is difficult to separate the relative influence of genetics from environment. If one parent has a depressive disorder, the risk of depression for the offspring is 27 per cent; with two affected parents the risk increases to 74 per cent (Aylward, 1985). There is also evidence that children who come from families with a history of alcoholism are at greater risk for depression (Strober, 1984).

Psychosocial factors also play a part in putting a child at risk for depression. Early trauma, self-blame, rigid family dynamics, a disturbance in mother-child relationships, or an unresolved loss experience have been reported to be precursors to depression (Valente, 1983). Any loss, such as the death of a loved one, rejection by a parent, a family move, divorce, abuse and maltreatment, or long-term hospitalization, puts a child at risk. Another contributing factor may be loss of self-esteem; learning disabilities, chronic illness, or physical deformity may affect a child's self-esteem (Aylward, 1985).

The study of biologic correlates in adults has recently been extended to children. These studies involve investigation of growth hormone secretion, cortisol hypersecretion, and level of norepinephrine secretion.

Debate continues about whether depression exists in childhood and if it does how to explain the phenomenon. Viewpoints within psychiatry include the following (Kazdin, 1987):

1. Depression in childhood is not possible because it is a phenomenon of the superego and the handling of aggression; the superego is not developed until adolescence.
2. Depression in childhood can exist, but its manifestations differ from those in the adult; in children it is "masked" by behaviors such as phobias, school refusal, tantrums, and others.
3. Symptoms of depression are part of normal development and are, therefore, transitory.
4. Depression is similar in children and adults; core features of depression are similar across the age spectrum, although there may be some variation in its expression according to developmental level.

The most widely adopted viewpoint is that depression has some core features and that it is expressed with some variation across the life span.

Clinical Manifestations and Assessment

According to the American Psychiatric Association (1987), the criteria to diagnose a major depressive syndrome in children are the same as for adults and are as follows:

A. At least five of the following symptoms have been present during the same two-week period and represent a change from previous functioning; at least one of the symptoms is either (1) depressed mood, or (2) loss of interest or pleasure. (Do not include symptoms that are clearly due to a physical condition, mood-incongruent delusions or hallucinations, incoherence, or marked loosening of associations.)
   1. depressed mood (or can be irritable mood in children and adolescents) most of the day, nearly every day, as indicated either by subjective account or observation by others
   2. markedly diminished interest or pleasure in all, or almost all, activities most of the day, nearly every day (as indicated either by subjective account or observation by others of apathy most of the time)
   3. significant weight loss or weight gain when not dieting (e.g., more than 5 per cent of body weight in a month), or decrease or increase in appetite nearly every day (in children, consider failure to make expected weight gains)
   4. insomnia or hypersomnia nearly every day
   5. psychomotor agitation or retardation nearly every day (observable by others, not merely subjective feelings of restlessness or being slowed down)
   6. fatigue or loss of energy nearly every day
   7. feelings of worthlessness or excessive or inappropriate guilt (which may be delusional) nearly every day (not merely self-reproach or guilt about being sick)
   8. diminished ability to think or concentrate, or indecisiveness nearly every day (either by subjective account or as observed by others)
   9. recurrent thoughts of death (not just fear of dying), recurrent suicidal ideation without a specific plan, or a suicide attempt or a specific plan for committing suicide

Clinical manifestations that vary with developmental level have not been clearly established during the early years. Depression can go unrecognized because it is masked. See Box 36-1 for a categorization of how depression may present at the various ages (Aylward, 1985).

The nurse needs to differentiate between normal periods of depressed moods, which are brief and fade away, and profound depression, which persists and tends to get progressively worse. A youth with this latter type of depression behaves noticeably in an irritable, tense manner and gives indications of lowered self-esteem. In identifying depression, the nurse will note that depression takes different forms. In some situations the depression will resemble adult depression. These youths may appear withdrawn; they may talk freely about feeling sad and lonely, rejected, and depressed; or, overwhelmed by feelings of despair and hopelessness, they may express suicidal thoughts. However, more often depression may take the form of somatic complaints such as changes in eating patterns ranging from anorexia to overeating, digestive complaints such as constipation, changes in sleeping habits ranging from insomnia to persistent fatigue, or changes in productivity such as slow speech, slow thought processes, or even school failure.

Behavioral changes may present in the form of destructive, disruptive, or aggressive acting-out behavior. The youth may become defiant, truant, or delinquent or may repeatedly run away from home. In attempts to deny depression, adolescents may resort to drugs, alcohol or sexual promiscuity.

Nurses should obtain a social-mental health history on all children to assess for the loss of some significant relationship. Loss is recognized as a primary etiologic agent in triggering the onset of depression. The

Box 36-1
Categorization of Depression at Various Ages

Infancy
(Biologic and deprivation syndromes)
Feeding problems and sleep difficulty
Affective disturbances (blank stare, apathy)
Excessive, irritability or lethargy
Failure to thrive or rumination

Early Childhood (3–4 years)
(Abnormal motor activity)
High levels of activity
Physical aggressiveness, protecting behavior, and demonstrations of anger
Enuresis, encopresis
Separation anxiety
Social withdrawal
Sleeping and eating problems
Sad or irritable, emotionally labile and clinging behavior

Middle Childhood (5–8 years)
(More observable episodes of sadness; child still not reflective)
Somatization disorders
Social withdrawal
Lying, stealing
Accident proneness
Physical aggression and oppositional behavior
Academic underachievement
Self-esteem problems (self-blame, guilt)
Perceived rejection by parents

Late Childhood (9–12 years)
(Involves low self-esteem and disappointment with self)
Social isolation, especially from peers
Obvious sadness
Apathy
Sense of helplessness
Irritability
Somatization disorders
Anhedonia (no pleasure in usual activities)
Psychogenic pain
Unable to concentrate
School problems
Self-endangering behavior
Suicidal ideation, and suicide attempts

Adolescence
Hopelessness and fear of the future
Looks at options in an inflexible all-or-none manner
Feels things will never change
Somatization disorders
Psychogenic pain
Anorexia nervosa
Drug abuse
Antisocial behavior
Social withdrawal
Verbalization of suicidal thoughts and suicidal attempts

nurse may find that there has been a death or divorce in the family, an alteration in some significant relationship with a friend, or loss of a loved pet. Sometimes the depression may stem from shifting adolescent boyfriend-girlfriend relationships or from more serious problems such as abortion or diagnosis of illness.

Depressive symptoms that persist for longer than 6 months, that are perceived to occur much more often in the patient than in peers, or that involve the child's serious consideration of suicide are of grave concern and require immediate further evaluation by a qualified professional.

Therapeutic Management and Nursing Strategies

Once the presence and severity of the depression are recognized, the nurse's role involves seeking appropriate referrals for the child so that a therapeutic treatment plan can be established. The treatment plan ideally is designed in consultation with a mental health professional. In addition to making referrals, the role of the pediatric nurse is to establish a trusting relationship with the depressed youth in which the nurse is seen as a caring professional. Early nursing interventions may include acknowledging how "down" the youth seems to be and aiding in the verbal expression of his or her feelings. Treatment methods vary and may range from short-term counseling regarding the development of coping strategies to individual or group psychotherapy, play therapy, or family therapy.

The depressed child's family may need support, especially during the period of diagnosis and early treatment. It is important for both the pediatric nurse and the psychiatric clinician to maintain contact with the family, using open, honest communication. Many of the youth's behaviors reflect a long-standing maladaptive behavior pattern. The nurse needs to assess the family's expectations about treatment and to help them realize that treatment may take time to succeed. Many experts believe it is essential for the family to be involved in the treatment plan in order to assist in identifying factors within the family that contribute to the child's problem.

Nursing interventions that help adults develop their parenting skills will foster healthy parent-child relationships. Promoting open communication between parent and child is a major area of concern for nurses. An assessment of mental health status is often overlooked in dealing with pediatric clients. Incorporating a brief mental health assessment in the nursing data base obtained for each child may result in increased recognition and treatment of depression. Specific teaching about stress coping strategies may help prevent serious outcomes of depression such as suicide.

Suicide

Current Centers for Disease Control statistics place suicide as the third leading cause of death in the 15- to 24-year-old age category (Valente and Saunders, 1987), preceded by accidents and homicide (Table 36-3). There is speculation that the actual numbers of deaths by suicide may be higher than reported figures. Since suicide produces tremendous guilt feelings in the survivors, death in which suicide is not clearly evident may be attributed to natural causes or labeled accidental. An example is the single-vehicle automobile accident in which a direct cause cannot be determined.

A difference exists between adolescent boys and girls regarding successful suicidal efforts. Although girls are more likely to attempt suicide, which should be interpreted as a cry for help, boys have a much higher suicide rate, up to four times that of girls. Another fact of importance is that with each succeeding attempt at suicide, success becomes more likely.

Suicidal methods also vary between the sexes. Girls are likely to use passive methods such as ingestion of pills. Boys, in contrast, resort to more quickly lethal methods such as hanging. The suicide rate below age 14 years is less than 1 death per 200,000 per year; it rises to 10 deaths per 100,000 per year in adolescents from 15–19 years of age (Mattsson, 1987).

Suicide attempts appear to have a direct relationship with the amount of stress experienced by the adolescent. Statistics reveal higher suicide rates among high school dropouts than among students in high school; college students have higher suicide rates than adolescents of the same age who are not in college. Other differences are noted in geographic locations. The Northern states show a higher suicide rate among black youths, whereas in the South the rate is higher among whites. A study of international statistics indicates that suicide is a relatively unimportant cause of death in developing countries (Barraclough, 1988).

Etiology

Causative factors related to adolescent suicide or attempted suicide are difficult to isolate. Suicide most likely results from the compounding of several factors. Retrospective research studies indicate that depression is a common preceding factor in many adolescent suicides. Loss of an important relationship in the child's life is an important risk factor for suicide, as it is for depression. Another commonly cited preceding factor is social isolation. Peck (1981) reports that a substantial number of suicides occur in males with isolated lifestyles and "loner" relationships. Adolescence seems to be a developmental period of increasing vulnerability for factors that have been associated with attempted and successful suicides. The task of gaining a sense of identity can lead to feelings of self-doubt and low self-esteem, particularly when adolescents compare themselves with their peers. Feelings of isolation result when adolescents perceive that their peers have greater independence, as interpreted from the social behaviors of the group. Modes of dress, interactions with the opposite sex, and independence in transportation and finance are but a few examples of social behaviors that have exaggerated importance in adolescence.

Assessment and Clinical Manifestations

Most victims of adolescent suicide have had a history of chronic childhood and family problems (Mattsson,

Table 36-3. Adolescent Suicide Incidence (Rate per 100,000)

	Age: 15–19 yr			20–24 yr		
Year	Males	Females	TOTAL	Males	Females	TOTAL
1955	4.0	1.3	2.6	8.8	2.6	5.6
1982	14.1	3.2	8.7	25.1	5.1	15.1
Per cent change	252	146	234	185	96	170

(From American Association of Suicidology, 1985.)

Box 36-2
Potential Suicide Risk Indicators

Depression
Expressed feelings of hopelessness
Lack of close friends
Feelings of isolation
Loss of a valued relationship
Feelings of sexual inadequacy
Poor self-image
Dependence on alcohol or drugs to alter mood
Disrupted family structure or communication with parents
School failure
School expulsion or suspension
Dramatic change in personality or behavior (e.g., marked change in sleep or eating patterns, disregard for personal appearance)
"Getting affairs in order" type of behavior, such as giving away valued personal possessions
Discussion of death thoughts
Threats of suicide

1987). Severe depression and suicide rarely occur spontaneously, but are preceded by emotional conflicts associated with the onset of adolescence. Potential suicide risk factors are listed in Box 36-2. Many suicidal adolescents have experienced the following warning signs for at least a month before the suicide or the attempt (Mattsson, 1987):

- decrease in school performance;
- withdrawal;
- loss of initiative;
- loneliness, sadness and crying episodes;
- appetite and sleep disturbance;
- verbalization of suicidal thoughts.

Days or weeks of loneliness precede the suicide attempt. This is often due to the loss of the few remaining relationships such as a close relative or friend.

Valente and Saunders (1987) cite the existence of a "ripple effect": bereavement and feelings of loss in response to the suicide of a friend influence other adolescents to attempt suicide.

Since pediatric nurses, especially school nurses, have daily contact with large numbers of adolescents, they have the opportunity to contribute to the prevention of suicide. Each individual needs to be assessed in terms of his or her mental health status. Assessment of mental health should be seen as an integral part of the nursing data base. Children and adolescents can be amazingly open in communicating death thoughts to a nurse in a confidential professional setting. Nurses need to be aware that many well-adjusted adolescents report thinking of death. However, such affirmative answers to the specific question "Have you ever thought about death or about killing yourself?" need to be explored in depth, with specific questions about when such thoughts occurred and about the frequency and duration of these types of thoughts. ***All threats of suicide need to be taken seriously by parents and nurses.*** Immediate referral to mental health professionals should be made ***whenever*** there is any question about the adolescent's intent.

In addition to assessing overall mental health status, pediatric nurses need to assess and teach personalized coping strategies. Coping techniques appropriate for children include actively seeking out friends, use of daily exercise and deep breathing as tension relievers, recognition of sources of stress and of one's own limitations, attempting to change stressful situations over which the youth has control or to change his or her own reactions to stressful situations over which the youth has no control. With guidance children can learn to focus on the positive aspects of stressful situations and to maximize their own coping abilities.

Therapeutic Management and Nursing Strategies

Professionals who work with suicidal youths believe that suicide is not a sudden decision, but the final result of repeated warnings given by the victims. Parents may fail to recognize behavioral changes signifying an altered emotional state. Parents may cope with such changes by denial. Nurses and teachers should be aware of the multiplicity of factors that influence adolescent behavior; they may be the first to detect significant deterioration in an adolescent's behavior and outlook. Valente and Saunders (1987) state that school and pediatric nurses "understand that many adolescents use physical complaints as a good reason to visit the school nurse to talk about their depressions, discouragements, disappointments and feelings that life may not be worth living."

The American Association of Suicidology* has been established to coordinate national suicide prevention centers and is a source of information and educational materials. The magnitude of the adolescent suicide problem has stimulated establishment of crisis intervention centers. One service offered through these agencies is a telephone hotline manned by professionals and trained volunteers. Callers are encouraged to talk through their concerns while the volunteer evaluates the immediate need of the caller. Crisis intervention techniques, along with referrals to appropriate agencies, constitute a large portion of services given by the telephone counselors. Telephone inter-

* American Association of Suicidology, 2459 South Ash, Denver, CO 80222; (303) 692-0985.

ventions have been successful in helping some, but major emphasis is still needed on education for prevention. Valente and Saunders (1987) report on the development of high school–based suicide prevention programs. Although their effectiveness is questioned by some researchers, their establishment reflects society's concern about suicide among adolescents. Adolescents need to be exposed to a comprehensive education program. They should know the scope of the suicide problem in their age group and the progressive stages of deterioration leading to suicide. Adolescent participation in prevention needs to be increased; that is, adolescents need to be granted permission through education to report the indications of potential suicide in their peers. Adolescents or adults who recognize signs or suspect a suicidal intention should never dismiss the idea, but should seek professional assistance immediately.

Warning signals include any threats of suicide or talk of personal death, such as questions about how many pills it would take to kill oneself or statements showing a belief that the family would be better off without the individual. Another danger signal may be a sudden upswing in mood in a previously depressed child or the sudden giving away of highly valued personal possessions. These behaviors can indicate that the adolescent has now actually made the decision to commit suicide. Any adolescent thought to be considering suicide should be asked about suicidal ideation. A referral to a mental health professional is required to evaluate the extent of the problem.

When an adolescent has attempted suicide, the safest course of action is hospitalization (Committee on Adolescence, 1988). Inquiry is made into the events that preceded the suicide attempt. Family members are also interviewed to determine the recent stresses and current problems of the adolescent. Intervention is individualized: some require brief, crisis-oriented intervention, whereas others show evidence of depression and psychiatric illness requiring long-term care. All adolescents who attempt suicide require carefully planned follow-up care.

Autism

Autism is a rare condition in which a child has severe problems in communication and behavior and an inability to relate to people in a normal manner. It seems to occur more frequently in males. It may be suspected as early as a few weeks or months after birth, or not until the child is 2 or 3 years of age.

Clinical Manifestations

The autistic child fails to develop normal social relationships. The child demonstrates ritualistic and compulsive behavior; changes in routines or surroundings may provoke tantrum-like rages. Detached, withdrawn, and unresponsive, the child appears to have disturbance of perception, speech, and language and sometimes mobility, as well as an inability to relate to people. This child does not react to either verbal commands or sounds; no response may be evinced to very loud, sudden noises. The child shows no reaction to new persons or objects in the environment and may walk into objects as if they are not seen. There is lack of response to tactile or painful stimuli. Eye contact is infrequent. Speech and language may be delayed, and echolalia (repetition of sounds) is common. The child frequently flicks, twirls, or spins toy objects rather than playing with them appropriately. There is little peer interaction and infrequent or delayed social smile. The child is disinterested in people and surroundings but has an unusual interest in inanimate objects. He or she is unable to perform two tasks simultaneously. Vision appears to be more peripheral than central. Frequently, the head is held to the side, and the child walks on the ball of the foot, frequently and habitually flapping the hands.

The American Psychiatric Association (1987) has established criteria to diagnose autism. It is classified as the most severe form of Pervasive Developmental Disorder.

Etiology

Little is known about possible causative factors or conditions preceding or accompanying autism. Conditions found to be associated with autism in some children include epilepsy (Deykin and MacMahon, 1979), mental retardation (Rutter, 1977), biochemical imbalance (Geller et al, 1982), and the fragile X syndrome (Christian, 1983). It is considered by some to be a neurologic abnormality (Connell, 1985). It appears to be biogenic rather than psychogenic in origin. There is some evidence that severe perinatal distress and autism are related (Finegan and Quarrington, 1979). Numerous investigations have searched for biochemical correlates such as hormones, amino acids, trace elements, and various metabolites. No biochemical marker has been identified (Volkmar and Cohen, 1986), although serotonin concentrations have been found to be elevated in one third of autistic individuals (Young et al, 1982). Although it is apparent that an abnormality in central nervous system function exists, the site or mechanism of dysfunction is not understood (Volkmar and Cohen, 1986).

Diagnostic Assessment

To establish the diagnosis, the child must have shown evidence of a failure to establish social relationships, retarded language development, and ritualistic and compulsive behaviors before 30 months of age (Connell, 1985). Other common characteristics, though not exclusive to autism, include abnormal motor activity, unexpected responses to sensory stimuli, and mood changes that occur without any obvious cause. The pathology may be idiopathic or be in conjunction with other diseases affecting the central nervous system.

Therapeutic Management and Nursing Strategies

A primary person should give care and attempt to help the child become person-oriented rather than object-oriented. The child and family need the help of educators skilled in the care of autistic children. The family undoubtedly will need special support, since there will be feelings of inadequacy, guilt, and low self-esteem. If there is no mutual agreement on discipline, there may be parental distance and family breakdown. Siblings become embittered or angry, and family members suffer fatigue and frustration. Mothers especially suffer from psychotic trauma because of the 24-hour responsibility of a disruptive child. The whole family will benefit from counseling and a relationship with an understanding and sympathetic significant person(s). Respite from care should be available periodically.

An autistic child is bewildering to parents, and it is difficult to get a developmental history because of periodic changes in symptoms. The head banging and similar bizarre behavior may lead to self-mutilation. Autistic children are not usually admitted to hospital for the condition, although they may be admitted for a diagnostic evaluation. As yet, there is no medication or treatment that alters the course of the condition. Previously, these children were institutionalized and did not have access to a stimulating environment or a warm, symbiotic relationship with a caring person.

The trend in management is to treat these children in community-based programs (Christian, 1983). The most effective management is a structured educational program and the environment of a special classroom (Connell, 1985). This should be begun as soon as the symptoms are recognized. Behavior modification is used in an attempt to change the child's autistic symptoms; however, the scientific value of this approach has not been established yet. Positive reinforcement in the form of food, affection, or activity (feeding the gerbils, water play) should be given immediately when the child responds appropriately. Accurate and detailed recording is necessary to note change in behavior. In a group setting, adverse conditioning such as a sharp "NO, Timmy!" or insisting that he sit on a chair removed from the group may eventually be effective. Any momentary awareness must immediately be rewarded to help draw the child from the world of fantasy and introversion into the world of reality.

Ideally, there should be an initial conference in the home to observe the child in the family setting. The attitudes of siblings and parents can best be evaluated in a nonthreatening setting. All family members can contribute to a discussion of the child's habits, routines, favorite objects and preferred foods. If specific things frighten the child, this should also be noted. The family should continue to be in close communication with the teacher to establish continuity of care and provide a consistent home environment. Parents are being trained to manage their children at home with the use of behavior modification techniques.

With the assistance of a warm, caring teacher, the child will receive guidance in impulse control, gross and fine motor coordination, and language development, as well as academic and social training. The diagnostic team evaluates the child's intellectual abilities as well as any physical contributing factors. Deafness and developmental aphasia must be ruled out. Intelligence of these children usually is in the functionally retarded range.

Consistent and structured care from a limited number of receptive people can allow the child to develop at her or his own speed in an individualized academic setting. Despite the intensive, individualized treatment that many children are receiving, approximately two thirds of autistic children remain autistic and need supervision and support for a life time (Volkmar and Cohen, 1986).

The National Society for Autistic Children* is dedicated to the education, welfare, and treatment of all children with severe disorders of communication and behavior. This is an active organization with annual national meetings and continued lobbying for the rights of autistic people. Parents may benefit from the suggestions and support of other parents who have children with similar problems.

Schizophrenia

The term *schizophrenia* describes the type of psychotic behavior characterized by a loss of contact with reality. The term *childhood* schizophrenia generally refers to psycotic disorders that appear after the first 5 years of life. In adolescents, this disease process is noted by a gradual disintegration in several areas of mental functioning. The youth's lack of integration in thought processes is manifested most often by disturbed behavior, emotions, and speech patterns.

The term childhood schizophrenia is no longer used in discussing mental disorders of childhood, since it is now recognized that children adapting to life experiences exhibit symptoms that in an adult would be characteristic of mental illness. Although children

* 1234 Massachusetts Avenue, Washington, DC 20005.

do incur a variety of emotional disturbances, their symptoms vary with each stage of development. Recent thinking has discouraged labeling these childhood problems with adult diagnostic labels. It is believed that an individual must at least attain the developmental stage of adolescence before the diagnosis of schizophrenia can be made. Some clinicians also differentiate between an adolescent schizophrenic reaction and adult schizophrenia, based partially on differences in outcome. Adolescent schizophrenic reaction is often limited to a few years and has an excellent prognosis for recovery, as opposed to the more chronic adult versions of schizophrenia.

Etiology

No one factor has been identified as the cause of schizophrenia. Some theories suggest a biologic etiology. This viewpoint attributes schizophrenia to deficiencies in metabolic or neural functioning or to genetic factors, citing studies that report a significantly higher incidence of schizophrenia among family members, especially twins. Other theories support a psychodynamic etiology, suggesting that disturbances in interpersonal relations are at the root of the illness. This viewpoint supports disturbed family relationships as the causative factor. Parents, especially mothers, have been characterized as being emotionally cold to the child, keeping her or him at a distance or confusing him by conveying inconsistent messages and by failing to acknowledge the validity of his own feelings. Parents themselves may behave inappropriately for their age and sex, acting out their own conflicts in their relationship with the child. Most likely many factors can be implicated.

Clinical Manifestations and Assessment

Nurses and other members of the health care team may be unaware of the adolescent's need for help until the youngster is confronted with a crisis situation. A number of factors may contribute to this lack of awareness. The youth may be unaware of anything but a growing sense of unhappiness. To an adolescent, asking for help is developmentally inconsistent with inner drives for mastery and control. Until recently, seeking professional help has also carried some social stigma. Nurses and other health professionals need to incorporate assessment of mental health status as part of adolescent health screening, since youth are particularly prone to emotional disturbances.

Psychotic behavior in a youth may be obvious from early childhood, or it may be triggered by a developmental crisis. For example, adolescent developmental tasks can overwhelm a youth with a shaky ego and heighten already existing fears, resulting in a loss of a sense of self. Feelings of ambivalence in the quest for independence, or hostility due to unmet dependency needs, is feared. These conflicting feelings and a poorly developed self-concept may lead to overt schizophrenic behavior characterized by delusions, hallucinations, and inappropriate emotional reactions. As the level of anxiety increases, it becomes more and more difficult for the adolescent to distinguish between fantasy and reality. The earliest symptoms may be noted as behavioral changes or alterations in habits. For example, the neat child becomes sloppy or the casual child begins to rigidly adhere to routine. In the early stages of this illness, the child may begin to exhibit overt signs of the struggle to maintain contact with reality by displaying rituals, phobias, or obsessive-compulsive behaviors. For example, a boy may fear germs to the point of refusing to touch door knobs, using a tissue to open a door or washing his hands repeatedly. As his personality structure continues to disintegrate, the youth exhibits obvious schizophrenic symptoms of paranoid delusions or hallucinations. He regresses to infantile behaviors, is unable to control impulses and may have activity changes varying from apathy to aggression. Depersonalization and motor and speech disturbance become apparent.

The nurse collects information from the parents about the history and progress of the illness. Observations of parent-youth interactions and the effectiveness of the child's interactions with the environment are documented. Other needed information may include the extent to which the adolescent is able to differentiate his or her body from the environment; the extent of impulsivity, regression or bizarre behavior; whether there is any self-mutilating or aggressive behavior; and whether the child can distinguish between reality and fantasy.

Therapeutic Management and Nursing Strategies

Caring for a schizophrenic adolescent in an acute care setting makes unusual demands on the nursing staff. The bizarre behavior may disrupt a unit designed primarily to serve medical needs. The nurse who reacts emotionally to the disturbed behavior cannot function therapeutically. For example, the nurse who gets angry and punishes one who hits her is responding nontherapeutically. Repeated episodes of disruptive, acting-out behavior can make members of the nursing staff feel they are losing control. Repeated attempts to help a schizophrenic young person may be rebuffed as he or she attempts to avoid any close interpersonal encounter. Such rejection of "helping" overtures can leave a nurse feeling helpless or inadequate. Nurses must recognize that the behavior is symptomatic of the illness. Group conferences with all health team members will help the nurse plan consistent therapeutic interventions.

The care of an adolescent with schizophrenia is a specialized area of practice; therefore, the reader is referred to texts in the field of psychiatry and psychiatric nursing.

References

American Academy of Pediatrics, Committee on Adolescence: Role of the pediatrician in substance abuse counseling. *Pediatrics* 1983; 72:251–252.

American Association of Suicidology: Incidence rate of suicide and percent change by adolescents (15–24 years old), 1955–1982. *Newslink* 11(4), 1985.

American Psychiatric Association: *Diagnostic and Statistical Manual of Mental Disorders* (DSM III). 3rd ed. Washington, DC, 1980.

American Psychiatric Association: *Diagnostic and Statistical Manual of Mental Disorders*—Revised (DSM III-R). Washington, DC, 1987.

Anders TF, Walton C: Psychotherapy with children. *In* Levine ML et al (eds): *Developmental-Behavioral Pediatrics.* Philadelphia, WB Saunders, 1983, 1058–1967.

Apter SJ, Conoley JC: *Childhood Behavior Disorders and Emotional Disturbance.* Englewood Cliffs, NJ, Prentice-Hall, 1984.

Aylward GP: Understanding and treatment of childhood depression. *J Pediatr* 1985; 107(1):1–9.

Babich, KS: *Assessing the Mental Health of Children.* Boulder, CO, Western Interstate Commission for Higher Education, 1982.

Bakwin H, Bakwin R: *Behavior Disorders in Children.* Philadelphia, WB Saunders, 1972.

Barraclough B: International variation in the suicide rate of 15–24 year olds. *Soc Psychiatr Psychiatr Epidemiol* 1988; 23:75–84.

Brook CG: Evidence for a sensitive period in adipose cell replication in man. *Lancet,* 1972; 11:624–627.

Brook, C: Obesity in childhood. *Practitioner* 1983; 227:213–219.

Brown MR, et al: A high protein, low calorie liquid diet in the treatment of very obese adolescents: long-term effect on lean body mass. *Am J Clin Nutr* 1983; 38:20–31.

Brownell KD, et al: Treatment of obese children with and without their mothers; changes in weight and blood pressure. *Pediatrics* 1983; 71:515–523.

Brownell KD, Stunkard AJ: Behavioral treatment of obesity in children. *Am J Dis Child* 1978; 132:403–412.

Bruch H: *Eating Disorders: Obesity, Anorexia Nervosa, and the Person Within.* New York, Basic Books, 1973.

Canadian Pediatric Society Nutrition Committee: Adolescent nutrition: 3. Obesity. *Can Med Assoc J* 1983; 129:549–551.

Cecere MC: PIP (positive image program): a group approach for obese adolescents. *Nurs Clin North Am* 1983; 18:249–256.

Christian WP: Childhood autism. *In* Levine ML, et al (eds): *Developmental-Behavioral Pediatrics.* Philadelphia, WB Saunders, 1983, 816–828.

Coe RM, et al: Patterns of change in adolescent smoking behavior and results of a one year follow-up of a smoking prevention program. *J School Health* 1982; 52:348–353.

Committee on Adolescence, American Academy of Pediatrics: Suicide and suicide attempts in adolescents and young adults. *Pediatrics* 1988 Feb; 81(2):322–324.

Connell HM: *Essentials of Child Psychiatry.* 2nd ed. London, Blackwell Scientific Publications, 1985.

Coolridge JC: School phobia. *In* Noshpitz J (ed): *Basic Handbook of Child Psychiatry.* Vol II. New York, Basic Books, 1977, 453–463.

Coupey SM, Schonberg SK: Evaluation and management of drug problems in adolescents. *Pediatr Ann* 1982; 11:653–658.

Crawshaw JP: Anorexia and bulimia: the earlier cues. *Patient Care* 1985; 19:80–95.

Dale S, et al: Middle childhood. *In* Hymovich DP, Chamberlin RW: *Child and Family Development: Implications for Primary Health Care.* New York, McGraw-Hill, 1980, 318–382.

Deykin EY, MacMahon B: The incidence of seizures among children with autistic symptoms. *Am J Psychiatr* 1979; 136(10):1310–1312.

Dietz WH: Childhood obesity: susceptibility, cause and management. *J Pediatr* 1983; 103:676–686.

Dietz WH, Gortmaker SL: Do we fatten our children at the television set? Obesity and television viewing in children and adolescents. *Pediatrics* 1985; 75:807.

Dworkin PH: *Learning and Behavior Problems of School Children.* Philadelphia, WB Saunders, 1985.

Epstein LH, et al: Effects of weight loss on fitness in obese children. *Am J Dis Child* 1983; 137:654–657.

Finegan J, Quarrington R: Pre-, peri- and neonatal factors and infantile autism. *J Child Psychol Psychiatr* 1979; 20:119–128.

Fleisher DR: Diagnosis and treatment of disorders of defection in children. *Pediatr Ann* 1976; 85:700–722.

Foman S: Factors influencing food consumption in the human infant. *Int J Obes* 1980; 4:348–350.

Foman SJ, Ziegler EE: Prevention of obesity. *In Nutritional Disorders of Children.* No. (HSA) 78-5104. Washington, DC, US Department of Health, Education and Welfare, 1976.

Forehand RL, Wells KC: Conduct disorders. *In* Hoekelman RA, et al: *Primary Pediatric Care.* St. Louis, CV Mosby, 1987.

Garn SM, et al: Effect of remaining family members on fatness prediction. *Am J Clin Nutr* 1981; 34:148–153.

Garn SM, Clark DC: Trends in fatness and the origins of obesity. American Academy of Pediatrics Ad Hoc Committee to Review the Ten-State Nutrition Survey. *Pediatrics* 1976; 57:443–456.

Geller E, et al: Preliminary observations on the effect of fenfluramine on blood serotonin and symptoms in 3 autistic boys. *N Engl J Med* 1982; 307(3):165–169.

Goodwin DW: Alcoholism and heredity. A review and hypothesis. *Arch Gen Psychiatry* 1979; 36:57–61.

Greenspan SI: *The Clinical Interview of the Child.* New York, McGraw-Hill, 1981.

Hagenbuch VEG: Obesity and the school-age child. *Nurs Clin North Am* 1982; 17:207–216.

Halmi K, et al: Binge eating and vomiting: a survey of a college population. *Psychol Med* 1981; 11:697–706.

Hasin DS et al: Cocaine and heroin dependence compared in poly-drug abusers. *Am J Public Health* 1988; 78(5):567–569.

Jellinek MS, et al: Pediatric Symptoms Checklist: Screening school-age children for psychosocial dysfunction. *J Pediatr* 1988 Feb; 112(2):201–209.

Jessor R: A psychosocial perspective on adolescent substance abuse. *In* Litt IF (ed): *Adolescent Substance Abuse. Report of the 14th Ross Roundtable on Critical Approaches to Common Pediatric Problems.* Columbus, OH, Ross Laboratories, 1983, 21–28.

Johnson LD, et al: Highlights from *Student Drug Use in America, 1975–1981.* Washington, DC, National Institute on Drug Abuse, US Department of Health and Human Services, 1982.

Johnson LD, et al: Drug use among American high school students, college students and other young adults. Rockville, MD, *US Department of Health and Human Services,* NIDA, 1986.

Johnson LD, et al: Drug use by high school seniors: The class of 1986. Publication (ADM) 87-1535. Rockville, MD, *National Institute of Drug Abuse.* 1987.

Kavanaugh JC, Mattsson A: Phobias. *In* Hoekelman RA, et al: *Primary Pediatric Care.* St. Louis, CV Mosby, 1987.

Kazdin AE: Depression. *In* Hoekelman RA, et al: *Primary Pediatric Care.* St. Louis, CV Mosby, 1987.

Kelly S, Liter S: Interpersonal process group: a psychodynamic/existential approach to the treatment of bulimia. Paper presented to the American Association for Counseling and Development, Houston, 1984.

Killen JD, et al: Depressive symptoms and substance use among adolescent binge eaters and purgers: a defined population study. *Am J Public Health* 1987; 77(12):1539–1541.

Kleber HD: Cocaine abuse: Historical, epidemiological and psychological perspectives. *J Clin Psychiatr* 1988 Feb; 49(2):3–6.

Knittle JL, et al: The growth of adipose tissue in children and adolescents. Cross-sectional studies of adipose cell numbers and size. *J Clin Invest* 1979; 63:238–246.

Langford RW: Teenagers and obesity. *Am J Nurs* 1981; 81:556–559.

Lansky D, Brownell KD: Comparison of school-based treatments for adolescent obesity. *J School Health* 1982; 52:384–387.

Levenkron S: *Treating and Overcoming Anorexia Nervosa.* New York, Charles Scribner's Sons, 1982.

Leventhal T, Sills M: Self-image in school phobia. *Am J Orthopsychiatr* 1964; 34:685.

Levine M: Children with encopresis: a descriptive analysis. *Pediatrics* 1975; 56:412–416.

Levine M: Encopresis. *In* Hoekelman RA: *Primary Pediatric Care.* St. Louis, CV Mosby, 1987.

Macdonald DI: Drugs, drinking, and adolescence. *Am J Dis Child* 1984; 138:117–125.

MacLeod S: The Art of Starvation. New York, Schocken Books, 1982.

Mansdorf IJ, Lukens E: Cognitive-behavioral psychotherapy for separation anxious children exhibiting school phobia. *J Am Acad Child Adol Psychiat* 1987; 26(2):222–225.

Mattsson A: Adolescent depression and suicide. *In* Hoekelman RA, et al: *Primary Pediatric Care.* St. Louis, CV Mosby, 1987.

Meyer EE, Neumann CG: Management of the obese adolescent. *Pediatr Clin North Am* 1977; 24:123–132.

Minuchin S, et al: *Psychosomatic Families: Anorexia Nervosa in Context.* Cambridge, MA, Harvard University Press, 1978.

Muscari ME: Identification and management of the early anorectic child. *J Pediatr Health Care* 1987; 1(4):196–203.

National Center for Health Statistics: *Vital Statistics of the United States, 1978.* Hyattsville, MD, 1982.

Nelson EC, et al: Weight reduction and maintenance for overweight, mentally retarded students ages 9–17. *J School Health* 1983; 53:380–381.

Neuman PA, Halvorson PA: *Anorexia and Bulimia: A Handbook for Counselors and Therapists.* New York, Van Nostrand Reinhold, 1983.

Pallikkathayil L, Tweed S: Substance abuse: alcohol and drugs during adolescence. *Nurs Clin North Am* 1983; 18:313–321.

Parcel GS: The pediatrician's role in drug education. *Pediatr Rev* 1982; 4:144–149.

Parke R, Slaby R: The development of aggression. *In Paul Mussen's Handbook of Child Psychology.* Vol 4. New York, John Wiley and Sons, 1983.

Parker L, Whitehead W: Treatment of urinary and fecal incontinence in children. *In* Russo DC, Varni JW (eds): *Behavioral Pediatrics: Research and Practice.* New York, Plenum Press, 1982, 143–174.

Patterson GR: *Coercive Family Processes.* Eugene, OR, Castalia Publishing, 1980.

Peck M: The loner: an exploration of suicidal subtype in adolescence. *Adolesc Psychiatr* 1981; 9:461–466.

Petchers MK, et al: Revalidation and expansion of an adolescent substance abuse screening measure. *Pediatr* 1988 Feb; 9(1):25–29.

Rames LK, et al: Normal blood pressures and the evaluation of sustained blood pressure elevation in childhood: the Muscarine Study. *Pediatrics* 1978; 61:245–251.

Rice MA, Kibbee PE: Review: identifying the adolescent substance abuser. *Am J Matern Child Nurs* 1983; 8:139–142.

Royal College of Physicians: Obesity. A report. *J R Coll Physicians Lond* 1983; 17:6–61.

Rutter M: Infantile autism and other childhood psychoses. *In* Rutter M, Hersov L (eds): *Child Psychiatry: Modern Approaches.* London, Blackwell Scientific Publications, 1977, 717–747.

Rutter M, et al: Research report: Isle of Wight Studies, 1964–1974. *Psychol Med* 1976; 6:313.

Schleicher IM: Teaching parents to cope with behavior problems. *Am J Nurs* 1978; 78:838–839.

Schmitt BD: Pediatric developmental-behavioral counseling. *In* Levine ML, et al (eds): *Developmental-Behavioral Pediatrics.* Philadelphia, WB Saunders, 1983, 1043–1057.

Selvini-Palazzoli M: Anorexia nervosa: a syndrome of an affluent society. *Transcult Psychiatr Res Rev* 1985; XXII:3.

Shestowsky BJ: Ego identity development and obesity in adolescent girls. *Adolescence* 1983; 18:551–559.

Shukla A, et al: Infantile overnutrition in the first year of life:

a field study in Dudley, Worcestershire. *Br Med J* 1972; 4:507–515.
Silber TJ, et al: Prevalence of PCP use among adolescent marijuana users. Clinical and laboratory observations. *J Pediatr* 1988 May; 112(5):827–829.
Smith MB: Hope and despair: keys to the socio-psychodynamics of youth. *Am J Orthopsychiatr* 1983; 53:388–399.
Strober M: Familial aspects of depressive disorder in early adolescence. *In* Weller EB, Weller RA (eds): *Current Perspectives on Major Depressive Disorders in Children.* Washington, DC, American Psychiatric Press, 1984.
Taitz LS: Infantile overnutrition among artificially fed infants in the Sheffield region. *Br Med J* 1971; 1:315–316.
Tashkin DP, Cohen S: *Marijuana Smoking and Its Effects on the Lungs.* American Council for Drug Education, Rockville, MD, 1981.
US Department of Health, Education and Welfare: *Ten State Nutrition Survey 1968–1970.* Washington, DC, Health Services and Mental Health Administration, 1972.
US Department of Health and Human Services, Public Health Service, Alcohol, Drug Abuse, and Mental Health Administration, National Institute on Alcohol Abuse and Alcoholism: *Sixth Special Report to the U.S. Congress on Alcohol and Health.* Publication (ADM) 87-1519. Rockville, MD, 1987.
US Morbidity and Mortality Weekly Report: Alcohol-related highway fatalities among young drivers. *MMWR* 1982; 31:641–644.
Valente S: Suicide in school-aged children: theory and assessment. *Pediatr Nurs* 1983; 9(1):25–29.
Valente SM, Saunders JM: High school suicide prevention programs. *Pediatr Nurs* 1987 Mar/Apr; 13(2):108.
Volkmar FR, Cohen DJ: Current concepts: infantile autism and the pervasive developmental disorders. *J Dev Behav Pediatr* 1986; 7(5):324–329.
Wagnaar A: *The Raising of the legal drinking age in Michigan and Maine.* Rockville, MD, National Institute on Alcohol Abuse and Alcoholism, 1981.
Walsh BT, et al: Bulimia and depression. *Psychosom Med* 1985; 47:123–131.
Waxman M, Stunkard AJ: Caloric intake and expenditure of obese boys. *J Pediatr* 1980; 96:187–193.
Webster-Stratton C: Recognizing and assessing conduct disorders in children. *MCN* 1983; 8(5):330–335.
Werry JS: The childhood psychoses. *In* Quay HC, Werry J (eds): *The Psychopathological Disorders of Childhood.* 2nd ed. New York, John Wiley & Sons, 1979, 43–89.
Weill WB Jr: Current controversies in childhood obesity. *J Pediatr* 1977; 91:175–187.
Wells KC, Forehand R: Conduct and oppositional disorders. *In* Bornstein PH, Kazdin AE (eds): *Handbook of Clinical Behavior Therapy with Children.* Homewood, IL, Dorcey Press, 1985.
Williams D: Substance use and abuse. *In* Howe J (ed): *Nursing Care of Adolescents.* New York, McGraw-Hill, 1980a, 161–195.
Williams D: Substance abuse treatment settings. *In* Howe J (ed): *Nursing Care of Adolescents.* New York, McGraw-Hill, 1980b, 427–439.
Wilson MH: Obesity. *In* Hoekelman RA, et al: *Primary Pediatric Care.* St. Louis, CV Mosby, 1987.
Wright GF, Nader PR: Schools as milieux. *In* Levine ML, et al (eds): *Developmental-Behavioral Pediatraics.* Philadelphia, WB Saunders, 1983, 276–283.
Ylitalo V: Treatment of obese school-children. *Acta Paediatr Scand* (Suppl) 1981; 290:1–108.
Young GJ, et al: Clinical neurochemistry of autism and associated disorders. *J Autis Dev Disord* 1982; 12:147–165.
Younger JB, Hughes LS: No-fault management of encopresis. *Pediatr Nurs* 1983; 9(2):185–187.

Bibliography

Brady MA, et al: Childhood depression: development of a screening tool. *Pediatr Nurs* 1984; 10(3):222–225.
Caddell A: Under the influence. *Nurs Times* 1983 Jun; 79(25):9–10.
Cohen MI: Marijuana—what is really known? *In* Litt IF (ed): *Adolescent Substance Abuse, Report of the 14th Ross Roundtable on Critical Approaches to Common Pediatric Problems.* Columbus, OH, Ross Laboratories, 1983, 10–16.
Dietz AJ: Amphetamine-like reactions to phenylpropanolamine. *JAMA* 1981; 245:601–602.
Finn PA: Self-destructive behavior in school-age children: a hidden problem. *Pediatr Nurs* 1986; 12(3):198–199.
Fond K, Brosman J: School phobia; the school anxiety syndrome. *Pediatr Nurs* 1980; 6(5):9–13.
Gierszweski SA: The relationship of weight loss, locus of control, and social support. *Nurs Res* 1983; 32:43–47.
Harding SE: Anorexia nervosa. *Pediatr Nurs* 1985; 11(4):275–277.
Hill JA, et al: The athletic polydrug abuse phenomenon. A case report. *Am J Sports Med* 1983; 11:269–271.
Horowitz JD, et al: Hypertensive responses induced by phenylpropanolamine in anorectic and decongestant preparations. *Lancet* 1980; 1:60–61.
Iveson JI: Barbiturates: a history of abuse. Forum 8, Drug Abuse. *Nurs Mirror* 1982 Aug; 155(7):viii.
McKerlie L, et al: Solvent abuse. Community Forum 10. *Nurs Mirror* 1983 Dec; (suppl).
Meller W, Lyle: Attention deficit disorder in childhood. *Primary Care* 1987; 14(4):745–759.
Nelms BC: Assessing childhood depression: do parents and children agree? *Pediatr Nurs* 1986; 12(1):23–26.
Percy EC: Drugs and athletics. *In* Smith NJ (ed): *Sports Medicine: Health Care for Young Athletes.* American Academy of Pediatrics, Committee on Sports Medicine, 1983, 176–183.
Whiting S: The problem of depression in adolescence. *Adolescence* 1981; 16:67–89.

Nursing Strategies: Pregnancy During Adolescence

Chapter 37

B. Helen Thomas
Alba Mitchell
M. Corinne Devlin

Adolescent pregnancy continues to be a serious problem in our society. In spite of a variety of interventions, the rates of pregnancy, particularly among those 17 years of age and younger, have not decreased appreciably. For this group, unintended pregnancy has numerous physical, psychologic, and social consequences, many of which can be negative and long term. These pregnancies also have ramifications for the adolescent father, the grandparents, the offspring, and society at large.

Since nurses may encounter pregnant and nonpregnant adolescents in different practice settings, they are in an ideal position to collaborate with other health professionals in the primary, secondary, and tertiary prevention of pregnancy. In schools, in the community, and in primary care settings these teens seek out accurate information, an opportunity to clarify their feelings about choices they have made, and ongoing support in their new roles. In pediatric or adolescent clinics, nurses may have many opportunities to work with pregnant adolescents: shortly after conception, throughout the pregnancy, and during postnatal follow-up care and well-baby visits. Adolescents are neither children nor adults. Successful intervention with them requires application of knowledge of their developmental stage and how it affects their behavior as well as skill in relating to this age group (Moore et al, 1984).

The purpose of this chapter is to provide nurses with an overview of the extent of the problem, and the factors that affect it. Following this, nursing strategies are described. The framework of prevention is used to outline specific nursing strategies. The focus is on interventions that a nurse in a pediatric primary care or institutional setting would be able to implement. Other nursing activities have been included to give the student a view of the overall needs of this group of clients, and an appreciation of the complexity of the challenge of preventing adolescent pregnancy.

Related Topics
Infant care, Chapter 5
Normal growth and development of adolescents, Chapter 9
Methods of contraception, Chapter 9
Nutritional requirements for the adolescent, Chapter 18
Promoting Healthy Sexuality, Chapter 22

Defining the Problem

Based on a study of teenage reproductive behavior in six developed countries, researchers reported that pregnancy rates (abortions plus live births) among adolescents 15 to 19 years of age vary from 96 : 1000 to 14 : 1000 for the United States and the Netherlands respectively. The rates for England, France, Canada, and Sweden fall between the two extremes and range from 45 : 1000 to 35 : 1000 (Jones et al, 1985).

Since the burden of adolescent pregnancy is greatest for those 17 years of age and younger, it is important to review the data for that group separately (Klein, 1978). According to Jones (1985) the pregnancy rates for 15 to 17 year olds are highest in the United States and Canada (62 : 1000 and 28 : 1000, respectively), followed by England and Wales (27 : 1000), Sweden (20 : 1000), France (19 : 1000), and the Netherlands (7 : 1000). Only two countries reported enough births among those younger than 15 years to calculate rates: the United States (5 : 1000) and Canada (1 : 1000).

Pregnancy, abortion, and birth rates are highest in the United States at all ages. Birth rates among young Canadian girls (14 to 16 years) are second only to the United States, and rise gradually with age. By the age of 17 to 18 years, rates in Sweden, England, Wales, France, and Canada are similar.

A comparison of U.S. pregnancy rates from 1976 to 1981 indicates that they have not significantly changed. In those 17 years and younger, the birth rates have declined and abortion rates have increased, reflecting somewhat easier access to abortion as a solution for unintended pregnancy (Public Health Service, 1981).

Unintended adolescent pregnancy (particularly in those 16 years of age or younger) is the cause of much human misery (Finkelstein et al, 1982), whether the mother decides to abort the pregnancy, give the child up for adoption, or raise the child.

Although abortion is a solution being chosen more frequently, the long-term cost of this in relation to emotional development of the adolescent is unknown. As well, in many states legislation has made therapeutic abortions difficult to obtain, especially for poor adolescents.

When carried to term, adolescent pregnancy has significant short-term and long-term health and social consequences for the pregnant teen, her partner, their families, their offspring, and society at large. There is general agreement that teenagers 16 years of age and older who receive early thorough prenatal care are at no greater risk for physical complications than women 20 years of age. However, girls younger than 16 years of age have an increased frequency of obstetrical complications (Clark et al, 1982). Some researchers have attributed this to the biologic immaturity of these adolescents (Zlatnik and Burmeister, 1977). Others believe that the increased rate of complications is a result of young teenagers not seeking prenatal care until late in the pregnancy, and other unhealthy lifestyle habits (McAnarney and Greydanus, 1981). The controversy is complicated by the fact that behaviors such as unprotected sexual intercourse (and resulting pregnancy) in early adolescence and the use of alcohol, tobacco, psychoactive drugs, poor diet and poor compliance with health care are highly interrelated (Loris et al, 1985). Furthermore, socioeconomic status (SES) and race appear to influence the development of complications even when age is taken into account. Complications of pregnancy occur more frequently at all ages in those of lower SES (Zlatnik and Burmeister, 1977). Hypertension during pregnancy is much more common in blacks than in those of other races.

Maternal mortality among teenagers is approximately 40 per cent greater than for 20 to 25 year olds due largely to the increased incidence of pre-eclamptic toxemia (hypertension, edema, proteinuria) (SOGC Bulletin, 1986). Cephalopelvic disproportion (CPD) is more common in young adolescents than in older women. This results in an increased rate of cesarean births for this age group, with the increased and attendant risks of anesthesia and major surgery.

Adolescence is a period of rapid growth, yet many adolescents have poor eating habits and subscribe to fad diets. Low weight gain and anemia during pregnancy may result from inadequate nutritional and caloric intake. Adolescents with a gynecologic age (age at conception minus age at menarche) of 2 years or less, who are most likely to still be growing fairly rapidly, are at increased risk for nutritional problems (Piechnik and Corbett, 1985).

In addition to the effects on physical development and the physical health hazards, adolescent pregnancy can profoundly influence normal psychosocial development of girls in this age group. The major task of adolescence, establishing an individual identity, is made more difficult by the fact that the teen must learn to accept her pregnant state and incorporate it into her personal self-concept. At this time, many teens have trouble accepting normal body changes. Incorporating additional changes caused by pregnancy can be overwhelming. These changes are not "normal" and are a major difference between the pregnant teen and her peer group.

Pregnancy can lead to social isolation. This isolation can be self-imposed or a result of peer rejection. Regardless of the cause, it hinders normal psychosocial development. Being isolated from peers not only retards the development of interpersonal social skills but also reduces the opportunities to discuss important issues with same-aged males and females—an important exercise in the process of values clarification. Rejection by the peer group can lead to a decreased sense of self-worth, which, in turn, may lead to a host of poor lifestyle choices that have long-term negative effects on the adult life of the adolescent.

At a time when most young people are seeking more independence from the nuclear family, a pregnant teen may find her family a major support system and may be unable to separate from them. Guilt about the sexual activity that led to becoming pregnant may compound the need to comply with parental wishes.

Pregnancy and motherhood may interrupt or alter educational goals and career choices. Increasing numbers of adolescents are choosing to remain single and to keep their offspring (Chilman, 1979). Pregnancy is the most common reason girls fail to complete high school in the United States: 50 per cent to 67 per cent of all female dropouts are pregnant or parents (Spivak, 1987). Lack of a high school diploma increases the probability that earning power will be lost or reduced, and increases the likelihood of a future life of poverty. The younger the mother at the time of birth, the greater the likelihood she will live in poverty and subsist on long-term public assistance (Lindsay, 1984).

Heterosexual relationships will also be influenced by unintended pregnancy. The pregnant teen's relationship with the father of the child may suddenly change. On learning about the pregnancy, teenage males are often frightened and unprepared to accept any responsibility. These young men may terminate the relationship. Others may wish to remain actively involved with the adolescent and infant and may or may not wish to live with/marry the girl. The outcome of this relationship either may teach the adolescent about the importance of caring support between a male and female, or it may reinforce her sense of being manipulated and exploited. Recognition of these possible negative attributes of relationships is important, but for successful adult living, the adolescent needs help to establish values that enhance a female-male relationship.

The effects of unintended pregnancy on the father have not been as well studied as those on the mother. Upon learning of the pregnancy, teenage males suffer many of the same emotions as the pregnant female: initial disbelief, fear of parental and peer reactions, and fear for the future. As well, many of these young men want to support and care for the pregnant adolescent, but they are unsure how to do it. Contrary to general belief, at least half of adolescent fathers either live with or visit their children regularly (i.e., daily or weekly) (Furstenberg, 1976; Rivara et al, 1985). Early marriages and the increased likelihood of marital problems and/or divorce are frequent stresses experienced by adolescent parents (Braverman, 1985). For those couples who select marriage, interrupted education leads to decreased family income and the increased likelihood of uncertain future employment and poverty.

Although many families of pregnant adolescents are supportive, initial reactions of guilt for having failed the teen, anger at their daughter and/or the father, disappointment that former ambitions for the girl may not be fulfilled, and embarrassment within the extended family and among social peers are not uncommon. As parents learn to live with the reality, they may become active in planning the future care of the unborn child. Particularly with young adolescents, parents may take over all the decision-making about the future for the adolescent and the infant. If the teen is not involved in these decisions, long-term resentment and feelings of inadequacy may result.

Being a "child-of-a-child" has numerous risks. Low birth weight and prematurity are much more common in offspring of young adolescents than in women aged 20 to 25 years (Dott and Fort, 1976).

Low birth weight appears to be related broadly to sociodemographic factors, inadequate nutrition, and other unsound health practices. Low socioeconomic status may account for inadequate nutrition in that the long-term diet of adolescents in this group is often missing essential nutrients either because of lack of knowledge, money, or both. Weight prior to pregnancy, weight gain during pregnancy, infant gestational age, and use of tobacco, alcohol, or other illicit drugs primarily account for infants with low birth weight (Zuckerman et al, 1983). The gynecologic age of the mother is also important in that optimal infant birth weight for adolescents 13 to 16 years of age is associated with a weight gain of 16 kg (35 lbs) as opposed to an 11 kg (24 lbs) weight gain for mothers aged 17 to 25 years (Frisancho et al, 1984).

The precise reasons for higher rates of premature births among this group of mothers are unclear. Some factors that have been suggested include frequent illicit drug use, the presence of sexually transmitted diseases (particularly gonorrhea), intercourse during the later part of pregnancy, and an immature reproductive system. Many of the above risk factors for the infants of adolescents can be dramatically decreased through early, effective prenatal care.

Long-term effects on the child of a young adolescent have also been documented. In one study which followed two groups of mothers and infants from the birth of the offspring to the time the child was age 12 years, significant differences between children of mothers aged 17 years or less at the time of the birth and those over 20 years were found (Hardy et al, 1978). There were significantly more low birth weight infants born to the 17 and younger group of mothers. Infants born to those under 20 showed significant disadvantages in development at all ages. In comparison with children of the older mothers, children of the adolescent mothers were performing less well academically and had repeated a school grade more frequently. Others have also noted that behavior problems, school problems, and low intellectual functioning are more common among children of adolescent parents.

The frequency of drug use and abuse among these teens also has devastating effects on their offspring. The incidence of fetal alcohol syndrome (FAS) (see Chapter 34), newborn drug addiction, and congenital sexually transmitted diseases is more common among infants of adolescent mothers than those of mothers in other age groups. Although child abuse appears more frequently with adolescent parents, the relationship of one to the other is unclear (Kinard and Klerman, 1980).

It is clear that the financial and resource costs of adolescent pregnancy to society are very high. Many adolescent mothers require long-term public assistance. Their lack of knowledge about infant development and care, coupled with sometimes limited social supports, makes this group of mothers and children frequent users of the health and social systems. The facts that the earlier teens conceive, the more children they are likely to bear, and that pregnancy in early adolescence occurs more frequently among offspring of mothers who were also pregnant very young, suggest that without effective primary prevention, adolescent pregnancy will continue to be a major health and social problem in our society (Shah and Zelnick, 1981).

Assessing the Problem: Factors That Influence Adolescent Pregnancy

The obvious cause of adolescent pregnancy is unprotected sexual intercourse. Herold et al (1978), Munz et al (1976), and Nadelson et al (1980) have concluded that sexual activity among adolescents is common, that contraceptive use is poor, and that the majority of adolescents are sexually active long before they seek contraception. Teens who become sexually active at the youngest ages are at the greatest risk for pregnancy and for greater numbers of pregnancies. Results of a nationwide survey indicate that of sexually active teens who did not use birth control, two-thirds became pregnant within two years (Zaben et al, 1979). A follow-up survey indicated that this probability was unchanged (Zelnik and Shah, 1983). Furthermore, half of American adolescent females aged 15 to 19 years report being sexually active. The mean age of first intercourse is dropping and is 15.5 years (Zelnik and Shah, 1983). Only about 10 per cent of adolescents regularly use a reliable method of birth control (most frequently, the pill). It is distressing to note that as a result of widespread publicity of the adverse effects of the pill, many of these young women are discontinuing its use and substituting withdrawal, which is leading to increased pregnancy rates (Zelnik and Shah, 1983).

Among adolescent girls who have been studied, about 10 per cent want to become pregnant and, therefore, do not use contraception. Reasons for wanting to become pregnant include: wanting someone to love, the perception that no other career choice is available, and peer approval for motherhood (Ryan and Sweeney, 1980).

For those adolescents whose pregnancy is unintended (the vast majority), common reasons for not using a reliable contraceptive method include:

- a misunderstanding of the fertility cycle;
- a belief that they are at low risk for pregnancy;
- unavailability of contraception;
- moral objection to the use of contraceptives;
- the belief that contraceptives interfere with the spontaneity and pleasure of sexual intercourse; and
- the unexpected nature of some sexual activity (Alan Gutmacher Institute, 1976; Zelnik and Kantner, 1979).

Unintended adolescent pregnancy appears to be the result of a combination of developmental factors, societal factors, and familial and peer influence (Schinke, 1984).

Developmental Factors

Although the process of physical sexual maturation is not complete until about 21 years of age, there is great variation in the beginning and rate of this process. Overall sexual maturation appears to be occurring earlier in both females and males. On average, female adolescents begin menstruating by 12 to 13 years of age. Regular ovulation and the resultant potential for pregnancy is usually present within several months of menarche.

By age 13, many adolescent males have experienced sexual arousal and/or nocturnal emissions. Since the semen in these emissions almost always contains sperm at this time, boys are physically capable of reproduction. The hormonal changes responsible for sexual maturation also cause mood alterations and an awakening libido (sexual drive).

At the same time that teens are becoming physically sexually mature at a younger age, young adults are postponing marriage until their mid-twenties. This means that adolescents can anticipate a decade of physical sexual maturity before they are likely to make long-term relationship commitments which will provide a family in which to bear and raise children.

Adolescents who receive education about pregnancy can intellectually understand the consequences of unprotected sexual intercourse. However, lack of knowledge is not the only influence on adolescent pregnancy. Adolescent behavior is affected by other cognitive and psychosocial developmental factors as well. Their belief in their individual uniqueness and indestructibility leads to "it will never happen to me" thinking. Adolescent behavior in all areas is strongly influenced by peer expectations and accepted normative behavior for the peer group. Perceived or real peer pressure to be sexually active often results in unplanned sexual intercourse and unintended pregnancy.

In the process of searching for an individual identity, adolescents often try a variety of behaviors, many of which are seen as rebellious by parents and other members of society. Experimentation with sexual activity, sometimes including sexual intercourse, can be one of these behaviors.

Use of contraception requires both acknowledgment of one's sexuality and planning. The infrequent, unexpected nature of much adolescent sexual activity makes planning difficult. However, the major issue is that teens, particularly in the early years, have difficulty accepting the fact that they are sexual beings. Denial of this fact, of course, results in lack of planning and unprotected sexual intercourse (Cvetkovich, 1975).

Societal Factors

The decision to engage in sexual activity and the decision whether to use contraceptive methods is also influenced by societal norms. The fact that many North American adults are unsure about adult values and norms for sexual behavior results in adolescents being faced with many behavior choices and little guidance. The increased rate of adolescent sexual activity in the last 20 years has led to its acceptance as normal by many segments of society. Sexual attractiveness and activity are promoted as desirable by the mass media—both print (magazines and books) and electronic (television programs and advertising and movies). Young adolescents are bombarded with messages such as, "Do your own thing," "Everybody's doing it," "You are in control of your body—use it," and the most powerful of all, "If you really loved me. . . ." Unfortunately, these messages are not balanced with the responsibility one must assume for the consequences of one's actions or the possible exploitation of others that can result from such egocentric behavior.

For adolescents who choose to be sexually active, access to both accurate contraceptive information and to the actual devices is limited. The quality and quantity of available services is variable and is influenced by geographic location, political empathy (which determines funding for public clinics), and the client's ability to pay for service. Although many clinics and health departments are equipped to handle adolescents, their service, based primarily on the medical model of care, is not very effective in promoting teenage cooperation in contraceptive use. To date, teen programs about contraceptive use have been directed almost singularly at females, reflecting another societal norm: Females should be responsible for preventing pregnancy. This is the prevailing attitude among adolescent males as well.

Only 13 per cent of sexually active teenagers approach private physicians for contraception (Chamie et al, 1982). Many adolescents (particularly minors) do not seek information from family doctors because they fear their parents will be informed. This fear is substantiated by the fact that, indeed, some physicians and family planning clinics will not prescribe contraceptives for adolescents without parental knowledge.

In response to the needs of the rising number of adolescent parents, welfare systems have been adapted to provide financial support for needy mothers and children. Although few would disagree that society has a responsibility to care for those who are unable to provide for themselves, some believe that the option of public support is a contributing factor to the growing number of adolescents who choose to keep their offspring.

An overriding concern for the quality of life of the adolescent and her offspring has led to removal of many of society's former sanctions. For example, pregnant girls are encouraged to continue going to school and day care centers have been established in some high schools to ease completion of the adolescents' education following delivery. In total, changing societal behavior and values have led to a much more permissive attitude toward the pregnant adolescent and teenage parenthood.

Family and Friends

Family and friends exert the strongest direct influence on adolescent behavior in general, including sexual behavior. Although adolescents are more strongly influenced by their peers than at any other stage in development, family values also continue to affect their behavior. Researchers have noted that teenage females who report having a good relationship with their mothers are less likely to be sexually active than those who do not (Fox and Inazu, 1980). Sexual activity among adolescents whose families have clear religious affiliations is lower than among those who do not. Most religious groups clearly disapprove of premarital sexual activity or intercourse and, therefore, adolescents in families belonging to these groups are presented with consistent behavior guidelines.

For those who may themselves be a product of a teenage pregnancy, and whose friends are sexually active or are teenage parents already, early sexual activity and pregnancy are much more acceptable than for those whose peers and family value personal development, maturity, career planning, and marriage before reproduction.

The increased frequency of both intended and unintended pregnancy among adolescents of low socioeconomic status has been explained by some investigators in the following way. Poverty breeds low self-esteem in that many poor children do not succeed at school and are not exposed to other activities in which they can do well. By adolescence, they do not believe that they can succeed and, therefore, have no career goals. This is often compounded by the fact that welfare is a "way of life" in their milieu, and they feel unable to change it. For many adolescent females caught in this trap, having a baby is seen as a way to both be creative and to achieve status and a meaningful role in life.

Even when socioeconomic status is taken into account, perceived or real peer pressure often results in sexual activity. The ability of peer pressure to influence behavior is, of course, dependent upon the self-esteem of the individual adolescent. Female sexual behavior has been shown to be particularly influenced by that of close girlfriends (Smith et al, 1985). As adolescents begin to engage in single couple dating, partners often have difficulty discussing their sexual relationships. Many of these teenagers, particularly younger ones, have not developed the communication skills necessary to discuss sexuality and behavior preferences with their partner. This lack of communication frequently leads to assumptions about behavioral expectations and to sexual behavior about which neither partner feels comfortable (Schinke, 1984; Cvetkovich, 1975).

The factors that influence adolescent pregnancy are summarized in Box 37-1.

Box 37-1
Factors Influencing the Incidence of Adolescent Pregnancy

DEVELOPMENTAL FACTORS

Early physical sexual maturation
Egocentrism
Personal fable (feeling that "it won't happen to me")
Responsiveness to peers' sexual activity
Independence from family
Denial of personal sexuality

SOCIETAL FACTORS

Variety of adult sexual behavior values
Implied acceptance of intercourse outside of marriage
Importance of involvement in heterosexual relationships stressed by the media
Inadequate access to contraception
Access to public financial support for teen parents and offspring

FAMILY AND FRIENDS

Difficult mother-daughter relationship
Lack of religious affiliation
Sexually permissive behavior norms of the larger peer group
Sexual permissive values and behavior of close friends
Inadequate communication in heterosexual relationships

Nursing Strategies

The factors influencing adolescent pregnancy are multiple. Their interactions are indeed complex and not fully understood. In order to systematically develop therapeutic strategies for intervention, it is necessary to recognize how adolescent development and behavior influence nursing strategies and to place the problem within a framework.

Adolescent Development: Its Implications for Intervention

The tasks of adolescent development, and relevant adolescent behavior with implications for effective nursing intervention in the case of pregnancy, are summarized in Table 37-1. The overall goal of adolescence is to reach the adult stage of physical, social-emotional, and cognitive development. Although some of the developmental tasks and behaviors overlap, they have been arbitrarily separated in Table 37-1 to improve clarity.

Furthermore, since adolescence refers to a stage beginning at 12 years and ending around 18 years,

Table 37-1. Adolescent Development: Implications for Nursing Strategies with the Pregnant Adolescent

Normal Adolescent Behavior	Implications for Nursing Strategies
Task: Increasing Independence From Family	
Rebellion against family rules and behavior norms	Adolescents may view the nurse as another authority figure and may be suspicious initially. This is normal behavior and should be treated as such.
Secretive about personal life	Nurse must establish the limits of confidentiality from the outset. Limits are influenced by • state laws about providing contraception/abortion to adolescents without parental consent; • practice setting regulations about confidentiality; and • clarification of personal values about adolescent sexual activity and pregnancy, so they do not interfere with professional therapeutic relationships.
Seek out adult role models	Adolescents do not come to nurses for peer support; they want a competent professional in whom they can have confidence. Consequently, nurses should adopt this demeanor.
Critical of family/social values	The nurse should appreciate this and allow the adolescent to verbalize these feelings. Adolescents are very aware of hypocrisy. To be effective, the nurse needs to like and respect adolescents and demonstrate this in a nonjudgmental, caring approach.
Ambivalent about independent decision-making	The adolescent may ask the nurse to make decisions for her related to telling significant others about the pregnancy and/or options for pregnancy outcome. It is more therapeutic for the nurse to: • provide clear, understandable information required for decision-making; • assist in exploring possible solutions and consequences; and • assist in implementing the decision selected by the teenage client.
Task: Establishing an Individual Identity 1. Physical	
Denial of normal physical changes by dressing to hide them	Adolescents require: • reassurance that there is a broad range of normal development and honest appraisal of whether theirs is normal; • accurage information about the normal sequence of physical development; • accurate information about the fertility cycle and their ability to reproduce.
Fad diets to "improve" physical appearance	For pregnant adolescents, adequate nutritional and caloric intake is essential
Decreasing intake to reduce weight gain so pregnancy will not be obvious to others	Careful assessment of dietary habits, explanation of an adequate diet, and rationale, particularly in relation to adolescent health, are important. Services of a nutritionist to plan intake that is both adequate and within the adolescent's lifestyle can be very valuable.
2. Sexual	
Experimenting with different sexual behaviors	Nonjudgmental approach that assists adolescents to clarify behavior with which they are comfortable. Nurses are sometimes the "other adults" adolescents seek out.
Discussing values/feelings, clarifying myths about sexuality with peers, parents, and other adults	A nonjudgmental approach that assists adolescents in: • expressing values/feelings about sexuality; • understanding that they have a choice about sexual behavior; • understanding the risks of sexual activity; • dispelling myths about fertility and fecundity; and • problem-solving about responsible sexual behavior.
3. Social/Emotional	
Behavior strongly influenced by peers (e.g., style, dress, academic attitude/success, extra-curricular activities, drug use/abuse, sexual activity)	Nurse requires a thorough social history to assess risk factors applicable to each client and to determine their strengths, which will facilitate treatment. Because peer approval is so important for

Table 37-1 *(continued)*

Normal Adolescent Behavior	Implications for Nursing Strategies
	adolescents, the use of peer groups in learning and decision-making can be very valuable.
Development of skills valued by peers (e.g., hobbies, sports, other activities, constructive communication skills), which enhances self-esteem Negative behaviors learned for peer approval include drug use/abuse and exploitation of others	Knowledge of these positive and negative attributes is essential to understand adolescent strengths and to assess those factors that will impede compliance with treatment plans. As well, it will clarify areas to be discussed with the adolescent in relation to desired methods for change.
Need for intimacy fulfilled by experimenting with behavior and one-to-one relationships in order to begin to identify the desirable characteristics in a future mate	Need to know the methods of communication used in these relationships, as well as the intensity of the relationship as perceived by both partners, to assess the potential role of the partner related to sexual activity, decisions about the pregnancy, and parenting.
4. Cognitive	
Career planning and academic/apprentice work necessary	Future plans are important for the nurse to know about, in order to assist the pregnant adolescent in long-term planning.
Egocentrism: concern of the pregnant adolescent may be only for herself and not include the fetus	Recognize that this is normal for adolescents and not react judgmentally. Support her concerns for herself. Encourage the adolescent to plan for the baby. Indicate the value of healthy behaviors to her personally as opposed to the value for the infant.
Idealism	Assess the level of this by asking where the adolescent expects to be in 5 years and how she will care for an infant, if that is her choice.
Concrete thinking as opposed to use of abstractions	When introducing a treatment plan, ensure the adolescent understands her role by having her demonstrate the expected behavior. Use of the cognitive-behavioral approach can be very effective (Schinke et al, 1979). (See Box 37-2 for an outline of the model.)

knowledge of the stage of development that an individual teenager has reached will be essential for determining the relevance of the implications for each client. This information can be obtained only through a thorough health history.

A *Theoretical* Perspective *for* Intervention

One perspective from which adolescent pregnancy can be viewed is that of prevention; primary, secondary, and tertiary. Pender (1987) has defined the three levels as follows:

- Primary prevention—activities directed toward decreasing the probability of encountering illness, including active protection against unnecessary stressors;
- Secondary prevention—organized, direct screening efforts or education of the target population to promote early case findings of individuals with the condition so that prompt interventions can be instituted to minimize complications and/or disability;
- Tertiary prevention—all those interventions necessary to help clients live full and productive lives, while successfully managing the limitations imposed by their condition.

This framework is particularly relevant in that the objectives of most programs directed at adolescent pregnancy relate directly to at least one level of prevention. Due to the complex nature of the problem and the proposed solutions, successful outcomes depend upon a team approach. The skills and knowledge of some professionals and community members are more useful in programs directed at one level of prevention than at another. However, some professions, including nursing, have a vital role to play at all three levels. A description of programs and nursing roles at each level of prevention follows.

Primary Prevention

All of the initiatives aimed at preventing unintended adolescent pregnancy from occurring can be designated as primary prevention. Controversy about whether primary prevention efforts should focus on sexual abstinence endeavors (e.g., return to "traditional" values or withdrawal of funding for birth control and abortion services), responsible sexual behavior, ready access to contraceptive methods and abortion, or a combination of these approaches is ongoing. Nevertheless, four types of programs which combine an emphasis on accurate knowledge acquisition, responsible sexual behavior, and access to contraception and abortion appear to be reducing adolescent pregnancy rates (Zaben and Hirsch, 1988).

The first type combines a school-based health clinic with access to contraceptive devices through a nearby hospital clinic staffed by the same professionals (Edwards et al, 1977). In a recent review of school-based clinics, Kirby (1985) suggests that these services are highly successful in reducing teenage pregnancy.

The second type of program combines all health care, including family planning, social services, vocational counseling, and legal aid resources, in one setting. The Door in New York City is a well-known example of an everything-at-one-site approach. Part of the success of these two types of programs lies in the fact that by providing a broad range of adolescent services, including sexuality counseling, they are seen as more acceptable by teens. Since use of the service can be for a variety of reasons, confidentiality is assured for those who want it.

A third type of approach combines standard birth control clinics with easy access to abortion. Since the effectiveness of this approach appears to be a result of the easy access to abortion, it may not be true primary prevention.

The fourth type of approach, known as the broadcast approach, is a comprehensive community action service. It includes regular use of the media to advertise contraceptive services, teen rap sessions, and educational programs within schools that address responsible sexual behavior as well as logical problem solving and decision making.

The range of professionals who provide these programs includes (primarily) nurses, physicians, and social workers. The scope and accessibility of such programs is somewhat determined by state and national funding and by legislation. Because of their knowledge and public credibility, nurses and other health and social service professionals are in an excellent position to advocate for such programs both locally and nationally. This advocacy may take the form of direct political pressure, or it may mean providing public information sessions to raise community consciousness of the severity of the problem and possible solutions or organizing community lobby groups.

Because of their knowledge and skills, nurses in adolescent clinics or community health can provide educational programs and rap sessions about sexuality for students in elementary and high schools and in community groups (e.g., church groups, Girl Scouts, Boy Scouts). There is ample evidence that students can learn the facts about sexual development and fecundity (Parcel and Luttman, 1981; Cull-Wilby et al, 1985). Unfortunately, knowledge gains alone do not appear to change attitudes toward sexual activity or actual sexual behavior. In a review of adolescent contraceptive behavior, Morrison (1985) has summarized several psychologic models that predict and explain these behaviors. Programs that allow active adolescent participation and discussion appear to be successful in assisting adolescents to take responsibility for their sexual activity. Programs based on the cognitive-behavioral model (Schinke, 1984) and the health belief model (Eisen et al, 1985) appear promising in decreasing adolescent pregnancy. These models are outlined in Box 37-2.

Introducing these programs sometimes generates considerable community discussion and dissension. Mitchell et al (1987) suggest the following guidelines, based on experience, to maximize community acceptance of such programs:

- Identify credible groups within the professional and lay community that are prepared to publicly support the program;
- Select the title of the program carefully, avoiding words that are likely to cause strong emotional reactions;
- Assure that all public presentations of the program are simple, clear, and concise;
- Be prepared to be flexible in those areas that are not crucial;

Box 37-2
Models for Use in Preventing Adolescent Pregnancy

THE COGNITIVE-BEHAVIORAL MODEL (Schinke, 1984)

The following learning steps constitute this approach

1. student access to relevant, accurate information;
2. demonstration that the knowledge has been correctly perceived, comprehended, and stored;
3. opportunity to practice decision-making based on personal values and new information;
4. development of skills required to implement decisions.

HEALTH-BELIEF MODEL (Champion, 1984)

This model states that an individual's behavioral response to a possible threat to health is influenced by the interaction of the following five concepts:

1. perceived susceptibility to the condition (i.e., pregnancy);
2. perceived seriousness of the condition;
3. perceived benefits of avoiding the condition;
4. perceived barriers to avoiding the condition; and
5. personal motivation.

- Consult an expert for coaching and feedback regarding interactions with the media; and
- Handle objectively public or private confrontations with opposition groups (often require prior strategy planning).

Nurses in primary care settings can play an important role in the primary prevention of adolescent pregnancy by using effective communications techniques that are developmentally appropriate for adolescents (see Table 37-1 for specific details). Adolescents who view the health care setting they used during childhood as open and understanding in the past will be more likely to use it when they have questions about sexuality. However, some teens are embarrassed to discuss such topics with professionals to whom they and their families are known. Others fear that their parents will be informed immediately. These settings could provide a useful service by making information about relevant clinics freely available to adolescents without their having to ask for it (i.e., placing pamphlets in the waiting room).

Nurses are equipped to function in the roles of adolescent advocate, educator and counselor in the primary prevention of adolescent pregnancy. These roles are summarized in Box 37-3.

> *Box 37-3*
> *Primary Prevention of Adolescent Pregnancy: Nursing Roles and Strategies*
>
> **As advocate for educational programs and accessibility to contraceptive devices:**
>
> Direct political lobbying.
> Community consciousness raising through public information sessions.
> Organization of community lobby groups.
>
> **As adolescent educator:**
>
> In office, clinic, and community settings provide:
> - accurate information about reproduction;
> - opportunities for the adolescent to develop and apply problem-solving and communication skills to decisions about sexual behavior.
>
> **As community educator:**
>
> Through sessions with groups of adolescent parents or other adults provide:
> - insight into the factors affecting adolescent sexuality;
> - opportunities to learn and practice effective communication techniques to be used with adolescents.
>
> **As adolescent counselor:**
>
> Use of age-appropriate communication techniques in encounters with adolescents.
> Provide information about relevant clinics (e.g., birth control) or other necessary referral services.

Secondary Prevention

All of the initiatives directed toward early detection of pregnancy and adequate health care of the affected adolescents are examples of secondary prevention. These strategies are crucial because many of the avoidable complications of adolescent pregnancy result from the lack of early prenatal care. Nurses and other health professionals can utilize several strategies to increase the probability that pregnant adolescents will seek health care early in their pregnancy. At a community level, they can assume an active role in assuring that information about the importance of early prenatal care and where to obtain it is easily accessible to adolescents. Such information can be posted in places where groups of adolescents congregate (e.g., school bulletin boards, youth centers, community centers).

Within the clinic, primary care, or institutional setting, the nurse can use a number of strategies to enhance early detection of pregnancy. Some common ones are:

1. Questions about sexual development and sexual activity should be included in all health histories of clients over 12 years of age.
2. Both male and female adolescents should be given the opportunity to ask questions about sexuality during appointments with health care professionals. Because most teens are embarrassed discussing sexuality, it is particularly important for the nurse to be sensitive to the adolescent's feelings. A comment like, "Many people your age are uncomfortable with the changes in their body and don't really understand what is happening. Do you have any questions or concerns in this area?" can assist in placing the adolescent at ease. Some adolescents are unsure of what to ask. A discussion about their stage of development and what they know about it will identify areas that require further discussion.
3. A written health questionnaire with a section on sexuality can be very useful. If a check list is used, adolescents can easily complete it before the interview. This allows adolescents to identify areas about which they want more information or discussion without feeling embarrassed. The results of the questionnaire can be used to direct the nurse's discussion.
4. Clear, honest answers should be given to questions. A nonjudgmental approach by the nurse is essential to establish a therapeutic relationship. Asking the adolescent to summarize the discussion at several points along the way assists the nurse to assess what

has been learned or focuses the need for further clarification. Use of plastic models to explain physiologic development can be an effective strategy, particularly for those whose thinking is still quite concrete. Providing written materials (pamphlets, books, articles) gives adolescents a long-term reference. They can be encouraged to discuss the information with parents. It can provide a focus for family discussion and may ease the initiation of such dialogue.

5. Questions about the possibility of pregnancy should be included in the history of any female teenager with vague physical complaints. Adolescents in early pregnancy may arrive at health care settings but be unable to state that they are pregnant. When directly questioned, however, they will be relieved to disclose the fact.

By implementing the five preceding strategies, important knowledge is provided to the adolescent. At the same time, an open, honest, therapeutic relationship is established. This increases the likelihood that should an adolescent become pregnant, the nurse and/or physician will be consulted for support and help in dealing with the pregnancy.

Once a pregnancy has been confirmed, support and patient advocacy are important nursing roles. The adolescent is faced with a number of choices both about the outcome and about telling her parents, boyfriend, and significant others. Although the decisions are the adolescent's to make, a skillful nurse can assist her in realistically assessing and appropriately using her social supports in decision-making (see Table 37-1).

Depending upon state laws, the adolescent usually has three outcome options: therapeutic abortion, delivery and adoption, or delivery and raising her offspring. It is the nurse's responsibility to explore all of these options and their implications with the pregnant teen. To do this effectively, the nurse must be aware of available community services and how to access them as well as how to enter into the health care system. The nurse must have clarified his or her own personal views and identified ways to keep personal values from interfering with therapeutic professional relationships.

National statistics indicate that therapeutic abortion (TA) is increasingly becoming the option of choice. Since TAs are usually performed before 16 weeks' gestation, the adolescent who has delayed in seeking health care for the pregnancy may have to make this choice very quickly, or it may be unavailable to her. The nurse can assist the adolescent in personal values clarification related to this choice. The methods of therapeutic abortion should be explained in a realistic, nonjudgmental way. This discussion should also explore professional and personal support systems available for the adolescent following the abortion (Howard, 1985).

A second alternative for the pregnant adolescent is bearing the infant and placing the baby for adoption. Musick et al (1984) have identified a steady decrease in the number of adolescents choosing to place their offspring for adoption. Although a number of factors appear to influence this, one relevant to nurses is that health care providers hesitate to suggest adoption as an alternative either because they are unaware of available community services or because they are uncomfortable with adoption (Musick et al, 1984). Responsible nurses must be able to present this alternative and its possible consequences for the adolescent and infant in an unbiased way. In fact, it should be readdressed as the pregnancy progresses. Another factor that reduces adoption as an option is the widespread belief that a girl who gets pregnant has a responsibility to have and keep the baby. Among black and Hispanic girls, adoption has never been widely accepted as an option. Among Caucasians, as well as other groups, there is little peer or family support for adoption. The fear that infants of minority groups might end up in foster homes, institutions, or with families of another culture is also a deterrent. Musick et al (1984) have recognized three crucial factors in this decision-making: (1) the ability of adolescents and, to a lesser degree, professionals working with them to view the choice from the unborn child's perspective; (2) the relationship between the reasons for becoming pregnant (e.g., to have someone to love) and the choices of outcome; and (3) the inability of adolescents to fully recognize the limitations on their future that will result from parenthood.

The third alternative, and one frequently selected by adolescents, is bearing the infant and raising the child. Often adolescents choose to bear the infant. However, it takes time to determine the most reasonable lifestyle for the mother and child. Consultation and ongoing assistance from a social worker can be very helpful for those adolescents and significant others having difficulty making a decision. Within the secondary prevention area, the role of the nurse is to assist the adolescent and her significant others in recognizing and evaluating the appropriateness of the various family constellations that can result.

The adolescent may choose to live with her parents and raise her child with their support. This option has several advantages. It usually provides the adolescent with financial support as well as ready access to people who have had experience with infant care. Often these families are prepared to take an active part in the care of the infant, freeing the adolescent both to return to school or work and also to carry on age-appropriate social activities. The success of this arrangement is determined largely by the ability of the teen and her family to clarify possible areas of friction and to negotiate mutually acceptable solutions.

When children bring an infant home to live with parents, potential areas of disagreement exist. First, the person who is going to take on the primary role and responsibility of mother must be identified. When the adolescent is young, the maternal grandmother may assume that she, not the mother, will be making all the decisions about the infant and the adolescent. This can lead to deep-seated resentment by the teenage mother. Second, in families in which the adolescent-parent relationship has been poor during the adolescent's childhood, the limits must be clearly stated and monitored to minimize decreasing the adolescent's self-esteem. Third, the adolescent and her parents must agree upon the nature of the relationship between the teen, her infant, and the infant's father. Finally, the effect of the presence of the adolescent and her infant on other family members must be examined.

In some cases, an adolescent chooses to live on her own with her infant. This may or may not be in conjunction with support from the extended family or the father of the child. Living alone offers the adolescent the opportunity to make independent decisions about her own lifestyle and the care of her infant. Some adolescents view this as a sign of their maturity. For many, however, the perceived advantages are overshadowed by the reality of the scope of the responsibility they have assumed. Frequently, their only source of income is public assistance, which restricts all areas of their life. Choices of accommodation are limited. Resources for child care are minimal, which inhibits the return to school or work, and results in long-term dependency. The restrictions of parenthood may isolate adolescent mothers from former friends; because of their young age, they are not always accepted by other mothers. They may have minimal experience with infant care and lack knowledge about how to access competent, helpful resource people. The overwhelming responsibility and increased infant demands are thought to be strong contributors to the fact that many adolescents who initially choose to keep their offspring relinquish them by the middle of the second year of life. Obviously, the amount of support these adolescents receive from their families, their friends, and the father can have a decisive influence on their own health and welfare as well as that of their offspring.

Other adolescents choose to live with the father of the infant. They may or may not be married. Sharing the responsibility of parenthood makes it easier, but many of these couples are faced with limited access to resources, financial and supportive, and limited knowledge and skill related to infant care and development.

In assisting the adolescent and her significant others to explore the possible alternatives, keep in mind the Implications for Nursing Interventions found in Table 37-1. The nursing roles in secondary prevention of adolescent pregnancy are outlined in Box 37-4.

Box 37-4
Secondary Prevention of Adolescent Pregnancy: Nursing Roles and Strategies

Early detection of adolescent pregnancy:

Include sexual development and activity in history taking of all clients 12 years of age and older.

Enhance the likelihood that pregnant adolescents will seek out early health care by:

- providing opportunities for them to ask questions about sexuality;
- answering questions honestly; and
- providing written information for future reference and family discussion.

Post information about community resources in areas where adolescents congregate.

Supportive advocate for adolescent after pregnancy:

Assisting adolescent in:

- telling parents and significant others;
- identifying and using available support systems;
- exploring pregnancy outcome alternatives; and
- supporting the adolescent's outcome decision.

Tertiary Prevention

As previously stated, tertiary prevention includes all those interventions necessary to help clients live full and productive lives while successfully managing the limitations imposed by their conditions. For pregnant adolescents this includes all the strategies used by the health care team and the teen to minimize complications of the pregnancy and delivery as well as those strategies that contribute to successful postnatal adjustment and decrease the likelihood of future unplanned pregnancies.

Providing optimum care for the pregnant adolescent requires a team effort among several health professionals, including nurses, physicians, social workers, and nutritionists. Although each team member has specific contributions, open, regular communication among the members is essential for provision of quality care to the adolescent and her significant others. In settings where the above services are not available, consultations with the necessary professionals at another agency may be arranged, or the nurses and physicians may provide all the care during the pregnancy.

Pregnant adolescents require the routine prenatal care that any pregnant woman requires. Students should consult an obstetrical nursing textbook to review the nurse's role in provision of such care. This discussion will address the unique aspects of care for adolescents who are pregnant.

Once a pregnancy has been confirmed and the adolescent has chosen to have the infant, data from the health and social history, laboratory results, and physical examination are compiled by the health care team and used to determine the "risk status" of the adolescent and her infant. It is important that this be done as soon as possible as it will guide the course of prenatal care. Adolescents are considered to be at high risk for complications if one or more of the following factors are present:

- age 16 years or less;
- anemia;
- poor physical state (e.g., obesity, low weight for height);
- any sexually transmitted disease;
- use of tobacco, alcohol, or street drugs;
- poverty;
- lack of social support; and
- prior medical conditions that pregnancy may complicate (e.g., diabetes mellitus, epilepsy, asthma).

The first step in effectively caring for a pregnant adolescent is to establish a therapeutic relationship based on trust. This will increase the probability that the adolescent will be honest and open about her problems and work at setting and meeting reasonable expectations for her health. It is important for the nurse to understand the adolescents' normal developmental needs and related nursing implications, as outlined in Table 37-1, in order to establish a relationship with a pregnant adolescent.

Common nursing diagnoses for pregnant adolescents, relevant nursing strategies, rationale, and expected outcomes are summarized in Table 37-2.

Tertiary prevention of adolescent pregnancy also includes nursing interventions following abortion or delivery. Postabortion support and counseling are services that nurses in clinics, the community, or the school are well suited to implement. For many adolescents, the nurse may be a major source of ongoing support and assistance because few others know about the abortion. The two major tasks involved are assisting the adolescent to (1) accept the fact that she has had an abortion, and (2) accept her own sexuality and planning for future responsible, realistic sexual behavior to prevent another unintended pregnancy (e.g., abstinence or use of a reliable method of contraception). These goals are best accomplished through two or three one-to-one sessions with the teen. In areas where contraceptive services are available to adolescents through clinics, the teen should be referred to the clinic for access to the selected method and ongoing monitoring of compliance.

The follow-up care of adolescents who place their offspring for adoption is similar to that of teens choosing abortion in that prevention of subsequent pregnancy is a major objective. However, another major component of care is supporting the adolescent who gave up her infant. Ambivalence about the decision, guilt, and peer or parental disapproval are difficult conflicts that require support and follow-up care.

Care of adolescents who keep their offspring is more complicated and long-term. They also require assistance in accepting their sexuality and planning to prevent subsequent unintended pregnancies. The other ongoing needs of adolescent mothers/parents include:

- knowledge of infant care, including safety, hygiene, nutrition, and treatment of minor childhood ailments (e.g., rashes, temperature elevation);
- knowledge about normal infant and child growth and development, including concrete, age-appropriate methods of infant stimulation, and the importance of mother-child interaction; and
- integration of the responsibilities of motherhood with those of adolescent development, particularly continuation of formal education but also provision of regular contact with peers, development of individual interests, and formation of positive heterosexual relationships (Howard et al, 1985).

Box 37-5
Tertiary Prevention of Adolescent Pregnancy: Nursing Roles and Strategies

Identification and implementation of nursing tasks within the care team:

Establishing/continuing a therapeutic relationship with the adolescent.

Assessing the risk status of the pregnant adolescent.

Identifying client problems (actual or potential) during pregnancy and negotiating client behaviors to minimize complications (see Table 37-2).

Assisting the adolescent in planning to prevent future unintended pregnancies.

Assisting the adolescent in learning about and practicing safe infant and child care.

Assisting the adolescent in integrating normal adolescent developmental tasks with those of parenthood.

Table 37-2. Nursing Care of Pregnant Adolescents

Nursing Diagnoses	Nursing Strategies	Rationale	Expected Outcome
***Potential for altered nutrition; less than body requirements,* related to:** • lack of adequate financial resources • lack of information about nutritional requirements for fetal growth	Accurate assessment of height and weight at first visit. Dietary history to assess adequacy of intake (see Chapter 18 for details)	Baseline from which to assess weight gain at subsequent visits	Under 16 years, 16 kg weight gain during pregnancy; 17–25 years, 11 kg weight gain during pregnancy
	Those with inadequate intake could benefit from ongoing nutritional counseling to improve their dietary status, in keeping with their socioeconomic status and cultural patterns	Establish and try to maintain caloric intake that allows for adequate fetal growth and avoids adolescent anemia	Adolescent uses nutritional information to improve her dietary status
	If the physician prescribes vitamins and/or iron, assure that the adolescent: • understands how they will affect her health • understands dose, frequency of administration, and side effects • has money/drug plan to cover their cost	Improve compliance	Adolescent can explain rationale. Drugs will be taken as prescribed
Potential for injury (of self and fetus),* related to:*chemical effects of drug use and abuse (including tobacco and alcohol)	Explain the effect of each on the adolescent, as well as the fetus	Information can be used by the adolescent to determine risk of continued behavior	Adolescent can state risks of drug use
	Assess social supports available to assist the adolescent in decreasing or stopping drug use	Accurate information can sometimes motivate behavior change if the risk is serious enough	Adolescent will identify desire and method for behavior change
	Provide ways to access community support groups for decreasing drug use		
***Fear,* related to:** • potential for pain upon physical examination (internal) • separation from support systems during a threatening procedure • unfamiliarity with procedure • unfamiliarity with health professional	Provide clear, honest explanation before doing procedures	Adolescent can understand the explanation	Teen relaxed during procedures
	When possible, the same person should do the history, physical, and internal examination	Reassuring for the teen and decreases embarrassment	
***Knowledge deficit* related to:** • body changes during pregnancy • fetal growth	Explain changes and fetal growth using plastic models and charts. Have adolescent summarize content of discussion	Clarify understanding of normal changes, increase acceptance of self, and improve body image	Adolescent can recognize changes during pregnancy and signs of possible complications
	Provide opportunity for the adolescent to hear the fetal heart, feel the fetus	Provides reality set about the infant. Encourages bonding	
***Potential for injury,* related to:** • presence of sexually transmitted disease (STD) • unwillingness of adolescent (diagnosed to have STD) to provide names and addresses of sexual contacts	Adequate history of sexual activity and prior STD	Screening for STD	
	Appropriate serum tests/swabs done at first visit		
	If any STD present, explain and initiate ordered treatment	Clarify treatment requirements. Encourage compliance with treatment	Adolescent will be able to explain treatment and how she will comply with it
	Have adolescent provide names and addresses of sexual contacts and report to the Public Health Department in accordance with state laws	Facilitate identification and treatment of other infected individuals. Prevent further spread of disease	Stop further spread of disease
	Explain methods to prevent/minimize future STD (e.g., consistent use of condoms during sexual intercourse)	Prevent reinfection	

continued

Table 37-2 *(continued)*

Nursing Diagnoses	Nursing Strategies	Rationale	Expected Outcome
Knowledge deficit, related to: • process of labor and delivery • lifestyle options for care of the baby • items needed for the baby	Assess adolescent's current knowledge about the topic Dispel myths Encourage teen to participate in prenatal classes, preferably a session for adolescents only, so it can be tailored to their level of development	Determine learning needs to establish an appropriate educational plan more likely to meet the needs of the adolescent	Adolescent can describe and use techniques taught during labor and delivery
	Review of rationale for lifestyle option after delivery and assessment of support for choice Adoption should be reintroduced as a choice	Assist adolescents in clarifying their choice	Ability to adapt to the selected choice
	Identification of items needed for care of a newborn baby and suggestions for ways to acquire them	Adolescent recognition of the need to prepare	Physical equipment will be in place before delivery
Ineffective individual coping, related to: • unrealistic estimate of short- and long-term implications of being a mother • multiple life changes associated with the care of a newborn baby	Assess short- and long-term goals of the adolescent. Assist in realistically clarifying these and planning to meet them. This may include referral to the services of several community agencies or programs	Realistic expectations for role changes after delivery will aid in adjustment to motherhood by giving the adolescent a sense of control over her life	Adolescents can set realistic goals and outline plausible ways to accomplish them
Potential noncompliance: failure to use appropriate contraceptives, related to: • lack of knowledge about contraceptive options • belief system of adolescent • cultural values	Begin early in pregnancy. Introduce the topic of responsible sexual behavior. Assist the adolescent in clarifying values around use of contraception in general and specific methods in particular. Explain advantages, disadvantages, and the effectiveness of the various methods. (See Chapter 9 for a discussion of contraceptive methods.) Have the adolescent summarize the information as it applies to her	Provide adolescents with the opportunity to explore the idea of being responsible for her sexual behavior and fecundity	No future unplanned pregnancy

A number of programs consisting of weekly group sessions for adolescent mothers or combinations of group and one-to-one sessions appear to address most of these needs, and improve the long-term outcome for the adolescents and their offspring. These programs have been implemented in schools (Delatte et al, 1985; McAfee and Geesey, 1984), within a pediatric-medical center as part of well-baby follow-up (Badger, 1985), and within community settings (Badger, 1985). Nurses, usually with postgraduate education, have been instrumental in developing and implementing these programs. For readers interested in the details of such programs, the cited references would be very informative.

The roles for knowledgeable, skilled nurses in the tertiary prevention of adolescent pregnancy are outlined in Box 37-5.

Effective prevention of adolescent pregnancy is a multifaceted, challenging, sometimes frustrating activity. Nurses who choose to develop the knowledge and skills to intervene with not-yet pregnant or pregnant adolescents, their partners, their offspring, or their other family members will be vital members of health care teams that are improving the health, in the broadest sense, of not only the target group but society at large.

References

Alan Guttmacher Institute: *Teenage Pregnancy: The Problem Hasn't Gone Away.* New York, 1986.

Alan Guttmacher Institute: *Eleven Million Teenagers: What Can Be Done About The Epidemic of Adolescent Pregnancies in the United States.* New York, Planned Parenthood Federation of America, 1976.

Badger E: Teenage mothers and their infants. *Clin Perinatol* 1985; 12(2):391–406.

Brann EA, et al: Strategies for the prevention of pregnancy in adolescents. *Adv Plann Parent* 1979; 14:68–76.

Braverman L: The phenomenon of teenage marriage. *Semin Adol Med* 1985; 1(3):189–194.

Chamie M, et al: Factors affecting adolescent use of family planning clinics. *Fam Plann Perspect* 1982; 14:126–135.

Champion VL: Instrumental development for health belief model constructs. *Adv Nurs Sci* 1984 Apr; 73–85.

Chilman CS: Teenage pregnancy: a research review. *Social Work* 1979; 24:492–498.

Clark JFJ, et al: Adolescent pregnancy: a twenty year review. *JAMA* 1982; 74:39.

Cull-Wilby BL, et al: The relationship between sex education and knowledge in grade eight students. *Can J Public Health* 1985; 76:163–166.

Cvetkovich G: On the psychology of adolescent use of contraception. *J Sex Res* 1975; 11:156–270.

Delatte JG Jr, et al: Project SCAN: counseling teen-age parents in a school setting. *J School Health* 1985 Jan; 55(1):24–26.

Dott AB, Fort AT: Medical and social factors affecting early teenage pregnancy. *Am J Obstet Gynec* 1976; 125(4):532–536.

Edwards LE, Steinman ME, Hakanson EY: An experimental comprehensive high school clinic. *Am J Public Health* 1977; 67(8):765–766.

Eisen M, Zellman GI, McAlister AL: A health belief model approach to adolescents' fertility control: some pilot program findings. *Health Educ Q* 1985; 12(2):186–210.

Finkelstein JW, et al: Teenage pregnancy and parenthood: outcomes for mother and child. *J Adol Health Care* 1982; 3:1–7.

Fox GC, Inazu JK: Patterns and outcomes of mother-daughter communication about sexuality. *J Soc Issues* 1980; 36(1):7–29.

Frisancho AR, Matos J, Bollettino LA: Influence of growth status and placental function on birth weight of infants born to young still-growing teenagers. *Am J Clin Nutr* 1984; 40:801–807.

Furstenberg FF: *Unplanned Parenthood: The Social Consequences of Teenage Childbearing.* New York, Free Press, 1976.

Hardy JB, et al: Long-range outcome of adolescent pregnancy. *Clin Obstet Gynecol* 1978; 21(4):1215–1232.

Howard JS: Adolescent mothers: self-perceived health education needs. *JOGNN* 1985 Sep-Oct; 399–404.

Howard T: Abortion: the teenage patient and the O.R. Nurse. *Can Nurse* 1985; 28–30.

Jones EF, et al: Teenage pregnancy in developed countries: determinants and policy implications. *Fam Plann Perspect* 1985; 17(2):53–63.

Kinard EM, Klerman LO: Teenage parenting and child abuse: are they related? *Am J Orthopsychiatry* 1980; 50(3):481–488.

Kirby D: *School-based Health Clinics: An Emerging Approaching to Improving Adolescent Health and Addressing Teenage Pregnancy.* Washington, DC, Center for Population Options, 1985.

Klein L: Antecedents of teenage pregnancy. *Clin Obstet Gynecol* 1978; 21(4):1151–1159.

Lindsay LW: *Teenage Marriage: Coping with Reality.* Buena Park, CA, Morning Glory Press, 1984.

Loris P, Dewey KG, Poirier-Brode K: Weight gain and dietary intake of pregnant teenagers. *J Am Diet Assoc* 1985; 85(10):1296–1305.

McAfee ML, Geesey MR: Meeting the needs of the teenage pregnant student: an in-school program that works. *J School Health* 1984; 54(9):350–352.

McAnarney ER, Greydamus DE: Adolescent pregnancy: A risk condition. *Semin Perinatal* 1981; 5:1–103.

Mitchell A, et al: Researching sensitive issues in the community: the case of adolescent pregnancy prevention. Unpublished manuscript, 1987.

Moore DS, Erickson PI, Wurgel M: Adolescent pregnancy and parenting: the role of the nurse. *Topics Clin Nurs* 1984 Oct; 72–82.

Morrison D: Adolescent contraceptive behaviour: a review. *Psychol Bull* 1985; 98(3):538–568.

Munz D, et al: Contraceptive knowledge and practice among undergraduates at a Canadian university. *Am J Obstet Gynecol* 1976; 124:499–505.

Musick J, Handler A, Waddill KD: Teens and adoption: a pregnancy resolution alternative? *Child Today* 1984 Nov-Dec; 24–29.

Nadelson CC, Notman TM, Gillon JW: Sexual knowledge and attitudes of adolescents: relationship to contraceptive use. *Obstet Gynecol* 1980; 55(3):340–345.

Nathanson CA, Becker MH: The influence of client-provider relationships on teenage women's subsequent use of contraception. *Am J Public Health* 1985; 75(1):33–38.

Parcel GS, Luttman D: Evaluation in sex education: evaluation research applied to program planning for sex education. *J School Health* 1981; 51:278–281.

Pender JN: *Health Promotion in Nursing Practice.* Norwalk, CT, Appleton-Century-Crofts, 1987.

Piechnik SL, Corbett MA: Reducing low birth weight among socioeconomically high-risk adolescent pregnancies. *J Nurse-Midwifery* 1985; 30(2):88–98.

Public Health Service: *Morbidity and Mortality Weekly Report.* (HHS Publication No. CDC 81-8017.) Atlanta, US Government Printing Office, 1981.

Rivara FP, Sweeney PJ, Henderson BF: A study of low socioeconomic status black teenage fathers and their non-father peers. *Pediatrics* 1985; 75:648–656.

Ryan GM, Sweeney PJ: Attitudes of adolescents toward pregnancy and contraception. *Am J Obstet Gynecol* 1980; 137(3):358–366.

Schinke SP: Preventing teenage pregnancy. *Prog Behav Modif* 1984; 16:32–64.

Shah R, Zelnik M: Parent and peer influence on sexual behaviour, contraceptive and pregnancy experience of young women. *J Marr Fam* 1981; 43:339–348.

Smith EA, Udry JR, Morris NM: Pubertal development and friends: a biosocial explanation of adolescent sexual behaviour. *J Health Soc Behav* 1985; 26:183–192.

Snyder JK, Fox GL: Maternal influence on the sexual behaviour of teenage daughters. *J Fam Issues* 1980; 1:81–102.

Society of Obstetricians and Gynecologists of Canada Bulletin 2. 1986 Mar-Apr; 15–16.

Spivak, H, Weitzman M: Social Barriers Faced by Adolescent Parents and Their Children, JAMA, Sept 18 1987, Vol 258, No. 11

Zaben LS, Hirsch M: *Evaluation of Pregnancy Prevention Programs in the School Context.* New York, Lexington Books, 1988.

Zaben LS, Kantner JF, Zelnik M: The risk of adolescent pregnancy in the first months of intercourse. *Fam Plann Perspect* 1979; 11(4):215–222.

Zelnik M, Kantner JF: Sexual activity, contraceptive use and pregnancy among metropolitan area teenagers: 1971–1979. *Fam Plann Perspect* 1980; 12:230–237.

Zelnik M, Kantner JF: Reasons for non-use of contraception by sexually active women ages 15–19. *Fam Plann Perspect* 1979; 11:289–296.

Zelnik M, Shah FK: First intercourse among young Americans. *Fam Plann Perspect* 1983; 15:64–70.

Zlatnik FJ, Burmeister LF: Low gynecologic age: an obstetrical risk factor. *Am J Obstet Gynecol* 1977; 128(2):183–186.

Zuckerman B, et al: Neonatal outcome: is adolescent pregnancy a risk factor? *Pediatrics* 1983; 71:489–493.

Zuckerman BS, et al: Adolescent pregnancy: biobehavioral determinants of outcome. *J Pediatr* 1984; 105(6):857–863.

Bibliography

Belsky S, Miller BC: Adolescent fatherhood in the context of the transition to parenthood. *In* Elster A, Lamb M (eds): *Adolescent Fathers.* Hillsdale, NJ, Erlbaum, 1986.

Cutrona CE, Troutman BR: Psychosocial outcomes of adolescent pregnancy. *Semin Adol Med* 1986 Sep; 2(3):235–242.

Haffner D, Casey S: Approaches to adolescent pregnancy prevention. *Semin Adol Med* 1986 Sep; 2(3):259–267.

Miller KA, Field CS: Adolescent pregnancy: critical reviews for the clinician. *Semin Adol Med* 1985; 1:195–212.

Yoos L: Perspectives on adolescent parenting: effect of adolescent egocentrism on the maternal-child interaction. *J Pediatr Nurs* 1987 Jun; 2(3):193–200.

Young M: Parenting during mid-adolescence: a review of developmental theories and parenting behaviors. *Matern Child Nurs J* 1988 Spring; 17(1):1–12.

Unit Seven

Nursing Strategies in Physiologic Alterations

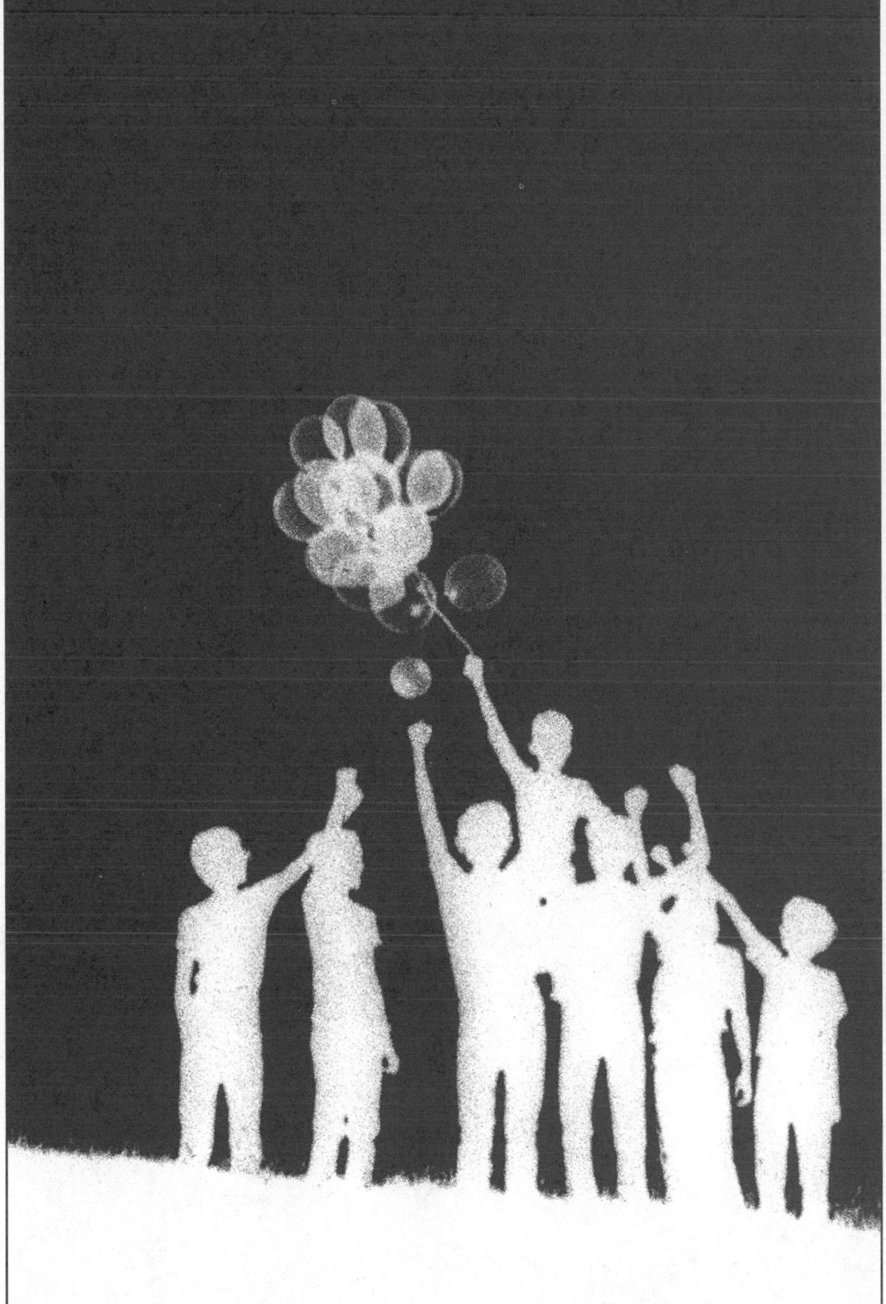

Nursing Strategies: Altered Respiratory Function

Chapter 38

Mabel Hunsberger

A continuous supply of oxygen is essential to carry out the vital processes of the human organism. One cannot "do without oxygen" for a little while as one does without food or water. The main function of respiration is to supply the body with oxygen and dispose of carbon dioxide. If the system fails, the cells die from oxygen starvation and accumulation of carbon dioxide. Alterations in the ability to consume oxygen and rid the body of carbon dioxide comprise a major segment of health problems in children. The problems discussed in this chapter cause varied degrees of distress to the family, depending on the suddenness, severity, duration, and outcome of the problem. The age of the child at the time of illness is a major variant in how a family copes and how the child is affected. Furthermore, many respiratory problems begin suddenly and frighten the child and family because of the difficulty in breathing.

Nurses need expert clinical skills to accurately assess the clinical status of children and the family's responses. Nurses also have a central role in the planning and administration of the therapeutic regimens, take responsibility for teaching children and families about their illness and how to prevent it, and provide emotional support during the illness.

This chapter presents the theoretical concepts of respiratory function applied to children, with a discussion of the most common health problems of infants and children. Nurses' roles in assessment and nursing strategies for each alteration are presented.

Many of the common respiratory alterations in children, particularly young infants, are life-threatening. For the nurse to respond effectively to the challenge of caring for children with respiratory problems, a basic understanding of respiratory function and the mechanisms of the various alterations is required.

Following is a review of the principles of altered respiratory physiology as they pertain to children and a discussion of diagnostic and therapeutic procedures that are common to respiratory problems in children. The most common alterations in children and adolescents are then discussed.

Principles of Altered Respiratory Function

To some degree, differences caused by the age of the child determine the type of problem that occurs and the degree of threat it presents, because of anatomic and physiologic differences.

Incidence and Etiology of Respiratory Dysfunction

Respiratory illness in children, both acute and chronic, is caused by intrinsic factors, extrinsic factors, or a combination of both. Intrinsic factors include congenital malformations of the airway, problems secondary to other organ defects (e.g., cardiac anomalies), and congenital, metabolic, or immunologic deficiencies. Extrinsic factors include infection, environment, pollution (including passive smoking), and aspirated foreign material (Strope and Stempel, 1984). Hyaline membrane disease and lung injuries during infancy and childhood are insults that have varied sequelae on long-term development.

Acute illness of the respiratory tract accounts for approximately 50 per cent of all illness in children under 5 years of age and 30 per cent in children between 5 and 12 years of age (Hughes, 1984). The primary cause of acute respiratory illnesses is viral infections; young children contract four or five per year. Viral infections result in a broad range of illnesses, from mild to life-threatening. Many deaths still occur from bacterial infection of the respiratory tract, although early use of antibiotic treatment has reduced the morbidity and mortality.

Chronic respiratory disease accounts for almost half of all childhood chronic diseases. One of every ten children is affected by asthma, cystic fibrosis, bronchopulmonary dysplasia, bronchiectasis, emphysema, or congenital bronchopulmonary disorders. Children with chronic lung disease are severely affected by air pollution and cigarette smoking, including passive smoking or second-hand smoke.

Passive smoking is defined as the inhalation of mainstream smoke exhaled by the smoker and sidestream smoke that goes directly into the air from the end of a burning cigarette, pipe, or cigar (Mohler, 1987). An association between parental smoking and

We appreciate the contribution by Margaret Crandall of the section on Asthma.

respiratory problems in children has been identified (Vedal et al, 1984; Ware et al, 1984; Burchfiel et al, 1986), especially in relation to bronchitis and pneumonia, with the greatest impact on the first three years of life (Fergusson et al, 1981).

Parental smoking also has been reported to be associated with frequent coughs in school-age children (Charlton, 1984) and to be a risk factor for recurrent otitis media, recurrent tonsillopharyngitis, and the need for tonsillectomy and adenoidectomy (Said et al, 1978). Decreased pulmonary function is also reported in children of parents who smoke (Vedal et al, 1984; Ware et al, 1984), and the annual rate of lung growth in children with parents who smoke is less than expected (Tager et al, 1983; Ware et al, 1984).

Age-Related Differences in Anatomy and Physiology of the Respiratory System

The process of respiration involves the same events in children as it does in adults. A basic physiology text should be reviewed to gain an understanding of the components of oxygenation, which include

- Pulmonary *ventilation* (exchange of gases between the external environment and the lung alveoli)
- *Diffusion* (exchange of oxygen and carbon dioxide between alveolar air and blood cells within the lung capillaries)
- *Transportation* of oxygen and carbon dioxide by the blood to the systemic tissue cells
- *Exchange* of oxygen and carbon dioxide between the blood and tissue cells throughout the body as blood flows through tissue capillaries

These physiologic processes are similar in adults and children, but some developmental differences have an impact upon the effectiveness and the vulnerabilities of the respiratory system in children. Important developmental differences in respiration that the nurse should understand are:

1. The predominance of diaphragmatic-abdominal breathing, normally present in the neonate, continues until around 5 years of age,
2. The chest wall is supple and very compliant, especially in infants. Because of this characteristic, when respiratory disease occurs and greater efforts at breathing are made the chest wall is easily sucked in (retractions),
3. Due to the small size of the airway, the infant is more susceptible to airway obstruction or collapse,
4. The respiratory rate of infants and children is higher than in adults, awake or asleep,
5. During the newborn and early infancy stage, the normal pattern of breathing is irregular, and:
6. Oxygen consumption is high in proportion to body size. The high proportionate surface area to body weight results in increased heat loss, requiring an increased metabolic rate.

The structure and function of an infant's or child's lungs that contribute to these differences are reviewed in the next section. Table 38-1 summarizes the differences.

Chest Wall and Respiratory Muscles. Chest expansion in the adult is accomplished by contraction of the diaphragm (which causes the diaphragm to descend) and contraction of the external intercostal muscles (which elevates the rib cage). A major difference in the infant's chest wall affecting expansion is the *position of the ribs.* In the adult it is the downward, lateral angle of the ribs that permits the elevation of the ribs (in a bucket handle action), which results in chest expansion. The ribs of an infant articulate with the vertebrae and sternum *horizontally,* allowing little leverage to increase the anteroposterior diameter of the chest. The infant's breathing is thus primarily diaphragmatic-abdominal. Normally the infant's chest and abdomen are raised together (synchronized). In respiratory distress, the chest falls on inspiration and rises on expiration—a symptom called paradoxic breathing. Furthermore, the abdomen moves in the opposite direction to the chest (falls on expiration and rises on inspiration), giving rise to the term *see-saw respirations.* This phenomenon is a result of the nonrigid (compliant) chest wall. The disappearance of the see-saw characteristic of breathing during respiratory distress is a result of the hardening of ribs/cartilage so that the framework is more stable.

The degree of stability of the chest wall affects the process of respiration. During inspiration the diaphragm contracts and descends, thus making the pleural pressure more negative (subatmospheric). The fall in pleural pressure is transmitted through the lung and causes a slightly negative intra-alveolar pressure. Airflow from the atmosphere to the alveoli occurs because of this pressure difference between the atmosphere and the alveoli.The amount of negative pressure in the intrapleural space (between visceral and parietal pleura) that is normally seen is −4 mm Hg (Guyton, 1987). The relatively rigid rib cage of an adult can be expanded and its shape maintained during this process. An infant, especially the premature infant, has a soft sternum and a less rigid rib cage. Consequently, inspiration may cause an inward movement of the rib cage because of the intrapleural subatmospheric pressure. This results in observable *retractions* (indrawing). Such retractions can occur in a mild form during normal breathing in the neonate, but in

Table 38-1. Developmental Differences in Structure and Function of the Respiratory System

Anatomy and Physiology	Significance
Chest Wall and Muscles of Respiration	
Ribs are horizontal in position. Intercostal muscles are immature, and the rib cage is supple. The neonate's diaphragm has very few fatigue-resistant muscle fibers.	Diaphragmatic-abdominal breathing is normal in infants. Retractions occur more readily in the event of large negative intrapleural pressures.
Airway	
Obligate nasal breather during first 3 weeks of life. Large tongue; U-shaped epiglottis; larynx is positioned 2–3 vertebrae higher than in an adult.	Oxygenation compromised if nasal obstruction occurs.
Airway diameter in absolute terms is smaller than the adult.	The potential for obstruction is increased.
Increased ventilatory dead space.	A larger increase in respiratory rate is required to increase alveolar ventilation.
Cartilage (trachea and bronchi) is present from birth but increases in first year of life and continues to develop to late school age.	Airway of young infant is more susceptible to collapse during expiration.
Less muscle is present in airways.	May be a decreased potential for bronchospasm in the very young child.
Mucous membranes of airways are highly vascular.	Susceptible to trauma, edema, and spasm.
Diameter of airway in infants and children is proportionately larger than in adults. Angle of right bronchus is reduced.	Increases potential for aspiration of foreign body (right side is most common).
Alveoli and Parenchyma	
Alveoli present at birth and fewer in number and smaller in size.	Although the number and size of alveoli are reduced, surface area is constant throughout life when expressed relative to body surface area.
Fewer intra-alveolar pores of Kohn and bronchoalveolar canals of Lambert.	Less able to achieve ventilation beyond obstructed units.
Surfactant is lacking in prematurity.	Absence of surfactant is the principal cause of respiratory distress syndrome.
Peripheral airways contribute a larger percentage of airway resistance than in the adult.	Respiration is severely compromised by illnesses that affect the peripheral airways.
Related Physiologic Factors	
Infants and young children have immature thermostatic control and proportionately large surface area when compared to adults.	Ability to adjust to temperature changes is decreased. Respiratory rate increases appreciably to meet metabolic demands.
Lymph tissues particularly active until child is 6 years of age. It then gradually becomes less active and atrophies after child is 12 years of age.	Infection and edema readily result in occlusion of the upper airway in a young child.
Development of accessory muscles is poor (head bobbing occurs in infants).	Reach point of respiratory insufficiency more quickly than adults.

the older infant and child they indicate that the negative intrapleural pressure required to distend the lungs is markedly below atmospheric pressure and is a sign of respiratory distress. The more marked the retractions, the greater is the negative intrapleural pressure being required to move the air from the mouth to the alveoli. This results from airflow obstruction or excessively stiff lungs. Retractions (indrawing) typically are intercostal, sternal, and paratracheal (tracheal tug). Retractions progressing from intercostal to sternal to paratracheal signify increasing respiratory distress and more negative pleural pressure.

Airways: Developmental Differences

The structure and components of the airway affect the ease with which air can move through the respiratory passageways. Infants are obligatory nose breathers. Therefore, intake of air is easily compromised in the event of a nasal obstruction such as a congenital anomaly or during therapeutic procedures (suctioning, tube feeding) when nares are obstructed. Most infants do not open their mouths to maintain an airway until approximately 3 weeks of age; however, air is taken in during crying.

The potential for edema and obstruction of the airway is enhanced owing to various anatomical differences when compared to an adult. The tongue is larger in proportion to the mouth, therefore occlusion of the airway is more likely. The larynx (epiglottis and glottis) of an infant or child has ciliated columnar epithelium below the glottis (vocal cord) that is loosely bound with areolar tissue, and there is greater vascularity of the mucous membrane. This area is highly susceptible to trauma, edema, and spasm. The infant epiglottis is large and U-shaped (the adult's is V-shaped), contributing to ease of obstruction. The cricoid cartilage is the narrowest part of the trachea, producing a funnel shape; a 1-mm increase in wall thickness from edema can compromise the airway 75 per cent (Mellins, 1971).

The airway diameter of an infant or child is in absolute terms smaller than that of an adult, increasing the potential for obstruction at all times. Proportionately, however, the diameter of the conducting airways is larger in the infant and child than in the adult. The proportionately large diameter increases the ratio of dead space (air that fills respiratory passages with each breath) to tidal volume (volume of air inspired or expired with each breath). This anatomic difference necessitates proportionately more air to be moved in and out of the lungs each minute (minute volume) to obtain a comparable amount of alveolar ventilation where gas exchange actually takes place. This possibly is one of the reasons infants breathe at a faster resting respiratory rate.

The airways change in structure and function throughout postnatal growth. During the first few months of extrauterine life, the diameter and length of the trachea and bronchi increase rapidly (Doershuk et al, 1975). At birth, cartilage, mucous glands, and goblet cells are all present. Cartilage in the trachea and bronchi increases during the first year of life, providing the rigidity that is required to keep the airways from collapsing. The epithelium of an infant's or child's airway contains almost twice the number of submucosal glands per unit surface as does the adult's (Doershuk et al, 1975). Muscle in the airway wall is present at birth in the same proportion as in adults, but it is located more predominantly in central than in peripheral airways (Wohl, 1983). The presence of smooth muscle throughout the lung from birth makes it possible for even a young infant to experience bronchospasms.

Growth of the airways in relationship to the vertebral column results in anatomic differences in the child. At birth the bifurcation of the trachea is at the level of the third thoracic vertebra, and by 12 years it is at the adult position, the sixth thoracic vertebra. The left main stem bronchus is larger in diameter than the right, and the normal angulation is sharper than that of the right. In the child, the proportionately large diameter of the airway, the proximity of the angulation, and the reduced angle of the right bronchus make the right bronchus the most prevalent site for foreign body aspiration.

Alveoli and Parenchyma

The developmental changes that occur in the alveoli and parenchyma during postnatal growth contribute to a gradual decrease in a child's vulnerability for obstruction and atelectasis. The newborn infant has only 20 million alveoli compared with 300 to 600 million in the adult. Furthermore, alveoli are smaller in size, and the terminal bronchioles have not completed their branching. The number of alveolar ducts and alveoli increase dramatically in the first few months and years of life. Growth by increase in the number of alveoli is thought to continue to about 8 years of age, after which it is primarily the result of an increase in size of units (Inselman and Mellins, 1981). The growth of the lung increases surface area for exchange of gases. The primary respiratory lobule is illustrated in the figure on this page.

The development of pulmonary surfactant within the lung is a principal factor in respiratory function at birth. Type II cells within the alveoli appear around 16 to 20 weeks' gestation, but secretion of surfactant does not occur until about 10 weeks later. Surfactant is a phospho-lipid-protein complex that lines the alveoli and has the ability to lower surface tension during expiration. Surface tension is a phenomenon in which liquid tries to minimize its surface area; for example, if water is dropped, it forms a sphere rather than a flat surface. Since the alveoli are really flat surfaces, the tendency of surface tension to form a sphere would result in collapse. A detergent-like substance such as surfactant causes the alveoli to remain open, resulting in less effort for the next inspiration. Surfactant enables the lung to remain air-filled at end-expiration; without surfactant, progressive diffuse atelectasis

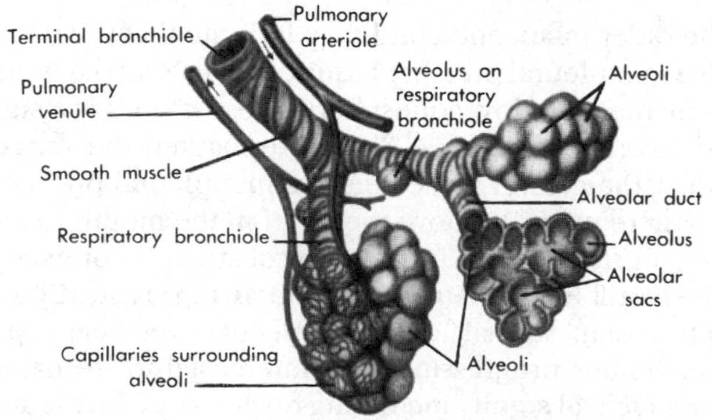

Primary respiratory lobule.

occurs shortly after birth because the alveoli collapse —that is, surface tension is high and pulls the surfaces together. Absence of surfactant in the neonate is the principal cause of respiratory distress syndrome (discussed in Chapter 5). See bronchopulmonary dysplasia in this chapter for a discussion of surfactant replacement therapy.

Collateral ventilation is another mechanism that can prevent atelectasis. In the adult, alveolar air can move from one acinus to another through holes in the alveoli (pores of Kohn) and through communications in terminal bronchioles (canals of Lambert). This mechanism prevents air from being completely absorbed (leading to atelectasis) in areas distal to an airway obstruction. The absence of collateral circulation in the infant and young child is a factor that contributes to the common phenomenon of patchy atelectasis in this age group.

Work of Breathing

During normal quiet respiration, respiratory muscles contract only during inspiration, whereas expiration is a passive process. The elastic recoil of the lung and chest wall completes the ventilatory cycle but it does not contribute to the "work of breathing." During inspiration, ***compliance work*** and ***airway resistance work*** take place.

Compliance work is required to expand the lungs and thorax against their elastic forces. We noted earlier that the neonate's rib cage is infinitely compliant. Neonatal lungs, however, are stiff and comparatively less compliant than in later life. Lung compliance in the full term infant increases during the first week of life and continues to increase through adulthood (Auld, 1975). However, when compliance is expressed per unit of lung volume (i.e., functional residual capacity, FRC), there is little change with age.

Airway resistance is many times greater in a neonate than in an older child or adult. The nasal passages contribute nearly half of total respiratory resistance, therefore retractions and labored breathing result when the nares are obstructed (Burgess and Chernick, 1982). Any reduction in the radius of the upper airway, such as even mild edema of the trachea or larynx, also poses a serious threat to the neonate because of the resultant increase in airway resistance.

The resistance to air flow produced by peripheral airways (bronchioles) is proportionately higher in children than in adults. Up to age 5 years, peripheral airways may contribute up to 50 per cent to the total airway resistance, compared with only 20 per cent after age 5 years. The infant and young child's respiratory status, therefore, is severely compromised by illnesses that affect peripheral airways (e.g., bronchiolitis), whereas after this period involvement of small airways may have minimal effect on overall airway resistance (Burgess and Chernick, 1982).

Related Physiologic Factors

The respiratory rate and pattern of infants and children under normal circumstances are observably different from that of adults. The respiratory rate is highest at birth and gradually decreases to the adult rate during early adolescence. Most of the decrease in respiratory rate takes place in the first few years of life. Awake and sleeping respiratory rates differ considerably during early infancy (up to 3 months of age). Normally the respiratory rate of an awake infant may be as high as 70 breaths per minute, yet the normal sleeping respiratory rate is less than 40 breaths per minute. An infant has a resting oxygen consumption and carbon dioxide output approximately twice that of an adult (based on kilogram of body weight). In the event of increased metabolic demands, as in elevated temperature, or compromised respiratory function, oxygen supply depletes more rapidly because of the high metabolic demands under normal circumstances.

A young child's immature thermostatic control and the proportionately large body surface area of infants causes difficulty in maintaining body temperature. These factors can result in increased oxygen consumption, putting stress on the respiratory system.

The young child's cardiac status and function affects the child's respiratory system. The child has a lower cardiac stroke volume, therefore the cardiac rate is higher than in the adult, to meet high metabolic demands. Consequently, when a child is in respiratory difficulty or has a fever, the pulse rate increases along with the respiratory rate in an effort to meet the metabolic demands.

Assessment of Respiratory Function

Assessment of the respiratory status of a child is one of the most frequently performed functions of a nurse. See Chapter 15 for the review of systems and how to perform a physical assessment of the chest and lungs (observation, palpation, percussion, and auscultation). This chapter expands the health history concerning respiratory function and reviews common clinical manifestations of respiratory difficulty.

Health History and Physical Assessment

Assessment of the child focuses on

- the child's physical, psychologic, and social environment pertaining to respiratory status to collect

Box 38-1
Historical Factors to Consider in Assessment of Respiratory Status

HISTORY OF PRESENT ILLNESS (if the illness presents with symptoms):

PAST HEALTH HISTORY

Allergies
Feeding history
Medications
Previous illnesses, injuries, or operations
Frequency of colds
Date of last chest examination

SOCIOECONOMIC AND FAMILY FACTORS

Stability of marriage and stress level in the home
Income level and ability to provide for food, clothing, shelter, and health care

PHYSICAL ENVIRONMENT

Presence of pets in the home
Exposure to cigarette smoking (parents, siblings, caretakers). Does client smoke?
Family dwelling location (proximity to industry, dump, or known source of air pollution)
Conditions of crowding
Cleanliness of home
Exposure level: day care, nursery school, elementary school, high school.

HEALTH PRACTICES

Routine immunizations
Handwashing—taught to children?
Health practices when family members have colds (covering of mouth when coughing or sneezing, disposal of tissues, avoidance of common eating and drinking utensils, and proper handwashing)
Protection from the elements (appropriate clothing)
Adequacy of diet, sleep, and exercise

REVIEW OF SYSTEM (see Chapter 15)

FAMILY PROFILE

A family health history is taken to determine presence of familial or hereditary disease

data for improvement of health status (health promotion) and prevention of respiratory illnesses;

- early identification of an existing unrecognized respiratory problem to facilitate early treatment; and
- assessment and evaluation of an existing respiratory condition to determine appropriate care.

It is important to recognize that all children, whether well or ill, should be assessed at the first two levels. Even though a child is first seen with a respiratory problem, the focus of assessment and care should include health promotion and prevention of illness and early detection components, as well as resolution of the immediate problem. Box 38-1 summarizes pertinent historical data to gather.

The nurse's understanding of the clinical presentation of a respiratory problem provides the base for independent decision making. Objective data and their significance are summarized in Table 38-2.

Accurate assessment of respiratory status helps the nurse make appropriate explanations to the child and parent. A respiratory alteration frequently is a frightening experience; the nurse can assist in the reduction of anxiety only by having accurate information.

Laboratory and Diagnostic Assessment

The nurse prepares the child and family for the various required diagnostic tests and procedures. The nurse must understand how the procedure is done and the purpose of the test in order to allay the anxiety of parents. In addition, an understanding of the developmental level of the child is required to give explanations appropriate for the child's age (see Chapter 27 for a discussion of the preparation of children for procedures).

Diagnostic procedures a nurse may encounter are summarized in Table 38-3. Radioisotope scanning, bronchoscopy, blood gas analysis, and pulmonary function testing are described next.

Radioisotope Lung Scanning

The preparation required for this depends on the type of scan that is to be done. Usually premedication is not necessary. When a ventilatory lung scan is done, a very young or uncooperative child may require sedation (Droske and Francis, 1981). A sedated child is kept NPO (nothing by mouth) for 4 hours preceding the procedure to prevent vomiting and aspiration of gastric secretions.

Table 38-2. Clinical Manifestations of Respiratory Alterations

Objective Data and Explanation	Clinical Significance
Restlessness, irritability, and an anxious expression Older Child: Restlessness and mental confusion Infants: irritability, poor activity, and seizures *Inability to breathe gives a sensation of strangulation and results in anxiety. A decrease in oxygen (hypoxemia) and an increase in carbon dioxide (hypercapnia) in arterial blood contribute to anxiety and restlessness*	A fatigued infant with labored breathing may suddenly become more active. This may indicate a general worsening of condition (i.e., respiratory failure). A $PaCO_2 > 45$ or a $PaO_2 < 60$ mm Hg in 50 per cent oxygen signifies failure
Cyanosis: Assess distribution, degree, duration, and response to oxygen *Cyanosis results from reduced alveolar ventilation, uneven distribution of oxygen relative to lung blood flow. An intrapulmonary shunt is the flow of blood past nonventilating alveoli, resulting in return of unoxygenated blood to the left side of the heart, and abnormality in diffusion. Cyanosis is seen when an excess of reduced Hgb is present (i.e., 5 or more grams of reduced Hgb/dl of blood)*	Cyanosis is difficult to assess if vasoconstriction has occurred (as in shock and acidosis). If a child is anemic, significant hypoxemia may be present without cyanosis because hemoglobin is insufficient to result in a reduced Hgb of 5 gm/dl of blood. On the contrary, in polycythemia cyanosis may be present when hypoxia is minimal. When oxygen is delivered to correct cyanosis and no improvement is seen, a right-to-left cardiac shunt is highly likely
Cough: Assess onset and duration; type (dry, hacking, moist); pattern (time of day, length of time, number of times a day); associated symptoms; and productivity *A cough is a normal protective mechanism to clear the tracheobronchial tree of irritants. Mechanical factors that induce coughing are cool or dry environment, irritation or inflammation, a foreign body, and accumulation of secretions*	The high intrathoracic pressures created during coughing can cause the child's airway to collapse. Children under 8 years of age cannot cough on demand, therefore a cough may need to be stimulated
Dyspnea: Observe rate and depth of respirations *Respiratory rate increases because of fever; drugs (central stimulation); stiff chest wall and/or lung; airway obstruction; stimulation of pulmonary receptors (i.e., in pulmonary edema); and weak muscles resulting in small tidal volume and faster rates*	Increased rates are associated with pneumonia, pleural effusion, and pulmonary edema. Respiratory rate can also be increased by other conditions associated with respiratory problems: fever, anxiety, acid-base imbalance
Tachycardia *Heart rate increases in response to reduced oxygen supply, or generalized increased sympathetic nervous system activity*	
Grunting *Signifies closure of the glottis, creating a positive expiratory pressure in order to stabilize alveoli and small airways. A compensatory mechanism: increases positive pressure in airway to prevent collapse of bronchioles and alveoli and prolong exchange of oxygen and carbon dioxide in the alveoli*	It is frequently associated with pneumonia. In the neonate it is associated with respiratory distress syndrome
Retractions: (nonrigid part of chest is drawn in during inspiration) Types include supraclavicular, intercostal, sternal, and paratracheal *Occurs whenever the respiratory muscles are working harder and creating a more negative pleural pressure to overcome the stiffness of the chest wall or lungs or airway obstruction. Air normally moves into lung when chest cavity is expanded; if airway entry resists, then accessory muscles are used. Retractions are common in infants and children due to their pliable rib cage. Airway resistance causes a greater-than-normal pressure difference between the atmosphere and the intrapleural space (i.e., greater than normal negative pressure). Because of the flexibility of the rib cage the greater-than-normal negative pressure draws soft tissues inward*	Slight intercostal depressions can be normal in the infant. Subcostal retractions seen at the lower anterior costal margin indicate a flattened diaphragm. This is seen in diffuse lower airway obstruction and in severe obstructive pulmonary disease
Intercostal bulging *A movement outward of the intercostal space is seen during expiration when effort is required to force air out of the lungs. When the lung is distended with trapped air and the intercostal muscles are active, bulging in the intercostal spaces occurs*	Occurs in asthma, bronchiolitis or cystic fibrosis. Retracting and bulging can occur together: retracting on inspiration and bulging on expiration
Stridor (A harsh sound owing to increased rate and turbulence of airflow in the larynx or trachea)	In younger children the larynx and trachea are soft and pliable. They can easily be compressed by the increased negative pressure

continued

Table 38-2 (continued)

Objective Data and Explanation	Clinical Significance
Obstruction to breathing in the larynx or trachea causes narrowing. There is an increased turbulence of air flow and an increased velocity. A greater negative intratracheal and intrathoracic pressure must be generated to overcome the obstruction. With upper airway obstruction, the child has stridor and has more trouble getting air in. *In lower airway obstruction, the child wheezes and has more difficulty getting air* out. *In severe cases both sites may produce noises on inspiration and expiration but the phase with the most trouble remains identifiable*	
Head bobbing: Head bobs forward in synchrony with each respiration	Is a sign of severe respiratory effort
Accessory muscles of inspiration (scalene and sternocleidomastoid) are contracted, resulting in flexion of the neck	
Flaring of the nares	Unilateral flaring indicates facial paralysis. The presence of bilateral nasal flaring indicates respiratory difficulty
Due to contraction of muscles in the nares (controlled by the facial nerve). These accessory muscles are used because of the increased work of breathing	
Clubbing (proliferation of tissue in terminal digits of fingers, causing lifting of the nail base) (see Figure 39-3)	Clubbing must be further investigated to search for problems other than respiratory (e.g., cardiac)
Occurs in response to prolonged hypoxemia or lung disease. The cause is unknown	
Chest pain	
Pain occurs in the chest wall, parietal pleura, bronchi, and trachea	Pain may be a complaint of older children but may also be present in the nonverbal child. Sneezing and coughing aggravate pleural pain
Breath sounds (see Chapter 15 for physical assessment of lungs and specific alterations in this chapter for explanation of breath sounds heard in various illnesses)	

Perfusion Scan. The only discomfort is the intravenous injection of the radiopharmaceutical. A perfusion scan usually takes approximately 20 minutes when multiple views of the lungs with a gamma camera are taken.

Ventilatory Scan. The child is requested to breathe a radioactive gas or aerosol through a mouthpiece with nose clips in place, or through a mask. Practice sessions of breathing with nostrils pinched should be performed before a ventilatory scan is done. The child should be told that the gas does not cause drowsiness or any unusual feelings. As the child breathes in the gas, or following inhalation if aerosol is used, scanning is begun. About 10 minutes are needed to complete a ventilatory scan with a gamma camera.

Postprocedural Care. Usually no special procedures are necessary after a perfusion or ventilatory scan, except that sputum from a productive cough should be disposed of in a closed container (Droske and Francis, 1981).

Bronchoscopy

The preparation required depends on the type of procedure and whether a general anesthetic is used. The type of scope varies in practice. The advantage of the rigid bronchoscope is that the child breathes *through* the hollow open tube. It is used when bleeding is present or for removal of a foreign body. The flexible fiberoptic bronchoscope is solid, therefore the child must breathe *around* the tube. Fiberoptic bronchoscope tubes are now available with an external diameter of 3.5 mm or less that can be used in younger children (Wood, 1984).

An infant is usually kept NPO at least 4 hours before the procedure; an older child from midnight prior to the procedure. A preoperative sedative and atropine are given prior to the examination. A sedative increases relaxation and helps alleviate coughing and gagging. Atropine decreases bronchial secretions, relaxes the bronchial smooth muscle, and reduces the risk of laryngospasm. Laboratory work performed preprocedurally usually includes platelet count, prothrombin time, PTT (partial thromboplastin time), and bleeding time, especially if a biopsy is to be done.

General Anesthesia. The child should be prepared by explaining the following:

1. preprocedural medication may be given intramuscularly,
2. child will be asleep during the procedure,
3. child will awaken with an IV line in the recovery room,
4. child will return to room when awake and the

Table 38-3. Diagnostic Procedures Used in Evaluation of Respiratory Alterations

Type of Procedure	Purpose	Comments
Radiology		
Posteroanterior (PA) and lateral chest radiographs	Visualize airways, lungs, heart, and great vessels	With maximal inspiration the chest radiograph shows nine to ten ribs above the diaphragm; the trachea should be straight. Since infants cannot cooperate to take a maximal inspiration, visualization of 10 ribs indicates hyperinflation and air trapping. Movement can cause blurring of the cardiothoracic structures that can resemble pulmonary infiltrates.
Lateral neck radiograph	Evaluate stridor. A swollen epiglottis is visible in epiglottitis; subglottic edema is evident in croup	
Fluoroscopy: An imaging method that records radiographic images rapidly. Images can be viewed on a television monitor	Assess regional ventilation and diaphragmatic excursion; also used during an esophagram	
Bronchography: An invasive procedure in which a radiopaque material is instilled into the trachea and bronchi	The entire tracheobronchial tree can be visualized by x-ray. Especially useful to visualize bronchi distal to area that cannot be visualized by bronchoscope	A small catheter is placed into the trachea and contrast media is instilled to provide a fine coating of the tracheobronchial tree. Performed under general anesthesia. These studies are rarely indicated.
Computed tomography (CT scan): A sequence of x-rays that produces a cross-section view of the thorax. Can also discriminate between changes in tissue density	Define lesions located anywhere within the chest wall, pleural space, mediastinum, or lung parenchyma. Often used to evaluate undiagnosed masses or to assess response of known lesion to therapy	Sedation or immobilization is usually necessary but general anesthesia is not recommended. Feedings are withheld 3–4 hours prior to the examination because IV contrast media is often given to opacify cardiac chambers and the great vessels.
Endoscopy		
Laryngoscopy: Direct inspection by inserting scope through mouth, or through nose if the newer type of small flexible fiberoptic bronchoscope is used	Evaluate stridor and local abnormalities	Indirect (mirror) laryngoscopy can be used for older children but direct laryngoscopy is usually necessary in infants and small children. General anesthesia is usually required. Topical anesthesia and mild sedation are used with the fiberoptic bronchoscope technique.
Bronchoscopy: Visualization of the tracheobronchial tree directly through a scope	For examination, for biopsy of mass lesions, to obtain specimens, and to remove foreign body or mucous plugs	Types of scopes: (1) Rigid bronchoscope: A laryngoscope is first passed, then the bronchoscope is passed through it. Child can breathe through the tube. (2) Flexible fiberoptic bronchoscope: Used in older children whose airway permits child to breathe around the tube (inserted through nose or through a special endotracheal tube). (3) Rigid scope with fiberoptic lens: Newer scopes are rigid with fiberoptic illumination and an improved telescopic lens system.
Nuclear Medicine		
Radioisotope scanning: Radioactive isotopes (radionuclides) are injected IV (perfusion scan) or inhaled (ventilation scan)	Identify defects in pulmonary arterial distribution and abnormal regional ventilation (e.g., asthma, foreign body aspiration)	Foreign body aspiration not noted within first 24 hours. (See text for discussion of preparation of the child.)
Specimen Collection		
Lung biopsy: An open thoracotomy is performed and pulmonary tissue is removed. (A closed procedure is not common in children)	Ensure an adequate specimen for histology and culture of microorganisms, and the lung can be inspected to choose the site of the biopsy	Done under general anesthesia. Requires chest tube postoperatively.
Lung puncture (percutaneous lung tap): A quick needle stab through a locally anesthetized intercostal space	Culture of microorganism Used when obscure interstitial pneumonia is present	Usually used only for critical cases when there is failure in response to therapy. No physical preparation for test. Complication of test is pneumothorax.

IV line will be removed when fluids are being tolerated, and

5. suctioning and postural drainage may be necessary.

Local Anesthesia. When local anesthesia is used for bronchoscopy, the nurse will want to keep these facts in mind:

1. Local anesthetic is sprayed into the mouth (cough and gag reflex are stimulated by this spraying).
2. After the spraying the tongue and throat begin to feel swollen, and there is a sensation of being unable to swallow (secretions are suctioned during the procedure).
3. Child should be reassured that he or she will be able to breathe while tube is in place.
4. Prepare the child by explaining that the room is dark and eyes will be covered to protect them.
5. Fluids will be given after normal swallowing reflexes return (usually approximately 2 hours after procedure).
6. Child will feel sleepy for about 2 hours because of the sedative.
7. Child may be placed in a mist tent to reduce laryngeal edema (child should have experience in the tent preprocedurally).
8. Child may need postural drainage.

Postprocedural Care. Following the procedure (general or local anesthesia), oral intake is withheld until the gag reflex has returned. Fluids help decrease throat soreness and liquefy secretions, therefore they should be given in small amounts after the gag reflex returns. The child should be assessed for the need to be suctioned and whether postural drainage is required. The child should be observed for complications, including hemorrhage and signs of respiratory distress (dyspnea, retractions, behavior change, change in vital signs, cyanosis). Also, the sputum should be observed for blood; slightly streaked sputum is normal following a biopsy. Following bronchoscopy the upper airway may be irritated, resulting in increased mucous production.

Arterial Blood Gas *Analysis*

A frequently performed diagnostic procedure to assess respiratory function is an analysis of arterial blood gases. Arterial blood gases (ABG) most commonly include values for PaO_2, $PaCO_2$, pH, and HCO_3. PaO_2 and $PaCO_2$ measurements are reported in millimeters of mercury (mm Hg). The "P" represents the partial pressure of the gas being measured. (Partial pressure of a gas is the force it exerts in a mixture.) The "a" refers to the mixture in which the gas is being measured, i.e., arterial. For example, PaO_2 is the pressure exerted by the small amount of oxygen that is dissolved in arterial blood. This oxygen is less than 2 per cent of the total oxygen content of the arterial blood. The remainder is bound to hemoglobin. Thus, the oxygen *content* of blood depends upon hemoglobin and its degree of saturation. Hemoglobin O_2 saturation (a number given in a percentage) represents the total oxygen-binding sites on the hemoglobin that are bound with oxygen. The percentage of hemoglobin saturated with oxygen depends on the PaO_2 (pressure being exerted by oxygen dissolved in the blood). In arterial blood, the relationship between PaO_2 and O_2 saturations is not a linear one and is represented by the oxygen-hemoglobin dissociation curve. The relationship depends on temperature and acidity of the blood (see Chapter 30 for further discussion of the oxygen-hemoglobin dissociation curve).

The value for $PaCO_2$ is an index of the amount of carbon dioxide in arterial blood. It is a measure of the degree of alveolar ventilation. Alveolar ventilation is the amount of "fresh" air* that reaches the alveoli and with appropriate blood flow exchanges oxygen and carbon dioxide across the alveolar-capillary membrane. The pH indicates the hydrogen ion concentration (lower than normal pH indicates the presence of *more* hydrogen ions and acidic blood). HCO_3 is the nonrespiratory component of the acid-base ratio and is altered when metabolic processes are disturbed. See Table 38-4 for normal values of blood gases. Acid-base balance and the interpretation of arterial blood gases are further discussed in Chapter 30.

Arterial blood sampling is the most reliable method of blood gas determination. "Capillary" blood gases underestimate PaO_2 but usually give reliable estimates of $PaCO_2$ and pH. New techniques that are noninvasive are being used increasingly: oximetry (ear and pulse) and transcutaneous monitoring of PO_2 and PCO_2.

Noninvasive Blood Gas Monitoring. Noninvasive electronic equipment that reflects reasonably accurate measures of oxygenation is commonly used in intensive care areas where continuous monitoring of blood gases is required. Noninvasive techniques are generally used in conjunction with direct arterial sampling. Continuous monitoring has the advantage of providing moment-to-moment information, whereas direct sampling of blood gives single readings at selected times.

Noninvasive monitoring is done by transcutaneous tension (PO_2) monitors and pulse oximetry. The transcutaneous monitor consists of a heated sensor (electrode) that is placed on the thorax or abdomen. (Extremities are generally not used in infants and young children because reliability depends on cutaneous perfusion.) Oxygen diffuses through the skin, so the

*"Fresh" air is newly inspired air on ventilation and is differentiated from "stale" air, which is the alveolar gas left in the conducting passages at the end of expiration.

Table 38-4. Normal Values for Blood Gases*

	Normal Range		Normal Range in International Units
PaO_2	First day	54–95 mm Hg	7.2–12.6 kPa
	Thereafter	83–108 mm Hg	11.0–14.4 kPa
$PaCO_2$	Infant	27–41 mm Hg	3.6–5.5 kPa
	Thereafter (M)	35–48 mm Hg	4.7–6.4 kPa
	(F)	32–45 mm Hg	4.3–6.0 kPa
pH	First day	7.29–7.45 mm Hg	35–51 mmol/L
	Thereafter	7.35–7.45 mm Hg	35–44 mmol/L
	(Must be corrected for body temperature)		
Bicarbonate (HCO_3^-)		21–28 mmol/L	21–28 mmol/L
Base Excess:			
	Newborn Infant	(−7)–(−1) mmol/L	(−7)–(−1) mmol/L
	Child	(−4)–(+2) mmol/L	(−4)–(+2) mmol/L
	Thereafter	(−3)–(+3) mmol/L	(−3)–(+3) mmol/L

* These values are normal at sea level. Normal values for high elevations may fall outside these ranges.

(From Behrman and Vaughan, 1987.)

diffused oxygen is measured by the electrochemical sensor. Heating the skin causes an increased amount of oxygen to diffuse through the skin, which compensates for the normal gradient between arterial (PaO_2) and transcutaneous oxygen (PO_2). The actual measurement, therefore, correlates well with PaO_2 (Carnevale, 1986).

Transcutaneous monitoring has some limitations. Frequent calibration periods are necessary, the heated electrode may cause burns, and some wide fluctuations that cannot be detected by intermittent arterial sampling have been noted (Jennis and Peabody, 1987).

A newer noninvasive method is the *pulse oximeter.* It measures the oxygen saturation (SaO_2) of arterial hemoglobin. Its accuracy in adults and children has been reported (Fanconi, et al, 1985), as well as its use in newborn infants who have no greater than 50 per cent fetal hemoglobin (Jennis and Peabody, 1987). The oximeter may be somewhat less accurate when used on dark-skinned or jaundiced patients because it measures SaO_2 on the basis of light absorption through the skin (Openbrier et al, 1988). The sensor is usually attached to a finger in children, or to a toe or foot in neonates. Pulse oximeters display a continuous arterial oxygen saturation reading; however, periodic measurement of arterial blood gases is done as with transcutaneous monitoring.

Pulmonary Function Tests

Pulmonary function tests evaluate adequacy of pulmonary function but they do not generally provide a diagnosis or an etiology. The primary uses of pulmonary function tests are to (1) assess the degree of pulmonary disease, (2) assess response to therapy, and (3) help distinguish between restrictive and obstructive disease. They are also useful to detect a respiratory limitation preoperatively and to establish a baseline of pulmonary function. The standard terminology is diagrammed and explained in Figure 38-1.

Pulmonary function tests include two categories of testing. The first evaluates the functions contributing to movement of air in and out of the respiratory tract and the distribution of air to the alveoli. These tests are called *ventilatory function tests* (tests of lung volumes, ventilation, and pulmonary mechanics). The second category measures the transfer of gas across the blood-gas barrier (diffusion) and the effectiveness of the vascular perfusion.

The most frequently used method of pulmonary function testing is spirometry. The simplest measurement obtained by a spirometer is a single forced expiration called forced expiration volume (FEV). This test can be done in the physician's office or clinic. After an inspiration of maximal volume (to total lung capacity) the child is instructed to exhale as hard and as completely as possible. The spirometer stylus marks a curve on graph paper that can be compared with a normal curve. A good expiratory curve starts with a steep slope that levels off near end-expiration. The volume exhaled in the first second is the forced expiratory volume within 1 second (FEV_1), and the volume exhaled within the first 3 seconds is FEV_3. The total volume exhaled is the vital capacity (VC). Note from Figure 38-1 that the vital capacity can be reduced by either a decrease in the total lung capacity (due to restriction of the chest wall or lung) or by an increase in the residual volume (due to airway obstruction and air trapping). The ratio of FEV_1 to VC (FEV_1/VC) is used to help differentiate between obstructive and restrictive airway disease. The ratio answers the question, "Of the total amount of air that can be expelled

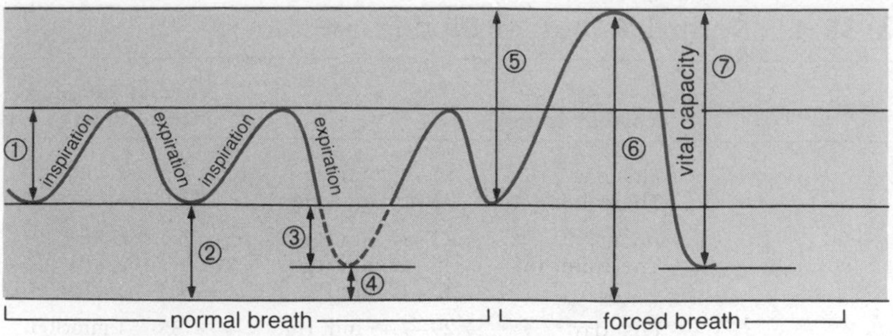

1. Normal breath—Tidal Volume
2. Air left in lungs—Functional Residual Capacity (FRC)
3. Air expelled *after* normal expiration—Expiratory Reserve Volume (ERV)
4. Air left after forced expiration—Residual Volume (RV)
5. Maximal inspiration—Inspiratory Capacity (IC)
6. Air in lungs at end of maximal inspiration—Total Lung Capacity (TLC)
7. Forced expiration after maximal inspiration—Vital Capacity (VC)

The graph depicts a normal breath and a forced breath to illustrate lung volumes and capacities. In a normal breath, the volume of gas inspired or expired during each normal respiratory cycle is called the *tidal volume*①. After a normal expiration, air remains in the lungs; this is the *functional residual capacity*② If additional effort is exerted at the end of a normal expiration, more air can be expelled; this is the *expiratory reserve volume*③. Even after a forced expiration some air remains in the lungs; this is the *residual volume*④. If at the end of a normal expiration no additional air is forced out but rather a maximal inspiration is taken, the total amount taken in from the level of normal expiration is called the *inspiratory capacity*⑤ (this includes the tidal volume). The amount of air in the lungs at the end of maximal inspiration is called the *total lung capacity*⑥ If air is expired after maximal inspiration, forcing it beyond the normal expiration point so that maximal expiration is performed, the total amount of air expelled is called the *vital capacity*⑦.

***Figure* 38-1.** Lung volumes and lung capacities: explanation of terminology.

from the lungs (VC), how much can I get out in the first second (FEV_1)?" The normal FEV_1/VC ratio is 0.8 (West, 1979) and varies slightly with age. In obstructive airway disease the ratio decreases (<0.8), whereas it is normal or increased in restrictive disease.

Of the two categories of pulmonary involvement (obstructive and restrictive), the obstructive pattern is seen most commonly in children—namely, bronchopulmonary dysplasia, bronchiolitis, bronchial asthma, and cystic fibrosis. The restrictive problems arise from deformities of the spine (e.g., scoliosis) or neuromuscular conditions that affect the muscles and structures involved in respiration.

Preparation of the Child for Pulmonary Function Testing. Pulmonary function tests are noninvasive but still can be frightening to children if they are unprepared. Children under the age of 5 years have difficulty accomplishing the tasks of blowing, pushing, and stopping respirations on command and require considerable practice. At ages 5 and 6 years, children can be tested without excessive difficulty, but they also require preparation.

During spirometry and other pulmonary testing, a mouthpiece is used in which the child is asked to blow according to the technician's instructions. The nares are obstructed by a nose clip, which is not painful but may be resisted by a fearful child. A child of any age should be permitted to practice the technique and receive information about the sounds and sensations associated with this procedure. Before the procedure, terms such as "take a deep breath," "hold your breath," "blow all the way out," "pant," and "breathe naturally" should be discussed and demonstrated. Although a firm and somewhat demanding approach is required to get the child's best effort, kindness and encouragement are essential to gain a child's cooperation. *No child should be forced to complete a test that is not being performed effectively but rather should be asked to return at a later time* (Doershuk and Orenstein, 1979).

Nursing Diagnoses

Table 38-5, Nursing Process Plan: The Child with Respiratory Tract Dysfunction, is designed for general care of the child with respiratory illness. It should be used to augment the discussions of specific nursing care for disease entities in this chapter.

Text continues on page 1183

Table 38-5
Nursing Process Plan: The Child with Respiratory Tract Dysfunction*

By Roxie Foster

I. Assessment of Physical Function

A. *Oxygenation*

Subjective Assessment

Chest comfort related to breathing, whether short of breath, past health history (see Box 38–1)

Objective Assessment

Respiratory rate, rhythm; breath sounds (air exchange); skin color; use of accessory muscles; nasal flaring, patency of nares; activity, emotional state; cough; heart rate and rhythm; shape of digits, shape of chest; blood gases; pulmonary function tests; cultures; chest radiograph

Analysis: Nursing Diagnosis 1

Ineffective airway clearance, related to

- *increased production and/or inadequate expectoration of secretions*
- *inflammation and edema of parts of the respiratory tract*
- *congenital obstruction*
- *pooling of secretions associated with immobility*

Defining Characteristics

Subjective: History of cough with or without expectoration; chest discomfort

Objective: Dyspnea, tachypnea, prolonged expiratory phase, crackles, wheezes, pallor or cyanosis, retractions, nasal flaring, nasal secretions and congestion, swollen turbinates blocking nasal passages, restlessness, irritability, tachycardia, alterations in pulmonary function tests (e.g., decreased vital capacity), chest radiograph indicative of obstructive changes

Analysis: Nursing Diagnosis 2

Impaired gas exchange, related to

- *changes in oxygen supply (e.g., ineffective airway clearance)*
- *changes in alveolar integrity*

Defining Characteristics

Subjective: Lethargy, decreased energy for activities of daily living

Objective: Dyspnea, tachypnea, decreased air exchange, pallor, circumoral cyanosis (especially upon exertion); moderate activity (e.g., feeding) results in pulse increase of 20 or more beats per minute and respiratory increase of 10 or more breaths per minute; lethargy/fatigue; anxiety/restlessness; tachycardia; increased anteroposterior chest diameter and clubbing of digits (if chronic hypoxia); alterations in pulmonary function tests; decreased PO_2 and SO_2, increased CO_2; cultures indicative of infection; chest radiograph indicative of tissue changes

* To be used with Table 31-2, Nursing Process Plan: The Hospitalized Child.

Continued

Client Goal/ Evaluation Criteria	Nursing Goals/Strategies (Selected Rationale)
1/2. The client will achieve optimal air exchange, as evidenced by: a. pulse and respirations within normal limits for age or at normal baseline for child b. breath sounds clear and equal c. color pink (or normal for race) d. absence of retractions and nasal flaring e. no abnormal increase in pulse or heart rate, nor unusual fatigue with activity that is appropriate to age f. arterial blood gases within normal limits	***Assess air exchange.*** Take vital signs and auscultate chest every 2–4 hours as dictated by respiratory distress and fluctuations in temperature. *Monitor for and immediately report to physician the signs of impending respiratory failure:* increasing pallor or cyanosis; fatigue; restlessness; significant tachypnea (>60 resp/min at rest for an infant) or an increase of ≥10 breaths per min at rest in an older child; tachycardia (>160–170 beats/min at rest for an infant) or an increase of ≥20 beats per minute at rest for an older child; $PO_2 < 70$mm Hg; decreasing breath sounds. ***Institute measures to facilitate air exchange.*** *Balance activity and rest* (to reduce metabolic O_2 needs). • Assess child's tolerance to activity by checking pulse, respirations, and color before, during, and after activity such as crying, feeding, bathing. • Allow time between activities for vital signs to return to baseline and for child to recover from fatigue. *Administer O_2 and respiratory treatments* as ordered, and *evaluate effects.* • Determine whether oxygen equipment is functioning properly, with correct setting, patent and intact tubing, and proper humidification. • Determine whether O_2 equipment, i.e., tubing, humidification bottle, has been replaced within the time dictated by hospital policy. (Bacteria may multiply within O_2 equipment that is not routinely replaced.) • By means of transcutaneous monitoring, pulse oximetry, or vital signs, assess whether oxygen setting is adequate, both at rest and during activity. Notify physician if PO_2 or SO_2 drop below prescribed limits, or if vital signs rise significantly during an activity like feeding. • Auscultate chest before and after chest physical therapy to determine therapeutic effects. • When administering chest physical therapy, pay particular attention to the involved lobes. • Evaluate whether the fatigue resulting from chest physical therapy outweighs the benefits of the amount of sputum expectorated. *Anticipate the need for suction equipment* and have at the bedside a suction machine, tubings, suction catheters, and an ear bulb syringe. • Suction following chest physical therapy and episodes of crying. (Crying will more fully inflate the lungs and displace secretions.) *Change the position of a small infant or immobile child every 1–2 hours* (to prevent pooling of fluid in the lungs). *Place the dyspneic child in a Fowler position and* slightly *hyperextend the neck* (to straighten the trachea, thereby opening

the airway, note that marked hyperextension will narrow the airway in a young infant with immature cartilaginous rings).

- An infant can be put in an infant seat; for an older child, the head of the bed or top of the crib mattress can be raised 30°. Place a small towel or blanket under the shoulders to straighten the airway.

Administer prescribed medications and observe for therapeutic effects versus side effects.

- Administer *antibiotics* and observe for therapeutic effects (decreased fever, increased respiratory function) and for side effects (phlebitis from IV administration, diarrhea, rashes).
- Yogurt given PO may help relieve diarrhea (by replacing lactobacillus organisms).
- Obtain specimens for culture before the first dose of antibiotic is given. (This will assure optimal colonies of the organism for culture growth.) If antibiotics have been administered, note this on the laboratory slip accompanying the specimen.
- If *theophylline* preparations are in use, monitor serum theophylline levels and signs of toxicity, especially agitation, vomiting, and tachycardia.
- Control continued elevations in temperature with *antipyretics* as ordered; only lightly clothe and cover the child; keep the room cool and well ventilated. (Fever increases metabolic O_2 needs and may predispose to febrile seizure.)

Institute isolation measures as ordered or as appropriate to culture results.

B. *Hydration*

Subjective Assessment

Thirst, parental report of number of wet diapers, or self-report of voiding frequency

Objective Assessment

Body weight; fluid intake versus urine output/output of liquid stool; moistness of mucous membranes; skin turgor; presence of tears; pulse; blood pressure; urine specific gravity and electrolytes; serum electrolytes; hematocrit

Analysis: Nursing Diagnosis 3

Potential fluid volume deficit, related to

- *increased insensible loss*
- *decreased fluid intake*

Defining Characteristics

Subjective: Thirst

Objective: Weight loss; increased urine specific gravity; dry mucous membranes; poor skin turgor; decreased urine output; absence of tears; increased pulse; decreased blood pressure; depressed fontanel; increased hematocrit; imbalance of serum electrolytes

Continued

Analysis: Nursing Diagnosis 4

Potential fluid volume excess, related to rapid administration of IV fluids

Defining Characteristics

Objective: Sudden weight gain; dyspnea; cough productive of frothy, pink-tinged sputum; tachypnea; rapid, weak pulse; pallor and cyanosis; moist basilar rales; full, tense fontanel; decreased specific gravity of urine

Client Goal/Evaluation Criteria

3/4. The client will maintain homeostatic fluid and electrolyte levels, as evidenced by:
   a. weight stable or gradually increasing as normal for age
   b. specific gravity <1.010 for an infant, <1.015 for an older child
   c. normal urine and serum electrolytes
   d. mucous membranes moist, skin turgor elastic, fontanel flat
   e. urine output normal for age: (neonate, 50–300 ml/24 hr; infant, 350–550 ml/24 hr; child, 500–1000 ml/24 hr; adolescent, 700–1400 ml/24 hr)
   f. pulse and blood pressure within normal limits for age
   g. absence of dyspnea, cough, adventitious lung sounds, tachypnea, tachycardia, pallor, and cyanosis

Nursing Goals/Strategies (Selected Rationale)

Ensure that the child is well hydrated (to facilitate expectoration of secretions, flush infectious products from the system, and maintain thermoregulation).*

- Weigh daily at the same time of day—usually before breakfast or the first feeding. (Weight loss usually indicates fluid loss; rapid weight gain in an ill child is usually a sign of fluid retention).
- Use the *same scale* for every measure of weight. (Scales may vary slightly, and variance of even a few grams may be significant in the young infant.)
- Institute I&O records as needed. (These records can be kept at the nurse's discretion and do not require a doctor's order.)
- Check specific gravity every shift if hydration is stable, or every void if hydration is suspect. (If there is a spectrometer on the unit, the nurse can check specific gravity prn without a doctor's order.)

Assess mucous membranes, skin turgor, skin color, and the anterior fontanel. (With significant dehydration, fluid will be drawn from the tissues into the intravascular compartment in order to maintain blood volume.† If dehydration progresses, low blood volume [poor perfusion] will present as pallor. The fontanel will be sunken in dehydration.)

Monitor laboratory values for urine and serum electrolytes.

Be alert for signs and symptoms of electrolyte imbalance.

Take precautions to prevent fluid volume excess (overhydration).

- Check vital signs and auscultate lungs every 4 hours, especially in the younger client. (When there is more intravascular fluid volume than the heart can handle, fluid may back up into the lungs. The younger the child is, the less capable the heart is of handling a volume overload.)
- Observe for a bulging fontanel and periorbital edema. (Periorbital tissue is very delicate and easily stretched; therefore, it is often the first tissue to show edema.)
- Administer IV fluids with an infusion pump when possible (to prevent accidental rapid infusion; changes in drip rate are

* See Chapter 30 for an in-depth discussion of fluid and electrolyte balance.

† Hypertonic dehydration is an exception to this principle; in this case the extracellular fluid volume is usually better preserved, and skin color may be flushed.

often associated with changes in body position when infusion is controlled by gravity alone).
- Always use IV tubing with a graduated fluid control chamber (to guard against accidental infusion of large volumes).
- Record infusion volumes hourly (to ensure adequate monitoring of parenteral intake).

C. *Nutrition*

Subjective Assessment	**Objective Assessment**
Appetite, nutritional intake	Weight, caloric intake

Analysis: Nursing Diagnosis 5

Potential altered nutrition: less than body requirements, related to anorexia associated with dyspnea and malaise

Defining Characteristics

Weight loss; refusal of liquids and/or solids; intake less than Minimum Daily Requirements (MDR) for an extended period

Client Goals/ Evaluation Criteria	**Nursing Goals/Strategies (Selected Rationale)**
5.1 The client will maintain adequate hydration during the initial period of anorexia as evidenced by: a. absence of dehydration (see nursing diagnosis 3)	
5.2 The client will experience no increase in respiratory distress related to mucus, as evidenced by: a. no observable increase in mucous production or dyspnea related to feedings	*Assess the effect of formula and dairy products on mucous production and adjust diet accordingly.* • Obtain order to dilute infant feedings to ¼ or ½ strength with water, if needed, to control mucus-related dyspnea. • Avoid dairy products in the older child and the infant who cannot tolerate even diluted feedings; offer *clear liquids* frequently. • *Suction nares with bulb syringe prior to feeding the infant or young child.* (Nasal obstruction will make sucking and chewing very difficult.)
5.3 The client will increase caloric intake appropriate to age as initial symptoms subside, as evidenced by: a. no further weight loss b. replacement of weight lost during initial phase of illness c. resumption of usual eating patterns	*Gradually increase normal caloric intake* (e.g., increase formula dilution from ¼ to ½ to full strength as tolerated). *Monitor progress;* weigh daily. *Make meal time as pleasant as possible.* • Encourage family to eat with the hospitalized child. • Counsel parents not to force the child to eat. (This may lead to a power struggle that will exaggerate feeding difficulties.) • Assure the family that decreased caloric intake can usually be well tolerated during the first 48 to 72 hours of the illness, provided hydration is maintained.

Continued

II. Assessment of Emotional/Social Patterns

Fear/Anxiety

Subjective Assessment

Child: Verbalization of anxiety about disease process/symptoms, family's interpretation of child's emotional behavior

Family members: Verbalized anxiety; child's verbalizations about anxiety of family members

Objective Assessment

Child: Alterations in pulse and respiratory rates, BP; presence of diaphoresis; voice quality

Family members: Alterations in level of activity; body posture; voice quality; eye contact; irritability; interactions with child

Analysis: Nursing Diagnosis 6

Fear/anxiety: client and/or family, related to dyspnea

Defining Characteristics

Subjective: *Client:* Verbalizes fear, e.g., "I get so scared when I can't breathe"; family members interpret behavior as related to fear of difficult breathing. *Family members:* Verbalize concern

Objective: *Child:* Anxiety increases with dyspnea; becomes agitated, irritable, with increase in symptoms; whine/tremors in voice. *Family members:* Frequent questioning about symptoms, treatment plan, test results, etc., or reluctant to interact with staff/poor eye contact; with increase in symptoms, family member becomes overly solicitous with child or withdraws, demands attention from staff and/or appears inappropriately cheerful/nonchalant, talkative, agitated or noticeably lethargic, displays marked muscle tightness in face/body; strain noticeable in voice; irritable with child, family and/or staff

Client Goals/ Evaluation Criteria

6.1. The client will experience reduced fear and anxiety related to dyspnea, as evidenced by:
  a. dyspnea less aggravated by anxiety
  b. decrease in agitation, irritability
  c. able to cooperate with treatment

Nursing Goals/Strategies (Selected Rationale)

Provide reassurance by frequent assessment.
- Keep infant or younger child near nurse's station to monitor for dyspnea.
- Stay with child during dyspneic episodes; comfort with calm manner, soothing voice, rocking or holding as appropriate.
- Instruct older child to ring call bell at onset of increased dyspnea and respond quickly. Provide comfort as appropriate to age.

Reinforce the child's sense of control and mastery whenever possible. (Fear and anxiety are reduced by a sense of adequacy.)
- Ask older child how you can best help relieve dyspnea and comply with appropriate suggestions. (This will increase the child's sense of control.)

Explain treatments to be instituted in simple, clear terms. (Anxiety makes comprehension more difficult.)

Maintain a firm but gentle manner. (Anxiety will decrease if the child senses the nurse is calm.)

6.2. The family member will experience less fear/anxiety related to the child's dyspnea, as evidenced by: a. responding to dyspneic episodes with appropriate treatment measures or by calling nurse at first sign of episode before anxiety rises b. ability to maintain calm, soothing interaction with child c. ability to verbalize concerns and feelings about illness to at least one staff member and to accept reassurance, information d. decrease in muscle tension e. less agitation/irritability	*Provide continuity of nursing care.* (Continuity will provide security and decrease the possibility of conflicting information that can lead to distrust.) *Teach family members intervention measures when appropriate and give reinforcement for their ability to manage dyspneic episodes.* (Feelings of adequacy decrease anxiety.) *Encourage physical contact between family members and the child.* • Facilitate this contact by demonstrating how the child can best be held without disturbing IV and O_2 tubings. • Appropriately reinforce family members' ability to comfort the child. (Anxiety is often decreased by the ability to relieve the suffering of a loved one.) *Be honest in relating information about the child to the family.* Information should be based on fact, not on conjecture or the nurse's desire to appear intelligent. (Honest interactions will enhance a trusting relationship and decrease anxiety.) *Encourage family members to share feelings/concerns* and acknowledge their right to these feelings. (This demonstrates a caring attitude and fosters a therapeutic relationship.)

Therapeutic Management and Nursing Strategies to Facilitate Respiration and Oxygenation

Maintaining adequate pulmonary function in some children requires constant vigilance and specialized nursing skills. The goal is to provide maximal benefits with the least possible energy depletion and trauma to the child. The various procedures should be planned with respect to the child's total nursing plan, trying not to interfere unnecessarily with feeding or nap schedules.

A child's developmental level is considered when formulating a plan of care. Young children may be unable to verbalize their difficulty in breathing and may be unable to produce a cough or to cooperate during these specialized procedures. A sense of fear when approached with equipment or placed in a tent may be expressed through inconsolable crying and resistive behavior. Respiratory procedures involving catheters for aspiration are particularly resisted with squirming, kicking, and body thrashing because of the irritating and choking sensations they produce. The more efficient and skilled the nurse is, the more effective is the treatment with less likelihood for trauma to the child.

Many of the procedures used to care for children are similar to those for adults. Procedures discussed in this section are the most commonly performed or require special adaptation when performed on children. For step-by-step instructions on how to perform various procedures, see texts on basic skills (fundamentals) of nursing.

Respiratory Therapy

Advances in understanding pediatric pulmonary physiology have resulted in an expanded repertoire of techniques for the support and monitoring of children with respiratory problems. The type of equipment and techniques used vary with the purpose of the therapy and the age and size of the child. An important factor is the child's ability to cooperate. Older children are more capable of understanding, but they are not without fear. The infant or young child, on the other hand, resists being separated from parents and struggles against restraint and having something placed on the face. Regardless of the technique used and the age of the child, an explanation precedes the procedure. The parent and child are better able to cooperate if they are shown the equipment. Observing a treatment being given to another cooperative child is often beneficial, and the treatment should always be followed by reassurance and praise. An infant or young child may benefit most when consoled by a parent who has been taught about the procedure.

The nurse's role in respiratory therapy varies according to the practice setting. Even when respiratory therapists take primary responsibility for therapy and for care of the equipment, it is imperative for a nurse to

Table 38-6. Methods of Oxygen Delivery

Type of Device	Developmental Considerations	Nursing Considerations
Isolette (Incubator)	Used during the neonatal period. Contact with infant is limited. Objects for visual stimuli can be placed on outside of clear Plexiglas	FiO_2* within incubator usually at 0.4 (40% oxygen concentration) or less. High flow rates can achieve between 40 and 85 per cent oxygen concentration if only O_2 (without room air) is allowed to enter Isolette. O_2 concentration can be analyzed inside the Isolette. An Oxyhood (see below) can be placed inside an incubator. Portholes must be kept closed and opened only briefly as necessary to prevent escape of O_2 from Isolette. Humidity and temperature controls are provided by an incubator
Oxygen Hood (Oxyhood). A clear Plexiglas dome placed over the infant's head. Gas is warmed and humidified; it should not blow directly on child's head (cold gas applied to a neonate's face may induce apnea)	The dome restricts movement and vision. Objects can be placed inside or outside the dome for visual stimulation. An infant's head is large in proportion to body, therefore gas must be warmed to reduce heat loss and resultant oxygen consumption	Oxygen entering the hood must be sufficient to prevent the accumulation of carbon dioxide (approximately 4–8 L/min). Oxygen is analyzed within the hood with an analyzer. Edges of hood must be carefully placed and frequently checked to prevent rubbing of the neck, chin, or shoulder. Vapor collecting on the inside of the dome should be wiped away to ensure unrestricted observation. Nursing care is difficult because of limited access to child's head. For an infant who cannot tolerate being out of oxygen for feeding, the child is held and oxygen delivered via cannula for that period of time
Nasal Cannula (Nasal Prongs)	Usually not tolerated by infants but sometimes useful for older children. Movement is not appreciably restricted; however, in very active and restless children dislodging of the cannula is probable	Provides low-to-moderate oxygen concentration (up to 40 per cent). Flow rates should not exceed 6 L/min since gastric distention and regurgitation can occur as a result of high flow rates. Also, high rates by this method can cause sinus headaches
"Blow-By" Nasal Cannula (without nasal prongs). A catheter placed below the nose and above the mouth, so that the holes in the catheter are matched with the nares (see Figures 38-2, 38-3, and 38-4)	Infants and children of all ages tolerate this reasonably well. Sensitivity of skin to tape must be taken into consideration and catheter changed accordingly (usually once a week if stoma adhesive is used)	Oxygen levels up to 30 per cent can be maintained; however, one cannot measure precise concentration
Nasal Catheter. A tube inserted into the nares and taped into place	Gives child mobility and unrestricted interaction with caretaker. Has been recommended when sending oxygen-dependent children home (Glassanos, 1980) but is increasingly being replaced by a nasal cannula placed across and under the nose (Voyles, 1981)	Cannot measure precise concentration of inhaled O_2 because end of catheter is inside nares. Tube must be changed every 8 hours, alternating between nares, to prevent nasal infection and necrosis. Provides an extremely variable FiO_2 (0.22 to 0.50). Flow rates should not exceed 6 L/min to prevent tissue irritation and gastric distention
Simple Oxygen mask†	Not well tolerated for continuous therapy. Older children may tolerate a mask for a short period, but young children pull them off	O_2 concentration is 35–55 per cent with 6–10 L/min of pure oxygen as room air is inhaled through side parts of mask. Used for short-term therapy but should not be used for comatose children because of danger of aspiration
Venturi Mask (Diluter Mask)†. Placed over child's mouth and nose	Young children may resist even short-term therapy, therefore they have to be held in place during aerosol therapy	Delivers between 24 and 50 per cent oxygen. Designed to deliver a specific oxygen concentration. Air entrainment ports (openings that permit room air to enter) vary in size and determine oxygen concentration. Not well tolerated for continuous therapy. Can be used for intermittent administration of O_2 with aerosol therapy

***Table 38-6** (continued)*

Type of Device	Developmental Considerations	Nursing Considerations
Tents. A canopy placed over a metal frame and placed on the bed *Types: Croup tent,* cooled by ice and cold water. *Ohio tent,* cooled by refrigeration system. No ice is required	For most children beyond infancy, tents are the preferred method for continuous delivery of O_2. Child can play in tent (toys inside). Safety precautions are necessary (plastic, sparks). Child resists separation from parents (see text for further discussion of developmental considerations)	Delivers oxygen and mist simultaneously and has a cooling mechanism. Approximate FiO_2 (0.4–0.5) can be provided by 6–10 L/min. Monitor temperature of infant (avoid overcooling). Check O_2 concentration. Keep edges of plastic tucked in well. Keep moisture off inside of tent for easy visibility. Parent teaching about the tent needed. Assess ongoing need for tent. Feeding can be done in the tent (see text for further discussion)

FiO_2 reading of 0.4 is the same as 40 per cent oxygen concentration; FiO_2 means "fraction of inspired oxygen."
† Flow rates to any mask must be sufficient to eliminate CO_2 accumulation (3–6 L/min depending on type of mask) (Burgess and Chernick, 1982).
(Sources: Burgess and Chernick, 1982; Glassanos, 1980; Voyles, 1981.)

understand the goals of therapy. In many settings, nurses are expected to handle aspects of respiratory therapy. The following techniques are common in most pediatric settings.

Oxygen Therapy

Oxygen is indicated when PaO_2 levels are significantly reduced (a decreased partial pressure of oxygen in arterial blood). Oxygen is frequently used in pediatrics because hypoxia develops early in most pediatric pulmonary problems. Its use is widespread in the treatment of most acute pediatric pulmonary problems (pneumonia, bronchiolitis, and asthma). Its use in chronic pulmonary disease is more complex. A lowered PaO_2 may be a significant stimulus for respiration, consequently the response to oxygen therapy may be a decrease in ventilation, resulting in a further rise in $PaCO_2$. However, significant increases in $PaCO_2$ in response to oxygen administration are unusual in adults and extremely rare in children. Although oxygen administration in chronic lung disease should be monitored by assessing the response of arterial $PaCO_2$, oxygen should never be withheld when needed. Only the amount of oxygen needed to maintain arterial oxygen tension at 60 mm Hg (90 per cent saturated) should be given (O'Brodovich and Chernick, 1983).

Oxygen has potential serious side effects and should be administered for the least amount of time and in the least amount of dosage that will effectively treat the condition. Although retinopathy of prematurity (retrolental fibroplasia) is now believed to be a multifactorial disorder, hyperoxia remains as one of the risk factors (Shapiro, 1986). Retinopathy of prematurity and the effects of oxygen are discussed in Chapter 51.

Oxygen in elevated concentrations is thought to be associated with bronchopulmonary dysplasia (BPD), but correlation is poor between the degree (concentration and duration) of oxygen exposure and the severity of the disease. Furthermore, infants who have received oxygen but have not required the use of mechanical ventilators have not developed BPD. The triggering events of BPD are thought to be oxygen-related injury and barotrauma (injury due to pressure from mechanical ventilation) in a susceptible infant with surfactant deficiency and respiratory distress syndrome (Sinkin and Phelps, 1987).

When oxygen is indicated, it is important to use the type of equipment that is most appropriate for the age of the child and that will deliver the percentage of oxygen needed without unnecessarily subjecting a child to excessive levels of oxygen. The use of oxygen blenders (a combination of oxygen and compressed air) facilitates selection and delivery of precise desired FiO_2. (See Table 38-6 for methods of oxygen delivery.)

Regardless of the type of equipment used to administer oxygen, some basic principles and nursing care considerations are common to all methods. Hospital oxygen is derived from compressed tank sources and is desiccated. If used directly, it would have a drying effect on the mucous membranes; therefore, it is humidified. In addition, dry oxygen induces bronchoconstriction and must be avoided. Whenever possible, oxygen is analyzed with an analyzer to determine the actual percentage of oxygen inspired. The number of liters at which the flow meter is set is adjusted to maintain the desired oxygen concentration for inhalation. When analyzing oxygen concentration, the measurement should be done at a position close to the child's mouth and nose (that is, the air the child is actually inhaling).

Care of the Child in a Tent. A popular method used to deliver a low-to-moderate concentration of oxygen is via a mist tent, known in pediatrics as a "croup tent." A tent is designed to provide an enclosed space in which a child can rest comfortably and breathe in air with a higher oxygen concentration than room air. Note, however, that a tent may be used to deliver oxygen *and* humidity or *only* humidity. If only humidity is required, then the tent is connected to an air outlet rather than to oxygen. When oxygen is required, the level of concentration that can be maintained is directly related to the number and length of times that a tent is opened. An environment of up to 50 per cent oxygen concentration can be maintained if leaks are minimized. Careful tucking-in of the canopy under the mattress on both sides and at the upper end of the crib is necessary to achieve a high concentration. Nursing care must be organized effectively to avoid repeated opening of the tent. Using the side zippers rather than lifting the tent is one way to prevent repeated escape of large amounts of oxygen. Excessive amounts of oxygen can accumulate, therefore the oxygen concentration should be routinely measured with an oxygen analyzer.

Numerous safety hazards accompany the use of oxygen tents. If a high-humidity environment is also desired, the presence of mist and droplets on the inside of the tent may interfere with the nurse's observation of the child's condition. If the mist cannot be reduced, then it may be necessary to wipe the inside of the tent periodically. A tent is usually cooled by the use of ice or a refrigeration unit, the goal being to maintain an environment cooler than room air. A small infant could easily be overcooled, therefore the child's temperature must be carefully monitored. If the baby's temperature drops, oxygen and mist can be continued but the refrigeration unit must be turned down; if a croupette with ice is being used, water is kept in the ice chamber but no ice is added. Because of the blowing effect of the oxygen and the dampness resulting from humidity, a child should be dressed when in a tent.

The usual safety precautions must be observed when oxygen is in use. No smoking is allowed in the room, and electrical devices like hair dryers and shavers should not be used inside the tent. Additionally, toys that produce sparks or "rev-up" toy trucks and cars should not be allowed inside the tent. The plastic canopy can be a hazard to young children, especially if they are agitated and try to get out of the tent. Keeping the tent tucked tightly under the mattress and tucking a folded sheet across the bottom of the tent helps keep the plastic away from the child's face. The potential exists for nurses, physicians, and parents to walk away from a crib without putting up side rails because the tent gives one the false impression that the child is enclosed even though the rail is down. Side rails must be put all the way up as for any other child. The nurse should monitor parents and other professionals closely to ensure that they do not leave a side rail down.

The willingness of a child to get into a tent varies according to the child's age, previous experiences, and the parents' reactions. The greatest source of discomfort that a tent creates is separation from parents. Additionally, an anxious parent contributes to the fear and distress that a child experiences when enclosed inside the plastic walls of a tent. Various techniques can be tried to get the child to stay in the tent. First, it is important to elicit the parents' cooperation. A brief explanation about the need for oxygen and mist should be given to the parents. The toddler and preschooler may be fearful about the noise the tent makes and need assurance that no part of the machine is hurtful. While the child is being placed into the tent, the parent is encouraged to remain at the bedside in the child's vision. Furthermore, the nurse and the parents reassure the child that the parent will stay, if this is possible. Permitting the child to take a favorite toy or blanket inside the tent can also provide some security. If a young child is screaming excessively after being put into the tent, the parent is encouraged to reach through the side of the tent and stroke the child's head or back. It is important not to keep taking the child out each time he or she cries. By doing so, the child is being rewarded for crying and is being conditioned to expect removal from the tent by crying long and hard. The nurse's collaboration with the parents is an important element in gaining the cooperation of the child. Parental suggestions of techniques to keep the child in the tent are elicited and used as appropriate.

When caring for a child in a tent, the nurse continues to evaluate the comfort of the child and the effectiveness of the therapy. To keep a child comfortable, the child is kept dry. Frequent changing of linens is necessary when high humidity accompanies oxygen administration. The proper functioning of the unit should be checked, ensuring that the desired oxygen concentration is maintained and that the temperature is cool but does not cause chilling. In the early stages of illness, it may be necessary to feed the child in the tent. The child can be assisted by an adult reaching into the tent or lifting the canopy up and leaning into the tent. The decision to begin feeding the child out of the tent is frequently made by the nurse in collaboration with the physician. It should be recognized that sucking requires energy and increases the demand for oxygen; therefore infants must be evaluated and monitored closely when taken out of the tent for feeding. As soon as the infant can tolerate being out of the tent, parents should be encouraged to hold and feed their child to re-establish the patterns of care that provide comfort and security to the infant.

Low Flow Oxygen Therapy. Low flow oxygen therapy is a method of oxygen delivery for infants and children who are oxygen-dependent for prolonged periods and do not require high oxygen concentration. Low flow oxygen is delivered by hood, by nasal cannula (a feeding tube inserted 1 to 2 cm into one or two nostrils), or by a catheter placed on the philtrum with-

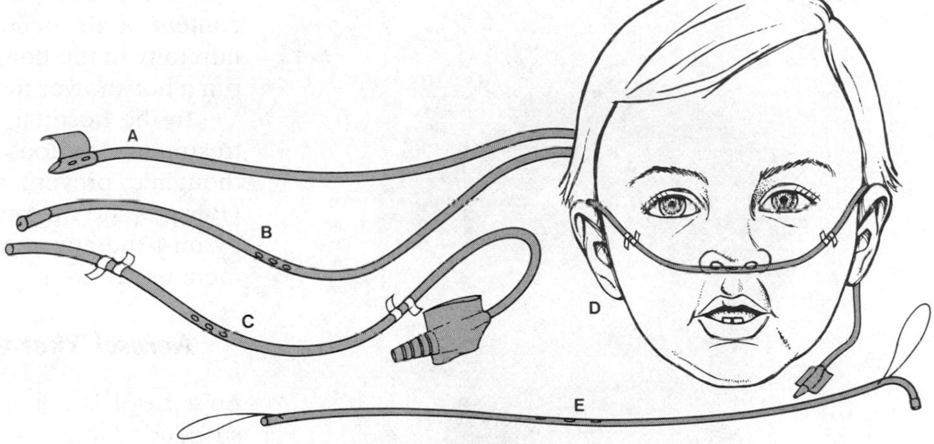

A. Occlude all the holes on a small feeding or suction catheter with tape.
B. Cut three to four small holes in catheter. Judge placement of holes by measuring from front of baby's ear to nares.
C. Place tape on cannula so that it can be attached to the baby's face. Make sure the holes point upward toward nares.
D. Paint area under tape with tincture of benzoin to protect the skin. Tape on one side of face, pull cannula tight, and secure on other side to prevent cannula from rolling over.
E. Attach umbilical or twill tape to the ends of the cannula and fit around the ears for an older child who is receiving long-term oxygen therapy.

***Figure* 38-2.** How to devise your own nasal cannula.

out entering the nares (catheter with two holes in a horizontal position below the child's nostrils) (Fig. 38-2). This is sometimes called a moustache catheter because of its position. Taping the catheter on the side of a baby's face may be problematic because of skin excoriation. The use of stoma adhesive, which needs to be changed only once a week, has been recommended as an effective alternative (Fig. 38-3) and for older children, a child's cap can be used to stabilize the cannula (Fig. 38-4).

Low flow oxygen is used when oxygen requirements are less than 55 per cent and when the infant weighs more than 1500 grams (Campbell et al, 1983). The difficulty in its use is that the exact amount of inspired oxygen is not known. When oxygen is delivered by hood or Isolette, oxygen concentration can be measured by using an oxygen analyzer. In the case of the nasal or moustache catheter, 100 per cent oxygen is delivered via a flow meter, and O_2 tubing is attached to the nasal catheter. The infant is breathing predominantly room air and the actual inspired oxygen concentration is unknown.

The danger of this technique is that the inspired oxygen concentration (FiO_2) may be unnecessarily high or too low in the infant whose oxygen requirements are greater than the inspired concentration. The recommended range of low flow oxygen reported by Campbell et al (1983) is from 0.05 to 0.5 L per minute if a nasal catheter is used. (These low flow rates require special flow meters as the usual hospital flow meter is inaccurate in these ranges.) When labial or moustache catheters are used, higher flow rates (1 to 3 L/min) are required and can be administered by the usual hospital

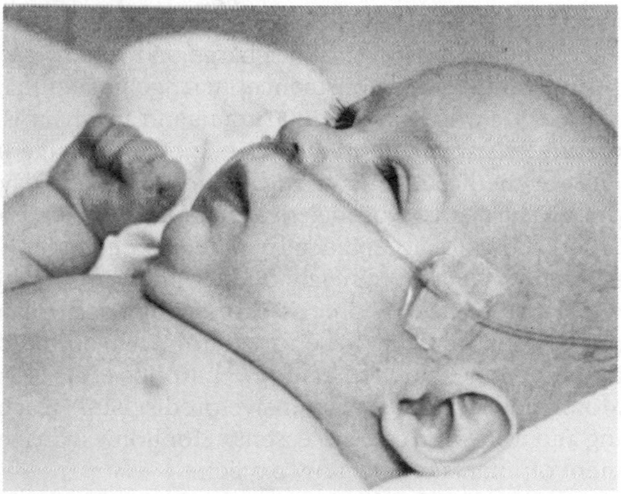

***Figure* 38-3.** Five-month-old boy with bronchopulmonary dysplasia illustrating the use of stoma adhesive to secure the cannula for continuous low flow oxygen therapy. The cannula is positioned on the philtrum without entering the nares. (From Koops BL, et al: Outpatient management and follow-up of bronchopulmonary dysplasia. *Clin Perinatol* 1984 Feb; 101–122.)

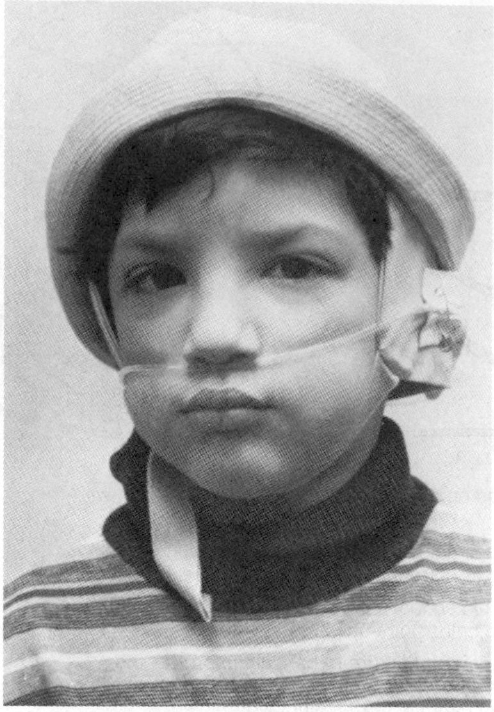

Figure 38-4. Four-year-old boy with bronchopulmonary dysplasia illustrating the use of a cap to secure the cannula for continuous low flow oxygen therapy. The cannula is positioned on the philtrum without entering the nares. (From Koops BL, et al: Outpatient management and follow-up of bronchopulmonary dysplasia. *Clin Perinatol* 1984 Feb; 101–122.)

flow meter. When hoods are used, the flow rate is also higher, with the flow meter being graduated from 3 to 10 L per minute (Monin and Vert, 1987).

Home Use of Low Flow Oxygen. Home care on low flow oxygen is widespread in current practice. Recommended criteria for discharge on low flow oxygen vary and include postconceptual age greater than 41 weeks, a weight above 2000 grams and an otherwise medically stable condition, absence of any change in FiO_2 or medications (diuretics) during the few days prior to discharge, absence of high pulmonary arterial blood pressure, acceptance by parents, a community support system (physician and community health nurse), a satisfactory home assessment by a health care professional, and the presence of more than one adult in the home (Campbell et al, 1983; Koops et al, 1984; Monin and Vert, 1987). Intensive predischarge teaching and follow-up care are essential for home management of infants on low flow oxygen.

Therapy to Increase Humidity

Humidity refers to the amount of water vapor present in a gas. Devices that add water vapor (humidity) to a gas are humidifiers. The amount of humidity that can be contained in a gas is proportional to the temperature of the gas. (As temperature increases, the water content of air increases.) A common way to provide humidity in the home is to use a room vaporizer or to run a hot shower in the bathroom.

In the hospital, mist tent therapy is used for the treatment of various respiratory problems. Humidity is thought to prevent water loss and mobilize secretions (Burgess and Chernick, 1982). The droplets produced by mist therapy vary according to the type of equipment used.

Aerosol Therapy

An aerosol is a fine particle (solid or liquid) that is suspended in a gas. The effectiveness of aerosol therapy is determined by the ability of the particles to reach the area of involvement. The major difficulty is that particles are deposited before they reach the lower airway. If the particles are larger than 3μ* in diameter, they do not reach the alveolar level; if they are less than 1μ in diameter, approximately 90 per cent is exhaled with expired air (Burgess and Chernick, 1982).

Aerosol therapy is delivered by use of a mechanical device called a nebulizer. Nebulizers are used for airway hydration or administration of aerosolized medication (small particles in a gas). It is important to observe the child closely for distress during aerosolization since any aerosolized substance may cause bronchospasm.

Aerosol therapy may be administered *continuously* or *intermittently*. Continuous aerosolization can be provided by a nebulizer device in a tent. Intermittent therapy can be administered via the aerosol mask. Such a device consists of a nebulizer attached to a mask. The aerosolization is produced by either a flow meter or a compressor. Hand-held devices, called metered dose inhalers, also can be used (see following section on Home Use of the Nebulizer).

An *ultrasonic nebulizer* is an electrically powered device that produces a vibration through the use of a transducer, resulting in a particle that averages approximately 3μ in diameter. It has been used in the treatment of illnesses like cystic fibrosis, in which secretions are thick and tenacious. Although this device is highly efficient, absorption of water and fluid overload are hazards in small infants and children. Mobilization of secretions via ultrasonic nebulization should be accompanied by attempts to evacuate the secretions in order to prevent their accumulation and resultant airway obstruction. This form of therapy can be delivered by tent (usually only at night to prevent overhydration) or by intermittent ultrasonic nebulization treatments every 4 to 6 hours. Administration by tent requires a canopy that drapes over the crib, but it does not require

*0.001 mm = 1 micrometer = 1μ, or micron.

tight tucking of plastic under the mattress. Therefore, physical contact with the infant is easy (Fig. 38-5).

Aerosol therapy is used in the treatment of upper and lower respiratory tract problems. The type of medication depends on the effect desired. Bronchodilators are the most common type. Also used are mucolytic agents (propylene glycol, Mucomyst), antibiotics, and expectorants.

The nurse collaborates with the respiratory therapist to ensure the safe and proper functioning of all equipment. A careful procedure for cleaning the equipment is important to decrease the potential for bacterial growth and transmission of pathogens.

Home Use of the Nebulizer. Older children can use the hand nebulizer, a device with a rubber bulb. When the bulb is compressed, the aerosolized medication is released and the child breathes in at the proper time. After inhaling the aerosol the child is instructed to hold the breath 5 seconds and then repeat the procedure. Various portable inert gas nebulizers are available to deliver a premetered dose of the aerosol. They all require coordination of breathing with release of the medication. Nebulizers with a rebreathing chamber are called aerochambers.. These are easier for children to use because they do not require breathing in coordination with release of the medication.

Chest Physical Therapy

Chest physical therapy (CPT) is a frequently used intervention in the pulmonary care of children when pulmonary secretions cannot be removed by the normal processes. It can include any or all of the following activities: deep breathing games or exercises, coughing, huffing, splinting, tracheal tickling, suctioning, postural drainage, percussion, and vibration. These

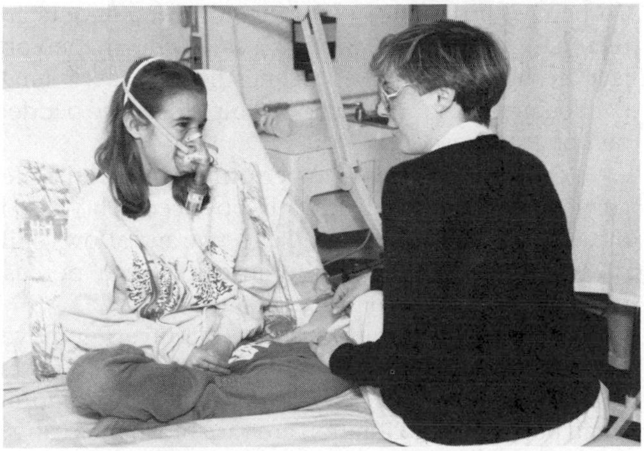

Intermittent aerosol therapy by mask is common for children hospitalized for respiratory conditions. This 11-year-old girl has cystic fibrosis and is very accustomed to this therapy.

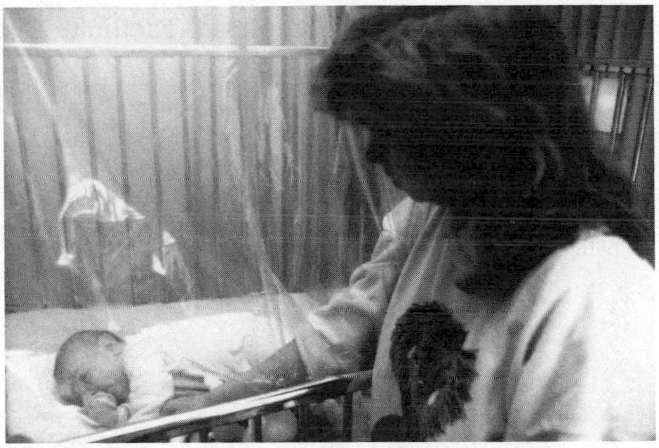

***Figure* 38-5.** If time is taken to explain the purpose of therapy, parents become very effective at calming their infant in a tent.

techniques are used singly or in combination in an effort to assist the infant or child in clearing excess or abnormal secretions from the lungs. The techniques in chest physical therapy often need to be modified for children because of their size and their inability to follow verbal instructions. Table 38-7 lists developmental considerations in breathing, coughing and suctioning.

Techniques for Chest Physical Therapy

Chest physical therapy involves a combination of techniques, including (1) positioning (postural drainage); (2) mechanical stimulation of the chest (percussion and vibration); and (3) suctioning.

Postural Drainage. In postural drainage, the child is placed in a series of positions so that gravity will assist in moving secretions from the periphery of the lung centrally toward the trachea. There are 18 lung segments and 12 classic postural drainage positions. In each classic drainage position, one or more segmental bronchi are perpendicular to the floor so that the force of gravity is optimal. Figures 38-6 and 38-7 show correlation of the segment being drained and the position of the child. The recommended positions used for a particular child will vary according to the lung segments most involved. Children are generally not able to tolerate more than four to six positions at one session; therefore, it may be necessary to rotate positions from one session to the next. For a young child, a comfortable position can be attained by placing him or her on a pillow while in bed or on the therapist's or parent's lap. A neonate in an Isolette can be positioned by using a rolled blanket and by raising and lowering the Isolette tray. With older children and adolescents, use of the knee gatch and pillows facilitates effective positioning for postural drainage. At home, an inverted chair, a home-made padded board,

Table 38-7. Nursing Strategies to Facilitate Deep Breathing, Coughing, and Suctioning

Developmental Considerations	Related Nursing Actions
1. Infants and young children do not cognitively understand the directions to take a deep breath or cough. 2. Even when the direction to take a deep breath and to cough is understood, child often needs to be encouraged to do so by being engaged in developmentally appropriate activities.	A cough can be stimulated by slowly passing a sterile catheter through child's nose until it reaches the pharynx or trachea. A natural cough reflex can be stimulated by exerting firm pressure over trachea at sternal notch during expiration. To facilitate deep breathing, the nurse can provide: • Balloons • Soap bubbles • Incentive spirometry • Pinwheels • Variety of blowing games. To facilitate an effective cough, the nurse should (a) Place child in an upright sitting position to provide for maximal expansion of chest and mechanical advantage for abdominal muscles. (b) Prepare child with appropriate pain medication and, in postoperative cases, splint the operative area with a pillow. (c) Demonstrate the desired cough and ask the child to imitate.
3. Mucous membranes are thin and easily traumatized; special precautions must be taken in technique of suctioning.	*Oral suctioning:* Insert catheter at each side of the mouth and advance to the back of the mouth. Gently rotate catheter; do not poke in and out of back of mouth. Suction each area once and then reassess the child and allow rest. Repeat procedure only if secretions are abundant. *Nasopharyngeal suctioning:* Catheter is measured by spanning it from tip of child's nose to earlobe. The measured distance on catheter is inserted through one nostril, then the other, smoothly and gently. On withdrawal, suction is applied and catheter is rotated between the fingers. Avoid a jerky in-and-out motion. Assess respiratory status and repeat procedure only if indicated. *Nasotracheal suctioning:* This potentially traumatizing procedure must be done with extreme caution (can result in laryngospasm and/or bradycardia). It is not a routine pediatric procedure but rather a specialized technique usually used for children in intensive care units.

or a stack of newspapers with couch cushions over them may be used.

Percussion. Percussion is performed intermittently during postural drainage to speed movement of the mucus. Percussion must always be comfortable for the child so that deep breathing can continue throughout the postural drainage treatment. To protect the skin from irritation, the child's chest should be covered with a light cotton shirt and no rings or bracelets should be worn by the therapist or the nurse. To percuss, the hand is tightly "cupped" (Fig. 38-8) and is "clapped" against the chest over the area being drained. (Percussion is also called "cupping" and "clapping.") This procedure should produce a hollow sound (not a slapping sound), indicating that air is being compressed between the therapist's hand and the child's chest wall. The compression wave is presumably transmitted to the bronchi, stimulating turbulence in the air the child is moving in and out with each breath. The turbulent air flow catches the secretions adherent to bronchial walls and moves the secretions in the direction of gravitational pull. Care should be taken to percuss only over lung tissue. In an infant the lower ribs cover liver and kidneys; therefore percussion even for the lower lobes should be performed two to three fingerbreadths above the lowest rib. When the size of the infant's chest does not accommodate the therapist's hand, other means of percussion are used. To percuss an infant's chest, two or three fingers are tented together (Fig. 38-9), or a small cup-shaped object can be used, such as an anesthesia mask, a small padded medicine cup, a padded nipple, or the padded bell of a stethoscope.

Percussion can also be performed by using a mechanical percussor, electrically powered. The use of these devices has been found effective and allows children to be independent because they can percuss many of the lobes themselves.

Vibration. Vibration is a rapid quivering movement of the therapist's arms and hands applied to the chest wall during the exhalation phase of respiration. Hand positions for vibration are variable; hands can be placed over each other, side by side, or on either side of the chest. To initiate the vibration the therapist contracts all the flexor and extensor muscles of the arm and shoulder. Because the infant's respiratory rate is so

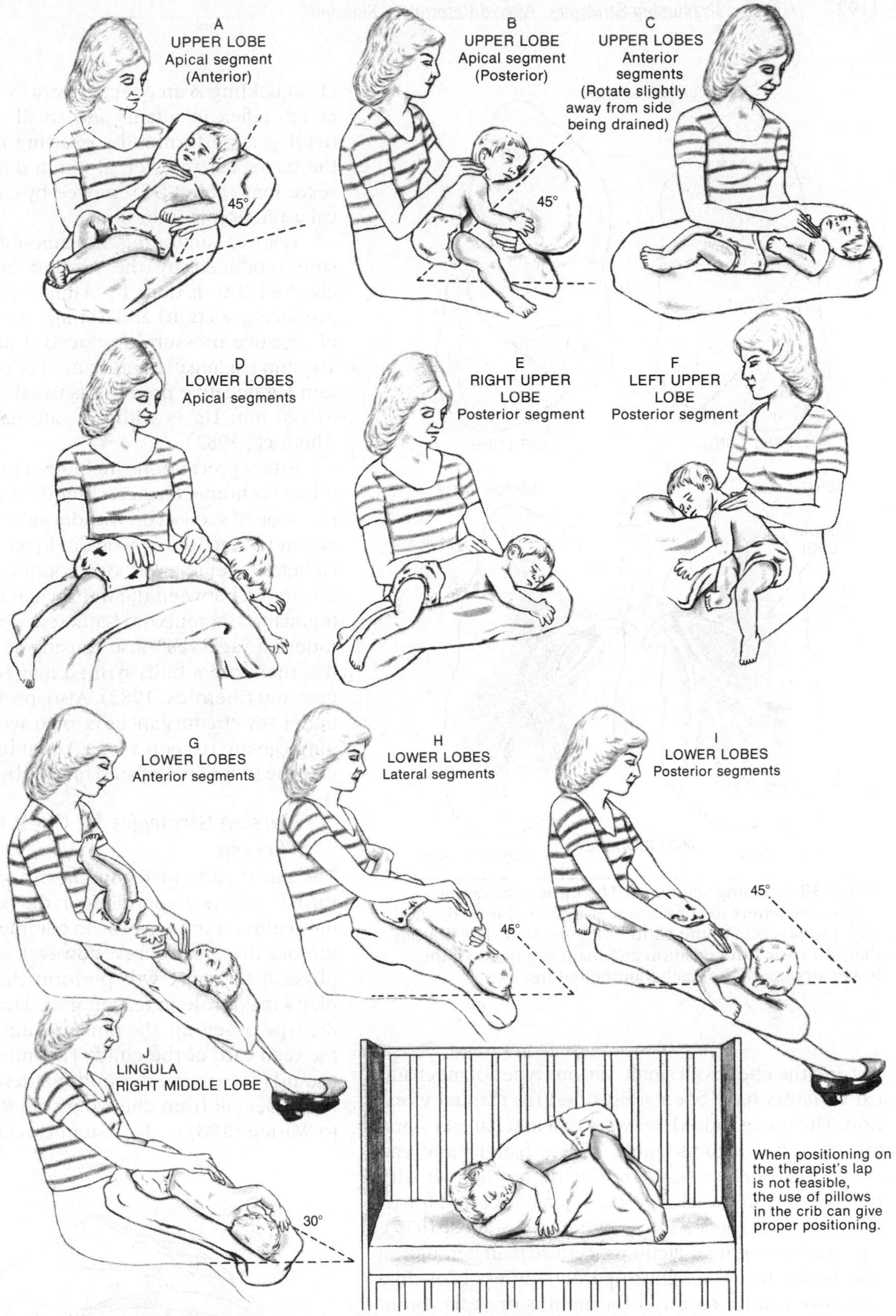

***Figure* 38-6.** Postural drainage. The positions for postural drainage are correlated with the segment being drained. See Figure 38-7. In positions *H* and *J*, the child is shown on the right side; however, the boy must also be turned to the left side to drain both lobes. (Adapted from materials used by the Chest Physical Therapy Department, Physical Therapy Division, Department of Physical Medicine and Rehabilitation, Hospital of the University of Michigan, Ann Arbor, MI.)

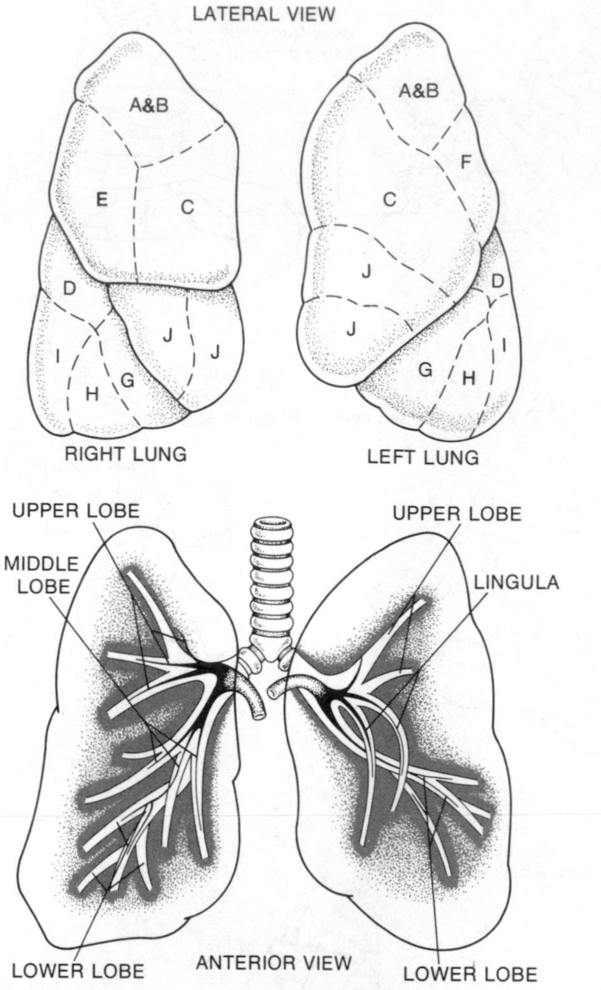

***Figure* 38-7.** Lung segments. The upper diagram is labeled by letters to correlate the segment being drained with the position of the child in Figure 38-6. The bottom diagram shows the position and main segments of the lower airways of the tracheobronchial tree.

fast and the chest wall small, various types of mechanical vibrators have been substituted for manual vibration. The nurse should be aware that mechanical vibrators may be uncomfortable to the patient and can produce bronchospasm. An electric toothbrush with the bristle portion padded has been suggested for vibration of neonates (Curran and Kachoyeanos, 1979). Vibration is a more difficult procedure than percussion and is not always taught to parents unless bronchial drainage will be required for months or years. Bronchial drainage with percussion and vibration is often fatiguing to the child; therefore, the areas of greatest involvement should be treated first.

Mechanical Aspiration. Removal of secretions completes the process of chest physical therapy. This is accomplished by coughing, suctioning, or both. Tracheal tickling is an effective way to stimulate a natural cough reflex in infants and small children. Tracheal tickling is performed by exerting firm pressure over the trachea at the sternal notch during expiration. If secretions cannot be removed by coughing, mechanical aspiration is indicated.

Prior to suctioning, the amount of negative pressure produced by the suction apparatus must be checked. This is done by clamping off the tubing (i.e., producing suction) and noting on the dial the amount of negative pressure produced. Infants require 80 to 100 mm Hg negative pressure. For older children, 100 mm Hg negative pressure is usually sufficient, but up to 120 mm Hg is within a safe range (Burgess and Chernick, 1982).

Safety precautions include (1) use of sterile technique (at home, clean technique is adequate), (2) application of suction on withdrawal only, and (3) gentle and quick suctioning to avoid hypoxia and apnea. The catheter is removed in one continuous motion as it is pill-rolled between the thumb and forefinger to avoid trauma to the mucosa. Catheters used on infants may induce a vagal response causing apnea and bradycardia; therefore a bulb syringe may be preferred (Burgess and Chernick, 1982). Also, prolonged suctioning under any circumstances is to be avoided without bagging (giving oxygen via an Ambu-bag) in between or else the lungs are deflated merely by aspirating the air.

Nursing Strategies for Chest Physical Therapy

The nurse participates in chest physical therapy in a variety of ways, depending on the patient's needs and the setting. Nurses may be in complete charge of carrying out the procedures; however, in many centers a physical therapist will perform the procedures and play a major role in teaching the family. Regardless of the type of setting, the nurse retains responsibility for the total care of the child. This means that the nurse should listen to chest sounds to identify any child who could benefit from chest physical therapy. According to Waring (1983), "Persistent crackles in a given seg-

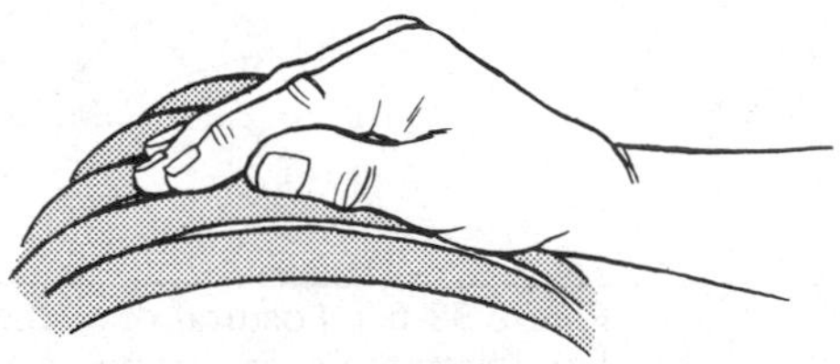

***Figure* 38-8.** Position of hand cupped for percussion. The wrist movement involves a brisk relaxed flexion and extension. The examiner should be careful not to use only the fingers or only the heel of the hand.

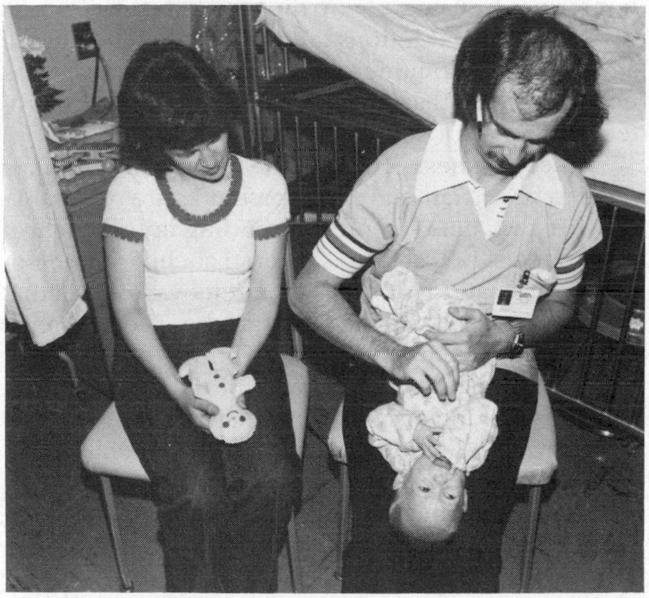

***Figure* 38-9.** Chest percussion of an infant. To percuss, two or three fingers are tented together. Parents can learn to perform the procedure at home by observing and practicing the technique.

ment or lobe constitute sufficient indication in themselves for drainage of the involved bronchi." The nurse evaluates the effectiveness of chest physical therapy and assists the physical therapist in teaching the family the necessary home program. Furthermore, the nurse checks that the chest physical therapy is being done and that it is being coordinated with other treatments the patient is receiving. Chest physical therapy is usually done two to three times a day and should be done before meals and at bedtime. Unless contraindicated, the child is encouraged to drink fluids to help liquefy pulmonary secretions.

The treatment is documented in the medical record by the nurse or physical therapist. Notes should include response to treatment, amount and type of secretions, duration of the treatment, the lung segments being drained, and a statement about the participation of the patient and parents.

Parents need to understand the purpose of each of the chest physical therapy procedures and the benefit their child can derive from them. The nurse and physical therapist involve the parents in the care of their child so that they learn to perform the chest physical therapy techniques effectively. If a home program is necessary, the parents are given written guidelines before discharge, including illustrations of the various positions. The nurse can also assist the family by demonstrating with puppets, dolls, horns, balloons, and bubbles. Parents of a critically ill child need information and support from the health care team, especially if the child is in pain or resistive to parts of the treatment program.

Incentive Spirometry

Incentive spirometry uses specially designed devices to effect maximal inspiration that results in optimal lung inflation. This technique is useful only in the treatment of older children because it requires the child's cooperation.

The devices that have been designed provide immediate feedback to the child and provide some entertainment as well. They have a preset volume that must be reached to accomplish the goal. The goal varies with the particular model of equipment used. In one device, the child's inspiration illuminates a clown's nose; in another one, it lifts a colored ball in a plastic column. The preset volume can be adjusted from time to time to increase the inspiratory flow required. The number of times that the child is asked to perform incentive spirometry varies according to the condition of the child. Performing the activity five to six times every 2 hours is usually tolerated. If the procedure is explained, and the child is not forced to the point of exhaustion, cooperation is usual. If this form of therapy is to be used postoperatively, the child should practice the maneuver before surgery.

Breathing Exercises

Breathing exercises can be taught to older children and are employed particularly in chronic lung problems (cystic fibrosis, asthma). The purpose is to promote a normal pattern of breathing through the correct use of the diaphragm and to avoid the use of the accessory muscles of respiration (scalene, intercostal, sternocleidomastoid, trapezius, and pectoralis). A common breathing exercise that is taught to children is diaphragmatic breathing. When teaching a child diaphragmatic breathing:

- Place child in semi-Fowler position with knees flexed.
- Place one hand on upper chest and one on abdomen to feel movement of air.
- Instruct child to breathe in gently.
- Instruct child to exhale through pursed lips (this produces back pressure on the airway and holds the airway open, allowing exhalation of air trapped in alveoli). Press gently with both hands during expiration.
- Emphasize relaxation of shoulders and upper chest throughout respiration.

Once the technique is mastered in the semi-Fowler position, it is practiced in other positions so that it can

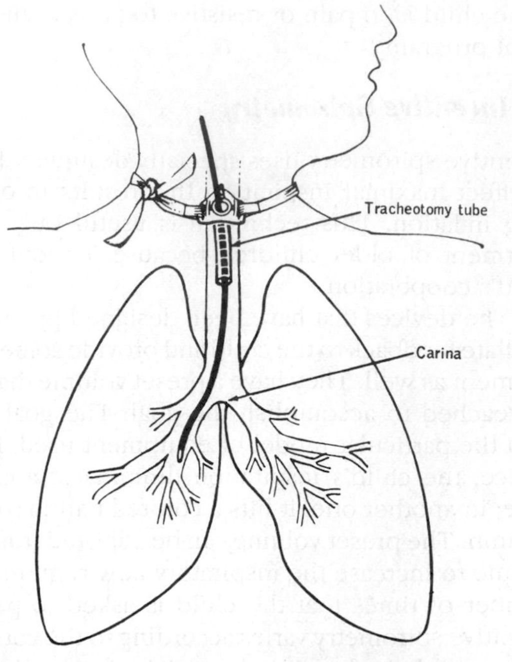

***Figure* 38-10.** Suctioning the tracheobronchial tree. In this procedure, the principles of general tracheotomy suctioning should be observed: gentle insertion and a continuous rotating motion during withdrawal with intermittent application of suction.

be performed while sitting or walking and especially during episodes of dyspnea.

Maintaining Airway of Child with Tracheostomy

A tracheostomy is a surgical procedure of cutting into the trachea through the neck. It is performed when an obstruction in the upper respiratory tract prevents adequate flow of oxygen through the trachea. An indwelling tracheostomy tube is placed to keep the artificial tracheal opening patent. See Figure 38-10.

Tracheal tubes are made of soft, pliable materials that comfortably conform to the contour of the trachea. Most tubes used for children today do not have an inner cannula. The inner cannula is unnecessary because the smooth plastic surface reduces collection of secretions and crust formation.

Maintaining Skin Integrity. Generally, it is not beneficial to place a gauze pad between the skin and the tube. If secretions are heavy, patting the area dry with gauze is preferred; gauze placed under the tube quickly becomes saturated and contributes to skin excoriation. The skin around the tracheostomy is kept clean and inspected for excoriation. Dip a Q-tip into a half-strength hydrogen peroxide (H_2O_2) solution, roll over the skin under the tube to remove crusted secretions, rinse by using a Q-tip dipped in clear water, and dry. Powders and lotions are not recommended, and any prescribed ointment is applied sparingly. It has been suggested that stoma adhesive is effective in protecting the skin (Kennedy et al, 1982).

Safety Issues. Infants and young children may need to be restrained (elbow restraints are preferable to wrist restraints) to prevent pulling at the tracheal tube. Special precaution is taken that children do not play with small toys or toys with removable parts that could be inserted into the tracheal tube. The tube must be protected from food spillage during mealtime by using a bib that fits the contour of the neck and has short ties. For infants with particularly chubby necks, a small towel rolled to support the neck prevents occlusion of the opening by skin folds.

A bath is permitted, but children are supervised to ensure that water does not enter the trachea. Showers are not recommended (Lichtenstein, 1986).

Humidification to Prevent Drying. The normal process of filtering, warming, and humidification of air by the upper airway is bypassed when a tracheostomy is necessary. Air can be humidified in a variety of ways, depending on the age and mobility of the child. A mist tent or a collar (special mask) is placed over the tracheostomy opening, or a mechanical ventilator may be used. Humidification prevents drying of the tissues and aids in loosening secretions.

Assessment for Signs of Obstruction. The nurse checks a child with a tracheostomy frequently to detect the need for suctioning. An increased pulse, restlessness, bubbling of secretions from the tracheostomy, changes in color (cyanosis or pallor), dyspnea, retractions, and noisy respirations are indications that the child's airway is being occluded with secretions. Infants and children require constant surveillance to identify these signs. Adults and older children have various means of summoning help. An infant or young child has only a cry to alert the caretaker of discomfort; with a tracheostomy, the cry is silent. Consequently, these children must be placed where the nurse can easily see their movements.

Emergency equipment, including an extra tracheostomy tube and equipment, a suction machine and suction catheters and obturator, is kept at the bedside. A hemostat, used to keep the trachea open in an emergency, is placed in a location where it is clearly seen.

Suctioning Through a Tracheostomy. A child's vulnerability to infection is great; therefore, sterile technique must be carefully observed and trauma to the tissues must be minimized. Bagging (giving oxygen via bag and mask) is done between repeated suctionings, otherwise the lungs are deflated merely by aspirating the air. Although the exact procedure may vary, the following guidelines can be used for suctioning infants and children:

1. Sterile technique is used to prevent secondary infection.
2. Normal saline, 0.5 to 2 ml, is instilled into the trachea just before suctioning to lessen secretions. (If a child requires bagging, saline is instilled just before bagging.) This may produce coughing or gagging.
3. After saline is instilled, the child should be suctioned with a sterile catheter moistened by saline.
4. The child's head is turned to the right side to suction the left bronchus and vice versa. This technique permits aspiration of the tracheobronchial tree beyond the carina (see Figure 38-10).
5. The suction catheter is inserted (without applying suction). Before applying suction, the catheter is pulled up 1 cm to avoid touching the tracheal walls (Lichtenstein, 1986). The catheter is then withdrawn in a continuous rotating motion while suction is applied intermittently. Withdrawing the catheter should take approximately 10 seconds in a child and 5 seconds in an infant.
6. The child is allowed to rest, the chest is auscultated to listen for air exchange, and the child's general condition is evaluated before repeating the procedure.
7. It also may be necessary occasionally to suction the oropharynx to remove accumulated secretions.
8. The suction tube and glove are discarded after each use.

Suctioning is done only as needed. Most commonly it is necessary in the morning, before meals, and at bedtime. The color, quantity, consistency, and odor of secretions are noted. Infection in the trachea or

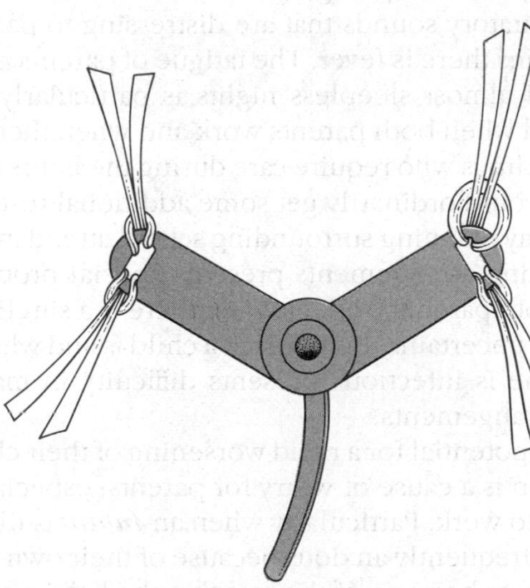

Figure 38-11. A lark knot.

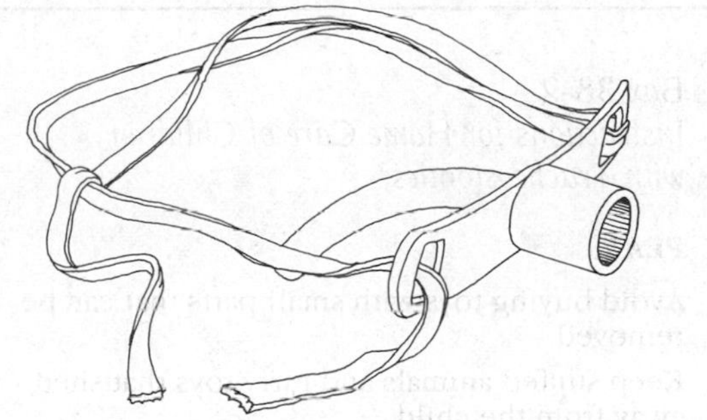

***Figure* 38-12.** Placement of tie for tracheal tube. (From Hughes W, Buescher E: *Pediatric Procedures.* Philadelphia, WB Saunders, 1980, 229.)

lungs results in a yellowish color change in the mucus and causes it to have an odor. Blood-tinged mucus can indicate that suctioning is done too frequently or with too great a negative pressure. Pressure is the same as for nasopharyngeal suctioning (80 to 100 mm Hg for infants and 100 to 120 for older children).

Changing the Tracheostomy Ties. The tracheostomy tube is kept in place by securing it with ties. Twill tape is attached to the wings of the tracheostomy tube and firmly secured around the child's neck. Various methods are used to attach the twill tape to the tube wings. Some recommend securing it with a lark knot (Kennedy et al, 1982) (Fig. 38-11), and others simply thread it through the tube wing holes (Hughes and Buescher, 1980) (Fig. 38-12). In both methods the free ends are secured with a square knot on the side of the child's neck. (Tying at the back of a child's neck may cause confusion with the ties of a gown or bib.)

Two people are required to change the ties. The child is positioned by elevating the shoulders slightly with a pad or blanket roll to expose the tracheostomy area. The old ties are slid to the upper edge of the tube wings (on both sides) so that new ties can be threaded through the wing holes using a lark knot (Fig. 38-11). The new ties are then secured with a square knot. One finger should fit snugly under the ties if secured correctly. It is advisable to alternate the placement of the knot from one side to the other each time the ties are changed to prevent development of a pressure area. With the new ties in place, the old ties are cut and removed.

Changing the Tracheostomy Tube. The most commonly used tracheostomy tubes are disposable. They are usually changed weekly, a procedure which parents are taught by a specifically prepared nurse or physician before discharge from the hospital. This is *not* a procedure routinely performed by nurses in the hospital.

The new tube to be inserted is prepared for insertion before the old tube is removed. The ties are at-

Box 38-2
Instructions for Home Care of Children with Tracheostomies

PLAY

Avoid buying toys with small parts that can be removed.

Keep stuffed animals and furry toys that shed away from the child.

Monitor play and play equipment use so that other children do not put toys, food, or other small objects into the tracheostomy tube.

FEEDING

A bib can be used to prevent food from entering tracheostomy (bib must be placed loosely to avoid occlusion).

Position infant on side after eating to prevent aspiration.

ENVIRONMENT

Stay with child when bathing or in a wading pool. The humidity collar can be used to protect the tracheostomy from water splashes.

Keep child away from irritants (hair sprays, perfume, smoke, and ammonia products).

Avoid exposure to extremely cold air (it causes tracheal spasm) and dust particles. The tracheostomy can be loosely covered with a scarf or light blanket (without fuzz) on extremely cold or dusty, windy days.

CLOTHING

Keep clothing away from airway, with the exception of the use of a light covering to prevent extreme cold, irritants, food, or dust from entering tracheostomy.

(Compiled from Kennedy, 1982; Leifer, 1982.)

tached through the trach wings, an obturator is inserted into the tube, and the tube's sterility is maintained for insertion. With the new tube ready for insertion, the old ties are cut and the tube removed. The new tube is then inserted, directing back, then down (Kennedy et al, 1982). The old tube is drawn out with one hand, and the new tube is in the other hand ready for immediate insertion. The old tube is inspected for any odor, mucous plugs, and any color change of mucus.

Closing a Tracheostomy. The tracheostomy tube is generally removed after daily insertion of a tube that is smaller than the previous one. Eventually the tube is plugged, after which it is left in place for 24 hours. If there are no apparent difficulties and the plug is well tolerated, the tube can be removed. Air leakage through the wound is not uncommon but generally ceases within 72 hours after removal of the plugged tube (Waring, 1983).

Home Care of the Child with a Tracheostomy

A child with a tracheostomy can be cared for by parents at home (Box 38-2). Parents require thorough teaching to prepare them for suctioning, use of humidity collar, changing trach ties and tube, and basic cardiopulmonary resuscitation. In some instances, a cardiorespiratory monitor is recommended, although this practice varies.

Emergency phone numbers should always be posted by the phone. If the airway becomes obstructed, parents are taught to attempt to clear it by suction, but if this is not successful a new tube must be inserted. The child's's breathing is evaluated by placing an ear over the tracheostomy and watching the chest for respiratory movements. If the child does not respond after a new tube is inserted, the child's nose and mouth are covered with one hand and four quick puffs of air are given by placing the mouth over the tracheostomy to form a seal. Cardiopulmonary resuscitation (CPR) is instituted, giving one breath to five compressions.

Impact of Respiratory Alterations on the Family

When a child is ill with a respiratory problem the entire family is affected. A respiratory problem usually represents nights of coughing, irritable behavior, and audible respiratory sounds that are distressing to parents; sometimes there is fever. The fatigue of parents after a series of almost sleepless nights is particularly pronounced when both parents work and when there are other siblings who require care during the hours that a parent would ordinarily get some additional rest. The day-to-day planning surrounding school attendance or baby-sitting arrangements presents special problems when both parents work or when there is a single parent. The uncertainty of how sick a child is and whether he or she is infectious presents difficulty in making these arrangements.

The potential for a rapid worsening of their child's condition is a cause of worry for parents, especially if they go to work. Particularly when an *infant* is ill, parents are frequently anxious because of their own inexperience or because of the fear that the baby's condition will worsen amd not be noticed by a babysitter. Some parents may be concerned that their infant will be a victim of the sudden infant death syndrome.

The overall discomfort associated with respiratory illness can range from minor problems to a high level of anxiety from the inability to breathe. Mouth breathing, skin excoriation, headaches, and cough are nuisances that children do not cope with particularly well. The more severe situation of severely compromised air exchange results in an element of panic and struggle for survival.

The generalized effect of struggling to breathe is externally obvious and brings about a panic response in those responsible for the child's care. Frequently there are audible symptoms associated with the exaggerated chest movements. The color changes and facial expressions that accompany these symptoms compound the stressfulness of the situation for the observer. The rapidity with which a child's appearance worsens is overwhelming to parents and can be the source of guilt feelings if immediate help was not solicited.

Respiratory problems often require some special form of therapy that can add an additional burden to the planning and organizing of family activities. The refusal to take medications and the resistance if inhalation or chest physical therapy is required add an additional burden to a stressed family. In the event of long-term respiratory problems, the use of special equipment like monitors, oxygen and mist therapy, and suction equipment restricts the family's time away from home and involvement in community activities.

Nursing strategies are presented for the various respiratory illnesses discussed in this chapter. In many instances the nurse can provide specific support through telephone counseling. The difficult decisions that parents must make can be made less stressful if they have access to counsel by phone.

When relating to parents, whether on the telephone or in a health care setting, it is important to recognize the multitude of stresses that parents endure when their child has a respiratory problem. Their anxiety, fatigue, and irritability require a nonjudgmental attitude and a willingness to respond sensitively to their needs. Often they require repeated explanations because they were too anxious to hear when told the first time. The plan of care is important to explain to parents because they urgently want to know what will be done for their child. The nurse permits the parents to stay near since they may still fear losing their child. Special attention to the fatigue of a parent is given by offering a comfortable chair and by assisting them to make arrangements to care for their own needs of rest and meals.

Malformations of the Respiratory Tract

Choanal Atresia

Pathophysiology

Each nasal cavity communicates with the nasopharynx by posterior nasal openings (choanae). Choanal atresia is an obstruction of one or both of these openings owing to the presence of a membranous or bony septum located between the nose and the pharynx. The atresia is located at approximately 2 to 3 cm anterior to the posterior margin of the hard palate. Congenital obstruction of the choanae is relatively common, with twice as many girls being affected as boys.

An infant with unilateral choanal atresia may be asymptomatic and require no treatment for a prolonged period of time. With bilateral choanal atresia, prompt provision of an adequate airway is essential.

Clinical Manifestations

Most newborn infants do not breathe through their mouths; therefore, when this anomaly is present, an infant develops varying degrees of respiratory distress depending on the degree of obstruction and whether it is unilateral or bilateral. Unilateral choanal atresia can be overlooked because the infant may be asymptomatic until the time of a respiratory infection. Signs of unilateral choanal atresia are nasal obstruction and nasal discharge from the involved side. Both these signs may be pronounced during a respiratory infection, giving the first diagnostic sign of choanal atresia.

Infants with bilateral choanal atresia usually develop severe signs of distress after the initial cry at birth. When the infant quiets and attempts to breathe through the nose, cyanosis and severe retractions follow. Vigorous attempts to inspire air are made by a sucking-in motion of the lips. The greater the sucking effort the more tightly the tongue is drawn against the pharyngeal wall. This distress can be relieved by opening the infant's mouth. Sucking is almost impossible in the presence of bilateral atresia.

Diagnosis of choanal atresia is considered if the dyspnea is increased by placing one's hand over the infant's mouth and if a firm catheter cannot be passed through the nostril. Instillation of a small amount of radiopaque dye into the affected side followed by a lateral x-ray of the nasal region documents the presence of an atresia (Bingham, 1987).

Therapeutic Management

An oral airway is mandatory to accommodate mouth breathing pending surgery. Once an oral airway is established, the infant can be fed. (See later discussion on nutrition.) Carbon dioxide laser-resection technology allows for definitive surgical repair, usually within the first month of life.

Major Nursing Diagnoses for Choanal Atresia

Ineffective airway clearance, related to congenital obstruction of one or both posterior nasal openings
Altered nutrition: less than body requirements, related to sucking difficulties associated with airway obstruction
Potential altered parenting, related to disrupted interactions associated with respiratory distress

Strategies for Nursing Care

Recognizing Ineffective Airway Clearance. The clinical signs of severe respiratory distress are cause to suspect bilateral choanal atresia and should be identified by the nurse. Unilateral choanal atresia should be suspected if, during suctioning of the nares, the nurse observes respiratory difficulty and cyanosis. As the uninvolved side is being suctioned, the only open airway is being blocked by the catheter; therefore, signs of respiratory distress may be manifested.

The nurse's astute observations in the first moments of life can lead to early recognition and management of this condition.

Providing Adequate Nutrition. Gavage feedings are administered until the infant learns to eat and mouth breathe without the assisted airway. Surgical correction of the anomaly can be deferred until much later, although some surgeons advise immediate operation when the atresia is bilateral (Boat, 1987). If it is postponed until the child is a year of age or older, cautious bottle and spoon feeding can be introduced after the initial period of gavage feeding.

Facilitating Parent-Infant Bonding. Parents are under considerable stress during the treatment process. The nurse must recognize that the respiratory distress manifested by the infant with bilateral obstruction is frightening for parents to see. The early feelings of closeness and satisfaction that feeding brings are delayed because of the need for gavage feedings and surgical intervention. The nurse intervenes by providing opportunities for the parents to have physical contact with their baby and to participate in the daily physical care, including holding the infant for gavage feedings.

Nursing Strategies for Follow-Up Care in the Home or Clinic

Assess respiratory status.

Weigh and measure the child and plot growth parameters on the growth curve to determine nutritional adequacy.

Determine the caregivers' level of comfort with care of the infant and feeding protocol.

Assess parent-infant bonding.

Congenital Laryngeal Stridor (Laryngomalacia)

Pathophysiology

The larynx is composed of three regions: supraglottis, glottis, and subglottis. It is a musculocartilaginous structure that provides for airway protection, clearance of secretions by a vigorous cough, and production of sound. The larynx is normally flaccid during infancy. When the laryngeal cartilage is especially soft and flaccid, the supraglottic structures are not well supported and collapse into the airway, causing a partial obstruction. The term *laryngomalacia* describes this excessively flabby larynx, which results in stridor (noisy breathing). In stridor caused by laryngomalacia, no underlying structural anomaly is present: it is an exaggeration of the normally flaccid infant larynx.

Incidence and Clinical Manifestations

Laryngomalacia is the most common congenital laryngeal abnormality, with boys affected twice as often as girls. It occurs in approximately 1:8000 births. The inheritance pattern is multifactorial, with a risk to siblings of less than 5 per cent.

The most characteristic sign is a noisy crowing sound on *inspiration* (stridor). Noisy breathing may be accompanied by retractions and is usually compounded by a supine position. When the child is in the prone position, the supraglottic structures fall away from the airway, causing less obstruction. The infant's cry is usually normal, cyanosis is uncommon, and weight gain is within normal limits.

Stridor may be present after the first few days of life, or it may not be noted until 2 months of age. In contrast, infectious croup (laryngotracheobronchitis) occurs late in infancy and is associated with low-grade fever.

Diagnostic Assessment

The nurse can assist in making a diagnosis by taking a thorough history: (1) duration and type of symptoms (intermittent, progressive, positional), (2) any association of symptoms with feeding, (3) worsening of symptoms with agitation, and (4) an incident of trauma or foreign body aspiration. A diagnosis of laryngomalacia can be made on direct laryngoscopy by the physician. Although no treatment is necessary if laryngomalacia is the cause of stridor, direct laryngoscopy is done to rule out other anatomic abnormalities that may require treatment.

Therapeutic Management

Congenital stridor caused by laryngomalacia is a self-limiting condition. The condition improves over 6 to 12 months as the supporting cartilage matures, and symptoms usually subside by 1 to 2 years of age. However, stridor without the presence of laryngomalacia during the first year of life may indicate a different and more serious condition and requires the attention of the nurse and physician for early identification.

Major Nursing Diagnoses for Laryngomalacia

Ineffective airway clearance, related to partial obstruction of the airway by supraglottic structures

Potential for injury: severe respiratory distress, related to increased oxygen demands associated with an upper respiratory infection

Anxiety: parental, related to

- *the infant's respiratory distress*
- *feelings of inadequacy in dealing with the clinical manifestations*

Strategies for Nursing Care

Promoting Optimal Airway Clearance. Stridor may be more pronounced during crying or feeding, therefore the nurse discusses these aspects of infant care with the parents. The prone position can be suggested as a means of easing the baby's respirations. Feeding slowly and allowing time for the baby to breathe between sucking is recommended.

Preventing Respiratory Distress Associated with Infection. Parents are encouraged to call for assistance if they note any changes in the respiratory status of their infant, because these changes may indicate an infection or other problems requiring treatment. Although the infant may be able to compensate physiologically for the partial airway obstruction, the added burden of a respiratory infection may lead to severe respiratory distress.

An infection may increase the body's demands for oxygen through such processes as fever, further airway obstruction from mucous secretions and laryngeal edema, and decreased lung area for gas exchange. Parents can be taught general techniques for infection control, notably good handwashing, proper cleansing of articles that enter the infant's mouth, and isolation of the infant from persons with an active infection.

Relieving Parental Anxiety. The nurse is an important resource to the family when their infant is a noisy breather. Parents are apprehensive about their baby's symptoms and need reassurance that the condition will resolve as their baby develops. The nurse should be prepared to answer repeated questions about the baby's symptoms and to offer suggestions for increasing the baby's comfort and reducing the parents' anxiety.

Nursing Strategies for Follow-Up Care in the Home or Clinic

Assess respiratory status, especially as it relates to

- the infant's positioning,
- evidence of an infectious process.

Assess growth parameters (height and weight) as an indication of adequate oxygenation.

Allow adequate time for parents to discuss fears and concerns. Provide information needed to facilitate their independent management of the infant's respiratory condition.

Infections of the Respiratory Tract and Related Structures

Respiratory infections of infants and children can cause serious illness requiring hospitalization and intensive therapy. Factors that contribute to an infant's or a young child's susceptibility to infection include: (1) immunologic immaturity, (2) a relatively small airway from the trachea to the end of the bronchioles, (3) accessory muscles that are not well developed, and (4) ineffectual coughing efforts. The net result is that even small amounts of secretions and edema within the lumen of the respiratory tract can cause obstruction and respiratory distress.

Prevention of respiratory illnesses by counseling families in proper nutrition, rest, and personal hygiene

Table 38-8. Clinical Manifestations of Respiratory Tract Infection

Clinical Manifestation	Developmental Considerations	Clinical Considerations
Fever	Neonates may have serious infections without fever Fever is associated with infection at 6 months to 3 years of age	Temperatures of 39.4–40.6°C (103–105°F) can occur with mild infections Fever often precedes other signs of infection, therefore a child with fever requires careful watching Behavior can be listless or irritable Elevated temperature occurs in both viral and bacterial infection May be accompanied by meningeal signs (headaches, pain and stiffness in neck, positive Kernig and Brudzinski signs)
Febrile Convulsions	Do not usually occur after 4 years of age	Convulsions result when there is a rapid change in temperature Only a small percentage of children with febrile convulsions later develop epilepsy
Anorexia	Infants and young children do not verbalize loss of appetite	May be demonstrated by refusal to suck, and lassitude May precede fever and other signs. Loss of appetite may continue through most of illness
Vomiting and Diarrhea	Fluid and electrolyte imbalance can occur in small children if vomiting or diarrhea continues throughout the course of illness	Vomiting usually occurs at the onset of illness but may continue throughout entire illness and become severe. Mild transient diarrhea is a common characteristic
Abdominal Pain	Children have difficulty explaining the source and character of pain	May be due to mesenteric lymphadenitis accompanying throat infection
Sore Throat	The elasticity of the tissues results in less pressure on sensitive nerve endings	Often the throat is inflamed but the child does not complain of a sore throat

(Based upon Hughes, 1984; Green, 1986; Behrman and Vaughan, 1987.)

is an important role of the nurse. When an infant has repeated respiratory infections, the nurse takes a careful history in search of underlying problems such as cystic fibrosis, foreign body aspiration, immunodeficiency, or allergies.

Infants and young children (birth to 3 years of age) are more susceptible to respiratory tract infection than older children and adults. Of particular concern is the neonate, especially if premature. The clinical manifestations of respiratory tract infection in infants and children can be more generalized and more severe than one expects in older children and adults (Table 38-8). A child that has any combination of these signs and symptoms can cause parents to become extremely anxious; in severe cases, parents may be in a state of panic. The onset of symptoms may be abrupt, often following a minor upper respiratory infection. This kind of situation has the potential to make parents feel guilty for not having sought treatment earlier. Although immediate life-saving measures are frequently necessary, the nurse should encourage parents to stay with their child and hold her or him as soon as the condition permits.

Nasopharyngitis (Common Cold)

The common cold is a self-limiting viral infection of the upper respiratory tract.

Incidence

Typically, three epidemic waves of the common cold occur annually. The greatest incidence seems to be during the fall with the opening of school, whereas the more severe cases with a greater tendency for complications tend to occur in midwinter. Another round of mild cases occurs in the spring. The common cold is, in fact, the most prevalent infectious disease among all ages, with older children and adults averaging two colds per year and children under 4 years, three to eight per year. Infants and toddlers can have severe responses to upper respiratory infections (URI) and more frequently develop complications.

Etiology and Epidemiology

The common cold is caused by a wide variety of viruses; however, rhinoviruses are the cause of approximately 90 per cent; there are about 100 rhinoviruses. These viruses have an incubation period of 2 to 4 days. During the latter part of the incubation period, the virus begins to spread and may continue to spread throughout the period of acute illness. The virus invades the mucous membranes of the upper respiratory tract and causes swelling and hypersecretion of mucus. Rhinoviruses are spread mainly by direct contact with nasal secretions whereas viruses that infect the lower respiratory tract are transmitted by air droplets resulting from coughs and sneezes (Shurin, 1983).

Other agents that cause the common cold include parainfluenza virus, respiratory syncytial virus, adenovirus, coronavirus, and enterovirus.

Clinical Manifestations

Symptoms usually last 2 to 10 days and in young children begin with fever. Excessively high fever, however, does not usually accompany the common cold and should raise one's suspicions that other disease processes or complications are present (Shurin, 1983). Neonates and premature infants often have no fever or may even show a reduction in temperature during infections. Older children and adults usually run a low-grade fever under 37.8°C (100°F) orally. Mucous membrane irritation by the virus results in rhinorrhea (a thin, watery nasal discharge), stuffy nose, and generalized nasopharyngeal congestion. The obstruction these symptoms pose to respirations causes the child to experience restlessness, malaise, and anorexia (because difficulty in sucking consumes energy and increases oxygen needs). The irritation to membranes also causes sneezing, increased lacrimation, and a raspy sensation in the back of the throat. Hypersecretion of mucus causes coughing, especially at night when secretions pool in the nasopharyngeal cavity. Viral enteritis may be present and account for an associated diarrhea. Bacterial superinfections of the tonsils, ears, sinuses, or lower respiratory tract are frequent, especially in infancy. Secondary dehydration and a mild degree of ketoacidosis can occur when fever is present. The crankiness and acetone breath so common in young children with minor infection is a result of this condition (Gellis and Kagan, 1984).

Diagnostic Assessment

Diagnosis is based on history and clinical manifestations. A culture of nasal discharge may be made to determine whether bacterial involvement exists. Allergic rhinitis must be differentiated from an infectious process. Allergic rhinitis is not accompanied by fever; nasal discharge generally is not purulent; and it is seen in combination with itching of the eyes and nose and nasal mucous membranes that are pale rather than inflamed. (See Chapter 43 for discussion of allergic rhinitis.)

Therapeutic Management

The common cold is self-limiting. Although it affects millions each year, its cure eludes medical science. Treatment, therefore, is symptomatic in nature, focusing on (1) general comfort measures, (2) procedures to relieve local irritation, (3) relief through use of antipyretics, and (4) prevention of the complications of dehydration, otitis media, and secondary bacterial infection. The most common complication is otitis media. No specific treatment exists for the common cold, and antibiotics are not thought to affect the course of illness or reduce the incidence of bacterial infection (Behrman and Vaughan, 1987).

Most of the discomfort is caused by the nasal obstruction and the effect of fever. Instillation of vasoconstrictive decongestant nose drops such as pseudoephedrine (Sudafed), phenylephrine (Neo-Synephrine) or phenylpropylmethylamine (Vonedrine) are commonly used in infants over age 3 months. They shrink congested nasal membranes, making breathing easier. In younger infants, sterile saline nose drops are used because a sympathomimetic decongestant may cause irritability and tachycardia. The addition of corticosteroids and antibiotics has not proved to be effective (Behrman and Vaughan, 1987).

Decongestant nasal sprays can be used by older children, but only with supervision. Any nasal medication should not be used for more than 4 to 5 days to prevent rebound engorgement from chemical irritation. With prolonged use of decongestants the involved capillaries lose their tone, resulting in a permanent state of nasal congestion (O'Grady, 1987). Orally administered decongestants are also widely used in older children to shrink engorged nasal mucosa.

Antihistamines are largely ineffective for treating the common cold although some studies report they are effective to relieve nasal congestion in children with acute nasopharyngitis (Behrman and Vaughan, 1987).

Acetaminophen is recommended for the first few days to reduce irritability, aching, and malaise. Aspirin is not prescribed for children with respiratory tract infections because when given to a child with influenza viral infection, the risk of developing Reye syndrome is increased (Behrman and Vaughan, 1987). Antitussives, if used, are used cautiously because they can depress the cough reflex, leading to aspiration. An antitussive may be desirable if coughing is paroxysmal or if needed at bedtime to facilitate adequate rest. Vitamin C is highly debated as an effective agent in treating a cold, but it has not been shown to have significant therapeutic or prophylactic value (Shurin, 1983; Gellis and Kagan, 1984). Furthermore, vitamin C in higher doses than required nutritionally (approximately 50 mg per day) may be toxic.

An antiviral agent, interferon, is being researched for intranasal use to prevent nasopharyngitis caused by the common cold viruses (Hayden et al, 1986).

Major Nursing Diagnoses for the Common Cold

Ineffective airway clearance, related to obstructed nares

Impaired tissue integrity: oral mucous membrane, related to
- *dehydration*
- *mouth breathing*
- *infection*

Hyperthermia, related to:
- *infectious process*
- *inadequate fluid intake*

Disturbance in sleep pattern, related to:
- *inability to breathe through nose*
- *paroxysmal cough*

Knowledge deficit, related to signs of complications of a common cold

Strategies for Nursing Care

Maintaining Effective Airway. Saline nose drops (1 teaspoon of salt in 1 pint of warm water) are usually satisfactory to clear secretions in young infants; in older children, decongestants may be used.

To administer nose drops, the child's head is lowered and turned to the side. Several drops are placed into the lower nostril and the position maintained for 1 minute; then the procedure is repeated in the opposite nostril.

Postural drainage facilitates loosening and drainage of secretions from the upper airway. A cold steam vaporizer also liquefies and loosens secretions of the upper airway as well as soothing irritated membranes and relieving coughing. Gentle removal of excessive mucous exudate with an infant aspirator or ear bulb syringe four to five times a day (especially before feeding) increases the effectiveness of nasal drops or vaporizer.

Placing the infant on the stomach facilitates drainage of nasal secretions and prevents fluid from draining via the eustachian tube to the middle ear during swallowing.

Maintaining Tissue Integrity. A vaporizer prevents drying of the mucosa. In addition, petroleum jelly or similar lubricants applied in a very thin film on chapped lips and irritated nose both soothe and prevent further excoriation. Excessive amounts are avoided as they can be aspirated.

Maintaining fluid intake promotes tissue integrity by liquefying secretions, preventing dehydration, and helping rid the body of the virus. Anorexia is often frustrating to the parent. Urging food often leads to vomiting or diarrhea, and forcing it may cause food aversions. Parents should be reassured that a brief interval without normal intake will not create malnutrition, but every effort is made to provide appealing fluids frequently and in small amounts. Diluting or temporarily eliminating formula, providing a liquid diet, and suctioning the nose with a bulb syringe to remove excess secretions prior to feedings are helpful suggestions for maintaining adequate intake.

Reducing Fever and Promoting Comfort. Rest in bed until the fever subsides helps reduce the likelihood of secondary complications. Bed rest is hard to achieve in the older infant, but a satisfactory compromise is quiet play in a playpen. Relief from the discomforts caused by fever is achieved by dressing the child in light clothing, keeping room temperatures somewhat cool, administering antipyretics, and sponging with tepid water when temperatures reach 39.5°C (103°F) or higher. Fever management and its various controversies are discussed in Chapter 27.

Acetaminophen is recommended for the acute phase of illness and is usually administered prior to sponging. Parents are taught the correct preparation and dosage of medication to be used. (See Chapter 27 for dosage and preparations.) Explain to parents that the use of aspirin in the presence of an influenza viral infection is associated with Reye syndrome.

Providing Information That Assists Family to Identify Complications. When a child under age 4 years is being treated for a cold at home, phone follow-up by the nurse is recommended. The nurse calls to assess whether the cold is resolving or complications are developing, since colds in young children often are a precursor to streptococcal infections. Parents should also be told to seek medical help if their child develops retractions, nasal flaring, or grunting; if nasal discharge becomes purulent, foul-smelling, thick, or bloody; when fever persists beyond 48 to 72 hours; or if the child has a cold without fever and fever occurs after 3 or 4 days, indicating bacterial involvement.

Otitis Media

Otitis media is an inflammation of the middle ear, which may occur with or without effusion. Middle ear effusion is the collection of a liquid in the middle ear space; the effusion may be serous (thin and watery), mucoid (thick and mucus-like) or purulent* (puslike). Otitis media is further defined by its temporal relation, using the terms *acute* (rapid onset lasting approximately 3 weeks), *subacute* (a 3-week to 3-month period during which an acute phase resolves), and *chronic* (persists longer than 3 months). These terms have been used inconsistently in the literature, leading to some confusion.

Acute otitis media (AOM) is the term used to describe otitis with *purulent* effusion (even though the word effusion is not used in its description). The collection of fluid in the middle ear is of infectious (purulent) etiology. Otitis media with effusion (OME) is the term that is usually used to describe a collection of fluid in the middle ear that is *not* infectious (nonpurulent), formerly called serous otitis media. (See Table 38-9 for terminology and definitions.) The distinction between purulent and nonpurulent cannot be clearly made either by otoscopic criteria or by the type of presenting symptoms (Marchant and Shurin, 1983). Table 38-10 compares OME and AOM.

Incidence

Otitis media is one of the most common infectious diseases of childhood. It is estimated that 50 per cent of all children will have had one episode of otitis media by 1 year of age and 76 per cent by 2 years of age (Mitchell, 1987). After age 5 years, the incidence and prevalence of otitis media decline.

Etiology and Pathophysiology

Otitis media is the most common complication of upper respiratory infections. Infants and children under 3 years of age are particularly predisposed because of their shorter, more horizontal, wider, and more distensible eustachian tube, which more readily allows passage of foreign matter up the tube. (See Chapter 15: Assessing Child Health.) The infant's humoral defenses are also less developed. The usual lying down position increases susceptibility because fluid pools in the pharyngeal cavity, hindering tube drainage. The abundance of nasopharyngeal lymphoid tissue normally present in infants and children is also thought to predispose to local infection and to eustachian tube obstruction (Paradise, 1980).

The primary factor causing recurrent otitis media is abnormal functioning of the eustachian tube. The three functions of the eustachian tube are (1) ventilation of the middle ear, (2) protection from nasopharyngeal secretions and sound pressure, and (3) drainage of secretions from the middle ear into the nasopharynx (Bluestone and Klein, 1988). Normally, the eustachian tube is closed and flat, opening only long enough to permit drainage of middle ear secretions. With blockage, drainage is impaired and a negative middle ear pressure is created. Causes of eustachian tube dysfunction are shown in Table 38-11. Normally the eustachian tube equalizes the pressure between the atmosphere and the middle ear and replenishes oxygen that has been absorbed. With obstruction, trapped air is absorbed during circulation and a vacuum is created. If this condition persists, secretions collect within the middle ear, resulting in otitis media with effusion (serous liquid). This is sometimes referred to as a sterile effusion.

When the eustachian tube is not totally obstructed, infectious organisms can enter the middle ear by aspiration owing to negative middle ear pressure and by insufflation during crying, nose blowing, and swallowing when the nose is obstructed. This results in acute otitis media (AOM). The most common offending organisms in AOM are *Streptococcus pneumoniae* (approximately 40 per cent) and Haemophilus influenzae (approximately 20 per cent). Additional organisms,

Table 38-9. Terminology and Definitions for Otitis Media and Related Disorders

Terms	Definition
Otitis media	An inflammation of the middle ear. This term does not make reference to etiology or pathogenesis
Middle ear effusion	Fluid resulting from otitis media. The fluid may be either: • serous (thin, watery) • mucoid (thick, viscid, mucus-like) • purulent (puslike)
Otorrhea	A discharge from the ear
Otitis media without effusion	Inflammation of the middle ear mucous membrane and tympanic membrane without evidence of middle ear effusion
Acute otitis media (AOM)	A rapid or short onset of signs and symptoms of inflammation in the middle ear. Other terms used are suppurative or purulent otitis media
Otitis media with effusion (OME)	Inflammation of the middle ear in which fluid has collected in the middle ear. Other terms used include nonpurulent, nonsuppurative, serous, secretory, or glue ear. Subdivisions are • acute (less than 3 weeks) • subacute (3 weeks to 2–3 months) • chronic (more than 2–3 months)

*Purulent and suppurative are used interchangeably.

Table 38-10. Comparison of Otitis Media with Effusion (OME) and Acute Otitis Media (AOM)

Type	Clinical Signs	Indicative Behaviors or Complaints
Otitis Media with Effusion (OME)		
Also called nonpurulent or nonsuppurative otitis media and serous, secretory, and glue ear *Pathology:* Nonpurulent middle ear effusion *Etiology:* Blocked eustachian tube causes retention of middle ear secretions	May be relatively asymptomatic. Light reflex obscured. Varying degrees of hyperemia; redness of tympanic membrane (eardrum). Bony landmarks are visible, with handle of malleus prominent and more horizontal; umbo is stark white. Fluid level (meniscus) sometimes visible through the eardrum. Membrane retracted, usually in posterosuperior region. Frequent otoscopic finding is opacification of the tympanic membrane. (Assessment of the type of effusion, whether serous, mucoid or purulent, is not possible then.) Pneumatic otoscopy reveals a retracted or convex tympanic membrane in which mobility is impaired	May be none. May have fullness in ear. May feel some pain in early stage. Snapping sensation when child swallows or yawns. Diminished hearing expressed by listlessness and general inattentiveness to voice in infant. May be restless. Signs and symptoms of acute infection (otalgia, fever) are lacking
Acute Otitis Media (AOM)		
Also called purulent or suppurative otitis media (AOM) *Pathology:* Purulent accumulation of exudate in middle ear *Etiology:* Bacterial or viral invasion of middle ear secretions often secondary to middle ear effusion (negative pressure draws infectious organisms in)	Light reflex obscured or absent. Fluid meniscus or bubbling visible through membrane; obscuring of bony landmarks. Membrane bulging and has limited or no mobility to pneumatic otoscopy, spontaneous rupture possible. Erythema of the eardrum is an inconsistent finding	Discomfort expressed when ear touched, or child pulls at ear. Acute onset of ear pain and fever. May have purulent ear drainage if eardrum ruptures. Inconsolable irritability and restlessness. Persistent crying. Anorexia, vomiting, or diarrhea. May have cervical lymph node involvement

each accounting for 5 per cent of the cases, are group A beta-hemolytic streptococcus, *Staphylococcus aureus*, and *Branhamella catarrhalis.* In addition, gram-negative enteric bacilli are found in neonates. Sterile effusions (nonpurulent) account for approximately 25 per cent of cases.

Clinical Manifestations

An upper respiratory infection with persistent fever always suggests otitis media. Although the distinction between suppurative and nonsuppurative (serous) otitis media cannot always be clearly made, some differentiating criteria can be helpful (see Table 38-10). If persistent or recurrent middle ear infection occurs, the tympanic membrane (eardrum) becomes stretched enough so that retraction or bulging does not create pain. Table 38-10 also describes the typical behavior or complaints and systemic signs that suggest otitis media.

Diagnostic Assessment

The tympanic membrane (eardrum) is usually easily visible on otoscopic examination, but its appearance varies. Table 38-9 describes the usual otologic manifestations in AOM and OME. Mobility of the eardrum is tested by applying negative and positive pressure with a pneumatic otoscope. An airtight seal is achieved by putting a piece of rubber over the tip of the speculum that is placed in the external auditory canal. Pressure (negative and positive) is applied by squeezing the bulb.

Nasopharyngeal cultures are not helpful in diagnosing purulent otitis media organisms, as the infectious agent of the ear is most often not the same one that is causing nasopharyngeal symptoms (Hughes, 1984). Any purulent ear drainage should be cultured for specific organisms.

If the mobility of the tympanic membrane is greater than normal, the drum is said to be *compliant* (i.e., it moves when even slight positive or negative external canal pressure is applied). In AOM and in OME, mobility is poor when either positive or negative pressure is applied. Mobility also can be examined by placing a soft rubber cuff over the external ear canal to achieve an airtight seal, at which time air pressure registers on an attached hand-held probe.

Electroacoustic impedance measurement, including tympanometry, is useful for screening OME to prevent hearing loss (see Chapter 51: Sensory and Communication Alterations, for further explanation of technique). See Chapter 15: Assessing Child Health, for further discussion of ear assessment.

Therapeutic Management

Management options for otitis media with effusion range from watchful waiting to aggressive surgical intervention. The option to wait and observe is based on the belief that, in most children, it will follow a benign course and resolve (Ghory, 1982).

Pharmacologic Therapy. Acute otitis media is treated with vigorous antibiotic therapy for 10 to 14 days. Oral ampicillin, 50 to 100 mg/kg/24 hour in four divided doses, or amoxicillin, 40 mg/kg/24 hour in three divided doses, is the recommended initial treatment (Bluestone and Klein, 1988). Amoxicillin is as effective as ampicillin and has fewer side effects, such as diarrhea. Trimethoprim-sulfamethoxazole (TMP-SMZ) or Cefaclor is also used because of the increasing prevalence of *H. influenzae* resistance to ampicillin and amoxicillin.

Decongestants to reduce edema and improve eustachian tube function and antihistamines have not been established as efficacious in the treatment of acute otitis media (Paradise, 1980; Bhambhani et al, 1983; Canilekin et al, 1983; Marchant and Shurin, 1983; Pelton and Whitley, 1983). However, these medications seem to provide some comfort and continue to be used. Analgesic and antipyretic drugs may be used to relieve earache and fever. Topical intranasal and systemic corticosteroids lack convincing evidence of their efficacy (Bluestone and Klein, 1988). Application of heat or cold to the affected ear region may relieve discomfort.

Young children should be watched closely for signs of secondary mastoiditis, meningitis (especially under 4 months of age), or hearing loss.

Aeration of the Middle Ear. This procedure has been recommended by some and can be taught to the older child. It is done by pinching the nose and forcing air into the ear by blowing up balloons or closing the lips while chewing sugarless gum (Kass and Beebe, 1979). The reason some object to this procedure is that bacteria may be blown from the nose to the middle ear. If allergy is contributing to serous otitis, its evaluation and treatment are important to prevent recurrent otitis involvement.

Myringotomy. Aspiration of fluid by surgical incision of the eardrum (myringotomy) or placement of tympanostomy tubes to facilitate drainage may be indicated if otitis media with effusion persists after nonsurgical methods of treatment have been tried. If myringotomy is elected and a general anesthetic is required, then a tympanostomy tube* is inserted at the same time. The incision allows for removal of the accumulated fluid, and tubes function as accessory eustachian tubes, allowing for air exchange between the middle and outer ear. The tubes work their way out in 2 to 9 months. A small amount of bloody drainage and slight pain are normal when the tubes work their way out.

The use of myringotomy with tube (M & T) insertion is not without some complications. Scarring (tympanosclerosis) and otorrhea may result, but they do not appear to have long-term sequelae (Pelton and Whitley, 1983). The major issue surrounding M & T is timing in relation to prevention of hearing loss. It is felt that children can tolerate effusion for around 3 months without significant hearing loss, and 90 per cent of such effusions will resolve if kept free from recurrent disease. The role of adenoidectomy continues to be unclear, but there is increasing evidence that removal of enlarged adenoids reduces the recurrence rate of otitis media with effusion (Paradise et al, 1987); however, some children do not improve after the procedure and others improve without undergoing the procedure.

Pneumococcal Vaccine. The use of pneumococcal vaccine continues to be experimental and is not routinely recommended for prevention of otitis media in children under 2 years of age. It may be of value, however, in children older than 2 years who suffer from recurrent episodes of acute otitis media (Bluestone and Klein, 1988).

Table 38-11. Causes of Eustachian Tube Dysfunction

Type	Cause
Functional	A decreased tubal stiffness related to immature development of cartilage, resulting in easy collapsibility
	An inefficient active opening mechanism
	An unrepaired cleft palate*
	Down syndrome*
Mechanical	
Intrinsic	Inflammatory mucosal edema of the tube related to allergy or infection
Extrinsic	Obstructive adenoids
	Nasopharyngeal tumors

* The reason for the dysfunction in these conditions is not clearly understood.

(Compiled from Bluestone and Klein, 1983; Paradise, 1980.)

Major Nursing Diagnoses for Otitis Media

Potential for (or actual) infection: middle ear inflammation, related to dysfunction of the eustachian tube, associated with:

- *anatomy of eustachian tubes in children under 3 years of age*
- *pooling of fluid in the pharyngeal cavity*

*Also called a pressure equalization (PE) tube.

- *abundant nasopharyngeal lymphoid tissue*

Altered comfort: pain, related to middle ear inflammation

Knowledge deficit, related to care of child with tympanostomy tubes

Strategies for Nursing Care

Preventing Middle Ear Infection and Promoting Its Resolution. To prevent middle ear infection, parents are taught to feed infants in the upright position and avoid laying them in their cribs with a bottle of milk. Children are taught to blow their noses properly during respiratory infections and not to hold one nostril closed while blowing.

In an infection requiring antibiotics, symptoms usually subside in 24 to 48 hours after instituting therapy. The nurse gives adequate explanations to parents so they understand that the full course of drug therapy is necessary to eradicate the infection, despite the child's apparent early improvement. A phone follow-up in 2 to 5 days after therapy is initiated is appropriate to determine whether symptoms are being relieved. The child should be re-evaluated at the end of the antibiotic course to determine whether the infection has resolved. Ideally, another check-up is done in 2 to 3 months to ensure that a chronic condition does not exist.

Relieving Pain and General Discomfort. Pain relief is necessary to reduce the severe earache that accompanies otitis media. Acetaminophen is used to reduce pain and is also effective for fever management. Either warm or cool compresses can be recommended, whichever provides the greatest comfort to the child. Care must be taken not to burn the child if a heating pad is used. In some instances, a pain-relieving prescription of ear drops may be ordered by the physician if pain cannot be managed effectively.

Preventing Dislodging of Tubes and Middle Ear Contamination. The child's activity around water when tympanostomy tubes are in place is controversial. Parents are instructed to plug the child's ears lightly with sterile cotton coated with petroleum jelly during baths or shampooing to keep water from entering the ear canal. Also, diving or swimming deeply under water is not permitted because it leads to contamination of the middle ear. Surface swimming can be permitted if ear plugs or specially designed ear defenders are worn, although some reports suggest that surface swimming without ear protection does not increase the risk for otitis media (Lounsbury, 1985).

Complications and Sequelae of Otitis Media

Hearing Loss. This is the most prevalent complication of otitis media. The presence of effusion or high negative pressure within the middle ear during each bout of otitis media is associated with temporary hearing loss. This episodic hearing loss is usually reversible, but permanent conductive hearing loss may develop owing to the complications of recurrent middle ear inflammation. Frequent episodes of otitis media and its related hearing loss may interfere eventually with the development of language and cognitive skills. The degree and duration of hearing loss necessary to interfere with development have not been defined.

Acute Mastoiditis. A frequent complication of suppurative otitis media in the past, this is now rare because of the availability of antibiotics. It does still occur in children with untreated otitis media or when the antibiotic course was inadequate in dose or duration of administration. The anatomic communication between the mastoid process and middle ear invites infectious exchange.

Clinically, mastoiditis reveals pain over the mastoid process, erythema, edema, and tenderness to pressure. Diagnosis may be difficult if the infection has been partially suppressed by antibiotics.

Once the condition is diagnosed, antibiotic therapy should commence immediately. Sedation may be necessary to allay restlessness until pain subsides. Pain is lessened by application of a cold compress or ice bag to the mastoid process. Fever is relieved with antipyretics. Mastoidectomy is indicated only if subperiosteal abscess occurs or if antibiotic therapy fails.

Acquired Cholesteatoma. A cholesteatoma is a saclike structure lined with squamous epithelial cells. It develops primarily in association with chronic otitis media. Impaired ventilation apparently is the primary factor leading to its development. A sustained high negative pressure in the middle ear and the loss of elasticity result in a flaccid and eventually atelectatic tympanic membrane. The most flaccid part of the tympanic membrane, the pars flaccida, is drawn inward to form a pocket. This pocket, called a retraction pocket, eventually adheres to the ossicles and surrounding structures. It fills with desquamated cells and forms a cholesteatoma. Shiny white pieces of debris collect that may have a foul-smelling discharge. On otoscopic examination, the flakes of debris will be observed through a large perforation or in a defect of the membrane in the involved area. The cholesteatoma is surgically excised to prevent destruction of the temporal bone and intracranial involvement. If the discharge is profuse, a preoperative antibiotic is administered.

Nursing Strategies for Follow-Up Care in the Home or Clinic

Assess ear canal and the tympanic membrane per otoscopy for clearing of inflammation. Note and record presence of tubes when applicable.

Obtain a tympanogram, if indicated, to assess mobility of tympanic membrane.

Assess nasopharyngeal cavities for signs of inflammation or allergy (see Chapter 15 for assessment guidelines).

Ask the parent and child about ear pain and about successful palliative measures.

Determine whether all prescribed doses of the antibiotic were taken.

Assess for signs and symptoms of complications:
- Screen for hearing loss of low, middle, and high tones through age-appropriate methods (see Chapter 15).
- Assess for indications of mastoiditis: pain over the mastoid process, erythema, edema, tenderness to pressure.
- Look for a perforation or defect in the tympanic membrane and a foul-smelling discharge, suggesting an acquired cholesteatoma.

Acute Pharyngitis

Incidence and Etiology

Acute pharyngitis is an inflammation of the structures in the pharynx, including tonsillitis and pharyngotonsillitis. It occurs at all ages, but the peak incidence is during the late preschool and early school-age years. At this time a child is more consistently exposed to infections outside the home. A natural hypertrophy of lymphoid tissue also develops at this time, shown in enlarged tonsils and adenoids.

The two most common causes of acute pharyngitis are viruses and group A beta-hemolytic streptococcus (referred to as strep throat). About 80 per cent of cases are caused by a virus, and 20 per cent or less are bacterial in origin. In children less than 3 years of age, the bacterium *Haemophilus influenzae* is common; streptococcal pharyngitis is rare before age 2 years. The most susceptible ages for acute pharyngitis are 5 to 15 years of age.

Clinical Manifestations and Diagnostic Assessment

Viral and streptococcal pharyngitis cannot be reliably differentiated by clinical manifestations. Some characteristics of each are summarized in Table 38-12, but even these overlap considerably. Streptococcal pharyngitis cannot be reliably diagnosed without a throat culture.

Therapeutic Management

Viral pharyngitis is treated symptomatically, whereas streptococcal infections require antibiotics to prevent complications (especially rheumatic fever and glomerulonephritis). In viral pharyngitis acetaminophen generally brings about a prompt reduction in fever, whereas in streptococcal infections, fever usually persists. On the other hand, antimicrobial therapy (penicillin) is so effective in streptococcal pharyngitis that fever does not usually persist longer than 24 hours after initiation of therapy.

The method of administering antibiotics varies. It is generally safe to wait for the results of the throat culture before instituting therapy (Widome, 1987). If

Table 38-12. Characteristics of Bacterial and Viral Pharyngotonsillitis*

	Streptococcal Pharyngotonsillitis		Viral Pharyngotonsillitis
	<2 Years of Age	>2 Years of Age	Any Age
Onset	Gradual or sudden	Sudden	Gradual
Presenting signs	Nasopharyngitis	Abdominal pain, vomiting, headache	Sore throat (often preceded by malaise and anorexia)
Fever	Slight to moderate (rarely, 39°C, 102°F), often irregular	Usually high (39.4–40°C, 103–104°F), but may be moderate	Slight to moderate, sometimes high
Tonsillar involvement	Little or none	May have any or all of following: follicular exudation, erythema of tonsils and pillars, petechial mottling of soft palate, lymphadenopathy; *or* mild-to-moderate tonsillar or pharyngeal inflammation	Similar to streptococcal, although petechial mottling is less common and erythema is often less
Clinical complaints	Anorexia, runny nose, listlessness, failure to thrive, vomiting	Sore throat	Sore throat, hoarseness, cough, rhinitis, conjunctivitis
Lab results	Leukocytosis	Leukocytosis	Leukocyte count normal to high

* In many children there is considerable overlap in symptomatology of viral and streptococcal disease.
(From Eichenwald, 1976.)

there is concern that a patient will not return for treatment, then therapy may be initiated sooner.

Penicillin is the drug of choice. It can be administered orally for 10 days or by one intramuscular injection. The advantage of intramuscular injection is that the patient who might not return is treated effectively, but this is a painful mode of treatment, and, unless streptococcal disease has been confirmed, it is thought to be unreasonable to subject a child to such therapy without proof of need (Eichenwald, 1976). If compliance is a problem and streptococcal infection is confirmed, one dose of benzathine penicillin is given intramuscularly to ensure adequate penicillin levels for a 10-day period. If the child is allergic to penicillin, the drug of choice is erythromycin for 10 days.

Strategies for Nursing Care

The nurse has an important role in obtaining a complete health history, giving particular attention to the history of the illness. The nurse also gathers sufficient data to recommend the mode of therapy (oral or intramuscular) that would be most appropriate for the particular family.

Promoting Compliance with Antibiotic Therapy. If the child is to receive a 10-day course of antibiotics, the nurse emphasizes the importance of continuing the medication even though the child feels well and is free of symptoms. If intramuscular penicillin is to be administered, both the child and parents are forewarned of the pain associated with the injection. Local measures can be suggested to provide relief at home, including warm baths and use of a warm water bottle.

Relieving Throat Discomfort. Additional symptomatic measures for sore throat include cool, bland liquids, acetaminophen (Tylenol), warm compresses to the neck, and warm normal saline gargles (if the child is able to gargle). Parents should be counseled not to force the child to eat and to avoid liquids and foods that are irritating to the throat, especially citrus and spicy foods. The nurse also advises the family to report similar symptoms in other family members. Recurrent streptococcal pharyngitis within the family is an indication for all family members to have throat specimens cultured.

Explaining the Need for Follow-Up Care. Viral pharyngitis is usually self-limiting, requiring only symptomatic treatment. Streptococcal pharyngitis, if adequately treated, generally results in complete recovery. Both nonsuppurative (rheumatic fever and glomerulonephritis) and suppurative (peritonsillar abscess, otitis media, mastoiditis, cervical adenitis, meningitis, osteomyelitis, pneumonia) complications can usually be prevented with prompt treatment. Follow-up practices for streptococcal infections vary. Many practitioners believe a reculture should be done 14 days after treatment with antibiotics. If the repeat culture is positive for group A beta-hemolytic streptococci, three possibilities should be considered: (1) the child did not complete the 14-day antibiotic therapy, (2) an organism that is resistant to the antibiotic is present, and (3) a new infection has been acquired (Castiglia and Aquilina, 1982). The question of whether the child is a carrier is also of concern. Most clinicians believe that a second course of antibiotics is warranted; however, if a third throat culture remains positive, one should consider that the child is probably a carrier. (It has been estimated that 15 to 20 per cent of healthy children might be carrying group A streptococci as normal flora) (Castiglia and Aquilina, 1982.)

Diseased Tonsils and Adenoids

In its common usage, the word tonsils refers to the two faucial tonsils (palatine) on either side of the opening of the oral cavity into the pharynx (see Figure 15-15 in Chapter 15). Adenoids (pharyngeal tonsils) are located superiorly in the midline of the posterior wall of the nasopharynx. Tonsils and adenoids, along with other lymphoid tissue, trap infection from the upper respiratory tract; tonsils also have the capacity to produce antibodies and have an important function in immunity. The size of lymphoid tissue increases to that of an adult when the child is around 6 years of age, almost doubles by age 10 years, then gradually shrinks to normal adult size by age 20 years. During early childhood lymphoid tissue (including tonsils and adenoids) responds to infection by becoming larger.

Close proximity of the palatine tonsils and the pharyngeal tonsils (adenoids) to the opening of the eustachian tubes has resulted in tonsillectomy and adenoidectomy as a treatment for recurrent otitis media. Removal of tonsils and adenoids is a subject of much controversy. Although the nurse may not play a primary role in the decision, an awareness of the nature of the controversy is helpful in discussions with the family. It is important for the nurse to have a clear understanding of the explanation that has been given to the family by the physician regarding the need for tonsillectomy and adenoidectomy (T & A).

The ultimate evaluation of T & A is made by weighing the potential benefits it can provide against potential risks. Some physicians still perform T & A to treat recurrent sore throats, whereas others recommend that it be done only in rare circumstances. Recently, a more conservative attitude is prevailing. The number of procedures done yearly has been reduced by more than half since the 1960s and 1970s (Kornblut, 1987). It is generally agreed that adenoidectomy alone may be indicated in children under 4 years of age and that tonsillectomy is preferably deferred until after 5 years of age. Removal of both tonsils and adenoids in very young children may stimulate hyperplasia of other lymphoid tissue in the oropharynx (Catlin, 1979). Some of the common indications with explanations for T & A are summarized in Box 38-3.

Surgical Management

Anesthesia may be given by endotracheal intubation or inhalation. Adenoidectomy by curettage is usually performed first, followed by the tonsillectomy. The tonsils are removed by surgical dissection, with the lower pole of the tonsil being severed by scissors or a snare. Tonsillectomy and adenoidectomy may also be done separately or in conjunction with myringotomy and tube insertion. Bleeding should be controlled before the child leaves the operating room. (See Box 38-3 for contraindications to T & A.)

Major Nursing Diagnoses for T & A

Anxiety: child and family, *related to scheduled tonsillectomy/adenoidectomy*
Potential for injury: physiologic, *related to the following contraindications for surgery:*

- *acute upper respiratory infection*
- *fever*
- *history of untoward reactions to anesthesia or bleeding tendencies*
- *evidence of a submucous cleft palate*

Potential for injury: postoperative complications, *related to:*

- *aspiration of oral secretions*
- *hemorrhage from the surgical site*

Altered comfort: throat pain, *related to surgical removal of pharyngeal tissues*
Knowledge deficit, *related to:*

- *lack of information about the postoperative course in the hospital*
- *lack of information about home care during the recovery period*

Strategies for Nursing Care

Relieving Anxiety Associated with Lack of Information About the Surgery. Once the decision has been made that removal of tonsils and adenoids is necessary, the nurse focuses on preparing the child and family for the surgical experience and providing optimal postoperative nursing care to prevent complications. Frequently the child is admitted to the hospital the evening before surgery, although some recommend that the child sleep at home the night before surgery and be admitted the morning of surgery. The child should be prepared for hospitalization and various procedures according to age.

Box 38-3
Indications and Contraindications for Tonsillectomy and Adenoidectomy (T & A)

TONSILLECTOMY

Indications

Recurrent tonsillitis. In the past, a specific number of these episodes has been given as an indication for surgery, but some recommend that surgery is justifiable for any patient if significant amounts of school attendance are lost (Kornblut, 1987).

Peritonsillar abscess. In the past, T & A was recommended. Paradise (1983) includes peritonsillar abscess as an indication for tonsillectomy only.

Cervical adenitis. Chronic (minimum of 6 months' duration) enlargement or tenderness of cervical lymph nodes, after trials of appropriate antibiotic treatment, is an indication for tonsillectomy.

Neoplasm. Unilateral removal of a tonsil is supported when a neoplasm is suspected and tissue is needed to establish a diagnosis.

ADENOIDECTOMY

Indications

Persistent nasal or airway obstruction. If adenoid enlargement results in obstructive sleep apnea, mouth breathing, and nasal congestion with discharge, adenoidectomy alone is indicated (provided symptoms are not due to allergy).

Recurrent otitis media secondary to eustachian tube obstruction. If tubes have been inserted at least once and ear infections are frequent, adenoidectomy alone may be indicated. Eustachian tube obstruction can result in middle ear effusion with hearing loss.

TONSILLECTOMY AND ADENOIDECTOMY

Indications

Hypertrophied tonsils. Enlarged tonsils alone in children (especially under 6 years of age) are not an indication for surgery. If swallowing and breathing difficulty, sleep apnea syndrome, or cor pulmonale exists, T & A are indicated.

Contraindications

Cleft palate (tonsils help reduce air escape during speech).

Under 3 years of age.

Acute infection (local inflammation increases risk of hemorrhage).

Blood dyscrasias (leukemia, purpura, aplastic anemia, hemophilia).

Uncontrolled systemic disease (diabetes, heart disease, seizure disorder).

(Compiled from Howard, 1983; Paradise, 1983; Kornblut, 1987.)

Preoperatively, the child and parents should be prepared for what the child will experience before and following surgery. Many hospitals have special programs, including a film or slide-tape, a prehospitalization tour, and a play program that provides an opportunity for the child to manipulate equipment and supplies that will be seen during the preoperative and postoperative experience.

Physical preparation of the child should also be explained to the child and family. Platelet count, prothrombin time (PT), and partial thromboplastin time (PTT) evaluations may be done in addition to routine admission laboratory tests of hemoglobin, hematocrit, and urinalysis. Foods and liquids are withheld for 8 hours before the operation to prevent vomiting with aspiration. Preoperative medication varies in type and method of administration.

Special attention is given to the child's understanding of the procedure. A young child may fear "being cut" and does not understand that the operation will be done through the mouth and that an incision is not made through the neck. The child and the parents should be prepared for the child's sore throat after surgery, including explanations of what will be done for it. (See Chapters 31 and 27 on Hospitalization and Preparations for Procedures and Table 27-7, Nursing Process Plan: Perioperative Care.) Nursing management of pain in children is discussed in Chapter 29.

Assessing for Contraindications to Surgery. The nurse performs a complete health assessment on admission, including a careful evaluation of the child's respiratory status. T & A should not be performed until several weeks after an upper respiratory infection has cleared. An elevated temperature should be reported to the surgeon. The child and the family are assessed to identify medication allergies, a history of bleeding tendency, an uncontrolled illness, or a family history of any reactions to anesthetics. In addition to these factors, a submucous cleft palate (soft palate with little or no muscle) is a contraindication for adenoidectomy. A submucous cleft palate may be recognized by hypernasal speech, a history of frequent cases of otitis media, a bifid uvula, and a palpable V-shaped notch in the posterior edge of the hard palate.

Preventing Postoperative Complications. Postoperatively, the bed is kept in a flat position, and the child is placed in a side-lying or abdominal position with the upper knee flexed and the head tilted slightly forward. This permits the tongue and jaw to come forward and secretions and vomitus to drain from the mouth, preventing aspiration. Vital signs are checked frequently beginning immediately after the child returns from the recovery room. The nurse should watch for tachycardia, pallor, and excessive swallowing. (Swallowing indicates that blood is trickling down the child's throat.) The throat is checked with a flashlight to assess for bleeding. Almost all cases of fatal bleeding occur within the first 24 hours postoperatively (Rasmussen, 1987).

On return to the ward, the child alternates between periods of sleep and restlessness owing to the effect of the anesthetic. When the child is fully awake and vital signs are stable, fluids are given cautiously. Small amounts of liquids should be given until the danger of vomiting has passed. Sucking through a straw produces a vacuum that could potentially stimulate bleeding; therefore drinking from a cup is recommended. A well-tolerated form of intake is a popsicle. Red-colored liquids are avoided during the postoperative period so that they are not confused with frank blood in secretions and vomitus.

Parents are encouraged to stay with their child. Having a parent quietly sit at the bedside is comforting to children as they periodically awaken. A suction machine should be immediately available in the event of obstruction from vomitus or secretions or if hemorrhage occurs.

Relieving Throat Pain. An ice collar wrapped in a soft material and applied to comfortably fit the contour of the child's neck may provide some relief of pain, but this varies. Analgesics need to be administered on the basis of the nurse's judgment rather than waiting for a child's verbal expression of pain. The first postoperative dose of analgesics should be administered routinely to keep the child from experiencing excessive throat pain. Children may resist taking the medication because it hurts to swallow but with encouragement and explanation will usually cooperate. It is important to explain the purpose of the medication and acknowledge the child's resistance and fears. A comfortable child is more likely to take fluids, which in turn promotes recovery and early discharge. Oral codeine or acetaminophen are the drugs frequently used for pain as needed. Aspirin should be avoided because of the risk of hemorrhage.

Promoting Effective Home Management. Most children can be discharged the next morning following surgery. Parents should be advised against giving their child hot, coarse, or spicy foods for 5 to 7 days; swimming is generally discouraged until the follow-up visit in 10 to 14 days; and any signs of bleeding should be reported promptly to the physician. A late hemorrhage (5 to 10 days after surgery) is associated with infection of the upper respiratory tract. Thus it is advisable during the recovery period to limit exposure to other children who are known to have colds. The hemorrhage occurs when the tissue (eschar) that normally forms over the raw surface separates prematurely during infection; parents should be aware of this. Analgesics may be necessary for the first few days after surgery for throat pain and referred pain to the ears, but pain should not persist beyond the first week. Many institu-

Box 38-4
Home Care of Your Child After Removal of Tonsils and Adenoids

DIETARY INSTRUCTIONS

First day

Avoid hot and highly seasoned foods

Encourage fluid intake by frequently offering water, bland fruit juices, gelatin, broth, etc.

Have child drink several glasses of water

Second day

Add soft foods as desired (gelatin, chocolate pudding, mashed potato, puréed vegetables, cottage cheese, etc.)

Third to fifth day

Gradually resume normal diet but avoid hot foods, potato chips, nuts, dry toast, and crackers until 1 to 2 weeks after surgery

GENERAL INSTRUCTIONS

The child should be kept relatively quiet for the first 3 days

Frequent coughing and clearing the throat should be avoided

Objectionable mouth odor is commonly observed and is relieved by abundant fluid intake

A gray membrane on the sides of the throat is normal and should disappear in 1 to 2 weeks

Earache or a slight fever is expected and may be disregarded unless condition worsens

Child may return to school 1 week after discharge

Do not use aspirin for 2 weeks; it increases the possibility of bleeding. Use acetaminophen (Tylenol) for pain

Avoid drinking orange juice, grapefruit juice, and tomato juice for 1 week after the operation as they will make the throat burn

The danger of serious bleeding is past after you leave the hospital. In about 2 per cent of patients there is some bleeding after 5 or 6 days. If this happens to you, do not become excited, for this bleeding is usually slight. Be quiet, lie down, and spit the blood out gently. Gargle gently with ice water and be quiet. If the bleeding does not stop promptly, call your doctor. If doctor is not available and bleeding continues, call the nearest emergency room

(Adapted from Rowe, 1982.)

tions have developed an instruction sheet to give parents (see Box 38-4 for an example).

Nursing Strategies for Follow-Up Care in the Home or Clinic

Assess retropharyngeal area for evidence of healing versus inflammation.

Palpate for enlarged lymph nodes in the head and neck that might signal a postoperative infection.

Measure the temperature and assess for any other evidence of an infectious process.

Determine whether any bleeding was noted after the child left the hospital.

Determine whether throat pain persists and whether the child has resumed a normal diet.

Allow adequate time for the child and parents to discuss the experience of hospitalization and surgery.

Retropharyngeal Abscess

Etiology and Pathophysiology

A retropharyngeal abscess develops when lymph glands located behind the posterior pharyngeal wall become infected. This may result from pharyngitis (group A hemolytic streptococcus) in which the infection extends to the lymph nodes via the lymphatic system. Purulent infection of contiguous areas (sinuses, adenoids, nasopharynx) causes the nodes to become infected, with resultant swelling and suppuration.

Clinical Manifestations

The illness usually follows an upper respiratory infection and produces an abrupt onset of fever, dyspnea, and difficulty swallowing. A typical response of the nurse may be to suction the nasopharynx to maintain the child's airway. This imprudent action could have disastrous results: rupture and aspiration of the contents of the abscess. If suctioning is necessary to prevent aspiration of oral secretions, it should be of the mouth only.

Diagnostic Assessment and Therapeutic Management

The diagnosis is established by a lateral radiograph of the neck and by digital palpation of a fluctuant mass on one side of the posterior pharyngeal wall. The child is placed in the Trendelenburg position for the digital examination to prevent aspiration. A suction apparatus must be immediately available in the event of rupture of the abscess during the examination.

A fluctuant abscess is treated by incision and drainage in conjunction with preoperative and postoperative antibiotic administration. Postoperatively, it is important to observe the child for signs of respiratory distress and frequent swallowing (a sign of bleeding), and keep the child in a prone position to facilitate drainage of secretions. Parents should be kept informed of the child's condition and be given explanations of how they can participate in the care.

Croup (Acute Laryngotracheobronchitis)

Croup is a syndrome characterized by a brassy, barking cough, a hoarse cry, inspiratory stridor, and varying degrees of respiratory distress. These symptoms are the result of laryngeal obstruction due to edema and spasm. *Croup syndrome* refers to infections of the epiglottis, larynx, trachea, and bronchi. Epiglottitis, although a form of croup, is discussed as a separate entity because of its uniqueness in presentation and management. The croup syndromes are summarized in Table 38-13. Acute viral larynyotracheobronchitis (LTB) is the most common form of croup and is discussed here.

Incidence and Etiology

Acute viral LTB, or croup, is most common in children between 3 months and 3 years of age. It usually follows an upper respiratory infection and is most often seen in late fall or winter, during the cold season. It tends to recur, but as the child grows attacks tend to disappear.

LTB is most commonly caused by the parainfluenza viruses. Other organisms include the adenoviruses and respiratory syncytial, influenza, and measles viruses.

Pathophysiology, Clinical Manifestations, and Diagnostic Assessment

The symptoms associated with croup occur primarily due to inflammation and edema with subsequent narrowing of air passages. The laryngeal airway is relatively smaller and mucous membrane is more loosely

Table 38-13. Differentiating Croup Symptoms

Common symptoms: Hoarseness; brassy, barking cough; inspiratory stridor; respiratory distress

Differentiating Features	Acute LTB*	Spasmodic Croup	Acute Epiglottitis	Aspirated Foreign Body
Age	<3 yrs	1–4 yrs	>3 yrs	Any age
History	Gradual onset; preceded by URI	Child awakens in night with symptoms	Sudden onset; symptoms worsen over a few hours	Sudden onset of symptoms; child playing or eating; environmental hazards present; adult supervision absent
Etiologic agent	Viral	Unknown	Bacterial *(H. influenzae)*	Foreign body
Symptoms	Fever (<40°C); mild-to-severe respiratory distress, worse at night	Afebrile; mild-to-moderate respiratory distress	Child's chin may be thrust forward; drooling; difficulty swallowing; epiglottis cherry-red; febrile (>40°C); child appears toxic	Mild-to-severe respiratory distress; afebrile; possibly clutching at throat
Comments	Most common	Sometimes relieved by vomiting; asymptomatic in day, symptoms recur during night	No attempt should be made to visualize child's epiglottis; child should be kept calm; emergency tracheotomy may be needed; high morbidity	Heimlich maneuver may help older child but not necessarily infants; emergency tracheotomy may be needed

* LTB, laryngotracheobronchitis.

Table 38-14. Subjective Assessment of Clinical Severity of Croup*

	0	1	2	3
Stridor	None	Mild	Moderate at rest	Severe on inspiration and expiration or none with markedly decreased air entry
Retraction	None	Mild	Moderate	Severe, marked use of accessory muscles
Air Entry	Normal	Mild decrease	Moderate decrease	Marked decrease
Color	Normal	Normal (0-score)	Normal (0-score)	Dusky or cyanotic
Level of Consciousness	Normal	Restless when disturbed	Anxious, agitated; restless when undisturbed	Lethargic, depressed

* Scoring system modified from Taussig LM, et al: Treatment of laryngotracheobronchitis (croup): use of intermittent positive pressure breathing and racemic epinephrine. *Am J Dis Child* 1975; 129:790–793.
(From Davis et al, 1981.)

attached and more vascular in children resulting in rapid compromise by edema and spasm.

As the infection extends down the respiratory tract, breathing becomes more difficult. Symptoms appear gradually, often initially in the evening, and worsen progressively. After several days of respiratory symptoms, there is a gradually increasing brassy or barking cough (like a seal's bark), a hoarse cry, and inspiratory stridor. Stridor is a harsh sound caused by increased rate and turbulence of airflow in the larynx or trachea. Stridor is predominantly inspiratory. Varying degrees of respiratory distress, including labored breathing, flaring of the nares, prolonged expiratory phase, and use of accessory muscles (substernal, intercostal, suprasternal retractions) accompany the typical cough and stridor of croup. Breath sounds may be diminished. Fever is generally present but not as severely as in epiglottitis.

Signs of increasing respiratory obstruction include increasing stridor and retractions at rest, respiratory rate above 60 per minute, tachycardia, cyanosis (circumoral and orbital), pallor, and restlessness. Restlessness and tachycardia are signs of increasing hypoxia. Diagnosis of viral croup is made on the basis of history and clinical manifestations and the exclusion of bacterial infection. An assessment of the severity of croup is summarized in Table 38-14.

Therapeutic Management

Medical treatment for croup focuses on maintenance of a patent airway. Initial medical assessment will determine whether the illness is so severe as to require emergency treatment. It is rare that sufficient obstruction occurs to warrant tracheotomy or nasotracheal intubation (Boat, 1987). If complete obstruction does occur, insertion of a large-bore needle into the trachea will provide a temporary airway; this procedure is to be followed immediately by tracheostomy. A No. 14-gauge intercatheter is ideal for this procedure since the needle can be withdrawn and the catheter left in place.

The child who has an adequate airway but who has stridor at rest will usually be admitted to the hospital. Therapy during the acute phase usually involves bronchodilating medications, racemic epinephrine by aerosol, cool mist administered within a croup tent, and intravenous hydration. Oxygen may be used to alleviate hypoxia, but the child must be observed particularly closely because cyanosis, a sign of impending obstruction, is masked. Sedatives are contraindicated because they mask restlessness, which is one of the principal clinical indications that the child's condition is worsening.

Corticosteroids are sometimes administered for their anti-inflammatory properties when croup fails to respond to conventional treatment. The most beneficial results from the use of steroid therapy have resulted when a single dose was given early in the course of illness (Davis et al, 1981). Because croup is of viral origin, antibiotics are not ordered unless a secondary bacterial infection exists.

Major Nursing Diagnoses for Croup*

Ineffective airway clearance, related to inflammation and edema of laryngeal, tracheal, and bronchial tissues
Potential fluid volume deficit, related to:

- *fever*
- *increased insensible water loss associated with increased respiratory effort*
- *decreased fluid intake associated with respiratory distress*

*To be used with Table 38-5, Nursing Process Plan: The Child with Respiratory Dysfunction.

Fear/anxiety (child), related to:
- *respiratory distress*
- *croup tent and other unfamiliar surroundings*
- *parental anxiety*

Knowledge deficit, related to care of child at home

Strategies for Nursing Care

Maintaining Airway Clearance. Maintenance of an adequate airway is central to the care of a child with croup, whether hospitalized or cared for at home. The child must be carefully and frequently observed for signs of increasing obstruction (see Table 38-17) and hypoxia (see Table 38-5).

Dramatic changes in the child's condition can occur quickly, and respiratory arrest from complete obstruction is always a possibility. Any progression of symptoms must be reported to the physician immediately. In the event of impending obstruction, giving humidified oxygen via positive pressure (Ambu-bag and mask) may force enough oxygen through the narrowing airway to maintain the child until the physician arrives. Equipment to perform intubations or tracheostomy should be kept at the bedside or in a place of immediate access when a child with severe croup is hospitalized.

The use of *cool mist* will relieve some of the distress of croup by decreasing laryngeal edema. If the child is hospitalized, a croup tent provides the ideal environment. A child may be frightened and resist staying in the tent at first. Parents should be nearby and encourage the child by distracting with toys or a game. The child's parents may have other suggestions as to how to keep their child in the tent.

Racemic epinephrine and 40 per cent oxygen may be administered in aerosol with or without intermittent positive pressure breathing (IPPB) to temporarily relieve moderately severe symptoms of airway obstruction. Racemic epinephrine by aerosol is administered over a 10- to 15-minute period. Thirty minutes is the minimum time that should be allowed between treatments.

Epinephrine is a potent adrenergic agent that is effective in croup because of its ability to increase oxygenation through bronchodilation and to decrease edema through vasoconstriction. When given by inhalation, epinephrine produces its effects very quickly, with onset at 1 minute and a peak of action at 3 to 5 minutes (Loebl and Spratto, 1986).

Epinephrine has yet another effect which is *not* advantageous for treatment of respiratory problems. It causes a marked increase in both heart rate and force of contraction. For this reason, it is essential that the pulse rate and quality be closely monitored during and after inhalation of racemic epinephrine. Depending upon institutional policy, administration of racemic epinephrine may be limited to an intensive care unit where electronic monitoring of cardiac status will be instituted.

It is important to recognize that not all children receive relief from this therapy, and repeated attempts should not be tried. In those children who do not respond to racemic epinephrine, the nurse should observe for a rebound effect. (A rebound effect is a worsening of symptoms in response to therapy.)

Maintaining Fluid Balance. Adequate hydration is important and is provided orally in cases of mild respiratory distress. Intravenous therapy is advisable when respiratory difficulty interferes with oral intake. As the child improves, clear fluids are gradually increased as diet is increased. Refer to Table 38-5, Nursing Process Plan: The Child with Respiratory Tract Dysfunction, for specific nursing strategies related to hydration.

Relieving Fear and Anxiety. A significant aspect of nursing management of croup is decreasing the child's and the family's anxiety. Croup is dramatic and frightening, and it usually worsens at night. Respiratory distress is aggravated by anxiety. Upsetting the child should be avoided. Unnecessary procedures or extensive examinations should be deferred until the child is in less distress. The child's perception of the situation will be significantly influenced by parental behaviors, therefore, the focus should be on helping calm parents. Parents can then be encouraged to remain with the child to hold and comfort. Rhythmic movements such as rocking and gentle touches will help calm the child. While in a croup tent, the child should assume a position of comfort and be able to maintain physical contact with the parents. Parents should be encouraged to reach in and touch the child to reassure and prevent feelings of isolation.

Parents who understand the purpose of cool mist therapy will be more likely to cooperate with treatment. They should know that the cool mist is effective in reducing fever, in liquefying secretions for easy expectoration, and in reducing edema of the affected portions of the airway. These effects will often be demonstrated within the first hours that the child is in the tent, and the results can be discussed with the parent.

When the child's condition begins to improve (i.e., when stridor and retractions have significantly decreased), attempts will be made to "wean" the child from the croup tent. In some institutions, physicians will make the decision for weaning; in others it is a nursing prerogative. Weaning from the croup tent is accomplished by allowing the child to be out of the tent for short periods that are gradually lengthened if the child tolerates room air without an increased respiratory effort. Periods out of the tent are first tried during the day rather than at night. After successful weaning from the croup tent, the child is usually discharged to finish recuperating at home.

Parents need to understand the course of illness and what to expect. Acute LTB lasts from several days to several weeks, sometimes with a persistent barking cough. The prognosis of acute LTB is excellent. Although it may recur during childhood, it eventually is outgrown as the child grows and airway dimensions increase.

Preparing Family to Care for Child at Home. Since croup tends to recur, once a child has an attack the nurse should provide the necessary information to parents for preventing future attacks or to minimize their stressful effects. Although there are no definite preventive measures, environmental control of temperature and humidity may be helpful. When a child has a cold, the possibility of an attack should be anticipated. Air passages should be kept clear and the child adequately hydrated.

Symptoms of croup at home can often be relieved by special techniques. A croup tent can be improvised by placing a sheet over the top of a crib or playpen and securing it. A vaporizer (warm or cool mist) is then directed into the crib. Safety precautions must be taken so that the child is not burned or otherwise injured by the equipment. Serious accidents can occur with warm humidifiers in the home. Plastic should not be used because of the possibility that the child might pull it down and smother. The child should be observed frequently while in a croup tent. If it is impractical to improvise a croup tent, the shower or tub water can be run in a bathroom with the door closed to provide an environment high in humidity to relieve the distress. The child should never be left alone under these conditions. Parents should be aware of signs of increasing obstruction and instructed to return the child to the hospital if the condition worsens. Exposure to the cold night air when taking the child to the hospital frequently has been reported by parents to give temporary relief.

Nursing Strategies for Follow-Up Care in the Home or Clinic

Assess vital signs and breath sounds, being particularly alert for signs of secondary bacterial infection.

Ask the parent/child whether coughing and upper respiratory congestion have continued to decrease since hospital discharge.

Discuss with the parent/child the possibility of recurrence and ensure the parent knows:

- the indications and techniques for cool mist therapy in the home
- the signs and symptoms of increasing respiratory obstruction

Epiglottitis (Supraglottitis)

Incidence and Etiology

Epiglottitis is an acute infection of the epiglottis with a potentially fatal outcome. The epiglottis is swollen, cherry-red in appearance, and surrounded by copious secretions. The infection occurs most commonly in children between 3 and 8 years of age and is almost always caused by *H. influenzae* (type B).

Pathophysiology

The epiglottis is a thin, leaf-shaped flap that covers the entrance to the larynx when a person swallows. It prevents food or liquid from entering the airway. Epiglottitis, an inflammation of this structure, generally occurs subsequent to an upper respiratory tract infection. The characteristically rapid and marked inflammatory response of the epiglottis and surrounding structures causes mechanical obstruction. The edematous epiglottis, like a ball valve, is pulled down into the larynx during inspiration. Inspiratory obstruction may occur because of the narrowing force that occurs with the negative intrathoracic pressure (Hall and Hall, 1987).

Clinical Manifestations

Symptoms of mild upper respiratory infection may or may not precede the sudden onset of the classic symptoms of epiglottitis. Over a period of several hours the child develops high fever and severe sore throat with dysphagia and rapidly progresses to a state of severe respiratory distress with some inspiratory stridor, a prominent respiratory snore, and retractions. The general appearance of the child is suggestive of the diagnosis: leaning forward with chin thrust out and mouth open with drooling that occurs because swallowing is too painful. The condition may worsen rapidly, with complete obstruction occurring within 6 to 12 hours from the time of onset.

Diagnostic Assessment and Therapeutic Management

A tentative diagnosis is based on the history and clinical presentation. Treatment is immediately instituted when there is clinical evidence that the child has epi-

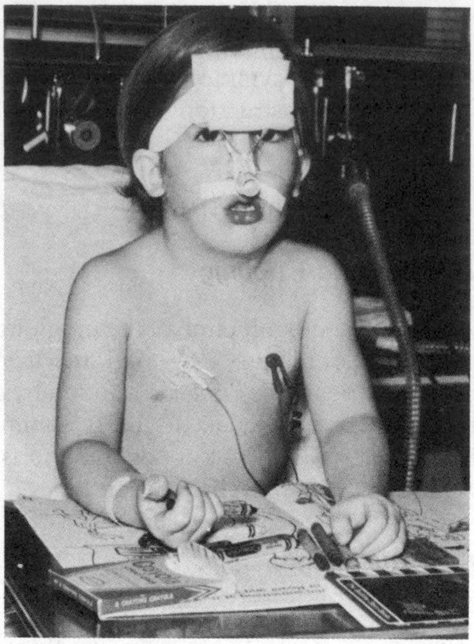

Figure 38-13. Young child with intubation treatment for supraglottitis. Nasotracheal tubes are well tolerated by most children. (From Barker G: Current management of croup and epiglottitis. *Pediatr Clin North Am* 1979 Aug; 576.)

glottitis. A throat swab should not be attempted before an airway is established. Placing the child in a recumbent position or using a tongue depressor may produce instant obstruction and is avoided until the child is moved to a facility in which skilled personnel have appropriate equipment to establish an airway. A lateral radiograph of the neck may show the swollen epiglottis. Radiographs are usually made with personnel in attendance who are capable of establishing an airway, and oxygen is administered on the way to the operating room.

A child diagnosed to have epiglottitis is treated immediately with an artificial airway. Until the early 1960s, tracheostomy was generally the accepted method of treatment, but because of the associated morbidity, mortality, and length of hospital stay, alternative methods have been investigated. Nasotracheal intubation has now become the preferred method and is performed in hospitals that have facilities to care for intubated children.

The child with an artificial airway requires respiratory care, including direct humidification of the airway, physical therapy, tracheal suctioning, and constant observation for signs of respiratory difficulty (increased pulse and respiration, retractions, restlessness, cyanosis). Mist can be delivered through a hood or a mist tent, whichever is most comfortable for the child. An intravenous line is required to deliver antibiotics and maintenance fluids, although these children are usually not dehydrated because they have been well until just before the rapid onset of symptoms.

Appropriate antibiotic therapy is initiated immediately and continued for 7 to 10 days. With increasing reports of infections from ampicillin-resistant *H. influenzae*, the recommended treatment is now combined therapy using chloramphenicol (50 mg/kg/24 hr) and ampicillin (200 mg/kg/24 hr) intravenously. Cefuroxine (100 mg/kg/24 hr) may also be effective (Boat, 1987). When results of antibiotic sensitivity testing are obtained, the specific effective antibiotic is continued and the other one discontinued. Racemic epinephrine and corticosteroids are not effective.

A nasotracheal tube is usually kept in place for a minimum of 24 to 36 hours (Fig. 38-13). After extubation, the child is observed in the intensive care unit in a mist tent for 24 hours, then transferred to a pediatric unit. One or two days later, the child is discharged on antibiotics. There is some evidence that racemic epinephrine and hydrocortisone facilitate extubation and are useful in the treatment of croup associated with extubation (Stern, 1983).

Major Nursing Diagnoses for Epiglottitis

Ineffective airway clearance, *related to progressive airway obstruction, associated with inflammation of the epiglottis*
Potential for injury: respiratory arrest, *related to accidental extubation*
Fear/anxiety, *related to acute respiratory distress*
Potential ineffective individual coping: posthospital behavior changes, *related to the fear and anxiety associated with epiglottitis*

Strategies for Nursing Care

Promoting Adequate Oxygenation. The nurse has an important role in the early management of epiglottitis. To avoid the catastrophe of bringing on obstruction of the airway, all team members must recognize the clinical presentation of epiglottitis. The nurse's ability to remain calm can reduce the child's and parent's anxiety during the emergency phase. The child is not left unattended even momentarily until an artificial airway is established. The child is allowed to assume a position of comfort and is not asked to lie down. The child is left undisturbed: no procedures are done that would cause crying or excitement. The nurse is an important member of the skilled team that intervenes immediately to establish an artificial airway. The nurse's familiarity with the equipment and the procedure can facilitate an efficient, skillful procedure.

Preventing Accidental Extubation. Accidental extubation must be prevented by applying appropriate restraints when the child is unattended; elbow restraints are usually sufficient. Taping of the endotracheal tube with regular adhesive tape or umbilical tape rather than clear plastic waterproof tape helps secure the tube. Use of excessive tape is avoided because secretions from the nose and mouth can seep between the layers of tape and cause the tube to slip, resulting in accidental extubation (Hazinski, 1984).

Positioning of an intubated child is done carefully to avoid movement of the tube. The head, neck, and shoulders must be rotated as one unit, and neck extension and flexion are prevented.

Preparing the Family for Potential Posthospital Behavior Changes. Epiglottitis seldom recurs, but the frightening experience is not easily forgotten by the child or the family. Because of the fear-producing experience that the child has been through, the nurse should prepare the parents regarding potential posthospital behavior changes according to the age of the child. (See Chapter 31 on Hospitalization.)

Nursing Strategies for Follow-Up Care in the Home or Clinic

Assess vital signs and breath sounds for evidence of residual disease.

Determine whether the entire course of antibiotics was completed as prescribed.

Allow time for the child and parent to talk about the frightening experiences of respiratory distress, intubation, and other aspects of the disease and hospitalization.

Determine whether posthospital behavior changes occurred and whether they have been resolved. Assure the parent that extra parental attention and understanding are usually all that are needed to resolve posthospital behavioral disturbances.

Bronchiolitis

Incidence and Etiology

Bronchiolitis, an inflammation of the bronchioles, is most frequently caused by respiratory syncytial virus (RSV). Other identified causative organisms include adenovirus and parainfluenza and influenza viruses. It rarely occurs after 2 years of age and has a peak incidence at 6 months of age, occurring most commonly during the winter and early spring months. Boys are affected more frequently than girls. It is primarily a condition treated on an outpatient basis, with only one of five children requiring hospitalization.

Pathophysiology

Inflammation of the bronchioles results in edema of the airway passages and eventual accumulation of mucus and exudate from cellular destruction. The bronchioles consequently become occluded; some are partially obstructed, and some may become totally obstructed. The alveoli are usually normal except those in the immediate vicinity of the inflamed bronchioles.

Under normal circumstances, expiration is an entirely passive process whereby relaxation and upward movement of the diaphragm move air out of the alveoli. Normally, the bronchial passages narrow during expiration, but when the lumen is further compromised by edema and exudate, air enters the alveoli and becomes trapped. Sufficient air is taken into the lungs, but there is difficulty in expelling the air, resulting in hyperinflation of the lungs and air trapping. When the obstruction is complete, the air is absorbed by the blood flowing in the pulmonary capillaries and the walls of the alveoli are pulled together, resulting in atelectasis. The impaired ventilation can result in hypoxemia and hypercapnia (carbon dioxide retention), leading to respiratory acidosis.

Clinical Manifestations

After a few days of serous nasal discharge and sneezing, diminished appetite, coughing, and a low-grade fever, an acute phase begins. The infant's condition worsens rapidly, with tachypnea (up to 80 per minute), chest retractions, and a paroxysmal wheezy cough. The infant may be irritable, appear anxious, and have some cyanosis, flaring of the nares, and wheezing, with a prolonged expiratory phase. ***It is important to know that when air exchange is severely compromised, a wheeze may not be heard because insufficient air is being exchanged.*** Fine crackles may be heard, especially on deep inspiration. When obstruction of the bronchioles is nearly complete, breath sounds are diminished. ***A sudden absence of breath sounds, cyanosis, pallor, and listlessness are signs of impending respiratory failure.***

Feeding is often a problem because of the difficulty of breathing experienced by the infant while sucking. The pulse rate is usually increased and body temperature may range from normal to as high as 41°C (105.8°F).

Diagnostic Assessment

Chest radiographs may be normal but usually show hyperinflation and occasional areas of atelectasis. Areas of consolidation on chest radiographs are thought to be due to atelectasis or inflammation. Certainty of diagnosis requires the use of virus isolation techniques. Immunofluorescent techniques applied to nasal aspirates are highly reliable (Wohl, 1983). Routine laboratory tests are not specific for the diagnosis of bronchiolitis. The age of the infant and the clinical manifestations in the face of an epidemic of respiratory syncytial virus in a community are highly suggestive of bronchiolitis.

Therapeutic Management

Most infants can be treated conservatively with rest, fluids, and high humidity. Careful handwashing and protection of other children is important because RSV continues to be shed for an average of 9 days in children less than 1 year of age (Wohl, 1983). The virus is transmitted by droplets; therefore, respiratory isolation is necessary. Mist therapy, combined with oxygen, loosens secretions and alleviates dyspnea and hypoxia. Clear fluids or hydration by intravenous therapy is provided, depending on the severity of illness.

A conservative approach is used in the administration of medications. Ribavirin (Virazole), an antiviral agent, is effective against RSV infection causing bronchiolitis if administered early in the illness (Boat, 1987). It is used in selected cases of severe infection or in children with underlying chronic illnesses.

Antibiotics generally are not indicated, and sedatives that depress respirations should be avoided. The role of bronchodilators remains controversial. Children under 18 months of age do not seem to respond to bronchodilators (Wohl, 1983). However, bronchodilators are frequently used in infants with *severe* bronchiolitis or when there is a positive family history of asthma. Although corticosteroids are not warranted in the usual cases of bronchiolitis, they may be used in the treatment of acute wheezing in infants. If antibiotics are used, it is in the case of small, acutely ill infants when there is uncertainty about the causative organism. Also, the fact that viral infection predisposes an infant to secondary bacterial invasion is sometimes used to justify administration of antibiotics (Wohl, 1983).

Major Nursing Diagnoses for Bronchiolitis

Ineffective airway clearance*, related to increased mucous secretion, associated with inflammation of the bronchioles (especially with RSV etiology)*

Impaired gas exchange*, related to air trapping in the alveoli, associated with narrowing of bronchioles by edema and exudate*

Potential fluid volume deficit*, related to:*

- *insensible fluid losses associated with tachypnea*
- *reduced fluid intake associated with feeding difficulties*

Potential ineffective family coping*, related to anxiety associated with the child's respiratory distress*

Strategies for Nursing Care

Promoting Adequate Oxygenation. The nurse gives careful attention to placing the infant where observation is easy and where other infants are not readily exposed. Constant surveillance is necessary to monitor respiratory status. Frequent assessment for tachypnea, retractions, flaring of the nares, cyanosis, and restlessness is necessary. Apnea monitoring is often indicated during the acute phase. A sudden increase in respiratory and cardiac rates and a dramatic increase in audible crackles are signs of cardiac failure. These findings should be reported immediately to allow rapid treatment by digitalization. Although uncommon, a small percentage (about 1 per cent) of hospitalized infants with bronchiolitis progress to respiratory failure and require intubation and ventilatory assistance.

The major consequence of inadequate ventilation is hypoxemia. Humidified oxygen is delivered via an Isolette, oxygen hood, or nasal catheter. An inspired oxygen concentration of 35 to 40 per cent is usually adequate to correct the hypoxemia (Wohl, 1983). The temperature within the device used for oxygen administration must be controlled to avoid increased oxygen consumption by the infant with hypothermia.

Mist therapy has not been proved to have a beneficial effect on the pulmonary problem. If mist tent therapy is used, a small particle mist delivered by an ultrasonic nebulizer is desired to aid in thinning secretions. (A large particle mist does not reach the lower respiratory tract.) These secretions can then be more readily removed through suctioning and postural drainage. Percussion and postural drainage may be ordered if moist crackles are present. Although treatments may be administered by the respiratory therapist, the nurse is also responsible for evaluating response to treatment. Frequently this procedure cannot be tolerated by the acutely ill infant.

Promoting Adequate Hydration. Some infants have dehydration and mild metabolic acidosis. Dehydration may occur as a result of insensible losses of fluid from tachypnea and because of reduced intake related to feeding difficulty. Intravenous fluids hydrate the child, resulting in thinner secretions, which enhances their removal. If intravenous fluids are administered, they should be given cautiously because unresolved bronchiolitis can eventually lead to heart failure. Specific gravity of urine can be monitored with the goal to maintain it not greater than 1.015.

Promoting Adaptive Family Coping. Parents are often anxious and fearful throughout the course of the illness. Therapy is supportive, and they may need help to understand that antibiotics and other medications are not indicated. The anxious appearance and respiratory difficulty of their infant are distressing to parents.

Nursing care provides maximal comfort for the infant and the parents. Care should be organized to avoid unnecessary disturbance of an infant who is already experiencing an energy deficit. Although infant-parent contact is hampered to some degree by an Isolette or mist therapy, touching, holding, and cuddling by parents should be encouraged as tolerated by the infant. When these anxious infants are extremely ill, the best sedative for them is provided by cuddling from their parents. It is the nurse's responsibility to help the parents feel sufficiently calm to provide that comfort.

Prognosis

Most infants improve within 3 to 4 days if given adequate supportive care, but usually 2 weeks are required to attain normal ventilation. However, in some cases, the clinical course is longer. Approximately 20 per cent of the infants develop persistent wheezing and hyperinflation of the lungs with abnormal gas exchange that may last for many months (Wohl, 1983). Abnormalities in respiratory function have been found in some children many years after an infection of the bronchioles. Also, there is a high incidence of asthma in children who have had bronchiolitis in infancy. It is unclear whether damage to the lungs from bronchiolitis predisposes these infants to asthma or whether the diagnosis of bronchiolitis was made when the first attacks of asthma were experienced.

Nursing Strategies for Follow-Up Care in the Home or Clinic

Plot height and weight on the growth curve to assess for overall adequacy of oxygenation.

Assess breath sounds for evidence of persistent crackles and/or wheezing.

Ask the parent whether the child's energy level has returned to normal or whether she or he continues to tire easily.

Determine whether feeding problems exist that may be linked to persistent nasal congestion or lethargy.

Emphasize the need for regular follow-up care and the need for medical intervention with recurrence of respiratory signs and symptoms.

Bronchitis

Bronchitis is a term that is inconsistently used to describe conditions in which the primary symptom is a cough. Chronic bronchitis is usually associated with an underlying disease and rarely exists as an isolated entity. This discussion is limited to acute bronchitis, a condition that can be transient or recurrent.

Acute bronchitis is an inflammatory process involving the lower trachea and upper bronchi. The terms *tracheobronchitis* and *bronchitis* are not clearly differentiated in the literature. In this discussion acute bronchitis is used, recognizing that bronchitis is usually accompanied by some degree of tracheitis.

Incidence and Etiology

Acute bronchitis affects children primarily during the first 4 years of life and is more common in boys (Loughlin, 1983). Attacks occur most commonly during the winter months, the peak season for respiratory viral illnesses. Acute bronchitis is usually associated with an upper respiratory tract infection of viral origin, most commonly rhinovirus. It can also be associated with pertussis, rubeola, diphtheria, influenza, scarlet fever, and pneumonia. Factors that may contribute to a child's susceptibility include allergy, environmental factors (climate, cigarette smoke, air pollution), and chronic upper respiratory infections (Stern, 1983). In some children with frequent or recurring bronchitis for whom an underlying cause is not established, it has been suggested that susceptibility may be genetically determined (Mellis, 1979).

Clinical Manifestations and Diagnostic Assessment

Acute bronchitis is usually preceded by a viral upper respiratory infection. After 3 to 4 days of common cold symptoms, the child is seen with a persistent, nonproductive, hacking cough that becomes loose and productive in a few days. The child is usually afebrile or may have a low-grade fever. As the illness progresses, coarse and fine crackles can be heard on auscultation. The cough usually subsides in 7 to 10 days unless it is a symptom of an underlying problem. Malaise may extend for a week or more after the cough has subsided.

Therapeutic Management

Most children do not require therapy and recover with palliative treatment. Cough suppressants are generally

Box 38-5
Causes of Chronic or Recurrent Cough According to Age

INFANCY (under 1 year of age)
Congenital malformations (e.g., tracheoesophageal fistula)
Infections [viral, bacterial (pertussis), chlamydial]
Aspiration (milk, gastric contents)
Asthma
Cystic fibrosis

TODDLER AND PRESCHOOLER
Aspirated foreign body
Infections (tonsillar and adenoid hypertrophy, bronchiectasis, pneumonia)
Asthma
Cystic fibrosis

SCHOOL-AGE TO ADOLESCENT
Cigarette smoking
Mycoplasma pneumonia
Asthma
Cystic fibrosis
Psychogenic cough
Sinusitis
Nasopharyngitis (postnasal drip)

(Adapted from Mellis, 1979; Eigen, 1982.)

avoided but may be used in severe cases when sleep is interrupted by cough. Antihistamines cause drying of secretions and are not recommended; the efficacy of expectorants is doubtful. Antibiotics should be reserved for conditions in which a bacterial organism is identified. There is some support for a trial of theophylline for those children with severe symptoms that disturb sleep and interfere with exercise and performance in school (Loughlin, 1983).

If the cough persists beyond 10 days, secondary bacterial infection or a complication such as pneumonia or atelectasis should be considered. A chest radiograph and sputum examination may be required for confirmation. Children with recurrent or chronic cough should be evaluated for an underlying cause (Box 38-5). Viral infections at the various levels of the respiratory tract are summarized in Table 38-15.

Strategies for Nursing Care

Maintenance of adequate fluid intake to liquefy secretions, humidification of inspired air, and chest physiotherapy help remove secretions. Adequate rest and avoidance of cigarette smoke are encouraged. If the child is afebrile, moderate activity helps free the secretions from the bronchial tree. General principles of care are provided in Table 38-5, Nursing Process Plan: The Child with Respiratory Tract Dysfunction.

Pneumonia

Pathophysiology

Pneumonia is a term to describe the presence of an acute inflammation of the lung parenchyma (tissue), including the smallest airways and alveoli. The lungs are involved in varying degrees, depending on the type of organism and the severity of the infection. The various forms of pneumonia are:

- Lobar—consolidation of all or part of a lobe or several lobes of the lung: exudate is chiefly within the alveoli. Bilateral involvement may occur (also called double pneumonia),
- Disseminated lobular—a patchy distribution of infectious areas in both lung fields, surrounding and involving the bronchi,
- Interstitial—a diffuse bronchiolitis and peribronchiolitis in both lung fields; inflammation is confined to the alveolar walls and the peribronchial and interlobular tissues.

Bronchopneumonia is a loose term used to describe a combination of disseminated lobular and interstitial pneumonia (Gordon, 1974). Lobar and lobular involvement are characteristic of bacterial pneumonia, whereas viral pneumonia is characterized by an interstitial inflammation.

Etiology

Pneumonia is most commonly caused by a virus or bacteria (see Tables 38-15 and 38-16), *Mycoplasma* (mycoplasma pneumonia), and in recent years *Chlamydia*, a bacteria-like organism. Certain causative organisms are more prevalent in certain age groups than others. Also, the same organism can result in varied clinical responses, depending on the age and general health of the child. The neonate and young infant are particularly vulnerable to serious consequences from pneumonia.

Pneumonia seen in infants and children can be acquired before birth, during birth, or after birth. Pneumonia acquired during birth (perinatal) is thought to be due to aspiration of infected amniotic fluid or secretions from the birth canal. Common organisms

Table 38-15. Viral Infections of the Lower Respiratory Tract*

Bronchitis† and Tracheobronchitis	Bronchiolitis	Viral Pneumonia
Definition		
Infection of upper bronchi and lower trachea	Inflammation of bronchioles	Inflammation of lung parenchyma
Organism		
Usually viral agents (paramyxovirus, respiratory syncytial virus, and adenovirus)	Respiratory syncytial virus (RSV); adenovirus (rarely)	Respiratory syncytial virus, parainfluenza and adenoviruses
Age		
Occurs most frequently during the first 4 years of life	Peak incidence at 6 months of age. Rarely occurs after 2 years of age	Can occur in any age group; most of the pneumonia caused by RSV occurs in the first 3 years of life
Onset		
Usually preceded by a viral upper respiratory infection, but it can also follow illnesses such as croup or pneumonia	Begins as a mild upper respiratory infection	Insidious or acute symptoms usually precede pulmonary illness
Clinical Manifestations		
Persistent nonproductive, hacking cough that becomes loose and productive in a few days; rhonchi and rales can be heard as illness progresses; cough subsides in 7–10 days	Tachypnea, chest retractions, and a paroxysmal wheezy cough; patient may be irritable, dyspneic, and have prolonged expirations. Rhonchi, wheezes, or rales throughout lungs. Diminished breath sound where obstructed. X-ray films show diffuse hyperinflation of lungs and peribronchial infiltrates suggestive of interstitial pneumonia. Scattered areas of consolidation are due to atelectasis or inflammation of alveoli	Cough, wheezing, coarse rhonchi, and frequently a high fever. Headache, malaise, and myalgia are present in older children
Treatment		
Cough suppression by medication is generally avoided (sometimes given in severe cases when sleep is interrupted by cough). Expectorants can be given. Mask inhalations of nebulized solutions and chest physiotherapy help raise secretions. Humidification of inspired air must produce small droplets to be effective. Hydration by increased oral fluids or intravenous fluids	Treated with rest, fluids, and humidified oxygen. Bronchodilators, sedatives, and corticosteroids not recommended. Antibiotics usually not indicated. Intravenous fluids for hydration, electrolytes, and pH balance are often necessary. Mist therapy delivering large droplets does not affect lower airway; therefore, ultrasonic nebulization is recommended	Symptomatic treatment. Antibiotics not used. Bed rest, analgesics, and antipyretics with adequate fluid intake and increased humidity. In severe illness, postural drainage and oxygen may be indicated. Ventilator assistance may be required
Nursing Considerations		
Counsel family against use of over-the-counter drugs to suppress cough; a vaporizer that produces a sufficiently small droplet is recommended	Most critical phase is the first 48–72 hrs. RSV highly contagious—isolate from other infants. Infant needs to be observed closely. Parent-infant contact extremely important because of infant's anxiety. Stress of parents must be reduced by frequent explanations of status of infant	RSV highly contagious—isolate from other infants

continued

Table 38-15 *(continued)*

Bronchitis† and Tracheobronchitis	Bronchiolitis	Viral Pneumonia
Complications and/or Prognosis		
Complications of otitis media, sinusitis, and pneumonia may occur in children who are undernourished or in poor health	Most improve within 3–4 days and in 2 weeks respiratory rate is normal, but in some instances illness is prolonged	Most recover in 7–10 days. Otitis media is common in children with RSV infections. Adenovirus can cause severe and fatal pneumonia in infants. There is some evidence that chronic lung disease in adulthood may be caused by viral pneumonia in childhood

* Also see Table 38-13 for Acute Laryngotracheobronchitis, which is a viral disease.
† Bronchitis is usually accompanied by some degree of tracheitis.

transferred are *Escherichia coli*, *Klebsiella*, group B beta-hemolytic streptococcus, herpes, and *Chlamydia*. Sources of infection of pneumonia acquired after birth (postnatal) include human contact and contaminated equipment (staphylococcal infections). See Table 38-15 for a summary of viral pneumonias and Table 38-16 for the various bacterial pneumonias.

Clinical Manifestations

Pneumonia during the neonatal period is predominantly bacterial in origin. Perinatal and postnatal infections are usually manifested by nonspecific signs of illness. Initially an infant has signs such as poor feeding, lethargy, and fever. Respiratory distress may develop at the onset of the illness or sometime later. When the pneumonia is acquired perinatally, illness manifests itself during the first several days of life, whereas pneumonia acquired after birth manifests itself during the first month of life (Klein and Mavey, 1976).

After the neonatal period, pneumonia in infants and children is predominantly of viral origin (see Table 38-15 for a summary of viral pneumonias). Although the majority of patients recover without sequelae, viral pneumonia cannot be viewed as a benign illness. Adenovirus can cause a particularly serious illness with potential fatality. Many infants and children can be treated at home, but severely ill patients should be hospitalized for intravenous fluids, oxygen, or in some cases ventilator assistance.

Bacterial pneumonia is often preceded by a viral respiratory disease. The lower respiratory tract is made more susceptible to bacterial pneumonia in the presence of a viral respiratory disease in the following ways: (1) secretions are increased, therefore aspiration of bacteria-laden fluid is more probable; (2) there may be temporary disruption of the ciliary activity, causing less efficient clearing of bacteria from the respiratory tract; (3) phagocytosis and bactericidal activity of alveolar macrophages may be decreased; and (4) the immune response may be reduced (Smith, 1983) (see Table 38-16 for a summary of various bacteria-caused pneumonias.)

Diagnostic Assesesment

Radiography. Chest films have limitations in their usefulness in establishing a diagnosis; they establish the location of involvement but do not verify etiology. However, certain findings are suggestive of specific organisms. For example, pleural effusion signifies a bacterial pneumonia, and the presence of empyema early in the illness is suggestive of pneumonia due to *Haemophilus influenzae* or staphylococcus (Eichenwald, 1976). Consolidation of a lobe or segment is suggestive of pneumococcal pneumonia. Consolidation is also seen in pneumonia caused by *Klebsiella*, but pneumococcal infections occur more frequently (Eichenwald, 1976).

White Blood Count. White blood counts are variable. In viral pneumonia the white blood cell (WBC) count is usually less than 20,000 per mm^3 or 20×10^9 cells/L. Bacterial pneumonia is generally associated with more extreme WBC elevations and the presence of many immature cells. The elevated WBC count is due primarily to an increase of polymorphonuclear cells. In severe illness, leukopenia may occur. Leukopenia, a poor prognostic sign, occurs when white cells leave the circulation faster than they are being produced by the bone marrow. (See Chapters 40 and 45 for further discussion of white blood cell counts during infection.)

Approaches to identify the causative organism in pneumonia include cultures and Gram stains of secretions in the posterior pharynx and of the blood, tests to detect bacterial antigen, and, when indicated, lung punctures. Throat cultures have been found not to correlate well with blood cultures and autopsy findings. Countercurrent immunoelectrophoresis (CIE) and

***Table* 38-16.** Bacterial Pneumonias Most Common in Infants and Children

Streptococcal*	Streptococcal (Group A)	Staphylococcal†	Pneumococcal‡	*Haemophilus Influenzae*‡
Organism				
Group B beta-hemolytic streptococcus	Group A beta-hemolytic streptococcus	*Staphylococcus aureus*	*Streptococcus pneumoniae*	*Haemophilus influenzae type B*
Age				
Occurs in neonates less than 5 days old (early onset) as an intrapartum infection or in infants up to 6 weeks of age (late onset). In early onset pneumonia is more common; in late onset meningitis predominates	Occurs most commonly in children 5–6 years of age through young adulthood	Occurs in infants more frequently than in older children. 30 per cent of patients under 3 months of age; 70 per cent under 1 year	Children under 4 years have a higher incidence. Children under 3 years with sickle cell disease have an attack rate of 20 per cent	Most frequent in children under 1 year. Gram-negative organisms account for only a small percentage of pneumonia in infants and children (after the neonatal period) but they are becoming increasingly prevalent
Onset				
History of prolonged rupture of membranes and low birth weight	Onset is extremely variable. Frequently associated with rubeola, varicella, or scarlet fever	History of mild upper respiratory infection (varies in duration from a few days to a week or sometimes longer)	In infants onset is abrupt, with a temperature of 39.5–40.6°C (103–105°F) and generalized convulsions; sometimes vomiting and diarrhea	Similar to pneumococcal but often with a more insidious onset. Most are preceded by a mild upper respiratory infection
Clinical Findings				
Apnea and shock within 24 hours of birth; hypoxia and hypercapnia. Pulmonary lesions may be patchy or extensive. Difficult to differentiate from respiratory distress syndrome of newborn	May be sudden with fever, chills, and pleuritic pain or may present with mild illness (low-grade fever and cough). Leukocytosis, increased ASO titer, diffuse bronchopneumonia and pleural effusion may be present. Pleural tap required for identification of organism	Extremely variable. Usually cough, high fever, abdominal distention, rapid grunting respirations. In more severe cases cyanosis and shock may occur. Chest auscultation may be misleading. In infants breath sound may be heard even with serious pneumonia. Progresses from a bronchopneumonia to consolidation of an entire lobe within hours. Pneumatocele, empyema, and pyopneumothorax are common	Rapid, shallow respirations with grunting, tachycardia, and circumoral cyanosis. Cough not usual. Abdominal distention and nuchal rigidity. Auscultatory findings not reliable. Patchy bronchopneumonia is most typical in infants. Lobar consolidation more common in older children	Cough almost always present (can be productive or nonproductive). Rales, fever, tachypnea, retractions, and nasal flaring; dullness to percussion. Can be either lobar or disseminated (bronchopneumonia). Empyema is often present. Pneumatoceles have been seen (difficult to differentiate from pneumococcal)
Treatment				
Penicillin G and intensive supportive therapy	Penicillin G (100,000 U/kg/24 hr). Initial dose is given parenterally followed by a 2–3 week course of oral administration. Erythromycin, clindamycin and cephalosporins are used in the event of a penicillin allergy	A penicillinase-resistant penicillin (methicillin) is used. If organism sensitive to penicillin G then methicillin is not used because of its nephrotoxicity. (Methicillin-resistant strains have also been reported.) Chest tube drainage of fluid or pus from pleural cavity. Blood transfusions for anemia may be necessary. Supportive therapy	Penicillin G is usual. Ampicillin is used for young children because it is effective for both pneumococcal and *H. influenzae*. If pneumonia is complicated by otitis media, medication is prescribed for a longer period than the usual course	Ampicillin and chloramphenicol. Ampicillin is required in large doses. Ampicillin-resistant strains occur; therefore, simultaneous chloramphenicol therapy is recommended

continued

Table 38-16 *(continued)*

Streptococcal*	Streptococcal (Group A)	Staphylococcal†	Pneumococcal‡	*Haemophilus Influenzae*‡
Specific Nursing Concerns				
Avoid inaccurate encouraging remarks about an illness with an extremely high mortality rate. These neonates are seriously ill; the mother is likely to be hospitalized in the obstetric department. Nurse caring for infant should facilitate communication with both parents	Compliance by family in administering full course of antibiotics. Early and vigorous chest physical therapy may be required to prevent complications	Nephrotoxicity of methicillin. Observe infection control procedure strictly. (Handwashing, gown and mask are required.) Long duration of hospitalization places entire family under severe stress	A pneumococcal vaccine is available that is recommended for persons 2 years of age or older who are especially vulnerable to high morbidity and mortality from pneumococcal infections	Observe for chloramphenicol side effects
Complications and/or Prognosis				
Mortality rate is 60–90 per cent	Bacteremia in 10 per cent. Empyema and septic foci (bones or joints)	Septic lesions outside the respiratory tract. Mortality rate is 10–30 per cent	Meningitis, otitis media, sinusitis, and purulent conjunctivitis. Empyema and pneumatoceles may develop. Mortality rate below 1 per cent	Frequent complications include bacteremia, pericarditis, cellulitis, empyema, meningitis, and pyarthrosis

* Since the early 1970s, the incidence of Group B beta-hemolytic streptococcus has increased as a cause of mortality and serious morbidity in neonates.

† Staphylococcal pneumonia has decreased in recent years.

‡ Beyond the neonatal period, pneumococcal and *H. influenzae* are by far the most common.

latex particle agglutination (LPA) are used on serum, urine, pleural fluid, and spinal fluid to detect specific bacterial antigens. The severity of the illness is suggested by the amount of antigen present, with an increased amount present in more severe illness. These tests are particularly useful in cases when no clinical response is obtained from the usual course of antibiotics. Lung punctures are recommended in some cases when immediate diagnosis is essential for prompt therapy (Smith, 1983).

In addition to radiographs, white blood counts with differential, and various cultures, the physician takes into account the child's age, the clinical manifestations, and existence of an epidemic in establishing a diagnosis.

Therapeutic Management

Medical treatment for pneumonia, as for many of the respiratory diseases, focuses upon improving oxygenation and preventing dehydration. For the child hospitalized with pneumonia, the physician usually will order oxygen as well as ultrasonic mist, and chest physical therapy. Antipyretics may be needed to control fever and intravenous hydration is usually instituted.

If the pneumonia is of bacterial origin, intravenous antibiotics will be used. Antibiotic regimens (types and dosage) change rapidly as resistant strains of organisms emerge. The physician's medication order will be based upon the most potent available antibiotic for the identified organism, with considerations for cost per dose, number of doses needed per day, and severity of potential side effects. (See Tables 38-14 and 38-15.)

In the event of fluid accumulation in the pleural cavity, drainage is accomplished either by continuous drainage by chest tube or numerous thoracenteses. Fluid accumulation is most common when pneumonia is caused by *Staphylococcus aureus.* Pain medications may be ordered on a prn basis to control the discomfort of invasive drainage procedures.

Major Nursing Diagnoses for Pneumonia*

Impaired gas exchange, *related to acute inflammation of lung parenchyma*
Ineffective airway clearance, *related to increased mucous production associated with the infectious process in the lungs*
Potential hyperthermia, *related to the infectious process*

*To be used with Table 35-5, Nursing Process Plan: The Child with Respiratory Tract Dysfunction.

Potential fluid volume deficit, related to:
- *fever*
- *increased insensible water loss associated with tachypnea*
- *decreased fluid intake associated with dyspnea*

Potential ineffective family coping, related to:
- *anxiety associated with the child's respiratory distress*
- *anxiety associated with treatment measures that are perceived as stressful for the child*
- *disruption in usual physical interactions associated with oxygen and intravenous therapy*

Potential altered comfort: pain, related to:
- *inflamed lung tissue*
- *invasive procedures to drain the pleural cavity*

Strategies for Nursing Care

Promoting Adequate Oxygenation. Various assessments and interventions are directed at assessing and promoting oxygenation.

Vital signs are checked frequently (initially every 2 hours); in serious illness, respiratory and cardiac monitors should be used. When assessing vital signs, the nurse checks the child's color, respirations, and breath sounds and observes for retractions, nasal flaring, and restlessness. When oxygen is administered via an Isolette, oxygen hood, tent, mask, or cannula, its concentration is measured by an oxygen analyzer.

Changing the child's position every 2 hours facilitates pulmonary drainage, helps prevent skin breakdown, and provides comfort. Respirations are generally eased by placing the child in a semi-Fowler position with the neck slightly hyperextended. Raising the head of the mattress 30 degrees and placing a small folded blanket or towel under the shoulders straightens the airway and facilitates respiration. Older children assume a position of comfort. Suction should be available whenever secretions are not being handled effectively by the child's respiratory system.

Promoting Clearance of Secretions. Clearance of secretions is accomplished through a combination of mist therapy and chest physiotherapy which loosens and removes secretions from the respiratory tract. Ultrasonic nebulizers are capable of producing a dense mist of the small particles that are more likely to reach the lower respiratory tract than are the large particles produced by a mist tent. Percussion, vibration, and postural drainage are usually done every 4 to 6 hours; times vary with the severity of the pneumonia and tolerance of the child. Chest radiograph reports can be used by the nurse to identify the lobes that need particular emphasis when chest physiotherapy is performed.

Parents should be taught to do percussion and postural drainage when their child is hospitalized. They should be given the opportunity to participate in the treatment and should be able to demonstrate the entire procedure at least once before their child is discharged. (See page 1189 for discussion of Chest Physical Therapy.)

Controlling Hyperthermia. Fever is closely monitored and treated to prevent convulsions. Antipyretics, fluids, and a cool mist environment are provided to reduce fever. A sponge bath with tepid water is recommended by some physicians for a rectal temperature of 39.4°C (103°F), although extended cooling is controversial. Cool mist moistens the airway and helps reduce fever, but chilling must be avoided. Acetaminophen (Tylenol) is prescribed to control fever and make the child more comfortable.

Promoting Adequate Hydration. The nurse also assesses for dehydration that is caused by high fever, insensible water loss from tachypnea, and poor fluid intake due to dyspnea. The nurse should monitor intake and output, check specific gravity of urine, and make ongoing assessments of hydration status. An elevated specific gravity indicates dehydration. Oral fluids are encouraged, but intravenous fluid therapy may be indicated when intake is poor. Infants in particular have difficulty maintaining an adequate intake because of dyspnea while sucking.

Promoting Adaptive Family Coping. The nurse should also respond to the stresses that parents experience because of the nature of the illness. The need for oxygen, mist, chest physiotherapy, intravenous fluids, and antibiotics is distressing to parents, especially when it interferes with their ability to hold their child. When a child can tolerate brief periods out of the oxygen tent or Isolette, the nurse can show parents how to properly handle the child to prevent intravenous infiltration or dislodgement. Parents should also be shown how to support and cradle an infant while feeding the child inside a tent. Providing for child-parent contact during all phases of the illness helps parents feel prepared to take their child home after discharge.

Before discharge the nurse should discuss the use of antipyretics, antibiotic administration and side effects, percussion and postural drainage, and signs of respiratory distress. A discussion of adequate fluids, rest, and diet for age will help parents take preventive measures in maintaining the health of their child.

Providing Optimal Comfort and Pain Relief. The nurse must be aware that inflammation of lung tissue often results in pain with the normal effort of breathing. Careful assessment is indicated to determine whether an analgesic should be administered. If pain is suspected and the physician has not ordered an analgesic, the nurse, in the advocate role, should request such an order.

An analgesic will almost always be warranted for relief of the discomfort associated with chest tubes and thoracentesis. The child in greatest comfort is more likely to obtain the rest needed for healing of infected tissues. Nonpharmacologic comfort measures can provide an effective adjunct to analgesic therapy. (See Chapter 29 for a complete discussion of pain control in children.)

Nursing Strategies for Follow-Up Care in the Home or Clinic

Assess vital signs and breath sounds for evidence of residual effects of pneumonia.

When applicable, determine whether the entire course of oral antibiotics was administered after hospital discharge.

Ask the child whether chest discomfort has subsided.

Inspect wounds from chest tubes/thoracentesis for signs of infection.

Encourage the child and parent to discuss questions pertaining to resumption of normal activity and measures to prevent recurrence.

Chlamydial Pneumonia

Chlamydia trachomatis is being implicated in an increasing spectrum of diseases affecting children and adolescents. It is the most common cause of ophthalmia neonatorum and is an important cause of pneumonia in infants in the first 3 months of life (Hammerschlag, 1981; Rettig, 1984). There is increasing evidence that *C. trachomatis* is the most prevalent sexually transmitted pathogen in adolescents (Fraser, 1983; Shafer, 1984). See Chapter 45 for a discussion of *Chlamydia* causing a sexually transmitted disease.

Incidence

The organism, present in the genitalia of males and females, causes urethritis in males and cervicitis in females. About 50 per cent of infants delivered vaginally to mothers infected with *C. trachomatis* acquire the infection. Conjunctivitis and pneumonia are the only illnesses of infancy that have been identified as associated with *C. trachomatis* infection (Beem et al, 1983). Not until 1975 was chlamydia reported as a cause of pneumonia in infants (Schachter et al, 1975). Our discussion focuses on the respiratory presentation of chlamydial infection in this age group.

Pathophysiology

Once thought to be viruses, chlamydiae are now recognized as having the characteristics of gram-negative bacteria. The organisms are intracellular parasites utilizing the nutrients of the cell. The life cycle of the organism includes an extracellular and an intracellular phase. The infectious particle (elementary body) attaches to the wall of the host cell, develops into a reproductive form (reticulate body), and eventually forms the characteristic cytoplasmic inclusion body (a compact, rigid, glycogen-like substance) of chlamydia. This substance displaces the host cell nucleus, leading to cell death. The entire cycle requires 48 hours after infection (Hammerschlag, 1981).

Etiology and Prevention

Chlamydial infection is transmitted through sexual contact from one adult to another and from infected mothers to infants during a vaginal birth. The eyes or nasopharynx serve as the portal of entry during birth, although rectal and genital shedding of the organism has also been reported in some infants (Schachter, 1979). Chlamydial conjunctivitis does not commonly extend to the respiratory tract, and not all infants who have nasopharyngeal (NP) infection develop pneumonia. A summary of epidemiologic studies shows that, of infants born to infected mothers, 30 to 40 per cent are likely to develop conjunctivitis; 10 to 20 per cent, pneumonia; and 20 per cent, asymptomatic NP infection (Hammerschlag, 1981). Since neonatal chlamydial infection is acquired perinatally, prevention aims at identification and treatment of sexually transmitted diseases in the adolescent and adult population (see Chapter 45).

Clinical Manifestations and Diagnostic Assessment

Chlamydial pneumonia is characterized by a gradual onset of upper respiratory tract signs in infants between 4 and 12 weeks of age. Nasal obstruction, with or without discharge, a gradually worsening cough, and tachypnea (40 to 80/min) are the predominant respiratory signs. The cough can become paroxysmal and cause vomiting and cyanosis. With lack of fever and only minor complaints of poor weight gain and malaise, the condition may exist for days or weeks before pneumonia is considered the cause. Conjunctivitis is present in about 50 per cent of infants with chlamydial pneumonia and usually occurs at 3 days to 3 weeks of age.

On auscultation, breath sounds are heard throughout the chest; crackles may be heard, but wheezing is uncommon. Chest radiographs show hyperexpansion of the lungs, with diffuse interstitial infiltrates. Because air exchange is good throughout the chest, careful assessment is required to identify the abnormalities. The absence of fever in combination with an abnormal chest film and crackles should raise one's suspicion of a chlamydial infection.

Pneumonia may be caused by various agents, therefore specific laboratory findings are essential to differentiate chlamydial infections from others. Isolation of the organism from the nasopharynx can be accomplished by aspirating secretions through a small feeding tube or by using a wire nasopharyngeal swab. A specimen from the conjunctiva should be obtained with a dry swab by rubbing firmly across the lower and upper tarsal conjunctivas. Although normal eosinophilic values are found in some patients, levels of more than 300 cells per mm^3 (300×10^6 cells/L) have been reported in these infants (Hammerschlag, 1981; Beem, 1983). Serum immunoglobulins IgM and IgG are usually elevated.

Although tissue culture is the definitive test, antigen antibody reaction tests such as ELISA (enzyme-linked immunosorbent assay) are less expensive and are processed more quickly (Marvin and Slevin, 1987).

Therapeutic Management

The most important element in treatment of chlamydial pneumonia is the administration of a systemic antibiotic. The recommended drugs are erythromycin (40 mg/kg/24 hr) or sulfisoxazole (150 mg/kg/24 hr) for a duration of 3 weeks. Although the infection may resolve without therapy, symptoms of cough, tachypnea, and weight loss may continue for as long as 2 months; with treatment, improvement is noted in 5 to 7 days.

Infants with chlamydial pneumonia can usually be treated at home, but for those infants who have respiratory distress and coughing spells that interfere with eating and sleeping, hospitalization may be appropriate. Apnea associated with coughing is particularly frightening to parents; therefore, an initial stabilization with apnea monitoring and supportive therapy in the hospital may be warranted. Coughing episodes can be diminished by supportive measures like physical therapy and suctioning. In serious cases, supplemental oxygen and parenteral fluids may be required.

Strategies for Nursing Care

The nurse facilitates the medical diagnosis by documenting the clinical findings. Chest assessments, eye assessment, documentation of lethargy, poor feeding, and paroxysmal cough are significant data. Proper handling of specimens is also important. Once obtained for culture, they should be transported immediately.

The nursing plan of care will be very similar to that discussed for acute viral and bacterial pneumonia and will draw upon the strategies detailed in Table 38-5.

Because improvement occurs in 5 to 7 days, parents may presume it is unnecessary to continue administering medication. Infants who are not adequately treated have been found to relapse, therefore it is important to advise parents of this and encourage them to administer the medication for the prescribed period of time.

The nurse's support of the infant and family varies according to the severity and stage of illness. During the frightening episodes of coughing and possible apnea, the nurse should remain with the infant and provide explanations and reassurance to the parents. Improvement will be noted in 5 to 7 days, and in 2 weeks the infant is usually asymptomatic and normal on physical examination.

Follow-up care is required for treatment of the mother and prevention of future cases of chlamydial infection (see Chapter 45).

Mycoplasma Pneumonia (Primary Atypical Pneumonia)

Incidence and Etiology

Mycoplasma pneumoniae is the organism causing the primary atypical pneumonia most commonly seen in school-age children. It is also an important cause of other types of respiratory illness in childhood, and it may affect other organ systems. Until 1960, *M. pneumoniae* was thought to be a virus, but it is now known to be a mycoplasm and is thought to be more like a bacteria than a virus. *M. pneumoniae* does not have a cell wall and is sensitive to certain antibiotics but resistant to penicillin (penicillin acts on the cell wall of an organism). Although it occurs predominantly in children 5 to 15 years of age, younger children are also infected but are not usually ill (Denny, 1983).

Epidemics of mycoplasmal pneumonia are long-lasting compared with the acute, short-lived nature of pneumonias caused by viral agents. Other family members frequently become ill after one member has been infected but not until weeks or months later. The incubation period is approximately 3 weeks, but varies. Over 50 per cent of infected children shed organisms (i.e., are communicable) for 4 to 6 weeks (Welliver and Wong, 1983).

Clinical Manifestations

Based on only clinical manifestations, a mycoplasmal pneumonia is difficult to differentiate from other pneumonias. The onset is usually gradual, with fever, headache, malaise, myalgia, cough, and sore throat.

The cough can increase in severity, taking on a hacking, paroxysmal nature, and is sometimes productive with blood-tinged sputum. These symptoms often indicate a very ill child, but a physical assessment may reveal only a reddened pharynx and slightly enlarged lymph nodes. Later in the illness, fine crackles are common, and chest radiography reveals interstitial pneumonia involving one or more of the lower lobes. The white blood cell count is usually normal.

Diagnostic Assessment

A diagnosis of mycoplasmal pneumonia is suspected when the symptoms occur in a school age child, especially with a worsening cough. Erythrocyte sedimentation rate (ESR) is usually elevated. The presence of cold hemagglutinins (greater than 1:64) supports the diagnosis, but these also develop when pneumonia is caused by other agents. Definitive diagnosis is based on isolation of the organism, or demonstration of a rise in titer of specific antibodies. The striking feature is the "relatively mild" clinical illness compared with the abnormalities on chest radiograph.

Therapeutic Management

The child can be made to feel more comfortable during the acute phase by supportive, symptomatic treatment. A school-age child will need to be encouraged to avoid strenuous activity and take adequate fluids. Humidity and postural drainage may be required to clear the secretions. Cough suppression by medication should be avoided. Fever over 38°C is treated and quiet activities are encouraged until the cough and myalgia subside. Erythromycin (50 mg/kg/24 hr in four daily doses for 7 days) is recommended for children younger than 9 years of age and tetracycline (25 to 50 mg/kg/24 hr in four doses) for children above 9 years of age.

Children with mycoplasmal pneumonia recover without complications, but there have been reports of fatalities. It has been suggested that this organism could possibly have some part in the development of chronic lung disease (Denny, 1983). The development of a vaccine against *M. pneumoniae* is not thought to be imminent in view of the incomplete understanding of the pathogenesis of the illness (Welliver and Wong, 1983).

Strategies for Nursing Care

For nursing strategies, see those preceding for Pneumonia and Chlamydial Pneumonia and Table 38-5, Nursing Process Plan: The Child with Respiratory Tract Dysfunction.

Chronic Alterations Affecting Respiratory Function

Asthma*

Asthma is a chronic pulmonary disease resulting from a wide variety of stimuli (pollen, dust, viruses), causing increased irritability of the tracheobronchial tree with varying degrees of airway obstruction. The condition is usually reversible either spontaneously or following therapy (Sly, 1985). Approximately 8 million children (12 per cent) in the United States experience at least one attack of bronchospasm in their lifetime; 5 per cent of children in the United States suffer from chronic asthma (Zieger, 1983; Friedman, 1984).

Asthma, also termed *reactive airway disease* (RAD), is most common in children, with onset usually before 3 years of age. During childhood, boys experience asthma more frequently than girls. Age is believed to affect the course of asthma. Young children (infants, toddlers, preschoolers), in comparison with adults, have anatomic and physiologic airway differences (see Table 38-1). Among these differences are smaller airways and compromised collateral ventilation. This makes young children more vulnerable to airway obstruction and makes the asthmatic attack more dangerous. Children may have severe symptoms, with acute attack symptoms progressing more rapidly and leading more often to respiratory failure. It is estimated that respiratory failure leads to death in 1 to 2 per cent of children with asthma. Pediatric deaths have occurred prior to therapy, during therapy, and from treatment complications (Friedman, 1984). This emphasizes the child's fragile respiratory state during acute episodes.

Etiology

Asthma is characterized by an extreme reaction of the trachea and bronchial tissues to chemicals released by the body in response to allergens, psychologic or physiologic stress, or infection. It is important to note that an asthmatic reaction occurs in some individuals in response to allergens but that in others allergic factors play little if any role.

Even when allergy is present, it rarely is the only important factor (Pearlman and Bierman, 1988). There is often, however, a family history of allergy when a child is diagnosed with asthma. Chapter 43 describes in detail the allergic response. As identified by Pearlman and Bierman (1988), the following factors can precipitate or aggravate an asthmatic episode:

*We appreciate the authorship of this section on asthma by Margaret Crandall.

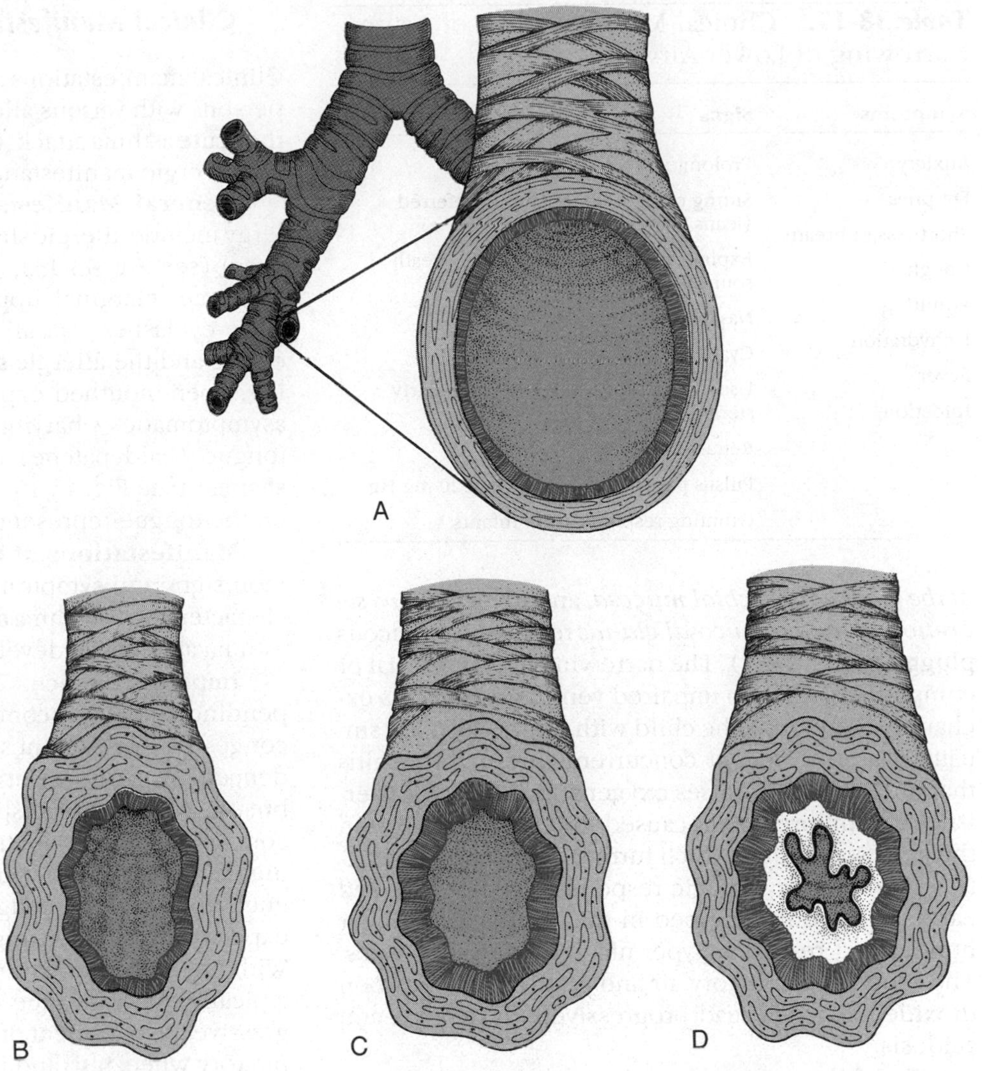

***Figure* 38-14.** Bronchial changes that decrease size of air passageway occur during an asthma attack. The narrowed bronchi increase airway resistance to the flow of inspired and expired air. *A*, Cross-section of a normal bronchus, with mucous membrane shown in color. *B*, Bronchospasm. The smooth muscle surrounding the bronchus contracts, causing narrowing of the airway. *C*, Edema of the mucous membrane further narrows the airway. *D*, Increased mucus secretion by the submucosal glands.

- *allergens,* including foods, animal allergens, mold spores, pollens, insects, infesting agents, and drugs
- *irritants,* including paint odors, hair sprays, perfumes, chemicals, air pollutants, active and passive cigarette smoke (also cigar and pipe smoke), cold air, cold water, coughing, and positive ions
- *weather changes* (atmospheric changes)
- *infections,* especially viral respiratory
- *exercise* that is strenuous and associated with breathlessness
- *emotional factors;* however, there is no evidence that psychologic factors are the *basis* for asthma
- *gastroesophageal reflux,* which is considered to be a cause of nocturnal asthma
- *allergic rhinitis, sinusitis,* and *upper respiratory tract inflammation,* related to irritation of the upper respiratory tract
- *nonallergic hypersensitivity* to drugs and chemicals, such as aspirin and nonsteroidal anti-inflammatory drugs and tartrazine (yellow food dye number 5)
- *endocrine factors,* including the menstrual cycle, birth control pills, and hyperthyroidism
- *interaction* of various of the preceding factors

The term *extrinsic* asthma is sometimes used to denote an atopic or allergic cause. *Intrinsic* usually refers to nonallergic factors. Regardless of the cause, the result of asthmatic triggers is bronchoconstriction, or narrowing of the airways.

Pathophysiology

The airway narrowing characteristic of an asthma attack (Fig. 38-14) is caused by three mechanisms: (1) *the contraction of the airway's smooth muscle,* (2) *edema*

Table 38-17. Clinical Manifestations of Acute Narrowing of Lower Airway

Symptoms	Signs
Anxiety	Prolonged expiratory phase
Dyspnea	Sitting or standing position preferred (leans forward)
Shortness of breath	Expiratory wheezing or silent "breath sounds"
Cough	Nasal flaring
Vomiting	Cyanosis
Dehydration	Use of accessory muscles, particularly sternocleidomastoid
Fever	Retractions
Infection	Pulsus paradoxus greater than 20 mg Hg
	Grunting respirations in infants

of the tracheobronchial mucosa, and (3) *excessive secretion of the submucosal glands* resulting in mucous plugging (Sly, 1985). The narrowing may be partial or complete, leading to impaired ventilation and gas exchange. Frequently the child with asthma also has sinusitis, nasal polyps, or concurrent chronic bronchitis that further compromises oxygenation. The characteristic mouth breathing caused by nasal congestion thickens secretions, which further aggravates obstruction. If these physiologic responses are not reversed early, air becomes trapped in the alveoli, causing air hunger and resultant hyperinflation of these tissues. The blocked inspiratory air and poor oxygen–carbon dioxide exchange lead progressively to hypoxia and acidosis.

The child's major physiologic problems from the nurse's perspective are therefore:

- (1) *ineffective airway clearance* related to bronchospasm, mucosal edema, hypersecretion of mucus, and tenacious bronchial secretions; and
- (2) *impaired gas exchange* related to air trapping in the alveoli.

During the early stage, the hypoxemia and metabolic acidosis may be offset by the child's increased respiratory rate. The fright and the vagal stimulation created by air hunger further aggravate the bronchospasm, increasing the severity of symptoms even more. As the disease progresses, there is a combined respiratory and metabolic acidosis. The respiratory acidosis is due to increased carbon dioxide retention; the metabolic acidosis is a result of both decreased oxygen and poor nutritional intake causing anaerobic metabolism, ketosis, and build-up of metabolites. If left untreated, the child can develop respiratory failure leading to irreversible brain damage or even death.

Clinical Manifestations

Clinical manifestations are either general, common to persons with various allergic conditions, or specific to the acute asthma attack. (Chapter 43 elaborates on general allergic manifestations.)

General Manifestations. Signs of chronic allergy include allergic shiners (discoloration below the eyes) (see Fig. 43-13), cobblestoned and boggy conjunctivae, marginal upper eyelid eczema, and long silky eyelashes. Nasal signs are a transverse nasal crease and the allergic salute (see Fig. 43-14). A gaping, open-mouthed expression, gingival hyperplasia, asymptomatic pharyngeal hyperemia, geographic tongue (bald patches of oval, round, or snakelike shapes) (see Fig. 43-15), and elevated, pearly margins on the tongue represent oral signs.

Manifestations of the Acute Attack. The common signs and symptoms of acute airway obstruction characteristic of asthma are outlined in Table 38-17. An asthma attack may develop slowly or begin abruptly.

Impending Attack. Early manifestations of an impending attack are complaints by the child of chest congestion or tightness, exercise intolerance evidenced by early onset of fatigue and shortness of breath, and increased sputum production, usually accompanied by a productive, paroxysmal cough. Vomiting may occur in the young child because of the tendency to swallow coughed-up mucus rather than expectorate it. Wheezing often is absent at this stage. Without intervention these symptoms may resolve, but typically they continue over hours or days with progressive development of acute respiratory distress, expiratory wheezing, and hypoxemia.

Progressive Distress. Wheezing is usually worse at night, may be sudden or gradual, and is often preceded by rhinorrhea. The child's cough, although it may be nonproductive, may sound loose due to an increase in secretions. Signs and symptoms indicating progressive or increased severity of airway obstruction are sternocleidomastoid contraction (indicating increased expiratory effort), supraclavicular retractions (indicating increased inspiratory effort), audible prolonged expiratory wheezing, and pulsus paradoxus greater than 10 mm Hg (Lockey and Bukantz, 1987; Mansmann et al, 1988). Subclavicular and intercostal retractions are common, as are nasal flaring and grunting respirations. Pallor occurs as oxygen saturation drops and the child becomes increasingly restless.

Pulsus paradoxus reflects a diminished left ventricular stroke output, indicating increasing resistance to blood flow into the lungs (through the pulmonary artery) because of airway obstruction. Pulsus paradoxus of 20 mm Hg or greater suggests moderate-to-severe airway obstruction. Pulsus paradoxus is usually obtained by subtracting the systolic blood pressure on inspiration from that on expiration. This can be done with older children, but infants, toddlers, and younger children, when distressed, have very rapid respiratory rates that make this technique difficult, if not impossible. A modified technique is utilized for younger children; the values correlate with the technique previously described. This technique involves measuring the systolic blood pressure at two points. The systolic pulse is measured when it becomes regular and again at its highest initial point when it becomes irregular. The first value is subtracted from the second value: the result is the pulsus paradoxus value (Galant et al, 1978). If the previously described symptoms persist for more than 2 hours and are unresponsive to the acute management regimen, status asthmaticus must be considered. Status asthmaticus is unresolved respiratory distress; it is described later in this section.

The child experiencing an acute attack may become dehydrated. Dehydration may occur from vomiting, decreased fluid intake, and increased insensible water loss with tachypnea and the work of breathing (Mansmann et al, 1988). See p. 899 for a discussion of signs and symptoms of dehydration.

Anxiety is a common symptom for both child and family. The child's chest is "tight" because of bronchoconstriction and airway narrowing from edema and mucus. This results in a feeling of not being able to get enough air. In addition, the child and family may be in a strange clinic or hospital with unfamiliar staff and unknown and painful procedures. Anxiety may also be a side effect of the prescribed medication. Parental fear of their child dying and feelings of helplessness and guilt that somehow they could have prevented the attack enhance parental anxiety. When the parent is anxious, the child often becomes more anxious and the attack may become more severe.

Impending Respiratory Failure. A child can mistakenly be thought to be improving if the wheezing decreases or stops. This does not always mean improvement. Decreased adventitious breath sounds actually may indicate respiratory obstruction, fatigue, and respiratory failure, with the child minutes away from having an arrest. Infants frequently present wheezing, tachypnea, and intercostal retractions that can very rapidly progress to respiratory failure. Therefore frequent chest auscultation for *air exchange* is critical.

Diagnostic Assessment

History

Because of features in the history and physical examination that children with asthma usually share in common, diagnosis often is possible from these alone. The history often includes eczema (atopic dermatitis), recurrent bouts of bronchitis, pneumonia, and persistent coughing with colds, or perhaps merely a chronic chest rattle throughout infancy and early childhood. Symptoms during these episodes historically have shown improvement after treatment with adrenergic drugs. Symptoms are also typically more severe at night or during early morning hours, with noticeable improvement through the daytime.

Episodes of coughing or coughing spells accompanied by expiratory wheezing are often reported. These episodes may clear spontaneously after 5 to 7 days. Observant parents or the child may even be able to identify "triggers," or factors that precipitate these episodes. The child's input to the history should be solicited, because children often can identify factors that parents have overlooked or misunderstood from the child's behavior. Documentation of any known allergies should also be made, as well as any family history of asthma or other allergic disorders.

Physical Examination

The physical findings will depend on the child's age, severity and chronicity of the asthma, and the timing of the assessment. Physical parameters for growth retardation may reflect a decrease in both weight and height, resulting from diminished appetite, and chronic hypoxemia or obesity associated with the side effects of steroids. Physical growth increases once the asthma is successfully managed.

Blood pressure should be recorded as a baseline for comparison after drug therapy for asthma has been initiated. (Steroids and adrenergic agents may cause elevations.) Respirations should be evaluated for rate, prolonged expiration, dyspnea, retractions or nasal flaring, and use of accessory muscles (shoulders rise). Use of neck muscles to facilitate inspiration is also called "tracheal tugging" or "chin lag." Skin color and capillary return of the nailbeds should be documented. A round shoulder posture indicates alveolar hyperinflation. If hyperinflation is marked, the liver will be pushed downward and will be palpable. The heart, too, will be displaced downward, shifting the location of the apical area for cardiac auscultation or point of maximal impulse (PMI). The lungs should be auscultated for unequal breath sounds, crackles that clear with coughing, and overt or latent wheeze produced with forced expiration. The child is asked to force expiration by taking deep breaths and breathing through the mouth during auscultation. Cardiac rate and rhythm should be carefully assessed, because asthma drug therapy can alter cardiac function. Assessment should be done for concomitant aggravating factors such as otitis media, the swollen turbinates and gray boggy nasal mucosa of sinusitis, and healed or active eczematous skin lesions.

Table 38-18. Laboratory Tests in Asthma

Test	Possible Abnormalities in Asthma	Comments
Complete blood count	Leukocytosis (occasionally)	Induced by infection, epinephrine administration, "stress" (?)
	Eosinophilia (frequently)	Varies with medication, time of day, adrenal function; not necessarily related to "allergy." (Often higher in "intrinsic" than "extrinsic" asthma)
Sputum examination White or "clear" and small yellow plugs	Eosinophils	In both "intrinsic" and "extrinsic" asthma
Nasal smear	Eosinophils	Suggests concomitant nasal allergy
	Lymphocytes, PMNs*, macrophages	Replace eosinophils in upper respiratory infections
	PMNs with ingested bacteria	Bacterial rhinitis or sinusitis
Serum tests	IgG, IgA, IgM	Often normal. May be abnormal—various patterns seen
	IgE	Sometimes elevated in "allergic" asthma. Often normal
	Aspergillus-precipitating antibody	Suggestive, not diagnostic of bronchopulmonary aspergillosis
Sweat test	Normal in asthma Perform to rule out cystic fibrosis	Cystic fibrosis and asthma can coexist
Chest radiograph	Hyperinflation, infiltrates, pneumomediastinum, pneumothorax Rule out tuberculosis	Indicated once in all children with asthma. Indicated on hospitalization for asthma
Pulmonary function tests	$\downarrow FEV_1$, $\downarrow FVC$, $\downarrow FEF_{25-75\text{ per cent}}$, $\downarrow$ PEFR;* $FEV_1/FVC < 75$ per cent	Useful for following course of disease, response to treatment
Response to bronchodilators	> 15 per cent improvement FEV_1; PEFR	Safest diagnostic test for asthma
Exercise tests	Decreased lung function after 6 minutes of exercise PEFR and $FEV_1 > 15$ per cent $\downarrow$ $FEF_{25-75\%} > 25\% \downarrow$	Useful to diagnose asthma in children. Often abnormal when resting lung function is normal
Methacholine inhalation test (Mecholyl test)	20 per cent fall in lung function with dose tolerated by "normal" subjects	Should be performed only by specialists
Antigen inhalation test	20 per cent fall in lung function immediately after challenge; may cause delayed response 6–8 hr later	Potentially dangerous; specialist only
Allergy skin tests	Identifies allergic factors that *might* be causative factors	Test only likely factors—selected by history
Serologic tests for IgE antibody (e.g., RAST)	Same significance as skin tests	More expensive than skin tests

* PMNs = Polymorphonuclear leukocytes.
FEV_1 = Forced expiratory volume; volume of air expired in one second.
FVC = Forced vital capacity; total volume of air released in one expiration.
$FEF_{25-75\text{ per cent}}$ = Forced expiratory flow; 25–75 per cent = maximal flow at midexpiration.
PEFR = Peak expiratory flow rate; an assessment of airflow through all airways.
(Modified from Pearlman and Bierman, 1988.)

Laboratory Tests

Table 38-18 summarizes the usual laboratory tests used in the differential diagnosis and ongoing evaluation of asthma. Blood tests indicate elevated eosinophils and serum IgE. Sputum cytology assesses for elevated eosinophils commonly associated with asthma. Pulmonary function tests evaluate lung volumes and flow rates. The most common and the easiest test to perform with children is the PER (peak expiratory flow rate). Most children can learn this technique by 3 years of age. The peak expiratory flow rate reflects the degree of airway obstruction. Pulmonary function tests aid in the diagnosis of asthma, provide information regarding the severity of an attack or disease, and evaluate the child's response to treatment or exercise. Exercise-induced asthma can be assessed this way. Sometimes a chest film is needed to assess the airway obstruction caused by atelectasis or the degree of obstruction based on lung hyperinflation. Skin testing or elimination diets may be indicated when allergic inhalants or ingestant allergens are suspected. The methacholine challenge test can be used to test the reactivity of respiratory tissues. The airways of children with asthma are 50 to 1000 times more sensitive to methacholine than in other children (Pearlman and Bierman, 1988).

Therapeutic Management

Asthma management is aimed at avoidance of specific allergens (if applicable) and at reducing hypersensitivity reactions by medication and immunotherapy (if indicated) (Bock, 1983; Sawley, 1983; Zieger, 1983; Zieger and Schatz, 1983).

Avoidance of Allergens. According to Sly (1986), the most effective treatment for allergy is the elimination of exposure to the antigen. Common house dust is the allergen most often identified in asthma. Mold, mildew, animal dander, and air pollution (notably cigarette smoke) are other common offenders. See Table 43-6 for allergy-proofing techniques involving reduction of common allergens. The subject of allergen avoidance is further addressed under management of allergy in Chapter 43, p. 1574.

Asthma in children can be classified as mild, moderately severe, or severe (Bierman and Pearlman, 1980). Mild asthma describes the child who has infrequent, intermittent attacks responsive to oral theophylline or adrenergics and who is symptom-free between attacks. The child with moderate-to-severe asthma may require medications around the clock (oral theophylline, oral adrenergics, or both or aerosol), and the chronicity of the disease has a much greater impact on the family. The latter condition interferes with activity, such as school, sports, academics, play, sleep, and family relationships, although with proper management these children may be symptom-free between attacks.

Pharmacologic Therapy. Pharmacologic management is complex and individualized; it is summarized in Table 38-19. The dosage of theophylline preparation is individualized for the infant and child because individuals vary widely in metabolism and clearance rates. Desirable blood therapeutic levels are between 10 and 20 μg/ml. To promote adherence to medication for the child with moderate-to-severe asthma, long-acting sustained-release preparations are prescribed to decrease the child's rapid clearance rate, improve compliance, and provide clinical control. Beaded sustained-release theophylline preparations such as TheoDur can be sprinkled on food; however, the beads must not be chewed. Beta-adrenergic aerosol treatments (e.g., albuterol, terbutaline) are preferred over oral preparations for children because they are faster and more effective in decreasing pulmonary obstruction and have fewer systemic side effects.

Cromolyn sodium, a mast cell stabilizer, prevents

***Table* 38-19.** Pharmacologic Treatment for Asthma

Drug	Drug Action	Nursing Implications
Adrenergic drugs (e.g., aerosolized albuterol)	Relaxation of bronchial smooth muscles; possible depression of the inflammatory response in the lungs	Aerosol medications provide good bronchodilating effects at a dose 10 to 20 times less than would be needed for oral or parenteral administration. Teach the child to use the inhaler after a normal expiration. The child should breathe the medication in slowly and hold the breath to a count of 10. Results are better if a few minutes elapse between inhalations
Theophylline	Bronchodilator; exact mechanism of action is unclear	Often administered in a sustained release capsule because it is excreted from the body rapidly when taken in liquid or uncoated tablet form. The family should know the child will need periodic blood tests for serum drug levels; concentrations >20 μg/ml are associated with toxicity. Classic manifestations of toxicity are irritability, marked restlessness, tachycardia, and vomiting
Cromolyn sodium	By an unidentified mechanism, cromolyn inhibits the release of chemicals that activate the inflammatory response. Also reduces the hyperreactivity of the airways	The family must understand that cromolyn is used exclusively for prevention of attacks; it will not open airways during an attack. It is an expensive medication that is inhaled. It is now available in a metered-dose inhaler. It is usually used in combination with adrenergic drugs
Glucocorticosteroids	Reduce the inflammatory and allergic responses and help dilate smooth bronchial muscles	New surface-active aerosol agents have been developed that produce bronchial steroid effects with relatively few systemic effects. The inhaler may be difficult for children under 5 years of age. The child must be taught to hold the canister outside the mouth rather than inside, to use the inhaler before meals, and to rinse the mouth and throat after inhalation. There is some concern that aerosolized glucocorticosteroids may damage the pharynx and airways in children

(Based on Lockey and Bukantz, 1987.)

the release of histamine. This medication can be inhaled and is useful to prevent cold-induced or exercise-induced asthma. Its pharmacologic action is effective only in prevention, not after an attack has started. Cromolyn is not an episode treatment but must be taken continuously to achieve optimum control. Corticosteroids enhance bronchodilator effects, decrease mucosal edema, and improve oxygenation (Fiel et al, 1983). Corticosteroids are used to prevent or treat status asthmaticus if asthma is unresponsive to bronchodilators. Corticosteroids are usually continued in daily doses for 4 to 10 days after the acute attack (Zieger, 1983).

Immunotherapy is sometimes given in inhalant-stimulated asthma, particularly when the specific inhalants are ones that cannot be eliminated from the environment or their elimination would require drastic lifestyle changes. Additional information about immunotherapy is located in Chapter 43.

Therapeutic Management of the Acute Attack

Management of the child's acute asthma attack begins at home. Prompt, effective treatment of early symptoms of an asthmatic attack significantly reduces the severity of the attack. When symptoms appear, the child and parent can intervene by having the child practice abdominal breathing and self-relaxation techniques along with prescribed oral bronchodilators or beta-adrenergic aerosol treatments (Voyles, 1981). If the child does not respond, an emergency visit to the clinic, doctor's office, or hospital emergency room is indicated.

The nurse receiving the child and family in an emergency situation needs to provide a calm, relaxed atmosphere. This type of encouragement and support can diminish the anxiety-related increase in oxygen consumption.

Upon arrival, the child is immediately provided oxygen because hypoxemia is a common consequence of airway obstruction. Although children may prefer nasal prongs to a mask, the prongs are effective only if the child is nose breathing and oxygen requirements are low. The child should be encouraged to assume a position of comfort. (Usually Fowler or semi-Fowler position is preferred, but no specific position should be forced.)

The child should be evaluated quickly for signs of hypoxemia (headache, anxiety, confusion, dizziness) or impending respiratory failure (drowsiness, diaphoresis, decreased oxygen saturation per pulse oximetry). Lung auscultation should be done to evaluate airflow. In severe bronchoconstriction, no wheezing will be audible or it will occur with inspiration—a sign of impending respiratory failure. In less severe episodes, wheezing is heard both on expiration and inspiration. Wheezing that clears with change of position or coughing is due to mucus that narrows large airways. Arterial blood gas levels are obtained to assess carbon dioxide and oxygen levels. The accumulation of carbon dioxide is a major problem in an acute asthma attack.

The assessment continues with evaluation of the child's hydration status and a family interview. Interview questions are presented calmly and focus on precipitating factors, duration of attack, course of previous episodes, medications taken, and known allergies. These questions assist in understanding how the child usually responds during an attack, how the child is currently reacting, and what treatments may be necessary to control the child's present attack.

Pharmacologic intervention with subcutaneous injections of epinephrine, or nebulized beta-adrenergics (e.g., albuterol) over a specified time, usually control the attack. If the child is responsive, stops wheezing, and the pulmonary function values return to baseline, the child is usually able to return home. If the child is not responsive, an intravenous line is then started for fluid and electrolyte maintenance* and for the administration of intravenous aminophylline and steroids. If response was poor to initial adrenergic drugs, oral or intravenous corticosteroid therapy may be initiated early in an acute attack to help reduce inflammation. The importance of early corticosteroid administration is based on the fact that 6 or more hours are required for the drug to take effect. Corticosteroids may prevent or reverse status asthmaticus.

An intravenous infusion pump should be used to ensure effective titration levels of the intravenous drug in the blood. Aminophylline is initially given in a loading dose, then a maintenance dosage is achieved by continuous infusion. Because aminophylline is a form of theophylline, serum theophylline levels need to be therapeutic to be most effective. Theophylline blood levels should be determined before the maintenance dosage is begun; the goal is to maintain theophylline blood levels at 10 to 20 μg/ml. Additional doses of inhaled adrenergic drugs may be given to control bronchospasm. Heart rate must be monitored because these drugs can cause tachycardia.

This therapy is continued until the patient has stopped wheezing and pulmonary function is stable. If after 4 to 6 hours there is no deterioriation, the child may be sent home; however, if there is deterioration or pulmonary clearing is incomplete, hospitalization for further evaluation is in order. Expectorants are occasionally prescribed to help bring up secretions but re-

---

* Urine specific gravities help establish hydration needs. Serum electrolytes should be used to determine the need for potassium replacement.

Box 38-6
Management of Status Asthmaticus

Hospitalization.

Be calm while continuing to monitor the child's respiratory, oxygen, mental, and hydration status.

Provide opportunity for the child to rest.

Administer oxygen.

Prepare the child and family for laboratory diagnostic work:

- arterial blood gases (to assess decreased PaO_2 and increased $PaCo_2$, O_2 saturation, and acid base balance)
- complete blood count (to assess for infection, hydration)
- urine specific gravity (to assess hydration)
- chest radiograph (may be needed to rule out pneumonia and assess air trapping)

Prepare child and family for intravenous fluids:

- need to rehydrate child
- need to provide intravenous medications

Administer prescribed medications to child. Explain actions, side effects to child (age-appropriate) and family. Medications commonly administered are:

- subcutaneous epinephrine or terbutaline
- intravenous aminophylline
- intravenous steroids (need to be started early to be effective therapy)
- *never* administer sedatives (may mask the signs and symptoms of impending respiratory failure)
- expectorants have not been shown to be effective
- continue with bronchodilator aerosol treatment with O_2

If child is unresponsive to previous treatment and displaying signs of respiratory failure, an isoproterenol (Isuprel) drip may be started *requiring pediatric intensive care monitoring.*

Institute intubation and respiratory ventilator support, if not responsive to Isuprel drip.

quire adequate hydration to be effective. If infection exists (this may be verified by an otoscopic examination, sputum culture, or chest film), an antibiotic will be prescribed.

During emergency care, questions to the child should be minimal and limited to those that can be answered yes or no. The parents should be permitted to stay with the child to offer reassurance and comfort. Likewise, any security item the child has brought along should remain as additional emotional support. Once the attack has diminished so that the child can swallow fluids without gasping, small but frequent drinks of liquid should be offered to help liquefy and bring up secretions. Chest physical therapy may be ordered to help remove secretions after the child has become stabilized.

Therapeutic Management of Status Asthmaticus

Status asthmaticus refers to the child who has continuing respiratory distress *not* responding to previous prescribed therapy, nor to subcutaneous epinephrine or aerosol bronchodilators. This child requires continuing observation, monitoring, and interventions to prevent respiratory failure and will, therefore, be hospitalized.

The nurse in the hospital setting encourages calmness and continues support of the child and parents. The child's history regarding previous therapy, previous course of therapy, and medications taken may be obtained from clinic records. If not available from past records, this information is obtained to aid in the child's treatment. Box 38-6 outlines common management techniques used in the treatment of status asthmaticus. Preparation of the child and family will diminish fears and anxieties regarding unexpected procedures or medications and help the child manage a very frightening situation. It is important to initiate steroids early as they enhance the aminophylline effects, improve oxygenation, and decrease edema. The nurse's observations for impending respiratory failure are critical throughout the child's treatment. Respiratory failure is determined by respiratory fatigue and deteriorating blood gases. Refer to Table 38-2 for signs and symptoms of impending respiratory failure.

Any child requiring an isoproterenol drip or intubation requires skilled pediatric intensive care personnel to provide cardiac and respiratory monitoring, because both therapies increase the potential for serious complications.

Major Nursing Diagnoses for Asthma

Ineffective airway clearance, related to
- *bronchospasm*
- *mucosal edema*
- *hypersecretion of mucus*

Impaired gas exchange, related to air trapping in the alveoli

Potential ineffective family and individual coping, related to the emotional, physical, and financial impact of asthma

Potential altered growth and development:
- ***emotional/social development, related to the stigma of a chronic illness***
- ***intellectual development, related to frequent school absences***

Knowledge deficit, related to management of asthma at home

Strategies for Nursing Care

The nurse has a primary role in the early identification of allergenic substances, referral to an allergy specialist, and support and education of the family to promote adaptive coping and effective home management. The nurse in the acute care setting is also directly involved with symptomatic relief of the acute attack. The first two nursing diagnoses deal with the pathophysiology of asthma, which governs specific therapy during an acute attack and which prompts the therapeutic regimen designed to prevent episodes of airway obstruction.

The five nursing diagnoses identified can provide the basis for a plan of care during an acute episode or during long-term home management. The Nursing Process Plan in Table 38-20 details nursing strategies for care of the child during an acute attack of asthma. The remainder of this section will consider nursing strategies for long-term management of asthma.

Promoting Home Management

The goal of nursing strategies with the asthmatic child and family is to provide information, education, and counseling to support the child's and family's self-management of asthma. The effects of self-management will lessen the disease's disruptive influence within the home, and foster the independence and development of both the child and the family.

Counseling regarding styles of discipline is frequently a family need. It is important to encourage consistency in the style of parental discipline. If parental discipline precedes an attack, the family is encouraged to continue to be consistent with their limit setting and to deal with the attacks as they occur. Parental love and attention when the child is well will help minimize the use of wheezing to gain attention.

The nurse involved in the community may identify ways to educate schoolteachers and the asthmatic child's peers. The nurse must provide information regarding

- participation in physical education activities,
- medications taken at school (including side effects),
- the possible hearing loss from otitis media,
- what to do if the child starts wheezing,
- the effect on the asthmatic child of having animals in the classroom
- foods the child can eat at school parties,
- the effect on the child from missing school for illness or doctor visits,
- ways to promote the child's strengths.

This information will facilitate an understanding and supportive environment for the child with asthma.

Long-term asthma management involves both the child and family. Family commitment is critical to promote adherence to the treatment protocol, to improve outcome, and lessen emergency room visits and hospitalization. The nurse can use therapeutic approaches to enhance family motivation and commitment.

Improving Airway Clearance and Gas Exchange

Involving the child and family in the child's asthma management is accomplished by

- providing information and discussions on environmental control to decrease contact with known antigens and reduce precipitating factors,
- teaching them to decrease the incidence of infections and administer asthma medications, and
- promoting self-management techniques in asthma-associated attacks.

Relaxation techniques may (1) reduce the frequency of asthmatic episodes, shorten their duration, and decrease their severity, provide physical conditioning that improves the child's stamina and (2) encourages school attendance and academics (McCaully, 1980; Schneider et al, 1980). Relaxation techniques and abdominal breathing techniques, if prescribed, can be accomplished by teaching the child to blow bubbles and by having the child learn to pretend to be a rag doll. These techniques are fun and can be practiced even by young children.

Avoiding Allergens and Reducing Precipitating Factors

Environmental factors known to precipitate or aggravate asthmatic attacks should be eliminated or avoided when possible, but not to the extent of inhibiting experiences valuable to the child's normal growth and development or to the degree that constant family discord is created. The nurse can help the family determine how vigorous to be in allergy-proofing techniques, and how to evaluate their utility.

Exercise-induced asthma in children is commonly caused by the activity of running. It can have crippling effects on the child's social development, affecting relationships with peers and having negative effects on self-image, if participating in certain sports or activities is perceived as critical to self-esteem. The child with exercise-induced asthma can use special techniques (Wolf, 1980; Shapiro and Bierman, 1983). Sports such as tennis and swimming do not have the same debilitating effects as running and provide alternatives for peer and social involvement. Inhaled cromolyn and bronchodilators before activity, along with a few minutes of warm-up exercise, have demonstrated their ability to control the reactive airway disease associated with exercise-induced asthma.

Preventing Infections

For the child with a chronic lung disease like asthma, infection is a double threat. Not only is there the usual concern about infectious illness, but that illness may trigger an asthmatic episode, especially if it involves the respiratory tract. Prevention involves promoting optimal general health and avoiding exposure to pathogens.

Children with asthma need careful attention to maintaining their general health at optimal levels with balanced nutrition, adequate rest, and a relatively routine, calm home and school environment. Consultation with the child's allergist will determine which immunizations may be safely given. The culture media for some vaccines are highly allergenic for some persons.

Avoiding pathogens is, of course, impossible in the literal sense, but the nurse can support the family's own common sense methods of keeping the child away from infectious persons. In addition, the nurse can teach the family about ways in which bacteria, viruses, and fungi are spread and can impress upon them the importance of good handwashing. The family can also consult with the allergist about the advisability of flu vaccine prior to flu season.

Achieving Compliance with Medication Therapy

Medications used to manage asthma play a major role in the child's life. Medications are a common cause for noncompliance with medical recommendations (Voyles and Menendez, 1983). The frequency of the medication dosage and social peer pressure are common reasons for nonadherence. The current long-acting theophyllines have improved medication adherence because the medication is required less frequently, usually only twice a day. In spite of the recent pharmacologic improvements, peer pressures and the social activities of school-age children and adolescents may result in irresponsible behavior regarding medications. Lack of compliance may result from fear of peer nonacceptance or an unconscious effort to avoid feelings of dependency or vulnerability.

For those children on round-the-clock medications, the schedule should be as convenient as possible. Ideally the schedule avoids school hours; when medication is necessary at school, arrangements should be made for the child to take the medication privately, with no undue attention.

Adequate information should be provided as growth and development progress to enhance the child's capability for self-management of the medical and environmental therapies. The dangers of attempting to manage asthma with unprescribed over-the-counter drugs advertised to relieve allergic symptoms should be emphasized. Parents should be cautioned that even under the most careful management, occasional asthmatic attacks may occur and should be reassured that these attacks are not evidence of parental failure.

Promoting Adaptive Coping and Optimal Development

The intermittent acute asthmatic attacks and the chronicity of a complicated, burdensome medical regimen have an emotional, physical, developmental, and financial impact on the child and family (Carty, 1977; Crummette, 1979; Carbary and Carbary, 1981; Clark et al, 1984; Friedman, 1984). The growing child faces many stresses associated with asthma, making it difficult to function independently.

Recognizing and Reducing the Impact of Illness on the Child. During acute attacks, the asthmatic child may have to cope with feelings of anxiety, irritability, sadness, and fears of suffocation and dying. The long-term consequences of this chronic condition create feelings of fear and uncertainty about future attacks, emergency visits, hospitalization, separation from family and peers, and painful or misunderstood procedures. The side effects of prescribed medications, along with the disease's behavioral aspects, may result in changes in psychologic functioning affecting school attendance and achievements and the child's participation in social activities (Khampolikit, 1983). Psychologic changes include central nervous system stimulation, inability to sleep, fatigue, decreased ability to concentrate, irritability, and anxiety.

Stress for the asthmatic child and parent at home usually involves fears of an attack that could occur when help and appropriate remedial treatment are not immediately available. The parents may fear sending the child to a day care center, leaving the child with a babysitter, and taking vacations very far from the local doctor or hospital. This leads to restrictions on family activity and overprotectiveness of the child, with resulting limitations on initiative and cognitive growth.

The child and family can deal with this insecurity by learning to give aerosol treatments for acute attack and prior to exercise to prevent exercise-induced asthma. After age 5 years, the child can be taught to use and carry an inhaler. With proper allergenic control, the symptoms will lessen and restrictions can be minimized. The greater responsibility the child takes for self-management, the greater the feeling of control with respect to the asthmatic symptoms. A sense of control will contribute to the child's self-confidence in mastering developmental tasks and in achieving an overall feeling of self-esteem and competence. Self-management must be linked, however, to developmental readiness. Parents must remain involved in care at least through the school-age years.

Some children with asthma have learned that wheezing behavior can manipulate others. Limit-setting should start early and remain consistent. The parent must be cautioned not to make threats that cannot be enforced. The child needs frequent assurance from health personnel and from parents that there is no cause for guilt, even though everyone involved sometimes feels frustration because of the asthma. Asthma is, in fact, something beyond anyone's control. Parents may need to be cautioned against using their child's asthma as a conversation topic. (Children react to overheard conversations about themselves long before they master language.) Some parents may need counseling if they persistently use the child's asthma as a convenient excuse for misbehavior.

An innovative teaching approach, the *I'm Breathing Easier* program, has been developed recently at the Children's Hospital of Michigan (Ramsey and Siroky, 1988). Hand puppets and family participation are employed to accomplish the program goals:

- removing the feelings of guilt about having asthma,
- introducing coping and decision-making skills to the individual child, and
- teaching the child and family members self-management skills.

If conflicts and anxieties in the family perpetuate the child's asthmatic episodes or the child frequently uses asthma behavior to express and meet emotional needs, counseling should be sought. Parents need help in developing in their child an increasing responsibility for self-care. The goal is to raise the child as normally as possible.

Recognizing and Reducing the Impact on Parents and Siblings. Parents may have the same experiences and feelings as their asthmatic child. Parents face physical fatigue from loss of sleep, anxiety, guilt, frustration, financial hardships, and restriction of family activities. Parental guilt may be compounded by financial constraints, such as not having enough money to allergy-proof their home. Interventions such as financial aid, finding a baby sitter qualified to care for the child in an emergency, and avoidance of precipitants that stimulate attacks may help diminish family stress.

Conflicts over dependency-independency needs often occur in families of children with asthma. Some parents experience difficulty both in separating from their school-age children and in encouraging independence and self-responsibility. Parental overprotection, rejection, neglect, and discipline issues may become evident (Mattson, 1975). Inconsistent limit-setting may become the parental style of discipline. The inconsistency and lack of structure can result from parental fears that discipline may precipitate an attack.

Parent groups led by qualified professionals help in solving day-to-day health and childrearing problems and emotional concerns. Suppressed parental anger about lifestyle changes can cause conflicts. Resolution of anger is essential to the management regimen. Parents who are in touch with their feelings about the chronic nature of asthma will be better prepared to support their child in the therapeutic regimen.

Siblings may exhibit behavior demonstrating resentment toward the "sick" child, or anxiety and overconcern for well-being. Sibling jealousy over preferential treatment given the child or restrictions on freedom imposed on the entire family may lead to suppressed anger. The angry younger child may benefit from toys such as modeling clay and pounding tables that allow release of pent-up emotions. Sibling rivalry is often reduced by ensuring that all children in the family share equally in family responsibilities. Sibling involvement in the family teaching and counseling is important for optimal family functioning. Through counseling parents and siblings can learn to identify and accept their feelings and to seek appropriate outlets.

The nurse can be supportive of the family by recognizing their need for intervention and by referring them to appropriate counseling and/or support groups. The nurse who has the opportunity for long-term follow-up with the family can be supportive by reinforcing effective problem-solving.

Nursing Strategies for Follow-Up Care in the Home or Clinic

Assess respiratory status, including the presence of adventitious lung sounds, and the child's general appearance with regard to color, signs of fatigue, and respiratory effort.

Obtain a blood sample, as indicated, for measurement of serum theophylline level.

Question the child and parent about the recent course of the illness.

Determine compliance with and effectiveness of routine and prn medications. Assess for side effects.

Encourage the child to talk about daily activities (both at school and at home) in order to assess developmental level and effects of asthma on daily living.

Encourage the parent to voice concerns and to identify any modifications instituted by the family in home management of the allergy.

Provide needed information, and reinforce the attempts of the child and parent toward effective self-management.

Text continues on page 1243

Table 38-20
Nursing Process Plan: The Child Hospitalized with an Acute Attack of Asthma

By Roxie Foster

Assessment of Emotional-Social Function

Fear/Anxiety

Subjective Assessment	Objective Assessment
Self-report or parental report of feelings about the acute attack	Nonverbal indicators of fear/anxiety: physical appearance, eye movement, behavioral response to diagnostic and therapeutic interventions

Analysis: Nursing Diagnosis 1

Fear/anxiety, related to
- *severe dyspnea*
- *hospital environment*

Defining Characteristics

Subjective: Self-report or parental report of being afraid. Pleading, telling nurse "I can't breathe." Crying in response to hospital personnel, equipment, therapies

Objective: Fearful expression associated with increased respiratory effort. Appearing "wild-eyed" and clinging to parent in response to attempts at diagnostic or therapeutic interventions

Client Goal/ Evaluation Criteria	Nursing Goals/Strategies (Selected Rationale)
1. The client will experience a reduction in fear and anxiety as evidenced by: a. more relaxed posture and expression b. verbalizing "easier breathing" c. less physical withdrawal from health care personnel, equipment, and interventions	*Quickly implement strategies to relieve hypoxemia and increase airway clearance and gas exchange.* (See nursing diagnoses 2 and 3.) • Restrict questions to the child as much as possible during the admission period (to reduce oxygen demands). *Implement strategies to reassure the child and parent and to reduce the threat of the unknown.* • Approach the family with a *calm, quiet, caring* attitude that establishes your competence. (Their anxiety will be reduced by a feeling that someone knows what to do to relieve the child's distress.) • Allow the child to assume a *position of comfort* and to sit on the parent's lap if desired. Approach the child with deliberate movements, *explaining* action. • If the child resists a necessary intervention, such as the oxygen mask or prongs, encourage the parent to help. If this technique fails, perform the action *quickly* despite the child's protests and without pleading or bargaining (which would delay therapy and cause prolonged protest behavior on the part of the child). Explain calmly why the action is necessary. (The child's anxiety will usually decrease as the parent's anxiety diminishes.)

Continued

Client Goal/ Evaluation Criteria	Nursing Goals/Strategies (Selected Rationale)
	• For additional measures to reduce anxiety of the child and parents, see Table 31-2, Nursing Process Plan: The Hospitalized Child

Assessment of Physical Function

(Airway/gas exchange/breathing)

Subjective Assessment

Self-report or parental report of increased respiratory effort, identification of possible allergens, and therapies administered at home before seeking medical intervention

Objective Assessment

Lung sounds; use of accessory muscles; presence of cough, skin color; vital signs, including systolic blood pressure on inspiration and expiration; signs of hypoxemia; urine specific gravity; arterial blood gases

Analysis: Nursing Diagnosis 2

Ineffective airway clearance, related to
- *bronchospasm*
- *mucosal edema*
- *hypersecretion of mucus*

Analysis: Nursing Diagnosis 3

Impaired gas exchange, related to air trapping in the alveoli

Defining Characteristics for Nursing Diagnoses 2 and 3

Subjective: Statements such as, "It's hard to breathe," "My chest feels so tight." Report of contact with known or suspected allergens. Report of ineffectiveness of home therapies (breathing and relaxation techniques, bronchodilators) to arrest the attack

Objective: Expiratory wheezing with occasional crackles (rales) and diminished airflow; retractions (especially intercostal); productive, paroxysmal cough; pallor with circumoral cyanosis; tachycardia, increased effort on expiration; hypoxemia indicated by arterial blood gases (decreased pH, decreased PaO_2, increased $PaCO_2$), and by fatigue from respiratory effort; increased urine specific gravity

Client Goals/ Evaluation Criteria	Nursing Goals/Strategies (Selected Rationale)
2/3. The client will experience increased airway clearance and increased gas exchange as evidenced by: a. increased air movement upon lung auscultation b. decreased retractions	*Assess air exchange.* • Take vital signs and auscultate lungs frequently, at least every hour initially (to ensure that any changes are noted promptly). • Assess carefully for changes in airflow, alerting the physician if diminished airflow is not resolved by change of position or coughing. (This could signal increasing airway obstruction and impending respiratory failure.)

c. expectoration of mucus
d. vital signs within normal limits for age
e. absence of headache, fatigue, confusion, dizziness
f. arterial blood gases within normal limits
g. urine specific gravity <1.015

- Assess for other signs of respiratory failure (see Table 38-2) and alert the physician should evidence indicate increasing airway obstruction

Teach and implement strategies to increase airway clearance and gas exchange.

- Reduce hypoxemia.
  Administer *oxygen,* as ordered, to ease the respiratory effort and resolve hypoxemia (related to the obstructive effects of mucus, bronchospasm, and edema).
- Reduce bronchospasm.
  Administer *bronchodilators,* as ordered, e.g., SC epinephrine, or SC terbutaline, IV aminophylline, nebulized beta-adrenergic agents (to relieve bronchospasm by relaxing smooth muscles).
  Monitor *blood* levels of *theophylline* during IV administration of and before administering the next oral dose of aminophylline. (Theophylline is the largest component of aminophylline; blood levels >20 μg/ml may lead to toxicity.)
  Use a *cardiorespiratory monitor* with IV aminophylline, if use of monitor is a nursing prerogative in the institution. (Aminophylline increases heart rate and force of contraction; high blood levels may lead to tachycardia.)
  Teach the cooperative child to inhale deeply on the nebulizer airway, hold the breath to a count of 10 (if possible) and exhale through pursed lips (to increase the penetration and effect of the medication on the bronchial tree).
- Reduce bronchial edema.
  Administer *corticosteroids* as ordered for severe asthma (to reduce pulmonary inflammation and edema, and to potentiate the action of β-adrenergic bronchodilators). Assure parents that short-term use of corticosteroids will not result in cushingoid effects or steroid dependency.
- Evaluate effectiveness of medications against evaluation criteria a–f.
- Promote expectoration of mucus.
  Keep the child well *hydrated* (to help liquefy secretions). (Calculate the child's fluid needs per kilogram of body weight [see Chapter 30] and ensure that the child receives at least this much fluid [IV + PO] every 24 hours.
  Measure urine specific gravity every shift. (If this is done with a spectrometer on the unit it does not need a physician's order.)
  After bronchospasm has resolved, perform chest physical therapy (CPT) as ordered, or, if this is a function of the respiratory therapy department, assist the therapist to evaluate the benefits of CPT in clearing the airway.

Continued

Assessment of Intellectual-Perceptual Function

(Anticipatory guidance and discharge planning)

Subjective Assessment

Replies to questions about knowledge of physical care; how to secure and operate equipment; necessary changes in diet, physical activity, school attendance; administration of and side effects of medications; signs and symptoms requiring medical attention

Objective Assessment

Return demonstrations of physical care, equipment operation, and medication administration

Analysis: Nursing Diagnosis 4

Knowledge deficit: child and/or parents, related to management of asthma at home

Defining Characteristics

Subjective and/or objective evidence of the need for further instruction

Client Goal/ Evaluation Criteria	Nursing Goals/Strategies (Selected Rationale)
4. The child and/or parents will display the knowledge and skills needed for home management, as evidenced by:	*Assure adequate time for learning home management.* • Begin discharge teaching on the day of admission. • Plan time for questions and clarification on the day of discharge. • Table 31-2 provides details of these strategies.
a. demonstrating effective physical care	*Ensure that the child and parent are aware of factors that may precipitate another attack.* • Discuss with them avoidance of allergens and irritants. As appropriate to the client, include house dust, animal dander, mold and mildew, seasonal pollens, particular foods, cigarette smoke, odors from paints and chemicals, weather and climatic changes, air pollution, exercise, infections, and/or emotional stress. *Ensure that the child and parents understand physical restrictions, if any apply.* • Discuss with them plans for exercise. Suggest these strategies to minimize the threat of bronchospasm (Sly, 1986): minimize intake of cold air by wrapping a muffler around the nose and mouth; precede physical exercise with a warm-up period; consider activities that do not require sudden bursts of activity, which increase air flow; consider using medications prior to exercise to increase tolerance.

	Request that the child and/or parents list signs and symptoms requiring medical attention: increased wheezing and difficulty breathing; increasing fatigue and lethargy; a respiratory infection; decreasing effectiveness of medications; and emotional dependency on prn inhalant bronchodilators. *Discuss with the family their plans for well child care.*
b. demonstrating effective operation of equipment	*Ensure that the child/parents can competently operate and clean necessary equipment such as a nebulizer.* • Institute self- or parental treatments with the equipment in question as soon as initial anxiety has decreased. (Repeated practice will increase competence.)
c. demonstrating safe medication administration and identifying side effects	*Provide verbal and written instructions about medication and allow self- or parental administration as often as possible.* • Provide information about the administration of *theophylline* products: common side effects: agitation, nausea and vomiting, tachycardia; may increase action of theophylline (by reducing clearance from body): large quantities of chocolate, coffee, tea, colas (Sly, 1986); may reduce action of theophylline (by increasing clearance rate): smoking tobacco or marijuana, ingestion of charcoal-broiled beef, high protein diet (Sly, 1986). • Provide information about metered-dose inhaler for *cromolyn* administration *Address the issue of compliance associated with feelings about being stigmatized.* • Encourage the child to voice feelings about taking the medications at home and at school. • Help the child identify feelings that may present a problem with regular administration. • Help the child plan ways to take the medications and still avoid unpleasant feelings about administration, e.g., taking the medications before and after school, going home for lunchtime therapies, taking the medications in the school nurse's office during a recess break. • Help the parents realize the benefits of self-management to the child's self-esteem. • Reinforce the family's efforts at the child's self-management.

Cystic Fibrosis

Cystic fibrosis (CF) is a multisystem disorder with the predominant characteristics of chronic pulmonary disease, pancreatic enzyme deficiency (resulting in digestive problems), and abnormally high sweat chlorides. The life span of children with cystic fibrosis continues to increase. The average age at death in the 1940s was 1 year; with the advent of antibiotics and various modes of treatment, CF children are now living to adolescence and early adulthood. Approximately 95 per cent live to the age of 16 years and approximately 50 per cent live to age 21 years.

Incidence and Etiology

Cystic fibrosis occurs equally in males and females, but affected males generally outlive females six to one by 20 years of age. It is the most common life-threatening genetic disease in caucasians. It occurs less commonly in blacks. It is estimated to affect 1 : 2000 and 1 : 17,000 white and black neonates, respectively, but this varies according to ethnic composition within a population.

The mode of transmission of cystic fibrosis is an area of continuing research, but it is thought to be transmitted by the autosomal recessive mode of inheritance. Evidence now suggests that the gene responsible for cystic fibrosis is located on chromosome 7 (Wainwright, 1985). This discovery enables families with a history of CF to determine whether they are carriers of the gene (Wells and Meghdadpour, 1988). It is estimated that 5 per cent of the white population are carriers (heterozygous) and that 1 in 400 marriages are between two individuals who are carriers of the disease (Hodson, 1983). When two individuals are carriers of the abnormal gene, there is a 1 : 4 risk with each pregnancy for their offspring to be a child with cystic fibrosis. The "normal" sibling of a child with cystic fibrosis has a 2 : 3 chance of being a carrier for CF. (See Chapter 4 for further discussion of patterns of inheritance.)

Pathophysiology

The exact cause of cystic fibrosis remains unclear; however, it is believed to involve a generalized dysfunction of the exocrine (mucous-producing) glands with varying degrees of severity. The basic problem is thought to occur at the cellular level, reflecting an alteration in a protein, possibly an enzyme, primarily affecting epithelial tissues. The *primary pathophysiology* is an abnormal accumulation of viscid mucus which leads to the obstruction and dilatation of many glands and organs. Although many organs may be affected, the pathology in the lung and the pancreas presents the greatest clinical problems. The degree of organ system involvement varies: digestive system involvement occurs in 75 to 80 per cent, whereas some degree of pulmonary involvement is eventually seen in most cases. However, a few patients have only enzyme deficiency without pulmonary disease (Gellis and Kagan, 1986).

Although the lungs are not exocrine glands, they are composed largely of epithelial cells. The lung usually appears normal at birth, but soon after birth obstruction of the airways with viscid mucus leads to infection and a chronic inflammatory process. At autopsy, the trachea and bronchi are generally filled with a mucopurulent material, the lungs are emphysematous with adhesions and areas of consolidation, and atelectasis is present. The mucopurulent material is thought to be a combined product of the tracheobronchial gland secretions and the infectious process (Schwachman, 1983).

Involvement of the pancreas is clinically important because of its effect on the digestive system. The exocrine glands of the pancreas, clogged with thick mucus, show dilatation of ducts and, in later stages, diffuse fibrosis associated with autodigestion from trapped proteolytic enzymes. Failure of the pancreas to secrete enzymes results in digestive disorders that are characterized by malabsorption, with excessive fat and protein in the stools.

The most consistent pathophysiologic observation is the presence of elevated chloride and sodium in sweat. It occurs in 98 to 99 per cent of affected children. This clinical finding is now thought to be related to a decreased absorption in the sweat glands associated with a decreased cellular permeability to chloride (Quinton and Bisman, 1983; Rosenstein, 1988).

A link may exist between thick mucous secretions and abnormal sweat electrolyte concentrations, or each may be the independent result of a more basic defect affecting secretory and transport mechanisms of cells (Schwartz, 1987). Other organs affected are paranasal sinuses, salivary glands, liver, intestine, the reproductive tract, and tear glands. The number and degree of organ involvement vary considerably from one child to another.

Clinical Manifestations

Since the two main organ systems involved in the disease are the respiratory and gastrointestinal tracts, the presenting signs and symptoms generally result in complications of these systems. Approximately 10 per cent of infants with CF show symptoms as early as the newborn period, with "meconium ileus" (an impaction of meconium). In the remaining children, symptoms of the disease are variable, differing in degree of severity; in fact, many are not readily apparent until quite late in life. The most common presenting signs are recurrent respiratory infections, poor weight gain with excessive appetite, persistent coughing with excessive mucus, and wheezing. Additional signs are salty taste of the skin, nasal polyps, and bulky, foul-smelling stools.

Respiratory Manifestations. Many affected children have a history of chronic pulmonary disease with onset as early as birth, but their condition often is not diagnosed for years. Initial symptoms include a dry, nonproductive cough, followed by obstruction of bronchioles, resulting in secondary infection and respiratory distress.

As the thick, tenacious mucus accumulates, obstruction occurs and the flow of air is impaired, with an increase in residual volume and subsequent decrease in the vital capacity of the lungs. Auscultatory findings may be normal in the early stages, but as the disease progresses, moist crackles and harsh breath sounds are heard. As the functioning alveoli become overaerated, the chest distends, resulting in a barrel shape. If ventilation is significantly impaired, clubbing of the fingers and toes and cyanosis are observed (see page 1279 for description of clubbing). The course of these symptoms follows a pattern of remissions and exacerbations. Major pulmonary complications include hemoptysis, pneumothorax, cor pulmonale, respiratory failure, and congestive heart failure.

Gastrointestinal Manifestations. Pancreatic involvement is apparent in approximately 85 per cent of children with cystic fibrosis. The earliest possible clinical manifestation is meconium ileus. Meconium ileus with intestinal obstruction is due to abnormal mucous secretion from the intestinal mucosal glands and the deficit of pancreatic enzymes (Huang and Palmer, 1981). Intestinal obstruction is a sign of meconium ileus, including abdominal distention, dehydration, vomiting, and absence of stools.

As cystic fibrosis progresses, children have a markedly impaired ability to digest food, resulting in malabsorption. Causes of malabsorption include obstruction of the pancreatic ducts and absence of the enzymes necessary for conversion of food into products that can be absorbed by the intestines. Since the enzymes (trypsin, lipase, and amylase) capable of breaking down fats and proteins are absent, the child characteristically has large, loose, foul-smelling stools caused by fat in the stool (steatorrhea).

Although the child has a voracious appetite, the nutrient loss from the intestinal tract causes the child to lose weight and appear malnourished, with a distended abdomen and thin extremities. A common gastrointestinal complication is rectal prolapse. Because of the inability to absorb fats, variable degrees of deficiencies of the fat-soluble vitamins A, D, E, and K can occur in children with CF; however, only occasionally do they have vitamin deficiency symptoms (Doershuk and Boat, 1987). Vitamin K, which is provided primarily through intestinal synthesis, may be deficient, causing hypoprothrombinemia requiring vitamin K supplementation.

Problems pertaining to reproduction are also frequent. In the male, the epididymis, vas deferens, and seminal vesicles are usually poorly developed or absent, resulting in most males being sterile. Sexual function is usually not impaired. Female fertility is low owing to plugging of the cervix with a thick mucus that is abnormal in physical and chemical properties and blocks entry of the sperm (Dushenko, 1981).

Diagnostic Assessment

Neonatal screening for CF remains unsatisfactory. The only reliable and valid diagnostic test for CF is the sweat test by pilocarpine iontophoresis, followed by Gibson-Cooke quantification of chloride concentration. This test is difficult to perform in the first few weeks of life due to the paucity of sweat and is ideally done after at least 1 month of age (Ad Hoc Committee Report, 1983). Furthermore, it is not known whether

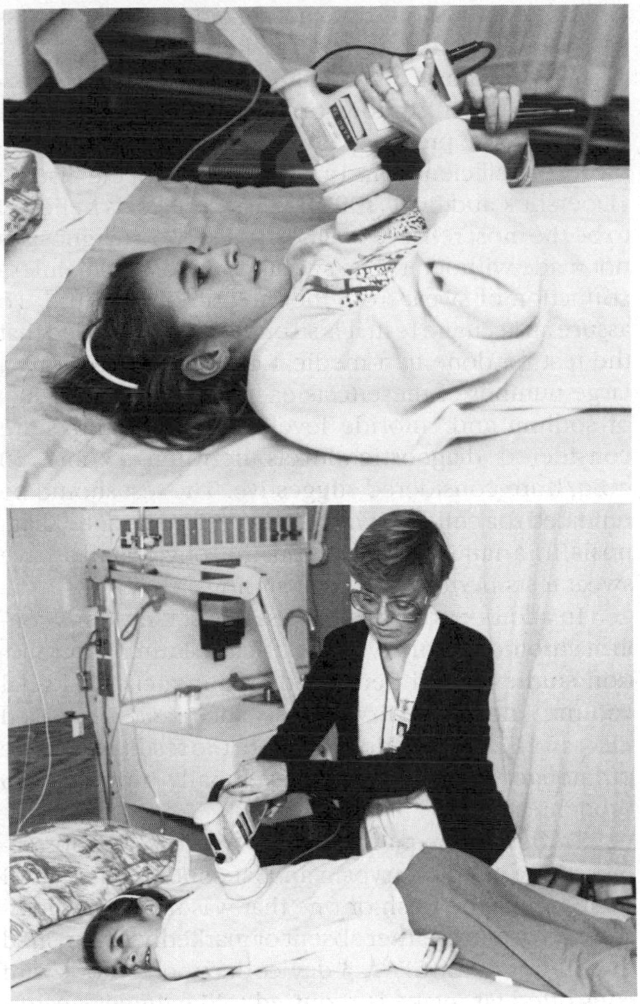

Hospitalized for cystic fibrosis, this 11-year-old girl performs parts of her own percussion. The nurse percusses the areas that the patient cannot reach. Mechanical percussion is now widely used, replacing manual percussion.

early treatment of an asymptomatic infant affects prognosis. The fact that a false-positive result could interfere with early infant-parent relationships is a serious concern. False-negative results also raise serious medical/legal issues.

Research continues in search of an appropriate screening test, including prenatal and postnatal tests. DNA analysis techniques can detect sibling heterozygotes or fetuses with cystic fibrosis when both parents and the sibling with CF are available (Doershuk and Boat, 1987). Evaluation of meconium for albumin content is not widely accepted. A relatively simple test—the dried blood immunoreactive trypsinogen (IRT) assay—continues to be studied. This assay measures a manifestation of the disease, deficient pancreatic enzymes, but has false-positive results and misses the 10 per cent of CF children with normal pancreatic function. The reliability and validity of this test has not yet been determined, and it is not recommended for mass screening (Ad Hoc Committee Report, 1983).

The diagnosis of cystic fibrosis is based on a positive sweat test in combination with one or more of the following: the presence of chronic lung disease, pancreatic insufficiency, and a family history of the disease (Doershuk and Boat, 1987). The sweat test is believed to be the most reliable diagnostic test and a diagnosis is not made without it. The sweat test involves a painless collection of sweat from the forearm of the child. To assure an accurate test, it is strongly recommended that the test be done in a medical center that performs a large number of these tests each year. Measurements of sodium and chloride levels above 60 mEq/L are considered diagnostic: levels between 45 and 50 mEq/L are considered suggestive. The test should be repeated for children with the latter finding. The diagnosis in a family should alert the physician to have sweat tests performed on all siblings.

In addition to the sweat test, chest x-ray films confirm chronic obstructive lung disease. Pulmonary function studies reveal decreased vital capacity and tidal volume, increased airway resistance, and decreased FEV_1 and FEV_1/VC ratio. These are the result of chronic pulmonary infection, which eventually progresses to bronchiectasis.

To determine pancreatic involvement, stool samples are studied for trypsin and fat content. (The stool sample must be fresh or one that was frozen immediately.) Trypsin is either absent or markedly diminished in children with CF. A 3-day collection of stool with controlled fat intake is required to document steatorrhea (fatty stools).

The nurse can help relieve some of the family's anxiety during the diagnostic period. Although the diagnostic tests are not traumatic, the child and the parents need to have a thorough explanation of the procedure and equipment involved. Encouraging a parent to stay with a child and even hold her or him during a procedure whenever possible are recommended. In the sweat test, a small electric current and the drug pilocarpine is placed on the forearm (thigh of infants) of the child to stimulate the sweat gland (iontophoresis). The sweat is then collected by overlying filter paper or gauze. A simple explanation of the procedure and allowing the young child to handle the apparatus are helpful in alleviating anxieties. The electrodes cause no discomfort, but the appearance of the apparatus may be frightening.

Therapeutic Management

Treatment is individualized and aimed at promoting an independent life as adolescence is approached. Promotion of good nutrition, prevention of pulmonary infection, and a healthy psychosocial adjustment to the disease by the child and family are the goals of therapy. A variety of treatments are used to deter the disease.

Digestive and nutritional therapy consists of pancreatic enzyme replacement, diet adjustment, and fat-soluble vitamin supplementation (in some instances) to promote growth, adequate nutrition, and normal bowel movements. A tablet or powdered form of animal pancreatic enzymes is taken orally whenever food is consumed, including snacks. The most frequently prescribed supplement is a capsule containing enterically coated microspheres that are designed to release the active enzyme in the duodenum. Infants under 12 months of age, however, may lack sufficient gastric acid to remove the enteric-coated microspheres (Lester and Rothberg, 1986), therefore, a powdered supplement is preferred.

The amount of extract will vary with the child's diet, activity level, number of bowel movements per day, and type of stool. If stools become large and bulky, more enzymes are required; if constipation is a problem, fewer enzymes may be required. Whenever a protein fluid such as a milkshake is consumed, enzymes need to be taken; if a high-fat meal is anticipated, enzymes should be increased. Since the enzymes are specific and only partially replace normal pancreatic function, a moderate-fat, high-protein, high-calorie diet may be prescribed to promote weight gain and digestion of foods. MCT oil, a dietary supplement of medium-chain triglycerides, is sometimes given to increase calories. Medium-chain triglycerides (MCT) are more readily digested and provide 8.4 cal per gm.

Because of the severe fat malabsorption, supplements of liposoluble vitamins in water-miscible liquid may be given to children with pancreatic involvement. When administered, vitamins A, D, and E are given in amounts double the usual daily dose. Vitamin K is given as necessary for infants with vitamin K deficiency and to older patients with hemoptysis and cirrhosis of the liver. The addition of vitamin B complex is usually recommended for patients receiving oral antibiotics. Iron is usually prescribed because pancreatic enzyme supplementation causes a reduction in iron absorption.

Salt is allowed in generous amounts to prevent salt depletion through sweating. Sweating complications usually do not occur except during excessive sweating when loss of salt can lead to dehydration and collapse; therefore, additional salt is usually taken during hot weather.

Pulmonary therapy is designed to prevent and treat pulmonary infection. Therapy aims to clear secretions from the airways, improve aeration, and reduce the intensity of pulmonary infection. It consists of chest physical therapy (CPT), breathing exercises, inhalation therapy, and antibiotic administration.

The purpose of *chest physical therapy* is to maintain good pulmonary hygiene. The lungs are drained by placing the patient in various positions and percussing and vibrating the chest. CPT is carried out two to four times daily prophylactically and more often during acute infections or bed rest.

Inhalation therapy liquefies mucus and prevents and treats infections. Intermittent aerosol therapy is usually done for 5 to 10 minutes prior to CPT to administer medications (bronchodilators, decongestants, or mucolytic agents) or water droplets to the lower respiratory tract. If thick, tenacious secretions are difficult to mobilize, direct inhalation from an ultrasonic nebulizer may help break up the mucus. With excessive amounts of sputum, and if the child can tolerate it, postural drainage before and after aerosol therapy may be necessary. Drainage before aerosol therapy allows the droplets to reach areas previously filled with secretions.

Mist therapy is used in an attempt to liquefy secretions and facilitate removal of mucus from the lung. Mist is sometimes used overnight to increase humidification, however, Mist tents are no longer routinely used for cystic fibrosis.

Breathing exercises help aerate the lungs to maximal capacity. These exercises are carried out daily before, after, or during postural drainage. Regular *exercise programs* are recommended for patients with CF as a means to improve breathing mechanics, posture, chest mobility, muscle strength, and aerobic fitness (Rose and Jay, 1986).

The *use of antibiotics* as a preventive measure is controversial. Many physicians prescribe antibiotic therapy only if there is an infection; others use it prophylactically. If used prophylactically, different antibiotics are given in rotation to prevent drug resistance. The most common organisms recovered in the sputum are penicillin-resistant *Staphylococcus aureus* and *Pseudomonas aeruginosa*. Two- to three-week courses of intravenous antibiotic therapy are given during acute exacerbations. Aerosol antibiotic therapy may be used in conjunction with systemic therapy.

Genetic counseling is an important component of care. A geneticist provides information to the family to assist them in decision making concerning reproductive plans. An interdisciplinary team may work together to provide the necessary guidance and support concerning these difficult decisions.

Major Nursing Diagnoses for Cystic Fibrosis

***Anticipatory grieving**, related to the diagnosis of a potentially fatal disease*
***Knowledge deficit**, related to lack of knowledge about the disease process and its management*
***Ineffective airway clearance**, related to thick mucus within the airways*
***Impaired gas exchange**, related to air trapping in the alveoli, associated with airways narrowed by tenacious mucus*
***Potential for infection: pulmonary**, related to chronic tenacious pulmonary secretions*
***Altered nutrition: less than body requirements**, related to impaired metabolism of nutrients and vitamins, associated with insufficient pancreatic enzymes*
***Potential ineffective individual/family coping**, related to the stress of a chronic and potentially fatal disease*

Strategies for Nursing Care

Nursing care is focused on promoting respiratory and gastrointestinal function, providing psychosocial support to the child and family, and preparing the family for effective home management.

Providing Support During the Period of Anticipatory Grief. *Emotional adjustment* to the diagnosis is often overwhelmingly difficult. The thought of a potentially fatal illness stimulates an acute anticipatory mourning reaction in family members, including feelings of denial, avoidance, shock, and disbelief, followed by information seeking. Anger is also a common manifestation of this stage, since parents see the doctor as having failed in not diagnosing the condition earlier. Often parents who have "known something was wrong" express ambivalent feelings about the diagnosis. They experience shock and guilt learning the poor prognosis but are relieved finally to have a diagnosis for their child's chronic condition (Mikkelson, 1978).

When parents are informed of the diagnosis, the nurse should make every effort to be with them to clarify it and to provide support, because the response and understanding of parents at this early phase can have long-lasting effects on the child's perception of self and the illness. Parents need careful explanation of the disease, information regarding the therapy involved, and additional support because they have been faced not only with the fatal outcome of the disease but also the treatment for which they must assume responsibility. It is also necessary to recognize that the ability of many parents to take in information regarding the disease during this early stage is limited. Reiteration and provision of written material are beneficial.

Counseling should also begin at the time of diagnosis. (See Chapter 50 for the Nursing Process Plan for Genetic Counseling.) A common response of parents is to become overprotective, creating anxiety and a poor self-image in the child. Knowing that children with cystic fibrosis are now living to adult life aids in decreasing parents' feelings of hopelessness.

Teaching to Facilitate Care in the Home. From the time of diagnosis, the goal is to involve the patient and family in self-care. Through education about the disease and the therapy required, the child and family are from the beginning prepared for discharge and home care. The National Cystic Fibrosis Foundation* has available many publications and educational aids for parents and for patients in their teens and twenties.

Preparation for home care includes teaching the parents and child how to carry out chest physical therapy, how to provide inhalation therapy by nebulizer, and how to give enzymes at home. To teach postural drainage correctly, it is necessary to demonstrate through pictures and to have parents practice the technique. (See page 1191 for illustrations of postural drainage.)

Care of the sick child at home, while demanding of a patient's time and energy, also may be very satisfying. The initial stage of care following diagnosis seems to present the most problems for parents, since they are attempting to learn as much as they can about their child's disease and their responsibilities. At the same time, it is not unusual for the child to rebel against changes in diet and the interference of routines and playtimes for postural drainage.

Promoting Optimal Respiratory Function. Chest physical therapy, breathing exercises, and inhalation therapy are central to the treatment plan. The nurse helps coordinate the various components of therapy with other activities and nursing care. If therapy is being introduced to a newly diagnosed child, it is important to explain the purpose of the various aspects of treatment. A respiratory therapist may perform the treatments, but the nurse participates in the overall assessment of the child's tolerance of the treatments and their effectiveness. The various positions for chest physical therapy and the equipment involved in inhalation therapy may be frightening to a young child. The nurse supports the child and family as they adjust to the newness of the routines and discomforts of therapy by answering questions and keeping the child as comfortable as possible.

Parents and the patient (when appropriate for age) are taught how to carry out the procedures since they must be done every day. Exercises can be taught to children to help oxygenation. In the young child, breathing exercises take on the form of a game, such as blowing soap bubbles or blowing out candles. Older children are encouraged to place their hands over the upper and lower portion of their chest to feel movement as they inhale and exhale.

Children with a chronic chest condition frequently develop poor posture. Daily exercises that help maintain good posture include back extension, shoulder exercises, and standing erect against a wall (Mallinson, 1978). Another important part of therapy for the child with CF is swimming or hydrotherapy. This type of exercise helps build the muscles of respiration while encouraging good breathing habits. Children and adolescents are encouraged to participate in sports and activities that promote good breathing habits.

When children with known CF are admitted to the hospital for care, it is important to let the child and parents adopt a routine that is similar to the one they usually follow at home. Letting the child and parents be responsible for as much of the treatments as possible is a way to foster independence and responsibility and avoid making them feel powerless.

Preventing Pulmonary Infection. The nurse ensures that the child and parents understand the importance of taking antibiotics for the prescribed course of treatment. During acute infections, antibiotics may be administered parenterally. The nurse may be involved in preparing families to administer intravenous antibiotics at home since this practice is generally gaining acceptance (Rosenstein, 1988).

Recurrent infections may result in frequent hospitalizations. Children may feel discouraged during bouts of pulmonary infection and need encouragement from the nurse to be cooperative in the full medical regimen. The usual treatments as done at home are continued, with an increase in the amount of percussion and postural drainage because of the decreased activity of the child. Mucolytic drugs may also be necessary to liquefy mucus during these periods of acute illness.

Measures to prevent pulmonary exacerbations are an important aspect of management. While unrestricted living style is the goal, some precautions should be taken to avoid exposure to respiratory infection. Avoiding large crowds during the flu season and avoiding contact with individuals who obviously have a respiratory infection may limit some exposure. Flu immunizations are strongly recommended on a yearly basis (Larter, 1981).

Promoting Optimal Nutrition. The underlying problem in children with cystic fibrosis is the inability of the pancreas to produce sufficient amounts of the enzymes to digest protein, fat, and carbohydrates adequately. Some cystic fibrosis centers are no longer imposing dietary restrictions. The rationale is to provide a better psychologic adjustment for the children, especially for those who are at an age when peer relationships and independence are important. The suggested

* National Cystic Fibrosis Foundation, 6000 Executive Blvd., Suite 309, Rockville, MD 20852.

alternative is to increase enzymes to match intake. Experience has shown that older children are able to determine for themselves what their systems can best handle and decide what needs to be eliminated. During acute illness, the child may become anorexic and the diet ordered may be restrictive. Ensuring adequate calorie intake is essential and usually requires the assistance of a nutritionist.

Enzymes should be mixed with carbohydrate foods (applesauce is often used) and administered at the beginning of the meal or snack. Enzymes are not mixed with protein foods because proteins would immediately be broken down and the mixture would become watery. Breakdown of skin can occur if enzymes remain on the lips or skin for an extended period of time.

MCT oil preparations are usually unpalatable to older children* but can be readily mixed into food or formula for infants.

Promoting Adaptive Individual and Family Coping. **Recognizing Common Stressors.** Major stresses are fears related to suffocation or dying while asleep, embarassment associated with odorous flatulence and stools, and the agony of engaging in the daily time-consuming activity of bronchial drainage (Dushenko, 1981). With the increasing life expectancy of these children, the family and the child will need additional support as adolescence is approached. The older school-age child and adolescent may require reevaluation for the need for more information. A child who grows up with a disease needs additional information as cognition expands and as new problems are encountered through the various developmental stages. The effect of the disease on physical appearance, the inadequacies surrounding sexuality, and the fear of diminished job opportunities become meaningful as the child matures. The shortened life expectancy and facts about the disease are reconsidered at this time. An adolescent may require individual or group therapy to cope successfully with the illness during this stage of development.

The family as a unit must adapt to the hardships imposed by the disease. The severe financial strain on the family budget, interruption of family routine, intrafamily communication breakdown, social isolation, sexual difficulties, and general depression are some of the usual problems. It has been found, however, that by the end of the first year after diagnosis, life becomes less stressful for the parents of CF children (Venters, 1981). Negative emotions subside, and a degree of reorganization in daily family activities is established.

* Recipes for using medium-chain triglyceride (MCT) oil are available from Mead Johnson and Company, Evansville, IN 47701.

Identifying Ways to Enhance Family Functions. The family is better integrated and functions more effectively when both parents are involved in the care of the child (Dushenko, 1981). Venters (1981) identified two coping strategies that strengthen family functioning throughout the years of coping with CF: "endowing the illness with meaning" and "sharing the burdens of the illness." A pre-existing religious or medical-scientific philosophy of life helped give meaning to the crises of CF and in addition such families viewed hardships with optimism (focused on the best qualities of the situation). Coping by "sharing the burdens of the illness" contrasts with the negative family response of social isolation. Families that shared the care of the CF child among family members and with someone outside the family demonstrated the highest level of family functioning. Health professionals therefore encourage families to share the care of their child.

Assessing the Impact of CF on Siblings. The impact of CF on siblings has received little study. The usual stresses of siblings are that attention to them suffers and that discipline is unequal, with the ill child favored. Siblings may feel guilty because of their resentment and jealousy. They may fear contracting the disease; they fear the death of their sibling and may feel guilty because they are healthy (Harder and Bowditch, 1982). Interviews of 19 siblings (aged 7 to 16) of CF patients revealed that there was also a potential for positive growth (Harder and Bowditch, 1982). None of the siblings believed that CF had caused their families to draw apart. On the contrary, some children reported that having a sibling with CF had helped them be less self-centered and had increased their ability to be more sensitive to people who are ill and to cope with difficult situations. The findings from this study emphasize the need for individual assessment of each family situation. The potential for a negative response from siblings is certainly present, but the potential for positive growth for many children must be considered and maximized.

Nursing Strategies for Follow-Up Care in the Home or Clinic

Plot height and weight on the growth curve and assess for steady progress.

Assess vital signs, breath sounds, and energy available to perform usual activities of daily living.

Determine effectiveness of expectoration with home chest physical therapy and inhalation therapy.

Ask the child and parent about gastrointestinal symptoms that would indicate inadequate enzyme replacement: bloating, abdominal cramping and distention, and diarrhea (Lester and Rothberg, 1986).

Have the child and parent record the dietary intake for the previous 24 hours to assess nutrient and caloric adequacy.

When appropriate, determine compliance with prescribed antibiotic therapy.

Encourage the child and parent to discuss psychosocial and developmental concerns and to ask questions about the technical aspects of home management.

Bronchopulmonary Dysplasia

Bronchopulmonary dysplasia (BPD) is an iatrogenic chronic lung disease that develops in premature infants following a period of intensive respiratory therapy. In the past, infants born prematurely either died or recovered fully during the first few days of life; few infants survived to develop residual lung disease. Improvement in the survival rate of very low birthweight infants has resulted in the emergence of respiratory insufficiency in the perinatal period, followed by chronic lung disease in subsequent years (Saigal and O'Brodovich, 1987).

Lifesaving measures and intensive therapy of these infants is confined to the specialty area of neonatal intensive care; long-term care is provided by nurses in clinics, on general pediatric inpatient units, through public health agencies, in schools, and in the child's home. The survival of these infants presents a new health care challenge.

Incidence

The wide variation in the reported incidence of BPD (5 to 68 per cent) is primarily due to the lack of consistency in defining BPD. Incidence is particularly high in premature infants treated with mechanical ventilation for respiratory distress. The more immature the infant, the more likelihood that chronic lung changes will occur (Brown, 1987).

Overall, the incidence of BPD has increased because of the increased survival rate of very low birthweight infants (Monin and Vert, 1987). However, it is not established that chronic lung disease is associated with hyaline membrane disease itself. The incidence of BPD in infants with respiratory distress syndrome (RDS) who receive intermittent positive pressure ventilation (IPPV) and survive varies between 10 and 20 per cent. The incidence of infants surviving with milder forms of chronic lung damage is much higher (Bancalari and Gerhardt, 1986).

Etiology/Pathophysiology

The triggering events of BPD are oxygen-related injury and barotrauma (trauma associated with mechanical ventilation) in an infant who is susceptible because of the surfactant-deficient state of the respiratory distress syndrome (RDS). Some evidence indicates that the presence of an endotracheal tube alone can cause mechanical damage to the tracheal epithelium (Sinkin and Phelps, 1987). Onset appears to be within minutes to hours after birth.

Other factors that place the infant at risk for BPD are meconium aspiration, persistent pulmonary hypertension, congenital pneumonia, pulmonary edema from a patent ductus arteriosus (PDA), excessive fluid administration, and any disorders that require prolonged mechanical ventilation in neonates.

The relative role of oxygen as a causative factor in BPD is debated in the literature and remains unclear (Sinkin and Phelps, 1987). Exposure of immature lungs to inhalation of high oxygen concentrations is thought to damage the protective system of the lungs. Existing alveolar Type I cells are damaged and replaced with poorly functioning Type II alveolar cells. This pathologic response results in an alveolar-capillary leak.

Edema and inflammation of the capillary bed and alveolar wall interfere with lung function. Some of the alveoli collapse while others are overinflated. Tissue cells in the lung are infiltrated with polymorphonuclear leukocytes that release free oxygen radicals and protease (a proteolytic enzyme). As a result of the collection of proteinaceous debris in the alveoli, any surfactant that is present is inactivated. (See page 1168 for discussion of the role of surfactant in the alveoli.)

The presence of edema and inflammation in the lungs makes the lung tissue more susceptible to barotrauma. Barotrauma causes alveolar rupture, leading to interstitial emphysema, pneumothorax, and airway damage. The combined effect of high oxygen concentrations and barotrauma thus damages the small airways and cells of the alveolar lining. This causes an increased capillary permeability and leakage of plasma proteins and fluid into the alveoli and interstitium.

Prolonged respiratory failure can lead to right heart failure secondary to pulmonary hypertension with cardiomegaly, hepatomegaly, and fluid retention. Right ventricular hypertrophy, cardiac enlargement, edema, and venous congestion are a consequence of pulmonary vasoconstriction (pulmonary vasocontriction is the result of hypoxemia). Cardiac involvement is also related to the presence of a patent ductus arteriosus (PDA) because of left-to-right shunting through a PDA and associated pulmonary edema.

Clinical Manifestations and Diagnostic Assessment

Clinical manifestations of BPD vary widely, with most infants exhibiting signs of respiratory distress such as wheezes, crackles, retractions, copious secretions, and cyanosis upon crying, agitation, or stress. The fussiness and irritability commonly seen in these infants is likely associated with the instability in arterial oxygen levels and transient hypoxia.

The diagnosis of BPD is based on clinical and radiographic characteristics, but no *specific* clinical signs or laboratory results confirm the diagnosis. It is characterized by hypoxia, hypercapnia, and oxygen dependence with a diagnostic chest radiograph. Stages of BPD have been described progressing from Stage I to Stage IV with mild, moderate, severe, and advanced-chronic phases. These stages were first described by Northway and colleagues (1967). Toce and colleagues (1984) have developed a BPD clinical scoring system including measures of gas exchange, respiratory distress criteria, growth parameters, and a chest radiograph assessment to be used at 21 days of age.

A variety of criteria are used to diagnose BPD:

- Intermittent positive pressure ventilation (IPPV) was required during the first week of life for at least 3 days.
- Clinical evidence of chronic respiratory distress persisting beyond around 30 days of age.
- Supplemental oxygen requirement for more than 28 days to maintain a PaO_2 over 50 mm Hg.
- An abnormal chest radiograph showing hyperinflation, dense linear opacities, and scattered hyperlucent foci (translucent cysts).

Other tests that contribute to the diagnosis are an electrocardiogram and an echocardiogram to confirm the diagnosis of hypertrophy of a ventricle, and pulmonary function tests to evaluate the degree of interference in lung function. Lung compliance and functional residual capacity (FRC) are found to be low and airway resistance is high (Scherf, 1985).

Therapeutic Management

Avoidance of the factors that contribute to BPD is the key to prevention. Precautions are taken to *prevent* respiratory distress syndrome and to *reduce* barotrauma and oxygen toxicity.

Prevention by Drug Therapy. Numerous research studies concerning prevention of BPD are underway. These include administration of dexamethasone to induce maturation of surfactant synthesis prior to premature birth (Roberts and Morrison, 1985; Avery, 1984), surfactant replacement therapy (Merritt et al, 1986; Avery, 1986), and the administration of antioxidants to reduce oxygen toxicity (i.e., vitamin E, N-acetylcysteine, and superoxide dismutase). Surfactant replacement therapy is a promising therapeutic approach that is being researched widely and has been shown to be beneficial in treating neonatal RDS (Notter and Shapiro, 1987). Formulation of synthetic lung surfactant that has negligible toxicity and is as effective as human lung surfactant is the goal of current research.

Monitored Ventilation and Oxygen Administration to Prevent BPD. Since barotrauma and oxygen toxicity contribute to the development of BPD, mechanical ventilation and oxygen administration are necessarily managed meticulously. The goal is to use the lowest inspired oxygen concentration and the lowest peak pressures and mean airway pressure that will maintain adequate gas exchange. Short inspiratory times (0.3 to 0.5 second) are recommended to reduce risk for BPD.

The acceptable range of blood gas levels to prevent BPD is to maintain $PaCO_2$ at 35 to 45 mm Hg and PaO_2 at 50 to 70 mm Hg. However, higher $PaCO_2$ levels may be acceptable to prevent excessively high inspired FiO_2 concentration and mean airway pressure.

New concepts in ventilation, introduced in the early 1980s, use greater-than-normal breathing frequencies. High-frequency oscillatory ventilation (rates of 300 to 800 per minute) and high-frequency jet ventilation are used in some cases with the aim to reduce mean airway pressure and tidal volumes and thus reduce barotrauma. These high-frequency methods have not yet demonstrated a reduced incidence of BPD despite encouraging results (Monin and Vert, 1987). (See Table 38-2.)

An infant must be weaned from the ventilator gradually, with careful monitoring of fluids to avoid pulmonary interstitial fluid and pulmonary resistance. Diuretics and intermittent mandatory ventilation (IMV) are often used during the weaning process. IMV means that mechanical ventilations are at slow rates, allowing for spontaneous respirations between the ventilator-driven breaths.

Bronchodilators (theophylline) and salbutamol (albuterol) may shorten the duration of ventilator weaning by decreasing airway resistance and increasing compliance. The ability of the infant to tolerate weaning is evaluated by the stability of pH, $PaCO_2$, and PaO_2 during the period of progressive reduction of ventilator settings.

Fluid Therapy. Fluid restriction may be required to reduce pulmonary congestion and prevent cardiac failure. Diuretic therapy may be beneficial in chronic lung disease. Frequently used diuretics include

- furosemide (Lasix), 1 to 2 mg/kg/day given in a single dose, IV or PO
- spironolactone (Aldactone), 3 to 6 mg/kg/day given in divided doses every 12 hours
- chlorothiazide (Diuril), 10 to 40 mg/kg/day given in divided doses every 12 hours PO

Chronic administration of furosemide requires monitoring as it results in urinary losses of calcium and can contribute to the development of osteopenia of prematurity (Monin and Vert, 1987) and renal calcification as a result of hypercalciuria. The use of chlorothiazide in combination with furosemide decreases urinary calcium excretion (Korones, 1988).

Adequate Oxygenation During Chronic Lung Disease. Adequate and stable oxygenation is required for the growth of the lung tissue and the healing process. Oxygen is administered in a variety of ways during the chronic phase, including Oxyhood, nasal cannula, or pharyngeal catheter (for FiO_2 above 35 per cent).

Nutrition. Very low birthweight infants have a functional limitation of the gastrointestinal tract, yet require a greater proportionate calorie intake compared to an older child. In the early phase of respiratory distress, calorie requirements are 50 to 70 cal per kg per day. These infants have a higher metabolic rate, secondary to BPD, therefore fluid overload may become a problem.

In the convalescent phase, the calorie needs are 120 to 130 cal per kg per day (Monin and Vert, 1987). Nutritional requirements are met through total parenteral nutrition (TPN) early in treatment and later on by nasogastric tube, gavage, and breast or bottle feedings.

Major Nursing Diagnoses for Bronchopulmonary Dysplasia

***Impaired gas exchange,** related to:*
- *alveolar-capillary membrane damage associated with oxygen toxicity and barotrauma*
- *atelectasis associated with surfactant deficiency*

***Ineffective breathing pattern,** related to:*
- *decreased lung expansion (compliance) associated with fibrotic changes*
- *fatigue and decreased energy associated with hypoxia*
- *inflammatory process associated with secondary respiratory infection*

***Potential for infection,** related to inadequate primary defense, associated with fibrotic lung changes of BPD*

***Altered nutrition: less than body requirements,** related to:*
- *25 per cent increase in metabolic rate associated with increased respiratory effort (Hodgman, 1986)*
- *feeding difficulties associated with dyspnea*
- *increased calorie expenditure associated with work of breathing*

***Potential altered fluid volume: excess,** related to increased work load of the right side of the heart, associated with increased pulmonary interstitial fluid*

***Altered cardiac output,** related to:*
- *cardiac failure associated with presence of a left-to-right shunt (in the presence of a PDA)*
- *cardiac failure associated with pulmonary vasoconstriction (pulmonary hypertension) due to hypoxemia*
- *cor pulmonale associated with pulmonary edema and right ventricular hypertrophy*

***Altered growth and development,** related to:*
- *reduced oxygenation associated with fibrotic lung changes*
- *overprotection from caretakers and significant others associated with BPD*
- *lack of adequate stimulation and developmentally appropriate activities*
- *prolonged and frequent hospitalization*

***Potential ineffective family coping: compromised,** related to:*
- *the stresses of long-term intensive management of BPD at home*
- *inadequate support systems*
- *inadequate information about the care of the infant*

Strategies for Nursing Care

Intensive care of the infant at risk for BPD is described in neonatal intensive care literature. The focus of this discussion is management of the infant with chronic lung disease.

Maintaining Adequate Oxygenation. Assessment of the infant's respiratory status is an important function of the nurse. Changes in the infant's clinical presentation are evaluated in relation to other diagnostic findings such as chest radiographs and blood gases.

As airway damage progresses, a barrel chest is apparent; oxygenation becomes more difficult and CO_2 retention increases. Careful assessment for increased signs of respiratory distress and close monitoring of blood gases are required. An increase in pulmonary vascular pressure is generally observed when arterial PaO_2 drops below 55 mm Hg (Monin and Vert, 1987). Special attention is also given to maintaining the infant's body temperature because hypothermia and hyperthermia increase oxygen consumption. During stress (feeding, crying, suctioning, and any procedures), oxygen may need to be temporarily increased. Home care issues concerning oxygenation are summarized in Box 38-7.

Preventing Infection. Children with BPD are at risk for lower respiratory tract infections. Parents are counseled to avoid close proximity with those who are known to have a respiratory infection and to seek early treatment of any signs of respiratory distress in their infant. Chest physical therapy and suctioning may be necessary for removal of secretions to prevent infections. See Box 38-7 for issues to discuss with parents regarding home care.

Maintaining Adequate Nutritional Intake. The nurse monitors the caloric intake of these infants to ensure adequate growth. Early in the phase of treatment, intake is parenteral. Because fluid overload complicates BPD, the required caloric intake cannot be easily achieved, therefore formula that contains 24- or 30-cal per ounce may be required. Home care issues to be raised with parents are summarized in Box 38-7.

Maintaining Fluid Balance. Fluid intake and output are monitored and infants are weighed daily because they are at risk for development of pulmonary edema. Caloric requirements must be met in the lowest volume of fluids possible. Any increase in respiratory or heart rate; retractions; cyanosis; change in chest sounds, such as the presence or increase of rales; or a

Box 38-7

Common Issues to Discuss with Parents Concerning Home Care Management of Child with Bronchopulmonary Dysplasia

MAINTAINING FLUID AND NUTRITIONAL BALANCE

Oxygen administration during feeding is usually necessary because of the work of breathing and sucking.

Infants with cardiac involvement may require fluid restriction.

Sometimes the use of MCT (medium-chain triglycerides) or 24- or 30-calorie per ounce formulas are required to meet caloric needs for growth.

Occasional gavage feedings may be necessary if baby is especially tired; therefore, parents may need to learn this type of feeding.

PREVENTING INFECTION

The usual preventive measures appropriate for a child with a chronic respiratory problem must be stressed: avoidance of smoking near the infant, avoidance of close proximity with those known to have a respiratory infection, and early treatment of signs of respiratory illness in the infants.

Careful feeding techniques to avoid aspiration are taught to parents as a way to reduce risk of infection.

Chest physical therapy and suctioning need to be increased for removal of secretions from the lungs to prevent lower respiratory infections.

Bronchodilators (by inhalation) for wheezing may be required, especially during respiratory infections. Parents must be helped to secure the equipment from a supply company and be taught proper administration.

MAINTAINING OXYGENATION

The oxygen-dependent infant or child usually can tolerate a cannula for oxygen administration. It can be taped to a stoma-adhesive patch (see Figure 38-3). This needs to be changed only once a week and protects the skin (Koops et al, 1984). A nasopharyngeal catheter is used for oxygen concentration of 35 per cent or greater.

Oxygen for home care is supplied by concentrates, tanks, or liquid oxygen systems. Of these, the concentrates seem to be preferred because no tank changing is necessary. However, the availability of liquid oxygen enables portability; therefore, it is usually also provided.

Chest physical therapy and suctioning may be required three to four times a day. Parents must have had supervised practice and demonstrate the necessary skills.

MAINTAINING FAMILY COPING

Even with excellent preparation for home care and the support of community resources, the family should be prepared for common problems, identified by Voyles (1981) to include:

Lack of identified support system. The nurse should encourage the family to find a few support people to help them during this period of adjustment.

The interruption of family life may sometimes lead to marital stress. A competent baby sitter should be taught how to care for the infant to allow parents to have time together and to themselves.

Parents should have an understanding about the illness, recognizing that respiratory infections may require readmission to the hospital but this does not mean they have failed.

decrease in breath sounds is an indication of increased respiratory difficulty and possible pulmonary edema.

Maintaining Adequate Cardiac Output. When an infant is in cardiac failure, fluid intake and output are very strictly monitored, as is the infant's weight. Episodes of stress are avoided by adopting a "minimal touch" policy organizing nursing care and tests to reduce interruptions of the infant's rest.

Fostering Normal Growth and Development. Prolonged respiratory dysfunction has been found to be associated with growth retardation (Markestadt and Fitzhardinge, 1981). Infants with BPD often have severe visual impairment, poor growth, recurrent respiratory infections, and frequent hospitalizations (Saigal and O'Brodovich, 1987). Parents need to understand the effects of BPD on growth and development to avoid the worry and self-blame that might occur if they feel these delays are related to their inadequate care. Parents are aided in providing adequate nutrition that will promote growth (see section on normal nutrition in Box 38-7). Although no controlled studies demonstrate the effectiveness of programs for sensory stimulation and movement and motor patterns, such interventions are prevalent in clinical practice. In one study, individualization of behavioral and environmental care for very low birthweight infants at risk for developing BPD has been shown to reduce the length of ventilation time and oxygen requirements and improve behavioral organization and mental development at 9 months of age (Als et al, 1986).

Whether a formal stimulation program is instituted or not, as soon after birth as possible nurses encourage parents to stroke, hold, and talk to their infant. Slow motor development, hypotonia or hypertonia, and asymmetry of movement frequently make it necessary for parents to perform specific exercises in the home; however, many of these children have normal development for corrected age, after some initial lag.

Promoting Adaptive Family Coping. The problems associated with BPD demand the services of a dedicated interdisciplinary team and care by a family that is able and willing to commit a large proportion of time and energy to their child. Multidisciplinary care begins immediately upon diagnosis, recognizing the scope and complexity of needs represented by these children and their families. Home management of a child with BPD often involves sending an oxygen-dependent child home, which presents a challenge to the nurse. Early involvement of the parents in the care of their infant, accompanied by ongoing teaching regarding the nature of the lung problem, is essential for successful management in the home.

Parents should be prepared for the extent of care that will be required of them at home. The preparation for discharge involves all team members and a coordination of efforts to facilitate consistency of instructions. An ongoing assessment of the parent's ability to care for the child and comfort in doing so provides the necessary information to determine readiness for discharge. Even after they realize the extent of care that is required, parents must still want to care for their child at home and demonstrate capability to do so.

Factors to be evaluated when home care is being considered include:

- Weight gain. A steady weight gain should be demonstrated, and the baby should weigh > 2 kg.
- Complexity of care (nurse should evaluate parents' ability to feed infant, frequency of feedings, number of medications, and need for chest physical therapy and suctioning).
- Percentage of supplemental oxygen required. Maintenance of transcutaneous oxygenation at 55 torr during care giving, feedings, and sleep is recommended.

The nurse collaborates with other health team members to evaluate the complexity of care and the realistic goals that can be set for home care. Some families are too overwhelmed to learn to care for their baby at home in the time that is expected by the health care team. The most important outcome is that parents will enjoy their child and establish a loving, trusting relationship with the baby (Koops et al, 1984). Consequently, a highly individualistic approach must be taken in assessing the appropriateness of home care for a child with BPD.

The first visit after discharge is recommended at 1 week and the second visit 1 to 2 weeks thereafter. Interdisciplinary care must continue to provide the necessary support and evaluation of progress. The anticipated problems encountered in children with BPD are summarized in Box 38-7.

Prognosis

With supportive care many of these infants seem to recover by growing new lung tissue. However, some infants with BPD continue to have poor health, with numerous hospital admissions for respiratory infections. Most studies show that infants with BPD have a higher incidence of neurodevelopmental disorders and developmental lag compared with other very low birthweight infants (Saigal and O'Brodovich), although they tend to improve after the first 2 to 3 years of life (Sauve and Singhol, 1985). Pulmonary problems also tend to decline during the first 2 to 3 years of life; however, the long-term pulmonary function of these infants remains to be determined (Markstad and Fitz-

Box 38-8
Definitions and Terminology for Apnea

APNEA

Cessation of respiratory air flow due to the following causes:

- central or diaphragmatic
- obstructive (usually upper airway)
- mixed

Central apnea of ≤ 15 seconds can be normal at all ages.

PATHOLOGIC APNEA

A respiratory pause that is 20 seconds or longer or is associated with the following:

- cyanosis
- abruptness
- marked pallor or hypotonia
- bradycardia

PERIODIC BREATHING

A breathing pattern in which there are three or more respiratory pauses of greater than 3 seconds' duration and which occur less than 20 seconds apart. Periodic breathing can be a normal event.

APNEA OF PREMATURITY

Periodic breathing with pathologic apnea in a premature infant. Apnea of prematurity usually ceases by 37 weeks' gestation but can persist for several weeks past term.

APPARENT LIFE-THREATENING EVENT (ALTE)

This event is frightening to the observer; it is characterized by some combination of the following:

- apnea
- color change (cyanotic, pale, or on occasion reddened)
- marked change in muscle tone (limpness usually)
- choking or gagging

Terminology such as "aborted crib death" or "near-miss SIDS" should not be used because these terms make an association between the event and SIDS that could be incorrect.

APNEA OF INFANCY

This term usually refers to infants greater than 37 weeks' gestation at onset.

An unexplained cessation of breathing for 20 seconds or longer or a respiratory pause of shorter duration but that is associated with the following:

- bradycardia
- cyanosis
- pallor and/or marked hypotonia

hardinge, 1981). The ultimate outcome of infants with BPD is unknown, since follow-up studies are few and none of these children have yet reached adulthood (Sinkin and Phelps, 1987).

Nursing Strategies for Follow-Up Care in the Home or Clinic

Weigh and measure the infant and plot parameters on a growth curve to assess respiratory and nutritional adequacy.

Assess progress on developmental tasks.

Assess vital signs, breath sounds, and energy for feeding and playing to screen for respiratory competency and for signs of infection.

Discuss with the parent the infant's tolerance of increased-calorie formula, i.e., retention versus loss through wet burps or increased stooling.

Encourage the parent to voice concerns regarding growth and development, technical management, and stresses upon family functioning. Refer to available social services support system as appropriate.

Apnea-Related Disorders

Apnea of Prematurity

Apnea of prematurity is differentiated from periodic breathing in Box 38-8. *Periodic breathing* is characteristic of premature infants and can be a normal event. When the pauses of periodic breathing are 20 or more seconds or when the pause is associated with other signs of distress (see Box 38-8), the episode is classified as *apnea of prematurity.* Apnea of prematurity usually is manifested at 1 or 2 days of age and resolves around 34 to 36 weeks' gestational age. Conversely, *apnea of infancy* occurs at or near term (onset of greater than 37 weeks' gestation) and is usually associated with serious causes (see Box 38-9 for the relation of apnea of infancy to apnea of prematurity).

As many as 25 per cent of all premature infants under 1800 grams (around 34 weeks' gestational age) will have at least one apneic episode. The incidence of apnea increases as gestational age decreases. Almost all premature infants under 30 weeks' gestational age will have occasional apneic spells.

Box 38-9
Relation of Apnea of Prematurity and Apnea of Infancy to Each Other and to Mortality in Infancy

No evidence exists that apnea of prematurity is an ***independent*** risk factor for infant apnea.

There is evidence that apnea of prematurity is ***not*** a risk factor of SIDS.

An ALTE is a risk factor for sudden death (including SIDS).

Infants with a history of ALTE or apnea of prematurity make up only a small proportion of total SIDS cases.

Etiology/Pathogenesis and Diagnostic Assessment

No single factor usually can be identified as the cause of apnea of prematurity. The respiratory control mechanisms and reflexes of the premature infant are immature, with characteristic responses, one of which is the response to hypoxia. Immature infants respond to hypoxia with an initial increase in respiratory effort, followed by periodic breathing, with eventual respiratory depression and apnea (Marchal et al, 1987). Hypoxia is thus suspected to be a primary factor that depresses the respiratory system, leading to apnea in the premature infant. As hypoxia increases, the ventilatory response to CO_2 decreases, a phenomenon which is the reverse of that of an older infant or an adult (Rigatto, 1982).

Stimulation of certain reflexes in the premature infant elicits responses different to those of an adult. Stimulation of receptors in the upper airway (especially laryngeal mucosa) produces apnea. This laryngeal reflex explains the apnea observed during tube feeding, upper airway suction, and gastric content regurgitation. Overheating or excessive cooling, poor positioning, and airway obstruction with mucus are additional stimuli that produce apnea.

The relationship of apnea to sleep is not entirely clear. Apnea is believed to be more common during REM (rapid eye movement) sleep and less common during quiet sleep and when waking. The more highly organized quiet state of sleep does not exist in the immature infant; the stimuli in an intensive care unit further disrupt a poorly organized circadian rhythm. Apnea in association with REM sleep may be due to an obstructive phenomenon associated with temporary loss of muscle tone in the upper airway structures (Corbet, 1983).

Apnea that persists without evidence of its cause is a perplexing problem. If apneic spells occur in the first few days of life, they are more commonly associated with an underlying disorder (Corbet, 1983), such as:

- Sepsis
- Metabolic disorders (hypoglycemia, hypocalcemia, hyponatremia)
- Anemia
- Patent ductus arteriosus
- Seizures
- Gastroesophageal reflux
- Central nervous system depression from drugs
- Intracranial hemorrhage
- Pulmonary disease

The diagnostic tests used vary according to the disorder being investigated. During the diagnostic phase, it is important for the nurse to carefully monitor and record apneic episodes, with a clear description of the degree of cyanosis and the degree of bradycardia, if any. It is also important for the nurse to note whether oropharyngeal secretions, gavage feedings, and suctioning are causing apneic spells. See next section on Apnea of Infancy for further discussion of diagnostic assessment.

Therapeutic Management

Premature infants considered to be at risk for apnea (those less than 32 weeks' gestational age or less than 1500 grams' birthweight) are placed on continuous cardiorespiratory monitors in neonatal intensive care units (Corbet, 1983).

Specialized nursing care is the major form of treatment for these infants, but if spells longer than 20 seconds occur more than three times a day, symptomatic therapy is instituted, including preventive stimulation, continuous positive airway pressure, and pharmacologic treatment.

Preventive stimulation can be provided in the form of cutaneous stimulation or by placing the infant on a water or rocking bed. Motion is thought to stimulate the labyrinthine passages and reduce apnea frequency (Marchal, 1987). *Continuous positive airway pressure (CPAP)* increases PaO_2, lung volume, and lung compliance and decreases the work of breathing, all of which contribute to reduced apneic episodes.

Pharmacologic therapy includes use of methylxanthines (oral theophylline or intravenous aminophylline). One of the ways that methylxanthines are thought to work is by increasing the ventilatory response to carbon dioxide; however, other mechanisms continue to be researched. Caffeine citrate also can be used to decrease the frequency of apneic episodes and may be less toxic (Aranda et al, 1983; Marchal, 1987).

Doxapram, a respiratory stimulant, may be useful if the treatment of apnea with other drugs is ineffective (Barrington et al, 1986). Home apnea monitoring may be indicated for some infants and is discussed in the next section, on Apnea of Infancy.

Major Nursing Diagnoses for Apnea of Prematurity

See Nursing Diagnoses and Nursing Strategies in the discussion that follows on Apnea of Infancy.

Apnea of Infancy

Incidence and Etiology

Apnea can also occur in healthy, full-term infants and is called *apnea of infancy.* Episodes of apnea that are frightening to the observer are called *apparent life threatening events (ALTE)* (see Box 38-8 for definition). Approximately 50 per cent of infants with apnea have diagnosable conditions; however, infants experiencing significant apnea without a known cause are thought to be at risk for *sudden infant death syndrome (SIDS)* (Spitzer and Fox, 1986). Apnea and SIDS have been linked because pathology findings suggest that SIDS infants have tissue changes consistent with chronic hypoxia. However, it must be understood that there are many other probable causes of SIDS and, conversely, apnea can be a symptom of many other underlying determinable conditions.

Diagnostic Assessment

The specific type of diagnostic testing is determined by the clinical indications and may include exploration of seizures, feeding problems, an infection, or other presenting clues to the etiology of apnea.

Detection of primary causes of apnea may require a period of hospitalization during which time the infant is placed on a cardiorespiratory monitor. A diagnostic workup may include a complete blood count, blood chemistry, chest film, electrocardiogram, and electroencephalogram. A specific test to evaluate for apnea is the pneumocardiogram, which simultaneously records heart rate and chest wall movements. However, these are not recommended as screening tools because their predictability has not been sufficiently documented.

Polysomnography (a sleep study) is a more elaborate study; it records brainwaves and movements of the eye and body, and measures oxygen. These tests, however, are not definitive for apnea of infancy.

Therapeutic Management

The most commonly used therapy for infants with apnea is home cardiorespiratory monitoring. Widespread controversy prevails about the indications for home monitoring. Certain circumstances clearly indicate the need for home monitoring. These include:

- Infants with one or more severe ALTEs requiring mouth-to-mouth resuscitation or vigorous stimulation.
- Symptomatic preterm infants.
- Siblings of two or more SIDS victims.
- Infants with certain diseases or conditions, such as central hypoventilation.

Situations in which the evidence is not conclusive include:

- Any sibling of a SIDS victim.
- Infants with less severe episodes of ALTE.
- Infants with tracheostomies.
- Infants with opiate- or cocaine-abusing mothers.

Before home monitoring is recommended, treatable causes of apnea are managed with appropriate therapy. In addition to home monitoring, a child with episodes of apnea or the preterm infant with apnea may require pharmacologic management (see section on Apnea of Prematurity for discussion of pharmacologic management).

The decision to discontinue home monitoring varies according to the individual circumstances. Box 38-10 lists the criteria used.

Major Nursing Diagnoses for Apnea

Ineffective breathing patterns, *related to*
- *a paradoxic failure in the premature infant to increase respirations in response to hypoxia*
- *recurrent cessation of breathing in the full-term infant associated with either known or unknown etiology*

Grieving, *related to the perceived loss of a healthy infant associated with the diagnosis of apnea*

Knowledge deficit, *related to*
- *the technical aspects of home apnea monitoring*
- *cardiopulmonary resuscitation*

Altered family processes, *related to*
- *anxiety associated with the threat of infant death*

Box 38-10
Criteria for Monitor Discontinuation in Apnea

Each of the following criteria are met:

- No life-threatening events requiring vigorous stimulation or resuscitation for 3 months OR no critical problems for 2 months following the present episode.
- No *real* monitor alarm for 2 months (with apnea setting at 20 seconds and heart rate at 60 beats per minute).
- Infant must have had an upper respiratory tract infection, or a DPT immunization, or another illness without a recurrence of apnea.
- Assessments (neurologic, developmental, and physical) must show that any initial reason for monitoring has resolved.
- No significant abnormalities on cardiorespiratory recordings.

(Adapted from Ariagno, 1984.)

- *feelings of inadequacy associated with home management*
- *difficulty in obtaining babysitters*
- *feelings of isolation and social deprivation*
- *difficulty in meeting the demands of other children*

Strategies for Nursing Care

Maintaining Effective Breathing Patterns. Nursing strategies to prevent and reduce the frequency of apnea during the acute phase of care are numerous. Precautions are taken in the method of handling and positioning of infants and the manner in which procedures are carried out. Hyperflexion of the neck is avoided to maintain maximal air entry. Placing infants in the prone position is associated with higher oxygen tension and shorter gastric emptying and reduces the frequency of regurgitation and aspiration.

Procedures that can produce apnea include suctioning and orogastric feedings. Pharyngeal suctioning is done gently and for the shortest time and least number of times possible. An orogastric tube must be carefully inserted; sudden gastric distention is avoided to reduce the likelihood of regurgitation (Marchal et al, 1987).

The environment should be maintained at a comfortable temperature, with avoidance of extremes. If oxygen is administered via a hood, it should be warmed to incubator temperature.

Supporting the Family in the Initial Period of Grief. Whenever an infant requires home monitoring, parents can be expected to go through a grieving process because they experience the loss of their perfect child. The dilemma that must be faced is that home apnea monitoring is potentially stress-producing for the family, yet its use is recommended even though there are no data from which to conclude that home monitoring reduces the incidence of SIDS (Weinstein and Steinschneider, 1983).

Teaching to Support Home Care. In view of the limitations of our knowledge about the effectiveness of monitors to prevent SIDS, the major task confronting the health team is assisting the family to accept the ambiguities surrounding the diagnosis of being "at risk" for SIDS. The decision to place the infant on a monitor must be explained to the family. The nurse participates in the process of providing the explanation and handles ongoing doubts and questions that are raised by parents.

It is a team responsibility to prepare the family for all aspects of home monitoring. Parents are taught to use the monitor, respond to an alarm, and perform cardiopulmonary resuscitation (CPR). Video tapes provide the opportunity for extended family members and baby sitters to also learn the technique.

In one study, the greatest reported concern of mothers about their preparation for home monitoring was their ability to get to the baby and intervene effectively (Dimaggio and Sheetz, 1983). Recognizing the anxiety and concern that parents have regarding performing CPR, the nurse encourages expression of these fears in preparing parents.

Promoting Effective Family Functioning. The long-term psychologic impact of home monitoring has not been studied. In a short-term follow-up by Cain and associates (1980), families reported being most anxious during the first week of home monitoring and stated that during this time they felt the greatest need for support. The inability to secure baby sitters for their infant, including family and friends, was a universal complaint. The greatest support was derived from spouses. Physicians and nurses in the community were reported to know "much about medicine but little about monitoring." In a study of 29 mothers by Dimaggio and Sheetz (1983), mothers emphasized that during the preparation for home monitoring the importance of learning to relax and reducing tension should be given priority. These mothers identified a variety of sources for their tension. They reported fears about the monitor malfunctioning, feelings of isolation and social deprivation, and difficulty in meeting the demands of their other children. They also had difficulty carrying out household tasks and taking care of themselves. It is also important to note that Cain and colleagues (1980) reported that 75 per cent of parents stated that home monitoring provided some relief from their anxiety and only 20 per cent reported that they remained anxious after the first month.

Heightened levels of anxiety have also been reported by Lyman and co-workers (1985), whereas McElroy et al (1986) did not find a difference in the anxiety of two groups of mothers at 12 weeks or 1 year after the birth of their infant who required home apnea monitoring.

Further research is required to understand the ongoing needs of families who monitor their infants at home. A thorough teaching approach to help parents learn how to operate the monitor, assess the infant, and perform CPR is essential. In addition to the technical aspects of preparation, responding to the psychosocial aspects of home monitoring, based on current research findings, should be considered. An *adequate support system* (family members and baby sitters) that can provide respite care, an *open communication system with a knowledgeable health care* team to discuss concerns and fears, and *contact with a parents' group* or telephone network with other parents who have monitored their infants should be incorporated. *Home visiting by a community health nurse* is essential to provide the necessary assessment of the family's adjustment to home monitoring. It is especially important that a health care professional intervene during the first week, when the highest level of anxiety is being experienced by the family. Ongoing assessments and interventions should focus on maintaining the infant's health status, restoring the mother's physical condition, establishing normal parent-infant relationships, and optimal family functioning.

Nursing Strategies for Follow-Up Care in the Home or Clinic

Perform a routine well-baby physical assessment (see Chapter 15), including plotting growth parameters.

Determine whether any apneic spells have occurred. Ask about their duration and whether stimulation (e.g., gentle shaking) was necessary to initiate resumption of respirations.

If in the home, examine monitoring equipment for proper function. Encourage the parent to discuss concerns about equipment operation. Act as a liaison with the equipment supplier as needed.

Encourage the parent to discuss family functioning in regard to apnea monitoring. Refer to parent support groups as available.

Sudden Infant Death Syndrome (SIDS)

Sudden infant death syndrome (SIDS) has been defined by the Second International Conference on Causes of Sudden Death in Infants as the sudden death of any infant or young child, which is unexpected by history, and in which a thorough postmortem examination fails to demonstrate an adequate cause for death (Bergman et al, 1970). Although sudden infant death syndrome (also called crib death or cot death) has only in recent years been described as a specific syndrome, its existence has been noted since biblical times. In spite of significant research advances, the cause of SIDS remains elusive. Research findings increasingly demonstrate that these infants as a group may be different from normal anatomically, histologically, chemically, and even physiologically (Valdes-Dapena and Steinschneider, 1983).

Incidence and Etiology

Approximately one third of all deaths occurring in infants from the ages of 1 week to 1 year are the result of SIDS. During the third and fourth months of life, the condition apparently accounts for more than one half of all infant mortality. The general risk is 2 : 1000 live births, but occurrence varies with ethnic background. Although American Indians and blacks are reported to be at greater risk for SIDS, the determining factor is believed to be socioeconomic status, not race (Valdes-Dapena and Steinschneider, 1983). The recurrence risk in siblings of SIDS is now thought to be 4 : 1000. Almost every study has shown a male preponderance.

A variety of epidemiologic factors have been investigated in relationship to the incidence of SIDS. Many theories emerge that are well publicized by the media—often prior to the completion of the scientific research. Parents of SIDS victims who are exposed to the publicity may grasp each theory as it comes along as an answer to questions regarding the death of their infant. It is essential that the nurses keep abreast of current research so that they can provide accurate information. Nurses must learn to discriminate between sensationalized reports that are essentially opinion sharing and sound, reproducible research findings.

No single predictive or diagnostic criterion can be employed to identify those at risk for SIDS. However, some demographic and environmental factors, and characteristics of the infant and mother, have been identified as probable risk factors.

Demographic and Environmental Risk Factors. SIDS can occur in any family but is more frequent in families who are poor or live in crowded housing. It is reasonable to suspect that maternal health and prenatal care are the critical factors underlying this association. The temporal distribution of SIDS shows a seasonal variation, with the peak incidence during the coldest months of the year and the fewest cases during the summer months. The SIDS event often occurs during the normal period of sleep. SIDS infants have been found in car seats or strollers, but most generally death occurs in the crib or parents' bed.

Characteristics of the Infant. SIDS babies are usually well developed and apparently normal and healthy. In some instances there is a history of preterm birth, low Apgar scores, the need for oxygen and resuscitation at birth, or intrauterine growth retardation. It has also been reported that infants in multiple births (especially if born second or third) are at greater risk for SIDS (Kelly and Shannon, 1982). Some evidence suggests that simultaneous deaths in twins occurs, but further research into this phenomenon must be conducted. Neonatal characteristics identified retrospectively that were found to be associated with SIDS include jitteriness and irritability, feeding difficulties, growth lag, and muscle hypotonicity. These risk factors and infant characteristics are present in vast numbers of infants who do not succumb to SIDS; furthermore, not all SIDS victims have had these problems.

Characteristics of the Mother. Some of the maternal risk factors associated with SIDS are related to fetal environment. Reported maternal risk factors include severe anemia, cigarette smoking, third trimester bleeding, and maternal sedation or anesthesia. Infants of mothers who use methadone (dolophine HCl) are at ten times the usual risk for dying from SIDS (Herbst et al, 1988). Maternal age is a risk factor, with the highest rate of SIDS occurring when mothers are less than 20 years of age. An inverse association of SIDS and maternal age may be an important clue to causation. Maternal nutrition during pregnancy has been suggested as an important direction for future research (Peterson, 1980).

Circumstances of the Event. There is no audible outcry at the approximate time of death. Even though death apparently occurs in silence, often evidence indicates activity prior to death. Often the parents find the infant face down, or with blankets pulled over the head, or wedged in a corner of the bed. Some infants are found face up with bedding clutched in their hands. These findings usually lead the caregivers to suspect suffocation and to feel guilty. The nurse must be aware of the developmental abilities of infants at various ages in order to reassure the parents and relatives of the unreasonableness of this hypothesis. The peak incidence of SIDS is 2 to 3 months of age, by which time the infant is able to reposition the head to maintain adequate ventilation. Also, evidence indicates that ordinary bedding is incapable of causing hypoxia to the point of suffocation. The suffocation hypothesis is also refuted by the fact that pathologic findings at autopsy are identical in SIDS cases regardless of the position in which the infant was found (Beckwith, 1978).

Theories of Causation. The conviction is growing that SIDS has multiple causes. It is difficult to stay abreast with the extensive research that is being conducted on causation. Parents may seek information or may have read in the popular literature or newspapers about the following causes of SIDS:

Feeding History. Early studies indicating that SIDS does not occur in breast-fed infants have since been refuted. Therefore, apparently no immunity to SIDS is passed to the infant from breast milk.

Infectious Disease. Because of the age distribution, the seasonal variations, the evidence of upper respiratory tract infections in SIDS victims, and the autopsy finding of mild inflammation, researchers are continuing to study this area of possible causation. A specific association has been identified between botulism and SIDS (4.3 per cent), but this requires further research (Arnon et al, 1978). Most studies exploring viral infections as a possible cause conclude that they do not *cause* SIDS but rather predispose the infant at risk (Shannon and Kelly, 1982).

Genetic Factors. No convincing evidence exists that SIDS is a genetic disease. Even though the risk of SIDS is increased four to ten times in the subsequent siblings of SIDS victims, genetic factors have not been shown to be the cause. It is suggested that intrauterine or extrauterine environmental deficits could be the associated factors of causation (Kelly and Shannon, 1982).

Apnea Hypothesis. The apnea hypothesis continues to be only speculative. It suggests that periods of apnea during sleep eventually may result in an apneic episode that results in SIDS. The question of carbon dioxide responsiveness of infants and parents has been evaluated in an attempt to identify a predictor for SIDS. The results of these studies have varied, but the majority of parents and siblings of SIDS victims have not shown an abnormal carbon dioxide responsiveness (Avery and Frantz, 1983).

A major body of research has developed in response to the belief that SIDS is associated with hypoxia and hypoxemia, a result of repeated apneic episodes. Naeye (1980) described subtle morphologic differences (seven tissue differences) between SIDS infants and control infants. These findings continue to be researched in an effort to understand the pathogenesis of SIDS.

The mechanism of the relationship between apnea and SIDS is not well substantiated. It is thought that a sleeping infant can become hypoxic with positional narrowing of the airway and respiratory inflammation. Additional factors such as autonomic-neurologic instability, the control of ventilation (Brady and McCann, 1986), and chemical factors such as pH balance, hypercalcemia, and others may place the hypoxic sleeping infant on the path toward obstructive apnea. The infant's floppy pharynx, the large muscular tongue, and neck flexion all may contribute to these obstructive episodes. The infant may either revert to normality after recuperating from an apneic episode or may die. The difficulty with this hypothesis is that infants who die from SIDS are almost invariably a "white" ashen color, not cyanotic as would be expected if obstruction were the cause.

Gastroesophageal Reflux (GER). Supporters of this hypothesis believe that reflux of gastric contents can cause a fatal reflex apnea. This hypothesis continues to be developed and researched (Walsh et al, 1981). The high incidence of GER in infants, however, makes this a difficult association to prove.

Prolongation of the Q-T Intervals. Disturbance in cardiac conduction (Q-T interval) has been researched by some investigators, but in a review of research findings the evidence supporting this hypothesis has been found to be inconclusive (Merritt and Valdes-Dapena, 1984).

Identification of Infants

Development of a profile of infants at risk for SIDS is receiving extensive study. Common SIDS characteristics have been identified but cannot be used as predictive or diagnostic criteria. Based on McClain (1985) and Black et al (1986), the following characteristics represent findings drawn from retrospective epidemiologic studies (Chan, 1987).

- boys 2 to 4 months of age
- black infants
- multiple births and/or low birthweight infants
- infants born to teenage mothers
- infant deaths in winter months
- time of death between 12 midnight and 8:00 A.M.
- lower socioeconomic status (despite normal development and adequate nourishment)
- maternal factors

Signs and Symptoms Found During Autopsy

External examination of the infant reveals the typical victim to be in a normal state of nutrition and hydration. Over half exhibit frothy fluids in the mouth and nostrils, indicative of pulmonary edema (Beckwith, 1978). Often this fluid is tinged with blood. The diapers usually are filled with urine and stool. These findings lead Beckwith to suspect that vigorous motor activity has occurred. Vomitus may be found on the face, and the hands may be clutching fibers of blanket materials.

Internal examination reveals intrathoracic petechiae. Typically, these dot the surfaces of lungs, pericardium, and thymus, and frequently they also involve the parietal serosal surfaces of the chest. Beckwith (1978) proposes that these petechiae may indicate intrathoracic negative pressure during the final moments of life. Typically, pulmonary congestion, edema, and inflammatory infiltrates in the upper airway and lungs are discovered. These findings, however, are not marked and do not provide an explanation for death.

Impact of SIDS on the Family

Following the SIDS event, severe stress is experienced by all members of the family, including parents, grandparents, and siblings. Friends of the family, including the baby sitter, also will be affected by the sudden unexpected death of an infant. This stress occurs without a noticeable precursor—the benefit of anticipatory grief is not experienced by the family.

The initial response to the child's confirmed death is extreme shock that produces varying degrees of confusion. This may be followed by outrage so intense that injury to self or others may occur. The absence of an explanation for the death increases the difficulty of resolving the loss. Family members commonly experience guilt either in the form of self-blaming or projecting the blame onto another family member (often the spouse). A typical psychologic reaction of parents is that they retrospectively review in their minds over and over every detail of the pregnancy, the birth, the life, and death of their child in search of a cause of the death (Zebal and Woolsey, 1984). These are the typical mixtures of responses experienced by all involved in the sudden death event. The nurse must be prepared to recognize these reactions.

During this critical period the parents of the SIDS infant need tremendous support. Reality orientation helps the family cope with their confusion and guilt. The first essential step in reality orientation is the physician's confirmation of the death to the family. This should not be done over the phone. Because of the extreme shock of sudden death, no family member should be told of the death without the presence of another family member, relative, or friend. Family members have less difficulty accepting the death and resolving their grief when they are permitted to view or even hold their dead infant. The family should always be prepared prior to seeing the dead infant. Stressful as it is, seeing or holding their child facilitates the family's acceptance of the death; however, no family member should ever by forced to have this experience.

The family needs an opportunity to sort their feelings and to begin to cope with their outrage. A place for the family to be alone affords them the privacy they need to regain composure and release feelings they do not wish to display publicly. An individual family member should never be left alone, nor should the family feel abandoned by the nurse. At this time the nurse serves as a therapeutic person by listening to fears and answering questions about the death.

Some families find that this event draws them closer together, whereas other families are immobilized to the extent that they are unable to support each other. Those families who are drawn apart are more likely to project their guilt. Providing the family with printed information about SIDS helps allay some of the blame-making and guilt.

Inadequate parenting, the infant's suffocation by blankets or choking on vomitus, or inability to mouth breathe, as well as parents' failure to take the infant to the physician in time to cure a slight cold, are false explanations for the death often voiced by parents. These misunderstandings must be dispelled at the first visit with the family (in the emergency room or wherever the nurse first has contact with the family members). The crucial piece of information that parents and relatives must have is that *the death was not preventable.*

Impact of SIDS on Siblings

The inability of parents to cope with the needs of their other children during the initial period of shock and confusion can cause stress for the remaining siblings. They are often temporarily housed with relatives or friends to "protect" them from the pain of the mourning process and the funeral events. Such actions do not recognize the need of siblings to remain with their parents during this intense stress or work through their own grief. Only their parents can continue to provide the security needed by the surviving children through this stressful time.

Young children may also develop their own explanations for the baby's absence from the family. They may experience intense guilt or anxiety associated with the baby's death. Sending the children away from home at this time further increases their anxiety, confusion, and sense of guilt. Although the parents are having an extremely difficult time supporting one another, they must somehow share in their children's grief as well. The nurse intervenes to provide information about childhood grief to the parents and facilitate the family's unique grief work. The use of play therapy with siblings may assist younger children to play out fears, guilty feelings, and anxieties. Older siblings may need time to talk about the death with the nurse or their parents. The nurse can facilitate their grief work by providing an opportunity for it to occur.

Intervention at the Time of SIDS Death

The National Foundation for Sudden Infant Death (NFSID) has advocated a management plan for SIDS. The four aspects of this program are

- Performance of autopsies on all infants dying suddenly and unexpectedly;
- Prompt notification of the results of that autopsy to the parents;
- Use of the term *sudden infant death syndrome* on the death certificate;
- Follow-up information and counseling for all families, provided by a knowledgeable health professional.

In the Home. Paramedical personnel are frequently the first persons called to the home when the nonbreathing infant is found. Therefore it is imperative that they possess adequate information about SIDS. They must be trained to deal with the death in an empathetic and nonjudgmental manner. Local police, county coroner, and other community officials are informed by the community health care personnel about the special needs of SIDS families at the time of death.

In the Emergency Room. Emergency room personnel may have an overwhelming reaction to the SIDS event. Because they are geared toward preservation of life, dealing with the family of a SIDS victim can be extremely difficult, so difficult that at times the family is left alone to deal with their grief and confusion. Emergency room personnel need assistance in dealing with their own feelings of grief so they can provide the kind of intervention needed by families at this critical time. Families need someone to stay with them and to reassure them that what has happened is not their fault. They need someone to listen to their pain, minister to their simple needs (get a cup of coffee for them), and help them make the important, immediate decision about an autopsy consent and perhaps organ donation. Parents also need to make funeral arrangements and deal with the reactions of siblings.

At Autopsy. According to Bergman (1970), autopsy serves two functions: in approximately 15 per cent of the cases a cause other than SIDS may be found, and the mysterious cause of death then may be clarified. Otherwise, families are left with doubt for the rest of their lives. It has been suggested that the member of the health team who provides this immediate information regarding the results of the autopsy be the pathologist or family physician. Following this information (preferably in person and within the first 24 hours after the death of the infant), a letter summarizing the cause of death should be sent. This letter is often viewed by the family as an official statement of their blamelessness (Miles, 1975).

Community Follow-Up

A community outreach program, including counseling at four critical periods, has been advocated. This program would include four steps: (1) when the baby is found dead, immediate intervention must be provided; (2) during the year following the death counseling must follow either in the form of one-to-one intervention or group intervention and support; (3) counseling is again critical at the time of subsequent pregnancy and birth; and (4) continued support is needed until the subsequent child's age passes that of the SIDS infant.

Every effort should be made to have contact with the family within the week following the SIDS event. Often a follow-up program involving community health nurses can be developed within the community health care network. Parents also need opportunities to draw support from other parents of SIDS infants if they so desire. During the first home visit the nurse must assess the family as to their level of understanding of the SIDS event. Information that has been misunderstood needs to be clarified at this time. Rather than commencing an involved discussion of etiologic theories, the nurse needs to focus on the family members' reactions to the SIDS event. During this time the nurse can provide continual reassurance that the parents could have done nothing to prevent, nor did they do anything to cause, the SIDS event.

During the next few months the nurse needs to be available to the parents through phone calls, letters, or visits. Assisting the family in their grief work is a prime function. Throughout this period the nurse must be aware that special days within the year—the child's birthday, Thanksgiving, religious holidays, the anniversary of the infant's death—have significance to the family members. The nurse should make every effort to prepare the parents for the extra stress that often exists on these days and see that they have support systems to lean on during these times. A subsequent pregnancy initiates a period of renewed anxiety and the nurse should be prepared to provide additional information, reassurance, and support. The issue of apnea monitoring must be faced and discussed at this time.

The support these families need is great and long-range. Support is often derived from a SIDS parents' group.* Films provided by these groups not only offer clarification of SIDS but also provide a focus for discussions about feelings and grief work. A unique relationship is shared among parents of SIDS infants. The strength of that relationship should not be underplayed by the health team.

Organizations that provide special information to health professionals and families include the following:

International Council for Infant Survival
9178 Nadine River Ct.
Fountain Valley, CA 92708
Phone: (714)968-7623 or (319)322-4870

National Center for the Prevention of Sudden Infant Death Syndrome
330 N. Charles St.
Baltimore, MD 21201
Phone: (301)547-8955; toll-free hot line is (800)638-7437

National Sudden Infant Death Syndrome Clearinghouse
8201 Greensboro Dr., Suite 600
McLean, VA 22102
Phone: (703)821-8955

National Sudden Infant Death Syndrome Foundation
2 Metro Plaza, Suite 104
8200 Professional Pl.
Landover, MD 20785
Phone: (301)459-3388; 24-hour answering service is (800)221-7437

* Information is available from the National SIDS Foundation, P.O. Box 2753, Landover Hills, MD 20784; phone: (301) 459-3388.

References

Introduction (Principles, Respiration and Oxygenation, Malformations)

Auld PAM: Pulmonary physiology of the newborn infant. *In* Scarpelli EM (ed): *Pulmonary Physiology of the Fetus, Newborn and Child.* Philadelphia, Lea & Febiger, 1975. 140–165.

Bingham WT: The neonatal airway: problems and management. *Can Fam Physician* 1987; 33:1467–1470.

Boat TF, et al: Congenital disorders of the nose. *In* Behrman RE, Vaughan VC (eds): *Nelson Textbook of Pediatrics.* Philadelphia, WB Saunders, 1987, 868–870.

Burchfiel C, et al: Passive smoking in children. *Am Rev Respir Dis* 1986; 133:966–967.

Burgess WR, Chernick V: *Respiratory Therapy in Newborn Infants and Children.* New York, Thieme-Stratton, 1982.

Campbell AN, et al: Low flow oxygen therapy in infants. *Arch Dis Child* 1983; 58:795–798.

Carnevale F: Transcutaneous oxygen monitoring: assessment techniques. *Dimens Crit Care Nurs* 1986; 5(5):264–269.

Charlton A: Children's coughs related to parental smoking. *Br Med J* 1984 Jun; 288:1647–1649.

Doershuk CF, et al: Pulmonary physiology of the young child. *In* Scarpelli EM (ed): *Pulmonary Physiology of the Fetus, Newborn and Child.* Philadelphia, Lea & Febiger, 1975. 116–182.

Doershuk CF, Orenstein DM: Pulmonary function and exercise testing. *In* Lough M, et al: *Pediatric Respiratory Therapy.* Chicago, Year Book Medical Publishers, 1979, 222–257.

Droske SC, Francis SA: *Pediatric Diagnostic Procedures.* New York, John Wiley and Sons, 1981.

Fanconi S, et al: Pulse oximetry in pediatric intensive care: comparison with measured saturations and transcutaneous oxygen tension. *J Pediatr* 1985; 107:362–366.

Fergusson DM, et al: Parental smoking and lower tract respiratory illness in the first three years of life. *J Epidemio Commun Health* 1981; 35:180–184.

Glassanos MR: Infants who are oxygen dependent—sending them home. *MCN* 1980 Jan/Feb; 42–45.

Guyton AC: *Human Physiology and Mechanisms of Disease.* Philadelphia, WB Saunders, 1987.

Holinger LD, Weiss KS: Diagnosis and management of airway obstruction in craniofacial anomalies. *Otolaryngol Clin North Am* 1981 Nov; 1015.

Hughes JG: *Synopsis of Pediatrics.* St. Louis, CV Mosby, 1984.

Hughes W, Buescher E: *Pediatric Procedures.* Philadelphia, WB Saunders, 1980.

Inselman LS, Mellins RB: Growth and development of the lung. *J Pediatr* 1981 Jan; 1–15.

Jennis MS, Peabody JL: Pulse oximetry: an alternative for the assessment of oxygenation in newborn infants. *Pediatrics* 1987; 79:524–527.

Kennedy AH, et al: An educational program for families of children with tracheostomies. *MCN* 1982, Jan/Feb; 7:42–49.

Leifer G: *Principles and Techniques in Pediatric Nursing.* Philadelphia, WB Saunders, 1982.

Lichtenstein MA: Pediatric home tracheostomy care: a parent's guide. *Pediatr Nurs* 1986; 12(1):41–48.

Lyman RD, et al: Psychological effects on parents of home and hospital apnea monitoring. *J Pediatr Psychol* 1985; 10(4):439–448.

McElroy E, et al: Emotional and health impact of home monitoring on mothers: a controlled prospective study. *Pediatrics* 1986; 78(5):780–786.

Mellins R, et al: *Respiratory Care in Infants and Children.* New York, American Lung Association, 1971.

Mohler SE: Passive smoking: a danger to children's health. *J Pediatr Health Care* 1987 Nov/Dec; 1(6):298–304.

O'Brodovich HM, Chernick V: The functional basis of respiratory pathology. *In* Kendig E, Chernick V (eds): *Disorders of the Respiratory Tract in Children.* Philadelphia, WB Saunders, 1983.

Openbrier DR, et al: Home oxygen therapy. Evaluation and prescription. *Am J Nurs* 1988 Feb; 88(2):192–197.

Said G, et al: Parental smoking related to adenoidectomy and tonsillectomy in children. *J Epidemiol Commun Health* 1978; 32:97–99.

Shapiro C: Retrolental fibroplasia: what we know and what we don't know. *Neonatal Network* 1986; 4(6):33–44.

Strope GL, Stempel DA: Risk factors associated with the development of chronic lung disease in children. *Pediatr Clin North Am* 1984 Aug; 31(4):757–771.

Tager I, et al: Longitudinal study of the effects of smoking on pulmonary function in children. *N Engl J Med* 1983; 309:699–703.

Vedal S, et al: Risk factors for childhood respiratory disease. Analysis of pulmonary function. *Am Rev Respir Dis* 1984; 130:187–192.

Ware J, et al: Passive smoking, gas cooking and respiratory health of children living in six cities. *Am Rev Respir Dis* 1984; 129:366–374.

Waring WW: Diagnostic and therapeutic procedures. *In* Kendig E, Chernick V (eds): *Disorders of the Respiratory Tract in Children.* Philadelphia, WB Saunders, 1983.

West JB: *Respiratory Physiology.* 2nd ed. Baltimore, Williams & Wilkins, 1979.

Wohl MEB: Age as a factor in respiratory disease. *In* Kendig E, Chernick V (eds): *Disorders of the Respiratory Tract in Children.* Philadelphia, WB Saunders, 1983, 135–141.

Wood RE: Spelunking in the pediatric airways: explorations with the flexible fiberoptic bronchoscope. *Pediatr Clin North Am* 1984; 31(4):785–799.

Infections of the Respiratory Tract

Ariagno L: Evaluation and management of infantile apnea. *Pediatr Ann* 1984 Mar; 240–247.

Beem MO, et al: Chlamydial infections of infants. *In* Kendig EL, Chernick V: *Disorders of the Respiratory Tract in Children.* Philadelphia, WB Saunders, 1983, 767–770.

Behrman RE, Vaughan VC (eds): *Nelson Textbook of Pediatrics.* 13th ed. Philadelphia, WB Saunders, 1987.

Bhambhani K, et al: Acute otitis media in children: are decongestants or antihistamines necessary? *Ann Emerg Med* 1983 Jan; 12(1):13–16.

Bluestone CD, Klein JO: Otitis media with effusion, atelectasis, and eustachian tube dysfunction. *In* Bluestone CD, Stool SE (eds): *Pediatric Otolaryngology.* Philadelphia, WB Saunders, 1983.

Bluestone CD, Klein JO: *Otitis Media in Infants and Children.* Philadelphia, WB Saunders, 1988.

Boat TF: An approach to recurrent or persistent lower respiratory tract symptoms in children. *In* Behrman RE, Vaughan VC: *Nelson Textbook of Pediatrics.* Philadelphia, WB Saunders, 1987.

Castiglia PT, Aquilina S: Streptococcal pharyngitis: a persistent challenge. *Pediatr Nurs* 1982 Nov/Dec; 377–382.

Catlin FI: Otolaryngologic disorders. *In* Ravitch MM, et al (eds): *Pediatric Surgery.* Chicago, Year Book Medical Publishers, 1979.

Curran CL, Kachoyeanos MK: The effects on neonates of two methods of chest physical therapy. *MCN* 1979 Sep/Oct; 309.

Davis HW, et al: Acute upper airway obstruction: croup and epiglottitis. *Pediatr Clin North Am* 1981 Nov; 859–880.

Denny FW: Infections of the respiratory tract due to *Mycoplasma pneumoniae.* *In* Kendig EL, Chernick V: *Disorders of the Respiratory Tract in Children.* Philadelphia, WB Saunders, 1983.

Eichenwald HF: Respiratory infections in children. Hosp Pract 1976 Apr; 81; Pneumonia syndromes in children. 1976 May; 89.

Eigen H: The clinical evaluation of chronic cough. *Pediatr Clin North Am* 1982 Feb; 67–68.

Fraser JJ, et al: Prevalence of cervical *Chlamydia trachomatis* and *Neisseria gonorrhoeae* in female adolescents. *Pediatrics* 1983 Mar; 333–336.

Gellis SS, Kagan BM: *Current Pediatric Therapy (11).* Philadelphia, WB Saunders, 1984.

Ghory J: OME: leading causes of preventable hearing loss. *J Respir Dis* 1982 Oct; 127–138.

Gordon S: Infectious diseases. *In* Wasserman E, Slobody LB: *Survey of Clinical Pediatrics.* New York, McGraw-Hill, 1974.

Green M: *Pediatric Diagnosis.* 4th ed. Philadelphia, WB Saunders, 1986.

Hall CB, Hall WJ: Epiglottitis. *In* Hoekelman RA, et al: *Primary Pediatric Care.* St. Louis, CV Mosby, 1987, 1591–1594.

Hammerschlag MR: Chlamydial infections. *Pediatr Rev* 1981 Sep; 77–84.

Hayden GF, et al: Prevention of natural colds by contact prophylaxis with intranasal alpha$_2$-interferon. *N Engl J Med* 1986; 314:71–75.

Hazinski MF: *Nursing Care of the Critically Ill Child.* St. Louis, CV Mosby, 1984.

Hoekelman RA, et al: *Principles of Pediatrics.* New York, McGraw-Hill, 1978.

Hughes J: *Synopsis of Pediatrics.* St. Louis, CV Mosby, 1984.

Hutchinson R: The common cold primer. *Nurs '79* 1979 Mar; 57.

Kass J, Beebe M: Serous otitis media. *Nurse Pract* 1979 Mar/Apr; 25.

Klein JO, Mavey M: Bacterial infections. *In* Remington JS, Klein JO (eds): *Infectious Diseases of the Fetus and the Newborn Infant.* Philadelphia, WB Saunders, 1976.

Kornblut AB: a traditional approach to surgery of the tonsils and adenoids. *Otolaryngol Clin North Am* 1987; 20:349–363.

Leifer G: *Principles and Techniques in Pediatric Nursing.* Philadelphia, WB Saunders, 1982.

Loebl S, Spratto GR: *The Nurse's Drug Handbook.* 4th ed. New York, John Wiley and Sons, 1986.

Loughlin GM: Bronchitis. *In* Kendig EL, Chernick V (eds): *Disorders of the Respiratory Tract in Children.* Philadelphia, WB Saunders, 1983, 275–283.

Lounsbury BF: Swimming unprotected with long-shafted middle ear ventilation tubes. *Laryngoscope* 1985; 95:340–343.

Marchant CD, Shurin PA: Therapy of otitis media. *Pediatr Clin North Am* 1983 Apr; 281–296.

Marvin C, Slevin A: Chlamydia—cause, prevention and cure. *MCN* 1987; 12:318–321.

Mellis CM: Evaluation and treatment of chronic cough in children. *Pediatr Clin North Am* 1979 Aug; 553–564.

Mitchell D: Otitis media in children. *Can Fam Physician* 1987 Jun; 33:1497–1499.

O'Grady MJ: Rhinitis: allergic and non-allergic. *Can Fam Physician* 1987; 33:1459–1463.

Paradise JL: Otitis media in infants and children. *Pediatrics* 1980 May; 917–943.

Paradise JL, et al: Efficacy of adenoidectomy for recurrent otitis media: results from parallel random and nonrandom trials. *Pediatr Res* 1987; 21:286A.

Pelton SI, Whitley P: Otitis media: current concepts in diagnosis and management. *Pediatr Ann* 1983 Mar; 207–218.

Rasmussen N: Complications of tonsillectomy and adenoidectomy. *Otolaryngol Clin North Am* 1987; 20:383–390.

Rettig PJ: Chlamydial infections in pediatrics: not for babies only. *J Pediatr* 1984 Jan; 82–83.

Rowe LD: Tonsils and adenoids: when is surgery indicated? *Primary Care* 1982 Jun; 355–369.

Schachter J, et al: Pneumonitis following inclusion blenorrhea. *J Pediatr* 1975 Nov; 779–780.

Schachter J, et al: Prospective study of chlamydial infection in neonates. *Lancet* 1979 Aug 18; 377–379.

Shafer M, et al: *Chlamydia trachomatis:* important relationships to race, contraception, lower genital tract infections, and Papanicolaou smear. *J Pediatr* 1984 Jan; 141–146.

Shurin PA: Inflammatory diseases of the nose and paranasal sinuses. *In* Bluestone CD, Stool S (eds): *Pediatric Otolaryngology.* Vol I. Philadelphia, WB Saunders, 1983, 781–790.

Smith MHD: Bacterial pneumonias: gram-negative. *In* Kendig EL, Chernick V (eds): *Disorders of the Respiratory Tract in Children.* Philadelphia, WB Saunders, 1983, 309–314.

Stern RC: Acute infections of the larynx and trachea. *In* Behrman RE, Vaughan VC (eds): *Nelson Textbook of Pediatrics.* Philadelphia, WB Saunders, 1983, 1034–1037.

Welliver RC, Wong DT: *Mycoplasma pneumoniae* infections of children and adolescents. *In* Moss AJ (ed): *Pediatrics Update.* New York, Elsevier Biomedical, 1983, 315–333.

Widome M: Pharyngitis and tonsillitis. *In* Hoekelman RA, et al: *Pediatric Primary Care.* St. Louis, CV Mosby, 1987, 1429–1433.

Wohl MEB: Bronchiolitis. *In* Kendig EL, Chernick V (eds): *Disorders of the Respiratory Tract in Children.* Philadelphia, WB Saunders, 1983, 283–294.

Chronic Alterations (Asthma, Cystic Fibrosis, Bronchopulmonary Dysplasia)

Ad Hoc Committee Task Force on Neonatal Screening, Cystic Fibrosis Foundation: Neonatal screening for cystic fibrosis: position paper. *Pediatrics* 1983 Nov; 741–745.

Als H, et al: Individual behavioral and environmental care for the very low birth weight preterm infant at high risk for bronchopulmonary dysplasia: neonatal intensive care unit and developmental outcome. *Pediatrics* 1986; 78:1123–1132.

Avery ME: The argument for prenatal administration of dexamethasone to prevent respiratory distress syndrome. *J Pediatr* 1984; 104:240.

Avery ME: Surfactant replacement. *N Engl J Med* 1986; 315:825–826.

Bancalari E, Gerhardt T: Bronchopulmonary dysplasia. *Pediatr Clin North Am* 1986; 33:1–23.

Bierman C, Pearlman D: *Allergic Diseases of Infancy, Childhood, and Adolescence.* Philadelphia, WB Saunders, 1980.

Bock S: Food-related asthma and basic nutrition. *J Asthma* 1983; 20:377–381.

Brown E: *In* Tawusch HW, Yogman MW: *Follow-up Management of the High-Risk Infant.* Boston, Little, Brown, 1987.

Carbary L, Carbary C: Asthma in children. *J Nurs Care* 1981 Apr; 14–21.

Carlsen K, Orstavik I, Leegaard J, et al: Respiratory virus infections and aeroallogens in acute bronchial asthma. *Arch Dis Child* 1984; 59:310–315.

Carty R: Some facts about allergy. *Pediatr Nurs* 1977 Mar/Apr; 3:7–9.

Clark N, Feldman C, Evans D, et al: Change in children's school performance as a result of education for family management of asthma. *J School Health* 1984 Apr; 54:143–145.

Crummette B: Maternal care of asthmatic children. *Matern Child Nurs J* 1979 Spring; 8:23–27.

Doershuk CF, Boat TF: Cystic fibrosis. *In* Behrman RE, Vaughan VC III (eds): *Nelson Textbook of Pediatrics.* 13th ed. Philadelphia, WB Saunders, 1987, 927–935.

Dushenko TW: Cystic fibrosis: a medical overview and critique of the psychological literature. *Social Sci Med* 1981; 15E:43–56.

Fiel S, Swartz M, Glanz K, et al: Efficacy of short-term corticosteroid therapy in outpatient treatment of acute bronchial asthma. *Am J Med* 1983 Aug; 75:259–262.

Friedman M: Psychological factors associated with pediatric asthma death: a review. *J Asthma* 1984; 21:97–117.

Galant S, Groncy C, Shaw K: The value of pulsus paradoxus in assessing the child with status asthmaticus. *Pediatrics* 1978 Jan; 61(1):46–50.

Harder I, Bowditch B: Siblings of children with cystic fibrosis: perceptions of the impact of the disease. *Child Health Care* 1982; 10:116–120.

Hodson ME: Cystic fibrosis in adolescents and adults. *Practitioner* 1983 Nov; 1723–1729.

Huang NN, Palmer J: Management of patients with cystic fibrosis. I: Clinical Manifestations. *Respir Ther* 1981, Jan/Feb; 49–53; II: Principles of Treatment. 1981 Mar/Apr; 65–74.

Jacobs J: Cystic fibrosis as it affects the patient and family. *Respir Ther* 1977 Nov/Dec; 52.

Johnson MP: Self-instruction for the family of a child with cystic fibrosis. *MCN* 1980 Sep/Oct; 345–348.

Khampolikit S: The interrelationship between the asthmatic child's dependency behavior, his perception of his illness and his mother's perceptions of his illness. *Matern Child Nurs J* 1983 Winter; 4:221–296.

Koops BL, et al: Outpatient management and follow-up of bronchopulmonary dysplasia. *Clin Perinatol* 1984 Feb; 101–122.

Korones SB: Complications. *In* Goldsmith JP, et al: *Assisted Ventilation of the Neonate.* Philadelphia, WB Saunders, 1988.

Larter N: Cystic fibrosis. *Am J Nurs* 1981 Mar; 527–532.

Lester LA, Rothberg RM: Cystic fibrosis. *In* Gellis SS, Kagan BM (eds): *Current Pediatric Therapy 12.* Philadelphia, WB Saunders, 1986, 225–231.

Lockey RF, Bukantz SC: *Principles of Immunology and Allergy.* Philadelphia, WB Saunders, 1987.

Loebl S, Spratto GR: *The Nurse's Drug Handbook.* 4th ed. New York, John Wiley and Sons, 1986.

Mallinson B: Seven rules of physiotherapy, Part 3. *Nurs Mirror* 1978 Aug 24; 18.

Mansmann HC, Bierman CW, Pearlman DS: Treatment of acute asthma in children. *In* Bierman C, Pearlman D: *Allergic Diseases of Infancy. Childhood, and Adolescence.* 2nd ed. Philadelphia, WB Saunders, 1988, 571–586.

Markestad T, Fitzhardinge PM: Growth and development in children recovering from bronchopulmonary dysplasia. *J Pediatr* 1981 Apr; 597–602.

Mattson K: Psychologic aspects of childhood asthma. *Pediatr Clin North Am* 1975 Feb; 22:77–88.

McCaully H: Breathing exercises as play for asthmatic children. *MCN* 1980 Sep/Oct; 5:340–344.

Merritt TA, et al: Prophylactic treatment of very premature infants with human surfactant. *N Engl J Med* 1986; 315:785–790.

Mikkelson C, et al: Cystic fibrosis: a family challenge. Child Today 1978 Jul/Aug; 22.

Monin P, Vert P: The management of bronchopulmonary dysplasia. *Clin Perinatol* 1987; 14:531–549.

Northway WH, et al: Pulmonary disease following respiratory therapy of hyaline membrane disease: BPD. *N Engl J Med* 1967; 276:357–368.

Notter RH, Shapiro DL: Lung surfactants for replacement therapy: biochemical, biophysical and clinical aspects. *Clin Perinatol* 1987; 14:433–479.

Pearlman D, Bierman C: Asthma (bronchial asthma, reactive airways disorder). *In* Bierman C, Pearlman D: *Allergic Diseases of Infancy, Childhood, and Adolescence.* 2nd ed. Philadelphia, WB Saunders, 1988, 559.

Quinton PM, Bisman J: Higher bioelectric potential due to decreased absorption in the sweat glands of patients with cystic fibrosis. *N Engl J Med* 1983; 308:1185.

Ramsey AM, Siroky AS: The use of puppets to teach school-age children with asthma. *Pediatr Nurs* 1988 May-June; 14(3)187–190.

Roberts WE, Morrison JC: Effects of maternal drugs on fetal pulmonary maturity. *In Lung Biology in Health and Disease.* New York, Marcel Dekker, 1985, 27.

Rose J, Jay S: A comprehensive exercise program for persons with cystic fibrosis. *J Pediatr Nurs* 1986; 1:323–334.

Rosenstein BJ: Cystic fibrosis: the outlook improves. *Patient Care* 1988; 22(2):30–44.

Saigal S, O'Brodovich H: Long-term outcome of preterm infants with respiratory disease. *Clin Perinatol* 1987 Sep; 14(3):635–650.

Sauve RS, Singhal N: Long-term morbidity of infants with bronchopulmonary dysplasia. *Pediatrics* 1985; 76:725–733.

Sawley L: Children with asthma. *Nurs Mirror* 1983 Oct; 157:27–29.

Scherf RF: Total patient care of the newborn infant who develops bronchopulmonary dysplasia. *Neonatal Network* 1985; 3:28–37.

Schneider M, Melton B, Reisch J: Effects of a progressive exercise program on absenteeism among school children with asthma. *J School Health* 1980 Feb; 92–95.

Schwachman H: Cystic fibrosis. *In* Kendig EL, Chernick V: *Disorders of the Respiratory Tract in Children.* Philadelphia, WB Saunders, 1983, 640–661.

Schwartz RH: Cystic fibrosis. *In* Hoekelman RA, et al: *Pediatric Primary Care.* St. Louis, CV Mosby, 1987, 1203–1210.

Shapiro G, Bierman D: Exercise-induced asthma. *J Asthma* 1983; 20:383–389.

Sinkin RA, Phelps DL: New strategies for the prevention of bronchopulmonary dysplasia. *Clin Perinatol* 1987; 14(3):599–620.

Sly RM: *Pediatric Allergy.* New York, Medical Examination Publishing Company, 1985.

Sly RM: Asthma. *In* Gellis SS, Kagan BM (eds): *Current Pediatric Therapy 12.* Philadelphia, WB Saunders, 1986, 630–637.

Toce SS, et al: Clinical and roentgenographic scoring systems for assessing bronchopulmonary dysplasia. *Am J Dis Child* 1984; 138:581–585.

Venters M: Familial coping with chronic and severe childhood illness: the case of cystic fibrosis. *Social Sci Med* 1981; 15A:289–297.

Voyles JB: Bronchopulmonary dysplasia. *Am J Nurs* 1981 Mar; 510–514.

Voyles JB: Asthma: reactive airway disease. *Am J Nurs* 1981 Mar; 522–524.

Voyles J, Menendez R: Role of patient compliance in the management of asthma. *J Asthma* 1983; 20:411–418.

Wainwright BJ, et al: Localization of cystic fibrosis locus to human chromosome 7 cen—q 22. *Nature* 1985; 318:384.

Wells PW, Meghdadpour S: Research yields new clues to cystic fibrosis. *MCN* 1988 May/Jun; 13:187–190.

Wolf S: Exercise, the asthmatic and PL 94-142. *Pediatr Nurs* 1980 Nov/Dec; 21–23.

Zeiger R: Special considerations in the approach to asthma in infancy and early childhood. *J Asthma,* 1983; 20:341–359.

Zeiger R, Schatz M: Immunologic approach to the management of asthma. *J Asthma* 1983; 20:391–409.

Apnea-Related Disorders (Apnea, SIDS)

Aranda JV, et al: Effect of caffeine on control of breathing in infantile apnea. *J Pediatr* 1983 Dec; 975–978.

Ariagno RL: Evaluation and management of infantile apnea. *Pediatr Ann* 1984 Mar; 210–217.

Arnon SS, et al: Intestinal infection and toxin produced by *Clostridium botulinum* as one cause of sudden infant death syndrome. *Lancet* 1978 Jun 17; 1273–1277.

Avery ME, Frantz ID: To breathe or not to breathe—what have we learned about apneic spells and sudden infant death? *N Engl J Med* 1983 Jul 14; 107–108.

Barrington KJ, et al: Physiologic effects of doxapram in idiopathic apnea of prematurity. *J Pediatr* 1986; 108:125–129.

Beckwith J: *The Sudden Infant Death Syndrome.* Washington, DC, US Department of Health, Education, and Welfare, DHEW Publication No. (HSA). 78-5251, 1978.

Bergman A, et al: Sudden infant death syndrome; Proceedings of the Second International Conference on Causes of Sudden Death in Infants. Seattle, University of Washington Press, 1970.

Black L, David RJ, Brouillette RT, et al: Effects of birth weight and ethnicity on incidences of sudden infant death syndrome. *J Pediatr* 1986; 108(2):209–214.

Brady JP, McCann EM: Control of ventilation in subsequent siblings of victims of sudden infant death syndrome. *J Pediatr* 1985; 106(2):212–217.

Cain LP, et al: Parent's perceptions of the psychological and social impact of home monitoring. *Pediatrics* 1980 Jul; 37–41.

Chan MM: Sudden infant death syndrome and families at risk. *Pediatr Nurs* 1987; 13(3):166–168.

Corbet A: Respiratory disorders in the newborn. *In* Kendig EL, Chernick V: *Disorders of the Respiratory Tract in Children.* Philadelphia, WB Saunders, 1983, 214–235.

Dimaggio GT, Sheetz AH: The concerns of mothers caring for an infant on an apnea monitor. *MCN* 1983 Jul/Aug; 294–297.

Herbst JJ, et al: New findings shed light on SIDS. *Patient Care* 1988 May; 22(9):61–76.

Kelly D, Shannon DC: Sudden infant death syndrome and near sudden infant death syndrome: a review of the literature. *Pediatr Clin North Am* 1982 Oct; 1241–1261.

Marchal F, et al: Neonatal apnea and apneic syndrome. *Clin Perinatol* 1987; 14(3):509–529.

McClain M: Sudden infant death syndrome: an update. *J Emerg Nurs* 1985; 11(5):227–233.

Merritt TA, Valdes-Dapena M: SIDS research update. *Pediatr Ann* 1984 Mar; 193–207.

Miles M (ed): *Mental Health Aspects of SIDS.* Report of a conference sponsored by the National Foundation for Sudden Infant Death and the National Institute of Mental Health. Kansas City, US Department of Health, Education and Welfare, July 30, 1975.

Naeye RL: Sudden infant death. *Sci Am* 1980 Apr; 56–62.

Peterson D, et al: Sudden infant death syndrome and maternal age. *JAMA* 1980 Apr 23; 2250–2257.

Rigatto H: Apnea. *Pediatr Clin North Am* 1982 Oct; 1105–1116.

Shannon DC, Kelly DH: SIDS and near-SIDS. *In* Kendig EL, Chernick V: *Disorders of the Respiratory Tract in Children.* Philadelphia, WB Saunders, 1983, 897–916.

Smith JC: Psychosocial aspects of infantile apnea and home monitoring. *Pediatr Ann* 1984 Mar; 219–224.

Spitzer AR, Fox WW: Infant apnea. *Pediatr Clin North Am* 1986; 33(3):561–581.

Valdes-Dapena M, Steinschneider A: Sudden infant death syndrome (SIDS), apnea, and near miss for SIDS. *Emerg Med Clin North Am* 1983 Apr; 27–44.

Walsh JK, et al: Gastroesophageal reflux in infants: relation to apnea. *J Pediatr* 1981 Aug; 99(2):197–201.

Weinstein S, Steinschneider A: The effectiveness of home

monitoring programs in preventing SIDS. *In* Tildon JT, Roeder LM, Steinschneider A (eds): *Sudden Infant Death Syndrome.* New York, Academic Press, 1983, 719–726.

Zebal B, Woolsey SF: SIDS and the family: the pediatrician's role. *Pediatr Ann* 1984 Mar; 13(3):237–261.

Bibliography

Introduction (Principles, Respiration and Oxygenation, Malformations)

Aradine C: Home care for young children with long-term tracheostomies. *MCN* 1980 Mar/Apr; 121.

Bailey BJ, Jones JK: Methods of examination. *In* Bluestone CD, Stool SE (eds): *Pediatric Otolaryngology.* Vol II. Philadelphia, WB Saunders, 1983.

Bose PK, Jones GP: Choanal atresia. *J Laryngol Otol* 1983 Aug; 711–717.

Boynton BR, et al: Combined high frequency oscillatory ventilation and intermittent mandatory ventilation in critically ill infants. *J Pediatr* 1984; 72:903.

Cameron TJ: Fiberoptic bronchoscopy. *Am J Nurs* 1981 Aug; 1462–1464.

Cardin S: Acid-base balance in the patient with respiratory disease. *Nurs Clin North Am* 1980 Sep; 593–601.

Crowley CM, Morrow AI: A comprehensive approach to the child in respiratory failure. *Crit Care Q* 1980; 3(1):27–43.

Doershuk CF: The respiratory system. *In* Behrman RE, Vaughan VC (eds): *Nelson Textbook of Pediatrics.* Philadelphia, WB Saunders, 1983, 991–999.

Frantz JD, Close RH: Alveolar pressure savings during high frequency ventilation in rabbits. *Pediatr Res* 1985; 19:162.

George DS, et al: The latest on retinopathy of prematurity. *MCN* 1988 Jul/Aug; 13:254–258.

Gerbeaux J, et al: *Pediatric Respiratory Disease.* 2nd ed. New York, John Wiley and Sons, 1982.

Gregory GA: *Respiratory Failure in the Child.* New York, Churchill-Livingstone, 1981.

Groeneveld M: Sending infants home on low-flow oxygen. *JOGN* 1986; 15:237–241.

Harper RW: *A Guide to Respiratory Care.* Philadelphia, JB Lippincott, 1981.

Hazinski MF: Pediatric home tracheostomy care: a parent's guide. *Pediatr Nurs* 1986; 12:41–48.

Hunter P: Bedside monitoring of respiratory function. *Nurs Clin North Am* 1981 Jun; 211–224.

Hurwitz ES, et al: Reye syndrome and aspirin. *JAMA* 1987 Apr; 257:1905–1911.

Kennelly C: Tracheostomy care: parents as learners. *MCN* 1987; 12(4):264–267.

Kenney MM: Hospital to home: care of the child with a tracheostomy. *Neonatal Network* 1987; 6(1):21–24.

Loper DL: Surfactant replacement therapy. *Neonatal Network* 1986; 4(5):14–17.

Lough MD: *Pediatric Respiratory Therapy.* Chicago, Year Book Medical Publishers, 1979.

McFadden R: Decreasing respiratory compromise during infant suctioning. *Am J Nurs* 1981 Dec; 2158–2161.

Montgomery JN, et al: Anesthesia for tonsillectomy and adenoidectomy. *Otolaryngol Clin North Am* 1987; 20:331–347.

Moser KM, Spragg RG: *Respiratory Emergencies.* St. Louis, CV Mosby, 1982.

Muller NL, Bryan AC: Chest wall mechanics and respiratory muscles in infants. *Pediatr Clin North Am* 1979 Aug; 503–516.

Nieves J: Avoiding spontaneous extubation of nasotracheal or oral tracheal tubes. *Pediatr Nurs* 1986; 12:215–218.

Riegel B, Forshee T: A review and critique of the literature on preoxygenation for endotracheal suctioning. *Heart Lung* 1985; 14:507–518.

Smith RJH, Catlin FI: Congenital anomalies of the larynx. *Am J Dis Child* 1984; 138:35–39.

Sprinkle PM, Sporck FT: Congenital malformations of the nose and paranasal sinuses. *In* Bluestone CD, Stool SE (eds): *Pediatric Otolaryngology.* Vol 1. Philadelphia, WB Saunders, 1983, 769–780.

Steele NF, Harrison B: Technology-assisted children: assessing discharge preparations. *J Pediatr Nurs* 1986; 1(3):150–158.

Winsatt R: Unlocking the mysteries behind the chest wall. *Nurs 85* 1985; 15(1):58–64.

Infections of the Respiratory Tract

Adams JL, et al: Diagnosing and treating otitis media with effusion. *MCN* 1984 Jan/Feb; 22–28.

Behrman RD: Acute Nasopharyngitis. *In* Behrman RE, Vaughan VC: *Nelson Textbook of Pediatrics.* 13th ed. Philadelphia, WB Saunders, 1987, 870–871.

Bluestone CD: Diagnosis of chronic otitis media with effusion: description, otoscopy, acoustic impedance measurements, and assessment of hearing. *Pediatr Infect Dis* (Suppl 5) 1982 Sep/Oct; 38–69.

Canilekin E, et al: Lack of efficacy of a decongestant-antihistamine combination for otitis media with effusion in children. *N Engl J Med* 1983 Feb 10; 297–301.

Centers for Disease Control: *Chlamydia trachomatis Infections: Policy Guidelines for Prevention and Control.* Washington, DC: US Government Printing Office, 1985.

Eigen H, et al: Recurrent pneumonia in children and its relationship to bronchial hyperactivity. *Pediatrics* 1982 Nov; 698–703.

Evans RT, Woodland RM: Detections of chlamydiae by isolation and direct examination. *Br Med Bull* 1983 Apr; 181–186.

Harkess CK: Clearing the occluded auditory canal. *Pediatr Nurs* 1982 Jan/Feb; 23–25.

Hobson D, et al: Chlamydial infections in neonates and older children. *Br Med Bull* 1983 Apr; 128–132.

Klein JD: Mycoplasma infections. *In* Gellis S, Kagan BM: *Current Pediatric Therapy.* Philadelphia, WB Saunders, 1984, 580.

Koren G, et al: Corticosteroid treatment of laryngo-tracheitis vs. spasmodic croup in children. *Am J Dis Child* 1983 Oct; 941–944.

Lewis K, et al: A protocol for management of acute epiglottitis. *Clin Pediatr* 1978 Jun; 494.

Long SS: Treatment of acute pneumonia in infants and children. *Pediatr Clin North Am* 1983 Apr; 297–321.

Paradise JL: Tonsillectomy and adenoidectomy. *In* Bluestone CD, Stool SE: *Pediatric Otolaryngology.* Vol II. Philadelphia, WB Saunders, 1983, 992–1012.

Peltola HC: Reactive protein in rapid differentiation of acute epiglottitis from spasmodic croup and acute laryngotracheitis: a preliminary report. *J Pediatr* 1983; 102:713.

Pinney M: Pneumonia. *Am J Nurs* 1981 Mar; 577–578.

Price SA, Wilson LM: *Pathophysiology: Clinical Concepts of Disease Process.* New York, McGraw-Hill, 1983.

Rowe LD: Airway obstruction in the pediatric patient. *Primary Care* 1982 Jun; 317–336.

Schwartz RH, et al: Use of a short course of prednisone for treating middle ear effusion: a double-blind cross-over study. *Ann Otol Rhinol Laryngol* (Suppl 68) 1980 May/Jun; 296–306.

Simkins R: The crises of bronchiolitis. *Am J Nurs* 1981 Mar; 515–516; Croup and epiglottitis. 519–520.

Sofer S, Chernick V: Increased need for tracheal intubation for croup in relation to bacterial tracheitis. *Can Med Assoc J* 1983 Jan 15; 160–161.

Wald ER: Throats small and sore. *Emerg Med* 1984 Jan 15; 226–238.

Widome MD: The common cold. *In* Hoekelman RA: *Primary Pediatric Care.* St.Louis, CV Mosby, 1987, 1194–1195.

Chronic Alterations (Asthma, Cystic Fibrosis, Bronchopulmonary Dysplasia)

Avery GD: *Neonatology.* Philadelphia, JB Lippincott, 1981.

Avery GD, et al: Controlled trial of dexamethasone in respirator-dependent infants with bronchopulmonary dysplasia. *Pediatrics* 1985; 75:106.

Berman B, MacDonnell K: *Differential Diagnosis and Treatment of Pediatric Allergy.* Boston, Little, Brown, 1981.

Cystic Fibrosis Foundation:
Guide to Diagnosis and Management of Cystic Fibrosis
Guide to Drug Therapy in Patients with Cystic Fibrosis
Parents' Handbook: Your Child and Cystic Fibrosis
Living with Cystic Fibrosis: A Guide for Adolescents
Teachers' Guide: A Child with CF Is in Your Class
Health and Nutrition Programs (informational pamphlet that addresses the economic aspects)
Available from Cystic Fibrosis Foundation, 6000 Executive Blvd, Suite 309, Rockville, MD 20852.

De Boeck C, et al: Cough versus chest physiotherapy. A comparison of the acute effects on pulmonary function in cystic fibrosis. *Am Rev Respir Dis* 1984 Jan; 182–184.

Desmond KJ, et al: Immediate and long-term effects of chest physiotherapy in patients with cystic fibrosis. *J Pediatr* 1983 Oct; 538–542.

Doershuk CF, Stein RC: Cystic fibrosis. *In* Gellis SS, Kagan BM: *Current Pediatric Therapy 10.* Philadelphia, WB Saunders, 1982, 207–218.

Drotar D, et al: Psychosocial functioning of children with cystic fibrosis. *Pediatrics* 1981 Mar; 338–342.

Dwyer JM: Scientific criteria for adopting health screening measures. *Pediatr Nurs* 1983 May/Jun; 195–197.

Fleming J: Common dermatologic conditions in children. *MCN* 1981 Sep/Oct; 6(5):346–354.

Gerrard J: Allergies in breastfed babies to foods ingested by the mother. *Clin Rev Allergy* 1984; 2:143–149.

Goldberg RT, et al: Rehabilitation with cystic fibrosis: from Utopia to reality. Rehabil Lit 1980 Sep/Oct; 218–227.

Guyton AC: *Human Physiology and Mechanisms of Disease.* 3rd ed. Philadelphia, WB Saunders, 1986.

Hanifin J, Lobitz W: Newer concepts of atopic dermatitis. *Arch Dermatol* 1977; 113:663–670.

Huang NN, Palmer J: Management of patients with cystic fibrosis. III. Treatment of pulmonary infections and complications. *Respir Ther* 1981 May/Jun; 81–91.

Kaliner M, Slater J: Allergic rhinitis: *In* Gellis SS, Kagan BM (eds): *Current Pediatric Therapy 12.* Philadelphia, WB Saunders, 1986, 628–630.

Logvinoff MM, et al: Bronchodilators and diuretics in children with bronchopulmonary dysplasia. *Pediatr Pulmonol* 1985; 1:198.

Mammel MC, et al: Dexamethasone in bronchopulmonary dysplasia. Acute effects and long-term outcome. *Clin Res* 1985; 83:114A.

Mansmann HC Jr: Treatment of acute asthma in children. *In* Bierman CW, Pearlman DS: *Allergic Diseases from Infancy to Adulthood.* 2nd ed. Philadelphia, WB Saunders, 1988, 571–586.

Marmon L, et al: Pulmonary resection for complications of cystic fibrosis. *J Pediatr Surg* 1983 Dec; 811–816.

Myer PA: Parental adaptation to cystic fibrosis. *J Pediatr Health Care* 1988; 2(1):20–28.

Nadler HL, Walsh MMJ: Intrauterine detection of cystic fibrosis. *Pediatrics* 1980 Nov; 690–692.

Newmark P: Testing for cystic fibrosis. *Nature* 1985; 318:309.

Pearlman DF, Bierman CW: Asthma (bronchial asthma). *In* Bierman CW, Pearlman DS: *Allergic Diseases from Infancy to Adulthood.* 2nd ed. Philadelphia, WB Saunders, 1988, 546–570.

President's Commission for the Study of Ethical Problems in Medicine and Biomedical and Behavioral Research: *Cystic Fibrosis: A Case Study. Screening and Counseling for Genetic Conditions; The Ethical, Social and Legal Implications for Genetic Screening; Counseling and Educational Programs.* Washington, DC, US Government Printing Office, 1983, 87–103.

Rosen F: Developmental immunology. *Clin Immunol Allergy* 1985 Jun; 5.

Rudolph A: *Pediatrics.* Norwalk, CT, Appleton-Century-Crofts, 1982.

Shaman D: Tots play games to beat asthma. *Am Lung Assoc Bull* 1982 May; 68:4–9.

Stullenbarger B, et al: Family adaptation to cystic fibrosis. *Pediatr Nurs* 1987; 13(1):29–31.

Apnea-Related Disorders (Apnea, SIDS)

Aranda J, et al: Pharmacologic considerations in the therapy of neonatal apnea. *Pediatr Clin North Am* 1981 Feb; 113–133.

Brown L: Home monitoring of the high-risk infant. *Clin Perinatol* 1984 Feb; 85–100.

Camfield P, et al: Infant apnea syndrome: a prospective evaluation of etiologies. *Clin Pediatr* 1982 Nov; 684–687.

Deal A, Bordeaux BR: The phenomenon of SIDS. *Pediatr Nurs* 1980 Jan/Feb; 48–50.

Dean PG: Monitoring an apneic infant: impact on infant's mother. *Matern Child Nurs J* 1986; 15(2):65–76.

DeForest J, Mitchell I: Home apnea monitoring in infancy. *Can J Nurs* 1984 May; 37–41.

DeFrain J, Ernst L: The psychological effects of SIDS on surviving family members. *J Fam Pract* 1978 May; 985.

Duncan JA, Webb LZ: Teaching families home apnea monitoring. *Pediatr Nurs* 1983 May/Jun; 171–175.

Glassanos MR: Management of newborn apnea. *Neonatal Network* 1983 Aug; 8–11.

Graber HP, Balas-Stevens S: A discharge tool for teaching parents to monitor. *MCN* 1984 May/Jun; 178–180.

Guilleminault C, et al: Five cases of near-miss sudden infant death syndrome and development of obstructive sleep apnea syndrome. *Pediatrics* 1984 Jan; 71–78.

Shannon DC: Pathophysiologic mechanisms causing sleep apnea and hypoventilation in infants. Sleep 1980; 3(314):343–349.

Southall D: Family and community factors associated with infant deaths that might be preventable. *Br Med J* 1983 Nov 12; 1469.

Special problems when sudden infant death strikes. *Patient Care* 1984 Mar 15; 1–12.

Stanton AN, Oakley JR: Pattern of illnesses before cot deaths. *Arch Dis Child* 1983; 58:878–881.

Swoiskin S: Sudden infant death: nursing care for the survivors. *J Pediatr Nurs* 1986; 1(1):33–39.

Webb LZ, Duncan JA: Selecting the right home apnea monitor. *Pediatr Nurs* 1983 May/Jun; 179–182.

Nursing Strategies: Altered Cardiovascular Function

Chapter 39

Elaine Daberkow

Nursing Process Plan
NPP: The Child with Congestive Heart Failure, page 1323

Related Topics
Genetic counseling, Chapter 4 and Table 50-3
Impact of chronic illness, Chapter 25
Nursing Process Plan: Perioperative Care, Table 27-7
Nursing Process Plan: The Hospitalized Child, Table 31-2
Organic failure to thrive, Chapter 35
Kawasaki disease, Chapter 43
Rheumatic fever, Chapter 43

When an infant is born with any type of birth defect, the parents' coping abilities are challenged. Because the heart is vital to human existence and is viewed by many as the "life force" of the human body, a defect of the cardiac structure may have heightened significance to the parents and family. The nurse caring for the child with a cardiac defect must help the parents cope with their feelings of grief and fear so that they are able to deal with the facts related to their infant's illness.

In the United States most alterations in cardiovascular function in children are the result of defects in the heart that are present at birth, or *congenital* heart disease. *Acquired* heart disease (e.g., rheumatic fever, arrhythmias, Kawasaki disease) occurs less than one-tenth as often as congenital disease.

An estimated 40,000 babies are born with congenital heart disease in the United States yearly. Of these, about one third become critically ill in the first year of life, one third develop problems later in childhood or as young adults, and one third never experience serious handicaps (Nadas, 1986). Management of congenital heart disease is primarily surgical. Usually cardiac catheterization, an invasive diagnostic procedure, precedes surgery.

This chapter deals with nursing strategies related to recognition and diagnosis of congenital cardiac anomalies, cardiac surgery, and long-term care. The impact of heart disease on the infant and family will be both acute and long-term. Because congestive heart failure (CHF) is a threat common to many cardiac disorders, nursing care for the child with CHF is detailed in Table 39-5.

Congenital Heart Disease

Incidence and Etiology

Approximately 1 in 100 infants has one or more congenital cardiovascular abnormalities (Moss, 1983). The risk of congenital heart disease occurring in offspring of an affected parent as well as the risk of occurrence in newborn siblings of an affected child varies widely depending upon the specific heart defect and the etiologic circumstance.

Ninety per cent of congenital heart disease is thought to be due to multifactorial inheritance, in which there is a genetic predisposition for congenital heart disease that interacts with an environmental trigger during a vulnerable period of gestation. Environmental triggers (Table 39-1) can be separated into three main categories: drugs, infections, and maternal conditions.

Development of the heart and great vessels takes place during the first 14 to 60 days of gestation. This is

Table 39-1. Environmental Triggers of Congenital Heart Defects

Environmental Triggers	Frequency (Per Cent)
Drugs	
Alcohol	25 to 30
Chemotherapy	5
Amphetamines	5 to 10
Hydantoin	2 to 3
Trimethadione	15 to 30
Lithium	10
Thalidomide	5 to 10
Sex hormones	2 to 4
Infections	
Rubella	35
Cytomegalovirus	?
Maternal Conditions	
Diabetes	3 to 5
Lupus erythematosus	?
Phenylketonuria	25 to 50

(From Daberkow and Washington, 1985.)

considered the vulnerable period of gestation for cardiac malformation. The specific type of cardiac malformation produced varies depending on the environmental trigger and its timing within the vulnerable period.

Approximately 8 per cent of congenital heart disease is associated with other abnormalities such as trisomies 21, 18, and 13, Turner syndrome, and Noonan syndrome. Approximately 2 per cent of congenital heart disease is thought to be due to environmental factors alone, not requiring a genetic predisposition. Alcohol, thalidomide, rubella, and possibly cytomegalovirus are environmental triggers in this category (Moss, 1983). Multiple environmental triggers have been identified in the last two decades, but many more have yet to be discovered. In most cases of congenital heart disease the specific cause cannot be identified. It is hoped that ongoing research in this area will delineate more clearly the full range of environmental influences that cause congenital heart disease. Box 39-1 outlines nursing strategies for prevention of congenital heart anomalies.

Anatomy and Physiology of the Circulatory System

In order adequately to assess and intervene for cardiac abnormalities the nurse must be aware of normal differences in structure and function that result from anatomic and physiologic immaturity. Table 39-2 summarizes these developmental differences. The remainder of this section describes fetal circulation and the physiologic changes that occur at birth. Knowledge of these cardiopulmonary changes provides a base for understanding congenital heart disease.

Fetal Circulation

A thorough understanding of fetal circulation and physiologic changes occurring in the neonate from birth through the first few weeks of life is important in order to understand congenital heart disease and its presentation. Fetal circulation (Fig. 39-1) differs from neonatal circulation in many significant ways. In the former, the placenta is the major route of gas exchange, excretion, and acquisition of essential fetal chemicals. The lungs are fluid filled and extract oxygen from the blood instead of providing oxygen for it. In addition, the pulmonary blood vessels are constricted and have a thick muscle coating, which offers a high resistance to blood flow. Therefore, in fetal circulation the right ventricle pumps against a higher resistance than the left ventricle. The left ventricle pumps against the low resistance of the placenta (Moss, 1983).

The three shunts present in fetal circulation—the ductus venosus, the foramen ovale, and the ductus arteriosus—enable the fetus to receive highly oxy-

Box 39-1
Congenital Heart Anomalies: Nurse's Role in Prevention

Assessing for children and families at risk

- Genetic counseling for parents with one child with CHD or a parent with CHD
- Screening infants of mothers with maternal rubella, diabetes, or lupus erythematosus
- Screening of premature infants
- Screening of infants with other congenital anomalies, or with chromosomal aberrations

Implementing preventive measures

- Rubella vaccine by 15 months of age
- Rubella titer on women with questionable history of rubella
- Genetic counseling of women over 35 years of age
- Maintaining a positive maternal environment
  1. no cigarette smoking
  2. no alcohol ingestion
  3. adequate nutrition, rest, and exercise
  4. prevention of illness during pregnancy
  5. no self-prescribed drugs

Table 39-2. Developmental Differences in Structure and Function of the Cardiovascular System

Anatomy and Physiology	Significance
Preterm	
Prostaglandin E_1: Preterm infants may have increased prostaglandin E_1 levels (in fetal life prostaglandin E_1 and decreased PO_2 maintain patency of the ductus arteriosus)	In the presence of lung disease (e.g., respiratory distress syndrome), which causes hypoxia, increased prostaglandin E_1 results in patent ductus arteriosus
Pulmonary vascular resistance and myocardial capacity: Preterm infants have a proportionately faster decline in pulmonary vascular resistance, leading to increased left to right shunting through anomalous connections in the heart. In addition their heart muscles are immature and poorly equipped to handle the increased volume that results with shunting	Preterm infants with congenital heart defects are more prone to congestive heart failure than are full-term infants
Full-Term Infant	
Pulmonary and cardiac pressures: Neonate retains increased pulmonary vascular resistance due to pulmonary vessel hypertrophy; this increases pressures on the right side of the heart	Detection of ASD and VSD may be delayed because increased right atrial and ventricular pressures decrease the left to right shunting
Stroke volume: Children have limited ability to increase stroke volume in response to decreased cardiac output	When cardiac output decreases the child will respond with tachycardia
Infants and Young Children	
Chest wall: Chest walls are thin in infants and young children because of the relative lack of subcutaneous and muscle tissue compared with older children	"Innocent" murmurs can be auscultated in structurally normal hearts because the normal turbulence is audible through the thin chest wall

genated blood from the umbilical veins and deliver it to the tissues with the highest oxygen demand, the fetal myocardium and the brain.* The *ductus venosus* shunts highly oxygenated blood from the umbilical veins to the inferior vena cava. The blood then enters the right atrium and most of it is directed through the *foramen ovale* into the left atrium. Here it mixes with blood returning from the lungs through the pulmonary veins and passes into the left ventricle. It then flows from the left ventricle into the aorta, perfusing the coronary, carotid, and subclavian arteries before entering the descending aorta and returning ultimately to the placenta. Blood returning from the head and upper limbs of the fetus enters the right atrium via the superior vena cava, passes into the right ventricle, and exits through the pulmonary artery. A small percentage of the blood flows to the left and right lungs via the left and right pulmonary arteries. The greatest percentage of blood, however, flows through the *ductus arteriosus* and into the descending aorta to return to the placenta. Blood flow through the ductus arteriosus is from pulmonary artery to aorta (right to left) because of the high resistance to flow in the lungs and the low resistance to flow in the aorta.

For normal development of the cardiac structure, including chambers, valves, and vessels, it is essential that blood flows in appropriate quantities unobstructed throughout the developing heart and great vessels. Lack of blood flow through a chamber or vessel results in hypoplasia of that chamber or vessel. For example, in tricuspid atresia with intact ventricular septum there is no forward blood flow to the right ventricle, and the right ventricle is usually very hypoplastic.

Changes in Circulation After Birth

Profound hemodynamic changes occurring immediately after birth allow the neonate to adapt to the external environment. With the first breaths, the alveoli expand and the resistance to blood flow in the lungs (pulmonary vascular resistance) decreases, allowing more blood flow to the lungs. The resistance to blood flow in the systemic circulation (systemic vascular resistance) and left ventricular pressure are greatly increased owing to removal of the placenta, which offered low resistance to blood flow (Merenstein, 1985). Systemic vascular resistance is now higher than pulmonary vascular resistance, and blood flow through the ductus arteriosus is therefore from left to right (from aorta to the pulmonary artery).

The volume of blood returning to the left atrium is greatly increased by two factors: 1) the decrease in pulmonary vascular resistance allowing for more blood flow to the lungs from the right heart, and 2) the shunting of blood from left to right through the ductus arteriosus to the lungs. The increased volume of blood returning to the left atrium distends the left atrium and increases left atrial pressure, which assists in closure of the foramen ovale. This takes place usually within the first few hours to days of life.

The ductus arteriosus closes anatomically within the first several days after birth; however, it does not

* In utero the umbilical artery carries the desaturated or unoxygenated blood from the fetus to the maternal circulation. The umbilical veins carry the highly oxygenated blood from the maternal circulation to the fetus.

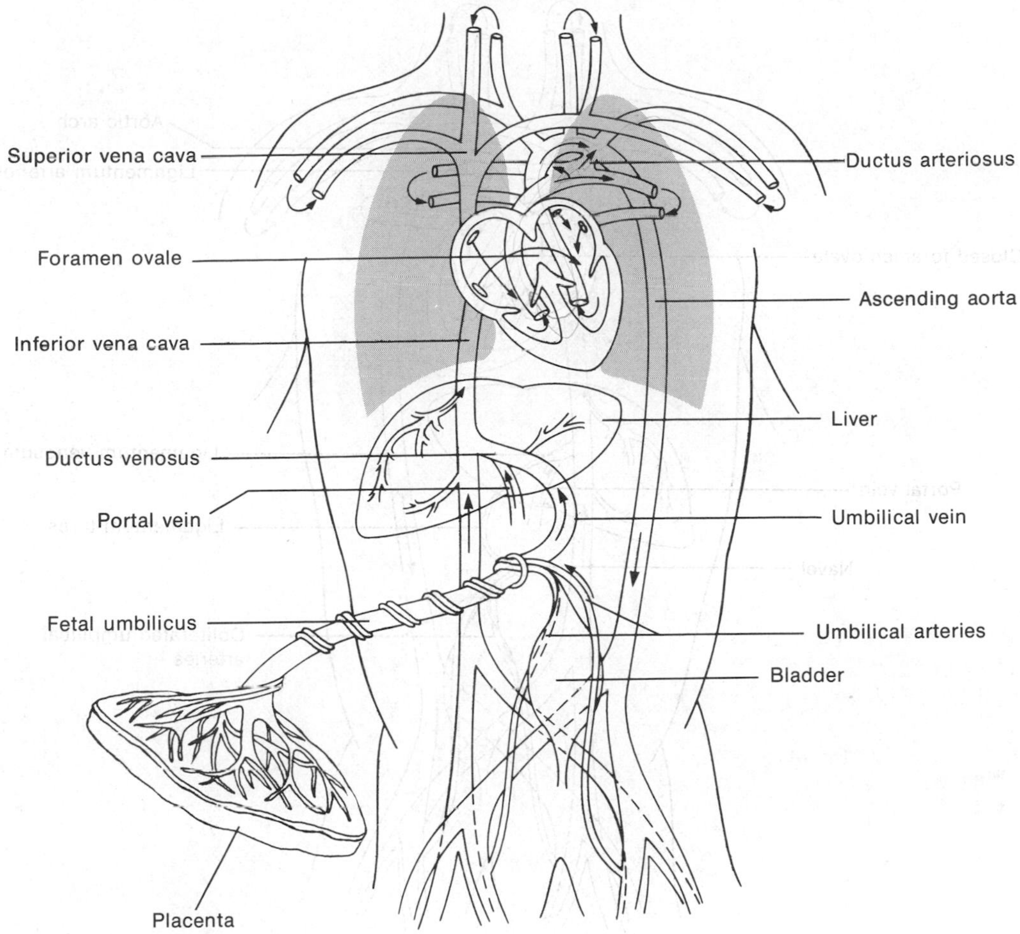

***Figure* 39-1.** Fetal circulation.

become obliterated until several months to a year later (Moss, 1983). The left to right shunt through the ductus arteriosus usually persists for 15 to 20 hours after birth or it may last for several days. The increased oxygen tension (PaO_2) in the neonate's arterial blood from increased pulmonary blood flow and oxygenation in the lungs initiates constriction of the ductus arteriosus. The umbilical veins, umbilical arteries, and ductus venosus no longer carry blood so the blood in these structures clots and they atrophy (Merenstein et al, 1985).

The neonate's circulation (Fig. 39-2) now resembles that of the adult in that desaturated blood returns from the body via the superior and inferior venae cavae to the right atrium and passes through the tricuspid valve to the right ventricle. From the right ventricle blood passes through the pulmonary valve into the main pulmonary artery, then into the left and right pulmonary arteries, and finally into the lungs, where oxygenation occurs. Saturated blood returns via the pulmonary veins to the left atrium and passes through the mitral valve into the left ventricle. From the left ventricle blood flows through the aortic valve into the aorta and the systemic arterial system. Neonatal circulation is unique, however, in that the newborn retains elevated pulmonary vascular resistance and elevated pressures in the right ventricle and pulmonary system owing to the hypertrophy of the pulmonary vessels. This hypertrophy slowly resolves, and the pulmonary vascular resistance and right heart pressures decrease to normal by 1 to 2 months of age (Merenstein et al, 1985). Adjustments in cardiopulmonary physiology at birth are summarized in Table 39-3.

Recognition of Congenital Cardiac Anomalies

Vital to the diagnosis of congenital heart disease is a thorough history and physical examination. A variety of other diagnostic procedures and tests may also be ordered. Diagnostic assessment is summarized in Box 39-2.

History

An infant who has symptoms of cardiac disease in the first few hours to days or weeks of life most likely has a significant defect. Complex lesions such as trans-

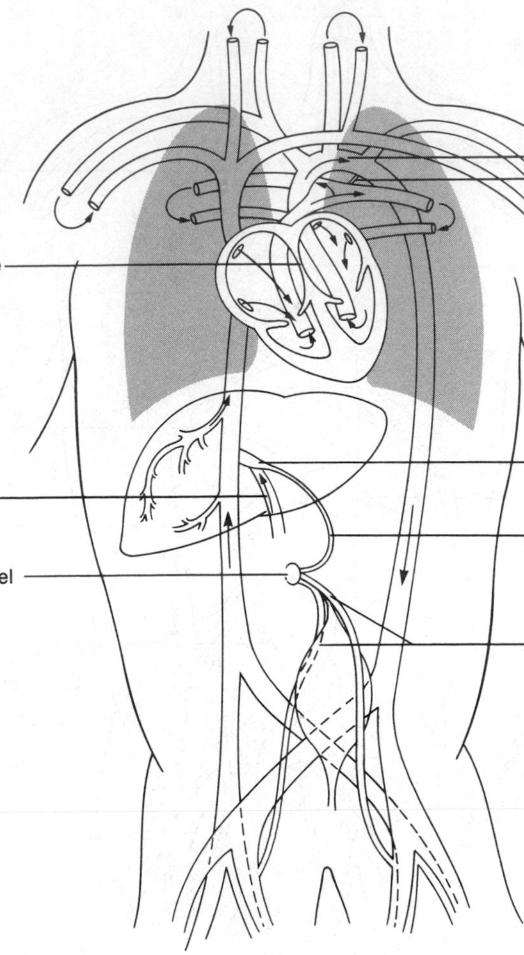

***Figure* 39-2.** Neonatal circulation.

position of the great arteries, tetralogy of Fallot, pulmonary atresia, hypoplastic left heart, coarctation of the aorta, and truncus arteriosus are likely to be diagnosed within the first 2 weeks of life.

Congenital heart disease may not be discovered while the infant is in the hospital. Parents may bring the infant to the physician's office with a number of concerns. During the history the parents may mention that the infant is having feeding problems. These problems may be characterized by profuse sweating or fatigue during feeding, tachypnea, irritability, reflux, and the desire to feed coupled with the inability to do so. Concern may be expressed that the infant has failed to gain weight appropriately. Parents should be asked to detail the infant's feeding behavior. How often does the infant eat? How long do feedings take? How does the infant act during the feedings? How much formula is taken during one feeding? How much formula is taken during 24 hours? How does the infant respond after a feeding? Is there any vomiting?

The toddler and the older child may be described as a "picky" or "slow" eater. The parents' main concern may be that the child has had poor weight gain.

Respiratory difficulties such as rapid respirations, difficulty breathing (retractions, nasal flaring, grunting, stridor, deep "sighing" respirations), anoxic spells, or respiratory infections may be reported by the parents. Parents should be asked to elaborate on any respiratory problems. Does the infant or child have a chronic cough or frequent choking episodes? If respiratory infections have been reported, how frequent have they been and of what severity? If the parents have been concerned about their infant having rapid breathing, it is important to discern how rapid the respirations have been and of what duration. Normal neonates often exhibit occasional periodic breathing with intermittent bursts of rapid respirations.

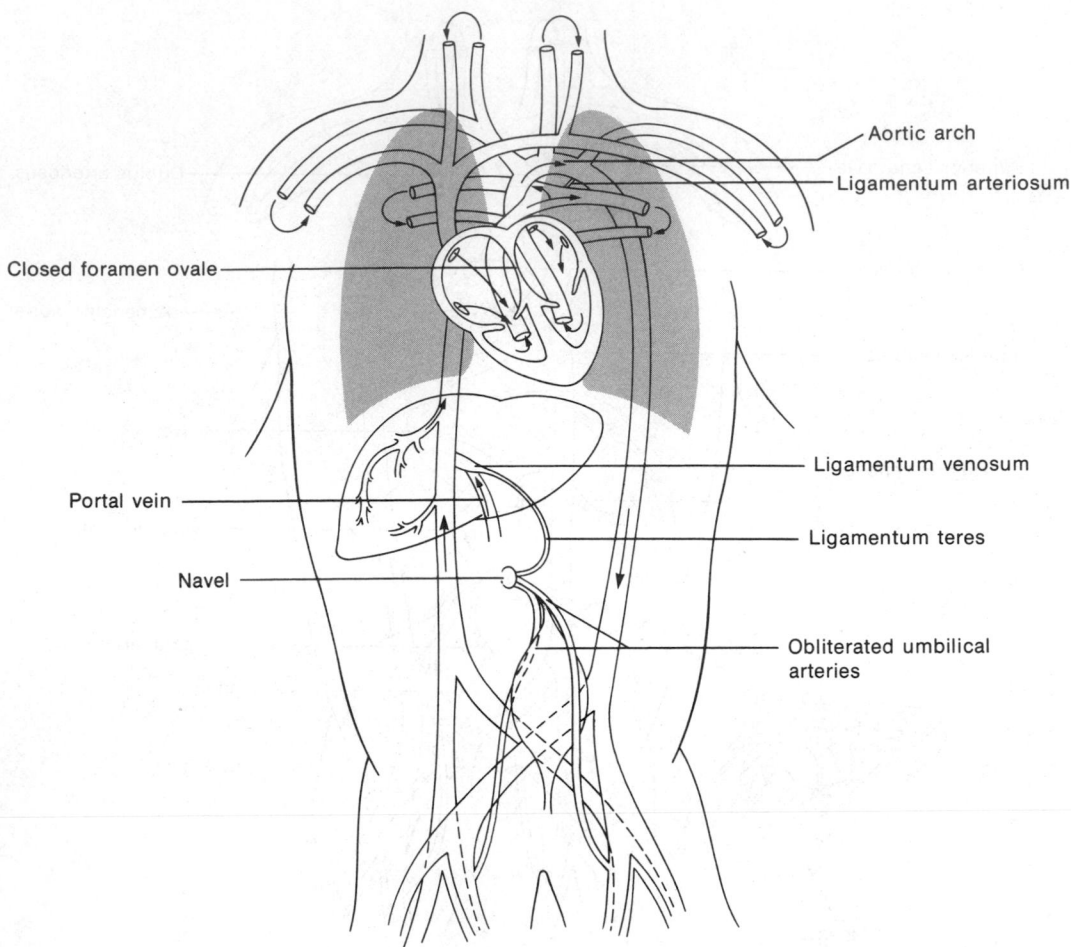

Parents may report pallor and a bluish cast (termed *cyanosis*) to the skin, mucous membranes, lips, nailbeds, and conjunctivae, either persistent or intermittent. Questions to ask include: Does the infant's color change when crying? when feeding? when defecating? when position is changed suddenly? Has the infant ever turned blue, and if so, under what circumstances and room temperature? For the toddler and older child, parents should be asked if the child's color

Table 39-3. Adjustments in Cardiopulmonary Physiology at Birth

Structure	Function Before Birth	Function After Birth
Placenta	Oxygen and carbon dioxide exchange	Eliminated from circulation: function assumed by lungs
Foramen ovale	Connects right and left atria. Oxygenated blood from the right atrium shunts directly into the left atrium, bypassing the right ventricle and pulmonary circuit	Functionally closes soon after birth and then undergoes obliteration by fusion of tissue margins during childhood
Lungs	Uninflated, pulmonary blood flow minimal	Fully aerated in about 2 wk. Pulmonary circulation provides for carbon dioxide and oxygen exchange
Ductus arteriosus	Bypasses the flow of blood through the lungs by shunting blood directly from the pulmonary artery to the descending aorta	Usually closes functionally soon after birth, and obliterates in the ensuing weeks
Aorta	Receives a mixture of oxygenated and nonoxygenated blood from the left ventricle and pulmonary artery	Carries only oxygenated blood from the left ventricle

changes during exercise, crying, respiratory infections, or rest.

Activity level or activity intolerance must be investigated. Parents may complain that their infant is continuously restless, becomes tired easily during feedings, or is lethargic and sleeps all the time. Parents should be asked to describe the position the infant usually assumes when asleep or resting. Often infants with cardiac problems sleep with the upper extremities flaccidly extended above the head or favor the knee-chest position. The parents may say that the infant is persistently "sweaty," especially during feedings but even while at complete rest. When asked to describe their toddler or older child's activity level, many parents may feel their child has normal exercise tolerance. Further questions can help clarify what "normal" means to them: What activities does the child perform? Are there siblings or other children the child plays with, so parents can compare his or her activity level with that of other children? Does the child keep up with other children at play or require frequent rest periods? Is there a tendency toward performing sedentary tasks? Does the child ever complain of headaches, dizziness, leg cramps, chest pain, or shortness of breath with exercise? Has he or she ever "passed out" or fainted? Does the child frequently squat during play or activities? Does the child feel palpitations (possibly described as a "funny" feeling in the chest or as chest pain) or a fast heart rate?

It is important to explore any other parental concerns. In addition, the school-age and adolescent child should be included in the interview and asked about his or her symptoms and concerns. It is important for the child to feel included and an integral part of the discussions. This will enhance the child's understanding, help to allay fears, and increase the child's sense of control.

The mother's history regarding the pregnancy, birth, and neonatal period should be elicited. Special inquiry should be made as to the maternal health history during the first trimester of pregnancy including rubella, viral infections, medications, and x-rays. Family history is obtained related to congenital heart disease as well as connective tissue disorders, hypercalcemia, and glycogen storage disease.

Physical Assessment

In addition to the concerns expressed by parents, the nurse may recognize signs indicative of congenital heart disease as evidenced by alterations in general appearance, skin, vital signs, chest, and abdomen. The nurse who performs a physical assessment of cardiac function will want to keep in mind those differences in cardiovascular structure and function that are related to development (see Table 39-2).

General Appearance

General body position and level of activity should be noted. Is the infant or child resting comfortably or is he or she fretful, agitated? Does the child respond to stimuli appropriately or appear flaccid and lethargic? What is the nutritional status? Is the child small for his or her

Box 39-2
Diagnostic Procedures and Their Purposes

NONINVASIVE

1. History

Identifies possible etiologic factors: checks on presence and character of symptoms to evaluate nature and severity of the cardiac defect

2. Complete physical examination

a. General: Reveals objective signs of congenital cardiac disease, such as cyanosis, clubbing of nails, increased respiratory effort; discloses features of syndromes that may be associated with congenital cardiac anomalies, such as Down syndrome, Turner syndrome, rubella
b. Vital signs: Determines respiratory and cardiac rates; reveals response of the child to cardiac disease; determines blood pressure in the arms and legs to detect coarctation of the aorta, as well as systemic hypertension
c. Thoracic: Reveals deformities of thorax and displacement of cardiac apex, which may reflect cardiomegaly
d. Lungs: Discloses pulmonary complications of congenital cardiac disease, such as pulmonary edema
e. Cardiac: Estimates cardiac size by palpating the apical impulse; identifies thrills reflecting loud murmurs; identifies cardiac rhythm and character of cardiac sounds by auscultation; identifies location and character of murmur
f. Abdomen: Identifies size of liver, which is enlarged in CHF, and size of spleen, which may be enlarged in infective endocarditis

3. Roentgenographic examination

a. Thoracic roentgenogram: Provides four types of information about the cardiovascular system: (1) cardiac size and size of specific chambers or great vessels; (2) cardiac contour; (3) status of pulmonary blood flow; and (4) status of lungs and other noncardiac tissue (e.g., size of thymus, rib notching, scoliosis)
b. Cardiac Fluoroscopy: Provides direct observation of the size, position, and contour of the heart, its chambers, and the venous and arterial trunks, and the motions of the heart, great vessels, lungs, and diaphragm

4. Electrocardiography

Records the electrical activity of the cardiac muscle from different sites and in different planes of the body. This electrical activity can be altered by myocardial damage, chamber enlargement, or hypertrophy, electrolyte imbalance, and pericardial disease. Also valuable in identifying cardiac arrhythmias

5. Echocardiography

Identifies and records, by means of reflected sound waves, intracardiac structures and their motion, whether normal or abnormal

6. Hemoglobin and hematocrit

Reflects magnitude of desaturation and cyanosis. Red blood cell count, hemoglobin, and hematocrit increase to compensate for decreased systemic arterial oxygen saturation (as in cyanosis). A high hematocrit (polycythemia) results in increased blood viscosity and may lead to cerebral thrombosis

INVASIVE

1. Heart catheterization

(Radiopaque catheters are inserted in veins or arteries and are advanced into the heart under fluoroscopy. This is usually done from the groin in children. Cutdown or percutaneous techniques may be used to insert the catheter. The venous catheter is used to probe the right side of the heart, and the arterial catheter the left ventricle in retrograde manner. The left side of the heart can often be entered with the venous catheter by way of the foramen ovale, especially in infants.)

Allows determination of oxygen saturation and pressure in the various cardiac chambers and vessels, thereby identifying obstructive lesions and shunting of blood from one side of the heart to the other. Cardiac output and vascular resistances can be calculated. The response of the heart to exercise and drugs can be evaluated using these data. Injection of dye is often used in evaluating cardiac anatomy

2. Angiocardiography

(Radiopaque media are injected into cardiac chambers or vessels and a record is made by means of serial x-ray films or movies. Usually included as a part of catheterization procedure.)

Provides visualization of cardiac chambers and vessels, demonstrating shunts, type of obstruction, and size and abnormal location of chambers or vessels. Constitutes a permanent record age? Does there seem to be adequate subcutaneous tissue or malnourishment? Are there any obvious features of syndromes that may be associated with congenital heart defects, such as Down syndrome?

Skin

Assess the infant's color for cyanosis or pallor or both. Cyanosis may be the only evidence of a cardiac lesion during the first weeks of life. With cyanosis there is a 3 g per cent of reduced hemoglobin in arterial blood or a 4 to 5 g per cent reduced hemoglobin in the peripheral capillary blood (Merenstein et al, 1985). This is best observed in the oral mucous membranes, lips, tongue, and gums, which have high vascularity and many superficial blood vessels. Mild cyanosis may appear as "high" or "ruddy" color, with unusually red cheeks, lips, and fingertips, all unrelated to the temperature of the environment.

Peripheral cyanosis is best demonstrated in the hands and feet, especially the nailbeds. It may be seen with those lesions causing right to left cardiac shunts as well as with conditions causing vasoconstriction and poor cardiac output. Clubbing, a broadening and thickening of the fingertips, can be seen in cyanotic patients by about 1 to 2 years of age (Fig. 39-3). Clubbing is a compensatory response to cyanosis. Capillary proliferation in the tips of the fingers and toes occurs as the result of decreased peripheral tissue perfusion. Accurate assessment of color requires good lighting. Also, the infant or child should be kept warm and assessed both while at rest and during activity. Because activity increases the body's requirement for oxygen, cyanosis will be more pronounced during activity. In dark-skinned children peripheral cyanosis is more difficult to assess; thus, these children should be assessed primarily by checking mucous membranes. Moistness of the skin should be observed. Diaphoresis may occur in children with left to right shunts.

Presence or absence of edema should be noted. Infants usually manifest fluid retention as weight gain; however, they may have facial, especially periorbital, edema. The toddler and older child may have generalized edema, noticeable in the face, hands, and feet.

Vital Signs

Respiratory status must be assessed. Respirations are counted for one full minute with the infant or child undressed and at rest. Observe for *tachypnea* (a resting respiratory rate greater than 60 respirations per minute in an infant up to 1 year of age, greater than 50 per minute in a 2-year-old, and greater than 35 per minute in a 3-year-old), expiratory grunting, stridor, nasal flaring, retractions (between and below the ribs), and dyspnea (Moss, 1983).

An apical pulse must be carefully assessed. A resting heart rate over 160 beats per minute in an infant,

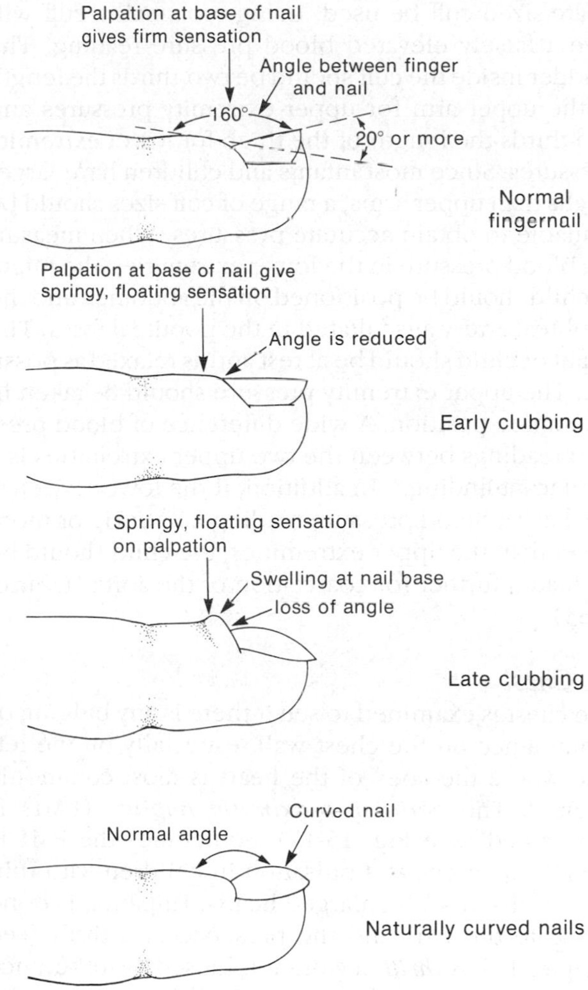

Figure 39-3. Clubbing in infant's fingers, caused by poor oxygenation.

over 120 beats per minute in a 1-year-old, and over 100 beats per minute in a 3-year-old is considered *tachycardia* (Moss, 1983). Fever and other existing illness must be taken into account when evaluating heart rate. The apical pulse is assessed for one full minute, with its character, regularity, and rate noted. Peripheral pulses are assessed simultaneously and any pulse deficit or other abnormalities are noted. Decreased or absent pulses in the lower extremities may be a sign of coarctation of the aorta. The following grades are commonly used to assess peripheral pulses:

0 = Absent pulse
1+ = Palpable
2+ = Normal
3+ = Full
4+ = Full and bounding

Blood pressure, another important parameter that the nurse must assess, should be measured in both upper extremities and one lower extremity. It is crucial in assessing accurate blood pressures that the appropriate-sized cuff be used. Using too small a cuff will give a falsely elevated blood pressure reading. The bladder inside the cuff should be two-thirds the length of the upper arm for upper extremity pressures and two-thirds the length of the thigh for lower extremity pressures. Since most infants and children have larger thighs than upper arms, a range of cuff sizes should be available to obtain accurate pressures. When measuring blood pressure in the lower extremities, the infant or child should be positioned on the abdomen and the popliteal artery auscultated in the popliteal fossa. The infant or child should be at rest and as relaxed as possible. The upper extremity pressure should be taken in the supine position. A wide difference of blood pressure readings between the two upper extremities is a significant finding.* In addition, if the lower extremities have a blood pressure reading 20 mmHg or more lower than the upper extremities, the child should be evaluated further for coarctation of the aorta (Uzarle, 1983).

Chest

The chest is examined to see if there is any bulging or prominence on the chest wall, especially on the left side where the apex of the heart is most commonly situated. The *point of maximum impulse* (PMI) is ascertained (see Fig. 15-17). Sometimes the PMI is visually apparent as a pulsation in children with thin chest walls or with enlarged hearts. Palpation is done to locate the PMI and the presence of a thrill (see Chapter 15). A *thrill* (a vibration caused by turbulence of blood flow in the heart) may be felt by placing the tips of the fingers on the anterior chest wall. The vibration has been described as like a purring kitten.

Auscultation of the heart using a stethoscope is done to check the quality, rate, and rhythm of the heart sounds and to identify murmurs. Murmurs are the most common means of identifying congenital heart disease. A *murmur* is a sound created by turbulent blood flow through the heart.

When assessing a murmur it should be described in terms of several parameters; its position in the cardiac cycle and its duration, configuration, pitch, intensity, quality, and response to exercise and movement. There are two categories of murmurs: innocent and organic. *Innocent murmurs* are not associated with any underlying pathology; the heart is structurally normal. Innocent murmurs represent the turbulence of normal blood flow through the heart and are commonly heard in infants and young children because of their thin chest walls. These murmurs increase in intensity with fever and exercise owing to increased heart rate and cardiac output. Innocent murmurs usually are no longer heard as the child reaches school age and adolescence. Parents require thorough explanations and reassurances that their child with an innocent murmur has a "normal" heart. *Organic murmurs* are associated with either acquired or congenital heart disease.

Heart murmurs are classified according to their loudness and the presence or absence of a thrill. Murmurs are graded from I (least severe) to VI (most severe) and are described as follows:

Grade I — Very faint, difficult to hear unless child is very quiet, may be heard faintly after a period of attentive listening
Grade II — Soft, though readily heard; louder than grade I
Grade III — Moderately loud; no thrill
Grade IV — Loud with a thrill
Grade V — Loud enough to be heard with a stethoscope barely on the chest wall; thrill is present
Grade VI — Can be heard without having the stethoscope on the chest wall; accompanied by a thrill

Abdomen

The abdomen should be palpated for hepatomegaly, defined as enlargement of the liver greater than 3 cm below the right costal margin (see section on congestive heart failure).

Diagnostic Tests

Electrocardiogram

An electrocardiogram (ECG or EKG) is a graphic tracing of the electrical activity produced by the heart muscle from different sides and from different planes of the body. The heart action that accompanies each phase of electrical activity is described in Figure 39-4. The ECG shows the sequence of electrical events in the heart, the heart rate and rhythm, damage to the heart muscle, and conduction disturbances. In addition, hypertrophy or enlargement of cardiac chambers can be determined from the ECG. Leads are placed on the extremities and the chest for recording of the ECG; this is a noninvasive technique.

Echocardiography

Echocardiography is a noninvasive technique using ultrasound (high-frequency sound waves) to obtain an image of the structure of the heart. It graphically records the position and motion of the heart walls and the internal structures of the heart and neighboring tissue by the echo obtained from beams of ultrasonic waves directed through the chest wall. M-mode echo-

* A 10 to 15 mmHg difference between the upper extremities can be found in normal individuals.

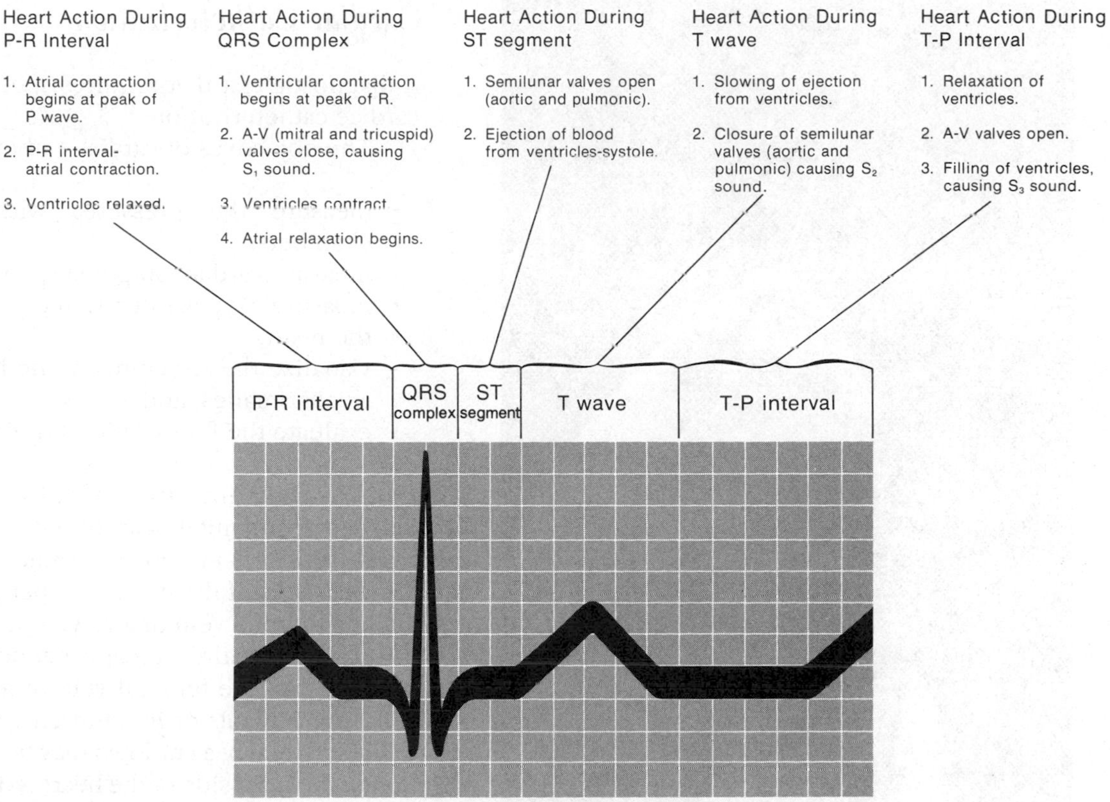
Heart Action During P-R Interval
1. Atrial contraction begins at peak of P wave.
2. P-R interval- atrial contraction.
3. Ventricles relaxed.
Heart Action During QRS Complex
1. Ventricular contraction begins at peak of R.
2. A-V (mitral and tricuspid) valves close, causing S_1 sound.
3. Ventricles contract.
4. Atrial relaxation begins.
Heart Action During ST segment
1. Semilunar valves open (aortic and pulmonic).
2. Ejection of blood from ventricles-systole.
Heart Action During T wave
1. Slowing of ejection from ventricles.
2. Closure of semilunar valves (aortic and pulmonic) causing S_2 sound.
Heart Action During T-P Interval
1. Relaxation of ventricles.
2. A-V valves open.
3. Filling of ventricles, causing S_3 sound.
P-R interval
QRS complex
ST segment
T wave
T-P interval

Figure 39-4. Electrocardiogram (ECG) with description of heart action in each phase of electrical activity.

cardiography provides a single-dimension view, whereas 2-D echocardiography gives a two-dimensional picture. When Doppler ultrasonography is used with 2-D echocardiography, the physician can measure the pressure on either side of valves in the heart and determine cardiac output and blood flow patterns within the heart and great arteries (Friedman, 1988). Color flow echocardiography adds the advantage of representing blood flow abnormalities in color. The advancement of these noninvasive techniques has reduced the necessity for cardiac catheterization and enhanced early diagnosis. However, echocardiograms may not always be totally accurate, owing to artifact (interference with the sound waves) or an inability to visualize specific areas of the heart. Further diagnostic procedures such as a cardiac catheterization are often necessary to define cardiac anatomy accurately.

Chest Roentgenogram

Chest roentgenograms provide information regarding the cardiac size and the size of specific chambers or great vessels, the cardiac contour, the status of pulmonary blood flow, and the status of the lungs and other noncardiac tissues (e.g., size of thymus, rib notching).

Although many of these diagnostic studies are noninvasive techniques that are not painful, careful explanation of each test must be given to the parents and to the child. The strangeness of the environment and the equipment is frightening; therefore, nursing intervention is aimed at informing the parents and the child to lessen their anxiety.

MRI (Magnetic Resonance Imaging)

Magnetic Resonance Imaging (MRI) has proved to be extremely useful in the diagnosis of coarctation of the aorta. It is a new, noninvasive imaging technique that gives high resolution tomographic images without either contrast injection or radiation. This is accomplished by the application of low-energy radio waves in combination with a strong magnetic field. The magnet aligns hydrogen atoms while the radio waves cause the protons to resonate and generate low-frequency signals. This, in turn, is translated into tomographic images.

As this technique is fairly new and the equipment costly, it is not available in all institutions.

Transcutaneous Pulse Oximetry

Transcutaneous pulse oximetry is an accurate, noninvasive means of assessing arterial oxygen saturation. It is an effective, nonthreatening way of evaluating suspected cyanosis in infants and children at rest and during rapidly changing circulatory states. See Chapter 38, page 1174.

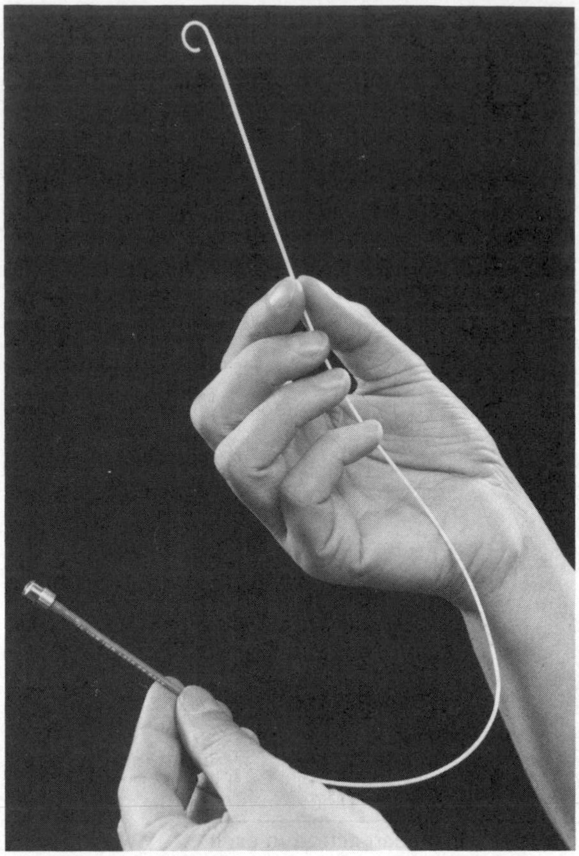

Figure 39-5. Catheter used for cardiac catheterization of an infant. This is called a pigtail catheter because of the curled end. This end has small holes out of which dye is injected into the heart chamber.

Hematologic Testing

Hematologic tests are done to help in the work-up and diagnosis of congenital heart disease. A complete blood count is ordered. The child with a cyanotic defect will usually show an increased hemoglobin and hematocrit. The tissue hypoxia associated with cyanosis stimulates the bone marrow to produce increased red blood cells (polycythemia) for additional oxygen carrying capacity. Polycythemia may lead to problems of clotting due to increased viscosity of the blood.

Arterial blood gases may also be ordered to determine the oxygen saturation of the arterial blood. In cyanotic newborn infants a shunt study is often ordered to determine if the cyanosis is due to congenital heart disease. A shunt study consists of obtaining arterial blood gases while the infant is breathing room air. The infant is then placed in 100 per cent oxygen for approximately 10 to 15 minutes and arterial blood gases are then redrawn. The infant's PaO_2 in 100 per cent oxygen should be greater than 150 (mmHg) and often it will rise as high as 250 (mmHg) to 300 (mmHg). If the infant's PaO_2 cannot be elevated to at least 150 (mmHg) then cyanotic heart disease is suspected (Moss, 1983).

Cardiac Catheterization

A diagnostic test that requires special nursing care is cardiac catheterization.

The objectives of cardiac catheterization are to:

- measure the pressures within the different chambers,
- measure cardiac output and function,
- measure oxygen saturation within the chambers of the heart,
- visualize the structures of the heart to determine any anomalies, and
- evaluate the flow of blood through the heart.

This is an invasive, definitive procedure used to diagnose congenital heart disease. It involves passing a thin, flexible, radiopaque catheter (Fig. 39-5) into the chambers of the heart via a peripheral vessel, usually the femoral vein or artery. A percutaneous needle puncture is usually all that is needed to introduce the catheter into the femoral vein or artery. However, in very small infants or in children with vessels that are difficult to reach, a cutdown may be done. Catheterization of the right side of the heart is done by passing the catheter into the femoral vein and advancing it through the inferior vena cava and into the right atrium, the right ventricle, and the pulmonary artery. Pressure measurements are recorded and saturations obtained. If the foramen ovale is patent or an atrial septal defect is present, the catheter may be advanced into the left atrium through this opening and the left side of the heart catheterized. If there is no atrial or ventricular level communication then the left side of the heart may be catheterized by passing the catheter into the femoral artery and into the descending aorta to the left atrium. The catheterization is usually done in combination with angiography. In this procedure a contrast medium is injected into a chamber of the heart and a video recording of the x-ray films is made. This allows for later replay and detailed examination of the cardiac structure.

Preparation of Child and Family

Psychologic preparation of the child and the family is an integral part of nursing care for the catheterization procedure. It is important to explain the procedure to parents and keep them informed of what will take place next (Box 39-3). For cardiac catheterization the infant or child may be admitted to the hospital for a 48-hour stay. The child is admitted the day before the procedure, during which time the physical examination, chest radiograph, ECG, and laboratory work are performed.

Laboratory work done will usually include a type

Box 39-3
Cardiac Catheterization—Parent Instruction Sheet

Your child will receive a local anesthetic (like a dentist gives), which will reduce feeling in the leg. When the local anesthetic is injected some slight discomfort and pressure will be felt, but everything is done to make this test as painless and comfortable as possible. During the procedure thin plastic tubes, called catheters, are inserted into a vein or artery in the leg. When the catheters are in place the cardiologist is able to learn the nature of your child's heart trouble by analyzing blood samples and by measuring blood pressures through these tubes. A special fluid that is visible on x-ray is injected into the heart chambers through the catheters. Heart malformations are identified by x-ray films as the fluid travels through the circulatory system.

The test usually takes approximately 2 hours. When it is over a bandage is placed over the area where the catheters were inserted. At times it is necessary to make a small incision to reach the vein or artery, instead of just through a needle stick. In this case the incision will be closed with several stitches which will be removed within a week.

Following the catheterization your child will return to the Day Surgery Unit and will most likely be very sleepy the remainder of the afternoon. Your child will need to keep his or her leg straight (and not bend the knees) to prevent bleeding from the catheterization site. You may hold your child in your arms if this is more comfortable; however, it is important to keep your child's leg straight while you are holding him or her. Your child may begin taking clear liquids soon after arriving in the Day Surgery Unit. If he or she can drink clear liquids without becoming nauseated or sick to the stomach regular food can be eaten. The nurses will be checking your child's pulses, blood pressure, temperature, and catheterization site frequently for the first hour. After 4 to 5 hours in the Day Surgery Unit if the cardiologist feels your child is ready, he or she may go home.

HOME CARE INSTRUCTIONS

Diet: Your child may return to a regular diet as soon as he or she reaches home. Once in a great while the effects of the catheterization may make a child lose appetite, in which case you should start with liquids and slowly return to solid foods over the next 24 hours. If nausea and vomiting do not stop, call your physician.

Cleanliness: It is best to keep the child out of the bathtub for 24 hours, using sponge baths instead. If there are stitches, it is better to use sponge bathing (staying clear of the wound) until the stitches are removed by your doctor.

Keep the catheterization site clean and dry. It is usually best to leave this area open to the air (without a bandage) after the child is home. The area may be gently cleaned with a wash cloth and air dried.

Activity: The child should be up and around the house playing quietly on the first day home. After the first day, he or she may return to previous activities. If there *are no stitches,* very active physical activities, such as gym, should be skipped for several days.

1. Check temperature once the evening after catheterization and twice the next day. Report to your doctor any reading over 101°F.
2. Watch the catheterization site for signs of infection, such as redness, swelling, or the presence of any drainage.
3. If bleeding should occur, it can be controlled by firm pressure directly over the wound applied for 3 to 4 minutes. If this does not stop the bleeding, bring the child to your physician, or the nearest general hospital emergency room.
4. If there is a slight bruise around the wound site, do not become alarmed, as this sometimes occurs and is not serious.
5. If there is pain at the catheterization site you may use acetaminophen (e.g., Tylenol); *please do not use aspirin.*
6. Your child may not be able to sleep for a short time after any hospitalization, particularly if an anesthetic has been given. This will go away with time and is not serious.

If your child has had an arterial as well as a venous puncture catheterization, watch the leg for pale color associated with pain or numbness. Call your doctor if paleness, pain, or numbness begin.

and cross match to ensure availability of blood should any bleeding occur during or after the procedure. Blood should not be drawn from the potential catheterization site.

The following day the catheterization is done; it lasts from 2 to 5 hours. The child is not allowed to eat or drink for 4 to 6 hours immediately before the procedure. Preoperative medications vary among institutions but they usually include an analgesic such as meperidine (1 mg/kg) or morphine (0.1 mg/kg) which is administered approximately 30 to 45 minutes before the catheterization to help the child relax. After the catheterization the child is observed closely overnight and is discharged the next morning.

Many institutions are now performing cardiac catheterization on an outpatient basis where the child is admitted the day of the catheterization and discharged, if stable, 5 to 6 hours after the catheterization. Outpatient catheterizations are only indicated in stable patients and parents require careful instructions (preferably written) regarding postcatheterization care and signs and symptoms of problems.

Preparing the Infant. Little can be done to prepare an infant psychologically for the procedure. Some security object such as a favorite blanket, toy, or pacifier can provide comfort, but the presence of parents provides the most security for an infant undergoing such a procedure. Comfort measures that may soothe the infant during the procedure are singing and talking to him or her, providing music, and stroking the baby. The parents are encouraged to hold and cuddle the infant and participate in the child's care as desired, before and after the procedure. The older child can understand explanations, but young children require special approaches to prepare them for this procedure. Whatever the age of the child, preparation for cardiac catheterization must be adapted to each child's individual level of understanding and emotional needs.

Preparing the Toddler. For the child 2 to 3 years of age, a simple explanation should be given on the morning of the procedure. The child should also be told that he or she will not receive breakfast. The parents and, in their absence, the nurse provide diversions such as play, taking the child for a walk down the hall, or reading to the child to keep him or her occupied during mealtime. If a parent will be there waiting when the child returns, explain this to the child.

Preparing the Young Child. The child 3 to 7 years of age is capable of understanding something about the inside of the body, and it is appropriate to give him or her simple explanations with a diagram or a doll. Fear of the unknown is reduced by allowing the child to play with a cap, mask, gown, and stethoscope and by taking the child for a ride on a stretcher. If possible, the child should be taken to the cardiac catheterization laboratory the day before the procedure and should meet the nurses and physicians who will be caring for the child. Many institutions have prepared movies or booklets for preparation of the child for cardiac catheterization, which will familiarize the child with the procedures and the surroundings. A child 3 to 7 years of age can understand why he or she cannot have breakfast; this should be explained to the child. When discussing the actual catheterization the nurse can show the child where the catheter will go by pointing to the place on a doll or the child. Institutions vary as to whether or not they use a general anesthetic agent during the catheterization. Therefore, the nurse needs to tailor the teaching to what the child will experience and that will depend on whether he or she is asleep or awake for the catheterization. Children who will be awake during all or portions of the catheterization need to have simple explanations as to what they will experience.

Describing the Experience. The first thing the child will experience will be premedication. This can be explained as an injection that will cause sleepiness, and that it will hurt but only for a minute or so. The child will usually ride on a stretcher or in the crib to the catheterization laboratory, which will be filled with many machines and strange equipment. These can be explained as being necessary to help the physicians and nurses look at the child's heart. In most catheterization laboratories, the physicians are dressed in green or blue, wear caps over their hair, and have masks covering their faces. The nurse can explain that everyone wants to keep things as clean as possible. A special table or bed that the child will be on moves from side to side and up and down. Children can be reminded that they will be safe on this bed because seatbelts will hold them firmly in place. While lying on the catheterization table (bed) the child will see many large x-ray cameras very close to his or her body. Children need to be reassured that this machinery will not fall on them.

The nurse should describe that the child's skin will be washed with a special soap, usually a thick brown liquid, after which he or she will be dried and covered with green towels to keep everything extra clean. The child will receive a small shot of medicine under the skin to put the leg to sleep. This small injection will cause a stinging sensation; however, within a very short period of time the area will be numb and the child will not feel the insertion of the catheters. The tubes (catheters) will then be inserted and the child will feel some pressure but can be reassured that it will not hurt. When the test starts the child will hear little clicking noises coming from the x-ray machines, and then if fully awake the child may look at the TV cameras and see a picture of his or her heart. The lights in the room will go off and on frequently because they need to be off when the x-ray pictures are being taken. When the contrast medium is injected the child will experience a warm flushed feeling for a minute or so. It is sometimes helpful to compare this feeling for the child to that of a hot summer day. When the tests are finished the catheter is removed from the child's leg. The leg should still be "asleep" so the child should not feel this. The child then is asked to lie very still for a while so that the physician can apply pressure at the catheterization site and place a pressure bandage there.

The child returns to the hospital room and, if the parents are waiting, is able to see them immediately. Both child and parents should be informed that the child will feel quite sleepy after the catheterization and may intermittently nap for the rest of the afternoon. The child needs to keep the leg straight, and the nurses will be checking vital signs, catheterization site, and pulses in the leg frequently following the catheterization.

Providing children with thorough explanations without making them so graphic they become frightened allows children to maintain some control when they go through the actual procedures because they know something of what to expect.*

Nursing Strategies During Intracatheterization

It is important to understand that in addition to preparation of the child prior to the procedure, it is the responsibility of the nurse to be supportive and informative during the procedure. Although many children sleep through the catheterization, the sedative is generally mild enough that the child is rousable during local anesthetic administration and occasionally during the procedure itself. One of the nurse's roles then is reinforcement of teaching with provision of emotional support.

Cardiac catheterization laboratories may vary as to the number of nurses present and their responsibilities. For the most part, though, technical responsibilities include setting up for the procedure, preparing and draping the patient, monitoring vital signs, intravenous fluids, and general status, assisting the physician, medication preparation, and generally overseeing the functioning of the laboratory. Specialized training is important, especially in sterile technique and in detection and treatment of dysrhythmias, as well as a thorough understanding of normal cardiac anatomy and physiology and congenital cardiac lesions.

Postcatheterization Nursing Care

From the moment the procedure is over and the child returns to the unit the nurse begins immediate, careful, systematic observations. The child must be observed closely for any complications. When moved from the stretcher to the bed, the child's color and level of consciousness are noted. The child will have a pressure dressing over the catheterization site, which must be checked to see that it is snug and that no bleeding is present. For infants, the diaper should be unfastened to allow for complete examination of the dressing on each assessment because blood can pool under the child. The pulse, color, temperature, and capillary refill of the extremity distal to the catheterization site should be checked, because arterial thrombosis and spasm of the vessels are the most frequent complications of the cardiac catheterization procedure. All of the vital signs are checked immediately on return from the procedure and monitored closely for several hours.

The child may have a transient *temperature elevation* due to physiologic dehydration from being without fluids for 4 to 6 hours before the procedure or from the contrast media, or both. (Many children have this very mild reaction to the contrast media.) If the fever persists, it may be due to the introduction of pathogens during the procedure.

The patient must be observed closely for signs of *bradycardia, tachycardia,* and *dysrhythmias.* The introduction of catheters into the cardiac chambers can cause irritation and/or stimulation of the myocardium, resulting in dysrhythmias. Usually any dysrhythmia, bradycardia, or tachycardia is temporary. However, occasionally it will persist and require therapeutic intervention. *Apnea, dyspnea with retractions, hypotension, and asymmetrical or decreased motion of the extremities* are also signs of complications. *Stroke* can occur from catheterization owing to thrombus formation on the catheter. Cyanotic children have an increased risk of stroke occurring from catheterization.

The extremity distal to the catheterization site must remain extended until the pressure dressing is removed, usually 6 hours after the catheterization. An older child will usually respond to instructions to keep the leg straight with frequent reminders to do so. For infants, attempt to position the leg in a position that is as extended as possible. Restraint of the leg should be avoided because it may actually increase the potential for *bleeding from the catheterization site* if the child pulls against this restraint. If the infant or toddler is awake and crying, it may be more beneficial to allow the parents to hold the child on a pillow on their lap or in their arms, keeping the leg as straight as possible. In addition, attaching a urine bag for urine collection helps prevent contamination of the catheterization site. It is important to note any urination following the test because it is possible that the bladder may have been perforated by the guide wire or catheter. The contrast medium is a hypotonic solution and tends, therefore, to diminish urine output as well.

Clear liquids are usually reintroduced immediately following the catheterization. If clear liquids are tolerated, the infant or child may advance to a regular diet. If nausea or vomiting, or both, should occur, the infant or child is kept on clear liquids until this ceases. The following morning the child is usually discharged from the hospital, provided there is a good pulse in the affected extremity, vital signs are stable, and the child is tolerating a regular diet. For children undergoing cardiac catheterization on an out-patient basis, the parent instruction sheet should be given to reinforce teaching about the procedure and about postprocedural care at home. A sample parent instruction sheet is found in Box 39-3.

Emotional and Social Impact of Heart Disease on the Infant and Family

The diagnosis of congenital heart disease in an infant has a tremendous impact on the family unit and those

* Explanations of what the child will feel during catheterization are adapted from "Todd's Heart Test" by Julie Scott, RN, University Hospital, Denver, 1983.

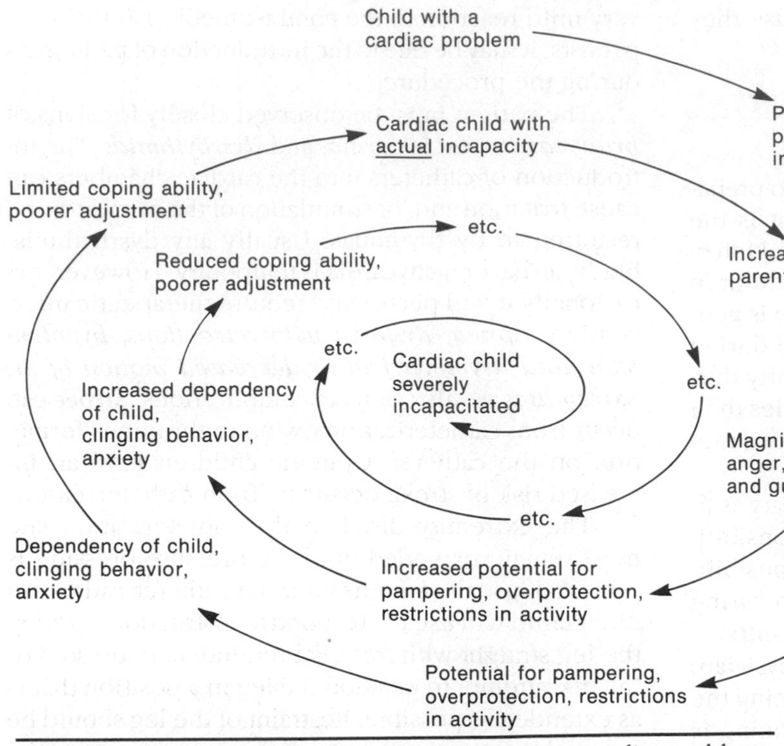

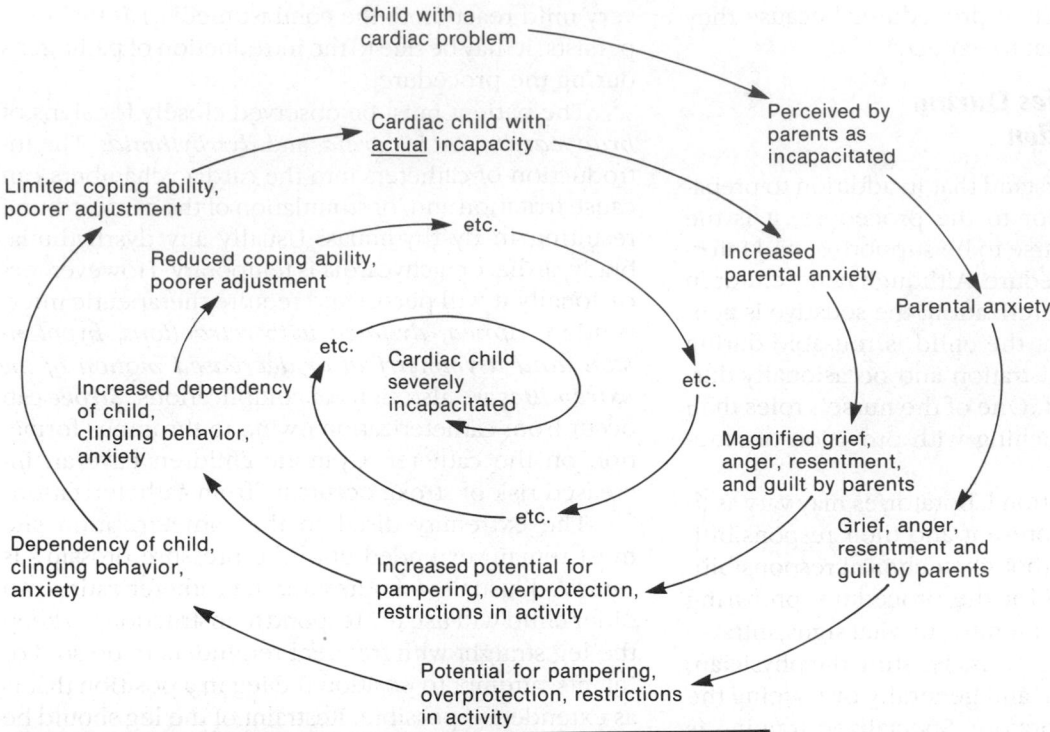

Figure 39-6. Cyclic pattern of parental responses in cardiac problems.

individuals involved in caring for the child in the community. These children not only must adapt to the physical stress of hospitalization, evaluative testing, and palliative and corrective surgery, but also may have to contend with an altered psychologic, social, and emotional environment.

Parents of the child with a congenital heart defect usually experience extreme stress, which may be compounded by guilt feelings and many fears. The family of this child requires support and practical guidance at the initial diagnosis and throughout the management of the disease to maintain and promote a healthy lifestyle for the child and the family's other members. Long-term psychologic outcomes for the child will depend on the family's response to the child. In turn, the family's response is greatly influenced by the health care team. *Effective nursing support can, therefore, directly influence the way in which heart disease affects a child and family.*

Studies have shown that parental anxiety is related to the presence rather than to the severity of the cardiac lesion (Linde, et al, 1966). Anxiety directly affects how parents relate to their children and rear them. In instances in which the parents demonstrate a high level of anxiety about their child's heart defect, the children have shown poor adjustment to their conditions. For example, the anxious parent may exhibit overprotective behavior and increased pampering, which fosters anxiety and dependency in the child (Fig. 39-6).

It has also been observed that parents may experience difficulty interacting with their infants who have congenital heart defects (Gundermuth, 1975). This may be due to parental perceptions of the infant's behavior—poor feeding, lethargy, restlessness. The parents may interpret these as reflections of poor parenting.

Parents of a child with congenital heart disease go through a grieving process. They must mourn the loss of their fantasized normal child before they are able to accept this child. Many parents block these feelings of loss and cope by denying the problem. Denial is especially prevalent in parents of asymptomatic children. These parents may exhibit behaviors such as refusal to discuss the diagnosis or to learn about the heart disease, pay little attention to plans for medical and/or surgical management, and fail to comply with the treatment plan for medications or follow-up visits. Anger may be displaced on the other parent (i.e., arguing or placing blame), the physician (i.e., distrust, discontinuance of care), or the nurse (i.e., hostility toward the nurse, angry complaints about care, interference with care). The nurse can help the parents express their feelings. Anger and resentment are normal feelings but they must be dealt with appropriately. Parents can be helped to deal with anger by calm acceptance of their outbursts followed by reassurance and a discussion of the feelings that prompted the behavior. Parents' anger and resentment may be expressed toward ill children by overprotective behavior leading to infantilization or by detachment from and decreased contact with the child.

Parents may go through a second grieving process

Box 39-4

Concerns of Parents About Their Infant with a Cardiac Condition and Nursing Interventions

What caused my child's heart defect? Am I responsible?

Tell parents: You are not responsible for the defect —we do not know the exact cause. (There are exceptions when the cause is known.) Heart development occurs in the first 2 months of gestation. Part of the heart sometimes fails to develop beyond this early stage. Many factors may be related, including maternal rubella during pregnancy, prematurity, chromosomal aberrations. The condition is not related to a family history of heart attacks

Why did it take so long to diagnose the problem?

Often a murmur is not heard until 6 weeks of age and it may not have been apparent at birth. Therefore, to identify problems early it is necessary to examine infants frequently in the first months of life

What causes the murmur? What is the defect?

Review flow of blood through normal heart. Using a diagram, explain the defect to parents. (This may have to be done 2 or 3 times.) Use the same terminology the physician has used (and explain it). Explain that the murmur is caused by abnormal flow of blood through the heart. Give diagram, name and definition of defect to the parents to keep at home for reference

What will my child look like when he gets sick?

Provide parents with a list of signs they may expect to see their child display: cyanosis, difficulty breathing, difficulty feeding, edema, perspiring, easy tiring, exhaustion, etc.

What does it mean to treat him normally?

Tell parents: Treat this child as you do your other children. Discipline and set limits for him. Physical education is ok unless physician advises against it. Infants usually limit their own activity. Give information on diet, usually a normal diet, rarely a salt-restricted diet. Instruct parents how and when to feed—small frequent feedings may prevent fatigue of infants. Allow parents ample time to feed and handle baby while in the hospital. Reinforce child's normal, desirable features: for example, remark on all normal aspects of the child when doing bath demonstration for parents

What is my child's future?

Outline the long range problems so that surprises in treatment are kept to a minimum: hospitalization, cardiac catheterization, surgical repair, if appropriate. Explain medications to be given, their purpose, name, dose, time, and side effects

What should I tell my child and my other children?

Explain that the child has a heart defect. Be honest with the other children. As the child grows older, explanations can go into greater depth

(Adapted from Garson et al, 1978.)

after the repair of the cardiac defect. During this grieving they mourn the loss of the defective child who now may be essentially normal. This is usually apparent in the children who are quite symptomatic and who, after repair, improve remarkably.

Box 39-4 summarizes the common concerns of families with children who have a congenital heart defect. Often parents are uncomfortable asking questions of health professionals and do not want to take up their time. These unanswered questions can add to the stress that parents experience. By giving parents some concrete and factual answers to their questions, the nurse can alleviate some of their anxiety and help them cope with the stress of the situation. Also, by supplying parents with factual information we aid them in becoming informed participants in their child's care and promote their increased self-esteem and competence as caretakers.

There are many things to keep in mind when teaching and working with parents of children with congenital heart disease. Parents and other family members will be shocked when they first hear the diagnosis and the two-way process of communication may suffer during this time of crisis. Parents must be allowed to grieve before they are taught to care for the child. Terminology used in explanations should be consistent with that used by other members of the health care team. Explanations of care must be built on current knowledge the parents have; therefore, ongoing assessment of parental knowledge is necessary. Information may need to be shared with parents repeatedly before they are able to take in and absorb the facts. Sharing information with parents makes them feel an integral part of the health care team. Referral to a community health nurse and school nurse while the child is hospitalized will supply some of the added support that is needed once the family returns to the community. Encouraging parental participation with a group of other parents with similar problems often is beneficial. It may help parents to feel less isolated in realizing there are many other parents who have children with congenital heart disease. Parent support groups can be a tremendous resource for these families. Talking with other parents who have been through the same experience, receiving a helping hand when needed, and having a place to turn for reassurance are all support services available through parent groups. However, parents are often too overwhelmed by the diagnosis of congenital heart disease to be able to seek out these resources on their own.

The nurse should know what support groups and resources are available in the community for these parents. Another valuable role support groups can play is offering the parent an outlet for action. Parents cannot change the fact that their child has congenital heart disease; however, they may be able to effect change through fund raising for research to prevent congenital heart disease or improved surgical and medical techniques. Parents may regain a sense of control through these types of positive activities.

Specific Congenital Heart Defects

This section provides detailed information about 14 specific heart defects. The discussion of each anomaly begins with the *incidence* and a *description* of the structural defect. *Pathophysiology* is discussed as it pertains to the altered hemodynamics (blood flow) and to potential complications of the altered flow (e.g., congestive heart failure). The section on *clinical manifestations* lists the signs and symptoms common to children with that type of congenital heart disease (CHD). In some cases these manifestations appear very early and are identified by the physician or nurse before the newborn infant leaves the hospital. In other disorders, the signs and symptoms may not appear for months or years.

The *diagnostic assessment* section for each disorder lists the specific results of the cardiac examination and three types of diagnostic tests described earlier (pages 1280–1281). Information in this section is quite technical and is not considered essential to a basic understanding of congenital heart disease. It is provided primarily for the reader who is trying to interpret test results from the child's chart or attempting to relate the pathophysiology of a specific disorder to a child's signs and symptoms.

Therapeutic management is described as it relates to both medical and surgical interventions. It is not necessary to memorize details of surgical procedures; they are provided for reference purposes. However, a rudimentary understanding of potential surgical techniques can give the nurse a base of knowledge to draw upon when helping the family understand explanations provided by the surgeon.

Often, congenital anomalies are corrected by surgery. Whenever possible, however, surgery is postponed until the child is beyond the neonatal period and can better tolerate the procedure. This means that for a period of months or years the family must manage the child's care at home. *Nursing care* during this period will occur most often in the home or clinic setting and will focus upon preparing the family to administer medications to improve heart function (e.g., digitalis), provide optimal nutrition, and conserve the child's limited energy. Congestive heart failure is a common complication of congenital heart disease in the period before surgical correction. Table 39-5 (page 1323) provides a nursing process plan for the child with congestive heart failure. Chapter 25 deals further with the impact of chronic illness on the child and family.

Nurses who practice in acute care settings will most often encounter children with CHD during the perioperative period. In planning perioperative care for the child undergoing heart surgery, the nurse builds upon knowledge of nursing care in any surgical procedure, as described in Table 27-7 (Nursing Process Plan: Perioperative Nursing Care, and care of the hospitalized child (Table 31-2, Nursing Process Plan: The Hospitalized Child).

In addition to knowledge of *general* perioperative nursing diagnoses and nursing strategies, the nurse who cares for the child with CHD must be aware of implications for care that are *specific* to heart surgery (see the section on perioperative nursing care later in this chapter) and to the specific type of heart defect. The major *perioperative nursing diagnoses* are listed for each disorder to identify potential problems that may result from either the defect itself or following surgical repair. They are designed to be used in conjunction with Table 27-7 and with the perioperative nursing strategies for CHD, which begin on page 1316.

Guidelines for Learning About CHD

Because of the amount of detailed information in this section, guidelines for learning are provided. If one learns the path of altered blood flow from each defect and the pathophysiology that prompts each flow pattern, the associated medical, surgical, and nursing interventions will follow quite logically. It is recommended, therefore, that the illustrations accompanying the description of the heart anomaly be used to locate the structural defect(s) and to trace the resulting alteration in blood flow. The following questions can help structure learning. (The answers that appear here for illustrative purposes apply to ventricular septal defect.)

- What is (are) the structural defect(s)?

  There is a hole between the ventricles.

- How does (do) the defect(s) change normal blood flow?

  Some oxygenated blood now flows from the left ventricle to the right ventricle.

- Why does blood flow in this direction (or in this manner)?

  Pressure is greater in the left ventricle than in the right (after the newborn period).

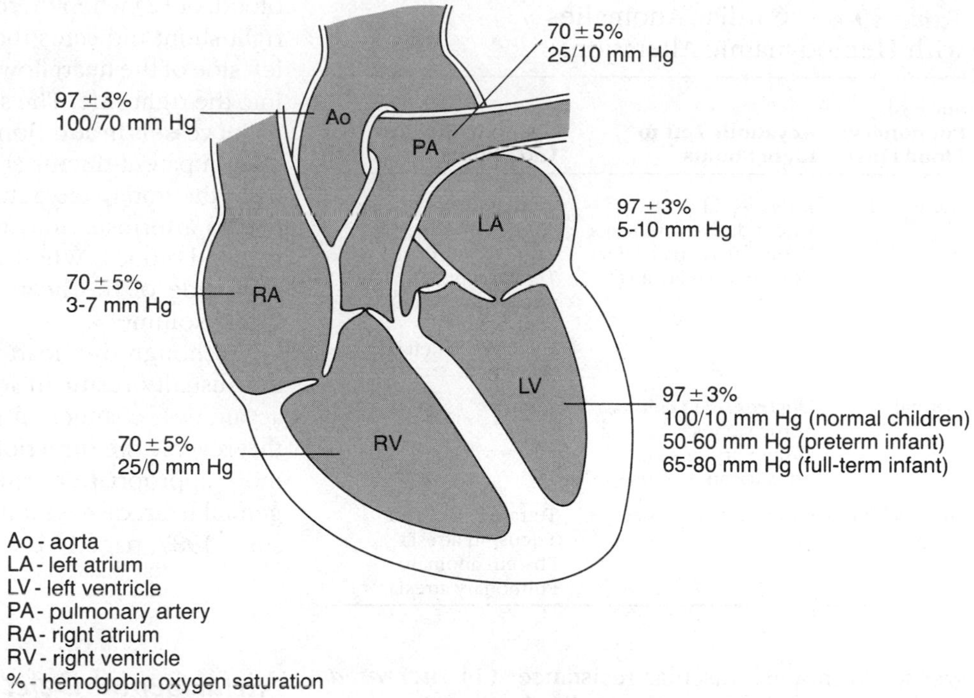

Figure 39-7. Normal pressures and oxygen saturations within the heart and great vessels.

- Does the altered flow result in increased work for any of the heart chambers? What are the associated complications?

  Both ventricles must deal with extra blood volume. Over time this can lead to congestive heart failure.

- Will the defect(s) affect the lungs? The peripheral circulation? How?

  The lungs will receive an increased volume of blood through the pulmonary artery that arises from the right ventricle. Over time, this can damage the pulmonary vessels.

- What are the special considerations for perioperative nursing care for a child with this disorder (i.e., in addition to general perioperative care)?

  Potential altered cardiac output: decreased; potential altered growth and development: failure to thrive; potential for injury: physiologic, related to damage to the pulmonary vessels, conduction abnormalities (dysrhythmias), and bacterial endocarditis.

Mastery of the answers to these questions for each of the major congenital heart defects will provide a sound basis for planning nursing care.

Hemodynamics of Congenital Heart Disease

For a better understanding of the hemodynamics of individual cardiac defects it is helpful to know the normal pressures and oxygen saturations within the cardiac chambers and great vessels.

In the heart and great vessels, blood will flow from an area of higher pressure to that of lower pressure (Fig. 39-7). Therefore, if abnormal communications exist between the left and right sides of the heart, the direction of blood flow through the communication will be determined by the relative pressures on the right and left sides of the heart.

Blood flowing from one chamber, artery, or vein to another, resulting in the mixing of oxygenated and unoxygenated blood, is called a shunt. Shunts are described in terms of the ratio of pulmonary blood flow to systemic blood flow (Qp/Qs). The amount of blood flow from the right ventricle to the lungs should be equal to the amount of blood flow from the left ventricle to the systemic circulation. The ratio should be 1 : 1. A left to right shunt of 3 : 1 would mean that three times as much blood would be flowing to the lungs as to the systemic circulation. This would be classified as an *acyanotic defect* because blood flow to the lungs is increased and no unoxygenated blood is reaching the systemic circulation. A right to left shunt exists when right heart pressures are greater than left, and unoxygenated blood flows from the right side of the heart to the left side and out to the systemic circulation, resulting in cyanosis. This would be classified as a *cyanotic heart defect.*

An important consideration with shunts is their effect on the pulmonary vasculature. Three stimuli can cause constriction of the pulmonary vessels and in-

Table 39-4. Cardiac Anomalies with Hemodynamic Alterations

State of Pulmonary Blood Flow	Acyanotic Left to Right Shunts	Cyanotic Right to Left Shunts
Increased	Atrial septal defect Patent ductus arteriosus Ventricular septal defect Atrioventricular canal defect	Transposition of great arteries Truncus arteriosus Total anomalous pulmonary venous connection Hypoplastic left heart syndrome
Normal	**Obstructive Lesions:** Aortic stenosis Pulmonary stenosis Coarctation of aorta	None
Diminished	Pulmonary stenosis	Tetralogy of Fallot Tricuspid atresia Ebstein anomaly Pulmonary atresia

crease pulmonary vascular resistance: (1) *increased pulmonary blood flow,* (2) *blood flow to the lungs under increased pressure,* and (3) *hypoxia.* If these stimuli persist individually or in combination irreversible damage can occur in the pulmonary vessels. Early changes in the pulmonary vessels such as medial hypertrophy and abnormal extension of muscle into small peripheral arteries are usually reversible. However, progressive damage such as occlusion of the vessels, fibrosis, and decreased number of vessels are irreversible resulting in permanently elevated pulmonary vascular resistance and pulmonary hypertension. *Eisenmenger syndrome* is the term used to describe the condition in which increased pulmonary blood flow secondary to left to right shunting has resulted in a progressive elevation in pulmonary vascular resistance and permanent damage to the pulmonary vessels. A reversal of the shunt and cyanosis result. Eisenmenger syndrome is a terminal condition.

Once pulmonary vessels are damaged irreversibly, the child becomes progressively hypoxic and dies (Moss, 1983). Therefore, medical management of any cardiac lesion must take into consideration the effects of the lesion on the pulmonary vasculature. Nursing care for children with different defects varies, depending upon the physiologic effects of the altered blood flow. This will be reviewed individually with each cardiac lesion. Various shunts and their effects on pulmonary blood flow are summarized in Table 39-4.

Acyanotic Heart Defects

Acyanotic defects are those which result (1) when there is no mixing of oxygenated and unoxygenated blood, or (2) when there is a *left to right* shunt. A left to right shunt indicates that oxygenated blood from the left side of the heart flows through the structural defect into the right side. The shunt may involve one or more major vessels in addition to heart chambers. Such is the case in patent ductus arteriosus in which blood flows from the aorta (oxygenated blood) through a patent ductus arteriosus into the pulmonary artery (unoxygenated blood). When a left to right shunt occurs, the right side of the heart must deal with an increased blood volume.

Although the heart defects discussed in this section usually result in left to right shunting (i.e., are acyanotic), changes in pressure gradients may occur that reverse the direction of flow. Therefore, it may be more appropriate to think of these disorders as congenital heart disease with "little or no cyanosis" (Gersony, 1987, page 981).

Atrial Septal Defect (Fig. 39-8)

Atrial septal defects (ASD) comprise about 15 per cent of all congenital cardiac defects and occur more frequently in girls than in boys (Guido, 1983). There are three common forms of ASD, ostium secundum* (the most common), ostium primum (also called a partial atrioventricular canal defect), and sinus venosus. Secundum ASDs located higher in the septal wall near the foramen ovale are usually not associated with other cardiac defects. However, primum ASDs located in the septum just above the tricuspid valve are associated with defects of the atrioventricular septum and the mitral valve. Sinus venosus ASDs, located adjacent to the superior vena cava, are commonly associated with anomalous connection of the right pulmonary veins to the right atrium or right superior vena cava (Borow and Braunwald, 1988).

Pathophysiology

In the presence of an ASD a portion of the oxygenated blood returning to the left atrium from the lungs crosses through the ASD to the right atrium and right ventricle and returns to the pulmonary circulation. The amount of left to right shunting depends on the size of the defect, its location and the difference in pressures in the right and left atria. The pressures in the atria are determined in part by the outflow resistances of the ventricles. In the early months of life right ventricular pressures are still elevated. As the pulmonary vascular

* Ostium secundum is an opening in the upper portion of the septum. Ostium primum is an opening in the lower part of the septum.

bed matures, pulmonary vascular resistance decreases and right-side pressures decrease. Shunting across the ASD is minimal until the decrease in right ventricular pressure occurs. Most ASDs are not diagnosed until after the neonatal period and may not be detected until the school-age years. The major stimulus to the pulmonary vasculature with an ASD is increased blood flow (see section on classification of defects, Effects on the Pulmonary Vasculature). Changes in the pulmonary vessels usually occur very slowly. Pulmonary hypertension and increased pulmonary vascular resistance do not usually occur until early adulthood, although they have been reported in the first and second decades of life (Moss, 1983).

Clinical Manifestations

Infants and children with secundum and sinus venosus ASDs are usually asymptomatic. Development of congestive heart failure is rare, and the only symptoms may be decreased exercise tolerance and dyspnea.

Diagnostic Assessment

Cardiac Examination. The increased flow of blood across the pulmonary valve produces a systolic ejection murmur heard best in the upper left sternal border. Fixed splitting of the second heart sound can usually be heard in older children. If the left to right shunt is large a diastolic murmur of increased blood flow across the tricuspid valve may be heard.

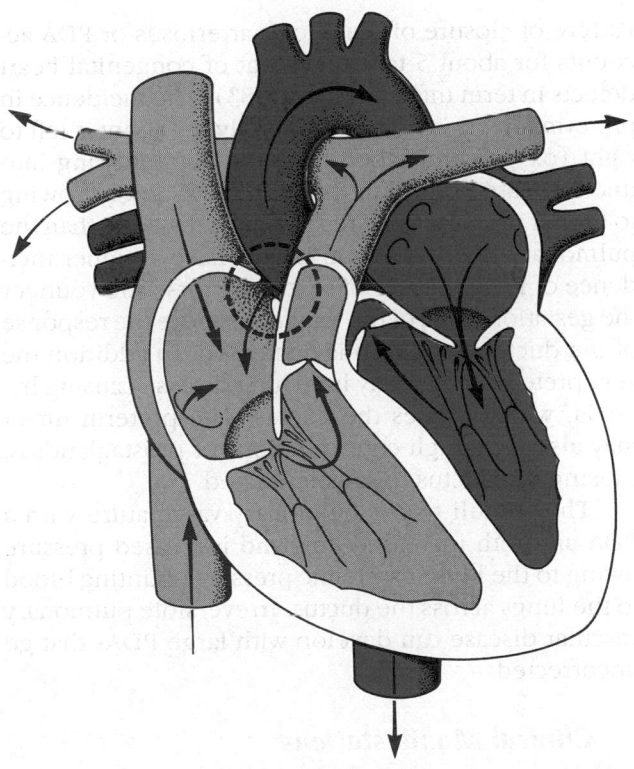

Figure 39-8. Atrial septal defect. The shunt is from left atrium to right atrium.

Electrocardiogram. Right ventricular hypertrophy and possibly atrial enlargement are usually present.

Chest Roentgenogram. Enlargement of the heart, a prominent pulmonary artery segment and increased pulmonary vascular markings are usually seen.

Echocardiogram. 2-D echocardiography can usually define the location and size of the ASD as well as dilatation of the atria and size and wall thickness of the right ventricle. In addition, color flow echocardiography can identify the presence of anomalous pulmonary veins.

Therapeutic Management

Small ASDs may occasionally close spontaneously, requiring no intervention. Surgical correction for significant ASDs is recommended between 2 and 4 years of age (Friedman, 1988). Earlier surgical repair may be done if the child is symptomatic. The surgical repair is most often done through a median sternotomy (an incision made along the midline of the sternum). Closure of the ASD can be accomplished by suturing the edges of the defect together, or with large ASDs, a pericardial or dacron patch is sewn over the defect. When anomalous pulmonary venus connection to the superior vena cava is present with a sinus venosus ASD, a tunnel is surgically constructed to divert the pulmonary venous flow through the ASD to the left atrium. Operative risk is usually minimal. Postoperative complications include cardiac enlargement, dysrhythmias, and mitral valve prolapse (Merenstein et al, 1985). Cardiology follow-up is required for the patient with the repaired defect since mitral valve prolapse may not occur until adolescence or adulthood.

Ostium primum ASDs or partial atrioventricular canal defects are associated with a cleft in the mitral valve and mitral valve insufficiency. These defects in infants are usually diagnosed early owing to the prominence of cardiac murmurs. The left to right shunt is usually large and the infant has a pulmonary flow murmur as well as a murmur of mitral insufficiency. These infants can present with congestive heart failure due to the combination of a large left to right shunt and mitral insufficiency. Growth failure, dyspnea, decreased exercise tolerance, and increased respiratory infections are common signs and symptoms. Surgical correction is usually performed earlier than with secundum ASDs and involves closure of the cleft in the mitral valve and patch closure of the ASD. Seven to 10 per cent of these infants will later require replacement of the mitral valve for residual mitral insufficiency (Moss, 1983).

Perioperative Nursing Diagnoses for Atrial Septal Defects*

Preoperative

The child with a left to right shunt through an atrial septal defect is usually asymptomatic. See the section on perioperative strategies for cardiac surgery later in this chapter for general preoperative nursing care.

Postoperative

Potential for injury: physiologic, related to

- *cardiac enlargement and dysrhythmias*
- *mitral valve prolapse*

Defining characteristics for cardiac enlargement: heart enlargement on chest roentgenography (as reported by radiologist)

Defining characteristics for dysrhythmias: rhythm alterations on ECG, heart monitor; sensation of heart skipping beats and then beating faster

Defining characteristics for mitral valve prolapse: often asymptomatic in children, may cause mid-systolic click and murmur; adolescents may experience precordial discomfort and dysrhythmias

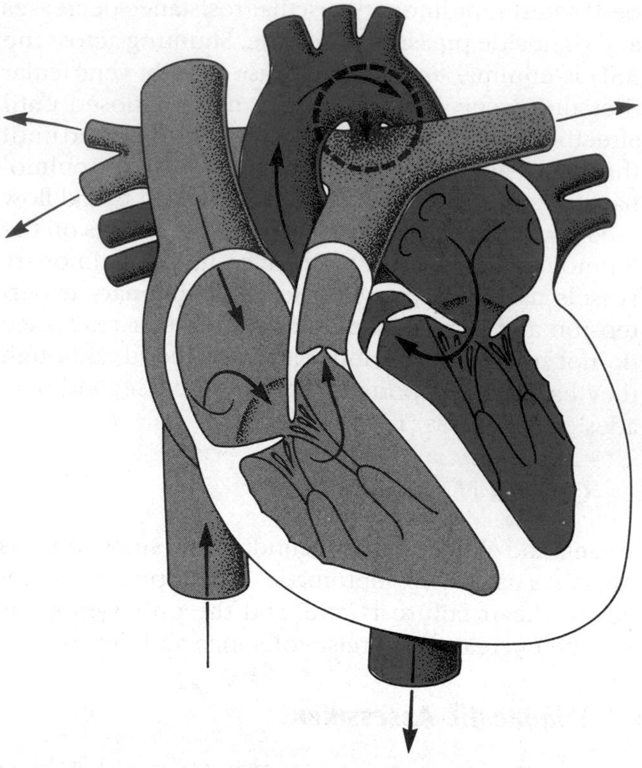

Figure 39-9. Patent ductus arteriosus. The shunt is from aorta to pulmonary artery.

Patent Ductus Arteriosus (Fig. 39-9)

The ductus arteriosus is a normal pathway in the fetal circulatory system. It is a large channel (roughly the same size as the descending aorta) between the pulmonary artery and the descending aorta that allows fetal blood to pass from the pulmonary artery to the descending aorta and ultimately to the placenta. Functional closure of the patent ductus arteriosus (PDA) usually occurs spontaneously during the first 10 to 15 hours after birth. Permanent closure occurs within 5 to 7 days in most infants but may take up to several weeks.

The exact mechanisms of closure of the ductus arteriosus are not fully understood. However, two major factors play an important role in ductal closure: the infant's arterial oxygen saturation (PO_2) and the presence of prostaglandins (PGE_1). Prostaglandins are produced in the placenta and are present in high concentrations in the fetus maintaining patency of the ductus arteriosus. At birth the placental source of prostaglandins is removed. With decreased prostaglandins the ductus arteriosus can close. Oxygen constricts the ductus arteriosus. After birth the infant ventilating on its own has a higher arterial oxygen concentration, which helps to constrict the ductus arteriosus.

Pathophysiology

Failure of closure of the ductus arteriosus or PDA accounts for about 5 to 10 per cent of congenital heart defects in term infants (Moss, 1983). The incidence in preterm infants is higher. Generally the shunt is left to right (oxygenated blood from the aorta flowing into unoxygenated blood in the pulmonary artery) owing to higher pressures and resistance in the aorta than the pulmonary artery. Preterm infants have a higher incidence of PDA because of several factors. The younger the gestational age of the infant, the more the response of the ductus to oxygen is decreased. In addition the very preterm infant may have lung disease causing hypoxia, which dilates the ductus. The preterm infant may also have high concentrations of prostaglandins, causing the ductus to remain dilated.

The stimuli to the pulmonary vasculature with a PDA are both increased flow and increased pressure owing to the higher systemic pressure shunting blood to the lungs across the ductus. Irreversible pulmonary vascular disease can develop with large PDAs that go uncorrected.

Clinical Manifestations

The clinical presentation of a PDA depends on the size of the PDA, the systemic and pulmonary vascular resistances, and the ability of the myocardium (the heart

* The sections on perioperative nursing care and nursing care for the child with congestive heart failure later in this chapter provide nursing strategies to support and supplement the diagnoses for each congenital heart defect in this section.

muscle) to handle the extra load. Preterm infants are usually symptomatic earlier. Because their pulmonary vascular resistance falls more rapidly, allowing more left to right shunting, and their myocardiums are immature and less able to handle the extra load, they go into congestive heart failure more readily. The symptomatology of the term infant is usually determined by the size of the ductus. Term infants with a small PDA are usually asymptomatic, whereas those with a large PDA may present in congestive heart failure. Any conditions that put extra demands on the heart for increased systemic flow will exaggerate the symptoms of cardiac failure. Such conditions include infection, poor nutrition, decreased hemoglobin, increased environmental temperature, and increased activity. Older children may be identified for the first time during a routine examination. They may have slight growth retardation and easy fatigability as their only symptoms.

Diagnostic Assessment

Cardiac Examination. Preterm and term newborn infants may or may not have a murmur. When present the murmur is usually systolic or continuous and is best heard in the second to third left intercostal space. The second heart sound is split normally and pulmonic closure is normal unless lung disease is present; then it may be accentuated. With large PDAs a diastolic rumble and a gallop may be heard. The older child may have the classic "machinery"-type murmur from blood flow across the PDA during systole and diastole. Pulses are usually described as bounding in any age group.

Electrocardiogram. The ECG is usually normal; however, it may show left ventricular hypertrophy and left atrial dilatation in the older child.

Chest Roentgenogram. The chest roentgenogram typically shows increased pulmonary vascularity with normal or increased heart size.

Echocardiogram. An M-mode echocardiogram may show increased left atrial size. With a color flow 2-D echocardiogram the PDA can be visualized, and with Doppler the amount of blood flow across the PDA can be estimated. 2-D echocardiography also helps to identify the presence or absence of other cardiac defects.

Therapeutic Management

Some PDAs will close spontaneously; however, preterm infants who are symptomatic and require increasing ventilatory support require early intervention. Surgical closure or closure with indomethacin, a prostaglandin inhibitor, is the treatment of choice (Friedman, 1988). By inhibiting prostaglandin, indomethacin allows the PDA to close. This agent is more effective in preterm than in term infants and should be administered before 10 days of age. It is given orally or intravenously at a dose of 0.2 mg/kg and may be repeated up to three times, 12 to 24 hours apart.

Surgical closure is indicated in the older infant or child and when indomethacin has been unsuccessful in young infants. Surgical closure is accomplished through a lateral thoracotomy. The ductus is either ligated with suture or divided completely. This is not an open heart surgery and is low risk. The presence of a PDA in an older infant or child, even if very small, is still an indication for surgery since operative risk is low compared with that of endocarditis in subsequent years. (See the section on endocarditis, page 1332).

Perioperative Nursing Diagnoses for Patent Ductus Arteriosus

Preoperative

Potential altered cardiac output: decreased, related to increased blood flow to the lungs
Defining characteristics: cardiac enlargement; tachycardia; tachypnea; gallop rhythm; decreased urine output; sweating; hepatomegaly; decreased exercise tolerance

Potential altered growth and development: failure to thrive, related to
- *feeding difficulties associated with respiratory distress*
- *increased basal metabolic rate*
- *decreased tissue perfusion*

Defining characteristics: Height and weight less than the 3rd percentile; developmental delays

Postoperative

Open heart surgery is not required; complications are rare. Nursing diagnoses and nursing strategies for postoperative care are found in the section on perioperative strategies for cardiac surgery later in this chapter and in Table 27-7.

Ventricular Septal Defect (Fig. 39-10)

Ventricular septal defects (VSD) are among the most common heart lesions, comprising 25 per cent of all congenital heart defects (Gersony, 1987). Often these defects are a part of other more complex defects such as truncus arteriosus, tetralogy of Fallot, and double outlet right ventricle; however, VSDs will be discussed here as isolated defects. VSDs are classified according to their size and location in the septum. Membranous VSDs beneath the aortic valve are the most common. Supracristal VSDs beneath the pulmonary valve comprise about 5 to 7 per cent of VSDs, atrioventricular canal type VSDs or posterior defects approximately 8 per cent. Muscular VSDs are frequently multiple and represent 5 to 20 per cent of VSDs (Moss, 1983).

Pathophysiology

In the presence of a VSD a portion of the oxygenated blood returning from the lungs to the left atrium and left ventricle crosses the VSD into the right ventricle and returns to the pulmonary circulation. The shunt is left to right. The magnitude of the shunt is determined by the size of the VSD and the amount of pulmonary vascular resistance present. High pulmonary vascular resistance will elevate pulmonary pressure (making it approximate left ventricular pressure) and decrease shunting across the VSD. In the newborn period pulmonary vascular resistance is still high; therefore, little shunting may occur at this time and the child may be asymptomatic. As pulmonary vascular resistance decreases at around 1 to 2 months of age, the child may become very symptomatic. The size of the VSD also plays an important role, with small defects having little shunting, and with moderate to large defects permitting unrestricted shunting in the presence of low pulmonary vascular resistance.

With a VSD, the blood vessels in the lungs receive increased blood flow and experience increased pressure. The combination of these stimuli with the moderate to large VSD can cause changes in the pulmonary vessels even within the first year of life. Irreversible pulmonary vascular changes usually do not occur before 2 years of age; although studies have shown irreversible changes as early as age 1 (Moss, 1983).

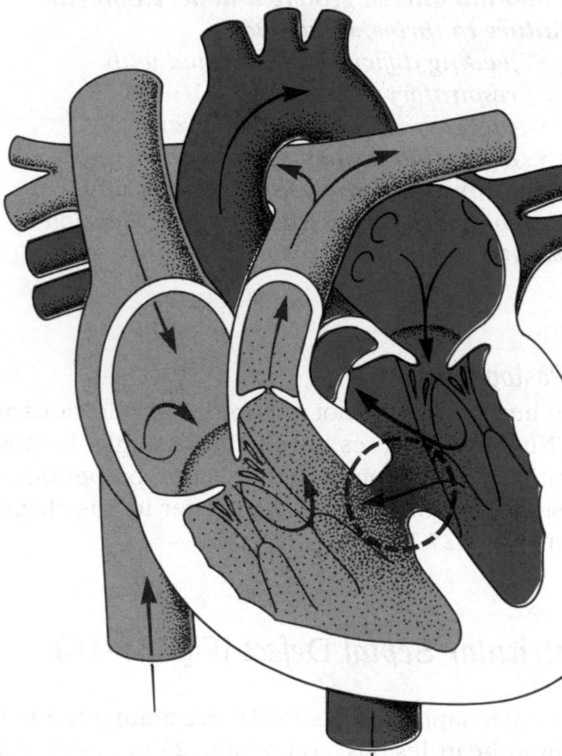

***Figure* 39-10.** Ventricular septal defect. Abnormal flow is from left ventricle to right ventricle.

Clinical Manifestations

Symptomatology depends on the size of the defect, the age of the child, and the pulmonary vascular resistance. With small VSDs there is little shunting and the infant or child is usually asymptomatic. In addition, there are rarely any changes in the pulmonary vasculature. With moderate to large VSDs and a large left to right shunt, the infant or child may experience failure to thrive and congestive heart failure (see Chapter 35 for failure to thrive and the section in this chapter on congestive heart failure for signs and symptoms). The child over age 2 may present with frequent respiratory infections and increased fatigue.

Diagnostic Assessment

Cardiac Examination. Blood flow across the VSD produces a systolic murmur that can be grade II to IV/VI,* heard best at the mid to lower left sternal border. In the presence of large left to right shunts (2:1 or greater) the increased blood flow returning from the lungs across the mitral valve produces a diastolic flow rumble. When increased pulmonary vascular resistance is present the second component of the second heart sound, P_2, will be accentuated.

Electrocardiogram. In the presence of small VSDs the ECG is usually normal. With moderate to large VSDs, left ventricular hypertrophy is usually present. Children with large VSDs may have left atrial enlargement, right ventricular hypertrophy, combined ventricular hypertrophy, or any combination of these.

Chest Roentgenogram. With small VSDs the chest roentgenogram is usually normal. With moderate-sized VSDs heart size and pulmonary vascular markings will be increased. With large VSDs heart size and pulmonary vascular markings will be increased and a prominent pulmonary artery segment will be present.

* Murmurs are often denoted in this manner to indicate both the grade of murmur and the scale on which it is based, e.g., II/VI means a grade II murmur on a scale where VI is the highest.

Echocardiogram. Color flow 2-D echocardiography is helpful in determining the size and location of the VSD as well as the presence of more than one VSD. The degree of left to right shunting and the pulmonary vascular resistance can also be assessed.

Therapeutic Management

Greater than 60 per cent of small VSDs and 5 to 10 per cent of large VSDs will spontaneously close, usually sometime during the first 2 years of life (Moss, 1983). Infants with small VSDs usually require no medical or surgical therapy except antibiotics to prevent endocarditis during susceptible periods. Infants with moderate to large VSDs who are symptomatic, showing signs of CHF and failing to grow are usually medically managed with a combination of digoxin and diuretics. If the infant continues to fail to thrive or continues to show signs of CHF, or both, then early surgical repair is indicated. Other indications for early surgical repair are increasing pulmonary pressures and frequent respiratory infections.

Infants or children with large VSDs who respond to medical management but have a persistent shunt of 2:1 or greater at 3 to 4 years of age usually undergo surgical repair. An important aspect of management for infants and children with moderate to large VSDs is careful assessment of pulmonary pressures and pulmonary vascular resistance. Surgical intervention is necessary before irreversible pulmonary vascular disease develops.

Surgical repair of VSDs is an open heart procedure; VSDs of children weighing less than 7 kilograms are usually repaired with the child in deep hypothermia with circulatory arrest (Merenstein et al, 1985). In larger children cardiopulmonary bypass is used. VSDs are closed through a median sternotomy and an incision in the right atrium rather than an incision through the left or right ventricle. The VSD can be closed by directly suturing the edges of the defect together or, with larger defects, a synthetic patch (e.g., of dacron) is used to close the defect. The patch is not rejected because it is an inert substance and cardiac tissue completely covers the patch within 6 months after surgery. Complications of surgical repair include residual VSDs and conduction abnormalities. Most conduction abnormalities are temporary because of edema and trauma to the conduction system; however, rarely, permanent interruption of the conduction system occurs, necessitating placement of a permanent pacemaker.

Pulmonary artery banding is a palliative procedure used to decrease pulmonary blood flow until total repair can be done. It is not an open heart procedure and is performed through a median sternotomy incision. This procedure is rarely used any more because the combined risk of pulmonary artery banding, debanding, and total repair is greater than total repair alone. A condition under which pulmonary artery banding is still used is when multiple VSDs exist and the infant is at too high a risk for total repair.

The surgical risk for any infant or child undergoing VSD repair is determined by the child's age, size, and condition, as well as the size and location of the VSD. Following surgical repair these children require continued antibiotic prophylaxis for endocarditis for certain procedures and continued cardiology follow-up.

Perioperative Nursing Diagnoses for Ventricular Septal Defects

Preoperative

Potential altered cardiac output: decreased, *related to volume overload*
Defining characteristics: see patent ductus arteriosus
Potential altered growth and development: *failure to thrive, related to increased metabolic demands of the myocardium*
Defining characteristics: see patent ductus arteriosus

Postoperative

Potential for injury: physiologic, *related to*
- *residual VSDs; Defining characteristics: murmur*
- *conduction abnormalities associated with temporary edema and surgical trauma; Defining characteristics: dysrhythmias, heart block*
- *bacterial endocarditis; Defining characteristics: fever, bacteremia*

Atrioventricular (AV) Canal Defect (Fig. 39-11)

Atrioventricular (AV) canal defect is also called "atrioventricular septal defect" and "endocardial cushion defect." Complete AV canal defects comprise approximately 2 per cent of all congenital heart defects and are often associated with Down syndrome (Sauer, 1983). The endocardial cushions are large projections of endomyocardial jelly that separate the atrioventricular canal into the atria and ventricles during fetal development. There are four cushions arising from the sides of the canal, with the posterior and anterior cushions contributing to most of the division. These two cushions also contribute to formation of the mitral and tricuspid

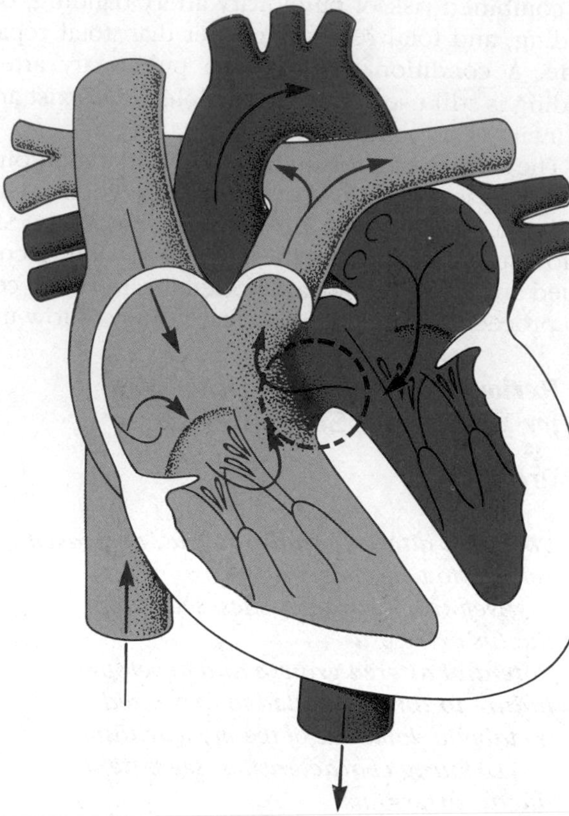

Figure 39-11. Great vessels are cut away to reveal the AV canal defect. The shunt is from left to right atria, left to right ventricle, and mitral regurgitation occurs from the abnormal mitral valve (not depicted in this figure).

valves. AV canal defects result from arrested or abnormal development of these cushions in utero. These defects are classified as complete or partial, each having varied clinical manifestations that depend on the size of the defect as well as the involvement of the atrioventricular valves.

The most common form of AV canal defect is partial AV canal or ostium primum septal defect, in which there is a large atrial septal defect, a cleft in the anterior mitral valve leaflet, and an intact ventricular septum. Complete AV canal defects involve a large atrial septal defect, a ventricular septal defect of varying size, and a common or single atrioventricular valve originating from both atria. Congenital heart lesions associated with AV canal defects include pulmonary stenosis and patent ductus arteriosus.

Pathophysiology

Blood flow resulting from this defect depends on the size of the septal defect as well as the degree of involvement of the atrioventricular valves. *Essentially, there is a large central hole in the heart.* Mitral regurgitation (the backward flow of blood from the left ventricle into the left atrium through an inadequate mitral valve), tricuspid regurgitation, and shunts—either left to right or right to left—may exist. The direction of the shunt is determined by pulmonic and systemic resistance and compliance of each chamber of the heart.

If a large ventricular septal defect exists, increased pulmonary vascular resistance and pulmonary hypertension may develop, causing the shunting to be bidirectional. The major stressors on the pulmonary vessels with an AV canal are increased pulmonary blood flow and increased pressure. This combination of stimuli may cause early pulmonary vascular changes and early onset of irreversible pulmonary vascular disease. In both partial and complete defects the atrioventricular node and the bundle of His may be interrupted or displaced, creating conduction abnormalities (altered transfer of electrical impulses through the heart) (Moss, 1983).

Clinical Manifestations

Patients with partial AV canal defects may present with symptoms similar to those with secundum atrial septal defects, depending on the degree of mitral regurgitation present. Clinical manifestations of complete AV canal defects are usually quite severe. The amount of atrioventricular valve regurgitation varies; however, most defects involve significant AV valve regurgitation. Symptoms develop in early infancy and include tachypnea, dyspnea, poor weight gain, and diaphoresis. Congestive heart failure and cardiomegaly (increased heart size) develop early. Cyanosis may result from bidirectional shunting. Usually these infants are pale and prone to recurrent respiratory infections.

Diagnostic Assessment

Cardiac Examination. Mitral regurgitation will produce a loud systolic murmur heard best at the lower left sternal border and at the apex. There may be an additional systolic murmur heard best at the upper left sternal border from increased blood flow across the pulmonary valve. A diastolic flow rumble may be present from increased blood flow returning from the lungs and flowing across the mitral valve. The first heart sound may be accentuated and, if pulmonary hypertension is present, the second component of the second heart sound (P_2) will be accentuated.

Electrocardiogram. With complete AV canal the ECG will demonstrate classic features of the counterclockwise rotation of the QRS loop, left axis deviation, and right ventricular hypertrophy. A prolonged PR interval is also frequently present.

Chest Roentgenogram. With complete AV canal there is an increased heart size, a prominent pulmonary artery segment, and increased pulmonary vascular markings.

Echocardiogram. Color flow 2-D echocardiograms are extremely helpful in identifying and classifying partial versus complete AV canal and in determining the AV valve structure.

Therapeutic Management

Infants with a complete AV canal defect who are symptomatic are usually medically managed with digoxin and diuretics early on. If medical management fails and the infant persists in congestive heart failure and fails to thrive or has pulmonary hypertension, early surgical repair is indicated. If the child grows well and does not develop pulmonary hypertension then surgical repair is performed electively before 2 years of age.

Surgical repair usually consists of total correction. Total repair is an open heart procedure requiring deep hypothermia and circulatory arrest, cardiopulmonary bypass, or both. It is performed through a median sternotomy. With total repair the common AV valve is divided into separate tricuspid and mitral valves, and a patch (usually dacron or teflon) is sewn over the VSD and ASD. The mitral and tricuspid septal leaflets are then attached to the septal patch. The most difficult part of this repair involves the AV valves. The surgeon must reconstruct the mitral valve to make it as competent as possible. Complications of the surgery include residual septal defects, conduction abnormalities, and AV valve regurgitation. A small percentage of these children will require a mitral valve replacement later in life. All of these children require life-long prophylaxis for endocarditis (see page 1332) and continued cardiology follow-up.

Perioperative Nursing Diagnoses for AV Canal

Preoperative

***Potential impaired gas exchange,** related to increased volume and pressure of pulmonary blood flow*
Defining characteristics: tachypnea, pallor, exercise intolerance and fatigability

***Potential altered cardiac output: decreased,** related to*
- *volume overload of the heart and lungs; Defining characteristics: cardiac enlargement; tachycardia; tachypnea; gallop rhythm; decreased urine output; decreased peripheral pulses; mottling of extremities; sweating; hepatomegaly; decreased exercise tolerance*

Postoperative

***Potential for injury: physiologic,** related to*
- *residual septal defects*
- *conduction abnormalities*
- *AV valve regurgitation; Defining characteristics: loud systolic murmurs, diastolic flow rumble*
- *bacterial endocarditis; Defining characteristics: fever, bacteremia*

Coarctation of the Aorta (Fig. 39-12)

Coarctation, a narrowing of the aorta, constitutes 7 to 8 per cent of all congenital heart defects (Nadas and Fyler, 1972). The narrowing can be either discreet or a long segment and can vary in severity from a mild constriction to total occlusion such as in interrupted aortic arch. The most common site of coarctation is juxtaductal, at the junction of the ductus arteriosus and

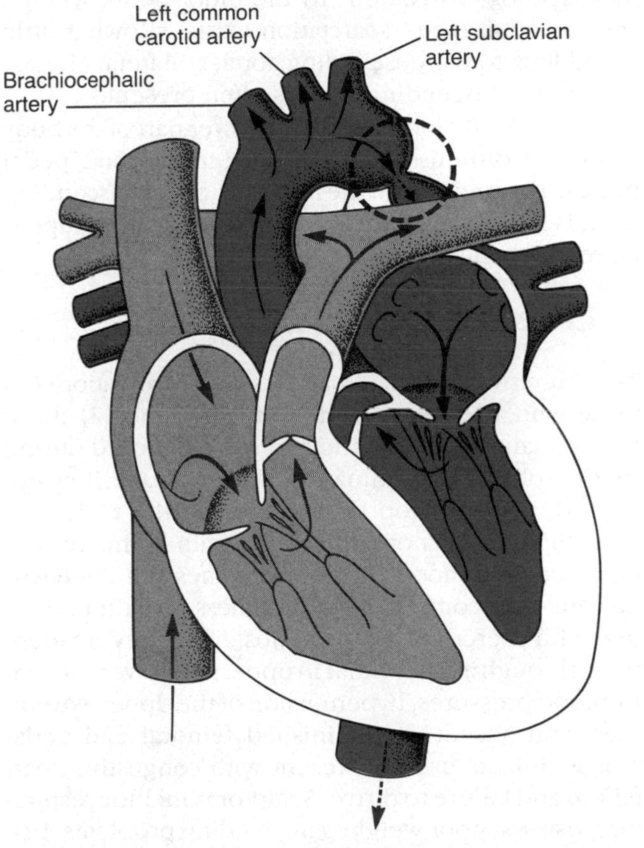

Figure 39-12. Coarctation of the aorta. Flow patterns are normal but are diminished distal to the coarctation. Blood pressure is increased in vessels leaving aorta proximal to the coarctation.

the aortic arch distal to the left subclavian artery. Bicuspid aortic valve is the most frequently associated anomaly (85 per cent). However, PDA, VSD, aortic stenosis, aortic regurgitation, mitral valve abnormalities, transposition of the great arteries, and double outlet right ventricle are also associated anomalies. Coarctation is the most common congenital heart defect found with Turner syndrome (Moss, 1983).

Pathophysiology

An important factor in coarctation, aside from the presence or absence of other cardiac defects, is the degree of isthmic narrowing. The isthmus of the aorta is that area of the aortic arch between the ductus arteriosus and the left subclavian artery. With long segment isthmic narrowing the ductus arteriosus is usually patent, and blood flow to the descending aorta is from the pulmonary artery through the patent ductus arteriosus. This type of coarctation is most often associated with severe cardiac defects, and infants are symptomatic early in life. With minimal isthmic narrowing blood flow to the descending aorta is from the left ventricle and ascending aorta. This has been referred to as "adult-type" coarctation. Infants can present with either type of coarctation. In the older child, when a severe "adult-type" coarctation exists, allowing little blood flow to the descending aorta, collateral circulation to the descending aorta is often present.

Decreased blood flow to the lower part of the body results in diminished or absent femoral and pedal pulses. The pressure in the left ventricle and ascending aorta is increased from the coarctation, causing upper extremity hypertension.

Clinical Manifestations

There are two groups of patients with coarctation: (1) those who are symptomatic in infancy and (2) those who remain asymptomatic and are diagnosed during routine physical examination in later years. If symptoms do not develop during infancy, the child will most likely grow normally and remain asymptomatic until later childhood. Occasionally these children will present with complaints of weakness or pain in their legs with exercise. However, most often they are identified through a differential in upper and lower extremity blood pressures, hypertension of the upper extremities, and absent or diminished femoral and pedal pulses. Infants usually present with congestive heart failure and failure to thrive. Symptoms include respiratory distress, poor weight gain, feeding problems, irritability, and tachycardia. Infants with coarctation and a PDA may have adequate blood flow to the lower extremities, good pedal pulses, and no differential in blood pressure. Once the PDA closes, however, they will have absent or diminished femoral and pedal pulses and a differential in upper and lower extremity blood pressures.

Diagnostic Assessment

Cardiac Examination. The first and second heart sounds are usually normal. There may be no murmurs present, or there may be a systolic murmur along the left mid to upper sternal border which radiates to the back. In addition, murmurs of associated cardiac defects such as a VSD may be heard. An additional systolic or continuous murmur may be present from collateral circulation. It is especially important to evaluate *both* upper extremity blood pressures and one lower extremity pressure with appropriate-sized cuffs. In the presence of a coarctation, upper extremity pressures will be at least 20 mmHg higher than lower extremity pressures. Femoral and pedal pulses are diminished or absent.

Electrocardiogram. Right ventricular hypertrophy is seen on ECG in the infant with coarctation. The older child may have left ventricular hypertrophy or a normal ECG.

Chest Roentgenogram. Increased heart size and increased pulmonary vascularity are often seen on the infant's roentgenogram. The older child may have a normal heart size but display such findings as rib notching and a prominent descending aorta.

Echocardiogram. The presence of a coarctation and the degree of isthmic narrowing, as well as the presence of other cardiac defects, may be determined by the echocardiogram.

Therapeutic Management

Infants presenting in congestive heart failure and with failure to thrive are stabilized with medical therapy (see section on CHF) and are surgically corrected once stabilized. If other cardiac defects, such as a VSD, are present, the coarctation is repaired first and if possible the other cardiac lesions are repaired when the infant is older. Coarctation may be surgically corrected using numerous approaches. The *end-to-end anastomosis* where the narrowed portion of the aorta is removed and the two parts of the aorta on either side of the defect are joined was the surgery of choice for many years. Unfortunately, when performed on infants this procedure resulted in a high incidence of recoarctation in later life. As the child grew, the site of the anastomosis did not. Introduction of the use of absorbable sutures and widening of the anastomotic site are thought by some to help eliminate future problems of recoarctation (Merenstein et al, 1985).

The *subclavian flap aortoplasty* is a procedure in which a longitudinal incision is made in the aorta across the coarctated site and continued to the end of the distally divided left subclavian artery. The left subclavian artery is used as a patch or flap to increase the diameter of the aorta. This procedure has been highly successful in relieving coarctation, especially in infants, and in providing for future growth of the aorta. If the coarctation is a very long, narrow segment, a *conduit* may be the surgical approach of choice with removal of the narrowed segment and placement of a conduit between the two ends of the aorta. *Patch aortoplasty* is still another technique, in which the coarcted area is excised and a patch graft placed on the aorta to widen the area.

If the child is asymptomatic, surgical repair is still recommended between the ages of 2 and 4. Delayed repair beyond 4 years of age may lead to prolonged or permanent hypertension, greater risk of premature death, and cardiovascular disease (Moss, 1983). Older children usually have an end-to-end anastomosis because there is less risk of recoarctation due to the size of the aorta. Surgical repair of coarctation is not an open heart procedure and therefore usually does not require cardiopulmonary bypass. It is performed through a lateral thoracotomy incision. Postoperative complications pertinent to nursing care include diminished or absent pulses in the left arm (with the subclavian flap aortoplasty) and persistent hypertension. Rebound hypertension immediately postoperatively is commonly present in patients regardless of the procedure and is treated with vigorous medical therapy. The severity of the hypertension and its duration are related to the child's age at the time of repair and the degree of preoperative hypertension.

Balloon aortoplasty, a special procedure in which a balloon catheter is introduced into the aorta during cardiac catheterization and inflated at the site of the coarctation to relieve the obstruction, has been tried in recent years with varying success. It appears to be a less successful procedure for infant coarctations or unrepaired coarctations in the older child. However, some success has been reported in relieving recoarctations in older children with this procedure.

Continued antibiotic prophylaxis for certain procedures is necessary, as is cardiology follow-up at least every 1 to 2 years. Without correction, coarctation can pose life-threatening dangers. Cerebral vascular accidents, aneurysms, and rupture of the aorta occur as a result of the increased pressure and formation of collateral circulation. If left untreated, calcification of the aorta, hypertension, and left ventricular hypertrophy develop.

Perioperative Nursing Diagnoses for Coarctation of the Aorta

Preoperative

Potential altered tissue perfusion: upper extremity hypertension, related to increased pressure in the left ventricle and ascending aorta associated with obstructed blood flow in the aorta

Defining characteristics: blood pressure in upper extremities greater than the 90th percentile for age

Potential altered cardiac output: decreased, related to decreased blood flow through the descending aorta

Defining characteristics: respiratory distress, irritability, tachycardia

Potential altered growth and development: failure to thrive, related to altered tissue perfusion, congestive heart failure, and feeding problems

Defining characteristics: height and weight less than the 3rd percentile; developmental delays

Postoperative

Open heart surgery is not required.

Potential for injury: physiologic, associated with

- *persistent hypertension*
- *Horner syndrome associated with sympathetic nerve trauma during surgical repair; Defining characteristics: unilateral ptosis of the eyelid and unequal pupil constriction*
- *bacterial endocarditis; Defining characteristics: fever, bacteremia*

Pulmonary Stenosis (Fig. 39-13)

Pulmonary stenosis, which exists in 25 to 35 per cent of all patients with congenital heart disease (Moss, 1983), is an obstruction that interferes with blood flow out of the right ventricle. The obstruction may occur below the pulmonary valve in the infundibular area (subvalvar), above the valve (supravalvar), or at the valve (valvar). Pulmonary stenosis is often associated with other anomalies such as tetralogy of Fallot, transposition of the great arteries, double outlet right ventricle defects, atrioventricular canal defects, VSD, ASD, and PDA. It is the most common defect found with Noonan syndrome and may also be found with rubella syndrome and William syndrome. Pulmonary stenosis with intact ventricular septum will be described in this section.

Pathophysiology

Pulmonary stenosis involves malformation of the cusps of the pulmonic valve that controls the flow of blood from the right ventricle into the pulmonary artery. It can vary in degree from mild to severe or critical. As the obstruction increases, right ventricular pressure increases and thickening of the right ventricular wall (hypertrophy) develops. If right ventricular hypertrophy is severe, as in critical pulmonary stenosis, right atrial pressure can increase, resulting in right to left shunting through the foramen ovale. The infant or child would then be cyanotic. However, most infants and children are acyanotic with mild to moderate pulmonary stenosis. When the obstruction is at the *valvar* level there is a "jetting" of blood through the stenotic valve, which dilates the main pulmonary artery. *Infundibular,* or subvalvar, stenosis may occur alone or in conjunction with valvar stenosis. There is a dynamic component to infundibular stenosis in that the infundibular muscle is thickened and is contracting more vigorously than the rest of the ventricle. This constricts the outflow portion of the right ventricle and decreases blood flow to the lungs. *Supravalvar* pulmonary stenosis can be an isolated constriction involving the main pulmonary artery, the left and right pulmonary arteries, and the smaller peripheral arterial branches.

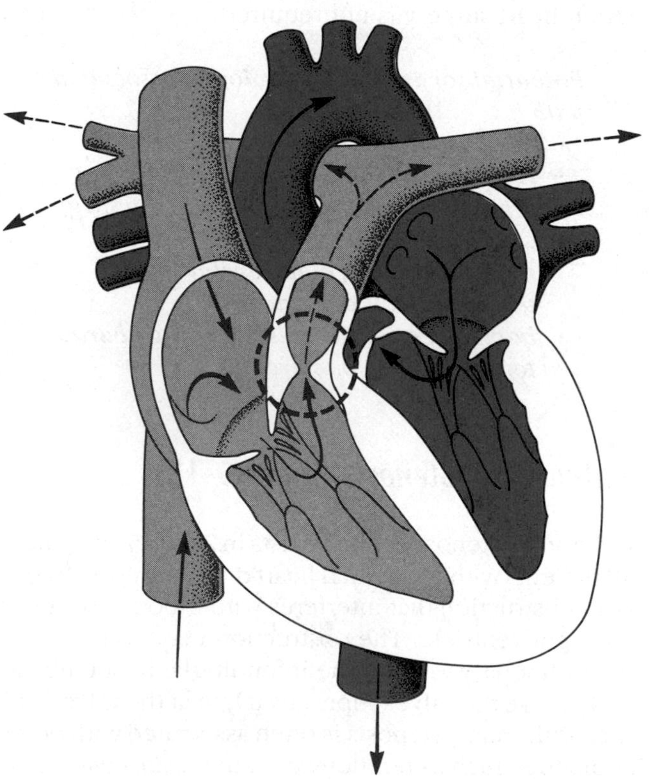

Figure 39-13. Pulmonary stenosis (valvar). Blood flow through the pulmonary artery is diminished, as illustrated by the broken arrows.

Clinical Manifestations

Symptomatology varies according to the degree of obstruction. With severe or critical pulmonary stenosis, heart failure may develop early in infancy. If the ductus arteriosus is patent, it will allow some pulmonary blood flow, but once it is closed symptoms increase. When the foramen ovale remains patent, cyanosis will be evident. The older child with severe pulmonary stenosis will have dyspnea and fatigability, even with moderate exercise. Strenuous exercise in these children may result in syncope or sudden death. Chest pain or epigastric pain, or both, may also occur. Children with moderate pulmonary stenosis are usually asymptomatic during the first 2 to 3 years of life, then may develop dyspnea on exertion and easy fatigability. Children with mild pulmonary stenosis are asymptomatic. The majority of children with pulmonary stenosis are asymptomatic and their cardiac defect is discovered on routine examination. Growth and development are usually normal.

Diagnostic Assessment

Cardiac Examination. This examination varies according to the degree and type of pulmonary stenosis. With valvar stenosis there may be a thrill palpable at the mid- to upper left sternal border and at the suprasternal notch. An ejection click is commonly heard with mild to moderate stenosis. A grade II–IV/VI harsh systolic murmur is present, which is loudest at the upper left sternal border but radiates to both axillae and can be heard throughout the chest. The first heart sound is normal. The second heart sound is usually normal; however, with severe pulmonary stenosis the murmur may be prolonged, obliterating a portion of the second heart sound. In this case the second heart sound would be a single sound. Diastolic murmurs are not typically present. The cardiac examination with infundibular stenosis is generally the same as with valvar stenosis, except that there is usually no ejection click. As with infundibular stenosis, supravalvar stenosis does not have an associated ejection click.

Electrocardiogram. With mild to moderate pulmonary stenosis the electrocardiogram may be normal or show right ventricular hypertrophy. In severe pulmonary stenosis the ECG almost always shows right ventricular hypertrophy.

Chest Roentgenogram. The heart size is most often normal, as is the pulmonary vascularity. With valvar pulmonary stenosis there is a prominent main pulmonary artery segment distinguishable on the chest roentgenogram. With infundibular and supravalvar pulmonary stenosis, the main pulmonary artery segment is not prominent.

Echocardiogram. Color flow 2-D echocardiography can demonstrate the size of the right ventricle and its outflow tract, the pulmonary valve, main pulmonary artery, and the left and right pulmonary arteries. The level(s) of obstruction can be visualized, as can the presence of other cardiac defects. With the addition of continuous wave Doppler measurements, the actual pressure gradient across the obstruction can be estimated.

Therapeutic Management

Symptomatic infants or older children with severe pulmonary stenosis need balloon valvuloplasty (dilatation of the stenotic valve with a balloon catheter) or surgical repair. When right ventricular pressures exceed left ventricular pressures the pulmonary stenosis is considered severe or critical. In newborn infants, prostaglandin E_1 has been used to maintain the patency of the ductus arteriosus, allowing adequate pulmonary blood flow until surgery.

Surgical intervention for valvar stenosis usually consists of a *valvulotomy.* However, the right ventricle and pulmonary arteries must be of adequate size. Pulmonary valvulotomies are usually performed through a median sternotomy and an incision in the pulmonary artery. The pulmonary valve commissures are incised, allowing the leaflets to open freely during systole. This procedure in neonates can usually be accomplished with inflow occlusion and circulatory arrest for 1 to 2 minutes (Merenstein et al, 1985). In older infants, cardiopulmonary bypass should be performed. If the valve annulus (the ring of tissue to which the leaflets are attached) itself is small, an incision into the annulus is made and a patch used to enlarge the annulus. When infundibular stenosis is present, resection of the hypertrophied muscle is performed and if necessary a pericardial or dacron patch is used to widen the outflow tract. For supravalvar stenosis, the area of obstruction is incised and a patch graft inserted to widen the area. Moderate pulmonary stenosis is not surgically repaired in infancy but rather followed throughout early childhood. If the stenosis increases, right ventricular hypertrophy increases, and/or the child becomes symptomatic the stenosis is repaired electively. Mild pulmonary stenosis does not need repair.

As an alternative to surgery for pulmonary valvar stenosis a technique called pulmonary balloon valvuloplasty has been utilized quite successfully in many institutions. In the procedure a balloon catheter is placed across the stenotic pulmonary valve during cardiac catheterization. The balloon is inflated, opening the stenotic valve and relieving the obstruction. This technique can only be used for valvar stenosis when the valve annulus is of adequate size. Balloon valvuloplasty is ineffective in relieving infundibular pulmonary stenosis. Some forms of supravalvar pulmonary stenosis have been successfully relieved by balloon valvuloplasty. The benefit of balloon valvuloplasty is obvious, in that it eliminates the need for a surgical repair. The long-term results of balloon valvuloplasty (e.g., degree of residual obstruction, rate and degree of reobstruction, rate and degree of pulmonary regurgitation) need further study. Residual obstruction, reobstruction, and pulmonary regurgitation are complications seen after both surgical repair and balloon valvuloplasty. Children with pulmonary stenosis require life-long antibiotic prophylaxis for endocarditis for certain procedures.

Perioperative Nursing Diagnoses for Pulmonary Stenosis

Preoperative

Potential activity intolerance, related to decreased blood flow to the lungs associated with pulmonary artery obstruction

Postoperative

Potential for injury: physiologic, related to

- *residual obstruction or reobstruction or both*
- *pulmonary valve regurgitation; Defining characteristics: diastolic murmur*
- *bacterial endocarditis*

Aortic Stenosis (Fig. 39-14)

Aortic stenosis (narrowing) constitutes about 5 per cent of all congenital heart disease (Gersony, 1987). The aortic valve controls blood flow between the left ventricle and the aorta. Aortic stenosis in infants and small children is always regarded as a congenital defect, whereas adults may develop aortic stenosis following rheumatic fever or from progressive atherosclerotic disease. Males have a much higher incidence of congenital aortic stenosis, especially the valvar type, than females. Other congenital heart defects asso-

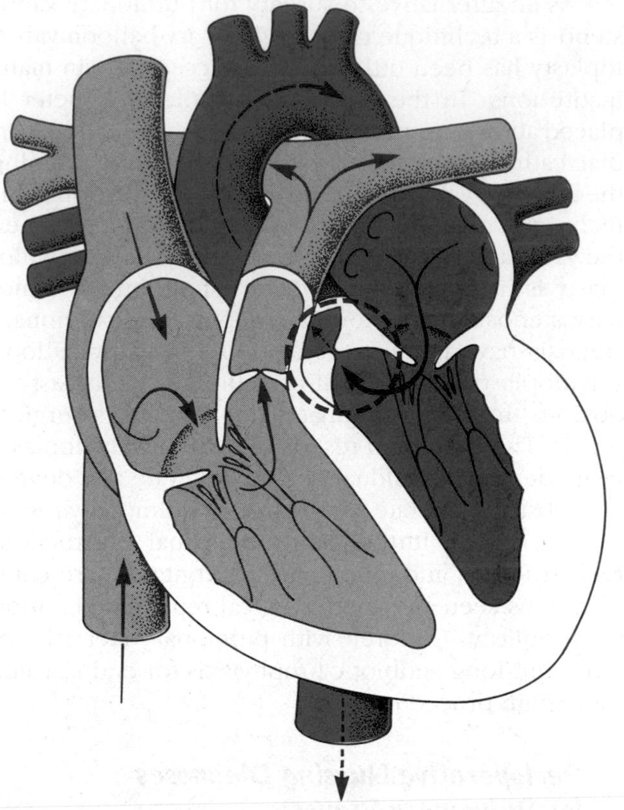

Figure 39-14. Aortic stenosis (valvar) with left ventricular hypertrophy. Flow patterns are normal, but blood flow into the aorta is diminished, as depicted by the broken arrows.

ciated with aortic stenosis are PDA, coarctation of the aorta, VSD, and pulmonary stenosis. Supravalvar aortic stenosis is commonly associated with William syndrome. Aortic stenosis is divided into three related types: (1) valvar, (2) supravalvar, and (3) subvalvar.

Supravalvar aortic stenosis occurs above the aortic valve. This type of stenosis is fairly uncommon and is usually associated with other defects such as mental retardation, defective dental development, abnormal facies, infantile hypocalcemia, and pulmonary stenosis. Discrete subvalvar stenosis (narrowing below the valve) results from a thin membrane or thick, fibrous ring in the subvalvar region of the aortic valve. Valvar aortic stenosis (stricture of the aortic valve) is the type most frequently encountered. The aortic valve may be unicuspid, bicuspid, or tricuspid. In most cases the valve is bicuspid and thickened.

Pathophysiology

In the presence of aortic stenosis there is obstruction to blood flow from the left ventricle. This results in thickening, or hypertrophy, of the left ventricle. The degree of obstruction varies from mild to severe or critical. With mild aortic stenosis there is minimal obstruction to blood flow from the left ventricle and consequently minimal, if any, left ventricular hypertrophy. With moderate to severe or critical aortic stenosis, however, the left ventricle is very hypertrophied and left ventricular pressure is quite high. Heart failure can develop due to the excessive workload placed on the left ventricle pumping against the obstruction. In severe cases, pulmonary edema may ensue as a result of increased left atrial pressure that may cause a backflow of blood into the lungs. In addition, blood supply to the heart muscle itself may be compromised. The hypertrophied left ventricular muscle must contract with stronger force over a longer period of time to eject blood from the heart. This increased workload in turn increases the heart muscle's need for oxygen. The coronary arteries often cannot keep pace with the increased oxygen requirement of the heart muscle and ischemia of the heart muscle results. This can occur at rest or during exercise. With ischemia chest pain, ventricular dysrhythmias, syncope, and sudden death can occur. Aortic stenosis, especially the subvalvar type, tends to become increasingly problematic without treatment.

Clinical Manifestations

The clinical manifestations vary according to the type and degree of stenosis. Most children are asymptomatic and their defect is discovered during routine physical examination. The murmur may be detected during infancy or not until the preschool period. Growth and development are usually normal. When symptoms do occur in the older child, those most commonly seen are fatigability, exertional dyspnea, chest pain, and syncope. Infants with critical aortic stenosis may present in heart failure in the newborn period or in the first few months of life. These infants will be irritable, pale, hypotensive, tachycardic, and tachypneic, and have decreased perfusion and pulmonary congestion.

Diagnostic Assessment

Cardiac Examination. The cardiac examination will vary with the degree and type of aortic stenosis. In general there will be a harsh systolic murmur, grade II–IV/VI, heard typically at the upper right sternal border radiating to the upper left sternal border and the neck. An ejection click may be heard at the apex and lower left sternal border. A suprasternal notch thrill is palpable.

Electrocardiogram. The ECG may be normal or demonstrate left ventricular hypertrophy. There is often very poor correlation between the ECG and the degree of aortic stenosis, i.e., in the presence of severe aortic stenosis the ECG may be normal or show only mild left ventricular hypertrophy.

Chest Roentgenogram. The heart size is most often normal, even when severe aortic stenosis is present. Dilatation of the ascending aorta may be seen with valvar aortic stenosis. Infants may have an increased heart size, especially if they are in heart failure.

Echocardiogram. With color flow 2-D echocardiogram, the type of aortic stenosis, as well as the presence of other cardiac defects, can be visualized. Left ventricular wall thickness and left ventricular function can also be evaluated. With the 2-D continuous wave Doppler an estimate of the pressure gradient across the obstruction can be made.

Therapeutic Management

Infants and children with mild to moderate aortic stenosis are usually followed clinically with no surgical intervention unless their aortic stenosis progresses. Infants with critical valvar aortic stenosis need surgical repair as soon as possible. Valvar aortic stenosis is repaired through a median sternotomy. The aorta is incised and the aortic valve commissures incised, permitting the leaflets to open freely during systole. The valve will never be normal, however, and residual obstruction is common as well as aortic regurgitation. If the aortic regurgitation becomes significant the child may require an aortic valve replacement at some time.

Supravalvar stenosis is repaired by incising the narrowed segment of the aorta and widening the area with a patch graft. Repair of discrete subvalvar aortic stenosis involves removing the obstructing membrane or fibrous ring below the aortic valve. Diffuse tunnel or muscular subvalvar aortic stenosis is a difficult lesion to repair. The traditional approach has been to remove surgically as much of the obstructing muscle as possible. However, residual obstruction is almost always present and the muscular obstruction most often progresses, necessitating further surgical repairs. Several surgical approaches have been devised to repair residual and/or recurring muscular subvalvar aortic stenosis. The Konno procedure is a surgical procedure that involves removing obstructing muscle, widening the outflow area of the left ventricle, including the aortic valve annulus, with a patch, and replacing the aortic valve with a larger valve. This procedure is relatively new but appears to be successful in relieving diffuse tunnel or muscular subvalvar aortic stenosis. Further studies are needed to evaluate the long-term effectiveness of this procedure.

When *replacing the aortic valve* there is a wide variety of valve types available. Three common types of valves are (1) tissue heterograft valves (porcine valves and bovine pericardium valves), (2) prosthetic valves, and (3) homograft valves (human donor valves). Porcine valves and bovine pericardium valves are used less often on the left side of the heart in infants and children because they tend to calcify rapidly and need to be replaced often. Prosthetic valves are commonly used on the left side of the heart because they seldom calcify. However, infants and children with a prosthetic valve require continuous anticoagulation to prevent clot formation on the valve. The third type of valve, the homograft, has been used relatively recently in most areas of the world. Preliminary results show minimal calcification of the valve and these children do not require continuous anticoagulation. Further studies are needed to evaluate the long-term effectiveness of the homograft valve. Another advantage to using the homograft valve is its flexibility and pliability during surgical insertion. In addition, it is possible to use a larger size in the homograft valve than can be used with a prosthetic or porcine valve. This allows the child a longer period of growth before a second valve replacement is required and in some children it is possible to place an adult-sized homograft, which would eliminate the need to replace the valve with a larger one later.

Aortic balloon valvuloplasty (see description of balloon valvuloplasty procedure under pulmonary stenosis) is a relatively new technique for relieving valvar aortic stenosis in infants and in older children. This procedure may carry a higher risk than pulmonary balloon valvuloplasty. The balloon catheter is inserted in the femoral artery, passed through the descending aorta, around the aortic arch and through the aortic valve into the left ventricle. The balloon is then inflated across the stenotic aortic valve. Dilatation of aortic valves with this technique has not been as successful as balloon dilatation of pulmonary valves. Complications of aortic balloon valvuloplasty include aortic aneurysms, rupture of the aortic wall, and tearing of aortic leaflets creating severe aortic regurgitation.

All children with aortic stenosis require antibiotic prophylaxis for endocarditis for certain procedures. These children also require close continued follow-up by a cardiologist for evaluation of progressive obstruction, development of aortic regurgitation, and other complications.

Perioperative Nursing Diagnoses for Aortic Stenosis

Preoperative

Potential altered cardiac output: decreased, related to obstruction of blood flow from the left ventricle

Defining characteristics: pallor, irritability, hypotension, tachycardia, tachypnea, decreased systemic perfusion, pulmonary congestion

Potential altered tissue perfusion: myocardium, related to inability of the left ventricle to meet metabolic demands of the myocardium

Defining characteristics: chest pain, ventricular dysrhythmias, syncope

Postoperative

Potential for injury: physiologic, related to

- *residual obstruction and aortic regurgitation*
- *bacterial endocarditis*

Cyanotic Heart Defects

The term *cyanotic heart disease* refers to mixing of unoxygenated blood with oxygenated blood and usually involves a right to left shunt. In this case, the blood perfusing the tissues contains less than the normal amount of oxygen. In mild cyanotic heart disease, the amount of unoxygenated blood may be negligible and result in no visible cyanosis or other manifestations. In more severe conditions, however, the heart is unable to supply the tissues with the oxygen needed for such common activities as feeding and crying. As in acyanotic heart disease, the direction of the shunt may reverse with changes in pressure gradients between right and left heart chambers.

Tetralogy of Fallot (Fig. 39-15)

Tetralogy of Fallot (TOF) accounts for 10 per cent of all congenital heart defects and is the most common cyanotic heart defect (Friedman, 1988). Described by Fallot more than 100 years ago, the anomaly has four components *(1) pulmonary stenosis, (2) VSD, (3) an over-riding aorta, and (4) ventricular hypertrophy.* The VSD is usually large and located high in the septum. The pulmonary stenosis may involve the infundibular region, the pulmonary valve, and/or the pulmonary arteries. Associated cardiac defects include PDA, ASD, and aortic regurgitation. The right ventricular hypertrophy results from the pulmonary stenosis.

Pathophysiology

A wide range of types and degree of pulmonary stenosis can be present in TOF. The degree of pulmonary stenosis determines the pattern of blood flow in the heart. With severe pulmonary stenosis right ventricular pressure is equal to or greater than left ventricular pressure. Unoxygenated blood therefore passes from the right ventricle through the VSD and out the over-riding aorta to the systemic circulation. These infants and children have a right to left shunt and are cyanotic. With mild pulmonary stenosis right ventricular pressure is lower than left ventricular pressure, which allows oxygenated blood from the left side of the heart to pass through the VSD and out the pulmonary artery to the lungs. This is a left to right shunt, and these infants and children will be acyanotic. TOF with mild pulmonary stenosis is often referred to as "pink" TOF.

The infundibular pulmonary stenosis associated with TOF usually increases in severity with time. These infants and children will become more cyanotic as pulmonary blood flow decreases. Even infants who are originally acyanotic or "pink" will eventually become cyanotic due to the progression in infundibular stenosis.

"TET" (from "tetralogy") or hypoxic spells may occur in children with TOF. *TET spells* are characterized by increased cyanosis, irritability, pallor, tachyp-

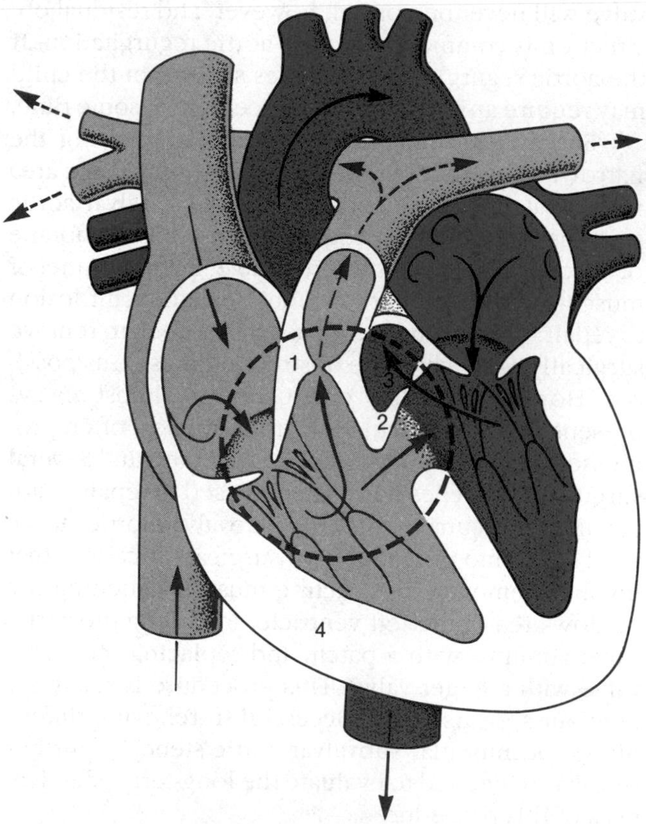

Figure 39-15. Tetralogy of Fallot, showing (1) pulmonary stenosis, (2) VSD, (3) over-riding aorta, and (4) right ventricular hypertrophy. Flow patterns are determined by the degree of pulmonary stenosis.

nea, flaccidity, and possible loss of consciousness. They commonly occur in the morning after a night's sleep and are most frequently precipitated by crying, defecation, and feeding, all of which cause an increased oxygen need. These spells may be the result of a transient increase in the obstruction of the right ventricular outflow tract (usually increased contraction of the muscular infundibular area). As the obstruction increases, more unoxygenated blood is passed through the VSD to the systemic circulation, causing severe hypoxia. TET spells can progress to seizures, cerebral vascular accidents, and death. *Treatment of TET spells* includes placing the infant or child in a knee-chest position and administering oxygen, propranolol, or morphine, or a combination of these agents. The knee-chest position enhances systemic venous return, which helps to dilate the right ventricle, decreasing the obstruction. Propranolol, usually administered at 1 mg/kg up to four times a day, aids in decreasing infundibular muscle spasm. Morphine 0.2 mg/kg suppresses the respiratory drive. These therapies are useful for halting TET spells. Propranolol is then commonly given on a routine basis to prevent further TET spells.

Clinical Manifestations

The symptoms present with TOF depend on the degree of pulmonary stenosis. Infants who are cyanotic in the first month of life usually have severe pulmonary stenosis. These infants commonly have TET spells, polycythemia, dyspnea on exertion, irritability, and poor exercise tolerance. In addition, poor growth and development is typical. If polycythemia becomes severe, cerebral vascular accidents and brain abscesses can occur.

Diagnostic Assessment

Cardiac Examination. A harsh systolic murmur of grade II–IV/VI is heard along the left sternal border. The second heart sound is single representing aortic valve closure. Pulmonic valve closure is usually not heard.

Electrocardiogram. Right ventricular hypertrophy is almost always present on the ECG.

Chest Roentgenogram. The heart size is usually normal, with a characteristic "boot-shaped" contour resulting from the small main pulmonary artery and the right ventricular hypertrophy. The pulmonary vascularity may be normal or decreased.

Echocardiogram. With color flow 2-D echocardiography and continuous wave Doppler, the VSD, the over-riding aorta, and the pulmonary stenosis can be visualized.

Therapeutic Management

Asymptomatic infants and young children require no surgical intervention until they become symptomatic. Infants who are severely cyanotic in the first few months of life require either a palliative procedure to increase blood flow to the lungs or a total repair. Total repair is not usually recommended in the neonatal period. The earliest age at which total repair is performed varies among institutions.

Palliative procedures for TOF consist of systemic to pulmonary shunts, and are indicated if the infant is too young for a full repair or if the pulmonary arteries are of small size. After a shunt procedure the pulmonary arteries hopefully will grow. The most common shunt used today is the *Blalock-Taussig shunt.* In this procedure the right or left subclavian artery is connected to the ipsilateral (on the same side) pulmonary artery. This allows for increased blood flow to the lungs. Although the Blalock-Taussig shunt increases blood flow to the lungs, the overall volume of blood reaching the lungs is still limited. Following the shunt procedure, the child will continue to be cyanotic but to a lesser degree. The Blalock-Taussig shunt is not an open heart procedure and is performed through a lateral thoracotomy incision. Complications of the Blalock-Taussig procedure include a diminished or absent pulse in the affected arm, congestive heart failure from too large a shunt or an inadequate shunt.

In instances when a Blalock-Taussig shunt cannot be performed, a Waterston shunt may be substituted. The *Waterston shunt* connects the ascending aorta to the right pulmonary artery. This shunt is less preferable because of the increased prevalence of pulmonary vascular disease and kinking and distortion of the pulmonary arteries associated with it (Moss, 1983).

Total repair of TOF consists of a patch (usually dacron) closure of the VSD and relief of the pulmonary stenosis. Resection of the infundibular muscle, a patch (pericardium or dacron) widening of the infundibular region, a pulmonary valvulotomy, and if necessary an extension of a patch across the annulus of the pulmonary valve to widen it may all be required to relieve the pulmonary stenosis. In some instances the pulmonary stenosis is severe and a pulmonary artery homograft conduit is placed from the right ventricle to the pulmonary artery to bypass the obstruction. The surgical approach is through a median sternotomy and it is an open heart surgery requiring cardiopulmonary bypass or deep hypothermia with circulatory arrest.

Complications of total repair include conduction abnormalities (heart block), a residual VSD, residual pulmonary stenosis, and pulmonary valve regurgitation.

Care for these infants and children *prior to surgi-*

cal repair should include special emphasis on (1) the provision of adequate iron intake (with hypoxia the need for increased oxygen carrying capacity requires increased iron for hemoglobin) and (2) scrupulous dental hygiene to reduce the risk of endocarditis.* In addition, when these infants and children have an intravenous line in place great care should be taken to avoid forceful unplugging of a clotted needle or other actions that could lead to air in the line. Because these infants or children are cyanotic with a right to left shunt, air or a clot may be transported directly to the systemic circulation causing a cerebral vascular accident. Life-long antibiotic prophylaxis for endocarditis for certain procedures is required by all children with TOF.

Perioperative Nursing Diagnoses for Tetralogy of Fallot

Preoperative

***Altered tissue perfusion: hypoxic (TET) spells**, related to insufficient oxygenated blood to meet metabolic needs*

Defining characteristics: increased cyanosis, irritability, pallor, tachypnea, muscle flaccidity, loss of consciousness, seizures, CVA

***Potential exercise intolerance**, related to polycythemia and hypoxia*

Defining characteristics: increased RBC, hemoglobin, and hematocrit; cyanosis; hyperemia of sclerae and mucous membranes; clubbing of the fingers

***Potential altered growth and development: failure to thrive**, related to insufficient oxygen to meet metabolic needs*

***Potential for injury: cerebrovascular accident**, related to polycythemia, or to a blood clot or air bubble introduced into the venous circulation, proceeding through the VSD into the left ventricle, and entering the systemic circulation*

Postoperative

***Potential for injury: physiologic**, related to the following complications of Blalock-Taussig procedure*

- *persistent cyanosis*
- *diminished or absent pulse in affected arm*

related to the following complications of total repair

- *heart block*
- *residual VDs*
- *residual pulmonary stenosis*
- *pulmonary valve regurgitation*
- *bacterial endocarditis (with all procedures)*

Complete D-Transposition of the Great Arteries (Fig. 39-16)

Complete d-transposition of the great arteries (TGA) is a cyanotic defect that accounts for about 5 per cent of congenital heart defects (Gersony, 1987). The aorta arises from the right ventricle and the pulmonary artery arises from the left ventricle, resulting in *two separate and parallel circulatory systems.* TGA occurs much more often in males than in females and usually in term infants (Moss, 1983). Cardiac defects commonly associated with TGA are PDA, ASD, VSD, and pulmonary stenosis.

Pathophysiology

With the great arteries transposed, the pulmonary artery, arising from the left ventricle, delivers blood to the lungs for oxygenation. This oxygenated blood returns to the left atrium and left ventricle and is recycled again through the pulmonary circulation. The aorta, arising from the right side of the heart, delivers unoxygenated blood to the systemic circulation. This blood then returns to the right atrium and ventricle and without being oxygenated, is circulated back to the systemic circulation via the aorta. The major physiologic abnormalities in TGA are an oxygen deficiency in the tissues and an excessive workload on the right and left ventricles. The only mixing of oxygenated and unoxygenated blood occurs in the presence of associated lesions (patent foramen ovale, ASD, VSD, PDA, or collateral circulation). The extent of the mixing depends on the number, size, and position of the anatomic communications, and the pressure differential between the two systems.

Clinical Manifestations

TGA is diagnosed in infancy. Cyanosis is always present and the degree will depend on the amount of intercirculatory mixing present. Cyanosis may be mild if the mixing occurs through a large VSD or PDA. Cyanosis is profound if the ventricular septum is intact or the PDA is closing, or both. Cyanosis will also be profound if significant pulmonary stenosis is present. Hy-

* Poor dental hygiene can result in swollen, bleeding gums. Bacteria in the mouth can enter the bloodstream through the gum lesions and cause endocarditis. See page 1332.

poxic spells may be frequent, especially during crying or exertion. Infants, especially those with a large VSD, may present in congestive heart failure. Clubbing (see page 1279) may be seen in older children.

Diagnostic Assessment

Cardiac Examination. Murmurs, if present, are usually those of associated cardiac defects such as a PDA or a VSD. The second heart sound is single and increased in intensity because of the aorta rising from the right ventricle (the anterior ventricle).

Electrocardiogram. The ECG may be normal or demonstrate right ventricular hypertrophy. Left ventricular hypertrophy or combined ventricular hypertrophy are uncommon.

Chest Roentgenogram. Heart size may be normal or moderately enlarged. The cardiac silhouette may assume the shape of an egg laying on a string and the pulmonary vascularity may be normal, increased, or decreased.

Echocardiogram. The color flow 2-D echocardiogram is extremely useful in establishing the diagnosis and evaluating the presence of associated cardiac defects.

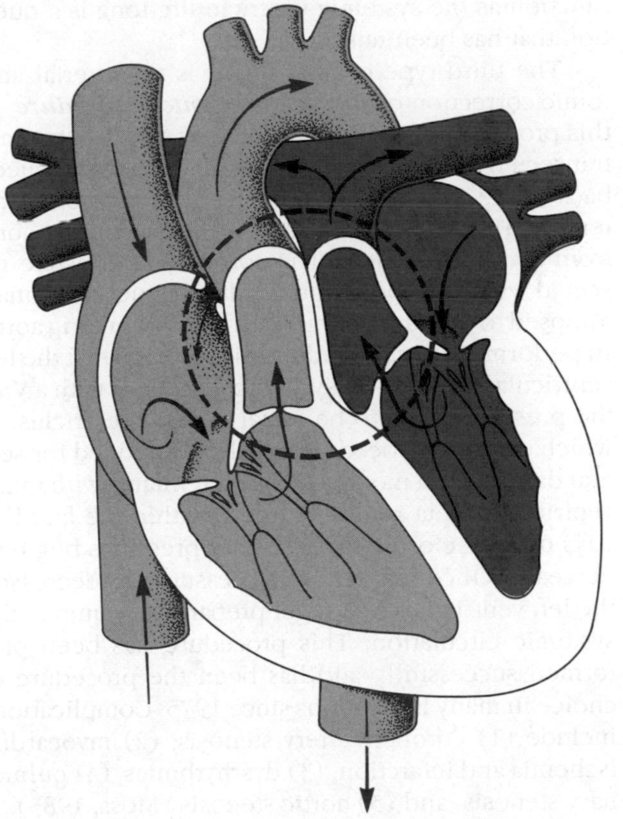

Figure 39-16. Complete D-transposition of the great arteries with an associated ASD. Blood flow exists as two parallel systems—one recirculating oxygenated blood, the other recirculating unoxygenated blood. Mixing occurs only through defects such as the ASD shown here.

Therapeutic Management

Oxygen therapy in the profoundly cyanotic neonate with TGA is of limited benefit. Only a certain amount of oxygenated blood is able to reach the systemic circulation, and administration of additional oxygen does not improve this situation. Enlargement of the interatrial communication by *balloon septostomy (Rashkind procedure)* during cardiac catheterization is critical in establishing adequate mixing of oxygenated and unoxygenated blood for these infants. A Rashkind procedure is performed by passing a balloon catheter through the foramen ovale, inflating the balloon, and pulling the catheter back to stretch open the foramen ovale and create a large opening between the two atria. Creation of an atrial septal defect or enlargement of the foramen ovale surgically is termed a *Blalock-Hanlon procedure.* Following these palliative procedures the infant will continue to be cyanotic, especially in times of stress (crying, feeding, or exposure to cold temperatures). However, oxygenation should be sufficient for the infant to thrive until the time for total repair.

Many surgical procedures exist for total repair of TGA; three of the most common will be discussed here. The most common surgical repairs for TGA are the Mustard, the Senning, and the arterial switch procedures. The Mustard and Senning procedures involve intra-atrial redirection of blood flow. With the *Mustard procedure* a new atrial septum is created by using pericardium to make a baffle. This baffle alters the blood flow by redirecting unoxygenated blood from the right atrium through the mitral valve to the left ventricle and out to the lungs via the pulmonary artery; oxygenated blood from the left atrium is redirected through the tricuspid valve to the right ventricle and to the systemic circulation via the aorta. The *Senning procedure* creates the same redirection of blood flow, but without the use of a pericardial patch. The atrial septum and a portion of the atrial wall are used to reroute the blood flow. Both the Mustard and the Senning procedures have been very successful, with a low mortality rate. Timing of repair varies among institutions; however, most commonly repair is recommended in the first year of life. Surgical repair should be performed before pulmonary vascular changes develop.

Complications of the Mustard and Senning procedures include (1) superior vena cava or inferior vena cava obstruction, (2) dysrhythmias, (3) tricuspid regurgitation, and (4) obstruction of the pulmonary veins (a severe complication requiring immediate correction). Whether the right ventricle can continue to function as the systemic ventricle life-long is a question that has been raised.

The third type of total repair is the arterial anatomic correction or the *arterial switch procedure*. In this procedure the pulmonary artery and the aorta are transected above the respective valves and "switched" back to the appropriate ventricles. The pulmonary artery then arises from the right ventricle and the aorta from the left ventricle. The coronary arteries are resected with a button of surrounding tissue and reanastomosed to the supravalvar area of the ascending aorta. In performing this procedure it is essential that the left ventricular pressure be systemic. In infants with a VSD the pressure tends to be equal in both ventricles, in which case this procedure may be postponed for several days or even months. However, infants with intact ventricular septa require surgery within the first few days of life before left ventricular pressures begin to decrease. Once left ventricle pressure has decreased the left ventricle is no longer prepared to pump to the systemic circulation. This procedure has been performed successfully and has been the procedure of choice in many institutions since 1975. Complications include (1) coronary artery stenosis, (2) myocardial ischemia and infarction, (3) dysrhythmias, (4) pulmonary stenosis, and (5) aortic stenosis (Moss, 1983).

The three total repair procedures described are all performed through a median sternotomy and are open heart procedures requiring cardiopulmonary bypass or deep hypothermia. Children with TGA require antibiotic prophylaxis for endocarditis for certain procedures and close cardiology follow-up. Without treatment 90 per cent of infants with TGA will die within the first year of life.

Perioperative Nursing Diagnoses for Complete D-Transposition of the Great Arteries

Preoperative

Altered tissue perfusion: systemic hypoxia, *related to oxygenated blood being recirculated through the lungs and unoxygenated blood being circulated through the body*

Defining characteristic: cyanosis, activity intolerance

Postoperative

Potential for injury: physiologic, *related to*

- *the following complications of Mustard or Senning procedures:*
  - *obstruction of the vena cavae*
  - *dysrhythmias*
  - *tricuspid regurgitation*
  - *obstruction of the pulmonary veins*
- *the following complications of the arterial switch procedure:*
  - *coronary artery stenosis*
  - *dysrhythmias*
  - *pulmonary stenosis*
  - *aortic stenosis*

Total Anomalous Pulmonary Venous Connection (Fig. 39-17)

Total anomalous pulmonary venous connection (TAPVC) represents approximately 2 per cent of all congenital heart defects (Moss, 1983). In TAPVC the pulmonary veins do not connect with the left atrium; rather they connect directly to the right atrium or one of the systemic veins. The presence of an ASD is necessary to allow blood to reach the left side of the heart. The four main types of TAPVC are (1) supracardiac (most common) in which the pulmonary veins drain into the superior vena cava through the innominate vein; (2) cardiac, in which the pulmonary veins drain into the coronary sinus or directly into the right atrium; (3) infracardiac, in which the four veins join behind the heart and travel through the diaphragm connecting to the portal venous system; and (4) mixed (Merenstein et al, 1985). Each of these types of anomalous connections can occur with or without obstruction of the pulmonary veins. Approximately 33 per cent of patients with TAPVC have other associated cardiac defects or a congenitally absent spleen.

Pathophysiology

In the presence of TAPVC blood flow depends on where the pulmonary veins connect and the presence or absence of pulmonary venous obstruction. In all varieties of TAPVC, both systemic (unoxygenated) and pulmonary venous (oxygenated) blood is returning ultimately to the right atrium. The only pathway for blood to reach the left atrium, left ventricle, and the body is through an ASD or patent foramen ovale. If there is no pulmonary venous obstruction then blood flow to the lungs is excessive and only mild cyanosis is present. These infants often present with heart failure. If pulmonary venous obstruction is present then blood flow to the lungs is limited and cyanosis is severe. In addition, pulmonary edema usually occurs owing to increased pulmonary venous pressure.

Clinical Manifestations

Infants with TAPVC without pulmonary venous obstruction may not exhibit symptoms until several weeks to months of life. These infants are usually only mildly cyanotic and present with tachypnea, feeding

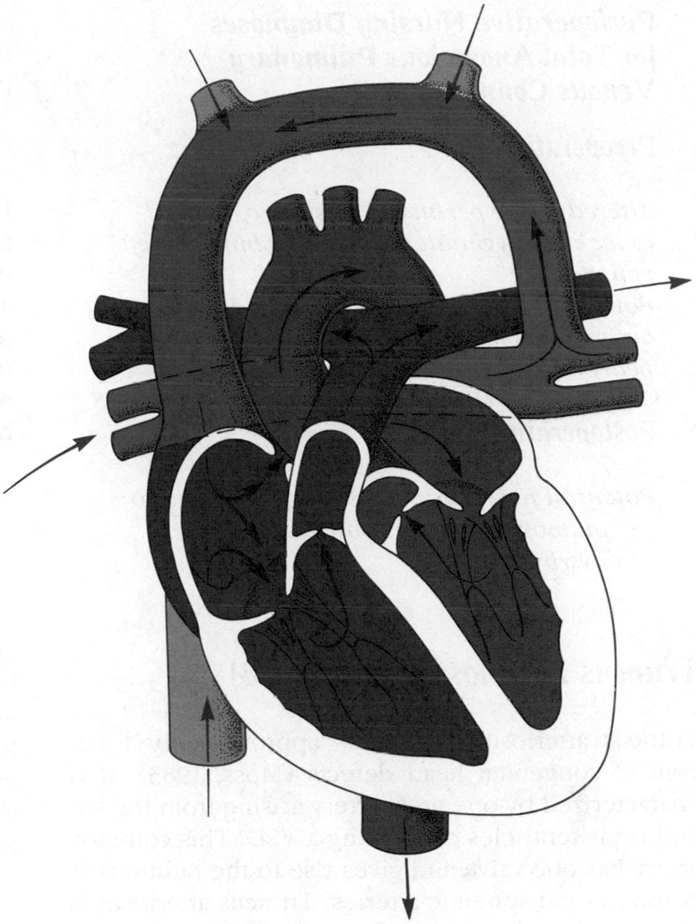

Figure 39-17. Total anomalous pulmonary venous connection (supracardiac, showing pulmonary veins connected to left innominate vein). The presence of an ASD is necessary to allow blood to reach the left side of the heart.

difficulties, failure to thrive, increased respiratory infections, and heart failure. Infants with pulmonary venous obstruction are symptomatic very early, usually at birth. Cyanosis, tachypnea, dyspnea, feeding difficulties, and heart failure are present within the first few days of life.

Diagnostic Assessment

Cardiac Examination. In patients without pulmonary venous obstruction the cardiac examination may be similar to that of a child with ASD including a systolic murmur, wide, fixed splitting of the second heart sound, and a tricuspid diastolic flow murmur. In patients with pulmonary venous obstruction there are usually no murmurs and the pulmonary component of the second heart sound is accentuated.

Electrocardiogram. The ECG may show right ventricular hypertrophy and right atrial enlargement.

Chest Roentgenogram. With pulmonary venous obstruction the heart size is usually normal; however, a pattern of pulmonary edema may be seen. Without pulmonary venous obstruction, heart size and pulmonary vascularity are both increased.

Echocardiogram. A color flow 2-D echocardiogram is helpful in determining the presence and type of TAPVC; however, it is difficult to visualize this cardiac defect on echocardiogram. A single large pulmonary vein can sometimes be seen draining into the superior vena cava or an extra cavity visualized behind the left atrium.

Therapeutic Management

Infants with obstructed pulmonary veins require surgical repair as soon as possible. Infants with unobstructed pulmonary veins may be treated medically for heart failure if necessary before undergoing surgical repair. The surgical repair will depend on the type of TAPVC present. Surgery is performed through a median sternotomy and is an open heart procedure requiring cardiopulmonary bypass or deep hypothermia with circulatory arrest. Supracardiac and infracardiac TAPVC require reimplantation of the pulmonary veins into the left atrium and closure of the ASD. Intracardiac TAPVC is repaired by realigning the atrial septum during closure of the ASD and directing the anomalous veins to the left atrial side.

Complications of surgical repair for all types of TAPVC are pulmonary venous obstruction and dysrhythmias.

Perioperative Nursing Diagnoses for Total Anomalous Pulmonary Venous Connection

Preoperative

Altered tissue perfusion: systemic, related to lack of oxygenated blood reaching the left ventricle
Potential altered cardiac output: decreased: activity intolerance, related to congestive heart failure and hypoxia

Postoperative

Potential for injury: physiologic, related to
- *pulmonary venous obstruction*
- *dysrhythmias*

Truncus Arteriosus (Fig. 39-18)

Truncus arteriosus represents approximately 1 per cent of congenital heart defects (Moss, 1983). It is characterized by one great artery arising from the left and right ventricles over-riding a VSD. This common artery has one valve and gives rise to the pulmonary, coronary, and systemic arteries. Truncus arteriosus is classified into three types depending on the origin of the pulmonary arteries.

Type I—A short, main pulmonary artery arises from the common trunk and divides into the right and left pulmonary arteries
Type II—The right and left pulmonary arteries arise directly from the posterior surface of the common trunk
Type III—The right and left pulmonary arteries arise directly from the lateral walls of the common trunk (Merenstein et al, 1985)

Commonly associated cardiac anomalies include a right aortic arch (30 to 35 per cent), an interrupted aortic arch, absent ductus arteriosus, PDA, ASD, unilateral absence of a pulmonary artery, and truncal valve regurgitation.

Pathophysiology

In the presence of truncus arteriosus the common trunk receives a mixture of unoxygenated blood from the right ventricle and oxygenated blood from the left ventricle. Blood flow to the lungs varies with the type of truncus but is usually increased and at systemic level pressure. When pulmonary blood flow is adequate or increased, minimal cyanosis is present. These infants with increased pulmonary blood flow (at systemic level pressure) are at high risk for developing early pulmonary vascular disease.

Clinical Manifestations

Infants may present in congestive heart failure shortly after birth or between 2 to 3 weeks of age. The presence of congestive heart failure will depend on the amount of pulmonary blood flow. The persistent high pulmonary vascular resistance in the first few weeks of life (see section on changes in circulation at birth) will decrease pulmonary blood flow and congestive heart failure may not be present. However, if the truncal valve is regurgitant then congestive heart failure will be present shortly after birth.

Diagnostic Assessment

Cardiac Examination. The first heart sound is normal. The second heart sound will be single and loud because of the single valve of the common trunk. A systolic ejection click may be heard. There may be a loud systolic murmur heard best at the lower left sternal border and radiating throughout the chest. If the truncal valve is regurgitant a blowing diastolic murmur may be heard.

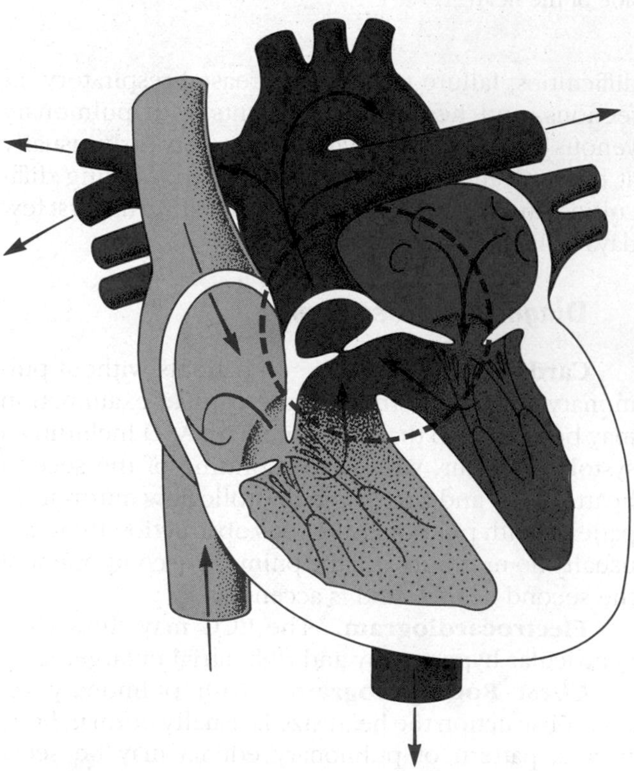

Figure 39-18. Type II truncus arteriosus. Blood flow is from both ventricles into a common great artery that over-rides a VSD.

Electrocardiogram. Combined ventricular hypertrophy and left atrial enlargement are most often seen. Right ventricular hypertrophy alone may be seen with normal or decreased pulmonary blood flow.

Chest Roentgenogram. Increased heart size and increased pulmonary vascularity as well as an absent pulmonary artery segment are typically found.

Echocardiogram. With a color flow 2-D echocardiogram and continuous wave Doppler the truncus arteriosus defect can be visualized and most often the type can be identified as well as the presence of truncal valve stenosis, regurgitation, or both.

Therapeutic Management

Infants with truncus arteriosus are treated medically if possible during the first few months of life. They generally require treatment for congestive heart failure. Surgical repair can either be palliative or a total repair. Palliative surgery consists of placing a band around the pulmonary artery or arteries to decrease pulmonary blood flow until full surgical repair can be performed. This procedure is thought to prevent pulmonary vascular damage until the child is older and can undergo a full repair. Pulmonary artery banding, however, is not always successful in preventing pulmonary vascular disease and can distort the pulmonary arteries. Full surgical repair consists of separating the pulmonary artery or arteries from the common trunk, closing the VSD with a patch (ensuring that the common trunk now arises from the left ventricle), and inserting a right ventricular-to-pulmonary artery valved conduit. The conduit may be of prosthetic material with a porcine valve or may be a homograft conduit. The surgical approach is through a median sternotomy, and full repair is an open heart procedure requiring cardiopulmonary bypass or deep hypothermia with circulatory arrest.

Complications and residual effects include residual VSDs, truncal valve regurgitation, conduit obstruction, and pulmonary vascular disease. These children require antibiotic prophylaxis for endocarditis for certain procedures, and continued follow-up with a cardiologist.

Perioperative Nursing Diagnoses for Truncus Arteriosus

Preoperative

Potential altered cardiac output: decreased: activity intolerance, related to congestive heart failure associated with increased cardiac workload and increased blood flow to the lungs

Potential impaired gas exchange, related to lungs receiving more blood at higher pressure

Postoperative

Potential for injury: physiologic, related to
- ***residual VSDs***
- ***truncal valve regurgitation/obstruction***
- ***conduit obstruction***
- ***pulmonary vascular disease***

Ebstein Anomaly (Fig. 39-19)

Ebstein anomaly represents approximately 0.5 per cent of congenital heart defects (Moss, 1983). It consists of an abnormally low placement of the tricuspid valve, resulting in a portion of the right ventricle being part of the right atrium. The remaining right ventricular cavity is small. Tricuspid regurgitation is present in varying degrees. Commonly associated cardiac defects are ASD (present in greater than 50 per cent), pulmonary stenosis, pulmonary atresia, and VSD. Ebstein anomaly occurs frequently in infants of mothers who have received lithium during their pregnancy.

Pathophysiology

The physiology and clinical manifestations of Ebstein anomaly vary widely depending on the size of the right

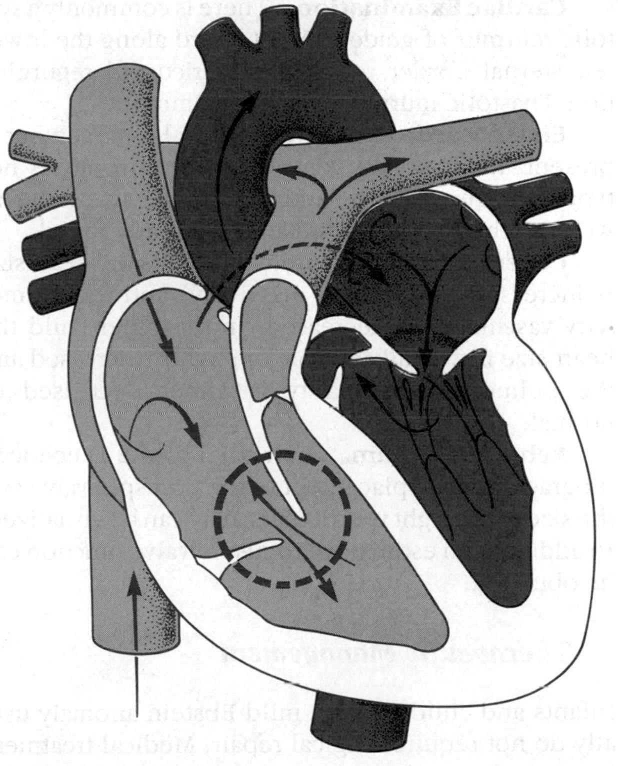

Figure 39-19. Ebstein anomaly with tricuspid valve significantly displaced downward in the right ventricle. Leakage occurs through the tricuspid valve back to the right atrium, and unoxygenated blood is shunted across the ASD into the left atrium.

ventricle and the degree of tricuspid regurgitation. If the tricuspid valve is only minimally displaced downward and mild regurgitation is present, then blood flow approximates normal and symptoms are absent. However, if the tricuspid valve is very displaced and moderate to severe tricuspid regurgitation is present, there is backflow of blood into the right atrium. This backflow of blood elevates right atrial pressure, causing unoxygenated blood to be shunted across the foramen ovale or ASD to the systemic circulation; cyanosis results. In addition, infants or children with Ebstein anomaly commonly have supraventricular tachycardia (25 per cent).

Clinical Manifestations

Infants may be asymptomatic or present with cyanosis, congestive heart failure, or tachycardic episodes, or some combination of these. The older child commonly has dyspnea on exertion, cyanosis, fatigue, and tachycardic episodes. Symptoms of tachycardic episodes include dizzy spells, fatigue, syncope, headaches, chest pain, and a sensation of palpitations or a "racing" heart.

Diagnostic Assessment

Cardiac Examination. There is commonly a systolic murmur of grade I–V/VI heard along the lower left sternal border representing tricuspid regurgitation. Diastolic murmurs are also common.

Electrocardiogram. Right atrial enlargement is present. Right or left ventricular hypertrophy is not typically seen. Wolfe-Parkinson-White syndrome as well as other dysrhythmias are commonly found.

Chest Roentgenogram. In infants the heart size is increased (sometimes massively) and the pulmonary vascularity is decreased. In the older child the heart size is typically normal or slightly increased and the pulmonary vascularity is either decreased or normal.

Echocardiogram. With color flow 2-D echocardiography the displacement of the tricuspid valve and the size of the right ventricular cavity can be visualized. In addition, an estimate of tricuspid valve function can be obtained.

Therapeutic Management

Infants and children with mild Ebstein anomaly usually do not require surgical repair. Medical treatment for supraventricular tachycardia or other dysrhythmias may be the only intervention needed. When surgical repair is indicated for more severe forms of Ebstein anomaly it is usually not performed in infancy. The surgical procedure involves repositioning and repairing the tricuspid valve to improve its competency. Sometimes the tricuspid valve needs to be replaced. In addition, plication (stitching folds or tucks in the wall) of the atrialized right ventricle (the portion of the right ventricle that is part of the right atrium) is performed to eliminate supraventricular tachycardias. The surgical approach is through a median sternotomy. This is an open heart surgery requiring cardiopulmonary bypass.

Antibiotic prophylaxis for certain procedures is necessary in these children to reduce the risk of endocarditis.

Perioperative Nursing Diagnoses for Ebstein Anomaly

Preoperative

Altered tissue perfusion: cerebral, related to tachycardic episodes
Defining characteristics: dizzy spells, fatigue, syncope, headaches

Postoperative

Potential for injury: physiologic, related to the following complications:
- *residual tricuspid regurgitation*
- *persistent dysrhythmias*
- *bacterial endocarditis*

Tricuspid Atresia (Fig. 39-20)

Tricuspid atresia represents approximately 3 per cent of all congenital heart defects (Moss, 1983). The tricuspid valve in this lesion is totally occluded and *no communication* exists between the right atrium and the right ventricle. The right ventricle is usually hypoplastic (small) and an ASD or patent foramen ovale is present. A VSD is also commonly present. The pulmonary arteries may be small or normal in size. Additional cardiac defects are present in 30 per cent of these patients, the most common being transposition of the great arteries, persistent left superior vena cava, coarctation of the aorta, and PDA.

Pathophysiology

In the presence of tricuspid atresia unoxygenated blood returning to the right atrium cannot pass into the right ventricle. It must therefore pass through an ASD or patent foramen ovale into the left atrium and left ventricle. From the left ventricle a portion of the blood flow passes through the VSD, if present, into the small right ventricle and the pulmonary circulation. The remaining blood flow goes to the systemic circulation. If no VSD is present then blood flow to the lungs is solely through the PDA.

Clinical Manifestations

Infants with tricuspid atresia are usually cyanotic at birth. If no VSD is present then the infant is totally dependent on the PDA for pulmonary blood flow. As the PDA closes the infant will become profoundly cyanotic, tachypneic, and acidotic. Infants with a large VSD may have excessive pulmonary blood flow and present in congestive heart failure. This, however, is uncommon. Older infants and children with a moderate-sized VSD and decreased pulmonary blood flow may have hypoxic spells, delayed growth, and clubbing.

Diagnostic Assessment

Cardiac Examination. Murmurs of associated heart defects such as VSD and PDA are usually present.

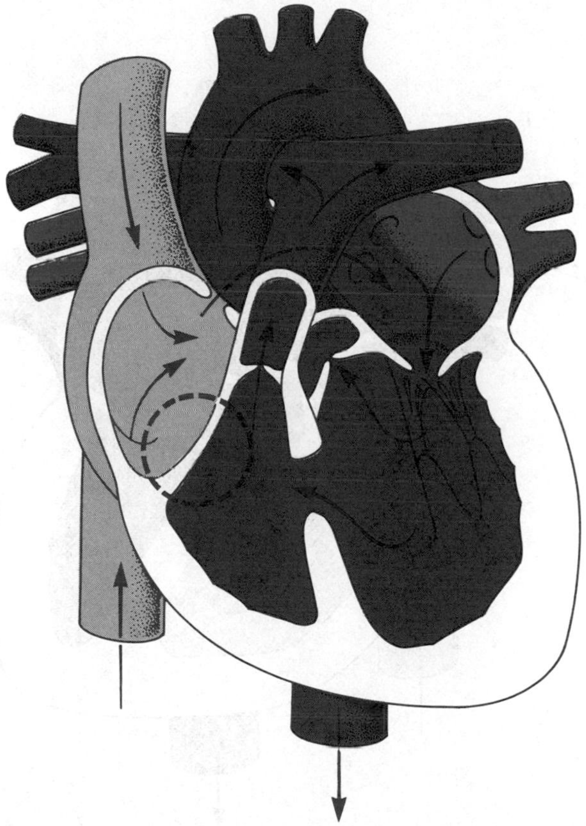

Figure 39-20. Tricuspid atresia, showing no communication between the right heart chambers. Blood is shunted through the ASD to the left atrium and through the VSD to the pulmonary artery.

Electrocardiogram. Right atrial enlargement, decreased or absent right ventricular forces, and left ventricular hypertrophy are typically found.

Chest Roentgenogram. The heart size can be normal or increased. The pulmonary vascularity may be decreased (most common), normal, or increased.

Echocardiogram. The absence of a tricuspid valve, the size of the right ventricle, and the presence of other cardiac defects such as a VSD can be identified with color flow 2-D echocardiography.

Therapeutic Management

Infants who are dependent on the PDA for pulmonary blood flow are given prostaglandin E_1 to maintain patency of the ductus arteriosus until a systemic to pulmonary shunt such as the *Blalock-Taussig shunt* (see previous description) can be performed. Prostaglandin E_1 is administered at dosages of 0.1 to 0.05 μg/kg/hr intravenously; *it must be administered with a continuous infusion pump.* Intermittent delivery of prostaglandin E_1 may allow the PDA to close. The infant must be continually monitored for signs of hypotension, a side effect of prostaglandin E_1. Appropriate agents to support blood pressure, if necessary, should be on hand. Another common side effect of prostaglandin E_1 is decreased respiratory rate and apnea. Intubation and ventilatory support may be needed (Merenstein et al, 1985).

A *balloon atrial septostomy* (see previous description) is commonly performed in the cardiac catheterization laboratory to ensure a large interatrial communication. This is vital to the infant's survival. The right atrium has no outlet other than through the interatrial communication. Infants with a VSD and adequate pulmonary blood flow do not require a systemic to pulmonary shunt.

The total repair for tricuspid atresia involves creation of a communication between the right atrium and the pulmonary artery or the right ventricle by direct anastomosis or a conduit. The ASD and VSD, if present, as well as any previous systemic to pulmonary shunts such as the Blalock-Taussig, are closed. This repair is typically referred to as the *Fontan procedure;* however, there are numerous variations of the procedure. The timing for total repair varies widely among institutions. The surgical approach is through a median sternotomy, an open heart procedure requiring cardiopulmonary bypass. Complications of surgical repair include congestive heart failure, pleural effusions, renal failure, residual VSD, conduit obstruction, and dysrhythmias. Children with tricuspid atresia require lifelong antibiotic prophylaxis for endocarditis for certain procedures.

Perioperative Nursing Diagnoses for Tricuspid Atresia

Preoperative

Impaired gas exchange, related to insufficient amount of blood reaching the lungs, associated with atresia of the tricuspid valve
Potential altered growth and development: *failure to thrive, related to inadequate oxygenation of blood to meet metabolic needs or to congestive heart failure*

Postoperative

Potential for injury: physiologic, related to
- *complications of Blalock-Taussig Procedure (see tetralogy of Fallot)*
- *complications of Fontan procedure:*
  - *congestive heart failure*
  - *pleural effusions; Defining characteristics: if small effusion, asymptomatic; if large accumulation: cough, dyspnea, retractions, tachypnea, cyanosis*
  - *renal failure; Defining characteristics: urine output less than 1 ml/kg/hr, rising BUN and creatinine*
  - *residual VSD*
  - *conduit obstruction*
  - *dysrythmias*

Pulmonary Atresia (Fig. 39-21)

Pulmonary atresia with intact ventricular septum represents approximately 1 per cent of all congenital heart defects (Moss, 1983). With this lesion there is *complete occlusion* of the pulmonary valve and usually a small right ventricle, though the right ventricle can be of normal size. A patent foramen ovale or an ASD is always present. The PDA varies in size and determines the amount of pulmonary blood flow.

Pathophysiology

The blood flow in the presence of pulmonary atresia is similar to that of tricuspid atresia. Unoxygenated blood returning to the right atrium bypasses the right ventricle, flowing through the interatrial communication to the left atrium and left ventricle. Some blood may enter the right ventricle through the tricuspid valve; however, as no outlet exists to the right ventricle, the blood then flows back through the tricuspid valve into the right atrium. The only pathway through which blood can reach the lungs is the PDA.

Clinical Manifestations

These infants become cyanotic and tachypneic shortly after birth. The degree of cyanosis depends on the amount of pulmonary blood flow through the PDA.

Diagnostic Assessment

Cardiac Examination. The second heart sound is single because the pulmonary valve closure component is absent. There may be systolic murmurs of either the PDA or tricuspid regurgitation.

Electrocardiogram. Right atrial enlargement is present, and typically left ventricular hypertrophy is found. However, infants with normal-sized right ventricles may demonstrate right ventricular hypertrophy.

Chest Roentgenogram. The chest roentgenogram may be normal or show an increased heart size and decreased pulmonary vascularity.

Echocardiogram. Color flow 2-D echocardiography can demonstrate the atretic pulmonary valve, the size of the main and branch pulmonary arteries, the size of the right ventricle, and the size of the ASD or foramen ovale.

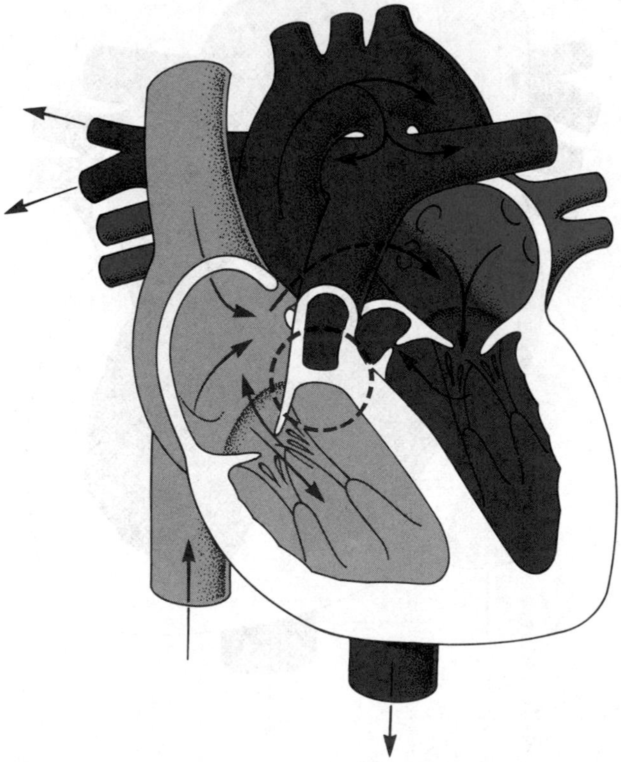

Figure 39-21. Pulmonary atresia with small right ventricle, ASD, and patent ductus arteriosus. Abnormal blood flow is from the right chambers through the ASD to the left side of the heart. Blood can reach the lungs only through a patent ductus arteriosus.

Therapeutic Management

These infants will be cyanotic shortly after birth and if the PDA closes they will become profoundly hypoxemic with severe cyanosis and acidosis progressing to death if no intervention is made. Prostaglandin E_1 infusions are used to maintain patency of the ductus arteriosus until a systemic to pulmonary shunt (most commonly the Blalock-Taussig shunt) can be performed. In addition a balloon atrial septostomy is performed in the cardiac catheterization laboratory to enlarge the interatrial communication from right to left atrium.

If the right ventricle is of adequate size some institutions perform a pulmonary valvulotomy or a pulmonary outflow patch procedure in addition to a shunt. This establishes an open pathway through the atretic valve area between the pulmonary artery and the right ventricle. Blood flow through the right ventricle and pulmonary artery will then promote growth of these areas.

Total repair of pulmonary atresia involves closure of any previous systemic to pulmonary shunts, closure of the ASD, and creation of a communication between the right atrium and the pulmonary artery or the right ventricle. As mentioned earlier, this is accomplished through a direct anastomosis or a conduit and is called the Fontan procedure. The timing of total repair varies among institutions. Complications of surgery include congestive heart failure, pleural effusions, renal or liver failure, conduit obstruction, and dysrhythmias. The Fontan procedure, performed through a median sternotomy, is an open heart procedure requiring cardiopulmonary bypass.

Life-long antibiotic prophylaxis for endocarditis when undergoing certain procedures is required by these children, as well as long-term follow-up by a cardiologist.

Perioperative Nursing Diagnoses for Pulmonary Atresia

Preoperative

Impaired gas exchange, related to the inability to pump an adequate amount of blood to the lungs, associated with obstruction of the pulmonary artery

Postoperative

Potential for injury: physiologic, related to

- *complications of Blalock-Taussig procedure (see tetralogy of Fallot)*
- *complications of Fontan procedure (see tricuspid atresia)*
- *bacterial endocarditis (with both procedures); Defining characteristics: fever, bacteremia*

Hypoplastic Left Heart Syndrome

Hypoplastic left heart syndrome (HLHS) represents approximately 7 to 9 per cent of all congenital heart defects (Moss, 1983). It is characterized by a range of left-sided heart defects including severe coarctation of the aorta, severe aortic valve stenosis or atresia, and severe mitral valve stenosis or atresia. The left ventricle and ascending aorta are usually small or hypoplastic. Blood flow to the coronary arteries is usually retrograde (having a backward flow) from the PDA.

Pathophysiology

Typically the small left ventricle is unable to sustain adequate cardiac output to the systemic circulation. In the presence of aortic or mitral atresia, or both, the only blood flow to the systemic circulation is through the PDA.

Clinical Manifestations

These infants may be cyanotic or have severe pallor and grayish skin. They may present in a state of vascular collapse with tachypnea, dyspnea, decreased blood pressures in all extremities, grunting, nasal flaring, and hypothermia. Heart failure is almost always present.

Diagnostic Assessment

Cardiac Examination. The second heart sound is single owing to the absence of the aortic valve closure component. A soft systolic ejection murmur is heard in most infants.

Electrocardiogram. Right atrial enlargement and right ventricular hypertrophy are usually present.

Chest Roentgenogram. The heart size is increased, and increased pulmonary vascularity as well as pulmonary edema are seen.

Echocardiogram. With 2-D echocardiography the size of the left ventricle, presence or absence of the aortic and mitral valves, and sizes of the ascending aorta, right ventricle, right atrium, and pulmonary artery can be visualized.

Therapeutic Management

Without surgical intervention approximately 95 per cent of these infants will die within the first month of life (Moss, 1983). However, the surgical repairs currently available are palliative procedures that have had very limited success. HLHS is a lethal heart defect that is considered by many institutions to be inoperable. Recently cardiac transplantation has been performed in some infants with HLHS. Cardiac transplantation in infants, however, is considered an experimental procedure.

The families of these infants require maximum support when taking their infants home to die. Public health nurses and community hospice programs can provide the family with daily support (if necessary) and long-term counseling. The infant may survive at home as long as several months. The family attempting to cope with this situation will be under enormous stress. Not all families are able to deal with the stress of having their infant at home. The family should always be given the option of hospitalization or of placing the infant in an alternative treatment facility. Regardless of whether the infant is in the home or at a treatment facility, the family will require ongoing support and help with the grieving process. After the death of the infant it is particularly important that the support be continued for as long as the family needs it.

Nursing Diagnoses for Hypoplastic Left Heart Syndrome

Altered cardiac output: decreased: pronounced activity intolerance, related to ineffective left ventricle

Defining characteristics: tachypnea, dyspnea, decreased blood pressure in all extremities, grunting, nasal flaring, hypothermia

Cardiac Surgery: Perioperative Nursing Strategies

Preoperative Preparation

Parents should start preparing their children for surgery approximately 3 to 5 days before coming to the hospital (older children may need a longer preparation period). Chapter 31 provides guidelines on preparation for hospitalization.

The child is usually admitted 1 to 2 days before surgery for physical and psychologic preparation. Physical preparation includes a complete history, thorough physical examination, laboratory studies (complete blood count, platelet count, hemoglobin, hematocrit, determination of clotting times, electrolyte levels, blood urea nitrogen, creatinine, calcium, type and cross match for 2 to 5 units of blood, and urinalysis), chest radiograph, ECG, echocardiogram, and results of a recent cardiac catheterization. The child will usually be kept NPO after midnight the evening before surgery; the time for fasting will be determined by the age and the scheduled time for surgery. It is important to post a sign on the door to the child's room and on the crib so that nothing is given by mouth before surgery. Preoperative medications vary considerably among institutions.

In the case of an older child, psychologic preparation for surgery must include both the parents and the child. It is ideal if the parents and the child can visit the hospital and the intensive care unit (ICU) before the operation to meet the nurses who will be caring for the child and to become more familiar with the environment. At this time a description of the equipment used postoperatively will be helpful. In some hospitals the nurses in the ICU visit the patients and their parents the evening before surgery to explain the care the patient will receive while in the unit.

It is most important that parents be prepared for the appearance of their child postoperatively because all the tubes and equipment can be frightening. It is helpful to use some type of visual aid (Fig. 39-22) such as a doll or a diagram to explain the purpose of the equipment, tubes, and nursing interventions. Parents also need reassurance that the nurses will be watching the infant or child closely and that medication will be given for pain. When teaching parents it is necessary to proceed slowly and discuss one aspect of care at a time. Parents should be told specifically how their child will appear postoperatively and forewarned that he or she will be asleep or heavily sedated for a period of time. Specific things to tell parents preoperatively and to review again immediately after the child enters the ICU follow:

1. An endotracheal tube is placed into the throat to aid the child's breathing. (An infant is unable to cry and an older child unable to talk while this tube is in place.)
2. A nasogastric tube is placed through the nose into the stomach to keep the stomach empty and free of air until digestive function is restored.
3. Three or four intravenous lines may be present to replace fluids and blood and to provide a means of checking pressures within the heart.
4. A dressing or tape (Steri-strips) or metal staples are placed across the incision.
5. Two or more chest tubes, one on either side of the chest, are required to remove air and blood that enters the chest during surgery.
6. A small plastic bag may be applied to the perineum to collect urine or a small tube may be placed into the bladder to drain the urine.
7. Disks with wires (cardiac leads) are put on the

child's chest to monitor the heart rate and observe the pattern of how the heart beats.

8. The nurse will be checking the status of the child at least every 15 minutes until his or her condition stabilizes.

Intraoperative Nursing Care

Open heart surgery is an extremely invasive procedure that requires opening the thoracic cavity and using an extracorporeal cardiopulmonary bypass machine (heart-lung machine). The most common approaches to opening the chest are the median sternotomy and the lateral thoracotomy. Open heart surgery is usually very lengthy. Following the cardiac repair the infant is taken either directly to the intensive care unit or to the recovery room. Immediate postoperative care through the first 24 to 72 hours will be in the recovery room or intensive care unit, or both. When the child returns to the general ward he or she will no longer require the acute care necessary in the immediate postoperative period. Constant observation by the nursing staff is done to monitor the child's vital functions, circulatory status, respiratory status, level of consciousness, and fluid and electrolyte balance.

Nursing Care in the Immediate Postoperative Period

On return from cardiac surgery the child will be admitted to a specialty unit. Nursing care during this period is highly specialized and requires additional training. This section provides an overview of care in the immediate postoperative period.

The child will be heavily sedated following surgery, and the level of consciousness should be noted frequently during the first 24 hours postoperatively. The infant will usually be without clothing for maximum observation and may be placed on a radiant heated table or Aqua K pad to maintain the body temperature. If hypothermia has been used during cardiac surgery (to reduce oxygen needs) the child's temperature may be unstable for a period of time. Vital signs should be checked every 15 minutes until they are stable. Signs of distress such as tachycardia, tachypnea, retractions, stridor, nasal flaring, expiratory wheezing, and grunting should be reported to the physician. The infant's skin should be observed for color, temperature, and diaphoresis. Cyanosis may be circumoral or circumorbital. The mucous membranes and tongue should always be checked for central cyanosis.

A monitor is attached to the infant to note the rate and rhythm of the heart. The central venous pressure (CVP) is monitored via a right atrial catheter, in order to measure cardiac output. Pacemaker leads may be left in place in case arrhythmias develop in the postoperative period. An intra-arterial line is placed to monitor blood pressure. This should be compared with the manual blood pressure reading obtained by cuff at the extremity.

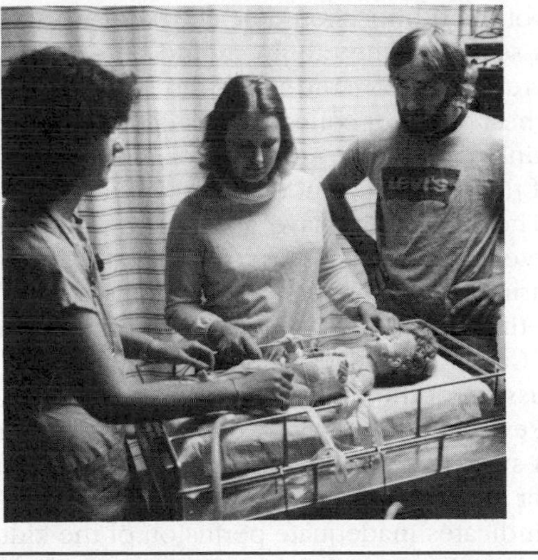

Figure 39-22. Preoperatively, a doll can be used to prepare parents for the appearance of their baby after the operation. This gives parents an opportunity to discuss their fears and concerns about the numerous machines and tubes.

To maintain a patent airway, an endotracheal tube will be in place. Percussion of the chest and application of suction via the endotracheal tube should be done every hour, or more often if necessary. If no endotracheal tube is in place, stimulation of a cough can be achieved by placing a suction catheter to the back of the pharynx. Suction return, amount, color, and mucous plugs should be noted and recorded. Oxygen concentration should be carefully assessed by use of an analyzer to ensure delivery as ordered. The infant may require the assistance of a respirator to maintain ventilation.

The nasogastric tube in the stomach is usually placed on straight drainage to keep the stomach decompressed; suction is usually not necessary. Normally the nasogastric tube is not irrigated; if plugged, the tube is replaced.

A dressing is in place over the chest incision. The incision site should be checked every 15 minutes during the first 24 hours for bleeding or hematoma formation. Two to three chest tubes are placed for drainage of fluid and air that entered the thoracic cavity during surgery. The chest tubes should be checked frequently for patency and should be stripped (milked) every hour.* The connections of the chest tube and every

* The policy regarding chest tube stripping varies among institutions.

inch of the tubing should be checked and all connections secured. The tubing should be carefully examined regularly from the site of insertion in the chest to the chest bottle or collection system to ensure that it is not kinked under the infant. Color, amount, and viscosity of the drainage is noted every hour.

The infant will have a urine bag on or a Foley catheter in place. Amount, color, and specific gravity of the urine is noted hourly. If the infant is not catheterized, the bladder may need to be emptied by massage (the Credé maneuver). (See Chapter 46 for further discussion of the Credé maneuver.)

Renal function may be depressed following open heart surgery. The expected urinary output for an infant or child is 0.5 to 1.0 ml/kg/hr. An output less than this indicates inadequate perfusion of the kidneys.

Accurate intake and output must be monitored every hour. Intravenous solutions and possibly blood will be given to make up for the blood lost during surgery. The hourly output includes chest tube drainage, urine, stool, nasogastric drainage, blood drawn, and drainage from the dressing. Usually the child will have an analgesic ordered for pain and prophylactic antibiotics. The child's weight is checked daily and a daily chest roentgenograph and ECG are done. Usually infants will be given nothing by mouth until they are alert, no longer require assisted ventilation, and bowel sounds are active. These children require good oral hygiene at least every 4 hours with either sponge-tipped applicators or lemon-glycerine swabs.

Ideally parents are allowed to visit frequently during the child's stay in the intensive care unit. The nurse can help parents express their feelings and can provide a supportive environment during this stressful period. Keeping the parents informed regarding how their child is doing and explaining the care helps to alleviate fears and gives parents some measure of control through better understanding (Fig. 39-23). One nurse on each shift should be assigned to the patient and family to provide for continuity of care. The primary nurse can facilitate a supportive climate by taking time to sit with and talk to the parents to assess their needs and concerns about their child. This assessment needs to be done daily to promote and maintain a healthy family environment.

Nursing Care Following Transfer from the Intensive Care Unit

After 2 to 3 days in the ICU, children return to the unit where they were before surgery. Children are hospitalized for an additional 5 to 7 days, during which normal daily activities are gradually resumed. Usually infants and toddlers resume activity on their own, whereas older children may need some encouragement. Fluids and foods are introduced gradually; occasionally fluid restriction may be necessary to prevent overloading of the cardiovascular system; however, fluid restriction is rarely used. The intake and output are carefully monitored and daily weight recorded. Accuracy in these nursing functions is crucial.

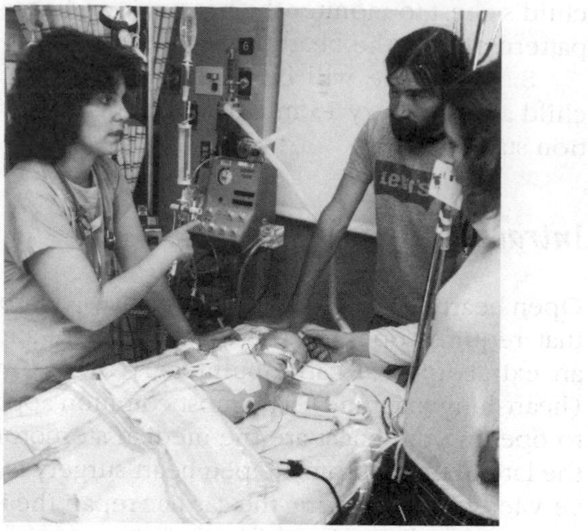

Figure 39-23. Keeping the parents informed of how their child is doing after the operation and explaining the care help to create confidence in the nursing staff.

Respiratory status continues to be watched closely and percussion and postural drainage is done every 4 hours while indicated. Nasopharyngeal suctioning may be done after postural drainage to remove secretions and to stimulate coughing. It is important for these children to cough and breathe deeply to aerate all lobes of their lungs fully.

For infants or toddlers who have had a thoracotomy, ***it is important not to pick them up under the arms*** because this puts stress on the suture line and may be painful. Nurses should put their arms under the children's shoulders and buttocks and lift them in this manner.

The incision should be carefully inspected for infection; integrity of the suture line should be ascertained, and redness, swelling, heat, tenderness, and presence of drainage should be assessed.

Medications ordered during the postoperative period may include digoxin, a diuretic, and an antibiotic. ***Before administering digoxin the apical pulse must be taken for 1 full minute. If the apical pulse is below 100 beats per minute in an infant, digoxin is usually withheld until the physician is notified.*** Digoxin strengthens the force of the heartbeat but also slows the rate.

Before discharge the parents should be given a written list of warning signs that will alert them to cardiac difficulty. This list should include the signs of problems specifically related to their child's cardiac defect and surgical repair. An example would be a list of signs of congestive heart failure for a child after repair of an AV canal: labored or rapid breathing, feeding difficulties, perspiration, swelling around the eyes, and irritability.

Parents should be taught wound care, cleaning any open areas with half-strength hydrogen peroxide and avoiding showers and baths until the wound is completely closed. *Parents should be cautioned to notify the physician should the child develop a fever, redness, or swelling around the incision; separation of the incision; or drainage from the incision.* Parents should demonstrate proficiency in giving medications before the child leaves the hospital. A list of medications, dosages, and a time schedule for administration, as well as a list of side effects, should be provided. Any activity restrictions should also be discussed before discharge.

The parents should be given a phone number to call for assistance, should any problems arise. A referral to a community health nurse is essential and provides the added support a family needs at such a stressful time. These infants require close follow-up and are usually seen for a return visit at the cardiology clinic or their private physician's office 2 weeks after discharge.

Nursing Strategies for Long-Term Care

The majority of children with congenital heart disease (CHD) will be able to lead normal lives. It is important that parents and family members see the child as a productive member of the family with individual strengths and weaknesses like every other member of the family. If the child with CHD is seen as a severely limited, handicapped child, then that is the self-image the child will have. Many families, because of their anxiety about CHD, overemphasize the cardiac condition and any limitations their child may have. They may even impose unwarranted limitations. These children may become very anxious about their cardiac condition and fearful of attempting physical activities, new experiences, and so forth. They may become very dependent and unfortunately may fail to develop to their fullest potential socially, physically, and emotionally. Parents should be encouraged to emphasize the positive. They should emphasize what the child *can* rather than cannot do.

At developmental stages throughout life individuals need to feel a sense of accomplishment and control over their environment. Helping their child with CHD progress through developmental stages successfully offers special challenges for parents. Adolescents, for example, must complete developmental tasks such as (1) accepting one's body, (2) expanding peer relationships to include both sexes, (3) gaining emotional independence from family members, (4) achieving economic independence, (5) selecting and preparing for a vocation, and (6) becoming socially responsible. The adolescent with CHD can accomplish these tasks with family support and guidance and a healthy perspective. Adolescents who are fearful of their cardiac condition, who feel different from their peers, and who feel inadequate to complete tasks or goals will be unable to achieve these developmental tasks. Acceptance of one's body and gaining emotional independence from family members are particularly difficult for these adolescents.

To foster a positive self-image and a sense of accomplishment, parents need to identify and emphasize what is uniquely special about their child. What talents and special skills does the child possess which can be developed further? If the child with CHD must be limited in exercise (uncommon) the family should emphasize another area of achievement. For many families, however, competitive sports and athletic activity are a priority. These families may have difficulty accepting and reacting in a positive manner to their child's physical limitations. These families in particular need special counseling regarding the influence they will have on their child's self-perception.

Exercise

Most children with CHD are not restricted in exercise. Rather they are usually allowed to self-limit, stopping when they are fatigued. Parents need to recognize early if their child will have a limited ability to tolerate strenuous physical activity. The child should then be encouraged to exercise as much as possible but not to be involved in competitive athletics. On the other hand children who have no limitations to physical activity should not be restricted because of their parents' anxiety about the cardiac condition. Parents need the guidance of the cardiologist in making decisions about their child's exercise. The cardiologist should provide specific exercise parameters for the family and child. Commonly when the child reaches school age an exercise stress test is performed to determine the child's exercise capabilities and physiologic response (such as ECG and blood pressure response) to exercise. Exercise stress tests have been very beneficial in identifying specific safe exercise parameters for these children. In addition, both the child and parents usually gain reassurance from the stress test and feel more comfortable regarding exercise.

School Environment

The school nurse is in a unique position to help the child with CHD in the school environment. The nurse should obtain information about the child's cardiac condition, any medications being given, and what the child's specific exercise parameters are. The nurse can then provide an optimum environment for the child by educating the teachers and others interacting with the child regarding his or her specific needs. Many teachers either "overprotect" or "overexert" these children owing to fears or misconceptions about CHD. The nurse, as the child's advocate in the school environment, can do much to influence how the child is treated.

For example, the child who is unable to participate in normal physical education classes should not view this as a "punishment." Taking an alternative class, acting as a teacher's assistant, or performing some enjoyable task should be offered in place of the physical education class. The child needs to see it as a positive experience. Open communication among parents, the cardiologist, and the school is important in providing an optimum home and school life for the child.

Occasionally children with CHD have additional needs that require special planning on the part of the school nurse. Two circumstances that would require additional planning would be (1) if the child had a pacemaker and (2) if the child were receiving anticoagulant therapy for a prosthetic valve.

Pacemakers. The child with a pacemaker may be totally pacemaker dependent or may need the pacemaker only as a backup in case of dysrhythmias. The location of the pulse generator (pacemaker battery pack) may be subxyphoid (most common in young children), abdominal, or in the right or left upper thorax. The pacemaker function is checked generally once a month by the cardiologist. This is done usually over the telephone (transtelephonic) from the child's home or school. The child will have a transmitter which is placed directly over the chest or connected by electrodes to the fingers. The cardiology office or pacemaker clinic is then telephoned and the mouthpiece of the telephone is placed over the transmitter. The receiver in the cardiology office or pacemaker clinic will print out an ECG and a digital readout of pacemaker parameters. In this way the cardiologist can monitor pacemaker function, and determine when reprogramming is necessary and when battery life is depleted. The school nurse may be called on to perform these pacemaker checks. *Precautions* for the child with a pacemaker in school include avoidance of hard blows to the chest, participation in contact sports such as football, jumping on trampolines or from heights (such as from trees or fences), or exposure to ungrounded electrical current and strong electromagnetic or radio waves (e.g., visiting a radio station). All of these activities or circumstances may cause damage to the pacemaker lead wires. Electrical current, strong magnets, and strong radio waves may actually change the pacemaker program and function. Vigorous physical activity is not contraindicated; it is the type of activity that is important. Swimming, running, bicycle riding, and baseball are all generally permitted because they do not involve extensive hard body contact or vigorous up-and-down jarring motion. More specific exercise parameters can be obtained from the cardiologist.

Signs and symptoms of pacemaker malfunction include dizziness, fatigue, pallor, syncope, and a pulse rate below the pacemaker's minimum heart rate setting. If pacemaker malfunction is suspected the child's pulse should be taken immediately and the physician notified.

A multitude of types of pacemakers are used today. The type of pacemaker a child will have depends on the underlying cardiac condition and reason for pacing. A ventricular demand (VVI) pacemaker was the standard pacemaker used most often in the past. With this pacemaker one (unipolar) or two (bipolar) lead wires are attached to the ventricle and deliver an electrical impulse to stimulate a heart beat if an intrinsic (the child's own) heart beat is not sensed. The heart rate is "fixed," in that the rate at which the pacemaker is set will be the child's heart rate unless the child's intrinsic heart rate is higher. Heart rate will not vary with exercise unless the child can increase his or her intrinsic heart rate.

A second type of pacemaker is the physiologic or atrial synchronous pacemaker. There are many varieties of this pacemaker; in general, it has atrial and ventricular lead wires that sense atrial and ventricular activity. If no atrial activity occurs an atrial beat is stimulated, followed by stimulation of a ventricular beat if no ventricular activity is sensed. The advantage to this type of pacing is the synchrony between atrial and ventricular contractions, allowing the ventricles time to fill. This type of pacing most closely simulates normal cardiac conduction and function.

A third type of pacemaker is the Activitrax, which is basically a ventricular pacemaker. It paces only the ventricle but at a variable, not a "fixed," rate. This pacemaker has the ability to sense large muscle activity and to increase the child's heart rate according to his or her activity. Therefore, depending upon how it is programmed the pacemaker will increase the heart rate when children are running and slow it down when they are resting. This rate-responsive pacemaker has improved exercise capacity for many children.

Anticoagulant Therapy. It is sometimes necessary to replace natural valves with prosthetic ones. Valves that are totally incompetent and cannot be repaired allow blood to regurgitate into the chamber from which it has come. Prosthetic valves come in various sizes and models. Perhaps the most often used is the St. Jude valve, which is made of carbonized steel. The child with a prosthetic metal valve should be educated with regard to lifestyle.

Children with prosthetic valves will be maintained on anticoagulants and require special precautions in the school and home environments. A list of instructions, signs and symptoms of bleeding, and emergency treatments should be provided the school and the family. Serum levels of anticoagulants such as Coumadin (warfarin) are significantly affected by the child's nutritional status and activity level. Wide swings in anticoagulant levels will occur, producing overcoagulation or undercoagulation if the child lacks a consistent, well-balanced dietary intake and consistent levels of activity. Vomiting, diarrhea, febrile illnesses, and medications also significantly affect anticoagulation levels.

Children receiving anticoagulants should refrain from taking any other medications without first checking with their cardiologist. In addition, loss of appetite, decreased exercise, and illnesses should be reported immediately, so that appropriate adjustments in anticoagulation therapy can be made.

Children receiving anticoagulant therapy should not bleed excessively from minor cuts and scrapes. Parents should be taught to hold pressure over the cut or scrape until the bleeding has stopped. The child may bleed longer than normal but the blood should clot. Frequent nosebleeds, blood in the urine or stool, excessive bruising, bleeding from an injury, or significant trauma such as hard blows to the chest or abdomen should be reported to the physician. Each child should wear a medical identification bracelet stating that he or she is on anticoagulants (blood thinners). If the child is in a car accident or suffers other physical trauma, an examination for internal bleeding by a physician is necessary. Signs of external bleeding may be absent, even when there are significant internal injuries. Safe, effective management of these children, which allows them the maximum of independence and activity, requires close cooperation and communication among parents, school personnel, and physician.

Congestive Heart Failure

Etiology

In the majority of cases congestive heart failure (CHF) is the result of a surgically correctable structural abnormality of the heart. CHF can also be caused by arrhythmias, anemia, myocardial disease (e.g., myocarditis), sepsis, or hypertension.

Pathophysiology and Clinical Manifestations

CHF is a clinical syndrome that reflects the inability of the heart to meet the metabolic needs of the body. *The following clinical manifestations of CHF therefore reflect the decreased cardiac output and decreased perfusion to various organ systems* (Merenstein et al, 1985).

Cardiac Enlargement. The heart will dilate or hypertrophy, or both, in the presence of a volume overload, pressure overload, cardiomyopathy, or dysrhythmias. Cardiac enlargement can be identified on chest roentgenogram.

Tachycardia. Tachycardia is a compensatory mechanism for increasing cardiac output and providing increased oxygen delivery to the tissues. Cardiac output can be enhanced through two mechanisms—increasing heart rate or increasing stroke volume (**CO = HR × SV**). Infants have very little ability to increase stroke volume, so they increase heart rate. The older child with a dilated heart from CHF also has limited ability to increase stroke volume and will become tachycardic.

Tachypnea. Inefficient emptying or overloading of the pulmonary system results in interstitial pulmonary edema. Tachypnea is the first clinical manifestation of pulmonary edema; however, as pulmonary edema progresses, alveolar and bronchiolar edema occur, resulting in intercostal retractions, grunting, nasal flaring, dyspnea, rales, cough, and possibly cyanosis.

Gallop Rhythm. A gallop rhythm is an abnormal filling sound heard as a triple heart sound on auscultation. It is related to dilatation of the ventricles.

Decreased Urine Output and Edema. Decreased perfusion to the kidneys results in decreased glomerular filtration. This is interpreted by the body as a decrease in intravascular volume so compensatory mechanisms such as vasoconstriction and fluid and sodium retention are initiated. Infants normally manifest this as weight gain or puffy eyelids. Edema of the face, hands, and feet can occur in the older child.

Decreased Peripheral Pulses and Mottling of the Extremities. Poor cardiac output results in a compensatory redistribution of blood flow to vital tissues. The resulting decreased peripheral tissue perfusion causes mottling of the skin, a grayish or pale skin color, and decreased pulses.

Sweating. Sweating represents an increased metabolic rate with CHF and probably increased activity of the autonomic nervous system. The increased metabolic rate is in response to the increased workload of the heart in failure.

Hepatomegaly. Hepatomegaly represents hepatic congestion due to elevated central venous pressure (CVP). In older children with an elevated CVP neck vein distention can also be seen. The right ventricle in CHF is less compliant and may not adequately empty, leading to elevated pressures in the right atrium, central venous system, and hepatic system.

Failure to Thrive and Feeding Difficulties. Failure to thrive and feeding difficulties result from multiple factors. Respiratory difficulties compromise the infant's ability to feed. The basal metabolic rate increases in infants with CHF, requiring a higher caloric intake (150 calories per kilogram per day or more). The infant must expend more energy to consume the calories but lacks the energy reserve to do so. In addition, the decreased tissue perfusion may curtail the infant's ability to grow. All of these factors lead to failure to thrive.

Decreased Exercise Tolerance. Infants may sleep a majority of the time; fall asleep during feedings; and be delayed in motor activities such as turning over, crawling, and sitting. The older child may show fatigue and decreased exercise tolerance owing to the decreased perfusion to peripheral tissues and the energy required by the heart in failure.

Diagnostic Assessment

Diagnosis of CHF will include pertinent findings from the history and physical examination, chest roentgenograms, an ECG, and results of arterial blood gases and electrolytes. In addition, echocardiography and radionuclide studies may be used to assess ventricular function (Gersony, 1987).

Therapeutic Management

Medical management of CHF takes into account the underlying cause. Since in the majority of cases the cause is a surgically treatable congenital anomaly, medical management comes into play before surgery and is often continued during the postoperative recovery period (Kaplan, 1986). The major goals of medical treatment are improvement of myocardial function (most often through the use of digitalis and diuretics) and the supply and conservation of energy (through nutritional support and prescribed rest).

Major Nursing Diagnoses in Congestive Heart Failure

Altered cardiac output: decreased, *related to the heart's inability to pump an adequate supply of blood to meet the body's metabolic oxygen needs*

Altered tissue perfusion: systemic, *related to decreased cardiac output*

Altered nutrition: less than body requirements, *related to*

- *anorexia associated with decreased perfusion of the gastrointestinal tract, medication side effects, or both*
- *decreased energy available for sucking/chewing*
- *increased metabolic demands associated with the increased workload of the incompetent heart*

Potential for infection: respiratory, *related to*

- *decreased immune competence associated with the stress of inadequate cardiac function*
- *compromised pulmonary function related to inefficient emptying or overloading of the pulmonary vasculature*

Altered growth and development, *associated with*

- *inadequate tissue perfusion to promote healthy tissue growth*
- *lack of energy to accomplish developmental tasks*

Strategies for Nursing Care*

The family of an infant or child in CHF needs detailed teaching and emotional support from the nurse. Explanation of the term *congestive heart failure* should be given early, as it is a frightening term for parents. The words "heart failure" often give rise to thoughts of a heart on the brink of stopping (American Heart Association, 1983). It is important that parents understand that stating a child is in heart failure does not imply that the child's heart is ready to stop. To decrease the family's anxiety, it is helpful to explain heart failure as any situation in which the heart shows signs of being unable to pump enough blood to meet all the needs of the body. Children in CHF have many specific needs requiring carefully structured nursing interventions. Table 39-5, Nursing Process Plan: The Child with Congestive Heart Failure, details additional nursing diagnoses and nursing strategies related to the emotional impact of CHF on the child and family.

Text continues on page 1328

* The section on nursing strategies for the child with CHF is adapted from Shor, 1980.

Table 39-5
Nursing Process Plan: The Child with Congestive Heart Failure

By Roxie Foster

Assessment of Physical Function

Activity/Exercise: Cardiac Output/Tissue Perfusion

Subjective Assessment

Self-report from child: presence of increased fatigue, rapid heart beat, shortness of breath, how well exercise tolerated, presence of edema. Parental report for infant or young child: feeding and sleep patterns, whether sweating with feeding or while sleeping, respiration patterns, how well exercise tolerated (i.e., feeding, crying)

Objective Assessment

Heart rate, respiratory rate; presence of adventitious heart sounds; peripheral pulses; skin color and temperature at rest and with activity; diaphoresis, presence of edema, neck vein distention; urine output; daily weight; placement on growth chart; developmental accomplishments; heart size, liver size

Analysis: Nursing Diagnosis 1

***Altered cardiac output: decreased,** related to the heart's inability to pump an adequate supply of blood to meet the body's metabolic needs*

Nursing Diagnosis 2

***Altered tissue perfusion: systemic,** related to decreased cardiac output*

Defining Characteristics for Nursing Diagnoses 1 and 2

Subjective: Self-report of lightheadedness, rapid heart rate, shortness of breath, fatigue with or without exercise. Parental report of infant's inability to take an adequate amount per feeding, falling asleep at feedings and spending little time awake, seeming short of breath with feeding and at rest, sweating with feedings and at rest, becoming pale, having a weak cry, not yet accomplishing developmental tasks expected for age, poor weight gain

Objective: Tachycardia, tachypnea; gallop rhythm, decreased cardiac output, decreased peripheral pulses; skin color pale and cool to touch, becoming mottled with increased oxygen demands (e.g., crying, feeding, playing); periorbital edema and edema of face, hands and feet; neck vein distention (in older child); urine output <1 ml/kg/hr; failure to thrive: $<$3rd percentile for height and weight on growth chart; cardiomegaly, hepatomegaly

Client Goal/ Evaluation Criteria	Nursing Goals/Strategies (Selected Rationale)
1/2. The client will balance energy demands with the cardiac output and the heart's ability to perfuse the tissues, as evidenced by: a. pulse and respirations within normal range for age	*Decrease unnecessary energy expenditure.* • Provide feeding, dry diapers, and tactile stimulation before infant cries. • Use a pacifier while preparing feedings, or during fussy times (crying increases energy expenditure). • Feed the infant frequently and in small amounts (large feedings tire the infant). • Allow frequent rest periods during feeding.

Continued

Client Goal/ Evaluation Criteria	Nursing Goals/Strategies (Selected Rationale)
b. peripheral pulses palpable c. skin color normal, mucous membranes pink, skin warm to touch d. urine output ≥1 ml/kg/hr e. able to maintain physical exercise (crying, feeding) for longer period without fatigue	• Use a soft nipple (to reduce the work of sucking). • Breastfed babies may need additional rest periods (Breastfeeding requires slightly more energy expenditure than bottle feeding.) • Limit feeding at breast to 8–10 min on the first side and 10–15 min on the second side (this will usually meet caloric needs; further sucking may burn more calories than it adds). • Some infants may require high-calorie formulas to increase the caloric intake per energy expenditure. • Continuous nasogastric drip formula feedings may be required to further decrease the work of feeding for the infant while providing optimum calories. • Ensure uninterrupted sleep/rest periods. • Schedule activities, such as bathing, after rest and at other than feeding times. • Maintain normal body temperature (to decrease energy demands of hyper- or hypothermia) by keeping the environment at a moderate temperature; preventing chilling during bathing; adjusting clothing and blanket coverings to the environmental temperature. *Decrease the cardiac workload.* • Facilitate O_2/CO_2 exchange in the lungs. Administer O_2 if ordered. Monitor O_2 saturation (per pulse oximetry or ABGs). Prevent respiratory infections by teaching the family good handwashing techniques and alerting them to the most common sources of pathogens (infection increases O_2 demands). • Administer digoxin as ordered (to increase ventricular contractility and decrease heart rate). Ensure safe administration by checking the dosage with another RN and by taking the apical pulse for 1 minute. Withhold the digoxin if the pulse is <100 for a neonate, <90 for a 1-yr-old, <85 for a 2-yr-old, <80 for a 4-yr-old, <75 for a 6-yr-old, <70 for an 8-yr-old, <60 for a 14-yr-old. Monitor for the therapeutic effects: decrease in pulse and respirations, increase in urine output (signaling better kidney perfusion), improvement in skin color and temperature (with better perfusion to the peripheral tissues). Monitor for the classic signs of digoxin toxicity: nausea (manifests as anorexia in the infant), vomiting, lethargy, bradycardia, and dysrhythmia (noted on ECG or cardiac monitor, and in irregular apical pulse). Monitor serum digoxin levels; levels >2.1 ng/ml may indicate toxicity.* Blood for digoxin levels should be drawn at least 6–8 hr after the last dose (to ensure equilibration between serum and tissue levels). • Administer diuretics as ordered (to decrease salt and water retention related to decreased renal perfusion and the resulting rise in ADH and aldosterone levels).

* Gersony and Steeg (1985) caution that elevated serum digoxin levels are not necessarily diagnostic of toxicity, but must be interpreted with the other clinical findings.

Monitor for therapeutic effects: increased urine output, decreased peripheral edema, decreased neck vein distention, clearing of lung sounds, and increased O_2/CO_2 exchange.
Monitor diuresis by recording input/output and by daily weights. (Weight is a sensitive indicator of fluid balance.) Weigh before breakfast or the first A.M. feeding. Weigh the infant and toddler nude; weigh the preschooler or older child with only a hospital gown.
Counsel the parents that the infant should wet at least 6–8 diapers per day to ensure adequate output.
Monitor for side effects: dehydration and electrolyte imbalance, especially hypokalemia (which potentiates digoxin and may lead to toxicity) (common symptoms: muscle weakness and cramping, decrease in peristalsis, dysrhythmia) and hyponatremia (common symptoms: muscle weakness, leg cramps, dry mouth, dizziness, and GI disturbances).

Nutrition/Metabolism

Subjective Assessment

Self-report of appetite; parental report of food intake

Objective Assessment

Weight, placement on growth chart, general nutritional status

Analysis: Nursing Diagnosis 3

Altered nutrition: less than body requirements, related to
- *anorexia* associated with decreased perfusion of the GI tract and/or the side effects of medications
- *decreased energy* available for sucking/chewing
- *increased metabolic demands* associated with the increased workload of the overloaded heart

Defining Characteristics

Subjective: Self-report of anorexia or of "being too tired to eat." Parental report of caloric/nutrient intake that is less than body requirements, falling asleep during feeding

Objective: Failure to maintain the weight percentile (and usually also the length percentile) on the growth chart established by the birth weight and length of the full-term infant

Continued

Client Goal/ Evaluation Criteria | **Nursing Goals/Strategies (Selected Rationale)**

3. The client will receive caloric intake to meet metabolic demands for growth and development as evidenced by:
   a. gradual increase in weight
   b. maintenance of or increase in weight/length percentiles on the growth chart

*Ensure caloric requirements per 24 hr period that equal or exceed these recommendations for the healthy child** (CHF increases metabolic needs).

Note: Infants in CHF require ≥150 kcal/kg/day to grow

Normal Requirements

0–6 mo	kg × 115 kcal
6–12 mo	kg × 105 kcal
1–3 yr	1300 kcal avg
4–6 yr	1700 kcal avg
7–10 yr	2400 kcal avg
11–14 yr	2200–2700 kcal avg for girls/boys
15–18 yr	2100–2800 kcal avg

- Consider gavage feeding if necessary (to ensure adequate intake and reduce caloric expenditure).
- Follow measures to decrease energy expenditure (see first goal in this nursing process plan).
- Administer 24 kcal/oz formula as ordered (to increase caloric intake per feeding). Monitor for therapeutic benefit (steady weight gain) versus intolerance (diarrhea and/or vomiting with weight loss).

   c. available energy to attempt developmental tasks

Encourage attainment of emotional, social, and cognitive tasks.
- Provide visual, auditory, and tactile stimulation appropriate to the child's age and energy level.
- Encourage loving and playful interactions with family members.
- Assure parents that most of the child's emotional, social, and cognitive tasks can be met despite the CHF, and that motor tasks will develop quickly once physical health improves.

Assessment of Emotional-Social Function

Self-Perception/Self-Concept, Fear/Anxiety, Parenting Patterns

Subjective Assessment

Verbalization by the client and/or family members pertaining to feelings about the illness and its impact on individual and family functioning, verbalization by parents of self-perception of parenting skills

Objective Assessment

Client: reaction to hospitalization and to diagnostic and therapeutic measures, appropriateness of interactions with family members, health care professionals, and peers. Family members: visiting patterns, appropriateness of questions, evidence of ability to ventilate feelings and begin problem solving

* See also Table 18-3.

Analysis: Nursing Diagnosis 4

Fear/anxiety: child and family, related to the potential for
- *lasting effects* of congestive heart failure on growth and development
- fear of being an inadequate caregiver
- *death*

Nursing Diagnosis 5

Altered family process, related to family role strain associated with financial, emotional, and time demands of the child's heart condition

Defining Characteristics for Nursing Diagnoses 4 and 5

Subjective: Verbalizations of client or family members of fears for the child's future, of concerns about the family's ability to manage the condition at home, of the possibility that the condition could result in death. Client or family frustration with the physical limitations imposed by CHF and the child's inability to "lead a normal life" and gain weight appropriately

Objective: Client cries and is irritable; appears withdrawn; has sleep disturbances; refuses food; declines opportunities for play; clings to caregiver. Parents hold infant very stiffly, tentatively; visit infrequently; fail to keep appointments for learning home care; are reluctant to express feelings about the child's heart condition and its effect on their lives; rarely ask questions about the diagnosis, the child's prognosis, or the treatment

Client Goal/ Evaluation Criteria	Nursing Goals/Strategies (Selected Rationale)
4/5. The child and family will demonstrate effective coping with the child's heart condition, as evidenced by:	
a. expressing feelings and emotions	*Encourage expression of feelings and emotions and identification of sources of anxiety.* • Determine the family's past experience with heart defects and diseases and their related health beliefs. • Convey that anxiety is normal and expected. • Encourage the parents to air guilt feelings about hereditary and perinatal factors; clarify misconceptions; refer to genetic counseling when appropriate. • Use leading statements such as, "Many parents tell me they feel inadequate when their baby won't take enough milk."

Continued

Client Goal/ Evaluation Criteria	Nursing Goals/Strategies (Selected Rationale)
	• Ask questions of the parent and the older child such as, "What frightens you most about caring for your child (being cared for) at home?" and "How do you visualize your child's (your) future?" • Make the family aware of support groups available through the hospital or local heart association that can bring them together with others who have experienced heart disease in their child. See Appendix 8.
b. indicating the need for information to facilitate problem solving	*Supply information needed for problem solving.* • Give clear, concrete answers to questions (anxiety decreases comprehension). • Explain every nursing care activity. (This will help the child and family relate to the treatment of CHF and will decrease their feelings of helplessness and hopelessness.) • Discuss the relationship between the physical problems and the child's behavior—e.g., poor sucking response, to help diminish frustration with the behavior. • Clarify misconceptions (effective problem solving is based on accurate information).
c. verbalizing individual and family strengths d. identifying sources of support e. setting realistic goals	*Assist the child and family to set realistic goals and possible methods of attaining them.* • Assist in identification of coping strategies that have been effective in the past. • Refer to external sources of support and counseling as these needs are identified.
f. verbalizing feeling a part of the health care team g. seeking participation in the child's care h. demonstrating the ability to make decisions	*Actively involve the child and family in the treatment plan.* • Invite participation in the nursing plan of care and in its implementation. (This will greatly help dispel feelings of powerlessness and increase self-esteem.) • Take every opportunity to reinforce with the family ways in which the child benefits by their participation. ("Doing for" a loved one can provide a healthy outlet for grief and frustration.)
i. discussing the roles of other family members in relation to individual roles	*Assist the family to explore ways to work together toward common goals.*

Major goals of nursing care for the child with CHF relate to the identified nursing diagnoses. The infant or child must be assisted to compensate for decreased cardiac output, increased nutritional demands with decreased energy for feeding, the potential for infection, and developmental delays.

Compensating for Decreased Cardiac Output. Compensation for decreased cardiac output involves (1) adequate rest so that the young patient can conserve energy and (2) medications to enhance cardiac function. In both instances the nurse has a vital role in family teaching as well as in direct care delivery during hospitalization.

Ensuring Adequate Rest. Identify the child's normal pattern for sleep, feedings, playtime, and so on. Often the best time for feeding is upon awaking. Infants with CHF quickly tire and become short of breath if allowed to cry with hunger; therefore, the infant should not be allowed to cry for extended periods. This does not mean that all crying should be prevented, but only that the infant should be soothed and satisfied before crying depletes his or her energy.

Baths should be given when the child feels relaxed and playful and should be a pleasurable interaction time for parent and infant alike. If the child is especially fatigued, skip the bath for that day.

Teach parents to recognize cues that indicate the infant or young child is ready for play and stimulation. Although the young patient may not have the energy for prolonged interaction, even short intervals of cuddling, playing, and stimulation are beneficial for bonding and developmental progress.

Administering Medications to Enhance Cardiac Function. The medications for the infant or child in CHF are determined by the child's symptomatology and the severity of CHF. Digoxin (Lanoxin) is a positive inotropic agent that improves myocardial contractility and slows the heart rate. As a side effect of improving cardiac function, the urine output will increase. Digoxin comes either as a lime-flavored elixir or in tablet form (Table 39-6 gives usual dosages).

Digoxin elixirs are administered via a calibrated dropper or an oral syringe. Have the parent practice drawing up the medicine. The infant's head and shoulders should be elevated (to prevent aspiration) as the digoxin is slowly dropped into the side of the mouth. The infant must be given time to swallow a few drops at a time. To ensure receiving the entire dose, never mix the medication with formula or food.

Occasionally the infant or child may have a little emesis after taking the medication. *Do not repeat* the dose. It is impossible to ascertain how much has already been absorbed. Serum levels of digoxin that are temporarily too high are more dangerous than those that are temporarily too low.

Digoxin is given at regular intervals, usually every 12 hours, to ensure uniform serum levels. The family needs to maintain the same schedule each day. If a dose is forgotten for more than 6 hours, advise the parents to skip that dose and continue with the next dose as scheduled. Should the forgotten dose be remembered in less than 6 hours, the parent can give the late dose and then adjust the following dose to be given somewhat later. After that they can return to regular times of administration.

Vomiting can often be decreased by giving the digoxin between meals, about 1 hour before feeding or 2 hours after. If the child vomits two or more consecutive doses of digoxin, the physician should be informed. The most common signs of digoxin toxicity are:

- Nausea and vomiting
- Anorexia
- Listlessness
- Dysrhythmias
- Bradycardia

The family must notify the physician at the first suspicion of digoxin toxicity. In addition, digoxin's effect on the heart may be altered by the loss of body

Table 39-6. Usual Dosages for Digoxin

Total Digitalizing Dose	Maintenance Dose
Prematures	
20 $\mu g/kg$	5 $\mu g/kg$ in divided doses
Less than 2 yr	
50 $\mu g/kg$	10–15 $\mu g/kg$ in divided doses
Greater than 2 yr	
25–50 $\mu g/kg$	5–10 $\mu g/kg$ in divided doses

fluids. Therefore, the physician should be notified any time the child has vomiting, diarrhea, or an elevated temperature.

Because the dose of digoxin is determined in part by the child's weight, an increase in dosage will usually be prescribed by the physician following a weight gain. Parents need reassurance that the increased dose is not related to increasing severity of the disease.

Digoxin is potentially lethal. It must be placed out of the reach of the ill child and the siblings. Box 39-5 summarizes answers to questions frequently asked about digoxin.

Diuretics such as furosemide (Lasix), chlorthiazide (Diuril), and ethacrynic acid (Edecrin) are used to decrease total body water and to increase urine output. Diuretics can deplete the potassium stores of infants and children. A potassium supplement may be prescribed to compensate for this loss or spironolactone (Aldactone), a diuretic that inhibits potassium excretion, may be used. Potassium supplements are usually poorly tolerated by infants and children. They have a disagreeable taste and tend to stimulate emesis. Because spironolactone has a weak diuretic effect when used alone it is usually prescribed in conjunction with a more powerful diuretic such as Diuril or Lasix.

Occasionally parents may experience difficulty complying with prescribed medication times. This problem is more likely to occur in a very busy household with several children or when the infant or child is receiving several drugs. These families may be helped by devising a daily check-off chart which may be placed, with an attached pencil, in a conspicuous spot.

Meeting Nutritional Needs. It can be difficult and frustrating to feed infants with CHF. They may have trouble sucking, swallowing, and breathing, simultaneously. They may need to rest frequently during a feeding, thus prolonging feeding time, and then may fall asleep exhausted before adequate intake is achieved. Older children may display an increasing loss of appetite and refuse food. To achieve optimal

Box 39-5
Answering Parents' Questions about Digoxin Administration

1. What if one dose is missed?
   Give the next dose on time. Do not double the dosage to make up for the missed one.
2. What if more than one dose is missed in a row or one dose is missed for several days in a row?
   Notify your physician of the number of doses missed and the times they were missed.
   It is helpful to make the administration of this medication part of your child's daily routine so that it will not be forgotten and to help with the child's acceptance of it.
3. How often is the medication given?
   Digoxin is usually given every 12 hours. It takes about 1 hour to take effect. It reaches its peak between 1 and 2 hours after it was given. The effects decrease over 24 to 35 hours.
4. What is the best time to give the digoxin?
   Digoxin is best absorbed when the stomach is empty because food may interfere with its absorption. For this reason it is best to give the digoxin 1 hour before or 2 hours after eating.
5. What if my child vomits after receiving the medication?
   The dose should not be repeated because some of the digoxin may have been absorbed. If your child continues to vomit notify your physician because this may be a sign of some other problem.
6. What shall I do if my child has the flu with vomiting, diarrhea, and fever?
   Your physician should be notified immediately. If your child becomes dehydrated through loss of fluid the effects of digoxin on the body may be altered. Continue to give the digoxin as prescribed and encourage fluids. The type of fluid will vary with the degree of illness.
7. Where should digoxin be stored?
   Digoxin, like any medication, should be stored in a secure place out of the reach of children. An accidental ingestion of digoxin could be fatal so it should not be kept at the bedside or in the child's room.
8. What should be done if a child accidentally swallows digoxin?
   Call your poison control center immediately. Have the bottle with you when you call. They will ask for age and size of the child who took the digoxin, when the incident occurred, and approximately how much digoxin was in the bottle. If you have ipecac (a medication that induces vomiting) they may recommend that you give one dose before going to your nearest emergency room. Time should not be wasted. If you do not have a car the police or fire department should be called or an emergency ambulance sent. Take the digoxin bottle with you to the emergency room.

(Adapted from Jackson, 1979.)

nutrition for the child the nurse will ensure that caloric intake is adequate, that energy is conserved, and that the parents receive support and encouragement.

Observe the infant feeding and watch parent-child interaction during the feeding. Each infant is different and any feeding plan must reflect individual needs. Include the parents in every aspect of nutritional planning and work together in developing an optimal feeding plan. Take into consideration the household schedule, presence or absence of other family members, food preferences, and ethnic background (see Chapter 1 for a discussion of intercultural communication and Chapter 2 for cultural assessment).

Anticipate the infant's hunger and provide feedings before energy is spent in crying. Smaller, more frequent feedings may help conserve energy and increase total intake. Position the infant in a semi-erect position in the parent's arms. If the infant tends to have "wet burps" or actual emesis after feeding, place him or her with head and torso semielevated for 30 minutes following each feeding. Burp the infant before, during, and after each feeding. Many babies with CHF have a poor suck and draw in large amounts of air with their food, which can result in colic. Burping the infant after every half ounce will help minimize this problem and will reduce the chance of emesis.

Never prop the bottle. Feeding the infant with CHF requires constant attention to feeding tolerance. Small infants do best with a soft, free-flowing (premature) nipple. This helps to ensure adequate intake in a shorter time with less energy expended in sucking. The nipple hole should be large enough to deliver the formula easily, but not so large as to increase the chance of aspiration. Infants with additional congenital disorders such as cleft lip or cleft palate may require special nipples and may need feeding appliances adapted to their individual needs.

Review formula preparation with the family. Most commercially prepared formulas contain 20 calories per ounce. Sometimes infants with CHF are placed on a formula containing 24 calories or more per ounce. This is aimed at increasing the caloric consumption without extra energy expenditure for additional feedings. Higher-calorie formulas are not always well tolerated, however. The infant may develop diarrhea, vomiting, or both. If this occurs the formula will be changed to a lower calorie preparation and then gradually the more concentrated form will be reintroduced. Gradual introduction of the higher calorie formula often increases tolerance. Low-salt formulas are rarely used for infants in CHF because they promote anorexia and may deplete normal sodium intake.

When an infant fails to grow, it is important to assess exactly how much intake he or she is receiving. Calculation of the formula consumed in 24 hours will help to determine whether or not the volume of formula is adequate.

Breastfeeding is slightly harder work for infants than bottlefeeding. Breast milk is, however, considered to be more easily digested than formula. In addition, breastfeeding can be a very special time for mother-infant bonding. The mother who chooses breastfeeding should be supported in her choice. The success of breastfeeding can be enhanced by following these guidelines:

- Encourage offering both breasts at each feeding, alternating the starting breast
- If the infant fatigues easily, limit the feeding time. Ninety per cent of the milk is ingested in the first 5 minutes of vigorous sucking at breast. Allowing 8 to 10 minutes on the first breast and 10 to 15 minutes on the second should provide adequate intake and satisfy the infant's sucking needs. Some infants may need to be fed as often as every 2 hours. Other infants may not need such frequent feedings, but the infant with CHF should never go longer than 4 hours between feedings
- If the mother's breasts become very engorged, it is difficult for the infant to grasp the nipple. Manual expression of a small amount of milk will soften the breast and decrease the sucking effort
- Nursing mothers use 600 to 1000 calories a day for breast feeding; therefore, they need to consume adequate calories and a nutritionally balanced diet
- The breastfed infant is receiving enough milk if there are 6 to 8 wet diapers per day, and if the infant feeds at least every 4 hours and is alert.

An important fact for families to understand is that many infants will not gain weight or will gain it very slowly regardless of the method of feeding, owing to their cardiac defect.

For the older child meals should be well balanced with small, attractive, and tasty portions. Empty calories, such as carbonated beverages, cookies, candy, and potato chips, should be avoided. Asking parents to keep a 7-day record of dietary intake helps to determine quantity and quality of nutrients taken in. It can also serve as a tool for nutritional counseling. Review with the parents the amount of milk the child is drinking each day. If large volumes of milk are being consumed, needed nutrients may be missing and iron deficiency anemia may occur.

Preventing Infection. Infants and children in CHF are much more susceptible to respiratory infections. Avoiding crowded public places during cold and flu season and asking friends and relatives not to visit when they have an active infection are sensible precautions. There is no point, however, in trying to isolate the infant or child: not only is this impossible, it is also inadvisable from the standpoint of the child's emotional development. Support the parents' efforts in caring for their ill child by advising them that it may be impossible to avoid the introduction of viral illnesses from siblings during the peak of flu and cold season. *Because tobacco smoke is particularly irritating for the child with CHF, smoking in the child's presence or home should be strongly discouraged.*

Encourage parents to provide good dental hygiene for the older infant and child with CHF. This helps to avoid the danger of bacterial endocarditis and other infections stemming from oral pathogens.

Promoting Healthy Growth and Development. Growth needs have been addressed with regard to conservation of energy, adequate nutritional intake, and enhancement of cardiac function. Developmental needs will be partially met by loving interactions between the family and the child. The family should be counseled, however, that some developmental delays are common and unavoidable because the infant's available energy will be used first for maintaining vital functions such as breathing and feeding, leaving little energy for pursuit of developmental tasks. They should be reassured that after the infant is stabilized by either medical or surgical treatment he will catch up to his peers.

Nursing Strategies for Follow-up Care in the Home or Clinic

Assess vital signs, peripheral pulses, capillary refill, skin color, urine output, and energy level for evidence of the heart's ability to supply the body's demands for oxygen.

Determine whether medications are being administered as prescribed and assess the child's tolerance for these drugs.

Weigh and measure the child and plot the measurements on the growth curve; determine the adequacy of nutritional intake and tolerance of prescribed formula.

Assess developmental stage and discuss with the family ways to enhance development without exceeding the child's energy limitations.

Encourage the parent (and verbal child) to talk about their concerns and feelings of success with regard to management of the illness at home.

Acquired Heart Disease

Infective Endocarditis

Other common terms used for infective endocarditis are "subacute" and "acute bacterial endocarditis." It is an inflammatory process resulting from infection of the valves, the endocardium, or the endothelium of the heart. The infectious agent may be bacterial (such as staphylococcus and streptococcus) or fungal (such as *Candida albicans*).

Pathophysiology

Congenital heart defects increase susceptibility to infections within the heart or blood vessels because of turbulent blood flow. Abnormal communications (VSD, ASD), stenotic valves, and so forth will produce turbulent blood flow which results in areas of tissue damage in the heart. Bacteria or fungi circulating in the bloodstream become entrapped at these sites and form vegetations. These vegetations can grow, interfere with cardiac function, and deteriorate valves (Fig. 39-24). In addition, vegetations can break off and become emboli causing cerebral vascular accidents and other infarcts. Infectious agents may be introduced into the systemic circulation during dental procedures such as teeth cleaning, cavity filling, tooth extraction, or any oral surgery. Other procedures at risk for introducing bacteria or fungi into the circulation are upper respiratory tract, gastrointestinal tract, and genitourinary tract operations (Committee on Rheumatic Fever and Infective Endocarditis, 1984). Postoperative intracardiac lines are also a potential source of bacterial contamination.

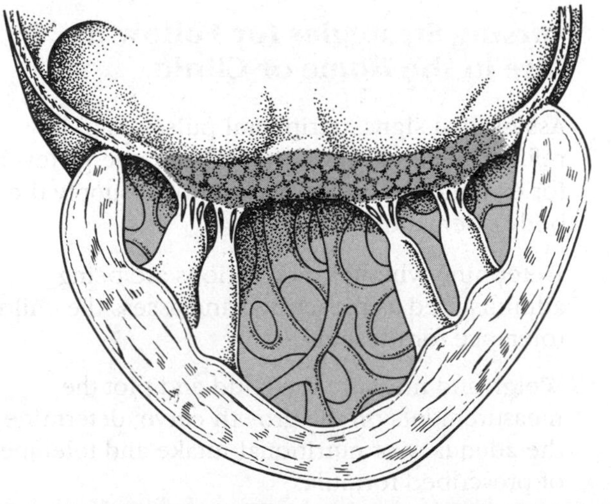

Figure 39-24. Endocarditis is characterized by the presence of vegetations (called Aschoff bodies) on the surface of the endocardium, most commonly the mitral valve.

Therapeutic Management

Infective endocarditis is a serious complication and must be treated vigorously. After culture identification of the infectious agent is made intravenous antibiotics are administered for up to 6 weeks or more. If the valves are extensively involved or significant emboli have occurred, surgery is usually needed. Infants or children who have had a previous valve replacement and who have a tissue or prosthetic valve in place may require replacement of that valve.

Strategies for Nursing Care

Nursing care of a child with infective endocarditis includes administration of prescribed medications, monitoring for fever and emboli, and providing information and emotional support for the child and family.

Administering Medication. Treatment of infective endocarditis will involve administration of intravenous antibiotics. It is important that the antibiotic be given on schedule to maintain therapeutic serum levels of the drug for maximum effect against the organism. Because antibiotics can be caustic to veins, the child must be monitored for signs of phlebitis with intravenous administration.

Monitoring for Fever. Temperature readings are recorded every 4 hours, and more often if the child has a fever. If the child remains febrile on antibiotics or becomes febrile after having been on antibiotics for several days or weeks, further cultures will be required to ascertain whether other organisms are involved that will require different antibiotics.

Monitoring for Emboli. Because emboli are a potential complication of infective endocarditis, the nurse's recording must reflect assessment for clinical manifestations. These include seizures, slurred speech, neurologic impairment, and asymmetrical movement of the extremities.

Providing Information and Support for the Child and Family. Teaching needs will include explanation of diagnostic procedures (such as blood tests and echocardiograms) and an explanation of the disease process, potential complications, and the treatment plan. Use of diagrams and a heart model can enhance teaching effectiveness.

Because of the serious nature of infective endocarditis and the prolonged hospital stay, the child and family will have a particular need for nursing support. The child's diversional needs may involve in depth planning with the recreational therapist and the family. Children of school age and older may benefit from having a large calendar in their room so that they can mark off the days of antibiotic therapy or the number of days until discharge. This can help to make the date of discharge seem more attainable.

Antibiotic Prophylaxis

Parents and the child require extensive teaching before discharge to prevent recurrence of infective endocarditis. Prevention consists of antibiotic prophylaxis for at risk procedures. Typically an oral dose of penicillin is given 1 hour before the procedure and a second dose 6 hours after the initial dose. Children who are allergic to penicillin may receive erythromycin (Committee on Rheumatic Fever and Infective Endocarditis, 1984).

Hypertension

Primary hypertension in adults is one of the greatest health risks facing our nation. Research indicates that hypertension may have its inception during childhood. Hypertension in children may be secondary to other conditions such as coarctation of the aorta, renal artery stenosis, renal disease, oral contraception, steroids, obesity, and adrenal disorders (Cushing disease, adrenogenital syndrome, primary aldosteronism). When a child is identified as being hypertensive, a secondary cause such as those just listed should be ruled out. If a secondary cause is indeed present, then treatment of the secondary cause will be initiated.

Some children will have primary hypertension with no apparent etiology. The exact incidence of this in the pediatric population is still being researched through long-term longitudinal studies on large populations of children. Geographical, ethnic, and racial differences in blood pressure readings in children are being investigated.

The child who is identified as having primary hypertension is usually followed closely with regular blood pressure checks and evaluation of serum lipids, serum cholesterol, and serum triglyceride levels. A careful family history is obtained to determine the presence of hypertension and coronary artery disease in other family members. The severity of the hypertension will dictate treatment. The definition of mild, moderate, and severe hypertension remains variable among institutions and in different areas of the world.

Mild hypertension is usually just monitored on a regular basis. Appropriate cuff size and measurement of blood pressure in children is discussed in the section on coarctation of the aorta. Treatment for moderate hypertension is usually close monitoring as well; however, some physicians institute medical therapy including sodium-restricted diets (no added salt) and occasionally the use of antihypertensive medications such as hydralazine and propranolol. Severe hypertension requires antihypertensive drug therapy and possibly dietary alterations. It is not yet known whether control of hypertension in childhood will have an effect on development of arteriosclerotic disease and hypertension in adulthood.

The role of the nurse in caring for a child with hypertension includes extensive teaching of the child and family. Life-long health habits such as diet, exercise, weight control, and attitudes toward smoking are established during childhood. The family as a whole must model a healthy lifestyle in order for the child to develop healthy patterns of living.

When teaching the child about exercise and healthy dietary practices, the information should be presented as a positive approach to life with enjoyable benefits such as feeling better with exercise, becoming more fit, being able to participate in more activities, and feeling a sense of accomplishment. Dietary restrictions and institution of an exercise routine should never be seen by the child as punishment for the hypertension. Family participation in lifestyle changes is particularly important so that the child will not feel singled out or punished. In addition, when the whole family participates, lifestyle changes tend to be more consistent and long-lasting. The nurse has an important role as a health advocate in teaching healthy lifestyles for the prevention of disease and the promotion of health.

Dysrhythmias

Normal Conduction System

Electrical conduction stimulates the muscular contraction of the heart. Disease processes and surgery may disrupt this system, producing a variety of results. In the normal heart, the impulse originates in the right atrium from the sinoatrial (SA) node located at the junction of the superior vena cava and the right atrium (Fig. 39-25). Cardiac cells are either of the pacemaker or the nonpacemaker type. Pacemaker cells have the ability to depolarize spontaneously (automaticity); nonpacemaker cells require an unusual stimulus (such as severe hypoxia) to depolarize spontaneously. Pacemaker cells with the highest rate of automaticity occur in the SA node. Therefore, the SA node functions as the pacemaker of the heart. Nerve centers in the brain control the release of impulses from the SA node by sympathetic fiber stimulation which increases the heart rate, and vagus (parasympathetic) nerve fiber stimulation which decreases it.

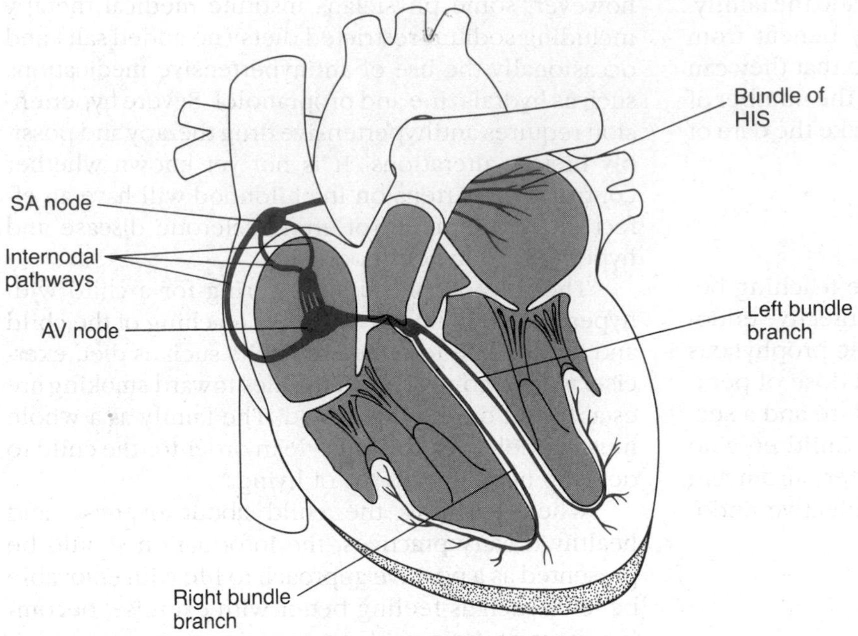

Figure 39-25. Internodal pathways.

Impulses originating in the SA node travel through the right and left atria via three internodal pathways to the atrioventricular (AV) node located at the lower atrial septum where there is a slight delay of the impulses. Impulses then continue from the AV node through the Bundle of His and bifurcate into the right and left bundle branches located in the ventricular septum. The impulses then continue through the Purkinje fibers in the myocardium and stimulate ventricular contraction (Fig. 39-26).

An ECG tracing shows the contraction of the atria (the P wave), the contraction of the ventricles (the QRS complex), and the recovery phase of the ventricles (the T wave). The PR interval represents the time for the original impulse to reach the ventricles and stimulate contraction. The ST segment represents the period between the completion of contraction and recovery of the ventricular muscle. Box 39-6 provides a detailed outline of fetal and neonatal dysrythmias. This detailed information is provided primarily for reference purposes.

Monitoring Dysrhythmias

The Holter Monitor. Infants and children suspected of having a dysrhythmia will usually undergo a Holter monitor evaluation. This is a 24-hour recording of the child's electrocardiogram. The Holter monitor itself is a portable device approximately the size of a transistor radio. The leads are attached to the child's chest and taped securely in place, and the recorder is turned on. The monitor itself is attached to the child's belt or carried in a small pouch or backpack. The de-

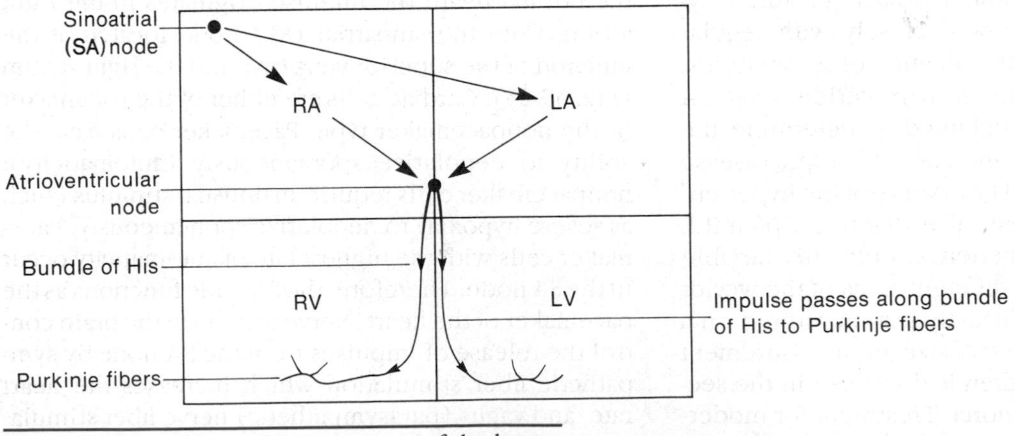

Figure 39-26. The conduction system of the heart.

Box 39-6
Fetal and Neonatal Dysrhythmias

FETAL DYSRHYTHMIAS

Fetal heart rate (HR) range is ~120–160

Estimated 1–2% incidence of dysrhythmias

Most dysrhythmias are supraventricular premature beats which disappear after birth

Serious dysrhythmias can occur, i.e., complete heart block (CHB) and supraventricular tachycardia (SVT)

Treatment in utero is limited to infants in congestive heart failure

CHB—delivery is induced if gestational age is appropriate, and a pacemaker is placed

SVT—Digoxin or propranolol have been used by giving the mother PO or IV doses

NEONATAL DYSRHYTHMIAS

Average HR of the newborn is ~130–145 with considerable variation (90–195).

Benign dysrhythmias:

1. Sinus bradycardia
   - repeated episodes of HR <80
   - up to 35% of normal premature infants have episodes of bradycardia
   - short episodes are associated with eating, defecating, hiccuping, and nasopharyngeal suctioning
   - most likely due to functional or developmental responses of the SA node
   - no intervention necessary
2. Sinus tachycardia
   - intermittent episodes of HR >195
   - associated with periods of increased activity, crying, fever, loud noise stimulation
   - can be associated with underlying problems, i.e., sepsis, congestive heart failure, hyperthyroidism
   - no intervention necessary unless treating an underlying problem
3. Sinus arrhythmia
   - phasic variation in HR with normal PR interval usually associated with respirations in the older child but not in neonates

PATHOLOGIC DYSRHYTHMIAS

1. Supraventricular tachycardia (SVT)
   - Clinical manifestations
     Most common tachyarrhythmia in neonates, greater incidence in males than females
     HR 210–350, HR is very consistent, little change in HR with activity or crying, generally no P waves are visible
     Infant is pale, gray, restless, fussy, feeding poorly, and/or vomiting
     With SVT of 24 hours or more duration, congestive heart failure develops
   - Etiology
     8–26% have congenital heart disease, i.e., Ebstein anomaly, corrected transposition, tricuspid atresia
     Myocarditis, cardiomyopathies, and myocardial tumors
     10% have Wolff-Parkinson-White (WPW) syndrome with an accessory pathway (bundle of Kent) present
     There is a classic short PR interval giving a delta wave with a wide QRS complex
   - Treatment *(done by specialist)*
     Vagal stimulation—gagging or carotid pressure—usually ineffective in neonates
     Ice bag to the face or facial immersion in cold water; occlude nostrils and immerse face in 5°C water for <5 sec. Causes bradycardia from parasympathetic stimulation
     Caution must be used to avoid aspiration or asphyxia
   - Drug Therapy
     Digoxin
     Digitalizing dose (initially, half the digitalizing dose is given, then in 6–8 hours one fourth of the digitalizing dose and in 12–16 hours one fourth of the digitalizing dose

Premature	20–13 μg/kg
Newborn	30–50 μg/kg
Infant	50–70 μg/kg

     Maintenance dose 10–25 μg/kg/day given BID
     Propranolol, verapamil, quinidine, and procainamide also used, although verapamil not used in neonates.
   - Cardioversion by Direct Current Countershock
     0.5–1.0 watt sec/kg
     Used if the infant in severe congestive heart failure or the SVT is long-term or does not respond to other management
     Maintenance drug therapy, i.e., digoxin, must be used following shock conversion to prevent recurrence
   - Prognosis
     Digoxin or drug therapy usually maintained for 1 year, after which SVT in most cases does not recur
     50% with WPW will persist with WPW pattern after 1 year; of these half will have recurrence of SVT despite maintenace therapy
     2–5% overall mortality
2. Atrial flutter
   - uncommon in neonates
   - atrial rate is 220–460, the atrial mechanism is regular, characteristic sawtooth pattern of flutter wave in leads II and III, usually some degree of AV block
   - degree of AV block determines ventricular rate. Variable AV block produces irregular ventricular rate

Continued

- may be associated with congenital heart disease,
- treatment
  cardioversion by direct current countershock
  Digoxin

3. Atrial fibrillation
   - rare in neonates
   - almost always associated with some form of congenital heart disease
   - ECG shows extremely rapid atrial depolarization and a rapid irregular ventricular rate, a chaotic appearing rhythm
   - neonate may have severe congestive heart failure with symptoms similar to those of SVT
   - treatment
     cardioversion by direct current countershock
     Digoxin
     Quinidine
4. Ventricular tachycardia
   - rare in neonates
   - usually associated with congenital heart disease, electrolyte disturbance, myocardial tumor, or myocarditis
   - treatment
     Cardioversion by direct current countershock
     Infusion of lidocaine, 0.5–1 mg/kg/hr
     Diphenylhydantoin (Dilantin), 3–8 mg/kg/dose
5. Heart block (AV block)
   - Uncommon in newborns
   - First degree AV block
     Prolonged PR interval, >0.12 sec in neonates
     One-to-one conduction ratio (every P wave is conducted through with a ventricular response)
     Most common cause is digoxin effect (does not necessarily mean digoxin toxicity)
     Can be caused by electrolyte abnormalities, i.e., hypokalemia or hyperkalemia
     No specific intervention is necessary except to watch digoxin levels or correct electrolyte imbalance
   - Second-degree AV block
     Not all atrial beats are conducted to the ventricle
     Type I (Wenckebach) is progressive lengthening of the PR interval until an atrial beat fails to be conducted and a dropped beat occurs; may be due to digoxin toxicity
     Type II is present when ventricular beats are dropped without preceding prolongation of the PR interval. Type II tends to progress to complete heart block
   - Third-degree (complete) AV block
     The ventricular rate is totally independent of the atrial rate with the ventricular rate being slower. The higher the level of block the higher the ventricular rate.
     Due to an anatomic discontinuity within the AV node or distal conduction system
     30% have associated congenital heart disease
     Associated with myocardial rhabdomyoma and endocardial fibroelastosis, infection, metabolic or vascular disorders, and maternal lupus erythematosus
     Clinically, the infant may be asymptomatic especially if the ventricular rate is 50–80. If the ventricular rate is <50, the infant may have CHF, dyspnea, tachypnea, peripheral cyanosis, cardiomegaly, and other arrhythmias (i.e., atrial flutter, PVCs, and bundle branch block)
     Treatment
       Not indicated in an asymptomatic, well infant with a ventricular rate >50. In symptomatic infants atropine or isoproterenol may be used until pacemaker insertion. Indications for pacemaker include CHF, underlying congenital heart disease, HR <50 especially if associated with syncope and wide complex QRS
     Prognosis
       Death can occur from infection, and cardiomyopathy despite adequate pacing.
       Good prognosis if the infant is asymptomatic, HR >50, and has a narrow QRS
       The ventricular rate tends to become slower as the infant gets older. Many children require pacemakers during school age or adolescence
6. Ectopic beats
   - common in healthy newborns: 31% incidence
   - supraventricular ectopic beats are more common and are identified by an abnormal P wave (abnormal configuration or timing). These are usually considered benign and no treatment is necessary
   - ventricular ectopic beats are characterized by a wide, bizarre QRS complex, not preceded by a P wave. These can be benign but bear close monitoring if multifocal, frequent, and/or paired

vice is worn for 24 hours, during which time the child should perform all normal activities, being as active as possible. A diary is kept by the parents or child and hourly entries indicate the type of activity the child is engaged in. Accurate diaries are very helpful in interpreting the Holter monitor recordings and determining what activities precipitate dysrhythmias. *Caution should be used while the monitor is on to avoid immersion in water, i.e., swimming, bathing, or showering.* At the end of 24 hours the Holter monitor is removed from the child and the tape deciphered and interpreted.

The TAM Monitor. At times a child's dysrhythmia occurs infrequently and does not occur while the Holter monitor is in place. For these children a portable dysrhythmia monitor (a TAM monitor) may be used. This monitor is placed over the child's chest (anywhere on the chest) only when the child is symptomatic. A button is pushed and a 38-second ECG is recorded automatically. The ECG is stored in the device and is then transmitted over the telephone by the parents to a receiver in the cardiologist's office. This particular monitor allows more flexibility in recording symptomatic episodes and in determining whether a dysrhythmia is occurring.

References

American Heart Association. *If Your Child Has a Congenital Heart Defect; A Guide for Parents.* Dallas, 1988.

Borow KM, Braunwald E: Congenital heart disease in the adult. *In* Braunwald E (ed): *Heart Disease; A Textbook of Cardiovascular Medicine.* 3rd ed. Philadelphia, WB Saunders, 1988, 967–1008.

Daberkow ED, Washington R: Congenital heart disease. *In* Merenstein G, et al: *Handbook of Neonatal Intensive Care.* St. Louis, CV Mosby, 1985.

Ehlers KH: Growth failure in association with congenital heart disease. *Pediatr Ann* 1978 Nov; 750.

Fink B: *Congenital Heart Disease.* Chicago, Year Book Medical Publishers, 1985.

Friedman WF: Congenital heart disease in infancy and childhood. *In* Braunwald E (ed): *Heart Disease; A Textbook of Cardiovascular Medicine.* 3rd ed. Philadelphia, WB Saunders, 1988, 896–975.

Garson A, et al: Parental reactions to children with congenital heart disease. *Child Psychiatry Hum Dev* 1978 Feb; 86.

Gersony WM: Congenital heart disease. *In* Behrman RE, Vaughan VC (eds): *Nelson Textbook of Pediatrics.* 13th ed. Philadelphia, WB Saunders, 1988, 962–1004.

Gersony WM, Steeg CN: (1985). Congestive heart failure. *In* Dickerman JD, Lucey JF (eds): *The critically Ill Child: Diagnosis and Medical Management.* Philadelphia, WB Saunders, 1985, 320–336.

Guido GW: *Septal Defects: Atrial and Ventricular. Unit 1 in Series 3. Cardiovascular Disease in the Young: Nursing Intervention.* Norwalk, CT, Appleton-Century-Crofts, 1983.

Gundermuth S: Mothers' reports of early experiences of infants with congenital heart disease. *Matern Child Nurs J* 1975 Mar; 155.

Jackson PL: Digoxin therapy at home: keeping the child safe. *MCN* 1979 Mar/Apr; 105.

Kaplan S: Congestive heart failure. *In* Gellis SS, Kagan BM: *Current Pediatric Therapy 12.* Philadelphia, WB Saunders, 1986, 132–135.

Linde LM, Linde SD: Emotional factors of pediatric patients in cardiac surgery. *Am Operating Room Nurs J* 1973 Jan; 95.

Linde LM, et al: Attitudinal factors in congenital heart disease. *Pediatrics* 1966 Jan; 92.

Linde LM, et al: Physical and emotional aspects of congenital heart disease in children. *Am J Cardiolo* 1971 Jun; 712.

Merenstein G, et al: *Handbook of Neonatal Intensive Care.* St Louis, CV Mosby, 1985.

Moss A: What every primary physician should know about the postoperative cardiac patient. *Pediatrics* 1979 Feb; 326.

Moss A, et al: *Heart Disease in Infants, Children and Adolescents.* Baltimore, Williams and Wilkins, 1983.

Moller J, et al: *Congenital Heart Abnormalities.* Columbus, OH, Ross Laboratories, 1976, pp 3, 56.

Nadas A, Fyler D: *Pediatric Cardiology.* Philadelphia, WB Saunders, 1972.

Nadas AS: Congenital heart disease. *In* Gellis SS, Kagan BM: *Current Pediatric Therapy 12.* Philadelphia, WB Saunders, 1986, 135–141.

Sauer SN: *Atrioventricular Canal. Unit 2 in Series 3: Cardiovascular Disease in the Young: Nursing Intervention.* Norwalk, CT, Appleton-Century-Crofts, 1983, 28.

Uzark K: *Obstructive Lesions: Pulmonic Stenosis, Aortic Stenosis, Coarctation of the Aorta. Unit 5 in Series 3: Cardiovascular Disease in the Young: Nursing Intervention.* Norwalk, CT, Appleton-Century-Crofts, 1983.

Bibliography

AIDS precautions changing practice, RNs agree; OSHA already moving to enforce CDC guidelines. *Am J Nurs* 1988 Mar; 88(3):372.

American Heart Association: *Caring for an Infant with Congestive Heart Failure: A Guide for Parents.* San Francisco, 1988.

Becker KL, Stevens SA: Get in touch and in tune with cardiac assessment. Part 1. *Nurs 88* 1988 Mar; 18(3):51–55.

Committee on Rheumatic Fever and Infective Endocarditis: A statement for health professionals: prevention of bacterial endocarditis. *Circulation* 1984; 70:1123A–1127A.

Cullen L, Laxson C: Ballooning open a stenotic valve. *Am J Nurs* 1988 Jul; 88(7):987–992.

DesRosier MB: Taking a baby. *Am J Nurs* 1988 Jan; 88(1):67.

Gellis SS, Kagan BM: *Current Pediatric Therapy 12.* Philadelphia, WB Saunders, 1986.

Gettrust KV, Ryan SC, Engelman DS: *Applied Nursing Diagnosis.* New York, John Wiley and Sons, 1985.

Gottsefeld I: The family of the child with congenital heart disease. *MCN* 1979 Mar/Apr; 101–104.

Higgins SS, Kashani IA: The cyanotic child: Heart defects and parental learning needs. *MCN* 1986 Jul/Aug; 11(4):259–263.

Horner MM, Rawlins KG: How parents of children with chronic conditions perceive their own needs. *MCN* 1987 Jan/Feb; 12:40–43.

Kashani IA, Higgins SS: Counseling strategies for families of children with congenital heart disease. *Pediatr Nurs* 1986 Jan/Feb; 12(1):38–40.

Keith JD, et al: *Heart Disease in Infancy and Childhood.* New York, Macmillan, 1978.

Loebl S, Spratto GR: *The Nurse's Drug Handbook.* 4th ed. New York, John Wiley and Sons, 1986.

McKeever P: Fathering the chronically ill child. *MCN* 1981 Mar/Apr; 6:124–128.

Miracle VA: Anatomy of a murmur. *Nurs 86* 1986 Jul; 16(7):26–31.

Ng L: *Complete "D"-Transposition of the Great Arteries. Unit 4 in Series 3: Cardiovascular Disease in the Young: Nursing Intervention.* Norwalk, CT, Appleton-Century-Crofts, 1983.

Pebler MA, et al: A cardiovascular risk assessment of high school sophomores. *Issues Compr Pediatr Nurs* 1987; 10(5–6):331–341.

Peterson M: Preparation of the cardiac child and the family for surgery. *Issues Compr Pediatr Nurs* 1979 Dec; 3:62–71.

Proia LM, et al: Assessment of cardiovascular risks in parents and their sons. *Issues Compr Pediatr Nurs* 1987; 10 (5–6):343–352.

Porterfield L, Porterfield JG: What you need to know about today's pacemakers. *RN* 1987 Mar; 44–49.

Rowe R, et al: *The Neonate with Congenital Heart Disease.* Philadelphia, WB Saunders, 1981.

Ryberg JW, Merrifield EB: What parents want to know. *Nurse Pract* 1984 Jun; 9:24–32.

Shor V: *Infants with Critical Heart Defects; Guidelines For Community Health Nurses.* Boston, 1980.

Smith J: Big differences in little people. *Am J Nurs* 1988 Apr; 88(4):458–462.

Smith K: Recognizing cardiac failure in neonates. *MCN* 1979 Mar/Apr.

Viger KH, et al: *Tetralogy of Fallot and Truncus Arteriosus. Unit 3 in Series 3: Cardiovascular Disease in the Young: Nursing Intervention.* Norwalk, CT, Appleton-Century-Crofts, 1983.

West CM: Ischemia. *In* Carrieri VK, et al (eds): *Pathophysiological Phenomena in Nursing. Human Responses to Illness.* Philadelphia, WB Saunders, 1986, 13–67.

Wolterman M, Miller M: Caring for parents in crisis. *Nurs Forum* 1985 Jan; 21:34–37.

Nursing Strategies: Altered Hematologic Function

Chapter 40

Marcia Sosnowski Leonard

Childhood blood disorders are a heterogeneous group of diseases with wide ranges of etiology, severity, treatment, and prognoses. This is due in great part to the complex structure and function of blood and to the independent functions of each of its components. Blood components affect every cell in the body. The constituents of blood are so vital to homeostasis that severe disorders or deficiencies may be incompatible with life, and even mild dysfunctions have systemic effects.

Related Topics
Genetic counseling, Chapter 4
Patterns of inheritance, Chapter 4
The impact of chronic illness, Chapter 25
Strategies for pain management, Chapter 29
AIDS, Chapter 43
Nursing Process Plan: The Family in Need of Genetic Counseling, Table 50-3.

Nursing care of children with blood disorders requires a sound knowledge of normal blood anatomy and physiology as well as an understanding of the inheritance patterns of genetic disorders, nutrition, and, as in all pediatric disorders, growth and development.

Anatomy and Physiology of Blood

Blood is composed of a liquid called *plasma* in which are suspended certain proteins (albumin, globulin, and the clotting factors) and the blood cells—*erythrocytes* (red blood cells, RBCs), *leukocytes* (white blood cells, WBCs), and *thrombocytes* (platelets). The constant movement of blood throughout the cardiovascular system keeps the cells suspended in the plasma, but when plasma is removed from the body and spun down in a centrifuge, it is possible to separate the solid components from the liquid plasma. The cellular components are quantified via a measurement called *hematocrit,* which represents the percentage of blood volume composed of blood cells. Because most* (about 97 per cent) of the cells in blood are red blood cells, the hematocrit is a reliable indicator of red cell population. It cannot be used to predict white cell or platelet levels, however.

* White blood cells and platelets are measured in thousands/cubic millimeter and red blood cells are measured in millions/cubic millimeter.

Red Blood Cells

Red blood cells are the most abundant cell component in the blood. Red blood cells have a biconcave disk form that easily adapts to small blood vessels. In fact, Guyton (1986) likens red blood cells to a "bag" because they can conform to almost any shape.

Production of Red Blood Cells

Red blood cells are produced in the marrow of bones. Essentially all bones are employed in red cell production during the first 5 years of life. After that time production in the shafts of the long bones (e.g., tibia, femur) is gradually reduced and replaced by hematopoietic action in the ribs, sternum, and vertebrae as well as the pelvis, skull, clavicles, and scapulas. The genesis of red blood cells is illustrated in Figure 40-1.

Red blood cell production is stimulated by decreased tissue oxygenation. That is, red blood cell production depends not upon the absolute numbers of red blood cells but upon their ability to carry oxygen and carbon dioxide. When tissue oxygenation decreases, the hormone *erythropoietin* stimulates stem

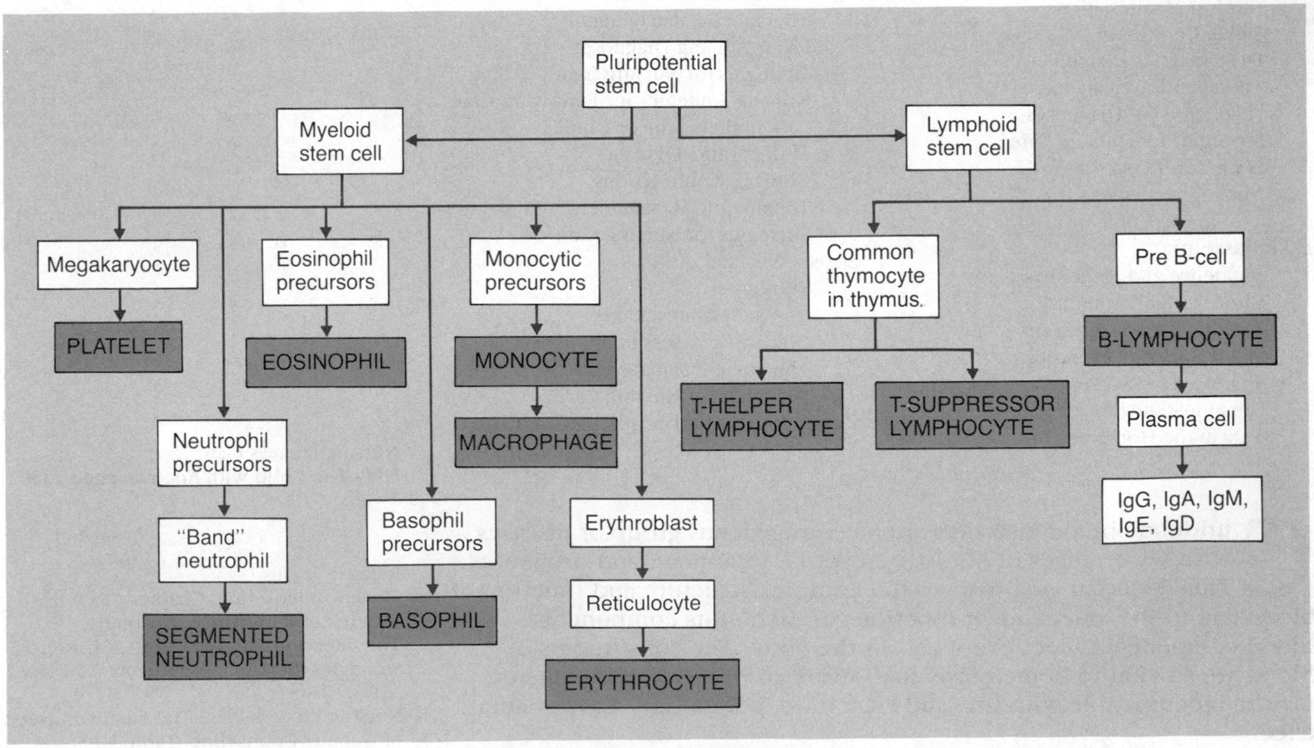

Figure 40-1. Genesis of blood cells.

cells in the bone marrow to progress to mature red blood cells. Whereas some erythropoietin is thought to be produced in tissues such as the liver and in macrophages, the majority (90 per cent) is produced in the kidney, probably either in or near the glomeruli (Guyton, 1986; Pearson, 1987). Therefore, kidney disease can affect the body's response to tissue hypoxia.

Red blood cells have a life span of about 120 days. As they become older, their membranes become more fragile and may rupture when the cells are required to squeeze through a small capillary. Many of the red cells fragment in the spleen where they must adapt to small spaces in the red pulp of that organ. When red cells burst, the hemoglobin is taken up by macrophages, to be released back into the blood for transfer to the bone marrow where it is used for production of new red blood cells. If no more iron is needed for that purpose, iron may be stored in the liver and other tissues in the form of ferritin (Guyton, 1986).

Function of RBCs

Red blood cells transport oxygen and carbon dioxide to and from the cells of the body, via a mechanism in which oxygen and carbon dioxide bind chemically to *hemoglobin* molecules, the major physiologic component of red cells.

Hemoglobin. Hemoglobin is a complex protein consisting of *heme* (iron-containing) molecules and globin molecules. It is capable of binding to oxygen and then releasing it at a tissue site. Oxygenated hemoglobin is bright red in color and gives arterial blood its characteristic color. Because most of the red cell weight is made up of hemoglobin, hemoglobin and hematocrit levels vary directly with each other (Fig. 40-2).

A secondary function of hemoglobin is its role in

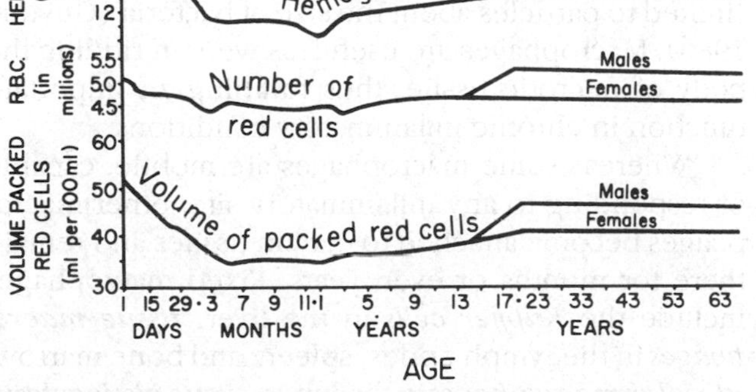

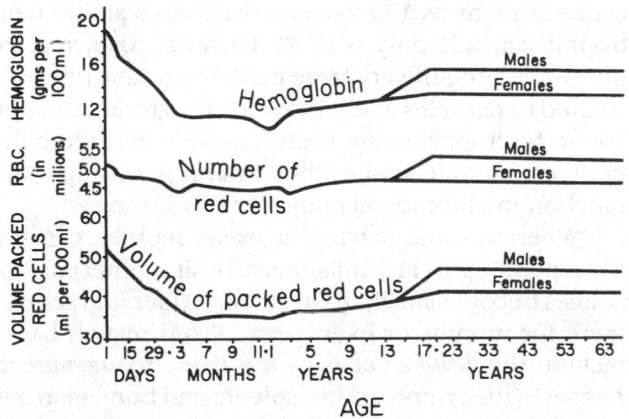

Figure 40-2. Relationship of age and sex to the hemoglobin content, red blood cell count, and volume of packed red cells (hematocrit) of the blood. (From Guyton AC: *Textbook of Medical Physiology.* 7th ed. Philadelphia, WB Saunders, 1986.)

the acid-base buffer system. Hemoglobin acts as a weak base to minimize the change in blood pH that occurs as oxygen is absorbed and carbon dioxide released in the lungs, and as oxygen is delivered and carbon dioxide taken up at the tissue level.

During intrauterine life the fetus receives oxygen indirectly, from the mother. To adapt to this lower oxygen tension, the fetus relies upon a different form of hemoglobin, called fetal hemoglobin (HgbF). HgbF efficiently binds oxygen and carbon dioxide at lower surface tensions. At 6 months' gestation, HgbF constitutes 90 per cent of the circulating hemoglobin. At birth, HgbF averages 70 per cent of the total hemoglobin but then declines rapidly so that by 6 to 12 months of age HgbF has been mostly replaced by adult hemoglobin (HgbA). Levels of 1 to 2 per cent of fetal hemoglobin persist throughout life, however.

Red Blood Cell Indices. Red blood cell indices indicate the size of the cells and their hemoglobin content. They are useful in differentiating types of anemias and are discussed in the section dealing with anemias.

Differences in RBC Concentration Related to Age, Gender, and Altitude

The number of red blood cells varies with age, gender, and the altitude at which a person lives. As illustrated in Figure 40-2, hemoglobin and hematocrit are higher at birth than ever again. The high levels at birth reflect the extra red blood cells and hemoglobin required in utero for oxygenation under conditions of lower oxygen tension. When the infant begins respirations at birth, the oxygen saturation rises from 45 per cent (normal fetal level) to 95 per cent (Pearson, 1987). This causes cessation of erythropoiesis and allows the neonate to enter a 6- to 12-week period of physiologic adaptation to extrauterine life. During this adaptive period, fetal red cells are destroyed, and hemoglobin and hematocrit levels drop to a low point called the *nadir.* The decline is commonly referred to as *physiologic anemia of infancy,* but as Pearson (1987) points out, this term is a misnomer since hemoglobin levels rarely fall below 9 gm/dl. Once hemoglobin reaches 9 to 11 gm/dl, erythropoiesis resumes to maintain hemoglobin at a mean of 12 gm/dl and hematocrit at a mean of 37 per cent during the first 6 years of life (Table 40-1).

At puberty, gender differences in red blood cell concentration become evident (Fig. 40-2). Males from that time throughout adulthood have higher mean values of RBCs, hemoglobin, and hematocrit.

Persons living at very high altitudes, where the quantity of oxygen in the air is significantly reduced, produce increased red blood cells (and consequently have higher hemoglobin and hematocrit levels). Nurses practicing in or near mountainous regions will

Table 40-1. Hematologic Values During Infancy and Childhood

	Hemoglobin g/DL		Hematocrit %		Reticu-locytes %	Leukocytes WBC/mm³		Differential Counts: Neutrophils %		Lympho-cytes %	Eosino-phils %	Mono-cytes %
Age	Mean	Range	Mean	Range	Mean	Mean	Range	Mean	Range	Mean*	Mean	Mean
Cord blood	16.8	13.7–20.1	55	45–65	5.0	18,000	(9–30,000)	61	(40–80)	31	2	6
2 wk	16.5	13.0–20.0	50	42–66	1.0	12,000	(5–21,000)	40		48	3	9
3 mo	12.0	9.5–14.5	36	31–41	1.0	12,000	(6–18,000)	30		63	2	5
6 mo–6yr	12.0	10.5–14.0	37	33–42	1.0	10,000	(6–15,000)	45		48	2	5
7–12 yr	13.0	11.0–16.0	38	34–40	1.0	8000	(4500–13,500)	55		38	2	5
Adult												
Female	14	12.0–16.0	42	37–47	1.6	7500	(5–10,000)	55	(35–70)	35	3	7
Male	16	14.0–18.0	47	42–52								

* Relatively wide range
(From Behrman and Vaughan, 1987.)

be aware that clients not only have higher RBC levels but also require these higher levels to function in their home environments. This means that resumption of functional Hgb and Hct (hematocrit) levels for these clients after blood loss or bone marrow suppression must be measured against their normal baseline values, not against norms calculated at sea level.

White Blood Cells

White blood cells can be classified into three major groups: lymphocytes, monocytes, and granulocytes. The white blood cell count or WBC (part of the complete blood count, CBC) expresses the total amount of all white cells in the blood. The white cell *differential* describes the types of white cells present (Table 40-1).

Production of White Blood Cells

Figure 40-1 illustrates the genesis of white blood cells. Pluripotential hematopoietic cells exist, from which any type of blood cell may be formed. These cells give rise to myeloid and lymphoid stem cells. Myeloid stem cells differentiate to precursors of monocytes and granulocytes. Monocyte precursors form monocytes, which are capable of becoming macrophages. Granulocyte precursors differentiate to form polymorphonuclear (segmented) neutrophils, eosinophils, and basophils. Lymphoid stem cells form T- and B-lymphocytes. Chapter 43 contains additional information on the immune functions of T-cells and B-cells. The relative percentages of lymphocytes and granulocytes among the white blood cells are shown in Table 40-1.

Polymorphonuclear cells and monocytes are normally formed in the bone marrow. Lymphocytes and plasma cells are produced in lymphogenous organs, including the lymph glands, the spleen, the thymus, the tonsils, and lymphoid tissue in the bone marrow, gut, and elsewhere (Guyton, 1986). White blood cells formed in the bone marrow, especially the granulocytes, are stored in the bone marrow until needed. Normally, the bone marrow has about a 6-day supply of granulocytes.

Function of White Blood Cells

An important function of white blood cells is to attack and destroy invading bacteria, viruses, fungi, and other foreign cells. This function falls primarily to the *neutrophils* and *monocytes.* Neutrophils are mature cells that attack and destroy bacteria and viruses both in the tissues and in the circulating blood. Monocytes, on the other hand, are immature cells and are of little help to the body's defense system in this form. When monocytes enter the body tissues, however, they develop into tissue macrophages, which are cells very effective in phagocytosis of microorganisms.

Macrophages are actually a more powerful defense than are neutrophils. A single macrophage can phagocytize as many as 100 bacteria, whereas a single neutrophil can kill only 5 to 20 bacteria. Also, macrophages can engulf very large particles; neutrophils are limited to particles about the size of bacteria (Guyton, 1986). Macrophages are useful, as well, in ridding the body of necrotic tissue, thus fulfilling an important function in chronic inflammatory conditions.

Whereas some macrophages are mobile, capable of responding to any inflammatory site, other macrophages become attached to certain tissues and remain there for months or even years. Fixed macrophages include the *Kupffer cells* in the liver, *tissue macrophages* in the lymph nodes, spleen, and bone marrow; *alveolar macrophages* in the lungs; *tissue histiocytes* in the subcutaneous tissues; and *microglia* in the brain. The combination of mobile and fixed tissue macrophages is called the *reticuloendothelial system* or the *tissue macrophage system* (Guyton, 1986).

Eosinophils function mainly in response to parasites and allergens. Eosinophils are mobile cells; they migrate to the tissues diseased by parasites where they attach to the invading organisms. They can kill immature forms of parasites by secreting chemicals the parasites find toxic. Eosinophils also appear in great numbers at sites of an allergic reaction (see Table 43-7, page 1573). They help mediate the untoward effects of the allergic response by deactivating substances such as histamine.

Basophils, like mast cells, secrete heparin into the blood stream to prevent blood coagulation and to facilitate the removal of fat particles from the blood after a fatty meal. Basophils are important to the inflammatory reaction and the allergic response because they release histamine, bradykinin, serotonin, and other substances into the injured tissues. See pages 1577–1578 for further discussion of basophils, mast cells, and the inflammatory response.

Stimulus for Production of Neutrophils and Macrophages

Tissue damage is the stimulus for increased production of neutrophils. Tissue damage may be related to an inflammatory response to infection, a malignancy, acute hemorrhage, poisoning, operative procedures, hemorrhage, or injection of foreign protein into the body (Guyton, 1986). In response to tissue damage, both the total white blood cell count and the proportion of neutrophils increase (Pearson, 1987). In its haste to supply neutrophils to fight bacteria (or another cause of tissue damage), the body often releases immature band cells or even less mature neutrophil precursors. This phenomenon is called a *"shift to the left."* Presumably the name reflects the fact that neutrophils are usually reported as the first column on the *left* of a differential count, and that a *shift* has taken place in which neutrophils now occupy a higher percentage of the total white blood cell population.

Whereas an increased number of neutrophils characterizes an acute infection or tissue damage, the response to a chronic infection is often an increase in monocytes rather than neutrophils. This results in an increased ratio of macrophages to neutrophils in the damaged tissue.

Age-Related Differences in Numbers of White Blood Cells

The proportion of neutrophils to lymphocytes changes with age (Table 40-1). Neutrophils predominate at birth but then decrease rapidly in the first weeks to reach a low point at 3 months that corresponds with the nadir of red cells. At about 5 years of age, neutrophils and lymphocytes are rather even in number. From that point neutrophils again increase in proportion until the adult mean of 55 per cent is reached at puberty. The significance of this for nurses is in interpreting values on laboratory reports. If the clientele of the laboratory is primarily children, as in a children's hospital, the forms on which the blood values are reported will often correct for age of the child. If this is not the case, however, the nurse will need to keep in mind the age-related differences in white blood cell components, especially in the young infant.

In general, younger children demonstrate a more pronounced *neutrophilia* (increased neutrophil count) in response to infection than do older children and adults. Younger children also tend to display greater numbers of immature neutrophils when neutrophil production is increased. This factor can make it difficult to evaluate an infectious process in a young child.

Platelets

Platelets are fragments of megakaryocytes (see Fig. 40-1). Megakaryocytes mature in the bone marrow where they eventually break up, each releasing some 5000 platelets into the blood (Andreoli et al, 1986). Platelets have a circulating life span of 7 to 10 days and are an integral component in blood *hemostasis* (prevention of blood loss). Among other hemostatic functions, platelets adhere to damaged blood vessel walls and aggregate, or clump together, to form plugs at the site of tissue injury. Blood flow can usually continue through the platelet plug so that the vessel remains functional. Platelet numbers normally remain stable, ranging from 150,000 to 400,000/mm³ throughout life.

Blood Clotting

Hemostasis is achieved by the following mechanisms: (1) vascular spasm, (2) formation of a platelet plug, (3) formation of a blood clot, and (4) formation of connective tissue, permanently closing the hole in the vessel (Guyton, 1986). The first three of these mechanisms are illustrated in Figure 40-3.

Vascular Spasm

A blood vessel responds to the trauma of being torn or cut by contracting for several centimeters along the vessel wall. This in turn reduces blood flow through the vessel and reduces the blood loss.

Formation of a Platelet Plug

Small holes in vessel walls can be repaired by platelet plugs. When platelets come in contact with damaged

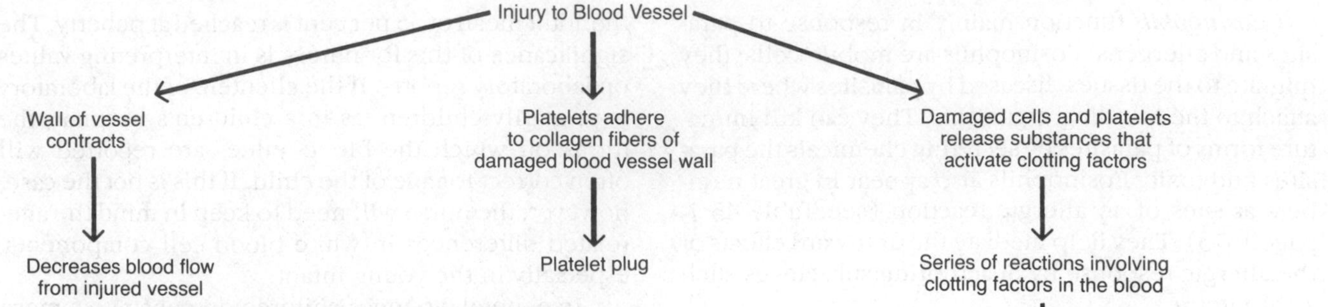
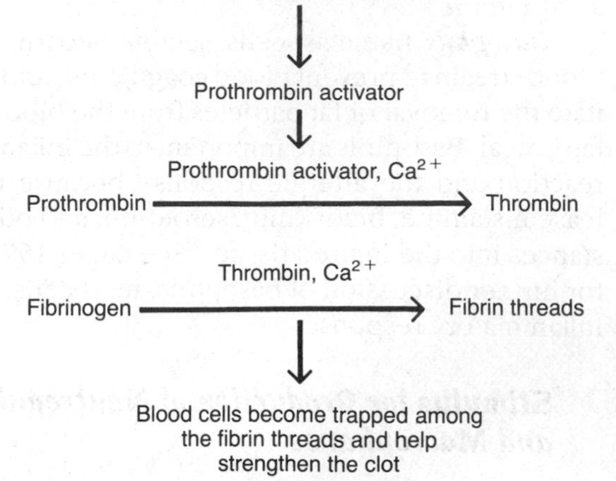

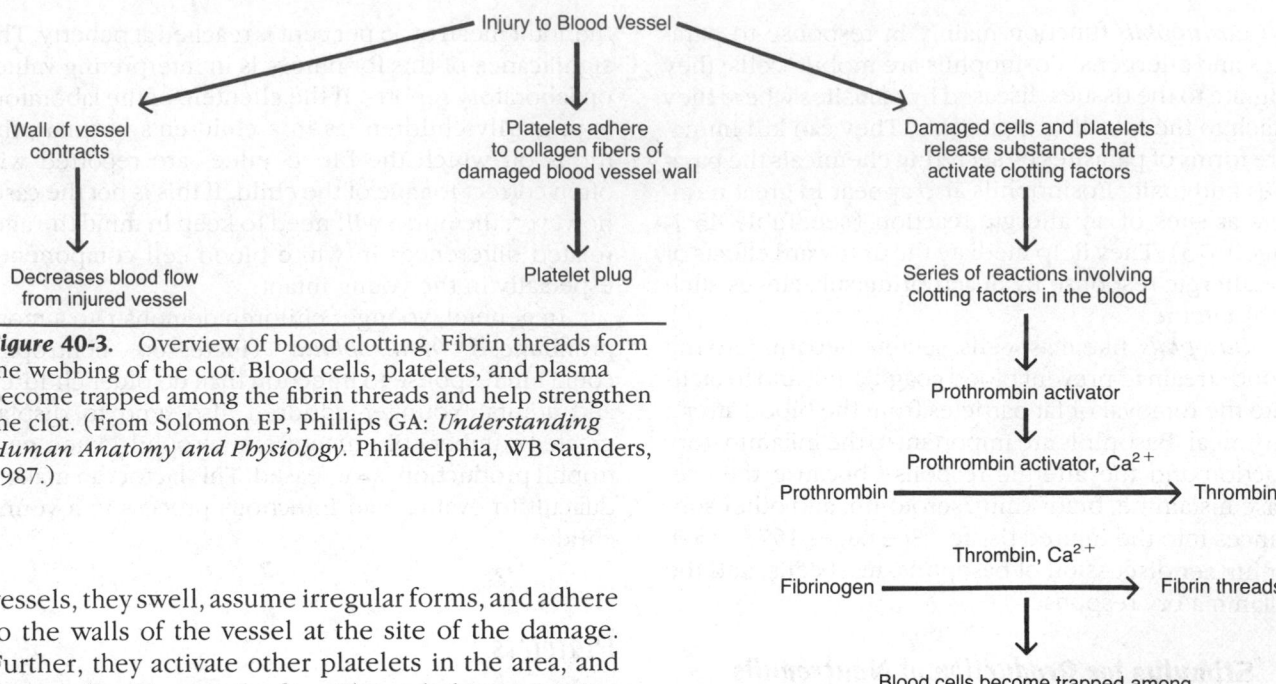

Figure 40-3. Overview of blood clotting. Fibrin threads form the webbing of the clot. Blood cells, platelets, and plasma become trapped among the fibrin threads and help strengthen the clot. (From Solomon EP, Phillips GA: *Understanding Human Anatomy and Physiology.* Philadelphia, WB Saunders, 1987.)

vessels, they swell, assume irregular forms, and adhere to the walls of the vessel at the site of the damage. Further, they activate other platelets in the area, and these cells adhere to the first. Through this succession platelets group together to "plug" the hole. The effect of decreased platelets *(thrombocytopenia)* can be seen in the multiple petechiae that occur when platelets are not available in sufficient numbers to plug the normally occurring holes in small blood vessels.

Formation of a Blood Clot

Clotting is generally agreed to occur in three steps: (1) the formation of prothrombin activator, (2) the conversion of prothrombin to thrombin, and (3) the conversion of fibrinogen into fibrin threads (Fig. 40-3). The first step is the most complex because it involves a group of clotting factors (involved in the intrinsic and extrinsic pathways). Each clotting factor depends upon the presence and activation of the one before it in the pathway, and in some cases, upon additional clotting factors as well. Table 40-2 lists the clotting factors and their synonyms.

Step One: The Formation of Prothrombin Activator. The *extrinsic pathway* is set in motion by trauma to the vascular wall and surrounding tissues. It involves conversion of factor X to activated factor X with the assistance of factor VII and chemicals released into the tissues at the time of injury (tissue factor). With the help of factor V, activated factor X forms prothrombin activator. Calcium ions are important for conversions all along the pathway.

The *intrinsic pathway* is stimulated by contact of factor XII and platelets with collagen in the wall of a damaged vessel. This pathway is even more complex, forming prothrombin activator only after a series of steps (sometimes called a "cascade") in which factors XII, XI, IX, and X are each activated in sequence. Factor VIII (which results in hemophilia when quantities are decreased) is also necessary for activation of factor X. Factor V also comes into play in the last phase of the process before prothrombin activator is formed.

Step Two: The Conversion of Prothrombin to Thrombin. Once prothrombin activator is formed it does just as its name implies and, with the assistance of calcium ions, activates available prothrombin. Pro-

Table 40-2. Clotting Factors in the Blood and Their Synonyms

Clotting Factor	Synonyms
Fibrinogen	Factor I
Prothrombin	Factor II
Tissue thromboplastin	Factor III; tissue factor
Calcium	Factor IV
Factor V	Proaccelerin; labile factor; Ac-globulin; Ac-G
Factor VII	Serum prothrombin conversion accelerator; proconvertin; SPCA; stable factor
Factor VIII	Antihemophilic factor: AHF; antihemophilic globulin; AHG; antihemophilic factor A
Factor IX	Plasma thromboplastin component; PTC; Christmas factor; antihemophilic factor B
Factor X	Stuart factor; Stuart-Prower factor
Factor XI	Plasma thromboplastin antecedent; PTA; antihemophilic factor C
Factor XII	Hageman factor
Factor XIII	Fibrin-stabilizing factor
Platelets	Thrombocytes

(From Guyton, 1986.)

thrombin is formed continually in the healthy liver, but in the event of liver disease or lack of vitamin K (needed for prothrombin formation), clotting may be impaired.

Step Three: The Conversion of Fibrinogen into Fibrin Threads. In the presence of thrombin and calcium ions, fibrinogen (also formed in the liver) is converted to fibrin threads. These threads form a fine meshwork across the damaged section of the vessel to trap blood cells, platelets, and plasma. These cells enmeshed in the fibrin strands form the blood clot and prevent further leakage through the damaged vessel wall. Within minutes after clot formation, clot retraction begins, pulling the sides of the damaged vessel closer together as the clot retracts. Platelets are essential to bonding of fibrin threads to form the meshwork for the clot. They also contribute to clot contraction.

Once formed, the clot can either form the base for new connective tissue or can undergo a process of lysis and dissipate. Often the clot is invaded by fibroblasts, and fibrous connective tissue is formed within 7 to 10 days (Guyton, 1986). If the clot is very large, however, such as a site of tissue hemorrhage, the clot itself secretes lytic enzymes (such as fibrinolysin) that digest the clot.

Diagnostic Assessment

The comon diagnostic tests to measure the type and number of blood cells and characteristics of blood clotting capacity are listed in Table 40-3. Normal values for these tests can be found in Table 40-1 and in Appendix Seven.

Disorders of Red Blood Cells

Anemias constitute the most common hematologic disorder in children. Anemia is defined as a decrease in either the total number of circulating red blood cells, a decrease in the concentration of hemoglobin, or both. Anemias can be classified on the basis of etiology or by the morphologic description of the red cells. Etiologic classification divides anemia into three categories:

- blood loss, which may occur from acute or chronic hemorrhage;
- excessive blood destruction, which may be due to structural defects of the RBC;
- decreased or impaired production, which originates in the bone marrow and may be acquired or constitutional.

The red blood cells indices reported on the CBC are measurements of the erythrocyte size and hemoglobin content. Indices tell whether the red cell size and shape is *microcytic* (small), *normocytic* (normal), or *macrocytic* (large) and whether the color is *hypochromic* (pale, indicating less than normal hemoglobin concentration) or *normochromic* (normal). The morphologically descriptive name may be used to define an anemia, for example "normochromic, microcytic," especially if the etiology has not been determined. The red blood cell indices are:

- *MCV*, the mean cell volume or size of an individual red blood cell;
- *MCHC*, the mean cell hemoglobin concentration; a measure of the hemoglobin concentration in 100 ml of red blood cells; and
- *MCH*, the mean cell hemoglobin or the hemoglobin concentration of each individual red blood cell. Table 40-4 correlates the indices with the descriptive terms.

Regardless of etiology or morphology, *tissue hypoxia* is the major consequence of anemia. The degree of hypoxia determines the severity of symptoms. Mild anemia is most often asymptomatic and may not be diagnosed except for the presence of another unrelated illness or routine screening. Severe anemia, on the other hand, affects virtually every organ system and, if untreated, will eventually result in death.

Iron Deficiency Anemia

Iron deficiency anemia is the most common nutritional deficiency during childhood. It is the most frequently encountered form of anemia in children in the United States and in the world. Nurses can play a major role both in the prevention and treatment of this disorder.

Pathophysiology

Hemoglobin synthesis is dependent on a constant supply of iron. In fact, 3.4 mg of iron is required to make 1 gm of hemoglobin (or 1 mg of iron is needed for every 1 ml of packed red cells). On the average, 0.5 mg to 1.5 mg of iron must be absorbed daily to maintain iron balance in the nonpregnant, nonbleeding adult (Lanzkowsky, 1980). In this adult population, the body's iron needs are normally met by absorption of iron from dietary sources. If an iron deficit occurs, the production of hemoglobin decreases and anemia develops, resulting in a reduced oxygen-carrying capacity of the blood.

Etiology

Infancy is the period of the greatest postnatal growth velocity in the life cycle. Infants normally triple their birth weight during the first year of life. Accompanying the weight increase is a corresponding increase in

Table 40-3. Common Hematologic Tests*

Test	Explanation
Complete blood count:	Frequently ordered for screening purposes
White blood count (WBC)	Total number of circulating white blood cells
Differential white count (Diff)	Percentage of the total WBC made up of neutrophils, eosinophils, basophils, lymphocytes, and monocytes
Red blood count (RBC)	Total number of circulating red blood cells
Hematocrit (Hct)	The percentage of red blood cells in a volume of whole blood
Hemoglobin (Hgb)	Measures the oxygen-carrying capacity of blood
Red blood cell indices	Define the size and hemoglobin content of RBCs
Platelet count	Total number of circulating platelets
Erythrocyte sedimentation rate	The rate at which RBCs settle out of unclotted blood in 1 hour
Hemoglobin electrophoresis	Identifies the types and percentages of hemoglobin in the blood; distinguishes between sickle cell trait and disease
Sickledex	Identifies the presence (but not the percentage) of sickle hemoglobin
Reticulocyte count	Numbers of immature RBCs (reticulocytes) compared to total RBCs: Indicates an increase in RBC production and/or an increase in RBC destruction
Stained red cell examination	Provides information about erythrocyte size, shape, structure, hemoglobin content, and staining properties. May indicate that cells are: • *normochromic*—have normal Hgb content and color; • *hypochromic*—decreased Hgb and color; • *normocytic*—normal size and shape; • *poikilocytic*—abnormal sizes and shapes, such as ***target cells*** (thinner than normal RCBs), *spherocytes* (small, round rather than biconcave), ***sickle cells*** (crescent or sickle shape), *schistocytes* (fragmented RBCs with bizarre shapes); • *microcytic*—abnormally small; • *macrocytic*—abnormally large
Partial thromboplastin time (PTT)	Time required for clotting of plasma; fibrin clot formation; assesses *Phase I* of clotting mechanism: adequacy of factors XII, XI, IX, and VIII
Activated partial thromboplastin time (APTT)	Same as for PTT but more sensitive and faster to perform
Prothrombin consumption test (PCT)	Determination of prothrombin in serum after coagulation of whole blood; tests for *phase I* factors
Thromboplastin generation test	A deficiency of any of the *Phase I* factors will lead to an abnormal generation of thromboplastin
Prothrombin time (Pro time, PT)	The time it takes plasma to clot after thromboplastin and calcium are added. Directly measures a defect in any of these *Phase II* clotting mechanisms: prothrombin, fibrinogen, factor V, factor VII, and factor X
Thrombin time	Time required for plasma to clot after the addition of bovine thrombin. Detects inadequate levels of fibrinogen; *Phase III*
Mean corpuscular volume (MCV)	Expresses the volume occupied by a single red blood cell. It indicates whether the red blood cells appear: • *normocytic*—of normal size; • *microcytic*—smaller than normal; • *macrocytic*—larger than normal
Mean corpuscular hemoglobin concentration (MCHC)	A calculated value, MCHC is an expression of the average concentration of hemoglobin in the red blood cells; i.e., the ratio of the weight of hemoglobin to the volume of RBCs
Mean corpuscular hemoglobin (MCH)	A measure of the average weight of hemoglobin in the red blood cell. Less accurate than the MCHC because it uses the red cell count in its calculation and that count may be inaccurate

* See Table 40-1 and Appendix Seven for normal values.

blood volume. During the first year of life, 150 mg to 200 mg of iron must be absorbed to provide enough iron to essentially double the total volume of red blood cells (and therefore hemoglobin). A daily iron absorption of 0.75 mg to 0.80 mg is required to meet this need (Lanzkowsky, 1980).

Full-term infants are born with some iron stores. The iron is stored at numerous sites but principally in the liver, bone marrow, spleen, and skeletal muscles. Essentially, all of this iron storage occurs during the third trimester of gestation, paralleling the period of greatest fetal weight gain. Premature babies miss this period of rapidly increasing iron storage and, therefore, are born with substantially less iron reserve. The

Table 40-4. Morphologic Description of Red Blood Cells Correlated with Red Blood Cell Indices

	MCV (mean cell volume, femto-liters)	MCH (mean cell hemoglobin, picograms)	MCHC (mean cell hemoglobin concentration, %)
Macrocytic	>94	35–40	>30
Microcytic	<70	12–29	<30
Normocytic	80–94	26–34	>30

(Modified from Klopovich, 1983.)

iron stores of the full-term infant will normally meet the baby's needs for 4 to 6 months. The premature baby's iron supply lasts significantly less time and is depleted by 2 to 3 months of age.

After complete utilization of the iron stores available at birth, the baby must rely solely on dietary sources to meet minimum daily iron requirements. Milk is the primary (and often the sole) source of nutrition for infants. Breast and cow's milk are poor sources of iron, containing only 0.5 mg to 1.5 mg iron per liter (Oski, 1981).

Not all the iron available in a food source is absorbed by the body. In fact, the "bioavailability" of iron from most food sources ranges from 1 to 20 per cent. Foods in the vegetable family rank on the lower end of the spectrum; meat sources are on the higher end. The average diet of combined food sources is generally believed to provide an iron absorption rate of 10 per cent. Infant formulas and cow's milk likewise provide only about 10 per cent iron absorption (Oski, 1981). In addition, the phosphate in milk binds with iron, removing it from the body. In other words, a food source containing 10 mg of iron per serving would have 1 mg (or 10 per cent) of iron actually absorbed by the intestine. A notable exception is breast milk which has an iron absorption rate of about 50 per cent (Oski, 1981).

To meet the daily requirement of 0.75 mg to 0.80 mg absorbed iron, the nonbreastfed infant requires a diet containing 7.5 mg to 8 mg of iron per day. If a diet consists of only nonfortified milk or formula, approximately two gallons per day are needed to meet the iron requirements! Consider that the recommended daily allowance for iron is the same for infants and adult males. These examples help illustrate why infants are at high risk to develop iron deficiency anemia.

Toddlers are also at risk because of their rapid growth during this period and the likelihood of inadequate iron intake. Milk is still a major food and caloric source at this age. Many high iron content foods are not preferred by picky toddlers. The high-bulk diet characteristic of some ethnic groups also reduces the body's utilization of iron because the foodstuffs are moved out of the gastrointestinal tract faster, resulting in less opportunity for iron absorption.

Causes of iron deficiency anemia other than dietary deficiency in toddlers are less common. Impaired iron absorption associated with conditions such as persistent or severe diarrhea or malabsorption syndromes may lead to iron deficiency anemia. This anemia may also be secondary to pica, lead poisoning, or intestinal parasite infection—all of which have a higher incidence during toddlerhood. Intestinal bleeding from cow's milk allergy may also cause anemia. Unless an iron supplement is given, children with chronic illness may have difficulty ingesting or utilizing adequate iron because of excessive need or poor absorption related to infection, the disease process, or iron absorption inhibiting effects of medications used to treat the chronic illness.

Incidence

Iron deficiency anemia can occur at any age but occurs most frequently between the ages of 6 months to 3 years and during adolescence. The child with small iron stores at birth (i.e., preterm infants) is at particular risk. Various surveys show that between 17 to 44 per cent of infants have some degree of iron deficiency anemia (Lukens, 1984). The disorder occurs most frequently in lower socioeconomic groups where both the knowledge of and ability to procure iron-rich foods may be limited but, of course, can occur in any child. The incidence of iron deficiency anemia in adolescents may range from 11 to 27 per cent (Lukens, 1984). The adolescent is experiencing a growth spurt, second in velocity only to the first year of life. The red blood cell mass of the adolescent is rapidly expanding to accompany the increased body mass. The increase in circulating hemoglobin mass is two times greater in adolescent males than in female counterparts. However, girls have the additional burden of blood loss during menstruation (20 mg of iron per menses) (Lukens, 1984). Both male and female adolescents are notorious for diets that are low in absorbable iron. Fast food, fad diets, and skipped meals all contribute to the development of iron deficiency anemia.

Clinical Manifestations

Children with slowly developing anemias may show no clinical symptoms even though their hemoglobin may be as low as 6 gm/dl. If signs and symptoms are present, they are likely to be vague and nonspecific. Symptoms of irritability and anorexia and signs such as pallor of skin and mucous membranes may have occurred insidiously; the parents are frequently unaware of their presence. Children with anemia of long duration may have some degree of growth retardation. Thirty to fifty-six per cent of iron deficient children are below the tenth percentile for weight at the time of diagnosis, but the heights of these children are normally distributed (Lukens, 1984). Exercise intolerance—impairing both performance and endurance—frequently occurs in iron deficient states, but once again, the onset is so gradual that caregivers may accept this as the child's norm. Often, a coincidental infection is the parent's sole reason for seeking medical help.

Diagnostic Assessment

The diagnostic process involves obtaining (1) a careful history and physical examination, (2) blood smear and red blood cell indices, and (3) serum iron and iron-binding studies. The nurse is often the first to notice symptoms suggestive of iron deficiency anemia and usually is responsible for gathering the history and conducting or participating in data collection, including physical examination and laboratory testing. The nurse should explain each procedure involved in terms the child and parent can comprehend. Parents should also be given enough information to understand the cause and meaning of the data in a manner that tactfully avoids accusations about their child care skills or ridicules their cultural beliefs or practices.

History and Physical Examination

The history must include information on the child's diet, activity, appetite, rate of growth, recent blood loss, and birth history. Physical examination should include evaluation of the child's oral, nasal, and conjunctival mucosa; the abdomen for splenomegaly; capillary refill of the nailbeds; auscultation for cardiac flow murmurs; general motor development; skin coloring; weight; and any evidence of infection. Mucosal and skin pallor and deficient capillary refill along with a history of iron deficient diet or pica are suggestive of anemia. (Pica involves repeated or chronic ingestion of inedible substances such as clay, plaster, paint, and earth.) Blood studies are indicated in the presence of significant history and physical findings.

Blood Studies

Tissue hypoxia, produced by the decreased supply of oxygen being carried by the blood as a result of decreased hemoglobin production, stimulates the bone marrow to continue producing red blood cells. Therefore, the RBC count is usually normal or only slightly reduced in anemia and typically is disproportionate with the decreased hemoglobin concentration. Hemoglobin is low because the iron required to form it is not available. Anemia is generally defined as hemoglobin less than 10 gm/dl. Since the red cells are not fully filled with hemoglobin when they are released into the blood, they are microcytic and hypochromic. The red cell indices in iron deficiency anemia shows MCV less than 80 femtoliters, MCH less than 27 picograms, and MCHC less than 30 per cent (Waskerwitz, 1983).

The diagnosis of iron deficiency anemia can most often be made from a standard blood smear and the clinical history. Additional studies may be required to distinguish iron deficiency anemia from other microcytic, hypochromic anemias and to re-examine patients with anemia who do not respond to iron therapy.

The three most useful additional studies are (1) serum ferritin, (2) transferrin saturation, and (3) free erythrocyte porphyrin (FEP). Ferritin levels increase or decrease proportionately to the levels of storage iron and are, therefore, a reliable indicator of the level of the body iron stores. One microgram (μg) of ferritin represents 8 mg of storage iron (Waskerwitz, 1983). Ferritin levels would therefore be reduced ($<$10 to 12 μg/ml) in iron deficiency anemia. Serum iron levels are decreased in iron deficiency anemia; however, the total iron-binding capacity (TIBC) is increased. TIBC is actually a measurement of serum transferrin, the substance that transports iron from storage sites to the tissues that synthesize it. Transferrin levels become elevated in iron-deficient states. Transferrin saturation is calculated by the following formula:

$$\frac{\text{serum iron}}{\text{TIBC}} \times 100 = \%\ \text{transferrin saturation}$$

Transferrin saturation is an indication of the adequacy of iron flow from blood to developing new cells in the bone marrow. Levels less than 7 per cent are definitive for iron deficiency anemia.

In developing red blood cells, substances called protoporphyrins chemically bind with iron to become heme. If iron is deficient, the protoporphyrins remain unbound and accumulate and can be measured in high levels in the blood. FEP levels greater than 10 to 11 μg/dl are characteristic in iron deficiency anemia.

Therapeutic Management

Iron deficiency anemia can be easily treated with oral iron therapy. However, unless permanent dietary changes are made, the child is in danger of repeated occurrence. The American Academy of Pediatrics Committee on Nutrition makes the following recommendations for infants:

- Iron supplements from one or more sources should start no later than at 4 months of age in full-term infants and no later than at 2 months in preterm infants.
- In formula-fed infants the most convenient and best sources of supplemental iron are iron-fortified formulas and 2 servings per day of iron-fortified cereal.
- The intake of supplemental iron should not exceed 1 mg/kg/day for a full-term infant and 2 mg/kg/day for preterm infants to a maximum intake of 15 mg/day.
- The maintenance of breastfeeding for 6 months or more should protect against the development of iron deficiency anemia in full-term infants, but preterm infants require ferrous sulfate drops after 2 months of age. Iron-fortified cereals should be given when solids are introduced.
- Commercially available infant formulas are preferable to fresh milk during the first 6 to 12 months of age. Excessive ingestion of fresh cow's milk may contribute to iron deficiency by causing increased gastrointestinal blood loss. (There is a substance in fresh cow's milk which, unless inactivated by heating, may induce protein-losing enteropathy and gastrointestinal bleeding in infants, probably on the basis of hypersensitivity or allergy [Oski, 1981].)
- If infants receive fresh cow's milk after 6 months of age, their total daily milk intake should not exceed three fourths of a quart (24 ounces). Infants who continue to receive formula after 6 months of age should receive no more than one quart (32 ounces) of formula per day in order to encourage the introduction of iron-rich solid foods and set the pattern for a more varied diet.

Daily administration of an oral iron supplement (usually Fer-In-Sol) is prescribed. The therapeutic dose is 6 mg/kg/day given in three divided doses. The elemental or ferrous form (ferrous sulfate) is normally used because it is better absorbed than the ferric form and is less likely to cause gastrointestinal irritation. It should be offered between meals when digestive acid concentration is highest in order to facilitate absorption. The supplement may be given with a citrus fruit or juice high in ascorbic acid to enhance its solubility and absorption.

Major Nursing Diagnoses for Anemia

***Activity intolerance**, related to reduced oxygen-carrying capacity of the blood associated with an iron deficit*

***Potential impaired tissue integrity: subcutaneous**, related to improper injection technique associated with parenteral iron injection*

***Potential for injury: poisoning: child or siblings**, related to accidental ingestion of iron supplement tablets*

Strategies for Nursing Care

Strategies pertaining to the nursing diagnosis of activity intolerance are common to any type of anemia and are addressed in Table 40-5 on the next page. The following additional strategies are specific to iron deficiency anemia.

Providing Dietary Sources of Iron. Guidelines for infant nutrition with regard to iron intake were listed previously. The nurse needs to be aware of iron sources for the older child. Children need iron-rich foods every day. Organ meats, dried legumes, shellfish, and muscle meats are the richest sources of iron and have the highest iron absorption rate. Other good iron sources include nuts, green vegetables, unsweetened chocolate, dried fruits, and whole wheat or iron-enriched flours and breads, but the iron in these food is less well absorbed than the iron from meats and legumes. The iron in eggs is poorly absorbed unless these are eaten with a good food source of vitamin C. Substantial sources of vitamin C are provided by citrus fruits, green vegetables, and liver.

Protein intake, especially from animal sources, and vitamin C intake should also be increased, as both of these enhance the intestinal absorption of iron from foodstuffs. If the previous diet was high in bulk, bulk intake should be reduced. Milk intake should be limited to a *maximum* of one quart per day, allowing calories to be provided by other food sources to lower phosphate levels, which inhibit iron absorption.

In presenting this nutrition education, the nurse must provide information that is realistic in terms of the family's economic resources, attitudes regarding food, and cultural practices. For example, if beef is not a practical source of iron and protein because of the family's finances or religious and cultural beliefs, the nurse might instead encourage increased intake of dried beans, peanut butter, or turkey, which also are iron-rich protein sources. The caretaker who plans meals and does the grocery shopping may need the nurse's assistance to learn how to plan balanced meals rich in vitamin C, protein and iron or how to shop for low-cost foods high in these nutrients. Parents unfamiliar with food sources with high iron content may appreciate recipes and preparation guidelines for these foods. Positive reinforcement of the caretaker's efforts and successes in providing the child with the proper nutrition to prevent or correct an iron-deficient diet should continue until these diet measures become habitual food practices. Often parents need simple instruction in basic nutrition before being taught

Table 40-5
Nursing Process Plan: The Child with Anemia

By Roxie Foster

Assessment of Physical Function

Activity/Exercise
Nutrition/Metabolism

Subjective Assessment

Fatigability in relation to activities appropriate to developmental age; report of child's progress on developmental tasks, especially as related to motor activity; client and family eating patterns

Objective Assessment

Pulse and respirations at rest and with activity; fever or other indication of infection; tissue perfusion (especially in the CNS and the periphery); observable developmental tasks; height, weight, status on growth chart; gastrointestinal integrity; color of skin and mucous membranes; diagnostic tests; complete blood count; blood smear; reticulocyte count; serum iron and iron-binding test; stool and urine for occult blood; serum bilirubin

Analysis: Nursing Diagnosis

Activity intolerance, related to reduced oxygen-carrying capacity of the blood

Defining Characteristics

For anemia regardless of etiology:

Subjective: Headache; vertigo; weakness; irritability; easy fatigability; anorexia

For chronic anemia:

Failure to progress normally on the growth chart; developmental delays; clubbing of the digits

For iron deficiency anemia:

Evidence of inadequate dietary intake of iron; (occasionally) blood loss in the stool; microcytic, hypochromic RBCs; RBC count normal or near normal; decreased serum ferritin and iron, increased iron-boinding capacity (TIBC) and free erythrocyte porphyrin (FEP)

For aplastic anemia:

Normochromic, normocytic RBCs in reduced numbers; leukopenia; thrombocytopenia

For anemia related to infectious processes:

Decreased RBC count; normochromic, normocytic RBCs; leukocytosis; possible fever and other evidence of infection

Objective: Tachycardia and dyspnea, especially with activity; pallor of skin and mucous membranes; hemoglobin <10 gm/dl and/or RBC <4 million /cu mm (Green, 1986)

For anemia associated with prematurity:

Nadir* at 1 to 3 months of age with hemoglobin at 7–8 gm/dl for infants weighing 1000–1500 gm at birth; 9.5 gm/dl for infants with birth weights between 2000 and 2500 gm (Green, 1986)

For hemolytic anemia:

Nausea; vomiting; diarrhea; abdominal pain; jaundice; hepatosplenomegaly (Green, 1986)

For anemia related to blood loss:

Normochromic, normocytic anemia; leukocytosis; reticulocytosis; possible evidence of blood in the urine and/or stool

* Nadir is that time in infancy when hemoglobin level is at its lowest; stores from the mother are depleted and bone marrow activity in the infant has not yet compensated.

Client Goal/ Evaluation Criteria	Nursing Goals/Strategies (Selected Rationale)
1. The client will balance metabolic demands for oxygen with the blood's ability to carry oxygen as evidenced by:	
a. pulse and respirations that return to normal limits within 15 minutes after increased activity (i.e., crying and feeding for the infant, loud crying and gross motor activity for the toddler and older child)	*Monitor pulse and respirations* before, during and after periods of activity (to assess the body's ability to compensate for the increased oxygen demand related to exercise). *Indicate the child's activity on the graphic record* each time routine vital signs are taken (to facilitate accurate comparison). *Utilize play therapy and visits from the family* to decrease the child's anxiety and irritability. (Fussing and agitation increase oxygen demands and increase fatigue.) Ensure that the family understands the relationship between activity and the body's demand for oxygen (to facilitate home care).
b. absence of signs and symptoms of congestive heart failure (CHF)	*Monitor for signs and symptoms of congestive heart failure* (related to the heart's inability to compensate, through tachycardia, for decreased oxygen-carrying capacity). *Monitor heart and lung sounds; report adventitious sounds.* If CHF is suspected, record weight daily. (Weight is a sensitive indicator of fluid rentention.)
c. adequate perfusion to the central nervous system and to the periphery	*Assess, monitor, and chart change in mental status, and color of skin and mucous membranes.*
d. absence of fever and infectious processes	*Measure temperature every 4 hours.* Monitor for prodromal signs and symptoms of illness such as irritability, malaise, nasal discharge, sore throat, dullness of the eyes. *Protect the child from nosocomial infection* by careful handwashing (especially in aplastic anemia because of the reduced lymphocytes). *Ensure that the family understands that fever and infection increase the metabolic demand for oxygen and that some infections interfere with the body's ability to produce RBCs.* Caution them about keeping the child away from crowds and ill people.
e. absence of fatigue in response to activity appropriate for age	*Plan and implement rest periods for the hospitalized child* that produce the desired outcomes.

special diet measures. Instruction should always include the reasons for and intended effect of these foods on the child's health state.

Teaching Parents to Administer Iron Supplements. The nurse has a major responsibility in educating parents to carry out the treatment regimen. This must be done tactfully and within the framework of the family's income, customs and food preferences. The nurse also has a role in helping parents overcome their feeling that they are to blame for their child's anemia and rebuilding the wavering confidence they have in their parenting abilities. Positive reinforcement of even minor efforts to comply with the treatment regimen, frequent pointing out of signs of the child's improved health state, and support through regular phone calls or home visits help restore feelings of parental adequacy. These feelings, in turn, yield greater cooperation for what needs to be done currently and on a long-term basis to resolve the child's anemia and prevent its recurrence.

Parents need to be aware of the differences between Fer-In-Sol Syrup and Fer-In-Sol Drops. Although both are forms of ferrous sulfate, the syrup contains only 6 mg/ml of elemental iron, whereas the drops contain 25 mg/ml. This significant difference in elemental iron content will obviously affect dosing instructions. The nurse should make sure that the parents understand whether drops or syrup have been recommended and that they realize the differing iron content of each.

Parents should be cautioned that liquid iron preparations may temporarily stain the child's teeth. Therefore, liquid iron should be taken through a straw or administered with a dropper to the back of the mouth. As an extra precaution, the child's teeth may be brushed after each administration. Parents should also be informed that the child's stool will turn a tarry green when adequate iron levels are reached. The nurse should assess for this occurrence periodically as an indicator of adequacy in administration or dose.

Although side effects are rare in children, oral iron does sometimes cause gastrointestinal irritation, nausea and vomiting, diarrhea or constipation, and anorexia. If gastrointestinal side effects do occur, the iron should be given with meals or right after meals. Sometimes the iron is initially prescribed with meals so the intestinal mucosa has time to build up some tolerance to the drug; after 3 or 4 days, the iron is administered between meals so that absorption is greater. Another alternative is to initially give lower doses of the iron, gradually increasing to a therapeutic dose within 3 to 5 days in an effort to avoid the adverse effects of the drug.

Hemoglobin and hematocrit levels begin improving immediately after oral iron therapy is begun. This can be observed or monitored via the reticulocyte count. Normally 1 per cent of the circulating RBCs are very immature forms called reticulocytes. In a child with iron deficiency anemia, 3 to 5 days of iron therapy will increase the production of red blood cells. The reticulocyte count will rise dramatically and reach maximum levels at 5 to 10 days. Lack of improvement is often attributable to inconsistent or inaccurate oral iron administration. If this is the suspected cause, a community health nurse may be assigned to administer the oral supplement or to teach, supervise, and support caretakers to gain their compliance with the prescribed regimen.

Normal hemoglobin values are usually attained 2 months after oral iron therapy begins. The iron preparation should be continued for at least 2 months longer to replenish the depleted iron stores. Children treated only until the anemia is corrected are likely to have recurrences of iron deficiency anemia.

Safely Administering Parenteral Iron. In some instances an anemic child cannot take an oral iron supplement because of the following reasons: severe intolerance, pre-existing gastrointestinal disorders that may interfere with intestinal absorption, acute surgery with anesthesia, or serious systemic infection concurrently. Under these circumstances, parenteral iron therapy may be ordered. The preferred route for parenteral iron (Imferon) is by intramuscular injection. The Z-track technique should be utilized to minimize skin discoloration and irritation. In addition, a fresh needle should be used to inject the medicine after drawing it from the vial, and a small amount of air should be allowed in the syringe. Both these actions will avoid tracking the medicine through the subcutaneous tissue.

Avoiding Accidental Ingestion of Iron Supplement. Iron poisoning has been known to cause death in children who have ingested as few as six iron tablets at one time (Pearson, 1987). Therefore, teaching parents to keep the medication out of the reach of children cannot be overstressed. No more than one month's supply of iron should be kept in the home.

Nursing Strategies for Follow-Up Care in the Home or Clinic

Obtain a blood sample as indicated for evaluation of hemoglobin and hematocrit.

Assess for signs of therapeutic action of the iron supplement: a gradual increase in activity, decreasing irritability, return of appetite, increased reticulocyte count within 3 to 5 days of beginning the iron supplement, and return of hemoglobin levels to normal limits after two months of therapy (Lukens, 1984).

Determine whether the child has been suffering GI upset from the iron preparation and suggest alternative administration methods.

Assess nutritional adequacy through a 24-hour recall.

Sickle Cell Anemia

Sickle cell anemia is a chronic disease resulting from a hemoglobin defect. Valine is substituted for glutamic acid in the sixth amino acid position of the β-globin chain of the hemoglobin molecule. The disease is transmitted genetically in an autosomal recessive fashion. The child with sickle cell anemia produces abnormal, sickle hemoglobin (Hgb S) rather than Hgb A. The child with *sickle cell trait* has inherited a sickle gene (Hb S) from one parent and a normal hemoglobin gene (Hb A) from the other parent. Sickle cell trait does not progress to sickle cell anemia. The child with sickle cell trait is a carrier of the disease, sickle cell anemia, and is almost always asymptomatic. Approximately 8 per cent of black Americans have sickle cell trait (Pearson, 1987).

Etiology

Sickle cell anemia results when the child inherits two abnormal recessive Hb S genes, one from each parent. (See the discussion of autosomal recessive inheritance, p. 145.) Children with sickle cell anemia have red cells that contain up to 80 to 100 per cent Hb S, the remainder being fetal hemoglobin (Hb F) and Hb A_2, a minor adult hemoglobin. Sickle cell anemia is a potentially fatal disease that occurs predominantly in the black race. The incidence is 1:625 births in American blacks (Gradolf, 1983).

The child with sickle trait also synthesizes Hb S, but because of the heterozygous state has the ability to produce HbA as well and usually does not experience symptoms. The red blood cells of children with sickle cell trait contain 30 to 40 per cent Hb S.

Pathophysiology

Hemoglobin S, sickle hemoglobin, is much less soluble than normal hemoglobin when deoxygenated. This is a direct result of the amino acid substitution in the hemoglobin molecule that occurs in this disorder. The decreased solubility of Hb S causes it to become more viscous and to crystalize, thereby deforming the shape of the cell. *Sickling* is the term used to describe the red blood cell change from the normal, round shape to a crescent or sickle shape. Sickling can occur in the red blood cells of persons with sickle cell anemia when oxygen tension or concentration is reduced or as a result of acidosis or other forms of stress (Figure 40-4).

Once sickled, RBCs are more rigid, fragile, and rapidly destroyed. They lose the ability to flow easily through tiny capillary beds; the sickled cells may become clumped, causing obstructions and impairment of blood flow beyond the obstruction. This results in severe tissue hypoxia and, subsequently, more sickling. As the hypoxia worsens, infarcts and necrosis may develop. The duration and size of the ischemic area will determine the extent of the injury. Conditions that predispose to sickling include infection, dehydration, hypoxia, fever, high altitudes, vigorous exercise, and emotional stress.

Clinical Manifestations

Clinical symptoms of sickle cell anemia are the results of (a) the decreased life span of the red cells—that is, hemolysis and the compensatory mechanisms evoked by the subsequent anemia and (b) the formation of thrombi in the small vessels of various organs as a result of sickling. General manifestations of sickle cell anemia include pallor, weakness, easy fatigability and jaundice as a result of hemolysis, and tissue hypoxia. Children with sickle cell anemia begin to demonstrate growth abnormalities around 7 years of age. Both

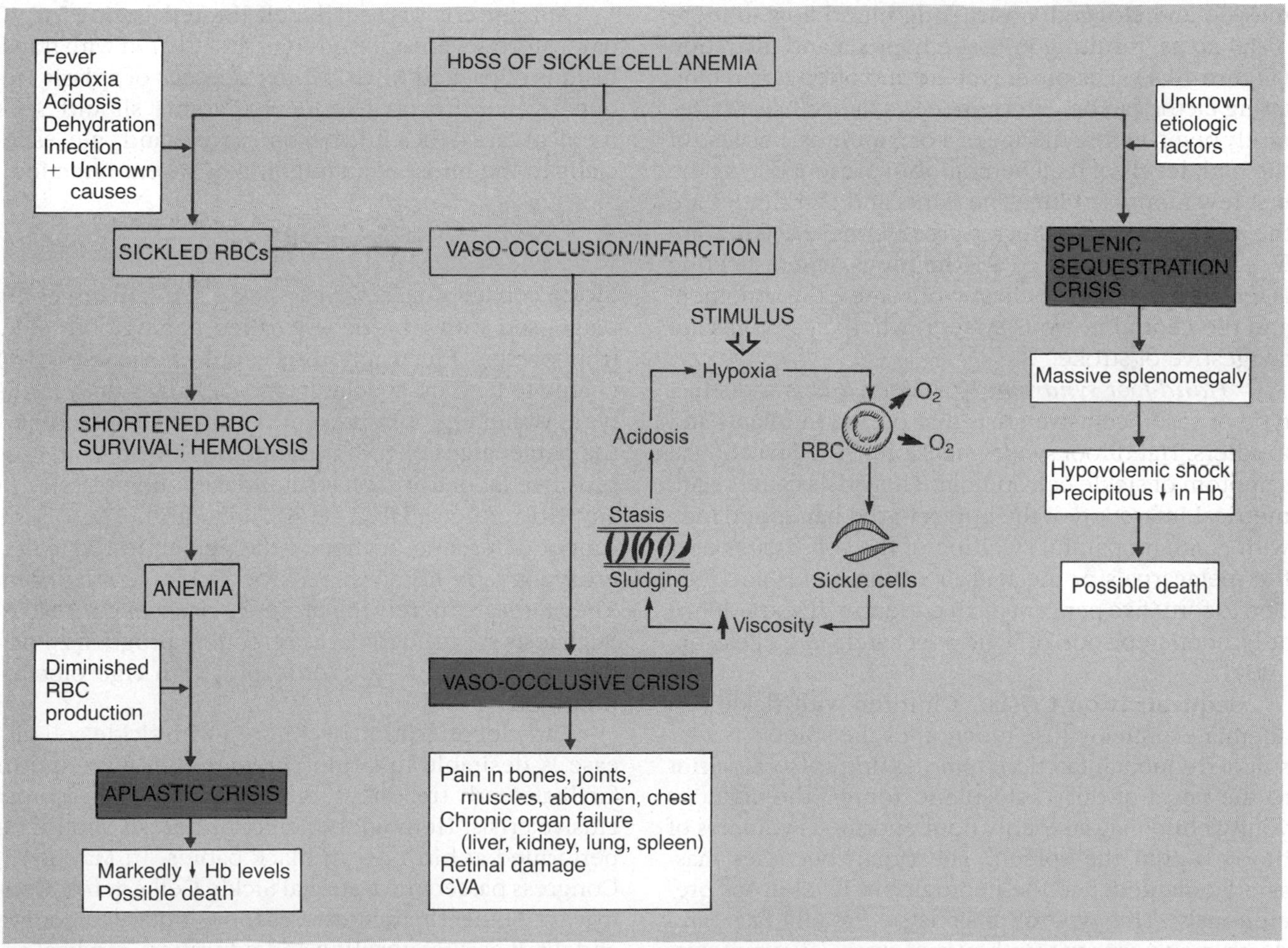

Figure 40-4. The pathophysiology of sickle cell anemia, including the three types of sickle cell crisis and the resulting clinical manifestations.

height and weight are below average, and puberty is usually delayed. The heart becomes progressively enlarged as a result of increased cardiac output associated with chronic anemia. The kidneys lose the ability to effectively concentrate urine as a result of renal medulla damage from tissue hypoxia, which results in enuresis and nocturia in 50 per cent of children with sickle cell disease. In addition microthrombi from clumped sickled cells cause progressive damage to multiple organs, including the eye, liver, and lungs.

Sickle Cell Crisis

A "crisis" is not a specific disease entity. Rather, it is an acute, painful event of various, sometimes unknown, etiology that occurs throughout the life of the person with sickle cell anemia. The frequency of these crises may range from an almost constant occurrence to a nearly asymptomatic life. Most patients fall in between these two extremes. The average child with sickle cell disease has 4 to 5 painful crises per year, one of which is severe enough to require hospitalization (Pearson, 1984). Crises can be classified into three main groups: (1) vaso-occlusive; (2) sequestration; and (3) aplastic.

Vaso-Occlusive Crisis. This is the most common, or classic, type of crisis. Sickled cells become massed and clogged, obstructing blood flow to more distal areas, resulting in tissue hypoxia and infarction (Figure 40-4). The onset is acute and often no precipitating factor can be determined. Vaso-occlusive crises rarely begin before the age of 4 or 5 months, because of the high levels of fetal hemoglobin present during the first few months of life. The joints and extremities are the most commonly affected areas. Other areas that are less frequently involved are the lungs, where sickling is referred to as "acute chest syndrome"; the abdomen; and the central nervous system, where symptoms are suggestive of stroke.

"*Hand-foot syndrome*" or *dactylitis* is a distinct type of vaso-occlusive crisis that occurs in infants and toddlers. Hand-foot syndrome is often the first clinical symptom of sickle cell anemia. This crisis causes symmetrical infarction of the bones in the hands and feet, with resultant painful swelling of the soft tissues over the metacarpals or metatarsals of the hands and feet. Ten to forty-five per cent of all patients will experience at least one episode of hand-foot syndrome (Pearson, 1984).

Sequestration Crisis. Children with sickle cell anemia eventually lose function of the spleen as a result of frequent infarction from sickling episodes. Prior to the onset of this "autosplenectomy," the infant or young child may suddenly pool enormous volumes of blood within the spleen. The organ becomes massively enlarged, and the hemoglobin level drops precipitously. This type of crisis is potentially fatal, and death may occur within hours of onset of symptoms. Parents must be instructed to bring their child to the hospital if sudden pallor, faintness, rapid breathing (signs of shock or deficient intravascular blood volume), and/or acute enlargement of the abdomen develops. Young children between the ages of 8 months and 2 years are at the highest risk.

Aplastic Crisis. The red blood cells of the child with sickle cell anemia survive only about 10 to 20 days in the circulation (Pearson, 1985). (Normal life span of RBCs is approximately 120 days.) Because red blood cells are destroyed so quickly, the child with sickle cell anemia is highly dependent on a strong compensatory mechanism that continually produces new RBCs at a rate five to eight times normal. Infections, especially of viral origin, can often cause a temporary cessation of bone marrow activity even in otherwise healthy persons. The need for new RBCs is so profound in sickle cell anemia that even a one-day arrest of bone marrow activity during an infection can cause a drop of 10 to 15 per cent in the hematocrit, resulting in aplastic crisis.

Aplastic crisis is characterized by a lack of reticulocytes in the blood. Platelet and white blood cell counts are usually not depressed. Hemoglobin may fall as low as 1 gm/dl; in this case, death often results from congestive heart failure (Pearson, 1985).

Aplastic crisis is usually self-limited, lasting 5 to 10 days. More severe aplastic crises are treated with transfusions of packed RBCs. Milder degrees of aplasia frequently require no treatment. Parents should seek medical care if the child becomes weak and pale, especially in the midst of an ongoing or recent infection.

Diagnostic Assessment

Sickle cell anemia as well as sickle cell trait are easily diagnosed with a blood test called hemoglobin electrophoresis. Electrophoresis applies an electrical charge to a blood specimen and separates the various types of hemoglobin present. This test also quantifies the percentages of various hemoglobins present. Less sensitive laboratory tests that indicate the presence of any Hb S are available (e.g., Sickledex). These tests cannot differentiate whether the person tested is heterozygous or homozygous for sickle hemoglobin. They indicate merely the presence or absence of Hb S. Such tests are used for large screening programs. Positive results require further testing with Hgb electrophoresis.

Early identification of children with sickle cell disease is desirable to begin parental education and to facilitate early treatment for sequestration or vaso-occlusive crisis. Hemoglobin electrophoresis should be performed at birth on all black babies. In May 1972, Congress passed the National Sickle Cell Anemia Control Act. Under this act services for voluntary screening and diagnosis, counseling and education, medical referral, follow-up, and research are mandated. Because sickle cell screening is available upon request and since sickle cell anemia and sickle cell trait are most prevalent in the black population, the nurse should discuss the importance and need for testing with parents of black infants. Genetic counseling should be offered to the parents of the child newly diagnosed with sickle cell anemia. (See Chapter 4 for a discussion of genetic counseling, and Table 50-3 for a nursing process plan for the family in need of genetic counseling.)

Accurate prenatal diagnosis of sickle cell disease is now possible, utilizing fetal blood obtained by placental aspiration or fetoscopy. Parents should be made aware of centers that provide this testing. The nurse must present this information in a sensitive manner, realizing that the decision to obtain prenatal screening for future pregnancies is highly emotional and personal. Parents should not feel pressured to obtain this service, nor be made to feel guilty if they refuse it.

Therapeutic Management

Currently there is no cure for sickle cell anemia. Treatment is palliative at best. The child and family are counseled to avoid the known "triggers" of sickle cell crisis: infection, dehydration, hypoxia, high altitude, vigorous exercise, and stress. Management of vaso-occlusive crisis includes adequate hydration, effective analgesia, and identification and treatment of any precipitating event (Vichinsky, 1987). Anemia associated with sequestration or aplastic crises is treated with transfusion of packed red blood cells.

"Hypertransfusion" programs describe regimens that provide routine PRBC transfusions to maintain hemoglobin levels greater than 12 gm/dl. Hemoglobin levels greater than 12 gm/dl shut down erythropoiesis, thereby preventing manufacture of Hgb S. Hypertransfusion programs may be used as treatment for life-threatening complications, especially cerebrovascular accidents. This treatment is usually very effective but carries the risks of possible hepatitis, and eventual iron overload (described later in the thalassemia section).

Major Nursing Diagnoses for Sickle Cell Anemia

Potential altered tissue perfusion: systemic, *related to*
- *occlusion of vessels by sickled cells (vaso-occlusive crisis)*
- *pooling of blood in the spleen (splenic sequestration crisis)*
- *temporary cessation of red blood cell production associated with effects of infectious agents on bone marrow function (aplastic crisis)*

Activity intolerance, *related to impaired oxygen-carrying capacity of the blood associated with hemolysis of red blood cells*

Potential altered comfort: pain, *related to tissue ischemia associated with vascular occlusion*

Potential for infection, *related to splenic dysfunction*

Potential disturbance in self-concept: body image, role performance, *related to*
- *physical restrictions associated with sickle cell anemia*
- *potential for transmission of the recessive trait to offspring*

Potential altered family process: sibling rivalry, *related to*
- *inadequate knowledge of the disease process and treatment plan*
- *jealousy associated with attention garnered by the ill child*

Knowledge deficit, *related to management of sickle cell disease at home:*
- *nature and course of the disease, including the signs and symptoms of crisis*
- *plan of treatment as it relates to infection, hydration, analgesia, and physical activity*
- *genetic counseling*

Strategies for Nursing Care

Strategies for the child with sickle cell anemia will be based upon the following principles related to (1) teaching self-management of the disease, (2) nursing management of sickle cell crises, and (3) techniques for facilitating family coping. Since the diagnosis of *activity intolerance* is common to all children with anemia, interventions for this diagnosis are addressed in Table 40-5.

Administering Transfusions to Increase Gas Exchange. The nurse is usually responsible for carrying out the regimen prescribed by physicians in the management of sickle cell anemia. Often this will entail transfusions of packed red blood cells (PRBCs). Other blood components may also be indicated. (See Table 40-6.) During aplastic crisis, the slow transfusion of PRBCs to increase the Hgb by 5 gm/dl is required (Pearson, 1984). During splenic sequestration, vigorous replacement of blood volume with whole blood or PRBCs and support of the child in shock is indicated. Box 40-1 lists guidelines for blood transfusion safety and transfusion reactions.

Should surgery be required for any reason, the anesthesia poses increased risk for the child with sickle cell anemia. Hypoxia, dehydration, circulatory stasis, acidosis, cold, and infections may result from the surgical procedure itself or as a result of general anesthe-

Table 40-6. Blood Component Transfusion

Blood Product	Description	Volume	Uses
Whole Blood		500 ml	Replace massive blood loss due to acute hemorrhage
PRBCs (Packed Red Blood Cells)	The RBCs extracted from 1 unit of whole blood Small amount of plasma and WBCs present	300 ml May be available in partial units (50–100 ml/unit)	Relieve symptomatic deficit of oxygen-carrying capacity
Spin Filter PRBCs	Blood is processed to produce a 50–60% reduction in WBCs	300 ml	History of documented significant febrile reactions to previous infusions
Washed PRBCs	Blood is processed to reduce WBCs by 80%	200 ml	History of severe, repeated, febrile reactions not relieved by spin filter process
Frozen Deglycerolyzed PRCBs	Process reduces number of WBCs by ~90%	200 ml	History of severe febrile reactions not ameliorated by washed RBC
Single Donor Plasma (SDP)	Plasma separated from 1 unit of whole blood Does not contain platelets or factors V and VIII	200–275 ml	Volume expander Replacement of stable coagulation factors or fibrinogen
Fresh Frozen Plasma (FFP)	SDP frozen within 6 hours to preserve factors V and VIII	200–275 ml	Factor V deficiency DIC
Platelet Concentrates (Random Donor)	Platelets harvested from 1 unit of fresh blood suspended in 50 ml of donor plasma	50 ml/unit (units can be pooled and concentrated to reduce volume for small children)	Relieve bleeding due to thrombocytopenia to increase platelet level over 20,000
Platelet Concentrates (Single Donor)	Obtained by platelet pheresis from one donor, equivalent to 6–8 units of random donor	250–350 ml (may be concentrated)	Patients refractory to random donor platelets
Granulocyte Contentrates (single donor)	1×10^{10} WBC obtained from donors must be ABO and RH compatible	250–350 ml	ANC <500 with proven bacterial sepsis unresponsive to antibiotics
Cryoprecipitate	Derived from the plasma from 1 unit of blood. Each bag contains ~100 u factor VIII and 170 mg fibrinogen	10 mg/bag	Factor VIII deficient patients DIC

Infusion Time

Rates should be ordered by physician for each individual case. The following are typical rates.

Whole Blood PRBCs Plasma	10 ml/kg typically can be transfused over 2 hours (No more than 2 ml/kg/hour for child in heart failure) Must be infused over 4 hours maximum
Platelets	Run in as rapidly as possible—concentrate units if volume is a problem.
Cryoprecipitate	Run in as rapidly as possible—concentrate units if volume is a problem. Wash bag with 10–15 ml of normal saline after empty to ensure complete usage
Granulocytes	Administer slowly over 2–4 hours. Premedication with acetominophen, Benadryl, or hydrocortisone is usually mandatory. Chills and fever frequently occur. Stop transfusion for high temperature, dyspnea, cyanosis, hypoxia. Use with caution in points also receiving amphotericin B.

sia. The child's hematocrit level must be increased prior to surgery. Direct transfusion of PRBCs can be performed to raise the hematocrit above 30 per cent. Preparation for surgery may require 10 days to 2 weeks. The process of transfusing PRBCs every few days results in suppression of the production of sickle cells, causing an overall decrease in Hgb S and a lower risk of crisis occurring due to the surgery or anesthesia.

Strategies for Vaso-Occlusive Crisis. Treatment of vaso-occlusive crisis is aimed at relieving symptoms and providing supportive care. It is important to ascertain that only a pain crisis is occurring and that there is no underlying cause or serious complication. Fluids, analgesia, and general comfort measures are the mainstay of sickle crisis therapy. Maintaining an adequate level of *hydration* is a primary intervention measure for the child in crisis, since the sickling process is enhanced by dehydration. Both oral and parenteral fluids are used to improve the level of hydration. Fluid intake should be increased to one and a half times normal maintenance, assuming cardiac function is adequate. The oral route of hydration maintenance is

Box 40-1
Blood Transfusion Safety

Determine patient's transfusion history. Assess nature of previous adverse reactions and notify physician and blood bank if there is a positive history

Always identify patient/blood product. Check ID wrist band and blood tag ask child to state full name if possible

The most severe and potentially fatal transfusion reaction—acute hemolytic crisis—is most often a result of patient/blood mix-up. You *must* double check this information with another person (hospital policy dictates appropriate personnel)

Be sure that the proper filter is in place for the product being infused

Be prepared to hang product immediately after received from the blood bank—if not possible send product back to the blood bank (once unrefrigerated for more than 30 minutes, the bank will refuse unit)

All IV lines should be primed with normal saline. This helps decrease hemolysis. PRBC transfusions can be assisted with the use of Y-tubing and normal saline

Never add medications to blood

Vital signs (temperature, pulse, respiration, and blood pressure) should be obtained prior to the start of the transfusion as a baseline. If abnormal, check with the child's physician before starting the infusion

Vital signs should be repeated frequently during the transfusion, usually every 15–30 minutes. However, close observation and inspection of child, especially during the first 15–30 minutes of the transfusion, is mandatory

Begin the transfusion slowly—the rate should not exceed 2 ml/minute during the first 15 minutes

Transfusion should last no longer than 4 hours

Most transfusions in children require an infusion pump to maintain proper rate. The IV site must be checked for infiltration frequently. If the transfusion is not being monitored on an infusion device, the following measures may help restore a proper rate if rate has slowed considerably and IV site is intact: raise the IV pole, use a pressure sleeve, agitate the blood bag frequently, change the filter or tubing

Blood warming devices are used with rapid transfusions that are infused through central lines (the cold blood may cause cardiac arrythmias). Blood warming is also required for exchange transfusions in infants

TRANSFUSION REACTIONS

Febrile

Extremely common, probably caused by host antibodies to white cells reacting with white cells in the transfused blood. Usually occur during or immediately after the transfusion. Symptoms include fever and chills

Allergic

Caused by reaction to foreign plasma protein. May occur during and immediately after transfusion. Symptoms include urticaria, hives

Acute Hemolytic Reactions

Transfused red blood cells react with circulating antibody resulting in intravascular hemolysis. Occurs most frequently when group O patients mistakenly receive group A, B, or AB blood. Usually occurs within the first 15 minutes of the transfusion. Occurs most often as result of error in blood/recipient. Symptoms include fever, chills, pain in lumbar region, chest pain, apprehension, hemoglobinura, dyspnea, burning along veins in which blood is being transfused

Delayed Hemolytic Reactions

Occurs 4–8 days after transfusion in patients that have developed antibodies previously, but the level is too low to be detected at the time of pretransfusion screening. Signs include falling hematocrit and positive Coombs' test. Most delayed hemolytic reactions are benign

If a Transfusion Reaction Occurs

Stop the infusion

Keep vein open with normal saline

Call physician

Monitor patient and vital signs closely. Follow hospital policy regarding blood and urine specimens and completing blood bank forms

Benadryl 1–2 mg/kg IM, IV, or PO may be ordered for allergic reactions. Aminophylline, 3 mg/kg IV over 20 minutes, may be ordered for wheezing in an allergic reaction

Antipyretics—aspirin or acetaminophen will be ordered for febrile reactions preferable, if possible. Parents can identify for the nurse the child's likes and preferences of various liquids. If IV fluids must be used, infants' and young children's sucking needs must be remembered; their preferred hand (or thumb) should be left free if at all possible or a pacifier offered if appropriate. The older child should be allowed some decision as to the site of the IV. The administration of packed red cells may occasionally be included in the immediate emergency care. The close monitoring of vital signs while the child is receiving hydration or blood products is critical. (See Box 40-1.) There is little evidence to support application of heat to areas of infarction for pain relief. Application of cold is contraindicated as this may enhance sickling.

Relieving Pain. Propoxyphene hydrochloride (Darvon), acetaminophen, or codeine-containing compounds may be useful for children during mildly painful episodes. Some physicians believe aspirin can increase acidosis, which enhances sickling, and should therefore be avoided. Others (Vichinsky and Lubin, 1987) recommended aspirin as an adjunct to narcotic analgesics. More potent narcotics may be required for children in severe pain. The nurse is responsible for pain assessment and drug administration during the course of each crisis. Most often the nurse must interpret the child's pain because analgesic orders are commonly written as prn. Pain medication should not be denied because a child does not ask for it. The pediatric nurse must observe nonverbal signs of pain and also realize that younger children may actually deny pain because they are afraid of the analgesics or the route required for administration. (See also Chapter 29.) The nurse may recommend that pain medication be ordered at regular intervals rather than prn as this may reduce the child's anxiety about asking for pain relief. This may also allow a drug of lower potency to be more effective because of consistent blood levels and eliminate the dulling side effects of more potent medications. Communication between child and nurse should be fostered so that the child becomes a partner in pain control. Increased participation allows the child a greater sense of control and decreased anxiety.

Teaching to Support Management of Sickle Cell Disease at Home. Parental teaching should always be specific rather than general. "Force fluids" gives no helpful guidelines to parents. Instead the nurse should calculate the required maintenance fluids for the child and provide the parents with the amount measured in common household terms. Lists of alternatives that provide high fluids (popsicles, soups, jello, etc.) and their equivalent liquid value should also be given. Parents need to be reminded to not withhold fluids at bedtime. This is often done in an attempt to control bedwetting which results from the damaged kidneys' loss of concentrating ability. Parental support and bladder training programs will be needed to manage the enuresis. Parents should be made aware that fluid restriction may precipitate other problems such as vaso-occlusive crisis.

Anticipatory guidance should be offered to parents both for normal developmental changes and for symptoms particular to sickle cell anemia such as short stature, delayed puberty, and cardiovascular limitations.

Maintaining the child's general health is an important preventive action. Comprehensive care of the child is indicated and is most optimally delivered from a sickle cell treatment center. The special needs of the child and family with sickle cell anemia should be addressed along with routine "well-child" management. Assessment of growth and development, routine immunizations, nutrition counseling, auditory and visual screening, and education should be available to families. Genetic counseling should be an integral part of family education. (See Chapter 4.)

Comforting the Child in Pain. The care of an infant in pain can be extremely frustrating to the family and the nurse because of the difficulty posed in managing the pain. Holding a younger child and providing a warm and caring environment will usually help the child maintain more control over feelings of anxiety associated with the pain. Gentle, slow movements when handling the child are essential. See Table 29-4, Nursing Process Plan: The Child in Pain, page 878, for additional pharmacologic and nonpharmacologic comfort measures.

If immobilization is necessary for parenteral infusions, the nurse must provide for the child's physical, psychosocial, and safety needs. Providing an infant seat may facilitate the comfort and safety of an infant. Restraints, if essential for safety, must be removed at least every 45 to 90 minutes.

All children with a painful crisis episode should be kept as free from stress as possible. The opportunity for rooming in is an essential component of basic care to the family. The caregivers' presence affords the child more security and should be permitted and encouraged in a manner that does not place guilt upon parent(s) unable to room in due to other family obligations. The presence of another person when the child is in pain is important; it gives the feeling that the pain is "shared." If the parents cannot stay with the child, it is helpful if nurses plan time to allow periods where they can sit with the child and offer support by their presence. Each nurse should make every effort to anticipate and provide for the needs of the sick child within the family. Parents should be provided with adequate information regarding the latest episode to facilitate their own problem solving and allow them to be supportive to the child.

Preventing Infection. The child with sickle cell disease is prone to serious bacterial infection because of splenic dysfunction. Young children (less than age 3 to 4 years of age) are frequently infected with *Pneumococcus* and *Haemophilus influenzae* organisms, and older children have a high incidence of *Salmonella* infection. Overwhelming sepsis is a frequent cause of death in young children with sickle cell anemia. The parents need information regarding common childhood illnesses and how to interpret the symptoms that may occur. The nurse should help parents learn the proper method of taking their child's temperature. They should be taught to recognize subtle changes in their child's behavior and to realize that picky eating or fussy behavior may be the first signs of infection. Many centers advocate the use of daily penicillin prophylaxis to help prevent acute overwhelming bacterial infections. The nurse should ascertain that parents understand the rationale for penicillin usage and should stress that its use does not imply that medical care is not needed at times of fever or illness. The need for immediate medical attention, regardless of time of day, cannot be overemphasized when a temperature of 101°F (38.3°C) develops. In addition, all children over the age of 2 should receive a pneumococcal vaccine (Pneumovax), the *Haemophilus* b vaccine and the meningococcal vaccine to reduce the incidence of infections with these organisms.

Promoting Self-concept by Normalizing the Environment. In all dealings with the child with sickle cell disease and the family, the nurse should strive to keep the emphasis on the normality of life. The child's painful crises can often be circumvented through prevention and early intervention; many episodes can be controlled at home by oral pain medication, increased fluids, and rest. The family should help the child to master various coping skills such as relaxation training and distraction at an early age to help reduce anxiety during crisis periods. (These techniques are taught in most comprehensive sickle cell programs.) The nurse, along with the parents, should appeal to the school system to permit the child with sickle cell disease to have rest periods, analgesia, and frequent fluids when needed. Undue absenteeism may be prevented by these measures thus allowing the child a greater chance for success in life. The availability of a homebound program should be explored when frequent crises prevent regular attendance.

Promoting Healthy Family Interactions. Siblings should be encouraged to play an active role in caretaking of their affected brother or sister. Depending on the sibling child's developmental level, factual explanations must be given for the repeated admissions to the hospital and the other events surrounding the management of the ill child's unique needs. Siblings should have an opportunity to participate in the child's care to the degree they wish. This may include accompanying the child to the doctor's office, clinic, or the hospital. Such visits can help clarify questions and help the sibling to understand the ill child's needs. It is not uncommon for siblings to experience feelings of concern for their ill brother/sister, and factual information will reduce the possibility of frightening fantasies. At the same time, siblings are likely to feel jealous and left out as their parents are forced to spend extra time with their ill brother/sister. They may direct their anger at their brother/sister or at their parents. Parents should be educated about the normal nature of these feelings and encouraged to spend "special time" with the healthy child to prevent him/her from feeling neglected. Special times need not be elaborate, planned events. Parents can take advantage of daily activities such as performing a household chore together, reading a bedtime story, having a bedtime chat, or accompanying the child on trips to the mail box or to the local store. Less frequent events like a special afternoon or a day trip can also provide "quality" interactions. (See Chapter 25 for further discussion on the impact of chronic illness on the family.)

Long-term Outcome

The child with sickle cell disease has a better prognosis today than previously. As adults, many affected individuals must make decisions regarding parenting. Women with sickle cell disease have been able to conceive and deliver normal children. However, early prenatal medical and nursing management are essential to foster a healthy outcome for both mother and newborn. Even though the prognosis has improved, it is believed that 20 to 30 per cent of children with sickle cell anemia die in the first five years of life. The high mortality is caused by overwhelming sepsis and sequestration crisis (Pearson, 1984). With close comprehensive health supervision that emphasizes parental education, these fatal complications should be largely preventable.

Nursing Strategies for Follow-up Care in the Home or Clinic

Assess the extremities for evidence of bone, muscle, and joint swelling and tenderness and for evidence of ulcers; urinary frequency for loss of renal concentrating ability; the CNS for signs of infarction; lung sounds and vital signs for evidence of infarction or infection; the liver and spleen for enlargement.

Determine if any of the child's activities of daily living appear related to the onset of crisis.

Discuss prevention and early signs of infection, alerting the family to current seasonal outbreaks of viral infections such as influenza and respiratory syncytial virus.

Determine compliance with prophylactic antibiotic therapy.

Determine the child's average fluid intake in a day. Discuss this with the family in relation to minimum requirements. Make sure they understand the need for increased fluids in warm weather.

Assess the child's and family's perception of their quality of life:

- Encourage expression of feelings about the lack of cure for the disease, the child's prognosis, the threat of recurring crises, their feelings about seeing the child in pain, and their feelings of adequacy to cope both physically and emotionally;
- Discuss with the child and family the adequacy of prescribed analgesics for mild crises; and
- Determine whether the family is aware of community services for genetic counseling and for social and financial support as needed.

β-Thalassemia

Incidence and Pathophysiology

Thalassemia major (Cooley anemia) is a disorder of hemoglobin synthesis resulting in a severe hemolytic anemia. Normal hemoglobin (Hgb A) is comprised of two polypeptide chains designated as α and β. Children with Cooley anemia have severe deficiencies or total suppression of the β chain synthesis. As a result, the circulating red cells are small and contain markedly reduced amounts of hemoglobin. The hemoglobin is severely compromised and is unable to support life for more than a few years. The disorder occurs mainly in persons of Mediterranean origin, especially persons with Greek or Italian ancestry, but the genes are distributed in the Middle East, India, Pakistan, Southeast Asia, Africa, and China.

The disease is inherited in an autosomal recessive pattern. The child who inherits only one gene for β-thalassemia is said to have "thal trait" or thal minor. Generally, the child with thalassemia trait is asymptomatic, however, a very mild degree of anemia may occur. This anemia may be misdiagnosed as iron deficiency anemia, as the red cells in both disorders are hypochromic and microcytic. Genetic counseling should be made available to parents of children with Thal trait and later to the children themselves. If the child later marries a person who also carries the thalassemia gene, the couple has a one in four chance of producing a child with thalassemia major. (See the discussion of autosomal recessive inheritance in Chapter 4.)

Clinical Manifestations

The child with β-thalassemia major is asymptomatic during the first 6 months of life due to the presence of Hgb F. Some children continue to produce high levels of Hgb F and may escape diagnosis until 2 to 3 years of age. Diagnostic presenting symptoms are those of anemia: pallor, listless or fussy behavior, poor appetite, and often frequent infections. Hemoglobin electrophoresis provides laboratory confirmation. As the child becomes older, the symptoms of anemia become more profound. The body attempts to overcome the anemia by increasing the production of RBCs. This compensatory mechanism in turn causes enlargement of the liver and spleen and hypertrophy of the bone marrow resulting in marked changes in the skeletal system. Older children with β-thalassemia have distinctive facial features as a result of the overstimulated bone marrow.

The typical child with "Cooley facies" has prominent forehead and cheeks, eyes that are slanted slightly downward, and an enlarged maxilla with poorly aligned and misshapen teeth. Growth retardation usually occurs as a consequence of severe anemia, and there is delayed or absent development of puberty and secondary sexual characteristics. Often cardiac enlargement occurs with a flow murmur. Other features include gallstones, pericarditis, and leg ulcers. Unfortunately, the compensatory activity of the marrow does not alleviate the severe anemia, because the defective gene does not allow for the production of useful hemoglobin. Without red blood cell transfusions, the child with β-thalassemia would die as a result of severe anemia.

Therapeutic Management

In the past, transfusion was delayed until clinical symptoms of anemia developed—generally at Hgb levels of 5 to 6 gm/dl. Since 1965, hypertransfusion—the maintenance of Hgb levels greater than 10 gm/dl, has become the accepted treatment. Hypertransfusion prevents many of the aforementioned bone marrow changes and stigmata as well as hepatosplenomegaly. The major drawback of repeated transfusions is the inevitable development of hemosiderosis, the accumulation of iron in body tissue from the breakdown of transfused RBCs. Iron overload is a well-described phenomena and causes endocrine dysfunction, liver failure, and cardiac abnormalities. Indeed, congestive heart failure, usually in the second decade of life, is the most frequent cause of death for these patients.

Agents that help mobilize (chelate) excess iron and allow for its excretion from the body have been developed. Only desferioxamine (Desferal, DF), an agent that is administered as a continuous subcutaneous infusion, appears to be effective with relatively low toxicity (Weatherall, 1983). The use of chelating agents early and continuously throughout life may prevent the side effects of hypertransfusion programs.

Hepatitis B infection remains a serious complication of frequent blood transfusions. In addition, there is risk of infection with hepatitis A; non-A, non-B hepatitis; and cytomegalovirus (Chapter 45). There is also some risk of HIV infection. (See Chapter 43 for a discussion of AIDS.)

The long-term outlook for β-thalassemia is poor. Death occurs no later than the third decade, most often from complications of iron overload.

Major Nursing Diagnoses for Thalassemia

Altered gas exchange, *related to significant decreases in size of RBCs and in hemoglobin levels associated with an autosomal recessive trait*

Disturbance in self-concept: body image, *related to*

- *development of "Cooley's facies" associated with compensatory hyperactivity of bone marrow*
- *growth retardation and delayed secondary sexual characteristics associated with inadequate oxygen to sustain normal cell growth*

Knowledge deficit, *related to home care:*

- *nature of the disease, including signs and symptoms of progressing anemia*
- *plan of treatment, including hypertransfusion, administration of chelating agents, and the relationship of activity to the body's need for oxygen*
- *genetic counseling*

Strategies for Nursing Care

Central to any plan of care is teaching specific to the identified knowledge deficit. Care of the child with β-thalassemia also involves management of blood transfusions to improve tissue perfusion and support of the child in relationship to altered physical appearance.

Teaching to Address the Knowledge Deficit. Nursing care for the child newly diagnosed with β-thalassemia must involve education and support of the parents. The nurse offers comfort to parents who may be grieving at the time of diagnosis. Repeated reinforcement of the physician's explanations of the treatment of β-thalassemia will be necessary but should be offered when the parents are emotionally ready to hear them. This may not be for several months in some families. Many parents feel overwhelming guilt at the time of diagnosis. The nurse should acknowledge this emotion but encourage parents to overcome it and focus their energies in a more positive area. Often, parents find comfort in support groups of families with chronically ill children. Information on the Cooley's Anemia Foundation should be given (address at the end of this chapter). The nurse should encourage all family members (grandparents, aunts, uncles, siblings) to be tested for the β-thalassemia trait.

As with all chronic diseases, care of the whole child must not be overlooked. Routine immunizations and health maintenance should be a priority.

Increasing Gas Exchange Through Transfusion. Transfusions for the child with β-thalassemia are best managed on an outpatient basis. This will disrupt the child's schedule the least and may help the child remain in school and in contact with the peer group. In later years transfusions may be complicated by increased sensitization to minor blood group antigens and development of antibodies to substances in blood. This results in increased difficulty in finding appropriate blood to transfuse and greater incidence of blood transfusion reactions. Cardiac involvement will require slower rates of transfusion as well. Parents and children (when they are old enough to understand) must be taught the correct and safe use of chelating agents. The importance of consistent usage cannot be overstressed. Desferal is infused into the subcutaneous tissue via a small needle and a portable infusion pump. The infusion is administered over 8 to 10 hours, usually during the night. Hard, painful lumps sometimes develop at the site of the infusion, rendering the site unusable for days or weeks. Compliance can become a serious problem when such difficulties ensue if the entire family is not highly motivated. The nurse should continually encourage and praise the child and family for their efforts if appropriate, while providing, at the same time, sympathetic acknowledgement of the inconvenience and frustration of the therapy.

Promoting a Healthy Self-Concept. Children and adolescents with β-thalassemia may feel extremely isolated. They are unlike peers in appearance and ability. In addition, they may have substantial feelings of guilt for placing such a burden on their family. Often they have no one with whom to share feelings of loneliness, fear, and despair. The nurse who consistently cares for the child or adolescent with β-thalassemia should provide the opportunity for sharing these feelings. Appropriate words of praise and encouragement can also mean a great deal to the young person.

Nursing Strategies for Follow-up Care in the Home or Clinic

Obtain blood samples as indicated for evaluation of hemoglobin and hematocrit.

Assess the adequacy of the child's rest/activity schedule.

Assess severity of signs and symptoms of anemia.

Assess for complications of hypertransfusion therapy: local inflammation at the Desferal injection sites and signs of hemosiderosis (congestive heart failure, endocrine dysfunction, and hepatomegaly.)

Assess the adaptation of the child and family to the limited prognosis. (See Chapters 25 and 26 on care of the chronically ill and terminally ill child.)

Ensure that the family has been referred for genetic counseling.

Acquired Aplastic Anemia

Aplastic anemia may be defined as bone marrow failure characterized by reduction or absence of the solid elements (red cells, white cells, platelets) of blood. The disease can be congenital (Fanconi anemia) or it can be acquired.

Approximately 1,000 new cases of the acquired form are diagnosed yearly of which 30 to 50 per cent have no established etiology (Miller and O'Reilly, 1984). Known agents capable of inducing aplastic anemia include chemicals such as benzene; drugs, most notably the antibiotic chloramphenicol; radiation; and viruses.

Clinical Manifestations and Therapeutic Management

Patients present with the typical symptoms of low blood count: bruises, petechia, and epistaxis as a result of decreased platelets, anemia, pallor, and fatigue from decreased RBCs, and often infections due to low white blood cell count. A bone marrow biopsy shows a marked decrease in all the normally present cells. Immediate treatment includes supportive care providing transfusions of the absent blood elements as needed. Treatment aimed at a cure includes androgen therapy, bone marrow transplantation, and in some centers immunosuppressive therapy. If a compatible donor is available, bone marrow transplantation is the preferred treatment of choice. This modality has a 3-year survival rate of 50 to 70 per cent (Miller and O'Reilly, 1984). Other modes of treatment offer very little hope for cure in severe aplasia.

Nursing care for children with aplastic anemia is similar to that administered to children with leukemia. Parental education regarding home care of the child with low blood counts is essential. Chapter 48 contains further information on bone marrow transplantation and care of the child with low blood counts.

Table 48-4 details a nursing process plan for the child undergoing chemotherapy. Chemotherapeutic drugs induce an aplastic anemia of sorts that is referred to as bone marrow suppression. This nursing process plan, therefore, addresses care of the child with decreased WBCs, RBCs, and platelets.

Congenital Aplastic Anemia: Fanconi Anemia

Congenital aplastic anemia, Fanconi anemia, is a rare disorder believed to be inherited by an autosomal recessive trait. Many patients are recognized at birth because of the associated congenital anomalies, although hematologic abnormalities rarely become evident before 17 months of age and may not develop until the second decade. Congenital anomalies include skin hyperpigmentation especially involving the neck, axilla, abdomen, umbilicus, and genitalia. Absence of thumbs and radii is associated, and other skeletal anomalies such as short stature (as a result of short trunk) may occur. Hypoplastic thumbnails have been frequently noted. Renal abnormalities may occur; these include horseshoe kidneys, hydronephrosis, or absence of one kidney. In addition, central nervous system (CNS) findings such as microcephaly, mental retardation, deafness, ptosis, nystagmus, and hyperreflexia are frequent. Treatment is similar to that for acquired aplastic anemia: supportive care, androgens, immunosuppressive therapy, and bone marrow transplantation. The majority of children with Fanconi anemia may have long-term disease remission (several years) with androgens and steroids alone, however, the potential for cure is very low.

Idiopathic Thrombocytopenic Purpura (ITP)

Incidence and Pathophysiology

Idiopathic thrombocytopenic purpura, commonly referred to as ITP, is an acquired blood disorder that is characterized by increased destruction of circulating platelets. The disorder occurs most frequently in the 2 to 5 year age range, although it can occur at any age. White children have a higher incidence than black children.

As its name suggests, the etiology of ITP is unknown. However, current theories of an autoimmune phenomenon are widely accepted (see Chapter 43 for a discussion of autoimmune mechanisms). For unknown reasons, platelets become coated with antiplatelet antibody, are recognized as foreign material, and are subsequently destroyed by the spleen.

Diagnostic Assessment

Signs and symptoms of ITP include the sudden onset of easy bruising and randomly distributed petechia and echymoses all over the body. Twenty to thirty per cent of children present with epistaxis or bleeding from other mucous membranes. About 70 per cent of children with ITP have a positive history of a recent febrile illness, usually a nonspecific upper respiratory infection, but rubella and rubeola have also been implicated (Pearson, 1987). It is of note that at presentation, despite their severely bruised appearance, these children do not look "sick." Careful assessment is indicated to differentiate the bruising of ITP from that of child abuse.

Laboratory studies show a reduced platelet count, usually below 20 to 30,000 mm^3/dl. A bone marrow aspiration should be performed to rule out malignant infiltration of the marrow; in ITP the aspiration is normal except for higher than normal levels of megakaryocytes—the parent cell of platelets. Laboratory tests that measure platelet function, specifically the bleeding time and tourniquet test, will be prolonged in children with ITP; all other blood studies are typically normal.

Therapeutic Management

A short course of steroids, usually prednisone, may be prescribed for treatment of ITP in some centers. Other physicians routinely do not use any treatment, allowing the disease to run its course. Platelet transfusions are of little value because the transfused platelets become coated with antibody and are destroyed as easily as autologous platelets. Transfusions may be indicated in life-threatening hemorrhage, such as an intracranial hemorrhage, but the incidence of such bleeding in ITP is less than 1 per cent (Bussel and Hilgartner, 1987). The majority of patients (80 to 90 per cent) recover spontaneously in 6 to 12 months; in fact, most of these within 8 weeks of diagnosis (Bussel and Hilgartner, 1987). By 12 months from diagnosis 90 per cent of these children have normal platelet counts and relapses are unusual (Pearson, 1987).

The unresponsive 10 per cent of cases are said to have chronic ITP. This form tends to occur more often in older children and females.

Treatment of chronic ITP is not clearly defined. Steroids, immunosuppressive therapy (Vincristine, cyclophosphamide), and high-dose gamma globulin have been used with varying success. Splenectomy may be performed after one year of refractory thrombocytopenia but should be reserved for children older than 5 years of age because of the potential for serious bacterial sepsis in splenectomized youngsters. The use of intravenous gamma globulin (IVGG) is gaining favor as a way to elevate the platelet count. Bussel and Hilgartner (1987) suggest that IVGG may be the least toxic and most effective approach to long-term therapy.

Major Nursing Diagnoses for ITP

Potential for injury: easy bruising and bleeding, related to autoimmune destruction of platelets

Fear/anxiety: family and individual, related to concerns that the child may have a life-threatening illness.

Knowledge deficit, related to management of ITP at home:
- *nature of the disease and the encouraging prognosis*
- *protection from bleeding*
- *signs and symptoms of CNS hemorrhage and emergency phone numbers*
- *administration of immunosuppressive medications, if ordered, including the child's increased susceptibility to infection during this therapy*

Strategies for Nursing Care

Preventing Unnecessary Bruising and Bleeding. Strategies will be directed toward limiting new petechiae and areas of ecchymosis and preventing prolonged bleeding. The child must be protected from either accidental or therapeutically induced trauma.

Invasive procedures such as intramuscular injections, suctioning, catheterization, or venipuncture must be performed by experienced, skillful clinicians. Aspirin and aspirin-containing products inhibit platelet aggregation and, therefore, should not be used. Inspect the child's entire body daily to check for new areas of petechia and purpura.

Allaying Unnecessary Fears. Nursing care of the child with ITP must include family education. Parents are often extremely frightened to discover their child suddenly covered with bruises. Most people have never heard of ITP, and parents of these children may assume the child has a life-threatening catastrophic disease such as leukemia. It may be difficult for parents to accept that "no treatment" may be the acceptable treatment. Frequent reassurance is indicated, with ample time provided for questions from the child and family.

Teaching to Support Management of the Disease at Home. Children with ITP are discharged from the hospital before the platelet count has returned to normal. Parents must be taught to help the child avoid injury. The child should avoid rough, injury prone activities such as contact sports, climbing up trees or jungle gyms, motorcycle riding, etc. Parents of younger children need to be reassured that the normal toppling over and frequent falls of a toddler just beginning to walk are not dangerous. They should be advised, however, to move furniture with sharp edges into nonobtrusive places and to remove throw rugs for the duration of the illness. A soft toothbrush is often advised to minimize bleeding from the gums.

Parents must be cautioned to avoid giving their child aspirin or aspirin-containing products. They need to read labels of over-the-counter preparations to ascertain that acetylsalicylic acid is not an ingredient.

If bruising appears to be increasing, or if bleeding from mucous membranes occurs, parents should notify the health center. In addition, if the child undergoes significant head trauma or if symptoms of CNS bleeding such as headaches, diplopia, projectile vomiting, lethargy, or sensorium changes occur the parents must immediately contact their doctor. Although rarely needed, the parent should be provided with a phone number that will provide telephone assistance 24 hours a day.

The child's platelet count is normally measured every 1 to 2 weeks following discharge. Once the levels are back to normal, parents should lift all restrictions and treat the child no differently than before. The incidence of recurrence is small, approximately 3 per cent (Gaady-Cohen, 1983).

Age-appropriate explanations should be given to the child and the parents. Children may be more apprehensive than is typical because of their parents' fears and also because of their dramatic body changes. The sight of blood panics many people, and children are no exception. Children need frequent reassurance that they probably will be better and back to normal in a short while. See nursing care of the child with thrombocytopenia related to leukemia (Ch. 48) for a summary of special considerations for planning nursing care.

Nursing Strategies for Follow-up Care in the Home or Clinic

Obtain a blood sample as indicated for a platelet count.

Assess for new areas of petechiae and purpura. Record the family's accounts of bleeding episodes.

Encourage expression of fears about the disease, treatment plan, and prognosis. Clarify misconceptions, provide information needed for adaptive problem solving.

Validate the family's understanding of safety precautions.

Disseminated Intravascular Coagulation (DIC)

Etiology

Disseminated intravascular coagulation, most commonly referred to as DIC, is in and of itself not a disease entity. Rather, it is the potential consequence of various pathologic conditions that may occur during the course of severe illness. The pathologic conditions that may predispose an individual to DIC include hypoxia, acidosis, tissue necrosis, endotoxic shock, and endothelial damage.

Disorders or diseases that may cause these altered states are numerous but can be broadly classified into the following: (1) infections, (2) neoplasms (e.g., promyelocytic leukemia), (3) immunologic disorders (e.g., blood transfusion reactions), (4) extensive tissue damage (e.g., burns, severe trauma), and (5) other disorders such as snake bites and giant hemagiomas.

Pathophysiology

The mechanism of DIC is complex and multifaceted. The DIC spectrum is triggered by the release of thromboplastic material such as snake venom, endotoxin, or leukemic or tumor cell content into the circulation, thereby activating the coagulation process. The continued release of coagulation-inducing substances causes abnormal levels of thrombin within the plasma. In addition to its key role in the coagulation cascade, thrombin is also essential to transform plasminogen into plasmin. Plasmin breaks down fibrinogen and fibrin clots in the normal functioning fibrinolytic system. Fibrin degradation products (FDP) are formed as a result of plasmin's action on a blood clot. In DIC the excess thrombin not only converts fibrinogen to fibrin at an accelerated rate, it likewise activates the fibrinolytic system. The FDPs have an affinity to bind with circulatory fibrinogen causing emboli to form. These emboli can be deposited in the microvasculature and may ultimately cause tissue necrosis. Bleeding ensues as the components required for hemostasis, the coagulation factors and platelets, are consumed by the ongoing intravascular coagulation process and are eventually depleted.

Clinical Manifestations

Clinical manifestations of DIC are often first noted by the nurse. Oozing from previous puncture sites and significant ecchymosis or purpura in a seriously ill child are the hallmarks of the disorder. Signs of circulatory failure (hypovolemia) are manifested by pallor, tachycardia, and decreased blood pressure; hypoperfusion of fingers and toes ensue secondarily. Laboratory confirmation of DIC demonstrates a decreased or falling platelet count, prolonged bleeding time, and significantly prolonged coagulation assays: PT (prothrombin time), PTT (activated partial thromboplastic time), and thrombin clotting time (TCT). The fibrinogen, factor V, and factor VIII levels are low, and, in addition, an assay of fibrin/fibrinogen degradation products (FDP) is significantly elevated.

Therapeutic Management

Treatment of DIC is aimed primarily at resolving the underlying disease responsible for triggering DIC. Supportive measures are necessary during the acute phase. Whole blood or packed red blood cells (PRBCs) are indicated for treatment of hypovolemia or shock. Fresh frozen plasma and/or cryoprecipitate may be used to help restore the previous homeostasis of the child's plasma, although this is often achieved by alleviating the underlying disease. Heparin therapy is controversial and is used mainly in cases where severe tissue or organ necrosis is present as a result of thrombi. The administration of heparin in a bleeding disorder seems paradoxical. Its use in DIC may be indicated, however, because "by its inactivation of thrombin and other clotting factors, heparin can interrupt the coagulation process and diminish fibrinolysis" (Flung and Karpatkin, 1985). With decreased fibrinolysis, bleeding and thrombus formation will also diminish. The overall prognosis of DIC is dependent upon the outcome of the underlying disease causing the coagulation disorder.

Major Nursing Diagnoses for DIC

Altered tissue perfusion: hypovolemia, *related to hemorrhage associated with disruption of the body's fine balance between clot formation and clot dissolution*

Fear/anxiety: child and family, *related to*
- *life-threatening nature of the disease*
- *sudden onset of severe illness*
- *blood product transfusions, including fear of transmission of hepatitis or AIDS*
- *intensive care setting*

Knowledge deficit: child and family, *related to*
- *nature of DIC and the suspected underlying illness*
- *treatment plan, including diagnosis and treatment of underlying disease, blood product transfusions, and possible heparin administration*

Strategies for Nursing Care

Children who do develop the full clinical picture of DIC are severely ill and should be managed in an intensive care setting. The nurse should make every attempt to keep the child informed of every action he or she is experiencing. At such times, the parents are often relegated to waiting rooms for long periods. When the parents are with the child, it is helpful for the nurse to volunteer information on any changes that have taken place since their last report. The nurse should point out any obvious equipment in use on or around the child. The parents often become very aware of the technical aspects of treatment and may seem to focus more on this than on their child. This may be the only means left for a parent to maintain some control of his/her child's life and parents should not be discouraged from doing so.

The nursing diagnoses identified will facilitate care planning for the nurse in the intensive care unit. Because DIC is managed in this specialized care setting, the nurse generalist will seldom be involved with direct nursing management. The principle responsibility of the nonspecialist is in recognizing disease states that may potentially lead to DIC and in astutely assessing and quickly reporting unusual signs of bleeding. Early medical intervention can often prevent the disease from becoming fulminant.

Hemophilia

Hemophilia as a term has a high index of familiarity to most people. The disease has many historic references and images of "bleeding to death from a pin prick" are common in the public's eye. In truth, children with hemophilia may experience prolonged troublesome bleeding from such minor events as tooth loss or nosebleeds, but these events are rarely, if ever, life threatening. Superficial cuts and scrapes do not require any further treatment than cleansing and pressure. Rather, *the hallmark of hemophilia is repeated oozing of blood into soft tissue, muscles, and, most frequently, joint capsules.* Indeed, the joint bleeding and subsequent limitations of movement and eventual crippling places hemophilia well within the scope of an orthopedic disorder.

Incidence and Etiology

Hemophilia occurs as the result of a deficiency in one of the clotting factors; all other aspects of coagulation are typically normal. The most common form of hemophilia is known as hemophilia A, which is also known as classical hemophilia or simply factor VIII deficiency. The second most frequent type is called hemophilia B, also known as Christmas disease or factor IX deficiency. Approximately 80 per cent of those affected have classical hemophilia. Although they are two separate diseases, both forms of hemophilia have similar symptoms, genetic rules, and treatment policies. For ease of writing, "hemophilia" will be generic for both disorders unless specifically noted.

Hemophilia occurs in 1 : 10,000 males born in the United States. The disease is transmitted in an X-linked recessive manner. The disease primarily affects males but can be rarely present in females. (See page 146 for further discussion of X-linked recessive inheritance.)

The nurse must fully understand and help explain the genetic rules of the disease to the parents and later to the child. It is crucial that parents understand that the overall risk is the same for each pregnancy regardless of what has occurred in prior births. Female relatives of the affected child can be tested for carrier status by a laboratory blood test with a fairly high rate of accuracy.

Diagnostic Assessment

In hemophilia A or B, factor VIII or factor IX, respectively, is present, but in a diminished capacity. The defective factor is unable to perform its function in the coagulation "cascade." The cascade sequence is halted and no fibrin clot can be formed. (Refer to section on anatomy and physiology of blood, page 1344.)

The severity of hemophilia is dependent on the percentage of the functioning factor present. Severely affected hemophilic individuals* have less than 1 per cent factor coagulant activity. Those moderately affected have 1 to 5 per cent and those with mild disease have 5 to 50 per cent coagulant activity. The person with mild hemophilia may be diagnosed only after surgery or major trauma. The child moderately affected may experience one to two bleeding episodes per year. The severely affected individual may have as many as two to three bleeding episodes per week, many of them "spontaneous" in origin (with no known trauma).

Hemophilia can be diagnosed at birth because maternal factor VIII is not transferred to the fetus. Diagnostic evaluation is likely to be done in families with a positive family history. Prenatal diagnosis has been performed with some success at several medical centers but is currently not a standard option. Laboratory confirmation of hemophilia would show a prolonged PTT, a normal PT, normal bleeding time, normal platelet count, normal factor VIII antigen (or factor IX), and low levels of factor VIII coagulant level (or factor IX in hemophilia B).

Thirty per cent of all new cases of hemophilia have no family history and are thought to be genetic mutations. These children may be diagnosed following prolonged bleeding after circumcision, but the majority of hemophilic boys will not have any substantial bleeding during the first year of life. Most will begin to have difficulty when they begin to walk and undergo subsequent bumps and falls. A common first injury in toddlers is oral mucous membrane bleeding following trauma to the tongue, frenulum, buccal mucosa, or gums.

Clinical Manifestations

Any part of the body has the potential to become the site of a bleeding incident. As stated earlier, young boys tend to have more oral bleeding and perhaps more bruises during the unsteady toddler period. Nosebleeds may be more frequent in young children, probably more as a result of "wandering fingers" than anything else (Helgartner and McMillan, 1984). Nosebleeds can generally be stopped with pressure alone and, although bothersome, do not present a significant health risk.

Central nervous system bleeding can occur at any age and most often follows trauma to the head but can be spontaneous in origin. CNS hemorrhage accounts for more deaths in hemophilic persons than any other bleeding.

Oozing of blood into soft tissue can occur and may appear as a nodular mass with definitive borders. No treatment is usually required unless the bleeding is in a critical area, such as the neck or wrist where obstruction from the blood-filled mass could result in serious injury from pressure on major vessels and nerves.

Bleeding may occur deep within a muscle belly, normally well supplied with blood vessels. This may result from blows, sudden twists, sprains, or deep intramuscular injections. The area is very painful, and the child may refuse to use an affected limb. Abdominal and retroperitoneal muscle bleeds may be indistinguishable from other serious abdominal conditions.

Bleeding into the joint spaces, *hemarthrosis,* is the most common site of injury in severe hemophilia. The knee is the joint most frequently involved, followed in frequency by the elbow, ankle, hip, shoulder, and wrist. The bleeding begins with a slight tear in the synovial tissue and, without treatment, will continue until the joint capsule is fully expanded and no more blood can leak into the capsule (Figure 40-5). Discomfort occurs at the onset of bleeding and progresses to severe pain and refusal to use the affected joint. Once the bleeding is stopped, the blood is gradually reabsorbed, however, with repeated "bleeds" into the capsule, progressive destruction of the joint occurs (Figure 40-6).

* In an effort to promote better self-concept, the National Hemophilia Foundation and hemophilia consumer groups advocate the use of the terms "hemophilic individual" or "person with hemophilia" rather than hemophiliac.

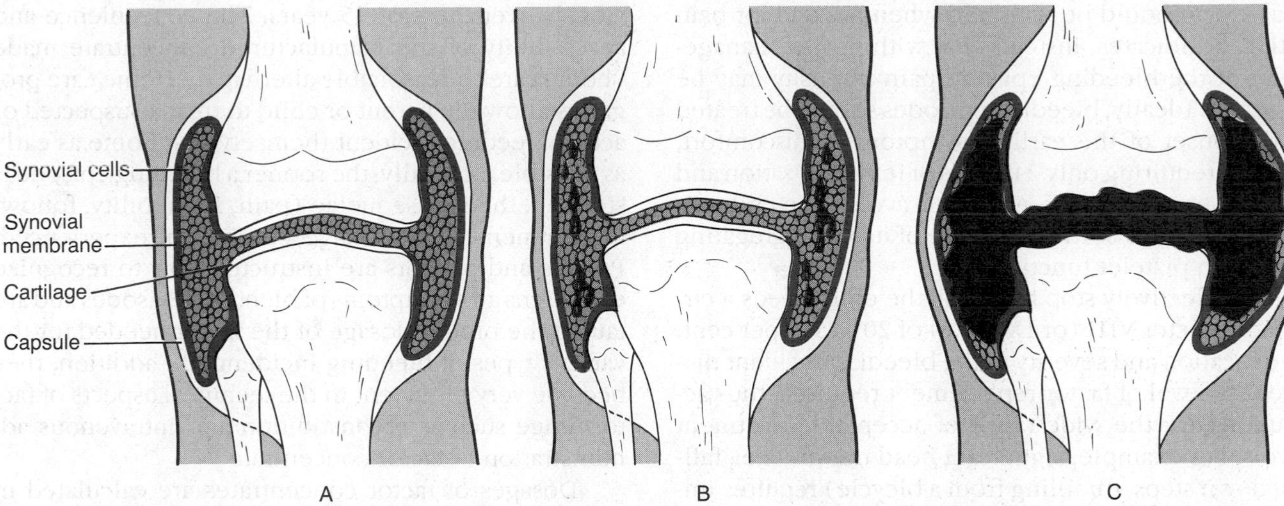

Figure 40-5. Hemarthrosis in hemophilia. *A*, Normal knee joint; *B*, bleeding; and *C*, joint capsule swollen with blood.

Therapeutic Management

In most cases, treatment of hemophilic bleeding consists of replacement of the deficient factor, local control measures—such as ice packs and elastic bandages—and analgesia if necessary. Immobilization is mandatory for comfort and to avoid further bleeding. Initially, the nurse should take care not to further aggravate the bleeding by moving the affected area, particularly a painful joint. Once the bleeding has been stopped—within 24 to 48 hours in most cases—the child's physician may order gentle, passive range of motion exercises several times a day to the affected joint. This is done to prevent stiffening and eventual contractures of the joint. It is not unusual for one particular joint to become especially troublesome for an individual child. The reasons for this are not clear, however, if the situation does occur it can be an extremely trying and frustrating time for both the child and family. To break the cycle of frequent bleeding the physician may order nighttime splints and "prophylactic" daily factor infusions with or without physical therapy. Surgery may eventually be required to remove the damaged synovial tissue that is responsible for repeated bleeding.

During the acute phase of hemarthrosis, pain can be quite severe. Pain control for the child with hemophilia must be an issue of concern to the comprehensive care team, the child, and the family. Pain medication should be used for severe bleeding but care must be exercised to avoid chronic use of strong analgesics—meperidine (Demerol), codeine, and propoxyphene (Darvon) for example—as tolerance and dependence may occur. This does not mean that narcotic

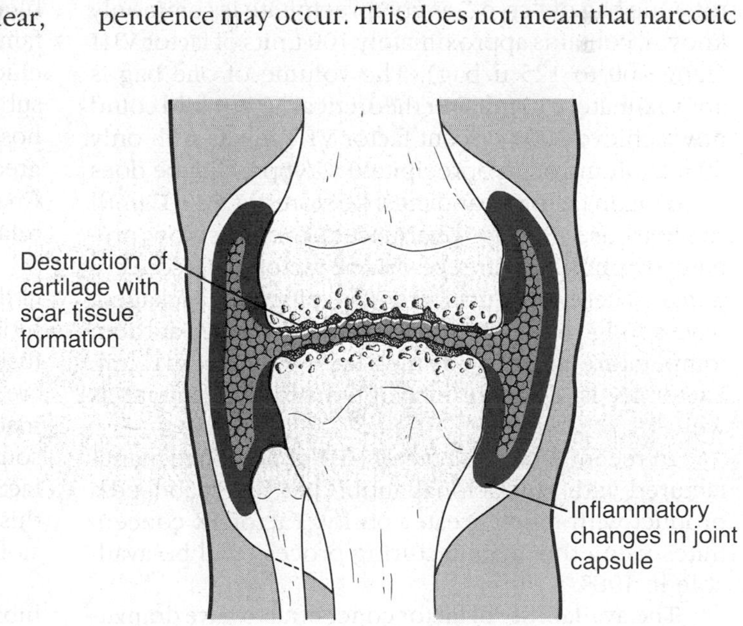

Figure 40-6. Hemophilic arthritis. Destructive effects of successive episodes of bleeding into the joint.

analgesics should be withheld when needed for pain relief! It indicates, instead, that with proper management of the bleeding episode pain intensity may be lessened. Ideally, bleeding episodes should be treated at the onset of the earliest symptom of discomfort, thereby requiring only 24 hours of immobilization and Tylenol for pain relief. Aspirin is avoided in children with bleeding disorders because of its antiaggregating effects on platelet function.

To effectively stop bleeding the child needs a circulating factor VIII (or IX) level of 20 to 100 per cent. The location and severity of the bleeding incident dictates the level of factor replacement required, thus accounting for the wide range of acceptable treatment levels. For example, significant head trauma (i.e., falling down steps, tumbling from a bicycle) requires immediate factor replacement to the 100 per cent level. On the other hand, bleeding into a joint capsule that is detected very early may be successfully treated with a 20 to 40 per cent level (Aronstram, 1980).

Factor replacement is achieved by infusion of plasma, cryoprecipitate, or factor concentrates. Fresh frozen plasma contains 1 unit of factor (VIII or IX) per ml. An infusion of 1 unit/kg of factor VIII (1 ml/kg plasma) will raise the factor VIII blood level by 2 per cent. Factor IX (1 unit/kg) will raise the blood level by 1½ per cent. To achieve 100 per cent replacement, a 10 kg child with factor VIII deficiency would require 50 ml plasma per kg or 500 ml. This large volume is impossible to give safely to a small child. Factor levels of 15 to 20 per cent are the highest levels possible with plasma treatment because of the volume required.

Cryoprecipitate is formed when fresh frozen plasma is thawed at 4°C. This substance is rich in factor VIII and fibrinogen as well as the von Willebrand factor. One bag of "cryo," as cryoprecipitate is commonly known, contains approximately 100 units of factor VIII (range 60 to 125 u/bag). The volume of one bag is approximately 10 ml. Our theoretical 10 kg child could now achieve 100 per cent factor VIII levels with only 50 ml volume of cryoprecipitate. Cryoprecipitate does not contain factor IX and must be stored at −20°C until ready to use. Several pharmaceutical firms now prepare lyopholized (freeze-dried) factor VIII concentrates. These products are conveniently packaged, have a long shelf life, can be stored or carried at room temperature, and provide high levels of factor VIII/ml. Factor IX is available in lyopholized concentrate as well.

In recent months, a factor VIII concentrate manufactured with monoclonal antibodies has produced a product with much greater purity. Factor IX concentrates using this manufacturing process will be available in 1989.

The availability of factor concentrates have dramatically improved the quality of care for hemophilic individuals over the past 15 years. The convenience and accessibility of the manufactured concentrate made "home care" a reasonable alternative. Home care programs allow the parent or child to treat a suspected or actual bleeding incident themselves at home as early as possible. Logically, the sooner a bleeding episode is stopped, the less sequelae (pain, immobility, follow-up treatments, joint damage, etc.) will be experienced. Parents and patients are instructed how to recognize early signs and symptoms of bleeding episodes and are taught the proper dosage of the factor needed for the various types of bleeding incidents. In addition, they become very proficient in the technical aspects of factor usage such as reconstitution and intravenous administration of factor concentrate.

Dosages of factor concentrates are calculated in the same manner as for plasma or cryoprecipitate. The desired percent of circulating factor must be decided by the patient's physician, then the following formula is utilized to calculate the dose (Agle et al, 1977):

$$\frac{\text{weight in pounds}}{4.4} \times \text{\% factor VIII or factor IX activity desired} = \text{\# of units of factor needed}$$

Almost all patients who require frequent factor infusions are on home care programs. Ineligible patients may include young children or babies with poor venous access, patients or parents with severe emotional problems, and in some treatment centers patients who have developed inhibitors (described in the following section on complications). It is not unusual for children enrolled in home care programs to receive all care as outpatients and to require infrequent hospitalization only for surgery or for treatment of a major bleed. Home care has meant a dramatic change for the families of children with hemophilia. The benefits include prompt treatment of bleeding episodes with subsequent decrease in serious arthropathy, decreased hospital time, increased school and work time, and greater sense of control by families and patients. (See Chapter 32 for a discussion of principles and strategies related to home care.)

Complications. Approximately 10 per cent of children with hemophilia will develop inhibitors. Inhibitors are circulating antibodies that render the infused factor VIII (or IX) molecule useless. Inhibitors are measured in terms of Bethesda units (BU). One BU inactivates the factor in 1 ml plasma. Hemophilic persons must have had at least one exposure to infused factor before they develop an inhibitor; however, at this time there is no evidence that frequent factor infusions predispose an individual to develop inhibitors.

The treatment of patients who have developed inhibitors is controversial. Some centers do not treat bleeding episodes in children with inhibitors unless they are life threatening. Other centers treat with massive doses of factor VIII. The number of units of factor that would be bound by the inhibitor is mathematically calculated, then units over and above this level are administered. In still other centers, a product that contains activated factor X (Xa) has been used with some success, as has therapy with high doses of prothrombin concentrates (Konyne, Proplex) which also contain appreciable levels of factor X. The high level of factor X is thought to "bypass" the need for factor VIII in the coagulation cascade. None of these methods has been highly successful and the last three methods are very expensive as well. The patient with an inhibitor is likely to spend more time hospitalized and is likely to have more severe joint disease.

Lyophilized factor products are produced from enormous amounts of pooled plasma, thus the risk of contamination with hepatitis virus is high. In fact, a high percentage of hemophilic patients have positive hepatitis antibody and elevated liver enzyme studies. The ultimate outcome of chronic liver irritation is as yet unknown. The newer manufacturing techniques have improved the quality and purity of factor concentrate.

AIDS (acquired immune deficiency syndrome) has recently come to the forefront as a risk to persons requiring frequent intravenous blood product infusions. As of July 1988, 3 per cent of hemophilic boys have the syndrome. The well-documented effects of untreated bleeding episodes versus the risk of AIDS has prompted the Medical and Scientific Advisory Council of the National Hemophilia Foundation to recommend continued aggressive early treatment of bleeding episodes with factor replacement. It is estimated that at least 70 to 80 per cent of the severely affected hemophilic males in the United States transfused between 1978 and 1985 are now HIV positive. During this time some of the country's factor supply was HIV positive. The next generation of hemophilic individuals should no longer be at risk for AIDS because of the improved donor screening, methods for HIV detection, and factor purification. The fate of those persons who are currently HIV positive remains uncertain. Currently the comprehensive hemophilic centers are teaching safe behavior of HIV-positive individuals to reduce spread of the disease. See Chapter 43 for further discussion of nursing strategies related to AIDS.

Major Nursing Diagnoses for Hemophilia

Potential for injury: localized hemorrhage, related to a significant decrease in clotting factor VIII (or IX) associated with a sex-linked genetic trait

Altered comfort: pain, related to hemarthrosis associated with trauma to a limb

Knowledge deficit, related to home care:

- *facts of hemophilia versus the myths*
- *signs and symptoms of bleeding within the GI tract, joints, muscles, soft tissue, and central nervous system*
- *appropriate first aid for nosebleeds and minor wounds*
- *administration of IV factor replacement*
- *risks of HIV infection from blood product infusion*
- *health promotion, including immunizations and dental hygiene*
- *provision of a safe but normal environment*
- *plan of treatment, including levels of activity, factor replacement, immobilization of joint following hemarthrosis, and emphasis on normalization of lifestyle*
- *where to obtain a Medic-alert tag*
- *availability of support groups and of genetic counseling*

Potential altered growth and development, related to

- *parental overprotection*
- *poor school attendance associated with treatment for bleeding episodes*
- *the stigma associated with a chronic disease and with physical restrictions*

Potential altered parenting: impaired patterns of discipline, related to

- *guilt associated with genetic transmission of the disease*
- *concern for the child's physical well-being*

Strategies for Nursing Care

Nursing interventions pertinent to the identified nursing diagnoses follow. Strategies for pain management are addressed under therapeutic management. Additional strategies for pain assessment and management can be found in Table 29-4, p. 878.

Administering and Teaching IV Factor Replacement. The nurse is often responsible for preparing and administering factor replacement to the hospitalized hemophilic patient. Detailed instructions for reconstitution accompany each bottle of factor concentrate. The unitage of each bottle varies, and this may sometimes cause confusion. The calculated factor replacement level should be approached as closely as possible without wasting any reconstituted factor. For example, if the physician calculates the required dose to be "500 units factor VIII" then any unitage *in that range* is acceptable. If the pharmacy or blood bank have only 550 unit vials available, then all the units should be given. At the same time, if only 480 unit vials

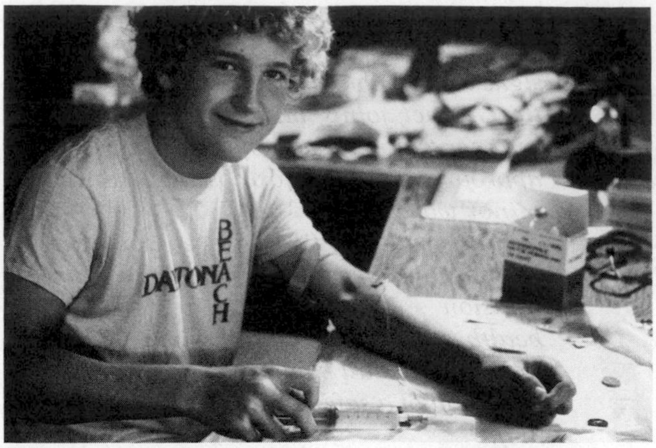

Self-infusion helps promote positive self-esteem and a sense of normality.

are available it would not be necessary to obtain an additional 20 units elsewhere. The calculated factor level should be regarded as an estimate.

The nurse should encourage the child and family to assist in mixing and administering the factor if they are not enrolled in a home care program. If the family is on home care, the nurse should not feel threatened by the family's desire to mix and perform venipuncture themselves. The nurse should encourage and reinforce this desire for independence. The child should be encouraged to participate in factor administration at an early age. He may begin by mixing the factor bottles or helping to push the plunger on the syringe. His responsibilities should increase gradually, and all boys should be using the self-infusion technique by their teenage years.

Teaching About the Risk of AIDS. The family must be given current information about the risk for AIDS infection related to transfusion of blood products. Updated information can be obtained from the Centers for Disease Control (1-800-342-AIDS or 1-800-342-7514). See Chapter 43, page 1590 for further discussion of AIDS.

Encouraging Health Promotion. The hemophilic child should receive his routine childhood immunizations. These shots are not deeply injected and firm pressure over the site or wrapping with an elastic bandage most often prevents muscle bleeding. Ice is probably of little benefit and must be used cautiously to prevent skin damage in young children. Other medications, such as antibiotics or pain medications, should be administered by oral or rectal routes if at all possible.

The nurse should reinforce the importance of a sound dental hygiene program. Preventive care will avoid an additional source of potential bleeding problems. Children should learn the proper technique of tooth brushing early. The child should be expected to brush at least twice a day with a soft-bristled brush. Visits to a dentist who is familiar with hemophilia should start at age 2 and should be maintained every 6 months. Dental anesthesia can be administered, but pretreatment with factor replacement is often necessary to prevent bleeding or hematoma at the injection site.

Providing a Safe, but Normal Environment. Parents are instructed to provide a safe environment for their child with hemophilia, but it is also important to normalize the environment as much as possible. The nurse can assist families by reviewing the various developmental and emotional stages of early childhood with the family and provide anticipatory guidance prior to each new stage.

Infancy is rarely a period of stress or bleeding problems. The infant is safely bundled and usually is not exposed to significant trauma. As previously stated, toddlerhood exposes the child to a whole new area of trauma, and it is at this time that most cases of hemophilia are diagnosed. In general, safety measures that should be employed for all children of this age are sufficient for the child with hemophilia. This includes gates or doors over stairs, locked cabinets, removal of dangling cords, removal of throw rugs, and placing obtrusive furniture in unobtrusive places as well as other well-described childproof measures. Padded clothing, padded furniture, helmets, and other similar measures are usually not recommended. These are largely ineffective in preventing hemophilic bleeding, and may psychologically ostracize the child. In addition, parents must be cautioned to not continually reprimand or remind the child with comments such as "Be careful," and, "Don't hurt yourself." It is inevitable that the child will hurt himself and will have bleeding episodes. The parents must realize early that this in no way reflects on their parenting ability. They must also be cautioned to never tell or even insinuate to their child that factor replacement is a form of punishment for participating in a forbidden activity.

Parents may have questions regarding appropriate toys for their children. Once again, age-appropriate and safe toys that would be used by any child are suitable. A Big Wheel tricycle may help prevent a few falls and subsequent bleeding because it is so low to the ground. A slightly longer period of training wheels on a new bike may also prevent some injuries. Working with scissors and later woodworking or similar shop type activities should not be forbidden as long as the child has been instructed in safe use and initially supervised.

The parents should be taught that physical activities and sports are vital to the child's muscular development and coordination as well as emotional well-being. Certain sports that predispose to injury and trauma such as football, soccer, ice hockey, karate, etc. must be avoided, but activities such as swimming, softball, running, hiking, and bicycling should be encouraged.

The nurse should inform all families of all new patients about the existence of the National Hemophilia Foundation (address listed at the end of this chapter). Nurses should encourage parents to avail themselves of the literature available through this group and to become involved in local chapters. Advice and support from a parent who has been through the same experience can be invaluable.

All children with hemophilia should wear Medicalert tags, even as infants. Young children should refrain from wearing necklaces for safety reasons, relying instead on bracelets or merely pinning the tag onto clothing.

Promoting Healthy Development. Stereotypes regarding the child with hemophilia as overprotected, timid boys with domineering guilt-ridden mothers or as risk-taking daredevils abound in the medical community. While this behavior may apply to some children and families, it is extremely unfair to label a population as such. In truth, until practical factor replacement became available, untreated joint bleeding with resultant severe pain and eventual crippling was the norm. Physicians urged families to protect their child from injury and expressly forbade any running, climbing, or other childhood activities.

Today, with the availability of factor replacement therapy, home care programs, and strong comprehensive hemophilia medical programs, families are encouraged to allow the child to run and play with friends, to attend regular classrooms, and, most importantly, to learn to set his own limits. Families and children require frequent interventions and counseling about psychosocial issues by the medical staff. The nurse who consistently cares for the child with hemophilia can develop a trusting relationship with the family. He or she may be the medical team member to whom the family feels most comfortable addressing their problems and concerns.

It is easy to understand why boys with hemophilia are at high risk of developing low self-esteem. The child may be thwarted in his attempts to achieve mastery of specific developmental tasks. The early wanderings and discoveries of toddlerhood may be restricted as may normal play activities when he gets older. School performance may be affected by poor attendance and by taunts or rejection by peers. Sadly, in some families the majority of the time that the child and parent spend together is medically related. The child can sense very early the burden he has placed on his family.

The family must be alerted to the subtle signs of overprotection that they may be giving their son. Constant admonishments to be careful, refusing to allow the child to participate in normal play activities, or not permitting the child to be away from home for extended periods lead the child to believe he is helpless and encourages a passive-dependent personality.

Promoting Healthy Patterns of Discipline. The boy with hemophilia needs lots of love and encouragement like any child, but he must not have ultraspecial status within the family. Allowing chronically ill children to "use" their disease to avoid discipline, household tasks, or homework must not be allowed. The same form of discipline should be used consistently with all children in the family, and the same expectations regarding achievements should be maintained. Allowing the child free reign of the home and school destroys his sense of industry and independence.

School personnel should be contacted by the medical team at the time of the child's entry into the system. Ideally, the nurse can make a school visit to facilitate the process. This can help correct misconceptions about the disease, and it helps teachers to develop a realistic approach with the child. The value of a good education cannot be overestimated for these children. This can best be achieved by early intervention with the school and open, honest communication among the school, family, and medical staff.

Nursing Strategies for Follow-up Care in the Home or Clinic

Assess for evidence of bleeding within the gastrointestinal, skeletal, and central nervous systems.

Assess the function of joints previously involved in hemorrhage into the joint capsule.

Monitor for complications of factor replacement therapy, especially hemolytic processes such as anemia and jaundice (Flug and Karpatkin, 1985).

Discuss with the child and family the child's progress on developmental tasks and encourage them to express their feelings about the effects of hemophilia on family functioning.

Facilitate self-management by acknowledging creative and/or adaptive responses of the child and individual family members.

von Willebrand Disease

von Willebrand disease is a complex, and as yet not fully understood, disorder of coagulation. It is usually inherited in an autosomal dominant fashion, although rarely it can be autosomal recessive (see Chapter 4 for a discussion of these inheritance patterns). The disease results in low levels of the factor VIII molecule and its component, the von Willebrand factor. Unlike classical hemophilia where the factor VIII molecule is present, but defective, the child with von Willebrand disease has diminished levels and, in very severe cases, complete absence of the entire factor VIII complex. The von Willebrand component of the factor VIII molecule is thought to be necessary for platelet aggregation (sticking together) to stop bleeding.

Clinical Manifestations

Clinical symptoms of von Willebrand disease vary greatly from person to person and may even vary within an individual's lifetime. Many children with the disorder escape diagnosis entirely unless routine coagulation studies are done prior to an unrelated surgery.

Children with severe disorders may present with frequent nosebleeds, bruising, gum bleeding, prolonged oozing of blood from minor wounds, and, in teenage girls, heavy and prolonged menses. Hemarthrosis, the bleeding most common in hemophilia, occurs very rarely in von Willebrand disease and only in cases where the factor VIII deficiency is severe.

Therapeutic Management

Most bleeding episodes in the child with classical von Willebrand disease will stop with conventional measures (i.e., pressure to the site of bleeding). The child requiring major dental extractions or surgery will require transfusions of cryoprecipitate or plasma and monitoring of the bleeding time and factor VIII levels prior to intervention. Commercially prepared factor VIII concentrates apparently do not contain the von Willebrand portion of the factor VIII molecule and, therefore, will not correct the bleeding defect, despite raising the factor VIII level. The bleeding defect in von Willebrand disease has responded to infusions of desmopressin acetate (DDAVP) (Lusher, 1984). DDAVP is a synthetic analog of the natural hormone arginine-vasopressin that is commonly used to treat diabetes insipidus. DDAVP causes immediate but transient release of factor VIII normally held in storage in the endothelium of blood vessels. The transient rise may be sufficient to protect a patient during minor surgery or dental work. DDAVP does not carry the risk of hepatitis or other blood product contamination and would be a preferred treatment if at all possible.

Menstrual periods may be quite a problem for young women with severe disease. Routine cryoprecipitate infusions may be necessary to control bleeding. A moderate degree of success has been achieved with hormonal modification of the menstrual cycle with anovulatory birth control pills. Pregnancy and childbirth can be safely achieved, but it is imperative that the young woman receive care from both obstetrician and hematologist. Cryoprecipitate infusions should begin prior to the delivery and should continue for several days postpartum.

The overall prognosis for the child with von Willebrand disease is very good. Those with mildly and even moderately decreased levels of factor VIII are apt to have no problems with routine activities. Children with severe disease are likely to be homozygotes (inheritance of gene from both parents), and the occurrence is uncommon. (The actual incidence is unknown.)

Strategies for Nursing Care

The family whose child is diagnosed with von Willebrand disease requires education about the disorder. Truthful reassurance is best for the parents of moderate or mildly affected children. Medic-alert tags should be worn by the child and physically demanding occupations should be discouraged. Children with von Willebrand disease are eligible for referral for services from the local and national Hemophilia Foundation.

Sepsis Neonatorum

Sepsis neonatorum, as the name implies, is an infection of the blood occurring in infants during the first month of life. The incidence is from 1 to 10 cases per 1,000 live births (McCracken and Freij, 1987).

Etiology

Although sepsis neonatorum may be caused by a variety of organisms, group B beta-hemolytic *Streptococcus* and *Escherichia coli* are by far the most prevalent. Infection may occur in utero by transplacental contamination from an infected mother, at the time of delivery (especially with aspiration of infected amniotic fluid or vaginal secretions), or after birth through contaminated articles or poor handwashing in the nursery or the home. The immature immune system of neonates makes them more prone to infection and less able to fight the organism once it has taken hold.

Clinical Manifestations

Although clinical manifestations vary somewhat depending upon the causative organism, the major signs and symptoms usually relate to thermoregulation and respiratory and gastrointestinal disturbances. Fever is less common than hypothermia, but either may result. Tachypnea and tachycardia are common, along with grunting respirations, cyanosis, intercostal and substernal retractions, and apnea. Gastrointestinal disturbances appear often as poor feeding, vomiting, abdominal distention, and diarrhea.

Meningitis may result from bacterial spread to the meninges. This is especially common with group B beta-hemolytic streptococcus infection. A bulging fontanel and a stiff neck are absent in the majority (at least 75 per cent) of neonates with meningitis, however (Overall, 1987).

Diagnostic Assessment

Suspicion of sepsis in the neonate will usually lead to a series of diagnostic tests to attempt to identify an organism in blood, urine, cerebrospinal fluid, and possibly other body secretions. Diagnosis is confirmed when an organism is isolated. Typically a "septic workup" includes a lumbar puncture to obtain cerebrospinal fluid for culture, a complete blood count with differential (preferably from a peripheral vein), a blood culture, a urinalysis and urine culture, and culture of any purulent drainage, as from the eye, umbilicus, or a surgical wound. Since hypoglycemia may also result from sepsis in the neonate, a blood sugar test is also frequently ordered.

Therapeutic Management

Immediately after cultures are obtained the neonate will be started on intravenous antibiotic therapy. The antibiotics ordered will vary with physician's preference, but therapy often involves ampicillin and gentamicin (Overall, 1987). Antibiotic therapy will be continued for 10 to 14 days or for at least 5 to 7 days after the signs and symptoms have resolved. Often, oxygen therapy is employed to ease the respiratory effort. The mortality rates for neonatal sepsis range from 10 to 40 per cent and increase to 15 to 50 per cent with meningeal involvement (Overall, 1987).

Strategies for Nursing Care

The major goals for nursing care are to maintain optimal blood levels of the antibiotic ordered, to conserve the neonate's energy so the little body can use all available resources to fight the infection, and to counsel and console the family.

Maintaining Optimal Blood Levels of Antibiotic. Maintenance of the intravenous line in a neonate requires a great deal of vigilance and ingenuity. The tiny vessels are fragile and infiltration is a common problem. See Chapter 30 for strategies related to protection of the intravenous site to prevent accidental dislodging of the needle or cannula. Inspect for infiltration and phlebitis before, during, and after each dose of antibiotic is given. Be alert to the neonate's comfort during drug administration in an effort to determine if the antibiotic is irritating the vein. The drip can sometimes be slowed somewhat or the drug can be further diluted to lessen irritation. This will not only make the infant more comfortable but will preserve the intravenous site for the optimum 72 hours.

Conserving Energy. When one considers the siege being waged against the newborn infant by the bacterial invasion and the potential for death if the neonate's body becomes overwhelmed by the infectious process, it helps to place this objective in perspective. Nursing care must be planned such that interventions deplete as little of the infant's energy reserve as possible. Attention must be given to thermoregulation, with the goal of keeping the temperature within normal limits. This includes not only intervening for fever but preventing unnecessary heat loss during baths and other procedures when the infant is uncovered.

Infants typically expend the most energy during crying and feeding. The infant may be too ill to cry as much as healthy neonates, but comfort measures are certainly an important consideration. Cuddling and rocking are often comforting, but the amount of time these infants are held must be based upon whether they rest better in the parent's (or nurse's) arms or in the crib (or isolette).

Feeding techniques must be geared toward maximum caloric intake for minimum energy expenditure. It may be advisable to use a "premie" nipple that delivers milk (formula or breast milk) with less sucking effort. The concern in using such a nipple is that the suck reflex will be diminished over time.

If the infant is receiving oxygen, it is helpful to use an oxygen monitor (e.g., transcutaneous or ear oximetry as detailed in Chapter 38). The monitor is an indirect measure of energy expenditure because oxygen saturation will diminish with increased effort in the infant with respiratory involvement. The nurse can then gauge such things as effort expended in feeding by the infant's ability to keep the blood saturated with oxygen. A decreasing saturation is an indication to allow the infant to rest.

Counseling and Consoling the Family. The family is likely to be very distraught at the sudden, severe illness of the newborn infant. The mother, often still recovering from childbirth, may be overwhelmed by feelings of sadness, concern, and guilt. The family may express frustration at not being able to "do" anything to help the infant and fear of diagnostic tests and treatments. The nurse who is available to inform, clarify, and console can be an invaluable ally at this time of crisis. See Table 31-2, p. 972 regarding crisis management with families of hospitalized children.

Resources Available for Information

Cooley's Anemia Foundation, 105 E. 22nd Street, Suite 911, New York, NY 10010, 800-221-3071.

National Hemophilia Foundation, 25 West 39th Street, New York, NY 10018, 212-869-9740.

National Association for Sickle Cell Disease, Inc. 34601 Wilshire Blvd., Suite 1012, Los Angeles, CA 90010.

See also Appendix Eight.

References

Agle DP et al: *Home Therapy for Hemophilia, A Physician's Manual.* New York, The National Hemophilia Foundation, 1977.

Andreoli TE et al: *Cecil Essentials of Medicine,* Philadelphia, WB Saunders, 1986.

Aronstram A et al: Double-blind controlled trial of three dosage regimens in treatment of hemarthrosis in hemophilia A. *Lancet* 1980 Jan 26; 169–171.

Behrman RE, Vaughan VC (eds): *Nelson Textbook of Pediatrics.* 13th ed. Philadelphia, WB Saunders, 1987.

Bussel JB, Hilgartner MW: Intravenous immunoglobulin therapy of idiopathic thrombocytopenic purpura in childhood and adolescence. *Hematol/Oncol Clin North Am* 1987 Sep; 1(3):465–482.

Flug F, Karpatkin M: Acquired disorders of homeostasis. *In* Zimmerman SS, Gildea JH (eds): *Critical Care Pediatrics.* Philadelphia, WB Saunders, 1985, 426–439.

Gaady-Cohen D: Idiopathic thrombocytopenia in children. *Issues Compr Pediatr Nurs* 1983 Sept-Dec; 6(5–6), 311.

Gradolf B: Sickle cell anemia in children. *Issues Compr Pediatr Nurs* 1983 Sept-Dec; 6(5–6):295–307.

Green M: *Green and Richmond Pediatric Diagnosis.* 4th ed. Philadelphia, WB Saunders, 1986.

Guyton AC: *Textbook of Medical Physiology.* 7th ed. Philadelphia, WB Saunders, 1986.

Helgartner M, McMillan CW: Coagulation disorders. *In* Miller D et al (eds): *Smith's Diseases of Infancy and Childhood.* 5th ed. St. Louis, CV Mosby, 1984, 868.

Klopovich P: An overview of anemia in children. *Issues Compr Pediatr Nurs* 1983 Sep-Dec; 6(5–6):281.

Lanzkowsky P: Iron deficiency anemia. *In Pediatric Hematology-Oncology.* New York, McGraw-Hill, 1980, 59.

Lukens J: Iron metabolism and iron deficiency anemia. *In* Miller DR et al (eds): *Smith's Diseases of Infancy and Childhood.* 5th ed. St. Louis, CV Mosby, 1984, 125, 131.

Lusher JM: Desmopressine Acetate (DDAVP): its use in disorders of hemostosis. *Thromb Hemost* 1984; 6(5).

McCracken GH, Freij BJ: Perinatal bacterial diseases. *In* Feigin RD, Cherry JD (eds): *Textbook of Pediatric Infectious Diseases,* Vol 1. Philadelphia, WB Saunders, 1987, 940–966.

Miller DR, O'Reilly RJ: Aplastic anemia. *In* Miller D et al (eds): *Smith's Blood Diseases of Infancy and Childhood.* 5th ed. St. Louis, CV Mosby, 1984, 523, 539, 542.

Oski F: Differential diagnosis of anemia. *In* Nathan D, Oski F (eds): *Hematology of Infancy and Childhood.* 2nd ed. Philadelphia, WB Saunders, 1981, 311–312, 328.

Overall JC: Infections of the newborn. *In* Behrman RE, Vaughan VC (eds): *Nelson Textbook of Pediatrics.* 13th ed. Philadelphia, WB Saunders, 1987, 422–435.

Pearson H: Sickle cell syndromes and other hemoglobinopathies. *In* Miller D et al (eds): *Smith's Diseases of Infancy and Childhood.* 5th ed. St. Louis, CV Mosby, 1984. 416, 422.

Pearson HA: Diseases of the blood. *In* Behrman RE, Vaughan VC (eds): *Nelson Textbook of Pediatrics.* 13th ed. Philadelphia, WB Saunders, 1987, 1033–1078.

Pearson HA: Sickle cell disease and its crises. *In* Dickerman JD, Lucey JF (eds): *Smith's the Critically Ill Child: Diagnosis and Medical Management.* 3rd ed. Philadelphia, WB Saunders, 1985, 229–241.

Vichinsky E, Lubin BH: Suggested guidelines for the treatment of children with sickle cell anemia. *Hematol/Oncol Clin North Am* 1987 Sep; 1(3):483–501.

Waskerwitz M: Iron deficiency anemia in children. *Issues Compr Pediatr Nurs* 1983 Sept–Dec; (5–6) 287–288.

Weatherall DJ et al: Editorial retrospective: iron loading in thalassemia—5 years with the pump. N Engl J Med 1983; 308:456.

Weetman RM, Boxer L: Childhood neutropenias. *Pediatr Clin North Am* 1980; 27:361–375.

Bibliography

AIDS Update. Hemophilia Information Exchange. New York, National Hemophilia Foundation, 1985 Mar.

Agle DP et al: *Psychological Factors in Hemophilia.* New York, National Hemophilia Foundation, 1980.

Carrai EB, Linney DR: *Employment Issues in Hemophilia: Questions and Answers.* New York, National Hemophilia Foundation, 1983.

Carroll PLF: Cyanosis. The sign you can't count on. *Nurs 88* 1988 Mar; 18(3):50.

Clements MJ, Mattison A: *Prevention of Social and Emotional Problems in Boys with Hemophilia.* New York, National Hemophilia Foundation, 1980.

Clements MJ: Patterns of impairment: Inherited hemostasis disorders. *In* Rose MH, Thomas RB (eds.): *Children with Chronic Conditions. Nursing in a Family and Community Context.* Philadelphia, WB Saunders, 1988, 213–244.

Fischbach FT: *A Manual of Laboratory Diagnostic Tests.* 2nd ed. Philadelphia, JB Lippincott, 1984.

Giver LN: New thinking about parenteral iron supplements. *Nurs '80* 1980 Aug.

Hubner C: Altered clotting. *In* Carrieri VK, et al (eds): *Pathophysiological Phenomena in Nursing. Human Responses to Illness.* Philadelphia, WB Saunders, 1986, 367–389.

Landier WC, et al: How to administer blood components to children. *MCN* 1987 May/Jun; 12(3):178–184.

Lipton J, Nathan D: Aplastic and hypoplastic anemia. *Pediatr Clin North Am* 1980; 27:217–235.

Lukens JD: Anemia of iron deficiency, blood loss, renal disease, and chronic infection. *In* Gellis SS, Kagan BM (eds): *Current Pediatric Therapy 12.* Philadelphia, WB Saunders, 1986, 243–246.

Martin M, Armstrong M: Busting the blood gas blues. *Am J Nurs* 1987 Oct; 87(10):1354.

Masoorli S, Piercy S: A lifesaving guide to blood products. *RN* 1984 Sep; 32–37.

National Association for Sickle Cell Disease, Inc. How to Help Your Child to "Take It In Stride." Los Angeles, 1974.

Querin J, Stabl L: Twelve simple sensible steps for successful blood transfusions. *Nurs '83* 1983 Nov; 36–42.

Rooney A, Hoveley C: Nursing management of disseminated intravascular coagulation. *Oncol Nurs Forum* 1985 Jan-Feb; 12(1):15–23.

Rozzell MS et al: The painful episode. *Nurs Clin North Am* 1983 Mar; 18(1).

Sergis-Davenport E et al: Overview of hemophilia. *Issues Compr Pediatr Nurs* 1983; 6(5–6):317–329.

Vichinsky EP et al: Sickle cell disease: basic concepts. *Hosp Med* 1983 Sep; 128–158.

Nursing Strategies: Altered Digestive Function

Chapter 41

Mabel Hunsberger
Robert Issenman

Nursing Process Plan
NPP: Care of the Child Following Abdominal Surgery, page 1394

Related Topics
Genetic counseling, Chapter 4
Promoting Healthy Dietary Practices, Chapter 18
Nursing Process Plan: The Child in Pain, Chapter 29
Principles of Fluid and Electrolyte Maintenance, Chapter 30
Nursing Process Plan: The Hospitalized Child, Chapter 31
Failure-to-Thrive, Chapter 35
Nursing Process Plan: The Family in Need of Genetic Counseling, Chapter 50

Digestive alterations can involve the gastrointestinal tract or its accessory organs, the liver, gallbladder, and pancreas. Such changes interfere with ingestion, transport, digestion, and absorption of nutrients. The child's growth and development may therefore be hindered, and chronic nutritional disturbances may occur. Although some alterations cause minor disruption, others, such as a diaphragmatic hernia or intestinal obstruction, can be life-threatening and require immediate treatment.

Disruptions that are caused by gastrointestinal anomalies, obstructive disorders, inflammatory illnesses, gastrointestinal dysfunction, malabsorption disorders, and liver disease are discussed in this chapter. Some of the alterations will be seen quite frequently by the nurse generalist in pediatrics; others have a much lower prevalence. Major nursing diagnoses and nursing strategies for follow-up care are included for those disorders that are encountered more frequently and for which nursing care is most complex.

Principles of Altered Digestive Function

The gastrointestinal system is responsible for breaking down fats, proteins, and carbohydrates into molecules that can be used by the cells as fuel. The gastrointestinal tract also defends the body against pathogens via lymphatic tissue in the small intestine (Peyer's patches), intestinal and gastric secretions containing immunoglobulins, and gastric acid in the stomach, which destroys pathogens because of its acidity. An alteration in the gastrointestinal system may affect the overall health of a child and can lead to fatal illness.

Developmental Differences Affecting Gastrointestinal Physiology

Developmental differences in absorption, immunity, membrane permeability, hepatic function, and type of gastric secretions affect gastrointestinal function of infants and children. In comparison with an adult, the newborn infant has a highly ineffective gastrointestinal system because function is still immature (see summary in Table 41-1).

By the first birthday, the major differences between the child and adult reflect the child's higher nutrient and energy needs for growth and a higher metabolic rate rather than inefficiency or immaturity of organ systems. Behavioral development also strongly influences the function of the gastrointestinal tract after the first year, and most problems of eating, digestion, and toileting can be traced back to this developmental aspect of childhood rather than to disease.

Differences in Intestinal Absorption

The loose stools of the newborn infant reflect a degree of malabsorption that would be thought pathologic for an adult. Lactose is incompletely absorbed because of lower lactase levels in the intestinal mucosa during the first three months of life. The normal infant absorbs only 90 per cent of ingested fat because of a smaller pool of bile acid. Less is known about protein diges-

Table 41-1. Developmental Differences in Structure and Function of the Gastrointestinal System

Anatomy and Physiology	Significance
Lactose Intolerance Decreased lactase levels in the intestinal mucosa	Lactose is incompletely absorbed, which can cause diarrhea
Fat Absorption Only 90 per cent of infant's ingested fat is absorbed because of decreased pool of bile acid	Fat in human milk is better absorbed owing to lipase (in mother's milk)
Immunocompromised* Immunoglobulin levels are generally lower. Anergic to skin tests (deficit in T-cell function)	Infants are immune compromised; however, human milk provides immunologic protective factors. Also, lactoferrin, a milk product, has an antibacterial effect
Intestinal Permeability to Whole Proteins An increased permeability facilitates uptake of immunoglobulin proteins	Cow's milk protein and other potential allergens also cross intestinal wall and may increase susceptibility to allergy
Physiological Jaundice Hepatic glucuronyl transferase levels not sufficient to conjugate water-insoluble bilirubin	Physiologic jaundice gradually clears as hepatic efficiency improves
Increased Gastrin and Stomach Acid May represent response to stress of birth or an adaptive response to help destroy ingested bacteria before breast feeding is established	High levels of secretion occur in first few days of life, which then gradually lower. Infants can develop stress ulcers

* See also Table 43-1.

tion. It is not clear whether this relative inefficiency serves some purpose or whether the newborn infant has insufficient resources to completely match the enormous metabolic demands that require 100 kilocalories per kilogram, compared with 30 to 40 kcal/kg characteristic of adult requirements.

However, certain relative deficiencies are compensated for by properties of human milk. Many studies suggest increased bioavailability of nutrients from human milk compared with cow's milk; for instance, fat in breast milk is more readily absorbed than the butterfat of cow's milk because of the activation of lipase present in mother's milk. Although iron levels are low in human milk, absorption is relatively complete.

Differences in Immune Competence

By most standards, the human infant is also immunocompromised. Immunoglobulin levels are generally lower, and infants are anergic (do not react) to skin tests, reflecting a relative deficit in T-cell function. Recently it has become known that human milk provides a variety of immunologically protective factors. Lactoferrin, a milk protein, has an antibacterial effect. Breast milk provides immunoglobulins, which may be surface active and are absorbed to a certain extent, possibly playing a role in systemic defenses.

Differences in Intestinal Permeability to Protein

Increased intestinal permeability to whole proteins, which facilitates uptake of protective immunoglobulin proteins, has been demonstrated in infants. However, the infant's system also allows cow's milk protein and other potential allergens to cross from the intestine into the bloodstream. This perhaps explains the young child's higher susceptibility to gastrointestinal allergic problems. The tendency toward these allergic responses decreases after 1 year of age, when the child's immunologic system becomes more like that of the adult.

Differences in Hepatic Function

Physiologic jaundice is one of the most consistent observations reflecting the unique metabolism of the newborn infant. For several days after birth, the child's hepatic glucuronyl transferase levels are incapable of conjugating all of the water-insoluble bilirubin created by the breakdown of old red blood cells. Consequently, most newborn infants have some degree of jaundice. This gradually clears as hepatic efficiency improves. For the same reasons, the liver of an infant has more difficulty metabolizing drugs. Consequently, medications must be given to infants in proportionately lower dosages or at longer intervals. (See Chapter 28 for further discussion on principles of pharmacology.)

Differences in Digestive Tract Secretions

Most secretory elements of the human digestive tract are present in lower amounts in the first few months after birth compared to later in life. However, some factors are produced in higher amounts. Serum gastrin and stomach acid, for instance, are produced in relatively high amounts in the first few days of life and then gradually decrease. This may represent a response to the stress of birth or an adaptive response to help kill ingested bacteria in the days before breast feeding is firmly established. However, the high levels of gastric hydrochloric acid may not be entirely beneficial, as certain infants develop stress ulcers. Such ulcers gradually resolve a few days after birth.

Box 41-1
Historical Factors to Consider in the Assessment of Gastrointestinal Alterations

PRESENTING SYMPTOM

PRENATAL AND PERINATAL HISTORY

Estimated gestation and birthweight
Prenatal care
Maternal nutrition
Polyhydramnios

PAST AND CURRENT HEALTH HISTORY

Prolonged jaundice at birth
History of gastrointestinal tract anomaly or surgery
Feeding history (ability to suck, episodes of aspiration or respiratory distress, frequency and amount of intake)
Regurgitation and vomiting
Gastric distention
General appetite
Bowel pattern (failure to pass meconium, diarrhea, constipation)
Abdominal pain
Weight gain or loss
Previous illness (inflammatory bowel disease, necrotizing enterocolitis)
Medications (related to gastrointestinal problem or other)

LIFESTYLE AND FAMILY FACTORS

Family history of anomaly, or gastrointestinal problem
Recent travel or move
Socioeconomic status
Health practices (food preparation, handwashing, general hygiene)
Stress within the family (social contacts, degree of isolation)
Individual stress for child

Assessment of Gastrointestinal Function

Health History and Physical Assessment

An assessment of the child with a gastrointestinal problem should begin with a standard history (see Chapter 15). The presenting symptom or symptoms should be assessed in depth and relevant areas that might be associated with gastrointestinal function should be explored. (See Box 41-1 for a summary of relevant historical information.)

A prenatal history, including a child's estimated duration of gestation and birthweight, yields important baselines to use when assessing growth patterns. Information about prenatal care should be gathered to determine any deficits or trauma during prenatal development.

Data from the neonatal and early infancy period are often relevant to gastrointestinal problems, which are often subtle and unrecognized in their early stages (such as feeding disturbances). Past and current history should therefore include a broad range of gastrointestinal system–related information. (See Past and Current Health History in Box 41-1) It is especially important to note whether a presenting symptom is associated in any way with a change in food or water intake. Information on recent travel or change of location is significant because of the potential for ingestion of contaminated food or water. Lifestyle and family factors are also explored. (See Box 41-1.) A family history should be obtained to seek a similar problem in other family members. Socioeconomic status and living conditions of the family should be considered because of their effect on general hygiene and health practices. The ability to provide an adequate diet and the presence of running water and indoor plumbing are often relevant factors. The number of children in the family and type of housing can affect the general health of children, especially in the case of infectious gastrointestinal problems. Finally, the stress, general happiness, and well-being within a family affect how children use food and relate to the experience of eating. Changes that have occurred in a child's life that might cause stress (e.g., starting to school, new sibling, death of a pet, a recent move) are particularly influential.

Because it is often a balance of intake and output that must be addressed when assessing gastrointestinal status, an important component in analyzing digestive function is a 24-hour nutritional history (see Chapter 18).

A complete physical examination is performed (see Chapter 15), including examination of the mouth for clefts, dental problems, or infections, and a thorough abdominal and rectal assessment for the presence or absence of clinical manifestations (see Table 41-2).

Laboratory and Diagnostic Studies

Gastrointestinal symptoms are often vague and frequently involve other body systems. Diagnostic tests are uncomfortable, require long periods of fasting, and may be both frightening and embarrassing to a child. Consequently, patients undergoing tests of gastroin-

Text continues on page 1382

Table 41-2. Clinical Manifestations of Gastrointestinal Problems

Clinical Manifestation	Clinical Significance
Regurgitation Lower esophageal sphincter is immature. Muscle is atonic (relaxed). Pressure on the fundus of the stomach exceeds that in the lower esophagus, resulting in spitting up	Many normal babies regurgitate one or more times a day. As long as normal weight gain progresses there is no cause for concern. Regurgitation usually disappears by 8 months of age but if it persists and is associated with failure to thrive, further evaluation is required
Vomiting Vomiting results from a coordinated sequence of abdominal muscle contractions and reverse esophageal peristalsis. It is usually associated with nausea except when projectile. Vomiting is classified as follows: *Mechanical:* secondary to an obstructive lesion. *Reflexive:* Due to gastrointestinal tract stimuli (e.g., infection, allergy). *Central:* 1. Central nervous system involvement (e.g., neoplasm, meningitis). 2. Caused by other than primary central nervous system involvement (e.g., abnormal metabolites, sepsis, psychogenic vomiting)	Vomiting is a common sign of gastrointestinal tract disturbance, but it also occurs in many other conditions. Character of vomitus is assessed to determine type of problem (see Box 41-2) and recognize clinical significance (see Box 41-3). Infants have immature cough and gag reflexes; therefore, they should be positioned on the side or abdomen to reduce aspiration. (See special positioning for Gastroesophageal reflux in Figure 41-22.) Note the onset, frequency, and severity (quantity, degree of forcefulness, presence of bile). Find out type of formula, amount ingested and amount expelled, feeding technique, and postfeeding position. Protracted vomiting may result in significant loss of hydrochloric acid, resulting in hypochloremic alkalosis. Urine is often paradoxically acidic because of intracellular deficits. Note associated symptoms such as fever, diarrhea, abdominal pain, bloody stools, and failure to thrive
Abdominal Distention Distention results from accumulation of fluid or gas (or both) within the gastrointestinal tract or peritoneal cavity	A young child's abdomen is normally rounded, thus making distention more difficult to evaluate. Also, children normally swallow air when eating or crying; therefore they have louder tympany. Palpation is easier because the abdominal wall is less developed. Gastrointestinal distention may be caused by congenital gastrointestinal tract malformations, constipation, hernia, gastrointestinal tract perforation, cirrhosis, or other problems, such as nephrosis, heart failure, or abdominal masses. Abdominal girth is measured at the umbilicus daily and marked with a pen
Abdominal Pain Abdominal pain may be acute, chronic, diffuse, or localized. It arises from the abdominopelvic viscera, the parietal peritoneum, or the capsules of the liver, kidney, or spleen. It is produced as a result of stretching or tension of the gut wall, traction on the peritoneum or mesentery, intestinal contraction, inflammation, ischemia, or sensory nerve irritation	Abdominal pain may herald an emergency; therefore, immediate assessment is required. Children cannot verbally describe pain as readily as adults and thus behavioral indices should be evaluated (grimacing, pulling legs up). Constant, steady pain may indicate organ perforation, ischemia, inflammation, or the presence of blood in the peritoneal cavity
Diarrhea Diarrhea is an increase in the frequency and fluidity of bowel movements. It may be *acute* as a result of infection, stress, a reaction to drugs, or fecal impaction, or *chronic* as a result of chronic infection, obstructive and inflammatory bowel disease, and malabsorption syndrome. Diarrhea may also result from food allergy, gastrointestinal tract anomalies or as a result of gastrointestinal surgery Diarrhea occurs when there is excess fluid in the small intestine. This occurs as the result of 1. stimulation of cyclic AMP by bacterial toxins or other factors, resulting in active transport of electrolytes into small intestine 2. disrupted integrity of small intestinal mucosa, impairing intestinal absorption 3. increased intestinal motility, resulting in decreased intestinal absorption	Note onset, duration, frequency, pattern, severity, and character of stool. Assess for associated gastrointestinal symptoms such as vomiting, abdominal pain, and anorexia. Systemic symptoms such as fever, coryza, weight loss, and reduced general activity are often associated with gastrointestinal disorders. Assess hydration, circulatory status, and mental status *Mildly ill:* Patient is alert, is active, appears well hydrated, and has normal urinary output *Moderately ill:* Patient may be lethargic, have ↓ tearing, dry skin, ↓ urine output *Severely ill:* Patient has altered mental status (irritability or lethargy), rapid pulse, poor skin turgor, delayed capillary refill, no tears. (See Box 41-4 for causes of diarrhea and associated symptoms)

Box 41-2
Character of Vomitus and Associated Symptoms in Common Gastrointestinal Disturbances

APPENDICITIS

May follow or accompany abdominal pain

GASTRITIS

Vomitus may contain mucus or blood and be associated with belching and pain. Slowly bleeding gastric or duodenal lesion can result in coffee-ground vomitus (digested blood)

GASTROENTERITIS

Vomitus often contains undigested food and is associated with diarrhea, hyperactive bowel sounds, fever, and abdominal pain

INTESTINAL OBSTRUCTION

Obstruction below pylorus (bile-stained or greenish vomitus). Intestinal obstruction or infarction (brown vomitus with fecal odor)

PYLORIC STENOSIS

Projectile vomiting associated with visible peristaltic waves across epigastrium

INTUSSUSCEPTION

Vomiting associated with bloody stools

Box 41-3
Clinical Significance of Character of Vomitus

UNDIGESTED FOOD

In a newborn infant, undigested food suggests esophageal atresia; in older children it suggests an obstruction or stricture at or above the cardia

ABSENCE OF BILE

Absence of bile suggests an obstruction proximal to the ampulla of Vater. In freshly passed vomitus bile may not be apparent because food and gastric juice may camouflage the yellow color of bile. On exposure to air, oxidation of bile causes it to turn green

BILIOUS VOMITING

A sign of intestinal obstruction

FECAL VOMITING

A sign of peritonitis or an obstruction of the lower bowel or colon

HEMATEMESIS

Bright red color indicates that the blood has not been in contact with gastric juices; therefore, acute bleeding must be occurring at or above the cardia or in the stomach

COFFEE-GROUND EMESIS

Vomitus that appears like coffee grounds indicates that blood has been altered by gastric contents and suggests slow bleeding from the esophagus, stomach, or duodenum

Box 41-4
Causes of Diarrhea and Associated Symptoms

MALABSORPTION

Occurs after meals. Diarrhea accompanied by distention, cramps, steatorrhea, anorexia, weight loss, fatigue

INFECTION

Is extremely watery and contains mucus. Is associated with pain, cramps, nausea, vomiting, and fever. May lead to dehydration, weight loss, and possibly blood in the stool

CROHN DISEASE

Patient may have 10 to 20 stools a day. Associated with crampy abdominal pain, nausea, fever, chills, weakness, anorexia, and weight loss

ULCERATIVE COLITIS

Bloody diarrhea and abdominal pain

INTESTINAL OBSTRUCTION

Partial obstruction increases intestinal motility, resulting in diarrhea, pain, nausea, and sometimes distention. Bloody stools may occur

IRRITABLE BOWEL SYNDROME

Diarrhea alternates with constipation or normal bowel function. Associated with pain, distention, dyspepsia, and nausea

LACTOSE INTOLERANCE

Diarrhea occurs after milk ingestion and is accompanied by pain and flatus testinal function require the nurse's attention and special support. Because many of these tests interfere with one another, the nurse must be clear about the order in which certain tests should be done, as well as how to prepare the patient.

In addition to physical preparation, the child and family should be given accurate explanations. During the test further explanations may be given, and steps are taken to reduce the discomfort and anxiety that accompanies these procedures. Because anxiety increases the perception of pain, sedation and analgesia are recommended for certain procedures even though they are not in themselves extremely painful.

Explanations and a supportive approach are especially important when the procedure is uncomfortable. Barium enema, sigmoidoscopy, and colonoscopy are generally uncomfortable and may be particularly embarrassing for a child or teenager. These tests should be performed as infrequently as possible in children and be done in a calm and gentle manner when they are necessary. It is important that someone be specifically assigned to remain at the patient's side (close to the head) while the tests are done. This could be a nurse, a parent, or ideally both. Every step in the procedure is explained. The child should first be allowed to touch the clean rectal glove to become familiar with the sensation encountered. A dab of lubricant is smeared on the patient's hand so that its coldness is not interpreted as pain before the procedure has begun. Similarly, the operator should first touch the anus with a gloved lubricated finger and ask the patient whether or not this is painful before inserting any instruments. Patients should be taught breathing techniques which give them some element of control to combat the intense feelings of vulnerability and powerlessness accompanying these examinations.

Following an examination, a child is given the opportunity to express his or her feelings about the experience and is encouraged to resume usual activities (unless physical activity is restricted by the medical condition).

Laboratory tests and diagnostic procedures commonly used to assess gastrointestinal alterations are summarized in Tables 41-3 and 41-4, respectively.

Nursing Strategies and Goals of Nursing Care

The overall goal of nursing care is to foster normal growth and development by maintaining a balanced nutritional state. The nurse's role is important because of the meticulous monitoring of nutritional intake and output that is needed and the clinical judgment that is required concerning feeding methods and approaches. The nurse's observations during feeding and assessment of the child's overall behavior and physiologic status provide important data on which management decisions are made. The nurse needs to understand the importance of precise monitoring, the use of a variety of nutrition and elimination procedures, principles of postoperative care and the psychosocial impact of gastrointestinal disturbances on the child and family.

Ensuring Precision in Monitoring and Measurement

Successful management of children with gastrointestinal problems rests primarily in the hands of those who calculate and record the daily nutritional and fluid balance data. Although these activities are easy to perform, if not done properly and consistently the nurse's efforts will be of little value. Inaccurate recording can actually present a danger to the patient because management decisions are then based on wrong information. A basic question to ask in any situation of measurement and calculation is, "Does this number make sense?" For example, if an infant's weight has dropped significantly but the intake has been maintained, the nurse should either search for an explanation (e.g., such as administration of a diuretic) or for an error in recording or calculation. ***Record-keeping thus involves, to a great extent, the process of analyzing and interpreting the meaning of what has been calculated and recorded.*** See Table 41-5 for a description of parameters frequently measured when caring for children with gastrointestinal problems.

Providing Altered Means for Nutrition and Elimination

Disruptions in digestive function frequently make it necessary to use alternative diets and feeding methods. When normal digestive processes are altered, intake is adjusted accordingly. Various types of dietary adjustments and nursing considerations are summarized in Table 41-6. Children with gastrointestinal problems require a variety of specialized procedures to re-establish and maintain digestive function. Following is a discussion on the care of children who require (1) a nasogastric tube; (2) an enema; and (3) a colostomy.

Caring for a Child with a Nasogastric Tube

Children require nasogastric tubes to provide a route for gavage feedings (given when a child is unable to

Text continues on page 1387

Table 41-3. Laboratory Tests Commonly Used to Diagnose Gastrointestinal Disturbances

Laboratory Test	Purpose or Use	Interpretation of Test or Other Information
Complete Blood Count (CBC)	Measures the hemoglobin (Hgb), hematocrit (Hct), and the red and white blood cell counts (RBC, WBC). Used to assess for infection, anemia, or hemorrhage	Low Hgb and Hct indicate blood loss, poor iron intake, or absorption. Hgb and Hct are elevated in dehydration because of vascular fluid volume deficit
Erythrocyte Sedimentation Rate	Measures the rate at which red blood cells settle to the bottom of a calibrated tube in the laboratory. Used to assess for inflammation	Reflects inflammation in the body but does not predict exactly where the problem lies. Useful as a screening test to indicate underlying disease such as Crohn disease
Serum Electrolytes (Na, K, Cl)	Serum sodium, potassium, and chloride are measured to assess electrolyte balance. Balance among electrolytes is critical to normal metabolism and cellular function	Disturbed by poor intake, metabolic disturbance, excess losses, or poorly regulated intravenous fluids
Liver enzymes:	A group of enzymes reflecting important liver functions	
Serum Glutamic Pyruvic Transaminase (SGPT) or Alanine Aminotransferase (ALT)	Elevated when damage to liver (or heart) cells has occurred	Reflects cell *integrity* rather than *function.* ALT (SGPT) and AST (SGOT) are similar. ALT (SGPT) is liver specific whereas AST (SGOT) is derived from other organs in addition to the liver; in most cases there are parallel rises
Serum Glutamic Oxaloacetic Transaminase (SGOT) or Aspartate Aminotransferase (AST)	Similar to SGPT	
Alkaline Phosphatase (Alk Phos)	Measures hepatic obstruction	Also raised by bone turnover, so it is always higher in the growing child (also in rickets)
Bilirubin	Increased with hemolysis or liver damage	Primary excretion product from the breakdown of red blood cells
Serum Ammonia	Measures impaired hepatic detoxification of protein	Measures liver *function* while other liver enzymes reflect liver *cell integrity*
Serum Amylase	An important pancreatic enzyme	One of the few measures of pancreatic function
Hepatitis Antigens	Measures components of the hepatitis B virus	Different components appear at different times in hepatic infection
Hepatitis Antibodies	Measures the immune response to infection	Can reflect present hepatic infection as well as past infection and immunity
Absorption Tests		
Xylose Tolerance Test	An indicator of intestinal mucosal function	Xylose, a passively absorbed sugar, is given by mouth after 8-hour fast. A blood level taken 1 hour later gives an index of intestinal absorption
Breath Hydrogen Test	Measures functioning of intestinal disaccharidase enzymes	Measured excretion of hydrogen in the breath reflects lactase, sucrase, or other sugar, depending on the sugar ingested. Breath samples are taken at ½ hour intervals after ingestion of the index sugar in solution
Carbohydrate Tolerance	Measures uptake of sugar into the bloodstream	Blood specimens are taken at ½ hour intervals to check serum glucose levels. Less a measure of absorption than of metabolic regulation
Stool Tests		
Reducing Substance	Measures certain sugars when they are not completely absorbed	Depends on which sugars are fed (lactose and glucose are reducing substances; sucrose is not)
Stool pH	Measures the acidity of the stool	Stool turns acid with the malabsorption of sugars
Stool Fat	Measured as a stain on a random sample or a 72 to 96-hour timed collection correlated to fat intake	Useful measure of malabsorption, as fat accounts for such a high proportion of ingested calories. The time when the test is initiated and completed should be carefully recorded. In children concurrent food intake over the same interval is recorded so that the dietitian can determine the fat content of the food ingested
Stool Trypsin	A random sample of the pancreatic enzyme	Normally found only in stools of infants; its absence may indicate cystic fibrosis
Stool Culture	Pathogenic bacteria are grown in the laboratory	Selective media are used to depress growth except the specific problem organisms. Hence samples may be taken from the diaper, the floor, and so forth

continued

Table 41-3 *(continued)*

Laboratory Test	Purpose or Use	Interpretation of Test or Other Information
Ova and Parasites	Parasites or their eggs are sought in the stool	Specimens must be freshly examined or preserved in fixative solution
Pinworm Test	Uses anal scotch tape imprint to locate the pinworm eggs	Tape is placed on the perianal folds as parasite emerges at night to lay eggs in the anal tissues. The sticky surface of tape is then placed on a slide. A commercially prepared swab with a sticky surface is also available
Occult Blood	A variety of tests are available, specifically developed to detect blood loss itself or minute traces, as in cancer	Denotes blood in the stool, indicating blood loss or inflammation

Table 41-4. Diagnostic Procedures Commonly Performed to Diagnose Gastrointestinal Disturbances

Diagnostic Procedure	Purpose or Use	Comments
Upper Gastrointestinal (UGI) Endoscopy	Direct examination of the esophagus, stomach, and duodenum using a fiberoptic endoscope	Usually accomplished by anesthetizing the throat and using sedation or general anesthetic
Colonoscopy	Direct endoscopic examination of the colon as far as the ileocecal junction	The colon must be entirely empty. Study done with sedation or general anesthetic
Sigmoidoscopy	Examination of the rectum and sigmoid colon using a rigid or flexible fiberoptic tube	A more limited examination than a colonoscopy. May only take 5 minutes. Sedation is used in infants and children especially if they are apprehensive
Upper Gastrointestinal (UGI) Radiography	Radiologic examination of the esophagus, stomach, and upper small bowel by use of a contrast agent (e.g., barium)	Patient must have taken nothing by mouth. Contrast medium is taken from a bottle or cup but is resisted by some children
Small Bowel Follow-through	Radiologic examination of the lower small bowel using contrast. Barium is followed by sequential x-ray films, as it progresses down the intestinal tract. Most useful to detect Crohn's disease or low small bowel lesions	Patient must have taken nothing by mouth. Test may take up to 90 minutes, depending on intestinal transit. Occasionally barium is introduced by tube. Sequential films are made and it is necessary to tilt the table in various positions
Barium Enema	Radiologic examination of the colon using contrast. May be used to diagnose Hirschsprung disease, causes of rectal bleeding, or polyps. Hydrostatic pressure can at times reduce an intussuception	Barium is run into the bowel from an enema bag. Sometimes air is introduced to give "double contrast" for greater detail. An uncomfortable test because cramps are felt when the colon is distended. Children will be asked to "hold" barium as the various x-ray films are taken
Flat Plate of Abdomen	Radiologic examination of the abdomen without contrast. Demonstrates air-fluid levels in obstruction, constipation, or stones	Can be done without bowel preparation. A simple x-ray of the abdomen
Three Views of Abdomen	Radiologic examination of the abdomen without contrast but includes a standing film and one with patient lying on the side	Moving the patient causes air to float to the top, and different features can be visualized
Duodenal-Jejunal Biopsy or Aspirate	These techniques are used to find parasites or to diagnose celiac disease	The child is sedated. A sample of tissue and fluid is taken from the upper small bowel either through an endoscope or through a sampling tube, which is passed down the alimentary canal until it lodges in the small bowel. Using a special capsule on the tube with a small cutting edge, the specimen is taken and removed for examination
Cholangiography Oral cholecystogram (OCG); Intravenous Cholangiogram (ICG); Endoscopic Retrograde Cholangiopancreatography (ERCP); Transhepatic Cholangeogram	Radiologic examination of the gallbladder and biliary tree	Contrast medium is administered orally. If more concentration is required, contrast agent may be given intravenously (ICG), or pushed into the biliary tree from an endoscope in the duodenum (ERCP), or injected directly through the liver (transhepatic)

***Table* 41-4** *(continued)*

Diagnostic Procedure	Purpose or Use	Comments
Liver Biopsy	Many liver diseases can be diagnosed only by examining the liver tissue	A sample of liver is obtained by putting a needle into the liver. It is done with sedation or a general anesthetic. Coagulation must be normal or corrected with vitamin K or plasma
Rose Bengal, Tech IIIDA, Tech BIDA (liver scan)	Nuclear imaging is used to track a radioactive tracer through the course of the liver. An abnormal test indicates obstruction	These tracers are injected intravenously and excreted much like bilirubin in the liver. The radioactive "tag" allows them to be recognized by the scanner. Involves less radiation than a chest radiograph
Ultrasonography of Abdomen	Uses sound waves to examine abdomen. Works best to view cysts, masses, and the gallbladder	Not an invasive test, but the patient must lie still. Helpful for a parent to accompany a small child
CT Scan of Abdomen	Multiple radiographs combined and interpreted by a computer. Contrast medium may be used	Can visualize "invisible" pancreas, adrenals, and blood vessels
Manometry or Motility	Measures the pressures in the esophagus and stomach through a tube. Can measure transmission of a peristaltic wave	Child must lie quietly despite presence of a nasal tube
24-hour pH Monitoring	Uses an "acid-sensitive" probe left in the esophagus and connected to a portable recorder to measure the number of times acid refluxes from stomach into esophagus. Most reliable test of acid reflux	Usualy done overnight as an inpatient or outpatient procedure
Meckel Scan	Uses radioactive-labeled technetium which is taken up in "ectopic" stomach tissue in the Meckel diverticulum to locate its presence	A non-invasive test but not always accurate
Rectal Biopsy	A small amount of tissue is removed from the rectum either by a direct incision, pinch biopsy, or suction biopsy. Special stains are used in processing the tissue to locate absence of nerves in Hirschsprung disease	Although the procedure does not cause pain, a child may be fearful because of the equipment and setting. Also, parents often think biopsy means looking for cancer

***Table* 41-5.** Parameters for Assessment of Gastrointestinal Status

Description	Nursing Implications
Calorie Count	
All food is measured and recorded. The nurse is not usually responsible for calculating calories; instead, the exact amount of food eaten is recorded (e.g., by teaspoons, tablespoons, or cups). The nutritionist then calculates caloric intake. Calorie-containing liquids must also be recorded	Parents can be taught to measure and record the amount of food eaten. Calorie count sheet should be kept at the bedside to facilitate recording after each meal and snack
Intake and Output Record	
Intake and output is recorded to assess fluid balance. All fluid intake orally, intravenously, or by other means is entered in separate columns and totaled. Similarly, urinary output is measured, as well as any other measureable liquid, (e.g., secretions from a nasogastric decompression tube). Stool is generally not measured unless accurate intake and output is required; however, the number, character, and color of stools is recorded. The number of voids for infants is generally counted unless accurate intake and output is required; then diapers are weighed	Foods such as Popsicles and gelatin can be calculated as a liquid when child is on liquid diet. ½ standard Popsicle = 50 ml

continued

Table 41-5 *(continued)*

Description	Nursing Implications
Accurate Intake and Output (Stool Collection, Diaper Weights, Emesis, Intravenous, and Nasogastric)	
All intake and output is measured, including food, liquid intake, urine output, stool, emesis, and body secretions. Stool can be measured by using a metabolic bed (a mesh stripped over frame of Isolette and collected into a funnel) or by taping a urinary bag over the anal area. This can only be done for a limited time period as skin breakdown occurs. If stool is well-formed the diaper can be lined with a plastic liner but again skin breakdown occurs with extensive use. Urinary output for infants can be measured by weighing diapers. Each diaper is weighed before use (weight of diaper is written on the diaper if disposable diapers are used) and again after it is wet. The difference is calculated in grams and converted to milliliters (1 gm = 1 ml). Vomitus is also calculated whenever it can be measured. If it is expelled on the linen it can be estimated. To estimate vomitus a liquid can be poured on the same linen at a different spot until an area of equal size is saturated. The actual amount of emesis is often less than one would estimate by observation only. Intravenous intake is calculated according to fluid in the chamber (not the intravenous bag). Additionally, any intravenous fluid that is used to administer medications is added to intake. Collection from a nasogastric tube is calculated as output, but any amount instilled to irrigate the tube must either be subtracted from the total collection or counted as input	When 72-hour stool is collected, the best method is to place a plastic bag over the anal area in order to keep stool and urine separate. To calculate accurate output diapers should be weighed individually to increase accuracy. Even disposable diapers in a single box may have different weights. Diapers must be weighed on the same scale before and after use. To increase accuracy they should be weighed as soon as possible after use as a diaper that has dried will not provide a correct measure of output
Daily Weight	
An infant is weighed with no clothes and no diaper. Weights should be done at the same time daily and *before* a feeding. The same scale should be used from day to day. If there is a large discrepancy in a weight compared to the previous weight it should be checked by two nurses for verification and charted accordingly	Scales should be moved as little as possible. Whenever possible the child should be brought to the scale. Struggling, kicking infants are difficult to weigh. The job can be made easier if the previous weight is known so that the actual weight can be found more quickly. Even when electronic scales are used, the previous weight should be known to be able to identify a discrepancy
Urine Specific Gravity	
Specific gravity of urine can be monitored by nurses on the unit by using a fractometer or a specific gravity set from the laboratory. Specific gravity range is normally as follows: 1.001 – 1.020 (neonate or infant) 1.001 – 1.030 (thereafter) 1.025 (after fluid restriction)	As specific gravity rises, the patient is becoming less hydrated. A low specific gravity occurs when patient has increased secretion of urine (diuresis)
Abdominal Girth	
The circumference of the abdomen is measured by placing a tape around the abdomen at the level of the largest diameter. The tape must be level from front to back	It is useful to mark the skin at two points (both sides or front and back) to indicate point of measurement from day to day. Use a tape that does not stretch (paper rather than cloth) and measure when patient is in same position from day to day (a lying down position is typical because the child who requires daily abdominal girth measurement is often too ill to be ambulatory)
Stool Chart	
When a stool chart is kept, descriptions of the stool should be included: (e.g., amount (scant, small, medium, large), color (yellow, green, brown, black, or combinations, such as yellowish-green), character (meconium, mucousy, watery, seedy, loose, solid or formed, hard pellets, greasy, bulky), odor (foul-smelling, musty, sour, or vinegar-like)	Interpretation of stool varies from one individual to another. To increase significance of assessment, it is beneficial if the same nurse can make the assessment from day to day on an individual patient. (Parents are helpful to provide continuity in assessment)

***Table* 41-6.** Nutritional Strategies and Nursing Considerations

Description	Nursing Considerations
NPO (Nothing By Mouth)	
Children frequently are not permitted to ingest anything by mouth because there is an anatomic abnormality (e.g., tracheoesophageal fistula), a digestive problem (e.g., Crohn disease), a temporary infectious process (e.g., gastroenteritis), or sucking inadequacy (e.g., low birthweight infants). Children also are put on NPO in preparation for diagnostic procedures and surgery and for a period of time postoperatively until postoperative ileus resolves.	Children who are not permitted to have anything by mouth should have a sign placed above their bed. It is also humane to take children from their rooms to the playroom when breakfast is served the morning of a procedure or surgery, if possible.
Clear Liquid Diets	
Clear liquid diets consist of water, gelatin-water, Popsicles, gelatin, broth, glucose water, flat sodas, and clear juice (apple or cranberry juice).	Liquids with high sugar content need to be kept to a minimum when treating conditions such as osmotic diarrhea (the high sugar content causes an influx of water into the small bowel and prevents absorption of water and electrolytes).
Thickened Feedings	
Thickened feeds are prepared by adding cereal to milk to a thickness that permits infant to take milk from bottle. These feeds reduce tendency for regurgitation.	This method of treatment is attempted with varying success. Be careful to avoid making the nipple hole so large that an infant would obtain too much too fast, causing aspiration.
Elemental Diet	
Elemental diets are used when regular food is not tolerated but the condition does not require total parenteral nutrition (TPN). Elemental diets are a complete nutritional regimen containing essential and nonessential amino acids, simple sugars, minimal fat, minerals, trace elements, and vitamins. These diets are nutritionally balanced, bulk- and residue-free, low in fat, and digested primarily in the upper jejunum. They are more rapidly absorbed than regular food.	Elemental diets are generally unpalatable; therefore, they are given by tube feeding. If they are taken orally, chilling increases palatability. Bolus feeding of these diets produces nausea, cramps, and diarrhea because of the high osmolarity. Feedings are started in one-fourth strength or one-half strength and increased in volume, then given in full concentration.
Positioning after Feeding	
Placing an infant on the right side during and after feeding facilitates emptying of the stomach because the pyloric sphincter muscle, which opens into the duodenum, is on the right side. Collection of fluid in the curvature of the stomach occurs more easily when the baby is placed on the left side. The danger of aspiration is reduced by placing infants on either side or on the abdomen. Elevation of the head slightly relieves the pressure of a full stomach on the diaphragm.	Placing infants into infant seats after feeding when there is a potential for vomiting can result in aspiration.

take nourishment by mouth), for abdominal decompression, or for lavage (washing out of the stomach). Regardless of the intended use, the principles for insertion are the same (Fig. 41-1). Insertion of this tube is a frightening experience and should be explained to the child and the parents. The parents should also be told how they may assist. The child is given descriptions of the sensations during and after the insertion. Parents should remain with the child during the insertion to provide comfort. The child is helped to sit quietly by the parents or a nurse during the insertion. A choking sensation occurs as the tube stimulates the gag reflex, but this will subside as the tube passes beyond the pharynx.

An older child may complain of a sore throat, earache, or dry mouth and lips while a tube is in place. Providing frequent mouth care and lubrication for the lips will lessen the discomfort. With the permission of the physician, a child can be allowed to suck on hard candy or ice chips to soothe the sore throat.

Nasogastric Tube Feeding. Nasogastric feeding may be given by a continuous drip feeding or an intermittent feeding. The formula and amount are prescribed by the physician. The continuous drip formula should be infused slowly to avoid distention or discomfort. If the patient complains of nausea, the feeding should be slowed or discontinued temporarily. The amount of formula that is hung should not exceed

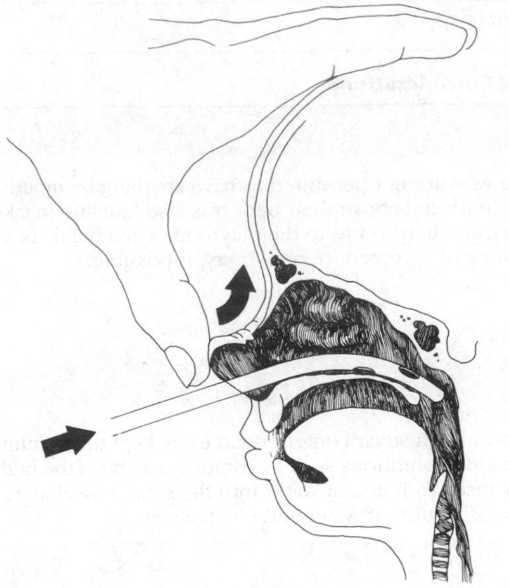

Figure 41-1. Nasal passage of tube. The tip of the nose is pressed slightly upward to enlarge the nasal opening. The tube is directed to slide along the base of the nose. If resistance is encountered, the tube must be withdrawn and redirected. (From Hughes WT, Buescher ES: *Pediatric Procedures.* Philadelphia, WB Saunders Co, 1980, p 246.)

that which will be used in 4 hours because the milk-based formula is an excellent medium for bacterial growth.

Previously used measurement techniques for the placement of gavage tubes have been found to be inaccurate when tested in premature infants. Measuring to a point midway *between* the termination of the xiphoid process and the umbilicus was compared to measuring *to* the xiphoid process. Both methods yielded incorrect placement rates (39.3 per cent and 55.6 per cent, respectively). Measurement to a point midway between the termination of the xiphoid process and the umbilicus yielded more accurate placement and is the current method in pediatric practice, although other placement methods are being explored (Weibley et al, 1987).

When administering a formula to an infant, provide the same stimulation that would be given if the feeding was taken orally. The infant should be held and talked to during the feeding. If it is not contraindicated, the infant may suck on a pacifier during the feeding. Loss of the suck reflex may occur in a short period of time if it is not stimulated in this way.

With intermittent feeding of infants, the tube may be inserted before each feeding and taken out after the feeding is completed. In this instance, the tube is usually inserted through the mouth rather than the nose. If a tube is to stay in place between feedings, it should be cleared with several milliters of water after the feeding is completed. To remove the tube, the procedure is explained to the child, as appropriate, and the tube is clamped and then gently withdrawn. Mouth care is provided, as soon as possible, following removal of the tube. (See Box 41-5 for summary of gavage feeding procedure.)

Decompression by a Nasogastric Tube. A nasogastric tube may be inserted to remove air and secretions from the stomach and intestines (decompression) preoperatively or postoperatively (or both) to prevent vomiting and bowel distention. Peristalsis is inhibited after abdominal surgery owing to handling of the abdominal organs, necessitating decompression by a nasogastric tube. Drainage is achieved by intermittent suction or by gravity drainage. Continuous suction is generally not used (except on very low suction) because it irritates the mucosal wall of the stomach.

When a child has a nasogastric tube for decompression, the amount, consistency, and color of drainage are observed and recorded. The drainage contains important electrolytes; therefore, it must be measured accurately to allow replacement. Drainage is replaced by giving an amount of intravenous fluids as ordered by the physician equal to the amount of drainage. (This is in addition to the daily 24-hour intravenous fluids.) Ensuring patency of the tube is accomplished by irrigating the tube with normal saline according to the physician's order.

The usual order is for irrigation with a specified amount of normal saline every 2 hours and as necessary. The diameter of the barrel of the syringe determines the degree of pressure that is being applied while irrigating. A very small barrelled syringe (i.e., TB syringe) produces an insufficient amount of force to effectively irrigate a nasogastric tube. Conversely, the barrel of a 10 cc syringe produces too great a force for a premature infant.

When irrigating, the saline is gently instilled with a syringe (without a needle) and then gently drawn back. The same amount that is instilled is withdrawn to ensure accurate calculation of the drainage. An alternative method is to reconnect the tube to suction after instilling saline, noting that the fluid is freely drawn back by suction. The amount of saline instilled each shift or each 24 hours must then be calculated and subtracted from the total amount of drainage to calculate the actual drainage. In either method, force is never used while instilling nor while drawing back because the stomach mucosa is easily damaged. The ease with which the tube irrigates and the consistency, color, and amount of the fluid returned at the time of irrigation are recorded. Bowel sounds should be checked whenever a child has a nasogastric tube for abdominal decompression.

Lavage by Nasogastric Tube. When a nasogastric tube is inserted as a consequence of poison ingestion, the child is positioned with his or her head to one

Box 41-5
Gavage Feeding Procedure

1. Warm formula and measure
2. Assemble:
   Feeding tube No. 5–8 French
   Syringes One 2-ml syringe for air insertion
   One 10- to 20-ml syringe (separate barrel from plunger) to hold formula
   Glass of water
   Tape
   Stethoscope
   Blanket
3. Explain procedure to parents
4. Change diaper if needed and wash hands
5. Wrap patient in blanket and position with head elevated
6. Measure tube:
   (1) From tip of nose to earlobe (or earlobe to tip of nose), then to a point between the xyphoid process and umbilicus for nasogastric insertion
   (2) From mouth to earlobe (or earlobe to mouth), then to a point between xyphoid process and umbilicus for orogastric insertion
   Mark tube at measured level with tape
7. Dip tip of tube into water (this step is often omitted in nasogastric insertion and is not necessary for orogastric insertion)
8. Insert tube:
   (1) Nasogastric:
   Inspect nostril and begin inserting tube into nostril at a slight downward angle. Nose may be pressed slightly upward. Do not force (see Fig. 41-1 for pathway)
   (2) Orogastric:
   hold infant's mouth open and direct tube to back of mouth. Insert gently, with a downward angle
   Insert to designated mark
   Observe for signs of distress during insertion
   Ask child to swallow during insertion (if age appropriate)
9. Check for proper position with air insertion
   Instill air into tube with a syringe. Premature infants receive 0.5 cc; full term infants receive 1–2cc. Listen with stethoscope for "whoosh." Withdraw the air
10. Secure tube with tape
    Do not tape on nose but rather directly below nose. Tube should not create pressure on the nares, as this may cause necrosis, especially in compromised infants
11. Check for gastric secretions
    The withdrawal of gastric secretions further verifies proper position
    When gavage feeding infants it is often advisable to check for residual formula (i.e., withdraw stomach contents and measure). Reinsert contents into stomach through tube to avoid loss of electrolytes (if excessively mucousy, small amounts may be discarded)
    Usually the amount of residual is subtracted from the amount to be fed
12. Attach syringe barrel to tube
    Clamp tube or hold tube below level of stomach
    Pour prepared formula into syringe
    Remove clamp and elevate tube above level of stomach
13. Begin feeding
    Insert plunger into tip of barrel and give one quick push of formula to begin flow. Remove plunger. Hold infant to feed and give pacifier (unless size or condition does not permit).
    Raise syringe only high enough to maintain flow by gravity. Keep refilling syringe and avoid letting syringe get empty until completed. Feeding should take 15 to 20 minutes
    Note: An orogastric tube becomes dislodged easily; therefore, it should be held in place between fingers while feeding
14. Ensure that formula in tube has run in by raising syringe
15. Remove by pinching tube and pulling it all the way out
    Pinching tube is done to avoid leakage of formula as it is pulled
    Flush with sterile water if it is to be left in place. This should be done before syringe is completely empty to avoid letting air enter
    Insert 1 to 2 ml of water, close end of tube, and burp infant (especially if pacifier used during feeding) or keep tube elevated and open for 30 minutes to provide a vent for air to escape
    Check that tape is secure

Note: Sometimes an infant is bottle-fed followed by a gavage feeding if the infant is unable to take the entire amount by bottle. In this case a nasogastric tube is inserted before the bottle feeding is begun to avoid stimulation of vomiting during the feeding side and slightly lowered to avoid aspiration in the event of vomiting. Suction should also be available for immediate removal of vomitus whenever stomach contents are removed by lavage. (See Chapter 52, p. 2063, for further discussion of lavage in the event of poisoning.)

Caring for a Child with a Gastrostomy Tube

A gastrostomy tube is a catheter that enters the stomach through a surgical incision in the abdominal wall. The tube that is inserted has either a "mushroom" or a balloon close to its tip, which remains snug against the inside wall of the stomach. The gastrostomy tube is used for temporary postoperative conditions or for long-term management of children who are unable to receive adequate nutrition through oral feedings.

The catheter is secured in place on the surface of the abdomen by using tape. The tape is wrapped around the tube and secured to the skin. The tube may also be secured by using a nipple. A slit is cut into a 4 × 4 gauze pad and placed around the tube. A hole is cut in the top of a nipple and small holes into the side. (The holes at the side are to provide for air circulation.) The tube is put through the hole in the top of the nipple. The nipple is then moved along the tube until it is firmly positioned on the gauze placed around the tube. Using 1-inch paper tape, the nipple and gauze are secured to the skin. Once granulation takes place around the tube, the nipple is no longer necessary.

The tube may come out regardless of the method used to secure it. If this happens with a child on tube feedings at home, the family should be instructed as follows:

1. Stomach contents may leak out; do not be alarmed.
2. Cover the opening with a diaper or other absorbent cloth.
3. Go to the emergency room of the local hospital or to the clinic of the hospital at which the tube was inserted. Do this before the next feeding time or within 2 hours.
4. Take the old tube with you; this will let the staff know the size of tube the child needs. You may have been given an extra sterile tube when the child was discharged. If you were, take this tube to the clinic or emergency room.

A family can, however, be taught to change a gastrostomy tube at home (Paarlberg and Balint, 1985).

A reddened area about the size of a quarter around the tube is normal. There may be a small amount of drainage around the tube, but if a bad odor develops, or if the drainage changes in any way, the site should be checked for possible infection. A fever may also indicate an infection. To keep the area clean, wash around the tube with soap and water or other mild antiseptic solution. The child can be bathed as usual.

During feedings, an infant should be held and cuddled; an older child can sit in a highchair. Type and amount of formula will be prescribed by the physician. The position of the tube can be checked by gently pulling until resistance is felt. To complete the feeding:

1. Wash your hands.
2. Check the temperature of the formula. It should be room temperature.
3. Attach the end of the tube to a syringe (10 to 50 cc, varying with size of the infant).
4. Clamp the tube.
5. Fill the syringe with formula.
6. Holding the tube above the height of the opening, unclamp the tube.
7. Add more formula to the syringe before it empties to prevent air from entering the stomach.
8. Follow the formula with one-half ounce of water to clear the tube.
9. Clamp the tube, fold it over, wrap it with a 4 × 4 gauze pad, and secure it with a rubber band.
10. Wash the materials in hot soapy water, rinse well, and store in a clean place.
11. The feeding should take approximately as long as a feeding by mouth.
12. Infants should be allowed to suck on a pacifier to satisfy normal developmental needs.

Medication may be given through the tube. Using the same syringe, give one-half ounce of water after the medicine to ensure that the medication has not remained in the tube.

The tube can be pinned to the child's undershirt or covered with soft, stretchy tube gauze. With a gastrostomy tube the child can resume regular play activities. Problems that might arise during the use of a gastrostomy tube are summarized in Table 41-7.

A new type of apparatus called the gastrostomy feeding button is gaining favor as an alternative to the traditional types of tubes. It is a small, flexible silicone device that has a mushroom-like dome on the end, which is inserted. A one-way valve inside the device prevents reflux of stomach contents. The external device (two small wings with an opening in the center) lies flat against the abdomen, thus eliminating the need for an external tube. Advantages, disadvantages, and use of this type of device have been reviewed by Huth and O'Brien (1987).

Caring for a Child Who Requires an Enema

An enema is used for the same purpose in children as it is in adults: (1) to facilitate defecation when normal physiologic processes of elimination are ineffective,

Table 41-7. Common Problems with Gastrostomy Tubes (G-tubes)

Problem	Possible Causes	Solution
Leaking around tube	1. Balloon of catheter has slipped away from wall of stomach.	1. Gently pull back on catheter or tube to ensure that balloon is snug against stomach wall.
	2. Balloon of catheter may have become somewhat deflated.	2. Reinflate balloon or change catheter.
	3. Tube is too small for size of stoma.	3. Consult physician to evaluate further. Placing larger catheter may only exacerbate the problem.
Blocked tube	1. Obstruction due to food or medication.	1a. Gently milk tube to dislodge obstruction. b. Use liquid medication when possible or well-suspended, finely ground medication. c. Change tube.
Erythema or drainage around tube or stoma	1. Some erythema or drainage is normal.	1. Clean area frequently with mild soap and water. Keep dressing dry.
	2. Skin irritation may result from dampness or gastric leaking around tube.	2a. Clean area more frequently. b. Karaya powder sprinkled on area and covered with dressing may heal area. c. Topical antibiotics are generally not indicated. d. Call physician if problem persists.
Vomiting or diarrhea* or both * *Note:* In each instance, consult the physician if vomiting or diarrhea persists.	1. In an otherwise healthy child, this may indicate that the tube has migrated into the stomach or beyond the stomach. a. Migration into the duodenum or jejunum may cause "dumping," resulting in liquid stool during or immediately following a feeding. b. Blockage or irritation of the pylorus by the G-tube may cause vomiting.	1. Gently pull back on the tube to assess tube position. Check tube position at each feeding.
	2. Vomiting may result from too rapid administration of a feeding.	2. Feed over a longer period of time.
	3. Vomiting may result from too large a feeding.	3. Smaller or more frequent feedings should be considered.
Bleeding around tube or stoma	1. Bleeding may occur during a tube change.	1a. Minimal bleeding is insignificant. b. The physician should be consulted if larger amounts of bleeding occur. c. Cauterization of the stoma may be necessary.
	2. The stoma may become irritated from movement of the tube in the stoma.	2a. Secure the tube to the child's shirt between feedings. b. Same as 1a, b, c.
Tissue build-up around G-tube	1. A small amount of epithelial tissue is normal and not painful.	1a. If tissue build-up is excessive and interferes with care, notify the physician. b. Cauterization may be necessary.

(From Paarlberg and Balint, 1985.)

and (2) to cleanse the bowel in preparation for surgery or diagnostic procedures. Specific differences between children and adults and related nursing actions to consider are discussed in Table 41-8.

There are three special considerations in giving an enema. First, comparing the sensation of the catheter tip insertion to the taking of rectal temperature is useful for some children, but the child should not be led to believe that an enema is "just like having your temperature taken." Second, a potty-trained child should be encouraged to expel the enema while sitting on a potty chair. Also, potty-trained children need special reassurance that it is alright if they do not make it to the potty chair to expel the enema. Third, preschoolers require special explanations and understanding because they do not clearly mentally separate rectal and genital regions of the body. Administration of an enema thus has the potential to arouse fears related to the genitalia.

Caring for a Child with a Colostomy

A colostomy is the surgical creation of an opening between the colon and the surface of the body. In many instances, a temporary procedure colostomy is done during infancy, with the definitive procedure being

Table 41-8. Procedure for Enema Administration to a Child*

Developmental Considerations	Related Nursing Actions
1. The child's bowel capacity and anal opening vary according to size. A young child's rectal mucosa is thin and easily traumatized.	Approximate normal saline* solution amounts according to age of child: • Infant, 150–250 ml • Toddler and preschooler, 250–350 ml • School-age, 300–500 ml • Adolescent, 500–750 ml Enema tips should be soft, well lubricated, and appropriate in size for age of child (French catheter No. 10-12 for young children). For older school-agers and adolescents, the standard enema tip can be used. The enema tip is inserted 1½ to 4 inches (3.7 to 10 cm), varying according to size of child.†
2. Young children are particularly vulnerable to fluid and electrolyte imbalances.	An isotonic (normal saline) solution (warmed) is used to prevent rapid fluid shift from bowel. Plain water is hypotonic and with repeated enemas water intoxication and fluid overload can result.
3. A child's bowel is more easily perforated under pressure.	The enema reservoir is elevated gradually until the solution begins to slowly flow by gravity. For young children, greater control of administration is achieved by using a 50 ml syringe attached to a catheter.
4. Young children do not have the cognitive or physiologic ability to "hold" the enema.	With child in supine position, head and back can be supported with pillow. The bedpan must be in position during administration because there is immediate return of the solution. After the solution has been administered, the buttocks can be gently pinched together to facilitate "holding" of the enema. A child who is old enough (school-age and adolescent) to understand the explanation "hold the enema" is positioned on the left side with right leg flexed and asked to hold the enema for 3–5 minutes.

* When instructions are given to administer an enema at home instructions should be given in cups (240 mm = 1 cup). A normal saline solution can be prepared by adding ½ teaspoon of table salt per cup of lukewarm water.

† Commercially prepared enemas are administered similarly. The tip is prelubricated. Warm the solution. The tip is inserted, then the enema container is gently squeezed; it is not usually possible to empty it completely.

performed at a later time (often when the child reaches 1 year of age). A colostomy may also be necessary for various reasons later in childhood. Parents and children, including siblings, benefit from explanations and demonstrations, using a doll or special models designed for teaching about a colostomy and colostomy care.

After surgery, the child and parents are encouraged to become familiar with the stoma (colostomy opening) and gradually increase their involvement in care of the child. Extra care is taken to provide an atmosphere that encourages them to discuss their concerns, fears, and feelings about caring for a colostomy. Adjustment by the child and parents is affected by the reason the colostomy is required and whether it is to be temporary or permanent. A child's adjustment also is determined by his or her particular developmental level and by how well the parents can accept their child's need for a colostomy.

As much as possible, nursing care should be provided by the same individuals to help the family learn and to ease their adjustment. Box 41-6 provides specific directions for care of an ostomy. A special hint to give parents is to make a pinhole near the top of the bag to release gas and then place a piece of tape over the hole to keep the odor inside the bag. The tape can be lifted whenever it is necessary to release gas.

Colostomy irrigation is performed before surgery to completely cleanse fecal material from the bowel. The equipment necessary for this procedure includes enema bag, warmed irrigation solution, a soft pliable catheter, a nipple, lubricant, and an intravenous pole. The irrigation solution is placed in the enema bag, and the tubing is filled with fluid. The pliable catheter is attached to the enema tubing. The tip of the enema tubing is cut off so that the irrigation solution will run continuously through both the tubing and the catheter. The catheter is inserted through the nipple. The catheter is then inserted into the stoma, followed by the nipple. The nipple is used to prevent leakage around the catheter as the enema is administered. The enema bag is placed 18 inches above the stoma, and the solution is administered gradually. This procedure should be done slowly. If the child complains of crampy abdominal pain, stop the solution for several minutes and then restart.

Caring for a Child After Abdominal Surgery

Postoperative care following abdominal surgery requires close monitoring by the nurse as for any other surgery. Depending on the type of surgical procedure, specific care, such as irrigation of abdominal wounds, shortening of incisional drains, care of colostomy, or irrigation of a nasogastric tube, may be required. General principles of care are presented in Table 41-9, Nursing Process Plan: Care of the Child Following Abdominal Surgery.

Text continues on page 1397

Box 41-6
Directions to Patients or Parents for Care of an Ostomy

PUTTING ON THE BAG

1. Wash your hands.
2. Have Karaya ring or Stomahesive (protective seal) ready to use. With clean scissors, cut openings in Stomahesive and bag. Guides are provided in the colostomy bag box. Cut hole in the Stomahesive slightly smaller than opening in bag so that Stomahesive fits closely around stoma. Cutting several at a time to have ready for future bag changes is easiest.
3. Remove the old Stomahesive or Karaya ring and bag, pulling gently. This is a good time to check to see that stoma is pink.
4. Wash skin with warm water. A tub bath may be taken at this time. Pat skin around stoma dry. Cover the stoma with Kleenex to prevent stool from leaking onto the skin.
5. Apply "Skin Prep" to skin around stoma and fan it dry.
6. Remove the white paper backing from the Stomahesive. Remove Kleenex from the stoma and place the Stomahesive or Karaya ring on the skin, centered around stoma. Push on one area at a time so it sticks to skin and has no wrinkles.
7. Remove white paper backing from bag. Put sticky side of bag onto the Stomahesive or Karaya ring; smooth it down to remove all wrinkles.
8. Roll bag up (turning edges to the outside) until you can see stoma, then sprinkle Karaya powder directly on the stoma. Then unroll bag.
9. If bottom of bag is open, fold bottom up twice horizontally, then fold it like a fan vertically. Use a rubber band to hold bag closed.
10. To dispose of old bag, rinse out in the toilet and then throw in the trash. Do not flush it down the toilet.
11. Wash your hands.

EMPTYING THE BAG

1. Remove rubber band from end.
2. Empty the stool into a container or right into the toilet if you can stand next to it.
3. Pour warm water into bag, gently washing water around in bag. For an infant or young child, bag can be rinsed by using a 50-ml syringe. Empty the water into the container or toilet.
4. Special deodorants are available to use if you wish.
5. Dry end of bag and close it again.

SKIN MAINTENANCE

1. Always use a protective seal over the skin (Stomahesive), placing it right up to stoma with bag placed on top ⅛ inch away from stoma.
2. Change bag promptly if any leakage occurs.
3. Avoid use of ointments or lotions around stoma.
4. Clean and dry skin area around stoma before applying bag.
5. If excoriation occurs, apply Mycostatin powder or Kenalog spray and dry the area with cool setting on hair blow dryer.

(Extracted from Sarahan T, et al: Ostomy Care for Infants and Children. *University of Michigan Printing Department, 1979, page 9. Additional sources for information on colostomy care: B. Bolinger, A Teenager's Ostomy Guide, Hollister Inc., 1978. Guide for the Colostonate. Coloplast Brand Ostomy Products, 1977. Managing Your Colostomy, Hollister Inc., 1971. Ostomy-Related Skin Problems, Hollister Inc., 1977.)*

Table 41-9
Nursing Process Plan: Care of the Child Following Abdominal Surgery*

by Roxie Foster

I. Assessment of Physical Function

Subjective Assessment

Level of comfort, pertinent sensations (e.g., tenderness around incision, stomach "rumblings"), ease of breathing, passage of flatus

Objective Assessment

Adequacy of systemic ventilation or perfusion, level of consciousness, status of breath sounds, effectiveness of cough, amount of spontaneous movement or turning, bladder distention, bowel sounds, passage of flatus, abdominal tautness or distention, placement and patency of intravenous lines, drains, catheters, and other tubes placed in surgery, status of dressings.

Analysis: Nursing Diagnosis 1

Altered tissue perfusion: systemic, related to hypovolemia associated with postoperative hemorrhage

Defining Characteristics

Restlessness; increased pulse and respirations; decreased blood pressure; decreased peripheral pulses; capillary refill greater than 3 seconds; decreased urine output; cool, pale skin; possible external evidence of bleeding

Analysis: Nursing Diagnosis 2

Ineffective airway clearance, related to poor cough effort associated with
- ***sedative effects of anesthesia and analgesics***
- ***incisional pain***
- ***inability to cooperate because of developmental level***

Defining Characteristics

Adventitious lung sounds, tachypnea, tachycardia, pallor of skin and mucous membranes

Analysis: Nursing Diagnosis 3

Urinary retention, related to
- ***effects of anesthesia on the bladder muscle***
- ***manipulation of the bladder during surgery***
- ***abnormal voiding position***

Defining Characteristics

See Table 27-7, Nursing Process Plan: Perioperative Care, for desired outcomes, evaluation criteria, and nursing strategies for Nursing Diagnoses 1, 2, and 3

Analysis: Nursing Diagnosis 4

Altered bowel elimination: decreased peristalsis, related to
- *manipulation of the bowel during surgery*
- *effects of anesthesia*
- *effects of morphine sulfate or codeine, or both*
- *immobility*

Defining Characteristics

Subjective: Complaints of crampy abdominal pain, feeling of "fullness," anorexia, absence of flatus, no "rumbling" or "gurgling" feelings or sounds in abdomen

Objective: Absent or only occasional bowel sounds; firm, distended abdomen; absence of flatus (nurse's observations of flatus may be only source of information in infant or young child); absence of bowel movement

Client Goal/ Evaluation Criteria

4. The client will regain peristalsis as quickly as possible† as evidenced by:
   a. return of normal bowel sounds (15–34 per minute in each quadrant)
   b. soft abdomen
   c. passage of flatus
   d. verbalization of decreased sense of fullness
   e. verbalization of abdominal comfort

Nursing Goals/Strategies (Selected Rationale)

Assess bowel status.
- Measure abdominal girth at the umbilicus preoperatively if possible, or immediately postoperatively (to establish a baseline). Then *record abdominal girth every shift* during the first 48–72 hours, or until normal bowel function has returned.
- Auscultate for bowel sounds every 4 hours, listening in all four quadrants. *Record actual number* of sounds per minute. (Using terms such as "decreased" or "increased" is too subjective to be of much value to the next evaluator.)
- Palpate the abdomen every 4 hours and record whether soft or firm, flat or distended.
- Listen for passage of flatus and ask the parent or older child about passage of flatus.
- Question the child about abdominal comfort.

Implement strategies to facilitate return of peristalsis and to decrease gaseous distention.
- Assist the child with frequent position changes.
- Ambulate as soon as and as often as ordered:
  1. Set specific ambulation goals for time and distance with the child and family and reinforce (verbally, with colored stickers, etc.) the child's progress in walking.
  2. Medicate the child for incisional pain *prior to ambulation,* planning the ambulation time during the medication's peak effect.
- Reduce air swallowing whenever possible.
  1. Reduce crying in the infant through pharmacologic and non-pharmacologic comfort measures.
  2. Ensure that the nipple is full of liquid (to prevent taking in air with feeding).
  3. Discourage gum chewing and sucking on hard candy. (These activities increase air swallowing.)

Continued

Client Goal/ Evaluation Criteria	Nursing Goals/Strategies (Selected Rationale)
	• Maintain patency of the nasogastric tube (if present). 1. Observe for withdrawal of fluid during intermittent suction. (Because the suction will usually be set at "low" intensity, fluid fluctuation in the tubing may not be dramatic, but it should gradually move toward the collection bag.) 2. Irrigate the nasogastric tube gently if it appears plugged and if orders have been written for irrigation. • Substitute non-narcotic analgesics for morphine sulfate and acetaminophen (Tylenol) with codeine once severe pain has subsided. This can usually be done after the first 48 hours without sacrificing the child's comfort. (Narcotics can decrease peristalsis.) • Differentiate between gas pain and incisional pain. (Ambulation and a rectal tube or flush-type of enema are appropriate strategies for gas pain. Narcotic analgesics will be counterproductive.) • Begin oral fluids slowly, assessing frequently for abdominal distention and discomfort. • As oral intake is advanced caution the child and parents about gas-forming foods: onions, cabbage, popcorn, carbonated beverages.

Analysis: Nursing Diagnosis 5

Potential for infection: peritonitis, related to release of intestinal contents into the abdominal cavity through:
- *rupture or penetration of a part of the bowel*
- *leakage through the bowel wall or suture line associated with the build-up of pressure within the bowel*

Defining Characteristics

Subjective: Severe abdominal pain and rebound tenderness

Objective: Fever; distention and "board-like" rigidity of the abdomen; absent or diminished bowel sounds; tachycardia; tachypnea; increased WBC

Client Goal/ Evaluation Criteria	Nursing Goals/Strategies (Selected Rationale)
5. The child will be free of peritonitis as evidenced by: a. increasing abdominal comfort after the first postoperative day b. soft, non-distended abdomen c. returning bowel sounds d. absence of fever, tachycardia, tachypnea e. WBC returning to normal levels	*Assess for evidence of peritonitis.* • Record vital signs, contour and tension of abdomen, bowel sounds, and level of comfort every 4 hours. • Monitor WBC reports. Report counts that are increasing or that fail to return to normal. *Implement strategies to prevent peritonitis.* • Prevent disruption of drains placed during surgery by restraining the infant or young child as needed. • Take measures to facilitate peristalsis and reduce gaseous distention. See strategies for Nursing Diagnosis 4.

If evidence of peritonitis occurs:
- *place the child in a semi-fowler's position* to localize pooling of intestinal contents.
- *alert the physician* immediately.

Analysis: Nursing Diagnosis 6

Impaired skin integrity, related to:
- ***leakage of abdominal fluids onto skin***
- ***tape associated with dressings***

Defining Characteristics:

Subjective: Verbalization of itching, tenderness

Objective: Erythema, excoriation, maculopapular rash

Desired Outcomes/ Evaluation Criteria	Nursing Strategies and Selected Rationale
6. The child will maintain skin integrity as evidenced by: a. verbalizing comfort of skin around incision, drains b. absence of erythema, excoriation, or rash	*Implement strategies to protect skin integrity.* • Ask the child and parent if allergies exist to tape. • Use Montgomery straps whenever possible (to reduce irritation from frequent tape removal). • Use *paper tape* (which is less adhesive and less irritating) when tape must be used. • Consider the use of tincture of benzoin to make skin less sensitive to tape and other irritants. • Cleanse skin of wound drainage (observing sterile technique) whenever dressings are changed. Keep skin as clean and dry as possible.

* This table is designed to detail care particular to the child after abdominal surgery. See the following sources for supporting information:
1. Table 31-2, Nursing Process Plan: The Hospitalized Child, for psychosocial concerns and discharge planning.
2. Table 29-4, Nursing Process Plan: The Child in Pain.
3. The beginning of this chapter for care of the child with a nasogastric tube.

† Realistic goals for return of peristalsis will depend upon the type and length of surgery, the amount of bowel manipulation, and the presence of peritonitis and may vary from 24 hours to several days.

This Nursing Process Plan is applicable regardless of the reason for the operation and, for the most part, can be used after most specific surgical procedures.

Impact of Gastrointestinal Alterations on the Child and Family

Although many of the alterations discussed in this chapter can be surgically corrected early in life, the extent of the disruption to the individual family can be great. Some disorders are life-threatening (e.g., diaphragmatic hernia, severe gastroenteritis), whereas many are chronic and require a lifetime of adjustment (e.g., Crohn disease and ulcerative colitis). Frequent hospitalizations and a series of surgical procedures are disruptive at any age and cause stress to both child and family.

Positive feeding experiences, nutritional intake, and the growth of children are evidence to parents that they have a normal child and that they themselves are succeeding as parents. Disturbances that interfere with these feelings of satisfaction and achievement can alter the normal growth of the family. Negative feelings may arise toward the infant if food is either rejected or regurgitated. Disturbances in nutritional intake and absorption also interfere with the infant's oral gratification and available energy for mobility. *The infant's and family's general sense of well-being is affected by interruptions in the normal process of feeding and the social exchanges that normally accompany these experiences.*

The early handling, touching, and human contact between infant and parent must sometimes be delayed because of surgical intervention. Frequently, gastrointestinal problems involve the use of tubes, appliances, and cumbersome equipment. Although parents become skilled at providing food through tubes and other apparatus, extensive adaptation is required. This adaptation can be aided by encouraging the parents to become involved when they are ready, which may not necessarily be at a time the nurse thinks they should be. The parent must first adjust and cope with the child's condition and then learn new skills in the care of their child.

Generally when eating habits and digestion are altered, a person's sense of well-being is disrupted. In some instances the alterations in nutritional state and in fluid and electrolyte imbalance become so severe that the individual does not feel well, and in some conditions even the appearance is altered. Need for a nasogastric tube, an ileostomy or colostomy, and the cachexic appearance associated with illnesses such as severe Crohn disease may lower the patient's self-esteem and acceptance among peers.

It is difficult for children and their families to accept a problem that concerns such a personal, private aspect of life as elimination. Parents often find it hard to explain to friends and other people the nature of their child's problem and therefore may need to discuss such feelings with health professionals. Particular problems that parents can anticipate, depending on the alteration, are problems in toilet training, resistance to participation in gym and in sports that involve changing clothes and sleepovers (especially if the child has a colostomy). In some instances children or parents, or both, can participate in a group conducted by a health professional or organized as a self-help group.

It is important that adequate time and attention be paid to providing information and teaching the child and family how to care for themselves. The initial step for the nurse is to accept patients' unwillingness to care for themselves. Recognizing that the child or parent is experiencing a loss by having to learn new techniques of care is part of this initial phase. Even though the procedure may be a temporary one, some resistance may develop because of the "abnormalcy" that it represents. Involving the child or parent gradually and consistently on a daily basis can eventually result in sufficient acceptance and support to initiate self-care. Many of the technical procedures discussed in the previous section are learned by children and parents. Regardless of the type of problem, the *individual* responses of children and their families must be explored and recognized. The nurse cannot predict any individual's response on the basis of how previous patients with similar disorders responded. Although the disruptions are similar from a physiologic viewpoint, the coping mechanisms, the support systems, and the person's perception of the disorder all determine adaptation in each specific situation.

Anomalies and Obstructions of the Digestive Tract

Disorders included in this section require surgical intervention ranging from facial surgery for cleft lip or palate to simple repair of an inguinal hernia to complex staged repairs of the intestines. In most instances of digestive tract surgery the infant's greatest source of gratification—eating—must be interrupted for a time. When an infant requires the withholding of oral feeding, other sources of comfort must be provided. Some parents may resist the use of a pacifier, but it is an appropriate option to suggest during this time, especially in an infant under 3 months of age, for whom the need to suck is particularly great.

Surgery on the gastrointestinal tract may affect toilet training. Because the majority of operations are done during infancy, the potential for normal bowel control remains in question for several years. These children may need extra time and support from parents to become continent.

The nurse has an important role in the early identification of gastrointestinal tract anomalies, most of which cause some degree of obstruction. Obstructive anomalies cause characteristic signs and symptoms that vary according to the level of the obstruction. Important observations to make are (1) clefts in the oral cavity; (2) presence of excessive secretions from the nose or mouth; (3) character of and color of vomitus, if present; (4) presence of abdominal distention and character of bowel sounds; (5) indications of abdominal pain and discomfort; (6) absence or diminished amount of meconium; and (7) character and color of stools.

Cleft Lip and Cleft Palate

Cleft lip, cleft palate, and combinations of these are the most common of all facial anomalies. Cleft lip (harelip) with or without cleft palate is more common in males. Cleft palate alone is more common in females. Males more commonly have a combined cleft lip and cleft palate, usually of more severe degree than in females.

Accurate incidence data are difficult to obtain, but it is generally believed that cleft lip with or without cleft palate occurs in 1:1000 births and cleft palate alone in 1:2500 births. The incidence varies by race, with a higher incidence rate in the Japanese (twice that of the white population), and a lower incidence rate in the black population (less than half as many as the white population).

Etiologic Factors and the Role of Genetics

A strong genetic component exists for cleft lip and cleft palate, yet environmental factors are likely as well (Owens et al, 1985). Available data indicate that cleft lip with or without cleft palate is etiologically and genetically distinct from isolated cleft palate (McWilliams et al, 1984; Aylsworth, 1985). Genetic factors are believed to be of greater significance in cleft lip with or without cleft palate than in isolated cleft palate. Children with isolated cleft palate have a greater incidence of associated anomalies than is noted in children with cleft lip with or without cleft palate.

Sometimes the family history reveals no previous occurrence of cleft lip or cleft palate. It is, however, possible for a small, non-detected cleft to have been present in a family; therefore, it is important not to falsely assure parents that there is no genetic basis present.

The role of non-hereditary factors remains unclear. Environmental studies in utero have been done primarily on laboratory animals; causative environmental factors in humans have not yet been clearly identified (McWilliams et al, 1984). However, some evidence has suggested that phenytoin (Dilantin) taken during pregnancy has possible teratogenic effects, such as formation of clefts (McWilliams et al, 1984).

The most widely accepted view is that the great majority of clefts are caused by multifactorial inheritance. Probably many genes contribute to clefting. Individually each is of minor importance, but their interaction together with negative environmental conditions may cause clefting (McWilliams et al, 1984).

Embryologic Development and Types of Clefting

Even though the embryologic development of the palate and lip takes place around the same time, it occurs independently; therefore, cleft lip and cleft palate may occur together or either defect may occur separately. The facial structures develop between 5 and 9 weeks after conception. The lips (primary palate) form at 7 weeks; the hard and soft palates (secondary palate) develop at 9 weeks. The lips are formed from three processes—a midline central nasal process and two wings of a branchial arch, which are called the maxillary processes. When fusion of the nasal process and maxillary processes does not occur, a clefting of the lip results.

Complete separation of the oral and nasal cavities normally results when the primary and secondary palates fuse to form a continuous structure. Early in development the tongue pushes into the nasal cavity, and two structures (palatal shelves) occur in a vertical position on either side of the tongue. During the seventh and eighth weeks the tongue drops, and the palatal shelves elevate into a horizontal plane and fuse. When fusion of the palate does not occur, a cleft palate results.

Diagnostic Assessment

Cleft lip and cleft palate appear in various forms. In some cases the defect is obvious but in others it is not. The cleft lip can be unilateral or bilateral (Fig. 41-2 and Fig. 41-3). Midline cleft lips are rare. The extent of clefting can vary from a slight indentation (incomplete) to a widely opened (complete) cleft. Varying degrees of nasal distortion usually accompany the cleft lip, and the defect may also involve supernumerary, deformed, or absent teeth.

The degree of deformity of the cleft palate also varies (Fig. 41-2). Because it is less obvious than the cleft lip, it may not be detected without a thorough assessment of the mouth. It can be identified by placing the fingers directly on the palate. The defect may involve only the uvula (incomplete cleft) or may extend to both the soft palate (posterior portion) and hard palate (anterior portion) (complete cleft). The isolated cleft palate occurs in the midline and may involve the uvula or extend to the soft and hard palates. Cleft palate associated with a cleft lip may take a variety of forms. It may involve the uvula and midline of the soft palate, and, if it extends into the hard palate, it may involve one or both sides (unilateral or bilateral cleft palate) (Fig. 41-2).

Therapeutic Management

Surgical repair of the cleft lip precedes repair of the palate and is done within the first 3 months of life (usually at 1 month) if the infant is gaining weight and is free of infection. Z-plasty, the most commonly performed surgical technique, utilizes a staggered Z-shaped suture line (Fig. 41-4). The goal is to approximate the vermilion border and minimize notching.

A Logan clamp (a curved metal bow taped down on both sides of the suture line over the lip) or a butterfly adhesive restraint is applied immediately after surgery to prevent tension on the suture line. The cosmetic

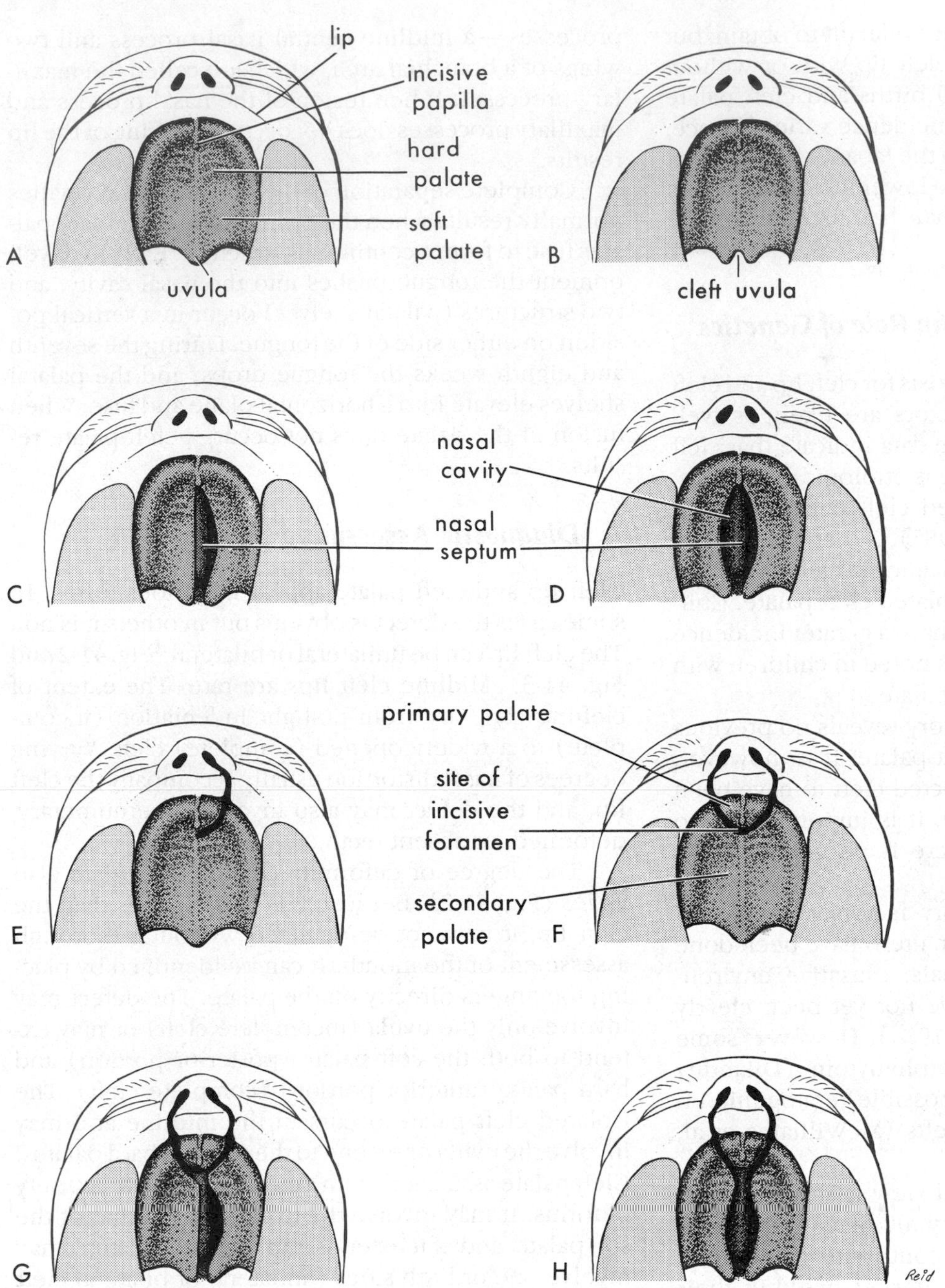

Figure 41-2. Drawings of various types of cleft lip and cleft palate. *A*, Normal lip and palate. *B*, Cleft uvula. *C*, Unilateral cleft of the posterior or secondary palate. *D*, Bilateral cleft of the posterior palate. *E*, Complete unilateral cleft of the lip and alveolar process of the maxilla with a unilateral cleft of the anterior or primary palate. *F*, Complete bilateral cleft of the lip and alveolar processes of the maxillae with bilateral cleft of the anterior palate. *G*, Complete bilateral cleft of the lip and alveolar processes of the maxillae with bilateral cleft of the anterior palate and unilateral cleft of the posterior palate. *H*, Complete bilateral cleft of the lip and alveolar processes of the maxillae with complete bilateral cleft of the anterior and posterior palate.

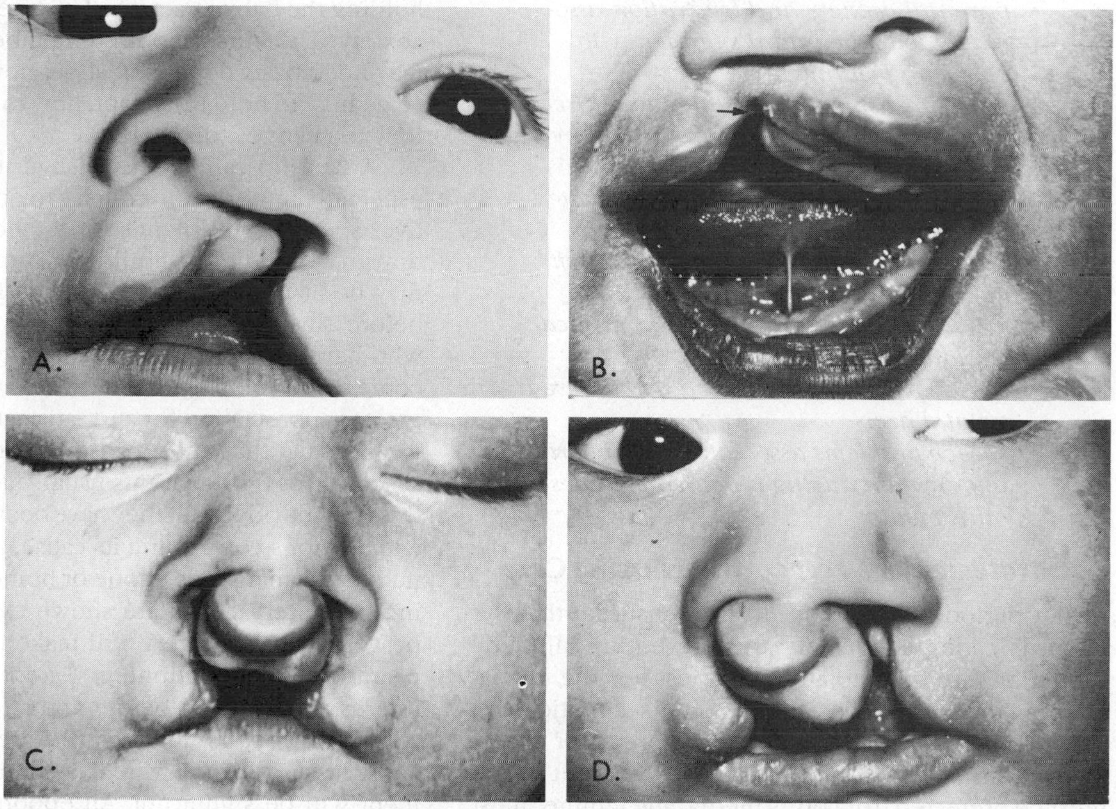

Figure 41-3. Photographs illustrating clefts of the lip. This malformation used to be referred to as "hare lip"; this is an inappropriate term because the hare's lip is divided in the median plane. *A* and *B*, Unilateral cleft lip. The cleft in *B* is incomplete; the arrow indicates a band of tissue (Simonart's band) connecting the parts of the lip. *C* and *D*, Bilateral cleft lip. (Courtesy of Dr. D. A. Kernahan, The Children's Memorial Hospital, Chicago.)

results of the surgery will depend on the extent of the original defect and the absence of infection or trauma. Additional surgery may be needed at a later age to improve the child's appearance.

The timing of cleft palate repair varies considerably. The initial repair may be done as early as 4 to 6 months. It may be done in one operation, as in the case of a soft palate defect, or may require several stages of repair, depending on the severity of the defect. Most surgeons prefer to close the palate before the age of 2 years in order to prevent the development of faulty speech habits (Lindsay, 1986).

Major Preoperative Nursing Diagnoses for Cleft Lip and Cleft Palate

Potential for ineffective family coping, *related to*

- *the shock of the newborn infant's facial or palatal anomaly*
- *altered feeding patterns*

Potential altered nutrition: less than body requirements, *related to*

- *sucking difficulties: ineffective suction on the nipple associated with the cleft*

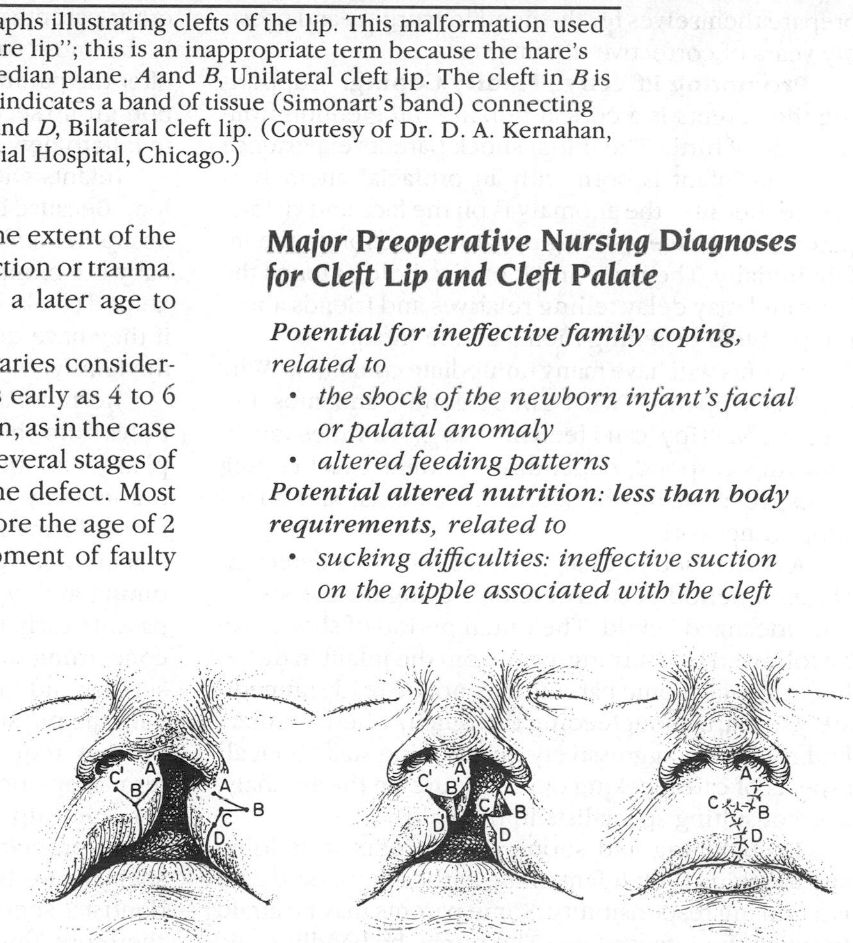

Figure 41-4. A procedure for cleft lip repair. The surgeon makes several incisions, then sutures the lip together. (From Fochtman D, Raffensperger J: *Principles of Nursing Care for the Pediatric Surgery Patient,* 2nd ed. Boston, Little, Brown & Co, 1976.)

- *parental anxiety and frustration associated with the infant's tendency to choke on feedings*

Potential for aspiration, *related to a direct pathway into the nasopharynx created by the cleft.*

Potential for infection: middle ear, *related to inefficient drainage of the middle ear associated with altered functioning of soft palate muscles*

Potential for impaired verbal communication, *related to*

- *speech problems associated with altered palatal arch*
- *speech problems associated with hearing impairment during repeated episodes of otitis media*

Strategies for Preoperative Nursing Care

In the period before cleft closure, ensuring that the infant is eating adequately and preventing injury by aspiration are immediate priorities for the nurse. Helping the family adjust to the infant's condition and teaching them how to feed the infant are other immediate priorities. In addition, infants with cleft palate must be protected from otitis media, and families must prepare themselves for the need for surgery and possibly years of corrective treatments.

Promoting Effective Family Coping. Supporting the parents is a critical nursing intervention from the time of birth. The initial shock parents experience when an infant is born with an orofacial anomaly is severe. Because the anomaly is on the face and visible, parents may have a strong negative reaction to the infant initially. They may find it hard to hold or touch the baby and may delay telling relatives and friends about the problem or letting them see the infant.

Parents will have many immediate concerns: "Why did this happen?" "What can be done?" and, most immediately, "How can I feed my baby?" Families vary in how they respond, depending on their usual coping styles, relationship between the parents, and social support network.

As discussed in Chapter 4, reaction to a defect includes a period of sorrow and grieving for the loss of the "idealized" child. The initial period of shock may be followed by a turning away from the infant in disbelief or denial. Some parents may not be ready immediately to learn about feeding the infant, whereas others find release in aggressively questioning staff about all aspects of care, seeking out literature on the anomaly, and consulting specialists in the field.

Encouraging and supporting parents in holding and touching their infant in the earliest hours and days is a nursing responsibility. Some parents may be afraid to touch the infant's face. The nurse, by handling and holding the baby in a natural manner, can lessen their anxiety. The nurse should remember that the parents may need basic education about newborn infant care, (e.g., how to hold the infant, how to wrap a blanket, or how to change a diaper).

A cleft lip can be very disfiguring; therefore, it is especially important for nurses to emphasize the positive aspects of the infant's appearance and express optimism about the possibility for correction. The infant may be at home with the parents for 1 to 2 months before surgical repair of the lip is initiated. Parents who have cared for their infant and have time to become comfortable with the deformity generally have a greater appreciation for and satisfaction about the surgical results than those whose infant's repair is done shortly after birth. Parents usually adjust fairly well to this cosmetic defect if they have been given reasonable explanations concerning its cause, are supported by a nurse who maintains phone or home visit contact during this interval, and are shown evidence of the improvement that surgery will make in their child's appearance and functioning. Parents are particularly interested in seeing before and after photographs of successful repairs. Photographs are more impressive and reassuring than verbal assurance that improvement will be significant. An opportunity to talk with other parents who have been through the experience is the most useful intervention the health team can offer the parents. Generally a hospital will have a support group service with names of other parents willing to talk to new parents.

Infants with cleft palate present a different problem. Because further growth of the secondary palate is desirable, definitive surgery may be delayed until the baby is 6 months to 18 months of age. Parents must be helped to take care of the child at home and counseled if they have difficulty in accepting the baby as part of the family.

Accurate and consistent answers to parents' questions from the first day are important. The treatment plan for an infant depends on the type and severity of the anomaly; therefore, the nurse should provide accurate information in conjunction with other professionals involved in immediate and long-term care. The timing and type of surgical repair are discussed with parents early to allow them to develop realistic goals concerning their family life. Financial concerns about surgery and long-term treatment need to be discussed with the physician, hospital, and social worker. A cleft lip may require early surgical treatment with short-term adaptations required of the family, whereas a severe cleft lip and cleft palate may necessitate a complete program of habilitation, requiring years of special care by physicians, surgeons, dentists, orthodontists, speech therapists, and social workers. It is therefore important that a team approach is established early, ensuring accurate, consistent information to the family.

Providing Adequate Nutrition and Preventing Aspiration. The difficulty of feeding an infant with a cleft lip or cleft palate varies according to the extent and type of cleft. Many infants born with a cleft of the lip only or with a very small cleft of the soft palate may have little or no difficulty sucking. An infant born with a cleft of the lip *and* palate or a complete cleft of the palate may have difficulty creating a seal to produce suction in the mouth. The usual bottle nipples frequently cannot be used for these infants. Large, soft nipples with large holes or long, soft nipples (lamb's nipples) seem to be most effective. Regular nipples can also be softened by boiling them. The nurse should be aware that feeding is initially a frightening experience for the parent because frequently in cleft palate, formula returns through the nose, accompanied by episodes of gagging and choking. Holding the infant in an upright position with head and chest slightly backward decreases the likelihood of aspiration. In this position, the natural cough reflex can more readily clear the airway. The nipple should be positioned firmly in the baby's mouth in a normal position (not in the cleft) and removed only to burp the child or when the coughing warrants removal. Continually removing the nipple each time the baby has a slight cough frustrates a hungry infant and increases the baby's distress. However, burping should be done frequently because these babies tend to swallow air readily.

If the infant has trouble with nipple feeding, a rubber-tipped medicine dropper or an Asepto syringe with a rubber tip can be used. The rubber piece should reach to the back and side of the mouth. Small amounts of formula are introduced to reduce the possibility of leakage through the nose. With some infants, spoon feeding may also work well.

Mothers who wish to breastfeed their infants should be encouraged to do so. In cleft lip alone, breastfeeding can usually be achieved with minor adjustments. If the baby has difficulty making a seal, the cleft in the lip can be filled with the mother's thumb or the breast can be molded to fill the gap. Breastfeeding can be made easier for the infant if the breast is massaged before nursing to bring the milk down. The local LaLeche League chapter may be able to help a new mother who would like to breastfeed her infant or express breast milk to save and feed the baby later. Assistance and support to discuss the alternatives is required from the health team during this time of adjustment.

Preventing Middle Ear Infection and Language Difficulties. Ear infections, speech difficulties, and hearing problems are common in children with cleft palate. Under normal conditions the muscles of the soft palate aid in proper functioning of the eustachian tube. In the presence of a cleft palate, involvement of these muscles results in inefficient drainage of the middle ear, resulting in a greater susceptibility to ear infections. Because ear and upper respiratory tract infections are frequent, precautions against infection should be taken. The pharyngeal opening of the eustachian tube is often in an abnormal position; consequently, the infant should not be fed in a lying-down position, nor should the baby be confined to a supine position for long periods. Good mouth care is also important in reducing infections. A milk feeding should be followed with a small amount of clear water to rinse the mouth. If an infection occurs and fluid accumulates, movement of the ear drum is inhibited, and a hearing loss may occur. Thus, when a child has a cleft palate, language acquisition may be hampered by inability to hear if careful attention is not given to early treatment of middle ear infections.

In many cases, myringotomy and placement of ventilation tubes is necessary. This surgery can be performed at the time of lip repair or in early infancy but can commonly be delayed until the time of palate repair (Trier, 1985). Another approach is to use a prosthesis that occludes the cleft palate. There is, however, no evidence such prostheses assist in feeding or lessen the amount of orthodontic work required (Trier, 1985). Before the child is sent for either of the surgical procedures, parents should be informed about postoperative care, especially the restraints that are necessary to protect the repair from self-inflicted injury.

Major Postoperative Nursing Diagnoses for Cleft Lip and Cleft Palate

Potential impaired tissue integrity, *related to*
- *rubbing of the surgical site*
- *suture line tension associated with sucking or crying*

Potential for aspiration, *related to ineffective positioning of the infant postoperatively*

Potential for infection: surgical site, *related to*
- *inadequate handwashing by persons coming in contact with the infant*
- *remnants of milk or formula that collect on the incision and form a culture medium for pathogens*

Altered comfort: pain, *related to surgical repair of the cleft*

Strategies for Postoperative Nursing Care

Preventing Disturbance of the Surgical Site After Cleft Lip/Palate Repair. The major emphasis in nursing care following cleft lip repair is on protecting the operative site. Arm restraints should be used to prevent the child from rubbing or otherwise disturbing the suture line, such as by thumbsucking or putting objects into the mouth. Children who are old enough to roll over will also need a jacket restraint to prevent them from rolling onto the abdomen and rubbing the face on the bed. (See Figure 27-13 in Chapter 27 for examples of arm restraints.) The arm restraints are removed periodically to exercise the arms and to check for skin irritation. Also, because the child is placed only on the back or side after repair, periodic positioning in an infant seat increases comfort and stimulation.

The watchfulness required to maintain the surgical repair of a cleft lip is demanding of the nurse and the parents. The parents require assistance in understanding the importance of keeping the baby's hands away from the face. Parents also need to be shown how to hold their baby safely and provide physical contact even though restraints are in place. Mobiles and toys with various sounds, colors, and textures are essential for these babies' developmental progress. Parents should be encouraged to participate in the provision of an appropriately stimulating environment.

Feeding methods postoperatively are similar to those used before surgery. Preoperatively, however, these methods were employed to reduce the threat of aspiration and to enhance sucking. Postoperative feeding methods are designed to reduce trauma to the surgical site. Some surgeons may permit the infant to breastfeed early in the postoperative period. Immediately postoperatively, a medicine dropper or Asepto syringe may be used. These should be placed in the mouth from the side to avoid the suture line, and care should be taken to prevent the infant from sucking. Because sucking would disrupt the suture line, a pacifier cannot be used until sufficient healing has taken place.

Following cleft palate repair, injury to the newly closed palate must be prevented. No sharp objects, such as spoons or forks, are permitted in the child's mouth. Liquids are given by mouth but straws are not used. Soft foods can be fed from the side of a spoon but self-feeding by a spoon could result in damage to the operative site.

Preventing Aspiration. Positioning of the infant postoperatively is critical to preventing aspiration of secretions. The position will vary depending on the surgical procedure. An infant who has had a cleft lip repair cannot be placed in a prone position without damaging the surgical site. Therefore, the position of choice for this infant is on either side, but well protected with sandbags or blanket rolls to prevent the child from turning onto the abdomen.

After cleft palate repair, the infant may be safely placed either on the abdomen or on the side; the palatal sutures will not be damaged by a prone position. A mist tent may occasionally be used to ensure that the secretions remain liquid.

Strategies for suctioning of secretions also differ depending upon the type of surgical repair. Although a bulb syringe may be used safely to gently suction secretions after a cleft lip repair, suctioning of any kind is contraindicated after surgery for cleft palate as introduction of a bulb syringe tip or a suction catheter may inadvertently damage the palatal suture line.

Preventing Infection. The importance of good handwashing should be impressed upon parents and other visitors who come in direct contact with the infant. Needless to say, the nurse's hands carry the greatest potential for cross contamination because of contact with other ill children and with contaminated surfaces. The nurse's careful handwashing is always a key to controlling iatrogenic infection.

Initial feedings will be of clear liquids as tolerated. When feeding with milk or formula resumes, the mouth should be gently rinsed with water after each feeding. This is particularly important after surgery for cleft palate as there is no other way to clean the suture line. After cleft lip repair, the suture line should be cleaned with a cotton-tipped applicator and half-strength hydrogen peroxide. Often the physician will order an antibiotic ointment as well. Protection and astute care of the suture line is essential to provide for optimum healing and cosmetic results.

Providing Optimal Comfort. The infant can be expected to have pain postoperatively from the surgical manipulation and suturing of tissues. Both analgesic medication and non-pharmacologic strategies should be considered. The provision of comfort is important not only for humane reasons, but also because crying will place pressure on delicate suture lines.

Acetaminophen (Tylenol) is often ordered for postoperative analgesia after such procedures. Tylenol can be effective in controlling pain if it is administered routinely (i.e., every 3 to 4 hours as ordered) during the first 24 hours or at the time when the infant can be expected to have the most pain. A single dose or widely spaced doses of a mild analgesic, such as Tylenol, will probably not accomplish the goal of providing optimal comfort.

Infants seem to derive a good deal of comfort from being held and cuddled after cleft lip or cleft palate repair. Physical closeness with their infant can also give parents an opportunity to express their love and concern and to assure themselves that the baby is alright. The nurse can facilitate this non-pharmacologic comfort measure by showing the parents how to prevent suture line disturbance and how to prevent aspiration of secretions while holding the infant.

Long-Term Outcome

Aside from surgical repairs, the complete program of habilitation for the child with a cleft lip or palate will require the care of other specialists, particularly with respect to dental corrections and the development of normal speech. A speech pathologist can help the child develop normal speech early in life and can assist parents in early speech training as needed.

Treatment is most effective when provided by a cleft palate team. The American Cleft Palate Association (ACPA) registers cleft palate teams and sets guidelines about team membership. A list of cleft palate teams or centers can be obtained from the ACPA National Office.* The Cleft Palate Foundation is an educational arm of the ACPA and is located at the same address. A 24-hour telephone service is available for referrals and information; call (800) 24-CLEFT.

Remarkable progress in the management of children born with a cleft lip or cleft palate, or both, has made it possible for these children to look like other children, speak like other children, and essentially live a normal life. The team approach provides the supportive care and coordinated treatment that is needed by these families. The nurse has an important role in helping families cope with the stress of having a baby with a defect and assisting them to understand and participate in the treatment and management program for their child.

Nursing Strategies for Follow-up Visits in the Home or Clinic

Plot height and weight on the growth chart to assess adequacy of nutritional intake.

Discuss with the parent any feeding concerns. Use every opportunity to appropriately reinforce parental competence. Parents can interpret feeding difficulties as a failure in their parenting role.

Preoperatively: If possible, observe the parent feeding the infant. Offer suggestions to improve suction and to decrease the risk of aspiration.

Postoperatively: Watch the child suck or drink from a cup. Determine if the child is making adequate adjustments to the alterations in the oral cavity after surgery.

Assess respiratory status for evidence of infection related to aspiration of formula (preoperatively) or secretions (postoperatively).

Assess the middle ear by otoscopy (when this falls within the nurse's role).

Listen for appropriateness of babbling speech sounds and closely observe tooth eruptions as the child develops If cleft palate is involved, ensure that the parent is aware of the probable need for speech therapy and regular dental examinations.

* The national office is located at:
The American Cleft Palate Association
1218 Grandview Avenue
University of Pittsburgh
Pittsburgh, PA 15211

Pyloric Stenosis

In pyloric stenosis there is an overgrowth (hypertrophy and hyperplasia) of the circular muscle of the pylorus, which results in obstruction of the pyloric sphincter. Although its cause is unknown, there seems to be a hereditary component, as a family history of the problem is present in about 15 per cent of cases. It is thought to be more common in males (1 : 150) than in females (1 : 750) and especially in firstborn males, although some authors believe these factors have been overemphasized (Filston and Izant, 1985).

Pathophysiology

The pylorus is the opening through which food passes from the stomach to the intestines. This opening is surrounded by a muscular ring called the pyloric sphincter. In pyloric stenosis the sphincter is in a state of spasm that causes hypertrophy of the muscle, resulting in a narrowed opening (Fig. 41-5). The stomach's peristaltic movements do not effectively move contents through the obstructed pylorus; consequently, the overworked stomach musculature hypertrophies. The stomach contractions increase in frequency and force as they attempt to push stomach contents through the elongated, partially obstructed pyloric canal.

Clinical Manifestations

Although the history may vary, typically at about 3 weeks of age the infant begins to regurgitate small amounts of milk immediately after a feeding. Within a week, the pattern and type of vomiting can change dramatically, becoming projectile in character (vomitus propelled distances of several feet) and occurring with almost every feeding. The vomiting usually occurs during the feeding or shortly thereafter, but in some instances may occur several hours later. The infant is hungry in spite of the vomiting and will usually

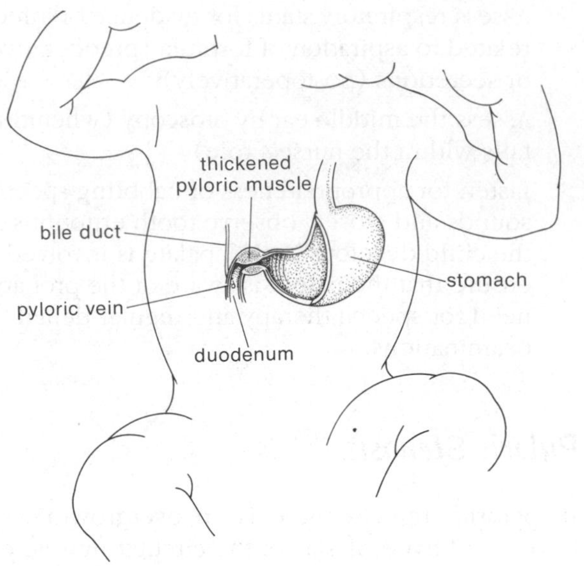

Figure 41-5. Pyloric stenosis. Hypertrophy, or thickening, of the pyloric sphincter blocks the stomach contents, causing the infant to regurgitate forcefully. Serious electrolyte imbalances ultimately occur and surgery is necessary to correct the condition.

take milk again. The vomitus contains no bile because the constriction is proximal to the ampulla of Vater, the site at which the common bile duct enters the duodenum.

Gastritis may occur owing to the irritation caused by stomach contents remaining in the stomach for prolonged periods. In gastritis the vomitus may be blood-tinged (brownish discoloration).

The initial pattern of regurgitation after feedings may not result in any decrease in the baby's weight, nutritional state, or fluid and electrolyte balance, but with continuous, progressive vomiting some serious alterations eventually develop. If untreated, the infant will lose weight. With eventual nutritional depletion the child will show signs of dehydration and become alkalotic. With excessive loss of gastric juices, the electrolytes sodium, potassium, and chloride are lost. Gastric juice contains more chloride than sodium; therefore hypochloremic alkalosis develops. As vomiting continues, a state of hypochloremia and hypokalemia results. Hydrochloric acid is lost, resulting in an increased pH and increased bicarbonate (carbon dioxide content) level. The fluid and electrolyte imbalance that results from excessive vomiting must be corrected before surgery is attempted.

Diagnostic Assessment

The nurse in a clinic or similar primary care setting may be the first to hear a parent's account of an infant who shows the beginning signs of pyloric stenosis. A careful history must be taken to differentiate this infant from the one who is vomiting owing to a poor feeding experience, such as might occur with an overly anxious caregiver or inadequate bonding. In 90 per cent of the infants with pyloric stenosis a mass (the hypertrophied pylorus) can be palpated in the right epigastrium under the edge of the liver. The mass feels hard and is movable and shaped like an olive. Successful palpation requires a relaxed abdominal muscle and an empty stomach. A nasogastric tube may be passed and placed on continuous suction to facilitate palpation. Abdominal muscle relaxation can be achieved by holding the infant to quiet him or her, offering a pacifier with sugar or a bottle of warm sugar water, and elevating the baby's feet or flexing the knees and hips. After feeding, peristaltic waves can sometimes be noted moving from left to right toward the pylorus.

Radiographs are indicated only when the mass cannot be palpated after several examinations. If pyloric stenosis is present, barium contrast studies reveal delayed gastric emptying and an elongated, narrow pyloric canal (string sign), which may appear as a small or double streak of barium. Frequently, the pyloric mass can also be identified on ultrasonographic examination of the abdomen. If the results of diagnostic studies are normal, other conditions must be considered. However, the infant may be examined again in a week or 10 days because it can take some time for the typical diagnostic findings to develop in the presence of pyloric stenosis (Colodny, 1978).

Therapeutic Management

In infants who are well hydrated and have no evidence of electrolyte and acid-base abnormalities, surgery is performed without delay. If an infant is dehydrated and has electrolyte imbalance, it is imperative that these conditions be corrected before surgery.

The stenosis is corrected by the Fredet-Ramstedt operation, which involves a longitudinal splitting of the hypertrophied muscle down to the mucosa so that the mucosa bulges between the split muscle. The mucosa and submucosa are left intact so that the lumen of the duodenum is not entered. The time for introduction of oral feedings varies.

Major Nursing Diagnoses for Pyloric Stenosis

Fluid volume deficit: preoperative, *related to persistent vomiting*
Fear/anxiety: parental, *related to the infant's impending surgery*
Potential fluid volume deficit: postoperative, *related to vomiting, associated with*

- *air swallowing with feeding*
- *vigorous activity after feeding*

Altered comfort: pain, *related to tissue trauma associated with abdominal surgery*
Knowledge deficit, *related to lack of information about infant care during the period of recuperation*

Strategies for Nursing Care

Rehydrating the Infant and Supporting the Parents Preoperatively. If the infant is dehydrated and experiencing an electrolyte imbalance, surgery may be delayed from 24 to 36 hours while the infant receives intravenous fluids containing potassium. The baby may be irritable and crying because of not receiving any oral fluids. It is disturbing to parents to see their tiny baby restrained and distressed; they should be encouraged to discuss their feelings. Parents are taught how to protect the intravenous site while holding their infant and are encouraged to be present during this period to hold, comfort, and talk to the baby.

Parents are prepared for the surgery and the postoperative period by being told what to expect. The operation is a short procedure (15 to 30 minutes), and the infant will probably return from surgery with an intravenous line. Parents are told about the potential for vomiting in the immediate postoperative period and the need for gradual reintroduction of fluids, with clarification about when breastfeeding can be resumed.

Preventing Postoperative Fluid Volume Deficit. For a bottle-fed infant, diluted formula is given postoperatively in small amounts, and gradually the quantity and strength of formula are increased. A basic rule to follow is not to change quantity and content of feeding at the same time (Filston and Izant, 1985). An infant who is breastfed can be allowed a gradual increase in the length of time at the breast.

Postoperative vomiting may occur for various reasons, and the nurse must make every effort to ensure that improper feeding technique is not the cause. These infants need to be fed using a firm nipple with a hole small enough so that milk is not taken too quickly. The nurse should emphasize that the nipple must be kept full of milk at all times to minimize swallowing of air and the infant should be burped at any sign of discomfort. Also, these infants are often hungry and should not be allowed to suck on an empty bottle. If the infant must be disturbed after feeding, he or she should be handled with extra care to prevent vomiting related to the activity.

Helping parents to feel at ease by staying with them, helping them feed the baby correctly, and reassuring them that they are playing an important part in the recovery of their infant gives them support and courage during this sometimes difficult period. Parents may easily become upset when vomiting recurs and may feel it is their fault. It is particularly discouraging if they have not been prepared preoperatively to expect this.

Providing Optimal Comfort. The infant can be expected to experience pain, especially in the first 24 to 48 hours after surgery. Because infants react to pain differently than do older children or adults, assessment is very difficult, and comfort measures often need to be instituted on the nurse's judgment that pain *must* be present. As always, both pharmacologic and non-pharmacologic strategies should be employed to ensure that the infant experiences no unnecessary distress. (See Chapter 29 for a discussion of pain assessment and management.)

Teaching to Facilitate Care at Home. Care of the surgical site includes observation for signs of drainage or inflammation. The infant can usually be bathed, but care is taken to avoid immersing the surgical site in water until it is completely healed.

Usually these infants can be discharged on the morning of the second postoperative day on an unrestricted diet. The incision is often sealed with collodion (a viscous liquid that is sprayed or applied with an applicator over an incision, which dries to form a strong, thin, transparent film) so that no dressing changes are required. Parents can resume their usual infant care routine and should be encouraged to plan their responsibilities in a way that will allow for a relaxed, quiet feeding environment. It is important that parents feel positive about the feeding experience at discharge; otherwise, preconditioned feelings of failure may again make feeding an unpleasant and unsuccessful experience.

The mortality rate is well below 1 per cent in infants whose conditions have been identified early and who have been properly prepared for surgery. The nurse, as a member of the health team, has an important role in both of these areas.

Nursing Strategies for Follow-up Care in the Home or Clinic after Surgery

Plot height and weight parameters on the growth chart to assess for resumption of adequate nutrition.

Record the infant's temperature and inspect the surgical incision to assess for postoperative infection.

Ask the parent about fluid intake (breast milk or formula) and whether there have been any episodes of vomiting since discharge.

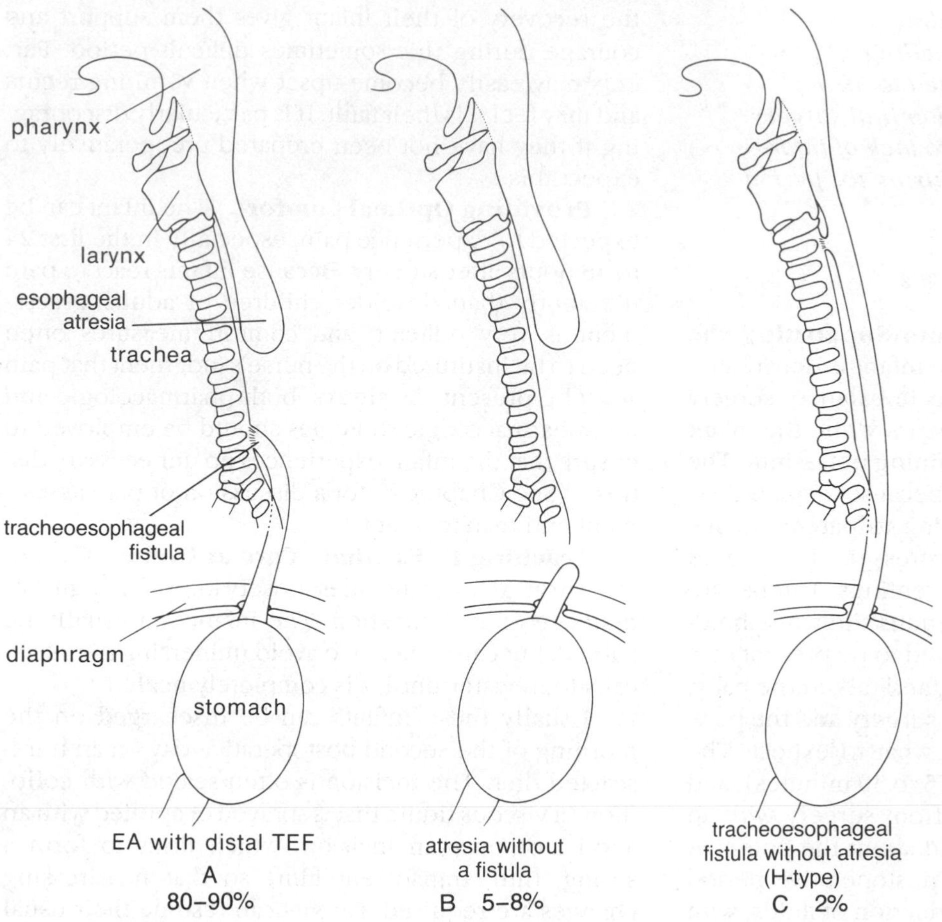

Figure 41-6. The three most common types of esophageal atresia and transesophageal fistula. *A*, Esophageal atresia with a distal fistula constitutes 80 to 90 per cent of all cases. *B*, Atresia without a fistula—5 to 8 per cent. *C*, Isolated tracheoesophageal fistula without esophageal atresia (H type)—2 per cent.

Encourage the parent to voice concerns about postoperative care of the infant. Reinforce appropriate care to increase the parent's self-confidence.

Esophageal Atresia and Tracheoesophageal Fistula

Esophageal atresia and tracheoesophageal fistula can each occur as a single entity, but usually they occur together. The reported prevalence of atresia (with or without tracheoesophageal fistula) is approximately 1 per 3000 live births. There are numerous types of esophageal atresia with or without tracheoesophageal fistula. Atresia with a distal fistula constitutes 80 to 90 per cent of all cases (Fig. 41-6*A*). In this type the upper (proximal) esophagus ends in a blind pouch and the lower (distal) esophagus exits from the stomach and joins the trachea instead of forming a continuous tube with the upper esophagus. The second most frequent type (Fig. 41-6*B*) is atresia without a fistula, accounting for 5 to 8 per cent of all cases. In this type there is a proximal dilated pouch and the distal end of the esophagus is narrowed and short. The third type, an isolated tracheoesophageal fistula without esophageal atresia, constitutes about 2 per cent of all cases. It is sometimes called the H-type because a fistula connects the trachea and esophagus in a way that resembles the letter H (Fig. 41-6*C*). Rare types occur in varying combinations of fistulas and atresia but will not be discussed here.

Clinical Manifestations and Diagnostic Assessment

Aspiration of secretions into the lungs has a major effect on prognosis. Aspiration can be prevented or diminished by early diagnosis and placement of a nasogastric sump tube in the proximal pouch to remove secretions.

Only a few clues can be relied on to identify an infant with esophageal atresia and tracheoesophageal fistula early. Prematurity and hydramnios (excess amniotic fluid) are two conditions that should alert the nurse to make further assessments. Eighty-five per cent of infants with atresia accompanied by fistula have a maternal history of hydramnios (Ashcraft and Holder, 1976). This suggests that effective swallowing and absorption of amniotic fluid in utero is prevented. Approximately one third of the affected infants are premature. When prematurity or hydramnios, or both, are present and the nurse suspects esophageal atresia or tracheoesophageal fistula, other signs to look for include excessive pharyngeal secretions, such as drooling or bubbling from the nostrils. Unfortunately, atresia is often first suspected when an infant coughs, chokes, regurgitates, or becomes cyanotic on feeding. In the H-type fistula, drooling does not occur (because this type does not consist of a proximal esophageal pouch), and choking and coughing on feeding are the first signs. Abdominal distention is noted with crying because air is shunted across the fistula.

When the fistula is small, the symptoms are not so obvious, but repeated pneumonia in the first few months of life should raise the suspicion of an H-type tracheoesophageal fistula. These episodes of pneumonia result from reflux of gastric secretions into the trachea.

When atresia is suspected, the presence of a blind pouch of the proximal esophagus can be confirmed by the inability to pass a radiopaque No. 8 to 10 French catheter into the stomach. Curling of the tube in the proximal esophagus is shown on radiographs. If a fistula is present, the radiographs will show air in the stomach and intestines because of the esophageal connection to the trachea. When there is no connection to the distal esophagus, neither air nor food enters the stomach. In these infants the abdomen is flat and scaphoid in appearance.

If a contrast medium is instilled to outline the blind upper pouch, it should be water soluble and given under fluoroscopic control. The contrast medium is then withdrawn to prevent overflow into the lungs. The procedure of choice for diagnosis is bronchoscopy with telescopic endoscopy. Other diagnostic methods are considered less accurate and introduce delay and the risk of aspiration (Filston and Izant, 1985).

In 30 per cent of cases of esophageal atresia, additional abnormalities are present, especially cardiac anomalies; therefore, a thorough physical examination and appropriate diagnostic studies in search of other anomalies are also done prior to surgery.

The parents are under a great deal of stress during the diagnostic period. If they witness the choking, coughing, and cyanosis produced by feeding, they may be particularly frightened; they need careful explanation of what the existing problem is and why their baby cannot be fed by mouth. Once the diagnosis is established, the family must be prepared for the necessary procedures and surgery that will follow.

Therapeutic Management

The goals of initial therapy are to prevent pulmonary complications and to ensure adequate nutrition (Gryboski, 1986). Preoperatively, the infant is placed in a position with head elevated (45 to 60°) to reduce the likelihood of regurgitation of stomach contents into the trachea. A sump tube* (usually a Replogle) will be placed in the proximal esophageal pouch to remove pooled secretions and to decrease the chance of aspiration. The infant's respiratory status is closely monitored. A gastrostomy tube may be placed to decompress the stomach, although this varies with the type of defect. The infant is placed in an Isolette, where oxygen, humidity, and thermoregulation can be provided.

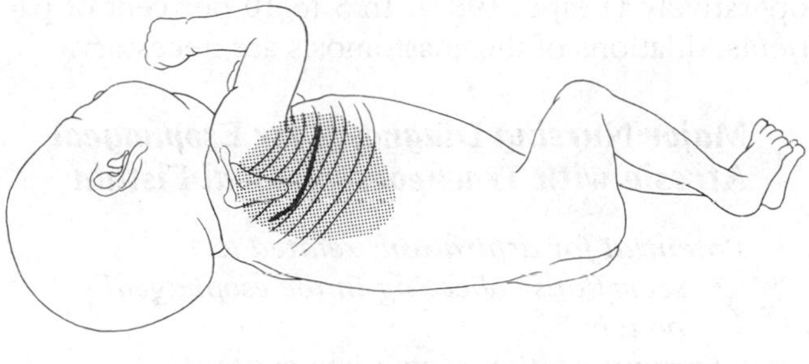

Figure 41-7. Incision for primary repair of tracheoesophageal fistula. (From Coran A: *Surgery of the Neonate.* Boston, Little, Brown & Co, 1979, p 48.)

Primary repair consists of ligation of the fistula and anastomosis of the upper and lower segments of the esophagus. This is done through a right posterolateral thoracotomy (Fig. 41-7). When the anastomosis is completed, the tube in the esophageal pouch is removed. At the end of the operation, a retropleural chest tube is placed through a stab wound. Primary repair may be delayed if the infant is at risk owing to low birth weight, pneumonia, or another congenital anomaly. In these cases, a gastrostomy is performed (Randolph, 1986).

Postoperatively, fluid and electrolyte balance is maintained by an intravenous line, and prophylactic antibiotics may be ordered. Intravenous overload and pulmonary congestion are avoided by keeping intravenous fluid volumes at low maintenance levels (Canty, 1986). Respiratory management is the major concern in the immediate postoperative period. Mechanical ventilation may be required during the first few days. Oral feedings are recommended by some to begin on the second day unless there is concern about the anastomosis (Leape, 1987). Other approaches of nutritional maintenance are total parenteral nutrition or gastrostomy feedings. The anastomosis is weakest at 5 to 7 days, therefore, if there is concern about the anastomosis, oral feedings are delayed until 10 days post-

* A sump tube has side holes over only the distal 1 inch of the tube. A standard nasogastric tube should not be used because it has side holes over the distal 2 to 3 inches. If a nasogastric tube is used in the pouch, too much available air would be suctioned from the pharynx.

operatively (Leape, 1987). In 5 to 10 per cent of patients, dilations of the anastomosis are necessary.

Major Nursing Diagnoses for Esophageal Atresia with Tracheoesophageal Fistula

Potential for aspiration, related to
- *secretions collecting in the esophageal pouch*
- *regurgitation of stomach contents through the fistula into the trachea*

***Fear/anxiety: parental,** related to the infant's diagnosis and impending surgery*

***Potential ineffective airway clearance: postoperative,** related to increased mucus production and edema associated with*
- *surgical trauma to the esophagus*
- *suctioning techniques*

***Potential impaired tissue integrity: surgical site,** related to*
- *improper suctioning techniques*
- *hyperextension of the neck*
- *pressure against the suture line associated with gastric regurgitation*

***Knowledge deficit,** related to infant care in the recuperative phase*

Strategies for Nursing Care: Esophageal Atresia with Tracheoesophageal Fistula

Preventing Aspiration. In the most common type of esophageal atresia (with fistula), the goals of preoperative care are to prevent aspiration of the secretions from the proximal esophageal pouch and prevent regurgitation of stomach contents through the fistula into the trachea. The latter condition is the more serious in that it causes chemical pneumonitis. Immediate nursing care includes allowing nothing by mouth and performing suctioning* of the nasopharynx until the pouch is drained via a sump tube. This tube requires frequent irrigation to ensure its patency.

The infant is positioned with head and chest elevated 45 to 60 degrees (Fig. 41-8). This accomplishes two goals: (1) secretions are pooled in the bottom of the esophageal pouch, facilitating withdrawal by constant suction, and (2) gravity counteracts gastric reflux into the trachea and lungs. In spite of this position, distention of the stomach during crying causes gastric regurgitation. Therefore, keeping the baby quiet by stroking and gentle handling are important measures during this period of frequent stimulation that occurs as a result of the required emergency care. Although use of a pacifier may increase salivation, once the sump tube is in the esophageal pouch the mucus is easily removed, and a pacifier will help to diminish crying and satisfy the infant's need to suck.

Easing Parental Anxiety. The family of a child with esophageal atresia experiences stress because of the immediacy and intensity of the care required. The nurse supports the parents prior to surgery by keeping them informed of the status of their infant. The need for suctioning, intravenous therapy, placement of a sump tube, and preparation for the impending surgery are distressing to parents and seemingly disruptive to the infant. They have not yet recovered from the shock of learning that something is wrong with their baby when they need to face yet another stress, the surgery itself. The nurse can be supportive by answering their questions about the purpose of the various procedures and kinds of equipment required. The careful monitoring their baby requires may actually make parents fear that something has gone wrong. The nurse makes ongoing explanations about the routine aspects of the infant's care to alleviate such fears and encourages parents to hold their infant as the condition improves.

Maintaining a Patent Airway and Preventing Trauma to the Surgical Site. Postoperatively, two of the nurse's most important goals are to maintain a patent airway and prevent trauma to the anastomosis. To meet both of these goals, a suction catheter is marked by the surgeon to the maximum length that it can be inserted when suctioning through the nares to ensure that it is not passed farther than a point just above the anastomosis. The nurse should place this premeasured catheter in a clearly visible location with careful instructions so that each person suctioning the infant will measure the catheter used against the premeasured catheter. The nurse carefully observes the infant for early signs of airway obstruction. An anxious expression on the infant's face is often the first sign, followed by an increase in respiratory rate, and, when there is serious trouble, the onset of retractions.

Suctioning technique is extremely important. It must be done gently to avoid trauma to the tissues, quickly to avoid oxygen deficiency, and frequently to maintain the airway. The nurse must use judgment regarding frequency of suctioning, realizing that it increases the edema that already exists from the operation. On occasion, endotracheal suctioning may be necessary. This is usually done by a physician under direct vision with a laryngoscope (Canty, 1986).

If ventilatory support is required because of prematurity or respiratory distress, the ventilator is kept at the lowest setting that will achieve adequate ventilation but avoid barotrauma to the lungs and the surgical areas.

Postoperatively, the infant is usually positioned with the head slightly elevated, in a warm, humidified environment. Hyperextension of the neck must be

---

* Suctioning may be necessary every 10 to 15 minutes but must be done gently to avoid traumatizing the mucosa and risk of edema.

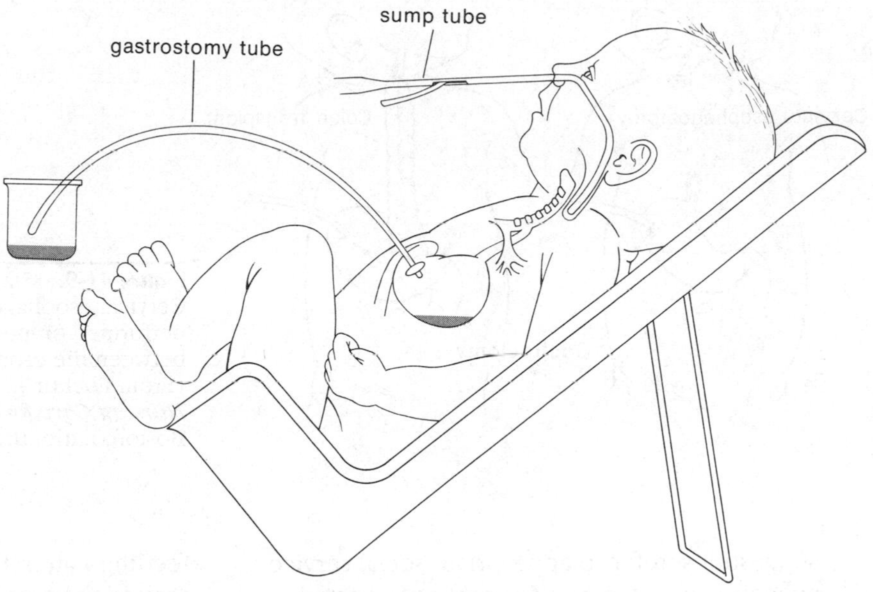

***Figure* 41-8.** Tracheoesophageal fistula preoperative position. Preoperative care is given with the child in the semi-Fowler's position with proximal sump drainage and gastrostomy decompression.

avoided to prevent pull on the sutured esophagus. In the immediate postoperative period, the upright position and placement of the gastrostomy tube (if present) on gravity drainage prevents gastric regurgitation, thereby decreasing pressure on the anastomosis. The infant's position should be changed from back to either side at least every 2 hours to prevent pneumonia and provide comfort. Percussion and postural drainage are also employed as preventive measures; for the first 3 to 4 days, only vibration is performed while the suture line heals (Cassani, 1984).

Oral feedings may be started by the second day or they may be delayed for 10 days. If the infant is NPO for 10 days, total parenteral nutrition is administered. If a gastrostomy has been done, it is placed on gravity drainage for 2 to 3 days then elevated. Gastrostomy feedings of formula or expressed breast are then administered, cautiously increasing volume and strength.

When oral feeding is begun, the nurse should immediately begin teaching the family effective feeding techniques. Extreme care must be taken to prevent the baby from swallowing large amounts of air that would potentiate regurgitation. If the infant is being fed gastrostomy feedings while awaiting primary repair, parents are taught the feeding procedure.

Teaching to Facilitate Home Care. The amount of family involvement varies with each institution and family situation. In many cases, parents can be helped to feed their baby after the first oral feeding has been given. Parents also readily learn the technique of gastrostomy feeding and are encouraged to feed their baby as they feel comfortable. If the family has been included in the infant's care during hospitalization, discharge preparation requires very little additional time by the nurse.

When the infant is discharged, the family should have had several experiences in feeding, positioning, and handling their infant. Parents should become familiar with signs of respiratory distress and be instructed to report any pronounced coughing, gagging, or dysphagia that may indicate anastomotic stricture. Parents should also be informed that the infant will have a raspy cough.

Frequently, referral is indicated for follow-up visits in the home, especially when special procedures are necessary. The parents should be made to feel that they can contact the hospital or home care nurses even for the smallest problem.

Nursing Strategies for Follow-up Care in the Home or Clinic

Assess growth parameters to determine if the infant is maintaining the percentiles established at birth.

Determine how many ounces of formula are being consumed daily and the extent to which the infant is tolerating oral feedings. Seek medical intervention immediately if the parent reports signs of esophageal stricture: inability to tolerate solid foods, increased drooling, frequent coughing and choking, and dysphagia.

Inspect the skin around the gastrostomy site for pronounced erythema and induration and for purulent drainage that would indicate an infection.

Encourage the parent to describe a typical day for the family and assess the major stressors associated with care of the infant at this stage of the recuperative process. Offer support and

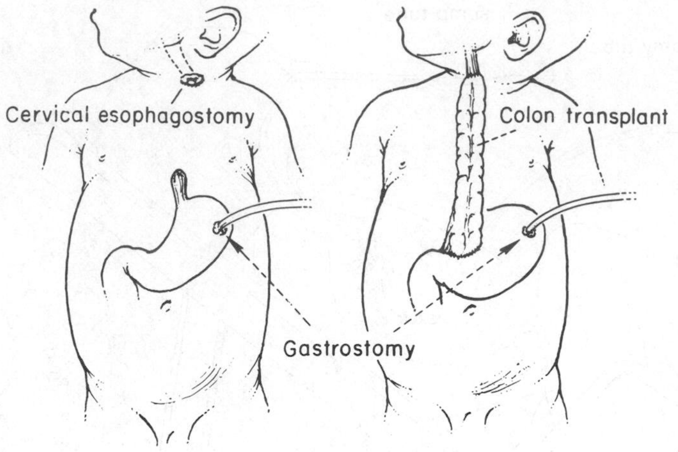

Figure 41-9. Stages in treatment of esophageal atresia. Cervical esophagostomy and gastrostomy, which are performed on newborns, and colon interposition between the esophagus in the neck and the stomach. (From Fochtman D, Raffensperger J: *Principles of Nursing Care for the Pediatric Surgery Patient,* 2nd ed. Boston, Little, Brown & Co, 1976, p 39.)

suggestions; refer to appropriate social service agencies (e.g., for respite care) as indicated.

Therapeutic Management and Strategies for Nursing Care: Esophageal Atresia Without Fistula

Cases of esophageal atresia without a fistula (see Fig. 41-6) will require some variations in treatment and care from those described for esophageal atresia with tracheoesophageal fistula. The presenting symptoms are similar, but radiographs demonstrate absence of gastrointestinal gas. Although stretching of the upper pouch has been tried, it is now recognized that waiting for the pouch to grow for 2 to 3 months is more effective (Randolph, 1986).

Meticulous nursing care is required in the interim to avoid aspiration of saliva and to assure adequate nutrition. Constant suction of the pouch by a sump tube is used and must be maintained at all times.

When anastomosis cannot be performed, cervical esophagostomy may be necessary. The proximal esophagus is brought to the exterior (opens on the neck above the left clavicle) to prevent aspiration of secretions from the blind pouch (Fig. 41-9). During this period, the infant is fed by gastrostomy tube, and sham*, oral feedings are offered to maintain swallowing reflexes and meet the infant's need to suck. These feedings take additional time and do not provide any nutritive value, but a nurse should not overlook the importance of meeting these normal developmental needs. Parents should be encouraged to give these feedings after their purpose is explained. The skin around the esophagostomy becomes easily excoriated from saliva, which contains digestive enzymes. A protective ointment can be applied or a pad of soft, absorbent material can be placed over the area and held in place by the infant's shirt. Tape should be avoided, as it increases skin breakdown. The pad must be changed frequently and the ointment removed daily to allow for thorough cleansing and drying of the skin.

The infant is maintained by gastrostomy feedings until a colon interposition is performed. A segment of the colon is mobilized from the abdomen and interposed in the chest to connect the proximal and distal ends of the esophagus (Fig. 41-9). This procedure is usually done after 6 months of age and before the child reaches 24 months of age.

Long-Term Outcome

Almost all full-term infants with esophageal atresia survive if no other serious anomalies are present (Filler, 1978). Pneumonia is a frequent complication in patients with tracheoesophageal fistula. Other complications are a leak at the anastomosis, recurrent fistula, and gastroesophageal reflux, but the most common late complication is stricture at the anastomosis (Coran et al, 1979). Parents, therefore, need to be informed about signs of stricture such as inability to tolerate solid foods, increased drooling, frequent coughing and choking, and dysphagia. It has been reported that from one to several dozen dilations are required in 50 per cent of patients until the esophagus is wide enough to permit passage of food (Coran et al, 1979). These dilations may be required over a period of weeks, months, or years. Therefore, the help the family needs from the professional team varies with the occurrence of complications and the type and length of follow-up treatment required.

* Sham feedings are any fluids given orally. These feedings drain immediately from the opening on the neck (esophagostomy) but provide a sucking experience for the infant. When such feedings are given at the time of gastrostomy feeding, the act of sucking is associated with the comfort of satiety.

Omphalocele

An omphalocele is a herniation of variable amounts of abdominal viscera through the open umbilical ring into the base of the umbilical cord. The size of the defect ranges from 2 to 15 cm. The herniated viscera are enclosed by a translucent membrane with the umbilical cord extending from its surface. A small sac may contain only one or two loops of bowel, but a large sac may contain the liver, spleen, and most of the bowel (Fig. 41-10). A peritoneal sac is always present in an omphalocele but may be ruptured during or after delivery.

Omphalocele occurs in approximately 1 : 5000 live births and is associated with many other anomalies. Almost all affected infants have malrotation and abnormalities in bowel fixation (Frentner, 1987).

Embryology and Pathophysiology

Between the fifth and tenth weeks of development, the midgut grows rapidly and projects from the abdomen through the umbilical ring into the umbilical cord. Herniation of the midgut into the umbilical cord in this period of embryonic life is a normal developmental process. The intestines thus grow outside of the abdominal wall for a portion of fetal life. As the midgut grows, it rotates counterclockwise within the cord. Reentry of the intestines into the abdominal cavity takes place around the eleventh week of fetal life. The intestines continue to rotate as re-entry takes place. If reentry fails to occur, a persistence of herniation of the intestines (omphalocele) exists, and the abdominal cavity remains small. (It is the presence of abdominal contents within the cavity that causes the cavity to grow and develop; consequently the larger the omphalocele, the smaller the abdominal cavity.)

Therapeutic Management and Strategies for Nursing Care

Protecting the Sac. The sac must be protected to prevent rupture and infection. Exposure of the sac is also dangerous to the infant because of hypothermia, which results from radiant heat loss. A variety of approaches are used to protect the sac preoperatively.

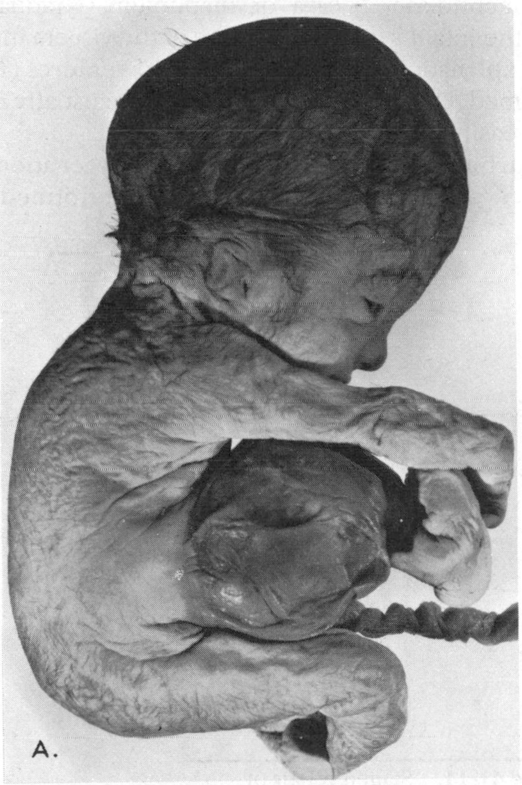

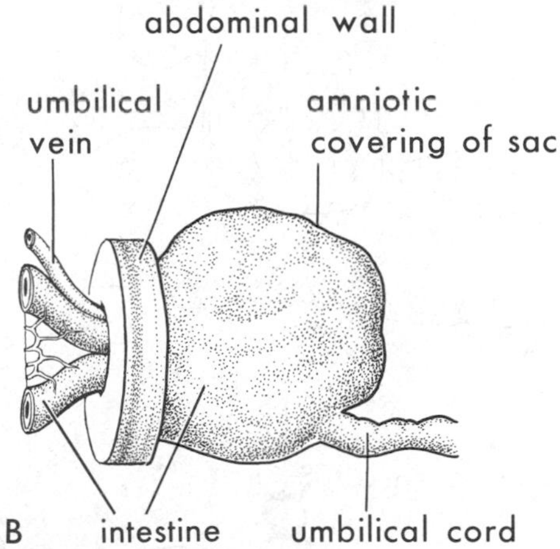

Figure 41-10. *A*, Large omphalocele in an immature 28-week fetus. Half actual size. *B*, Drawing illustrating the structure and contents of the hernial sac. The protruding mass of intestine is covered by a transparent, bilaminar membrane composed of peritoneum and amnion. Occasionally, these membranes rupture prior to or during birth. In this case, the eviscerated intestine lies freely around the gaping defect in the abdominal wall.

The sac can be covered with warm, sterile, moist saline gauze. A bowel bag (a large plastic bag covering the lower half of the baby's body) is also used and often is preferred because it protects the sac and helps to prevent hypothermia by interfering with radiant heat loss (Frentner, 1987).

Care of the omphalocele is done with sterile gloves and without placing undue pressure on the omphalocele. A nasogastric tube must be inserted and placed on low suction to prevent distention of the stomach and intestines. The infant is kept in an incubator and prepared for immediate surgery, including fluid therapy, administration of antibiotics, and overall stabilization.

Supporting the Family. The family will be shocked by the appearance of their infant. When the omphalocele is large, the parents may feel repulsed by the gross abnormality. It may be difficult for them to comprehend that an anomaly of this magnitude can be corrected with excellent results when there are no associated anomalies. They may be pessimistic about the surgery and show little interest in their infant. It is the nurse's role to encourage parents to talk about their infant and help them express what they are experiencing. The nurse needs to be patient with the parents who do not seem to hear or believe that their child can be helped. In this early phase of bonding, the infant's appearance may be a drawback. Even with explanation and encouragement, parents feel overwhelmed. Once the abdomen is closed, the nurse can more easily help them make contact with their infant by touching and holding when possible.

Surgical Repair. The ideal form of treatment is primary closure. The sac is excised, the bowel and abdominal organs are examined, the abdomen is stretched, and the abdominal contents are returned to the abdominal cavity, followed by abdominal wall closure. Although this technique may cause pressure within the abdomen and compromise the diaphragm, it is now the most common approach because ventilatory support is highly advanced in neonatal care units. For those infants in whom primary closure is not feasible, a staged repair is done (Frentner, 1987).

In a staged repair, the omphalocele is encased in a Silastic mesh sac. The mesh is sutured in place all around the defect to create a tall cylindric silo, which is then tied with umbilical tape or other device to form a pouch over the defect (Fig. 41-11). The contact area between the skin and the mesh is susceptible to infection and can be protected by wrapping the silo with gauze that has been saturated with half-strength Betadine solution. The top of the silo is loosely supported by attaching it to a flexible device suspended from the top of the incubator. This is done to prevent it from falling to one side.

The viscera are moved gradually into the abdominal cavity without causing undue pressure on the vena cava or diaphragm. Gradually, the surgeon gently pushes more of the viscera into the abdomen and ties a new tape at the lower level (Fig. 41-11). Within 5 to 10 days, the viscera are usually reduced into the abdominal cavity.

Maintaining Oxygenation Postoperatively. When a primary repair is performed, the enclosed abdominal

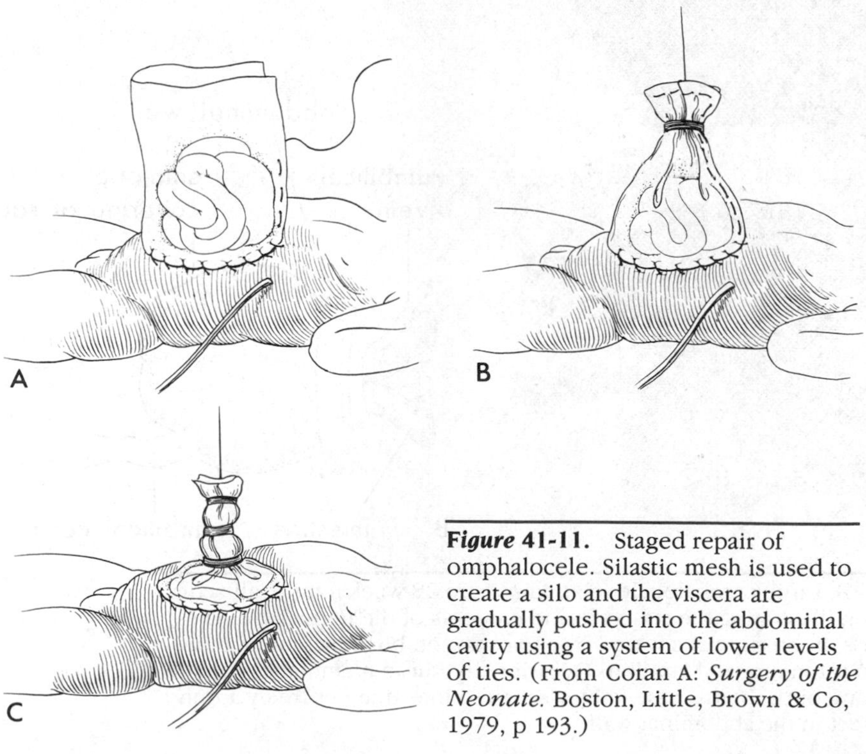

***Figure* 41-11.** Staged repair of omphalocele. Silastic mesh is used to create a silo and the viscera are gradually pushed into the abdominal cavity using a system of lower levels of ties. (From Coran A: *Surgery of the Neonate.* Boston, Little, Brown & Co, 1979, p 193.)

contents cause pressure on the diaphragm. These infants are commonly placed on a ventilator for 7 to 10 days. As third space fluids* cause increasing intra-abdominal pressure, ventilator settings are increased to maintain oxygenation.

If the infant has a staged repair, the bowel is reduced gradually. As the intestines are gradually pushed back into the abdominal cavity, there is increased pressure on the inferior vena cava. This can result in circulatory overload problems manifested by edema in the lower extremities, and the incision must be inspected carefully for signs of dehiscence. After reduction of the viscera is complete, the infant must be returned to surgery for closure of the abdomen.

Maintaining Fluid Balance. The type of fluid and method of feeding vary with the severity of the defect. Total parenteral nutrition, gastrostomy feedings, or nasogastric feedings are approaches that are used during the postoperative period, depending on the infant's needs.

A colloid, such as albumin, is generally required to increase osmotic pressure, which will re-establish equilibrium and interstitial spaces by pulling fluid back into the vascular compartment. During the postoperative period, the nurse keeps careful intake and output records and assesses the infant for symptoms of hypovolemia, including tachycardia, decreased urinary output, increased urine specific gravity, and decreased blood pressure.

Teaching to Ensure Prompt Treatment of Complications. The potential complications after surgery include the development of intestinal obstruction or malabsorption. Parents should alert the physician if any of the following signs occur after discharge (Kenner et al, 1988):

1. Poor appetite
2. Vomiting
3. Abdominal distention
4. Constipation or diarrhea

Gastroschisis

Pathophysiology

Gastroschisis differs in appearance from omphalocele, but the operative management of the two anomalies is similar. Gastroschisis is a herniation of bowel to the right of the midline beside the umbilicus (Fig. 41-12), whereas in an omphalocele herniation is into the base of the umbilical cord. Gastroschisis is thought to be due to a rupture of the base of the umbilical cord caused by atrophy of the right umbilical vein (Filston and Izant, 1985), although other embryologic explanations have also been given. Infants with gastroschisis tend to be small for gestational age and often premature. The large exposed surface area leads to rapid extensive fluid and heat loss.

* Third space fluids are fluids lost from the intravascular space to the interstitial space because of capillary permeability associated with the trauma of surgery. As proteins are lost from the intravascular space, fluids also shift.

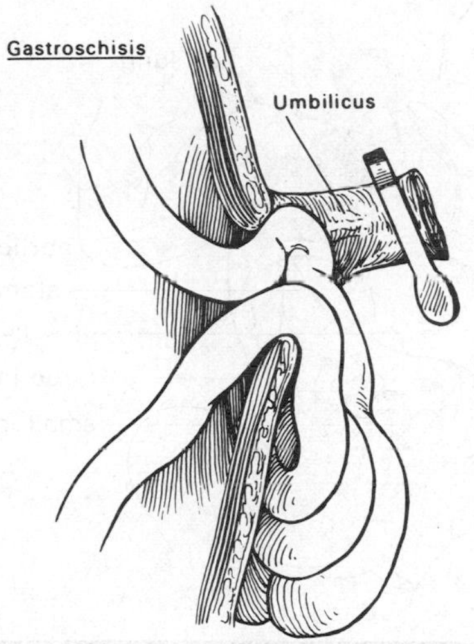

Figure 41-12. Gastroschisis: a defect in the abdominal wall that allows the intestines to protrude from the abdomen in utero. (From Schwartz, et al: *Principles of Surgery.* New York, McGraw-Hill Book Co, 1979, p 1653.)

Therapeutic Management and Strategies for Nursing Care

In gastroschisis the bowel is not protected by a sac, as in omphalocele. The bowel is irritated by amniotic fluid, and there is considerable inflammation and edema, which interfere with normal bowel activity after surgical repair. The infant should be positioned on the side to permit the bowel to rest on a surface and avoid creating a pull on the bowel as it exits from the abdominal wall defect. Broad-spectrum antibiotics are initiated preoperatively and nasogastric tube decompression is begun to avert aspiration pneumonia and to decompress the bowel to allow as much bowel as possible to be placed into the abdomen during surgery.

Treatment varies with the amount of bowel outside the abdomen. The bowel should be protected with warmed, saline-soaked sponges and a bowel bag. The intestines can be placed into the abdomen and closed (primary repair) or, for some cases of gastroschisis that are excessively large, a staged repair as for omphalocele is done.

Postoperatively, the infant is managed in a similar way to the infant with omphalocele (see previous discussion). Most of these infants survive and lead normal lives.

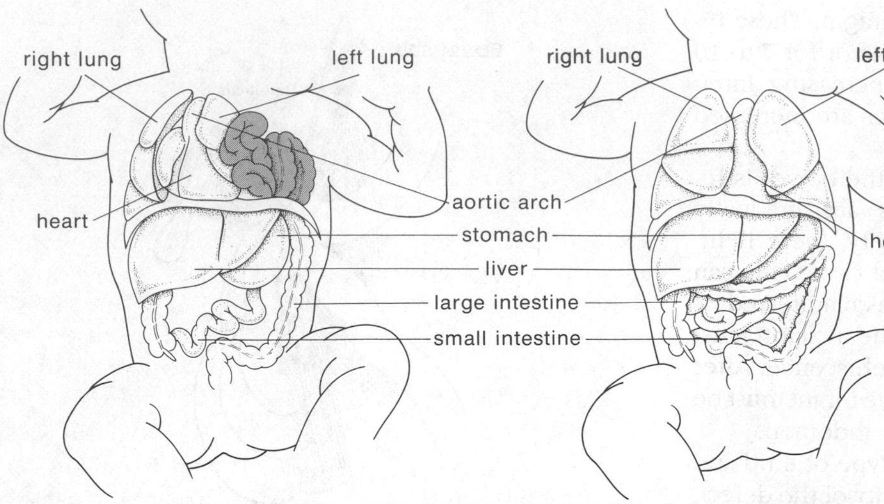

Figure 41-13. Diaphragmatic hernia; on the right is shown the normal relationships of the heart, lungs, and diaphragm. When an abnormal hole exists in the diaphragm (left), abdominal contents can crowd the lungs. Respiratory embarrassment can result, with severity of symptoms depending on the amount of bowel displaced into the thorax.

Diaphragmatic Hernia

A diaphragmatic hernia is an opening in the diaphragm through which abdominal contents herniate into the thoracic cavity.

Pathophysiology

Normally, the strong musculature of the diaphragm prevents entrance of abdominal viscera into the chest. When defective embryonic development occurs, an aperture persists in the posterior lateral segment of the diaphragm, located most often on the left side (foramen of Bochdalek). Abdominal contents protrude through the defect and cause a group of symptoms that nurses should be able to recognize as indicative of diaphragmatic hernia. Abdominal contents in the left thorax compress the lung on the left and displace the heart to the right (dextrocardia) (Fig. 41-13). Congenital hypoplasia of the lung is usually present on the affected side; it has also been observed on the opposite side. There is also an increased muscularity of small pulmonary arteries that may contribute to increased pulmonary resistance and hypertension (Behrman, 1987). Respiratory acidosis, hypoxemia, and hypercapnia occur as a result of inadequate exchange of oxygen and carbon dioxide. Metabolic acidosis rapidly develops as peripheral tissues are inadequately perfused. These infants are highly susceptible to developing persistent pulmonary hypertension (PPH) (severe pulmonary hypertension with a pulmonary artery pressure that is equal to or greater than systemic pressure). Right-to-left shunting then occurs through a patent ductus arteriosus and foramen ovale. A knowledge of the physiologic alterations allows the nurse to help identify this condition and contribute to the care of these infants.

Clinical Manifestations

The nurse should expect to find diminished or absent breath sounds on the affected side and listen carefully for bowel sounds that may be audible over the chest. The apical heartbeat will be heard at a point to the right of the usual position owing to dextrocardia. A barrel chest and scaphoid abdomen result, depending on the degree of visceral displacement into the thorax. Usually, respiratory distress develops soon after birth. As the infant begins to breathe, the negative intrathoracic pressure causes increasingly more bowel to be drawn into the chest. Further compression of the heart occurs as the infant cries and swallows air, causing the bowel loops within the chest to become increasingly distended (Burrington and Powers, 1985).

The severe respiratory embarrassment that results from compression and hypoplasia of the lungs causes dyspnea, cyanosis, nasal flaring, tachypnea, and chest retraction that may constitute an acute emergency. These symptoms vary with the amount of bowel that is displaced into the thorax and the degree of lung hypoplasia present.

If the hernia is less severe and symptoms are not present at birth, soon after birth the infant has mild respiratory distress and later in life may develop indigestion, severe colic, vomiting, or hiatal hernia.

Diagnostic Assessment

A typical radiograph shows fluid and air-filled loops of the intestine in the chest and a shift of the mediastinum to the unaffected side. The presence of bowel sounds in the chest, a scaphoid abdomen, and a typical radiographic film are indications for surgery (Coran et al, 1979).

Therapeutic Management

The potential for cardiorespiratory collapse and severe acidemia makes diaphragmatic hernia one of the most *urgent neonatal surgical emergencies.* Nasogastric intubation with intermittent or low continuous suction is begun as soon as the diagnosis is suspected. The amount of air entering the intestines is thereby reduced, and respirations are less compromised. The infant may also require respiratory assistance through endotracheal intubation and positive pressure ventilation to maintain adequate blood gas levels. The lungs are fragile and easily ruptured; therefore, assisted ventilation is done cautiously, recognizing the risk of pneumothorax.

Metabolic acidosis is corrected by the administration of bicarbonate, and ventilatory insufficiency is corrected through positive pressure ventilation. In patients with an increased CO_2 level, metabolic acidosis is corrected with tromethamine (THAM) (Williams, 1982).

The surgical procedure involves repositioning the abdominal contents into the abdomen and closing the defect. In most cases, malrotation of the intestines accompanies a diaphragmatic hernia and is also corrected. A gastrostomy tube is inserted through a separate stab wound. In some instances, the peritoneal cavity is too small to contain the abdominal contents; therefore, it is necessary to leave the fascia open and close only the skin. This results in a ventral hernia that is repaired several months after the initial surgery.

The lung on the affected side (usually the left) is hypoplastic and may require days or weeks for expansion to occur. Postoperative pharmacologic intervention to counteract pulmonary vascular resistance is often required. This may include digitalis derivatives, diuretics, and pulmonary vasodilators. The most important postoperative therapy is ventilatory management.

Arterial oxygenation (PaO_2) above 100 torr, $PaCO_2$ at 30 to 35 torr, and pH between 7.45 and 7.50 (a slightly alkalotic state) are desirable values to prevent vasoconstriction of the hypoplastic lung (Filston and Izant, 1985; Leape, 1987). Close monitoring of blood gases and periodic evaluation of electrolyte, hematocrit, and blood glucose levels are required.

Survival rate is about 50 per cent for severely affected infants diagnosed within the first 24 to 72 hours (Williams, 1982). When resuscitation and surgery have been managed optimally the prognosis still depends on three factors: (1) the size of the defect, (2) the degree of hypoplasia of the lung, and (3) the condition of the lung on the unaffected side. In general, the earlier symptoms appear, the poorer the prognosis. The final determinant of success is the total amount of pulmonary function available for gas exchange. Many infants who do not survive are found to have associated severe congenital anomalies (especially of the heart).

Strategies for Nursing Care

Relieving Respiratory Distress. The nurse can improve the infant's condition by instituting some immediate nursing measures: (1) placing the infant in semi-Fowler position reduces intrathoracic pressure and facilitates downward position of the abdominal viscera, and (2) placing the infant on the affected side aids in expansion of the good lung. Facilitating rapid and efficient treatment to relieve respiratory distress is an important nursing role. Progressive distention of the intestines is prevented by maintaining suction and patency of the nasogastric (N-G) tube. Heat loss increases oxygen demands and compounds the acidosis. Minimal handling and careful thermoregulation are essential strategies to reduce respiratory distress.

Supporting the Family. The nurse must be attentive to the stress that the parents are experiencing during these emergency procedures. Although little time is available to explain the emergency treatment in any detail to parents, briefly telling them what is being done while the baby is being treated is appreciated. Before surgery, the family should be told about the procedure and the postoperative appearance of the infant.

In the postoperative period, parents will continue to feel anxious because of the constant threat of respiratory complications and fear of the equipment needed to maintain their infant. *Extreme caution is taken in the handling of these infants.* No holding, touching, or stimulation is permitted by parents because the infant is at risk for developing PPH. Nurses can intervene by helping the parents understand the reason for this restriction. They also must be kept informed of the general status of their infant.

Monitoring Nutritional and Respiratory Status. Careful monitoring of intravenous fluids and respiratory assessment are nursing responsibilities. If mechanical ventilation is necessary, precautions against pneumothorax must be taken (i.e., low ventilation pressures). Poor lung function continues to be a threat during the postoperative period. Frequent position changes, nasopharyngeal suction, endotracheal suction if the child is intubated, and chest physiotherapy require constant nursing attention.

Teaching to Support Home Management. The family should feed the infant for at least several days before discharge. After surgery, the infant may be lethargic, and coaxing him or her to eat may cause vomiting or gagging. Parents should be taught to burp the infant frequently and not to force the baby to eat when there is disinterest in feeding. Parents should report to the physician:

1. An increase in respiratory rate or effort,
2. Cyanosis, whether it occurs during feeding or at rest,
3. Feeding intolerance: vomiting or refusing to eat (Kenner et al, 1988).

Hiatal Hernia

Hiatal hernia is the intermittent or constant displacement of the proximal segment of the stomach through the esophageal hiatus of the diaphragm. This protrusion causes a displacement of the esophagogastric junction and portions of the proximal part of the stomach through the esophageal hiatus into the mediastinum, resulting in the regurgitation of food and fluid. As a consequence, the child may experience recurrent emesis severe enough to result in failure to thrive, aspiration pneumonia, or septic esophagitis with anemia due to gastrointestinal bleeding. Hiatal hernias are rare in the neonatal period, but the frequency increases after the first few months of life.

A hiatal hernia is manifested by symptoms similar to the condition known as gastroesophageal reflux (chalasia). Documentation of the frequency, volume, and presence of bile or blood in the emesis and respiratory symptoms such as coughing, wheezing, or short apneic periods facilitates diagnosis. It is important to determine the adequacy of weight gain by referring to the child's placement on a growth chart.

In addition to the history, diagnosis involves a barium swallow, which will demonstrate reflux from a segment of the stomach situated above the diaphragm into the esophagus.

Management is similar to that for gastroesophageal reflux, including a period of conservative medical management followed by a Nissen-Hill fundoplication if reflux does not resolve after several months of therapy. (See discussion in section under dysfunctional disorders in this chapter.)

Umbilical Hernia, Inguinal Hernia, and Hydrocele

General Pathophysiology

A hernia is the protrusion of a part of the bowel, ovary, or testis through an abnormal opening in the containing walls of the abdomen. It consists of three parts: the sac or outpouching of the peritoneum, the coverings of the sac that are derived from the abdominal wall, and the contents of the sac—bowel, ovary, or testis. The most frequent locations for hernias are the umbilical and inguinal regions. Although congenital, the hernia may not appear until the infant is several months old.

Pathophysiology of Umbilical Hernia

During fetal development the intestines return to the abdominal cavity around the eleventh week of fetal life. Failure of the umbilical ring to close completely as the intestine returns to the abdominal cavity leaves a fascial defect at the base of the umbilical cord. An umbilical hernia is the protrusion of the intestines at the umbilicus through this fascial defect.

Diagnostic Assessment and Therapeutic Management for Umbilical Hernia

Diagnosis is made by observation and palpation of the defect. Parents should be advised that 90 per cent of these hernias resolve on their own. It is rare for an umbilical hernia to become incarcerated. (If the hernia has not resolved by age 5 years, surgery is scheduled, usually on an outpatient basis.) Parents should be advised not to use binders, tape, or other materials to compress the hernia. It has never been documented that these remedies aid in the closure of the defect, and they can cause infection.

The umbilical hernia is repaired through a transverse incision, which is made within the fold of the inferior aspect of the umbilicus. The incision is then carried through the subcutaneous fat and areolar tissue to the linea alba at the inferior rim of the umbilical ring. A plane is dissected around the ring at the level of the linea alba, and the sac is dissected away from the umbilical skin. The sac is then transected and closed along with the fibrous umbilical ring in one to two layers. The incision is coated with a protective sealant, and a compression dressing is applied for 7 days.

Strategies for Nursing Care: Umbilical Hernia

Teaching to Support Postoperative Care at Home. The child is ready for discharge from the recovery room within 2 hours. The parents are requested to sponge bathe the child and to maintain the compression dressing for a week. It is important that the parents attempt to limit the child's physical activities for several weeks, although this is not easy to accomplish. Otherwise, there are no dietary or activity restrictions. The child is seen 1 week after surgery and the dressing is removed. The parents should be advised that edema will still be present and that this will decrease over time.

Pathophysiology and Diagnostic Assessment of Inguinal Hernia

An inguinal hernia is the protrusion of bowel into the groin region (Fig. 41-14*B*). In the male, the testis descends from the abdominal cavity into the scrotum. The testis carries the parietal peritoneum with it, thus

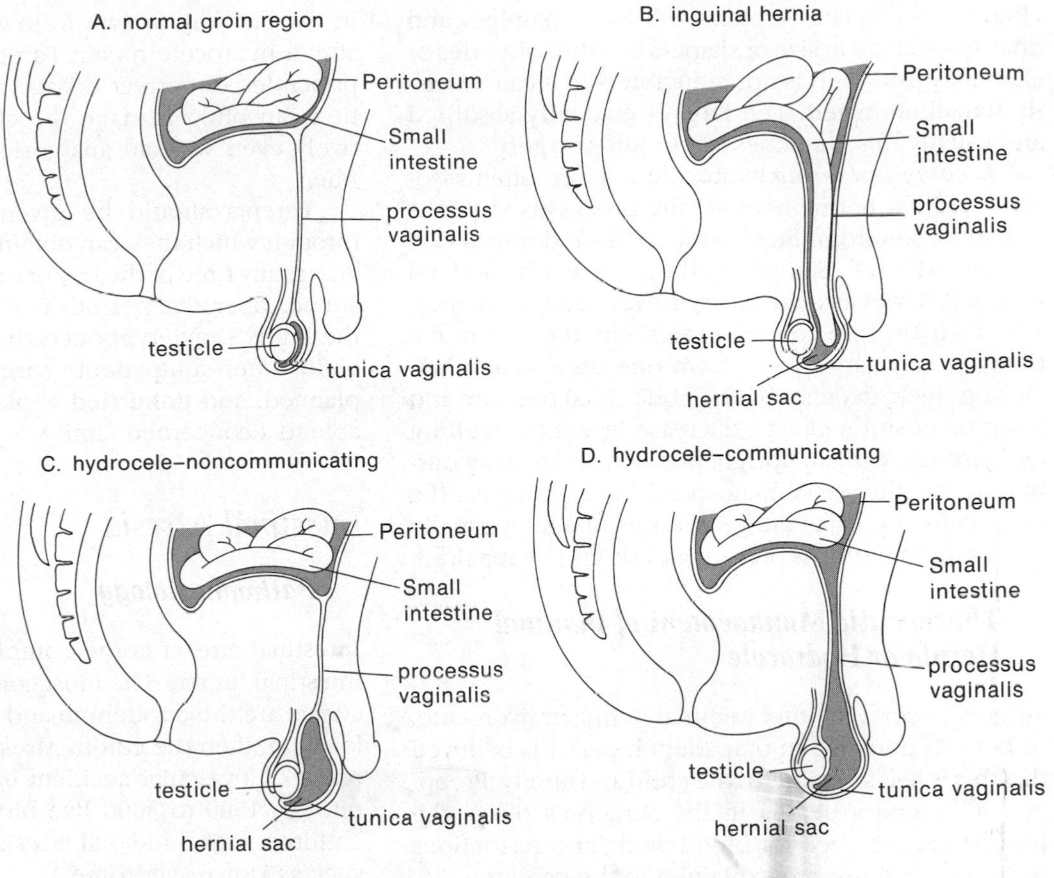

Figure 41-14. Hydroceles and hernias. *A*, Groin region of the normal male infant. *B*, An *inguinal hernia* is the protrusion of bowel into the groin region. *C*, A *hydrocele* is a collection of fluid within the processus vaginalis. In a *noncommunicating hydrocele*, the scrotal swelling does not change in size or shape because there is no connection with the abdominal cavity. *D*, In a *communicating hydrocele*, the processus vaginalis remains open from the scrotum to the abdominal cavity, and scrotal swelling may vary in size during the course of an infant's day.

forming a tube (processus vaginalis) from the abdomen to the scrotum. Normally, the processus vaginalis will close spontaneously during development; if not, the descent of the intestine into the patent processus produces an inguinal hernia.

In the female, the round ligament extends from the uterus through the inguinal canal to its attachment in the labia majora. Weakness of the tissue around the round ligament together with increased abdominal pressure produces an inguinal hernia.

Diagnosis of inguinal hernia is made by observation and palpation of a bulge in the groin area. Frequently, the diagnosis must be made on the basis of a history of a bulge in the groin that a parent has noted while the infant was crying or straining to defecate. During the examination, it is important to check that both testes are in the scrotal sac and to determine the presence or absence of a scrotal or cord hydrocele (a collection of fluid in the tunica vaginalis of the testicle or along the spermatic cord). See Chapter 15 for assessment strategies.

The hernia causes the infant little discomfort unless it becomes incarcerated. There is a high frequency of incarceration of an inguinal hernia in the first 3 months of life. Parents must be advised to watch for redness in the area of the hernia, increased swelling of the hernia, and an inability to reduce the hernia. Under any of these circumstances they should be advised to contact their pediatrician immediately.

Pathophysiology and Diagnostic Assessment of Hydrocele

A hydrocele is a collection of fluid within the processus vaginalis. Hydroceles are most commonly seen in males. The type seen at birth presents as a soft scrotal swelling. In this type the upper portion of the processus vaginalis is obliterated, but the portion within the scrotum (tunica vaginalis) remains open. Peritoneal fluid is trapped within the tunica vaginalis. There is no communication with the peritoneal cavity—thus it is referred to as a *noncommunicating* hydrocele

(Fig. 41-14*C*). The scrotal swelling is painless and does not change in size or shape when the baby cries or changes position. It is not reducible, but it can be easily transilluminated. The fluid is gradually absorbed and usually this type does not require surgery.

A *communicating* hydrocele is more often associated with a hernia because the processus vaginalis remains open from the scrotum to the abdominal cavity (Fig. 41-14*D*). Scrotal swelling may not be noticed until a few weeks after birth or even later in infancy. When a hydrocele communicates with the abdominal cavity it may vary in size from one time to another. During sleep, decreased intra-abdominal pressure and a supine position effect a decrease in scrotal swelling by morning. With an upright position and activity during the day the scrotum again gradually enlarges. If a hydrocele is present after 3 months of age, it usually means that a hernia is present and should be repaired.

Therapeutic Management of Inguinal Hernia or Hydrocele

Surgery to correct either inguinal hernia or hydrocele, or both, is done on an outpatient basis. It is believed that this is less stressful for the child and family. Preoperative teaching begins in the surgeon's office: the procedure, the need for blood work, and restrictions for food and fluids are explained to the parents.

All inguinal hernias should be promptly repaired to avoid incarceration. Surgical treatment is rarely indicated for a hydrocele (90 per cent resolve spontaneously). If surgery is indicated (i.e., large, symptomatic, or one that does not disappear by age 5 years) the procedure is the same as for inguinal hernia: ligation of the processus vaginalis.

Parents should be advised that the scrotum may become edematous and appear bruised. This is due to the manipulation of the testis during the operation and should resolve in 1 to 3 weeks after the operation. The incision is coated with a protective sealant, and no dressing is applied.

Strategies for Postoperative Nursing Care: Umbilical Hernia or Hydrocele

Teaching to Support Care at Home. The major concern for home care of the child after surgery for umbilical hernia or hydrocele is protection of the incision. Parents should be advised to change diapers frequently and to gently remove feces from the skin with soap and water. Sponge baths (versus tub) should be given for 1 week. In an older child, parents should attempt to limit physical activities for several weeks. Otherwise, the child has no restrictions.

The nurse should make sure that the family receives a prescription for an analgesic before discharge. The infant or young child is likely to be uncomfortable in the first day or two following surgery, especially after a hydrocele repair. Parents who understand the principles of correct dosage and regular administration can often manage the child's discomfort effectively even with an analgesic as mild as acetaminophen.

Parents should be given a telephone number through which they can obtain nursing or medical advice at any time of the day or night during the immediate postoperative period. The nurse should anticipate the family's anxiety about caring for the infant or young child after outpatient surgery. Confident, well-planned, and unhurried explanations can be invaluable to a concerned family.

Intestinal Atresia

Pathophysiology

Intestinal atresia is the complete obliteration of the intestinal lumen. The most common sites of intestinal atresia are the duodenum and ileum, followed by the jejunem, then the colon. Atresia is believed to be the result of a vascular accident in utero. It occurs about once in 1500 to 3000 live births. A large number of children with duodenal atresia have other anomalies such as Down syndrome.

Clinical Manifestations

Polyhydramnios (excess amniotic fluid) should raise the suspicion that esophageal or duodenal atresia is present. The clinical manifestations of atresia are signs of intestinal obstruction that include bilious vomiting, jaundice, abdominal distention (more pronounced in ileal atresia), and failure to pass meconium. Distention of the abdomen causes an elevation of the diaphragm, necessitating close observation for respiratory distress.

Diagnostic Assessment

Atresia is documented on an abdominal radiograph by evidence of dilated loops of bowel and air-fluid levels. Ileal atresia can be differentiated by noting dilated proximal loops of bowel and small unused distal bowel. In duodenal atresia, an upright abdominal film will document a distended stomach with the appearance of a "double bubble." This strongly suggests that the obstruction is in the duodenum. The two distinct bubbles are formed by the air that rises to the top of the duodenum and to the top of the stomach. The rest of the abdomen is devoid of gas. A barium enema is performed to distinguish between small and large bowel distention, to determine if the colon is functional or nonfunctional, and to locate the position of the cecum in order to rule out the presence of an abnormal rotation of the cecum and duodenum. It is important to obtain results of these tests quickly. The infant is at risk of developing a volvulus (a twisting of the bowel upon itself).

Therapeutic Management and Strategies for Nursing Care

Many times the parents are able to see the infant only briefly before he or she is taken to the operating room or is transferred to another hospital. It is essential to spend time with the family, to answer their questions, and to encourage involvement in the infant's care.

Preoperatively the infant is maintained in the incubator, and a nasogastric tube is inserted through the mouth or nose in order to decompress the abdomen and prevent further vomiting and gaseous distention. It is essential that this tube remain patent; this may require irrigation with air or water once every 4 to 6 hours. Baseline laboratory studies (complete blood count and electrolytes) are done, and the infant is maintained on intravenous hydration. Broad-spectrum antibiotics are administered; and fluid and electrolye deficits must be corrected prior to surgery.

During the surgical procedure, the entire bowel is inspected for evidence of malrotation, volvulus, and atresia. Various types of anastomosis (side-to-side, end-to-end) are performed between the proximal and distal segments of the bowel. A gastrostomy may be performed if early recovery is not anticipated. In some instances, an end-to-end anastomosis is not possible because of the size disparity of the two ends. In these circumstances an ostomy is performed with a nearby fistula (Burrington and Powers, 1985). The two ends can be anastomosed at a later time.

Postoperatively, gastric decompression is maintained until there is evidence of gastric emptying and bowel sounds are heard. Parenteral nutrition may be required, depending on the speed of recovery. Oral or gastrostomy feedings are begun in small amounts and are increased in volume and strength gradually. It is important to document the consistency and number of stools per shift.

Ninety per cent or more of the infants operated on for duodenal atresia survive the operation; the major complication is anastomotic strictures. Malabsorption may be a problem in jejunal or ileal atresia, because of an inadequate intestinal surface for absorption. Parents need encouragement during the period of waiting for intestinal adaptation (sometimes 1 to 2 years).

Malrotation and Volvulus

A volvulus is the twisting of the intestine upon itself (Fig. 41-15). Malrotation is an abnormal rotation of the cecum and duodenum.

Pathophysiology

During early fetal development the abdominal cavity is unable to accommodate the rapidly developing intestine; therefore, a large portion of it herniates into the umbilical sac outside the abdomen. The position of the

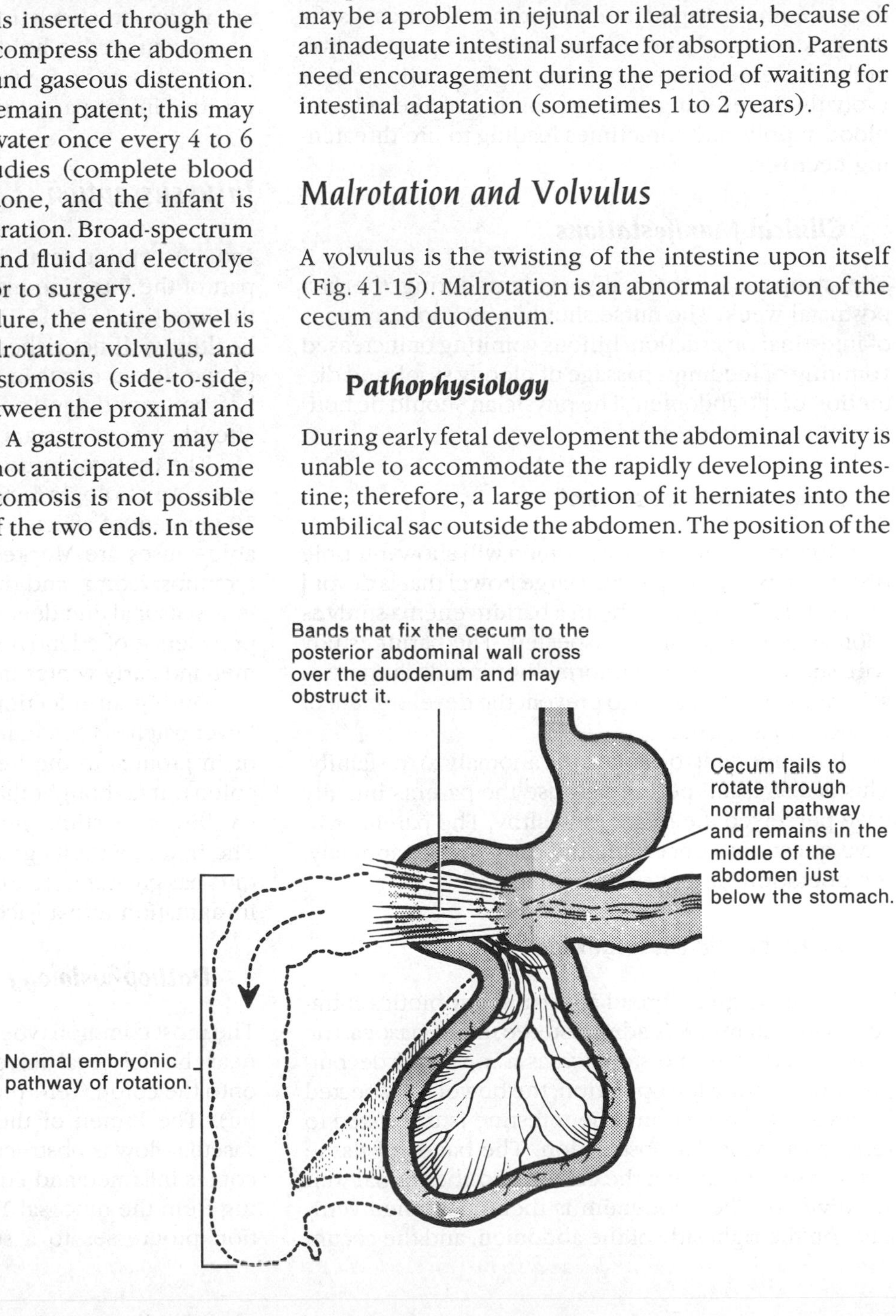
Bands that fix the cecum to the posterior abdominal wall cross over the duodenum and may obstruct it.
Cecum fails to rotate through normal pathway and remains in the middle of the abdomen just below the stomach.
Normal embryonic pathway of rotation.

Figure 41-15. Malrotation of the intestine. (From Nixon H, O'Donnell B: *The Essentials of Pediatric Surgery.* Philadelphia, JB Lippincott Co, 1961.)

intestine at this time is reversed from its later normal position; the ascending colon at this time is on the left instead of its later normal position on the right. Around the eleventh week of gestation, the intestinal loops return to the abdominal cavity. As the bowel moves into the abdomen, it rotates until the colon is in its normal position in the lower right quadrant, and the mesentery of the ascending colon fixes to the posterior abdominal wall. Three abnormalities can occur during this process: malrotation of the colon, volvulus of the midgut, and formation of adhesive bands that constrict the duodenum.

If rotation of the bowel is incomplete the mesentery cannot attach in its usual position. The duodenum then becomes trapped behind peritoneal bands that fix the abnormally placed cecum. The inadequate fixation of the mesentery allows twisting of the small intestine (volvulus), resulting in compromise of the bowel's blood supply, and sometimes leading to life-threatening necrosis.

Clinical Manifestations

The symptoms are usually evident during the first postnatal week. The nurse should watch for any signs of intestinal obstruction: bilious vomiting or increased vomiting of feedings, passage of bloody stool, and distention of the abdomen. The physician should be notified of any of these signs.

Diagnostic Assessment

A radiographic film of the abdomen will show multiple distended bowel loops and a large bowel that is devoid of gas. It is essential to obtain a barium enema study as soon as the diagnosis is suspected. The barium study will show the cecum abnormally placed. Surgery is scheduled immediately to prevent the development of intestinal gangrene.

It is important to explain the anomaly to the family. This is a stressful period because the parents initially have perceived the infant as healthy. The parents will have questions concerning the cause of the anomaly, the operation, and postoperative care.

Therapeutic Management

The infant is given broad-spectrum antibiotics intravenously, vitamin K is administered, and a nasogastric tube is placed in the stomach as a means of decompression. During the operation, the bowel is inspected for areas of obstruction. The intestine is untwisted to relieve the vascular obstruction. The bands of tissue (Ladd bands) between the cecum and abdominal wall are divided. The duodenum is then positioned vertically on the right side of the abdomen, and the cecum is placed in the left lower quadrant. An appendectomy is also performed. If a large portion of the bowel is compromised, it will be necessary to perform a bowel resection and a jejunostomy or ileostomy (a portion of the small bowel is brought out to the skin to provide an outlet for defecation).

Strategies for Nursing Care

The child is maintained on intravenous hydration postoperatively. If stooling does not occur by the third or fourth postoperative day, parenteral hyperalimentation should be considered. Once the infant has begun to defecate, oral feedings are initiated. The feedings are increased slowly in volume and strength. Parents are encouraged to hold, feed, and care for their infant during this period, which will help them establish a positive infant-parent relationship.

Intussusception

Intussusception is an invagination or telescoping of part of the intestine into an adjacent distal portion of the intestine (Fig. 41-16). It occurs most commonly in healthy, well-nourished male infants around 6 months of age. It can occur in children of any age but is rare before 3 months and occurs with decreasing frequency after the age of 3 years.

The cause of intussusception is unknown in most cases. An etiologic factor is determined in fewer than 10 per cent of afflicted children. Some of the identifiable causes are Meckel diverticulum, an ileal polyp, lymphosarcoma, and duplication of the bowel. There is a seasonal incidence that has been linked to the prevalence of adenovirus infections in the early summer and early winter months.

During an infection, there is hypertrophy of the Peyer patches (configuration of lymph nodules, single or in groups, in the ileum near its junction with the colon). It is thought that the presence of the resultant swelling may stimulate peristalsis (Shandling, 1983). The ileum, with its greater number of Peyer patches, thus has greater potential to become the lead point for invagination into adjacent bowel.

Pathophysiology

The most common type of intussusception begins at or near the ileocecal valve, pushing into the cecum and onto the colon (referred to as ileocecocolic or ileocolic). The lumen of the bowel is compromised, and vascular flow is obstructed. The involved intestine becomes inflamed and edematous, with eventual bleeding from the mucosa. The initial incomplete obstruction progresses to a state of complete obstruction,

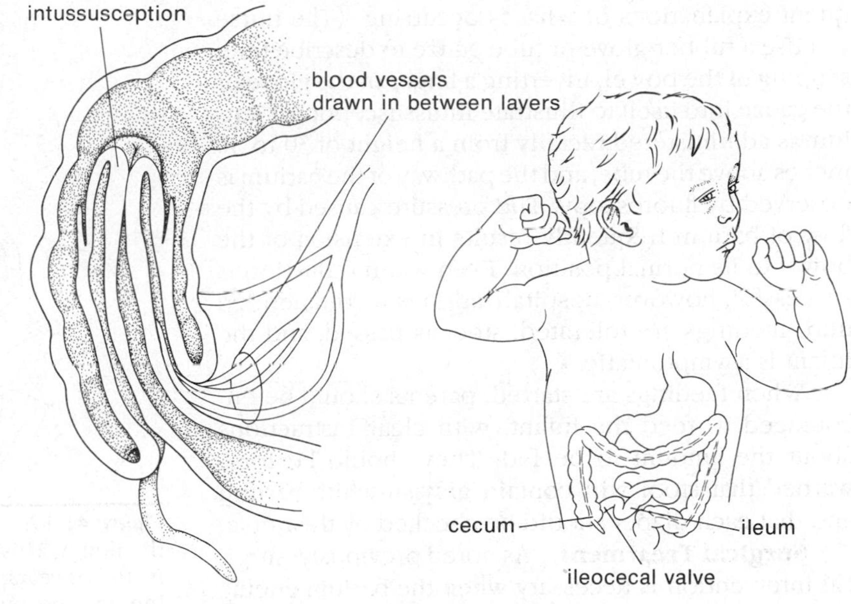

Figure 41-16. Intussusception. The most common type begins at or near the ileocecal valve, pushing into the cecum and onto the colon. At first, the obstruction is partial, but as the bowel becomes inflamed and edematous, complete obstruction occurs.

producing distention and vomiting. Strangulation of the bowel can result, although this does not usually occur in the first 24 hours (Shandling, 1983). Intussusception, if untreated, can lead to intestinal gangrene, peritonitis, and death.

Clinical Manifestations

The infant with intussusception has symptoms that are frightening and disturbing to parents. A healthy infant suddenly shows symptoms of severe abdominal pain, which recurs at frequent intervals. The infant draws the legs up sharply with a piercing cry. The infant usually vomits, becomes extremely restless, and often appears diaphoretic and pale. Normal stool may be passed during the initial phase. The attack then subsides, and the infant shows no abnormal signs between the severe attacks of abdominal pain.

As the condition worsens, the infant becomes lethargic and progressively weaker. Vital signs reflect a shock-like state, vomitus may now be bile-stained, and abdominal distention is apparent. There will be either no stool or a stool characteristically described as currant jelly–like in appearance owing to the presence of blood and mucus as a result of intestinal irritation. This type of stool occurs in about 50 per cent of cases (Filston and Izant, 1985). Blood usually appears in the stool within 12 hours of the onset of symptoms. Between attacks of pain, in some cases a sausage-shaped mass can be palpated in the right upper quadrant of the abdomen. A barium enema study confirms the diagnosis and in many cases can successfully treat the intussusception through hydrostatic reduction.

The nurse must be able to give accurate guidance when parents initially report symptoms. Because the infant may sleep and is comfortable between attacks, the seriousness of the symptoms can be overlooked by a nurse who is not familiar with the characteristic pattern of their onset. Nurses must advise the family to seek immediate medical attention and explain to them that, even though the baby seems normal between attacks, the condition may change rapidly.

Therapeutic Management and Strategies for Nursing Care

Three types of treatment are used for intussusception: (1) reduction by the hydrostatic pressure of a barium enema, (2) reduction by surgical manipulation, and (3) surgical resection of a nonreducible involved intestine.

Reduction by Barium Enema. During the first 24 hours of symptoms, the intussusception can be reduced by hydrostatic pressure. The success rate varies, but in one review, it was found to be 70 per cent (Liu et al, 1986). Contraindications for reduction by barium enema are (1) a complete mechanical obstruction, and (2) a high temperature, vomiting, and signs of peritonitis, sepsis, or shock (Welch, 1978).

The infant must be prepared for a barium enema as though surgery will follow, because if reduction by barium enema is unsuccessful, the infant undergoes an operation immediately. The family must understand the purpose of the barium enema and must realize that surgery may be necessary. Preparation for the barium enema includes giving the infant nothing by mouth, insertion of a nasogastric tube to prevent aspiration during the barium enema, and administration of intravenous fluids. Preparation for such treatment occurs rapidly and may leave parents stunned. They can be helped to calm the infant if the nurse attends to their need for a description of the problem and gives frequent explanations of what is occurring. (The nurse can use a rubber glove or tube gauze to describe telescoping of the bowel, inverting a finger of the glove or the gauze into itself to illustrate intussusception.) Barium is administered rectally from a height of 30 to 36 inches above the tube, and the pathway of the barium is observed by fluoroscopy. The pressure caused by the flow of barium frequently results in extension of the bowel to its normal position. Even when reduction is successful, however, hospitalization is recommended until feedings are tolerated, stool is passed, and the infant is asymptomatic.

When feedings are started, parents should be encouraged to feed the infant, with clear instructions about the amount to be fed. They should be forewarned that stool will contain grayish-white barium and that each diaper should be checked by the nurse.

Surgical Treatment. As noted previously, surgical intervention is necessary when the barium enema is not successful in reduction and when there is clinical evidence of intestinal obstruction with abdominal distention. The intussusception is reduced surgically by milking the intestine (distal to proximal) to move the invaginated portion back to its normal position. (Attempts lasting longer than 10 minutes are not recommended.) If this is not successful, intestinal resection and anastomosis may be necessary. Postoperatively, the nurse must help the family cope with the stress of caring for the infant, who is not allowed to eat, requires frequent position changes, and needs to be restrained to prevent dislodging of the nasogastric tube and intravenous needle or catheter. Also, the nurse must frequently assess the infant's vital signs (particularly a high fever), blood pressure, bowel sounds, sutures and dressing, proper functioning of the nasogastric tube, and accurate infusion of intravenous fluids. (See also Table 41-9, Care of the Child Following Abdominal Surgery.)

Spontaneous reduction occasionally occurs. When an intussusception is reduced by barium enema there is a recurrence rate of 5 to 10 per cent. Recurrence is also possible after surgical reduction; it is least common after intestinal resection. The length of time that elapses between onset and reduction of the intestines affects prognosis. Prognosis is excellent if the condition is treated within 12 to 24 hours and grave in the event of strangulation.

Meckel Diverticulum

Meckel diverticulum is a congenital anomaly characterized by an outpouching of the ileum. This outpouching is caused by a persistent duct that in early embryonic development connected the primitive gut to the yolk sac (omphalomesenteric duct). Failure of the duct to atrophy results in a Meckel diverticulum.

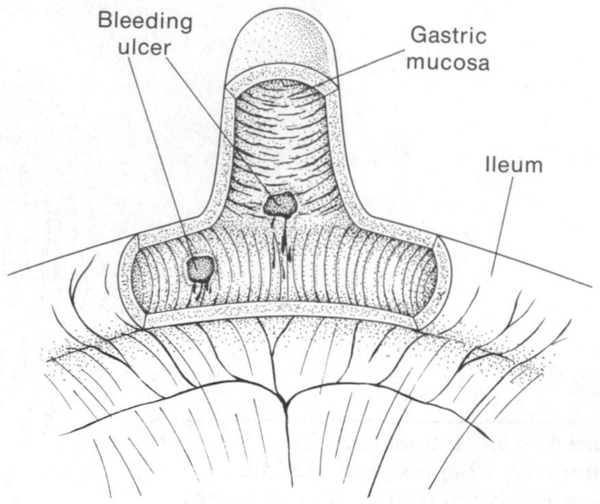

***Figure* 41-17.** Meckel diverticulum is an outpouching of the ileum. This congenital anomaly may remain asymptomatic for years, may become a source of intestinal bleeding, may become inflamed and lead to perforation, or may become the focal point for intussusception, obstruction, or volvulus.

Pathophysiology

The condition may be asymptomatic for many years and may be found only in the course of abdominal surgery. It is the most common gastrointestinal anomaly and is present in 1 to 2 per cent of the population. It is usually asymptomatic. Meckel diverticulum may manifest itself at any age, but the majority of symptomatic cases become apparent before the child reaches 2 years of age. This anomaly is significant because it can cause intestinal obstruction, massive bleeding, perforation, and peritonitis. The diverticulum may be attached to the anterior abdominal wall directly or by a fibrous cord. Most often it is free from the abdominal wall. The band may compress another loop of intestine and cause obstruction, or it may be the focal point of a volvulus (twisting of the intestines). The free outpouching ileum can act as a lead point for intussusception, with resulting symptoms.

Clinical Manifestations

Bleeding occurs because the tip of the outpouched ileum frequently contains ectopic gastric mucosa rather than ileal mucosa (Fig. 41-17). The gastric secretions are an irritant to the surrounding tissue. Eventually there is severe ulceration of the ileal mucosa at the base of the diverticulum or within the adjacent ileum to which it is connected. The eroded area hemorrhages, resulting in painless rectal bleeding, the most common sign in children. Rectal bleeding is dark red or bright red and is usually passed without stool. Less frequently, the diverticulum becomes inflamed and may perforate.

Diagnostic Assessment

Meckel diverticulum is generally not demonstrated on radiographs. Diagnosis is made by the history and on clinical manifestations, i.e., massive rectal bleeding. A technetium scan shows an area of radioactivity suggestive of gastric mucosa in the diverticulum but is negative in about half of symptomatic patients.

Therapeutic Management and Strategies for Nursing Care

The immediate concern is to remove the lesion surgically to prevent hypovalemic shock from bleeding. When a peptic ulcer is present in the adjacent ileum, excision of the involved bowel is necessary. Postoperatively, the child has a nasogastric tube and requires the usual postoperative care indicated for bowel surgery. Postoperative nursing responsibilities are to maintain patency of the nasogastric tube, administer intravenous fluid, check vital signs and bowel sounds, calculate intake and output until eating is resumed, and provide for the early resumption of a normal level of activity. (See also Table 41-9.)

It is frightening to parents when their otherwise healthy child develops massive rectal bleeding and requires immediate surgery. The family needs frequent reassurance that the child is recuperating satisfactorily. The nurse can reduce the stress the child and family have experienced by keeping parents informed and ensuring that their questions are answered.

Hirschsprung Disease (Congenital Aganglionosis or Aganglionic Megacolon)

Hirschsprung disease is a congenital abnormality in which obstruction is caused by reduced motility in the colon. It occurs in 1 in 5000 full-term births and predominantly affects males. it has been associated with other anomalies, such as Down syndrome and genitourinary abnormalities. Usually it is diagnosed in infancy.

Pathophysiology

Hirschsprung disease is also referred to as congenital megacolon (large colon present since birth). The anomaly is characterized by partial to complete obstruction associated with the distal alimentary tract (Fig. 41-18*A*). The absence of intramural ganglion cells (nerve cells) involves both the submucosal and intermuscular nerve plexuses. This may involve as small an area as the lower rectum (short-segment Hirschsprung disease) or as large an area as the entire colon (long-segment Hirschsprung disease). The lack of ganglion cells prevents the bowel from transmitting the coordinated peristaltic waves that normally enable fecal material to pass through the alimentary tract. The internal sphincter is unable to relax; evacuation of solids, liquids, or gases is prevented. Thus the patient has a mechanical intestinal obstruction.

Clinical Manifestations and Diagnostic Assessment

The onset of symptoms is usually noted in the first 24 to 48 hours of life. The nurse should consider Hirschsprung disease as a possible diagnosis for any infant who does not pass meconium within the first 24 hours of life and alert the physician. The nurse should watch the infant closely for passage of meconium or for bile-stained vomitus and abdominal distention. In older infants, the initial symptom is constipation or overflow diarrhea or both. In addition, abdominal distention is present, and a large fecal mass may be palpated. Anorexia, malnutrition, muscle wasting, nausea, and lethargy are manifestations of more advanced involvement.

The history the nurse obtains should include a detailed documentation of family members with stooling difficulties. A genetic factor has been associated with Hirschsprung disease in 3 to 5 per cent of all cases. There is an 18 per cent frequency for brothers of females with long aganglionic segments to also have the disease and a 0.6 per cent frequency for sisters of males with short segments to likewise be affected. This is an important consideration for genetic counseling. (See Chapter 4 for a discussion of genetic counseling.)

The rectal examination may raise the suspicion of Hirschsprung disease. A tight sphincter is frequently evident, and the examination produces explosive, watery, foul-smelling diarrhea. During the diagnostic period, the nurse must be aware of any signs of enterocolitis, an inflammation of the small intestine and colon. The physician should be notified of fever, bloody diarrhea, and vomiting.

A barium enema study documents radiologically the retention of barium and any evidence of a transition zone. The transition zone represents the abrupt change from dilated proximal intestine (ganglionic bowel) to narrowed and frequently spastic-appearing bowel (aganglionic bowel) (Fig. 41-18). The dilation of the proximal intestine is due to the peristaltic activ-

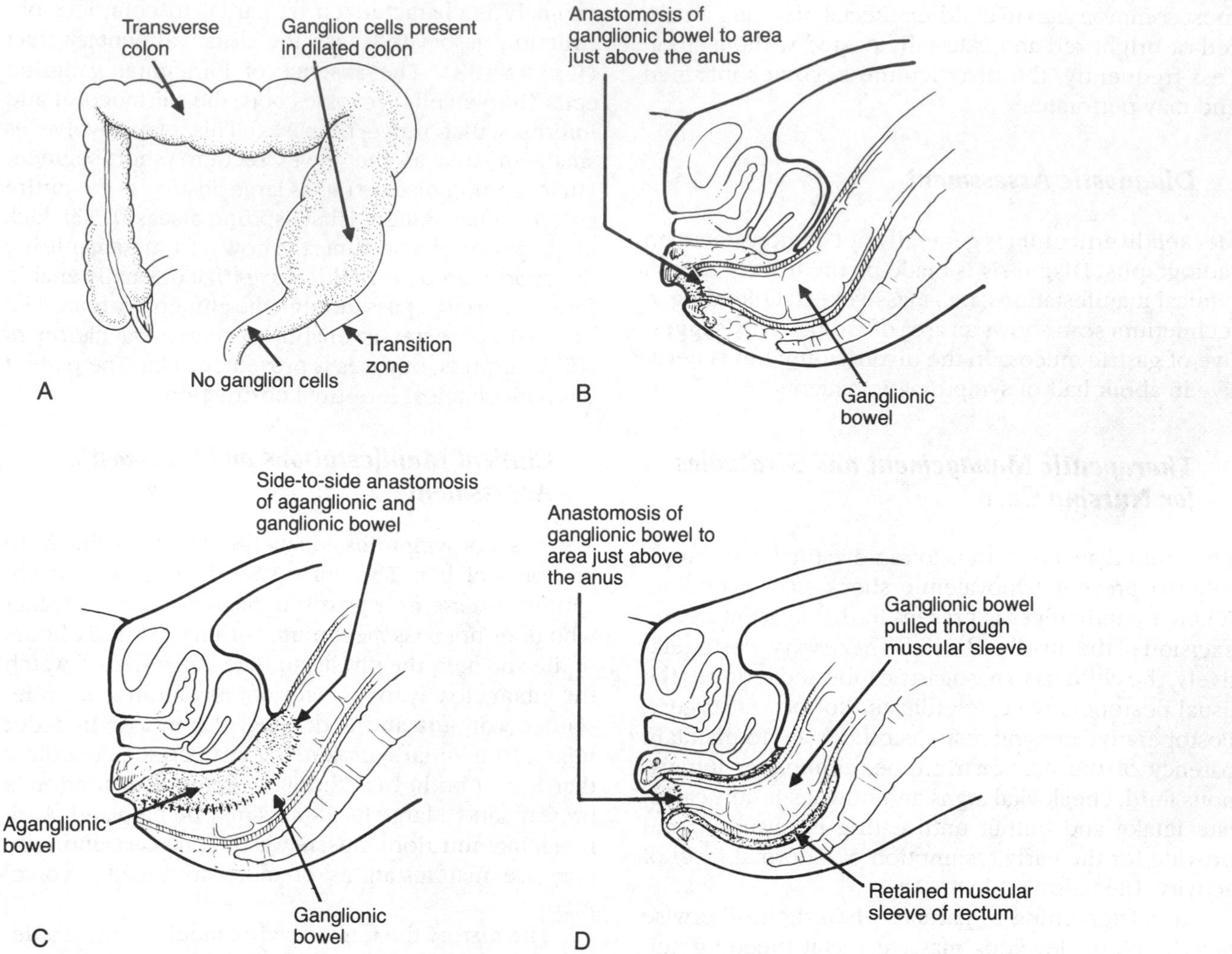

***Figure* 41-18.** Hirschsprung disease and surgical procedures for repair. *A*, Lack of ganglion cells in a segment of the colon prevents the transmission of normal peristaltic waves and results in an intestinal obstruction. *B*, Swenson procedure. Aganglionic bowel is completely resected and ganglionic bowel is anastomosed to anus (see Box 41-7 for further description). *C*, Duhamel procedure. Ganglionic bowel is anastomosed side-to-side to aganglionic bowel and to the anus. *D*, Soave procedure. Ganglionic bowel is brought through a retained muscular sleeve of the rectum and anastomosed to the rectum.

ity above the affected area which results in edema and hypertrophy of the bowel.

The definitive diagnostic study is a rectal biopsy. In Hirschsprung disease there is an absence of ganglion cells in Meissner and Auerbach plexuses and an increase in nerve fibers (Martin and Torres, 1985). A punch or suction rectal biopsy is usually performed without anesthesia. Parents should be forewarned that a biopsy can result in a small amount of rectal bleeding that disappears in a day.

Absence of ganglion cells in the specimen documents the presence of the disease. If the biopsy is negative for Hirschsprung disease (does reveal ganglion cells), further testing by a full-thickness biopsy may be necessary to rule out the disease (Kenner and Breuggemeyer, 1984).

Therapeutic Management *of* Initial Phase: *Temporary* Colostomy

If the submucosa does not contain ganglion cells, surgery is scheduled. The infant is prepared for surgery by placing a nasogastric tube to low suction for abdominal decompression, administration of broad-spectrum antibiotics and vitamin K, and initiation of intravenous fluids with electrolytes. A cleansing isotonic enema is given to empty the bowel.

Once the infant has been anesthetized, the surgeon must determine where the junction of aganglionic and ganglionic bowel lies. This is accomplished by obtaining multiple specimens for histologic evaluation. It is important to explain to the parents that this can be time-consuming, thus lengthening the time of the operation. A temporary colostomy (an opening of the colon through the abdominal wall) is created just above the determined level of ganglionic bowel.

The colostomy is created to provide the infant with the means to defecate and to allow the distended bowel to become normal in size. Because loop colostomies tend to prolapse in infants, an end-colostomy is preferred. The bowel is resected, the distal end is closed, and the proximal end is sutured to the abdominal wall to create a colostomy. The point in the bowel at which the colostomy is created is individualized according to the extent of aganglionosis. It is preferred to place it sufficiently proximal (i.e., ascending colon) so that a large amount of ganglionic bowel is available below that point for definitive surgery (a pull-through) later. (Otherwise the colostomy must be taken down and a new colostomy created at that time.) Postoperatively, the distal colon is irrigated with saline to remove remaining feces and barium (Leape, 1987).

Major Nursing Diagnoses for Hirschsprung Disease: Temporary Colostomy Phase

These diagnoses are meant to be used with those listed in Table 41-9, Nursing Process Plan: Care of the Child Following Abdominal Surgery.

Altered bowel elimination, related to temporary colostomy
***Knowledge deficit**, related to colostomy care*
***Potential impaired skin integrity**, related to skin contact with stool associated with ostomy drainage*
***Potential altered parenting**, related to difficulty accepting the infant's altered appearance and bowel function*

Strategies for Nursing Care: Temporary Colostomy Phase

The infant remains on intravenous hydration and antibiotics for 3 to 5 days. The nasogastric tube is discontinued after defecation through the colostomy has begun, usually on the third postoperative day. It is important for the parents to hold and comfort the infant during this period so they can develop a relationship with the baby. (See Table 41-9 for detailed strategies for postoperative care.)

Teaching to Support Care at Home. Initially, the parents should be advised that the stoma will decrease in size. The bowel has a good vascular supply and few nerves, so parents can be assured that they will not hurt the infant when they touch the stoma. The infant can be placed on the abdomen and can be held on the shoulder without pain.

Postoperative teaching of ostomy care is the primary responsibility of the nursing staff. Many hospitals have enterostomal therapists who can help the nurse and family in selection of the appropriate equipment for proper care of the ostomy. Parents should be given time initially to adjust to the physical appearance of the infant with an ostomy and then to become more involved in the actual care of the ostomy.

Parents must be taught to empty, cleanse, and change the ostomy bag. Skin care is essential because the stool is irritating. (See Box 41-6 for a description of ostomy care.) The nurse can establish a discharge teaching plan cooperatively with the parents. Because ostomy equipment is expensive, in appropriate cases parents should be referred to a social worker for financial assistance. A community health nurse referral provides continued help for the family after discharge.

Supporting Effective Parenting

When a trusting relationship has been established, the nurse can aid parents in voicing their perceptions of their infant and in working toward an acceptance of the baby and the condition. Although body image is not an issue for the infant, it is for the parents who must care for the child with an ostomy. Also, when they are provided with an atmosphere of support, participation, and understanding, the family will be prepared when the infant is medically ready for discharge.

Nursing Strategies for Follow-up Care in the Home or Clinic

Carefully plot growth parameters and alert physician if infant slips below height or weight percentiles established at birth.

Inspect skin around colostomy for irritation. Discuss with the parent usual colostomy care, encouraging questions and reinforcing appropriate techniques. Refer to an enterostomal therapist for additional teaching.

Assess for signs and symptoms of enterocolitis: sudden abdominal distention, disinterest in feeding, vomiting, foul diarrhea, high fever (Sieber, 1986). Alert the physician immediately if enterocolitis is suspected.

Box 41-7
Corrective Surgical Procedures for Hirschsprung Disease

SWENSON'S PULL-THROUGH OPERATION

After resection of the aganglionic segment from just above the anus, the normal bowel is brought down and a direct end-to-end anastomosis of the proximal colon just above the rectum is performed

DUHAMEL PROCEDURE

The aganglionic rectum is left in place and the ganglion-containing colon is brought through the pelvis behind the retained rectum. A side-to-side anastomosis between the ganglion-containing colon and the aganglionic rectum is performed

SOAVE PROCEDURE

The rectum is retained but the mucosa is removed. The aganglionic colon above the rectum is resected. The outer layer of the rectum then forms a conduit through which the aganglionic bowel is pulled until it reaches the anus. The ganglionic bowel is then sutured to the anal opening. The sphincters (muscles of continence) in the rectal region are preserved

(Adapted from Martin and Torres, 1985; Leape, 1987).

Determine if the family is able to meet the financial costs of ostomy care. Refer to a social services agency for financial assistance, if appropriate.

Therapeutic Management for the Final Phase: Corrective Surgery

The ostomy is maintained until the infant weighs approximately 20 pounds or is around 1 year of age. A pull-through operation is then done. This involves removal of the aganglionic segment and anastomosis of normal ganglionic bowel to the rectum or anus.

The child is admitted several days prior to the operation so the bowel can be cleansed adequately to prevent contamination during the operation. The child is immediately placed on a clear liquid diet. The day before surgery, antibiotics are usually started and the ostomy is flushed with a neomycin-based irrigation solution to cleanse the bowel of bacteria. (See section on care of a child with a colostomy in this chapter for a discussion of colostomy irrigation.) The physician may also order rectal irrigations to dislodge any stool in the distal limb of the intestine.

The procedures used to attach ganglionic bowel to the rectum or anus are Swenson, Duhamel, or Soave procedures. (See Box 41-7 for descriptions of each.) After the pull-through procedure is completed, a Penrose drain is placed between the anus and the pulled-through bowel to prevent any collection of serous fluid in that area. This is helpful in reducing the possibility of infection. The temporary colostomy is left in place another 3 months until complete healing of the definitive surgery has taken place. If the temporary colostomy must be taken down to complete the repair, then a new colostomy is created; it is closed approximately 3 months after the definitive repair.

Major Nursing Diagnoses for Hirschsprung Disease: Pull-Through Phase

These diagnoses are meant to be used with those listed in Table 41-9, Nursing Process Plan: Care of the Child Following Abdominal Surgery.

Potential impaired tissue integrity: surgical site, related to mechanical trauma to rectal tissues (e.g., taking rectal temperature, rectal examination)
Impaired skin integrity: buttocks, related to frequent acidic stools

Strategies for Nursing Care

Providing Effective Postoperative Care and Preventing Trauma to Rectal Tissues. Postoperatively, the child is fed intravenously, a nasogastric tube is inserted to prevent distention of the abdomen,* urinary output is measured through a Foley catheter, and a Penrose drain provides for drainage of serous fluid through the rectum. The child is restrained to prevent dislodging the various tubes. The nasogastric tube is placed to intermittent suction in order to decompress the stomach. It should be irrigated routinely (every 4 hours) with air or saline to ensure its patency. The Penrose drain is removed by the physician within the first 48 hours postoperatively. The child should be turned every 2 hours. This can be done in conjunction with postural drainage, with cupping and clapping or nasopharyngeal suctioning. These nursing measures are important to prevent atelectasis or pneumonia. *It is essential that rectal temperature not be taken and rectal examinations not be done postoperatively.*

* The stomach and upper gastrointestinal tract continuously secrete digestive juices. The nasogastric tube allows these juices to be drained, which reduces the child's feeling of nausea and prevents vomiting. It also prevents pressure of the distended abdomen on the new suture line.

When the child begins to pass flatus (usually on the third postoperative day), intermittent suction of the nasogastric tube is no longer necessary and the nasogastric tube is placed on dependent drainage (drained by gravity). Once the child has begun to pass stools, the nasogastric tube is removed. The Foley catheter is removed on the third to fifth postoperative day. It is important to obtain a urine culture after removal of the catheter to identify any possible source of infection. Diet is slowly advanced from clear liquids to full liquids and eventually to a regular diet. Intravenous antibiotics are given for 5 days or as indicated.

Maintaining Skin Integrity in the Diaper Area. On the tenth postoperative day, the surgeon performs a rectal examination to assess the sphincter tone and the site of anastomosis. The child is then medically ready for discharge. The parents must understand that the child may have 5 to 15 stools per day. Excoriation of the skin of the buttocks is the major concern before and after discharge. The stool lacks consistency and is very acidic, causing excoriation.

The reason for the excoriation should be explained to the parents before discharge. They should be encouraged to apply an ointment as prescribed with each diaper change and to air-dry the area whenever possible. Skin excoriation can be a problem for 2 to 3 months after the operation. Parents need to be supported and their diligent care of the skin acknowledged.

Follow-up Care

After discharge, the infant is followed closely according to need. A rectal examination is done at each clinic visit. The purpose of this is to dilate and assess the patency of the anastomosis site. The segment of intestine that has been pulled through may undergo stricture, and it is essential that it remain patent and functioning. The rectal examinations are upsetting and uncomfortable for the child. There is usually a moderate amount of bloody discharge from the rectum for about 24 hours after the examination.

After the initial postoperative period, the child has rectal examinations in the clinic every 6 months. It is important to emphasize to the parents that the child may be difficult or slow to toilet train but that the infant will defecate normally after the definitive operative procedure is performed. They are encouraged not to attempt toilet training until the child is over 2 years of age. Once toilet trained, the child is followed on a yearly basis to monitor the stooling patterns.

This disease process affects the functioning of the family primarily for the first year or two of the child's life. During the adjustment phase support is provided through community health services.

Nursing Strategies for Follow-up Care in the Home or Clinic

Plot growth parameters and assess for signs and symptoms of enterocolitis as outlined for the temporary colostomy phase of Hirschsprung disease. Enterocolitis may occur immediately after a temporary colostomy or as long as 6 to 8 years after surgical correction (Sieber, 1986).

Anticipate that the child will be afraid of health care professionals and of the clinic because of the frequent rectal examinations.

- Allow the parent to hold the child during as much of the examination as possible.
- Provide the child with a rectal examination glove and lubricant and encourage the child to "act out" the procedure on a doll.
- Provide other toys and distractions to make the visit less threatening.
- Take care that the child who is seen in a clinic is not left waiting in the examining room any longer than absolutely necessary as this will escalate anxiety.

Talk with the parent about the child's bowel control and plans for toilet training.

Anorectal Malformations

Congenital anomalies of the anus and rectum occur in various forms with or without fistulas. They occur in approximately 1 : 3000 to 4000 live births and are more common in males.

The various anorectal malformations occur as a result of abnormal separation of the cloaca (caudal hindgut). Normally the cloaca divides into the rectum dorsally and the urogenital sinus ventrally, as a result of inward migration of mesoderm from the lateral sides of the cloaca at around the seventh week of gestation. The ridges created on either side of the cloaca meet in the midline. Malformations occur when this process is impeded in any way. Whenever the passage of fecal material is obstructed by a structural anomaly of the anus and rectum, the anus is described as imperforate.

Imperforate Anus

There are four main types of imperforate anus: (1) anal stenosis, (2) imperforate anal membrane, (3) anal agenesis, and (4) rectal atresia (Fig. 41-19).

Type I

Congenital anal stenosis is a narrowing of the anorectal canal that may occur at any point or extend its entire length. Diagnosis can be established by digital and

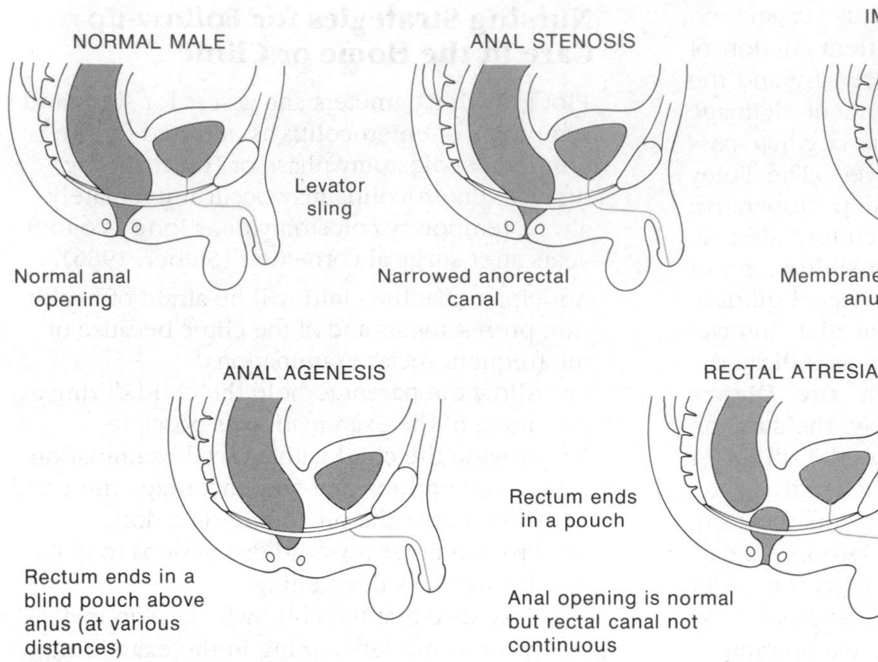

Figure 41-19. Normal anal anatomy and four main types of imperforate anus. Type I, Anal stenosis. Type II, Imperforate anal membrane. Type III, Anal agenesis (this is the most common type, occurring in about 80 per cent of cases of imperforate anus). Type IV, Rectal atresia.

endoscopic examination. Manual dilatations can often correct this type of malformation.

Type II

In imperforate anal membrane atresia, a thin cutaneous membrane persists across the anal opening. Meconium fills the rectum and can frequently be seen as a discoloration of the membrane. Treatment consists of incision or excision of the membrane followed by anal dilations until bowel function is normal.

Type III

In anal agenesis the terminal end of the rectum ends in a blind pouch at variable distances above the anus. This type accounts for approximately 80 per cent of anorectal malformations. Most of these infants have associated fistulas of various types. Treatment is surgical and varies with the type of lesion and fistula.

Type IV

In rectal atresia there is a normal anus but the rectal canal is not continuous. The lower rectal pouch can be identified by careful digital examination. Usually a complete block is encountered when examining with the little finger. This rare anomaly is corrected by anastomosis through an abdominoperineal approach.

Because 80 per cent of anorectal malformations are type III (anal agenesis), the remainder of this discussion covers anal agenesis.

Anal agenesis is described as high if the blind pouch of the rectum lies above the levator sling. (The pubococcygeal and puborectalis muscles constitute the levator sling.) For rectal continence to be accomplished, the rectum must be placed within the sling. A line drawn from the tip of the coccyx to the symphysis pubis would approximate the level of the levator sling. If the blind pouch lies below this line it has theoretically transversed the levator sling and is referred to as a low lesion. Most males have high lesions, whereas most females have low lesions. Fistulas occur in 80 to 90 per cent of patients with anal agenesis.

The specific variations of anal agenesis are as follows.

Anal Agenesis in Females: Pathophysiology and Therapeutic Management

Females usually have larger fistulas than males; therefore it is not necessary for surgery to be done immediately. A larger fistula permits stool to be expelled, therefore, the child does not become obstructed.

Low Lesions

The terminal end of the rectum forms a fistula that opens in the perineum anterior to the normal site of the anus (rectoperineal fistula) (Fig. 41-20*B*), or a fistula connects the rectum to the vagina (rectovaginal

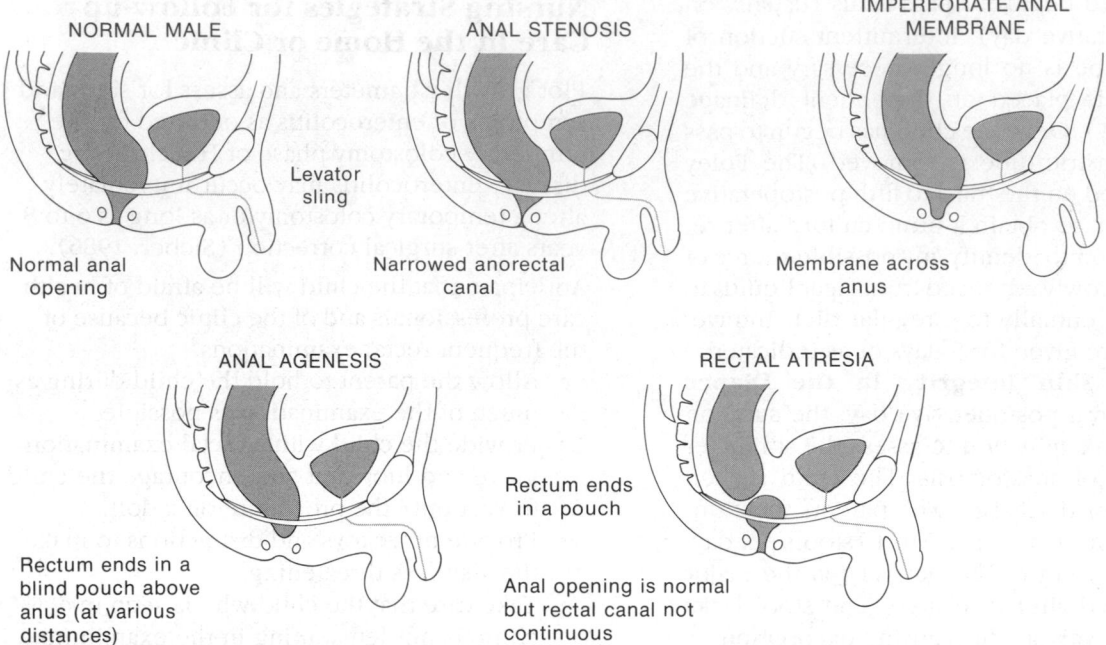

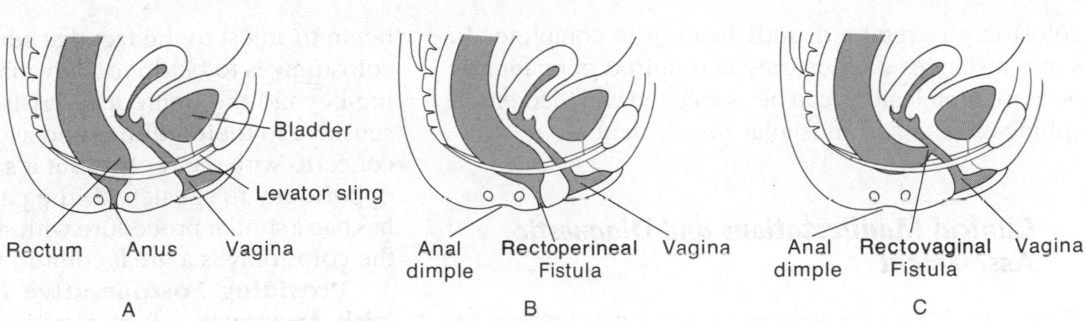

Figure 41-20. Anal agenesis in females. *A*, Normal configuration. *B*, A low lesion in which the terminal end of the rectum opens in the perineum in front of the normal site of the anus (termed *rectoperineal fistula*). *C*, A low lesion in which the rectum is connected to the vagina *(rectovaginal fistula)*. The openings are large enough for stool to be expelled through the fistulas.

fistula) (Fig. 41-20*C*). A dimple may be present at the normal anal site, and stool will pass through the fistula anterior to the dimple or through the vagina. These anomalies can be corrected by anoplasty (creation or enlargement of the anus) in the newborn period, but 3 to 6 months of age is recommended as the optimal time for repair.

High Lesions

High lesions are not common in females, but when they exist a fistula is usually associated; this opens into the proximal portion of the vagina (rectovaginal). Anomalies of the spine are commonly associated with high lesions in females. To correct the anomaly, a sigmoid loop or divided colostomy is done when the diagnosis is confirmed and a pull-through is deferred for 6 months to 1 year or until a weight of 8 to 10 kg is attained. The colostomy is retained until healing is complete.

Anal Agenesis in Males: Pathophysiology and Therapeutic Management

Low Lesions

Low lesions are not common in males but when they exist there is usually a fistula to the perineum, opening at a point anterior to the normal anal site (Fig. 41-21*B*). These lesions are corrected by perineal anoplasty followed by dilations.

High Lesions

High lesions exist almost exclusively in males and almost always have an associated urinary fistula (usually rectourethral) (Fig. 41-21*C*). These infants are initially treated by a sigmoid loop or divided colostomy, followed by a pull through* at 6 to 12 months of age. The

* Pull-through is the terminology used to describe corrective surgery in which the rectum is brought through the muscles of control (i.e., puborectalis, levator ani, and external sphincter).

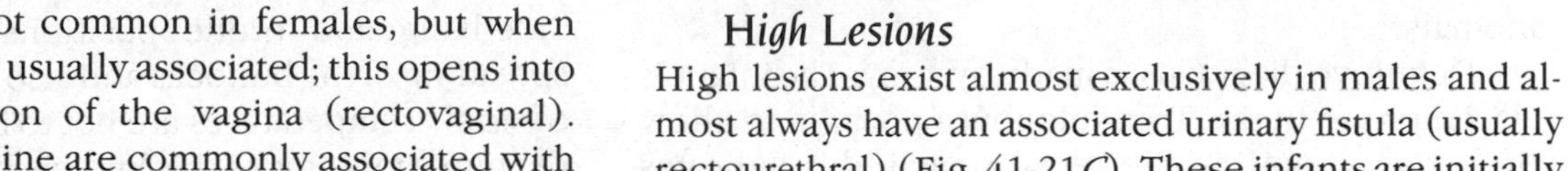

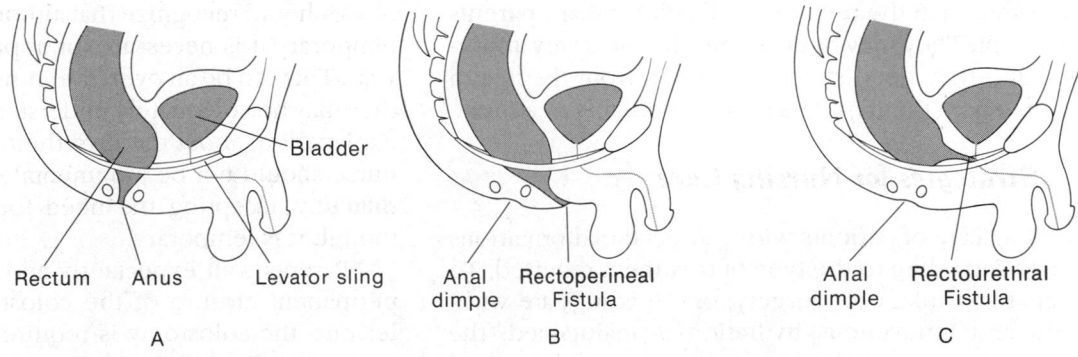

Figure 41-21. Anal agenesis in males. *A*, Normal configuration. *B*, A fistula to the perineum, with the opening anterior to the normal anal opening. *C*, A high lesion in a man, in which there is a connection between the rectum and the urethra.

colostomy is retained until healing is complete. In some instances a colostomy is required permanently because high lesions can be associated with decreased sphincter tone and muscular impairment.

Clinical Manifestations and Diagnostic Assessment

When checking temperature rectally on a newborn infant the nurse should always inspect the anus to be sure the thermometer is being inserted into the anus and not into a perineal fistula. The anal area should always be inspected for a dimple as a clue to imperforate anus. The nurse must carefully check that there is a normal anal opening and that there is no membrane present.

An understanding of the various anorectal malformations assists the nurse to make accurate observations. If meconium is not passed the perineum, urethra, and vagina are inspected for a speck of meconium. Fistulas may not be apparent at birth, but usually during the first 24 hours of life meconium is gradually forced through the fistula by peristalsis and is seen as a tiny speck at the opening of a fistula. Each voiding must be inspected for meconium, which may have passed via a rectourethral fistula (most common in males). Also, abdominal distention observed by the nurse could lead to the diagnosis of an undetected anorectal anomaly.

Definitive diagnosis is made by x-ray. The infant is placed prone in the Trendelenburg position to allow air to rise to outline the rectal pouch; this indicates whether a high or low lesion exists. A retrograde urethrocystogram will usually confirm the presence of a rectourethral fistula. Other anomalies are common and the infant should be inspected for their presence. The nurse should be in communication with the physician about the various procedures to be done. It is a comfort to parents when the nurse is informed and can reinforce explanations given by the physician. Also, the fact that stool can be expelled from any body orifice other than the rectum is difficult for many parents to accept. They may believe their infant is very abnormal and they need special attention from the health team to help them understand the available treatment.

Strategies for Nursing Care

Nursing care of patients with anorectal malformations varies according to the type of treatment required. To prepare an infant for surgery, oral feedings are withheld and intravenous hydration is maintained; the nurse continues to observe for any signs of abdominal distention. When stool is expelled it should be gently wiped from the opening of the fistula with cotton balls and soap and water.

The nurse must be available to parents as they begin to adjust to the fact that surgery is required. If a colostomy is to be done, they may have difficulty seeing beyond the immediate crisis. The nurse must be sensitive to their feelings and avoid discounting their concerns with the reply, "But it's only temporary." An opportunity to speak with the parents of a child who has had a similar procedure with subsequent closure of the colostomy is a great comfort to these parents.

Providing Postoperative Care for the Child with Anoplasty. Postoperative nursing care varies according to the type of lesion corrected. When an anoplasty is done for low lesions, the diaper is left off to expose the perineum to air to promote healing. The suture line should be kept clean by removing stool from the anoplasty with a soft cloth and mild soap and water. Care must be taken to avoid disrupting the sutures; a material that will not catch on the sutures should be used for wiping. After the stool has been removed, meticulous cleaning can be done with cotton-tipped applicators and water or a solution as ordered by the physician. Urine generally does not come in contact with the surgical site (i.e., rectal area) when the infant is in a prone position. If the surgical area becomes contaminated with urine, it is cleansed in a similar way as for stool (i.e., cotton-tipped applicators). In the event of excoriation of the skin, a bland ointment may be used to promote healing. Generally the baby is allowed to assume a position of comfort. Side-lying and prone positions prevent excessive spreading of the buttocks and also permit easy removal of stool. Temperatures are not to be taken rectally and the nurse must make this known, by way of written and verbal communication, to the family and all team members who care for the infant. Regular diet is resumed as soon as peristalsis returns. Dilations may be required for several months after anoplasty, and parents are taught to perform them daily.

Providing Postoperative Care for the Child with a Colostomy. When a colostomy is performed for high lesions, parents are taught how to care for the colostomy (see Box 41-6 for colostomy care). The nurse should recognize that although the colostomy is temporary it is necessary for approximately an entire year. This can be an overwhelming thought to parents; they may not adequately understand, in spite of careful explanation, about the care their infant requires. The nurse should not be judgmental of parents who have difficulty accepting the need for a colostomy, even though it is temporary.

Parents wait expectantly and with great hope for permanent closure of the colostomy. In some high lesions, the colostomy is required permanently. It is irresponsible of the nurse to give false hope to these families. Fecal continence varies according to the type of lesion and surgical technique; therefore, specific information should be given by the surgeon and reinforced by the nurse.

Normal or near-normal bowel control is achieved in 85 to 90 per cent of the infants with low lesions because the rectum has traversed the main muscle of continence, the levator sling. When the rectum must be placed within the muscles of continence, a lesser success rate is achieved. In children with high lesions only 50 to 65 per cent will be continent at all times (Coran et al, 1979).

Parents may need assistance in later years when toilet training is necessary. The parents must be made aware of the normal stresses of toilet training and should be encouraged to maintain a relaxed attitude. Repeated failures may be due to physiologic reasons or to stress within the family. Encouraging the family and the child during this stressful time is an important nursing role.

Alterations Associated with an Inflammatory Process

Disorders caused by an inflammatory process occur at any age. Some may result from a known infectious disease, whereas others are not associated with any recognized infection. The cause of the non-infectious inflammatory disorders remains obscure. Inflammatory (infectious and non-infectious) alterations discussed in this section include necrotizing enterocolitis, ulcerative colitis, Crohn disease, peptic ulcer, appendicitis, and gastroenteritis.

Necrotizing Enterocolitis

Necrotizing enterocolitis (NEC) continues to be the most serious and most frequently seen gastrointestinal disorder in neonatal intensive care units (NICU) (Walsh and Kliegman, 1986). In this condition a diffuse or patchy necrosis of the mucosa or submucosa occurs in the large and small bowel. Intestinal perforation, peritonitis, and shock are potential outcomes of this disturbance. It is primarily a disease of low birthweight infants (usually less than 34 weeks' gestation) but can also occur in full-term infants. Reported frequency varies, ranging from 1 to 5 per cent of all admissions to the NICU. In the very low birthweight (less than 1500 gm), frequency approaches 12 per cent (Walsh and Kliegman, 1986).

Pathophysiology

Currently no single explanation is generally accepted for the pathogenesis of NEC. Most investigators believe that NEC is a multifactorial disease. Mechanisms thought to be important in the pathogenesis of NEC are summarized in Box 41-8. The best hypothesis that can

Box 41-8
Probable Mechanisms in the Pathogenesis of Necrotizing Enterocolitis (NEC)

GASTROINTESTINAL AND IMMUNOLOGIC IMMATURITY

There is some evidence that enteral feeds may be the critical element that initiates intestinal maturation. It is unknown whether prolonged periods without enteral feedings or the effect of timed bolus feedings by nasogastric tube contributes to the pathogenesis of NEC. Immunologic immaturity may also be a factor in the development of NEC. Infants fed exclusively human milk (which contains many immunoactive components) have, however, not been protected against developing NEC.

HYPOXIC-ISCHEMIC INSULT TO THE BOWEL

Intestinal hypoperfusion with ischemia of the bowel is thought to occur as a result of events associated with high-risk premature infants (e.g., perinatal asphyxia, respiratory distress syndrome, shock, localized vasospasm, or thromboembolic phenomena). The "diving reflex" phenomenon, in which blood is shunted away from the intestines during systemic hypoxia with selective perfusion of the brain and heart, has been proposed as an explanation for bowel ischemia. Additionally, clinical factors such as umbilical arterial catheterization (because of the potential for large vessel thromboemboli) and neonatal polycythemia (because of sluggish gastrointestinal blood flow) continue to be studied as potential causes of bowel ischemia.

BACTERIAL INVASION OF THE BOWEL

Infection is thought to play a prominent role in NEC. The initial precipitating event preceding infection remains unclear but could be related to hypoxemia, sepsis, low cardiac output or hypertonic feeding. NEC occurs endemically and epidemically. Organisms associated with outbreaks of NEC include *Escherichia coli*, *Klebsiella*, *Enterobacter*, *Pseudomonas*, *Salmonella*, *Clostridium* species, coronavirus, rotavirus, and enteroviruses. Intestinal mucosa is thought to allow passage of intraluminal bacteria through the wall into the bloodstream.

SUBSTRATE FOR BACTERIAL REPLICATION THROUGH EXCESS FEEDING

Conflicting opinions exist regarding the role of enteral feeding in the development of NEC. Ninety to 95 per cent of all infants who develop NEC have been fed enterally. The mechanism by which excess feeding may contribute to NEC remains obscure. It has been postulated that excess formula may be malabsorbed and pass to the colon, where it may serve as a substrate for the bacterial flora in the colon.

(From Walsh and Kliegman, 1986; Klaus and Fanaroff, 1986.)

be formulated at this time is that NEC results as a response of the immature gastrointestinal system to multiple potentially injurious factors and may be caused by their producing synergistic damage (Walsh and Kliegman, 1986).

Clinical Manifestations and Diagnostic Assessment

Over 90 per cent of patients develop symptoms within the first 5 days of life and the remainder usually within 2 weeks after birth. Almost all infants that develop NEC have been fed formula or breast milk. Systemic manifestations that raise the nurse's suspicion include temperature instability, lethargy or irritability, apnea, or bradycardia. Signs and symptoms associated with feeding and gastrointestinal function include difficulty with feedings, increased pregavage residuals (feeding retained in the stomach or from the previous feeding), abdominal distention, inability to defecate (may indicate a developing ileus), and occult blood in emesis or stool (Holzman and Brown, 1986). The infant can be tolerating feedings and requiring decreasing amounts of oxygen and then unexpectantly develops this disease. The changes can occur quite rapidly and must be dealt with immediately; however, it is essential that explanations and support for the parents be provided.

The earliest radiologic sign is segmented distention of the small bowel. The cardinal sign of the disease is pneumatosis intestinalis, which is the presence of air pockets within the intestinal wall caused by invading bacteria that can result in the perforation of the bowel. This most commonly affects the terminal ileum and right colon, but it can be much more extensive.

Therapeutic Management

Medical Management

Nonoperative treatment is successful in a high percentage of infants with NEC if therapy is instituted before there is extensive bowel necrosis. A sump tube (a nasogastric tube attached to suction) can be used to decompress the abdomen. The infant is given nothing orally; hydration and nutrition are maintained via peripheral or central parenteral nutrition for approximately 2 weeks, although the timing of the reinstitution of feeding is controversial. After blood, urine, stool, and spinal fluid cultures are taken, antibiotics are administered, both intravenously and orally. The use of oral antibiotics also is controversial. If they are administered, it is to decrease the risk of septicemia and reduce intestinal colonization (Holtzman and Brown, 1986). Blood studies are carried out to monitor the infant's electrolyte and blood gas levels and to obtain complete blood count and platelet count. Intubation of the infant may be necessary if respiratory compromise develops.

Abdominal radiographs are taken every 8 to 12 hours to look for distention of bowel loops, pneumatosis intestinalis (air in the intramural wall of the intestines), pneumoperitoneum (air in the peritoneum), or air in the hepatic vein. The only absolute indication for surgery is intestinal perforation. The challenge in management is to "avoid operating on the infant with NEC who does not have necrosis yet not delay operating on the infant who does" (Leape, 1987).

Surgical Management

If surgery is performed the entire bowel is examined for perforations and necrotic tissue. Only the *obviously* necrotic intestine is removed (Leape, 1987). Intestinal diversion is performed by creating an enterostomy (opening into the intestine and creating a stoma on the abdomen). The final stage of treatment is removal of the ostomy and reanastomosis of the two ends of the intestine. When the majority of the intestine appears to be necrotic, massive resection leads to a short-bowel syndrome, but *not* resecting it is fatal.

Postoperative management requires a qualified intensive care team. These infants may require ventilatory support, large amounts of fluids, and repeated infusions of platelets and clotting factors to correct disseminated intravascular coagulation (DIC).

Strategies for Nursing Care

Providing Nutrition Postoperatively. Postoperatively, the infant is maintained on parenteral nutrition. Nasogastric low-osmotic feedings are begun gradually. Breast milk or predigested formula in small amounts and diluted strengths is used for feedings. The infant must be watched closely for residuals before feedings and for diarrhea and bloody feces, which would signify further irritation or necrosis of the bowel.

As the infant continues to improve, attempts are made to give feedings via the nipple. The infant is given the opportunity to take a designated amount by mouth and the remainder is given via gavage.

Supporting Care at Home. Necrotizing enterocolitis is a debilitating disease that results in prolonged hospitalization with the potential of at least two major operative procedures for the infant. This places added stress on the family and on the bonding process between the infant and parents. The nursing staff can minimize family members' anxieties by establishing a trusting relationship with them. This is done through honestly answering their questions and being available to hear their concerns. This relationship will foster the exchange of information and support the development of plans for discharge. These families have been under a great deal of stress and usually require referral to community resources, such as a visiting nurse, to facilitate adjustment to home care of the infant.

The nurse should explore with the mother the possibility of breastfeeding her infant who is at risk for NEC. *Fresh* breast milk contains lymphocytes, macrophages, and lactoferrin, which aid the infant's natural defenses against bacterial invasion of the intestinal mucosa; however, NEC is known to also occur in breastfed infants. (Protective elements of breast milk are lost when breast milk is stored.) Many hospitals have breast pumps that can be utilized during the infant's long hospitalization to aid the mother to continue to feed her baby. Resource groups such as La Leche League may be supportive referrals.

Inflammatory Bowel Disease (Ulcerative Colitis and Crohn Disease)

Ulcerative colitis and Crohn disease are two diseases of the bowel not caused by recognizable infection. They are viewed as distinct but related diseases whose common features are described by the term inflammatory bowel disease (IBD). The causes of ulcerative colitis and Crohn disease are unknown. Many potential etiologic factors continue to be investigated, including heredity, environmental and infectious agents, immunologic mechanisms, and psychogenic factors. Both are diseases of young people and frequently arise in the second decade, with a peak incidence in the twenties. They occur more frequently in whites than in blacks and are particularly common among persons of Jewish descent. About 20 per cent of patients will have a first degree relative with one or the other of these diseases.

Pathophysiology and Clinical Manifestations

Inflammatory bowel disease (IBD) has become an important entity in pediatrics. Early recognition of IBD can lead to earlier treatment and can substantially influence the quality of life for affected children and adolescents. The similarities between these diseases have led to the use of the common term IBD; however, there are distinguishing features that the nurse should understand when caring for these children (see Table 41-10).

Diagnostic Assessment

The assessment should include a complete history and physical examination. (See Chapter 15 for nursing history and physical examination.)

The presenting symptoms are explored, including a search for historical factors that might contribute to the development or exacerbation of IBD (see Table 41-10 for presenting symptoms of each disease). The family history in particular is reviewed to search for other similar problems in other family members, not necessarily diagnosed as IBD. Stresses in the home, in school, or on the job (for an adolescent) are potential aggravators of the disease.

The history should rule out other causes of symptoms, such as infectious diarrhea and allergy. Details of travel, source of drinking water, and recent changes in food intake may provide important clues. If growth retardation is present, a review of height and weight since birth should be included. During the assessment phase, an environment is promoted in which the child or parent feels comfortable in describing the symptoms. Fear and embarrassment about bloody bowel movements may lead the child to conceal the problem from parents. Once the condition is diagnosed the child or adolescent will often minimize the description of symptoms to avoid visits to the doctor or further medical tests. Appreciating the feelings that are associated with the symptoms are an important aspect of the communication process during assessment.

Laboratory data provide supportive evidence but generally do not provide a definitive diagnosis. Findings that may be present are anemia because of blood loss and malnutrition, electrolyte imbalance (especially hypokalemia), reduced serum protein levels because of losses through diarrhea and inadequate protein intake, and an elevated white blood cell count and sedimentation rate because of inflammation and blood in the stool.

Diagnostic studies used include a barium enema and upper gastrointestinal series with small bowel follow-through, and sigmoidoscopy or colonoscopy. (See Table 41-10 for summary of their use and findings in each disease.)

Supporting the Child and Family During Assessment

Health professionals must realize that the diagnostic investigations performed for IBD engender great anxiety. Parents and relatives may be even more fearful than the patient because most adults associate the use of barium enema, endoscopy and especially biopsy with the possibility of cancer. This fear is seldom spoken and should be specifically addressed. Ulcerative colitis and Crohn disease both have a tendency to relapse and remit and the course is highly variable from individual to individual. An acquaintance will often tell patients and families about those IBD victims who have had the most severe disease and complications. Families should be warned about this in advance. Similarly, all chronic incurable diseases sooner or later be-

Table 41-10. Comparison of Pathophysiology and Diagnosis of Ulcerative Colitis and Crohn Disease

Ulcerative Colitis	Crohn Disease
Location	
Primarily a disease of the rectum and distal colon but in children usually involves the entire colon. The most severe disease occurs distally.	The distal small intestine (terminal ileum) is most frequently involved (80% of cases), but it may involve any area of the alimentary tract.
Character	
An inflammation of the colonic mucosa. Vascular engorgement of the mucosa and submucosa is present with increased leukocytes. The lesion rarely extends beyond the mucosa into deeper layers. Acute edema and inflammation result in thickening of the bowel.	Inflammation is characterized by transmural or deep-bowel-wall involvement. Lesion penetrates bowel wall. Thickened intestinal wall, mucosal fissures, and fistulas are typical. Granulomas occur in 50% of cases.
Pattern	
Lesion is continuous. When a lesion develops it spreads to adjacent areas without skipping healthy bowel.	Lesion occurs as a skip lesion (i.e., diseased bowel is separated by normal bowel).
Long-term Changes and Complications	
As the disease becomes chronic the bowel takes on a lead-pipe appearance (i.e., shortening of colon, loss of mucosal folds, loss of haustral folds [scalloped appearance of colon], and the development of fibrous tissue and linear strictures). Complications include toxic megacolon, in which the colon suddenly dilates and perforates, spreading infection into the abdominal cavity and bloodstream. This is a rare complication.	Chronic inflammation is characterized by the presence of granulomas, scarring, and formation of fibrotic strictures. Strictures can eventually cause bowel obstruction. The transmural nature of the lesion results in fistula formations, but the inflammation and engorgement on the serosal surface inhibits perforation. As a result, spillage of intestinal contents into the peritoneal cavity is rare.
Presentation of Illness	
The most frequent manifestations are bloody diarrhea and abdominal pain. Blood loss can be profound. Patients experience cramping sensations (tenesmus) with bowel movements, which frequently come on with a sense of urgency. Extraintestinal manifestations (skin rash, arthritis, iritis) are rare in children but occur in adolescents and young adults. Occasionally anorexia, nausea, fever of undetermined origin, anemia, and dehydration accompany the presenting symptoms. Physical examination reveals a tender and distended abdomen with signs of peritoneal irritation.	Crampy abdominal pain is the most common initial complaint. Many have diarrhea, and constitutional symptoms are characteristic of the disease. These include fever, malaise, and anorexia. Pain is most frequent in the right lower quadrant. Abscess formation is common; therefore, a spiking fever and leukocytosis may be noted. Failure to thrive is the reason for seeking care in 20–30% of children with Crohn disease (Gryboski and Hillemeier, 1980). Extraintestinal symptoms often accompany the disease and include mouth ulcers, iritis, arthritis, arthralgia, or skin rashes.
Making the Diagnosis	
A barium enema reveals the characteristic lead-pipe appearance of a previously inflamed bowel. A barium enema also identifies the extent of ulcerative colitis. Direct examination of the large bowel by sigmoidoscopy or colonoscopy will reveal friability and ulceration confirmed by characteristic changes in the biopsy specimens taken during the procedure.	As the symptoms are often non-specific and difficult to localize in the intestinal tract, the diagnosis may not be made for months to years after the onset of symptoms. A small bowel follow-through study or barium enema is initially done to allow the entire colon to be visualized. A colonoscopy may be used to document the extent of disease. The presence of skip lesions on radiographs or colonoscopy is confirmed by finding granulomata in the biopsy specimens.
Effect of IBD on Growth and Development	
Inflammatory Bowel Disease (IBD) results in growth retardation. Growth is retarded if a child falls below the third percentile on standard growth charts in height and fails to develop sexually at the normal rate. Growth retardation is considered a common occurrence in IBD. Originally it was believed that growth retardation was due to low levels of growth hormone, but it is now thought it is due to inadequate intake or poor intestinal absorption of nutrients with large doses of corticosteroids as a contributing factor (Grand et al, 1977). After puberty the chances of recovery from growth retardation are reduced. The potential for growth retardation to be minimized is related to child's age, duration of illness, calorie depletion, and nutritional replacement therapy (Kelts et al, 1979).	

come the subject of sensational media reports of miraculous cures. Parents and grandparents should be encouraged to bring these items in to be discussed openly so that a foundation of trust is maintained. It is the nurse's responsibility to ensure that patients are informed and prepared for the various procedures that are required to arrive at a diagnosis. The tests required during the diagnostic phase are uncomfortable and may be embarrassing to some children or teenagers. The nurse's role during this phase involves a sensitive response to the child's and family's particular reactions.

Therapeutic Management

Pharmacologic Management. The treatment of IBD remains limited. The medications available include sulfasalazine (Salazopyrin), mesalamine (5-ASA) (a newer, more purified form of sulfasalazine), and corticosteroids. Salazopyrin and 5-ASA are most useful in the treatment of disease involving the colon, whether in Crohn disease or ulcerative colitis. Occasionally a patient with Crohn disease of the small bowel seems to respond to these drugs despite the findings of the National Collaborative Crohn's Disease Study, which suggested they would be ineffective (Summers, 1979).

Corticosteroids may be used in the form of prednisone, cortisone, or methylprednisolone. They will usually induce a remission but will not halt progression of the disease despite making the patient feel much better. Corticosteroids must be used judiciously because of the multitude of side effects that can be produced. These include weight gain, moon face, dowager's hump, acne, cataracts, muscle weakness, salt retention, hypertension, glycosuria, osteomalacia, aseptic necrosis of the hip, increased susceptibility to infections, and euphoria. However, used in the smallest effective dose with monitoring for side effects, they can be very safe. The nurse must be sure the parents understand the side effects and dangers to be watched for. Monitoring for side effects should be part of the nursing care plan for both inpatients and outpatients. Patients should acquire a medical alert bracelet indicating corticosteroid use and the possibility of adrenal suppression in the event of severe illness or accident. Alternate-day corticosteroids are used more frequently in children with Crohn disease than in adults because they stimulate appetite and promote a sense of well-being, thus encouraging normal growth and development while minimizing side effects. See also Table 45-2, Nursing Process Plan: The Child on Corticosteroid Therapy.

Nutritional Management. Nutritional management is becoming increasingly important in IBD. Most patients with Crohn disease will go into remission on total parenteral nutrition or elemental feeding. Elemental feeding may be provided at home by nasogastric tube given overnight. Most teenagers prefer to remove the tube in the morning and reinsert it in the evening rather than go to school with a tube in the nose. Elemental diet by tube feeding is used most often to correct growth failure in Crohn disease. For most patients, a relapse of the disease can be expected several months after the elemental feeding regimen is stopped. These techniques are not effective for ulcerative colitis, although total parenteral nutrition (TPN) may be necessary to prepare a chronically malnourished patient for surgery.

Surgical Management. Neither of these bowel diseases can be cured medically, although operative removal of the entire colon will cure ulcerative colitis. Colectomy and subsequent ileostomy is understandably resisted by patients and families until they have experienced the full ravages of the disease. However, the severity of the disease in young people and the increasing chance that cancer will arise in the colon after 10 years of disease means that most young patients with ulcerative colitis will eventually have the colon removed surgically. Consequently, there is great enthusiasm for the techniques that produce the "continent ileostomy" or ileoanal continuity so that the patient can go to the bathroom in the normal fashion. These newer techniques are rarely done immediately after the removal of the colon, particularly if surgery was performed because the patient had been acutely ill.

Major Nursing Diagnoses for Inflammatory Bowel Disease

Altered bowel elimination: diarrhea, *related to intestinal inflammation*
Potential for injury: physiologic, *related to untoward effects of prescribed medications*
Altered comfort: pain, *related to*

- *abdominal cramping associated with intestinal inflammation and ulceration*
- *excoriation of skin around the anus*

Potential for injury: complications of IBD, *related to chronic inflammation and ulceration of the bowel*
Altered nutrition: less than body requirements, *related to poor absorption of essential nutrients associated with chronic inflammation of the bowel*
Potential altered growth and development: failure to thrive, *related to poor absorption of essential nutrients*
Potential activity intolerance: acute phase,

related to the tendency for exercise to increase intestinal motility
***Impaired skin integrity**, related to frequent and prolonged contact of the skin with feces*
***Potential ineffective individual coping**, related to the ongoing alterations in daily living associated with chronic inflammatory bowel disease*
***Altered family process**, related to the stress of long-term illness of a child*

Strategies for Nursing Care

Nursing care of patients with IBD focuses on several major problems associated with the manifestations and management of the disease. The major problems of elimination (diarrhea) and associated discomfort (abdominal pain and cramping) are the most apparent difficulties faced by these patients. Additionally they suffer from nutritional deficits and fluid and electrolyte imbalances because of malabsorption. This overall depleted nutritional state interferes with usual activities of daily living, and during acute phases activity is restricted to decrease intestinal motility. Skin breakdown, fistulas, and abscesses are problems that frequently arise and require special nursing care. Finally, a knowledgeable nurse who provides sensitive nursing care can foster an understanding of the disease and psychologic adjustment by these patients.

Controlling Diarrhea. The usual recording of stools is supplemented with a notation of any relationship of the diarrhea to types of food, emotional stress, or activity.

Antidiarrheal drugs such as diphenoxylate (Lomotil) or anticholinergics should be given as ordered and their effectiveness evaluated. These medications reduce cramping as well as diarrhea. The nurse and the family must monitor for side effects of the medications used in the management of IBD. The preceding section on pharmacologic management includes nursing strategies to address potential untoward effects of medications.

The problem of diarrhea is often embarrassing to patients and is associated with abdominal discomfort and problems of skin irritation. Maintaining an odor-free environment by promptly removing linens, supplying appropriate pain medication, using comfort measures, and carefully cleansing the perineal area are important nursing interventions. When severe skin irritation is present, application of a thin film of protective ointment may prevent further irritation.

Providing Optimal Comfort and Assessing for Complications. Pain management involves administration of pain medication, repositioning, alleviation of anxiety through supportive conversation, and quiet diversional activities.

Pain of increased intensity that is not responsive to therapy should be monitored closely as this may indicate a complication (obstruction, peritonitis, or hemorrhage). Careful documentation of the character and pattern of pain and its relationship to meals is important.

Providing Essential Nutrients. Dietary management of IBD may involve TPN, elemental feeding by mouth or tube, a low-residue bland diet, or, in some cases, a regular diet. Care of the patient with TPN is discussed in Chapter 30.

Instruction in tube placement and feeding techniques is usually done by the nurse. The timing of education is important. After the therapy has been discussed and the technique is explained it is important to proceed with the placement of the tube. Delaying its use for days or weeks simply gives the child or adolescent time to experience increased anxiety.

Elemental diets are nutritionally balanced, bulk- and residue-free, and low in fat. They are digested mainly in the upper jejunum and are relatively nonstimulating, allowing the bowel to rest. *Any signs of intolerance* (abdominal distention, diarrhea, nausea, vomiting) *to the feedings that occur should be consistently documented by the nurse.* Children who are required to receive an elemental diet by tube feeding need the support of parents and relatives. Preparation for therapy at home should include the counsel of a nutritionist. The nurse should be involved, devising the plan for home care with the goal of providing the parents and child with adequate information and supervision to carry out the procedure at home.

Dietary counseling for maintenance of nutritional status is provided. The nurse spends time with the child to identify which foods may aggravate symptoms. Sometimes children need to be persuaded to eat because they associate pain and diarrhea with eating. Foods that cannot be tolerated should be eliminated, but involvement of the child in these decisions may increase overall intake and satisfaction with the diet. Keeping an accurate record of food and fluid intake and output provides important information for management during acute phases. Management at home is more relaxed, and usually measurement of intake and output is unnecessary.

Monitoring Physical Activity. During the acute phase physical activity is usually kept to a minimum to decrease intestinal motility. Patients on parenteral nutrition can be encouraged to exercise if they are feeling strong enough and free of symptoms. Exercise is in these cases promoted to use the dextrose and protein supplied in parenteral nutrition to build muscle tissue (Simmons, 1984).

Preserving Skin Integrity. Skin breakdown in the form of fistulas and fissures is common in Crohn disease. Patients with ulcerative colitis and Crohn disease suffer from excoriation of the anal region owing to diarrhea. Sitz baths, meticulous skin care, and medicated wipes such as Tucks provide some relief. Care around a draining fistula site is important to prevent further breakdown. Small fistulas can be cared for by using a small, sterile saline packing, which is changed every 4 to 6 hours; for excessively large fistulas, a stoma adhesive around the fistula can provide a skin barrier. A pouch can be attached to the stoma adhesive and accurate drainage measured (Simmons, 1984).

In acute phases when a patient is on bedrest the usual measures to prevent skin breakdown must be instituted, including use of sheepskin, a foam mattress, or a waterbed; repositioning; and gradual ambulation.

Supporting Adjustment of the Child and Family to IBD. Inflammatory bowel disease considerably disrupts the patient's life. The way he or she can participate in society and the impact on daily life must be appreciated by the nurse who cares for these individuals and their families. During active disease, considerable restrictions are placed on the type of food that can be eaten, the extent to which the patient can socialize, and how far the patient can venture from a restroom. Disruption in education, career, and family life must be tolerated and adjustments made to fulfill responsibility.

The nurse should be preapred to cope with behaviors of a chronically ill patient. Anger, denial, and often perfectionism are behaviors that are expressed during illness. Loss of control over bowel function, eating, and daily activities arouses feelings of frustration and anger. Having the patient identify those aspects that are providing the greatest burden may be helpful. Additional information about the treatment plan, drugs, and feedings may correct or expand the patient's understanding.

Careful attention should be given to how patients can participate and gain some control in their own care. Nonverbal messages are of particular importance during the care of an ostomy, cleaning up soiled linens, and bedpans. Patients are particularly sensitive to any signs of disgust or revulsion.

Adjustment can be facilitated if expression of the patient's fears and frustrations is encouraged. Questions should be answered honestly and in collaboration with other health team members. Demands on nursing time may become extensive if not controlled. Those patients who repeatedly call for the nurse should be recognized as persons who have fears or unanswered questions. Gradually these fears and questions should be dealt with by the professional team.

Assistance from specialized nurses called "stomal therapists." should be sought for preparation of the patient before surgery and for management of the ostomy after surgery (see Box 41-6). Patients with ostomies require counseling concerning sexual issues, an area that requires specialized support. The United Ostomy Association* has pamphlets available on sex, courtship, and pregnancy for male and female ostomy patients. Information concerning fertility and sexuality can be obtained from the National Foundation for Ileitis and Colitis.†

Long-Term Outcome

The prognosis for both these diseases is surprisingly good considering the trouble they cause when they are active. Both are compatible with a full life, including employment, marriage, and childbearing. Young patients with ulcerative colitis often have sporadic school attendance. The combination of embarrassment and a tendency for symptoms to worsen under stress often leads to school avoidance. School attendance and well-being should be checked at every visit. Similarly, patients with Crohn disease frequently do not feel well even though objective signs and symptoms of disease are not apparent. If the child or adolescent is not active in school and participating in sports and activities or not growing, some element in the program should be adjusted. The nurse plays a critical role in these assessments because patients frequently confide their true feelings and complaints to a sympathetic nursing professional. This sense of trust is necessary to the effective understanding and management of the young person with IBD.

Nursing Strategies for Follow-up Care in the Home or Clinic

Plot growth parameters and alert the physician if the child fails to maintain previously established percentiles for height and weight.

Determine the average number and quality of stools per day and whether or not they are associated with cramping.

Gently palpate for abdominal distention and inspect for excoriated skin areas. Reinforce teaching about skin care as needed.

Assess nutritional intake in the previous 24 hours. (See Chapter 18 for details of a 24-hour recall.)

Discuss with the parent and child ways to increase intake of essential nutrients without creating a power struggle between the child and family over the issue of eating (e.g., eliminate

* United Ostomy Association, 201 Beverly Road, Los Angeles, CA 90052

† National Foundation for Ileitis and Colitis, Dept. N-80, 295 Madison Avenue, New York, NY 10017.

low-nutrient "junk food" from the home, allow the child to choose favorite foods from a list of nutritional foods, allow the child to help shop and plan menus for the family, and reinforce with the child that good nutrition is important for all the members of the family to decrease any feelings of being a martyr on the part of the child).

Assess for side effects of medications and reinforce the family's responsibility for monitoring the effects of medications.

Assess the child's developmental level and sense of self-esteem. (See Chapters 15 and 16.)

Encourage the child to discuss the ways in which he or she manages the symptoms of IBD. Verbally reinforce adaptive coping to enhance the child's sense of control.

Peptic Ulcer

A peptic ulcer is a general term describing any erosion of the mucosal wall of the stomach (gastric ulcer) or duodenum (duodenal ulcer). Peptic ulcers are more common in adults; however, now that fiberoptic technology has made endoscopy practical for infants and children, the diagnosis is increasingly encountered in pediatric patients. No firm prevalence figures exist, but peptic ulceration is encountered in 1 to 2 per cent of hospitalized pediatric patients. Males are affected more often than females. Peptic ulcers are more common in late school-age children and adolescents than in younger children.

Etiology and Pathophysiology

The exact cause of peptic ulcers is unknown. In most instances, the ulcers arise as a complication of the stress of other diseases. These secondary ulcers typically are multiple and superficial. They may occur equally in the stomach and duodenum. They are associated with more serious insults, such as head injury, multiple trauma, or severe burns (Curling ulcer). However, they may also accompany sepsis and respiratory, renal, or hepatic failure.

"Primary ulcers" are usually deeper and solitary and are most often found in the gastric antrum or duodenum. These ulcers occur in genetically predisposed individuals with a strong family history of peptic ulcer disease. Recent research has indicated two mechanisms as possible causes: (1) increased gastric acid secretion, or (2) impaired mucosal defense against back-diffusion of acid. In addition, stress is thought to be an important contributing factor in the development of peptic ulcers. A spiral bacterium, *Campylobacter pylori,* has been identified as a possible etiologic factor in peptic ulcers and gastritis in both adults and children. A brief review of these findings can be found in an article by Nord (1988).

Clinical Manifestations

Bleeding is the most common presentation of peptic ulceration. This may take the form of *hematemesis*—the vomiting of blood from the stomach, which usually gives the appearance of coffee grounds because of the interaction of blood and stomach acid. Bright red blood is more likely vomited from the pharynx or the esophagus. Parents are usually more alarmed by the appearance of recognizable blood. Some reassurance can be offered that the problem is rarely as dramatic as it appears. By contrast, the vomiting of large amounts of coffee-ground material may not worry parents but should be recognized by professionals as an alarming sign.

When blood is passed in the stools, they take on a tarry black appearance known as melena. A characteristic foul metallic odor is present.

Diagnostic Assessment

Differential diagnosis includes any of the causes of acute upper gastrointestinal tract bleeding. Parents should be questioned about all possible factors when a child has bleeding. Hematemesis is often the result of blood ingested from a posterior nose bleed. Individuals with a bleeding tendency may bleed more easily from this and other causes. These conditions are exacerbated by aspirin ingestion, which impairs platelet function. Forceful vomiting accompanying gastritis may tear the esophageal mucosa, a condition known as a Mallory-Weiss tear. Erosions of the esophagus, stomach, and duodenum result from the ingestion of corrosives. These may be caused by lye, the residue from automatic dishwasher soap, or medications such as aspirin. Rarely, upper gastrointestinal bleeding results from esophageal varices, a complication of chronic liver disease in both children and adults.

Chronic abdominal pain or even weight loss may be the only sign of chronic primary peptic ulcer disease. This is seen most often in children and adolescents with a strong family history of ulcers but may occur acutely after unusual stress. Abdominal pain may be nonspecific, particularly in younger children, but epigastric pain, especially if it penetrates to the back and is relieved temporarily by eating, points to the possibility of an ulcer. Most children with abdominal pain have no serious organic process, but complaints which are very specific are more suggestive of pathology (Appley, 1975). Presence of anemia or occult blood in the stool is a strong indication for further investigation for peptic ulcer disease.

In adult patients, upper gastrointestinal tract (UGI) barium studies are probably as effective as endoscopy in making a diagnosis of ulcer. (See Table 41-4.) However, it is difficult for infants and children to cooperate fully during the radiographic techniques that make reliable diagnosis possible. Accordingly, endoscopy is preferable in infants and children. This can now be performed in most children without the need for general anesthesia. However, very few children with nonspecific abdominal pain will be found to have ulcers and are spared endoscopy unless there are specific signs pointing to the diagnosis. If UGI bleeding is present, endoscopy will most frequently lead to a diagnosis.

Therapeutic Management

As in most conditions, the best treatment for ulcer disease is prevention. Children at risk for the development of secondary ulcers should be treated prophylactically. The intensive care unit (ICU) patient with an indwelling nasogastric tube should be given sufficient liquid antacid to keep gastric acid pH above 5 as measured at the bedside. This may require 10 to 30 ml of antacid instilled every 1 to 2 hours. Alternatively, one of the histamine H_2 receptor antagonists, such as cimetidine or ranitidine, can be very effective in blocking secretion of stomach acid. Again, the effect on gastric pH is checked and the dose adjusted, because metabolism of these drugs varies considerably in severely ill patients. In the presence of mucosal erosions, sucralfate is used. This is a medication that combines with fibrin to form an occlusion over the ulcer site to protect it from the effects of acid and digestive enzymes and allow healing. Antacids interfere with the action of sucralfate, so they should not be administered concurrently.

Treatment of a chronic ulcer relies on use of the same medications. It is now appreciated that in adult patients one or two doses of H_2 antagonist medication daily are as effective as more doses given frequently. Liquid antacids are equally effective, but they must be given in relatively large doses four times daily for 4 to 6 weeks. Most parents have difficulty complying with treatment lasting this long, so use of the H_2 antagonists has become increasingly popular. Because ulcers are relatively rare and abdominal pain is so common in children, it is probably unwise to use these medications unless diagnostic tests verify that an ulcer is present.

Major Nursing Diagnoses for Peptic Ulcer

Potential for impaired tissue integrity:* *erosion of gastric or duodenal wall, related to
- *increased gastric acid secretion*
- *impaired mucosal defense of the wall from the acid*

Altered comfort: pain,* *related to ulceration of gastric or duodenal tissues

Altered health maintenance,* *related to inadequate knowledge of etiologic and preventive factors associated with peptic ulcer

Strategies for Nursing Care

Assisting in Diagnosis. The nurse plays an important role in all phases of care. During diagnosis, careful use of Hematest tablets or Hemoccult paper to test for occult blood in the stool, and accurate documentation facilitate early recognition. Helping to identify the child at risk for secondary peptic ulcer disease is an important nursing responsibility as well.

Teaching to Control Symptoms and to Promote a Healthier Life Style. The nurse's role in teaching includes the areas of medication, stress management, and dietary management. Medications both aid in healing and help to control the pain associated with a peptic ulcer. The child (when old enough) and family should be thoroughly familiar with the use of prescribed medications and should be given written instructions to refer to as questions arise during home management.

Stress management deals with both illness-related stressors and chronic stressors encountered as the result of individual and family lifestyles. Nursing strategies to minimize the stress of acute illness and hospitalization are detailed in Table 31-2, Nursing Process Plan: The Hospitalized Child. Chapter 23 deals with the general topics of stress, coping, and related nursing strategies.

Most parents think that peptic ulcers should be treated by diet. There are few dietary regimens that are truly necessary, however. The family is asked what they believe about the relation between diet and ulcers. It has recently been appreciated that milk products probably cause more harm than good in ulcer patients. Initially milk buffers the acid and provides symptomatic relief. However, the high levels of calcium present in milk are potent stimulators of acid secretion and result in a rebound effect, which produces more stomach acid. Alcohol, caffeine, and cigarettes are also potent stimulants to acid secretion and should be particularly avoided by the adolescent patient. The nurse should encourage the patient to eat a normal well-balanced diet for age, and relatives should be counseled to avoid aggravating the patient at mealtime with unnecessary suggestions about food.

Healthy dietary patterns are also encouraged. Striving to maintain a regular mealtime schedule, avoiding overeating, and eating a small snack between meals are preventive measures.

Prognosis

The prognosis for "secondary ulcers" depends on effective treatment at the time they occur and the course of the underlying disease. Once the acute phase is over, the ulcers are unlikely to recur and the antiulcer medications may be discontinued within days. Primary ulcers in children follow the well-described adult pattern. The tendency to ulcer formation is a chronic condition and in about one half of patients they will recur. These may have a seasonal pattern, flaring in the spring or fall or coming on at times of stress. In adults, prophylaxis for 4 to 6 weeks with one half the therapeutic dose of antiulcer medications can prevent recurrence. This has not been tested in children. However, with the availability of modern diagnostic and therapeutic approaches, few children will require surgery because of recurring ulcers. Despite this, many myths about the origin and treatment of ulcers persist. It is up to the nurse as part of the health care team to inquire about the family's attitude toward the disease and to guide them to remedies.

Nursing Strategies for Follow-up Care in the Home or Clinic

Test available feces or vomitus for occult blood.

Obtain a blood sample for determination of hemoglobin and hematocrit as appropriate.

Question the child who is old enough to talk about appetite and epigastric discomfort. Make these subjective assessments for the younger child by discussing with the parent feeding and sleeping behaviors and other indicators of the child's comfort.

Caution the parent to seek immediate medical attention if symptoms recur.

Appendicitis

Acute appendicitis is the most common surgical emergency in children and, although the mortality rate has declined steadily, this condition is still the cause of many preventable deaths. The disease tends to occur slightly more often in boys.

Pathophysiology

The appendix is located at the end of the cecum and has no apparent function. The cause of appendicitis is an obstruction of the appendiceal lumen, usually by a fecalith (hardened feces). Secondary obstruction may result from inflammatory changes of blood-borne or enteric infections or from parasites, stenosis, or kinking. The obstruction causes inflammatory changes in the mucosal wall, which becomes edematous and filled with leukocytes. This distention relays pain via stretch receptors through visceral nerve fibers so that pain is first perceived in the periumbilical region. Inflammation of the appendix leads to vomiting and fever, and with increased inflammation the pain localizes to the right lower quadrant. Distention also compromises the blood supply. Gangrene and perforation may result. Perforation of the appendix allows bacteria to escape and produces a generalized peritonitis or a localized abscess (confined by the adjoining omentum).

Clinical Manifestations and Diagnostic Assessment

Appendicitis has a wide variation in onset and pattern of symptoms; however, symptoms usually do not come to the attention of a health professional until they are acute. It is not uncommon for the child with appendicitis to appear in the school nurse's office complaining of severe abdominal pain. Many children will not be comfortable standing upright and will attempt to lessen discomfort by bending over and guarding the abdomen with their hands. It is difficult to assess the location of pain because the child is fearful of anyone touching the abdomen. However, the nurse can ask the child to show "where it hurts" and avoid palpation. *The presence of low-grade fever, periumbilical or right lower quadrant pain (at McBurney's point), and vomiting should alert the nurse to seek immediate medical assistance for the child.* In young children (toddlers and preschool-age children), appendicitis does not necessarily present with the classic symptoms of pain, vomiting, and fever. The first symptoms may be irritability or listlessness, followed by vomiting. Diarrhea is more common and more extensive than in the older child. Nausea and vomiting occur after the onset of pain, whereas in gastroenteritis the reverse is true. This is an important difference in differentiating appendicitis from gastroenteritis (Leape, 1987).

Pain elicits fear; therefore during the examination the nurse calmly explains what is going to be done and that parents will be contacted. The child should be told why it is necessary to see a physician.

Because appendicitis is an emergency, there is little time available to prepare the child adequately for the diagnostic work-up. If at all possible, parents should be encouraged to stay with the child. Letting the parents know that the nurse is aware of their concern and will answer their questions helps them cope with their anxiety.

The abdomen is palpated to assess for rigidity and

tenderness. Adequate preparation will decrease the child's tendency to tense the abdominal muscles. Sedation (sodium pentobarbital [Nembutal], 2 mg/kg) can be used to allay the child's anxiety and overcome voluntary guarding without masking the underlying process (Kottmeier, 1986).

The examination is started in an area opposite the suspected region of the inflamed appendix. Bowel sounds during the early acute phase of appendicitis are usually normal or occasionally may be high-pitched. Advanced inflammation and perforation result in diminished or absent bowel sounds. Tenderness at McBurney's point (right lower quadrant) is the most important finding on physical examination. With progressive inflammation, involuntary spasm is present, and with the onset of peritonitis rebound tenderness is noted. Rebound tenderness is elicited by applying deep pressure to the abdomen followed by a quick release of pressure. Pain (localized or general) felt upon release of pressure indicates peritoneal irritation. If the inflammation is located in the pelvic area, the abdominal examination may be negative. A rectal examination should be done last. School-age children are particularly modest and it is important to explain the need for rectal examination and to provide privacy. Although the rectal examination is questioned as a diagnostic tool, it remains an essential part of the examination to rule out other causes (Kottmeier, 1986).

Diagnostic tests will include blood studies, urinalysis, and radiographs of the chest and abdomen. A leukocytic count of 14,000 to 16,000 cells per mm^3 and pus cells present in the urine are significant findings. Radiographs will aid in excluding the possibility of pneumonia and may show the presence of a fecalith. The physician must also rule out other possible causes of acute abdominal pain, including severe constipation, urinary tract infection, acute gastroenteritis, pelvic inflammatory disease, and discomfort associated with ovulation.

Therapeutic Management

Perforation occurs frequently in children, so when a diagnosis of appendicitis is made an emergency appendectomy is scheduled. Contraindications to immediate surgery include the presence of a high fever, dehydration, or sepsis, all of which must be controlled before the child is anesthetized.

Preoperatively the patient usually receives sedation to relieve anxiety if the child was not sedated during the physical examination. The use of prophylactic antibiotics preoperatively has been shown to lower postoperative wound infection (Winslow et al, 1983). Prophylactic antibiotics are also given for 24 hours postoperatively in nonperforated appendicitis and 10 days for perforated or gangrenous appendicitis.

Strategies for Nursing Care

If perforation did not occur and there was no abscess, the child usually remains in the hospital for 3 to 4 days. Nursing care includes monitoring the intravenous fluids and vital signs; assessing the incision at dressing changes; encouraging ambulation, deep breathing, and coughing; and observing for signs of abscess formation (increased pain, restlessness, irritability, and a decrease in ambulation). Table 41-9 details an appropriate plan of care for the child following appendectomy.

The child will experience pain from the incision, and pain medication should be offered. Many children hesitate to ask for medication because they are afraid of a "shot." The nurse should obtain an order for oral medication to be given as soon as the child can tolerate liquids, usually 24 hours after surgery. Intravenous analgesia is another alternative.

The child with an abscess or perforated appendix will return from surgery with an intravenous line, a Penrose drain in the incision, and a nasogastric tube. The child will be given parenteral antibiotics for the period of hospitalization, usually 10 days. The child is acutely ill and needs intensive nursing care during the immediate postoperative period.

The child without peritonitis recovers rapidly and may return to school a week or two after surgery. Strenuous exercise should be curtailed for several weeks, however. School personnel will need to be informed of these restrictions to ensure the child's recovery.

Acute Infectious Diarrhea

Diarrhea is a frequent symptom of illness in infants and young children. Causes of diarrhea are numerous, one of which is the presence of infectious organisms. When diarrhea is presumed or known to be due to an infection, the terms infectious gastroenteritis and acute infectious diarrhea are used. Gastroenteritis can be mild or severe and is caused by a virus, bacteria, or parasite. It is an alteration of the gastrointestinal tract resulting in increased motility and rapid emptying of the intestinal contents. This rapid excretion interferes with the absorption of necessary nutrients, electrolytes, and water.

In children, infectious gastroenteritis is second only to upper respiratory tract infections as a cause of illness. Although the illness is generally benign and self-limited, it accounts for 3 to 5 per cent of pediatric hospital admissions. In developing countries it remains the largest single cause of death because of the prevalence of malnutrition, parasites, and poor hygiene (Silverman and Roy, 1983).

Etiology

The majority of acute diarrheal illnesses in infants and young children are of viral origin (Barnett, 1983). *Rotavirus* is the major cause of viral diarrhea and has been consistently associated with 50 to 70 per cent of wintertime gastroenteritis in children (Barnett, 1983). Rotavirus may cause a prolonged illness because of its ability to cause a secondary lactose malabsorption or monosaccharide intolerance (Davison, 1986). The Norwalk-like viruses are thought to be the etiologic agents in about one third of the epidemics of diarrhea (Davidson, 1986).

Organisms responsible for bacterial diarrhea are many and vary according to environmental factors. *Campylobacter* and *Yersinia* have recently been isolated more frequently because of improved culture techniques. *Shigella, Salmonella, Staphylococcus aureus, enterotoxigenic Escherichia coli* (ETEC), and pathogenic *E. coli* are other pathogens that cause bacterial diarrhea. *Giardia lamblia* and *Dientamoeba fragilis* are the most common parasitic agents affecting children.

Pathophysiology

The pathogenic mechanism of viral infection is not well understood. The infection damages or destroys some of the epithelial cells lining the intestinal tract. Recovery entails regeneration of epithelial cells and their associated enzyme systems. Illness continues while this regeneration occurs (48 to 96 hours).

Bacteria may act upon the intestinal mucosa, causing (1) enterotoxin production, (2) mucosal invasion and destruction, or (3) penetration.

Enterotoxin Production (Non-inflammatory)

In this mechanism the organism does not invade the mucosal epithelium but rather multiplies in the small intestine, then adheres to the mucosa, and releases an enterotoxin. The interaction between the toxin and the epithelium activates adenyl cyclase in the cell membrane, leading to an increase in cyclic adenosine monophosphate (cyclic AMP), which causes active electrolyte and water secretion. Diarrhea resulting from this process is called *secretory diarrhea* (Silverman and Roy, 1983). Action of the enterotoxin reduces the absorptive function of the surface area in the upper small bowel. The organisms that cause this reaction are cholera, enterotoxigenic *Escherichia coli* (predominates in infants), and certain strains of *Shigella* (e.g., *Shigella dysenteriae* I). In addition, food poisoning caused by the enterotoxins of *Staphylococcus aureus* or *Clostridium perfringens* is associated with this type of diarrhea. Diarrhea associated with these organisms is profuse and watery, leading to dehydration and acidosis, particularly in children under 2 years of age.

Invasion and Destruction of Epithelial Cells (Inflammatory)

In this process enterocytes (cells in the epithelium) are invaded by organisms, which results in mucosal inflammation and destruction. On histologic examination bacterial organisms are seen within epithelial cells where they multiply, causing superficial mucosal ulcerations (Silverman and Roy, 1983). Organisms that cause an inflammatory reaction in this way include *Shigella, Campylobacter jejuni, Salmonella,* certain strains of *E. coli* (e.g., enteroinvasive *E. coli*) and antibiotic-associated *Clostridium difficile* (Guerrant et al, 1986). The inflammatory nature of this type of infection often results in high fever and tenesmus associated with blood, mucus, and pus (leukocytes) in the stool on microscopic examination. Superficial ulcerations of the mucosa occur as a result of the inflammatory process.

Penetration and Systemic Invasion

This type of process involves penetration of the gut wall (often through Peyer's patches in the ileum) followed by multiplication of organisms intracellularly. Eventually the organism may reach the systemic circulation. Organisms causing infection in this way include *Salmonella typhi, Yersinia,* and *Campylobacter fetus.* Clinical symptoms include a febrile illness that often begins without diarrhea and is diagnosed by blood, bone marrow, or involved lymph node culture (Guerrant et al, 1986).

The pathophysiology of *Giardia lamblia* is currently under investigation. *Dientamoeba fragilis* has recently been identified and its pathophysiology is not yet understood.

Clinical Manifestations

The major complication from gastroenteritis, regardless of cause, is dehydration and accompanying electrolyte imbalance. Signs of dehydration are not always apparent to parents. These signs are depressed fontanels, sunken eyes, loss of skin turgor, oliguria, or concentrated urine. Parents should be informed of these signs and should report them. A decreased urinary output, indicated by fewer than six wet diapers per 24 hours or a period of longer than 4 hours without urination, is significant in an infant. Skin turgor can be checked by pinching the skin on the abdomen. If the skin returns to normal after being released, there is no loss of skin turgor. Skin that remains elevated after being released signifies loss of subcutaneous fluid and is indicative of dehydration. Other signs for parents to watch for are the absence of tears, increasing lethargy or irritability, and dry lips and tongue.

Potassium and sodium are normally lost through stool but replaced through oral intake. During diarrheal disease, these losses are greater than can be replaced by normal oral intake. Sodium losses in turn create additional extracellular fluid loss, compounding the problem of volume deficit. Potassium losses cause muscle weakness, abdominal distention, and possible electrocardiographic changes.

Transmission of Organisms

Children are particularly at risk for infections because subclinical infection in an adult may be transmitted to a child. Most organisms that cause diarrhea are spread by the fecal-oral route. When an organism can be spread by a relatively low dose or inoculum, person-to-person contact may be sufficient to transmit the disease. For example, *Shigella, Giardia,* and possibly *Campylobacter* are spread by direct contact. Transmission through contaminated food or water usually requires a larger dose or inoculum. An example is *Salmonella,* which is ingested with milk, meat, or eggs contaminated by the organisms during preparation or storage. The contamination may occur in the home or in commercial preparation. Staphylococcal gastroenteritis is caused by ingestion of *Staphylococcus.* Frequently, the foods affected are dairy products that have been stored improperly.

Diagnostic Assessment

Diagnosis is made largely by history. Parents report a large number of watery stools. These stools are frequently green from the excretion of bile. Stools resulting from bacterial infection may contain pus and, infrequently, blood. The child often has a history of vomiting and a low-grade fever. An accurate history is important in differentiating normal stool changes, which occur with age and diet changes, from diarrhea, which reflects pathology.

Routine total and differential white blood cell counts are of little value in identifying the causative organism. The total white blood cell count may be normal, increased, or decreased. Over 50 per cent of children with infectious diarrhea have an increased percentage of band forms (immature white blood cells) (Feigin and Stoller, 1987).

Laboratory studies include microscopic examination of the stool for leukocytes, examination for occult blood by the guaiac test (Hemoccult), stool culture and sensitivity, and stool virology. Stool pH of 5.5 or less and a positive Clinitest (0.5 per cent glucose or greater) suggest impaired carbohydrate utilization, which may be due to a non-infectious process or be found in children with acquired lactase deficiency that follows persistent infectious diarrhea (Feigin and Stoller, 1987). The presence of fat and neutrophils suggests steatorrhea or an inflammatory process. A stool that is positive for polymorphonuclear (PMN) cells is usually sent for cultures for *Salmonella, Shigella,* and *Campylobacter.* A fresh stool specimen is required when ova and parasites are suspected (which must be delivered to the laboratory immediately), or the stool can be put into a fixating solution for transport.

Therapeutic Management

The management of infectious gastroenteritis has three components: (1) to maintain or restore fluid and electrolyte balance, (2) to restore the bowel to normal functioning, and (3) to prevent the infection of others in contact with the child. Mild cases of the disease can be treated at home by the parents. While the child is actively vomiting, little is given by mouth for 2 to 6 hours. Fluids recommended for parents to use at home are various soft drinks or clear juices and flavored gelatin water.

The parents should be informed of specific minimal fluid intake required for the individual infant. Controversy exists over how to reintroduce the oral feedings. Most often small frequent feedings are given, yet larger quantities offered less frequently may be recommended owing to the fact that frequent feedings have the potential to induce peristalsis. Also, the timing of advancing from clear fluids is debated. Early reintroduction of feeding has generally replaced the concept of "resting the bowel." Feeding after 24 to 36 hours may provide a surge of diarrhea, yet the children recover more quickly.

Breastfed infants with mild diarrhea are able to remain on breast milk. The diarrhea will usually resolve when the infant takes nothing orally for several hours and then continues with breastfeeding. Other infants advance from clear fluids to a lactose hydrolyzed milk or soy substitute after 24 hours and toddlers to a bland milk-free diet. Bananas, rice, applesauce, and toast (known as BRAT) or rice, applesauce, and bananas (known as RAB) are diets that have traditionally been prescribed for children following diarrhea and continue to be used.

Infants and children with severe diarrhea, those with symptoms of dehydration, and those in whom vomiting accompanies diarrhea are usually hospitalized for observation and fluid and electrolyte therapy. Medical treatment during hospitalization is aimed at restoring normal fluid and electrolyte balance and allowing the bowel to resume normal function. This is accomplished by the use of normal saline intravenous feeding with potassium and bicarbonate added as necessary. Before intravenous potassium is added, kidney function must be established.

It has recently been demonstrated that dehydration from diarrhea can also be treated effectively using a glucose-electrolyte oral solution (Tolia and Dubois, 1985; Listernick et al, 1986). The new oral rehydrating solution provides a 2 per cent glucose solution, which enhances sodium transport in the small intestine (glucose-coupled sodium transport is the physiologic basis of oral rehydration therapy). If sufficient sodium is provided, water will follow the osmotic gradient produced by the sodium transport, thus maximizing the absorptive potential of the gut.

Oral rehydrating solutions have been evaluated in developed and developing countries. The composition of the oral rehydration solution recommended by the Diarrhea Disease Control Program of the World Health Organization contains sodium, 90 mM/L; potassium, 20 mM/L; chloride, 80 mM/L; bicarbonate, 30 mM/L; and glucose, 111 mM/L (2 per cent) (Robson, 1987). The amount and rate of oral rehydration vary according to the patient's condition. The purpose is to meet maintenance requirements, replenish previous losses, and meet ongoing requirements. Vomiting that occurs in the first 2 hours of rehydration is not a contraindication to continue therapy.

As with the child treated at home, the hospitalized child gradually advances to a more solid diet. The introduction of milk may cause the child's diarrhea to begin again because of possible disaccharidase deficiency. For this reason, formula may be introduced at a lower strength, with slow advance to full strength. In some instances it may be necessary to give the infant a soy formula until the deficiency is corrected naturally. It has, however, increasingly been recognized that steadily advancing the diet hastens recovery and prevents iatrogenic malnutrition.

Major Nursing Diagnoses for Acute Infectious Diarrhea

Altered elimination: diarrhea, *related to*
- *the secretory action of enterotoxin upon the intestinal mucosa*
- *inflammation of epithileal cells in the intestine*
- *penetration and systemic invasion of pathogens*

Potential for injury: electrolyte and hydrogen ion imbalance, *related to*
- *loss of Na^+, K^+, and HCO_3^- in diarrheal stools*
- *increased production of keto acids associated with starvation and dehydration*
- *increase in lactic acid associated with decreased tissue perfusion*
- *retention of non-volatile H^+ associated with decreased urine output*

Knowledge deficit, *related to care of the child with mild acute infectious diarrhea*

Altered comfort: pain, *associated with abdominal cramping*

Potential for infection: transmission of gastroenteritis to others, *related to*
- *inadequate handwashing*
- *inadequate disinfecting of contaminated articles*

Impaired skin integrity, *related to repeated perineal contact with acidic stools*

Strategies for Nursing Care

Acute infectious diarrhea may sometimes be avoided by instituting basic hygiene measures. The nurse functioning in a variety of settings is in an excellent position to teach families and children correct methods of storage and preparation of meat and dairy products. Discussing the importance of handwashing after diapering, after using the toilet, and before food preparation and feeding is an important measure in decreasing the frequency of gastroenteritis. In addition, good handwashing and proper disposal of contaminated articles by personnel within institutions will discourage the spread of the disease.

Teaching to Support Care at Home. During the course of an illness, specific instructions are needed by parents who are managing gastroenteritis at home. Detailed dietary guidelines must be given. Other important information includes handwashing technique and proper disposal of soiled articles. Families should also be familiar with the signs of dehydration and instructed to seek additional assistance if these signs are present or if the diarrhea continues beyond a few days.

When giving soft drinks to the child with diarrhea, the parents should be told to allow the drink to become "flat" by stirring until the carbonation is no longer present. Gelatin water is made by mixing two tablespoons of flavored gelatin powder in eight ounces of water. It is important to inform parents that the child's stools will be the color of the gelatin water, and this is not cause for alarm. Liquids should be offered at room temperature because cold liquids increase bowel motility.

Monitoring Fluid, Electrolyte, and Hydrogen Ion Status. The child with dehydration and electrolyte and hydrogen ion imbalances will usually be hospitalized for intravenous therapy. Nursing responsibilities include administration of intravenous fluids and electrolytes and, with the physician, evaluation of this therapy.

Monitoring of fluid balance necessitates accurate daily weights, recording of intake and output, and close monitoring of specific gravity. The most accurate assessment of fluid loss is through body weight. Weight is the basis for assessing the success of management during the acute phase of the disease, and weighing must be done on an accurate scale with the child completely undressed. The child is weighed on admission, and all subsequent weighings should be done on the same scale. A precise record of oral and parenteral intake and of output is important. Stool and urinary output is most easily measured by weighing the diapers dry and again after soiling. This eliminates the difficulties associated with attempting to maintain a urine collection bag on a small child. Urine specific gravity (USG) is done to measure the state of hydration; measurement can easily be done on the unit with a fractometer. The USG reflects the density of the urine: the higher the reading, the more concentrated the urine. A USG of 1.025 or greater is indicative of dehydration, with a reading of approximately 1.015 indicating normal hydration. As intravenous fluids are begun, the USG will decrease. During the acute phase of hospitalization USG should be checked every 4 hours.

Monitoring electrolyte and hydrogen ion status entails assessment for signs of imbalance. See Tables 30-2 and 30-3 in Chapter 30 for clinical manifestations of hyponatremia, hypokalemia, and metabolic acidosis. In addition, the nurse can monitor results of serum electrolyte studies.

Providing Comfort. During the acute phase of excessive stooling, the infant or child can be expected to experience discomfort from abdominal cramping. In addition, lack of oral intake will be frustrating to most infants and small children. These discomforts are best addressed by non-pharmacologic means.

During periods without oral feedings, the infant's need to suck is not decreased; not being able to do so is often a source of great frustration to the child. Offering a pacifier or allowing the child who normally sucks the thumb to continue to do so often relieves some of the frustration.

Although the child's activity is more limited if an intravenous line is used, restrictions are minimized by using catheters rather than needles. Normalization of activity enhances the young child's motor coping patterns and reduces frustration. Parents can be shown safe positions in which to hold an infant without disturbing the intravenous line, thus providing security and comfort.

Preventing Transmission of Organisms. Hospitalized children with gastroenteritis are in enteric isolation. Proper handwashing and disposal of soiled articles will prevent the spread of the disease. Parents need to be instructed in these techniques and on the rationale for their use. (See Chapter 27 for further discussion of principles of isolation.)

Preventing and Treating Perineal Excoriation. The stools in diarrhea are acidic and irritating to the skin around the perineum. If the child is not cleaned promptly after defecation, the skin quickly becomes excoriated. To prevent this, the area should be gently cleaned immediately with soap and water and dried thoroughly. Excoriation frequently responds quickly to air-drying; the area can simply be cleaned and then left uncovered to the air. The area is very painful and the child will be uncomfortable during diaper changes. Applying a protective ointment to the area will keep the diaper from sticking to the skin area and also prevent contact of the skin with stool.

Gastrointestinal Dysfunctional Disorders

Children who have gastrointestinal dysfunctional disorders are generally healthy children with chronic digestive symptoms. Although only a few of the problems are life-threatening, they can cause considerable personal stress and interruption in family life. Accurate delineation of the problem and early prescription of an effective strategy can allay anxiety and may well prevent a brief interlude of dysfunction from developing into an entrenched maladaptive problem.

The following conditions are categorized as dysfunctional: (1) colic; (2) gastroesophageal reflux (chalasia); (3) irritable bowel syndrome; and (4) chronic constipation.

Colic

Colic is characterized by vigorous crying and drawing the legs up to the abdomen as if the baby were in severe pain. It occurs in infants under 3 months old and rarely persists past 6 months of age, although parents cannot be guaranteed of this. It usually begins in the first 3 weeks of life and is suspected to be the result of paroxysmal abdominal cramping, although a specific cause is rarely uncovered. Crying is intermittent, occurring one or more times a day, with each episode lasting from 30 minutes to 2 hours (Schmitt, 1986). Gas may rumble in the stomach, and temporary relief seems to occur if this is passed. Some infants can be quieted with handling but will cry incessantly as soon as they are put down. Colicky babies are healthy and between crying spells are usually happy. If the crying is continuous, other causes should be suspected.

Pathophysiology and Etiology

Factors thought to be associated with colic include the absorptive immaturity of the gastrointestinal tract, food allergy, maternal factors, infant characteristics, and feeding practices.

Absorptive Immaturity. In comparison with the adult, the normal term infant has malabsorption of many nutrient classes. Virtually all infants have some degree of lactose malabsorption (Balistieri et al, 1983). This gradually improves until maximum efficiency is achieved by 3 to 4 months of age (Maclean and Fink, 1980). Similarly, most term infants fail to absorb as much as 15 per cent of ingested fat from formula, in contrast to the adult's normal malabsorption of 5 per cent. Part of this is due to a reduced bile acid pool. (Balistieri et al, 1983). The delayed appearance of colic may be related to an infant's arousal state as described by Carey (1972) and Brazelton (1972). As the infant develops, the state of arousal is more prominent, at which time there may be the "sudden appearance of pain" starting at 2 to 3 weeks.

Allergy. The extent to which food allergy contributes to colic continues to be studied and debated. It is speculated that the ability for whole protein to cross the mucosal barrier in the intestinal tract of a newborn renders the infant more susceptible to allergy (Jakobsson and Lindberg, 1978). Jakobsson and Lindberg (1983) have published a series of studies which suggest that up to two thirds of colicky infants are allergic to cow's milk proteins. Only 18 per cent improved on a soy formula, but 53 per cent were colic-free on a hydrolyzed casein formula (Nutramigen). These studies have, however, been criticized because of a selection bias. Furthermore, allergy is questioned as a cause because colic occurs with equal frequency in bottlefed and breastfed infants.

Maternal Factors. If the mother's pregnancy or delivery was particularly arduous, if perinatal complications have developed, and if the mother has been sleep deprived, her ability to tolerate a crying infant may be limited. Although early studies by Paradise (1966) failed to pinpoint the maternal personality as the cause of colic in the infant, in many instances it appears that parental frustration and anger following the appearance of colic may aggravate symptoms or at least affect the family's tolerance of it. The physical demands made of the mother or the amount of support she is receiving may well contribute to the likelihood of the baby's being viewed as colicky by the mother.

Infant Characteristics. The infant's temperament also influences the degree to which colic will affect the child. The average infant cries about 2 hours daily at 2 weeks. This increases to 3 hours at 6 weeks, with some infants crying for close to a mean of 4 hours (Brazelton, 1972). In careful studies, Brazelton has documented earlier observations that infants are born with different temperaments. These differences may also be indicated in utero by fetal activity levels.

Sometimes a parent's main concern is differences observed between a first child and the second with the first child's characteristics being viewed the norm. If the first child was particularly placid, the second baby's greater irritability may be labeled as "sick." Certain infants as a group are particularly difficult to console; these include infants born small for gestational age and others with some element of neurologic impairment.

Feeding Practices. Occasionally colic can be connected with improper feeding techniques or inadequate burping, but this cause is not nearly as prevalent as was once thought, as changes in diet or burping and feeding methods rarely eliminate colic. Rapidly growing infants who require very large volumes of milk may experience discomfort.

Diagnostic Assessment

The vast majority of infants with symptoms of colic have a self-limiting syndrome of multifactorial causation. The distinction from diseases requiring investigation or remediation begins with a careful history.

Careful determination of the timing and volume of feeds provides helpful clues concerning overfeeding, underfeeding, or chaotic schedule, all of which may be contributing to the child's symptoms. Colic associated with improper feeding methods, although rare, is readily halted by teaching better technique. Caregivers should be asked to demonstrate the feeding process to rule out this possible source of colic. A detailed history of daily events helps establish any pattern to the colic attacks or any precipitating factors and to document caregiver reactions and efforts taken to relieve the crying.

On physical examination, comparison of height, weight, and head circumference with the norms is the single most valuable tool. If the infant's development is normal and the child is well nourished, most concerns for underlying disease can be eliminated.

Therapeutic Management and Strategies for Nursing Care

Despite the fact that colic disappears spontaneously and is frequently given only minor attention by health care professionals, it often has a strong emotional impact on the family. Any family that has lived through only a few days of the crying episodes of an infant who is unresponsive to any efforts to comfort or console, feels extremely exhausted and emotionally drained. This is especially true for the main caregiver. The disruption that a crying, irritable infant causes to family relationships and routines produces a vicious cycle of fatigue, frustration, anger, and helplessness. This can be destructive to the functioning of the family unit if empathetic intervention is not begun early and maintained until the colicky period is outgrown.

Intervention should have three foci: (1) emotional support to family members, especially the primary caregiver; (2) efforts to maintain healthy attachment; and (3) efforts to reduce or prevent colic episodes.

Providing Emotional Support. Emotional support involves reassurances to the caregiver that despite the crying and pain, the infant is gaining weight and developing normally. Regular emphasis should be placed on the fact that colic is not the result of poor mothering, and that maternal feelings of inadequacy, anger, or periodic dislike of the baby and of mothering are universal. The caregiver should be offered regular opportunities to talk about feelings and be encouraged to do so. Some communities have parental stress hot lines (COPE, CALM), of which parents of colicky infants should be informed. They should be encouraged to keep the phone number available even if they never need to use it. Some parents find solace just in knowing there are resources in case the stress becomes too much.

The caregiver should be urged to spend time away from the colicky infant on a fairly regular basis. Some relief from constant full responsibility makes most caregivers better able to handle themselves when they are "on duty." Some parents need help to overcome guilt feelings associated with "getting away" for awhile.

Recognizing those times when it is harder to cope helps some parents achieve better control or think of ways to circumvent total responsibility for infant care at those times. Situations that are commonly more stressful include the dinner hour, premenstrual days, holidays, and days when routine is disrupted.

Fostering Attachment. Fostering attachment is important, as frequent negative feelings can eventually disrupt development of a healthy parent-child attachment. Pointing out the infant's desirable features and signs of normal development regularly helps the parents view the child more positively, which encourages attachment feelings. Acknowledging and praising good interaction between parent and infant as well as helping the parent notice how the infant responds to parental overtures also nurture healthy bonds.

Preventing or Reducing Episodes of Colic. Efforts to prevent or reduce colic episodes require experimentation, as the success of a given method is highly individualistic. Some infants respond to measures that stimulate peristalsis. This may be achieved by carrying the infant close,* placing the baby prone over a warm towel or warm water bottle, or giving the infant a few ounces of warm diluted tea. Much caution should be used with a warm water bottle, as burns can occur with too much heat. The infant's skin does not tolerate as much heat as that of older children or adults. The warm water bottle should be securely closed and covered with a towel before placing the baby on it. The infant's skin should be checked frequently to ensure that overheating of the skin does not occur. Another suggested approach is walking and placing the infant over the caregiver's arm, which provides gentle pressure on the abdomen (Gillies, 1987).

Other infants show improvement when their position is changed often, when they are burped using the shoulder method and with massaging rather than patting, and when smaller feedings are offered more frequently. Taking time to relax and play with the baby before beginning feeding and placing the baby in an

* An infant carrier allows the caregiver to keep the infant close in either a chest or back position while leaving the hands free to carry out other activities.

Box 41-9

Adaptation of Caregiver's Response to Reduce Colic

HOLD THE BABY FOR ALL FUSSY CRYING EPISODES

Taubman (1984) reduced crying by 70 per cent by advising parents not to let their baby cry. Letting the colicky baby "cry himself to sleep" is thought to perpetuate and worsen the problem. A prompt response, gentle motion, and touching (i.e., by using a front infant carrier) are recommended. Front carriers are preferred over backpacks because eye contact can be maintained and the infant can hear the maternal heart beat and be cushioned by the mother's breasts.

CARRY THE BABY 3 HOURS PER DAY WHEN HE IS NOT CRYING

This practice of supplemental carrying has been found to reduce total crying by 50%.

DISCOURAGE DAYTIME SLEEPING FOR MORE THAN 3 CONSECUTIVE HOURS

Colicky periods at night should be shifted to daytime hours by adjusting sleeping times. Nighttime sleeping can also be encouraged by not permitting the infant to sleep between 8:00 P.M. and 10:00 P.M.

DISCOURAGE OVERFEEDING

Advise parents not to feed the infant unless 2½ hours have elapsed (2 hours for breastfed babies) since the last feeding. A bloated stomach can cause discomfort; therefore, the stomach should be allowed to empty between feedings.

URGE THE CAREGIVER TO ENLIST HELP AND GET ADEQUATE REST AND RELAXATION

(From Schmitt, 1986.)

infant seat for at least 30 minutes after feedings are sometimes effective in reducing colic episodes. The caregiver's response to crying and management of sleep patterns can also be adjusted to reduce colic. (See Box 41-9.)

Glycerine suppositories (child size) or digital stimulation of the rectum with the little finger to relieve flatus may be effective in infants whose colic episodes seem to be associated with abdominal distention (Rowell, 1978).

Some infants can be distracted successfully from their colicky episodes with brightly colored wrapping paper, pictures of varying complexity and depth, or music of varied rhythm and loudness. Some colicky infants respond to the rhythm of an automatic infant swing or to being placed (with proper securement and continued presence of the caregiver) on top of a running clothes dryer. (In this case it may be the sound, vibration, or warmth that quiets the baby.)

In some circumstances management includes a change of formula. The rationale for making more than a single formula change is highly questionable. In severe cases a trial of casein hydrolysate formula (Nutramigen) may be contemplated, although it is prohibitively expensive (Eastham et al, 1983). Similarly, elimination of cow's milk protein from the diet of breastfeeding mothers may help a small number of infants. In either case, a milk challenge with recurrence of symptoms is required before cause and effect can be presumed.

In cases refractory to the approaches outlined above, the judicious use of a mild sedative for the infant may carry a family through the most difficult period. This may include the use of phenobarbital elixir or one of the antihistamines, such as hydroxyzine Atarax) or diphenhydramine (Benylan). The efficacy of proprietary preparations such as Gripe Water likely derives from the alcohol content. Antispasmodics such as dycyclamine hydrochloride (Bentyl) are widely used. However, there is increasing reluctance to use either antihistamines or antispasmodics because of a concern about their association with infantile apnea. Atropine-like agents should be avoided, as they frequently give rise to constipation by immobilizing the gut, which relies on increased transit to compensate for some of its other immaturities.

The most effective tool available to the family with a colicky infant is professional support. Scheduled weekly visits or telephone calls can contribute to their growth as confident caregivers during this difficult period.

Gastroesophageal Reflux (Chalasia)

Gastroesophageal reflux (GER) occurs as a result of relaxation or incompetence of the lower esophageal sphincter, permitting reflux of gastric contents into the esophagus. This condition may exist with or without a hiatal hernia. Its cause is not known. Although many infants have some degree of incompetence of the lower esophageal sphincter, in more severe cases the infant is threatened because of chronic esophageal inflammation or pulmonary aspiration. Failure to thrive may also result, requiring intervention.

Pathophysiology

The advent of newer diagnostic techniques has confused the once simplistic picture of gastroesophageal reflux. A physiologic high-pressure zone of 1 to 3 cm of the distal esophagus is termed the lower esophageal sphincter (LES). Pressures in this zone increase steadily from birth to 2 months of age in healthy infants. However, competence of the valve depends upon coordinated relaxation and closure. The entrance of the esophagus into the stomach at an acute angle enhances effectiveness of closure. Delayed gastric emptying is associated with reflux (Hillemeir et al, 1981).

Some reflux of gastric contents has been shown to occur even in healthy subjects. Total number and duration of episodes of reflux, documented by prolonged pH monitoring, seem to be important determinants in the development of esophagitis (Herbst, 1981). This in turn may affect the functioning of the LES. Shortened esophagus is likely a consequence of chronic esophagitis from chronic reflux rather than the cause. Likewise, a demonstrable hiatus hernia is probably an associated factor rather than a causative one.

Most infants will improve spontaneously. In healthy infants regurgitation should have stopped by the time the child begins to walk at 10 to 12 months. Neurologically impaired children have a much higher prevalence of significant reflux. In fact, some authors distinguish two groups of children, those with simple reflux and those in which it occurs in association with other significant problems. Many of these are older children (Herbst, 1981).

Clinical Manifestations

Signs of GER usually appear in the first week of life and most commonly consist of chronic vomiting or regurgitation. There are usually no signs of discomfort or gastrointestinal dysfunction, and the infant readily eats again if given the opportunity after vomiting. Vomiting is usually quite forceful and does not contain bile. Because of a possible significant loss of calories the infant may show weight loss and eventually failure to thrive. A variety of cardiorespiratory symptoms may accompany the vomiting. Reflux into the pharynx predisposes to aspiration and may cause respiratory symptoms, including apnea, bradycardia, SIDS (sudden infant death syndrome), severe aspiration episodes, recurrent upper respiratory infections, and aspiration pneumonia. Repeated reflux of gastric acid can cause irritation of the esophagus leading to esophagitis and esophageal bleeding, manifested as hematemesis or melena (blood in stools).

Diagnostic Assessment

The presence of reflux is evaluated through use of a barium esophagogram. Because reflux is an intermittent phenomena, it may not occur at the exact time that the barium esophagogram is done. Therefore, the sensitivity of this method is in question (Johnson et al, 1981). Reflux can also be evaluated by using the Tuttle test, in which a probe is inserted (2 to 3 cm proximal to the esophageal sphincter) to measure reflux of acid from the stomach. With an indwelling electrode, reflux episodes can be evaluated before, during, and after eating with the child placed in varying positions (Filston and Izant, 1985). Ambulatory pH monitoring systems are available, making home monitoring an acceptable alternative (Petersen, 1986).

Medical Management. Medical management of the infant with GER is aimed at reducing the likelihood of reflux and its consequences. This is done by use of (1) cereal-thickened formula, (2) small-volume feedings, (3) slow feedings; (4) burping during feedings (after each 1 to 1½ ounces) and after each feeding; and (5) an upright (30° angle) prone position after feeding.

It has been demonstrated that the use of a slant board and prone position (Fig. 41-22) is superior to the use of the traditional infant seat (Orenstein et al, 1983). Propping against pillows and setting an infant upright in a standard infant seat may in fact cause an increase in intra-abdominal pressure because the baby tends to slide down into a slumped position (Kurfiss-Daniels, 1982). The prone, slant position is used for one to several hours after each feed, depending on the severity of the problem. Antacids between feeding are sometimes required to treat esophagitis. Symptoms and weight gain are monitored carefully during this trial period of conservative medical management.

The length of conservative treatment varies. GER resolves in most infants by 18 months of age if treated medically with good positional therapy. However, it is recommended that children with an esophageal stricture or be treated surgically.

Surgical Management. Unsuccessful medical therapy of 6 to 8 weeks usually warrants re-evaluation and often surgical intervention (e.g., Nissen-Hill fundoplication), depending on the severity of complications. In this procedure the distal esophagus is wrapped with the adjacent gastric fundus and secured with plicating sutures to create a new gastroesophageal junction and thereby curtail reflux. During the immediate postoperative period, gastric decompression by nasogastric tube is necessary to prevent tearing of the sutures. A gastrostomy is not performed unless there is a particular feeding problem.

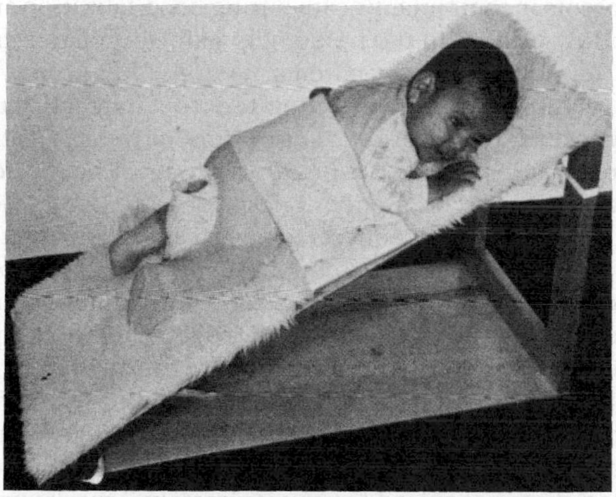

***Figure* 41-22.** Positional treatment for gastroesophageal reflux. The child is straddled on a padded peg on the board and restrained in this position. (From Behrman RE, Vaughan VC (eds): *Nelson Textbook of Pediatrics.* 13th ed. Philadelphia, WB Saunders, 1987.)

Strategies for Nursing Care

Nurses participate in all phases of care. Assisting parents to promote the child's normal development and helping them understand the treatment modalities are important nursing roles.

Nursing Strategies Related to Medical Treatment. Management during conservative medical therapy requires careful monitoring and documentation of nursing observations. Confinement of the infant to the prone, slant position requires specialized nursing care. Pressure areas around the straddle bar that keeps the infant from slipping downward must be well padded. Also, these infants tend to develop edema of the feet and legs; therefore, they should be exercised by elevating and lowering them before feedings. Torticollis should be prevented by frequent turning of the child's head from side to side if the child tends to turn to only one side (Kurfiss-Daniels, 1982).

Of great concern are the restrictions imposed by this position and its interference in the normal growth and development of the child. Appropriate toys and activities must be made available at eye level, and a special play time should be planned before feedings. Cuddling and caressing can be done while the baby is on the board by putting arms around the infant and bringing the face close to the infant.

Parents may resist this form of therapy because they feel it is hurting the infant. Reassurance and repeated explanations about the purpose of the therapy will often be necessary. Ongoing involvement of the parents in their infant's care during hospitalization and follow-up care in the home help gain acceptance and faster cooperation by parents.

Nursing Strategies Related to Surgical Management. A major focus of postoperative care is the preservation of good respiratory function. The surgical procedure is commonly done prior to the age when cooperation with requests to cough and deep breathe is possible; therefore, frequent suctioning and repositioning every 2 hours are necessary. An additional important measure is postural drainage. This should be done prior to feedings to prevent regurgitation.

Gradually small amounts of oral feedings are given and the child is observed for any signs of intolerance such as distention, vomiting, or discomfort. A blenderized diet is required for approximately 2 weeks until the operative swelling has subsided.

It is essential that older children be encouraged to chew their food thoroughly when they eat. Parents should be advised that the child may complain of a bloated sensation after eating. This is due to delayed gastric emptying. Hiccuping may also be occasionally seen but gradually resolves. Parents are advised to see the surgeon for follow-up care and further evaluation.

Irritable Bowel Syndrome (IBS)

Irritable bowel syndrome is characterized by intermittent episodes of large, loose stools or crampy abdominal pain. Although there is an increase in numbers of stools per day there is no evidence of malabsorption or impaired growth. In the toddler, recurrent diarrhea is the common presentation of irritable bowel syndrome, whereas school-age children usually have recurrent, abdominal pain.

Etiology and Pathophysiology

The cause of this condition is unknown. Explanations for the phenomenon include disordered motility, rapid transit, artificial sweeteners, dietary factors, emotional factors, and family dysfunction. An explanation for toddler diarrhea has been given by Cohen and associates (1979), who noted resolution of symptoms in infants put on a high-fat diet in preparation for a 72-hour stool collection for fat analysis. A retrospective analysis of the clinic population by these authors showed that many of the toddlers had been on diets with calories derived from fat accounting for less than 27 per cent of total caloric intake. When put on 4 grams of fat per kilogram per day the stool pattern returned to normal in 80 per cent of the patients. The postulated mechanism was the effect of fat in delaying gastric emptying time and thus influencing transit through the small bowel.

Another cause has been suggested by Greene and Ghishon (1983), who have identified a group of children with excessive fluid intake, which has overwhelmed their intestinal capacity for absorption of fluid or solute. Children in this group were drinking an average of 196 ml/kg compared with an observed pattern of 91 ml/kg for the normal child of this age. Restriction of fluid to normal amounts restored most patients to an acceptable bowel pattern.

An excessive number of children are considered allergic and placed on progressively more restrictive diets as an ever widening selection of food groups appear to be responsible for the essentially random nature of the loose stools (Lloyd-Still, 1979). Often the child with irritable bowel syndrome has a parent with the same condition, and in some instances children with irritable colon had colic as an infant. No sex difference is noted until adolescence, when females outnumber males.

Undoubtedly, some of these children's symptoms result from previous infection with subclinical damage to the small bowel. Examining intestinal mucosa by scanning electron microscopy, Poley (1983) noted evidence of excessive bacterial adherence to the mucosal surface, increased cell shedding associated with more surface mucus, and damage to the brush border. Disturbed fat absorption follows viral infection, possibly as a result of impaired bile acid uptake. However, it is possible that initial fat intolerance eventually resolves and a state of chronic diarrhea persists because of prolonged fat deprivation.

Clinical Manifestations and Therapeutic Management

Clinical manifestations vary according to the age of the child, as does management. The presentation and management of IBS in the toddler and school-age child are therefore presented separately.

Toddler

Recurrent diarrhea is the common presentation of irritable bowel syndrome in toddlers. The definition relies on the observation of an increased number of loose movements lasting greater than 3 weeks without evidence of malabsorption or impaired growth. The usual onset occurs at 6 to 18 months. The problem starts insidiously. The parent describes three to eight stools per day, which initially are slightly formed but become progressively watery throughout the day (Jonas and Dever-Haber, 1982). The child often has an intense thirst. Toddlers generally do not become dehydrated, nor do they lose weight unless their diet is markedly restricted. Infants with diarrhea or dietary restrictions are more easily affected adversely.

The goal of management is to have the child on a diet that does not have excess fluid and contains sufficient fat. This may be accomplished easily by suggesting that the child have some form of fat with every meal, such as formula or homogenized milk, peanut butter, bacon, margarine, or butter. A maximum of 8 oz per day of juice and sweetened drinks should be allowed, with the rest of the desired fluid offered as water. Some children should no longer be given the "bottle" as this fosters habitual excessive fluid intake. The rare person with a strong family history of the irritable bowel syndrome may respond to the judicious inclusion of increased fiber in the diet. By contrast, some toddlers seem exquisitely sensitive to large morsels of chewed food, such as raisins or carrots, which may be eliminated from the diet or pureed.

School-Age Child

Recurrent abdominal pain (RAP) is described as repeated complaints of nonspecific stomachaches. When RAP occurs at least three times over a period of 3 months and the pain is severe enough to interfere with normal functioning, it is considered RAP. The pain is usually periumbilical, although location is variable. It usually is not associated with eating, a bowel movement, or any particular experience. The stool varies in consistency, and constipation may occur. Other symptoms, such as headaches, dizziness, blurred vision, and dysuria or frequency, may also be present. On abdominal palpation there is often vague tenderness but without muscle guarding.

Common personality traits in children with RAP are heightened sensitivity, lowered self-image, and an intense concern for friends and family suggestive of a sense of insecurity in the child (Barbero and McKay, 1983). Management of these children calls for open supportive communication with the family. Antispasmodics may benefit some children, but many respond to increased dietary fiber and supportive open communication.

Strategies of Nursing Care

Nurses can provide supportive counseling for families who are faced with trying to alter their basic approach to a child's dietary habits. It is difficult to change a toddler's habits because of the ritualism in this phase of development. Parents can be encouraged to replace the bottle and the usual sweet juices with water from a cup and simultaneously engage the toddler in favorite activities to divert attention from the habit.

Families with school-age children can benefit from the nurse's support and encouragement as they cope with their child's pain and vague symptoms. The pain should be accepted as real, and strategies to strengthen the child's self-image and sense of security are used. (See Chapter 13 on parenting and Chapter 16 on self-esteem.) The nurse can help the child and parents identify environmental factors that might be exacerbating the symptoms. The child's school situation and relationships with friends and family may be stressful and should be discussed. Interviewing the child separately from the parents is often appropriate.

The nurse should recognize that some families may need additional professional counseling and should make an appropriate referral to community resources.

Constipation

Some infants and children have recurrent or chronic constipation during which stool is passed infrequently or, if passed daily, consists of hard, small masses. Often the cause is a diet that contains too much milk or insufficient amounts of fluids or bulk-forming foods.

Etiology and Therapeutic Management

Conditions that make defecation painful may promote constipation, as the child withholds feces to avoid pain. The most common condition is anal fissures that have developed during the previous passage of hard stool. Inspection of the anus to identify fissures is done by placing a thumb on either side of the anus and retracting the anal tissues laterally. Until healing is complete, an anesthetic ointment and stool softener may be prescribed to relieve defecatory distress.

Mechanical obstruction may also precipitate constipation. Rectal stenosis and Hirschsprung disease are occasional etiologic factors. Rectal stenosis can be confirmed by digital examination. The little finger will be difficult to insert into the anus, and it will seem to meet with resistance in the presence of stenosis. The stenosis is corrected by frequent dilation of the anal canal with the finger until the stenosis is eliminated. Hirschsprung disease and rectal malformations are discussed earlier in this chapter.

In older infants and children, constipation may be due to a chronic misuse of laxatives by apprehensive parents or a psychologic response to faulty toilet training, producing poor bowel evacuation habits.

Regardless of the cause of constipation, measures may be taken to promote adequate defecation while the etiologic factor is being remedied. If medications are used, docusate sodium (Colace) is a frequent first choice as a stool softener. Stimulant laxatives stronger than senna glycerides (Senokot) should not be employed. (There is a common tendency to use glycerine suppositories excessively in young infants.) Accordingly, suppositories should be recommended only with caution against their overuse. If impaction exists, an isotonic enema solution (1 level teaspoon of salt to a pint of water) may be administered to clear the bowel. It should be stressed, however, that most constipation in infancy is readily managed by diet alone.

Strategies of Nursing Care

An important role of the nurse in the prevention of constipation is to counsel parents about elimination patterns and dietary habits during well child visits. After 6 months of age, infants can have some foods that are finely chopped rather than puréed to increase bulk. Corn syrup or molasses may be added to milk for infants who are prone to constipation, although there has been some concern about botulism spores in these products. Nurses can advise parents to offer prunes or prune juice regularly to infants who have hard stools. Providing fluids in addition to milk is an important preventive measure at all ages.

Diets adequate in fiber constitute another preventive measure to encourage for older children. There can be no doubt that the greatest deficiency in the standard North American child's diet is the absence of fiber. This is probably the biggest problem of the so-called "junk" foods. Even the much maligned "fast foods" probably provide sufficient vitamins, minerals, and protein, but they consistently lack a significant amount of fiber. High-fiber diets have not been well studied in infants, however, and there is concern about binding of essential nutrients if high-fiber diets are given to infants (Cummings and Stephen, 1981).

Parents may also need information about the normal variations in bowel habits among children. Excessive attention and coerciveness about toilet training should be avoided (see Chapter 6 for a discussion of toilet training).

Any treatment approaches to be carried out at home should be explained (i.e., suppository, other medication, an enema). Both verbal and written instruction should be given to parents regarding treatment measures to be conducted at home. One or two demonstrations should also be given if parents seem unsure of instructions or if the nurse judges it necessary.

Malabsorptive Alterations

Intestinal malabsorption in a mild and transient form may produce only temporary indigestion. If it is severe and persistent, it can, however, lead to serious consequences, such as nutritional deficits and clinical starvation. Malabsorption occurs when there is a disruption in any step of the digestive process that interferes with the absorption of water and electrolytes, vitamins, minerals, carbohydrates, proteins, and fats. Malabsorptive alterations have diverse causes, including inadequate production of digestive juices, growth of organisms, inflammation of the lining of the intestines, disturbed lymphatic or vascular flow, loss of surface area of bowel, such as in surgical resection, lactose intolerance, and mild malnutrition. Common causes of malabsorption in infancy and childhood discussed in this section include celiac disease and lactose intolerance. Infectious and inflammatory disorders are discussed earlier in this chapter. Cystic fibrosis is discussed in Chapter 38 and milk allergy in Chapter 44.

Gluten-sensitive Enteropathy (Celiac Disease)

Gluten-sensitive enteropathy (GSE) is second only to cystic fibrosis as the most common cause of malabsorption in children. The exact prevalence of the disease is unknown, as treatment is not sought for many asymptomatic children. Prevalence is higher in parts of Europe and in Canada than in the United States. The highest frequency of GSE (1:597) has been found in west Ireland (Silverman and Roy, 1983). Peak frequency is between the age of 9 and 18 months. There is some indication that the incidence of celiac disease is declining. Some attribute this decline to the delayed introduction of solid foods, but the relationship is not clear.

Pathophysiology and Etiology

The mucosa of the small bowel is damaged by gluten-containing foods, resulting in nutrient malabsorption. Gluten is a form of protein contained in wheat, barley, rye, and oats. The toxicity of gluten derived from wheat and rye is more clearly established than for barley and oats. The gluten itself consists of two protein fractions, glutenin and gliadin. Of these, gliadin appears to be the causative agent. The exact means by which gluten damages the mucosa of the small bowel remains obscure. However, two explanations currently exist. In the first, an enzymatic insufficiency (intestinal) is thought to cause an accumulation of toxic gluten peptides. However, because this deficiency appears to be reversed by dietary management, it may be a consequence of the disease rather than a cause (Silverman and Roy, 1983). It may well be that the peptidase deficiency is secondary to the epithelial damage (Gryboski and Walker, 1983). A second theory, which is now gaining increasing support, holds that the gluten toxicity results from an alteration in immunologic response. Gliadin is thought to play the role of an antigen that causes an injurious immune response. This theory is supported by the striking response to corticosteroid therapy.

Normally the intestinal mucosa is lined with tall villi whose function is the absorption of nutrients. In celiac disease sensitivity to the undigested gluten causes the villi to gradually flatten out, resulting in a reduced absorptive surface area. Digestion of fats is affected primarily, but there is also some interference with carbohydrate and vitamin absorption.

Clinical Manifestations and Diagnostic Assessment

The resulting malabsorption, if untreated, leads to chronic diarrhea with large amounts of digested but unabsorbed fats being excreted (steatorrhea). The stools are characteristically bulky and foul smelling. As the disease progresses, absorption of proteins, carbohydrates, calcium, iron, and vitamins D, K, B_{12}, and B_6 (folic acid) is greatly impaired. Abdominal distention develops, and the child appears malnourished. Owing to the failure to utilize ingested calories, wasting is seen in normal areas of fat distribution, particularly the buttocks. Vitamin D malabsorption can cause bone changes, and rickets or tetany may develop. Anemia may be present owing to malabsorption of iron or vitamins B_{12} or B_6, or of all three, and bleeding disorders may result from vitamin K deficiency.

Symptoms may begin at any time after the introduction of gluten into the diet, usually at the time cereals are first given. Affected children often have a history of digestive disturbances starting at 6 to 12 months of age.

The disease is insidious, marked by poor weight gain and failure to grow, which may persist throughout childhood without notable gastrointestinal symptoms. Other children with the disease may, however, be well during childhood and not manifest symptoms until adult life.

Certain changes in behavior often correlate with the presence of celiac disease. These changes include irritability, lack of cooperation, and eventually apathy. However, 30 per cent of children do not exhibit behavioral changes (Hamilton, 1983).

The child with celiac disease may initially appear irritable and anorexic, with chronic diarrhea, failure to thrive, a pot belly, and muscle wasting. The child may first come to medical attention in a state of celiac crisis. This is an acute episode of watery diarrhea and vomiting leading to severe electrolyte imbalance and dehydration, which may progress to metabolic acidosis. The crisis may be precipitated by infection, alteration in diet, or use of anticholinergic drugs, commonly for preoperative medication. Because celiac disease may have a genetic basis, the nurse should be aware of significant family history when gathering assessment data. This would include information on family members who may have had obscure complaints of digestive problems, intermittent diarrhea, or failure to thrive and gain weight. The child's dietary history should be reviewed to ascertain at what age new foods were introduced.

In evaluating the physical status of a child who is not thriving, the nurse should observe for body distribution of fat. A protuberant abdomen in conjunction with frequent, foul-smelling, fatty stools that float in the toilet bowl lends credence to the diagnosis. Although the family and child must make adaptations to the disorder, celiac disease is usually quite well controlled by strict adherence to the dietary regimen, and in other respects a normal life-style can be maintained.

Although a jejunal biopsy is mandatory to make the diagnosis, malabsorptive screening tests can be carried out before the biopsy is performed (Gryboski and Walker, 1983). The serum D-xylose absorption test is used as a screening test to assess upper small bowel surface area. Following the ingestion of D-xylose a serum level of 20 mg/dl at 1 to 1½ hours suggests reduced small bowel surface area (Gryboski and Walker, 1983). A 72-hour stool test for fat is done to confirm the presence of steatorrhea. Prior to the intestinal biopsy, blood clotting function should be assessed. A complete blood count, platelet count, prothrombin time and partial thromboplastin time should be obtained. The nurse should know the results of clotting function tests before biopsy and identify any abnormalities. After a 6- to 8-hour fast and appropriate sedation, the biopsy is done.

Atrophy of the villi demonstrated by biopsy coupled with a dietary history consistent with the disease supports the diagnosis. Serum protein and immunoglobulin levels may be low owing to the protein-losing enteropathy. Radiologically, bone age may be retarded, and osteoporosis and osteomalacia are often present. If the child responds favorably to a withdrawal of gluten from the diet and subsequently the condition is exacerbated in response to gluten challenge,* the diagnosis is confirmed.

Therapeutic Management

The treatment of celiac disease centers on correct dietary management. This involves the institution and maintenance of a lifetime diet free of gluten. Corn and

* Gluten challenge means the reintroduction of gluten (usually in 10 to 30 gm daily amounts) to the diet under controlled conditions. This may be continued for 2 to 3 weeks if symptoms are absent. Patients with true celiac disease develop steatorrhea and have decreased xylose absorption.

rice as well as soybean flour may be substituted for the grain portion of the diet. Health food stores are a good source for many appropriate foods. Care must be taken in purchasing *all* foods, as grains are frequently used as fillers or thickeners. Labels must be read carefully to avoid ingestion of grains. Foods labeled "with hydrolyzed vegetable protein" or "vegetable protein added" must be avoided. Because of the suppression of disaccharidase activity, a lactose-free diet is advocated initially to help lessen the diarrhea. A nutritionist is involved from the beginning of treatment to assist the family with careful dietary management.

If the diet is followed carefully and consistently, a dramatic response is seen. Within the first few days the child's disposition improves; he or she becomes less irritable and less apathetic. A progressive improvement in muscle tone and lessening of diarrhea and decreased abdominal distention are seen.

Those seriously ill children who are in crisis may need replacement therapy with intravenous fluids, parenteral nutrition, and vitamin administration. A dramatic improvement has been seen in crisis when corticosteroid therapy is initiated to decrease the inflammation of the bowel. A nasogastric tube may be passed to decrease abdominal distention and should be attached to intermittent suction. When the crisis is resolved, the child returns to diet therapy for maintenance.

Prior to the child's discharge, parents should understand what precipitates a celiac crisis and have a good knowledge of the dietary regimen. Other members of the health care team who may be required to treat the child should be made aware of the celiac disease status so that anticholinergic drugs will not be prescribed to treat the symptoms.

Within 6 months to 1 year after beginning the diet, the child with celiac disease should be within normal weight for age. Height and bone age take somewhat longer to become normal, usually 2 years. Relapses occur whenever the child eats gluten-containing foods.

The possible correlation between celiac disease and intestinal lymphoma and other forms of gastrointestinal cancer is a sufficient reason to remain on a gluten-free diet for life, and this should be brought to the parents' attention.

Major Nursing Diagnoses for Celiac Disease

***Altered nutrition: less than body requirements**, related to nutrient malabsorption associated with gluten toxicity in the small bowel*

***Altered family process**, related to*
- *diagnosis of a condition requiring lifelong dietary alterations*
- *concern about a genetic basis*
- *irritability of the child in the acute phase*
- *financial burden of a gluten-free diet*

Strategies for Nursing Care

Nursing responsibility involves care during diagnosis and crisis, dietary management and instruction, facilitating the adaptation to a modified diet, and stimulation of appropriate emotional and developmental responses.

Assisting with Diagnosis. Nursing responsibility during the diagnostic period is diverse. The nurse assists in collection of 72-hour stool specimens to be examined for fecal fat and coordinates collection of hematologic specimens for evaluation of anemia, protein and prothrombin levels, and electrolyte imbalance. Radiographic studies may be done to determine bone age and lower gastrointestinal tract function. While coordinating these procedures, the nurse should be aware of the importance of timing. If possible, tests should be scheduled so that they do not interfere with mealtimes. Honest, concise explanations should be given to the child, without exaggeration. These are best given immediately before the procedure to avoid increasing the young child's anxiety level. This is particularly important to ensure cooperation in the future. The comfort and safety needs of the child should be met prior to, during, and after each procedure.

Enhancing the Family's Adjustment and Home Management. The nurse responds to the family's needs throughout all diagnostic procedures. Because of the slow, insidious onset of the condition, the parents' abilities to cope with the situation may be severely altered. Parents will be extremely worried about their child and may question their own abilities to provide adequate care. Every effort should be made to give them as much information as they are able to absorb and allow time for them to express their fears and concerns.

The child with celiac disease may be irritable, anorexic, unsociable, and withdrawn during the diagnostic phase and may be difficult for the parents and the nurse to deal with. The parents may be on the verge of exhaustion and occasionally need opportunities to have time out from the stress of this situation. They should also be informed that the child's irritability will quickly disappear once the diet is initiated and the intestinal tract becomes normal.

As is true for many other situations, the parents initially have to adjust to the potential changes in their own lives as well as feelings of guilt, and they may not readily absorb large amounts of information. Parents will not necessarily adjust at the same pace. Explanations may need to be detailed, and repeated and frequent feedback sessions are helpful to determine the parents' level of understanding.

Careful explanation of the role of gluten in the disease as well as a copy of the diet and recipes to bring variety to meals should be given to the family. The family just learning of this diagnosis can contact another family with more experience in dealing with this disease, who can share methods of coping that have worked for them. This will also provide an opportunity to ask for recipe ideas. Suggestions are helpful for making special treats and favorite foods for the child, such as gluten-free cookies, birthday cakes, and pizza. Appropriate snack foods such as fruit chunks, cheese, and carrot sticks are suggested for between-meal snacks. The nutritionist also can provide specialized information that helps the family adjust to the restrictions of the disease.

A special diet is expensive and may place an added financial burden on a family. Means of rebudgeting or working out a more economical method of preparing the diet may need to be explored. Incorporating low- or no-gluten foods into the family diet may be beneficial, as cooking special foods for one individual is more expensive and will set the child apart.

As the child's condition improves, appropriate physical, social and intellectual activities should be initiated. Children with celiac disease learn early that their diet will always be a little different, and if they also learn at an early age to make the correct decisions, they will adapt well throughout life. The normality of their lives should be stressed. In essence, celiac disease is a dietary problem, and with correct dietary control other limitations on lifestyle are not major.

Nursing Strategies for Follow-Up Care in the Home or Clinic

Plot height and weight on the growth chart and alert the physician if the child fails to make steady progress toward the 50th percentile range for weight within the first 6 months. (Height should approximate normal percentiles within 2 years.)

Observe for reduction of abdominal protuberance and the appropriate appearance of body fat in the buttocks.

Obtain a blood sample for evaluation of serum protein level if appropriate.

Determine the frequency and nature of the child's stools.

Ask the parent and child about the child's usual mood and activity level.

Question the parent and child about usual food intake to assess for the adequacy of nutrition in the absence of gluten-containing foods. Refer for nutritional counseling as needed.

Encourage the child and parent to share ways in which they cope with the dietary alterations. Reinforce creative solutions (to enhance their self-esteem and sense of control).

Caution the parent and child to contact the physician if the child should develop an infection or accidentally ingest foods containing gluten. These events (as well as ingestion of an anticholinergic drug), can precipitate a celiac crisis.

Lactose Intolerance

Lactose intolerance is the result of a lack or deficiency of the enzyme lactase, which is present within the border of the intestinal villi and is required to hydrolyse (or reduce) the disaccharide lactose into the monosaccharides glucose and galactose. The term lactose intolerance is used interchangeably with lactase deficiency. Milk allergy, however, is a sensitization to one of the milk proteins and should not be confused with lactose intolerance. (See Chapter 43 for a discussion of food allergy.)

Lactose intolerance occurs as a familial, congenital, late-onset, or secondary disorder. The *familial type*, which is thought to be an autosomal recessive condition, is a rare and severe disorder. It is often fatal and is characterized by vomiting, failure to thrive, and dehydration acidosis (Gryboski and Walker, 1983). A small intestinal biopsy reveals normal lactase activity; therefore, a defect in the stomach is believed to be the cause of abnormal transport of lactose into the system (Gryboski and Walker, 1983). Elimination of lactose from the diet is helpful to many infants, but some continue to vomit and may die.

Congenital lactose intolerance is also a rare form of the disorder and is genetically determined. Normal intestinal mucosa is found on small bowel biopsy, but lactase activity is markedly diminished or absent, resulting in malabsorption. At birth the infant appears normal but after one or two feedings of milk, irritability, and abdominal distention develop with explosive, watery, frothy stools having a sour or vinegar-like

Table 41-11. Disorders Associated with Secondary Lactase Deficiency

Infection	Viral gastroenteritis Bacterial enteritis Giardiasis
Inflammation	Protein-induced enteropathy Chronic inflammatory bowel disease Immunodeficiency Eosinophilic gastroenteritis Nonspecific enterocolitis
Reduced Surface Area	Short bowel syndrome Malnutrition Hypoxia Radiation enteritis

smell. Vomiting is not as common as in the familial type of disorder.

Late-onset lactose intolerance occurs after infancy. Prevalence of the disorder in Jews, Indians, Asians, and blacks range between 50 and 90 per cent (Gryboski and Walker, 1983). The frequency of this disorder increases with age as lactase activity is known to be maximal during infancy. As part of normal development, up to 70 per cent of the world's population gradually loses lactase activity beginning at age 4 years (Wald et al, 1982), at which time symptoms begin to be more prominent. Up until age 4 or 5, the only symptom may be an aversion to milk. Some children have complaints that may mimic appendicitis, including recurrent abdominal pain and flatulence. Diarrhea often does not begin until months after repeated episodes of abdominal pain.

Secondary (acquired) lactose intolerance develops when the maturation of gastrointestinal epithelial villi becomes disrupted. Reductions in activity are associated with disorders of infection and inflammation and with conditions that reduce the intestinal surface area (see Table 41-11 for a list of common conditions associated with secondary lactase deficiency).

Pathophysiology

The mucosal enzyme lactase splits lactose, a disaccharide, into the monosaccharides glucose and galactose for absorption. Inadequate levels of the enzyme lactase (disaccharidase) on either a congenital or an acquired basis results in the presence of unabsorbed lactose in the gut. Unabsorbed lactose remains osmotically active, drawing water into the intestinal lumen, which in turn stimulates intestinal motility and shortens transit time. When the unabsorbed lactose reaches the distal intestine and colon the sugar is fermented to hydrogen, carbon dioxide, and organic acids (especially lactic acid). As a result, osmotic activity increases, the pH of the stool drops to below 5.5, and there is reduced absorption of water and electrolytes from the colon. Some of the sugars are not fermented and can be found in stools as reducing substances.

Clinical Manifestations and Diagnostic Assessment

Symptoms are produced as a result of ingestion of lactose-containing foods (especially milk). In infants, lactose intolerance produces severe diarrhea, acid stools, dehydration, and failure to thrive. After infancy, symptoms are less dramatic. The gas generated from the fermentation of sugar may produce a sensation of bloating or belching and flatulence. This may be associated with abdominal pain, watery stools, and urgency.

Lactose intolerance can sometimes be identified by the presence of symptoms after ingestion of lactose-containing products and the absence of symptoms after withdrawal of these foods. Laboratory tests can be used to diagnose lactose intolerance. In infants a high level of reducing sugars in the stool (above 0.5 per cent glucose using a Clinitest tablet) and an acid pH (below 5.5) are seen in the presence of lactose intolerance. Another test, breath hydrogen testing, is performed to identify increased levels of hydrogen in expired air after lactose ingestion. Hydrogen production increases during the fermentation of the disaccharide and therefore its presence in expired air also increases. A biopsy of a segment of the small intestine will also identify lactase deficiency. The breath hydrogen test for lactose has the advantage of being relatively inexpensive, non-invasive, and applicable throughout childhood.

Therapeutic Management

Elimination or reduction of lactose intake is the initial approach depending on whether the deficiency is partial or complete. After 6 months of age or more, many infants can tolerate diets containing low levels of lactose, whereas some cannot tolerate even the smallest amount. For infants a lactose-free formula such as Isomil, Soyalac, or Prosobee is prescribed; however, older children rarely find these palatable. Elimination of lactose from the diet entails exclusion of milk and milk products. Milk products are ingredients in many unexpected substances; therefore, labels must be checked

Table 41-12. Milk Protein or Lactose-Free Diet

Foods Allowed	Foods Not Allowed
Milk: None (exception: use of LactAid additive to predigest lactose).	All milk and milk drinks—including whole, skim, low fat, dried, evaporated, and condensed milk; human breast milk. Yogurt—any type. Cream—sweet or sour. Infant formulas other than those permitted. Ice cream sodas, milk shakes.
Beverages: Powdered, fruit-flavored drinks, ginger ale, tonics.	Any made with milk, such as milkshakes, eggnog, hot chocolate.
Eggs: As desired	Eggs made with milk—use specific formula. Do not prepare with butter.
Meats: Any baked, broiled, roasted, or boiled, except those to be avoided.	Creamed or breaded meat, fish, or poultry. Prepared meats that may contain dried milk solids, including bologna and cold cuts, frankfurters, salami, commercially prepared fish sticks, and some sausage.
Cheese: Although made from milk, some cheeses are lactose-free and may be permitted. These are Camembert, brick, cheddar, Edam, Provolone, Swiss, pasteurized processed American.	All types of cheese and cheese dishes not listed as allowed.
Breads: Only breads made without milk such as French bread, Italian bread, water bagels, or "parva" breads.	Made with any form of milk. Any baked product made with milk. Muffins, biscuits, waffles, pancakes, doughnuts, sweet rolls, commercial mixes.
Cereal: Any made without milk, cooked or ready to eat. Macaroni, spaghetti, pasta, rice—all prepared without milk or cheese.	Any prepared cereal that contains dry milk solids.
Vegetables and Potatoes: All—cooked, canned, frozen, or fresh.	Any vegetable prepared with milk, butter, milk solids, bread, or bread crumbs. No cheese or cream sauces.
Fruits: All.	All are allowed.
Desserts: Any made without milk or milk products, such as gelatin desserts, fruit crisp, snow puddings, fruit and water sherbets, pie with fruit filling, angel cake.	All commercial cake and cookie mixes, ice cream, custard puddings, junket, ice milk, or sherbets that contain milk. Frosting made with milk or butter, dessert sauces, cheese cakes.
Soup: Any prepared without milk or milk products. Homemade or canned, e.g., chicken rice.	All creamed soups, chowders.
Fats: Milk-free margarine or "parva"margarine. Oils, nuts, peanut butter.	Butter, margarine, some commercial salad dressings (check labels).
Sugar and Seasonings: Sugar, honey, molasses, maple syrup, corn syrup, jelly and jam, hard candy, gum drops, marshmallows, hard peppermints, fondant. Salt, pepper, spices, herbs, condiments, vinegar, catsup, relish, pickles, olives, tomato sauce, coconut, wheat germ. Artificial flavoring and extracts.	Any product made from milk, butter, cream, chocolate, toffee, cream mints, caramel candy, candy with cream centers.
	Miscellaneous: Medications that may contain lactose as filler or bulk agents; party dips; nonprescription vitamins; spice blends; Easter egg dyes. Dietetic foods and foods advertised as "high protein" sometimes contain lactose or dry milk solids.
	Check all labels carefully.

This diet is for the patient who must eliminate *all* sources of lactose from the diet. Lactose is the sugar found in milk, so all foods containing milk are to be excluded from the diet.

Read the label carefully. Avoid any food containing *milk, nonfat milk solids, skim milk, butter, cream, lactose, casein, caseinate,* or *sodium caseinate.* Some children sensitive to milk protein may not tolerate beef products.

(From Gryboski and Walker, 1983.)

carefully. When milk is excluded from an infant's diet, adequate calcium and vitamins must be provided in the formula or by supplementation. A commercially prepared lactase (LactAid) in powder form can be added to milk to predigest lactose. Some areas have access to commercial milks with lactose predigested or fermented. A lactose-free diet is summarized in Table 41-12.

Hepatic Alterations

Biliary Atresia

Biliary atresia, a congenital defect in which an infant is born with fibrotic or absent bile ducts, occurs once in every 10,000 live births.

Neonatal hepatitis and biliary atresia are now considered to be two parts of a single prenatal disease, with neonatal hepatitis involving the intrahepatic ducts and biliary atresia the extrahepatic major ducts (Filston and Izant, 1985). The cause of biliary atresia is unknown. Research has focused on the possibility of a viral infection, with reovirus type 3 being the most commonly cited virus believed to cause biliary atresia (Morecki et al, 1982). Rubella virus, cytomegalovirus, hepatitis A and B virus, and prenatal infection by *Listeria monocytogenes* have also been associated with biliary atresia (Oski, 1984; Oellrich and Cusmano, 1987). Prevalence is higher in females than in males.

Pathophysiology

Normally, the liver secretes bile, which passes through the bile ducts in the liver to the hepatic duct. The hepatic duct joins with the cystic duct from the gallbladder to form the common bile duct, which empties bile into the duodenum. Atresia may occur in any part or all of this duct system. Intrahepatic atresia occurs when the liver has no internal duct system. This is a defect for which there is no treatment other than supportive care for the infant with a terminal illness. Extrahepatic atresia is the most common type. It involves defects of the hepatic or common bile duct and can be corrected surgically with varying success rates. Both types create build-up of bile in the liver because it lacks a passageway to enter the intestines. Untreated, this condition eventually causes cirrhosis. Since the introduction of the Kasai procedure, previously "inoperable" types of atresia can be corrected, but surgery continues to be only marginally successful (Kasui et al, 1968).

Diagnostic Assessment

Diagnosis is based on the history of jaundice at 3 to 4 weeks of age, the physical examination, and laboratory and diagnostic tests. Conjugated serum bilirubin, serum alkaline phosphatase, and cholesterol levels are elevated, indicating blockage of the bile ducts; however, these and other tests are not specific for biliary atresia. Biochemical studies are helpful in ruling out other disease entities, but making a diagnosis requires more specific tests, such as ultrasonography and nuclear imaging.

A liver biopsy provides a definitive result and is reliable in approximately 90 per cent of the cases. A core of liver tissue is obtained under local anesthesia by inserting a special needle (Menghini needle) into the liver. The tissue sample is sent for laboratory examination. *Hemorrhage* is the most frequent and serious complication of this procedure. Adequate immobilization of the infant's abdomen during the biopsy by holding the infant securely on the examining table is an important assistive nursing intervention. Moderate pressure is maintained over the biopsy site for 5 to 10 minutes after the procedure. Both of these nursing actions minimize the chance of hemorrhage.

Therapeutic Management

The infant with biliary atresia has no chance for survival without surgical correction. Parents must deal initially with the news that their infant has a congenital defect that is usually fatal within 18 months. They can be told that there is a chance for cure by surgical correction but that the surgery may not be successful.

The surgical success rate is greatest when the operation is performed within the first 2 months of life. After this time, the liver is permanently damaged by the trapped bile. The operation consists of using a portion of the small intestine (jejunum) to replace the blocked or fibrotic ducts. A bile duct is reconstructed using jejunum and is anastomosed to the dissected porta hepatis at the base of the liver to create a pathway for bile to exit the liver and enter the intestines.

Anastomosis of a Y-shaped portion of the jejunum (called Roux-en-Y)* to the dissected porta hepatis will result in a hepatojejunal fistula between the intrahepatic ducts at the hilum of the liver and the intestine (Filston and Izant, 1985). The newly constructed bile duct is then brought out onto the infant's abdomen to form a conduit by way of a double-barreled enterostomy. This is known as the portajejunostomy (Kasai operation). Initially, the bile flows from the liver into a collection bag on the infant's abdomen. It is then injected back into the intestine via the distal loop of the conduit. The enterostomy decreases the frequency of postoperative bile duct infection, a major surgical complication. Usually, within a year, when normal bile flow is established, the enterostomy is closed and bile flows from the liver into the intestine through the reconstructed bile duct. Variations of the original Kasai operation have evolved to help reduce its major complication of cholangitis. Cholangitis is the result of bacteria ascending from the intestine to the newly constructed bile duct.

If surgical correction is not possible or is unsuccessful, liver transplantation has been carried out for

---

*In the Roux-en-Y procedure, the distal end of the divided jejunum is anastomosed to the bile duct. The proximal end of the divided jejunum is implanted into the side of the distal jejunum below the point where the distal portion is anastomosed to the bile duct.

infants with biliary atresia. Liver transplantation may become increasingly more successful with the wider use of the immunosuppressive drug cyclosporin A (Starzl et al, 1982).

Strategies for Nursing Care

Nursing intervention for the parents under stress during this time requires active listening and the development of a supportive relationship. Loss and grief are predominant themes for the parents.

Supporting the Family. Preparation of the parents for the infant's surgery and appropriate support while they cope with the postoperative course are the mainstays of nursing care for the family. Preoperatively, the infant may be irritable and uncomfortable. The physical closeness of the parents will comfort the infant and will help the parents prepare for the reality of the surgery.

Teaching to Support Care at Home. Questions concerning the surgical procedure and the anticipated postsurgical course should be answered by the surgeon. Nurses should also be informed about the expected outcome and participate in preparing the family to care for the child at home. Parents need to learn how to maintain skin integrity around the enterostomy and to apply the collection device properly. Signs and symptoms of infection should be reviewed, and parents should demonstrate competence in taking and interpreting the results of rectal temperatures. The reduced bile salts in the intestine may lead to poor uptake of the fat-soluble vitamins A, D, E, and K. Vitamin K is frequently given by injection if the possibility of hemorrhage is great, so parents must learn how to administer intramuscular injections to the infant.

A special diet, which includes predigested fats and water-miscible vitamins, is prescribed for 6 to 12 months after surgery. A formula such as Portagen or Pregestimil may be used. Such a formula is a high-calorie one, but it contains fats (medium-chain, fatty acid) that can be digested without the need for bile and contains water-miscible vitamins. Parents should feel comfortable with the dietary regimen before the infant returns home. Plans for the necessary long-term medical follow-up are made with the parents before they leave the hospital. (See discussion on cirrhosis of the liver in the next section.)

Cirrhosis

Cirrhosis is an alteration in hepatic lobular structure and function which is the result of injury to the hepatocytes (liver tissue cells). Hepatocytes have a remarkable capacity for regeneration. Therefore, injury to cells results in a process of destruction and regeneration, which eventually leads to permanent scarring of the liver tissue.

Table 41-13. Type of Cirrhosis

Type	Cause	Pathology
Postnecrotic cirrhosis	Previous acute viral hepatitis	Replacement of liver tissue with nodules of fibrous tissue
Biliary cirrhosis	Chronic biliary infection and obstruction	Scarring around bile ducts and the lobes of the liver
Portal or Laennec cirrhosis	Chronic alcoholism	Scarring around the portal area

Etiology

Cirrhosis is the result of a variety of diseases with varying mechanisms of injury. It is believed that hepatic injury must be prolonged and repeated for cirrhosis to develop (Hughes and Griffith, 1984). Injury to hepatocytes occurs as a consequence of metabolic diseases, toxins, biliary obstructions, infections, and vascular conditions. See Table 41-13 for a description of the three types of cirrhosis and related pathology.

Some of the more common causes of cirrhosis in infancy, childhood, and adolescence are cystic fibrosis, alpha$_1$-antitrypsin deficiency, biliary atresia, and hepatitis. The adolescent population is at particular risk for cirrhosis as hepatitis B becomes more widespread among teenage illicit parenteral drug users.

Pathophysiology

When hepatocytes suffer an insult, a regeneration process is initiated by the activation of fibroblasts. Although in some instances, regeneration can lead to repair, a continuing process of destruction and regeneration results in excessive growth of fibrotic tissue. The fibrotic process compounds cellular damage because it interferes with blood flow to the cells.

Hepatic dysfunction causes major alterations in the body because of interruption in the important functions of the liver, including synthesis and storage of glycogen, deamination of amino acids and synthesis of proteins, biotransformation of bile pigments, synthesis of fibrinogen and prothrombin, destruction of bacteria, storage of vitamin B and fat-soluble vitamins, and lipid metabolism. Hepatic function leads to a group of interrelated pathophysiologic processes resulting in jaundice, portal hypertension, ascites, impairment of fat digestion, reduced clotting mechanisms, encephalopathy, and renal dysfunction.

Jaundice occurs because damaged parenchymal hepatic cells fail to conjugate and excrete bilirubin into the bile. Instead, it accumulates in the blood resulting in yellowing of the skin, dark-colored urine, and clay-colored stools. The clay color of feces is caused by the lack of stercobilin. Normally bilirubin is excreted into the biliary tree and then into the gastrointestinal tract, where it is converted to urobilinogen and then to stercobilin. Retained components of bile salts can also cause pruritus; however, the degree of itching is not related to the degree of hyperbilirubinemia (Balistreri, 1987).

Portal hypertension occurs because the hepatic fibrotic process obstructs blood flow through the liver, causing a back pressure into the portal system. Normally the hepatic portal vein carries blood *to* the liver from the abdominal portion of the gastrointestinal tract, pancreas, and spleen. In the presence of portal hypertension, collateral flow around the liver increases with the development of varices (particularly esophageal) and spider angiomata as a result of dilated abdominal wall veins. Hypersplenism can also occur, resulting in a diminished production of platelets.

Ascites, an accumulation of serous fluid in the peritoneal cavity, commonly occurs with cirrhosis. The mechanism of its formation is poorly understood. A major contributing factor is the reduced amount of albumin that is synthesized by an injured liver. The resultant hypoalbuminemia reduces vascular osmotic pressure, thereby contributing to fluid loss from the vascular space. Portal hypertension further contributes to ascites because of increased vascular hydrostatic pressure. Another explanation is that lymph is formed in the hepatic sinusoids in excess of what can be drained by the thoracic duct; therefore, lymph accumulates in the peritoneal cavity as ascites (Balistreri, 1987). An alternative explanation is that the kidney retains sodium, causing a plasma volume expansion which is lost to the peritoneal cavity as ascites.

Impairment of fat digestion occurs because there is a decrease in intestinal bile salts. Furthermore, decreased fat digestion interferes with the absorption of the fat-soluble vitamins A, D, E, and K. The vitamin K deficiency that results contributes to the bleeding tendency seen in advanced cirrhosis.

Reduced clotting mechanisms occur because of altered synthesis of the clotting factors fibrinogen and prothrombin and altered production and function of platelets in the presence of hypersplenism (Balistreri, 1987).

Encephalopathy in hepatic dysfunction is thought to occur because a primary *inhibitory* neurotransmitter is not cleared from the blood and crosses the blood-brain barrier to inhibit brain activity (Balistreri, 1987). Also, ammonia is thought to have a role in hepatic encephalopathy. Increased serum ammonia levels interfere with metabolism within the brain. Ammonia levels increase because there is a reduction in the ability of the liver to convert ammonia to urea for excretion by the kidney. Ammonia (which is formed in the intestine) is also allowed to bypass the liver and enter the general circulation because of the collateral circulation that develops in the presence of portal hypertension.

Renal dysfunction may be caused by the same systemic disease or toxins that affect the liver. Liver and renal dysfunction are closely related. Renal alterations include impaired concentrating ability, altered potassium metabolism, and alterations in sodium and water retention.

Diagnostic Assessment

A diagnosis is made by gathering historical information, doing a physical examination, and performing selected laboratory tests and diagnostic procedures. A history of loss of appetite, nausea and vomiting, and prior liver disease such as hepatitis may contribute to making a diagnosis. In the adolescent population, information that might reveal drug and alcohol abuse should be sought. A physical examination will reveal clinical manifestations as discussed earlier, although symptoms may be vague. In biliary atresia, jaundice is usually evident, whereas in cirrhosis from other causes, an insidious onset can be expected. Laboratory tests used for diagnosis of cirrhosis are included in Table 41-4.

Definitive diagnosis is made by liver biopsy if coagulation is normal or corrected. A high-carbohydrate, low-fat, and moderate-protein diet is given to maintain high energy, at the same time trying not to exacerbate the problems of poor fat digestion and avoiding an excessive protein load on the diseased liver. Deficiencies in fat-soluble vitamins A, D, E, and K are replaced parenterally or orally with water-soluble derivatives depending on the child's condition. If deficiencies in water-soluble vitamins exist, they are supplemented with twice the recommended dose.

Therapeutic Management

Pruritus is a troublesome problem in cirrhosis. If there is any degree of patency of the bile duct, phenobarbital, 5 to 10 mg/kg/day, or bile acid binders such as cholestyramine (Questran), 8 to 16 gm/day, are given. Cholestyramine can be administered to stimulate bile flow and inhibit reabsorption of bile salts through the normal route of enterohepatic circulation (bile salts are normally reabsorbed from the intestine to the liver via the enterohepatic circulation). Cholestyramine is given with caution because it can decrease absorption of fats and fat-soluble vitamin as well.

Gastrointestinal hemorrhage, which can be due to gastritis, peptic ulcer, or esophageal varices, is managed according to its cause. Blood transfusions, fluid and electrolyte replacement, administration of vitamin B complex and vitamin K, stomach gavage with iced solutions, vasoconstrictive agents such as vasopressin, and a Sengstaken-Blakemore tube are therapeutic approaches that are used. Additionally, esophageal varices are increasingly being treated by sclerosis during endoscopy.

Ascites is controlled by restricting dietary salt to 0.5 gm/day. If urinary output is adequate, it is not usually necessary to restrict fluid intake. Diuretics are administered and serum and urinary electrolyte levels are monitored. A shunt may be created surgically in which the portal vein is anastomosed to the inferior vena cava, resulting in blood by-passing the liver. In advanced chronic cholestasis liver transplantation may be performed, but there is a scarcity of donors of livers for small patients.

The child's prognosis depends on the cause of the cirrhosis and the severity of the hepatic damage. The major complications of cirrhosis are hemorrhage, ascites, and hepatic encephalopathy.

Strategies for Nursing Care

Nursing care is directed toward reducing the potential for further damage to the liver, keeping the child comfortable, and helping the child and family cope with the child's current condition and to plan for the future realistically.

The child's *activity level* is kept to a minimum during the acute phase to conserve energy. A child with cirrhosis is usually tired and weak and should be cautioned against strenuous exercise.

Adequate nutrition is difficult to maintain when a child has nausea and vomiting. The dietary restrictions of limited salt, fat, and protein can further decrease the appetite of a child who does not feel like eating. Tube feeding may become necessary, particularly if the child is being prepared for liver transplantation.

Skin assessment is an important function of the nurse. Hyperbilirubinema is assessed by checking the skin for jaundice, the child's sclera for increased yellow staining, the urine for a dark color, and stool for clay color. If pruritus is present, warm baths can be used without soap followed by application of a lotion.

Assessments for signs of bleeding are made by checking gums for bleeding (especially during tooth brushing), assessing the skin for signs of bruising, and testing stool and urine for occult blood.

Nursing care varies according to the therapeutic regimen that is instituted and consists of accurate assessment of the child's status and effect of therapy. The family and child (as appropriate for age) are kept informed of the purpose of the various procedures being performed and the child is kept comfortable. Parents are also encouraged to express their feelings of loss and fear surrounding the uncertainty of their child's illness.

References

Appley J: *The Child with Abdominal Pain.* 2nd ed. New York, Blackwell Scientific, 1975.

Ashcraft KW, Holder TM: Esophageal atresia and tracheoesophageal fistula malformations. *Surg Clin North Am* 1976; 56:299.

Aylsworth AS: Genetic considerations in clefts of the lip and palate. *Clin Plastic Surg* 1985; 12:533–542.

Balistreri WF: Liver and biliary system. *In* Behrman RE, Vaughan VC (eds): *Nelson Textbook of Pediatrics.* 13th ed. Philadelphia, WB Saunders, 1987, 821–849.

Balistreri WF, et al: Immaturity of the enterohepatic circulation in early life: factors predisposing to "physiologic" maldigestion and cholestasis. *J Pediatr Gastroenterol Nutr* 1983; 2:346.

Barbero GJ, McKay RJ: Irritable bowel syndrome. *In* Behrman RE, Vaughan VC: *Nelson Textbook of Pediatrics.* Philadelphia, WB Saunders, 1987.

Barnett B: Viral gastroenteritis. *Med Clin North Am* 1983; 67:1031–1058.

Behrman RE: Peritoneum and allied structures. *In* Behrman RE, Vaughan VC (eds): *Nelson Textbook of Pediatrics.* 13th ed. Philadelphia, WB Saunders, 1987, 850–853.

Bell MJ, et al: Antimicrobial prophylaxis in pediatric surgical patients. *Communication AAP Committee on Infectious Disease*, 1983, 1–7.

Brazelton TB: Crying in infancy. *Pediatrics* 1972; 29:579.

Broder H, Trier WC: Genetic counseling: psychological and surgical perspectives. Annual meeting of the American Cleft Palate Association, Seattle, May 22, 1984.

Burrington J, Powers L: Pediatric surgery. *In* Merenstein GB, Gardner SL: *Handbook of Neonatal Intensive Care.* St. Louis, CV Mosby, 1985, 373–393.

Canty TG: Esophageal atresia and tracheoesophageal fistula. Aspects of respiratory care. *Perinatology-Neonatology*, 1986 Jul/Aug; 42–47.

Carey WB: Clinical applications of infant temperament measurements. *J Pediatr*, 1972; 81:823.

Cassani VL: Tracheoesophageal anomalies. *Neonat Network* 1984; 3(2):20–26.

Cohen SA, et al: Chronic non-specific diarrhea. Dietary relationships. *Pediatrics* 1979; 64:402.

Colodny AH: Pyloric stenosis and antral web. *In* Hoekelman, RA et al (eds): *Principles of Pediatrics.* New York, McGraw-Hill Book Co, 1978.

Coran AG, et al: *Surgery of the Neonate.* Boston, Little, Brown & Co, 1979.

Coran AG, Weintraub WH: Modification of the endorectal procedure for Hirschsprung's disease. *Surg Gynecol Obstet* 1976 August; 143:277.

Cummings JH, Stephen AM: The role of dietary fibre in the human colon. *Can Med Assoc J* 1981; 123:1109.

Davidson GF: Viral Diarrhea. *Clin Gastroenterol* 1986; 15:39–53.

Doershuk CF, Boat TF: *In* Behrman RE, Vaughan VC: *Nelson Textbook of Pediatrics.* Philadelphia, WB Saunders, 1987, 926–935.

Eastham EJ, et al: Antigenicity of infant formulas and the induction of systemic immunological tolerance by oral feeding: cow's milk versus soy milk. *J Pediatr Gastroenterol Nutr* 1983; 1:23.

Fanaroff AA, Kliegman RM: Necrotizing enterocolitis. *In* Klaus MH, Fanaroff AA: *Care of the High-Risk Neonate.* Philadelphia, WB Saunders, 1986.

Feigin RD, Stoller ML: Diarrhea. *In* Behrman RE, Vaughan VC: *Nelson Textbook of Pediatrics.* Philadelphia, WB Saunders, 1987, 553–555.

Filler RM: Esophageal atresia and tracheoesophageal fistula. *In* Hoekelman RA, et al (eds): *Principles of Pediatrics.* New York, McGraw-Hill Book Co, 1978.

Filston HC, Izant RJ: *The Surgical Neonate,* 2nd ed. New York, Appleton-Century-Crofts, 1985.

Frentner S: Abdominal wall defects: omphalocele and gastroschisis. *Neonat Network.* 1987; 6(3):29–40.

Gillies C: Infant colic: is there anything new? *J Pediatr Health Care* 1987; 1(6):305–312.

Grand RJ, et al: Reversal of growth arrest in Crohn's disease. A new approach. *Abstr Pediatr Res* 1977; 11:444.

Greene HL, Ghishon FK: Excessive fluid intake as a cause of chronic diarrhea in young children. *J Pediatr* 1983; 102:836–846.

Gryboski JD: Disorders of the esophagus. *In* Gelles SS, Kagan BM (eds): *Current Pediatric Therapy 12.* Philadelphia, WB Saunders, 1986, 178–181.

Gryboski JD, Hillemeier C: Inflammatory bowel disease in children. *Med Clin North Am* 1980; 64:1185–1202.

Gryboski J, Walker WA: *Gastrointestinal Problems in the Infant,* 2nd ed. Philadelphia, WB Saunders, 1983.

Guerrant RL, et al: Acute infectious diarrhea. I. Epidemiology, etiology, and pathogenesis. *Pediatr Infect Dis* 1986; 5:353–359.

Hamilton JR: Celiac disease. *In* Behrman RE, Vaughan VC: *Nelson Textbook of Pediatrics,* 1983. Philadelphia, WB Saunders Co, 933–934.

Herbst JJ: Gastroesophageal reflux. *J Pediatr* 1981; 98:859.

Hillemeier AC, et al: Delayed gastric emptying in infants with gastroesophageal reflux. *J Pediatr* 1981; 98:190.

Holtzman IR, Brown DR: Necrotizing enterocolitis: a complication of prematurity. *Semin Perinatol* 1986; 10(3):208–216.

Hughest JG, Griffith JF: *Synopsis of Pediatrics.* 6th ed. St. Louis, CV Mosby, 1984.

Huth MM, O'Brien ME: THe gastrostomy feeding button. *Pediatr Nurs* 1987 Jul/Aug; 13(4):241–245.

Jakobsson I, Lindberg T: Cow's milk protein causes infantile colic: a double blind crossover study. *Pediatrics* 1983; 71:268.

Johnson DG, et al: Gastroesophageal reflux in infants and children: recognition and treatment. *Surg Clin North Am* 1981; 61:1101–1115.

Jonas A, Diver-Haber A: Stool output and composition in chronic non-specific diarrhea syndrome. *Arch Dis Child* 1982; 57:35.

Kasai M, et al: Surgical treatment of biliary atresia. *J Pediatr Surg* 1968; 3:1968–72.

Kelts D, et al: Nutritional basis of growth failure in children and adolescents with Crohn's disease. *Gastroenterology* 1979; 76:720.

Kenner C, et al: *Neonatal Surgery.* Orlando, FL, Grune & Stratton (Division of Harcourt-Brace-Jovanovich), 1988.

Kenner C, Breuggemeyer A: Hirschsprung's disease: current trends and practices. *Neonat Network* 1984; 3(1):7–16.

Kirschner BS: Inflammatory bowel disease in children. *Pediatr Clin North Am* 1988; 35(1):189–208.

Korones SB: *High-risk Newborn Infants,* 4th ed. St. Louis, CV Mosby, 1986, 364–392.

Kottmeier PK: Appendicitis. *In* Welch KJ, et al: *Pediatric Surgery,* 4th ed, Vol 2. Chicago, Year Book Medical Publishers, 1986.

Kurfiss-Daniels D: Positioning as treatment for infant gastroesophageal reflux. *Am J Nurs* 1982; 82:1535–1537.

Leape LL: *Patient Care in Pediatric Surgery.* Boston, Little, Brown, 1987.

Lindsay WK: Cleft lip and cleft palate. *In* Welch KJ, et al: *Pediatric Surgery,* 4th ed, Vol 2. Chicago, Year Book Medical Publishers, 1986.

Listernick R, et al: Outpatient oral rehydration in the United States. *Am J Dis Child* 1986; 140:211–215.

Liu KW, et al: Intussusception—current trends in management. *Arch Dis Child* 1986; 61:75–77.

Lloyd-Still JD: Chronic diarrhea of childhood and misuse of elimination diets. *J Pediatr* 1979; 95:10.

Maclean WC, Fink BB: Lactose malabsorption by premature infants. Magnitude and clinical significance. *J Pediatr* 1980; 97:383.

Martin LW, Torres AM: Hirschsprung's disease. *Surg Clin North Am* 1985; 65:1171–1180.

McWilliams BJ, et al: *Cleft Palate Speech.* St. Louis, CV Mosby, 1984.

Morecki R, et al: Biliary atresia and reovirus type III infection. *N Engl J Med* 1982; 307:481.

Nord KS: Peptic ulcer disease in the pediatric population. *Pediatr Clin North Am* 1988; 35:117–140.

Oellrich RG, Cusmano MM: Biliary atresia. *Neonat Network* 1987; 5(5):25–35.

Orenstein SR, et al: The infant seat as treatment for gastroesophageal reflux. *N Engl J Med* 1983; 309:760–763.

Oski F: Obstructive jaundice due to biliary atresia and neonatal hepatitis. *In* Avery ME, Taeusch HW: *Schaffer's Diseases of the Newborn.* Philadelphia, WB Saunders, 1984, 637–643.

Owens J, et al: Epidemiology of facial clefting. *Arch Dis Child* 1985; 60:521–524.

Paarlberg J, Balint JP: Gastrostomy tubes: practical guidelines for home care. *Pediatr Nurs* 1985 Mar/Apr; 99–102.

Paradise JJ: Maternal and other factors in the etiology of infantile colic. *JAMA* 1966; 197:123.

Petersen M: Esophageal pH monitoring. *J Pediatr Nurs* 1986; 1(5):354–357.

Pickering LK, et al: Occurrence of *Giardia lamblia* in children in day care centers. *J Pediatr* 1984; 104:522–525.

Poley JR: Chronic non-specific diarrhea, investigation of the surface morphology of small bowel mucosa utilizing the scanning electron microscope. *J Pediatr Gastroenterol Nutr* 1983; 2:71.

Radl S: *Mother's Day is Over.* New York, Warner Books, 1974.

Randolph JG: Esophageal atresia and congenital stenosis. *In* Welch KJ, et al: *Pediatric Surgery.* 4th ed. Vol. I. Chicago, Year Book Medical Publishers, 1986, 682–693.

Robson AM: The pathophysiology of body fluids. *In* Behrman RE, Vaughan VC: *Nelson Textbook of Pediatrics.* Philadelphia, WB Saunders, 1987, 172–207.

Rowell P: Infantile colic: reviewing the situation. *Pediatr Nurs* 1978 May/Jun; 20.

Schmitt BC: The prevention of sleep problems and colic. *Pediatr Clin North Am* 1986; 33:763–774.

Shandling B: Congenital anomalies of the gastrointestinal tract and intestinal obstruction. *In* Behrman RE, Vaughan VC: *Nelson Textbook of Pediatrics.* Philadelphia, WB Saunders, 1983.

Shah C, Wong D: Management of children with cleft lip and palate. *Can Med Assoc J* 1980; 122:19.

Sieber WK: Hirschsprung's disease. *In* Gellis SS, Kagan BM (eds): *Current Pediatric Therapy 12.* Philadelphia, WB Saunders, 1986, 206–207.

Silverman A, Roy CC: *Pediatric Clinical Gastroenterology,* 3rd ed. St. Louis, CV Mosby, 1983.

Simmons MA: Using the nursing process in treating inflammatory bowel disease. *Nurs Clin North Am* 1984; 19:11–25.

Starzl TE, et al: Liver and kidney transplantation in children receiving cyclosporin-A and steroids. *J Pediatr* 1982; 100:681.

Summers RW, et al: National Cooperative Crohn's Disease Study: Results of drug treatment. *Gastroenterology* 1979; 77:847.

Tolia VK, Dubois RS: Update on oral rehydration: its place in treatment of acute gastroenteritis. *Pediatr Ann* 1985; 14(4):295–303.

Trier WC: Primary palatoplasty. *Clin Plast Surg* 1985; 12:659–675.

Wald A, et al: Lactose malabsorption in recurrent abdominal pain in children. *J Pediatr* 1982; 100:65.

Walsh MC, Kliegman RM: Necrotizing enterocolitis: treatment based on staging criteria. *Pediatr Clin North Am* 1986; 33:179–201.

Weibley TT, et al: Gavage tube insertion in the premature infant. *MCN* 1987; 12:24–27.

Weissbluth M: Dicyclomine hydrochloride in management of infant colic. *J Pediatr* 1984; 104:951.

Welch KJ: Intussusception. *In* Hoekelman RA, et al (eds): *Principles of Pediatrics.* New York, McGraw-Hill, 1978.

Williams R: Congenital diaphragmatic hernia: a review. *Heart Lung* 1982; 11:532–538.

Winslow RE, et al: Acute nonperforating appendicitis. Efficacy of brief antibiotic prophylaxis. *Arch Surg* 1983; 118:651–655.

Bibliography

Adams DA, Selekof JL: Children with ostomies: comprehensive care planning. *Pediatr Nurs* 1986; 12(6):429–433.

Aquilina SS: Gastroesophageal reflux: problem or nuisance? *J Pediatr Health Care* 1987; 1(5):233–239.

Brown KH, et al: Effect of continued oral feeding on clinical and nutritional outcomes of acute diarrhea in children. *J Pediatr* 1988; 112(2):191–200.

Day DW: Accurate diagnosis and assessment of growth in patients with orofacial clefting. *Birth Defects* 1985; 21:1–14.

Ghory MJ, Sheldon CG: Newborn surgical emergencies of the gastrointestinal tract. *Surg Clin North Am* 1985; 65:1083–1098.

Issenman RM: Management of diarrhea in infants and children. *Can Fam Physician* 1987; 33:1261–1264.

Issenman RM: Toddlers: chronic diarrhea, constipation, diet and supplements. *Mod Med Can* 1985; 40(3):15–19.

Kapp-Simon K: Self-concept of primary-school-age children with cleft lip, palate or both. *Cleft Palate J* 1986; 1:24–27.

Kirschner BS: Inflammatory bowel disease in children. *Pediatr Clin North Am* 1988; 35(1):189–208.

Koldovsky O: Perinatal adaptation of gastrointestinal functions in man. *Perinatology-Neonatology* 1987; 11(1): 31–39.

Lynn MR: Use of infant seats for gastroesophageal reflux. *J Pediatr Nurs* 1986; 1(2):127–129.

McInerney TG: Cleft palate repair. Surgical procedure and nursing care. *AORN J* 1985; 42:516–534.

Ostertag SG: Early enteral feeding does not affect the incidence of necrotizing enterocolitis. *Pediatrics* 1986; 77:275–280.

Pizarro D: Oral rehydration therapy: its use in neonates and young infants. *J Pediatr Gastroenterol Nutr* 1986; 1:6–8.

Postuma R, Moroz SP: Pediatric Crohn's disease. *J Pediatr Surg* 1985; 20:478–482.

Ryan NM: Recurrent abdominal pain among school-aged children. *MCN* 1986; 11:102–107.

Scheuerle J, et al: A survey of nursing care for parents and infants with cleft lip and palate. *Cleft Palate J* 1984; 21:110–114.

Simstein N: Congenital gastric anomalies. *Am Surgeon* 1986; 52:264–268.

Strauss RP, et al: Interdisciplinary team care of cleft lip and palate: social and psychological aspects. *Clin Plast Surg* 1985; 12:543–551.

Tanner MS, Stocks RJ: Neonatal gastroenterology: contemporary issues. *Intercept* 1984 Apr.

Tobiasen JM: Psychosocial correlates of congenital facial clefts. A conceptualization and model. *Cleft Palate J* 1984; 21:131.

Welch KJ, et al: *Pediatric Surgery*, 4th ed, Vol 2. Chicago, Year Book Medical Publishers, 1986.

Nursing Strategies: Altered Genitourinary Function

Chapter 42

Susan N. Van Cleve
S. Elizabeth Baldwin

Genitourinary disorders in children encompass a wide range of problems, from common ones such as enuresis or cystitis to rare ones such as exstrophy of the bladder. Congenital anomalies affect a significant percentage of children with sequelae that may be minor or life-threatening. Urinary tract infections are fairly common and constitute one of the most frequently seen bacterial diseases in children.

The role of the nurse includes the assessment, planning, intervention, and evaluation of children with disorders of the genitourinary system. Because these disorders have such a wide variety of manifestations and treatment plans, the nursing role is diverse and requires a sound knowledge base. In order to better understand genitourinary disorders, a review of the anatomy and physiology of the genitourinary system is presented. Common laboratory and diagnostic studies including pertinent nursing interventions are discussed. A comprehensive description of genitourinary system disorders and anomalies, including the nursing role and current modes of therapy, is included.

Anatomy of the Urinary System

Overview of the System

The genitourinary system comprises the *kidneys, ureters, urinary bladder,* and *urethra.* Urine is formed by the kidneys and transported outside the body by the remainder of the system (Fig. 42-1).

The kidneys are located retroperitoneally to the right and left of the lumbar spine. Each kidney is supported by fascia, covered by a tough capsule, and surrounded by a cushion of fat. The right kidney is displaced by the liver and lies lower than the left kidney.

The production of urine takes place in the kidney. From the kidney, the urine flows through the ureters to the urinary bladder. The ureters are a pair of mucosa-lined tubes that have no sphincters but use peristalsis to transport the urine. The ureters join the bladder at an oblique angle, which helps to prevent the occurrence of reflux (backflow) when the bladder empties.

The urinary bladder is a hollow, muscular sac that is located in the pelvis posterior to the pelvic bones. The urethral orifice is located at the inferior portion of the bladder, joining the bladder to the urethra.

The urethra is a hollow tube that leads to the urinary meatus. In males the urethra is long (approximately 20 cm in the adult male) and in females it is relatively short (3 to 5 cm in the adult female). In children, the length of the urethra is proportionately shorter according to their growth and age.

The Kidney

Three general regions may be identified within the kidney: the *renal cortex,* the *renal medulla,* and the *renal pelvis* (Fig. 42-2).

The renal cortex is the outer section of the kidney. This section arches over the renal pyramids of the medulla. The sections that extend inward between the pyramids are called the *renal columns.*

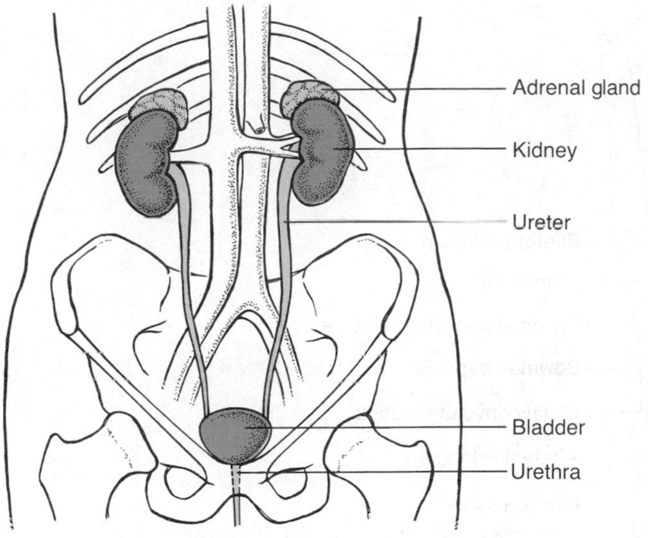

Figure 42-1. Components of the urinary system.

The renal medulla is composed of approximately 18 to 20 triangular wedge-shaped masses called the *renal pyramids.* Each pyramid projects centrally toward the renal pelvis to form a *papilla.* The papilla has a number of openings that allow urine to flow into the cup-shaped extension *(calyx)* of the renal pelvis.

The renal pelvis is a funnel-shaped sac that receives urine from all parts of the kidney via the calyces. The renal pelvis is attached to the ureter. Urine collects in the renal calyces and pelvis and drains into the ureters, from which it is transported by active peristalsis to the bladder.

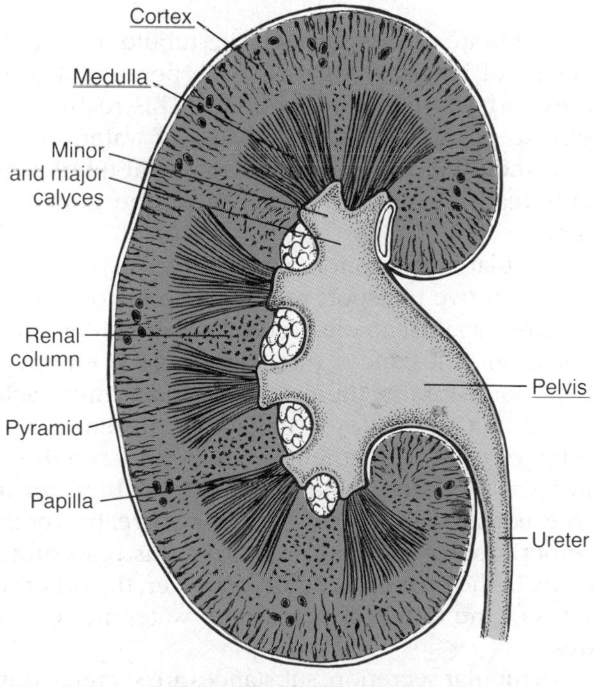

Figure 42-2. Cross-section of the kidney.

The Nephron

The basic functional unit of the kidney is the nephron. There are approximately 1 to 1.5 million nephrons in each kidney. Each nephron consists of a renal tubule and a renal corpuscle.

The renal corpuscle is made up of the *glomerulus* and encased by *Bowman capsule.* The glomerulus is a network of capillaries that lie between the afferent and efferent arterioles. The *afferent arteriole* transports blood to the glomerulus where it divides into up to 50 capillary loops inside the structure. These loops join to form the *efferent arteriole* that carries blood away from the glomerulus to the *peritubular capillaries.* The peritubular capillaries and hairpin loops called the *vasa recta* surround the tubule of the nephron (Fig. 42-3). The diameter of the afferent arteriole is twice that of the efferent arteriole; it also has a more substantial layer of smooth muscle compared with the efferent arteriole.

Bowman capsule serves two purposes: to filter materials in and out of the glomerulus and to act as the beginning point for the renal tubule. The renal tubule begins its course at Bowman capsule and ends at the collecting tubule. The tubule changes names as it progresses through the nephron—the *proximal convoluted tubule;* the *loop of Henle;* and the *distal convoluted tubule.* The collecting tubule passes through a renal pyramid and joins other collecting tubules or ducts to form one of the papillary ducts that opens into a calyx. Several nephrons drain into each collecting tubule.

The renal corpuscles of the nephrons lie within the renal cortex. The renal corpuscles of *cortical nephrons* are located in the outer two thirds of the cortex. These nephrons usually have small glomeruli and short loops of Henle. The nephrons that remain within the inner third of the cortex are called *juxtamedullary nephrons.* These nephrons have long loops of Henle that extend downward in variable distances to the medulla.

Physiology of the Urinary System

The kidneys are major body organs that serve many functions: the detoxification of the blood and elimination of metabolic wastes such as urea, creatinine, uric acid, phosphate, sulfates, potassium, nitrates, and phenols; the regulation of volume, electrolyte concentration of body fluids, and acid-base balance; the regulation of blood pressure through the release of renin and prostaglandins; the release of erythropoietin to stimulate new red blood cell production; and the regulation of calcium balance through vitamin D metabolism.

The production of urine by the kidney provides the body with a mechanism to excrete waste products,

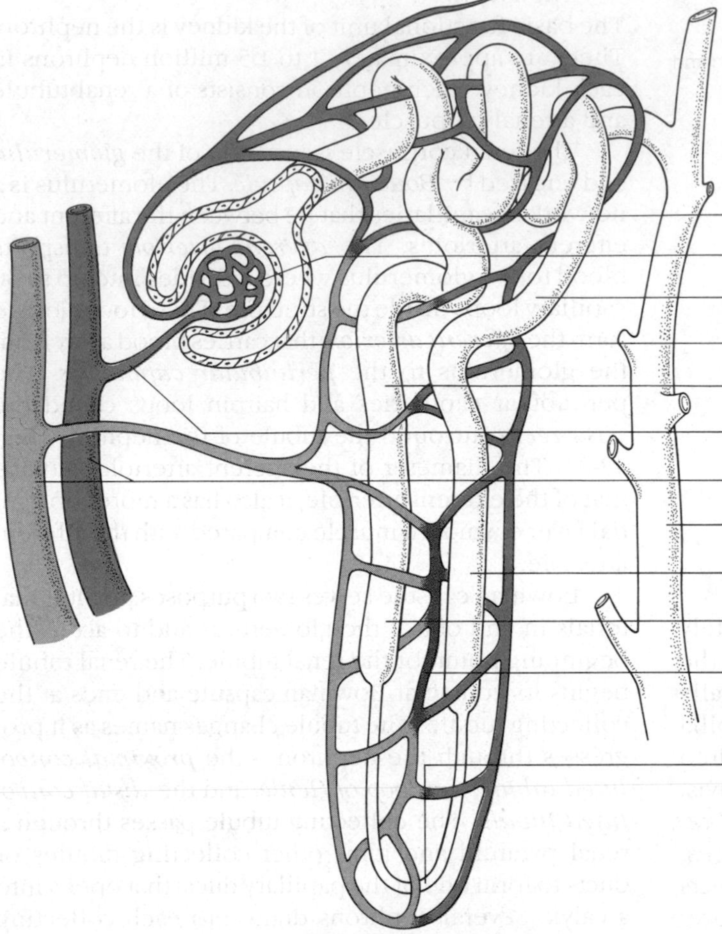

Figure 42-3. The nephron.

to clear foreign substances, and to detoxify substances. The processes involved in urine formation are glomerular filtration and tubular reabsorption and secretion.

Glomerular Filtration

The blood entering the glomerulus through the afferent arteriole is at a high pressure. The force of this pressure creates a difference between the glomerular capillary pressure, the colloidal osmotic pressure and the capsular pressure. The difference in these pressures is called *net filtration pressure.* The net filtration pressure forces substances of a small molecular weight across the glomerular membrane into the lumen of the surrounding Bowman capsule. However, large molecules such as proteins are unable to pass and are retained in the blood.

The glomerular filtration rate (GFR) is determined by the blood pressure, the effective filtration pressure, and the permeability of the capillary walls. If abnormalities in any of these exist, the GFR will be altered. The GFR in children is calculated according to the child's age and body size.

Tubular Reabsorption and Secretion

As the filtrate passes through the tubule a large percentage of it is reabsorbed by the peritubular capillaries and returned to the plasma. This reabsorption helps to prevent an excessive loss of water, electrolytes, and other necessary solutes. Renal tubules normally reabsorb up to 99 per cent of the glomerular filtrate.

Tubular reabsorption or secretion can be active or passive. Active transport requires energy to move the substance against an electrochemical gradient or concentration. Substances that require such energy include potassium, sodium, glucose, and amino acids. Passive transport takes advantage of present concentration or osmotic gradients and does not require any energy. Water, urea, chloride, and some bicarbonates represent substances that are passively reabsorbed by the peritubular capillaries. Most of this reabsorption occurs in the proximal tubule; however, the other segments of the tubule also reabsorb water and electrolytes.

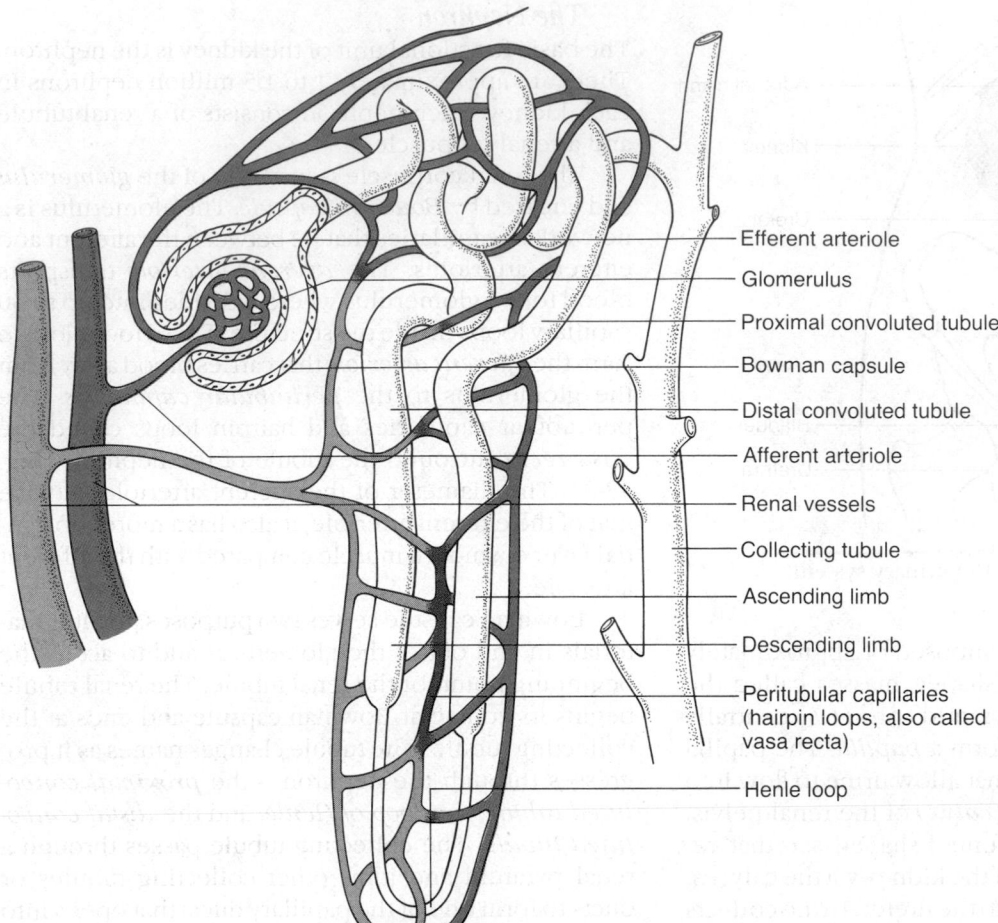

In tubular secretion, substances are secreted out of

the peritubular blood into the lumen of the renal tubule by active transport or passive diffusion. Such substances include ammonia, uric acid, potassium, hydrogen, exogenous substances, and other wastes.

The ability of a child's kidneys to adjust the excretion of urine and solute (i.e., dilute or concentrate) in response to the body's demand for water and electrolyte balance is normally adequate but is less adaptable than an adult's kidneys in times of emergency. Infants gain the ability to dilute their urine on approximately the 14th day of life and the ability to concentrate urine during the third month of life (deWardener, 1985). After a 12-hour fluid deprivation period the infant beyond the age of 2 months should be able to concentrate urine to about 900 mOsm/l, or a specific gravity of 1.024 (Bergstein and Michael, 1987).

Anatomy of the Genitalia

Female Genitalia

The female genitalia involve both internal and external structures. The internal organs include the ovaries, fallopian tubes, uterus, and vagina. The reader is directed to a textbook of gynecologic and obstetric nursing for a description of the complex hormonal physiology of these internal structures.

The external genitalia include the mons pubis, labia majora, labia minora, clitoris, vestibule, and Bartholin's and Skene's glands. The labia majora and labia minora form the outer and inner lips of the female genitalia or vulva. (See Figure 15-19.) The inner surfaces of the labia contain many sebaceous glands, which become active at puberty. The perspiration from these glands predisposes some young women to vulvar irritation; such individuals may need to be counseled to bathe and change underwear more frequently.

Formed of erectile tissue, the clitoris is the homologue of the penis. Because of its structure the clitoris can be mistaken for the urethral opening by an inexperienced practitioner. The clitoris joins the anterior folds of the labia minora while the urethral and vaginal openings are found in the vestibule, the cleft between the labia minora.

Skene glands, which surround the urethral meatus, are the homologues of the male prostate gland. Bartholin glands are found near the vaginal opening and, although usually not palpable, may at times present as small, round bumps. Bartholin glands are believed to provide vaginal lubrication during coitus.

Male Genitalia

The penis and the scrotum constitute the major structures of the male genitalia. (See Figure 15-20.) The urethra is positioned ventrally within the shaft of the penis and the normal meatal opening in the glans penis. The prepuce, or foreskin, is the retractable fold of the skin that covers the glans penis in uncircumcised males.

The scrotum contains the testes, the epididymis, and a portion of the vas deferens. The testes are palpable as smooth, firm, olive-shaped structures within each scrotal sac. Spermatic cords suspend each testis and are composed of blood vessels, nerves, and the vas deferens. Because the right spermatic cord is shorter, the left testis hangs somewhat lower than the right.

The vas deferens carries sperm from the testis to the ejaculatory duct formed by the union of the vas deferens and the vesicles. The semen is propelled from the ejaculatory duct into the urethra. The prostate gland is located within the abdominal cavity, and surrounds the urethra and the ejaculatory ducts. Abnormalities of the prostate gland are rare before adulthood.

Diagnostic Assessment of Genitourinary Function

Because the kidneys play a major role in maintaining homeostasis in the body, an impairment of genitourinary functioning has the potential to affect other body systems. Therefore, a wide range of signs and symptoms must be considered related to the potential for or presence of genitourinary dysfunction.

The child's age and level of maturation in assessment are important. The type of disorder and the incidence of its occurrence may be more significant to a child of one age group than another. For example, the implications for an infant with a urinary tract infection differ vastly from those for a sexually active female adolescent with the same problem.

The components of the assessment are the history and physical examination. If the child is young, the presence of the parents is helpful in obtaining the information and in gaining the child's cooperation.

The History and Physical Assessment

Assessment of genitourinary function should be included in every history. Many genitourinary disorders may have only subtle manifestations in their early stages, with ensuing serious complications if not detected early. Therefore, a comprehensive history is imperative. Although a previous history or physical examination, or both, may not reflect a genitourinary disorder, this should not deter the nurse from assessing for a subtle abnormality. Table 42-1 summarizes normal differences in structure and function of the genitourinary system according to development.

Table 42-1. Developmental Differences in Structure and Function of the Genitourinary System

Anatomy and Physiology	Significance
Urine Concentration	
Infants do not gain the ability to concentrate urine until about 3 mo of age	• A low specific gravity for the young infant is not necessarily indicative of adequate hydration • The lack of concentrating ability makes the young infant particularly prone to dehydration
Urine Dilution	
While the infant's capacity to dilute urine is comparable to that of an adult, the infant kidney is less well-equipped to process a sudden large quantity of fluid (Drummond, 1983)	• The infant is more prone to fluid volume excess; IV fluids must be carefully monitored to prevent volume overload
External Genitalia of Newborn Female	
Labia: The labia minora may be relatively prominent and protrude beyond the labia majora in preterm and some fullterm infants. In addition, the edges of the labia minora are typically darkly pigmented at birth. Swelling of the external genitalia may be present in the first days of life. *Vaginal discharge:* In the first 2 wk of life alterations in circulating hormones may produce a grayish or milky, thin or mucoid discharge, which may also be blood-tinged	• The nurse who recognizes normal developmental immaturity from anatomic and physiologic anomalies can reassure parents about their baby's health and can appropriately refer signs and symptoms of concern
External Genitalia of Newborn Male	
The nonerect newborn penis is typically 2–3 cm in length. Transient penile erection is common in the infant and small child. At birth the testicles often appear large for the infant's size	• The nurse can reassure parents about the normalcy of their son's anatomy
The uncircumcised foreskin is usually difficult to retract during the first 2–3 mo, becoming more easily retractable at 4 mo, and fully retractable at 4 yr of age	• The private physician's advice should be followed regarding whether or not to routinely retract the uncircumcised foreskin in early infancy; practices and opinions vary

When a child presents with a genitourinary disorder, a comprehensive nursing history should be performed as explained in Chapter 15. In assessing a child with a genitourinary disorder, specific factors should be assessed that will be pertinent to the nursing care and treatment (Box 42-1).

The goal of physical assessment is to identify abnormalities—specifically those associated with genitourinary disorders. A complete physical examination should be performed as described in Chapter 15.

Box 42-1
Nursing History for a Child with a Genitourinary Disorder

HISTORY OF PRESENT ILLNESS

1. Identify complaint
2. Identify duration, location, severity, past and current treatment of the genitourinary problem

BIRTH HISTORY

1. Presence of polyhydramnios or oligohydramnios during the pregnancy
2. Number of umbilical vessels at birth
3. Presence of congenital anomalies
4. What were the neonatal voiding patterns?

PAST HEALTH HISTORY

1. Previous serious illnesses
2. Exposure to nephrotoxic agents
3. Exposure to potentially nephrotoxic drugs
4. Previous bladder infections or obstructions
5. Has the child ever had headaches, irritability, seizures, visual disturbances (suggestive of hypertension)?
6. Has the child ever been fatigued, anorectic, had failure to thrive, or stopped growing (suggestive of chronic renal failure)?

DEVELOPMENTAL HISTORY

Has the child reached developmental milestones (i.e., toilet training)?

What words does the child use for elimination?

HABITS

Diet

Alterations in feeding or changes in fluid intake

Alterations in the child's appetite

Elimination

Bowel: Identify the child's bowel patterns, consistency of stool, frequency of elimination

Bladder—child's voiding pattern: Is there any frequency, change in volume, dysuria, alterations in urinary stream, dribbling, pain in the genital area, urgency? Color and odor of urine

Presence of daytime or nocturnal enuresis

Sleep

Alteration in the sleeping pattern

Behavior

Does the child fatigue easily?

Is the child irritable?

Table 42-2. Clinical Manifestations of Genitourinary Alterations

Clinical Manifestation	Clinical Significance
Headaches, irritability, visual disturbances, seizures	Indicative of hypertension, acidosis or alkalosis
Paleness of conjunctivae, skin, and mucous membranes	Indicative of anemia
Breath odor may be ammoniac or urine-like	Indicative of uremia
Heart murmur, arrhythmia or pericardial friction rub	Cardiovascular abnormalities may result from anemia, hypertension, or fluid overload
Tachypnea, rales, rhonchi, Kussmaul's respirations. Infant may have nasal flaring, retractions	Respiratory alterations may indicate fluid overload, metabolic acidosis
Abdominal masses, abdominal or flank pain, palpation of enlarged kidneys	Indicative of hydronephrotic kidneys, tumor, presence of infection
Urine color, odor, urinary stream, pain on urination, hematuria, frequency. *In younger children:* child may complain of abdominal pain, cry with urination. *In older children:* child may have enuresis, complain of dysuria	Alteration may indicate presence of infection, obstruction, or dehydration
Skin color—pale, sallow, or jaundiced	Indicative of obstruction, anemia, or uremia
Edema, weight gain	Indicative of fluid retention
Growth retardation	Indicative of chronic infection or renal failure
Congenital anomalies: low-set ears, widely spaced nipples, absence of abdominal musculature (prune belly syndrome), spina bifida, abnormalities of the external genitalia	These anomalies are associated with genitourinary disorders

Common clinical manifestations seen in children with genitourinary disorders may be identified during this examination (Table 42-2).

Laboratory and Diagnostic Studies

Children with genitourinary disorders frequently undergo numerous laboratory tests or diagnostic procedures. These children and their families can benefit from careful teaching and reassurance prior to the performance of these tests and procedures. Procedures associated with the genitalia or with the function of urination usually produce a great deal of anxiety in families. Some of the procedures are intrusive and painful or uncomfortable. Preparation for discomfort can help the child and family members cope more effectively with the procedure and feel more in control of themselves and their situation.

Chapter 27 outlines procedures for urine specimen collection in children. Laboratory tests and diagnostic procedures in children are frequently more difficult to do than they are in adults secondary to the child's anxiety and limited ability to understand and cooperate during specimen collection procedures.

Tables 42-3 and 42-4 outline common laboratory tests and diagnostic procedures performed in children with genitourinary disorders. Test results in children are frequently different from those in adults and are noted in these tables, as well as in the anatomy and physiology section of this chapter.

Strategies for Nursing Care of a Child with a Drainage Device

Understanding the Purpose of Catheters, Stents, and Drains

Children who have had urinary tract surgery frequently return from the operating room with multiple appliances that require expert nursing knowledge and care. These appliances fall into three main categories: catheters, stents, and drains. *Catheters* transport urine from any part of the urinary tract to a drainage bag and are named according to the anatomic part they drain, e.g., nephrostomy tube (kidney), ureterostomy tube (ureter). Because the bladder can be drained in several ways, bladder catheters are named according to the route of drainage: urethral catheter (through the urethra), suprapubic tube (through the bladder and abdominal walls), or perineal urethrostomy (through the middle portion of the urethra).

Stents are very thin catheters that serve also as internal splints for surgical sites within the urinary tract. They promote tissue healing and, by draining urine, prevent pressure on the surgical site from the build-up of fluid. The terms "ureteral tube" and "ureteral stent" are frequently used interchangeably. Stents usually exit the body through the urethra or through an incision in the abdominal wall.

Drains are placed outside the urinary tract to allow urine that has leaked from surgical sites to reach the outside of the body, thereby preventing infection and scarring caused by urine build-up in the tissues surrounding the urinary structure. When the child has more than one drainage tube or catheter, the nurse must carefully label the tubes according to their origin within the body. The volume of urine from each catheter or tube should be recorded separately.

Parents can become disconcerted upon seeing their child return from surgery with multiple tubes and bandages and, as a result, may have difficulty support-

Text continues on page 1477

Table 42-3. Laboratory Tests: Urine and Blood

Test	Normal Values	Interpretation
Routine Urinalysis		
Appearance	Clear	Cloudy: bacteria, white blood cells, phosphates
Color	Pale amber to yellow	*Reddish:* beets, blackberries, certain cold drink and food dyes, certain drugs, urates, bile, hemoglobin and myoglobin *Blue/green:* oxidation of bilirubin in poorly preserved specimen (Wallach, 1983)
Specific gravity (SG)	1.010–1.030	Provides information about hydration status and the kidney's ability to concentrate/dilute urine *Increased:* dehydration, nephrosis (secondary to proteinuria), excretion of IVP contrast medium *Decreased:* glomerulonephritis, severe renal damage
pH	4.6–8.0 (depends on time of day and freshness of specimen) average = 6.0	Affected by medications and diet Alkaline urine (pH 7.5) can develop in presence of urea-splitting bacteria (e.g., *Proteus*)
Glucose	Negative	Positive in diabetes mellitus or in any condition causing decreased ability of renal tubules to reabsorb glucose May be positive in 25% of normal premature infants and infants up to the third day (deWardener, 1985)
Protein	Negative–trace (trace protein may or may not be normal)	Positive in a variety of acute and chronic renal diseases (e.g., nephrotic syndrome) May be positive in 25% of normal premature infants and infants up to the third day (deWardener, 1985)
Ketones	Negative	Increased in conditions resulting in acidosis (e.g., diabetes mellitus, starvation, fever, high-fat diet)
Red blood cells (RBC)	1–2	Increased in menstrual flow, lower urinary tract infection, glomerulonephritis, pyelonephritis, renal trauma
White blood cells (WBC)	1–2	Increased in nearly all urinary tract diseases
Casts	Negative	Specific types of casts are frequently associated with certain renal disorders (but can vary) *Hyaline casts:* serious renal disease *Granular/waxy casts:* chronic renal failure, renal transplant rejection *WBC casts:* pyelonephritis *RBC casts:* glomerulonephritis (McConnell and Zimmerman, 1983)
Other Urine Tests		
Creatinine	1.0–1.6 g/24 hr(15–25 mg/kg of body weight/24 hr)	Based on 24-hr urine collection and comparison with serum creatinine levels Reflects GFR Decreases when GFR decreases secondary to disease process (e.g., glomerulonephritis)
Osmolality	500–1200 mOsm/kg water Usual urine:serum ratio = 4:1	More accurate than specific gravity in evaluating renal concentrating mechanisms because does not vary with diet or changes in urine content Compared with serum osmolality Decreases with diabetes insipidus, chronic renal disease
Volume	**Age** — **(ml/24 hr)** Neonate — 30–60 1–7 days — 100–300 10–60 days — 250–450 2–12 mo — 400–500 1–3 yr — 500–600 3–5 yr — 600–700 5–8 yr — 650–1000 8–14 yr — 800–1400 Adults — 600–1600	

Table 42-3 *(continued)*

Test	Normal Values	Interpretation
Blood Tests		
Creatinine	0.6–1.5 mg/dl	Increased with impaired renal function Glomerular filtration rate must be reduced by at least 50% before a significant increase in serum creatinine occurs
Blood urea nitrogen (BUN)	5–25 mg/dl	Increased with impaired renal function, obstruction of the urinary tract, or in any condition causing reduced renal blood flow (e.g., shock, salt and water depletion, cardiac failure) Decreased with overhydration, low-protein diet, liver failure In chronic renal disease, BUN correlates better than creatinine with symptoms of uremia

Table 42-4. Diagnostic Procedures

Description	Nursing Strategies
Intravenous Pyelogram (IVP) (Excretory Urogram)	
Intravenous injection of radiopaque contrast medium Excretion of medium through kidneys with concentration in the collecting tubules allowing visualization of calyces, renal pelvis, ureters, and bladder 20–30 min radiograph series One post voiding radiograph (total time: approximately 45 min) Useful in the diagnosis of hydronephrosis, renal scarring, cysts, tumors, pyelonephritis, reflux and calculi	***Preprocedural Care*** 1. Explain purpose and procedure to parents and, if appropriate, to child. Prepare child for feelings associated with injection of contrast medium: general feeling of warmth, burning at IV site, nausea. Avoid use of word "dye" as this may frighten younger children (may confuse with "die") 2. Verify that child has had no past allergic reactions to radiopaque contrast medium 3. Restrict diet prior to test as indicated by institution 4. Administer cathartics/enemas as indicated 5. Assure that a supportive family member or a familiar nurse will be with child during procedure ***Postprocedural Care*** 1. Be alert for allergic reaction to contrast medium (pruritus, sneezing, wheezing, dyspnea, flushed skin). Allergic reactions usually occur within first few minutes after injection of contrast medium 2. Encourage fluids and a few hours of rest after procedure 3. Expect urine to have high specific gravity for up to 24 hr after the procedure (secondary to dehydration and excretion of contrast medium) 4. Notify physician if urine output decreases. Renal failure is an uncommon but serious complication of IVP
Voiding Cystourethrogram (VCUG)	
Catheterization and filling of the bladder with contrast medium Series of radiographs before, during, and after voiding (total time: approximately 15 min) Useful in the diagnosis of vesicoureteral reflux, urethral valves, and strictures	1. Explain purpose and procedure to parents and, if appropriate, to child. Prepare child for the feeling of having to go to the bathroom as the bladder is filling with the special liquid—contrast material. Explain to child that he or she will be a little sore the first few times going to the bathroom after the procedure, but reassure that the soreness will go away soon 2. Ensure that a supportive family member or a familiar nurse will be with child during procedure *Note:* Radiology department may request that a pediatric physician or nurse catheterize child for procedure
Abdominal/Renal Ultrasound	
Sound waves bounced off anatomic structures resulting in an electronic image of structures Application of lubricant to abdomen and/or flank and movement of transducer over the area (total time: approximately 15 min) Useful as a complementary procedure in the diagnosis of congenital anomalies, hydronephrosis, reflux, renal tumors, cysts, calculi, and abscesses. Increased use predicted as procedure becomes perfected	1. Explain purpose and procedure to parents and, if appropriate, to child. Reassure them that procedure is painless 2. Ensure that a supportive family member or a familiar nurse will be with child during procedure 3. Administer sedation if ordered

continued

Table 42-4 *(continued)*

Description	Nursing Strategies
Plain Film or Flat Plate of Abdomen (KUB—Kidneys, Ureters, Bladder)	
Routine radiograph of abdomen and bladder Older child may be asked to hold breath for a few seconds Useful in diagnosis of gross structural abnormalities. Can be used to determine size, shape, and placement of kidneys	As for routine radiograph
Cystoscopy	
General or local anesthesia Insertion of thin tube-like cystoscope into the urethra and visualization of the urethra and the interior of the bladder Useful in the diagnosis of bladder wall anomalies, urethral valves, and strictures	***Preprocedural Care*** 1. Explain purpose and procedure to parents and, if appropriate, to child 2. Nothing orally as ordered 3. Premedication as ordered ***Postprocedural Care*** 1. Reassure parents and child that urination after procedure is frequently uncomfortable. Having child urinate in a tub of warm water may be helpful 2. Encourage fluids 3. Monitor urine volume and character for 24 hr after procedure. Very small amounts of bleeding within normal 4. Monitor temperature carefully. Bacteremia can occur after instrumentation of the urinary tract. Notify physician if temperature over 101°F (38.4 degree C) 5. Administer prophylactic antibiotics if ordered, prior to procedure and for several days afterward

Box 42-2
Guidelines for Care of Catheters and Drainage Devices

1. Always wash hands before and after doing catheter care.
2. Position child carefully to prevent kinking or looping of tubing. Infants and very young children may need gauze mittens or restraints to keep them from pulling at the catheter.
3. Prevent movement of the catheter by taping it to the thigh/flank/abdomen and allowing some slack in the tubing.
4. Keep a careful record of urine output and character (e.g., clear, cloudy, blood-tinged, clots) from each catheter. Prepare parents and child for appearance of drainage postoperatively (watery and bright red 24 hours after surgery, progressing to reddish-brown with small clots, to clear within 4 to 7 days). Notify physician if significant amount of bleeding occurs at any time.
5. Watch for signs of obstruction: no output for more than an hour, urine leaking around the catheter, bladder distension, large blood clots, or tissue shreds inside the catheter. If no external obstruction (e.g., kinks) can be found, gently "milk" the tubing and/or irrigate with sterile normal saline, if ordered. Notify physician immediately if not successful with preceding procedures.
6. Always keep the collecting bag below the level of the child's bladder to facilitate gravity drainage of urine. Never fasten bag to bed siderails as it could inadvertently become caught when siderails are raised or lowered.
7. Carefully cleanse catheter entry site at least twice a day according to institutional policy. Apply antimicrobial ointment and/or dressing if indicated.
8. Maintain sterile closed drainage system. Open the system only for irrigation or collection of specimens as ordered. Always thoroughly cleanse site where system will be opened before and after opening.
9. Administer comfort measures and pain medication as ordered for bladder spasms. Check for kinking or obstruction of tubing as cause for pain.
10. Encourage adequate oral intake.
11. After catheter removal, prepare parents and child for some discomfort over next 24 hours. Keep careful record of intake/output; notify physician if child does not void within 6 hours after catheter removal.

ing the child. The nurse should prepare parents and children preoperatively for postoperative appearances and procedures, using words that can be understood by both. In preparing the child, the catheter can be described as a "tube"; surgery can be described as "fixing." Indiscriminate use of frightening words like "cut" or "bleed" should be avoided.

Box 42-2 outlines general principles of catheter care that apply to all categories of drainage devices.

Teaching Clean Intermittent Catheterization

Clean intermittent catheterization is most frequently used in children with neurogenic bladder dysfunction. It is based on the theory that the bladder is resistant to infection as long as it is emptied frequently and does not become overdistended. Catheterization is done at least every 3 to 4 hours; the frequency depends on the type of neurogenic bladder dysfunction, bladder capacity, sphincter function, and fluid intake.

The nurse's assessment of the parent's and child's willingness and ability to perform routine frequent catheterizations is of the utmost importance. Serious urinary tract infections can result if the bladder is not routinely emptied and becomes overdistended. Box 42-3 outlines the procedure for clean intermittent catheterization. Under Public Law 94-142, the law mandating certain educational services for handicapped children, clean intermittent catheterization is a mandated school health service. For children who cannot catheterize themselves, school personnel, ideally the school nurse, must be available to perform the procedure (Stauffer, 1984). The hospital or clinic nurse can work with school personnel to ensure their understanding of the child's health care needs. A private area with a sink, a place to store equipment, and a change of clothing are all necessary.

Box 42-3
Directions for Clean Catheterization

1. Wash hands with soap and water or with a towelette, if possible. Because the avoidance of bladder overdistension is so important, catheterization should be done even if unable to wash.
2. Preferably, catheterization is done with the child sitting on the toilet or standing beside it. However, any position that is comfortable, including lying, is acceptable.
3. Lubricate catheter (optional for females).
4. Insert catheter.
   A. *Male:* Grasp penis, holding on sides and hold it erect, then insert catheter slowly.
   B. *Female:* Separate labia and insert catheter. A mirror may be helpful while learning but child can usually learn to locate meatus by palpation.
   Note: Catheter sizes range from 8 to 14 French. A clear plastic No. 8 feeding tube may be used to catheterize infants and young children.
5. Insert 1 to 2 inches farther than point at which urine begins to flow.
6. Allow urine to flow into a cup or other container until flow stops.
7. Remove catheter slowly; hold catheter tip up after withdrawal to avoid spilling urine.
8. Wash catheter in soap and water; rinse and dry. Store in dry clean bottle, plastic bag, or other small container.
9. Replace catheter once a month.

Impact of a Genitourinary Disorder on the Child and Family

Families of children with genitourinary disorders face a number of unique stressors. Because of the close association between the urinary tract and the reproductive system, genitourinary disorders may cause significant, frequently unspoken, concerns about virginity, future fertility, and sexual functioning, even for parents of very young children. Procedures for diagnosis and treatment of urologic disorders are invasive, frequently are painful, and focus attention on body parts and functioning that are usually not discussed openly in our society. Loss of renal function, prior to the advent of hemodialysis and renal transplants, in the past was synonymous with death and still may be for many children. In addition, dialysis and kidney transplants carry with them the family burdens of any chronic illness. The nurse caring for the child with a genitourinary problem needs to recognize the stressors that are unique to this group of disorders and needs to know how best to support the family and child during the diagnosis, treatment, and rehabilitation phase of the child's illness.

Nursing intervention begins with a thorough assessment of each family, and its individual members' roles, strengths, and coping mechanisms. If the disorder was inherited, parents may be dealing with feelings of guilt and will need support in working through these feelings. If discussion of the genitals or body functions is taboo within a given family, it may be difficult for family members to express fears that their child may never be able to have children or be sexually active. Parents may have seen their child masturbating or involved in sex play and fear that these activities somehow contributed to their child's current problem. The nurse needs to clarify family perceptions and educate family members about their child's disorder and its real impact on functioning. Careful, honest explanations should be provided and time for verbalization of fears and anxieties allowed. The nurse needs to remember that all family members, including the child's siblings, are affected by the illness. Many parents benefit from thoughtful advice on how to discuss genitourinary problems with their children.

In addition to having an impact on the overall family system, genitourinary illness may affect the individual child's psychosocial and emotional development. It is the nurse's role to be aware of such an impact. If the disorder interrupts the child's achievement of a developmental milestone, a temporary cessation of development could result. In some cases, the interruption may cause the child to regress.

Table 42-5 outlines the potential impact on children of varying ages. The nurse should be knowledgeable about these developmentally vulnerable times so that nursing strategies may be used to foster healthy coping in children and their families.

Congenital Anomalies of Genitourinary Function

Genitourinary tract anomalies range from those that are visible at birth to those that are not easily detected but cause progressive damage to the urinary tract. The nurse plays an important role in facilitating the early identification of urinary tract anomalies at birth and throughout childhood and adolescence. Urinary tract anomalies may have a considerable effect on the child and family. The nursing role is vital in assessment, planning, and intervention in order to minimize the impact of the disorder.

Table 42-5. Impact of Genitourinary Disorder on Child's Development

Stage of Development	Developmental Tasks	Impact on Development
Newborn Klaus and Kennell: Maternal-infant bonding	Attachment and bonding occurs between child and parent(s)	Congenital anomalies may cause prolonged hospitalization Visible anomaly and parental grief over loss of "perfect child" may hinder attachment and bonding
Infant Freud: Oral stage Erikson: Trust vs mistrust	Child receives gratification from sucking, eating, rooting Feels secure with caregiver (parent) May develop stranger anxiety	Hospitalization may interfere with sucking needs Painful procedures do not foster trust in others Separation from parent(s) may strain security and trust
Toddler Freud: Anal stage Erikson: Autonomy vs shame/doubt	Has dependent-independent behavior Negativism Temper tantrums Toilet training Developing ability to hold on/let go	Hospitalization or painful procedures may threaten independence Separation from parent(s) may be poorly tolerated Surgery in genital area may cause regression in toilet training
Preschool Freud: Phallic stage Erikson: Initiative vs guilt	Development of conscience/guilt Vivid imagination Enjoys accomplishing tasks Castration complex (boys) Electra complex (girls) Both sexes curious about genitals	Painful procedures or hospitalization may be interpreted as punishment Procedures or surgery in genital area may increase castration anxiety or create guilt about masturbation and normal sex play Normal sexual curiosity of this age may be heightened by care providers' focus on genitals
School-age Freud: Latency stage Erikson: Industry vs inferiority	Masters new skills Carries tasks to completion Has same sex orientation Plays well with others, likes competition Develops modesty about nudity	If hospitalized or has chronic illness, may be unable to complete school work If physically handicapping condition, child may feel inferior to peers Embarrassment may result from physical exam of the genitals
Adolescent Freud: Genital stage Erikson: Identity vs identity diffusion	Developing identity Body image is very important Peer group has great influence Sex role identity develops	If physically handicapping condition exists, body image will be affected Chronic disease may prevent conformity to peer group Genitourinary manipulation may cause concerns about future fertility, virginity, or sexual functioning Embarrassment may result from focus on genitourinary functioning by care providers of the opposite sex

Nursing care in the perioperative period specific to that anomaly is included with the discussion of each disorder. The strategies that are included should be considered *in addition to* the general perioperative care detailed in Table 27-7.

Hypospadias

Hypospadias is the most common anomaly of the penis, occurring in about 8.2 out of every 1000 live male births (Belman, 1985). Genetic factors are thought to contribute to hypospadias, although the mode of inheritance is unclear.

Pathophysiology

This disorder results when the urethral folds fail to fuse in the midline, and the urethral meatus opens on the ventral surface of the penis. The prepuce (foreskin) is smaller ventrally and presents as a hood or flap. Classification of hypospadias is based on the position of the urethral opening. The types of hypospadias are glandular (urethra opens at the base of the glans penis); coronal (urethra opens at the junction of the glans and the penis); distal, mid, or proximal shaft (urethra opens on the shaft between the glans and the scrotum); penoscrotal (urethra opens at the junction of the penis and scrotum); scrotal; or perineal (urethra opens on the perineum) (Fig. 42-4).

A ventral curvature of the penis, chordee, is present in almost all forms of hypospadias. This curvature is caused by tough, fibrous bands that extend ventrally behind the urethra to the glans. The chordee will vary in severity and is generally proportional to the degree of hypospadias.

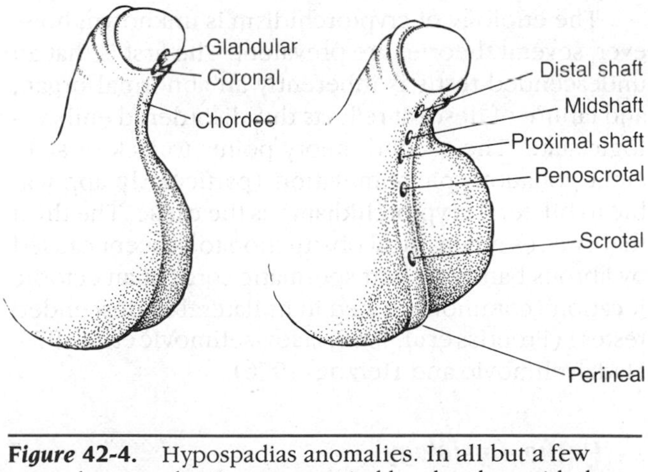

Figure 42-4. Hypospadias anomalies. In all but a few cases, hypospadias is accompanied by chordee, with the curvature proportional to the severity of hypospadias. It is best to classify hypospadias severity according to the site of the proximally displaced meatus, as shown here, rather than by imprecise quantification of "degrees of hypospadias."

Diagnostic Assessment

The nurse can assist in the identification of hypospadias by performing a genital examination on all newborns. Mild degrees of hypospadias may be missed on casual examination. A thorough examination is essential because if any degree of hypospadias is present circumcision should not be performed without urologic consultation. Urinary incontinence is not usually manifested, since the urethral abnormality in this condition occurs distal to the urinary sphincter.

After the newborn period, the nurse should continue to assess for mild degrees of hypospadias in all males. Often, less severe cases of hypospadias are missed in early infancy and diagnosed later. Thus, inspection of the position of the urinary meatus and examination for penile curvature should be included in routine physical assessments.

The anomaly most commonly associated with hypospadias is undescended testes (cryptorchidism) (see discussion of cryptorchidism later in this chapter). If hypospadias occurs with one or both testes not palpable, the child may have ambiguous genitalia. In this situation, an extensive investigation should be done to determine the appropriate assignment of the infant's sex. When ambiguous genitalia are present, the assignment of gender may be delayed for several days while tests such as chromosome analysis and cystography are performed. The family needs the help and support of the entire health team in order to cope with their anxiety and stress during this period. The nurse can be particularly helpful to the family in dealing appropriately with inquiries of relatives and friends. An indepth discussion of ambiguous genitalia is presented in Chapter 49 (endocrine alterations).

Hypospadias, as either an isolated anomaly or part of a more complex syndrome, may be difficult for the family to understand and accept. The nurse with other health team members can help the family understand the condition, its long-term implications, and methods of management.

Therapeutic Management

Surgical repair of hypospadias should occur before the child is of school age, but the ideal age, technically and psychologically, has not been universally agreed on. The surgery may be performed during infancy or during the preschool period, depending on the degree of abnormality present and the preference of the surgeon. Belman (1984) cited a trend in recent years toward earlier surgical intervention. Because body image begins to develop in infancy and is influenced by parental attitudes, Belman proposed that both the infants and their parents suffer less psychologic trauma when the repair is undertaken in the first year of life.

The goal of surgical management is to normalize the appearance and function of the penis. To achieve this, the fibrous bands and skin adhesions causing the ventral curvature must be completely released, and a urethral tube must be created to allow the urethra to terminate in its expected location. The surgery may be performed in two stages, separated by an interval of 6 to 12 months, or it may be completed in a one-stage procedure.

Strategies for Nursing Care

No special physical preparation is required prior to surgery for hypospadias. Psychologic preparation varies according to the age of the child. The preschooler will not necessarily verbalize his fears, nor will he completely understand what is happening to him. He may experience castration anxiety and fear that his penis will be cut off; therefore, an attempt must be made to prepare him in order to diminish his fears as much as possible. He should be told that the opening on his penis will be moved to a position from which he can urinate more easily; telling the child that surgery will make his penis "look better" should be avoided as it suggests that he does not currently appear normal. The child should be reassured that the penis will *not* be cut off, that only the opening will be located differently. Preoperatively the child can be given a simple explanation about the dressing and the catheter that will be in place postoperatively. The family should be made aware of the hospitalization procedures as well as what they may reasonably expect during the preoperative and postoperative periods.

Following the operation, a pressure dressing is often used to reduce bleeding and tissue swelling. The tip of the penis should be checked frequently to be sure that it is pink and viable. The dressing is usually left in place for several days to encourage healing of the grafted skin flap. Thereafter it is changed by the surgeon and should not be removed unless this has been ordered. Some form of urinary diversion such as a suprapubic catheter is often used to enable the urine to temporarily bypass the operative site. Early ambulation is encouraged, often the same day as surgery.

After catheter removal (usually by the 7th to 10th postoperative day), urinary infection, dysuria, hematuria, or frequency may develop. Parents should be cautioned about symptoms of infection so that they can report them early. Discomfort upon initial voiding after catheter removal is common; children and parents usually manage this well if they have been prepared for the temporary discomfort.

The most common complication of hypospadias repair is a fistula in which an opening forms between the urethra and the skin of the shaft. If the fistula is small, it may close spontaneously; larger fistulas may require further surgical intervention. Persistent chordee, meatal stenosis, urethral stricture, stenosis, and urethral diverticula are other complications of hypospadias repair; all require additional surgical intervention.

Epispadias

While hypospadias is a common congenital anomaly, epispadias is rare. It involves location of the urethral orifice along the dorsal surface of the penis. The severity of epispadias varies from a mild anomaly, in which the meatal opening is proximal to the glans penis, to the severe epispadias that is associated with exstrophy of the bladder (see the discussion of exstrophy of the bladder earlier in this chapter). Epispadias can be surgically repaired. The goals of treatment and strategies for nursing care are similar to those discussed for hypospadias.

Cryptorchidism

Cryptorchidism refers to a condition in which a testis has not descended into the scrotal sac but has been arrested in descent at some point between the kidneys and the scrotal sac. The incidence of cryptorchidism is higher in premature male infants (approximately 33 per cent) than in term male infants (approximately 3 per cent). Spontaneous descent of the testes may occur during the first 6 to 12 months after birth, so that the incidence of true cryptorchidism is really only 0.7 to 0.8 per cent (Kogan, 1985).

The etiology of cryptorchidism is unknown; however, several theories are prevalent. The first is that an undescended testis is inherently an abnormal organ, and failure of descent reflects this disordered embryologic state. The second theory points to lack of sufficient gonadotropic stimulation (particularly applicable to bilateral cryptorchidism) as the cause. The third theory cites mechanical obstruction to descent caused by fibrous bands, a short spermatic cord, or an ectopic location (commonly noted in unilateral undescended testes) (Prentiss et al, 1960; Hadziselimovic et al, 1975; Hadziselimovic and Herzog, 1976).

Pathophysiology

The classification of undescended testes is based on whether the testes are palpable or impalpable on clinical examination. Impalpable testes are totally absent from the body or located in a position where they are never palpated by a clinician. Palpable testes are divided into three categories: retractile, ectopic, or truly undescended testes within the canal.

Retractile testes are most commonly found in the groin, but may be palpated at any level along the line of descent. These testes are normally descended but have been pulled back into an extrascrotal position because of a hyperactive cremasteric reflex, which retracts the testes into the upper part of the scrotum or into the inguinal canal in response to cold, pain, fear, or touch. Retractile testes may be manually drawn into the scrotum, where they will remain.

The second type of palpable cryptorchid testis is the *ectopic* type. An ectopic testis is one that has deviated from the normal path of descent after emerging from the inguinal canal. The testis may be located in the superficial inguinal pouch, the perineum, over the pubic bone, or in the femoral region.

Truly undescended testes, the third category of palpable undescended testes, are intermittently palpable to the clinician and may be palpated in the abdomen, scrotal canal, or inguinal ring. In truly undescended testes, the spermatic vessels are felt to be shorter, thus preventing the testes' normal descent into the scrotum.

Diagnostic Assessment

Accurate documentation of the position of both testes immediately after birth and during well-baby examinations is an essential part of medical and nursing assessment. Before the child reaches 6 months of age the scrotal contents are easily examined and the cremasteric reflex is absent or rudimentary. After 6 months of age, the cremasteric reflex becomes quite active and may simulate the empty scrotum of cryptorchidism in up to 50 per cent of boys (retractile testes). A reassuring attitude and thorough explanation of what the child or parent should expect will facilitate the examination. If examination of the inguinal and scrotal regions in the upright and supine positions suggests an undescended testis, it is often helpful to repeat the examination if the child is able to be seated with his knees drawn up to his chest. This will diminish the cremasteric reflex. Early documentation of a testis in its normal scrotal position (4 cm below the pubic tubercle) eliminates confusion in later years. Whenever a nurse is unable to palpate a testis in the scrotum he or she should bring it to the attention of a physician for further examination. If upon repeated examination a testis is not palpable in its normal position by the time the child reaches 1 year of age, the diagnosis of cryptorchidism can be made and appropriate management instituted.

When cryptorchidism is suspected, the child by age 1 year should be referred to a surgeon skilled in pediatric urologic procedures.

Therapeutic Management

Cryptorchidism should be treated before puberty, but there is controversy about the best age of treatment. It is generally agreed that no therapeutic intervention should take place before the first birthday because of the possibility of spontaneous testicular descent during the first year of life (Rezvani, 1987). Therapy is usually initiated before 5 years of age (Pinch et al, 1979), often at 2 years. The toddler period may be a psychologically advantageous time for therapy because the child is not experiencing castration anxiety at this point in his stage of development.

Medical therapy using hormones that may stimulate testicular descent may be attempted as the first intervention. Human chorionic gonadotropin (hCG) has been used to cause testicular descent by stimulating testosterone synthesis; however, this therapy remains controversial. HCG may be an effective treatment in approximately 20 per cent of patients with undescended testes (Rezvani, 1987). The success rate is somewhat better in children with bilateral rather than unilateral cryptorchidism. HCG may be given by injection from 10 days to 3 weeks. The child should be examined within a few days after completion of the hCG course to determine whether testicular descent has occurred. If medical therapy with hCG is not successful, surgical placement of the testes in the scrotum (orchidopexy) is performed.

To perform an orchidopexy, a small transverse incision is made in the lower abdominal skinfold and the testes and spermatic cord are freed from surrounding tissues. A hernia sac is present in up to 90 per cent of cases, although it is not usually detectable preoperatively and only occasionally symptomatic. After an adequate length of spermatic cord is obtained, an incision is made through the skin of the lower portion of the scrotum, a pouch created, and the testis is pulled down into the pouch and then sutured to the inner wall of the scrotum. Subcutaneous sutures that do not require removal are used to close the skin incisions. The child may be discharged on the afternoon of surgery or the following morning and may resume normal activities as tolerated. Tub bathing is usually withheld for several days; showers, however, are permitted.

The potential for reduced fertility and the long-term risk of testicular malignancy should be discussed with the patient and his parents. Although the physician plays the primary role in this discussion, the nurse should have sufficient knowledge to participate effectively in counseling these families. It is important for the nurse to be present when the physician discusses these issues with the family so that he or she is aware of specific information that has been given by the physician. The nurse is then prepared to be supportive of family members as they deal with the effects of this information.

Specific information given to a family will vary; however, there are some facts that will assist the nurse in understanding the approach to management of cryptorchidism. Spermatogenesis may be significantly impaired in undescended testes. Although orchidopexy improves the situation, the fertility rate among these patients, even when only one testis is undescended, is reduced in comparison to that of unaffected men. Additionally, the risk of developing a malignant testicular tumor is increased 20 to 44 per cent in the third or fourth decade of life. Males who remain untreated for intra-abdominal cryptorchidism or those who had corrective surgery during or after puberty are at greatest risk (Gonzalez and Michael, 1987).

Strategies for Nursing Care

The nurse, working together with other members of the health care team, can play a central role in the management of these children. Early examination and documentation of the position of the testes by the nurse may obviate a false diagnosis later in life, thus eliminating needless anxiety, costly examinations, and unnecessary testing. Discussions with the patient and his family on the importance of long-term follow-up for development of tumor and for evaluation of fertility are essential. Additionally, instructing the patient in the method and importance of self-examination of the testes to check for tumor is critical because of the length of time between surgery for undescended testes at 1 to 5 years of age, and the possible development of a tumor at about 30 to 40 years of age.

Exstrophy of the Bladder

Exstrophy of the bladder is a rare congenital malformation that occurs in 1 of 30,000 live births (Duckett and Caldamone, 1985). It affects males three times more than females and is rarely familial.

Clinical Manifestations

Exstrophy of the bladder results from a deficiency in the development of the anterior abdominal wall, the symphysis pubis, the bladder, and the urethra during gestation. When the child is born, the bladder appears in the suprapubic region as a protruding red mass that constantly seeps urine. There is a wide separation in the symphysis pubis, and the hip sockets are rotated posterolaterally. These abnormalities cause the child to have difficulty walking, perhaps exhibiting a waddling gait. In the female, the clitoris is often bifid, the labia are widely separated, and the vaginal opening is tilted slightly anteriorly. Bilateral inguinal hernias and undescended testes in males may accompany exstrophy of the bladder. The penis is often epispadic, points upward, is short and stubby, and has an open urethral strip on the dorsum. The exposed mucosa is very sensitive to touch because the parasympathetic nerves are intact. Repair of the epispadias often involves cosmetic and functional reconstruction of the penis and urethra and is usually done after the other repairs are complete.

Therapeutic Management

Various surgical treatment modalities and philosophies are used in the management of exstrophy of the bladder. The success of the intervention depends on the severity of the defect. The major goals for treatment are to prevent and treat any infection, avoid trauma to the bladder, and promote the child's growth and development.

Current recommendations for treatment of exstrophy of the bladder (Duckett and Caldamone, 1985) are to intervene surgically during the neonatal period, usually before 3 days of age. Surgical closure of the defect and repair of the abdominal wall creates a closed system. By surgically intervening during the newborn period, the bladder has an opportunity to grow and expand safely, without trauma, during the first few years of life. This intervention closes the symphysis pubis and enables the urine to pass through the ureteral orifice; however, the child remains incontinent after this procedure.

When the child is 3 to 4 years old, the second stage of the repair, called the bladder neck tightening procedure, is done. This involves reconstruction of the bladder neck and reimplantation of the ureters. The goal of this procedure is to help the child gain urinary control and prevent reflux from the ureters. However, it may take months or years before the child gains complete urinary control.

Urinary Diversion

If surgical closure of the defect is not possible, some type of temporary urinary diversion will be performed, such as a *bilateral ureterostomy,* an ileal conduit, or a ureterosigmoidostomy. A bilateral ureterostomy involves attaching the ureters directly to the abdominal wall, where urine is passed into two collecting appliances. The child with bilateral ureterostomy is at risk for ascending infection because of the short length of the ureters.

The creation of an *ileal conduit* involves resecting a small section of the colon or ileum and attaching one end of the resected bowel to the distal ends of the ureters and the other end of the bowel to a small opening (stoma) in the lower abdomen. This conduit provides transport for the urine from the ureters to the stoma. The child wears an ileostomy appliance over the stoma to collect the continuously flowing urine.

Ureterosigmoidostomy involves the anastomosis of

the ureters to the sigmoid portion of the colon, thus permitting urinary excretion through the bowels. This form of urinary excretion occurs without the use of an abdominal stoma, enhancing the child's body image and continence. Because the urine is passed with the stool, complications may result from ascending bacteria or reflux. Common problems that are associated with a ureterosigmoidostomy include recurrent pyelonephritis, hyperchloremic acidosis due to the absorption of chloride, hypokalemia, and growth impairment.

Major Nursing Diagnoses for Exstrophy of the Bladder

Altered family process: ineffective bonding, *related to*
- *grief associated with loss of the expected "perfect infant"*
- *disruptions in physical closeness associated with the need to protect the exposed bladder*
- *prolonged hospitalization for surgical procedures*

Potential impaired tissue integrity: bladder mucosa, *related to irritation and trauma*

Potential for infection, *related to*
- *contamination of bladder mucosa and ureteral openings*
- *irritation of exposed bladder tissue*

Impaired skin integrity, *related to leakage of urine from the incompetent bladder*

Knowledge deficit, *related to home care:*
- *specialized care of skin, ostomies, and appliances*
- *signs and symptoms of urinary tract infections*
- *normalization of infant activities*

Strategies for Nursing Care

The major goals of nursing care are to promote parent-infant bonding, protect the bladder mucosa, prevent infection, maintain skin integrity, and provide information and guidance that will support home care. Table 27-7 provides a general nursing process plan for perioperative care.

Promoting Parent-Infant Bonding

Parents of a child born with exstrophy of the bladder experience grief related to loss of the "perfect" child. The birth of a defective child may create anxiety, guilt, and much stress within the family. Because this defect is physically obvious and not well known to the general public, parents of children with exstrophic bladders have an added burden.

Parents and family members will need emotional and physical nursing support during the neonatal period in order to attach and bond to the infant. They will need information about the defect and about treatment options, as well as much encouragement for providing physical care for the child. Because the defect is friable and visible, parents will need to learn how to safely bathe, feed, and diaper the infant.

Protecting the Bladder Mucosa

The bladder mucosa is easily irritated and susceptible to trauma from rubbing or friction. The exposed mucosa should be covered with sterile gauze that is impregnated with Vaseline. A cloth or disposable diaper may then be carefully fastened around the child but should not fit snugly or rub harshly against the bladder. The diaper and gauze should be changed every 2 hours during the day in order to minimize irritation.

Preventing Infection and Maintaining Skin Integrity

The bladder mucosa and surrounding skin are prone to infection from the accumulation of stagnant urine and irritation. The bladder should be cleansed daily with a moist cloth and patted dry with a soft towel. The surrounding skin will benefit from exposure to air, sunlight, or artificial light. Daily exposure to air will help to prevent skin breakdown and irritation.

If the child has a collecting appliance from an ileostomy or ileal conduit, the skin surrounding the stoma must receive meticulous skin care including frequent washing, air drying, and changing the collection appliance as needed.

Teaching to Support Home Care

The family of the child with exstrophy of the bladder should be encouraged to have physical contact with the child from birth on (Fig. 42-5). Physical caring enhances parents' ability to bond with the infant. Parents may also need encouragement to allow their child freedom of mobility during the later months of infancy. They may fear that the child may cause trauma to the bladder before corrective surgery by falling or banging objects against themselves. As long as the bladder is protected by the Vaseline, gauze, and a thick diaper, the child should be encouraged to participate in normal infant activities.

The child will require many tests, procedures, and possible surgical repairs during the first few years of his or her life. The family will need information, guidance, and support concerning the care of their child. They will need to know the signs and symptoms of urinary infections (e.g., fever, malodorous urine, and hematuria). If the child has had a ureterosigmoidostomy, the parents will require information about the symptoms of hypokalemia and acidosis that may result from the ostomy. Skin breakdown in the genital area

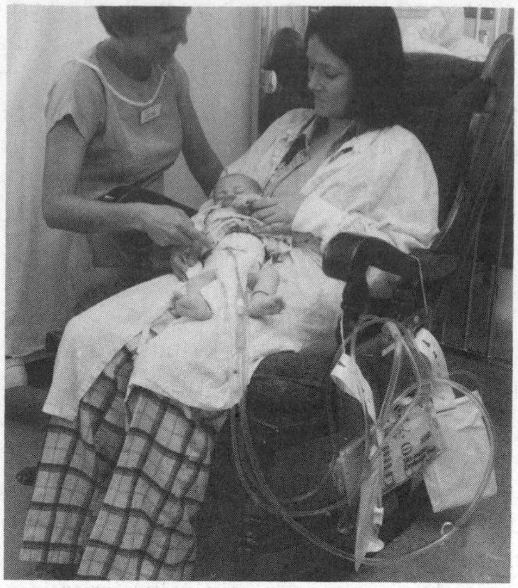

Figure 42-5. An important role of the nurse after an infant has urologic surgery is to help parents become comfortable in holding their baby in spite of the cumbersome tubes and urinary bags.

should be prevented by changing diapers frequently and by periodically exposing the area to air.

Although reconstructive surgery has improved the prognosis for children with exstrophy of the bladder, the child will still require multiple hospitalizations, tests, and frequent health care visits. The psychologic, social, and physical impact of this anomaly are felt by the child and family throughout the child's life. The nurse is important in physically and psychologically supporting and guiding the parents and child throughout the course of this unusual but serious anomaly.

Nursing Strategies for Follow-Up Care in the Home or Clinic

Assess for signs and symptoms of urinary tract infection: fever, irritability, foul urine odor, anorexia, vomiting, or diarrhea.

- Obtain a urine specimen if initial bladder closure has been accomplished.
- Alert the physician to any evidence of infection.

Inspect skin exposed to urine drainage from the exstrophied bladder or from urinary diversion devices. Reinforce teaching about skin care as needed.

Assess closely parent-infant interactions and parental comfort with necessary alterations in care. Reinforce adaptive coping to enhance the parent's sense of competence and control. Refer to community support groups when available.

Assess the child's accomplishment of developmental milestones (see Chapter 15).

Assist parents to plan ways to normalize development despite necessary safety precautions and repeated hospitalizations.

Encourage the verbal child to discuss issues of body image and peer response to altered urinary function.

Urachal Anomalies

Urachal anomalies are rare, occurring in boys twice as often as girls. The urachus is a structure that extends from the anterior bladder to the umbilicus. If this structure fails to undergo normal obliteration it persists as a tubular structure at birth.

Pathophysiology and Clinical Manifestations

Urachal anomalies present as four basic disorders. A *patent urachus* is a communication between the bladder and umbilicus (Fig. 42-6*B*). It often presents as a persistently wet umbilicus or umbilical granuloma in the neonatal period. A patent urachus is associated with incidence of prune-belly syndrome* and obstruction in the lower urinary tract.

The second type of urachal anomaly is the *urachal cyst* (Fig. 42-6*C*). This cyst usually develops in the lower third of the urachus and symptoms are not often present until late childhood or adult life. The symptoms of this anomaly include suprapubic pain and tenderness and a palpable abdominal mass (Duckett and Caldamone, 1985).

In the third instance a small cyst becomes chronically infected and results in an external urachal sinus (opening) into the bladder or umbilicus, or both. Symptoms may include fever, tenderness, periumbilical pain, umbilical inflammation, granuloma formation, and persistent umbilical drainage.

The fourth type of urachal anomaly is the *vesicourachal diverticulum,* which occurs when the urachus fails to obliterate at the bladder apex, and a pouch, or diverticulum, forms. The diverticulum is usually asymptomatic and will not require any treatment. It is associated with prune-belly syndrome and lower urinary tract obstruction.

Diagnostic Assessment

A nursing history should be obtained to assess for presence of fever, pain, umbilical drainage, and prune-belly syndrome or lower urinary tract infection.

---

* Prune-belly syndrome is a congenital anomaly that varies in severity and presentation. Typical manifestations include a deficiency in the abdominal musculature, cryptorchidism, and nonobstructive dilatation and dysplasia of the urinary tract.

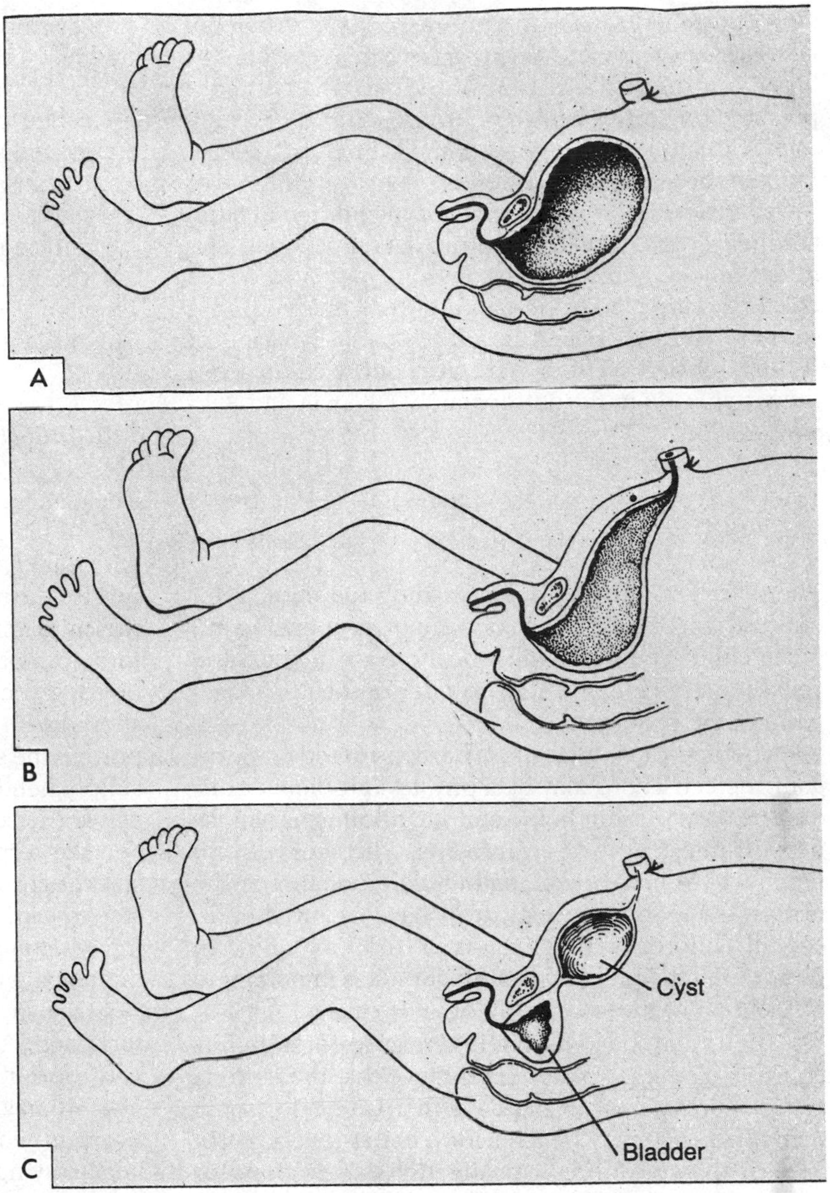

Figure 42-6. Midline abdominal masses. *A*, Normal structure. *B*, Patent urachus. *C*, Urachal cyst. (From Koff S: Clues to neonatal genitourinary problems. *Postgrad Med* 1977; 95.)

An abdominal examination should determine the presence or absence of tenderness, masses, and umbilical drainage or granuloma. Diagnostic evaluation is necessary to ascertain the location and extent of the urachus. This may include a voiding cystourethrogram, cystoscopy, and ultrasound.

Therapeutic Management

With patent urachus, spontaneous closure of the urachus may occur. However, if persistent drainage exists, it may result in recurrent urinary tract infection, stone formation, or excoriation of the umbilicus. This situation requires early surgical intervention to excise the urachal tract. When a urachal cyst is involved, surgical intervention is aimed at excision of the cyst or sinus. If infection is present, surgery will be done after the infection is under control.

The Child with Enuresis

Enuresis is defined as the involuntary passage of urine by a child over the age of 3 years (Parker and Whitehead, 1982). It can occur during the day *(diurnal enuresis)*, during the night *(nocturnal enuresis)*, or at both times. A child who has never been totally continent is said to have *primary enuresis*. A child with *secondary enuresis* has experienced a period of dryness of at least 3 to 6 months after toilet training was completed.

From 4 to 25 per cent of all children between the

ages of 6 and 12 years have enuresis. For children between 13 and 17 years, the prevalence ranges from 1 to 9 per cent (Gross and Dornbusch, 1983). It is more prevalent in children with neurologic disorders, such as myelomeningocele (Parker and Whitehead, 1982). Enuresis occurs more frequently in boys, in children of lower socioeconomic classes, and in children of large families. Friman (1986) reported data supporting a familial tendency toward enuresis: 77 per cent of the children with 2 enuretic parents were enuretic. In a study of children raised in a kibbutz, 44 per cent of siblings of bed wetters were also bed wetters, even though they were raised separately (Bakwin and Bakwin, 1972).

Etiology

There are several theories regarding the etiology of enuresis. All or part of each one might be operating in a given child. The nurse must be aware of the possible causes of enuresis in order to offer optimal management of the problem.

The first cause that must be considered is an organic defect. There may be a physical problem or disease process present in the child. Dribbling urine may be a manifestation of an infection, diabetes, or epilepsy. There may be an anatomic abnormality of the urinary tract. Some investigators have reported enuresis in children with a history of food allergies. In performing the physical examination it is important to rule out all of these possible organic causes.

There may be a psychologic cause for a child's enuresis. Some practitioners believe that the child is using enuresis to "get back" at the parents for some "unfairness." It may be a reaction to too-strict control or to the parents' unrealistically high expectations for the child's behavior and performance. Parental response to the enuresis may perpetuate this problem. Use of shaming or punishment techniques gives the child further reason for "getting even." In children with secondary enuresis having a psychologic component, a threatening event or anxiety-producing situation, such as the birth of a sibling or threatened school failure, usually precipitates the bed wetting.

There is good support for the theory that enuresis is caused by a developmental or maturational delay in the child. Some studies have shown that the child with enuresis has a smaller functional bladder capacity (FBC) than a nonenuretic child (Parker and Whitehead, 1982). This means some children are not physically ready for full control of urinary function at the time considered "average." They may also have an immature arousal mechanism from stages 3 to 4 (non-REM) sleep (Shelov, 1984). They do not have adequate bladder size or sphincter control to last an entire night without voiding. Support for this theory is seen in the fact that enuresis spontaneously disappears in many children as they get older.

Some children have only diurnal enuresis; environmental stresses are most prevalent in these cases. Some causative factors in this situation may be (1) nervous tension in a given situation such as school; (2) the child's shyness in front of classmates in having to ask the teacher to leave the room to urinate; or (3) reluctance of some children, particularly girls, to use unfamiliar toilets (Bakwin and Bakwin, 1972).

Diagnostic Assessment

The management of a child with enuresis begins with a careful history. It serves not only as the principal tool with which to collect data but also offers the opportunity for the nurse to establish a caring relationship with the child and parents. This history should be obtained in a comfortable environment, with the information being given by the parents and the child. The nurse should maintain a calm, nonjudgmental attitude, supporting the strengths of the family. Many times parents simply need to vent their feelings regarding the enuresis and to sort out the approaches they have attempted and the respective results. The nurse should emphasize the fact that the family has sought help as a positive step toward eliminating the enuresis. The history-taking session itself can be an important intervention in the management of enuresis.

In many instances, the enuresis has been present for months or years; therefore, it is important to know why the family has sought assistance *at this particular time.* It may be that the enuresis had not been viewed as a problem by the parents until friends or relatives began saying that the child is "not normal." Or perhaps the enuresis has become a social problem for the child. "Sleeping over" at a friend's house, a popular activity, may cause the child to fear humiliation at wetting the friend's bed. Many practitioners think that enuresis should not be treated until it limits the normal activities of the child. It is believed that since so many children spontaneously stop enuresis, putting them through the regimen required to manage the problem might be more traumatic than wetting the bed.

The family history contributes to the management of enuresis. Determining that one or both parents was enuretic can help allay some of the child's concerns about the future, particularly in the area of marriage. Knowing that a parent had the same problem and was able to overcome it helps the child deal with this problem. A family history of urinary tract problems may give direction for defining the etiology of this child's enuresis, suggesting that enuresis might be a symptom of an organic problem.

The past medical history of the child should be reviewed. A history of urinary tract infections may contribute to the cause of this child's enuresis. The prenatal history should be reviewed for any possible neurologic complications in the child prenatally or during birth that might contribute to incontinence. The allergic history of the child and family helps rule out allergies as the cause of enuresis. Developmental milestones should be discussed in order to assess the child's progress.

Methods used by parent and child for handling enuresis are significant. Enuresis is an emotional issue and the nurse needs to know the attitudes and feelings of all involved. Knowledge of past attempts to deal with the problem gives important insight into management issues. *Shaming and punishing the child the next morning are of no value; in fact, these approaches are harmful.* They compound the child's existing feelings of inadequacy and "differentness." All attempts made at controlling the enuresis should be discussed, including the child's response to each attempt and the degree of success achieved with each effort.

The history should include the number of bedwetting episodes per week, the approximate amount of urine passed (at night and during the day), and the frequency with which the child urinates during the day. These facts can provide a clue as to whether the child's functional bladder capacity is small. Some practitioners feel that the enuretic child sleeps more deeply than the normal child; depth of sleep can be assessed by inquiring about the difficulty with which the child is aroused from sleep. It is important to know if the enuretic episodes are becoming more or less frequent and whether they can be related to any stressful event in the child's life. It should be determined whether the child has ever been continent, and if so, for how long.

Data collection should include a general physical examination with special attention to the genitourinary function. Color, stream, and odor of the urine should be assessed. Frequency, dribbling, dysuria, or hesitancy in beginning urination should be noted to rule out organic causes. The neurologic system should be reviewed with parents and child for any abnormal behavior or activity. The child's height and weight should be noted, and blood pressure should be checked for evidence of renal disease. The abdomen should be palpated for masses or tenderness. External genitalia should be examined for any gross abnormalities. Observations as to cleanliness and hygiene should be made and any signs of allergic manifestations noted.

Laboratory testing of urine should include a check of specific gravity and evaluation for glucose, protein, and blood. If a urinary tract infection is suspected, a urine culture should be done.

Therapeutic Management

In planning a management program, it is important to have the cooperation of the child and the parents; otherwise, success is unlikely. The child can assume a large role in affecting cure, but parental support and reinforcement is essential. Similarly, if the parents seem eager to work on the problem and the child is indifferent, positive results will not occur. This must be a joint venture. Contemporary therapies include waiting for the child to outgrow the condition, retention-control training, drug therapy, urine-alarm treatment, and behavior modification.

Waiting for the Child to Outgrow Bedwetting. Many health care providers will not start a program with children of age 5 or 6, owing to the high incidence of spontaneous resolution of the enuresis in a child of this age. Shelov (1984) recommends that, if the child is between 3 and 4 years of age, the health care provider should try to reduce the family's anxiety by informing them that it is a self-limited problem. Friman (1986) cautions, however, that this period of waiting should be accompanied by the assessment and support of health care professionals to prevent physical, social, and emotional problems that may result from the waiting approach. The potential for victimization of the child cannot be overlooked.

Retention-Control Therapy. If a small functional bladder capacity is diagnosed, efforts to enlarge the bladder may be attempted. These include having the child drink a large amount of fluids during the day and wait to urinate until discomfort is felt at least once each day. Restriction of fluids after dinner (or after 6 P.M.) may yield positive results. The child should void just before bedtime. There is some controversy as to the effectiveness of having parents wake the child to urinate when they retire. Some think this is beneficial, since nocturnal urine production is highest in the early hours of sleep. Others believe that it contributes to enuresis since the child does not really wake up at this time and that it teaches the child to urinate in his or her sleep. Shelov (1984) points out that bladder-stretching exercises have not been found to be uniformly valuable, but are harmless. The procedure for these exercises is as follows: (1) have the child drink fluids and then hold the urine as long as possible, (2) measure the amount when the child voids, and (3) mark the amount on a calendar in order to keep track of progress.

Drug Therapy. Some physicians prescribe medication for children with enuresis. Imipramine is the drug of choice. The exact mechanism of this drug is not agreed upon by practitioners. It does produce improvement in many children, but the long-term result with its use is not significantly better than in those cases that spontaneously resolve (Friman, 1986). In addition, the use of imipramine is not without danger to the child; neurologic side effects and overdoses are potential problems. Use of imipramine is considered inappropriate before other treatments have been employed.

Urine-Alarm Treatment. Another method of treating children with enuresis involves use of a mechanical device installed on the child's bed. An alarm goes off if the child begins to wet the bed, thus waking the child so he or she can finish urination in the toilet. In principle, this should condition the child to wake up when urination begins. These devices have varying degrees of success. Their strength seems to be with older children; however, the relapse rate is quite high, up to 50 per cent (Friman, 1986). Success depends on several variables: (1) proper functioning and installation of the device, (2) proper placing of the sleeping child directly on top of the device, so the urine touches the sensing mechanism, (3) the child waking up, and (4) the child not disconnecting the apparatus. Rashes on the buttocks are a complication of this treatment. Before going to bed, the child should (1) set the alarm, (2) void completely, (3) trigger the buzzer to be sure the alarm is working, (4) have a light or flashlight near the bed, and (5) say to him- or herself that urinating will stop when the alarm goes off. Once awakened by the alarm, the child should (1) get up, go to the bathroom, and finish voiding; (2) dry off the electrodes; and (3) reset the alarm before going back to bed (Shelov, 1984).

Behavior Modification. Behavioral modification techniques, including the principles of positive reinforcement and shaping, are also used in the treatment of enuresis. These approaches, either with or without the urine alarm, have been found to be more effective than using the alarm alone (Azrin and Thienes, 1978).

Whichever plan of treatment is chosen, the method of reinforcement is critical. None of the plans will work if the child does not receive positive reinforcement from the parents for dry nights. Special activities can be used as positive reinforcers. The reward must be meaningful to the child and must be consistently given.

Another factor to be considered is the provision of a warm, convenient place for the child to urinate. A child who must go down a long, dark hallway to the bathroom will not be as likely to get up in the middle of the night to void. A warm bathroom with a night light is much more conducive to night-time use.

Strategies for Nursing Care

Both the child and parent(s) will need ongoing support to overcome enuresis. Parents should be encouraged to share frustrations of failed or only partially successful therapies with the nurse. In this way, the nurse can help put the treatment in perspective and suggest modifications. Parents who can share frustrations with health care professionals may be less likely to vent their feelings upon the child. They must be reminded that punishment is ineffective and potentially very harmful to the child's developing self-concept. They should also be reminded that children with enuresis do eventually outgrow the condition.

The Child with Infection

Urinary Tract Infection

The diagnosis of urinary tract infection encompasses a broad range of bacterial infections of the urinary tract. Infection may be limited to the urethra *(urethritis)* or the bladder *(cystitis),* or may involve the kidney *(pyelonephritis).* In young children it is often difficult to establish whether infection is present only in the lower urinary tract (the urethra and the bladder) or has spread to the upper tract (the ureters and the kidneys).

In the newborn period, urinary tract infections occur most frequently in males, possibly because of the higher incidence of anatomic abnormalities in male neonates. Recent evidence suggests that urinary tract infections also may be directly linked to whether or not the male infant is circumcised. Uncircumcised infants seem to have significantly more urinary tract infections than circumcised infants (Wiswell et al, 1985, 1987). By 4 months of age, urinary tract infections are 10 times more common in girls than in boys (Kroovand and Perlmutter, 1983; Durbin and Peter, 1984). This increased incidence in girls continues throughout childhood and into adulthood.

In infancy, bacteria frequently enter the urinary tract through the blood and cause infection (hematogenous). After infancy, nearly all urinary infections occur when bacteria enter the urethra and ascend into the urinary tract. Females are therefore especially at risk for infection because the female urethra is much shorter than the male urethra. The female urethra is also more subject than the male urethra to contamination because of its proximity to the anal opening.

Escherichia coli causes approximately 75 to 90 per cent of all urinary tract infections in females. No one fully understands why and how bacteria that are normally found in the stools invade the urinary tract and cause infection. It seems, however, that the ability of some bacteria to adhere to the cells of the genitourinary tract may be linked to their ability to cause infection. However, congenital anomalies of the urinary tract, neurogenic bladder dysfunction, vaginal foreign bodies, and indwelling urethral catheters all predispose an individual to urinary tract infection. Other factors such as sexual intercourse, use of bubble bath, and constipation have also been suggested as contributing factors in the development of urinary infections; however, scientific evidence that supports these factors as causal is limited.

Pathophysiology

In an acute, uncomplicated infection, inflammation is usually limited to the bladder (cystitis). Urinary urgency and frequency develop when the inflammation causes irritability and spasm of the bladder wall. Bleeding secondary to inflammation may result in the appearance of blood in the urine (hematuria).

Repeated infection of the bladder and chronic inflammation may lead to changes in the bladder wall, especially at the site where the ureters enter the bladder (the vesicoureteral valves). Damage to these valves can allow urine to reflux into the ureters, especially during voiding. The ureters may become dilated. Urine and bacteria then have easy access to the kidneys, and kidney infections (pyelonephritis) may result (see discussion of vesicoureteral reflux later in this chapter).

Pyelonephritis may interfere with the normal concentrating and filtering mechanisms of the kidney. With chronic infection, scarring and loss of renal tissue may also result. The development of scarring in association with reflux appears to occur primarily in children under 5 years of age. Identification of urinary tract infections in this age group is therefore especially crucial.

Clinical Manifestations

The nurse must know signs and symptoms associated with urinary tract infection in children of all ages. Although the majority of the time no specific etiology will be found, the infection may point to an underlying problem. Renal anomalies are found in 5 to 15 per cent of children with urinary tract infection (Durbin and Peter, 1984). Renal scarring occurs in as many as 20 per cent of children with urinary tract infection, especially in children with significant reflux (Smellie, Normand, and Katz, 1981). The challenge is to detect the infection early. To do this, the nurse must have a high index of suspicion for a variety of signs and symptoms.

In neonates and infants, nonspecific symptoms predominate and include vomiting, diarrhea, irritability, lethargy, poor feeding, slow weight gain, and unexplained jaundice. Fever or hypothermia can be present. The prevalence of urinary tract infection in infants who have fever, failure to thrive, jaundice, and other nonspecific symptoms ranges from 4 to 20 per cent (Spencer and Schaeffer, 1986). Specific urinary signs such as a weak urine stream, frequency, and foul-smelling urine may be present but difficult to document. In older children, dysuria, urgency, fever, abdominal or flank pain, and enuresis prevail.

Urinary tract infections are frequently missed because the diagnosis is not considered. Urine cultures should be obtained whenever possible in ill children, especially if any of the aforementioned signs and symptoms are present.

Up to two thirds of children with urinary tract complaints may not have a documented infection. Alternative explanations for dysuria are numerous and include vaginitis, urethritis (secondary to bubble bath, masturbation, sexual intercourse, pinworms, or diaper rash), or falsely negative urine culture results.

Diagnostic Assessment

Specimen Collection for Laboratory Studies

One of the most important responsibilities of the nurse is the correct collection and transportation of the urine specimen for culture. The diagnosis of urinary tract infection rests on the detection of significant amounts of bacteria in the urine. Urine for culture can be collected in one of three ways: (1) clean-voided (preferably midstream) specimen, (2) catheterization, or (3) suprapubic aspiration. The method of collection determines, in part, the interpretation of the urine culture results.

Clean-voided urine specimens can easily become contaminated with bacteria from stool and vaginal secretions, despite cleansing of the external genitalia before collection. Contaminated urine, however, usually contains fewer than 10,000 (10^4) bacterial colonies per milliliter. Frequently, two or more species of organisms will grow in culture when there has been contamination. In contrast, truly infected urine usually contains over 100,000 (10^5) colonies/ml, usually of only a single organism. When culture results are equivocal (between 10,000 and 100,000 colonies/ml) the urine culture may need to be repeated.

The above guidelines for bacterial counts apply only to urine collected as a clean-voided specimen. Urine obtained by suprapubic aspiration with more than 1000 colonies/ml indicates infection. Likewise, urine obtained by catheterization which contains more than 10,000 colonies/ml indicates infection (Durbin and Peter, 1984).

In addition to contamination from the external genitalia, delays in getting the collected urine to the laboratory and storing the urine at a warm room temperature give false-positive results because these practices allow bacteria to proliferate. False negative results can occur with a very dilute urine (low specific gravity), a low urine pH, the presence of antibacterial drugs (possibly for the treatment of another infection), or inappropriate culture techniques (Wallach, 1983).

Radiographic Studies

Once a urinary tract infection is diagnosed, decisions must be made about the need for radiographic studies. An intravenous pyelogram (IVP) and a voiding cystourethrogram (VCUG) should be performed in (1) all boys with their first urinary tract infection, (2) all girls under age 3 with their first urinary tract infection, and (3) all children with pyelonephritis. Some physicians now recommend that a renal ultrasound replace the IVP because ultrasound is a safe, seemingly accurate diagnostic study that is less traumatic to most children than the IVP (Johnson et al, 1986). Girls between the ages of 3 and 12 may also be candidates for radiographic studies if they have a history of an abnormal pattern of urination, poor physical development, elevated blood pressure; an abnormal flank, abdominal, or genital examination; previous urinary tract infection; or a poor response to antibiotic treatment for infection (Durbin and Peter, 1984). The nurse should compile a careful history of the child's past health. Up to 40 per cent of urinary tract infections may be asymptomatic or may have been mistakenly diagnosed as respiratory or gastrointestinal infections. What seems to be a first infection may actually be a recurrent infection.

IVP and VCUG are usually done 4 to 6 weeks after diagnosis because transient inflammatory changes of the urinary tract are at times difficult to distinguish from permanent abnormalities. Children may be given prophylactic antibiotics in the interim to prevent recurrent infection. Radiographic studies at the time of diagnosis are indicated if the child has any sign of urinary obstruction, abdominal masses, or poor response to antibiotic therapy.

Tables 42-3 and 42-4 outline common urologic tests and procedures and their nursing implications. The nurse needs to be knowledgeable about the various diagnostic tests and procedures in order to appropriately prepare the child and family for them. Children under ages 3 to 4 years may benefit from explanations using dolls. Simple drawings of the urethra, bladder, ureters, and kidneys can be used with parents and older children.

Therapeutic Management

Management of urinary tract infections is aimed at achieving three goals: (1) cure of the infection, (2) identification and correction of any factors that predispose the child to infection, and (3) prevention of recurrent infections. Treatment approaches for three categories of infection are discussed next.

Acute, Uncomplicated Infection (Cystitis)

A child with an acute, uncomplicated urinary tract infection typically is school-age and has no symptoms of kidney infection (fever, flank pain); lower urinary tract symptoms (dysuria, frequency, urgency) predominate. Antibiotics that are most effective against the infecting bacteria are chosen to treat the infection. Because approximately 80 per cent of all urinary tract infections are caused by *E. coli,* a 7- to 10-day oral course of amoxicillin, sulfisoxazole (Gantrisin), or trimethoprim-sulfamethoxazole (Bactrim) is usually given, although single-dose therapy is currently being studied in some institutions. At times, a urinary analgesic such as phenazopyridine hydrochloride (Pyridium) is also given to relieve the pain of dysuria. Parents and children should be warned that this medicine turns urine an orange-red color.

Recurrent Infections

A recurrent urinary tract infection is one that occurs after a previous infection has been successfully treated. Recurrent infections are frequently caused by organisms different from those that caused the previous infection. Therefore, antibiotics should be chosen based on culture and sensitivity reports. Indications for radiographic studies with recurrent urinary tract infections were discussed earlier. Children who have normal urinary tracts but have had three or more infections frequently are given prophylactic antibiotics to prevent recurrent infection. Trimethoprim-sulfamethoxazole or nitrofurantoin given daily in half the usual dose are the drugs of choice. The nurse needs to be knowledgeable about possible side effects of long-term antibiotic therapy.

Complicated Infections

Complicated urinary tract infections are those in which the child is febrile, less than 3 years of age, or a male of any age. They are classified as "complicated" because of the high likelihood of renal infection (pyelonephritis) or structural abnormalities of the urinary tract, or both. *Proteus, Klebsiella, Pseudomonas,* and *Enterococci* are the most common infecting organisms. These children are frequently hospitalized and treated, at least initially, with intravenous antibiotics. Ampicillin, gentamicin, and cefamandole are the usual drugs of choice.

Major Nursing Diagnoses for Urinary Tract Infection

Potential for injury: urinary tract, related to inadequately treated or recurrent infections

Potential for injury: chronic renal disease, related to inflammatory changes associated with severe or recurrent pyelonephritis

Strategies for Nursing Care

Ensuring Adequate and Safe Administration of Antibiotics. The nurse needs to work with the child and family to ensure that the correct amount of the antibiotic will be given at the correct time. Medication names, dosages, and administration times, as well as follow-up instructions, should be given to the family in writing. Families frequently need to be encouraged to complete the full prescribed course of the medicine, even though the child is feeling better. If the child does not feel better within 24 to 48 hours the parents should call their health care provider. If the child is in school, the school nurse should be contacted about the prescribed medicine, and any required forms for the administration of medication in school should be completed.

Teaching Families the Importance of Follow-Up Care. The diagnosis of a urinary tract infection necessitates a number of follow-up urine cultures. A culture should be done 2 days after the initiation of antibiotic treatment to ensure that the antibiotic is working effectively. Urine is usually sterile after 48 hours of antibiotics. Routine follow-up urine cultures should be obtained 2 to 3 days after the cessation of treatment, then at monthly intervals for 3 months, at 3-month intervals for 9 months, and finally annually thereafter (Thomas, 1982; Durbin and Peter, 1984). Families often become discouraged with the number of health care visits required for follow-up, especially when the child feels healthy. The nurse can explain to the family that one third (males) to two fifths (females) of children will have a recurrent urinary tract infection. Two thirds of these recurrent infections will be during the first year after the initial infection—especially during the first 3 months. As these infections are frequently asymptomatic, close follow-up through urine cultures is vital.

Teaching Preventive Measures. The nurse needs to work with the child and family to prevent recurrent infection. Adequate fluid intake and regular emptying of the bladder (every 3 to 4 hours) may be beneficial. All girls should be taught to wipe themselves from front to back after using the bathroom. Other preventive measures include avoidance of tight-fitting and potentially irritating nylon underwear, bubble baths, and constipation. Adolescent girls who seem to develop urinary tract infections in association with sexual activity can be encouraged to urinate both before and immediately after sexual intercourse to wash away any bacteria that may have entered the urethra.

The actual effectiveness of these preventive measures is poorly documented. Nurses can conduct and participate in research to facilitate the development of preventive interventions.

Assessing for Signs and Symptoms of Chronic Renal Disease. When pyelonephritis is present, in addition to urine culture follow-up, other indices of renal function including urine concentration (specific gravity), blood urea nitrogen (BUN), and serum creatinine must be assessed periodically. The development of elevated blood pressure and growth failure may also indicate chronic renal problems. The nurse assists in the assessment of the child with a complicated urinary tract infection through careful monitoring of temperature, blood pressure, weight, input and output, and routine urine dipsticks to test for blood or protein in the urine.

Vesicoureteral Reflux

Vesicoureteral reflux is the regurgitation of urine from the bladder into the ureters and the kidneys. Experts estimate that the prevalence of vesicoureteral reflux in healthy children is less than 1 per cent. Vesicoureteral reflux is found, however, in 29 to 50 per cent of children with urinary tract infections and is the most common radiographic abnormality associated with urinary tract infections in children. Development of reflux may be, at least in part, genetically determined. Siblings of children with vesicoureteral reflux are 10 times more likely to have reflux than other children (Levitt and Weiss, 1985). Some researchers recommend that all siblings of children with reflux, whether symptomatic or asymptomatic, should have a screening cystourethrogram (van den Abbeele, 1987).

Pathophysiology

Normally, the ureters enter the musculature of the bladder at an oblique angle and travel through the bladder mucosa before opening into the interior of the bladder (Fig. 42-7). When bladder pressures rise, during voiding and during the accumulation of urine, the length of this submucosal segment of ureter becomes compressed and acts as a valve to prevent urine from refluxing back into the ureter and the kidney. This valvular mechanism malfunctions when the submucosal ureter is either congenitally abnormally short (primary reflux) or has been damaged by chronic infection or increased pressures caused by bladder outlet obstruction (secondary reflux).

The ultimate danger of reflux is the development of chronic renal infection and scarring (reflux nephropathy). Urine that has backed into the ureters returns to the bladder and remains there until the next

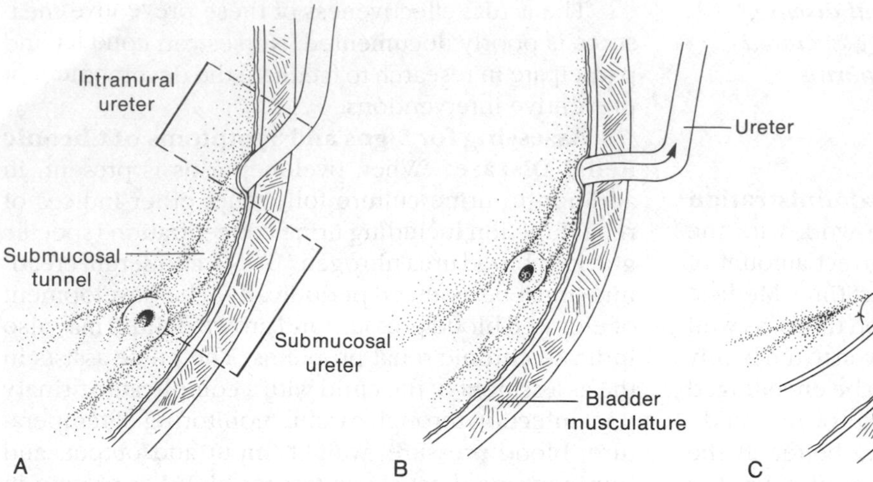

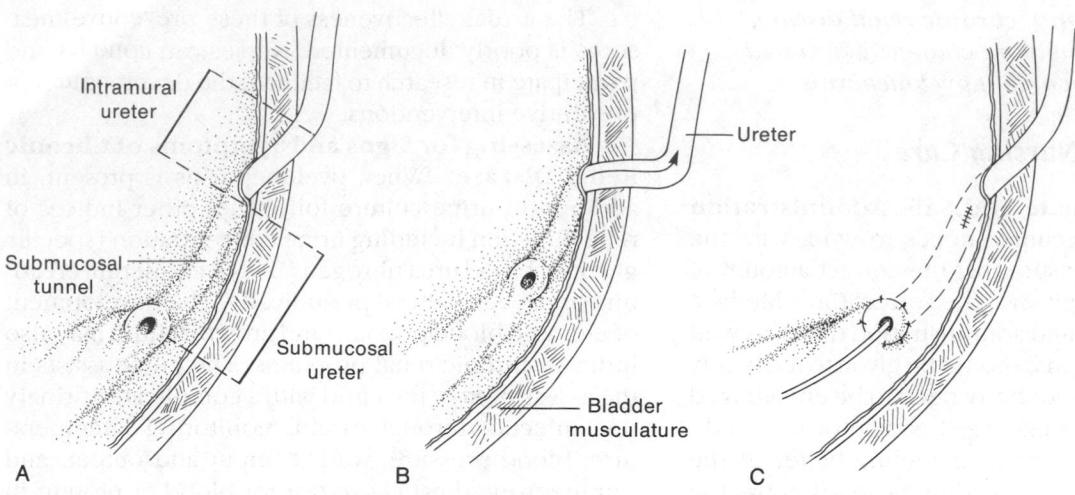

Figure 42-7. Reimplantation of ureters. *A*, The ureter enters the bladder at an oblique angle to form a normal ureterovesical junction. Normally, as pressure in the bladder rises, the angled position of the ureter causes a temporary closing off of the lumen, preventing urine backflow (reflux). *B*, In vesicoureteral reflux the ureter enters the bladder at an acute angle and the submucosal tunnel is shortened. As pressure in the bladder rises, urine is directed up the ureter (reflux). *C*, Reimplantation of the ureter is done to correct the ureterovesical angle and lengthen the submucosal tunnel to prevent reflux.

time the child voids. This residual urine serves as an excellent medium for bacterial growth. Bladder infections can swiftly lead to renal infections when infected urine refluxes from the bladder into the kidneys.

Diagnostic Assessment

The diagnosis of vesicoureteral reflux is made by VCUG (see Table 42-4 for a discussion of the procedure and nursing interventions). Classification of reflux depends on the degree of filling and dilation of the ureter and renal pelvis (Fig. 42-8). Grading is usually based on a scale of 1 through 5, with 1 being reflux into the ureter with no dilation and 5 being gross reflux and dilation of the ureter, renal pelvis, and calyces (International Reflux Study in Children, 1985).

Therapeutic Management

The ultimate goal of treatment is to protect the kidneys from scarring and allow them to grow as normally as possible. Factors predisposing the child to reflux (e.g., bladder outlet obstruction, neurogenic bladder dysfunction) must be identified. Reflux can be treated either medically or surgically.

Medical Management

Medical management is based on the assumption that mild to moderate reflux without infection is not harmful. Studies have documented spontaneous resolution in 60 to 85 per cent of cases of mild reflux (Bellinger, 1985). In an attempt to prevent infection, continuous low-dose prophylactic antibiotics are administered to the child until resolution of the reflux is documented. Commonly used antibiotics are nitrofurantoin, short-acting sulfonamides, or trimethoprim-sulfamethoxazole (Anderson and Smey, 1985). Antibiotics must be taken daily, often for years; frequent urine cultures are

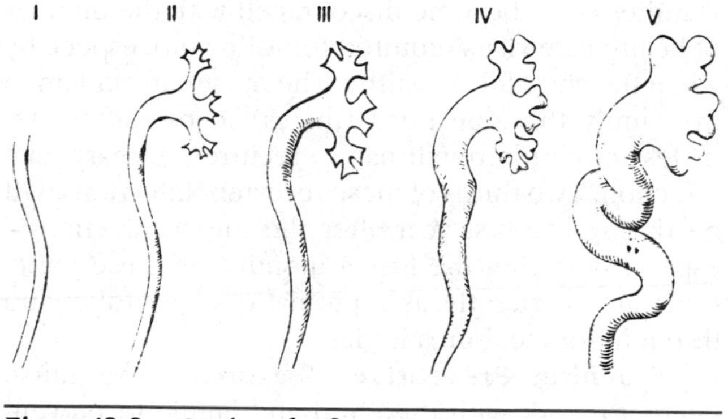

Figure 42-8. Grades of reflux—International Study Classification. *I*, Ureter only. *II*, Ureter, pelvis, and calyces. No dilatation, normal calyceal fornices. *III*, Mild or moderate dilation and/or tortuosity of ureter and mild or moderate dilatation of renal pelvis, but no or slight blunting of fornices. *IV*, Moderate dilatation and/or tortuosity of ureter and moderate dilatation of renal pelvis and calyces. Complete obliteration of sharp angle of fornices but maintenance of papillary impressions in majority of calyces. *V*, Gross dilatation and tortuosity of ureter. Gross dilatation of renal pelvis and calyces. Papillary impressions are no longer visible in the majority of calyces. (From Anderson GF, Smey P: Current concepts in the management of common urologic problems in infants and children. *Pediatr Clin North Am* 1985; 32(5):1145.)

also needed to screen for breakthrough infection. The child and family need support and encouragement during this long-term treatment period. Nursing interventions aimed at the prevention of urinary tract infections are outlined in the urinary tract infection section of this chapter.

Surgical Management

Surgical management of reflux is indicated when there is: (1) recurrent infection despite prophylactic antibiotics; (2) noncompliance with medical management; (3) ureteral obstruction in association with reflux; (4) no submucosal ureteral segments; or (5) persistent severe reflux (Levitt and Weiss, 1985). The corrective surgical procedure is called ureteroneocystostomy, or reimplantation of the ureter. A variety of different surgical techniques are used, but they all focus on lengthening the submucosal segment of ureter and/or moving the site where the ureter opens into the bladder closer to the bladder neck, thereby correcting the angle at which the ureter enters the bladder (see Fig. 42-8).

Major Nursing Diagnoses for Vesicoureteral Reflux

Potential for injury: surgical site, related to pressure exerted upon site of reimplantation by
- *tension on the stent*
- *obstruction of urinary drainage devices*

Potential for infection: urinary tract, related to introduction of pathogens by
- *surgical intervention*
- *contamination of urinary drainage devices*

Altered comfort: pain, related to
- *bladder spasms*
- *inflammation and edema associated with surgical manipulation*

Strategies for Nursing Care

Surgery is rarely performed on initial presentation of reflux; therefore, the child and family have usually had multiple contacts with health care providers and have some understanding of the management of reflux before surgical intervention becomes a necessity. Assessment of the family's knowledge of the disorder will clarify the need for teaching. Close collaboration with the urologist will ensure that the family does not receive conflicting information.

Preventing Trauma to the Surgical Site. The child will usually return from surgery with either a suprapubic or a urethral catheter. In addition, stents may be placed in the ureters to maintain patency and divert urine while healing occurs. Stents are very small, soft, supple catheters with multiple perforations along their length. They exit the body through small incisions in the lower abdomen and are attached to drainage tubing and collection bags. Stents do not occlude the ureters and therefore some urine drains around them and into the bladder.

In order to prevent trauma to the site of ureteral reimplantation it is important that the stent(s) be free of tension and that all catheters are patent. Tubing attached to stents must be taped to the child's leg and a stress loop (a loop of tubing that is taped or otherwise secured below the first taping site) should be formed in the tubing for additional protection. Securing the drainage tubing will protect against accidental trauma to the ureter that could occur with tension on the stent. Wrist restraints for unattended children may sometimes be necessary to prevent a child from pulling upon the drainage tubings.

Patency of drainage devices is essential to prevent back pressure of urine upon the surgical site. Urine flow should be checked and recorded hourly for the first 24 hours, and at least every 4 hours thereafter.

Preventing Infection. Antibiotics to suppress infection will be ordered postoperatively and will usually be continued for several weeks to 3 months. Teaching in preparation for discharge must include the importance of continuous administration of the antibiotics. The family needs to be aware of signs and symptoms of side effects of long-term antibiotic therapy so that early medical intervention may be sought.

Nursing responsibility for postoperative infection control includes meticulous care of drainage devices to ensure their sterility. Box 42-2 shows specific care strategies.

Providing Pain Relief. In addition to general postoperative discomfort, painful spasms of the bladder and involved ureter(s) are common after reimplantation. Physicians' orders frequently include antispasmodics or sedatives as well as narcotic pain relievers. The informed nurse will be aware that antispasmodics may be more effective than narcotic analgesics for relief of pain associated with smooth muscle spasms. Antispasmodics are designed to relieve spasticity of smooth muscles (such as those of the bladder and ureter); narcotic analgesics may actually increase the tone and spasms of these organs and may delay bladder emptying. In addition, narcotics stimulate the secretion of antidiuretic hormone, further decreasing urinary output. Nursing strategies for pain relief must therefore focus on careful assessment of the source and type of pain experienced. If the pain is primarily from spasms an antispasmodic is indicated; if the pain is related to general postoperative discomfort a narcotic analgesic may be more appropriate.

As always, appropriate nonpharmacologic measures should also be employed. Parents should be encouraged to institute (and to share with nurses for inclusion in the care plan) any appropriate comfort measures that have been beneficial to the child in the past. These might include close physical contact with parents and significant others, diversionary activities, gentle massage, and music of the child's choice.

Adequate rest will increase the child's ability to cope with postoperative discomfort and will enhance rapid healing. It is the nurse's responsibility to schedule some rest periods for the child that are uninterrupted by procedures, medications, and visits by other health care professionals.

Long-Term Outcome

Surgery for vesicoureteral reflux is highly successful, with elimination of reflux in over 95 per cent of cases. Follow-up radiographic studies (usually VCUG) are performed 3 to 6 months, 18 months, 3 years, and 5 years from the time of surgery (Kelalis, 1985). Persistent reflux and obstruction at the vesicoureteral junction are the most common complications.

Nursing Strategies for Follow-Up Care in the Home or Clinic

Obtain a specimen for urinalysis or urine culture or both (see guidelines for specimen collection earlier in this chapter).

Measure vital signs and alert the physician to fever or to elevations in blood pressure.

Assess for signs and symptoms of urinary tract infection:

- *Infants:* vomiting, diarrhea, irritability, lethargy, poor feeding, slow weight gain, unexplained jaundice, fever, or hypothermia
- *Toddler or older child:* dysuria, urgency, fever, abdominal or flank pain, and enuresis
- *All children:* weak urine stream, frequency, foul-smelling urine

Determine compliance with prophylactic antibiotic therapy. Share innovations for remembering to administer each dose.

Discuss with the child and parent(s) their reactions to the last radiographic diagnostic procedure. Be alert to possible interventions that could reduce the stress of these repeated tests.

Vulvovaginitis

Vulvovaginitis is the most common gynecologic problem in female children. The diagnosis subdivides into inflammation of the vulva (vulvitis) and inflammation of the vagina (vaginitis). Primary vulvitis with secondary inflammation of the outer portion of the vagina occurs most frequently in children, has a nonspecific cause 85 per cent of the time and is usually linked with lack of adequate perineal cleansing. In contrast, primary vaginitis with secondary inflammation of the vulva is more likely to be linked with a specific causal organism and necessitates careful evaluation. Frequently, however, it is difficult to distinguish between primary vulvar and primary vaginal inflammation.

> Box 42-4
> *Causes of Vulvovaginitis in Children*
>
> Bacterial infections
> - Nonspecific, mixed bacteria
> - Specific (e.g., *Neisseria gonorrhoea, Haemophilus vaginalis, Chlamydia trachomatis, Shigella, group A β-hemolytic Streptococcus)*
>
> Other infectious organisms (e.g., *Candida albicans, Trichomonas vaginalis,* pinworms)
>
> Sexual abuse
>
> Foreign body (most frequently toilet paper)
>
> Trauma
>
> Contact dermatitis from irritating clothing, chemicals
>
> Allergic reactions
>
> Vulvar skin disease (e.g., atopic dermatitis, psoriasis, lichen sclerosis)
>
> Systemic illnesses (e.g., measles, chickenpox, scarlet fever)
>
> Neoplasms
>
> Urologic problems (e.g., ectopic ureters, enuresis, prolapsed urethra)

Girls are susceptible to vulvovaginitis for a number of reasons. The vulva of a child is relatively exposed compared with that of an adult; the vulvar fat pads are undeveloped, the labia minora are small, and there is no pubic hair. The vaginal wall is especially vulnerable to infection because it is thin, warm, and moist and has a neutral rather than an acidic pH. Children also tend to wipe from back to front after bowel movements, play in soiled underwear, and touch their genitals with dirty hands. Therefore, it is not surprising that the most common cause of vulvovaginitis in young girls is infection with nonspecific, usually normal, bacterial flora. Box 42-4 lists common causes of vulvovaginitis in children. Sexually transmitted diseases are discussed in Chapter 45.

Pathophysiology

The infant's vagina is sterile prior to birth and becomes colonized only when she passes through her mother's vagina during the birth process. A physiologic vaginal discharge is frequently present during the first week of life as a result of exposure to maternal estrogens during gestation. This discharge is white, mucoid, nonirritating, and odorless. It may become slightly blood-tinged as the infant withdraws from maternal estrogen stimulation. Temporary colonization with *Lactobacillus* causes the pH of the vagina to be acidic (4.0 to 5.0). Within 2 to 3 weeks, without further estrogen stimulation, the vaginal mucosa thins, dries, and becomes reddened. The lactobacilli fail to survive and the vaginal pH rises to 6.5 to 7.5, where it will stay until adolescence. This neutral or alkaline pH due to the lack of estrogen effect on the vaginal mucosa is thought to be responsible for survival of bacteria rarely encountered in the postpubertal female. A number of bacterial species including *Staphylococcus epidermidis*, *β*-hemolytic streptococci, *Escherichia coli*, and *Bacteroides fragilis* may be found as part of normal vaginal flora in healthy, asymptomatic prepubertal girls (Altchek, 1984).

The second occurrence of physiologic vaginal discharge begins in the year prior to the onset of menstruation. This discharge, often called leukorrhea, is viscous, gray-white, non-irritating, and odorless. It normally contains a few white blood cells but no pathogenic bacteria. This normal discharge will continue throughout the woman's reproductive years but is frequently the cause for alarm among young adolescent girls who are unprepared for its appearance. The nurse can teach parents of newborn girls and young adolescents about physiologic vaginal discharge and reassure them of its normal occurrence.

Diagnostic Assessment

Vulvovaginitis typically presents when a mother brings her daughter in for evaluation of vaginal discharge, burning with urination (without frequency), pruritus, or redness of the vulva. The infant or young child who is unable to verbalize complaints may be irritable, walk awkwardly, cry during urination or when touched, or repeatedly rub or scratch her vulva. The vulva may be reddened, edematous, and macerated. Vaginal discharge or discrete lesions, or both, may be visible.

The nurse assists with history taking and the physical examination. Parents frequently feel embarrassed discussing genital complaints. The nurse can help make parents feel more at ease by speaking matter of factly and using the correct anatomic terminology for body parts. Children and parents may use alternative names for the genitals; the nurse needs to find out what these names are, teach parents and children the correct names, yet still be able to use the alternative names when talking with the child if it makes the child feel more comfortable.

A thorough history includes a description of the symptoms, any associated illnesses or events, and treatments tried. Past medical history (similar problems, allergies, rashes), family social history (who is living at home, family relationships), and family medical history (allergies, skin disorders, pinworms, vaginitis) are also important. As a screening question for sexual abuse, *every* child should be asked, preferably without the parent(s) present, if anyone has ever touched his or her genitals.

The physical examination should also be approached matter of factly (see Chapter 15 for examination protocol). A pediatric gynecologic text can be consulted for more specific details. The child's response to examination of her genitals depends upon her age, her family environment, her previous experiences, and the examiner's approach. Parents should be encouraged to stay with their child unless she is an adolescent or the parents are extremely anxious. Younger children frequently enjoy playing with gloves, like the gloves worn by the examiner, during the examination. The presence of a supportive nurse can also be reassuring. History and inspection of the external genitalia are frequently all that is needed for diagnosis. Infrequently, a more thorough inspection of the vagina is needed. The nurse assists in the proper handling of cultures obtained from any vaginal discharge or from vulvar lesions.

Therapeutic Management and Strategies for Nursing Care

The nurse assists the parents and child to understand the diagnosis and treatment. Children with nonspecific vulvovaginitis are typically treated with wet compresses of Burow solution, normal saline or plain water for 20 to 30 minutes several times a day. Sitz baths with normal saline, plain water, colloidal oatmeal (Aveeno), or baking soda are an alternative treatment. The nurse works with the parents to devise ways of keeping the child occupied during treatments and demonstrates how to make wet compresses or set up sitz baths. Healing is enhanced if the vulva is kept clean and dry. A soothing cream (sometimes a mild steroid cream) may also be prescribed. Recurrent nonspecific vulvovaginitis suggests the need for further evaluation.

To prevent vulvovaginitis the nurse must teach parents and children the basics of good perineal care. The vulva should be kept as clean, cool, and dry as possible. Daily cleaning with a nonmedicated, unperfumed soap and thorough rinsing is important. Patting, rather than rubbing, the vulva dry can decrease tissue trauma. Children should be taught to wipe from front to back after they have had a bowel movement. Underpants should be thoroughly rinsed after being washed. Loose-fitting, white cotton underpants are best. Pantyhose, leotards, and tight blue jeans should be avoided, especially when the child has an acute infection. The nurse may need to work with the adolescent, especially, to encourage alternative forms of dress.

Vulvovaginitis caused by specific organisms is treated with appropriate medication. Nonsexual transmission of gonorrhea, chlamydia, herpes simplex virus, and trichomonas is not well documented, and careful evaluation for sexual abuse should always ensue when these organisms are present (Neinstein, Goldenring, and Carpenter, 1984).

The Child with an Alteration in Filtration

Nephrotic Syndrome

Nephrotic syndrome is an alteration in renal function that may be congenital, idiopathic, or secondary to another disease. It is the most prevalent disorder associated with glomerular injury in children, with an incidence of 16 per 100,000 population (Kim and Grupe, 1986).

Pathophysiology

This disorder is characterized by massive proteinuria, hypoproteinemia, oliguria, generalized edema, and hyperlipidemia (Fig. 42-9). In nephrotic syndrome, proteinuria occurs owing to a defect in the glomerular basement membrane that allows protein to pass freely into the urine. Hypoproteinemia may result if the liver is unable to synthesize enough protein to compensate for the loss of protein in the urine. Generalized edema occurs in nephrotic syndrome in two ways. First, there is a reduction of plasma colloid osmotic pressure in response to a decrease in circulating serum protein. This reduction in pressure causes fluid to leave the intravascular spaces and fill the interstitial spaces, resulting in edema. As a result of this fluid shift, there is a reduced blood volume. Second, there is an increase in the reabsorption of sodium and water in response to the decreased blood volume. This reabsorption further compounds the edema. The mechanism for the hyperlipidemia is not clearly known but is believed to occur secondarily to the hypoproteinemia.

Although pathogenesis is not clearly understood, it is thought that the kidney may be impaired in nephrotic syndrome as the result of an undefined immunologic response. The majority of the cases of nephrotic syndrome (approximately 90 per cent [Bergstein and Michael, 1987]) are classified as idiopathic or as minimal change nephrotic syndrome (MCNS). MCNS may occur at any age, but usually between the ages of 2 and 7 with a peak incidence between 2 and 3 years of age (Drummond, 1983). This condition is seen twice as frequently in boys as in girls

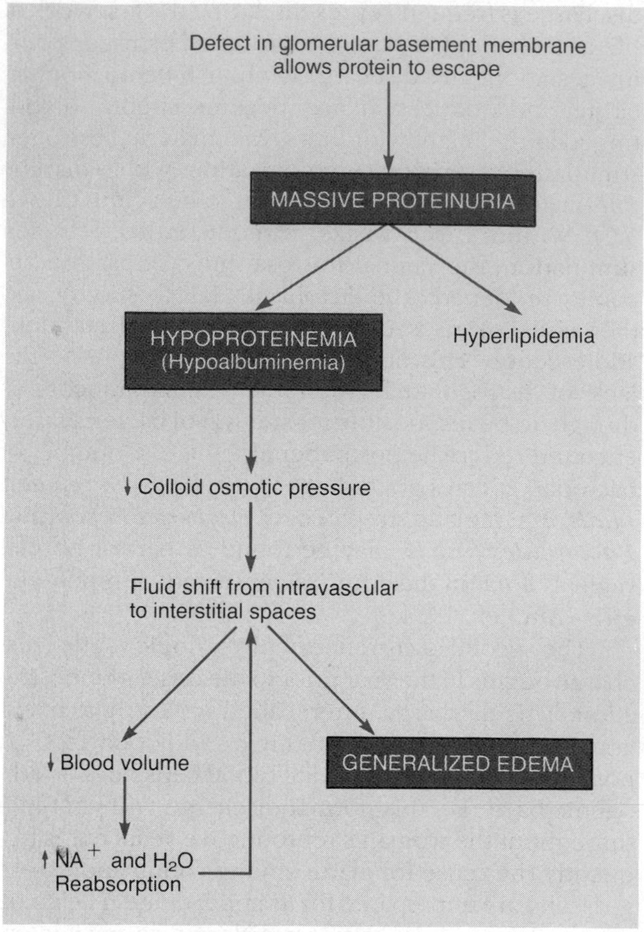

Figure 42-9. Pathophysiology of minimal change nephrotic syndrome.

until adolescence, when they are affected equally. In MCNS, the glomeruli appear essentially normal under routine microscopy. However, electron microscopy reveals a change in the outer surface of the basement membrane. This form of nephrotic syndrome is readily responsive to corticosteroid therapy, with eventual clearing of proteinuria and reversion to normal status.

The congenital form of nephrotic syndrome is rare. Infants born with this disorder are small for gestational age and have proteinuria and edema. They usually fail to respond to corticosteroid or cytotoxic drug therapy and die within the first or second year of life. Renal transplants have been tried in children with congenital nephrotic syndrome with limited success.

The secondary form of nephrotic syndrome develops during the course of a diverse group of diseases including systemic lupus erythematosus, acute or chronic glomerulonephritis, syphilis, diabetes mellitus, malaria, Alport syndrome, and anaphylactoid purpura. It may also occur secondary to systemic infections (infected atrioventricular shunt, subacute bacterial endocarditis) or as the result of drug toxicity.

Diagnostic Assessment

Congenital Nephrotic Syndrome

Congenital nephrotic syndrome may be seen first by the nurse working in a neonatal nursery or in a well-baby screening clinic. This form of nephrotic syndrome is commonly associated with toxemia of pregnancy, an enlarged placenta, and prematurity. The presence of other clinical signs such as proteinuria, distended abdomen, and atypical facies with wide-set cranial sutures, low-set ears, and a small snub nose should alert the nurse to the possibility of nephrotic syndrome. Astute observation in the delivery room for identification of infants at risk is essential.

Careful screening and developmental assessment throughout infancy will help in making the diagnosis of nephrotic syndrome. These children may fail to gain weight as they should despite conscientious efforts to help them feed. Nursing investigation may identify other members of the family with renal disease since the congenital form of nephrotic syndrome is believed to be transmitted by an autosomal recessive gene. (See Chapter 4 for a discussion of patterns of inheritance.) The child should be observed for an edematous abdomen, which may be indicated by an arched-back position and increases in abdominal girth measurements.

Minimal Change Nephrotic Syndrome (MCNS)

Children with MCNS will usually present with insidious edema that has developed over a period of several weeks. Parents may report that the child has periorbital edema upon arising, which diminishes throughout the day. They may also indicate that it is difficult to find clothes and shoes that fit properly and that ankle and pedal edema seem to develop in the later hours of the day. Volume and frequency of urination are decreased, and the urine is foamy and dark in color. Hematuria is uncommon. The edema is more prevalent where subcutaneous tissues are loose, such as around the eyes, neck, and genitalia. Ascites and pleural effusion may be present.

Respiratory difficulty may occur if ascites produces sufficient pressure on the diaphragm. With an increase in edema, the child may become anorexic and lethargic. It is essential for the nurse to interview the parents carefully and document the pattern of the edema, any prior infection, and the child's pattern of development. Changes in behavior and eating patterns may also be valuable clues. It is important to note that the blood pressure is usually normal or slightly decreased; only in 5 to 10 per cent of cases is it elevated.

Nursing Strategies

In making the diagnosis the nurse must draw or assist with the drawing of blood specimens, as well as collecting and examining repeated urine specimens. The nurse must understand the child's fear of undergoing repeated assaults on his or her body. A simple explanation of what is going to take place should be given immediately before the procedure. Blood can be difficult to draw from the edematous child because veins are more difficult to find. Rest periods may be indicated if efforts are repeated. The child who is placed in a supine position for blood collections should be watched closely for respiratory difficulty.

Urine specimens must be screened frequently for the presence of protein. Because of the decreased urinary output this may be difficult. The child who is toilet trained should be regularly encouraged to void in an appropriate container. If a urine collection bag is necessary, apply it to clean skin and remove it very carefully to avoid injury to edematous tissues.

Renal biopsy may be done to examine glomerular tissue. However, usually a trial test of prednisone is given first to assess response to corticosteroids. If the response is favorable, steroid treatment is usually continued and the biopsy is deferred. If a renal biopsy is done, the child must be prepared for a surgical procedure with appropriate play techniques and simple explanations. (See Chapter 27 for age-appropriate teaching strategies.) Parents will also need to be assured that the procedure is necessary and will require an explanation of its methodology.

Parents will want to know about nephrotic syndrome and its cause, and to be reassured that there was nothing they could have done to keep their child from getting it. The nurse should be available to answer these questions and to participate with other team members in the explanation given to parents about the long-term course of the disease.

Therapeutic Management

Treatment with pharmacologic agents should be initiated as soon as possible. Bed rest may be instituted to bring about a mild spontaneous diuresis, but generally ambulation is encouraged. The male child may find comfort in a scrotal support during periods of ambulation.

The diet should be high in protein, with the elimination of highly salted foods. A low-salt diet is encouraged in order to prevent further retention of sodium and subsequent increases in edema. Care must be taken not to severely restrict salt because this may make food unpalatable just at a time when an increase in protein intake is desired. Occasionally diuretics are ordered. Fluids are not usually restricted unless edema progresses despite sodium restriction.

Corticosteroids will usually induce remission in children with MCNS. A daily dose of 2 mg/kg of prednisone is given. Remission is usually induced in 6 to 14 days and is indicated by an abrupt diuresis and the absence of urinary protein. Care must be taken to observe the child for side effects of the steroids. An increase in weight and appetite, an elevation of blood pressure, obesity, moon facies, and striae may occur. Serious infections may be masked, and growth in height may be decreased. (See Table 43-2.) As soon as feasible, steroids are gradually tapered and only reinstituted in cases of relapse.

Patients who fail to respond to prednisone after 4 weeks of therapy are considered steroid resistant and are treated with cyclophosphamide (Cytoxan) in combination with the steroid. Cyclophosphamide is an oral alkylating agent that has proven effective in reducing the incidence of relapse. The severe side effect of cyclophosphamide is leukopenia, which will drastically increase the child's susceptibility to infection. Hair loss results from cyclophosphamide and may be a distressing problem to children who are already experiencing body image concerns because of the edema. Because chemical cystitis may occur if the drug precipitates in the bladder, increased fluid intake is indicated.

Major Nursing Diagnoses for Nephrotic Syndrome

Fluid volume excess: extracellular (edema), *related to massive proteinuria possibly associated with an immune response*
Potential impaired tissue integrity, *related to edema*
Potential sensory-perceptual alteration: visual, *related to marked periorbital edema*
Potential altered nutrition: less than body requirements, *related to anorexia and lethargy*
Disturbance in self-concept: body image, *related to marked edema*
Potential for injury: falls, *related to altered coordination associated with marked edema*
Potential for infection, *related to altered immune response associated with corticosteroid therapy*
Knowledge deficit, *related to*

- *signs and symptoms requiring medical attention*
- *importance of follow-up care*
- *urine testing for protein*

Strategies for Nursing Care

Nursing care for the child with nephrotic syndrome centers primarily on care of the child and family during the acute phase and preparation of the family for assuming care in the home setting.

Administering Corticosteroids. Corticosteroid administration to address the disease process requires that the nurse be alert for associated fluid retention (which would aggravate existing edema), hypokalemia, gastric irritation, hyperglycemia, and neurologic changes. Table 43-2, Nursing Process Plan: The Child on Corticosteroid Therapy, provides detailed strategies for nursing care.

Protecting Edematous Body Surfaces. Careful attention and meticulous cleansing of touching skin surfaces is essential; skin creases should be padded with a soft material. Supporting edematous areas with pillows may provide a measure of comfort. The child should be turned, positioned, and gently massaged frequently. A bed cradle may be helpful in lifting bed covers off the child's skin and allowing air to flow.

Reducing Periorbital Edema. Edema about the eyes may interfere with sensory perception and comfort. The use of eye irrigations or ophthalmic creams may be indicated. Allowing the child to sleep with the head elevated on a pillow may prevent the eyes from swelling closed and eliminate the fear associated with this.

Encouraging Adequate Nutritional Intake. As the edema diminishes the child's malnourished appearance may become visible. Getting the child to eat may become a challenge. The nurse should make meals as attractive as possible, and smaller portions should be offered more frequently. Using a small glass with a small amount of fluid will help gain the child's cooperation to drink. The child should be weighed on a daily basis to monitor the edema and diuresis.

Promoting a Positive Body Image. Body image is just beginning to emerge in the younger child. During the edematous phase, the child may become concerned when parts of his or her body are no longer visible. Boys need reassurance that their penis is still there, even if edema conceals it from their view. Opportunities should be provided for the child and family to express their fears and concerns about the rapid changes in body size.

Ensuring Safety from Falls. Safety must be constantly monitored, as changes in body size may alter the child's ability to move and maintain position. Bed siderails are usually necessary, and are absolutely essential for the younger child. Parents should be made particularly aware of the need for safety as they prepare to take the child home.

Protecting the Child from Known Sources of Infection. Because infection is the leading cause of death in nephrosis (Kim and Grupe, 1986), the nurse's role is critical in protecting the child from known sources of infection. The child's resistance to all infections is lowered and compromised by corticosteroid therapy. Whether hospitalized or at home, the child should be protected from exposure to other children with infections. Appropriate handwashing is an emphasis for family teaching.

Providing Information and Support for Home Care. Care of the family focuses on support and education. The protracted course of the disease with remissions, relapses, and occasional admissions to the hospital may place severe stress on the family. Although outpatient treatment is usually practical for children with moderate edema, parents must be taught the signs and symptoms that need prompt medical attention and the importance of complying with a regimen of regular office or clinic visits. Parents will also need instruction regarding the testing of urine for protein; practice sessions should be initiated as soon as their level of readiness is deemed appropriate.

Long-Term Outcome

The prognosis of children with nephrotic syndrome is generally quite good. Although relapses are common, most children respond to treatment. For children with lesions other than minimal change disease the outlook is less optimistic, with progression to renal failure necessitating dialysis or transplantation.

Nursing Strategies for Follow-Up Care in the Home or Clinic

Collect a urine specimen for protein analysis.

Assess for fever and other signs and symptoms of infections that may follow nephrotic syndrome —especially pneumonia, bronchitis, peritonitis, cellulitis, urinary tract infection, and septic arthritis (Kim and Grupe, 1986).

Weigh and measure the child. Compare weight with that upon hospital discharge to assess fluid retention. Alert the physician to significant increases or decreases in weight and to delays in linear growth.

Inspect edematous body areas for skin irritation and excoriation. Reinforce teaching begun in the hospital concerning skin care.

Determine whether the child is receiving precise dosages of corticosteroids as ordered. Share with the family innovations for remembering to administer the medication.

Encourage the child to talk about the "chubby parts" of his or her body. Reinforce the temporary nature of these edematous changes.

Reinforce the importance of regular follow-up care to ensure early medical intervention in case of relapse.

Acute Poststreptococcal Glomerulonephritis

Glomerulonephritis is an inflammation of the glomeruli of the kidneys. The diagnosis represents a number of different disease processes, some causing glomerular inflammation as the primary disorder and others in which glomerular inflammation is only one manifestation of an overall systemic disease. Acute poststreptococcal glomerulonephritis is the most common form of glomerulonephritis in children and typically follows a streptococcal infection of the throat or skin.

Acute glomerulonephritis associated with pharyngeal streptococcal infections is most common in temperate or cold climates; it occurs 8 to 14 days after the pharyngitis and has a peak incidence during the winter and spring months (Jordan and Lemire, 1982). Early school-age children are most frequently affected, boys twice as often as girls for unknown reasons.

In contrast, glomerulonephritis associated with streptococcal infections of the skin (e.g., impetigo) is most common in hot, tropical climates; this form occurs 14 to 21 days after the skin infection and has a peak incidence during the late summer and early fall (Jordan and Lemire, 1982). Preschool children, with equal distribution to both sexes, are most often affected.

If one family member develops acute poststreptococcal glomerulonephritis, other family members are at high risk for developing the same disease. Second attacks of acute glomerulonephritis rarely occur in the same individual (Bergstein and Michael, 1987).

Pathophysiology

The glomeruli initiate the formation of urine by filtering the blood as it passes through the kidneys. Glomerulonephritis results when immune complexes (antigen-antibody complexes) formed during the streptococcal infection become entrapped in the glomerular membrane and cause inflammation. White blood cells, specifically polymorphonuclear leukocytes, collect in the glomeruli; the cells of the membrane proliferate, become edematous, and occlude the affected glomeruli. The glomerular filtration rate decreases, resulting in sodium and water retention and eventual circulatory congestion and edema. Those parts of the glomerular membrane that are not occluded malfunction and allow large amounts of protein to leak into the glomerular filtrate (proteinuria). Red blood cells may also pass into the filtrate if the membrane ruptures (hematuria) (Fig. 42-10). Permanent damage of the glomeruli, although rare, can occur with severe disease.

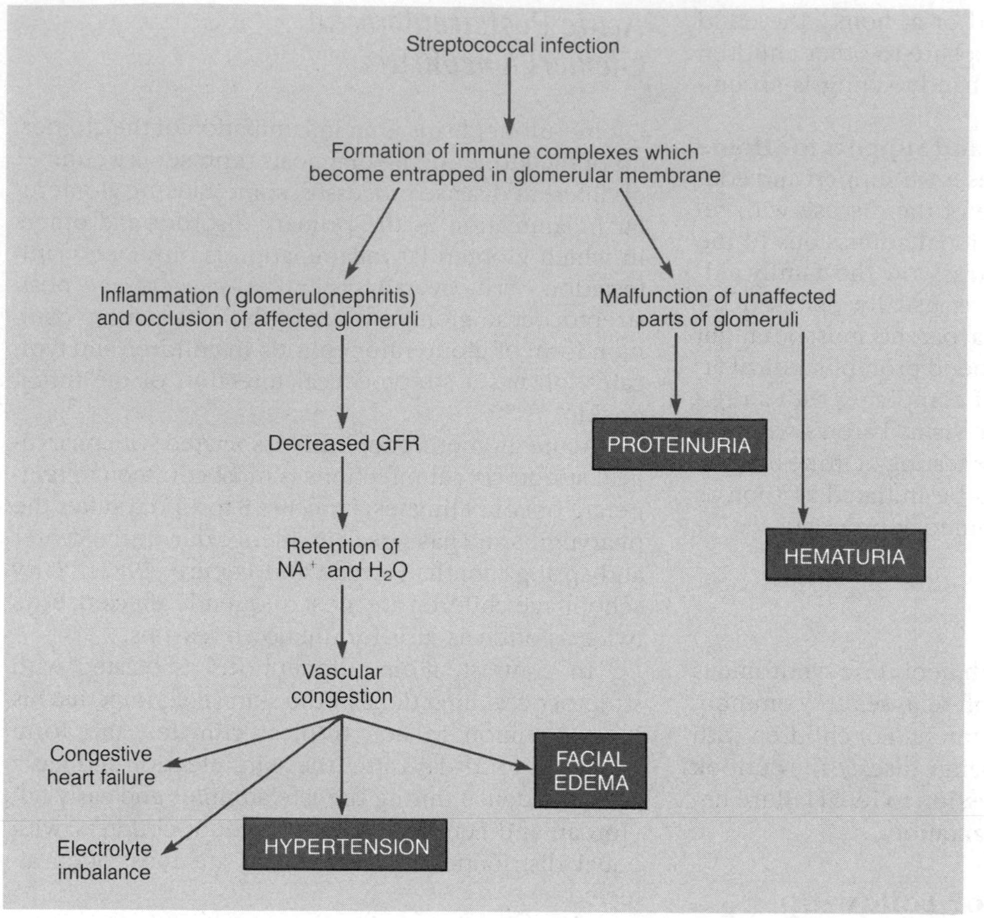

***Figure* 42-10.** Pathophysiology of acute poststreptococcal glomerulonephritis.

Etiology

Only certain types of group A beta-hemolytic streptococci cause acute poststreptococcal glomerulonephritis. The most common nephritogenic strains are types 12 and 49, associated with streptococcal infections of the pharynx and skin, respectively (Bergstein and Michael, 1987).

As streptococcal infection of the upper respiratory tract or the skin frequently precedes acute poststreptococcal glomerulonephritis, the nurse must elicit a careful history to determine if such an infection in fact did occur 1 to 3 weeks prior to the present symptoms. Documented prior infections will not always occur, however; viruses, parasites, and bacteria other than streptococci have also been implicated in the development of acute glomerulonephritis.

Early diagnosis of acute poststreptococcal glomerulonephritis is especially important because prevention does not seem possible. Early antibiotic treatment of streptococcal infections as a method of preventing the subsequent development of glomerulonephritis is not well supported, although it may be somewhat effective in reducing the severity of the disease. Because there may be a familial incidence of infection with nephritogenic strains of streptococci, family members of a child with acute poststreptococcal glomerulonephritis should have throat cultures done; those with streptococcal infections should be treated with antibiotics prophylactically (Bergstein and Michael, 1987). Routine screening throat cultures of all children, however, are not indicated because healthy, asymptomatic individuals can have nonnephritogenic streptococci cultured from their throats. Appropriate treatment of insect bites, cuts, and abrasions may inhibit the development of streptococcal impetigo. If impetigo does develop, systemic antibiotics are superior to local antibiotic creams and ointments for treatment.

Clinical Manifestations

Signs and symptoms are acute in onset and range from very mild to extremely severe. A puffy face (edema) and discolored urine (hematuria) are the two most common presenting complaints. Edema frequently involves the periorbital area and is usually confined to the face, except in severe disease when it may be more generalized. Gross hematuria, often described as cola- or tea-colored, rusty or reddish-brown, occurs in 30 to 50 per cent of children hospitalized with acute glomerulonephritis (McCrory, 1983). Microscopic he-

Table 42-6. Comparison of Minimal Change Nephrotic Syndrome and Acute Poststreptococcal Glomerulonephritis

	Nephrotic Syndrome	Glomerulonephritis
Etiology	Probably autoimmune responses leading to changes in glomerular membrane	Streptococcal infection leading to autoimmune response, which produces changes in glomerular membrane
GFR	Normal	Decreased
Proteinuria	Massive	Usually moderate
Hematuria	Rare	Often grossly evident
Fluid volume	Hypovolemia (fluid shifts to interstitial spaces)	Hypervolemia (fluid remains in intravascular compartment)
Blood pressure	Usually normal	Hypertensive
Edema	Pronounced—systemic	Usually confined to face

maturia is present in nearly all children with the disease (Jordan and Lemire, 1982). A decreased urine output, flank or abdominal pain, anorexia, weight gain, pallor, and low-grade fever are other symptoms that the nurse may detect.

Hypertension is a frequent complication; it is usually mild to moderate (120–180/80–120 mmHg), asymptomatic, and found only by checking blood pressure. Occasionally, hypertension can be severe enough to cause headaches, visual disturbances, sleepiness, coma, or seizures. Other signs of circulatory overload such as dyspnea, tachypnea, and cough may also be present. Table 42-6 compares the etiology and clinical manifestations of glomerulonephritis and minimal change nephrotic syndrome.

Diagnostic Assessment

The diagnosis of acute poststreptococcal glomerulonephritis rests upon (1) evidence of injury of the glomeruli (hematuria and proteinurea); (2) identification of a nephritogenic type of group A beta-hemolytic streptococcus; and (3) the sequential occurrence of a streptococcal infection, a 1- to 3-week latent period, and a subsequent rise in streptococcal antibody titers.

A number of laboratory findings document glomerular injury. The urinalysis will usually show an increased specific gravity (>1.030), positive blood, and positive protein. White blood cells and red blood cell casts will frequently be present on microscopic examination of the urine and are strongly associated with acute glomerular inflammation (Madaio and Harrington, 1983). The BUN and creatinine may be elevated because of impaired glomerular filtration. Hyponatremia secondary to retained fluid and hyperkalemia can occur. Retained fluid may also cause a mild dilutional anemia (Hb 10 to 11 mg/dl). Children with clinical symptoms of circulatory overload should have a chest radiograph to rule out cardiac enlargement and pulmonary congestion.

Appropriate throat and skin cultures should be done to attempt to document infection with nephritogenic streptococci. Antibody responses to streptococcal products including increased antistreptolysin-O (ASO), antistreptokinase (ASKase), antihyaluronidase (AHase), and antideoxyribonuclease-B (ADNase-B) titers also provide indirect evidence of a previous streptococcal infection. Decreased hemolytic complement activity and complement-3 levels are seen in 90 to 100 per cent of children with poststreptococcal glomerulonephritis (Jordan and Lemire, 1982). A mild increase in the white blood cell count and an elevated erythrocyte sedimentation rate (ESR) are other laboratory signs of inflammation. Renal biopsy is rarely needed for diagnosis.

The nurse assists in making the diagnosis by helping the child and family cope with the frequently frightening and painful diagnostic laboratory procedures. Doll play and age-appropriate explanations can help gain cooperation and decrease anxiety for both the child and the parents.

Therapeutic Management

The acute phase of glomerulonephritis usually lasts 1 to 2 weeks; however, the severity of the illness is unpredictable, and ranges from very mild to life-threatening. Children who have normal blood pressure, an adequate urine output, and very mild symptoms may be managed carefully as outpatients. Parents can be taught how to check their child's blood pressure, weight, and urine output daily. A visiting nurse may intervene to support parents during their child's illness. Children who develop hypertension, oliguria, or acute weight gain secondary to fluid retention will need to be hospitalized. Criteria for admission will vary with the institution.

The major danger during the acute phase of glomerulonephritis is renal failure with subsequent hypertension and circulatory congestion. Nursing and medical intervention focus on preserving renal function and preventing circulatory overload. Children who are sick generally restrict their activities according to how they feel; therefore, enforced bed rest is usually not needed unless severe hypertension or edema is present.

Fluid restrictions and diets high in carbohydrates and fats and low in sodium, potassium, or both, may be implemented. Antihypertensives and diuretics may be ordered if the diastolic pressure is 100 mmHg or greater. Antibiotics may be prescribed if the child still has a positive streptococcal culture.

Diuresis occurs after the initial 1- to 3-week edematous phase of the illness. Hospitalized children can be discharged when they have normal weight, normal blood pressure, and require no antihypertensives. Weekly to monthly follow-up visits for blood pressure and urinalysis are indicated until the urine returns to normal. Microscopic hematuria will resolve within 6 months in 90 per cent of children with acute poststreptococcal glomerulonephritis. Proteinuria may persist in 60 per cent of patients for more than 1 year and in 36 per cent for 2 or more years (Jordon and Lemire, 1982). Exacerbations during the months following the illness are uncommon. If they do occur, they are usually preceded by an acute respiratory illness, are manifested primarily by hematuria, and resolve without specific treatment. However, the nurse should discuss with parents the importance of keeping follow-up appointments to ensure that any exacerbation requiring treatment is diagnosed before kidney injury occurs.

Major Nursing Diagnoses for Acute Poststreptococcal Glomerulonephritis

Fluid volume excess: intravascular, *related to decreased glomerular filtration rate associated with inflammatory changes in the glomerular membrane*
Potential for injury: renal failure, *related to glomerular inflammation*
Knowledge deficit, *related to*
- *measurement of blood pressure, weight, intake and output*
- *administration of prescribed medications*
- *identification of evidence of congestive heart failure, electrolyte imbalance, and renal failure*
- *expected course of the disease*

Strategies for Nursing Care

The nursing diagnoses direct the nursing goals: monitoring and reducing excess intravascular fluid volume, assessing for evidence of renal failure, and providing information and guidance needed to support home care. Strategies to meet these goals are discussed subsequently.

Monitoring Fluid Volume. The child hospitalized with acute glomerulonephritis will require careful monitoring of fluid balance. An accurate intake/output record will be needed, as well as daily weights and blood pressure measurement at least every 4 hours. The physician must be alerted to increasing oliguria, weight gain, or increasing hypertension.

The oliguric state (inadequate excretion) may predispose to electrolyte imbalances — most notably, hyperkalemia. The nurse can monitor for this complication by checking laboratory reports and by assessing for muscle weakness, bradycardia, hyper-reflexia, flaccid paralysis, malaise, nausea, shallow breathing, and intestinal colic and diarrhea (see also Chapter 30). Intravascular congestion may also lead to congestive heart failure. Careful assessment for classic signs and symptoms of this complication is an important nursing responsibility (see Table 39-7, Nursing Process Plan: The Child with Congestive Heart Failure).

Reducing Intravascular Volume. Nursing interventions can assist in reducing intravascular volume. Antihypertensives and diuretics may be ordered if hypertension becomes severe. Correct administration, patient and family teaching, and evaluation of the drugs' therapeutic effects are among nursing responsibilities. In addition, the nurse will be the one to explain and enforce fluid and dietary restrictions. The child and family will be more cooperative if they are aware of the reasons for the restrictions and are allowed to exercise as much control as possible within the prescribed guidelines. The nurse can help stimulate the child's already decreased appetite by working with the parents to plan a diet that appeals to the child, serving small portions, and encouraging family members to be there to eat with the child at meal times. Fluid restriction is less obvious to the child if liquids are served in small, rather than large, cups.

Assessing for Evidence of Renal Failure. Because renal failure is the major threat to the child with glomerulonephritis nursing assessment for this complication cannot be overemphasized. The section on acute renal failure later in this chapter provides a complete list of clinical manifestations.

Providing Information and Guidance Needed to Support Home Care. The nurse must be sensitive to what this illness means for the child and family. Facial edema and dark-colored urine can be frightening for the child. The nurse can help by listening to these and other concerns and by stressing the temporary nature of these bodily changes.

Kidney disease sounds frightening to parents and often is associated with the words "dialysis" and "kidney transplant." Parents will cope better with their child's illness if they are given information about acute glomerulonephritis and its treatment. Children can be told that their "kidneys are sick but will get better."

Long-Term Outcome

The expected outcome for children with acute glomerulonephritis is excellent. A few children, however, will develop chronic glomerular disease. Most experts believe that the severity of the initial illness correlates with the development of chronicity. Documentation of this belief is difficult because chronic glomerulonephritis develops through a variety of different disease processes. The disease may go undetected for years; therefore, it is seen primarily in adolescents and adults. The signs and symptoms of the illness reflect progressive renal failure as the glomeruli gradually become replaced with fibrous tissue. Treatment is predominantly symptomatic; hemodialysis or renal transplant may ultimately be needed.

Nursing Strategies for Follow-Up Care in the Home or Clinic

Obtain a urine specimen for urinalysis.

Measure blood pressure and weight and compare both with baseline measurements and with postdiagnosis measurements. Alert the physician to increasing hypertension or abnormal weight gain.

Determine whether the child is voiding in "usual" (i.e., adequate) amounts.

Encourage the child and parents to discuss their concerns about the disease process and about home therapy. Reinforce earlier teaching.

Hemolytic-Uremic Syndrome

Hemolytic-uremic syndrome is an acute disease characterized by renal failure, hemolytic anemia, and thrombocytopenia. The syndrome predominates in whites and affects males and females equally. In its most common form in North America, it will affect children under 5 years of age following an enteric illness (Fong et al, 1982). This disease predominates also in certain geographic areas in the world, including the western United States, Argentina, Southern Africa, and the Netherlands.

Etiology

The frequency of gastroenteritis as a predecessor has marshalled medical research to look for enteric pathogens related to hemolytic-uremic syndrome. Recent findings suggest that the majority of cases of idiopathic hemolytic-uremic syndrome are associated either with *Escherichia coli* or *S. dysenteriae* (Cleary, 1988). The specific type of *E. coli* implicated with this disease is spread by both person-to-person contact and by contaminated food (typically beef or unpasteurized milk). Familial factors are thought to be present in some cases.

Pathophysiology

In hemolytic-uremic syndrome, the glomeruli and arterioles are damaged. The actual process by which *E. coli* and *S. dysenteriae* produce the cell damage remains unknown. It is known, however, that this damage directly alters the endothelial barrier of the arterioles and leads to coagulation of fibrin strands in the capillary walls. As platelets and red blood cells pass through these abnormal capillary walls, they fragment and are damaged. The red blood cells become anisocytotic or helmet-shaped and eventually are trapped by the spleen. This reduction and damage to the red blood cells results in severe hemolytic anemia. Thrombocytopenia occurs from the platelet aggregation within the damaged vessels or from the damage occurring to the platelets as they pass through the capillary walls.

Clinical Manifestations

Hemolytic-uremic syndrome usually follows a gastroenteritis or viral illness within several days to 2 weeks. The onset of this disorder is acute, characterized by extreme pallor, lethargy, irritability, anorexia, bruising, and a decreased urine output. The child may have associated problems with hypertension, edema, mild jaundice, splenomegaly, seizures, and symptoms of circulatory congestion. The urine may remain amber or be brownish-red in color.

Diagnostic Assessment

The diagnosis of hemolytic-uremic syndrome is made by identifying the presence of hemolytic anemia, renal failure, and thrombocytopenia in the child. In order to confirm the diagnosis, numerous blood and urine tests are done. A complete blood count with differential and reticulocyte count will confirm the presence of anemia and hemolysis. Often, the hemoglobin will be 5 to 7 g/dl and there will be an elevated reticulocyte count. The platelet count will initially be normal but decreases during the first few days of the illness. Serum electrolytes, blood urea nitrogen, and creatinine values will be consistent with renal failure. Uric acid concentrates will be elevated. Urinalysis will reflect renal damage, manifested by hematuria, proteinuria, and the presence of urinary casts.

The role of the nurse during the diagnostic phase is to assist with the collection of specimens, ensure the child's comfort and safety, monitor the child's vital signs, and observe for alterations in skin integrity, neurologic status, and renal and cardiovascular functioning. The child will usually be catheterized so that the urine output may be carefully monitored. As each test or procedure is done, the parents and child should be informed about the purpose of the test and what is involved in carrying it out.

The physician will make the final diagnosis of hemolytic-uremic syndrome and communicate information to the parents about the course of the disease and expected medical interventions. The nurse should be available during this phase to provide added information about this disease to the family. Because hemolytic-uremic syndrome is relatively uncommon, yet serious, the family will require much information and support during the diagnostic phase of the illness.

Therapeutic Management

The acute phase of hemolytic-uremic syndrome usually lasts for 1 to 2 weeks with gradual improvement over 1 to 2 months. In more severe cases, the acute phase may lead to chronic renal failure or death. Drugs such as corticosteroids, anticoagulants, or antiplatelet agents have not been found to be effective and are not used in the treatment of hemolytic-uremic syndrome.

During the acute phase of the illness, therapeutic measures are aimed at alleviating complications associated with the anemia, thrombocytopenia, and renal failure. Peritoneal dialysis is often necessary to alleviate problems associated with renal failure.

If the child experiences a severe anemia, transfusion with fresh-washed, packed red blood cells may be necessary. If bleeding occurs secondary to the thrombocytopenia, the child may be transfused with platelets. If the child is acutely ill, a nutritional diet should be provided through nasogastric feedings or hyperalimentation.

Strategies for Nursing Care

The nurse generalist will seldom be involved in the initial care of the child with hemolytic-uremic syndrome. Specialized care is usually necessary and is often provided in an intensive care setting. Goals of nursing care will be similar to those detailed later in this chapter for acute renal failure.

The nurse may be responsible for administering blood transfusions, monitoring intravenous fluids, assessing for evidence of hypertension and pulmonary edema, monitoring hourly urine output, and monitoring for signs and symptoms of electrolyte imbalance and uremia. Nutritional support may be unusually challenging because of associated anorexia. If oral intake is not sufficient to prevent tissue catabolism, parenteral nutrition may be ordered. Neurologic involvement occurs in most cases (Novello, 1986) and requires careful nursing assessment and seizure precautions.

Long-Term Outcome

The expected outcome for the child with hemolytic-uremic syndrome is fairly good, with the majority of the patients surviving the acute phase. Approximately 15 per cent of the patients have adverse sequelae, including hypertension, proteinuria, and azotemia. Approximately 10 per cent of the children with hemolytic-uremic syndrome develop end-stage renal disease.

The Child with Renal Calculi

Urolithiasis (renal calculi) is an uncommon pediatric disorder among children in the United States. This condition, however, has been found to be endemic among children from low socioeconomic classes who live in Asia and is the most common pediatric urologic problem in that part of the world. Urolithiasis occurs more often in males and affects children with equal frequency between the ages of 1 and 15 years (Malek, 1985).

Etiology

The etiology of renal calculi is either *idiopathic* or *secondary* to disorders such as urinary tract infections, hypercalciuria, or a variety of metabolic disorders.

Idiopathic calculi are composed of calcium oxalate. Children with idiopathic calculi have a genetic predisposition. The symptomatology of calculi, however, usually will not occur until the child is between the ages of 10 and 15 years.

Secondary calculi may form in children with frequent urinary tract infections as a result of urease, which is produced by bacteria. Urease converts urea to ammonia; this increases the alkalinity of the urine, favoring the formation of calculi. These calculi are mostly composed of magnesium ammonium phosphate. They usually form in the upper collecting system and may be associated with congenital structural anomalies.

Calculi resulting from hypercalciuria are created by an increased deposit of calcium in the kidneys. Hypercalciuria is a disorder that results from several conditions, including hyperparathyroidism, uncontrolled renal tubular acidosis, Cushing's syndrome, neoplasms, and prolonged immobilization.

Metabolic abnormalities may cause renal calculi and account for 10 per cent of urolithiasis in children.

The main symptoms of urolithiasis include colicky flank or abdominal pain, hematuria, and sepsis. Spontaneous passage of the stone may occur without previous symptomatology. Less commonly, patients with renal calculi may exhibit enuresis, polydipsia, and urethral obstruction. If an underlying disease or infection exists, symptoms of this disorder may also be present.

Diagnostic Assessment

During the acute phase, the nursing assessment should include a family history; the child's medical history; an assessment of the child's growth and development; a diet history, including the use of vitamins; and an assessment of exposure to medical or surgical procedures. This information will help determine if a predisposition to renal calculi exists.

The nurse will need to assist with several urine and blood tests, including a urinalysis and a urine culture. The urine may indicate the presence of infection. The serum calcium, phosphorus, alkaline phosphatase, and uric acid levels may be elevated in children who have renal calculi. The child may undergo a CT scan or intravenous pyelogram to evaluate the location and presence of stones.

Therapeutic Management

Surgical intervention during the acute phase of urolithiasis is usually unnecessary, unless emergency conditions such as complete obstruction or hemorrhage exist. As mentioned, some renal calculi will pass spontaneously. If this does not occur, the acute phase will be managed supportively. The decision to intervene surgically in the event of renal calculi will be made on an individual basis and will be determined by the size and location of the calculi.

Strategies for Nursing Care

The primary goals for nursing care are to (1) dilute the urine, (2) administer analgesics for colicky pain, (3) monitor urine output for passage of the stone, and (4) provide information and guidance to support home management. A high intake of dilute fluids is almost always recommended, to ensure a reduction in the concentration of crystalloids. The nurse will be responsible for maintaining specific gravity of the urine within the prescribed limits (usually under 1.005). In order to prevent increased specific gravity of urine during the night it may be necessary to give large amounts of fluid at bedtime and to awaken the child in the night to give additional fluids. Parents may need support to abandon temporarily attempts to toilet train the child during this period.

Adults who have experienced renal colic will attest to the excruciating pain that may be associated with the body's attempt to pass a renal stone. The nurse is responsible for pain assessment and for providing optimal comfort through pharmacologic and other supportive means. (See Table 29-4, Nursing Process Plan: The Child in Pain.)

Urine must be strained in order to determine when the stone is passed. This can be accomplished by stretching a piece of fine mesh gauze over the urine collection bottle before it is emptied. Signs should be prominently posted in the child's hospital room and bathroom to prevent a well-meaning visitor from emptying urine that has not been strained.

If the cause of the stone can be determined treatment may include medications to reduce the particular crystals that caused the problem. Parents will need to be advised of appropriate medication techniques and of potential side effects. Prevention of recurrence will almost always involve a continued high fluid intake.

The Child with Acute Renal Failure

Acute renal failure (ARF) is an abrupt deterioration or cessation of renal function. The onset of ARF is characterized by oliguria (a decrease in urine output) or anuria (no urine output over 24 hours); electrolyte and acid-base disturbances; and impaired excretion of substances such as urea, creatinine, and phosphate. ARF develops in response to a variety of conditions and is classified according to the mechanism that causes the disturbance in renal function: prerenal; intrinsic renal; or postrenal. (See Box 42-5.)

Pathophysiology

Prerenal Failure. In prerenal ARF an impairment of renal perfusion (a marked decrease in blood flow to the kidneys) occurs, leading to decreased glomerular filtration and increased proximal tubular absorption. The urine sodium concentration remains low, while the urine osmolality, urea, and creatinine concentrations are high. Acute prerenal ARF is often readily reversible when the cause of the renal hypoperfusion is corrected.

Intrinsic Renal Failure. The second type of ARF is intrinsic renal failure. The renal cortex and medulla are the principal sites damaged in intrinsic ARF, resulting in an oliguric or anuric state.

Postrenal Failure. Postrenal ARF, a relatively rare condition in children, results from obstruction of urine flow at a point within the pelvicalyceal collecting system or in the ureters. Renal calculi, a tumor, or a congenital malformation may cause this obstruction.

Clinical Manifestations

The clinical manifestations of ARF may be overshadowed by the precipitating disorder; therefore, the cli-

Box 42-5
Major Causes of Renal Failure in Children

PRERENAL FAILURE

Hypovolemia and hypotension caused by:
- Dehydration
  - Vomiting
  - Diarrhea
  - Febrile illness
  - Massive reduction in colloid oncotic pressure (protein-losing enteropathy, nephrotic syndrome)
  - Septic shock
  - Congestive heart failure
  - Hemorrhage
  - Hyponatremia

INTRINSIC RENAL FAILURE

Acute tubular necrosis
- Prolonged secondary hypotension
  - Vomiting
  - Diarrhea
  - Shock
  - Nephrotoxins
  - Organ perfusion
- Glomerulonephritis
  - Primary
  - Secondary

Interstitial nephritis
- Primary
- Secondary
  - Drugs
  - Toxins

Vascular
- Venous thrombosis
- Cortical necrosis
- Disseminated intravascular coagulation

Pigmenturia (myoglobinuria, hemoglobinuria)

POSTRENAL OBSTRUCTION

Urethral obstruction
- Stricture
- Posterior urethral valves
- Diverticulum

Ureterocele

Solitary renal unit with ureterovesical or ureteropelvic juncture obstruction

Extrinsic tumors compressing bladder outlet

Intrinsic urinary tract tumors

Neurogenic bladder

(From Osofsky and Lewy, 1985.)

nician must be astute to recognize the symptoms of ARF. *The principal manifestation of ARF is oliguria or anuria.* Other common symptoms include edema, drowsiness, tachypnea, and laboratory abnormalities. The urine may contain red blood cells, protein, casts, and tubular cells. The urine sodium may be low or elevated, depending on the type of ARF. Blood abnormalities that are the hallmark of ARF include an elevated BUN, creatinine, and uric acid concentration.

Diagnostic Assessment

The condition causing ARF must be determined immediately because the treatment for prerenal, intrinsic, and postrenal failure will vary according to the precipitating problem. The nursing role during the diagnostic phase involves history taking, monitoring the child's vital signs, recording intake and output, obtaining needed laboratory tests, and assisting in diagnostic procedures. Throughout this phase, the child and family will need emotional support and information pertaining to the multiple tests and procedures.

In order to determine the cause of ARF the following interventions are needed: a complete history; a thorough physical examination, including weight, blood pressure, and evaluation of hydration; placement of a Foley catheter to obtain the urine volume, a urinalysis, a urine culture, osmolality, and pH; blood studies, including BUN, creatinine, uric acid concentration, electrolytes, phosphorus, calcium, bicarbonate, complete blood count, and platelet count; and an ECG to evaluate any dysrhythmias. Ultrasonography may be used to assess for the presence of obstruction. Radiographs of the chest and abdomen may be indicated to determine the presence of congestive heart failure, pulmonary edema, or renal calculi.

Therapeutic Management

If intrinsic ARF is suspected, the immediate approach will be to infuse a bolus of normal saline intravenously over 1 hour. If the child responds to this intervention with an increased urinary output, then hypoperfusion of the kidney, or intrinsic ARF, is the likely diagnosis. This therapy is not attempted if the child manifests symptoms of fluid overload, such as congestive heart failure.

ARF can be reversed or may lead to chronic renal failure or death. Prompt and aggressive treatment of ARF and the underlying disorder will minimize mortality. The three major goals of treatment of ARF are to correct the cause of ARF, to manage the complications of renal failure, and to support the child until the tubular epithelial cells regenerate and normal renal function returns.

Reversible ARF progresses through three phases:

oliguric; early diuretic; and late diuretic. The *oliguric phase* may last from 7 to 21 days. During this phase, BUN levels will be elevated and oliguria will be present. The child will require intensive nursing care and may require dialysis at this time. Dialysis is described later in this chapter.

The second phase, *early diuresis,* may last up to several weeks. During this phase, the urine volume may be high and the BUN level ceases to rise.

The *late diuretic phase* may last from several months to 1 year. During this stage, the BUN level and urine output begin to return to normal. The tubular epithelium begins to regenerate and normal renal function will return.

Major Nursing Diagnoses for Acute Renal Failure

Potential altered fluid volume: excess, *related to oliguria/anuria associated with*
- *decreased renal perfusion*
- *damage to renal tissue*
- *obstruction of urine flow*

Potential for injury: metabolic imbalance, *related to*
- *electrolyte and hydrogen ion imbalance associated with impaired excretion or intravascular dilution*
- *elevation of urea and creatinine associated with decreased excretion*

Potential impaired gas exchange, *related to anemia associated with*
- *decreased production of erythropoietin by the diseased kidney*
- *hemolysis*

Potential for infection, *related to altered immune responses associated with serious illness*

Fear/anxiety: child and family, *related to the serious nature of ARF*

Strategies for Nursing Care

Although the initial care of the child with ARF will usually take place in a specialty unit, the nurse generalist will often be involved with care of the child before hospital discharge. The nursing diagnoses and goals of care are directed by the fact that ARF renders the kidneys unable to maintain their usual functions of excreting nitrogenous wastes and maintaining fluid, electrolyte, and acid-base balance. Both medical treatment and nursing care are focused, then, on assisting the body to maintain these functions until the kidneys recover.

Monitoring Urine Output. Since decreased urine output is the hallmark of ARF, knowledge of hourly urine output (and hourly fluid intake) is essential for many medical and nursing decisions. A special collection system will be attached to the catheter when hourly output is to be recorded. The catheter will drain into a small, graduated plastic chamber. After the hour's output is recorded the contents of the chamber can be released into an attached, larger collection bag. Some systems include ports through which a sterile needle may be inserted to collect a urine specimen for analysis.

Weight may be recorded as often as every 12 hours to help determine fluid balance. Because of the critical nature of these measurements, it is essential that all extraneous variables (scales, clothing, relation to meals) be held constant so that any differences in measures reflect actual changes in fluid balance.

Monitoring and Reducing Complications of Fluid Excess. Complications of excess intravascular fluid include hypertension, edema, and pulmonary edema. *Hypertension* is usually the direct result of sodium and water retention. Nursing responsibilities include judgments related to frequency and techniques of blood pressure measurement. In order to ensure the most accurate measurement, the blood pressure should always be taken with the child in the same position (to avoid alterations related to position change), in as restful a state as possible (to avoid temporary increases in systolic pressure), and with the same equipment (to avoid alterations associated with cuff size and manometer settings). Strategies to reduce the risk of hypertension (and other complications of fluid overload) include careful regulation of intravenous fluids. See Table 27-7, Nursing Process Plan: Perioperative Care, for detailed strategies related to monitoring of intravenous fluids.

Edema may result from vascular overload. It may present as periorbital, pretibial, or pedal edema; ascites; or pleural or pericardial effusion. Nursing assessment for edema should be reflected in the chart. If edema is present particular care will be needed to prevent skin breakdown.

Pulmonary edema, a very serious complication, results when vascular fluid backs up in the lungs because the heart is unable to deal with the increased vascular load. Pulmonary edema presents with tachypnea, tachycardia, rales (crackles), rhonchi (wheezes), and increased respiratory secretions. Expert nursing assessment is essential to aid in early diagnosis and treatment.

Monitoring and Reducing Metabolic Imbalances. Metabolic imbalances include electrolyte disturbances, metabolic acidosis, and azotemia. The most common electrolyte disturbances in acute renal failure are hyperkalemia (resulting from decreased renal excretion and release of potassium by injured tissues), hyponatremia (resulting from dilution of body fluids), hyperphosphatemia (related to reduced renal excretion), and hypocalcemia (which occurs in response to hyperphosphatemia). The nurse must be alert for physical evidence of electrolyte imbalance (see Chapter 30 for clinical manifestations). Serum electrolytes will be measured frequently in renal failure. Because the nurse may often be the first to see the laboratory report, it is important that he or she be able to evaluate the findings and alert the physician appropriately.

Hyperkalemia is a life-threatening imbalance because potassium levels that approach 6 mEq/l cause cardiac conduction abnormalities (Schact, 1985). The child with renal failure should have a cardiorespiratory monitor to aid in detection of cardiac dysrhythmias. Kayexalate, a cation-exchange resin, may be given orally or by enema to reduce serum potassium levels.

Dietary potassium will usually be restricted. Restrictions in diet commonly include sodium as well, in order to prevent the sodium from drawing additional fluid into the vascular compartment. Table 42-7 lists common foods that are high in sodium and potassium and can guide the nurse in monitoring the child's diet.

Metabolic acidosis may result from decreased renal excretion of nonvolatile hydrogen ions and from catabolism of body protein. Kussmaul respirations are a common sign of this disorder (see Chapter 30 for additional manifestations). Sodium bicarbonate or sodium lactate may be given orally or intravenously to control the acidosis.

Azotemia denotes accumulation of nitrogenous wastes in the blood. It is reflected by BUN levels greater than 20 mg/dl and elevated creatinine levels. As noted in Table 42-3, glomerular filtration rate must be decreased by at least 50 per cent before creatinine level is affected. If the child is not oliguric fluid therapy will be ordered to optimize urinary output and thereby reduce serum accumulation of nitrogenous wastes.

Urea also rises in response to catabolism and is reflected in an increased BUN. The goal of dietary management will be to meet the child's metabolic demands for calories, usually 40 to 60 cal/kg/day (Schact, 1985). Failure to do so will cause catabolism of body protein and a resultant rise in BUN. Protein intake will be restricted to 0.5 to 1 g/kg/day and will be chosen on the basis of essential amino acids to reduce the nitrogenous wastes from nonessential protein catabolism (Schact, 1985). A diet high in carbohydrates will further reduce the body's burning of endogenous protein.

Reducing Metabolic Demands for Oxygen. Anemia may occur as a complication of acute renal failure because of decreased production of erythropoietin by the diseased kidney and through hemolysis. Hemoglobin and hematocrit values must be closely monitored. Blood transfusions will usually be contraindicated for all but the most extreme cases of anemia because of the danger of circulatory overload. Nursing strategies are therefore essential to help the

Table 42-7. Foods High in Sodium and/or Potassium

Food Source	Sodium (mg)	Potassium (mg)
Fruits		
Apricots, dried, 17 lg halves	26	*979**
Banana, raw 1 med	2	*550*
Dates, domestic, 10 med, pitted	1	*648*
Watermelon, 1 slice 6 × 1½ in	6	*600*
Meats		
Beef, ground chuck, 3½ oz	60	*370*
Beef, dried, chipped, 3 oz	*3660*	170
Chicken, light meat, fried, 3½ oz	68	*434*
Ham, 1 slice, 60 g	*518*	239
Hot dog, 1 avg	*542*	108
Lamb, loin chop, 3½ oz	49	*466*
Liver, calf, fried, 3½ oz	118	*453*
Pork chop, loin 1 chop, 68 g	41	*386*
Salami, dry, 1 oz slice	*540*	102
Turkey, light meat 3½ oz	82	*411*
Vegetables		
Artichoke, raw, 1 lg bud	86	*860*
Asparagus, frozen, in butter sauce, 1 cup	*747*	270
Avocado, ½	10	*574*
Beans, canned with pork and tomato, ½ cup	*579*	263
Beans, frijoles, 1 serving	*1102*	*693*
Beans, green, canned ½ cup	*565*	227
Spinach, raw, 3½ oz	159	*795*
Potato, white, baked without skin, 3¼ in diameter	6	*755*
Potato, dehydrated flakes 3½ oz	80	*1600*
Potato chips, 3½ oz	*1130*	197
Seaweed, kelp, raw 3½ oz	*3007*	*5273*
Squash, winter, baked, ½ cup	1	*461*
Squash, acorn ½ baked squash	2	*749*
Tomato, canned, 1 cup	*1000*	*1060*

Table 42-7 *(continued)*

Food Source	Sodium (mg)	Potassium (mg)
Miscellaneous		
Hershey bar	24	*456*
Meat tenderizer, 1 tsp	*1745*	Trace
Meat tenderizer, low-sodium, 1 tsp	1	*2392*
Milk, whole, 1 cup	120	*370*
Peanuts, roasted, salted, 3½ oz	*460*	*700*

* The values in italics represent the high electrolyte content for that food source.

(Extracted from Pennington and Church, 1980.)

child's body cope with the reduced capacity to supply oxygen for metabolic demands. Table 40-5, Nursing Process Plan: The Child with Anemia, details these strategies.

Reducing the Risk of Infection. As discussed in Chapter 43, page 1532, significant physical and psychologic stress can alter immune processes. In addition, immune function may be impaired by the disease that caused ARF, such as glomerulonephritis. Add to this increased risk of infection the probability for invasive diagnostic and therapeutic procedures, and *potential for infection* becomes an important nursing diagnosis.

The strategies involved with reducing the risk for infection may seem repetitious and mundane until one considers that infection is a major cause of death in acute renal failure. *The nurse's responsibility for reducing the risk of infection is critical to a favorable outcome for the child.* The importance of handwashing before each contact with the child cannot be overemphasized. Instruct family members about proper handwashing. Posting signs can be helpful and is often less threatening than a verbal reminder. Health care professionals who know they have an infectious condition should refrain from caring for children with ARF.

Urinary and central venous catheters are potential avenues for pathogens. These will be removed as quickly as possible, but while in place aseptic technique and assessment for signs of infection are imperative. Intermittent straight catheterization may sometimes be used instead of an indwelling Foley catheter. Cultures should be obtained from suspected infection sites.

Policies governing care for central venous catheters are set by each institution. However, it is interesting to note that in a recent review of studies related to central venous catheter infections, Decker and Edwards (1988) concluded that iodophor ointment, applied to the insertion site with sterile technique, is the topical agent of choice to reduce infection. Further, they recommend that the cannula be secured at the insertion site to reduce movement and irritation, and that dressing changes be done every 72 hours. Central venous catheters require less meticulous care once the granulation tissue forms around the cannula at the insertion site and reduces risk of pathogen entry. Catheters are often at this stage when families are responsible for the care at home.

Antibiotics are rarely used prophylactically and those prescribed for infection should be the least nephrotoxic. When administering any medication to the child with renal failure, particularly if the child is oliguric, the nurse must be aware of the drug's mechanism for elimination from the body. Pharmacologic agents and their metabolites that rely upon glomerular filtration for excretion (e.g., digitalis) will be retained by the body. The physician may alter the dose or time interval between doses to offset some of these effects. The nurse, who is in constant attendance, can provide valuable assessments for evaluating the child's response to medications.

Supporting the Child and Family. The child with ARF is seriously ill and requires multiple tests and procedures. Throughout all phases of the disease, the child and family will require emotional support to deal with this crisis. Because the course of ARF covers several months, the child and family will require repeated information and reassurance about the child's progress. Table 31-2 provides detailed strategies for guidance and support of the hospitalized child and the family.

Care During the Diuretic Phase. Careful management of fluid and electrolyte balance will extend through the diuretic phase of ARF. If the glomerular filtration rate improves faster than function of the tubules a fluid balance deficit may result. Nursing assessment of intake and output, urine specific gravity, and evidence of dehydration are important in this phase of recovery from ARF. Medication dosages will be adjusted in accordance with increased glomerular filtration.

Nursing Strategies for Follow-Up Care in the Home or Clinic

Obtain blood and urine samples for analysis as appropriate.

Weigh the child and compare with weight upon hospital discharge. Altert the physician to abnormal weight gain that may signal fluid retention.

Ask the child and parents about voiding patterns, i.e., number of wet diapers per day, approximate number of voidings (if toilet trained), and whether voided amounts seem normal.

Assess appropriately for evidence of remission of

the original cause of the acute renal failure (e.g., glomerulonephritis, urolithiasis).

Assess for signs and symptoms of infection (secondary to altered immune responses in ARF).

Reinforce teaching to prevent further renal disease (related specifically to the cause of ARF and the child's history).

The Child with Chronic Renal Failure

In chronic renal failure (CRF) a reduction in renal function occurs over time in response to *irreversible* damage to the nephrons. This alteration in renal function decreases the glomerular filtration rate (GFR) and causes metabolic, biochemical, and clinical disturbances. However, the onset of CRF is insidious, and the symptoms are often present only after severe damage to the kidneys has occurred.

Etiology

CRF is caused by several conditions. Glomerular diseases are responsible for 40 per cent of the cases of CRF, and developmental abnormalities of the kidneys and urinary tract with or without obstruction comprise 20 per cent of the cases. Hereditary renal diseases and pyelonephritis with reflux nephropathy constitute 15 per cent each, and miscellaneous disorders make up 10 per cent of the cases of CRF.

Conditions that are highly associated with CRF vary with age. Children up to age 5 years with congenital anomalies of the kidney or urinary tract (particularly renal hypoplasia and severe bilateral vesicoureteral reflux) make up the greatest number of children with CRF. During the school-age and adolescent years, glomerulonephritis is responsible for the majority of the cases of CRF.

Clinical Manifestations

The signs and symptoms of CRF are vague and nonspecific in the early stages and progress to affect every body system in the final stages of the disease. CRF progresses in three stages: decreased renal reserve, renal insufficiency, and end-stage renal disease (ESRD). During the decreased renal reserve stage, the child is asymptomatic and BUN and serum creatinine levels are normal. In renal insufficiency, more than 75 per cent of the nephrons have been destroyed and the GFR is approximately 25 per cent of normal. The BUN and serum creatinine levels begin to rise and nocturia or polyuria may occur.

In ESRD, or uremia, 90 per cent of the nephrons are destroyed and the GFR is 10 per cent of normal or less. The serum creatinine and BUN levels rise sharply and the child becomes oliguric. The kidneys cease to function effectively and dialysis or kidney transplant must be considered.

Most children with CRF do not come to the attention of the health care personnel during the decreased renal reserve stage but are diagnosed after the damage to the kidney is quite severe. They may have vague complaints of anorexia, polyuria, easy fatigability, and poor growth that go unnoticed. Often, the renal failure is detected only when the child manifests symptoms of edema, symptomatic hypertension, or gross hematuria, or develops a urinary tract infection.

During the renal insufficiency phase, the child may have nocturia, bone or joint pain, growth retardation, skin dryness or itchiness (uremic frost), muscle cramps, and signs of motor or sensory neuropathy. Physical findings include a pale or sallow complexion, growth retardation with bony deformities (osteodystrophy), diastolic and systolic hypertension, uremic breath (uremic fetor), and signs of neuropathy and retinopathy. Signs of circulatory overload may be present, manifested by tachycardia, tachypnea, cardiomegaly, and a systolic ejection murmur.

In the later stages of the disease, the child may have vomiting, bloody diarrhea, confusion, edema, bruising, headache, seizures, and a decreasing urine output. Symptoms of cardiac failure may be present.

The electrolyte, metabolic, and chemical manifestations of CRF are quite complex and are described in Table 42-8.

Diagnostic Assessment

The diagnostic criteria used in acute renal failure can be applied to the evaluation of a child with CRF (see section on ARF earlier in this chapter).

Therapeutic Management

The treatment of CRF demands an understanding of the complex physiologic disturbances that occur and an appreciation of the impact this disease process has on the child and family. CRF affects all aspects of a child's life and impedes the child's activity level, school participation, and peer and family relationships. The child faces dietary and activity restrictions and experiences altered elimination patterns. Children with CRF may have varying degrees of growth retardation that can affect the development of body image and self-esteem. The child's daily routine includes medications, multiple visits to the hospital or physician, invasive procedures, and often dialysis.

The family members also face multiple stressors. The financial burden of multiple tests, hospitalizations, and perhaps dialysis can be overwhelming. Knowing that the child has a life-threatening illness creates anxiety and may cause conflict among family relationships.

Table 42-8. Clinical Manifestations of Chronic Renal Failure

Clinical Manifestation	Pathophysiology	Symptoms	Nursing Strategies
Sodium and Water Retention	Renal insufficiency prevents sodium excretion and leads to retention of sodium and water	Edema, hypertension	Restriction of sodium and water intake Administer diuretics as directed Monitor weight Monitor vital signs frequently Monitor electrolyte values
Cardiac Irregularities from Hyperkalemia	Renal insufficiency causes decreased renal excretion of potassium. Acidosis and catabolism also increase extracellular potassium	Arrhythmias, high serum potassium levels	Provide adequate caloric intake Provide low-potassium diet Monitor vital signs Monitor electrolyte values Administer Kayexalate as directed Monitor ECG, observe for prolonged P-R intervals and peaked T waves
Metabolic Acidosis	Occurs in response to reduced hydrogen in excretion	Respiratory symptoms (tachypnea)	Monitor respiratory status Administer bicarbonate as directed
Glucose Intolerance	Plasma insulin levels are elevated which cause an inhibition of cellular glucose uptake (Lemire and Fine, 1985)	Hyperglycemia, abnormal glucose tolerance test	Monitor urine and blood glucose levels
Dehydration or Fluid Overload	The renal diluting and concentrating mechanism is frequently absent	Dehydration or pulmonary edema	Administration and careful monitoring of intravenous or oral fluids as ordered Insert Foley catheter or accurately monitor urine output
Anemia	Reduction of red blood cell production from a lack of renal erythropoietin. Sequestration of red blood cells by spleen may contribute to anemia	Pallor, fatigue, low hemoglobin and hematocrit	Provide diet high in iron and folic acid Administer supplementary iron as ordered Administer red blood cells as ordered
Hypertension	Salt and water retention causes hypovolemia which increases blood pressure. Overproduction of renin by kidney may also cause hypertension	Increased blood pressure, headaches, dizziness, flushing	Monitor vital signs including blood pressure Provide low-sodium diet Restrict fluids as directed Monitor output Administer hypertensives as ordered
Cardiac Dysfunction	Hypervolemia and hypertension may cause congestive heart failure. Pericardial effusion may be associated with severe uremia	Tachycardia, gallop heart rhythm, poor peripheral perfusion, dyspnea, tachypnea, hepatomegaly, edema	Restriction of sodium and fluid intake Monitor vital signs and cardiac function Transfuse packed red blood cells as ordered Administer diuretics and digoxin as prescribed
Hypocalcemia and Hyperphosphatemia (Renal Osteodystrophy)	The diseased kidney produces a decreased amount of vitamin D resulting in decreased calcium absorption. Reduced GFR and excretion of inorganic phosphates cause elevated plasma phosphate	Growth arrest or retardation, osteomalacia, valgus deformities of lower extremities	Administration of phosphate binders, vitamin D, and calcium supplements Reduction of protein and milk
Growth Retardation	Etiology unknown. Factors affecting growth include age of onset of renal disease, etiology of primary disease, acidosis and presence of renal osteodystrophy	Retardation of height, bone growth	Monitor child's height, weight, and growth velocity and plot on growth chart Provide child with nutritional caloric intake Supportive measures around body image

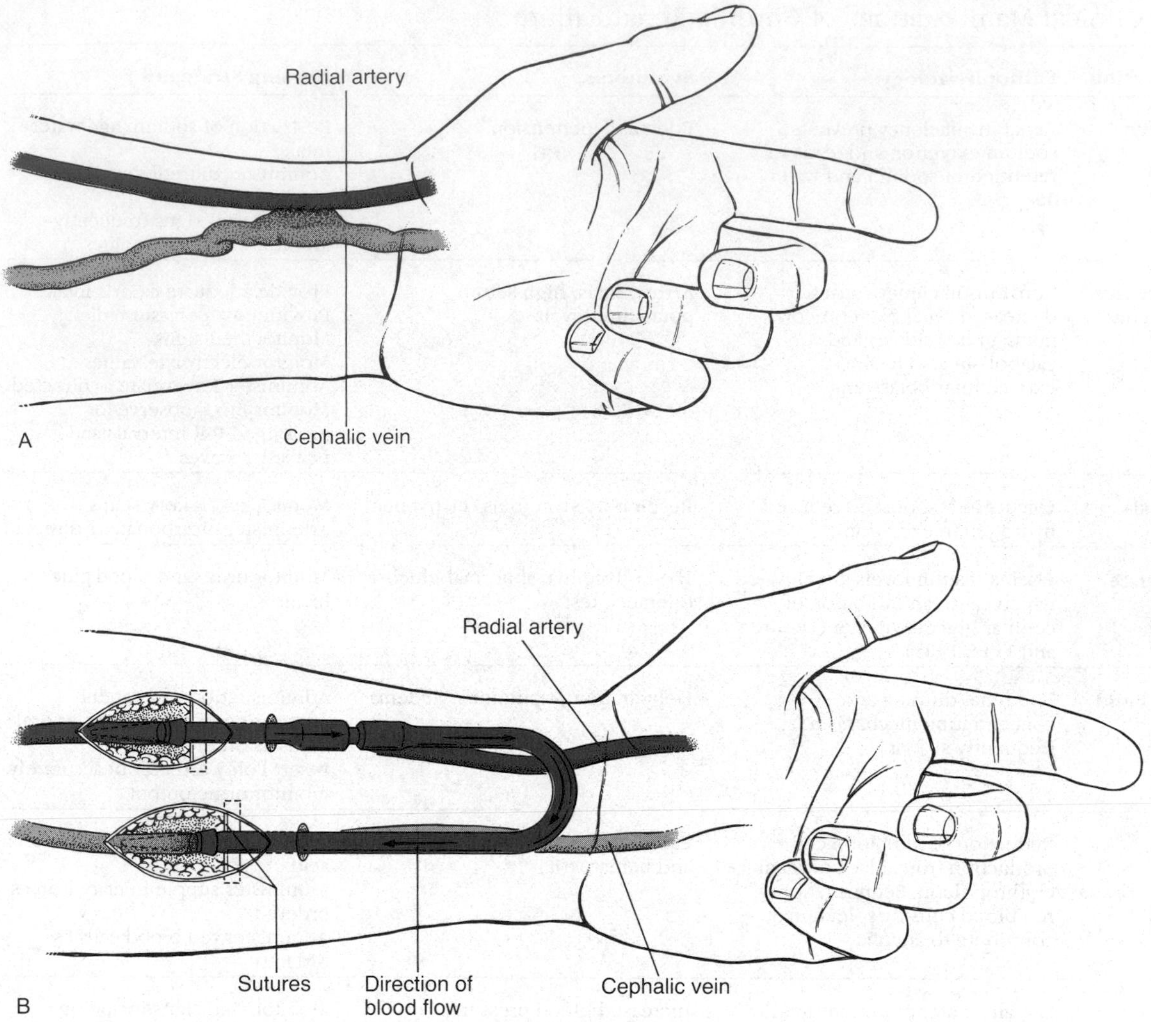

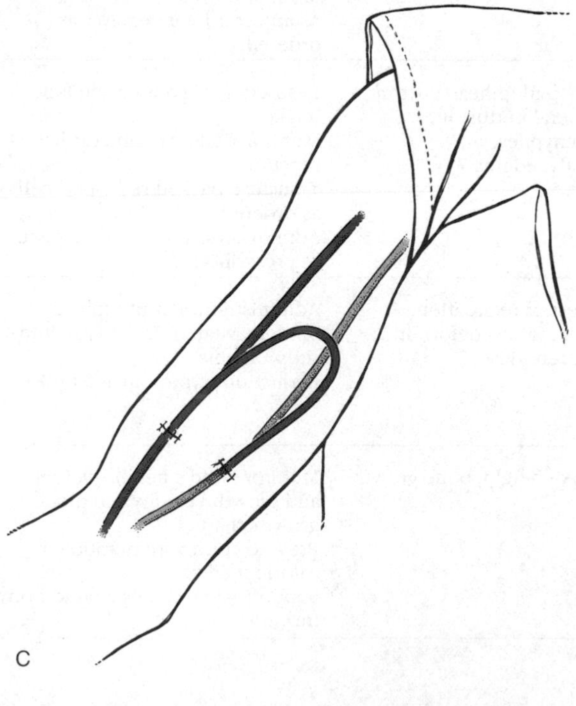

***Figure* 42-11.** *A*, Arteriovenous fistula. *B*, External arteriovenous shunt. *C*, Subcutaneous vascular prosthesis, synthetic graft. Although blood vessels are colored gray and red here for illustrative purposes, there is, of course, significant mixing of unoxygenated and oxygenated blood proximal to the fistula, shunt, or graft.

Many children with acute or chronic renal failure may be treated with drug, dietetic, and supportive therapy to combat the metabolic and chemical imbalances of renal failure. However, when conservative management becomes ineffective in permitting the child to function normally in his or her environment or in preventing the symptoms of uremia, then dialysis or kidney transplant, or both, should be considered. End-stage renal disease requiring dialysis or transplantation develops in 2 to 3.5 children per million population per year.

Dialysis

The decision to institute dialysis will be made by the child and family in collaboration with the health care team. All dialytic options as well as transplantation should be evaluated. The long-term problems that are associated with dialysis in children should be considered in making a decision about treatment. These problems include the impact on the child's social and emotional development, growth retardation, and technical difficulties in obtaining access sites because of the child's smaller size.

Indications for Dialysis

The decision to institute dialysis should be made prior to the need for it so that the necessary surgical procedure can be performed while the child is in an optimum clinical state. Fine (1985) has described six absolute indications for initiating chronic dialysis: uncontrollable hypertension, congestive heart failure, pericarditis, peripheral neuropathy, renal osteodystrophy, and bone marrow depression. The options for dialysis include hemodialysis, intermittent peritoneal dialysis, continuous ambulatory peritoneal dialysis, and continuous cycling peritoneal dialysis. These may be conducted in a treatment center or at home.

Hemodialysis

Hemodialysis relies upon the passage of the child's blood through a shunt or fistula to an artificial semipermeable membrane (dialyzer), which allows the removal of solute and water by diffusive and convective transport. The child's blood must circulate at a high rate in order for the solute to clear. When embarking on hemodialysis for a child, special consideration should be given to obtaining vascular access and the child's compliance with the prescribed therapeutic regimen.

Hemodialysis requires permanent access to the child's bloodstream, which is accomplished by the creation of a shunt, a fistula, or a vascular prosthesis. Three vascular connections are considered: the arteriovenous fistula (anastomosis usually between the radial artery and the cephalic vein), the arteriovenous shunt (an external plastic tube connecting an artery to a vein), and the subcutaneous vascular prosthesis or synthetic graft that connects the artery and vein (Fig. 42-11). If immediate access is needed dialysis can be performed through a central venous catheter that is especially designed for that purpose (Fig. 42-12). However, central venous access is only a temporary solution for vascular access.

When a vascular connection is made between an artery and vein, a saphenous vein autograft, a bovine arterial heterograft, or a synthetic pediatric cannula is used to create the fistula or shunt. These connections are thicker and tougher than normal vascular walls and withstand the frequent needle insertions necessary in hemodialysis.

Once vascular access is established, the child will undergo hemodialysis approximately three times per week for 3 to 5 hours per dialysis. During this time, the child must be attached to the dialyzer and closely monitored. Hemodialysis may be performed at home or in a hospital center as long as qualified people are present to monitor the child during the procedure. A

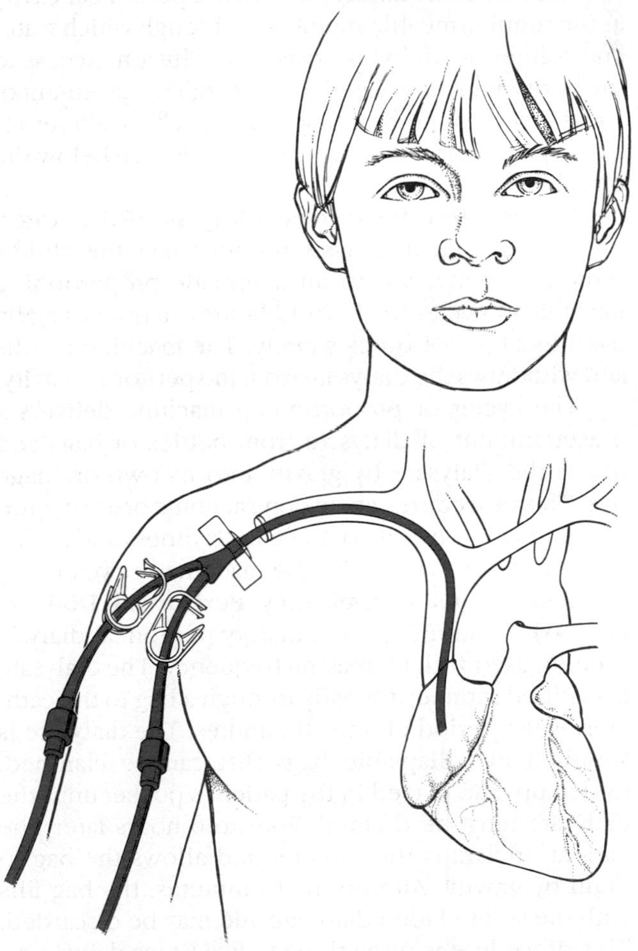

Figure 42-12. Central venous catheter for dialysis access.

text on hemodialysis can supply additional information about this procedure.

Dietary restrictions must be quite severe in children receiving hemodialysis in order to prevent metabolic imbalances, hypertension, or episodes of congestive heart failure. The child should adhere to a fluid intake of 400 ml/m² per day plus urinary output restriction. The child's diet should be low in sodium, potassium, protein, and phosphorus. Adherence to these restrictions will be quite difficult for the child because many "favorite" foods must be limited (e.g., soda, chocolate) (see also Table 42-7).

The child and family will require much counseling, support, and guidance concerning hemodialysis. The need for repetitive needle insertions and the strict diet may create anxiety in the child and family. The dialysis sessions are lengthy and require that the child remain somewhat immobile during the procedure. This may cause the child to be socially isolated and limit educational opportunities.

Peritoneal Dialysis

Peritoneal dialysis is used to treat children with acute and chronic renal failure. It uses the peritoneal cavity as the semipermeable membrane through which water and solutes move by osmosis and diffusion. Access to the peritoneum is created by the surgical placement of a catheter into the peritoneal cavity. This catheter remains permanently in place in the abdomen below the umbilicus.

Intermittent Peritoneal Dialysis (IPD). Intermittent peritoneal dialysis requires that the child's catheter be attached to an automatic proportioning machine or cycler for 10 to 12 hours at a time (usually overnight) 3 to 4 times weekly. The machine instills and withdraws the dialysate from the peritoneal cavity.

The cycler or proportioning machine delivers a preset amount of dialysate from bottles or bags and drains the dialysate by gravity into its own drainage bag. This procedure can be done at home or at a center, depending on severity of the child's illness and ability of the family to work with the machine or cycler.

Continuous Ambulatory Peritoneal Dialysis (CAPD). Continuous ambulatory peritoneal dialysis is being used with increasing frequency. The dialysate is instilled intraperitoneally through a bag to the catheter over a period of 5 to 10 minutes. The dialysate is supplied in collapsible bags that can be clamped, folded up, and placed in the patient's pocket until the dialysate must be drained. Four to 6 hours later, the patient unclamps the catheter and allows the bag to drain by gravity. After 10 to 15 minutes, the bag fills with the solute-laden dialysate and may be discarded. This procedure is done three to five times daily.

CAPD is often preferred in children for several reasons. It provides a more continuous control of uremia and salt and water balance. This permits the child's diet to be more liberal and gives the child "machine-free" mobility. Because of the simplicity of the procedure, the child and family may be able to perform the procedure outside the hospital. The child can participate in more activities at school and with his or her peers.

Continuous Cycling Peritoneal Dialysis (CCPD). Continuous cycling peritoneal dialysis combines the techniques of IPD and CAPD. A cycler is used for dialysis every night and a small amount of solution is left in the abdomen during the day. This solution is then drawn off in the first cycle when the machine is reattached (Binkley, 1984).

The complications of peritoneal dialysis include recurrent peritonitis secondary to faulty sterile technique, obstruction of the catheters, or metabolic consequences of glucose absorption from the dialysate. Over time, the efficiency of the peritoneum to act as a dialyzer may diminish. Chronic dialysis therapy has resulted in only variable improvement in growth in children. The primary cause for growth retardation among these children is unknown but continues to affect children receiving dialysis.

Renal Transplantation

Renal transplantation is considered to be the optimal choice of treatment for children with end-stage renal disease, particularly with respect to restoration of the child's growth and rehabilitation. With renal transplant, the child may attain normal or near normal renal function. The problems associated with long-term dialysis (chronic uremia, frequent invasive procedures, restricted diet) are avoided and the child is able to lead a relatively healthy life.

Criteria

The selected criteria used for performing renal transplants in children are quite liberal but vary with institutional policies. In general, children are excluded from renal transplant if they have severe mental retardation, psychoemotional problems, or active malignancy (Fine and Ehrlich, 1985). The presence of a lower urinary tract abnormality (e.g., obstructive uropathy), of primary renal disease (e.g., nephrotic syndrome), or of systemic disease (e.g., diabetes mellitus or systemic lupus erythematosus) does not contraindicate transplantation. Each child must be individually evaluated and the effect of the underlying disease considered.

Renal transplantation in children less than 10 kg has not been proven to be uniformly successful (Fine and Ehrlich, 1985). These children present technical and management problems because of their small size. If possible, the transplant will be deferred until the child grows, and dialysis or supportive management meanwhile used.

Donor Selection

Children with end-stage renal disease who are eligible candidates for a renal transplant may receive the kidney from a live donor or from a cadaver (a donor who died a few hours earlier). Immunologically, the transplant has a higher survival rate if the donor is a relative to the child. Twin siblings are often the best donors because the tissue typing is almost identical. Siblings, parents, aunts, and uncles are also optimal donors.

If a relative is not available as a donor, a cadaver source may be used. The cadaver kidney is closely matched in terms of tissue type and ABO grouping to minimize rejection.

Procedure

The transplanted kidney is usually placed retroperitoneally in the anterior iliac fossa. However, in small children who weigh less than 20 kg, a transperitoneal incision is used with intraperitoneal placement. If a congenital anomaly of the lower urinary tract exists, a urinary conduit may be necessary in order to prevent reflux to the new kidney and allow for urinary drainage.

The recipient's kidneys are usually left in place. However, a bilateral nephrectomy is indicated if the kidneys are harmful to the child, as in cases of severe hypertension, persistent massive proteinuria in nephrotic syndrome, or persistent clinical pylonephritis.

Large adult kidneys that are transplanted into children will function adequately, although they are quite large initially. Over time, the kidney will decrease in size. Conversely, cadaveric kidneys from small children that are transplanted into adolescents will hypertrophy and increase in function. The nursing considerations and care in working with a child during the perioperative transplant period are highly specialized and beyond both the purview of this text and the role of the nurse generalist.

Management After Transplant

The management of caring for a child after transplant is aimed at preventing and treating rejection of the kidney and infection. Immunosuppression therapy is used to minimize the immune response of the recipient. Drugs that are used to prevent rejection include corticosteroids and azathioprine. Other agents used include cyclosporine and antilymphocyte globulin.

Opportunistic infections may occur in the child who is undergoing immunosuppression. Children with renal transplants are particularly vulnerable to herpes group viruses, especially within the first 3 months after the transplant (see Chapters 43 and 48 for a discussion of immunosuppression and related nursing care).

Growth retardation is one of the most important complications for children following a renal transplant. The etiology of growth failure results from the persistence of metabolic acidosis and phosphatemia after the transplant, the bone age or presence and/or degree of bone disease at the time of transplantation, and the use of corticosteroids. Children older than age 7 at time of transplant seem to have poor growth during their preadolescent and adolescent growth spurt (Topor, 1981), whereas children younger than 7 years of age at the time achieve a normal height for age. Growth retardation has long-term implications in that the child may have problems with body image, peer group acceptance, and social relationships.

Rejection of the transplanted kidney is the most common cause of transplant failure. Rejection may occur immediately after the transplant, within the first few days to 1 to 2 years after the transplant, or as a chronic rejection over time.

If rejection occurs immediately after the transplant, it is related to the inability of the recipient's antibodies to accept the foreign organ. The child will manifest symptoms of fever, abdominal discomfort over the graft site, hypertension, and a decreased urine output. Serum creatinine and BUN levels will increase, reflecting the diminishing renal function. In an attempt to prevent rejection intravenous methylprednisolone should be administered.

Chronic rejection occurs gradually and reflects diminishing renal function. The child may manifest hematuria or proteinuria, or both, and may develop symptoms of chronic renal failure. Inevitably, the loss of the transplanted kidney will occur.

Strategies for Nursing Care

Goals for nursing care of the child with CRF are similar to those for the child with ARF. They include monitoring fluid, electrolyte, and acid-base balance, and reducing the risks of complications such as anemia and infection. In addition, the child with chronic renal failure faces the possibility of dehydration (from alteration in the kidney's ability to concentrate urine), glucose intolerance, and growth retardation. The clinical manifestations and related nursing strategies are summarized in Table 42-8.

When the child with chronic renal failure reaches end-stage renal disease dialysis or kidney transplantation will be necessary. There is a national trend to allow home dialysis for children whenever possible. The nurse's role in providing information and guidance to support the family's home management of the child on dialysis is critical to a favorable outcome. Table 42-9 presents an appropriate nursing process plan for the child receiving dialysis either in a treatment center or at home.

Text continues on page 1520

Table 42-9
Nursing Process Plan: The Child Undergoing Dialysis Secondary to Chronic Renal Failure*

by Roxie Foster

Assessment of Physical Function

Subjective Assessment

Comfort of access site (hemodialysis) or of abdomen (peritoneal dialysis), malaise, comfort of abdomen upon palpation, presence of nausea, comfort of dialysis procedure; report of bowel function/stool character

Objective Assessment

Vital signs, presence of bruit and thrill over arteriovenous connection; character of blood visible in external shunt tubing; appearance of access site; skin temperature of limb with access site or of abdominal insertion site; appearance of effluent; amount of dialysate returned; abdominal palpation; height and weight; muscle mass of limbs; laboratory reports on effluent; culture reports of wound drainage; BUN

Analysis: Nursing Diagnosis 1

Potential for injury: complications of hemodialysis:
- ***infection**, related to repeated cannulation of the vascular access site*
- ***vascular obstruction**, related to blood clots or vascular damage associated with repeated cannulation*
- ***hemorrhage**, related to leakage or accidental disconnection of external shunt*
- ***seizures**, related (probably) to cerebral edema associated with the response of cerebral tissue to rapid shifts in extracellular fluid osmolality*

Defining Characteristics

Infection: Redness, swelling, pain, warmth, drainage, fever, malaise, increased WBC
Vascular obstruction: Absent or diminished bruit and thrill, decreased pulse below arteriovenous connection, decreasing redness and warmth of blood in external tubing (if an external shunt)

Hemorrhage: Frank bleeding from connection site
Seizures: Seizure activity during or after hemodialysis

Client Goals/ Evaluation Criteria	Nursing Goals/Strategies (Selected Rationale)
1.1. The client will be free of infection related to the site of venous access as evidenced by: a. normal skin color b. warm skin temperature c. absence of swelling d. absence of pain e. absence of drainage f. absence of fever g. WBC within normal limits	*Assess for evidence of infection* • Assess insertion site and associated limb every 4–8 hr. • Ask child and family to report immediately any changes in sensation, warmth, comfort, or appearance of the site • Monitor blood values for WBC count *Initiate strategies to prevent infection* • Use and teach meticulous aseptic technique when connecting and disconnecting tubings† • Arteriovenous fistula cannulation sites should be covered with small dressings until the puncture sites are well occluded • Swimming and tub-bathing are contraindicated for the child with an external shunt

	• Teach child and family to assess frequently for cracks or leaks in an external shunt • Ensure that the child, family, and other health care professionals know that the limb with the access site is not to be used for IVs or for venipunctures
1.2. The client will maintain patency of the arteriovenous connection as evidenced by: a. bruit heard over site b. thrill felt over site c. normal pulse below access site d. warm, red blood in external shunt tubing	*Assess for patency of the arteriovenous connection* • Auscultate for a bruit and feel for a thrill over the site • Check radial (or pedal) pulses bilaterally (in order to detect a decrease in arterial flow below the site) • Inspect the character of blood visible in external shunt tubing. Leave part of the tubing exposed when dressing the site *Initiate strategies to reduce the incidence of obstruction* • Monitor BP carefully. (A decrease in BP can cause clotting or collapse of the vein [Alt, Balduf, and Thompson, 1986]) • Alert family to the need for medical attention if child is at risk for dehydration (e.g., with vomiting and diarrhea). Explain need for adequate fluids during warm weather (within fluid restrictions) • Monitor closely for orthostatic hypotension if new antihypertensive is begun. Teach child to change positions more slowly in the first several days after beginning drug • Ensure that child, family, and other health care professionals know that BP should *never* be measured in the limb containing the access site • Instruct child not to lie upon the limb containing the access site
1.3. The client will be free of bleeding from the external shunt	*Assess the integrity of the shunt tubing and connections* • Teach child and family to assess for leaks and cracks, and how to ensure connections are firmly in place after disconnecting the tubings from home hemodialysis equipment • Ensure that the child understands the consequences of accidentally disconnecting the tubing • Keep two bulldog clamps attached to the shunt dressing or the child's clothing for ready access in case of accidental disconnection. Ensure that the child and all family members know how to use them
1.4. The child will suffer no preventable seizures during or after dialysis	*Assist in prescribed measures to reduce the threat of seizure* • Administer prescribed dialysate solution (to decrease rapid clearance of urea) • Administer prescribed IV mannitol during dialysis (to reduce cerebral edema) • Administer prescribed phenobarbital (to decrease risk of seizures
1.5. The client will suffer no injury from unpreventable seizures	*Institute seizure precautions to reduce the risk of injury (see Chapter 46)*

Analysis: Nursing Diagnosis 2

Potential for injury: complications of peritoneal dialysis:

- ***peritonitis,*** *related to repeatedly connecting and disconnecting the peritoneal catheter*
- ***tunnel infection,*** *resulting from pathogen invasion along the insertion site of the peritoneal catheter*

Continued

Table 42-9 (continued)

Nursing Diagnosis 2

- *pain, related to*
  peritoneal irritation associated with initial dialysis treatments
  infusion of cold dialysate
  stretching and irritation of the diaphragm
- ***insufficient return of dialysate,*** *related to constipation*
- ***protein deficiency,*** *related to loss of protein to the returning dialysate*
- ***blood in returning solution,*** *related to peritoneal or intraabdominal irritation from the catheter or to other intraabdominal lesions*

Defining Characteristics

Peritonitis: Fever, rebound tenderness, nausea, general malaise, cloudy output, CAPD effluent (dialysate return) with WBC >100, IPD or CCPD effluent with WBC >300 (Binkley, 1984)
Tunnel infection: Fever, malaise, warmth, redness, drainage at insertion site; increased WBC, positive wound culture
Pain: Report of discomfort associated with inflow or "dwell" stages of dialysis
Insufficient return of dialysate: Failure after the first month of therapy to return most of the dialysate; palpable bowel; infrequent, hard stools that fail to achieve evacuation
Protein deficiency: Growth delay, wasting of muscle tissue
Blood in returning solution: Effluent positive for blood on visual inspection or upon hematest

Client Goals/ Evaluation Criteria	Nursing Goals/Strategies (Selected Rationale)
2.1. The client will be free of peritonitis as evidenced by: a. absence of fever b. absence of nausea or rebound tenderness c. usual energy level d. clear effluent e. WBC of CAPD effluent <100 f. WBC of IPD or CCPD effluent <300	*Assess for evidence of peritonitis* • Assess and record each shift/visit: vital signs, abdominal comfort, energy level, character of effluent • Obtain effluent specimen for periodic analysis *Initiate strategies to reduce the risk of peritonitis* • Ensure that child, family, and other health care professionals understand that child is at risk for entry of pathogens *every* time peritoneal catheter is connected and disconnected • Use and teach meticulous aseptic technique in connecting and disconnecting tubings • Use and teach use of any of the following techniques as appropriate and as the family can afford the cost (Binkley, 1984): a Betadine block (Betadine in the distal, clamped portion of the catheter after dialysis) an in-line filter a Sterile Connection Device (SCD) (Abbott Laboratories device for forming a heat weld between dialysate bag and the catheter) an ultraviolet light (developed by Travenol Laboratories to irradiate the conduction assembly before the dialysis bag is connected)

2.2. The client will remain free of tunnel infection as evidenced by: a. absence of fever b. absence of warmth, redness, or drainage at insertion site c. WBC within normal limits d. negative wound culture	*Assess the insertion site for evidence of infection each shift/visit* • Culture any wound drainage • Obtain a blood specimen for analysis as appropriate *Institute strategies to reduce the risk of tunnel infection* • Instruct the child to shower (rather than bathe) and to avoid swimming (to reduce concentration of bacteria at insertion site) • Keep insertion site clean and dry. Apply Betadine or other antiseptic according to treatment center protocol
2.3. The client will be free of pain associated with insertion or retention of dialysate as evidenced by: a. verbal report b. usual activity and behavior	*Assess for pain associated with dialysis. Provide comfort measures* • Assure the child and family that discomfort associated with inflow on initial treatments is not uncommon and usually subsides within the first 2 weeks (Binkley, 1984) • Prewarm the dialysate before instilling it • If pain exists between the shoulder blades it may be referred from diaphragm and may be an indication to decrease amount of dialysate instilled (Binkley, 1984)
2.4. The client will remain free of constipation as evidenced by stool number and character normal for age	*Assess and record adequacy of bowel evacuation* • Ask child/parent about stool patterns • Palpate abdomen for evidence of full bowel *Initiate strategies to reduce the risk of constipation* • Ensure that child receives a diet adequate in natural fiber and fluids (within prescribed limits) • Encourage exercise appropriate to age and physical condition • Consult physician about use of dark syrup or mineral oil in the diet to facilitate evacuation
2.5. The child will not suffer a protein deficiency as evidenced by: a. consuming the prescribed mg/kg of protein per day b. steady (although often slow) growth c. maintenance of muscle mass	*Assess protein intake* • Ask family to keep a food diary for a week • Weigh and measure child monthly and plot growth curve • Assess muscle mass of limbs *Assist in increasing inadequate protein intake* • Share with family high-protein recipes and lists of protein foods that might be palatable to child • Consult with physician or nutritional clinical specialist about supplemental nutrition such as N/G tube feedings while child sleeps
2.6. The client will obtain early diagnosis and treatment for significant intra-abdominal bleeding	*Assess for blood in the returning dialysate* • Instruct the family to notify the physician of visible bloody return • Obtain periodic samples of effluent to test for occult blood • Monitor hemoglobin and hematocrit levels

II. Assessment of Emotional-Social Function

Subjective Assessment:

Self-report or parental report of feelings about self, and about self in relation to others

Objective Assessment:

Posture, eye contact, presence of fidgeting, attachment behavior (physical contact with parent), choice of clothing, personal hygiene

Continued

Table 42-9 (continued)

Analysis: Nursing Diagnosis 3

Disturbance in self-concept: body image and self-esteem, related to
- ***dependency upon a dialysis machine***
- ***possible inability to wear fashionable clothing because of urinary diversion tubings and collection bags***
- ***short stature associated with chronic renal disease***
- ***delayed appearance of secondary sexual characteristics***

role performance, related to difficulty in achieving developmental tasks associated with the physical and social restrictions of dialysis

Defining Characteristics

Subjective: Verbalizes feelings of inferiority, negativity, pessimism, boasts about achievements, declines opportunities for social activities, new experiences

Objective: In group situations tends to watch rather than participate, acting out behavior, poor impulse control, poor sportsmanship, takes little pride in appearance

Client Goal/ Evaluation Criteria	Nursing Goals/Strategies (Selected Rationale)
3.1. The client will display self-valuing behaviors as evidenced by: a. describing the self positively b. displaying more happy than unhappy behavior c. talking about realistic plans for the future d. displaying more autonomy and faith in self than guilt and shame	*Assess the child's self-concept* (see Box 16-2) *Institute strategies to enhance self-concept* • Discuss with family ways they can facilitate healthy development of self-concept. See Table 16-1 • Ensure that family receives physical and emotional support for their needs so they can, in turn, meet the child's needs Assess the family's support system (see Table 12-6, section II) Refer to appropriate agencies and support groups for financial, physical, and emotional support

* This plan is appropriate for inpatient care or home care (see Chapter 32 to modify this care guide for use by the family or other lay caretakers).

† Treatment centers will vary somewhat on techniques used. Institutional policy records should be consulted.

The nursing role in working with a child undergoing a renal transplant is complex and long-term. The child will require intensive nursing care during the transplant as well as supportive care in the years following the transplant. Because the children often receive long-term corticosteroid therapy, they suffer the physical side effects of retarded growth, Cushing syndrome, cataracts, and peptic ulcers. The child and family require an intradisciplinary approach to the child's health care for several years. The staff must be sensitive to the medical, psychologic, educational, social, and emotional needs of the children and their families.

To care for a child with CRF the nursing role is demanding. The child requires many nursing and medical procedures and constant assessment of all body systems. Because the disease is chronic and life-threatening, there are multiple stressors on the family and child. The nurse must be supportive of the child and family, encouraging as normal a lifestyle as possible for the family. Families will require information about numerous medications, procedures, and symptoms so they can be involved and informed about the child's care.

Nursing Strategies for Follow-Up Care in the Home or Clinic

Strategies for follow-up care for the child with CRF in the predialysis phase will be very similar to care of the child with ARF (see strategies for follow-up care for ARF earlier in this chapter). In addition the nurse should obtain a specific gravity of the urine, test the urine for sugar and acetone, and assess thoroughly for physical evidence of uremia.

Strategies for care of the child undergoing hemodialysis or peritoneal dialysis are detailed in Table 42-9. This nursing process plan can easily be modified to provide a guide for parents as well as for health care professionals (see Chapter 32 for an example of family guidelines for care).

Follow-up care for the child after renal transplantation involves collecting blood and urine specimens for analysis and assessment for the effects of long-term immunosuppression. See Table 43-2, Nursing Process Plan: The Child on Corticosteroid Therapy, for strategies specific to immunosuppressive therapy.

References

Alt D, Balduf R, and Thompson E: When a vascular access site complicates care. *RN* 1986 Oct; 36–39.

Altchek A: Pediatric vulvovaginitis. *J Reprod Med* 1984; 29(6):359–375.

Anderson GF, Smey P: Current concepts in the management of common urologic problems in infants and children. *Pediatr Clin North Am* 1985; 32(5):1145.

Azrin NH, Sneed TJ, and Foxx RM: Dry bed training: rapid elimination of childhood enuresis. *Behav Res Ther* 1974; 12:147–156.

Azrin NH, Thienes PM: Rapid elimination of enuresis by intensive learning without a conditioning apparatus. *Behav Ther* 1978; 9:342–354.

Bakwin H, Bakwin R: *Behavior Disorders in Children*. Philadelphia, WB Saunders, 1972.

Behrman RE Vaughan VC (eds): *Nelson Textbook of Pediatrics,* 12th ed. Philadelphia, WB Saunders, 1987.

Bellinger MF: The management of vesicoureteric reflux. *Urolog Clin North Am* 1985; 12(1):23–29.

Belman AB: Early surgery for hypospadias. *Hospital Pract* 1984 Mar; 192–198.

Belman AB: Urethra. *In* Kelalis PP, King LR, and Belman AB (eds): *Clinical Pediatric Urology,* 2nd ed. Philadelphia, WB Saunders, 1985.

Bergstein JM, Michael AF: Nephrologic diseases. *In* Behrman RE, Vaughan VC (eds): *Nelson Textbook of Pediatrics.* 13th ed. Philadelphia, WB Saunders, 1987, 1111–1146.

Brink RE: How serious is the child's behavior problem? *MCN* 1982; 7:33–36.

Brundage DJ: *Nursing Management of Renal Problems,* 2nd ed. St Louis, CV Mosby, 1980.

Cleary TG: Cytotoxin-producing *Escherichia coli* and the hemolytic uremic syndrome. *Pediatr Clin North Am* 1988 Jun; 35(3):485–502.

Cohen M: Enuresis. *Pediatr Clin North Am* 1975 Aug; 545.

Decker MD, Edwards KM: Central venous catheter infections. *Pediatr Clin North Am* 1988 Jun; 35(3):579–612.

deWardener HE: *The Kidney,* 5th ed. New York, Churchill-Livingstone, 1985.

Doleys DM, Dolce JJ: Toilet training and enuresis. *Pediatr Clin North Am* 1982 Apr; 29:297–313.

Duckett JW, Caldamone AA: Bladder and urachus. *In* Kelalis PP, King LR, Belman AB (eds): *Clinical Pediatric Urology,* 2nd ed. Philadelphia, WB Saunders, 1985.

Durbin WA, Peter G: Management of urinary tract infections in infants and children. *Pediatr Infect Dis* 1984; 3(6):564–574.

Fine RN: Acute and chronic renal failure in children. *In* Kelalis PP, King LR, Belman AB (eds): *Clinical Pediatric Urology,* 2nd ed. Philadelphia, WB Saunders, 1985.

Fine RN, Ehrlich RM: Renal transplantation in children. *In* Kelalis PP, King LK, Belman AB (eds): *Clinical Pediatric Urology,* 2nd ed. Philadelphia, WB Saunders, 1985.

Fong JSC, et al: Hemolytic-uremic syndrome: current concepts and management. *Pediatr Clin North Am* 1982; 29:835–856.

Friman PC: A preventive context for enuresis. *Pediatr Clin North Am* 1986 Aug; 33(4):871–886.

Fritz GK, Armbrust J: Enuresis and encopresis. *Psychiatr Clin North Am* 1982 Aug; 5(2):283–296.

Ginsburg CM, McCracken GH: Urinary tract infections in young infants. *Pediatrics* 1982; 69(4):409–412.

Gross RT, Dornbusch SM: Enuresis. *In* Levine, et al: *Developmental-Behavioral Pediatrics.* Philadelphia, WB Saunders, 1983, 573–586.

Gualtieri C: Imipramine and children: a review and some speculations about the mechanisms of drug action. *Dis Nerv Syst* 1977 May; 38(5):368–375.

Hadziselimovic F, et al: Surgical correction of cryptorchidism at 2 years. *J Pediatr Surg* 1975 Feb; 10(1):19–26.

Hadziselimovic F, Herzog B: The meaning of the Leydig cell in relation to the etiology of cryptorchidism. *J Pediatr Surg* 1976 Feb; 11(1):1–8.

Hellerstein S, et al: Consensus: Roentgenographic evaluation of children with urinary tract infections. *Pediatr Infect Dis* 1984; 3(4):291–293.

International Reflux Study in Children: International system of radiographic grading of vesicoureteric reflux. *Pediatr Radiol* 1985; 15:105–109.

Johnson CE, et al: Renal ultrasound evaluation of urinary tract infections in children. *Pediatrics* 1986; 78(5):871–878.

Jordan SC, Lemire JM: Acute glomerulonephritis: diagnosis and treatment. *Pediatr Clin North Am* 1982; 29(4):857–873.

Kelalis PP: Renal pelvis and ureter. *In* Kelalis PP, King LR, Belman AB (eds): *Clinical Pediatric Urology,* 2nd ed. Philadelphia, WB Saunders, 1985.

Kelalis PP: Surgical correction of vesicoureteral reflux. *In* Kelalis PP, King LR, Berman AB (eds): *Clinical Pediatric Urology,* 2nd ed. Philadelphia, WB Saunders, 1985.

Kim MS, Grupe WE: The nephrotic syndrome. *In* Gellis SS, Kagan BM (eds): *Current Pediatric Therapy 12.* Philadelphia, WB Saunders, 1986, 366–369.

Koff S: Clues to neonatal genitourinary problems. *Postgrad Med* 1977 Sep; 62(3):95.

Kogan SJ: Cryptorchidism. *In* Kelalis PP, King LR, Belman AB: (eds): *Clinical Pediatric Urology,* 2nd ed. Philadelphia, WB Saunders, 1985.

Krabbe S, et al: High incidences of undetected neoplasia in maldescended testes. Lancet 1979 May 12; 1, 999.

Kroovand RL, Perlmutter AD: Acute post-streptococcal glomerulonephritis. *In* Behrman RE, Vaughan VC (eds): *Nelson Textbook of Pediatrics.* 12th ed. Philadelphia, WB Saunders, 1983, 1330–1334.

Kroovand RL, Perlmutter AD: Urinary tract infections. *In* Behrman RE, Vaughan VC (eds): *Nelson Textbook of Pediatrics.* 12th ed. Philadelphia, WB Saunders, 1983, 1367–1372.

Kunin CM: *Detection, Prevention and Management of Urinary Tract Infections.* Philadelphia, Lea and Febiger, 1979.

Levitt SB, Weiss RA: Vesicoureteral reflux. *In* Kelalis PP, King LR, Belman AB (eds): *Clinical Pediatric Urology,* 2nd ed. Philadelphia, WB Saunders, 1985.

Madaio MP, Harrington JT: The diagnosis of acute glomerulonephritis. *N Engl J Med* 1983; 309(21):1299–1302.

Malek RS: Urolithiasis. *In* Kelalis PP, King LR, Belman AB (eds): *Clinical Pediatric Urology,* 2nd ed. Philadelphia, WB Saunders, 1985.

McConnell EA, Zimmerman MF: *Care of Patients with Urologic Problems.* Philadelphia, JB Lippincott, 1983.

McCracken GH: Recurrent urinary tract infections in children. *Pediatr Infect Dis* 1984 May-Jun; 3:528–530.

McCrory WW: Glomerulonephritis. *Pediatr Rev* 1983; 5(1):19–25.

Neinstein LS, Goldenring J, Carpenter S: Nonsexual transmission of sexually transmitted diseases: An infrequent occurrence. *Pediatrics* 1984; 74(1):67–76.

Novello AC: Hemolytic-uremic syndrome. *In* Gellis SS, Kagan BM (eds): *Current Pediatric Therapy 12.* Philadelphia, WB Saunders, 1986, pp 383–385.

Osofsky SG, Lewy JE: Acute renal failure. *In* Dickerman JD, Lucey JF: *Smith's The Critically Ill Child: Diagnosis and Medical Management.* 3rd ed. Philadelphia, WB Saunders, 1985, 288.

Parker L, Whitehead W: Treatment of urinary and fecal incontinence in children. *In* Russo DC, Varni JW (eds): *Behavioral Pediatrics: Research and Practice.* New York, Plenum Press, 1982, pp 143–174.

Pennington, JAT, Church HN: *Bowes and Church's Food Values of Portions Commonly Used.* 13th ed. New York, Harper and Row, 1980.

Pinch L, et al: Cryptorchidism: A pediatric review. *Urolog Clin North Am* 1979; 1:573.

Prentiss R, et al: Undescended testis. *J Urology* 1060 May; 83:686.

Rezvani I: Cryptorchidism: a pediatrician's view. *Pediatr Clin North Am* 1987; 34(3):735–746.

Schact RG: Acute renal failure. *In* Zimmerman SS, Gildea JH (eds): *Critical Care Pediatrics.* Philadelphia, WB Saunders, 1985, pp 313–327.

Schmitt BD: Nocturnal enuresis. *Primary Care* 1984 Sep; 11(3):485–495.

Shelov SP: Nocturnal enuresis. *In* Shelov SP, et al (eds): *Primary Care Pediatrics: A Symptomatic Approach.* Norwalk, CT, Appleton-Century-Crofts, 1984, pp 308–316.

Smellie JM, Normand ICS, Katz G: Children with urinary infection: A comparison of those with and those without vesicourelateral reflux. *Kidney Int* 1981; 20:717–722.

Spencer JR, Schaeffer, AJ: Pediatric urinary tract infections. *Urol Clin North Am* 1986; 13(4):661–672.

Stauffer D: Catheterization: A health procedure schools must be prepared to provide. *J School Health* 1984; 54(1):37–38.

Thomas CK: Childhood urinary tract infection. *Pediatr Nurs* 1982; 8(2):114–119, 142.

Topor M: Chronic renal disease in children. *Nurs Clin North Am* 1981 Sep; 16(3):587–597.

van den Abbecle AD, et al: Vesicoureteral reflux in asymptomatic siblings of patients with known reflux: radionuclide cystography. *Pediatrics* 1987; 79(1):147–153.

Wallach J: *Interpretation of Pediatric Tests.* Boston, Little, Brown, 1983.

Wiswell TE, et al: Decreased incidence of urinary tract infection in circumcised male infants. *Pediatrics* 1985; 75(5):901–903.

Wiswell TE, et al: Declining frequency of circumcision: implication for changes in the absolute incidence and male to female sex ratio of urinary tract infections in early infancy. *Pediatrics* 1987; 79(3):338–342.

Bibliography

Allen TD: Cryptorchidism. *Pediatr Rev* 1984; 5(1):317–319.

Altcheck A: Vulvovaginitis, vulvar skin diseases and pelvic inflammatory disease. *Pediatr Clin North Am* 1981; 28(2):397–432.

Barta MA: Correcting electrolyte imbalances. *RN* 1987 Feb: 30–34.

Binkley LS: Keeping up with peritoneal dialysis. *Am J Nurs* 1984; 84(6):729–733.

Brundage DJ: *Nursing Management of Renal Problems.* 2nd ed. St. Louis, CV Mosby, 1980.

Calloway C: When the problem involves magnesium, calcium, or phosphate. *RN* 1987 May: 30–36.

Chaffee EE, Lytle IM: *Basic Physiology and Anatomy.* 4th ed. Philadelphia, JB Lippincott, 1980.

Chambers JK: Fluid and electrolyte problems in renal and urologic disorders. *Issues Compr Pediatr Nurs* 1987 10(3):815–826.

Chenevey B: Overview of fluids and electrolytes. *Nurs Clin North Am* 1987 Dec; 22(4):749–759.

Chesney RW, Novello AC: Forms of nephrotic syndrome likely to progress to renal impairment. *Pediatr Clin North Am* 1987; 34(3):609–627.

Emans SJH, Goldstein DP: *Pediatric and Adolescent Gynecology.* Boston, Little, Brown, 1982, 45–58.

Fine RN: Acute and chronic renal failure in children. *In* Kelalis PP, et al (eds): *Clinical Pediatric Urology.* 2nd ed. Philadelphia, WB Saunders, 1985.

Frank A, Murray SM: A no-guess guide for urinary color assessment. *RN* 1988 Jun: 46–51.

Ghiotto DL: A full range of care for nephrostomy patients. *RN* 1988 Apr; 72–77.

Guyton AC: *Human Physiology and Mechanisms of Disease.* 3rd ed. Philadelphia, WB Saunders, 1982.

Hahn K: The many signs of renal failure. *Nurs 87* 1987 Aug; 17(8):34–41.

Kroovand RL, Perlmutter AD: Anomalies of the testis. *In* Behrman RE, Vaughan VC (eds): *Nelson Textbook of Pediatrics.* 12th ed. Philadelphia, WB Saunders, 1983.

Lancaster LE: Renal and endocrine regulation of water and electrolyte balance. *Nurs Clin North Am* 1987 Dec; 22(4):761–772.

Lebowitz RL: Pediatric uroradiology. *Pediatr Clin North Am* 1985; 32(6):1353–1362.

LePontois J, et al: Family adjustment to pediatric ambulatory dialysis. *Am J Orthopsychiatr* 1987; 57(1):78–83.

Lerner J, Khan Z: *Mosby's Manual of Urologic Nursing.* St. Louis, CV Mosby, 1982.

Neff EJA: Nursing the child undergoing dialysis. *Issues Compr Pediatr Nurs* 1987 10(3):173–185.

Nova G: Dialyzable drugs. *AJN* 1987 Jul; 87(7):933–942.

Nurse's Clinical Library: *Renal and Urologic Disorders.* Springhouse, PA, Nursing '84 Books, 1984.

Poyss AS: Assessment and nursing diagnosis in fluid and electrolyte disorders. *Issues Compr Pediatr Nurs* 1987; 10(3):773–783.

Rivers R: Nursing the kidney transplant patient. *RN* 1987 Aug; 46–53.

Ruge CA: Catheter-related U.T.I.s. What's the best way to prevent them? *Nurs 87* Dec; 17(12):50–51.

Schwartz MW: Potassium imbalances. *Am J Nurs* 1987 Oct; 87(10):1292–1300.

Smith J: Big differences in little people. *Am J Nurs* 1988 Apr; 88(4):458–462.

Stark JL: A quick guide to urinary tract assessment. *Nurs 88* 1988 Jul; 18(7):57–58.

Stevens MS, Reinitz M: Nursing care through exstrophic bladder reconstruction surgery. *MCN* 1980; 5:265–270.

Strangio L: Believe it or not . . . peritoneal dialysis made easy. *Nurs 88* 1988 Jan; 18(1):43–46.

Tarr PI, Hickman RO: Hemolytic uremic syndrome epidemiology: a population-based study in King County, Washington, 1971 to 1980. *Pediatrics* 1987; 80(1):41–45.

Topor M: Chronic renal disease in children. *Nurs Clin North Am* 16(3):587–597.

Toto KH: When the patient has hypokalemia. *RN* 1987 Mar: 38–42.

Toto KH: When the patient has hyperkalemia. *RN* 1987 Apr: 34–38.

van Diemen-Steenvoorde R, et al: Growth and sexual maturation in children after kidney transplantation. *J Pediatr* 1987; 110(3):351–356.

Weiss RA, Edelmann CM: End-stage renal disease in children. *Pediatr Rev* 1984; 5(1):295–303.

Nursing Strategies: Altered Immune Function

Chapter 43

Ann Harkins
Margaret Crandall
Roxie Foster

The immunologic system is designed to protect the body through the mechanisms of defense, homeostasis, and surveillance (Bellanti, 1985). It defends against invasion by microorganisms, promotes homeostasis by removing cellular wastes and worn-out cells, and monitors for and destroys abnormal cells (e.g., tumor cells) that may arise within the body. Considering the importance of these functions, it may seem curious that the immune system has remained relatively obscure. Whereas even elementary school children can recite the basic functions of the heart and lungs, the functions of such immune system organs as the thymus and spleen may puzzle considerably more sophisticated students. Although theories of cellular and humoral immunity were postulated in 1908, not until the 1930s were functions of specific antibodies identified; not until the 1960s did the role of the thymus become better understood; in the 1980s the role of heredity became central to the understanding of the immune response (Bellanti, 1985). Research in the next decade promises to further explain individual differences in the ability of the immune system to protect the body from pathogens, to eradicate mutant cells arising within the body, and to differentiate between *self* and foreign proteins.

Although normally protective in function, the immune system is subject to physiologic alterations that can be quite harmful to the host. The immune elements that defend against invading organisms may react inappropriately, leading to *hypersensitivity* (allergy), or underreact, resulting in *hyposensitivity* (immunodeficiency disorders). The homeostatic mechanisms that catabolize cellular wastes may malfunction and selectively destroy healthy tissues, a phenomenon termed *autosensitivity* (autoimmune disease). The surveillance mechanism may fail to identify and dispose of cell mutations, the proliferation of which may lead to malignant disease. This chapter presents the normal immune response and the alterations in that response that lead to (1) certain autoimmune or chronic inflammatory diseases, (2) allergy, and (3) immunodeficiency. Malignant diseases are discussed in Chapter 41.

The Normal Immune Response

Anatomy and Physiology of the Immune System

The organs and tissues that comprise the immune system are spread diffusely throughout the body. Lockey and Bukantz (1987a) defined the nature and function of the immune system according to primary and secondary components. Lymphocytes designated as T-cells and B-cells develop in the primary (or central) organs and then migrate to secondary (or peripheral) organs where they reside in their mature form. The primary organs and tissues of the immune system are the thymus and bone marrow. The secondary organs and tissues are the spleen, lymph nodules and nodes (e.g., tonsils, Peyer patches), gut-associated lymphoid tissue (GALT), bronchus-associated lymphoid tissue (BALT), skin-associated lymphoid tissue (SALT), and the blood (Fig. 43-1). These organs and tissues are important to immunity because of their relationship to both nonspecific and specific immune mechanisms.

Both T- and B-lymphocytes originate from the same type of stem cell (Fig. 43-2), but they are prepared for their unique immune functions in different organs. T-lymphocytes further differentiate in the thymus, and B-lymphocytes mature in the bone marrow.

The spleen functions as a filter for blood and lymph. It screens out foreign particles and organisms, along with worn-out blood cells, to allow phagocytosis by the many macrophages that reside in splenic tissue. Children who sustain splenic injury resulting in splenectomy, or who have a disease that leads to splenic atrophy, are at increased risk for infection without this protective mechanism.

The lymph nodes and nodules (including the tonsils and Peyer patches of the intestine) are filters within the lymphatic drainage system that remove particulate matter and microorganisms. Lymphatic channels are found in all body tissues except for the cornea and the central nervous system; the CNS is protected by the lymphocytes within its rich blood supply (Lockey and Bukantz, 1987a).

The gut-associated lymphoid tissue (GALT), bronchus-associated lymphoid tissue (BALT), and skin-associated lymphoid tissue (SALT) represent conceptual "subdivisions" of the immune system, which emphasize the importance of the gastrointestinal and respiratory tracts and the skin as defenses between the body and foreign antigens. All these subsystems contain macrophages. In addition, the GALT and BALT are protected by IgA, a class of antibodies which are secreted by mucous membranes.

Because the immune system is designed to protect the body from foreign proteins, it is essential for immunologic cells to differentiate between the body's own healthy tissues and the foreign proteins that they seek to destroy. This differentiation is based upon a

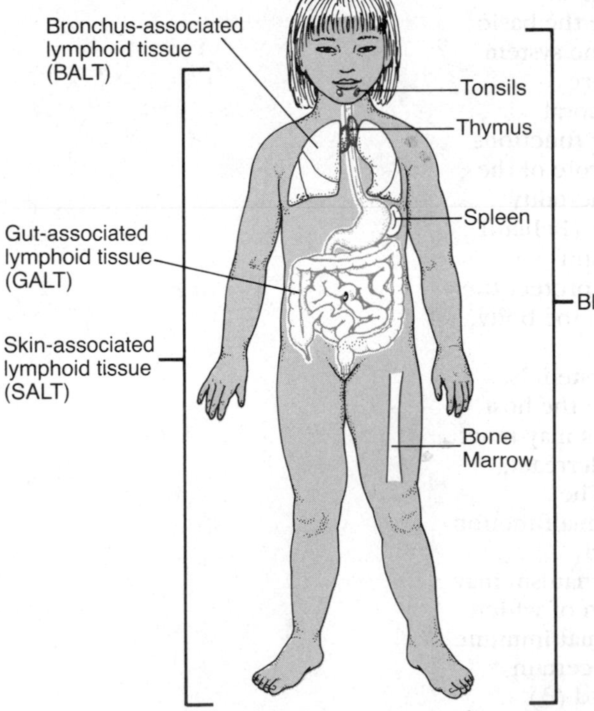

Figure 43-1. Organs and tissues of the immune system.

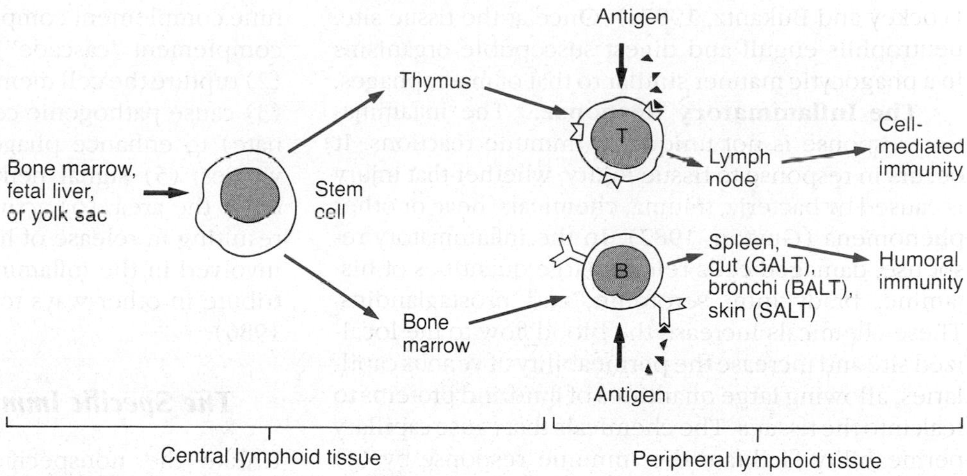

Figure 43-2. Development of the lymphoid system. (Modified from Bellanti JA: *Immunology: Basic Processes.* Philadelphia, WB Saunders, 1985, 33.)

genetic code that determines cell surface protein configurations for body cells.

Human Leukocyte Antigen (HLA)

Cells of the immune system identify foreign proteins according to a "self" versus "not-self" scheme of recognition that is determined by the arrangement of genes on the short arm of the sixth chromosome. This chromosomal region is referred to as the major histocompatibility complex (MHC) or, more specifically, as the *human leukocyte antigen (HLA).* HLA designates the configuration for proteins on leukocyte cell surfaces.* The unique arrangement of surface proteins that results from the HLA blueprint acts as a signal for immune cells. Cells with surface proteins in a configuration matching that individual's HLA are recognized as "self"; proteins configured in any other way are identified as "foreign." Foreign proteins are dealt with in one of three ways:

- (1) a state of *tolerance* develops in which the body fails to respond to that protein (for example, as when repeated small doses of an antigen are injected to desensitize an allergic individual to that antigen),
- (2) a nonspecific immune reaction occurs involving phagocytosis and inflammation, or
- (3) a specific immune response occurs with involvement of cellular and humoral mechanisms.

Tolerance is further discussed in the section on allergy. A description of the nonspecific and specific immune responses follows.

* The configuration of cell surface proteins is also pertinent for cells other than the leukocyte. Leukocytes, however, are the cells that have been most thoroughly studied at this time, and that is why HLA configurations are frequently denoted in the genetics literature. As cell surface mapping is completed on other types of cells, scientists will begin using those designations as well.

The Nonspecific Immune Response

The nonspecific immune response is the first immune reaction to a foreign protein, such as a bacterium or a virus. Phagocytosis, the inflammatory response, and the complement system comprise this primary immune response.†

Phagocytosis. The major phagocytes are monocytes (which become macrophages) and neutrophils (also known as polymorphonuclear leukocytes, or PMNs). Both monocytes and neutrophils are produced from nonlymphoid stem cells in the bone marrow. Monocytes circulate in the blood for only a brief time before they migrate to the body tissues and develop into macrophages. Tissue *macrophages* can respond very quickly to infectious organisms because they are already present in the tissue. The macrophages are highly specialized to engulf and destroy certain bacteria, damaged or worn-out body cells, neoplastic cells, colloidal materials, and macromolecules such as antigen-antibody complexes (Bellanti, 1985).

Neutrophils, unlike tissue macrophages, remain in the circulating blood until they are signaled by an infectious or inflammatory process to enter the tissues. Chemicals released within injured tissues during the inflammatory process facilitate the escape of neutrophils through the vascular walls. These chemical mediators and others stimulated by encounters of microorganisms with the complement cascade (described below) provide a directional signal for neutrophils to follow as they migrate to the area of tissue injury

† The complement system also comes into play as a result of the antigen-antibody reaction within the specific immune response.

(Lockey and Bukantz, 1987a). Once at the tissue site, neutrophils engulf and digest susceptible organisms in a phagocytic manner similar to that of macrophages.

The Inflammatory Response. The inflammatory response is not unique to immune reactions. It occurs in response to tissue injury, whether that injury is caused by bacteria, trauma, chemicals, heat, or other phenomena (Guyton, 1987). In the inflammatory response, damaged cells release large quantities of histamine, bradykinin, serotonin, and prostaglandins. These chemicals increase the blood flow to the localized site and increase the permeability of venous capillaries, allowing large quantities of fluid and proteins to leak into the tissues. The chemicals that cause capillary permeability facilitate the immune response by (1) allowing entry of phagocytic neutrophils into the tissues and (2) drawing the neutrophils to the site of greatest antigen concentration. This "drawing" power is termed *chemotaxis* and is essential to phagocytosis. Chemotaxis is augmented by the complement system.

The *cardinal signs of inflammation* are redness, heat, swelling, and pain. It is important to remember that despite these unpleasant effects of the inflammatory response, *inflammation is a protective mechanism* that facilitates phagocytosis and limits spread and replication of at least some organisms (Fulginiti, 1987). Increased blood flow manifests as erythema and heat; the local heat and characteristic systemic fever of microbial invasion are thought to inhibit multiplication of microbes. The inflammatory exudate which develops from the fluids that escape the blood stream provides a medium for the phagocytic process.

Pain associated with inflammation may occur for several reasons. Endogenous chemical substances such as bradykinin, serotonin, histamines, and prostaglandins are known to have an irritating effect upon the tissues. The tissue tension/pressure exerted by the edema also may be a source of pain. Pain in itself is protective, however, by alerting the host to the infective process.

The Complement System

The complement system involves at least 20 plasma proteins that circulate in an inactive form until activated either by an antigen-antibody reaction or by direct encounter with a microorganism. Although the complement system is often activated by an antigen-antibody reaction (thus making it secondary to the specific immune response), it can also be activated without the mediation of an antigen-antibody reaction. This "alternate pathway" for complement activation makes the complement system one of the first lines of defense against an invading organism (Guyton, 1986).

Once activated, the proteins grouped within the nine complement components work sequentially (the complement "cascade") to (1) activate phagocytosis, (2) rupture the cell membranes of invading organisms, (3) cause pathogenic cells to stick together (agglutinate) to enhance phagocytosis, (4) inactivate some viruses, (5) signal neutrophils and macrophages to enter the area, (6) activate mast cells and basophils, resulting in release of histamine and other chemicals involved in the inflammatory response, and (7) contribute in other ways to local inflammation (Guyton, 1986).

The Specific Immune Response

Unlike the nonspecific immune response, which occurs in a general way to any foreign protein, the specific immune response is highly discriminatory. The specific immune response occurs not because it senses that "something" foreign is present, but because a *particular* antigen is recognized. The specific immune response is characterized by specificity, memory, mobility, replicability, and cooperation.

Specificity is the ability to distinguish one antigen from another. Once lymphocytes of the specific immune system have initial contact with an antigen and become sensitized to it, they *remember* that antigen and, upon subsequent exposure, react more swiftly and effectively to eliminate it. The elements of the specific immune system are mobile; they travel throughout the body. They also frequently reproduce, or *replicate,* when activated. The nonspecific and specific immune responses interact *cooperatively* to rid the body of potentially harmful proteins. There is constant interaction among lymphoid and nonlymphoid cells, antibodies, and secretory chemical mediators.

Lymphocytes are the essential element of both cellular and humoral immunity. Cellular and humoral immunity began as separate theories proposed by different immunologic researchers. The emphasis of the cellular theory was upon the "biologic effects of intact cells involved in the host's response to foreignness" (Bellanti, 1985, page 4), whereas the humoral theory emphasized the study of chemical products produced by cells. Subsequent research has recognized the *interaction* of cellular and humoral elements and has built upon and expanded the hypotheses of these early researchers.

Cellular Immunity. Cellular (or cell-mediated) immunity is based upon the action of *T-lymphocytes,* which are capable of *direct action* upon foreign proteins. T-lymphocytes are formed from lymphoid stem cells identical to those that produce B-lymphocytes but are differentiated during their pathway through the thymus (Fig. 43-2). T-cell development begins early in fetal life; the newborn infant has a fully formed (though small) thymus containing T-cells at various stages of development.* It is not yet clear whether the newborn thymus contains all the stem cells necessary to supply T-lymphocytes throughout life or whether stem cells continue to be supplied to the thymus by the bone marrow via the blood stream (Lockey and Bukantz, 1987a,; Stutman, 1985).

T-lymphocytes are not a single cell type but a family of cells with different effector and regulatory functions. *Effector T-cells* recognize and destroy foreign proteins (antigens) without the aid of antibodies. The two types of effector T-cells are cytotoxic (Tc) cells and delayed hypersensitivity (Tdh) cells. Cytotoxic cells act directly upon a virus-infected cell. In killing the virus, however, the host cell is usually killed as well. Delayed-type hypersensitivity cells, as their name implies, are responsible for delayed hypersensitivity (allergic) reactions like contact dermatitis. Tdh cells are activated directly by an antigen and secrete chemical mediator substances, lymphokines, which produce localized inflammation and enhance phagocytosis.

Regulator T-cells help regulate the actions of B-lymphocytes. They include T-helper cells (Th) and T-suppressor cells (Ts). T-helper cells are so named because they help activate B-lymphocytes. T-suppressor cells secrete chemicals that decrease the action of B-lymphocytes, leading to "down-regulation" of immune activity (Lockey and Bukantz, 1987a).

Humoral Immunity. Humoral immunity depends upon the antibody-producing properties of B-lymphocytes. B-lymphocytes originate in the bone marrow and are activated in response to antigen. Upon activation, these lymphocytes mature into plasma cells that synthesize immunoglobulins (antibodies) specific to the presenting antigen. The major classes of immunoglobulins (Ig) are IgM, IgG, IgA, IgD, and IgE. These classes contain various antigen-specific antibodies. Their functions are listed below (Young and Geha, 1985; Lockey and Bukantz, 1987a,b; Miller, 1988):

IgM	First line of defense, first antibody formed in response to an antigen, activates complement
IgG	Major antibody against bacteria and viruses; neutralizes toxins and enhances phagocytosis. Activates complement. The only antibody to cross the placenta; the basis for passive immunity in the first 3 to 6 months of life
IgA	Protects mainly secretory surfaces of mucous membranes where antigen contact is nonvascular; found in saliva, tears, bronchial mucosa, nasal mucosa, mucous secretions of the small intestine, vagina, and breast milk
IgD	Functions remain largely unknown. May have a role in the differentiation of B-cells
IgE	Responsible for stimulating mast cells to release chemical agents that cause allergic reactions; effective against parasitic infections and may defend against antigens penetrating the mucosa of the skin and the GI and respiratory tracts. Appears to be involved in some viral infections such as RSV (Ch. 38) and to be instrumental in potentiating the inflammatory response

* The thymus reaches adult size at about 12 years of age.

To this point the various elements of the immune system have been discussed separately. To understand the complex protective immune functions, however, it is necessary to consider the ways in which these elements interact. The reactions that occur upon initial and prolonged or subsequent antigen invasion are described next.

Initial Immune Response to an Antigen

The body's response to a new antigen is nonspecific. The foreign protein (antigen) activates the immune system in one of two ways: either by activating the complement cascade (which promotes both the inflammatory response and phagocytosis) or by direct contact with tissue macrophages. Activated macrophages secrete chemicals that, in turn, stimulate activation and proliferation of both T- and B-lymphocytes. More specifically, activation of lymphocytes involves

- "presentation" of the antigen to a T-cell by a macrophage,
- activation of the T-cell by the encounter with the antigen and by the chemicals secreted by the macrophage,
- activation of B-cells by T-helper cells, and
- production (by B-cells) of antigen-specific antibodies.

This process of lymphocyte activation requires some time, and several days pass before a rise in serum antibodies can be detected (Lockey and Bukantz, 1987a). Because of this lag time in enlisting the help of lymphocytes, phagocytosis and the cell-killing effects of complement are the major weapons in the initial immune response.

The invading protein may be contained and killed by phagocytosis that occurs within the inflammatory

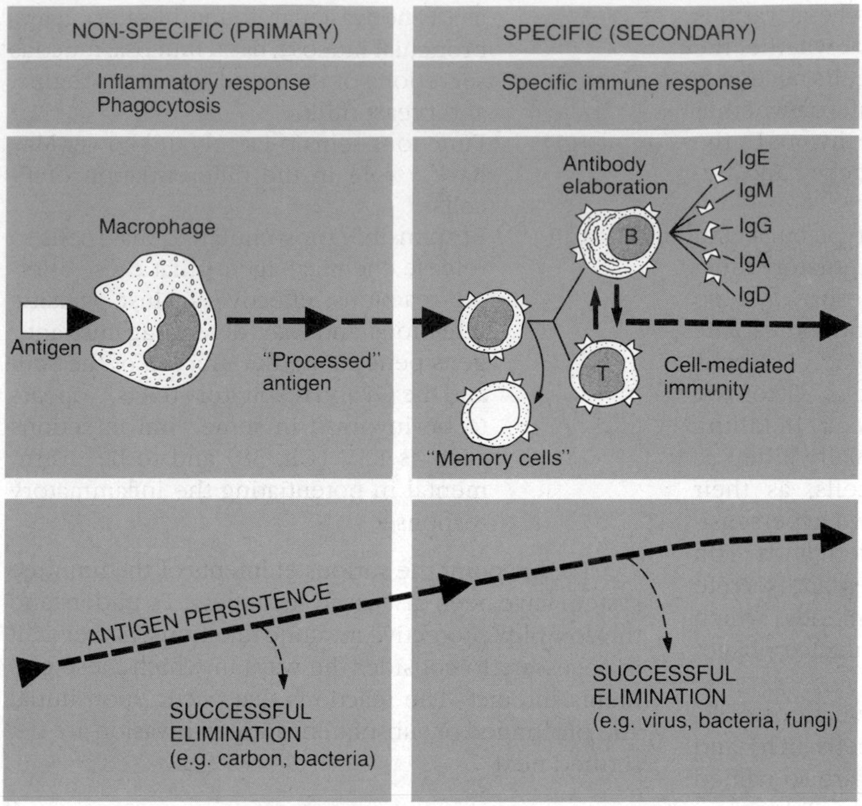

Figure 43-3. Schematic representation of the nonspecific and specific immune responses. (From Bellanti JA: *Immunology: Basic Processes.* Philadelphia, WB Saunders, 1985, 187.)

exudate or by the attack of late-acting proteins of the complement system upon the foreign cell membrane. This initial response may, however, be unsuccessful either because of characteristics of the antigen (i.e., large quantities of antigenic cells or antiphagocytic properties of the cells) or because of an immature or unhealthy immune system (Fig. 43-3). When the antigen persists despite the initial nonspecific immune response, the outcome of the attack is governed by the efficiency of the specific immune response (T- and B-lymphocytes).

Immune Response to Prolonged or Subsequent Encounters with an Antigen

In prolonged or subsequent encounters with an antigen, the specific immune response becomes the major protective mechanism. The specific response *does not replace* the actions of the nonspecific immune elements but rather enhances phagocytosis and adds the cell-killing effects of cytotoxic T-cells. A subsequent response to the antigen results in a shorter lag period, a more rapid rise in serum antibodies (with IgG predominating), and a higher antibody affinity for the antigen (i.e., greater binding power) (Lockey and Bukantz, 1987a).

An antigen that survived the nonspecific response is now attacked additionally by cytotoxic T-cells and is covered with antibodies that enhance phagocytosis by breaking down antiphagocytic capsules and promoting the binding (and subsequent engulfment and destruction) of the antigen with macrophages and neutrophils. Antigen-antibody reactions also activate the complement system.* If the specific immune response fails to contain the invader, drugs (e.g., antibiotics) may be given to assist the body in eliminating the microorganism.

Factors That Affect the Immune Response

Considering the important protective properties of the immune system, it seems pertinent to consider factors that enhance or limit immune competence. Because immunology is a relatively new field, there remain more questions than answers in relation to maintaining a healthy immune system. Several areas, however, have been examined for their effect upon immune competence; these include genetic, age-related, nutritional and metabolic, environmental, anatomic, microbial, physiologic, and stress factors.

* When complement is activated by an antigen-antibody response, the "classical pathway" for activation is said to have been used. If complement is activated by properties of the antigen itself (during the nonspecific response), the process is termed the "alternate pathway."

Genetic Factors

The entire immune system is under genetic control (Bellanti, 1985). Genes control the body's ability to respond to antigens, as well as the level and duration of the response. Genetic defects in immune elements result in an increased susceptibility to disease. One example is the increased susceptibility to infection that is characteristic of children with Down syndrome (see Chapters 4 and 34). Although the mechanisms are poorly understood, children with this genetic disorder have deficits of both cellular and humoral immune elements (Anderson, 1987).

Alterations in human leukocyte antigen (HLA) have been associated with increased incidence of certain inflammatory, autoimmune, and endocrine disorders. The exact mechanisms of this predisposition remain poorly defined. Recent research suggests that other genetic factors related but not linked to HLA may be partly responsible for this predisposition (Stastny, 1987).

Age-Related Factors

At birth, the immune response is compromised by the immaturity of phagocytic cells, T-lymphocytes, and complement proteins, as well as by decreased levels of immunoglobulins (antibodies). Premature infants possess considerably less immunocompetence than full-term babies. Table 43-1 details developmental differences in structure and function of the immune system.

Nutritional and Metabolic Factors

Malnutrition has been linked with

- diminished secretory IgA, which decreases the effectiveness of the mucous membrane barrier to infection
- depression of complement proteins, and
- depletion of T-lymphocytes (although B-lymphocytes remain at normal levels) (Feigin and Garg, 1987).

Breast milk supplies the infant with additional IgA that protects secretory surfaces of mucous membranes. Breast feeding, therefore, has been associated with a decreased incidence of upper respiratory, ear, and gastrointestinal infections.

Increased susceptibility to infection is associated with hypoadrenal and hypothyroid states. Steroid administration also alters the immune response by inhibiting the secretion of interleukin-1, and thus decreasing replication and development of "killer" (cytotoxic) T-cells (Fuller, 1985).

Environmental Factors

Environmental factors concern conditions in which exposure to pathogens is increased. These conditions include feeding contaminated formula, poor handwashing among caregivers (including health care professionals), repeated exposure to siblings or adults with frequent infections, day care in settings that allow attendance of infectious children, infrequent bathing, use of contaminated linens and clothing, mouthing of dirty toys, and so on. In addition, climate, weather, air pollution, and other environmental factors are known to affect the presentation and aggravation of allergic symptoms. (See the following section on allergy.)

Anatomic Factors

Breaks in the skin and mucous membranes decrease the competence of these anatomic barriers to infection. This principle underlies the need for extra precautions to prevent infection in children with burns, eczema, and other tissue damage.

Microbial Factors

The normal body flora (nonpathogens) help protect the body from pathogenic organisms. To gain entry into the body, invading bacteria must first "dislodge" the normal flora at a given site, thus when normal flora are present in sufficient numbers it is more difficult for pathogens to gain entry (Fulginiti, 1987). Treatment with broad-spectrum antibiotics, however, is known to kill normal flora along with pathogenic organisms and thereby to depress this protective mechanism. Staphylococci and yeast organisms are particularly likely to invade while normal flora are depressed.

Physiologic Factors

Many physiologic factors provide protection against foreign antigens. Gastric juice is known to kill certain bacteria. The ciliary action of the respiratory tract and the cough reflex help remove organisms and other particles that enter through the upper respiratory tract. Normal urine flow flushes pathogens from the urinary tract. The blood contains bactericidal substances sometimes referred to as "natural antibodies" (Bellanti, 1985). In addition, normal flow of phagocytic cells from the circulation to tissues and onto endothelial surfaces provides a broad surveillance for foreign proteins (Fulginiti, 1987).

Table 43-1. Developmental Differences in Structure and Function of the Immunologic System

Structure and Function	Significance
Organ Structure	
The premature and neonate's skin is thinner and more permeable.	Thinner skin is more vulnerable to skin breakdown, thus destroying the body's first line of passive defense, which places this age group at great risk for infections.
In later childhood lymphoid tissue mass increases.	The increased mass size of tonsils and adenoids is a normal physical finding in the school-age child.
Nonspecific Response	
Neonate demonstrates immaturity of inflammatory response; phagocytic cells have less effective chemotactic (cell movement) activity with immature phagocytic (cell-ingesting) ability. The neonate's complement system is deficient.	Diminished responses of the nonspecific immune system place the neonate at greater risk for infection and allow for more rapid spread of infection leading, potentially, to sepsis. The lessened inflammatory response masks the more common signs and symptoms of infection (i.e., fever), making clinical diagnosis more difficult.
Cell-Mediated Immunity (T-Cell)	
Altered T-cell activity with neonates and stressed infants, i.e., small for gestational age (SGA) and prematures.	Immature and inexperienced immune cells place the neonate and stressed SGA infant at greater risk for viral/bacterial infections. The premature is more vulnerable to infection for a longer time and is less able to mount an appropriate response. Altered T-cell activity may affect neonates' responsiveness to immunizations (i.e., pneumococcal vaccine) Immature or inexperienced cell-mediated responses to certain antigens during first few years of life affect the reliability of delayed hypersensitivity skin reactions. The reliability is influenced by the infants' immature skin and inflammatory response. Therefore the test is not routinely used with infants.
Humoral Immunity (B-Cell)	
IgM, IgE, IgA, IgD, IgG normally at low levels at birth. IgM, IgE, IgA, IgD do not cross the placenta. The immunoglobulins reach adult levels at different ages (Miller, 1988): Immunoglobulin — Age at which serum concentration reaches ≥80% adult level IgM — 9–11 years IgG — 3–5 years IgE — 10–15 years IgA — 12–16 years	Lower immunoglobulin levels place infant and young child at greater risk for bacterial infections. As child's exposure and response to specific antigens become more experienced, the child will develop higher levels and be less vulnerable. Lower IgE level may account for lack of immediate hypersensitivity type allergies in the first 2–3 months of life (Bierman et al, 1988).
IgG crosses placenta and provides protective transmission to infant from mother.	Passive, placental transfer may affect infants' response to active immunization, i.e., pertussis and/or diphtheria. Because of transplacental IgG, most immunodeficiency diseases do not become apparent until 1 month of age (Regelmann et al, 1987). Prematures born less than 30 weeks gestation receive very little IgG from mother and are unable to produce own. This enhances the infection risks for fatal outcomes.

Stress Factors

In recent years both the popular and professional literature have made numerous references to the notion that stress alters immune function and predisposes individuals to such disorders as infection, cancer, and autoimmune diseases. Reviews of relevant research by Fuller (1983) and by Dorian and Garfinkel (1987) support the premise that stress alters immune function. In light of studies showing that immune responses may be either depressed or enhanced at different times in relation to a stressor, Dorian and Garfinkel concluded that stress tends to exert *dysregulatory* effects on immune function. The implication for clinical nursing is that persons under increased physiologic and psychologic stress are likely to experience periods of increased susceptibility to organisms.

Nursing Strategies Related to Factors That Affect Immune Function

To enhance immune function, assessment and analysis of factors that potentiate immunity must be made.

Immune function is compromised when genetic defects, immaturity, nutritional deficiencies, environmental hazards, anatomic and physiologic alterations, depression of normal body flora, or significant physiologic or psychologic stress is present. When the body's own protective responses malfunction or are overtaxed, the plan of care should include the diagnosis *Potential for infection* with implementation of appropriate precautionary measures to reduce transmission of microorganisms.

Altered Immune Response: Autoimmune and Immune-Related Inflammatory Disorders

Autoimmunity is an immune response launched by lymphocytes against the body's own healthy tissues. It represents a failure in the body's ability to recognize "self" versus "nonself." Although several hypotheses have been postulated to account for this untoward immune reaction, the mechanisms resulting in autoimmunity remain largely unexplained. The diseases presented in this section are all thought to be related to altered responses of the immune system.

The disorders in this section are also grouped together because they all involve inflammation of connective tissue. Connective tissue is a fibrous type of tissue that is spread throughout the body. It supports and connects internal organs, forms bones and the walls of blood vessels, attaches muscles to bones, and makes up the scar tissue formed after an injury. Connective tissue contains a protein called collagen, thus disorders of connective tissue are also termed collagen diseases.

Because connective tissue is found everywhere within the body, inflammatory diseases of connective tissue usually involve many tissues and organs and exhibit systemic symptoms. The tissue and organ involvement described in the following disorders varies, but these diseases often involve arthritic involvement of joints, inflammation of blood vessels, and damage to organ tissues.

Systemic Lupus Erythematosus (SLE)

Systemic lupus erythematosus (SLE) is a complex, chronic inflammatory disorder characterized by circulating autoantibodies that affect connective tissue. Because connective tissue is present in the body as fibroelastic, reticular, adipose, and elastic tissue, as well as bone, cartilage, synovial membrane, and the vascular system tissue, multiple systems of the body (including the skin, joints, pleural and pericardial membranes, kidney, and hematologic and nervous systems) may be affected. See Figure 43-4. There seem to be

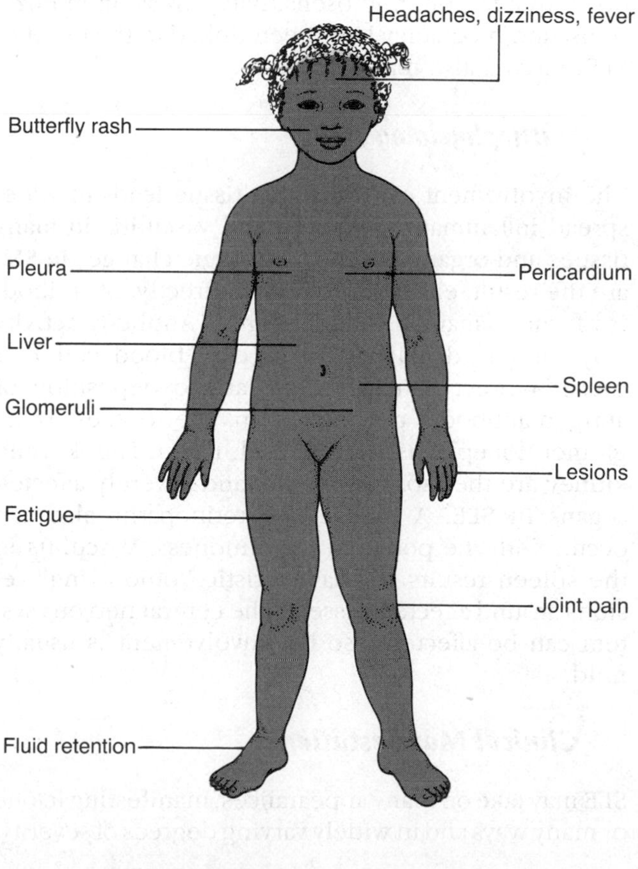

Figure 43-4. Symptoms and sites of pathologic changes in systemic lupus erythematosus.

several different types of lupus, therefore the disease may appear as a trivial problem in one child while in another it is catastrophic (Miller et al, 1986). Typically, remissions and exacerbations occur, and death can result from cardiovascular, renal, or neurologic complications or overwhelming bacterial sepsis.

Affecting approximately 500,000 patients in the United States, lupus is most commonly seen in the second and later decades of life. Twenty per cent of cases of SLE occur in childhood, however, predominantly in females over 8 years of age (Behrman and Vaughan, 1987). All races are affected, but the incidence is approximately three times greater in dark-skinned females (i.e., blacks, Latin Americans, and some native Americans).

Etiology

The etiology of systemic lupus erythematosus is thought to be multifactorial with involvement of immunologic, genetic, environmental, and infectious factors. SLE is considered the prototype for immune complex disease because of the significant defects in both humoral and cell-mediated immunity and in the complement system (Lockey and Bukantz, 1987b).

Support for the genetic theory of cause is found in the high rate of occurrence of SLE in both persons of a pair of monozygotic twins. Environmental causes include medications such as procainamide, hydralazine, anticonvulsants, oral contraceptives, and some antibiotics. In addition, photosensitivity, stress, immunizations, and pregnancy have been linked to the onset of SLE. Viruses also may be a factor.

Pathophysiology

The involvement of connective tissue leads to widespread inflammatory changes and vasculitis in many tissues and organs. All the pathologic changes in SLE are the result, either directly or indirectly, of antibodies formed against "self-antigens." Antibody activity may directly damage tissues (e.g., blood cells) or cause indirect damage secondary to deposition of antigen-antibody complexes in the tissues (e.g., glomerulonephritis) (Miller et al, 1986). The skin and kidney are the most frequently and severely affected organs in SLE. A progressive retinopathy also can occur, with the potential for blindness. Vasculitis in the spleen results in characteristic "onion ring" lesions around affected vessels. The central nervous system can be affected also but involvement is usually mild.

Clinical Manifestations

SLE may take on many appearances, manifesting in one or many ways and in widely varying degrees of severity. As a chronic process, unpredictable exacerbations and remissions of one or more of these manifestations are common.

Although symptoms vary widely, general systemic complaints are frequent at first. A typical presentation for a child with SLE is arthralgia or arthritis, fever, and rashes. Myalgia, malaise, fatigue, and/or weight loss may also occur. During the course of the disease, symptoms may vary in appearance, location, and intensity. A discussion of specific manifestations follows.

Joints/Musculoskeletal. Joint disease is the most common manifestation, appearing in approximately 95 per cent of patients with SLE. In fact, joint discomforts may be the first symptom of active SLE, preceding other signs or symptoms, and may be migratory or rheumatoid-like. The child may have complaints of pain on movement or tenderness, and these complaints may be out of proportion to physical findings. Involvement is symmetric and occurs most commonly in the proximal interphalangeal joints, knees, wrists, and metacarpophalangeal joints. Effusions also may be seen. Rheumatoid nodules may appear with disease exacerbations and disappear when disease activity is suppressed. Deformities of fingers may appear, but permanent joint changes are rare.

Myalgias (muscle pains) are seen in about 25 per cent of patients with SLE. When they occur, they are most common in proximal muscles. Muscle weakness also may be noted, but this is relatively rare.

Skin. Skin and mucous membranes are frequent targets of SLE. The lesions include rashes, erythematous macules, photosensitivity, oral ulcerations, and alopecia. The skin of the patient with SLE typically is photosensitive; exposure to bright sunlight and other sources of ultraviolet radiation, especially if prolonged, can precipitate skin eruptions and serious vital organ involvement.

The classic butterfly rash was first described by Hebra in 1845. It is an erythematous rash distributed across the bridge of the nose and cheeks, seen in approximately 50 per cent of patients (Fig. 43-5). A similar rash may appear on the palmar surface of the hands and the soles, as well as on the chest.

Discoid lesions occur in approximately 15 per cent of patients. Beginning as a small area of erythematous plaque or a papule, the lesions spread outward and leave a hyperkeratotic area with follicular plugging and atrophy.

Vasculitic lesions with ulceration, purpuric lesions, and subcutaneous nodules also may be seen on the hands and arms. Vasculitis may be found as periungual (around the nails) erythema and spider hemorrhages. Livedo reticularis (a mottled discoloration of the skin) is common in these patients, especially when exposed to cold. Other cutaneous lesions less frequently observed include periorbital edema, bullous lesions, and ulcerations of the buccal mucosa.

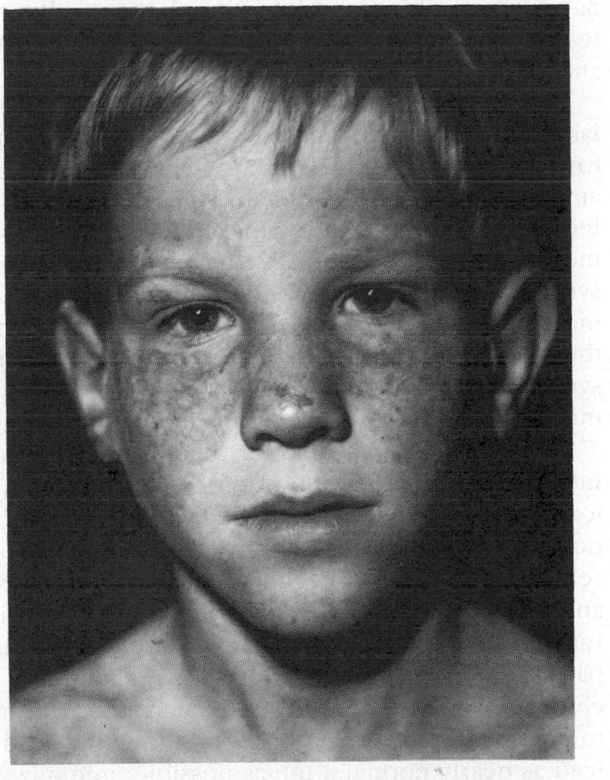

Figure 43-5. Discoid lupus erythematosus with typical butterfly distribution, atrophy, and depigmentation of skin. (Courtesy of Dr. L. Schweich. From Kelley W, et al: *Textbook of Rheumatology.* Philadelphia, WB Saunders, 1981.)

Alopecia (loss of hair) is a common feature of patients, occurring in about 65 per cent of patients with SLE, particularly in periods of active systemic disease. This occurs as patchy losses rather than total loss. Hair may become thin and brittle, prone to breaking.

Renal. Renal involvement is present in 50 to 70 per cent of children with SLE and is potentially the most life-threatening complication. Nephrotic syndrome and glomerulonephritis (see Chapter 42) are the forms of renal disease typically seen. Symptoms are usually noted early in the disease and include microscopic hematuria, proteinuria, and increased urinary sediment. These may vary from one urine specimen to the next and do not necessarily accurately reflect disease activity. Increased serum creatinine and decreased creatinine clearance reflect renal insufficiency. Other manifestations of renal disease include edema (secondary to sodium and water retention), weight gain, and hypertension.

Gastrointestinal. Recurrent abdominal pain is a common complaint in children with lupus; its cause is often unclear. Pancreatitis and serositis may be responsible for some of this discomfort, but it also may result from irritation caused by medications. Sepsis must be considered if these complaints occur with fever.

Pulmonary. Pleurisy and pleural effusion are the most common pulmonary manifestations of SLE. Pulmonary function tests are characteristically abnormal. The child may be dyspneic due to the pain associated with breathing. Effusions are not usually large and on chest films usually are seen as streaky lesions at the base of the affected lung. Because of defective immunologic function, as well as the immunosuppressive medications prescribed, pneumonia is relatively common. Symptoms include a nonproductive cough, fever, and rales.

Cardiac/Cardiovascular. Cardiovascular symptoms are seen in more than 50 per cent of lupus patients. Pericarditis, the most frequent cardiac manifestation, occurs in approximately 25 per cent. Its presence may vary from a transient friction rub to a pericardial effusion. The child may complain of substernal or precordial pain. Murmurs, persistent tachycardia, and transient dysrhythmias may be noted. Pleural and pericardial effusions may be seen repeatedly when disease activity flares. Congestive heart failure may be the presenting indication of myocarditis.

Cardiovascular manifestations may present in a number of ways. Raynaud syndrome may be seen; in this condition vasoconstriction occurs in peripheral vessels in response to cold or emotional stress. Distal portions of fingers and toes may appear blue while proximal portions appear to have more normal circulation. Gangrene may result from decreased circulation, possibly with loss of digits.

Hematologic. Nearly all children with SLE have one or more hematologic abnormalities, including anemia, leukopenia (neutropenia and most commonly lymphopenia), and thrombocytopenia. A prolonged partial thromboplastin time (PTT) may be found, as a result of antibodies to phospholipid antigens. Circulating lupus anticoagulants also cause a false-positive test for syphilis. Other hematologic findings, in varying frequency of occurrence, include positive LE cells, antinuclear antibodies (ANA), and rheumatoid factor (RF).

Eye. Conjunctivitis is frequently an initial symptom. Other parts of the eye affected by inflammation include the sclera, uveal tract, and the retina. Fundoscopic examination may reveal cytoid bodies (white fluffy patches) in the retina. These inflammatory processes are usually associated with the acute disease and do not result in visual impairment.

Central Nervous System. CNS symptoms can be divided into three groups: organic disorder secondary to CNS lupus, toxic disorder secondary to medications, and behavioral disorder as a reaction to the diagnosis.

Organic Disorder. Symptoms include irritability, depression, headache, lethargy, dizziness, seizures, hallucinations, loss of orientation to time and place, ataxia, cranial nerve palsies, chorea, and, rarely, coma.

The headache may be one of the presenting symptoms and generally subsides as disease activity remits. Like a migraine, these headaches may begin with a visual aura. In general, headaches in lupus are not cause for concern. However, it must be determined that they are not an indication of hypertension, increased intracranial pressure, or an adverse effect of medication.

Toxic Disorder. Corticosteroids are part of the primary treatment regimen for SLE. However, they lower the threshold for seizure and may also precipitate personality changes, depression, or euphoria. It is important to determine whether these occur because they are medication-induced behavior changes or CNS changes resulting from disease activity.

Behavioral Disorder. Depression may be a reaction to being told one has SLE. Denial also may be a compensatory coping mechanism.

Lymphoid System. Hepatomegaly is common in children with SLE. This is not directly correlated with disease activity, as is the more prominent splenomegaly. Generalized lymphadenopathy may also occur.

Diagnostic Assessment

The criteria established in 1971 by the American Rheumatism Association were designed to classify or identify patients with a diagnosis of SLE more clearly. New serologic systems were recognized, indicating the need for the revisions made in 1982 (Box 43-1). Serologic tests that reveal LE cells or antinuclear antibodies (ANA) provide a clear-cut diagnosis since these are relatively specific for lupus. However, SLE rarely makes a dramatic presentation with all or a majority of symptoms present at any given time. Rather, the symptoms usually unfold episodically over time. Therefore, diagnosis is based on a group of overt symptoms and confirmed by serologic, histopathologic, and other laboratory findings. As indicated in Box 43-1, patient identification is made if any four or more of the 11 diagnostic criteria are present, serially or simultaneously, during any period of observation.

Therapeutic Management

Death is no longer a "given" expectation when a diagnosis of SLE is made. Although a significant portion of the patients have systemic involvement and do die, advances in early diagnosis, intervention, and ongoing care have made it possible to anticipate a relatively normal lifestyle, albeit with restrictions, precautions, and monitoring. The goals of the care are control of symptoms, minimizing or preventing exacerbations of systemic symptoms and complications, and promotion of as nearly normal a lifestyle as possible. With coordinated efforts of a broad interdisciplinary health care team and the cooperation and compliance of the child and family, this goal is not unrealistic.

There is no "protocol" for treating the diagnostic label SLE. Treatment must be flexible and directed toward specific problems of a specific patient during any given time of disease activity. The intensity and length of therapy depend on the clinical and laboratory measures of disease. The patient with mild or no overt symptoms of active SLE may be managed with regular monitoring but no medication. At the other extreme, the child with gradually increasing or sudden onset of symptoms must be treated quickly and aggressively to minimize the potential for permanent tissue damage.

The components of drug therapy include anti-inflammatory and immunosuppressive agents, cytotoxic drugs, and antimalarial medications. Prophylactic measures for managing aspects, such as photosensitivity and general health measures, including rest and diet, are important. Patient and family education (as a medical-nursing ongoing team effort) is a critical part of the management of lupus. A regimen that includes any or all of these components must be geared to control the disease in order to allow the child to lead as nearly normal a life as possible, minimize or prevent scarring, which can result from extensive inflammation, and minimize or prevent serious side effects of the medications.

Aspirin and other nonsteroidal anti-inflammatory drugs (NSAIDs) are used to control arthritis and arthralgias, serositis, and fevers. When a fever occurs, great caution must be taken in ruling out the possibility of infection as a cause of the fever. If aspirin is ineffective in reducing or eliminating these symptoms or is poorly tolerated, other NSAIDs can be selected, such as ibuprofen and tolmetin.

If rash or other cutaneous lesions occur that are not responsive to aspirin therapy, antimalarial drugs such as hydroxychloroquine may be used. Because of its ability to diminish penetration of ultraviolet light, this is the drug of choice for the child who is photosensitive as well. Regular eye examinations every 6 to 8 months are important for the child on antimalarial agents because of the progressive retinopathy that may be induced by these drugs.

For patients who do not respond to aspirin, NSAIDs, or antimalarial drugs, or who have involvement of other major organ systems (e.g., hematologic, CNS, renal), steroids are necessary. These have both anti-inflammatory and immunosuppressive functions. Dosage and route may vary, from maintenance doses of prednisone every other day to high-dose steroids in divided doses several times a day, to "pulse" doses (high-dose intravenous administration) to interrupt or control severe exacerbations. When symptoms have been controlled and the child has been asymptomatic

Box 43-1
*The 1982 Revised Criteria for Classification of SLE**

1. MALAR RASH:

Fixed erythema, flat or raised, over the malar eminences, tending to spare the nasolabial folds

2. DISCOID RASH:

Erythematous raised patches with adherent keratotic scaling and follicular plugging: atrophic scarring may occur in older lesions

3. PHOTOSENSITIVITY:

Skin rash as a result of unusual reaction to sunlight, by patient history or physician observation

4. ORAL ULCERS:

Oral or nasopharyngeal ulceration, usually painless, observed by a physician

5. ARTHRITIS:

Nonerosive arthritis involving two or more peripheral joints, characterized by tenderness, swelling, or effusion

6. SEROSITIS:

a) Pleuritis—convincing history of pleuritic pain or rub heard by a physician or evidence of pleural effusion
OR
b) Pericarditis—documented by ECG or rub or evidence of pericardial effusion

7. RENAL DISORDER:

a) Persistent proteinuria greater than 0.5 gram per day or greater than 3+ if quantitation not performed
OR
b) Cellular casts—may be red cell, hemoglobin, granular, tubular, or mixed

8. NEUROLOGIC DISORDER:

a) Seizures—in the absence of offending drugs or known metabolic derangements; e.g., uremia, ketoacidosis, or electrolyte imbalance
OR
b) Psychosis—in the absence of offending drugs or known metabolic derangements, e.g., uremia, ketoacidosis, or electrolyte imbalance

9. HEMATOLOGIC DISORDER:

a) Hemolytic anemia—with reticulocytosis
OR
b) Leukopenia—less than 4000/mm^3 total on two or more occasions
OR
c) Lymphopenia—less than 1500/mm^3 on two or more occasions
OR
d) Thrombocytopenia—less than 100,000/mm^3 in the absence of offending drugs

10. IMMUNOLOGIC DISORDER:

a) Positive LE cell preparation
OR
b) Anti-DNA: antibody to native DNA in abnormal titer
OR
c) Anti-Sm: presence of antibody to Sm nuclear antigen
OR
d) False-positive serologic test for syphilis known to be positive for at least 6 months and confirmed by *Treponema pallidum* immobilization or fluorescent treponemal antibody absorption test

11. ANTINUCLEAR ANTIBODY:

An abnormal titer of antinuclear antibody by immunofluorescence or an equivalent assay at any point in time and in the absence of drugs known to be associated with "drug-induced lupus" syndrome

* For the purpose of identifying patients in clinical studies, a person shall be said to have systemic lupus erythematosus if any 4 or more of the 11 criteria are present, serially or simultaneously, during any interval of observation.
(From Tan et al, 1982.)

for a period of time, a carefully designed "tapering" schedule can begin. Attention must always be given to the possibility of infection that may be masked by steroid administration. Table 43-2 is a Nursing Process Plan for the child on corticosteroid therapy (see page 1597).

Cytotoxic drugs, particularly azathioprine, may be given to intervene in progressive renal disease. These drugs, especially in combination with steroids, have been shown to delay or interrupt lupus nephritis. When disease progression has been stabilized, these drugs may be tapered to minimal maintenance doses.

Major Nursing Diagnoses for SLE

Potential impaired physical mobility, *related to joint inflammation*
Potential altered cardiac output: decreased, *related to inflammation of the pericardium*
Potential altered tissue perfusion: peripheral, *related to abnormal vasoconstriction*
Potential altered patterns of urinary elimination, *related to inflammatory changes in glomerular capillaries*

Potential altered thought processes, *related to*

- *organic changes associated with inflammatory processes of the central nervous system*
- *behavioral changes associated with the impact of the diagnosis*
- *toxic changes associated with steroid therapy*

Potential impaired skin integrity, *related to*

- *rash*
- *discoid lesions*
- *impaired circulation*
- *photosensitivity*

Potential for injury: physiologic, *related to untoward effects of medications*

Potential for infection, *related to alterations in humoral and cell-mediated immunity and in complement proteins*

Disturbance in self-concept: body image, self-esteem, role performance, *related to*

- *physical signs and symptoms*
- *social/emotional impact of the disease*
- *changes in physical appearance associated with administration of corticosteroids*

Potential ineffective coping: individual/family, *related to the impact of a chronic and potentially debilitating disease*

Knowledge deficit, *related to home care*

Strategies for Nursing Care

Physical, psychologic, and emotional assessments and interventions are essential to quality nursing care of the child with SLE and of the child's family. Ongoing teaching and support at a level commensurate with the child's stage of growth and development are equally vital components of care, with the goal of increased knowledge about the disease, its management and prognosis, relief of unrealistic fear, and promotion of participation in and compliance with the regimen of care.

Managing Joint Inflammation

Painful and swollen joints are one of the most frequent presenting symptoms. As therapy is begun and therapeutic serum levels of aspirin or other NSAIDs are obtained, any objective or subjective changes should be noted. Effectiveness of medications can be monitored by changes of comfort levels with movement of fingers, elbows, ankles, and toes. Early signs of exacerbations may be noted by increases in discomfort or swelling. A physical therapist can help develop an exercise program that includes range-of-motion exercises, positioning of joints to prevent contractures, and activities to maintain strength and endurance. As the most consistent contact in the health care team, the nurse can help the child practice and reinforce these "routines," explain their rationale, and encourage the child and/or family to participate actively in this aspect of maintaining "normality."

The nurse may also ask an occupational therapist to recommend appropriate activities to facilitate a physical therapy program. Such a program will accommodate any decrease in energy level and increased need for rest, while being responsive to the needs and tasks appropriate to the child's stage of growth and development.

A medication regimen should be developed to maximize effectiveness of medications while minimizing interruptions in rest times or activities (both therapeutic and recreational). In addition, warm baths may be helpful in reducing pain associated with inflamed joints.

Assessing Cardiovascular/Peripheral Vascular Status

Cardiovascular assessments should detect possible indications of carditis, which has a potential for permanent damage. Tachycardia, possible dysrhythmias, pericardial rub, complaints of chest pain, lethargy, and perhaps dyspnea all suggest a change in cardiac status. As noted, changes in cardiac function can lead to congestive heart failure. Daily weight measurements may provide early indication of congestive failure. If cardiac function changes significantly, the pumping action of the heart and, subsequently, vascular sufficiency may be compromised. The picture may be further complicated if Raynaud phenomenon is present. Therefore, thorough cardiovascular and pulmonary assessments are important components of routine evaluations of the child with SLE. These should include heart sounds, rate, and rhythm; breath sounds and respiratory rate; and evaluation of the vascular status of the extremities. Hands and feet should be protected from the cold to facilitate circulation.

Monitoring Renal Function

Deterioration of renal function is the most significant potential complication. Early detection of renal compromise is essential to minimize or prevent permanent renal damage and, ultimately, failure. A 24-hour urine collection for creatinine clearance will indicate adequacy of or changes in renal function. Routine evaluations of urine should include tests for hematuria, proteinuria, increased urine sediment, and casts—all measures of adequate kidney function. Other symptoms of renal involvement are hypertension and weight gain. Nursing assessment for adequate renal function, therefore, should include monitoring blood pressure, intake and output, daily weight, and laboratory reports, in addition to routine evaluations of urine specimens. Patients with SLE are also more susceptible to urinary tract infections, which present as increased frequency and pain or burning on urination. If infection is severe, hematuria may be seen. One of the adverse effects of cytotoxic drug therapy is hemorrhagic cystitis. If hematuria is noted, therefore, its cause must be identified and treated.

Managing CNS Alterations

Central nervous system involvement can be a very frustrating and depressing aspect of SLE for the patient. Although the etiology of the headaches, anxiety, mood swings, mental confusion, disorientation, personality changes, chorea, or seizures may be either organic or psychologic, steroid therapy is usually effective management. However, if the patient is already on steroids, it may be difficult to distinguish between exacerbation of the illness with CNS involvement and a steroid-induced psychiatric disorder. It is important for the nurse to assess and document actions and interactions carefully, particularly as they relate to medication administration, environmental factors, or other symptoms that might signal increased disease activity (see also Table 43-2).

Both the patient and family need to be helped to understand that once the systemic illness is under control, the symptoms will most likely disappear. However, these are frightening symptoms for the child (especially if he or she is an adolescent) and family; building and encouraging an ongoing, trusting relationship between members of the health care team and the child and family is an important aspect of care.

Regular assessment of neurologic status is important. Appropriate precautions should be taken for any indication of seizures. Chorea also may occur as one of the neurologic symptoms. The child with chorea needs to be protected from injury and given physical assistance with whatever basic tasks may be difficult or impossible to perform. Both the child and family need to hear that these uncontrollable movements are not permanent nor do they impair intellectual abilities.

Preventing Injury to Integument

Skin integrity may be compromised as a result of rashes (especially if pruritic, causing the child to scratch) or discoid lesions or as a result of impaired circulation to extremities. Monitor any increase of rash or lesions and further decreases in vascular competence. Fingers and toes will become numb and painful if exposed to cold. Socks, gloves, and warm, layered clothing will help encourage peripheral circulation and provide warmth and protection. Tight clothing should be avoided. The nurse must be alert to early evidence of infections either in lesion sites or as the result of scratching. If erythema, induration, or pustules occur, the physician is informed and treatment begun

Monitoring Medication Therapy

The effects of medication, both therapeutic and adverse, are also important assessments. Some are effective in a brief time, whereas others (e.g., hydroxychloroquine) require several weeks to take effect. As a mainstay of therapy, aspirin may have adverse effects such as gastritis, tinnitus, or increased bleeding when platelet competency may be already compromised by the disease process. Documentation of the positive effects of steroids must be made, but the nurse needs to be aware of their side effects, some of which may be difficult to distinguish from the disease manifestations. Hypertension, irritability, capillary fragility, and depression may be characteristic of both. Therefore, awareness of both the individual child's symptoms as well as any changes, especially as they relate to possible undesired responses to medications, is important.

Preventing Infection

Any child with an altered immune response has an increased potential for infection. Susceptibility for the child with SLE is related specifically to genetic, anatomic, physiologic, metabolic, and microbial factors. It is thought that at least some of the immune defects of cellular and humoral immunity are linked to genetic inheritance. Anatomically, the child is at risk during periods of skin involvement that cause a break in this barrier to infection. Physiologically, the decreased B-cell function may affect the normal antibody protection of the genitourinary system, and renal complications may alter normal urine flow that tends to flush out bacteria. Metabolic factors include steroid administration, which further alters the immune response. Microbial factors may be involved during periods of antibiotic administration for systemic infection. The nurse (and family) must be alert to signs and symptoms of overgrowth of nonsusceptible bacteria.

The child's immune competence can be bolstered by insurance of adequate calories consumed in a balanced diet. The importance of good handwashing in reducing the spread of infection cannot be overemphasized. The child and all family members should be taught proper handwashing techniques. In addition, the family will need guidance about the mode of transmission of common cold and flu viruses so that they can adequately protect the child without being unduly restrictive.

Teaching to Support Home Care

The overall goals for teaching and support are to help the child and family gain confidence in their abilities to manage this chronic illness and to know when to "call for help."

Understanding the Disease Process. Patients and families need to learn about SLE, its cause(s), its course and prognosis, therapeutic aims, and general health care. General knowledge and expectations about the course of SLE have changed a great deal in the last several years. Many people may know little or nothing about the disease; others may have distorted, outdated knowledge that carries with it an overwhelming hopelessness. Some aspects of the disease process may be frightening; some are frustrating because there are no definite answers. Therefore, it is important to assess the levels of knowledge and stress and begin teaching at a level where the child and family can hear and understand. An important first step is for the child and family to *begin* to verbalize their fears and anxieties, as well as their knowledge and self-confidence in their abilities to manage this chronic illness.

Administering Medications. Explaining clearly the types and doses of medications prescribed, their purpose, side effects that might be anticipated, and an appropriate schedule is important. Indeed, maximal efficacy of any drug program depends on a general knowledge base, and the more understanding there is, the greater the likelihood of compliance. The child and family must know the side effects of medications and realize that some of these are difficult to distinguish from symptoms of the disease process. They should be instructed to inform their physician of any of these unusual occurrences rather than try to determine cause and effect themselves. They should also be reminded that if antimalarials are part of the medication regimen, regular eye examinations are important, even after the medication has been discontinued. Discussion of the administration procedure for steroids will help the patient and family understand dosage variations and the rationale for a dramatically increased dosage with subsequent slow tapering. Steroids also may be used topically for skin and scalp lesions. (See also Table 43-2.)

Testing Urine. When renal involvement is a component of the disease process, steroids will most likely be part of the medication regimen. Diet, then, becomes an important issue for teaching for both these factors. Fluid retention occurs in patients taking steroids. With renal compromise and fluid retention due to medications, the child and family need to be taught the need for low-sodium, low-protein foods. A dietitian may be helpful as a resource and facilitator.

Monitoring renal involvement requires that the child and family be instructed about urine testing. Simple observation may be all that is necessary if kidney disease is not a current issue. Any changes in appearance (e.g., increased sedimentation) or amount that cannot be directly attributed to fluid intake should be reported to the physician. If monitoring for proteinuria or hematuria is indicated, the nurse can teach the child and family to use and read one of the commercial dipsticks for urine testing. Weekly weights (or more often if there is concern) are a good indicator of renal ability to regulate body fluid. Any sudden weight gain needs to be reported.

Limiting Exposure to Ultraviolet Rays. Photosensitivity may not be a problem at the time of diagnosis, but it may appear at any point so is an issue for discussion with the patient and family. Exposure to sunlight is not necessarily totally avoided, but because of the potential for serious systemic exacerbations caused by ultraviolet rays, exposure should be limited. To minimize exposure, the patient should be fully clothed (including a hat) when outdoors in bright, intense sunlight and should use sunscreening lotions or ointments containing para-aminobenzoic acid (PABA) on exposed skin surfaces.

Obtaining Adequate Rest. Rest is a significant component of care for the child with SLE. Unfortunately, it is frequently either forgotten or ignored. Energy levels are usually much lower when a child is ill, and this is also true of the child with SLE. *Increased fatigue, stress, and anxiety can trigger exacerbations* of the disease process; therefore, the nurse helps the child and family formulate a schedule that allows for adequate uninterrupted rest. It should also be remembered that inflexible adherence to such a schedule also may create anxiety, which is counterproductive. It is important to encourage reasonable flexibility for plans and expectations.

Recognizing Potential Complications. Some symptoms are "signals" for concern that the child and family need to know about. When the child has a fever; chills; abdominal, chest, or joint pain; urine changes; or undue fatigue, the physician should be notified. Doubts or concerns should be shared with either the nurse or the physician for validation.

Discussing Family Planning. For the adolescent patient, some discussion of the relationship between SLE, contraceptives, and pregnancy may be indicated. Because female sex hormones appear to accelerate autoimmune disease (Miller et al, 1986), mechanical modes of contraception are recommended instead of oral contraceptives. Pregnancy is not absolutely contraindicated in the patient with SLE, especially if the disease is quiescent. However, pregnancy and delivery can precipitate a flare, including nephritis, which can present an unpredictable hazard for both mother and child. Therefore, the anticipation of pregnancy should be discussed in depth, and progress through it should be closely monitored by a physician who is aware of the disease process and its potential hazards. For the nurse, the patient, and the family, these discussions may be difficult and uncomfortable. But they are important aspects of the teaching process for adolescent patients as they anticipate these steps of growth and development.

Enhancing Self-Concept. Unsightly rashes, joint pain, fatigue, changes in body weight distribution, and a cushingoid appearance that may result from medications all may affect self-image. In addition, photophobia may inhibit many outdoor activities. Some suggestions the nurse can make to enable the child or adolescent to feel like one of the crowd and acceptable to self are use of hypoallergenic cosmetics to cover rashes, pacing of activities to keep fatigue at bay, choosing various styles of clothing that can help camouflage some weight gain, and structuring outdoor activities in early morning or evening hours.

Promoting Adaptation

Ongoing emotional support, in sickness and in health, for the child and family will be an important aspect of nursing care. They will likely have many questions, fears, anxieties, angers, and frustrations. The nurse is a primary source for information, comfort, and care and can respond to many of the physical, emotional, and educational needs that exist and will continue to evolve for these patients and families. The nurse can also refer them to community resources and support groups. Some of these include the Arthritis Foundation, the American Lupus Society, and various published materials (videos and written) for patients and families. (See Appendix Eight.)

Nursing Strategies for Follow-up Care in the Home or Clinic

Assess musculoskeletal integrity for evidence of joint involvement.

Assess cardiovascular status, including peripheral pulses. Determine whether there have been recent changes in the child's stamina.

Determine whether urinary output (number of wet diapers, number of voids per day) has changed. Obtain a urine sample, as indicated, for evidence of glomerular changes or infection.

Assess mental status with age-appropriate techniques (see Chapter 15).

Assess skin integrity. Determine incidence of photosensitivity and counsel about limiting exposure to the sun.

Determine compliance with medication therapy and assess for side effects.

Encourage the child to talk about activities of daily living, including social interactions, to assess self-concept. Ask the parents about the child's self-esteem, body image, and comfort with role.

Encourage the child and parents to express their feelings about the disease and the ways in which it interferes with individual and family functioning.

Supply information needed for problem solving. Refer for additional support.

Juvenile Arthritis

Juvenile rheumatoid arthritis (JRA) is the term applied to inflammatory arthritis in children. Since 1977, there has been controversy about the title given this disorder. In 1973, a committee was appointed by the Arthritis Foundation to review the criteria for nomenclature and classification of arthritis found in children. This committee determined that the title JRA should be retained. However, this disorder is *not* simply a childhood version of the rheumatoid arthritis found in adults. Based on studies and the accumulation of statistics reported from centers where these children are diagnosed and cared for, there is only a 5 to 6 per cent correlation (clinically and serologically) between arthritic children and adults with *rheumatoid* arthritis. We join the movement to designate this childhood inflammatory process as simply juvenile arthritis (JA) and will so designate this disorder within this chapter.

Arthritis is defined by the American Rheumatology Association as joint swelling or restriction of motion, with pain, tenderness, or heat. Pain and tenderness alone are not enough to diagnose JA. Juvenile arthritis is a systemic disorder of connective tissue, joints, and viscera and includes several arthritis-like manifestations that are designated into three onset types: systemic onset, pauciarticular onset, and polyarticular onset. The onset type is determined by the manifestations during the first 6 months of illness. Although symptoms resembling another type may appear later, the type that was present during the initial 6 months remains the designated type of JA for a particular patient. The course of the disease is marked by remissions and exacerbations.

Each subtype of juvenile arthritis has its defining characteristic and prognosis.

- Systemic-onset JA is defined by the presence of a recurrent intermittent high fever (103°F and above). The rheumatoid rash and other organ involvement may or may not also be present.
- Pauciarticular-onset JA is defined by the presence of arthritis in fewer than five joints.
- Polyarticular-onset JA is defined as the presence of arthritis in more than four joints.

Patients whose diagnosis is systemic-onset JA are excluded from the latter two types.

Although the cause of juvenile arthritis remains unknown and there are no criteria for accurate prediction of outcome in an individual patient, the outlook for most children with this disorder is good. For some children the condition will be chronic. But approximately 75 per cent of children emerge 10 to 15 years after onset to lead normal lives without crippling (Brewer, 1986). In addition, studies have shown that these young adults fare as well as or better than their siblings in educational level, marriage, childbearing, and income (Miller, 1982).

Etiology and Incidence

Research studies continue to identify causes for juvenile arthritis, but the etiology remains unclear. Several theories have been postulated, including the relationship among JA, infections, and an autoimmune response. Although their relationship to JA remains unclear, several factors, including upper respiratory infections and trauma, may precipitate this inflammatory process. Genetic factors (HLA type) are also suspected (Bellanti, 1985).

Statistics are incomplete but, based on those available, the prevalence of juvenile arthritis appears to be approximately 0.5 per 1000 children. Oriental children seem to be less affected than Anglo-American children. It appears that fewer black than white children are affected.

Objective onset of juvenile arthritis may occur as early as 6 weeks of age; however, in general, the age of onset occurs between the ages of 2 and 16 years. Each of the onset types appears to have its own characteristic incidence, just as it has its own characteristic areas of symptoms and degree of involvement (Table 43-3). Thirty per cent of children with JA have systemic-onset JA. It occurs often around 10 years of age; girls are affected slightly more often than boys. Approximately 25 per cent of children with JA have polyarticular-onset JA. In this group more than twice as many girls as boys are affected, and symptoms usually appear after 10 years of age. The remaining 45 per cent of children with JA have the pauciarticular-onset type and are most commonly girls under age 10 years (Brewer, 1986).

Pathophysiology

The inflammatory process of juvenile arthritis may begin insidiously, being almost unnoticeable, or may appear as sudden joint swelling that might cause one to suspect trauma. Swelling is caused by inflammation of the synovial membranes and the adjacent joint capsule. Inflammation of the synovial tissues causes increased secretions of joint fluids. As this fluid volume increases it causes swollen, boggy joints and is termed *joint effusion*. The joints are edematous and feel warm to the touch. The normally clear joint fluid becomes cloudy as it is infiltrated with lymphocytes and plasma cells. Pain and stiffness result from the pressure on sensory nerves in the area. In later stages of JA, stiffness and limited mobility may result from joint destruction or contractures.

Villi of the inflamed synovium may begin to protrude into the joint spaces. As this process spreads, they may adhere to and subsequently erode the articular cartilage. Children may have long periods of synovitis before permanent joint damage occurs. "Once joint

Table 43-3. Classification of Juvenile Arthritis

	Incidence		
Mode of Onset	Age (Years)	Sex F:M	Prognosis
Systemic (30% of all JRA cases)	10	1.5:1 F:M	All JA mortality is in this group (1%–2% of all JRA patients); 40% evidence of joint destruction
Polyarticular (>4 joints) (<25% of all JRA cases)			Mortality—0; duration longer; more crippling; 25% remission
Subtype 1. (RF+)	>10	mostly female	
Subtype 2. (RF−)			Less crippling than RF+
Pauciarticular (<5 joints) (45% of all JRA cases)	<10	6:1 F:M	Continuous—25%. Arthritis rarely erosive, 5-year remission 60%
Subtype 1. (iritis)	<10	almost all girls	10%—functional blindness 55%—acute 45%—chronic
Subtype 2. (HLA-B27+)	>10	1:9 F:M	Possible juvenile ankylosing spondylitis later
Subtype 3. (Arthritis only)			Best outlook for recovery

(From Brewer, 1986)

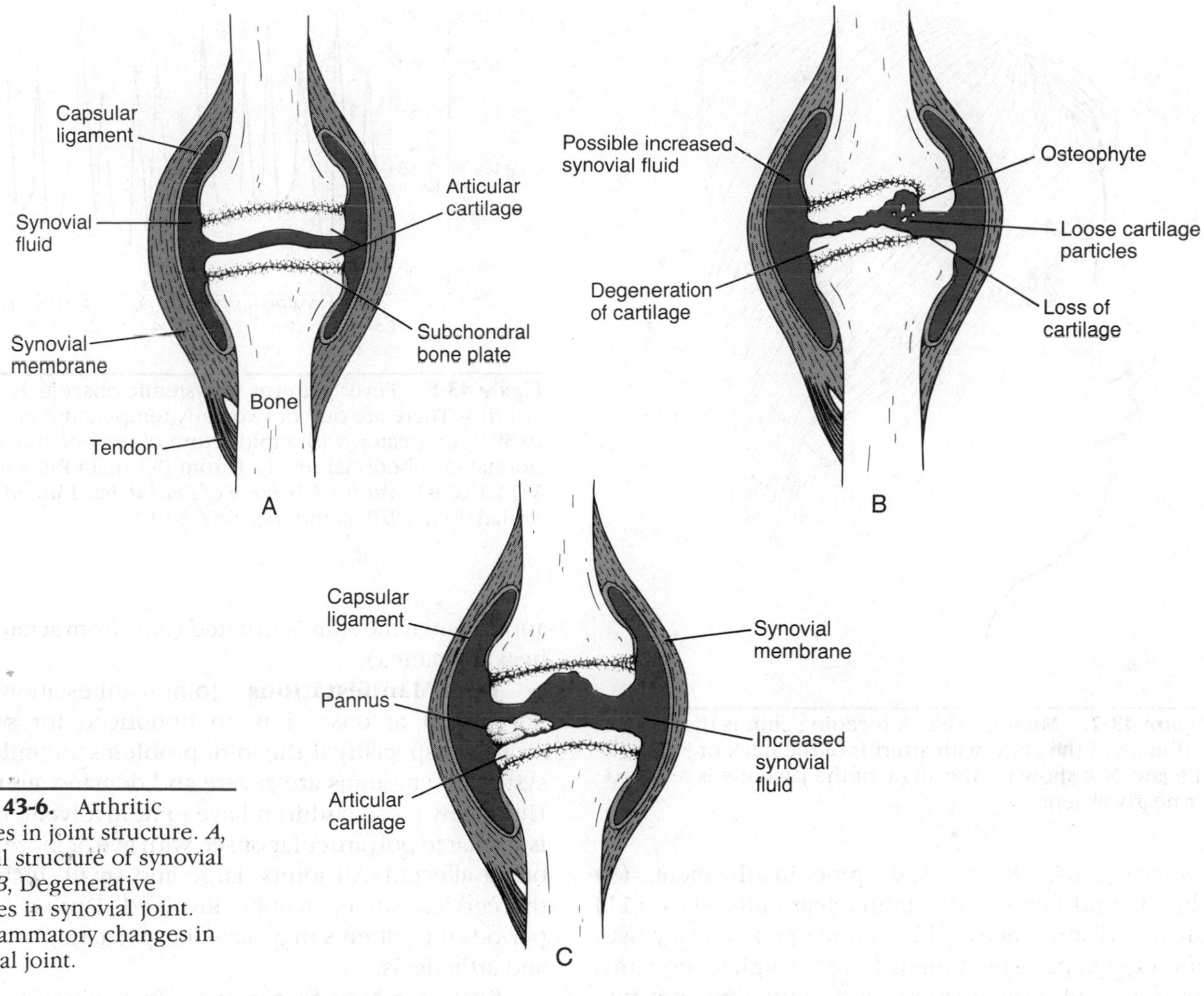

Figure 43-6. Arthritic changes in joint structure. *A,* Normal structure of synovial joint. *B,* Degenerative changes in synovial joint. *C,* Inflammatory changes in synovial joint.

destruction has commenced, erosions of subchondral bone, narrowing of the joint spaces (loss of articular cartilage), destruction of fusion of bones, and deformity, subluxation, or ankylosis of joints may result" (Schaller and Wedgwood, 1983). See Figure 43-6.

Other pathologic changes which may occur as the result of the inflammatory process include serositis of the pleura, pericardium, and peritoneum. The rash that may be seen in systemic-onset juvenile arthritis occurs as the result of a mild vasculitis in the subepithelial tissues. Fever, loss of appetite, weight loss, fatigue, and generalized weakness also may be associated with systemic inflammation.

Inflammation of the iris and ciliary body of the eye, termed anterior uveitis or iridocyclitis, may occur. Uveitis is a serious and frequent complication in young girls with pauciarticular onset. Typically this inflammatory process is asymptomatic, but eye pain and diminished vision have been reported. Whereas some cases of iridocyclitis are acute in nature and respond to topical corticosteroids or are self-limiting, about 70 per cent of children with this type of inflammation have a chronic relapsing course with resulting visual impairment (Petty, 1987).

Growth disturbances may result from generalized growth retardation associated with chronic childhood illness, including overgrowth or undergrowth around the affected joints, localized effects of inflammation on the epiphyseal growth, and growth failure of the mandible (micrognathia, Fig. 43-7).

Clinical Manifestations

Arthritis may be a manifestation of many different diseases, including systemic lupus erythematosus, rheumatic fever, and dermatomyositis. However, each of these has its own characteristic rash and diagnostic laboratory data. No specific diagnostic laboratory tests are available for juvenile arthritis. Tests such as rheumatoid factor, antinuclear antibodies, and HLA antigens can be used to help classify the different types of JA. However, the diagnosis of JA is made only after many other diseases have been ruled out.

JA has many signs and symptoms. Some are general and occur in all three types whereas others are characteristic of one specific onset type. The signs and symptoms include (1) fever, (2) rash, (3) iridocyclitis, (4) cardiac involvement, (5) nodules, (6) stiffness, (7)

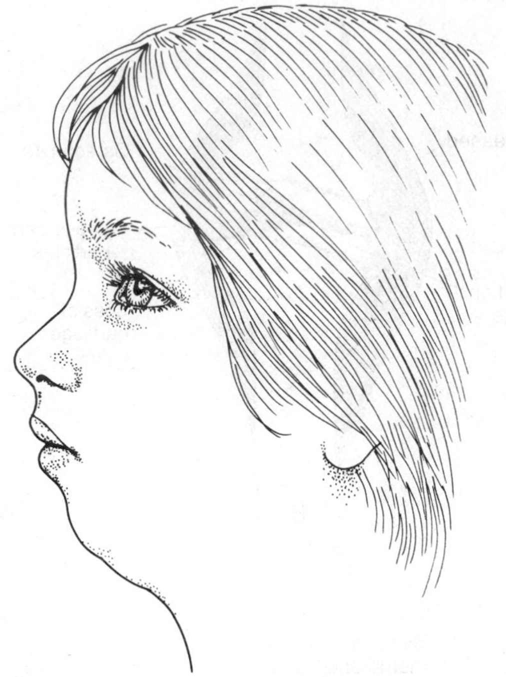

Figure 43-7. Micrognathia. A receding chin is the hallmark of the child with arthritis of the neck or joints of the jaw. Not shown—the angle of the jawbone is reduced or nearly absent.

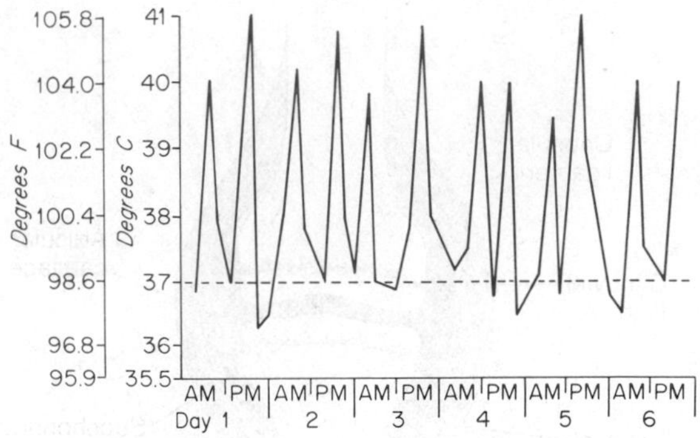

Figure 43-8. Fever patterns in systemic-onset juvenile arthritis. There are one or two daily temperature elevations to 39°C or greater, with rapid return of temperature to normal or subnormal levels. (From Behrman RE, Vaughan VC III (eds): *Nelson Textbook of Pediatrics.* 13th ed. Philadelphia, WB Saunders, 1987, 520.)

tenosynovitis, (8) cervical spine involvement, (9) rheumatoid factor, (10) antinuclear antibodies, (11) growth disturbances, (12) anemia and leukocytosis, and (13) hepatosplenomegaly and lymphadenopathy. As indicated, exacerbations and remissions of symptoms are common. Accurate diagnosis and optimal management depend on an understanding of these symptoms and their association with each type of JA.

Systemic-Onset JA *(Still Disease)*

Systemic-onset juvenile arthritis (previously known as Still disease) is characterized by fever, rash, joint involvement, and other systemic manifestations. Laboratory data most often will show an elevated erythrocyte sedimentation rate, leukocytosis with a significant percentage of polymorphonuclear leukocytes, and anemia.

Fever. Fever occurs intermittently, usually in a diurnal pattern with spikes to at least 39.5°C (103°F). Between spikes the child's temperature is usually normal or below (Fig. 43-8).

Rash. The rash associated with juvenile arthritis is most commonly seen in children with systemic-onset JA. This rash is an evanescent, pale red, nonpruritic, macular rash. The macules frequently coalesce. It will most often decrease or disappear during afebrile periods, but when present is usually seen on the trunk and extremities (except soles and palms). In addition to appearing during periods of fever, the rash may also appear when the skin is irritated (e.g., from scratching, heat, or trauma).

Joint Manifestations. Joint manifestations may be present at onset but go unnoticed for several months, especially if the joint problems are mild and systemic symptoms are severe and demand attention. Ultimately these children have joint involvement that is similar to polyarticular onset, with five or more joints being affected. All joints, large and small, including the cervical spine, may be involved. During febrile periods the patients may have incapacitating myalgias and arthralgias.

Systemic Manifestations. In addition to fever and rash, other systemic manifestations are common: hepatosplenomegaly and/or lymphadenopathy, pleuritis and/or pericarditis, leukocytosis, and severe anemia. These signs and symptoms may occur over a period of months, fluctuate through periods of remission and exacerbations, and then abate, but rarely continue into adulthood. Articular symptoms may follow a similar course, but they may also persist as chronic arthritis.

Polyarticular-Onset JA

The polyarticular-onset type of juvenile arthritis is defined as involvement of more than four joints. The type is further broken down into those patients who have positive tests for IgM rheumatoid factor (antibodies that react with gamma globulin) and those who are negative for the factor. The child with rheumatoid factor–negative polyarticular JA has the same characteristic signs and symptoms as one with systemic-onset JA except that according to the American Rheumatism Association, the fever is below 39.5°C (103°F). Fever, rash, anemias, fatigue, anorexia, and failure to gain weight will be present.

Joint Manifestations. Generally speaking, children with polyarticular-onset juvenile arthritis have

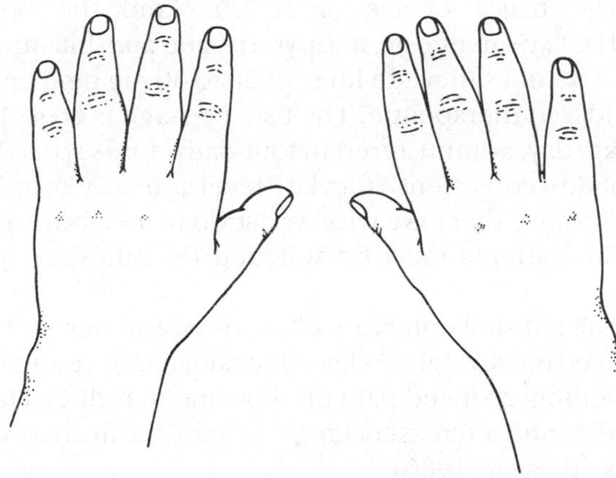

Figure 43-9. Arthritic involvement of the hands and wrists. The fingers of children with arthritis become fusiform in shape, with fat central portions around the swollen near (proximal) joint and pointed toward the tips. The joint nearest the fingertip (distal) is rarely involved.

fewer systemic manifestations, so attention is focused on the articular manifestations. The joints most commonly affected include wrists, knees, ankles, elbows, and feet. Affected joints are often symmetric but may also be asymmetric or even unilateral. Occasionally, polyarticular-onset JA can affect the large joints such as the cervical spine, hips, and shoulders. Regardless of location, the joints usually become swollen and tender. If joints of the feet are involved, the child may walk with a shuffle to avoid putting pressure on the joints of the distal foot. If the cervical spine is involved, neck pain with limitation of extension and lateral rotation of the neck is common. When the finger joints are involved, the fingers are fusiform (Fig. 43-9). In an effort to protect their joints, children assume a position of comfort, that of flexion. Flexion contracture deformities can occur quickly.

Systemic Manifestations. Although the emphasis in this type of juvenile arthritis is upon joint involvement, systemic manifestations are present in the majority of patients. Malaise, low-grade fever, organomegaly, adenopathy, anemia, and growth retardation or weight loss are commonly found.

Variations in Clinical Manifestations by Subtype. In polyarticular-onset juvenile arthritis, it is important to distinguish between those children who have rheumatoid factor–positive and rheumatoid factor–negative JA because the probable manifestations as well as the prognosis of each differ significantly. Rheumatoid factor–positive JA closely resembles adult-onset rheumatoid arthritis. Children with positive rheumatoid factor tests are more likely to develop severe chronic arthritis than children with negative rheumatoid factor. Rheumatoid nodules and rheumatoid vasculitis are likely to occur in rheumatoid factor–positive JA patients. There is a strong correlation between this type of JA and a genetic etiology.

Pauciarticular-Onset JA

As the prefix *pauci* implies, this type of juvenile arthritis affects only a few joints within the first 6 months of the disease. Onset can be either abrupt or insidious and involves joints as well as other connective tissues.

Joint Manifestations. The knees are the most common joints affected; however, ankles and hips also may be affected. Involved joints may be asymmetric and spotty. Joints may appear swollen and warm but are seldom red.

Systemic Manifestations. Children with pauciarticular-onset JA are frequently irritable and tired, with poor appetite and poor weight gain. Chronic eye inflammation may be seen, presenting as an inflammatory process of the anterior uveal tract with few signs and symptoms; early detection is possible only by slit-lamp examination. Several terms are used to identify this eye inflammation, including uveitis, iritis, and iridocyclitis. Iridocyclitis is often chronic and, since it is insidious, has great potential for damage (including cataracts and glaucoma) and vision loss or blindness.

Variations in Clinical Manifestations by Subtype. Pauciarticular juvenile arthritis is frequently divided into types or subsets according to age of onset, sex, presence of rheumatoid factor, presence of antinuclear antibodies, and certain HLA-B27* characteristics. Of these, three subsets are significant: ANA-positive girls, HLA-B27–positive older boys, and rheumatoid factor–positive patients. The first of these subsets is primarily girls with age of onset at 5 years or less, who have a high incidence of iridocyclitis. The second significant subset is that of boys for whom the age of onset is generally after 8 years of age and who have a greater incidence of HLA-B27 than do JA patients in general. These boys tend to develop changes typical of ankylosing spondylitis. The third subset is a small group of pauciarticular-onset patients who have a positive rheumatoid factor. These children tend to follow a polyarticular course and may develop erosive disease.

Diagnostic Assessment

The JA subcommittee of the American Rheumatism Association has proposed the following criteria for diagnosis of JA:

- (1) Objective evidence of arthritis (defined as joint swelling or joint limitation of motion with heat, pain, or tenderness) in one or more joints.

* HLA, human leukocyte antigen, is the major human histocompatibility complex. The letter B represents one genetic locus on the short arm of chromosome 6; the number 27 represents the allele at that site. See also the previous discussion of HLA, page 1527.

(Pain or tenderness alone are not sufficient for a diagnosis of arthritis.)

- (2) Persistence of arthritis for at least 6 weeks in a given joint.
- (3) Exclusion of other specific diseases that may cause or be associated with arthritis (Brewer, 1977).

This differential diagnosis may include ruling out such childhood disorders as malignancies, other inflammatory disorders (e.g., rheumatic fever, ankylosing spondylitis, systemic lupus erythematosus), infections of bacterial or viral origin, "growing pains," or congenital anomalies.

Laboratory Tests. No specific laboratory data are absolutely diagnostic for juvenile arthritis, but some tests and values are characteristically associated with JA. The sedimentation rate (ESR) is usually elevated; anemia is common; the white blood cell count is frequently elevated; any or all of the serum immunoglobins may be elevated; and antinuclear antibodies are found in 25 per cent of children with rheumatoid factor–negative JA, 75 per cent of children with rheumatoid factor–positive JA, and about 60 per cent of young girls with pauciarticular arthritis. Rheumatoid factors (antibodies that react with gamma globulin) are not specific for rheumatoid arthritis. They are found in other rheumatic diseases such as lupus erythematosus and scleroderma and in association with certain infections and malignancies.

Therapeutic Management

Drug therapy and physical therapy are the bases for treatment of juvenile arthritis. The goals of therapy include reducing inflammation, relief of symptoms of active disease, and maintenance or restoration of joint position, function, and strength. Accomplishment of these goals may require a concerted, well-orchestrated interdisciplinary effort; frequently it is the nurse who can or must coordinate such an endeavor.

Drug Therapy. The drugs used are the same as those for treatment of adult rheumatoid arthritis, some of which have not been specifically approved for use in children. The first-line drug is aspirin.

Aspirin (ASA). Aspirin administration in children has come under scrutiny because of its possible relationship to Reye syndrome. In addition, dental caries have been linked to the chewing of baby aspirin (Brewer, 1986). Despite these concerns, aspirin remains the drug of choice for juvenile arthritis. It is more effective than any other single nonsteroidal anti-inflammatory drug (NSAID)* and costs significantly less (Brewer,1986).

The major effects of aspirin (and the other NSAIDs) are analgesic, antipyretic, and anti-inflammatory. A serum salicylate level of 20 to 30 mg per cent is considered therapeutic. The usual dosage is 60 to 100 mg/kg/day, administered in four daily doses spread to maintain a consistent salicylate level as nearly as possible. Because there is a wide variation in metabolism of aspirin, patients must be watched for salicylate toxicity.

The anti-inflammatory effect of aspirin may not be achieved for several weeks. It is evaluated by reduction in swelling, reduced pain on movement, reduced tenderness, and increased range of motion in involved joints (Brewer, 1986).

Other Nonsteroidal Anti-inflammatory Drugs (NSAIDs). In recent years, the development of new nonsteroidal anti-inflammatory drugs has provided a significant alternative or adjunctive drug treatment for all types of arthritis. Most of these drugs, however, have not yet been approved for use in children and are still being studied. In general, they are considerably more expensive than aspirin but have the advantages of fewer gastrointestinal side effects and less frequent administration.

Indomethacin is an older NSAID that is recognized as one of the most effective drugs for treating severe forms of systemic juvenile arthritis, particularly if the child is not doing well on aspirin alone. If the child is started on a NSAID because of toxicity to aspirin, the nurse must be alert for signs of toxicity to the new drug. Patients who react to one NSAID have a 50 per cent chance of developing toxicity to another drug within this classification and often show similar toxic symptoms (Brewer, 1986).

Slower-Acting Antirheumatic Drugs (SAARDs). Another classification of drug therapy is the slower-acting antirheumatic drugs (SAARDs). These drugs are used for their effect upon the immune system but do not have anti-inflammatory properties. SAARDs include gold (Myochrysine, Solganal) and antimalarials (penicillamine, hydroxychloroquine). They are generally administered in conjunction with aspirin and other NSAIDs when these two types of drugs cannot effectively control the disease after a 4- to 6-month trial.

Of the SAARDs, gold is the treatment of choice. It is given by intramuscular injection. Prior to administering a therapeutic dose, test doses may be given to assess for allergic response. The gold preparation is usually given weekly for 20 weeks, subsequently tapering administration to every 2 to 4 weeks. A response to gold will probably not be seen for at least 2 to 6 months. The effects, if present, will be long-lasting.

Toxicities, including oral ulcerations, proteinuria, and alterations in polymorphonuclear white blood cell or platelet counts, are not uncommon. These may be

* Despite the tendency to think of aspirin as being in a class by itself where arthritis is concerned, it is actually classified as a nonsteroidal anti-inflammatory drug.

mild and reversible, or they may be severe, requiring complete cessation of the medication. Therefore, it is necessary to monitor blood counts, urine, and transaminases prior to each injection. Auranofin is an oral preparation of gold that has been used in doses of 0.1 to 0.15 mg/kg/day. However, it too has significant side effects that must be monitored, including diarrhea, gastrointestinal bleeding, hematuria, and anemia.

Hydroxychloroquine (Planquenil) and penicillamine are oral agents that are also slow acting; their effects may not be seen for several weeks or months after their initiation. Side effects of hydroxychloroquine may include visual complications, bleaching and loss of hair, anorexia, abdominal discomfort, and neuromuscular weakness. Therefore, it is important for the child taking this drug to be examined by an ophthalmologist once every 6 months. Side effects of penicillamine are similar to those associated with gold, and monitoring of blood counts, urine, and platelets, as well as liver function, is important.

Steroids. The use of steroids for children with juvenile arthritis is usually inappropriate. While they are the most potent anti-inflammatory drugs available and can dramatically suppress symptoms, there are few indications for their use. They neither alter the overall course of the disease nor prevent joint destruction. Furthermore, their side effects, particularly that of growth impairment, make them undesirable. However, they may be indicated in life-threatening situations, e.g., myocarditis, pericarditis, and progressive iridocylitis, or in children who are immobilized by severe debilitating disease that does not respond to other anti-inflammatory medications. In children with pauciarticular-onset JA in which only one or two inflamed joints are involved, intra-articular injection of steroids may control inflammation for 4 to 6 weeks, facilitating exercise and rehabilitation. This is a painful procedure, however, and repeated injections can result in steroidal damage to the cartilage and bone necrosis.

Immunosuppressive Drugs. Immunosuppressive drugs are being used experimentally in children with juvenile arthritis whose disease simply will not respond to any other medical treatment. These include cyclophosphamide (Cytoxan), chlorambucil (Leukeran), azathioprine (Imuran), and methotrexate. Each of these has serious potential side effects, including bladder inflammation, infertility, and severe immunosuppression predisposing to malignancy. As a result, their use is controversial and is limited to extreme cases.

Physical Therapy. Drug therapy is only one aspect of care for the patient with juvenile arthritis. A balanced program of medication, rest, and a regular schedule of exercise that includes physical therapy is necessary in most cases. Goals often include (1) increasing or maintaining strength and range of motion, (2) promoting independence in ambulation and other activities of daily living, and (3) controlling pain (Scull et al, 1986).

Considerations for Rest and Exercise. Rest has long been acknowledged as an effective treatment for joint swelling and heat. In fact, casting has long been used to facilitate periods of rest. However, muscle atrophy quickly occurs with this type of immobilization. Therefore, for the body as a whole as well as for individual joints, rest must be balanced with exercise.

Exercise for the child occurs both in normal play activities and in directed school activities. It is tempting (particularly for the parents) to consider this "normal activity" adequate exercise for the child with juvenile arthritis. But a formal program that takes all affected areas of the body through maximum active range-of-motion exercises is essential to maintain function. This is usually done twice a day, but the frequency can be decreased if exercise results in increased pain or swelling. Exercises such as swimming or bicycle riding may be helpful if the child is not cooperative or if joints are actively inflamed. Only at the time of acute exacerbations is a passive exercise program acceptable since excessive exercise will increase inflammation.

Early morning stiffness may make normal activities as well as range-of-motion exercises extremely painful and difficult. Heat, which may be applied in a variety of ways, often provides pain relief and facilitates movement. Warm baths or warm packs are simple methods for heat application. Warm packs are more practical when only a few joints are involved. Carefully controlled paraffin baths also may be helpful for improving function in older children.

The use of splints provides benefits of both rest and exercise. While helping protect joints from deformity by maintaining a position of function, splints also allow for resting from otherwise normal movement and activity, thereby reducing pain. However, splints do not *prevent* deformities. The splints should be made from a lightweight material by an experienced occupational therapist or orthotist and should be as comfortable as possible. To absorb moisture, they can be lined with leather, or stockinette can be applied before putting the splint on. Hand splints that include support for the hand and fingers can be used at night, and splints that allow for finger movement while still providing support and rest for the wrist and hand can be used during the day. If contractures have begun, serial casting may be necessary.

Surgical Intervention. Surgery may be necessary for some patients with juvenile arthritis. Contractures that do not respond to splinting, exercise, or other therapies should be released before cartilage destruction makes them immovable. Joint replacements in children continue to be controversial. Hip, knee, wrist, and shoulder replacements are done but must be postponed until late adolescence or until bone growth has ceased. Surgical interventions present other problems, including lack of motivation by the child to participate actively in rehabilitation and anesthesia for the child who has temporomandibular or cervical spine disease.

The primary goal of care is to facilitate social, physical, and emotional growth that is as nearly normal as possible. This is accomplished through drug and physical therapy that is aimed at preventing deformities and blindness. Promoting a lifestyle and interactions that encourage the child and family's growth and development is equally important.

Major Nursing Diagnoses for JA

Impaired physical mobility, *related to chronic joint inflammation*

Altered comfort: pain, *related to joint inflammation*

Potential altered growth and development, *related to*

- *overprotective behavior of parents*
- *physical limitations associated with joint involvement and systemic symptoms*
- *irregular school attendance*

Potential self-esteem disturbance, *related to the reactions of significant others to the physical limitations*

Potential ineffective family coping, *related to the impact of an illness that is chronic and potentially debilitating*

Knowledge deficit, *related to home care*

Strategies for Nursing Care

Overview of Nursing Goals. Juvenile arthritis frequently involves physical, functional, and adaptational alterations as well as alterations in comfort (Fig. 43-10). Nursing goals include coordinating all aspects of care (including community care) so that the lives of the child and family members are normalized to the extent possible. This implies an honest, sensitive, trusting, cooperative relationship between the child, the family and a broad multidisciplinary team of health care professionals to ensure continuity and consistency of care.

Coordinating Care. The acute care nurse may encounter the child during acute exacerbations of the disease. The child will be hospitalized (1) when the disease process "flares" and intensive occupational therapy/physical therapy (OT/PT) are required, (2) when medications need to be re-evaluated, or (3) when operations are required (synovectomies, muscle/tendon releases for treatment of contracture, serial casting, joint replacements). The acute care nurse begins management responsibilities which, upon the patient's discharge, become the domain of the home care nurse. These include facilitating and monitoring the involvement of the parent and child in the therapy regimen, assessing the psychologic impact of illness on an ongoing basis, making referrals for counseling as needed for promoting positive attitudes toward school and psychosocial development, intervening with community resources (school, OT, PT), and recognizing needs for teaching. Teaching needs include aspects such as medications, physical assessment, appropriate activities, nutrition, availability of community resources, use of orthoses, and utilization of community resources.

Management of the child with juvenile arthritis occurs primarily in the home. The child and family will benefit from a disciplined daily routine that balances time for individual and collective needs for therapies, rest, relaxation, pleasure, school, adequate nutrition, and normal or routine family activities. This balance may be delicate and precarious, but it is essential for facing the challenges of juvenile arthritis and promoting the most positive passage through each stage of growth and development. Therefore, the role of the nurse may be extremely broad, encompassing that of caregiver, teacher, advocate, and coordinator.

Managing Medication Therapy. Nursing responsibilities for medications include administration when the child is hospitalized, evaluation of effectiveness, and teaching and support of the patient and family for medication administration at home.

If the child is on aspirin therapy, it is important to monitor for evidence of gastritis or gastric ulcers (including blood in the stool). Since small children rarely complain of tinnitus, an apparent hearing loss may be an early clue of salicylate toxicity. Parents may be concerned about the side effects of aspirin and inquire about acetaminophen. It is necessary for parents to understand that acetaminophen does not have anti-inflammatory properties.

The risks of aspirin administration during flu season and during outbreaks of chickenpox cannot be ignored in light of the probable link among these infections, ASA, and Reye syndrome. Parents should be cautioned to contact the physician for potential changes in medication at these times.

If aspirin therapy and other nonsteroidal anti-inflammatory drugs are ineffective in controlling the disease process, immunosuppressive drugs may be necessary. This presents another concern for the nurse, both when the patient is hospitalized and at home. The child will be more susceptible to infectious diseases because of the immunosuppression. The child and family should be counseled to avoid large groups or enclosed public areas during flu season to prevent unnecessary exposure to infection. The child also is at risk for septic conditions that may be masked by the

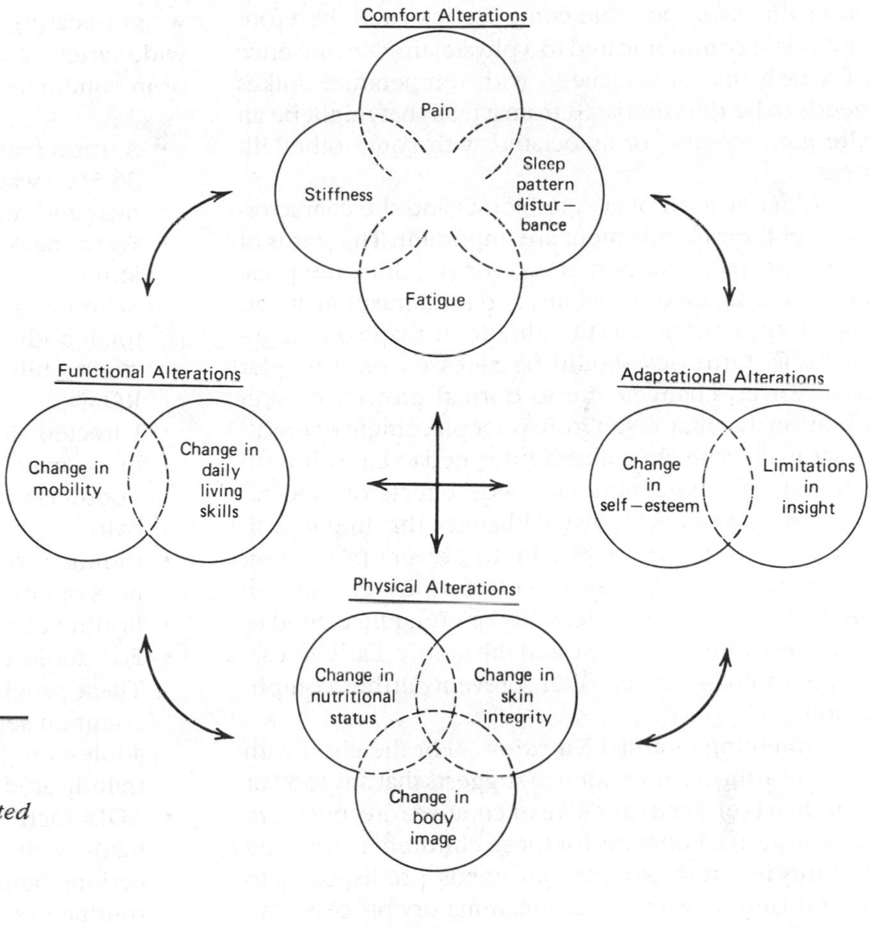

Figure 43-10. Frequently occurring problems of patients with rheumatic diseases. (Redrawn from Pigg JS, et al: *Rheumatology Nursing: A Problem-Oriented Approach.* New York, John Wiley & Sons, 1985.)

steroids. This possibility must always be considered when the patient has otherwise nonspecific symptoms. When the immunosuppressed child is hospitalized, room assignment must reflect the need to protect the child from a nosocomial infection. (See Table 43-2.)

Teaching to Support Home Care. The goal of patient and family teaching is to assist the child and family to be active, knowledgeable, and responsible participants in disease assessment and management. Teaching should include the child in age-appropriate ways. The child's ability to participate in the management of the disease depends in large measure on understanding the illness and its management. Accordingly, the family's ability to cope/adjust and progress through their individual and collective stages of growth and development will reflect the education, understanding, and support they receive throughout the course of the disease process.

Teaching Techniques for Administration of Medications. The nurse is often responsible for patient and family instruction regarding medications, their purpose, appropriate dosage and potential adverse effects. Aspirin therapy is the most common form of treatment. Instruction must include the therapeutic dosage that has been calculated specifically for the child. Brushing the teeth after chewing baby aspirin will reduce the chance for cavities associated with residual aspirin packed into indentations on chewing surfaces. Aspirin should be administered with food or milk to reduce gastric irritation. Antacids should be discouraged except as recommended and monitored by the physician since they interfere with medication absorption.

Parents should be reminded that aspirin and all medications should be kept out of reach of children who are too young to be responsible for their own medication administration. Overdoses of aspirin can cause gastrointestinal bleeding and severe acid-base disturbances in children. (Chapter 28 provides detailed strategies related to age-appropriate administration of medications.)

Other aspects of teaching for which the nurse may be responsible include discussion of assessments that need to be made by the child or parents, such as temperature patterns, rashes, changes in mobility or ability to function, and use of orthoses (splints or braces).

Teaching Assessment Skills. The purpose of teaching disease-specific assessment skills is to provide the family with a framework for judgments. For example, the child and family need to be aware of any pattern of fevers so that they can feel comfortable with differentiating between what may be normally associated with the disease process and what indicates other illness or possible complications and therefore should be communicated to a physician. The presence of a rash that is associated with temperature spikes needs to be differentiated from a rash that might be an allergic response or associated with some other illness.

Identification of affected joints and the characteristics of their involvement are important. The status of and changes in warmth and color of joints, the presence or absence of effusions, and joint position are all significant assessments that should be made on a regular basis. Orthoses should be assessed on a regular basis for fit, changes due to normal growth, or skin irritation that may result from poor placement or unsatisfactory fit. The child and family need to know how to evaluate the therapeutic and side effects of medications. Assessments for visual changes that might indicate iridocyclitis are important to prevent permanent visual impairment. Assessments for any changes in physical and emotional stability or endurance need to be made by both the nurse and the family. Early assessments/evaluations can often prevent further complications.

Promoting Optimal Nutrition. For the child with juvenile arthritis, no evidence suggests that any food or vitamin has either a causative or curative role, but there are nutritional concerns for these children. Decreased mobility may reduce metabolic needs, predisposing to weight gain. However, the inflammatory process coupled with anemia may increase metabolic needs, leading to weight loss or inadequate weight gain. Obesity is a concern for the child with JA because excessive weight places more stress on already inflamed joints and because the overweight child tends to be less active and, therefore, stiffer. Being too thin is a problem as well if caloric intake is insufficient for normal growth. Recognizing the potential for calorie intake that either exceeds or fails to meet nutritional needs and incorporating nutritional aspects into teaching can prevent unnecessary physical and emotional stress for the child.

Maintaining Mobility. A well-developed, integrated physical therapy program will maintain mobility by (1) invigorating physical activities that strengthen muscles and daily put joints through full range of motion, and (2) promoting a positive attitude about physical capabilities. A major challenge is the development of a program that is interesting and stimulating and that will encourage compliance. Such a program will need to be a well-planned, coordinated effort between the two disciplines of occupational and physical therapy and may also involve school nurses and teachers.

It is important to carefully and cleverly select *activities that maintain mobility/range of motion (ROM) but do not strain inflamed joints,* particularly weight-bearing strain, which aggravates synovitis. A wide variety of such activities may be used individually or in combinations.

- A warm bath or shower or soaking in warm (32 to 36.5°C) water can help reduce early morning stiffness and relax muscles prior to exercises.
- Warm packs may enhance mobility of individual joints.
- Swimming is particularly good because it provides total body exercise and protects joints against strain while strengthening muscles and improving ROM.
- Directed slow movements imitating birds or animals may be effective for younger children. Toddlers may enjoy kicking a balloon or soft beach ball.
- Riding a tricycle or bicycle can help reduce stiffness of knees and hips.
- Rolling clay exercises hands and wrists.
- For adolescents, t'ai-chi routines can be used. These progressive resistive exercises be used with common sense and reasonable caution, when the adolescent is free of pain. However, they are contraindicated when joints are inflamed and painful.
- ADLs (activities of daily living) are natural, automatic sources of activities and ROM. Dressing, bathing, and grooming activities provide natural, routine exercises that are also therapeutic. Adaptations of both function and equipment may be necessary to facilitate these activities and allow more independent self-care while protecting joints from excessive strain.

Activities that are "in harmony with" the natural or acquired interests or inclinations can be used or modified to meet individual needs. Running, jumping, and prolonged walking should be avoided, however, if active lower extremity synovitis is present. Long periods of reading or watching television weaken muscles and cause fixed joint deformities.

Occupational therapists can develop appropriate orthoses. When joints are inflamed and painful, splints may provide comfort and rest. The child may object to wearing the splints, but they are important in maintaining function and reducing the possibility of deformity. The most frequently used splints are night-time knee splints prescribed to prevent knee flexion (or contracture) and to improve knee extension. Splints for wrists are also commonly used to improve wrist dorsiflexion.

A home visit may be necessary to determine the need for assistive devices or the presence of factors in the home that may be a problem for the child or the family. A bathroom not wheelchair accessible, or multiple steps into or within the home, are examples of problems that make daily living difficult for the family and the child and must be resolved for the goal of normal living. Adaptive devices for the bathroom for toileting and bathing are relatively easy to obtain and can make these intimate aspects of daily living possible on a more independent basis. The nurse can assess the need for these and other aids and provide information and assistance in locating these resources.

Reducing Pain. Pain control should incorporate physical care, such as application of heat, positioning, and limitation of activities. Although it is not clear how they work, cutaneous application of menthol ointments may provide temporary relief of joint pain. Such techniques as distraction and relaxation can be effective. Redirection of attention by story-telling, singing, or other areas of concentration may be helpful. Relaxation techniques may be more effective in the older child and may vary from meditation to breathing exercises to relaxing with music. The use of imagery or self-hypnosis also has been shown to be effective in pain relief for children with JA and may enhance the child's sense of mastery and control (Olness and Gardner, 1988). Benefits of the techniques listed include reducing anxiety, easing of muscle tension, promoting rest (may be as effective as napping), and increasing effectiveness of other interventions used for pain relief.

Reducing Fatigue. Many children with juvenile arthritis experience increased fatigability. The demands of school and routine ADLs may be very tiring. Excessive emotional and physical fatigue may trigger exacerbations of JA. Younger children usually respond more appropriately to feelings of fatigue, pacing physical activities and rest time. School-age children and adolescents who tend to get caught up in peer activities and possibly job responsibilities may need encouragement to allow themselves extra rest. Rest, relaxation, leisure activities, and relief from emotional distress may relieve fatigue and reduce exacerbations and therefore become an important aspect of management.

Promoting Normal Development. The key to promoting normal development is normalization of the environment to the extent possible. This can often be accomplished by focusing upon the *abilities* of the ill child rather than upon the limitations. For example, assignment of appropriate household chores and responsibilities fosters a sense of normality, acceptance, and accomplishment for the child and promotes more normal family functioning. Attention to normal development also includes the enhancement of self-esteem and promotion of regular school attendance. (See Chapter 25 for additional strategies related to normal development for the child with a chronic illness.)

Promoting Regular School Attendance. School is an integral part of growth and development, and regular attendance should be encouraged. Some adjustments may be necessary, however, to accommodate some of the limitations imposed by JA. Climbing stairs or walking long distances may be difficult or impossible, and access to classes may need to be arranged. Early morning stiffness may make getting to school difficult. Because of the child's increased fatigability, the school day may need to be shortened by temporary withdrawal from less-essential classes. Social interactions in the school setting are an important part of normal development, so part-time school attendance or home tutoring on a regular basis is discouraged. Tutoring, however, occasionally may be advisable to allow the child to "keep up" when mobility is further restricted by disease exacerbations or surgery. The individual child's needs may change frequently, depending on the course of the disease. Medications may need to be given during the school day and the school nurse may be required to administer them. Therefore, extensive ongoing communication and cooperation are essential among the health care provider, the patient and family, and the school personnel.

It is important for the nurse to portray a positive attitude about the child's potential for normal development. Research summarized by King and Hanson (1986) supports optimism. They concluded that children with JA did not have unique personality traits, nor were they socially maladjusted. Further, the majority of children with JA are expected to achieve educational levels at or beyond the average for the population as a whole.

Enhancing Self-Esteem. The limitations imposed on the child by inflamed joints and by any permanent limitations and disfigurements can significantly alter the child's perception of both abilities and worth. Assessment of what is real or accurate in these perceptions is an important role of nurses. They should assist the child to a realistic perception and expectation while affirming the positive characteristics and abilities of the child, thereby affirming his or her worth.

Children, as well as parents, must have an accurate perception of the disease process in order to understand which aspects of the process can be altered by their interventions and which are beyond their control. This understanding will help assuage guilt feelings that somehow they are getting worse because of failure to comply with prescribed therapy. The child (particularly the preschooler) also needs to be absolved of guilt by understanding that the illness was not caused by thinking "forbidden" thoughts or by "naughty" behavior.

Nurses can also enhance the child's self-esteem by pointing out age-appropriate accomplishments, attractive physical features (lovely smile, beautiful hair), a caring, gentle personality, or special cognitive abilities. They also can remind the family of the child's need for this reinforcement. Studies have shown that a child's interactions with peers are significantly affected by visible signs of impairment such as deformity, splints, or a wheelchair. Because the child's self-perception is greatly influenced by the behavioral and verbal response of peers, the school nurse or parent can ask to speak with teachers and students in the classroom. Again, it will be important to emphasize the ways in which the child with JA is just like peers, as well as to explain some fundamentals of the disease process.

For the adolescent, juvenile arthritis presents concerns about vocational preparation, heterosexual interactions, and realistic expectations for marriage and family. Adolescent support groups are one way of providing a safe environment for exchange of ideas, concerns, frustrations, and feelings.

Supporting Adaptive Coping. Diagnosis of juvenile arthritis may be a long and tedious process requiring more than one physician to complete the diagnostic work-up. The anxiety associated with the child's discomfort and the fear and frustration of the diagnostic process can take an incredible toll on the whole family. The fears and frustrations of the parents are further increased when the child is unable to either understand or articulate discomforts.

An additional anxiety-producing experience is the hospitalization of the child for "flares," control of fevers, acute joint inflammation, or complications such as pericarditis or myocarditis. The nurse may be the single most consistent person in the large interdisciplinary health care team and, as such, must function as a resource/comfort/support person throughout all these periods.

Siblings of the ill child often require special consideration by parents and health care professionals. It has been observed that siblings often have a lower self-esteem than does the child with juvenile arthritis. Siblings should be allowed to vent their feelings of guilt, frustration, and anxiety during the long, tedious, physically and emotionally draining course of the illness. Support groups for these family members can provide education, encouragement, and understanding. In addition, organizations such as Crippled Children's Service and the American Juvenile Arthritis Organization, which is sponsored by the Arthritis Foundation, may provide educational materials, specialized services, and financial aid to qualified families.

Nursing Strategies for Follow-up Care in the Home or Clinic

Assess the progression of the disease process by determining which joints are currently involved, assessing the function and comfort of involved joints, and discussing whether activities that were formerly tolerated are now causing increasing fatigue.

Evaluate the child's/family's satisfaction with drug therapy, physical therapy, orthoses (if any), and prescribed pain control measures.

Encourage the child to describe a typical day, evaluating the response for evidence of (1) balance of rest/activity, (2) normal peer relations, (3) regular school attendance, and (4) positive self-image.

Reassess the adequacy of the home physical environment as the child's condition changes.

Determine whether the family is aware of sources of emotional, educational, and financial support through community agencies and organizations.

Dermatomyositis

Juvenile dermatomyositis is one of a group of multisystem inflammatory disorders. As its name implies, it affects skin and muscles. It has been thought to be a form of polymyositis. There is controversy, however, concerning the histopathology and immunogenetic factors, and this causes confusion in establishing consistent terminology. In general, juvenile dermatomyositis is considered a distinct entity that exhibits clinical, histopathologic, and epidemiologic characteristics distinguishing it from other forms of polymyositis.

Dermatomyositis is less common than juvenile arthritis or systemic lupus erythematosus. It occurs primarily between the ages of 5 and 14 years. Manifestations include symmetric weakness of striated muscles accompanied by cutaneous involvement, which may range from a relatively mild, self-limiting illness to rapidly disabling contractures, muscle atrophy, and even death. Vasculitis and calcinosis (defined below) are also significant manifestations.

Etiology

Although the cause of dermatomyositis is not known, several infectious agents have been suggested as possible origins, including viral agents such as influenzas A and B and Coxsackie. There is also evidence of an autoimmune response of T-lymphocytes against the patient's own muscle cells (Lockey and Bukantz, 1987b).

Pathophysiology

Major pathologic abnormalities occur in the blood vessels of the connective tissue of the skin, gastrointestinal tract, muscles, fat, and small nerves. The evidence, on biopsy, suggests that abnormal antigen-antibody complexes are laid down on the walls of blood vessels. Capillaries, venules, and small arteries are damaged, with loss of muscle capillary network. This causes inflammation and occludes blood flow to tissues. Both focal and diffuse degeneration of muscle fibers results. A direct attack on muscle cells by abnormal T-lymphocytes may also destroy muscle tissue. Calcinosis is the development of calcifications under the skin and in muscles. It occurs in a high percentage of patients and may be the most debilitating consequence of juvenile dermatomyositis.

Cardiac abnormalities may also occur as the result of small vessel disease. The abnormalities may include all degrees of heart block, dysrhythmias, pericarditis, or focal and diffuse inflammatory infiltrates, necrosis, or fibrosis.

Gastrointestinal (GI) involvement probably occurs to some degree in all children with dermatomyositis and may progress to GI perforation. Again, necrotizing vasculitis, which involves the small vessels of the bowel wall, generally is thought to be the causative factor. This results in thrombosis and ischemia, which may progress to infarction and perforation at one or more sites.

The clinical course of juvenile dermatomyositis is variable. Before steroid therapy was available, a significant percentage of children died of complications associated with vasculitis or with progressive muscle disease, including the cardiopulmonary musculature. A similar percentage were severely handicapped as a result of permanent muscle weakness or contractures; the remainder recovered to near functionally normal. Although a few children may still die from intractable muscle weakness, sepsis, vasculitis, or pneumonias secondary to immobility, most children with dermatomyositis are now expected to respond to drug therapy and return to normal or near-normal states of health. In a few cases of incomplete response to therapy, the progression of disease can lead to immobility and handicapping when muscles scar, contract, and become stiff. Drugs used to stabilize or reverse the inflammatory process and its effects may be weaned to minimal maintenance doses or may be stopped completely. However, relapses of the disease process *may* occur for many years following disease onset.

Clinical Manifestations

Juvenile dermatomyositis may present as an insidious onset of weakness of the major proximal muscles (specifically, shoulder and pelvic girdle). Initially symptoms may be fatigue and malaise. These children may have difficulty climbing stairs or getting up from the floor. (The signs are similar to those of Duchenne muscular dystrophy, Chapter 47.) Muscle groups are symmetrically involved. A sensitive early indicator of muscle involvement is neck flexion weakness. This can be assessed by asking the child to lift the head up from a pillow. (This weakness may also be the last to resolve.) Muscle weakness makes ordinary activities difficult: getting up from a squatting position, push-ups, walking on toes or heel, and knee bends can be difficult or impossible.

Skin rashes related to vasculitis may vary from limited to extensive. Most commonly this rash appears as a reddening, shininess, and dry scaling over the knees, elbows, knuckles, and tips of fingers. The rash also appears on the face, neck, and chest (Fig. 43-11). Edema, particularly periorbital, is usually seen in association with the rash. Swelling may occur on the backs of hands and the feet. In addition, most children develop the characteristic lilac discoloration of the eyelid (heliotrope). Calcinosis (deposits of calcium salts) are common over heels, elbows, and knuckles, and occasionally may be more diffuse. Calcinosis appears as knobs or plates of calcium that protrude through the skin and may crack with movement.

The children may have muscle weakness in the upper airways and throat. As a result, they may aspirate food or saliva, causing aspiration pneumonia. Upper airway weakness may be evidenced by nasal speech and inability to pronounce *k*, *b*, or *r*.

Diagnostic Assessment

Five major diagnostic criteria are applied to juvenile dermatomyositis: the presence of progressive symmetric weakness of the limb and girdle muscles and anterior flexor muscles of the neck; a muscle biopsy that shows evidence of necrosis of certain types of muscle fibers; elevated serum levels of skeletal-muscle enzymes (CPK); an abnormal electromyogram (EMG); and the characteristic rash.

Therapeutic Management

Medical treatment includes early, aggressive treatment with corticosteroids. The long-term prognosis is directly related to the rapidity of diagnosis and treatment. High-dose steroid therapy relieves inflammation and reduces the muscle enzyme levels. As inflammation is relieved, muscle strength improves. The dose of steroids is tapered slowly as muscle strength is regained. Relapses of the disease may occur as the medication is being tapered. However, these exacerbations generally respond well to treatment. Some medication may be required for many years.

Other drugs may be prescribed if the child responds poorly to the administration of corticosteroids. These may include cytotoxic or immunosuppressive drugs like methotrexate, azathioprine, and chloram-

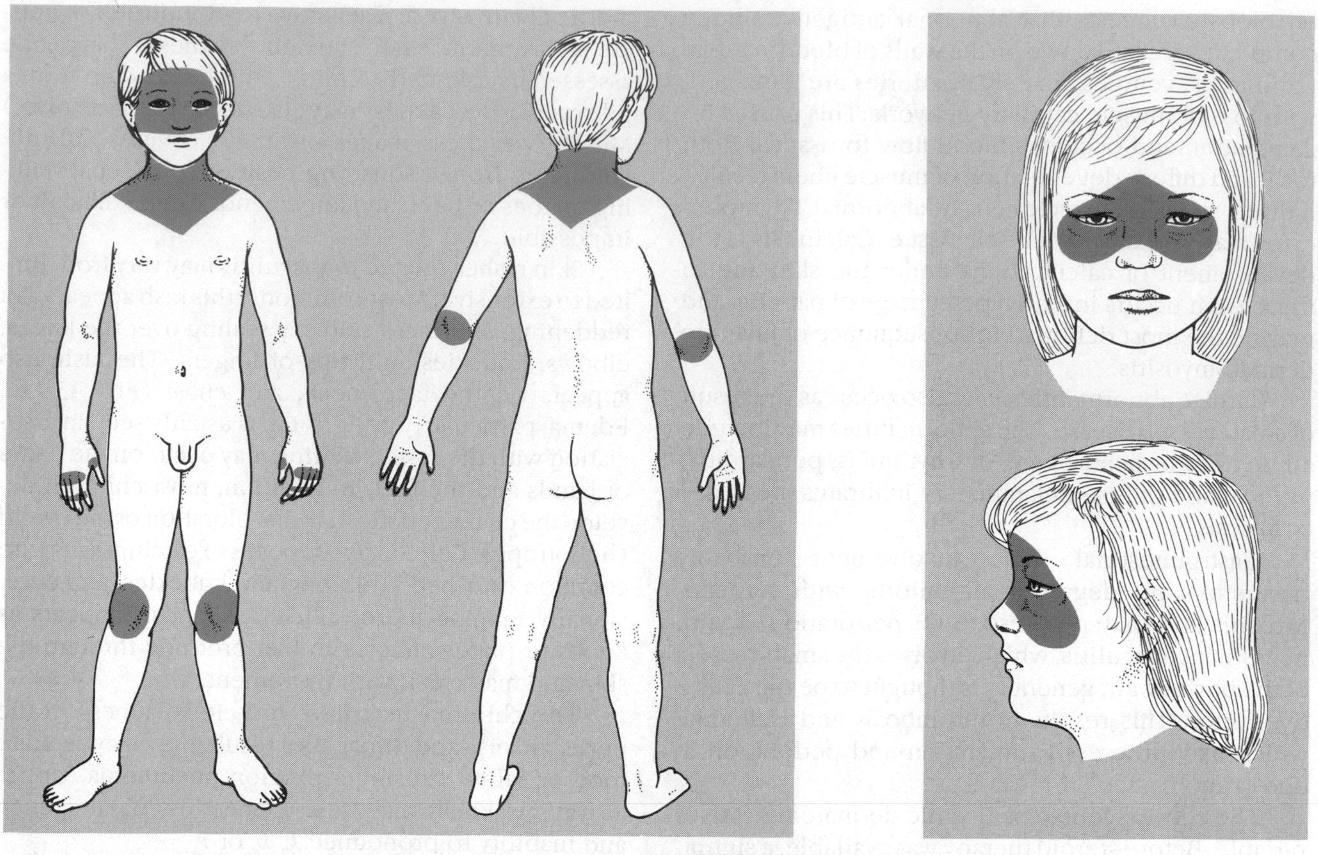

Figure 43-11. The characteristic distribution of rash in dermatomyositis: cheeks and forehead, "shawl" area, elbows, knees, knuckles, fingertips. The rash on the face may be widespread, but it is usually localized to the cheeks and central portion of the forehead. The eyelids are often swollen and discolored, with a characteristic "heliotrope" (violet) hue.

bucil. For local skin care, a regimen of Burow soaks, sunscreens, and Eucerin cream may be used to relieve the pain associated with areas of calcinosis. Diphenylhydramine can be given to relieve itching.

Supportive therapy includes bedrest during the acute phase. Physical therapy is also an important part of the child's treatment to prevent contractures and increase muscle strength. Bracing and splinting may be helpful for maintaining correct positioning and alignment and preventing contractures.

Major Nursing Diagnoses for Dermatomyositis

***Impaired physical mobility,** related to muscle weakness, associated with degeneration of muscle fibers*
***Potential altered tissue perfusion: cardiac and gastrointestinal,** related to inflammatory changes in the microvasculature*
***Impaired skin integrity: rash, calcinosis, and discoloration of eyelids,** related to inflammatory changes in the dermis and epidermis*
***Potential for infection: pneumonia,** related to*
- *decreased immunocompetence*
- *stasis of secretions associated with decreased mobility*
- *aspiration associated with dysphagia*

***Knowledge deficit,** related to home care*

Strategies for Nursing Care

Nursing care of the child with dermatomyositis must address physical aspects of the disorder, which include care of skin, pulmonary function, joints and muscles, gastrointestinal integrity, and cardiac stability, as well as psychologic and social aspects. These should be tailored appropriately to the child's stage of growth and development.

Minimizing Muscle Damage. Attention to insidious progression of muscle weakness is essential. (Careful assessment and recognition can lead to the appropriate level of medical therapy.) Temperature and blood pressure should be carefully monitored for early indications of physiologic changes that may be either an undesirable effect of steroid therapy or an exacerbation of the disease process.

Exercise, both passive and active, is an important aspect of therapy. Because exercise may be painful, it may be resisted. Gentle, passive range-of-motion exercises may be done by a physical therapist. As the child progresses toward recovery, the nurse and physical therapist should develop a plan that encourages the child to do exercises independently. The child and parents should be taught how to develop an effective program of exercises, as well as the importance of routinely following that program for most effectively maintaining muscle strength and joint flexibility. Activities of daily living should be encouraged but also should be paced to avoid undue fatigue.

Assessing Cardiovascular Function. The nurse must be particularly alert for evidences of cardiac abnormalities. While not as common in children as in adults, these can occur as a result of myocardial infarctions and degenerative changes due to small vessel disease. Involvement can include dysrhythmias, pericarditis, various degrees of heart block, and other signs and symptoms as noted earlier.

Assessing Gastrointestinal Function. Gastrointestinal function is an important part of frequent assessment. GI dysfunction may range from bowel immobility to intestinal perforations. Nursing assessment includes auscultation for bowel sounds, monitoring of stools for presence of blood, and noting any change in vital signs that might indicate localized infection or sepsis from abscess.

Reducing Skin Breakdown. Skin condition is assessed for evidence of breakdown or infection where cracks may have occurred in areas of calcifications. If the child is confined to bed for any length of time, good skin care is essential as skin damage can result in scarring. (The scarring is similar to that which can occur in the muscles.) Skin also should be assessed carefully when splints and braces are applied.

Preventing Respiratory Infection. The nurse must be alert for signs and symptoms of pulmonary compromise. Children with severe disease of muscles and skin may be virtually immobile; this may lead to pulmonary deterioration. In addition, the nurse must guard against possible aspiration pneumonia, which could result from the child's decreased ability to swallow food or secretions.

Teaching to Support Home Care. Teaching is an integral part of care for the child and family: information about the disease process, medications (their indications and side effects), activities and the limitations being imposed, and expected outcome for the child with this disorder.

Psychologic disturbances, neurologic dysfunction, and functional disability all have been reported as sequelae of dermatomyositis. Children may experience anger and depression as a result of the limitations produced by the disease. Patients and families should be encouraged to express feelings and fears. Counseling may be desirable to help the patient and family address issues that surround this illness.

Following the acute stage of disease, return to school may also be a problem. Participation in general activities may be tolerated. However, falling is a common problem because the weakness does not allow the child to regain balance to prevent a fall. Therefore, physical education program expectations may be unrealistic. Noncompetitive activities that promote mobility and increase strength should be encouraged.

Nursing Strategies for Follow-up Care in the Home or Clinic

Assess muscle strength (see Chapter 15 for detailed technique).

Assess for the presence of blood in the stool (related to bowel perforation associated with necrotizing vasculitis, or to GI ulceration from steroid therapy).

Assess cardiovascular and respiratory status for complications resulting from inflammation of the microvasculature.

Assess for skin breakdown related to areas of calcification and to decreased vascular integrity.

Remind the child and parents that physical activity may produce muscular ischemia and pain if the activity raises the metabolic demands for oxygen above the level that can be supplied by the diseased vasculature.

Coordinate client teaching efforts with the physical therapy staff to eliminate conflicting instructions.

Determine the effectiveness of the child's and family's social support system in providing an outlet for emotional responses and guidance for problem solving.

Rheumatic Fever

Rheumatic fever, named for its joint involvement and increased temperature in the acute stage, is a systemic inflammatory disease of childhood that can involve the heart, joints, central nervous system, skin, and connective tissue.

Although the incidence of rheumatic fever has decreased in the Western world, it is still considered the most common cause of heart disease in people under 40 years of age. The natural history of the disease has been altered by environmental as well as medical factors. Industrialization, urbanization with improved socioeconomic conditions, the advent and increasingly widespread administration of antibiotics, as well as improved health care practices, and better criteria for identification are all factors that have contributed to this reduced incidence.

Rheumatic fever has not been eradicated, however. An estimated 100,000 cases occur each year in the United States, and studies have shown an increased incidence in New York City (Lockey and Bukantz, 1987b).

It is more often found in school-age children between 6 and 15 years old, with a peak incidence at about 8 years of age. It also appears to be more commonly seen in cold, humid climates. Statistics suggest that there may be an increased familial incidence, but it is not known whether this is due to heredity, environment, or other factors. Rheumatic fever is known to recur.

Etiology

Rheumatic fever is a potential sequelae of Group A beta-hemolytic streptococcal infections and may occur after such illnesses as strep tonsillitis or pharyngitis. A direct relationship between a Group A beta-strep infection and the occurrence of rheumatic fever has been firmly established, but the exact pathologic mechanism responsible for development of rheumatic fever is still unknown. It has been documented, however, that when a beta-hemolytic streptococcal infection (e.g., pharyngitis, scarlet fever, or middle ear infection) occurs, antibodies are formed against the toxin released by the streptococci. The antibodies formed in this immune response react with tissue antigens and can cause damage in different tissues of the body (an autoimmune response), specifically the heart, joints, glomeruli of the kidney, central nervous system, and skin. Some tissues are more susceptible to damage than others, particularly the heart. The fact that only 3 per cent or fewer (Behrman and Vaughan, 1987) of children with strep infections contract rheumatic fever suggests, however, that undefined genetic or other factors may be operating.

Pathophysiology

The acute stage of rheumatic fever is characterized by inflammation of connective tissue in the heart, joints, and skin. The acute stage usually lasts 2 to 3 weeks and is followed by a proliferation phase that involves primarily the heart. During this second phase, Aschoff bodies (large, multinucleated cells) may accumulate on heart valves weakened by inflammation. (Figure 39-24 in Chapter 39 illustrates this phenomenon.) Cardiac valve injury, the most serious complication, occurs as the valve leaflets become scarred. The extent of resulting valvular stenosis and regurgitation depends on the degree of the initial insult and any added damage with recurrence of rheumatic fever. The mitral valve is the most commonly affected, followed by the aortic valve.

Clinical Manifestations

As indicated, rheumatic fever characteristically follows a group A beta-hemolytic streptococcal infection. The initial infection may have occurred a few days to 6 weeks earlier. The entire episode of rheumatic fever lasts from 1 to 3 months and is self-limiting. The Jones Criteria for guidance in the diagnosis of rheumatic fever have identified major and minor manifestations of the disease (Table 43-4). The sequence of signs and symptoms is fairly predictable, with inflammation of joints, heart, and erythematous rash appearing and often associated with a temperature of 38°C (100.4°F) or higher. The major manifestations identified in the revised Jones Criteria are discussed next.

Arthritis. The onset of rheumatic fever may be insidious, with the child merely appearing tired and apathetic. One of the first complaints may be that of joint tenderness. The area may appear swollen, red, and warm. However, these complaints may seem out of proportion to evidence of arthritis. The joints most frequently affected by these arthritic changes are the large joints: knees, elbows, and wrists. Other joints that may be affected are shoulders, ankles, and finger joints. These arthritic pains, usually migratory, generally last from 1 to 4 weeks and rarely cause permanent

***Table* 43-4.** Jones Criteria (Revised) for Guidance in the Diagnosis of Rheumatic Fever*

Major Manifestations	**Minor Manifestations**	
	Clinical	Laboratory
Carditis Polyarthritis Chorea Erythema marginatum Subcutaneous nodules	Previous rheumatic fever or rheumatic heart disease Arthralgia Fever	Acute phase reactants: Erythrocyte sedimentation rate, C-reactive protein, leukocytosis Prolonged P-R interval
Supporting Evidence of Streptococcal Infection		
Increased titer of antistreptococcal antibodies, ASO (antistreptolysin O), others		
Positive throat culture for Group A streptococcus		
Recent scarlet fever		

* The presence of two major criteria, or of one major and two minor criteria, indicates a high probability of acute rheumatic fever, **if supported by evidence of preceding Group A streptococcal infection.**

(Data from Committee on Rheumatic Fever and Bacterial Endocarditis, American Heart Association, Dallas, 1982.)

deformities. Three fourths of children with rheumatic fever experience arthritic symptoms (Behrman and Vaughan, 1987).

Carditis. Carditis (cardiac inflammation) is the most severe manifestation of rheumatic fever and occurs in a majority of children with the disease (Griffiths, 1986). It may involve the myocardium, endocardium, and pericardium as well as the heart valves, most commonly the mitral and aortic valves. The other signs and symptoms of the acute illness will disappear, but children who have had carditis may suffer some degree of residual valvular damage.

The mildest cases of carditis may not exhibit signs and symptoms. Indeed, on radiography, the chest may appear normal. The first indication may be a new systolic murmur. If pericarditis is present, a pericardial friction rub may be heard. Conduction abnormalities (prolonged P-R intervals or atrial fibrillation) may be seen on electrocardiogram (ECG).

Other signs of carditis may include tachycardia (particularly a persistent increase in the sleeping pulse rate), shortness of breath with exertion, muffled heart sounds as a result of pericardial effusion, edema of the face, abdomen, or ankles as a result of increased cardiac workload or cardiac insufficiency, pericardial friction rub, and enlargement of the liver. As the inflammation resolves, scarring or fusing of the leaflets of the valves can result in valvular stenosis, which may subsequently lead to left-sided heart failure. Changes in electrical conductivity of the heart (prolonged P-R interval) may be seen in a significant number of patients, but this alone is not diagnostic or prognostic of rheumatic carditis.

Erythema Marginatum. Erythema marginatum is a rare skin manifestation found in fewer than 5 per cent of children with rheumatic fever (Markowitz, 1983). It is characterized by an erythematous, nonpruritic, macular rash with a circular pattern on the trunk, buttocks, and proximal limbs. It blanches when pressed and is accentuated with heat. It may occur in the acute phase of illness but may come and go for several months. Erythema marginatum usually occurs in patients who also have carditis.

Subcutaneous Nodules. These are usually visible nodules that are found on the flexor surfaces of the joints and bony prominences, such as feet, hands, scapula, scalp, and vertebrae. They are small, firm, nontender swellings that occur during the febrile stage of illness and persist for a relatively long period of time, eventually resolving with no permanent damage. This manifestation also usually occurs in patients with carditis.

Chorea. Chorea is also known as Sydenham chorea, St. Vitus dance, and encephalitis rheumatica. It is an infrequent manifestation of rheumatic fever and its cause is unknown. It is rare in children under 3 years and over 15 years of age. As the incidence of rheumatic fever declines, so does this unusual associated symptom.

Like erythema marginatum and subcutaneous nodules, chorea appears in patients with carditis; however, it may have a later occurrence than other sequelae. Its occurrence also varies with age relative to the appearance of other major manifestations.

Chorea is characterized by involuntary movements of facial muscles as well as muscles of the limbs, particularly upper extremities. Signs and symptoms may be insidious and nonspecific, beginning with irritability and emotional lability. Indeed the child may at first be thought to have behavioral problems, such as being fidgety and showing altered school performance. This process may progress to the point of interference with normal activities of daily living through uncontrollable jerky movements that interfere with voluntary control. Slurred speech may be present.

The central nervous system changes typically occur 2 or more months after the initial streptococcal infection or after the other symptoms of rheumatic fever have subsided. There may be electroencephalogram (EEG) abnormalities; however, these usually return to normal. The symptoms may persist for as little as a week or for as long as 1.5 to 2 years. Chorea is generally a benign and self-limited aspect of rheumatic fever, and full recovery is expected.

Less significant manifestations of rheumatic fever include abdominal pain, pleurisy, and rheumatic pneumonitis. Figure 43-12 summarizes the major and minor manifestations of rheumatic fever.

Diagnostic Assessment

The revised Jones Criteria for diagnosing rheumatic fever have been significant for differentiating this disease from other illnesses with which it may be confused. Diagnosis depends on recognition of the classic symptoms and a detailed patient history. Most children with an acute pharyngitis have a viral rather than a bacterial infection. A throat culture, therefore, is important for determining the presence of Group A beta-hemolytic streptococcus. It should be noted that rheumatic fever may follow a streptococcal infection anywhere in the body; the risk is not limited to pharyngitis.

Although no diagnostic laboratory tests are specific for rheumatic fever, elevations in the erythrocyte sedimentation rate (ESR), C-reactive protein (CRPA), and white blood count (WBC) will usually be seen, indicating the presence of an inflammatory process. A mild anemia is also common and is due to suppressed erythropoiesis during inflammation. Cardiac enyzmes may be increased if severe carditis occurs. If the pharyngitis has resolved within the previous 2 months, the

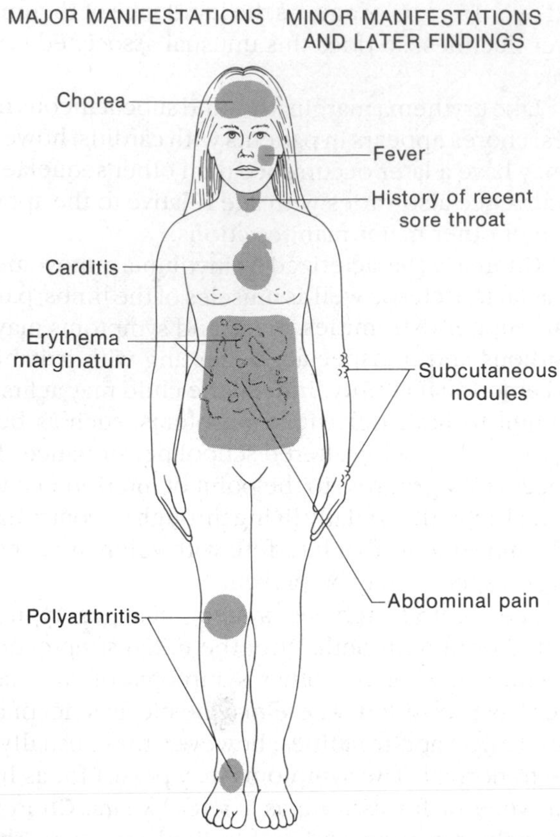

Figure 43-12. Manifestations of rheumatic fever.

presence of an increased strep antibody titer will indicate the preceding infection. The test for identifying strep antibodies is the antistreptolysin O (ASO) test. Streptolysin O is a streptococcal extracellular byproduct that causes lysis of red blood cells. ASO titers indicate the presence of antibodies to these products within the blood. Echocardiography and cardiac catheterization can identify and evaluate valvular damage and ventricular function.

Therapeutic Management

Prevention of rheumatic fever is the best "treatment." Effective management of beta-strep infections can prevent development of rheumatic fever. Early recognition of strep symptoms and appropriate treatment can also prevent recurrence of rheumatic fever, which then reduces the chance of permanent cardiac damage. The goals of treatment are (1) eradication of the streptococcal infection, (2) prevention of permanent cardiac damage, (3) suppression of tissue inflammation, and (4) palliation of symptoms associated with the various manifestations.

If the child has a positive strep culture from the throat, impetigo lesions, or elsewhere at the time of inflammatory symptoms, the active streptococcal infection will be treated.

The treatment of choice to eradicate beta-strep is penicillin, usually in the form of an intramuscular injection of benzathine penicillin G. This form of penicillin is a long-acting drug, and, therefore, treatment may be limited to a single injection. Other penicillins may be administered parenterally or in a combination of parenteral and oral doses.

During the acute phase of the disease, bed rest is recommended to decrease the workload of the heart. The duration of bed rest will depend upon the severity of the disease (Table 43-5).

Salicylates are often administered in the acute phase. These help control inflammation, particularly in the joints. They also provide analgesia for palliation of other symptoms. In cases involving severe carditis, steroids may be prescribed for their anti-inflammatory properties. However, there is still controversy about the long-term benefits of steroids in preventing rheumatic heart disease and their advisability in view of the significant potential side effects (Behrman and Vaughan, 1987). Follow-up care is important.

Residual heart disease is the most destructive long-term complication of rheumatic fever; the incidence is proportional to the degree of carditis. If valvular or other cardiac damage is present, the physician will be alert for subsequent signs of congestive heart failure. (See Chapter 39 for management of congestive heart failure.)

Cardiac valvular damage increases the susceptibility to bacterial endocarditis, particularly if procedures are carried out that could cause septicemia (e.g., dental procedures that may cause entry of mouth bacteria into gum lesions). Prophylactic antibiotics are therefore ordered, usually throughout childhood and adolescence, or for at least 5 years in the older adolescent, even in patients with no residual heart disease. If valvular heart disease is present, lifelong prophylaxis may be recommended. (See Chapter 39 for further discussion of bacterial endocarditis.)

Table 43-5. Guide for Bed Rest and Ambulation in Patients with Acute Rheumatic Fever

Cardiac Status	Management
No carditis	Bed rest for 2 wk and gradual ambulation for 2 wk even if on salicylates
Carditis, no enlargement	Bed rest for 4 wk and gradual ambulation for 4 wk
Carditis, with enlargement	Bed rest for 6 wk and gradual ambulation for 6 wk
Carditis, with heart failure	Strict bed rest for as long as heart failure is present and gradual ambulation for 3 mo

(From Behrman and Vaughan, 1987.)

Major Nursing Diagnoses for Rheumatic Fever

Activity intolerance, related to
- *inflammation of joints*
- *carditis*

Potential diversional activity deficit, related to prolonged bed rest

Altered comfort: pain, related to arthritis/arthralgia

Potential impaired skin integrity, related to
- *erythema marginatum*
- *prolonged bedrest*

Potential altered growth and development, related to
- *social isolation associated with prolonged bed rest*
- *chorea associated with central nervous system involvement*

Potential altered nutrition: less than body requirements, related to anorexia associated with inflammation and immobility

Knowledge deficit, related to home care

Strategies for Nursing Care

Overview of Nursing Goals. The goals of nursing care for the patient who has rheumatic fever are closely correlated with those of medical care, but strategies will differ as nurses focus on appropriate assessments, patient/family teaching, and comfort measures and attend to the needs significant to the child's stage of growth and development. Care of the child with rheumatic fever now primarily occurs in the home rather than in the hospital. In general, interventions will be manifestation- or symptom-specific. Referral likely will be made to a community health nurse who can both assess and anticipate the needs of the child and the family. The nurse will be instrumental in helping the family secure needed supplies. Supplies for home care may include a bed cradle, bedside table and commode, wheelchair, and footboard. In addition, when the child is well enough, arrangements should be made for tutoring.

Family support is also an important aspect of care. The nurse should encourage expression of anger, guilt, frustration, fears, and concerns. The nurse can act as a liaison between the family and community resources (e.g., Crippled Children Commission and American Heart Association), which can provide information and possibly financial assistance.

An important responsibility of the nurse is participation in screening programs aimed at preventing rheumatic fever. Community health nurses as well as school nurses should be alert to children who exhibit signs and symptoms of Group A beta-hemolytic strep infections, particularly if these children live in "at risk" environments. Upon diagnosis of a strep infection, emphasis is placed on completion of antibiotic therapy to ensure eradication of the bacteria. Compliance with this regimen will reduce the risk of rheumatic fever.

The following section discusses nursing strategies for the identified nursing diagnoses. Because management of rheumatic fever commonly occurs in the home, the diagnosis of knowledge deficit will be addressed first.

Teaching to Support Home Care. Included may be all or part of the following areas:

- the disease and its treatment (characteristics and progress of the illness, possible complications, expected outcome, and potential effects of noncompliance with prescribed therapy;
- relationship of exercise to cardiac workload;
- rationale, side effects, and expected length of administration of each medication;
- psychologic and physical preparation for procedures (purpose of the test, the procedure itself, and any follow-up);
- importance of minimizing contact with other infections, particularly respiratory;
- recognition of signs of recurrent strep infections and the importance of seeing the physician for prompt treatment of sore throat after the initial recovery period;
- reassurance that, except for possible valvular damage, all other symptoms are temporary.

Aspects of teaching are incorporated throughout the plan of care, but special attention to administration of medications is warranted here. Medication therapy is important in eradicating any remaining streptococcal organisms, in providing anti-inflammatory and analgesic relief during the acute phase, and in prophylaxis against recurrence.

Managing Medications. Penicillin to eradicate strep is often given by injection, and is therefore the responsibility of the nurse, rather than the family. Intramuscular injections of benzathine penicillin G must be administered with care. Gluteal injections can cause vasospasms and sciatic nerve damage if injected into the neural area. To prevent potential tissue ischemia and nerve damage, the midlateral thigh is the recommended site for injection. If oral penicillin is prescribed instead of, or in addition to, the injection, the family must realize the importance of administering all of the pills.

Alertness to signs of an allergic response to medications is essential. In the initial assessment, the nurse should inquire about any previous adverse reactions to penicillin, and the child should remain in the clinic for 20 minutes following the injection in case an anaphylactic reaction occurs. Epinephrine must be available for this emergency. The child and parents should be taught the side effects of oral penicillin (or erythromycin), including any indications of hypersensitivity (rash, pruritus, chills, dyspnea, and so on).

Aspirin (ASA) and steroids may be used to minimize the inflammatory process. Fever, arthritis, arthralgias, and myalgias are generally controlled well with ASA. Children's ability to tolerate aspirin is variable. Side effects of aspirin include gastrointestinal disturbances, decreased platelet count, tinnitus, headaches, and possible mental disturbances.

Steroids, which may be prescribed if the child has an associated carditis, have significant anti-inflammatory properties but also have serious side effects. See Table 43-2 for the nursing process plan related to steroid administration.

Digoxin may be added to the medication regimen. It slows conduction (and therefore the heart rate) and strengthens the contractions of the myocardium, thereby improving cardiac efficiency. If there are changes in pulse rate or quality, particularly if there is a significant decrease in rate, the digoxin should not be administered and the physician should be notified. (See Chapter 39 for additional information on administration of digoxin.)

Promoting Compliance with Bed Rest and Activity Restrictions. Maintaining bed rest for the child with rheumatic fever may prove to be one of the greatest challenges for the nurse and the family. Because the child may not feel ill, bed rest may seem unreasonable or unnecessary. The parents and child need to understand that to feel well does not mean that the body has recovered. Explaining the reason for activity restrictions often helps the child and family cope with the frustration and inconvenience.

Explaining the Relationship Between Exercise and Cardiac Workload. The child who is old enough to understand and incorporate the information should be included in an explanation of the activity intolerance associated with rheumatic fever. The discussion should explain the relationship between activity and cardiac workload, thus providing a rationale for activity restrictions. The school-age child and adolescent will be able to understand the importance of the heart as a vital organ. This may make activity restrictions somewhat more tolerable. (See Chapter 27 for detailed information about age-appropriate teaching strategies.)

Clarifying the Restrictions. The child and family will need clarification of the physician's intent for activity. The nurse can clarify what the specific expectations of "bed rest" are (i.e., does this include bathroom privileges, activities of daily living such as out of bed to dress, eat meals, and ambulation, or does this mean strict or absolute bed rest?).

Encouraging Self-Management. Once it is clear why extra rest is needed and exactly what the activity restrictions are, the nurse can talk with the family about allowing the child some self-management responsibilities. The child who is allowed to exercise some autonomy is usually more willing to follow the prescribed treatment. Self-management may include participation in developing a schedule that includes appropriate activities and planned rest periods. An activity list with related expenditure of energy will help with planning. During follow-up visits, the nurse can reinforce the child's sense of accomplishment for self-management by commenting on appropriate choices and evidence of good judgment. A gradual increase in activities can be anticipated as the sedimentation rate returns to normal, inflammation subsides, and any cardiac involvement stabilizes.

Encouraging Expression of Feelings. Despite explanations and promises of being able to normalize activity after a few weeks, restrictions may cause the child to feel angry, frustrated, frightened, and anxious. The nurse can be supportive by communicating understanding and by providing a safe environment for sharing of these feelings and concerns. Gradual resumption of normal activities should be seen as indications of improvement and provide encouragement for all concerned.

Managing Associated Carditis. The presence of carditis with its associated potential for permanent cardiac damage requires careful follow-up and management. Often the child with mild-to-moderate carditis can be treated in the home. Severe carditis usually involves congestive heart failure and will require hospitalization.

A change in the quality of the pulse may be the first indication of cardiac involvement. Nursing assessment on follow-up visits will therefore include careful respiratory and cardiac assessment. The pulse parameters and the rate and rhythm of the apical pulse will be compared with the child's baseline at the time of diagnosis. Any irregularities or significant changes must be referred to the physician for diagnosis.

The administration of oxygen may be indicated with carditis, to reduce the workload of the heart. The nurse can facilitate home oxygen therapy by serving as a liaison between the family and the company supplying the equipment. The family will need a 24-hour-per-day phone number in case of questions or malfunction of the equipment.

If oxygen is required, a nasal cannula provides the most accurate method of administration. Children also consider it the least restrictive. Appropriate explanation of the rationale and benefit of oxygen is important to promote compliance with therapy and reduce anxiety for both parents and child.

Vital signs (particularly heart rate and blood pressure) are good indicators of progress or status of cardiac function. As the acute stage resolves, the heart rate should be more nearly normal for age, and decompensation with activities should be less significant (i.e., the heart rate returns more quickly to normal).

Promoting Diversional Activity. Boredom becomes a problem for the child confined to bed. The child can be encouraged to participate in development of a daily schedule, which should include as many of the usual activities as possible, e.g., getting dressed, eating meals with the family, attending to studies, and so on. All the activities must be geared to decrease boredom while conforming to the limits imposed by the degree of restrictions, expectations, and implications of "bed rest." Age-appropriate diversional activities can be encouraged or provided (for example, quiet games, art activities, books, video recordings, or television). Family and friends can be encouraged to write, call, or visit (after being screened for upper respiratory infections or other illnesses). When the child's condition permits, a tutor should be provided to help keep the child current with school assignments.

Alleviating Discomfort. Discomforts occur throughout the course of rheumatic fever as a result of fever, arthritis, and arthralgias. Analgesics (aspirin and acetaminophen) are given to reduce the fever and discomfort. Equipment such as bedcradles can be used to lift linens and reduce pressure on sensitive skin and joints. Bedrails (which can be rented from a home care supply service) can aid the child in moving in bed and also prevent falls. Care should be organized to minimize handling of the child. Massage, manipulation of joints, and heat or cold may aggravate discomforts. Proper body alignment will help reduce joint discomfort.

Preventing Skin Breakdown. Erythema marginatum is a transitory skin manifestation that leaves no residual tissue damage. The child and family will often need reassurance, however, that recurrence of the rash does not signal a relapse of the disease. Because the rash is nonpruritic, the skin requires no special care other than the hygiene indicated to prevent breakdown.

Because of fever, discomfort associated with movement, joint pains, and stiffness, skin breakdown is a potential problem. Breakdown can be avoided by regular repositioning, and making sure that the skin is kept clean and well lubricated, that linens are clean and wrinkle-free, and that bony prominences are well lubricated and protected from irritation and pressure.

Promoting Normal Development. Emotional and social development may be temporarily interrupted because of prescribed bed rest that takes the child out of the classroom and away from normal peer activities. When the disease is complicated by the occurrence of chorea, development is further obstructed. The nurse can alert the family to age-appropriate developmental tasks and help them normalize the child's environment as much as possible. When chorea is present, the family will need reassurance of its temporary nature, and practical advice for management.

Reducing Social Isolation. The child may feel isolated if confined to bed away from normal activities of the family. The nurse can clarify that "bed rest" need not mean "in the bedroom." The child can be kept near the family activities by lying on a cot in the kitchen or on a sofa in the living room. At times when the child is alone in a bedroom, anticipation of needs may help reduce feelings of isolation. Some means should be provided (e.g., a bell) to allow the child to indicate the need for assistance or attention. Family pets can be wonderful companions, and a telephone can provide an important link to peers and extended family.

Supporting Family Management of Chorea. Children with uncontrollable body movements related to chorea are usually frightened and frustrated, as are their families. Even the most basic tasks of growth and development may be difficult or impossible to perform. Fine motor activities may be impaired. The child may experience mood swings and outbursts of anger. To cope with this unusual behavior the child and family need consistent, supportive assistance and care.

The child and family will need reassurance that this is only a temporary disorder and that while it is a neurologic phenomenon, the child's intellect is not affected. It may be necessary to intervene with teachers and perhaps students to explain the child's problem and to assure all concerned that this is not a behavioral or learning disorder. With family support, interruptions in development encountered during chorea need not result in significant delays.

Caregivers should anticipate that the child will probably need assistance with such basic care as feeding, toileting, and bathing. In addition, the child must be protected from injury related to uncontrollable movements. Persons who assist with feeding should be reminded that sudden choreic movements of the head make use of a fork or a straw dangerous. Plastic (rather than glass) is advised for plates and drinking glasses. The child's bed should have rails (or some other protection) that prevent falling out of bed. Rails or protective barriers should be padded to prevent injury. Mittens and head covering may be indicated at times. Toys and games should be assessed for sharp edges.

Choreiform movements disappear during sleep; therefore sedatives may be prescribed. In the acute phase of chorea the child may rest better in a room where stimulation is minimized. However, as the condition improves, the child may become more anxious when isolated and may benefit from the company of other children and family members.

Promoting Optimal Nutrition. The child with rheumatic fever often experiences an increased metabolic rate associated with fever and inflammation. However, immobility, boredom, and discomfort may lead to anorexia. In addition, aspirin and steroids can cause gastric irritation, further diminishing appetite. The additional need for calories, coupled with anorexia, can lead to insufficient intake.

During convalescence, the diet should have adequate protein and calories to meet the recovery needs of the body, especially when fever or infection is present. (It is also important, however, to avoid excessive weight gain.) Fluid intake should be monitored to prevent either dehydration or overhydration. The febrile patient needs additional fluids, but hypervolemia increases the workload of the heart. Medications should be taken with milk or food to minimize stomach upsets. Parents should be encouraged to be tolerant when the child's appetite is poor, offering small frequent meals in lieu of large meals. Intake may increase if the child is allowed some control by selecting from choices of nutritious foods for meals and snacks.

Nursing Strategies for Follow-up Care in the Home or Clinic

Assess vital signs, lung sounds, and heart sounds for evidence of carditis or respiratory infection.

Weigh the child to assess for fluid retention.

Assess the neurologic status for evidence of chorea.

Determine whether anti-inflammatory and analgesic medications are effective in reducing joint pain.

Obtain a blood specimen, as indicated, for determination of sedimentation rate.

Assess nutritional adequacy by asking the child to recall the intake for the previous 24 hours.

Reinforce the necessity of avoiding exposure to other infections during the convalescent period.

Discuss with the child and family ways in which developmental tasks may be addressed during the period of activity restriction.

Following recovery, determine compliance with prophylactic antibiotic therapy during dental procedures involving gingival bleeding and for surgical techniques predisposing the child to recurrent carditis.

Discuss with the child and family the importance of throat culture for any subsequent sore throat symptoms.

Kawasaki Disease

Kawasaki disease (KD) is the name currently given to the syndrome previously known as mucocutaneous lymph node syndrome. It is a febrile, multisystem disorder in which vasculitis is the most potentially dangerous characteristic. Generally considered a self-limiting disease, KD can also be fatal if aneurysms or myocardial infarction occurs.

Etiology

It is generally agreed that Kawasaki disease is not a new pathologic entity. In the past, KD was probably misdiagnosed as other types of vasculitis before criteria were established to clearly define it from other disease processes. Kawasaki appears to be occurring more frequently, sporadically and in clusters, than at the time it was first described by Kawasaki in 1967. However, this may be due to more accurate diagnosis or reporting.

Kawasaki disease may be seen at any age, but is virtually restricted to prepubertal children. It is most common in boys younger than 2 years and in persons of Japanese ancestry (Hicks and Melish, 1986). Genetics has been suggested as a possible explanation for a higher incidence among Japanese children, but the evidence to support this is inconclusive. Kawasaki disease has a seasonal pattern, with a significantly greater number of cases in the winter and spring months.

Although the etiology of Kawasaki disease remains unknown, several possible causes have been proposed. Environmental factors (e.g., rug shampoo) have been implicated but remain unconfirmed. When "epidemics" have occurred, the affected children have had a significantly higher-than-average occurrence of mild respiratory upset. No specific etiologic organism was identified, however, and no person-to-person infectious tendency was found. This suggests that hypersensitivity or an altered immune system may play a role in the pathogenesis of KD. Melish (1987) summarized studies that have shown a sharp rise in antibody production in the first 4 weeks of the disease (probably related to depression of T-suppressor cells) and then a subsequent fall in all the immunoglobulins. The rise in immunoglobulins supplies additional antibodies for reaction with antigens, and circulating immune (antigen-antibody) complexes are frequently detected in Kawasaki disease. It is thought these immune complexes may bind directly to the vascular endothelium, causing inflammation of the vessels.

Pathophysiology

The most common and potentially dangerous effect of the Kawasaki disease process is vasculitis, which can result in occlusive or ischemic manifestations during the acute disease process or at a later period in life. Over the course of illness, any or all parts of the vascular system can be involved, beginning with the microvessels (arterioles, capillaries, and venules) and progressing to involve small and medium-sized vessels.

The inflammatory process begins in the perivascular tissues and moves into the other layers of vascular tissue. The combination of vascular inflammation and the typically increased thrombocyte count may result in clot formation (thrombi). The vascular changes in the heart muscle and the coronary arteries are of most concern since they can lead to lifelong morbidity or mortality.

Clinical Manifestations

Typically, the child with acute Kawasaki disease has an unexplained fever of 38.9 to 41.1°C (102 to 106°F) that does not remit with administration of analgesics. Additionally, a pruritic, polymorphic rash; a marked cervical lymphadenopathy; dry, red, cracked lips; a "strawberry" tongue; bilateral conjunctivitis; and striking erythema (perhaps with desquamation) of the palms and soles are likely. The child is also likely to be irritable and lethargic.

The clinical course of the disease occurs in three phases. Symptoms appear and resolve in a typical pattern. In the acute phase (the first 8 to 10 days), fever, strawberry tongue, cracked/fissured lips, rash, erythema and edema of the palms and soles, and lymphadenopathy are seen. In the subacute period (10 to 35 days), desquamation of the toes, feet and fingers, and palms occurs. The child will likely continue to be irritable and anorectic and have conjunctival injection. Also during this period arthritis, thrombocytosis, and cardiac and vascular manifestations occur. The recovery phase is said to continue until the erythrocyte sedimentation rate becomes normal (perhaps as long as 10 weeks after onset).

Diagnostic Assessment

Criteria developed for diagnosis require that the child meet five of the following six criteria and that other diseases are ruled out: (1) abrupt onset of fever unresponsive to antibiotics, (2) bilateral conjunctivitis, (3) changes in the mouth: dry, chapped, fissured or reddened lips; strawberry tongue; or reddened mucosa, (4) changes in the extremities: reddened palms or soles, indurative edema of hands or feet, or desquamation (peeling skin) from the fingertips or toes, (5) rash on the trunk, and (6) enlargement of cervical lymph nodes (Hicks and Melish, 1986).

Laboratory Tests. Laboratory data used for diagnosis are fairly nonspecific. Complete blood count (CBC) with differential, erythrocyte sedimentation rate (ESR), and platelet count are the tests most commonly used for both diagnosis and monitoring the course of the disease. A markedly elevated ESR is common in the early stages of illness and helps distinguish this illness from viral illnesses that otherwise might be suspected. The white blood count is significantly elevated (leukocytosis), with a shift to the left (a high percentage of polymorphonuclear cells). A marked thrombocytosis (increased platelet count) occurs 10 to 12 days after onset of the fever. In the early period of illness, abnormal liver function tests may be seen in a slightly elevated level of transaminase.

Therapeutic Management

Therapy for Kawasaki disease continues to be controversial. Aspirin has been the primary means of therapy for both its anti-inflammatory and antiplatelet effects (i.e., to counteract thrombocytosis). In the acute period, dosages of at least 100 mg/kg/day of aspirin are prescribed for the anti-inflammatory effect. For unexplained reasons, therapeutic aspirin levels are difficult to achieve in the acute period. The most widely accepted explanation for this is a markedly impaired absorption of aspirin. Serum aspirin levels of 20 to 25 mg/dl appear to be adequate to achieve an anti-inflammatory effect, abolish the high fever, and reduce the incidence of further cardiac involvement. As the course of disease progresses into the subacute phase, the aspirin dose can be reduced because there is improved absorption and therefore higher serum levels. In addition, at this point the indication for aspirin becomes its antiplatelet effect rather than its anti-inflammatory effect, and this effect can be gained at a much lower serum level (10 mg/dl). Accordingly, aspirin levels must be regularly monitored to assure that appropriate therapeutic levels are achieved to accomplish the specific purpose while preventing toxicity.

Low-dose aspirin is continued until the child's platelet count and sedimentation rate return to normal. This therapy may also be continued as long as coronary artery dilatation persists. If the child has difficulty taking aspirin (gastritis), other anti-inflammatory preparations may be prescribed.

Recent studies indicate that aspirin has not been shown to reduce the occurrence of coronary artery abnormalities. High-dose intravenous gamma globulin given in conjunction with aspirin, however, appears to be effective in rapidly reducing fever as well as having a rapid, generalized anti-inflammatory effect (Newburger, 1986; Melish, 1987). In addition, as shown on echocardiogram, the number of children with coronary artery abnormalities was greatly reduced.

Major Nursing Diagnoses for Kawasaki Disease

Altered tissue perfusion: cardiac and peripheral, *related to*

- *inflammation of blood vessels, associated*

probably with binding of immune complexes to vessel walls
- *thrombocytosis*

***Hyperthermia,** related to the disease process*

***Impaired skin integrity,** related to erythema and possible desquamation of the palms and soles*

***Altered comfort: pain/pruritus,** related to edema and skin irritation*

***Potential altered nutrition: less than body requirements,** related to anorexia associated with*
- *malaise*
- *gastritis*
- *involvement of oral mucous membranes*

***Fear/anxiety: child/parents,** related to*
- *prognosis*
- *diagnostic tests*

Strategies for Nursing Care

Nursing care must be multifaceted, involving assessment and monitoring for complications and strategies for teaching and supporting the child and family.

Assessing Cardiovascular Status. Assessment of cardiac status is critical. A cardiopulmonary monitor is indicated. Tachycardia, gallop rhythm, chest pain, and ECG changes (depressed ST segment) suggest myocarditis. Tachypnea or dyspnea, rales or other noisy respirations, costal retractions, nasal flaring, orthopnea, distended neck veins, and edema are all signs and symptoms of congestive heart failure. Unusual dysrhythmias may indicate impairment or disruption of the electric conduction system of the heart. Signs of cardiac tamponade may be similar to those of congestive heart failure. This also may present as distant heart sounds, narrowing of pulse pressure, and/or presence of pulsus paradoxus.

Careful assessment of the circulatory status of the extremities is important, particularly in the subacute phase of illness when thrombi are more likely to cause circulatory impairment that could contribute to progression of infection or necrosis of fingers or toes.

Monitoring Fever. Because the fever associated with Kawasaki disease tends to be high and unrelieved by medication, careful monitoring is indicated. Management for a high fever includes increased fluid intake and the removal of clothing and blankets. Sponging at times may be indicated, but it is a controversial intervention and must be done carefully to avoid injury. See Chapter 27, page 825, for detailed information about sponging.

Promoting Optimal Skin Integrity. It is important to note the presence and status of rash and edema. As the desquamation occurs, the skin condition should be assessed to note early signs of infection that might occur. Keeping the skin clean, dry, free of irritation from linens and clothing, and well lubricated will help preserve the integumentary barrier to infection and will make the child more comfortable as well. Protect edematous areas from friction and prolonged pressure. Gentle handling of the child is indicated in light of altered skin integrity but does not override the child's need for physical comfort.

Maintaining Adequate Nutrition. Adequacy of the nutritional status may be difficult to maintain, and ongoing assessment of intake and output (both fluids and solids) is important. The discomfort of the mucous membranes may be one deterrent to adequate nutrition. Pain that results from gastritis or other organ involvement may also decrease appetite and willingness to eat and drink and requires intervention. Application of petroleum jelly or other ointment to lips, cleaning of the mouth with a soft sponge saturated with dilute hydrogen peroxide, and perhaps a topical anesthetic applied at eating time can provide comfort and a sense of control and independence.

Reducing Discomfort. Edematous hands and feet may be painful because of the pressure exerted on tissues by the inflammatory exudate. There is also discomfort associated with the pruritic rash. Systemic antipruritic medications may be used to reduce itching. The aspirin administered for anti-inflammatory and antiplatelet properties will also provide analgesia. Nonpharmacologic comfort measures of holding, rocking, singing, reading stories, and other distraction techniques should also be included in the plan of care.

Reducing Fear and Anxiety. The vascular and potential cardiac involvement associated with Kawasaki disease often causes fear for the child's prognosis. Some children may have coronary artery aneurysms, suffer infarctions (which may occur in any organ system or part of the body), or die in the acute, subacute, or recuperative phase of the disease process, but families should be reassured that 95 to 99 per cent of patients with KD totally recover without any sequelae.

The child and family need preparation and emotional support for several procedures. These may include frequent blood tests, possible intravenous infusions, lumbar puncture, echocardiogram, cardiac monitoring, collection of urine specimens, and perhaps angiograms. Support for anxious parents can be provided by regular updates on the child's status and information regarding the symptoms which are present. Parents can participate in the child's care to support their needs for parenting as well as the comfort needs of the child.

Nursing Strategies for Follow-Up Care in the Home or Clinic

Assess cardiovascular status for evidence of cardiac involvement or systemic thrombosis.

Obtain a blood specimen, as indicated, for determination of platelet count and sedimentation rate.

Assess skin integrity. Remind the child and parent to keep areas of skin rash and desquamation clean and dry and to protect edematous areas.

Determine compliance with aspirin therapy (which will be at low dosages during Stages II and III to decrease platelet aggregation).

Prepare the child for an electrocardiogram or echocardiogram, as indicated, using age-appropriate teaching techniques to allay anxiety.

Stevens-Johnson Syndrome

Stevens-Johnson syndrome (SJS), first reported in 1922, is classified as a severe form of erythema multiforme. Of diverse etiology and affecting many systems, it is characterized by distinctive skin lesions, mucosal involvement, and often severe systemic symptoms. Unless it is quickly and carefully treated, SJS can be fatal.

SJS is an uncommon disease seen most frequently in children and young adults; boys are affected more often than girls, and it is more often seen in the winter months.

Etiology

The exact etiology remains unknown, but it is generally considered to be a hypersensitive-immunologic reaction to one or more of many different stimuli, including diverse disease states and drugs. Viral, bacterial, and fungal infections, as well as collagen diseases, some vaccines, foods, and contactants, have been implicated. When drugs are suspected as an etiologic factor, symptoms may appear within hours up to 3 weeks after administration. Barbiturates, penicillins, sulfonamides, and many others have been identified as possible causes of SJS; the penicillins appear to be more frequently associated with this syndrome than the others. A significant number of patients who develop SJS are noted to have chronic or recurring infectious processes, suggesting a possible immune deficiency. Exactly what the relationship or role any of these agents play is not clear, and each may, in fact, be only one of several interacting factors.

Pathophysiology

In SJS, a split occurs in the dermal-epidermal junction and an inflammatory response develops in the dermis. Tissue damage occurs and skin actually peels off the body.

Complications are of significant concern in Stevens-Johnson syndrome. The most common complications are those associated with the eye. Acute lesions or conjunctival scarring can lead to permanent visual impairment. Tear duct atrophy, corneal ulceration, and adhesions also may occur. Gastrointestinal problems that may occur include esophageal strictures resulting from esophagitis. Respiratory complications are also common. Upper airway involvement and different types of pneumonias, particularly that caused by *Mycoplasma pneumoniae,* are frequently seen. As with burn patients, when skin damage is severe, complications such as fluid and electrolyte imbalances and sepsis are the significant concerns. Mortality rate can be as high as 10 per cent in the acute phase, especially if there is respiratory involvement (Schaller and Wedgwood, 1987).

Clinical Manifestations and Diagnostic Assessment

Diagnosis is made upon the following minimum characteristics: target lesions, bullae, vesicles, involvement of two or more mucous membranes, purulent conjunctivitis, and systemic toxicity. A prodromal phase may be seen in which there is fever, sore throat, cough, and malaise. Differential diagnosis must rule out contact dermatitis, Reiter disease, chickenpox, impetigo, and herpes simplex.

Laboratory Tests. Laboratory data are not likely to be helpful in making a diagnosis. Not only are there no specific laboratory tests for SJS, the most common abnormal hematologic criteria—elevated sedimentation rate and leukocytosis—are too general to be of value in making a diagnosis. To complicate the picture even further, there are some contrasting reports (Westley and Wechsler, 1984; Ruiz-Maldonado, 1985) of marked reduction in leukocytes which has yet to be explained. In fact, when this occurs and does not improve within 5 to 7 days, the prognosis appears to be grave.

Description of Skin Lesions. A description of skin lesions is difficult because they evolve and change appearance throughout the course of the disease. Typical early lesions look like an insect bite with an erythematous papule. A blister may develop or a central area of epidermal necrosis may occur without a blister. These are known as "target" or "iris" lesions. These lesions may progress from fine maculopapular lesions to confluent areas of erythema to toxic epidermal necrosis, which is a massive denudation (peeling) of the epidermis. Skin pigmentation may also affect the appearance of the lesions. Lesions commonly appear over a 3- to 5-day period, but new eruptions may occur for up to 2 weeks. Depending on the severity of the mucosal damage, the course of the disease process from eruption to healing may take up to 6 weeks, not including recurrent lesions.

Distribution of Skin Lesions. The distribution of lesions is commonly symmetric on the extremities, spreading to the trunk, but it is extremely variable. Mucosal involvement is frequently present; these lesions are characteristically found in the mouth and eyes but may also be accompanied by genital, pharyngeal, and upper respiratory lesions. Serious sequelae or morbidity results from damage to the mucous membranes. Itching, burning, and pain may be associated with mucosal lesions. Systemic symptoms associated with the disease process include fever, myalgias, and prostration.

Therapeutic Management

Treatment should be supportive and appropriate for symptoms that occur. This includes maintenance of fluid balance, debridement of crusted lesions, and aggressive pulmonary care to limit or prevent pulmonary complications. Mouth care is important to treat stomatitis (oral mucous membrane lesions). Warm saline mouthwashes and topical anesthetics may provide relief. Any eye involvement must be closely monitored. Irrigations, application of warm compresses, and topical steroids may be helpful. If the eye lesions are severe, it may be necessary to instill artificial tears solution.

A method of management of severe cutaneous involvement that seems to be most effective in minimizing complications and reducing mortality has been to use a regimen similar to that followed in caring for burn patients. This appears to reduce the incidence of septicemia and fluid and electrolyte imbalances.

Despite a variety of management philosophies and methods, the outcome for the patient with Stevens-Johnson syndrome is unpredictable. Severe skin involvement or continuous leukopenia usually indicates poor prognosis. Although many children recuperate without residual problems, some permanent disabilities can result, including corneal and conjunctival scarring, dermal scarring secondary to infections, prolonged gastric ulceration, and esophageal strictures. Respiratory compromise resulting from an initiating factor of *Mycoplasma pneumoniae* infection may contribute further to this mortality rate. Aggressive, meticulous care, and careful monitoring of status may minimize or prevent complications and death.

Major Nursing Diagnoses for SJS

Impaired skin integrity, related to dermal tissue damage, associated probably with a hypersensitive immune response
Potential fluid volume deficit, related to increased insensitive loss through denuded skin
Potential for infection, related to
- *loss of skin defense against pathogens associated with denudation*
- *altered immune response*

Altered comfort: pain, related to skin lesions
Potential altered nutrition: less than body requirements, related to
- *painful stomatitis/esophagitis*
- *general discomfort/malaise*

Potential for injury, related to development of the following complications:
- *permanent visual impairment*
- *esophageal strictures associated with esophagitis*
- *urinary retention associated with inflammation of the genitalia*

Fear/anxiety, related to
- *hospitalization*
- *altered appearance*
- *social isolation*

Knowledge deficit, related to home care during the recuperative phase

Strategies for Nursing Care

Nursing care must cover a broad scope of physiologic systems, including the integumentary, respiratory, and digestive systems; the eyes; fluids; laboratory data including electrolytes, CBC, and cultures of lesions; nutrition; and the child's emotional status.

Assessing and Treating Lesions of Skin and Mucous Membranes. Frequent, thorough observations should be made and any changes in the status of the lesions documented. This includes the appearance of new lesions and changes in eye lesions. Record the type and amount of drainage from the eyes.

Soothing soaks may be ordered, which, for the young child, can be administered like a bath in a tub that has been meticulously disinfected. Bath toys can decrease fear of this procedure. Ointments may also be ordered and are usually scheduled to follow soaks. Application of the ointment with a sterile glove can help prevent transfer of organisms from caregiver to child and increases comfort by reducing friction with the denuded skin.

Maintaining Fluid and Electrolyte Balance. Fluid requirements will increase as larger surface areas become denuded. Attention to intake and output records and to urine specific gravity will aid judgments related to administration of fluids. The nurse must also monitor for urinary retention, which can be associated with inflammation of the genitalia. Intake that is significantly greater than output and a palpable bladder are signs of urinary retention.

Preventing Infections. The presence of open or draining lesions presents an inviting medium for sepsis. If leukopenia occurs as a part of the disease process, immune status is compromised. Good handwashing technique, meticulous management of intravenous lines, monitoring of visitors to screen for infectious disease, and instructions for visitors regarding interactions and contact with the child are important physical concerns.*

Thorough assessments of respiratory status are critical. With the high incidence of *Mycoplasma pneumoniae* as a precipitating factor of this disease, continuous monitoring, documentation, and aggressive management are essential.

Providing Comfort. Comfort measures are important when lesions are pruritic or painful. Careful administration of antihistamines and analgesics can provide relief. However, because of the high correlation between medications and SJS, nonessential drugs should be avoided. Most comfort measures will be nonpharmacologic, although rocking and cuddling may cause additional discomfort to denuded areas of the skin. The nurse who collaborates with the parent and other family members concerning potential nonpharmacologic measures will be more successful in comforting the child.

Managing Nutritional Intake. Lesions in the mouth and mucous membranes of the gastrointestinal tract may necessitate nasogastric (NG) feeding. Adequate nutrition is essential for replacement of lost fluids and for healing of what may be a large percentage of the cutaneous and mucocutaneous surfaces. Maintaining a nasogastric tube in these children, however, presents a special challenge. If there are esophageal lesions, insertion (and replacement) may be irritating and quite painful. Maintaining correct placement of the tube can be difficult if there are lesions on the face and nose, making tape a contraindication. Nursing ingenuity is often essential in safeguarding tube placement. Careful recording of intake and output must be maintained to determine nutritional adequacy.

Providing Emotional Support. Thoughtful, appropriate explanations of procedures should be made before they are done. Time should be allowed for listening to the child's concerns. Diversional activities consistent with the stage of growth and development and appropriate for the limitations imposed by the disease process can help the child cope with the stress of the illness. The child must be assured that the skin will heal and that the itching and discomfort will then be gone.

Teaching to Support Home Care During Recuperation. Because of the potential severe complications of Stevens-Johnson syndrome, care during the acute phase will occur in the hospital. The recuperative phase of the illness, however, will be managed primarily on an outpatient basis and parents will need information and support for home management. Anticipating that the child will be maintained on salicylates or steroids, the nurse can begin teaching early in the hospitalization about administration techniques and side effects of the drugs.

The child's activities may also be curtailed during the recovery phase, and the nurse can use the interactions with family during the period of hospitalization to facilitate planning of appropriate, quiet activities, including a rationale for the activity restriction, and perhaps including a consultation with the play therapist. Care of skin lesions at home will follow techniques used during hospitalization, and, once again, it will be advantageous to involve the parents in this therapy early in the hospitalization. The family also will need instruction in preventing skin and systemic infections.

Nursing Strategies for Follow-up Care in the Home or Clinic

Assess respiratory status. Alert physician immediately if infection is suspected.

Assess skin integrity. Culture any suppurative lesions, as indicated.

Test the child's vision in an age-appropriate way (see Chapter 15).

Ask the child/parent to recount nutritional intake in the last 24 hours to assess for nutritional adequacy and evidence of residual painful mucosal lesions or esophageal strictures.

Determine the child's current level of activity, compared to usual ADL, to assess level of comfort and energy.

* In the past, "reverse" isolation or "protective" isolation practices were used with an immunocompromised child. This involved donning various combinations of gown, gloves, and mask to protect the child from the caregiver. Reverse and protective isolation procedures have been discontinued in most institutions (Kirkis and Grier, 1988) because they provided a false sense of security and led to breakdown in certain strategies (such as handwashing) that have proved effective in reducing the spread of microorganisms.

Altered Immune Response: Allergy (Hypersensitivity)

The term *allergy* brings to mind sneezing, wheezing, itching, general discomfort, and even life-threatening anaphylaxis. Despite this well-deserved connotation, allergy is largely a protective function. In all cases, allergic reactions occur in response to a cell that the body recognizes as foreign (i.e., an antigen). The problem is that, for genetic or other undefined reasons, the immune response in these instances occurs with such intensity (i.e., *hypersensitivity*) that host tissues are damaged in the process.

Allergy is a general term for a broad group of disorders. To help in classifying these disorders, Gell and Coombs proposed the four (now classic) types of allergic response (Box 43-2). The first three of these hypersensitivity reactions involve the humoral immune response (antibodies); the fourth is mediated by the cellular immune response (delayed hypersensitivity T-cells, Tdh). This section begins with a general overview of assessment and management of allergy in childhood and nursing strategies to promote effective family coping with chronic allergy. Allergic disorders are then presented, which represent two of the four types of allergic reactions, Type I and Type IV. Categorized as Type I reactions are allergic rhinitis, conjunctivitis, atopic dermatitis, urticaria and angioedema, insect sting allergy (may also be Type IV), and food allergies. Contact dermatitis is presented as an example of the Type IV reaction. Box 43-2 lists chapters dealing with certain of the Type II and Type III disorders.

Assessment of Allergic Disorders

Assessment of the child for a suspected allergic disorder involves a careful history, physical findings, and diagnostic laboratory data. A thorough history is the first and most significant aspect in identifying an allergy. See Box 43-3.

History

The history includes the child, family, and environment as essential components. Many children with atopic allergies have a family history of allergies. Assessing the family provides information of the child's genetic predisposition and assists in ruling out allergic manifestations associated with immunologic disorders. Assessment of the child's chief complaint focuses on three basic questions. They reflect the *when, where* and *what* of the child's symptom state as well as symptom-free state (Korenblat and Wedner, 1984)

Box 43-2
Classification of Allergic Reactions

TYPE I — **IMMEDIATE HYPERSENSITIVITY (ANAPHYLACTIC REACTIONS)**

Features antigen interaction with IgE (and possibly some IgM molecules) bound to a mast cell or basophil. The cell releases histamine and other chemical mediators to produce a local inflammatory reaction. Reactions include hayfever, allergic rhinitis, allergic asthma, many urticarias, and anaphylaxis.

TYPE II — **ANTIBODY-MEDIATED CYTOLYSIS**

Involves lysis of the cell membranes of foreign-appearing blood cells. Lysis occurs as the result of antigen binding to IgM or IgG antibodies on the cells and initiating complement activation. Reactions include blood transfusion reactions (see Chapter 40); hemolytic disease of the newborn; drug-induced hemolytic anemia, leukopenia, and thrombocytopenia (see acquired aplastic anemia, Chapter 40); and hyperacute kidney transplant rejection.

TYPE III — **IMMUNE COMPLEX – DEPENDENT TISSUE INJURY**

Certain circulating antigen-antibody complexes (immune complexes) deposit within tissues such as the kidneys, choroid plexus, joints, skin, or lungs. Chemical mediators are released that stimulate inflammation (with phagocytosis) and activate the complement system. Phagocytosis and complement reactions cause injury to the tissues containing the immune complexes. Reactions include serum sickness, systemic lupus erythematosus (page 1533), glomerulonephritis (see Chapter 42), and juvenile arthritis (see page 1541).

TYPE IV — **DELAYED HYPERSENSITIVITY**

This response is *not* antibody-related. Caused by interaction of antigen with certain T-lymphocytes (delayed hypersensitivity T-cells, Tdh), which release lymphokines, causing inflammation and tissue injury. The response is usually well localized. Reactions include contact dermatitis, organ rejection, and graft-versus-host disease. May play a part in resistance to certain tumors.

(Based on the classic Coombs and Gell classification, 1975; Lockey and Bukantz, 1987a,b; and Bierman et al, 1988.)

Box 43-3
Historical Factors to Consider in Assessment of Allergic Disorders

HISTORY OF PRESENT COMPLAINT

Assess when, what, and where of child's symptom state and symptom-free state

When refers to time of day, week, month, and year

What refers to what child and family assess the cause is

Where refers to place or geographic location

PAST HEALTH HISTORY

Pulmonary manifestations

Nasal, ear, sinus symptoms

Dermatitis, urticaria

Gastrointestinal symptoms

Irritability, fatigue, headache (tension-fatigue syndrome)

Drug reaction(s)

Feeding history

SOCIOECONOMIC AND FAMILY FACTORS

Family history of allergies (Family Profile)

Stability of family members' relationships and stress level in home

Income level and ability to provide food, clothing, shelter, and health care

PHYSICAL ENVIRONMENT

Structural description of home (air/heating system, carpets, cellar, plants, etc.)

Description of child's toys, bedroom, bedding, other rooms of the house where child spends waking hours (e.g., TV room)

Presence of pets in home

Exposure to irritants and/or pollutants (cigarette smoking, proximity to industry, dump or known source of air pollutions, household cleaning supplies)

Cleanliness of home

Exposure level: baby sitters, relatives, day care, school

HEALTH PRACTICES

Routine immunizations

Child's daily routine, including adequacy of eating, activities, rest, sleep

REACTION TO COMMON ALLERGENS

See Box 43-4

FAMILY PROFILE

A family history taken to determine presence of immunologic or allergic disorder(s)

(Box 43-3). Additionally, any present or past history of the following should be documented:

- bronchial manifestations
- nasal and sinus symptoms
- skin disorders
- gastrointestinal symptoms
- recurrent periods of inactivity or lassitude
- colic or irritable behavior
- dietary history
- drug reaction history
- environmental reaction history
- exercise history

The presence or absence of symptoms in all these areas should be noted. The source of this information (often parents) is important because valid recall of times and events associated with symptomatology is critical in providing clues to the causal antigen as well as in establishing the diagnosis. Box 43-4 contains a list of common allergens.

Physical Examination

The physical examination is a systems approach that takes into consideration the child's age and understanding (Table 43-6). Infants and toddlers may cry

Box 43-4
Common Allergens

INHALANTS

Pollen
Mold
House dust
Animal dander
Fabric fiber
Feathers
Dyes
Chemicals

INJECTANTS

Vaccines
Injected drugs
Animal serum
Animal saliva
Animal venom
Insect stings

BACTERIAL INFECTANTS

VIRAL INFECTANTS

INGESTANTS

Food
- Cow's milk
- Eggs
- Wheat
- Chocolate
- Cola products
- Fish, pork, chicken
- Corn, legumes
- Citrus fruits, strawberries, nuts

Drugs
- Aspirin
- Antibiotics
- Barbiturates

Food additives

CONTACTANTS

Plants
Topical drugs
Resins
Metals
Cosmetics
Dyes
Chemicals

OTHER ENVIRONMENTAL FACTORS

Sunshine
Temperature changes
Air pollution

Table 43-6. Physical Assessment for Allergic Disorders

Signs/Symptoms	Explanation for Clinical Manifestations
Skin	
rash/hives dryness, scaliness itching involves cheeks, forehead, extensor or flexor surfaces nails buffed from rubbing skin contact dermatitis involves exposed area	Elevated IgE levels suggest allergy. Mast cells and basophils release histamine, resulting in inflammation, rash, and itching. Chronic itching causes buffed nails, skin breakdown, and dryness. Reason for anatomic location of rash unknown with the exception of contact reaction. In these situations exposed area in contact with allergen elicits a rash.
Eyes	
conjunctivitis itching, burning, excessive lacrimation puffiness of eyelids allergic shiners (dark circles under eyes) (Fig. 43-13) deep transverse crease, lower eyelid Dennie folds—lines progressing from the inner eye, slanting downward and ending in slight swing located in the lower orbitopalpebral grooves	Chemical release of histamine from sensitized IgE mast cells and basophils causes swelling, itching, and excessive lacrimation (conjunctivitis). Dennie folds and allergic shiners are associated with swelling and discoloration of tissue located below the lower eyelid (orbitopalpebral groove).
Nose	
broadened nose bridge (chronic nasal allergy) nasal salute, with transverse nasal crease above tip of nose from nose rubbing (Fig. 43-14) persistent nasal discharge mucosa pale, swollen, congested external irritation from chronic discharge paroxysmal sneezing	Chemical release of histamine by nasal mucosa mast cells causes vascular dilation and swelling, hypersecretion, and itching. This involves frequent wiping of nasal discharge (nasal salute) with subsequent nasal crease and broadened nose bridge if allergic response is chronic. Nasal swelling is associated with nasal obstruction and inability to breathe through the nose (check obstruction by having child sniff from each nostril with other nostril closed)

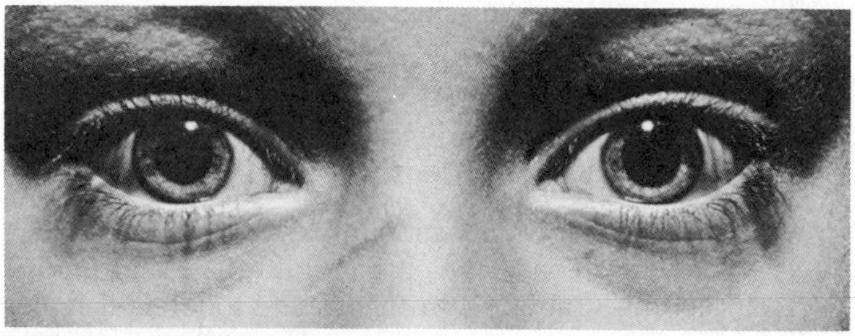

***Figure* 43-13.** Allergic shiners.

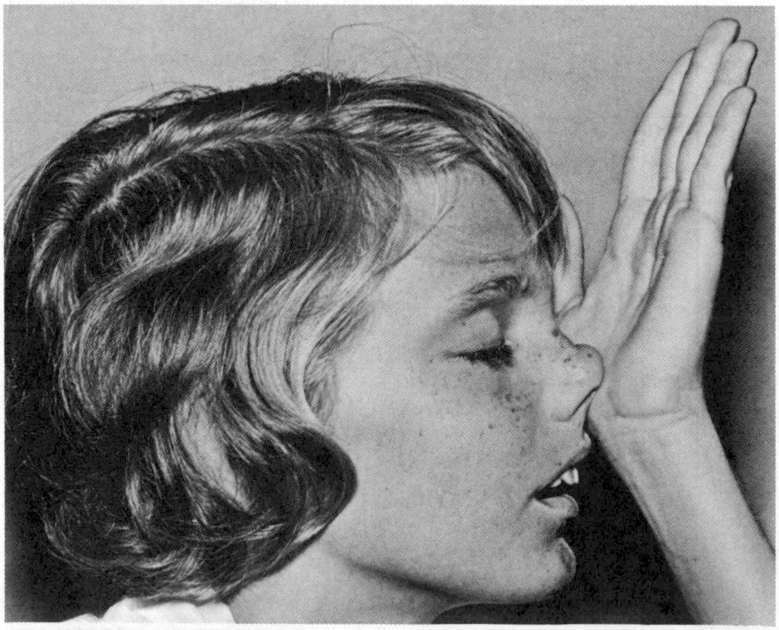

***Figure* 43-14.** Allergic salute.

Signs/Symptoms	Explanation for Clinical Manifestations
Mouth	
mouth breathing high-arched palate geographic tongue (Fig. 43-15) throat clearing continuous	Nasal swelling and obstruction associated with allergic rhinitis leads to mouth breathing. Mouth breathing is associated with oral dryness. Geographic tongue involves red patches with gray margins. Red patches result from desquamation of tongue epithelium. Gray area is thickening of tongue epithelium. Chronic oral breathing is believed to be associated with the development of a high-arched palate. Increased nasopharyngeal mucus leads to frequent attempts to clear the throat.
Ears	
otitis media pain, drainage hearing loss	Swelling and fluid accumulation is medium for infection (otitis media) and affects hearing ability. Pain is a common symptom with otitis media. Chronic ear infections may result in hearing loss.
Chest/respiration	
accessory muscle use increased breathing rate prolonged inspiration or expiration, shortness of breath wheezing pear-shaped chest barrel-shaped chest increased mucus chronic cough	Increased pulmonary mucus production, edematous airway walls, and bronchospasm result in increased respiratory work effort, air trapping, and more resistance to air movement. Increased respiratory effort results in accessory muscle use (retractions) and faster breathing rates. Obstructed airways cause the wheezing sound. The anatomic appearance of pear/barrel chest is associated with air trapping (Chapter 15).
Gastrointestinal	
diarrhea, vomiting, stomachaches, flatulence, cramps colic food intolerances	Antigenic substances from food can pass the intestinal mucosa despite mucous barrier and IgA. IgE-mediated reaction may occur with submucosal edema, dilated blood vessels, and smooth muscle spasm. These pathologic findings are associated with diarrhea, stomachache, cramps, and flatus.
Central Nervous System	
tension-fatigue syndrome irritability tiredness depression headaches	No clear etiology is identified for symptoms of tiredness, irritability, depression, and headache.

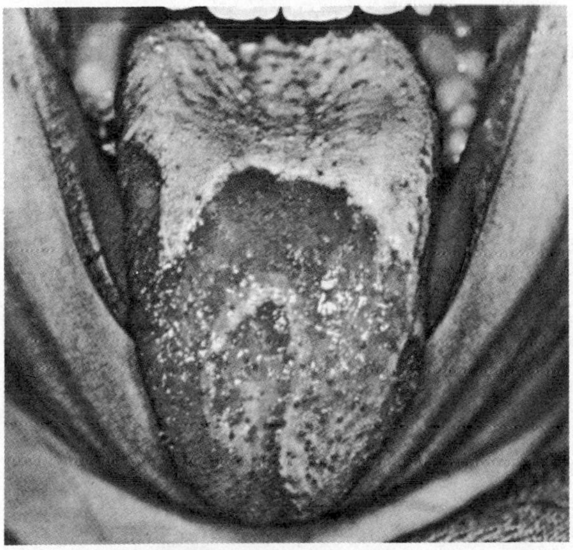

***Figure* 43-15.** Geographic tongue.

(Figures from Marks M. Stigmata of Respiratory Tract Allergies. *Upjohn, 1977.)*

during the examination, therefore it may be best to assess their lungs and respirations before they become upset. In all cases, the child's weight and length are measured and plotted on appropriate growth charts to assess for long-term effects of the allergic condition or medications (steroids), resulting in growth failure.

Laboratory and Diagnostic Studies

Laboratory and diagnostic studies may be necessary. The need to perform these studies is based on the child's history, physical assessment, and inability to control the allergic reaction by elimination or avoidance measures. (Elimination procedures can be invaluable in the improvement of symptoms and diagnosis of allergies.) Skin testing and the serum radioallergosorbent test (RAST) are useful diagnostic methods to identify specific antigen(s) or causative agent(s). There are many variations of this test (e.g., MAST, FAST, ELISA), each of which uses different carriers for antigen (Shapiro, 1988).

Skin Testing

The skin test procedure involves skin exposure through scratch, prick, or intradermal injection (Fig. 43-16) of minute quantities of suspected allergens followed by observation for the type of skin reaction. This test is useful because there is usually a high correlation between antibodies in the skin and those in the blood and respiratory tract (Shapiro, 1988). See Box 43-5 for details of allergy skin testing.

When allergens are introduced to an allergic individual, the allergen commonly interacts with the IgE molecule attached to the mast cell, triggering histamine release (Wasserman, 1988). The histamine release causes a wheal or flare to develop around the tested area. The skin reaction may be immediate (occurring within 15 to 30 minutes) or delayed (occurring up to 48 hours after testing). Skin testing is less often performed with infants because the skin response is usually delayed or incomplete. This is due to a slower rate of IgE synthesis and a less responsive immunologic system.

The RAST Test. The RAST test is a blood test for specific IgE antibodies to pollens, animal danders, house dust, mites, foods, molds, penicillins, and stinging insect bites. The RAST blood test quantifies the amount of specific IgE present in serum. RAST testing, instead of skin testing, is used to identify allergens in infants, pregnant women, children with dermatitis, and asthmatics in whom a severe reaction to skin testing is suspected or who are wheezing. This test is easier and safer to perform, but it is much more expensive and is believed to be less sensitive (and therefore less accurate) than skin testing for identifying the antigen (Sampson and Albergo, 1984; Shapiro, 1988). Both skin testing and the RAST are used as aids in the development of environmental control and as a guide to immunotherapy with those allergens that cannot be avoided.

Other Diagnostic Tests. Patch tests are done when the child is suspected of having a contact allergy. The suspected material is taped to the skin for 1 to 2 days. The test is then read and scored.

Echograph, using the technique of ultrasound, is a new diagnostic tool to assess the presence of sinusitis in children with rhinitis. This quick and noninvasive tool causes little discomfort.

When food allergies are suspected, removal of the suspected food from the diet may provide definite diagnosis of the child's adverse reaction to the food.

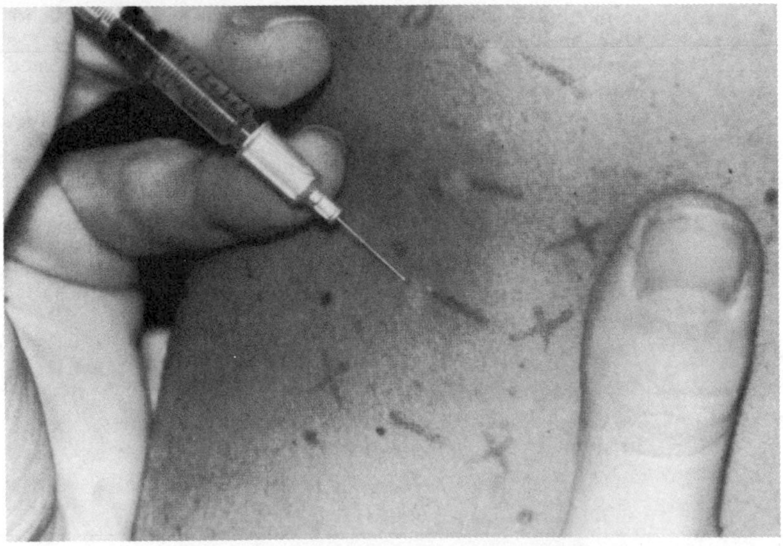

Figure 43-16. Intradermal skin testing for allergy. A 27-gauge needle is used for the intradermal injection of a small amount (0.2 ml) of allergen extract. (From Bierman CW, Pearlman DS: *Allergic Diseases from Infancy to Adulthood.* 2nd ed. Philadelphia, WB Saunders, 1988, 236.)

Box 43-5
Allergy Skin Testing

Allergy skin testing involves the use of extracts from numerous common antigens. Scratch, prick, or intradermal injection are the common techniques used. Prick testing involves dropping the extract onto the skin through which a light puncture is made. Scratch testing is very similar, except that small scratches (1/3″ long) are made. The intradermal method constitutes injecting a small amount of allergens just under the skin. Which antigen extracts are tested is determined by the child's age and size, geographic and environmental exposure, history, and physical findings. The extracts are injected in rows, in a specific pattern, and a control substance is injected for comparison. The usual test site is the back or arm. The back is commonly used for scratch or prick testing. The forearm is most desirable for intradermal testing since it is more accessible to a tourniquet should an extreme allergic response occur to one of the antigen extracts. No antihistamines should be given to a child within 96 hours of testing.

Preparation of the child for skin testing is based on the child's cognitive development. The testing is often scary and uncomfortable because of the itching associated with positive reactions. Intradermal (ID) testing involves a pinching sensation as the needle is inserted under the skin. Children who fear needles may find the repeated ID injections very traumatic. Preparation of the child and family includes explanation of the possible itching and swelling of the tested area, the reaction appearance, length of time for testing, and methods the child and parent can use to assist the child in holding still during the procedure. Sitting on the parent's lap and distractions such as reading stories, imagery, or music may comfort and support the child.

A child is never to be left alone during the testing procedure or in the following period when reactions may occur. Reactions will occur within 10 to 30 minutes after exposure if the child is allergic. The tests are usually read in 15 to 20 minutes and scored according to the skin reaction. A positive reaction is evidenced by erythema and wheal information at the site. In the prick or scratch test, once a reaction occurs the area should be immediately wiped off to prevent further reaction. All the extracts should be removed in approximately 30 minutes after the testing. Reactive manifestations may persist for 8 to 12 hours. The family should be instructed to report delayed reactions (occurring 24 to 48 hours later). The tester monitors the child closely for any systemic reactions during the testing procedure. Since false-negative reactions can occur, skin testing results should be interpreted in conjunction with the history, physical examination, and laboratory findings.

When multiple foods are suspected, a systematic blind approach to removing foods from the diet is often the only way to sort out the actual allergen(s).

Challenge testing involves administering the suspected allergen and observing the child's response. This testing may be done for diagnosing food allergy or causes of asthma. Challenge testing, particularly bronchial challenge testing for identifying causative allergens for asthma, can be very dangerous and must be carried out in a controlled setting.

Additional serum testing may be performed to assist the diagnosis of allergy. Elevated serum IgE and total eosinophil counts are associated with allergic disorders and may have a predictive value in determining later allergy development in infants. Eosinophils may be measured from body secretions to assist diagnosis of allergic rhinitis, conjunctivitis, and food allergies (Sly, 1985). See Table 43-7 for specimen collection.

Table 43-7. Eosinophil Collection and Results Indicative of Allergic Disease

Test	Obtaining Specimen	Significant Results
Mucous cytology (Rhinitis)	Infant: aspirate nasal secretions in bulb syringe. Older child: blow nose into wax paper	10%+ eosinophils
Conjunctival cytology (Conjunctivitis)	Swab (sterile) inner canthus of conjunctiva	10%+ eosinophils
Bronchial secretion cytology (Asthma)	Infant: aspirate bronchial secretions by suctioning; seldom done. Older child: rinse mouth several times with mouthwash, then cough sputum into sterile container	10%+ eosinophils
Stool mucus (Food allergy)	Stool specimen with mucus (if present)	10%+ eosinophils
CBC	Peripheral blood smear from finger, earlobe, or heel prick	7–25% eosinophils

Box 43-6
Home Allergy-Proofing Techniques and Environmental Controls

FOR MILD ALLERGY:

House dust (focusing on child's bedroom)

Vacuum and dust frequently

Damp mop to reduce dust

Change filters monthly on central air conditioner/furnace

Use bedroom for sleeping; close door during the day

Keep pets out of bedroom

No smoking in the house

FOR SEVERE ALLERGY:

House dust (focusing on child's bedroom)

Bed

- Plastic mattress cover with zipper for mattress and box springs
- Washable synthetic blankets and bedspread and nonallergenic (not foam or feathers) pillows

Washable toys in bed at night

Washable curtains

No carpeting or scatter rugs

Cover heat ducts with cheesecloth to reduce dust circulation. Tape cloth to floor or ceiling. Wash and change at least every 2 weeks. Do not place bed directly under, over, or beside duct

Avoid using closet as storage area. Avoid keeping extra materials on floor or shelves. Clean with rest of room

Keep organization of room simple. Avoid having open shelves and dust-gathering collections (planes, cars, stuffed toys, dolls) or books. Keep toys in storage box

Keep doors and windows closed if using an electrolytic furnace filter

Wood or linoleum floor recommended. Damp mop. If carpeting present, vacuum daily

MOLD, MILDEW

Eliminate plants and aquariums from child's bedroom and play area; keep to minimum throughout home

Avoid use of cellars as play or living area

Clean bathroom and tile areas with antimold agent (e.g., Lysol) regularly

Always clean water jar on vaporizers or humidifiers with vinegar solution (2 parts vinegar/3 parts water) before filling. Have vinegar solution run through machine for 15–20 minutes. Follow with a water rinse. Dry with clean cloth. Clean a minimum of three times per week

Use dehumidifier in humid or damp areas

Clean drip pans under frost-free refrigerators at least monthly

Prevent mold and mildew by airing tennis shoes and boots. Teach children not to put damp towels with other laundry

DANDERS, FEATHERS

Find new homes for pets or limit to outdoors

Avoid stuffed animals and upholstered furniture; including clothing stuffed or insulated with feathers (down)

CONTACTANTS

Buy no wool clothing

Wash all new clothing and linens before using

Double-rinse infant's clothing and diapers

Wash baby articles in mild soap

Use mild soap to bathe baby and rinse well

Avoid use of perfumed lotions, powders, oils

Avoid tobacco smoke

Therapeutic Management

Three basic goals in the treatment of allergic children are to (1) identify and remove the allergen, (2) relieve the symptoms, and (3) control severity of future attacks. Treatment is provided while helping the child and family achieve an environment supportive of the child's growth and development.

Removing the Allergen

When proper diagnosis and identification of causative allergen(s) is possible, elimination or removal of the allergen is the most logical step to take. For example, if the antigen is from animal dander or from cow's milk, removal or avoidance will relieve the allergic symptoms. Success with removal or avoidance of the allergen depends on the family's willingness to adhere to recommendations. This may be particularly difficult when the family pet is to be avoided. Keeping the pet outdoors may be more acceptable to the family than giving the pet away. Home allergy-proofing techniques and environmental controls are valuable information to the child and family (Box 43-6). This information may help the family eliminate causative agents and have some control over the effects the allergy has on their child.

Relieving the Symptoms

If avoidance or removal of causative agents cannot be achieved, symptomatic relief is indicated. Medications commonly used for relief of symptoms are antihista-

Table 43-8. Drugs for Treatment of Pediatric Allergy

Drug Group	Treatment Action	Side Effects
Antihistamines		
Route: Oral; Nasal spray	Antagonist to most actions of histamine (once histamine released), thus decreasing severity of allergic reaction. Antagonizes histamine-induced bronchospasm. Decreases edema by vasoconstriction and by reducing capillary permeability. Prevents pruritus by suppressing stimulant action on nerve endings. Nose spray effective for short-term use (no more than 72 hours)	Common but with marked variation in individuals. Drowsiness, sedation, headache, tinnitus. GI complaints. Dry mouth. Dizziness, blurred vision. Depression, nervousness, hypotension. Polyuria, dysuria. Repeated nasal spray use leads to irritated and tender nasal mucosa (rhinitis medicamentosa)
Bronchodilators		
Theophylline (Methylxanthine) • Slophylline • Somophylline • Theodur • Slobid	Relaxes bronchial smooth muscles. Vasoconstriction of mucosal blood vessels, reducing congestion of mucous membranes. General relief of allergic symptoms	Agitation, nausea, vomiting, tachycardia, palpitation, hypertension. Tremors. Headache. Insomnia
Route: Oral (give with food); IV		
Adrenergics		
(Sympathomimetics) • Epinephrine • Bronchosol • Alupent • Albuterol • Terbutaline	Same as above, except uses different pathway. Therefore, can be used together. Potentiates effects of theophylline	Similar to above; decreased side effects with inhalation
Route: Oral; IV; Subcutaneous; Inhaled		
Corticosteroids		
Route: Oral; Inhaled; Nasal spray; IV	Anti-inflammatory, antiallergic effect. Enhances effect of bronchodilators	Oral and inhaled—when inhaled, rinse mouth after use to avoid overgrowth of Candida (thrush). Short courses without dangerous side effects. Suppression of linear growth with long-term therapy. Electrolyte imbalance. Cushing syndrome symptoms. Depression of immune response to infections. Alternate-day steroids do not affect growth like daily doses do.
Respiratory Inhalant		
Cromolyn sodium • Intal • Nalcrom • Nasalcrom • Opticrom • Rynacrom	Acts locally on lung mucosa to prevent release of histamine and slow-reacting substance of anaphylaxis. No antihistaminic, anti-inflammatory, or bronchodilator effects. Used for prophylactic treatment of severe asthma and for prophylaxis of exercise-induced asthma	Bronchospasm, cough, dizziness, drowsiness, headache
Route: Oral; Inhaled		

mines and bronchodilators (Table 43-8). Antihistamines are the most frequently used drugs for the treatment of allergies. Antihistamines are most effective when taken before or early in an allergic reaction.

Immunotherapy. When removal or avoidance of the allergen is not possible, immunotherapy or hyposensitization is also an option. Bierman and colleagues (1988) caution, however, that immunotherapy "is an adjunct to allergic management, not a substitute for it" (page 283). Patients should understand that this treatment can help control symptoms but does not cure the allergy.

Immunotherapy provides an estimated 75 per cent reduction of signs and symptoms associated with seasonal pollen (Korenblat and Wedner, 1984). Once the allergen is identified, it is given subcutaneously in the form of a dilute extract at weekly or more frequent intervals with a gradual increase in strength over succeeding doses. The strength is increased until the child develops *tolerance* to the allergen (i.e., the immune system becomes *desensitized* to that antigen). The strength that accomplishes tolerance becomes the maintenance dose. The injections are received one or two times weekly until the maintenance dose is reached. (This may take 2 months to a year or longer.) The maintenance dose is then administered on a regular basis at 2- to 4-week intervals.

The immunotherapy may be given preseasonally (before the time of year when the antigen is present in quantity) or perennially (throughout the whole year), which is the most common approach. The goal of this therapy is desensitization to the antigen. The series of regularly injected antigen stimulates development of IgG antibodies. IgG has a higher or greater affinity to the allergen than does IgE. Therefore, the allergen binds with the IgG first, preventing the antigen-antibody IgE reaction from occurring, and therefore preventing the Type I hypersensitivity reaction that releases histamine. The allergen is subsequently destroyed by phagocytosis or complement proteins.

For the child receiving frequent injections, it will be necessary to rotate the injection site and document the dosage and injection site reactions. *Monitoring of the child is critical during and for at least 20 minutes after the antigen injection because anaphylaxis may occur that requires emergency intervention.* Emergency equipment and supplies (epinephrine, oxygen) must be readily available. Local reactions can be treated with cold compresses and oral antihistamines. If a dose causes a systemic response or creates local erythema or edema the size of a nickel or larger, the next dose should not be given until an allergist is consulted.

Preventing Future Attacks

The risk for the infant of developing an allergic disorder is 70 per cent if both parents have allergies and 54 per cent if one parent has allergies (Johnstone, 1988). Therefore, it is recommended that allergic parents consider breastfeeding their infant because human milk contains fewer antigens to which the infant may become sensitized. The breastfeeding mother is advised to eliminate highly allergenic foods from her diet to further reduce the infant's exposure to allergens (Buscinco and Cantani, 1984).

Reduction of allergens in the home can also help protect the allergy-prone infant. Exposure should be reduced as much as possible to house dust, house dust mites, indoor mold, animal allergens, and cigarette smoke (Johnstone, 1988).

Potential for Ineffective Family Coping

The chronicity and periodic crisis of the allergic child's illness impact emotionally, socially, and financially on the child and family (Bridgewater and Voignier, 1978; White and Owsley, 1983).

Impact of Allergy on the Child

The child with an allergic illness may experience complicated treatment, daily medication(s), lack of sleep from acute asthmatic attacks, intense itching from atopic dermatitis, loss of school, and diminished involvement in social activities. The demands of the chronic illness may result in anxiety, fatigue, poor self-esteem, nonadherence to the medical regime, and feelings of guilt that somehow the child is responsible for the illness. During an acute asthmatic attack, feelings of suffocation and death have been described by children.

Impact on the Parents

Parents have similar emotional and psychologic reactions to their child's allergic disorder. Both parents and children experience uncertainty about future emergency hospital admissions and frequent visits to the clinic or doctor. In addition, they experience feelings of separation from home and friends, they may not fully understand medical procedures, and they live with the effects of the allergy on family activities, leisure, trips, and school attendance. Parents may experience fear, helplessness, and self-blame for their child's illness. These feelings can result in alterations in parenting behavior. The resulting impact may affect the child's growth and development, the quality of support for the child, and, therefore, the child's ability to cope with the allergy.

Impact on the Siblings

Siblings are also affected by the allergy. Feelings of resentment and anger may develop, based on their perception that their parents are always spending time with the "sick" child. Feelings of guilt and self-blame for their sibling's illness may occur, if the well siblings perceive themselves as responsible for causing the allergy. They may also be afraid of developing the same disorder.

Financial Impact on the Family

The financial impact on the family may be tremendous. The cost for medications; special allergy-proofing of the home; frequent doctor, hospital, and clinic visits; time lost from work or perhaps the necessity for one parent to quit work to provide special care for the child puts a tremendous financial strain on the family. The monetary and time commitment by the parents may contribute to feelings of resentment, anger, and anxiety.

Nursing Strategies to Enhance Family Coping

Nursing strategies with the allergic child need to focus both on minimizing future allergic exacerbations and supporting the family's strengths so they can adapt and manage the allergic disorder.

Supporting the Family in the Health Care System. Family support involves orienting the child and family to new environments, clarifying the role of the nurse, and involving the parent and child in the care and ongoing follow-up. For example, the child receiving immunotherapy for the first time in the clinic may be anxious and uncooperative. As part of the family's preparation, the nurse can provide information to both the child and caregiver about the play area, restrooms, what they can do while waiting, who will be giving immunotherapy, and what the procedure involves. Informing the child and family of examinations, procedures, and care usually diminishes their anxiety, enhances their sense of control, and assists them in coping with the medical demands of the allergy.

Supporting the Family in the Community. Community follow-up is based on the nursing assessment of the family's functioning and resources. The school nurse can be an invaluable resource to the child and family by supporting the child's transition from home to school and meeting the child's health needs in the school system.

Collaborative planning strengthens the family unit's resources and coping. A family-centered approach to counseling and education is critical for the child to adhere to medical treatments and medications. These actions reinforce the child's and family's strengths. Collaborative problem solving with the child and parent regarding timing of medications, treatments, and social/daily activities individualizes the physical, psychologic, and developmental care of the child and parent, thus promoting commitment and adherence to recommended care. An example of collaborative planning is a school-age child with asthma who required bronchodilator aerosol treatment three times a day to manage acute seasonal attacks. The nurse who interviewed the child and parent discovered that the child received only two treatments a day, which did not control his wheezing. Both parents worked outside the home and the school nurse was not always available to provide the treatment. Through problem solving with the family, it was recognized that the child's baby sitter could be taught to provide the third treatment. In fact, the youngster participated in the teaching of his baby sitter. The listening and collaborative problem solving provided effective options for treatment.

Supporting the Family Through Teaching. Education involves information regarding causes, management, and prognosis of allergic disorders. The discussion will focus on environmental control, medications, and treatments. The goal of education is to promote parental responsibility with the infant and young child and self-care for the older school-age child and adolescent. The preparation of a child with an allergy is as important as the parents' understanding. When assessing the child's understanding, the child's coping style and cognitive level are considered. Written information reinforcing the teaching is provided to both parents and older children to improve understanding of home care needs and adherence to treatment (Kruger and Rawlings, 1984).

The following sections describe specific allergic disorders that fall within the Type I and Type IV classifications. (See Box 43-2 for an overview of the four types of allergic reactions.) Type II responses often result in blood dyscrasias, such as those described in Chapter 40. Type III responses include systemic lupus erythematosus and juvenile arthritis, discussed earlier in this chapter.

Type I Allergic Disorders

Pathophysiology of the Type I Response

Type I allergic responses result in the signs and symptoms most often associated with the word "allergy." Among those manifestations are sneezing, watery eyes, nasal congestion, hives, and anaphylaxis. The Type I allergic response is mediated primarily by IgE antibodies. IgE is known for its extremely high binding capacity with tissue mast cells and blood basophils; any open receptor sites on these cells tend to be filled by available IgE molecules. The significance of this binding action is that when the mast cell (or basophil) carrying IgE antibodies on its surface encounters an antigen, the mast cell releases a sudden burst of histamine and other chemical mediators into the tissues (or, in the case of a basophil, into the blood stream) (Fig. 43-17). These chemicals may cause a variety of allergic responses, including local or systemic anaphylaxis, asthma, allergic rhinitis, urticaria, and angioedema (Buckley, 1988).

Histamine is the chemical most commonly associated with Type I allergic reactions. It is known to

- contract smooth muscles of the bronchial tree (with resultant wheezing as air passes through narrowed passages)
- contract smooth muscles of the gastrointestinal tract (leading to nausea, cramping, diarrhea, and other GI symptoms)
- enhance vascular permeability (leading to release of inflammatory elements, neutrophils and plasma, into the tissues)
- cause constriction of pulmonary vessels (decreas-

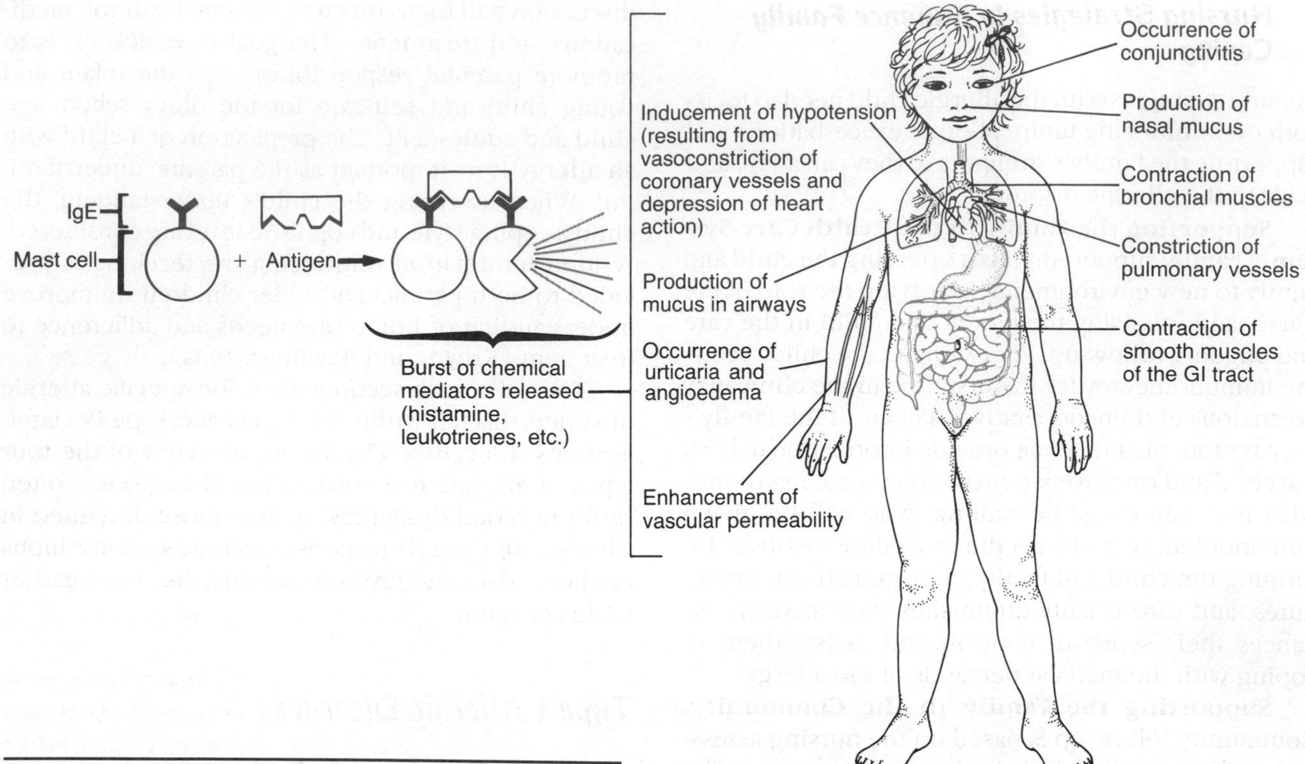

***Figure* 43-17.** Type I systemic hypersensitivity reaction.

ing the capacity for oxygen exchange and leading to shortness of breath)

- stimulate nasal mucous production (Wasserman, 1988)

Histamine released from cutaneous mast cells can cause urticaria and angioedema (Fineman, 1987). It may also cause inflammation of the conjunctiva of the eye.

Leukotrienes (formerly called slow-reacting substance of anaphylaxis, or SRS-A) are among the other chemicals released by the mast cell or basophil. These substances have several actions in common with histamine. In addition they increase mucous production in the airways (leading to reduced diameter of airways, wheezing, and coughing), induce hypotension (resulting in symptoms of faintness or light-headedness), produce localized wheal and flare responses (urticaria and angioedema), and may inhibit lymphocyte function (Wasserman, 1988).

The Type I allergic disorders discussed in this section are allergic rhinitis, allergic conjunctivitis, atopic dermatitis, urticaria and angioedema, insect sting allergy, and food allergies.

Allergic Rhinitis

Allergic rhinitis is the most common allergic disorder, occurring in 10 per cent of all children (Korenblat and Wedner, 1984). Although the condition can occur at any age, it is most common in children over 5 years of age. Allergic rhinitis may be seasonal, commonly referred to as hay fever, or perennial (chronic), in which symptoms are present throughout the year. Common causes of chronic rhinitis are house dust and dander. In the winter, the chronic symptoms may become worse because the child spends more time indoors. Seasonal pollens, molds, or foods can result in either seasonal or chronic symptoms.

Etiology

Rhinitis is an inflammation of the nasal mucosa resulting from the chemical release of histamine by the mucosal mast cells. The histamine causes local vascular dilation, edema, sneezing, and hypersecretion from stimulation of nerve fibers (Sly, 1985). This Type I hypersensitivity reaction (local anaphylaxis) is responsible for the mild-to-moderate nasal eosinophilia counts supporting the diagnosis.

Clinical Manifestations

The symptoms of allergic rhinitis may vary in duration, severity, and pattern, based on the child's hypersensitivity to the antigen or allergen and the extent of exposure. Common symptoms are nasal congestion, clear watery discharge (a change in color may mean infection or extreme abundance of eosinophils), sneezing, and itching. Children may also complain of an itchy throat or of headache. The child may become irritable

Box 43-7
Clinical Manifestations of Chronic Allergic Rhinitis

Allergic shiners

Dark circles noted around the eyes from chronic nasal and sinus congestion. (See Fig. 43-13 in Table 43-6)

Allergic salute

Upward brushing of the nose tip to allay pruritus and open nasal passages; a white crease across bridge of nose may be present. (See Fig. 43-14 in Table 43-6)

Allergic gaping

Open mouth breathing, particularly during times of rest; often accompanied by a high, V-shaped palate and aseptic red throat

Transient hearing loss with immobile or scarred tympanic membrane

Results from chronic serous otitis media associated with persistent (allergic) rhinitis and blockage of the eustachian tubes

Abnormal nasal mucosa

Pale or blue and swollen, with gray, boggy, enlarged nasal turbinates

Conjunctivitis

Common finding with allergic rhinitis. Itching, excessive lacrimation, eye vessels look hardened

Hypernasal voice

Vowels are heard to be muffled during episodes of seasonal rhinitis

and experience both lack of appetite and decreased ability to smell. Box 43-7 summarizes characteristic symptoms of the child with chronic rhinitis. Complications may result, including sinus infection, tonsil or adenoid hypertrophy, epistaxis, serous otitis, otitis media, and oral-facial abnormalities resulting in malocclusion.

Diagnostic Assessment

Diagnosis is based on previously described physical findings and history. Nasal eosinophil counts may support the diagnosis; skin testing will assist in identifying causative allergens. An echogram of the sinuses is frequently done to rule out sinusitis, a common complication.

Therapeutic Management

Treatment involves avoidance or elimination of causative allergens, immunotherapy if indicated, and pharmacologic interventions. Common drugs used in management are antihistamines and decongestants. Topical steroids have been found useful with severe cases. Cromolyn sodium spray is sometimes effective in preventing and managing symptoms associated with allergic rhinitis (Sly, 1985). Nasal irrigations with saline nose drops can also be helpful.

Major Nursing Diagnoses for Allergic Rhinitis

Ineffective airway clearance: upper respiratory system, related to nasal congestion and discharge associated with increased nasal mucous production produced by antigen-triggered histamine
Knowledge deficit, related to management of symptoms at home

Strategies for Nursing Care

Teaching the Family to Manage Symptoms at Home. Nursing support focuses on teaching the child and family about environmental control of the allergen, medication administration, and, if indicated, immunotherapy procedures. Side effects of commonly used antihistamines include fatigue, insomnia, anorexia, and nausea or vomiting. Knowledge of side effects will assist both the child and parent to deal more competently with the impact of the allergic disorder. The family should be aware that over time tolerance to medications develops and a particular antihistamine may become less effective in controlling symptoms. This is the time to contact the physician who can order another medication. One might wonder about the alternative when the child has been through all the commonly prescribed antihistamines. The good news is that, for most persons, tolerance is not permanent, and a medication previously used may be effective later.

The nurse can also instruct about supportive measures such as those suggested by Kaliner and Slater (1986). A stuffy nose may be relieved by saline nose drops that help reduce discomfort and promote mucous draining. For best results the child should remain in a position with the head back (neck hyperextended) for a few minutes after the drops are instilled. (See Chapter 27 for detailed techniques of nose drop administration.) Distraction techniques can help accomplish this positioning in the infant and toddler. Tell children they may feel and taste the salty drops running down the throat and explain how the drops get from the nose to the throat. Assure the child that this feeling will be temporary and that this will not reduce the effectiveness of the saline drops.

Because of chronic irritation and frequent nasal drainage, nasal passages tend to become dry, irritated, and prone to small painful cracks in the mucosa. Humidification of the air can help maintain moist mucous membranes in a dry climate or during winter months when the home is heated. If the family does not own and cannot afford a central humidification system, a portable humidifier can be effective. Even a cool mist vaporizer operated in the child's room during hours of sleep will help reduce nasal dryness and stuffiness.

Exercise and an upright position cause nasal vasoconstriction and thus help relieve stuffiness. Because nasal congestion is often most severe upon arising in the morning, a regimen of morning exercise may increase comfort.

With the realization that allergic rhinitis will probably be a lifelong condition, it is advisable for the family to begin assigning responsibility for management to the child as soon as feasible. The child who controls symptoms through self-management is likely to develop a more positive self-image and to feel less debilitated by the symptoms.

Nursing Strategies for Follow-up Care in the Home or Clinic

- Assess for classic signs and symptoms: nasal congestion and/or drainage, pale, boggy turbinates, swelling of periorbital tissue, injection of conjunctiva and sclera, watery discharge from the eyes, headache, tenderness over frontal and maxillary sinuses, scratchy, red throat, evidence of retropharyngeal drainage, sneezing, mouth breathing, "allergic shiners."
- Assess for common complications of allergic rhinitis:
  - Inspect the nares and septum for lesions and inquire about nose bleeds, particularly if steroidal inhalants are being used.
  - Inspect the ears for evidence of otitis media.
  - Inspect the tonsils for unusual hypertrophy and listen for evidence of adenoidal hypertrophy in the child's speech.
- Inquire about the effectiveness and any side effects of currently prescribed therapies.
- Encourage the child and parent to talk about the experience of the allergy; reinforce adaptive coping and effective management.

Allergic Conjunctivitis

Etiology and Clinical Manifestations

Conjunctivitis is the inflammation of the delicate membrane that lines the eye and is associated with a discharge. Allergic conjunctivitis is a common finding associated with allergic rhinitis and is believed to result from chemically mediated release of histamine from sensitized IgE mast cells, usually in response to environmental allergens such as pollen (Sly, 1985). Common physical findings are itching, excessive lacrimation, and edema of the eyelids and periorbital tissues. These findings may affect the child's attention span, ability to read, and participation in classroom activities or sports.

Therapeutic Management

Treatment consists of topical vasoconstrictors, Opticrom (cromolyn sodium for optical use), and oral antihistamines to relieve the swelling and itching. In rare instances, topical steroids are used to decrease the inflammation and swelling. It has been documented that frequent acute reactions may result in corneal changes and abnormal tear patterns (Bierman and Pearlman, 1988). Wetting agents to help lubricate the eye may be needed. Cold water compresses may be soothing and reduce swelling.

The family may require instruction in ophthalmic medicine administration (Chapter 27) and the effect of conjunctivitis on the child's behavior. For example, the child with conjunctivitis may appear inattentive and uncooperative with learning activities. The itching, edema, and excessive tearing may make it very difficult for the child to concentrate or focus on tasks demanding visual attentiveness.

Atopic Dermatitis (Eczema)

Atopic dermatitis is a chronic, severely pruritic skin disorder. It is a relatively common allergic skin response in children between 2 months and 5 years of age, usually developing in the first year of life. Although some children will outgrow this disorder, for many others it becomes a lifelong malady. At least 50 per cent of children with atopic dermatitis at age 2 years will have it into adulthood (Jacobs and Goldsobel, 1988).

Etiology

The term *atopic* refers to the hereditary predisposition to develop some form of allergy. Seventy per cent of children with atopic dermatitis have a family history of allergy (asthma, hay fever, or allergic conjunctivitis) (Paller, 1987a). The exact mode of genetic transmission has not been established. Although the susceptibility to atopic dermatitis is inherited, environmental factors greatly influence if and how the tendency for dermatitis will be expressed.

Pathophysiology

When allergens do gain entry, they are thought to interact with IgE molecules to produce the Type I allergic reaction previously described. The skin of affected children, however, has been shown to release twice as much histamine as that of normal children. The inflammatory response that follows histamine release causes erythema and edema, which aggravate the pruritus.

Skin lesions resulting from frequent scratching are prone to infection. It is notable that children with atopic dermatitis have an increased susceptibility to viral, fungal, and staphylococcal infections (Jacobs and Goldsobel, 1988). Therefore, herpes simplex and impetigo are commonly associated with exacerbations of eczema.

Clinical Manifestations

Clinical manifestations vary with the age of the child. In infancy, a red, papular rash often appears first on the cheeks and spreads to the forehead and scalp and down the extensor surfaces of the arms and legs. Eventually it may cover the entire body. In older children, the rash is more commonly on the flexor surface of the elbows and knees, the neck, sides of the face, eyelids, and dorsum of the hands and feet (Nicol, 1987). The pruritus is intense and the child scratches the lesions, causing excoriation of the skin. Jacobs and Goldsobel (1988) quote the old axiom, *"Atopic dermatitis is not a rash that itches but an itch that rashes."* The trauma of scratching plays a major role in the occurrence and progression of the dermatitis. The child with atopic dermatitis has a higher-than-normal colonization of *Staphylococcus aureus* on the skin, and secondary infection is common. Infection leads to the typical vesiculation, oozing, and crusting (Jacobs and Goldsobel, 1988) (Fig. 43-18). As the crusts heal they fall off, leaving healthy new epithelium.

Diagnostic Assessment

If atopic dermatitis develops, the parents are usually concerned about the facial rash and seek medical attention as it spreads and becomes excoriated by the child's scratching. The diagnosis is made based on the positive family history, the character and distribution of the lesions, the intense pruritus, and the pattern of exacerbation and remission of the condition. As with all the dermatitides,* a thorough history is imperative to an accurate diagnosis (see Box 43-3).

Physical examination of the child with eczema often reveals an array of several types of dermatitides in varying stages of healing. The child's discomfort and fatigue are usually apparent in a forlorn, sallow appearance.

* Dermatitides is the plural of dermatitis.

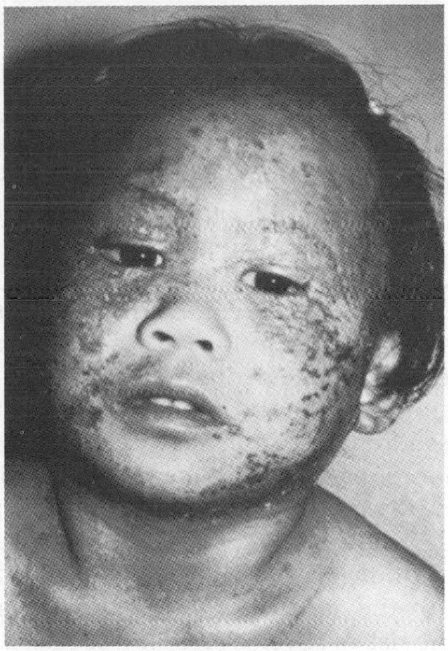

Figure 43-18. Three-year-old child with severe atopic dermatitis. (From Bierman CW, Pearlman DS: *Allergic Diseases from Infancy to Adulthood.* 2nd ed. Philadelphia, WB Saunders, 1988, 393.)

Therapeutic Management

The goals of therapeutic management are hydration, control of pruritus, prevention of secondary infection, and identification and removal of allergens.

Hydration. Hydrating the skin through the use of bathing, wet wraps, and occlusive creams or ointments is now thought to be the key in relieving the cycle of drying, cracking, itching, and scratching (Nicol, 1987). Nursing strategies related to these techniques are detailed in Table 43-9, page 1603.

Controlling Pruritus and Preventing Secondary Infection. Arm and hand restraints may be needed for the infant or small child to prevent scratching. Fingernails should be kept short and clean. The young infant's hands can be covered with long socks that are then taped or pinned to the shirt sleeves. This allows free movement of the arms while reducing scratching.

Consideration of the adverse effect of increased environmental temperature and humidity on itching is important. In particular, overheating aggravates itching. Dressing the infant in lightweight cotton or cotton-blend garments will help minimize this effect. The same amount of clothing that is comfortable for an adult is appropriate for the child.

Care of the skin is important in minimizing itching. In the acute exudative phase, a carefully followed topical skin regimen as described for the management of contact dermatitis can control the symptoms.

Inflammation is controlled by the application of a steroid cream or ointment following the hydrating bath or wet soaks. A fluorinated steroid cream is never used on the face because it causes unsightly acne-like eruptions and capillary dilation. A 1 per cent hydrocortisone cream or ointment is most often used on the face. Other local steroids often used on the rest of the body include Kenalog Cream 0.1 per cent, Cordran Cream 0.05 per cent, Synalar Cream 0.025 per cent, and Valisone Cream 0.1 per cent. During the acute exudative phase, a cream or lotion base is used to avoid the occlusive effects of an ointment. Applied to large areas, steroids may be absorbed in quantities sufficient to depress adrenal function. Parents are taught to apply thin applications of steroid cream twice daily. Small areas may be wrapped with a plastic film (Saran Wrap) or, as suggested by Nicol (1987), with wet Kerlex dressings followed by bandages to enhance the effectiveness of the medication. Since this practice increases the risk of adverse systemic effects, large body areas should not be wrapped. Another teaching point related to topical therapy is that steroids have a tendency to mask infection. The skin must be inspected carefully for subtle signs of bacterial and yeast infection. Increased inflammation, pain, or pruritus may indicate infection. Systemic antibiotics such as erythromycin are prescribed for infection. The antibiotic dosage and administration schedule should be thoroughly discussed with parents to promote compliance with treatment.

Atopic dermatitis can be controlled but not cured. By 2 years of age, 50 per cent of children may undergo permanent remission. They have little scarring, and the changes in pigmentation that occur after inflammation are temporary. Not reassuring is the fact that half of the remaining infants with atopic dermatitis develop asthma or hay fever later in life. For those in whom there is not a permanent remission, a childhood stage of atopic dermatitis usually appears during the preschool years. It is characterized by less redness and beginning lichenification (thickening of the dermal and epidermal skin layers). The third stage, the adult stage, is characterized by dermatitis on the face, neck, and flexural spaces such as the antecubital and axillary areas. Popliteal lichenification is common.

Eliminating Allergens. Elimination of identified or common allergens is an approach that may be used in treating infants with atopic dermatitis. Allergy-proofing the home may be recommended (see Box 43-6). The results, however, are often disappointing. Although foods have sometimes been identified as antigens in atopic dermatitis (Paller, 1987b), many authorities now believe that unless a specific allergy to a specific food can be demonstrated, the trial elimination diet (discussed in the following section on food allergies) is of questionable value.

Major Nursing Diagnoses for Atopic Dermatitis

See Table 43-9, Nursing Process Plan for the child with atopic dermatitis.

Strategies for Nursing Care

Teaching the family about home management of eczema will involve hydration and skin care, symptomatic control of pruritus to prevent scarring and secondary bacterial infection, and ensuring that the caregivers can recognize the signs and symptoms of secondary infection. In some cases identification of allergens will be pertinent. Because the eczematous rash can be unsightly and often involves the head and face, the child and family will need a great deal of support in dealing with the very visible and frustrating exacerbations of the illness during childhood. Learning methods to control pruritus and, subsequently, to prevent scarring can help the family gain a sense of control. Appropriate reinforcement for good management techniques and assurance that new lesions are usually not the result of inadequate care can further increase the confidence of caregivers. Additional nursing strategies for the child with atopic dermatitis are detailed in Table 43-9.

Nursing Strategies for Follow-up Care in the Home or Clinic

See recommendations under contact dermatitis, page 1587; also:

Determine whether the child's activities prior to the onset of another exacerbation may provide clues to allergens.

Assess respiratory status in the older child for signs and symptoms of hay fever or asthma.

Urticaria and Angioedema

Etiology

Urticaria (hives) is easily recognized and may occur either alone or with angioedema. Both skin conditions result in interstitial edema and dilated blood vessels (Korenblat and Wedner, 1984). Reactions are acute and are believed due to Type I hypersensitivity reaction (Sly, 1985). Table 43-10 compares urticaria and angioedema. Some of the causes of angioedema and urticaria involve drugs, especially penicillin; food; blood products; insect stings or bites; inhalants; physical factors (cold, heat) emotional factors; parasitic infections; and exercise. Special attention must be paid to allergic urticaria reactions to medications. The rein-

Table 43-10. Comparison of Urticaria and Angioedema

	Urticaria	Angioedema
Onset	Acute (usually occurs within minutes)	Subacute (may develop more slowly)
Location	Dermis	Deeper layers of skin, including subcutaneous tissue
Clinical Manifestations	Multiple reddened lesions that look like wheals Itching	Usually single lesion Lesions smaller in size, with less itching and redness Lesions evolve more slowly Stinging, tingling, or burning feeling Commonly involves face, extremities

troduction of the drug may cause a more severe reaction or systemic anaphylaxis. The medication should be avoided along with similarly structured drugs. Inhalant urticaria is less common and may be seen with seasonal exacerbations of rhinitis, conjunctivitis, or asthma (Bierman and Pearlman, 1988). A complication associated with urticaria and angioedema is systemic anaphylactic shock involving upper airway obstruction. If untreated, this can lead to death.

Pathophysiology

Although urticaria and angioedema can also be caused by Type II and Type III hypersensitivity reactions, Type I is the most common. The reaction is believed to be the result of antigen contact with IgE-bearing cutaneous mast cells.

Diagnostic Assessment

Diagnosis results from a careful history, physical assessment of lesions, and laboratory work. The cause of urticaria often is easily recognized due to the acute reaction. Serum eosinophils are occasionally elevated. Allergy skin testing and an elimination diet may be helpful in diagnosing possible allergens. The elimination diet involves either removing the suspected allergen or restricting the child's diet and slowly reintroducing the suspected foods. Both approaches require careful monitoring by the parents. The dietary challenge is conducted in a controlled setting if there is the potential for an anaphylactic reaction (life-threatening respiratory distress usually followed by vascular collapse and shock). Stool collection for laboratory analysis for ova and parasites is valuable if parasitic infection is suspected. In spite of these tests, the child's history and physical assessment are the most helpful in establishing a diagnosis.

Therapeutic Management

Treatment for urticaria and angioedema is avoidance of the causative agents. Epinephrine injections may be necessary to prevent life-threatening angioedema or severe urticaria. Antihistamines are effective in controlling skin lesions but must be given soon after the onset of symptoms to be effective.

Urticaria and angioedema are usually transient conditions. Both are usually more frightening and bothersome than they are serious.

Strategies for Nursing Care

Nursing interventions include educating the family about procedures for avoiding allergens, administration of medication, screening of children for drug allergies, and the monitoring and organizing of emergency supplies and equipment in hospitals, clinics, and doctors' offices to prevent systemic anaphylaxis. Parents will need to carry and learn to use an emergency kit containing epinephrine.

Insect Sting Allergy

Etiology and Clinical Manifestations

Honeybees, bumblebees, wasps, hornets, yellow jackets and fire ants are responsible for most insect hypersensitivity reactions. These insects are of the Hymenoptera order (Sly, 1985). Refer to Table 52-3 in The Injured Child chapter for further information about insect bites and stings.

Insect stings cause 40 to 50 deaths each year. Reactions vary from local to systemic. A normal reaction occurs even without a hypersensitivity to the venom, because pharmacologic properties in the venom do cause skin responses of pain lasting for a few minutes, followed by local erythema and a pruritic wheal that disappears within a few hours. Cellulitis has been known to develop after wasp and yellow jacket stings because these may transmit bacteria. A local reaction involves edema confined either to a small area or involving an entire extremity. The edema may persist for several days. Multiple stings may result in a toxic systemic reaction with vomiting, diarrhea, fever, headache, or convulsions.

Type I hypersensitivity reaction (systemic anaphylaxis) may also occur with an onset within minutes of the sting or at any time up to 6 hours and cause death from angioedema progressing to upper airway obstruction (Sly, 1985). Delayed reactions (Type IV) may occur several days after a sting. Some findings associated with delayed reaction are bloody diarrhea, thrombocytopenic purpura, and nephrotic syndrome. Diagnosis is based on reported history from the child or parent, physical findings, and skin testing.

Therapeutic Management

Treatment is available to children with sting or bite reactions that cause large local reactions, that are increasing in severity from repeated stings, or that produce systemic reactions. Treatment involves avoidance (Box 43-8) and emergency measures. Emergency management includes airway maintenance, administration of oxygen, and, often, administration of epinephrine. A short course of corticosteroids may be administered after anaphylactic episodes (McLean, 1987). Although some authorities recommend immunotherapy with insect venom only for adults (Yunginger, 1988), other clinics report successful results with this form of treatment in children.

Strategies for Nursing Care

Table 52-3 details nursing strategies appropriate to an insect sting in a child for whom there is no immediate danger of anaphylaxis. When the child is allergic to the venom, additional teaching is indicated. The nurse helps the family obtain a Medic-Alert bracelet, indicating the child's hypersensitivity, and acquire an emergency kit containing oral antihistamines and a prefilled epinephrine syringe. They should, of course, be taught the technique of subcutaneous injection. A medication emergency kit may be kept at several areas (school, home, baby sitters). Additional instructions on how to handle emergency situations need to be provided to other people involved in the child's care. A child experiencing systemic reactions with or without administration of medication should be seen at an emergency facility.

Box 43-8
Avoiding Stinging Insects

Avoid loose fitting clothes outdoors (may entrap bee).

Avoid brightly colored clothes. White is least likely to attract bees.

Avoid scented cosmetics, hairsprays, deodorants, and perfume.

Avoid going barefoot outdoors.

Avoid areas harboring stinging insects (i.e., flower beds, orchards, garbage cans, picnic grounds).

Have a professional exterminator destroy wasp nests or beehives near the home.

Keep automobile windows closed.

Keep windows and doors closed unless screens are available.

When away from home, take an insecticide spray.

Food Allergies

Etiology

Certain physiologic and immunologic intestinal properties provide barriers to food proteins (antigens) that have the potential for causing food allergies in children (May and Block, 1978; Sly, 1985). The intestinal physiologic and immunologic properties are the low pH of secretions; the intestinal mucus, secretory IgA on the intestinal lining, and Peyer patches. These patches possess the capacity to impede the absorption or digestion of the food antigen. If this is not accomplished, the antigen may penetrate the mucosa, enter the circulation, and stimulate the allergic response in sensitive children. Food allergies may occur at any age, although infants are at greater risk for developing them. The infant's immature digestive system and immune capability allow for an easier absorption of larger amounts of incomplete catabolized proteins that can be antigenic (Bierman and Pearlman, 1988; Buscinco and Cantani, 1984). Also, infants may develop food sensitivities from intrauterine sensitization or from antigens ingested from their mother's breastmilk. Another reason why food allergy is common in infants is because this is the time when the child is introduced to many new (and potentially antigenic) foods. In addition, diarrhea or other inflammation of the intestinal lining may enhance the absorption of antigens, causing an allergic reaction to certain foods in some children.

Common Food Allergens. Any food can produce allergic symptoms, but some foods are considered highly allergenic. The most common food allergens in children are cow's milk, eggs (largely due to egg white), wheat, corn, chocolate, cola, citrus fruits, legumes, and shellfish. Allergy to legumes and shellfish is not outgrown as often as allergy to other foods. Occasionally vitamins and drugs (e.g., antibiotics) with lactose fillers will also cause gastrointestinal allergic responses.

Cow's milk is the most common allergic food, with a 2 to 7.5 per cent incidence in childhood. Three fourths of the children with cow's milk allergy show allergic signs and symptoms within the first few months of life, most likely owing to the infant's immature digestive and immunologic systems. Any infant on cow's milk with a history of colic, irritability, or repeated bouts of respiratory infection is suspect. Metabisulfites, which are preservatives used on fruits and vegetables, have demonstrated food sensitivity in asth-

Box 43-9
Clinical Manifestations of Food Allergy

INTEGUMENTARY

Eczema
Urticaria
Angioedema
Geographic tongue

GASTROINTESTINAL

Vomiting
Diarrhea
Abnormal pain or colic
Colitis
Malabsorption — iron deficiency
failure to thrive

RESPIRATORY

Rhinitis
Otitis media
Wheezing, asthma

NEUROLOGIC

Fatigue
Irritability
Drowsiness
Inability to concentrate
Headache
} Tension-fatigue syndrome

SYSTEMIC

Anaphylactic shock

matic children. These preservatives have provoked signs and symptoms of bronchoconstriction, flushing, weakness, urticaria, and angioedema (Sly, 1985).

Clinical Manifestations

Clinical features have been shown to involve the gastrointestinal tract, skin, respiratory system, and nervous system (Hill et al, 1984). Infants experiencing acute reactions to cow's milk within a few hours after ingestion may exhibit metabolic acidosis, gastroenteritis, or septicemia-like features. Delayed reactions in infants are manifested as failure to thrive, chronic cutaneous eruption, anemia, and food malabsorption.

As with allergic reactions from cow's milk, the child sensitized to other foods may experience reactions that are mild or severe. The reaction may occur immediately after ingestion, leading to anaphylaxis, or be delayed, occurring 48 to 72 hours after ingestion. The child's allergic symptoms may be diverse and multiple (Walker, 1980; White and Owsley, 1983). Clinical manifestations are presented in Box 43-9. An immediate response is usually due to the food substance itself, whereas a delayed response is usually caused by some product formed during the digestion of the food.

Diagnostic Assessment

Diagnosis of food allergies is focused primarily on the child's nutritional history, the family's history, and the child's response to dietary elimination of a suspected food. Dietary elimination is done by removing the suspected food from the diet for approximately 3 weeks, followed by reintroduction of the food (Sly, 1985). Diagnosis is confirmed after two more elimination food trials. Diagnosis is made more difficult if the offending antigen is in a food that is eaten only occasionally, or is only antigenic under certain conditions (e.g., causes a reaction only when eaten raw). Sometimes certain food combinations or certain quantities of a food produce the reaction, or the food may produce a reaction only when ingested during certain seasons or with exercise. In this situation, the infant or child will be placed on a restricted diet eliminating the more highly allergenic foods. Foods that are removed are reintroduced one at a time, with 3 days allowed between each food added back to the diet.

Food challenges are not recommended for children who have histories of severe anaphylaxis. Food challenges involve the introduction of the suspected food(s) into the child's restricted diet. One suspected food at a time is introduced to avoid confusion. When the suspected food is introduced, the amount is slowly increased while the child is closely monitored for signs of an antigen reaction. Children who experience severe anaphylaxis are extremely vulnerable to this test. In this case, skin testing or RAST provides the best alternative in diagnosing the allergen(s). Skin testing (in contrast to the RAST) is believed to be more accurate in predicting allergies to wheat and milk. As mentioned earlier, infants usually are not responsive to skin testing. Therefore, when the infant's history suggests there may be a systemic anaphylaxis, food challenge needs to be performed in a controlled environment, such as a hospital.

Therapeutic Management

Treatment involves the dietary elimination of the allergic food(s) while maintaining and supporting the child's nutritional needs for growth. Infants with cow's milk allergy may be switched to a soybean formula, only to discover an intolerance to soy (Hill et al, 1984). In this situation, the diet is changed to an alternative formula such as Pregestimil or Nutramigen or an elemental formula (Vivonex) (Table 43-11). When the breastfeeding infant develops sensitivities to foods ingested by the mother and secreted in the breastmilk, an elimination diet or restricted diet may be necessary for the mother in order to control her infant's food sensitivities. If the maternal elimination diet is unsuccessful, the infant may need to be switched to a milk-free or elemental formula.

Symptomatic relief of gastrointestinal reactions

Table 43-11. Common Alternatives to Cow's Milk Formulas*

Formula	Kcal/Oz	Protein Source	Carbohydrate Source	Fat Source	Indication
Infant Formulas					
Human milk	22	Lactalbumin, casein	Lactose	Human milk	Cow's milk protein allergy (CMPA), soy allergy
Isomil (Ross)	20	Soy protein	Sucrose, corn syrup solids (lactose-free)	Coconut oil, soy oil	CMPA, lactose intolerance, galactosemia
Prosobee (Mead Johnson)	20	Soy protein	Corn syrup solids (lactose-free, sucrose-free)	Soy oil	CMPA, lactose intolerance, galactosemia, postgastroenteritis
Nutramigen (Mead Johnson)	20	Casein hydrolysate	Modified tapioca, sucrose	Corn oil	CMPA, lactose intolerance, soy allergy, multiple food allergies, galactosemia
Portagen (Mead Johnson)	20	Sodium caseinate	Corn syrup, solids, sucrose	Corn oil, MCT oil (86%)	Steatorrhea in cystic fibrosis, intestinal resections, pancreatic insufficiency, celiac disease, biliary atresia
Pregestimil (Mead Johnson)	22	Casein hydrolysate	Modified tapioca, corn syrup solids	Medium chain triglyceride (MCT) oil (40%), corn oil	CMPA, soy allergy, multiple food allergies, disaccharidase
Elemental Formulas					
Precision (Doyle Pharmaceutical)	30	Egg albumin, sodium caseinate	Glucose oligosaccharides, sucrose	Vegetable oil	Multiple food allergies, disorders of digestion and absorption
Vital (Ross)	30	Partially hydrolyzed whey, soy and meat protein, free amino acids	Glucose oligosaccharides, glucose polysaccharides	MCT oil, safflower oil	Multiple food allergies, disorders of digestion and absorption
Vivonex (Norwich Eaton)	30	Amino acids	Glucose, glucose oligosaccharides	Safflower oil	Multiple food allergies, disorders of digestion and absorption

* Formulations change frequently; to ensure updated information, it is best to contact the company representative.
(From Grant and Kennedy-Caldwell, 1988; Krause and Mahan, 1984.)

may be initiated until the reaction subsides or the causative food is identified and eliminated. An antihistamine may be used to control intestinal spasms or abdominal pain (colic). Reducing the spasms and pains usually results in eliminating other complaints such as nausea, diarrhea, or constipation.

Preventive Aspects of Management. In highly allergic families, prevention may start during pregnancy with the maternal elimination of highly allergenic foods. This hypoallergenic diet is maintained during breastfeeding. Infants who develop acute gastroenteritis would benefit from the restriction of suspected allergens (thereby limiting the possible absorption of allergenic antigen during this vulnerable period when the intestine is inflamed).

Prevention of allergy by beginning appropriate teaching before the child is born, especially when a strong family history for allergy exists, cannot be overemphasized. Avoiding introduction of solid foods until after the infant is 6 months old also helps reduce the likelihood of food allergy. See detailed strategies for anticipatory guidance related to introduction of solid foods, Chapter 5, page 239. These actions by the nurse can aid significantly in reducing the incidence of food allergy in infancy.

The prognosis is good for children with food allergies. Children whose food allergies start during the first 3 years of life are likely to be allergy-free within a few years.

Major Nursing Diagnoses for Food Allergy

Altered nutrition: less than body requirements, related to physiologic intolerance of one or more foods associated with an allergic reaction

Potential altered parenting: overprotection, related to fear of anaphylaxis associated with allergen contact
Knowledge deficit, related to management of food allergy at home

Strategies for Nursing Care

Helping the Family Reduce Overprotective Tendencies. Home management of a food allergy requires a great deal of vigilance on the part of the parent and other caregivers (such as the baby sitter, day care center, and extended family). It is not uncommon for a child with a food allergy to react violently to a food antigen just from *touching* the food. One child we know who is allergic to wheat flour developed a significant reaction (with hives and marked facial edema) from holding a soda cracker someone had "kindly" given her while she was in the church nursery. Such accidental encounters with allergens, despite unusual vigilance, may cause the parent to feel that overprotection is not only justified, but imperative. The nurse can be instrumental in helping the family cope with the threat of allergen contact and balance that threat with the child's developmental needs for independence. One strategy is to help the family separate actual threats from those that are only perceived, and then to assist them with problem solving to protect the child. Another strategy is to discuss with them the child's developmental tasks and then help them balance the benefits of meeting tasks for independence against the threat of time away from the primary caregiver. (See the discussion on Phenylketonuria in Chapter 50 for further suggestions about avoiding contact with forbidden foods.)

Teaching to Support Management of Food Allergy at Home. Teaching methods to avoid allergens involves, first of all, clarifying exactly what the allergen is. If the allergy is reported to be to wheat flour, does that mean barley flour is all right? Is the wheat flour found in canned soup really off limits, or is it allowed because "there can't be much of it"? When this clarification has been made, the problem has been identified and a plan can be formulated. Parents must be alerted to read labels carefully to be sure the eliminated food(s) are not contained in other products. This can be as confusing as it is time consuming. The nurse or nutritionist can be helpful in providing for the parent a list of other names for the food; for example, milk products may be listed as whey or lactose. In some cases, the parent will need to prepare special foods. A list of health food stores and other suppliers of ingredients (such as rye flour) can be an invaluable resource.

Another resource can be a family who is experiencing similar management problems. The nurse is often in a position to provide support links among families, for both emotional and informational help. For example, families may be able to share special recipes and cookbooks.

Children can benefit from family support groups as well. It is helpful for them to know they are not alone in dietary restrictions. As children get older and begin assuming more self-management, their support group of peers with food allergies can help them with problem solving, such as ways to avoid "feeling different" and ways to avoid pressure from other friends to "have one just this once."

Nursing Strategies for Follow-up Care in the Home or Clinic

Measure height and weight (and head circumference in the infant); plot on the growth chart. Notify the physician of any delay in growth parameters that could signal inadequacies in the diet.

Assess for related allergic disorders such as eczema, allergic rhinitis, or asthma.

Encourage the child and parent to talk about the experience of home management. Assist them with ongoing problem clarification and problem solving.

Type IV Allergic Disorders

Type IV allergic disorders are characterized by the response of delayed-hypersensitivity T-cells. The general pathophysiology of Type IV allergic disorders is summarized in Box 43-2, page 1568. The pathophysiology of allergic contact dermatitis illustrates one specific example of this type of allergic response.

Allergic Contact Dermatitis

Etiology

Allergic contact dermatitis is an acquired immune reaction resulting from skin contact with allergens. Common sensitizers in children include poison ivy, shoes, metals, preservatives, and topical medications. (See Chapter 52 for additional nursing care strategies for the child with poison ivy.) Boys show a greater tendency for this allergy than do girls. It occurs more often in infants and toddlers, usually beginning around 3 to 4 months of age. Susceptible children tend to have unusually dry skin from birth and a family history of allergy.

Pathophysiology

Allergic contact dermatitis begins with penetration of the skin by small antigenic particles (called haptens).

Once inside the stratum corneum, they combine with other proteins in the skin to form a complete antigen. This antigen is then processed by skin macrophages (Langerhans cells) and presented to T-lymphocytes. Only a few T-cells need be present at the skin site to trigger the sensitization process. After the initial antigen–T-cell contact, lymphokines are released that cause further activation and proliferation of T-cells. The T-cells then migrate from the epidermis to area lymph nodes where they proliferate into large numbers of T-effector and T-memory cells. Clones of these effector and memory cells circulate in the blood to reach all parts of the lymphatic system. Circulation of the sensitized cells is a key component of the Type IV reaction in allergic contact dermatitis. It means that subsequent skin contact with that antigen, anywhere on the body, will result in T-cell recognition of the antigen and the activation of a cell-mediated immune response (Parker, 1988).

Allergic sensitization in this manner generally takes 7 to 10 days after the allergen is first contacted, but it is not uncommon for sensitization to occur over a period of many years. Once sensitization (allergy) develops, all future contacts with the allergen will result in an inflammatory reaction at the contact site, usually within 24 to 72 hours. Contact allergies tend to persist indefinitely (Parker, 1988).

Clinical Manifestations and Diagnostic Assessment

The inflamed skin area may be configured to match the antigen contact with the skin. The exposed skin area is erythematous, edematous, and pruritic. Papules and vesicles form, which weep, ooze, and crust if scratched. Lichenification (hardened, leathery skin) develops if the dermatitis becomes chronic.

A history of dry skin, family members with allergies, and ready skin blanching (tendency toward vasoconstriction of cutaneous vessels), coupled with localized inflammatory configuration and distribution, are evidence of contact dermatitis. Diagnostic evaluation usually includes patch testing to identify the cause. Suspected allergens are applied to the back on adhesive strips. After 48 hours the strips are removed and the skin is observed for reactions. A positive reaction usually appears as vesicles on an edematous, red base and exactly outlines the area covered by the adhesive patch (Parker, 1988).

Therapeutic Management

Because this allergic disease is self-limiting, treatment is primarily symptomatic. In most cases topical treatment is sufficient. Steroid creams such as Kenalog or Valisone may be used during the acute phase. Antihistamines may be necessary to control itching. The physician will also usually order cool wet dressings; these may be soaked in a soothing solution such as Burow's. Burow solution not only cools and soothes the skin but helps clean and dry the lesions.

Because secondary bacterial infection is common, a wound culture will be obtained if purulent lesions, fever, and/or increased erythema develop. Antimicrobial drugs will be ordered to combat identified organisms.

Major Nursing Diagnoses for Contact Dermatitis

***Impaired skin integrity: circumscribed inflammation**, related to direct contact with an allergen*
***Altered comfort: pruritus**, related to skin inflammation*
***Potential for infection: secondary**, related to entry of pathogens through skin lesions*
***Disturbance in self-concept: body image**, related to unsightly skin lesions*
***Knowledge deficit (child and family)**, related to*

- *management of allergic contact dermatitis at home*
- *prevention of future skin breakdown*
- *treatment for pruritus and other accompanying symptoms*
- *prevention of secondary infection*

Strategies for Nursing Care

Teaching to Address Knowledge Deficit. Preparing the family for home management of allergic contact dermatitis will include both preventive strategies and treatment of symptoms. Preventive management involves keeping the skin lubricated, clean, and healthy to increase its resistance and to minimize infection secondary to allergic response. Daily tepid baths without soap and lasting 15 to 20 minutes, followed by application of a bland lubricant (e.g., Eucerin creme) while the skin is still wet, are usually sufficient to maintain general integumentary health and to promote absorption of topical agents. Use of a humidifier in the home during dry months also helps combat an infant's dry skin condition. Daily cleaning of the humidifier is recommended to prevent aerosolizing mold and bacteria that can colonize this device.

Preventing Antigen Contact. Once the antigen is identified, its elimination, if possible, prevents further bouts of contact dermatitis. If the allergy can be traced to an allergen like perfume, a metal, a detergent, or a type of fabric, elimination may be manageable. If, however, the allergen is something like the dichromate used in leather processing or a chemical compound found in printer's ink, the task will be more difficult. Desensitization therapy is hardly ever successful in managing this dermatitis, although it may decrease the severity of reaction if the antigen is a plant source that cannot be eliminated. In these cases it is usually used preseasonally for a few weeks.

Relieving Pruritus and Preventing Secondary Infection. Relief of pruritus will greatly reduce the incidence of secondary infection. The nurse must demonstrate to parents how to mix Burow solution in the correct concentration and how to apply the compresses. Compresses are usually applied at room temperature with a thoroughly soaked cloth one layer thick. They remain on the affected areas for 20- to 30-minute periods and are resoaked every 10 to 15 minutes to prevent drying and sticking. This routine is repeated three to four times a day. During the soaks, parents can divert the child with brightly colored toys, books, or music. Wearing a plastic apron for protection will enable the parent to also hold and rock the child. Discomfort severe enough to disturb sleep should be controlled with temporary use of antihistamines or steroid ointments administered at bedtime. In some cases sedatives may be prescribed.

Emotional distress increases susceptibility to allergic response and intensifies reaction severity. Once the dermatitis is present, such distress increases the pruritus experienced. Therefore, a calm environment void of as much friction and emotional pressure as possible is of utmost importance to the child.

Nursing Strategies for Follow-up Care in the Home or Clinic

Assess for clearing of the lesions and integrity of the unaffected skin. Reinforce teaching about keeping the skin clean and well lubricated.

Assess for secondary bacterial infection: note fever, unexpected changes in the lesions with accompanying odor or purulent drainage, lingering rash or lesions, lethargy, lymphadenopathy.

Culture suspicious lesions.

Assess status of immunizations.

Altered Immune Response: Immune Deficiency

As newsworthy as immune deficiency is today, it is interesting to note that the first identified immune deficiency disease, agammaglobulinemia, was not described until the 1950s. Since that time many other immunodeficiency disorders have been identified. These disorders can involve any part of the immune system, including T- and B-lymphocytes, phagocytes, complement proteins, or organs of the immune system (Lockey and Bukantz, 1987a,b). Whereas some immune deficiencies have been related to genetic causes (e.g., X-linked agammaglobulinemia), others are acquired (e.g., AIDS). The exact etiology of many of these disorders remains unknown. What is known is that immune deficiency leaves the body without adequate protection from microorganisms, and persons afflicted with these diseases suffer repeated, and often life-threatening, infections. Neutropenia is one common example of immune deficiency. It is usually considered more a sign of another disorder than a disease in itself. Neutropenia is discussed briefly here. Pertinent nursing strategies also can be found in Chapters 40 and 48, Table 43-9, and Table 48-4. The remainder of the section deals with acquired immunodeficiency syndrome (AIDS).

Neutropenia

Neutropenia is a reduction in the number of neutrophils in the blood. It may occur alone or in combination with reductions in other blood cell components. Neutropenia can be congenital, drug induced, or the result of other diseases such as leukemia and vitamin B_{12} and folate deficiencies (Altman, 1988). At times neutrophil destruction is related to autoimmune processes. In autoimmune neutropenia, circulating antineutrophil antibodies (ANAs) bind to and destroy neutrophils faster than the bone marrow can replace them.

Recalling the function of neutrophils in the immune system (page 1527), it is not surprising that children with neutropenia are particularly susceptible to infection. Infection sites are most often the lungs, oral cavity, and perianal area. The depressed immune response that results from decreased neutrophils allows the infectious process to progress more quickly than normal. The danger of infection in the child with neutropenia is that the remaining immune mechanisms may fail to contain the infection at the local level, allowing it to spread to the bloodstream (septicemia).

Diagnostic assessment will rely upon history and physical findings as well as blood tests to measure the total WBC, the differential leukocyte count, the absolute neutrophil count (see page 1589), and ANA titers. In some cases a bone marrow aspiration may be necessary to determine the cause. Management will be determined by the cause and the neutrophil count. When neutrophil counts range between 100 and 500 cells/μl, therapy may be instituted. If neutropenia is the result of chemotherapeutic drugs (as is frequently the case), doses of these drugs may need to be lowered to allow the bone marrow to replace leukocytes.

Strategies for Nursing Care

Nursing care for the child with neutropenia will be directed at reducing the potential for infection and monitoring for infectious processes. See Table 48-4, page 1884, which details nursing strategies for the child undergoing chemotherapy. The section that deals with leukopenia is pertinent to care of the child with neutropenia regardless of cause. (See also Table 43-9.)

Acquired Immunodeficiency Syndrome (AIDS)

Acquired immunodeficiency syndrome is an irreversible, fatal disease of the immune system. The first official case of AIDS in a child was reported in November, 1982, about 18 months after the first reported adult case (Rogers et al, 1987). Since that time AIDS in childhood has been steadily increasing. Between June, 1981, and July 18, 1988, 1079 children were diagnosed as having AIDS (Centers for Disease Control, 1988). This number is mediated by the fact that persons older than 13 years of age are classified as adults by the AIDS guidelines issued by the Centers for Disease Control. As of December, 1986, 17 cases of AIDS in children had been reported in Canada (Understanding AIDS, 1988).

Despite public education efforts, the incidence of AIDS in adults and children continues to increase. The major risk factors in children are (1) having a mother who is HIV positive or is at risk for AIDS, and (2) receiving a transfusion of blood or blood products (Edmundson, 1988). It is estimated that the percentage of children with the disease will rise even higher as more women of childbearing age contract the disease (Rubinstein and Bernstein, 1986).

Etiology and Transmission

AIDS is caused by infection with the human immunodeficiency virus (HIV). The virus is carried in the body secretions of an infected person, particularly in blood and semen; HIV is transmitted when it enters the bloodstream of another person. Eighty per cent of the cases of AIDS in children appear to be transmitted to the infant in utero through the placenta (Rubinstein and Bernstein, 1986). Of the 1079 cases on record as of July 1988, 77.5 per cent were born to parents at risk for AIDS, almost 6 per cent were children with hemophilia who contracted the disease through transfusion of blood products, another 12.8 per cent of the cases were linked to blood transfusions, and 3.6 per cent were listed as undetermined etiologies (Centers for Disease Control, 1988). Not every infant with an infected mother will develop the virus. At least one case has been reported in which one identical twin contracted AIDS and the other (at age 3 years) was still healthy (Menez-Bautista et al, 1986). The mechanism that protected one twin and that protects some other infants in utero remains a mystery.

Box 43-10
Children at Risk for AIDS

Mother or father an intravenous drug user
Mother having sexual relations with persons at risk for AIDS
Father bisexual
Parent has had multiple drug transfusions
Parent recent immigrant from Haiti or central Africa
Infant/child exposure to contaminated blood:
(1) at time of delivery
(2) through transfusion of blood or blood components (e.g., children with hemophilia)

Most of the children who contracted HIV through transfusions did so prior to HIV antibody screening of blood beginning in May 1985. However, the CDC estimates that 1 in 40,000 units of blood will be contaminated until antigen testing is perfected. Currently, screening techniques test for *antibodies* to HIV, not to the virus itself. Therefore, a person who donates blood soon after exposure to HIV, before antibodies have been formed, can transmit the virus in an undetectable state. The child with hemophilia remains at greatest risk for exposure because as many as 1000 units of blood may be needed to extract the required concentration of clotting factor for one transfusion. New screening techniques on the horizon promise to further decrease the risk of transfusion through antigen testing, that is, testing for the AIDS virus itself.

The immature immunologic systems of premature and newborn infants make them especially susceptible to contaminated transfusions (Rubinstein and Bernstein, 1986). The AIDS virus has also been identified in breast milk. Although research is limited, breastfeeding may therefore be an additional source of transmission (Ziegler et al, 1985). The risk factors for AIDS in children are summarized in Box 43-10.

Pathophysiology

The virus thought to cause AIDS produces abnormalities in both T-cell function (cellular immunity) and, indirectly, in B-cell function (humoral immunity). The initial attack is upon the T-lymphocytes, leading to a marked depression of the T-helper cells that regulate B-cell function (Lockey and Bukantz, 1987a). Depression of T-helper cells reverses the usual ratio of T-helper to T-suppressor cells. Although antibodies

(IgG, IgA, and IgM) are typically increased in the serum of persons with AIDS, the T-suppressor effect on B-lymphocytes renders the B-cells incapable of forming antibodies to new microorganisms. Thus the patient is somewhat protected against those microorganisms to which antibodies have previously been formed but cannot defend against newly introduced pathogens. Because children have had fewer exposures to pathogens, they have fewer circulating antibodies than do adults. In addition, phagocytic macrophages in the AIDS victim have a decreased ability to process and kill antigens and to interact with T-cells (Ammann, 1987). All this means that the child (or adult) with AIDS is extremely susceptible to infection, and, once infected, has little defense against the invading organism.

Clinical Manifestations

Infants infected in utero or at birth tend to remain symptom-free for a period of time. Rubinstein and Bernstein (1986) reported that 6 months was the average age between exposure and onset of symptoms, with a range of from 6 weeks to 23 months. Another study reported incubation periods of between 9 months and 5 years (Ammann, 1987). Children most often had recurrent bacterial infections with sepsis, persistent oral thrush, and failure to thrive. Later manifestations of the disease were identified as lymphadenopathy, hepatosplenomegaly, chronic or recurrent diarrhea, and enlargement of the salivary glands.

Other clinical manifestations associated with AIDS include failure to thrive, developmental delays, neurologic disease, dysmorphic syndrome, and thrombocytopenia. Failure to thrive and developmental delays are quite common among children with AIDS. Although chronic diarrhea would seem the obvious reason for failure to thrive, Rubinstein (1986) reported that growth retardation occurs in the absence of diarrhea, and that HIV also appears linked to small gestational age of neonates. The mechanism by which the virus retards growth remains unknown. Developmental delays may relate to psychosocial factors, such as the adaptation of the family to the diagnosis. Failure to meet developmental milestones has also been linked with neurologic disease, common in children with AIDS. Because neurologic damage has been documented by CT scan in the first weeks of life, there is concern that HIV may produce brain damage in utero (Rubinstein, 1986).

Dysmorphic syndrome (dysmorphic meaning abnormal in form), characterized by severe growth failure and craniofacial anomalies, has been found in some infants born to mothers with AIDS (Marion et al, 1986). The exact mechanism by which the HIV affects the embryo or fetus is unknown. Another of the poorly understood actions of HIV is a reduction in platelets. Thrombocytopenia is found in both adults and children with AIDS.

Diagnostic Assessment

Antibodies for HIV can be detected through serum tests, which can indicate exposure to the virus. One type of diagnostic blood test is the enzyme-linked immunosorbent assay (ELISA). Considered somewhat more reliable is the Western blot test. Newer methods that increase reliability involve detection of the AIDS virus in lymphocytes and tissues.

Unfortunately, none of these diagnostic tests can discriminate between an acute infection and a carrier state (Coulis and DiSiena, 1987). They simply confirm that antibodies have been formed to the AIDS virus. Therefore diagnosis also depends upon physical findings and is structured according to the Centers for Disease Control (CDC) criteria for AIDS, which specify either that an opportunistic infection* be diagnosed or that lymphocytic interstitial pneumonitis be documented by lung biopsy. If the condition fails to meet one or more of the CDC criteria, the child will be classified as having AIDS-related complex (ARC). The term ARC is being replaced with the term HIV-positive (as distinguished from actually having AIDS). Adults with ARC may live symptom-free lives for years, but children do not fare as well. Very few children with positive antibody tests are asymptomatic beyond age 3 years (Rubenstein, 1986).

Therapeutic Management

Management of AIDS in children parallels that for adults. It involves:

- treatment of infections,
- reduction of viral replication within the T-lymphocyte (and therefore reduction of T-lymphocyte destruction),
- immunopotentiation (Rubinstein,1986).

Prevention of infection and suppression of HIV activity in children who are HIV positive or who have AIDS is most often addressed through periodic intravenous doses of gamma globulin. Although this therapy will not prevent infection indefinitely in the child with AIDS, it has shown the ability to reduce illness and prolong life in current clinical trials (Gupta et al, 1986; Rubinstein, 1986; Ammann, 1987; Fischer, 1988).

Once diagnosed, infections are usually treated with bactericidal agents. Prophylactic antimicrobials may be continued for extended periods.

---

* The term *opportunistic* refers to the fact that the person with AIDS is so immunodeficient that pathogens that do not usually cause disease may result in an infection.

Efforts have also been made to enhance the failing immune system through thymic hormones or thymic transfers. Unfortunately, research with these methods has resulted in increased HIV activity within the cells and has therefore been abandoned pending the development of further control agents (Rubinstein, 1986). Stimulation of T-cell lymphocytes within the thymus is being attempted with thymosin fraction (Iazetti, 1986). This drug remains investigational in nature.

Suramin, an antiviral agent, is one of 200 drugs that have been screened for potential effectiveness against AIDS (Bennett, 1986). Azidothymidine (AZT) has been useful in prolonging the lives of some AIDS patients. Research continues in quest of an AIDS vaccine and drugs that may be effective against AIDS.

Major Nursing Diagnoses for AIDS

Potential for infection, *related to HIV attack on T-lymphocytes and the subsequent suppression of antibody function*

Potential for altered growth and development:

- *failure to thrive, related to unknown mechanisms associated with AIDS*
- *developmental delays, related to chronic infection, alterations in attachment associated with a terminal prognosis, and central nervous system involvement*

Potential for injury: allergic reaction, *related to intravenous gamma globulin*

Potential for ineffective family coping, *related to*

- *parental feelings of guilt*
- *terminal prognosis of one or more family members*
- *loss of social support associated with fear of AIDS transmission*

Knowledge deficit, *related to management of AIDS at home*

Strategies for Nursing Care

Protecting the Nurse. The nursing plan of care must address the safety of the nurse as well as that of the child. The facts about AIDS transmission are that although HIV has been found in blood, semen, saliva, and tears, the disease has only been known to be transmitted sexually, perinatally, and by direct inoculation (Lilleyman, 1986; Blattner, 1987; US Public Health Service, 1988). The concern for health care professionals, then, is to prevent the last-named; i.e., to ensure that body secretions, especially blood, from the patient do not enter the bloodstream of the caregiver.

Universal Precautions. In August, 1987, the Centers for Disease Control published a document entitled "Recommendations for Prevention of HIV Transmission in Health-Care Settings." It was recommended that blood and body fluid precautions be consistently observed for ALL patients regardless of their diagnosis or bloodborne infection status. The extension of blood and body fluid precautions to all patients has come to be known as *universal precautions.* Under universal precautions, blood and certain body fluids for any patient are considered potentially infectious for HIV, hepatitis B virus (HBV), and other bloodborne pathogens. (See Box 43-11.) *The implementation of universal precautions is intended to supplement, not replace, other category- or disease-specific isolation precautions.* (General isolation guidelines are discussed in Chapter 27.)

Blood and Body Fluid Precautions. Specific policies for *blood and body fluid precautions* will vary somewhat among institutions. However, most institu-

Box 43-11
Universal Precautions for Prevention of Transmission of HIV, Hepatitis B Virus, and Other Bloodborne Pathogens in Health-Care Settings*

ALWAYS use blood and body fluid precautions for these substances:

Blood†
Body fluids containing visible blood†
Semen
Vaginal secretions
Tissues
Cerebrospinal fluid
Synovial fluid
Pleural fluid
Peritoneal fluid
Pericardial fluid
Amniotic fluid

Universal precautions do not apply (unless visible blood is present):

Feces
Nasal secretions
Sputum
Sweat
Tears
Urine
Vomitus
Saliva

* NOTE: The implementation of universal precautions does not eliminate the need for other disease-specific or category-specific precautions as outlined in Chapter 27.

† These are the only sources of HIV and HBV (hepatitis B virus) that have been implicated in transmission of infection from patient to health care worker. Semen and vaginal secretions have been associated with sexual transmission of bloodborne organisms but not with patient-to-nurse transfer. The other fluids listed in this column are potential sources of infection and are the subject of ongoing epidemiologic studies.

tions have adopted policies similar to the guidelines outlined by Kirkis and Grier (1988):

- Put the patient in a private room if hygiene is poor or if the environment is likely to become contaminated with blood.
- *Wash hands* thoroughly before and after patient care and after handling contaminated articles. *Handwashing is the most cost-effective, practice-effective method to reduce the spread of infection.*
- Always wear *gloves* when touching blood or body fluids.
- Wear a *mask* only if aerosolization of secretions is likely (e.g., suctioning).
- Wear a *gown* only if soiling of clothes is likely.
- Discard contaminated disposable articles; bag and send reusables for reprocessing.
- Avoid needle-stick injuries. Handle needles and sharps carefully.
- Clean up blood spills promptly with a solution of bleach diluted 1 : 10 with water.

The Centers for Disease Control recommend that needles not be recapped, bent, removed, or otherwise manipulated, because this increases the risk of accidental puncture. Syringes with needles attached should be disposed of, intact, in a metal container in the room. If an incident of contamination occurs (i.e., needle stick, breaking the skin with a contaminated sharp object, splash contamination) report it immediately to the employee health service department for that institution. Tests will be conducted to determine whether the patient carries antibodies for hepatitis or AIDS. Follow-up testing of the nurse for AIDS or provision of hepatitis B immune globulin will be carried out as indicated.

The precautions for hospital personnel exceed the precautions recommended for families in home care. The reason is because of the repeated risks of exposure for these professionals, and because of the danger to other patients from spread of the virus by the contaminated hands of the nurse.

Exemption Policies. The practice of providing exemption for the pregnant nurse from care of persons with AIDS, cytomegalovirus (CMV), and certain other communicable diseases is becoming much less prevalent. In part this is due to the nursing shortage and the fact that staffing patterns are becoming less flexible. In a more humane sense, however, it is also the direct result of CDC recommendations for universal precautions. It is becoming increasingly evident that nurses and other health care professionals are at greater risk for exposure from the patient presumed free of infection (but who may in fact be infectious) than from the patient with a diagnosed communicable disease for whom appropriate precautions are observed. If blood and body fluid precautions are consistently followed for all patients, regardless of health status (universal precautions), the risk of exposure is greatly reduced for all members of the staff.

Preventing Infection and Caring for the Child with Opportunistic Infection. AIDS destroys the body's natural defenses against bacterial, viral, and fungal infections, making it imperative that precautions be taken to protect the child from pathogens. Despite precautions, however, it can be expected that some opportunistic infections will develop. The infections common in children vary somewhat from those found in adults with AIDS. The body organs most often attacked by opportunistic infections are the lungs and the skin; chronic bacterial infections are an additional concern.

Pneumocystis carinii pneumonia is the most frequent opportunistic infection in children (Ammann, 1987). Less frequently, *Mycobacterium avium* or *Candida albicans* may be the cause of lung infection.

Recognizing the child's tendency toward lung infection, the nurse can meticulously assess for changes in pulmonary status and can teach and implement good pulmonary hygiene. Assessment findings of concern are fever, increased pulse and respirations, adventitious lung sounds, a cough, pallor on exertion, and retractions or other signs of increased respiratory effort.

Preventive hygienic measures include assuring that the child's lungs are fully inflated at regular intervals, and that secretions have no opportunity to pool within the lung because of immobility. Young children with AIDS who are feeling well enough to play usually meet these criteria for pulmonary hygiene on their own through running, jumping, yelling, and other activities that stimulate movement and deep breathing. The child hospitalized with a serious infection may need some innovative nursing help to accomplish this goal, however. The nurse can draw upon techniques used to promote turning and deep breathing after anesthesia. Gentle oral suctioning may be warranted if the child is unable to expectorate secretions.

Another important preventive measure is to ensure that the child is not needlessly exposed to pathogens. Research has shown that the most effective way to prevent spread of infection is through good handwashing. When the child is hospitalized, nurses and other health care professionals must remember that *the child is in more danger of contracting an infection from the nurse than the nurse is in peril of contracting AIDS from the child.* Parents, siblings, and the ill child should be taught proper handwashing techniques and counseled about avoiding exposure to crowds and to persons with active infections of any kind.

Infections of the integument in children are frequently either oral thrush (candidiasis) or chronic herpes simplex. Thrush is considered an opportunistic infection in children when it also involves the esophagus (Rubinstein, 1986). Because thrush causes discomfort, comfort measures like normal saline rinses are in order (Iazzeti, 1986). In severe cases, oral antiseptic rinses may be needed in order for the child to eat or drink without pain.

Herpes simplex is more common in children than in adults (Rubinstein, 1986). The blisters may occur in the perianal region as well as orally. Perianal lesions are in danger of secondary infection from fecal contamination, so gentle cleansing is needed after bowel movements. Severe infections may involve hospitalization and treatment with acyclovir.

Kaposi's sarcoma, although not common among children with AIDS, may be found in adolescents with the disease. The raised, purple tumors may be seen through the skin or mucous membranes. They are disfiguring because of their dark color but are usually not painful or irritating unless they involve the mucous membranes of the intestinal tract, where they often cause malabsorption and chronic diarrhea (Schietinger, 1986).

Nurses are often the persons responsible for teaching and implementing assessment and preventive measures for skin care. Parents can be taught to check the child's body daily for evidence of rashes, redness, bruises, blisters, or other unusual findings. Evidence of abrasions, such as "skinned" knees, will mean extra precautions to prevent secondary infection until a protective scab is formed. Usually such "scrapes" can safely be treated with half-strength hydrogen peroxide three to four times per day and protected with an ointment such as Neosporin. When in doubt, check with the attending physician regarding a specific protocol for each child. Preventing infections of the skin and mucous membranes involves keeping the skin clean, dry, and well lubricated and reporting the first evidence of an infectious process before a full-blown infection occurs.

Bacterial infections are common among children with AIDS (Ammann, 1987). It is important to alert parents that common childhood illnesses, such as ear aches, gastroenteritis, and impetigo, can become serious illnesses in the child with AIDS because of the lack of usual body defenses. Adolescents should be advised that opiates, alcohol, and marijuana can act as immunosuppressants and therefore may increase the susceptibility to infection (Dhundale and Hubbard, 1986).

Teach families that milk or formula is an excellent medium for bacterial growth. Infants should not be put to bed with a bottle which may be only partially consumed before sleep and finished hours later. Baby food, too, can become a culture medium. Teach parents not to feed directly from the babyfood jar; bacteria from saliva can contaminate remaining food. Fruits and vegetables should be washed and peeled or cooked before eating (Berry, 1988).

If a gastrostomy tube or nasogastric tube is required for supplemental feeding, it should be rinsed with water following feedings and clamped to avoid regurgitation. Strict aseptic technique is indicated in the care of central venous catheters to reduce the risk of localized infections or sepsis. Signs of sepsis include marked changes in temperature of the skin or body, tachycardia, hypotension, weak peripheral pulses, mottling, and altered mental status (Iazzeti, 1986). Prompt assessment and treatment of infection and compliance with prophylactic antimicrobial therapy are the best protection we currently can offer the child with AIDS.

Monitoring Growth and Development. While some part of growth retardation and developmental delays seems attributable to actions of the AIDS virus, enhancement of growth and development is still an attainable goal. Why should one be concerned about growth and development in a child with an incurable disease? Because it is the position of the scientific community that AIDS *is* curable and that it is only a matter of time until those cures are found. Drug research continues. Currently, intravenous gamma globulin is proving effective in preventing infections in children and prolonging their lives. Care must be structured to ensure that those children who will benefit from chemotherapeutic and other advances in AIDS treatment will have the capacity to lead normal lives and not be scarred by early neglect of well-child practices.

Height and weight should be assessed and plotted regularly and developmental milestones should be traced and recorded. Neurologic assessments are important as a basis for interpreting developmental progress. Significant delays in growth and development should be reported to the physician.

Growth can sometimes be enhanced through nutritional supplements. Children may be placed on enteral feedings or hyperalimentation, especially if chronic diarrhea or frequent vomiting is present. Monitoring of these therapies will include assurance that enteral feedings are being digested (that is, little residual feeding is left in the stomach when the next feeding is due and no increase in diarrhea is evident) and that hyperalimentation is not producing glycosuria or ketonuria (i.e., negative Clinitest and Acetest).

Older children and adolescents may be encouraged to supplement their diets with nutritious foods such as fruit, vegetables, milk shakes, and so on. They should be cautioned to eat only peeled or cooked fruit and vegetables to avoid infectious organisms and to make sure their milk products are pasteurized (Dhundale and Hubbard, 1986).

Development will be affected by frequent infections and the child's lack of energy to achieve new tasks. Hospitalizations that involve separation from parents and siblings also may have detrimental effects. The nurse who is aware of these hazards can discuss with the family the child's current tasks and plan with them ways to help the child master them despite illness. In the severely ill child, developmental delays may have to be accepted, but continuing to work with the child at his or her own pace will usually enhance the quality of life.

Administering Intravenous Gamma Globulin. As outlined by Iazzeti (1986), certain precautions should be observed when administering intravenous gamma globulin. The vial containing gamma globulin should not be shaken or rotated because bubbles may form in the solution. Gamma globulin is compatible *only* with a 5 per cent dextrose intravenous solution. No other medications or solutions should be administered through the same line.

Assessment for side effects of gamma globulin is similar to that for a transfusion reaction. Vital signs, including temperature, should be taken immediately before, and frequently during, administration. The most common side effects are skin rash, urticaria, fever, and dyspnea. If any of these signs or symptoms occur, stop the transfusion. Keep the line open with 5 per cent dextrose, record the vital signs and physical assessment, and alert the physician.

Supporting Family Coping. To begin to understand the impact of the diagnosis of AIDS in a child, one must consider the most likely family environment. Since most children with AIDS contract it in utero, the diagnosis may accentuate the fact that the mother, and possibly other family members, are seropositive for AIDS. Further consider that AIDS in women is most prevalent among intravenous drug abusers, prostitutes, and those whose husbands are bisexual. The adolescent diagnosed with AIDS is likely to be homosexual, to have a bisexual lover, or to be an intravenous drug user. Statistically, the family environment is likely to have multiple stressors and to be one in which a great deal of intervention is indicated. The nurse who is aware of this likelihood will be prepared to involve social service agencies early and to collaborate with them in providing support for the family as a whole.

Families must deal with feelings of guilt about the child's condition as well as with their grief over the terminal prognosis. Compounding the crisis is the fact that they may lose essential support from friends and family because of the fear of "catching" the disease. The nurse can be instrumental in separating the facts of transmission from the public panic about AIDS. Referral to AIDS support groups within the community can provide a valuable resource. Hospitals, physicians' offices, public health departments, The American Red Cross, the Centers for Disease Control in the United States (1-800-342-AIDS) and the Ontario Public Education Panel on AIDS (1-800-268-6066) are some sources of information.

Perhaps the most important attributes for the nurse who desires to support the family of an AIDS victim are the abilities to base practice on the facts about transmission versus the emotional fears of transmission, and refrain from judging the personal values and practices that led to exposure. This is a family in crisis, a family with needs that may go unmet unless professional practice can rise above public hysteria.

Teaching to Support Home Care. Teaching the family to manage the care of the child or adolescent with AIDS includes information about transmission of the virus, normalization of the child's lifestyle, protection of the child from infection, and protection of the adolescent's sexual partners or fellow drug-users. Care of the child in relation to infectious processes was discussed under the section dealing with the first nursing diagnosis.

Transmission of the Virus. The family will be relieved to know that there are *no* reported cases of transmission of the virus by *casual* contact between family members (Berry, 1988). The one reported case of a mother contracting AIDS from her child involved extensive, unprotected exposure to the child's blood (Centers for Disease Control, 1986). Studies such as the one conducted by Rubinstein (1986) involved not-so-casual contact. In many homes children shared beds, toothbrushes, toys, and food and lived under crowded conditions without transmission of HIV. Although these practices are not recommended, the study gives credence to the safety of family members. In the words of the U.S. Surgeon General, "We would know by now if AIDS were passed by casual, non-sexual contact" (Koop, 1987).

It is recommended that precautions be taken to protect family members. The nurse can counsel the family to avoid the mixing of the ill child's body secretions and excretions with their own. That means having separate linens, a separate toothbrush, a separate razor for the adolescent, and not sharing eating utensils between washing them. Linens and clothing can be washed with detergent (and for extra protection with 1 cup of bleach or Lysol per load) and dried in the dryer. Dishes are considered properly disinfected if washed with detergent in hot water or in the dishwasher.

More stringent precautions are indicated for blood and body excretions. Gloves should be worn to change dressings. Spills of blood or excretions can be disinfected with a 1:10 bleach solution (Dhundale and Hubbard, 1986; Schietinger, 1986). Trash can be kept in closed plastic containers for normal trash pickup (Berry, 1988). Feces, urine, and other body fluids or secretions can be flushed down the toilet. The nurse can help the family obtain a safe container for needles or sharps. This container should be taken to the hospital for proper disposal or picked up by the needle vendor.

Normalizing the Child's Lifestyle. Normalization necessarily begins with understanding of the disease process and of child behavior. As expressed by Schietinger (1986), "having a life-threatening illness yet feeling healthy can be confusing" (page 1021). It can also be confusing for the family to see the child active and playing one day and hospitalized with an overwhelming infection a few days later. The fact that the child will look and act quite well between infections can lead to denial of the illness and doubt about the diagnosis. The nurse can be instrumental in helping the family understand the disease process. The family must also come to understand that "children with AIDS can be touched, hugged, and loved" (Berry, 1988, page 344).

Because this child is first of all a child, and only secondly an AIDS victim, normalization of the lifestyle to the extent possible will greatly enhance the quality of life for the child and for the entire family. Normalizing efforts begin with attention to growth and development, as previously discussed. Discipline practices and family interactions should be no different for the child with AIDS than for siblings. Well-child care is important; the nurse can help the family understand the value of keeping these appointments.

Immunizations will not proceed on a normal schedule because of the risk of giving a live virus vaccine to an immunodeficient child. AIDS patients should not receive oral polio vaccine or measles, mumps, or rubella vaccines. Killed vaccines are recommended exclusively in children with AIDS (Rubinstein, 1986). The child with AIDS who is exposed to a communicable disease should be referred to medical care immediately since prompt intervention will often be needed to prevent an overwhelming infection.

School attendance has received national press coverage for some children with AIDS. The issue is a grave one. Mills and associates (1986) believe that "AIDS poses the most profound issues of constitutional law and public health since the Supreme Court approved compulsory immunization in 1905" (page 931). Standards, such as those set by the Centers for Disease Control, consider the risks and benefits to both the infected child and to others in the school. Authorities in both the United States and Great Britain, however, believe that the benefits of public education for the child with AIDS far outweigh the risk of acquiring infection (Education and foster care, 1985; Lilleyman, 1986). The school nurse and community health nurse can be instrumental in helping the public sort the facts about transmission of AIDS from the fears (Hughes and Bailey, 1987). As stated by the Centers for Disease Control, "It should be emphasized that any theoretical transmission would most likely involve exposure of open skin lesions or mucous membranes to blood and possibly other body fluids of an infected person" (Education and foster care, 1985, page 519).

Protecting the Child from Infection. In addition to protection measures discussed previously, the child at home may be in danger of infection from household pets. Avoid contact between the ill child and young animals that may bite or scratch. Because children often have responsibility for pet care, certain precautions, as outlined by Dhundale and Hubbard (1986), should be discussed with the family. If the family cat is allowed out of doors at all, the child should wear gloves and a mask when cleaning the litter box, to protect against toxoplasmosis. Gloves and mask should also be worn when cleaning the bird cage, to protect against psittacosis. Because of the danger of mycobacterial infection, the child should *never* clean the fish tank.

Protecting the Adolescent's Friends from AIDS. Since AIDS in adolescence is most likely to be acquired by sexual or intravenous drug practices, the adolescent must take responsibility for protecting friends from the disease. The nurse's rapport with the adolescent will play a large part in whether there is compliance with the teaching.

As reported by Bennett (1986), transmission of AIDS appears to be dose-related—that is, semen is more likely to transmit HIV than is simple contact with vaginal or rectal mucosa. Rectal intercourse is particularly contraindicated because even small breaks in the mucosa provide a direct route to the blood stream. Heterosexual transmission has been reported, however, with only vaginal intercourse. The key to safe sexual practice is to avoid the mixing of body secretions. This means using a condom and diaphragm for intercourse in addition to a water-soluble lubricant with 5 per cent nonoxynol 9 (Dhundale and Hubbard, 1986). In addition, great care should be taken not to damage rectal or vaginal mucosa.

Drug users should avoid sharing needles or syringes with friends. Further, they should be taught aseptic technique so that they if they are unable to stop drug use, they can at least do it with less risk of infection.

Nursing Strategies for Follow-up Care in the Home or Clinic

Assess for subjective and objective evidence of infection.

Allow time for the child and family to ask questions, voice concerns, and obtain needed information and support.

Inform the family of local epidemics and provide appropriate precautionary information.

Culture draining or purulent lesions, as indicated.

Assess growth and development parameters.

Inquire about family coping and determine whether additional resources are indicated.

Table 43-2
Nursing Process Plan: The Child on Corticosteroid Therapy

by Roxie Foster

I. Assessment of Physical Function

Subjective Assessment

Self-report or parental report of appetite, history of gastric distress, thirst, number of voids/day or changes in voiding pattern, perceived susceptibility to infection, history of persistent headache, muscle cramps, paresthesias or muscle weakness

Objective Assessment

Weight, length/height percentile compared with own baseline; evidence of edema, infectious process; intake versus output; eye grounds; vision; cranial nerve function; GI function, facial contour, muscle strength, urinalysis, fasting blood sugar, serum potassium, occult blood in body secretions

Analysis: Nursing Diagnosis 1

Fluid volume excess, related to mineralocorticoid activity associated with the prescribed corticosteroid

Defining Characteristics

Objective: Increase in weight and blood pressure, palpable edema, intake significantly greater than output

Client Goals/ Evaluation Criteria	Nursing Goals/Strategies (Selected Rationale)
1. The client will experience a minimal amount of edema, as evidenced by: a. absent or only slight edema of the extremities b. BP within normal range for age c. no sudden increases in weight d. output balanced with intake	*Monitor for edema.* • Assess for edema of extremities and sacrum every shift and record findings. • Measure I&O • Weigh daily on same scale with only diaper or underwear • Measure BP every shift with child under like conditions (i.e., preferably with child at rest, not crying or protesting). • Monitor any elevations in BP: recheck in 1–2 hr; correlate with weight, urinary output. • Report to physician elevations judged to be associated with fluid retention. *Teach and implement strategies to control fluid retention.* • Teach parent/s and child how to assess for edema (to support home management). • Implement a "no-added-salt" diet for the child prone to fluid retention. • Discuss with parent the need for regular follow-up care. Explain that if edema becomes significant, physician may change to different corticosteroid (with a weaker mineralocorticoid activity).

Analysis: Nursing Diagnosis 2

Potential for injury: physiologic, related to increased excretion of potassium associated with corticosteroid therapy

Continued

Table 43-2 (continued)

Analysis: Nursing Diagnosis 2

Defining Characteristics

Subjective: Muscle cramps, nausea, paresthesias

Objective: Diarrhea, vomiting, tetany, dysrhythmias, potassium <3.5 mEq/L

Client Goal/ Evaluation Criteria	Nursing Goals/Strategies (Selected Rationale)
2. The client will not experience hypokalemia, as evidenced by: a. serum potassium between 3.5 and 5 mEq/L b. absence of muscle cramps, nausea and vomiting, paresthesias, diarrhea, tetany, and dysrhythmias	*Assess for hypokalemia.* • Question client about classic signs and symptoms. • Monitor laboratory reports for serum potassium level. • Assess cardiac status carefully. Monitor apical pulse for 1 full minute, being alert for dysrhythmia. Institute use of a cardiorespiratory monitor if indicated. *Teach and implement measures to avoid hypokalemia.* • Avoid potassium-depleting diuretics. • Increase potassium-rich foods in the diet.

Analysis: Nursing Diagnosis 3

Altered comfort: pain, related to gastric irritation, associated with ulcerogenic effects of corticosteroids

Defining Characteristics

Subjective: Nausea, anorexia, epigastric pain that may or may not be relieved by eating or antacids

Objective: Heme-positive stools or vomitus

Client Goal/ Evaluation Criteria	Nursing Goals/Strategies (Selected Rationale)
3. The client will be free of gastric irritation, as evidenced by: a. denying epigastric distress b. usual appetite (or slight increase) c. absence of blood in vomitus or stool	*Assess for gastric irritation.* • Ask the child about comfort level. Use measures designed to assess pain in children; see Chapter 29. • Note appetite; if intake is decreased, determine whether related to medication or to other factors. • Routinely test vomitus and stool for blood. • Alert parents to contact the physician if evidence of gastric irritation occurs. *Teach and implement measures to prevent gastric irritation.* • Administer corticosteroid with food or milk. • Avoid known gastric irritants—aspirin and other nonsteroidal anti-inflammatory drugs, alcohol. • Limit intake of caffeine in chocolate, coffee, tea; (caffeine increases gastric acidity).

Analysis: Nursing Diagnosis 4

Potential for injury: physiologic, related to hyperglycemia, associated with promotion of gluconeogenesis and decreased glucose utilization effects of corticosteroids

Defining Characteristics

Subjective: Hunger, thirst

Objective: Polyuria, glycosuria, increased blood sugar

Client Goal/ Evaluation Criteria	Nursing Goals/Strategies (Selected Rationale)
4. The client will not experience a hyperglycemic reaction, as evidenced by: a. Absence of unusual hunger or thirst b. absence of polyuria c. absence of glucosuria d. fasting blood sugar <120 mg/dl	*Assess for hyperglycemia.* • Monitor for polydipsia, polyuria, polyphagia. • Measure urine sugar and acetone every shift during initial therapy, periodically thereafter. • Monitor laboratory reports of serum glucose. • Teach child and parents symptoms of hyperglycemia and how to test blood or urine for sugar. • Alert the family to contact the physician if evidence of hyperglycemia occurs. *Caution the diabetic client to obtain regular follow-up care.* More insulin may be needed while on corticosteroid therapy.

Analysis: Nursing Diagnosis 5

Altered growth and development: linear growth, related to protein catabolism and inhibition of growth hormone associated with corticosteroid therapy

Defining Characteristics

Objective: Failure to maintain height and weight at pretherapy percentiles on the growth chart

Client Goal/ Evaluation Criteria	Nursing Goals/Strategies (Selected Rationale)
5. The client will maintain pretherapy percentiles for height and weight on the growth chart	*Assess growth parameters.* Measure and plot height and weight at every follow-up visit. *Encourage a high protein diet* (to help offset the effects of protein catabolism). *Alert the physician to the first evidence of growth failure.* (It may be possible to use an alternate-day dosage schedule that minimizes protein catabolism.)

Continued

Table 43-2 (continued)

Analysis: Nursing Diagnosis 6

Potential for infection, related to altered immune function, associated with corticosteroid therapy

Defining Characteristics

Subjective: "I seem to catch every virus that goes around"

Objective: Evidence of infectious process (although not necessarily with the typical signs)

Client Goal/ Evaluation Criteria	Nursing Goals/Strategies (Selected Rationale)
6. The client will remain free of avoidable infections	*Teach the child and family principles of infection control:* transmission of organisms, meticulous handwashing, maintenance of general health *Alert the family to the contraindication for immunization with live virus: TOPV, MMR* (because of immunosuppressive effects of corticosteroids). *Explain the necessity to seek medical advice for wounds that are slow to heal, persistent inflammation, or persistent malaise* (because of immunosuppression and the potential of corticosteroids to mask other illness).

Analysis: Nursing Diagnosis 7

Impaired physical mobility, related to muscle weakness, associated with the protein-catabolizing effects of corticosteroids

Defining Characteristics

Subjective: Report of decreased muscle strength

Objective: Decreased strength of extremities evident upon physical examination

Client Goal/ Evaluation Criteria	Nursing Goals/Strategies (Selected Rationale)
7. The client will maintain muscle strength, as evidenced by: a. denying changes in muscle strength b. exhibiting normal and equal strength in extremities upon examination	*Assess muscle strength* both subjectively and objectively at each follow-up visit. *Teach child to promote muscle strength through* regular exercise and a high-protein, high-calcium diet (Wiener and Pepper, 1985).

Analysis: Nursing Diagnosis 8

Potential for injury: neurologic, related to untoward reaction to corticosteroids

Defining Characteristics

Subjective: Headache

Objective: Papilledema, oculomotor or abducens nerve paralysis, visual loss (Loebl and Spratto, 1986).

Client Goal/ Evaluation Criteria	Nursing Goals/Strategies (Selected Rationale)
8. Client will not experience neurologic effects of corticosteroids, as evidenced by: a. absence of papilledema or vision changes b. absence of nerve paralysis c. absence of persistent headache	*Assess for evidence of neurologic reactions.* • Alert the physician to evidence of neurologic effects (because this signals an untoward reaction to the corticosteroid). *Assure the client and family that the syndrome is reversible.*

Analysis: Nursing Diagnosis 9

Knowledge deficit, related to safe administration of corticosteroid

Defining Characteristics

Subjective or objective indication of being unfamiliar with corticosteroid actions and potential side effects

Client Goal/ Evaluation Criteria	Nursing Goals/Strategies (Selected Rationale)
9. The client (family) will be knowledgeable about safe administration practices for corticosteroid, as evidenced by: a. discussing plans to implement appropriate criteria for administration b. suffering no avoidable untoward effects c. demonstrating safe usage over time	*Teach and implement safe administration.* • Inject IM corticosteroids deeply into approved site with largest muscle mass (to avoid tissue atrophy at site).* • Avoid SC injection or reuse of injection site. • Explain that morning administration, before 9 A.M., will minimize immunosuppression. • Instruct the family that the child should receive no over-the-counter drugs without consulting the physician. • Consult the physician should severe infection, injury, or other significant stress occur (that may necessitate an increased dose of corticosteroid). • Explain that the corticosteroid should not be stopped abruptly; (withdrawal syndrome and hypoadrenalism may occur). • The child on long-term corticosteroids should wear a Medic-Alert bracelet to inform emergency personnel of the medication.

*Corticosteroids are rarely ordered for children by the IM route. However, when this route is chosen careful technique is indicated.

Continued

Table 43-2 (continued)

II. Assessment of Emotional-Social Function

Subjective Assessment	Objective Assessment
Report of feelings about self and self in relation to others	Signs of Cushing syndrome

Analysis: Nursing Diagnosis 10

Disturbance in self-concept: body image, related to Cushing syndrome, associated with prolonged high corticosteroid dosages

Defining Characteristics

Subjective: Report of feeling "different" from peers, embarrassed about appearance, being teased about appearance, avoiding social interactions

Objective: Moon facies, hirsutism, acne, muscular weakness, cervicothoracic hump, hypertension, osteoporosis, amenorrhea, striae, thinning of hair and nails, ecchymosis

Client Goal/ Evaluation Criteria	Nursing Goals/Strategies (Selected Rationale)
10. The client will demonstrate an adaptive attitude toward change in appearance, as evidenced by: a. discussing plans to manage aspects that can be manipulated b. initiating social relationships c. reporting "feeling better about self"	*Assess for evidence of Cushing syndrome.* • Report concerns to physician for consideration of dose adjustment. *Promote adaptive behavior.* • Encourage the client to express feelings about changes in appearance and facilitate problem solving. • Suggest the use of depilatories for hirsutism. • Counsel the client with acne about skin care; see Chapter 44. • Suggest the use of artificial nails and full or partial wigs (especially for the female adolescent). • Counsel the client about the need to prevent injury. Help the client think of suitable alternatives for activities that must be sacrificed, e.g., tennis or track versus football. (Bone demineralization associated with corticosteroid therapy makes one more prone to injury.)

Table 43-9
Nursing Process Plan: The Child with Atopic Dermatitis

by Roxie Foster

I. Assessment of Physical Function

Skin Integrity

Subjective Assessment

Parental and/or client report of degree of skin comfort/discomfort, changes in skin comfort relative to seasonal and climate variations, known allergens, family history of allergy (e.g., asthma, hay fever, eczema)

Objective Assessment

Texture of skin, presence of scaling or "goose bumps," skin integrity with respect to excoriation and lesions

Analysis: Nursing Diagnosis 1

Impaired skin integrity: cutaneous dryness, related to the inability to hold moisture in the stratum corneum

Analysis: Nursing Diagnosis 2

Altered comfort: pruritus, related to:
- *dry skin*
- *external irritants (e.g., scratching, woolen or synthetic clothing, secondary infection)*
- *low threshold for itching*

Defining Characteristics for Nursing Diagnoses 1 and 2

Subjective: Complaints of dry, itching, chapped skin; seasonal variation in symptoms

Objective: Skin dry, with some scaling evident; erythema and excoriation present from scratching; gooseflesh appearance of skin; accentuated skin folds under the eyes; see Nursing Diagnosis 3 for signs of infection

Client Goals/ Evaluation Criteria	Nursing Goals/Strategies (Selected Rationale)
1/2.1. The client will experience reduced dryness and skin irritation as evidenced by: a. verbalizing increased skin comfort b. decreased scaling c. decreased excoriation from scratching	*Institute and teach strategies to promote skin hydration.* • Bathe at least once every day, soaking for 15 to 20 minutes in warm, not hot, water. Bathe more often when signs and symptoms increase. (Bathing in warm water allows water to enter the pores and hydrate the skin.) • Apply hypoallergenic creams or ointments *immediately* after bathing (to help seal in moisture). Avoid perfumed lubricants and bubble baths (that may trigger an allergic skin response). • Use a topical preparation like Eucerin cream, Moisturel cream, or Aquaphor ointment. (Creams and ointments seal better than lotions.)

Continued

Table 43-9 (continued)

Client Goals/ Evaluation Criteria	Nursing Goals/Strategies (Selected Rationale)
	• Avoid extremes in temperature and humidity. Use a humidifier, especially in dry climates and in winter months when heating lowers humidity indoors. If the family cannot afford a humidifier, a cool-mist vaporizer used in the child's room will help. • If a humidifier or vaporizer is used, ensure the family understands the necessity of cleaning before each water refill (to avoid aerosolization of mold or bacteria).
1/2.2. The client will experience a decrease in pruritus, as evidenced by: a. verbalizing increased comfort b. decreased restlessness during napping/sleeping c. decrease in observed and reported scratching d. decreased excoriation from scratching	*Institute and teach strategies to reduce external irritants.* • Break the scratch-itch-scratch cycle by keeping skin clean and well lubricated, keeping fingernails short, putting mitts on small infants, and administering topical steroids, antipruritics, antihistamines, or sedatives, if needed. These measures are especially important at naptime and at night (because pruritus caused by atopic dermatitis typically increases at night). • Apply wet compresses of Burow solution as ordered (to dry weeping lesions, rehydrate skin, and cool inflammation through evaporation). 1. Use material for compresses that is soft, lightweight, and loosely woven, such as a single thickness diaper or Kerlix. 2. Use solution at room temperature or heat just until tepid. (Extremes of temperature increase pruritus.) 3. Wet compresses thoroughly but avoid dripping (since solution that runs off the body is of no value). 4. Keep soaks wet; do not allow to dry on skin. • Use *soft cotton clothing* when possible. Avoid clothing with rough fibers, tightly woven fibers (that prevent natural evaporation from the skin), and wool (which may cause an allergic skin response). • Avoid exposure to *potential allergens.* Do not let the child crawl on a wool carpet. Stuffed animals and fuzzy toys may also be suspect. It is best to avoid exposure to dogs and cats. (See Boxes 43-3 and 43-4.) • Wash new clothing and sheets before use (to remove formaldehyde and sizing). Avoid strong detergents and fabric softeners. Rinse clothing thoroughly. • Administer *systemic antibiotics* to alleviate secondary bacterial infection. (Topical antibiotics are of no value and their use on excoriated skin may cause the child to become allergic to the drug [Jacobs and Goldsobel, 1988]). Assess for therapeutic and side effects. • Reduce sweating (which increases pruritus). 1. Avoid excessive clothing and high environmental temperatures when possible. 2. The child of preschool age and older should be alerted that physical activity may increase itching. • Reduce anxiety (which also increases pruritus). Table 31-2 discusses anxiety reduction for the hospitalized child and the family. Parents who are aware of the relationship between anxiety and pruritus often can increase comfort measures and teach the child appropriate coping strategies.

Analysis: Nursing Diagnosis 3

Potential for infection: secondary, related to:
- *skin excoriation*
- *decreased resistance to cutaneous viral, fungal, and staphylococcal organisms*

Defining Characteristics

Subjective: Pruritus, loss of sleep, irritability

Objective: vesicles in various weeping and crusted stages

Client Goal/ Evaluation Criteria	Nursing Goals/Strategies (Selected Rationale)
3.1 The client will experience a reduction in infectious lesions, as evidenced by absence of erythema with vesiculation, exudation, and crusting	*Assess for evidence of infection.* Teach parent/s the signs of infection; ensure that they understand that presence of these signs indicates the need for medical intervention. *Teach the relationship between scratching and infection.* Encourage appropriate skin care techniques, as discussed earlier. *Institute and teach proper administration of antibiotics.* • Explain the virulence of the identified pathogen (usually staph) and emphasize the importance of administering the medication according to schedule and until gone. • Ensure that caregivers realize the need for re-evaluation with each outbreak of pustular lesions and that they do not attempt to use "left-over" medication.

II. Assessment of Emotional-Social Function

Self-Concept

Subjective Assessment

Self-report or parental report of feelings about self, and self in relation to others

Objective Assessment

Attachment behavior, social development

Analysis: Nursing Diagnosis 4

Disturbance in self-concept: body image, related to
- *skin lesions*
- *response of significant others to appearance*

Defining Characteristics

Subjective: Verbalizing feelings of inferiority, negativity, pessimism; reporting few friends, limited social interactions

Objective: Delayed social development, absence of expected comfort response in interactions with significant others.

Continued

Table 43-9 (continued)

Client Goal/ Evaluation Criteria	Nursing Goals/Strategies (Selected Rationale)
4.1. The child will exhibit a positive self-concept, as evidenced by: a. displaying social development appropriate to age b. expressing feelings of importance, self-worth c. enjoying interpersonal interactions	*Explain to parent/s that the young child's self-concept is closely related to the responses of significant others.* Encourage parent/s to explain to others that eczema is not contagious unless severely infected (it may otherwise be mistaken for impetigo or as an indication of uncleanliness). • Encourage family members to express their feelings about the child's appearance and the chronic nature of eczema. (Unidentified fears and concerns may hinder the relationship of parents and siblings with the child.) • Assure parents that it is not uncommon to experience occasional feelings of rejection toward the child because of skin lesions and the fussing and crying that tend to accompany the pruritus of an acute exacerbation. (Acknowledging and understanding these feelings can help allay guilt that might otherwise interfere with adaptive coping.) *Teach family members ways to enhance the child's self-concept.* • *Reinforce* the child's sense of *identity.* Encourage the expression of caring among the child and significant others. Talk to the child about ways in which he or she excels. • *Reinforce* the child's sense of *personal competence.* Encourage self-management of eczema as appropriate for age. Ensure that the child understands that controlling scratching will greatly reduce lesions. Allow the child to make age-appropriate decisions about when to use palliative measures such as wet soaks.

III. Assessment of Intellectual-Perceptual Function

Health Perception
Knowledge of Illness/Health Management

Subjective Assessment

Child's and parents' perception of the illness; health beliefs and cultural values; knowledge of the disease process, home management, and well child care

Objective Assessment

Return demonstration of physical care and medication administration

Analysis: Nursing Diagnosis 5

Knowledge deficit, related to
- *identification and alleviation of allergens*
- *control of dry skin and pruritus*
- *secondary infection: assessment, prevention, and treatment*
- *well child care*

Defining Characteristics

Subjective: Asking questions, requesting demonstration of procedure(s)

Objective: Inability to demonstrate physical care behaviors or to verbalize what was previously taught

Client Goal/ Evaluation Criteria	Nursing Goals/Strategies (Selected Rationale)
5.1. The family will be able to identify and eliminate allergens, as evidenced by: a. identifying the relationship between contact with certain substances and an increase in cutaneous signs and symptoms b. compliance with hypoallergenic diet (if prescribed) c. allergy-proofing the home (if indicated)	*Teach the family about the allergy regimen prescribed.* • Ensure that they realize hypoallergenic diets and allergy-proofing do not cure eczema and may provide only limited control. (If they do not understand this, they may feel that increased eczematous symptoms are the fault of their inadequate management.) • If a hypoallergenic diet is prescribed, teach parents to read food labels carefully for alternate names of prohibited ingredients. *Support the family's efforts to control allergen contact.* • Acknowledge the time and energy involved in controlling possible allergens. • Because allergy-proofing requires rather drastic measures to reduce dust in the home, help the family assess the resources available to enforce this regimen. • Reinforce the family's attempts to identify possible allergens by commenting upon accurate assessment of signs and symptoms.
5.2. The family will demonstrate an understanding of strategies to control dry skin, pruritus, and secondary infection, as evidenced by: a. verbalizing understanding b. demonstrating techniques of care c. listing signs and symptoms of secondary infection	*Teach the family strategies to control the chronic skin irritation.* See strategies for Nursing Diagnoses 1, 2, and 3. *Assist the family to evaluate the outcome of their interventions and to modify home management as necessary.* Take into account the perceptions, health beliefs, and cultural values identified in assessment.
5.3. The family will recognize the importance of usual well child care, as evidenced by: a. discussing the developmental tasks pertinent to this child b. indicating their plan to normalize the child's environment c. verbalizing a plan for regular follow-up care	*Teach the family about the developmental tasks* pertinent to this child and assist them in planning ways to help the child accomplish those tasks. *Discuss with parents and siblings ways to normalize the child's life* despite the chronic nature of eczema. *Reinforce the importance of regular follow-up care* to ensure health assessment, immunizations, and an opportunity to evaluate the effectiveness of home treatments previously prescribed.

References

Altman LC: Overview of autoimmune and immune mechanisms. *In* Bierman CW, Pearlman DS: *Allergic Diseases from Infancy to Adulthood.* 2nd ed. Philadelphia, WB Saunders, 1988, 761–778.

American Academy of Pediatrics: *Pediatric Nutrition Handbook.* Evanston, IL, 1979.

Ammann AJ: Pediatric acquired immunodeficiency syndrome. *In* Feigin RD, Cherry JD (eds): *Textbook of Pediatric Infectious Diseases.* 2nd ed. Philadelphia, WB Saunders, 1987, 1044–1049.

An AIDS pill that offers hope. *US News World Report* 1986; 101(13).

Anderson DC: Infectious complications resulting from phagocytic cell dysfunction. *In* Feigin RD, Cherry JD (eds): *Textbook of Pediatric Infectious Diseases.* 2nd ed. Philadelphia, WB Saunders, 1987, 41–78.

Araujo OE, Flowers FP: Stevens-Johnson syndrome. *J Emerg Med* 1984; 2:129–135.

Behrman RE, Vaughan VC III (eds): *Nelson Textbook of Pediatrics.* 13th ed. Philadelphia, WB Saunders, 1987.

Bellanti JA: *Immunology: Basic Processes.* 2nd ed. Philadelphia, WB Saunders, 1985.

Bennett JA: What we know about AIDS. *Am J Nurs* 1986; 86(9):1016–1021.

Berry RK: Home care of the child with AIDS. *Pediatr Nurs* 1988 Jul-Aug; 14(4):341–344.

Bierman CW, Pearlman DS: *Allergic Diseases of Infancy, Childhood, and Adolescence.* Philadelphia, WB Saunders, 1980.

Bierman CW, Pearlman DS, Berman BA: Injection therapy for allergic diseases. *In* Bierman CW, Pearlman DS: *Allergic Diseases from Infancy to Adulthood.* 2nd ed. Philadelphia, WB Saunders, 1988, 279–293.

Blattner WA: Human retroviruses. *In* Feigin RD, Cherry JD (eds): *Textbook of Pediatric Infectious Diseases.* 2nd ed. Philadelphia, WB Saunders, 1987, 1795–1810.

Brewer EJ: Collagen vascular disease. *In* Gellis SS, Kagan BM (eds): *Current Pediatric Therapy 12.* Philadelphia, WB Saunders, 1986, 353–357.

Brewer EJ, et al: Current proposed revision of JRA Criteria. Arthritis Rheum 1977; 20(Suppl 2):195.

Brewer EJ, et al: *Juvenile Rheumatoid Arthritis.* 2nd ed. Philadelphia, WB Saunders, 1982, 120.

Bridgewater S, Voignier R: Allergies in children: teaching. *Am J Nurs* 1978 Apr; 620–621.

Buckley R: Advances in asthma/allergy. *Pediatr Nurs* 1979 Mar/Apr; 5:39–45.

Buckley RH: IgE antibody in health and disease. *In* Bierman CW, Pearlman DS: *Allergic Diseases from Infancy to Adulthood.* 2nd ed. Philadelphia, WB Saunders, 1988, 75–94.

Buscinco L, Cantani A: Prevention of atopy—current concepts and personal experience. *Clin Rev Allergy* 1984; 2:107–123.

Centers for Disease Control: Apparent transmission of human T-lymphotropic virus type III/lymphadenopathy–associated virus from a child to a mother providing health care. *Morbid Mortal Weekly Report* 1986 Feb; 35(5):76–77.

Centers for Disease Control: *AIDS Weekly Surveillance Report—United States.* Atlanta, CDC, Jul 18, 1988.

Coombs RRA, Gell PGH: Classification of allergic reactions responsible for clinical hypersensitivity and disease. *In* Gell PGH, et al (eds): *Clinical Aspects of Immunology.* 3rd ed. London, Blackwell, 1975.

Coulis PA, DiSiena JJ: AIDS immunodiagnosis: questions and answers about screening tests. *AIDS Patient Care* 1987; 1(1), 25–27.

Dhundale K, Hubbard PM: Home care for the AIDS patient: safety first. *Nurs 86* 1986; 16(9):34–36.

Dorian B, Garfinkel PE: Stress, immunity and illness—a review. *Psychol Med* 1987; 17:393–407.

Edmundson KS: Acquired immune deficiency syndrome in the neonate. *Neonatal Network* 1988 Feb; 7–12.

Education and foster care of children infected with human T-lymphotropic virus type III/lymphadenopathy–associated virus. *Morbid Mortal Weekly Report* 1985; 34(34):517–520.

Feigin RD, Garg R: Interaction of infection and nutrition. *In* Feigin RD, Cherry JD (eds): *Textbook of Pediatric Infectious Diseases.* 2nd ed. Philadelphia, WB Saunders, 1987, 17–27.

Fineman SM: Urticaria and angioedema. *Immunol Allergy Clin North Am* 1987; 7(2):265–276.

Fischer GW: Therapeutic uses of intravenous gamma-globulin for pediatric infections. *Pediatr Clin North Am* 1988 Jun; 35(3):517–533.

Fulginiti VA: Immunologic responses to infection. *In* Feigin RD, Cherry JD (eds): *Textbook of Pediatric Infectious Diseases.* 2nd ed. Philadelphia, WB Saunders, 1987, 28–40.

Fuller BF: Using research in practice: Some beneficial effects of stress. *West J Nurs Res* 1983; 5(1):99–104.

Fuller BF: Organ graft rejection. The biological process. *AORN J* 1985 Apr; 41(4):738–745.

Grant JA, Kennedy-Caldwell C: *Nutritional Support in Nursing.* Philadelphia, Grune & Stratton, 1988.

Griffiths SP: Acute rheumatic fever. *In* Gellis SS, Kagan BM (eds): *Current Pediatric Therapy 12.* Philadelphia, WB Saunders, 1986, 167–169.

Gupta A, et al: Restoration of suppressor T-cell functions in children with AIDS following intravenous gamma globulin treatment. *AM J Dis Child* 1986; 140(2): 143–146.

Guyton AC: *Textbook of Medical Physiology.* 7th ed. Philadelphia, WB Saunders, 1986.

Guyton AC: *Human Physiology and Mechanisms of Disease.* 4th ed. Philadelphia, WB Saunders, 1987.

Hicks RV, Melish ME: Kawasaki syndrome. *Pediatr Clin North Am* 1986 Oct; 33(5):1151–1175.

Hill D, et al: A study of 100 infants and young children with cow's milk allergy. *Clin Rev Allergy* 1984; (2):125–142.

Hughes RB, Bailey FK: AIDS from a school health perspective. *Pediatr Nurs* 1987 May-Jun; 13(3):155–156.

Iazzeti L: Nursing management of the pediatric AIDS patient. *Issues Compr Pediatr Nurs* 1986; 9(2):119–129.

Jacobs AH, Goldsobel AB: Atopic dermatitis. *In* Bierman CW, Pearlman DS: *Allergic Diseases from Infancy to Adulthood.* 2nd ed. Philadelphia, WB Saunders, 1988, 385–404.

Johnstone DE: Prevention of allergic diseases. *In* Bierman CW, Pearlman DS: *Allergic Diseases from Infancy to Adulthood.* 2nd ed. Philadelphia, WB Saunders, 1988, 294–299.

Kaliner M, Slater J: Allergic rhinitis. *In* Gellis SS, Kagan BM (eds): *Current Pediatric Therapy 12.* Philadelphia, WB Saunders, 1986, 628–630.

King J, Ziegler S: The effects of hospitalization on children's behavior: a review of the literature. *Child Health Care* 1981 Summer; 10:20–28.

King K, Hanson V: Psychosocial aspects of juvenile rheumatoid arthritis. *Pediatr Clin North Am,* 1986 Oct; 33(5):1221–1237.

Kirkis EJ, Grier M: *Nurse's Guide to Infection Control Practice.* Philadelphia, WB Saunders, 1988.

Koop CE: Surgeon general report. *Prof Nurs Q* 1987 Fall; 2(3).

Koren GK, MacLeod SM: Difficulty in achieving therapeutic serum concentration of salicylate in Kawasaki disease. *J Pediatr* 1984:105(6):991–995.

Korenblat P, Wedner H: *Allergy Theory and Practice.* Orlando, FL, Grune and Stratton, 1984.

Krause MV, Mahan LK: *Food, Nutrition and Diet Therapy.* 7th ed. Philadelphia, WB Saunders, 1984.

Kruger S, Rawlings P: Pediatric dismissal protocol to aid the transition from hospital to home care. *Image* 1984 Fall; 16(4):120–125.

Lilleyman JS: Haemophilia, blood transfusion, and the AIDS virus. *Arch Dis Child* 1986; 61:105–107.

Lockey RF, Bukantz SC: *Fundamentals of Immunology and Allergy.* Philadelphia, WB Saunders, 1987a.

Lockey RF, Bukantz SC: *Principles of Immunology and Allergy.* Philadelphia, WB Saunders, 1987b.

Loebl S, Spratto GR: *The Nurse's Drug Handbook.* 4th ed. New York, John Wiley & Sons, 1986.

Marion RW, et al: Human T-cell lymphotropic virus type III (HTLV-III) embryopathy. A new dysmorphic syndrome associated with intrauterine HTLV-III infection. *Am J Dis Child,* 1986; 140(7):638–640.

Markowitz M: Rheumatic fever. *In* Behrman RE, Vaughan VC (eds): *Nelson Textbook of Pediatrics.* 12th ed. Philadelphia, WB Saunders, 1983, 588–594.

Marvin JA, et al: Improved treatment of the Stevens-Johnson syndrome. *Arch Surg* 1984 May; 119:601–605.

May C, Block S: A modern clinical approach to food hypersensitivity. *Allergy* 1978; 33:166–188.

McLean DC: Stinging insect allergy. *Immunol Allergy Clin North Am* 1987; 7(2):277–283.

Melish JE: Kawasaki syndrome: a new infectious disease? *J Infect Dis* 1981; 143(3):317–324.

Melish ME: Kawaski syndrome: a 1986 perspective. *Rheum Dis Clin North Am* 1987 Apr; 13(1):7–17.

Menez-Bautista R, et al: Monozygotic twins discordant for the acquired immunodeficiency syndrome. *Am J Dis Child* 1986; 140(7):678–679.

Miller JJ: The social function of young adults who had arthritis in childhood. *J Pediatr* 1982 Mar; 100(3):378–382.

Miller ME: The immune system. *In* Bierman CW, Pearlman DS (eds): *Allergic Diseases from Infancy to Adulthood.* 2nd ed. Philadelphia, WB Saunders, 1988, 1–19.

Miller ML, et al: The immunologic basis of lupus. *Pediatr Clin North Am* 1986 Oct; 33(5):1191–1219.

Mills M, et al: The acquired immunodeficiency syndrome. Infection control and public law. *N Engl J Med* 1986; 314(14):931–936.

Newburger JW, et al: The treatment of Kawasaki syndrome with intravenous gamma globulin. *N Engl J Med* 1986; 315(6):341–347.

Nicol NH: Atopic dermatitis; The (wet) wrap-up. *Am J Nurs* 1987; 87(12):1560–1565.

Olness K, Gardner GG: *Hypnosis and Hypnotherapy with Children.* Philadelphia, Grune & Stratton, 1988.

Paller AS: Allergy and atopic dermatitis. *Immunol Allergy Clin North Am* 1987a Aug; 7(2):255–264.

Paller AS: Allergy in atopic dermatitis. *Primary Care* 1987b Sep; 14(3):491–501.

Parker F: Contact dermatitis. *In* Bierman CW, Pearlman DS (eds): *Allergic Diseases from Infancy to Adulthood.* 2nd ed. Philadelphia, WB Saunders, 1988, 405–414.

Petty RE: Current knowledge of the etiology and pathogenesis of chronic uveitis accompanying juvenile rheumatoid arthritis. *Rheum Dis Clin North Am* 1987; 13(1):19–36.

Public Health Service, Department of Health and Human Services: Immunization of children with HTLV-III/LAV infection. *Prof Nurs Q* 1987 Fall; 2(3).

Recommendations for preventing transmission of infection with human T-lymphotropic virus type III/lymphadenopathy-associated virus during invasive procedures. *Morbid Mortal Weekly Reports* 1986; 35(14):221–223.

Regelmann WE, et al: Immunology of the newborn. *In* Feigin RD, Cherry JD (eds): *Textbook of Pediatric Infectious Diseases.* 2nd ed. Philadelphia, WB Saunders, 1987, 921–939.

Rogers MF, et al: Acquired immunodeficiency syndrome in children: report of the Centers for Disease Control National Surveillance, 1982 to 1985. *Pediatrics* 1987; 79(6):1008–1014.

Rubinstein A: Pediatric AIDS. *Curr Prob Pediatr* 1986; 16(7):367–409.

Rubinstein A, Bernstein L: The epidemiology of pediatric acquired immunodeficiency syndrome. *Clin Immunol Immunopathol* 1986; 40:115–121.

Ruiz-Maldonado R: Acute disseminated epidermal necrosis. Types 1, 2, and 3: study of sixty cases. *J Am Acad Dermatol* 1985 Oct; 13(4):523–535.

Sampson H, Albergo R: Comparison of results of skin tests, RAST, and double blind, placebo controlled food challenges in children with atopic dermatitis. *J Allergy Clin Immunol* 1984; 74:26–33.

Schaller JG, Wedgwood RJ: Juvenile rheumatoid arthritis. *In* Behrman RE, Vaughan VC (eds): *Nelson Textbook of Pediatrics.* 12th ed. Philadelphia, WB Saunders, 1983, 564–574.

Schietinger H: A home care plan for AIDS. *Am J Nurs* 1986; 86(9):1021–1028.

Scull SA, et al: Physical and occupational therapy for children with rheumatic diseases. *Pediatr Clin North Am* 1986 Oct; 33(5):1053–1077.

Shapiro GG: Diagnostic methods for assessing the patient with possible allergic disease. *In* Bierman CW, Pearlman DS: *Allergic Diseases from Infancy to Adulthood.* 2nd ed. Philadelphia, WB Saunders, 1988, 224–238.

Sly M: *Pediatric Allergy.* New York, Medical Examination Publishing Company, 1985.

Stastny P: HLA and the role of T cells in the predisposition to disease. *Rheum Dis Clin North Am* 1987 Apr; 12(1):1–6.

Stutman O: Ontogeny of T cells. *Clin Immunol Allergy* 1985; 5(2):191–234.

Tan EM, et al: The 1982 Revised Criteria for the classification of systemic lupus erythematosus. *Arthritis Rheum* 1982: 25(11):1271–1274.

Understanding AIDS and HIV Infection. Information for Hospitals and Health Professionals. Ontario, Canada, Queen's Printer for Ontario, 1988.

US Public Health Service: *Understanding Aids.* HHS Publication No. (CDC) HHS-88-8404. Rockville, MD, 1988.

Virant FS, et al: Multiple pulmonary complications in a patient with Stevens-Johnson syndrome. *Clin Pediatr* 1984 Jul; 23(7):412–414.

Voyles J, Menendez R: Role of patient compliance in the management of asthma. *J Asthma* 1983; 20:411–418.

Walker J: Childhood gastrointestinal allergy: forbidden fruits. *Nurs Mirror* 1980; 151:32–36.

Wasserman SI: Chemical mediators of inflammation. *In* Bierman CW, Pearlman DS: *Allergic Diseases from Infancy to Adulthood.* 2nd ed. Philadelphia, WB Saunders, 1988, 65–74.

Westley ED, Wechsler HL: Toxic epidermal necrolysis. *Arch Dermatol* 1984 Jun; 120:721–726.

White J, Owsley V: Helping families cope with milk, wheat and soy allergies. *MCN* 1983 Nov/Dec; 8(6):423–428.

Wiener MB, Pepper GA: *Clinical Pharmacology and Therapeutics in Nursing.* 2nd ed. New York, McGraw-Hill, 1985.

Young MC, Geha RS: Ontogeny and control of human IgE synthesis. *Clin Immunol Allergy* 1985; 5(2):339–349.

Yunginger JW: Insect allergy (adults and children). *In* Bierman CW, Pearlman DS: *Allergic Diseases from Infancy to Adulthood.* 2nd ed. Philadelphia, WB Saunders, 1988, 678–683.

Ziegler JB, et al: Postnatal transmission of AIDS-associated retrovirus from mother to infant. *Lancet* 1985; 1:896–897.

Bibliography

AIDS—caring in the community. *Nurs Stand* 1987 Feb 5; 3:482.

American Academy of Pediatrics Committee on Infectious Diseases: Health guidelines for the attendance in day-care and foster care settings of children infected with human immunodeficiency virus. *Pediatrics* 1987 Mar; 79(3):466–471.

Amman AJ, Levy J: Laboratory investigation of pediatric acquired immunodeficiency syndrome. Clinical Immunology and Immunopathology. 1986; 40:122–127.

Arisaka O, et al: Chorea as in initial manifestation of systemic lupus erythematosus. *Clin Pediatr* 1984; 23(5):298–300.

Avery G: *Neonatology.* Philadelphia, JB Lippincott, 1981.

Baum J: Juvenile arthritis. *Am J Dis Child* 1981; 135(6):557–560.

Beales JG, et al: Children with juvenile chronic arthritis: their beliefs about their illness and therapy. *Ann Rheum Dis* 1983; 42:481–486.

Beales JG, et al: The child's perception of the disease and the experience of pain in juvenile chronic arthritis. *J Rheumatol* 1983; 10(1):61–65.

Bell DM, et al: Kawasaki syndrome in the United States. *Am J Dis Child* 1983; 137:211–214.

Beringer TR: Hypercalcemia during resolution of calcinoses in juvenile dermatomyositis. *Br Med J* 1984 May 5; 288:1345.

Berman B, MacDonnell K: *Differential Diagnosis and Treatment of Pediatric Allergy.* Boston, Little, Brown, 1981.

Bleck EE, Nagel DA (eds): *Physically Handicapped Children: A Medical Atlas for Teachers.* 2nd ed. New York, Grune & Stratton, 1982.

Bowler J, et al: Kawasaki syndrome presenting as pyarthrosis of the hip. *J Bone Joint Surg* 1986; 68-A(3):467–468.

Brown ML: AIDS and ethics: concerns and considerations. *Oncol Nurs Forum* 1987; 14(1):69–73.

Calabro JJ, et al: Preventing coronary involvement in Kawasaki disease. *JAMA* 1986 Jan 10; 255(2):200.

Crowe WE, et al: Clinical and pathogenic implications of histopathology in childhood polydermatomyositis. *Arthritis Rheum* 1982 Feb; 25(2):126–139.

Dhanaraj M: Sodium valproate in Sydenham's chorea. *Neurology* 1985 Jan; 35:114–115.

DiSciascio G, Taranta A: Rheumatic fever in children. *Am Heart J* 1980 May; 99(5):635–654.

Dumas R: Lupus nephritis. *Arch Dis Child* 1985; 60:126–128.

FDA finds zidovudine effective against AIDS. *Am J Nurs* 1987 May; 88(5):593–594.

Feigin RD, Barron KS: Treatment of Kawasaki syndrome. *N Engl J Med* 1986 Aug 7; 315(6):388–390.

Fisher P, Shigeoka A: Familial occurrence of SJS. *Am Dis Child* 1983 Sep; 137:914–919.

Fleming J: Common dermatologic conditions in children. *MCN* 1981 Sep/Oct; *Am J* 6(5):346–354.

Gerrard, J: Allergies in breastfed babies to foods ingested by the mother. *Clin Rev Allergy* 1984; 2:143–149.

Glidden RS, et al: Systemic lupus erythematosus in childhood: clinical manifestations and improved survival in fifty-five patients. *Clin Immunol Immunopathol* 1983; 29:196–210.

Hallett M, Kaufman C: Physiological observations in Sydenham's chorea. *J Neurol Neurosurg Psychiatr* 1981; 44:829–832.

Halliburton P: Impaired immunocompetence. *In* Carrieri VK, et al (eds): *Pathophysiological Phenomena in Nursing. Human Responses to Illness.* Philadelphia, WB Saunders, 1986, 319–342.

Hartnett SM: A hospital-wide AIDS education program. *J Cont Educ Nurs* 1987 Mar:Apr; 18(2):64–67.

Haugen MS, Lynch PA: Diagnostic tests in pediatric rheumatology: Application for nurses. *Pediatr Nurs* 1987 Nov-Dec; 13(6):389–393.

Hickling P, et al: *An Outline of Rheumatology.* Bristol, England, John Wright & Sons, 1984.

Hogue EE: Pediatric nurses' obligation to AIDS patients. *Pediatr Nurs* 1988 Jul-Aug; 14(4):339–340.

Horne EM: AIDS: informing patients and clients. *Prof Nurse* 1987 Feb; 2(4):144–146.

Huff JC, et al: Erythema multiforme: a critical review of characteristics, diagnostic criteria and causes. *J Am Acad Dermatol* 1983 Jun; 8(6):763–775.

Infantile polyarteritis nodosa. *Dev Med Child Neurol* 1984; 26:814–821.

Investigational AIDS vaccine. *Am J Nurs* 1987 Dec; 87(12):1540.

Jackson MM, et al: Why not treat all body substances as infectious? *Am J Nurs* 1987 Sep; 87(9):1137–1139.

Jacobs JC: *Pediatric Rheumatology for the Practitioner.* New York, Springer-Verlag, 1982.

Katzin I: New drugs; Hands-on experience. Part 1. *Am J Nurs* 1988 May; 88(5):648–653.

Kinrade LC: Typhlitis: A complication of neutropenia. *Pediatr Nurs* 1988 Jul-Aug; 14(4):291–295.

Klug RM: AIDS beyond the hospital: children with AIDS. *Am J Nurs* 1986 Oct; 86(10):1126–1131.

Koffler D: Systemic lupus erythematosus. *Sci Am* 1980 July.

Koren GK, et al: Kawasaki disease: review of risk factors for coronary aneurysms. *J Pediatr* 1986; 108(3):388–392.

Korkis JA, Stillwater LB: An unusual otolaryngological problem: Mucocutaneous lymph node syndrome (Kawasaki syndrome); case report. *J Otolaryngol* 1985; 14(4):257–260.

Koutras A: Myositis with Kawasaki's disease. *Am J Dis Child* 1982; 136(1):78–79.

Krener PG: Impact of the diagnosis of AIDS on hospital care of an infant. *Clin Pediatr* 1987 Jan; 26(1):30–34.

Kunkel HG: The immunopathology of SLE. *Hosp Pract* 1980 Nov; 47–56.

Lachat MF: An update on acquired immune deficiency syndrome (AIDS): report on the international conference. *Midwifery* 1987 Mar; 3(1):46–50.

Larson E: Kawasaki disease. *West J Med* 1984; 140(6):929–930.

Lillard J, et al: Acquired immunodeficiency syndrome (AIDS) in home care: maximizing helpfulness and minimizing hysteria. *Home Healthcare Nurs* 1984 Nov/Dec; 11–16.

Lindsey AD, Carrieri VK: Stress response. *In* Carrieri VK, et al (eds): *Pathophysiological Phenomena in Nursing. Human Responses to Illness.* Philadelphia, WB Saunders, 1986, 301–318.

Lockshin MD: Systemic lupus erythematosus: problems in management. *Comp Ther* 1982; 8(4):7–10.

L'Orange C: Werner-McCullough M: Kawasaki disease: a new threat to children. *Am J Nurs* 1983; 83(4):558–562.

Marion RW, et al: Fetal AIDS syndrome score: correlation between severity of dysmorphism and age at diagnosis of immunodeficiency. *Am J Dis Child* 1987 Apr; 141:429–431.

Markowitz MM: The decline of rheumatic fever: role of medical intervention. *J Pediatr* 1983; 106(4):545–549.

Miller DS: Intravenous immune globulin for treating primary immunodeficiency diseases. *MCN* 1987 Jul/Aug; 12(4):244–248.

Miller JJ: Juvenile arthritis. *In* Gershwin ME: Musculoskeletal Diseases of Children. New York, Grune & Stratton, 1983.

Nass T: Helping the patient who has lupus. *RN* 1987 Oct: 69–74.

Nausieda PA, et al: Sydenham chorea: an update. *Neurology* 1980 Mar; 30:331–334.

Nordin J: Recurrence of rheumatic fever during prophylaxis with monthly benzathine penicillin G. *Pediatrics* 1984 Apr; 73(4):530–531.

Nursing Grand Rounds: Supporting the mother and infant at risk for AIDS. *Nurs 87* 1987 Nov; 17(11):44–47.

Pachman LM, Maryjowski MC: Juvenile dermatomyositis and polymyositis. *Clin Rheum Dis* 1984 Apr; 10(1).

Pachman LM, et al: Immunogenic studies of juvenile dermatomyositis—III. Study of antibody to organ-specific and nuclear antigens. *Arthritis Rheum* 1985 Feb; 28(2):151–155.

Phillips A: Are blood transfusions really safe? *Nurs 87* 1987; 17(6):63–64.

Pigg JS, et al: *Rheumatology Nursing: A Problem-Oriented Approach.* New York, John Wiley & Sons, 1985.

Pisetsky DS: Systemic lupus erythematosus. *Med Clin North Am* 1986; 70(2):337–353.

Price J: Kawasaki syndrome. *Br Med J* 1984; 288:262–263.

Reckling JB, Neuberger GB: Understanding immune system dysfunction. *Nurs 87* 1987 Sep; 17(9):34–41.

Robinson CA: Systemic lupus erythematosus. *In* Lichtenstein LM, et al: *Current Therapy in Allergy, Immunology, and Rheumatology.* St. Louis, CV Mosby, 1985.

Rodman G, et al (eds): *Primer on the Rheumatic Diseases.* 8th ed. Atlanta, Arthritis Foundation, 1983.

Rosen F: Developmental immunology. *Clin Immunol Allergy* 1985 Jun; 5.

Roth SH, et al: *Rheumatic Therapeutics.* New York, McGraw-Hill, 1985.

Rowe RD, Rose V: Kawasaki disease: Canadian update. *Can Med Assoc J* 1985; 132(1):25–28.

Salyer J, et al: AIDS: holistic home care. *Home Health Nurs* 1987 Mar-Apr; 5(2):10–21.

Second AIDS vaccine approved for testing. *Am J Nurs* 1988 Mar; 88(3):282.

Senter SB: Use of topical steroids in children. *Pediatr Nurs* 1988 Jul-Aug; 14(4):337.

Shulman S, et al: Prevention of rheumatic fever—a statement for health professionals by the committee on rheumatic fever and infective endocarditis of the council on cardiovascular disease in the young. *Circulation* 1984 Dec; 70(6):1118–1121.

Silber TJ, et al: Psychiatric manifestations of systemic lupus erythematosus in children and adolescents. *Clin Pediatr* 1984; 23(6):331–335.

Smith AM: Alternatives in AIDS homecare. *AIDS Patient Care* 1987 Jun; 1(1):28–31.

Stein H, et al: Systemic lupus erythematosus—a medical and social profile. *J Rheumatol* 1986; 13(3):570–576.

Stein MT: Kawasaki syndrome in office pediatrics. *West J Med* 1984; 141(4):519–521.

Thompson LM: Dealing with AIDS and fear: would you accept cookies from an AIDS patient? *South Med J* 1987 Feb; 80(2):228–232.

Tibulski JA: The true odds of getting AIDS from a patient. *RN* 1988 May; 64–70.

Trumble T, Fitch RD: Kawasaki disease—a cause of vasculitis in children. *J Pediatr Orthop* 1986; 6(1):92–95.

Walton J: The inflammatory myopathies. *J Roy Soc Med* 1983 Dec; 76:998–1010.

White JF: Teaching patients to manage systemic lupus erythematosus. *Nurs 78* 1978; 8(9):27–34.

Wickinson VA: Juvenile chronic arthritis in adolescence: facing the reality. *Int Rehab Med* 1981; 3(1):11–17.

Winkel MF: Juvenile rheumatoid arthritis—Parent support group: Do parents perceive a need? *Pediatr Nurs* 1988 Mar/Apr; 14(2):131–132.

Yanagihara R, Todd JK: Acute febrile mucocutaneous lymph node syndrome. *Am J Dis Child* 1980; 134:603–612.

Ziegler GC: Systemic lupus erythematosus and systemic sclerosis. *Nurs Clin North Am* 1984; 19(4):673–695.

Nursing Strategies: Altered Skin Integrity

Chapter 44

Roxie L. Foster

Related Topics

Newborn acne, Chapter 4
Birthmarks, Chapter 4
Immune response, Chapter 43
Contact dermatitis, Chapter 43
Atopic dermatitis (Eczema), Chapter 43
Poison ivy, Chapter 43, Chapter 52
Thrush, Chapter 45
Measles, chickenpox, Chapter 45
Burns, Chapter 52
Frostbite, sunburn, topical exposure to poisons, Chapter 52
Cuts, scrapes, punctures, lacerations, Table 52-12
Prevention, identification, and management of stings and bites, Table 52-13

The skin is often underrated for its service to the body. "Skin" may bring to mind the softness of a baby's hand, the rosiness of a preschooler's cheek, or the emotional upset caused by a teenage blemish. Less often are the skin and mucous membranes credited for their vital function as *the body's primary physical barrier* against a rather inhospitable environment. As Lookingbill and Marks (1986) observed, it is the integumentary system which keeps *us* within and the world without.

This chapter discusses the structure and function of the skin, including developmental differences for infants and children; factors that affect the skin's ability to protect the body; assessment and identification of primary skin lesions, principles of topical therapy, and the impact of integumentary disorders on children and families. Skin disorders covered in this chapter include certain dermatitis conditions, bacterial and viral skin infections, and acne.

The Structure and Function of the Skin

The skin serves several important functions (Table 44-1). The epidermis provides a barrier against physical injury, light, and infectious organisms. The dermal layer supplies a support structure for body tissues. The skin facilitates temperature regulation, provides for touch sensation, insulates from cold and trauma, and serves as a calorie reservoir. In addition the skin is important to one's appearance. Skin disorders in childhood and adolescence can greatly influence the development of self-concept.

Table 44-1. Skin Functions

Function	Responsible Structure
Barrier	Epidermis
Physical	Stratum corneum
Light	Melanocytes
Immunologic	Langerhans cells
Tough, flexible foundation	Dermis
Temperature regulation	Blood vessels Eccrine sweat glands
Sensation	Nerves
Grasp	Nails
Decorative	Hair
Unknown	Sebaceous glands
Insulation from cold and trauma	Subcutaneous fat
Calorie reservoir	Subcutaneous fat

(From Lookingbill and Marks, 1986.)

The Epidermis

The epidermis is composed of four layers—stratum corneum, stratum granulosum, stratum spinosum, and the basal cell layer (Fig. 44-1). Together these layers provide the physical protective barrier for the body.

Stratum Corneum

The stratum corneum is the outermost layer of skin. It is composed of dead skin cells that are tightly joined to form an almost impenetrable barrier against microorganisms. The stratum corneum tends to be somewhat dry and the dead cells "shed" during bathing and rubbing of the skin. A continual supply of cells is needed to replace those that are sloughed. The other three layers of the epidermis are the source for those cells.

Basal Cell Layer

Epidermal cells originate as basal cells. Here they divide and begin to migrate upward through the layers of epidermal tissue. *Melanocytes* are found within the basal cell layer. They produce the pigment that provides skin color. Skin pigment helps to protect the body from ultraviolet rays of the sun. Thus, persons with darker skin (more pigment) are less likely to sustain skin damage that results in sunburn or skin cancer. Skin tanning occurs because exposure to sunlight stimulates the melanocytes to produce more pigment and to disperse it more widely.

Stratum Spinosum

By the time the basal cells reach the stratum spinosum they have differentiated into keratinocytes, cells that produce the fibrous keratin that is a major component of the stratum corneum. Within this layer are the *Langerhans* cells, skin macrophages that mount a phagocytic response to microorganisms that manage to penetrate the stratum corneum. The importance of these

We appreciate the contributions of Jo Joyce Anderson and Noreen Heer Nicol in preparation of this chapter.

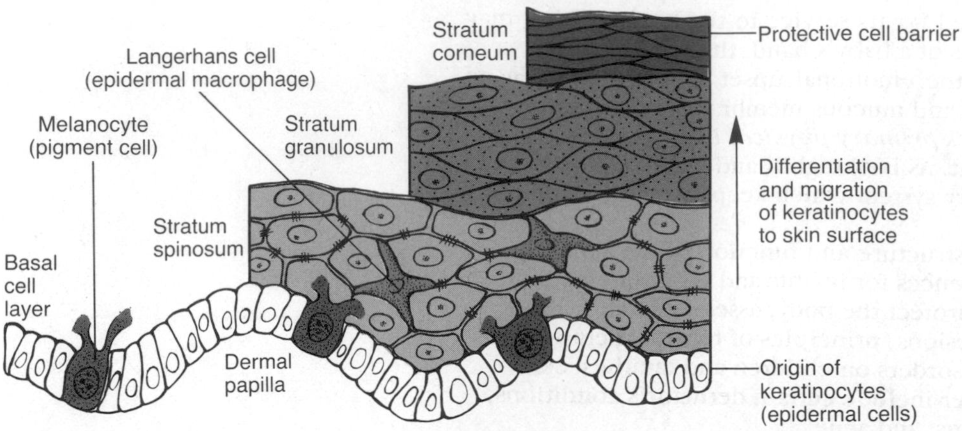

Figure 44-1. Structure of the epidermis.

macrophages and the normal skin flora (nonpathogenic microorganisms that discourage pathogenic invasion) has been given increasing recognition in recent years and is now designated the skin-associated lymphoid tissue (SALT) (see Chapter 43 for further discussion).

Stratum Granulosum

Within this layer the differentiation of epidermal cells is completed. The cells are degraded by enzymes and pushed upward to form the stratum corneum, the top layer of skin.

The Dermis

The dermis underlies the epidermis and provides a tough, elastic support structure for body tissues (Fig. 44-2). The dermis contains connective tissue, elastic fibers, and a ground substance that facilitates movement of fluids and inflammatory cells. Nerves and blood vessels in the dermis have protective functions. The nerves provide the protective sensations of touch, temperature, and pain. The blood vessels help to regulate temperature. Increased blood flow to the skin (the flush of fever) helps to cool the body, whereas diminished blood flow helps to decrease heat loss (the pallor associated with being cold). The blood vessels supply both the dermis tissue and the nonvascular epidermis with nutrients and oxygen.

Subcutaneous Fat

The layer of fat below the dermis has achieved so much infamy for its "pinch-an-inch" characteristics that its protective functions often go unheralded. This layer helps to insulate the body from cold (as witnessed by the decreased thermoregulatory ability of the premature infant and the neonate who have not yet formed a functional fat layer and of the elderly person who has lost much of this layer). In addition the subcutaneous fat provides a cushion that absorbs trauma. It also serves as a calorie reserve for the body.

Skin Appendages

Skin appendages include nails, hair, sebaceous glands, and sweat glands. Except for the nails, all of these are located in the dermis.

Nails, Hair and Sebaceous Glands

Nails and hair are made of keratin. The pink color of the nail is due to the highly vascular dermis underneath. That is why depressing the nail (blanching) and

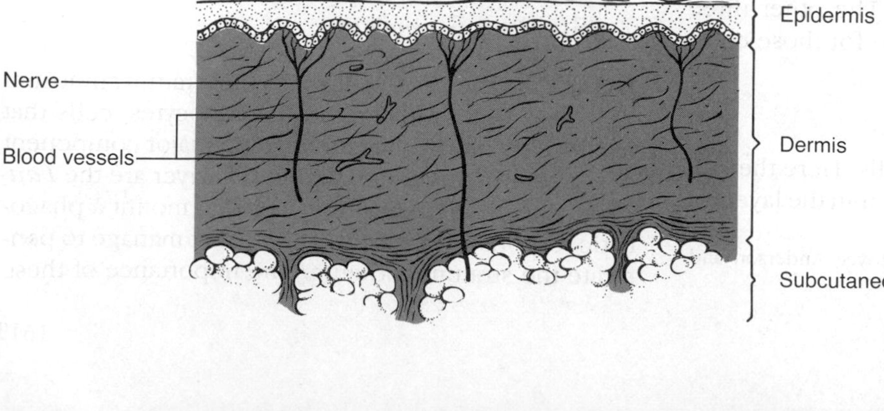

Figure 44-2. Structure of the dermis. (From Lookingbill DP, Marks JG: *Principles of Dermatology.* Philadelphia, WB Saunders, 1986, p 5.)

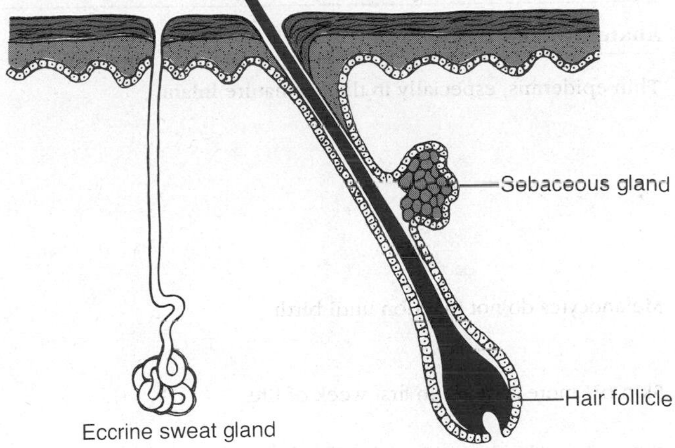

Figure 44-3. Normal hair follicle, sebaceous gland, and eccrine sweat gland. (From Lookingbill DP, Marks JG: *Principles of Dermatology.* Philadelphia, WB Saunders, 1986, p 6.)

awaiting return of color is an indication of peripheral circulation.

Hair grows from a hair follicle in the dermis and receives its color from melanocytes in the bottom of the hair follicle (Fig. 44-3). The fine hair of the neonate is replaced by coarser and sometimes more darkly pigmented hair as the child grows. Genital hair growth is stimulated by hormones and does not develop until puberty.

Sebaceous glands are attached to hair follicles. They secrete their oily, fatty product, sebum, into the hair follicle, from which it progresses to the epidermal surface. Sebaceous glands are located everywhere except on the palms, soles, and dorsa of the feet and perhaps on the lower lip. The highest concentrations, however, are on the face, chest, and back, as evidenced by the skin areas prone to acne (Hurwitz, 1981).

Sweat Glands

Eccrine sweat glands are distributed over the entire body and fulfill a thermoregulatory function by producing sweat, which helps to cool the body as it evaporates from the skin surface. Eccrine glands are stimulated by heat, exertion, nausea, fever, and certain drugs (e.g., alcohol, pilocarpine) (Kahn, 1988).

Apocrine sweat glands appear to have no useful function. Although apocrine sweat is odorless when first secreted, the action of body bacteria produces body odor. These glands are located in the axilla and anogenital region and are stimulated primarily by emotional factors.

Developmental Differences in Structure and Function

Like most of the body systems, the integumentary system is not mature at birth. Therefore, it is not as effective a barrier to physical elements or microorganisms at birth and in infancy as it is later in childhood (Table 44-2). These limitations in skin protection make infants and young children more prone to infection.

Factors that Affect the Skin's Protective Function

Skin function is affected by genetic inheritance and hormonal factors and by cleanliness, hydration, and nutrition.

Genetic Factors

Skin cells are affected by their genetic blueprint just as other body cells are. Alterations in skin integrity that are thought to be genetically inherited include albinism (a defect in pigment production), neurofibromatosis (which results in multiple café-au-lait spots), atopic dermatitis (which predisposes the skin to persistent dryness and pruritus), and psoriasis (which manifests as scaling plaques).

Hormonal Factors

Skin is affected by both increased and decreased hormone production. The classic example of hormone-induced skin problems is acne, which may result from pubertal androgens. Increased glucocorticoids also can cause acne, along with hirsutism, atrophy, purpura, and moon facies. Decreased secretion of glucocorticoids (Addison's disease) leads to hyperpigmentation of the skin. Hyperthyroidism results in a warm, moist skin while hyposecretion of the thyroid gland causes the skin to be dry and cool. Effects of hormone secretion on the skin are further discussed in Chapter 49.

Table 44-2. Developmental Differences in Structure and Function of the Skin

Anatomy and Physiology	Significance
Thin epidermis, especially in the premature infant	Absorption through the skin is dramatically increased. Most compounds placed on the skin of premature infants can be found in the urine and saliva in a matter of minutes. No topical ointments or other skin preparations should be used without a physician's order. The thin epidermis is fragile and requires careful handling The thin epidermis blisters easily. The younger the child the more easily the skin will blister. This characteristic makes it more difficult to assess the trauma that caused blistering
Melanocytes do not function until birth	Soon after birth skin pigmentation changes with darkening first in the nipples, face, and genitalia. This is the reason for a light complexion in a black neonate
Skin pH more alkaline in first week of life	A more acidic skin surface discourages microorganisms. The neonate is therefore more susceptible to infection
IgA secreted by the epithelial cells of mucous membranes does not reach adult levels until age 2–5 (Vogler and Lawton, 1985)	Diminished ability to produce these antibodies reduces the mucosal resistance to organisms. Objects "mouthed" by infants need to be cleaned frequently, and young children should be taught good handwashing as early as possible since their hands are often in contact with their mouths, noses, and other vulnerable surfaces
Sebaceous glands well developed at birth owing to stimulation by maternal hormones; become inactive after birth and do not begin producing the oily "sebum" secretion until age 8–10. Continue to develop throughout adolescence	Newborn "acne" may result from androgen stimulation of sebaceous glands in utero. Evaporation of sebum helps to lower skin pH, thus increasing skin resistance to infection in later childhood. Teenage acne is related to function of the sebaceous glands. Without lubrication by sebum the skin is more prone to dryness and chapping, making hydration precautions important in infancy and early childhood
Eccrine glands begin to function at 2–5 days of life and reach mature function by 2–3 years of age	The ability to perspire freely, gives the toddler and older child better thermoregulatory function than is possessed by the infant. The evaporation of eccrine sweat lowers skin pH and thus increases resistance to microorganisms
Apocrine glands become functional at age 8–10	Because axillary sweating begins a few years before puberty its appearance can be a sign of normal progress toward the pubertal stage
Premature and newborn infants possess limited subcutaneous fat	They are more sensitive to changes in environmental temperature because they are less well "insulated" than older infants and children. The lack of subcutaneous fat provides better conduction, however, when monitoring transcutaneous oxygen

(Based on Kahn, 1988.)

Cleanliness and Hydration

Skin that is clean and well hydrated is less prone to breaks in its integrity. Dirt and body secretions (e.g., urine and feces) not only have the potential to cause skin irritation, but also may "seal" microorganisms against the skin, thus prolonging their contact and increasing the chance for penetration of the stratum corneum.

Skin must be well hydrated, however, as well as clean. Dry skin is prone to irritation and cracking. If soap is used it should be a mild preparation such as Keri, Purpose, Neutrogena, Oilatum, or Dove. Among the harshest soaps are Ivory, Lowila, Zest, and Irish Spring (Kahn, 1988).

Baths can actually help to hydrate dry skin if the skin pores are allowed time to absorb the water (15 to 20 minutes) and are then quickly sealed against evaporation. Skin (preferably still damp) should be sealed after the bath with an occlusive application such as petrolatum ointment or a good moisturizing cream or lotion (Nicol, 1987).

Nutritional Factors

The skin is a rapidly dividing tissue, and therefore has a high demand for nutrients (Table 44-3). Vitamins A and C are particularly important to healthy skin. Vitamin A regulates the process of keratinization (differentiation and migration of epidermal cells toward the surface). Vitamin A deficiency leads to skin dryness and scaling. Vitamin C is necessary for normal development of connective tissue within the dermis. Vitamin C deficiency delays wound healing (scar tissue is primarily connective tissue), and leads to skin fragility and easy bleeding (Lookingbill and Marks, 1986).

Table 44-3. Nutritional Factors in Skin Integrity

Deficiency	Cutaneous Manifestations
Vitamin A	Dry eyes—corneal scarring Generalized scaling with hyperkeratosis
Vitamin B	
Niacin (pellagra)	Dermatitis in sun-exposed areas
Biotin*	Dermatitis with desquamation Alopecia
Vitamin C (scurvy)	Impaired wound healing Perifollicular purpura Red, swollen, bleeding gums
Zinc*	Seborrheic dermatitis-like rash Alopecia
Amino acids (glucagonoma)	Glossitis Dermatitis with superficial epidermal necrosis
Essential fatty acids*	Scaling rash starting in flexural folds—then generalized Alopecia

* Has been associated with total parenteral nutrition.
(From Lookingbill and Marks, 1986.)

Emotional Factors

Emotions also affect the skin. Emotions stimulate itching, flushing, and sweating, and stress can exacerbate acne, possibly through the increased glucocorticoids associated with the stress response.

Skin as a Mirror of Health

Skin is often a mirror of one's health and one's lifestyle. Skin characteristics change with circulation and oxygenation (e.g., cyanosis), with altered excretion of body wastes (e.g., jaundice), with fatigue (e.g., circles under the eyes), with nutrition (e.g., scaling), with hydration (e.g., loss of turgor, maceration), with changes in environmental temperature (flushing, pallor, goose flesh), with response to antigens (e.g., hives), with hormonal cycles (e.g., blemishes with menstruation), with emotions (e.g., blushing, sweating, itching), with caloric intake (e.g., amount of subcutaneous fat), and with the loss of collagen in aging. Since these and so many other physiologic and psychologic processes are "written" on the skin, it is little wonder that the skin is so important to diagnostic assessment.

Skin assessment is included throughout the chapters of this unit as it relates to assessment of the various body systems. In the following section skin assessment is discussed as it relates to alteration of the integument itself.

Diagnostic Assessment of Skin Lesions

History

The nurse is often the one who first recognizes signs of skin breakdown or to whom parents and teachers bring their concerns about a child. Therefore, the nurse's assessment skills in identifying and differentiating various skin lesions and in associating them with other symptoms are important to proper management of these conditions. Recognition is as much dependent on a thorough history as it is on assessment of physical factors. A history should cover three areas: (1) local, systemic, or prodromal symptoms, (2) exposure to causative agents, and (3) risk factors (Box 44-1).

Symptomatic History. The nurse will want to determine (1) where the skin lesions started, (2) whether they have changed in appearance since the onset, (3) whether they "bother" the child (i.e., burn or itch), (4) whether there are systemic signs or symptoms, (5) what home remedies and over-the-counter medications have been tried, and (6) what makes the condition better or worse.

Many infectious diseases of childhood have a prodromal phase of systemic symptoms that precedes the skin lesions. Of particular significance are any symptoms reported within the past 7 to 10 days. Common manifestations involve enlarged lymph nodes, respira-

Box 44-1
Considerations in Obtaining a History of the Integumentary System

SYMPTOMATIC HISTORY

- Time of onset and changes in lesions
- Whether lesions itch or burn
- Systemic signs and symptoms
- Home treatment
- What makes conditon better or worse
- Prodromal symptoms in the last 7 to 10 days

HISTORY OF EXPOSURE IN THE LAST MONTH

- Environmental irritants
- Infectious organisms
- Local epidemic or pandemic disease patterns

RISK FACTORS

- Immunization status
- History of infectious disease
- Immunosuppressive and other drugs
- Genetic predisposition
- Family lifestyle

tory complaints (e.g., sniffling, nasal stuffiness), fever, anorexia, malaise, or various neurologic complaints. Prodromal symptoms are often near resolution by the time the nurse has contact with the child, making the nurse dependent on the child's or parent's recall of the symptoms and their onset. See Chapter 45 for a further discussion of childhood infectious diseases.

Exposure History. The child and parent(s) should be questioned regarding exposure within the past month to environmental irritants or infectious organisms that might cause integumentary diseases. Inquiry should be made as to recent changes in environment, recent exposure to a crowd or large numbers of people, or recent illness of family members, playmates, or others with whom the child has regular contact. The nurse should also be familiar with any epidemic (regional outbreak) or pandemic (widely spread) disease patterns in the locale, particularly within the schools.

Risk Factors. Because many of the integumentary disorders are preventable with immunizations, knowledge of the child's immunization status is imperative to a thorough assessment. Ask whether the child has had any of the childhood infectious diseases involving the skin (e.g., measles, chickenpox).

Medications that the child is taking or has just finished should be noted. Sensitivity to antibiotics and other drugs may result in a rash. Children who are taking immunosuppressive drugs (e.g., Imuran, prednisone) as the result of organ transplant or a malignancy are at increased risk for infection because of diminished immune response to microorganisms.

A family history is pertinent to determine genetic predisposition to skin disorders. Atopic dermatitis, for example, is more common in the child whose parents have a history of allergies. In addition, aspects of the family's lifestyle and living environment should be explored for the potential of various parasitic conditions. Questions should include whether the family has recently visited another country and whether children routinely walk barefoot outside. Chapter 45 presents further information on parasitic infections.

Physical Assessment

Inspection and palpation are the primary assessment techniques for skin disorders. The child should be clothed in an examination gown to provide visual access to all areas of the skin. The diaper should be removed when that area of the body is examined. Be sure to observe the privacy of the child who has begun to develop modesty (some preschoolers and all school-age children). Mucous membranes, scalp, hair, and nails should be included in inspection of the integumentary system (see Chapter 15). Adequate lighting is necessary.

Lesions should be described according to (1) exact placement, (2) number and distribution (i.e., whether discrete or *confluent,* running together), (3) shape, (4) size in centimeters, (5) color, (6) elevation, (7) texture (soft, hard), (8) tenderness, and (9) odor. Figure 44-4 gives examples of common skin lesions.

Laboratory and Diagnostic Tests

Microscopic examinations, cultures, biopsy, and patch tests may be helpful in diagnosing skin disorders. Skin scrapings, exudate from vesicles and pustules, and even mites can be examined microscopically to identify causative bacteria and viruses, or, in the case of mites, to confirm the suspicions of the naked eye. Cultures can be done with skin scales, exudate from vesicles or pustules, or tissue obtained from a deep punch biopsy. Bacteria and fungi can be identified by culture. Skin biopsies are also examined under an electron microscope to determine the origin of cells.

When collecting an exudate specimen for culture, obtain material from an intact vesicle or pustule whenever possible. The exudate within an intact lesion will contain the highest concentration of organisms. The top of the lesion can be carefully removed with a sterile scalpel and a swab inserted to obtain exudate. If there are no intact lesions, carefully remove crusted exudate (by soaking and gentle debridement) to obtain the liquid material underneath.

Immunofluorescence tests of biopsied tissue or of serum can identify the type of antibodies being produced in response to the microorganism. Patch testing is used to determine antigens producing a delayed (type IV) allergic response. (See Chapter 43, page 1568, for further information about the type IV response.) Antigenic test materials are placed on the upper back or forearm under occlusive patches and removed 48 hours later. The sites are then assessed for local inflammation at 48, 72, and 96 hours and sometimes again 1 week after patch removal.

Upon diagnosis of the type of skin disorder and its cause, therapeutic management is instituted. Often treatment will be carried out at home and success of the therapy may depend upon the nurse's skill in teaching the child and family the rationale and techniques of the prescribed regimen.

Therapeutic Management: Principles of Topical Therapy

Management of many skin disorders will involve symptomatic treatment of pruritic, scaling, weeping, and/or crusting lesions. Topical medications and soothing baths or soaks are often prescribed. The child and family will need to know (1) how the skin lesions

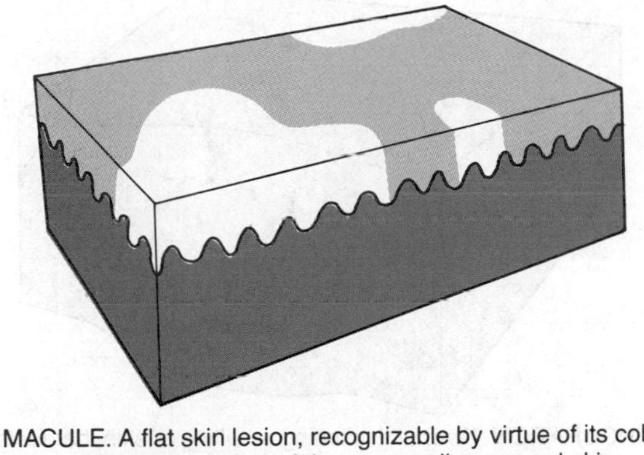

MACULE. A flat skin lesion, recognizable by virtue of its color being different from that of the surrounding normal skin. The most common color changes are white (hypopigmented), brown (hyperpigmented), and red (erythematous and purpuric). *Example:* Measles

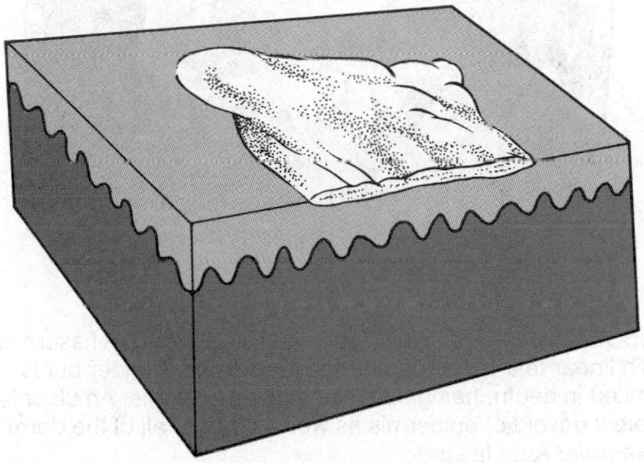

PATCH. A macule with some surface change—either color or texture. *Examples:* Café-au-lait spot, Mongolian spot

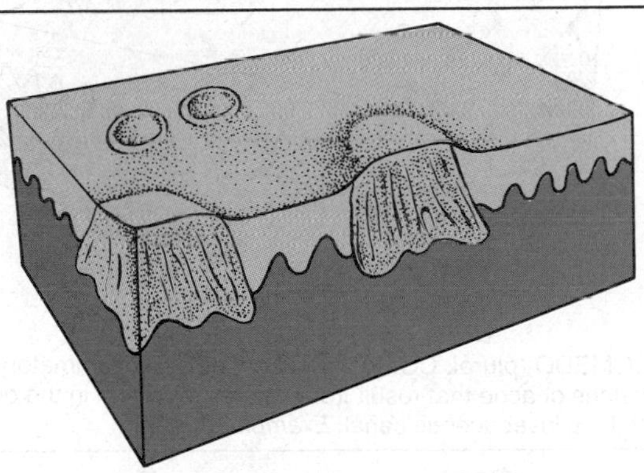

PAPULE. A small, elevated skin lesion, less than 0.5 cm in diameter. *Example:* Diaper dermatitis from *Candida albicans*

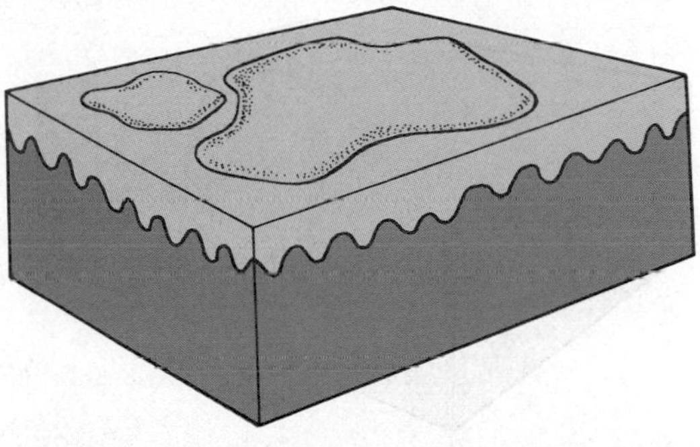

PLAQUE. An elevated, "plateau-like" lesion greater than 0.5 cm in diameter but without substantial depth. *Example:* Psoriasis

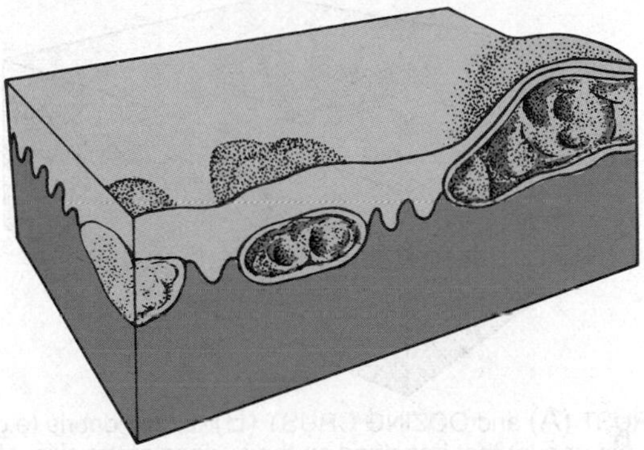

NODULE. An elevated "marble-like" lesion greater than 0.5 cm in both width and depth. *Example:* Subcutaneous nodules of juvenile arthritis

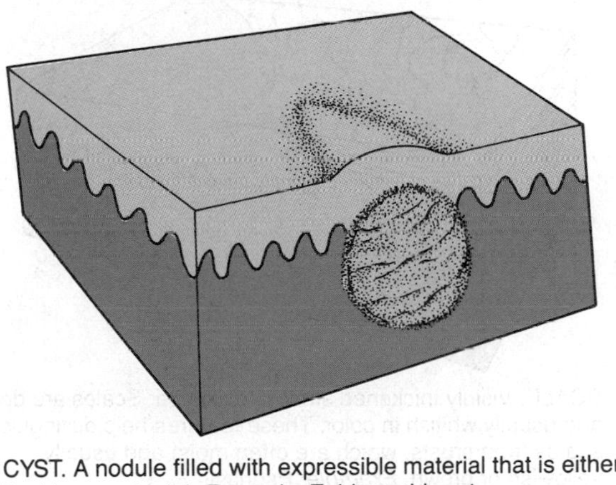

CYST. A nodule filled with expressible material that is either liquid or semisolid. *Example:* Epidermoid cyst

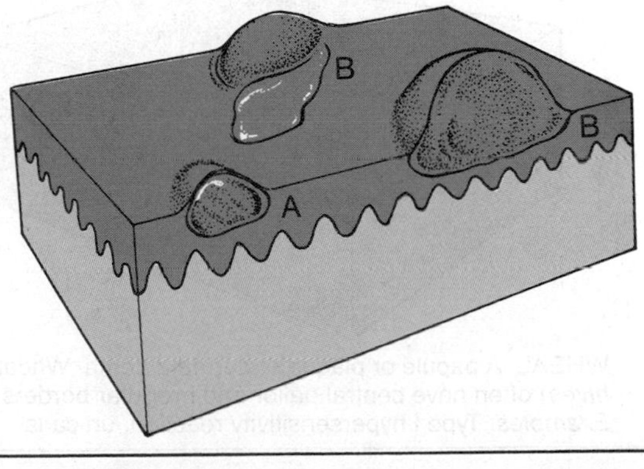

VESICLES (A) and BULLAE (B). Blisters filled with clear fluid. Vesicles are less than, and bullae greater than, 0.5 cm in diameter. *Examples:* Second degree burn, chickenpox, herpes simplex

Figure 44-4.

Illustration continued on following page

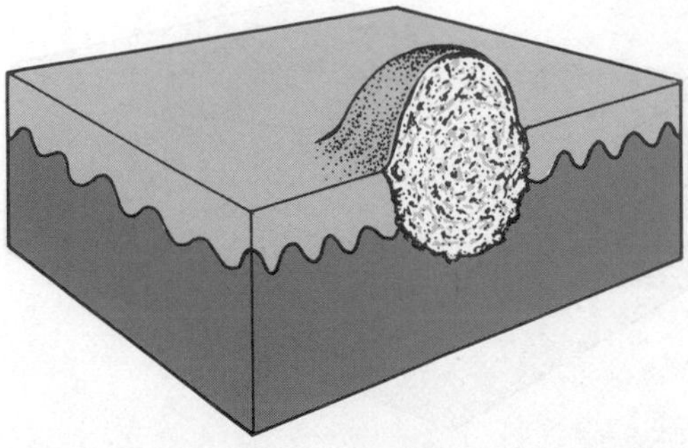

PUSTULE. A vesicle filled with cloudy or purulent fluid. *Examples:* Infectious lesion of atopic dermatitis, acne

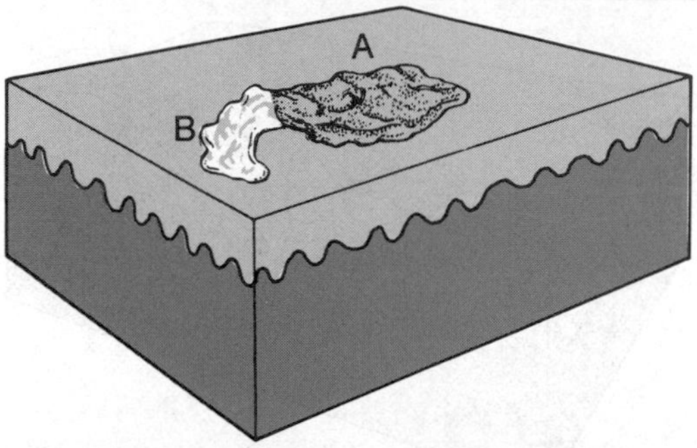

CRUST (A) and OOZING CRUST (B). Liquid debris (e.g., serum or pus) that has dried on the surface of the skin. Most frequently crusts result from breakage of vesicles, pustules, or bullae. *Examples:* Impetigo, atopic dermatitis

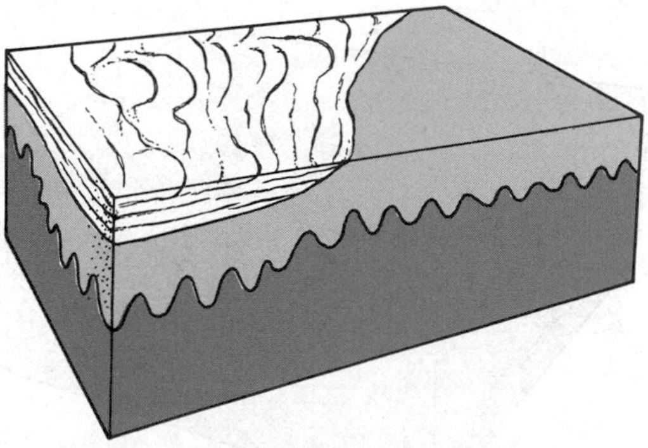

SCALE. Visibly thickened stratum corneum. Scales are dry and usually whitish in color. These features help distinguish scales from crusts, which are often moist and usually yellowish or brown. *Example:* Psoriasis

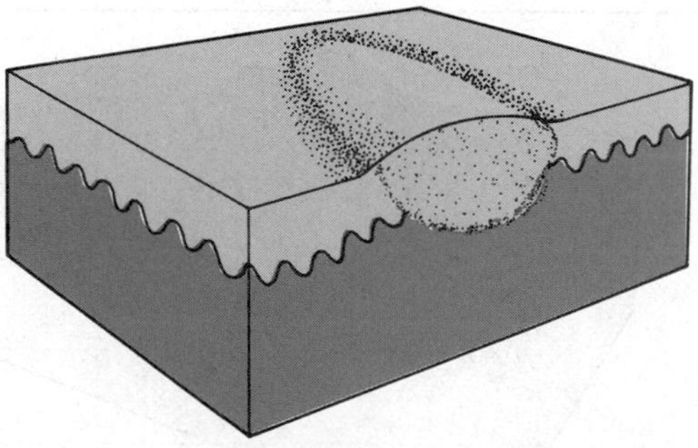

WHEAL. A papule or plaque of dermal edema. Wheals (or *hives*) often have central pallor and irregular borders. *Examples:* Type I hypersensitivity reaction, urticaria

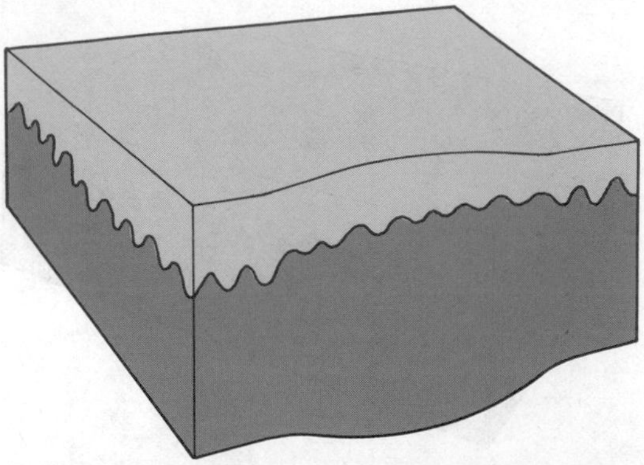

INDURATION. Dermal thickening resulting in skin that *feels* thicker and firmer than normal. *Example:* Poorly approximated edges of an inflamed wound

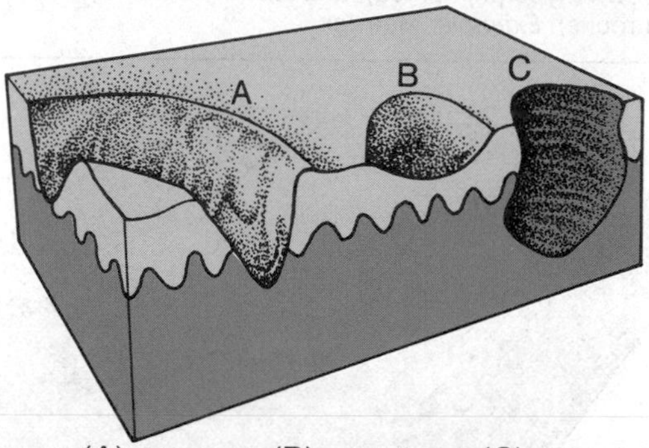

FISSURE (A), EROSION (B), and ULCER (C). A fissure is a thin linear tear in the epidermis. An erosion is wider but is limited in depth, being confined to the epidermis. An ulcer is a defect devoid of epidermis as well as part or all of the dermis. *Example:* Anal fissure

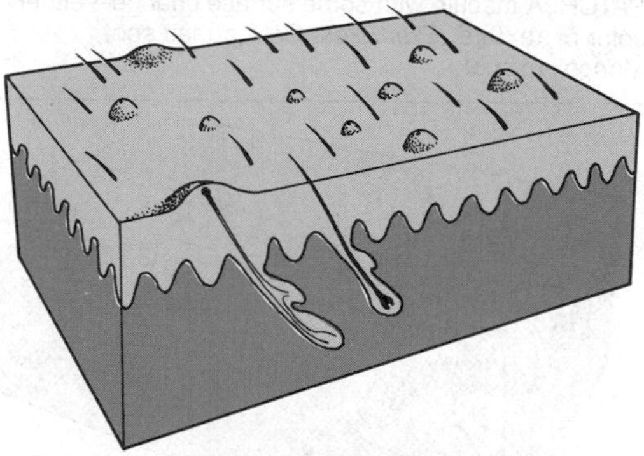

COMEDO (plural, COMEDONES). The noninflammatory lesions of acne that result from keratin impaction in the outlet of the pilosebaceous canal. *Example:* Acne

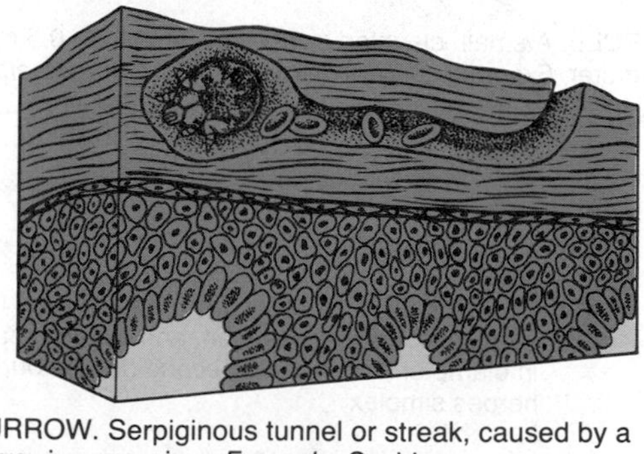

BURROW. Serpiginous tunnel or streak, caused by a burrowing organism. *Example:* Scabies

Figure 44-4 *Continued*

Table 44-4. Properties of Topical Preparations

Preparation	Properties	Nursing Implications
Cream (e.g., Eucerin, Unibase, Plastibase, Polysorb, Hydrosorb, Keri, Lubriderm)	Water-based, semisolid emulsion of *oil in water;* white, non-greasy	Not occlusive; rubs completely into skin. Can be made into a lotion by adding water. Contains several preservatives to prevent the compound from becoming rancid; may rarely cause allergic reaction. For use on oily, moist, opposing skin surfaces and on weeping eruptions
Ointment (e.g., Petrolatum, Aquaphor, lard, Crisco, Albolene)	Oil-based emulsion of *water in oil;* clear, greasy	The most occlusive vehicle for medication; does not easily rub off or wash off. Petrolatum considered by some to be the standard ointment of dermatologic therapy; inexpensive and hypoallergenic. Ointments often used on dry and lichenified skin when absorption otherwise limited
Lotion (e.g., Calamine)	Suspension of powder in water	More drying than creams and ointments. Relieves itching by cooling effect as water evaporates; leaves protective powder on skin. Shake before using to suspend powder evenly in the liquid. Often effective on scalp lesions
Tincture, aerosol spray	Suspension of active ingredient in alcohol	Alcohol evaporates, cooling skin, reducing itching, and leaving active ingredient on skin. Sprays are especially useful for hairy areas
Gel	Transparent, colorless, semisolid emulsion	Nonocclusive; liquefies when applied to skin. May be used in place of cream

(Based on Lookingbill and Marks, 1986.)

will change as they heal (e.g., from vesicles to oozing lesions to crusts and finally to clear skin), (2) signs of secondary infection (increased erythema, pustules, fever, malaise), (3) how to apply topical medication, and (4) how to decrease itching and discomfort.

The absorption of topical medication is affected by the quality of the skin on which it is placed and by the vehicle in which the medication is suspended (e.g., cream, ointment). The barrier capacity of the stratum corneum is lowest in warm, moist skin, so absorption is

Table 44-5. Therapeutic Use of Dressings and Baths

Treatment	Nursing Implications
Nonadherent (Dry) Dressing (e.g., petroleum gauze, semipermeable plastic membrane)	Used to prevent disruption of new tissue. Should not stick to wound when removed. Preserves skin moisture, which enhances healing
Adherent (Dry) Dressing (e.g., absorbent gauze-type dressing, fine mesh gauze)	Used to debride moist wounds. When removed, dressing pulls off dead tissue and dried secretions, which adhere to it. Fine mesh gauze often used to prevent cotton fibers sticking to lesions. Removal is painful; check with the physician to see if dressings may be soaked to ease removal. Prepare the child by administering analgesia, and allow the child as much control as possible during dressing changes (to decrease feelings of anxiety, helplessness, hopelessness); e.g., allow child to pull off old dressings, apply new tape
Wet to Dry Dressings (e.g., gauze [usually fine mesh] soaked in saline, water or an antiseptic solution, covered by dry gauze dressings/pads)	Used to debride crusts, dead tissue. Allow to dry, then remove (see debridement comments under adherent dressings)
Wet Dressings (e.g., gauze, cotton-filled pads or towels soaked and kept wet with water, astringent such as Burows solution, or antimicrobial solution such as povidone iodine	Used to treat acute inflammation. They soothe, cool, and dry skin by evaporation. Help to remove crusts and exudate. Towels, wash cloths, or wet clothing can be just as effective as expensive gauze material. Cover with dry clothing to prevent chilling. Skin may become macerated if plastic wrapping is used to keep soaks wet. Plastic wrap also a safety hazard for young child. Tubular bandage retainer (Surginet, Spandage) can secure soaks even to the face if holes are cut for the eyes, nose, and mouth (Nicol, 1987). Soaks are often best tolerated by the young child during naptime. Child can be rocked or otherwise lulled to sleep as the soaks begin to provide comfort; child may then associate treatment with comfort rather than the frustration of immobility and "wet towels"
Therapeutic Baths Tar emulsions, colloidal oatmeal, baking soda	Used for acute eruptions that crust and weep. Soothe, clean, relax, decrease itching

(Based on Lookingbill and Marks, 1986, and on Kahn, 1988.)

usually best when a cream or ointment is applied after a bath. Occlusive vehicles (e.g., petrolatum) generally deliver the highest concentration of medication because they increase local skin temperature and resist being rubbed from the skin. Table 44-4 details the properties of common topical preparations. Table 44-5 describes the use of dressings and therapeutic baths.

Noninfectious Skin Disorders of Childhood

Diaper Dermatitis

Contact dermatitis is an inflammatory skin reaction either to allergens (Chapter 43) or to external irritants. Diaper dermatitis (diaper rash) is the most common form of nonallergic, irritant contact dermatitis in infancy. The irritation in diaper rash is usually from urine ammonia but may also be caused by inadequate cleansing of the diaper area, by acidic urine, or by residual antiseptics, soaps, or detergents in the diapers. Diaper rash tends to exacerbate with heat, moisture, friction, and tight clothing (Sternbach and Callen, 1985).

Clinical Manifestations

Diaper rashes involve inflammatory response in areas normally covered by a diaper (Fig. 44-5, 44-6). They are extremely common in infants and untrained toddlers. Intertrigo, a dermatitis that develops in skin-

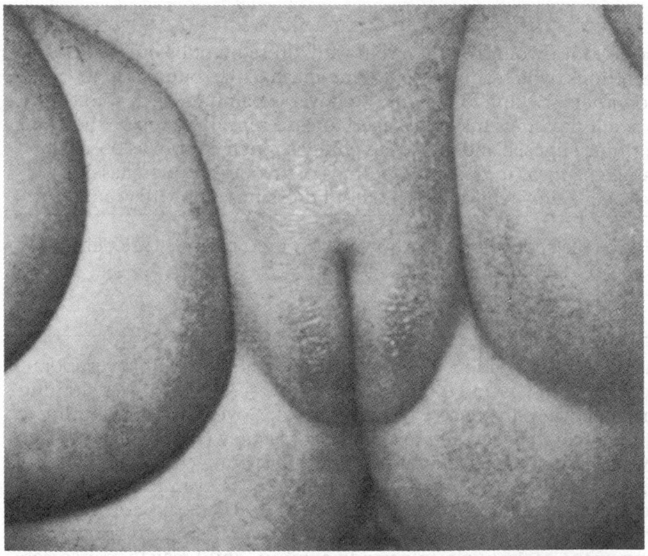

Figure 44-5. Primary irritant contact dermatitis (ammoniacal). Note involvement of convex surfaces but not the folds. (From Jacobs AH: Eruptions in the diaper area. *Pediatr Clin North Am* 1975 May; 212.)

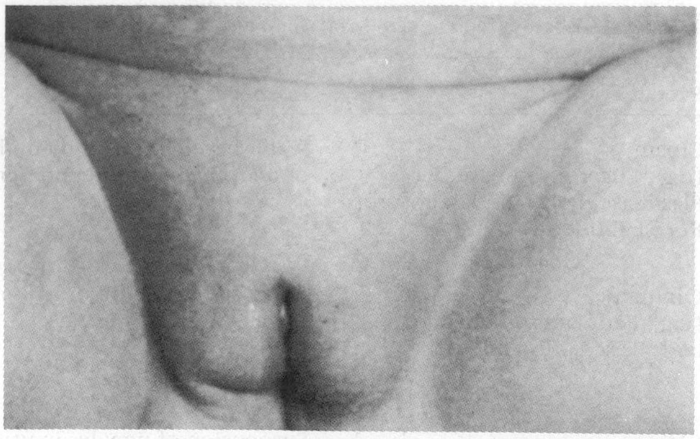

Figure 44-6. Early intertrigo. Note the erythema in the folds with sparing of the convex surfaces. (From Jacobs AH: Eruptions in the diaper area. *Pediatr Clin North Am* 1975 May; 213.)

folds, is also fairly common in toddler and preschool girls who forget to wipe after voiding or who do so inadequately. Table 44-6 describes the most frequent diaper eruptions, their characteristic appearance, and specific treatments. Diagnosis is readily made by inspection of the rash characteristics and the area involved.

Major Nursing Diagnoses for Diaper Dermatitis

Impaired skin integrity: inflammation and rash, *related to irritation of the diaper area by*
- *Urea and ammonia salts*
- *Feces*
- *Detergent left in cloth diapers*

Knowledge deficit (caregiver), *related to*
- *Cause of rash and prevention of recurrence*
- *Symptomatic treatment*

Strategies for Nursing Care

Relieving Diaper Area Irritation. General treatment of any of the diaper rashes requires basic diaper and skin care. The goal is "clean and dry." Prompt, thorough cleansing of the diaper region with a mild soap and water or mild baby wipes after each defecation or voiding is imperative to rid the skin of irritant byproducts and reduce the pathogen population. The caretaker should be instructed to check every hour for elimination in the newborn and young infant and every 2 hours in the older infant.

Teaching to Address Knowledge Deficit. Compliance is more likely when the caretaker(s) understands the reasons for the diaper rash and is given a clear explanation of how adequate skin hygiene and cleansing of diapers will help prevent or eliminate

Table 44-6. Clinical Manifestations and Therapeutic Management of Diaper Rashes

Area Involved	Source	Treatment	Comments
Primary Irritant Contact Dermatitis: Parchment-like erythema (similar to scald)			
Convex area of buttocks, medial thighs, mons pubis, and scrotum, but not the folds Occurs at age 3 mo or older	Ammonia (urine) and putrefactive enzymes (feces) interact to create byproducts. In older infants the contact dermatitis may be an allergic response to enzyme detergent or rubber	Topical glucocorticoid cream (1% hydrocortisone or triamcinolone). add 1 cup of vinegar to last diaper rinse and let soak ½ hr before spinning (acidifies urine); basic diaper and skin care	Allergic contact dermatitis of diaper area is similar but does not usually occur in infancy
Intertrigo: Red macerated area of sharp demarcation			
Area where skin surfaces are in opposition, particularly groin folds Occurs at any age	Heat, moisture, and sweat retention combine to irritate and macerate the skin	Basic diaper and skin care. Teach appropriate wiping to child being potty-trained	Bacterial populations grow with maceration, increasing risk of secondary infections
Seborrheic Dermatitis: Characteristic salmon-colored greasy lesion with yellowish scale, found primarily in intertriginous areas; nonpruritic (differentiates it from eczema)			
Presence of intertrigo in groin and in other skin folds (neck or axilla) plus cradle cap indicates seborrheic dermatitis Occurs at age 3 wk–4 mo	Inborn physiologic trait	Same as for contact dermatitis	May spread to entire diaper region after initial appearance in folds; highly susceptible to secondary yeast or bacterial infection; subsides spontaneously
Miliaria: Small, sterile, clear vesicopustules			
Anywhere that heat and moisture accumulate, especially diaper area Occurs at any age	Reaction to concentrated heat and humidity	Basic diaper and skin care	Also known as heat rash or prickly heat
Primary Candidiasis: Small red papules with peripheral scaling			
Sharply marginated area, usually involving the anterior thighs, and abdomen, as well as the diaper area Occurs at any age, usually after age 2 wk	*Candida albicans* from GI tract or an untreated infected caretaker	Topical antimonilial (e.g., Vioform, Nilstat, Mycostatin, Micatin); severe cases may benefit from wet soaks with tap water or Burow solution. Oral Nilstat or Mycostatin is often indicated; basic diaper and skin care	Often secondary to seborrheic dermatitis; usually occurs following oral thrush. Do not use cornstarch on rash as it may be metabolized by microorganisms, promoting disease

diaper rash. The region should be air dried and exposed to the air at additional frequent intervals to promote faster healing. Because diaper rash is exacerbated by heat, moisture, and the friction and restriction of a diaper, exposing the skin surface to air helps to soothe irritation and dry any lesions present. In severe cases use of a heat lamp may be prescribed in addition to the air exposure as detailed in Table 44-6.*

Topical steroid cream or ointment may sometimes be ordered. Usually, however, a protective ointment such as Desitin or zinc oxide is used after inflammation is reduced, or prophylactically. An antibiotic may also be prescribed if secondary infection exists. Suggesting that the diaper and ointment be removed when the infant is resting or sleeping and that ointment and a loosely applied diaper be put on when the child is up or being held may be helpful to the caretakers.

Rubber pants and disposable diapers should be avoided either during bouts of diaper rash or continuously in very susceptible infants. Parents need explanations that the rubber and plastic prevent evaporation, thereby increasing maceration from urine breakdown. Even though disposable diapers are advertised to reduce wetness by pulling the urine toward

* In some hospitals lamps are used only if ordered by a doctor. They should be used with great care. Never use a lamp until any medication or ointment has been completely removed, because moisture causes burning. Never leave the infant unattended while the lamp is on. The lamp should *not* be left at the bedside when not in use.

the liner and away from baby's skin, the urea and ammonia salts that cause the breakdown are left behind as a residue on the diaper surface touching the child's skin, just as they are in cloth diapers. Parents need to know that the "wicking" action of disposable diapers does not eliminate the need to change them frequently.

Healing of diaper rashes involving skinfolds is facilitated by frequent applications of unmedicated powder, which helps reduce moisture and irritation. (Talcum powder can cause irritation and should be avoided. Cornstarch should be avoided as well; it encourages the growth of bacteria and fungi.) The previous application of unmedicated powder should be completely washed off before each new application. A new application should be applied at each diaper change. Wet powder forms little balls, causing irritation. Powder wet from urine also holds ammonia against the skin.

If diaper laundering has been inadequate or the parent has never used cloth diapers before, instruction should be given to launder them separately, using a mild soap and a *double rinsing.* Soaking rinsed, soiled diapers in a quaternary ammonium compound such as Diaparene helps to disinfect them.

Seborrheic Dermatitis

Etiology and Pathophysiology

Seborrheic dermatitis (cradle cap, seborrheic eczema) is an inflammatory skin disease thought to be related to a dysfunction of the sebaceous glands (Hurwitz, 1981). It usually appears shortly after birth when hormone levels are high, disappears after several weeks even without treatment, then reappears at adolescence when hormone levels again rise (Hurwitz, 1981). This dermatitis occurs most often on the scalp (cradle cap)

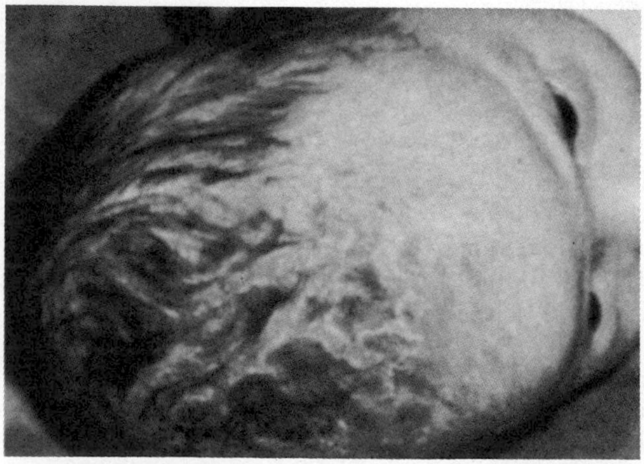

Figure 44-7. Cradle cap, a seborrheic dermatitis of the scalp, is extremely common in young infants. (From Jacobs AH: Eruptions in the diaper area. *Pediatr Clin North Am* 1975 May; 214.)

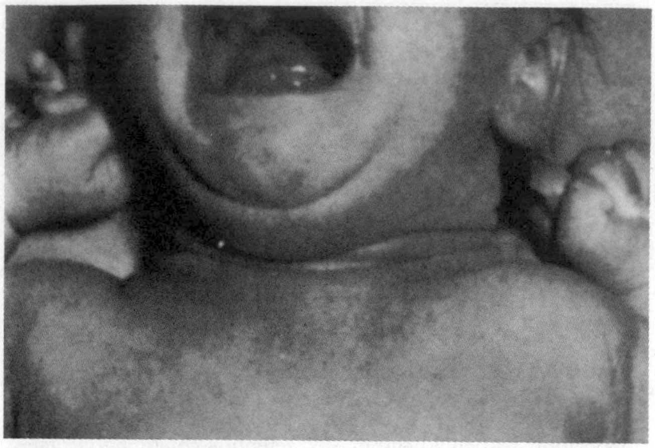

Figure 44-8. Seborrheic dermatitis may involve the axillae and neck folds. (From Jacobs AH: Eruptions in the diaper area. *Pediatr Clin North Am* 1975 May; 214.)

(Fig. 44-7) although it may also involve the eyelids and eyebrows (blepharitis), the external ear canal (otitis externa), the postauricular region (behind the ears), the axillae, and neck folds (Fig. 44-8), and the inguinal region (seborrheic diaper dermatitis). The lesions appear as thick, greasy crusts of a salmon color or as waxy yellow plaques with large scales. Transient alopecia may be present over the area of the crusty or scaly patches.

Clinical Manifestations and Diagnostic Assessment

Seborrheic dermatitis is similar to eczema in appearance and is, in fact, frequently referred to as seborrheic eczema, but it differs in several recognizable ways. Unlike eczema, cradle cap can and usually does occur in the first month of life. The lesion surfaces of seborrhea are pink or yellow, compared with the obvious red lesions of eczema. Seborrhea is not usually accompanied by a positive family history of allergy (Jacobs and Goldsobel, 1988). Lichenification of lesion areas does not occur in cradle cap. While infantile eczema often begins on the cheeks, seborrhea usually presents on the scalp, eyelids, or ear folds. Seborrhea also responds rapidly to treatment. The most significant difference, however, is the fact that seborrhea is not pruritic, while eczema produces extreme pruritus. Diagnosis is based upon the characteristic appearance of the crusts and the absence of pruritus.

Strategies for Nursing Care

Preventive and symptomatic intervention is essentially the same. The most important aspect is adequate and frequent scalp hygiene measures. The scalp should be shampooed vigorously and thoroughly every other day. Parents usually have some reservations about vigorous scalp hygiene because of misconceptions about the durability of the "soft spots," or fontanels. They should be informed that these spots are as durable as the skin anywhere else on the body and will not be punctured by the pressure required for vigorous scrubbing. For some families, a demonstration shampoo may be more convincing than verbal descriptions. The "no tears" shampoos or those containing salicylic acid or coal tars are most effective, with two applications of shampoo used each time.

Measures may be taken to soften and remove some of the crusts prior to shampooing. Slightly warmed mineral oil or petrolatum can be massaged into the scalp 15 to 20 minutes before shampooing. A soft brush or fine-toothed comb can then be used during the shampoo to loosen and remove crusts and scales. Two to three treatments of this sort may be needed to clear the scalp but scrubbing should be limited to once a day to prevent scalp irritation.

If lesions are extensive or inflamed, topical corticosteroids are effective in producing remission. Secondarily infected lesions, although infrequent, may require treatment with either topical or systemic antibiotic or antifungal therapy. Parents should be cautioned to avoid getting these ointments in the infant's eyes.

Although the lesions are of concern to parents and the crust-softening techniques somewhat bothersome, the child's behavior is generally unaltered by this disorder because it produces little if any discomfort. Seborrhea is a self-limiting disease in infancy and often clears by 8 to 12 months, even without treatment (Hurwitz, 1981). Parents can generally institute the prescribed treatment without difficulty, however, once given adequate instruction. Recurrence can be prevented by regular shampooing.

Psoriasis

Psoriasis is a chronic, inflammatory rash with scaling. It may begin at any age, with onset before 15 years of age in 27 per cent of patients. In the childhood form, males are affected twice as often as females (Hurwitz, 1981). Although the exact etiology is unknown, there is a family history of psoriasis in 35 per cent of the cases (Lookingbill and Marks, 1986).

Pathophysiology

Psoriasis is a disease of the stratum corneum in which the usual differentiation and migration of keratinocytes through the layers of epidermal tissue is dramatically accelerated. Ordinarily it takes 28 days for a cell to travel from the basal cell layer to the stratum corneum. In psoriasis, cells make that transition in 3 to 4 days. The problem results when the outer layer of skin fails to shed the cells as quickly as they are produced. Cells of the stratum corneum then accumulate with resulting scales and inflammation of the dermal layer (Lookingbill and Marks, 1986).

Clinical Manifestations

The word "psoriasis" is derived from the Greek word for itching, and the pruritus accompanying this disorder ranges from mild to severe. The scales of psoriasis are distinctive for their silver "mica-like" color and the fact that they attach at the center rather than at the periphery. If scales are removed they leave a small bleeding point associated with a ruptured capillary (Hurwitz, 1981). Classically the lesions begin as tiny, red papules covered by scales. They grow together (coalesce) to form plaques that may measure several centimeters in diameter. The lesions are most common on the scalp, knees, and elbows and between the gluteal folds. Nails may be involved with the appearance of small depressions or pits in the nail plate. Diagnosis is often made on signs and symptoms and a family history of the disease. Cell studies can be done to confirm the diagnosis.

Therapeutic Management

Because psoriasis cannot be cured, management focuses on control of the recurrent exacerbations. Specifically, therapy seeks to decrease both the dermal inflammation and the proliferation of cells in the stratum corneum. Topical steroids, topical tar preparations, and ultraviolet light have proven effective.

Major Nursing Diagnoses for Psoriasis

Impaired skin integrity, related to
- *rapid proliferation of cells in the outer epidermal layer*
- *inflammation of the dermal layer of skin*

Potential for infection: secondary staphylococcal, related to
- *scratching associated with characteristic pruritus*
- *characteristic staphylococcal colonization of the skin in persons with psoriasis*

Potential disturbance in self-concept: body image, related to chronic and unpredictable skin outbreaks

Strategies for Nursing Care

Teaching the Child and Family Topical Skin Care. The child and family will need some knowledge of the nature and usual course of psoriasis to manage the disease effectively at home. They should be aware that outbreaks are unpredictable and seemingly without cause; otherwise they may become frustrated with the prescribed treatment or blame themselves unjustly. Parents and child should understand that prescribed steroid and tar preparations do more than just "soothe." They actually reduce the rapid cell division and decrease the dermal inflammation to help bring about a remission. Tar preparations are available for baths (e.g., Polytar Bath, Zetar Emulsion) and may be an acceptable alternative for young children who insist upon rubbing off topical compounds.

Ultraviolet light is beneficial, the most effective and most practical form being sunlight. Children will often be happy to hear that playing outdoors is part of the "prescription" and adolescents are frequently pleased to further their suntans. Precautions are necessary, however, to avoid overexposure. A sunburn can damage tissue enough to bring about an exacerbation of the disease. In climates or seasons where sunlight is not plentiful, ultraviolet light treatments can be administered by a dermatologist. The young person must be warned to protect the eyes with specially made goggles or with moist cotton balls to avoid damage to the corneas and, again, to avoid overexposure.

Preventing Infection. Secondary infection in psoriasis results for the same reason as it does in many of the other inflammatory skin disorders—pruritus leads to scratching, which results in breaks in the skin barrier and penetration by bacteria. Proper use of the prescribed topical gel, cream, or ointment can reduce pruritus significantly. Young children should always have short, smooth fingernails and should be taught techniques such as applying pressure over the pruritic area rather than scratching it. Strange as it may sound, gently rubbing the opposite limb in the corresponding spot may help relieve itching (McCaffery, 1972). Infants may need to wear mits during naptime or when the caretaker cannot distract them from scratching. Children should be taught proper skin care, with attention to cleanliness, hydration, and good nutrition (see factors that affect skin function in the first part of this chapter). Skin that is generally healthy will recover more quickly from exacerbations of psoriasis and will be better able to resist infection.

Promoting a Positive Body Image. Psoriatic lesions can be a very real source of embarrassment for the child and adolescent. Their peers may express concerns of "catching" the skin lesions or may taunt and tease. In early childhood the child may look upon each new outbreak as retribution for some real or imagined wrongdoing (see Chapter 7 on cognitive development of preschoolers.) The preschooler will need reassurance that the new outbreak of lesions was unpreventable.

Children who are allowed age-appropriate self-management may feel somewhat more in control and less frustrated. They may find that prompt application of the prescribed topical preparation can limit the spread of a new attack and thus feel that there is, after all, something they can do about the disorder. Support and understanding of the parent and the nurse can be invaluable in helping the youngster build a positive body image. Focusing upon strengths and refusing to "generalize" the limitations of this skin disease to other aspects of the child's personality are effective strategies.

Nursing Strategies for Follow-up Care in the Home or Clinic

Inspect the skin thoroughly for new lesions; assess healing of prior lesions and evidence of secondary bacterial infection. Do not neglect inspection of the scalp and gluteal skin folds.

Ask about use of prescribed topical preparations and determine if the child and parent feel the preparation is helpful. Individual response to therapy may vary greatly and the child should be referred to the physician for alternate therapy if the current one is ineffective.

Ask the child about involvement in age-appropriate activities with peers and other favorite pastimes to assess body image.

Conversation with the child will also help affirm his or her "importance" in the nurse's eyes, and thereby enhance self-esteem.

Acne Vulgaris

Acne vulgaris, the classic skin eruption of adolescence, is also seen in 40 per cent of children between the ages of 8 and 10 years and may persist into adulthood (Lookingbill and Marks, 1986). Caused primarily by androgen stimulation of pilosebaceous units (hair follicle/sebaceous gland structures) in the skin, acne occurs in nearly all males and in 80 per cent of females in their teenage years (Strauss, 1987). Although the term "acne vulgaris" sounds as though it must refer to a severe type of this disorder, it actually describes ordinary acne. The word "acne" is derived from a Greek word meaning eruption on the face and "vulgaris" comes from the Latin for common or ordinary.

Pathophysiology

The pathophysiology of acne involves three mechanisms: (1) androgenic hormones, (2) obstruction of follicles, and (3) bacteria. Secretion of *androgens* during puberty leads not only to development of secondary sexual characteristics but to an increase in the size of sebaceous glands and increased production of sebum. This change in itself does not lead directly to

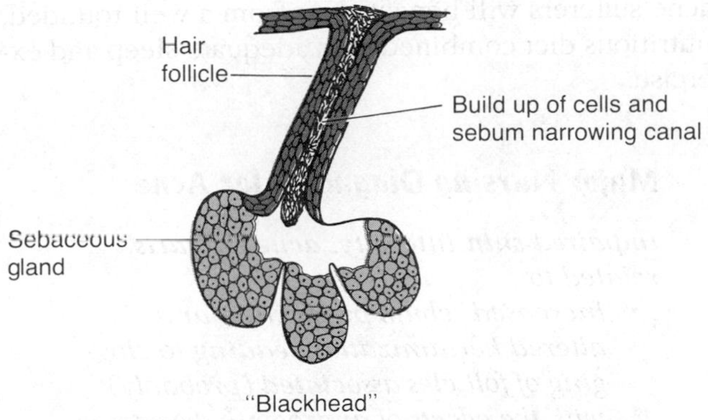

Figure 44-9. Open comedo with widely dilated follicle opening.

acne. As long as sebum is secreted into an open follicle it flows out onto the skin and evaporates. In acne vulgaris, however, follicles tend to *obstruct.* Epithelial cells, keratinocytes, accumulate within the follicle and seem to adhere to the follicular lining, thus clogging the channel through which sebum would normally be excreted. It is thought that this accumulation of cells may also be the result of androgen stimulation (Lookingbill and Marks, 1986). *Propionibacterium acnes (P. acnes)* are ordinarily harmless *bacteria* that live within the hair follicles. When follicular contents become stagnant, however, these bacteria appear to increase the inflammatory process, possibly by secreting chemicals that attract neutrophils (Lookingbill and Marks, 1986) (see Chapter 43 for the role of neutrophils in the inflammatory response).

Clinical Manifestations

Acne lesions begin as noninflammatory lesions called comedones ("blackheads" and "whiteheads"), which may progress to inflammatory pustules, papules, and nodules. When sebum accumulates within a follicle it first forms a comedo. Open comedones are called blackheads. These are widely dilated follicles (pores) clogged with thick secretions of keratin and lipid (Fig. 44-9). The black color is not entirely understood but it is not the result of poor hygiene. It may be related to oxidation of the keratin substance at the skin surface or to the production of melanin within the follicle (Hurwitz, 1981). Blackheads, although unsightly, do not progress to inflammatory lesions unless squeezed and manipulated.

Closed comedones are termed whiteheads, a term that is not to be confused with a white pustular lesion. These "whiteheads" are small, nonerythematous papules (bumps) just under the skin surface. The closed comedone is essentially that—a closed follicle that prevents sebum and other accumulations from escaping to the skin surface. Without treatment to help open the pore, closed comedones become inflammatory lesions (Fig. 44-10). As cells and sebum continue to accumulate they apply pressure that eventually ruptures the follicular wall. The follicular contents spill into the dermis, causing an inflammatory reaction. The lesion that results depends upon the size of the ruptured follicle and upon the location of the rupture within the dermis (Hurwitz, 1981). If the rupture was high in the dermis the lesion will be a pustule, pushing out against the thin epidermis and disclosing the white inflammatory exudate underneath. If the rupture was deeper within the dermis the lesion will present as a larger papule or firm nodule. Nodular lesions are especially bothersome because of the intense feeling of pressure from the deep inflammation. Squeezing in an attempt to "pop" the lesion and relieve the pressure is useless, however, since there is no channel through which the inflammatory contents can exit. This sort of manipulation increases tissue injury, further increasing the inflammation and predisposing to secondary infection through breaks in the epidermis.

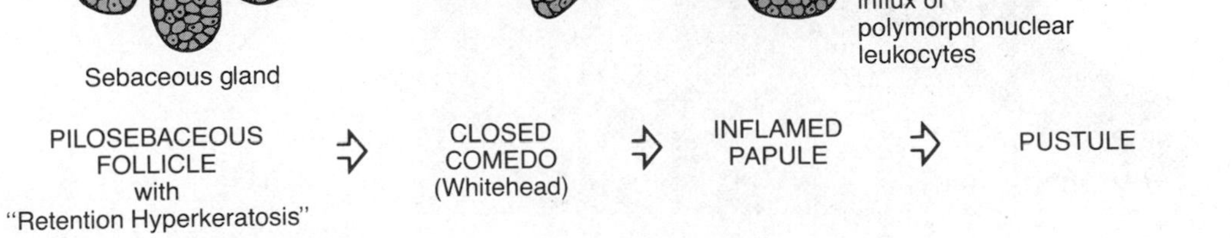

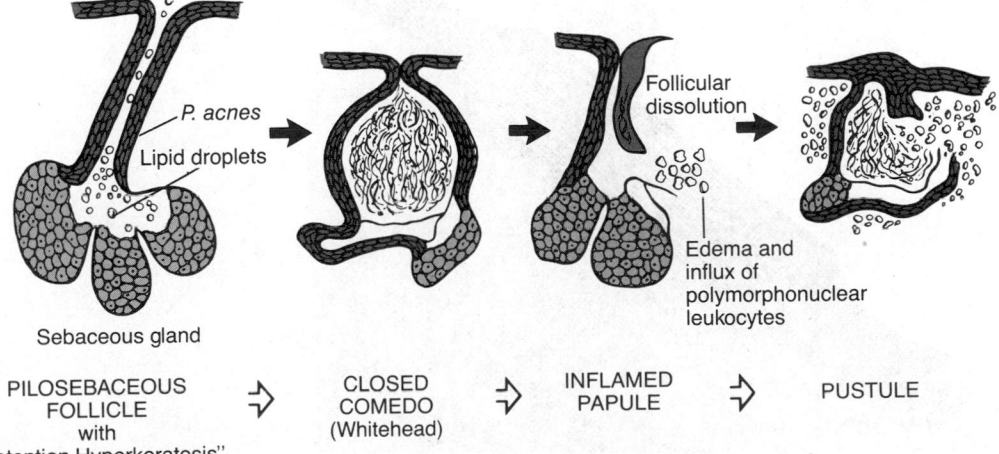

Figure 44-10. The development of an inflammatory acne lesion. (Adapted from Hurwitz S: *Clinical Pediatric Dermatology.* Philadelphia, WB Saunders, 1981, p 108.)

Therapeutic Management

Therapeutic management is aimed at (1) normalizing keratinization within the follicle, (2) decreasing sebum production, (3) inhibiting *P. acnes,* and (4) producing an anti-inflammatory effect. These aims are accomplished primarily through drug therapy (Strauss, 1987). Drugs that affect *keratinization* include topical vitamin A acid (tretinoin [Retin-A]), benzoyl peroxide, topical salicylic acid, and oral retinoids (isotretinoin [Accutane]). Drugs that decrease *sebum* production include oral estrogens, low-dose corticosteroids, and oral retinoids. The actions of *P. acnes* are inhibited by topical benzoyl peroxide, topical and oral antibiotics, and oral retinoids. *Anti-inflammatory* drugs include locally injected corticosteroids, oral corticosteroids, and oral retinoids.

Therapy may also include removal of lesions with a comedo extractor (Fig. 44-11). It forces the contents of the follicle out through the hole in the center of the extractor by applying uniform pressure on the tissue around the lesion. Comedo extraction is done most often to alleviate closed comedoes, which are the precursors to inflammatory lesions. Some dermatologists will allow their clients or someone in the family to use the comedone extractor at home. Usually, however, this is done by the physician in the clinic because improper use can lead to damage of dermal tissue and scarring.

Whereas a decade ago adolescents deprived themselves of chocolate, cola drinks, refined sugars, milk, ice cream, fried foods, potato chips, shellfish, and iodides in an attempt to "clear their complexions," it is now thought that diet has little effect on acne. For the occasional person who can relate skin eruptions to particular foods, dietary restrictions are in order. Most acne sufferers will benefit most from a well-rounded, nutritious diet combined with adequate sleep and exercise.

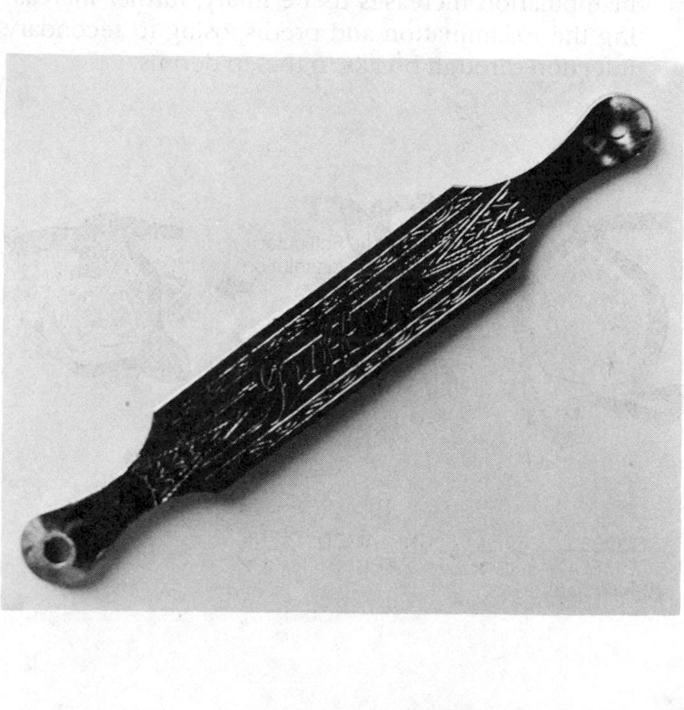

Figure 44-11. The comedone extractor is effective in nontraumatic removal of acne lesions.

Major Nursing Diagnoses for Acne

Impaired skin integrity: acne vulgaris, *related to*
- *increased sebum production and altered keratinization leading to clogging of follicles associated (probably) with the effects of androgenic hormones*
- *the action of* P. acnes *on the contents of clogged follicles*

Disturbance in self-concept: body image, *related to*
- *comedones, pustules, and nodules*
- *scarring associated with chronic pustule or nodule formation*

Knowledge deficit, *related to*
- *proper skin care*
- *safe use of prescribed medications*

Strategies for Nursing Care

Addressing the Disturbance in Self-Concept. Acne should never be dismissed as an inevitable fact of growing up that must simply be tolerated and ignored to the extent possible. Such attitudes on the part of parents or health professionals lead to unnecessary physical discomfort and possibly disfigurement associated with permanent scarring. Even more destructive is the injury to self-concept as a result of the embarrassment and self-consciousness acne causes at a time when identity development is crucial.

Although treatment does not cure acne, reasonable management can control the severity of the inflammatory process, reduce scarring, and improve appearance.

No one treatment regimen seems to adequately achieve these aims in all individuals. Self-treatment with over-the-counter benzoyl peroxide may be effective for mild acne. Reasons for poor success, whether the treatment is self-prescribed or professionally prescribed, are the adolescents' tendency to be inconsistent in compliance with the treatment, their lack of understanding of this long-term disease process that often causes them to experiment with a multitude of commercial products, and their possibly erratic emotional state. These factors define the first step needed to manage this disease.

Teaching to Address Knowledge Deficit. Whatever treatment regimen is tried, health professionals intervening need to begin by educating the adolescent about the pathophysiology and etiology of acne. Myths and fears need to be replaced with factual information. Youths need to understand that treatment will be lengthy and will not totally prevent or cure their acne state. They must be impressed with the importance of faithfully complying with the treatment regimen, despite a seeming lack of improvement, if successful results are eventually to occur. Understanding of these facts by parents is also important to their cooperation with and reinforcement of the plan of care. Therefore, they should either be included in these initial discussions or provided the same information in a separate session before specific treatment is initiated. The nurse may also see the need during this session to increase the parents' understanding of what acne means to their teen.

These interventions by the nurse are often desirable actions to motivate the youths or their parents to follow through on the referral recommendation to a dermatologist. Once treatment is prescribed the nurse can help interpret the therapy as specific and practical actions the adolescent can understand. Nurses can periodically monitor teens' compliance and help them to see the gradual improvement of their condition. (Color snapshot close-ups every 3 to 6 months provide visual evidence of the steady changes in their skin condition that go unnoticed under daily observation.) Nurses can tactfully remind parents not to use nagging as a means to keep their child compliant. The nurse may also be the one who instructs the teen in the use or application of the treatment modalities. During each interaction with youths, nurses should attempt to positively reinforce their self-image and self-confidence.

Teaching Appropriate Skin Care. Appropriate skin care involves attention to external occlusive agents, cleanliness, and picking of lesions. Hair follicles may be occluded externally by oil from the hands or from hair that touches the face. Avoiding resting the face in the hands and altering hair style to pull hair away from the face and forehead can be helpful. Cosmetics also can be occlusive. Many dermatologists will suggest that cosmetics not be used, but this must be balanced with the benefits of cosmetics in hiding acne breakout and thereby improving self-concept. Nurses can counsel adolescent girls to buy only *water-based* cosmetics, to apply them sparingly, and to remove them at night.

The adolescent should know that acne is not the result of uncleanliness and therefore washing the face repeatedly throughout the day will not cure the problem. Clients should understand that the value of facial cleansing is in removing oils and external irritants from the face that may externally occlude hair canals. Cleansing two to three times per day is sufficient for that purpose; more frequent cleansing may dry and further irritate the skin. The face should be washed with lukewarm water and a mild soap such as Dove, Aveenobar, Neutrogena, or Purpose. If a washcloth is used is should be employed gently, not abrasively.

One of the nurse's greatest challenges will be to convince the adolescent not to pick the lesions. The temptation is almost overwhelming! The young person should know, however, that much of acne skin damage is self-inflicted. When one understands the cause for lesions and realizes that pushing against lesions to extract their contents causes a good deal of damage to the surrounding tissues, that temptation may be somewhat abated. Another teaching technique is to have the adolescent conduct a bit of personal "research." If they find they simply must pick one lesion, have them keep track of the days between eruption and complete healing of that lesion versus a similar one that they do not pick. Demonstrating that healing progresses faster without the additional inflammation caused by squeezing the skin can be a convincing argument.

Teaching Appropriate Use of Topical Agents. The most frequently used topical agents are benzoyl peroxide and Retin A (in cream, gel, or solution). Retin A is often considered the treatment of choice for noninflammatory disease, open and closed comedones. (Benzoyl peroxide is the agent of choice for inflammatory lesions because it has antibacterial properties (Strauss, 1987).) However, benzoyl peroxide is also often used to treat mild-to-moderate acne with comedones, and for patients with both types of lesions both preparations may be prescribed. The two agents are chemically incompatible, however, and should not be used together. They will be prescribed either on alternate days, or one for use in the morning and the other at night.

Both Retin A and benzoyl peroxide are potentially irritating to the skin, especially in fair-complexioned individuals. Imagine the frustration of the adolescent who enthusiastically applies the new "answer" to his or her acne problem only to be rewarded by a bright red face. Every client should be aware of this possibility and instructed that the best insurance against such a happening is to follow the dermatologist's instructions to the letter. *Overuse will not result in faster results.* Hurwitz (1981) suggested that irritation could be further minimized by delaying application of the topical agent for 30 minutes after washing the face, to be sure that the skin is completely dry. This waiting period is especially helpful for Retin A. Generally, treatment will begin with the least irritating form of the agent (e.g., Retin A cream versus gel), gradually increasing in strength until the desired effect is produced without skin irritation. Minor irritation experienced with the start of topical therapy usually dissipates after 1 or 2 weeks of use (Lookingbill and Marks, 1986).

Persons using Retin A must be warned that this agent makes them particularly prone to sunburn. A sunscreen should be used when there is prolonged exposure to the sun.

Teaching Safe Use of Oral Antibiotics. Antibiotics may be prescribed to control inflammatory lesions. Tetracycline is often the drug of choice because of its low cost, effectiveness, and relative safety (Lookingbill and Marks, 1986). Erythromycin also is commonly used for acne. The adolescent taking tetracycline must be taught to take it on an empty stomach because food, particularly dairy products, interfere with absorption. Persons with asthma or other disorders who also take theophylline preparations should know that tetracycline potentiates the action of theophylline. Patients should call their doctor if they experience symptoms of theophylline toxicity: nausea, a feeling of agitation, or a racing pulse.

Teaching About Other Oral Agents. Accutane has been found extremely effective in inducing remission of severe acne but should only be used when all other methods have failed. It tends to normalize follicular keratinization, inhibits sebaceous gland activity, inhibits the growth of *P. acnes,* and has anti-inflammatory effects. Although it has dramatic effects on acne, Accutane is reserved for use in cases of severe cystic acne because of its significant side effects. Strauss (1987) commented that "for all practical purposes, every patient who is treated with isotretinoin develops some side effects that are associated with chronic hypervitaminosis A" (p. 174). These effects include cheilitis, dry skin, pruritus, skin eruptions, drying of the mucous membranes, conjunctivitis, and nosebleeds. The most disturbing side effect of Accutane, however, is its ability to cause *birth defects.* Male patients are in no danger since there is no effect upon sperm. Female patients who are sexually active must be warned to use effective contraception and to consult a genetic counselor should they become pregnant during the course of Accutane administration. The risk of serious birth defects is so great that some physicians will not prescribe Accutane unless the patient signs an agreement that should she become pregnant while on the medication, she will seek a therapeutic abortion.

Estrogen may be administered to females in the form of certain birth control pills to reduce hyperfunction of sebaceous glands. Because of the risks associated with high doses of estrogen, however, it is restricted to cases of acne resistant to other forms of therapy (except Accutane) (Dobson, 1984).

Nursing Strategies for Follow-up Care in the Home or Clinic

Assess the adolescent's expectations for the treatment protocol and encourage expression of feelings about the condition and about the therapy.

Determine if there are factors in the young person's physical, mental, or spiritual well-being that are contributing to the acne.

Assess for dry, peeling, or irritated skin that would indicate overly vigorous cleansing practices, improper use, or adverse effects of topical agents.

Assess for therapeutic effects and side effects of oral medications.

Assess for evidence (subjectively and objectively) of picking of lesions.

Ask the adolescent whether he or she feels the skin condition is improving and why or why not.

Allow the adolescent as much input into the treatment regimen as possible to increase sense of control and enhance compliance.

Infectious Skin Disorders of Childhood

The integumentary disorders discussed in this section are all associated with streptococcal or staphylococcal bacterial agents. Therefore, a discussion of specific bacterial immunity seems appropriate here. In early bacterial infection, host reactions are nonspecific— fatty acid secretions of the skin can inactivate bacteria, and lysozymes present in tears, saliva, and blood can break down the cell wall of gram-positive organisms. These bacteria, because of their capsular structure, are phagocytosis resistant. Thus, specific antibody mediators are necessary to enable phagocytic activity. Primary infection stimulates IgM class antibody formation, which aids phagocytic activity early in the infection process. If the infection progresses or reinfection occurs, IgG antibodies are available to assist phagocytosis, but they are not as effective as IgM antibodies in facilitating phagocytosis, particularly in staphylococcal infection (Stiehm and Fulginiti, 1980). Unfortunately, this same bacteria also becomes easily resistant to antibiotics.

Diagnostic Assessment and Therapeutic Management

Diagnosis of each of the integumentary infections discussed in this section is made by visual recognition of the characteristic lesion and by culture of the exudate to establish staphylococcal or streptococcal origin.

Management similarities also exist in that warm wet soaks may be applied to bring the infection to a head and to provide relief from pain or tenderness. Typically a topical and/or systemic antibiotic is prescribed to facilitate resolution of the infectious process.

Conscientious hygiene is important both in preventing the development of these skin infections and in reducing the likelihood of spread or transfer of the infectious organisms.

The effect of integumentary infections on the child and family members is related to three factors primarily: (1) the unpleasant appearance of the lesions that occur primarily on the face; (2) the potential transfer of the infection to other members, and (3) hygienic implications.

Education and teaching and reinforcing meticulous hygiene measures are the most appropriate nursing interventions to facilitate physical resolution of the infection and to minimize the psychosocial effects on the child and family members. Parents, siblings, and peers should be urged to continue to communicate acceptance and to avoid making derogatory statements or teasing the child about his or her appearance. This is especially imperative for the adolescent for whom appearance is developmentally bound to self-concept.

Hygienic practices that emphasize cleanliness and frequent handwashing, careful cleansing of wounds and insect bites, and individual use of bath and bed linens should be taught to all children from the time they are toddlers. These practices should be reviewed and re-emphasized when skin infections do occur.

Impetigo

Etiology

Impetigo is the most common skin infection in children (Melish, 1987). Also known as pyoderma, this highly contagious skin infection often locates around the mouth and nose, but is occasionally found on the extremities. It results when group A beta-hemolytic streptococci (or, rarely, staphylococci) come in contact with a broken skin area or an insect bite. The incubation period is 2 to 10 days. Impetigo is endemic in the southern United States but is seen commonly during warm, humid summer months in northern climates.

Clinical Manifestations and Diagnostic Assessment

The lesions begin as intact, erythematous papules. Within hours a pruritic vesicle or pustule forms. Eventually the vesicle ruptures and a thick, honey-colored crust forms (Fig. 44-12). These lesions have a rapid peripheral spread so that the nurse typically will see a group of lesions forming a circle or arc. The lesions are highly contagious for as long as they exist. Diagnosis is generally possible based on the characteristics of the lesions. Regional lymph nodes may be enlarged. A vesicle culture is not generally needed unless the child fails to respond to conventional therapy.

Therapeutic Management

Although topical antibiotics were formally used for impetigo, current management involves systemic antibiotics administered either orally or parenterally. Typically, one dose of benzathine penicillin is given intra-

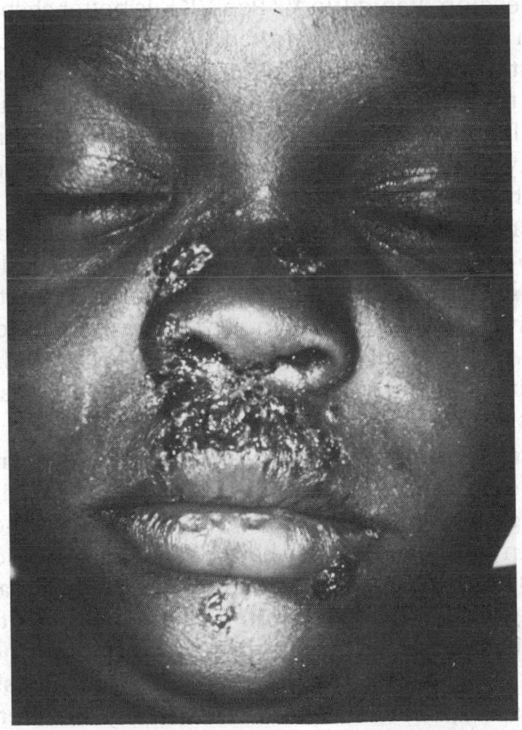

Figure 44-12. The characteristic distribution of impetigo is about the nose and chin. (From Green M, Haggerty RJ: *Ambulatory Pediatrics.* 2nd ed. Philadelphia, WB Saunders, 1977.)

muscularly, or 10 days of an oral preparation such as erythromycin or penicillin V is prescribed (Melish, 1987). Antibiotic therapy is important to limit the continued spread of the disease in the child and to prevent family members and playmates from contracting impetigo. Antibiotic therapy does not prevent the onset of acute glomerulonephritis, the most serious sequela of impetigo.

Major Nursing Diagnoses for Impetigo

Impaired skin integrity: vesicles, pustules, and crusts, *related to streptococcal infection of a skin lesion or insect bite*
Knowledge deficit, *related to*

- *antibiotic administration*
- *preventing spread of the infection to family members and playmates*
- *care of lesions*
- *signs and symptoms of acute glomerulonephritis*

Strategies for Nursing Care

Teaching Antibiotic Administration. The family must be instructed how often to give the antibiotic and impressed with the importance of giving the child all of the medication in properly spaced doses so that an antibiotic-resistant strain of streptococci will not develop. Penicillin V (Pen VK), is better absorbed when taken after a meal than on an empty stomach. Question the child and parent about previous reactions to penicillin or other medications. Instruct them to call the physician should any signs of drug hypersensitivity result: rash, fever, hives, pruritus, or difficulty breathing.

Erythromycin may be ordered if the child is allergic to penicillin. It is less effective in an acid medium; pills that have been crushed or chewed will be partially inactivated by stomach acid. Erythromycin should not be given with fruit juice. Generally, it is best to administer it on an empty stomach, 1 hour before meals or 3 hours after.

Preventing Spread of Impetigo. Parents should be cautioned that impetigo lesions are highly contagious. Children in school or in day care should remain at home until they have been taking antibiotics for 48 hours and/or the lesions are dry. Contamination among siblings can be limited by frequent and thorough handwashing and by encouraging the child not to touch the lesions. The infected child should not share towels and washcloths with other family members.

Teaching Care of Lesions. The crusts may be softened by application of a warm, wet washcloth. Crusts that loosen can then be gently removed. Parents and the child should know that removing the crusts too early will simply result in recrusting and will prolong healing rather than enhance it. Scratching the lesions may result in secondary infection despite the administration of antibiotics. Mits may be necessary for the infant. The toddler is best discouraged from scratching by distraction and comfort techniques.

Recurrence of impetigo is best prevented by regular bathing and attention to minor wounds and insect bites. Minor breaks in the skin integrity should be washed with soap and water and a topical antibiotic preparation applied to any minor wound that begins to appear infected (inflamed).

Alerting the Family to Signs and Symptoms of Acute Poststreptococcal Glomerulonephritis. In geographic areas where impetigo often leads to acute glomerulonephritis, a urinalysis should be performed at the time of diagnosis and the child should be followed for at least 7 weeks following healing of the lesions (Hurwitz, 1981). Parents should alert the physician if the child's urine output significantly decreases (decreased wet diapers or voiding) or if the urine changes color. (Acute glomerulonephritis is covered in Chapter 42.)

Nursing Strategies for Follow-up Care in the Home or Clinic

Assess compliance with antibiotic therapy.

Inspect the skin for healing of lesions versus eruption of new vesicles.

Inquire if other family members have lesions that might be impetigo.

Assess for the onset of acute glomerulonephritis. Measure the child's blood pressure. Obtain a urine specimen for analysis if appropriate.

Cellulitis

Cellulitis is a bacterial infection of the subcutaneous tissue and the dermis. The most common causative organisms are staphylococci, group A beta-hemolytic streptococci, and (in children under 5 years of age) *Haemophilus influenzae,* type b (Melish, 1987). The infection usually occurs at or near the site of a wound or previous trauma. Often, the initial wound is so minor it was overlooked.

Clinical Manifestations

In the classic course of cellulitis, a red, tender, warm swelling appears within a day or two of the original skin trauma. The swelling rapidly increases to produce a large, firm area of edema. The child experiences pain as a result of the intense pressure of the inflammatory exudate on skin tissues.

Therapeutic Management

Whereas mild cases of cellulitis may be treated with oral antibiotics at home, children are often admitted to the hospital for intravenous antibiotics. Intravenous therapy is continued until there is a noticeable reduction in the redness and edema.

Strategies for Nursing Care

The antibiotics given for cellulitis (e.g., methicillin) are frequently quite irritating to veins, and special attention must be given to the onset of phlebitis. The child with venous irritation will often complain of burning during administration, the site of intravenous injection will be especially tender, and the redness may begin creeping up the vein. Irritation can be lessened by reducing the rate of administration and by mixing the drug to the maximum dilution. If more than one antibiotic is being administered, the nurse must check whether the drugs can be safely administered through the same intravenous line.

The child with cellulitis will often be irritable from the discomfort of the edematous area and from fear of or discomfort from the intravenous therapy. Palpation of the edematous area is especially painful and assessment of this nature should be held to the minimum needed to ensure that edema is not increasing. A mild analgesic such as acetaminophen (Tylenol) can significantly decrease pain, and the child can be further comforted by rocking, being distracted with toys for quiet play, and the presence of a parent or family member. Warm soaks may also help to relieve pain and may enhance healing by increasing blood circulation (and thereby circulation of antibiotic) to the area.

Herpes Simplex Virus, Type I

There are four types of human herpes viruses: herpes simplex virus (HSV, types 1 and 2), cytomegalovirus (CMV), Epstein-Barr virus (infectious mononucleosis), and varicella-zoster virus. With the exception of herpes simplex virus type 1, these forms are covered in Chapter 45. With all types of herpes virus, the immune status of the host determines whether and to what degree the virus will be manifested.

HSV type 1 is classically the "oral" type of herpes ("cold sores," "fever blisters") and type 2 has been known as the "genital" type. Clinical distinction between the two types has become less clear, however, with increasing practices of oral-genital sex and it is now known that either type can affect any given region of the body (Kohl, 1987). This discussion will be confined to the type 1 virus, which is not classically passed through sexual contact.

Incidence and Etiology

Exposure to herpes virus is widespread. Among young children from a lower socioeconomic environment, 40 to 60 per cent are seropositive by the age of 5 years. Most of these children will, by adulthood, exhibit HSV-1 antibodies. The incidence is somewhat less in higher socioeconomic populations, with only about 30 per cent of university students showing serologic evidence of HSV infection.

Herpes simplex virus is transmitted by infected body fluids such as saliva coming in contact with microscopic or larger breaks in the skin or mucous membranes. Newborn infants may acquire HSV in passage through an infected birth canal. Nurses and other health care workers can (and do) transmit HSV between patients when handwashing protocols are overlooked. Children especially susceptible to HSV are those with burns, infants with diaper rash or eczema, and those immunosuppressed by illnesses or drug therapy (e.g., children with leukemia or other cancers) (Kohl, 1987).

Pathophysiology

In most cases HSV-1 infection occurs at the site of entry on the skin or mucous membranes. HSV shows particular affinity for tissues that arise from the ectoderm (epidermis, hair, nails, cutaneous and mammary glands, anterior pituitary gland, tooth enamel, inner ear, lens of the eye, and nervous tissue) (Moore, 1983). The infected cells swell and degenerate leading to local inflammation (nonspecific immune response) and subsequent formation of antibodies (specific immune response). Vesicles form, become infected by resident bacteria on the skin, form pustules, ooze, dry, and crust. Lesions on mucous membranes usually present as shallow ulcers. HSV-1 lesions are superficial and do not leave scars, although following pronounced lesions, skin color under the lesion may be altered for a few weeks. The incubation period between contact with the virus and appearance of infection is 2 to 20 days.

After once being infected with HSV the virus remains latent, probably within nerve cells innervating that portion of the skin originally infected (Kohl, 1987). HSV can be reactivated by several factors, including fever, emotional upset, exposure to sunlight, menstruation, and immunodepression.

Clinical Manifestations

The most common form of HSV-1 in children is gingivostomatitis, herpes infection of the mouth. It is most common in children between 10 months and 3 years of age. Vesicular lesions can be found on the lips, gums, tongue, and hard palate. The breath may have a particularly foul smell (fetor oris). Cervical and submental lymph nodes are usually enlarged. As the vesicles break, shallow gray ulcers are left which are extremely painful. The child usually refuses to eat or drink and dehydration becomes a concern. Resolution of the lesions occurs spontaneously within 10 days to 2 weeks. In adolescents HSV-1 may present as pharyngitis with painful, ulcerative lesions on markedly swollen tonsils.

Therapeutic Management

Management of oral herpes is usually symptomatic and can be handled in the home unless fear of dehydration results in hospitalization for administration of intravenous fluids. Intravenous or topical acyclovir (Zovirax) may be effective in severe cases but has had little testing in children (Kohl, 1987).

Strategies for Nursing Care

Gingivostomatitis is a particularly distressing illness for both the child and the family caretaker. The child will be extremely irritable because every swallow of saliva brings intense pain from oral lesions and, perhaps, from lesions in the throat. Attempts to swallow even bland liquids meet with the same pain, and the child is generally a little bundle of misery. The fetid breath is unpleasant for caretakers and even if one can convince the child to swish with a diluted mouthwash (e.g., quarter-strength hydrogen peroxide) or gently brush the teeth, the odor returns almost immediately. Parents become exhausted because comfort measures and other care is often necessary throughout the night. Attempting to swallow during sleep may cause the child to awaken with a cry.

The nurse who is aware of the discomfort associated with this disorder can provide the family with a good deal of support and reassurance. In addition, the nurse can advocate prescription of oral anesthetics and analgesics to reduce the pain.

Parents will need to be reassured that the child will not be harmed by a few days without solid food. They must realize the necessity of fluids, however. Minimum fluid requirements to prevent dehydration should be calculated on the basis of body weight (see Table 30-6) and translated for the parent into household measures. The nurse may suggest keeping a chart to mark down the sips of fluid taken and suggest that "success" be measured by the ability to entice the child to take one sip at a time throughout the day and night. Fluids must be bland, and parents will need an explanation of that term, i.e., no fruit juices or salty liquids. Milk-based fluids (including pudding), noncarbonated or "flattened" soft drinks, gelatin, and Kool-aid preparations are often best tolerated. Parents should know that the first overt sign of dehydration will be decreased urination with increased color and odor to the urine. The physician should be contacted at the first sign of dehydration. Guidelines for care that are as specific as possible can help to relieve unnecessary anxiety. If the nurse works in a setting that allows time to do so, a phone call to the family can support their efforts and answer questions that have arisen since diagnosis.

Chalazion

Clinical Manifestations

A chalazion is caused by chronic granulomatous inflammation of sebaceous glands in the eyelid. Although the chalazion may begin in childhood, it often does not become pronounced until adolescence. It is most prevalent in adolescent girls when they begin wearing eye make-up.

The granulomatous cyst remains localized as a firm, nontender swelling that is covered by freely moving skin. It can be diagnosed by visual examination or, if the cyst is draining, by a culture of the exudate.

Strategies for Nursing Care

Management involves application of local heat to bring the cyst to a head and application of a topical antibiotic to eliminate the source of the infection. The teen should also be encouraged to reduce or discontinue her use of eye make-up or, if she will not avoid the make-up, to at least thoroughly remove it daily and cleanse the eyelids with a mild soap and water. If the chalazion persists despite these actions, surgical drainage of the cyst is indicated, and the client should be referred back to the physician.

Hordeolum (Stye)

Clinical Manifestations

A stye is the result of an acute infection of the glands on the margin of the eyelid that produces a small abscess. There will be pain and redness, localized on the lid margin, with preauricular lymph node enlargement. The lid around the area may become tender and swollen. Superficial abscesses come to a head, rupture spontaneously, and heal completely without treatment.

Strategies for Nursing Care

If the abscess does not either reabsorb or come to a head (point) on its own within 1 to 2 days, treatment consists of localizing the abscess by applying warm, wet compresses for 20 to 30 minutes four to six times a day, followed when necessary by application of a topical antibiotic or sulfa ointment. If the condition does not improve, a culture and sensitivity test may be necessary to find an effective medication. Children who have repeated styes should have their vision checked because, although styes have nothing to do with vision problems, children with a refractive error do a lot of rubbing, which can contribute to the development of styes. If styes tend to occur in crops, underlying staphylococcal infection usually exists, requiring both local and systemic antibiotic treatment. Rarely, incision and drainage of the abscess by a physician may be required.

Furuncles (Boils) and Carbuncles

Pathophysiology and Etiology

A furuncle, or boil, is an acute localized perifollicular staphylococcal abscess of the skin and subcutaneous tissue that undergoes necrosis and suppuration.

Development of a furuncle results from obstruction of a sebaceous gland or ingrowth of a hair follicle. Typically, a furuncle is preceded by a superficial staphylococcal folliculitis. A small pustule enlarges around the hair follicle, becoming firm, red, and tender. The lesion becomes fluctuant and will eventually drain purulent material, allowing healing to occur in 1 to 2 weeks. Furuncles may occur at any age. In children, they are most commonly seen in staphylococcal carriers and those with chronic nutrition problems, immunodeficiency states, and other debilitating diseases (Demis et al, 1979).

Carbuncles represent a more severe and extensive skin infection than furuncles. The incidence of carbuncles is greater in males and is seen most often in children with diabetes, hypogammaglobulinemia, and other resistance-lowering diseases. This perifollicular abscess affects adjacent hair follicles and drains through multiple openings in the skin; thus, carbuncles are often described as multiple furuncles. The neck, back, and thighs are common sites for abscess development. The simple pustule develops slowly, enlarges to the size of an egg or an orange, and causes extensive pain. When carbuncles drain, the entire center lesion may slough off a large amount of necrotic material, leaving a large ulcerated area. The ulcer will granulate in several weeks, but a scar is usually present.

Diagnostic Assessment and Therapeutic Management

Furuncles occur most commonly in the neck, buttocks, extremities, perineum, axillae, and face. The child may initially experience itching but usually will ignore the pustule until it enlarges and causes pain. Malaise and an elevated temperature (38.3 to 38.9°C or 101 to 102°F) are other presenting symptoms. Diagnosis is made by isolation of *Staphylococcus aureus* from the purulent drainage. Simple furuncles can be treated with heat alone. Referral to a physician is warranted if the child is experiencing intense pain and the lesion does not drain spontaneously. Large boils are carefully incised and drained and treated with topical antibiotics. Occasionally a systemic antibiotic is ordered, depending on the results of culture and sensitivity tests.

Children with carbuncles will usually experience general malaise, fever, and chills and complain of severe pain. The nurse will easily recognize a carbuncle from its large size, red color, and tenderness. Any child presenting with this skin condition should be referred to the physician for diagnosis and immediate treatment. Management usually includes systemic antibiotics, rest and warm, moist compresses. Analgesics may be needed if the pain is severe.

Major Nursing Diagnoses for Furuncles and Carbuncles

Impairment of skin integrity: inflammation of hair follicle(s), related to staphylococcal infection

Disturbance in self concept: body image, *related to*
- *draining lesion*
- *scarring from the lesion (carbuncle)*

Altered comfort: pain, *related to pressure of enlarging abscess upon nerve endings*

Knowledge deficit, *related to*
- *treatment*
- *prevention of spread of the staphylococcal organism to other breaks in skin integrity or to other persons*
- *hygiene practices to prevent recurrence*

Strategies for Nursing Care

Nursing care for home management of a boil includes careful instruction on good handwashing, a daily bath and shampoo, avoiding hand contact with the pustule, and disposal of drainage in a closed container. Fingernails should be kept short and clean. The child's towels, washcloths, sheets, and clothing should be separated from those used by the rest of the family and should be washed daily.

The application of warm, moist compresses may alleviate some of the child's discomfort. Children with draining lesions may attend school if bandages are used to cover the area. Clean, dry gauze is placed over the area but may need to be changed while the child is in school. The nurse can help change the bandage and evaluate whether further treatment is necessary. This is also an opportunity for the nurse to demonstrate proper handwashing and disposal of the soiled dressing. Also assess the child's discomfort, if pain is severe, attendance at school should be evaluated. The school nurse can contact the child's teacher and arrange for make-up work to be done at home. Children with furuncles will benefit from knowing that the skin infection is only temporary and there will be no residual scarring.

Nurses working with children identified as "at risk" should facilitate early treatment by teaching the signs and symptoms of furuncles. When teaching good skin care to children, they should include a description of furuncles, and children should be cautioned against "picking" at infected hairs. Recurring furuncles may require checking family members for staphylococcal carriers.

Recurrence of carbuncles is common, and children prone to development of this skin condition should avoid skin irritation from constrictive clothing.

Occasionally excision of the carbuncle is necessary to promote drainage. The nurse should prepare the child and parents for the excision in these ways: (1) describe the procedure and equipment to be used, (2) describe possible pain the child may feel, and (3) discuss whether the child wants to have his or her parents present during the treatment. Adequate preparation for treatment enhances the child's coping abilities and promotes parental support.

Nursing Strategies for Follow-up Care in the Home or Clinic

Obtain nasal swab cultures of family members for *Staphylococcus aureus* if repeated infections occur in the child.

If culture results are positive, instruct all family members to instill the prescribed antibiotic cream or ointment into the anterior nares daily.

Reinforce teaching to prevent recurrence, especially in children at risk for chronic furunculosis (those who are obese, have poor hygiene, or have excessive perspiration).

References

Demis D, et al (eds): Furuncles and carbuncles. *In Clinical Dermatology.* New York, Harper and Row, 1979.

Dobson R: An interview with the president of the American Academy of Dermatologists. *In* Stress Tied to Problems With Skin. *St Louis Post Dispatch* 1984 Aug; 19.

Green M, Haggerty RJ: *Ambulatory Pediatrics.* 2nd ed. Philadelphia, WB Saunders, 1977.

Hurwitz S: *Clinical Pediatric Dermatology.* Philadelphia, WB Saunders, 1981.

Jacobs AH, Goldsobel AB: Atopic dermatitis. *In* Bierman CW, Pearlman DS (eds): *Allergic Diseases from Infancy to Adulthood.* 2nd ed. Philadelphia, WB Saunders, 1988, 385–404.

Kahn G: Principles of diagnosis and treatment of skin disorders. *In* Bierman CW, Pearlman DS (eds): *Allergic Diseases from Infancy to Adulthood.* 2nd ed. Philadelphia, WB Saunders, 1988, 377–384.

Kohl S: Postnatal herpes simplex virus infection. *In* Feigin RD, Cherry JD (eds): *Textbook of Pediatric Infectious Diseases.* 2nd ed. Philadelphia, WB Saunders, 1987, 1577–1601.

Lookingbill DP, Marks JD Jr: *Principles of Dermatology* Philadelphia, WB Saunders, 1986.

McCaffery M: *Nursing Management of the Patient With Pain.* Philadelphia, JB Lippincott, 1972.

Melish ME: Bacterial skin infections. *In* Feigin RD, Cherry JD (eds): *Textbook of Pediatric Infectious Diseases.* 2nd ed. Philadelphia, WB Saunders, 1987, 861–872.

Nicol NH: Atopic dermatitis: the (wet) wrap-up. *AJN* 1987 Dec; 87(12):1560–1563.

Sternbach G, Callen JP: Dermatitis. *Emerg Med Clin North Am* 1985 Nov; 3(4):677–692.

Stiehm R, Fulginiti V: *Immunologic Disorders in Infants and Children.* Philadelphia, WB Saunders, 1980.

Strauss JS: Update on acne. *Primary Care* 1987 Mar; 14(1):167–176.

Bibliography

A case of candidiasis. *Am J Nurs* 1986 Feb; 86(2):120, 125.

Bryant RA: Saving the skin from tape injuries. *Am J Nurs* 1988 Feb; 88(2):189–191.

Dunn ML, et al: Treatment options for psoriasis. *Am J Nurs* 1988 Aug; 88(8):1082–1087.

Feldman AL, Aretakis DA: Herpetic gingivostomatitis in children. *Pediatr Nurs* 1986 Mar/Apr; 12(2):111–113.

Fischer RG: Topical corticosteroid preparations. *Pediatr Nurs* 1986 Mar/Apr; 12(2):133–134.

Kronmiller JE: Oral soft tissue abnormalities in children. *Pediatr Nurs* 1987 May/Jun; 13(3):161–165.

Nicol NH, Clark RAF: Current therapy for atopic dermatitis. *Med/Sci Update* 1987 Jun; 6(6):1–6.

Nicol NH, Clark RAF: Atopic dermatitis. *In* Provost TT, Farmer ER (eds): *Current Therapy in Dermatology 2.* BC Decker, Inc, CV Mosby, 1988.

Once-a-day topical steroid. *Am J Nurs* 1988 Jan; 88(1):16.

Sterile Vaseline on scrubbed hands? Why not? *Am J Nurs* 1988 Jan; 88(1):14–15.

Nursing Strategies: Infectious Disease

Chapter 45

Jo Joyce Anderson
Roxie Foster

Related Topics
Isolation strategies, Chapter 27
Developmental delays, Chapter 34
Other respiratory infections, Chapter 38
Infective endocarditis, Chapter 39
Pinworms, Chapter 41
Other gastrointestinal infections, Chapter 41
Other genitourinary tract infections, Chapter 42
Neurologic infections, Chapter 46

During an individual's lifetime a multitude of microbial contacts are experienced. Infants and children generally experience successive exposure to a variety of viruses and bacteria. Healthy children rarely experience devastating illness from these infections, and upon recovery the immunologic response that has occurred with the microbe often renders the child immune to further infection due to that particular microbe. For some of these diseases the child can acquire immunity without experiencing the disease, through specific vaccinations.

This chapter deals with certain of the viral and bacterial infectious diseases that are not covered in the body systems chapters. Additionally, diseases that are caused by parasites, fungi, rickettsia, and protozoa are covered. The sexually transmitted diseases and vaginal infections are addressed in the final section.

Specific Immune Responses

The general immune response is detailed in Chapter 43. Specific responses to viruses, bacteria, parasites, and fungi are addressed here.

Viruses

Viruses are pathogens that have the capacity to penetrate healthy cells. They possess a special coating that makes them seem benign until they are internalized. When the body cell tries to digest the virus, however, the protective coating is destroyed, releasing viral nucleic acid that takes over the function of healthy cells. Instead of serving the purpose for which it was created, the diseased body cell puts most of its energy into the replication of the virus.

Immune mechanisms that protect against viruses are (1) the anatomic and physiologic barriers (intact skin and mucous membranes, intact cellular layers of the respiratory and gastrointestinal tracts); (2) phagocytes that engulf and destroy viruses; (3) interferon that renders noninfected cells resistant to the virus; and (4) the specific immune response, including macrophages, T-cells, and antibodies. The barrier effect of intact skin and mucous membranes is enhanced by IgA antibodies, which neutralize many viruses (Fulginiti, 1987).

Bacteria

Intact skin and mucous membranes protect against bacteria as well. Tissue macrophages that reside in the liver, spleen, bone marrow, kidney, and lung help remove bacteria before they gain hold in the body. Bacteria stimulate both T-cell and B-cell responses, and antibodies produced by B-cells (as well as complement components) destroy bacteria. One component of the immune attack against both bacteria and viruses is the inflammatory response, which manifests as fever and malaise in the infected individual.

Parasites

The immune mechanisms against parasites are very poorly understood. Parasite antigens are complex and elicit a host of responses, which may or may not play any role in immunity. The primary antigens of helminths appear to be secreted by the worm itself. It is known that certain of the helminthic antigens stimulate mononuclear inflammatory cells in the host (Fulginiti, 1987).

Fungi

Fungi gain hold primarily in hosts who are immunocompromised. Fungal diseases that act on the surface of the body (e.g., *Candida albicans* and tinca) produce a localized infection that results in little if any immune response. These surface fungi are transmitted to areas within the body via indwelling vascular catheters, endotracheal tubes, and artificial organ parts, especially when antimicrobial therapy is being administered. Antimicrobials alter the normal bacteria that protect against fungi colonization. Fungal invasion of body organs can be lethal, especially in the immunosuppressed child, making prevention imperative.

The next section deals with certain viral infections and with tuberculosis. Subsequent sections address parasitic, fungal, rickettsial, and amebial infections. Sexually transmitted diseases and vaginal infections are covered in the last sections.

Diseases of Viral and Bacterial Origin

Childhood Infectious Diseases

Diagnosis of the various childhood communicable diseases is made from visualization of the characteristic lesions and their location and by history of exposure and prodromal symptoms.

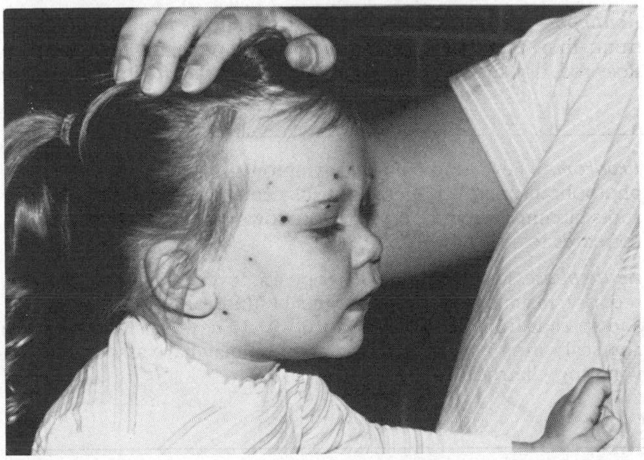

Figure 45-1. Chickenpox lesions must be crusted before the child returns to preschool or day care. At this stage, the child is no longer infectious.

The commonalities of treatment are those interventions related to comfort from fever and/or pruritus and to helping the child and family members adjust to the temporary isolation measures.

Generally, the childhood communicable diseases are not highly stress-producing for either the child or family members as long as comfort measures are understood and employed. The greater concern for the nurse is to help parents take responsibility for preventing most of the childhood communicable diseases by ensuring current and complete immunization of their children (see Chapter 14 for additional information about immunizations). Table 45-1 gives specific information about each of the childhood infectious diseases and other commonly known viral and bacterial infections.

Cytomegalovirus Infection

Etiology

Cytomegalovirus (CMV) infection, cytomegalic inclusion disease (CID), cytomegaly, and salivary gland disease are synonymous. Cytomegalovirus belongs to a unique group of viruses, the herpes family, in which the primary infection is followed by a latent form that may reactivate in the body at any time. All ages may be affected by CMV, beginning even before birth. It is the most common cause of intrauterine infection. Most infections take place during the childbearing years, between 15 and 35.

There are three types of CMV infections: congenital, perinatal, and other acquired forms. The congenital form is caused by a primary infection in the mother. The virus crosses the placenta and infects the fetus, causing inflammation and necrosis, especially of the central nervous system, resulting in brain damage and mental deficiency. Fetuses of mothers infected during the second trimester are most at risk for developing symptoms.

Clinical Manifestations

Ninety per cent of congenitally infected infants are healthy and asymptomatic at birth. The other 10 per cent of these infants exhibit symptoms. A small percentage of these infants present with "classic" newborn cytomegalic inclusion disease. Perinatally acquired CMV is transmitted at birth through contact with maternal cervical secretions, and the infant experiences mild transient illness. Other acquired forms of the disease are generally asymptomatic. During the early months of life the infection may be acquired from

Text continues on page 1646

Table 45-1. Characteristics of Commonly Known Infectious Diseases

Disease (Agent)	Clinical Manifestations
CHICKENPOX (Herpesvirus; also called varicella-zoster) **Epidemiology:** Highly contagious *Transmission:* contact, air *Incubation:* 10–21 days *Infectious period:* From 1–2 days before lesions appear until all lesions are crusted (usually 5–6 days from onset) (see Fig. 45–1) *Most common:* Late winter, early spring *Immunity:* Usually lifelong after illness but second occurrences have been reported	*Prodromal:* Low-grade fever, malaise, anorexia, occasionally accompanied by a scarlet uniform rash *Acute phase:* Lesions begin as red maculopapular rash, which turns almost immediately to vesicles, each on an erythematous base. Vesicles ooze and crust. New crops of vesicles continue to form for 3–5 days, spreading from the trunk to the extremities. *Pruritus* is an outstanding symptom. Mucous membranes of the mouth and genitalia may be involved, and these lesions may be quite painful. Disease course varies from mild with a few lesions to severe with hundreds of lesions and a high fever *Immunosuppressed child:* Lesions may continue to erupt with fever of up to 40.5°C (105°F) up to 7–10 days from onset. The mortality rate in progressive varicella is 20 per cent.
HERPES ZOSTER (Herpesvirus hominis; also called shingles) A latent infection produced by same virus that causes chickenpox **Epidemiology:** *Transmission:* Contact, air *Incubation:* 4–24 days; person with shingles may give chickenpox to someone who has never had the disease *Infectious period:* As for chickenpox *Immunity:* Second attacks occur in fewer than 1%	*Prodromal:* Pain and itching along ganglion lines for 1–5 days before lesions erupt. Pain is burning, stabbing, worse at night and with movement *Acute phase:* Lesions located along the ganglion of peripheral nerve roots, most commonly in the thoracic area. Always unilateral eruption that does not cross midline. Successive crops of vesicles for 1–4 (or up to 7) days. Eruptions clear in 7–14 days
MUMPS (Paramyxovirus; also called parotitis) **Epidemiology:** Only slightly less contagious than rubella and measles *Transmission:* Contact, air, fomites* contaminated by saliva, possibly urine *Incubation:* 12–22 days (usually 16–18 days) *Most common:* Late winter, early spring *Immunity:* Considered lifelong from clinical or subclinical infection, although rarely a second case occurs	*Prodromal:* Rare, but possibly fever, muscular pain, headache, malaise *Acute phase:* Unilateral or bilateral swelling of parotid glands (lymphocyte infiltration of glands with cell necrosis and blockage of openings) and/or other salivary glands; ⅔ of cases symptomatic; ⅓ subclinical. Swelling peaks by 3rd day, returns to normal by 10th day. Chewing and sour liquids or foods aggravate the earache-like pain
RUBELLA (Rubivirus; also called 3-day measles, German measles) **Epidemiology:** *Transmission:* Air, transplacental *Incubation:* 14–21 days *Infectious period:* From up to 7 days before rash until rash disappears *Immunity:* Permanent immunity from disease or vaccine	*Prodromal:* Young children: none, except for possible lymphadenopathy Older children: lymphadenoapthy, low-grade fever, anorexia, mild conjunctivitis, runny nose, sore throat *Acute phase:* Begins on face and hairline and as it clears moves to trunk, then extremities. Also pinpoint rose-red spots on soft palate. Rosy red, dry, maculopapular rash, diffuse configuration, lasts 3 days
MEASLES, Rubeola (Paramyxovirus; also called hard measles, red measles, regular measles) **Epidemiology:** *Transmission:* Air, hand-to-nose after direct contact *Incubation:* 8–12 days *Infectious period:* From 7 days after exposure until 5 days after rash appears *Immunity:* Permanent from vaccine or disease	*Prodromal:* Fever and cold-like symptoms, conjunctivitis, photophobia, nasal congestion, hacky cough. Koplik spots (white spots circumscribed in red, opposite lower molars). Fever increases to about 39.5°C (103°F) *Acute phase:* Rash begins as fever peaks, fever then subsides. Dark red, dry, maculopapular rash begins behind ears and at hairline and spreads from head to feet. Lasts 10–15 days. Rash turns brown and scaly after 5–6 days. Young children may have associated vomiting, diarrhea or otitis media

* Fomites are any substances to which infectious agents adhere; e.g., articles of personal grooming, clothing, linens, and so forth.

Complications	Nursing Strategies for Family Teaching	Prevention
Secondary skin infection with staphylococcus or streptococcus, especially with poor hygiene and increased temperature and humidity. CNS: postinfectious encephalitis most common, also aseptic meningitis, Reye syndrome **Therapeutic Management:** Supportive: antihistamines, antipruritics, mild analgesia (Tylenol, *not* ASA), calamine lotion. Acyclovir for immunosuppressed child	Avoid use of aspirin or aspirin-containing products (because of link with Reye syndrome). Cut nails to decrease irritation from scratching. Cool sponge bath without soap; light, loose-fitting clothing; fluids for fever. Avoid cornstarch soaks (may increase chance for infection). May use paste of baking soda and water on lesions to control itching. Alert family that premature removal of crusts by scratching may cause permanent scars. Frequent handwashing by child and caregiver. Avoid excessive contact with siblings; successive cases in the same family may be more severe because of overwhelming exposure to virus	Vaccine now available for children at high risk (e.g., children with leukemia). Used with caution in general population because of risk of latent disease and untoward effects of the herpesvirus in later life. Passive immunity with IM immune serum globulin (ISG) or zoster immune globulin (ZIG) within 3 days after exposure to children at high risk for complication or fatality. Isolation of high-risk children from known cases
Rare. Encephalitis, secondary bacterial infection. **Therapeutic Management:** As for chickenpox. May employ soaks of Burow solution to aid drying of lesions. Analgesia for pain. Acyclovir or vidarabine to retard viral activity.	Avoid use of aspirin. Cut nails to decrease irritation from scratching. Frequent handwashing. Attention to comfort—both pharmacologic and nonpharmacologic; plan diversion for child whose mobility is limited by zoster lesions	Isolate from those who have not had varicella
Meningoencephalitis; orchitis, epididymitis (especially in adolescents) with atrophy of the affected testes occurring in 30–40%, impaired fertility in 13%; pancreatitis, nephritis; thyroiditis; myocarditis; mastitis, deafness; visual complications, arthritis **Therapeutic Management:** Symptomatic	Liquid or soft bland diet as tolerated; bed rest with testicular support for orchitis. Tylenol for pain. Warm or cold compresses for swelling, whichever increases comfort.	Vaccine (with measles, rubella; MMR) given at or after 15 mo of age. Permanent immunity with vaccine or disease, whether or not disease symptomatic
Postinfectious encephalitis, arthritis, thrombocytopenia. Virus crosses placenta in pregnancy causing birth defects, especially if mother exposed in first trimester. Congenital rubella may lead to deafness, visual anomalies, congenital heart defects, musculoskeletal defects, CNS anomalies, immunologic defects **Therapeutic Management:** Supportive	Self-limiting activity, Tylenol for fever or headache	Vaccine (with mumps, rubeola; MMR) at or after 15 mo of age. *Isolate from pregnant females*
Otitis media, laryngotracheitis, pneumonia, encephalitis, appendicitis **Therapeutic Management:** Supportive for uncomplicated cases: Tylenol, antitussives	Bed rest or quiet activities as tolerated during febrile period, then very gradual return to normal activity. Increased fluids during fever, sponge baths for comfort, room humidification for cough, dimly lit room or sunglasses for photophobia, cleanse eyes to remove crusts, discourage rubbing of eyes, pharmacologic and nonpharmacologic comfort measures, diversionary activities	Vaccine (with rubella, mumps; MMR) at or after 15 mo of age

continued

Table 45-1 *(continued)*

Disease (Agent)	Clinical Manifestations
ROSEOLA INFANTUM (numerous viruses; also called exanthem subitum, pseudorubella, exanthem criticum, sixth disease, 3-day fever) **Epidemiology:** Most cases in children 6–18 mo of age *Incubation:* Unknown *Infectious period:* Unknown	Sudden onset high fever—39.4–41.2°C (103–106°F), possibly with slight irritability and mild cold-like symptoms. Fever falls rapidly on the 3rd–4th day and a macular or maculopapular rash appears on the trunk, spreading to the rest of the body. Rash fades within 24 hr
ERYTHEMA INFECTIOSUM (Human parvovirus; also called fifth disease) **Epidemiology:** *Transmission:* Air *Incubation:* 7–28 days (commonly 16 days) *Infectious period:* Uncertain; probably only during prodrome; no longer infectious when rash appears, therefore isolation not required	*Prodromal:* headache, chills, muscle aches, malaise, then free of symptoms for about 7 days before acute phase *Acute phase:* 3 rash stages. Stage 1 rash: bright red cheeks (slapped cheek appearance) with circumoral pallor; fades in 1–4 days. Stage 2 rash: red, symmetrical, maculopapular; begins 1 day after stage 1 rash disappears. Starts on trunk, then extremities and buttocks. Lasts 2–40 days (average 11 days). Frequently pruritic; headaches common. Stage 3 rash: periodic recurrence, especially with exercise, environmental temperatures, emotional upset, or skin irritation. Fades from center in lacy appearance
PERTUSSIS (*Bordetella pertussis;* also called whooping cough) **Epidemiology:** Highly contagious *Transmission:* Air, direct contact with nasopharyngeal secretions, contact with contaminated fomites *Incubation:* 6–20 days (average, 7 days) *Infectious period:* From catarrhal stage through the 4th wk *Immunity:* Vaccine provides limited immunity (wanes with age); antibody for pertussis does not cross placenta—newborn has no protection; permanent immunity with disease	*Catarrhal stage:* Lasts 1–2 wk. URI-like symptoms, headache, low-grade fever, sneezing, irritating cough, anorexia *Paroxysmal stage:* Lasts 4–6 wk. Cough worsens, developing to spasms and ends with prolonged inspiration (crowing or "whoop" sound). Cough spasm often followed by vomiting of large amounts of thick, stringy mucus; may appear to be strangling during paroxysm. Paroxysms initially occur several times per hour, decrease to 3–4 per day. Attacks triggered by yawning, sneezing, eating, drinking, exertion. *Not* all children will have whoop-type cough. Young infants in particular tend not to *Convalescent stage:* Lasts 1–2 wk, although cough may persist for months. Any intercurrent respiratory infections may result in cough, vomiting. Cough gradually decreases, vomiting stops, appetite and strength return
DIPHTHERIA *(Corynebacterium diphtheriae)* **Epidemiology:** Transmission: Air, direct contact *Incubation:* 1–6 days *Infectious period:* 2–4 wk without therapy, 1–2 days after start of therapy; until child no longer harbors organism (determined by 3 consecutive negative cultures) *Immunity:* Vaccine may not always give complete protection; disease gives immunity for 50% of children for 1 yr or more, but immunization needed after recovery	Depends on site of diphtheritic membrane: *Nasal:* Most common in infants. Mild cold-like symptoms, few systemic signs. Nasal discharge becomes serosanguineous, then mucopurulent, excoriates upper lip. Foul odor; white membrane on nasal septum *Tonsillar/pharyngeal:* Initially anorexia, malaise, low-grade fever, pharyngitis. White or gray adherent membrane covers tonsils, pharyngeal surfaces, possibly into larynx, trachea; bleeding results if membrane disturbed; possible cervical lymphadenopathy. In mild cases membrane sloughs in 7–10 days followed by recovery. In severe cases cardiopulmonary collapse may occur *Cutaneous:* Ulcerative skin lesions on a membranous base

Complications	Nursing Strategies for Family Teaching	Prevention
Febrile seizures, rarely: encephalitis, hemiplegia, permanent paresis, mental retardation **Therapeutic Management:** No specific treatment. Tylenol for fever	Often child not diagnosed until fever crisis is over and rash beginning. If seen at this time, reassure parent that the rash will fade quickly and child will soon feel well. If seen during febrile period teach regarding temperature measurement and methods to safely lower temperature	None at present because of multiple viruses linked to cause
Arthralgia to arthritis (less than 10% of children), transient hemolytic anemia, encephalitis **Therapeutic Management:** No specific treatment, analgesics for joint involvement	Parents may need help in explaining disease to school personnel. School attendance allowed. Saline baths or calamine lotion for pruritus, Tylenol for joint aches or headache. Prepare family for prolonged nature of rash and recurrence in stage 3	No vaccine available
Pneumonia responsible for >90% of deaths from pertussis in children < 3 yr old. Otitis media, seizures, ulcer of the frenulum of the tongue, epistaxis, melena, subconjunctival hemorrhages, rupture of the diaphragm, umbilical or inguinal hernia, rectal prolapse, dehydration, CNS and nutritional disturbances **Therapeutic Management:** Erythromycin to shorten period of communicability (to 3–4 days from start of administration). Supportive care with oxygen, hospitalization in early stages	During hospitalization. *Maintain patent airway* through gentle suction during paroxysms; monitor respiratory and cardiac effort per noninvasive oxygen monitor and cardiorespiratory monitor. *Maintain hydration* via PO and IV fluids as ordered; monitor urine specific gravity, skin color and turgor. Small, frequent feedings; often best tolerated immediately after a vomiting episode. *Conserve energy:* cool room with good ventilation, antipyretics and decreased clothing to control fever; calm, supportive manner to comfort child during paroxysms; plan for uninterrupted naps when possible; plan care to avoid tiring infant/child. *Monitor for signs of pneumonia. Support family in home care during convalescent stage.* • Teach to use and clean room humidifier; keep room free of dust, smoke, temperature extremes • Encourage tepid liquids often; small frequent feedings after vomiting • Teach to suction as necessary to relieve strangling effects of mucous expectoration during paroxysms • Teach signs of impending respiratory distress (see p 1178). • Teach signs of pneumonia, otitis media. Encourage follow-up care	Vaccine (with diphtheria, tetanus; DPT). Despite risk of neurologic sequelae from vaccine, children are at *much* greater risk for neurologic damage, pneumonia, and death if they contract the disease. Siblings and others <7 yr exposed to disease who have not completed 4 doses of DPT or who have not received DPT within 3 yr of exposure should receive DPT vaccine; oral erythromycin may also be given to close contacts
Respiratory obstruction leading to death, myocarditis, neurologic complications, paralysis of eye muscles or diaphragm, gastritis, hepatitis, nephritis **Therapeutic Management:** Intravenous antitoxin to neutralize free toxins; skin or conjunctival test for sensitivity to horse serum must precede administration. Antibiotics; bed rest for 2–3 wk to reduce risk of myocarditis; tracheostomy for laryngeal obstruction	Initial care will be in the hospital. Maintain patent airway. Maintain hydration by PO and IV fluids as ordered. High-calorie liquid or soft diet. Suction excess secretions. Monitor quality of voice, gag reflex. Gavage feedings for pharyngeal or palatal paralysis. Place on cardiorespiratory monitor; auscultate chest regularly. Alert parents to need for follow-up care and regular immunizations after recovery	Vaccine (given with pertussis and tetanus; DPT). No permanent immunity; must be maintained through boosters (Td) at 10-yr intervals

Continued

Table 45-1 *(continued)*

Disease (Agent)	Clinical Manifestations
TETANUS *(Clostridium tetani)* *C. tetani* is a spore-forming bacillus. Spores are harmless until body conditions are right for their conversion to vegetative forms that multiply. The clinical symptoms are caused by toxins from the vegetative cells **Epidemiology:** *Transmission:* Introduced into an area of injury from contaminated soil or intestinal contents *Incubation:* 1 day to several months (commonly 3–21 days) *Immunity:* Vaccine gives time-limited immunity; second attacks after disease are rare	Classically trismus (lockjaw), spasm of the masticatory muscles with difficulty opening the jaw. Also irritability, restlessness, stiff neck, dysphagia, rigidity of the abdominal or thoracic muscles. Tonic spasms may also involve the neck, back, and abdomen, leading to opisthotonus. Generalized seizures triggered by very slight external stimuli
POLIOMYELITIS (Poliovirus) **Epidemiology:** *Transmission:* Air, contact (fecal-oral) *Incubation:* 14–21 days *Infectious period:* Virus in throat for 1 wk after onset, in feces intermittently for 3–4 wk	*Abortive type:* Brief febrile illness—fever seldom >39.5°C (103°F) along with one or more of the following: malaise, anorexia, nausea, vomiting, headache, sore throat, constipation, abdominal pain *Nonparalytic type:* As for abortive, but headache, nausea, becoming more intense with muscle stiffness of neck, trunk, limbs. Progresses to nuchal and spinal rigidity, changes in reflexes *Paralytic type:* As for nonparalytic, plus weakness of one or more skeletal or cranial muscle groups progressing to paralysis, including paralysis of bowel and bladder muscles and paresis of respiratory muscles. Vital signs reflect damage to medullary centers
SCARLET FEVER (Group A beta hemolytic streptococcus; also called scarletina and septic sore throat) **Epidemiology:** *Transmission:* Air, direct contact *Incubation:* 1–7 days (average, 3 days) *Infectious period:* Variable, until 1–2 days after start of therapy	Abrupt high fever, abdominal pain, vomiting, sore throat, headache, malaise. In early days, tongue has white coat through which edematous red papillae project (white strawberry tongue); white coat sloughs, leaving prominent papillae (strawberry tongue). Rash appears within 12–48 hr of onset: red, papular; appears first in axillae, groin, neck, but then becomes generalized; fades on pressure, almost always leads to desquamation. Flaking begins on face, spreads to entire body
INFLUENZA (Orthomyxoviruses of 3 types—A, B, C—and multiple subtypes) **Epidemiology:** *Transmission:* Air, direct or indirect contact *Incubation:* 1–7 days (commonly 2–3 days) *Infectious Period:* Influenza A—6 days before onset of symptoms until 1 wk after onset Influenza B—1 day before onset of symptoms to 2 wk after recovery *Immunity:* Persists *for that type of virus* for several years after natural infection in older children but is probably of shorter duration in infants and young children. Immunity from vaccine is time-limited and restricted to viruses in the vaccine	*Influenza A:* Sudden onset with systemic symptoms of fever (>38.9°C or 102°F) and chills, headache, anorexia, malaise, muscle aches, cervical adenopathy. Respiratory symptoms of cough, runny nose, sore throat, sputum production, hoarseness; sometimes accompanied by abdominal pain, vomiting, nausea, diarrhea *Influenzas B and C:* Similar signs and symptoms but less severe and of shorter duration

(Compiled from Behrman and Vaughan, 1987; Feigin and Cherry, 1987; Farrar and Lambert, 1984; Lookingbill and Marks, 1986.)

Complications	Nursing Strategies for Family Teaching	Prevention
Lethal glottal and laryngeal spasms, hyperpyrexia, tachycardia, hypotension, cardiac arrest, death in 45 to 55% **Therapeutic Management:** Administration of tetanus antitoxin; surgical removal of the site of entry of the organism (to eliminate the toxin "factory"); sedatives, muscle relaxants, neuromuscular blocking agents, penicillin; close monitoring of fluid, electrolyte, and calorie balance	Because of the extremely serious nature of this disease the child will be cared for in an ICU. Nursing strategies, for the nurse generalist, pertain to prevention	Vaccine(given with diphtheria and pertussis; DPT) as a basic series in childhood with follow-up boosters, and every 10 yr in the adult. ***The importance of vaccination is underscored by the fact that the portal of entry in 80% of cases is an insignificant wound!*** The environment of the tissue is optimal for tetanus to develop in the following wounds: burns, injuries induced by blank cartridges, deep punctures, furunculosis, dental extraction, embedded splinters, decubitus ulcers, hypodermic injections, compound fractures complicated by chronic active osteomyelitis
Paralytic Polio: Intestinal erosion, hypertension, cardiac irregularities, acute pulmonary edema, pulmonary embolism, skeletal decalcification, renal calculi **Therapeutic Management:** *Abortive:* Supportive treatment at home with analgesics, sedatives, bed rest until fever is normal for several days. Antibiotics and immune globulins not effective. Careful follow-up *Nonparalytic:* As for abortive *Paralytic:* Hospitalization with attention to airway maintenance, maintenance of joint and muscle function, bowel and bladder programs	*Abortive:* Teach regarding use of analgesics, nutritious diet, emphasize need for bed rest with very gradual return to activity; need for follow-up care *Nonparalytic:* As for abortive with addition of application of hot packs or warm tub baths for stiff muscles, firm bed, footboard *Paralytic:* In hospital: total care as for paralysis from other causes (see Chapter 46)	Vaccine (OPV)
Extension of streptococcus: otitis media, pneumonia, peritonsillar abscess, rheumatic fever, acute glomerulonephritis **Therapeutic Management:** Hospitalization for IV penicillin; bed rest during febrile stage, analgesics for comfort	Initial care in hospital. Maintain IV site to ensure optimal blood level of antibiotic. Monitor fever, antipyretics as needed. Monitor heart sounds. Maintain bedrest; provide diversion. Cool mist humidification; liquid or soft diet for sore throat. Alert family to need for follow-up care. Instruct regarding signs and symptoms of complications	Throat cultures for suspected strep; administration of *all* of antibiotic ordered
Pneumonia, otitis media, sinusitis most common. Also acute myositis, Reye syndrome, neurologic disease, pericarditis, myocarditis, glomerulonephritis, sudden death **Therapeutic Management:** Symptomatic: bed rest, adequate oral hydration, control of fever and muscle aches with Tylenol, nasal decongestants, humidified air, cough suppressants for persistent cough during convalescence	Teach caregiver to take the child's temperature and appropriate methods for temperature control. Talk with the family about the amount of fluid that should be ingested in 24 hr and suggest age-appropriate measures to encourage this consumption. Alert them to signs of dehydration (e.g., significant decrease in number of wet diapers). Teach signs and symptoms of impending airway obstruction so that family may seek medical assistance before an emergency arises. Teach caregiver how to suction nares with bulb syringe to relieve mucus plugging in infant and small child. Encourage follow-up care to rule out secondary infection or other complications	Vaccine for high-risk children (chronic illness or immunosuppression). Keep child away from crowds during flu season

the mother's breast milk. Table 45-2 lists the clinical manifestations and prognosis of CMV.

Diagnosis

Both congenitally infected infants and those affected perinatally or postnatally excrete large amounts of the virus in the throat and urine, often for many months or years. Diagnosis of CMV depends on isolating the virus from the throat, body fluids, or blood. In the congenitally infected neonate, an elevated IgM (specific CMV antibody) correlates with active disease. In acquired CMV, significantly rising antibody titers are usually sufficient for diagnosis.

Other diagnostic signs that may be found on surface appraisal or in monitoring the child's health status include a petechial rash on the first day after birth, failure to thrive, or repeated respiratory infection with a high incidence of chronic interstitial pneumonia during infancy.

Therapeutic Management

No effective treatment of CMV is known; therefore, preventive measures must be stressed. Recent attempts have been made to treat affected neonates with cytosine arabinoside and adenine arabinoside (metabolic inhibitors that interfere with in vitro synthesis of CMV), and although urinary excretion of the virus was suppressed, the long-term beneficial effects need further study before such drugs can become widely available. Treatment with interferon inducers and various antiviral agents has to date produced minimal effects.

A live vaccine is under active investigation. Research suggests that it is possible to prepare a vaccine that is well tolerated and antigenic and that results in both neutralizing and complement-fixing antibodies. Further work needs to be undertaken specifically in relation to mothers and infants. The safety of widescale use of this vaccine has not been established. Whether the vaccine would increase the potential for neoplastic disease and increase susceptibility to infection, and whether giving the vaccine to pregnant women will also afford immunity to the fetus are questions that remain unanswered.

Strategies for Nursing Care

During the hospitalization of the child with CMV, isolation procedures are instituted, since infants excrete the virus in saliva for approximately 6 months and in urine for 4 months or more. The degree of thoroughness of isolation practices is controversial, varying from careful handwashing to strict isolation. Pregnant women and also children are prohibited from rooms as a preventive measure.

Since the disease seems to occur more commonly in conditions of poor sanitation and overcrowding, the nurse may help families to ensure adequate sanitation.

Complications of congenital CMV often result in spastic quadriplegia, mental retardation, obstructive hydrocephalus, or acute respiratory problems. There-

Table 45-2. Description of Cytomegalovirus Infections

Classification			Clinical Manifestations	Prognosis
Congenital		-90% asymptomatic	Normal development	Occasional mental retardation
	10%	Symptomatic	Transient jaundice Purpura Respiratory illness Hepatosplenomegaly Failure to thrive	High recovery Some with brain damage and mental retardation
		Symptomatic Classic	Severe jaundice Thrombocytopenia Chorioretinitis Hepatosplenomegaly Pneumonia Encephalitis	High mortality Survivors have severe brain damage, mental retardation, microcephaly
Acquired		Perinatal	Mild transient illness with symptoms similar to those of congenital symptomatic CMV	CNS damage may become evident at school entry
		Neonatal and early childhood	Asymptomatic Occasionally: Respiratory symptoms → pneumonia Hepatosplenomegaly Petechial rash	CNS damage may become evident at school entry
		Late childhood and adult	Mononucleosis-type symptoms	

fore, management of the child must be individualized and long term. The nurse is especially helpful in coordinating the efforts of the health team and community services involved. Most parental concerns result from the child's failure to attain developmental milestones. Support, understanding and proper referral to agencies designed to work with children with development delays are important.

The families of children with CMV may be socially isolated due to the stigma attached to the child who will be excreting the virus over many months. Although the virus is believed to be contagious only on intimate contact, encouraging good hygiene and proper disposal of diapers is imperative in such families. Discussing the rationale for protection of pregnant women and of children may alleviate anxieties.

Infectious Mononucleosis

Infectious mononucleosis is a viral disease often attributed to the dating years. In actuality, it can occur at any age, although rarely before age 2 or after age 40, when most adults are immune. The overall incidence is 50 : 100,000 population per year, rising to about 1 : 1000 per year in adolescents and young adults (Plotkin and Henle, 1987).

Etiology

Infectious mononucleosis is caused primarily by the Epstein-Barr virus (EBV), a member of the herpesvirus group. In Western countries 60 to 80 per cent of ado lescents are seropositive for EBV, the more affluent being somewhat less likely to have been exposed. Seroconversion increases with age until in the United States nearly all adults test positive for the virus (Plotkin and Henle, 1987). Other infectious agents associated with mononucleosis include cytomegalovirus, *Toxoplasma gondii,* adenoviruses, rubella, and hepatitis A virus (Brown, 1987).

Clinical Manifestations

The cardinal symptoms of infectious mononucleosis are fever, sore throat, malaise, and fatigue, accompanied by tonsillitis and lymphadenopathy. Frequently there is a 2- to 5-day prodromal period of malaise and fatigue, with or without fever. Fever in the acute phase may be quite high but usually resolves within 2 weeks. Pain may be significant, owing to tonsillitis and pressure from enlarged lymph glands. Swallowing may be impaired, and the adolescent and family caregivers should be alerted to the possibility of pharyngeal occlusion so that they will seek care before a medical emergency arises. Splenomegaly develops in about 50 per cent of cases and hepatomegaly in about 10 per cent (Brown, 1987). Organomegaly usually resolves within 3 months. Other possible clinical signs include a rash, petechiae of the soft palate, bilateral edema of the eyelids, and jaundice. Neurologic complications and aplastic anemia are potential sequelae.

A particularly unpleasant aspect of mononucleosis may be the development of acute ulcerative gingivitis (Vincent infection). The gum margins become swollen with areas of bacterial invasion and necrosis. The breath takes on a persistently fetid odor. Treatment of this infection may be complicated by the contraindication of antibiotics during mononucleosis, especially ampicillin, which causes a rash in persons with mononucleosis.

Diagnostic Assessment and Therapeutic Management

Laboratory analysis usually reveals lymphocytosis (at least 50 per cent lymphocytes), a mild to moderate rise in liver enzymes, and a positive mononucleosis test (e.g, Mono-Test, Mono-Diff, Mono-Spot).

Treatment is primarily supportive, as no effective chemotherapeutic agent has been found other than interferon, which is scarce and very costly. Adenine arabinoside has little activity against EBV, and acyclovir is typically reserved for immunosuppressed patients because it is effective only in very high concentrations (Brown, 1987). Several experimental drugs are currently being tested for their clinical efficiency and safety for use against the Epstein-Barr virus.

Strategies for Nursing Care

The young person may be diagnosed in the prodromal phase of the disease and leave the clinic or physician's office feeling no worse than if he or she had a common virus. The onset of the acute phase of the disease may proceed in this same mild fashion, with only moderate curtailment of activities necessary, or it may result in severe prostration. The adolescent and the family should be alerted to the latter possibility. The severely affected young person should observe bed rest during the acute phase, and will often need supportive care from family members. In case of a severely sore throat, an anesthetic gargle can be prescribed to increase comfort. Tylenol may also help for sore throat, fever, and muscle aches.

Fluid intake must be preserved despite the sore throat to offset the dehydrating effects of the fever. Bland, thin liquids or puddings may be best tolerated. Fluid intake should be nutritious as well because significant weight loss may occur from tissue catabolism in relation to the virus.

Once the acute phase resolves, adolescents will need guidance about their return to normal activities. School attendance on a half-day basis is one way to ease back into activities until the student feels stronger. Vigorous athletic activities and contact sports should be avoided until organomegaly has resolved. Whereas recovery may be prompt for some individuals, it is not unusual for a return to full vigor to require several months. If this should be the case, adolescents may need repeated support and encouragement that they will indeed recover.

Hepatitis

Hepatitis (inflammation of the liver) is a viral disease of three distinct types: hepatitis A, hepatitis B, and non A, non B hepatitis. In the United States there are estimated to be 70,000 cases of hepatitis yearly (Brunell, 1987).

Hepatitis A and hepatitis B were for a long time referred to as infectious hepatitis and serum hepatitis, respectively, because of a recognized oral-fecal mode of transmission in A and parenteral mode of transmission in B. However, research has shown that both types can be transmitted parenterally and nonparenterally so that the names serum hepatitis and infectious hepatitis are no longer meaningful. Hepatitis A refers to clinical disease with a short incubation period and hepatitis B to clinical disease with a long incubation period. Non A, non B hepatitis refers to clinical disease resembling hepatitis B, but in which tests do not confirm hepatitis A or B antigens. Table 45-3 summarizes the similarities and differences in characteristics of each of the hepatitis forms.

Pathophysiology and Clinical Manifestations

Characteristic liver changes in hepatitis are liver cell damage, spotty necrosis, and inflammatory infiltrate. The clinical course of hepatitis varies considerably from one infected person to another. In more than 50 per cent of cases the disease is subclinical or very mild (Aach, 1987). Children and young adults are particularly likely to have a subclinical response. In a small number of individuals, however, hepatitis is severe, develops rapidly, and may lead to death from liver failure.

Ordinarily hepatitis is a self-limiting illness, but in some cases, it becomes chronic. Both the type of hepatitis and the age of infection play a part in the predilection to chronic hepatitis (see Table 45-3, which compares the three types). Infants who contract hepatitis B in the first 12 months of life have about an 80 per cent

Table 45-3. Characteristics of Hepatitis A, Hepatitis B, and Non A, Non B Hepatitis

Characteristic	Hepatitis A (Short-Incubation Hepatitis)	Hepatitis B (Long-Incubation Hepatitis)	Non-A, Non-B Hepatitis
Agent	Hepatitis A virus (HAV virus)	Hepatitis B virus (HBV virus; HB Ag)	Unknown; more than one agent
Mode of transmission (Direct or indirect transmission possible in all 3 types)	Primarily fecal-oral secretions (stool, urine, semen, tears, menses) and in contaminated food (especially shellfish), breast milk, and water. Transmitted rarely, if at all, by blood transfusion. Virus will cross placental barrier in third trimester	Primarily parenteral route via serum, blood and blood products; also detected in saliva, semen, vaginal secretions, and even breast milk. Virus will cross placental barrier in 3rd trimester	Parenteral route (accounts for approximately 90% of post-transfusion hepatitis). Other routes suspected but not well defined. Perinatal transmission is rare
Incubation period	15–50 days	60–180 days	14–115 days
Recovery time	Average 28–30 days	Average 90 days	Average 45 days
Carrier state	No	Yes (persistence of HB_sAg† in blood for years or life)	Yes
Seasonal variation	Greatest incidence in winter; rare in summer	None	None
Pre- or post-exposure prophylaxis	IG* 80–90% effective; may cause long-lasting natural immunity	HBIG†† or IG effective for 3–4 mo; hepatitis B vaccine gives long-lasting immunity	Unknown; effectiveness of IG unproved

* IG, Immune globulin.
† HB_sAg, Hepatitis B surface antigen.
†† HBIG, Hepatitis B immune globulin.
(Adapted from Brunell, 1987; Aach, 1987.)

chance of chronic infection, whereas children from 1 to 10 years of age have a 40 per cent chance. The percentage decreases with age and is less than 10 per cent for adults (Aach, 1987).

Hepatitis A is generally considered to be a milder illness than hepatitis B or non A, non B. The clinical manifestations are indistinguishable between types, however.

Clinical (or symptomatic) hepatitis may be categorized as icteric or anicteric. The term *icteric* designates the presence of jaundice. *Anicteric* hepatitis is more frequent than the icteric type, especially among children and young adults.

The major preicteric symptoms experienced by 65 to 95 per cent of persons with clinical hepatitis are severe anorexia, lassitude, weakness, fever, headache, abdominal discomfort or pain, and nausea, often accompanied by vomiting (Aach, 1987). Other manifestations include cold-like symptoms of cough, sore throat, and runny nose, with diarrhea or constipation. Persons with the anicteric variety of hepatitis usually experience less intense symptoms for a shorter duration.

Commonly, lessening of the preicteric symptoms heralds the appearance of the icteric phase—jaundice, dark urine, and light stools. These signs correspond with increased blood bilirubin from obstruction of biliary flow and damage to liver cells. Absence of bilirubin in the bile leads to light or clay-colored (acholic) stools. Conjugated bilirubin in the urine leads to a brownish urine color. Deposition of bile pigments in the skin produces the characteristic deep yellow of jaundice and may lead to pruritis.

Jaundice deepens rapidly over a period of days and then begins to fade. Urine and stool color typically return to normal before skin color. The average duration of jaundice in children with hepatitis A who are younger than 15 years is 10 days, with full recovery within 3 weeks from the onset of jaundice. The icteric phase and recovery times are somewhat longer for hepatitis B and non A, non B.

Diagnostic Assessment

The diagnosis of hepatitis may be made upon a history of possible contact and laboratory evidence of liver damage. Direct and indirect serum bilirubin are elevated with or without jaundice. (Icteric signs do not occur until plasma bilirubin values are greater than 2 mg/dl.) The serum transaminases (SGOT and SGPT), released in response to liver damage, often exceed 1000 units, peaking about the time jaundice appears. Lactate dehydrogenase (LDH) is also elevated but offers little additional information to that provided by the transaminases. Serum alkaline phosphatase is elevated but rarely exceeds two to three times the normal value. The prothrombin time and other clotting parameters are normal unless the hepatitis is of the severe fulminating variety or malnourishment is involved.

Therapeutic Management

Management of hepatitis is supportive, usually involving care at home unless the child has severe fulminating or subacute varieties of hepatitis. Limited activity is advised although complete bed rest is not deemed necessary (Brunell, 1987). Children should not return to school until jaundice has resolved and the serum enzymes are no more than twice the upper limits of normal. Children need not be isolated from other family members but good handwashing is imperative. Parents should be cautioned about giving the child any over-the-counter medications without the physician's advice since most medication is detoxified in the liver. Adolescents should be warned to avoid alcoholic beverages during the illness and recovery period.

Household contacts of a child infected with hepatitis A will be given immune globulin (IG), which is 80 to 90 per cent effective in preventing hepatitis A if given within 2 weeks of exposure. The degree of protection IG offers for persons exposed to hepatitis B is less certain. Persons exposed to non A, non B hepatitis may be given IG as well, although the extent and duration of protection remain unclear.

Hepatitis B vaccine is recommended prophylactically for persons at high risk of exposure. Persons exposed to hepatitis B may be given hepatitis B immune globulin to provide passive protection for the current exposure, and at the same time may begin a three-dose series of hepatitis B vaccine to obtain longer lasting immunity.

If the child with hepatitis is hospitalized, isolation precautions will be part of the plan of care. Although hospital policies differ among institutions, most hospitals now observe the ***universal precautions*** recommended by the Centers for Disease Control. Under universal precautions, blood and body fluid precautions are consistently observed for ALL patients regardless of their diagnosis or blood-borne infection status. That is, blood and certain body fluids for any patient are considered potentially infectious for HIV, hepatitis B virus (HBV), and other bloodborne pathogens. (See Chapter 43, page 1592, for further discussion of universal precautions and blood and body fluid precautions.) *The implementation of universal precautions is intended to supplement, not replace, other category- or disease-specific isolation precautions.* (General isolation guidelines are discussed in Chapter 27.)

Major Nursing Diagnoses for Hepatitis

Activity intolerance, related to decreased metabolism of carbohydrates, proteins, and fats associated with liver disease

Altered nutrition: less than body requirements, related to anorexia and the increased nutrient demands associated with the infectious process
Potential altered comfort: pruritus, associated with jaundice
Potential for infection: close contacts of ill child, related to transmission of hepatitis virus in blood, urine, or feces

Strategies for Nursing Care

In uncomplicated hepatitis the majority of nursing care will involve teaching the child and family to care for the illness at home.

Limiting Activity. Although bed rest is no longer prescribed for hepatitis, limited activity is advised to decrease the metabolic workload of the diseased liver. Quiet play indoors or play confined to a sandbox or other small area outdoors can be advised to discourage running and other strenuous activities. Care at home will certainly lessen the diversionary problems that arise for hospitalized children with activity restrictions, but planning for additional quiet activities can reduce the frustration for both child and caregiver.

Optimizing Nutrient Intake. Anorexia is a major problem for children with hepatitis. When children feel ill and out of sorts and are confined to their home for several weeks, eating is one of the few things over which they have much control. When the caregiver is urged to ensure the child consumes nutritious food to help in the healing process, the stage is set for a power struggle at meal time. The nurse can be helpful in alerting the parent to the possibility of this scenario and working with the family to circumvent some of the problems.

The physician will usually prescribe a diet low in fat and high in protein for the child. The nurse can talk with the parent about foods the child likes that fit that distinction and suggest that these be offered in several small meals or snacks throughout the day rather than in normal portions. Nausea may be less a problem in the morning and breakfast may be a time when nutritious foods are better tolerated. In the long run, it is usually advisable to set the desired food before the child in small portions and then let the child choose whether or not to eat. Generally, the child's intake will be sufficient with this method as long as non-nutritious snacking is not allowed.

Relieving Pruritus. Only about one third of children with icteric hepatitis experience pruritus, but for those who do, it can be quite uncomfortable. Suggest to the family that they try cool tub baths or emollient baths (e.g., Aveeno) and apply creams such as Eucerin to the skin immediately after bathing to reduce dryness. A cool environment will reduce perspiration, which potentiates itching. Teach the child to apply firm pressure to areas that itch rather than to scratch them. Keep the child's nails short to minimize skin irritation from scratching. Administer antihistamines and antipruritic lotions as ordered. Alert the family, however, that these drugs are rarely effective by themselves and that nonpharmacologic measures should be used as well.

Preventing Spread of Infection. Depending on the type of hepatitis, the child and family should be educated about the transmission of the virus and taught to protect themselves and others. They should be provided with a box of disposable gloves and taught to use them when in contact with bodily secretions from the infected child (especially blood, urine, and feces). Family members should avoid sharing linens, drinking glasses and utensils, toothbrushes, and other personal articles. Teach the family to make a 1 : 10 solution of household bleach in water for the purpose of disinfecting contaminated surfaces. Encourage family members to follow through with appointments for administration of immune globulin and hepatitis B vaccine, as appropriate.

Nursing Strategies for Follow-Up Care in the Home or Clinic

Obtain a blood sample (as appropriate) for determination of liver enzymes.

Palpate for adenopathy, and enlarged liver and spleen. Measure temperature. Note skin color and integrity. Inquire about color of urine and stools.

Ask about the child's appetite and intake in the last 24 hours.

Ask how the child's energy compares with normal levels, and discern whether activity restrictions are being met.

Inquire as to potential signs and symptoms of hepatitis among other family members.

Encourage regular follow-up care until liver enzymes return to normal.

Rabies

Etiology

Rabies is a disease of the central nervous system that is transmitted to humans in the saliva of infected wild animals such as squirrels, skunks, and bats, as well as domestic cats and dogs. It is caused by a neurotropic virus, which travels from the peripheral nerves to the central nervous system. Preschool children are more frequently bitten by cats and dogs. They are losing their fear of animals and think of even wild animals as potential pets but do not yet understand that certain animals can transmit serious disease. Older children, particularly teens, who participate in camping or hunting are more likely to be bitten by infected wild animals. The incidence of rabies is steadily increasing in the United States.

In dogs the incubation period is 3 to 8 weeks, while in humans it is 2 to 6 weeks but may be as long as 2 years. A rabid animal does not usually behave like a healthy animal; it staggers and runs blindly and is more aggressive. It may drool and hide after biting another animal or a human, since rabid animals seek seclusion for death. A rabid animal can transmit the disease by licking abraded skin or mucosa. If the animal doing the biting has been properly immunized against rabies, it will probably not transmit the rabies virus even if it was bitten by a rabid animal.

Clinical Manifestations

The disease has three stages. The first is the *prodromal* stage, which lasts about 2 to 4 days and is characterized by itching, tingling, or burning at the area of the bite. This is followed by fever, headache, nausea, sore throat and irritability or restlessness. Increased salivation, diaphoresis and sensitivity to bright lights and noises are also evidenced during this stage.

The next stage is the excitement (or furious) stage. The child becomes increasingly excitable and apprehensive; muscle twitching and generalized convulsions occur. Throat spasms occur when the child tries to eat or drink and even when the sound of running water is heard. The name *hydrophobia* (morbid fear of water) comes from this symptom. There is also spasm of the respiratory muscles and, at times, continuous tonic convulsions. The temperature frequently is from 39.5° to 40.5°C (103° to 105°F). This stage lasts 1 to 3 days, and many patients die at this time.

If the child survives the excitement stage, the third stage, called the *paralytic,* or *terminal,* stage, occurs. There is increasing paralysis and coma, and then death. Only one documented case of a person surviving rabies has been reported, and that child was treated vigorously for each symptom before the symptom developed (Vella, 1977).

Therapeutic Management

Prevention of the disease is of major importance. Most communities have ordinances requiring immunization of pets. Leash laws should be enforced, and all stray dogs and cats should be picked up for confinement or destruction. Children should be taught early to treat pets kindly and to avoid stray or sick animals, whether tame or wild. Programs should be instituted to control wildlife population during rabies epidemics. When a child is bitten by *any animal,* tame or wild, or licked by *any unimmunized* or *wild animal,* the site should be washed immediately and flushed with copious amounts of soap and water, followed by an application of 70 per cent alcohol or povidone iodine. In an emergency, any alcoholic liquor of 86 per cent proof or greater can be used. The child should then be evaluated by a physician to determine what, if any, prophylactic treatment should be initiated. The wound should be cleaned again in the doctor's office. Suturing, if necessary, should not be done immediately, since it is believed that closing the wound may cause the virus to spread.

History taking is very important, especially if the child was alone at the time of the bite. The child is asked to describe the animal, since he or she might not know what the animal was. Keeping a picture book of animals available for the small child to pick out the kind that caused the bite can be helpful.

Children are asked to describe what they were doing when the animal bit them. Unprovoked attacks are more likely to be from rabid animals. Many children provoke animals such as cats and dogs, without realizing it, while hugging the animal or helping it to eat. A bite from a familiar animal that is healthy does not usually produce rabies; however, the parent should be sure of the animal's immunization status and the animal should be confined for 10 days to be observed for signs of rabies. If the animal is unknown, all efforts should be made to locate it. If it cannot be located or if the animal is a bat, regardless of the bat's condition, rabies treatment should be instituted. If the animal has been killed or found dead, the head should be packed in ice and sent to the state Department of Public Health or to a competent veterinarian for examination. Any time a domestic animal that has been confined develops symptoms of rabies, it should also be killed and the head sent for examination.

Rabies treatment utilizes a rabies vaccine in conjunction with rabies serum (Table 45-4). The vaccine allows the child to develop his or her own active immunity. Human diploid cell vaccine (HDCV) is now the only vaccine licensed in the United States. It replaces previous vaccines that required 14 to 21 doses. HDCV is usually given in five intramuscular doses: on the day of exposure, and at 3, 7, 14, and 28 days.

Passive immunity is provided in the form of equine antiserum or human rabies immunoglobulin. This provides protection from rabies until the body can make antibodies in response to the vaccine.

The child and parents will need substantial psychologic support and preparation to cope with the treatment as well as the gravity of the situation. Instruction should be given regarding the side effects and their relief. Reassurance should be offered as to

Table 45-4. Postexposure Antirabies Treatment Guide

Animal	Evaluation of Animal at Time of Exposure*	Treatment of Exposed Human
Wild Skunk Fox Raccoon Coyote Bat	Regard as rabid unless brain negative for rabies virus	HRIG + V†
Domestic Dogs and cats	Healthy	None‡
	Escaped (unknown)§	HRIG + V
	Rabid or suspected rabid	HRIG + V†
Other		Consult veterinary public health authorities

These recommendations are only a guide. They should be used in conjunction with knowledge of the animal species involved, circumstances of the bite or other exposure, vaccination status of the animal, and presence of rabies in the region.

V = rabies vaccine; HRIG = human rabies immune globulin.

* An exposure is considered to be a bite, a scratch with claws, or contamination of mucosal surfaces or skin that has been cut or abraded with saliva.

† Discontinue vaccine if fluorescent antibody tests of the animal are negative.

‡ Begin HRIG + V at first sign of rabies in biting dog or cat during holding period (10 days).

§ If the behavior of the animal is suspect or if rabies is constantly present in the animal community in the area.

(Modified from Public Health Service Advisory Committee Recommendations by Feigin and Cherry, 1987.)

the satisfactory results obtained by prophylactic antirabies treatment in preventing this dreaded disease.

Tuberculosis

Tuberculosis (TB) is a long-term, communicable disease caused by a bacillus, *Mycobacterium tuberculosis.* In developed countries the morbidity and mortality rates for this disease have dramatically declined in the last 50 years. However, in many countries tuberculosis remains a leading cause of death.

Children are the most vulnerable to this infection during their first 3 years of life and again in the years immediately before, during, and after puberty. Many factors have contributed to decline in the incidence of TB in children. Earlier diagnosis and treatment of infected adults, who are a primary source of infection for children, has been accomplished by comprehensive public health screening programs. These programs identify and test all known contacts of people diagnosed with active tuberculosis. Another important factor in declining incidence has been the discovery and use of new, effective antituberculin drugs. Public health nurses making field visits to patients' homes have succeeded in effecting an increased compliance with drug therapy. Under current laws, food handlers and all school employees are required to receive annual TB screening tests for detection of exposure to the bacillus. Routine screening by simple skin testing of babies between the ages of 12 and 18 months has also contributed to the control of tuberculosis in children.

Etiology and Pathophysiology

The usual mode of communicability is inhalation of aerosolized sputum (cough spray) from another infected human. The spread of tuberculosis *(Mycobacterium bovis)* by drinking milk from an infected cow has almost been eliminated in the United States owing to mandatory pasteurization of commercial milk.

Once a susceptible child inhales bacilli, organisms begin rapid multiplication in lung tissue, alveoli, or lymph glands draining lung areas. Following an incubation period of 2 to 10 weeks, the child will demonstrate a systemic hypersensitivity as evidenced by a positive skin test. In this test bacilli are injected immediately under the epidermis, forming a wheal. If the child has been exposed to TB and subsequently formed antibodies, a local induration will develop at the injection site. This simple skin test can be used as a screening tool to detect exposure to TB.

Most children exposed to inhaled *M. tuberculosis* mobilize a defensive inflammatory reaction. As a part of this defensive reaction, white blood cells, especially macrophages, are deployed to attack and kill invading bacilli. As further defense, the body walls off small infected areas by the formation of tubercles. Caseous or fibrous tubercles prevent the further spread of infective organisms. Unfortunately, tuberculosis bacilli possess remarkable abilities to remain dormant in this necrotic tissue for many years. If at some later date the child's resistance is decreased, bacilli may begin to multiply, causing active disease.

The term *primary lesion,* or *focus,* denotes the original site of infection. The *primary complex* includes the primary lesion and any nearby lymph nodes that have been invaded. In many children, once the primary lesion is contained in tubercles, subsequent healing will occur through a process of calcification. Although these calcified tubercles may later be visible on roentgenography, they do not indicate active disease. In older children the healed primary lesion is visualized as a scar or shadow. In both cases it is important to explain to parents the distinction between these findings and active tuberculosis.

In some children the body's defense mechanisms fail to successfully control the primary lesion. After inhalation the bacilli may continue to multiply and spread by direct extension into nearby tissues. Or the bacilli may enter the blood and circulate to other sites, setting up multiple foci of infection, resulting in *miliary tuberculosis.*

In summary, following the primary lesion, possible subsequent outcomes are (1) complete healing, (2) persistent quiescent lesions, (3) direct extension of infection at the original site, (4) spread of infection via the circulatory system to sites outside the lungs, or (5) possible reactivation of the lesion at a later date should the patient become debilitated.

Clinical Manifestations and Diagnostic Assessment

The communicability of TB is increased by conditions of poverty and crowding, which foster poor hygiene. Factors such as malnutrition and fatigue can lower resistance to tuberculosis. There is a higher incidence of TB among nonwhite and Indian Americans and in large urban poverty areas that house transient peoples arriving from areas in which TB is widely disseminated.

In assessing whether a child is at risk for TB, the nurse must recognize that children are usually infected by adults with progressive cavitary lesions. These adults discharge droplets containing infective organisms into the air. Droplet residue remains in the air for long periods of time. However, prolonged contact is usually necessary before a child develops active disease.

Periodic testing of children to determine whether they have been exposed can be done by the nurse using any one of several skin tests (see Chapter 14 for a discussion of tuberculosis skin testing).

If a positive skin test results from the screening, the nurse may assume the major responsibility for explaining the significance of a positive skin test to parents and to the child. At this time the nurse obtains a health history for each family member in an attempt to identify the source of the infection. All contacts are listed so that they may be screened also. The nurse provides information about further diagnostic measures and arranges for treatment. Family members need counseling as well as information. Many adults view TB not only as a serious threat to life but also as a threat to the integrity of their family unit.

Children with positive skin reactions receive chest roentgenographs to determine the presence and extent of active lesions. A diagnosis of active disease is documented if sputum smears show the presence of bacilli. Gastric washings to obtain swallowed sputum are sometimes done. A child may be hospitalized for this procedure; he or she receives nothing to eat during the night and until test completion. In the morning a nasogastric tube is inserted and stomach contents are lavaged and removed for microscopic examination. Obtaining sputum from a young child can be extremely difficult. Physicians often prefer to waive such tests rather than submit the child to a period of hospitalization, placing him or her on medication instead.

In some countries a BCG (bacille Calmette-Guérin) vaccination is given to produce immunity to the bacillus. This artificial immunity is effective for at least 10 years. Widespread use of BCG vaccine has not been adopted in the United States, primarily because it would eliminate skin testing as an effective case finding tool.

There is a dangerous trend away from routine TB screening. Failure to implement screening programs may result in subsequent failure in diagnosing TB in its early stages. The effect will necessarily be an increase in incidence and also an increase in serious complications such as miliary TB and TB meningitis. Such complications are largely preventable with early diagnosis and treatment.

The majority of children found to have tuberculosis have a noncomplicated pulmonary primary focus and are not infectious. The organisms are confined to a small area of the lung and the child has little or no coughing. However, if a child (usually a teenager) develops a cavitary lesion and is coughing up sputum containing bacilli or if the child has direct drainage from an infected site, he or she is a potential source of infection. Isolation precautions for all items contaminated with organisms and respiratory isolation precautions are required.

Most children will not have any symptoms and will be unaware of their tuberculosis until diagnosis. Knowing that symptoms in children are minimal, the nurse observes for low-grade fever, slight cough, history of fatigue, weight loss or anorexia. Recognizing age and risk factors can assist the nurse in case finding, but mass screening is the key to early identification.

Therapeutic Management

Management stresses four major interventions: (1) general supportive measures such as adequate rest, gradual resumption of activities, diet, prevention of other infection; (2) drug therapy; (3) emotional support; and in some cases (4) surgery.

Rest, Activity, and Diet. Ensuring that an active youth follows the treatment prescription for adequate rest can present difficulties. Fortunately, bed rest is required only when miliary TB has affected the child's weight-bearing structures. Bed rest may be desired on occasions when the child is feeling particularly ill and should be enforced during bouts of fever.

There are no restrictions on physical activities during treatment for active TB except that participation in competitive sports is discouraged. Nurses should counsel the youth and parents about the need to avoid excessive fatigue, and recommend brief rest periods during the day. Sports that do not require strenuous physical activity may appeal to youths.

A nutritionally balanced diet is also part of the treatment program. Nurses cannot assume that children are receiving an adequate diet. A diet history should be obtained by collecting a 24-hour food intake diary kept by the youth. This diary can be an effective tool for both evaluation and teaching. Infected persons usually have reduced retention and utilization of nutrients; therefore, the youth's diet should be carefully planned so that what is taken in is highly nutritious and particularly rich in foods supplying protein and calcium.

Intercurrent infections encourage the spread of tuberculous processes and retard their healing. The additional stress caused by such infections seems to suppress inflammatory response and decrease allergic responsiveness. Youths should limit their exposure to crowds and to infected persons until active disease has been controlled. This requires observant screening of family members, relatives, and friends during the period of active disease.

Drug Therapy. The American Academy of Pediatrics advocates that all infants, children, and adolescents with positive skin tests be treated with isoniazid (INH) for 12 to 18 months. When there is evidence of active tuberculosis such as demonstrable lesions on a chest roentgenograph, a combination of two antituberculosis drugs is often prescribed. Standard therapy for tuberculosis in the United States and Canada is a 9-month regimen of isoniazid and rifampin, usually supplemented in the initial phase with ethionamide, streptomycin, or pyrazinamide (Committee on Chemotherapy, 1985). Table 45-5 lists antituberculosis drugs for children.

Surgery. Whether surgical intervention is desirable depends on the site, nature, and extent of the active tuberculosis focus and the degree of compliance with and effectiveness of drug therapy. Vigorous antibiotic therapy is usually continued despite surgical removal of the involved organ or body tissue to help ensure subsequent healing.

With adequate treatment the incidence and complications of TB should continue to decline.

Strategies for Nursing Care

Offering information about the side effects of medication and the importance of faithfully taking drugs each day for the entire 12 to 18 months is a crucial nursing action. Explanation of the serious consequences of failure to take medication as prescribed is an appropri-

Table 45-5. Drug Treatment of Tuberculosis

Drug	Daily Dose (per 24 hr)	Possible Toxic Effects	Nursing Implications
Isoniazid (INH) *Route:* PO, IM or IV	10–25 mg/kg (up to 300–500 mg total) *Duration:* 6–12 mo	Peripheral neuropathy, hepatotoxicity	INH syrup in sorbitol is unstable at room temperature; must be refrigerated. Tablets may be crushed and given with food but must not be put in nursing bottle or offered in liquid because of uncertainty of amount ingested
Rifampin (RIF, RMP) *Route:* PO	10–40 mg/kg (up to 600 mg) *Duration:* 6–9 mo	Hepatotoxicity	Turns urine and tears red; will stain contact lenses; interferes with oral contraceptives
Ethionamide (ETA) *Route:* PO	10–20 mg/kg *Duration:* 9–12 mo	Gastric irritation, liver damage, peripheral neuritis	Give after meals to minimize gastric irritation
Streptomycin (STM) *Route:* IM	20 mg/kg (up to 1 gm) *Duration:* 2–3 mo	Ototoxicity, vestibular damage	Administer deep into muscle mass to minimize pain and local irritation
Pyrazinamide (PZA) *Route:* PO	20–40 mg/kg (up to 1.5 gm total) *Duration:* 2 mo	Gout, hepatotoxicity	Assess for fatigue, poor appetite, weakness, irritability, signs of anemia and prodromal signs of hepatitis
Ethambutol *Route:* PO	15–25 mg/kg *Duration:* 9–12 mo	Optic neuritis	Schedule for frequent vision checks while on therapy
Para-aminosalicylic acid (PAS) *Route:* PO	200–300 mg/kg (up to 12 gm) *Duration:* 12 mo	Gastric irritation, fever, rash, jaundice	Principal companion to INH for many years; withdrawn from market in US

(Adapted from Smith and Marquis, 1987; Loebl and Spratto, 1986.)

ate part of the education. Family members, especially parents, are sometimes upset that a child has to take medication for such a long period of time.

Other family members, especially those of the grandparents' generation, tend to remember the time when tuberculosis was greatly feared. They may have an inaccurate understanding of current treatment and prognosis, as well as incorrect opinions about diet and the amount of activity that should be permitted. If family members are to be actively involved with caring for the infected child, they must also be given information currently available about the disease and its management.

Nursing functions in regard to population screening and seeking out contacts, especially for the purpose of locating the source of the infection, have already been described. Another role of the nurse is to help implement the prescribed treatment program to prevent further spread of the disease. Teaching children and their families about the disease may serve to facilitate their adaptation. The child may not be future oriented but should still be reassured that tuberculosis will not adversely affect most of the goals he or she will eventually have.

Nurses must be willing and able to meet the physical, intellectual, and emotional-social needs of each child. Specific care measures are determined by the extent and type of tuberculosis. The plan of care must be appropriate for the child's level of understanding and development and take into consideration the child's particular coping ability. Assisting youths to assume responsibility for some of their treatment and rehabilitation goals is a nursing intervention that may ensure their cooperation.

Some youths may feel that a stigma is attached to the diagnosis and may respond by withdrawing from friends and activities. Even during the time that the initial nursing history is requested, youths may feel constrained when asked to list all their recent contacts. They may think their friends will resent being named or being exposed to this disease. If the source of the infection turns out to be one of their friends, this can cause some friction. If the source is one of the youth's own parents, the youth may experience some negative feelings toward that parent. Tuberculosis, like most other long-term illnesses, tends to increase or prolong dependency. This may be resented and contribute to the youth's feelings of discouragement.

Nurses can help the child structure outlets for energy or aggressive feelings. Support groups are becoming popular. Such groups allow children with long-term illnesses to ventilate their feelings and also provide peer support for members. Nurses need to recognize that anger is often expressed as rebellion against treatment orders or boredom and lack of interest in activities or school work. Fears about never again being completely well should be anticipated by the nurse and dealt with by frank discussion of the optimistic outcome for successful treatment of tuberculosis. Older children usually respond positively to visits from friends. Occasionally, however, a youth may try to avoid these contacts, fearing that the friends will be afraid of catching TB.

Youth with active TB are frequently treated on an outpatient basis and may return to school when their sputum is negative for bacilli. Although there is some controversy about allowing children with infective TB in school, returning them to school and their peer group as soon as is safely possible may motivate them to comply with the drug regimen. Until a return to school is feasible, specific plans to avoid disruption of intellectual achievements may include a hospital or homebound teacher.

Another stressor deserving consideration is when a child with tuberculosis is from a family whose members are not citizens. These families may fear having their child's tuberculosis reported, which may result in deportation of any family members who are illegal aliens. An ethical question must be faced by nurses and medical personnel caring for families of illegal aliens. If the family thinks that medical caregivers will report the tuberculosis to government officials and deportation will result, they will be reluctant to seek treatment, may not follow up with treatment, may fail to identify all their contacts, or may drop out of the community, thereby curtailing treatment efforts.

Parasitic Infections

Parasitic infections are much less common in the United States, because of better sanitation and the greater emphasis on hygiene, than in the Third World. However, the nurse who works with migrants from temperate climates, with immigrants to the United States (Vietnamese, Cubans) or with impoverished Americans, especially in the southern states, is likely to have regular acquaintance with parasitic infections. These infections can occur in any age group with fairly equal incidence; however, because of the greater tendencies of the toddler and preschooler to engage in spontaneous hand-to-mouth activities without handwashing, to play on the ground and go barefoot, and to investigate dirt with their hands, mouth, and feet, these younger children are at greater risk for contracting parasitic infection.

Helminthic Infections

There are a variety of helminthic infections, but this discussion will cover only three of the most common

Table 45-6. Summary of Basic Features of Three Helminthic Infections

Features	Roundworm	Tapeworm	Hookworm
Causative agent	*Ascaris lumbricoides*	*Taenia saginata* or *solium*	*Necator americanus*
Mode of transmission	Ingestion of ova in dirt contaminated by human feces. Hand contamination from infested household dust	Ingested from handling or eating infested beef or pork	Penetration of bare feet. Ingestion through contaminated water
Clinical manifestations	May be asymptomatic. Fever and malaise; restless, disturbed sleep. Abdominal distention and discomfort; vomiting. Anemia. Infested stools; steatorrhea; intestinal obstruction. Peritonitis	Varied symptoms: Abdominal cramping or pain, nervousness, insomnia, anorexia, weight loss. Sometimes asymptomatic	Severe anemia. Occult blood in feces. Abdominal colic, malnutrition, intestinal or bile duct obstruction. Intestinal mucosa and liver damage
Diagnostic findings	Positive stool culture for ova and parasites	Positive stool culture for ova and parasites	Positive stool culture for ova and parasites
Drug treatment	Piperazine or mebendazole	Niclosamide	Tetrachloroethylene or mebendazole; supplemental iron

ones: roundworm, tapeworm, and hookworm. Table 45-6 describes the main characteristics, the definitive diagnostic findings, and the primary medical treatment of each. Pinworm, another common helminth, is discussed in Chapter 41.

A careful environmental and economic history is helpful in establishing the diagnosis and in determining the most realistic approach to nursing intervention in treating and preventing recurrence of these infections. Nursing intervention in the helminthic infections requires strict adherence to enteric isolation and nursing measures to relieve accompanying symptoms. The nurse's more critical role, however, lies in educating the child and family regarding the cause of the infection and the measures that can be taken to prevent further infestations. Teaching about handwashing and personal hygiene is a first step. Community health nurse involvement to explore the family's environment and to identify the source(s) of infestation is usually essential to planning and motivating appropriate change so that the child is not reinfested. Because lack of sanitation facilities and overcrowding are frequently factors in the etiology, government involvement also becomes necessary and may require prompting from nurses and other health and social providers who can exert united political pressure.

Roundworm (Ascariasis)

Pathophysiology and Etiology. Occurring mostly in the southern United States, ascariasis can be a chronic infection of the small intestine. Ova are usually ingested from hands that have contacted contaminated dust or soil or from inadequately cleansed raw fruits or vegetables. The ova live in the small intestine and, when the larvae stage is reached, penetrate the intestinal villi and enter the portal circulation. Reaching the lungs, the larvae rise to the oropharynx and are swallowed, settling in the small intestine to mature to adult worms. Enough adult worms (measuring 15 to 35 cm × 3 to 4 mm) may accumulate to cause intestinal obstruction, or they may migrate to the appendix, causing perforation and peritonitis.

Therapeutic Management. Treatment includes anthelminthic drugs, enteric isolation, and relief of symptoms. Prevention involves careful washing of raw fruits and vegetables, regular hygiene and handwashing, and improvement of sanitation facilities or practices or both.

Tapeworm

Pathophysiology and Etiology. A nonfatal parasitic infection, tapeworm results from the ingestion of the tapeworm larvae in improperly cared for or inadequately cooked beef or pork. The encysted larva settles in the small intestine and lengthens by generating segments. It is regurgitated to the stomach and migrates from there to the brain or eye to form cysts.

Therapeutic Management. Treatment consists of oral anthelminthic medications. Prevention involves careful handwashing after handling meat and thorough cooking of the meat before eating it.

Hookworm

Pathophysiology and Etiology. This worm thrives in the warm, sandy soil of the southern United States, especially where sanitation is inadequate. Infestation occurs through penetration of the skin or by drinking contaminated water. The worms penetrate the bare feet, causing a local dermatitis that may go unnoticed. Traveling through the lymph and blood systems to the lungs, the worm migrates to the throat, is swallowed, and attaches to the walls of the small intestine. After sucking blood from the intestinal walls for several weeks, ova are produced.

Therapeutic Management. Treatment is provided for the entire family and includes an anthelminthic, a diet high in protein and iron to correct the associated anemia, and improvement of sanitary conditions. Prevention includes routine personal hygiene, avoidance of going barefoot, and adequate sanitary facilities and practices.

Major Nursing Diagnoses for Helminthic Infections

***Potential for injury: physiologic,** related to the physical effects of helminthic infestation*

***Fear/anxiety (child and family),** related to visualization of regurgitated worms or of worms or worm segments in the stool*

***Knowledge deficit,** related to:*

- *transmission of microscopic eggs or larvae*
- *methods of and need for enteric isolation practices*
- *handwashing methods and personal hygiene practices to prevent recurrence*
- *specific treatment, including anthelminthic medication and sterilization of contaminated clothing, linens, and other fomites**
- *signs and symptoms of complications (e.g., intestinal obstruction from roundworm)*

Strategies for Nursing Care

Nursing strategies in common among the parasitic diseases involve teaching the correct use of the appropriate medication, instruction regarding hygienic measures to rid fomites of parasites, and preventive education of children and adults.

Panic and anger are typical responses of parents and school officials when parasitic infection is discovered. The nurse or school nurse often receives the brunt of their reaction and must learn to accept this response syndrome without taking it personally. Preventive education as well as eduction as to the cause, transfer, and treatment of the parasitic disease prior to any major occurrence may help allay some of these negative reactions. When a diagnosis is made, feelings of guilt, shame, and uncleanliness are usually provoked in the child or the caregivers or both. Constant reassurance offered by the nurse that the child is not unclean because he or she contracted parasites and that parents cannot be responsible if their child uses other children's possessions or comes in close contact with other children during play often produces better cooperation and reduces parental aggressive responses. School or community funds may be required to make treatment possible for children of low-income families who cannot afford the costs involved in treatment. Involvement of community health nurses may be necessary if a family's cooperation is questionable or if infestation is widespread in the community.

* Fomites are inanimate objects such as combs or clothing that serve to transfer infectious organisms from one person to another.

Nursing Strategies for Follow-Up Care in the Home or Clinic

Allow the child and family to express fear, guilt, shame, anger, and other emotions related to this health crisis.

Determine family compliance with anthelminthic therapy.

Assess for effectiveness of the anthelminthic: negative stool culture for ova and parasites (roundworm, hookworm, tapeworm).

Reinforce teaching regarding avoidance of recurrence.

Pediculosis Capitis (Head Lice)

Approximately three million cases of head lice are diagnosed annually in the United States alone. Females are affected twice as often as males. Pediculosis is 20 times more prevalent in whites than in other racial groups, presumably because of the difference in the makeup of the hair shaft. The peak incidence is in preschool and early school-age youngsters, with a steady decline after that age until about sixth grade, when the incidence again rises somewhat.

Etiology

The bloodsucking louse lives its entire life (nit or egg to nymph to adult louse) on the head of the child it infests. The eggs, called *nits,* attach to the hair shaft by a cement-like substance and hatch within a week (Fig. 45-2). The hatched nymph matures into a mature louse

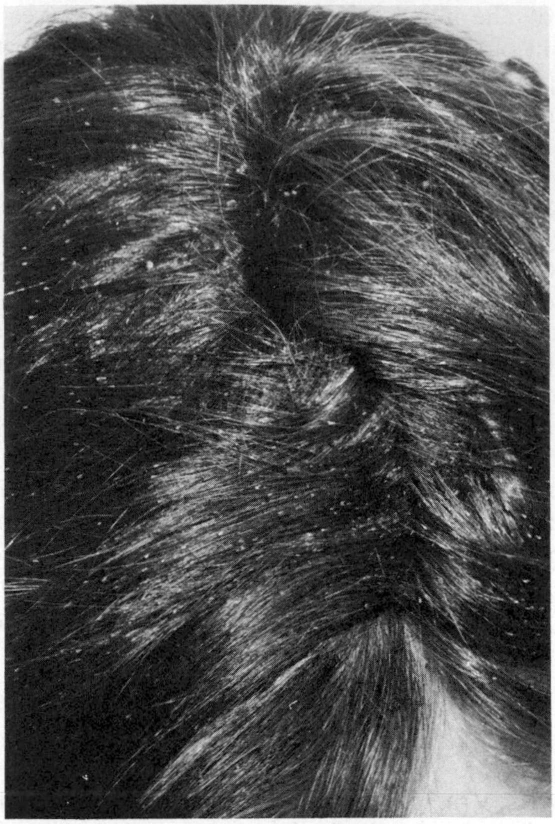

Figure 45-2. Nits on scalp hair.

in another week to 10 days and punctures the scalp with its hook-like claws to suck blood. It remains attached until it is dislodged or dies (about 1 month).

A child is infested either by direct contact or from fomites (comb, headgear, play wigs, clothing). Human head lice do not jump from head to head unless there is direct contact, nor are they transferred from one person to another in the breeze. The nits are not communicable; only the hatched louse is. These insects avoid light or perspiration.

Clinical Manifestations

A week after the child is bitten, he or she develops an allergic response evidenced by a mild fever, malaise, intense scalp itching, and enlarged cervical and occipital nodes. After a prolonged exposure, the body's sensitivity is diminished and the child becomes oblivious to the bites, i.e., asymptomatic. Occasionally a child will develop focal alopecia due to the allergic response. The nits can be seen as silvery or grayish-white, smooth and glistening specks resembling dandruff but securely attached to the hair shaft near the scalp. (Prominent locations are behind the ears and the nape of the neck.) The adult louse can be seen as a minute black speck that moves and jumps on the scalp and hair. The child's scratching during the period of allergic reactivity may result in secondary infections.

Medical Diagnosis

Diagnosis is made by identification of the nits and lice using a magnifying glass and strong direct lighting or a Wood lamp. Microscopic examination differentiates the head louse from the body louse or from aphids, which can carry other diseases. Examination of the scalp is done by parting the hair in several places (especially in the region behind the ears and nape of the neck) with two applicator sticks, moving systematically from side to side and front to back. The magnifying glass or Wood lamp is then used to inspect the exposed scalp and hair for nits and lice.

Major Nursing Diagnoses for Pediculosis Capitis

Impaired skin integrity: scalp infestation, related to direct scalp contact with live lice
Altered comfort: pruritus of scalp, related to an allergic response associated with lice bites
Potential infection: secondary, related to scratching of the scalp
Knowledge deficit: (child and family), related to:

- *corrective treatment, including medicated shampoo, nit removal, and disinfection of contaminated articles*
- *enteric isolation procedures during, and until 24 hours after, treatment*
- *expected duration of scalp pruritus*
- *prevention of recurrence, including avoiding contact with possible fomites, and keeping hair short and clean*

Strategies for Nursing Care

Addressing the Knowledge Deficit. Treatment is both preventive and corrective, necessitating that families be taught how to avoid contact with contaminated fomites as well as treatment to rid the scalp of lice. Specific teaching activities are identified throughout this section.

Preventing Scalp Infestation. Preventively, children should be taught not to exchange combs, brushes, headgear, or clothing with other children. Keeping hair short and clean may also help prevent infestation. At home and in settings in which a group of children are gathered, individually assigned hooks or lockers for wraps and possessions help decrease the incidence and spread of the louse. (The adult louse may survive 1 to 2 days away from the scalp.)

Children found to be infested should be confined at home until 24 hours after treatment is complete to minimize spread to others. It is generally recommended that all family members be treated simultaneously; often louse infestation is so widespread that entire classrooms or schools of children are encouraged to undergo treatment. (The treatment may actually be carried out at school with parental approval.)

Treating Scalp Infestation and Pruritus. Corrective treatment involves three activities: (1) using medicated shampoo, (2) disinfecting fomites, and (3) examination of contacts. Nonprescription shampoo (RID [includes a fine-tooth comb]; Triple X) or prescription shampoo with a pyrethrin or benzene derivative may be used and should be applied exactly according to directions. The child prone to eczema may have an allergic response to the shampoo. The parent or child must understand that the shampooing must be done vigorously to be effective. After the shampoo, the hair is combed (teasing backward) with a fine-tooth comb, preferably outdoors, to remove any remaining nits. All the nits must be removed. Sometimes dipping the comb in vinegar helps to loosen tightly attached nits. Itching may continue for three or four days after the insecticide shampoo, but if pruritus lasts longer than this, it is evidence of more nits and lice requiring retreatment.

All contactable items should be laundered in hot water and dried in sunlight or a clothes dryer (20 minutes on high) or ironed. Nonlaunderable items may be soaked in 2 per cent Lysol or one of the pediculocidal shampoos for an hour or heated in water (65°C) for 5 to 10 minutes.

All the child's contacts should be examined and treated if necessary. Family members must be treated simultaneously with the child to prevent immediate reinfestation.

Nursing Strategies for Follow-Up Care in the Home or Clinic

Inspect the scalp and hair with a magnifying glass for visible lice or nits.

Ask the child if the scalp still itches; inspect for evidence of secondary infection from scratching.

Assess the compliance of family members with examination for infestation and with prescribed treatment.

Scabies

Scabies is an infectious skin condition most common in school-age children, causing a vesicular or papulovesicular eruption. There are several forms of scabies. The most common "classic scabies" is transmitted by direct contact with a person infested with the *Acarus scabies (Sarcoptes scabiei),* or itch mite.

Etiology

The adult female itch mite, approximately the size of a grain of sugar, digs into the superficial stratum corneum of the epidermis and forms a burrow, leaving debris and feces. Each day for approximately a month burrowing continues a few millimeters and the female mite lays two to three eggs. The adult mite then dies and the eggs mature to an adult form in 10 days. The skin of the infested person reacts in an allergic fashion and small vesicles and papules form.

Identification of scabies is difficult and often it is misdiagnosed in children. Although it is often classified as a "social disease," it occurs in all socioeconomic levels, and cleanliness is not necessarily a protection. Children who bathe regularly will remove many of the mites, and the burrows may be impossible to detect. The nurse may use an ink pen to trace the burrows to the vesicle (mite hill) in an attempt to visualize the lesion (Fig. 45-3). Because scabies is transmitted by direct contact, it is imperative that all family members be treated for scabies regardless of the presence of lesions. Because the mite will survive only 2 to 3 days away from human skin, disinfection of fomites is usually confined to those articles with which the child is repeatedly in contact.

Clinical Manifestations

Children infested with the itch mite will first experience nocturnal itching. Pruritus is increased with the warmth of the bed and occurs only after sensitization to the mite and debris, usually a month after infestation. Scabetic lesions will usually be present on the sides or webs of the digits of hands and feet, extensor surface of the elbows, anterior axillary skin folds, glans penis, scrotum, and abdomen (Fig. 45-3). The nurse will rec-

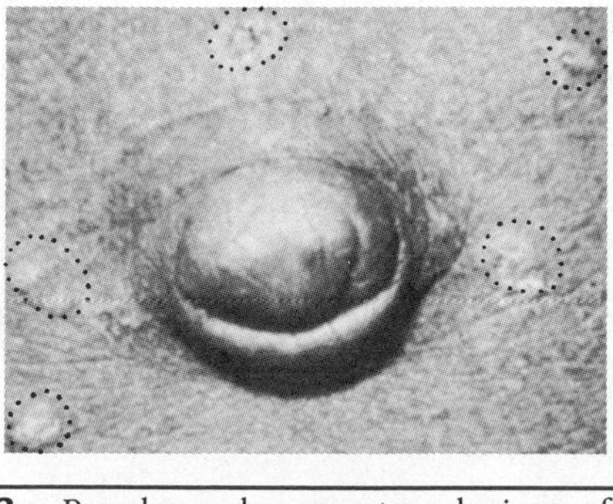

Figure 45-3. Papular and eczematous lesions of the abdomen are usually present in a "spokelike" periumbilical arrangement in classic scabies. (From Orkin M: Scabies in children. *Pediatr Clin North Am* 1978 May; 373.)

ognize initial lesions as small erythematous, excoriated papules. These may appear eczematous if the child has had pruritus and scratching resulted.

Diagnostic Assessment

The diagnosis of scabies must be made microscopically by identification of the mite from skin scrapings. It is imperative that the nurse provide factual information regarding the transmission of the mite in an attempt to alleviate guilt feelings of the parents and child. Notification of local health authorities is not required with individual cases, and parents will be relieved to know that confidentiality will be maintained. Examination by a physician is imperative for appropriate treatment.

Therapeutic Management

Gamma benzene hexachloride (GBH) is the usual treatment for scabies. Sulfur and Crotamiton are recommended for infants and young children because of the possibility of central nervous system toxicity with GBH (Garcia, 1987).

Strategies for Nursing Care

The infected child and all family members should initially bathe, towel dry, and then apply the scabicide from the neck down, being especially careful to apply between the fingers and toes and in the genital area. Bathing should be repeated 12 to 24 hours after application of the scabicide. One application is usually sufficient, although some physicians may recommend a second treatment in 1 week. Clothing in direct contact with the skin should be washed in hot water and dried. Underclothes and bed linens should be changed with each bath.

Treatment is usually very effective if instructions are followed correctly. Symptoms may continue for several days after treatment due to hypersensitivity to mite antigens. This should not be confused with treatment failure (Minster, 1980).

Allowing the child an opportunity to ventilate feelings and providing basic information about the disease and treatment will be a major role for the nurse. Older children with scabies may feel ashamed or guilty. An understanding of the condition will help the child cope and maintain a positive self-image.

Toxoplasmosis

Toxoplasmosis is a parasitic disease that may be either congenital (transmitted from an infected mother) or acquired. Acquired infection is transient and only mildly symptomatic. Congenital infection is more common and has severe consequences, with 23 to 38 per cent of infected infants experiencing severe central nervous system impairment, ocular damage, or death. Once infected, a woman has a lasting immunity, which means future offspring will not be affected.

Etiology

The *Toxoplasma gondii* parasites can be acquired from two primary sources: (1) the handling or ingestion of raw or undercooked fresh meat that contains a specific cyst, and (2) direct contact with the feces of an "infected" common house cat (in cat litter box or vegetable garden).

Clinical Manifestations and Diagnostic Assessment

Manifestations of acute active disease in congenitally infected infants include jaundice, petechiae, enlarged liver or spleen, chorioretinitis (inflammation of the choroid and retina), cerebral calcifications of damaged areas, encephalitis, and convulsions. These infants often die within the first month. Survivors are usually mentally retarded, with psychomotor impairment and varying degrees of blindness.

Third trimester infections result in subacute symptoms. Infants with a subacute form of congenital toxoplasmosis usually have no symptoms at birth, although chorioretinitis may be present. During the first year, subacutely infected infants may develop hydrocephaly, chorioretinitis, intracerebral calcification, and psychomotor disturbances.

In those children or adults who acquire the disease after birth, the only symptom is usually swollen lymph glands behind the ears. The presence of toxoplasmosis is diagnosed through serologic examination.

Therapeutic Management and Strategies for Nursing Care

Congenital Toxoplasmosis. Treatment of congenital toxoplasmosis is unsatisfactory, but daily doses of pyrimethamine (Daraprim) and sulfadiazine for 4 to 8 weeks is sometimes effective. Folinic acid is given to stop adverse actions on the bone marrow by the sulfonamide drugs. Since Daraprim is an antifolic agent, blood counts should be monitored biweekly to prevent leukopenia, thrombocytopenia, or anemia. In infants with the severe form of the disease, corticosteroids are often given to reduce inflammation, as in chorioretinitis.

The progressive nature of the disease suggests that

treatment should begin whether the infection is clinically apparent or not. Early treatment may prevent further tissue invasion and may arrest progression of the disease. Treatment of asymptomatic infants is undertaken in order to prevent later sequelae.

In the severely affected infant with congenital toxoplasmosis, the nurse's role primarily consists of palliative treatment for the infant and support to the parents of this critically ill child. Infants with the subacute form of the disease are generally hospitalized for the duration of drug therapy due to the near toxic level of the dosages. Nursing care needs to consist of monitoring the child for signs and symptoms of drug toxicity, leukopenia, thrombocytopenia, and anemia.

Acquired Toxoplasmosis. The disease is self-limiting in children and adults; thus, the only significant intervention is prevention. Simple preventive measures include (1) proper cooking of meat and cleaning of raw vegetables; (2) handwashing following handling of raw meats and vegetables coupled with avoidance of contact with mucous membranes while handling these items; (3) daily discarding of cat litter box contents, avoiding of litter box contact by pregnant women or handling only with disposable gloves; and (4) covers placed on sand boxes to prevent their use by cats to deposit feces. Public education and prenatal and child health maintenance counseling should teach these precautions. Cats that are kept indoors and are not fed uncooked meat are considered to pose no threat (Feldman, 1983). If a rise in the titer occurs during the first trimester in pregnant females, decision must be made regarding termination of the pregnancy. While maternal infections frequently do not result in infection of the fetus, the fetus appears to be at greatest risk when the mother contracts toxoplasmosis early in pregnancy (Feldman, 1983).

Fungal Infections

More than 60 fungi are known to be pathogenic in humans. This discussion is limited to those causing thrush, ringworm, and histoplasmosis. Permanent resistance is not developed to fungal infections; therefore, the nurse is likely to see mycoses (fungal disease) often in his or her practice.

Although immune responses to specific fungi are demonstrable, they are not well understood. Skin fatty acids, gastric acids, and intestinal enzymes help inhibit the growth of fungi. Serum antibodies are present and help establish presence of active disease but play little role in protection or recovery from most fungal infections. Cell-mediated immunity is believed to have some effect in recovery from fungal infection, particularly candidal fungi.

Thrush (Moniliasis)

Pathophysiology and Etiology

Thrush involves a stomatitis, particularly of the tongue, buccal membranes, and pharynx, caused by a yeast-like fungus, *Candida albicans.* Five per cent of all newborns contract thrush during descent through an infected birth canal, evidencing symptoms 7 to 10 days later. Infection with *Candida* may also result from prolonged antibiotic therapy or be transmitted by contaminated hands, bottles, or nipples. The incidence is greater in females, in infants with immunologic deficiencies, in infants of diabetic mothers, and in infants with oronasal anomalies. It is much less common after the neonatal period.

Candida is normally present in the mouth, gastrointestinal tract, and vagina. However, the circulating anticandidal factor present in normal serum that keeps most individuals asymptomatic is reduced or virtually absent in the serum of newborn infants. This factor is present, but in reduced levels during the first 6 months of life, and in the serum of persons with hematopoietic disorders.

Clinical Manifestations and Diagnostic Assessment

Moniliasis is characterized by white or gray-white patches in the oral cavity, which are slightly elevated and closely resemble curdled milk (Fig. 45-4). When an attempt is made to scrape off the patch, the underlying mucosa is seen to be raw and may bleed. Inspection alone is usually adequate to diagnose thrush, although the plaque may be cultured for *Candida albicans.*

Therapeutic Management

Upon diagnosis of thrush the physician will order a topical fungicide. The diaper area will also be assessed for a monilial rash, as *Candida* is common throughout the gastrointestinal tract. Characteristics of this type of rash can be reviewed in Table 44-6. A fungicide ointment such as nystatin will be used to treat the diaper area.

Major Nursing Diagnoses for Thrush

Impaired tissue integrity: stomatitis,
related to infection with Candida albicans
associated with

- *passage through an infected birth canal*
- *overgrowth of nonsusceptible organisms secondary to antibiotic therapy*

- *direct transmission from improper handwashing, mother's infected breast, or improper cleansing of bottles and nipples*

Knowledge deficit (parents), related to:
- *etiology of the infection*
- *administration of antifungal medication*
- *treatment of breasts if breastfeeding*

Strategies for Nursing Care

Treating the Stomatitis. Thrush is eventually self-limiting, but it should be treated with good hygiene and application of a fungicide to prevent spread into the upper respiratory or gastrointestinal tracts.

Nystatin is a fungicide that is effective against *Candida* when applied to the oral cavity four times a day for 1 week. Parents should be directed to complete the 7-day regimen even if the lesions have cleared. Nystatin can be swallowed to treat any moniliasis of the gastrointestinal tract, and should be applied after feedings. It must be given slowly, with some applied to each side of the mouth before it is swallowed to ensure adequate exposure of the oral mucosa to the medication. Typically, 1 ml of nystatin is ordered, with 0.5 ml to be used in each cheek. A cotton swab can be used to ensure contact of the medication with the buccal membrane, but this often results in much of the medication being absorbed in the cotton. A more effective method is for the nurse or the parent to gently rub a gloved finger inside the cheek after the nystatin has been inserted with an oral syringe. A disposable rubber glove will not absorb the medication. Application of 3 per cent hydrogen peroxide may also be effective treatment and promotes debridement of the affected membranes.

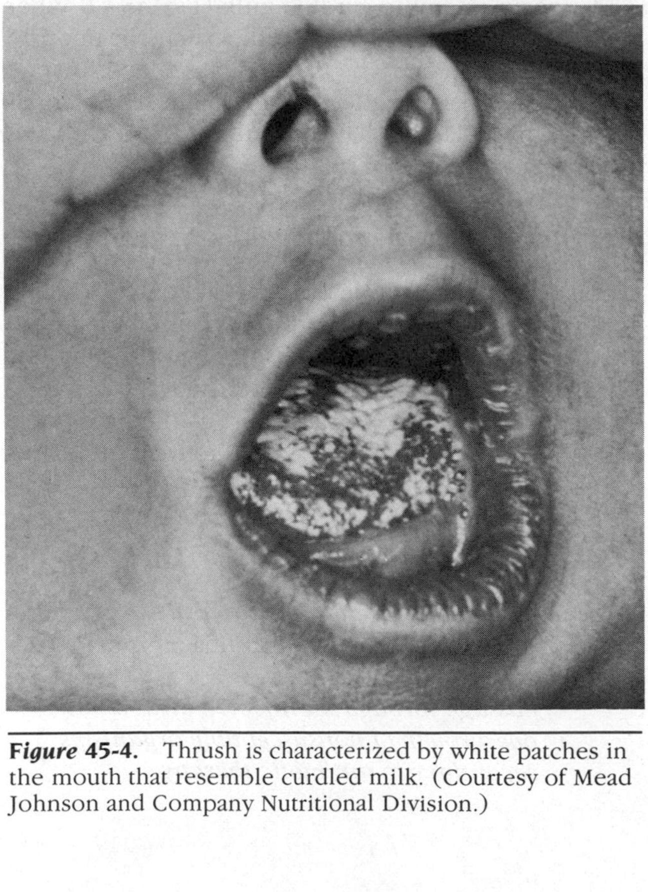

Figure 45-4. Thrush is characterized by white patches in the mouth that resemble curdled milk. (Courtesy of Mead Johnson and Company Nutritional Division.)

Addressing the Knowledge Deficit. The parents must understand the etiology of the infection in order to combat it effectively. If the mother is breastfeeding it is usually necessary for her to treat her breasts with an antifungal ointment to prevent reinfection between her breasts and the infant's mouth. Instruction regarding administration of medication to the infant's oral mucous membranes should include a return demonstration by the parent, as it is unlikely that the parent has had practice with this type of administration previously.

Preventing future infections with this organism involves careful washing of bottles and nipples (boiling or washing in a dishwasher is often recommended), following feedings with plain water (since small amounts of formula left in the buccal cavities provide an excellent bacterial medium), and use of good handwashing techniques. The parents should be aware that antibiotic treatment may also precipitate another infection and must be alert for the white patches should the infant require antibiotic therapy.

Nursing Strategies for Follow-Up Care in the Home or Clinic

Assess for clearing of the white oral lesions.

Assess the diaper area for a monilial rash which may occur with GI involvement: erythematous, circumscribed rash with confluent papules and pustules.

Determine whether the full course of medication was administered.

Assess infant feeding patterns and weight.

Ringworm

Several different closely related fungi are known to cause ringworm, which is a general term for mycotic disease of the keratinizing areas (nails, scalp, skin) of the body. Tinea capitis, tinea corporis, tinea cruris, and tinea pedis are described here.

Tinea Capitis (Scalp Ringworm)

Etiology. Ringworm of the scalp is an ancient disease with worldwide incidence. The greatest susceptibility is in young boys (rare after puberty) from urban areas. The fungus is transferred from infected animals or humans and from contaminated fomites (combs, hats).

Clinical Manifestations. The infection begins with a pimple and spreads to form a round, sharply outlined area in which hairs exist but have dried and broken off just above the skin. One or several such lesions may exist. The scalp varies from being mildly erythematous and slightly scaly to being affected with a painful, deep, boggy, and swollen inflammation called a *kerion.* The child's condition is communicable as long as the lesion(s) exists.

Diagnostic Assessment. Diagnosis is positive if a Wood light shone on the scalp results in fluorescence of tinea capitis organisms or if a microscopic examination of scales or hairs treated with 10 per cent KOH reveals the fungi. A culture is required to determine the specific species of fungus causing the infection.

Strategies for Nursing Care. Table 45-7 describes the management of the infection and associated symptoms. The nurse's approach to the child and family is crucial to the feelings they experience. Careful explanation of the cause helps diminish parents' feelings that they have not kept their child clean enough. Their cooperation should be enlisted to help identify the source of the infection. Animals the child has contact with should be carefully inspected for evidence of ringworm lesions. The child's playmates and siblings should also be examined since children tend to share personal articles during play, making transfer more likely. The nurse and parents together can teach and reinforce that personal articles such as combs, brushes, barrettes, and headgear are not playthings and should not be interchanged among siblings or playmates.

Tinea Corporis (Body Ringworm)

Etiology and Clinical Manifestations. Body ringworm also has a higher incidence in young boys and is more prevalent in rural, humid climates. This fungus infects nonhairy skin surfaces. The lesions are usually asymptomatic and appear in a flat, annular, or arcuate shape. There is scaling and erythema of the border with a clear central area; the border may also contain vesicles. The lesions are contagious as long as they exist.

Diagnostic Assessment and Nursing Strategies. Diagnosis is by microscopic examination and culture of scales or scabs. As with tinea capitis, parents should be approached in a nonaccusing manner that does not suggest they are inadequate parents, and their help should be solicited in finding the source. (See Table 45-7 for a discussion of treatment.)

Tinea Cruris (Jock Itch)

Etiology. Jock itch is a ringworm infestation of the groin that occurs primarily in pubescent males and adult men. Two ringworm fungi *(Epidermophyton floccosum* and *Tinea rubrum)* invade the medial proximal aspects of the thighs, the crural folds, and the scrotum, living off the dead keratinized skin and hair tissues of that area. Individual susceptibility is poorly understood, but poor hygiene, heat, friction, maceration in the groin area and obesity are predisposing factors. Direct contact with the organism when any of these conditions exists makes the young man a potential host to the fungus.

Clinical Manifestations and Diagnostic Assessment. The fungal invasion is characterized by round, sharply delineated lesions, with the pubic hairs

Table 45-7. Management of Ringworm and Associated Symptoms

Tinea Capitis	Tinea Corporis	All Ringworm Forms
1. Clip hair short and thoroughly wash daily	1. Bathe thoroughly daily, removing scabs or crusts before applying medication	1. Exclusion from gym, public showers and pools
2. Do not use towel more than once before laundering	2. Avoid heat, moisture and trauma during treatment, as these cause increased inflammation and pruritus	2. Apply an antifungal agent containing haloprogin, toinaftate, or salicylic acid after shampooing or bathing (e.g., Tinactin or Viaform ointment). Do not apply to highly inflamed lesions. Usually prescribed for 1 to 3 wk
3. If a pillow is used, change pillowslip daily	3. Change towels, clothing and linens daily	3. For extensive or topical resistant ringworm, give 6 wk course of oral griseofulvin (antifungal antibiotic). Should be given after meals, which should be high in fat content. Child should not be given phenobarbital. Blood anticoagulating action is decreased by griseofulvin
4. Avoid use of headgear till lesions healed	4. Wear nonocclusive clothing until lesions healed	
5. Apply cold compresses to any oozing or swollen lesions	5. Distract child from scratching or picking at lesions	

of that region broken off. These pruritic lesions vary from a scaly, red area to a painfully edematous, boggy one. Diagnosis is confirmed by presence of the fungi on direct microscopic examination of the scales.

Therapeutic Management and Nursing Strategies. Management involves comfort measures such as wet compresses or sitz baths to relieve the itching and swelling, eradication of the fungi with local applications of tolnaftate liquid (Tinactin) or a similar antifungal preparation, and education regarding personal hygiene and management of other predisposing factors. The youth also needs reassurance that this temporary condition in no way alters his sexuality, since any infections of the involved body region are typically perceived by young men to be somehow affiliated with venereal diseases such as syphilis or gonorrhea (there is actually no association). His parents, if they have awareness of their son's ailment, may need similar assurance and education to correct misconceptions they may hold about the disease.

Tinea Pedis (Athlete's Foot)

Etiology. Tinea pedis (dermatophytosis), more commonly known as athlete's foot, is also a fungal disease. Although tinea pedis is not frequent in the young school-age child, its incidence increases near puberty. *Trichophyton rubrum, T. mentagrophytes,* and *E. floccosum* are the usual causative organisms.

Clinical Manifestations. The appearance of tinea pedis can range from an acute inflammatory vesiculobullous eruption to a dull erythema and scaling (Fig. 45-5). An acute episode initially involves the intertriginous area of the fourth and fifth toes and extends to the plantar surface of the foot. Skin maceration, scaling, vesicles, and fissures result. The absence of vesiculation and the presence of moccasin-like scaling occurs in chronic tinea pedis and is usually limited to a small area between the toes.

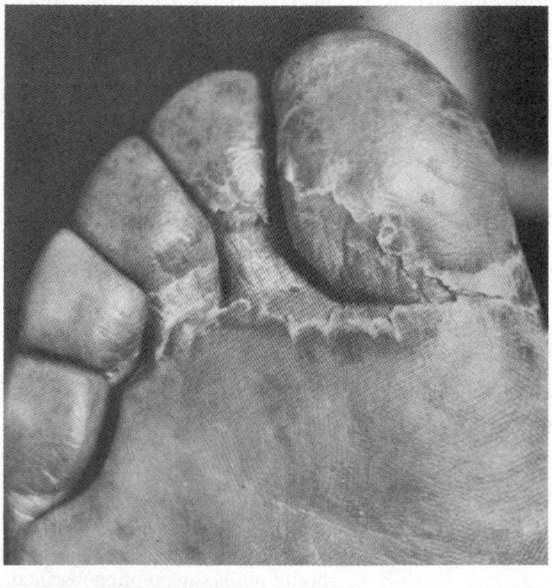

Figure 45-5. Tinea pedis.

Diagnostic Assessment. Children complaining of itchy feet with signs of scaling or vesicle formation should be referred to a physician for diagnosis and treatment. Diagnosis can usually be made clinically; however, tissue scrapings examined under a Wood lamp will confirm suspicions. Some children experience discomfort and burning from the vesicles. A child unable to walk probably has a secondary infection in conjunction with acute tinea pedis.

Therapeutic Management and Nursing Strategies. Management of tinea pedis involves both preventive and treatment measures. Prevention of tinea pedis is virtually impossible because the organisms are present on most people. However, proper foot hygiene is an important health consideration for all children. Instruction should include the importance of daily bathing and careful drying between all toes. Many children now wear nonventilated shoes, which provide an excellent growth medium for fungus, especially during the summer months when their feet are warm and moist. Nurses should encourage older children to go barefoot when appropriate or to wear sandals, which allow the feet to stay dry. Early treatment of a fungus-infected toenail may prevent an episode of tinea pedis and complications from secondary infections.

Treatment for acute tinea pedis is somewhat involved, and parents will need specific written instructions. Systemic treatment is with oral griseofulvin and a broad-spectrum antibiotic. Parents and child need to be shown how to apply wet compresses to the foot for 20 minutes four times a day. Local treatment of the vesicles with wet compresses is continued until the blisters heal, and then topical antifungal agents are used. The child with tinea pedis should be instructed to wear cotton socks and to alternate between pairs of shoes to allow complete drying. Parents and siblings need to be informed that the skin condition is not contagious; however, the exchange of socks and bath towels should be prohibited. If the child is not in acute distress, arrangements should be made to allow him or her to continue with school. The child with a severe case of acute tinea pedis may feel some resentment at having to temporarily curtail ambulatory activities, particularly physical education or athletics that stimulate foot perspiration. The school nurse should discuss the child's condition with the teacher so that the child's discomfort and lack of participation in some activities will be understood. The teacher responsible for gym classes should be informed so that attention is given to proper hygiene.

Chronic tinea pedis may be treated with nonprescription topical antifungal medications such as Tinactin or Whitfield's ointment. Application of the ointment must be continued for 3 to 4 weeks after healing has occurred.

Histoplasmosis

Etiology Common to All Forms

Caused by *Histoplasma capsulatum,* a fungus found predominantly in soil with a high organic content (e.g., chicken coops, composts) in the central United States, histoplasmosis can occur in persons of all ages. This fungus is not transmitted from human to human; airborne spores are inhaled in dust contaminated by the fungus and settle in the lungs. The disease may be (1) asymptomatic and benign, (2) symptomatic but benign, or (3) acute, progresssive, and disseminated, producing serious systemic disease.

Forms of Histoplasmosis

Asymptomatic Benign Histoplasmosis. This form of the disease is detected only by a positive histoplasmin test. The primary lung lesions created by the fungus calcify without causing any symptoms. No treatment is indicated.

Symptomatic Benign Histoplasmosis. Symptoms are general and may appear as mild respiratory illness or temporary general malaise. The child may complain of some weakness and chest pain. A low-grade fever and dry or productive cough are usually present. Recovery is slow but spontaneous. Treatment involves symptomatic relief of fever and cough.

Acute Progressive Disseminated Histoplasmosis. This form of the disease is most prevalent in infants and toddlers. The course is rapid and, left untreated, the disease is fatal. Symptoms include a high sepsis-related fever, prostration, hepatosplenomegaly, skin ulcers and mucosal purpura, atypical pneumonitis, and often anemia.

Diagnostic Assessment

Diagnosis is tentative when a serologic test for serum antihistoplasma antibody (histoplasmin test) is positive. Diagnosis can be made quickly when the fungus can be seen in Giemsa- or Wright-stained smears of sputum, bone marrow, blood or ulcerative exudate. Definitive diagnosis depends on culturing the fungus from these smear sources, but a longer time is required to learn the findings from culture than from the serologic test, so treatment is usually begun before the results of the report of the culture findings are known.

Therapeutic Management

Management usually involves hospitalization so the course of the disease can be closely monitored. Wound isolation is initiated and amphotericin B (Fungizone) or a triple sulfonamide suspension or both are administered. All family members should be evaluated and infected members treated. Treatment of symptoms is also initiated. With prompt treatment recovery does occur.

Strategies for Nursing Care

Parents will need emotional support as they learn the cause and potential seriousness of their child's disease. They should be educated as to the etiology of the disease and encouraged to take preventive precautions such as wearing a mask while inside chicken coops, periodically cleaning and spraying the coop and surrounding soil with 3 per cent formalin spray to reduce dust, and fencing in compost areas. Parents should be urged to keep their infant or toddler, who is more susceptible to the serious form of the disease, away from these sites of potential contamination.

Rickettsial Infections

Two fairly common rickettsial infections—Q fever and Rocky Mountain spotted fever—are discussed. These diseases can affect all ages; young children are susceptible because they tend to spend a lot of time crawling, sitting, and playing on the ground, making them readily accessible to infected ticks, which are a major source of rickettsial disease.

Q Fever

Etiology

This is an acute febrile disease of sudden onset. Major reservoirs from which humans contract this disease are ticks, farm animals or raw milk from them, and dust.

Clinical Manifestations and Diagnostic Assessment

There is much variability in the severity and duration of symptoms, which include chills, diaphoresis, headache, and malaise. Pneumonitis symptoms of cough and chest pain exist without any upper respiratory involvement. Diagnosis is made from a positive complement fixation or agglutination test.

Therapeutic Management and Strategies for Nursing Care

Oral tetracycline is given for this disease and is continued for 7 to 10 days after the fever dissipates. A person who has had Q fever develops permanent immunity. Immunization is also available and should be given to those at high risk for exposure. Prevention is an important aspect of nursing care in areas where Q fever seems to be prevalent. Preventive action should include education regarding sources of the rickettsiae and concerning the practice of appropriate hygienic measures in potential reservoir areas (e.g., animal barns and sheds). Parents should be cautioned not to give their children unpasteurized milk.

Rocky Mountain Spotted Fever

Etiology

This disease is caused by *Rickettsia rickettsii* and is transmitted to humans via tick bite. The incidence is highest in the Kentucky mountains, the Carolinas, and the Cape Cod area during spring and summer. However, in recent years as many as 15 or 20 cases have been documented in each of the midwestern states. Persons who contract this disease may be asymptomatic or seriously ill; there is a 20 to 50 per cent mortality in untreated cases.

Clinical Manifestations and Diagnostic Assessment

The clinical picture is a sudden onset of symptoms that include fever (lasting 2 to 3 weeks), headache, chills, conjunctivitis, and severe myalgia (muscle pain) of wrists, ankles, and forearms that precedes a rash by 2 to 4 days. The rash, if recognized, can be life saving. Typically it begins with macular and papular lesions that are pink and blanchable. These progressively cover the palms, soles, trunk, and face within 24 hours. After 24 hours the rash turns red and is palpable, and petechiae are visible in the rash. By the fourth day the rash is no longer blanchable, has progressed to purpuric vesicles (small blood-filled sacs or wheals) and has extended to involve the scrotum or vulva. If treatment has not been initiated by this time, ulcers and gangrene can develop on the fingertips, nose, and earlobes.

Aside from identification of the characteristic rash, diagnosis is made from a positive Weil-Felix test. However, it takes 24 to 48 hours to obtain results of this test. Treatment should be initiated if the clinical picture suggests this disease rather than waiting for test results, since waiting could prove fatal.

Therapeutic Management

Treatment involves five days of oral tetracycline or chloramphenicol or both. Penicillin is ineffective and sulfonamides worsen the symptoms. Begun early in the course of the disease, treatment favors a good prognosis; if extreme vasculitis involving the brain, heart, or kidneys or all these has evolved, treatment is unlikely to be effective. Persons who survive the disease have permanent immunity.

Strategies for Nursing Care

Because of the critical factor of identifying this disease early, nurses should play a major role in educating the public regarding the clinical manifestations and the incidence in their locale. Preventing children from playing in high reservoir areas is a significant preventive action. When the disease is contracted, parents need much help from the nurse to work through the guilt feelings they are likely to experience and to cope with the potential seriousness of the disease. They should be kept continuously informed of their child's status and involved in his or her care as much as possible.

Nursing Strategies for Follow-Up Care in the Home or Clinic

Assess for therapeutic effects of treatment: absence of fever and clearing of the rash, increased appetite, and increased energy for play.

Remind the family that the child has a permanent immunity to the disease.

Teach the family to protect other members from the disease:

- Children and their pets should frequently be inspected for ticks, especially after playing in wooded areas.
- If a tick is found, induce it to back out voluntarily so that the head is removed intact. This may be accomplished by covering the tick with a substance that prevents it from receiving oxygen, e.g., nail polish, mineral oil, or petrolatum. Sometimes the tick will simply die, partially imbedded in the skin, rather than backing out. At this point it is best to seek medical attention for removal.
- Anyone who has been bitten by a tick should seek medical attention; treatment may be instituted before symptoms begin.

Amebic and Shigella Infections

Amebiasis

Etiology

Amebiasis, or amebic dysentery, is a disease of the large intestine as a consequence of mucosal invasion by pathologic protozoa. Reservoirs of transfer to humans include flies, contaminated water or raw vegetables and fruits, and hand-to-mouth transfer from contact with an infected person's stool. The disease occurs primarily in underdeveloped areas when sanitation is lacking and in temperate climates.

Clinical Manifestations

Symptoms vary depending on the degree of mucosal necrosis. The disease may be asymptomatic and resolve spontaneously after several days or remain at a carrier level. Carriers may fail to gain weight and be slightly anemic. Symptoms may be relatively mild, with diarrhea and mild cramping that alternates with constipation and bloating, accompanied by alternating anorexia and ravenous appetite, each lasting a few hours or days. A more severe picture appears in some children who experience an amebic enteritis characterized by colic and foul, watery stools containing blood and pus. If these stools reach a frequency of from 15 to 30 during 24 hours, true amebic dysentery exists. A serious complication of this disease is extension of the protozoa directly or via the bloodstream to cause abscesses of the liver, lungs, or brain.

Therapeutic Management and Strategies for Nursing Care

Diagnosis is made by identifying cysts in a fecal or lesion exudate smear. Various amebicides may be used to treat amebiasis, common ones being tetracycline, Milibis, or Flagyl. The child is infective until the organism no longer appears in the feces, which is usually within 72 hours after therapy is initiated. Complete cure usually takes a couple of weeks; however, fecal smear should be repeated for 3 months to ensure elimination of the organism. The remainder of treatment is symptomatic and supportive. Preventive measures include personal hygiene education, pest control, adequate sanitation, and chlorination of water supplies.

Shigellosis

Shigellosis, or bacillary dysentery, is an acute bacterial disease of the large intestine. Two thirds of cases occur in children under 10; it is especially prevalent in toddlers. The incidence is greater in the summer. Persons from lower socioeconomic areas, in institutions or who practice poor personal hygiene are at greater risk.

Etiology

Caused by any one of four groups of Shigella organisms, the disease is transmitted by the fecal-oral route, hence the lay term "hand-to-mouth disease." The organisms may be passed as a result of direct contact with an infected patient or carrier or indirectly from contact with flies or objects contaminated with infected feces, or by consuming fecally contaminated food or water.

Clinical Manifestations

The severity of symptoms varies widely, ranging from asymptomatic disease to serious illness. Mild disease results in daily passage of a few more stools than normal, lasting only a couple of days. The onset may be characterized by sudden fever, anorexia and gastrointestinal upset, followed hours later by diarrhea. The diarrhea is at first watery and green, then changes to bloody, mucous stools; their frequency increases to 10 or 20 a day. Dehydration and electrolyte imbalance can occur quickly, progressing to renal failure if not treated promptly. Untreated, symptoms persist 2 to 3 weeks, then subside. Severe cases are manifested by sudden high fever, convulsions and delirium, and meningitis-like symptoms. Stools contain blood, pus, and mucus and are explosive.

Diagnostic Assessment

Diagnosis is made from the symptomatic history, environmental history, and culturing of the Shigella organism from a stool specimen. All cases must be reported to local health departments so that contact follow-up (epidemiologic investigation) may be conducted.

Therapeutic Management

Treatment involves killing the organisms with antibacterial drugs; ampicillin is usually given until the specific organism has been identified by culture. The drug is given orally in mild disease but intramuscularly or parenterally in more acute disease. Fluid and electrolyte replacement is necessary in all but mild cases of the disease. Oral intake of food and fluid is contraindicated for the first 24 to 48 hours, then gradually progressed through the typical diarrhea diet routine (see Chapter 41). Strict isolation is maintained until cultures are negative for the Shigella organisms, which is generally 5 to 7 days. Treatment of symptoms is also initiated.

Strategies for Nursing Care

This extremely uncomfortable, isolated child will need the supportive presence of the parents and a primary nurse. Toddlers who have just mastered toilet training will need reassurance that their bowel incontinence is from the disease and is not their fault, and that it will eventually stop. If possible, young children should be able to observe their caretakers (parents, nurse, doctor) from a window before they put on isolation attire and watch them while they put on the gown, mask, and gloves. This reassures them that they are not strange monsters, but rather people they know.

Preventive education involves proper sanitary and hygiene practices and instruction in clean, safe ways to handle food. Environmental improvement of sanitary facilities, pest control, and water purification are also necessary to prevent Shigella epidemics in communities.

Sexually Transmitted Diseases

Teaching Preventive Measures

The nurse plays a major role in helping young people understand sexually transmitted diseases (STD). Teenage girls need to be taught that only two types of vaginal discharge — menstrual flow and a clear vaginal secretion at the time of sexual excitement — are normal, and that sexually transmitted diseases can be transmitted to a fetus during pregnancy or birth.

Both prevention and prompt treatment of any genitourinary symptoms are the individual's responsibility to his or her own body. Several preventive measures can be taken by the teenager who chooses to become sexually active, including (1) using a condom to reduce the likelihood of genitourinary disease and pregnancy, (2) washing the perianal region well with soap and water after sexual contact, (3) urinating after intercourse (more effective for males), and (4) being selective in sexual behavior, by avoiding contact with persons at risk for infection.

Although these are simple preventive measures, they are often unrealistic in terms of adolescent sexual activity. A teen's sexual activity is often sporadic, casual, or unplanned — a consequence of sexual curiosity and experimentation. Thus the teen is unlikely to begin the sexual contact prepared with a condom or with thoughts about the possibility of the partner being infected; nor are restroom facilities likely to be readily available for prompt use after sexual activity.

What should be stressed is that the burden of DISPROOF rests with both partners where sexually transmitted diseases are concerned. DISPROOF means that both partners can give evidence that they are free of the signs and symptoms of disease:

- Discharge (from the vagina or penis)
- Itching (around the genitals or anus)
- Soreness or swelling (around genitals or lymph nodes)
- Pain (on intercourse, in joints, in abdomen, in the genitals)
- Rash (anywhere on the body)
- Odor (from the genitals)
- Organisms (things moving around that one can see)
- Fever and fatigue

The problem is that sexually transmitted diseases are often asymptomatic; the absence of signs and symptoms does not ensure absence of disease.

Teaching About Resources

Nurses working with teen populations should make sure that literature about these diseases is readily available to teens and that information about recommendable clinics for the diagnosis and treatment of these communicable diseases is visibly posted (hours, locations, fees, client conditions). Most states now permit physicians to treat minors for sexually transmitted disease without parental consent.

Nurses involved in educating teens about sexuality or the sexual diseases must evaluate their own sexual attitudes. The nurse's personal sexual attitudes do not matter to the teen being taught or counseled, but the nurse's ability to be comfortable with the teen and to discuss the issues in an environment in which both nurse and teen respect each other as individuals with responsibility for their own decisions and behaviors is imperative to gaining the teen's attention and cooperation. "Rap sessions" in which a group of teens and young adult leaders (nurses, for example) discuss feelings and facts about a problem and devise practical solutions are still a popular mode for educating teens about sexually transmitted diseases.

A nonjudgmental approach and the assurance of confidentiality are the minimal essentials to whichever method is used to teach or counsel adolescents in sexual matters. The counseling role of the school nurse-teacher is especially worthy of attention because of the tendency of youth to trust and consult a school nurse rather than other adults in their environment. The school nurse can also be politically influential in helping identify inadequate health services for teens in the community and in arousing public support for provision of readily available and adequate health care.

The epidemic of STD, primarily among teens and young adults (peak ages 15 to 24 years), has made this the number one group of communicable diseases in our nation. Despite the discovery of penicillin to treat gonorrhea and syphilis and widespread education efforts, these two diseases — plus chlamydia, genital herpes, and genital warts — persist and increase yearly. The nurse plays a vital role in preventive education regarding sexually transmitted diseases as well as in casefinding and encouraging prompt treatment. Table 45-8 summarizes the features of these diseases as well as the treatment currently recommended for them.

Nursing Strategies for Follow-Up Care in the Home or Clinic

Encourage expression of feelings about the diagnosis; assess the patient's ability to accept responsibility for his or her sexual behavior.

Evaluate the effectiveness of problem-solving behaviors related to the disease (i.e., coping with the feelings of family members; contacting sexual partners to alert them to the need for examination; verbalizing a plan for preventing further STDs).

Assess for remission of symptoms.

Ensure that the follow-up visit reinforces:

- Availability of health care professionals for supportive, nonjudgmental, and confidential counseling on matters of sexual hygiene
- The need for adolescents to accept responsibility for their sexual behavior
- Measures to prevent recurrence:
  1. Use of a condom
  2. Adequate knowledge of the sexual partner to predict the likelihood of STD in that individual
  3. Urinating after intercourse
  4. Careful cleansing of the genital region before and after intercourse
  5. Avoiding intercourse during times of genital irritation (when one is more prone to infectious processes)
- Signs and symptoms by which the patient would recognize other STDs.

Pelvic Inflammatory Disease (PID)

Pelvic inflammatory disease is the leading cause of infertility in young women (Wilfert and Gutman, 1987). It is the most serious complication of sexually transmitted disease. Vaginal infection progresses to the fallopian tubes and may disseminate through the pelvis, with purulent infection and scarring during healing. It is estimated that 15 per cent of teenagers who develop gonorrhea will progress to PID (Wilfert and Gutman, 1987).

Pelvic inflammatory disease is diagnosed on the basis of lower abdominal pain, fever, leukocytosis, an elevated sedimentation rate, and the presence of an adnexal mass on abdominal ultrasonography. Treatment usually includes hospitalization with aggressive intravenous antibiotic therapy. It is thought that the outcome for fertility is enhanced by prompt and vigorous therapy.

Vaginal Infections

Vaginitis

Vaginitis, an inflammation of the vagina, is one of the most common gynecologic complaints of females of all ages, but particularly once menarche is reached. The most frequently associated agents are *Trichomonas vaginalis, Candida albicans,* and *Gardnerella vaginalis.* These vaginal infections frequently occur together.

Etiology

Vaginitis may result from physiologic causes related to elevation in estrogen or progesterone (pregnancy, premenstrual and preovulatory hormonal changes, contraceptives, emotional stress), which lowers vaginal pH, rendering the person more susceptible to pathogens. Chemical causes — too frequent douching or sensitivity to feminine hygienic products or to contraceptive or prophylactic preparations — may also increase susceptibility to vaginitis. Foreign bodies such as tampons or irritation from intercourse may also increase susceptibility. Exposure to a variety of viruses, bacteria, fungi, or protozoa not normally in the vaginal canal may also result in vaginitis.

Diagnostic Assessment and Therapeutic Management

A commonality of symptoms — vulvar pruritus or pain, offensive odor, and vaginal discharge — prompts the patient to seek medical attention. Management involves determining the cause, whether a hormonal fluctuation, a chemical irritation, a foreign body or other mechanical irritation, a pathogenic organism, or simply poor hygiene. Inspection, vaginoscopy, micro-

Table 45-8. Characteristics of the Sexually Transmitted Diseases

Disease (Pathogen)	Transmission	Incubation	Clinical Manifestations	Diagnostic Tests	Therapeutic Management
Gonorrhea *(Neisseria gonorrhea)*	Direct contact, usually sexual May be contracted by infant during delivery	2–14 days (average 3–5)	*Early signs:* Copious mucopurulent discharge from phagocytosis, vaginal in female and urethral in male; pharyngeal if oral sex. Pain and frequency of urination from urethritis. 90% of females and 10% of males are asymptomatic *Other possible signs:* Cervicitis, salpingitis, peritonitis, PID, and abscesses of Skene's or Bartholin glands in females. Eipdidymitis and abscess of prostate glands in males *Late signs:* Arthritis, endocarditis, sterility	Culture of discharge for gonococcal growth (GC smear) positive. Visualization of discharge on physical exam	Oral amoxicillin or ampillicin or intramuscular injection of penicillin or ceftriaxone. The first 3 drugs (not ceftriaxone) are accompanied by oral probenecid. Oral tetracycline or doxycycline is given concurrently. This regimen addresses the fact that chlamydial infection coexists in up to 45% of cases of gonorrhea
Syphillis *(Treponema pallidum)*	Direct contact, usually sexual, during infective stage Transfusion of contaminated blood May be transmitted to fetus across placenta	Primary stage 10–90 days (average 3 wks)	*Primary—Infectious:* Chancre (painless, indurated ucler) that heals spontaneously in 2–6 weeks. Located at site where pathogen entered *Secondary*—very infectious: Skin and mucous membrane rash, lymphadenitis, fever, headaches, sore throat that disappears spontaneously. Lasts few months to several years *Early latent*—may be infectious: No physical symptoms *Late latent*—blood infectious: No symptoms *Late active:* Not all clients experience this stage. Gummas (nodular or ulcerative lesions) of skin, bones, liver, stomach	RPRCT (nontreponemal rapid plasma reagin card test) or ART (automated reagin test) commonly used. Rapid, inexpensive, and determine level of disease activity. FTA-ABS (fluorescent treponemal antibody-absorption) test may be used to detect antibodies from early through late stages	Early syphilis (≤1 yr duration): 2,400,000 U benzathine penicillin G, IM Oral tetracycine, 500 mg qid for 15 days may be given if client has penicillin allergy Later syphilis (>1 yr duration): 2,400,000 U benzathine penicillin G IM once a week for 3 wk If allergic to penicillin, oral tetracycline 500 mg qid for 30 days

			CNS involvement • 10% optic atrophy, deafness • General paresis • Insanity Cardiovascular involvement in 80% of cases • Aortic insufficiency or aneurysm • Endarteritis		
Genital herpes simplex *(Herpesvirus hominis* [HSV-2])	Direct contact, usually sexual May be contracted by newborn during delivery	3–7 days	*Symptomatic phase:* Contagious. Minor itching or extensive rash of genital region followed by a cluster of blister-like lesions that then rupture and ulcerate; these are pruritic and painful, especially during intercourse. Painful urination, inguinal lymphadenitis and pain, fever, malaise Symptoms disappear spontaneously after 2–6 wk Many cases asymptomatic *Dormant phase:* Symptoms absent but reappear with emotional or physical stress during which person again is infectious; once a person is infected, virus is harbored for life, though recurrences are less severe and last about 2 wk Cervical cancer 8 times more likely in women with HSV-2 virus	Viral culture of lesions. Scraping and staining of ulcer tissue with Papanicolaou solution demonstrates characteristic giant cells and viral inclusion bodies. Antibody blood titer of HVH-2 21 or more days after infection	Incurable. Treatment aimed at pain relief, fostering healing of lesions and preventing other infections. • Pain medication • Use of condom during intercourse to reduce likelihood of spread of HVH-2 or of infection with other pathogens; no intercourse when sores are present • Keep lesions clean and dry • Acyclovir PO or IV shortens duration of the first episode and may reduce systemic symptoms. First episode treatment with Acyclovir does not affect the subsequent risk, rate, or severity of recurrences Cesarean birth in all pregnancies if active sores exist at time of delivery
Chlamydia trachomatis	Direct contact, usually sexual. May be contracted by infant during delivery	1–5 wk	Symptoms often mild, nonspecific; great majority are asymptomatic. Dysuria, frequency, slight white or clear discharge, cystitis, cervicitis, urethral itching	Tissue culture; also stained smear of epithelial cell scrapings, fluorescent antibody examination of direct smear (direct smear FA), enzyme immunoassay (ELISA)	Oral tetracycline HCL or doxycycline hyclate for 7 days
Genital warts, also known as *Condylomata acuminata* (human papilloma virus)	Direct contact; usually but not always sexual	Up to several weeks	Rapidly growing, irregular, confluent masses with a cauliflower-like appearance; found commonly on labia majora, shaft of penis, or perianal region	Inspection	Cryotherapy (liqid nitrogen or dry ice), or successive podophyllin applications, or electrosurgery or surgical removal

(Adapted from Centers for Disease Control, 1985; Johnson, 1987; Kalter and Rosen, 1985; Lutz, 1986; 1988 Canadian Guidelines, 1988.)

scopic examination of vaginal secretions, and culture are the common diagnostic strategies.

Treatment is aimed at the specific cause and includes the relief of pruritus and inflammation. Oral Flagyl and/or vaginal preparations will be ordered for infectious processes, depending on the causative organism. A topical corticosteroid ointment may be ordered to control intense vulvar pruritus. Table 45-9 details specific symptoms, diagnosis, and treatment for trichomoniasis, *Gardnerella vaginalis* vaginitis, and candidiasis.

Diagnosis and treatment of vulvovaginitis in a child includes considerations different from those in a sexually active adolescent. In the young child a high or microperforate hymen may trap drops of urine or mucus that become infected with fecal organisms (Friedlander, 1986). If this becomes a source of recurrent infection, removal of some hymen tissue may be considered. Sexual abuse must also be considered a potential cause of vulvovaginitis. See Chapter 35 for assessment strategies pertinent to sexual abuse.

Foreign bodies trapped within the vagina are another cause of vaginitis in young children. Often the foreign object has become trapped in the vagina accidentally, such as with toilet paper or some dried stool, but small children are also prone to exploring body

Table 45-9. Differentiating Vaginitis

Causative Agent	Transmission	Symptoms	Diagnosis	Treatment
Trichomoniasis (*Trichomonas vaginalis,* a protozoan) Incubation period 4–20 days	Direct contact with discharges during sexual intercourse or to infant as it passes through the vaginal canal at birth. Organism survives 24 hr in urine and on wet linens, tampons, douch equipment, or sponges. Onset and recurrences commonly associated with menstruation, probably due to increased pH during flow	Harbored asymptomatically in men and in 25% of infected women. Vulvar pruritus is only symptom in another 25% of infected females. Remainder of infected females experience: • Thin, foamy, profuse yellowish discharge with foul odor • Itching, burning and chafing of vulvovaginal and anal areas • Dysuria and frequency • Vulvar and vaginal edema and erythema • Cervical erosion	Microscopic examination of organism in discharge (no douching 24 hr before exam). Monthly recheck after menstruation for 3 mo recommended to ensure cure	Oral Flagyl (single dose or 7 day dose) is 95% effective in curing the disease, especially if male partner also treated. Lactating women should not breastfeed for 24 hr after ingestion of Flagyl. First trimester pregnant women should be treated with clotrimazole intravaginally for 7 days and Betadine or vinegar douch for symptomatic relief, instead of with oral Flagyl. Use condom during and for 24 hr after treatment of both partners
Gardnerella vaginalis vaginitis/nonspecific vaginitis (*Gardnerella vaginalis,* a gram-negative bacillus, is speculated to be the causative agent) Incubation period less than 10 days	Direct contact during sexual intercourse. Other modes of transmission also suspected but undefined currently	Moderately profuse grayish, thin, malodorous discharge. About 50% of women complain of slight pruritus. Mild inflammation of vaginal wall	Microscopic examination. pH <5.5. Potassium hydroxide test—a drop of 10% solution on smear gives off a "fishy" odor	Oral Flagyl or sulfonamide vaginal cream or Terramycin vaginal tablets, or oral ampicillin (recommended during pregnancy)
Candidiasis (*Candida albicans,* a yeast-like fungus)	Direct contact during sexual intercourse. Contamination from mouth, rectum, contaminated fingers or fomites.	Harbored asymptomatically in 40% of women with flare-ups only during pregnancy, hormonal or antibiotic therapy, or emotional stress. Intense, intolerable vulvovaginal itching. Profuse, watery discharge or thick, white cheesy discharge. Erythematosis or excoriated vulva	Culture of microscopic exam of vaginal discharge	Various, equally effective treatments are used. Vaginal tablets, foams, or creams of fungicidal agents (Nystatin, Monostat, Gyne-Lotrimin) applied bid for 7–10 days

(Adapted from Hume, 1983; Feigin and Cherry, 1987.)

orifices and depositing therein any small object that will fit, such as a bean or a small part from a toy. Pelvic radiography may sometimes be used in diagnosis. Removal of the object and cleansing of the vagina with warm water is usually sufficient to relieve the irritation (Friedlander, 1986).

Major Nursing Diagnoses for Vaginitis

Impaired skin integrity: inflammation of the vaginal mucosa, related to:
- *hormonal fluctuations*
- *chemical irritation*
- *mechanical irritation*
- *pathogenic organisms*
- *sexual abuse*

Situational low self-esteem, related to:
- *the embarrassment of a genital disorder*
- *feeling "unclean" because of vaginal discharge and odor*
- *feelings of shame associated with perceived wrongdoing*
- *fears about possible long-term effects*

Altered comfort: pruritus, associated with irritation of the vaginal and vulvar mucosa

Knowledge deficit, related to:
- *etiology*
- *treatment*
- *prevention of recurrence*

Strategies for Nursing Care

Treating Vaginal Inflammation. Nursing strategies for treating vaginal inflammation will depend on the cause. If the etiology involves a noninfectious process, teaching will focus on eliminating the source of irritation and on initiating good hygiene to reduce the risk of infection. If an infectious organism is identified, the patient will need instruction about medication administration.

When infectious vaginitis is diagnosed, the pediatric patient is most often an adolescent. Many medications for vaginitis are dispensed in the form of vaginal creams or suppositories. The nurse should take into consideration that the teen may never have used a tampon or douche and may not know exactly where the vaginal opening is or how to insert medication into it. Furthermore, the patient will often be too embarrassed to ask questions. It is usually safe to assume that the young person will need detailed instructions. Mannequins can be valuable teaching aids in that they can help to decrease the adolescent's embarrassment by shifting the focus from her body to that of the dummy.

Compliance with vaginal preparations is often compromised because symptoms subside within the first few days of the regimen, and because the preparations tend to leak from the vagina, causing a damp and uncomfortable feeling. The adolescent must understand the consequences of failing to complete the course of medication: in most cases a prompt recurrence of the infection. The teen must know that she should continue the medication even if her menstrual period begins.

Reducing Pruritus. Pruritus that is unrelieved by medication or that is of chemical or mechanical etiology may respond to efforts to keep the area clean and dry. It is important that the patient (and parent, in the case of the young child) understand the etiology of vulvar or vaginal pruritus. Females who are prone to genital inflammation are advised to exclude contact with perfumes and dyes, and to avoid prolonged perineal dampness. Both preventive and symptomatic care, therefore, dictate using only nonperfumed soaps, avoiding bubble baths and perfumed douches, wearing loose-fitting panties with a white cotton crotch, wiping (always from front to back to avoid fecal contamination) with white, nonperfumed toilet paper, avoiding sitting for long periods in tight-fitting jeans, and changing sanitary pads or tampons frequently.

Adolescents who are sexually active should be advised to use a water-soluble lubricant during periods of frequent intercourse to reduce mechanical irritation. They need also to be advised of the importance of medical assessment and treatment of their sexual partner(s) if the vaginitis involves an infectious organism.

Addressing the Disturbance in Self-Concept. The child's or adolescent's perception of vaginitis may be quite different from the actual diagnosis. She may feel she is being punished for masturbation or for sexual activity. She may fear that the vaginitis will affect her ability to become pregnant or her future children. The odor and discharge associated with an infection may make her feel "dirty" and fear that others will guess her "condition." The nurse who anticipates these responses can often establish an empathetic rapport that will allow assessment of feelings, and a frank discussion of what vaginitis is and what it is not. Teaching preventive measures that allow the older child and adolescent a sense of control will also enhance self-concept.

Nursing Strategies for Follow-Up Care in the Home or Clinic

Assess for decreased discharge and pruritus.

Assess compliance with the medication protocol as applicable.

If sexual partners are involved, determine if they are being treated.

Encourage the patient to verbalize a plan of prevention.

References

Aach RD: Viral hepatitis. *In* Feigin RD, Cherry JD (eds): *Textbook of Pediatric Infectious Diseases.* 2nd ed, Vol I. Philadelphia, WB Saunders, 1987, pp 718–741.

Brown NA: The Epstein-Barr virus. *In* Feigin RD, Cherry JD (eds): *Textbook of Pediatric Infectious Diseases.* 2nd ed, Vol II. Philadelphia, WB Saunders, 1987, pp 1566–1577.

Brunell PA: Hepatitis. *In* Behrman RE, Vaughan VC (eds): *Nelson Textbook of Pediatrics.* 13th ed. Philadelphia, WB Saunders, 1987, pp 684–688.

1988 Canadian Guidelines for the Treatment of Sexually Transmitted Diseases in Neonates, Children, Adolescents and Adults. *Can Dis Wkly Rep* 1988 Apr; 14S2.

Centers for Disease Control: Chlamydia trachomatic infections. Policy and guidelines for prevention and control. *MMWR* 1985 Aug; 23:34(3S).

Centers for Disease Control: 1985 STD treatment guidelines. *MMWR* 1985 Oct; 18:34(4S).

Committee on Chemotherapy of Tuberculosis: Standard therapy for tuberculosis 1985. *Chest* 1985 Feb(Suppl); 87:117S–184S.

Feldman Y: Kaposi's sarcoma and opportunistic infections. *Dermatol Clin* 1983 Jan; 131–136.

Friedlander L: Vulva and vagina. *In* Gellis SS, Kagan BM (eds): *Current Pediatric Therapy 12.* Philadelphia, WB Saunders, 1986.

Fulginiti VA: Immunologic responses to infection. *In* Feigin RD, and Cherry JD (eds): *Textbook of Pediatric Infectious diseases.* 2nd ed., Vol I. Philadelphia, WB Saunders, 1987, pp 28–40.

Garcia LS: Parasitic diseases. *In* Feigin RD, Cherry JD (eds): *Textbook of Pediatric Infectious Diseases.* 2nd ed. Vol II. Philadelphia, WB Saunders, 1987, pp 2007–2137.

Johnson J: Sexually transmitted diseases in adolescents. *Prim Care* 1987 Mar; 14(1):101–120.

Kalter DC, Rosen T: Sexually transmitted diseases. *Emerg Med Clin North Am* 1985 Nov; 3(4):693–716.

Kazura JW, Mahmoud AAF: Helminths. *In* Behrman RE, Vaughan VC (eds): *Nelson Textbook of Pediatrics.* 13th ed. Philadelphia, WB Saunders, 1987, pp 739–743.

Loebl S, Spratto GR: *The Nurse's Drug Handbook.* 4th ed. New York, John Wiley and Sons, 1986.

Lutz R: Stopping the spread of sexually transmitted diseases. *Nursing 86* 1986 Mar; 47–50.

Minster J: Nursing management of patients with scabies and lice. *Nurs Clin North Am* 1980 Dec; 747.

Plotkin SA, Henle W: Infectious mononucleosis. *In* Behrman RE, Vaughan VC (eds): *Nelson Textbook of Pediatrics.* 13th Ed. Philadelphia, WB Saunders, 1987, pp 670–673.

Smith MHD, Marquis JR; Tuberculosis and other mycobacterial infections. *In* Feigin RD, Cherry JD (eds): *Textbook of Pediatric Infectious Diseases.* 2nd ed, Vol I. Philadelphia, WB Saunders, 1987, pp 1342–1387.

Vella E: Research in rabies. *Nurs Times* 1977 Mar; 17:37.

Wilfert C, Gutman L: Sexually transmitted diseases. *In* Feigin RD, Cherry JD (eds): *Textbook of Pediatric Infectious Diseases.* 2nd ed, Vol I. Philadelphia, WB Saunders, 1987, pp 595–608.

Bibliography

Burke PJ: Adolescents' motivation for sexual activity and pregnancy prevention. *Issues Compr Pediatr Nurs* 1987; 10(3):161–171.

Cornell C: Tuberculosis in hospital employees. *Am J Nurs* 1988 Apr; 88(4):484–486.

Dirubbo NE: The condom barrier. *Am J Nurs* 1987 Oct; 87(10):1306–1309.

Genital herpes: Who should take oral acyclovir? *Nurse's Drug Alert* 1987 Jul; 11(7):951.

Gurevich I: How to make every culture count. *RN* 1988 Aug: 49–55.

Kirkis EJ, Grier M: *Nurse's Guide to Infection Control Practice.* Philadelphia, WB Saunders, 1988.

Kuffel J: Treating a child with head lice. *RN* 1987 Sep; 32.

Lewis HR, Lewis ME: What you and your patients need to know about safer sex. *RN* 1987 Sep; 53–58.

Loucks A: *Chlamydia:* The unheralded epidemic. *Am J Nurs* 1987 Jul; 87(7):920–922.

Marvin C, Slevin A: *Chlamydia*—Cause, prevention, and cure. *MCN* 1987 Oct; 12(5):318–321.

McElhose P: The "other" STDs. As dangerous as ever. *RN* 1988 Jun; 53–58.

Muscari ME: Obtaining the adolescent sexual history. *Pediatr Nurs* 1987 Oct; 13(5):307–310.

Orshan SA: The pill, the patient, and you. *RN* 1988 Jul; 49–53.

Pachter A: Should nurses receive the hepatitis B vaccine? *Nurs 88* 1988 Jun; 18(6):51.

Stewart DC: Sexuality and the adolescent: Issues for the clinician. *Prim Care* 1987 Mar; 14(1):83–99.

Two new vaccines against whooping cough. *Nurse's Drug Alert* 1988 Aug; 12(8):1104–1105.

Zack R: What to do if your patient has lice. *RN* 1987 Sep; 30–31.

Nursing Strategies: Altered Neurologic Function

Chapter 46

Jennifer Disabato
Judy Wulf

Nursing Process Plan
NPP: The Child with Increased Intracranial Pressure, page 1713

Related Topics
Patterns of inheritance, genetic counseling, Chapter 4
Impact of Acute Illness, Chapter 24
Impact of Chronic Illness, Chapter 25
Febrile seizure (management of fever), Chapter 27
Neonatal sepsis, Chapter 40
Malignant brain tumors, Chapter 48
Nursing process plan for the family in need of genetic counseling, Table 50-3

Any adult who has ever watched an infant learn to walk, a toddler teetering on a counter top, a preschooler climb a tree, a school-age child wield a bat, or an adolescent on a motorcycle has entertained an urge to reach out to protect them from harm — and with good reason. The concept of altered neurologic function in the child brings to mind shattered dreams for the child and family and an uncertain future. Fortunately, nature provided children (especially the infant and young child) with a skull that withstands trauma much better than does the head of an adult, and many potentially dangerous mishaps result in minor bumps and scrapes. Unfortunately, nature also makes mistakes, and some children suffer from congenital and chronic neurologic abnormalities linked to causes such as incomplete development in utero and heritable traits. By virtue of their susceptibility to organisms such as

Haemophilus influenzae, children also develop infections of the neurologic system.

This chapter is designed to prepare the nurse generalist to care for the more common alterations in neurologic function. The chapter begins by describing the differences in structure and function of the neurologic system by developmental age, details assessment and interventions for nursing care common to many neurologic problems, and then proceeds to a discussion of specific conditions grouped by congenital and chronic abnormalities, neurologic infection, and neurologic injury.

Age-Related Differences in Structure and Function

A thorough understanding of the anatomy and physiology of the nervous system is necessary in caring for children with alterations in neurologic function. Recognition of the spatial relationships that the structures have to each other becomes crucial in acute dysfunctions to better understand and anticipate potential problems. Figure 46-1 and Table 46-1 provide a review of the anatomy and physiology of the *central nervous system.* For a review of the structure and functions of the *peripheral nervous system,* see Figure 46-2 and Table 46-2. The focus of this section is the differences in structure and function of the nervous system at different ages.

Size, Shape, and Physical Characteristics

At birth the brain is one quarter of adult size; at one year of age it becomes about one half of adult size; and by age 5 it has attained 90 per cent of its total growth. This growth in the brain places pressure on the bones of the skull, specifically at the suture lines which respond by depositing new bone at the suture edges thus increasing the circumference of the head (Stewart, 1978). Review of head circumference growth charts (Appendix Three) should serve to reinforce the knowledge of tremendous growth, especially in the first year of life and in early childhood. The increases in horizontal skull girth occur during the first 2 years of life and account for much of the expansion in head circumference (Conway, 1977). Two conditions that can affect the size of the brain and skull are microcephaly and macrocephaly.

Microcephaly is a rare condition characterized by a small skull and severe mental retardation because of lack of brain growth. Primary microcephaly is caused by arrested brain growth in utero. The brain is not formed to the usual size, resulting in diminished skull growth. Secondary microcephaly occurs after injury and is accompanied by neurologic manifestations.

In primary microcephaly, the congenital pathology is an embryologic defect and may be caused by an autosomal recessive disorder or a chromosomal abnormality. Other suspected causes are maternal rubella in the first trimester, toxoplasmosis and maternal exposure to repeated roentgenography. There is no increased intracranial pressure in primary microcephaly because the brain has stopped growing. The criterion for microcephaly is a head circumference of 33 cm or less in a 6-month-old infant and 43 cm or less in an adult. The head must be disproportionately small in comparison to the rest of the body. Primary microcephaly can be recognized in a newborn with a small and conical skull shape, receding forehead, and flattened occiput. Face and ears may appear normal. Physical growth is delayed and many children have spinal curvatures and visual defects.

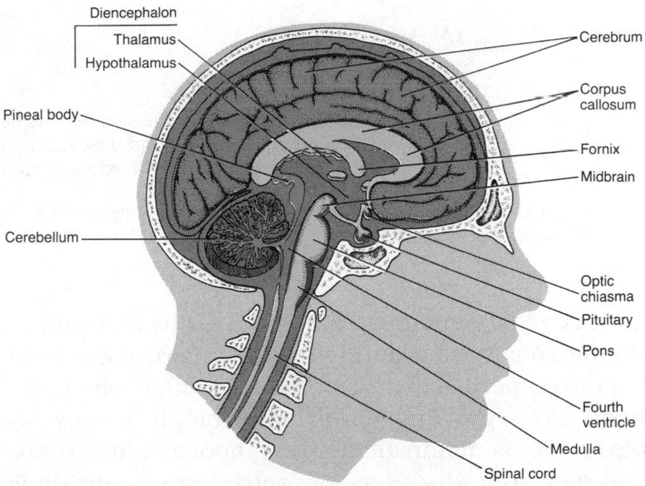

Figure 46-1. A midsagittal section through the brain. Note that in this type of section half the brain is cut away so that the structures normally covered by the cerebrum are exposed.

Table 46-1. Divisions of the Brain

	Description	Functions
Medulla	Most inferior portion of the brain stem; continuous with spinal cord; its white matter consists of nerve tracts passing between the spinal cord and various parts of the brain; its gray matter consists of nuclei; the anterior portion consists mainly of the pyramids; contains nuclei of cranial nerves IX through XII;* its cavity is the fourth ventricle	Contains vital centers (within its reticular formation) that regulate heartbeat, respiration, and blood pressure; contains reflex centers that control swallowing, coughing, sneezing, and vomiting; relays messages to other parts of the brain
Pons	Consists mainly of nerve tracts passing between the medulla and other parts of the brain; forms a bulge on the anterior surface of the brain stem; contains a respiratory center and nuclei of cranial nerves V through VIII	Serves as a link connecting various parts of the brain; helps regulate respiration
Midbrain	Just superior to the pons; cavity is the cerebral aqueduct; posteriorly, tectum consists of corpora quadrigemina; within midbrain are nuclei of cranial nerves III and IV	Corpora quadrigemina mediate visual and auditory reflexes; cranial nerves III and IV control certain eye movements
Diencephalon	Consists of two parts: *Thalamus*—located on each side of the third ventricle; consists of two masses of gray matter partly covered by white matter and contains many important nuclei	Main relay center conducting information between spinal cord and cerebrum; incoming messages are sorted and partially interpreted within the thalamic nuclei before being relayed to the appropriate centers in the cerebrum
	Hypothalamus—forms ventral floor of third ventricle; contains many nuclei; optic chiasma mark the crossing of the optic nerves; infundibulum connects the pituitary gland to the hypothalamus	Contains centers for control of body temperature, appetite, and water balance; regulates pituitary gland and links nervous and endocrine systems; helps control autonomic system; involved in some emotional and sexual responses
Cerebellum	Second largest part of brain; superior to the fourth ventricle; consists of two lateral cerebellar hemispheres	Responsible for smooth, coordinated movement; maintains posture and muscle tone and helps maintain equilibrium
Cerebrum	Largest, most prominent part of the brain; longitudinal fissure divides the cerebrum into right and left hemispheres, each containing a lateral ventricle; each hemisphere is divided into six lobes; frontal, parietal, occipital, temporal, limbic, and insula	Center of intellect, memory, language, and consciousness; receives and interprets sensory information from all sense organs; controls motor functions
Cerebral cortex	Convoluted, outer layer of gray matter covering the cerebrum; functionally divided into:	
	(1) Motor areas	Control voluntary movement and certain types of involuntary movement
	(2) Sensory areas	Receive incoming sensory information from eyes, ears, touch, and pressure receptors, and other sense organs; sensory association areas interpret incoming sensory information
	(3) Association areas	Responsible for thought, learning, language, judgment, and personality; store memories; connect sensory and motor areas
White matter	Consists of fibers that connect the two hemispheres and fibers that are part of ascending and descending tracts; basal ganglia are located within the white matter	Links various areas of the brain

* Cranial nerves are discussed in more detail in Table 15-8.
(From Solomon and Phillips, 1987.)

Secondary microcephaly is caused by an insult to the nervous system during the latter part of the third trimester, perinatally, or postnatally, after which the brain stops growing normally. Etiologic factors include anoxia, traumatic delivery, neonatal infections, and metabolic disorders. Secondary microcephaly is first recognized by symptoms of neurologic impairment that vary depending on the age of the child when the insult or damage occurred. The degree of mental retardation that occurs depends on the degree of injury.

Macrocephaly, an unusually large brain and skull, may be caused by either a primary congenital developmental error, in which there are cellular and structural defects in the brain tissue, or by a secondary progressive, destructive process seen in demyelinating disease such as Schilder disease and in the leukodystrophies (Conway, 1977). Clinical findings include accelerated head growth, delay in fontanel closure, mental and physical retardation and seizures, but no increased intracranial pressure. This needs to be differentiated from two other conditions affecting head

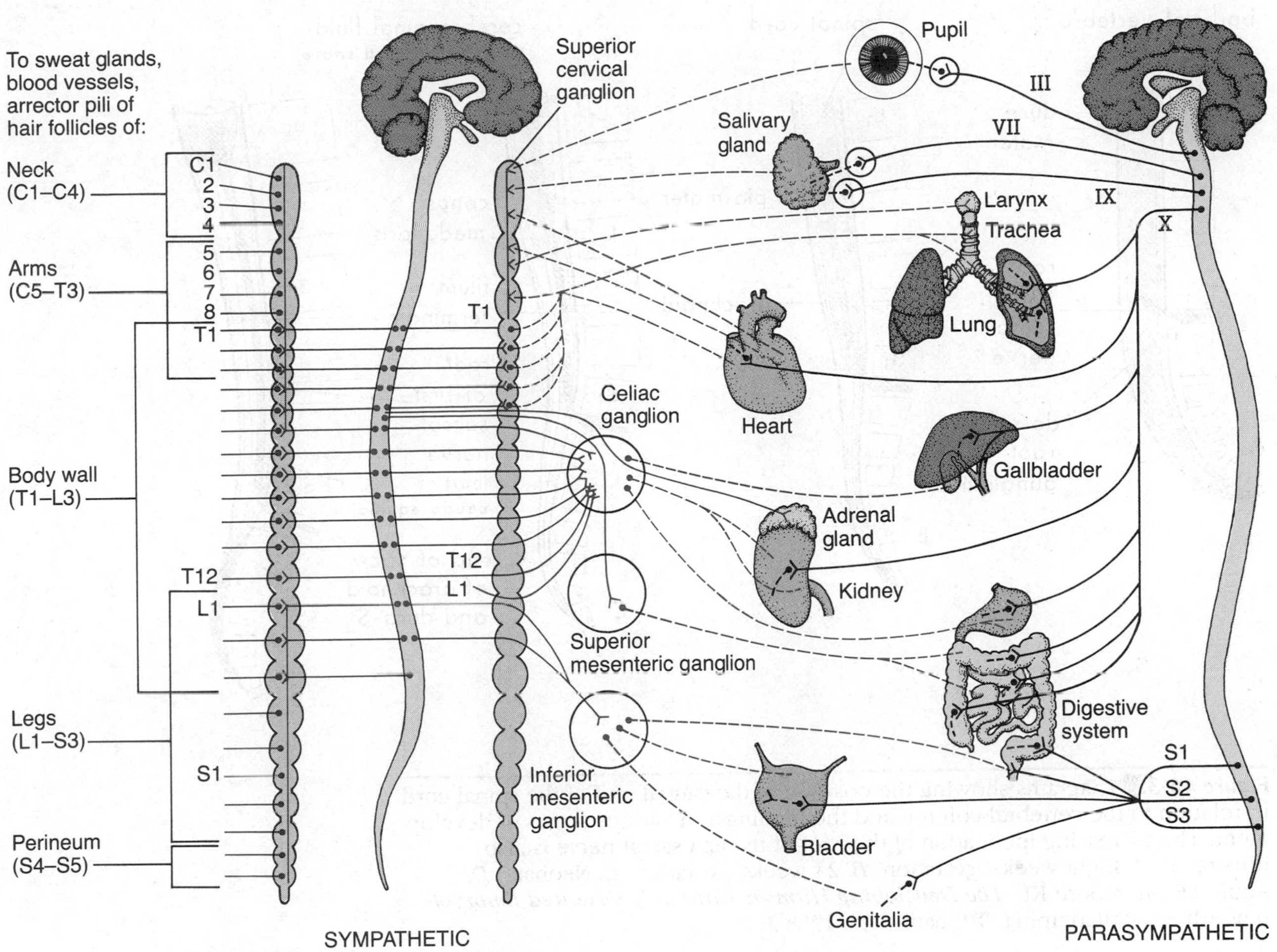

***Figure* 46-2.** Sympathetic and parasympathetic nervous systems. For clarity, peripheral and visceral nerves of the sympathetic system are shown on separate sides of the cord. Complex as it appears, this diagram has been greatly simplified. (Colored lines represent sympathetic nerves, black lines represent parasympathetic nerves, and dotted lines represent postganglionic nerves.)

***Table* 46-2.** Comparison of Sympathetic and Parasympathetic Actions on Selected Effectors

Effector	Sympathetic Action	Parasympathetic Action
Heart	Increases rate and strength of contraction	Decreases rate; no direct effect on strength of contraction
Bronchial tubes	Dilates	Constricts
Iris of eye	Dilates (pupil becomes larger)	Constricts (pupil becomes smaller)
Sex organs	Constricts blood vessels; ejaculation	Dilates blood vessels; erection
Blood vessels	Generally constricts	No innervation for many
Sweat glands	Stimulates	No innervation
Intestine	Inhibits motility	Stimulates motility and secretion
Liver metabolism	Stimulates glycogen breakdown	No effect
Adipose tissue	Stimulates free fatty acid release from fat cells	No effect
Adrenal medulla	Stimulates secretion of epinephrine and norepinephrine	No effect
Salivary glands	Stimulates thick, viscous secretion	Stimulates profuse, water secretion

Note that many other examples could be added to this list.
(From Solomon and Phillips, 1987.)

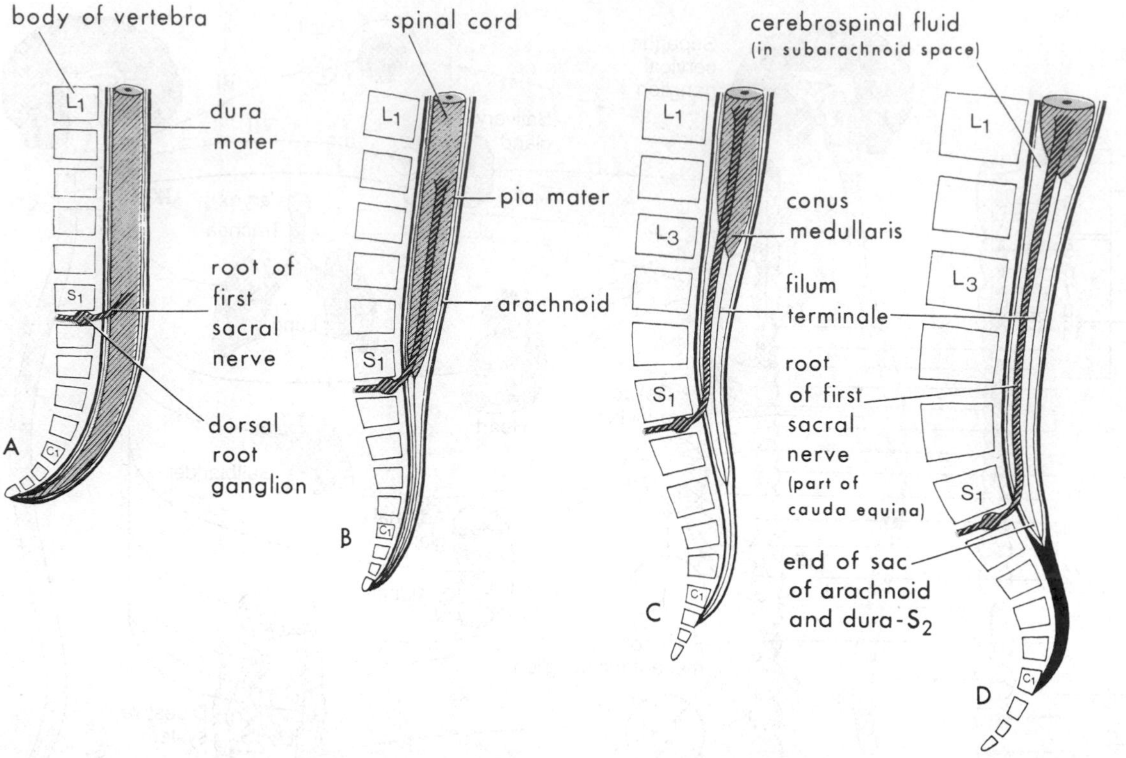

Figure 46-3. Diagrams showing the position of the caudal end of the spinal cord in relation to the vertebral column and the meninges at various stages of development. The increasing inclination of the root of the first sacral nerve is also illustrated. *A*, Eight weeks' gestation. *B*, 24 weeks' gestation. *C*, Neonate. *D*, Adult. (From Moore KL: *The Developing Human: Clinically Oriented Embryology*. 4th ed. Philadelphia, WB Saunders, 1988.)

size: familial macrocephaly and hydrocephalus. Familial macrocephaly results in a large head size that follows the shape of the growth curve, appears genetically determined, and does not result in any developmental problems. Hydrocephalus results in an abnormally enlarging head because of defects in the production, absorption, or flow of cerebral spinal fluid in the ventricular system, resulting in increased intracranial pressure.

The spinal cord, cranial, and peripheral nerves elongate during the growth of childhood. The termination of the spinal cord and its relationship to the lumbar vertebrae change inversely, so that in newborn infants the cord terminates at L3 and in adults it terminates at L1–2 (Moore, 1988) (Fig. 46-3). This has implications for the location of needle insertion for tests such as lumbar puncture.

Ossification, Calcification, and Fontanel Closure

Skull ossification begins in infancy and continues into adulthood. Ossification occurs most rapidly in young children and then begins to slow in early school age. Prior to age 7 sutures may spread as a sign of increased intracranial pressure; after this age however, separated sutures are more uncommon as a strong fibrous joint develops (Conway, 1977). The pineal gland, a useful landmark in neurodiagnostic studies because of its midline position, becomes calcified sometime during adolescence.

The six fontanels, or soft spots, in the infant vary in the time of closure depending on location and relationship to various suture lines. The first fontanels to close (around 2 months of age) are the posterior fontanel, which is formed by the intersection of the sagittal and lambdoidal sutures, and the two anterolateral fontanels, which are formed by the intersection of the frontal, parietal, temporal, and sphenoid bones. The last fontanels to close are the anterior fontanel formed by the intersection of the coronal and sagittal sutures (closes between 12 and 18 months), and the two posterolateral fontanels, formed by the intersection of the parietal, occipital, and temporal bones (close by 24 months of age).

Timing of fontanel closure is important. For example, premature or early fontanel closure and suture ossification in a normally developing brain could restrict a plane of growth, risk brain damage, and result in craniosynostosis (discussed later in this chapter).

Physiologic Differences

Cerebral Spinal Fluid

Cerebral spinal fluid (CSF) formation, flow and absorption in children is comparable to that in adults. The difference is in rate of formation and in volume. Comparisons available in the literature are of infants and adults, the assumption being that children of other ages would fall somewhere between the two. The rate of formation for a newborn is about 1 ml/hr or 25 ml/day, as compared with that for the adult which is 20 ml/hr or 500 ml/day (Swaiman and Wright, 1982). Total CSF volume in the newborn is 6 to 8 cc, in the adult 110 to 140 cc (Bell and McCormick, 1978). Comparison of the rate of formation to volume notes that there is a constant production and absorption of CSF resulting in a changeover of CSF approximately five times per day. This has implication for how rapidly symptoms can change with increases in intracranial pressure due to dysfunction in the ventricular system.

Cerebral Function

Probably the most striking neurologic achievements in children are the attainment of developmental milestones including gross and fine motor, speech and language, perceptual and integrative, personal, social, and cognitive skills. Further information in this area can be found in Unit Two. Information on changes in developmental reflexes throughout infancy and childhood are also detailed in that unit.

Neurons

Neurons are the structural and functional units of the nervous system. Neurons are specialized to be excitable and to conduct impulses. This is important when considering the role of early experience and environmental stimulation on the development and further specialization within the nervous system.

The cerebral cortex is formed by migrating cells that pass through previously formed layers in the third fetal month. By the sixth fetal month, six layers of cell bodies and their processes are evident (Conway, 1977). The ultimate growth of these layers is not completed until middle childhood or early adolescence. The neuron and its neighboring cells have variable functions depending on their location, most likely highly influenced by neurotransmitters and other substances (Swaiman, 1982). It is important to have an understanding of the specific regional and topographic localization of the brain as well as the lateralization, in order to appreciate how neurologic function can be altered by processes that can occur at various ages of childhood (Fig. 46-4).

Transmission of Impulses in Unmyelinated Nerves. The reader needs to have a basic understanding of the transmission of the impulses by neurons as this is a major function that can be triggered by chemical, mechanical, thermal, and electrical stimuli (Fig. 46-5). Changes in electrical charges within the cell occur as a result of a stimulus. The stimulus effects

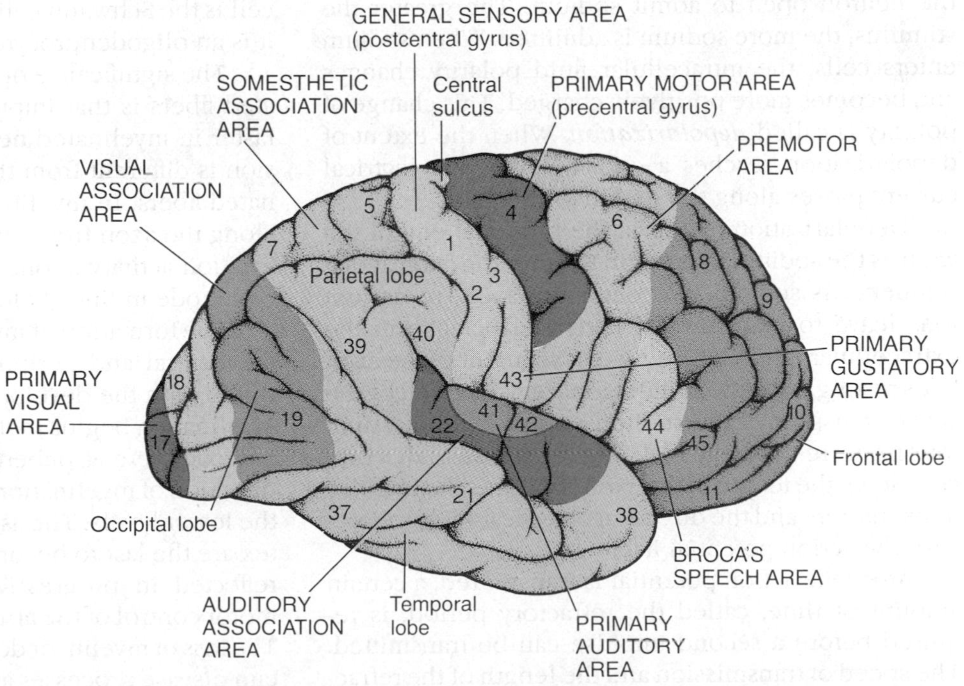

Figure 46-4. Map of the lateral surface of the cerebral cortex, showing some of the functional areas. Areas 4, 6, and 8 are motor areas; areas 1, 2, 3, 17, 41, 42, and 43 are primary sensory areas; and areas 9, 10, 11, 18, 19, 22, 38, 39, and 40 are association areas.

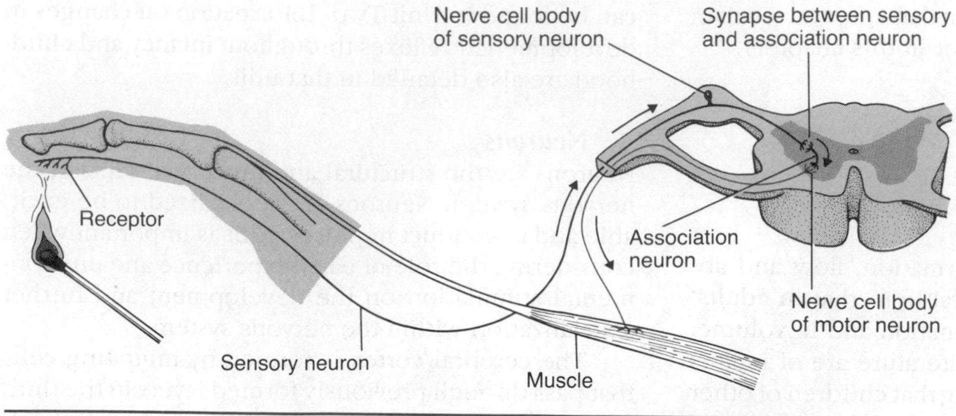

Figure 46-5. The withdrawal reflex shown here involves a chain of three neurons. A sensory neuron transmits the message from the receptor to the CNS, where it synapses with an association neuron. Then an appropriate motor neuron (shown in color) transmits an impulse to the muscles that move the hand away from the flame (the response).

change at the synapse, where there is a release of neurotransmitter substance which changes the permeability of the cell membrane in the adjoining cell. It is these changes in the cell that are responsible for the transmission.

The cell membrane is only permeable to certain substances and differences exist between the extracellular and intracellular ion concentrations. The extracellular fluid components provide a positive ion balance. The intracellular fluid components provide a negative balance. When the cell is at rest the extracellular fluid contains more positively charged ions than does the intracellular fluid (Fig. 46-6). When a stimulus of sufficient intensity excites the cell, tiny pores in the neuron open to admit sodium. The greater the stimulus, the more sodium is admitted. When sodium enters cells, the intracellular fluid polarity changes and becomes more positively charged. This change of polarity is called *depolarization.* When the extent of depolarization reaches a critical level, an electrical current passes along the length of the axon.

Depolarization begins at the proximal end of the axon as the sodium ions begin to enter the axon at that segment. As sodium ions enter the axon, potassium ions leave to maintain the electrical balance in the extracellular fluid. Returning that segment of the axon to its resting state, the sodium ions leave the cell by the active transport of the sodium pump, and potassium ions freely re-enter the cell. The repetition of this process down the length of the axon produces the impulse transmission, and the direction of ionic flow correlates with the action potential itself.

After one action potential is transmitted, a certain amount of time, called the refractory period, is required before a second impulse can be transmitted. The speed of transmission and the length of the refractory period varies with the diameter of the axon and the presence or absence of a myelin sheath, as well as the stimulus intensity. Both axon diameter and degree of myelination change with age (Snyder, 1983).

Impulse Transmission in Myelinated Nerves. Whereas unmyelinated fibers are abundant in the autonomic nervous system, myelinated nerve fibers occur predominantly in the cranial and spinal nerves and compose the white matter of the brain and spinal cord. The lipid substance myelin, which forms the sheath around these nerve fibers, gives the whitish color to the white matter of the brain. The myelin sheath is formed from a glial cell that wraps around the axon (Fig. 46-7). In the peripheral nervous system the glial cell is the Schwann cell; in the central nervous system it is an oligodendrocyte.

The significance of myelinated versus nonmyelinated fibers is that impulses travel hundreds of times faster in myelinated nerves. The process of transmission is different from that just described for unmyelinated fibers. In myelinated nerves the impulse jumps along the axon from one node of Ranvier to the next. The ion activity at one node serves to depolarize the next node in line (Solomon and Philips, 1987).

The formation of myelin around neuronal axons in the central and peripheral nervous systems is associated with the development of functional capacities. Myelination begins in the third fetal month and is usually complete at puberty (AANN, 1984). The general direction of myelination begins in the cervical spine to the lower levels. The association areas of cerebral cortex are the last to become myelinated. This process is reflected in progressive development as voluntary motor control of the arms precedes control of the legs. The loss of myelin, or demyelination, that occurs in certain disease processes alters transmission of impulses.

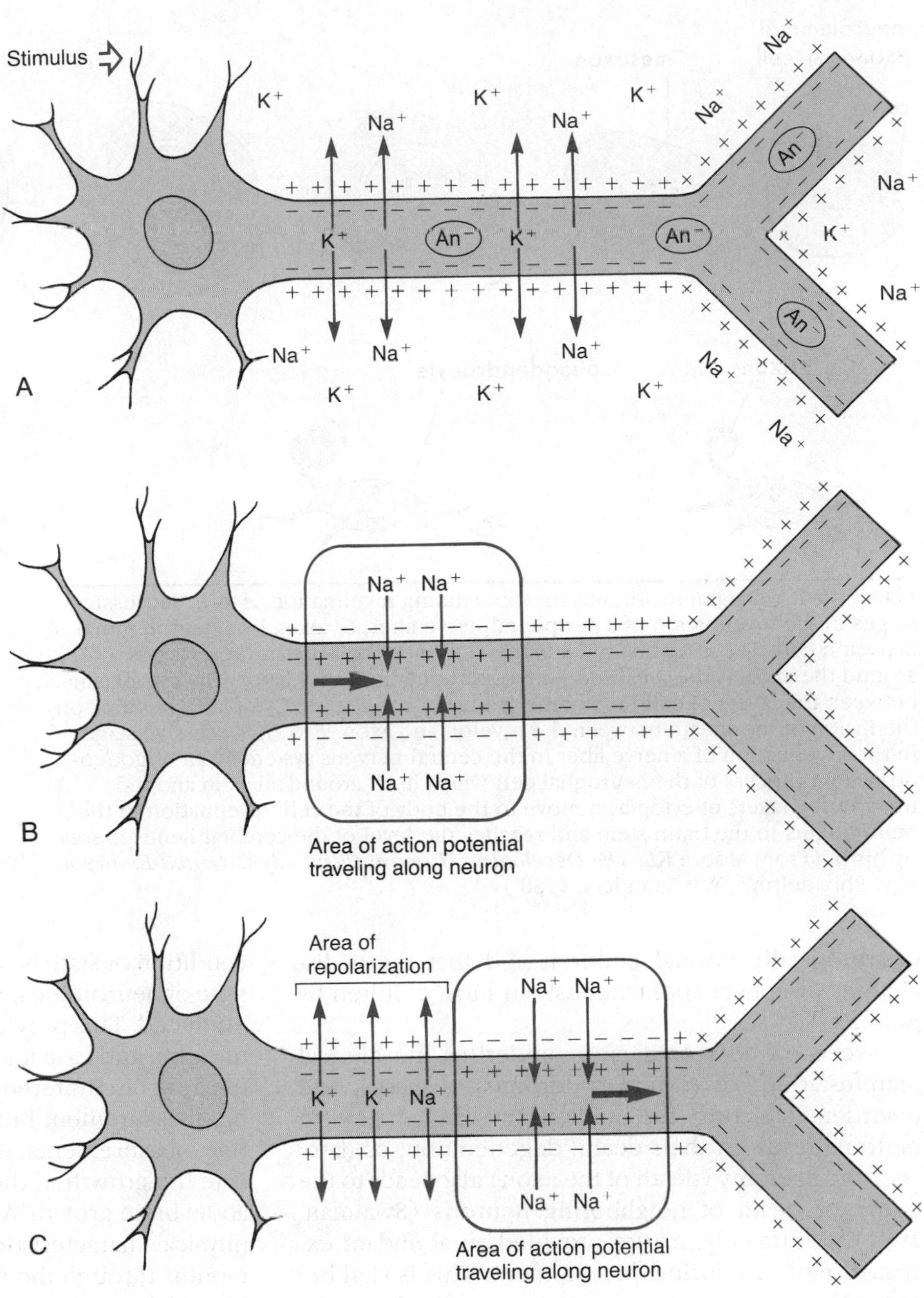

Figure 46-6. Transmission of an impulse along an axon. *A,* The dendrites of a neuron are stimulated sufficiently to depolarize the cell membrane to firing level. The axon shown is still in the resting state and has a resting potential. *B* and *C,* An impulse is transmitted as a wave of depolarization that travels down the axon. At the region of depolarization, sodium ions diffuse into the cell. As the impulse passes along from one region to another, resting conditions are quickly re-established. (Na^+, sodium ions; K^+, potassium ions; An^-, large ions within the neuron.)

Brain Waves

The gross electrical activity of the brain during wakefulness and sleep, as measured by the electroencephalogram (EEG), shows gradual changes in wave amplitude, frequency, and distribution with normal brain growth and development. In an extremely general sense the waves become more organized and rhythmic, and are of increased frequency and decreased amplitude. The age of the child is of importance when interpreting the findings on EEG. For example, while the predominance of theta rhythms (4 to 8 cycles per second) and delta rhythms (1 to 4 cycles per second) may be normal for a young child, their predominance for an adolescent would be read as abnormal and indicate a slowing of electrical activity, compared with same-age peers. Sometimes these EEG findings correlate with clinical symptoms of developmental delays or other diffuse processes affecting the brain. At other timcs these findings may be nonspecific (Ferry et al, 1986). Children may show some focal or localized electrical discharges on EEG that would be viewed as abnormal for an adult, such as 2 to 3 cycle per second rhythms during drowsiness (Ferry et al, 1986). Cavazuti and coworkers (1980) noted in a longitudinal study that some epileptiform or seizure-like discharges may be present in as many as 3.4 per cent of

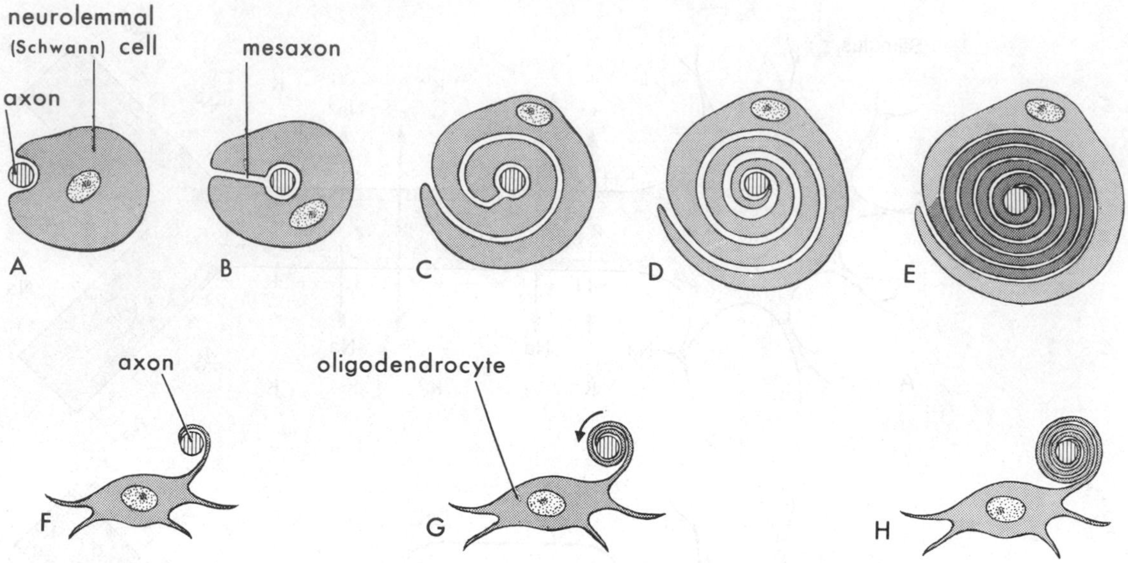

Figure 46-7. Diagrammatic sketches illustrating myelination. *A* to *E*, Successive stages in the myelination of a peripheral nerve fiber, or axon, by a neurolemmal or Schwann cell. The axon first indents the cell; then the Schwann cell rotates around the axon as the mesaxon (site of invagination) elongates. The cytoplasm between the layers of cell membrane gradually condenses. Cytoplasm remains on the inside of the sheath between the myelon and axon. *F* to *H*, Successive stages in the myelination of a nerve fiber in the central nervous system by an oligodendrocyte. A process of the neuroglial cell wraps itself around an axon and the intervening layers of cytoplasm move to the body of the cell. Myelination in the brain begins in the brain stem and reaches the level of the cerebral hemispheres by birth. (From Moore KL: *The Developing Human; Clinically Oriented Embryology.* Philadelphia, WB Saunders, 1988.)

neurologically normal children and that these discharges disappear spontaneously in most children by puberty.

Neuronal loss or damage underlies the clinical manifestations of clinical syndromes, diseases, and disorders affecting the nervous system. Injury to neurons result in their death, degeneration, or damage, and axotomy (death of the axon) also leads to the injury or death of neighboring neurons (Swaiman, 1982). Fortunately, nature provided an abundant excess of neurons during development. This is vital because the cerebral cortex contains neuronal populations that are incapable of dividing or regenerating after full differentiation by the end of the second trimester of life (Swaiman, 1982). The implications of either localized or diffuse damage at various ages can effect the outcome and potential recovery.

Nursing Implications of Developmental Differences

The nursing implications of the age-related differences in structure and function are numerous. During assessment for actual or potential problems the nurse should realize that not only will the child's present condition or state be assessed, but also that the overall state of neurologic maturation or development will be evaluated. This provides an opportunity for early identification and case finding. For example, assessment of the head circumference should involve more than simple measurement but include comparison with baseline measurements, when available, to be able to evaluate the growth of the head and provide indirect data about brain growth. Assessment of the size, shape, and physical characteristics of the skull during the first few months through the first 2 years of life assists in early identification of problems and prompt treatment.

The assessment of infants and young children is limited by their developmental level. It is important to be aware that neurologic status can appear to change rapidly because of the limits of assessment and because open sutures and fontanels help to compensate for increases in intracranial pressure. Neurologic signs may be apparent, or they may manifest themselves in more subtle ways such as lack of interest in eating or irritability. School-age children and adolescents are more similar to adults in the area of neurologic assessment, physiologic responses, and compensatory mechanisms.

Age-related differences in structure and function are also important for the interpretation of diagnostic tests and in the nursing care related to monitoring of neurologic function. Having a solid understanding of the principles of neurologic function and an appreciation for how different types of damage can affect the brain at different stages of development is useful in instructing, reinforcing, and clarifying information the physician has given the family. It is important to realize those times when some prediction of outcome may be possible and those situations in which prognosis is uncertain. Care must be taken neither to remove all hope nor to set totally unrealistic expectations when talking with a child and family about disease outcome.

Assessment of Neurologic Function

This section will discuss factors that guide and influence the type of assessment, factors that should be included in the health history, and factors that affect the assessment of children of different ages. This section will expand upon the basic neurologic assessment presented in Chapter 15.

As previously mentioned, neurologic assessment of children is a two-part process. It includes evaluation for actual and potential problems at the time of assessment, and also provides an evaluation of the rate of maturation of the nervous system. The purpose is to determine how the dysfunction or alteration has affected or may affect the child's and family's self-care, daily living, and ability to cope. This assessment will provide direction for patient and family care planning, teaching, and counseling and should become the beginning of the rehabilitative or adaptive process.

Factors Influencing Assessment

Rate of Change

Criteria that guide the assessment of a neurologic problem include the rate of change, severity of the problem, and its nature or location. The rate of change has implication for the speed, organization, and frequency of assessment that may be needed. For example, a child comes home from the playground late and is irritable for 3 hours, then suddenly becomes listless and is only arousable to loud voices and displays "fending off" behavior and inappropriate conversation. Assessment of an acute situation like this would focus on quickly establishing baseline function of level of consciousness; pupil responses; motor responses; protective reflexes such as blink, swallow, gag, and cough; respiratory pattern; and vital signs (AANN, 1984). The time required for this assessment may be several minutes, and depending on the patient's acuity, reassessment may be necessary every 1 to 2 hours. Let us suppose that this child subsequently undergoes surgery to evacuate a subdural hematoma. If the child is alert in the postoperative period, the nurse may take time for a more comprehensive and orderly assessment. The frequency of subsequent assessments might then be daily or several times a day, depending on the child's status.

The rate of change also has some diagnostic implication as to the general cause of the problem (Swaiman and Wright, 1982). Changes occurring over minutes to a day may indicate a vascular or traumatic cause. Changes occurring over several days may indicate such processes as infections, electrolyte imbalances, or toxic poisoning. Changes occurring over days to weeks or months may give indication of causes that could be neoplastic, metabolic, or degenerative.

Severity of the Problem

The severity of the problem, whether static (unchanging), or progressive, also influences the assessment. The manner in which the nurse might assess the child who has been delayed in development since birth will differ from the assessment of another child whose parents give a history suggesting a loss of certain motor skills previously acquired.

Nature and Location of the Problem

The nature and location of the problem also affects the assessment. Level of consciousness may be altered and the assessment may need to be carried out frequently if the nature of the problem is unknown. Problems are frequently referred to as being focal (attributable to a discrete neuroanatomic area), multifocal (several areas affected), or diffuse (widespread, affecting the majority of the brain). This also may have some general diagnostic implication in that focal problems may have causes that are more frequently of vascular, neoplastic, or traumatic origin while multifocal or diffuse problems are more frequently of toxic, metabolic, infectious, congenital, degenerative, and unknown origin.

Various Types of Assessment

Nurses may use different types of assessment depending on their judgment, the patient's needs, and the medical plan of care. The three most common examples are the *acute neurologic check,* the *screening examination,* and the *comprehensive examination.* The screening and the comprehensive examinations are usually used upon first contact with the patient, while the acute neurologic check is used primary for acute monitoring of the patient during the hospitalization. During practice the nurse may find that a combination of the different assessments are actually being used, which may allow for screening gross assessments in those areas without suspected problems and more indepth comprehensive evaluation in problem areas. Whatever the method used, the focus is upon nursing diagnosis, intervention, and evaluation.

Acute Neurologic Check

The components of the acute neurologic check usually include assessment of

- level of consciousness
- pupil size and reactivity
- eye movements
- motor function
- respiratory pattern
- vital signs

The organization of these components and importance given a specific component may vary depending on the type of problem the patient may be experiencing and certainly on the age of the patient. The purpose of the acute neurologic check is to identify significant changes in neurologic function that may indicate deterioration or improvement, provide early detection of potentially life-threatening problems, and provide the means for early interventions that can further prevent complications and may positively influence outcome. The frequency of the assessment is determined by the patient's level of consciousness, acuity level, nature and location of the problem, nursing assessment, and physician's orders. The following section details the components of the acute neurologic check.

Level of Consciousness. Plum (1980) defines level of consciousness as an awareness of self and environment that includes two components: content and arousal. *Content* includes processes such as perception, attention, memory, and judgment. *Arousal* is described as wakefulness. ***In assessing infants and young children assessment of level of consciousness primarily involves assessing arousal.*** The neuroanatomic correlates of consciousness are in the cerebral cortex and the reticular activating system of the brainstem.

It is important in assessing level of consciousness to use the least amount of stimulation necessary to evoke the best response. Note both the quality of the response and the degree of arousal. Medical conditions that may alter arousal include those that interfere with cerebral blood flow, alter cerebral metabolism, affect synaptic transmission with the brain, or produce increased intracranial pressure (Snyder, 1983). To begin, move into the child's visual field and speak his or her name. If no response is observed, add a light touch with the name and note the quality of the response. If there is still no response, call the child's

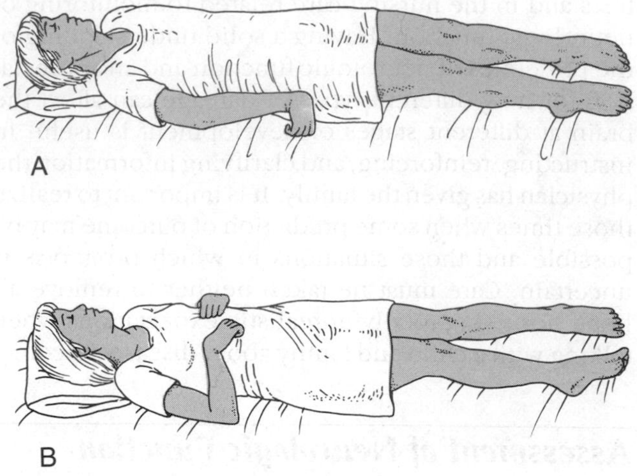

Figure 46-8. Pathologic posturing occurring in severe brain injury. *A*, Extension posturing (decerebrate rigidity). *B*, Abnormal flexion (decorticate rigidity).

name loudly, and use firm touch; note the quality of the response. If these strategies fail to elicit a response, then painful stimulation is used. The assessment of motor responses can be combined with this assessment of consciousness.

When assessing level of consciousness and using noxious or painful stimuli note whether the patient can localize the stimuli, merely withdraws from the stimuli, has a generalized response through decreased or increased activity, has a reflex response with decerebrate or decorticate posturing (Fig. 46-8), or has no observable response to noxious stimuli. Although an institution may have defined terms for the patient's level of consciousness, there are no universally accepted terms. A description of the stimuli required and the patient's response should be recorded. Alterations in arousal indicate alterations in either one or both areas: the cerebral cortex or the reticular activating system in the brain stem.

Pupil Responses and Eye Movements. The technique for assessing both direct and consensual pupil responses to light, comparing pupil size, and assessing eye movements are described in Chapter 15, page 525. Pupil responses are mediated by the interaction between two cranial nerves: the optic and the oculomotor. Pupil responses can be affected by damage to the eye itself, cranial nerves, and upper brainstem, by both the local and systemic effects of certain drugs; by seizure activity; and by anoxia (Box 46-1). Pupil responses may be spared in metabolic alterations affecting the brain.

Pupil size is determined by the input of the sympathetic nervous system which dilates the pupil (such as during anxiety and pain) and the parasympathetic nervous system, mediated by the oculomotor nerve, which constricts the pupil. Pupil size will normally vary with age. Newborn infants and the elderly commonly have very small pupils, while toddlers and adolescents may have very large pupils.

Eye movements may not be assessed in the acute neurologic check unless there is an alteration in the level of consciousness. Neuroanatomic structures involved with voluntary, spontaneous, and reflex conjugate eye movements are the oculomotor, trochlear, and abducens nerve; the medial longitudinal fasciculus (MLF) tract of the midbrain and pons; and the vestibular system. Observe the eye movements through all planes as described in Chapter 15. Observe whether they are conjugate, indicating intact cranial nerve and upper brainstem structures, or dysconjugate and/or fixed, reflecting localized damage to cranial nerve(s) and/or the vestibular system. Spontaneous, random, roving eye movements may be characteristic of patients with a depressed level of consciousness and in patients who are blind.

Assessment of eye movements in a patient with depressed level of consciousness may include assessment of the oculocephalic (doll's eye) reflex if there are no contraindications to rapid head and neck rotation. It is important to understand that this reflex is only elicited when there is depressed level of consciousness. The oculocephalic reflex is tested by holding the patient's eyelids open while briskly rotating the head laterally in one direction and observing the eye movements. A normal response is for conjugate eye deviation to the opposite direction of head turning with a return of the eyes to the resting position in a few seconds. This normal response indicates intact cranial nerves and MLF tract function. An abnormal response would be for the eyes to move in the same direction as the head turning or for the movements to be dysconjugate. The oculocephalic reflex is carried out in both lateral directions and can also be tested using neck flexion and extension for assessment of vertical movements. Assessment of vertical movements using flexion and extension may not be done in infants and young children because of the risk of airway injury due to hyperextension.

The testing of the oculovestibular reflex (ice water calorics) is not considered a part of the acute neurologic check and is usually performed by the physician. It will be briefly mentioned here because it also is a method for assessing extraocular movements in patients with depressed level of consciousness and gives data on brainstem function. The test involves slowly irrigating the external auditory canal with a small amount of ice water and observing the eye movements. A normal response indicating brainstem integrity is a tonic conjugate nystagmus or deviation of the eyes toward the stimulated ear. An abnormal response would be dysconjugate eye deviation or no response at all.

Motor Responses. The assessment of motor responses in the acute neurologic check involves observation of the patient and all extremities for spontaneous movements, and movements in response to command, and, in patients with depressed levels of consciousness, all extremity movements in response to tactile and then noxious stimuli if necessary. Observe for abnormal reflex posturing and the assessment of protective reflexes such as blink, gag, and swallow. It is important to assess whether movements are purposeful or nonpurposeful and symmetrical or asymmetrical, and to compare muscle strength, tone, and reflexes for symmetry.

Assessment of motor responses in infants includes testing Moro, grasp, and Babinski reflexes for symmetry. Toddlers may be able to reach your finger with their hands and to kick your hand with their feet. Older children may be able to cooperate with testing grip strength and the major flexors and extensors. Testing of pronator drift in older children by asking them to hold their arms extended with palms upward in front of their body while they sit or stand with their eyes

Box 46-1
Significance of Pupil Signs

1. No pupil response to direct light; indicates problem with optic nerve (II) or oculomotor nerve (III); proceed to check for consensual reaction
2. No pupil response to direct light and appears more dilated
   a. Opposite pupil has a consensual reaction; this indicates problem with oculomotor nerve in dilated eye
   b. Dilated pupil has a consensual reaction; this indicates problem with optic nerve in dilated eye
3. No pupil response to direct light
   a. Opposite pupil does not have a consensual reaction; this may indicate blindness (amaurosis) in that eye, if other eye has a direct response to light and there is good consensual reaction in first eye tested
4. Both pupils appear dilated (mydriasis, parasympathetic lesion); this may be indication of hypoxia, drug effect, or increased intracranial pressure
5. Both pupils appear constricted (miosis, sympathetic lesion); if there is some reaction to light, may indicate problem with diencephalon (e.g., thalamus); if there is no reaction to light, it may indicate problem with brain stem; if only one pupil is constricted, it may indicate a Horner syndrome where there is unilateral sympathetic nervous system injury

closed may disclose subtle weakness in one arm if the arm drifts slightly downward and pronates during this test. This can sometimes be an early sign of deterioration. Motor tone can be assessed by completing range of motion in each limb.

In patients with depressed levels of consciousness motor responses can be assessed by lifting the arms up to equal height while the patient lies supine, then dropping the limbs simultaneously to the bed. This technique can also be used to assess motor responses in the lower extremities. If there is weakness in an extremity it appears to fall more rapidly and in a limp manner. Again, in using tactile stimuli to evoke motor responses, one uses the least amount of stimuli possible. Digital pressure using the thumb and forefinger to squeeze all of the extremity nailbeds can be used. Digital pressure to both Achilles tendons and the trapezius muscles could be used in place of nailbeds. Generally more noxious stimuli such as sternal massage and supraorbital pressure are not used routinely by nurses, in order to avoid possible sternal injuries and possible vasal vagal responses. These types of noxious stimuli may be used selectively by physicians. It is important that pinching not be used, to avoid unnecessary injury to the skin.

Reflexes. The patient with a depressed level of consciousness should also be observed for abnormal reflex posturing. If present, note if it is unilateral or bilateral, and if bilateral whether or not it is symmetrical. *Decorticate posturing* (Fig. 46-8) involves adduction of the arm with flexion of the arm, wrist, and fingers, and extension, internal rotation, and plantar flexion in the lower extremity. When present it indicates dysfunction located between the motor cortex and the midbrain. *Decerebrate posturing* (Fig. 46-8) involves rigid extension, adduction, and hyperpronation in the arms, and rigid leg extension with plantar flexion. The presence of decerebration indicates dysfunction located between the midbrain and the pons.

Assessment of *protective reflexes* (corneal, gag, and swallow reflexes) is important in the acute neurologic check if the nurse suspects any difficulty with suck and swallow, increased intracranial pressure, potential for masses or lesions in the posterior fossa, or depressed level of consciousness. It is important to note whether these normal protective reflexes are present and if so whether they are symmetrical. The corneal reflex is checked by lightly touching the outer aspect of each cornea with a wisp of sterile cotton. The normal response is a prompt bilateral blink, except in infants, in whom the blink may be prompt but asymmetric. An absent response may indicate dysfunction with the trigeminal nerve in perceiving the sensation, or dysfunction in the pons. The implication for nurses in the absence of this response is to protect the eyes and corneas from injury. Interventions such as use of artificial tears and taping the eyelids closed may be necessary.

Gag and swallow reflexes are difficult to test and observe in infants and younger children. If the oral cavity can be entered and observed using a small spoon or tongue depressor, either place firm pressure on the tongue or, using a cotton swab, stroke the posterior wall of the pharynx. Either of these techniques should elicit a gag reflex. It should be noted that after tonsils and adenoids are removed the palatal movements may appear asymmetric. It is important that when gag, swallow, and cough reflexes in children appear inadequate, fluids and feedings be withheld until further data are available.

Respiratory Pattern and Other Vital Signs. Of the vital signs, respiratory patterns are the most sensitive indicators of neurologic change, especially change in the brainstem. Keep in mind that changes in respiratory patterns due to neurologic dysfunction do not occur until there are problems either deep in the cerebral hemispheres or in the brainstem. Neuroanatomic structures involved in respiration include the medullary respiratory center which innervates the muscles of inspiration and expiration, the apneustic center and the vagus nerve in the pons which control inspiratory efforts, the pneumotaxic center in the pons which terminates inspiratory activity, and the cerebral cortex and diencephalon which provide influence over the brainstem structures (AANN, 1984).

Respiratory patterns, as well as respiratory rate, effort, and adequacy of respiration are important in assessment of the neurologically impaired patient because hypoxia and hypercapnia can both have significant effects on neurologic function. Posthyperventilation apnea may be a useful test for detecting early changes in respiratory pattern. This test can be done only with an alert child who is able to follow directions, and involves having the child take five deep breaths, then closely observing subsequent respirations. A normal response is for the patient to resume normal breathing. An abnormal response is for a brief period of apnea to occur because the carbon dioxide in the blood ($PaCO_2$) has been reduced, followed by the resumption of normal breathing after the $PaCO_2$ level returns to normal. Posthyperventilation apnea is seen when there is bilateral diffuse dysfunction affecting the brain.

Temperature regulation is under neurologic control via the hypothalamic nuclei and the sympathetic nervous system. Both hyperthermia and hypothermia affect cerebral metabolism. Hyperthermia increases cerebral metabolism and increases the consumption of glucose and oxygen. Hypothermia decreases cerebral metabolism and decreases consumption of glucose and oxygen. Extremes of temperature may be life threatening. Temperature may sometimes be altered as a means of treatment. It is important when interpreting body temperature to look at the trends: whether the change is sudden or gradual, the environmental conditions, the general condition of the patient, treatment modalities, and the nature and location of neurologic dysfunction (AANN, 1984). Hyperthermia can occur with increases in intracranial pressure and with central nervous system infections. Hypothermia can be seen in dysfunction involving the hypothalamus, pituitary, and toxic and metabolic disease. It can be the result of immobility due to coma, profound retardation, and problems affecting mobility, such as cerebral palsy and cervical cord injuries. It can also be the result of treatment modalities such as drug-induced coma, drug paralysis, drug toxicity, and induced hypothermia.

Cardiovascular function is also under neural control. Pathways from the cerebral cortex, diencephalon, and brainstem integrate cardiovascular responses; descending pathways from the hypothalamus affect the sympathetic stimulation of the heart, resulting in increased heart rate and coronary artery dilation. Brainstem centers, including the pons and medulla, control peripheral vascular resistance by descending pathways; the medulla and vagus nerve produce parasympathetic stimulation of the heart to slow heart rate (AANN, 1984). Recognition of cardiovascular alterations is important for two reasons, first, for diagnostic purposes as evidence of neurologic dysfunction, and secondly and most importantly, for the purpose of management to optimize cerebral blood flow and perfusion and to prevent cardiovascular arrest.

Changes in blood pressure and pulse (Cushing reflex) are considered late signs of increased intracranial pressure, usually before this the patient has manifested other signs and symptoms of deterioration. In the early compensatory state the blood pressure increases and heart rate decreases; later in the decompensatory stage the blood pressure falls and the pulse becomes irregular and thready; dysrhythmias may also occur. Dysrhythmias may occur as well with lesions in the posterior fossa and following posterior fossa surgery.

Nursing Implications of the Acute Neurologic Check

It is important to compare changes in the acute neurologic check with other data about the patient's condition and to take prompt action if necessary. When assessing level of consciousness remember to arouse the child fully. Children do not always follow adult manifestations of neurologic dysfunction. In children wakefulness may not always reflect the integrity of the nervous system; that is, they can remain wakeful in spite of progressive neurologic deterioration until compensatory mechanisms have been expended; then they appear to change rapidly. Because of this it is important to use all the components of the neurologic check as carefully and thoroughly as possible.

The baseline developmental level of the child should guide the nurse in making the neurologic check more appropriate and useful. For example, spending time asking children their name may be inappropriate if they were unable to say their name when asked before the problem developed. Usually by age 3 children can tell you their name if they so desire. Preschoolers may be able to answer questions of place and person, but assessing full orientation to time, place, and person is usually not appropriate before school age.

Take care when doing the neurologic check to protect the safety and well-being of the child. If tactile stimuli must be used in assessing consciousness and motor responses remember to use the least noxious first. Use of the proper techniques will avoid injury to the skin and other body structures. If the child is experiencing alterations in neurologic function take the opportunity to provide developmentally appropriate interventions for security, safety, and psychologic support.

Parents and family members may need repeated explanations for the frequency of these checks, the need to use various types of stimuli, and some explanation of the patient's responses. Family members often interpret all movements or responses the patient makes as being voluntary, and may need considerable support to understand the patient's condition. Remember to let family members know if the condition appears stable, is improving, or is becoming worse. When it appears the nurse has once again found no change or improvement in the patient, it can sometimes be an extremely anxiety producing, frustrating, and depressing experience for the family members. Provide them an opportunity to ask questions and express their feelings.

Some institutions use the Glasgow Coma Scale (GCS) developed by Teasdale and Jennett in 1974 in addition to the acute neurologic check to assess patients with depressed levels of consciousness. The GCS scores the patient's best eye opening, motor, and verbalization responses (Table 46-3). A total can be plotted from this system with 15 points maximum and 3 points minimum. The GCS was designed to detect change for patients who had severe head injuries, and does indicate early changes in arousal. It is used primarily for patients with head injuries. The GCS is not specific enough and does not have enough gradations and descriptors to be used alone in evaluating neuro-

Table 46-3. Glasgow Coma Scale

Parameter	Score
Eye Opening (E)	
Spontaneous	4
Responds to speech	3
Responds to pain	2
Nil	1
Best Motor Response (M)	
Obeys commands	6
Localizes pain	5
Withdraws	4
Abnormal flexion	3
Extensor response	2
Nil	1
Best Verbal Response (V)	
Oriented	5
Confused conversation	4
Inappropriate words	3
Incomprehensible sounds	2
Nil	1

The Glasgow Coma Scale is designed as a standardized assessment of the patient with disturbed consciousness. The tests can be performed serially to determine the patient's progress. The coma scale (E + M + V) = 3 to 15. All combinations equal to 7 or less define coma. Approximately 50 per cent of scores that equal 8 also define coma. Patients achieving a score of 9 or more are noncomatose.

logic status and in determining care needs. Table 46-4 shows a modification of the GCS that facilitates assessment of verbal response in infants.

Another scale frequently used in assessing consciousness is one that was developed by the staff at the Rancho Los Amigos Rehabilitation Center in Downey, California. This scale grades consciousness into five levels (Box 46-2). This may be useful in addition to the neurologic check for planning care of the older child but the nurse needs to remember its limitations in children of different ages. Using this scale the *normal* infant is at a level 4, the older infant and toddler are at a level 3, and older children normally fit into portions of levels 2 and 1. Usually by middle school age and older, the normal child is at a level 1.

Neurologic Screening Assessment

A screening examination may become necessary at times when there is a lack of adequate time for the nurse to do a comprehensive assessment. It allows evaluation of some basic functions that can serve as a starting point when the nurse can later add to the depth of the evaluation (Mitchell et al, 1984). Table 46-5 shows a sample screening examination for an adult, which could be used for adolescents and older school-age children. These components can be modified for screening various-age children. Modification would also be necessary in screening children who have baseline neurologic alterations.

Comprehensive Neurologic Assessment

Comprehensive assessment of neurologic function is covered in Chapter 15. This section will present additional information to be included with the health history.

Health History. In discussing the present illness it is important to develop a clear understanding of the progression of symptoms and the period of time over

Table 46-4. Glasgow Coma Scale for Verbal Response in Infants

One Month	1. None 2. Crying to stimuli 3. Crying spontaneously 4. Blink when eyelashes touched 5. Throaty noises
Two Months	1. None 2. Crying to stimuli 3. Shuts eyes to light 4. Smiles when caressed 5. Babbles—single vowel sounds
Three Months	1. None 2. Crying to stimuli (moans) 3. Stares to response and looks at environment 4. Smiles to sound stimulation 5. Coos, chuckles, *vowels* in a prolonged way
Four Months	1. None 2. Crying to stimuli (moans) 3. Turns head to sound 4. Smiles spontaneously or when stimulated, laughs when socially stimulated 5. Modulating voice and perfect vocalization of vowels
Five and Six Months	1. None 2. Crying to stimuli (moans) 3. Localizes general direction of sound 4. Discriminates family members 5. Babbles to people, toys
Seven and Eight Months	1. None 2. Crying to stimuli (moans) 3. Recognizes familiar voices and family 4. Babbles 5. "Ba," "Ma," "Da"
Nine and Ten Months	1. None 2. Crying to stimuli (moans) 3. Recognizes (smiles or laughs) 4. Babbles 5. "MaMa," "DaDa"
Eleven and Twelve Months	1. None 2. Crying to stimuli (moans) 3. Recognizes—smiles 4. Babbles 5. Words (specifically "Mama" and "Dada")

(Courtesy of Dr. Kenneth Shapiro, Department of Neurosurgery, Albert Einstein College of Medicine, New York, New York.)

Box 46-2
Scale for Assessing Consciousness

Level 1: ***oriented to self and surroundings,*** oriented to time and place

Level 2: ***responsive to environment,*** purposeful activity, follows commands

Level 3: ***localized response to sensory stimuli,*** visual focusing, blinking, following objects, movement of extremities localized

Level 4: ***generalized response to sensory stimuli,*** startles, responds to stimuli with increased or decreased activity, responds to pain with reflex response

Level 5: ***no response to stimuli,*** complete absence of observable change in behavior to visual, auditory, tactile, or pain stimuli

(Developed by Rancho Los Amigos Rehabilitation Center, Downey, California.)

which these changes occurred. Are the symptoms progressively worsening, plateauing, or remitting? Is there any change in the frequency of the symptoms related to the time of day? Are there any factors that the child or parents can identify that influence the symptom(s), either improving or worsening? Are there any symptoms from any other body systems that may be affecting the neurologic symptoms?

It is important in discussing the aforementioned problems to develop an understanding of the family and child's perceptions, the child's strengths and weaknesses, how they are currently coping or compensating with the problem, how their daily life is affected, the immediate and future concerns, the support and resources available to the child and family, and the character of the home environment. This information assists in planning present care and in promptly beginning rehabilitation if it is needed.

A review of systems is located on page 513. Additional inclusions for a child who may be experiencing an alteration in neurologic function would include:

- *Skin*—decubiti
- *EENT*—visual change or loss, diplopia, dizziness, vertigo, voice change, difficulty with swallowing, choking, history of aspirations
- *CV/Resp*—syncope, fainting, palpitations, history of apnea or aspirations
- *GI/GU*—recent loss of ability to remain continent of stool and urine
- *Neuro*—areas of decreased/increased or altered sensation, alteration in memory or thinking, change in muscle tone (either more rigid or floppy), any loss of skills that the child was able to perform consistently.

Neurologic Assessment. Mitchell and associates (1984) developed an alternative organizational framework for incorporating neurologic assessment into nursing practice, using functional categories. Table 46-6 uses Mitchell's organizational categories to show the tests that might be used for assessment of infants, toddlers, preschoolers, and school-age children.

Important factors in infant and toddler assessment include head size, shape, and symmetry; motor and social landmarks; presence, absence, and symmetry of developmental reflexes; abdominal examination; and vision and hearing examinations. The important factors to include in the assessment of preschoolers and older children are categories that are similar to those in the adult examination but would also include developmentally appropriate skills for a given age. This may include mentation, movement (musculoskeletal and cranial nerves), gait and balance, coordination, reflexes, and sensory abilities (Droske and Francis, 1981).

Text continues on page 1696

Table 46-5. Screening Examination of Neurologic Function

Examination Stimulus	Function or System Tested
1. Observe gait, symmetry	Motor, cerebellar, position sense
2. Ask: why are you here, has your ability to take care of yourself changed?	Perception, expectations, orientation, self-care change, coping
3. Read headline, tell meaning, recall later	Seeing, recall, language
4. Take glass of water, swallow, hand back to examiner (or any act across midline, with three components)	Swallow, right-left orientation, concentration sensory, coordination
5. Dress or undress	Motor, sensory cerebellar
6. Simultaneously observe language, eye movement	Language, seeing

Note: If no abnormality is present, this entire examination can be performed in 5 minutes.
(From Mitchell, 1984, page 17.)

Table 46-6. Neurologic Assessment by Age Group

Infant Assessment

Screening Questions

1. How do they respond to their name?
2. How long do they pay attention to something they like?
3. How do they regard familiar faces and objects?
4. What kinds of vocalizations do they make?
5. Do they recognize familiar faces?
6. Can they control their head, smile, roll, sit alone, crawl, pull to stand?
7. Do you (parent) think that they see and hear? What are the smallest objects that they can see and retrieve?

Consciousness	
Arousal	Describe their response to stimuli once they are wakeful, or describe how much stimuli is required to keep them wakeful, describe sleep and wake cycles
Mentation	
Attention Thinking and language Remembering	Describe their response to their name, describe if any differential response between nurse and parent, describe regard for and play with objects, describe their participation in eating and drinking (hold bottle, fingerfeed), describe any vocalizations, describe behavior
Movement	
Eye movements Eating Expressing facially Speaking Moving Head Trunk Arms Legs Coordination Reflexes	Test tracking to bright object (may have dysconjugate gaze in first month; after 6 wk may indicate blindness, nystagmus may be present until 3 mo), observe drinking from bottle, cup or feeding, observe facial expression during assessment, hold object out of their reach while sitting or lying; place them supine or prone; pull them to a sit or stand and observe their movements for quality, symmetry, and developmental appropriateness, (fine tremors and infrequent involuntary movement normal to 2 mo), tone will depend on activity, observe hand position in grasping, test Moro, tonic neck or parachute reflex depending on age, test protective reflexes such as gag and swallow if appropriate
Sensory	
Blinking Seeing Hearing Tasting Feeling Touch Pain	Test blink to visual threat (newborn slower and may have asymmetric blink), place small edible item within their reach and observe vision, observe response to unexpected sounds (clap) (6 mo should be able to localize sound), test taste after 3 mo when expulsion reflex has disappeared and can note infant acceptance or rejection of new food tastes placed in mouth, note infant responses to tactile stimuli with examination, if lack of speech need to investigate for hearing problem
Integrated Regulatory Functions	
Breathing Circulation Temperature Ingestion/Digestion Elimination Bowel Bladder	Assess respiratory pattern, rate, quality, and effort, assess heart rate and rhythm, blood pressure, color in face; trunk and extremities, note extremity nailbed color, assess axillary or rectal temperature, note skin temperature in hands and feet, note strength and coordination to suck, swallow, and chew, if there are problems with elimination assess abdomen and perineum
Head Circumference, Fontanels	Measure head circumference; palpate fontanels for size, fullness

Toddler Assessment

Screening Questions

1. Can they tell you their first name?
2. How long do they play with something they like?
3. How do they respond to their name and to no?
4. Do they use words appropriately (never, sometimes, most of the time)?
5. How many words do they use together at a time?
6. Do they know some body parts?
7. Do they remember where things are? Unpleasant situations?
8. Do they eat with fingers or utensil, do they eat by themselves?
9. Do they undress, pull on some clothes?

Table 46-6 (continued)

10. Can they walk alone, throw, kick, jump?
11. Do you (parent) have any concerns about their sight or hearing? Can they see and find small objects from across the room?

Consciousness	
Arousal	Describe their response to stimuli once they are wakeful, or describe how much stimulus is required to keep them wakeful, describe sleep/wake cycles. Older toddlers may be able to tell you their name, and identify family members by name
Mentation	

Attention
Thinking/Language
Remembering
Gnosis
  Body parts
Praxis
  Eating
  Undressing
	Observe attention span during assessment, usually 1–3 min, ask to locate/name body parts and common objects, describe words used and any combinations, assess ability to follow 1 step commands, observe drinking, eating, and undressing, play hide and seek with an object; note short-term memory; describe behavior

Movement	

Eye movements
Eating
Expressing facially
Speaking
Moving
  Head
  Trunk
  Arms/Hands
  Legs/Feet
Fine motor
Gait
Coordination
Reflexes
	Test tracking of an object in all directions, note visual fields by confrontation, note convergence, cover/uncover test, observe eating and drinking, test gag and swallow if necessary, note facial expressions for symmetry during assessment; older toddlers may be able to stick out tongue and show you how they blow, and should be speaking words that are largely intelligible; note gait and throw in younger toddler, add kick and jump for older toddler, note balance, coordination, strength, and symmetry in these movements, observe for hand preference, note gait (is wide based until 2 yr), test reflexes if there are any problems with movement, tone, or strength

Sensory	

Blinking
Seeing
Hearing
Tasting
Feeling
  Touch
  Pain
	Test blink to visual threat or by stroking lashes, place small toy/block on floor across room to retrieve, ask younger toddler to localize quiet sounds out of their visual field, ask older toddler to repeat words whispered in each ear, ask child to close eyes, touch each extremity and then ask toddler to point to where they were touched; this usually takes practice

Integrated Regulatory Functions	

Breathing
Circulation
Temperature
Digestion
Elimination
  Bowel
  Bladder
	Assess respiratory pattern, rate, quality, and effort, assess heart rate and rhythm, blood pressure, color in face, trunk, and extremities, assess nailbed color and blanching, assess axillary or rectal temperature, note skin temperature in hands and feet, note strength and coordination in drinking, chewing, and swallowing, ask if the child gives indication or awareness of elimination and need to eliminate

Head Circumference	

Preschooler Assessment

Screening Questions

1. Can they tell you their full name?
2. Do they know day from nighttime?
3. Can they tell you where they live?
4. How long can they stay with an activity they enjoy?
5. Give some examples of how they use words together in sentences?
6. Can they identify specific body parts and colors? Can they count to 10?
7. Do they remember daily routines, situations?
8. Are they able to feed self neatly, and dress? Are they toilet trained?
9. Tell me about the most complicated or difficult movement activities that the child can do with arms, legs, whole body.
10. Do you (parent) have any concerns with vision or hearing?

continued

Table 46-6 *(continued)*

Consciousness	
Arousal Content	Describe their response to stimuli once they are wakeful or how much stimuli is required to keep them wakeful, describe sleep/wake cycles, ask them their full name, ask them where they live and if where they are is their house, ask if it's day or night-time, ask them to name family members
Mentation	
Attention Thinking/language Remembering Gnosis Body parts Right/left Figure copying Stereognosis Graphesthesia Praxis Eating Undressing/dressing Toileting Bathing	Observe attention span during assessment, usually 10–15 min, observe for full vocabulary and speech in longer more complex sentences, can count to 10, identify coins and colors, define objects by how they are used, correctly follow two-step commands, identify specific body parts, copy circle and cross, know right from left, identify coin from a key when placed in hand with eyes closed, identify circle from cross or "x" when drawn with finger on their palm with their eyes closed, may be able to repeat 3 or 4 numbers when asked to recall, can repeat a familiar song or story, observe ability to dress with zipper and buttons, ask about ability to toilet by self, bathe with guidance; understands concepts like up/down, big/little, short/long
Movement	
Eye movements Eating Expressing facially Speaking Moving Head Trunk Arms/hands Legs/feet Fine motor Gait Coordination Reflexes	Test tracking of finger all directions, observe or ask about them eating and drinking neatly, ask for different facial expressions (show teeth, blow a kiss, imitate a grouch face), note pronunciation and intelligibility, stick out tongue and wiggle it, observe balance and hopping for each leg, catch a ball or object, walk heel to toe, observe with scissors or thumb/forefinger rapid touching with each hand, finger to nose touching, observe gait note quality, symmetry and coordination in all movements, observe hand preference, test reflexes if any problems with movement, tone or strength
Sensory	
Blinking Seeing Hearing Tasting Feeling Touch Pain Temperature Smelling	Test blink to visual threat and by stroking lashes, test each eye separately by holding up a small object from across the room for them to identify, test visual fields by asking them to point to wiggling finger, ask them to repeat words whispered in each ear or with closed eyes to identify when they hear a ticking watch, ask to localize both unilateral and bilateral touch, if concerns of sensation arise can test sense of hot/cold, up/down position sense, and soft/sharp touch, may be able to recognize familiar smells
Integrated Regulatory Functions	
Breathing Circulation Temperature Ingestion/digestion Elimination Bowel Bladder	Assess respiratory pattern, rate, quality, and effort, assess heart rate and rhythm, blood pressure, color in face, trunk, and extremities, assess nailbed color and blanching, assess oral or axillary temperature, note skin temperature in hands and feet, note strength and coordination in drinking, chewing, and swallowing, note their ability to carry out toileting independently
Head Circumference	
School-Age Assessment	
Screening Questions	

1. Can they tell you their address and phone number?
2. Can they tell time?
3. Do they know the date and year?
4. How long can they pay attention to an activity they enjoy?

Table 46-6 *(continued)*

5. Can they print, write, read?
6. What areas are difficult in school? Is the child in any special classes? What areas of strength does the child have in school?
7. Tell me about the most complicated or difficult movement activities that you can do with arms, legs, whole body. Are you right- or left-handed?
8. Do you (parent) have any concerns about the child's vision or hearing?

Consciousness	
Arousal Content	Describe their alertness, ask them to tell you their full name, address and determine orientation to time, date, year, and present place
Mentation	

Attention
Thinking/language
Remembering
Gnosis
  Figure copying
  Stereognosis
  Graphesthesia
Praxis
  All ADLs
	Observe attention span during assessment, usually 15–20 min, ask them the months of the year and days of the week, ask them to describe several objects in the room and to follow a three-step command, ask their phone number and to solve some simple math problems, ask to draw a person and copy a 3-dimensional cube, identify a dime from a nickel placed in each hand with eyes closed, identify any letters or numbers drawn on either palm with eyes closed, observe abilities to undress and dress, and in completing other ADLs

Movement	

Eye movements
Eating
Expressing facially
Speaking
Moving
  Head
  Trunk
  Arms/hands
  Legs/feet
Gait
Coordination
Reflexes
	Observe eye movements by testing tracking of finger in all directions, ask to take a drink of water with left hand; transfer to right hand and hand back to examiner (observe memory, swallow, movements, coordination, right-left orientation) observe symmetry of facial movements throughout assessment and ask for different facial expressions, observe clarity of speech, observe balance during gait and when walking forward and backward heel to toe on a straight line, observe speed, accuracy and coordination when touching thumb to each finger in succession, test reflexes if any problems with movement, tone, or strength

Sensory	

Blinking
Seeing
Hearing
Tasting
Feeling
  Touch
  Pain
  Temp
  Position
  Location
Smelling
	Test blink to visual threat and lash stroke, test visual acuity of each eye with reading from book or using pocket Snellen, test visual fields by identifying moving finger, ask them to repeat words whispered in each ear, with eyes closed ask to localize unilateral and bilateral simultaneous touch stimuli, if there are concerns regarding sensation test sharp/dull, hot/cold, up/down position sense, also test (with eyes closed) recognition of objects that are placed in each hand (coins, button, key) and identification of numbers and letters that are drawn on the palm of the hand, should be able to identify smells such as mint, cinnamon, coffee, lemon

Integrated Regulatory Functions	

Breathing
Circulation
Temperature
Ingestion/digestion
Elimination
  Bowel
  Bladder
Sexuality
	Assess respiratory pattern, rate, quality, and effort; assess heart rate and rhythm, blood pressure; face, trunk and extremity color; assess nailbed color and blanching; assess temperature; note skin temp in hands and feet; note drinking, chewing and swallowing abilities; assess any problems with toileting or elimination; observe for secondary sex characteristics; ask about menarche characteristics and any concerns regarding sexuality

By Judy Wulf.

Noninvasive Diagnostic Tests

CT (*Computed Tomography*) Scan

Noninvasive tests (unless contrast enhancement is used) involve radiation that allows a three-dimensional look at normal and abnormal structures. These tests are performed to visualize the brain, blood vessels, and cerebral spinal fluid (CSF), and to follow the progression or improvement of disease. The CT scan (also called CAT scan for computed axial tomography) is effective for visualizing hematomas, and tumors; it is less effective for picking up cranial defects such as linear skull fractures or for use immediately after a cerebral vascular accident (CVA) (Smith et al, 1983).

The CT scan differentiates tissue by their densities and uses about the same amount of radiation as a skull series or 1 to 2.5 rads (Swaiman, 1982). The patient, with the head immobilized, lies supine on a movable table that slides into the scanner. The x-ray beam and detector rotate around the head measuring densities in a series of cross-sectional scans The computer averages the densities for each point in the brain and makes pictorial representations of the absorption measurements taken. On the scan, densities with lower coefficients (the lowest being air) appear darker in color, densities with higher coefficients (the highest being bone) appear lighter in color. The use of contrast enhancement (which involves intravenous injection of an iodine-type contrast medium) provides for better viewing of blood vessels, well-vascularized lesions, and local alterations in the blood brain barrier.

Nursing Strategies. No physical preparation is required for regular CT scan. Psychologic preparation involves teaching children to lie completely still and preparing them for sensations they may experience. The child can be told that the table will feel hard, and the room cool, that the head will be stabilized with cushions or a strap, and that the machine will move around and make some sounds. If coronal views are needed, the patient will need to extend the head while lying on the back. The child can be assured that the CT scan does not hurt, and should know that it takes about 20 minutes.

The use of contrast enhancement necessitates intravenous injection of a contrast media. Sensations experienced include a warm rushing feeling when the contrast is given. The child must be observed during and after the scan for possible allergic reactions to the contrast media. Tables 46-7 and 46-8 describe care both before and after the contrast procedure.

In a younger or uncooperative child sedation or general anesthesia may be required. Although sedation may not require any change in care, the use of anesthesia may require consent, NPO status, and observation of pre- and post-procedure vital signs.

MRI (*Magnetic Resonance Imaging*) *Scan and* NMR (*Nuclear Magnetic Resonance*) Scan

The MRI or NMR scan is a new type of imaging without radiation that has the capacity for imaging body tissues or organs in action, and for spectroscopy, a technique that examines the chemistry of individual cells in health and disease (Rudy, 1985). NMR has appeared to be especially effective in imaging the brain and identifying necrotic tissue, areas of ischemia, malignancies, degenerative diseases, and problems near the bony fossae of the brain such as posterior fossa lesions, acoustic neuromas, and spinal cord tumors. Because of its potential safety, the study appears effective in following the progress or course of children with hydrocephalus who are shunted and require repeated scans.

During this study the patient lies on a sliding table with a shield that is placed around the head and shoulders. The table is slid within a strong magnetic field. A computer processes the measurements taken during the study and presents it in a cross-sectional pictorial representation.

Nursing Strategies. No physical preparation is required. Patients do need to be screened carefully for objects that could cause potential hazards during the study. These objects include ferromagnetic metallic devices or implants and electronic equipment that could be affected by the magnetic field: cardiac pacemakers, metal vascular clips, metal prostheses used in joint replacements, bone pins, plates, and screws, artificial heart valves, cerebral surgical clips. The study is also contraindicated during pregnancy until more information becomes available. No risks have been identified with NMR at this time for patients who are free of any potential hazards as mentioned earlier. Most centers use a consent form for this type of testing.

Psychologic preparation includes instructing the patient that there is no discomfort or pain associated with the study, that they will need to lie still for 60 to 90 minutes, and that the machine will surround them and makes a loud banging sound similar to a washing machine. Older patients may complain of boredom, difficulty lying motionless for the time required, and feelings of claustrophobia and confinement. Parents or supportive staff who have been screened for any potential hazards may accompany the patient to provide psychologic support, to read or sing songs to the patient.

Sedation may be required for children under age 5 and for uncooperative children. General anesthesia is not possible if sedation is unsuccessful because of the limited accessibility to patients when they are in the scanner.

Table 46-7. Basic Preprocedure Care for Noninvasive and Invasive Studies

Nursing Diagnosis	Nursing Strategies
Fear/anxiety, related to uncertainty of what the diagnostic test will be like	Adjust teaching as appropriate to the child's developmental level and condition
	Explain purpose of pre- and post-test care
	Clarify misinformation and reinforce that physician has encouraged patient/family to express fears, concerns, and so on. Explain expected sensations and reactions, have practice test with a doll. If there is discomfort during the test, let children know what they can do to cope and how long it will last
	Identify a support person (family member or staff) to accompany the child and provide reinforcement, reassurance, and support
	Avoid delays by prearranging adequate transportation and coordinating the time to give the sedation
	Explain to child the necessity of lying still so that the study is completed as quickly as possible. Have the child practice lying still for the prescribed amount of time
	Provide premedication as ordered
	Communicate any special needs the patient may have to the diagnostic team staff
Potential for injury: physiologic, related to inadequate physical preparation for the procedure	Obtain or assist physician in obtaining consent (usually required for anesthesia, invasive procedures, or contrast enhancement)
	Encourage good night's sleep and daytime naps prior to the test. Obtain baseline vital signs and neurologic check. For angiograms, assess and mark distal pulses, depending upon whether a femoral or brachial approach will be used. For angiograms involving a carotid approach, measure the neck circumference
	Provide skin prep as ordered
	Encourage the child to void before giving preprocedural medications or before leaving the unit for the test
	When the study involves contrast enhancement, check renal function tests for normal values (BUN, creatinine); the contrast medium is excreted through the kidneys
	Encourage fluids or liquids until NPO
	Administer sedative medications, anticholinergics as ordered
	Remove earrings, barrettes, jewelry, and so on, from the body area involved with the procedure
	Dress the child in a cotton hospital gown for invasive tests and those involving contrast enhancement
Potential for injury: physiologic: hypersensitivity related to allergy to iodine or other contrast media components	Ask child and parent about history of allergy or allergic reaction to previous contrast studies (e.g., CT scan, IVP, angiogram) or to iodine. Notify physician and diagnostic team of any allergy
	Give steroids and/or antihistamines as ordered prior to procedure, usually 24 to 72 hours
	Ensure that emergency equipment and medications are immediately available
	Accompany child during transfers to and from unit

(Adapted from AANN, 1984.)

Table 46-8. Basic Postprocedure Care Following Invasive and Contrast Studies

Nursing Diagnosis	Nursing Strategies
Anxiety, related to misconceptions and unresolved feelings about the diagnostic test	After the study is finished and the child has rested, if appropriate allow the child to express or play out the experience, allow time to clarify misconceptions with the child, provide time for the child to work through feelings. Older children may want to write a story or draw a picture about the test, or let the child talk into a tape recorder and tell about the experience. (Collaborate with the Child Life therapist)
	Provide praise for appropriate coping behavior during the test
Altered tissue perfusion: peripheral, related to hematoma at site of invasive procedure	Check and record the condition of the site; for an angiogram check and record the quality and symmetry of both distal pulses: • Pedal pulses following femoral access • Radial pulses following brachial access • Temporal pulses following carotid access
	After carotid access also note airway and respiratory effort, check neck circumference and facial color
	Apply manual pressure and ice pack to minimize bleeding as appropriate. Monitor vital signs
	Limit and then advance patient activities as appropriate
Potential for injury: physiologic, related to physiologic response to diagnostic procedure	Perform and record neurologic check frequently and compare with prestudy baseline
	Check and record vital signs. During study BP often increased, after study may be hypotensive secondary to dehydration
Altered comfort: nausea and vomiting, related to anesthesia or medications associated with the diagnostic test	If ordered, observe NPO or clear liquid restriction pretest
	Administer anticholinergics and antiemetics as ordered
	Slowly increase oral intake amounts, and advance as tolerated (do not just let the child decide)
	IV therapy if vomiting persists
	Minimize anxiety
Potential fluid volume deficit, related to postprocedure vomiting or diuresis associated with dilution of contrast media	Encourage fluids postcontrast unless otherwise ordered
	Monitor intake and output if vomiting persists
	Specific gravity of urine may increase secondary to contrast excretion
	IV therapy if diuresis or vomiting persists
Potential for injury: physiologic, related to allergic reaction to contrast media used	Monitor vital signs, skin, respiratory quality, and general condition 30 and 60 minutes after study
Defining Characteristics: ***Itching, watery eyes, nasal congestion, hives, rash, bronchospasm, pulmonary edema, renal failure, cardiopulmonary collapse, death***	Have emergency medications available (antihistamines, epinephrine and antidysrhythmics, steroids)
	Treat symptomatically
Potential ineffective family coping: compromised, related to psychologic response to the test results	Be present when physician explains test results to family, to be able to reinforce test results, clarify misconceptions or misunderstandings, provide opportunity for patient/family to express feelings and concerns
	Depending on test results, common feelings may include relief, grief, shock, confusion, anger, and so on
	Assist patient/family to consider their options and alternatives regarding treatment alternatives
	Provide anticipatory teaching as appropriate

(Adapted from AANN, 1984.)

EEG (*Electroencephalogram*)

This study provides a graphic record of the electrical activity across large areas of the brain's cortex. It is important to remember that this electrical activity represents the sum of synaptic activity across millions of neurons. This study is useful in the management of seizure disorders or epilepsy, as well as in patients with a head injury, stroke, encephalopathy, or metabolic coma. It is also used in psychiatric illness and in the determination of brain death. Different types of electroencephalograms have evolved in recent years. The EEG is interpreted for both the quality and characteristics of the background or ongoing electrical activity as well as for any abnormal electrical discharges. This study also requires correlation with other findings.

The routine EEG is still the most common and takes 45 to 60 minutes to complete. The method involves gluing 17 to 21 electrodes to specific locations on the scalp and then filling the cup electrodes with a conductive jelly. The electrical signals are transmitted through the electrodes to the machine, where the difference in electrical activity between two electrodes is displayed in graphic form on the moving paper. During the study several different recording systems or montages are used as the machine is briefly stopped and switches change the way that the electrodes pair up electrically. Usually some activation procedures are used, such as photic stimulation (flashing a light in the eyes at various frequencies) or voluntary hyperventilation in hopes of precipitating a seizure for the purpose of diagnostic recording. When the recording is finished the electrodes are removed, and the hair will require some care to remove all the glue and jelly.

Another technique that may precipitate certain types of seizure discharges is sleep deprivation. This involves keeping the patient awake all or a part of the night before the EEG is to be done, and then, depending on the physician's order, either letting the patient sleep or keeping him or her awake during the study.

Video EEG and EEG telemetry follow the same set-up procedure but may only involve one recording system or montage and usually use no activation procedures. These tests may be available through more specialized EEG labs where there may be an epilepsy center. The video EEG may last from several hours to days, and patients are usually confined to an area because they are cabled to the machine. This technique combines an ongoing videotape with EEG recording to allow better diagnosis and classification of a given type of seizure.

The EEG telemetry may last for several days and is useful when seizures occur infrequently. The patient's electrodes are connected to a transmitter and battery pack, allowing the patient to be mobile in the general range of the receiving antennas.

Nursing Strategies. No physical preparation is required, unless the patient is to be sleep deprived or requires sedation. Hair elastics and barrettes are usually removed, and unless the hair is dirty or oily it does not require washing prior to the test.

Psychologic preparation involves instruction about the test procedure. Children may fear that the machine will deliver some kind of electrical shock or that it may be able to read their minds or is some type of a lie detector test. Most children find the smell of the glue noxious and should know it will feel cold and wet on their head. A small pen-like air compressor is used to blow dry the glue and the sound of this may be startling. When the conductive jelly is placed inside the electrodes with a syringe children may fear an injection, and find that the surface rubbing or scratching is annoying and uncomfortable. From the child's point of view, the set-up and removal of the electrodes is usually the most disliked part and may require very frequent support and reassurance to be tolerated. The study often seems rather mysterious to parents. They may misinterpret normal and abnormal findings, view it as a highly objective study, and not realize the limitations of the test.

The same care is required for video EEG and EEG telemetry except that the child will require supportive care to occupy him- or herself during the duration of the study and continuous seizure observation.

After the test is finished the child will require some special attention to the hair in order to remove all of the glue and jelly, to avoid scalp irritation and sores. Excess glue can usually be removed with acetone or can be combed out. Hair care products that reduce snarls and tangles may also be quite useful.

Skull and Spine Radiography

The purpose of these studies is to identify fractures, anomalies, tumors, and calcifications, and to note indirect evidence of increased intracranial pressure by suture widening in a younger child or skull erosion in an older child. Care should be taken in positioning or moving the child for this study in cases of suspected fracture or dislocation.

Nursing Strategies. No physical preparation is required. Hair elastics, pins, and barrettes should be removed for skull radiography. For spine films the child is dressed in an "x-ray" or patient gown.

Psychologic preparation involves explaining the procedure of proper positioning and holding still briefly while the x-ray film is taken. Let the child know that the test does not hurt, and explain why other people stand back or wear shields or aprons during the test. Explain that the machine will make some noises.

EMG (*Electromyogram*) *and* Nerve Conduction Velocities

The purpose of the EMG is to analyze the electrical events that are associated with the contraction of skeletal muscle fibers. This includes (1) insertion potentials, as the needle is inserted into the muscle and measures the brief electrical discharges that are produced by this mechanical stimuli; (2) spontaneous potentials, that may occur as fibrillations from single muscle fibers or fasciculations from groups of fibers; and (3) motor unit action potentials as the electrical activity is studied during voluntary muscle contraction (Swaiman, 1982). Nerve conduction velocities measure the muscle contraction that is evoked by the electrical stimulation along a peripheral nerve such as motor and sensory nerves. These velocities increase with age during the first few years of life and reach the lower end of the adult norms by 3 years of age (Swaiman, 1982). Nerve conduction velocities can also slow down with decreased body temperature. These tests may assist in defining types of muscle disease involving the lower motor neuron or muscle, locating nerve lesions, and quantitating nerve regeneration and muscle recovery (Snyder, 1983).

The method for EMG involves some discomfort as needle electrodes are placed into the muscle to be examined and there is a momentary prick. If the needle needs to be repositioned this may produce a slight dull ache in the muscle. Patients will be asked periodically to contract and relax their muscles. Nerve conduction velocities may follow the EMG and involve the proximal and distal stimulation of a motor nerve and then the distal stimulation of a sensory nerve. The stimulations may produce a muscle twitch or contraction or a tingling sensation, depending on the type of nerve that is stimulated.

Nursing Strategies. There is no physical preparation involved in this study unless sedation has been ordered for the patient. Psychologic preparation involves explaining what the test involves and letting children know what they will be expected to do. It may be helpful to plan some things that the child can do during some of the uncomfortable parts of the study. If serum enzyme studies are ordered as well for the child, these should be completed before the study, as these values will be elevated following the study. After the study is finished observe the needle insertion sites for possible hematoma.

Evoked Potentials

Several types of evoked potential studies are available: brainstem auditory evoked responses (BAERs also called BAEPs for evoked potentials), somatosensory evoked responses (SERs or SEPs), visual evoked responses (VERs or VEPs), and multimodality evoked responses (MMERs or MMEPs).

These studies are used for pre-, intra-, and postoperative monitoring of the integrity of various sensory pathways near the surgical site. They can also assess brain activity during drug overdose, drug-induced coma, or coma due to brain damage; and determine the integrity of sensory pathways in diseases such as multiple sclerosis, spinal cord injuries, hearing loss, or in children (especially neonates) who will be receiving long-term aminoglycoside antibiotic and diuretic therapy, which may be known for ototoxic side effects (AANN, 1984; Giubileto and Metcalf, 1984; Clochesy, 1955).

The multimodality evoked potential is used for diagnostic purposes in localizing areas of lesions and in the evaluation of prognosis, since both the BAER and SER are unaffected by arousal, anesthesia, CNS depression, or drug-induced coma.

Nursing Strategies. Box 46-3 reviews patient information for the visual, brainstem, and somatosensory evoked response or potentials study. The visual evoked responses do usually require a certain amount of cooperation to keep the patient's visual attention focused on a specific area. In young children and infants the visual evoked responses may utilize a flashing strobe light rather than an alternating checkerboard as the stimulus. Sometimes sedation may be ordered for young children and infants in order to minimize movement artifact.

Echoencephalogram

This screening study uses a pulsed ultrasonic (Doppler) beam in order to locate midline brain structures for the diagnosis of intracranial abnormalities such as supratentorial masses, which would displace the third ventricle. A probe is placed against the side of the head, a beam is emitted and, as it encounters structures in its path, is reflected back to the transducer also in the probe. The waves are displayed on a screen, pictures can be made and measurements taken. The structures in the measurement are the two tables of the skull and the third ventricle. In a normal study the third ventricle is found in the midline between the tables of the skull. A finding of the third ventricle more than 2 to 3 mm away from the midline is considered abnormal and would require other studies such as the CT scan for further definition (AANN, 1984).

Nursing Strategies. No physical preparation is required for this study. It is important that the patient lie still for the study. This study does not involve any pain or discomfort. As the Doppler transducer is placed against the skin the only sensation felt is the

Box 46-3
Patient Information Tool

PATIENT INFORMATION: VISUAL EVOKED POTENTIALS STUDY

What is a VEP?

1. A VEP is a written record of the brain's response obtained by stimulating the retina with a pattern of light.

2. An instrument registers this activity in the form of a wavy line written on a computer screen. This study is a part of the total neurologic examination your physician may order. Your physician may use this test to determine more precisely your diagnosis and treatment.

Preparation for study

1. There are no restrictions prior to this test. You can eat your routine diet and take usual medications.

2. The study is pain free.

Examination

1. An escort will accompany you to the examination room via wheelchair.

2. Once you are in the examination room and seated on a comfortable chair, the technician will review the purpose of this procedure with you.

3. The technician will apply 3–6 small electrode discs to your scalp, attaching them with a sticky substance.

4. The room will be dimmed and the door closed. You will be instructed to watch the dot in the center of a screen with one eye.

5. Your test will be over when each eye has been tested twice. The complete study takes 20 minutes.

6. You will be accompanied back to your room via wheelchair and may resume your normal activities.

After the study:

1. There are no activity restrictions.

2. The sticky substance used to apply the electrodes can be washed with soap and water.

3. Your physician will give you the results of the study.

PATIENT INFORMATION; BRAIN STEM AUDITORY EVOKED POTENTIALS STUDY

What is a BAEP?

1. The BAEP is a written record of the brain's response to a sound stimulus.

2. An instrument registers the brain's response to the sound stimuli in the form of a wavy line written on a computer screen. This study is a part of the total neurological examination your physician may order. Your physician may use this test to determine more precisely your diagnosis and treatment.

Preparation for study:

1. There are no restrictions prior to this test. You can eat normal meals and take usual medications.

2. The study is pain free.

Examination:

1. An escort will accompany you to the examination room via wheelchair.

2. Once you are in the examination room and lying on the bed on your back, the technician will review the purpose of this procedure with you.

3. The technician will apply 3–4 small electrode discs to your scalp attaching them with a sticky substance. Electrodes will be applied (1) to the top of your head, (2) to the side of your head, and (3) to each of your earlobes.

4. The room will be dimmed and the door closed. You will be instructed to shut your eyes, lie quietly and avoid talking. The door is closed to block extraneous outside noises. The technician will stay in the room with you at all times.

5. Earphones will be placed on your head. You will hear clicks at the lowest possible sound level necessary for conducting the test.

6. The technician will be at the controls of the computer screen which is adjacent to the bed.

7. All you have to do is rest. Throughout the exam, all you will hear through your earphones is repetitive clicks.

8. The complete study takes between 45–90 minutes.

9. Following the exam, the technician will remove the earphones and electrodes.

10. You will be accompanied back to your room via wheelchair and may resume your normal activities.

After the study:

1. The sticky substance used to apply electrodes can be washed with soap and water.

2. There are no activity restrictions.

3. Your physician will give you the results of the study.

PATIENT INFORMATION; SOMATOSENSORY EVOKED POTENTIALS STUDY

What is a SEP?

1. The SEP is a written record of the nerve pathways between the brain and spinal cord.

2. An instrument registers this activity in the form of a wavy line written on a computer screen. This study is a part of the total neurological examination your physician may order. Your physician may use this test to determine more precisely your diagnosis and treatment.

Preparation for study:

1. There are no restrictions prior to this test. You can eat normal meals and take usual medications.

2. The study is pain free.

Continued

Examination

1. An escort will accompany you to the examination room [explain exactly where it is] via wheelchair.
2. Once you are in the examination room and seated on a comfortable chair, the technician will review the purpose of this procedure with you.
3. The technician will apply 6–8 small electrode discs to your scalp, neck, and arm and/or 6–8 electrodes to your scalp, back, and leg.
4. The room will be dimmed and the door closed.
5. You will be instructed to relax.
6. The electrode applied to a specific nerve on your arm will create an involuntary twitch of your thumb.
7. The test is performed twice for each extremity.
8. The study takes approximately 1 hour.

After the study:

1. There are no activity restrictions.
2. The sticky substance used to apply the electrodes can be washed with soap and water.
3. Your physician will give you the results of the study.

(From Giubilato and Metcalf, 1984, page 246.)

cold wet conductive gel against the skin. The child should know that the machine will make some sounds and that the test may take about 15 minutes.

Brain Scan

This scan may often be confused in labeling with the CT scan. This test is quite different from the CT scan as it usually involves the injection of a tiny amount of radioactive isotope to measure the tissue uptake throughout the brain. These substances may have increased uptake in areas of vascularity and permeability. Under normal circumstances the blood-brain barrier prevents passage of the isotope into brain tissue. When a lesion is present in the brain the isotope may pass through the barrier to the site of the lesion to appear as an area of increased density on the scan or of darker color compared with surrounding tissue. Some of the uses of the scan are in screening for and following the course of primary brain tumors: cerebral metastasis, cerebral vascular disease, and benign brain tumors (Snyder, 1983).

Nursing Strategies. No physical preparation is usually required, unless sedation is ordered. Psychologic preparation involves instructing the patient regarding the test procedure. Patients must hold their head very still as they lay supine on a table for about 45 to 60 minutes. Some discomfort is experienced with the venipuncture to inject the isotope (usually ^{99m}Technetium); however, there is no other discomfort associated with this study. Patients should be reassured that they are not radioactive, because of the small amount and short half-life of the isotope used. During the test a radiation detector moves back and forth above the patient's head to complete the study.

Tables 46-7 and 46-8 show basic preprocedure and postprocedure care plans for neurologic diagnostic studies (AANN, 1984).

Invasive Diagnostic Tests

LP (Lumbar Puncture)

This study consists of inserting a spinal needle into the subarachnoid space between the lower lumbar vertebrae. In infants this occurs between L3–L4 and in children between L4–L5. There are two purposes for performing an LP: (1) *diagnostic*—to note the CSF pressure, to obtain CSF fluid for analysis, to test CSF dynamics for a block in the circulation, or to inject substances for x-ray studies; and (2) *treatment*—to inject medications, to induce spinal anesthesia, and to remove foreign contrast media. The LP is usually contraindicated if there is suspicion of greatly increased intracranial pressure or expanding mass lesions (especially in the posterior fossa) because of the risk of brainstem herniation, respiratory arrest, and death secondary to a sudden decompression in intracranial pressure. At these times it would be performed only to rule out subarachnoid hemorrhage or meningitis. Other risks involve infection (e.g., meningitis) if aseptic technique is not followed; and transient low back pain and nerve root irritation (Snyder, 1983). The most common problem following the LP is a headache, which appears positional and disappears when the patient lies flat. This is thought to be caused by the slightly lower CSF pressure which may put traction on some of the pain-sensitive structures or due to a slow leak of CSF through the dural puncture site which may take a couple of days to heal (Snyder, 1983).

The LP procedure involves assisting the patient to

a sidelying position, with hips and legs flexed. Using aseptic technique the skin is prepped over the site and drapes are used. A topical and/or local anesthetic is used. The needle is inserted between the vertebrae until it enters the subarachnoid space, the stylet is removed, and a column is attached for CSF pressure readings. Following this several drops of CSF are put in test tubes, a closing pressure may be determined, the needle is withdrawn, gentle pressure is applied to the site and a sterile dressing is applied.

Nursing Strategies. There is no physical preparation for this test. The test may be performed in the office examination room, in the treatment room, or at the bedside. Consent is usually obtained. Correct positioning is important for the test. This can be attained by positioning children on their side with their face toward the nurse and their back positioned as close to the far edge of the table as possible (Fig. 46-9). The neck is gently flexed forward and the knees drawn up toward the chest. The nurse should hold the child securely but avoid placing any weight on the child. Older children should be instructed to avoid any movement and be advised of the importance of lying very still. The nurse should monitor respirations during and after the procedure.

When a CSF pressure reading is to be measured, only slightly relax the flexion of the child's hips but retain a secure hold on the child. This is because marked hip flexion increases intracranial pressure. After the needle is correctly inserted, attempt to comfort and reassure the child that the test will soon be finished as ICP will be elevated with crying and struggling.

An alternate position that may be used with infants is the sitting position. This position utilizes the effects of gravity to distend the dural sac slightly to ease the insertion of the needle into the subarachnoid space. This positioning involves securely holding the infant in the same position, with the buttocks at the edge of the table and with neck and hips flexed and stabilized.

After the procedure, if there are no specific orders, the nurse should monitor and record neurologic checks and vital signs every 15 minutes the first hour, and periodically thereafter depending on the patient's stability. The LP site should be checked and recorded for CSF leakage and any redness at the puncture site. To reduce post-LP headache encourage intake of fluids and have the patient lie flat for the first few hours after the test, gradually elevating the head and allowing resumption of activities as tolerated. Younger children may not be able to follow this instruction and will determine their own position of comfort. The headache usually will disappear upon lying flat. If this does not relieve the headache, if it is severe, or if it is accompanied by an increased temperature contact the doctor immediately, as these may be symptoms of either the primary CNS infection or an infection secondary to the LP.

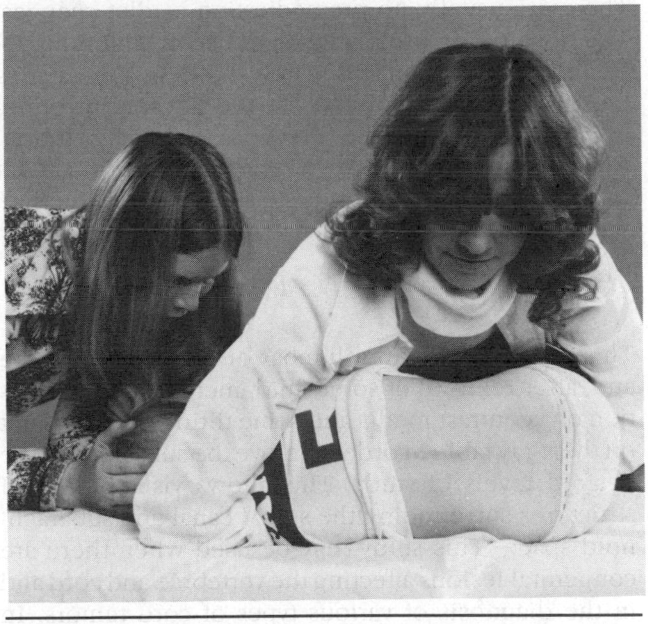

Figure 46-9. Lumbar puncture. If parents are present for this procedure, they can be supportive by focusing on the child rather than the procedure.

Cisternal Puncture

The cisternal puncture is similar to the LP but involves inserting the needle into the cisterna magna at the level of C2. This study is used to identify an upper level block in the CSF circulation, to perform a tap when there are lesions or infections present at the lumbar site, and to inject substances for diagnostic or treatment purposes.

Subdural Tap

The subdural tap is another similar study that is generally restricted to infants or young children with fontanelles. It is used to identify subdural effusions and subdural hemorrhage, to withdraw CSF for culture, to instill medicines, or to reduce temporarily the volume of CSF. The study may be performed together with craniotomy or separately. It involves the use of a local anesthetic followed by the insertion of a spinal needle through the opening at the junction of the anterior fontanelle and the coronal suture, to the subdural space, followed by removal of the stylet and then removal of CSF. No more than 30 to 35 ml is removed, to avoid cranial decompression with its risk of herniation, respiratory arrest, and death. A sterile dressing is applied at completion. This test usually takes about 20 to 30 minutes.

Nursing Strategies. Consent is usually obtained. Physical preparation may include a betadine shampoo.

There are usually no premedication or diet changes. The positioning usually involves use of a mummy restraint with the nurse securely holding the infant's head. The physician may shave the site and surrounding area and cleanse the site with a betadine solution. Nursing care may also involve keeping the infant flat for several hours, with frequent assessment of the site, neurologic checks, and vital signs.

Myelogram

This test begins with a lumbar or cisternal puncture and, after removal of some fluid, includes the instillation of a contrast media and some tilting of the patient on the x-ray table in order to move the substance to the desired levels of study. This allows visualization of structures surrounding the spinal canal and subarachnoid space. This study may be used when there are congenital lesions affecting the vertebrae and cord and in the diagnosis of various types of cord tumors. In adults it is most commonly used in the study of vertebral disc disease; however, this is uncommon in children. This test often takes 2 hours.

Three types of contrast media are used:

1. Air and gases may be used if there is blood in the subarachnoid space, if the person is allergic to other contrast, and in cases when positioning may be difficult because of a fracture.
2. Pantopaque may be used. This is an oily preparation that must be removed at the end of the procedure.
3. Metrizamide, a water-base preparation, may be used. It may or may not be removed at the end of the procedure. Metrizamide is absorbed by the body and excreted by the kidneys, exerting a large molecule diuretic effect (AANN, 1984).

Complications are similar to those for LP, with the addition of arachnoiditis, an inflammation in the arachnoid membrane, and cord compression that could lead to progressive neurologic deficits usually seen in cases in which there is spinal block.

Nursing Strategies. This requires consent, and in general requires care similar to that for lumbar puncture. Sedation is usually used together with an anticholinergic drug. The child may be NPO if sedation will be used. Activity related to having the head elevated or lying flat depends on whether metrizamide or Pantopaque is used, respectively. Postprocedure positioning is usually ordered by the physician. Patients who have received metrizamide need positioning so that their head remains above their heart for 6 to 8 hours after the test to prevent the contrast material from migrating up the subarachnoid space to irritate the cortex of the brain and possibly cause seizures. Fluid intake should also be encouraged for the excretion of the contrast media.

Cerebral Angiography

This invasive study involves the injection of contrast media into an artery to visualize both the intra- and extracranial vessels and to examine the arterial, capillary, and venous phases of the cerebral circulation. It helps identify vascular deficits such as aneurysms, arteriovenous malformations, and other developmental anomalies. It also allows a more precise view of the vessels' lumens. It may precede craniotomy to assist the neurosurgeon in determining the surgical approach. This test usually takes 1 to 2 hours. The test may be contraindicated if there is renal insufficiency, history of allergy to the contrast material or to iodine, blood dyscrasias, or previous thrombotic or embolic events. Persons receiving anticoagulant therapy would require special care, usually discontinuing anticoagulants several hours to days before the test, depending on the anticoagulant's clearance.

Consent is required. The method involves aseptic technique. The skin is prepped with Betadine and drapes are placed. The femoral artery is punctured and the catheter is inserted and, using fluoroscopy, is threaded through the vessels to one of the carotid arteries. Less commonly the brachial artery may be used or there may be direct insertion into one of the carotid arteries. Multiple injections of the contrast media into each vessel occur, while a rapid sequence of films is taken. Then the catheter is withdrawn slightly and advanced into the other carotid artery. After this similar studies of the two vertebral arteries may also be done. Finally, the catheter is removed and manual pressure is maintained on the puncture site, after which a pressure dressing is applied. It is common for an intravenous pyelogram (IVP) to be completed following this test, as the contrast material is excreted by the kidneys.

Nursing Strategies. Physical preparation involves sedation before the test and NPO restrictions. Some physicians may require a skin prep prior to the test. Because the contrast media will be excreted through the kidneys and has been known to cause renal failure in dehydrated patients, it is essential that the patient be well-hydrated before the test. The patient should wear a hospital or x-ray gown and must remove jewelry and any hair ornaments. The patient should void, and the nurse should record the baseline neurologic check and vital signs.

Psychologic preparation for the angiogram involves knowledge of sensations that the patient will experience and instruction about the procedure as appropriate. The room itself will be dark and the patient will be positioned on a hard table with the head secured to a headrest. Equipment for assessing blood pressure and pulse will be applied, the skin prep will feel cold and wet, and some pain will occur with the injection of the local anesthetic and to a lesser extent with the arterial puncture. When the contrast is injected most patients experience very brief hot, burning, flushing sensations in their face, head, and behind their eyes. They may also experience nausea and headache. During the injections and the rapid sequencing of films the machine will make loud "kaboom" noises.

Care after the study involves checking the site and pressure dressing along with vital signs and neurologic checks every 15 minutes for 1 hour; every 30 minutes for 4 hours; every hour for 4 hours; and then every 2 to 4 hours for 24 hours, depending on the patient's condition (see Table 46-8 for care related to the arterial puncture and injection of contrast material [hematoma, edema, vasospasm, thrombosis, embolism, allergic reaction]). Transient and permanent alterations in speech, motor and sensory functions, and consciousness have been reported as a result of cerebral emboli with carotid studies, and visual loss and signs of brainstem damage may occur with vertebral studies (Snyder, 1983). The patient is usually kept on bed rest for 12 to 24 hours to reduce clot dislodgement and hematoma formation. Postprocedure hydration is important and the patient should begin with sips of fluid every 15 minutes, increasing the volume as tolerated. Intravenous hydration is usually maintained until the patient is able to maintain a well-hydrated state. Intake and output records for the first 24 hours help the nurse quickly to identify a patient experiencing renal problems.

Digital Subtraction Angiography

Another technique in cerebral angiography is digital subtraction angiography. This technique is similar to that just described except for the much larger volume of contrast media that is usually injected venously. This procedure may be used only with older children and adolescents, as the patient must remain motionless during the study (even swallowing may impair the quality of the films) and because of the larger volume of contrast material given with potential circulatory overload. However, this study involves less risk than a regular angiogram because of the venipuncture, and produces improved clarity of image with reduced artifact.

Nursing Strategies. Physical preparation is the same as cerebral angiography. Adequate pre- and postprocedure hydration is very important with this technique because of the very large volume of contrast material to be excreted by the kidneys. During and immediately after this study the patient must be assessed for symptoms of circulatory overload. The remainder of the nursing care is similar to that described for cerebral angiography, except that the patient does not need to remain immobile as long with the venipuncture as with the arterial puncture angiogram.

Pneumoencephalogram

This invasive study begins with a lumbar puncture followed by injecting gas (oxygen) into the subarachnoid space and tilting the patient to allow the gas to rise and fill the various ventricles, cisterns, and subarachnoid spaces. This test may be indicated when there is obstruction in the CSF pathways, in order to better define and diagnose the problem; it is used only when less risky procedures cannot be done. Prior to the availability of the CT and NMR scans this test was also used in identifying mass lesions and cerebral atrophy. The risks involved with this study are seizures, air embolism, and various types of brain herniations. The test is contraindicated if signs of greatly increased intracranial pressure are present (because of the increased risk for herniation), if there is infection at the puncture site, and if the patient is receiving anticoagulant therapy.

The child sits securely strapped in a special chair that rotates in any position and an LP is performed. After the opening CSF pressure is recorded a small volume of gas is injected into the subarachnoid space and films are taken. The films are taken with the child in an upright position; then the chair is rotated horizontally to visualize fully all the ventricular structures. If any problems develop during the study such as severe hypotension or altered neurologic function, the study is terminated. At the completion of the procedure the needle is removed, manual pressure is used, and a sterile dressing is applied.

During and after the procedure headache accompanied by nausea and vomiting is common. This can last from 12 to 36 hours or longer and is thought to be due to the withdrawal of CSF and the presence of the gas in the ventricular system (Snyder, 1983). A stiff neck and a slightly elevated temperature may also be experienced. If the fever is prolonged and temperature markedly elevated it may indicate a possible meningitis secondary to the study.

Symptoms of autonomic dysfunction may occur after the study because of irritation by the gas: chills, sweating, cool skin, drooling, hypotension, and bradycardia. These will usually subside within a few hours and may be prevented to some extent by premedicating with a sedative and an anticholinergic agent.

Nursing Strategies. Consent is required for this invasive study, and aseptic technique is used. Physical preparation includes NPO restrictions and premedication with both a sedative and an anticholinergic drug.

The child is dressed in a hospital gown with baseline neurologic signs and vital signs established. Jewelry and hair ornaments are removed.

Psychologic preparation involves explaining the procedure appropriate to age using simple terms. The injection of gas will be heard by the patient as a sloshing, wave-like sound in their head until all of the gas is finally absorbed. Explaining what will be involved in assessing neurologic checks and vital signs after the study and practicing these may help the child comply with these tasks after the procedure.

During the study the patient should be closely monitored (neurologic checks and vital signs) every 5 to 10 minutes. Caring for the child after this study involves close monitoring for any signs of complications. Neuro checks and vital signs may be done every 30 minutes for the first hour or two, every hour for the next 4 hours, then every 2 to 4 hours for the next 24 hours depending on the child's condition. Making the child comfortable and minimizing headache is the next priority. Keeping the child flat and relatively immobile for the first 24 hours and making turns and movements very gradually seem to reduce the headache. An ice bag or cool compress to the head may also afford some relief. In addition keeping the room lights down and the room quiet may be beneficial. Administer analgesics as ordered, but avoid giving antipyretics as these can minimize symptoms of infection. Low-grade temperatures are not uncommon for several days after the study. Fluids should be given orally or intravenously unless the patient has a restriction because of increased intracranial pressure.

Laboratory Tests

Laboratory tests which may be used in the diagnostic process include chromosome studies, which may assist in identifying genetic disease. Other tests include those designed to screen for inborn errors of metabolism, degenerative disease, and abnormalities in carbohydrate, lipid, protein, or urea cycle metabolism. Tests for toxicity include urine metabolic screen, serum amino acids and organic acids, urine amino acids and organic acids, and serum lactate and pyruvate. Examination of WBC with electron microscopy and screening for heavy metals may also be conducted.

Therapeutic Interventions

This section will discuss some basic knowledge areas that span care for children with various alterations in neurologic function. This will include care for the child experiencing increased intracranial pressure (ICP) or with potentially increased ICP, care of children experiencing craniotomy, care of children experiencing seizures or at risk for seizures, and care of children with altered levels of consciousness.

The Child with Increased Intracranial Pressure

A sound knowledge base in this area is important in order to identify those who could be at risk for developing increased ICP, and early recognition of those with symptoms of increased ICP.

Pathophysiology of ICP

The ICP inside the skull depends on the volumes and pressures exerted by three components: brain, blood, and cerebral spinal fluid (CSF). After fontanels have closed and sutures are fused the skull forms a rigid, unyielding container with a fixed volume capacity. Any increase in the volume of one of the components (brain, blood, or CSF) would be accompanied by a decreased volume in the other components in order to maintain a constant volume-pressure relationship. Once there is an imbalance in the volume-pressure relationship increased ICP develops.

In infants and younger children, in whom the fontanels may still be open or the sutures not completely fused, the skull, in the case of acute and markedly increased ICP, is still a rigid box but it is a box with some expandability. This is important because it relates to the various signs and symptoms of both acute and chronic increased ICP for infants and young children.

Compensatory Mechanisms. The brain has several initial compensatory mechanisms that can help to balance the volume-pressure relationships and maintain equilibrium of ICP without apparent damaging effects on the brain. These occur primarily with the decrease in CSF and cerebral blood volume.

Although the CSF is produced at a fixed rate the rate of absorption across the arachnoid villi can be increased if ICP is increased. At the same time the sac of subarachnoid space at the distal end of the spinal cord can distend; CSF may be squeezed through the ventricular system into this area. Some shifting of cerebral blood flow may occur with increased venous outflow into the venous sinuses and slight reduction in arterial perfusion, although this has not been well proven.

Cerebral Blood Flow. Cerebral blood flow is essential for oxygenation in the brain and the transportation of metabolic nutrients to and from the cell. Cerebral blood flow influences and is influenced by ICP via the arterial blood gases, cerebral perfusion pressure, and the autoregulation of blood flow. Carbon dioxide

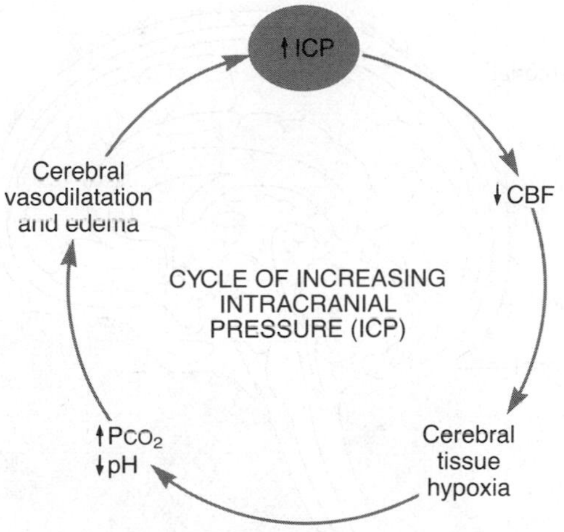

***Figure* 46-10.** Dynamics of increased intracranial pressure (ICP). CBF, Cerebral blood flow; PCO_2, serum carbon dioxide.

is a potent vasodilator of cerebral blood vessels. Vasodilatation causes increased blood volume, which can increase ICP. Reducing $PaCO_2$ by controlled hyperventilation causes vasoconstriction of blood vessels, which in turn reduces blood volume delivered and reduces ICP. This is the basis for using controlled hyperventilation in the management of increased ICP. Oxygen content also affects ICP but to a much lesser degree than $PaCO_2$. Conditions of profound hypoxia (PaO_2 <50 mmHg) can cause cerebral vasodilatation. This has implication for the attention paid to the airway, adequate oxygenation, and normal levels of PaO_2.

Autoregulation. Autoregulation describes the mechanisms in the cerebral blood vessels to maintain a constant cerebral blood supply despite fluctuations in the arterial blood pressure. This is accomplished by constriction and dilatation of the cerebral blood vessels. When arterial pressures are elevated vasoconstriction occurs, and when arterial pressures fall there is vasodilatation. This has implication for the understanding that either extreme of arterial pressure—an arterial pressure less than 50 mmHg or greater than 150 mmHg—may increase or decrease cerebral blood flow, respectively, and thus affect ICP (Swaiman, 1982). Autoregulation of blood flow can also be impaired by cerebral edema, cerebral acidosis associated with ischemia, serious injuries of the brain that cause disseminated intravascular coagulation, extreme changes in blood pressure within an area of decreased regional cerebral blood flow as a result of CVA, with most severe arteriographic changes such as vasospasm, and impairment of cardiac function.

Cerebral Perfusion Pressure. The relationship between ICP and systemic arterial pressure in blood flow is the cerebral perfusion pressure. Cerebral perfusion pressure, under conditions of normal autoregulation, can be estimated by subtracting the mean intracranial pressure from the mean systemic arterial pressure. Cerebral perfusion pressure can then be increased by lowering ICP or by raising the systemic arterial pressure, or by a combination of these. When autoregulation is impaired cerebral perfusion pressure and cerebral blood flow become passively dependent on systemic arterial pressure, cerebral blood flow may not increase with an increase in cerebral perfusion pressure, and cerebral blood flow may be reduced at relatively normal levels of cerebral perfusion pressure (AANN, 1984). Figure 46-10 shows the dynamics occurring with increased ICP.

Herniation Syndromes

With continued increased ICP or intracranial hypertension, the brain begins to decompensate and herniate. This involves a physical displacement of a portion of the brain through or around other brain structures, usually because of the increase in volume in an area of the brain, blood, or CSF. There are many types of herniation syndromes (Fig. 46-11) and all of these are life threatening unless they are recognized early and treated. The best treatment is to prevent a situation in which herniation syndrome could occur. The most common type of supratentorial (above the tentorium) herniation is uncal herniation (Fig. 46-12). As the uncus of the temporal lobe pushes into midline structures it compromises the oculomotor nerve and thereby causes pupil dilation with poor direct response to light on the same side as the lesion.

Figure 46-13 shows the two directions that the cerebellum in the infratentorium (beneath the tentorium) can herniate. These types of herniation can occur with expanding masses or blood in the cerebellum

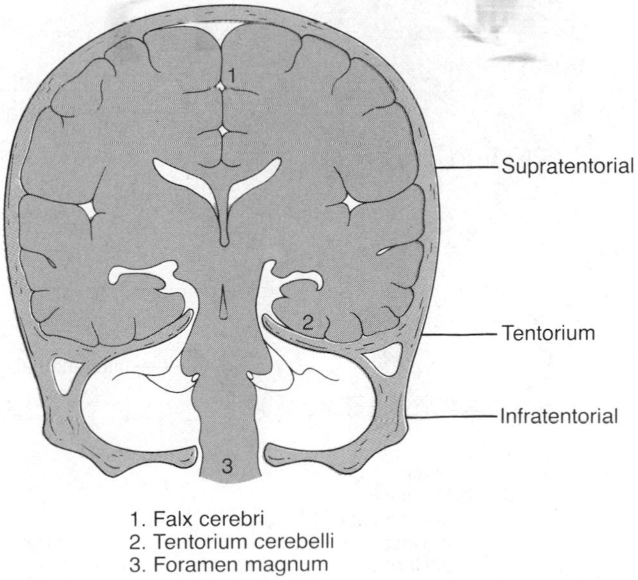

***Figure* 46-11.** A normal coronal section showing potential sites of brain herniation.

where the cerebellum pushes either upward against upper brainstem structures, causing symptoms of oculomotor and trochlear nerve involvement, or downward against the medulla portion of the brainstem, causing rapid deterioration of respiratory and circulatory efforts or arrest.

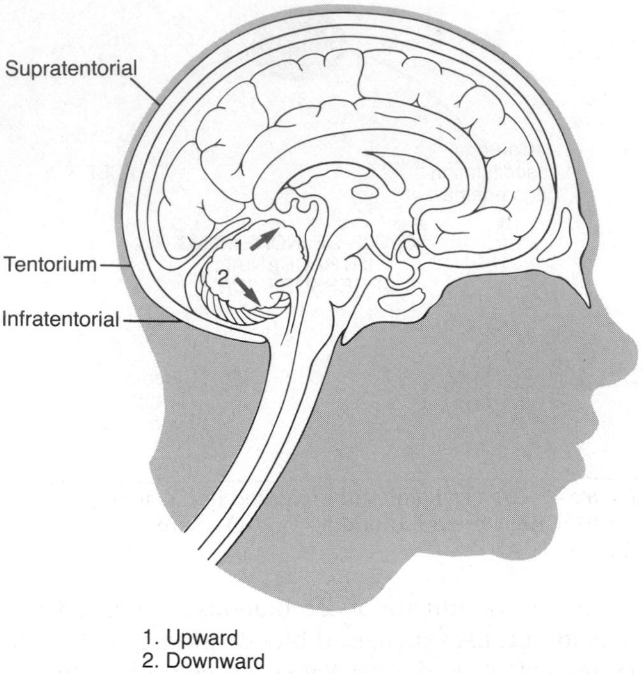

Figure 46-13. Infratentorial herniation.

Clinical Manifestations

Table 46-9 lists the clinical manifestations of increased intracranial pressure. Differences in signs and symptoms are related to open fontanels and unfused sutures in infants with some expandability for compensation, compared with children in whom the skull is less accommodating. Early recognition of these symptoms can lead to prompt treatment of increased ICP with better outcome.

Diagnostic Assessment

Increased intracranial pressure can be diagnosed by the presenting symptoms. Diagnostic studies may be obtained to identify the specific cause. This may include skull roentgenography, CT and NMR scans, cerebral blood flow studies, EEG, evoked potentials, and laboratory tests.

ICP Measurement

Intracranial pressure is measured in millimeters of mercury (mmHg) or in centimeters of water (cm H_2O). Various devices are available for monitoring, ranging from a noninvasive transducer that may be placed over a fontanelle to more commonly used invasive devices such as an epidural transducer, a subarachnoid bolt or screw, and an intraventricular catheter that is connected to an external transducer.

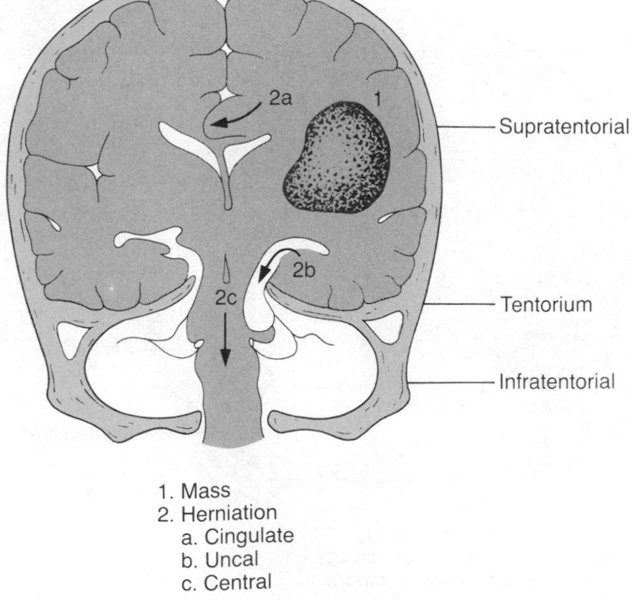

Figure 46-12. Schematic drawing of supratentorial herniation sites.

Nursing care for patients on ICP monitoring focuses on assessment of intracranial pressure, maintaining monitoring system integrity, and assessing the patient for signs of infection, hemorrhage, and risk of CSF leakage secondary to and depending on the type of ICP device (Jones and Cayard, 1982). Normal ICP ranges from 0 to 15 mmHg. The ICP is usually quite stable although temporary elevations as high as 100 mmHg can occur with activities like coughing and straining (AANN, 1984). Increased ICP may be considered moderately elevated (20 to 40 mmHg) or severely elevated (greater than 40 mmHg).

Mechanisms that Increase ICP

With respect to the three main components inside the skull, Table 46-10 lists some of the mechanisms known to influence or effect intracranial pressure. Mechanisms that increase brain mass can include the edema from head injury and postoperative brain surgery as well as infectious and inflammatory diseases such as encephalitis and Reye syndrome. Cysts and tumors as well as intracerebral hemorrhage, aneurysm rupture, and large arteriovenous malformations also increase brain mass. Mechanisms that increase ICP by increasing cerebral blood volume are numerous and include many factors that are influenced by nursing care. Increased CSF as a mechanism for increasing ICP can

Table 46-9. Clinical Manifestations of Elevated Intracranial Pressure

Bulging anterior fontanel	Full, tense, bulging above bone and firm enough to cause difficulty distinguishing bone/fontanel junction; closure delayed in chronic increase of ICP
Increased head circumference	Greater than 2 cm/month in first 3 months of life, greater than 1 cm/month in the second 3 months, and greater than 0.5 cm/month for the next 6 months (Fenichel, 1988)
Headache	May be generalized or localized; often present upon awakening and standing up in the morning. Pain increased by Valsalva maneuver: coughing, sneezing, straining at stool, holding breath, and straining to turn in bed
Altered mental state	Irritability, fatigue, altered consciousness, memory loss
Vomiting	In the absence of nausea, especially upon arising in the morning
Altered vital signs	Elevated blood pressure, decreased pulse and respiration
Altered vision	Diplopia (double vision), strabismus, results from pressure on one or both abducens nerves; "setting sun" sign (especially with hydrocephalus); restricted visual fields; papilledema

include hydrocephalus which may be from increased production of CSF as in choroid plexus tumors, decreased absorption as may occur as a complication of meningitis due to debris clogging the arachnoid villi, or just obstructions in the system that are idiopathic, caused by neural tube defects or the presence of some type of space-occupying lesion. When caring for patients with any of these potential mechanisms the nurse should observe carefully for symptoms of increased ICP. Children with head injuries should all be cared for as though they have increased ICP until a definitive diagnosis is established.

Therapeutic Management

The treatment of increased ICP may involve medical and/or surgical methods (Table 46-10). Passive hyperventilation is helpful to decrease ICP provided $PaCO_2$ is not brought below 25 mmHg while maintaining PaO_2 between 80 and 100 mmHg.

Another common treatment is the use of intravenous mannitol which stays in cerebral blood vessels increasing the osmotic pressure, causing water to move from the brain through the capillary walls into the blood. It also has an effect on reducing the production of CSF, which again further reduces ICP. The use of mannitol can sometimes lead to a secondary increase in ICP, or "rebound," however.

Pentobarbital or barbiturate therapy is used mainly with moderate and severe increases in ICP that have not responded to the usual medical treatment. Other treatments of increased ICP also include the use of diuretics. Furosemide is probably most common; however, others may include acetazolamide and ethacrynic acid. Diuretics decrease total body water, thereby reducing brain water and decreasing ICP, although the exact mechanism has not been defined. The use of diuretics such as furosemide is associated with significant potassium depletion.

Adjunctive measures include the use of other med-

Table 46-10. Mechanisms Known to Increase Intracranial Pressure and Related Treatment

Mechanisms That Increase ICP	Treatment
Increased brain mass	
Edema from head injury, brain surgery, infectious and inflammatory diseases (e.g., meningitis) Increased mass resulting from growths (cysts, tumors), leakage of fluid (hemorrhage), and large arteriovenous malformations	Surgery Corticosteroids Osmotic diuretics (mannitol, glycerol)
Increased cerebral blood volume	
Vasodilation (e.g., with oxygen deprivation resulting in increased $PaCO_2$, decreased PaO_2) Decreased venous outflow (e.g., head position restricting jugular venous flow) Increased thoracic pressure (Valsalva, positive end-expiratory pressure) Increased systemic blood pressure	Hyperventilation Elevating head of bed Maintaining alignment of head and neck Hypothermia Pentobarbital coma Diuretics (furosemide, acetazolamide, ethacrynic acid) Pancuronium to decrease muscular response to stimuli Thorazine to decrease restlessness
Increased cerebrospinal fluid (CSF) volume	
Increased CSF production (e.g., from choroid plexus tumors) Decreased CSF absorption (e.g., from debris clogging arachnoid villi in meningitis) Obstruction to CSF flow (e.g., infratentorial tumor)	Surgery Shunting

ications to reduce posturing, normal, and abnormal physiologic responses that may increase ICP. Pancuronium decreases muscle responses to voluntary, central, and environmental stimuli that may be reflected in decerebrate and decorticate posturing, or in fighting the ventilator. Thorazine may be useful in some patients for decreasing restlessness and shivering, which can be a problem if hypothermia is used.

Invasive and operative interventions for the treatment of increased ICP may include supdural tap, ventriculostomy with controlled drainage, epidural evacuation, placement of a ventricular shunt, decompressive craniectomy, and surgery to remove an expanding mass lesion such as a tumor.

Strategies for Nursing Care

The components of nursing care for actual or potential increases in intracranial pressure include (1) prompt recognition and institution of treatment; (2) prompt recognition and treatment of hypercapnia and hypoxia; (3) maintenance of normothermia; (4) maintenance of optimal head, neck, and body positions; (5) protective nursing care; and (6) administration of medications and monitoring for medication effectiveness and side effects.

Early Recognition and Treatment of Increased ICP. This begins with assessment of factors in the patient's history that could put the patient at risk. In general, situations that may cause increased ICP include head injury, intracranial tumors, hydrocephalus, neural tube defects, infectious disorders such as meningitis and encephalitis, and metabolic disorders. Assess the history for concerns of altered mental state such as decreased alertness or responsiveness, and history of headache or vomiting.

After neurologic baseline is established, the nurse should monitor neurologic checks and vital signs with the frequency determined by the patient's condition and the nursing and physician orders. This may be as frequently as every 15 minutes, for a patient who seems unstable or whose condition appears to be changing, to several times daily for a more stable patient (see the previous section on neurologic assessment).

If the patient's ICP is being monitored the goal should be to keep the ICP at less than 15 mmHg, the mean arterial systemic pressure greater than 70 mmHg, the cerebral perfusion pressure greater than 50 mmHg, and temperature less than 38.5°C in order to prevent secondary brain damage. If sudden increases occur in intracranial pressure or if abnormal wave forms develop, the nurse should quickly assess what may have caused the increase: (1) further neurologic deterioration with decompensation and herniation; (2) head and neck position interfering with cerebral blood flow; (3) partially obstructed airway with inadequate respirations; (4) recent care activities that could have caused the increase; (5) hyperthermia; or (6) increased patient movements, posturing, or restlessness caused by problems with nasogastric tube, intravenous site, urinary catheter, or other factors (Zeidelman, 1980). The nurse needs to remember that ICP devices are no replacement for good clinical assessment, as they can malfunction and it is possible to get low readings in spite of increased ICP.

Recognition and Treatment of Hypercapnia and Hypoxia. This involves assessment of the patient for a patent airway and adequate ventilation, which entails assessment of airway and auscultation of breath sounds regularly, and at least daily arterial blood gas determinations. Both hypercapnia and hypoxia markedly alter cerebral blood flow and may affect the development of increased ICP and add to preexisting problems. When brain tissue is compromised or has shifted there may be alteration in respiratory rate and patterns, or respiratory arrest.

Suctioning may be necessary to maintain the airway and prevent hypercapnia and hypoxia. Suctioning should be limited to not more than 15 seconds in duration in patients with increased ICP, to prevent suctioning-induced hypoxia (Shapiro, 1975). Suctioning appears to be a factor for increased ICP secondary to the tracheal stimulation involved rather than increased Pa_{CO_2} or decreased Pa_{O_2} secondary to the procedure (Fisher et al, 1982). The nurse should take this into account when arranging periodic suctioning with other nursing care activities.

Patients with increased ICP, nonpatent airway, and/or hypoventilation that cannot be controlled may require intubation or mechanical ventilator support, or both, for more precise control to maintain hypocapnia with the Pa_{CO_2} between 25 to 30 torr, and Pa_{O_2} greater than 80 torr. These ranges should avoid increases in intracranial blood volume. Positive end-expiratory pressure (PEEP) may be used to manage pulmonary hypoxia and this may present problems for a trauma patient with mixed injuries to the head and chest. PEEP may increase ICP by increasing the intrathoracic pressure and decreasing return of cerebral venous blood. Patients with increased ICP requiring PEEP should use moderate levels of PEEP, should have close monitoring of arterial and intracranial pressures to detect any changes, and should be gradually weaned from PEEP to avoid rebound increases in systemic blood pressure.

Hyperventilation may be used as a short-term treatment for increased ICP because it has an immediate effect, does not lead to a secondary increase or rebound of ICP, and does not potentiate bleeding. An Ambu bag and 100 per cent O_2 should be available at the bedside for emergency manual hyperventilation in a child not receiving ventilator support. Manual hyperventilation should be performed cautiously because of lack of adequate control (AANN, 1984). Generally, if hyperventilation has not reduced the ICP in 15 minutes, other measures are taken.

Maintenance of Normothermia or Temperature Regulation. Assessment of temperature is one aspect of monitoring the patient's vital signs. Normothermia is maintained by keeping body temperature at 36.5° to 38.0°C (97.7 to 100.4°F) without using cooling devices or antipyretics (Snyder, 1983). A study with adults found that for every degree centigrade of temperature elevation the brain demanded 7 per cent more oxygen (Hindfelt, 1976). The presence of fever causes vasodilation, thus increasing cerebral blood flow.

Maintenance of normothermia involves patient assessment as well as monitoring temperature and laboratory and diagnostic tests for the cause of the fever. Dressing the patient in cool clothing and using light bed covers are beneficial. Providing adequate hydration is usually another intervention for maintaining normothermia but may not be possible in a patient with increased ICP who may have fluids restricted. Administering antipyretics as ordered and instituting tepid water sponge baths or using cooling devices may be necessary.

Hypothermia may be used as a treatment modality for increased ICP in children. Hypothermia produces vasoconstriction, which reduces cerebral blood flow, which in turn reduces ICP. For example, reducing body temperature to 32°C reduces cerebral metabolism by 35 to 40 per cent (AANN, 1984). Advantages to using hypothermia include no risk of ICP rebound or intracranial bleeding (Swaiman, 1982). Hypothermia is usually accomplished using a cooling blanket. The nurse should be familiar with the instructions of the particular unit to be used.

Consequences of hypothermia may include cardiac arrhythmias with temperatures less than 32°C, hypercoagulopathies due to increasing hematocrit, decreased systemic arterial perfusion, reduced renal perfusion with reduced urine output, and frostbite and burns.

Careful monitoring with frequent nursing care can minimize and prevent many untoward effects of hypothermia. It is important to cool the patient slowly to prevent shivering. A rate of temperature reduction commonly used is not more than 1°C per 15 minutes. If a cooling blanket is used continuously body temperature will begin to decrease within the first hour of use, with the effect peaking in 2 to 3 hours. A downward drift of body temperature from 2 to 10°C usually continues after hypothermia is discontinued. This should be anticipated to avoid lower body temperatures than desired to help prevent cardiac arrhythmias.

Patients need to be turned and positioned slowly to avoid rushing chilled blood back into the heart, which can cause ventricular fibrillation (AANN, 1984). Monitoring vital signs, laboratory tests such as CBC, and intake and output help to measure the patient's response to the treatment and to identify rapidly potential problems.

Good skin care is essential with applications of Vaseline to all bony prominences, and wrapping of hands, feet, and genitals to prevent frostbite and burns. Intramuscular and subcutaneous injections are usually contraindicated because of reduced peripheral circulation and the potential for abscesses to develop.

Shivering can increase requirements for oxygen and glucose and quickly exhaust glycogen stores, producing acidosis. This can be minimized by cooling the patient slowly and by administering medications (such as chlorpromazine) as ordered.

Careful monitoring is also required when the hypothermia is to be discontinued. The patient should be rewarmed over 24 to 48 hours in order to prevent shock and to minimize acidosis and pulmonary edema secondary to the increased circulatory volume being presented to a depressed heart.

Maintaining Optimal Head, Neck, and Body Positions. Head and neck position should be kept neutral with regard to the shoulders and upper trunk. Nurse researchers have found that neck flexion and head rotation appear to increase intracranial pressure (Mitchell 1980; Mitchell et al, 1981; Snyder, 1983; Parsons and Wilson, 1984). Mitchell and co-workers (1981) postulate that changes in head position in patients with existing increased ICP may completely or partially obstruct basal cisterns, decreasing collateral venous outflow, thus leaving more venous blood and CSF in the cranium to increase ICP.

The following measures are used by the nurse to maintain neutral head and neck positions. Pillows should be avoided when the patient is supine, but may be required for neutral positioning in sidelying positions. The patient's head should be supported in a neutral position during turning and lifting. The head of the bed should be kept elevated at 30 degrees at all times, which means that the patient should be kept from sliding down in bed in order to benefit from this position. In patients with severe closed head injury ICP is increased and remains increased both during and 1 minute after activities such as head flexion, lateral head rotation to either side, and changing the head of bed either higher or lower than 30 degrees (Parsons, 1984). The patient's head therefore should remain elevated even during transport and when measuring pulmonary artery wedge and CVP pressures (adjustments in measurement must be considered).

Increases in intracranial pressure have also been seen in response to lateral and prone positioning (Mitchell et al, 1981; Snyder, 1983). A more recent study noted that with lateral positions and increases in

ICP, ICP returned to baseline 1 minute after the turn (Parsons, 1984). It is important for the nurse to recognize the problem in flexion and lateral rotation of the head in sidelying positions, as this can account for sustained increases in ICP. The prone position should be avoided in patients with increased ICP. This position appears to increase intrathoracic and intra-abdominal pressures, which increases blood pressure, decreasing venous outflow and increasing cerebral blood volume and ICP (Mitchell, 1980). Patients who are lucid should be encouraged to allow passive turning to avoid Valsalva maneuvers and to decrease isometric contractions which can increase ICP (Mitchell, 1980).

Practice Protective Nursing Care. The nurse should arrange care in ways least likely to increase ICP and should be alert for situations and other problems that may increase ICP. For example, Mitchell and associates (1981) found that ICP increased with cumulative activities but did not increase when those activities were spaced 1 hour apart. This is exactly the opposite of the usual way nurses try to organize care activities in clusters when working with a patient. The nurse should prioritize needed care activities and space them appropriately. Critical ICP patients may be better managed on a pressure-distributing device, avoiding turning altogether. If a patient receiving ICP monitoring is noted to have increased ICP while in a certain position, then during subsequent similar turns it may be prudent to consider eliminating that position if possible (Mitchell et al, 1981).

Other patient activities that have been noted in research studies to increase ICP, presumably by increasing the systemic blood pressure during the Valsalva maneuver, include hiccoughing, coughing, straining with constipation, reflex posturing, isometric contractions, and psychosocial stressors such as emotionally charged conversation about the condition and prognosis, and invasive or painful procedures (Mitchell, 1980; Mitchell et al, 1981; Bruya, 1981; Zegeer, 1982; Snyder, 1983). The nurse may want to instruct or coach the more responsive older patient in how to avoid Valsalva maneuvers, may instigate a bowel program to avoid constipation, may obtain medication orders if necessary to suppress coughing, and may institute measures to minimize emotional upset.

Several studies have noted reductions in ICP with the use of touch (Bruya, 1981; Walleck, 1980). The nurse may want to encourage frequent visits from the family and use touch in an effort to decrease ICP.

Administration of Medications. The nurse administering medications in the management of increased ICP will monitor for beneficial and deleterious effects. When using steroids the patient usually receives antacids every 2 hours to minimize the side effects that include stress ulcers and gastrointestinal bleeding. All stools should be tested for blood. If the patient receiving antacids is also taking an anticonvulsant drug, then the two medications should be given at different times as the antacid may decrease the absorption of the anticonvulsant.

The administration of mannitol, an osmotic diuretic, requires frequent monitoring of ICP and neurologic assessment, and assessment for symptoms of dehydration and hypovolemic shock secondary to the diuretic effect. Close monitoring of intake and output and serum osmolality is essential. The effects last only 3 to 8 hours, and it is important to remember that the drug may become less effective after 48 hours of use. Rebound effects with sharp increases in intracranial pressure can occur. Mannitol causes cerebral hyperemia and can actually increase intracranial pressure if used too early when a child has vasogenic rather than cerebral edema (Zeidelman, 1980).

Pavulon may be used to help decrease reflex posturing and responses to environmental stimuli, and also to enable controlled mechanical ventilation. Pavulon induces complete paralysis of voluntary muscles so the patient has no response to stimuli. Complete physical care is required. The patient needs to have a neurologic evaluation every hour, with the assessment consisting primarily of vital signs and pupil size and reactivity. The nurse should also provide meticulous skin care, frequent turning with passive range of motion, and application of artificial tears with the eyes taped shut in order to minimize potential complications or injuries. It is very important when Pavulon is used to provide psychologic support, as the patient is still able to hear and needs to be touched to promote comfort and reassurance (Zeidelman, 1980).

In some centers barbiturate therapy may be used to treat patients with intractable increased ICP. Its use is controversial in terms of overall effectiveness. Barbiturates are thought to decrease cerebral metabolism and to have some protective effect on the brain. They are usually given in hourly doses or by intravenous drip to maintain a consistent serum level. During this treatment complete physical care, as well as ventilatory support, is required.

As the patient responds to treatment or as ICP becomes stabilized and under control, or both, each treatment is withdrawn gradually one at a time. If no further problems develop ICP monitoring devices and lines can be removed.

Table 46-11 provides a nursing process plan for the child with increased intracranial pressure. Because increased intracranial pressure is common to so many neurologic problems, this nursing process plan is applicable for a number of the disorders discussed in this chapter.

Table 46-11
Nursing Process Plan: The Child with Increased Intracranial Pressure

by Roxie Foster

Assessment of Physiologic Function and Intellectual-Perceptual Function

Activity-Exercise
Nutrition-Metabolism
Pain
Sensory-Perceptual Alterations

Subjective Assessment

Level of consciousness/responsiveness, mood, level of comfort, level of energy, memory; ask about GI and visual disturbances

Objective Assessment

Fontanels, head circumference, height, weight, vital signs, vision, intracranial pressure, reports of skull roentgenograms, CT and NMR scans, cerebral blood flow studies, EEG, evoked potentials (as applicable)

Analysis: Nursing Diagnosis 1

Altered tissue perfusion: cerebral, related to increase in volume of one or more of the intracranial components:

- *brain tissue mass*
- *cerebral blood volume*
- *cerebrospinal fluid volume*

Defining Characteristics

Subjective: Headache, pain increased by coughing, sneezing, straining at stool; irritable; fatigued; memory loss; report of vomiting in absence of nausea, especially upon arising in morning; double vision

Objective: Fontanel full, tense, bulging above skull; elevated BP; decreased pulse, respirations; restricted visual fields; papilledema; failure to thrive; ICP >15 mm Hg; diagnostic reports consistent with pathology leading to increased ICP

Client Goal/ Evaluation Criteria	Nursing Goals/Strategies (Selected Rationale)
1.1 The client will regain adequate cerebral perfusion, as evidenced by: a. reduced headache, irritability, fatigue, vomiting, visual disturbances b. fontanel(s) soft, lightly pulsating, slightly depressed c. vital signs within normal limits; temperature <38.5°C (101.3°F) d. ICP <15 mm Hg e. mean arterial systemic pressure >70 mm Hg	*Monitor neurologic status closely.* • Perform neurologic check every 1 to 2 hours or as condition dictates; (level of consciousness/responsiveness, pupil size and reactivity, eye movements, motor function, respiratory patterns and vital signs, protective reflexes) • Palpate fontanel(s) with each neurologic check • If ICP monitor in place, watch effects of child's behaviors on ICP *Inform physician of indications of increasing ICP.* *Implement strategies to reduce or at least prevent further elevation of ICP.* • Elevate head of bed 30° and keep head/neck in straight alignment (to facilitate venous outflow from brain by gravity and through patent neck veins)

Continued

Table 46-11 (continued)

Client Goal/ Evaluation Criteria	Nursing Goals/Strategies (Selected Rationale)
f. cerebral perfusion pressure >50 mm Hg g. arterial blood gases within normal limits	• Maintain patent airway (to avoid hypercapnia, which dilates cerebral vessels) (1) Remind child to deep breathe and change position every 1 to 2 hours unless position change increases ICP. Prevent flexion and lateral rotation of head in side-lying position. Avoid prone position (which increases intrathoracic and intra-abdominal pressure) (2) Clear mucus from nasal passages and oropharynx as necessary. Hyperventilate with Ambu bag and 100% O_2 before suctioning; (suctioning decreases PaO_2) (3) Elevating head of bed will also facilitate lung inflation. Monitor air exchange through frequent chest auscultation • Maintain temperature <38.5°C (101.3°F) (1) Administer antipyretics to reduce fever (2) Use tepid sponge baths or cooling blanket as necessary, being careful not to reduce temperature faster than 1°C every 15 minutes • Administer diuretics as ordered (1) Measure and record intake and output and daily weight to help evaluate results (2) Notify physician of urine output <1 ml/kg/hr or >2 ml/kg/hr • Maintain fluid restriction as ordered (to decrease central, and therefore, cerebral blood volume). Maintain IV fluid rate with a mechanical pump and a small fluid chamber (to minimize the risk of accidental fluid overload) • Reduce crying and agitation (which increases ICP) (1) Administer analgesics (2) Enlist parent's help to provide nonpharmacologic comfort measures (3) Encourage presence of family member (4) Explain all procedures carefully (5) Encourage use of a security object • Explain to child (if lucid) how to cooperate with treatment by limiting coughing and straining activities (1) Teach child to exhale with movements (e.g., turning) to avoid Valsalva (2) Administer stool softeners to prevent constipation • Plan for uninterrupted periods of rest/sleep • Avoid too many nursing activities with child at one time • Prevent infection (fever leads to cerebral vasodilation) (1) Observe, and teach family, meticulous handwashing techniques (2) Observe sterile technique when indicated (3) Avoid contact with child when one is potentially infectious • Use an Ambu bag and 100% O_2 to reduce temporary elevations in ICP, e.g., after uncomfortable procedures. NOTE: Manual hyperventilation must be done under the supervision of an experienced nurse!

Table 46-11 (continued)

- Administer medications as ordered
  (1) Monitor for GI bleeding with steroids: Hematest stools and vomitus
  (2) Children on Pavulon or barbiturates need total patient care; see section in this chapter on care of the child with altered responsiveness
  (3) Remember that children on Pavulon have lost motor function, not sensory function. Provide relief from pain and attend to psychosocial comfort measures to help overcome their fear and frustration at the drug-induced paralysis

Craniotomy/Craniectomy

This section will describe general care for a child having brain surgery involving supratentorial craniotomy and infratentorial craniectomy (to review general information on basic pre- and postoperative care, see Chapter 27 and the Nursing Process Plan for perioperative care.

Craniotomy involves removing and replacing a part of the skull to allow access for surgery on the brain. *Craniectomy* refers to the removal of skull without replacement, which may be done in posterior fossa surgery in which the neck muscles provide protection for the brain. Sometimes a craniectomy is done to treat patients with increased intracranial pressure after head trauma; this is called a decompressive craniectomy. Craniectomy may be required after depressed skull fractures. If a large skull defect is left after surgery, a helmet should be obtained to protect the brain from external injuries. *Cranioplasty* refers to the repair of a cranial defect, or replacement of a bone flap, usually with a molded plastic material.

The procedures of craniotomy and craniectomy both require that the head be shaved. Usually this involves the entire head but in some cases may only be partial, as in infratentorial craniectomy, in which only the back of the head may be shaved. The shave and the skin prep are usually done after the child is anesthetized.

The head position is usually secured with clamps and pins, and various operative positions may be used, depending on the nature and location of the surgery. The scalp is incised, muscles are stripped, and usually 4 to 5 burr holes are drilled in the corner points of the skull. A saw or craniotome is used to cut across the bone and lift off the skull. After the skull is opened the meninges are excised. Hemostasis must be meticulously completed during cranial surgery because even small hematomas are not tolerated in the brain.

Following the surgical procedure all anatomic layers, starting with the meninges, are closed. During a craniotomy the skull is sutured back into place. Scalp layers are closed and a pressure dressing is applied for 2 to 3 days, along with a head dressing. A drain may be used for the first 24 hours. Following this brief period the dressings may be removed by the neurosurgeon.

Preoperative Care

In addition to providing the general preoperative care required before surgery, the nurse should include and be aware of some of the differences involved with neurosurgical procedures on the brain.

Preoperative anxiety and fear of mutilation can be related to shaving the hair and worry about visible scars. It needs to be understood that the reason for the shave is to decrease wound contamination and prevent infection. The patient and family need to understand that the hair will grow back, and to consider the use of a wig, scarf, or cap after the surgery. Some persons may fear visible scars, and they need to know that the incisions are usually made within the hairline on the scalp and are not visible on the face. Often the child and family understand the reasons and simply need support, reassurance, and time to express their feelings or to begin an anticipatory grief process.

Because potential complications, surgical outcomes, and the irreversible nature of neurosurgery can have a major impact on the quantity and/or quality of the child's life and because decisions must be made quickly, often during an acute crisis, parents expend considerable effort during the preoperative period or during an operative wait reviewing all the events and identifying questions. Again, sensitivity to these needs with an opportunity to ask questions and time to reinforce previously given information can be very helpful.

Care should also include information about the head shave, incision, head dressing, and whether or not the patient will be transferred to an ICU. Preoperative teaching may not include coughing; especially in cases with increased ICP, but generally includes deep breathing and turning. Knowledge of routine postoperative orders is useful, such as the frequent neurologic checks. The nurse should review the fact that postoperative cerebral edema with a worsening in the patient's condition, usually 24 to 96 hours after surgery, may occur (this can be frightening to the family if they are not prepared for it).

Accurate and well-documented preoperative neurologic assessment becomes essential when monitoring the child's postoperative functioning for potential complications. In addition to specifics on the preoperative neurologic check of responsiveness and consciousness, describe the location of any focal neurologic deficits such as decreased movement, sensation, and weakness, and describe any alterations in speech, vision, and hearing. It is helpful to share basic information about the child's normal developmental level of functioning and abilities, so that postoperative assessments can be meaningful.

Preoperative assessment for the child experiencing an infratentorial craniectomy should also include documentation of the function of cranial nerves VII, VIII, IX, X, XI, and XII, especially the quality of gag and swallow reflexes, and the rate, pattern, and quality of respirations (see Table 15-8).

If the patient has seizures preoperatively the events should be well described, and siderails of the cart may be padded to prevent injuries. If the patient is receiving anticonvulsant agents, these are usually given in spite of or rescheduled around the NPO orders, so that serum levels remain constant.

Postoperative Care

The nursing role after brain surgery involves frequent assessment to monitor the patient for any potential complications and interventions to prevent problems. This often includes neurologic and vital sign checks, assessment of airway and ventilation, monitoring blood gases, electrolytes, intake and output, dressing and drainage checks, and keeping the patient safely positioned with the head of the bed elevated 30 degrees.

Potential Structural Complications. Cerebral edema begins to peak 24 to 96 hours after surgery with a corresponding decrease in alertness and responsiveness. It is important during this time to recognize promptly and seek early treatment for increased ICP, hypoxia and hypercapnia, and hyperthermia; to maintain optimal head, neck, and body positions; to practice protective nursing care; to administer medications as ordered; and to explain what may be happening to the family. The highest incidence of intracranial bleeding occurs in the first 24 hours after surgery. This is usually characterized by (rapid) neurologic deterioration with symptoms dependent on the location of the bleed and the age of the child. The complication of acute hydrocephalus may occur after surgery but may also be present preoperatively. Signs and symptoms are similar to increased ICP. Paralysis of upward gaze may occur after posterior fossa or infratentorial surgery if expanding masses exert pressure on the pretectal area and on the sylvian aqueduct. Cerebral vascular accidents occur less commonly in children than in adults as a postoperative complication.

Be vigilant for subtle concerns raised by the parents, as these could be indicators of early neurologic change. Upon early recognition of signs and symptoms, provide clear documentation and present facts to the physician in a clear and logical way.

Potential Metabolic Complications. Potential metabolic complications involve wound infections, hypoxia, fluid and electrolyte disturbances, hypotension, and seizures. *Wound infections* increase metabolic demands, increase oxygen requirements, lengthen hospitalization, and increase the risk for osteomyelitis and further complications. The incidence of wound infection after craniotomy is 1.7 to 7.3 per cent, with wound contamination the most important risk factor (Vlahov, 1984). Temperature elevations in the first 24 to 48 hours usually are related to hypoventilation atelectasis. Incisional redness and drainage with temperature elevations several days after surgery may indicate wound infection. It is important to remember that surgery near the third ventricle and hypothalamus may also disturb temperature regulation. Temperature elevations may also result from drug reactions and from aseptic meningitis following subarachnoid hemorrhage and infratentorial surgery. Focal infections from intravenous sites, central venous pressure and arterial lines, urinary catheters, and ventriculostomies may also occur.

Drainage from the nose or ears after surgery and also after traumatic injury to the head is always treated as a suspected CSF leak until it is otherwise identified. Cerebral spinal fluid can leak into the ears or nose if there is a tear in the dura close to these structures. Suspected drainage should be collected in a sterile test tube for lab evaluation. The patient should be discouraged or instructed not to touch the drainage. Drainage from the nose should not be picked at or blown; likewise, a draining ear should not be picked at. These areas should not be packed, suctioned, or disturbed until the drainage has been identified in order to minimize sources of infection. The patient should be encouraged to remain quiet.

Nursing care oriented toward reducing the risk of infection includes

- handwashing before and after contact with the child
- using aseptic technique for procedures
- inspecting dressings and incision
- cleaning and trimming patient fingernails
- administering antibiotics as ordered
- monitoring WBC and culture reports
- culturing any questionable sites
- maintaining the integrity of tubings, drainage systems, and lines

Avoid the use of any creams, lotions, or powders near the incision, and check with the neurosurgeon regarding when the patient's hair may be washed.

Hypoxia after cranial surgery is the most common cause of altered level of consciousness. Hypoxia can also be caused by an altered level of consciousness, or by the effects of anesthesia. Nursing care to detect and prevent hypoxia includes observation of face color and peripheral filling in nailbeds, assessing adequacy of the airway, noting any change in secretions, and assessing respiratory rate, rhythm, and quality. Assess breath sounds more frequently for a child with altered levels of consciousness or when cough and gag reflexes are decreased or absent; suction as needed. Place a humidifier at the bedside and perform chest physiotherapy to loosen secretions, turning and positioning every 2 hours. Monitor arterial blood gases.

Fluid and electrolyte disturbances after surgery can include hypoglycemia and endocrine disturbances. The patient is at increased risk for these problems after subarachnoid hemorrhage, head trauma, or surgery near the pituitary and hypothalamus; during periods of fluid restrictions; and whenever osmotic diuretics are used. The nursing care required to detect or prevent these disturbances includes monitoring serum osmolality, electrolytes, hematocrit, urine output compared with fluid intake, urine specific gravity, assessment of skin and mucous membranes, and administering medications and parenteral fluids as ordered (Box 46-4).

Hypotension due to cardiovascular instability can occur, secondary to elevating the head of the bed or to hypovolemia. Nursing care includes monitoring blood pressure and apical pulse to maintain adequate systolic pressures to ensure sufficient cerebral blood flow. Also assess urinary output and hematocrit, and administer vasopressors as ordered.

Seizures may be a complication in the postoperative period. Seizure activity increases metabolic demands, increases systolic blood pressure, increases cerebral blood flow, and depletes energy stores. At increased risk for postoperative seizures are patients

Box 46-4
Risk Factors and Causes in the Development of Postoperative Metabolic Complications

INFECTIONS

Wound contamination
Atelectasis
Drug reactions
Aseptic meningitis
Localized infections
Immunosuppression

HYPOXIA

Anesthetic agents
Cerebral edema
Acid-base imbalances
Pulmonary embolism
Anemia
Disseminated intravascular coagulation
Fat embolism
Air embolism

WATER AND ELECTROLYTE DISTURBANCES

Hypo-osmolar states
- Syndrome of inappropriate antidiuretic hormone (SIADH)
- Excess free water loads (i.e., DSW)

Hyperosmolar states
- Excess fluid loss
- Diabetes insipidus
- Hyperglycemia
- High-protein tube feedings with insufficient water
- Hyperalimentation
- Osmotic diuretics

Hypercalcemia
Hypoglycemia

ENDOCRINE DISTURBANCES

SIADH
- Post-traumatic head injury
- Post-op pituitary/hypothalamic surgery
- Pituitary/hypothalamic lesions

Diabetes insipidus
- Post-op pituitary/hypothalamic surgery

Adrenal failure or insufficiency
- Abrupt discontinuation of steroids

SEIZURES

Pre-existing seizure history
Post-op cortical resection
Cerebral abscess
Meningiomas
AV malformations
Hypoxia
Hypoglycemia
Hyponatremia
Hypoosmolarity

(Adapted from Arsenault, 1985.)

who have resections of the cortex, surgery near the sensorimotor strip, cerebral abscess, meningiomas, and arteriovenous malformations. Seizures can also be precipitated by metabolic factors such as hypoxia, hypoglycemia, hyponatremia, and hypoosmolarity (Arsenault, 1985). The incidence rate in a study by Matthews (1980) noted that if there was no preceding history of seizures there is a 12 per cent incidence of seizures in the first postoperative week, with only 3 per cent of those recurring. If there was a preoperative history of seizures there is a 35 per cent incidence in the first week, with 20 per cent recurring.

Nursing care related to seizures includes assigning the child to a room closer to the nursing station for observation, frequent observations to detect any seizure activity, asking family members about any unusual activities, thorough documentation of any observed seizures, padded siderails if seizures have occurred or there is a history of seizures, and administering antiepileptic drugs as ordered. After the initial seizure the patient may receive a loading dose of the antiepileptic drug with the expected consequence of sedation. Following this a regular maintenance dose is given and adjusted for seizure control, side effects, and serum drug levels.

Other Postoperative Problems. Headaches postoperatively need to be carefully investigated. Headaches that coincide with stiff neck, fever, irritability, photophobia, and other symptoms of complications need to be brought to the attention of the physician immediately. Comfort measures are important, such as subdued lighting, soft music, touch, relaxing massage, and quiet play activities such as reading or telling stories. Analgesics can be given as ordered, with the effects or results documented. Narcotics are usually avoided because of their depressant effect on level of consciousness and respirations.

Infratentorial Cranial Surgery

This type of cranial surgery below the tentorium or in the posterior fossa may be done for patients with posterior fossa tumors such as cerebellar astrocytomas (see Chapter 48). Rhodes and Grosser (1983) state that because of the position of anatomic structures and location of vital centers, manipulation of the brainstem and cerebellum during posterior fossa surgery may predispose the patient to a greater degree of danger than surgery in the cerebral hemispheres.

After infratentorial or posterior fossa craniectomy patients may experience muscle soreness in their shoulders and neck secondary to the effects of surgical positioning and the surgical incision. Mild massage and administering analgesics as ordered can assist in reducing pain. The patient usually has temporal pin sites that need observation in the immediate postoperative period for signs and symptoms of infection. The temporal pins are used in the operating room for positioning and stabilization of the head. Sometimes nausea and vomiting after surgery can occur with sudden turning and movement. If this occurs space apart activities of turning and feeding to minimize nausea and vomiting.

Nursing Strategies

Nursing care after surgery involves careful patient monitoring for the following potential problems:

Potential for Altered Levels of Responsiveness Related to Cerebellar Herniation as Manifested by Increased Intracranial Pressure. The monitoring of neurologic and vital signs, especially respiratory patterns, for any deteriorating changes is crucial. It should also be noted that respiratory arrest without warning of impending cerebellar herniation is also possible. Sidelying positions of the patient after surgery are preferred to supine to avoid exerting pressure on the surgical site. Pillows are also usually avoided, unless needed in a sidelying position to avoid lateral rotation and flexion of the head. Any hiccoughing should be reported to the physician, as this symptom may be related to irritation of the medulla.

Potential for Injury Related to Cranial Nerve Dysfunction. Here again a solid knowledge of cranial nerve function and location, together with knowledge of the location and nature of the surgery in the posterior fossa, greatly assist the nurse to anticipate potential problems that the patient may have. Most posterior fossa surgery can involve cranial nerves IX, X, XI, and XII. Infratentorial surgery in the cerebellopontine angle may also involve cranial nerves VII and VIII. Gag and swallow reflexes in the immediate postoperative period should be completely assessed before any drinking or eating occurs. Suction equipment should be available at all times. If the child's gag and swallow abilities are absent, suctioning and mouth care may be needed frequently, and nourishment and fluids via a nasogastric tube may be considered. If problems of dysphagia are mild, consults to dietary and speech therapy may assist in development of a feeding plan. This may include feeding the child in an upright position, using thickened liquids and foods that are easy to swallow, using cold and warm foods, and always staying at the child's side during mealtime and drinks in case choking occurs.

Other symptoms of dysfunction may include nasal speech, hoarseness or other change in voice characteristics, increased salivation, tachycardia, regurgitation, vomiting, coughing, dysarthria, loss of ability to shrug shoulders, loss of blink, and reduced hearing. These problems should be brought to the physician's attention immediately. Children experiencing dysarthria need to have an alternative means of communication, such as pointing, picture or alphabet board, or writing. Patients who have absent blink responses must have immediate care with artificial tears and taping of the eyelids. Corneal abrasion and damage can occur within 4 to 6 hours in a patient whose eyelids remain partially or fully opened (Arsenault, 1985).

Potential for Altered Mobility Related to Cerebellar Dysfunction as Manifested by Ataxia. Patients who experience ataxia need reminding to slow down their movements, get up slowly, and ambulate with assistance. Sitting balance may improve if they can have their feet on a stool or step to increase sensory input to the posterior columns to assist in orientation in space. Occupational and physical therapy may be consulted.

Seizure Observation/First Aid

Seizures may occur for many reasons and are not necessarily related to epilepsy. (Epilepsy is discussed later in this chapter.) This section will discuss the care of a child experiencing a seizure, regardless of circumstance, cause, and seizure type. This will include definition, incidence, seizure recognition, appropriate first aid, observational interactions, seizure documentation, and status epilepticus. More detailed information regarding etiology, seizure classification, treatment, and management of seizure disorders/epilepsy and febrile seizures can be found later in this chapter.

A seizure can be defined as a paroxysmal, uncontrolled episode of behavior that results from an abnormal electrical discharge from the brain. This may affect the person in any one or a combination of the following: (1) altered responsiveness, (2) altered sensation or perception or both, and (3) altered movements, mobility, or tone. What happens to the person during the seizure depends on the characteristic of the abnormal electrical discharge and what part of the brain is involved. Children may have a single seizure perhaps related to a febrile illness or an electrolyte imbalance. Some children may continue to have repeated seizures for an unidentifiable reason and some because of acquired cause.

According to the DHEW 75 per cent of seizures will occur before the age of 18 years (Commission for the Control of Epilepsy and Its Consequences, 1977). About 5 per cent of children experience one or more seizures before they reach adulthood (Huttenlocher, 1987).

Other paroxysmal events that occur in childhood can be mistaken for seizure activity. The nature of these can range from rather benign events to those of a life-threatening nature. The nurse should also be familiar with these in order to evaluate health history information, and to aid in observation and assessment to help the patient obtain the most appropriate treatment. Box 46-5 provides an overview of paroxysmal events that can be mistaken for seizure activity (Dreifuss, 1983; Ferry, 1986). There are no incidence statistics for these various paroxysmal events. Because seizures and paroxysmal events can occur frequently in childhood, the pediatric nurse should maintain skills in observational assessment and first aid.

Box 46-5
Paroxysmal Events that may be Misinterpreted as Seizure

- Nonepileptic episodes
- Breath-holding spells
- Hyperventilation
- Benign syncopal attacks
  - Vagal hypersensitivity reactions
  - Postural hypotension
- Cardiogenic syncope
  - Aortic stenosis
  - Mitral valve prolapse
  - Sick sinus syndrome
  - Prolonged QT interval
- Migraine
  - Basilar artery
  - Hemiplegic
- Hypoglycemic attacks
- Sleep disorders
  - Night terrors
  - Nocturnal myoclonus
  - Somnambulism
- Motor spells
  - Benign infantile myoclonus
  - Acute dystonic reactions
  - Tourette syndrome
  - Choreiform movements
  - Shuddering attacks
- Periodic syndromes of childhood
  - Benign paroxysmal vertigo
  - Cyclic vomiting
- Gastrointestinal attacks
  - Gastroesophogeal reflux
  - Intestinal obstruction
  - Hiatal hernia
- Masturbation

(Adapted from Dreifuss, 1983; Ferry, 1986.)

Seizure Recognition

One of the difficulties with first aid and seizure observation is the prompt recognition that a seizure is occurring. This is more of a problem when there is no preexisting history of seizures and when the nurses are relatively inexperienced observers of seizures. Seizures are paroxysmal events and for the most part occur without warning. For example, the nurse may enter the child's room to find the patient staring and unresponsive, yet sitting in the bed holding a puzzle piece. Thinking that the child is simply day-dreaming, the nurse may continue and check the IV. It may not be until the nurse is almost ready to leave that he or she may be concerned about the child's lack of responsiveness. The nurse may question the event as a possible seizure, but repeated observations may be needed.

In another example, the nurse may hear a crash coming from the playroom and enter to find the child lying on the floor in a rigid posture. This time, event recognition may be immediate and allow for prompt first aid and observation of the event. Sometimes the nurse may be interacting with the child when the event occurs, allowing for assessment at the onset.

First Aid

Seizure activity often involves the diagnosis of potential for injury, physical and psychosocial. The potential for injury can be minimized with first aid measures. Basic first aid can be divided into four parts, regardless of the seizure type:

1. Remain calm and stay with the child so first aid and observations can be done.
2. Protect the child from additional injury as necessary.
3. Provide time to recover and reorient if necessary.
4. Reassure and provide psychosocial support to the child and others to minimize negative stigma.

Protecting the child from injury during an event depends on the seizure events. Individuals experiencing only altered responsiveness may not require any particular first aid other than standing by to see that they do not fall or lose their balance. Speak softly, if at all, to the child with altered responsiveness. Shouting and shaking serve no purpose, as it is the seizure activity that is causing the altered responsiveness not an attentional or hearing problem. If speaking appears to agitate or confuse the child, it may be better to remain silent.

If the patient is having altered sensations or perceptions, these should be acknowledged and the child reassured that everything is okay and that it will be over soon. It is not helpful to ignore, refute, or worry considerably with the child about these phenomena.

If altered tone, movements, or mobility occurs, it is important not to restrain or restrict the patient's movements but to move any harmful objects out of the way. If the child is walking, allow this and observe. If headed for a dangerous situation (e.g., open stairs) attempt to steer the child in a new direction, while realizing that this may be resisted or increase agitation. Avoid the use of force. If the person is having altered tone and movements in a standing position it may be prudent to assist or move the child to a lying position on the floor and when the event is finished to turn him or her in a semiprone or sidelying position with head turned toward the floor. This will avoid choking and aspiration on saliva that has pooled in the mouth during the seizure.

If the child is lying on the floor it may be helpful to place a soft material under the head for protection from injury. Any restrictive clothing around the neck should be loosened. If the child is in a sitting position when the event occurs use good judgment in deciding whether the child is safe in that position or whether he or she needs to be moved to the floor. No objects should be inserted into the mouth, nor should anything be given to eat or drink until the individual has clearly recovered from the event.

Patients experiencing combinations of altered responsiveness, perceptions, sensations, and movements will need various combinations of first aid in order to prevent additional injury.

Children need to have someone with them until they have recovered from the event if this is a first-time occurrence, in order to continue observation and any necessary first aid. The need and frequency for direct supervision of patients having recurring events will depend on the situation. Children will vary in how they will respond after an event. The recovery time after a seizure can also be extremely variable.

Reassurance and psychosocial support during and after a seizure or event are quite important both for the child and for others who may have also observed the event. After recovery, it is important that the child be reassured, "You just had a seizure and it's over now; everything is okay." Let the child's questions determine whether more information is needed. Children who have missed information because of altered responsiveness during a seizure may need to have instructions repeated when they have recovered from the seizure.

Seizure activity is unexpected, and often startles and may frighten other people. Simple statements such as "It's okay, he's having a seizure; it will be over soon" can be tremendously reassuring if delivered in a calm, confident manner. Young children may think that the child is dying, having a tantrum, choking,or misbehaving. Surprisingly, adults often consider the same possibilities. Again, simple explanations are helpful. Let adults standing by know if there is anything that you need their help with. Generally, children and adults will take their cues from the nurse. A calm and accepting manner will reduce negative stigma toward the child. Parents need instruction on seizure recognition and the appropriate physical and psychosocial first aid measures.

It is rarely necessary to call for emergency help during a seizure as the event is self-limited and does not injure the person. The following situations indicate times when emergency help should be contacted: (1) the person does not start breathing after the seizure and mouth-to-mouth resuscitation is initiated; (2) the seizure activity does not subside and has continued for 5 minutes; (3) the person has one seizure after another without a return of consciousness in between; or (4) the person has sustained serious injuries. If this is the patient's first seizure the physician should be contacted. Diagnostic tests may be indicated and treatment may be considered.

When seizures recur other safety measures may be needed to prevent possible injury. Box 46-6 is a list of safety measures that may be considered for home, hospital, or school. In developing any plan with the child and family, the nurse considers the child's situation and the possible risks and benefits associated with activities.

Seizure Observation

One purpose of observation is to provide an accurate account of what happened. This assists the physician in accurate diagnosis, seizure classification, and antiepileptic drug selection. Another purpose is to monitor the clinical efficacy of antiepileptic drug treatment. Many persons approach seizure observation as a rather passive process, not understanding the value and importance of their observations. Good seizure observation is an interactional process. Wulf (1986) noted that among nursing staff observing five different seizures, the most frequent observations were focused on the location and description of movement and how long the event lasted. Observational responses were less frequent for altered responsiveness, sensations, and perception. Box 46-7 is a list that can be used to enhance and expand observation and documentation repertoire.

Response to Stimuli. When assessing responsiveness the nurse should attempt an interaction using various stimuli and describe the child's response rather than to describe the child as being conscious, having impaired consciousness, or being unconscious. On appearance alone children may appear to be unresponsive but in another domain they may be able to respond. For example, one nurse recounted that a child was having jerking movements that were rather asymmetric involving the right arm and leg to a greater degree than the left arm and leg. The child made no eye contact and did not appear aware of the nurse. When the nurse asked the child to touch her finger, the child was able to do so with the left hand but not with the right. Without this interaction the nurse may have mistakenly described the patient to be unconscious during the seizure. This child was able to perceive auditory stimuli appropriately and had motor control of the left hand.

Movements and Tone. When assessing movements and tone it is important to identify if one extremity or one or both sides of the body are affected. Children with altered tone can be assessed using motor commands and a gentle attempt to take all extremities through their range of motion in order to compare their tone.

Repetitive Movements. When assessing repetitive movements it is important to determine whether they are interruptable, and goal directed and purposeful. Generally, the repetitive movements or automatisms of seizure activity are (1) not interruptable and only subside when the seizure ends, and (2) are not goal directed or purposeful. In some children it may prove difficult to distinguish self-stimulating behaviors from seizure automatisms. Circumstances, duration of the event, and whether or not the event is interruptable may prove helpful.

For example, consider a child who had cognitive deficits, self-stimulating behaviors, and seizures consisting of altered responsiveness and automatisms. This girl was observed making repetitive movements

Box 46-6
*Safety Measures to Consider for Recurring Seizures**

Seizure Related Falls and Injuries
- Helmets—extra protection where likely to strike head, consider least restrictive helmet possible
- Stairs with supervision, instruct to use rail, consider elevator
- Chairs with arms to prevent falls off chair
- Safe environment, carpeting, protected stairs, remove breakable glass

Water safety
- Bathing with supervision (showers preferable, tub in few inches of water, consider foam protectors for fixtures, for teens bathe when someone aware in house, keep bathroom doors unlocked)
- Swimming with direct supervision (pool safer than lake)

Sleeping safety
- Consider room changes rather than sleeping with parents or parent sleeping with child
- Siderails, or place mattress on floor, remove nearby furniture
- Avoid use of pillows and numerous stuffed animals
- Protect open stairways

*Needs will vary depending on seizure type(s).

Box 46-7
Considerations for Seizure Observations/Documentations

A. Describe the Beginning
1. What were the circumstances?
2. Were there any precipitating factors?
3. Was the seizure onset observed?
4. Did the child state or give any indication that the seizure was beginning? (An aura is the beginning of the seizure: expressed before altered responsiveness occurs.)
5. Did they attempt to continue, stop or slow down in their activities?
6. What happened first? Then describe in order, how the rest occurred.

B. Assessing Responsiveness
1. Description of patient's observed response to you, self, environment.
2. Describe whether responses were rote or more complex, and how much they were affected (partially,totally, etc.).
3. Assess response to tactile stimuli (blow on face, light touch, tickle, a mild shake of an extremity, ice, attempt to open eyes or move extremities).
4. Assess response to auditory stimuli (clap hands, call name, give a command, state a word, and ask for recall later).
5. Assess response to visual stimuli (check pupil reactions, note visual flinch, throw an object to them unexpectedly).

C. Assessing Movements, Mobility, or Tone
1. Was there any movement or change in posture? Give location and description, be as specific as possible. Consider a head to toe approach.
2. Did this affect one or both sides of body? If both sides involved, did they look the same or different?
3. Assess whether tone is increased (tonic, spastic, rigid), decreased (flaccid, limp), or normal.
4. Were there any automatisms (repetitive, purposeless movements)? Were there any purposeful movements?

D. Assessing Sensation and Perception
1. What does the child describe or state? Ask them during or after seizure for as detailed description/location possible.
2. Are there any autonomic signs and symptoms (e.g., skin temperature change, change in color, sweating)?
3. Did they say or do anything strange (mumbling, speaking inappropriately, cursing, wandering, climbing up or under objects, fumbling, resisting or combating touch, agitation, and so on)?

E. Assessing Postictal Responses
1. What were they like after the seizure? Describe their behavior.
2. How long did it take before resumption of previous activities?
3. Could they recall the event in general or remember what happened at the beginning or throughout the seizure?
4. Were there any temporary deficits (memory loss, aphasia, paresis)?
5. Was there any confusion or disorientation? Describe and give duration.

By Judy Wulf

of tipping her head backward, with shaking and rocking of the trunk forward and backward when in a sitting position. This occurred during quiet times with a duration of 5 to 15 minutes when uninterrupted. The movements could be interrupted, however, by introducing a novel stimulus such as a hand clap or assisting the child to a standing position. Contrast that with her movements consisting of head and trunk tipped forward with repetitive blowing movements of the mouth and picking movements of the hands, duration 45 seconds. Attempts to interrupt these activities generally produced some motor resistance but did not abolish the movements. The first example of repetitive movements represents self-stimulating behaviors; the second example seizure activity.

Altered Sensation or Perception. When assessing the child for altered sensation or perception the nurse needs to attend to the child's statements and evaluate the appropriateness of the responses to various stimuli. Patient statements preceding observable activity may actually be the beginning of the seizure. Verbal children may state they feel sick, are going to have a seizure, or feel scared. Sometimes the sensations are specific, such as a tingling in a part of the body; at other times they are more vague. Young children may go to an adult before observable activity begins. Continued observation may provide subtle evidence that the seizure may begin with a sensation that the child cannot express, other than to seek out another person. Perceptions may be altered during seizure activity, accounting for peculiar statements or inappropriate motor and verbal responses.

Identifying the End of the Seizure. Another area of difficulty in seizure observation can be identifying when the seizure ends. Although most are easy to determine by the cessation of altered movements, mobility, and tone, or by an immediate resumption of previous activities, others are less distinct. Sometimes the end of the seizure may be evident by a return of facial expression or a cessation of previous behaviors.

Here again, evaluating the child's responses to stimuli, commands, and orientation can be useful.

Postictal Responses. A variety of postictal (after the seizure) responses are possible. Some children are fully oriented and can immediately resume activities right where they left off. Others may seem confused, disoriented, dazed, and so on, and require some quiet time and reorientation during their recovery. Some may begin sleeping, with varying levels of arousability. Moods may vary depending on the event, the child, and how surrounding adults are behaving. This can range from laughing and silliness to crying, fearfulness, and acting-out behaviors. Some children may have difficulty speaking and organizing thoughts, and may even experience a temporary motor paresis in part of the body (Todd's paresis).

Frequent and Subtle Seizures. The last problem encountered in seizure observation is how to observe the child who has extremely frequent and brief or subtle seizures. Often observations made jointly with the parent or other provider who is familiar with the child are helpful when learning to identify the seizures. Parents who are spending more time with the child may also provide additional feedback about the child's seizure frequency.

Observing seizure frequency is a difficult task, as the frequency may be inconsistent and variable throughout the day and from one day to the next. Seizure observation may become an index of how much time was spent observing the child. For example, one day shift the child may be noted to have 60 seizures during several intervals of direct observation, totaling 90 minutes. The next day during the same shift, the child may be noted to have 10 seizures, but this time only two intervals, totaling 30 minutes of direct observation, were used. What conclusion can be drawn from this? Had the child's seizure frequency improved, worsened, or remained the same? In this case because sampling periods with direct observation were different, it would be difficult to know. Children experiencing numerous seizures each day may be better observed by using a consistent number of random sampling intervals each day.

Seizure Documentation

Documentation of these events should include a description of the circumstances, any precipitating factors, a chronologic account of what happened, and a description of the patient's postictal responses. Circumstances include the date, time of day, and a description of what the child was doing (e.g., sleep, wake from sleep, wakeful time, before meal, physical activity, change in body position, unusual positions or postures, Valsalva maneuvers with elimination, time of discipline, and extreme fear or fright). Sometimes the circumstances and precipitating factors assist the physician in determining whether or not a seizure occurred.

Precipitating factors may be those events or circumstances that consistently increase the likelihood that a seizure may occur. It is important to understand that precipitating factors are not the cause of the seizure. Precipitating factors may include irregular use of medicines and drug interactions, fever, illness, fatigue, stress, hyperventilation, repetitive flashing light, excessive fluid intake, and certain times of the menstrual cycle. It is important to ask parents about this, as they may have identified other precipitating factors for their child. Some precipitating factors may allow for management strategies.

It is important to distinguish whether or not the onset was observed in the written description. If it was observed this should be described in detail; if not, then the description should state that onset was not observed. The details surrounding the onset may be very important in seizure classification as to type. If it is difficult to remember what happened after the event was over, memory aids, such as the guide listed in Box 46-7, may be of some help.

When patients have recurring seizures, it is helpful to have the patient or parent record seizure frequency data and descriptions of seizure activity and postictal responses in a diary or calendar, to assist in the continued evaluation and treatment with the health care provider. Parents need to report change in the frequency, severity, type, and characteristic of seizures.

Status Epilepticus

Status epilepticus can be defined in two ways: (1) continuous seizure activity which does not stop, and (2) seizures that occur in succession without a return of consciousness between them. The length of time required before a seizure is considered status epilepticus varies in the literature between 5 and 30 minutes (Browne, 1983; Pellock and Myer, 1983). In this discussion, status epilepticus is considered to be *an unremitting seizure lasting longer than 5 minutes, or two or more seizures occurring without regaining consciousness between them.* Either of these two situations should alert nurses, family, and lay persons to seek emergency care.

Incidence statistics on status epilepticus indicate that 20 per cent of patients have this as their initial seizure presentation (Gumnit, 1983). In this group an idiopathic cause is uncommon, so this usually warrants a full diagnostic work-up. The incidence of status epilepticus among those with epilepsy is 1.3 to 6.6 per cent, with the cause most likely related to antiepileptic drug withdrawal and poor drug adherence (Pellock and Myer, 1983).

Box 46-8
Physiologic Changes Secondary to Status Epilepticus

- Hypertension initially (later hypotension)
- Elevated venous pressure
- Hypoxia
- Hypercapnia
- Increased cerebral blood flow (later decreased cerebral blood flow)
- Hyperglycemia initially (later hypoglycemia)
- Hyperkalemia
- Lactic acidosis
- Increased metabolic rate
- Hyperpyrexia later

(From Pellock and Myer, 1983, page 191.)

Status epilepticus is considered a medical emergency. There are many types of status epilepticus depending on the seizure type. Generalized tonic and/or clonic status epilepticus is life threatening; other types such as absence or complex partial status epilepticus also require treatment but are not immediately life threatening. The overall mortality rate of status epilepticus is 10 to 15 per cent (Pellock and Myer, 1983). Left untreated, many persons will die. The prognosis of status epilepticus will vary, depending on the cause of the disorder and the patient's response to treatment. Structural alterations are thought to occur when seizure activity lasts longer than 30 minutes (Pellock and Myer, 1983). Among persons having seizures lasting longer than 60 minutes, 67 per cent will have sequelae consisting of epilepsy, mental retardation, and other neurologic deficits (Pellock and Myer, 1983). Patients with status epilepticus secondary to severe hypoxic brain insults usually have poor responses to treatment (Gumnit, 1983).

Pathophysiology

The pathophysiology of status epilepticus is unclear. Pellock and Myer (1983) summarize that neuronal metabolism is unable to keep up with the continual demand, which causes cerebral hypoxia and acidosis leading to cellular damage. In Box 46-8 the physiologic changes that are seen in status epilepticus are noted. The causes can range from acute central nervous system disorders to idiopathic or unknown factors. Acute CNS disorders may include hypoxia, infections, head injury, subarachnoid hemorrhage, subdural hematoma, metabolic encephalopathy, toxin exposures, tumors, degenerative disease, and cerebrovascular accidents. Again, the most frequent cause of status epilepticus for a patient with a history of epilepsy or seizure disorder is acute antiepileptic drug withdrawal. Status epilepticus may be idiopathic, or may result from an acute illness in which fever or medications may have reduced the blood levels of antiepileptic drugs.

Therapeutic Management

The child experiencing status epilepticus is usually brought to emergency care, and may be admitted to the hospital for treatment, monitoring, and stabilization. The management of the disorder involves basic life support, controlling seizure activity, and the diagnosis and treatment of any underlying cause.

Almost simultaneously in an emergency setting, an airway is secured, cardiac status is evaluated, vital signs are measured, an intravenous line is established, blood is drawn, antiepileptic drugs are given, and diagnostic tests are completed. Blood is usually drawn for a Dextrostix test, CBC, SMA12, and antiepileptic drug levels (if appropriate). If blood glucose is low or a Dextrostix test is not available a 1 ml/kg bolus of 50 per cent glucose is usually administered intravenously (Ferry et al, 1986).

The treatment of status epilepticus is usually completed simultaneously with an investigation for the cause. The goal of treatment is to terminate seizure activity rapidly with the least depression of consciousness and cardiopulmonary function. This is accomplished with the intravenous or rectal administration of antiepileptic drugs—primarily diazepam, phenytoin, phenobarbital, lorazepam, and paraldehyde. In the acute state of treatment there is a variety of antiepileptic drugs to choose from. When status epilepticus is caused by acute drug withdrawal the treatment of choice is to reinstitute that drug; however, this is not always feasible when, for instance, the particular drug formulation is not available or when drug withdrawal has been ordered in a hospital setting.

Ferry and co-workers (1986) state that the single most common mistake in treating status epilepticus is the failure to give a sufficient amount of the drug *early*. Typically, intravenous diazepam is the initial drug given, followed by phenytoin. If seizures persist, an infusion of phenobarbital may be started. If there is still no response, an infusion of paraldehyde may be used (Rowe, 1987). After early aggressive treatment has brought status epilepticus under control, maintenance therapy is initiated. Further information on maintenance antiepileptic drug therapy can be found in the section on epilepsy. If seizure activity does not respond to initial treatment efforts, the diagnosis may need re-evaluation as the cause may be as life threatening as the seizure (Gumnit, 1983). If status epilepticus persists beyond 6 hours the use of a barbiturate-induced coma may be recommended (Gumnit, 1983).

Strategies for Nursing Care

Nursing care of the patient experiencing status epilepticus includes seizure first aid and seizure observation and documentation as explained previously. The focus is on prompt recognition of status epilepticus with immediate contact of the physician. The nurse has interdependent functions with the physician in basic life support: maintaining adequate cardiopulmonary function, controlling seizure activity; administering medications and monitoring the patient's response to the treatment, and assisting with diagnostic tests and treatment; participating in the physical and psychologic preparations; as well as post-test monitoring for any complications. Other nursing strategies in the care of a patient experiencing status epilepticus address the nursing diagnoses: *potential for injury, self-care deficit, knowledge deficit,* and *fear.*

Reducing the Potential for Injury. This may include seizure-related falls and injuries, aspiration pneumonia, hyperthermia, and drug side effects. Patients with seizure-related falls and injuries may have fractures, dislocations, lacerations, and hematomas. Children may have seizure-related injuries at the onset or be at risk for injuries secondary to continued seizure activity. Nursing care includes continuous observation, using siderails with adequate protective padding, applying soft waist restraints, and avoiding the use of extremity restraints that may restrict movement. Remember to scan visually and remove from the bedside and surrounding area harmful objects that children with altered responsiveness could harm themselves with. Health care providers should never force open a clenched jaw to insert an endotracheal tube; injuries may occur.

Aspiration pneumonia can occur during status epilepticus secondary to choking on something in the mouth or vomiting stomach contents. Nursing care may include suctioning as needed, adequate positioning in a semiprone or sidelying position, monitoring vital signs and lung sounds, and maintaining NPO status until the patient has recovered from status epilepticus and from acute side effects of antiepileptic drugs, and has adequate gag and swallow reflexes.

Hyperthermia may occur as a symptom of an underlying cause of status epilepticus such as CNS infection, or it may occur as a result of continued seizure activity—especially those involving motor symptomatology. Nursing care may include keeping the patient in minimal light clothing, giving tepid sponge baths, monitoring temperature, and using cooling devices. Antipyretics may be withheld in order to monitor the natural course of temperature.

Common dose-related side effects of the antiepileptic drugs used in the treatment of status epilepticus involve altered level of responsiveness, ineffective breathing patterns, and ineffective airway clearance. Less common but more serious reactions may include allergic and other idiosyncratic responses. The nurse may administer or assist in administering the medications, monitor the child's response to these medications, and provide early identification and treatment of side effects. Nursing care involves monitoring serum levels; seizure activity; laboratory tests of CBC, liver, and kidney function; inspecting skin; monitoring vital signs and lung sounds; assessing the adequacy of breathing patterns and airway clearance. The use of the supine position with the head flexed with pillows should be avoided to minimize aspiration and airway problems.

Self-Care Deficit. The level of self-care deficit depends on the type of status epilepticus and how consciousness and responsiveness are affected. For example, status epilepticus of the generalized tonic-clonic or absence seizures type will involve total self-care deficits, and status epilepticus of the partial seizures type may vary from partial to total self-care deficits depending on how consciousness and responsiveness are affected. Nursing care may include provision of adequate fluids and nutrition (i.e., NPO status, intravenous fluids, and NG feeds until the patient recovers, then progressing to oral food and fluids as tolerated). The patient may also require attention for skin care, turning and positioning, hygiene related to urine and bowel incontinence, eye care if lids do not shut, and oral hygiene.

Knowledge Deficit. The deficit may include knowledge about status epilepticus, antiepileptic drugs, diagnostic tests, cause, seizure recognition, and first aid. The nurse becomes involved with knowledge assessment, and provision and evaluation of instruction. Parents need basic information about the definition of seizure and status epilepticus, and their cause if known. They need to know the name of the drug and have a basic understanding of how it works. They should understand why the medicine must be given consistently and why it cannot be stopped abruptly, as well as basic information about common and uncommon side effects and what to do if these occur. It may not be known whether or not seizures will recur. In either case, it is usually appropriate to discuss briefly seizure recognition, first aid, and what the parents should do. Written materials can be helpful so that the parent can read them at home to reinforce verbal information.

Fear. In many situations, the parents' fear relates to the possible death or potential disability of the child. They may be afraid and worry about the cause of the status epilepticus. Even the family of a child who has a pre-existing history of seizures may be uncomfortable with a seizure that does not stop. Parents should be encouraged to verbalize their feelings; these fears need to be acknowledged and parents need to be given realistic information about their child.

Nursing Care of the Child with Altered Responsiveness

For the purposes of nursing care, it is helpful to consider the child with an altered level of *consciousness* to be experiencing an altered *responsiveness.* This distinction allows one to focus on the child's state of arousal in a way that more clearly defines the problem and facilitates planning and implementation of nursing strategies.

Human responsiveness to the world within and around us is related to the integration of information obtained from external and internal stimuli: input, throughput, and output (Snyder, 1983). *Input* is the process of selecting and prioritizing the stimuli to which one responds. This process requires conscious awareness, attention span, orientation, and the ability to focus beyond oneself. *Throughput* is defined as the processing, analysis, and integration of input. It is the "mental processing" of selected stimuli. *Output* is considered the end product or response to stimuli. This can be expressed as thought, facial or body expression, movement, or change in mood or behavior. In children responsiveness (input, throughput, and output) is affected by the developmental age or current level of maturity in the nervous system.

Altered responsiveness may involve loss of one or more of the components just discussed. For example, input may be altered in a child with congenital blindness or deafness by decreasing the availability of external stimuli. Throughput may be altered in a child with a perceptual problem such as a visual motor deficit or in a child who experiences delays in processing time after severe head injury. Output is altered in a child who experiences paralysis, sensory motor deficits, or speech impairment.

Altered responsiveness may present as an acute process for one child (e.g., following head injury) and may be a daily reality for others (e.g., inoperable brain tumor). If the child is immobilized because of decreased responsiveness hazards of immobility also become a problem. The mobile child with sensory and perceptual deficits is at increased risk for physical injury.

The nursing care provided will vary according to the nature of altered responsiveness. In general, goals for nursing care are to (1) continue assessment for health care problems, especially those of a life-threatening nature; (2) protect the child from additional injury; and (3) assist the family in adapting to the child's care needs. This commonly involves the following nursing diagnoses: *self-care deficit, potential for injury, knowledge deficit,* and *altered family process.*

Self-Care Deficit

The degree of self-care deficit will depend on the child's age and level of responsiveness. In this section nursing care will be discussed for the unresponsive child who has a complete self-care deficit—that is, needs total nursing care. Emphasis is placed on preventing the hazards of immobility. When the child recovers from the neurologic injury, will he or she have a body that is capable of supporting ongoing growth and development or will the hazards of immobility have claimed one or more of the other body systems? It is important to note that all of the nursing strategies listed in this section are within the *independent* domain of nursing. There can be little excuse for failing to include these precautions in the plan of care.

Preventing Respiratory Complications of Immobility. The bedridden child has a decreased lung capacity because (1) inspiratory muscles are not aided by gravitational pull, (2) chest expansion is limited by the weight of the body against one aspect of the chest, and (3) when in a horizontal position, abdominal contents push against the diaphragm. Further, there is little stimulus for fully expanding the lungs when there is little or no muscular activity. Pooling of secretions within the lungs and exposure to microorganisms may lead to serious respiratory infection.

Although pulmonary toilet for the unresponsive child cannot include voluntary deep breathing and coughing, turning from side to side at least every 2 hours will help expand different areas of the lungs and reduce pooling of secretions. Elevate the head of bed periodically as tolerated. Positioning in a sitting position for short periods may also be an alternative. Careful handwashing and avoidance of persons with active respiratory infections is imperative.

Attention to gentle suctioning of nasal and oral secretions and to hygiene of oral and nasal mucous membranes will further help to prevent infection. Mucous membranes should be kept free of dried secretions and lubricated to prevent breaks in membrane integrity. Oral care is often complicated by the bite reflex in children with neurologic damage. The nurse should never insert fingers in the child's mouth, and care should be taken not to insert anything that will cause damage to the teeth or gums should the child's jaws close suddenly.

Preventing Musculoskeletal Complications of Immobility. Muscles that are not used lose strength, tone, and mass very rapidly. Likewise, contractures may form at unused joints, permanently limiting musculoskeletal function. Passive range of motion exercises (unless contraindicated by volatile intracranial pressure) and attention to body alignment when positioning the child can prevent these complications. The heavier the child, the more care will be needed in positioning because the weight of limbs pulls against major joints, causing strain on muscles, ligaments, and tendons. Pillows placed under arms and between legs can greatly minimize this stress. Remember to protect the hands and feet. Washcloths (or small gauze rolls for the infant and young child) can help to keep fingers in functional alignment. A footboard is necessary to prevent footdrop.

When the child begins to recover, weight bearing should be reinstituted as soon as possible. Physical therapy regimens including a tilt table, and parallel bars will help gradually to restore weight bearing and active range of motion.

Preventing Gastrointestinal Complications of Immobility. Oral feedings will not be attempted unless the gag and swallow reflexes are intact.The unresponsive child is usually fed through a nasogastric tube or a gastrostomy tube (see Chapter 41 for further information about gastrostomy feedings). Posturing or seizures during feeding can cause food to reflux through the tubing. If a nasogastric tube is being used, elevating the head of bed during feeding may help to prevent aspiration of the liquid feeding should reflux occur. Caloric needs must be carefully calculated to be sure that the child receives adequate nutrition to prevent muscle wasting, but because metabolism decreases with inactivity, care must also be taken not to overfeed. Irritability and crying may be related to the neurologic condition instead of to hunger. Infants who retain a sucking reflex should be given a pacifier during gavage feedings. The suck reflex is lost rapidly if it is not stimulated.

Infants and small children can often be held for feedings to preserve the social contact and caring interactions they have previously associated with feeding. Holding, rocking, and other caring interactions with family and nursing staff are equally important for older children. Remember that their inability for "output" does not necessarily rule out their ability for "input" and "throughput." If the child's condition contraindicates being held, techniques such as massage (tactile stimulus), singing to the child (auditory stimulus), and frequent contact that keeps one's face in the child's line of vision (visual stimulus) may be appropriate.

Bowel function can be monitored by auscultating bowel sounds in all abdominal quadrants and by maintaining a record of bowel movements. Both diarrhea and constipation are common and may alternate because of variable peristaltic action. Diarrhea may accompany a change in the feeding regimen and is a sign that the feeding is not being tolerated. Management of the diarrhea may therefore involve adjustments in oral intake.

Constipation, on the other hand, may be a sign of inadequate fluid intake (as well as of sluggish peristalsis related to immobility). Abdominal palpation for firm, full intestines can help to confirm suspicions of inadequate bowel evacuation. With prompt assessment of this condition, the nurse can request an order for a laxative or cleansing enema before impaction results.

Preventing Urinary Tract Complications of Immobility. Bladder tone and bladder emptying are also affected by immobility. Catheterization is usually instituted for the unresponsive child. Urine specific gravity and urine output provide an indication of whether fluid intake is adequate to maintain a healthy urinary tract. Meticulous catheter care will help to prevent unnecessary infections (see Chapter 42).

Maintaining Skin Integrity During Immobility. Bed rest is a major assault to the integumentary system. Constant rubbing on bed linens, body pressure against wrinkled garments, the pressure of body weight on delicate tissues, reduced blood flow in pressure areas, mechanical irritation from tubings, and chemical irritation from wet and soiled diapers—all add up to the need for nursing vigilance. General body hygiene will be much easier to provide for the infant than for the heavier school-aged child or adolescent. Obtain help as needed for bathing, washing the hair, and positioning for skin massage. Cleanse the perineum after each diaper change (older children who are unresponsive often are diapered as well).

Protect the skin from mechanical irritation. Use an egg crate mattress or flotation mattress as available. Keep linen wrinkles to a minimum and be very careful that no small objects (e.g., plastic sheaths from disposable needles) are left in the bed. Protect opposing skin surfaces and pressure points with pillows and foam supports. Inspect the skin thoroughly every shift for areas of decreased perfusion. Reposition and massage to increase blood flow to these areas immediately.

Unresponsiveness sometimes includes the loss of motor function of the eyelids. In this case eyelids may be taped closed to moisten corneas. During periods when the eyes are allowed to remain open, liquid tears and lubricating ointments can be applied to protect the cornea.

Potential for Injury

The child with altered responsiveness must be protected against further physiologic injury, including additional neurologic complications, and against physical injury from falls.

Monitoring Neurologic Status. Monitoring for changes in neurologic status that may signal either progress toward recovery or deterioration of the child's condition includes routine neurologic checks (see previous section on neurologic assessment) and observation for evidence of increasing ICP. Assess arousal, pupil size and reactivity, eye movements, motor function, respiratory pattern, and vital signs. In the responsive child note changes in mental status such as irritability which may indicate headache pain from increasing ICP. Other signs of increasing ICP include a bulging fontanel, rapidly increasing head circumference, visual deficits, altered vital signs, and vomiting (see Table 46-9). Table 46-11 details nursing goals and strategies for the child with increased intracranial pressure.

Preventing Injury From Falls. Physical safety is a concern for the child with altered responsiveness. Keep siderails up at all times to prevent falls from the bed. Even in the unresponsive child, involuntary movements or seizures can lead to falls. When the child is positioned in a chair for time out of bed, ensure that comfortable restraints will help to maintain the upright position and that there is no danger of the child slipping from the chair to the floor. Even with these precautions, children positioned out of bed must always be closely monitored. The mobile child may be prone to falls because of altered spatial perception and altered motor ability. Altered mental processing can lead to impulsive behavior. Football helmets can be used to protect the mobile child's head from further injury. Toys and equipment should be confined as much as possible to allow a clear path for walking. Gates can be used to protect the child from wandering near stairs or into medication rooms and other areas.

Knowledge Deficit

In some children altered responsiveness will be a long-term or permanent condition. The parents must then consider how to care for the child after hospital discharge. Discharge teaching should begin as soon as possible. Involving the parent (or the family members who will care for the child at home) as early as possible will help to ensure that they have time to learn new care procedures and become comfortable with them before they resume the role of primary caretaker. The child should be included in teaching and in self-care to the extent possible.

The family will need explanations of diagnostic tests, treatment modalities, the normal anatomy and physiology of neurologic processes, and the disruption of these that led to the child's condition. An understanding of responsiveness in terms of input, throughput, and output may help the family understand and cope with alterations in response as well as to recognize the capabilities for response that have been retained.

Differentiating the child's reflex movement from voluntary movements, so that such involuntary acts as posturing are not mistaken as purposeful responses, will require practice on the part of the family. A list of signs and symptoms indicating the need for medical intervention is necessary also, to enable the family to know when to call the physician.

Special care techniques the family may need to learn will be dictated by the child's condition. They include such things as feeding through a nasogastric tube, tracheostomy care, eye care, oral care, positioning, use of various types of equipment (e.g., suction machine), passive range of motion exercises, skin care, and safety concerns. Parents often appreciate discussing with the nurse appropriate discipline for the mobile child with altered responses.

Altered Family Process

By NANDA definition, altered family process is the state in which a family that normally functions effectively experiences a dysfunction. When one considers the tremendous impact on the family charged with care of a child with altered responsiveness, there is evident need for sensitive and knowledgeable nursing support. Family members may need to deal with the loss of closeness that results from altered ability to communicate and to respond to affection. They may question the child's ability to hear or feel in the absence of normal "output" responses. They often will have concerns about the prognosis and questions about whether to seek additional opinions. Discussion of these aspects calls for particular sensitivity on the part of the nurse. It takes time for the family to come to terms with the reality of a neurologic deficit, whether temporary or permanent. The nurse can assist in this process by explaining facts about the child's condition and refraining from offering personal opinion. When the facts are not known, state that this is the case and tell the family you will answer the question after obtaining the facts. Even minor inconsistencies in information obtained from health care professionals can cause the family to feel they are "getting the runaround" or that "the doctors and nurses here just don't know what's going on." A trusting relationship is built on honesty, not on always knowing the answer.

The family will also need information about the availability of physical and financial support for care after discharge. They should be counseled about the tremendous physical and emotional burden associated with full-time care of the disabled child. Family members should be encouraged to take advantage of respite care offered by friends and relatives (see also Chapter

25, which details the impact of chronic illness on the child and family).

Congenital and Chronic Neurologic Conditions

The remainder of this chapter deals with specific neurologic conditions. In the first section, several congenital and chronic disorders are discussed. Following are sections dealing with neurologic infections and neurologic injuries.

Craniosynostosis

Craniosynostosis is either the absence of or the premature fusion of one or more of the cranial sutures that join the bones of the infant skull. The skull deformity that results from this developmental aberration can range from mild, as in cases of single suture synostosis, to severe, as seen in cases of multiple suture synostosis evident in children with certain genetic syndromes and other anomalies. The term "craniostenosis" is often used interchangeably with "craniosynostosis." Craniostenosis refers to the actual deformity that results from absence or early fusion of the sutures, while craniosynostosis refers to the inherent process of early suture closure (Tessier, 1971). At present, the latter term is more commonly accepted and will be used in this chapter.

When diagnosed, craniosynostosis is classified as primary, secondary, or syndromic. *Primary craniosynostosis* may be either simple or compound. Simple synostosis refers to the obliteration of one suture, while compound refers to the absence or early fusion of two or more of the cranial sutures. The majority of cases of primary craniosynostosis are also referred to as isolated because they occur without any association to other developmental anomalies (Cohen, 1986).

In *secondary craniosynostosis*, suture obliteration occurs as a result of a known disorder. Various metabolic and hematologic disorders may lead to early fusion of the cranial sutures. Hyperthyroidism and thalassemia are examples of known causes of secondary craniosynostosis. The failure of brain growth that occurs in microcephaly may also lead to early closure of the cranial sutures. It is important to remember that craniosynostosis resulting from these other known disorders is very different from the more common primary type of craniosynostosis described earlier (Cohen, 1986).

In contrast to isolated craniosynostosis, *syndromic craniosynostosis* occurs in conjunction with other morphologic syndromes or developmental anomalies. There are many genetic syndromes that are associated with craniosynostosis, the two most common being Apert and Crouzon syndromes. Apert syndrome is characterized by craniosynostosis, midfacial malformations including bulging (proptotic), wide set (hypertelorie) eyes, and recessed chin, as well as syndactyly of the hands and feet. Children with Crouzon syndrome have somewhat similar facial characteristics, but do not exhibit the characteristic limb malformations seen in Apert syndrome. All but 3 per cent of children with Crouzon syndrome will exhibit normal intelligence, while many children with Apert syndrome will exhibit mental deficiencies (Cohen, 1986).

The incidence of primary isolated craniosynostosis in the United States is approximately 0.4 to 1.0 per 1000 live births. This varies slightly depending upon which data are used (Cohen, 1986). Winston (1985) states that the true occurrence is probably higher; just as many mild cases likely go unreported because of the considerable variation in the severity of the cosmetic manifestations of craniosynostosis. Since the late 1970s, Colorado is reported as having an incidence of primary isolated craniosynostosis two to three times greater than the national average with clusters of cases identified from various regions throughout the state. At present, no direct cause for this dramatic increase has been identified, although many factors are currently being explored, including diagnostic criteria, referral patterns, and environmental factors (Freisleben, 1987).

Etiology

The etiology of primary isolated craniosynostosis is unknown. It is generally agreed that there is likely not one isolated cause but rather a multifactoral basis for this disease. Although the majority of cases of simple craniosynostosis occur sporadically, some familial instances have been reported. Hunter and Rudd (1976, 1977) reported a 2 to 8 per cent familial occurrence of primary craniosynostosis of one suture.

Pathophysiology

The embryologic development of cranial sutures and the abnormality in this development that results in craniosynostosis have been the center of much attention in recent years. To understand abnormal head shape resulting from suture obliteration, knowledge regarding normal cranial growth is paramount. In the introductory section of this chapter, ossification and fontanelle closure are addressed, particularly regarding age-related differences in structure and function. A review and further clarification of these concepts will be presented here in the context of this disease process.

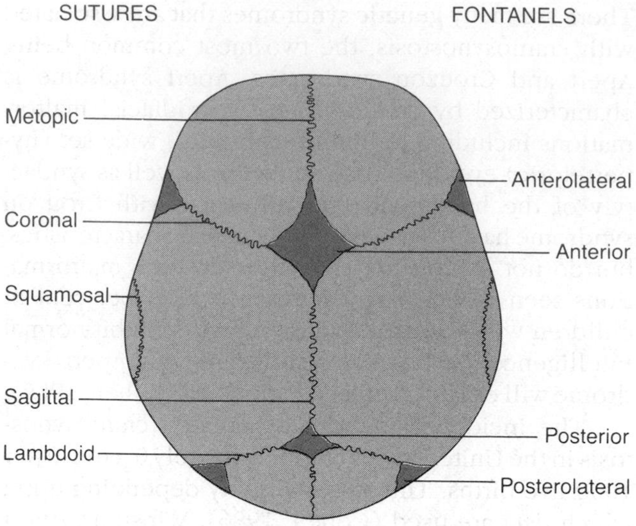

***Figure* 46-14.** Superior view of normal infant skull, showing sutures and fontanels.

Figure 46-14 shows a superior view of the normal infant skull. Five cranial sutures (three—the coronal, lambdoidal, and squamosal—are paired) allow the rapidly developing brain to grow at a normal rate. The anterior and posterior fontanels close at approximately 12 to 18 months and 2 to 3 months, respectively.

Development of the Cranial Bones. The cranial bones originate as a series of ossification centers that emerge from the fibrous embryologic cerebral capsule. At a later point in this stage of development, the cerebral capsule actually develops into the outer and inner layers of the dura mater. In early fetal life, the brain and cranial bones expand rapidly, although their borders (eventual suture sites) are widely separated. When the rate of brain growth slows down later in fetal life, the bones become more closely approximated, allowing for the eventual formation of a suture (Kokich, 1986). The suture itself is not thought to have potential for actual cell proliferation, but rather acts as a site of adaptation during growth by allowing for new bone generated from the cerebral capsule to be deposited and resorbed in a continuous and progressive fashion. In essence, the sutures grow in response to the changes and needs of the developing brain, particularly its fibrous covering (Koski, 1968).

Premature Suture Synostosis and Head Shape. In adulthood, all sutures are eventually obliterated by bone. If this occurs before the functional need for adaptation is complete, it is referred to as premature synostosis or fusion. Kokich (1986) and others question whether "premature synostosis" is actually the correct terminology since, in many cases, the fibrous, adaptive ligament that is referred to as a suture never even begins to form, thus allowing two adjacent cranial bones to merge. Whether the underlying pathology is referred to as "suture agenesis" or "premature synostosis," the outcome in terms of abnormal head shape is essentially the same with some potential for variation in the actual severity of the deformity.

The cranial bones grow in a perpendicular fashion to each of the cranial sutures. For example, the sagittal suture allows for growth of the parietal skull bones in a lateral fashion adding to the width of the skull. When this suture is absent or closed, growth is inhibited in the lateral direction, and instead growth occurs parallel to the ossified suture. The classic appearance of an infant or child with sagittal synostosis is one of a very long and narrow head, or *scaphocephaly.*

The *rule of thumb* that is helpful in remembering how head shape will appear in craniosynostosis is that growth is inhibited at right angles to the fused suture with compensatory expansion occurring at the sutures that are functional. To help clarify this concept, think of the following scenario. A child presents with a left coronal suture that is fused. Growth of the skull is inhibited perpendicular to the left coronal suture, so that the forehead appears recessed and the left eye may appear to bulge slightly. Because the brain needs to continue to expand, it is forced to grow in the direction of the open cranial sutures. In this situation, the brain expands along the right coronal suture, giving the appearance of a prominent right forehead and a sunken right eye in contrast to the left eye. This characteristic asymmetry of the skull is also referred to as *plagiocephaly.* The open sutures in a sense "work overtime" to allow the brain to expand. Figure 46-15 depicts schematic drawings of the various forms of craniosynostosis and outlines of the corresponding cranial shapes, including the accepted Greek terminology. Although this nomenclature continues to be commonly used, Cohen (1986) emphasizes that, regardless of the classification system or terminology used, the most important information is a ". . . clear description of which suture or sutures are involved and the extent of involvement . . . (p. 11)."

In summary, the ultimate head shape in the diagnosis of craniosynostosis depends on which sutures are synostosed, and the order in which they obliterate. The earlier in fetal or infant life synostosis occurs, the more dramatic the effect on cranial growth and appearance; the later synostosis occurs, the less dramatic the outcome (Cohen, 1986).

Diagnostic Assessment

The presence of craniosynostosis may be suspected either at birth or in later visits to health care providers for well child care. In cases when it is not evident at birth, parents are often the individuals who first notice the unusual head shape developing, especially when there are siblings with whom to make comparisons.

Initially, when craniosynostosis is questioned, a thorough "hands on" assessment of the cranium is called for. Palpation of the head for suture location and mobility is essential. Bony ridges along suture lines and any facial and/or cranial asymmetry are noted. Asymmetry can be evaluated by comparing the location of the external ear canals and outer canthi of the eyes from right to left. This comparison is best elucidated with the examiner looking down on the infant or child from the superior view. It is important for the examiner to pull the hair back from the forehead during the examination, especially when synostosis of the metopic or either coronal suture is suspected.

Along with palpation, measurement of the child's head circumference (HC) is vital. Many infants with craniosynostosis will present initially with a mild to moderate fall-off in this measurement. Height and weight parameters need to be assessed simultaneously with HC to ensure that the child is not failing to grow on all parameters for other reasons. A thorough neurologic and developmental examination is necessary to assess for other abnormalities, or the possibility of any genetic or syndromic basis for craniosynostosis.

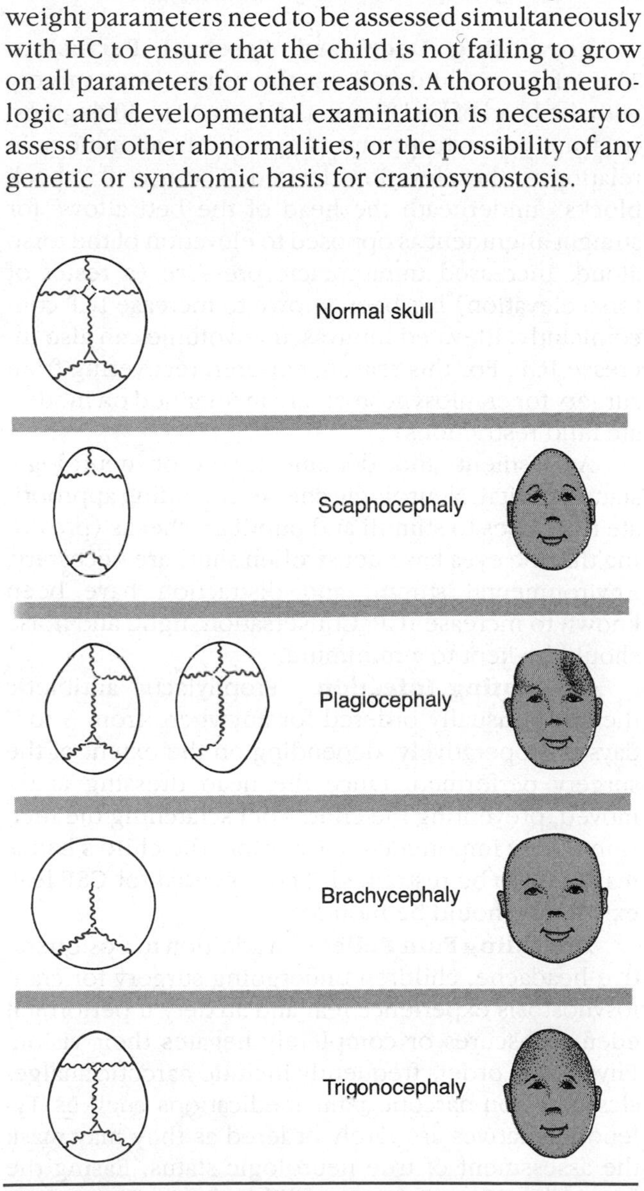

Figure 46-15. Normal skull and variations that occur in single or compound craniosynostosis.

Table 46-12. Suggested Aspects of Diagnostic Assessment for Craniosynostosis

Clinical evaluation	Complete history and physical • Palpation of sutures • Asymmetry • Head circumference • Neurologic examination
Radiographic evaluation	Skull roentgenograph CT scan, including bone windows
Developmental evaluation	Cognitive function Gross and fine motor Social/emotional Speech and language Genetic or syndromic findings

Generally, once the pediatrician or other health care provider suspects a diagnosis of craniosynostosis, a referral is made to a neurologist or neurosurgeon. In some instances, the primary physician will order radiographic studies to be taken prior to the consultation visit and given to the referring physician for review. These will include plain x-ray films of several different views of the skull. A computed axial tomography (CAT) scan with bone windows is also performed. "Bone windows" refers to the computerized mechanism for shading out the contours of the brain, producing a picture showing only the inner and outer contours of the skull bone. If these radiographic studies have not been done prior to referral, they are ordered by the consulting physician.

As well as a complete neurologic examination—including checking for sensory and motor function, cranial nerve findings, and evidence of chronic increased intracranial pressure—the neurologist or neurosurgeon does an assessment of the families' concerns regarding the unusual head shape. Because craniosynostosis can range from very mild, requiring no intervention, to very severe, requiring several surgical procedures, parental concerns may vary widely.

Table 46-12 contains an overview of suggested assessment for children with a diagnosis of craniosynostosis.

Therapeutic Management

The goals of modern surgical management of craniosynostosis are to prevent the development of increased intracranial pressure that may result in serious neurologic damage and to correct the cosmetic deformity that may result in long-term psychologic sequelae for the affected individual (Marchac and Renier, 1982). The decision to correct craniosynostosis surgically is based on the severity of the deformity, the number of sutures thought to be synostosed, and the child's present neurologic and developmental condition. There is an ongoing controversy in the area of surgical management as to whether primary neurologic findings are a result of craniosynostosis or whether they are intrinsic aspects of abnormal brain development (Camfield and Camfield, 1986). A question also exists as to whether mild chronic increases in intracranial pressure really cause impairment of intellectual function (Renier et al, 1982). Nonetheless, for children in whom more than one suture is synostosed or in whom symptoms of increased ICP exist, or both, surgical correction is almost always attempted.

Surgical Techniques

The choice of the surgical technique employed to correct craniosynostosis depends primarily on the individual surgeon and his or her philosophy and experience. Sometimes, strips or wide portions of bone around, or including, the affected sutures are removed, cut into various pieces, and rewired together to attain a more normal shape. In other instances, synthetic materials are placed along cut bone edges around the affected suture to prevent reclosure after operations. Acrylic onlays to correct an asymmetric appearance of the skull visually and plication or incision of the dura mater in an effort to reshape the underlying brain are also techniques that may be used at various centers across the country. Recently, there has been a trend toward a union of neurologic and plastic surgery techniques and the formation of multidisciplinary craniofacial teams to provide care for children with craniosynostosis. More specific information regarding surgical techniques can be found in neurosurgical textbooks. Regardless of the procedure chosen, the ultimate goals of allowing for brain growth and correcting the cosmetic deformity are maintained.

Therapeutic postsurgical management includes close monitoring of neurologic status, which may be affected by cerebral edema. This can, in turn, affect fluid and electrolyte balance, and put the child at risk for further edema if not managed properly. As with any neurosurgical procedure, risk of infection and bleeding are present and must be followed. Respiratory complications may ensue as a result of the lengthy anesthetic time needed for the more extensive procedures.

Major Nursing Diagnoses for Postoperative Care of the Child with Craniosynostosis

Altered tissue perfusion: cerebral, *related to postoperative edema as evidenced by:*
- *changing level of consciousness*
- *signs and symptoms of increased intracranial pressure*

Potential for infection: incisional, bone or meningeal, *related to introduction of pathogens by:*
- *surgical intervention*
- *postoperative wound contamination*
- *postoperative CSF leak*

Altered comfort: pain, *related to:*
- *facial and intracranial edema associated with surgical intervention*
- *pressure of postoperative pressure dressing to head*

Ineffective family coping, *related to anxiety about surgery in a vital area resulting from:*
- *inadequate information*
- *lack of familiarity with hospital setting and surgical techniques*

Strategies for Nursing Care

Preventing Decreased Cerebral Perfusion. The infant or child will usually return from surgery with the head of bed elevated at least 20 to 30 degrees. It is important to ensure proper body alignment in relation to the elevation desired. The use of "shock blocks" underneath the head of the bed allows for straight alignment as opposed to elevation of the torso alone. Increased intrathoracic pressure (a result of torso elevation) has been known to increase ICP concomitantly. Elevated intravascular volume can also increase ICP. For this reason, children recovering from surgery for craniosynostosis are maintained on moderate fluid restrictions.

Assessment and documentation of neurologic status are vital. Neurologic checks, including appropriate responses to stimuli and pupillary checks (providing that the eyes have not swollen shut) are necessary. Environmental stimuli and distraction have been known to increase ICP. Conversation, light, and noise should be kept to a minimum.

Preventing Infection. Prophylactic antibiotic therapy is usually ordered for anywhere from 3 to 7 days postoperatively, depending on the extent of the surgery performed. Once the head dressing is removed, preventing the child from scratching the incision is very important. On occasion, the child's hands may need to be restrained. The potential for CSF leak exists and should be monitored.

Providing Pain Relief. In addition to postoperative headache, children undergoing surgery for craniosynostosis experience fear and anxiety if periorbital edema obscures or completely negates their vision. Physicians' orders frequently include narcotic analgesics and non-narcotic pain medications such as Tylenol. Sedatives are rarely ordered as they may mask the assessment of true neurologic status. Easing the fear and anxiety of a young child who cannot see is a true nursing challenge. Often parents are the experts at the nonpharmacologic measures that help their child cope. Maximizing use of the senses of touch, taste, smell, and hearing is usually the best way to assure the infant or child that their familiar and comforting world has not disappeared. Adequate periods of rest are also extremely vital even as the child appears to be getting back to normal activity.

Supporting Family Coping. Many families have difficulty understanding the procedures necessary to correct craniosynostosis, and often appear baffled. It is hard for the parent of an otherwise healthy appearing child to consent to a surgery of this magnitude even when the child is obviously deformed. Often what parents need most is someone to listen to their concerns and provide positive reinforcement for their participation in, and coping with, hospitalization. In some circumstances other families who have been through the surgery are helpful. Anxiety on the part of the parents is often sensed by the child and contributes to their fear. Family members may feel guilty if they leave the child's side. They need to be encouraged to spend time away from the child, so that their time with the child is a helpful rather than a draining experience. For all of these reasons, a family-centered approach to the nursing care of these children is essential to the creation of a positive hospitalization experience.

Discharge teaching is a large part of the nurse's responsibility in the hospital setting. Instructions are given in regard to incision care, activity, use of a protective helmet, positioning, and follow-up visits. It is helpful if this information is in a written format, so parents can refer to it when necessary.

Long-Term Outcome

The degree of severity of the deformity and which sutures are affected usually determine the ease with which craniosynostosis is surgically corrected. Long-term outcome depends greatly on the function of the child prior to the surgery, and whether the classification is isolated or syndromic craniosynostosis. Children who experience symptoms of increased ICP prior to surgery will likely experience relief of symptoms postoperatively and benefit from a more aesthetic appearance as they grow older.

Nursing Strategies for Follow-up Care in the Home or Clinic

Depending on the surgery performed, some children go home with the initial surgical dressing intact. Important aspects of caring for these children in the home and clinic settings:

In the first week, discuss the use of acetaminophen (Tylenol) for general irritability or fussiness.

Observe the incision for any areas of redness, infection, or CSF leak.

Assess the home for safety hazards and the parents' ability to assure a safe environment.

Assess the fit of the protective helmet and the parents' ability to enforce compliance in helmet use.

Review positioning strategies for sleeping, eating, and activities of daily living with parents (these will vary depending on the surgical procedure performed).

In circumstances when the clinic or home health care nurse encounters a child who will undergo surgery for craniosynostosis, preoperatively, the following interventions would be appropriate:

If offered, refer the family to the hospital for a preoperative tour to begin familiarizing themselves with the hospital setting.

Discuss postoperative appearance and activities, so that the family can plan any necessary changes for the home environment.

Myelodysplasia

Myelodysplasia refers to defective development of any part of the spinal column in embryonic life. In the clinical context, this term is often used interchangeably with the term *spinal dysraphism* or *spina bifida*, which refers to incomplete closure of the primary neural tube. Cranium bifidum refers to incomplete closure of the rostral end of the neural tube, resulting in abnormal development of the brain, meninges, and/or skull bones. At a more basic level, all of the congenital malformations involving the neural tube are also often referred to as *neural tube defects (NTD)*. If defective closure occurs in the area of the developing embryonic head, anencephaly or encephalocele may result, and if defective closure occurs lower in the spinal column, spina bifida occurs. These malformations constitute the greatest number of neurologic developmental disorders (Passo, 1980).

The most commonly seen neural tube defects are listed and defined as follows in order of decreasing severity.

- *Anencephaly*: Absence of brain tissue above a rudimentary brain stem and basal ganglia. This is often listed under the family of defects called cranium bifidum. Sustained extrauterine life is virtually impossible in these children.

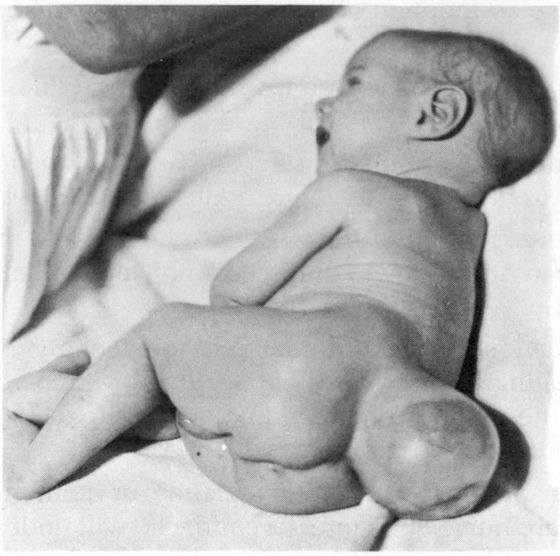

Figure 46-16. Infant with spina bifida cystica. Handling this infant requires exteme care so that the sac incurs no tension or pressure. The infant's head and the spine above the sac should be supported at all times, as well as the lower extremities when the child is held.

- *Encephalocele*: Another type of cranium bifidum that presents as an external sac or mass that may occur at any point over the vertex or base of the skull. May be covered either with scalp or a transparent membrane.
- *Spina Bifida Cystica*: The incomplete fusion of one or more of the vertebral laminae, resulting in an external protrusion of the spinal tissue (Fig. 46-16). This open type of defect occurs most commonly in the lumbosacral area. There are two classifications of spina bifida cystica.

  Myelomeningocele: This more severe open NTD involves a protruding sac-like structure that contains meninges, spinal fluid, and neural tissue. The spinal nerve roots may terminate at the sac, ending motor and sensory function below that point. The most severe and rarest form of myelomeningocele is called *myeloschisis*, in which the neural folds fail to meet and fuse, causing the spinal cord to become a flattened mass of nervous tissue with no dural covering.

  Meningocele: This less common open NTD contains only meninges and CSF. Neurologic complications can occur but are less severe than with myelomeningocele.
- *Spina Bifida Occulta*: The incomplete fusion of the vertebrae at one level that may be signaled only by an overlying dimple or tuft of hair. The majority of these defects occur without any evidence of neurologic or musculoskeletal disorders. Some will present with symptoms in late childhood and require eventual surgical intervention if clinical deterioration is present. Dermoid cysts, fibrous bands, or lipomas (fatty tumors) are the most common etiologies for this diagnosis (Humphreys, 1985).

Figure 46-17 depicts three of these congenital malformations of the spine.

Embryology

All of the developmental anomalies involving the neural tube are best understood through consideration of the normal embryologic development of the brain and spinal cord. At about 18 days of gestation, the nervous system begins to develop from a thickened area of embryonic ectoderm called the *neural plate.* By the 22nd day of gestation, the neural plate begins to fold into the *neural tube* (See Figure 46-18). This folding initially occurs centrally, and then proceeds in a somewhat irregular fashion superiorly and inferiorly. The cranial end opening of the neural tube is called the *rostral neuropore*, while the lower spinal opening is called the *caudal neuropore.* The neuropores close on the 25th and 27th days of embryonic life, respectively. The central lumen of the neural tube eventually becomes the ventricular system of the brain, superiorly, and the central canal of the spinal cord, inferiorly (Moore, 1988).

Malformations of the neural tube usually involve malformations of the laminae and pedicles of the vertebral column as well (Moore, 1982). The formation of the bony vertebral column occurs simultaneously with the formation of the neural tube, except that it originates from mesodermal, rather than ectodermal, cells. If the neural tube either fails to close properly on either end or becomes overdistended and ruptures after initial normal closure, then a neural tube defect of the varieties described earlier will occur.

Etiology

The incidence of neural tube defects varies considerably depending on geographic location. In the United States the frequency is 1 to 2 per 1000 live births. In certain areas of Ireland and England, the frequency is as high as 8 to 9 per 1000 live births. Some countries, like Japan and Finland, have frequencies less than 0.5 per 1000 live births. Incidence also varies by race, with Orientals and blacks having the lowest occurrence rates, and Irish and Moslems having the highest occurrence of NTDs (Mortimer, 1980). Because many of these children are spontaneously aborted early in gestation or stillborn, true incidence rates may actually be higher than estimated (Cohen, 1987).

Unfortunately, there is no one identified etiology for neural tube defects. The exact reasons for abnormal closure of the neural tube have remained unclear at

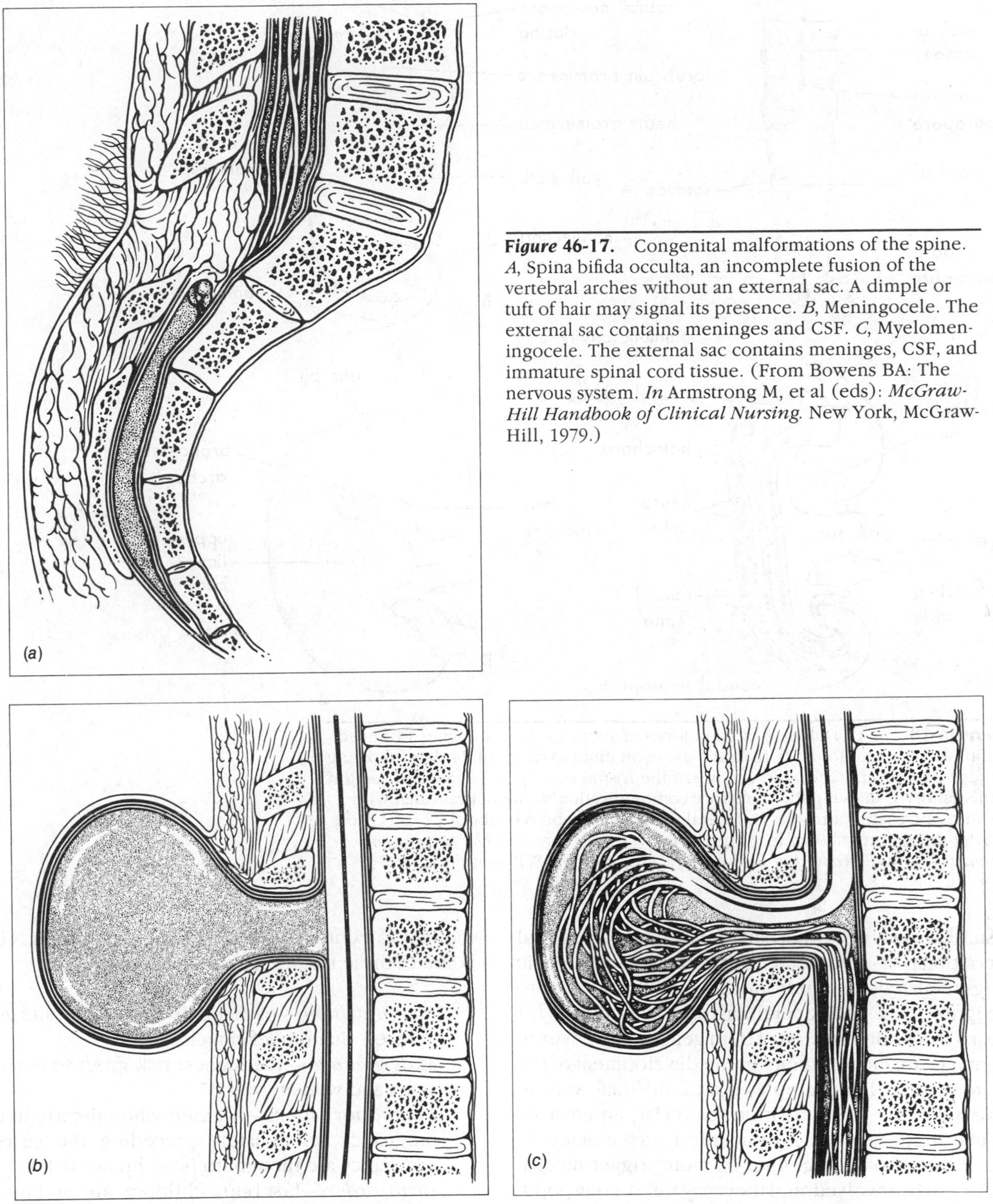

Figure 46-17. Congenital malformations of the spine. *A*, Spina bifida occulta, an incomplete fusion of the vertebral arches without an external sac. A dimple or tuft of hair may signal its presence. *B*, Meningocele. The external sac contains meninges and CSF. *C*, Myelomeningocele. The external sac contains meninges, CSF, and immature spinal cord tissue. (From Bowens BA: The nervous system. *In* Armstrong M, et al (eds): *McGraw-Hill Handbook of Clinical Nursing.* New York, McGraw-Hill, 1979.)

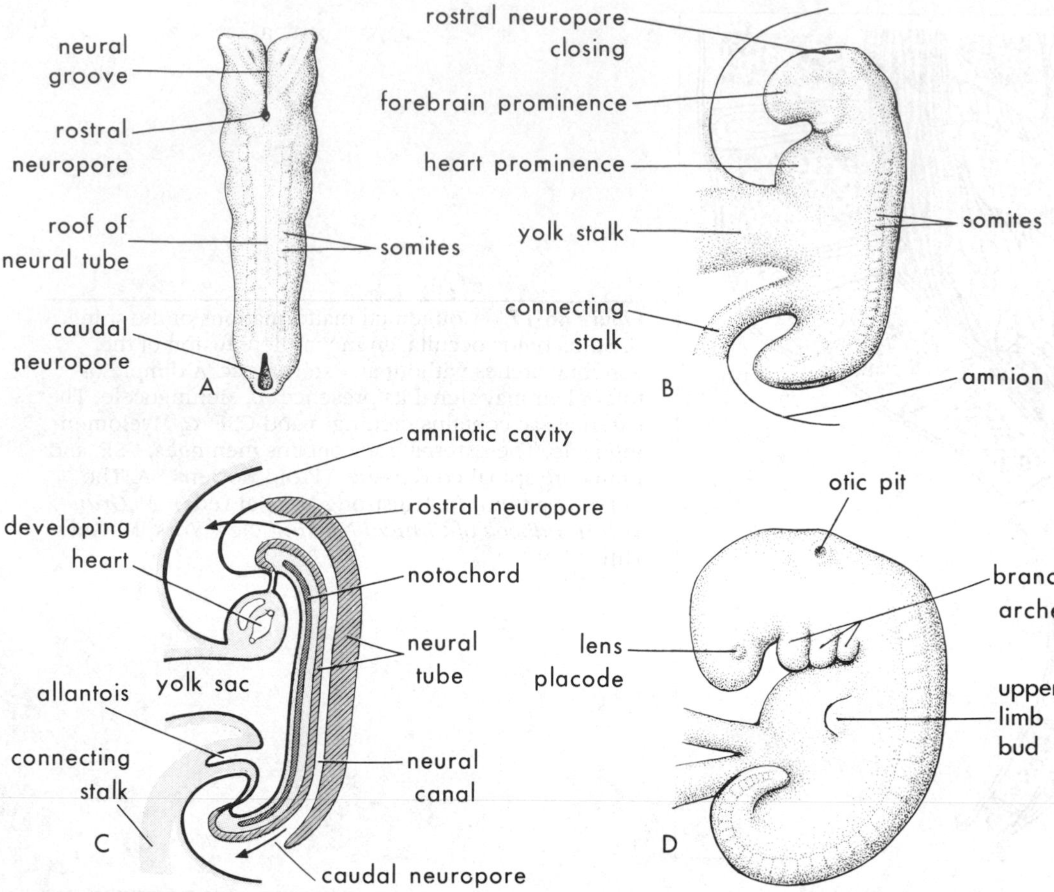

Figure 46-18. *A*, Dorsal view of an embryo of about 23 days, showing advanced fusion of the neural folds. *B*, Lateral view of an embryo of about 24 days, showing the forebrain prominence and closing of the rostral neuropore. *C*, Sagittal section of this embryo, showing the transitory communication of the neural canal with the amniotic cavity (arrows). *D*, Lateral view of an embryo of about 27 days. Note that the neuropores shown in *B* are closed. (From Moore KL: *The Developing Human: Clinically Oriented Embryology.* Philadelphia, WB Saunders, 1988.)

best. NTDs may occur as a part of various chromosomal aberrations or after fetal exposure to teratongenic drugs. Isolated, nonsyndromic neural tube defects are recognized as having multifactoral causation. This means that a combination of both genetic and environmental factors may interact in the development of the malformation. For example, if an individual were to have a genetic predisposition for NTDs, an environmental trigger could act to manifest such a defect in that person's offspring. One or more trigger mechanisms can be involved, and they may vary among populations. Genetic and environmental components are considered to be additive, increasing a particular couple's risk for producing a child with a NTD (Cohen, 1984). Many epidemiologic studies have been carried out in an effort to identify etiologic agents and promote prevention of these defects. In a summary of various epidemiologic observations noted in the literature, Cohen (1987) points out the variety of factors thought to contribute to the development of a NTD. Some of these factors are summarized here:

- *Poor nutrition*—particularly zinc, folate, and generalized vitamin deficiencies
- *Maternal age*—the highest risk groups are teenagers and women over 35
- *Pregnancy history*—women who miscarry in the pregnancy immediately preceding the current pregnancy are thought to be at higher risk
- *Birth order*—first-born children are at highest risk; second-born children at lowest risk
- *Socioeconomic status*—frequency of NTDs higher in low socioeconomic groups; may be related to nutrition

It should be noted that even though a family history of NTDs increases the risk of subsequent NTD births, between 90 and 95 per cent of infants with

NTDs are born to couples with negative family histories of the same (Cohen, 1987).

Pathophysiology

The degree of functional impairment associated with the various types of myelodysplasia depends on the level and extent of the defect. Neurologic findings correlate with the particular myotomes (muscle groups) that are innervated by affected spinal cord segments. Dysfunction can range from complete paralysis to minimal involvement but is most often somewhere in between. A lesion at the middle thoracic level causes total paralysis of lower extremities. The more common lumbosacral lesions generally leave the child with some degree of hip, knee, or ankle flexion, allowing for walking with either braces and crutches or minimal assistive devices, depending on the functional level of the lesion. The closed or nonvisible lesions (spina bifida occulta) often go undiagnosed until later childhood and frequently are not associated with any degree of impairment.

In the majority of lumbosacral lesions, the muscles of the legs are affected and the electrical responses of these muscles may vary. Sensory disturbances are usually symmetric and determined according to the affected dermatomes (areas of skin). Club feet, scoliosis, contractures, and dislocated hips are very common in children born with lesions of the lumbosacral area (Conway, 1977). Bowel and bladder dysfunction are almost always apparent because the nerves that supply these organs are located in the sacral area. Bowel problems commonly include constipation or incontinence. The neurogenic bladder can make the child prone to retention and resultant urinary tract infections, or the child may have problems with incontinence (Passo, 1980). The nursing assessment and care strategies will be addressed separately, following the discussion of therapeutic management. The pathology associated with all of the myelodysplastic lesions is only as clear as the diagnostic assessment of functional capacity. As in most instances of congenital CNS disorders, the true extent of dysfunction is often only apparent as the child grows and a clearer assessment of ability is obtained.

Diagnostic Assessment

With the use of modern ultrasound and laboratory technology, prenatal diagnosis of open neural tube defects is now possible. In the early 1970s, an association between an elevated serum alpha fetoprotein (AFP) level and the presence of an open NTD was discovered. Henceforth, many health care providers have relied on AFP levels drawn between 16 and 18 weeks of gestation as a screening tool for open NTDs. The test is not foolproof, as many other congenital anomalies can cause increases in AFP levels, and there are other maternal factors known to cause false-positive and false-negative results with this test. Nonetheless, AFP levels have become a useful screening tool for open NTDs (Passo, 1987). Although prenatal screening has added a dimension to anticipatory guidance of families with myelodysplastic children, the discovery of this anomaly in the delivery room continues to be a common occurrence. The importance of an honest and compassionate approach with the grief-stricken family cannot be overemphasized.

The initial diagnostic assessment of the newborn infant who presents with a NTD is multifaceted. As well as the appropriate delivery room routines, care is taken to protect the spinal or cranial lesion from injury and infection. As soon as possible, the infant is brought from the delivery room to the specialty care nursery to be monitored closely and examined by a neonatologist or pediatrician. A complete physical examination with attention to the NTD itself, presence or absence of hydrocephalus, and motor and sensory functional capacities is carried out. The defect is examined in regard to size, level, and nature of tissue covering. Any leakage of CSF is noted. Palpation of the cranial sutures and fontanelles and a measurement of head circumference are performed. Development and movement of upper and lower extremities are assessed. Infants with thoracic or high lumbar lesions are often born with atrophied lower extremities. An initial evaluation of bowel and bladder function is also carried out. Once an assessment of the infant is completed, a discussion with the family in regard to long-term prognosis should take place. According to Conway (1977), the four primary prognosticating factors are the degree of neural involvement, the size and location of the sac, the presence of other anomalies, and any complications that occur.

Therapeutic Management

Decisions as to whether or not surgical closure of the lesion is appropriate can be controversial and difficult for families and health care providers alike. Criteria for nonclosure advocated by Lorber (1971) and used widely today included paralysis at L2 or above, marked hydrocephalus, kyphosis, and the presence of other major congenital birth anomalies. Still, others believe that lesions of all children should be closed, as it is not a given that those who are left untreated will die quickly. Freeman (1973) suggests that children who survive nontreatment become significantly more impaired than if they had been operated upon early. In either case, Humphreys (1985) stresses that it must be clear to the family that the surgery is not to repair the faulty spinal cord which has never matured, but to limit the possibility of meningitis and preserve what neurologic function the child has.

Surgical Management. The goals of early operative care of spina bifida cystica are to preserve all neural tissue, provide a normal anatomic barrier, and control early progressive hydrocephalus. A sterile, constantly moistened saline dressing is maintained on the sac until the surgery is performed. The surgical procedure involves dissection of the exposed sac and closure of the dura mater and skin over the preserved neural tissue. When the defect is large, the assistance of a plastic surgeon for skin grafting over the lesion is called for. If hydrocephalus is present at birth, a ventriculo-peritoneal shunting device may be placed at the time of initial closure. If the clinical features of hydrocephalus are not apparent initially, the child is assessed for this condition frequently. Eighty per cent of children with myelomeningocele will eventually develop hydrocephalus (Humphreys, 1985). Surgical repair of spina bifida occulta, regardless of the specific anomaly, is usually undertaken soon after diagnosis. The primary surgical aim in these cases is to free up the tethered or tied spinal cord, so that progressive deterioration of function is arrested.

In cases of encephalocele, the timing of surgical intervention may vary depending on the size, location, and extent of nervous tissue involvement. In severe cases, early death is common, usually related to complications of hydrocephalus, infection, or actual rupture of the encephalocele (Conway, 1977). In any or all of the aforementioned cases, when surgery is performed, the primary concerns of the neurosurgeon relate to wound integrity, prevention of infection and CSF leaks; and timely healing of the repair. Meticulous postoperative care is essential, and will be covered in the nursing care sections to follow.

Medical Management. Once the neurosurgeon has repaired the cranial or spinal defect and placed a ventriculoperitoneal shunt (if necessary), the neonatologist or pediatrician assumes the bulk of the postoperative management. Cardiopulmonary function and adequate nutrition are essential to wound healing. The child must lie prone for several days postoperatively to avoid pressure on the wound and possible CSF leaks inviting infection. Once the infant is less restricted in positioning and allowed to be supine, orthopedic, rehabilitation, and urologic consults are obtained allowing for a better understanding of the child's functional capacity. Hip and spine roentgenographs, renal ultrasound, electrical muscle testing, and auditory testing are commonly done before discharge. Close follow-up of fontanel size and head circumference are also important. Normal well child care routines and infant development are followed as they would be for any child, and should not be overshadowed by the special care requirements of these children. As the child heals from the surgery and discharge is planned, an assessment of the family's coping skills and available resources is essential to ensuring a successful transition to home. It is normal for parents to still be grieving the birth of a defective child at this point, and referral for supportive counseling may be necessary.

Major Nursing Diagnoses for Myelodysplasia

Most children born with a neural tube defect face chronic health problems for a lifetime. Depending on the age of the child, the level or type of defect and the setting in which the child is encountered, certain diagnoses may or may not be applicable at any given point in time. Obviously the more severe the cranial or spinal defect, the more interface the child and family will have with the health care delivery system. Comprehensive care of the child with any type of neurodevelopmental anomaly calls for a multidisciplinary approach. The nurse is often the key individual in coordinating and understanding the complex care of these children. In an effort to clarify the important nursing issues with these children, major nursing diagnoses will be presented in two categories: newly diagnosed infant and long-term follow-up of the child.

Nursing Diagnoses for the Infant Born with a Neural Tube Defect

***Potential for infection: meningitis,** related to*
- *an open membranous sac*
- *surgical intervention*
- *possible CSF leak from incomplete closure of the dura*

***Potential for injury: neurologic trauma,** related to:*
- *possible rupture of the sac*
- *exposed nervous tissue*

***Altered tissue perfusion: cerebral: increased intracranial pressure,** related to hydrocephalus often associated with neural tube defects*

***Altered skin integrity,** related to*
- *sensory neurologic deficits*
- *limited mobility*
- *nature of neonatal skin*

***Altered elimination: bowel and bladder dysfunction,** related to poor or absent motor or sensory innervation*

***Altered parenting: grief and shock,** related to*
- *birth of a defective infant*
- *unexpected lengthy hospitalization*

Nursing Diagnoses for Long-Term Follow-Up of the Child With a Neural Tube Defect

Potential for infection: urinary tract, *related to:*
- *chronic retention of urine*
- *repeated catheterizations*

Altered nutrition, more than body requirements, *related to decreased metabolic needs as a result of*
- *immobility*
- *little exercise*

Impaired physical mobility: orthopedic and neurologic problems, *related to neuromuscular and sensory deficits*

Potential for injury: increased intracranial pressure, *related to malfunctioning VP shunt, associated with physical growth or mechanical failure of the shunt*

Altered bowel elimination: neurogenic bowel, *related to:*
- *decreased mobility*
- *neurologic deficits*

Disturbance in self-concept: body image, *related to:*
- *chronic illness*
- *altered physical capabilities*
- *lifestyle changes*

Strategies for Nursing Care

The strategies for nursing care discussed here follow the major nursing diagnoses listed previously. The individual applicability of these strategies to each child will vary according to the type and level of the lesion. When appropriate, variations within specific diagnoses are addressed. Because of the inherent complexity of this disease entity, only the major diagnoses and strategies will be covered, although there may be others that are individually applicable.

Preventing Initial Infection of the Spinal or Cranial Defect. Care of the protruding sac is extremely important. In the case of an encephalocele, if the defect is covered with skin, positioning of the infant is done to avoid pressure on the lesion. If the encephalocele is in the occipital area, a foam donut may be useful. The more common lumbosacral spinal myelomeningoceles are usually only protected by a thin membrane. A sterile, saline soaked dressing is applied after the sac is examined for gross tears or leakage. Rather than change the dressing frequently, it is usually kept moist with a sterile saline solution at regular intervals. The infant is placed on prophylactic broad spectrum antibiotics and meticulous care is taken to avoid any contamination of the sac by stool and urine. Signs and symptoms of meningitis include irritability, fever, feeding intolerance, and seizures. The physician should be alerted if any of these symptoms become apparent.

Postoperatively, the wound is treated aseptically and the prone position is maintained for several days to avoid pressure on the incision and CSF leak. A protective barrier drape is used to prevent contamination by stool or urine and must be changed when necessary. Figure 46-19 depicts the use of a barrier drape. The surgical dressing should be changed if soiled with stool. Frequent diaper changes may be necessary, as these children may stool and void continuously.

Preventing Injury or Neurologic Trauma. Rupture of the fluid-filled sac could lead to immediate death as a result of sudden decompression of CSF from the cranial cavity. Correct positioning for children with spinal lesions is either prone or sidelying, depending on the function of the lower extremities. A low Trendelenburg position is also favored to decrease the pressure in the sac. Several cloth rolls underneath the infant's hips in the prone position are helpful in creating the head down position and allowing for both proper alignment of the lower extremities and a downward flow of stool and urine away from the open lesion.

Watching for Signs and Symptoms of Hydrocephalus. Between 80 and 90 per cent of children with spinal defects manifest clinically significant hydrocephalus (Passo, 1980; Humphreys, 1985). Hydrocephalus as an individual disease entity is discussed later in this chapter. In any event, the nurse should closely monitor fontanel size, sutures, and head circumference daily. Teaching the family about signs and symptoms of shunt malfunction or infection should begin once the shunt is in place and the parents appear ready to learn.

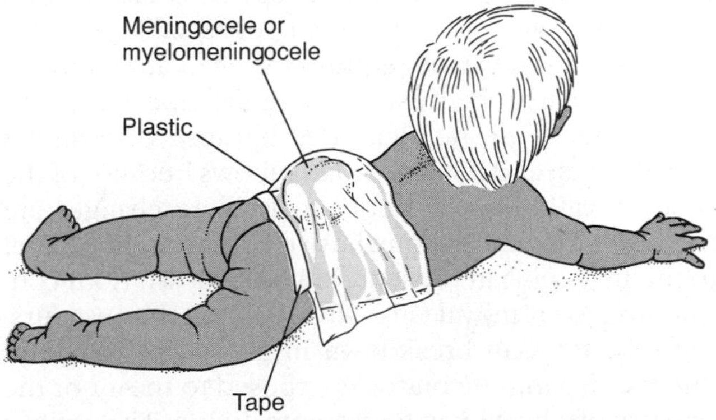

Figure 46-19. Use of ordinary kitchen-variety plastic wrap to protect a spinal defect from contamination.

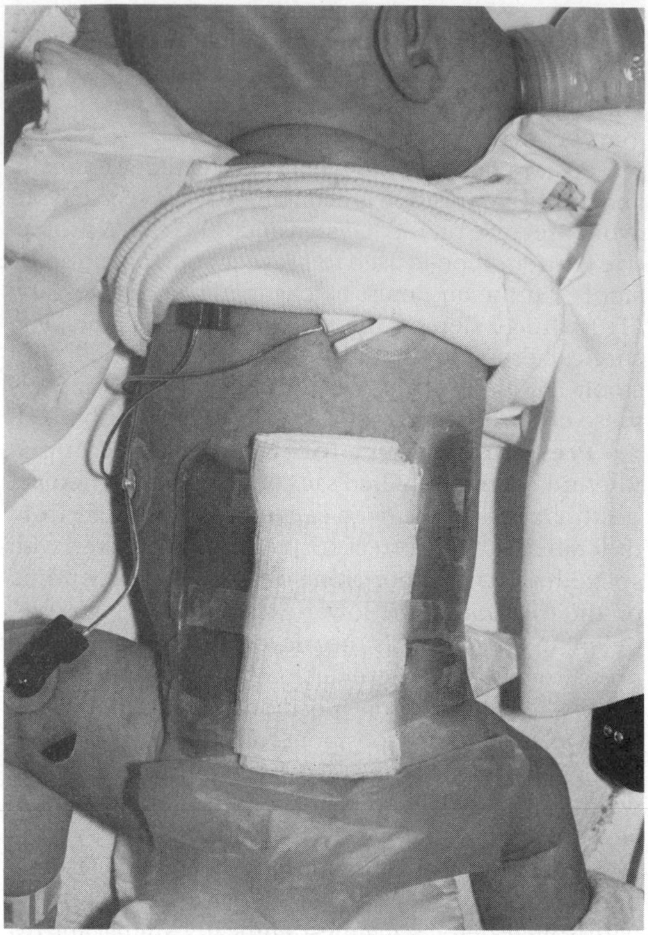

Figure **46-20.** Use of stomahesive to prevent skin breakdown in children with myelomeningocele. The plastic below the dressing is the barrier drape, which has been pulled down to reveal the dressing. Note the shunt visible as a raised line along the back of the head.

Avoiding Skin Breakdown. Children with myelomeningocele experience absence of sensation below the level of the defect. Nursing care strategies are geared toward optimizing skin integrity and avoiding pressure sores. This can be especially challenging in the neonate since the skin is especially prone to breakdown. The areas requiring special attention are the wound area, because of continual tape and dressing changes; the perianal area because of frequent loose stools; and the knees and elbows because of the prone positioning. If frequent dressing changes are required, the use of stomahesive in two strips parallel to the incision can prevent skin breakdown from continuous tape removal (Fig. 46-20). Often the best nursing care for skin breakdown in the anal area is frequently leaving the buttocks exposed to the air or the safe use of a heat lamp to promote drying. The use of a waterbed, sheepskin, or clear, nonocclusive dressing may prevent breakdown to the knee and elbow areas. Frequent range of motion exercises and infant massage may also promote blood flow to the skin and aid in preventing breakdown. Another important factor in healthy skin integrity is adequate nutrition. Nursing care should incorporate any or all of the above strategies as they apply individually. Any redness, warmth, or early signs of skin breakdown should be documented and appropriate nursing measures instituted to avoid further breakdown.

Maintaining Adequate Bowel and Bladder Elimination. Even children with small insignificant-appearing spinal lesions may experience bowel and bladder dysfunction because the nerves that supply these organs are in the sacral area (Passo, 1980). Urinary problems are those of both incontinence and retention. Intermittent dribbling can cause skin breakdown and psychosocial problems when the child is past diaper-wearing age. Retention can lead to urinary reflux into the ureters and kidneys, predisposing the child to urinary tract infections and nephritis. The nurse can teach the parents the Credé maneuver prior to discharge. This consists of applying somewhat firm hand pressure from the umbilicus toward the symphysis pubis to manually express urine from the bladder (Fig. 46-21). Other nursing strategies include teaching parents to keep their infant well-hydrated and to note any foul-smelling or dark, sedimented urine and report it to their physician. Problems with bowel elimination will be addressed in a future section.

Promoting Parental Coping. Macedo and Posel (1987) state that nursing has the responsibility of preventing maladaptive family coping patterns. The initial crisis following the birth of a "not-perfect" child must be effectively resolved if the family is to function well as a unit. Appropriate nursing strategies include allowing the parents to grieve by being with them and listening. An example of a phrase that might be helpful in getting at some of their feelings is "This really isn't what you expected, is it?" or "This whole event must be so overwhelming to you." The family also needs to have honest information about the most immediate aspects of medical care—specifically, closure of the defect or potential for ventriculo-peritoneal shunting, or both—if a procedure is to be done imminently.

The nurse is often the one person who has the knowledge, skill, and time to clarify any misconceptions, repeat any information that is necessary, and assess family values and perceptions in regard to neural tube defects. Another important nursing strategy is to assess the family's support system and availability of resources (Macedo and Posel, 1987). Parents may need assistance in mobilizing resources to help them care for a special needs infant. Upon discharge from the nursery, the parents need to have practiced, and to feel comfortable, caring for their infant. The infant's primary nurse should have a checklist of discharge teaching activities that need to be accomplished prior

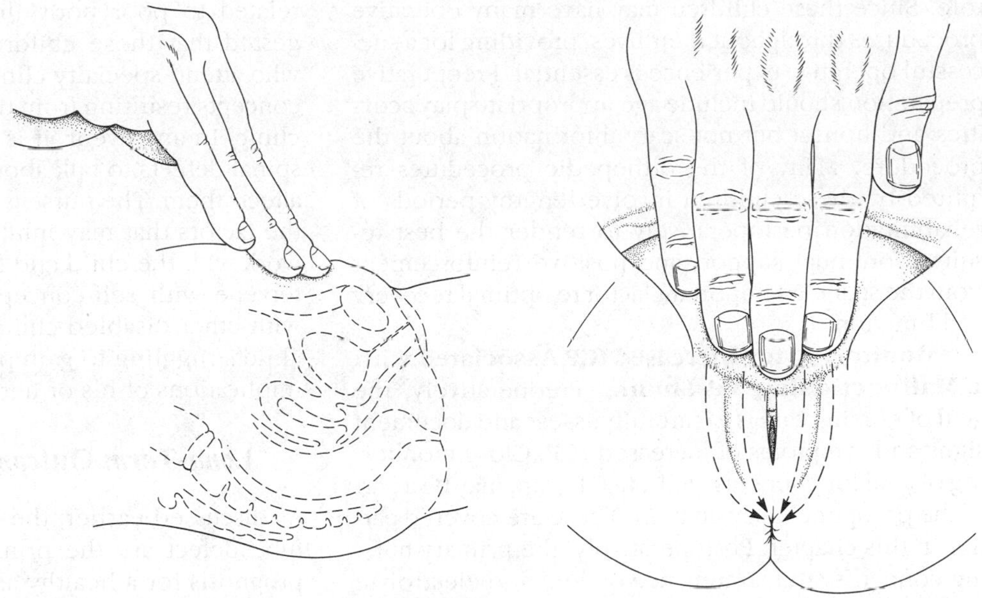

Figure 46-21. The Credé maneuver, in which external manual pressure is used, with the fingertips of one hand (for infants) pressing inward and downward over the abdomen, starting over the umbilicus and moving down below the pubis as urine is eliminated. The Credé method permits manual emptying of the bladder and is an important part of the bladder training program.

to discharge. Box 46-9 is an example of a discharge teaching checklist that is helpful in organizing and planning for nursing care.

The remaining goals and strategies are based upon the nursing diagnoses identified for long-term follow-up.

Preventing Urinary Tract Infection. Urinary tract infections (UTIs) are usually managed with a bladder program that includes the Credé maneuver, a program of intermittent catheterization, or in more severe cases, surgical diversion to protect the upper urinary tracts from infection. As children approach school age, they are taught to catheterize themselves. Nursing strategies include teaching children and their parents how to recognize UTIs, and administration of appropriate antibiotics. Even when the child is on a self-clean-catheterization program at home, the routine is adapted to a more sterile procedure in the hospital because of the threat of nosocomial infection. Odorous or malappearing urine, pain on urination, and hematuria are common symptoms. Because of frequent catheterization, normal urinary tract flora for these children may vary. It is the nurse's responsibility to educate the child and family in regard to the long-term effects of frequent UTIs—specifically, renal failure, and, ultimately, death.

Encouraging Proper Nutrition and Exercise. Nurses can promote healthy eating habits in accordance with the child's activities of daily living at an early age. Obesity is a common problem, particularly in adolescents with spina bifida. Involvement in wheelchair sports activities should be encouraged. Activities geared toward improving self-esteem may have a direct impact on the child's desire to maintain a normal weight. It is paramount that the nurse involve the whole family in these activities, since a program of weight maintenance or reduction will need to be a family-centered project to be truly successful.

Promoting and Supporting Mobility. Many of the hospitalizations the child with a spinal defect will encounter relate to the musculoskeletal deformities that result from neuromuscular and sensory deficits. The ultimate goal of any orthopedic devices or treatments is to provide for the most independent function possible for the individual child. Most of these children spend many hours in physical therapy sessions and on specific exercise programs at home. When surgery is required, preoperative preparation and discharge teaching are important aspects of the nurse's

Box 46-9

Discharge Teaching Check List for Parents of Infants with Spina Bifida

Wound care and dressing changes (if necessary)
Feeding
Bladder Credé maneuver
Diapering (with barrier drape if necessary)
Positioning
Skin integrity examination
Physical therapy/range-of-motion exercises
Normal infant development and stimulation
Possible complications
- Signs and symptoms of hydrocephalus or VP shunt malfunction
- Infection of wound or shunt
- Urinary tract infection

role. Since these children may have many operative procedures throughout their lives, providing for a successful operative experience is essential. Preoperative preparation should include age-appropriate play activities and honest but not scary information about the procedure. Many of the orthopedic procedures required by these children involve lengthy periods of rehabilitation postoperatively to render the best results. Continual support and positive reinforcement from the staff is an important factor to optimal recovery and function.

Monitoring for Increased ICP Associated with a Malfunctioning VP Shunt. Preoperatively, the goal of nursing care is to carefully assess and document signs and symptoms of increased ICP. Close monitoring of vital functions, as well as a CT scan, may be a part of the preoperative evaluation. These are covered earlier in this chapter. Postoperatively, the primary nursing concerns are maintenance of fluid and electrolyte balance, pain control, and assessment of neurologic functions and vital signs. The nurse should observe for redness or swelling along the shunt path, fever, and any other change in the neurologic assessment that is not consistent with the child's baseline status. Older children may suffer alterations in body image when hair has to be shaved to replace the proximal end of the shunt.

Promoting Optimal Bowel Elimination. Incontinence, diarrhea, and constipation are the three major problems experienced by children with myelomeningocele (Coffman, 1986). Two different bowel patterns can occur. The spastic bowel is one in which the external anal sphincter functions well enough to keep the anus closed.These children become constipated and need daily rectal suppositories or stimulation. Children with a flaccid bowel have a weak or absent anal sphincter, causing frequent diarrhea and bowel accidents. A bowel program is generally instituted about the time the child is a toddler. A well-balanced diet, high in fiber and low in carbohydrates, will help regulate the consistency of the stools. The regimen usually includes the use of a suppository shortly before meal time, incorporated with techniques to help evacuate the bowel, like abdominal massage or digital stimulation. It is very important that the hospital nurse follows the family's home regimen whenever possible, to provide continuity for the child. Impaction, when it occurs, can be removed with the use of a cleansing enema. It is the nurse's responsibility to ascertain the child's normal routines from the child or family and ensure compliance. If the child is not on a bowel program, but would benefit from one, the nurse should begin assessing the family's readiness, to determine if initiating a program is possible.

Promoting a Positive Self-Concept in Children With Neural Tube Defects. Any child with a chronic debilitating disease may be at risk for low self-concept related to poor body image. MacBriar (1983) suggested that those children with myelomeningocele who attend specialty clinics may have enhanced self-concepts resulting from the treatment approach of the clinic. In any event, it is important for children with spinal defects to talk about their disability and how it affects them. The nurse is in a prime position to assess the factors that may inhibit positive self-concept and work with the child and family to understand and intervene with self-concept issues. Activities planned with other disabled children are often helpful to the child struggling to gain perspective on the long-term implications of his or her disability.

Long-Term Outcome

As discussed earlier, the extent and level of a neural tube defect are the primary factors that impact the prognosis for a healthy and productive life. Children afflicted with spina bifida occulta may lead completely normal lives, while those with myelomeningoceles may always struggle with their functional limitations. It is important to remember that those children who have grown up with a positive attitude regarding their capabilities are much more likely to lead a full life than those children who have always viewed their handicap in a negative light.

Nursing Strategies for Follow-up Care in the Home or Clinic

Assess surgical wound healing.

Examine VP shunt site (if appropriate) and rule out signs and symptoms of shunt malfunction.

- Measure and plot head circumference
- Assess fontanel (if still open)
- Assess for lethargy irritability, vomiting, and fluid around shunt or along shunt pathway.

Discuss bowel and bladder patterns with parents.

Assess movement and sensation of lower extremities, including skin integrity and existence of pressure sores.

Ensure proper feeding techniques, nutrition, and growth.

Assess parental coping, problem-solving, and availability of resources.

Hydrocephalus

The term "hydrocephalus" is derived from the Greek terms "hydro," meaning water, and "cephalo," meaning brain. Hydrocephalus in simplest terms is an imbalance between the rate of production and rate of absorption of cerebrospinal fluid in the brain. This imbalance results in an excessive amount of CSF that ultimately causes increasing head growth (if the sutures are open), or signs and symptoms of increased intracranial pressure, or both. If not alleviated, chronic increased intracranial pressure can cause long-term neurologic sequelae, including blindness. The discovery of hydrocephalus in infancy or later childhood may vary considerably depending on the underlying disease process. In all cases the enlarged ventricles are caused by excess CSF that is unable to be absorbed at a rate equal to that of its production.

Etiology/Pathophysiology

In order to understand fully the various mechanisms that lead to hydrocephalus, a basic knowledge of CSF physiology and circulatory dynamics is essential. A thorough review of these concepts is located at the beginning of this chapter. Briefly, CSF is primarily manufactured in and secreted by the choroid plexus. This structure lines the floor of the lateral ventricles and the roof of the third and fourth ventricles. CSF is produced at the approximate rate of 0.3 to 0.4 ml per minute or 25 ml per hour (Milhorat, 1978). From the paired lateral ventricles, CSF is propelled in a pulsatile fashion through the foramen of Monro to the third ventricle and then through the aqueduct of Sylvius into the fourth ventricle. From the fourth ventricle the CSF flows through the foramen of Magendie and the paired foramina of Luschka into the subarachnoid space around the brain and spinal cord. The CSF is then reabsorbed by the arachnoid villi located in the dural sinuses, which are the large blood vessels draining the venous blood from the head. Small amounts of CSF are absorbed in the cells lining the ventricles and through the lymphatic system of the spinal cord. Figure 46-22 illustrates the normal flow of CSF in the brain.

There are two different ways in which hydrocephalus has historically been classified. The terms "communicating" versus "noncommunicating" hydrocephalus have been used to describe the location of obstruction in CSF flow, the latter being described as obstruction outside the ventricular system (in the cisterns or subarachnoid space), and the former being an obstruction actually located within or between the lateral and fourth ventricles. Since this classification system was somewhat confusing, a more descriptive classification system has become popular. Basically, hydrocephalus is classified as either congenital or acquired.

Congenital hydrocephalus occurs in approximately 3 to 4 per 1000 live births and is usually readily apparent at birth or in the first 2 to 4 months of life. Congenital malformations include the following: Chiari II malformations, congenital arachnoid cysts, congenital atresia of the foramina of Luschka and Magendie (Dandy-Walker cyst), and other intracranial masses including congenital tumors. Stenosis or

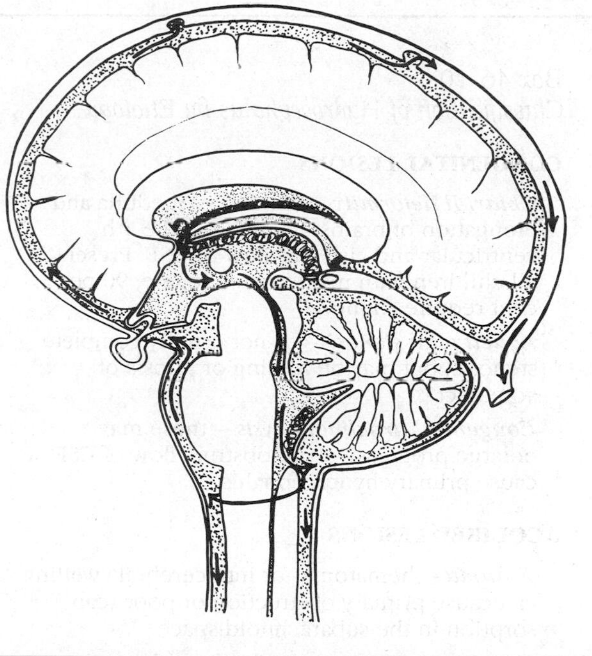

Figure 46-22. Schematic representation of cerebrospinal fluid circulation. (From Behrman RE, Vaughan VC (eds): *Nelson Textbook of Pediatrics.* 13th ed. Philadelphia, WB Saunders, 1987.)

"forking" of the aqueduct of Sylvius is a common congenital malformation that also results in hydrocephalus (Milhorat, 1978).

Acquired hydrocephalus is primarily the result of one of three processes. Infection, trauma (including hemorrhage) and neoplasms (tumors) can all result in blocked CSF passageways and ultimately hydrocephalus (O'Briens, 1982). Acquired lesions in infancy are more commonly a result of intracranial bleeding or meningitis, or both, resulting in fibrosis of the meninges preventing the reabsorption of CSF by the arachnoid villi (Milhorat, 1985). Box 46-10 outlines the various etiologies of congenital versus acquired hydrocephalus. Essentially the two primary causes of congenital or acquired hydrocephalus are (1) a blockage of the flow of CSF or (2) impaired venous absorption of CSF in the subarachnoid space. A third and extremely rare cause is the overproduction of CSF caused by a tumor identified as a choroid plexus papilloma. In any or all of the aforementioned scenarios, it is important to remember that the clinical manifestations of this disease vary with the precise cause and duration of hydrocephalus, the age of the child, and the ability of the skull to expand (Milhorat, 1985).

Diagnostic Assessment

Clinical Manifestations

Table 46-9 shown earlier in this chapter describes the signs and symptoms of increased ICP in infants and children. An abnormal increase in head circumference that goes above the established growth curve or begins

Box 46-10
Classification of Hydrocephalus by Etiology

CONGENITAL LESIONS

Chiari II deformity—kinking of medulla and elongation of brainstem obstruct the 4th ventricular and cisternal flow of CSF. Present in all children with myelomeningocele; 90 per cent require shunting

Aqueductal stenosis—is not usually complete stenosis, but may be forking or gliosis of aqueduct

Congenital arachnoid cysts—these may enlarge progressively to obstruct flow of CSF or cause primary hydrocephalus

ACQUIRED LESIONS

Trauma—hematomas or intracerebral swelling can cause primary obstruction or poor reabsorption in the subarachnoid space

Neoplasm—tumors commonly in the posterior fossa can cause obstruction of CSF flow in the 3rd and 4th ventricles

Inflammatory process

Infection: purulent exudate from meningitis may cause thickening of dural membranes and poor absorption of CSF from arachnoid villi

Hemorrhage: ventricular system is often unable to absorb products of blood breakdown leading to ventricular blockage

above the 95th percentile at birth should always raise suspicion. A full or bulging fontanel, especially one that is nonpulsatile, indicating high pressure should be noted. Other clinical signs and symptoms that become apparent as hydrocephalus progresses include increased motor tone, irritability, poor feeding, high-pitched cry, and cranial nerve palsies resulting in the classic "sunset" (or "setting sun") eyes appearance wherein the sclera are visible above the iris and the infant is unable to look upward with the head facing forward (Fig. 46-23). Distended prominent scalp veins may also be evident (Hausman, 1981).

In the older child with a fused cranium, signs and symptoms of hydrocephalus may be more worrisome. Signs of increased ICP in these children include frontal headache, and nausea and vomiting that may be projectile. If these symptoms occur upon awakening or actually wake the child, a definite suspicion of hydrocephalus should be raised. While asleep, the child retains CO_2 which in turn dilates cerebral vasculature. Upon awakening, the child's symptoms are exacerbated. Once awake and CO_2 has decreased, the symptoms may subside temporarily. Other signs and symptoms include diplopia, restlessness, personality change, and ataxia. In later stages bradycardia and/or altered respirations and seizures can become life threatening if not attended to (O'Briens, 1982).

Radiographic Findings. After a thorough neurologic examination, radiographic evidence of hydrocephalus is sought. The most widely used test is the CT scan. Besides being simple and painless it provides an excellent view of ventricular size and often shows the apparent cause of ventricular blockage. Skull roentgenographs may show signs of pressure with a "beaten silver" appearance characteristic of chronic increased ICP. Other radiographic tests include isotope cisternography or ventriculography to obtain a better assessment of how CSF flows in the brain.

Therapeutic Management

Once hydrocephalus is identified, treatment is directed to resolving the cause of obstruction. Of course, in cases of congenital hydrocephalus, this may be impossible. When hydrocephalus is acquired as an older child, the lesion causing obstruction (most frequently neoplasm) can be removed, allowing the flow of CSF to return to normal. There are cases, however, in which even complete resection fails to re-establish normal pathways, and the insertion of a mechanical shunting

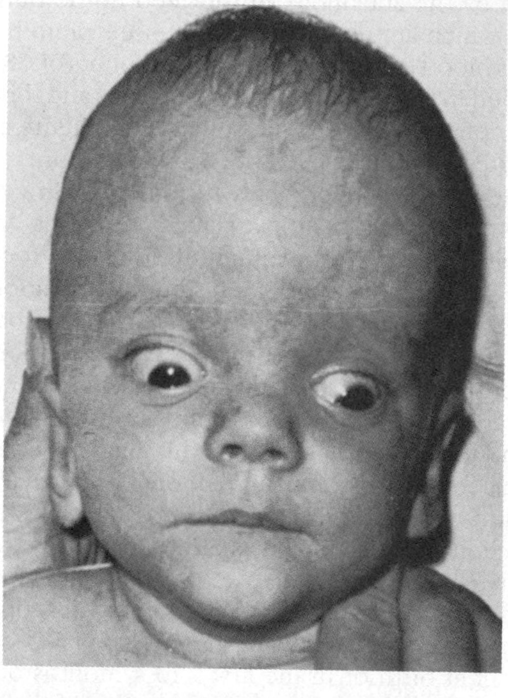

Figure 46-23. Marked hydrocephalus with "setting sun" sign and divergence of the eyes. (From Youmans JR: *Neurological Surgery.* 2nd ed. Philadelphia, WB Saunders, 1982.)

device is necessary. The only real treatment for persistent hydrocephalus is the surgical insertion of such shunting devices. Historically, shunts have been placed in nearly every body cavity. The most commonly chosen shunt today is the ventriculo-peritoneal shunt, followed by either atrial or direct cardiac shunts and, less frequently, by pleural shunts.

The three main components of mechanical shunting devices are (1) ventricular catheter, (2) reservoir and pumping device (placed directly under the scalp on the skull bones) with a one-way flow valve, and (3) distal tubing with a slit valve to regulate the flow of CSF. Newer pressure-regulated valves are now available as well. As in all mechanical devices, malfunction can and does occur. Blockage from choroid plexus or proteinaceous CSF can occur at the proximal end. The distal end can be blocked by fatty plugs or CSF pseudocysts. In any of these cases, signs and symptoms of shunt malfunction depend on the duration and extent of blockage. As expected, they do mimic signs and symptoms of increased ICP. Shunt infections although rare can be serious and difficult to eradicate. Besides several weeks of antibiotics, the shunt must be removed and replaced. A more extensive background on shunts and shunt problems is left for more specialized medical and nursing texts. The three most common locations will be addressed briefly here.

Ventriculo-peritoneal (VP) Shunt

This is the choice location for most mechanical shunts (Fig. 46-24). After insertion of the ventricular tube through a cranial burr hole, the length of the shunt is tunneled subcutaneously to the upper quadrant of the abdomen. A small incision is made and the shunt is guided into the peritoneal cavity with plenty of extra tubing to allow for growth. Specific risks of this procedure include bowel perforation and ascites if the CSF is poorly absorbed.

Ventriculo-atrial (VA) Shunt

This procedure is chosen if for some reason a concurrent abdominal problem exists precluding the insertion of a VP shunt. This shunt can be inserted into the right atrium of the heart via passage through the jugular vein or, in more extensive cases, directly into the heart. Specific risks include catheter movement, dysrhythmias, and operative risks associated with more extensive surgery.

Ventriculo-pleural Shunt

Used infrequently, this procedure is one of choice if either peritoneal or cardiac access is unobtainable. Specific risks include pleural effusion resulting in respiratory compromise or infection, or both, from stasis of respiratory secretions.

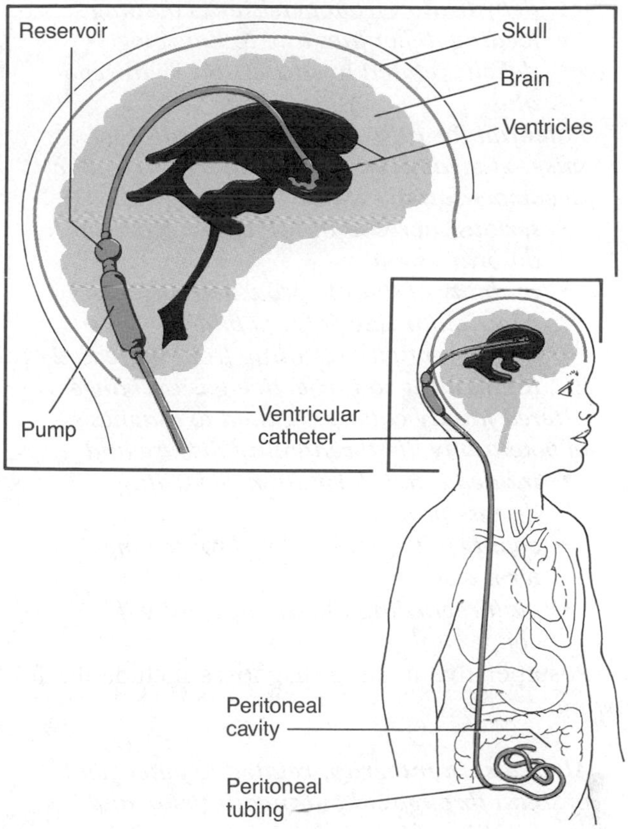

Figure 46-24. Placement of the ventriculo-peritoneal shunt.

Major Nursing Diagnoses for Hydrocephalus

Children may come to the acute care facility with signs and symptoms of hydrocephalus either before initial diagnosis or with an acute shunt malfunction, both of which require expert nursing assessment and intervention. The nurse may also care for the child postoperatively following the insertion of a ventricular shunting device. Major nursing diagnoses addressing both of these situations will be covered here.

Preoperative nursing diagnoses include the following:

Altered tissue perfusion; cerebral, *related to increased ICP as a result of hydrocephalus caused by*
- *excessive accumulation of CSF*
- *inadequate absorption of CSF*
- *lesion causing obstruction of ventricular flow*

Altered nutrition: less than body requirements, *related to*
- *decrease in appetite related to nausea and vomiting from increased ICP*

- *dehydration from persistent vomiting*
- *feeding difficulties due to neurologic deficits related to congenital hydrocephalus*

Potential for injury: neurologic compromise, *as evidenced by respiratory or cardiac decompensation related to*

- *serious increase in ICP causing pressure on brain stem*
- *inability of skull to grow with increasing ventricular size (older child)*
- *seizure activity resulting from increased ICP leading to ineffective gas exchange*

Altered family coping, *related to diagnosis of potentially life-threatening disease and*

- *inadequate information regarding disease process*
- *coping with potentially chronic long-term disease*
- *guilt regarding illness, especially if congenital*

Postoperative nursing diagnoses include the following:

Altered skin integrity, *related to placement of shunt through subcutaneous tissue and*

- *fragility of infant skin*
- *immobility after surgery*

Altered comfort: pain, *related to operative manipulation*

Potential altered tissue perfusion: cerebral, *as evidenced by subdural hematoma related to too rapid shunting of CSF*

Potential for infection, *related to*

- *insertion of foreign body into cranium*
- *poor skin integrity*

Disturbance in self-concept: body image, *related to*

- *hair loss required for operation*
- *visibility of shunt*
- *possible restrictions on activities*

Strategies for Nursing Care

Assessing and Intervening in the Event of Increased ICP. Once the nurse has identified the child with increasing ICP from hydrocephalus, many interventions can take place prior to surgery to alleviate the pressure. The head of the bed should be elevated to 30 degrees. Measuring head circumference for infants once or twice daily is important, to document any acute increase in head size. This measurement as well as an assessment of the size and bulging or flatness of fontanels should be recorded regularly. Intravenous hydration may be necessary if the child is vomiting. This should be administered at a rate of no greater than 75 to 80 per cent maintenance fluid requirements. Other nursing interventions include decreasing external stimuli and having O_2 and suction ready at the bedside. Preoperative teaching and preparation with the child and family should begin as soon as the decision to place a shunt has been made.

Ensuring Adequate Nutrition. Small frequent feedings may be necessary to ensure nutrition preoperatively. Feeding the child in a manner that allows for the least movement after the feeding may also decrease vomiting. The most effective resolution to this problem is to alleviate the cause of the problem by surgically shunting the enlarged ventricles. Electrolytes should be monitored in cases of prolonged emesis.

Preventing Neurologic Compromise. Frequent vital signs and neurologic checks are important in monitoring subtle changes that may lead to impending deterioration. Assessment of pupil size, equality, and reaction time as well as overall level of consciousness and responsiveness should be noted. Irregular respirations or bradycardia or both should be reported to the physician immediately. A cardiorespiratory monitor and oxygen with a bag and mask should be readily available. If apparent, seizure activity should be monitored and documented closely and the physician notified. Most importantly, the nurse needs to be certain that neurologic assessments are done, even if it means waking the child from a sound sleep to do so.

Promoting Family Coping. This nursing diagnosis is appropriate for all neurologic disorders. For children with hydrocephalus, families must cope with the thought of a mechanical device in their child's head for a lifetime. Guilt regarding activities during pregnancy may also be apparent, especially if the child is born with a large head. The nurse is in a prime position to provide clear and concise information to the family and offer support and referral to other resources as necessary. If a shunt is required, showing the family a child who already has one in place may ease their anxiety about the size and appearance of the device.

The remaining goals and strategies relate to nursing diagnoses for postoperative care.

Preventing Skin Breakdown. Many children who require ventricular shunting have fragile infant skin. Nursing interventions include avoiding cardiac lead patches, temperature probes, or unnecessary tape over the shunt site. Careful attention should be given to the scalp as it is often stretched and more prone to breakdown. The use of a foam donut in which to place the child's head is helpful, particularly when a long period of immobility is called for. Frequent repositioning or light massage to bony prominences, or both, is also helpful.

Providing Pain Relief. Both pharmacologic and

nonpharmacologic comfort measures should be employed to keep the child comfortable in the postoperative period (see Table 29-4). Analgesics should be carefully titrated to provide relief, while allowing for adequate neurologic assessment.

Assessing for Decreased Cerebral Perfusion or Subdural Hematoma. Children who experience a rapid decrease in intracranial pressure and ventricular size are prone to develop brain sag and subdural fluid collections. This is assessed by watching for signs of increasing neurologic deterioration after initially appearing better, or signs of slow and incomplete recovery. Any of these overall trends should be reported to the physician so that appropriate radiographic tests can be ordered.

Preventing Infection. The nursing interventions for this diagnosis are similar to those for promoting skin integrity. The nurse must pay close attention to the integrity of the surgical incisions and make sure that the child keeps his or her hands away from the fresh incision. A stockinette cap may be a useful aid. Appropriate administration of antibiotics is essential as well.

Promoting a Healthy Body Image. Older children undergoing neurosurgery for a shunt frequently are very focused on the issues of hair loss and the visibility of the mechanical device. Dealing with these issues openly and allowing these children to express their fears is helpful. Encouraging them to talk about how they normally cope with stressful events can often help them identify and capitalize on their personal strength. Introducing them to other children with similar problems can also be a useful intervention as they can relate to their peers on the same level.

Long-Term Outlook

With the improvement of shunting devices and techniques for surgical management of hydrocephalus, the long-term survival of these children has been greatly enhanced. The morbidity of children with hydrocephalus is often related to the success of the shunting procedure, the need for revisions, and the underlying disease process (O'Briens, 1982). In general, the long-term neurologic sequelae of hydrocephalus are directly related to the underlying disease process and its association with other congenital defects or problems. For example, children with straightforward hydrocephalus from aqueductal stenosis may lead a completely normal life after shunting is accomplished.

Nursing Strategies for Follow-up Care in the Home or Clinic

Educate parents as to signs and symptoms of shunt malfunction.

Observe and help parents in their handling of the infant with a shunt.

Assess adequate safety in the home and review any potential restrictions for the child set forth by the physician.

Review follow-up needs and when to call the physician regarding problems.

Perform a neurologic assessment of the child and compare with baseline.

Examine shunt incisional areas for redness, swelling, or exudate.

Chiari II Malformation (Arnold-Chiari Malformation)

Since the late 1800s, the term "Arnold-Chiari malformation" has been used to describe a developmental anomaly of the structures at the junction of the brain and spinal cord. This anatomic area is often referred to as the cervicomedullary junction. Oakes (1985), after investigating the historic aspects of this anomaly, determined that very little insight to the problem was actually added by Arnold to Chiari's original descriptions of the various degrees of hindbrain herniation. Even though two of Arnold's colleagues coined the term "Arnold-Chiari malformation" in 1907, it is not truly representative of the contributions of various individuals, and therefore is slowly being replaced with the term "Chiari II malformation" (Oakes, 1985). Chiari actually described four different types of hindbrain anomalies; however, the type II anomaly is the one most commonly seen in the pediatric population, specifically in children with myelodysplasia. Therefore, it will be the only one discussed here.

Two other diagnoses that should be mentioned in conjunction with Chiari malformations are *syringomyelia*, or *syrinx*, and *hydromyelia*. The former describes a cavity lying outside the central canal area of the spinal cord that is not lined by ependymal cells, while the latter is a cavity within the spinal cord that is partially or completely lined with ependyma. All three of these diagnoses are frequently discussed in conjunction with each other because of their similar clinical presentations and their probable common pathophysiologic development (Oakes, 1985).

Etiology and Pathophysiology

Chiari II deformities are nearly always associated with myelodysplasia. There are several theories related to the pathogenesis of this malformation. Initially it was thought that the downward traction on the spinal cord caused by an open NTD pulled on the brain stem and cerebellum causing malalignment of the cervical

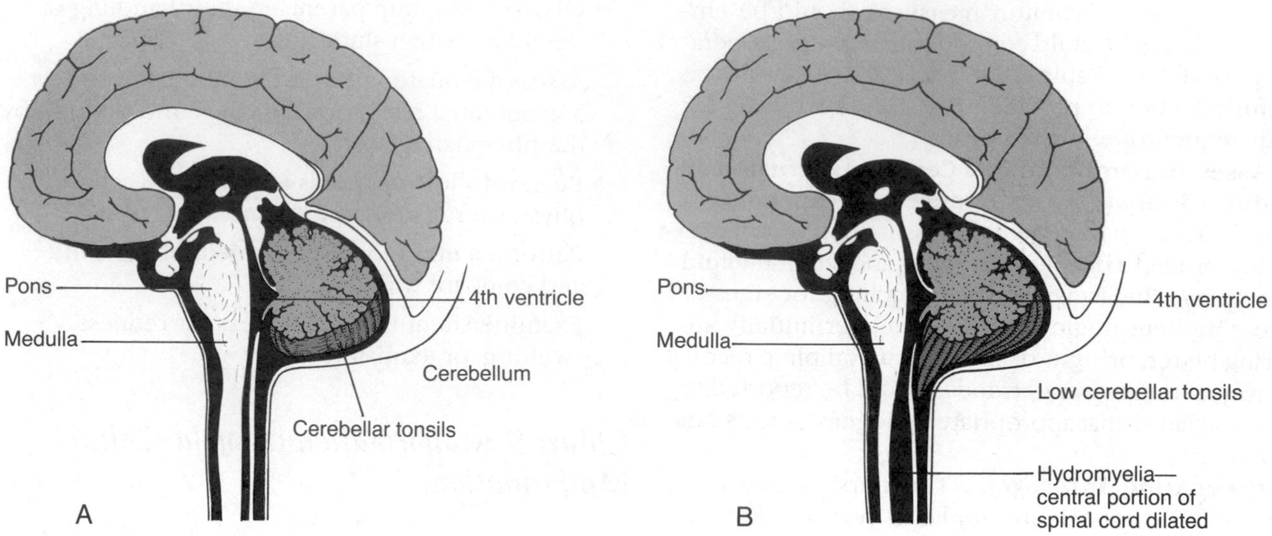

Figure 46-25. *A*, Anatomy of the normal posterior fossa. *B*, Arnold-Chiari malformation with hydromyelia.

nerve roots. Later theories have discredited this early view and attribute the malformation to actual dysgenesis of the brain stem, causing it to elongate into the cervical canal. Caudal displacement of the cerebellum and brain stem results. Still another theory points to alterations in cerebrospinal fluid (CSF) dynamics at the craniospinal junction. Although all of these theories have led to a better understanding of the problem, there is yet to be a universally accepted concept for this disease (Guin, 1985).

What occurs in the Chiari II malformation is that the cerebellar tonsils and medulla are displaced downward through the foramen magnum. This causes elongation of the fourth ventricle, which may obliterate the foramina of Magendie and Luschka, thereby causing hydrocephalus. The cranial nerves (particularly those that originate on the medulla) become stretched, and are the cause of many of the signs and symptoms. Figure 46-25 shows the anatomic aspects of this deformity.

Although the majority of children with myelodysplasia are born with the Chiari II deformity, no more than one third of these children will develop Chiari II symptoms in infancy. Most of these infants will eventually improve on their own after 6 to 12 months of age. Many will develop apneic spells and associated problems leading to death before the age of 2 (Oakes, 1985).

Diagnostic Assessment

The two main components of the diagnostic assessment are the clinical examination and roentgenographic studies. The clinical examination focuses on the most common signs and symptoms of the Chiari II malformation. These include the following: nystagmus, nuchal rigidity, poor suck reflex, drooling, difficulty swallowing, vomiting, weak or absent cry, and inspiratory stridor when agitated. In more severe cases, episodes of apnea may be reported by the parents. In older children, decreased strength in upper extremities with increased tone and exaggerated deep tendon reflexes may also be present.

Radiographic techniques are used to demonstrate the type and extent of the lesion, including the presence of hydromyelia or hydrocephalus. Plain roentgenographs of the skull and spine are taken. A myelogram is also performed to identify the anatomy of the upper spinal cord. In some cases, an angiogram is helpful in identifying the peculiarities of blood flow to the cervicomedullary junction. Today the use of magnetic resonance imaging is beginning to replace the use of more invasive techniques. MRI is particularly useful to identify the anatomy in this area and to provide for accurate diagnosis without the need for many other procedures (Guin, 1985).

Therapeutic Management

Initially, if signs and symptoms are not life threatening, a conservative approach may be advocated in the hope that the child will stabilize and outgrow the symptoms. When more severe problems like apnea or frequent aspiration pneumonia are apparent, surgery must be undertaken. The surgical procedure of choice is called a posterior fossa decompression. It involves removing the posterior aspect of the foramen magnum and excision of the upper cervical vertebral arches. This decompression alleviates the pressure on the fourth ventricle and the affected cranial nerves, hopefully allowing for an arrest of symptom progression. With some children, there is only little objective improvement. In these cases, the preoperative deficits may be permanent (Guin, 1985). In rare instances where a ventriculoperitoneal shunt is not already in place, it may be placed in conjunction with, or instead of, the posterior fossa decompression (AANN, 1984).

Major Nursing Diagnoses for Chiari II Malformation

These may relate to preoperative care, postoperative care, or both. They will be designated as such here.

Potential for infection: respiratory, *related to aspiration pneumonia caused by (preoperative and postoperative):*
- *absent or weak gag reflex or swallow reflex or both*
- *relative inactivity and inability to clear respiratory secretions*

Ineffective breathing pattern: episodic apnea, *related to:*
- *compression of cranial nerves and medulla (preoperative)*
- *operative swelling or effects of anesthesia (postoperative)*

Altered comfort: pain, *related to surgical intervention (postoperative):*
- *lengthy operative course*
- *failure to maintain adequate blood levels of analgesia*

Potential ineffective family coping, (pre- and postoperatively, *related to:*
- *further treatment for already chronically debilitated child*
- *depleted family financial and emotional resources*
- *inadequate knowledge about the disease process*

Strategies for Nursing Care

Preventing Respiratory Infection. Infants or children with poor gag and swallow reflexes should be fed slowly, and placed in an upright position after feeding to avoid aspiration and recurrent pneumonia. Solids may be difficult to swallow for these children, so food may need to be pureed. Postural drainage or chest physiotherapy may need to be instituted when aspiration has occurred. Nurses caring for children with Chiari II malformations should plan daily activities so that feedings are uninterrupted, and activities that may induce vomiting or aspiration take place just prior to feeding rather than immediately after.

Avoiding Respiratory Distress. A complete and thorough baseline neurologic assessment is essential for these children. Frequent examination and preparedness for resuscitation are important aspects of nursing care. Placing the child on an apnea monitor and having oxygen and suction available at the bedside may be necessary. Documenting consistent changes in the respiratory pattern, and alerting the physician to any significant changes, is also of vital importance. The effects of various nursing interventions on overall neurologic status should be documented in the care plan, so that trends in patient status can be easily recognized.

Managing Postoperative Pain Effectively. Adequate control of postoperative pain in these children is a difficult nursing challenge. Care should be taken to avoid overmedication, thereby negating the use of a neurologic assessment to signal changes or decline in patient status. Even when the child is resting comfortably after medication, neurologic assessments should be done as ordered, or more frequently, if indicated. A good blood level of analgesics should be maintained, so that the child is not experiencing periods of excruciating pain requiring large amounts of narcotic analgesics at one time. Nursing care should always incorporate nonpharmacologic methods of pain control into the patient care plan.

Promoting Family Coping. Families of children with chronic health problems need continual support from the nursing staff through their many hospitalizations. The importance of continuity of nursing staff and primary nursing cannot be overemphasized. Parents may see the hospitalization as a break from their daily care routines, and need to spend time away from the hospital. The nursing staff should give them permission to do so, while identifying which aspects of care the parent(s) would like to participate in and supporting them in their participation. Well siblings may also need some extra attention during hospitalization. Nurses can be advocates for the siblings and the ill child, and provide overall support for family cohesion.

Nursing Strategies for Follow-up Care in the Home or Clinic

Assess and document neurologic baseline, and any changes in examination.

Assess risk for potentially serious respiratory problems.

Postoperatively, assess incision for healing, redness, or irritation.

Assess need for occupational therapy to adapt feeding or stimulation programs to meet child's functional capacity.

Offer support and encouragement to family, assessing the need for resources and assistance.

Epilepsy

A seizure is a sudden, involuntary, time-limited alteration in function occurring as the result of an abnormal discharge of neurons in the central nervous system (Holmes, 1987). The terms "seizure" and "epilepsy" are not synonymous. Epilepsy is a *chronic* condition characterized by seizures. There are many types of seizures that do not fall under the classification of epilepsy. Box 46-11 contains examples of nonepileptic seizures.

Although epilepsy indicates a chronic seizure disorder it does not necessarily mean the disease will last the patient's entire lifetime. Remissions of childhood epilepsy occur quite frequently (Holmes, 1987). Epilepsy is not a single disease entity but rather represents any number of conditions with underlying brain dysfunction.

Incidence and Etiology

Holmes (1987) reported that various studies have shown the incidence of epilepsy to range from 11 to 49 cases per 100,000 population. Incidence for developing epilepsy appears to be highest in the first year of life. There are multiple causes of epilepsy, depending on the nature of the underlying brain pathology. Although the exact genetic components have not been identified there is known to be a familial predisposition to epilepsy.

Pathophysiology

In normal brain activity certain groups of neurons are active (firing) in the process of thinking, hearing, moving, or other activities, while other groups of neurons are less active and still others are inactive at that moment. During a seizure, for reasons poorly understood, groups of neurons all activate at the same time, causing a sudden burst of electrical activity in the brain and disrupting normal brain function. In a partial seizure this burst of activity is confined, initially, to one hemisphere of the brain and effect on brain function is limited or "focal." In a generalized seizure, however, the abnormal electrical activity occurs throughout the brain and all cortical functions are disrupted (Friedman, 1988).

Clinical Manifestations of Epileptic Seizures

Because epilepsy comprises a group of varied disorders characterized by chronic seizures, classification of the types of epileptic seizures is difficult. Various systems have been used in the past but the one most frequently used in the current medical and nursing literature is the International Classification of Epileptic Seizures (Dreifuss, 1981). According to that classification, there are two types of partial seizures (simple and complex) and four types of generalized seizures (generalized tonic-clinic, absence, myoclonic, and atonic) (Box 46-12).

"Clonic" and "tonic" are terms frequently used to describe seizure activity. *Clonic* refers to alternate involuntary muscular contraction and relaxation that occurs in rapid succession, such as a rapid patting action of the hand or jerking movements. *Tonic* (as in muscle *tone*) refers to stiffening or rigidity of muscle groups.

Box 46-11
Common Causes of Seizures in Different Age Groups

NEONATAL (BIRTH TO 28 DAYS)

Asphyxia
Intracranial hemorrhage
- subarachnoid hemorrhage
- periventricular-intraventricular hemorrhage
- subdural hemorrhage

Hypocalcemia
Hypomagnesemia
Hypoglycemia
Hyponatremia/hypernatremia
Infection
- intrauterine
- postnatal

Congenital CNS malformations
Inborn errors of metabolism
Drug withdrawal
Accidental injection of anesthetic

INFANCY TO ADOLESCENCE

Chronic conditions continuing from neonatal period
Infection
- meningitis
- encephalitis

Trauma
Neoplasms
Degenerative disorders
Idiopathic
Genetic disorders

(From Holmes, 1987.)

Partial Seizures

In partial seizures the group of neurons involved in abnormal firing is initially confined to one hemisphere of the brain. The abnormal electrical activity may spread to involve the entire brain. Partial seizures are further classified according to whether consciousness is lost during the attack. In a simple partial seizure consciousness is not impaired, whereas a complex partial seizure involves altered consciousness or awareness.

Simple Partial Seizures. Simple partial seizures are usually brief, often lasting less than a minute (Holmes, 1987). Clinical manifestations are determined by the area of the brain involved (Figure 46-4). For example, if the neuronal burst occurs in the occipital region, vision will be altered. Motor involvement is the most common type of partial seizure; in fact, this type of seizure was formerly called a focal motor (or jacksonian) seizure. Clonic seizure activity is typically limited to one muscle group (such as the fingers) or a contiguous group of muscles (as in an arm or leg). Involvement may spread from this initial site to involve all the muscles on one side of the body, a phenomenon formerly labeled "jacksonian march." Transient paralysis of the involved muscle groups (lasting up to 24 hours) may follow a simple partial seizure, especially in young children.

Simple partial seizures which begin in the parietal lobe are associated with sensory symptoms such as a "needles and pins" sensation or a feeling of numbness. Autonomic symptoms, which may occur with either simple or complex partial seizures, include vomiting, pallor, flushing, sweating, dizziness, erection of body hairs, pupillary dilation, tachycardia, incontinence, and other autonomic functions (Holmes, 1987).

Complex Partial Seizures. Complex partial seizures originate in a temporal lobe, the seat of memory and emotion. Some children with complex partial seizures experience a *prodrome*; that is, they are aware of an impending seizure days or hours before it occurs. A prodrome differs from an aura in that a prodrome is not part of the actual seizure (*ictal*) event. An *aura* is an ictal phenomenon; it is part of the actual seizure activity. It is that portion of the seizure that occurs before consciousness is lost and for which memory is retained when consciousness is regained (Holmes, 1987). Auras vary considerably among individuals; children may experience sensory (e.g., visual, auditory, olfactory, gustatory) symptoms, visceral sensations, or complex subjective experiences such as fear, embarrassment, or dizziness. Following the loss of consciousness various types of automatic behavior (automatisms) may occur such as chewing, gagging, choking, lip smacking, spitting, waving, clapping, scratching, masturbatory behavior, walking, skipping, running, screaming, crying, or laughing. Because of the bizarre behavior associated with this type of seizure it was formerly termed a psychomotor seizure. Upon regaining consciousness (the *postical* period) the child often feels tired and falls asleep. If the attack is brief, however, normal alertness may return almost immediately.

Box 46-12
Classification of Partial and Generalized Seizures

Partial Seizures (initial changes confined to one hemisphere)
- Simple partial seizure (formerly called focal motor or focal sensory seizure)
  No impairment of consciousness
- Complex partial seizure (formerly called psychomotor seizure)
  Altered consciousness (i.e., altered responsiveness, altered awareness)

Generalized Seizures (disturbance involves entire brain; loss of consciousness occurs)
- Generalized tonic-clonic seizure (formerly called grand mal seizure)
- Absence seizure (formerly called petit mal seizure)
- Myoclonic seizure (infantile spasms are a type of myoclonic seizure)
- Atonic seizure (formerly called drop attacks)

Generalized Seizures

Generalized seizures affect the entire brain. They may begin with generalized electrical bursts or spread from what were initially localized sites. Although children with generalized seizures always lose consciousness, the loss may be so brief as to go unnoticed.

Generalized Tonic-Clonic (GTC) seizures. Generalized tonic-clonic seizures were formerly called "grand mal seizures." These seizures may be preceded by both a prodromal phase and an aura. If an aura is experienced it indicates that the seizure began focally (as a partial seizure) and then spread throughout the brain. Typically GTC seizures involve five recognizable phases: flexion, extension, tremor, clonic, and postical (Holmes, 1987).

Consciousness is lost during the brief (5-second) *flexion* phase. It usually begins in the face with the eyes rolling upward and the mouth opening with jaw muscles rigid. Flexion of the extremities follows. The *extension* (tonic) phase (lasting 10 to 30 seconds) begins with extension of the back and neck and includes extension of the legs. The jaws clamp together tightly and tongue biting can occur. Apnea may begin with the rigid extension of thoracic and abdominal muscles and persist through the clonic phase. The *tremor* phase (5 to 10 seconds) marks the transition between the tonic and clonic phases. Fine tremors usually begin in the extremities and spread proximally. The *clonic* phase may last 30 to 50 seconds. The char-

Table 46-13. Properties and Toxic Reactions of Commonly Used Anticonvulsants

Drug	Serum t½* (hours)	Therapeutic Blood Level (μg/mL)	Starting Dosage (mg/kg/Day)	Daily Doses	Days to Attain Steady State Blood Level	How Supplied	Life-Threatening Side Effects	Other Side Effects
Phenobarbital	36–72	10–30	2–3	1 or 2	14–21	Elixir: 4 mg/mL; tablets: 15, 30, 60, and 100 mg	Stevens-Johnson syndrome (rare); blood dyscrasias (rare)	Hyperkinesis; drowsiness; drug rash
Primidone	6–18	5–10	5	2 or 3	4–7	Tablets: 50 and 250 mg; Suspension: 50 mg/mL	Same as phenobarbital	
Phenytoin	15–45	10–20	5–7	2	7–21	Tablet: 50 mg; Capsules: 30 and 100 mg	Stevens-Johnson syndrome (rare); acute hepatic necrosis (rare); blood dyscrasias (rare)	Drug rash (10% in first 2 weeks), gingival hyperplasia, lymphadenopathy, hirsutism, acromegaloid facies, ataxia, nystagmus, vomiting, dystonic reaction, rickets, folate deficiency, embryopathy (fetal hydantoin syndrome) if used during pregnancy
Carbamazepine	8–20	5–10	10–15	2 or 3	5–10	Tablets: 100 and 200 mg	Leukopenia, thrombocytopenia, aplastic anemia (rare)	Drowsiness, abdominal distress
Valproic acid	6–14	40–80	10–20	3 or 4	4	Capsules: 250 mg; Syrup: 50 mg/mL	Acute hepatic failure (Reye syndrome-like)	Hyperammonemia, drowsiness, alopecia, abdominal discomfort
Ethosuximide	24–36	40–80	10–20	2	5–8	Capsules: 250 mg; Syrup: 50 mg/mL	Blood dyscrasias (very rare)	Drowsiness, nausea
Clonazepam	20–32	0.015–0.04	0.04–0.05	2	10–14	Tablets: 0.5, 1, and 2 mg	Blood dyscrasias (very rare)	Drowsiness (common)
Acetazolamide	4–10	—	10–20	2 or 3	3	Tablets: 125 and 250 mg	Blood dyscrasias (very rare)	Metabolic acidosis, paresthesias, anorexia, weight loss

* t½ = half-life
(From Behrman and Vaughan, 1987.)

acteristic rhythmic jerking is orchestrated by rapid contraction and relaxation of opposing muscle groups. The jerking decreases in frequency as this phase nears completion. Apnea frequently lasts through the clonic phase, causing increasing cyanosis. Secretions pool in the mouth and throat, leading to noisy respirations. This can be a difficult stage for observers because the child appears in great distress, yet nothing can interrupt the seizure. After the last clonic jerk the bladder sphincter relaxes and incontinence may occur. In the immediate *postical* phase the child will still be unconscious, but relaxation of muscles will result in a flaccid posture. Cyanosis resolves as breathing returns to normal, but pallor often lingers. The child may either gradually awaken or progress directly into a sleeping state.

Absence Seizures. This type of generalized seizure was formerly called "petit mal." Occurrence of these seizures is uncommon. It consists of a sudden, brief (usually no longer than 30 seconds) arrest of motor activity accompanied by a blank stare and loss of awareness. Posture is maintained. At the end of the seizure the child returns to the activity that was in progress as though nothing had happened. Interruption of mental activity may be incomplete, allowing the child to continue simple or automatic behavior during the lapse of full mental function. There is no memory of the seizure but the child may be aware of a "time loss."

Myoclonic Seizures. The term "myoclonus" means a quick movement of a muscle. Myoclonic seizures, then, are characterized by sudden, brief jerks of muscle groups. Flexor muscles are often involved on both sides of the body, resulting in sudden falls for older children or *infantile spasms* for infants. Consciousness is lost for only about 5 seconds, and may therefore go unobserved. Myoclonic seizures may occur in clusters, either several in a row or several during a day's time.

Atonic Seizures. Atonic seizures involve a sudden loss of muscle tone and loss of consciousness. With a brief attack the head may drop suddenly or the child may fall. More prolonged attacks may begin with a fall but then continue with the child lying limp and unresponsive for seconds or minutes (Huttenlocher, 1987). Longer attacks are usually followed by a period of postictal drowsiness.

Therapeutic Management

Therapeutic management of chronic seizure activity includes anticonvulsant drugs, education of the family and child and attention to associated emotional or learning disabilities. The goal of drug therapy is to control the seizures with as few drug side effects as possible.

The drug of choice for absence seizures is ethosuximide (Zarontin). The major anticonvulsants for the other forms of epilepsy are phenobarbital, phenytoin (Dilantin) carbamazepine (Tegretol), and valproic acid (Depakene) (Huttenlocher, 1987). The properties and toxic reactions of these and other commonly used anticonvulsants are listed in Table 46-13. Drug treatment typically begins with one anticonvulsant agent, with the dosage increased gradually either until seizures are controlled, clinical manifestations of toxicity are experienced, or serum drug levels reach the high end of the therapeutic range without controlling seizures. If the first drug proves ineffective, a second will be added or another drug tried. During this process it is essential that the child and family be aware of the need to report changes in sensation and behavior that may signal a toxic reaction and that they understand the importance of close follow-up care. Serum blood levels will be drawn frequently until it is determined how a particular drug is metabolized by a particular child.

Anticonvulsant therapy is usually continued until the child has been seizure free for 2 to 3 years (Holmes, 1987). In the young child anticonvulsants may be discontinued earlier than this because rapid brain development has the potential to raise the seizure threshold. In any case, anticonvulsant drugs are always tapered in dosage to the point of complete withdrawal; the drug should not be stopped suddenly.

Strategies for Nursing Care

Nursing care is focused on the physical and mental attitude of the child and family. Today's child with epilepsy is more fortunate than such children even 50 years ago, since there is now a healthier attitude toward seizure disorders. With more information available to the public, some of traditional stigma attached to the disease is lessening. School-age children with epilepsy have a complex problem, since they have a strong need for peer approval and acceptance. Physical changes and stress may trigger a seizure and they may resent having to take medication, or they may not want their peers to know about their condition for fear of rejection.

Nursing care of an epileptic child hospitalized for the disease must be given objectively, with an adequate understanding of the disease and its treatment. Since the first exposure to a seizure is a frightening experience, the nurse should seek opportunities to view films or to observe a child having a seizure before caring for such a child. Seizure activity is bizarre and nurses must be comfortable with their own feelings about it.

Not all children who have seizures are hospitalized; it is only for further diagnostic evaluations and control of lengthy seizure activity that hospitalization is required. Diagnostic tests include skull roentgenographs, brain scans, pneumoencephalograms, and EEGs. Electroencephalograms record the cyclic changes in the brain and help localize involved areas. Interpreting EEGs in children is much more difficult than in adults because of the wide ranges of normality in children. This study is informative but is not a substitute for further types of diagnostic evaluation. It is imperative that the nurse explain procedures to the child and any other significant persons. Coloring books and cartoons are available to help inform the child about various diagnostic tests as well as the disease itself. Children should be allowed to express their feelings through conversation or drawings. Questions must be answered simply and honestly. Assure the child that many people with epilepsy are able to lead quite normal, productive, happy lives.

Epilepsy cannot be cured, but most seizure activity can be controlled by medicine. Various medications are effective for different types of epilepsy. The nurse must understand the function of the medication and its side effects and must be sure to record any suggestive symptoms. Medication must be given regularly.

Some drugs have the potential for creating an adverse effect on the hematopoietic system, liver, and kidneys. This may become manifest through symptoms such as fever, sore throat, enlarged lymph nodes, epistaxis, and petechiae. It is the nurse's responsibility to know the medication and be alert to the action of the drug and its possible toxic effects. This information must be shared with the family.

Encourage the family to allow the child to engage in competitive sports if the child so desires, and to minimize their comments on the child's epilepsy. If the disease is accepted matter of factly and explained in terms peers will understand, the child will more likely be accepted and social stigma can be avoided.

Siblings are a vital part of the team. Their social life should not be affected because there is epilepsy in the family. They play a vital role in helping the affected child find acceptance in school. After the child is diagnosed as being epileptic, the school nurse or teacher should prepare the students for the child's return by explaining the pathology of epilepsy. This will greatly lessen the child's anxiety. The school-age child is especially at risk for absenteeism if seizures are not controlled. This can hinder academic achievement. Some epileptic children are also mentally retarded, but the majority are of average intelligence. In general, intelligence is more apt to suffer if (1) seizures begin at a young age, (2) the child has symptomatic (versus idiopathic) epilepsy, and (3) seizures are of the following type: atypical absences, infantile spasms, or tonic seizures (Holmes, 1987).

A staff conference at school, including the physical educator, can be a means to define the child's needs. The staff should know the type of medication the child is taking and any side effects. Encourage the family to provide a Medic-Alert* identification bracelet for the child to wear at all times. There is a tendency for school personnel to either pamper the child or restrict activities unduly. If the child has akinetic seizures, a helmet might be needed when the child is engaged in physical activity, since this type of seizure is difficult to control. The helmet should be removed during sedentary activity to minimize the child's being labeled as "different."

Parents' acceptance of this condition can never be hurried. The nurse should allow the parents to stand away and watch the child's activity during a seizure with someone else helping the child. Explain what is happening, and encourage calmness and confidence. Involve the family in the plan of care during a seizure. Assure them that the most important intervention is to prevent the child from injury and to maintain a patent airway. Nothing can be done to stop the seizure. No attempt should be made to hold the child or resist seizure activity. If the child is in bed, the siderails or crib sides should be padded. Clothing should be loosened and toys that could injure or suffocate the child removed. If possible, have the child lie on a side to aid breathing. Do not attempt to put anything in the child's mouth. If seizures are extreme, a suction machine or oxygen may be necessary. If the child is at home and seizures are extreme, he or she should be brought to the hospital by ambulance. After the seizure, accurate reporting should include the activity of the child before the seizure, length of seizure in minutes, the part(s) of the body involved, site where contracture or twitching began, type of movement, posture of body, and any incontinence before or after seizure activity. (See the earlier section on seizure management for more detailed nursing strategies.)

The manner and attitude of the family is very important to the child. If a seizure is handled calmly, the child will have less fear. After a seizure (or convulsion) is over, the child is frequently confused and embarrassed. Assure the child that all is well. Care is directed toward the child and not the seizure.

Long-Term Outcome

If the child is properly medicated, seizures can be controlled in over 50 per cent of cases. In an additional 30

*Medic-Alert bracelets are available at drug stores, jewelers, or the Medic-Alert Foundation, Turlock, CA 95380.

per cent, seizure activity can be reduced so that persons with epilepsy can lead normal, productive lives.

One major effort toward prevention is better postnatal care. Because of modern medical skills and technology, many high-risk infants are saved, but at the expense of some form of irreversible damage. They may have epilepsy as a secondary effect. Since there is a hereditary element in some forms of epilepsy, genetic counseling is recommended for their siblings.

The Epilepsy Foundation of America has a bibliography of literature available. Most states have an epilepsy foundation, and many communities have local chapters. Parents and families can gain strength through contacts with other parents. The foundation makes medication available at a reduced rate. Speakers are available for school or community groups. It also provides individual and group counseling.

Neurocutaneous Syndromes

The most frequently occurring neurocutaneous syndromes are collectively called *phakomatoses.* These diseases are characterized by their tendency toward tumor formation in the central nervous system, skin, and visceral linings of various organ systems and their recognizable cutaneous manifestations. Because of the rarity of these diseases, only the three most common will be addressed here. They are tuberous sclerosis, neurofibromatosis, and Sturge-Weber disease.

Pathophysiology

Tuberous sclerosis is an autosomal dominant disease affecting many organ systems. (See Chapter 4 for a discussion of patterns of inheritance.) A wide variety of clinical findings are associated with this disease, the most common being mental retardation, seizures, and adenoma sebaceum. The major organ systems that may be affected in tuberous sclerosis are the brain, skin, kidneys, heart, lungs, and bone. Growths called "tubers" may invade the brain and retina. Other types of tumors may invade the heart and kidneys (Berg, 1982).

Neurofibromatosis is also referred to as von Recklinghausen disease, so named for the man who identified it. Like tuberous sclerosis, neurofibromatosis is an autosomal dominant trait disease. Its main characteristics are areas of increased skin pigmentation (café-au-lait spots), central and peripheral nervous system tumors, and other skeletal, endocrine, and vascular findings. This disease is characterized by multiple tumors called neurofibromas occurring in a few or many organ systems of the affected child. Peripheral nerve tumors are the most common, and a higher incidence of brain tumors in these children has also been documented. Neurofibromatosis is more common in males. The first symptoms are usually cutaneous changes rather than the neurologic symptoms that often occur in later stages of the disease (Berg, 1982).

Sturge-Weber Disease (encephalofacial angiomatosis) is the only phakomatosis without a recognizable hereditary pattern. The characteristic features are a port wine stain (facial nevus), focal or generalized seizures, intracranial calcification, hemiparesis, and often, mental retardation. Abnormalities of the dura mater over the occipital lobe are common, as are calcification and necrosis of underlying brain tissue. The facial nevus is usually apparent at birth, and often it is associated with congenital glaucoma. Seizures usually begin before one year of age, and are difficult to treat. Behavior problems, mental retardation, and hemiparesis can also occur (Berg, 1982). A thorough discussion of all the neurocutaneous diseases, including many too rare to be discussed here, can be found in *The Practice of Pediatric Neurology*, 2nd edition, by Swaiman and Wright, published in 1982.

Diagnostic Assessment

The diagnosis of neurocutaneous diseases is often made on the characteristic clinical findings of each disease. A thorough genetic and family history is helpful in the diagnosis of tuberous sclerosis and neurofibromatosis. In both of these diseases, a confirmed diagnosis is made through a tissue sample of one of the characteristic lesions or tumors. Because of the wide variability of manifestations of these diseases, the diagnostic assessment may range from minimal to extensive. Some possibilities include the need for an EEG, CT scan, MRI, skin biopsy, ophthalmologic examinations, and various other tests, depending on the organ systems involved.

Therapeutic Management

Medical and/or surgical management of neurocutaneous disease in childhood is aimed at alleviating symptoms, as there are no cures for these conditions. When seizures are present, various anticonvulsant regimens may be tried until control is achieved. In some cases of Sturge-Weber disease, surgical removal of the lobes of the brain causing seizures is attempted. Any lesions of the brain (tumors, tubers, or neurofibromas) may be surgically excised, especially if they cause increased ICP. Various other orthopedic and/or plastic surgery procedures may be indicated (Berg, 1982). However, in most cases, medical care is geared toward helping the family cope with the diagnosis and the provision of expert genetic counseling to assess the probability of future children manifesting such abnormalities.

Major Nursing Diagnoses for Neurocutaneous Syndromes

Nursing care for these children is extremely individualized and depends on the clinical characteristics of the specific disease. The following nursing diagnoses, although broad in nature, may be applicable:

Potential for injury, related to:
- *uncontrolled seizure activity*
- *mental retardation or behavior problems*

Ineffective family coping, related to the magnitude of the disease:
- *possible hereditary factors*
- *limited resources to care for a chronically ill child*
- *possible multiple hospitalizations*

Knowledge deficit: family, related to:
- *denial of child's problems*
- *hereditary possibilities*
- *complexity of disease processes*

Strategies for Nursing Care

Protecting the Child from Injury. Because many neurocutaneous diseases manifest with convulsive disorders, when children with these diseases are hospitalized seizure precautions may be necessary. Such precautions include padding siderails and ensuring the availability of oxygen and suction, if necessary. It is no longer necessary to pad a tongue blade to place it in the child's mouth. Nurses caring for these children should be aware of appropriate anticonvulsant levels and possible side effects of drugs administered. Safety may also be threatened when a child displays difficult to control behavior or an element of mental retardation. It is the nurse's responsibility to assess the patients' individual potential for injury and to plan interventions to avoid possibly dangerous situations.

Promoting Effective Coping. Families facing these seemingly unexplainable and incurable diseases require ongoing support. This is especially true when the family is faced with many hospitalizations. In some instances, the nurse may need to encourage the family to explore long-term resources. With the wide variety of symptoms with these diseases, an individual assessment of each family is necessary, as some children may have few outward signs of illness. A nurse may interface with the same child several times during many hospitalizations. Continuity of nursing care can promote trust and a more positive view of the health care system for the child.

Expanding the Family Knowledge Base. Information given to families needs to be geared toward their level of understanding. Nurses may need to rely on principles of teaching and learning to plan a teaching strategy for parents. It is important to accept the initial denial and guilt that may manifest shortly after diagnosis, and to allow for its expression. Parents may need information about the genetic basis of the disease, and they should be referred for genetic counseling.

Nursing Care Strategies for Follow-Up Care in the Home or Clinic

Assess symptomatic problems:
- Seizures
- Visual deficits
- Orthopedic problems

Assess parental knowledge base in regard to the disease process. Give information as appropriate.

If neurosurgery has occurred, check for signs and symptoms of infection or increased intracranial pressure.

Identify the need for genetic counseling and make appropriate referrals.

Neurodegenerative Disorders

The large and diverse group of diseases characterized by progressive loss of central neurologic function are collectively referred to as neurodegenerative diseases. The occurrence and correct diagnosis of these disorders during infancy and childhood is a common and challenging clinical problem. The diversity of the numerous diseases in this category and the lack of definitive knowledge regarding their etiology have lead to some confusion among health care professionals, and ultimately among families and children facing these diagnoses (Dyken and Krawiecki, 1983). For the purposes of this text, basic definitions and categories will be discussed with the most common disease entities listed. Generalized nursing diagnoses applicable to many or all of the neurodegenerative disorders will be identified. Nursing care should be individualized to the specific disease process and overall needs of the child and family.

Etiology/Pathophysiology

There are many possible causes of neurologic deterioration in children that must be ruled out before a diagnosis of neurodegenerative disease is made. Some of these include neoplasms, infection, trauma, or vascular disorders (Allen et al, 1982). Once other possibilities are ruled out, disorders of myelination are consid-

Table 46-14. Classification of Neurodegenerative Diseases in Infancy and Childhood

General Classification	Disease Name	Comments
Polioencephalopathies *Anatomic location:* Cerebral cortex	*Genetic* Neuronal ceroid lipofuscinoses (NCL) Hereditary poliodystrophy *Nongenetic* West disease Hypoxic degenerative polioencephalopathy with spasms Idiopathic sporadic polioencephalopathy	All genetic polioencephalopathies are referred to as poliodystrophies
Leukoencephalopathies *Anatomic location:* Subcortical white matter	*Genetic* Adrenoleukodystrophy Metachromatic leukodystrophy *Nongenetic* Subacute sclerosing panencephalitis (SSPE) Schilder encephalitis periaxalis diffusa Disseminated sclerosis (multiple sclerosis)	All genetic leukoencephalopathies referred to as leukodystrophies Usually early adult onset (20–30 yr)
Corencephalopathies *Anatomic location:* Deep telencephalic, diencephalic, or mesencephalic structures, including both gray and white matter, the extrapyramidal system, and the upper brain stem	*Genetic* Huntington disease Familial deteriorating extrapyramidal syndrome Ataxia telangiectasia *Nongenetic* Idiopathic subcortical degeneration with extrapyramidal symptoms	All genetic corencephalopathies referred to as cordystrophies
Diffuse Encephalopathies *Anatomic location:* Diffuse anatomic involvement or unclear anatomic localization	*Genetic* Tuberous sclerosis with degeneration *Nongenetic* Idiopathic degenerative encephalopathy Hypoxic degenerative encephalopathy with spasms	Also covered under neurocutaneous disorders. The more severe cases are considered neurodegenerative diseases
Spinocerebellopathies *Anatomic location:* Pons, medulla, cerebellum, and spinal cord	*Genetic* Hereditary spastic paraparesis Familial Werdnig-Hoffman disease Friedrich ataxia *Nongenetic* Sporadic Werdnig-Hoffman disease Acute cerebellar ataxia	

(Adapted from Dyken and Krawiecki, 1983.)

ered. As noted earlier in this chapter, the process of myelinization is associated with the development of functional capacity in childhood. There are two types of myelin disorders. *Demyelinating* disease refers to an inflammatory process that destroys normal, healthy myelin. The inflammation may be with or without a known infectious component. *Dysmyelinating* disease describes a process of destruction to myelin that is already abnormally constituted because of genetic mechanisms. It is important to recognize that a considerable amount of overlap exists with regard to how children with either of these specific disorders present clinically. With the exception of a few diseases wherein the etiology is known to be the deficiency of an enzyme necessary to make the lipid and protein myelin sheath, there is no certain or known cause for neurodegenerative disease. As a result it has been suggested that classification of these diseases be based primarily on anatomic criteria. There are well over 600 identified neurodegenerative diseases that can be classified into the following five groups: *polioencephalopathies, leukoencephalopathies, corencephalopathies, diffuse encephalopathies, and spinocerebellopathies.* The number of disorders that have been shown to have a genetic predisposition varies within and between groups (Dyken and Krawiecki, 1983). Table 46-14 identifies the most commonly seen disease entities in each of the above classifications, the anatomic area affected, and the genetic predisposition of the selected disorders.

Another method of classification for neurodegenerative diseases involves differentiating whether they are disorders primarily of the white matter or of the gray matter. The majority of neurodegenerative diseases are of the white matter, as by definition it consists of primarily axons with (whitish-color) myelin sheaths. There is no absolute differentiation between the clinical signs and symptoms of white matter disease and of gray matter disease although it is a means of classifying the multitude of disorders (Allen et al, 1982). Whether classified anatomically or by white/gray matter differentiation, each disease has a distinct pathologic process at the cellular level, even though the diagnostic assessment and clinical presentation may be similar. In all of the degenerative disorders, the incorrectly formed myelin or the breakdown of once normal myelin prevents the accurate transmission of impulses through the axon and results in slow but progressive neurologic deterioration until death. The actual symptoms will depend on the location of the degenerating myelin within the central nervous system and the rate and type of degeneration (i.e., acute versus sporadic versus diffuse).

Diagnostic Assessment

The type and extent of diagnostic assessment will depend on the signs and symptoms leading to the initial need for medical evaluation. When signs and symptoms of neurologic compromise exist, various radiographic studies will be performed. These may include a computed tomogram (CT), skull roentgenographs, arteriogram, nuclear brain scan, or a combination. An EEG study may be helpful in distinguishing between focal and diffuse cerebral degenerative processes. However, the EEG can be totally normal in the presence of disease depending on the location and extent of demyelination. Because examination of the CSF may be helpful in diagnosing certain disorders, a lumbar puncture may be done. Biopsy of the actual brain tissue is controversial and rarely attempted (Allen et al, 1982).

Probably the most important aspect of diagnostic assessment is a thorough and complete history, physical, and detailed neurologic examination, done by an experienced pediatric neurologist. Depending on the actual disease, progression of symptoms may be rapid or consist of periodic exacerbation and remission as in multiple sclerosis. In either case, frequent and serial assessments of neurologic function are important.

Therapeutic Management

Medical care for neurodegenerative disorders consists of symptomatic and supportive care. Hospitalization may be required for diagnostic work-up and involvement of various health care professionals. If seizures are present, a regimen of one or more anticonvulsant medicines will be instituted. Frequently physical and occupational therapy will be helpful in increasing adaptive capabilities. Progressive loss of sensory functions may require the need for visual or auditory adaptation. Psychologic and emotional adjustment of the family to a chronic and life threatening disease must be addressed. Unfortunately there is no real cure for these disorders. If the degeneration is slow, good quality of life may be attainable for some period of time with the appropriate support and resources.

Major Nursing Diagnoses for Neurodegenerative Disease

Potential for Injury, related to:
- *possible seizure disorder*
- *ataxia, unsteady gait*
- *visual or auditory difficulties*
- *cranial nerve deficits*

Disturbance in self-concept: body image, *related to:*
- *progressive neurologic dysfunction*
- *change in appearance*
- *inability to communicate well with peers*

Ineffective family coping, *related to:*
- *stress of having child with deteriorating function*
- *impending death of child*
- *guilt, especially if disease is genetically predisposed*
- *limited community resources for education and support*

Strategies for Nursing Care

Preventing Injury. There are many reasons why children with neurodegenerative disorders may be more prone to injury including loss of coordination and of sensory and cognitive function. These children may need to wear a protective helmet. Teaching the child to wear the helmet, particularly during high-risk activities, is vital. Those children with known seizure disorders should understand the importance of routine times to take their medications as well as the signs and symptoms of toxicity. It is the nurse's responsibility to help the child and family discuss their functional limitations openly so that adaptive mechanisms can be initiated and ultimately safety can be ensured.

Promoting Effective Coping With Body Image. Children with obvious neurologic disorders will feel "different" from their peers. Open discussion about body image should be encouraged by the nurse caring for these children. If necessary, a referral to a counselor specializing in work with disabled children should be made., One way of helping a young child cope with altered body image is to encourage the child to meet and socialize with others who have similar handicaps. In some instances handicapped sports programs also have a positive effect on self-esteem and body image.

Enhancing Parental Coping. The most frustrating aspect of parental coping with the diagnosis of neurodegenerative disease in infancy or childhood is often the lack of a known etiology for the disease. The questions of "why" and "how" often do not have answers. Parents may display a myriad of grief reactions as they cope with the reality of the loss of a normal child. A referral should be made for genetic counseling early on. The nurse needs to offer empathy, support, and education. Knowledge regarding what to expect can help parents identify strengths and weaknesses in their coping styles and may alert them to the need for outside counseling. The nurse should be able to identify resources like support groups or volunteer organizations that may offer services and support.

Nursing Strategies for Follow-up Care in the Home or Clinic

Perform a thorough assessment of functional ability and safety hazards.

Identify any new or progressive neurologic deficits.

Assess child and family's emotional and psychologic state and need for referral for more extensive support.

Identify when the family's ability to care for a debilitated child in the home necessitates the need for potential placement into a long-term health care facility or hospice.

Identify the need for genetic counseling and make appropriate referrals.

Central Nervous System Infections

This section contains discussions of bacterial meningitis, neonatal meningitis, viral or aseptic meningitis, encephalitis, Guillain Barré syndrome and Reye syndrome. Of these infections, bacterial meningitis will be most frequently encountered by pediatric nurses.

Bacterial Meningitis

Bacterial meningitis is a serious central nervous system infection caused by an invasion of the meninges by bacteria. Bacterial meningitis is a significant health problem for infants and young children because of the mortality rate associated with the disease and the incidence of severe, long-term neurologic sequelae.

Incidence and Etiology

Bacterial meningitis is most frequent in infants and children below the age of 5 with an incidence of 26 to 40/100,000 children per year (Swaiman and Wright, 1982). It occurs infrequently in children between 5 and 10 years of age, and is rare in children above the age of 10. The disease is usually caused by one of three pathogens: *Haemophilus influenzae* type B (H. flu meningitis), *Neisseria meningitis* (meningococcal meningitis), or *Diplococcus pneumonia* (pneumococcal meningitis). Other pathogens less commonly seen may include *Streptococcus, Staphylococcus,* Myobacterium tuberculosis, *Escherichia coli, Klebsiella pneumoniae, Listeria monocytogenes,* and *Treponema pallidum.*

The mortality rate associated with bacterial meningitis beyond the neonatal period is from 1 to 5 per cent (Feigin, 1987). Antibiotic therapy is largely responsible for improving the prognosis of this disease in recent years.

Pathophysiology

The pathogens responsible for meningitis disseminate from a distant site into the meninges, most commonly following an upper respiratory infection or with bacteremia of otitis media, sinusitis, and mastoiditis. Pathogens can also enter through penetrating wounds such as skull fractures or operative incisions or via the skin in the presence of a structural defect such as a meningomyelocele (Gaddy, 1980). Once the pathogen has implanted, it proliferates and spreads into cerebral spinal fluid (CSF) and through perivascular channels and meningeal folds to brain parenchyma. Later clumps of purulent exudate collect around the base of the brain causing obstruction of CSF with possible hydrocephalus and cranial nerve palsies. Blood vessel walls and endothelium become involved and cerebral perfusion may be compromised, leading to cerebral edema. Vasculitis associated with thrombosis can cause infarctions (strokes), seizures, and focal deficits. Continued necrosis of cells in the brain cortex and hydrocephalus can lead to permanent damage, increased ICP, and even death.

The risk of hospital personnel contracting meningitis after exposure to a child with the disease is very slight. However, there is some risk that a young sibling may be infected. The use of prophylactic antibiotics for young children is controversial; in any case parents should be advised to seek medical help promptly if other young children develop symptoms.

Table 46-15. Cerebrospinal Fluid in Bacterial Meningitis Compared with Normal Findings in Children (after the Neonatal Period)

Condition	Pressure	Leukocytes	Protein	Sugar
Normal CSF	60–160 mm H_2O	≤5/mm³	10–30 mg/dl	40–80 mg/dl
Bacterial meningitis	↑, avg 300 mm H_2O	↑, up to 60,000/mm³, polymorphonuclear cells predominate	↑, 100–500 mg/dl	↓, often <40 mg/dl

(Adapted from Behrman and Vaughan, 1987; Feigin and Cherry, 1987.)

Clinical Manifestations

Inflammation of the meninges and the pain-sensitive structures surrounding them is thought to be responsible for the nuchal rigidity (stiff neck) and headache which are the most striking symptoms of meningitis in older infants and children. Classically these children also have a high fever and appear very ill. Kernig sign (the inability to fully extend the legs when lying supine) and Brudzinski sign (flexion of the hips when the neck is flexed from a supine position) are frequently present. An infant may have less striking symptoms. The parents may notice only the infant's resistance to being cuddled or diapered, irritability, and mild fever. The infant may have a high-pitched cry, a transient vacant stare, and anorexia. A bulging tense fontanel is a frequent symptom and may indicate increased ICP. Meningococcal meningitis is associated with rapidly spreading petechiae. Any parent inquiring about a "purple rash," especially if associated with other symptoms, should be advised to have the child seen by a physician immediately.

Major factors in predicting the outcome of bacterial meningitis are the age of the child and the interval between onset of symptoms and the initiation of therapy. The sequelae appear to be worse in very young infants less than 2 months of age or if there is a delay in treatment. Sequelae are less frequent in cases of meningococcal meningitis (Swaiman and Wright, 1982). Neurologic sequelae are common in children who have had meningitis compared with their siblings. These sequelae can range considerably from mild learning disabilities to severe physical and mental handicaps. Alterations in vision and hearing may result. Seizures occur in about 60 per cent of all meningitis patients, presumably in response to cerebral edema, fever, or cortical irritation and damage.

Other complications can include cranial nerve dysfunctions, peripheral circulatory collapse, arthritis (especially after meningococcal meningitis), arteritis, phlebitis, and abscess (Krugman and Katz, 1981). Subdural effusion and empyema should be suspected in infants who do not respond to treatment and have prolonged fever, bulging tense fontanelles, increasing head circumference, seizures, and other focal deficits (Krugman and Katz, 1981).

Diagnostic Assessment

When meningitis is suspected, lumbar puncture to examine spinal fluid is indicated. This is not performed in children in whom fontanelles have closed or in adults, until optic fundi have been examined and papilledema has been ruled out (Snyder, 1983). Cloudy fluid indicates pathology but the pathogen and the cause may not be determined until further testing is completed. Cerebral spinal fluid upon microscopic examination shows increased white cells, primarily polymorphonuclear. Glucose is usually lowered and protein elevated. Table 46-15 shows CSF parameters in children with meningitis compared with normal fluid findings. The fluid is cultured in order to identify the specific pathogen, so that appropriate antibiotic therapy can be promptly initiated.

Other laboratory tests may include cultures of blood, urine, nasopharynx, and any CSF leaks to identify the source of septicemia. Complete blood cell counts may show an increase in total WBC with an increase in immature granulocytes and a shift to the left; however, peripheral WBC are not helpful to distinguish viral from bacterial meningitis (Swaiman and Wright, 1982). Electrolytes, glucose, BUN, and creatinine may identify other imbalances often present. Other tests used can include the Mantoux test, VDRL, clotting studies, immunoglobulins, electrocardiogram, sinus and mastoid roentgenographs, EEG, and CT scan.

Therapeutic Management

Treatment involves the administration of antibiotics intravenously for 10 days, according to the type of pathogen. The patient is usually hospitalized, and may be placed in isolation from 24 to 48 hours after the antibiotic therapy has begun. Supportive care includes management of fever and dehydration, and monitoring response to treatment. Supportive care may also include recognition and treatment of seizures, cerebral edema, hydrocephalus, and subdural effusion and empyema. The children should be closely followed with periodic developmental screening for a period of 1 year at 3- to 4-month intervals. Careful follow-up with developmental testing and information regarding appropriate infant stimulation is advisable. Early detection of delays will allow for intervention for the infant at a young age and assist in minimizing the effects of such delays. Rehabilitation may be needed for sequelae, which affect nearly 50 per cent of children with the disease. These sequelae include hearing loss from damage to the eighth cranial nerve, mental retardation, and arthritis.

Preventive measures for bacterial meningitis include prompt treatment for upper respiratory infections, otitis media, sinusitis, mastoiditis, and other infections, especially in younger infants and children. Immunization with *Haemophilus influenzae* vaccine promises to reduce occurrence of the disease in children after 18 months of age (Feigin, 1987). Family members exposed to H. flu meningitis may be administered rifampin prophylactically. This antibiotic stains the urine, sweat, and tears orange; contact lenses may be permanently stained by the drug. The drug is contraindicated in pregnancy.

Major Nursing Diagnoses

Potential for injury: secondary brain injury, related to
- *increased intracranial pressure*
- *the infective process associated with bacterial meningitis*

Altered comfort: pain, related to
- *headache associated with increased intracranial pressure*
- *nuchal rigidity associated with meningeal irritation*
- *intravenous infusion of antibiotics*

Potential for injury: physiologic, related to complications of bacterial meningitis:
- *seizures*
- *hearing loss*
- *muscular weakness, arthritis*
- *stress ulcer*

Fear/anxiety: child and family, related to diagnosis of a serious disease affecting brain function

Strategies for Nursing Care

Reducing Intracranial Pressure. The nurse can monitor changes in intracranial pressure through frequent assessment of neurologic signs and vital signs. Palpation of the anterior fontanel (in infants) and attention to vomiting are important aspects of neurologic assessment in meningitis. Daily head circumference measurement is another diagnostic aid (see previous sections on neurologic assessment and increased intracranial pressure for additional information and specific nursing strategies). Intracranial pressure can be reduced by providing a calm, quiet atmosphere for the child: darken the room, close the door to noise (when this action will not limit observation of the child), and provide comfort measures as suggested further on. Intracranial pressure is also related to fluid volume.

Preventing Fluid Overload. The child with bacterial meningitis will usually be NPO initially to reduce the chance of aspiration from vomiting and to better measure and control the fluid volume. Fluids will often be restricted at this stage to reduce central blood volume (thereby reducing cerebral blood volume and ICP). However, fluid administration must also ensure a blood volume adequate for brain perfusion because cerebral hypoxia would result in cerebral edema (and increased ICP). This means that fluid requirements will be carefully calculated on the basis of the child's body weight and intravenous administration of fluids should be maintained at a constant rate. A volume pump can help to ensure a constant drip rate, but careful monitoring by the nurse will still be required. If fluid administration lags behind the prescribed level there is a risk for dehydration (and a potential for cerebral hypoxia). If fluids are administered too quickly, volume overload may increase ICP to dangerous levels.

Fluid overload may also result from inappropriate secretion of antidiuretic hormone, which causes fluid retention. Indications of this syndrome are increasing body weight, decreased concentrations of serum electrolytes, decreased urine output, and increased urine specific gravity. Nursing implications, then, are for daily weights, monitoring of laboratory values, accurate recording and thoughtful analysis of intake and output, and assessment of urine specific gravity every shift (if there is a spectrometer available on the unit).

Controlling the Infective Process. Intravenous antibiotics will usually be ordered for a period of about 10 days. Timely administration will ensure that serum drug levels stay at the optimum level to eliminate the causative organism. Maintaining a patent infusion site in a small child for that period of time requires nursing vigilance and ingenuity (see Chapter 30 for suggested ways to secure the infusion site). Assess the site carefully before, during, and after drug administration. The antibiotics prescribed will be quite potent, and phlebitis is not uncommon. If the needle or cannula becomes dislodged, tissue irritation may result from infiltration of fluid containing antibiotics.

Fever associated with bacterial meningitis is persistent in some cases, lasting or recurring for 8 to 9 days or more. Sometimes this is a sign of concomitant viral infection (usually contracted in the hospital setting) but it may also signal complications such as septic arthritis, subdural or pleural empyema or pericarditis, and the physician should be notified (Feigin, 1987).

Reducing Pain. If one were to ask a seasoned pediatric nurse for one word to describe a child acutely ill with bacterial meningitis the answer might be "irritable." Considering the probability of severe headache from increased ICP and the pain associated with meningeal irritation, these children have good reason to be out of sorts.

Physicians differ in their practice of prescribing pain medication for these children. Some believe that medication will mask evidence of neurologic changes and refrain from ordering any analgesia at all. Most, however, will prescribe a mild analgesic such as acetaminophen. Nurses will usually find that a mild analgesic decreases crying and fretting (which raises intracranial pressure) and allows the child to rest more easily without altering the ability for arousal. Nonpharmacologic measures are effective as well. Try offering a security object, encourage the loving attention of a parent, rock the child, stroke the skin, and employ any measures that the child finds comforting at home.

If the child cries and indicates pain at the site of the intravenous infusion the site should be inspected carefully for phlebitis or infiltration. In the absence of these findings the discomfort can sometimes be allayed by slightly decreasing the rate of drug infusion. If infiltration occurs or the child pulls the intravenous line out of the vein, inflammation at the site can be reduced with warm, moist soaks. The small child may best tolerate a warm washcloth on the arm while being held or when asleep.

Monitoring for Complications. Assess for evidence of seizure activity. Keep the siderails on the bed up at all times and allow only soft toys in the bed. Consider padding siderails for the child at increased risk for seizures (the younger the patient and the more seriously ill, the greater the risk for complications). The family should be alerted to report any brief repetitive behaviors such as sudden changes in arousal; alteration in movement, mobility, or muscle tone; or repetitive behaviors (see previous section on nursing care for seizures).

Hearing loss from pressure on the eighth cranial nerve is a relatively common side effect of bacterial meningitis. Often, auditory testing will be done before discharge and again a few weeks later.

Muscular weakness and arthritis can also result. Nursing assessment should include attention to gait in the child who walks, to determine if both legs are bearing weight equally. Younger children can be assessed by noticing use of legs and arms as they pull to stand at the crib rail and their reaction to hip movement with diaper changes. Muscular weakness, if observed, may be transient and gradually improve with the child's overall condition.

Stress ulcers have been noted in some children with bacterial meningitis. Monitor laboratory values for hemoglobin and hematocrit levels. If unexplained decline occurs, test stool and emesis for evidence of occult blood. Report findings to the physician.

Reducing Parental Fear and Anxiety. The period of diagnosis, although usually brief, is very frightening for families. They are aware that the child is seriously ill and often associate the diagnosis of meningitis with times when treatment was less effective and mortality was much greater. Keeping the parents informed of the child's status, explaining diagnostic and treatment regimens, and allowing the child to be with the parents as much as possible will help to allay some of this anxiety. Assess the family's understanding of meningitis, the cause, and the risk to other family members. Reinforce their knowledge and clarify misconceptions as appropriate.

Nursing Strategies for Follow-up Care in the Home or Clinic

Assess ease of neck movement. Note any residual resistance to normal range of motion or discomfort with movement.

Assess neurologic status and vital signs against preillness baselines (if available) and against status at hospital discharge. Ask the parent whether there has been persistent irritability. Record the results of testing of muscle strength with the neurologic assessment to document whether muscle weakness exists as a sequelae of meningitis. Assess joint function and note whether pain is present on movement.

Note results of audiometry testing before discharge and schedule another testing time if appropriate.

Assess progress on developmental tasks and compare with last recorded assessment to determine if there is reason to suspect mental retardation as a complication of meningitis.

Encourage the verbal child and the parent to talk about the illness experience and the hospital stay.

Neonatal Meningitis

This type of meningitis occurs within the first month of life. The incidence varies from 1 in 1000 full-term infants per year to 1 in 450 preterm infants per year with a mortality rate that can range from 40 to 80 per cent (Gaddy, 1980). *Escherichia coli* and group B Streptococci are responsible for 66 per cent of the cases of neonatal meningitis in North America (McCracken and Freij, 1987).

Pathophysiology

The dissemination of pathogens to the meninges is similar to the process described for bacterial meningitis. In neonatal meningitis the modes of transmission and risk factors expand to include maternal infections, prolonged membrane rupture, complications of labor and delivery, premature birth, and low birth weight (Gaddy, 1980). Sepsis in the first month of life may place infants at risk; 25 to 30 per cent of those infants will develop meningitis (Swaiman and Wright, 1982).

Clinical Manifestations

Recognition of the infection is difficult because neonates may respond nonspecifically to infection. This often delays identification and thus initiation of treatment. In neonates the symptoms of infection and meningeal irritation may be minimal or absent. Presenting symptoms may include poor acceptance and decreased quantity of feeding, grimacing, decreased activity level, and irritability with position changes such as cuddling or diapering. Sometimes symptoms of shock may be the only indication of meningitis in the infant, and the staff should be prepared to cope with this possibility (Conway, 1977). Neurologic sequelae may occur in 50 per cent of cases with neonatal meningitis (Swaiman and Wright, 1982). The most frequent sequelae is communicating hydrocephalus with only one third of those infants surviving (Swaiman and Wright, 1982).

Diagnostic Assessment

Diagnosis of neonatal meningitis is hindered by the difficulty in interpreting cerebrospinal fluid values in newborn infants. Cerebrospinal fluid in neonates normally contains more white blood cells than CSF in older infants and children. Protein and glucose levels are increased at this time as well. Several new sophisticated laboratory tests may aid diagnosis. These include counterimmunoelectrophoresis (CIE), latex particle agglutination (LPA), and the limulus lysate test (McCracken and Freij, 1987).

Therapeutic Management

Treatment for neonatal meningitis, as for bacterial meningitis, employs intravenous antibiotics. The course of antibiotic therapy is typically longer (at least 3 weeks) for neonates, however, to prevent relapse after the drug is discontinued.

Strategies for Nursing Care

Nursing care for the neonate with meningitis is similar in focus to that for the older infant or child with bacterial meningitis. Neurologic assessment will be more difficult because of the developmental age. Attention to slight changes in behavior and vital signs is therefore important, with careful monitoring to see if these parameters return to normal or continue to worsen. Decreased sucking strength and desire may be an important indication of neurologic changes in the neonate. In general, the younger the infant, the more frequently assessment is necessary.

Parents will need a great deal of support to deal with this serious diagnosis in their newborn infant. Provide time to clarify facts and encourage parents to express their concerns and questions. Allow parents to spend time with and hold their neonate as the infant's condition allows. Encourage their involvement in care; this will facilitate bonding and provide comfort for the infant as well.

Aseptic or Viral Meningitis

Viral meningitis is frequently referred to as aseptic (without bacteria) meningitis. Identifiable viruses associated with viral meningitis include enteroviruses (the most frequent cause), coxsackievirus, echovirus, and mumps virus. Inflammation of the meninges may also be associated with exanthematous conditions such as varicella, herpes, measles, and roseola. Less common pathogens may include arborvirus, lymphocytic choriomeningitis, herpes simplex, chlamydia, Epstein-Barr virus, cytomegalovirus, and amoeba. Aseptic meningitis is generally a benign self-limiting illness with complete recovery usually occurring in 3 to 10 days and few fatalities reported (Krugman and Katz, 1981).

Pathophysiology

Enteroviruses are probably transmitted by the enteric-oral pathway and have the greatest incidence during the summer months. Lymphocytic choriomeningitis virus is transmitted by the bite of infected mice or by vectors such as mosquitos and ticks that transmit the virus to humans. Other viruses gain access to the central nervous system through systemic circulation or cranial or peripheral nerves. They enter cells in the meninges for obligatory growth and reproduction, causing inflammation and localized edema.

Clinical Manifestations

The clinical manifestations are similar to those of bacterial meningitis but do not progress as rapidly. Initial symptoms in a neonate or young infant may be confined to fever, lethargy, and irritability when handled. Older children may have headache, fever, vomiting, malaise, muscle aches, and nuchal rigidity. Seizures are seen less frequently in aseptic meningitis than in bacterial meningitis (Cherry, 1987).

When aseptic meningitis results from echovirus, the child may have a discrete, red, maculopapular rash on face and trunk that does not itch and appears during the first 5 days. When coxsackievirus is the offending pathogen, symptoms may also include the appearance of vesicles and ulcers on the soft palate, paroxysmal pain in the intercostal muscles due to the irritation of pleural surfaces, and symptoms of pericarditis. If aseptic meningitis is caused by mumps virus, parotitis and orchitis may also occur.

Diagnostic Assessment and Therapeutic Management

Diagnosis is made on the basis of history of exposure and examination of CSF to differentiate this condition from bacterial meningitis. Cerebrospinal fluid in aseptic meningitis usually contains a greater amount of white blood cells than normal, but fewer than in bacterial disease. Glucose in the CSF is normal in aseptic meningitis. Protein may be elevated as well, but not as dramatically as in bacterial meningitis (Fenichel, 1988).

Therapy is primarily symptomatic, as the disease will not respond to antibiotics. The child may be hospitalized if symptoms are severe or if dehydration is a concern. Reducing external stimuli and encouraging rest helps to control headaches. Antipyretics may be ordered for fever and also for their analgesic effect.

Although some etiologic agents (e.g., tuberculous meningitis) result in a guarded prognosis for this disease, children usually recover completely from meningitis caused by enterovirus and other viral agents. Language development may be altered if the disease is contracted in early infancy, however (Cherry, 1987).

Encephalitis

As the name implies, encephalitis is an inflammation of the brain. Commonly, however, it involves the meninges as well as brain tissue (Fenichel, 1988). Once quite common as a complication of measles, mumps, and rubella, the advent of vaccine for those childhood infections has significantly reduced its incidence. The pediatric nurse is much more likely to encounter a child with bacterial meningitis than with encephalitis.

Enteroviruses are the most frequent cause of encephalitis in the United States, followed by arboviruses (Cherry and Shields, 1987). Encephalitis may follow chickenpox, herpes zoster, and infectious mononucleosis. It is more common in children who are immunosuppressed.

Pathophysiology

It is thought that the central nervous system is usually involved secondary to an infectious process elsewhere in the body. The virus or other agent enters the lymphatic system, and subsequently infects the blood. Extensive viremia (proliferation of viruses in the blood) develops, and the central nervous system is infected in this way (Cherry and Shields, 1987).

Clinical Manifestations and Diagnostic Assessment

Manifestations of encephalitis may vary greatly from one child to another, and the course of the disease is also extremely variable. As noted by Cherry and Shields (1987), one child may seem to be just mildly affected only to suddenly lapse into a coma and die, whereas another child may present with high fever, violent convulsions, bizarre movements, and hallucinations, then recover with relatively few sequelae.

Most commonly the initial symptoms resemble a simple viral illness with fever, headache, pronounced irritability, gastrointestinal distress, and possibly mild respiratory symptoms. As the temperature increases, however, involvement of the central nervous system is manifested through such signs as changes in arousal, nuchal rigidity, and seizures.

Diagnosis involves a careful history of exposure; a physical examination; culture of CSF, blood, feces, and throat secretions; and analysis of CSF. The number of white blood cells in the fluid and the protein content may range from normal to elevated; the glucose level is initially normal. The presence of insect bites can be of diagnostic value when arbovirus is the causative agent.

Therapeutic Management

Treatment is primarily supportive with hospitalization for close monitoring of neurologic status. Severely ill children will be admitted to the intensive care unit for cardiac and intracranial pressure monitoring. Cardiac and respiratory arrest are potential outcomes of this disease. Anticonvulsants may be ordered and dexamethasone may be given intravenously to reduce cerebral edema.

The prognosis related to outcome and sequelae of encephalitis is guarded, with young infants having the poorest prognosis. Herpes simplex viruses generally carry a worse prognosis than do the more commonly encountered enteroviruses (Cherry and Shields, 1987). Sequelae may involve the central nervous system or any other body system.

Strategies for Nursing Care

Nursing care for encephalitis is very similar to that detailed for bacterial meningitis. Because seizures are more common in patients with encephalitis, extra precautions should be observed (see the previous section on nursing care for seizures). The course of the disease may be more frustrating and more frightening to the family, however, than bacterial meningitis. The fact that there is a specific treatment (antibiotic therapy) for bacterial meningitis makes it somewhat easier for many families to deal with. Encephalitis must be left to run its course with only supportive care available. The nursing diagnosis, *Powerlessness,* is often an appropriate consideration for interaction with family members.

Guillain-Barré Syndrome

Guillain-Barré syndrome, also known as postinfectious or idiopathic polyneuritis, is a disease affecting nerve roots or peripheral nerves, causing varying degrees of motor and sensory disturbances. Although relatively uncommon, it may affect children of both sexes at any age from early infancy.

In GBS, nerve fibers undergo demyelination from an inflammatory process. With the decline in poliomyelitis, GBS is the primary cause of acute, severe paralysis (Glaze, 1987). Although it typically occurs several weeks after an upper respiratory or gastrointestinal infection, it can also follow immunizations and surgery. The chronic demyelinating neuropathies like GBS are considered to be immune-mediated, although the exact mechanism is unknown (Fenichel, 1988).

Clinical Manifestations

Typically, signs and symptoms occur several days after an identifiable infection. Children may hesitate to walk or run because their legs "feel funny." Peripheral neuritis usually starts bilaterally in the legs with weakness and numbness that extends up to the arms and hands. The progressive paralysis usually peaks at 3 weeks. Deep tendon reflexes are decreased or absent and the child may complain of muscle tenderness or cramping pains upon examination. Assessment of paresthesia (altered sensation of the limbs) is very important but may be difficult in the young child. The child's vague complaints should be taken seriously.

Cranial nerve involvement occurs in 46 to 75 per cent of individuals, especially of nerves VII, IX, and X, causing facial weakness and swallowing difficulty (Glaze, 1987). Ten to 20 per cent of affected persons will have sufficient involvement of the abdominal and thoracic muscles to cause respiratory insufficiency. Some will require mechanical ventilation.

Diagnostic Assessment

There is no specific diagnostic test for GBS. Diagnosis is based upon clinical features (especially progressive motor weakness of more than one limb, and areflexia), and upon other findings such as an elevated CSF protein, electrophysiologic changes, and pathologic changes of the peripheral nerves. The physician will need to rule out the presence of viral and infectious diseases, especially those altering muscle function such as poliomyelitis. It is extremely stressful for parents and siblings to observe a child with signs of paralysis. Helplessness at not being able to do anything and guilt that help may not have been sought early enough are paramount. The family will need reassurance that everything possible is being done to help the child. Having someone to answer questions, explain procedures, and listen to concerns is therapeutic.

A lumbar puncture is required to assess the cerebral spinal fluid for an increase in protein and cell count. This test is usually frightening to the parents and child. The nurse should thoroughly explain the procedure, including why it is necessary, what it feels like, how long it takes, and what position the child needs to assume during the procedure. If parents do not feel comfortable staying with the child during a lumbar puncture, they should be assured that the nurse will be present to comfort the child and hold him or her in position.

Although an electroencephalogram (EEG) is a painless procedure, preparation of the child is needed to alleviate fear and ensure cooperation. Findings may show denervation and decreased nerve conduction velocity.

Clinical signs of a symmetrical ascending paralysis and the positive findings from the lumbar puncture and the EEG are important to diagnosis of Guillain-Barré syndrome. As soon as the diagnosis is made the parents and child should be given an explanation of the disease and treatment.

Therapeutic Management

There is no specific treatment for GBS. Treatment is primarily supportive, with hospitalization for skilled nursing care. Since the majority of deaths are related to respiratory failure, pulmonary embolism, and autonomic dysfunction, particular attention is given to respiratory and cardiac function. Endotracheal intubation with mechanical ventilation is necessary for children who have significant involvement of abdominal and thoracic muscles. Physiotherapy and other measures, such as elastic stockings, will be instituted to prevent pulmonary embolism. Electrocardiogram and blood pressure are monitored as parameters of autonomic function within the cardiovascular system. Serum electrolytes will be carefully monitored to assess for hyponatremia, which sometimes develops. Although some physicians recommend prednisone in the treatment of GBS (Fenichel, 1988), others report that steroids have little effect on this disease (Glaze, 1987).

Strategies for Nursing Care

Nursing care during the acute stage is supportive and consists of promoting the child's comfort, preventing deformity, and assessing respiratory and cardiac status. The threat of cardiopulmonary complications makes nursing assessment and analysis a vital part of therapeutic management. Vital signs and chest auscultation are indicated every 4 hours, with comparison to baseline values and careful recording of findings.

Irritability, restlessness, and pain from nerve root involvement may be present. Both pharmacologic and nonpharmacologic comfort measures are indicated. An indwelling catheter for urinary retention or incontinence may be needed. Meticulous technique is needed in catheter care to avoid urinary tract infection. Maintaining adequate nutrition and hydration is important. Parenteral or enteral fluids may be given to prevent aspiration if there is involvement of the ninth or tenth cranial nerve. Respiratory paralysis will necessitate transfer to the intensive care unit for mechanical ventilation.

Prevention of contractures is a primary need during the entire disease process, and physical therapy with passive range of motion to all extremities is needed at least every 4 hours. Repositioning the child every 1 to 2 hours will help prevent deformity and skin breakdown.

Care during recovery will involve several health professionals. The occupational therapist and the physical therapist will help the child recover muscle strength and motor abilities. Bracing or splinting may be needed for the child with residual muscle weakness. The activity or play therapist has an important role in providing the child with appropriate energy-releasing activities. Immobilized children often express a wide range of behaviors, including withdrawal, aggression, noncompliance, and loneliness. The nurse who understands this will be able to accept some aggressiveness and noncooperation. However, providing the child with outlets for aggression and frustration through therapeutic play, physical exercise within the limits of the disease, and verbalization of feelings can minimize the behaviors and facilitate healthy coping. (See Chapter 21 for further information about therapeutic play.)

The long recovery period can be emotionally and financially draining for the entire family, and a medical social work referral is useful. Discharge planning should include a community health nurse referral to assist with home management and arrangements for a home-bound teacher to help the child with school work. The long-term outlook is good, with 95 per cent of these children having complete recovery.

Reye Syndrome

Reye syndrome was first described by Reye and associates in 1963 as acute encephalopathy associated with fatty degeneration of the viscera affecting mainly the liver, brain, and kidney.

Incidence and Etiology

Reye syndrome occurs equally in both sexes, is more prevalent in white children, rarely occurs after age 18, and is more likely to strike rural and suburban than urban children (Keating, 1987). Studies between 1980 and 1985 confirmed a relationship between aspirin administration during viral illness and the onset of Reye syndrome (Hurwitz et al, 1985). Since that time both the use of aspirin for relief of fever and discomfort of viruses and the incidence of Reye syndrome have decreased markedly (Fenichel, 1988). Reye syndrome is now an uncommon disease.

The detrimental effects of salicylates on mitochondria are but one theory to explain Reye syndrome. Others include the possibility of a hereditary enzyme deficiency or environmental toxins. Investigation of these and other possible etiologies continues.

Clinical Manifestations

The history generally reveals that the child was ill with flu-like symptoms for approximately a week, healthy for a few days and then developed repeated episodes of vomiting that lasted for 2 or more days, accompanied by an altered state of consciousness that progressed. Upon examination the child appears healthy, although possibly agitated, confused, or combative. Signs include slight tachycardia, normal blood pressure, and normal temperature or low-grade fever. Neurologically there is no evidence of increased intracranial pressure. Pupils are generally reactive and no papilledema is evident; nuchal rigidity is absent although hyper-reflexes are characteristic. The liver is generally not palpable and there is no evidence of jaundice. Initial electroencephalogram is generally abnormal and shows a pattern unique, but not exclusive, to Reye syndrome.

The clinical course in Reye syndrome can be divided into four predictable stages, occurring in rather rapid succession if there is no intervention (Fenichel, 1988):

- Stage I: Vomiting, confusion, and lethargy
- Stage II: Agitation, delirium, decorticate posturing, and hyperventilation
- Stage III: Coma and decerebrate posturing
- Stage IV: Flaccidity, apnea, and dilated, fixed pupils

The clinical manifestations in Stages I and II represent increasing encephalopathy, including metabolic dysfunction and cerebral edema. Stages III and IV indicate generalized increased intracranial pressure and herniation. Outcome is variable. Generally, the prognosis is better for children who contract the disease after infancy. Children who progress to Stages III and IV have a higher mortality rate; if they survive they often suffer neurologic impairment.

Diagnostic Assessment

After other diseases that present similar signs and symptoms (such as diabetes mellitus, drug overdose, salicylism, meningitis, encephalitis, or acute hepatic failure) have been ruled out, Reye syndrome is suspected. The more promptly the diagnosis is made, the better the prognosis.

Laboratory tests used in making the diagnosis of Reye syndrome include blood glucose levels, serum ammonia, liver function tests, and prothrombin time. If the laboratory report shows normal or low blood glucose levels, elevated ammonia levels (80 per cent of affected individuals have this), elevation of SGOT and SGPT to twice normal levels, and increased prothrombin times, a diagnosis of Reye syndrome is confirmed. The need for hepatic tissue to confirm the diagnosis of this syndrome is controversial. A liver biopsy may be indicated when deviations from the typical clinical picture are found. Microvesicular fat droplets found on liver biopsy are diagnostic of the syndrome.

Therapeutic Management

Because Reye syndrome develops quickly and progresses rapidly, treatment must be instituted immediately. The recommended first step is to begin intravenous administration of 100 per cent glucose as soon as blood samples are drawn in an attempt to prevent coma. The child will be cared for in a pediatric intensive care unit. Care will be directed at airway maintenance, tissue oxygenation, and control of cerebral edema. Whereas mechanical hyperventilation was once commonly used to control intracranial pressure in Reye syndrome, this practice has become controversial (Keating, 1987). Management may involve a variety of treatments, including exchange transfusion, peritoneal dialysis, bowel sterilization, and barbiturate coma.

Strategies for Nursing Care

Initial nursing care for the child with Reye syndrome will occur in the intensive care unit. Discussion of this highly technical care is beyond the scope of this text and not pertinent to the role of the nurse generalist. The transition to the general pediatric unit and expected behavior patterns are of interest, however.

Weeks (1976) described a behavioral pattern unique to children with Reye syndrome that occurs upon their awakening from a comatose state; knowing about this aids in providing care. At first the children appear withdrawn and disoriented, capable of responding only to basic questions about physical needs. They cannot remember past events in the ICU and become quite anxious and upset when procedures are unexplained. Like all children, they are upset by separation from their parents and feel powerless in the events and decisions that are affecting their lives. The feeling of powerlessness can be observed in their lack of resistance to procedures and treatments. The goal of the ICU nurse needs to be that of reorienting and restructuring the child's environment so that he or she comprehends procedures and is allowed the opportunity to make choices and exert control over the environment, regardless of how insignificant this may seem. Parents also need to be encouraged to bring familiar things from home and spend as much time as possible with their child.

Once the child is moved out of ICU (24 to 48 hours after awakening), it is important for the ICU nurse to provide the pediatric staff with information regarding the child and family's physical, social, and emotional needs. Recovery is generally rapid in those who survive. The direction and support received by the child and family during the period of hospitalization will strongly influence their acceptance and resolution of the condition. Referral and follow-up care are crucial for families in such circumstances.

Neurologic Injury

Head Injuries

Head injury in the pediatric population is one of the most common causes of death and disability. Nearly 250,000 children are admitted annually to United States hospitals for evaluation and/or treatment of minor or major head trauma. The spectrum of injury can range from minor concussion requiring a few hours of observation to major trauma necessitating heroic efforts and resulting in a dismal long-term outcome for the child (Rosman and Herskowitz, 1982).

The male incidence of head injury in childhood is twice that for females. The age group affected most frequently is the adolescent population. Head injuries occur most frequently in the spring and summer, on weekends, and in the late afternoon or early evening (AANN, 1984).

This portion of the chapter will focus on general concepts regarding various types of head trauma. (In-depth coverage of concepts related to management of increased ICP from cerebral edema is located earlier in this chapter.) Management of minor head trauma will be addressed here under therapeutic management.

Etiology and Pathophysiology

The causes of head injury vary somewhat among age groups and developmental stages. Infants may have minor head trauma as a result of a difficult delivery with forceps or a prolonged traumatic labor and delivery. Infants or toddlers may sustain a head injury from a fall out of a caretaker's arms, from a loft or balcony, in walkers, out of windows, or down stairs. These children are also at the age when they may be victims of child abuse. Preschool children may be hurt in a vehicular accident as either a passenger or a pedestrian. The preschooler is prone to being injured while playing or climbing outside. School-age children may be hurt in playground accidents or, more commonly, in accidents involving bicycles, skateboards, or athletic activities. Vehicular accidents and athletic injuries are the most common causes of head trauma in adolescent age groups (Bakay and Glasauer, 1980). Other factors that may predispose a child to head injury are seizure disorders, gait instability, and alcohol or drug ingestion (Rosman and Herskowitz, 1982).

The pathophysiology of head injuries is complex in that the extent of the visible injury may not be at all indicative of the extent of actual brain injury. A head injury may involve any or all of the cranial and skull layers, including scalp, skull, dura, brain, and blood vessels, as well as neurons and supportive glial cells. Injuries can be classified as primary, meaning resulting from the actual traumatic event; or secondary, indicating that the damage is caused by pathologic processes (such as cerebral edema or anoxia) that occurred as a result of the initial injury.

There are several mechanisms of injury in pediatric head trauma. An injury may be blunt or nonpenetrating causing the distortion of brain tissue and shearing of neurons even without outward evidence of injury or trauma. Penetrating or open injuries can produce either focal or diffuse injuries depending on the velocity and type of penetration. Compression injuries are the result of the skull being compressed between two forces causing the brain integrity to be crushed (AANN, 1984). Other commonly used terms are "coup" (pronounced "coo") and "contrecoup" injuries. These are used to describe an injury to brain tissue that results when a blow to the head causes the brain to hit the skull at the location of impact (*coup*), then rebound to the opposite side of the skull where injury can also occur (*contrecoup*) (Fig. 46-26).

"Head injury" is in effect the general term used to describe several different types of injury. Scalp injuries, skull fractures, concussions, contusions and lacerations, vascular injuries and hematomas, and cranial nerve and diffuse brain tissue injuries will each be addressed individually in this portion of the chapter.

Scalp Injuries. The scalp is composed of a tough fibrous layer and a vascular layer. Together these layers offer tremendous protection to the skull. Scalp injuries include both abrasions and lacerations, both of which are handled by suturing in an aseptic fashion. The presence of CSF is indicative of a more serious injury and deserves further investigation.

Skull Fractures. The human skull is composed of two layers — the inner and outer tables — separated by a spongy tissue called the diploic space. During a head injury, the fracture may occur at the site of impact or in areas of the skull with less tensile strength (Yanko, 1984). There are five types of skull fractures. Nearly 70 per cent of skull fractures are *linear.* Linear fractures appear and feel like a line on the skull. In the majority of cases, they are benign and treated only by observation and by allowing time for the cracked bone to heal. Danger arises when the fracture crosses a place in the skull that houses a blood vessel (Gurdjian and Gurdjian, 1980).

Depressed skull fractures are usually associated with scalp lacerations. The one case in which this is not true is with "ping pong" type fractures of the infant skull. Skull fractures that are depressed beyond 2 cm or are causing obvious intracranial damage or shift of structures will need to be surgically elevated. Often depressed fractures are also *comminuted,* or broken into several fragments (Yanko, 1984).

Diastatic skull fractures occur along the suture line. The separation is usually visible on skull roentgenograph. These fractures often do not occur at the site of impact.

The most serious type of skull fracture is a *basilar skull fracture.* These fractures involve a break in the basal portions of the frontal, ethmoid, sphenoid, temporal or occipital bones. Two classic associated findings are the Battle sign and "raccoon eyes." The first is the presence of bruising or ecchymosis behind the ear caused by leakage of blood into the mastoid sinus. "Raccoon eyes" are caused by blood leaking into the frontal sinuses and causing an edematous and bruised periorbital area. These fractures may also present with

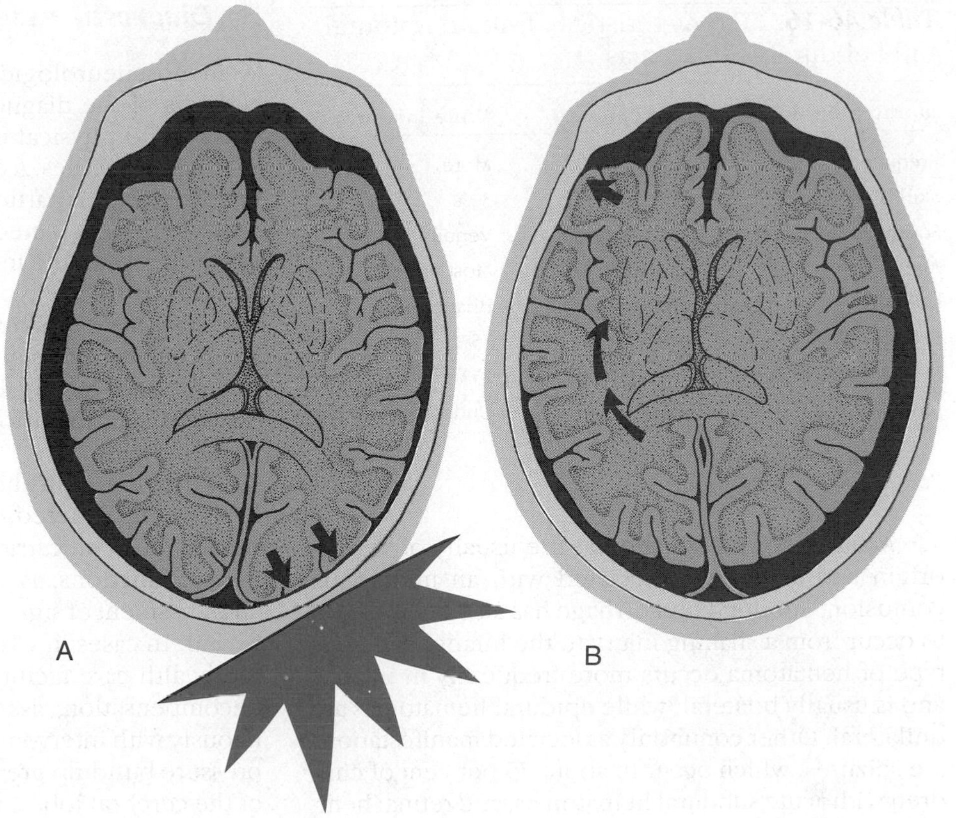

***Figure* 46-26.** Because the brain is surrounded by cerebrospinal fluid, it may move within the skull upon impact, causing damage in more than one area. The *coup* is the point of impact. The brain is forced against the skull in the area of the blow *(A)*. The brain then rebounds *(contrecoup)* off that point and strikes the skull wall opposite the injuring blow *(B)*. Some twisting of the brain stem (concussion) may occur with the contrecoup movement.

CSF leakage from the nose or ears. In either of these cases, close observation is necessary as there is a potential for meningitis (Rosman and Herskowitz, 1982).

Concussions. A concussion by definition is a period of unresponsiveness or loss of consciousness immediately following a head injury. Other key aspects of concussion include various types of memory impairment, which usually disappears by 24 hours postinjury. Concussion tends to occur when the head is in a position of movement after impact rather than in a fixed position (Rosman and Herskowitz, 1982).

Postconcussion Syndrome. When posttraumatic amnesia occurs for a longer period of time or a long period of unconsciousness (over 2 weeks) persists after initial injury, or both, cognitive loss often accompanies the severe physical disabilities. Postconcussion syndrome is defined by Stevens (1982) as "a series of temporary somatic and cognitive dysfunctions experienced for several weeks to one year after head injury" (page 240). These complaints include headache, fatigue, vertigo, emotional lability, loss of judgment, and photophobia, among others. Often communication skills, attitudes, and behaviors all seem to be affected. Another aspect of this syndrome to cause concern is termed "posttraumatic stress reaction." Basically this is the tendency for pretraumatic unresolved problems to be exacerbated postinjury. Both of these problems are major barriers to the resumption of a "normal" life for the child and family postinjury (Stevens, 1982).

Contusions and Lacerations. Bruising or crushing injuries of the brain are considered contusions, while actual discontinuity of brain tissue is referred to as a laceration. Contusions are usually caused by blunt trauma, lacerations by penetrating wounds. The area of brain tissue surrounding a contusion site is generally composed of small areas of perivascular hemorrhage. A laceration can result in focal swelling with intracranial bleeding and eventual herniation and death if not attended to (AANN, 1984).

Vascular Injuries and Hematomas. Subdural and epidural hematomas occur in about 6 to 7 per cent of pediatric head injuries. The shearing force created by the impact can cause the tearing of bridging vessels that supply blood to the various layers of the dura mater (AANN, 1984). Epidural hematomas are more likely to be of an acute nature and usually are the result of a tear in an artery, although 25 per cent of epidural hematomas are of a venous origin. The child will usually have a short period of unconsciousness followed by a period of lucidity wherein he or she is believed to be recovered; then, within 4 to 8 hours, the child will begin to experience a rapid decline in neurologic function causing severe cerebral shift and eventually death if the condition is not treated (AANN, 1984).

Table 46-16. Characteristics of Acute Epidural and Subdural Hematomas

Supratentorial	Acute Epidural	Acute Subdural
Frequency	Less	More
Skull Fracture	75%	30%
Source of hemorrhage	Usually arterial	Venous
Age	Most over 2 yr old	Most under 1 yr old
Laterality	Unilateral	Bilateral
Seizures	Under 25%	75%
Retinal hemorrhages	Under 25%	75%
Mortality	25%	Under 25%

(Adapted from Rosman, 1986.)

Acute subdural hematomas are usually of venous origin and are often associated with an underlying contusion. Subdural hemorrhage has also been shown to occur from a shaking injury to the infant head. This type of hematoma occurs more frequently in infancy and is usually bilateral, while epidural hematomas are unilateral. Other commonly associated manifestations are seizures, which occur in about 75 per cent of children with acute subdural hematomas, and retinal hemorrhages, which is also a hallmark of the shaken infant (Rosman and Herskowitz, 1982). Table 46-16 compares the characteristics of epidural and subdural hematomas.

Chronic subdural hematomas are quite different in that they may not be associated with a history of significant head trauma, but rather are usually discovered after head growth has been shown to be accelerating. The characteristic symptoms are irritability, full nonpulsatile fontanel, failure to thrive, and low hematocrit levels.

Cranial Nerve and Brain Tissue Injury. Trauma to the head can injure cranial nerves by several mechanisms. Compression, stretching, or a basilar skull fracture near the areas where the nerves exit the skull are all possible. The most common cranial nerve injuries are to CN I (loss of smell), CN VII (facial paralysis), CN V and VI (eye movements), CN II (optic fields), and CN VIII (hearing) (Yanko, 1984).

Injury to actual brain tissue occurs in the form of a concussion, contusion, or laceration as discussed earlier. At a more basic level, injury to the tissue can occur from shearing of neuronal cells, particularly at the axons. Since white and gray matter have different densities, the impact on the skull may cause the less dense areas to move while the more dense area remains stationary. The shearing of these areas across each other produces injury to the cells and alters their ability to transmit impulses effectively (Yanko, 1984).

Diagnostic Assessment

As in most neurologic disorders, the two primary components of the diagnostic assessment are a thorough history and physical examination and appropriate radiographic studies. A complete history of the traumatic event or injury is particularly important in cases of head injury. The actual mechanism of injury or state of consciousness after the injury, or both, can be a useful tool in diagnosing the type of trauma. Another important aspect of history taking is determining whether there has been post-traumatic amnesia as in concussion injuries. A history of any CSF leaks prior to hospitalization is useful. Family history of bleeding disorders should also be noted.

Once the family history and the history of the event have been gathered, a complete neurologic assessment should be carried out. Testing of cognitive and mental functions, as well as cranial nerve testing and an assessment of signs and symptoms of increased ICP, is vital. In cases in which the injured child presents to the health care facility in a state of rapid neurologic decompensation, assessment is often done simultaneously with interventions. If there is any evidence of a pressure build-up great enough to threaten herniation of the cerebral lobes, immediate action must be taken to alleviate the pressure. A more indepth coverage of this type of assessment and management is found in the section on increased intracranial pressure.

Radiographic studies for head injury are basically skull and cervical spine films as well as computed tomography (CT scan). If the injury is minor and the child appears neurologically intact, a CT scan may not be necessary, although plain skull films are usually done to rule out a skull fracture.

If there has been seizure activity after the injury, an EEG will be necessary. Injuries involving the cranial nerves may be followed with brain stem auditory evoked responses (BAER) or visual evoked responses (VER), or both. A child with long-term cognitive deficits may require a neuropsychologic evaluation to assess functional, learning, and vocational abilities.

Therapeutic Management

There is a broad spectrum of medical and surgical interventions on the continuum of head injury ranging from mild to severe. The treatment for mild head injury is generally a conservative observational approach that may involve following the clinical manifestations for several hours before discharging the patient. Most nondepressed skull fractures heal over time. A moderate head injury may involve a prolonged hospital stay and the employment of methods to decrease ICP short of mechanical hyperventilation. Some children may need to stay hospitalized to follow cranial nerve functions and ascertain that there is not a worsening disease process. Children with severe injuries necessitate a critical care environment with close monitoring of vital functions. The insertion of an ICP measuring device by the neurosurgeon may be necessary to monitor changes in ICP and initiate medical therapy based on these changes. Medical therapy for increased ICP is covered in an earlier section of this chapter.

Surgical management of head injury is necessary in a few instances. The elevation of a depressed skull fracture and the removal of an acute epidural or subdural hematoma are the most common reasons for surgical intervention in the head injured child. Chronic subdural hematomas may require mechanical shunting to the peritoneal space. In the majority of cases, aggressive medical and pharmacologic management is the therapy of choice for moderately to severely injured children.

Major Nursing Diagnoses for Head Injury

Sensory-perceptual alteration: altered level of consciousness, related to:
- *concussion, contusion, laceration or hemorrhage*
- *secondary cerebral edema causing increased ICP*

Altered tissue perfusion: cerebral, related to aforementioned mechanisms and resulting in
- *cell anoxia, edema and death*
- *deteriorating neurologic function*
- *potential for seizure activity*

Ineffective airway clearance, related to
- *decreased level of consciousness*
- *possible lower cranial nerve deficits leading to poor gag and cough reflexes*
- *relative immobility*

Potential for infection, related to
- *tear in the dura from the injury*
- *basilar skull fracture resulting in CSF ottorhea or rhinorrhea*
- *invasive procedures*
- *immobility and nutritional deficits*
- *immunosuppression from use of steroids, if applicable*

Potential for injury, related to
- *possible seizure activity*
- *restless or combative state*
- *poor judgment, motor, and/or perceptual deficits*

Ineffective family coping, related to:
- *family denial, anger, guilt*
- *lack of understanding regarding potential outcomes*
- *stress of hospitalization and possible change in family roles*

Strategies for Nursing Care

Assessing and Responding to Changes in Level of Consciousness. An assessment of neurologic function including alertness, orientation, eye movements, and responsiveness should be done every 1 to 2 hours. The nurse caring for a patient with a diminished level of consciousness should monitor cardiovascular and pulmonary function to ensure that adequate oxygenation is provided to brain tissue. It is the bedside nurse's responsibility to document and report any changes that occur and do more frequent assessments if the child's condition warrants it. The nurse should always be prepared for emergency diagnostic procedures and any drastic changes in the child's status.

Promoting Optimal Cerebral Tissue Perfusion. Nursing care for the child with threatened cerebral tissue perfusion requires frequent and ongoing assessment of vital signs, including blood pressure and pulse. Overall perfusion status can be assessed by monitoring fluid status including urine output. Following the child's hematocrit is also important. Blood products may need to be administered. The nurse should always be aware of the potential for seizures and administer anticonvulsants as ordered. An awareness of the signs and symptoms of anticonvulsant toxicity is another important nursing responsibility (see Table 46-14).

Ensuring A Patent Airway. Elevating the head of the bed is important for decreasing ICP and is also useful in promoting good airway position. Very slight hyperextension can be achieved by putting a roll under the child's shoulders after checking that there has not been a cervical spine injury. Oral and deep suctioning should be done every 2 hours or as needed. Oxygen should be readily available; especially a bag and mask for "bagging" if necessary. If alert or semialert, the child should be encouraged to cough and deep breathe or at least should be repositioned every few hours. Nursing care should be geared around the concept that increased intrathoracic pressure also increases ICP (see Table 46-11).

Preventing Infection. Any leaks of possible CSF from the nose, ears, or scalp lacerations should be quantified and reported to the physician as soon as possible. Antibiotics will most likely be administered prophylactically when the scalp has been lacerated or there is an open injury. If and when steroid medicines are ordered, the nurse should be aware of the potential for opportunistic infections. Frequent oral care should be given and extra special care given to incisions. Other measures for preventing infection in neurologically impaired or postoperative patients have been addressed elsewhere.

Preventing Injury. With the head-injured child, a major component of nursing care may be helping them make better judgments in their daily activities. Comprehensive rehabilitation programs that involve a component of behavior modification are usually effective in beginning to help children become aware of their own safety. A protective helmet will often be necessary.

Promoting Adaptive Family Coping. The biggest task facing the family with a severely brain injured child is the grief of losing the child they once had. Frequently the personality changes are dramatic and disturbing. The entire structure of the family will likely change. Initially, when progress seems to occur daily, families have a lot of hope for a complete recovery. As time wears on and the family realizes their loss, depression can set in. Stress also has its effect on the marital and sibling relationships. The nurse's role is to offer realistic expectations to the family and support through their grief work. Referring the family for further counseling is also an important role. The family needs to be encouraged to take part in their child's care but also be given permission to take occasional breaks.

Long-Term Outcome

The sequelae from a head injury in the pediatric years can become a lifetime burden. Seizure activity becomes post-traumatic epilepsy. Postconcussion syndrome can be apparent for a year or more postinjury. Hydrocephalus can occur as the result of an infectious process. The most difficult aspects of long-term outcome are the ensuing personality and behavior changes that can prevent a completely independent lifestyle. Persistent physical difficulties may impact independence as well. In light of the often dismal long-term outcome, it is important to remember that most pediatric head injuries are minor occurrences that require no hospitalization and engender no long-term damage.

Nursing Strategies for Follow-up Care in the Home or Clinic

If the injury was minor, do pertinent assessment of neurologic function appropriate to the child's age.

In infants, follow head circumference and hematocrit carefully.

Assess the safety of the home, especially if the child has some persistent cognitive or perceptual deficits.

Follow-up with parents' awareness of prevention techniques, especially if the injury was easily preventable.

Assess the progress of child and family on developmental tasks.

Identify the need for additional resources and make appropriate referrals.

Spinal Cord Injury

Although acute spinal cord injury (SCI) is an infrequent occurrence in the general pediatric population, the incidence of these injuries does increase significantly in middle and late adolescence. The most common causes are vehicular accidents, falls, athletic injuries, or violent penetrating wounds. Young males between the ages of 18 and 30 comprise nearly 80 per cent of the victims of acute SCI (AANN, 1984). The emotional and psychologic sequelae of these potentially devastating injuries is overwhelming. The need for excellent acute care management and comprehensive long-range planning for these children and their families cannot be overstated. The changes affecting a family after an SCI are significant and long-lasting.

Classification of Spinal Cord Injuries

Spinal cord injuries are classified in many different ways. The simplest classification is by *level of injury*, with cervical injuries being the most common and thoracic injuries the least common. Often classification is according to the actual *mechanism of injury*. Feuer (1976) describes four major mechanisms resulting in trauma to the vertebral column and spinal cord: flexion-dislocation, hyperextension, vertical compression, and rotation. Flexion-dislocation injuries occur in head-on collisions where unrestrained passengers are thrown forward with their head hyperflexed to their trunk. Hyperextension injuries are the more commonly termed "whiplash" injuries that frequently occur during falls by elderly people or from being hit in a motor vehicle from the rear. Vertical compression injuries are often the result of diving or trampoline mishaps. Each of these three types of injury can occur with or without rotation.

Another common classification method is the determination of the *degree of functional impairment* of the spinal cord. This is usually done by designating a lesion as complete or incomplete. Complete spinal cord injuries are those in which sensory, motor, and autonomic disruption below the level of the lesion reflect irreversible spinal cord damage. *Quadriplegia* results from an injury to the cervical region, and is a complete loss of leg function with variable, but usually limited, use of arms. *Paraplegia* results from thoracic or high lumbar injuries and is characterized by loss of leg function alone. Incomplete lesions of the spinal cord involve variable degrees of motor and sensory loss below the level of injury. The six types of incomplete lesions will not be detailed in this chapter except to discuss the most common ones, referred to as the *central cord syndrome.* This syndrome is characterized by various degrees of sensory loss and bladder dysfunction with motor loss in upper extremities greater than motor loss in lower extremities reflecting sparing of certain tracts (AANN, 1984). The last form of classification of these traumatic injuries is by *spinal cord segmental level.* This involves assessing functional loss by spinal cord segments. The functional level of the injury may not correspond to the actual vertebral level of the injury (Donovan and Bedbrook, 1982).

Pathophysiology

Several factors may influence the severity of the actual injury to the spinal cord. The fact that the spinal cord exists in a very small space surrounded by bone tends to make it less adaptable to even small physiologic changes. Children have an advantage in that their relatively wider spinal canal allows the cord more space to move without compression. For this reason, fewer children with cervical spinal injuries become quadriplegic (AANN, 1984).

The four primary mechanisms of injury to the spinal cord are concussion, contusion, laceration (including partial or complete transection), and compression. These entities range from mild disturbance lasting no longer than 24 to 48 hours, as in cases of concussion, to severe laceration of the cord, often seen in more violent injuries. Compression injuries are frequently caused by spinal epidural or subdural hematomas that can occur after trauma. If pressure from the hematoma is not alleviated early on, permanent damage can result (Rosman and Herskowitz, 1982).

The edema that occurs after the initial spinal cord injury produces further impairment of capillary circulation and venous return. If circulation is impaired for a significant length of time, the spinal tissue is deprived of necessary oxygen and ischemia can occur as a result of compression from the edema. A common physiologic consequence of spinal cord injury is a phenomenon referred to as *central cord necrosis.* As further edema and ischemia develop, vascular stasis and thrombosis occur, propagating the vicious cycle, with the eventual outcome being necrosis of gray matter.

This necrosis also affects the individual neurons, resulting in a neurophysiologic cessation of nearly all of the reflexes below the level of the injury. This state is known as *spinal shock.* Spinal shock can last anywhere from 2 days to several months. The appearance of involuntary spastic movement indicates that spinal shock is resolving. In summary, irreversible cord damage is ultimately the result of ischemia associated with edema, hemorrhage, vascular congestion, and vasospasm all contributing to cell death and loss of function (AANN, 1984).

Diagnostic Assessment

After immediate stabilization of respiratory and circulatory systems has occurred, a detailed neurologic examination of the child should be carried out. The precise level of sensory and motor injury should be determined. The spine should also be examined for overt injury or tenderness, or both. Once the clinical examination has been carried out, a thorough roentgenographic examination should be made. Anteroposterior, lateral, and oblique views of the spine down to where the injury is suspected are obtained. Routine films of the spine and pelvis below the level of the injury are necessary to rule out any other hidden fractures. Spinal CT scans, magnetic resonance imaging, and myelography may each be useful, depending on the type of injury and information desired (Donovan and Bedbrook, 1982).

Therapeutic Management

Treatment of acute SCI begins immediately. Initial management at the scene of the trauma should include stabilization of the spine, as well as the establishment of an adequate airway. Other appropriate medical measures during the acute phase include the administration of intravenous dexamethasone to reduce swelling around the spinal cord, and aggressive pulmonary hygiene measures to prevent pneumonia. Stress ulcer is common, and is often prevented with the use of antacids. Frequent repositioning is ordered, and the patient may be placed in a special frame or bed for turning. Urinary catheterization is also necessary until a determination of bladder function can be made and the Credé maneuver or other measures instituted.

The role of surgery in the acute phase of treatment has been somewhat controversial (Donovan and Bedbrook, 1982). Those who advocate surgery believe in the importance of restoring spinal alignment and decompressing the neural tissue as soon as possible. Others who advocate conservative medical management counter with many arguments, the first and most important being that good evidence to suggest that surgery improves outcome is lacking, and secondly, that in some cases loss of function has resulted from early surgical intervention (Feuer, 1976). There are times when surgery is clearly indicated. The two most frequent instances are failure to reduce a fracture to acceptable alignment by closed methods, and progressive neurologic deficit ascending beyond two segments above the initial level of injury (Donovan and Bedbrook, 1982).

Throughout the acute care phase, rehabilitative measures are instituted in an effort to ensure the best possible outcome for each individual. Safe and early mobilization is attempted through the use of a variety of stabilizing devices. Cardiovascular complications include *orthostatic hypotension* and *autonomic hyper-reflexia* (also called dysreflexia). The latter occurs when there is an uncontrolled increase in sympathetic activity that cannot be inhibited because of the SCI. It is usually caused by overdistention of the bladder or bowel, and it can be a serious complication if it is not attended to.

There are many important aspects of medical care during the rehabilitative phase following acute SCI. These children are at risk for thromboembolism and respiratory compromise. Many children will require a tracheostomy to wean them from the ventilator slowly. Bowel and bladder care need to be adapted as mobility increases. A bladder program geared toward prevention of UTI is vital. Prevention of skin breakdown is a task that is taken on by all who provide care for the spinal cord injured child. Physical, occupational, and speech therapy, as well as an assessment of learning, nutritional, and psychosocial needs, are extremely important. The complex and emotional medical care of these children is best dealt with in a multidisciplinary rehabilitative center. Reintegrating the disabled child into the family requires a group of individuals committed to the ultimate goal of providing the child with the best possible quality of life.

Major Nursing Diagnoses for Spinal Cord Injury

There are many nursing diagnoses applicable to the complex care of children with traumatic spinal cord injuries. Loss of function in the spinal cord leads to altered function of nearly every other body system. Nursing care needs to be broad based, so that the interrelatedness of the many problems experienced by these children is recognized. The nursing diagnoses listed subsequently overlap each other. Although this listing is not exhaustive, it establishes a good base from which to provide comprehensive nursing care for the child and family facing a spinal cord injury.

Potential for infection: respiratory or urinary, related to:
- *decreased movement of chest wall, allowing for pooling of pulmonary secretions and potential for pneumonia*
- *stasis of urine in the bladder, or presence of a Foley catheter, or both*

Ineffective airway clearance, related to:
- *decreased innervation to diaphragm, causing frequent shallow breaths, which are ineffective in clearing the airway*
- *long-term ventilator dependence, creating weak respiratory musculature*

Altered skin integrity, related to:
- *decreased or absent mobility*
- *poor nutrition resulting in decreased ability to heal*

Altered elimination: bowel and bladder, resulting from altered innervation from the spinal cord, related to:
- *spasticity or flaccidity of bowel, bladder, or both*
- *physiologic changes that occur between the time of acute injury and the rehabilitative phase*

Potential for ineffective coping, related to:
- *immense emotional adjustment to injury*
- *immediate lengthy hospitalization*
- *realization of long-term outcome*

Other appropriate diagnoses include those related to safety, cardiovascular function, nutrition, perceptual disturbances, and dysreflexia.

Strategies for Nursing Care

Preventing Infection. Respiratory care of children with SCI should be meticulous and frequent. Ensuring that chest physiotherapy is done in a timely fashion and that frequent turning, deep breathing (if possible), and suction are done is important. Following temperatures and results of routine chest roentgenographs is also necessary. If the child does develop pneumonia, the administration of antibiotics is important to prevent systemic spread of the infection.

Microorganisms may be introduced into the bladder via an indwelling or intermittent catheterization program. Meticulous catheter care and prevention of stool near the catheter is vital. Once a program of intermittent Credé maneuver or catheterization is begun, urinary stasis can provide a perfect medium for bacterial growth. Nursing responsibilities include an assessment of signs and symptoms of UTI and administration of antibiotics, as well as teaching the child and family all aspects of prevention. These include adequate hydration, proper catheterization technique, and complete bladder emptying.

Promoting Effective Airway Clearance. Children suffering paresis or paralysis of their diaphragm, intercostal, or abdominal muscles, or a combination of any of these, may have difficulty clearing normal airway secretions. Other factors influencing this nursing diagnosis include shock lung, chest trauma, and/or pulmonary edema. Consistent monitoring of respiratory parameters at least every 2 hours is necessary. Other nursing interventions include encouragement of deep breathing and incentive spirometry to prevent atelectasis. Any evidence of respiratory insufficiency, dyspnea, air hunger, or abnormal arterial blood gases should be reported to the physician immediately (AANN, 1984).

Preserving Skin Integrity. Immobility, circulatory impairment, and poor nutrition all contribute to the potential for skin breakdown. Nursing care for this diagnosis should focus on prevention. Skin should be inspected daily for any beginning areas of redness. An eggcrate mattress or sheepskin or both should be used as appropriate. In all repositioning, foam pads should be used to cushion bony prominences. Preventing any kind of moisture on the skin and providing light massage during skin care are basic but necessary nursing interventions. (For further elaboration on nursing care related to immobility, see the section on nursing care of the child with altered responsiveness earlier in this chapter.)

Dealing With Bowel and Bladder Dysfunction. Loss of voluntary bladder control requires the insertion of an indwelling urinary catheter to evaluate fluid status and renal function. As soon as possible, intermittent catheterization should begin, to promote reflex bladder emptying. In either case, asepsis and proper technique are essential. An intermittent catheterization program involves slowly decreasing the number of catheterizations while simultaneously recording the amounts of residual urine. If the child is school age or older, teaching of self-catheterization should begin if a readiness to learn is displayed.

Initially, paralytic ileus may hinder bowel function. Maintenance of a nasogastric tube to low suction may be ordered. Assessment of the abdomen, including palpation and auscultation, should be done regularly. Abdominal girths should be recorded every 4 to 6 hours. At some point, a bowel program should be initiated with the use of a stool softener and digital stimulation. Once a pattern has been established, the stool softener may be discontinued and regularity maintained with diet and digital stimulation alone.

Supporting the Child and Family. A traumatic injury to the spinal cord has lifelong implications for the child and family. Since many of these injuries occur in adolescence, there may be pre-existing tension between the parent and child depending upon the nature of the injury. The denial, anger, and fear need to be addressed as the child recovers. The nurse is often the key in supporting and promoting family cohesiveness and recognizing when other subspecialties need to be involved. Family adjustment to this illness should never be taken for granted, but rather continually re-examined and discussed.

Nursing Strategies for Follow-up Care in the Home or Clinic

Coordination of the many disciplines involved in the care of the child and family when appropriate.

- Physical/occupational therapy
- Rehabilitative medicine
- Psychologist or social worker, or both
- Urology care
- Nursing Specialists

Assess for infection of any type: skin, respiratory, or bladder.

Assess psychologic state for depression or maladaptive coping.

Perform a thorough assessment of skin integrity and begin early prevention of pressure breakdown.

Assess child's and family's progress on developmental tasks. Discuss ways to meet these tasks in spite of altered family processes.

Identify the need for additional resources and make appropriate referrals.

References

Allen RJ: Degenerative disorders of the central nervous system. *In* Swaiman KF, Wright FS (eds): *The Practice of Pediatric Neurology*, Vol 2. St Louis, CV Mosby, 1982, pp 881–957.

American Association of Neuroscience Nurses: *Care Curriculum for Neuroscience Nursing.* Park Ridge, IL, AANN, 1984.

Arsenault L: Selected postoperative complications of cranial surgery. *Neurosurg Nurs* 1985; 17(3):155–163.

Bakay L, Glasauer F: *Head Injury.* Boston, Little, Brown, 1980.

Baldridge J: Arnold Chiari malformation. *J Neurosurg Nurs* 1982; 14:162–165.

Behrman RE, Vaughan VC (eds): *Nelson Textbook of Pediatrics.* 13th ed. Philadelphia, WB Saunders, 1987.

Bell W, McCormick W: *Increased Intracranial Pressure in Children.* 2nd ed. Philadelphia, WB Saunders, 1978.

Berg BO: Neurocutaneous syndromes. *In* Swaiman K, Wright F: *The Practice of Pediatric Neurology.* 2nd ed. Vol II. St. Louis, CV Mosby, 1982, 914–934.

Browne T, Feldman R: *Epilepsy; Diagnosis and Management.* Boston, Little, Brown, 1983.

Bruya M: Planned periods of rest in the intensive care unit: nursing care activities and intracranial pressure. *J Neurosurg Nurs* 1981; 13(4):184–194.

Camfield PR, Camfield CS: Neurologic aspects of craniosynostosis. *In* Cohen MM (ed): *Craniosynostosis: Diagnosis, Evaluation, and Management.* New York, Raven Press, 1986; pp 215–226.

Cavazuti G, et al: Longitudinal study of epileptiform EEG patterns in normal children. *Epilepsia* 1980; 21:43.

Cherry JD: Aseptic meningitis and viral meningitis. *In* Feigin RD, Cherry JD (eds): *Textbook of Pediatric Infectious Diseases.* 2nd ed. Philadelphia, WB Saunders, 1987, pp 478–484.

Cherry JD, Shields WD: Encephalitis and meningoencephalitis. *In* Feigin RD, Cherry JD (eds): *Textbook of Pediatric Infectious Diseases.* 2nd ed. Philadelphia, WB Saunders, 1987, pp 484–496.

Clochesy J: Problems in interpreting abnormal auditory brainstem responses in comatose patients. *J Neurosurg Nurs* 1985; 17(4):253–255.

Cloward RB: Acute cervical spine injuries. *Clin Symp* 1980; 32(1):1–32.

Coffman S: Description of a nursing diagnosis: alteration in bowel elimination related to neurogenic bowel in children with myelomeningocele. *Iss Compr Pediatr Nurs* 1986; 9(3):179–191.

Cohen FL: *Clinical Genetics in Nursing Practice.* Philadelphia, JB Lippincott, 1984.

Cohen FL: Neural tube defects: epidemiology, detection, and prevention. *JOGNN* 1987; (2):105–115.

Cohen MM: *Craniosynostosis: Diagnosis, Evaluation, and Management.* New York, Raven Press, 1986.

Commission for the Control of Epilepsy and Its Consequences: Plan for Nationwide Action on Epilepsy. US DHEW, DHEW Publ No 78–276, 1977.

Conway BL: *Pediatric Neurologic Nursing.* St Louis, CV Mosby, 1977.

Donovan WH, Bedbrook SF: Comprehensive management of spinal cord injury. *Clin Symp* 1982; 34(2):1–36.

Dreifuss FE: Proposal for revised clinical and electroencephalographic classification of epileptic seizures. *Epilepsia* 1981; 20:489–501.

Dreifuss FE: *Pediatric Epileptology.* Boston, John Wright, 1983.

Droske S, Francis S: *Pediatric Diagnostic Procedures.* New York, John Wiley and Sons, 1981.

Dyken F, Krawiecki N: Neurodegenerative diseases of infancy and childhood. *Ann Neurol* 1983; 13(4):351–364.

Feigin RD: Central nervous system infections. *In* Feigin RD, Cherry JD (eds): *Textbook of Pediatric Infectious Diseases.* 2nd ed. Philadelphia, WB Saunders, 1987, pp 439–516.

Fenichel GM: *Clinical Pediatric Neurology. A Signs and Symptoms Approach.* Philadelphia, WB Saunders, 1988.

Ferry P, et al: *Seizure Disorders in Children.* Philadelphia, JB Lippincott, 1986.

Feuer H: Management of acute spine and spinal cord injuries: old and new concepts. *Arch Surg* 1976; 111:638–645.

Fisher D, et al: Increase in intracranial pressure during suctioning-stimulation vs. rise in $PaCO_2$. *Anesthesiology* 1982; 57:416–417.

Freeman JM: To treat or not to treat: ethical dilemmas of treating the infant with a myelomeningocele. *Clin Neurosurg* 1973; 20:134–146.

Freisleben LA: Craniosynostosis data compared in Colorado and Atlanta. *The Craniosynostosis Newsletter,* Colorado Department of Health, 1987.

Friedman D: Taking the scare out of caring for seizure patients. Nursing 88 1988 Feb; 18(2):53–59.

Gaddy D: Meningitis in the pediatric population. *Nurs Clin North Am* 1980; 15(1):83–97.

Giubilato R, Metcalf J: Evoked potentials: nursing perspectives. *J Neurosurg Nurs* 1984; 16(5):241–247.

Glaze DG: Guillain-Barré syndrome. *In* Feigin RD, Cherry JD (eds): *Textbook of Pediatric Infectious Diseases.* Vol I. 2nd ed. Philadelphia, WB Saunders, 1987, 507–516.

Guin PR: Arnold Chiari malformation—a closer look. *J Neurosurg Nurs* 1985; 17:45–52.

Gumnit RJ: *The Epilepsy Handbook. The Practical Management of Seizures.* New York, Raven Press, 1983

Gurdjian ES, Gurdjian E: Acute head injury: a review. *Surg Ann* 1980; 12:223–241.

Hausman KA: Nursing care of the patient with hydrocephalus. *J Neurosc Nurs* 1981; 13(6):326–332.

Hindfelt B: The prognostic significance of subfebrility and fever in ischemic cerebral infarction. *Acta Neurol Scand* 1976; 53:72–79.

Holmes GL: *Diagnosis and Management of Seizures in Children.* Philadelphia, WB Saunders, 1987.

Hummelgard A: Prognostic value of brainstem auditory evoked potentials in head trauma. *J Neurosurg Nurs* 1984; 16(4):181–187.

Humphreys RP: Spinal dysraphism. *In* Wilkins RH, Rengachary SS (eds): *Neurosurgery.* Vol 3. New York, McGraw-Hill, 1985, pp 2041–2053.

Hunter AG, Rudd NL: Craniosynostosis I. Sagittal synostosis: its genetics and associated clinical findings in 214 patients who lacked involvement of the coronal suture(s). *Teratology* 1976; 14:185–193.

Hunter AG, Rudd NL: Craniosynostosis II. Coronal synostosis: its familial characteristics and associated clinical findings in 109 patients lacking bilateral polysyndactyly or syndactyly. *Teratology* 1977; 15:301–310.

Hurwitz ES, et al: Public health service study of Reye's syndrome and medications. JAMA 1987; 257:1905.

Huttenlocher PR: The nervous system. *In* Behrman RE, Vaughan VC (eds): *Nelson Textbook of Pediatrics.* 13th ed. Philadelphia, WB Saunders, 1987, pp 1274–1330.

Jones C, Cayard C: Care of ICP monitoring devices: a nursing responsibility. *J Neurosurg Nurs* 1982; 14(5):255–261.

Keating JP: Reye syndrome. *In* Feigin RD, Cherry JD (eds): *Textbook of Pediatric Infectious Diseases.* Vol II. 2nd ed. Philadelphia, WB Saunders, 1987; 1845–1848.

Kokich VG: The biology of sutures. *In* Cohen M (ed): *Craniosynostosis: Diagnosis, Evaluation, and Management.* New York, Raven Press, 1986; pp 81–103.

Koski K: Cranial growth centers. *Am J Orthodont* 1968; 54:566–582.

Krugman S, Katz S: *Infectious Diseases of Children.* 7th ed. St Louis, CV Mosby, 1981.

Lorber J: Results of treatment of myelomeningocele: an analysis of 524 unselected cases, with special reference to possible selection for treatment. *Dev Med Child Neurol* 1971; 18:279–303.

MacBriar BR: Self-concept of pre-adolescent and adolescent children with a meningomyelocele. *Issu Compr Pediatr Nurs* 1983; 6(1):1–11.

Macedo A, Posel LF: Nursing the family after the birth of a child with spina bifida. *Issues Compr Pediatr Nurs* 1987; 10(1):55–65.

Marchac D, Renier D: *Craniofacial Surgery for Craniosynostosis.* Boston, Little, Brown, 1982.

McCracken GH Jr, Freij BJ: Perinatal bacterial diseases. *In* Feigin RD, Cherry JD (eds): *Textbook of Pediatric Infectious Diseases.* 2nd ed. Philadelphia, WB Saunders, 1987, pp 940–966.

Milhorat TH: *Pediatric Neurosurgery.* Philadelphia, FA Davis, 1978.

Milhorat TH: Hydrocephalus, pathophysiology and clinical features. *In* Wilkins RH, Rengachary SS (eds): *Neurosurgery.* Vol 3. New York, McGraw-Hill, 1985, 2135–2140.

Mitchell P: Intracranial hypertension: implications of research for nursing care. *Journal of Neurosurg Nurs* 1980; 12(3):145–154.

Mitchell P, et al: Moving the patient in bed: effects on intracranial pressure. *Nurs Res* 1981; 30(4):212–218.

Mitchell P, et al: *Neurological Assessment for Nursing Practice.* Reston, VA, Reston Company, 1984.

Moore KL: *The Developing Human.* 4th ed. Philadelphia, WB Saunders, 1988.

Mortimer EA: The puzzling epidemiology of neural tube defects. *Pediatrics* 1980; 65:636–638.

Narayan R, et al: Improved confidence of outcome prediction in severe head injury. *J Neurosurg* 1981; 54(6):751–762.

Oakes WJ: Chiari malformations, hydromyelia, syringomyelia. *In* Wilkins RH, Rengachary SS (eds): *Neurosurgery,* Vol 3. New York, McGraw-Hill, 1985; pp 2102–2115.

O'Briens MS: Hydrocephalus. *In* Youmans JR (ed): *Neurological Surgery.* Vol 3. Philadelphia, WB Saunders, 1982; pp 1381–1422.

Open neural tube defects. *Genet Pract* 1(2):1.

Parsons L, Wilson M: Cerebrovascular status of severe closed head injured patients following passive position changes. *Nurs Res* 1984; 33:68–75.

Passo S: Malformations of the neural tube. *Nurs Clin North Am* 1980; 15(1):5–21.

Pellock J, Myer E: *Neurologic emergencies in infancy and childhood.* New York, Harper and Row, 1983.

Plum F: *The Diagnosis of Stupor and Coma.* 3rd ed. Philadelphia, FA Davis, 1980.

Renier D, et al: Intracranial pressure in craniostenosis. *J Neurosurg* 1982; 57(3):370–377.

Rhodes M, Grosser B: Complications of posterior fossa craniotomy. *J Neurosurg Nurs* 1983; 15(1):9–12.

Rosman NP, Herskowitz J: Trauma to the brain and spinal cord. *In* Swaiman KF, Wright FS (eds): *The Practice of Pediatric Neurology,* Vol 2. St Louis, CV Mosby, 1982, pp 958–997.

Rowe PC: *The Harriet Lane Handbook* 11th ed. Chicago, Year Book Medical Publishers, 1987.

Rudy E: Magnetic resonance imaging: new horizon in diagnostic techniques. *J Neurosurg Nurs* 1985; 17(6):331–337.

Shapiro H: Intracranial hypertension: therapeutic and anesthetic considerations. *Anesthesiology* 1975; 43:445.

Smith K, et al: CAT scans: what do they tell us? *J Neurosurg Nurs* 1983; 15(4):222–227.

Snyder M: *Relationship of nursing activities to increase in intracranial pressure. J Adv Nurs* 1983; 8:273–279.

Solomon EP, Phillips GA: *Understanding Human Anatomy and Physiology.* Philadelphia, WB Saunders, 1987.

Stevens M: Post-concussion syndrome. *J Neurosurg Nurs* 1982; 14(5):239–244.

Stewart R: Craniofacial malformations. *Pediatr Clin North Am* 1978; 25(3):485–515.

Swaiman K, Wright F: *The Practice of Pediatric Neurology.* 2nd ed. St Louis, CV Mosby, 1982.

Tessier P: Relationship of craniostenoses to craniofacial dystoses and to faciostenosis, a study with therapeutic implications. *Plast Reconstruct Surg* 1971; 48:224–237.

Walleck C: Head trauma in children. *Nurs Clin North Am* 1980; 15(1):115–127.

Weeks H: What every ICU nurse should know about Reye's syndrome. *MCN* 1976 Jan; 231.

Winston K: Craniosynostosis. *In* Wilkins RH, Rengachary SS (eds): *Neurosurgery.* Vol 3. New York, McGraw-Hill, 1985, pp 2173–2191.

Wulf J: Effects of observer variables and seizure attributes on seizure observation and documentation. *Epilepsia* 1986; 27(5):632.

Yanko J: Head injuries. *J Neurosurg Nurs* 1984; 16(4):173–180.

Zegeer L: Nursing care of the patient with brain edema. *J Neurosurg Nurs* 1982; 14(5):268–275.

Zeidelman C: Increased intracranial pressure in the pediatric patient: nursing assessment and intervention. *J Neurosurg Nurs* 1980; 12(1):7–11.

Bibliography

Abe H, et al: Functional prognosis of surgical treatment of craniosynostosis. *Child Nerv Sys* 1985; 1(1):53–61.

Adams M, et al: Trends in clinical characteristics of infants with spina bifida—Atlanta 1972–1979. *Am J Dis Child* 1985; 139(5):514–517.

Adams M, et al: Survival of infants with spina bifida—Atlanta, 1972–1979. *Am J Dis Child* 1985; 139(5):518–523.

Amacher A, Wellington J: Infantile hydrocephalus: long-term results of surgical therapy. *Child Brain* 1984; 11(4):217–229.

Ammann A, et al: Pediatric acquired immune deficiency syndrome. *Ann NY Acad Sci* 1984; 437:340–349.

Arsenault L: Delayed onset symptomatic hydrocephalus related to aqueductal stenosis. *J Neurosurg Nurs* 1983; 15(5):291–298.

Austin J, et al: Parental attitude and adjustment to epilepsy. *Nurs Res* 1984; 33(2):92–96.

Beller LC, Neunaber KL: The "simple" Valsalva. *Am J Nurs* 1986 Apr; 98(4): 398–399.

Bowens B: Injury to the brachial plexus. *J Neurosurg Nurs* 1985; 17(5):293–300.

Britton C, Miller J: Neurologic complications in acquired immune deficiency syndrome. *Neurol Clin* 1984; 2(2):315–339.

Carlson C: Psychosocial aspects of neurologic disability. *Nurs Clin North Am* 1980; 15(2):309–320.

Coffman S: Description of a nursing diagnosis: alteration in bowel elimination related to neurogenic bowel in children with myelomeningocele. *Issues Compr Pediatr Nurs* 1986; 9(3):179–191.

Conway-Rutcowski B: *Carini and Owens' Neurological and Neurosurgical Nursing.* 8th ed. St Louis, CV Mosby, 1982.

Derechin ME: Pediatric head injury. *Crit Care Nurs Q* 1987; 10(3):12–24.

Dieter J (ed): *Epilepsy, Pregnancy and the Child.* New York, Raven Press, 1982.

Davenport-Fortune P, Dunnum L: Professional nursing care of the patient with increased intracranial pressure: planned or 'hit and miss'? *J Neurosurg Nurs* 1985; 17(6):367–370.

Eggleston C, Cruvant D: Review of recovery from intracerebral hematoma in children and adults. *J Neurosurg Nurs* 15(3):128–135.

Ellenberg J, et al: Age at onset of seizures in young children. *Ann Neurol* 1984; 15(2):127–134.

Epstein F: How to keep shunts functioning, or the 'impossible dream.' *Clin Neurosurg* 1985; 32:608–631.

Fisher J: What you need to know about neurological testing. *RN* 1987 Jan: 47–53.

Fode NC: Subarachnoid hemorrhage from ruptured intracranial aneurysm. *Am J Nurs* 1988 May; 88(5):673–680.

Foy P, et al: The incidence of postoperative seizures. *Acta Neurochir* 1981; 55:253–264.

Frank J, Fischer RG: Drug interactions with carbamazepine. *Pediatr Nurs* 1987 Jan/Feb; 13(1):54–55.

Friedman D: Taking the scare out of caring for seizure patients. *Nurs 88* 1988 Feb; 18(2):53–60.

Gapen P: Neurological complications now characterizing many AIDS victims. *JAMA* 1982; 248(22):1941–1942.

Gastaut H: *Dictionary of Epilepsy, Part 1: Definitions.* Geneva, World Health Organization, 1973.

Grant L: Hydrocephalus: an overview and update. *J Neurosurg Nurs* 1984; 16(6)313–318.

Griebel R, et al: CSF shunt complications: an analysis of contributory factors. *Child Nerv Sys* 1985; 1(2):77–80.

Griswold K, et al: An approach to the care of patients with Guillain-Barré syndrome. *Heart Lung* 1984; 13(1):66–72.

Guin P: Arnold-Chiari malformation—a closer look. *J Neurosurg Nurs* 1985; 17(1):45–52.

Hanno R, Beck R: Tuberous sclerosis. *Neurol Clin* 1987; 5(3):351–360.

Hayden P: A longitudinal study of shunt function in 360 patients with hydrocephalus. *Devel Med Child Neurol* 1983; 25(3):334–337.

Hinkle JL: Treating traumatic coma. *Am J Nurs* 1986 May; 86(5):551–556.

Hobdell EF: Infantile spasms. *Pediatr Nurs* 1988 May/Jun; 14(3):207–209.

Hunt A: Tuberous sclerosis: a survey of 97 cases, I: seizures, pertussis, immunization, and handicap. II: physical findings. III: family aspects. *Dev Med Child Neurol* 1983; 25(3):346–357.

International League Against Epilepsy: Proposal for revised clinical and electroencephalographic classification of epileptic seizures. *Epilepsia* 1981; 22:489.

Jess LW: Assessing your patient for increased I.C.P. *Nurs 87* 1987 Jun; 17(6):34–41.

Kennedy R, et al: Guillain-Barré syndrome: a 42 year epidemiologic and clinical study. *Mayo Clin Proc* 1978;53:93.

LaFerla G, et al: A simple method of assessing intracranial pressure in hydrocephalic patients with shunts. *Dev Med Child Neurol* 1984; 26(6):732–736.

Lipe H: Prevention of nervous system trauma from travel in motor vehicles. *J Neurosurg Nurs* 1985; 17(2):77–82.

Lundgren J: *Acute Neuroscience Nursing: Concepts and Care.* Boston: Jones and Bartlett, 1986.

Marida M: Regional cerebral blood flow: patient correlations. *J Neurosurg Nurs* 1982; 14(6):309–314.

Marshall J: A teaching plan: ventriculoperitoneal shunting procedure. *AORN J* 1984; 40(6):847–851.

Marshall J, Ross J: Hydrocephalus: ventriculoperitoneal shunting in infants and children. *AORN J* 1984; 40(6):842–846.

Matthew E, et al: Seizures following intracranial surgery: incidence in the first postoperative week. *Can J Neurol Sci* 1980; 7:285–290.

Mauldin R, Coleman L: Intracerebral herniation. *J Neurosurg Nurs* 1983; 15(5):287–290.

Messner R, et al: Neurofibromatosis: a familial and family disorder. *J Neurosurg Nurs* 1985; 17(4):221–229.

Miezio P: *Parenting children with disability.* New York, M. Dekker, 1983.

Millar S: *Methods in Critical Care.* Philadelphia, WB Saunders, 1980.

Miller J, Arsenault L: Reye's syndrome. *J Neurosurg Nurs* 1983; 15(3):154–164.

Mills N, Plasterer H: Guillain-Barré syndrome: a framework for nursing care. *Nurs Clin North Am* 1980; 15(2):257–264.

Mitchell P: Decreased adaptive capacity, intracranial: a proposal for a nursing diagnosis. *J Neurosci Nurs* 1986; 18(4):170–175.

Moore PC: When you have to think small for a neurologic exam. *RN* 1988 Jun: 38–44.

Nelson C, Miner M: Brain injury disseminated intravascular coagulation and fibrinolysis syndrome in children. *J Neurosurg Nurs* 1983; 15(2):72–76.

Neveling E, Truex R: External obstructive hydrocephalus: a study of clinical and developmental aspects in ten children. *J Neurosurg Nurs* 1983; 15(4):255–260.

Nurse's hotline helps the spinal cord-injured. *Am J Nurs* 1987 May; 87(5):720-721.

Passo S: Malformations of the neural tube. *Nurs Clin North Am* 1980; 15(1):5-21.

Pinyerd B: Siblings of children with myelomengocele: examining their perceptions. *Matern Child Nurs J* 1983; 12(1):61-70.

Post E: Currently available shunt systems: a review. *Neurosurgery* 1985; 16(2):257-260.

Rainer J, Hollis J: Evaluation of the comatose patient. *J Neurosurg Nurs* 1983; 15(5):283-286.

Remington P, et al: Decreasing trends in Reye's syndrome and aspirin use in Michigan, 1979 to 1984. *Pediatrics* 1986; 77(1):93-98.

Riccardi VM: Neurofibromatosis. *Neurol Clin* 1987; 5(3):337-349.

Richardson K, et al: Biofeedback therapy for managing bowel incontinence caused by meningomyelocele. *MCN* 1985 Nov/Dec; 10(6):388-392.

Rogers M, et al: National Reye's syndrome surveillance, 1982. *Pediatrics* 1985; 75(2):260-264.

Romeo JH: The critical minutes after spinal cord injury. *RN* 1988 Apr; 61-67.

Romeo JH: Spinal cord injury: Nursing the patient toward a new life. *RN* 1988 May; 31-35.

Rosman NP, Herskowitz J: Trauma to the brain and spinal cord. *In* Swaiman KF, Wright FS (eds): *The Practice of Pediatric Neurology*. Vol 2. St Louis, CV Mosby, 1982, pp 958-997.

Santilli N, Tonelson S: Screening for seizures. *Pediatr Nurs* 1981; 7(2):11-15.

Scherer P: Assessment: The logic of coma. *Am J Nurs* 1986 May; 86(5):542-550.

Scherz R: Fatal motor vehicle accidents of child passengers from birth to 4 years of age in Washington State. *Pediatrics* 1981; 68:572-575.

Simpson J: Neurological disorders with autosomal dominant transmission. *J Neurosurg Nurs* 1984; 16(5):262-269.

Slota M: Pediatric neurological assessment. *Crit Care Nurs* 1983 Nov/Dec; 106-112.

Smith J: Big differences in little people. *Am J Nurs* 1988 Apr; 88(4):458-462.

Snider W: Neurological complications of acquired immune deficiency syndrome: analysis of 50 patients. *Ann Neurol* 1983; 18(4):403-418.

Snyder M: Effect of relaxation on psychosocial functioning in persons with epilepsy. *J Neurosurg Nurs* 1983; 15(4):250-254.

Tse AM: Seizures and societal attitudes: A teaching tool for children, siblings, classmates, parents, and classroom teachers. *Issues Compr Pediatr Nurs* 1986 9(5):299-303.

Vlahov D, et al: Neurosurgical wound infections: methodological and clinical factors affecting calculations of infection rates. *J Neurosurg Nurs* 1984; 16(3):128-133.

Wong D: Changing what children hear in the ICU can lower intracranial pressure. *Am J Nurs* 1988 Mar; 88(3):279-280.

Wong J, et al: Care of the unconscious patient: a problem oriented approach. *J Neurosurg Nurs* 1984; 16(3):145-150.

Nursing Strategies: Altered Musculoskeletal Function

Chapter 47

Stephanie Wright

Nursing Process Plan
NPP: The Child at Risk for Neurovascular Impairment Associated with Trauma, Traction, or Casting, page 1786

Related Topics
Genetic counseling, Chapter 4
Patterns of inheritance, Chapter 4
The impact of chronic illness, Chapter 25
The impact of death and dying, Chapter 26
Strategies for pain management, Chapter 29
Juvenile arthritis, Chapter 43
Bone tumors, Chapter 48
The injured child, Chapter 52

Musculoskeletal problems in children are extremely common, often associated with the rapid growth of their skeletal frame and their normal physically active state. Providing nursing care to children with orthopedic conditions often brings the nurse into long-term contact with the child and family, since musculoskeletal problems often require long-term treatment. Many musculoskeletal conditions are temporary alterations of health, and caring for children who will return to robust good health and activity is a joyous experience. Among children with musculoskeletal problems are a group with permanent physical disability. The pediatric nurse has the privilege of watching these children develop their potential in other areas and learn to cope with their handicaps.

While this chapter includes many of the commonly encountered musculoskeletal problems of children, the reader is also referred to Chapter 43 for a discussion of juvenile arthritis and Chapter 48 for a discussion of bone tumors in children.

Growth and Development of Bone

Embryology

The musculoskeletal system arises from the mesodermal layer of the embryo, which appears during the second week of embryonic life. From the mesoderm appear 43 pairs of somites, blocks of tissue from which the skeletal, muscular, and certain dermal structures will develop. The three primitive segments separate from the somite, migrate, and differentiate into specialized cells.

Sclerotomal cells migrate around the neural tube and notochord and begin establishment of the vertebral column. The bones of the skull develop from the mesodermal structures surrounding the brain. The bones of the extremities develop from the mesodermal layers in the limb buds.

Formation of bone occurs by two processes: intramembranous and endochondral ossification. Intramembranous ossification occurs in the thin flat bones of the skull, while endochondral ossification occurs in the axial skeleton and the appendicular skeleton. In intramembranous ossification the mesodermal cells form a layer or membrane. Some of the mesodermal cells differentiate into osteoblasts and begin deposition of bone-like tissue.

In endochondral ossification, bone forms within a cartilage model that is developed from mesodermal tissue at that site. Cartilage is destroyed and bone is laid down within the model, beginning in the center or the diaphysis of a long bone. This is the primary ossification center of the bone. Figure 47-1 illustrates how

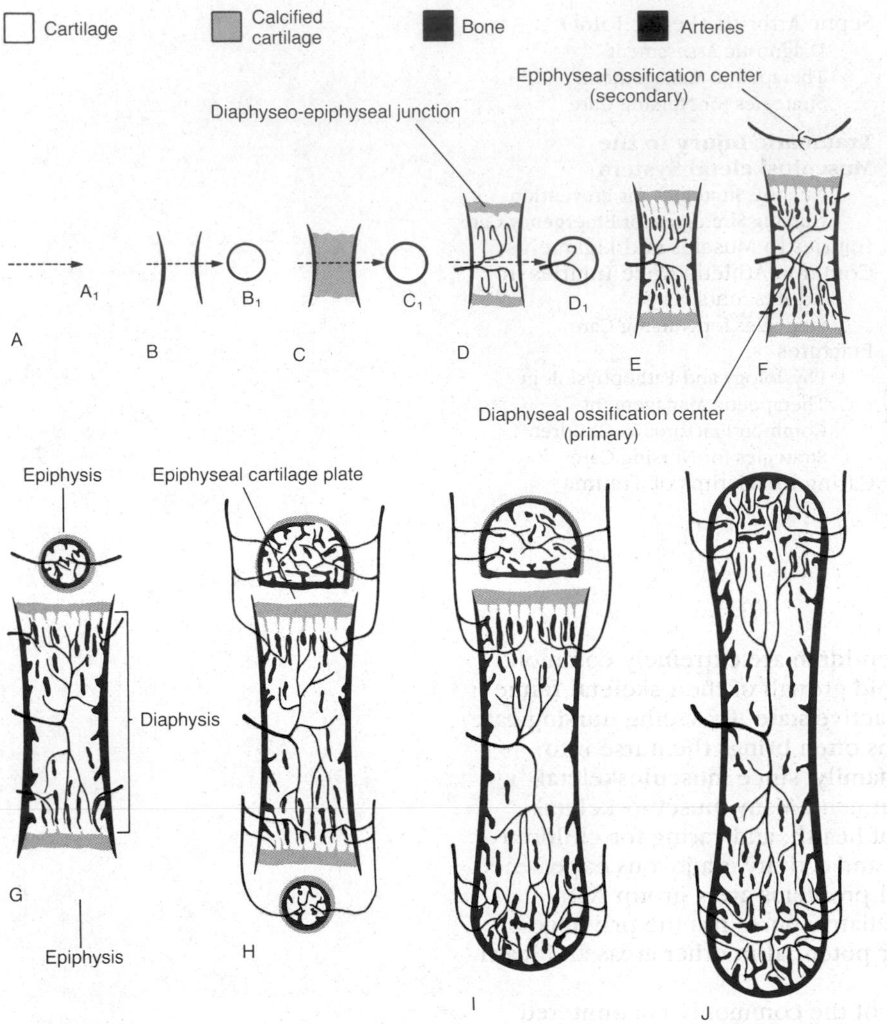

Figure 47-1. Schematic diagrams illustrating intracartilaginous, or endochondral, ossification and the development of a typical long bone. *A* to *J* are longitudinal sections, and *A* to *D* are cross-sections at the levels indicated. *A*, Cartilage model of the bone. *B*, A subperiosteal ring of bone appears. *C*, Cartilage begins to calcify. *D*, Vascular mesenchyme enters the calcified cartilage. *E*, At each diaphyseo-epiphyseal junction, there is a zone of ossification. *F*, Blood vessels and mesenchyme enter the superior epiphyseal cartilage. *G*, The epiphyseal ossification center grows. *H*, A similar center develops in the inferior epiphyseal cartilage. *I*, The inferior epiphyseal plate is ossified. *J*, The superior epiphyseal plate ossifies, forming a continuous bone marrow cavity. When the epiphyseal plates ossify, the bone can no longer grow in length. (Modified from Bloom W, Fawcett DW: *A Textbook of Histology.* 11th ed. Philadelphia, WB Saunders, 1986.)

this occurs. Ossification begins as early as 8 weeks after fertilization and continues throughout gestation and childhood, so that at birth the diaphyses of the long bones are well ossified. Ossification of the ends of the long bones occurs separately and later with a secondary ossification center developing there. A few secondary centers develop late in fetal life, but most appear postnatally.

The joints begin as loosely woven fibrous connective tissue between the epiphyses of two developing adjacent bones. As the connective tissue thins out, the joint cavity is formed. Even after secondary centers of ossification appear, the articulating surfaces of the bones continue to be covered with cartilage, providing a smooth surface for articulation. Voluntary muscle develops from the myotomes or from mesodermal cells in the limb buds. Table 47-1 summarizes musculoskeletal development in utero.

Bone Growth and Ossification

The process of bone growth and ossification, begun in utero, continues after birth with the ossification of long bones continuing as depicted in Figure 47-1. Bone growth occurs in two dimensions: increase in diameter and increase in length. Bone growth occurs on the external surfaces of the bone rather than from within. Growth in diameter occurs by the laying down of new bone directly on the surface of the bone cortex by specialized cells of the periosteum.

Growth in length occurs at the epiphyseal plate where the two ossification centers meet. The epiphyseal plate is a vascular area of active cell division. On the epiphyseal end of the plate, new cartilage is laid down and, as it passes through the zones of the epiphysis, is converted to bone at the metaphyseal end of the plate. The growing cells of the epiphysis are highly sensitive to the hormonal influences of growth hormone, estrogen, and testosterone. Growth hormone increases the cell reproduction and synthesis. Estrogens slow down activity in the epiphysis and tend to narrow the epiphyseal plate, while testosterone has the opposite effect (Lovell and Winter, 1978). Nutrition has a direct effect on cells of the epiphyseal plate.

The epiphyseal plate is present from birth until adolescence, at which time it too is converted to bone and growth stops. The age at which this occurs differs

Table 47-1. Timetable of Musculoskeletal Embryology

Ovulation Age	Event
2nd Week	Appearance of germ layers
3rd Week	Somites develop from mesoderm
4th Week	Arm buds appear
5th Week	Leg buds appear
6th Week	Fingers and toes appear
8th Week	All major bones present in cartilaginous skeleton
	First primary ossification centers appear
12th Week	Fetus capable of some movement
	Ossification of vertebral bodies apparent
	Nails appear
16th Week	Most bones have begun ossification and would appear on roentgenograph
	Movement may be detected by mother
20th Week	Sternum ossified; fetal movements strong
36th–40th Weeks	Some secondary ossification centers appear

from one adolescent to another, with epiphyseal closure generally occurring earlier in girls than in boys.

The presence of the epiphyseal plate has significance when dealing with children with musculoskeletal problems. It represents an area of weakness in bone structure and is subject to injury by fracture, crushing, or slippage. Injury to the epiphysis always carries with it the risk of affecting future growth, and all treatment modalities must be considered in light of their effect on the future growth of the bone. Considering the tremendous change in bone length that occurs between birth and adolescence, injury to one epiphysis can have disastrous effects on overall length of the limb. Each of the major long bones has two epiphyseal plates, and growth at one plate will tend to compensate for altered growth at the opposite end of the bone. However, this ability to compensate is limited and cannot correct great discrepancies in bone length.

Bone Healing and Remodeling

Healing of bone in children follows the same process as in adults (Fig. 47-2). A hematoma forms at the site of injury and fracture. The bone ends that have had their blood supply interrupted become necrotic and die. The hematoma is gradually reabsorbed and, through the action of the osteoblasts (specialized cells), a bridge of connective tissue develops between the two bone ends. This initial connective tissue is callus. Callus formation occurs more rapidly in children than in adults, greatly reducing the time needed for immobilization (see section on fractures, p. 1840). Callus is then converted to bone over a period of weeks or months.

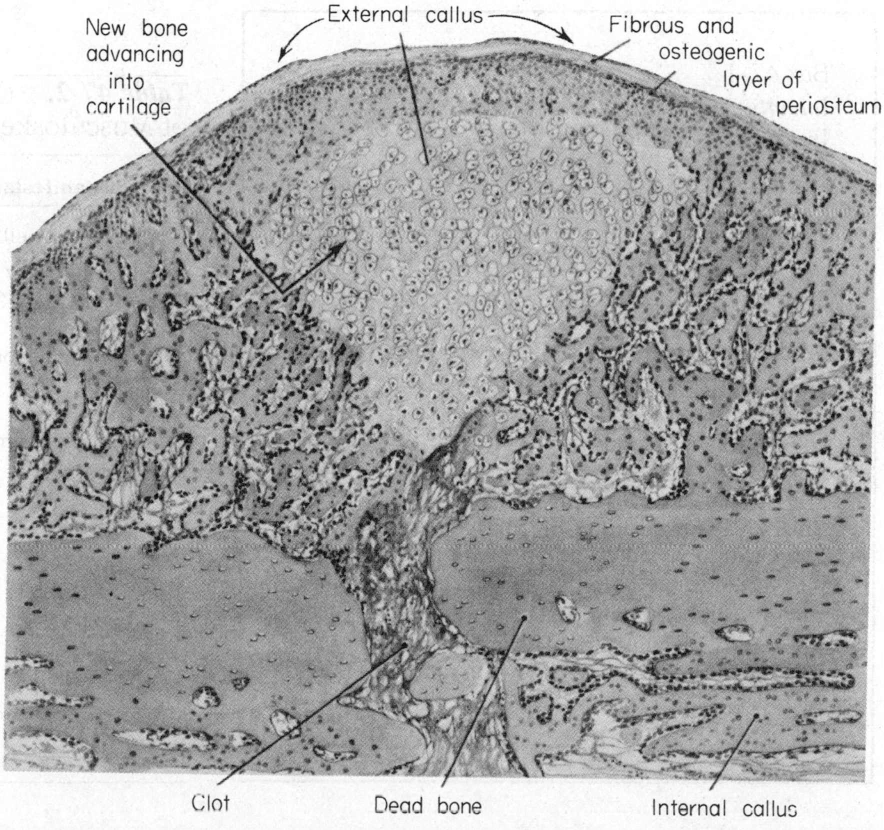

Figure 47-2. Drawing of part of a section cut from a rabbit's fractured rib that has healed for 2 weeks. This drawing illustrates the external callus to advantage and shows that the cartilage in it is being replaced by bone along a V-shaped line. Some clot, still unorganized, can be seen. (From Ham AW, Harris WR: *In* Bourne GH: *The Biochemistry and Physiology of Bone.* 2nd ed. New York, Academic Press, 1972.)

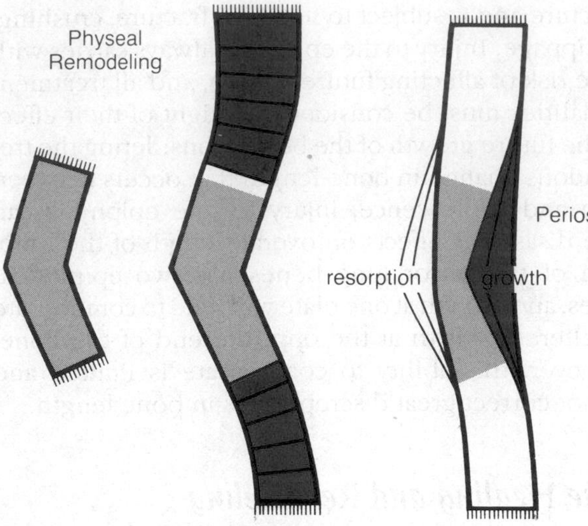

Figure 47-3. The basis of fracture remodeling. (From Rang M: *Children's Fractures.* Philadelphia, JB Lippincott, 1983.)

Due to their continued growth, children are capable of actually remodeling or straightening some bony deformities that occur as a result of injury or treatment. Figure 47-3 illustrates how remodeling occurs. The more rapid the rate of growth, the more rapidly healing and remodeling occur. Both of these processes tend to decline with age. Box 47-1 summarizes the developmental differences in the musculoskeletal system.

Box 47-1
Important Musculoskeletal Differences and Implications (Children versus Adults)

Epiphyseal plate present:
Area of weakness
Injury may disrupt growth, cause overgrowth, or deformity
Dislocations/sprains less common (epiphysis gives way first)
Treatment method may differ from adult

Bones growing:
Remodeling potential great
Deformity may progress with growth

Bones more plastic:
More force required to fracture
Bones may bow but not fracture
Force produces different types of fractures

Periosteum thicker and more active:
May remain intact with fracture
Produces callus more quickly
Healing occurs more quickly

Abundant blood supply:
Rapid healing

Assessment of Musculoskeletal Problems

Initial Physical Assessment

As part of the initial assessment of the musculoskeletal system, the nurse obtains a complete history of problems pertaining to these body systems. The child should supply as much of the subjective data as possible. Adolescents should be encouraged to be responsible for the majority of the assessment interview.

The interviewer obtains a complete history of all problems related to movement and musculoskeletal function, including physical limitations and alterations in lifestyle imposed by the problem, and any mobility aids that are being used. Elicit detailed information on the circumstances under which any clinical manifestations described might appear.

If the interview is problem-oriented around musculoskeletal dysfunction, the interviewer will focus on this problem but should also include a general health history and assess any other identified problem areas. Both the interview and general assessment should follow the guidelines in Chapter 15 on Health Appraisal. Assessment of the musculoskeletal system begins on page 547. Measurements of height and weight are of particular significance in many musculoskeletal disorders and should be included whenever feasible. During examination the nurse should be alert for any of the manifestations described in Table 47-2.

Table 47-2. Clinical Manifestations of Musculoskeletal Problems

Clinical Manifestation	Significance
Pain, redness, swelling	May indicate injury or disease
Asymmetry of body parts, length discrepancies	May indicate growth disturbance, injury, or disease in one extremity
Abnormal turning or rotation of body part	May indicate abnormal development or growth disturbance
Limitation of joint motion	May indicate abnormal relationship between articulating parts, contracture due to disease, disuse, or immobilization
Crepitus	May indicate joint disease or injury
Weakness	May indicate muscular problem due to disease or disuse of body part
Limp or other abnormal gait	Indicates weakness, pain, or deformity of the lower extremity

Assessment of Neurovascular Status

The greatest hazard of trauma to the musculoskeletal system, whether accidental or part of some therapeutic treatment plan, is that the trauma, the swelling that accompanies it, or the compression of cast or traction may interfere with circulation or damage the nervous system. Either can cause irreparable and permanent damage and disability. **One of the key responsibilities of the nurse caring for the patient with musculoskeletal problems is the intermittent assessment of neurovascular status to ensure that no deterioration in neurologic function or circulatory compromise has occurred.**

Assessment of neurovascular status includes evaluation of the following eight areas. In each case, the affected extremity should be compared with the unaffected extremity whenever possible.

1. Color—Normal skin color is the ideal. Some redness often accompanies swelling. Of particular concern is pallor or cyanosis, which can indicate interference with blood supply. Following application of a cast, the dampness may cool the extremity and cause some color change.
2. Temperature—Warmth indicates good circulatory perfusion. Coolness of an extremity warrants close observation. Coolness can be due to exposure in a cool environment or cooling due to evaporation from a wet cast. Temperature changes from a wet cast are most pronounced in the first 12 to 24 hours.
3. Sensation—Normal sensation should be present. Children may not be reliable descriptors of sensation. Checks of sensation should always be done out of the child's sight. The examiner must ask definitive questions, avoiding the common "Can you feel this?" A better indicator may be elicited by "Wiggle each finger (toe) as I touch it." Note any numbness or tingling described by the patient and its location and boundaries.
4. Motion—The extremity should be capable of normal motion or whatever is possible within the confines of immobilization. The child should be able to wiggle fingers or toes of the affected extremity. This motion should not cause extreme pain. Some discomfort with motion is not uncommon.
5. Pain—Pain is a normal accompaniment to trauma or surgery. The pain experienced by the child should be appropriate to the injury and relieved by usual amounts of medication. Excessive pain may be a sign of neurovascular compromise.
6. Pulse—A normal pulse should be present distal to the injury, cast, or traction.
7. Capillary Filling—By pressing on each nailbed, releasing, and observing the return of color, the assessor can estimate the amount of circulatory compromise. Capillary filling of the affected extremity should be rapid and comparable to that of the unaffected extremity.
8. Edema—Swelling is often present but needs to be assessed and controlled to avoid compression of nerves and blood vessels. Swelling is usually controlled by elevation of the extremity. Elevation above the level of the heart is most effective.

Assessment of neurovascular status (NVS) is part of the initial assessment of the child when first contact is made. This provides a baseline for future neurovascular assessments. If first contact is following the trauma or procedure, one can often use an unaffected extremity as a partial guideline or obtain information on prior NVS from emergency department personnel or the physician.

How frequently neurovascular status is assessed depends on the diagnosis or extent of injury. A good general rule is hourly until normal, then every 4 hours (Table 47-3).

Documentation of NVS assessments should be clear and precise. The terminology used should be descriptive in nature, and judgmental terms (e.g.,

***Table* 47-3.** Neurovascular Assessment

Problem	Items to Assess	Frequency
Fracture/surgery with cast	Extremity distal to cast	Hourly for 24 hours,* then every 4 hours
Fracture/surgery with continuous traction	Extremity distal to traction	Hourly for 24 hours,* then every 4 hours
Intermittent skin traction	Extremity distal to traction	Half hour after each application, then every 4 hours
Hip spica cast	Both lower extremities, perineal area	Hourly for 24 hours,* then every 4 hours
Body casts	All four extremities	Hourly for 24 hours,* then every 4 hours
Halo traction or cast, cervical/Tongs	All four extremities, cranial nerve functions	Hourly for 24 hours, then every 4 hours
Cervical traction	All four extremities	Hourly for 4 hours, then every 4 hours

* Or until neurovascular status (NVS) has returned to normal. Any deterioration in NVS indicates a continuation or resumption of hourly assessments.

Table 47-4
Nursing Process Plan: The Child at Risk for Neurovascular Impairment Associated with Trauma, Traction, or Casting

by Roxie Foster

Assessment of Physical Function

Activity/Exercise: Neuromuscular Integrity

Subjective Assessment

Sensation in extremity distal to site of surgery or trauma compared with other extremity.

Objective Assessment

Vascular perfusion and motor ability of extremity distal to site of surgery or trauma compared with other extremity.

Analysis: Nursing Diagnosis 1

Potential for injury: physiologic, related to neurovascular impairment associated with pressure exerted on blood vessels and nerves secondary to:

- *bleeding into a muscle compartment*
- *edema of soft tissues within a constricting cast*
- *malalignment of the traction force*
- *improper position of traction apparatus (e.g., ropes, spreader bar)*

Defining Characteristics

Subjective: Verbalization/vocalization of altered sensation in digits of affected extremity: numbness, tingling, pain that increases with movement and is not relieved by analgesics.

Objective: Perfusion in affected extremity: decreased or absent pulse(s); skin cool and pale; capillary refill >3 seconds. Neuromuscular integrity in affected extremity: child unable to distinguish which digits are being touched; decreased ability (or unable) to flex and extend digits; evidence of tissue swelling within a closed compartment (i.e., muscle compartment, cast) or of pressure over a major nerve.

Client Goals/ Evaluation Criteria	Nursing Goals/Strategies (Selected Rationale)
1. The client will maintain neurovascular integrity of the affected extremity as evidenced by: a. verbalization of equal sensation in the affected and unaffected extremities b. absence of severe pain in the affected extremity c. pulses palpable and equal in the affected and unaffected extremities d. capillary refill time <3 seconds	*Monitor neurovascular status (NVS) upon first contact with the child to establish a baseline for future assessments.* Thereafter monitor NVS at least every 4 hours (see Table 47-3). *Ensure accurate assessment data by:* • Assessing for sensation in the digits in such a way that the child cannot see which digit is being touched • Assessing all 5 fingers or toes (digits innervated by different nerves) • Acknowledging the pain experienced upon movement of the digits, but encouraging the child to demonstrate flexion and extension to the fullest ability • Being alert to irritability in the preverbal child and making more frequent NVS assessments to compensate for decreased subjective data

e. skin color and warmth equal in affected and unaffected extremities
f. ability to flex and extend digits of the affected extremity

- Telling the verbal child to alert the nurse if numbness, tingling or pain occurs at any time
- Assessing skin warmth, color, and pulses in both extremities at the same time

Ensure accurate interpretation of the data by:
- Reassessment of alterations and comparison with the unaffected extremity
- Comparison with last recorded findings
- Consideration of the effects of a drying cast upon skin temperature

Institute and teach the child and family measures that will prevent alteration in NVS in the immediate post-trauma period:
- Monitor the child with musculoskeletal trauma for signs of shock (that would indicate possible bleeding into a muscle compartment).
- Splint musculoskeletal injuries before transport to avoid additional soft tissue trauma.

Institute and teach the child and family measures that will prevent alteration in NVS related to casting:
- Avoid indentations in a wet cast (a plaster cast dries in 10–72 hr, a synthetic cast in 5–30 min [Wise, 1986]): handle with palms, not fingertips; cushion with pillows instead of placing wet cast on firm mattress; facilitate drying by turning the child every two hours and by leaving the cast uncovered. Once the cast is dry, keep it dry.
- Prevent swelling inside the cast: elevate the extremity on pillows (to facilitate venous return); use ice packs around the cast, with physician's order. Assess the cast for tightness by making sure a finger can be inserted between the cast and the skin at all points. Be especially alert to reports of "tightness" over bony prominences (a window may need to be cut in the cast to relieve localized pressure over a nerve).
- Prevent foreign objects from entering the cast. Brush away plaster, petal the cast edges. Do not allow the infant or young child to play with objects that are small enough to fit inside the cast. Monitor finger foods and pieces of food that may spill into the cast at mealtime. Insert fabric or soft cotton between the skin and cast when the child is eating and remove afterward (so it does not get pushed into a firm ball and become lodged inside the cast). Do not allow the child to scratch the skin inside the cast with a coat hanger or similar objects (this action pushes the cotton lining inside the cast into lumps that can form pressure points). Avoid powder inside the cast (it forms small "balls" on contact with moisture). Control itching by blowing cool air from a hair dryer inside the cast or by scratching the opposite extremity.

Institute and teach the child and family measures that will prevent alteration in NVS related to traction:
- Maintain traction in proper alignment. Children often move about so that alignment is altered. A child of preschool age or older may be able to cooperate by agreeing to stay within a boundary of colored tape on the bottom sheet. Place the telephone and the child's belongings within easy reach and instruct them to use the call bell for objects out of reach
- Assess frequently for pressure exerted over major nerves by traction apparatus, especially over the bones of the ankle, elbow, and wrist

Table 47-5. Diagnostic Procedures in Musculoskeletal Disease

Test	Purpose/Description	Comments
Roentgenography (X-ray)	Visualize bony structures for detection of bone/joint abnormalities or to determine bone age	Young children require immobilization. Prepare adequately to insure cooperation. No dietary restrictions indicated
CT scan	Visualize bony structures and some soft tissue areas. Contrast material may or may not be used	Length of time required necessitates sedation of young children. CT tunnel frightening to child. If IV contrast used, prepare child for injection and keep NPO for 4 hours
Bone scan	Roentgenograph following injection of radioactive tracer to detect tumors, infection, or inflammation	Child needs preparation for discomfort of injection. May need immobilization or restraint. Increase fluid intake between injection and scan to facilitate excretion of isotope
Bone or muscle biopsy	Direct examination of abnormal area, gross and microscopic	Surgical procedure with general anesthesia. Operative preparation needed
Arthrogram	Improved roentgenographic visualization of joint through use of injected air or contrast media to diagnose joint disorders	Preparation should include local anesthetic and injection into joint. No dietary restrictions. Not often needed in young children. Prepare for post-test swelling and pain
Arthroscopy	Direct visualization of joint, most commonly knee, through arthroscope to detect abnormalities. Biopsy or surgery may be performed through scope	Surgical procedure—requires surgical preparation and anesthesia. Prepare for post-test swelling, pain, pressure dressings
Joint aspiration	Withdrawal of fluid from joint for analysis, usually to detect infection or inflammation	Local anesthetic used, but some discomfort may be expected during and following procedure
Electromyogram	Measures electrical potential in a muscle via inserted needle to delineate neuromuscular disorders	Requires much cooperation from patient; needle insertion uncomfortable and frightening. Requires detailed preparation and support during procedure

(Adapted from Hilt and Cogburn, 1980; Hamilton, 1981.)

good, poor) should be avoided as they do not convey accurate information. Nursing care of the child who is at risk for impairment of neurovascular status is detailed in Table 47-4.

Diagnostic Procedures

The usual diagnostic procedures used in children with musculoskeletal problems are described in Table 47-5. Many others may be used in the diagnosis of individual conditions or complications. Roentgenographs are by far the most common procedure and may be required frequently to assess injury and healing.

Therapeutic Interventions

Immobilization

Immobilization is an integral part of the treatment regimen of many musculoskeletal disorders. Advances in surgery and other treatment methods have greatly reduced the time of immobilization required for many problems, but proper alignment and healing of bones still requires immobility for a period of time. Immobility may be a side effect of the disease itself owing to pain or weakness, rather than a treatment modality. In either situation, immobilization has specific effects and creates definite problems for the nurse to address.

Physiologic Effects. Immobilization has multisystem effects, and the extent of these effects depends on the degree and duration of immobility. Generally, young children have a physiologic resilience that makes them less prone to some of the effects of immobilization than older persons, but when immobilized for an extended period of time, they too will begin to show the effects of inactivity.

With inactivity the heart rate and circulation slows. Venous return, normally assisted by the contraction of skeletal muscle in the extremities, becomes sluggish. The patient is prone to clot formation, particularly in the lower extremities, and has an increased risk of pulmonary embolus. Young children, even when immobilized in bed, are frequently active enough that this problem is not of great concern. Adolescents need to be taught to develop an exercise program for their feet and legs (dorsiflexion and plantarflexion of the feet) to prevent venous stasis.

With lowered metabolic rate and less oxygen consumption, respirations slow and become more shallow. A supine position encourages the accumulation of secretions, and the patient runs the risk of developing a hypostatic pneumonia. Frequent change of position is helpful when possible. Every immobilized child needs to be instructed in a deep-breathing routine. Blowing balloons or pinwheels are good diversionary activities that encourage lung expansion.

Appetite decreases as bodily caloric needs drop, and peristaltic activity slows with decreased activity and decreased food intake. Children, particularly those of school age and adolescents, may find using a bedpan or being assisted with elimination very embarrassing. Constipation is one of the most frequently encountered effects of immobilization. It should be anticipated and prevented through the use of a high-fiber diet, adequate fluid intake, and appropriate use of stool softeners. Providing the child with as much privacy as possible will aid relaxation and elimination.

Fluid needs decrease because the insensible fluid loss is less, the metabolic rate is lowered, and kidney filtration rate slows. Stasis of urine is more likely to occur, making immobilized patients more prone to both urinary tract infections and the formation of renal calculi. Calcium salts are present in the urine in greater quantities when osteoporosis due to disuse is occurring; the presence of these salts provides a situation in which precipitation can more easily occur. Increased fluid intake prevents stasis of urine and dilutes the calcium salts. One can easily ascertain what fluids the child enjoys and provide these in generous quantities.

The absence of the normal stresses on the skeletal system produces a gradual decalcification of the bones and increased bone fragility. Any physical activity will slow this process, but returning to weight bearing as soon as possible is of premium importance.

Skin breakdown is of continued concern when nursing patients with orthopedic problems. Pressure from body weight, cast, or traction apparatus on any skin surface can rapidly produce ischemia and breakdown. Change of position, if possible, is the most effective preventative. Reducing pressure by providing an egg-crate mattress, sheepskin, or other padding will also be beneficial. Of greatest importance is a continuous diligence in providing skin care and careful observation for signs of pressure.

Muscle atrophy begins as soon as muscle contraction stops. The muscle becomes weak and incapable of usual activity, and muscle mass decreases. When held in place or allowed to assume a continuous position, some muscle groups will become contracted. Both effects are easily seen upon removal of a cast. When immobilization of a body part is necessary for healing, this atrophy is unavoidable. The patient needs to be prepared for the weakness of disuse atrophy and anticipate that a gradual program of restrengthening will be necessary.

When bed rest is required, the aim is to prevent all disuse atrophy and contracture that is not mandated because of the treatment regimen. A regular exercise program can be established to provide full range of motion and stimulation to any muscle group able to be exercised. A physical therapist may provide this service. If this is not available, the nurse can easily establish a program. Of particular concern are three lower extremity contractures that develop rapidly and may seriously interfere with reambulation. First, footdrop with resulting contracture of the calf muscles will occur in any unsupported foot and can be prevented by a footboard and regular dorsiflexion of the foot. When skeletal traction is applied to a lower extremity, a cast may be applied to the foot for purposes of foot support (see Fig. 47-9). Second, knee flexion contractures occur when continuous support behind the knee is provided. Pillow supports for the knee should be used with caution. Third, hip flexion contractures develop from a continuous sitting posture. Both the knee and hip must regularly be placed in full extension.

General weakness and decreased endurance are seen after even 1 day of bed rest. For the child or adolescent who has been recumbent for a period of time, this will be accompanied by postural hypotension when an upright position is attempted. Reambulation must be attempted very gradually and as tolerance permits. Children are often unaware of these effects and need to have a reambulation program carefully explained.

Emotional/Social Effects. Most children are by nature extremely active beings. Interfering with their normal activity is not without consequences. Immobilization for musculoskeletal conditions may involve physical restraint and discomfort. Immobilizing a child for an extended period of time interferes with usual methods of dissipating frustrations and anxieties while imposing many new frustrations and reasons to be anxious. The inability of young children to understand the reason for what has happened leads them to their own conclusions about their predicament. Not unusually, one of these conclusions is that they are being punished. To counter this, all treatment regimens must be explained in age-appropriate language with diagrams, roentgenographs, or both, and with explanations of their benefit to the child's health.

Although many musculoskeletal conditions are reversible in nature, many also require long-term treatment. Adults, adolescents, and some older children are able to comprehend a month or longer plan of treatment, but the perception of this timeframe in young children is absent and in many older children may be distorted. When progress is slow, children need frequent reassurance that they are getting well and that the time in cast or traction is limited.

Children who are immobilized are socially isolated from their usual world and have limited peer contact. Sensory deprivation easily occurs in a hospital room. Children in our culture are normally exposed to daily sensory and intellectual stimulation at school or preschool and at home.

Normalizing the environment as much as possible is the aim. The child and family should be encouraged to create a home-like atmosphere in the patient's surroundings. Change of surroundings is always beneficial when not medically contraindicated. Visiting of siblings and peers is to be encouraged. The child needs to be provided with the diversions and activities that are normally found pleasurable. Children immobilized in traction often resort to hours of television viewing because activity is so limited. This can be avoided by providing other diversions. Of course, a tutor must be provided to continue school work.

Patterns of Adaptation in Children and Families. A few maladaptive patterns are seen among children and families in this situation; the nurse needs to respond to these situations in a therapeutic fashion to help establish a more healthy pattern of interaction.

Demanding Child/Indulgent Parent. The child responds to the anxiety and anger at his or her situation by becoming extremely demanding of both the parents and the nursing staff. The parents respond to their concern and guilt over the child's condition by indulging every whim. The parents may simultaneously become very resentful of their child's demands. The child may become increasingly anxious over the lack of usual limits upon behavior. The nurse can intervene by establishing definite limits with children in a nonthreatening fashion, assuring them that their needs will not be neglected. Parents need an opportunity to discuss their feelings. The nurse can provide reassurance and support that it is acceptable to establish limits and discipline for children, even while they are incapacitated, and that they will feel more secure if this is done.

Perfectionism. The child's lack of control over the world and an attempt to regain some control may surface in attempts to establish rigid standards and procedures for how care is delivered: the bed must be made in a certain way, arrangement of the child's belongings are rigidly specified, and food must be exactly to his or her choosing. Within limits, this behavior should be respected if it gives the child some semblance of control. Simultaneously, the nurse might concentrate on eliciting the child's feelings about his or her helplessness, vulnerability, and lack of control.

Submissiveness/Pleasing Behavior. Some children will respond to their extremely vulnerable position by being afraid to misbehave in any way or express the normal negative emotions of anger, frustration, and fear. They are model patients. The nursing personnel may be delighted, while the parents may express disbelief that the child is not reacting in a more appropriate fashion. The family and staff can reinforce the acceptability of nonviolent expressions of anger and frustration and the universality of such feelings. Suppression of these feelings during hospitalization may be a temporarily effective coping mechanism but may be followed by some repercussions for the family once a safe home environment is reached.

Depression/Withdrawal. The child may feel totally overwhelmed by the situation and choose to withdraw. Expression of feelings must be encouraged. The family and staff can look for ways to give the child some control and involvement in decision making regarding his or her care. The need for repeated explanations and reassurance that this time will pass cannot be overstressed.

When maladaptive responses do not resolve, family or psychiatric counseling may be indicated. Most children have resilient coping mechanisms and will master the crisis of immobilization and hospitalization if love and support are provided.

Casts

Casts are applied to hold position and provide protection after reduction of a fracture or to correct deformity, as when serial casting is used in the correction of clubfoot. The most commonly used casting materials are plaster of Paris and fiber glass. Both are applied by wetting the impregnated bandaging material and wrapping the extremity after it has been covered with stockinette or one of a variety of other wrapping materials. As the casting medium is applied, it is simultaneously molded to the extremity. Plaster, the more traditionally used material, has the advantage of conforming somewhat more readily to the shape and form of the body part but is heavy and deteriorates if wet. Fiber glass is lighter and not harmed by water.

Types of casts commonly used are illustrated in Figure 47-4. The majority of children in casts will have these applied on an outpatient basis and will be cared for at home. The nurse must be comfortable and knowledgeable about cast care in order to convey this knowledge to the family of the child.

Strategies for Nursing Care

The nurse has an important role in preparing the child for cast application. If time permits, the nurse can demonstrate the procedure on a doll or show the child a picture of the type of cast to be used. The child should always be prepared for how the cast is applied and what its purpose is. When plaster of Paris is applied, heat is generated as the plaster sets. The child needs to be prepared that the cast will feel quite warm but will not burn.

During cast application, the nurse may assist with the cast application and explain to the child each step of the procedure.

After the cast has been applied, nursing care will involve two components: (1) care to ensure drying of

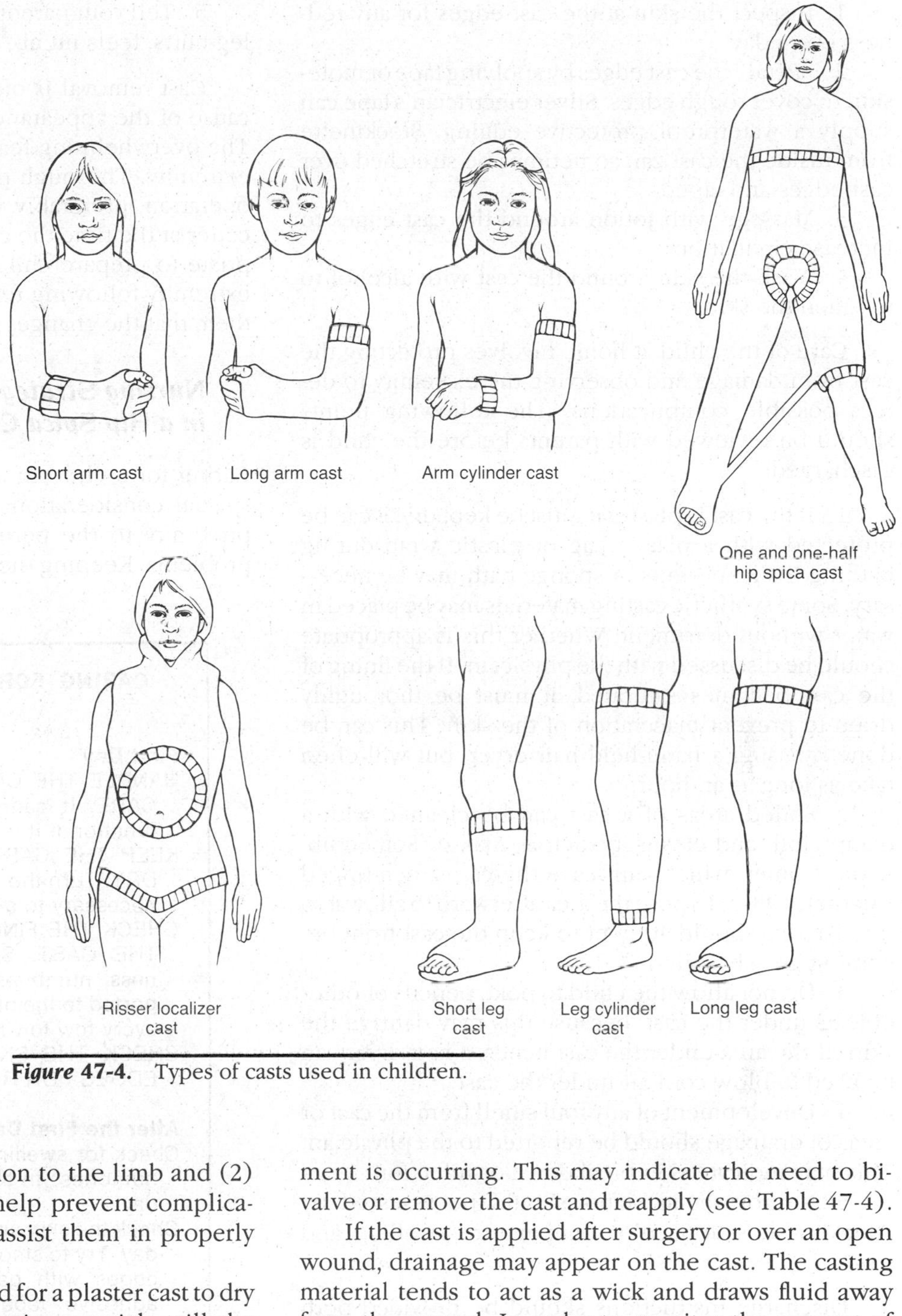

Figure 47-4. Types of casts used in children.

the cast and adequate circulation to the limb and (2) instructions to the family to help prevent complications of cast application and assist them in properly caring for the cast.

About 24 hours are required for a plaster cast to dry completely. The newer synthetic materials will dry more quickly. During this drying period, the exposure of the cast should be changed frequently so that all surfaces are exposed and evaporation may take place. This may require turning or repositioning the patient in some circumstances. The cast should remain uncovered during this time.

Elevating the affected limb with pillows after cast application will help prevent swelling. Neurovascular status of the affected extremity should be assessed frequently as previously discussed. Any change in the neurovascular parameters should be carefully recorded and reported to the physician if serious impairment is occurring. This may indicate the need to bivalve or remove the cast and reapply (see Table 47-4).

If the cast is applied after surgery or over an open wound, drainage may appear on the cast. The casting material tends to act as a wick and draws fluid away from the wound. In order to monitor the amount of drainage, it is helpful to draw a circle around the area with a pen and note the time on the cast itself. Because of the wicking action of the cast, the drainage is often distributed over a large surface area, making it difficult to estimate the amount of drainage. Any question about the appropriateness of the amount of drainage on the cast should be addressed to the physician. During this period vital signs should be observed closely to monitor for significant bleeding leading to hypovolemic shock.

To prevent skin breakdown resulting from the cast, several steps may be taken:

1. Inspect the skin at the cast edges for any redness every day.
2. "Petal" the cast edges by applying tape or moleskin to cover rough edges. Silver electrician's tape can supply a waterproof protective edging. Stockinette from inside the cast can sometimes be stretched over cast edges and taped.
3. Massage with lotion around the cast edges to increase circulation.
4. Wash the skin around the cast with alcohol to toughen the skin.

Care of the child at home involves protecting the cast from damage and observing the extremity to detect possible complications. The following points should be reviewed with parents before the child is discharged:

1. If the cast is plaster it must be kept dry; it can be protected with a plastic bag or plastic wrap during bathing if size permits. A sponge bath may be necessary. Some synthetic casting materials may be placed in water without detriment. Whether this is appropriate should be discussed with the physician. If the lining of the cast becomes saturated, it must be thoroughly dried to prevent maceration of the skin. This can be done by using a hand-held hair dryer, but will often take as long as an hour.
2. Soiled areas of a cast can be cleaned with a damp cloth and cleanser, such as Ajax or Soft-Scrub. Avoid Comet, which can leave the cast green-tinged (Mather, 1987). Expose the area afterward to allow it to dry. Parents should attempt to keep the cast from becoming grossly soiled.
3. Do not allow the child to poke pencils or other objects under the cast, because this may damage the skin. If the area under the cast itches, a hair dryer can be used to blow cool air under the cast.
4. Development of any foul smell from the cast or areas of drainage should be reported to the physician. This may indicate skin breakdown or infection.
5. Neurovascular status should be assessed by checking sensation, color, temperature, swelling, and pain.

Discharge instructions should be provided both verbally and in writing to the child and parents. An example of simple discharge instructions for a child with a cast is shown in Figure 47-5. Most children adapt very well to limitations in their activity resulting from the cast. Discharge instructions to the child should include the following:

1. Do not bang or hit your cast.
2. Do not let the cast get wet (unless appropriate material).
3. Do not put anything inside the cast.
4. Do not scratch underneath the cast.
5. Tell your parents or another adult if your arm or leg hurts, feels numb, tingles, or looks different.

Cast removal is often frightening to children because of the appearance and noise of the cast cutter. The overwhelming fear is that it will cut or harm the extremity. Thorough preparation is necessary for cooperation, preferably with demonstration of the cast cutter at the time the cast is applied. It may be appropriate to prepare children for the appearance of the extremity following removal of the cast and to assure them that the changes to the skin are only temporary.

Nursing Strategies for Care of a Child in a Hip Spica Cast

Caring for a child in a hip spica cast requires some special consideration. The size of this cast and the proximity to the perineal area create some special problems. Keeping the cast clean and dry becomes an

CARING FOR YOUR CHILD IN A CAST

First Day

HANDLE THE CAST WITH REASONABLE CARE. It cannot perform its intended function if it is cracked.

KEEP THE CAST EXPOSED TO AIR TO DRY. Turn the child from front to back if necessary to allow all sides to dry.

CHECK THE FINGERS OR TOES BELOW THE CAST. Swelling, blueness, coldness, numbness or pain should be reported to the nurse or doctor. Check this every few few hours.

CHECK THE SKIN AROUND THE CAST EDGES FOR REDNESS.

After the First Day

Check for swelling, coldness, blueness or numbness in the fingers or toes twice a day.

Check the skin around the cast edges each day. Try to smooth or pad any sharp cast edges with gauze or small pieces of adhesive tape placed over the cast edges in this fashion.

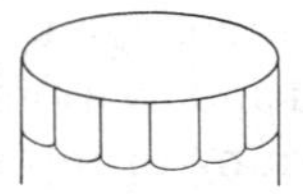

Keep the cast clean and dry. If the cast becomes wet, soft, or should crack, it should be replaced as soon as possible.

Figure 47-5. Discharge instructions for cast care.

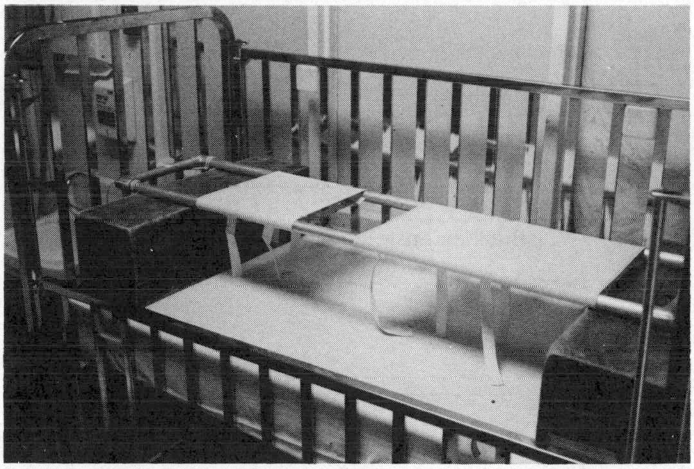

Figure 47-6. A split Bradford frame being set up in a crib. (Photograph by Stephanie Wright.)

important goal. It is not difficult, but requires diligence.

Commonly used for hospital care is a split Bradford frame (Fig. 47-6). The frame is often made of metal covered with padding and canvas. Although the frame may also be used for immobilization purposes, its most common use is for caring for a child in a spica cast who is not toilet trained. The child is positioned either prone or supine on the frame and secured with a drawsheet or other restraining device with the perineal area over the split. Several pieces of heavy plastic sheeting are tucked into the cast's perineal opening so that all the cast edges are covered. The plastic sheets are funneled into a bedpan on the bed under the frame. Urine and feces drain into the bedpan without soiling the edges of the cast. It is important that the head of the frame be elevated slightly so that urine cannot run up inside the cast. The perineal area needs to be washed several times a day and the plastic sheeting changed to minimize odor and prevent skin problems.

Bradford frames are available for rental by parents taking home a child in a spica cast. At home the frame may be used in a crib or bed, or placed in a wagon so the child may be wheeled from room to room. When the child is not on the frame, half a disposable diaper may be tucked inside the cast opening. These are rapidly saturated and must be changed frequently in order to keep the cast dry. A combination of a sanitary napkin and a disposable diaper may be used effectively for more absorbency (Black, 1979).

Older children who are toilet trained need assistance and special precautions during toileting to prevent wetting and soiling the cast. The same method of covering the cast edges with plastic and funneling them into a bedpan works in this situation as well. Older children may also be taught crutch walking and encouraged to be up and about as soon as they are able, to reduce the hazards of immobility.

Parents need generous amounts of time and practice to learn to care for a child in a spica cast and to feel confident upon discharge. Parents should be urged to begin planning for discharge early in hospitalization, as there are often some adaptations that need to be made to accommodate the child at home in these circumstances.

Traction

Traction is the application of pull or force to a body part. This may be accomplished through the use of weights and pullies or through the use of distracting bars. Traction is used for the following purposes:

- Correction of deformities
- Gradual correction or improvement of joint contractures
- Treatment of dislocations
- Reduction of fractures
- Treatment of disease processes of the musculoskeletal system
- Preoperative and postoperative positioning and alignment
- General immobilization of specific areas of the body

The pulling force of traction decreases muscle spasm in many of these situations, making the patient more comfortable. Countertraction is the opposing force or pull that is necessary for traction to be maintained on a body part. This is frequently provided by the body weight alone, but may need to be aided by the use of restraining devices. The main disadvantage of traction is that it usually requires hospitalization and prolonged bed rest.

Equipment used varies according to the orthopedist, the age of the child, the condition being treated, and the type of traction. Most situations will require a

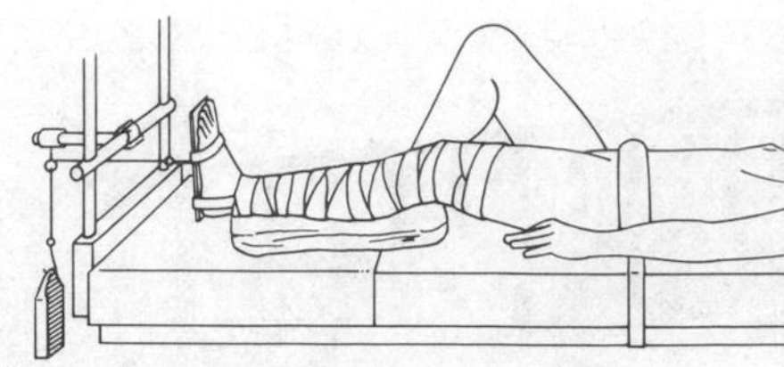

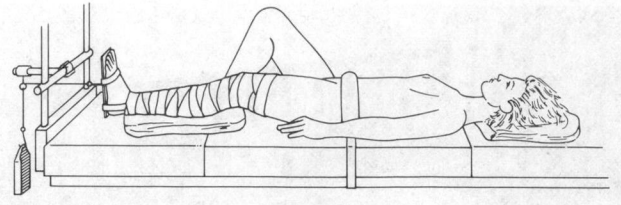

Figure 47-7. Buck extension traction.

bed with an overhead frame for attachment of the traction apparatus and a firm mattress or the use of a bedboard to prevent flexion contractures. An overhead trapeze should be used whenever possible to aid in providing nursing care.

Types of Traction. Traction may be continuous or intermittent. Continuous traction is used for reduction and can be of the skeletal or skin traction type. Intermittent traction may be used to correct deformity or to overcome muscle spasm in a body part.

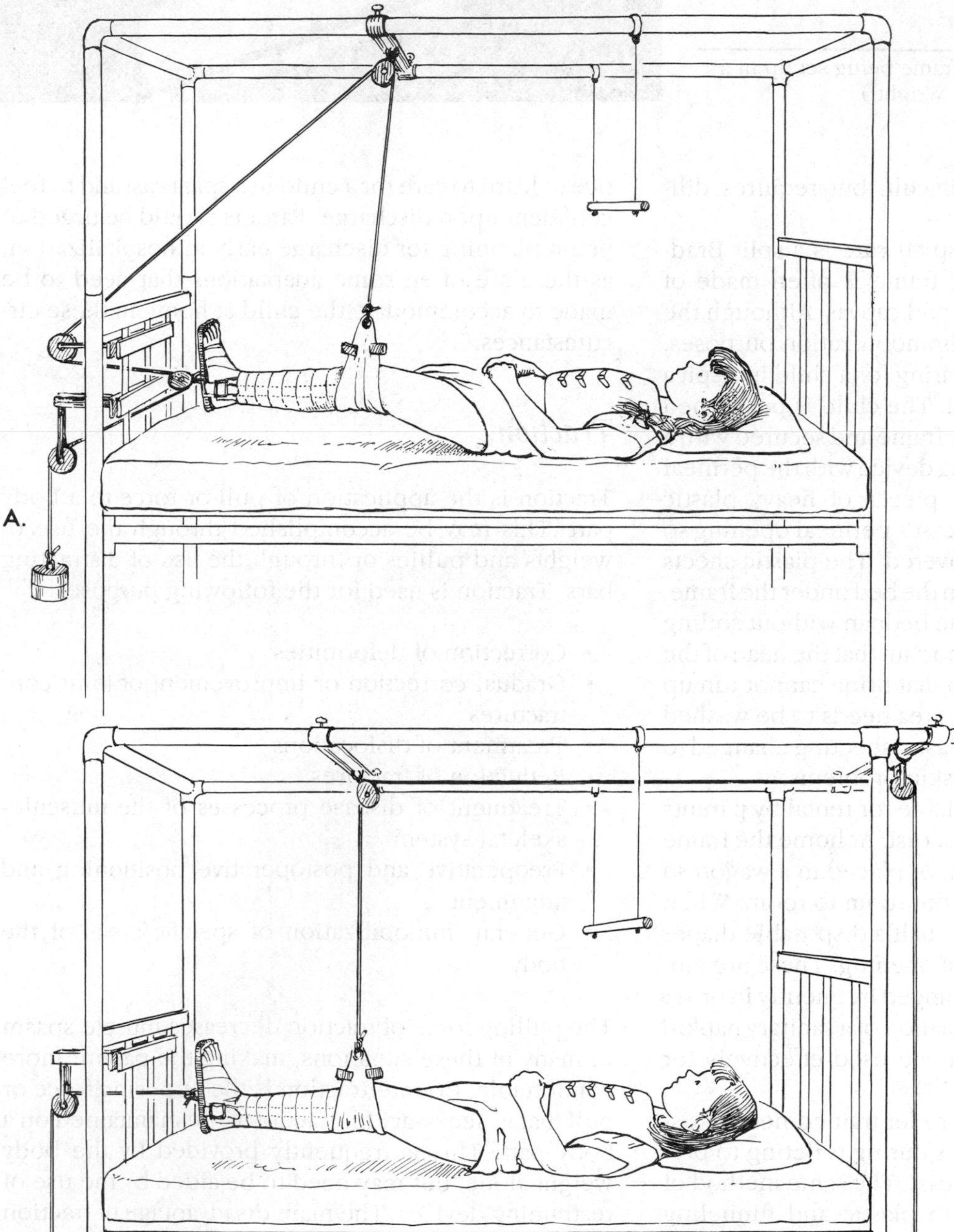

Figure 47-8. *A*, Russell skin traction. *B*, Split Russell traction.

Skin traction is applied directly to the skin, usually with adhesive strips of some type if the traction is to be continuous. If intermittent, it will be secured with Ace bandages or with one of various special boots or other apparatus designed specifically for this purpose. The amount of traction that can be applied is limited when using skin traction because of the friction it produces on the skin and the potential for skin breakdown.

Skeletal traction is applied directly to a bone by use of a Steinman pin or Kirshner wire inserted into a bone, or Crutchfield tongs inserted into the skull. More pull can be applied when skeletal traction is used because the force is applied directly to the skeleton.

Manual traction is the term used when a person's hands maintain pull on a body part, usually used when a cast or traction is being applied.

Buck Extension. Buck extension, a type of skin traction is obtained by applying straps to the child's extended legs and connecting these to weights at the foot of the bed (Fig. 47-7). Countertraction is provided mainly by the body, but some additional countertraction may be needed to keep the child from sliding toward the end of the bed.

Russell Traction. In Russell traction, a sling is added behind the knee while the legs are in Buck extension. The traction pull is in two directions, from the knee sling and from the footplate (Fig. 47-8). The knee sling and footplate may be incorporated into one weight system or separated, in which case it is called split Russell traction. The child must be in a supine position. Countertraction can be increased by raising the foot of the bed.

90-90 Skeletal Traction. A common type of skeletal traction used for fractures of the femur is 90-90 traction (Fig. 47-9). A wire or pin is inserted through the distal femur or proximal tibia and traction applied directly to the bone. A short leg cast is often used to provide suspension of the lower leg and foot support.

Balanced Suspension Traction. Balanced suspension is often used in conjunction with other traction devices for older children and adolescents. Support of the hip and knee is provided by a metal frame (the Thomas splint) with flexion of the lower leg provided by a jointed attachment (the Pearson attachment) (Fig. 47-10). The leg is supported by canvas. As the child moves, the suspension apparatus adjusts without disturbing the traction pull. This allows the child greater movement and is helpful in long-term treatment.

Bryant Traction. Bryant traction is a form of skin traction used to treat fractured femurs in children under age 2 who weigh less than 14 kg (30 lb). It is not used on larger children because of the danger of impairing circulation to the legs. Both legs are suspended above the child at a 90-degree angle of flexion from the hips (Fig. 47-11). The child's buttocks are raised slightly off the bed to provide the countertraction of the child's own weight. Both legs are always suspended, even if just one is broken.

Sidearm or Dunlop Traction. Sidearm or Dunlop traction is used for supracondylar fractures of the elbow. The upper arm is abducted and the forearm is placed in a 90-degree angle from the plane of the child (Fig. 47-12). Pull is obtained in two directions, one in line with the upper arm and one in line with the lower arm. Sidearm traction may use either skin or skeletal

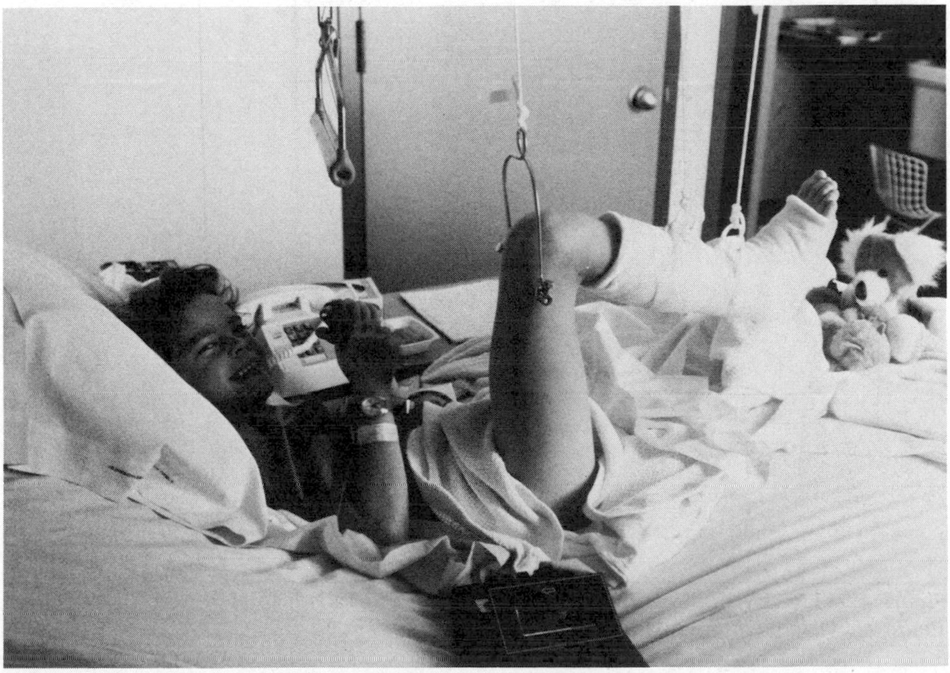

***Figure* 47-9.** Child with fractured femur in skeletal 90-90 traction. (Photo by Stephanie Wright.)

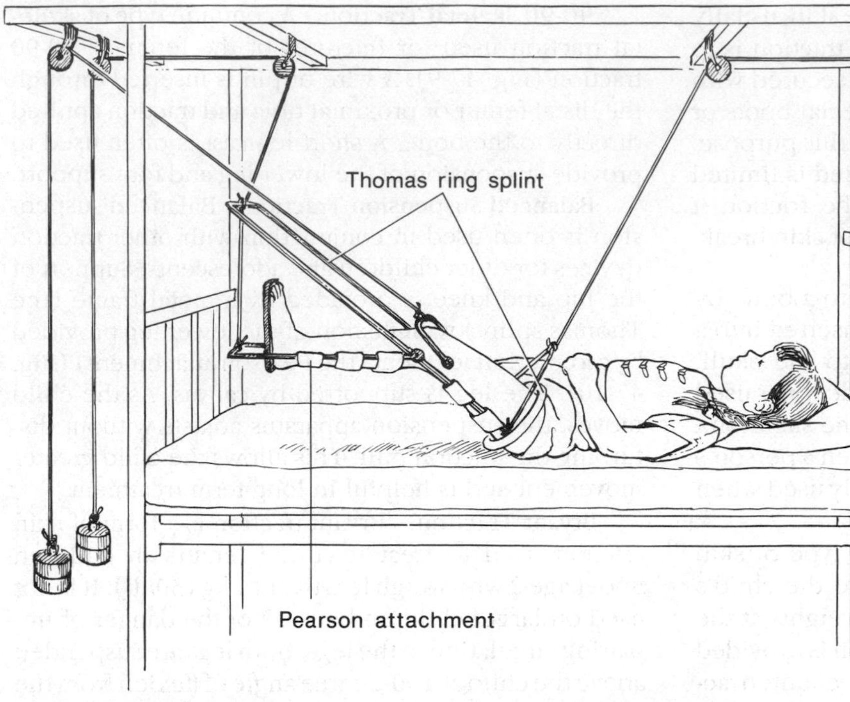

Figure 47-10. Suspension traction with wire through the distal femur with Thomas splint and Pearson attachment. (Drawing modified from Tachdjian M: *Pediatric Orthopedics.* Philadelphia, WB Saunders, 1972.)

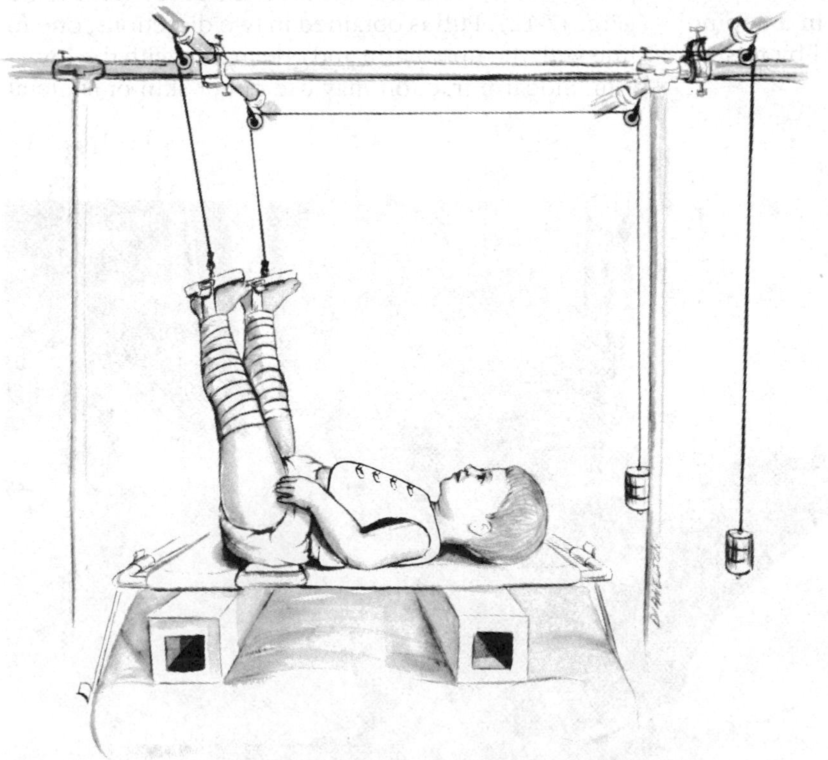

Figure 47-11. Bryant direct overhead traction. (From Tachdjian M: *Pediatric Orthopedics.* Philadelphia, WB Saunders, 1972.)

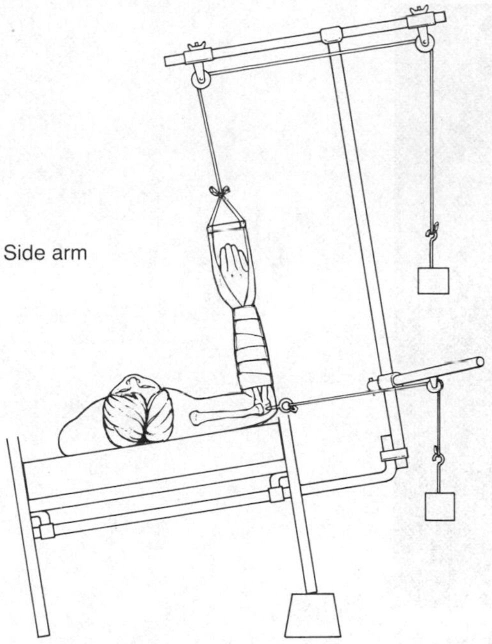

***Figure* 47-12.** Sidearm skeletal traction.

traction. Additional countertraction may be provided by raising the side of the bed on blocks.

Overhead Skeletal Arm Traction. Overhead skeletal arm traction (see Fig. 47-40, page 1842) may also be used to treat supracondylar fractures of the humerus. The traction force is applied to a pin in the distal humeral fragments.

Cervical Traction. Cervical traction is used either for cervical injuries or to overcome muscle spasm. It can be applied by the use of a head halter (Fig. 47-13) or cervical tongs inserted into the skull.

Halo Traction. Halo traction is a type of skeletal traction utilizing a halo ring around the head which is fastened to the skull by pins (Fig. 47-14). Countertraction is provided by the use of pins into the femurs (halo-femoral traction) or the pelvis (halo-pelvis traction). Halo traction is used for treating severe scoliosis or cervical injuries.

Nursing Care of the Child in Traction. The child in traction requires skilled and creative nursing care to maintain physical and emotional health. Maintenance of traction and proper alignment will be a primary concern to ensure that the traction can perform its intended function in the shortest possible period of time. Careful observation of the traction includes the following:

- Weight should be the correct ordered amount
- Weights should hang free
- Ropes should be in good condition
- Ropes should be in the center of the pulley track
- All traction equipment should be properly tightened
- Child should be in the body position to provide the correct line of pull; i.e., the traction pull should align the bone ends. Coordination with the orthopedist is essential to ensure that the nursing plan of care includes detailed instructions for maintaining the line of pull in the intended direction.

Maintaining correct body alignment and sufficient countertraction may require the use of restraints to prevent the child from being pulled toward the end or side of the bed. It is important that children do not view these restraints as punishment for activity but rather as a necessary part of the treatment regimen. They are a "reminder" to the child to stay in a certain position. A Bradford frame may be used to immobilize younger children very effectively by restraining the child to the frame (see Fig. 47-6).

Countertraction is important to proper alignment because once any part of the child's body rests against the bed frame, in the direction of the traction pull, the force of traction is significantly altered. In addition to

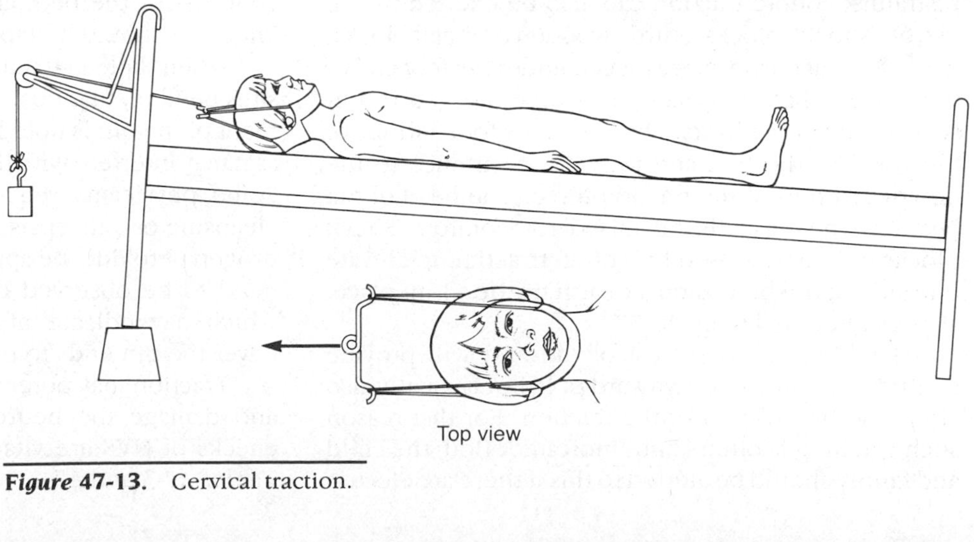

***Figure* 47-13.** Cervical traction.

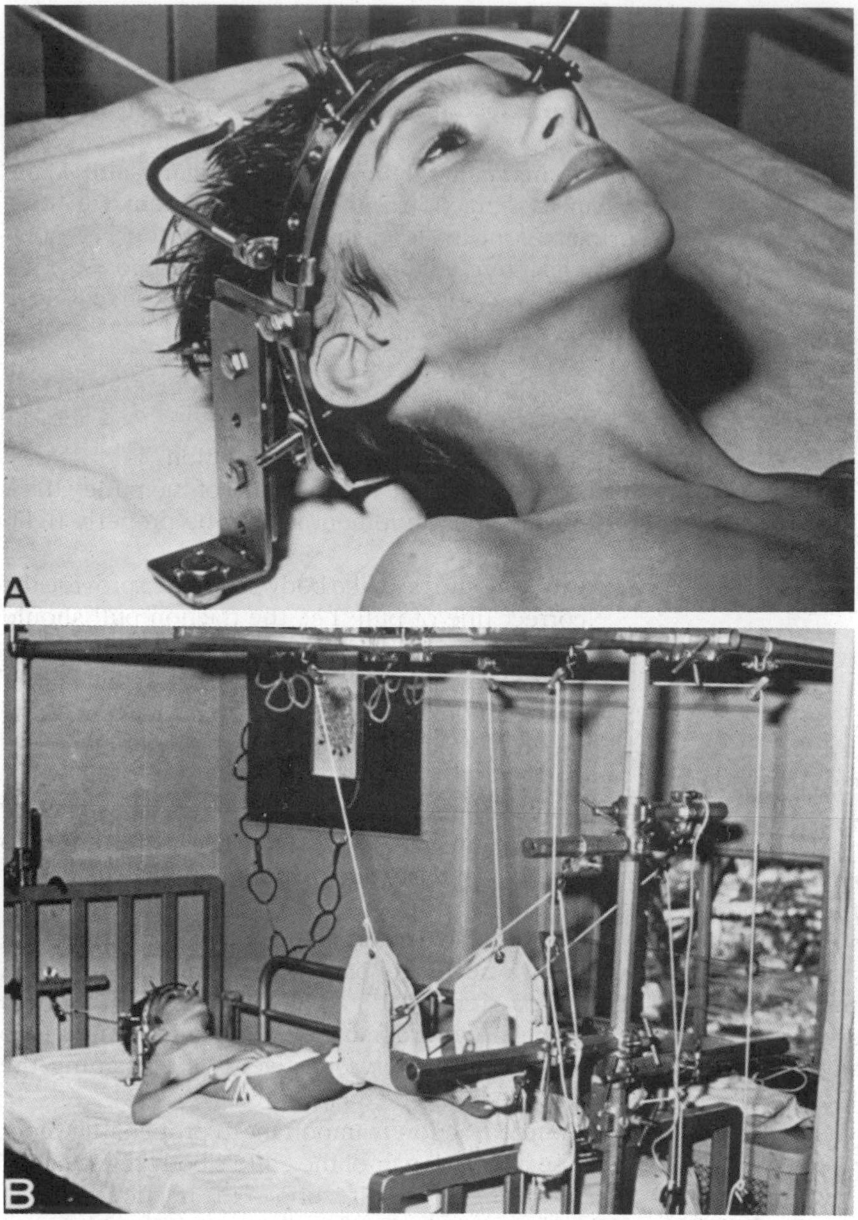

Figure 47-14. Halo–femoral traction. *A*, Halo; *B*, traction. (From Ferguson AB: *Orthopedic Surgery in Infancy and Childhood.* Baltimore, Williams and Wilkins, 1981.)

restraints, countertraction can also be exerted by the use of "shock" blocks. Sturdy wooden or metal blocks, made for that purpose, are placed under the foot end of the bed so that the casters on which the bed roll fit securely into the blocks. This raises the foot end above the head of the bed and provides resistance to the downward pull of the traction force. The head of the bed can then usually be raised for comfort. Shock blocks can also be used for countertraction to elevate one side of the bed when sidearm traction is in place, as illustrated by Figure 47-12.

Gatching the knee rest of the bed will provide countertraction for a downward pull, but it usually also alters the line of pull of the traction. For that reason such gatching is often contraindicated. Both the child and family should be alerted to this if there are electric controls for the bed, and the button controlling the knee rest should be taped as a reminder.

When skeletal traction is applied, the pin insertion sites need regular observation. Any slippage or movement of the pin is noted and reported to the physician as it may interfere with the effectiveness of the traction. Some physicians request that a regular routine of cleansing or antisepsis, such as with half-strength hydrogen peroxide, be applied to the pin sites. Pins sites need to be observed daily for redness or drainage, which may indicate infection. Corks are often used to cover the pin ends to prevent accidental injury.

Traction may potentially interfere with circulation and damage the neuromuscular apparatus. Regular checks of NVS are vital, following the guidelines of Tables 47-3 and 47-4.

Children in traction are radically immobilized and are subject to the development of all the emotional and physical complications of immobilization previously discussed. Plans to counteract these effects should be addressed in the nursing plan of care.

Congenital and Hereditary Musculoskeletal Conditions

There are numerous congenital anomalies involving the musculoskeletal system. Three common ones are congenital clubfoot, metatarsus adductus, and congenital dislocation of the hip. Early diagnosis is the critical factor that determines whether these conditions can be corrected. The nurse's recognition of each is extremely important in increasing case findings. When the condition is recognized early, the treatment period is also dramatically shortened. Although the prognosis is good, the treatment course brings some special stresses on the family. In many cases, most of the physical care and the implementation of the treatment regimen will be the parents' responsibility. Their education will ensure good results and greater comfort for the child. The ability to communicate with the parents concerning all aspects of treatment and care is the nurse's primary tool.

The Impact of Physical Deformity

Birth of a child with a physical deformity represents for every parent a loss of the perfect child they had expected. The grief process will ensue with a period of grieving necessary before acceptance of the problem will occur. Parents have individual grief patterns, influenced by the meaning of the particular defect to them. Most parents will search for a cause or explanation as a method of dealing with their feelings of guilt and helplessness.

The one element that most musculoskeletal defects have in common is that most are very obvious to the casual observer. Although physical disability presents many problems for the child and family, parents often find this type of disability easier to accept than mental or emotional disability, and express this openly. Musculoskeletal deformity often requires treatment with surgery and casts, which may not be easily hidden from the curiosity of onlookers. The parents' acceptance of the problem and treatment will determine their response to the reactions of others. As these children mature, they will model the attitudes of those around them. For children with physical disability and deformity, developing normal relationships is often as great a challenge as coping with their own physical limitations.

In their manner of handling and approach to newborn infants with physical deformity, nurses provide a model for parents. The ability to hold and fondle the baby despite the deformity or the impediment of a cast is important in reinforcing acceptance of the child and condition and providing necessary tactile experiences for the infant.

Clubfoot

Incidence and Etiology

Clubfoot is a congenital anomaly involving bones, muscles, and tendons of the foot. The most common form of clubfoot is talipes equinovarus, in which the forefoot is adducted, along with inversion and equinus (plantarflexion). A typical clubfoot is shown in Figure 47-15. Congenital clubfoot occurs in about 1 of every 1000 live births and is more common in males. It can occur unilaterally or bilaterally (Lovell and Winter, 1978). Incidence is increased in families who already have one child with clubfoot.

The etiology of congenital clubfoot remains unknown. Whether it is a primary germ plasm defect originating in either bones or muscles or whether the intrauterine environment contributes to the development of this problem is unclear.

Clinical Manifestations

True clubfoot is an anatomic deformity that prevents the foot from being manipulated into a normal position. It varies in severity. The severe forms are easily recognized, but the milder forms can go undetected. Some infants are born with a positional deformity of

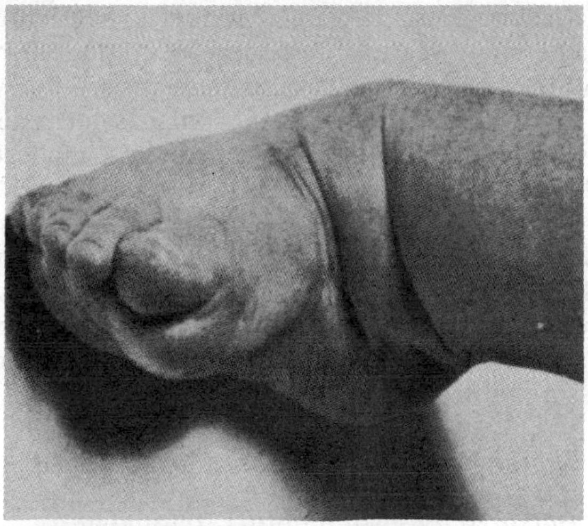

Figure 47-15. Typical clubfoot deformity. (From Delp M, Manning R: *Major's Physical Diagnosis.* Philadelphia, WB Saunders, 1981.)

the foot resembling clubfoot. If the foot can be manipulated into a normal position, there is no bony deformity. Positional deformities, usually treated with a passive exercise program, are readily corrected.

Diagnostic Assessment

The diagnosis is made by examination, manipulation, and roentgenograph. Since the defect is often quite apparent at birth, parents may become aware of it in the delivery room. Usually some explanation of the nature of the problem and the usual methods of treatment is given to them at this time. The retention of this information varies, since the parents are experiencing considerable stress at this time.

Therapeutic Management

Treatment is usually begun within a few days after birth. The longer treatment is delayed, the more pronounced the soft tissue changes become and the more difficult correction becomes. Serial casting is the usual method of treatment. The foot is gradually manipulated toward a normal anatomic position and a short leg cast is applied to hold the correction. Casts are usually changed at weekly intervals. With each cast removal, the foot is manipulated and recasted. With this method the foot is gradually corrected over a period of months. Once correction is obtained, some method of maintaining correction is used in conjunction with stretching to be performed by the parents. Bivalved (split) casts or corrective shoes attached to a Denis-Browne bar may be used to maintain correction. The Denis-Browne bar is a metal bar attached to the soles of the shoes that maintain the feet in a prescribed position. Whichever splinting method is used, it is worn continuously until the child is ready for walking and then only at naptime or bedtime. Stretching exercises may be prescribed and may need to be continued for a period of years. Unless surgery is required, treatment is completed on an outpatient basis.

For the child, the treatment course is not a painful one. Children are often frightened by cast application and removal, but this is in reaction to the wetnes and warmth generated by the plaster application, the noise of the cast cutter, and the physical restraint. Distraction with a pacifier or some visual stimulus will often work quite well to quiet an infant. The parent should be present to provide comfort during cast changes and be reassured that it is not painful.

Major Nursing Diagnoses for Clubfoot

Impaired physical mobility, *related to congenital adduction, inversion, and plantarflexion of one or both feet*
Potential altered parenting: impaired attachment behavior, *related to:*
- *parental reaction associated with the fear, concerns, and stigma of the anomaly*
- *difficulty in holding the infant with one or both feet in casts*

Potential for injury: neurovascular impairment, *related to casting*
Knowledge deficit (parents), *related to:*
- *anatomic aspects of clubfoot*
- *chance of clubfoot deformity with successive pregnancies*
- *correctional treatment (including casting, splinting, possible surgery)*
- *cast care (see Fig. 47-5 and Table 47-4)*
- *prescribed stretching exercises for home therapy*
- *need to provide appropriate stimulation for infant whose impaired mobility limits normal opportunities for assimilation of the environment*
- *how to contact families who have been through this treatment regimen and are willing to offer support and counsel*
- *expected outcome of the treatment plan and esthetic appearance of affected extremities*
- *need for follow-up throughout childhood because of the chance of recurrence*

Strategies for Nursing Care

Promoting Healthy Parenting. The meaning of the defect to the parents must be ascertained as part of the initial nursing assessment. Medical personnel often view clubfoot as a minor health problem to be resolved. The parents, however, may see only a very nonfunctional-appearing foot and may be thinking about long-term repercussions for the child. In some families, physical prowess and athletic ability may be highly valued; for them this type of physical anomaly will be more difficult to accept.

Factual information can help to dispel fears and misconceptions and provide the parent(s) with answers to questions from friends and relatives. The sensitivity of the nurse in anticipating that the family may view clubfoot as a serious anomaly can create an atmosphere in which they feel free to ask questions and express concerns. Understanding the rationale for treatment can also make them more comfortable in physical interactions with the child by dispelling concerns about holding and playing with the infant in a normal fashion.

Preventing Neurovascular Impairment. With each cast change, there is the possibility of circulatory compromise or neurologic impairment, or both, from the manipulation of the foot or from the cast itself. The NVS should be checked hourly for the first 4 to 6 hours following application and then several times a day. The nurse should check the NVS immediately after cast application and before the family takes the child home. Checking neurovascular status can be easily demonstrated to parents; this should be followed by a return demonstration. Any unusual or extreme fussiness on the part of the child is an indication to have the cast checked. Written instructions on cast care and checking neurovascular status (see Fig. 47-5) should be supplied to parents.

Teaching to Address Knowledge Deficit. The cast must be kept clean and dry. With a small infant, keeping a short leg cast clean is usually relatively easy. The main change in routine will be the bath. A tub bath will not be possible until after the casts have been removed.

The skin proximal to the cast edges needs special attention. After the cast is applied and before the child is taken home, any obviously rough edges should be trimmed away. The cast edges cannot be covered with adhesive petals when the cast is still damp, but can be done later at home. The skin around the cast edges should be checked daily for redness. With a short leg cast, the most common area for skin abrasion and breakdown is behind the knee. The cast edge may need to be trimmed or smoothed with adhesive or moleskin to prevent this problem. When the cast is removed for cast change, the skin surfaces under the cast should be inspected for signs of pressure or abrasion.

The cast is heavy and may limit the normal kicking of the infant and impede his or her early efforts to turn over. Since major treatment is often completed within the first few months of life, any effects on physical development are rapidly corrected as the child develops normally. Attention should be given, however, to ensuring adequate stimulation for this less mobile infant.

The vast majority of infants with clubfoot will have good correction with serial casting and will develop a normal foot without limitations. However, the possibility of recurrence later in childhood requires careful follow-up. Some clubfeet are more resistant to treatment and will require surgical intervention in the form of tendon transfers or releases and a longer treatment period. This may be apparent at the onset of the treatment or may not become apparent until later.

Nursing Strategies for Follow-up Care in the Home or Clinic

Assess for potential injury related to casting or splinting (neurovascular integrity, skin impairment visible when cast removed).

Assess parental attachment behaviors.

Assess infant's progress on developmental tasks.

Allow parents ample time to express feelings and ask questions; determine understanding of and compliance with the treatment plan.

Ask the parents to perform an assessment of NVS (especially after a new cast has been applied).

Provide a referral for genetic counseling if desired by the parent(s).

When appropriate, put the parent in touch with another parent who has been through a similar treatment protocol with a child who has clubfoot.

Assess for recurrence throughout childhood.

Metatarsus Adductus

The most common congenital foot deformity, this condition occurs in both sexes and is usually bilateral (Fig. 47-16). It is one of the three deformities present

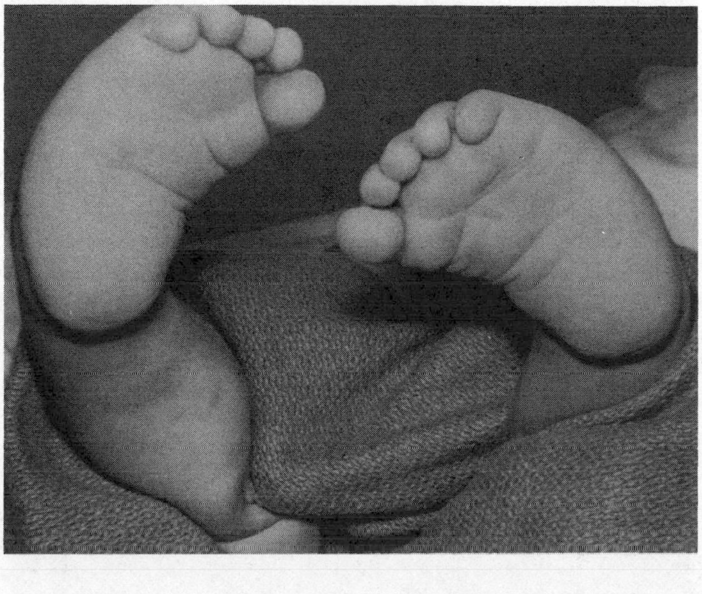

Figure 47-16. Infant with a metatarsus adductus deformity. (Photograph courtesy of Mead Johnson Nutritional Division.)

in clubfoot and is frequently associated with internal tibial torsion and flatfeet. Abnormal intrauterine position is thought to be the etiology. Mild cases will resolve spontaneously. When deformity is rigid (resists being turned to a normal position) or severe, it is likely to persist into adulthood if untreated.

If the deformity is mild or apparent at birth, parents can be taught to manipulate the foot by stabilizing the heel with one hand and massaging the forefoot medially with the other hand. This should be done several times at each diaper change. In addition, parents should be encouraged to put the infant to sleep on the side or back. If correction is not achieved by 4 months, a cast that immobilizes the foot in a corrected position is applied for 2 to 4 weeks.

Some orthopedists prescribe that casting be followed by reverse last (outflared) shoes for a few months to maintain correction. If internal tibial torsion accompanies the metatarsus adductus, a Denis-Browne night splint may be needed.

Strategies for Nursing Care

If the child is casted, parents should be encouraged to hold the infant frequently and provide extra sensory and motor experiences, since the child's own ambulatory exploration may be temporarily interrupted. Parents will also need instructions in skin care, cast care, and checking NVS (see the nursing strategies for clubfoot).

Congenital Dislocation of the Hip

Congenital dislocation of the hip (CDH) is one form of a group of hip problems often described collectively as congenital hip dysplasia. Hip dysplasia includes hips that are unstable or capable of being dislocated, subluxed (the femoral head has moved upward and laterally in the hip socket), or actually dislocated (out of the hip socket). At birth the hip joint is largely cartilage. As ossification of the hip structures proceeds during infancy, the head of the femur must be properly located within the acetabulum for the correct configuration of the hip to develop. If the head of the femur is outside the acetabulum or improperly located within it, the hip joint will develop abnormally. As ossification proceeds, correcting the deformity becomes more and more difficult. Once the child begins walking, the added stresses to the hip joint will worsen the deformity that occurs.

Etiology

The etiology of this disorder is not clearly understood. There is a familial tendency. The condition is more prevalent in females, at a ratio of eight females to one male. Incidence ranges from 4 to 7 per 1000 live births. There appears to be some relationship between relaxation of the hip capsule associated with increased estrogen levels and hip dislocation. Position in utero also has some effect on this problem. Congenital hip dislocation is much more prevalent in babies carried in the breech position. Rapid or forceful extension of the hips immediately following birth may precipitate dislocation in an unstable hip. Infants should be allowed to hold their legs in the normal partially flexed position.

Diagnostic Assessment

Early diagnosis is the greatest problem encountered when dealing with congenital dislocation of the hip. Every newborn infant must be carefully checked for signs of dislocation or instability of the hip joint. The three commonly described signs of dislocation are (1) *unequal skinfolds on the thighs and buttocks,* (2) *limitation of abduction on the affected side,* and (3) *unequal knee height* (Fig. 47-17). Although these signs can be easily checked as part of an initial assessment, they are often not present in newborn infants because their presence depends on muscular changes that usually occur only after the hip has been dislocated for some time. Therefore, these three "classic" signs are more likely to be seen in an infant who is several months old.

A more accurate diagnostic method involves an attempt to either reduce or dislocate the hip manually. One hand grasps the femur and, with the hip and knee flexed, abducts and lifts the thigh. In a child with CDH, the hip can be heard and felt to reduce as the head of the femur enters the acetabulum (Ortolani sign). If this procedure is reversed and the leg is adducted and some downward pressure applied, the hip may be felt to dislocate as the femoral head leaves the acetabulum (subluxation test of Barlow). This is an examination that is not difficult to perform but requires some practice and training. *This procedure should not be attempted by the novice.* Most unstable hips in neonates will be diagnosed with these two maneuvers. Roentgenographs may or may not confirm the diagnosis. The newborn hip is largely cartilage and not radiopaque. Roentgenographs are more likely to be diagnostic in infants several months of age. Once diagnosis is made, parents need a thorough explanation of the problem at hand. Their child's condition is not visible and presents no current difficulty for him or her. A thorough understanding of the repercussions of neglect of the problem is necessary to ensure compliance with the proper treatment regimen.

Therapeutic Management

No matter what degree of dysplasia exists, treatment should be begun immediately. Treatment in early in-

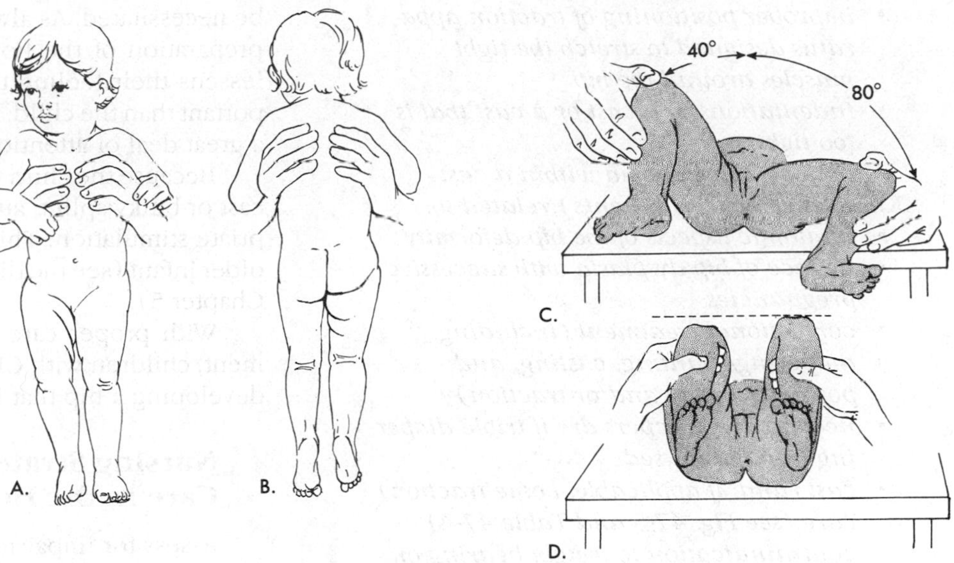

Figure 47-17. The three "classic" signs of CDH: *A* and *B*, unequal skin folds, *C*, limitation of abduction, and *D*, unequal knee height. (From Tachdjian M: *Pediatric Orthopedics.* Philadelphia, WB Saunders, 1972.)

fancy (up to 2 to 3 months) consists of placing the head of the femur within the acetabulum and keeping it there by maintaining the legs in position of flexion and abduction. There are a variety of methods to accomplish this. For infants in whom the hip is not actually dislocated, use of triple diapers or a Frejka pillow (Fig. 47-18) may suffice. In infants in whom the hip is capable of being dislocated, diapers or a pillow will not be satisfactory because they will be removed at each diaper change and the hip may dislocate at this time (Chung, 1986).

Various splints (abduction devices) are used to maintain proper placement of the hip continuously,

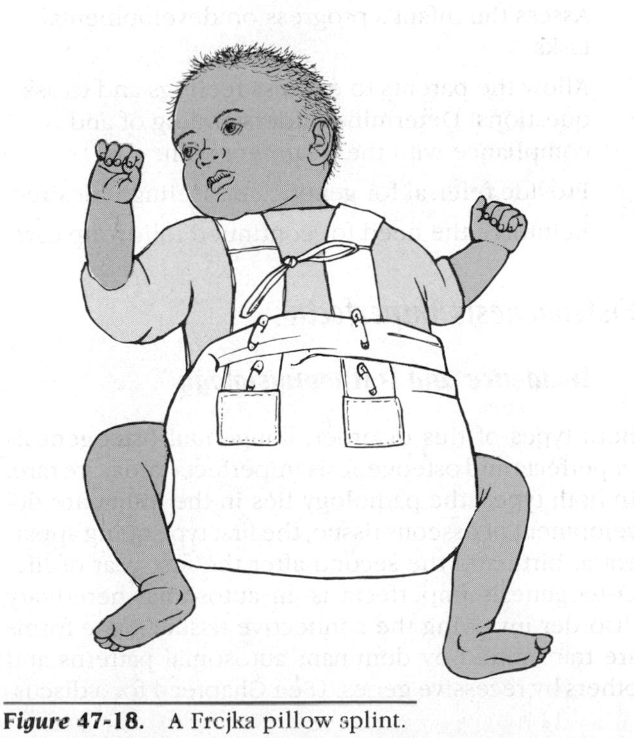

Figure 47-18. A Frejka pillow splint.

including during diapering. The length of time an infant will have to wear an abduction device depends on the age at which diagnosis is made. When diagnosis is made in a newborn infant, treatment may be completed in 2 to 4 months. Treatment is continued until the hip is stable and can often be completed on an outpatient basis.

When CDH is not diagnosed until after 2 or 3 months of age, changes in hip structure may have occurred that prevent the hip from being reduced. Traction, either skin or skeletal, may be used to pull the head of the femur down to a position where it is opposite the acetabulum. This may require several weeks of hospitalization, although some centers have experimented with home traction. The period of traction is followed by a closed reduction of the hip, usually with the child anesthetized, and the application of a hip spica cast with hips in the abducted position. The cast maintains the proper position of the hip for the period of treatment. The child is usually cared for at home and returns to the hospital periodically for cast changes.

Surgical Treatment. When traction and closed reduction cannot reduce the hip, surgery may be required. This may take the form of an adductor tenotomy to allow for more movement of the hip. An open reduction of the hip may be required to correct some problem that is preventing the head of the femur from entering the acetabulum. These surgical procedures will be followed by immobilization in a hip spica cast.

Major Nursing Diagnoses for CDH

***Impaired physical mobility,** related to congenital instability or altered placement of the head of the femur within the acetabulum, either unilaterally or bilaterally*

***Potential for injury: neurovascular impairment,** related to:*

- *improper positioning of traction apparatus designed to stretch the tight muscles around the hip*
- *Indentations in a cast or a cast that is too tight*
- *Postoperative edema within a cast*

Knowledge deficit (parents), related to:

- *anatomic aspects of the hip deformity*
- *chance of hip dysplasia with successive pregnancies*
- *correctional treatment (including diapering/splinting, casting, and possible surgery and/or traction)*
- *need to keep diapers dry if triple diapering treatment used*
- *cast (and, if applicable, home traction) care (see Fig. 47-5 and Table 47-4)*
- *contraindication to weight bearing on the affected side*
- *implications of failure to correct hip dysplasia before the child begins walking*
- *need to provide appropriate stimulation for infant whose impaired mobility limits assimilation of the environment*
- *names and phone numbers of parents who are willing to offer support by sharing similar experiences*
- *necessity of continued treatment (e.g., cast changes) and follow-up until the hip is stabilized*
- *expected outcome of the treatment plan*

Strategies for Nursing Care

Strategies will be aimed at postoperative care, should surgery be necessary, and at teaching the family about home care. General postoperative care is detailed in Table 27-7, a nursing process plan for the child in the perioperative period. In addition, the child must be protected from neurovascular injury related to casting after surgery (see Table 47-4). Of course, precautions related to neurovascular injury apply whether or not the child had surgery before casting.

Teaching to Enhance Care of the Child at Home. A teaching plan can be patterned after the points listed under the nursing diagnosis, *knowledge deficit*. Parents need to be involved in the care of the child as early as possible so that, upon discharge, they have confidence in their ability to care for him or her at home. Alterations of home care routines should be thoroughly discussed before discharge so that any necessary physical adaptations in the home can be anticipated.

Parents should be encouraged to prepare siblings for the appearance of their brother or sister in a splint or cast and the adaptations in family routines that will be necessitated. As always, participation of siblings in preparation of the home or in the care of the child lessens their feeling that they are somehow less important than the child, who is necessarily the subject of a great deal of attention during treatment.

Because the child will be less mobile in a hip spica cast or bulky splint, attention must be given to appropriate stimulation. This is especially pertinent for the older infant (see the discussion of infant stimulation in Chapter 5).

With proper care and early diagnosis and treatment, children with CDH have an excellent chance of developing a hip that is functionally normal.

Nursing Strategies for Follow-up Care in the Home or Clinic

Assess for impairment of neurovascular status related to casting or traction (see Tables 47-3 and 47-4).

Assess home traction apparatus by systematically checking each aspect of the system, from traction source (e.g., Ace wrap of leg) to the weight applied, to ensure it complies with the desired treatment.

Ask the parents to demonstrate neurovascular assessment of the involved extremities whether the child is in traction or in a cast.

Assess for skin impairment when a cast is removed; wash the area that was under the cast to remove dead skin and to stimulate circulation. Massage skin with lubricant before recasting.

Assess parental attachment behaviors.

Assess the infant's progress on developmental tasks.

Allow the parents to express feelings and to ask questions. Determine understanding of and compliance with the treatment plan.

Provide referral for genetic counseling if desired.

Reinforce the need for continued follow-up care.

Osteogenesis Imperfecta

Incidence and Pathophysiology

Both types of this disorder, congenital osteogenesis imperfecta and osteogenesis imperfecta tarda, are rare. In both types, the pathology lies in the immature development of osseous tissue, the first type being apparent at birth and the second after the first year of life. Osteogenesis imperfecta is an autosomal hereditary disorder involving the connective tissue; some forms are transmitted by dominant autosomal patterns and others by recessive genes. (See Chapter 4 for a discussion of autosomal inheritance.) Since there is defective osteoblast formation, immature bone structure results. This is a systemic disease in which the mesenchyme and some of its derivatives such as the sclera, bones, and ligaments are defective, resulting in inadequate cellular formation. The condition is considered an inborn error of metabolism.

In congenital osteogenesis imperfecta, fractures may be incurred during the birth process, or evidence of intrauterine fracture may be present. Because of the defective periosteal bone formation, the shafts of the long bones have reduced cortical thickness. The infant may be born with a deformed spine because of intrauterine fractures. Those children who survive may suffer fractures from any slight trauma and may never learn to walk because of frequent falls. The limbs may have angulations, and there may be growth retardation because of epiphyseal trauma. The child may also develop kyphosis or scoliosis if the vertebral bones are involved.

Osteogenesis imperfecta tarda is transmitted as a dominant hereditary trait (see Chapter 4). Frequently, more than one family member may have the condition. It usually develops after the first year of life and is not as severe as the congenital type. There may be fewer fractures after puberty. It is very difficult to make a clear distinction between the two.

Clinical Manifestations

In both types the symptoms are the same. Because of the disturbed formation of periosteal bone, the cortex is thin and immature. The mesenchyme is halted in its development of connective tissue, and the sclera appears blue and thin. The skin has a transparent look, giving the child a delicate and fragile appearance. These children are usually short, owing to frequent fractures. Because of the involvement of the osseous labyrinth, there may be auditory dysfunction. Cataracts also occur frequently. The child bruises easily, and a tendency for frequent epistaxis may be present. There may be immature and deformed dentition. The child may experience pain at the fracture site, with resultant redness, heat, and swelling, although pain may be lessened somewhat because the fragile bone usually breaks so easily that it causes little soft tissue damage.

Therapeutic Management

Prevention of fractures and of deformity is the primary aim. Stainless steel or alloy rods may be inserted into the long bones of severely affected children to prevent further fractures. Because bone healing is slow, proper healing of fractures may require long periods of immobilization, which will further compromise mineralization of the bones. Adequate nutrition is vital, and calcium, magnesium, and vitamin supplements may be given in an attempt to strengthen the bone structure.

Major Nursing Diagnoses for Osteogenesis Imperfecta

Potential for injury: fractures, *related to fragility of the bones associated with an inherited defect in osteoblastic activity.*

Altered family process, *related to the overwhelming nature of the disease and the long-term intensity of care required by the child*

Potential for altered growth and development: physical, intellectual, and emotional/social, *related to:*
- *frequent immobilization for fracture treatment*
- *physical restrictions imposed by protective parents and siblings, (and, later in childhood, self-protective restrictions)*
- *decreased assimilation of the environment associated with physical restrictions*
- *time spent out of the classroom because of hospitalizations for fracture treatment*
- *decreased peer contact associated with frequent hospitalizations and with the stigma of the disease*

Disturbance in self-concept: body image, self-esteem, role performance, personal identity, *related to the significant limitations imposed by osteogenesis imperfecta on the child's physical activities and on aspirations for marriage and parenthood*

Knowledge deficit, *related to:*
- *implications of defective formation of bones and of connective tissue*
- *the need for and availability of genetic counseling*
- *home care of the child with osteogenesis imperfecta*
  1. *Need for a firm mattress*
  2. *Adaptation of clothing to prevent accidental fracture with dressing*
  3. *Review of normal infant/child/adolescent safety implications with modifications for the child with high potential for fracture and bruising, (who may also have sensory impairment)*
  4. *Assessment for and first aid for fractures*
  5. *Cast care and assessment of neurovascular status*
- *ways to normalize the child's (and family's) environment despite the implications of the disease*

- *ways to facilitate the child's progress on developmental tasks without compromising physical safety*
- *the need to include siblings in important family roles to ensure them of their worth and importance at a time when the focus may be on the affected child*
- *names and phone numbers of families who can provide help and support through shared experiences*

Strategies for Nursing Care

Protecting the Child from Unnecessary Fractures. As the nurse listens to the child's physical history and the family history, he or she may assist in restructuring the child's life to attempt to avoid fractures. There is no effective treatment for the condition other than adequate nutrition and good physical and orthopedic care.

Physical care of these children requires constant awareness of the stresses placed on body parts. Extreme gentleness is needed when handling or moving these children, combined with frequent examination for signs of fracture.

Promoting Healthy Family Process. The most beneficial intervention that may be made is to assist the child and the family to accept the condition. The family values and the members' relationships with each other are evidenced in the child's acceptance of his or her handicap. Sibling competitiveness should be discouraged and the child allowed to develop his or her own individuality despite the handicap. A broken personality could be a greater handicap than the actual disease. Family members should be referred for genetic counseling.

Promoting Healthy Development and a Positive Self-Concept. The child will undoubtedly have repeated hospitalizations and be in traction frequently. Both the hospitalizations and the restricted physical activity can cause anger and resentment. Immobilization is a threat to the child's need for independence. The frequent disruption of schooling and limited social activity can cause feelings of inadequacy and bring about withdrawal and personality changes.

The family needs the support of a caring nurse who can give anticipatory guidance about areas in which the child can function independently and still be alert to the need for protection from trauma. If the child enjoys physical competitive sports, he or she may need to accept more sedentary roles such as umpire or scorekeeper. These children frequently find satisfaction in spectator sports or enjoy reading or studying.

The first tendency of the family is to overprotect the child, but this can cause emotional crippling. The child and the family can be helped to see that most people are handicapped in some way. Since physical skills are limited, the child should be encouraged to develop leadership skills that will allow him or her to continue to be a part of a peer group. Hobbies should be encouraged. The child must have as much involvement as possible with his or her peers. The condition should be explained to friends, who should be encouraged to accept the child for whatever he or she can contribute.

The child may be absent from school frequently. The teacher should keep in close communication with the child. If possible, academic work should be continued in the hospital or home if the child is immobilized. If the parents have not arranged for this, the nurse should initiate a contract through the parents. Children who cannot achieve physically often achieve academically.

Teaching to Enhance Care of the Child at Home. The nursing diagnosis *knowledge deficit* details a list of considerations for teaching that is suitable to use as a guideline in working with families affected by osteogenesis imperfecta. In addition to those areas covered previously in this section, the family should be encouraged to watch for and report signs of sensory impairment resulting from involvement of connective tissue. Cataracts may form, limiting vision, and involvement of the bony labyrinth may lead to hearing difficulties. Care for the child with a sensory impairment is discussed further in Chapter 51. Dental involvement may lead to frequent caries and loss of fillings. Frequent dental check-ups are indicated with a dentist who understands osteogenesis imperfecta.

Because some fractures will be unavoidable, family members must be well coached in first aid for fractures (see p. 1840) and in care of the child in a cast (see the previous discussion of cast care).

Genetic counseling is indicated for the parents and, at the appropriate time, for the affected child and the siblings. Chapter 4 contains further information on genetic counseling and Table 50-3 presents a nursing process plan that details the role of the nurse in support of the family in genetic counseling.

Nursing Strategies for Follow-up Care in the Home or Clinic

Assess status of healing fractures and current musculoskeletal integrity.

Assess for cataracts and hearing loss.

Assess progress on the child's and family's developmental tasks.

Allow the child, parents and siblings to express feelings about the experience of the disease and assess their adaptation. Make referrals as appropriate to social services agencies and other sources of support.

Muscular Dystrophy

Muscular dystrophies constitute one of the most prevalent muscle diseases in childhood. They are hereditary diseases characterized by gradual onset in early life, with atrophy and weakness of the proximal muscles. Although the etiology is unknown, a defect in metabolism of creatine is suspected owing to increased serum levels in affected individuals.

There are three major types of muscular dystrophy: (1) Duchenne muscular dystrophy, (2) the fascioscapulohumeral form, and (3) the limb-girdle type. The various forms of these dystrophies are presented in Table 47-6, which describes pattern of inheritance, age of onset, and progressive involvement. Since Duchenne muscular dystrophy is the most common type in childhood, it is presented here in greater detail.

Duchenne Muscular Dystrophy (Pseudohypertrophic)

The most common type of muscular dystrophy in childhood, Duchenne muscular dystrophy (DMD), is transmitted as an X-linked recessive disorder in which males primarily are affected. The onset is between 2 and 6 years of age, with death resulting between the

Table 47-6. The Primary Myopathies of Muscular Dystrophy

Primary Myopathies Muscular Dystrophy (Major Types)	Type of Inheritance	Initial Symptoms	Progression	Treatment
Pseudohypertrophic (Duchenne) *Clinical Onset:* Early childhood	Sex-linked recessive, transmitted through unaffected females. There is a 50% probability that male offspring will be afflicted, and a 50% probability that female offspring will be carriers	Swayback, a waddling gait, and difficulty in rising from the floor and climbing stairs, due to pelvic girdle muscle weakness. Fat deposits replace wasting muscle tissue in the calves	Rapid, ultimately involving all the voluntary muscles. Death usually occurs within 10–15 years of clinical onset	None. Physical therapy may delay atrophy of disuse of healthy muscles and antibiotics control secondary illnesses, but neither halts the dystrophic process
Facioscapulohumeral (Landouzy-Dejerine) *Clinical Onset:* Early adolescence, occasionally in the 20's	Autosomal dominant, transmitted by either parent to children of both sexes, with a 50% probability of incidence	Lack of facial mobility, difficulty in raising arms over head, forward slope of shoulders, due to initial weakness of face and shoulder girdle muscles	Very slow, often with intervals in which the disease marks time. Average life span rarely shortened, despite considerable disability	None. Physical therapy may delay atrophy of disuse of healthy muscles and antibiotics control secondary illnesses, but neither halts the dystrophic process
Limb-girdle (includes juvenile dystrophy of Erb) *Clinical Onset:* Any time from the 1st to the 3rd decade of life	Autosomal recessive, transmitted to children of both sexes **only** when both parents carry the defective gene. 25% may then be disabled, and up to 50% carriers	Usually weakness of the proximal muscles of both the pelvic and the shoulder girdles	Variable, sometimes slow and sometimes fairly rapid. Disability may remain slight and some patients live to old age	None. Physical therapy may delay atrophy of disuse of healthy muscles and antibiotics control secondary illnesses, but neither halts the dystrophic process
Muscular dystrophy of late onset *Clinical Onset:* 4th or 5th decade of life	Not known to be hereditary. Affects both sexes	Weakness of the proximal muscles of the pelvic girdle	Variable	None. Physical therapy may delay atrophy of disuse of healthy muscles and antibiotics control secondary illnesses, but neither halts the dystrophic process
Polymyositis *Clinical Onset:* Any time of life	None	Proximal muscle weakness not connected with any identifiable systemic disorder	Variable, may be mild and chronic, severe and chronic, or rapidly fatal. Occasional periods of remission	Corticosteroid therapy brings marked improvement in many cases
Dermatomyositis (See also Chapter 43) *Clinical Onset:* Any time of life	None	Similar to polymyositis symptoms, with the addition of a reddish skin eruption on face and upper trunk	Similar to polymyositis	Corticosteroid therapy brings marked improvement in many cases

(Adapted from chart of Differential Diagnostic Characteristics of the Primary Diseases Affecting the Neuromuscular Unit. Made available through the Muscular Dystrophy Associations of America, Inc.)

ages of 15 and 25 from cardiac complications or respiratory infections. It is a relatively common disease with an incidence of about 1 in 25,000 (Menkes, 1974).

Clinical Manifestations

The course of the disease is gradual, with initial symptoms often overlooked. Presenting symptoms include bilateral involvement of the pelvic girdle with later progression to the shoulder girdle. Parents or playmates often notice initial signs of the disease in the young child. They may note that the boy is clumsy, has a waddling gait, frequently falls, and has difficulty climbing stairs, riding a tricycle, or rising to a sitting position. An early sign of pelvic weakness is the manner in which affected children rise from the floor. The child positions himself on all fours, then extends his knees and climbs up his thighs with his hands *(Gower sign)*. As the disease progresses muscle atrophy is noted. In spite of the atrophy, pseudohypertrophy of the calves, thighs, and upper arms results from fatty infiltration of the muscle fibers. Contractures and joint deformities are not uncommon. Walking is generally possible until approximately 12 years of age. Occasionally mental deficiency is observed in these children. Involvement of the diaphragm, myocardium, and auxilliary respiratory muscles does not occur until the final stages of the disease.

Diagnostic Assessment

Diagnosis is based on the clinical features of the disease, family history, and measurement of serum enzyme levels. Serum creatine phosphokinase (CPK) and serum glutamic-oxaloacetic transaminase (SGOT) levels are increased until late in the disease. Electromyography (EMG) reveals a disease of striated muscles with low voltage action potentials. Muscle biopsy is used to detect degeneration of muscle fibers and fatty infiltration.

Confirming the diagnosis of muscular dystrophy is often a frightening and anxiety-producing period for parents. A young boy may not understand the meaning of the diagnosis, but as he approaches adolescence he must deal with the threat of impending death.

Preparation for muscle biopsy and EMG varies with the age at diagnosis. The onset is usually in the preschool years; a child of that age should be told that he will be asleep for the biopsy and that a small cut will be made and a tiny piece of muscle removed. Vital signs and drainage from the incision will need to be monitored following the procedure. In preparation for the EMG, parents and child both need to be informed that small needles are placed in the child's muscles to record contractions. For the young child needle play prior to the procedure is appropriate; for an older child an opportunity is provided to ask questions, and clear explanations must be given. Regardless of the age of the child, the nurse should plan to be present during the procedure.

Therapeutic Management

Although no treatment exists for arresting the course of the disease, several activities must be carried out to maintain optimal levels of functioning. Therapy needs to be symptomatic, preventive, and supportive, focusing not only on the pathophysiology of the disease but also the emotional and social needs of the child and family, which change as the child develops and the disease progresses.

Major Nursing Diagnoses for DMD

Impaired physical mobility, *related to muscle weakness, contractures and joint deformities associated with DMD*

Altered growth and development: physical and emotional/social development, *related to:*

- *development of muscle weakness in the toddler or preschool period before refinement of motor skills*
- *impairment of normal social activities associated with decreased motor ability*

Potential for infection: respiratory, *related to weakness of the pulmonary musculature*

Altered nutrition: more than body requirements, *related to decreased calorie expenditure associated with muscle weakness*

Disturbance in self-concept: body image, self-esteem, role performance, personal identity, *related to:*

- *the diagnosis of a disabling, chronic disease that is expected to significantly limit life expectancy*
- *muscle weakness that limits even ordinary physical activity*

Knowledge deficit, *related to:*

- *the course and manifestations of the disease*
- *the beneficial effect of regular exercise on muscle strength*
- *the susceptibility of the child, in later stages of the disease, to respiratory infections, and the methods of prevention*
- *the need to balance nutrient intake with caloric expenditure*
- *ways to normalize the child's and family's lifestyle despite the devastating aspects of the disease*
- *the need for and availability of genetic counseling and testing to determine carriers*
- *registration with the Muscular Dystrophy Association for support services*

Strategies for Nursing Care

Promoting Healthy Development. Symptomatic treatment requires that the nurse assess the patient and his family for their understanding of the disease process, attitudes toward the condition, and coping abilities. Normal development of the child or adolescent can be delayed because exercise and activity are limited. A priority of nursing care is an activity-exercise program that allows for independence to promote maximum development (see Figure 47-20 on page 1813). Through childhood to adolescence and young adulthood, active exercise aids in improving muscle strength, and passive range of motion exercises and physiotherapy help prevent contractures. Strenuous exercises, however, may increase muscle atrophy. If for any reason the patient is on bed rest, it is very important that range-of-motion exercises be performed to maintain muscle strength.

Preventing Respiratory Infection. Respiratory infections and aspiration pneumonia are fairly common in these children. Avoidance of crowds, good nutrition, and optimal rest will put the child in the best position to resist infection. Prompt treatment of respiratory symptoms is required because these children are unable to cough effectively, resulting in pooling of mucus in the lungs. Postural drainage and antibiotic therapy are generally helpful.

Preventing Obesity. Prevention of obesity, a common problem in the presence of muscular dystrophy, is paramount. Since obesity leads to premature loss of ambulation, nutritional status of the patient needs to be assessed. Caloric intake should be adjusted in accordance with his level of activity. A balance between rest, activity, and adequate nutrition is necessary for the prevention of fatigue and obesity.

Promoting a Healthy Self-Concept. The muscle weakness and progressive physical limitation of muscular dystrophy make it difficult for children to accomplish developmental tasks and feel good about their abilities. Encouraging the family to concentrate on the things the child can do instead of on the limitations is often helpful. Children will learn to value what the parent values; a parent who values and supports the child will contribute significantly to that child's positive self-concept. Therefore, nurses who value and support the role of the parent can indirectly benefit the child.

Teaching to Support Care of the Child at Home. Teaching parents and patients the importance of exercise and the danger of immobility promotes a more positive attitude toward the disease. Knowing that they have a role and can participate in therapy often provides the stimulus needed for parents to become involved in their child's care, reducing anxieties or fears. The parents' role in helping build their child's self-esteem aids immeasurably in reinforcing his attitude of cooperation in maintaining an exercise program.

In addition to teaching, assessment of the home environment for possible problems is important. It is essential to provide equipment that may aid in therapy and to help the family solve everyday practical problems that arise when a child is handicapped. Such help may range from aiding parents in determining the best way to alter a stairway to accommodate a wheelchair to helping them modify the patient's environment to encourage his independence. Children with muscular dystrophy encounter difficulties dressing, bathing, and eating, which must be modified to help the child or adolescent gain fullest potential.

Supportive care is the most demanding intervention in this disease. Although the family of a child or adolescent with muscular dystrophy will have many problems to deal with, the nurse can help allay fears, anxieties, and misunderstandings of the disease through teaching, active listening, and coordination of the patient's care.

Provision of genetic counseling for the immediate and extended family is one of the primary approaches to muscular dystrophy. Simple serum enzyme levels of CPK determine carrier status.

Parents should be strongly encouraged to register with the Muscular Dystrophy Association, since the association has a number of services to offer patients and their families. Providing information on camp programs and parent groups will help parents lead less isolated social lives.

Nursing Strategies for Follow-up Care in the Home or Clinic

Assess the child's musculoskeletal integrity for changes from the last documented baseline; include muscle strength, coordination, and current abilities in fine and gross motor developmental tasks.

Assess the heart and lung sounds, peripheral perfusion, and vital signs for evidence of cardiopulmonary disease. Ask the child about changes in energy level or difficulty in breathing.

Weigh the child and provide nutritional counseling as needed.

Determine the current level of self-care and the family's ability to normalize the child's environment. Provide encouragement for their efforts and be sensitive to their level of adaptation. Make referrals for additional support services as needed.

Encourage the parents to involve siblings in the child's care to reinforce their worth and role within the family at times when the attention may be focused on the ill child.

Encourage siblings to discuss the experience of having a chronically ill brother or sister.

As the child's condition deteriorates help the child, parents, and siblings to explore with one another their feelings about death.

Cerebral Palsy

Incidence and Etiology

Cerebral palsy (CP) is a neurologic problem with musculoskeletal consequences. The primary disorder involves a lack of motor control of voluntary muscles owing to a lesion in the brain that has occurred prenatally, at birth, or shortly thereafter. It is a collective term that indicates paralysis of the pyramidal motor system, which consists of the motor cortex, cerebellum, and basal ganglia. The most common cause is hypoxic or anoxic insult to the brain at birth. Cerebral palsy is not genetic or hereditary, but rather the result of external factors that injure the brain. *The condition is not progressive.* While not always immediately apparent, the deficits involved are most often present at birth or in the neonatal period. The neuromuscular symptoms may be accompanied by seizure disorders or vision, speech, or hearing problems. Children with cerebral palsy may have normal or superior intelligence, although damage to the cognitive area of the brain is frequent. Incidence of CP may be as high as 6 in 1000 live births (Lovell and Winter, 1978). Because of advances in neonatology, more premature infants and infants with problems at birth are being saved. Predictably, this has led to an increase in the number of children with handicapping conditions, among them cerebral palsy. Box 47-2 lists some of the causes of the brain insult that produces cerebral palsy.

Box 47-2
Causes of Cerebral Palsy

Intrauterine Factors
- Rh or ABO incompatibility
- Rubella in first trimester
- Maternal toxoplasmosis infection
- Maternal diabetes

Complications at Birth
- Prematurity
- Precipitate delivery
- Anoxia
- Toxemia
- Asphyxia from cord around neck
- Trauma during delivery

Postnatal Period
- Infections (meningitis, encephalitis)
- Trauma
- Poisonings
- Cerebral vascular accidents

Types of Cerebral Palsy and Their Pathophysiology

Cerebral palsy is usually classified according to the clinical manifestations seen in the muscular system and subclassified according to the distribution of these symptoms. The following types are present in most classification systems. It is not unusual for a child to have more than one type of cerebral palsy, in which case it is classified as *mixed.*

Spastic. Children with *spastic* cerebral palsy have muscles that are in a state of increased tension with an exaggerated stretch reflex. This exaggerated muscle response is particularly evident with rapid passive movement. The increased muscle tension has been attributed to a loss of the normal inhibiting functions of the cerebral cortex on the anterior horn cells. Spastic cerebral palsy is further subdivided by distribution of spasticity into spastic hemiplegia, diplegia, quadriplegia, monoplegia, or triplegia. Some muscle groups are more commonly affected than others, resulting in certain characteristic deformities in children with spastic cerebral palsy. The spastic type accounts for 50 to 60 per cent of all cerebral palsy (Tachdjian, 1974).

Athetoid. The child with *athetoid* (dyskinetic) cerebral palsy has damage to the basal ganglia. Athetosis is characterized by uncontrolled and involuntary movements. Movements are usually intensified by emotional stress or tension and disappear during sleep. Facial grimacing may be present.

Ataxic. The affected child with *ataxic* cerebral palsy has damage to the cerebellum and loses coordination, equilibrium, and kinesthetic sense. There is an unsteady, staggering gait that resembles alcoholic intoxication. If one side is affected, there may be deviation or falling to one side only.

Rigid. The child with *rigid* cerebral palsy has resistance in both flexor and extensor muscles and is in a constant state of muscle tension.

Clinical Manifestations

Commonly seen clinical manifestations include the following:

- Obvious spasticity or uncontrolled movements of the extremities

- Delayed developmental milestones
- Poor muscle tone
- Persistence of primitive reflexes
- Disturbances of gait, particularly ataxia or walking on toes
- Abnormal posturing
- Disturbances of hand function

Any of these manifestations would make an observer suspicious that the child might have cerebral palsy. Clinical manifestations occur in all degrees, ranging from very mild to severely disabling.

Therapeutic Management

All treatment aims at maximizing the child's capabilities. In treatment of the musculoskeletal problems, therapy is directed toward attaining locomotion and using the upper extremities in a functional pattern. Surgical treatment is helpful in children with spasticity. Spastic children are particularly prone to development of equinus deformity owing to shortening of the heel cord (Fig. 47-19). Achilles tendon lengthening is an extremely common surgical procedure performed to improve function of the foot. Scissoring of the legs in children with spasticity may be treated with an adductor tenotomy. Muscle transfer procedures may improve function of the wrist or other joints.

Many children with CP have multiple handicaps. The most common are speech and hearing impairment, mental retardation, oculomotor impairment, and convulsive disorder. Assistance should be available through interdisciplinary teams consisting of a speech and hearing therapist, a pediatrician, a nurse, a social worker, an occupational therapist, a physical therapist, a neurologist, an orthopedist, and a family member.

Major Nursing Diagnoses for CP

Impaired physical mobility, *related to lack of motor control of voluntary muscles.*
Possible altered thought processes: mental retardation, *related to the brain lesion associated with cerebral palsy*
Potential sensory-perceptual alteration: visual, auditory, kinesthetic, *related to the particular type of brain lesion responsible for the cerebral palsy*
Potential altered nutrition: less than body requirements, *related to:*

- *dysfunction of the muscles of mastication and swallowing*
- *increased caloric needs with increased involuntary muscle movements and muscle tension*
- *decreased ability to feed self associated with muscular incoordination*

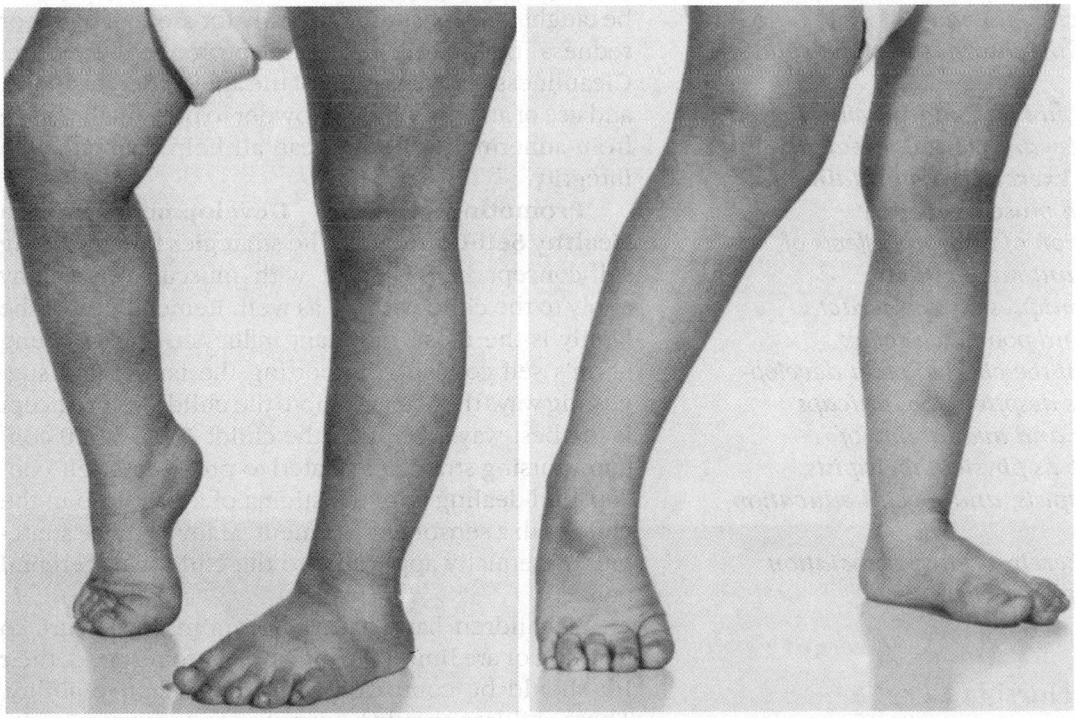

Figure 47-19. Right spastic hemiplegia showing equinus deformity. (From Tachdjian MO: *Pediatric Orthopedics.* Philadelphia, WB Saunders, 1972.)

Potential impaired skin integrity, *related to friction between a brace and the skin*

Altered growth and development: physical, intellectual, emotional/social, *related to:*

- *limitations in environmental stimulation related to motor deficits*
- *lack of coordination for learning motor skills*
- *inability to flex the muscles needed to perform such tasks as rolling and sitting*
- *limited social play opportunities associated with speech and motor deficits*

Disturbance in self-concept: body image, self-esteem, role performance, personal identity, *related to:*

- *physical deformities associated with spasticity*
- *spastic or athetoid movements*
- *tendency for the public to generalize the physical deformity to include intellectual and emotional/social functioning*
- *personal frustration with difficulty in motor and speech behaviors*

Potential altered parenting: impaired attachment behavior, *related to:*

- *the inability of the infant to "mold" to the caregiver when held*
- *feelings of the parents associated with the strong social stigma of a disorder that often involves intellectual as well as physical dysfunction*

Knowledge deficit, *related to:*

- *the cause of the disorder and the child's prognosis*
- *the fact that not all children with cerebral palsy are mentally retarded*
- *therapeutic exercises to maintain joint mobility and muscle integrity*
- *administration of and side effects of anticonvulsant medications*
- *feeding techniques to counteract dysphagia and poor suck reflex*
- *ways to assist the child to meet developmental tasks despite the handicaps*
- *the need for and availability of resources such as physical therapists, speech therapists, and special education centers*
- *the United Cerebral Palsy Association and the support it offers*

Strategies for Nursing Care

Nursing care needs to be highly individualized for the age of the child and the degree of pathologic involvement. Children who have CP are usually treated at home unless surgery is required. When hospitalized for orthopedic procedures, the care of their orthopedic problem is no different from that of any other child having orthopedic surgery. It may be the attendance to activities of daily living that will challenge the nurse.

Supporting the Child with Mental Retardation or a Sensory-Perceptual Alteration. Additional information on mental retardation and associated nursing strategies can be found in Chapter 34. Chapter 52 details care of the child with alterations in vision, hearing, and communication.

Promoting Optimal Nutrition. Motor deficits of the muscles of the mouth and throat may present special problems with eating and speech. Because muscle tension increases caloric needs, these children are given a high-calorie diet. Proper positioning in a fitted chair with sturdy foot support is needed. The child's head and trunk must be well controlled. Swallowing may be difficult and may be assisted by stroking of the throat. Maintaining adequate fluid intake is important but may be difficult due to poor sucking and swallowing. Most children with CP are highly motivated toward independence and should be taught early to develop independent feeding skills.

Maintaining Skin Integrity. Since many children with CP wear braces, the nurse must be alert for skin problems, especially when the child is nonverbal. Wearing a t-shirt between the skin and the brace can help if the shirt does not ride up under the brace and cause pressure points from wrinkles. Parents should be taught to inspect the skin daily for areas of pallor or redness that would indicate prolonged pressure. Cleanliness, daily massage of the area under the brace, and use of an unperfumed powder to prevent the brace from adhering to the skin can all help maintain skin integrity.

Promoting Optimal Development and a Healthy Self-Concept. The strategies for enhancing self-concept in the child with muscular dystrophy apply to the child with CP as well. Remember that the family is the most important influence on the young child's self-concept. Supporting the family and suggesting ways they can promote the child's self-concept is the best way to support the child. Table 51-10 contains nursing strategies related to promoting self-concept and dealing with the stigma of a handicap in the child with a sensory impairment. Many of those strategies are equally applicable to the child with cerebral palsy.

If children have had only minimal exposure to learning or are limited in their ability to respond, their IQ should be compared with their adaptive ability. These children should be exposed to new experiences and given opportunities for learning. Educational opportunities, including transportation to classes, are now the right of the handicapped. If feasible, children should attend regular classes with their peers. If needed, speech therapy or physical therapy should be provided as part of their school experiences. Mainstream school experiences help these children to minimize their differences from other children. Summer camps for handicapped children or Special Olympics can help these children see that they are not alone in their particular handicap, and they can gain strength from healthy relationships. Parents and siblings may have community support systems available to them as well. The United Cerebral Palsy Association is a source of information, guidance, and treatment in many communities.

Promoting Healthy Parenting. The nurse must be sensitive to the impact of CP on the family. Chapter 25 details strategies for helping the child and family deal with the diagnosis and with the often overwhelming care responsibilities of a chronic disorder. The parenting role will be enhanced as the parent receives the support needed for personal coping.

Teaching to Support Care of the Child at Home. Depending on the type and severity of cerebral palsy, exercises may be prescribed to preserve muscle tone and joint function. Often these will be taught by the physical therapist, but the nurse as well should be aware of the proper technique so that he or she can answer questions and evaluate the child's progress.

Anticonvulsants are frequently prescribed. Parents should receive a written list of potential side effects so that they will know when to alert the physician. Anticonvulsants and strategies for care of the child experiencing seizures is discussed further in Chapter 46.

One of the most important aspects of quality nursing care is the emotional support given to the child and family. The interdisciplinary team aids the family through periods of grief and adjustment and helps them accept the child and put the disease in perspective.

Feeding the Child with Cerebral Palsy

Feeding difficulties result from:

1. Persistence of infantile reflexes (tongue thrust)
2. Weak or absent suck
3. Muscular spasms during swallowing
4. Difficulty controlling tongue and lips
5. Inability to coordinate chewing activity
6. Inability to fully close jaw and lips
7. Hyperactive bite and gag reflex

NURSING STRATEGIES

1. Use a Teflon-coated spoon to minimize trauma due to bite reflex; Never use plastic eating utensils, as the child may bite down and break the plastic.

2. Children tolerate soft and semi-soft food the best.

3. Proper positioning is essential: Place child in a specially adapted chair rather than holding during feedings. Sit child upright with head, back, and arms well supported. Feet should be on solid surface, arms positioned forward and head slightly flexed and facing straight ahead. Prevent neck hyperextension.

4. Place food on center of tongue, pressing down gently with spoon. Prevent spoon from excessively touching lips; this encourages tongue thrust.

5. To encourage the child to close his or her mouth, chew and swallow food, use jaw control:

Sitting facing child: Place middle finger under chin which helps to close jaw. Position thumb on chin just below lower lip which promotes opening of the mouth. Rest index finger just below cheek bone for support (Fig. 47-20).

Standing behind child: Place an arm around back of the child's neck. Place middle finger under chin just behind bone and position index finger lengthwise on chin.

6. Gentle upward stroking of the neck will facilitate swallowing.

Courtesy Lynn E. Kelly, R.N., M.S.N.

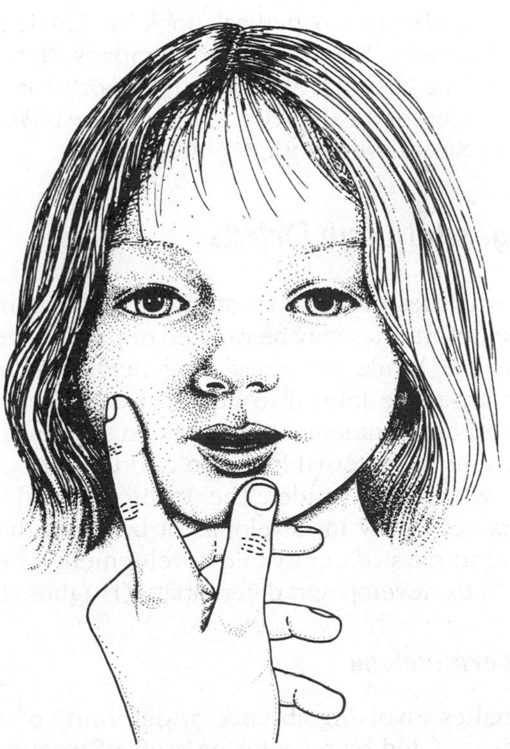

Figure 47-20. Feeding management: three-finger jaw control.

Nursing Strategies for Follow-up Care in the Home or Clinic

Assess muscular strength and joint range of motion, comparing it with the recorded baseline. Determine if home care exercises are being performed to prevent further loss of function.

Encourage expression of feelings; support adaptive coping strategies and effective parenting behaviors.

Assess progress on developmental tasks; instruct the parents and siblings on ways to facilitate mastery of the next appropriate tasks. Realize that progress will be slow and that the family will need continued reassurance and encouragement to help the child develop to potential.

Assess for appropriate weight gain and provide nutritional counseling as needed.

Assess for commonly related impairments: seizure activity and vision, and hearing impairments.

Assess for signs of respiratory infection associated with the tendency toward aspiration.

Remind the family of the importance to the child's self-esteem of their love, acceptance, and encouragement.

Recommend available sources of support as appropriate:

- *Handling the Young Cerebral Palsied Child at Home,* a paperback book by Nancie R. Finnie (E.P. Dutton and Company, New York)
- The National Association of Sports for Cerebral Palsy, UPCA, Inc., 66 East 34th Street, New York, NY 10016

Congenital Limb Defects

Abnormalities in limb formation are not uncommon. These deformities may be isolated or part of a general syndrome. While the cause is generally unknown, some types are known to be genetic. Some are the result of environmental influences on the developing limb, such as maternal infection or drug ingestion, as seen with thalidomide. The environmental insult occurs very early in development between the 27th and 42nd days of embryonic development when the limb buds develop and differentiate (Hughes, 1980).

Terminology

Anomalies involving absence or deformity of a limb are surrounded by a confusing array of terminology. Some commonly used terms are

- *Amelia* or *ectromelia*—Complete absence of a limb
- *phocomelia*—absence of some segment of an extremity so that the distal portion is attached to a proximal portion with some intervening part missing
- *Hemimelia*—Absence of half an extremity
- *Meromelia*—All limb deficiencies other than complete absence

Defects may further be subdivided as transverse or longitudinal, and terminal or intercalary. Transverse refers to absence extending across the width of a limb and longitudinal to absence extending parallel with the long axis of the limb. Terminal refers to absence of all distal segments. Intercalary refers to absence of middle parts (Swinyard, 1969). Complete absence of a hand would be a transverse terminal defect. Absence of a radius would be a longitudinal defect. Phocomelia with the hand attached to the shoulder would be an intercalary defect.

Limb defects, of which there is a wide variety, are usually quite obvious at birth. These defects range in severity from very mild anomalies, such as extra digits to very severe ones, such as complete absence of a limb. One longitudinal type of defect, radial clubhand deformity, is illustrated in Figure 47-21.

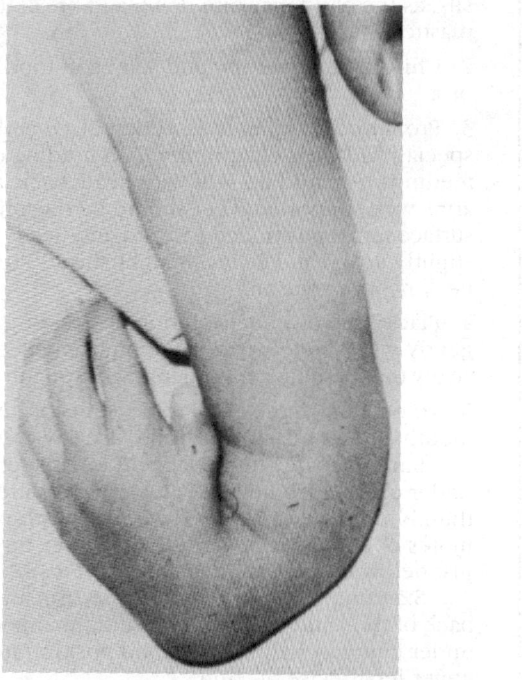

Figure 47-21. Radial clubhand deformity. (Courtesy of Drs. James Hunter and Lawrence Schneider, Thomas Jefferson University Hospital, Philadelphia. *In* Gartland JH: *Fundamentals of Orthopaedics.* 4th ed. Philadelphia, WB Saunders, 1986.)

Therapeutic Management

The main concern with children with limb deformity is the development and maintenance of functional extremities: a prehensile hand and a weight-bearing lower extremity. Of secondary concern is the appearance of the defect, although this may not be secondary to the family or the child. The rapid advances in prosthetics offer great hope for persons with limb deformities. Much of this progress is due to the thalidomide tragedy and the large numbers of affected children born at that time in Europe.

Surgical procedures of various types are used to increase function and improve appearance. These might include muscle and tendon transfers and plastic procedures. Occasionally amputation of a part might be necessary in order to allow for proper fitting and use of a prosthetic device.

Strategies for Nursing Care

Helping these children meet the challenges of activities of daily living and maintain normal development is the aim of parents and caregivers. When disabling limb defects are present from birth, children often make remarkable adaptations to them, having known no other life experience. Children with amelia of both upper extremities are examples of this, as they are able to develop extreme prehensile agility with their feet.

Interactions with children with limb defects are best begun with the assumption that they are normal and capable of normal activities since attitudes of normality are extremely important in helping these children feel accepted. If amputation is necessary, the child will grieve for loss of a deformed part just as one would for any body part.

Growth-Related Musculoskeletal Disorders

Developmental Leg Problems

Torsional deformities of the tibia or hip or both, also known as bowlegs (genu varum) and knock-knees (genu valgum), respectively, are common findings that affect the lower extremities of growing children and become particularly noticeable when the child begins walking. Although the vast majority of these orthopedic problems are part of normal physiologic development and are self-corrective as the child grows, it is important to differentiate the physiologic conditions from those that may be pathologic, requiring additional evaluation and treatment (McDade, 1977). The nurse is often the first to suspect orthopedic problems during well-child assessments. The following discussion is intended to help the nurse recognize when medical or orthopedic referral is advisable.

Torsional Deformity

Torsional deformity (malrotation or twisting of the femur or tibia) is the most common orthopedic problem. The torsional deformity may occur anywhere between the foot and hip; identifying precisely the location of the deformity becomes important in managing the problem correctly.

Etiology and Pathophysiology

Prenatally the fetal lower limbs normally rotate internally to bring the great toe to midline; therefore, the infant seems to be pigeon-toed. During infancy external rotation of the femur and tibia gradually occurs, steadily diminishing the child's pigeon-toed appearance. By adolescence the normal stance of slight external rotation of the tibia and femur is established.

If, owing to environmental or genetic factors, this gradual external rotation is restricted, an internal rotation deformity persists. Two major etiologies have been attributed to perpetuation of internal tibial rotation, producing intoeing. Sometimes internal tibial torsion is a consequence of the intrauterine position. A deformity with this etiology usually improves spontaneously unless a predominantly prone sleeping posture causes it to persist. Heredity is sometimes a factor in femoral torsion. Table 47-7 lists the characteristics of torsional deformities.

Table 47-7. Characteristics of Torsional Deformities

Direction: Intoeing	Direction: Out-Toeing
Hip	
Femoral torsion as estimated by internal hip rotation: 70°–80° rotation—mild 80°–85° rotation—moderate 85°+ rotation—severe	Normal physiologic position (i.e., internal hip rotation less than 70%)
Tibia	
Internal tibial torsion indicated by thigh-foot angle: −10°—mild −20°—moderate −30°—severe	External tibial torsion (thigh-foot angle greater than +30°)

(From Staheli, 1977.)

Clinical Manifestations and Diagnostic Assessment

Torsional deformities are primarily structural (resulting from bone position), although they may occasionally arise from abnormal abduction of the great toe muscle (dynamic deformity). Torsional deformities are almost always bilateral.

When a torsional deformity is suspected from routine physical examination or family history, a detailed medical history of the condition should be obtained that covers the progression of the deformity, any previous diagnosis and treatment, and parental response to the condition. Evaluation involves an estimate of hip rotation and tibial rotation.

Measurement of hip rotation is done with the child in a comfortable prone position. The lower legs are raised and permitted to fall outward; this puts the hip into full internal rotation. The angles formed by an imaginary line drawn vertically from the hip joint to the knee and another drawn from the knee to the great toe are measured to estimate the degree of internal hip rotation (Fig. 47-22). The lower leg is then allowed to fall inward. This puts the hip into full external rotation while the examiner or parent holds the pelvis against the examination table. The angles formed by imaginary lines drawn vertically from the hip joint to the knee and from the knee to the small toe are measured to determine the degree of external hip rotation (Fig. 47-23). The angles of internal and of external hip rotation are measured for each leg.

The normal angle of hip rotation varies according to the child's age. External rotation of the hip is greatest (about 90 degrees) during early infancy. By the time the child is walking alone, internal and external hip rotation are about equal. External hip rotation supersedes internal rotation in the adolescent male, whereas internal and external hip rotation are still equal or internal rotation is slightly greater in the adolescent female (Staheli, 1977).

The sum of the internal and external hip rotation angles approximates 100 degrees normally, with the internal rotation angle comprising 70 degrees or less. Increased internal hip rotation is almost always evidence of femoral torsion. Table 47-7 correlates rotation with severity of a deformity when internal rotation exceeds 70 degrees.

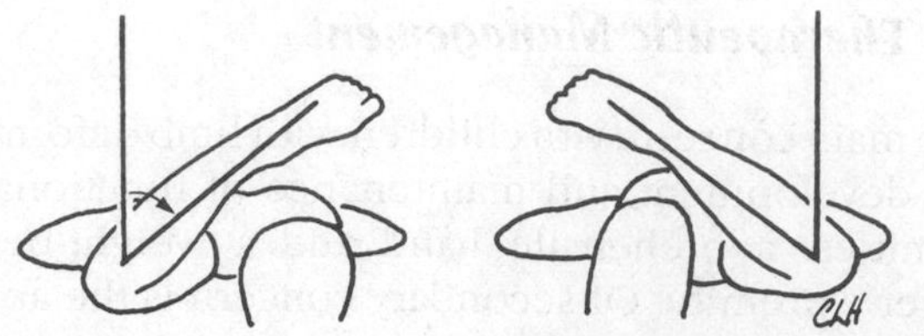

Figure 47-23. Assessment of external hip rotation. (From Staheli L: Torsional deformity. *Pediatr Clin North Am* 1977 Nov; 803.)

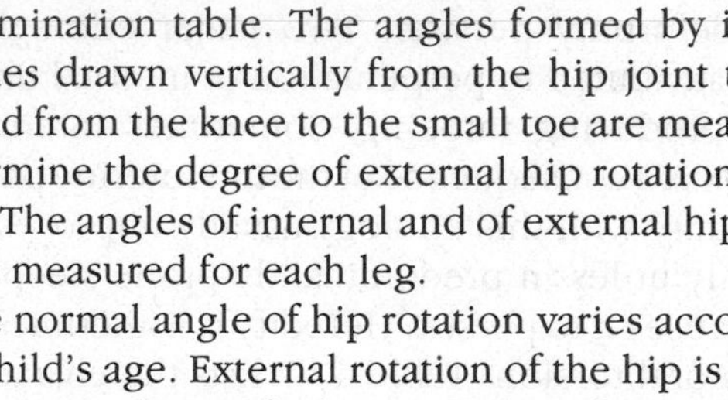

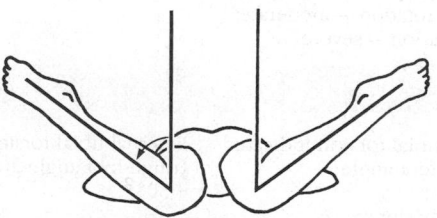

Figure 47-22. Assessment of internal hip rotation. (From Staheli L: Torsional deformity. *Pediatr Clin North Am* 1977 Nov; 803.)

Tibial rotation is determined by measuring the angular difference between an imaginary line drawn vertically down the back of the thigh and another line drawn vertically across the axis of the foot sole (Fig. 47-24), called the "thigh-foot angle." This is most easily done by placing the child in a prone position and flexing the knee to 90 degrees. When the foot sole line is being made, the foot is depressed across the toes with one finger to place the ankle into weight-bearing position. Medial (thigh-foot angle turned inward) rotation beyond infancy, noted in negative degrees, indicates internal tibial torsion; external rotation of the tibia (0 to +30 degrees thigh-foot angle) is normal by toddlerhood.

A profile of the factors just discussed determines the presence of and type of torsional deformity, its severity, and whether it is bilateral or unilateral. Correct diagnosis is critical in establishing the proper management.

Internal Tibial Torsion

The most common torsional defect, this deformity is usually recognized at the onset of toddlerhood. Most of these deformities disappear by the time the child is

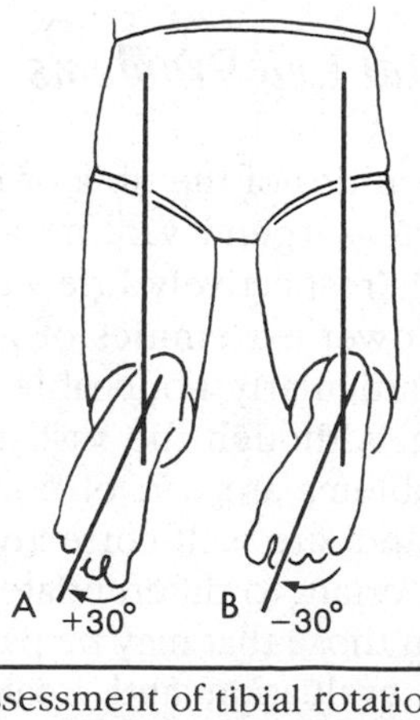

Figure 47-24. Assessment of tibial rotation. *A*, External tibial rotation; *B*, internal tibial rotation. (From Staheli L: Torsional deformity. *Pediatr Clin North Am* 1977 Nov; 809.)

18 months old; if not, a corrective night splint may be necessary. The "clamp-on" splint consists of a bar the width of the pelvis (2 to 4 inches longer if the child is bowlegged) that is attached to the child's high-topped, stiff-soled shoes at night to maintain the feet in external rotation of 30 to 35 degrees (Staheli, 1977). If the deformity is unilateral, the normal foot is set at 10 to 15 degrees external rotation. Usually correction is achieved in a year; the child should be checked every 3 months and treatment discontinued when the involved foot shows a 10- to 15-degree external rotation (Staheli, 1977). Parents may need support to continue use of the night splint despite their toddler's obvious resistance. They should be reassured that, if they persist, their child will adjust to the splint and cooperate after a few nights. To help ensure the parents' cooperation in using the brace in spite of their child's rebellion, the nurse should make certain they understand the importance of the splint and how it works to correct the defect. After age 3, correction other than by surgery is seldom satisfactory.

Internal Femoral Rotation

This is a common cause of intoeing in late toddler and preschool years. It is sometimes familial, is more common in girls, and is rarely unilateral. Unless the internal hip rotation is severe, treatment is usually not recommended, since the deformity is eventually compensated and does not result in functional disability in adulthood.

Whatever treatment is prescribed, parents' involvement and cooperation in carrying it out is imperative if it is to be successful. The nurse must be sure the parents understand their responsibility in the treatment regimen by providing adequate explanations of the deformity and the purpose of treatment and by teaching them the skills required to carry out the treatment. Progress should be shared with the parents at each follow-up visit, and their efforts to comply with the regimen positively reinforced. If financial assistance is needed, the nurse may refer the family to a local crippled children's program for help. If parental compliance is doubted, the community health nurse is an appropriate adjunct to the treatment team.

The child will need age-appropriate explanations of the treatment and an opportunity to handle and investigate equipment used in the treatment. If the parents continue to relate to the child in a positive and consistent fashion, he or she will feel secure and cooperation is more likely.

Strategies for Nursing Care

The nurse plays a major role in educating the family as to the pathophysiology and the physiologic recovery typical of mild and moderate torsional deformities. Reassurance offered at each health visit, as well as sharing of measurements indicating progress in resolution of the deformity, helps to relieve parental anxiety.

Genu Varum and Genu Valgum

Bowlegs (genu varum) and knock-knees (genu valgum) usually are features of normal physiologic development that resolve as growth progresses. Studies of large numbers of children have shown that bowlegs are characteristic until 1½ to 2½ years of age, followed by knock-knees until around 4 to 6 years of age, at which time the lower extremities straighten to represent the normal adult stance (McDade, 1977). Physiologic varus is accentuated by the internal tibial torsion that is characteristic of the infant and young toddler. Conversely, valgum also seems more extreme than it is because of the external tibial torsion characteristic of the toddler and preschool years. Sleep position, obesity, and posture may also accentuate physiologic varus and valgus.

Therapeutic Management

Physiologic varus and valgus do not require any intervention other than periodic follow-up to assess the progressive resolution of each as the child develops. Roentgenographs are not necessary, although the observations discussed earlier to determine the degree of femoral and tibial rotation may be conducted to ensure that lower extremity alignment is within normal limits for the child' age. A family history should be obtained at this time. Whether the deformity is bilateral or unilateral should be established, since unilateral deformities often require treatment. Likewise, leg symmetry should be determined so that asymmetrical deformities may also be treated. Parents may need reassurance that the deformity they perceive is normal and will resolve as the child grows.

Nonphysiologic or Extreme Varus

Bowlegs (Fig. 47-25) that are unilateral, asymmetrical, or that persist after 2 years of age are often pathologic. Extreme varus has a greater incidence in black children. Etiologically it may be congenital or familial. It may also be associated with Blount's disease (a growth disturbance of the proximal tibia creating extreme internal tibial torsion) or rickets (a disturbance of calcium and phosphorus metabolism causing inadequate bone calcification during skeletal growth).

Therapeutic Management. Any toddler in whom varus is not resolving by 18 to 24 months and

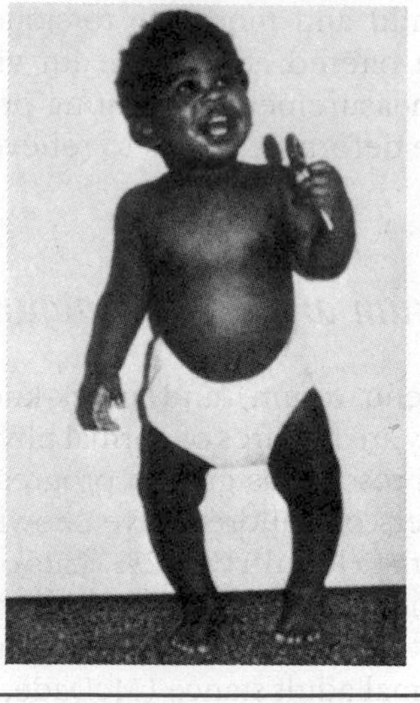

Figure 47-25. The "extreme variation," a 15-month-old boy with bowlegs. (From McDade W: Bowlegs and knock knees. *Pediatr Clin North Am* 1977 Nov; 833.)

who has a tibiofemoral angle (bowing of tibia and femur) on roentgenograph of 25 degrees or more of varus should be braced day and night for correction. A brace is usually required for 1 to 2 years. If the brace has not achieved correction of the varus by 3 years of age, osteotomy may be recommended some time during the preschool years (McDade, 1977).

Strategies for Nursing Care. The nurse may need to maintain frequent contact with the family via phone calls or home visits initially to encourage and reinforce the family's compliance efforts. The brace may be removed twice a day for 30 to 45 minutes to relieve the pressure from the brace and provide skin care. Parents should be informed of the importance of daily skin care of the extremities to prevent skin breakdown from the pressure and tension exerted by the brace.

Children should be allowed and encouraged to participate in their usual activities to the extent possible to maintain their normal developmental progress. For example, consideration should be given to providing extra time for them to walk to reduce adults' temptation to carry them.

Nonphysiologic or Extreme Valgus

A condition of excessive knock-knees (Fig. 47-26) as established by a tibiofemoral angle on roentgenograph of more than 15 degrees of valgus, by leg asymmetry, or by a shortened stature, requires intervention to achieve correction. Likewise, a severe valgus deformity that has not corrected to at least a mild valgus by age 10 will also need intervention.

Knock-knees may be congenital, familial, or associated with obesity, polio, rickets, or trauma or infection of the proximal tibial epiphysis. Girls tend to be more susceptible to extreme valgus deformity, probably because of their wider pelvis and more relaxed musculature.

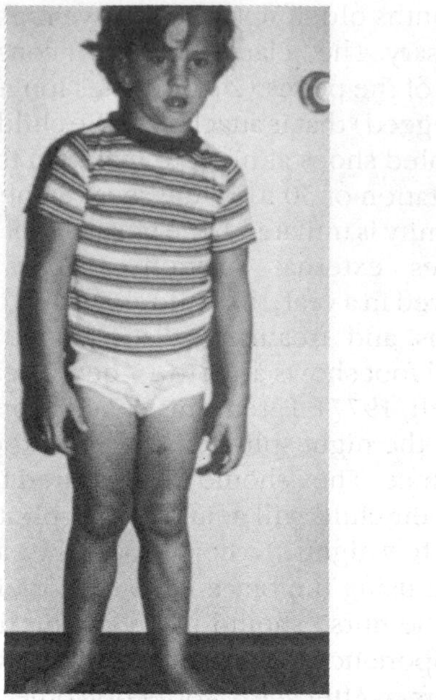

Figure 47-26. A 5-year-old boy with knock-knees. (From McDade W: Bowlegs and knock knees. *Pediatr Clin North Am* 1977 Nov; 831.)

Extreme genu valgum, left uncorrected, contributes to gait awkwardness, which increases the child's risk for sprains and fractures as he or she gets older, particularly during active or contact sports. The deformity also causes easy fatigability and joint pains.

Therapeutic Management. If resolution of symmetric knock-knees is not in progress by 7 years of age, day and night braces are usually prescribed to correct the deformity. Any correctable underlying etiology is also treated. When the valgus is asymmetric, braces may be recommended earlier. If bracing is not successful by 10 years of age in girls or 12 years in boys, or if the condition is not diagnosed before this time, osteotomy is recommended to correct the angular deformity.

Strategies for Nursing Care. The prognosis for the torsional deformities and genu varum or valgum is excellent if the conditions are followed closely and treatment is initiated promptly when spontaneous resolution does not occur. The critical factor in treatment rests upon parental cooperation and compliance with prescribed interventions. The nurse has an important responsibility in helping parents understand the condition and its treatment sufficiently to cooperate and in providing the support and reassurance necessary to maintain that cooperation.

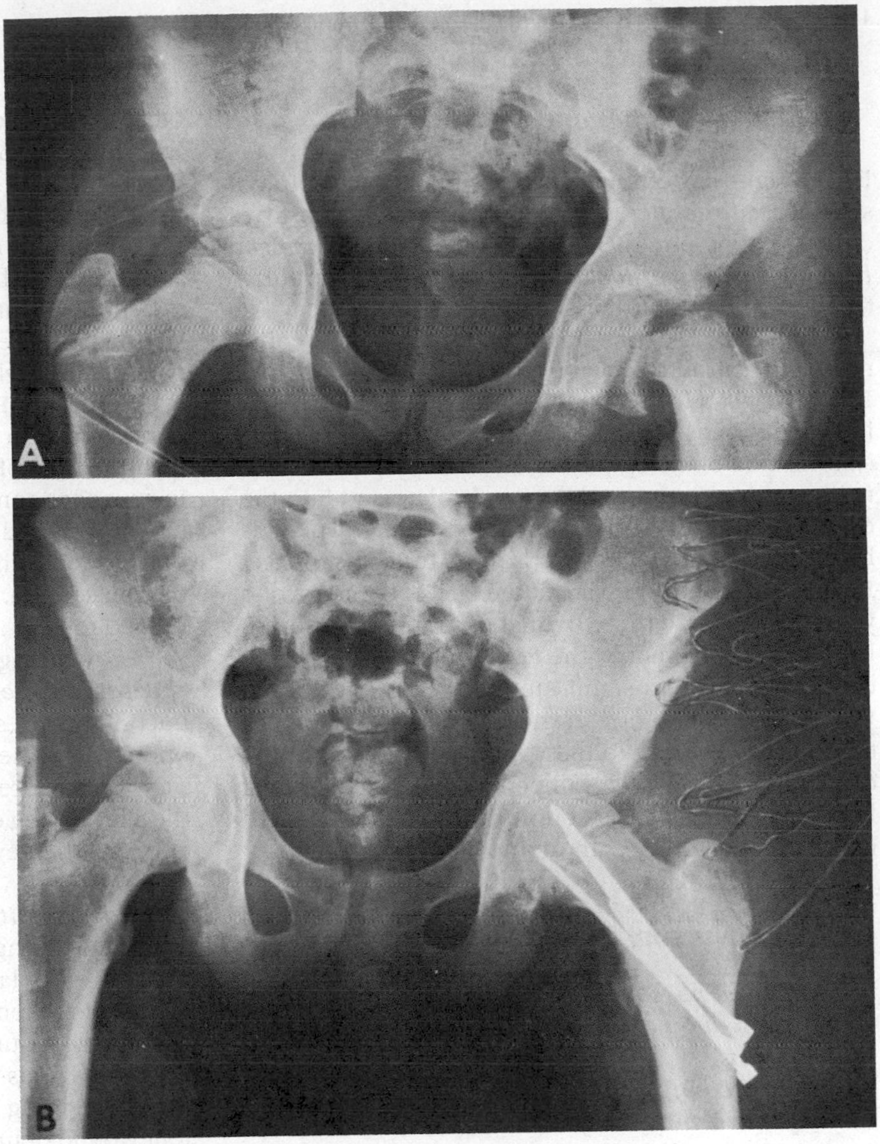

Figure 47-27. *A*, Complete slip of capital femoral epiphysis of left hip. *B*, Same patient after operative replacement of the epiphysis, bone pegging of the growth line, and fixation with metallic pins. (Courtesy of Dr. John Dowling, Lankenau Hospital, Philadelphia. *In* Gartland JH: *Fundamentals of Orthopaedics.* 4th ed. Philadelphia, WB Saunders, 1986.)

Slipped Capital Femoral Epiphysis (SCFE)

Slippage of the head of the femur at the proximal epiphyseal line occurs generally between 10 and 17 years of age. It is much more common in males, outnumbering females with slipped epiphysis by 5 to 1 (Ferguson, 1981). It tends to occur in girls at a younger age, probably related to their earlier growth spurt.

Etiology

The etiology of this problem is unknown, but its rarity in younger children has led to the assumption that the epiphyseal changes associated with a rapid growth spurt or endocrine changes, or both, may predispose an adolescent to SCFE. The condition frequently occurs in two types of children: the overweight child and the tall, thin child who has recently had a growth spurt (Hilt and Cogburn, 1980).

Pathophysiology and Clinical Manifestations

Slippage may be acute and associated with trauma but is more commonly chronic, with a history of increasing pain and disability beginning weeks or even months earlier. The epiphyseal head typically slips downward and posteriorly. The epiphysis remains partially attached to the femoral neck by periosteum and fibrous tissue (Ferguson, 1981). The child complains of hip or knee pain, often associated with a limp. There may be adduction and external rotation of the femur with limitation of motion. On roentgenograph, the earliest sign is a widening of the epiphyseal line (Gartland, 1979). Actual slippage is clearly visible on roentgenograph (Fig. 47-27).

Therapeutic Management

Early diagnosis before large movement of the epiphysis has occurred increases the likelihood of a positive outcome. As soon as SCFE has been diagnosed, *weight bearing should be stopped immediately* to minimize the possibility of further slippage.

Buck or Russell traction may be used to overcome muscle spasm and make the patient more comfortable. It may be used in conjunction with non–weight bearing in mild cases. However, in most cases, surgical stabilization of the epiphysis will follow. One or more nails are driven across the growth plate and into the epiphysis. This results in closure of the growth plate as healing occurs, which will prevent further slippage. Because these children are at the end of their growing years and because the proximal epiphysis contributes less than 30 per cent to the total length of the femur, there is usually no significant shortening of the leg (Gartland, 1979). Interference with blood supply to the epiphysis owing to the condition or its treatment can produce an avascular necrosis of the epiphyseal head. Symptoms of this complication include limited range of motion and pain on movement.

Major Nursing Diagnoses for SCFE

Impaired physical mobility, *related to displacement of the head of the femur at the epiphysis*
Altered comfort: pain, *associated with displacement of the femoral head and with manual realignment of the leg with traction*
Potential for injury:
- ***neurovascular impairment,*** *related to preoperative traction*
- ***osteomyelitis,*** *related to surgical opening of the hip joint*

Knowledge deficit, *related to:*
- *anatomy of the head of the femur, results of epiphyseal slippage, and treatment techniques (including no weight bearing, traction, and probable surgery)*
- *expected outcome of the treatment process*
- *signs and symptoms of postoperative infection*
- *need for follow-up to assess for involvement of the other leg*

Strategies for Nursing Care

These adolescents are usually admitted for treatment immediately after diagnosis, so the admission may be on very short notice. SCFE is considered an emergency, and weight bearing is stopped in the physician's office. The patient may have had little time to assimilate information about the condition. Roentgenographs provide the most enlightening explanation of what is happening for the patient and family. The treatment regimen needs to be carefully outlined, as the adolescent will undoubtedly have many unanswered questions about the treatment, the length of hospitalization, and the repercussions of this episode on the patient's lifestyle.

Relieving Pain. Typically, a good deal of pain is associated with slippage of the epiphysis and with the manipulation of the hip joint required to place the leg in proper alignment for traction. The nurse should anticipate this and talk with the child or adolescent about options for pain relief, both pharmacologic and nonpharmacologic. See Chapter 29 for specific strategies related to pain assessment and pain relief.

Preventing Complications. Assessment of *neurovascular integrity* is appropriate both in relation to traction before surgery and in relation to edema postoperatively. The client will return from surgery with an incision and dressing on the lateral hip. Assess NVS of the affected leg every hour immediately following surgery and then every 4 hours (see also Tables 47-3 and 47-4).

Osteomyelitis is a potential complication of the surgical opening of the hip joint (see the discussion of osteomyelitis later in this chapter). Observe sterile technique when changing surgical dressings or contacting the wound in any way. Instruct the patient to wash the hands well before touching the area. Assess for the defining characteristics of this infection: purulent wound drainage, redness and tenderness over the incisional area, fever, and increased white blood count. The patient and family also should be made aware of these signs of infection, in case they develop after discharge.

Teaching to Support Care of the Child/Adolescent in the Home. The young person and family will need a good deal of support to cope with the suddenness of the diagnosis and treatment. Simple but thorough explanations and willingness to repeat information are important. The patient and family should know that crutches may be prescribed for several months so that closure and stabilization of the epiphysis can occur before resumption of weight bearing on the affected limb. They should know as well that bilateral involvement occurs in approximately 20 per cent of cases. Follow-up care is therefore important.

Nursing Strategies for Follow-up Care in the Home or Clinic

Assess the surgical site for healing/infection.

Assess for understanding of and compliance with the order for no weight bearing on the affected leg.

Assess for level of comfort (increase in pain might signal complications).

Assess comfort level and range of motion of the other hip; involvement may be bilateral.

Spinal Abnormalities

Spinal abnormalities such as kyphosis, lordosis, and scoliosis are commonly identified and treated during the adolescent growth spurt that begins sometime between the ages of 10 and 15 years. These abnormalities are exaggerations of the natural spinal curves that may occur as a result of organic or structural vertebral changes or as a result of persistent poor posture. *Kyphosis* (humpback or hunchback) is an exaggerated angulation forward (convexity) or a natural vertebral curve, most commonly the thoracic curve. Exaggerated inward (concavity) spinal curvature, usually of the lumbar spine, is called *lordosis* (swayback). Lateral deviation of the spine, creating a side-to-side or S-shaped curvature, is *scoliosis*. Prior to adolescence children display developmental spinal curve exaggerations to accommodate the changes in their center of gravity. By adolescence normal adult curvature should be attained.

Kyphosis and Lordosis

Kyphosis (Fig. 47-28) may be congenital, neuromuscular, postural, or the result of Scheuermann disease. Congenital kyphosis is the result of anomalous vertebral bodies. It may be apparent at birth or not until the adolescent growth spurt. Progression of the kyphosis usually continues until growth is completed. Congenital kyphosis usually requires spinal fusion. Scheuermann disease is a disturbance of the epiphyses of the thoracic vertebrae and is discussed under osteochondroses.

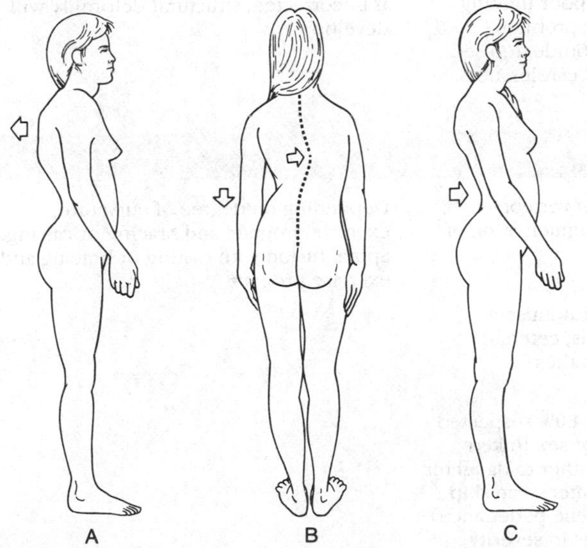

Figure 47-28. Skeletal abnormalities of adolescence. *A*, Kyphosis; *B*, scoliosis; and *C*, lordosis.

The vast majority of cases of kyphosis seen in youth are caused by habits of posture. This postural form is particularly common in the female adolescent, probably because of the round-shouldered slouch that she assumes during prepubertal and pubertal years to "hide" breast development and to make her seem less noticeably taller than her male peers, whose growth spurt comes later. An exercise program that emphasizes proper sitting and standing, along with measures to increase the girl's self-esteem, usually brings about successful correction of postural kyphosis, although a Milwaukee brace is occasionally necessary if the kyphosis does not resolve within 2 to 3 years.

Lordosis (Fig. 47-28) is almost always a compensatory curvature associated with kyphosis or scoliosis. It is a normal compensatory curve of young children that corrects itself slightly earlier in males. Any lordosis that persists after 8 years of age should be evaluated for the underlying cause. Treatment is the same as for kyphosis.

Because of the characteristic uncooperativeness of many adolescents in doing things that they "have to do," very few will want to do the daily exercises required for spinal correction, especially if these exercises are being overseen by a parent. Better success is achieved if the exercise program is supervised by a competent physical therapist who can relate to the emotional stresses of growing up. Exercises are supervised on a weekly basis initially, the frequency decreasing as the adolescent incorporates the exercises into a daily routine. The program will also be more successful if built around postural sports (weightlifting, track, dancing, or swimming) that strengthen shoulder, abdominal, and lumbar muscles. Success depends on the adolescent's motivation and the relationship achieved between the youth and the parent or therapist supervising the exercise program.

Scoliosis

Scoliosis is the most common skeletal deformity of adolescence, being manifested in about 15 per cent of youth between the ages of 10 and 21; it occurs predominantly in girls. Although the deformity has usually been present before puberty or adolescence, the rapid vertebral growth that occurs during this period causes it to progress faster, making the characteristic C- or S-shaped curvature more apparent. If the deformity progresses very much, the physical changes can result in impaired cardiopulmonary function, neurologic damage as a result of tethered nerves, and development of an unhealthy self-image.

Etiology

Scoliosis may be either nonstructural (postural or functional) or structural (Table 47-8). Structural scoliosis is further classified as congenital, idiopathic, or neuromuscular, according to etiology (Table 47-9). Idiopathic scoliosis, the most common type, is more severe near puberty. It has three forms: infantile, juvenile, and adolescent. This classification is based on the age of the child at diagnosis. Variations in the degree of severity occur in any of the scoliotic forms.

Pathophysiology

The basic pathophysiology of scoliosis is a lateral deviation (most often a right thoracic curvature) of the spinal column from midline that may or may not involve rotation or deformity of the vertebrae (Fig. 47-28). The deviation is a consequence of weakened muscle strength from any one or a variety of genetic, environmental, or physiologic factors. During progression of the curvature that occurs at the growth spurt, pressure exerted on the vertebrae cause them to become wedged. If structural changes begin occurring early, when extensive spinal growth is taking place, a more severe curvative abnormality will be created. Correctional prognosis is best when the curvature is identified and treated while still mild. Because idiopathic adolescent scoliosis is the most prevalent type, the remainder of this discussion will deal with that class of scoliosis.

Diagnostic Assessment

The importance of early identification of scoliotic curvature cannot be overemphasized, because early intervention greatly improves the prognosis and diminishes the length of time needed for treatment and the accompanying emotional trauma. The procedures to diagnose scoliosis are simple and take little time, yet several factors tend to impede early diagnosis in youth. The child between 10 and 15 years of age (the peak ages for incidence) is usually healthy and, as a consequence, frequently does not have a yearly physical examination. Even when a physical examination is included in health maintenance for a child this age, a back examination may be overlooked or inadequately done. In addition, the vertebral changes of scoliosis often progress slowly and may go unnoticed. The adolescent, whose identity and self-concept are so easily threatened, may not report a deviation even when it is noticed. The majority of parents do not see their teen-

Table 47-8. Classification of Scoliotic Deformities

Clinical Manifestations	Etiology	Usual Management
Nonstructural		
No specific vertebral changes or rotation Flexible curve, easily corrected by bending forward or toward convex side of curve C-shaped curve	From outside spine: 1. Malnutrition 2. Muscle spasms from injury 3. Pain 4. Poor posture related to poor lighting, vision problem, hearing problem, negative psychologic attitude, too sedentary lifestyle, postural carelessness, chronic fatigue	Active and passive exercises Correct etiological factor(s) causing curvature If uncorrected, structural deformity will develop
Structural		
Visible vertebrae, bony changes and fixed rotation toward the convexity	Congenital malformation of vertebrae (hemivertebra, failure of segmentation of vertebra, rib fusion)	Depending on degree of curvature, exercise program and bracing or casting. Spinal fusion with casting or bracing and exercise program
Inflexible or rigid curve, not corrected by bending. Bending produces a rib hump that is the result of vertebral rotation and muscle distortion	Neuromuscular asymmetrical muscle paralysis (neurofibromatosis, cerebral palsy, various muscle anomalies)	
S-shaped curve results from a major curve (usually thoracic) and compensatory minor curves above and/or below the major curve	Idiopathic with at least 70–80% suspected to be the result of dominant sex-linked inheritance (passed from father to daughter and mother to son or daughter); can skip generations (incomplete gene penetrance) and, when expressed, varies in severity (variable gene expressivity)	

Table 47-9. Etiologic Classification of Structural Scoliosis

Etiology and Pathophysiology	Diagnostic Assessment	Therapeutic Management
Congenital scoliosis		
Embryologic malformation of spine during third to fifth embryonic week Localized or generalized deformity: hemivertebra (only half-formed), failure in segmentations (vertebra segments do not fully separate) and rib fusion are typical anomalies Thoracic curves most common	Anteroposterior and lateral roentgenographs verify curvature and identify anomalous vertebrae Usually other congenital anomalies coexist; urinary tract anomalies most prevalent Secondary neurologic symptoms from long-term spinal cord tethering Secondary signs: short trunk; sacral area hair tufts; unequal leg length; cafe-au-lait markings	Early treatment essential; usually spinal fusion before preschool age to stabilize progressive curves Complete evaluation for any other anomalies; intravenous pyelogram recommended as a minimal screening
Neuromuscular (Paralytic) Scoliosis		
Secondary to neuropathic or myopathic disease (polio, cerebral palsy, muscular dystrophy, neurofibromatosis, myelomeningocele) that results in muscle imbalance Initially flexible, becoming rigid as it progresses; tends to progress after skeletal growth completed: Long C curve—generalized neuromuscular disease with severe muscle weakness S curve similar to idiopathic scoliosis—result of localized muscle imbalance	Presence of primary neurologic or muscular disease Anteroposterior and lateral roentgenographs verify curvature Rib hump may or may not be present, depending on flexibility of curve	Occasionally bracing stabilizes progression if no structural changes Spinal fusion usually necessary if structural change present
Idiopathic Scoliosis		
Dominant X-linked inheritance in 70–80% of cases justifies evaluation of all family members when one is diagnosed S-shaped curvature most common with vertebrae changes and rotations See below for individual forms	See below for individual forms	See below for individual forms
Infantile Idiopathic Scoliosis		
Occurs in first years of life; often associated with intrauterine position More in males, rare in US, common in Britain Usually left thoracic curve	Occurs before 4 years of age Verification of curve with anteroposterior and lateral standing and side-bending roentgenographs	50% resolve spontaneously 50% rapidly progressive and require spinal fusion
Juvenile Idiopathic Scoliosis		
Occurs in middle childhood, usually around 6 years Usually right thoracic curve Sexes are equally affected	Occurs between 4 and 10 years of age Standing and side-bending roentgenographs verify curve severity	Will not resolve spontaneously Bracing or Orthoplast jacket usually adequate Spinal fusion indicated if rapidly progressive or curve is severe (55 to 60 degrees)

continued

Table 47-9 *(continued)*

Etiology and Pathophysiology	Diagnostic Assessment	Therapeutic Management
Adolescent Idiopathic Scoliosis		
Occurs between age 10 and skeletal maturity Most prevalent in US; seven times more common in females May or may not progress during growth spurt Various curves possible *Lumbar curve* (T11 to L5) Fairly common Majority are left Seldom any compensatory curves Minimally deforming but does become rigid, causing arthritic pain during childbearing and old age *Right thoracic curve* (T4 to L1) Very common Severe cosmetic defect and cardiopulmonary impairment if untreated Usually compensatory left minor curves above and below major curve Much vertebral change and rotation *Double major curves* Right thoracic and left lumbar prominence most common combination *Thoracolumbar curve* (T4 to L4) Very common Long curve Moderate cosmetic deformity May cause rib and flank distortions *Cervicothoracic curve* (C5 to T4) Rare Usually to left Shoulder asymmetry only cosmetic problem	Occurs after age 10 Positive screening test findings: Scapular prominence Rib hump Shoulder asymmetry Spinal curves Hip asymmetry Deeper creasing on one side of waist Torso malalignment when standing erect Anterior rib and breast asymmetry Suggestive signs: unequal hemline, back pain, poor posture, attached earlobes, cavus (high arch) feet	Will not resolve spontaneously Exercise program alone ineffective Milwaukee brace or Orthoplast jacket or spinal fusion with/without instrumentation (cast or traction may be used preoperatively or postoperatively)

age daughters undressed, and visualization of the bare back is necessary to observe early curve deformity.

Two practices are currently improving early identification of scoliosis, and nurses can actively endorse these or initiate them in their own community. One practice initiated in several states is statewide school scoliosis screening for all school-age youth as a part of the school health program. The other is the screening of all siblings in families in which a case is diagnosed. This practice has been initiated by many nurses, physicians, and orthopedists as a result of the research that has revealed a genetic etiology of the condition.

Screening for scoliosis involves observing the child while walking, standing erect, and bending forward. Figure 47-29 describes the specific observations that are included in a thorough screening evaluation.

A child suspected of having scoliosis after screening should be referred for further evaluation by the nurse to the family physician or to a competent orthopedist experienced in treating scoliotic deformities of adolescence. The teen and parents should be informed of the possibility of a deformity and of the importance of early intervention (ideally between 12 and 15 years of age) to avoid possible surgery or cosmetic deformity. The nurse can also inform the family that the evaluation does not involve any painful or lengthy procedures but includes a thorough history and complete physical examination and roentgenographs of the spine and chest. Families who hesitate to initiate diagnostic evaluation or treatment measures because of their costs may be reassured that finances from crippled children's services (as part of local social services or health departments) may be available.

The nurse may be involved in collecting the history data and accompanying the teenager during the physical examination. Pertinent history includes the child's age, the age at which deformity was first noticed or suspected, and the parents' and youth's impression of the curve's progression since it was first noticed. Age at onset of sexual development, a history of dental development, rate of growth through infancy and childhood, and any subjective complaints (e.g., fatigue, pain) should also be documented for the orthopedist's evaluation. The nurse involved in initial

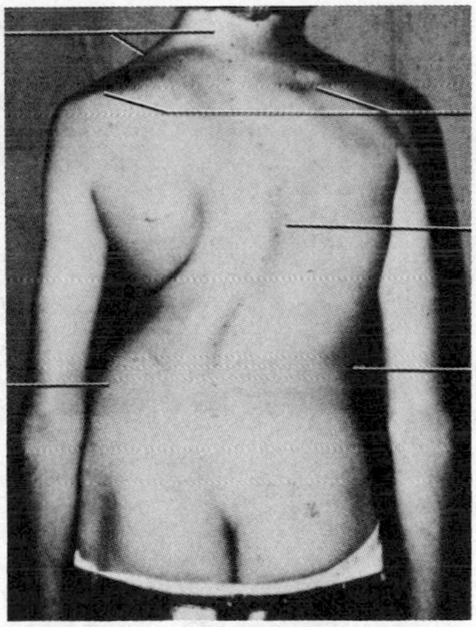

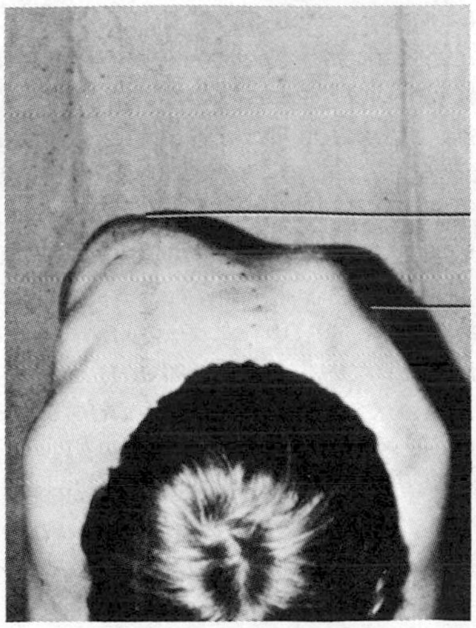

Screening of youth 9–15 promotes early detection of scoliosis. Adequate screening requires complete exposure of back, chest and hips.

Observe child from front while he or she is standing erect, assessing for:
- Shoulder asymmetry (shoulder elevated on convex side of scoliotic curve).
- Anterior rib asymmetry.
- Breast asymmetry (one breast may appear higher, larger or more protruding than the other).
- Hip asymmetry (one hip may protrude).

Observe youth from side and back while standing erect, assessing for:
- Shoulder asymmetry.
- Scapular asymmetry (scapula on convex side of curve higher).
- Rib cage asymmetry (rib cage prominent on convex side of curve).
- Waist asymmetry (waist fuller, more creased on convex side of curve).
- Hip asymmetry.
- Drop a plumb line (tape measure) from occiput to check for trunk malalignment—indicated when plumb line does not pass through gluteal fold. (If line passes through gluteal folds but curves are visible, compensation is indicated.)
- Malalignment of spinous processes. (Mark each process with a marker pen. Line formed is not straight in malalignment).

Observe youth from back while bending over, feet together until back is parallel to floor and arms dangling freely (forward bending test), assessing for:
- Thorax asymmetry (posterior rib hump may appear on convex side of curve).
- Hip asymmetry.

Run measuring tape from anterior superior iliac spine to medial malliolar at ankle, assessing for:
- Asymmetry in leg length.

Figure 47-29. Screening procedure for scoliosis.

screening or the nurse working with the orthopedist often becomes the liaison among the teen, family, orthopedist, and many other team members, ensuring that follow-up of screening and diagnostic recommendations occurs.

Roentgenographs of the anteroposterior and lateral views of the spine are required to determine whether the curvature is structural or functional and the extent of vertebral changes and rotation, as well as to estimate the correctability of the deformity.

Therapeutic Management

Treatment of scoliosis is a long, tedious process that requires a great deal of cooperation from the teen and parents to perform the treatment regimen consistently and to keep follow-up appointments. Both of these are essential to successful correction of the scoliotic deformity. The nurse has a critical role in motivating the family to seek medical advice and to practice treatment measures and in supporting them through the years required for correctional therapy.

Two modes of treatment have been successful in correcting scoliosis: bracing and spinal fusion. Each requires adherence to a daily exercise program if maximal success is to be achieved. This program can be supplemented by activities of interest to adolescents (swimming, weightlifting, dancing, track) that strengthen back, shoulder, and abdominal muscles. It cannot be overemphasized that an exercise program alone has been shown by data from years of research to be ineffective in stopping or correcting scoliotic progression.

Electrospinal orthosis is an alternate method of therapy being used in some treatment centers. Electrodes are applied to the skin at the apex of the curvature. They are operated from a battery pack and send low-voltage electrical stimulation to the paraspinal muscles. The device is used only at night, thus avoiding the inconvenience of bracing (Bunnell, 1986).

Major Nursing Diagnoses for Nonsurgical Management of Scoliosis

Impaired physical mobility, *related to abnormal curvature of the spine*
Knowledge deficit, *related to nonsurgical management of scoliosis*
Disturbance in self-concept: body image, self-esteem, personal identity, *related to:*

- *asymmetric body contour*
- *alterations in posture associated with abnormal spinal curvature*
- *the attention called to bulky braces or casts worn for corrective purposes*
- *concern for limitation of breast development within a Milwaukee brace or body cast*
- *concern for physical/sexual attractiveness during lengthy treatment period superimposed upon the adolescent task of developing heterosexual relationships*

Ineffective family coping: compromised, *related to guilt and concern associated with diagnosis and treatment for scoliosis*

Strategies for Nursing Care Related to Nonsurgical Management

The nonsurgical treatments employed to treat scoliosis include the Milwaukee brace, the Orthoplast jacket, and various casting and traction methods (mostly used preoperatively to improve spinal flexion or postoperatively to maintain alignment during fusional correction, or at both times). Table 47-10 describes each of these methods, including when each is indicated, potential problems, and general nursing care required. Figure 47-30 shows a Milwaukee brace, Figure 47-31 an Orthoplast jacket, Figure 47-32 the Turnbuckle cast, and Figure 47-33 a localizer cast.

Teaching to Support Home Management of Scoliosis Therapy. Before the selected form of nonsurgical intervention is begun, parents and the teen need indepth preparation to maintain correct management at home and to understand the importance of their long-term compliance with the regimen. Anderson (1979) outlines a basic teaching program for parents and children in terms of behavioral objectives. Teaching, of course, must be tailored to the individual

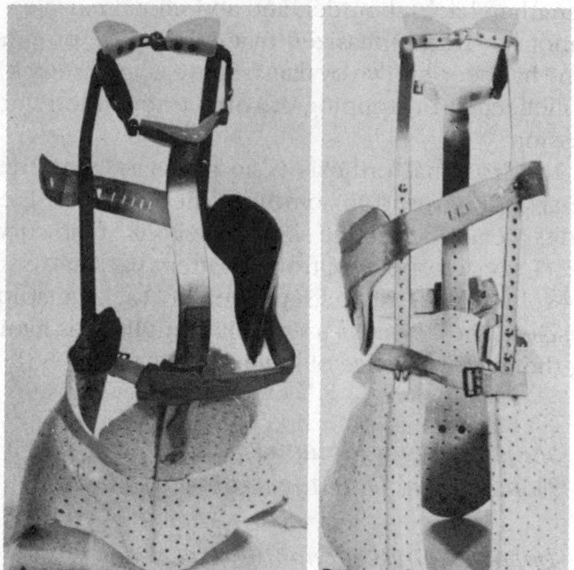

Figure 47-30. Milwaukee brace; *(A)* front and *(B)* back views. (From Tachdjian M: *Pediatric Orthopedics.* Philadelphia, WB Saunders, 1972, p 1210.)

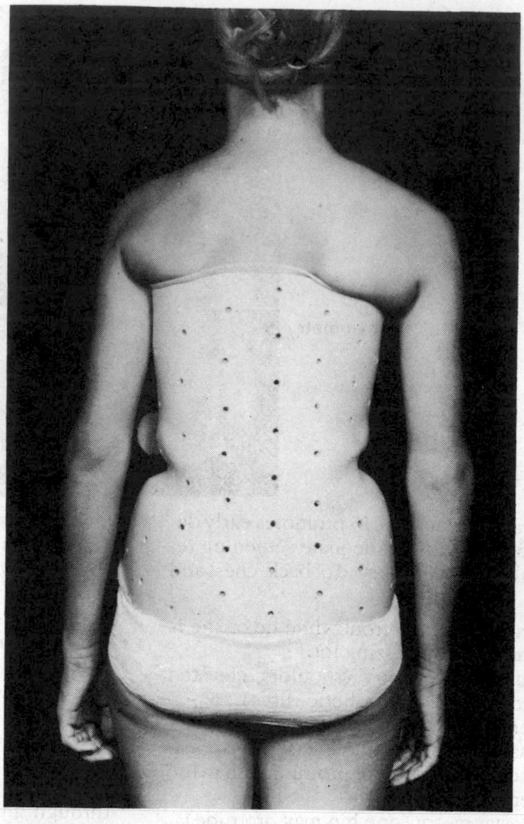

Figure 47-31. Orthoplast jacket. (From Hungerford D: Spinal deformity in adolescence. *Med Clin North Am* 1975 Nov.)

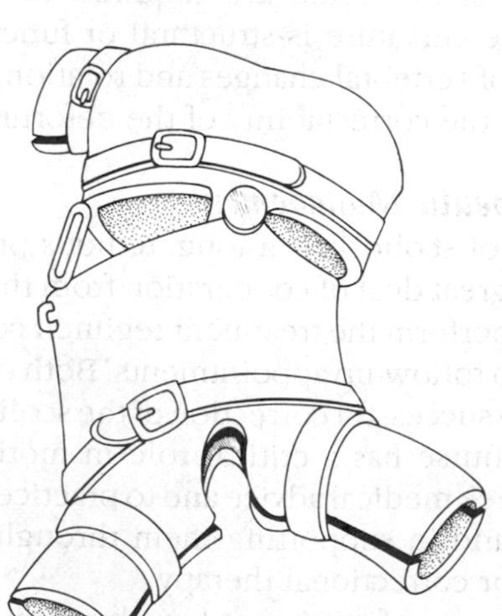

Figure 47-32. Turnbuckle cast.

Table 47-10. Nonsurgical Management of Scoliosis

Therapeutic Management	Indications	Related Nursing Strategies
Observation		
Frequent measuring of curves and roentgenographic evaluation to monitor improvement, stabilization or progression of curves	Mild curves of less than 20°	Emphasize that further intervention will be required if curve progresses and that cardiopulmonary compromise may occur
Usually an exercise program also prescribed		Emphasize that checkups every 3 months are essential to effectively monitor status of curve
		Teach exercise program or refer to physical therapy for such instruction
EXTERNAL BRACING		
Milwaukee brace		
A combination of straps, pads, and metal struts are used to straighten the spine and hold it in position	Curve of 20°–40° in skeletally immature spine	Instruct and demonstrate and require return demonstration of the following: • Brace application and removal (imperative to prevent skin breakdown) • Brace maintenance and cleaning • Exercises
Brace may be removed for 1 hour for personal hygiene; the brace is worn continuously otherwise	Sometimes indicated in greater than 40° curve if patient a poor surgical risk	
May have daily exercises prescribed additionally		
The patient is gradually weaned from the brace over a 1–2 year period when spinal maturity is nearly complete		Instruct in proper skin care: • Daily bathing • Undershirt under brace to absorb perspiration and protect skin from brace • Tincture of benzoin, moist tea bags (tannic acid), or alcohol daubed on skin areas where brace rubs or creates pressure to toughen skin and decrease skin breakdown • Wear underpants over brace for easier toileting
Low profile (Pasadena) brace is available, which is similar to Milwaukee brace but does not require neck ring		Endorse all activity except horseback riding, driving and contact sports
		Work in collaboration with school personnel and school nurse to coordinate adjustments of school program
		Counseling • Frequent follow-up evaluations imperative • Psychological adjustments to brace and altered body image
Orthoplast jacket		
Plastic jacket similar to Milwaukee brace but less aesthetically distracting	Same as for Milwaukee brace	Same as for Milwaukee brace
Costs considerably less than Milwaukee brace		
CASTING		
Turnbuckle		
Full body cast with wedges cut over convexity of curve; adjusted periodically to cause progressive, gradual curve correction	Seldom used today Rigid curves	Teach cast care Assure patient the cast will not alter breast development
Involves lengthy hospitalization and immobilization		See the section on hazards of immobility in this chater
Localizer cast (Risser)		
Full body cast that immobilizes the spine in alignment	Preoperatively to stretch curve and tissues During surgery to maintain alignment Postoperatively to maintain correction until healing is progressed	Same as for turnbuckle cast

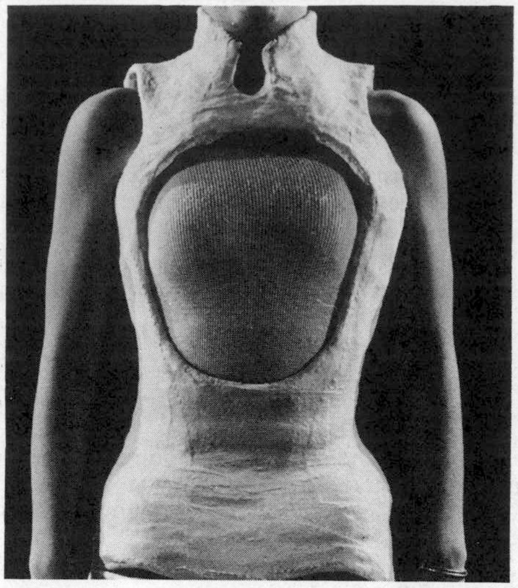

Figure 47-33. Localizer cast. (From Rothman R, Simeone F: *The Spine.* Philadelphia, WB Saunders, 1975, p 376)

situation, but the following guidelines can help the nurse plan the topics to be covered:

1. Normal anatomy of spine; terminology involved
2. Causes of spinal deformities
3. Causal factors in specific person involved, when known
4. Various approaches to nonsurgical management (observation, exercise, casting, bracing, traction)
5. Reasons that specific management program was selected for that person
6. Course of management program to be expected
   a. Sequence of events
   b. Anticipated outcome
   c. Frequency of check-ups
   d. Purpose of procedures during management (measurements, roentgenographs, sequential photography)
7. Self-care activities
   a. Application of brace (or other device)
   b. Skin care
   c. Appliance care and cleaning
   d. Clothing selection
   e. Exercise and maintenance of activities
8. Potential problems (e.g., advancement in curve, pressure sores)
   a. How to recognize
   b. How to prevent
9. Psychosocial impact of management program
   a. Self-image of adolescent undergoing treatment
   b. Peer acceptance
   c. Fears, anxieties, need for control
   d. Concerns about normal adolescent sexual development
10. Responsibilities of parents during child's treatment program
    a. Care activities
    b. Psychologic support of adolescent
    c. Financial responsibilities

As with all other procedures, the youth needs thorough explanations of what is involved in brace or cast application, what sensations can be experienced, what can be done to assist, and the rationale for wearing the appliance or cast. Before casting is done, the nurse should discuss the sensations that will be experienced in being balanced prone on straps in midair and of having a body stockinette covering one's body from head to toe. (Most patients complain of a suffocating feeling.) Reassurance that the nurse will be with the youth throughout the procedure and that a parent or best friend may be present, if this is preferred, provides some security.

Promoting a Healthy Self-Image. These nonsurgical techniques attack three major areas in which the adolescent may be vulnerable: self-image, developing sexuality, and peer acceptance. The adverse cosmetic effect of the brace or cast can be extremely threatening to the sensitive self-image of the adolescent. The teen must learn how to handle the reactions and curiosity of other people and at the same time to incorporate the brace or cast into his or her self-image. The school nurse can be invaluable as a listener during the early adjustment period; a phone call or invitation to stop by the health center every few days is greatly appreciated by most teens during the first days back in school. The teen and family members should be encouraged to handle public and peer curiosity with honest confrontation ("I see you are curious about my brace. Would you like me to tell you about it?")

A part of the teenage girl's self-identity is the development of a sense of femininity and sexuality. That the brace or cast hides the developing feminine figure is a source of anxiety to the adolescent. She fears that boys will find her unattractive, that the appliance will hinder breast development, and that with the brace she cannot compete with her female peers in attractiveness. Reassurance should be offered that breast development is in no way diminished by the appliance. Attention and hugs received from male relatives and family friends often provide the reassurance the girl needs to retain her sense of feminine attractiveness. During evaluation examinations, or during casting, the nurse should make every effort to preserve the teen's privacy, because being observed in her underwear does not hold the same meaning for the teen that being observed at the beach in a bikini does.

Nonsurgical techniques also impinge on the teen's feelings of peer acceptance. The brace or cast makes it difficult for her to wear the halters, bikinis, and filmy fabrics so popular among teens and so important to "being one of the crowd." The appliance represents visible evidence that she is different from her peers at a time in her development when it is important to conform to peer norms and standards; including those of appearance.

Facing school and peer reactions the first day is one of the hardest tasks the girl with scoliosis must confront. Her adjustment can be eased tremendously when the school nurse has prepared the teacher(s) and classmates ahead of time for her return. The nurse may plan with the girl to teach her peers about scoliosis and her treatment and to answer their questions on her first or second day back with the assistance and presence of the school nurse. This has been cited by many scoliotic youths as the most helpful activity in their adjustment back into school and their peer group. Teen activities such as camp or slumber parties also help to desensitize the girl to her brace or cast.

Nonsurgical techniques may also be perceived by the teen or her parents to place constraints on her independence and social life. Most teens are surprised and reassured to learn that they may participate in any activity they choose except for aggressive contact sports (sometimes horseback riding and skiing are also excluded). However, even with this knowledge the teen must still deal with the fact that the brace or cast must be worn for several years and with the problems of fatigue and overheating induced by the appliance. The nurse should help ensure that the teen has some say, whenever possible, in her treatment, and that an effort is made to show the girl at each evaluation the progress being made as a result of the treatment (compare roentgenographs from one visit to the next, or take postural photographs at each visit to compare). Reassurances about not needing surgery should not be made at any time, however, as surgery always remains a possibility.

Many teens wearing a brace have found that for study at home an adjustable drafting table relieves some of the muscle tension created by sitting and that a beanbag chair is the most comfortable for reading, resting, or watching television. Avoiding carrying anything heavy or bulky and avoiding carrying things for long periods of time helps reduce fatigue. Overheating, the result of having little skin surface exposed to the air, is a real problem even in cool weather. Talcum powder and an undershirt help absorb the moisture. Frequent application of body deodorant and a midday change of perspiration-saturated clothing helps to maintain a sense of freshness. The importance of a daily shower or bath is obvious.

As with any other health problem that persists over time, the most effective support system is contact with others who have the same problem. The nurse should be able to find or organize a support group for newly diagnosed adolescents with scoliosis and their parents.

Helping to Allay Parental Guilt and Concern. Parents will need reassurance to relieve the guilt feelings they experience when their child is diagnosed as having scoliosis, especially when they discover the genetic etiology of this condition. Overcoming these guilt feelings is important to their ongoing participation in management of the teen's condition and to the prevention of an overprotective response. They need reassurance that they will eventually be able to look at their teen without noticing the brace or cast that causes feelings of surprise and sorrow, and that the need to protect their child from the sometimes tactless public will pass. Whether parental counseling takes place with the adolescent present or separately, parents need to be taught as much information about intervention effectiveness as does the teen. They also need the listening ear of the nurse and an opportunity to be supported by other parents who have been through or are currently going through the same experience. Assistance and referral should be offered to help offset the costs of equipment and its upkeep and of follow-up evaluations, special furniture, and the clothing that wears out so fast because of the appliance.

Strategies for Nursing Care Related to Surgical Management

The most commonly used surgical management is now a one-stage spinal fusion (arthrodesis) procedure. (Table 47-11 contains a description of surgical interventions.) The procedure is done under general anesthesia and usually involves about 1 week of hospitalization, after which the teen is discharged, sometimes in a localizer cast (Risser). When the fusion is supported by Harrington rods, the patient is ambulatory shortly after casting. The cast, if used, is applied either at the end of the surgical procedure or several days postoperatively. It is changed 3 months after surgery so that roentgenographs can be taken to assess early fusion and maintenance of correction. The cast is worn for another 6 to 9 months before being removed permanently. Follow-up evaluations are necessary every 3 to 6 months for 3 to 5 more years to ensure maintenance of correction. Restrictions on horseback riding, skiing, and skating activities are necessary until the cast is removed; restriction on heavy-contact sports continues until follow-up is no longer necessary (3 to 5 years later).

Spinal fusion may be done alone or in conjunction with either Harrington or Dwyer instrumentation or the use of Luque wires (Table 47-11). The Stryker frame may be used for the patient with Harrington instrumentation. The teen should be given an explana-

Table 47-11. Surgical Management of Scoliosis

Therapeutic Management	Indications
Spinal Fusion (Arthrodesis) One-stage procedure. The paraspinal muscles are stripped from the lamina of the vertebrae to be fused. The vertebrae are fused and a bone graft (usually autogenous from one iliac crest), which is broken into matchstick pieces, is placed along one entire fusion area to promote bone formation	Curve progression despite bracing or casting. Many paralytic and some congenital curves do this. Thoracic scoliosis with associated lordosis seldom responds to bracing Physiologic cardiopulmonary compromise Progressive pain and fatigue despite nonsurgical measures Must be done prior to skeletal maturity for maximum correction Lumbar scoliosis of 30 degrees with associated lordosis often causes such imbalance that surgery is indicated
Harrington Rod Instrumentation Posterior approach by which a series of rods and hooks are implanted on the concave side of curve to apply traction and/or on the convex side of curve to apply compression to the posterior spinal elements	Harrington factor of 5+ (obtained by dividing number of vertebrae involved in the curve into the degree of the curve) and spinal fusion indications
Dwyer Instrumentation Anterior approach by which spine is exposed from the front and bolts are inserted transversely through each vertebral body. The bolts are attached to a cable that is applied to the convexity of the curve. The intervertebral discs between adjacent vertebrae are removed and the vertebrae are pulled together	Same as for Harrington procedure; adds stability
Luque Wires Posterior approach in which thin, flexible wires are threaded around vertebrae and secured to flexible rods resting on the transverse processes. Provides transverse traction on each vertebrae	Same as for Harrington procedure; adds stability

tion of the frame and a chance to practice manipulating it before surgery. Immobilization in bed is required after the Dwyer procedure.

In addition to preoperative teaching begun 2 days before surgery that prepares the youth for what to expect during and after the operation, the patient should be given a chance before surgery to practice voiding in a supine position and to eat horizontally. If casting will not be done until several days postoperatively, "logrolling" should be explained and practiced. Honest, open communication should be maintained between the teaching nurse and the teen throughout the preoperative period to ensure that the youth's anxieties and questions are dealt with. The youth should be informed that the surgery involves an incision from T1 to the sacrum at midline. In understandable terms, the teen should receive a description of the procedure and be told when the cast will be applied and how it is done.

Teaching regarding the postoperative period should emphasize the teen's participation in recovery. Box 47-3 outlines the typical postoperative period and can be used as a guide to prepare the teen and parents for what to expect. Psychologic care during the postoperative period is extremely important. The teen will experience periods of depression and withdrawal. Diversions in which the teen's specific interests are involved are extremely helpful during this time, as are visits from peers, family, and other teens with scoliosis.

After discharge the family takes the responsibility of helping the teen do things she cannot do for herself. They should be provided with a resource person whom they may consult 24 hours a day. Periodic home visits from a community health nurse are supportive to the family and facilitate evaluation by the health team as to the adequacy of management and compliance at home. The school nurse should become involved in assisting the teen to adjust to return to school.

Nursing Strategies for Follow-up Care in the Home or Clinic

Assess for complications of surgery and casting: neurovascular impairment, infection, altered skin integrity.

Assess psychologic adjustment to the bulky cast and allow ample time for the adolescent to ventilate feelings about necessary alterations in clothing and activities. Compliment the youth's appearance when it can be done sincerely.

Collaborate with the school nurse to insure optimal support from health care professionals during the postoperative period of casting.

Determine the adolescent's and family's understanding of assessment of neurovascular status, and the need for frequent follow-up until the cast is removed and 2 to 4 times per year after cast removal to assure stability of the fusion.

Box 47-3
Postoperative Nursing Strategies Following Spinal Fusion

First 24–48 hours

Sometimes patient stays in ICU until stable.

Monitoring of vital signs, circulation and neurologic status of extremities every 1–2 hours, more often if indicated.*

Cough and deep breathe, IPPB, or spirometer every hour for several days, frequency gradually decreased depending on pulmonary function test results.*

Catheterization if no voiding by 12 hours postop.

IV fluids and antibiotics; monitor I & O.

Patient kept NPO with nasogastric tube until peristalsis resumes (usually 2–4 days).

Large frequent doses of narcotic given to relieve bone pain and muscle tension in spine.

Patient may have assisted ventilation, especially if preop pulmonary function tests were 30% or less of expected function.

Meticulous skin care and hygiene practiced.*

Chest tubes, Hemovacs used to facilitate drainage from chest and graft site.

Cardiac and central venous monitoring done.

Patient turned every 2 hours (rolled pillow support to supine/side-lying positions; firm, flat bed.)*

By the 2nd–3rd day

Turning every 1–2 hours continued.

Nasogastric tube and Foley catheter removed.

Diet high in protein, vitamin C, thiamine, iron, and bulk; low in calories.*

Daily bowel evacuation of feces and flatus. (Suppositories, laxatives, and diet may facilitate.)

Push fluids to maintain hydration and prevent renal calculi; monitoring of intake and output continues; IV may be stopped.

Encourage diversional activities; prism glasses allow reading and TV watching, long tongs help adolescent feel independent in reaching bedside items.*

Fitted for brace, if applicable.

Teaching begun for family about cast care and other skills required for home care.

By the 4th day

Begin ambulation.

May have hair washed.

Usually on oral pain medications.

By 5th–6th day postop

Assumes activities of daily living as feasible.

Has progressive ambulation; discharge when patient can walk and climb stairs independently.

---

* Intervention continued from time initiated throughout hospitalization.

Osteochondroses

The osteochondroses are a group of self-limiting disorders that involve the epiphyses of the growing child or adolescent. The conditions involve an avascular necrosis of the epiphysis. The cause of the interruption of blood supply is unknown, but the results are a softening and absorption of the bone. The articular cartilage surrounding the bone remains intact. Over a period of time, revascularization occurs and new bone forms.

Legg-Perthes Disease

Legg-Perthes disease, Legg-Calvé-Perthes disease, coxa plana, and Perthes disease are all synonyms for osteochondrosis of the femoral head. The condition is four times more common in boys than in girls, with the usual onset between 4 and 8 years of age (Gartland, 1979).

Pathophysiology

The disease process is self-limiting; three stages occur over a 12- to 36-month period. Stage 1 is aseptic necrosis, with radiopacity of the epiphysis. Stage 2 is revascularization; the epiphysis is mottled and fragmented. Reossification with gradual reformation of the femoral head is stage 3.

Diagnostic Assessment

The usual method of confirming the diagnosis is the visualization of the aforementioned changes on roentgenograph (see Figure 47-34). Occasionally, a bone scan may be used to differentiate Legg-Perthes disease from toxic synovitis of the hip, septic hip joint, or osteomyelitis. Without treatment, the femoral head will flatten and deform permanently.

The nurse's early identification of affected children will aid in treatment, although it will not necessarily ensure a better prognosis. The disease process has usually reached the second stage before signs and symptoms become apparent. These children may be limping on the affected leg. They have pain in the groin that may be referred to the thigh or knee. Pain increases with activity and decreases with rest. Inspection of the affected leg may show atrophy of the buttock or thigh muscles and a decrease in range of motion.

Therapeutic Management

The goal of treatment for Legg-Perthes disease is to prevent deformity of the femoral head from the stress of weight bearing. Treatment plans include methods to keep the femoral head within the joint capsule so that the normal configuration of the femoral head will

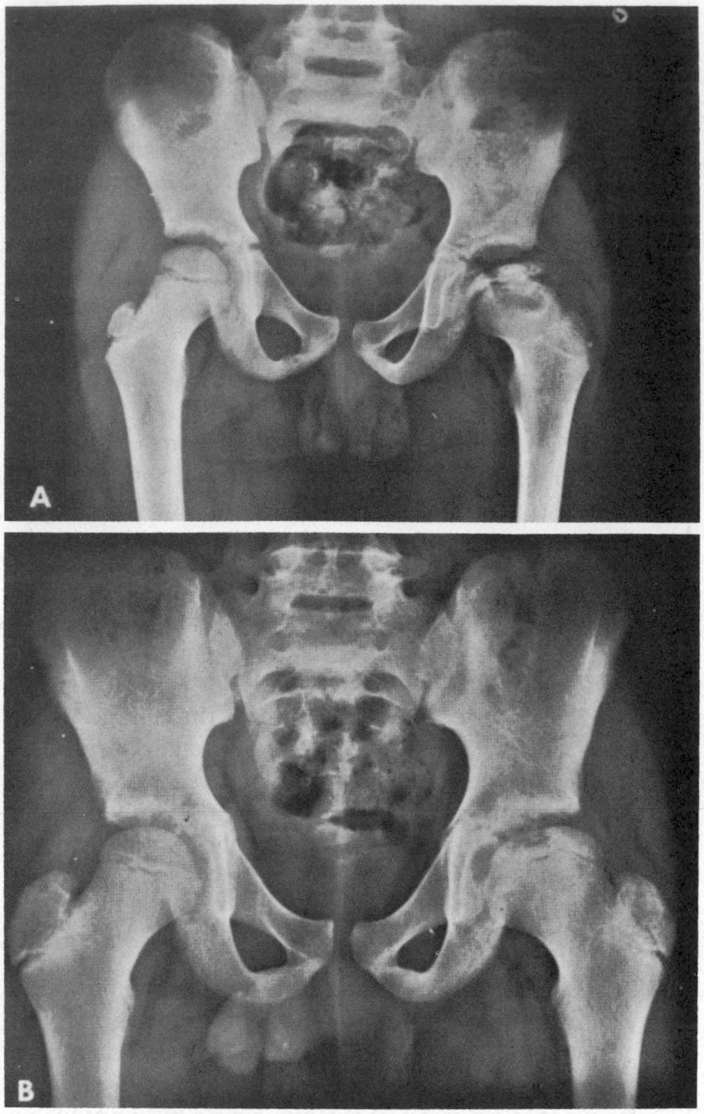

Figure 47-34. *A*, Legg-Perthes disease of left hip. Capital femoral epiphysis is undergoing necrosis and fragmentation. *B*, Same hip, 5 years later, showing residual flattening of femoral head. (From Gartland JH: *Fundamentals of Orthopaedics.* 4th ed. Philadelphia, WB Saunders, 1986.)

be retained as it regenerates. Complete bed rest with Buck or Russell traction for lengthy periods of time was historically the treatment of choice. This method obviously puts an inordinate amount of stress on the child and family. Most physicians now recommend a period of bed rest and traction in abduction to reduce pain and regain range of motion. The child will be hospitalized for this period of time, then will be fitted with a non–weight bearing brace device or harness that prevents weight bearing on the affected side (Fig. 47-35). The child must use crutches, but mobility is greatly increased. Some physicians do not believe that weight bearing is detrimental as long as the femoral head remains in the acetabulum; they suggest use of long leg casts with an abduction bar (Larson and Gould, 1978; Watts, 1987). Atrophy of the extremity is prevented with non–weight-bearing exercises. Surgery may also be used to maintain the femoral head within the acetabulum.

Major Nursing Diagnoses for Legg-Perthes Disease

Impaired physical mobility, related to decreased perfusion to the femoral head
Potential for injury:

- ***deformation of the femoral head,*** *related to weight bearing during the period of avascularization and softening*
- ***neurovascular impairment,*** *related to:*
  1. *Improper alignment of traction*
  2. *Pressure exerted by the non–weight-bearing brace over a peripheral nerve*
  3. *Crutch paralysis associated with prolonged pressure on the nerves in the axilla by improperly fitted or improperly used crutches*
- ***falls,*** *related to ambulation with a non–weight-bearing brace and crutches*

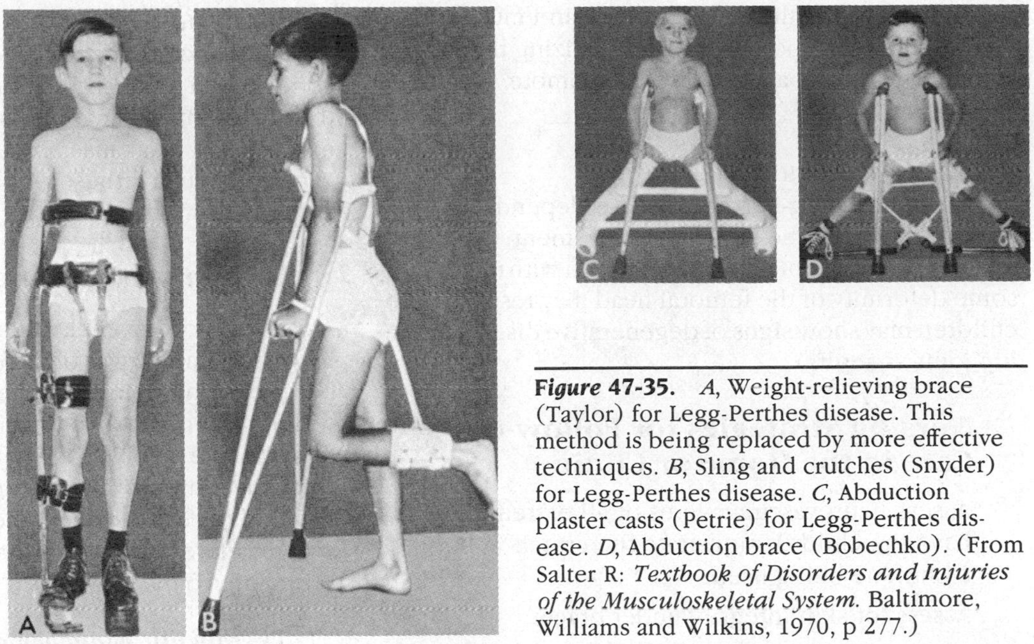

Figure 47-35. *A,* Weight-relieving brace (Taylor) for Legg-Perthes disease. This method is being replaced by more effective techniques. *B,* Sling and crutches (Snyder) for Legg-Perthes disease. *C,* Abduction plaster casts (Petrie) for Legg-Perthes disease. *D,* Abduction brace (Bobechko). (From Salter R: *Textbook of Disorders and Injuries of the Musculoskeletal System.* Baltimore, Williams and Wilkins, 1970, p 277.)

Potential for alteration in skin integrity, *related to:*

- *Buck or Russell traction (both skin traction)*
- *impaired mobility during traction*
- *friction between the brace and the skin*

Disturbance in self-concept: body image, self-esteem, *related to imposed physical restrictions at a time when physical agility is very important to peer relationships*

Knowledge deficit, *related to:*

- *anatomy of femoral head and the disease process*
- *assessment for neurovascular impairment associated with traction, brace, crutches*
- *reason why the child must not bear weight on the affected extremity (if that is the case)*
- *non-weight-bearing exercises to prevent muscular atrophy of the affected leg*
- *need to alter the home environment to prevent falls*
- *need for follow-up until the condition has resolved*

Strategies for Nursing Care

Preventing Injury and Complications. Neurovascular assessment will be important during therapy with traction and throughout the course of treatment (see Tables 47-3 and 47-4). Skin care is equally important and includes reducing friction between the skin and traction equipment, cast, or brace. The child should have an opportunity to become comfortable with crutch walking before leaving the hospital. It is important that the client understand that the palms of the hands, not the axillae, are to support the body weight. Falls during crutch walking are of concern both within the hospital and at home. Making the home environment safe may include removing loose rugs and rearranging furniture to allow for the space required to ambulate with the brace and crutches. The major responsibility for preventing falls rests upon the affected child. It is important to look at where the crutches and unaffected foot are landing, and to avoid daredevil activities.

Promoting a Healthy Self-Concept. Liaison with the school nurse can facilitate the child's return to school. The school nurse can help to prepare the child's teacher(s) and classmates and can be an important source of support during the treatment period. It is important that the child continues with as many of the usual activities as possible, despite the limitations in mobility. For example, rather than just leaving the softball team, perhaps the child can help the coach with scorekeeping. Continued contact with peers will help the child achieve age-appropriate developmental tasks.

Teaching to Promote Care in the Home. Whereas the initial period after diagnosis is likely to be spent in the hospital in traction, the majority of the treatment will occur after discharge with prolonged bracing or casting. It is important, therefore, that the child and family understand the rationale for treatment, correct use of a prescribed brace, how to assess for and prevent neurovascular injury and muscular atrophy, and the importance of normalizing the child's activities as much as possible to promote a positive self-image.

Long-Term Outcome

Prognosis for Legg-Perthes disease depends entirely on the severity of the femoral involvement, the age of onset, and treatment compliance. Even with treatment, some deformity of the femoral head may result. These children may show signs of degenerative disease of the hip joint as adults.

Nursing Strategies for Follow-up Care in the Home or Clinic

Assess neurovascular status of all extremities; have the child demonstrate the crutch-walking technique being used.

Assess for skin integrity under brace.

Assess level of comfort in affected hip (increased pain might signal a relapse).

Have the child demonstrate the non–weight-bearing exercise routine being used at home.

Assess muscle bulk and strength on the affected side.

Encourage the child to talk about home and school activities and assess the adjustment to the brace and crutches.

Collaborate with the school nurse to assure optimal support for the child from health care professionals.

Osgood-Schlatter Disease

Traditionally thought of as an osteochondrosis, this affliction results in pain and swelling in the area of the tibial tubercle, just below the knee. Again the etiology is not clear, although it is more common in adolescent males engaged in athletics (Smith, 1977). If this is truly an osteochondrosis, then disruption of the blood supply to the tibial tuberosity and subsequent fragmentation will occur. Repetitive stress of the tibial tuberosity by a tight quadriceps muscle may contribute to the problem.

Therapeutic Management

Osgood-Schlatter Disease usually responds well to rest. Mild cases may only require activity restriction, particularly kneeling, running, stair climbing, and bicycle riding. More severe cases may require immobilization in long-leg cylinder casts for a period of weeks. Activity is gradually resumed. The problem ceases when growth stops. The only permanent impairment may be an enlargement of the tibial tuberosity.

Strategies for Nursing Care

Since Osgood-Schlatter disease is a fairly common condition in adolescents, nurses need to be aware of the symptomatology. Even though this problem is a mild one, it can cause some great distress to adolescents, particularly those who are athletic and for whom athletics is an important part of his or her self-esteem.

Scheuermann Disease

A cause of adolescent kyphosis, Scheuermann disease is an osteochondrosis of the epiphyses of the vertebral bodies of the spine. As the epiphyses soften, body weight will cause an anterior wedging and some flattening of the involved vertebrae. If wedging occurs to a sufficient number of vertebral bodies, kyphosis will develop. Scheuermann disease is most commonly seen in adolescent girls between 12 and 16 years of age (Hilt and Cogburn, 1980).

Therapeutic Management

Usual treatment is immobilization with a brace or cast to allow for revascularization and healing. A Milwaukee brace is commonly used. Immobilization may be required for a year or longer.

Strategies for Nursing Care

The adolescent with Scheuermann disease faces the same problems and frustrations as those with scoliosis. Compliance with treatment is an important determinant of outcome.

Inflammatory/Infectious Problems of the Skeleton

Toxic Synovitis of the Hip

Toxic or transient synovitis of the hip is a very common disorder in children. It occurs between 2 and 12 years of age and is more common in males (Lovell and Winter, 1978). The child experiences pain, either in the hip or knee, and will limp. Very young children may suddenly refuse to walk. The child may hold the hip in a position of flexion. Upon examination, there is a limitation of hip motion and the child may have a low-grade fever.

Pathophysiology

The inflammation of the synovial membrane is nonsuppurative and self-limiting. There is frequently a history of recent upper respiratory illness in children presenting with toxic synovitis although the association between the two events is not clearly understood. There may be a slight rise in the erythrocyte sedimentation rate.

Diagnostic Assessment

Since toxic synovitis is a self-limiting disorder, the most important aspect of diagnosis is to distinguish it from more severe problems, particularly Legg-Perthes disease and septic arthritis of the hip. Roentgenographs of the hip are normal. Aspiration of the hip joint may be done to rule out septic arthritis of the hip. Occasionally, in severe cases, a bone scan may be used as an aid to differential diagnosis.

Therapeutic Management

Resting the hip is the only treatment needed. Symptoms usually resolve within two weeks. Children with severe pain may benefit from Buck or Russell traction to overcome muscle spasm. The incidence of Legg-Perthes disease is higher in children with a history of toxic synovitis. This could represent a relationship between the two conditions or a failure to identify early symptoms of Legg-Perthes. For this reason, these children are often followed for several months after resolution of the symptoms.

Strategies for Nursing Care

Most cases of toxic synovitis are treated at home, with a few children hospitalized for treatment and observation. The entire purpose of traction in this situation is to relieve spasm and increase range of motion, and its effectiveness and length of application should be evaluated in this light. Nonadherent skin traction requires frequent rewrapping to avoid discomfort and constriction. The general guidelines for caring for a child in traction should be followed. Analgesics may be administered to decrease pain. The child and family need reassurance of the transitory nature of the problem.

Osteomyelitis

Osteomyelitis is a rapidly developing bacterial infection of the bone and its marrow. The metaphyseal area of the long bones in the legs and arms is affected. The disease commonly occurs in rapidly growing children, with males affected 2.5 times more than females (Syriopoulou and Smith, 1987).

Etiology and Pathophysiology

Osteomyelitis is a localization of infectious organisms that proliferate from either an endogenous or an exogenous source. Primary endogenous sources include skin and respiratory infections. Exogenous sources include trauma and surgical techniques. *Staphylococcus aureus* is the causative organism 80 to 90 per cent of the time. Inflammation with hyperemia and edema begins in the spongy tissue and marrow of the metaphyseal region of the bone. This causes an increase in intraosseous pressure and local pain, because the bone is unable to expand. Pus forms and interferes with circulation. Eventually there is thrombosis, leading to necrosis and bone death. The area of dead bone separates, forming a separate area called a sequestrum. The infection spreads via the bloodstream, causing septicemia. It also spreads laterally under the periosteum, causing abscess formation. If the epiphyseal plates remain intact there is no direct spread of the infection; however, the presence of septicemia may allow an infection to develop in another bone.

Prevention

Primary prevention includes eliminating factors that lower one's resistance to infection. Adequate nutrition, rest, and maintenance of skin integrity are important in avoiding infections. Health education programs should teach children how to stay healthy, as well as teaching basic first aid for skin cuts and abrasions. Appropriate treatment of all skin lesions and infections is essential in the prevention of osteomyelitis.

Clinical Manifestations

A sudden fever and local tenderness and pain are the first signs of osteomyelitis. The child hesitates or refuses to use the involved limb (more commonly the lower limb) because of severe pain (Syriopoulou and Smith, 1987). Upon examination the nurse may see evidence of a cutaneous infection or injury. Early treatment is imperative and any child with the symptoms described should receive immediate medical attention. School nurses should suspect osteomyelitis in any child with musculoskeletal complaints and pain.

Diagnostic Assessment

Diagnosis involves (1) obtaining a careful history of recent infections or local injuries or both; (2) clinical signs of fever, severe pain, and point tenderness at the end of a long bone; and (3) an elevated sedimentation rate, leukocytosis, and a positive blood culture.

Bone roentgenographs are not diagnostic, because bone destruction will not be evident until 10 to 21 days after the onset (Syriopoulou and Smith, 1987). Early osteomyelitis can be detected by bone scan.

Therapeutic Management

Signs of septicemia are usually apparent 24 hours after the onset of fever. The child is acutely ill and needs bed rest with analgesics. Blood cultures are drawn immediately and parenteral antibiotic therapy begun.

The usual course of treatment lasts 3 to 4 weeks. A nutritious, high-calorie diet facilitates bone healing.

If the child shows no signs of improvement within 24 hours, surgery is done to decrease pressure within the muscle compartment and allow drainage of the pus. Antibiotics may be instilled into the infected area during surgery. Surgical incision and drainage of the area followed by instillation of antibiotics may be repeated several times in the course of therapy. Management of this infection is complicated by the significantly reduced blood supply in the area of the infection, which decreases the blood-borne antibiotics that reach the site. Children with severe infection may have a continuous irrigation system placed to continue instillation of antibiotic postoperatively. After bone surgery, it is imperative that aseptic technique be followed during dressing changes. Wound irrigations, likewise, must be strictly aseptic to avoid the introduction of other organisms.

Major Nursing Diagnoses for Osteomyelitis

Impaired physical mobility, *related to an infectious process in the metaphysis of a long bone with resultant necrosis*

Potential for injury, *related to:*

- ***phlebitis,*** *associated with administration of intravenous antibiotics*
- ***neurovascular impairment,*** *associated with increased pressure within a muscle compartment resulting from edema and suppurative secretions*
- ***reinfection,*** *associated with improper handwashing (child, family, health care professionals), or break in sterile technique during dressing changes or irrigation procedures*
- ***hazards of immobility,*** *associated with bed rest*

Altered comfort: pain, *related to interosseous pressure associated with the infectious process*

Knowledge deficit, *related to:*

- *the disease process and treatment (including bed rest, intravenous antibiotics, and possible surgical incision and drainage)*
- *activity restrictions after discharge*
- *administration schedule and side effects of oral antibiotics to be continued at home*
- *home care of a central venous catheter for continued intravenous antibiotics (if applicable)*
- *ways to facilitate optimal perfusion to involved limb*
- *activity restrictions after discharge*
- *prevention of reinfection of this wound or osteomyelitis at another site*
- *nutrition to promote tissue healing (high-protein, high-calcium, high–vitamin C)*
- *need for follow-up care*

Strategies for Nursing Care

The major goals of nursing care are to prevent complications, relieve pain, and teach the child and family about the disease process and the treatment.

Preventing Complications. Parenteral antibiotic therapy is often required for weeks to completely eradicate the infection. After the acute episode is past, the most challenging nursing task will be the maintenance of intravenous infusion sites. Observation for phlebitis and infiltration should occur every few hours. Protecting sites will help preserve their use for a maximal 72 hours, so that the child is not subjected to intravenous insertion any more often than is absolutely necessary. Some of these children are candidates for outpatient intravenous therapy programs and this should be considered, if available, to decrease length of hospitalization.

Neurovascular impairment may occur from increased pressure within a muscle compartment as a result of edema and pus formation. The hazards of immobility associated with bed rest are also of concern, as is reinfection. Nursing vigilance is required in prevention. Specific strategies related to neurovascular assessment and the hazards of immobility are detailed in Tables 47-3 and 47-4, and on p. 1788. Reinfection is best prevented with attention to handwashing by *everyone* who comes in contact with the wound, and meticulous attention to sterile technique for dressing changes and other procedures.

Wound isolation techniques should be observed as well; that is, not only must the child be protected from pathogens, but also those coming in contact with wound secretions must be protected from the organism responsible for the osteomyelitis. Dressings should be put immediately into a bag for disposal, as should the sterile gloves used for the dressing change. Depending on the causative organism, a gown and mask may be required for dressing changes.

Relieving Pain

Pain is intense and children will be afraid to have anyone touch them or the bed. Before the child is moved for any reason, an explanation is given of what will be done and how the painful area will be protected. It is usually necessary to use two people, one to support the joints above and below the affected area, and one to move the child's body. Splints or traction are sometimes used to immobilize the extremity and promote comfort. Nursing assessment and intervention for pain is discussed further in Chapter 29.

Teaching to Enhance Care in the Home. The diagnosis may precipitate parental feelings of guilt for not having prevented the infection, and the nurse should be supportive in allowing the parents to verbalize these feelings. Taking time to explain the infection and the treatment regimen will help allay some anxiety.

Both the parents and child will need thorough instructions on activity restrictions after discharge. It is necessary to avoid falls and jerky movements; therefore, the child will need to continue with quiet play activities until the physician recommends otherwise. Siblings usually are happy to have their brother or sister home again with the hope that their lives may regain some normalcy; however, the child will not be able to share in household responsibilities for some time, and siblings may resent this. Therefore, they should be included in the discharge planning discussion and helped to view the situation realistically.

Long-Term Outcome

The prognosis for complete recovery is good if effective antibiotic treatment was initiated early. However, the possibility of chronic osteomyelitis exists and the child will need to be monitored closely by the physician. Fortunately, mortality rates from septicemia have decreased with the use of antibiotic therapy.

Nursing Strategies for Follow-up Care in the Home or Clinic

Assess the involved extremity for adequate perfusion, swelling, pain, and for motor and sensory function.

Assess (if applicable) the peripheral or central venous catheter for patency and signs of infection.

Assess for side effects of antibiotic therapy.

Obtain blood samples for culture as necessary.

Encourage the child and family to express feelings about the illness and its treatment. Determine adaptation status and make referrals for additional support as necessary.

Collaborate with the school nurse to assure optimal support for the child and family from health care professionals.

Reinforce the need for follow-up care.

Septic Arthritis (Septic Joint)

Septic arthritis in children begins as a blood-borne infection just as osteomyelitis does. A septic joint may in fact be an extension of a developing osteomyelitis. The most common joint involved is the hip, although it not uncommonly occurs in knees and elbows. The problem encountered with septic joints as compared with osteomyelitis is that the bacteria and purulent exudates will break down and destroy the articular cartilage, which is not capable of regeneration. A septic arthritis is considered a surgical emergency because permanent damage to the joint and life-long disability can occur within a very short time.

A child with septic arthritis has severe pain and will resist any attempt to move the joint. Elevation of temperature is significant, except in infants. The white blood count and erythrocyte sedimentation rate are elevated.

Diagnostic Assessment

Roentgenographs may show some joint swelling. As with osteomyelitis, a bone scan will show increased uptake of the radioisotope in the areas of infection. Aspiration of the joint is the main tool for confirming diagnosis. The joint fluid will contain pus, and culture will confirm the causative organism.

Therapeutic Management

If joint aspiration is positive, surgical opening and drainage of the joint is indicated immediately to prevent further damage. Continuous joint irrigation is often employed in infants and children with septic joints. Salicylates may be used to decrease inflammation.

Strategies for Nursing Care

Nursing care centers on patient comfort, maintaining intravenous access for the administration of antibiotics, and wound irrigation and care, all previously discussed. The ultimate outcome will depend on the extent of joint damage that has occurred.

Traumatic Injury to the Musculoskeletal System

Falls on playgrounds, pedestrian and bike accidents, and casualties of participation in sports all contribute to the high incidence of skeletal and muscle trauma in children. Children spend a great deal of time in activities that develop their musculoskeletal abilities. Their need to investigate and their lack of inhibition often lead to risk taking. It is impossible to protect a child from all injuries; to do so would severely limit the development of their potential.

Nursing Strategies for Prevention

Nurses can help prevent childhood injury by discussing with children and parents the importance of safety education. Every child should learn safety rules for home, school, and athletic activities. Parents are often unaware of the hazards of some of the usual childhood activities. Nursing strategies related to teaching safety are detailed in Chapter 17.

Nursing Strategies for Emergency Care

Any injured child should be thoroughly assessed by the nurse before being moved. Establishing an open airway is the first priority, and tilting of the head or artificial respiration may be needed. Bleeding must be controlled, which may necessitate applying direct pressure proximal to the fracture. Open wounds should be covered with a sterile dressing to help prevent infection. Pain and local hemorrhage from fracture may cause shock; pallor, tachycardia, and hypotension are its early signs. The child should be kept lying still and covered for warmth. Back or neck injuries are always a possibility, so the child should never be moved until it is determined that no injury exists. Before being examined, the child should be offered an explanation of what will be done. Talking to them usually helps children to relax; they can then be asked to give an account of what happened.

Pain that increases upon movement of the affected limb is the most obvious symptom of fracture. Other signs include swelling over the fracture site, ecchymosis, decreased mobility of the affected limb and deformity. (Deformity may be minimal with greenstick fractures.) In some children the thick periosteum will stabilize the fracture enough to allow weight bearing or limited use, so movement does not immediately rule out a fracture. The area distal to the fracture may feel cool, appear discolored, and have a decreased or absent pulse. These are signs of vascular impairment and indicate the need for careful splinting and immediate medical attention.

Suspicious musculoskeletal injuries should be treated as if fracture exists, until proved otherwise. Splinting is necessary to support the joints above and below the site and to prevent damage to vessels and tissues. The extremity must be immobilized before moving the victim. Commercially available standard splints consist of a padded board that is bandaged to the extremity; an air splint is zipped over the extremity and inflated by blowing air into the intake valve. In emergencies, improvised splints made with magazines, newspapers, boards, pillows, or the victim's own body can be utilized. Pillow splints can be used for fractures of the foot, ankle, tibia, or knee. For elbow or forearm fractures, instruct the child to cradle the arm close to the body or use a sling. (The reader may refer to the American Red Cross First Aid Manual for specifics on splinting.)

When immobilization is completed the child should be taken to the emergency department for treatment. Emergency rooms are noisy, frightening, and completely foreign to most children, and the parents or nurse should stay with the child for support. A history of the accident is important but often difficult or impossible to obtain from an apprehensive child. The nurse on duty should try to obtain a description of what happened from the person who transported the child. Roentgenographs of the involved part are needed before treatment. In children it is difficult to diagnose trauma to unossified bone and a roentgenograph of the opposing limb may be used for comparison. An undisplaced epiphyseal plate injury will not be evident on the roentgenograph; therefore, the physician should carefully assess the area for tenderness before eliminating the possibility of a fracture. Blood and urine tests will be needed if the child is in shock or has multiple injuries.

When children are struck by motor vehicles, the nurse needs to be alert for signs of Waddell triad: a combination of fractured femur, abdominal injury, and head injury. The child's femur is injured when struck by the bumper, abdominal injury is sustained from the fender, and head injury occurs when the child is thrown and lands on the skull.

Injuries to Muscles and Ligaments

Injuries to muscle and ligaments may be categorized as contusions, strains, or sprains. *Contusion* results from a direct blow and produces soft tissue hemorrhage into subcutaneous, adipose, and muscle tissue (Hilt and Cogburn, 1980). It will usually heal spontaneously, although the area may be quite painful.

A *strain* is an overuse injury to a muscle. The muscle body is overstretched, causing injury to the muscle tissue. It may cause acute pain or chronic soreness. Treatment consists of rest, cold application to control swelling, and later heat application to relieve soreness, increase circulation, and promote healing. When children have chronic strain, the degree of involvement in athletics should be examined.

Sprains are tears of ligaments or joint capsules. Ligamentous injury is uncommon in young children. Prior to the end of skeletal growth the weakest area of the musculoskeletal system is the epiphyses, and this area will give way first when stress is applied. Injury to ligaments is not a common problem until adolescence.

Sprains can be either incomplete or complete tears of ligaments, also called ruptures. Ligaments may be stripped from their attachment to the bone with an associated avulsion of a piece of bone. Ligamentous injury is often the result of a twisting or rotational stress having been applied to the joint. Sprains are characterized by pain, swelling, tenderness, and limitation of joint motion. Complete tears or ruptures may also result in joint effusion, hemarthrosis, or joint instability. Roentgenographs will be normal, except for soft tissue swelling, unless bone avulsion has occurred at an attachment site.

Treatment is based on the extent of the tear. All ligamentous injury can be treated with cold and elevation to control swelling. Most incomplete tears will respond to rest and support with bandaging or taping, and may occasionally require further immobilization with splint or cast. Complete tears require surgical repair in order to heal without excessive scar formation and to stabilize the joint.

Common Athletic Knee Injuries in Adolescents

Figure 47-36 illustrates the normal anatomy of the knee. The knee is vulnerable to excessive stress in many types of athletics; therefore, knee injuries are extremely commonplace in adolescents.

Ligament injuries can occur to the medial collateral and lateral collateral ligaments, often caused by a blow to the side of the knee. Injury to the anterior cruciate ligament may occur as a result of hyperextension of the knee. Treatment is based on the extent of ligamentous damage.

Injuries to the medial or lateral meniscus may occur from rotational stress to the knee. The patient may experience clicking or locking of the knee joint from a torn meniscus. Treatment depends on the extent of the tear and the symptoms and disability experienced by the patient. Partial or complete meniscectomy may be performed, either through an arthroscope or by arthrotomy.

Recently, the FDA approved two artificial ligaments for limited use in treatment of torn knee ligaments—the Gore-Tex ligament and the Ligament Augmentation Device (LAD). The artificial ligaments are implanted through arthroscopy procedures (Peters and Fox, 1988).

Dislocation of the patella may occur and produce knee instability. It may be treated with immobility, but in some cases will progress to a condition of chronic subluxation or dislocation which will require surgical stabilization.

Strategies for Nursing Care

Nurses need to be aware of the principles of first aid treatment for injury to muscles and ligaments. Rest,

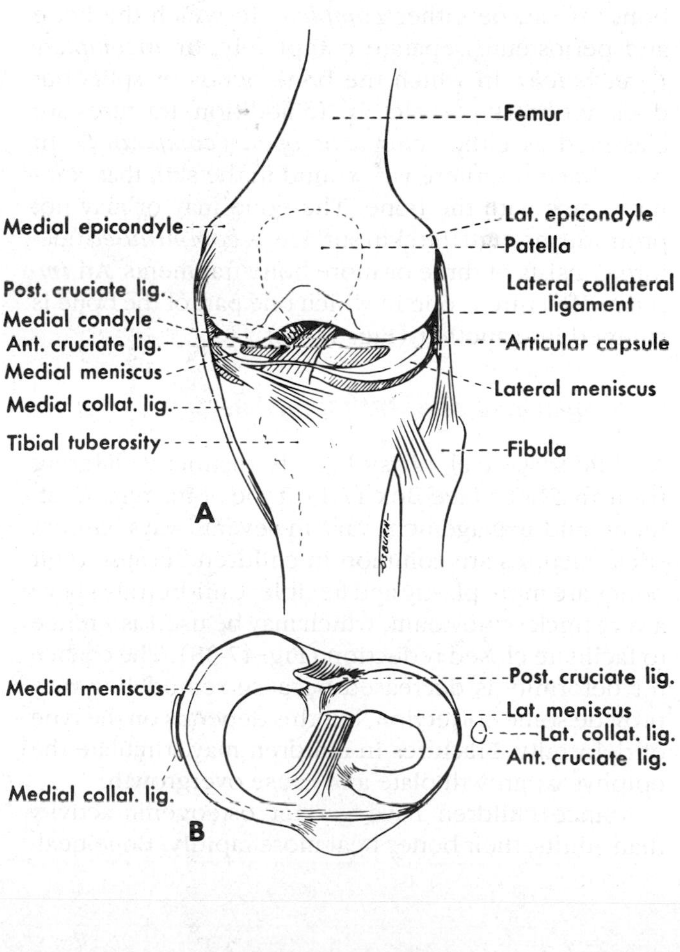

Figure 47-36. Anatomy of the knee joint. (From Gartland JH: *Fundamentals of Orthopaedics.* 4th ed. Philadelphia, WB Saunders, 1986.)

ice, and elevation may be universally applied. Splinting or support and immobilization are indicated. Assessment of neurovascular status should continue until the extent of injury is known. When dealing with knee injuries, special attention is paid to the peroneal nerve, as swelling of the knee may compress it. A simple check for intact function may be performed by asking the patient to dorsiflex the foot. Analgesics will be required during the acute phase of the injury.

Knee injuries may require arthrogram, fluid aspiration, arthroscopy, or arthrotomy for purposes of diagnosis and treatment. Postoperative care for adolescents having arthroscopy or arthrotomy would include frequent assessment of NVS, including dorsiflexion of the foot and assessment of pain, swelling, drainage, and condition of the wound.

With knee injuries, maintenance of function of the quadriceps is extremely important for remobilization. Patients with knee immobilization should routinely be taught quadricep setting and straight leg raising.

Many adolescents with knee injuries will be crutch walking for a period of weeks. Correct gait training, according to weight-bearing instructions, must be taught, practiced, and reinforced.

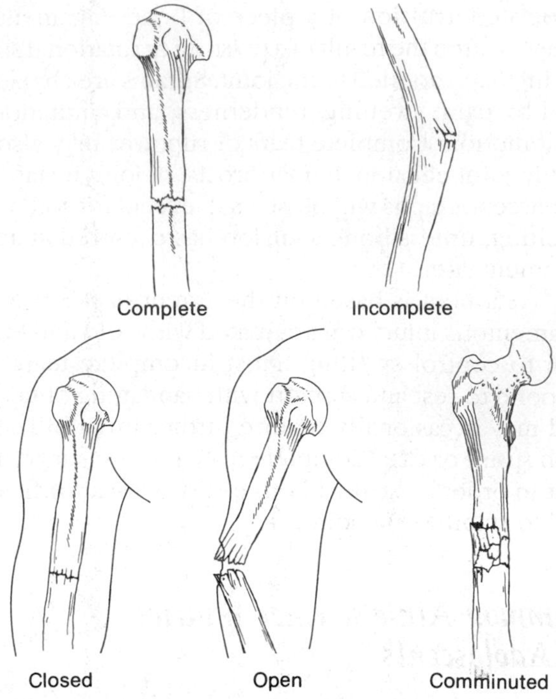

***Figure* 47-37.** Types of fractures.

Fractures

A fracture is defined as a break in the continuity of bone. It can be either *complete,* in which the bone and periosteum separate completely, or *incomplete (greenstick),* in which the bone bends or splits but does not break completely. In addition, fractures are classified as either *closed* or *open (compound).* In open fractures, there is a wound in the skin that communicates with the bone. The bone may or may not protrude through the skin surface. A *comminuted* fracture consists of three or more bone fragments. An *impacted* fracture is one in which one part of the bone is jammed into another (Fig. 47-37).

Physiology and Pathophysiology

A child's skeletal physiology is distinctly different from an adult's (see Box 47-1). Type of fracture, treatment, and management vary in several ways. Greenstick fractures are common in children because their bones are more plastic and flexible. Children also have a very thick periosteum, which may be used as a hinge to facilitate closed reduction (Fig. 47-38). The chance for deformity is decreased because remodeling may provide some correction, but this depends on the type of deformity. Fractures in children may stimulate the epiphyseal growth plate and cause overgrowth.

Since children have greater osteogenic activity than adults, their bones heal more rapidly. Bone healing is discussed on page 1783. The length of time required for complete healing varies greatly with age. A fractured femur in an infant may require 3 weeks in traction before callus formation is sufficient for casting. A similar fracture in an adolescent will commonly require 6 weeks of traction before sufficient callus is present.

Therapeutic Management

Setting or reduction of a fracture involves bringing the fracture fragments into proper alignment so that healing will occur with the bone in its normal contour and capable of normal function. In children, some over-

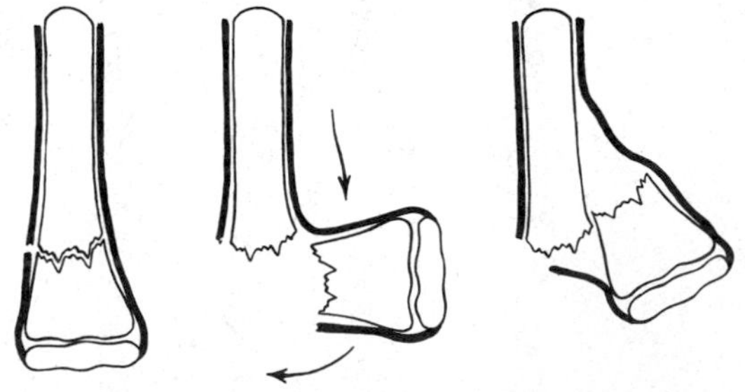

***Figure* 47-38.** The periosteal hinge. *Left,* A fracture with an intact periosteum on one side. The other drawing illustrates the manner in which this should be used to reduce the fracture, using the hinge to prevent overcorrection of the deformity. (From Salter R: *Textbook of Disorders and Injuries of the Musculoskeletal System.* Baltimore, Williams and Wilkins, 1970.)

riding of the fracture fragments is sometimes desirable, as overgrowth may occur in the injured extremity (Hilt and Cogburn, 1980). In many cases, reduction is achieved through the application of manual traction and manipulation, following which the fragments are held in place by a cast. The ease or difficulty of reduction is often determined by the amount of muscle pull on the fracture fragments. Muscles may pull in opposing fashion and encourage displacement of the bone fragments (Fig. 47-39). Spasm of the individual muscles may make it impossible or difficult to set the fracture and maintain position. In this situation, traction or internal or external fixation devices are required to hold the fracture fragments in place. Fractures of the femur usually require traction because of the powerful displacement effects of the large muscles of the thigh.

Reduction of a fracture may be closed, as described earlier, or open (operative). Some fractures require operative intervention in which the fracture is exposed and fixation achieved through the use of pins or screws. Generally in young children, there has been a tendency to use nonoperative methods of reduction because of their remodeling capability and because operative placement of fixation hardware risks trauma to the epiphyses.

External fixation devices (Hoffmann and Wagner devices), frequently used for adult fractures, are occasionally used in children. They maintain fracture position through the use of pins placed proximal and distal to the fracture site with placement maintained by distraction bars connecting the pins. Hoffmann devices may be used when traditional reduction methods fail or when the fracture is open or associated with skin loss (Tolo, 1983). These devices allow for treatment of skin wounds while the position of the bone is maintained.

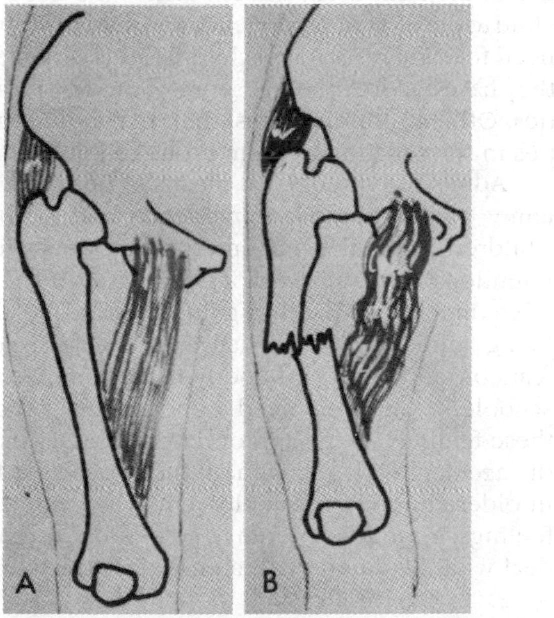

Figure 47-39. *A,* Normal muscle tension pull on bone. *B,* After fracture, muscle tension pull may displace the bone fragments. (From Gartland JH: ***Fundamentals of Orthopaedics.*** Philadelphia, WB Saunders, 1986.)

Complications. Malunion is always a possibility as healing occurs, even with the advantage of remodeling. If malunion is severe, operative repair will be required.

Interference with neurovascular status is always a risk, either due to the injury or the treatment of the injury, and can cause permanent disability. Compartment syndrome occurs when the swelling of the muscles (often produced or aggravated by ischemia) is sufficient that the blood vessels within the fascia compartment are further compressed producing severe ischemia to the extremity. The patient experiences severe pain, often unrelieved by analgesics, in addition to signs of neurovascular impairment. Treatment is a fasciotomy in which the fascia is surgically opened until swelling has subsided.

Growth disturbances will not be evident until sometime later. Shortening of a fractured extremity can occur as a result of injury to the epiphyseal plate. Overgrowth may occur as a response to injury. Angulation of a bone may result from partial damage to the growth plate or overgrowth of one bone or area.

Common Fractures in Children

Fractures of the clavicle, elbow, radius, ulna, tibia, fibula, and femur are all common injuries in children.

Fractures of the clavicle commonly occur as a result of a fall on an outstretched arm or shoulder, or at birth. In infants, the only sign may be lack of movement of the upper extremity on the affected side. Older children will complain of pain. The fracture is treated in newborn infants by immobilizing the arm on the fracture side. In older children, the shoulders are held back by bandaging or bracing to prevent over-riding of the bone fragments.

Most simple fractures of the radius and ulna result from falls and can be treated with closed reduction and casting. Fractures in the area of the elbow require careful evaluation because either the injury or the swelling subsequent to the injury may damage or compress the brachial artery or the radial or median nerve. Supracondylar fracture of the humerus is the most common elbow fracture in children. These fractures may require traction for varying amounts of time to allow for reduction of swelling and to maintain alignment of the bone fragments. Either sidearm traction (see Fig. 47-12) or overhead arm traction (Fig. 47-40) is used.

The neurovascular status of the hand must be carefully monitored, as permanent loss of hand function can occur within 24 hours if circulatory compromise

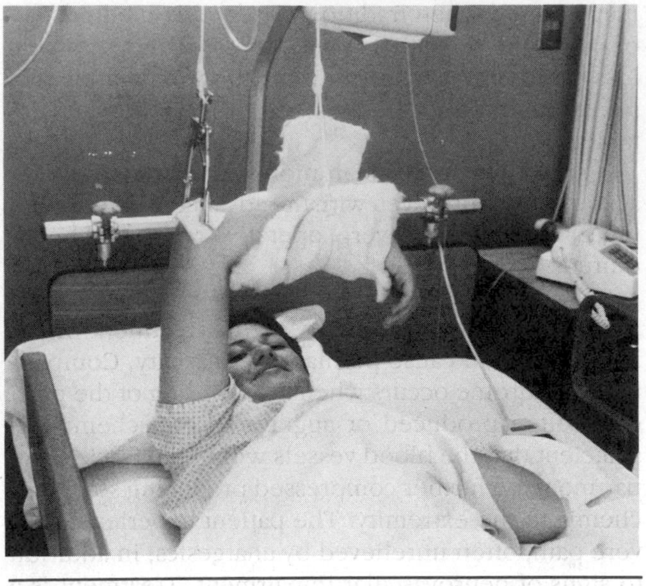

***Figure* 47-40.** Child with supracondylar fracture in overhead skeletal arm traction. (Photograph by Stephanie Wright.)

and nerve compression go undetected (Volkmann ischemic contracture). Compartment syndrome is not uncommon in the forearm. Checks of NVS should include an assessment of the radial pulse and the ability to extend the fingers. If extension of the fingers, either passive or active, produces pain, the physician must be notified.

In the lower extremity, simple fractures of the tibia and fibula are often treated with closed reduction and casting. Femoral shaft fractures usually require traction: Bryant traction (see Fig. 47-11) for very young children, 90-90 traction (see Fig. 47-9) or skeletal traction with balanced suspension (see Fig. 47-10) for older children.

Strategies for Nursing Care

Emergency care should be administered as previously discussed on page 1838. Children and parents will need a thorough explanation of and preparation for whatever treatment is selected. Closed reduction is usually painful, and children require sedation or tranquilization plus physical restraint during this procedure.

Following reduction and casting or placement of traction, children will have pain and will need regular analgesia for the first few days. The extremity should be handled with extreme care; bumping or jarring of the extremity, or of the bed if the child is in traction, will cause pain. Muscle spasm may be a problem for the child in traction and should be treated separately from the pain of the fracture. Frequency of neurovascular assessments depends on the individual situation, injury, and treatment. It is commonly done hourly until the examiner believes that the situation is stable; then it is done every 4 hours.

The child will require appropriate application of the nursing interventions previously discussed pertaining to immobilization and application of cast or traction.

Preparation for discharge from the hospital or emergency facility should include cast care instruction, careful delineation of amount and nature of activity permitted, signs and symptoms of complications, crutch-walking instruction as needed, and discussion of adaptations in home and school routines needed to accommodate recovery of the injury.

Caring for Victims of Trauma

In most persons, accidental injury evokes feelings of uncertainty and anxiety about the nature of the world in which we live. For adults, this includes questioning about why this accident has occurred. For parents, this involves attempts to eradicate the tremendous guilt feelings they have whenever a child is injured. Parents need numerous opportunities to discuss how and why the accident occurred and to speculate on how it might have been prevented. Parental conflict may surface if one parent was responsible for the child when the accident occurred.

Any suggestions on how the injury might have been avoided must be carefully timed to avoid increasing the parents' burden of guilt. Parents may be asking the permission of those around them to be human, to know that all parents make errors in judgment. Parents constantly have to make decisions about the capabilities of their children, and to balance the need for the child to develop independence and autonomy with the need for safety. For some children, this is not difficult; they have a more inherent sense of their own capabilities. Others continually test their expanding capabilities in ways that make them prone to injury.

Adults use intellectual means to deal with uncertainty; they understand incidence and probability. Children do not; they may interpret accidental injury as intentional. They may experience guilt if they were operating beyond parental guidelines and feel they are being punished. Accidental injury may exacerbate fears of mutilation and bodily harm common in preschoolers. Children need opportunities to express these feelings in age-appropriate ways. Discussion of the accident with and without their parents is helpful in older children and adolescents who can verbalize feelings. Younger children need play opportunities to deal with the emotional trauma of accidental injury.

References

Am J Nurs 1978 Jan; 54.

Anderson B: The patient with scoliosis. *Am J Nurs* 1979 Sept; 1592.

Avery ME, Taeusch HW: *Schaeffer's Diseases of the Newborn.* Philadelphia, WB Saunders, 1984.

Black Y: Spica cast care in the infant with a CDH. *Orthoped Nurs Assoc J* 1979 Nov; 439.

Boos ML: A program of home traction for congenital dislocation of the hip. *Orthoped Nurs* 1982 Mar-Apr; 11.

Bunnell WP: Spinal deformity. *Pediatr Clin North Am* 1986 December; 33(6):1475–1487.

Chung SMK: Diseases of the developing hip joint. *Pediatr Clin North Am* 1986 Dec; 33(6):1457–1464.

Ferguson AB: *Orthopedic Surgery in Infancy and Childhood.* Baltimore, Williams and Wilkins, 1981.

Gartland JJ: *Fundamentals of Orthopedics.* Philadelphia, WB Saunders, 1979.

Hamilton H (ed): *Diagnostics.* Springhouse, PA, Intermed Communications, 1981.

Hill P, Romm L: Screening for scoliosis in adolescents. *MCN* 1977 May/Jun; 156.

Hilt NE, Cogburn SB: *Manual of Orthopedics.* St Louis, CV Mosby 1980.

Hughes S: Cause unknown. *Nurs Mir* 1980 Oct; 16.

Keim H: Back deformities. *Pediatr Clin North Am* 1977 Nov; 871.

Knittel G, Staheli L: The effectiveness of shoe modification for intoeing. *Orthoped Clin North Am* 1976 Jul/Aug; 1019.

Larson C, Gould M: *Orthopedic Nursing.* St Louis, CV Mosby, 1978.

Lovell WW, Winter RB: *Pediatric Orthopedics.* Philadelphia, JB Lippincott, 1978.

McDade W: Bowlegs and knock-knees. *Pediatr Clin North Am* 1977 Nov; 825.

Mather MLS: The secret to life in a spica. *AJN* 1987 Jan; 87(1):56–58.

Menkes J: *Textbook of Child Neurology.* Philadelphia, Lea and Febiger, 1974.

Peters JV, Fox JM: Knee surgery clears a hurdle. *RN* 1988 July: 20–25.

Schmeisser G: *A Clinical Manual of Orthopedic Traction Techniques.* Philadelphia, WB Saunders, 1963.

Smith JB: Knee problems in children. *Pediatr Clin North Am* 1977 Nov; 845.

Staheli L: Torsional deformity. *Pediatr Clin North Am* 1977 Nov; 799.

Swinyard C: *Limb Development and Deformity.* Springfield, IL, Charles C Thomas, 1969.

Syriopoulou VPh, Smith AL: Osteomyelitis and septic arthritis. *In* Feigin RO, Cherry JD (eds): *Textbook of Pediatric Infectious Diseases.* 2nd ed. Philadelphia, WB Saunders, 1987, 759–779.

Tachdjian M: *Pediatric Orthopedics.* Philadelphia, WB Saunders, 1974.

Tolo VT: External skeletal fixation in children's fractures. *J Pediatr Orthoped* 1983 Sep; 435.

Watts HG: The bones and joints. *In* Behrman RE, Vaughan VC (eds): *Nelson Textbook of Pediatrics.* Philadelphia, WB Saunders, 1987, 1343–1360.

Wise LB: A comparison of orthopedic casts: breaking the mold. *MCN* 11(3):174–176.

Bibliography

Behrman RE, Vaughan VC (eds): *Nelson Textbook of Pediatrics.* Philadelphia, WB Saunders, 1987.

Cochran S: Action stat! Open fracture. *Nursing 87* 1987 May; 17(5):33.

Conway-Rutowski BL: *Carini and Owens' Neurological and Neurosurgical Nursing.* St Louis, CV Mosby, 1982.

Crelin ES: Development of the Musculoskeletal System. *Clin Symp* 1981.

Cruess RL: *The Musculoskeletal System: Embryology, Biochemistry, and Physiology.* New York, Churchill-Livingstone, 1982.

Eliason MJ, Richman LC: Psychological effects of idiopathic adolescent scoliosis. *Dev Behav Pediatr* 1984 Aug; 5(4):169–172.

Francis EE: Lateral electrical surface stimulation treatment for scoliosis. *Pediatr Nurs* 1987 May/Jun; 13(3):157–160.

Gamron RB: Taking the pressure out of compartment syndrome. *AJN* 1988 Aug; 88(8):1076–1080.

Garrick JG: The sports medicine patient. *Nurs Clin North Am* 1981 Dec; 759.

Gellis SS, Kagan BM: *Current Pediatric Therapy 12.* Philadelphia, WB Saunders, 1986.

Gurnham RM: Adolescent compliance with spinal brace wear. *Orthop Nurs* 1983 Nov/Dec; 13–17.

Heppenstall RB: *Fracture Treatment and Healing.* Philadelphia, WB Saunders, 1980.

Hilt NE: Screening for congenital dislocation of the hip. *Orthop Nurs* 1982 Mar/Apr; 22–24.

Hoyt NJ: Infections following orthopaedic injury. *Orthop Nurs* 1986 Sep/Oct; 5(5):15–23.

Karn MA, Ragiel CA: The psychological effects of immobilization on the pediatric orthopedic patient. *Ortho Nurs* 1986 Nov/Dec; 5(6):12–16.

Kylberg HK: Descriptions of growth disturbances in children with osteomyelitis at different ages. *Orthop Nurs* 1983 Nov/Dec; 28–32.

Lieber MT, Taub AS: Common foot deformities and what they mean for parents. *MCN* 1988 Jan/Feb; 13(1):47–50.

Linley JF: Screening children for common orthopaedic problems. *AJN* 1987 Oct; 87(10):1312–1316.

McCullough FL, Evans LM: Assessment of neurovascular status in children. *Orthop Nurs* 1985 Jul/Aug; 4(4):19–25.

Moore KL: *The Developing Human.* Philadelphia, WB Saunders, 1987.

Ogden JA: *Skeletal Injury in the Child.* Philadelphia, Lea and Febiger, 1982.

Rang M: *Children's Fractures.* Philadelphia, JB Lippincott, 1983.

Spickler LL: Knee injuries of the athlete. *Orthop Nurs* 1983 Sep/Oct; 11–19.

Swanson AB: Congenital limb defects. *Clin Symp* 1981.

Taft LT: Cerebral palsy. *Pediatr Rev* 1984 Aug; 6(2):35–44.

Wilson JB (ed): *Fractures and Joint Injuries.* New York, Churchill-Livingstone, 1982.

Nursing Strategies: Aberrant Cell Growth

Chapter 48

Mary J. Waskerwitz
Ruth M. Heyn

Nursing Process Plan

NPP: The Child Undergoing Chemotherapy, page 1884

Related Topics

Impact of chronic illness, Chapter 25
Impact of death and dying, Chapter 26
Total parenteral nutrition, Chapter 30
Nursing care of the hospitalized child, Chapter 31
Principles and strategies of home care, Chapter 32
Blood components and their normal function, Chapter 40
Normal and abnormal immune function, Chapter 43
Thrush (moniliasis), Chapter 45
Care of the child with neurologic sequelae, Chapter 46

Cancer, a word that in the past has been synonymous with death, in this generation has become associated with chronic illness and, not infrequently, with cure. This increased potential for a normal lifespan for the child with cancer is due largely to advances in drug treatment (chemotherapy), radiation treatment (radiotherapy), and refinement of surgical techniques. National research studies, such as the Children's Cancer Study Group (CCSG), have facilitated the rapid advances in cancer treatment by pooling data on patients from across the country and thereby arriving more rapidly at findings upon which to base subsequent practice.

These therapeutic advances, however, do not negate the fact that the diagnosis of cancer remains a devastating event for the child and family. Treatment usually involves long-term treatment with surgery, chemotherapy, radiation therapy, or some combination of these modalities. For the family this often means adapting to repeated hospitalizations, seemingly endless clinic visits, possible changes in the child's appearance, financial concerns, and, always, the unsettling possibility of the child's untimely death. Nurses who care for children with cancer and their families are called upon to understand not only the body's reaction to aberrant cell growth, but how to monitor and intervene for the often severe side effects of cancer treatments and to somehow foster the child's normal growth and development in the midst of this health crisis.

This chapter deals with the common forms of cancer in childhood. Leukemia, because it is the most prevalent form of childhood malignancy, is detailed as a prototype. Another prototype for nursing care is found in the nursing process plan for the child undergoing chemotherapy (see Table 48-4).

Overview of Cancer in Childhood

Incidence of Childhood Malignancy

Most people think of cancer as a disease of the elderly. Cancer, however, is the leading cause of death from disease in children over 1 year of age (Leventhal, 1987). The most common malignancies in children in the United States are, in order, leukemia, brain tumors, lymphomas (including Hodgkin disease) neuroblastoma, Wilms tumor, soft tissue sarcomas (including rhabdomyosarcoma), bone tumors (Ewing sarcoma and osteogenic sarcoma), and retinoblastoma. Figure 48-1 graphically illustrates the common pediatric malignancies by percentage occurrence. From a review of 834 patients with these diagnoses who were treated at the University of Michigan from 1962 to 1978, the percentage distribution of children according to age group is presented in Figure 48-2.

Etiology

"What causes cancer in children?" is a question that remains unanswered. Potential environmental carcinogens such as smoking, diet, and industrial pollutants are difficult to link to the etiology of pediatric malignancies because children have had such little time for exposure. Other epidemiological factors such as family history, prenatal exposures, and the pre-existence of certain constitutional disorders may be significant. In fact, children with chromosomal disorders form the largest group of children who have a higher than normal incidence of cancer. Researchers continue to investigate links between immunodeficiency states and the development of malignancy, and to search for possible oncogenic viruses.

Pathophysiology

A cancer is a cellular tumor, a malignant neoplasm. A neoplasm is any tumor (benign or malignant) arising from new and abnormal cell growth. Malignant neoplasms are progressive growths in which there is a loss of differentiation of cells; that is, the cells no longer perform their intended function. Malignant cells undergo changes in deoxyribonucleic acid (DNA) leading to transmission of faulty information for cellular development and subsequent uncontrolled growth

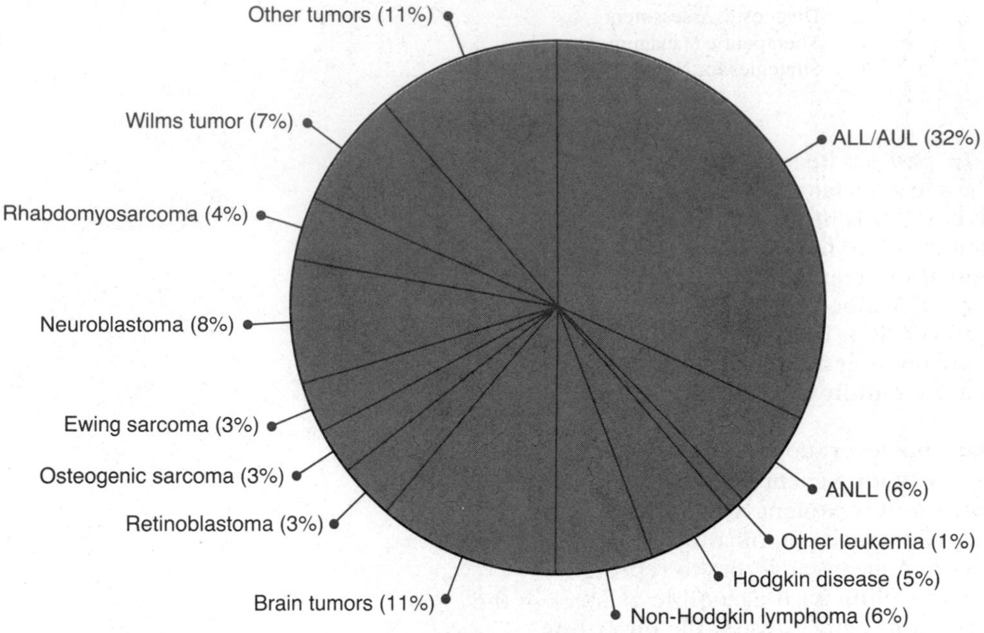

Figure 48-1. Approximate per cent distribution of common pediatric malignancies, using patient registration of the Children's Cancer Study Group.

and loss of normal cellular function. Proliferation of these abnormal cells can be viewed as a failure of the surveillance function of the immune system (Bellanti, 1985).

Although research continues, it is currently thought that failure of the immune system to provide adequate surveillance is linked to the development of malignancy. A healthy immune system identifies and destroys aberrant cells. When the immune system is less competent, however, it may fail to perform adequate surveillance and allow proliferation of malignant cells. Incompetence may result because of chemically induced suppression (e.g., corticosteroids and other immunosuppressant drugs), suppression as the result of prolonged or frequent viral infections, or congenital or acquired immunologic disease (e.g., AIDS). (Chapter 43 further details functions of the immune system.)

Malignant cells probably do not kill healthy cells directly* but rather compete with them for nutrients and blood supply to sustain growth. They eventually starve and replace the healthy cells in the involved tissue, resulting in the loss of function of that organ or tissue. Cancerous tumors are classified histologically (according to cell type) but also differ by location, growth rate, metastatic patterns, response to treatment, and prognosis.

* Although it has been postulated that cancer cells may release toxins that kill healthy cells to open pathways by which the malignancy can spread to other tissues, there is currently little support for this hypothesis (Groenwald, 1987).

Classification of Malignant Neoplasms

Malignancies can be classified according to histogenesis, anatomic site, and degree of differentiation (Rubin, 1983).

Histogenesis. Histogenesis denotes whether the tumor is benign or malignant and the tissue from which the tumor originates. Most tumors, whether benign or malignant, end in the suffix *-oma,* which means "tumor." Further, the tumor is named for the tissue from which it arises. For example, *carcinoma* refers to a malignant tumor of epithelial tissue, whereas *sarcoma* refers to a malignant tumor of connective tissue.

Cancers in childhood tend to attack different tissues than do cancers in adults. Although most adult tumors are carcinomas (i.e., involving epithelial tissues), many pediatric tumors are *sarcomas,* involving connective tissue. It is thought that this difference in tissue sites occurs because children have had a relatively shorter exposure to environmental carcinogens (causing many carcinomas) than have adults. Another prevalent form of cancer in children is tumors of embryonal origin. *Embryomas* contain tissue that does not develop beyond the stage of fetal tissue and therefore fails to differentiate into functional cells.

Anatomic Site. In naming the tumor, the anatomic site is often linked with the type of tissue involved. For example, *osteogenic* sarcoma is a malignant tumor of the connective tissue of the bone. A tumor of striated muscle tissue is preceded by the prefix meaning "striated muscle;" that is, *rhabdomyo*sarcoma. An embryonal tumor is designated by the term

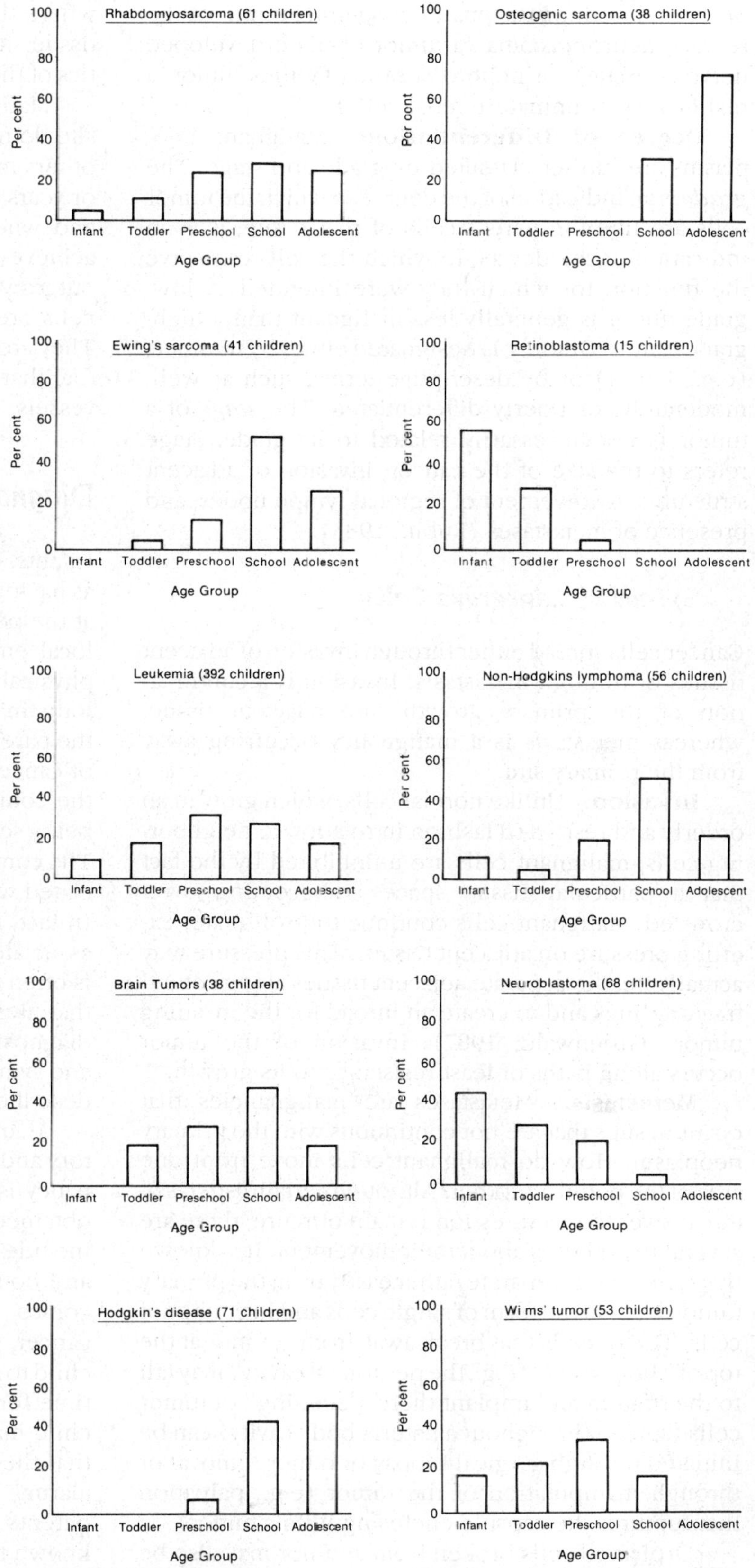

***Figure* 48-2.** Distribution of cancer by age at diagnosis. (Distribution in percentages of 834 children treated at the University of Michigan over 16 years, by age at diagnosis, using age distribution defined by this textbook.)

blast, as in retino*blast*oma (a congenital tumor of the retina), neuro*blast*oma (a tumor of underdeveloped nervous tissue), or nephro*blast*oma (Wilms tumor, a malignancy of immature renal cells).

Degree of Differentiation. Malignant neoplasms are further classified by grade and stage. The *grade* is an indication of the degree to which the tumor cells are like the parent cells of that tissue; it is an indication of the degree to which the cells can serve the function for which they were intended. A low-grade tumor is generally less malignant than a high-grade tumor. Grading is designated either by numbers (e.g., 1 to 4) or by descriptive terms, such as well, moderately, or poorly differentiated. The *stage* of a tumor is not necessarily related to its grade. Stage refers to the size of the cancer, invasion of adjacent structures, involvement of regional lymph nodes, and presence of metastases (Rubin, 1983).

Spread of Cancerous Cells

Cancer cells spread either through invasion of adjacent tissues or through metastasis. Invasion is a continuation of the primary growth into adjacent tissue, whereas metastasis is a malignancy occurring away from the primary site.

Invasion. Unlike normal cells, which grow in an orderly and restricted fashion in relation to neighboring cells, malignant cells are uninhibited by the fact that a particular tissue space is becoming overcrowded. Malignant cells continue to proliferate, exerting pressure on adjacent tissues. This pressure may actually help to separate adjacent tissues along natural fracture lines and to create an inroad for the invading tumor (Groenwald, 1987). Invasion of the tumor occurs along paths of least resistance to its growth.

Metastasis. Metastases are malignancies that occur in sites that are not continuous with the primary neoplasm. How do malignant cells move from one area of the body to another? Although certain aspects of the answer to that question remain obscure, there are several hypotheses about their movement. It is known that cancer cells separate rather easily from the primary tumor, both in the form of single cells and in clumps of cells. Tumor cells that break away from a tumor at the top of a body cavity (e.g., the peritoneal cavity) may fall to the bottom and implant there. "Seeding" of tumor cells (spread throughout a natural body cavity) can be initiated through surgical biopsy or tumor removal or through manipulation of the tumor (e.g., palpation that ruptures the capsule enclosing Wilms tumor).

Orphaned cells broken from a tumor may also be picked up in the lymph and subsequently make their way into the blood stream. Other malignant cells reach the blood stream through direct invasion of capillaries and veins. Once in the blood or lymph flow, it is postulated that malignant cells "stop" and implant in tissues where they are most likely to survive and that those tissue sites depend, in part, upon certain characteristics of the tumor cells themselves (Groenwald, 1987).

Malignant cells that migrate to a secondary tissue site do not necessarily begin to grow. Many cells die; others may become dormant, only to activate months or years after the primary tumor has been removed. If and when the tumor cells do proliferate, they can achieve a size of only a few millimeters before they outgrow the area's blood supply. Unfortunately, tumor cells are well prepared for this temporary setback. They are able to secrete a chemical (angiogenesis factor) that stimulates the formation of additional blood vessels.

Diagnostic Assessment

Infants, children, and adolescents who are diagnosed as having some form of cancer usually present initially at the pediatrician's office, child health care clinic, or local emergency room with signs and symptoms or physical findings that either have been present for a long time or have just been brought to the attention of the parents or themselves. Occasionally the diagnosis of cancer is first suspected by the practitioner during the course of an examination of a well child who is being seen for a routine health maintenance check-up. The complete list of signs and symptoms that are associated with childhood malignancies is immeasurable. In fact, many of these findings are the same as those associated with other common childhood illnesses. It is often the persistence and intensity of these findings that alert the skilled clinician to the possibility of a diagnosis of cancer. Box 48-1 is a summary of the signs and symptoms of the common pediatric malignancies described in this chapter.

If, upon completion of a careful and complete history and physical assessment, the diagnosis of a malignancy is suspected, various preliminary tests may be obtained at the local clinic or hospital. These tests may include blood studies, radiographs, and scans (e.g., CT and bone scans). As the local primary physician becomes increasingly convinced that a patient has cancer, he or she will likely transfer the care of the child to a pediatric cancer center. This is a very difficult time for parents, who understand and fear that their child may have cancer yet continue to hope and pray that the findings may turn out to be merely a "false alarm." Providing emotional support while supplying parents with honest information regarding what is known thus far is imperative.

At the cancer center, completion of the battery of studies needed to make a specific diagnosis of cancer and to document the extent of disease may take several days. Parents, of course, must provide consent for these special studies to be carried out. Nurses should

Box 48-1
Common Signs and Symptoms Associated with Pediatric Cancers

Leukemia
Bleeding, bone pain, bruising, fever, hepatomegaly, infection, lymphadenopathy, malaise, pallor, petechiae, splenomegaly

Brain Tumors
Anorexia, ataxia, changes in behavior and personality, clumsy gait, cranial nerve dysfunction, diffuse or focal nerve dysfunction, diplopia, headache, irritability, lack of weight gain or continuing development, motor dysfunction, nystagmus, papilledema, seizures, strabismus, torticollis, urinary retention, vomiting, weakness

Hodgkin Disease
Fever, lymphadenopathy, night sweats, weight loss

Non-Hodgkin Lymphoma
Abdominal distention, mass, or pain, ascites, cough, diarrhea, dyspnea, epistaxis, lymphadenopathy, nasal congestion, rhinorrhea, tonsillar mass, vomiting, wheezing

Neuroblastoma
Abdominal mass, anemia, fever, hypertension, irritability, neck mass, orbital ecchymosis, pain, proptosis

Wilms Tumor
Abdominal mass, anorexia, fever, hematuria, hypertension, malaise

Rhabdomyosarcoma
Chronic otitis media, cranial nerve palsies, dysphagia, dysuria, epistaxis, eyelid swelling, facial nerve palsy, hearing loss, hematuria, hoarseness, nasal discharge, proptosis, sinusitis, soft tissue mass, urinary retention

Osteogenic Sarcoma
Bone pain, mass, or swelling

Ewing Sarcoma
Mass, pain

Retinoblastoma
"Cat's eye reflex," loss of vision, pain, and redness at orbit

be prepared to explain the significance of each study to the child and to describe exactly how each test is done and any degree of discomfort that the child may experience. Box 48-2 lists the studies that are usually obtained to diagnose the common pediatric cancers. Table 48-1 describes how these studies are performed. A tissue sample of the tumor is necessary for the pathologist or oncologist to make the diagnosis of a specific malignancy. Appropriate treatment can begin as soon as the diagnosis is known and appropriate studies for the extent of disease are completed.

Box 48-2
Special Tests That Diagnose Pediatric Cancers

Leukemia
complete blood count
bone marrow aspiration
lumbar puncture

Brain Tumors
CT scan of the brain
myelogram
lumbar puncture

Hodgkin Disease
chest radiograph
CT scan of chest and abdomen/pelvis
bone scan
bone marrow biopsy
staging laparotomy

Non-Hodgkin Lymphoma
chest radiograph
bone marrow aspirate and biopsy
lumbar puncture
bone scan
abdominal CT scan or ultrasound

Neuroblastoma
abdominal CT scan or ultrasound
chest radiograph
bone survey
bone scan
bone marrow aspirate and biopsy
24-hour urine collection for catecholamines
intravenous pyelogram

Wilms Tumor
CT scan
intravenous pyelogram
chest radiograph

Rhabdomyosarcoma
radiographs
CT scans
nuclear scans

Osteogenic Sarcoma
bone survey
bone scan
chest radiograph
chest CT scan

Ewing Sarcoma
CT scan of chest and bone
bone scan

Retinoblastoma
CT scan of head
skull radiograph
bone scan
lumbar puncture
bone marrow aspiration

Therapeutic Management

The treatment of children with cancer may involve surgery, radiation therapy, and chemotherapy, and

Table 48-1. Tests Commonly Performed on Pediatric Oncology Patients

How Test Is Performed	How Child Is Prepared; Comments
Bone Marrow Aspiration	
Aspiration of marrow into syringe but is obtained through heavy, wide-gauge needle with stylet that is inserted into marrow space through skin, subcutaneous tissue, and bone cortex using rotary motion; the anterior or posterior iliac crest is the bone marrow site most often chosen for aspiration in children	The child is most often held tightly in a prone or supine position on a treatment table. Local anesthesia is injected to the site to provide some analgesia, but the actual aspiration of marrow into the syringe, which is often done over a period of a few seconds, is usually very painful and not amenable to the local anesthesia premedication. The entire procedure usually takes a few minutes.
Bone Scan	
Scan of skeletal system after an injection of intravenous radionuclide that within a few hours localizes in the bone, with increased focal accumulation of tracer in areas of bone disease	The child must be still on a hard surface, for up to an hour after intravenous injection of the radionuclide, while the larger scanner passes over the body.
CT Scan	
Computed transverse tomography that allows noninvasive evaluation of various body parts; it produces anatomic cross-sectional images of specific body parts that readily demonstrate organ structures and lesions, easily discriminating among soft tissue variations that are too subtle for simple radiographs	The child must lie still on a firm surface for the duration of the scan, sometimes for up to an hour, while large machinery passes over the body. Sometimes IV or oral contrast material is administered prior to the test to enhance the quality of film produced.
Intravenous Pyelogram	
Radiograph that is obtained after intravenous contrast medium is injected and then concentrated and excreted by the kidney, delineating the urinary tract	The child must be held still for the radiograph, after the intravenous injection. The films are obtained in less than an hour.
Lumbar Puncture	
Injection of needle into lumbar spine interspace to obtain sample of cerebrospinal fluid	The child must be held in a flexed-spine position (curled on the side) for a few minutes.
Liver-Spleen Scan	
Scan of liver and spleen after an injection of intravenous radionuclide that localizes in those organs, with increased focal accumulation of tracer in abnormal tissue sections	The child must lie still on a hard surface, for up to an hour, while the large scanner passes over the body.
Lymphangiogram	
Radiograph of trunk after injection of radiopaque substance into feet dorsum to demonstrate retroperitoneal lymph nodes	Generally this test can be performed only on larger children (minimum about 5–10 years of age). The injection is very uncomfortable, so often patients are premedicated with a sedative or an analgesic. The test often takes more than 1 hour to perform.
Ultrasound	
Photograph of internal structures made through use of high-frequency sound waves: the reflected sound wave patterns vary with tissue density and sound travels fastest through the most compact molecules—abnormalities in tissue density can be visualized	The child must hold still for an ultrasound but there is no pain involved in the test. The test is performed in less than an hour.

these three treatment modalities are often used in combination. Surgery was the only treatment available for patients with solid tumors until radiation therapy and chemotherapy became appropriate adjunctive therapies. Leukemia, the most common malignancy in children, is treated primarily with chemotherapy, and it was for this disease that chemotherapy was first used successfully in children.

Of necessity, children with cancer may be cared for by more than one medical specialist. Pediatric surgeons and other subspecialty surgeons, radiotherapists, and pediatric oncologists all play a role in the team caring for the child with cancer, but the pediatric oncology team is responsible for overall patient management. The nurses who are assigned to care for children with cancer must assist parents in assimilating their child's complex health care system. The nurses who are at the child's bedside each day can lend great support to parents by providing consistent and intelligible explanations of treatment plans and procedures.

Surgery

A surgical procedure is almost always employed to diagnose cancer in children with solid tumors. Biopsies of tumors establish an accurate diagnosis by supplying the pathologist with tissue samples of the tumor. For some tumors it is preferable to attempt complete surgical excision. Complete surgical excision is not always possible for large tumors that are adjacent to vital structures and may not be indicated if it leaves the child with a mutilated or grossly disfigured appearance. Some treatment plans make use of radiation therapy and chemotherapy to reduce the size of large tumors preoperatively, allowing for either a complete excision or less radical surgical procedure at a later time.

Radiation Therapy

Radiotherapy is the treatment of malignant disease with roentgen rays or other radiant energy. When tissue is exposed to ionizing radiation, radiation fragments are absorbed and their energy is deposited within that tissue. Ionization produces changes within the cell molecules that result in biologic damage. Normal cells have a greater capacity for subsequent repair when exposed to radiation than do malignant cells. Hence radiotherapy is used as a cancer treatment because it is capable of killing tumor cells.

Newer techniques allow for very precise direction of radiotherapy beams to the tumor, sparing the surrounding normal tissues. Different tumors show varying degrees of radiosensitivity, as do normal tissues. Different organs tolerate specific limited doses of radiation before the normal function of that organ is impaired.

Radiotherapy is most often employed in combination with surgery or chemotherapy in the treatment of leukemias, lymphomas, and solid tumors. It may also be used alone to achieve palliation of symptoms caused by tumor masses.

Most courses of radiation therapy are given as one treatment daily for 5 out of each 7 days. A specific dose is given each day depending on the tumor being treated and its site. A total course may take several weeks since all tissues have a limited daily tolerance.

It is usually frightening for children to begin radiation therapy treatment since they are left alone in rooms with large machines. Members of pediatric radiotherapy departments are experienced in working with children under these circumstances, and even young children often become less resistant and more accepting of the procedure after a few days. Radiotherapists, radiation therapy nurses, and other staff members work together to allay the child's anxiety before and during each treatment session, which may last only a few minutes. Babies and young children may need restraints or sedation to lie still for radiation treatments.

Parents of children who receive radiotherapy need careful, repeated explanations of the principles of radiotherapy. They must understand the immediate as well as the late side effects caused by the treatment. Symptoms are usually confined to the body site receiving radiation. For example, cranial radiation may cause alopecia, whereas abdominal radiation may cause gastrointestinal symptoms of diarrhea, nausea, or vomiting. Late effects are primarily those of growth impairment in the irradiated site and disturbance in the normal function of treated tissues. Secondary malignant tumors are also known to occur in previously irradiated sites. Radiation therapy nurses are prepared to develop special nursing and home care plans for children undergoing radiation therapy treatments.

Chemotherapy

Treatment with chemotherapy involves the use of drugs that kill or interfere with the proliferation of fast-growing malignant cells. Chemotherapeutic drugs are also called *antineoplastic* agents; that is *against* (anti-) *new, abnormal cell growth* (neoplastic). Most antineoplastic agents affect cells in the process of dividing to make new cells. But normal cells, particularly those known to grow rapidly— *bone marrow, hair follicle cells, gastrointestinal epithelial cells, and cells of the gonads*— will be affected to varying degrees. To understand the rationale for administration of chemotherapy, it is helpful to review the cell cycle.

Cell Cycle

Cells, whether normal or malignant, go through four cell cycle phases (Fig. 48-3). The first phase is *G_1*, or the gap stage between mitosis and DNA synthesis. In

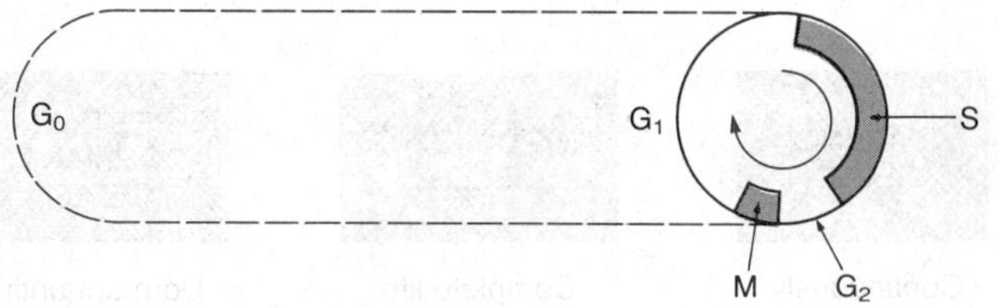

Key: G_1 = Gap 1, preparation for synthesis
S = Synthesis of DNA; concludes when DNA has doubled
G_2 = Gap 2, preparation for mitosis (synthesis of RNA, proteins)
M = Mitosis, cell division into two daughter cells
G_0 = Some cells may be called into this dormant phase until needed by the body, whereupon they re-enter at G_1

Figure 48-3. Cell cycle.

this phase the cell produces enzymes needed for DNA synthesis. The synthesis phase (*S*) denotes the period during which DNA doubles in preparation for mitosis. G_2 is the second gap phase; at this time RNA and proteins are synthesized that are necessary for mitosis. The last phase, mitosis (*M*), is completed with the division of the parent cell into two daughter cells. Cancer cells may divide into several new cells, instead of the normal two cells, at this phase (Ziegfeld, 1987).

It is hypothesized that cell populations contain, at any given time, three categories of cells: cycling cells, nondividing cells, and resting cells (Groenwald, 1987) (Fig. 48-4). Cycling cells are those that continuously divide; these are the rapidly growing cells most affected by antineoplastic drugs. Nondividing cells divide for a time but then differentiate into functional cells that complete their life cycles without further division. Resting cells leave the cell cycle after mitosis to remain dormant until called back into action at the G_1 phase of the cell cycle. It is further speculated that cycling cells and resting cells divide into stem cells and nonstem cells (Groenwald, 1987). Stem cells are precursor cells, or "mother cells"—those cells necessary to maintain the cell line. Stem cells ensure the survival of that particular cell population. As long as there are dormant malignant stem cells (in the G_0 phase), there is the threat of regrowth of the tumor when the resting cells reactivate.

The Action of Chemotherapeutic Agents. Chemotherapeutic agents can be classified according to activity exerted on the tumor cells (Table 48-2). *Cell cycle–specific* agents are those that exert their maximum cytotoxic (cell-killing) effect during a particular phase of the cell cycle. These agents are most effective against rapidly dividing cells. As tumors grow in mass, the length of time between each phase of the cell cycle increases, thus decreasing the effect of cell cycle–specific agents (Groenwald, 1987). *Cell cycle–nonspecific* agents are effective against both dividing and resting cells. Cells affected by these drugs have difficulty dividing or repairing themselves (Ziegfeld, 1987).

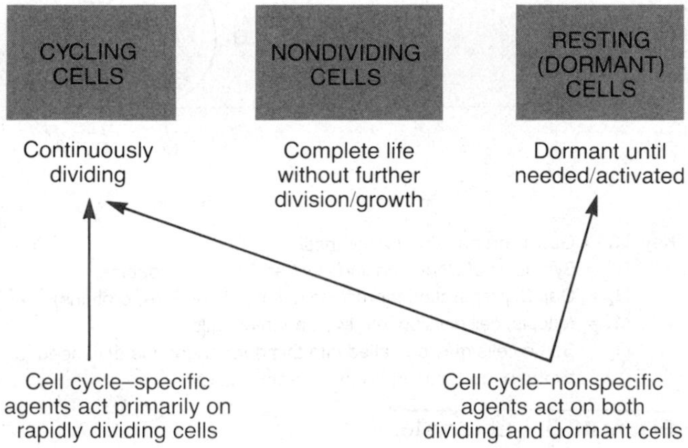

Figure 48-4. Cell populations of normal and malignant tissues: action of chemotherapeutic agents.

Table 48-2. Actions of Chemotherapeutic Agents

Drug Classification	Major Action
Alkylating agents	Interfere with the replication of DNA; most are cell cycle–nonspecific
Vinca alkaloids	Interfere with cell division and inhibit RNA and protein synthesis; cell cycle–specific agents (M phase)
Antimetabolites	Interfere with DNA synthesis; cell cycle–specific agents (S phase)
Synthetic hormones	Interfere with protein synthesis and alter cell metabolism (cell cycle–nonspecific)
Antibiotics	Interfere with nucleic acid (both RNA and DNA) synthesis; cell cycle–nonspecific
Enzymes	Inhibit certain cell metabolites, interfere with protein synthesis

(Based upon Groenwald, 1987; Ziegfeld, 1987.)

Chemotherapeutic agents can be classified according to activity exerted on the tumor cells. *Alkylating agents* are compounds that interfere with the structure and function of DNA, combining chemically with DNA so the cell becomes damaged. *Alkaloids* disorganize the mitotic spindle to arrest cell division. *Antimetabolites* are substances similar to natural body substances that act falsely to incorporate into DNA. *Synthetic hormones* alter normal hormonal balance in patients to modify the growth of cancers arising from tissues that are particularly susceptible to hormonal influence, preventing effective cell proliferation. *Antibiotics* used in cancer therapy are chemicals produced by living bacteria that interfere with cell metabolism. *Enzymes* can inhibit certain cell metabolites and prevent protein synthesis. Table 48-3 summarizes the most commonly used agents, their generic and brand names, classification, route of administration, and major side effects. Table 48-4 on page 1884 provides a Nursing Process Plan for the child undergoing chemotherapy.

Combination Chemotherapy. Treatment with a combination of antineoplastic drugs optimizes the

Table 48-3. Chemotherapy

Name	Route	Classification	Major Side Effects
actinomycin-D	IV	antibiotic	Bone marrow suppression, nausea and vomiting, anorexia, diarrhea, stomatitis, alopecia, severe soft tissue damage with extravasation, hepatotoxicity
L-asparaginase	IM	enzyme	Hypersensitivity reaction, hyperglycemia and transient diabetes mellitus, hepatotoxicity, pancreatitis, bone marrow suppression, coagulation and protein abnormalities, local reaction at injection site
5-azacytidine (5-AZA-C)	IV	antimetabolite	Bone marrow suppression, especially leukopenia; nausea and vomiting, diarrhea
bleomycin	IM, IV, SQ	antibiotic	Progressive pulmonary toxicity, cutaneous toxicity, hypersensitivity reactions
CCNU	PO	antimetabolite and alkylating agent	Bone marrow suppression, nausea and vomiting
cis-platin	IV	heavy metal compound	Bone marrow suppression, nausea and vomiting, ototoxicity, renal toxicity
cyclophosphamide (Cytoxan)	IV, PO	alkylating agent	Bone marrow suppression, nausea and vomiting, anorexia, alopecia, hemorrhagic cystitis, amenorrhea, testicular atrophy, SIADH
cytosine arabinoside (ARA-C, Cytosar)	IV, SQ	antimetabolite	Bone marrow suppression, nausea and vomiting, anorexia, alopecia, hepatotoxicity, fever
dacarbazine (DTIC)	IV	alkylating agent	Bone marrow suppression, flulike syndrome, nausea and vomiting, anorexia, local pain and burning at injection site, alopecia, soft tissue damage with extravasation
daunorubicin (Daunomycin)	IV	antibiotic	Bone marrow suppression, nausea and vomiting, stomatitis, alopecia, severe soft tissue damage with extravasation, chemical phlebitis at injection site, red-colored urine, cardiotoxicity
dexamethasone (Decadron)	PO	adrenocorticosteroid	Electrolyte imbalance, hypertension, fluid and salt retention, increased appetite, weight gain, esophagitis, cushingoid manifestations, glucosuria, immunosuppression
doxorubicin (Adriamycin)	IV	antibiotic	Alopecia, nausea and vomiting, stomatitis, bone marrow suppression, red-colored urine, severe soft tissue damage with extravasation, chemical phlebitis at injection site, cardiotoxicity
etoposide (VP-16)	IV/PO	alkaloid	Leukopenia, thrombocytopenia, nausea and vomiting, alopecia, hypotension and bronchospasm with rapid infusion
6-mercaptopurine (6MP)	PO	antimetabolite	Bone marrow suppression, hepatotoxicity
methotrexate	IV, IM, IT, PO	antimetabolite	Bone marrow suppression, nausea and vomiting, diarrhea, stomatitis, hepatotoxicity, rashes, leukoencephalopathy, renal impairment
nitrogen mustard	IV	alkylating agent	Bone marrow suppression, nausea and vomiting, phlebitis, alopecia, severe soft tissue damage with extravasation, amenorrhea and impaired spermatogenesis
prednisone	PO	adrenocorticosteroid	Electrolyte imbalance, hypertension, fluid and salt retention, increased appetite, weight gain, esophagitis, cushingoid manifestations, glucosuria, immunosuppression
procarbazine	PO	alkylating agent	Bone marrow suppression, nausea, rashes
thioguanine (6TG)	PO	antimetabolite	Bone marrow suppression
vinblastine (Velban)	IV	alkaloid	Bone marrow suppression, alopecia, neurotoxicity, severe soft tissue damage with extravasation
vincristine (Oncovin)	IV	alkaloid	Neurotoxicity, alopecia, fever, severe soft tissue damage with extravasation, constipation

cell-killing properties of the drugs while minimizing the side effects. Because the drugs have various actions, particular combinations can deliver a wide variety of assaults to the malignant cell. Because certain chemotherapeutic agents have additive and synergistic effects, individual drug dosages can be decreased, thus reducing their side effects.

All chemotherapeutic agents are immunosuppressive to varying degrees (they suppress the function of normal lymphocytes in the immune system), so patients must not receive live virus immunizations while on treatment and they must be cautioned to avoid exposure to common contagious viral diseases. They will, likewise, mount poor antibody responses to vaccines containing proteins from killed organisms. If an immunosuppressed child contracts a viral disease or receives one of these immunizations, he or she could develop a serious form of the disease because of this inability to mount a proper antibody response to the virus.

Supporting the Child and Family during Diagnosis

When cancer is diagnosed in a child, the parents may already have suspected the child's symptoms and condition could represent cancer. Nonetheless, when the diagnosis is actually made, the parents are immediately terrified that the child will die. The nurse should be present when the parents are told the diagnosis. As the physician tells the parents that their child has cancer, they may become instantly withdrawn. They often fail to recall any of the details of initial conversations with the physicians and nurses. The nurse should take an active role in helping parents to deal with the reality of the diagnosis by offering frequent explanations of the disease and its treatment in the ensuing days.

After the initial shock, the parents will have numerous questions. Each question must be addressed and answered with gentle honesty. The parents are depressed about the possibility of their child's death. They may feel guilty about not having sought medical attention sooner. They are angry that this is happening to them and their child. They are in a state of shock and disbelief. Since most children with cancer are referred to pediatric oncology centers, the parents may not know any of the members of the medical or nursing team and thus may not be ready to openly share their feelings. The health team must be there, however, ready to offer support when the parents are ready to verbalize.

The initial hospitalization of a child with cancer may be the parents' first experience with hospitals and complicated treatments. Even the simplest procedures must be explained to the child and his or her parents. The nurse must keep abreast of the diagnostic plan to be able to prepare the child and the parents for each step. The nurse can help the child and family develop trust and feel more secure during this frightening period by communicating an attitude of caring and by giving accurate information about the illness, diagnostic tests, and treatments. These nursing functions can relieve some of the overwhelming stress that the child and family experience at this time.

At the time of diagnosis of cancer, the child often does not feel well. He or she may be irritable and in pain but typically is not especially worried because he or she has felt sick before and has always gotten better. Children do begin to worry, however, as soon as they can sense uneasiness, anxiety, and sadness in their parents. As soon as the parents can speak calmly with the child, he or she must be told something about why he or she is in the hospital and undergoing many tests and painful procedures.

Young children do not need and will not benefit from a detailed description of their disease. They should be told the name of the disease to avoid embarrassment or fears later when they are in public and exposed to persons who may freely use diagnostic terms. They will probably be satisfied with the information that this is an illness that requires special care from special doctors and nurses. They should know that at times some of the special treatments may hurt them for a while but that all the treatments will eventually make them feel better and will help them to get better. It is very important for the parents to tell the child that they will always be there and that they love the child.

Interactions and discussions with older children and teenagers must be open and honest, enhanced by the ever-present support and love of their parents. Adolescents must be presented with the basic facts about their diagnosis and its proposed treatment. Even direct questions such as "Will I die?" must not be ignored. That question can be answered with gentle honesty by relaying information that yes, children with cancer have died but that today's improved treatments work well and that everyone is going to work together so that they will not die. Teenagers vary in their desire and need to learn details about their disease and its treatment. Some want to learn a great deal and to make decisions independently. Others pursue more passive roles, relying on parents and staff to take care of them. They are happier not talking or learning about their disease in depth. These varying patterns of behavior need to be accepted by the health care team.

The entire family unit immediately centers all its emotional energies on the child with cancer. It is easy for the mother and father to overlook the need for sharing their anxiety and comforting each other. As soon as the child's condition is stable, parents will probably need to be told to get away from the hospital for a while just to be alone together. They may need reassurance from the nurse that their child will be well cared for in their absence. Likewise, parents must remember the special needs of the siblings at home.

Brothers and sisters are usually frightened about what is happening at the hospital. As soon as possible, the siblings must receive an age-appropriate explanation of the child's diagnosis. They need reassurance about their own health. For a while the parents may not have much time to spend with the siblings, but it is particularly important for them to know and feel the love of their parents. A warm, comfortable home environment is crucial at this time when parents cannot be at home. If possible, a familiar relative or friend should be in the home with the siblings. They should be encouraged to visit their brother and sister in the hospital to allay fears of the unknown about the child, the illness, and the hospital. Siblings are often frightened; the parents should talk with them about their fears and the seriousness of the diagnosis.

The parents may wish to have the physician or nurse describe the illness to relatives and friends who are important to them. This may relieve some of the burden on the parents, who may also feel responsible for supporting the anxieties and reactions of these other people.

Reaction of Child and Family to Treatment

Cancer treatment begins almost immediately after the diagnosis is made. To the young child, this translates to "pokes and pains." The child will soon learn to associate white coats with painful experiences. The child may cry at the mere sight of someone in white. A consistently kind and pleasant attitude from doctors and nurses will lead the child to trust in these special individuals who are providing care.

Older children and teenagers deal with the emotional stress and tension at their own pace. They may need time alone to think, cry, or scream. They may be afraid to be alone and seek the constant presence of parents, friends, and staff. Others may want to deny the gravity of the situation for a while and try to laugh off what is going on. Many teenagers are too proud to show depression or dependence. They must be allowed to take charge with some degree of independence. Older children and teenagers may react in any or all of these ways. The nurse must recognize clues in verbal and nonverbal behavior and allow patients to express themselves as they feel most comfortable.

Children of all ages may initially show signs of developmental regression or immaturity. That reaction is understandable, considering the seriousness of the situation and the demands that are placed on them. With consistent kindness, parents must continue to maintain some standard of discipline and expectations of acceptable behavior. Fortunately, most children with cancer seem to withstand the emotional and physical strain, growing up with the strength of having faced and weathered very serious problems at an early age.

Most children's hospitals have rooming-in programs for parents, and parents are encouraged to participate in treatments, usually as hand-holders. Procedures must be explained fully before they are performed. Even though the child and family have been told about the procedure by their physician, the nurse should again give a brief explanation. This provides an opportunity for them to ask questions and clarify their understanding.

Children must feel comfortable and safe before a threatening procedure is performed. A parent's presence in the treatment room can provide that feeling of safety. Young children may squirm and fight a procedure even after it has been explained. Thus the kindest thing to do is to speak to the child quietly and calmly, hold the child gently and firmly, and complete the procedure quickly. The nurse can be particularly effective by talking to the child and offering encouragement in enduring the procedure. Physicians and nurses must also be sure that local anesthesia is adequate before a procedure is done. Although these painful procedures must be done as part of the treatment, perhaps some fun can be associated with the painful ordeal, such as picking a trinket from a toy box after each visit to the treatment room. Hypnotherapy is a new venture which may be successful if appropriate staff such as psychologists, social workers, or nurses trained in this area are available (Olness and Gardner, 1988).

Home Care

When the child is well enough for discharge, the parents become the primary caregivers. The nurse plays a major role in preparing parents for this responsibility from the first day of hospital admission. (See Chapter 32 for further discussion of principles and strategies of home care.) To care for their child at home, parents must understand the disease, its treatment, and its possible complications. They must be comfortable and confident in their ability to care for their child. There is a great deal of new information for them to remember. The nurse can provide a written explanation of the disease and related articles or booklets as ready reference for parents to use at home. Sometimes it is hard to give specific guidelines for home care, but general hints in writing are helpful. The nurse can design calendars of the treatment plan for parents to follow. They should have phone numbers for 24-hour medical assistance, and they should be encouraged to call if any specific questions or concerns arise. Most children with cancer receive chemotherapy. The nurse should provide lists of the drugs in writing, with their possible side effects. Most chemotherapy drugs will cause low blood counts. Parents should understand the different levels of blood counts so that when the child is home they can plan activities according to any specific limitations dictated by test results. Many parents like to keep diaries of what has been happening to the child between clinic visits. These help them to feel more comfortable as historians on the child's interim medical condition.

When the child is home, getting back into the normal family routine is very important. The child with cancer will need special medical treatment, hospitalization, and frequent clinic visits, but this must not totally disrupt family life or fulfillment of the needs of each family member. Sibling rivalries can arise out of jealousy for the sick child's special treatment and attention. Parents and friends must remember the needs of all children in the family. Each member needs special attention and loving from the others. This does not mean material gifts but rather time spent with a child or parents. Offering to stay with children at home when the patient goes to the clinic or hospital is a caring gift, for example. It can be easy for the mother engrossed in caring for the child with cancer to forget her obligations to the rest of the family. The father may feel "left out" because he must be at work and cannot be present at many clinic visits. The nurse should assess how the family is coping with these typical stresses and suggest that they make the clinic visits a family affair when possible.

Maintaining as much normality as possible is imperative for the child with cancer. It is important for the nurse to support and foster a quick return to normal activities, especially schooling. Since most teachers have never dealt with cancer in their classroom, the nurse should communicate directly with teachers, explaining the diagnosis and its treatment. Classmates likewise need a formal group explanation of what is going on to allay any of their fears and misconceptions.

Clinic visits need not mean only pain and treatment to the young child. The presence of a play therapist and toys in the clinic can add some fun to the day. A stop at a favorite restaurant after each visit can provide something for the child to look forward to. The nurse can also suggest that the parents occasionally bring the child to visit the hospital or clinic just for fun, when no treatment is given. Older children and teenagers often develop great trust and strong friendships with their oncology nurses. Just being there, talking, and showing a sincere interest in their lives provides the patients with an atmosphere that makes them truly feel that they will be "okay." With careful, thoughtful nursing interventions, the hospital and clinic may gradually be viewed as more comfortable, supportive, and friendly.

The Nurse's Role in Supporting Parents

As time goes by, the parents tend to become more relaxed, but they still realize each day that their child has cancer. Years ago if children had cancer, they would almost surely die. Now there is great variability in prognosis, depending on the diagnosis and stage of disease. Statistics can be offered parents, but they are difficult to apply to an individual child. The fact that much time has elapsed following the initial diagnosis does not mean that the child no longer has cancer or that the parents can cease to be concerned that the child will die. The nurse has a major responsibility in helping parents through this difficult time; fears and feelings of anger and despair must be expressed. Parents need the opportunity to tell another caring person how it feels to be threatened by a loss of the joys that their child brings. The nurse can offer tremendous support by being available to the family for that purpose. The nurse should also help the family find additional community and support resources. In many cities support groups have been formed of parents of children with cancer; these are excellent sources of information and emotional sharing. There are also national organizations for parents of children with cancer. There are many good publications and newsletters that help parents realize that other families have similar problems and concerns. They also offer information about progress in research and current treatment reports.

Having a child with cancer can be a tremendous financial burden to a family. Even if the family has good medical insurance, there are still many nonmedical expenses, such as transportation to the clinic, meals at the hospital, and babysitters for siblings while the parents are away. Parents must be aware of all available resources in their area, such as state aid for chronically ill children, the American Cancer Society, and various leukemia foundations. Ronald McDonald houses have been built near many major children's hospitals to provide families with inexpensive housing while they are away from home.

The Child Who Dies

Although the statistics for children with cancer have been improving, nearly 45 per cent of children with cancer died in the reporting period between 1977 and 1980 (Leventhal, 1987). When it becomes obvious that a child has reached a terminal state, he or she will sense a change in the mood of the family. The child will have many scary feelings about what is happening. He or she may have many questions. Chapter 26 is devoted to discussions of children and death. The nurse should help parents understand their child's views of the situation. Parents should be encouraged to answer questions honestly. Children and teenagers may not be able to put their feelings into words. The child may need to express his or her inner feelings in some way. The child needs reassurance. Children of all ages need to know that their parents will always be there with them, and parents must know that all medical means will be used to prevent undue pain and suffering for their child.

Most parents will know when the child's fight for survival has become futile. They may never before have experienced the death of a loved one. They may have many questions about the actual event of death. A staff member who is close to the family should talk about these things with the parents. It is not morbid to talk about funeral arrangements before the child dies, so that at that time of death parents will be spared some of the agonizing chores. This concrete discussion of death will often initiate mourning, which may reduce despair at the time of death. Parents need one or two special staff members to support them more than at any previous time.

There is an increasing trend for parents to have the child die at home where he or she is most comfortable. This possibility should be explored with parents. If they do wish the child to be at home, the nurse or other special staff member should prepare them for any emergency that may arise. They should have 24-hour support available to them by phone. Visiting nurses can make regular visits to check on physical abnormalities and help with their management. Parents should be prepared for common preterminal events such as changes of consciousness, alteration of respirations, loss of bowel or bladder continence, and emesis.

During this terminal stage the needs of other family members must not be forgotten. Siblings need every opportunity to release their emotions and express their fears. Contact with their dying brother or sister should be maintained as long as communication is possible, to allay regrets about not having said last words or last goodbyes. A brother or sister may feel responsible for the sibling's death because of an old argument or fight. These concerns must be addressed even when they are not expressed openly by the siblings. The dying child will look and feel very sick, so the amount of time that the children spend with the child is a personal decision for the child and parents to make. It is up to the professional team members to be aware of all these family needs and to help the parents to be aware of them.

It is emotionally very difficult for nurses to face death in any patient. The death of a child can be particularly difficult to understand and accept. Sometimes it is hard for nurses to become involved with children whom they know will die. The nurse's important role is to provide warmth and kindness, with every attention given to the child's comfort. Table 31-2, the nursing process plan for the hospitalized child, specifies alterations in nursing strategies for a child who is terminally ill. If nurses can know that they helped a short life to be a more comfortable one, they will be rewarded inwardly and embraced outwardly for their care by the grateful families of these children.

The family that has come to rely on the persons in the cancer center cannot be forgotten once the patient has died. A social worker or community health nurse can help families get through these difficult times. The child may be dead, but he or she will never be forgotten and will be a part of the parents' and siblings' everyday life for a long time. Many parents realize the bond of friendship that has grown between them and the health team during the child's illness. As a sign of this friendship, parents should be urged to come back to see the team members at any time. It is rewarding to know that a large number of parents return to visit frequently, and some have been willing to talk with other parents and continue to be active in parent groups.

The Association of Pediatric Oncology Nurses (APON), which was founded in 1976, is a nursing organization that is devoted to fostering high-quality care for children with cancer. Its annual meetings, quarterly journal, and other publications provide means of sharing ideas and support among pediatric oncology nurses.

Survivors of Childhood Cancer

As more and more children survive cancer, issues concerning their subsequent state of physical and emotional health are being addressed. In fact, childhood cancer survivors may face health hazards that are in part caused by the same therapy that allowed them to live. "Late effects" is the colloquialism used to describe the range of posttherapeutic disabilities that are seen in survivors of pediatric cancer. The exact nature, timing, and severity of the development of late effects depend on (1) the extent and location of the cancer, (2) the modalities and intensity of treatment, and (3) the age and developmental stage of the child at the time of treatment.

Late effects can involve any organ system. Findings can range from clinically insignificant laboratory abnormalities to serious, life-threatening complications. The time interval to the onset of late sequelae is unpredictable. The following areas are of particular concern in the survivor population:

1. *Damage to the central nervous system: psychosocial, neurologic, and intellectual.* The milieu of stress, anxiety, and dependency that surrounds children with cancer can leave them unprepared to face adult life. Treatment that was directed to the central nervous system, such as cranial radiation and intrathecal chemotherapy, has in many cases caused documented damage to the brain with related subnormal intelligence and neurologic dysfunction.

2. *Impaired growth and development.* Growth and development can be impaired in any child with a chronic illness. Some children treated for cancer have

added direct insults to growth that include, most significantly, radiation to the pituitary gland and other growing bones and organs.

3. *Gonadal development and reproduction aberrations.* Systemic chemotherapy with alkylating agents and gonadal radiation can affect gonadal development and function of children treated for cancer. Some children will need hormonal replacement to artificially produce advancement to normal adult gonadal development.

4. *Oncogenesis.* For reasons that are unclear, childhood cancer survivors are at a greatly increased risk of developing a second, perhaps totally unrelated, malignancy within a relatively short time after their initial diagnosis. This oncogenicity may be related to the cancer treatment, immune disturbances induced by the disease or its treatment, or the individual's own genetic susceptibility.

5. *Disruption of function in other organ systems.* Chemotherapy, surgery, and radiation can cause acute toxicity to specific organ systems such as the heart, kidneys, liver, lungs, bone, and gastrointestinal tract. That acute toxicity has the potential to develop into chronic, lifelong health problems.

This overview is by no means complete. Late effects in childhood cancer survivors is an issue that has been granted increasing attention in recent years. It is acknowledged that quality of survival is just as important as survival itself. Research now documents the imperative need for close, continued follow-up and monitoring of childhood cancer survivors. Early recognition and prompt management of sequelae may, in some cases, lessen the severity of residual problems.

Malignant Diseases in Childhood

The remainder of this chapter deals with specific malignant diseases that occur in childhood. Because chemotherapy is common to the treatment of many of these malignancies, the nursing process plan for this chapter details nursing strategies for the child undergoing chemotherapy (Table 48-4).

Leukemia

Leukemia is the most common form of childhood cancer. Although leukemia may have its onset at any age, its peak incidence is between the ages of 3 and 5 (Steinherz, 1987). Leukemia is a proliferation of abnormal white blood cells in the body. Death comes from secondary complications resulting from the presence in vital tissues of these abnormal cells. To understand why children with leukemia die and how the leukemic cells affect the body, it is important to have a basic understanding of the origin and function of normal blood cells.

Normal Blood Components

Whole blood is composed of plasma and cells. *Plasma* is the fluid portion of the blood. The solid, or cellular, portion is composed of red cells, white cells, and platelets circulating in the plasma. Red cells carry oxygen to the body tissues from the lungs. Oxygen provides tissues with a vital ingredient of all cell metabolism. *Hemoglobin* is the oxygen-carrying protein of red blood cells and imparts a pink or red appearance to the skin, lips, and nails. Normal hemoglobin from the age of 2 to 5 is about 12 to 13 gm/dl. *Platelets* are the tiny cells that promote clotting and prevent bleeding. A normal platelet count is 200,000 to 400,000/mm^3. The white blood cells form the body's defense against infection. Normal total white blood count is 5000 to 10,000/mm^3. The three major types of white blood cells are *granulocytes, lymphocytes,* and *monocytes.* In addition, there are three major types of granulocytes: *neutrophils, eosinophils,* and *basophils.* (See also Chapter 40, page 1342, and Figure 40-2.)

While caring for children with malignant disease it is important to know about white blood cells and their specific functions. Table 48-5 summarizes the kinds of white blood cells, the proportion of these cells in the normal white blood count (WBC), and their major function. When a differential count is done, the percentage of each type of white cell is reported.

Words used to describe the most mature neutrophils are *segmented,* or *segs, polymorphonuclear (polys),* or *bands,* and *stab cells* (*stabs*). The absolute

Table 48-5. Categories of White Blood Cells and Their Functions

White Cell Type	Mean* Per Cent in Normal WBC	Function
Granulocytes		
Neutrophils	55	Ingest and digest bacteria during bacterial infection
Eosinophils	2	Summon antigen-antibody response in allergic reactions
Basophils	1	Specific action unknown
Lymphocytes	38	Effect cellular and humoral immunity; produce specific antibodies against viruses, bacteria, and other proteins
Monocytes	5	Act as phagocytes in bacterial infections and are an integral part of normal immune response

* Relatively wide range.

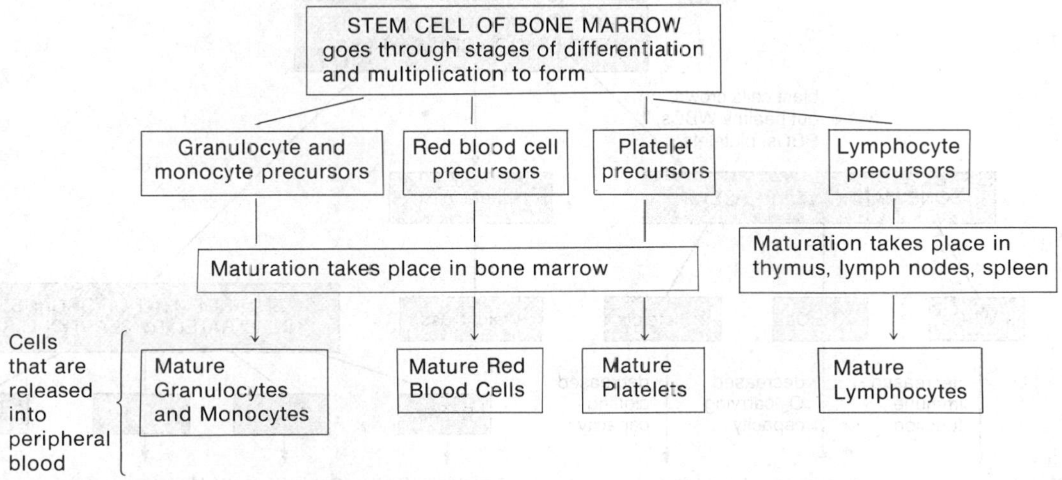

Figure 48-5. Blood cell production in the body.

neutrophil count (ANC) is the total (or absolute) number of neutrophils in the blood. ANC is found by multiplying the percentage of functional neutrophils (segs and bands) in the differential by the total white count. Thus if the WBC is 8000/mm^3 and the differential lists 40 per cent segmented forms, the ANC is 40 per cent of 8000, or 3200/mm^3. Since neutrophils are very important in protecting against infection, the ANC is a guideline of the body's ability to fight bacterial disease. Serious bacterial infection may occur when the ANC is less than 500/mm^3. Knowing normal values and those that are associated with increased risk of infection is very helpful in developing guidelines for caring for the child with cancer, since chemotherapy, radiotherapy, and leukemia itself are often associated with low neutrophil values.

Blood cells are produced in the *bone marrow,* the soft material located in the cavities of bones. All blood cells arise from a common cell called the *stem cell.* Under genetic control, stem cells in the marrow differentiate to form red blood cells, white blood cells, and platelets. Once a cell has differentiated into the parent cell of a red cell, a granulocytic white cell, or a platelet, it continues to undergo division while maturing into a functional cell ready to work for the body. In the normal state the bone marrow releases only these mature, functional cells into the peripheral blood. Lymphocytes arise from the stem cell, but as soon as the commitment to this cell takes place, further maturation occurs in the thymus, lymph nodes, and spleen. The exact site of monocytic maturation is unknown. Figure 48-5 illustrates the process of blood cell production.

Pathophysiology

With the information that leukemia is a proliferation of abnormal white blood cells, and relating that information to knowledge of the normal blood, two statements about leukemia can be made: (1) The abnormal white blood cell continues to divide but may not mature beyond the blast state. It is released into the peripheral blood as a blast. Leukemic blasts have no normal functional capabilities. (2) As the abnormal white blood cells increase in number, fewer and fewer normal cells are made, so that at the time of diagnosis the percentage of abnormal cells in the marrow is usually 80 to 100 per cent of the cells present. The lack of normal cells accounts for the symptoms seen in leukemia and, in large part, accounts for death from the disease. The pathophysiology in acute leukemia that leads to clinical manifestations is diagrammed in Figure 48-6.

Etiology

The etiology of leukemia is unknown. It is known that a few cases of leukemia in adults have been linked to exposure to environmental factors such as radiation or chemicals. The role of inheritance in the development of leukemia is demonstrated by the enhanced incidence of leukemia in identical twins. If an identical twin has leukemia, the twin has a 1 in 4 chance of developing leukemia (Steinherz, 1987). Leukemia in nontwin siblings is extremely rare.

Several genetically determined diseases have also been associated with an increased incidence of leukemia. Children with Down syndrome, Fanconi hypoplastic anemia, agammaglobulinemia, and Bloom syndrome have shown a higher incidence of leukemia (Fochtman et al, 1982). However, even though incidence is increased, the majority of children with genetic predisposition for leukemia remain free of the disease (Steinherz, 1987). Several of the genetic defects listed are associated with immune deficiencies. Although the Ebstein-Barr (EB) virus has been associated with Burkitt lymphoma and nasopharyngeal carcinoma, no other specific virus is known to be causally

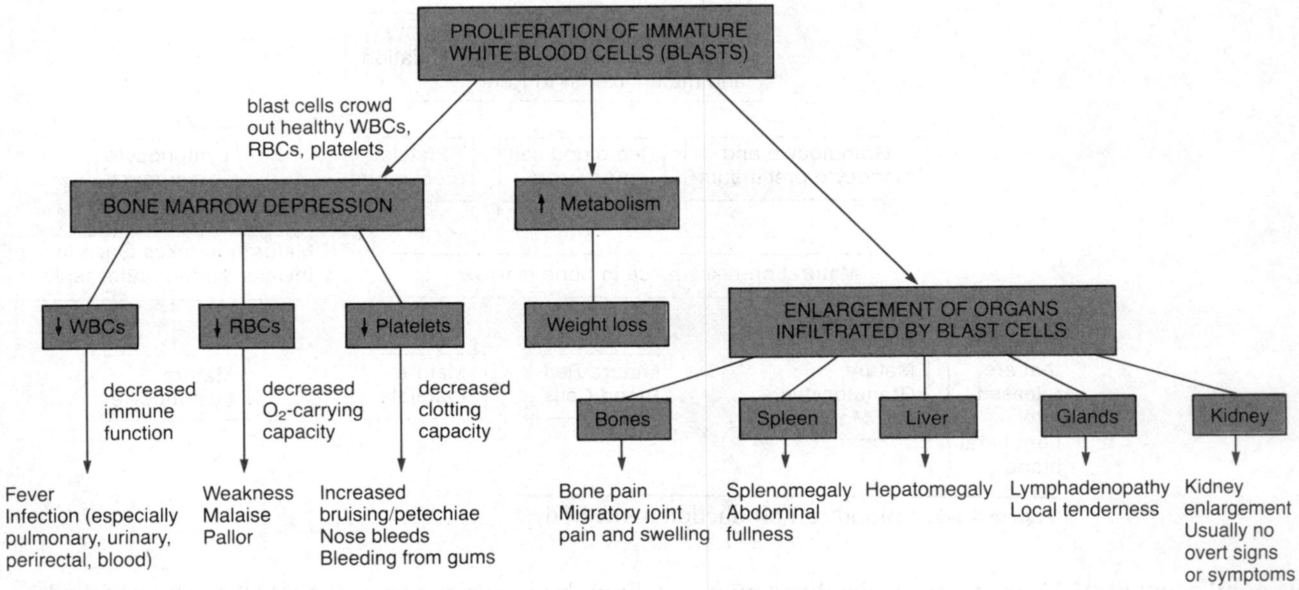

Figure 48-6. Pathophysiology leading to clinical manifestations in acute leukemia.

related to the development of leukemia or other malignancies, with the exception of the human T-cell leukemia virus, which is etiologically related to adult T-cell leukemia. Research seeking an answer to the etiology of leukemia continues with the investigation of carcinogens, viruses, genetics, and other potential etiologic factors.

Types of Leukemia

There are several different types of leukemia, classified on the basis of the course of disease and the morphology of the cells. Each type is associated with a different prognosis and characteristics, making it important for the nurse to know what kind of leukemia each child has.

Whereas leukemia in adults is more often chronic, most childhood leukemia has an acute course (97 per cent). Acute leukemia has a short history of symptoms and, without treatment, a rapidly declining course to death within 3 to 6 months. Chronic leukemias have a more gradual onset and a course extending over two or more years. Chronic granulocytic leukemia is rarely seen in children; chronic lymphocytic leukemia does not occur in children.

The morphology of the white blood cells involved in the disease also varies. The most common childhood leukemia (80 to 85 per cent) is acute lymphoblastic leukemia (ALL), which results from malignant change of the lymphocyte or its precursors and is acute in onset (Maguire, 1987). Less common in childhood are acute granulocytic leukemia (AGL) and acute monocytic leukemia. Because the cells in the granulocytic and monocytic types are so varied, they are collectively referred to as acute nonlymphocytic leukemia (ANLL). When the cells resemble neither myeloblasts nor lymphoblasts, the diagnosis of acute undifferentiated leukemia (AUL) is applied. Once classified as a separate category of leukemia, it is now most commonly listed as a subtype of acute nonlymphocytic leukemia (Gale and Foon, 1986; Hakami and Monzon, 1987). Tables 48-6 and 48-7 list the two major types of acute leukemia in children, their subtypes, and their prognosis.

Long-Term Outcome

The outlook for a child with leukemia depends upon many prognostic variables, not the least of which is the primary histology. With present-day treatment options a child with ALL has a 95 per cent chance of obtaining an initial remission and a 75 per cent chance of surviv-

Table 48-6. Subtypes of Acute Lymphocytic Leukemia (ALL)

Subtypes in Order of Incidence	Prognosis
Null-cell	Most favorable prognosis; approximately 95% will enter remission, 75% of those will be in remission 5 years from the onset of therapy; majority will achieve cure
Pre B-cell	Although 95% achieve remission, only about 60% will be in remission 5 years from the start of therapy
T-cell	Curable in a minority of patients
B-cell	Rarely curable

(Based on Leventhal, 1987.)

Table 48-7. Subtypes of Acute Nonlymphocytic Leukemia (ANLL)

Subtypes	Overall Incidence and Prognosis
M1, Undifferentiated myelocytic M2, Myelocytic M3, Promyelocytic M4, Myelomonocytic M5a, Monoblastic M5b, Differentiated monocytic M6, Erythroleukemic M7, Megakaryocytic	The great majority (70–90%) of cases of ANLL are made up of M1, M2, and M4. Overall, 60–80% will obtain a remission; 15–20% will die of infection and/or hemorrhage during induction. About 50% of those who obtain remission sustain it, with a 30–40% cure rate overall. Children with M4 and M5 variants appear to have a higher incidence of CNS involvement

(Based on Gale and Foon, 1986; Hakami and Monzon, 1987; Leventhal, 1987.)

ing 5 years or more (Leventhal, 1987). By contrast, a child with ANLL has a 75 to 80 per cent chance of obtaining an initial remission; about 50 per cent of children who obtain remission stay in remission after therapy is stopped (Hakami and Monzon, 1987; Leventhal, 1987). ANLL is less responsive to available chemotherapeutic agents than is ALL even when aggressive therapy is used. Although leukemia relapses can occur after 5 years, present data support the fact that most children who survive 5 years are continuing in prolonged remission. Up to 80 per cent of children with ALL are achieving a cure and 30 to 40 per cent with ANLL can be cured (Leventhal, 1987; Gale and Hoffbrand, 1986).

Studies of ALL involving large numbers of children have identified prognostic factors that indicate how children with leukemia will fare with their disease. Most children who at diagnosis are 2 to 10 years of age and have total white blood counts of less than 10,000/mm³ may have up to a 90 per cent chance of being alive 5 years after diagnosis and are called "good risk." Children with high white blood counts (greater than 50,000/mm³), infants less than 1 year of age, and children with large bulky disease at diagnosis are considered to be at high risk and have an unfavorable prognosis (Steinherz, 1987).

It is important to note the continually improving prognosis for children with leukemia. In 1948 the first drug to effect a remission in leukemia was used. Before that time every child who developed leukemia died. Today the outlook for children with leukemia is continually changing as improved treatment plans are developed. Today's intensive treatment programs for children with both ALL and ANLL show great promise of improving the survival data included in this text.

Clinical Manifestations

Recalling that leukemic blasts crowd out normal cells in the bone marrow, it is obvious that the child may present with bone marrow depression (decreased numbers of mature white blood cells, red blood cells, and platelets). The child may have fever or obvious infection due to decreased numbers of normal white blood cells (neutropenia). A decrease in red blood cells and hemoglobin (anemia) causes weakness, malaise, and pallor. Decreased platelets may be associated with increased bruising, petechiae, or bleeding from the nose and gums. The spleen, liver, lymph nodes, thymus, and kidneys may become enlarged because of an infiltration of these tissues with blast cells. Bone pain (often accompanied by limping) is common and is due to infiltrates in the cortex of bone or the subperiosteal area. Figure 48-6 summarizes the clinical manifestations.

Diagnostic Assessment

Leukemia is suspected when a child presents with the symptoms just described. If a complete blood count (CBC) is taken, the decreased numbers of normal red blood cells, white blood cells, and platelets may be evident. This condition is known as *pancytopenia.** (Although pancytopenia occurs in the majority of children with leukemia, some children have an elevated WBC count at the time of diagnosis [Steinherz, 1987].) Leukemic blasts may be seen in the blood smear. The definitive diagnosis is made after examining a sample of bone marrow (see Table 48-1). To obtain a bone marrow specimen in the child, an area of accessible marrow, usually the anterior or posterior iliac crest or vertebral spine, is treated with local anesthesia. A small skin wheal and a small amount of anesthesia in the periosteum is necessary. A heavy, wide-gauge needle with a stylet is inserted into the marrow space and the marrow is aspirated with a syringe. To the naked eye, bone marrow looks like blood, but when put onto slides and studied under a microscope it has characteristic histologic features. Normal marrow contains less than 5 per cent of normal stem cells *(hemocytoblasts).* Most leukemic patients at diagnosis will have about 90 per cent abnormal leukemic blasts (immature white blood cells) in their bone marrow.

* Pancytopenia is the abnormal depression of all blood cells, i.e., WBCs, RBCs, and platelets.

Therapeutic Management

Remission is the term used to describe an absence of detectable leukemic cells in the marrow following treatment. A *relapse* is the reappearance of leukemic cells in a marrow that has been in remission. Once relapse has occurred, a second remission can be achieved, but this tends to be more difficult. Remission is of shorter duration with each successive relapse. Thus *the major aim of initial treatment is to achieve a primary remission that lasts without relapse.*

Treatment protocols are highly individualized and follow complex guidelines. In general, however, treatment can be considered in three stages: induction, central nervous system (CNS) prophylaxis, and maintenance.

Induction. Induction is the term used for the initial treatment period of chemotherapy that induces or brings about remission. Remission occurs when leukemic cells have been reduced to undetectable levels (less than 5 per cent bone marrow blast cells). Vincristine, prednisone, and L-asparaginase, with or without an agent such as doxorubicin or daunorubicin, are often used in induction treatment in ALL. In ANNL, drugs to induce remission include daunorubicin and doxorubicin, cytosine, etoposide, and 5-azacytidine (Hakami and Monzon, 1987). Induction treatment is the most intensive and potentially the most life-threatening because of the bone marrow depression associated with antineoplastic drugs. The child is at risk for bleeding and infection during the period of drug treatment, and until the bone marrow can resupply healthy blood cells.

CNS Prophylaxis. CNS prophylaxis is instituted to prevent development of leukemia within the central nervous system. Normal cerebrospinal fluid contains less than $5/mm^3$ white blood cells, and these are usually lymphocytes or monocytes. Leukemic cells are thought to enter the central nervous system from meningeal capillaries when the peripheral blood contains blasts. The blast cells can remain in nongrowth phases for variable periods of time before increasing in number and causing symptoms. The usual symptoms are those of increased intracranial pressure and include headache, nausea, and vomiting. Cranial nerve palsies, especially of the 6th and 7th nerves, are not uncommon, and occasionally seizures may occur. CNS leukemia can also be asymptomatic. A complication of leukemic cells in the spinal fluid is their ability to extend along nerve roots through the vertebral foramina. The child who has this problem can have variable motor weakness depending on the degree of root compression.

Most drugs given systemically do not cross the blood-brain barrier to a very great extent, so that CNS treatment must consist of administering drugs directly into the cerebrospinal fluid. This is done by injecting a limited number of chemotherapeutic agents directly into the spinal fluid via lumbar puncture (intrathecal). Methotrexate has been used most often for this purpose, but cytosine arabinoside, hydrocortisone sodium succinate, and other agents can also be given. The three drugs may be used in combination intrathecally. The second form of therapy that is effective in treating CNS leukemia is radiotherapy directed to the brain and spinal cord. Radiotherapy is limited by the total dose that can be tolerated by the CNS tissue.

Early studies showed that more than 50 per cent of children with leukemia would develop CNS leukemia during their disease course. Treatment to prevent CNS involvement is now given as part of the standard initial therapy so that any cells present will be eradicated at the same time that the marrow and other tissues are cleared of blasts. Most investigators have referred to such treatment as "prophylactic," in that it is given when children are asymptomatic and the cerebrospinal fluid is normal. However, some children develop CNS leukemia in spite of such "prophylaxis." CNS leukemia can occur without bone marrow relapse (that is, leukemic cells can be found in the spinal fluid when bone marrow is free of disease).

Most practitioners use a combination of cranial radiation and intrathecal methotrexate for CNS prophylaxis. Children who are thought to be at low risk for leukemic relapse may receive intrathecal methotrexate during maintenance therapy in lieu of prophylactic cranial radiation, in hopes of avoiding late sequelae thought to be caused by CNS radiation. Children who receive cranial radiation may be at risk to develop long-term problems involving memory and cognitive learning, although these changes are often subtle.

Children with resistant CNS disease may be given chemotherapy intracranially via a special reservoir. The Ommaya reservoir is a permanent mechanical reservoir and catheter that is implanted in the ventricular system to facilitate the instillation of drugs. It thus expedites the process whereby drugs reach the brain. Various types of vascular access ports (e.g., Medi-port, distributed by Cormed) are also being used. These devices are implanted subcutaneously and connected to a catheter that provides access to the circulation or to body cavities (Hagle, 1987).

Maintenance. Maintenance therapy provides chemotherapy to maintain the remission. Maintenance treatment is usually given for 2 to 3 years, although the optimal duration of therapy for ALL has not been clearly defined. Standard maintenance therapy in ALL often involves daily oral 6-mercaptopurine, weekly methotrexate, and monthly vincristine and prednisone (Steinherz, 1987). Additional agents may be given to children who require more than conventional therapy. These agents are similar to those described for induction therapy. Because treatment for ANLL remains less effective than for ALL, the duration of chemotherapy and optimal combinations of drugs for maintenance therapy are less well established (Hakami and Monzon, 1987).

Relapse

Children with ALL who relapse after discontinuing chemotherapy usually do so within the first year off the drugs. Those who relapse within 6 months have a significantly poorer prognosis. Relapse may occur at any time, however, even after 9 years or more of continuous remission. There is currently no way to predict which children will sustain remission and which will not (Steinherz, 1987). Children with ANLL relapse more frequently than children with ALL. With either type of leukemia, the prognosis becomes increasingly more grave with each relapse.

Diagnosis of relapse may occur as a result of evidence of increased blast cells in the bone marrow or elsewhere in the body, such as leukemic cells in the cerebrospinal fluid or in the testicles. Relapse is treated with "reinduction" of antineoplastic agents and, in some cases, with additional radiotherapy and bone marrow transplant.

Testicular Leukemia. The male testis is the second most common site of extramedullary (leukemia cells present outside of the bone marrow) relapse after CNS leukemia. It occurs in 8 to 33 per cent of boys with ALL (Steinherz, 1987), but is rare in boys with ANLL. The sign of overt testicular leukemia is a firm, enlarged testis. It may also be discovered in the occult stage (undetectable by physical examination) with testicular biopsy. This complication may occur without marrow relapse, but it is often a predictor of future marrow change. It is most apt to occur in males who present with high-risk prognostic factors at the time of diagnosis. Treatment of testicular leukemia includes testicular radiation and systemic reinduction therapy.

Bone Marrow Transplantation

Bone marrow transplantation is an alternative form of therapy for children with leukemia. Currently it may be employed as the treatment of choice for newly diagnosed patients with ANLL in remission and for relapsed patients with ALL who are in a second or third remission.

The purpose of a bone marrow transplant is to provide the child with healthy bone marrow that can produce functional blood cells. A bone marrow transplant can thus reverse the effects of severe bone marrow depression. A bone marrow transplant can make it possible to use higher, and potentially curative, doses of chemotherapy and radiation because the child can be "rescued" from life-threatening bone marrow depression by the transplanted marrow cells. Additionally, there is evidence that immune cells in the transplanted marrow may help to kill remaining leukemic cells in the host (Gale and Champlin, 1986).

There are three types of bone marrow transplants: autologous, syngeneic, and allogeneic. *Autologous* transplants infuse bone marrow cells previously harvested from the child. Autologous transplants in leukemia, however, carry the risk of relapse because the bone marrow is the site of origin of the disease (Vega et al, 1987). If the bone marrow for transplant is not the child's own, it must be donated by a person who is histocompatible with the patient. Histocompatibility is the degree of immunologic likeness between donor and recipient; a good match reduces the likelihood of graft-versus-host disease, discussed below. A *syngeneic* transplant is bone marrow donated by an identical twin. In an *allogeneic* transplant, the donor is not genetically identical but compatible, such as a sibling. A full sibling has a one in four chance of matching a brother or sister. Parents and other relatives have only a remote chance of matching the child.

Prior to a bone marrow transplant, most children receive a short course of intensive chemotherapy (such as high-dose cyclophosphamide) and total-body irradiation. This therapy is termed "conditioning" and is delivered for three purposes: (1) to eradicate leukemic cells to the extent possible and thereby decrease the chance of posttransplant relapse, (2) to suppress the host's immune response to the transplanted tissue, and (3) to create space in the bone marrow to allow the newly transplanted stem cells to generate healthy blood components (Vega et al, 1987).

Bone marrow is harvested from the donor by multiple bone marrow aspirations from the iliac crest. This procedure is conducted under general anesthesia. The donated bone marrow is then processed and transfused into the host intravenously. It takes time for transfused marrow to implant and produce new blood cells. The child will remain myelosuppressed (bone marrow suppressed) for an average of 3 weeks after transplant. Transfusions of packed red blood cells and platelets are usually required during the first month. During this period of bone marrow suppression, the child is at risk for infection and bleeding (Vega et al, 1987).

Graft-versus-Host Disease. Graft-versus-host disease (GVHD) is a serious complication of allogeneic bone marrow transplants. GVHD occurs when T-lymphocytes in the donated bone marrow react against tissues in the host. About 10 per cent of children under 10 years of age develop acute GVHD within 3 to 4 months after transplant (typically between the 2nd and 10th weeks). In older patients the incidence rises to 30 to 50 per cent (Vega et al, 1987). Clinical manifestations of acute GVHD begin with a maculopapular rash on the palms and soles that may spread to the entire body. The liver may be involved, as evident by a rise in serum bilirubin and alkaline phosphatase. Gastrointestinal manifestations include nausea, abdominal pain, and diarrhea.

Chronic GVHD may follow the acute disease or develop without acute involvement. It may develop up to a year or more after transplant. Again, the skin is involved, with dryness, pigmentation abnormalities, and lichenified lesions or plaques. Gastrointestinal involvement is common, and immunologic function may be impaired by abnormal T-cell and B-cell function. (See Chapter 43 for a discussion of T-cell and B-cell functions.)

GVHD is treated with corticosteroids and other immunosuppressive drugs with varying degrees of success. The best "treatment" is still prevention. Pre- and posttransplant immunosuppressive therapy is used in an attempt to reduce the incidence of GVHD. Depletion of T-lymphocytes from donor marrow is another approach, although this therapy remains somewhat controversial (Gale and Champlin, 1986).

Survival statistics for children who have undergone bone marrow transplantation are promising. As reported by Vega and colleagues (1987), a study of children with ANLL in first remission showed a greater than 50 per cent survival rate post-bone marrow transplantation. Another study they reviewed showed a 33 per cent survival rate for children with ALL in second remission, with a median duration of remission of 19 months. Six months was the median duration of remission for a control group of similar patients treated with chemotherapy alone.

Bone marrow transplant centers are limited in the United States, so many families must relocate for 1 to 3 months. It is very important for the nurse at the primary hospital to prepare the child and the family for the transplant procedure and to maintain contact with them throughout their stay at the transplant center. The child and the family need unlimited support to meet the stress and anxiety imposed by the transplant procedure.

Major Nursing Diagnoses for Leukemia

***Potential for injury: physiologic, related to bone marrow suppression, associated with** the proliferative production of blast cells and the resultant decrease in normal levels of mature blood cells:*

- *decreased RBCs (anemia)*
- *decreased WBCs (neutropenia/leukopenia)*
- *decreased platelets (thrombocytopenia)*

***Fear/anxiety,** related to:*

- *diagnosis of a life-threatening disease*
- *invasive diagnostic and therapeutic procedures*
- *hospital environment/disruption of usual activities and schedules*
- *separation from family and peers*

***Disturbance in self-concept: body image, related to expected alopecia and cushingoid** features associated with chemotherapy and radiation therapy*

***Knowledge deficit (child and family),** related to:*

- *normal function of WBCs and the systemic effects of the proliferation of immature blast cells*
- *significance of diagnostic tests and procedures*
- *signs and symptoms of relapse*
  (a) resumption of presenting signs and symptoms
  (b) bone pain
- *side effects of medications (see also Table 48-3)*
- *child's developmental capability to understand and deal with the diagnosis*
- *ways to facilitate the child's coping with the emotional and physical trauma of painful, invasive procedures (see also Table 48-4)*

Strategies for Nursing Care

Special care for the child with leukemia should include emotional support for the child and the family, provision of maximal physical comfort, and management of problems that relate to low blood values and to drug side effects. Table 48-4 provides a comprehensive guide for care of the child undergoing chemotherapy and addresses the major nursing diagnoses identified for the child with acute leukemia.

Initial supportive care depends on the blood counts at diagnosis and the complications present. Nurses caring for children with leukemia should be aware of the child's current hematologic status. Such knowledge is necessary for the nurse to remain alert to the many potential problems that may arise when counts are low or abnormal. Nurses should also be familiar with each child's specific treatment plan, especially the drugs the child is receiving. The primary nurse will likely be the main source of emotional support for the child and family. (Discussion on the family's needs and the support the nurse can offer is included later in this chapter.) It is the nurse who has the skill and is ever present to respond to the fears and distress that a child and family experience during the course of illness and treatment of leukemia.

Children with very low hemoglobins (anemia) must be observed for increasing fatigue, increasing heart rate, increasing respiratory rate, and irritability. Red blood cell transfusions can be given to correct the anemia. Children with low neutrophil counts (ANC less than 1000/mm³) must be observed for fever or other signs of infection. If a patient with a very low neutrophil count develops infection, he or she will require antibiotic therapy to help combat the infection. Children with low platelet counts (less than 20,000/mm³) must be careful to avoid traumatic injury. Epistaxis and gum bleeding are common in children with very low platelet counts. The child may require platelet transfusions to control bleeding.

The goal of treatment is to achieve and maintain a remission. The doses of chemotherapy used are derived by experience and calculated on the basis of the patient's body weight or surface area. The calculated dose may not always be tolerated; therefore, close surveillance is necessary. Drug doses are decreased when defined toxicity occurs. A child in remission on maintenance therapy often has a normal blood count and at these times is not at additional risk for bleeding. But even with a normal white blood count the child is always at some risk for infection because of the immunosuppressive effect of the majority of the chemotherapeutic agents used. These agents decrease the functional capabilities of normal lymphocytes.

Nursing Strategies for Follow-up Care in the Home or Clinic

Allow time for the family members and the child to express feelings and ask questions about:

- the physical experience of leukemia and its management
- the current visit (if in the clinic, often for a physical exam, repeat lumbar puncture, bone marrow aspiration, and/or intravenous chemotherapy)
- disruptions in family structure and personal/family activities

Assess for signs and symptoms of relapse and for side effects of medications.

Provide a supportive milieu in which the family may wait for test results.

Reinforce, with the child and family, the physicians' explanation of test results.

Assess the child's ability to cope with invasive procedures without suffering undue loss of self-esteem.

Allow opportunities for therapeutic play in which the child, using actual equipment, administers the diagnostic procedures to a doll.

Discuss with the family the child's progress on developmental tasks.

Determine if the family is receiving adequate physical and emotional support to manage successfully this phase of the child's care at home.

Reinforce previous teaching about: (1) administration of oral chemotherapeutic agents at home, and (2) care of the child who has bone marrow suppression associated with chemotherapy.

Brain Tumors

Brain tumors represent the most common solid tumor in children, accounting for about 20 per cent of childhood malignancies (Walker, 1982) and are the second most common type of cancer in children and adolescents (Finlay et al, 1987). They most often occur in the school-age years, but they can occur at any age from infancy to adulthood. Brain tumors are classified according to histology and location. About two thirds of intracranial tumors are infratentorial (below the tentorium), occurring in the posterior third of the brain, and about one third are supratentorial (above the tentorium), occurring in the anterior two thirds of the brain (Hausman, 1979) (Fig. 48-7). (The tentorium is the dura mater located between the cerebrum and cerebellum supporting the occipital lobes.) This section describes the common types of brain tumors that present in childhood.

Clinical Manifestations

The signs and symptoms of brain tumors in children are diverse and relate to the location of the tumor in the brain, the rate of tumor growth, the child's age, and the child's developmental stage. Symptoms include signs of increased intracranial pressure—most commonly headache and vomiting, seizures, diffuse or focal neurologic dysfunction, changes in behavior and personality, lack of weight gain or continuing development, and torticollis. Because many of the early symptoms of intracranial tumors are similar to those of common childhood illnesses—nausea, vomiting, headache, and irritability—early diagnosis is usually difficult. Changes in behavior in school such as decreased performance and irritability or fatigue may be attributed to school phobia or some problem that the child "will outgrow." It is usually not until significant physical changes have occurred that medical assistance is sought.

Diagnostic Assessment

If a brain tumor is suspected, one or more special studies are done. Foremost of these is a CT scan (computerized tomography). The CT scan is a noninvasive radiologic procedure that produces multiple serial pictures

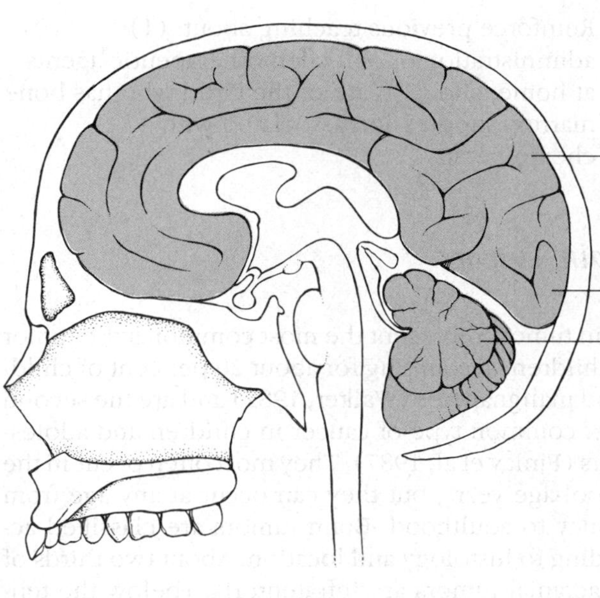

Figure 48-7. Location of supratentorial and infratentorial tumors.

of cross sections of the brain. If a contrast-enhancing isotope is given intravenously at the time of the scan, most tumors will take up the isotope and the site of the tumor is "enhanced," providing more precise definition of the tumor's size. CT scans have become the single most important study for the diagnosis of brain tumors. Additionally, magnetic resonance imaging (MRI) is now available in many medical centers. MRI is a noninvasive nuclear procedure that has proven effective for early diagnosis of some types of brain tumors and for monitoring tumor growth. Other studies may include cerebral angiography, myelogram, electroencephalogram, and lumbar puncture. Depending on the site, surgical removal or biopsy is performed.

Although these diagnostic examinations may have been explained to parents, the nurse must assess the parents' and child's need for further information or repeated information as the testing proceeds. During the diagnostic phase, the family is usually anxious and distraught once they recognize the possibility that their child may have a brain tumor. The nurse must assist the family during this phase by continually reassessing the family's ability to cope with the medical information and procedures to which they are being exposed. It is imperative that the nurse be able to provide information regarding the actual procedure to be performed, what the child can expect to feel and see during the procedure, what is expected of the child, and what the results of each test will contribute to the management of the child's care.

The parents should be permitted and encouraged to accompany the child to each procedure and to stay with the child throughout the procedure if feasible. The nurse should provide support to the child in the absence of the parents during a procedure. Parents must not be made to feel guilty if they choose not to remain with their child during a procedure.

Therapeutic Management

The treatments utilized for brain tumors are surgery, radiation therapy, chemotherapy, or combinations of these modalities.

Surgery. Ideally, surgical resection is the treatment of choice for brain tumors. Surgical resection is limited, however, to those tumors that occupy areas that can be safely resected and the extent to which the tumor invades normal surrounding brain tissue. Some tumors can only be biopsied, and in some instances biopsy itself is considered too hazardous to perform. Needle biopsies done under CT scan may be performed rather than a craniotomy. These procedures are best utilized for tumors presenting in inoperable areas.

Radiation Therapy. Radiation therapy may be employed in combination with surgery or it may be used alone as primary treatment. The success of radiotherapy depends on the tumor being treated. Some tumors are highly responsive and can be cured by this modality alone. However, many that respond to radiotherapy initially may recur after variable periods of time.

The child undergoing radiation therapy has unique needs that must be addressed in terms of nursing management. Short-term goals involve assisting the child and family to understand how successful this treatment is expected to be. The nurse must assess the level of fear and anxiety associated with the treatment. The family needs information regarding side effects during therapy, such as hair loss, nausea, and anorexia, and the potential need for a ventricular shunt should intracranial pressure increase in spite of steroid therapy with dexamethasone. (See Chapter 46 for further information about ventricular shunts.)

Information regarding the length of treatment and how it is given must be provided and understood. Very young children may require sedation for each therapy session, and many will need a plaster cast, made to help children hold perfectly still.

Chemotherapy. The role of chemotherapy in the treatment of brain tumors still requires definition. Many studies have shown several chemotherapeutic agents or combinations of agents to be effective in recurrent tumors by causing either regression of symptoms or tumor regression as measured by CT scans.

Chemotherapy has limited usefulness, in part because of the "blood–brain" barrier, which interferes with the concentration of systemic drugs in the CNS. Drugs that are lipid soluble such as nitrosoureas and steroids most effectively penetrate the blood–brain barrier. Additional controlled studies are necessary to evaluate further the potential role of chemotherapy in the treatment of children with brain tumors.

Major Nursing Diagnoses for Brain Tumors

Disturbance in self-concept: body image, *related to cutting/shaving of hair associated with brain surgery*

Potential for injury: physiologic: depression of autonomic function, *related to postoperative edema affecting the brain stem associated with removal of posterior fossa (infratentorial) tumors*

Altered tissue perfusion: cerebral: increased intracranial pressure, *related to*

- *edema of brain tissue associated with surgery*
- *postoperative intracranial bleeding*
- *malfunctioning of ventricular shunt (infratentorial tumors)*

Altered comfort: nausea and vomiting, *related to*

- *prolonged anesthesia required for neurosurgery*
- *shifts in intracranial fluid volume associated with release of pressure through tumor removal and/or shunting*

Potential for injury: physiologic: subdural hemorrhage (infratentorial tumors), *related to rapid decompression of cerebral ventricles associated with rapid drainage of cerebrospinal fluid through the ventricular shunt*

Potential for infection: postoperative, *related to*

- *preoperative administrative of corticosteroids*
- *leukopenia/neutropenia associated with chemotherapy and/or radiation therapy*

Potential for injury: physiologic: seizures, *related to postoperative edema associated with removal of a supratentorial tumor (especially in the temporal lobe)*

Altered comfort: pain, *related to*

- *operative incision*
- *headache associated with changes in intracranial fluid pressure*

Potential for injury: physiologic: bone marrow depression, *related to chemotherapy/radiation therapy*

Strategies for Nursing Care

Nurses in acute care settings will encounter children with brain tumors primarily in the perioperative period. Preoperative teaching should address the fact that the child will spend the first 2 to 3 days in the intensive care unit, will have an IV line, will probably experience some nausea and vomiting, and may have a headache. Chapter 29 contains questions pertinent to preoperative assessment of the child's concept of pain and what the child would like the nurse to do when pain is experienced. Often this part of the preoperative teaching is less anxiety-producing for the child than for the parent, who may be better able to conceptualize the postoperative period. There is an aspect of the preoperative information, however, which even most preschoolers find upsetting. That is the news that they will have to have a portion of their head shaved for the surgery.

Being Sensitive to Changes in Body Image. The nurse's sensitivity to this assault upon the child's body image can help to minimize the trauma somewhat. The child should know exactly which area must be shaved and which areas will be spared. Girls may find some comfort in suggestions for pulling the hair on the sides of the head back into a pony tail to cover shaving of the posterior fossa area, or pictures of how other children have used scarves and wigs to conceal hair loss until regrowth occurs. Young children will need to be assured that their hair will grow back. Boys can decide whether they want their entire head shaved to "match" the surgical site, a short haircut to minimize the difference in hair length, or to preserve hair everywhere but at the surgical site.

Postoperatively, children will usually spend the first 48 to 72 hours in the intensive care unit to permit careful monitoring of vital signs and neurologic signs. (See also Table 27-7, page 835, a Nursing Process Plan for perioperative care.) Postoperative care will vary somewhat among children, depending on the tumor site.

Providing Postoperative Care for Children After Removal of an Infratentorial Tumor. Care of the child following removal of an infratentorial tumor differs from postoperative care for a supratentorial tumor. Surgery in the posterior fossa often necessitates decompression of enlarged ventricles and creates concern for postoperative edema affecting the brain stem.

Monitoring Autonomic Function. Children with tumors of the posterior fossa are at risk for depression of autonomic function postoperatively because edema at the operative site may cause pressure on the brain stem. Arterial pressure, heart rate, and respiration are therefore monitored carefully. Children considered to be at increased risk for depression of these vital functions (e.g., because of tumor placement, operative trauma) will be intubated and placed on ventilatory support in the immediate postoperative period. Cranial nerve function is affected by pressure on the brain stem as well, and monitoring of eye movement, facial symmetry, and swallow and gag reflexes is especially important. Because the child with an infratentorial tumor often presents with cranial nerve dysfunction at the time of diagnosis, it is important to know the child's baseline to detect progression of cranial nerve involvement in the postoperative period.

Monitoring for Increased Intracranial Pressure (ICP). In addition to tissue edema, increased ICP may result from intracranial bleeding or malfunction of the ventricular shunt. Classic signs of increasing intracranial pressure include a change in alertness, changes in vital signs (elevated blood pressure, decreased pulse and respiration), changes in pupil reaction, and vomiting. Table 46-11 provides a comprehensive Nursing Process Plan for care of the child at risk for increased intracranial pressure.

Nausea and vomiting are common postoperatively because the child has often been under anesthesia for 6 to 8 hours. Vomiting causes increased intracranial pressure, and antiemetics should be administered to the child who vomits repeatedly.

Maintaining a Slow, Steady Rate of Ventricular Decompression. Children with an infratentorial tumor often have an associated hydrocephalus that requires decompression through either an external drainage system or a ventricular shunt. Initial decompression will occur preoperatively in the hours or days before surgery. (See the section on hydrocephalus in Chapter 46.) Because of the continued drainage of cerebrospinal fluid postoperatively, the child must be monitored for changes in intracranial pressure.

The child will be carefully positioned to control the rate of decompression of ventricles (that is, the rate of drainage of cerebrospinal fluid). Positioning will depend upon the degree of dilation of the ventricles preoperatively. The greater the hydrocephalus, the more slowly drainage must take place to reduce the risk of subdural hemorrhage from rapid shifts in fluids. If the ventricles were greatly dilated, the child may be placed flat in the immediate postoperative period. Typically, however, the head of the bed will be elevated 10 to 20 degrees for the first 24 to 48 hours. A CT scan will often be done to ensure the absence of subdural hemorrhage before slowly increasing the elevation of the head of the bed.

Preventing Infection. Children with posterior fossa tumors may have received corticosteroids preoperatively to relieve cerebral edema (and thereby potential pressure on the brain stem). Although administered for the anti-inflammatory effect in this case, corticosteroids have immunosuppressive properties that must be considered as well. Children who have been on oral or parenteral corticosteroids preoperatively are at increased risk for infection postoperatively. This vulnerability is compounded by the need to keep the child quite flat postoperatively, a position that limits bladder emptying and lung expansion. Adequate fluid intake and meticulous catheter care will help to decrease the chance of urinary tract infection.

The nurse who is alert to the potential for respiratory infection can institute frequent turning, even in the immediate postoperative period. The child can be turned from side to side, and sometimes the supine position can be used as well, with a foam donut to relieve pressure on the infratentorial surgical site. The nurse must become familiar with each neurosurgeon's preferences for postoperative positioning. Coughing in the immediate postoperative period will increase intracranial pressure and result in a severe headache. Deep breathing is not contraindicated, however. After the first 48 to 72 hours the child can be started on an incentive spirometer to reduce the risk of atelectasis.

Providing Postoperative Care for Children After Removal of a Supratentorial Tumor. Children with supratentorial tumors rarely have associated hydrocephalus, therefore eliminating the risk of subdural hemorrhage associated with ventricular decompression after infratentorial surgery. Positioning following supratentorial surgery often begins with a 30-degree elevation in the head of the bed and progresses gradually to 90 degrees over the first 48 to 72 hours as tolerated.

There is also much less danger of pressure on the brain stem because of the higher surgical site. Although vital signs and neurologic signs are carefully monitored postoperatively, they tend to be more stable. Further, children with supratentorial tumors are less likely to have been on corticosteroid therapy preoperatively and therefore do not incur the extra risk of immunosuppression unless preoperative chemotherapy or radiation therapy was involved.

Monitoring for Seizure Activity. Surgery in the supratentorial area of the brain, particularly in the temporal lobes, incurs the risk of seizures. Children at high risk for seizures will often be placed on anticonvulsant therapy prophylactically. Seizures are most likely to develop during the first 48 hours when the child is in the intensive care unit. (See Chapter 46, Boxes 46-6 and 46-7, for further nursing strategies related to seizures.)

Monitoring for Increased Intracranial Pressure. As with infratentorial tumors, intracranial pressure may rise postoperatively in response to tissue edema or intracranial bleeding. Careful monitoring of vital signs and neurologic signs (page 1686) is imperative. Antiemetic therapy to reduce vomiting is also important. (See also Table 46-10.)

Relieving Pain. Regardless of tumor site, pain relief will be a necessary concern in the postoperative period. Pain relief is made somewhat more difficult following neurologic surgery because of the need for the child's cooperation in assessing neurologic integrity. Doses of medication in excess of that needed to keep the child comfortable may result in a child who is difficult to arouse and therefore difficult to assess. Withholding medication is also of concern because pain will increase intracranial pressure by increasing the tendency for breath holding during turning and other procedures and by increasing crying. The nurse who is knowledgeable about the recommended therapeutic ranges for analgesics and the actions of these drugs can usually achieve that fine middle ground between too little and too much analgesia. This requires calculation of the dose of analgesic ordered in relation to the recommended therapeutic dose (Chapter 29), a sensitivity to the child's unique reaction to each analgesic administered, and incorporation of feedback from the child and parent in relation to both pharmacologic and nonpharmacologic methods for obtaining comfort.

Providing Supportive Care for Bone Marrow Depression. The child with a malignant brain tumor will usually undergo chemotherapy and/or radiotherapy, with the resulting effects of bone marrow depression. In this case the nursing strategies detailed in Table 48-4 become an important aspect of quality care.

Nursing Strategies for Follow-up Care in the Home or Clinic

Assess neurologic function for changes from the baseline documented at discharge.

Assess for the potential side effects of medications and other treatment modalities.

If an intraventricular shunt was inserted:

- assess for its patency (absence of signs and symptoms of increased intracranial pressure)
- assess for shunt infection (increased intracranial pressure, increased WBCs, fever)

Allow the family and the child adequate time to express what the child's brain tumor means to them—their fears, their insights, their perceptions of life since the diagnosis.

- Use this information to determine the adequacy of their physical and emotional support systems.
- Make appropriate referrals to social services agencies and to local and national support groups for children with cancer, their parents, and siblings.

Assess the child's progress on developmental tasks. Memory deficits, selective attention deficits and sensorimotor problems are potential late effects of therapy (Finlay et al, 1987).

Encourage the family and the child to ask questions. Reinforce teaching that was begun during the child's hospitalization.

Medulloblastoma

Medulloblastoma is an infratentorial tumor that is characteristically found in the area of the fourth ventricle and cerebellum. It is the brain tumor most commonly found in children. It occurs about twice as often in boys as in girls. The peak incidence occurs in children under 6 years of age (Huttenlocher, 1987).

Clinical Manifestations

The child with medulloblastoma usually has a history of 1 to 3 months of headache, vomiting, ataxia, and cranial nerve or motor dysfunction. Deterioration of the child's condition can be documented, for example, as he or she goes from being able to walk to being unable to stand unassisted. Later, the child may be unable to sit unassisted or to hold up the head. Nucchal rigidity and head tilting can occur. Papilledema is usually present.

Therapeutic Management

Surgical removal of most of the tumor decreases symptomatology and re-establishes unobstructed flow of cerebrospinal fluid (CSF) and subsequently decreases intracranial pressure. Total resection of the tumor has become increasingly more feasible using microsurgery aided by the precise delineation that CT scans afford the neurosurgeon. Craniospinal radiation is given postoperatively. The efficacy of chemotherapy in treating medulloblastoma has been the subject of several studies. Although early findings were inconclusive, Finlay and colleagues (1987) reported that a study conducted by the Children's Cancer Study Group (CCSG) showed chemotherapy to be of benefit to children with extensive local tumor or metastatic disease.

With surgery and radiotherapy, the 5-year survival rate is about 50 to 60 per cent. Prognosis is poorer for younger patients, patients with large tumors, and those with tumor cells in the spinal fluid.

Ependymoma

This tumor originates from ependymal cells that form the lining of the spinal cord and the cavities of the brain. Therefore this tumor may be found either supratentorially or infratentorially. The peak incidence of occurrence is around 2 years of age (Hausman, 1979).

Clinical Manifestations

The child with an ependymoma usually has a 1- to 3-month history of vomiting, clumsy gait, and headaches. Clinical signs of papilledema, ataxia, and incoordination of the hands are usually noted. The clinical presentation is very similar to that of the child with a medulloblastoma; until surgery and pathologic identification, the tumors may be indistinguishable.

It has been found that when this tumor occurs infratentorially it is benign, although it does invade the brain stem (Hausman, 1979). Compromised cardiorespiratory function may be noted if the onset is acute (less than 1 month). Limited range of motion of the neck may signal extended growth of the tumor. If an ependymoma is located supratentorially, the frontal and parietal lobes are most frequently affected. Metastasis to the surrounding brain tissue can occur. These tumors may grow quite large before any signs or symptoms are noted by the parents. There may be a gradual change in personality, making the child irritable, fatigued, or sluggish.

Therapeutic Management

The treatment of choice is surgical removal, but usually complete tumor resection is not possible. Craniospinal radiation is given postoperatively but has not improved the 5-year survival rate very substantially. Chemotherapy trials for children with ependymoma have shown that occasional tumors may have limited response to multiagent therapy. However, there are few long-term survivors (Huttenlocher, 1987).

Cerebellar Astrocytoma

This infratentorial tumor is often cystic in nature and is usually located in one lobe of the cerebellum. It later expands to the midline, especially to the pons, the midbrain, and the medulla. It does not "seed" along the CSF pathway as other tumors, such as medulloblastoma, are apt to do. The peak incidence of occurrence is around 8 years of age (Walker, 1982).

Clinical Manifestations

The child with cerebellar astrocytoma usually has a 3- to 6-month history of morning headache, vomiting, and anorexia. Ataxia of gait and hand incoordination appear much later than do the overt signs of increased intracranial pressure. The child may gradually become irritable and lethargic, but this is usually so subtle in onset that parents may not be able to indicate just when the behavioral changes began. The child may develop a squint and complain of double vision. Ophthalmologic examination reveals papilledema. An increased head circumference with separation of the sagittal suture may be noted on radiographs.

Therapeutic Management

Because of its location, complete surgical resection of this tumor is often possible. Surgery results in long-term survival for nearly 90 per cent of children. Radiation therapy is reserved for cases in which the tumor recurs or is not completely resectable (Huttenlocher, 1987).

Brain Stem Glioma

This infratentorial tumor is located in the brain stem and presents with severe neurological signs and symptoms before any sign of increased intracranial pressure is noted. The tumor appears as a growth on the external surface of the brain stem. It is fast growing and is usually diagnosed within 2 months of onset of symptoms and signs. Peak incidence of occurrence of this tumor is in children 6 years of age (Walker, 1982).

Clinical Manifestations

Neurologic signs, including ocular palsies, nystagmus, ataxia, diplopia, squint, difficulty in swallowing and talking, lack of hand coordination, facial and limb weakness, drooling, and urinary retention, are noted. Because of difficulty with swallowing, aspiration of both food and fluids may occur with subsequent bronchopneumonia. Progressive urinary retention can lead to urinary tract infections.

Therapeutic Management

Surgery is limited to biopsy because critical vital centers of the brain would be compromised by surgical excision of the tumor. Radiotherapy, although merely palliative, does extend the survival from a few months to a few years. Certain combinations of chemotherapeutic agents have caused regression of symptoms but are not curative (Walker and Allen, 1983; Huttenlocher, 1987).

Cerebral Astrocytoma

These supratentorial tumors are usually invasive solid tumors that can grow to be very large. The frontal lobe is most often involved, with extension into midline structures, basal ganglia, and the thalamus. The peak age of the occurrence of this tumor is 9 years (Walker, 1982).

Clinical Manifestations

Children with cerebral astrocytomas usually have symptoms such as headache, vomiting, and apathy. These are all indicators of increased intracranial pressure. Other neurologic signs may be seen, such as diplopia, focal seizures, ataxia, and incoordination. Weakness of limbs contralaterally is sometimes noted.

Therapeutic Management

Complete surgical resection is rarely possible. Radiation is palliative and is sometimes used in conjunction with chemotherapy. The prognosis is poor, with the average survival being about 1 year with radiotherapy and surgery alone. The prognosis for children with high-grade cerebral astrocytoma may be enhanced with adjuvant chemotherapy, employing agents such as vincristine and CCNU (Ertel et al, 1984).

Optic Nerve Gliomas

These slow-growing, supratentorial tumors are found with five different presentations:

- confined to the nerve in one orbit,
- extending from the optic chiasm to the eyeball,
- diffuse involvement bilaterally of the optic nerves and the chiasm,
- bilateral involvement of optic nerves and chiasm with extension into the adjacent cerebral tissue, and
- obstructing the entire third ventricle.

Peak incidence of diagnosis is around 5 years of age (Walker, 1982).

Clinical Manifestations

Neurologic signs such as strabismus and nystagmus may be noted. Decreased visual acuity, diabetes insipidus, and obesity may also occur. If the tumor invades the third ventricle, signs of increased intracranial pressure may exist. Proptosis (forward and downward displacement of the eyeball) is often an early symptom. In infants, failure to thrive may be noted, with general growth retardation. Café-au-lait spots are sometimes seen in patients with this tumor because of its frequent association with neurofibromatosis.

Therapeutic Management

Surgical excision is sometimes possible when only one of the optic nerves is involved. With more extensive disease there is less likelihood for total resection. At times a total enucleation of the eye is necessary. Invasion of vital centers is usually the cause of death. Radiation therapy may be either curative or palliative, depending upon the extent of the invasion. If the optic chiasm is involved, radiation therapy is the only treatment available. Chemotherapy for optic nerve glioma has not yet proved to be useful, but trials with multiagent therapy continue.

Hodgkin Disease

Hodgkin disease is a malignant lymphoma characterized by the presence of Reed-Sternberg cells and neoplastic proliferation of lymphoid tissue. It presents most commonly in one or more lymph node sites. Other tissues that may be involved are the spleen, lung, liver, and bone.

Hodgkin disease is rare before 5 years of age but peaks from age 15 to 34 years and again at age 50. It is almost twice as common in boys as in girls (Leventhal, 1987).

Clinical Manifestations

Most often the adolescent with Hodgkin disease has painless lymph node enlargement (lymphadenopathy), usually in the supraclavicular or cervical area. The disease commonly spreads from one lymph node area to others via the lymphatic pathway, but regions adjacent to the primary site of disease may be bypassed. Constitutional symptoms of fever (> 38°C [100.4°F]), drenching night sweats, splenomegaly, anorexia, malaise, weight loss in excess of 10 per cent of body weight, and pruritus may be evident (Sullivan, 1987).

Some evidence suggests that Hodgkin disease may be associated with abnormalities in T-cell lymphocytes, with resultant impairment in cellular immunity (Skarin et al, 1978). The exact etiology of the disease is still unknown.

Diagnostic Assessment

Frequently a peripheral lymph node biopsy is obtained initially to establish the presence of Reed-Sternberg cells and nodal changes consistent with the diagnosis of Hodgkin disease. Although the Reed-Sternberg cell is essential to the diagnosis of Hodgkin disease, diagnosis cannot be made upon this finding alone since this abnormal cell is also seen in other diseases, such as infectious mononucleosis (Groenwald, 1987). Four histologic patterns are seen: nodular sclerosing, mixed cellularity, lymphocyte predominant, and lymphocyte depleted. The subsequent evaluation includes a variety of studies necessary for determining the extent of disease.

Radiographic examination of the chest demonstrates mediastinal adenopathy in over half the patients with cervical adenopathy (Sullivan et al, 1984). CT scan of the chest and abdomen is useful in delineating disease in the mediastinum, hilar areas, lungs, and para-aortic areas. Pedal lymphangiography outlines the appearance of involved retroperitoneal nodes. Bone scan and bone marrow biopsy are necessary for investigating disease involvement in those areas.

A staging laparotomy may be included as part of the initial workup of Hodgkin disease. Its purpose is to detect abdominal disease that is not evident through noninvasive tests. At laparotomy, splenectomy, liver biopsy, lymph node biopsies, and bone marrow biopsy are performed. Children who undergo splenectomy are rendered susceptible to serious infections with bacteria that have polysaccharide capsules, such as pneumococcus, streptococcus, and *Haemophilus influenzae.* Some protection postsplenectomy is offered by immunization with pneumococcal vaccine prior to surgery and long-term daily oral penicillin.

Staging. Following the diagnostic procedures, the patient's disease is staged based on the degree of disease present (Fig. 48-8). Staging assists in the selection of therapy to be used. The staging system used for Hodgkin's disease is as follows:

Stage I: Disease limited to one anatomic region or to two contiguous anatomic regions on the same side of the diaphragm.

Stage II: Disease in more than two anatomic regions or in two noncontiguous regions on the same side of the diaphragm.

Stage III: Disease in lymph node regions on both sides of the diaphragm but not extending beyond involvement of lymph nodes or spleen.

Stage IV: Involvement of extralymphatic organs (for example, bone marrow, lung, pleura, liver, bone, skin, or gastrointestinal tract).

All patients are also subclassified A or B to indicate the presence or absence of one or more constitutional symptoms. These symptoms include unexplained weight loss of more than 10 per cent of body weight, unexplained fever with temperature above 38°C, and night sweats. Children with any of these symptoms have a less favorable prognosis than children who are asymptomatic.

Therapeutic Management

Children with Hodgkin disease are treated with radiation therapy and often with chemotherapy or a combination of these modalities. The exact treatment plan is largely determined by the stage of disease at diagnosis. Children with Stage I or IIA disease receive radiation therapy, usually to an "extended" field that includes all nodal sites on the involved side of the diaphragm. Children with Stage IIB or III disease usually receive radiation therapy, either to limited or extended fields,

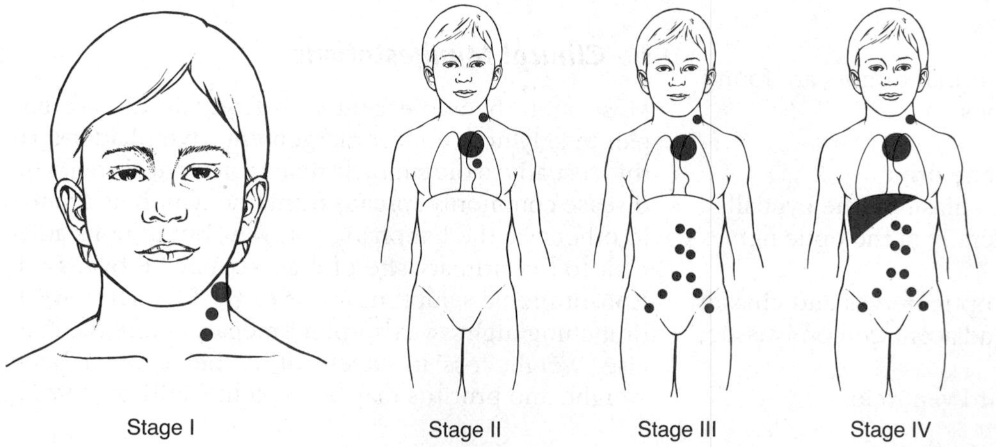

Figure 48-8. The Ann Arbor Staging System for Hodgkin disease.

and combination chemotherapy. Children with Stage IV disease receive combination chemotherapy.

The first combination chemotherapy used to treat Hodgkin disease successfully consisted of nitrogen mustard, vincristine (Oncovin), prednisone, and procarbazine, and became known as MOPP. Most programs utilize MOPP therapy for 6 months. Further maintenance courses of MOPP have not enhanced remission duration. Clinical trials evaluating other effective chemotherapy programs have discovered two other effective drug combinations: ABVD (Adriamycin, bleomycin, Velban, and DTIC) and CCNU (Velban, procarbazine and prednisone). Clinical trials are presently attempting to select the most efficacious combinations of chemotherapy and radiotherapy that will give the best disease-free survival rate with the fewest sequelae. Identified late sequelae include the occurrence of second malignancies and, in children, problems with growth in radiated areas.

Both MOPP and ABVD are associated with moderately severe nausea and vomiting. Children and teenagers who receive this chemotherapy need much support and encouragement to understand and deal with the treatment and its annoying toxicity. It is important for the nurse to work closely with them. Together they can identify the best antiemetic regimen that will enable the patient to accept and tolerate the chemotherapy.

Hodgkin disease is now managed with several different regimens, with a cure rate of approximately 90 per cent. Radiation therapy alone is considered curative only in unilateral high cervical or inguinal Stage I disease. With all other forms of Hodgkin disease, radiotherapy and chemotherapy are used together (Sullivan, 1987).

Major Nursing Diagnoses for Hodgkin Disease

Potential for infection, *related to the impairment of immunity associated with dysfunction of the lymphatic system and with both chemotherapy and radiation therapy*

Fear/anxiety, *related to*
- *diagnosis of a malignant disease*
- *diagnostic and therapeutic modalities, including laparotomy, chemotherapy, and radiation therapy*

Altered comfort: nausea and vomiting, *related to side effects of MOPP and ABVD combination chemotherapy*

Disturbance in self concept: body image, self-esteem, role performance, and personal identity, *related to*
- *the diagnosis of a life-threatening illness in the adolescent years*
- *alopecia, cushingoid features, and other alterations in appearance associated with treatment modalities*

Knowledge deficit, *related to*
- *normal function of the lymphatic system and the changes in function associated with the disease*
- *diagnostic and treatment modalities (see also Table 48-4)*
- *transmission of infective organisms and preventive actions*
- *community support groups for adolescents with cancer, and for their siblings and parents*

Strategies for Nursing Care

Nursing strategies for the child or adolescent with Hodgkin disease center on three major goals: (1) providing psychosocial support in the diagnostic period, (2) minimizing the hazards of bone marrow depression and the discomfort of systemic symptoms during chemotherapy and/or radiation therapy, and (3) monitoring for advancing disease and for late effects of treatment during follow-up visits. The nurse can use the guidelines for psychosocial support of children and families that were provided earlier in this chapter. The impact of the disease upon adolescents will be especially devastating, however, in light of their developmental tasks of establishing an independent identity. The nurse who is sensitive to this conflict can be instrumental in helping the adolescent express fears and frustrations and in suggesting ways to reach out to friends and family for needed support.

Table 48-4 contains the strategies appropriate to the support of young people involved in chemotherapy. Nursing considerations for radiation therapy were also addressed earlier in this chapter. The next section lists strategies to consider during follow-up care.

Nursing Strategies for Follow-up Care in the Home or Clinic

Assess for signs and symptoms of infection associated with cancer of the lymphatic system (and with splenectomy if this was done).

Assess for bone marrow suppression associated with chemotherapy and radiation therapy.

Allow the adolescent and the family to express their feelings about the meaning that Hodgkin disease and its treatment has for each of them, and the effects of the disease upon usual roles within the family and community. (As with all serious diseases, determine whether the family's psychologic and physical support systems are adequate and make referrals as necessary.)

Assess for long-range side effects associated with chemotherapy and radiation therapy for Hodgkin disease (Gellis and Kagan, 1986):

- secondary oncogenesis (classic signs of cancer elsewhere in the body)
- growth impairment
- breast atrophy
- immune suppression (fever and infection)
- sterility (if pelvic irradiation was involved)

Non-Hodgkin Lymphoma

Non-Hodgkin lymphoma is a highly malignant neoplasm of lymphoid tissue. Several histologic (cell type) patterns are seen in children, including lymphoblastic, undifferentiated (Burkitt and non-Burkitt or pleomorphic), and large cell lymphoma. Common sites of primary disease in children are lymphoid tissue in the abdomen, anterior mediastinum, neck, and nasopharynx. Bone marrow and the CNS are the most frequently involved extralymphatic sites. Although non-Hodgkin lymphoma can occur at any age, a peak incidence is evident between the ages of 5 and 15 years (Gardner and Graham-Pole, 1983).

Clinical Manifestations

Signs and symptoms of non-Hodgkin lymphoma relate to sites of disease. Abdominal masses, diarrhea, distention, vomiting, episodic colicky pain, ascites, and intussusception are suggestive of intra-abdominal disease. Cough, wheezing, and dyspnea may be present with mediastinal disease. Enlarged lymph nodes, tonsillar masses, nasal congestion, rhinorrhea, epistaxis, and loosening of teeth may be signs of head and neck disease. The kidneys may be involved, with infiltrative disease causing renal dysfunction.

Diagnostic Assessment

A diagnosis of non-Hodgkin lymphoma is made by surgical biopsy of an involved tissue site. Studies to determine extent of the disease include abdominal ultrasound and CT scan, gallium scan, bone scan, and bone marrow aspiration (Magrath, 1987). In addition, a lumbar puncture is done to evaluate the CSF. The diagnostic workup must be done with expediency, since the disease may progress rapidly.

Therapeutic Management

Treatment for non-Hodgkin lymphoma is primarily chemotherapy, with radiotherapy used only in adjunctive fashion. Occasionally, radiotherapy is useful in reducing bulky disease such as in the mediastinum when respiratory distress is present. Non-Hodgkin lymphoma is very sensitive to combination chemotherapy, often resulting in an initial rapid breakdown of tumor cells. Renal function must be evaluated, since the kidneys can be involved with disease. Adequate hydration and alkalinization of the urine, combined with allopurinol therapy, must be instituted before therapy is begun. Following initial chemotherapy, diligent monitoring of fluid, electrolyte balance, and kidney function is necessary. In the presence of extensive disease, kidney involvement, or renal dysfunction, hemodialysis may be necessary because of uric acid nephropathy and deteriorating renal function.

Drug combinations used to treat non-Hodgkin lymphoma are determined by the histologic diagnosis. Lymphoblastic lymphoma is best treated with a multidrug regimen resembling therapy for acute lymphoblastic leukemia. One of the most commonly used combinations utilizes cyclophosphamide, prednisone, vincristine, methotrexate, and daunomycin for induction therapy. A consolidation period follows using L-asparaginase, cytosine arabinoside, and other agents. Maintenance therapy includes repeated cycles of the same drugs. The other histologies (undifferentiated and large cell lymphoma) respond best to a combination of cyclophosphamide, vincristine, prednisone, and methotrexate used for induction and subsequent maintenance courses (Gardner and Graham-Pole, 1983). Intrathecal chemotherapy is included "prophylactically" in most children because of the relatively high incidence of CNS disease. Treatment is generally given for 6 to 18 months.

Prior to the time when chemotherapy was introduced as the primary treatment for non-Hodgkin lymphoma, only about 10 to 25 per cent of children with the disease survived. The use of chemotherapy and the knowledge of the importance of supportive care precautions during induction therapy have increased the overall survival rate for children with non-Hodgkin lymphoma such that nearly all children with limited overt disease survive, as well as 50 to 75 per cent of children with extensive disease (Magrath, 1987).

Strategies for Nursing Care

Nursing care of the child with non-Hodgkin lymphoma involves supportive care for signs and symptoms related to disease sites (e.g., respiratory, gastrointestinal) and monitoring for kidney involvement. The strategies related to chemotherapy (Table 48-4) are central to the nursing plan of care. As with all the malignant diseases, the need for psychosocial support of the child and family cannot be overemphasized. The nurse who can interpret the medical regimen to the child and family and give them a written list of signs and symptoms to watch for provides them with knowledge needed to cope with day-to-day care after hospital discharge. This is but another situation in which primary care can be beneficial; having one particular nurse who is knowledgeable and supportive can quite literally be a lifeline for the family during the diagnostic and treatment crises.

Neuroblastoma

Neuroblastoma is a malignant neoplasm that develops in cells of neural crest origin that give rise to the adrenal gland and the sympathetic nervous system. It occurs in 500 children in the United States each year (Finklestein, 1987). The etiology of neuroblastoma is unknown.

The majority of children with neuroblastoma are under 5 years of age, with a peak incidence at 2 years (Evans et al, 1976). The sites of the primary tumor (site of origin) in the body vary. Over half the primary tumors occur in the abdomen (Voute, 1984). Most of these are in the adrenal gland. Other primaries arise in sympathetic ganglia in the cervical, thoracic, and pelvic regions. Neuroblastoma commonly metastasizes to bones (especially skull, pelvis, femur, and humerus), bone marrow, liver, and lymph nodes. Infants less than 1 year of age tend to have either localized tumors or metastatic disease in sites such as liver, bone marrow, and skin. These three metastatic sites constitute a special stage and are known to be favorably responsive to treatment with either chemotherapy or radiotherapy. Two thirds of patients have metastases at diagnosis (Hayes and Green, 1983).

Clinical Manifestations

Children with neuroblastoma may look and feel very sick. The chief signs and symptoms include an abdominal mass, fever, irritability, pain from bone metastases, and orbital ecchymosis or proptosis (displacement of the eyeball, causing it to protrude) from skull metastases. Since the primary tumors are retroperitoneal, they often extend posteriorly and may invade the spinal canal through vertebral spaces or foramina, producing symptoms of cord compression.

Diagnostic Assessment

Diagnostic studies focus on the principal sites of primary or metastatic disease. Physical examination may reveal a palpable, firm mass in the abdomen. Tumors at other sites, such as the chest, may be impossible to detect on physical examination. The tumor cells secrete increased amounts of catecholamines and other tyrosine metabolites, which are excreted in the urine. Analysis of the urine for catecholamines is imperative, since this provides an excellent means of following tumor presence. Neuroblastomas also produce other metabolic products. One of these is an enzyme, neuron-specific enolase, which can be used prognostically, since infants under 1 year of age with low values usually have a good prognosis (Zellzer et al, 1983). Lactic dehydrogenase (LDH) is commonly elevated during active tumor growth. Serum ferritin may also be elevated in some patients (Hann et al, 1983). These latter metabolites may be measured in serum samples.

Collecting complete and accurate urine samples can be difficult in a child who is not toilet-trained. Immobilization devices and secure urine bags or Foley catheterization is usually required. The nurse should be particularly sensitive to the stress that immobilization causes for the child and family. Special efforts should be taken to provide quiet diversional activities for the child during this period. The urine is kept in bottles that contain hydrochloric acid as a preservative. Ninety five per cent of all neuroblastoma patients have one or more elevated catecholamines at diagnosis (Voute, 1984).

Specific x-ray films are made to define the primary disease and extent of metastases, if present. Chest radiograph, abdominal ultrasound or CT scan, and intravenous pyelogram (IVP) with inferior venacavagram (IVC) are used to elaborate intrathoracic and intra-abdominal extent of disease. Small calcified deposits may be seen in the primary tumor and occur when areas of tumor undergo necrosis and become calcified. Skeletal radiographs may show lytic lesions in bones. Nuclear bone scans and liver scans may detect subtle disease in the liver and bones. Bone marrow aspiration and biopsy are performed to check for infiltrates of tumor cells in the bone marrow. As many as half of all patients have disease that has spread to the bone marrow (Groncy and Finklestein, 1978). Bone marrow disease may be reflected in the blood count, but the most common finding is anemia, which is not dependent upon tumor involvement of the marrow. The diagnosis of neuroblastoma is made upon examination of tissue histology. This must be made from a biopsy of primary or metastatic tissue. If the bone marrow is abnormal and elevated catecholamines are present, tissue biopsy is not necessary for diagnosis.

Staging. Extent of disease is described in a staging system. Stage I is represented by a localized primary tumor that has been completely resected. Stage II disease extends beyond the primary tissue involved but does not cross the midline of the body and is grossly resectable. Disease classified as Stage III is localized to the primary site but extends across the midline. Stage IV involves distant metastases. Stage IV-S is a special classification in which metastatic disease is limited to liver, bone marrow, or skin.

Therapeutic Management

Treatment varies with extent of disease. Stage I or II disease is treated with surgical removal of the primary tumor. Stages III and IV tumors are frequently too extensive for complete or safe surgical removal. When residual tumor is present, radiation therapy may be used for Stages II and III. Radiation therapy is useful in Stage IV disease for treatment of symptomatic metastatic sites or for primary tumors when chemotherapy has controlled metastatic sites. The role of chemotherapy in Stage II disease is questionable. It is necessary in Stage III and IV disease because of the inoperability and poor outcome of Stage III tumors and the widespread disease found in Stage IV. No drug regimen or combination has been found that effectively treats many cases of Stage III and Stage IV neuroblastoma. Cyclophosphamide, vincristine, dimethyltriazenoimidazole carboxamide (DTIC), doxorubicin, cis-platin, VM-26, and melphalan are drugs that are presently used in various combinations and schedules.

Long-Term Outcome

The prognosis for children with neuroblastoma depends on the age of the child at diagnosis and the stage of the disease. Very young children have the best prognosis; infants under 1 year of age usually have either localized or Stage IV-S disease. Children with Stage I tumors have almost a 100 per cent survival, whereas those with Stages II, III, and IV-S have a 50 to 80 per cent survival. Children with Stage IV disease have a dismal prognosis: less than 10 per cent. Older children with neuroblastoma tend to have Stage IV disease (Voute, 1984).

Although children with localized neuroblastoma do fairly well, those whose disease is Stage III or IV may have a devastating course and fatal outcome. Children who die with widespread neuroblastoma often have severe pain and growth of tumor masses in multiple sites. The terminal stages of this disease are very difficult for a family to accept, since the child's body can become grossly disfigured. When a child with neuroblastoma is dying, the child and family are very dependent on the nursing staff for much of their support and comfort.

Strategies for Nursing Care

Care of the child with neuroblastoma will involve psychosocial support of the child and family in light of the grave prognosis for children with advanced disease. The strategies detailed in Chapter 26 will assist the nurse in providing support to the family with a dying child. The nurse must be sensitive to the child's changing body image related to disfiguring tumors.

Postoperative care will be dictated by the tumor site. Strategies for perioperative care (Table 27-7), care of the child following abdominal surgery (Table 41-9), and care of the child undergoing chemotherapy (Table 48-4) and radiation therapy are likely to be pertinent to the plan of care. Collection of urine samples for analysis of catecholemines is another nursing responsibility. Intervention for pain will be necessitated by pressure of the neuroblastoma against tissues and organs; the nurse should take the initiative to develop and institute a comprehensive comfort protocol of both pharmacologic and nonpharmacologic measures to improve the child's quality of life.

Wilms Tumor

Wilms tumor is a malignant neoplasm of the kidney that most often affects young children. The median age of incidence is 3 1/2 years (Belasco et al, 1984), but Wilms tumor also occurs in adolescents and, rarely, in adults. In 40 per cent of cases, the tumor is of genetic origin (Ganick, 1987). Children with Wilms tumor may have congenital anomalies such as aniridia (a congenitally absent iris), renal anomalies, skeletal anomalies (e.g., clubfeet), or genitourinary malformations (Ganick, 1987).

Clinical Manifestations

The child with Wilms tumor is usually a well child in whom an abdominal mass has been seen or felt. Sometimes parents are the first to notice increasing abdominal girth when belts or waistbands become tight. Less common presenting signs and symptoms are abdominal pain, malaise, anorexia, fever, gross hematuria, and hypertension. The primary tumor mass may be discovered on palpation of the abdomen during a routine check-up.

Diagnostic Assessment

The initial workup for these patients is designed to define the renal mass and search for areas of metastases. Wilms tumor may metastasize to lung, liver, lymph nodes, or bone. Intravenous pyelogram and inferior venacavagram delineate the area of the tumor involvement in the kidney and, very importantly, show the status of the other kidney. Although abdominal ultrasound and CT scan are also useful, all three studies are not necessary. About 5 per cent of Wilms tumors are bilateral at initial diagnosis (Belasco et al, 1984). Chest radiograph, liver/spleen scan, and a complete skeletal survey are done to evaluate for metastatic disease.

Tumor Classification. The National Wilms

Tumor Study (NWTS), which began in 1969, has provided excellent data for staging and prognosis in this tumor (Belasco et al, 1984). Wilms tumor is classified in a staging system based on extent of disease. Stage I disease is confined to the kidney and is completely resected by nephrectomy. Stage II disease extends beyond the kidney but can be completely removed at the time of nephrectomy. Stage III represents regional spread of disease beyond the kidney with incomplete resection or completely resected disease involving regional lymph nodes. Also included are those tumors that are ruptured either before surgery or at surgery, spilling tumor contents into the peritoneal cavity. Stage IV represents blood-borne spread of disease to lung, liver, bone, or distant lymph nodes. Stage V Wilms tumor involves both kidneys.

More important than staging is the histology of Wilms tumor. Children with tumors that show a defined degree of anaplasia or are sarcomatous in pattern make up the majority of those succumbing to this disease. Those with "favorable" histology have an excellent prognosis. Favorable histology includes blastemal and epithelial kidney tissues.

Therapeutic Management

Treatment for Wilms tumor includes all modalities of cancer treatment: surgery, radiation therapy, and chemotherapy. Surgery is performed as soon as the diagnosis is suggested by physical examination and radiography. A nephrectomy is performed, with removal of all regional lymph nodes and any resectable regional tumor. Stage I disease is not treated with radiotherapy and has an excellent prognosis with limited chemotherapy for 6 months or less. Children with Stage II and III disease may receive radiotherapy to the original tumor site combined with chemotherapy, using two or three drugs, for 15 months. When intra-abdominal disease is extensive or tumor contents have spilled into the peritoneal cavity, radiotherapy is given to the whole abdomen. Stage IV disease is treated with a combination of intensive chemotherapy and radiotherapy to metastatic sites (Belasco et al, 1984). The drugs that are commonly used today for Wilms tumor include actinomycin D, vincristine, and doxorubicin. Occasionally surgical removal of resistant lung or node metastases is warranted.

Long-Term Outcome

When patients are adequately treated, the long-term survival in Wilms tumor is about 90 per cent (Belasco et al, 1984). The patients who do the best are the youngest children with Stage I or II disease with favorable tumor histology. Since the outlook for children with Wilms tumor is good, the quality of survival is of great concern. These children are left with only one kidney, so they must always be treated adequately for urinary tract infections. Routine urinalysis, blood pressure readings, and kidney function tests are part of quality long-term follow-up care.

Major Nursing Diagnoses for Wilms Tumor

Potential for injury: physiologic, *related to rupture of the tumor capsule and seeding of malignant cells throughout the peritoneal cavity*

Fear/anxiety (child and family), *related to*
- *diagnosis of a malignant disease*
- *impending surgery, chemotherapy, and/or radiation therapy*

Potential for injury: physiologic, *related to the following complications after a nephrectomy:*
- *hypovolemic shock associated with blood loss during surgery and inadequate postoperative fluid replacement*
- *pneumothorax associated with surgical manipulation or with malfunction of chest tubes after a thoracic surgical approach*

Disturbance in self-concept: body image, *related to the loss of a kidney*

Knowledge deficit, *related to*
- *usual function of the kidney and changes brought about by the tumor*
- *diagnostic and treatment modalities (see also Table 48-4)*
- *home management of the child who has had a nephrectomy and who has bone marrow suppression associated with chemotherapy and radiation therapy*
- *ways to maintain health of the remaining kidney*
- *community support groups for clients with cancer, their siblings, and parents*

Strategies for Nursing Care

Preventing Rupture of the Tumor Capsule. It is imperative that nurses avoid palpation of the tumor and caution the child and parents not to poke at or massage the region. If the tumor capsule ruptures, malignant cells may seed throughout the peritoneal cavity. Although the time between diagnosis and surgery will be minimal, it is often advisable to post a sign on the child's bed indicating "No Abdominal Palpation."

Providing Information to Reduce Fear and Anxiety. The sudden diagnosis of a malignant tumor in an otherwise healthy child is a shock for the child and family. Sensitivity to the emotional adjustments and the practical arrangements that must be made in relation to sudden surgery can make the nurse a valuable resource. Information will be needed for cognitive coping, but the stress of surgery following closely upon the diagnosis will reduce the ability to understand and remember the information related. Patience is essential in repeating information as necessary. Making oneself available for questions and clarification of information will be greatly appreciated by the family.

Monitoring for Complications of Nephrectomy. Postoperative care following nephrectomy will be quite similar to care following any abdominal surgery (Table 41-9). However, the plan of care must also include monitoring for hypovolemic shock and pneumothorax, which are potential complications of nephrectomy. The nurse who is aware of these possibilities is best equipped to make judgments about the seriousness of changes in vital signs and breathing patterns.

Promoting a Healthy Body Image. Because children affected with Wilms tumor are usually very young, the loss of a kidney may mean something quite different to them than adults realize. Exploring the child's perception of the surgery and of what is now "missing" from his or her body through play therapy, drawings, and so on can help determine whether the child has a realistic understanding or whether the fantasy is much worse than the actual situation. As children progress through new developmental crises, the loss of a kidney may again be examined in light of their expanding cognitive abilities. Nurses who see the child for follow-up visits can facilitate the child's coming to terms with the former surgery by encouraging expression of feelings and clarifying information as appropriate.

Teaching to Support Management at Home Following Nephrectomy. The family who understands normal kidney function will be better able to protect the child from urinary tract infections and unnecessary trauma that may put the remaining kidney at risk. The signs and symptoms of urinary tract infection should be written out for them, as well as the preventive measures of adequate fluid intake, cleanliness of the genital area, teaching little girls to wipe from front to back after voiding and defecating, and avoiding irritation from nylon underwear and perfumed bubble baths. (See also the discussion of urinary tract infection in Chapter 42.) Fluid intake and frequent voiding will be particularly important postoperatively if chemotherapy involves agents known to precipitate in the urine and cause chemical irritation of the bladder.

The family will need intensive and extensive teaching regarding the side effects of chemotherapy and ways to minimize the effects of bone marrow suppression. See Table 48-4.

Nursing Strategies for Follow-up Care in the Home or Clinic

Allow the child and family members to verbalize feelings about the loss of a kidney, the prognosis of the disease, and the effects of the disease and its treatment on individual and family functioning. (Make appropriate referrals if it is determined that the family does not have an adequate physical and psychologic support system to maintain home management during this phase of the treatment process.)

Assess the status of the surgical incision.

Assess for signs and symptoms of urinary tract infection and for function of the remaining kidney. Obtain blood and urine samples for tests of kidney function, and check blood pressure readings against the child's baseline.

Determine retention of and compliance with predischarge teaching about ways to maintain health of the remaining kidney.

Assess the child's progress on developmental tasks.

Rhabdomyosarcoma

Rhabdomyosarcoma (a malignancy of skeletal muscle tissue) is the most common soft tissue tumor diagnosed in children. Primary tumors are most often found in the urogenital tract, head, neck, and extremities. The trunk and abdomen are other less common primary sites. Metastases occur early in the course of the disease, often to the lungs or regional lymph nodes. The tumor can occur at any age in childhood but has age incidence peaks among toddlers and adolescents (Van Wezel-Bolen, 1982).

Clinical Manifestations

Rhabdomyosarcoma is associated with signs and symptoms related to the primary tumor site. A soft tissue mass may be evident visually or palpated on physical examination. Orbital tumors may result in proptosis or lid swelling. Neck tumors may cause hoarseness and dysphagia. Nasopharyngeal tumors may create airway obstruction, sinusitis, epistaxis, or dysphagia. Children with tumors of the paranasal sinuses may have sinusitis, nasal discharge, epistaxis, or obstruction. Middle ear tumors may present as chronic otitis media, a facial nerve palsy, or hearing loss. Bladder or prostate primary tumors may cause dysuria, urinary retention, constipation, or hematuria. In addition, tumors of head and neck areas may be locally invasive to the CNS, resulting in cranial nerve palsies and meningeal symptoms.

Diagnostic Assessment

Pretreatment studies for children with rhabdomyosarcoma include tests to assess the extent of disease. Radiographs, bone marrow aspiration, CT scans, and nuclear scans appropriate for the involved site will be among the selected studies. A chest CT scan to check for lung metastases should be done on all patients. Lumbar punctures are performed on children with head and neck tumors that may invade the CNS. Myelograms should be done when the primary tumor is in the paraspinal region.

Therapeutic Management

Multimodality treatment for most children includes surgery, radiotherapy, and chemotherapy. The ideal surgical procedure is complete tumor excision, but that is not always possible or feasible. For example, complete removal of some primary tumors such as orbital tumors leaves marked facial disfigurement, and resection of pelvic tumors may commit a child to lifelong urinary diversion and/or colostomy. Radiotherapy to the primary tumor site provides good local control in most tumors, but it must be combined with chemotherapy to treat micrometastatic disease for total tumor control. Chemotherapy is given in various multidrug combinations depending on the stage and often includes vincristine, actinomycin D, cyclophosphamide, and Adriamycin. Children with metastatic disease or those with histologic patterns known to be associated with a poor prognosis may receive more intensive chemotherapeutic regimens.

Children and adolescents with rhabdomyosarcoma now have a 60 to 65 per cent survival rate when treated with multimodality therapy. Patients with favorable histologic (cell type) features and either complete resection or only microscopic disease after surgery have an 80 to 85 per cent probability of long-term survival (Ruymann, 1987).

Strategies for Nursing Care

Nursing care for the child with rhabdomyosarcoma is primarily dictated by the tumor site. The child and family may need to be prepared for major lifestyle changes, such as a permanent colostomy after the tumor is removed. This information, coupled with impending surgery, radiotherapy, and chemotherapy, can certainly be overwhelming. The role of the nurse in providing caring and knowledgeable support cannot be overstated. Table 48-4 outlines care for the child during the period of chemotherapy. Chapter 26 addresses strategies for care pertinent to the child with a poor prognosis.

Osteogenic Sarcoma

Osteogenic sarcoma is an osseous tumor of the bone that arises in the mesenchyme. It is seen predominantly during the time of bone growth spurts and in areas that demonstrate rapid growth, such as the distal femur, the proximal tibia, and the proximal humerus. Metastases most commonly occur in the lungs, but other bones, the lymphatic system, and the liver may also be involved. Because areas of rapid bone growth are most often affected, it is rare to see osteogenic sarcoma before the preadolescent period of development. Osteogenic sarcoma is the most common malignant bone tumor seen in childhood.

Diagnostic Assessment

The primary symptom in a child with osteogenic sarcoma is localized pain that becomes increasingly frequent and more severe. A mass or swelling associated with the pain is usually a late finding and indicates longstanding tumor growth. The pain may be mild or transient, dull or aching. Referred pain to the leg or knee may be noted if the primary lesion occurs in the hip area. The child often describes a fall or an accident that preceded the onset of pain, but trauma merely elicits pain from the tumor that was already present. A radiograph of the painful site, or of the pelvis when pain is in the thigh or knee, should be made immediately.

If a bone tumor is suspected on plain radiograph, the patient must undergo a series of diagnostic tests. Most important of these are evaluations of the chest and primary site with CT scans and a nuclear bone scan.

A surgical biopsy is critical in determining the diagnosis of osteogenic sarcoma. As soon as a definitive diagnosis is made and the initial extent of disease evaluated, a treatment plan can be devised. Ideally, specialists such as a pediatric orthopedic surgeon, a diagnostic radiologist, a pediatric oncologist, and a pediatric pathologist help establish the plan of therapy together.

Although the medical necessity of performing the diagnostic examinations may have been explained to the adolescent and the family, the nurse must assess their need for further information or repeated information as the testing proceeds. Since the shock experienced initially may alter the family's ability to comprehend the information presented, the nurse must continually assess their level of understanding. The nurse must be prepared to provide exact information regarding the procedure to be performed, know whether the procedure will be painful or not, and tell the patient what will happen during the procedure. If possible, the nurse should accompany the child and parents to the test, particularly if the adolescent indicates a high level of anxiety about the procedure. Information provided before the procedure will assist the adolescent in coping before, during, and after it is over.

The diagnostic period is a time of fear and tension as decisions are awaited. The patient and the family will rely on the nurse for explanations of what is going on. Honesty is imperative, and it is important that information not be withheld from the family in an attempt to reduce stress. Likewise, providing hope and support is essential. Once the diagnosis is confirmed, new needs emerge and more help is necessary for the family to understand the treatment selected for their child.

Therapeutic Management

The treatment for osteogenic sarcoma depends on the primary tumor site and its extent and the presence or absence of metastatic disease. Some osteogenic sarcomas arise in bones that cannot be completely resected. These include the skull, the mandible, vertebrae, and certain sites in the pelvis. Most of the extremity lesions can be removed by appropriate amputation at the joint proximal to the lesion. In recent years "limb salvage" operations have been offered to a chosen group of adolescents whose tumors are confined within periosteal margins with very little soft tissue extension. Candidates for these procedures must have completed their adolescent growth spurt. In such patients a prosthetic replacement or cadaver bone is inserted following the removal of all or part of the involved bone. These replacements have been most successful in humeral and femoral lesions. Limb salvage procedures are almost always preferable for upper-extremity lesions since no prosthetic device is yet available to match human hand function. Patients need to know that limb salvage procedures are not without problems, and in some patients amputation may need to be performed later for secondary complications such as infection or recurrent tumor.

Radiotherapy offers little more than transient palliation for pain associated with osteogenic sarcoma. Certain chemotherapeutic agents, however, have shown striking tumor response in a limited number of patients. These agents include "high-dose" methotrexate with citrovorum rescue and the combination of cis-platin and Adriamycin. About 40 to 50 per cent of patients will have complete tumor response or have only microscopic foci of viable tumor remaining when the tumor is removed following preoperative chemotherapy. A similar response is seen when cis-platin and Adriamycin are employed preoperatively. Unfortunately, there is currently no way at diagnosis to differentiate between those patients who will respond to chemotherapy and those who will show little effect. Other chemotherapeutic agents have been used with less response in osteogenic sarcoma, including the combination of bleomycin, cyclophosphamide, and actinomycin-D. Present therapy study programs are attempting to sort out the efficacy of preoperative chemotherapy and adjuvant chemotherapy used postoperatively.

Strategies for Nursing Care

Providing Support During Chemotherapy. The chemotherapy regimens described above may be accompanied by severe acute toxicity or chronic toxicity, the most significant of which is renal tubular damage, which can be caused by high-dose methotrexate and cis-platin. Meticulous management of fluid and electrolyte balance before, during, and after infusions of these agents is necessary so that kidney function measurements do not gradually deteriorate. High-dose methotrexate must be followed by citrovorum factor rescue to avoid lethal effects of such doses on the bone marrow and epithelium of the oral mucosa and bowel. Citrovorum factor supplies folinic acid, which is prevented from being formed when the enzyme tetrahydrofolate reductase is inhibited by methotrexate.

These intensive chemotherapy regimens are poorly accepted by most adolescents. The anxiety over the potential loss of an extremity is still acute when highly toxic chemotherapy regimens are introduced. The nurse can be of great support during this period by assessing the adolescent's understanding of the treatment and teaching about the drugs and the reason for using them in the fashion in which they are administered.

The amount of physical discomfort associated with the use of chemotherapy must be described clearly to the patient and the family before treatment begins. Toxic effects of drugs must be discussed, as well as the means available to counteract complications. Medications that will be available for the control of pain, nausea, and vomiting must be described. The nursing care plan, which is written and determined in conjunction with the entire oncology health team, the adolescent, and the family, can serve as a form of contract between the nurse and the patient.

Clarifying Information About Surgical Options. Decisions regarding the type of surgical management present another dilemma to the patient and the family. Adolescents need extremely sensitive care during this very stressful time. They need information before the surgery about the choice of amputation versus limb-salvage surgery and why one or the other procedure is recommended. It is the physician's responsibility to provide this information, but the nurse is responsible for helping the client and family comprehend the information so that they can reach an informed decision.

The positive aspects of life with prosthetic limbs need to be stressed so that parents know their child can lead an active life following amputation. Most amputees can swim, dance, ski, participate in gymnastics, and do many other less demanding activities. The degree of function possible with prosthetic implants must also be addressed. Adolescents with prosthetic implants may be required to wear braces for a long period after surgery. They may likewise be instructed to avoid physical activity that could cause injury to the limb, such as contact sports.

The independent lifestyle that most teenagers envision rapidly disintegrates when decisions such as these are being made. Will they be able to drive a car? Will anyone want to dance with them? How can they wear bathing suits or shorts? Who will want to engage in sexual activity with them now? These questions need to be answered positively and can be most vividly presented by a successful amputee who had the same type of tumor. Adolescents need an accepting person to listen to their rage and fear. Their behavior at this time should be viewed by the nurse and family as an attempt to cope in the best way possible.

Promoting Successful Ambulation Postoperatively. A primary goal for the adolescent who undergoes a lower-extremity amputation is early ambulation. The earlier the return to ambulation, the earlier the adolescent will regain independence. Immediate postoperative stump care includes measures to shrink and shape the stump in preparation for prosthetic fitting. This is done through use of a plaster cast or by wrapping the stump 24 hours a day with an Ace bandage. The proper technique for wrapping the stump is to wrap in "figure eights" with tightness distally and a looser fit proximally to prevent compromised circulation. Physical therapists should become involved in the preoperative phase in the cases of all potential amputees. They may suggest that the patient meet with another amputee to discuss future options regarding prosthetic fitting and change in lifestyle. Physical therapy goals to be met before hospital discharge include:

- independent ambulation with crutches
- independent home exercise program
- independence in stump wrapping
- availability of all necessary home equipment

Many patients experience "phantom pain" or "phantom sensation" (feelings sensed as if they were in the patient's limb) for a long time after their amputations.

Long-Term Outcome

Although definite increases in the 5-year survival rates for osteogenic sarcoma have been made in the past decade, continuing clinical research programs are in progress. The adolescent who has osteogenic sarcoma must deal with the ever-present possibility and fear of recurrent tumor and death. The disease-free survival rates for the child with osteogenic sarcoma who has been treated with the combined modality approach appear to be greater than 50 per cent at 5 years (Rosen, 1984).

Ewing Sarcoma

Ewing sarcoma is a bone tumor characterized by anaplastic cells of small round cell type. It occurs predominantly in patients under the age of 20 years, with peak incidence during the period of adolescence (Nesbit et al, 1984). Ewing sarcoma is even rarer than osteosarcoma, with fewer than 200 new cases per year in the United States (Meyers, 1987).

The primary tumor may be in almost any bone of the body, but about half the tumors occur in the femur, tibia, or humerus (Jaffee et al, 1978). Metastases may appear in the lungs, viscera, other bones, and bone marrow. At times, pathologic fractures occur; the site and extent of the fracture dictate the severity of symptoms.

Diagnostic Assessment

Children with Ewing sarcoma generally have pain at the site of their tumor. Evaluation for suspected Ewing sarcoma includes x-ray films and CT scans of the primary tumor and the chest in addition to a bone scan and skeletal survey.

Therapeutic Management

Treatment of Ewing sarcoma includes surgery, radiation therapy, and combination chemotherapy. Complete surgical excision of the primary tumor is desirable but is rarely possible. Primary tumors in the ribs and fibula and relatively small lesions in the ilium are sites that can be removed surgically without amputation. Large tumors, such as those in the pelvis, are usually unresectable. Radiation therapy and chemotherapy may reduce tumor size to the extent that a surgical resection is possible later.

Radiation therapy is the primary treatment for Ewing sarcoma lesions, especially if they are unresectable. The aim of this treatment is destruction of the tumor and retention of adequate function. Children who receive high doses of radiotherapy to an extremity lesion before that bone has completed its growth will encounter long-term problems related to growth retardation and weakness of the bone.

Multidrug chemotherapy is used in a series of cycles administered over 1 or 2 years. Agents that are effective in combination for Ewing sarcoma include Adriamycin, cyclophosphamide, actinomycin-D, and vincristine. Chemotherapy is started at the time of the primary therapy. The role of chemotherapy is to treat micrometastases in lungs and in other sites that are undetectable at diagnosis.

Long-Term Outcome

Before the advent of chemotherapy and radiotherapy, the prognosis for a child with Ewing sarcoma was grim. Today, control of local disease is achieved in about 90 per cent of patients. The overall survival rate for patients with Ewing sarcoma is approximately 55 to 60 per cent (Nesbit et al, 1984).

Strategies for Nursing Care

Although treatment for Ewing sarcoma rarely involves amputation, the serious effects of the tumor and the late effects of radiation therapy and chemotherapy involve extensive nursing care and long-term follow-up. Nursing strategies related to the perioperative period and to care of the adolescent during radiation therapy and chemotherapy will not differ from those discussed previously in this chapter. Follow-up care, however, must take into account the potential for growth retardation and weakness of the affected bone after radiation therapy and the potential for lung metastasis. The family must be encouraged to faithfully keep follow-up visits to assure that any recurrence or metastasis is discovered as early as possible.

Retinoblastoma

Retinoblastoma is the most common tumor of the eye in infancy and childhood. It is a congenital malignant growth derived from embryonal retinal cells. Although the tumor may be present at birth, the average age at the time of diagnosis is 13 months, with the majority of children diagnosed before 3 years of age (Abramson, 1982).

Etiology

Although the mechanism of transmission is not fully understood, retinoblastoma is thought to result from both somatic and germ cell mutations. Somatic mutations are not hereditary. They result in unilateral involvement and account for the majority of all retinoblastomas. Germ cell mutations, on the other hand, are inherited and transmitted by the autosomal dominant mode of inheritance. (The parent has the trait but not the disease.) The majority of germinal mutations are bilateral, with about one third resulting in unilateral movement. Children of parents with unilateral retinoblastoma have a 15 per cent risk of having retinoblastoma if the tumor is not multifocal (Abramson, 1982). That risk increases to 50 per cent when the parent has bilateral involvement or a unilateral multifocal tumor. Because the incidence with a positive family history is significant, it is extremely important for siblings of an affected child to have an adequate ophthalmologic examination at birth and at frequent intervals until 3 years of age. Likewise, children of patients with histories of retinoblastoma must have similar ophthalmologic evaluations.

Clinical Manifestations

The tumor arises as one or more white lesions in the retina that grow at variable rates, eventually causing retinal detachment or formation of a mass protruding anteriorly from the retina. The tumor cells may spread via the optic nerve into the brain and subarachnoid space, producing CNS symptoms, or into the choroid and lymphatics with potential metastases to bones, bone marrow, and other tissues.

The most common presenting sign of retinoblastoma is a white reflex of the pupil, known as the "cat's eye reflex." A white spot on the retina seen on ophthalmoscopic examination is usually diagnostic of this tumor mass. If the tumor is small and located near the macula of the retina, the initial sign may be strabismus. Whenever strabismus is observed in an infant, a thorough ophthalmologic examination is required to rule out retinoblastoma. Loss of vision and redness or pain with or without glaucoma may be observed. The child may be irritable, or the parent may note changes in behavior indicative of decreased vision (bumping into objects, poor coordination). Because young children may not complain of loss of vision and the defects may not be apparent on superficial appraisal, the practitioner needs to carefully check the eyes for red reflexes, abnormal protrusions of the eyeball, atrophy, or venous congestion.

Diagnostic Assessment

CT scans of the head are particularly useful in determining the extent of the tumor within the orbit and brain and to help plan therapy. CT scans and skull radiographs are also obtained to document calcifications within the eye that aid in making the initial diagnosis of retinoblastoma. Bone scan, lumbar puncture, and bone marrow aspiration are done before treatment to detect the presence of metastatic disease.

Therapeutic Management

The size of the tumor and its location dictate the type of treatment. Radiation is often effective in destroying small, localized tumors of unilateral retinoblastoma, thereby preserving vision. Other treatment options for small, localized tumors include the use of cobalt plaque applicators (implantation of a cobalt applicator on the sclera to aid in delivering radiation to the tumor), cryotherapy (destruction of tumor blood vessels by freezing), and photocoagulation (destroying the blood vessels that lead to retinal lesions). Infants and little children require sedation in order to hold still for each treatment. In advanced cases with unilateral involvement, removal of the affected eye (enucleation) is necessary and greatly reduces the likelihood of metastasis. In bilateral cases, the eye with the more advanced tumor may need to be removed, and, if possible, the other eye is treated with radiation. In cases of advanced disease in both eyes, bilateral enucleation is indicated. Since metastasis can spread along the optic nerve pathway, a long optic nerve stump is removed with the eye to encompass tumor that may already have invaded or surrounded the optic nerve. The size and location of the tumor at the time of removal will provide staging information indicative of prognosis.

If the tumor has metastasized, chemotherapy may be used in conjunction with radiation. Early diagnosis is important because the stage of the disease at the time of diagnosis is most significant in determining outcome. If the tumor is detected at an early stage and adequate treatment is carried out, the prognosis is good. The patient survival rate is greater than 90 per cent, and vision is preserved in 75 per cent of treated eyes that have not been enucleated (Abramson, 1982). Once the tumor has metastasized out of the eye into the orbit, the chance of survival is greatly decreased.

Strategies for Nursing Care

The nursing care of the child with retinoblastoma and the family will depend on the child's age at diagnosis, the treatment required, and whether an inheritance factor is involved. If a family has a positive history of the disease, additional feelings of guilt may evolve. The nurse must consider all these factors in devising a care plan with the family.

Once the decision to perform an enucleation has been made, the parents must be prepared for their child's appearance following surgery. The child will initially have an eye patch in place that will be changed regularly by the ophthalmologist. Postoperatively the face may be edematous. Fittings for a prosthesis do not take place until the edema subsides. It is important to explain to the parents that the surgery will not result in a cavity in the skull; the periorbital area will appear quite normal because a sphere is surgically implanted to replace the eyeball until a prosthesis is available. Unless complications arise, such as infection, hemorrhage, or prolonged edema, the child is fitted with a prothesis within 3 weeks of surgery. Teaching the parents how to care for the prosthesis is critical. Techniques for insertion, removal, and cleaning of the prosthesis must be understood.

Once the diagnosis has been made, it is imperative that the risk of retinoblastoma in subsequent children be discussed with the parents and genetic counseling obtained. It is also critical to have the eyes of other children in the family examined as early as possible. In addition, both parents must have ophthalmologic examination even if their vision is normal and there is no prior history of disease, since in a small number of families one parent may have an obvious tumor scar that healed by spontaneous regression.

Text continues on page 1895.

Table 48-4
Nursing Process Plan: The Child Undergoing Chemotherapy

By Roxie Foster

I. Assessment of Physical Function

A. *Activity/Exercise* (associated with RBC, WBC, and platelet function)

Subjective Assessment

- RBC function: activity/exercise tolerance—breathing patterns upon exertion, energy level
- WBC function: symptoms of infection anywhere in the body
- Platelet function: bleeding tendencies

Objective Assessment

- RBC function: RBC count; hemoglobin and hematocrit; pulse and respirations at rest and with exertion; color of skin and mucous membranes
- WBC function: WBC and differential; temperature; cultures of blood and/or secretions to determine source of infection if one is suspected
- Platelet function: Platelet count; tests for occult blood; coagulation tests; visualization of stool and body secretions

Analysis: Nursing Diagnosis 1

Potential for injury: physiologic: bone marrow suppression, related to the side effects of chemotherapeutic medications

Defining Characteristics

Subjective: Shortness of breath with exercise; fatigue; weakness; dizziness; report of symptoms of infection (e.g., runny nose, sore throat); chills; headache and feeling of warmth associated with fever; prolonged bleeding from a cut; client observed red streaks in emesis or sputum and black, tarry stools

Objective: Decreased RBC, decreased hemoglobin and hematocrit; tachycardia, tachypnea, especially with mild exertion; skin and mucous membranes pale; decreased WBC (possibly with differential increase in remaining neutrophils or lymphocytes); fever; signs of infectious process; positive culture results; decreased platelet count; prolonged coagulation indicated by abnormal values on such measures as prothrombin time, activated partial thromboplastin time, thrombin time, platelet aggregation, platelet count, and bleeding time; positive results of tests for occult blood; petechiae, bruising; stools black and tarry; streaks of red blood evident in emesis/sputum

Client Goals/ Evaluation Criteria	Nursing Goals/Strategies (Selected Rationale)
1.1. The client will balance metabolic demands for oxygen with the blood's ability to carry oxygen, as evidenced by:	

a. pulse and respirations that return to normal limits within 10 minutes after increased activities (i.e., crying and feeding for the infant, loud crying and gross motor activity for the toddler and older child)	*Monitor pulse and respirations* before, during, and after periods of activity (to assess the body's ability to compensate for the increased oxygen demand related to exercise). *Indicate the child's activity* on the graphic record each time routine vital signs are taken (to facilitate accurate comparison).
b. adequate oxygenation to the central nervous system and to the periphery	*Assess, monitor, and chart signs and symptoms* of central nervous system hypoxia (changes in mental status, dizziness); color of skin and mucous membranes.
c. absence of fatigue in response to activity appropriate for age	*Plan and implement rest periods* for the hospitalized child that produce the desired outcomes. *Assess whether the anemia will necessitate alteration of the child's usual rest activity* patterns at home and discuss this with the family. *Utilize therapeutic play and family visitors* to decrease the child's anxiety and irritability. Insure that the family understands the relationship between activity and the body's demand for oxygen (so that they can more fully participate in the treatment plan).
1.2. The client will remain free of infection associated with leukopenia/neutropenia, as evidenced by:	
a. absence of fever	*Record temperature* every 4 hours.
b. absence of signs and symptoms of infection	*Record baseline assessments every shift* that include the status of each body system. Be alert for changes in the baseline that would indicate an infectious process. Watch for development of thrush (a common opportunistic infection during chemotherapy). *Administer prophylactic antifungal and antibiotic medications.* *Monitor WBC and differential counts.* Calculate the Absolute Neutrophil Count: $ANC = (\%\ Neutrophils + Bands) \times WBC$. If ANC <500, institute established unit policies to protect child who is at increased risk for infection. *Use meticulous handwashing techniques* at all times (there is an increased potential for infection with neutropenia even when the ANC is >500). Teach the child and family the major routes of transmission of organisms and the importance of good handwashing. *Teach the child and family the importance of lessening exposure* by avoiding crowds and persons with known infections. *Health care professionals must stay away from the oncology unit during times of illness.* Herpes simplex ("cold sore" or "fever blister") and childhood diseases caused by viruses (e.g., chickenpox or measles) are particularly dangerous for the child with bone marrow suppression (because there are fewer lymphocytes to fight the disease and few drugs currently available that are effective against viruses).*

* Although drugs such as Symmetrel (amantadine hydrochloride) have demonstrated antiviral properties, they are effective against a limited number of organisms.

Continued

Table 48-4 (continued)

Client Goals/ Evaluation Criteria	Nursing Goals/Strategies (Selected Rationale)
	Implement measures to reduce the risk of infection: • urinary tract: insure an adequate fluid intake to keep specific gravity between 1.002 and 1.020; avoid bubble baths and nylon panties (which may irritate the urethra); instruct girls to wipe from front to back. Use meticulous sterile technique if catheterization is necessary. • respiratory tract: encourage inflation of the lungs through activities such as balloon blowing; encourage avoidance of cigarette smoke and other irritants. • skin: wash even small cuts thoroughly with soap and water; then cleanse at least once per shift with hydrogen peroxide, or other solutions as ordered, to reduce pathogenic organisms. • central venous catheter: use and teach child and parents meticulous techniques for catheter care as prescribed by hospital/agency protocol. • keep the immunocompromised child in a private room if possible.
1.3. The client will minimize bleeding associated with thrombocytopenia, as evidenced by:	
a. skin and mucous membranes free of additional bruises and petechiae	*Document carefully the condition of skin and mucous membranes* on admission to form baseline data. *Caution the child and family members to prevent bumps, falls, and cuts.* Monitor toys for sharp edges; monitor child during play activities, especially if a tricycle, scissors, or other potentially harmful toy is involved. Avoid putting blankets and other potentially slippery articles on the floor; wipe up wet spills immediately. Discourage climbing and tumbling in play; encourage quiet activities such as listening to music, watching videos, coloring, finger painting, board games, and talking to friends on the phone. Large muscle exercise may be achieved through beanbag games, "impressionistic" movement to music, and monitored play of games such as "Twister." *Use a bubble top or crib net* for the toddler. Keep adult-sized bed in the lowest position. *Avoid overinflation of the cuff* when taking blood pressures. *Caution the child and family to make sure the child is in a seat belt or car seat* when riding in the car. *Ask the child and parents whether a written note from the MD or RN will be needed* to excuse the child from contact sports and regular physical education activities at school.
b. absence of frank bleeding, such as prolonged bleeding from wounds, hematomas, bleeding gums, epistaxis (nose bleeds), bright red blood in stools	*Avoid injections* when possible. When a needle must be used, use the smallest gauge possible (e.g., 25 gauge). Apply gentle pressure for 3–5 minutes following the injection. *Supply a soft toothbrush* and instruct the client and family on its proper use. *Caution the child not to blow the nose forcefully* and not to sneeze with both the nose and mouth closed.

Avoid constipation by insuring adequate fluids and fiber in the diet and adequate exercise, and by administration of stool softeners as appropriate; (constipation may lead to hemorrhoids and fissures that predispose the child to bleeding).

Avoid rectal temperatures and enemas; if suppositories are indicated (e.g., antiemetics) lubricate them well and insert carefully. (The fragile and vascular rectal muscosa is easily damaged.)

Avoid the use of aspirin and nonsteroidal anti-inflammatory drugs. Teach the child and parents how to recognize aspirin in product labels. (Aspirin and the NSAIDs are antiplatelet drugs.)

c. absence of hypovolemia associated with hemmorrhage

Take vital signs every 4 hours and as needed. Monitor for signs of hypovolemia: significant drop in B/P accompanied by an increase in pulse; pale, diaphoretic skin; decreased urine output; restlessness or confusion.

Monitor RBCs, hemoglobin, and hematocrit.

Teach child and parents the signs and symptoms of hemorrhage to be reported immediately. In addition to the aforementioned are hemarthrosis (bleeding into a joint, which causes pain and swelling) and intracranial bleed (sudden severe headache followed by changes in mental status).

B. Nutrition/Metabolism and Elimination

Subjective Assessment: Comfort of mucous membranes, appetite, GI symptoms, foods eaten in last 24–48 hours; number of wet diapers or voiding in the last 24 hours; recent bowel elimination patterns

Objective Assessment: Status of mucous membranes; weight compared to baseline; hydration status

---

Analysis: Nursing Diagnosis 2

Impaired skin integrity: ulceration of oral mucosa, related to the effect of cytotoxic drugs on the rapidly dividing mucosal cells

Defining Characteristics

Subjective: Pain in the mouth and throat; refusal of food and fluids

Objective: Drooling of saliva; white mucosal lesions with red borders; leukoplakia

---

Client Goal/ Evaluation Criteria — **Nursing Goals/Strategies (Selected Rationale)**

2.1. The client will experience a reduction in ulcerated areas, as evidenced by:

a. fewer ulcerations visible

Carefully document ulcerated areas to form a baseline for future assessment.

b. decreased oral pain

c. increased intake of food and fluids

Implement measures to relieve the pain of stomatitis:

- Instruct child to "swish and spit" a solution of warm saline, or half-strength hydrogen peroxide (to increase healing). Avoid commercial mouthwashes and lemon-glycerin swabs (they may further irritate the mucosa).

Continued

Table 48-4 (continued)

Client Goal/ Evaluation Criteria	Nursing Goals/Strategies (Selected Rationale)
	• Administer prescribed topical anesthetic agents such as viscous xylocaine before meals. • Instruct the child and parents to avoid foods and fluids that are very hot or cold, that are spicy or rough in texture, and that are acidic.

Analysis: Nursing Diagnosis 3

Altered nutrition: less than body requirements, related to:
- *increased metabolic rate associated with rapidly dividing malignant cells*
- *utilization of available nutrients by malignant cells resulting in insufficient nutrients for normal cells*
- *dysphagia associated with stomatitis*
- *anorexia associated with nausea and vomiting from the disease process and from chemotherapeutic agents*

Defining Characteristics

Subjective: "I'm not hungry;" "Take it away;" "It makes me feel sick;" "It hurts when I swallow"

Objective: Weight loss; oral intake less than minimum daily caloric requirement; ulcerated mucosa; vomiting associated with oral intake

Client Goal/ Evaluation Criteria	Nursing Goals/Strategies (Selected Rationale)
3. The client will maintain an adequate nutritional status, as evidenced by:	
a. weight returning to baseline and increasing in accordance with percentile for height	*Weigh daily* during hospitalization and with each follow-up visit to document progress toward goal. *Implement and teach measures to improve oral intake:* • Plan meals and snacks carefully to avoid food with little nutritional value. • Encourage high-protein, high-calorie foods that will not irritate mucous membranes. • Institute measures to decrease the incidence and effects of stomatitis (see Client Goal 2.1). • Take care to avoid making food an issue for power/control with the child. (This may be one of the few things the child can control in the therapeutic environment). Offer small portions of food, attractively prepared, frequently throughout the day but avoid insisting that the child eat or offering undue praise for foods consumed. • Counteract nausea by (1) avoiding food with distinctive smells (for this reason cold food is often better tolerated); (2) avoiding water, caffeine (found in cola and chocolate), and red meat (these foods are usually poorly tolerated by the client who has nausea and vomiting associated with chemo-

	therapy); (3) serving liquids between meals instead of with meals.
b. normal BUN and serum albumin	*Monitor BUN and serum albumin levels.* (Decreased levels reflect insufficient dietary protein.)

Analysis: Nursing Diagnosis 4

Fluid volume and electrolyte deficit, related to
- *inadequate fluid intake associated with stomatitis and anorexia*
- *loss of fluid associated with diarrhea and vomiting*

Defining Characteristics

Subjective: "I don't want to drink;" "I feel sick when I drink;" report of diarrhea and vomiting

Objective: Specific gravity >1.020 in an infant or young child, >1.035 in an older child or adolescent; dry mucous membranes; poor skin turgor; urine output <1 ml/kg/hr for an infant or child up to 30 kg and <30 ml/hr for the child over 30 kg; decreased BP and tachycardia (if dehydration has progressed to hypovolemia); observation of vomiting and/or of frequent, water-loss stools

Client Goals/ Evaluation Criteria	Nursing Goals/Strategies (Selected Rationale)
4.1. The client will maintain adequate hydration, as evidenced by:	
a. Urine output ≥ 1 ml/kg/hr for the child up to 30 kg and ≥ 30 ml/hr for the child over 30 kg	*Record intake and output,* including diaper weights for infants, during hospitalization.
b. Intake $\geq$ maintenance fluid requirements: • 100 ml/kg for the first 10 kg of body weight • 50 ml/kg for the next 10 kg of body weight • 10 ml/kg for each succeeding kg of body weight	*Calculate the maintenance fluid requirements* and determine the amount of fluid to be given during each hospital shift or at various hours of the day when the child is at home. • Offer fluids frequently and in small amounts. • School-age children and adolescents may find incentive in recording their own intake (thus demonstrating their ability to meet fluid requirements). *Record specific gravity each shift* if a spectrometer is available on the unit.
c. Specific gravity <1.020 in an infant or young child; <1.035 in an older child or adolescent	
4.2. The client will maintain acid-base balance, as evidenced by:	
a. normal serum electrolytes	*Monitor serum electrolyte levels.* In metabolic acidosis, the pH and serum CO_2 will be decreased, and base excess will be negative. In metabolic alkalosis, the pH and serum CO_2 will be increased, and base excess will be positive.

Continued

Table 48-4 (continued)

Client Goals/ Evaluation Criteria	Nursing Goals/Strategies (Selected Rationale)
b. absence of signs and symptoms of metabolic acidosis	*Monitor for metabolic acidosis* in the presence of diarrhea (the loss of bicarbonate ion leads to acidosis). Record and report changes in mental status, tachypnea, headache, nausea, and vomiting.
c. absence of signs and symptoms of metabolic alkalosis	*Monitor for metabolic alkalosis in the presence of vomiting (the loss of NaCl and HCl* leads to alkalosis). Record and report dizziness; agitation; bradypnea; tingling of the fingers, toes, and circumoral area; muscle twitching; or seizure activity. *Implement and teach measures to prevent vomiting and diarrhea.* • See Client Goal 3. • Avoid foods that stimulate peristalsis, will be poorly digested, or cause gas: fats (including dairy products), fiber (whole grains, fresh fruits and vegetables), cabbage, popcorn, beans, caffeine, hot and cold foods. • Provide small, frequent meals instead of large meals (a bolus of food is more likely to stimulate peristalsis).

II. Assessment of Emotional-Social Function

A. Self-Perception/Self-Concept
B. Coping/Stress/Tolerance Patterns
C. Spiritual Health

Subjective Assessment:

Verbalization of the following: fears and anxieties, perceptions of self, feelings about the disease and the treatment modalities, ability to manage invasive procedures, changes in family and social responsibilities

Objective Assessment:

Signs of fear and anxiety, nonverbal behavior that indicates feelings about self and others, observation of parenting patterns, observed coping patterns of child and family members

Analysis: Nursing Diagnosis 5

Fear/anxiety (child and family), related to
- *diagnosis of a malignant and life-threatening disease*
- *the administration and side effects of chemotherapy*
- *the pain of invasive diagnostic and therapeutic measures*

Defining Characteristics:

Subjective: Verbalization by child and family members of fears related to the prognosis and to the length of prescribed chemotherapy and its effects upon the child

Objective: Body posture indicating anxiety; child and/or family members actively seeking comfort in the nurse's touch and presence; tearful behavior; actively withdrawing from health care professionals when they enter the room; verbally, vocally, and/or physically protesting both invasive and noninvasive treatment and diagnostic measures

Client Goals/ Evaluation Criteria	Nursing Goals/Strategies (Selected Rationale)
5. The child and family will experience decreased fear and anxiety, as evidenced by: a. verbalization of being less afraid b. relaxation of body posture, less tearful behavior, less protest of nonpainful procedures c. verbalization of an understanding of the prognosis and procedures associated with the treatment	*Encourage verbalization* of the fear/anxiety (to facilitate identification of the actual sources of the fear). *Express both verbally and nonverbally the client's right to the feelings.* (Denying or belittling the fear by comments such as, "There's no reason to be afraid," only adds to the anxiety and frustration.) Assuring the client that many other children or parents have expressed similar concerns may be comforting. *Implement direct care with confidence.* (It is important for the child and family to believe the nurse is knowledgeable and in charge of the situation.) *Explain procedures and other aspects of care carefully and repeatedly,* as necessary. (The unknown is usually more anxiety-producing than the known.) *Always conduct painful or unpleasant procedures in the treatment room.* (Children's fear will be reduced if their room is a "safe" place.) *Always answer questions as honestly as possible.* Do not hesitate to say, "I don't know" when that is the case. (The child and family do not expect the nurse to know everything, but their confidence will be enhanced and their anxiety reduced if they can count on an honest response.) *Include the child and family in every possible aspect of care planning, delivery, and evaluation.* (Fear and anxiety will decrease as their sense of control increases.) *Explore the concept of death with the child* and dispell unwarranted fears as appropriate. Determine whether the concept of death and major fears are typical for the age. Explain developmental norms to the family.

Analysis: Nursing Diagnosis 6

Disturbance in self-concept: body image, self-esteem, role performance, personal identity, related to

- ***alopecia associated with many chemotherapeutic agents***
- ***cushingoid features associated with the use of prednisone for its cytotoxic properties***
- ***the potential for sterility associated with cytotoxic drugs***

Defining Characteristics

Subjective: Verbalization of concern about how peers and others will react to body changes, unwillingness to receive visitors or to leave the room, verbalization of feelings of worthlessness, unwillingness to dress and perform usual grooming activities, unwillingness to discuss return to school, unwillingness to assume self-care or to learn aspects of procedures for home care

Objective: Flat affect, malaise, avoidance of social contact and of personal responsibility

Continued

Table 48-4 (continued)

Client Goal/ Evaluation Criteria	Nursing Goals/Strategies (Selected Rationale)
6. The client will demonstrate acceptance of changes in appearance and renewed self-esteem, as evidenced by: a. expressing feelings about the body changes and the potential for sterility b. beginning problem-solving activities, such as asking the family to buy a wig or bring in a favorite baseball cap c. renewed interest in personal appearance d. resumption of normal interest in peer relationships e. verbalization of plans to make up school work missed during hospitalization f. asking questions about the potential for sterility and the possible treatment	*Encourage verbalization of feelings.* (Ventilation of emotion is often preliminary to problem-solving activity.) *Maintain an attitude of confidence in the child.* (Nonverbal communication of an attitude is often more convincing than words.) *Assist the child to identify strengths* and to capitalize on them. *Encourage supportive peer contacts.* *Help the child to plan for activities* that will provide an incentive for discharge. *Facilitate contact with other children of similar age* who have experienced these same body changes. *Assure the child and family that hair loss is not permanent.* *Encourage family contact with other parents and siblings* who have been through a similar experience. *Discuss the child's and family's fears about sterility* and explain appropriate alternative ways to become a parent. *Encourage family members to express their need for the child to return to former responsibilities within the family* (to reinforce self-worth and role within the family).

Analysis: Nursing Diagnosis 7

Spiritual distress (child and family), related to:
- *worry associated with the prognosis and potential reactions to therapy*
- *a search for the meaning of the illness*
- *feelings of guilt associated with the etiology or delay between onset of the disease and diagnosis*
- *powerlessness associated with the uncertainty of the prognosis and the need to undergo therapies that have potentially harmful side effects*

Defining Characteristics

Subjective: Verbalization of concern, worry, insomnia; verbalization of guilt and frustration; parental statements like "If only it were me instead of my child;" child's questions of "Why did this happen to me?" "Did I get this because I was naughty?"; verbalization of anger and resentment

Objective: Distracted behavior; daydreaming; irritability; sad and woeful appearance; acting-out behavior; restlessness; decreased attention span; sleeping for prolonged periods, or insomnia

Client Goal/ Evaluation Criteria	Nursing Goals/Strategies (Selected Rationale)
7. The client will demonstrate renewed strength of spirit, as evidenced by: a. resumption of more normal affect and activities b. verbalization of having more "peace of mind" c. expression of a philosophic purpose for the disease	*Encourage verbalization* and listen with empathy and a nonjudgmental attitude. Encourage the child and family to seek out persons (e.g., clergy) who have been helpful in helping them find meaning in other situations. *Assist the client to correct misconceptions,* but do not attempt to solve the client's problem. (No one else can do that but the client. Expression of feelings with an empathetic listener will help the client gain perspective needed for problem solving.) *Explore with the client the activities that are usually the most enjoyable* and produce a feeling of happiness and lightheartedness. Facilitate and encourage these activities, as permitted, in the hospital setting and at home. (Activities that have produced this effect in the past carry a great potential for facilitating the client's emotional self-healing.)

III. Assessment of Intellectual-Perceptual Function

A. Knowledge of the Illness
B. Health Perception/Management (associated with compliance with treatment regimen)
C. Pain (associated with diagnostic and therapeutic procedures, e.g., lumbar puncture, intrathecal injections, and intravenous infusions)

Subjective Assessment:

Questions about the disease and its management; verbalization of understanding or lack of understanding; verbalization of health beliefs and attitudes; verbalization of pain.

Objective Assessment:

Return demonstration of procedures necessary for home care management (e.g., care of central venous catheter); willingness to participate in teaching sessions; willingness or reluctance to hold child or physically demonstrate affection during procedural periods (e.g., during intravenous infusions); activity indicative of pain.

Analysis: Nursing Diagnosis 8

Knowledge deficit, related to
- *the disease process*
- *the course and side effects of chemotherapy*
- *laboratory values and the relationship of diagnostic procedures to the chemotherapy protocol*

Defining Characteristics

Subjective: Verbalization of lack of understanding, questions about various aspects of the disease and therapy

Objective: Demonstration of insufficient knowledge to (1) perform necessary procedures for home management, (2) administer medications and recognize major side effects, (3) understand the need for and significance of follow-up visits.

Continued

Table 48-4 (continued)

Client Goal/ Evaluation Criteria	Nursing Goals/Strategies (Selected Rationale)
8. The client and family will demonstrate knowledge of the disease process and therapeutic measures necessary to maintain home care management upon discharge, as evidenced by: a. verbalizing the signs and symptoms of relapse and of medication side effects b. verbalizing care for the child who has bone marrow suppression c. verbalizing a willingness to comply with the therapeutic plan d. demonstrating direct care measures that will be needed in the home e. identifying sources of physical and emotional support	*Provide appropriate support and teaching.* See previous nursing diagnoses for teaching measures. • Begin discharge teaching upon admission. (Teaching is much too involved and important to be left until late in the hospital stay or until the day of discharge.) • See specific discharge planning strategies in Table 31-2, page 972.

Analysis: Nursing Diagnosis 9

Altered comfort: pain, related to
- *proliferation of blast cells within the intramedullary cavities of bones and within abdominal organs*
- *administration of intrathecal and intravenous chemotherapy*
- *side effects of cytotoxic agents*

Defining Characteristics

Subjective: Verbalization and vocalization of pain

Objective: Alteration in usual activity patterns; eyes dull in appearance; skin cool and pale; possible increase in pulse, decrease in blood pressure

Client Goal/ Evaluation Criteria	Nursing Goals/Strategies (Selected Rationale)
9. The child will maintain a level of comfort without significant pain, as evidenced by: a. resumption of usual activities b. eyes brighter in appearance c. vital signs within normal limits d. skin warm and without pallor	*Assess pain:* • Note activity level. (Children in pain are often much quieter than usual but may also show a marked increase in activity. Dullness of the eyes and lethargy often accompany pain.) • Assess and interpret vital signs for their relation to pain versus other physiologic activity. (Increase in pulse, decrease in blood pressure, along with cool, clammy skin, indicate the neuroendocrine response to the stress of pain.) • Analyze carefully the child's subjective response to questions about comfort. (Children may deny pain because they dislike the treatment for pain.)

e. verbalization of comfort	• Use adjunctive measures to assess pain, such as those detailed in Chapter 29. *Allow the child control over pain medication,* as appropriate to developmental age; e.g., allow the child to choose from the analgesics ordered, which medication to take and how many tablets or capsules. (Control will decrease the anxiety associated with pain and will make the pain more manageable.) *Implement and teach the child and family adjunctive measures for pain relief,* such as muscle massage, a warm tub bath, distraction and relaxation techniques (Chapter 29 details adjunctive therapies.) *Prior to painful invasive procedures, assess how the child usually copes with acute pain, and which of the strategies is most adaptive.* Reinforce the useful coping behavior and teach additional coping strategies, such as relaxation techniques. (New coping behavior must be practiced repeatedly before the painful experience, otherwise, the child will revert to familiar, even though possibly less effective, strategies, when faced with the stress of the moment.) *When planning and teaching new coping strategies, keep in mind that motor and emotional coping strategies (being allowed to pound with one hand or to cry and scream) are extremely useful* for young children who have poorly developed cognitive coping abilities.

References

Abramson D: Retinoblastoma: diagnosis and management. *CA* 1982; 32(3):2–12.

Allen J, et al: The value of adjuvant chemotherapy in the management of newly diagnosed medulloblastoma, malignant astrocytoma, and brain stem glioma: results from the Children's Cancer Study Group. XIX Canadian Congress of Neurological Sciences, 14, 1984.

Belasco JB, et al: Wilms tumor. *In* Sutow W, et al: *Clinical Pediatric Oncology.* St. Louis, CV Mosby, 1984.

Bellanti JA: *Immunology; Basic Processes.* 2nd ed. Philadelphia, WB Saunders, 1985.

Ertel I, et al: Adjuvant chemotherapy of high grade astrocytomas in children: radiation therapy with or without CCNU, vincristine, and prednisone. *Proc Am Soc Clin Oncol* 1984; C-309.

Evans A, et al: Diagnosis and treatment of neuroblastoma. *Pediatr Clin North Am* 1976 Oct; 161.

Finklestein JZ: Neuroblastoma: The challenge and frustration. *Hematol/Oncol Clin North Am* 1987 Dec; 1(4):675–694.

Finlay JL, et al: Progress in the management of childhood brain tumors. *Hematol/Oncol Clin North Am* 1987 Dec; 1(4):753–776.

Fochtman D, et al (eds): Nursing Care of the Child with Cancer. Boston, Little, Brown, 1982, page 83.

Gale RP, Champlin RE: Bone marrow transplantation in acute leukaemia. *Clin Haematol* 1986 Aug; 15(3):851–872.

Gale RP, Foon KA: Acute myeloid leukaemia: recent advances in therapy. *Clin Haematol* 1986 Aug; 15(3):781–810.

Gale RP, Hoffbrand AV: Acute leukemias: Biology and treatment. *Clin Haematol* 1986 Aug; 15(3):567–571.

Ganick DJ: Wilms' tumor. *Hematol/Oncol Clin North Am* 1987 Dec; 1(4):695–719.

Gardner RV, Graham-Pole J: Non-Hodgkin's lymphoma. *Pediatr Ann* 1983 Apr; 12(4):322–335.

Gellis SS, Kagan BM: *Current Pediatric Therapy 12.* Philadelphia, WB Saunders, 1986.

Ghavimi F: Rhabdomyosarcoma. *Pediatr Ann* 1983 May; 12(5):395–401.

Groenwald SL: *Cancer Nursing; Principles and Practice.* Boston, Jones and Bartlett Publishers, 1987.

Groncy P, Finklestein J: Neuroblastoma. *Pediatr Ann* 1978 Aug; 7(8):73–89.

Hagle ME: Implantable devices for chemotherapy: Access and delivery. *Semin Oncol Nurs* 1987 May; 3(2):96–105.

Hakami N, Monzon CM: Acute nonlymphocytic leukemia in children. *Hematol/Oncol Clin North Am* 1987 Dec; 1(4):567–575.

Hann HL, et al: Serum ferritin levels as a guide to prognosis in patients with Stage IV neuroblastoma. *Proc Am Soc Clin Oncol* 1983; 2:C-282.

Hausman K: Brain tumors in children. *J Neurosurg Nurs* 1979 Mar; 8.

Hayes FA, Green AA: Neuroblastoma. *Pediatr Ann* 1983 May; 12(5):366–373.

Huttenlocher PR: Neoplasms of the brain. *In* Behrman RE, Vaughan VC (eds): *Nelson Textbook of Pediatrics.* 13th ed. Philadelphia, WB Saunders, 1987, 1319–1330.

Jaffee N, et al: Integrated multidisciplinary treatment for pediatric solid tumors. *In Cancer: A Manual for Practi-*

tioners. Massachusetts Division, American Cancer Society, 1978, 279.

Johnson FL, Thomas ED: Treatment of relapsed acute lymphoblastic leukemia in childhood (letter). *N Engl J Med* 1984; 310(4):263.

Kaplan HS: *Hodgkin's Disease.* Cambridge, MA, Harvard University Press, 1974.

Leventhal BG: Neoplasms and neoplasm-like structures. *In* Behrman RE, Vaughan VC (eds): *Nelson Textbook of Pediatrics.* 13th ed. Philadelphia, WB Saunders, 1987, 1079–1109.

Maguire M: Leukemia. *In* Ziegfeld CR: *Core Curriculum for Oncology Nursing.* Philadelphia, WB Saunders, 1987, 173–192.

Maurer HM, Ragab AH: Rhabdomyosarcoma. *In* Sutow W, et al: *Clinical Pediatric Oncology.* St. Louis, CV Mosby, 1984.

Miller D: Acute lymphoblastic leukemia. *Pediatr Clin North Am* 1980 May; 27(2):269–291.

Myers PA: Malignant bone tumors in children: Ewing's sarcoma. *Hematol/Oncol Clin North Am* 1987 Dec; 1(4):667–673.

Nesbit ME, et al: Round cell sarcoma of bone. *In* Sutow W, et al: *Clinical Pediatric Oncology.* St. Louis, CV Mosby, 1984.

Olness K, Gardner GG: *Hypnosis and Hypnotherapy with Children.* 2nd ed. Philadelphia, Grune and Stratton, 1988.

Rosen G: Spindle cell sarcoma—osteogenic sarcoma. *In* Sutow W, et al: *Clinical Pediatric Oncology.* St. Louis, CV Mosby, 1984.

Rubin P (ed): *Clinical Oncology. A Multidisciplinary Approach.* 6th ed. The American Cancer Society, 1983.

Ruymann FB: Rhabdomyosarcoma in children and adolescents. *Hematol/Oncol Clin North Am* 1987 Dec; 1(4):621–654.

Skarin A, et al: Malignant lymphomas. *In Cancer: A Manual for Practitioners.* Massachusetts Division, American Cancer Society, 1978, 249.

Steinherz PG: Acute lymphoblastic leukemia of childhood. *Hematol/Oncol Clin North Am* 1987 Dec; 1(4):549–566.

Sullivan MP, et al: Hodgkin's disease in Children. *In* Sutow W, et al: *Clinical Pediatric Oncology.* St. Louis, CV Mosby, 1984.

Sullivan MP: Hodgkin's disease in children. *Hematol/Oncol Clin North Am* 1987 Dec; 1(4):603–620.

van Eyes, J: Malignant tumors of the central nervous system. *In* Sutow W, et al: *Clinical Pediatric Oncology.* St. Louis, CV Mosby, 1977.

Van Wezel-Bolen G: Rhabdomyosarcoma. *In* Fochtman D, Foley G: *Nursing Care of the Child with Cancer.* Boston, Little, Brown, 1982.

Vega RA, et al: Bone marrow transplantation in the treatment of children with cancer. Current status. *Hematol/Oncol Clin North Am* 1987 Dec; 1(4):777–800.

Voute PA: Neuroblastoma. *In* Sutow W, et al: *Clinical Pediatric Oncology.* St. Louis, CV Mosby, 1984.

Walker MD: Tumors of the central nervous system. *In* Levine AS: *Cancer in the Young.* New York, Masson Publishing USA, 1982.

Walker RW, Allen JC: Pediatric brain tumors. *Pediatr Ann* 1983 May; 12(5):383–394.

Zeltzer P, et al: Elevated serum neuron specific enolase in metastatic neuroblastoma. *Proc Am Soc Clin Oncol* 1983; 2:C-307.

Ziegfeld CR: *Core Curriculum for Oncology Nursing.* Philadelphia, WB Saunders, 1987.

Zwaan FE, Jansen J: Bone marrow transplantation in acute nonlymphoblastic leukemia. *Semin Hematol* 1984 Jan; 21(1):36–41.

Bibliography

Battista EM: Education needs of the adolescent with cancer and his family. *Semin Oncol Nurs* 1986 May; 2(2):123–125.

Blotcky AD: Helping adolescents with cancer cope with their disease. *Semin Oncol Nurs* 1986 May; 2(2):139–141.

Cohen DG: Future perspectives in adolescent oncology. *Semin Oncol Nurs* 1986 May; 2(2):75–83.

Cohen DG, et al: Growing up differently: An adolescent's perspective. *Semin Oncol Nurs* 1986 May; 2(2):84–89.

Doyle MA: Whole body hyperthermia: Making things too hot for cancer. *RN* 1987 Aug: 39–40.

Frank-Stromborg M, et al: Carcinogens: Are some risks acceptable? *Am J Nurs* 1986 Jul; 86(7):814–817.

Grant M: Nausea, vomiting, and anorexia. *Semin Oncol Nurs* 1987 Nov; 3(4):277–286.

Green M: *Pediatric Diagnosis.* 4th ed. Philadelphia, WB Saunders, 1986.

Harris LC, et al: Implantable infusion devices in the pediatric patient: A viable alternative. *J Pediatr Nurs* 1987 Jun; 2(3):174–183.

Hilton A: Approaches for feeding the young child with anorexia. *J Pediatr Nurs* 1987 Feb; 2(1):45–49.

Kobrinsky NL, et al: Acute nonlymphocytic leukemia. *Pediatr Clin North Am* 1980 May; 27(2):345–359.

Kramer RF, Moore ID: Childhood cancer: Meeting the special needs of healthy siblings. *Cancer Nurs* 1983 Jun: 213–217.

Lauer ME, et al: Children's perceptions of their sibling's death at home or hospital: The precursors of differential adjustment. *Cancer Nurs* 1985 Feb: 21–27.

Leonard MA, Waskerwitz MJ: Late effects in adolescent survivors of childhood cancer. *Semin Oncol Nurs* 1986 May; 2(2):126–132.

Lind J, Bush NJ: Nursing's role in chemotherapy administration. *Semin Oncol Nurs* 1987 May; 3(2):83–86.

Mahon SM: Taking the terror out of amphotericin B. *Am J Nurs* 1988 Jul; 88(7):961–964.

Maul-Melott SK, Adams JN: *Childhood Cancer: A Nursing Overview.* Boston, Jones and Bartlett Publishers, 1987.

Mayer DK: Alpha interferon: Reinforcing the body's anticancer arsenal. *RN* 1987 Aug: 40–41.

Meeske K, Ruccione KS: Cancer chemotherapy in children: Nursing issues and approaches. *Semin Oncol Nurs* 1987 May; 3(2):118–127.

Moeller KL, Swartzendruber EJ: Suppressing the risks of bone marrow suppression. *Nurs 87* 1987 Mar; 17(3): 52–54.

Moore J, et al: The late psychosocial consequences of childhood cancer. *J Pediatr Nurs* 1988 Jun; 3(3):150–158.

Nelson T: Current cancer information for you and your patients. *RN* 1987 Aug: 43.

The new immunology. Helping the body heal itself. *Am J Nurs* 1987 Apr; 87(4):455–473.

Nirenberg A, Bridgewater CF: Malignancies in adolescents. *Semin Oncol Nurs* 1986 May; 2(2):75–83.

Nuscher R, et al: Bone marrow transplantation. *Am J Nurs* 1984 Jun; 84(6):764–772.

Shea MC, Dragone N: Active specific immunotherapy: Turning cancer cells into anticancer agents. *RN* 1987 Aug: 38–39.

Smith CE, et al: Content analysis of interview using a nursing model: A look at parents adapting to the impact of childhood cancer. *Cancer Nurs* 1983 Aug: 269–275.

Spies C: Giving amphotericin B in the home. *Am J Nurs* 1988 Jul; 88(7):965–966.

Rahr V: Giving intrathecal drugs. *Am J Nurs* 1986 Jul; 86(7):829–831.

Ruccione K: The role of nurses in late effects evaluations. *Clin Oncol* 1985 Jul; 4(2):205–221.

Shalet SM: The effects of cancer treatment on growth and sexual development. *Clin Oncol* 1985 Jul; 4(2):223–228.

Sherman DW, et al: Comforting the terminally ill leukemia patient. *Nurs 88* 1988 Jun; 18(6):53–57.

Sullivan L: Photodynamic therapy: Flashing a red light at cancer. *RN* 1987 Aug: 42–43.

Van Dongen-Melman JEWM, Sanders-Woudstra JAR: Psychosocial aspects of childhood cancer: A review of the literature. *Child Psychol* 1986; 27(2):145–180.

Vargo NL: The skin cancer success story. *RN* 1987 Jul: 50–57.

Wofford LG: "Cured!". . . Now what? *Pediatr Nurs* 1987 Jul/Aug; 13(4):252–254.

Young CM: Intraoperative radiation: Taking a clear shot at cancer. *RN* 1987 Aug: 41–42.

Chapter 49

Nursing Strategies: Altered Endocrine Function

Deborah Coody
Bonnie Stevens

Nursing Process Plan

NPP: The Child with Diabetic Ketoacidosis, page 1956

Related Topics

Genetic counseling, Chapter 4
Patterns of inheritance, Chapter 4
Strategies to assess and enhance self-esteem, Chapter 16
The impact of chronic illness, Chapter 25
NPP: The Family in Need of Genetic Counseling, Chapter 50

The endocrine system consists of a group of specialized tissues with one vital function in common: These tissues produce and secrete the major chemical regulators of the body called hormones. Hormone secretion significantly affects such important body functions as growth, fluid and electrolyte balance, the stress response, sexual characteristics, and glucose metabolism. If a hormone is either oversecreted or undersecreted, those organs whose actions are "programmed" by that hormone respond with disturbing, and sometimes life-threatening, changes in function. This chapter is concerned primarily with altered secretion of endocrine glands and the nursing strategies that relate to the child's experience of endocrine dysfunction. Nursing strategies related to disorders of the pituitary gland, the thyroid gland, the parathyroid glands, the adrenal glands, and the gonads are presented first. Altered function of the pancreas resulting in diabetes mellitus, the most common endocrine disorder in childhood, follows and is covered in depth.

Structure and Function of the Endocrine System

The endocrine system (also known as the hormonal system) is composed of a diverse group of tissues that produce and secrete chemical substances (hormones), which stimulate actions of other tissues. The body tissues sensitive to the effects of hormones are called target tissues. Seven glands are included in the endocrine system: pituitary, thyroid, parathyroid, adrenal, pancreas, ovary, and testis (Fig. 49-1). Table 49-1 reviews the basic functions of these glands and their target tissues, each of which will be discussed at length in this chapter. *Endocrine glands are unique by virtue of the fact that their secretions are released directly into the bloodstream for distribution throughout the body rather than passing through ducts into localized areas.* Secretions released into ducts are termed exocrine, and glands such as the salivary glands and sweat glands of the skin are exocrine glands.

Hormones act in a catalytic manner by stimulating a physiologic response in a target site without being directly involved in the target site's biochemical reactions. Many hormones act by becoming bound to a special receptor site on the target cell membrane. This binding initiates synthesis of cyclic adenosine monophosphate (AMP), which acts as a second messenger to produce cellular enzyme activity changes and thus the hormone's physiologic effect (Fig. 49-2). Other hormones are believed to enter the target cell's nucleus to induce the formation of messenger ribonucleic acid (mRNA), which then enters the cytoplasm to increase the synthesis of specific cellular proteins (Watts and

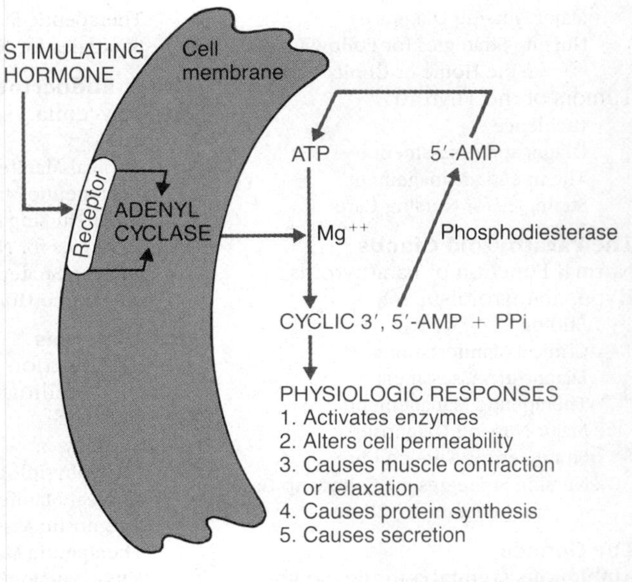

Figure 49-2. The cyclic AMP mechanism, by which many hormones exert their control of cell function. (From Guyton AC: *Textbook of Medical Physiology.* Philadelphia, WB Saunders, 1986.)

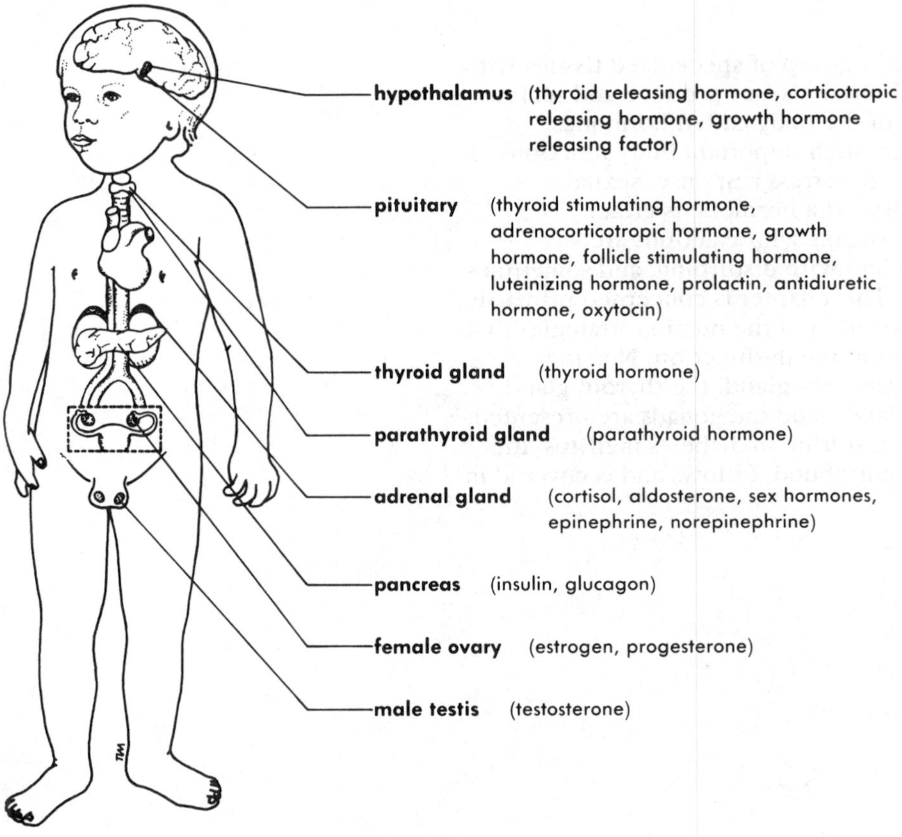

Figure 49-1. The endocrine glands. (Courtesy of Deborah Coody, RN, MS, PNP, The University of Texas Medical School at Houston, Department of Pediatrics.)

Table 49-1. Endocrine Glands: Secretion, Target, and Actions

Gland	Hormone	Target	Basic Action
Pituitary gland			
Anterior lobe	Somatotropin (growth hormone)	Bones, muscles, organs	Retention of nitrogen to promote protein anabolism
	TSH (thyroid stimulating hormone)	Thyroid	Promotes secretory activity
	FSH (follicle stimulating hormone)	Ovaries, seminiferous tubules	Promotes development of ovarian follicle, secretion of estrogen, and maturation of sperm
	LH (luteinizing hormone) ICSH (interstitial cell stimulating hormone in male)	Follicle, interstitial cell	Promotes ovulation and formation of corpus luteum, secretion of progesterone, and secretion of testosterone
	Prolactin (luteotropic hormone)	Corpus luteum, breast	Maintains corpus luteum and progesterone secretion; stimulates milk secretion
Posterior lobe	ADH (antidiuretic hormone)	Distal tubules of kidneys	Reabsorption of water
	Oxytocin	Uterus	Stimulates contraction
Thyroid	Thyroxine	Widespread	Regulates oxidation rate of body cells and growth and metabolism; influences gluconeogenesis, mobilization of fats, and exchange of water, electrolytes, and protein
	Calcitonin	Skeleton	Calcium and phosphorus metabolism
Parathyroids	PTH (parathyroid hormone)	Bone, kidney, gastrointestinal tract	Essential for calcium and phosphorus metabolism and calcification of bone
Adrenal gland Cortex	Mineralocorticoid (aldosterone)	Widespread, primarily kidney	Maintains fluid and electrolyte balance; reabsorbs sodium chloride; excretes potassium
	Glucocorticoids (cortisol)	Widespread	Concerned with food metabolism and body response to stress; preserves carbohydrates and mobilizes amino acids; promotes gluconeogenesis; suppresses inflammation
	Sex hormones (testosterone, estrogen, and progesterone)	Gonads	Ability to influence secondary sex characteristics
Medulla	Epinephrine	Widespread	Vasoconstriction with increased blood pressure; increased blood sugar via glycolysis; stimulates ACTH production
	Norepinephrine	Widespread	Vasoconstriction
Pancreas	Insulin	Widespread	Increased utilization of carbohydrate; decreased lipolysis and protein catabolism; decreased blood sugar
	Glucagon	Widespread	Hyperglycemic factor; increases blood sugar via glycogenolysis
Gonads			
Ovaries	Estrogen	Widespread	Secondary sex characteristics; maturation and sexual function
	Progesterone	Uterus, breast	Preparation for and maintenance of pregnancy; development of mammary gland secretory tissue
Testes	Testosterone	Widespread	Secondary sex characteristics; maturation and normal sex function

(From Krueger and Ray, 1976.)

Keffer, 1982). The response of a particular target tissue to a hormone may be immediate or delayed. The magnitude of the response is altered by the rate of synthesis and secretion of the hormone into the blood, the rate of transport in the blood, and the rate of inactivation and excretion in the body.

Hormones are secreted cyclically and in response to certain body and environmental rhythms. For example, there are a diurnal variation in adrenocorticotropic hormone (ACTH) secretions and monthly variations in a woman's estrogen and progesterone secretion. In addition, the endocrine glands are interdependent, and the release of one hormone influences the release of other hormones. It is this interdependence, as well as neurologic and chemical control, that helps maintain hormonal levels in homeostasis.

Hormonal Control of Homeostasis

Interaction Between the Hormonal and Nervous Systems

Many interrelationships exist between the hormonal and nervous systems, because integration of both is necessary to maintain homeostasis. Both systems synthesize and release chemicals that are transported

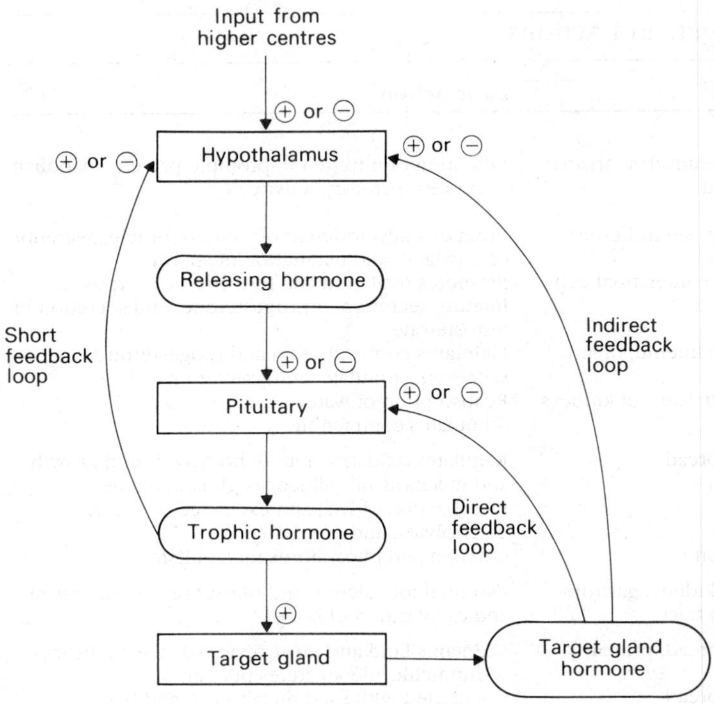

Figure 49-3. A schematic representation of hormonal interactions. (From O'Riordan JL, Malan PG, Gould RP: *Essentials of Endocrinology.* Boston, Blackwell Scientific Publications, 1982.)

throughout the body. Hormones tend to act more slowly over longer periods of time, whereas nervous mechanisms bring about rapid but short-lasting responses. When the central nervous system reacts to various external and internal stimuli, it transmits a message to the hypothalamus. The hypothalamus can, in response, manufacture and release several releasing or inhibiting factors that are conveyed to the anterior pituitary, thereby stimulating or inhibiting the release of specific pituitary, or trophic, hormones. When released, these trophic hormones stimulate the appropriate endocrine glands to produce hormone at a faster rate (Guyton, 1982; O'Riordan et al, 1982). For example, emotional or physical stress (stimuli) can lead to hypothalamic production of corticotropin releasing factor (CRF), which in turn stimulates the pituitary release of ACTH. Increased levels of ACTH lead to increased cortisol production by the adrenal gland (Fig. 49-3).

Chemical Control of Hormone Production and Secretion

Chemical control of hormone production and secretion is best understood in terms of *feedback control.* Negative feedback, or feedback inhibition, occurs when the rising concentration of a hormone inhibits the system which releases that particular hormone. Thus, an increased secretion of a hormone from a target gland generally leads to a decrease in the secretion of the stimulating pituitary hormone. For example, an increased secretion of thyroxine hormone (T4) from the thyroid gland (target gland) leads to a decrease in the pituitary secretion of thyroid stimulating hormone (TSH).

Endocrine disorders result from a disruption in the neurologic or chemical control of hormone secretion. Such a disruption may be caused by neurologic, glandular, or target organ malfunction. The cause may be congenital, infectious, necrotic, neoplastic, autoimmune, or idiopathic (Krueger and Ray, 1976). Nurses caring for children with endocrine disorders must understand the altered physiologic states in order to assess, plan, and deliver effective patient care. The discussion that follows is organized according to the particular gland that is affected: the pituitary, adrenal, thyroid, parathyroid, gonads (ovary and testis), and pancreas. Clinical manifestations and diagnostic tests are grouped similarly according to a specific gland. Assessment data that the nurse uses to identify endocrine alterations are summarized in Tables 49-2, 49-4, 49-6, 49-8, and 49-10. During the assessment phase the nurse will also be involved in planning with the family and health care team to carry out diagnostic tests. A summary of relevant tests appears in Tables 49-3, 49-5, 49-7, 49-9, and 49-11.

The Pituitary Gland

Normal Pituitary Functions

The pituitary gland lies in a bony cavity, the sella turcica, at the base of the brain. Composed of two parts physiologically, the anterior lobe and the posterior lobe, the pituitary secretes hormones that control major target organ functions. The anterior lobe secretes growth hormone, thyroid stimulating hormone, follicle stimulating hormone, luteinizing hormone, ACTH, and prolactin. The posterior lobe secretes antidiuretic hormone and oxytocin. These hormones, their specific functions, and target tissues are listed in Table 49-1. Clinical manifestations involving the pituitary gland are summarized in Table 49-2. Many factors influence the production and release of hormones from the pituitary, including genetic aberrations, developmental and degenerative lesions, hyperplasia or tumor formation, hormone structural abnormalities, and target organ defects. Furthermore, an understanding of the various diagnostic tests permits the nurse to participate in the teaching and preparation of the child and family for these tests. Diagnostic tests used to identify pituitary alterations are summarized in Table 49-3. A child who experiences a deficiency of a single specific pituitary hormone or selected combinations of hormones is described as having hypopituitarism.

Growth Hormone Deficiency

Growth hormone (GH) is a potent anabolic (protein-building) agent that affects most of the tissues of the body, causing growth by promoting both increased cell size and increased cell number. It does not act on its target organs directly but generates another factor called somatomedin that mediates its effects on the peripheral tissues. In general, somatomedin activity tends to parallel that of growth hormone secretion. For example, high levels of growth hormone secretion lead to greater production of somatomedin by the liver and possibly kidneys (Watts and Keffer, 1982). *Growth hormone affects the metabolic processes of the body by enhancing the rate of protein synthesis, impairing carbohydrate utilization, and increasing fat mobilization and utilization.*

Etiology and Clinical Manifestations

Deficiency of growth hormone leads to growth failure, or dwarfism. The causes of growth hormone deficiency are classified generally as congenital, acquired, or idiopathic. The majority of cases are idiopathic (no cause detected) (Root, 1972). Infants with idiopathic growth hormone deficiency usually have normal birthweight and length, yet impairment of linear growth occurs within the first year or two of life. A characteristic finding related to growth hormone deficiency is the development of hypoglycemia. *Growth hormone is one of the hormones responsible for maintaining normal blood sugar levels.* When growth hormone is absent or levels are inadequate, blood glucose concentration may drop to low levels in fasting states. Parents may notice that their baby demands feedings every few hours and shows signs of low blood sugar (paleness, shakiness, irritability, sweatiness, hunger) if feedings are not given promptly. Children may require large bedtime snacks and often awaken in the morning with signs of hypoglycemia. Prolonged severe hypoglycemia can even lead to seizures, coma, and brain damage.

Growth hormone deficiency may be discovered only after parents seek medical attention for their child's problem with hypoglycemia. Growth hormone deficiency leads to abnormal rates of development of the facial bones, resulting in protrusion of the frontal bones and poor development of the nasal bridge. Children appear physically immature and much younger than their stated ages. Dental eruption and closure of the anterior fontanel may be delayed, and delay of skeletal maturation and of puberty is almost universal. The hair is thin and nail growth is poor. The voice may be high pitched. The penis is often quite small, and its small size is accentuated by truncal obesity. Intelligence is normal, although school performance may suffer owing to decreased self-esteem.

Brain tumors, primarily those of the midline, such as craniopharyngiomas and optic gliomas, are the second most frequent cause of growth hormone deficiency in children. Younger children may develop the more typical signs of increased intracranial pressure with craniopharyngiomas, but in older children growth impairment may be the only symptom. The third most frequent cause of growth hormone deficiency in children is septo-optic dysplasia, a congenital malformation of the midline brain. The factors responsible for development of this anomaly are not known. The endocrine deficiencies involve several hormones of both the anterior and posterior pituitary, yet growth hormone deficiency is the most frequent abnormality. Infants with septo-optic dysplasia experience hypoglycemia, prolonged jaundice, apnea, and hypotonia in the newborn period. Hepatomegaly, psychomotor retardation and receding mandible have also been described.

Diagnostic Assessment

The nurse has an important role in early detection of delayed growth. It is vital for the pediatric nurse to assess height and weight gains on all patients at least once a year. Data should be recorded on growth charts and compared with standardized norms. Growth recorded over many months or years is a better indicator of disrupted patterns than single measurements. Most cases of delayed growth or growth failure will be attrib-

Table 49-2. Clinical Manifestations of Common Pituitary Alterations

Clinical Manifestations	Reason for Clinical Manifestations	Significance to the Nurse
Growth Hormone Deficiency		
Growth Failure	Poor protein synthesis leading to decreased linear growth of bones	The nurse can detect growth failure only by assessing linear growth at regular intervals (at least once a year after age 1)
Delayed closure of fontanel Delayed dentition Immature facies Thin hair Poor nail growth	Poor protein synthesis	Child may be late in cutting or losing primary teeth; child appears younger than he or she really is; should be treated age-appropriately
Truncal obesity	Growth hormone has a lipolytic effect; deficiency leads to increased fat storage	
Hypoglycemia • shakiness • sweating • tachycardia	Enhanced insulin sensitivity leads to hypoglycemia	Recurrent episodes of hypoglycemia may cause permanent brain damage or seizures. Episodes of hypoglycemia should be documented (i.e., time, severity of symptoms, time of last meal)
Small penis Delayed puberty	Believed to be due to deficiency of growth hormone itself	
Growth Hormone Excess		
Excessive Growth • bones • soft tissues	Excessive growth hormone levels prior to growth plate fusion leads to a rapid rate of growth; if growth plates are fused, height remains the same yet bones thicken and soft tissue growth occurs (extremity enlargement)	"Acromegalic" is a term used to describe the classic feature of acral (extremity) enlargement in pituitary giants
Joint pains	Bone thickening, ligament lengthening	
Headache	Brain tumor leads to increased intracranial pressure	Often accompanied by vomiting without preceding nausea
Visual disturbances	Brain tumor obstructs optic pathways	
Polyuria; polydipsia	Brain tumor destroys the area in the pituitary that secretes antidiuretic hormone	Easily confused with signs of diabetes mellitus
Delayed, absent sexual development	Brain tumor destroys the area of the pituitary that secretes LH, FSH	
Antidiuretic Hormone Deficiency		
Polydipsia Polyuria (up to 4–10 liters)—clear, unconcentrated urine	Area of the pituitary that secretes antidiuretic hormone is affected	Symptoms usually occur abruptly Iced water preferred
Enuresis, nocturia		Enuresis occurs in a previously toilet-trained child
Antidiuretic Hormone Excess		
Headache Anorexia Irritability Personality change Severe: Vomiting Confusion Convulsion	Cerebrospinal fluid retention and swelling secondary to water intoxication	
Gonadotropin Deficiency		
Absent signs of secondary sexual characteristics	LH, FSH surges are necessary to stimulate production of sex hormones Sex hormones are necessary for growth	Children may appear younger, less mature than chronologic age
Delayed pubertal growth spurt		
Gonadotropin Excess (precocious puberty)		
Boys Testicular enlargement Penile enlargement Pubic hair before 9.5 years of age	Increased levels of testosterone (produced by testes)	Encourage parents to treat child according to chronologic age rather than appearance

Table 49-2 *(continued)*

Clinical Manifestations	Reason for Clinical Manifestations	Significance to the Nurse
Girls		
Breast development before 7.25 years of age Vaginal mucosa changes • walls appear pearly pink rather than bright red • increase in vaginal mucosa Increased body fat Menses before 9.25 years of age	Increased levels of estrogen stimulate breast development, vaginal mucosa changes and increased body fat When estrogen levels rise and fall in a cyclic pattern with progesterone levels, menses begin	Reassure parents that libido is not increased Parents may need guidance in discussing pubertal changes with their child
Both boys and girls		
Accelerated growth	Estrogen, testosterone, and adrenal sex steroids all cause a growth spurt	Precocious growth spurt causing stunting of final adult height owing to premature bone maturation and closing of growth plates
Pubic hair Axillary hair Acne	Androgen production by adrenal glands (testosterone, DHEA) causes virilization in females Androgen production by the testes (testosterone) causes virilization in males	Children may be embarrassed to undress in front of friends Encourage parents to discuss situation with physical education teacher if necessary
Mood swings	The combined effect of sex steroids leads to mood swings	Counsel parents that mood swings are a part of the pubertal process

uted to factors other than pituitary deficiency. Genetic factors, such as the growth patterns and final adult stature of a child's family members, must be considered. The child's general state of physical and emotional health, as well as past history of chronic illness, is also considered. Renal failure, congenital heart disease, cystic fibrosis and other genetic diseases, celiac disease, chronic vomiting or diarrhea, and malnutrition can lead to growth impairment. Skeletal anomalies, chromosomal abnormalities, and intrauterine growth retardation are often associated with growth disturbances. Growth failure can also be seen in infants and children who are psychosocially deprived. A child with a history of trauma, surgery, or radiation to the skull warrants careful periodic growth assessments. A child who demonstrates a consistent pattern of growth well below expected norms should be referred to a pediatric endocrinologist for further evaluation. Refer to the end of this chapter for recommended readings regarding growth.

Testing for growth hormone deficiency can be divided into screening tests and definitive tests. (See Table 49-3 for a summary of diagnostic tests.) Screening tests include an x-ray of the hand and wrist for skeletal age. Significant skeletal age delay is associated with growth hormone deficiency, yet it can also be seen in hypothyroidism, Turner syndrome, renal disease, pituitary tumors, or regional enteritis (Kaplan, 1982). Depending on clinical signs and symptoms, tests to rule out disorders other than growth hormone deficiency may be done. Because secretions of growth hormone occur in a series of irregular bursts through the day and night, concentrations in the blood plasma are variable and often below levels of detection. Therefore, random sampling of the blood for measurement of growth hormone levels is of little value as a screening tool. Somatomedin levels are stable throughout the day and reflect growth hormone levels. Therefore, a single measurement of serum somatomedin may be drawn in the screening process.

Definitive testing for growth hormone deficiency involves "stimulation tests," which entail extensive serial blood sampling after appropriate stimulation of growth hormone secretion. The goal of such testing is to assess whether the pituitary gland is capable of secreting growth hormone. Agents that stimulate growth hormone secretion include intravenous insulin, intravenous arginine, oral clonidine, oral levo-dopa, and oral propranolol; exercise also stimulates secretion. A particular agent is administered to the patient, and blood samples are drawn every 15 to 30 minutes to measure growth hormone levels.

The nurse involved in the diagnostic workup of a child with growth delay or growth failure can offer understandable information to the parents regarding the complex issue of hormonal interactions. During the stimulation tests, the nurse must carefully assess the child for side effects of specific stimuli and intervene when necessary. Throughout the testing period, parent-child interactions can be observed for disturbances that may contribute to psychosocial growth failure, although psychosocial neglect or abuse is difficult to evaluate and document in a hospital setting.

Therapeutic Management

Treatment with growth hormone is generally limited to children with well-documented growth hormone

Table 49-3. Diagnostic Tests for Pituitary Alterations

Diagnostic Test	Purpose	Comments
Growth Hormone Alterations		
Blood studies		
Somatomedin-C	Indirect reflection of growth hormone	Random growth hormone levels are not useful when deficiency is suspected as growth hormone is secreted in spurts throughout the day
Random growth hormone level		Done only when excessively high levels are expected (gigantism); usually done in early morning
Stimulation tests		
Insulin (intravenous)	Leads to hypoglycemia, which stimulates growth hormone secretion	Maximum hypoglycemia occurs at 20 minutes after intravenous insulin. Severe hypoglycemia can lead to seizures and coma. If child becomes unarousable during test, give intravenous solution of 50 per cent glucose and terminate test
Levodopa (oral) Propranolol (oral) Arginine (intravenous) Clonidine (oral)	All agents listed stimulate growth hormone secretion	Levodopa and propranolol can cause nausea and vomiting Clonidine can lead to hypotension; blood pressure must be monitored frequently during test Trendelenburg position plus increased intravenous fluids if hypotension occurs
Radiography		
Skull radiograph	Identifies erosion of the sella turcica (bony structure which encases the pituitary)	Pituitary tumors often cause erosion of sella turcica
CT scan of brain	Identifies brain tumor	
Bone age radiograph (hand and wrist)	Assesses maturation of bones	Delayed maturation seen in growth hormone deficiency
Gonadotropin Alterations		
Blood studies:		
Luteinizing hormone (LH) Follicle stimulating hormone (FSH)	Indicate whether the pituitary has initiated puberty	LH, FSH levels high at a young age in central precocious puberty, low in gonadotropin deficiency
Estradiol (girls)	Assess how much estrogen the ovaries are producing	Estradiol levels high in girls, testosterone levels high in boys with precocious puberty
Testosterone (boys)	Assess how much testosterone the testes are producing	
Human chorionic gonadotropin (HCG)	HCG levels are determined when a gonadotropin-secreting tumor is suspected	High HCG levels are indicative of a tumor
Bone age radiograph (hand and wrist)	Assesses maturation of bones	High levels of sex steroids mature the bones excessively, leading ultimately to stunted final adult height Low levels of sex steroids secondary to gonadotropin deficiency lead to delayed bone maturation
Skull radiograph	Identifies erosion of the sella turcica (bony structure which encases the pituitary)	Pituitary tumors usually cause erosion of the sella turcica
CT scan of brain	Identifies brain tumor	The CT technician should be told that a pituitary tumor is suspected so that special attention can be paid to that area
Radiograph of long bones	Done only if polyfibrous dysplasia is suspected	
Antidiuretic Hormone Alterations		
Urinalysis with specific gravity (SG), osmolality	Evaluates body's ability to concentrate urine	Urine SG and osmolality very low
Serum electrolytes Serum osmolality		Serum osmolality high in ADH deficiency, low in ADH excess
Water deprivation test	Designed to stimulate secretion of ADH, causing decreased and concentrated urine output	Patients with diabetes insipidus do not decrease or concentrate urine output Monitor vital signs and hydration status at least every 30 min during test; dehydration and vascular collapse can occur quickly
Skull radiograph or CT scan of brain	Identifies brain tumor	

deficiency. The hormone is given by intramuscular or subcutaneous injections three times weekly. Until recently, growth hormone was available solely from human pituitaries obtained at autopsy, and the demand greatly exceeded the supply. Production of synthetic growth hormone by recombinant DNA technique is hoped to alleviate this shortage. Very few side effects are associated with growth hormone administration. Local tenderness and allergic reactions have been reported but are rare. Antibodies to growth hormone can develop, but they rarely rise to sufficient titers to inhibit the action of the administered hormone.

Growth hormone is very effective in the first year of treatment, yet with each successive year the growth response may diminish. Anabolic steroids are sometimes given to older children to enhance the effect of growth hormone. If they are used, careful attention is paid to advancement of skeletal age, and their use is discontinued or modified if excessive skeletal maturation occurs. Growth hormone therapy is continued until the growth plates fuse, which may occur as late as the early twenties in patients with significantly delayed skeletal ages.

Major Nursing Diagnoses for Growth Hormone Deficiency (Dwarfism)

Altered growth and development: linear growth, *related to decreased anabolic activity associated with insufficient growth hormone*

Potential altered nutrition: hypoglycemia, *related to insufficient growth hormone*

Knowledge deficit (child and parents), *related to*

- *etiology and disease process*
- *administration of growth hormone, including injection technique*
- *methods for financing growth hormone therapy*
- *realistic expectations of therapy*

Disturbance in self-concept: body image, self-esteem, role performance, and personal identity, *related to*

- *reactions of peers and significant others to short stature*
- *handicap of short stature associated with certain motor skills*
- *need for long-term therapy that makes child different from peers*

Potential altered growth and development: developmental delay:

physical, *related to inability to achieve age-appropriate motor development*

intellectual, *related to decreased stimulation associated with decreased mobility for exploration of environment*

emotional/social, *related to*

- *poor self-concept*
- *parental "protection" from emotional trauma*
- *social stigma of physical appearance suggestive of storybook characters*
- *tendency of adults to treat child appropriate to size rather than age*

Strategies for Nursing Care

Nursing strategies, which are derived from the major nursing diagnoses for dwarfism, relate primarily to support of the child and family during the prolonged treatment phase. In addition to administration of growth hormone for impaired linear growth, the family must be taught to recognize signs of hypoglycemia. (See clinical manifestations of growth hormone deficiency.)

Providing Information to Support Home Care. Treatment with human growth hormone necessitates a major readjustment period for the child and family. Initially, the parents must deal with apprehension and possibly guilt associated with administering injections to their child. Apprehension often stems from lack of knowledge regarding correct hormone reconstitution, injection technique, and side effects of treatment. Thorough teaching and written instructions regarding each aspect of therapy help to alleviate much apprehension. Health professionals must present up-to-date information to parents as it evolves and must be willing to openly discuss risks of side effects versus benefits of treatment. Parents must be aware that the cost of human growth hormone is extremely high. The cost of treating a 30-kg child for 1 year exceeds $10,000, and the cost increases as the child grows. Treatment is usually covered by group medical insurance plans if there is well-documented growth hormone deficiency.

As treatment progresses, parents may begin to feel the need to redefine their relationship with their child, especially if their present relationship fosters age-inappropriate dependency. The child must also adjust to a changing self. Anticipated and real growth provokes the child to reorganize his or her defenses and attitudes toward the outside world. This movement toward "normalcy" may prove to be distressing, as patterns of thoughts and behavior must often be restructured (Money and Pollit, 1966).

In spite of accelerated growth with human growth hormone treatment, children and parents sometimes perceive the treatment to be a failure relative to their expectations. Although the final adult height of children receiving growth hormone treatment is usually within normal and acceptable limits, it may not reach the full predestined genetic potential (Burns et al, 1981). There is often a disparity between expectations of health professionals, who consider the treatment successful, and those of the children or parents, who do not. Nearly 80 per cent of growth delayed children and families have unrealistically high expectations of human growth hormone therapy (Grew et al, 1983). Disappointment and grief can result when expectations are not met, leading to further feelings of anger, pessimism, and guilt. The parents may lose confidence in the physician prescribing the treatment, yet may be unable to openly discuss their feelings. The child is usually well aware of the financial burden that treatment places on the parents, and perceived or real failure of treatment can intensify the significance of this burden. The nurse must be aware of the disparity between patient or parent expectations and realistic growth achievement. Specific, concrete, and clear expectations of a child's growth must be delineated during treatment. Open communication is essential during the entire treatment period.

Enhancing the Child's Self-esteem and Achievement of Developmental Tasks

Height, a relative attribute based on comparison of self to others, is a vital ingredient to a child's development of body image and total self-concept. School-age children are acutely aware of their size in relation to classmates and friends. They also quickly learn that physical size often influences potential despite chronologic age and maturity. A short child is "different" in a way that is very obvious to the child and others, and this difference often becomes more difficult for the child to cope with as he or she grows older and tries to master developmental tasks appropriate for age. Thus, short stature places the child at risk for social, academic, and psychologic difficulties. An understanding of these potential difficulties enables the clinician to design care approaches to facilitate the child's adaptation.

Recognizing Potential Threats to Self-esteem and Healthy Development. Short children tend to exhibit social behaviors that may accentuate the discrepancy between their chronologic age and physical stature. They may become withdrawn and isolated from peers or may seek out the company of younger children. Certain children even assume the role of clown or mascot. Gordon and colleagues (1982) found that children with short stature have significantly more behavior problems than children with normal height. Parents of children with short stature were found to have a less strict approach to childrearing than that used by parents of children with normal height. They tended to set fewer clear limits on behavior, and there was a lower level of cooperation and effective communication in the families. Indices of self-esteem were lower in the short stature group, and children more often saw themselves as unhappy and unpopular.

Stabler and coworkers (1980) found that short children exhibit less ability to perceive, organize, and integrate logical sequences of cause-and-effect relationships in social situations. They are less able to anticipate the outcome of social interpersonal encounters, which often leads to poor relations with peers.

Children with hypopituitary short stature typically perceive less adaptive, mature solutions to frustrating situations than do peers of average stature (Drotar et al, 1980). They tend to emphasize obstacles rather than solutions to frustrating situations. From their earliest years they are likely to encounter a series of frustrations secondary to their small size, including skills such as climbing, exploring, and various sports. Physical environments of school (desks, drinking fountains, chalk boards, stair railings) and playgrounds (monkey bars, ladders) are geared to their taller peers. Small children are often helped and protected too much, teased, and discouraged from age-appropriate, assertive solutions to frustrations. Nicknames like "shrimp," "shortstuff," and "midget," and comments like "How's the weather down there?" and "You can stand up now" only reinforce the size discrepancy between these children and their peers. When choosing sides for a team, whether for baseball, relay races, or playing jump rope, the small children are often picked last, and this becomes a clear message regarding their perceived potential. Differences in size and strength between them and their peers of the same age may cause anxiety about assertive behavior and encourage withdrawal from such frustrating situations.

Several studies suggest that because short children experience more interpersonal anxiety and have greater sensitivity to their interpersonal environment than do normal children, they may be unable to respond positively to competitive challenge (Money et al, 1966; Krims, 1968; Lindley, 1972) and are deficient in assertive and aggressive characteristics (Money and Pollit, 1966; Kusalic et al, 1972). Their inability to respond to the competitive challenge of school often interferes with academic achievement. Despite normal IQ scores, school performance may be unsatisfactory.

Treating the Child Appropriately for Age. Children who begin treatment at younger ages make a better overall psychosocial adjustment than older children (Kusalic and Fortin, 1975). This is attributed to a lesser and shorter awareness of their situation and to their earlier stage of personality formation. *In successful adjustment to growth hormone treatment, the degree of psychologic maturation may be related not so* *much to the actual growth achieved as to the ability of the parents and other adults to treat the child according to age instead of size.* Emphasizing positive areas of achievement may also help contribute to the child's positive self-concept and adjustment.

Setting the Child Up for Success. Children with short stature often choose activities and sports that are unsuited to their physical size. The nurse can encourage short children to develop interest in areas in which they can succeed and to choose sports activities in which size is not necessarily a factor to compete. By choosing activities in this fashion, children set themselves up to be winners and frustrations are minimized.

Minimizing Psychosocial Trauma Through Liaisons with Other Professionals. Nurses can offer suggestions to school teachers and counselors on ways to minimize psychosocial trauma of short stature in their students. They can be encouraged to line children up by another method than "smallest to tallest" and to choose teams for sports by methods that avoid having the smaller children picked last. They should also be encouraged to treat their short students according to age rather than size. Teachers and parents often ask about the advisability of holding a child back in school because of short stature. Academic placement should not be altered on the basis of height alone, but children who experience emotional distress or social immaturity because of their size may benefit from changes in school placement.

Nursing Strategies for Follow-up Care in the Home or Clinic

Measure height and weight and plot measurements on growth curve to determine effects of therapy.

Encourage questions and comments about therapeutic protocol, including any misgivings about the value of expensive treatments.

Question the child and family about any signs and symptoms of hypoglycemia.

Assess development; note any delays and counsel parents about ways to facilitate age-appropriate physical, intellectual, and motor or social development.

Help redefine problems and alter solutions as perceptions change throughout the developmental process of child and family.

Pituitary Gigantism

Pituitary gigantism is caused by growth hormone excess and is associated with tumors of the anterior pituitary. Children are termed "giants" when their height and weight exceed three standard deviations above the mean (Job and Piersin, 1981). This disorder is very rare in children.

Clinical Manifestations

The signs and symptoms of growth hormone excess depend on the age at which excessive secretion occurs. If it occurs before growth plates fuse, linear growth may continue in excess of 220 cm (86.5 inches). A famous giant (the Alton giant) was over 9 feet tall at the time of his death at age 24 years. The most common manifestations of pituitary gigantism are enlargement of the extremities, soft tissue growth, headache, visual impairment, and excessive perspiration (Kaplan, 1982). Delay or lack of sexual development is also common. There may be carbohydrate intolerance, galactorrhea, polyuria, and polydipsia. The bones are thick, and joint pains, kyphosis, and osteoporosis occur frequently. Organ enlargement, hypertension, and heart failure may lead to death.

Diagnostic Assessment

Radiologic signs of pituitary gigantism include enlargement of the sella turcica and paranasal sinuses and marked elongation of the mandible. The teeth become separated by large spaces. Bony overgrowth of the joints lead to osteoarthritis. Fasting growth hormone levels are elevated.

Therapeutic Management

Treatment of growth hormone–secreting pituitary tumors is usually surgical excision. Prognosis for recovery after removal of such tumors is uncertain because so few have been described in children in recent years. Hormonal replacement may be necessary depending on the degree of damage to the pituitary during surgery.

Strategies for Nursing Care

Nursing strategies for care of the child with pituitary giantism are closely aligned with strategies for the child with pituitary dwarfism. Because this disorder is rare, however, families may experience even less social support than do families with children suffering from growth hormone failure. The child and family are therefore particularly dependent upon the support of health care professionals in dealing with the psychologic sequelae of the disorder.

In addition, the family will need information pertaining to the perioperative care for excision of a pituitary tumor and instruction about hormone replacement, should it be necessary postoperatively. Follow-up care for the child after pituitary surgery will include assessment for pituitary insufficiency: hypothyroidism, growth hormone deficiency, hypogonadism, hypoadrenalism, and diabetes insipidus.

Diabetes Insipidus

Antidiuretic hormone (ADH), a hormone secreted by the posterior pituitary, controls the body's water excretion rates by altering the permeability of the tubules and collecting ducts of the kidneys. The amount of hormone secreted is proportional to body need. *Higher levels of ADH secretion lead to water conservation; lower levels lead to diuresis.* Diabetes insipidus is characterized by deficient ADH secretion leading to diuresis, an inability to concentrate urine and conserve body water.

Etiology

Tumors of the hypothalamus, most frequently craniopharyngiomas, are the most common cause of diabetes insipidus. Surgically induced trauma during removal of a tumor in the hypothalamic area is also a major cause of diabetes insipidus (Kaplan, 1982). Other etiologic factors include histiocytosis, tuberculosis, encephalitis, meningitis, aneurysms, and defective synthesis of vasopressin.

Clinical Manifestations

The symptoms of diabetes insipidus in children vary and are influenced not only by the extent of ADH deficiency but also by diet, renal function, and preservation of the thirst mechanism. Most children experience an abrupt onset of symptoms. Polyuria, nocturia, and enuresis in a previously toilet-trained child are common presenting complaints. The excess water lost from polyuria leads to dehydration and secondary polydipsia. The excessive thirst that these children have is not life-threatening, but it does interfere with their play, learning, and sleep. The urinary output of a child with diabetes insipidus can be between 4 and 10 liters a day. Children often prefer iced water, are thirsty during the night, and become irritable if fluid is withheld. Their urine color is clear even upon the first morning void. Anorexia and poor weight gain are common. A history of associated ocular abnormalities or growth failure, or both, can be suggestive of a mid-brain tumor.

Diagnostic Assessment

The diagnosis of diabetes insipidus is confirmed when inappropriately dilute urine is excreted in the presence of high serum sodium levels. Initial screening studies may include urinalysis with determinations of specific gravity and serum sodium, potassium, calcium, and glucose levels to rule out renal insufficiency or diabetes mellitus as the cause of polyuria. A skull x-ray may be done to screen for an intracranial tumor or histiocytes (macrophages). A measurement of random serum sodium concentration and osmolality tends to be elevated in children with diabetes insipidus owing to decreased blood volume. Tests designed to increase the serum osmolality, thereby stimulating secretion of ADH, are done to evaluate a child with possible diabetes insipidus. A water deprivation test is the most commonly used test. Water deprivation in normal individuals leads to serum hyperosmolality, causing release of ADH. This ADH release leads to body water conservation through decreased and more concentrated urine output. Restriction of oral fluid intake in an ADH-deficient individual results in rapid depletion of body fluid volume, a rise in plasma osmolality, and weight loss. Urine output is neither decreased in volume nor concentrated in these individuals.

It is best to carry out water deprivation tests during the day when the child can be carefully observed, as polyuria, dehydration, and collapse may occur after only a short period of water deprivation (Hung et al, 1983). Careful hourly monitoring of hydration status, including assessment of blood pressure, pulse, skin turgor, mucous membranes, temperature, urine specific gravity, and weight, is done. The fluid is usually withheld until weight loss is 3 to 5 per cent of the child's total body weight. A compulsive water drinker without diabetes insipidus will concentrate urine during this test and will not usually have significant weight loss. If the child's pulse increases significantly or if the blood pressure drops in the presence of dehydration, the physician should be notified. A toddler or young child may become highly irritable and inconsolable during a water deprivation test and the parents may feel guilty in denying liquids. The nurse can provide emotional support to the child as well as the parents and can explain the importance of restricting fluids.

Therapeutic Management

Treatment of diabetes insipidus includes identifying and removing the cause when possible. Although diabetes insipidus is rarely life-threatening in itself, it can signal the presence of a serious underlying disorder (DiGeorge, 1987). The drug of choice for symptomatic control of diabetes insipidus is DDAVP (1-deamino-8-D-arginine vasopressin).

Major Nursing Diagnoses for Diabetes Insipidus

Fluid volume deficit, related to diuresis associated with insufficient ADH secretion

Potential altered fluid volume: excess, related to improper administration of synthetic ADH (DDAVP)
Knowledge deficit: child and parents, related to
- *etiology and disease process*
- *intranasal administration of DDAVP, including indications for administration, precise measurement of the drug according to the graduation marks on the soft plastic nasal tube, and effects of increased nasal mucus upon absorption*
- *resources to assist with cost of DDAVP*
- *the need for medical consultation any time the child's fluid intake is significantly altered*
- *signs and symptoms of fluid volume deficit and fluid volume excess*

Fear/anxiety: child and parents, related to the diagnosis of a chronic disease

Strategies for Nursing Care

Providing Information to Support Home Care

DDAVP is delivered intranasally through a small insufflator once or twice daily. Dosage and frequency of administration vary from child to child and according to the state of hydration, with the goal of treatment being to eliminate polyuria except during short periods just prior to the next dose (DiGeorge, 1987). The child should be taught to take a dose of DDAVP only when urine output begins to increase noticeably. This precaution reduces the risk of low urine output and fluid overload. In children who require only a single daily dose of DDAVP, the hormone should be given in the evening so that breakthrough polyuria prior to the next dose will not interfere with sleep or school. The child and parents should be aware that an increase in the dosage of DDAVP will not significantly raise the urinary concentration but will prolong the drug's duration of action. The child and family should be instructed that during respiratory infections and allergic rhinitis, excess nasal mucus may interfere with hormone absorption, and they may notice that polyuria prior to the next dose occurs sooner than usual. They may need to contact their physician for advice on altering the hormone dose on those days. The therapy of diabetes insipidus has to be adjusted under conditions that either demand high fluid intake for coverage of caloric need or prohibit drinking entirely, as in the postoperative period. Infants and children requiring surgery must be closely followed by a pediatric endocrinologist.

One disadvantage of DDAVP is the expense. Treatment of a school-age child for 1 year can easily exceed $1000. DDAVP is also difficult to obtain in local pharmacies and may need to be specially ordered. The nurse should forewarn the parents about the cost and limited availability so that they can make necessary arrangements prior to discharge from the hospital for its purchase. At least 80 per cent of the cost of DDAVP is usually covered by group medical insurance plans and Medicaid.

Reducing Fear and Anxiety

As with the diagnosis of any chronic illness, the family undergoes an emotional adjustment period when a child is diagnosed with diabetes insipidus. The parents may feel responsible for the illness and may feel guilty for delaying medical attention. The nurse can provide an opportunity for them to discuss their fears and feelings and can offer assurance that the child has a treatable problem.

Nursing Strategies for Follow-up Care in the Home or Clinic

Assess hydration status, including measurement of weight, skin turgor, status of mucous membranes, blood pressure, pulse, temperature. Ask parent how many diapers child wets per day. Ask child how many times per day he or she urinates. Measure specific gravity of urine.

Assess for early signs of water intoxication: drowsiness, headache, vomiting.

Evaluate family's perception of the value of treatment, and determine compliance with suggested protocol.

Encourage the child and family to discuss their fears and concerns. Appropriately reinforce adaptive coping and innovative management.

Panhypopituitarism

Etiology and Clinical Manifestations

Panhypopituitarism refers to a generalized state of hypopituitarism. Complete absence of all pituitary hormones is rare; partial deficiencies occur more frequently. Congenital abnormalities, pituitary tumors, infections, vascular abnormalities, cranial irradiation and trauma have been identified as causes of panhypopituitarism. Symptoms can include those related to hypothyroidism, growth hormone deficiency, hypogonadism, hypoadrenalism, and diabetes insipidus. Specific symptoms and diagnosis of each of these disorders are discussed elsewhere in this chapter.

Therapeutic Management

Treatment of panhypopituitarism depends on the cause. Pituitary tumors are treated with surgery or radiation therapy, or both. Both of these treatments can lead to even further pituitary damage and more hormone deficiencies. Appropriate hormone replacement is vital to the treatment of panhypopituitarism. The child may require thyroid hormone, growth hormone, cortisol, and ADH replacement. In addition to these hormones, the adolescent requires estrogen (female) or testosterone (male) replacement. The child and family must be instructed about the importance of administering hormone replacements as ordered. They must be aware that proper growth depends on proper doses of thyroid, cortisol, and growth hormone replacement. If one hormone is not given consistently, growth can be impaired. Periodic medical follow-up and blood studies to evaluate the adequacy of hormonal replacement is very important in the growing child.

Strategies for Nursing Care

Because inconsistent administration of hormone doses can be dangerous to the child's health and may impair growth and development, family and patient teaching is critical. The nurse should recommend that the child with panhypopituitarism wear a medical alert tag that specifies the required doses of hormones. Such a tag may save a child's life if he or she should sustain major trauma away from relatives.

Precocious Puberty

Precocious puberty is an abnormally early appearance of secondary sex characteristics (Frasier, 1980). Breast development before the age of 7.25 years or menses before the age of 9.25 years is considered precocious in girls, and pubic hair growth before the age of 9.5 years is considered precocious in boys (Kaplan, 1982; Hung et al, 1983).

Normal puberty in girls is a process in which the ovaries begin producing estrogen and the adrenal glands begin producing androgens (testosterone, dehydroepiandrosterone sulfate [DHEAS]). The elevated estrogen levels lead to breast development, vaginal maturation, and the onset of menses. The elevated androgens cause axillary and pubic hair growth, adult body odor, and acne. Normal puberty in boys is a process in which the testes enlarge and begin producing testosterone. High levels of testosterone cause penile enlargement, axillary and pubic hair growth, adult body odor, acne, accelerated growth, and voice changes. The main difference between normal puberty and precocious puberty is the age at which the changes occur.

It is important to distinguish between true precocious and pseudoprecocious puberty. In true precocious puberty, maturation is complete, with both pubic hair and breast development in girls and pubic hair, testicular enlargement, and penile growth in boys. A growth spurt typically occurs as well. In pseudoprecocious puberty, maturation is incomplete, with only one or some of the sexual characteristics developing early. Premature adrenarche (early pubic hair growth) and premature thelarche (early breast development) are discussed in other areas of this chapter.

Incidence and Etiology

The overall incidence of true precocious development is not known, although it is two to three times more common in girls than in boys (Frasier, 1980). Boys are more likely to have a specific demonstrable cause for early puberty than are girls. True precocious puberty may be caused by a wide variety of processes or may be idiopathic (no discernible cause). Congenital anomalies of the central nervous system, especially those leading to hydrocephalus, brain tumors, and a variety of inflammatory processes, may affect the pituitary, leading to abnormally early production of gonadotropins (luteinizing hormone [LH] and follicle stimulating hormone [FSH]). This situation is described as "central precocious puberty." In children with a normal pubertal sequence, gonadotropin levels begin to rise gradually after 8 years of age. In children with central precocious puberty, the gonadotropin levels rise quickly at an early age. The high levels of LH and FSH stimulate the gonads, leading to sex hormone production and early development of secondary sexual characteristics. Embryonal tumors located in the gonad, abdomen, or central nervous system often secrete gonadotropins, usually human chorionic gonadotropin (HCG) or LH. The HCG and LH from these tumors stimulate gonadal and adrenal sex hormone secretion, which in turn stimulate development of secondary sexual characteristics. McCune-Albright syndrome is a triad of polyostotic fibrous dysplasia of the bone, unilateral café-au-lait spots, and various endocrine abnormalities, the most common of which is precocious puberty. In 90 to 95 per cent of girls and 40 to 50 per cent of boys with precocious puberty, there is no demonstrable underlying cause (Frasier, 1980). These children are considered to have idiopathic precocious puberty, in which the timing of events leading to sexual maturation is advanced for unknown reasons.

Clinical Manifestations

Girls with true precocious puberty have breast development, growth of the internal and external genitalia, pubic and axillary hair growth, estrogenic stimulation of the vagina (the vaginal walls appear pearly pink rather than bright red), and precocious menstruation.

These manifestations are accompanied by an acceleration of both linear growth and bone maturation. Boys have bilateral testicular enlargement, scrotal pigmentation, penile growth, and the appearance of both pubic and axillary hair. Later changes include acne and deepening voice. Acceleration in linear growth and bone maturation can also be seen.

Diagnostic Assessment

True central precocious puberty owing to early maturation of the hypothalamic-pituitary-gonadal system is characterized by high levels of LH, FSH, and sex steroids (estrogen, testosterone, DHEAS). Serum chorionic gonadotropin levels are checked if a gonadotropin-secreting tumor is suspected. A bone age x-ray is usually done to evaluate the bone maturation. X-rays of the skull and long bones may be obtained to look for polyostotic fibrous dysplasia. Skull x-rays and computed tomographic (CT) scans of the brain may be done, especially if there is clinical evidence of neurologic changes.

Therapeutic Management

Therapy for precocious puberty is directed at the underlying cause. The only permanent complication of idiopathic true precocious puberty is short stature, as the excessive sex hormone production in the first 10 years of life causes early bone maturation and premature growth plate closure. Several drugs have been used with variable success in treating precocious puberty, including danazol and cyproterone acetate. Antagonists to the hypothalamic hormone gonadotropin releasing hormone (GnRH), which stimulates pituitary secretion of LH and FSH, are being evaluated for safety and effectiveness. GnRH antagonists inhibit GnRH release from the hypothalamus, thereby inhibiting LH and FSH release from the pituitary. Lack of stimulation by LH and FSH leads to decreased gonadal sex hormone production.

Major Nursing Diagnoses for Precocious Puberty

Altered growth and development: early development of secondary sexual characteristics, *related to premature production of gonadotropins*

Knowledge deficit: parents and child, *related to*
- *etiology*
- *facilitating the child's mastery of age-appropriate tasks despite the early maturation of secondary sexual characteristics*
- *administration of medications and their potential side effects*

Disturbance in self-concept: body image, *related to*
- *early sexual development*
- *short stature associated with premature epiphyseal closure*

Ineffective family coping, *related to difficulty in*
- *accepting the changes in the child's body*
- *explaining puberty to a younger child*

Strategies for Nursing Care

Providing Information to Support Home Care

The child and family will be best prepared for home management of precocious puberty if they understand the cause and the actual effects of the disorder. Because precocious puberty may involve sensitive issues for a family, the nurse's expertise in therapeutic communication will be especially important. Communication can be enhanced by listening carefully for indications of fears and concerns that the child or parent may be afraid or embarrassed to voice. Stressing the normalcy of the puberty process (even though it is occurring early) is often helpful. If medications are prescribed, the family will need instructions about administration and potential side effects.

Enhancing the Child's Self-Concept and Promoting Effective Family Coping

The nurse can help the child and family cope with the psychologic difficulties associated with early physical maturation. Parents should be encouraged to respond to their child in a manner appropriate to chronologic age rather than to physical appearance. Similar encouragement must be given to teachers and school personnel.

Parents may have difficulty relating to a physically precocious child and must understand the importance of accepting the normal physical contact appropriate for the child's age. Their child does not have increased sexual interest and activity beyond that appropriate for chronologic age. Many children with precocious puberty withdraw because they feel different from their peers. They may seek older friends who appear more similar physically, yet they often find it difficult to keep up with these friends' intellectual and social maturity. *It is important to reassure parents and the child with idiopathic sexual precocity that the child is simply going through a normal process early.* Many parents feel uninformed and confused about their own sexuality and find that discussing the puberty process with their own child is very difficult (Gilbert and Bailes, 1980; Aquilino and Ely, 1985). They may need assistance in clarifying their own mores, conflicts, and inhibitions before they can be comfortable discussing sexual topics with their child. Refer to the bibliography at the end of the chapter for books and pamphlets that are helpful in explaining sexual development and precocious puberty.

Nursing Strategies for Follow-up Care in the Home or Clinic

Measure height and weight and plot measurements on the growth chart.

Assess physiologic reaction to medications.

Assess the child's understanding of body changes. Encourage verbalization of feelings.

Evaluate parent-child communication patterns.

Assess the child's progress on age-appropriate developmental tasks.

The Adrenal Gland

Normal Adrenal Functions

The adrenal glands consist of the inner cortex and outer medulla. The cortex secretes glucocorticoids and mineralocorticoids, both of which are fundamental to metabolic regulation and stress adaptation. Sex hormones are also produced in the cortex but represent only a small portion of the total body sex hormones. The medulla secretes epinephrine and norepinephrine.

Glucocorticoids, notably *cortisol,* perform important regulating functions in the body. The most outstanding effects are on glucose, protein, and fat metabolism; stress reactions; and inhibition of inflammatory processes. The overall effect is to conserve the body's glucose supplies. Cortisol production is regulated by plasma ACTH levels. ACTH secretion by the pituitary is governed by negative feedback control, biologic rhythms, and stress. Low plasma cortisol levels stimulate ACTH release, which in turn stimulates the rate of cortisol biosynthesis. Alternatively, high plasma cortisol levels inhibit ACTH production. Pituitary adrenal rhythms are governed by a biologic clock. ACTH secretions are higher in the morning in people with regular nightly sleep habits. They decrease throughout the day and are at a minimum the few hours before sleep. Alterations in sleep habits can change the pituitary adrenal secretion cycle. Stress appears to act directly to stimulate pituitary ACTH production, which in turn stimulates adrenal cortisol secretion. Stresses include trauma, sepsis, anesthesia, acute anoxia, acute dyspnea, hypothermia, and emotional states such as acute anxiety (Krueger and Ray, 1976).

Mineralocorticoids, the most important being *aldosterone,* are responsible for maintaining extracellular fluid volume and blood pressure. Aldosterone functions by increasing sodium, chloride, and water conservation and potassium excretion by the kidney. Its secretion is mainly under control of the renin-angiotensin system. In this system, nephrons of the kidney respond to blood volume, pressure, and sodium concentrations. Decreases in any of these stimulate production of the kidney enzyme renin, which ultimately leads to stimulation of adrenal aldosterone secretion. Increased aldosterone production leads to higher levels of angiotensin, which ultimately increases the body's blood pressure. Clinical manifestations involving the adrenal gland are summarized in Table 49-4. Tests used to diagnose alterations of the adrenal gland appear in Table 49-5.

Congenital Adrenal Hyperplasia

Incidence

Congenital adrenal hyperplasia is transmitted as an autosomal recessive trait, and the frequency varies throughout the world. In the United States the occurrence of CAH is 1 in approximately 80,000 to 100,000 live births (Kaplan, 1979). The most common form of CAH is due to a 21-hydroxylase deficiency.

Pathophysiology

Congenital adrenal hyperplasia (CAH) is a genetic disorder involving a deficiency of one or more enzymes required for normal synthesis of cortisol and at times aldosterone (Bongiovanni, 1978).

The adrenal cortex produces cortisol, testosterone, and aldosterone from the basic cholesterol structure (Fig. 49-4). Cholesterol goes through many chemical changes leading up to the final product of cortisol, and each of these changes relies on specific enzymes for its completion. If an enzyme is absent or deficient, the chain of chemical changes is stopped at that point in the pathway. The compound prepared to undergo its next change is unable to do so and it "backs up" much like water at a dam. Eventually, many of the precursor compounds begin a stockpiling effect and are shunted to another pathway to produce testosterone instead of cortisol. Because cortisol synthesis is impaired, the feedback message to the pituitary is for more cortisol to be produced. Therefore, production of ACTH by the pituitary rises. Elevated ACTH levels stimulate the adrenal gland, leading to hyperplasia, causing even further excess in production of testosterone.

Aldosterone, like cortisol, is produced from the basic cholesterol molecule but through another pathway. Certain enzyme deficiencies lead to impediment of aldosterone formation. Children with inadequate cortisol production and excessive precursor production are also believed to be resistant to the effects of

Table 49-4. Clinical Manifestations of Adrenal Alterations

Clinical Manifestations	Reason for Clinical Manifestations	Significance to the Nurse
Cortisol Deficiency		
General weakness	Decreased cortisol	
Anorexia		
Weight loss		
Dehydration		
Shock secondary to relatively mild illness	Inadequate cortisol production in response to stress	Intramuscular or intravenous cortisone must be given if shock occurs
Increased pigmentation of skin, buccal mucosa		
Cortisol Excess		
Obesity (face, trunk, abdomen)	Fat mobilized from lower part of body and deposited in thoracic region	Body image is often altered significantly
Plethoric skin of face		
Purplish atrophic striae of abdomen, arms, thighs	Diminished collagen fibers in the subcutaneous tissues due to protein catabolism	
Muscular weakness and wasting	Increased protein catabolism	
Ecchymoses		
Acne	Secretion of adrenal androgens is often increased in Cushing's disease	
Excessive hair growth on face, limbs, pubis (hirsutism)		
Slowed growth		
Osteoporosis	Lack of protein deposition in the bones	
Hypertension	Sodium and water retention	Patient should be instructed to limit salt intake
Edema		
Irritability, emotional outbursts		
Gastric burning		Small, frequent meals often reduce gastric burning
Aldosterone Deficiency		
Hypotension	Hyponatremia	Intravenous access is a priority when hypotension occurs
Dehydration		
Shock		
Salt-craving		Child craves dill pickles, chips, salt from salt shaker Monitor blood pressure closely
Aldosterone Excess		
Hypertension	Hypernatremia	Monitor blood pressure, urine output closely
Edema		
Catecholamine Deficiency		
Catecholamine deficiency in children is extremely rare		
Catecholamine Excess		
Hypertension	All signs and symptoms due to effect of increased epinephrine, norepinephrine, dopamine on target tissues	Both systolic and diastolic blood pressure increased
Tachycardia		
Headache		
Perspiration		
Emotional lability		
Anxiety		
Tremors		
Adrenal Androgen Deficiency		
Delayed development of pubic, axillary hair in females	Adrenal gland is sole source of androgens in females; testes produce androgens in males	

continued

Table 49-4 *(continued)*

Clinical Manifestations	Reason for Clinical Manifestations	Significance to the Nurse
Adrenal Androgen Excess		
Virilization in female • clitoral enlargement • labial fusion • increased labial pigmentation	Excess androgen production leads to virilization in females; male infants appear normal	A female infant may appear with ambiguous genitalia and must be evaluated immediately for gender identity and underlying cause of ambiguity
Excessive development of external genitalia Increased muscularity Rapid growth Adult body odor Early development of facial, axillary, and pubic hair	Excess androgen production	
Advanced bone maturation Stunted final adult height	Excess androgen levels lead to excessive bone maturation and early closure of growth plates	Treatment to decrease androgen levels prevents excessive bone maturation, allowing for more growth prior to closure of epiphyses

Table 49-5. Diagnostic Tests for Adrenal Alterations

Diagnostic Test	Purpose	Comments
Blood studies		
AM, PM cortisol AM ACTH	Detects abnormally high levels of cortisol or ACTH	Excessively high ACTH levels are indicative of a pituitary tumor
Serum glucose	Detects hyperglycemia	Excessive cortisol can lead to impaired carbohydrate metabolism and hyperglycemia
17-Hydroxyprogesterone (17-OHP) Androstenedione	Evaluates whether there are excessive "backed up" precursors in cortisol production pathway	These values are elevated in congenital adrenal hyperplasia; they are suppressed with adequate treatment
Plasma renin activity (PRA)	Assesses the degree of dehydration secondary to salt loss	The greater the dehydration, the higher the PRA
Dehydroepiandrosterone (DHEA) Testosterone Aldosterone	Detects altered production	High levels of adrenal androgens are indicative of congenital adrenal hyperplasia, adrenal tumors
Serum epinephrine, norepinephrine	Detects high levels secondary to tumor	High levels may indicate pheochromocytoma, neuroblastoma
Urine studies		
24-hour collection for corticoids, free cortisol, urinary glucose, urinary vanillylmandelic acid (VMA)		High urinary corticoid levels are indicative of Cushing disease Often positive in Cushing disease
Dexamethasone suppression test	Determines whether cortisol production can be suppressed	Dexamethasone should suppress ACTH, thereby suppressing cortisol production If cortisol remains high after ACTH suppression, this is suggestive of an adrenal tumor
Metyrapone test	Assesses ACTH and cortisol production	Metyrapone is given every 4 hours for 6 doses, after which 11-deoxycortisol level is determined Metyrapone blocks cortisol production, causing a rise in ACTH and 11-deoxycortisol (intermediate compound in cortisol pathway)
Buccal smear	Chromosome analysis	Allows the clinician to distinguish between a virilized female and an inadequately virilized male newborn infant
Abdominal CT scan	Detects adrenal hyperplasia, tumor	
Abdominal ultrasonography	Detects adrenal hyperplasia, tumor	
Lateral skull radiography	Detects erosion and enlargement of sella turcica	Enlarged and eroded sella turcica is indicative of pituitary tumor
CT scan of brain	Detects pituitary tumor	
Bone age radiograph	Determines degree of exposure to increased levels of androgens	Advanced bone age is indicative of prolonged or significant exposure to androgens

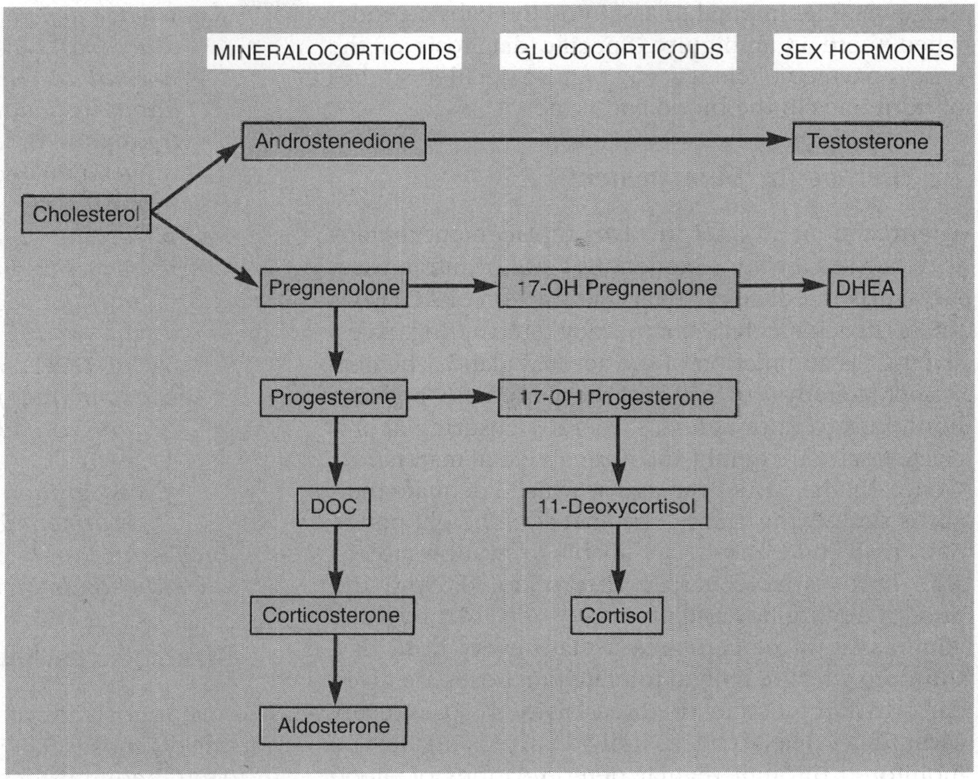

Figure 49-4. Adrenal cortex hormone production.

aldosterone even if adequate amounts are produced. The precursors of cortisol, notably progesterone and 17-hydroxyprogesterone, are aldosterone antagonists. Children with poor aldosterone production or utilization are termed "salt losers" and have difficulty maintaining extracellular fluid volume.

Clinical Manifestations

The excess androgen sex hormones in children with CAH produce virilization and development of secondary sex characteristics. The newborn girl with the disorder usually has enlargement of the clitoris, varying degrees of labial fusion, and often increased labial pigmentation. In rare instances, masculinization may be so complete that a penile urethra is formed. The newborn boy appears normal but may present with sexual precocity in early childhood. Many male infants are first diagnosed only after they are admitted to hospitals in shock secondary to a relatively minor illness. Their inability to produce adequate cortisol in response to the stress of an illness leads to shock. In untreated pubertal children, there is excessive development of external genitalia, increased muscularity, rapid growth, and early development of facial, axillary, and pubic hair. Final adult height may be stunted owing to early closure of the bone epiphyses. Children with inadequate aldosterone utilization have the propensity to lose salt and water, often leading to dehydration and vascular collapse.

Diagnostic Assessment

Laboratory studies in the newborn infant or child who is suspected of having congenital adrenal hyperplasia include determination of 17-hydroxyprogesterone level, one of the "backed-up" precursors in the cortisol production pathway. This level is usually elevated. A plasma renin activity (PRA) level may be determined to assess whether the child is a salt loser. The kidney is extremely sensitive to any degree of blood volume and sodium depletion. When blood volume and sodium levels decrease, renin production increases, leading to increased blood pressure. Children who lose salt through the urine decrease their blood volume in an attempt to compensate for and normalize serum sodium levels. The decrease in blood volume leads to increased renin production by the kidney. Therefore, the higher the PRA level, the greater the degree of dehydration.

Aldosterone levels may or may not be abnormally low in these children, depending on the cause of the problem. A buccal smear for sex chromosome analysis is done when a newborn infant presents with ambiguous genitalia. Sex chromosome analysis enables the clinician to determine whether an infant is a virilized female or an inadequately virilized male. This information is fundamental to assigning the baby's gender when there is ambiguity. Specific diagnosis of the exact enzyme deficiency may require detailed studies of hormones in the blood and urine.

Therapeutic Management

The treatment of CAH involves replacement therapy with corticosteroids. Exogenous (oral or intramuscular) cortisol reduces pituitary production of ACTH via the feedback mechanism, thereby interrupting excessive ACTH stimulation of the adrenal gland. The goal of such therapy is to suppress the abnormally high sex hormones to normal levels, thereby ensuring appropriate final adult height and normal sexual maturation. Generally the earlier the age at which adequate therapy is started, the greater the final adult height potential. Small children who are unable to swallow tablets, who have variable gastric absorption, or who frequently regurgitate usually receive an intramuscular administration of cortisone acetate every third day. Children who are able to tolerate oral doses are given daily hydrocortisone in three divided doses every eight hours. The dosage is individualized and must be monitored through regular determinations of blood levels of specific hormones (usually 17-hydroxyprogesterone or androstenedione) and regular determinations of height, weight, blood pressure, and bone age (Hung et al, 1983). Overtreatment can cause a decrease in linear growth and retardation of bone age.

For children who are salt losers, a salt-retaining agent such as deoxycorticosterone acetate (DOCA) or fludrocortisone (Florinef) is given. DOCA in 125-mg pellets may be implanted subcutaneously in infants. Usually one or two pellets are implanted and last 9 to 12 months before they are replaced. Infants receiving DOCA therapy require one-fourth teaspoon salt daily in their formula. The older infant and child can be treated with Florinef, a synthetic mineralocorticoid in tablet form.

Major Nursing Diagnoses for Congenital Adrenal Hyperplasia

***Altered growth and development: virilization and early development of secondary sexual characteristics,** related to excess testosterone production associated with stimulation of ACTH secretion by low levels of serum cortisol*

***Potential for injury: acute adrenal crisis,** related to insufficient cortisol and aldosterone to meet physiologic demands of stress*

***Fluid volume deficit,** related to hyponatremia associated with insufficient production of aldosterone*

***Knowledge deficit,** related to*

- *autosomal recessive etiology*
- *normal adrenal function and alterations associated with the disorder*
- *treatment, including:*
  - *a. need for regular administration of corticosteroids*
  - *b. alteration in dosage of corticosteroids required during stress*
  - *c. need for regular follow-up care*
  - *d. salt requirement for children receiving DOCA therapy*
  - *e. techniques for intramuscular injections and blood pressure measurement*
  - *f. recognition of and emergency treatment for acute adrenal crisis*

***Ineffective family coping,** related to birth of a child with ambiguous genitalia*

Strategies for Nursing Care

The major goals for nursing care are directed by the nursing diagnoses. They include (1) teaching the family to safely administer medications and to monitor the child for hypertension and adrenal crisis, and (2) helping the family cope with the birth of a child with ambiguous genitalia.

Providing Information to Support Home Care

Children receiving DOCA or Florinef may develop hypertension and blood pressure determinations must be taken frequently. The nurse can teach parents to take home blood pressures, to interpret their readings, and to notify their primary health care provider if readings rise above acceptable levels. Plasma renin activity levels are monitored in conjunction with the other necessary studies in these children.

During physical stress, there is a deficiency of glucocorticoids in children with congenital adrenal hyperplasia. Parents must be thoroughly instructed in the management of illness in their child. During illness, the dosage of oral steroids is doubled for several days. If the child has vomiting or diarrhea and is unable to tolerate oral treatment, he or she may require an intramuscular preparation of cortisone. Parents must be taught how to give intramuscular injections. They should also receive an emergency kit list, including a vial of hydrocortisone 21-sodium succinate (Solu-Cortef), syringes and needles, and written instructions on how and when to use them. The nurse should recommend that they notify their primary health care provider for advice when their child is ill.

In acute adrenal crisis secondary to physical stress, there may be deficiency of both glucocorticoids and mineralocorticoids as well as dehydration. Dehydration and hypotension can lead to shock if untreated. Treatment includes hospitalization for intravenous therapy of isotonic fluids and high doses of soluble hydrocortisone. Intravenous or intramuscular DOCA may also be given. Throughout the treatment of adrenal crisis, the nurse should closely monitor pulse, blood pressure, and hydration status, including urinary output, skin turgor, and mucous membrane integrity. Electrolytes may be ordered frequently, and the results, especially the serum sodium level, should be monitored closely. If serum sodium levels drop below 130 mEq/liter, the physician should be notified so that more sodium can be added to the intravenous solution. If the intravenous line becomes nonfunctional for any reason, another one must be started immediately, as dehydration can quickly occur without fluid and salt replacement.

Promoting Adaptive Family Coping

The diagnosis of CAH can be devastating emotionally for the parents. The birth of an infant with ambiguous genitalia is considered a psychosocial emergency and is discussed in detail under the section "Ambiguous Genitalia." The family may require extensive psychosocial support, and the nurse must create an atmosphere of acceptance that encourages full expression of feelings. The parents may be very confused about the cause and may feel guilty for transmitting the disorder to their child. The nurse can help explain the disorder in understandable terms. This is a difficult task, requiring a simple discussion of a somewhat complicated topic. Referral to appropriate sources, including genetic counseling, is indicated. The nurse can reassure the parents that, with appropriate treatment, their child will live a normal life without restrictions. For boys, normal pubertal development and fertility can be expected, and for girls, secondary sexual development is usually normal, although amenorrhea and irregular menses may occur. Parents may express concern that their "masculinized" female infant will develop body image and sexual identity problems later on in life. Studies indicate that the majority of virilized infants grow up to develop a female sexual identity and normal sexual function (Kaplan, 1982). The ambiguous external genitalia of the infant girl with CAH often requires surgical correction, and this is usually done in the first year of life to avoid psychological trauma at an older age.

Nursing Strategies for Follow-up Care in the Home or Clinic

Obtain a blood sample for analysis of hormone levels as indicated.

Measure height, weight, and blood pressure.

Assess hydration status.

Monitor for side effects of medications.

Determine parents' comprehension of the disorder and of rationale for treatment.

Assess individual and family coping patterns and adaptation to the disorder.

Refer for genetic counseling.

Cushing Disease

Cushing disease is the result of excessive cortisol levels in the body, whether produced endogenously or administered exogenously. The disease is variable, with either an abrupt or gradual onset, a short or long course, and signs that can be subtle or very obvious.

Etiology

Cushing disease is rare in childhood but can occur at any age, even in early infancy. Causes of Cushing disease include pituitary tumors, adrenal hyperplasia, adrenal tumors, or exogenous administration of glucocorticoids in the treatment of various diseases, such as autoimmune disorders and cancer. During infancy and in the first few years of life, the cause is usually a tumor of the adrenal gland. After the age of 6 or 7 years, the cause is usually pituitary secretion of high levels of ACTH secondary to a pituitary tumor with resulting bilateral adrenal hyperplasia.

Clinical Manifestations

Clinical findings include an obesity affecting the face, trunk, and abdomen. The child is often described as being "moon-faced" with "buffalo obesity" (Kaplan, 1982). The skin of the face is often plethoric, and skin in other areas may have a purplish pigmentation with atrophic striae of the abdomen, arms, and thighs. Ecchymoses and acne may be seen, and an excessive growth of hair may occur on the face, limbs, and pubis. Hair growth is not associated with other signs of virilization. In older children there is a slowing of growth velocity and muscular weakness. Hypertension, with elevation of both systolic and dystolic pressure, and osteoporosis are common. There is frequently carbohydrate intolerance as indicated by high serum glucose levels and sugar in the urine.

Diagnostic Assessment

Laboratory tests may include determination of total 24-hour urinary corticoids, urinary free cortisol, and a morning and evening serum cortisol level. If a pituitary tumor is suspected, morning serum ACTH levels are determined. Abnormally high levels suggest a pituitary tumor. Additional, more sophisticated suppression blood studies may be done to distinguish between an adrenal tumor and other causes of Cushing disease. An abdominal CT scan and ultrasonography may be done to detect an adrenal tumor, and a lateral skull x-ray and CT scan of the brain may be obtained to detect a pituitary tumor.

Therapeutic Management

Treatment of Cushing disease attributable to an adrenal tumor is primarily surgical. High doses of steroids are given before, during, and after surgery until the function of the residual tissue is determined. Pituitary tumors are treated with either surgery or radiation therapy. A variety of methods have been used to treat adrenal hyperplasia, including complete and subtotal adrenalectomy and drug therapy. These various methods are still being compared for effectiveness.

Major Nursing Diagnoses for Cushing Disease

Altered fluid volume and electrolytes: water and sodium excess, *related to increased levels of cortisol and aldosterone associated with*

- *increased endogenous production*
- *exogenous administration of glucocorticoids*

Potential for injury:

- ***gastric ulcers,*** *related to the effects of increased cortisol on the gastric mucosa*
- ***transient diabetes mellitus,*** *related to impaired glucose transport associated with high cortisol levels*
- ***infections,*** *related to the immunosuppressive action of increased cortisol*
- ***hypertension,*** *related to increased blood volume associated with water and sodium excess*

Ineffective individual coping, *related to emotional lability associated with increased cortisol levels*

Disturbance in self-concept: body image, *related to moon facies, redistribution of fat to the trunk with resultant wasting of extremities, and weight gain associated with increased appetite and fluid retention*

Potential altered tissue perfusion: systemic, *related to inadequate blood volume associated with postoperative adrenal insufficiency*

Strategies for Nursing Care

The nursing diagnoses just described detail the physical and emotional problems for the child with Cushing disease. Nursing goals relate to management of physical sequelae in the pre- and postoperative phases and psychosocial support of the child and family.

Monitoring for Physical Complications

The child with Cushing disease is at risk for several potential problems, including sodium and water retention, gastric ulcers, transient diabetes mellitus, infections, personality changes, and altered body image. The nurse must monitor for hypertension, edema, and excessive weight gain and should instruct the child and family on the importance of limiting oral salt intake. Small, frequent feedings and antacids may be required to prevent gastric discomfort. The urine should be checked daily for glucose and acetone. Signs and symptoms of infection should be monitored closely and antibiotics given as ordered should infection occur.

Helping the Family Cope with Emotional Lability and Enhancing Body Image

Parents often find that their child becomes irritable with highly labile emotional outbursts. The nurse can offer emotional support by facilitating expression of feelings by both the child and parents and by pointing out that emotional lability is a common problem in children with Cushing disease. Altered body image adds even more psychologic stress to the child. He or she should be told that many of the physical changes are reversible, including the obesity, facial roundness, excessive hair growth, acne, and bruising. The skin striae, however, are usually permanent.

Monitoring for Hypovolemia Postoperatively

The major postoperative complication of adrenalectomy is shock. Vital signs must be monitored closely, and the physician should be notified immediately if there is a significant increase in pulse or decrease in blood pressure. Intravenous fluid replacement must be adequately maintained, and urine output should be assessed frequently. (See also Table 27-7, a nursing process plan for the perioperative period.)

Nursing Strategies for Follow-up Care in the Home or Clinic

Preoperative visit:

Assess weight, blood pressure.

Monitor for complications:

- gastric ulcers: ask about blood in emesis, epigastric pain
- transient diabetes mellitus: assess for polydipsia, polyuria, polyphagia, fatigue, weight loss
- infections: presence of fever, discomfort, lymphadenopathy

Postoperative visit:

Assess for healing of surgical site.

Assess weight, blood pressure, and blood sugar as an indication of adrenal function.

Encourage questions about postoperative home care.

Premature Adrenarche

Premature adrenarche is a condition involving the isolated development of sexual hair at a young age.

Etiology

Premature adrenarche is caused by early secretion of adrenal sex hormones (androgens). The adrenal gland normally begins producing sex hormones during puberty, yet little is known about what initiates and controls the timing of hormone secretion. In the pubertal female, the adrenal androgens are responsible for development of sexual hair; in the pubertal male the influence of adrenal androgens is obscured by the more obvious influence of testicular testosterone secretion.

Clinical Manifestations

Prepubertal children with premature adrenarche develop pubic and axillary hair but undergo no other pubertal changes. In girls, there is no breast development and in boys the penis and testicles remain prepubertal in size. The amount of sexual hair in children with premature adrenarche usually increases very slowly.

Diagnostic Assessment

The diagnostic evaluation of the prepubertal child with sexual hair is usually not extensive, yet it involves identifying the cause of androgen hormone production. Precocious puberty, congenital adrenal hyperplasia, and adrenal tumors are usually ruled out on the basis of history and clinical examination. Laboratory studies in the evaluation of premature adrenarche may include determination of serum dehydroepiandrosterone (DHEA) level and levels of pituitary gonadotropins (LH and FSH). The concentration of DHEA, an adrenal androgen, is often elevated in children with premature adrenarche, and the pituitary gonadotropin levels remain in the low, prepubertal levels. Increased growth rates and advanced bone maturation can be seen in this condition, and a bone age x-ray is usually obtained.

Strategies for Nursing Care

No medical treatment is necessary for premature adrenarche, as it is a physically harmless condition. The child, however, may suffer body image problems, requiring psychosocial intervention. The nurse should reassure the child and parents that the condition is not a disease, but a "timing" variation of the adrenal clock, and that normal puberty at about the average time can be expected. Hair growth will not progress to other parts of the body.

Adrenal Tumors

Adrenal tumors in children can arise from the cortex or medulla. Symptoms differ greatly depending on the location. Tumors of the cortex are usually associated with an increased production of sex hormones, whereas tumors of the medulla are associated with an increased production of catecholamines.

Tumors of the adrenal cortex are seen from birth into adolescence. They are of various types, and the clinical manifestations depend upon the nature of the hormone or hormones secreted. They are usually virilizing, producing masculinization in girls and pseudoprecocious puberty in boys. In tumors with mixed hormone production, cushingoid symptoms as well as virilization may occur. In both sexes there is an increase in growth rate and advancement of skeletal maturation.

Diagnostic Assessment

A child with inappropriate virilization may undergo many laboratory evaluations in an effort to differentiate an adrenal virilizing tumor from congenital adrenal hyperplasia. Serum levels of testosterone, DHEA, and 17-hydroxyprogesterone are determined. Urinary 17-ketosteroid levels are also evaluated. Abdominal ultrasonography and CT scan are done to localize a suspected tumor.

Therapeutic Management

Treatment of a virilizing tumor is surgical excision. Corticoid treatment is given during and for several days after surgery until it can be determined that sufficient functioning adrenal tissue is present. Chemotherapy and radiation therapy are rarely employed unless there is metastasis at diagnosis or recurrences. The hormones found to be present at elevated concentrations at diagnosis are monitored at least every 6 months after surgery to detect recurrences. More than 50 per cent of these tumors recur, and chemotherapy is usually used as the next treatment of choice. The child with a virilizing adrenal tumor is at risk for body image problems and postoperative complications. The parents undergo severe emotional stress owing to the diagnosis itself, the changes they have seen in their child, the surgery, and the prognosis. The family requires intensive psychosocial support from all members of the health care team. Depending on the degree of virilization in perceived body image alterations, the child may be a candidate for individualized psychiatric counseling. The parents may require counseling to work through feelings of anger, fear, disbelief, and guilt. As with other adrenal surgeries, the major postoperative complications after removing an adrenal cortex tumor is shock. Vital signs are monitored closely, and the physician is notified if the pulse increases and the blood pressure decreases significantly.

Tumors of the adrenal medulla include neuroblastomas and pheochromocytomas. Refer to Chapter 42 for a discussion of neuroblastomas.

Pheochromocytoma

The pheochromocytoma is a rare tumor in childhood, is usually benign, and is most commonly found in the right adrenal medulla. The incidence in pediatric patients peaks between the ages of 9 and 12 years. Familial pheochromocytomas have been reported many times either as a single disorder or as part of a multiple endocrine disorder.

Clinical Manifestations. The clinical manifestations are caused by the effects of norepinephrine and epinephrine, which are produced in large quantities by the tumor. The systolic blood pressure may reach levels as high as 250 mm Hg, with corresponding increases in diastolic pressure. Headache, sweating, nausea and vomiting, visual disturbances, and weight loss are the most common symptoms. The child may appear anxious, pale, and weak and is often emotionally labile. Tremors and tachycardia may also be present.

Diagnostic Assessment. Laboratory studies include 24-hour urinary samples to detect levels of vanillylmandelic acid (VMA) and normetanephrine-metanephrine, which are metabolites of epinephrine and norepinephrine. Nearly all patients with the tumor have an abnormally high urinary output of these metabolites. Epinephrine and norepinephrine levels may also be determined when metabolite concentrations are abnormally high. Intravenous pyelogram, CT scan, and abdominal ultrasonography are used for localizing a suspected tumor. Arteriography may be used in select cases.

Therapeutic Management. Treatment of pheochromocytomas is surgical excision. The patient is given alpha-adrenergic blocking agents 2 or 3 weeks prior to surgery to lower the blood pressure. Patients with serious tachycardia often require treatment with beta-adrenergic agents prior to surgery.

Strategies for Nursing Care. Nursing care during and after surgery includes close monitoring of blood pressure and pulse. Hypertension may be present for 24 to 36 hours after surgery, yet if it persists, another tumor or renal vascular disease may be present. Transient hypoglycemia has been reported postoperatively, and frequent evaluations of blood glucose levels may be ordered. Symptoms of sudden shakiness, hunger, anxiety, and increased sweating warrant a blood glucose evaluation. The nurse must reinforce that continued follow-up medical care is important, because although the tumor is benign, it may recur years later.

The Thyroid Gland

Normal Functions of the Thyroid Gland

The thyroid gland exerts widespread effects on metabolic processes throughout the body. *Thyroid hormone regulates body metabolism,* thereby affecting body temperature, growth, cardiovascular function, gastrointestinal motility, neurologic reflexes, muscle tone, and respiratory rate.

The thyroid gland traps iodine from ingested food to produce the thyroid hormone thyroxine (T4), and, as with other hormones, the amount produced is dependent upon a negative feedback mechanism. Decreased levels of thyroid hormone in body fluids stimulate pituitary secretion of thyroid stimulating hormone (TSH) in two ways: (1) by a direct effect on the pituitary itself; and (2) by an indirect effect acting through the hypothalamus. The hypothalamus produces thyrotropin-releasing hormone (TRH) that stimulates the pituitary to produce TSH. The TSH stimulates the thyroid gland to produce thyroid hormone. The thyroid gland traps circulating iodide, oxidizes the iodide to iodine via a peroxidase enzyme, and binds the iodine to a tyrosine residue on thyroglobulin to form monoiodotyrosine (MIT) and diiodotyrosine (DIT). MIT and DIT couple to form T3; DIT and DIT couple to form T4. The thyroid hormones are then released into the circulation (Coody, 1984) (Fig. 49-5). Clinical manifestations of thyroid alterations are summarized in Table 49-6. Tests used to diagnose thyroid alterations appear in Table 49-7.

Congenital Hypothyroidism

Congenital hypothyroidism is a condition resulting from inadequate thyroid hormone production to meet an infant's needs. From fetal life through the first 2 years, thyroid hormone is crucial for growth and development of the skeletal and nervous systems. Untreated hypothyroidism in the first few years of life can result in poor linear growth and irreversible mental retardation.

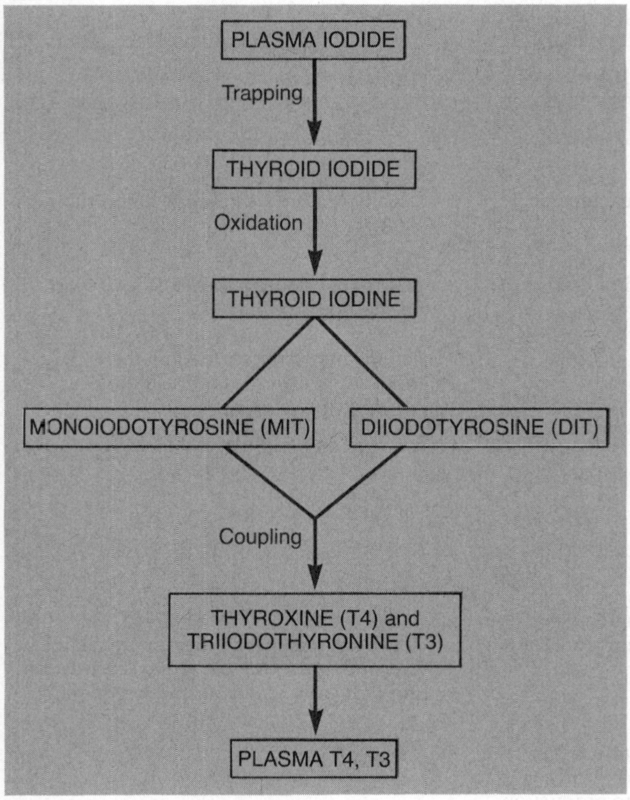

***Figure* 49-5.** Thyroid hormone synthesis.

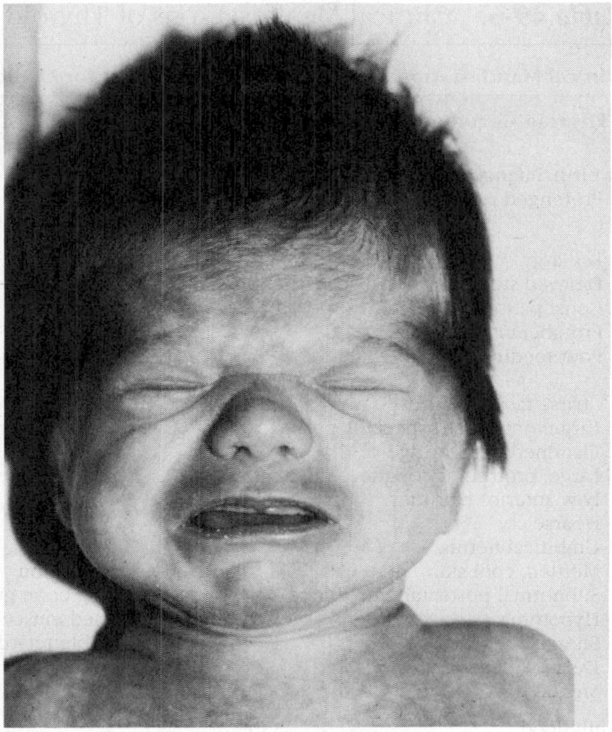

***Figure* 49-6.** A 21-day-old infant with congenital hypothyroidism. Note the subtle clinical findings of puffy face with low anterior hairline, flattened nasal bridge, and mottled skin.

Incidence and Etiology

The incidence of congenital hypothyroidism is approximately 1:4000 newborn infants. There is an unexplained female-to-male ratio of between 2.5:1 and 3:1 (Kaplan, 1982). Thyroid dysgenesis, or improper development of the gland, accounts for 80 per cent of the known cases. Inborn errors of thyroid hormone synthesis, secretion, and utilization are autosomal recessive hereditary enzyme deficiencies that account for 10 to 15 per cent of the cases. Transient congenital hypothyroidism may occur when pregnant women with hypothyroidism receive antithyroid medication. The drugs cross the placenta and disrupt fetal thyroid hormone production. Less frequent causes of congenital hypothyroidism include low levels of dietary iodine (endemic goiter) and hypothalamic-pituitary disorders associated with septo-optic dysplasia, microcephaly, and anencephaly.

Clinical Manifestations

The clinical signs of congenital hypothyroidism are usually absent or subtle at birth and may not appear for several months, depending on the severity of the hormone deficiency. Unfortunately, irreversible damage to the central nervous system may occur before clinical manifestations suggest the diagnosis. Screening programs for newborn infants have greatly improved the prognosis for infants with congenital hypothyroidism through early recognition and treatment of the disorder. Infants with congenital hypothyroidism tend to have prolonged gestation and high birthweights, although they may have normal birth lengths and head circumferences. Decreased gastrointestinal motility may delay stooling after birth for over 20 hours. These infants often have feeding difficulties, prolonged physiologic jaundice, lethargy, and constipation. Parents often describe their babies as good, quiet babies who sleep a lot, seldom cry, and are difficult to keep awake while feeding. On physical examination, a minority of the hypothyroid newborns have the classic "cretinoid" findings: puffy face with coarse features; wide fontanels and sutures; flattened nasal bridge; large, protruding tongue; low anterior hairline; hoarse cry; protuberant abdomen with an umbilical hernia; cool and mottled skin; hypotonia; and sluggish reflexes (La Franchi, 1980) (Fig. 49-6).

Table 49-6. Clinical Manifestations of Thyroid Alterations

Clinical Manifestations	Reason for Clinical Manifestations	Significance to the Nurse
Thyroid Hormone Deficiency		
At birth/infancy:		
Prolonged jaundice	Slow metabolism, slow clearance of bilirubin	Usually require treatment with bilirubin light
Lethargy		
Delayed stooling at birth (over 24 hours)	Decreased gastrointestinal peristalsis	Newborns should pass first stool within first 24 hours of life
Constipation		
Protuberant abdomen		
Poor feeding	Decreased appetite	Parents may find that feeding their newborn is difficult and frustrating
Coarse facial features		
Large fontanels (especially posterior)	Delayed skeletal maturation	
Flattened nasal bridge		
Large, protruding tongue		
Low anterior hairline		
Hoarse cry		
Umbilical hernia		
Mottled, cool skin	Poor circulation	
Subnormal postnatal growth rate	Poor long bone growth	
Hypotonia	Decreased muscular strength	
Sluggish reflexes	Irreversible retardation in maturation of nervous system	Newborn screening programs are aimed at preventing irreversible mental retardation through early detection and treatment
Delayed development		
Mental retardation		
Childhood		
Goiter (swollen thyroid)	Gland swells owing to autoimmune inflammatory process or to gland trying to compensate for inadequate production	
Slow growth	Poor long bone growth	
Decrease in appetite, energy level	Slow metabolism	Symptoms may be very subtle and may develop over months
Constipation	Decreased gastrointestinal peristalsis	
Cold intolerance	Poor circulation	
Poor school performance	Decreased ability to concentrate, decreased level of alertness	
Thyroid Hormone Excess		
Hyperactive behavior	Hypermetabolism; affects all body systems	Many children with thyrotoxicosis are treated for simple behavior and academic problems without success prior to the diagnosis
Nervousness, tremor		
Emotional lability		
Poor school performance		
Insomnia		
Fatigue, poor endurance		
Heat intolerance		
Thin, velvety, moist skin		
Tachycardia, palpitation		
Flushed, sweaty skin		
School problems	Easy distractibility, poor concentration	
Exophthalmia, stare	Believed to be due to an autoimmune process; poorly understood	There is no correlation between degree of proptosis and severity of thyrotoxicosis; following therapy the eyes often improve, but 25% of the patients have no change. Patient or parent should be taught to instill methylcellulose eyedrops at night to protect cornea
Lid lag		
Impaired peripheral vision		
Dryness of eyes in morning		
Enlarged thyroid gland	Thyroid stimulating immunoglobulins (TSI) stimulate the gland to hyperfunction and enlarge	

Table 49-7. Diagnostic Tests For Thyroid Alterations

Diagnostic Test	Purpose	Comments
Serum levels		
Thyroxine (T4) Thyroid stimulating hormone (TSH) T3 radioimmunoassay Thyroid binding globulin (TBG)	Detects actual level of circulating thyroid hormone, binding proteins, and TSH	T4 level is low and TSH level is usually high in hypothyroidism; T4 level is high and TSH level low in hyperthyroidism
Thyroid releasing hormone (TRH) stimulation test	TRH stimulates TSH production; evaluates pituitary reserve	
Thyroid stimulating immunoglobulins (TSI)	Done when Graves disease suspected	Positive in Graves disease patient
Radioactive iodine-123 (^{123}I) uptake and scan	Identifies location and size of gland; assesses function of gland Differentiates between an absent gland, a small dysplastic gland, and a gland of normal size that is over- or underfunctioning	Infant swallows ^{123}I; thyroid gland uptake of ^{123}I is measured at 2, 4, 6 and 24 hours after ingestion of ^{123}I Verify that patient is not allergic to iodine prior to test
Technetium scan	Identifies location and size of gland; does not assess function of gland	Requires an intravenous line for injection of technetium, which is incorporated into thyroid gland Scan is done immediately after injection of technetium
Knee radiograph	Assesses skeletal maturation in infants	Delayed bone maturation on knee film indicates that low levels of thyroid hormone were present during gestation
Bone age radiograph (hand and wrist)	Assesses skeletal maturation in children	Delayed bone age in children is seen in hypothyroidism

Diagnostic Assessment

The initial screening test for congenital hypothyroidism is usually included in a panel of screening tests for newborn infants, including those for phenylketonuria (PKU), galactosemia, and homocysteinuria or sickle cell disease (or both). This screening test usually indicates a low T4 level and high TSH level, yet further testing is necessary to determine the exact cause of the deficiency. Repeat blood studies are done to verify thyroid hormone levels obtained on initial screening tests. A radioactive iodine-123 (^{123}I) uptake and scan are performed to identify the location, size, and function of thyroid tissue. The infant swallows a small amount of ^{123}I isotope, and uptake of the isotope into the neck area is measured at several intervals over a 24-hour period. A low uptake of the iodine isotope in the neck indicates that either a very small amount of thyroid tissue is present or that a normal amount of tissue is not trapping iodine properly. A technetium scan, which identifies only size and location of the thyroid gland and not function, is done if an ^{123}I scan cannot be done owing to scheduling or supply constraints. Knee radiographs are often obtained in infants with suspected hypothyroidism. Delayed bone maturation indicates that low levels of thyroid hormone were present during gestation. A thyroid releasing hormone (TRH) stimulation test is done in infants with low T4 *and* low TSH levels. Usually, if the T4 level is low, the TSH level increases to stimulate the gland to produce more T4. The TRH stimulation test is performed to determine if the pituitary can make TSH.

Therapeutic Management

The treatment of choice for hypothyroidism during infancy and childhood is oral levothyroxine. Dosage is adjusted by weight to achieve desired serum levels of levothyroxine without inducing hyperthyroidism. Signs and symptoms of excessive levothyroxine include fussiness, disturbance of sleep, excessive food and fluid intake with poor weight gain or weight loss, jitteriness, increased stooling with or without diarrhea, and diaphoresis (Foley, 1986).

Major Nursing Diagnoses for Congenital Hypothyroidism

Potential altered growth and development:
- ***impaired growth of skeletal and nervous tissue,*** *related to congenital insufficiency of thyroid hormone*
- ***impaired intellect,*** *related to deprivation of thyroid hormone in early infancy*

Ineffective family coping, *related to the potential for mental retardation*
Knowledge deficit: parents initially, child later, *related to*

- *cause of disorder and function of thyroid hormone within the body*
- *administration of levothyroxine*
- *signs and symptoms of hypo- and hyperthyroidism*
- *need for genetic counseling*
- *methods to facilitate development of the mentally retarded child*
- *need for lifelong follow-up*

Strategies for Nursing Care

Supporting the Family in the Initial Diagnostic Period

Parents may become very frightened when they learn that their baby has congenital hypothyroidism. They may have no idea where a thyroid gland is or what it does. They may feel guilty that somehow they did something to cause their child to be born with an absent or abnormal thyroid gland, or that they ignored the subtle signs of hypothyroidism. It is important to reassure parents that their child's disorder did not result from anything they did or did not do during pregnancy. They should also be reassured that only a minority of the infants with congenital hypothyroidism are detected by clinical findings, and that the majority of infants do not exhibit clinical symptoms at birth. Many parents believe that congenital hypothyroidism results in cretinism and irreversible mental retardation. They must be reassured that early screening, diagnosis, and treatment of their infant's disorder can prevent these problems.

Providing Information to Support Home Care

Treatment of congenital hypothyroidism is synthetic thyroid hormone (levothyroxine), started at a dose of 0.025 mg to 0.05 mg daily. The nurse teaches the parents to crush and mix the tablet with a teaspoon of water or formula, and to administer the mixture through an eye dropper or a 5 ml syringe. The tablets have no taste of their own and have no side effects if given at the appropriate dosage. The nurse explains the importance of giving the thyroid replacement every day and should instruct the parents that if they do forget to give a dose one day, twice the dose should be given the following day. The tablet should not be dissolved in the baby's formula bottle, as a full dose will not be received if the baby does not finish the bottle. The parents must be aware that their child will always be on thyroid replacement. They may ask if giving more thyroid hormone than is recommended will help their child grow faster or become smarter. Just as too little is harmful, too much thyroid hormone will speed up body metabolism to a dangerous level. Extra thyroid hormone does not make babies grow faster, nor will it make them smarter. After treatment is started, parents may notice an improvement in their baby's appetite, an increase in activity and interest in the environment, and even a tendency to be more demanding of attention.

Parents often express concern about the occurrence of congenital hypothyroidism in future children. The probability of siblings' being affected depends on the cause of the disorder, and genetic counseling is appropriate after an accurate diagnosis is made. Thyroid dysgenesis usually occurs sporadically, and siblings of children with the disorder are not at a significantly higher risk of being affected than are persons in the general population. Inborn errors of thyroid hormone synthesis are autosomal recessive in inheritance, and siblings of a child with such a disorder have a 1 : 4 chance of being affected.

As infants grow, their need for thyroid replacement increases. Parents must be aware of the importance of close medical follow-up, especially during the first few years of life. Blood thyroid levels should be checked every 3 months for the first year, every 6 months during the second year, and every year thereafter through adulthood. Infants with congenital hypothyroidism whose condition is detected and who are treated before 3 months of age are expected to have normal linear growth, bone maturation, and sexual development. Mental development, however, is much less predictable. In general, the more profound the deprivation of thyroid hormone in the early months of life, the poorer the prognosis for mental development. The earlier the disorder is detected and treated, the better the intellectual outcome. Refer to the bibliography at the end of this chapter for recommended readings regarding congenital hypothyroidism.

Nursing Strategies for Follow-up Care in the Home or Clinic

Assess for therapeutic effects of thyroid replacement therapy: improved appetite; increased physical, cognitive, and social behavior.

Obtain blood sample for thyroid level.

Assess developmental level to screen for:

- evidence of mental retardation
- adjustment to chronic condition

Acquired Hypothyroidism

Incidence and Etiology

The incidence of acquired hypothyroidism in children is estimated to be 1 : 500 to 1 : 1000 (Kaplan, 1982). The most common cause is chronic lymphocytic thyroiditis, an autoimmune disorder in which the thyroid gland is incorrectly recognized by the body to be foreign and is destroyed. Goitrogens, substances that decrease thyroid hormone production, can also lead to hypothyroidism. Goitrogen-induced hypothyroidism may be seen in children ingesting iodine-containing expectorants for asthma or cystic fibrosis or antithyroid drugs for hyperthyroidism. Hypothyroidism may follow radioactive iodine treatment for hyperthyroidism as well as partial or total thyroidectomy. Hypothalamic or pituitary disease as a result of tumors, trauma, infection, or radiation therapy can lead to hypothyroidism owing to a deficiency of either TRH or TSH. Finally, hypothyroidism may occur in certain diseases such as cystinosis or histiocytosis owing to infiltration or destruction of the thyroid gland or pituitary gland.

Clinical Manifestations

The child with acquired hypothyroidism may experience slow growth, generalized puffiness, decreased appetite, constipation, a swollen thyroid gland, lethargy, a drop in school performance, and cold intolerance (Kaplan, 1982). Acquired hypothyroidism due to chronic lymphocytic thyroiditis is often insidious in onset, and the most common presentation is a decrease in the growth rate, which may be accompanied by a goiter. The child whose condition produces subtle signs usually presents with a decrease in growth rate and developmental delay or poor school performance. On physical examination the child may have short stature, a dull, placid expression, slow pulse, decreased blood pressure, pale and thick skin, cool hands and feet, goiter, delayed dental maturity, delayed puberty, mild obesity, protuberant abdomen, coarse hair, flabby muscles with pseudohypertrophy, and delayed deep tendon reflexes.

This disorder emphasizes the importance of complete and accurate growth charts on all patients whom the nurse follows. A child who has grown well in the past but suddenly reaches a growth plateau should be brought to the physician's attention. A careful interim nursing history may elicit much information about subtle changes in appetite, energy level, bowel habits, and school performance. Poor growth may be very difficult emotionally and socially for the child, especially in early or preadolescence.

Diagnostic Assessment

Laboratory studies in suspected hypothyroidism include determinations of serum T4, T3 resin uptake, and TSH concentration. Primary hypothyroidism is confirmed by a low serum T4 level and T3 resin uptake and an elevated serum TSH concentration. Hypothalamic-pituitary hypothyroidism is diagnosed by a low serum T4 level and a normal serum TSH level.

Therapeutic Management

The treatment for acquired hypothyroidism is levothyroxine, and the dosage is individualized on the basis of clinical and biochemical response. The goals of treatment are to achieve normal growth and development and normal results of blood studies.

Strategies for Nursing Care

The nurse should reassure the child and parents that if hypothyroidism develops beyond age 2 or 3 years, there does not appear to be a risk of permanent intellectual impairment, and all changes seen in the child should be reversible. However, it should be pointed out that children with long-standing hypothyroidism may miss out on important learning experiences, and that their genetically predestined height potential may not be fully attained. The nurse should emphasize the importance of taking the thyroid replacement doses as ordered, explaining that symptoms of hypothyroidism will recur within a few weeks if treatment is discontinued. Levothyroxine is inexpensive, is readily available in pharmacies, and is available in a form that can be chewed and swallowed by children who cannot swallow whole tablets.

Graves Disease

Graves disease, or juvenile thyrotoxicosis, is characterized by an accelerated metabolism of all body tissues secondary to an increased production of thyroid hormones.

Incidence and Etiology

The increased production of thyroid hormones is caused by an autoimmune process that may have a genetic as well as immunologic base. Although Graves disease may occur at any age, it is very rare in infants and young children. The incidence increases with age, and the majority of cases occur during adolescence (Buckingham et al, 1981). It is more common in females in a ratio of approximately 4:1, and there is frequently a family history of thyroid disease.

Clinical Manifestations

The clinical manifestations of Graves disease include nervousness, emotional lability, increased appetite, weight loss, school problems, proptosis, sleep disturbances, and heat intolerance. Fatigue and poor endurance in physical activities are common complaints. The thyroid gland is enlarged two to four times in size and is usually firm, smooth, and nontender. There may be tachycardia and increased blood pressure. The skin may be flushed, with a smooth texture, and the hair is sometimes thinned. Prominence of the eyes as well as lid lag is commonly seen. Hyperactive behavior is common, and a tremor in the hands is seen when the patient extends the arms and spreads the fingers.

Diagnostic Assessment

The diagnosis of Graves disease is frequently missed for months, as the symptoms usually develop over time. Teachers may complain of the child's poor attention span, failure to complete work, and emotional lability. The symptoms are frequently thought by parents to be part of a normal adolescence process, and they may feel guilty about having delayed medical attention for their child.

Laboratory studies show an increase in serum T4 and T3 levels with a normal or low TSH concentration. Thyroid stimulating immunoglobulins (TSI) are found in nearly 100 per cent of patients with Graves disease. (See Chapter 43 for further discussion of autoimmunity.) A radioactive iodine uptake test shows very high uptake of iodine owing to overactivity of the gland.

Therapeutic Management

Three modes of therapy are currently used for the treatment of Graves disease: (1) antithyroid drugs to block the synthesis of thyroxine; (2) destruction of the thyroid by radioiodine; and (3) subtotal thyroidectomy. Most children under 18 years of age are treated initially with antithyroid drugs (propylthiouracil or methimazole) (Cooper, 1984). If the drug is properly administered, a patient will usually develop normal thyroid hormone levels within 6 weeks. Treatment with antithyroid drugs is safe and inexpensive, but it requires taking pills three times a day. The more common side effects of the drugs include pruritus (itching), skin rash, urticaria, and joint pains. Most reactions are mild and necessitate either reducing the dosage or changing drugs. Therapy is usually continued for 1 to 3 years, after which the patient is reevaluated for remission.

The use of radioactive iodine is not advocated in children because of risk of inducing thyroid carcinoma, leukemia, thyroid nodules, or genetic mutations. Surgery is effective and safe when performed by a highly skilled surgeon under optimal conditions. Complications of surgery include transient hypocalcemia, hypoparathyroidism, damage to one or both recurrent laryngeal nerves, wound infections, hemorrhage, keloid formation, and recurrence of hyperthyroidism.

Graves ophthalmopathy includes exophthalmia, lid retraction, stare, mild itching of the eyes, and lacrimation. The cause is unknown but is believed to have an autoimmune base. However, there is no correlation between the degree of eye involvement and the severity of thyrotoxicosis. Following therapy, the eyes often improve, but one fourth of the patients have no change.

Major Nursing Diagnoses for Graves Disease

Altered growth and development: accelerated metabolism, related to increased production of thyroid hormones

Disturbance in self-concept: body image, related to disease-induced changes in emotions, weight, skin, hair, and eyes

Knowledge deficit: child and parents, related to
- ***cause of the disease and normal thyroid function***
- ***treatment, including side effects of antithyroid drugs***
- ***postoperative home care***

Potential for injury, related to the following complications of thyroid surgery:
- ***hemorrhage***
- ***laryngeal nerve damage***
- ***transient hypocalcemia***

Strategies for Nursing Care

Nursing care for the child with Graves disease will be influenced by the type of treatment prescribed. Major nursing goals will always include family support and teaching and management of symptoms. Should surgery be necessary, postoperative care and teaching will be a major nursing focus.

Supporting a Healthy Body Image

The physical and emotional changes associated with hypersecretion of thyroid hormones can be troubling for any client, but especially so for the adolescent who is already sensitive to changes in body image as the result of normal development. The nurse will be challenged to assist the adolescent with maintenance of a healthy body image by teaching symptom control through environmental manipulation.

The nurse can be an effective liaison person with the school in helping to decrease preventable stresses in the young client's daily routine. Nervousness and emotional lability often respond to increased rest, a quieter environment, and decreased demands. School personnel will usually be quite cooperative when they realize specific ways in which they can help before drug or surgical interventions can afford symptom relief.

Young persons with Graves disease may be quite concerned about emotional lability and wonder if they are "going crazy." The nurse's reassurance about the temporary nature of these episodes along with support for both the child and family can be invaluable in restoring normal family relations.

If ophthalmopathy is present as the result of Graves disease, the young client and the family should know that these changes in eye appearance usually improve with therapy. Provided that the use of eye make-up is congruent with family values, the adolescent girl can be shown how to enhance attractive facial features and downplay the effects of ophthalmopathy.

Providing Information to Support Home Care

The child and family may need advice about nutritious ways to increase the child's caloric intake to meet increased metabolic needs. They should be advised that this is a temporary measure, which will no longer be necessary once control is achieved through drug therapy or surgery.

Heat intolerance can be eased by commonsense measures, such as loose-fitting cotton clothing, adequate ventilation, and attention to body hygiene. The family may need to be reminded that the child's intolerance for heat is legitimate, however.

Monitoring for Postoperative Complications

Should surgery be necessary, postoperative assessment will include the major risks of hemorrhage, laryngeal nerve damage, and transient hypocalcemia. Postoperatively, the patient should be carefully observed for hemorrhage at the operative site, swelling, dyspnea, and cyanosis. Occurrence of any of these signs demands immediate medical attention. Suction equipment and tracheostomy trays should be available at the bedside.

Damage to a recurrent laryngeal nerve results in hoarseness that usually improves, but damage to both nerves may result in severe stridor and may also require tracheostomy. The patient should be checked for hoarseness and for pitch and tone of voice every hour for the first 24 hours after surgery.

Signs of hypocalcemia (numbness, tingling, twitching, tetany) usually appear 24 hours following surgery. The patient should be assessed for the Trousseau and Chvostek signs. *Trousseau sign* includes carpal spasms of the fingers and hands following application of a pressure cuff to the arm. *Chvostek sign,* spasms of the facial muscles elicited by tapping the face in front of the ear, indicates hyperirritability of the facial nerve. Mild hypocalcemia can usually be controlled with oral calcium, and several weeks may be required to determine if the condition is permanent. Hypothyroidism, should it occur, usually develops within 1 year of surgery.

Nursing Strategies for Follow-up Care in the Home or Clinic

Assess healing of incision.

Monitor for evidence of hypothyroidism within the first year postoperatively, and for recurrent hyperthyroidism.

Tumors of the Thyroid

Tumors of the thyroid gland are very rare in children, and they differ from those in adults in that they tend to be more benign.

Incidence

Of all children presenting with a nodule in a thyroid, approximately one third will have a malignant carcinoma and one third will have a benign adenoma (Kaplan, 1982). The remaining lesions that cause nodularity include thyroiditis, thyroid abscess, cysts, absence of one lobe, and multinodular goiter.

Benign adenomas are well-encapsulated solitary tumors that do not metastasize to distant sites. The tumor is smooth and firm upon palpation. Treatment is usually surgical removal of the nodule. Malignant carcinomas often cause a firm, irregular, nontender nodule or a woody-hard enlargement of the lobe or part of the lobe. Lymph node metastasis is common, but metastasis to lung and bone may occur.

Diagnostic Assessment

The discovery of the thyroid nodule warrants immediate medical attention. The patient's neck is examined for size and consistency of the nodule and for tenderness and presence of enlarged lymph nodes. Tenderness may suggest thyroiditis rather than a tumor. Enlarged lymph nodes may indicate local invasion. Laboratory tests include routine thyroid function tests and thyroid antibody tests. There are reports of hyperthyroidism resulting from functional nodules; however, the nodules are usually nonfunctioning. Antibody tests are usually positive with thyroiditis and are negative with tumors. An x-ray of the chest and neck is carried out to identify metastases. A thyroid scan with ^{123}I is one of the most important tests in the diagnosis of thyroid nodules. The presence of a "cold" or inactive nodule in an otherwise normal gland suggests an adenoma or carcinoma. Ultrasonography and CT are helpful in determining whether thyroid nodules are solid or cystic.

Therapeutic Management

Treatment of thyroid tumors is usually surgical removal of the involved lobe and lymph nodes. The prognosis for the great majority of thyroid tumors is excellent.

Strategies for Nursing Care

Nursing management of the child with a thyroid tumor involves psychosocial support and effective pre- and postoperative care. The child and parents undergo severe emotional stress owing to the diagnosis, and the nurse must be available to listen to their feelings and offer support. Because of excellent prognosis of thyroid tumors, the health care team can offer very optimistic projections about the tumor's course. Pre- and postoperative care is discussed in the section on Graves disease in this chapter.

The Parathyroid Glands

Normal Function of Parathyroids

The four parathyroid glands, embedded in the thyroid tissue, produce parathyroid hormone (PTH), which plays a vital role in the metabolism and balance of calcium and phosphorus in the body. Hypocalcemia stimulates and hypercalcemia suppresses PTH synthesis and secretion. The major target organs of PTH are kidney and bone. In the kidneys the hormone promotes renal excretion of phosphate by decreasing tubular resorption, thereby producing a low serum phosphorus level. A decrease in the concentration of phosphate ion allows for larger amounts of calcium to exist in solution. Therefore, calcium is mobilized from bone. *PTH acts directly on the bone tissue to cause increased osteoclastic activity,* resulting in increased calcium release from the bone (Habener and Potts, 1978).

Clinical manifestations of parathyroid alterations are summarized in Table 49-8, and relevant diagnostic studies are noted in Table 49-9.

Hypoparathyroidism

Hypoparathyroidism is a condition in which there is a lack of production of parathyroid hormone. Pseudohypoparathyroidism (PSH) is a condition in which there is increased production of parathyroid hormone but deficient target organ responsiveness to the hormone. The two conditions are contrasted in Figure 49-7.

Etiology

Hypoparathyroidism can be primary or secondary. Primary disease is usually idiopathic (no cause detected). Transient neonatal hypoparathyroidism and syn-

Table 49-8. Clinical Manifestations of Parathyroid Alterations

Clinical Manifestations	Reason for Clinical Manifestation	Significance to the Nurse
Parathyroid Hormone Deficiency		
Muscle cramps, twitching Tetany Paresthesias Chvostek, Trousseau signs	Hypocalcemia leads to increased muscle irritability, decreased relaxation	Child may require intravenous calcium gluconate; keep at bedside
Brittle hair Thin nails	Decreased incorporation of calcium into teeth, hair, nails	
Respiratory stridor		Keep tracheostomy tray at bedside; position head with pillow to facilitate breathing
Dry, coarse skin Maculopapular skin rash Dermatitis Short stature (PSH) Thickset build (PSH) Round facies (PSH) Short fingers, toes (PSH)	Hypocalcemia	
Mental retardation		Developmental evaluation indicated to help in school placement
Parathyroid Hormone Excess		
Renal colic Bone pain, masses Osteoporosis	Hypercalcemia	Very rare in children

Table 49-9. Laboratory and Diagnostic Studies for Parathyroid Alterations

Laboratory or Diagnostic Test	Purpose	Comments
Blood studies Serum calcium Serum phosphorus Plasma parathyroid hormone (PTH)	Assesses production of PTH by gland	Serum calcium levels low, phosphorus levels high in hypoparathyroidism; PTH levels low in idiopathic hypoparathyroidism, high in pseudohypoparathyroidism
Skeletal radiograph	Assesses calcium deposition into bone	Osteoporosis seen in hyperparathyroidism

dromes of congenital absence of parathyroids occur early in life. The average age of onset of idiopathic hypoparathyroidism is 16 years, and the average age of onset of pseudohypoparathyroidism is 8.5 years (Bronsky et al, 1958). Pseudohypoparathyroidism is an inherited disease that affects females approximately twice as often as males. Familial instances of idiopathic hypoparathyroidism are uncommon. Secondary disease may occur after thyroid surgery, as the parathyroids are vulnerable to injury or accidental removal.

Clinical Manifestations

In both idiopathic hypoparathyroidism (IHP) and pseudohypoparathyroidism (PSH), clinical manifestations are secondary to hypocalcemia and include tetany, seizures (generalized tonic-clonic, absence seizures, and simple partial seizures), carpopedal spasms, muscle cramps or twitching, paresthesias, and respiratory stridor. The skin can be dry and coarse; maculopapular skin eruptions and eczematous derma-

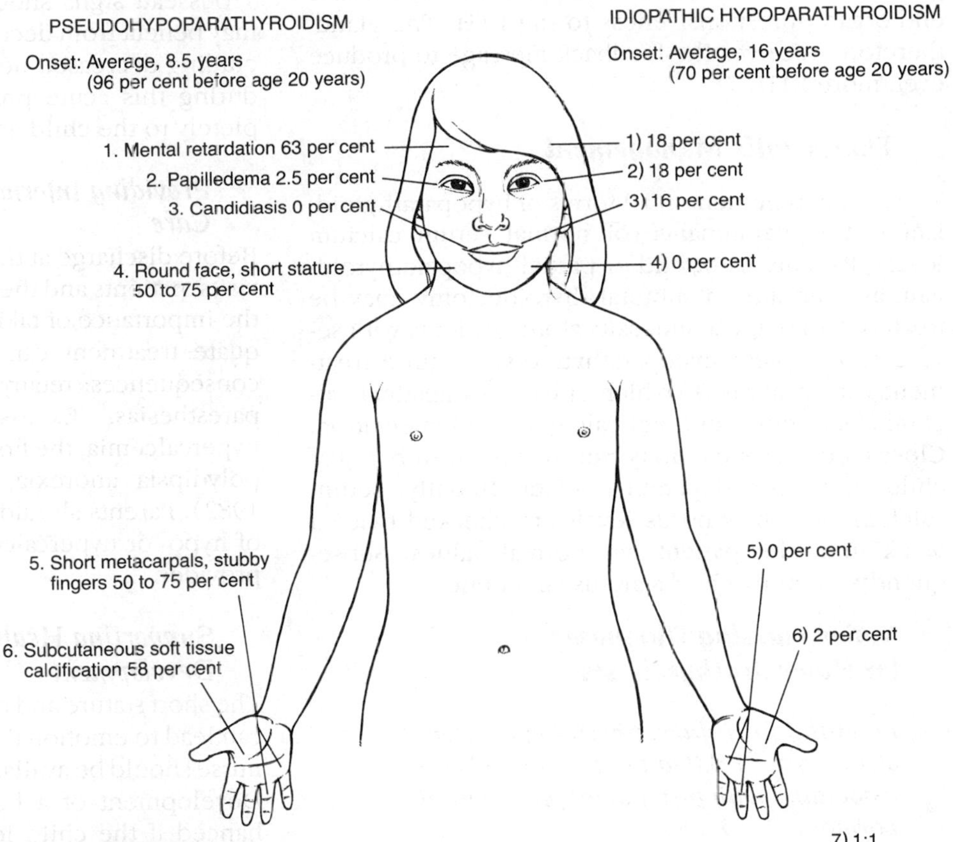

Figure 49-7. Comparison of effects of pseudohypoparathyroidism and idiopathic hypoparathyroidism.

titis can occur. The hair is often brittle, with areas of alopecia. The nails are thin and brittle, and there is dental and enamel hypoplasia.

Children with PSH are short and thickset and have round facies and short, thick necks. The fingers and toes are short and stubby, with dimpled skin over the knuckles. Subcutaneous soft tissue calcification is common. Mental retardation is a more prominent feature of PSH than of IHP. Swings of emotion, loss of memory, depression, and confusion can occur.

Candidiasis of the nails and mouth occurs in IHP but is rare in PSH. In addition, papilledema, presumably related to increased intracranial pressure, may occur in IHP but is rare in PSH.

Diagnostic Assessment

The diagnosis of hypoparathyroidism is made from signs and symptoms in association with decreased serum calcium and increased serum phosphorus concentrations. Idiopathic hypoparathyroidism appears to be a more severe biochemical disorder than pseudohypoparathyroidism. Plasma PTH levels are low in idiopathic hypoparathyroidism because production by the gland is low. Plasma levels of PTH are high in pseudohypoparathyroidism. As stated earlier, the gland produces adequate levels of PTH, but there is end-organ unresponsiveness to the PTH. The gland, therefore, receives the feedback message to produce even more PTH.

Therapeutic Management

The goal of treatment in all forms of hypoparathyroidism is the maintenance of normal serum calcium levels. Patients with mild or partial hypoparathyroidism, as seen after a subtotal thyroidectomy, may be treated with oral calcium salts alone. Patients with severe or complete hypoparathyroidism require treatment with vitamin D (which enhances intestinal calcium absorption) and oral calcium supplementation. Close medical follow-up is crucial to the well-being of children with hypoparathyroidism. Initially, serum calcium and phosphorus levels are checked twice a week until the patient has normal values. Subsequently, monthly checks are usually done.

Major Nursing Diagnoses for Hypoparathyroidism

Potential for injury: physiologic: altered electrolytes, *related to increased phosphorus associated with insufficient parathyroid hormone*

Potential ineffective airway clearance, *related to tetany of the muscles of respiration associated with hypocalcemia*

Knowledge deficit: child and parents, *related to*
- *etiology and normal parathyroid function*
- *treatment, including calcium replacement and signs and symptoms of hypocalcemia and hypercalcemia*
- *need for close medical follow-up*

Potential altered growth and development:
- ***short stature and round facies,*** *associated with pseudohyperparathyroidism*
- ***mental retardation,*** *associated with pseudohyperparathyroidism*

Strategies for Nursing Care

Maintaining a Patent Airway

During episodes of acute hypocalcemia, the patient's vital signs should be monitored and the airway should be evaluated for stridor and hoarseness. Positioning the head with a small pillow under the neck may facilitate breathing. A tracheostomy tray and calcium gluconate should be kept at the bedside. The child may require intravenous calcium during episodes of acute tetany. The patient should be evaluated frequently for tingling, stiffness, cramps, and tremors. Chvostek and Trousseau signs should also be checked. The child may benefit from decreased environmental stimuli, including decreased noise and soft lighting. Treatment during this acute phase should be explained completely to the child and parents.

Providing Information to Support Home Care

Before discharge at time of diagnosis and at follow-up visits, patients and their families must be instructed on the importance of taking treatment as ordered. Inadequate treatment can lead to hypocalcemia and its consequences: tetany, seizures, muscle cramps, and paresthesias. Excessive treatment can lead to hypercalcemia, the first signs being nocturia, polyuria, polydipsia, anorexia, and constipation (Bacon et al, 1982). Parents should be advised to report symptoms of hypo- or hypercalcemia to the primary health care provider.

Supporting Healthy Growth and Development

The short stature and round facies associated with PSH can lead to emotional difficulties for the child, and the nurse should be available for the child to vent feelings. Development of a healthy body image will be enhanced if the child learns to focus upon his or her strengths. The family's attitudes toward the child's appearance is critical to the child's self-esteem. The nurse has an opportunity to make a positive impact upon the child's life by helping the family to understand their role in the child's development of self-esteem.

A child with PSH who has mental retardation may benefit from a complete developmental and intellectual evaluation so that appropriate school placement can be made. Parents of a child with PSH may desire genetic counseling because it is an inheritable disease.

Nursing Strategies for Follow-up Care in the Home or Clinic

Obtain a blood sample for measurement of serum, calcium, and phosphorus levels.

Assess for evidence of hypo- or hypercalcemia.

Refer for genetic counseling if family desires.

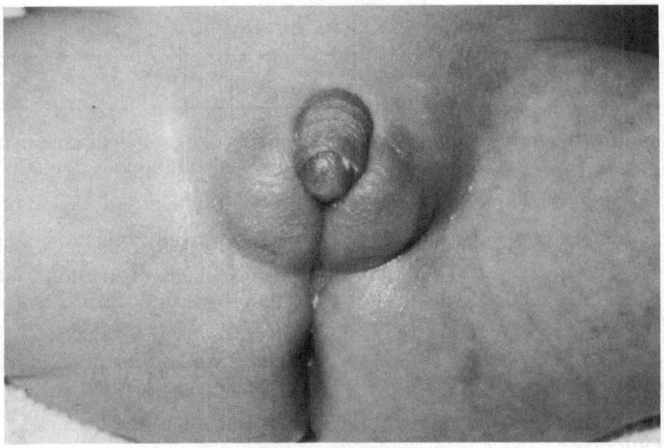

Figure 49-8. Ambiguous genitalia in a newborn girl with congenital adrenal hyperplasia.

The Gonads

An alteration in sexual development may be discovered at birth or at a later time in life when expected development does not occur. When such an abnormality is identified, clear information must be provided to facilitate the best possible adjustment. Some alterations require only minimal intervention, whereas others require long-term therapy. Clinical manifestations of gonadal alterations are presented in Table 49-10 and related diagnostic tests in Table 49-11.

Ambiguous Genitalia in the Newborn Infant

The neonate's external genitalia are described as ambiguous if there is (1) a structure that appears either as an enlarged clitoris or as a small penis with hypospadias, (2) a partial fusion of labioscrotal skin that appears as an incompletely formed scrotum, and (3) absence of gonads or a single gonad in an incompletely formed scrotum (Mazur, 1984) (Fig. 49-8). The presence of ambiguous genitalia in the newborn infant is considered a psychosocial emergency, and further diagnostic evaluation is performed as quickly as possible.

Etiology

Ambiguous genitalia can be caused by chromosomal abnormalities, congenital adrenal hyperplasia, placental transfer of masculinizing agents (females), and defective sex hormone synthesis (males).

Diagnostic Assessment

Recognition of ambiguous genitalia often occurs in the delivery room when the doctor or nurse finds it difficult to judge whether the infant is a boy or a girl. The

Table 49-10. Clinical Manifestations of Gonadal Alterations

Clinical Manifestations	Reason	Significance to the Nurse
Ambiguous genitalia in newborn infant	Masculinized female or undermasculinized male	Considered a psychosocial emergency; pediatric endocrinologist must see infant immediately
Breast development in girls under age 7 years	Increased estrogen production by ovary or oral ingestion of estrogen	Ovarian production of excess estrogen can be caused by a tumor or cyst
Breast development in boys (gynecomastia)	Imbalance of testosterone-estrogen levels during early puberty; sex chromosome disorders; drug exposures	Breast tissue must be differentiated from fat padding in obese boys
Delayed secondary sexual characteristics	Decreased levels of sex steroids	

Table 49-11. Diagnostic Tests for Gonadal Alterations

Diagnostic Test	Purpose	Comments
Serum 17-hydroxyprogesterone	Identifies congenital adrenal hyperplasia in infants with ambiguous genitalia	
Serum testosterone	Assesses testicular production of testosterone	
Serum estradiol	Assesses ovarian production of estrogen	Levels are high in ovarian tumors, pubertal females
Serum testosterone-estradiol ratio	Evaluates whether estradiol level is high in relation to testosterone in boys with gynecomastia	Testosterone is normally converted to estrogen in pubertal boys; sometimes there is an imbalance and too much estrogen is produced
Chromosomal studies (blood or buccal smear)	Identifies genetic sex of child with ambiguous genitalia, gynecomastia	
Bone age (left hand and wrist) radiograph	Assesses maturation of bones	High levels of estrogen mature bones quickly
Human chorionic gonadotropin (HCG) stimulation test	Stimulates testosterone production	HCG given by intramuscular injection
Pelvic or abdominal ultrasonography	Assesses ovaries for size, masses, cysts	

diagnostic evaluation involves questions based on the physical examination. It is important to ask whether the appearance of the genitalia is consistent with partial male virilization along a normal pathway. Is this a genetic male infant who did not completely virilize or is it a genetic female who is virilized? It is essential to assess whether gonads are palpable. Two scrotal or inguinal gonads suggest that the infant is an undermasculinized genetic male. A single, palpable gonad suggests mixed gonadal dysgenesis, in which the single gonad is abnormal. Mixed gonadal dysgenesis is associated with abnormal chromosome patterns. A single, palpable gonad may also be found in hermaphroditism, a condition in which both ovarian and testicular tissue are present.

An infant with ambiguous genitalia requires chromosomal studies. A 46,XY (female) karyotype in an infant with palpable gonads is suggestive of hermaphroditism. A diagnosis of true hermaphroditism requires histologic examination of gonadal tissue and recognition of both ovarian and testicular elements. A 45,X/46,XY karyotype is suggestive of mixed gonadal dysgenesis. Diagnosis of mixed gonadal dysgenesis requires demonstration of a unilateral testis and a contralateral absent, or streak, gonad. The single testis is structurally and functionally abnormal, and masculinization of the external genitalia is usually incomplete.

Because congenital adrenal hyperplasia can lead to varying degrees of masculinization in the female, blood studies (17-hydroxyprogesterone) are done to rule out this disorder. In the undermasculinized male, blood studies are done to detect whether the infant is able to produce testosterone. A human chorionic gonadotropin (HCG) stimulation test is done, in which HCG is administered to the infant to stimulate testosterone production. Infants with testosterone biosynthesis abnormalities are unable to produce increased levels of testosterone after stimulation by HCG. These infants are unable to produce adequate levels of testosterone to lead to masculinization.

Therapeutic Management

Treatment is based on the cause of the ambiguous genitalia. In infants with hermaphroditism and mixed gonadal dysgenesis, management involves choosing an appropriate gender assignment, maximizing the potential for adult sexual function, and minimizing psychosocial problems. Depending on the gender assignment chosen, surgical intervention is done as quickly as possible and the child receives hormonal replacements at puberty. Treatment of congenital adrenal hyperplasia is discussed elsewhere in this chapter. Male infants with defective testosterone biosynthesis are treated with testosterone injections to complete the masculinization process and receive testosterone in their teenage years and adulthood to initiate puberty and to sustain adult masculinization.

Strategies for Nursing Care

The nurse must be available to offer emotional support, explanations of the condition, and information about the necessary medical, surgical, and hormonal treatments. Information should be provided in a manner that fosters both parental confidence in rearing the child and the development of a positive self-image in the child.

When an infant is born with ambiguous genitalia, factual information is presented to the parents (Baker, 1981). They should be told that their infant's sex organs are "unfinished" or "underdeveloped," and that when external sex organs are underdeveloped, the internal ones may also be underdeveloped. After an evaluation by a specialist is completed, a sex assignment or reassignment is made. A decision is often very complex and difficult for the professional as well as the family. Parents may require guidance or actual assistance in talking with their other children and family members. They may also require professional counseling to recognize, confront, and discuss their feelings. Refer to the bibliography at the end of the chapter for recommended readings that are helpful in explaining sexual development.

Premature Thelarche

Etiology

Premature thelarche is the isolated appearance of breast development in girls at an early age.

The cause of premature thelarche is not clear, but it may be due to transient secretion of estrogen by the ovary. It may also be seen in girls who have accidentally ingested oral contraceptives or estrogen preparations. Typically, girls with premature thelarche are between 6 months and 2 years of age (Bacon et al, 1982).

Clinical Manifestations

Premature thelarche must be differentiated from neonatal hyperplasia of the breast, which can occur in either sex and generally subsides spontaneously within a few weeks or months after birth. Breast development in premature thelarche is only modest and often regresses over several months to a year, but it may persist even until the onset of normal puberty. Menses do not start until the usual age.

Diagnostic Assessment

Diagnosis of premature thelarche is made on a clinical examination. A bone age x-ray is often done to investigate whether there is excessive maturation of the bones secondary to estrogenic stimulation. Serum total estrogen or estradiol level may be determined to detect excessive hormone production from the ovaries.

Therapeutic Management

Premature thelarche without accelerated growth, high estrogen levels, or other pubertal changes is harmless and does not require treatment.

Strategies for Nursing Care

Although premature thelarche is a harmless condition, parents may experience emotional difficulty in adjusting to their daughter's body changes. They can be reassured that the breasts will not continue enlarging significantly and may even possibly regress in size. They should see no personality changes, growth spurt, facial acne, pubic hair, or axillary hair. If they do, their physician should be notified immediately. Puberty should begin at a normal age.

Gynecomastia

Gynecomastia is the growth of breast tissue in boys, observed most commonly in neonatal, prepubertal, and adolescent males. It is usually a benign condition.

Gynecomastia is relatively common during the neonatal period, but it is extremely rare between the newborn period and the onset of puberty. It occurs in varying degrees in 70 per cent or more of boys during adolescence. It is usually transient but may persist for 2 or 3 years.

Etiology

Neonatal gynecomastia is transient and is attributed to maternal hormones transmitted to the fetus during gestation. Adolescent gynecomastia most often results from a transient imbalance of testosterone and estrogen levels in the body. This imbalance is normal and relatively common during puberty. Prepubertal gynecomastia is associated with several disorders, including sex chromosome disorders, adrenal hyperplasia, hyperthyroidism or hypothyroidism, certain drug exposures (estrogens, testosterone, marijuana), and various types of tumors.

Diagnostic Assessment

The evaluation of gynecomastia includes an extensive history, including growth rate, rapidity in time and onset, drug exposure, and familial incidence. The patient is examined for height, extent of sexual development, size and contour of breasts, and whether the gynecomastia is unilateral or bilateral. Gynecomastia must be distinguished from the fat padding that frequently looks like breast tissue in obese individuals. Depending on the history and physical findings, hormone studies may be done. Skull x-rays or CT may be done if a brain tumor is suspected, and chromosome studies are done if Klinefelter syndrome (XXY karyotype) is suspected. (See Chapter 4 for additional information about Klinefelter syndrome.)

Therapeutic Management

The majority of boys with gynecomastia receive no treatment. In certain severe cases, plastic surgery is recommended. Research is currently being conducted on hormonal treatment of gynecomastia. Because obese boys tend to have a more noticeable problem, they are counseled to lose weight. In patients with associated disorders, the disorders are treated.

Strategies for Nursing Care

Parents are often shocked to see that their newborn has enlarged breasts. The nurse can alleviate fears by discussing the effect of maternal hormones on the fetus and by assuring them that the gynecomastia is transient. Gynecomastia can lead to varying degrees of psychological difficulties for adolescent boys. Patients may wonder if they are transforming into females, and the boys may be too embarrassed to remove their shirts during physical education class, during sports, or while playing with friends. The body image alterations can affect social interactions with peers, especially girls, during a time when interacting is already difficult.

The nurse can offer emotional support to the child by listening to his concerns. Certain clients may benefit from professional counseling. If the diagnostic studies indicate that the patient has transient pubertal gynecomastia, the nurse can reassure him that the problem is temporary. If the patient is referred for surgery, he must be aware that there will be scarring from the procedure.

Other Endocrine Disorders

Hypoglycemia

Hypoglycemia is not a disease; it describes a condition in which blood glucose level falls below the acceptable range for the patient's size and age. In the neonate hypoglycemia is defined as two blood glucose values less than 30 mg/dl in full-term infants, or less than 20 mg/dl in infants who are premature or small for gestational age. After the newborn period, hypoglycemia is diagnosed for blood glucose levels below 40 mg/dl (Sperling, 1987).

Hypoglycemia is not uncommon in newborn infants. It affects 4 in 1000 live-born full-term infants and 16 in 1000 premature infants (Schwartz, 1987). After the neonatal period, however, hypoglycemia is relatively rare.

Etiology

Approximately 50 per cent of neonates with hypoglycemia have an asymptomatic transitional form. The low blood sugars tend to occur during the first 6 to 12 hours of life, often in association with perinatal distress, delayed feedings, or diabetes in the mother. Symptomatic, transient hypoglycemia is seen in infants who are small for gestational age, with males predominating in a ratio of 2.5 : 1. If symptoms persist or fail to clear completely after correction of hypoglycemia, a search is made for another underlying or associated abnormality. Such abnormalities include sepsis, hydrops fetalis, congenital heart disease, hypothyroidism, asphyxia, drugs given to the mother, or central nervous system defects or infections (Kaplan, 1982). Approximately 35 per cent of infants with neonatal hypoglycemia have other associated disease states. In rare cases (1 to 2 per cent of all newborns with hypoglycemia) in which symptoms persist or recur in spite of treatment, specific primary causes must be investigated. These causes include an excess production of insulin, hereditary defects of carbohydrate or amino acid metabolism, or pituitary hormone deficiencies.

In the first year of life, an excess production of insulin accounts for over 50 per cent of cases of hypoglycemia. The second most frequent cause is liver enzyme deficiencies, leading to an inability of the liver to transform glycogen into glucose. In the toddler and preschool age group, ketotic hypoglycemia is the most common form of hypoglycemia. The child usually experiences hypoglycemia in the early morning after a small supper and long sleep. The child may be small and underweight and may have an associated isolated or combined hormone deficiency. Another cause of persistent hypoglycemia in a child of any age is a pancreatic islet cell tumor. Causes of acute isolated episodes of hypoglycemia include inappropriate periods of fasting for age, alcohol ingestion, oral hypoglycemic agent ingestion, and severe illness such as Reye syndrome.

Clinical Manifestations

The symptoms of hypoglycemia in the infant range from localized or generalized seizures to simple irritability. Episodes of cyanosis, limpness, apnea, or irregular respirations are common, and difficulty in feeding and abnormal cry and apathy have been described. The older infant and young child may experience a headache, nausea, anxiety, hunger, pallor, staring, listlessness or irritability, motor incoordination, ataxia, inattention, coma, or convulsions.

Therapeutic Management

Neonates with asymptomatic or symptomatic transient hypoglycemia are treated with an intravenous infusion of glucose until the blood glucose values are restored to normal. If symptoms persist or fail to clear completely after correction of hypoglycemia, a search is made for an associated abnormality. Treatment of the underlying disorder usually alleviates the hypoglycemia.

Major Nursing Diagnoses for Hypoglycemia

Potential for injury: neurologic, related to insufficient serum glucose to meet cerebral metabolic needs
Knowledge deficit: parents, related to
- *etiology and pathophysiology*
- *technique for performing Chemstrip testing at home*
- *treatment of hypoglycemic reactions with carbohydrate foods, intramuscular glucagon, or buccal glucose preparations*
- *need to avoid products containing alcohol*

Strategies for Nursing Care

Assisting with Detection

Because half of the neonates with hypoglycemia are asymptomatic, the nurse must accurately perform Dextrostix or Chemstrip testing on each newborn to detect the problem. Technique is crucial to the accuracy of the readings, and low readings should be verified by laboratory analysis. Bilirubin in plasma and isopropyl alcohol applied to the skin may significantly reduce the apparent glucose value obtained with Dextrostix (Fox and Redstone, 1976; Grazaitis and Sexson, 1980). If a full-term infant has a blood glucose level below 30 mg/dl, a physician is notified and an intravenous line is started immediately for glucose administration. The infant is assessed closely for symptoms and blood glucose levels are evaluated for response to treatment. If the infant is unresponsive to treatment, the nurse assists in coordinating studies to detect associated abnormalities.

Providing Information to Support Home Care

The nurse caring for the toddler and young child must be knowledgeable about the symptoms of hypoglycemia in order to discuss them with parents. A history of repeated clusters of hypoglycemic symptoms should be clarified for frequency, usual time of day of onset of symptoms, association with eating patterns, and severity. Obtaining a blood glucose level at the time of symptoms is critical, and parents can be taught to accurately perform Chemstrip testing at home. Urine testing for ketones may also be indicated in toddlers and preschool-age children suspected of having ketotic hypoglycemia. Parents should be instructed on the use of the Acetest or Chemstrip UK test for urinary ketones. If hypoglycemia is documented, the parents are instructed to feed the child immediately to prevent worsening of symptoms. A glass of milk or orange juice is often readily available and effective. If the child becomes disoriented or comatose, the parents should be instructed on the use of intramuscular glucagon as a means of increasing the blood glucose level. Monogel and Glutose (glucose gels) also increase blood glucose levels and can be used by squeezing them between the cheek and gum of the mouth. The buccal mucosal capillaries absorb the glucose into the bloodstream.

Parents should be instructed at well child visits that alcohol ingestion in toddlers and young children can lead to hypoglycemia. Commercially available mouthwashes contain ethanol, with concentrations ranging from 14 per cent in Cepacol to 26.9 per cent in Listerine. Listerine may be potentially lethal if 5.7 ounces are consumed by a 12 kg, 2-year-old child (Weller-Fahy et al, 1980). Alcoholic drinks should be discarded after parties in households with young children, and "tasting" of alcoholic beverages by youngsters should not be permitted. As with any other medications, oral hypoglycemic agents, often found in grandparents' homes, should be placed where children cannot reach them.

Nursing Strategies for Follow-up Care in the Home or Clinic

Obtain blood glucose measurement.

Determine frequency of hypoglycemic episodes, exact signs and symptoms, and response to treatment.

Encourage expression of feelings and concerns and determine family adaptation to the condition.

The Pancreas

Normal Function of the Pancreas

The pancreas is situated behind the stomach in a horizontal position with its head firmly attached to the duodenum by the pancreatic duct (duct of Wirsung) and its tail reaching to the spleen. The pancreas is made up of two distinct types of tissues: (1) the acini, which excrete digestive juices through ducts into the duodenum, and (2) the islets of Langerhans, which secrete insulin (from the beta cells) and glucagon (from the alpha cells) directly into the bloodstream. The pancreas, therefore, is both an exocrine (duct-type) and an endocrine (ductless) gland.

Pancreatic juice, excreted through the pancreatic ducts into the duodenum, is important to the digestion of carbohydrates, fats, and proteins. The hormones insulin and glucagon play an important role in carbohydrate metabolism.

Diabetes Mellitus

Diabetes mellitus (DM) is the most common endocrine disease of childhood. Although DM has been diagnosed for centuries, the causes, prevention, and cure still remain obscure. The word "diabetes" originates from the Greek language and means *siphon* or *flow through,* relating to the increased loss of body fluids with increased urination. The word "mellitus" means *sugary* or *honey-like* in Latin and differentiates DM ("sugar diabetes") from diabetes insipidus ("bland diabetes"). The latter is a disease of the posterior pituitary gland.

Incidence

Owing to several difficulties in obtaining exact statistics, published estimates of both the prevalence and incidence of DM vary. In the United States the incidence is approximately 16 newly diagnosed cases of type I (insulin-dependent) per 100,000 population yearly in children younger than 19 years of age. Although the incidence may be as high as 30 per 100,000 in some parts of Scandinavia, prevalence and incidence of insulin-dependent diabetes in Great Britain, Sweden, and Australia are similar to those reported in the United States (Sperling, 1987).

In the United States the incidence for blacks is only about 66 per cent of the incidence for whites (Sperling, 1987). The incidence of insulin-dependent DM is the same across a population of boys and girls, but the incidence increases with increasing age (i.e., a child is more likely to be diagnosed as having DM at 16 years of age than at 5 years). Type I DM is most common in the 10- to 14-year-old age group.

According to the National Diabetic Commission Report, in 1980 there were 10 to 12 million people with diabetes in the United States: between 5 and 6 million diagnosed diabetics (approximately 2.5 per cent of the population), and about the same number of undiagnosed cases. The National Diabetes Commission (1980) and Harris (1980) estimate that the prevalence of the disease is increasing at approximately 3 to 6 per cent per year, indicating that *diabetes is one of the most prevalent serious chronic illnesses in today's society.*

Nurses most often encounter children with diabetes in the hospital or clinic during the diagnostic phase or in the clinic or home for follow-up care. The emphasis, in these instances, is on providing information and support for self-care management. Acute care nurses also encounter children hospitalized for diabetic ketoacidosis and for other complications of diabetes mellitus. If hospitalization is related to complications of diabetes, the emphasis is on quickly reestablishing metabolic control and on teaching to prevent recurrence. In all cases, the nurse's command of information regarding normal versus abnormal pancreatic function and glucose metabolism will provide the basis for effective nursing care.

DM is not a single disease entity but rather a syndrome or group of diseases differing etiologically but having many common clinical signs and symptoms. Because a variety of ambiguous definitions and inconsistent terminology have been used in the past, the National Institutes of Health (1979) appointed an international committee (National Diabetes Data Group, 1979) to develop a classification system and universal terminology. The various types of diabetes were divided into (1) diabetes mellitus, (2) gestational diabetes, and (3) states of altered carbohydrate metabolism. Table 49-12 further details the classification of diabetes mellitus types, subgroups, and previous terminology. Because most children develop type I DM, this chapter will concentrate primarily on that category.

Etiology

Diabetes mellitus results from either a relative (type II) or an absolute (type I) deficiency of pancreatic insulin. This results in chronic high blood sugar and other problems with carbohydrate and fat metabolism.

The causes of type I DM are not completely understood, but increasing research (over the past decade) has produced a much clearer understanding of how the beta cell in the pancreas is destroyed. Many investigators have thought that type I DM has a genetic component, but the mode of inheritance is still not well defined. There is some evidence that genetic predisposition is an important factor to consider, but the disease is generally not considered to be inherited.

Some epidemiologic studies and animal experiments indicate that environmental factors may play a role in the cause. Notkins (1979) suggests that viral infection may be a significant antecedent, on the basis of the following findings: (1) increased levels of coxsackie B_4 virus in newly diagnosed children; (2) increased seasonal diagnosis in the winter months; and (3) onset of DM after mumps infections. The viral theorists suggest that certain genetic factors (HLA configurations [see Chapter 43]) can make an individual more susceptible to viral infections. However, confirmation of the role viruses play in human diabetes is still uncertain. Still other investigators (Nemchik, 1982) suggest that a genetic predisposition and HLA-directed response to viral infections lead to beta cell destruction and consequently to the development of type I diabetes in children.

It is now fairly well accepted that the autoimmune response is involved in some way in beta cell destruction. Research has revealed the presence of minor abnormalities in the islet cells of the pancreas, resulting

Table 49-12. Classification, Types, and Previous Terminology of Diabetes Mellitus

Classification	Types and Subgroups	Previous Terminology
Diabetes mellitus	Type I: Insulin-dependent diabetes mellitus (IDDM)	Juvenile diabetes mellitus; ketosis-prone diabetes; unstable or brittle diabetes
	Type II: Non-insulin-dependent diabetes mellitus (NIDDM)	Adult diabetes mellitus; maturity onset diabetes mellitus
	Obese: Insulin requiring	
	Non-insulin requiring	
	Non-Obese: Insulin requiring	
	Non-insulin requiring	
	Other types:	Secondary diabetes
	1. Pancreatic causes	
	2. Hormonal causes	
	3. Drug-induced causes	
	4. Receptor site abnormalities	
	5. Other syndromes	
Gestational diabetes		Class A diabetics
Asymptomatic state of carbohydrate intolerance	Impaired glucose tolerance Previously impaired glucose tolerance Potential abnormality of glucose tolerance	Asymptomatic diabetes; chemical diabetes; borderline diabetes; latent diabetes

(Adapted from National Diabetes Data Group, 1979.)

in islet cell antibodies (ICAs), which are present in about 70 per cent of newly diagnosed diabetics (Lendrum et al, 1975). Islet cell antibodies are sometimes present in relatives of people with type I diabetes, making ICA a possible indicator of an individual's potential to develop DM. Other factors, including diabetogenic drugs, gross pancreatic disease (in chronic illnesses such as cystic fibrosis), and obesity can also cause diabetes.

Pathophysiology

Glucose is the primary source of energy for all body cells, with the brain cells utilizing approximately 25 per cent of the total body supply. Small amounts of glucose can be stored as triglycerides in fat tissues and as glycogen in muscle or liver cells. However, *because glucose can only be stored in small amounts, the blood glucose level must be maintained at least at a minimum fasting level (approximately 60 to 110 mg/dl or 3.3 to 6.2 mmol/liter) sufficient to meet central nervous system demands.*

Insulin is a hormone secreted by the beta cells of the pancreas. *The primary function of insulin is to regulate blood glucose levels by controlling the rate at which blood glucose is taken up by the body cells.* Insulin is often referred to as the "key" that opens the door to the various body cells. Insulin is also necessary for the maintenance of the enzyme mechanism required for the utilization of glucose within the cell.

In addition to manufacturing and storing insulin, the beta cells of the pancreas act as a sensor to determine blood glucose levels. When the levels of carbohydrates in the blood increase, the beta cells are stimulated to release a small amount of insulin, thus acting as a feedback mechanism. Pancreatic insulin is secreted into the portal circulation, where it is carried to the liver and then distributed by peripheral circulation to the body cells.

Insulin has various functions in different body cells. In fat cells, insulin promotes the uptake of glucose and the storage of triglycerides. In muscle cells, insulin increases the transport of glucose and amino acids into the cell. In liver cells, insulin enhances conversion of glucose into glycogen and also inhibits the release of glucose from the liver. As well, insulin enhances protein synthesis. Insulin is excreted by the kidney in the urine.

Inadequate secretion of insulin results in (1) decreased glucose transport from the bloodstream into the cells, thus leading to high blood glucose levels; (2) metabolism of triglycerides into free fatty acids, which are converted into ketoacids by the liver and are used for energy during the shortage of glucose; and (3) glucagon secretion leading to production of glucose from liver stores of glycogen (glycogenolysis) and from amino acids (gluconeogenesis), further raising blood sugar levels. As glucose levels reach 180 mg/dl (approximately 10 mmol/liter) of blood, the renal tubules are unable to reabsorb the glucose (renal threshold), and glucose spills into the urine (glucosuria). The excreted glucose acts as an osmotic diuretic, causing the loss of large amounts of water, sodium, potassium, and bicarbonate salts.

Clinical Manifestations

Clinically, the diabetic patient is left dehydrated and thirsty *(polydipsia)*. In attempts to quench this thirst, the individual consumes large quantities of fluid, which leads to increased urination *(polyuria)*. In addition, the patient may also feel hungry and eat large amounts *(polyphagia)* in response to the body's hunger for glucose, and he or she may be fatigued owing to decreased energy production. These symptoms—polydipsia, polyuria, polyphagia, and fatigue—are known as the "classic" symptoms of diabetes mellitus, although not all patients will develop all of these clinical manifestations. Weight loss, attributable either to dehydration or to the mobilization of fat stores and liberation of triglycerides, may also be present in some individuals. Byproducts of triglyceride breakdown are free fatty acids, which are then converted to ketones by the liver.

The ketone bodies are made up of acetoacetic acid, β-hydroxybutyric acid, and acetone. If high blood sugar levels persist (indicating inadequate glucose transport), the production of ketones for energy rapidly increases. Although small amounts of ketones can be removed from the body by the kidneys, large amounts cannot. As keto acids accumulate, *ketoacidosis* develops.

Excretion of keto acids by the kidneys is the second important mechanism in the development of ketoacidosis. Bicarbonate is lost in the urine during the excretion of keto acids, thus further decreasing the serum pH. Ketoacidosis can pose a serious threat to the body's delicate balance and may lead to coma and possibly death if not treated.

However, treatment with insulin, water, and appropriate electrolyte replacement therapy reverses the catabolic state created by the insulin deficiency. The blood sugar levels will then decrease and the utilization of glycogen stored in fat and liver cells decreases. Ketones will no longer be produced, and pH and bicarbonate and electrolyte levels will return to normal.

Box 49-1
*Criteria for Diagnosing Diabetes Mellitus**

NORMAL GLUCOSE TOLERANCE:

- Fasting blood sugar (FBS) <115 mg/dl *and* . . .
- 2-hour postprandial <140 mg/dl *and* . . .
- No FBS or 2-hour postprandial value >200 mg/dl

IMPAIRED GLUCOSE TOLERANCE (after glucose load of 1.75 gm/kg body wt):

- FBS <140 mg/dl *and* . . .
- 2-hour postprandial >140 but <200 mg/dl *and* . . .
- At least one FBS value or 2-hour postprandial value >200 mg/dl

DIABETES MELLITUS:

- FBS >140 mg/dl on at least two occasions *or* . . .
- Random glucose ≥200 mg/dl with classic signs and symptoms of diabetes (polydipsia, ketonuria, polyuria, weight loss) *or* . . .
- FBS <140 mg/dl and 2-hour postprandial >200 mg/dl, with at least one value >200 mg/dl after a glucose load of 1.75 gm/kg

* Established by the National Diabetes Data Group of the National Institutes of Health.

(From Christman and Bennett, 1987; Travis et al, 1987.)

Diagnostic Assessment

The diagnosis of type I diabetes in children is not usually difficult. Box 49-1 lists detailed diagnostic criteria.

Therapeutic Management

Factors Influencing Treatment

A glucose tolerance test (GTT) is rarely required in the diagnosis of type I diabetes. Management of the illness at diagnosis will depend on several factors, which may include (1) severity of illness at diagnosis, and (2) management style, which encompasses such factors as (a) the experience and philosophy of health professionals and (b) financial constraints, such as health insurance coverage.

Severity of Illness. The severity of the child's condition on arrival in the doctor's office or the hospital emergency department will greatly influence the initial management. For DM, three types or stages of presentation are seen, with specific symptoms (or clinical manifestations) and management for each. The three stages of severity of illness include diabetic ketoacidosis (DKA), diabetic ketosis, and hyperglycemia. These stages, their clinical manifestations, and medical and nursing responsibilities are outlined in Table 49-13.

Management Style or Philosophy. Because there remain many unanswered questions about the cause, cure, and prevention of diabetes, many aspects of managing diabetic children and their families are arbitrary. Generally, there are two diverse schools of thought concerning initial management, with many compromises available. These two approaches include initial hospitalization management or initial outpatient management.

If the child is hospitalized at the time of diagnosis, the goals of hospitalization are usually geared to stabilizing the child's blood glucose level and insulin regulation, and reducing the child's and parents' anxiety. Education of the child and family may be (1) totally accomplished while the child is an inpatient, (2) started while the child is an inpatient and completed as an outpatient, or (3) performed totally on an outpa-

***Table* 49-13.** Symptoms, Medical Management, and Nursing Management of Newly Diagnosed Diabetic Patients

Clinical Manifestations	Therapeutic Management	Strategies for Nursing Care
Diabetic Ketoacidosis (DKA) (Acute Stage)		
Hyperglycemia, glycosuria, ketones Dehydration Electrolyte imbalance (serum potassium ↑ or ↓, total body potassium ↓, serum sodium ↓, BUN ↑, plasma bicarbonate ↓, serum pH ↓) Kussmaul respirations Abnormal laboratory values (↑ WBC, RBC and WBC, ↑ in urine) CNS depression → coma, vascular collapse and death	Treatment with frequent doses of regular insulin (IV, SC, or IM) (common dosage: 0.1 unit/kg stat; 0.1/kg/hour) Fluid and electrolyte therapy Careful monitoring of glucose levels in blood and urine, electrolyte and abnormal laboratory values Informing both the family and the child of what is happening	Careful observation of patient receiving IV insulin and child's reaction to insulin Accurate intake and output Constant observation of child's neurologic and vital signs Basic comfort measures of the child and family
Diabetic Ketosis		
Hyperglycemia Glycosuria Ketones (in both blood and urine) Possible dehydration	Treatment with regular insulin Careful assessment of serum glucose levels, glycosuria, and ketones Careful monitoring of electrolytes and fluids Information/education of the child and parents	Assessment of child's response to insulin, vital signs Careful monitoring of intake/output Begin to encourage self-care when appropriate
Hyperglycemia		
Polyurea, polydipsia, polyphagia, fatigue Glycosuria No ketones	Careful assessment of insulin requirements (may require the addition of or ↑ regular insulin) Careful assessment of serum glucose levels and glycosuria Encourage usual diet and activities Assess and plan education of the child and family	

tient basis. However, by far the most popular treatment of newly diagnosed diabetic children is initial hospital admission.

If the child is not in diabetic ketoacidosis (DKA) and possibly not hospitalized at the time of diagnosis, the tasks of metabolic stabilization, insulin regulation, and the education of the patient and family must all be completed on an outpatient basis. To be successful, this second method of management demands (1) responsibility, motivation, and proximity to the treatment center on the part of the child and family; and (2) adequate staffing and comfort in allowing families to be maximally involved in their child's care early in treatment on the part of the health team.

As well as differences in the location of the newly diagnosed child's initial management, there are two major options in the insulin-dependent diabetes mellitus therapy. These two options are conventional or intensive treatment (Kaye, 1984). Kaye describes conventional treatment as usually including one or possibly two injections of insulin per day. Blood glucose monitoring at least twice a day is now also considered a part of conventional treatment. Intensive treatment, as its name suggests, encompasses a more rigorous therapeutic regimen, including more frequent home blood glucose monitoring, insulin adjustment (on the basis of blood glucose level results), and two or more injections of insulin daily or continuous subcutaneous infusion of insulin using an insulin pump.

Whatever the management philosophy of the health care team, the goals of treatment for the child with type I diabetes and family usually are similar. These goals include (1) metabolic control of the child's diabetes, (2) self-care by the child or family through education about illness management, and (3) normal growth and development of the child and family.

Achieving Metabolic Control

Shortly after the discovery of insulin, an ongoing debate focused on whether complications of diabetes would be prevented if good metabolic control prevailed. Good metabolic control means that blood glucose levels in diabetics would be as close as possible, over time, to their nondiabetic counterparts. By keeping blood glucose levels close to normal, many occurrences of acute problems (i.e., hypoglycemic and hyperglycemic reactions) can be prevented. The importance of good metabolic control in relation to long-term complications has not been definitely established, but this topic is one of the most debated and important issues in diabetes management (Ingelfinger, 1977) and is the basis for large multicenter collaborative studies (Kroc Collaborative Study Group, 1984). Criteria for good metabolic control for the child vary, but usually include

1. a desirable pattern of urine or blood glucose results (i.e., few episodes of hypoglycemia or hyperglycemia).
2. evidence of normal growth and development.
3. infrequent occurrence of mild hypoglycemic reactions.
4. few (diabetes-associated) school absences.
5. generally feeling well with no related signs or symptoms.
6. ability to participate in social and recreational activities with peers.

Urine testing and blood glucose monitoring assist the child and family in managing diabetes on a day-to-day basis. Long-term metabolic control, however, is measured by the hemoglobin A_{1C} (HbA_1, HbA_{1C}, glycosylated hemoglobin) blood test, which is a powerful retrospective index of glucose control (Bunn, 1981). Hemoglobin A constitutes approximately 90 per cent hemoglobin in the erythrocyte, and hemoglobin A_{1C} is the most important of the minor components, accounting for 3 to 6 per cent of hemoglobin in nondiabetic persons. Hemoglobin, when manufactured in the bone marrow, has no glucose attached. As the red blood cells (RBCs) circulate throughout the body during their approximately 120-day life cycle, an interaction between glucose and the hemoglobin occurs. Because turnover of RBCs is constant, the percentage of the total RBC pool that has glucose attached to it will reflect the average level of blood glucose throughout the life span of the RBC or the average daily blood glucose level. In this way, the HbA_{1C} test can be viewed as an indication of the blood glucose level over time or as the degree of metabolic control in diabetes patients, although there is some variation in how these values are used. Box 49-2 correlates test values and degree of metabolic control.

HbA_{1C} values may vary with the time of day drawn, the temperature, and the method of analyzing the specimen; therefore, only changes of 10 to 25 per cent or more are clinically significant (Ehrlich, 1982). HbA_{1C} values are measured approximately every 2 to 3 months or on regular visits to the physician or clinic. These measurements are particularly useful in patients on tight control regimens, noncompliant patients, patients doing urine testing with unknown renal thresholds, or patients suspected of falsifying home blood glucose monitoring or urine test results. If the HbA_{1C} level is elevated and metabolic control is deemed poor, the results may need to be reviewed with the child and family, and the treatment program may need to be modified.

Box 49-2
HbA_{1C} Test Values and Metabolic Control

DEGREE OF CONTROL	APPROXIMATE HbA_{1C} VALUES
Excellent	<8.5
Good	8.5–9.5
Fair	9.5–10.5
Fair to poor	10.5–12
Poor	>12
Nondiabetic individual	5.2–8.3

Insulin Therapy. Insulin was discovered in Toronto, Canada, in 1921 by Banting and Best. Insulin is a hormone or protein substance that is produced by the beta cells of the pancreas in the normal healthy person. This pancreatic insulin is often referred to as endogenous insulin. When type I diabetes develops, children lose their ability to produce endogenous insulin. Because insulin is a hormone essential to life, another, or exogenous (manufactured outside the body), source must be found. The most common source of exogenous insulin used by humans is a mixture of insulin extracted from the pancreata of cows and pigs. More purified forms of pork insulin are also available. The newest type of insulin on the market is human insulin, which is not extracted from humans but is made in a laboratory from a specially programmed bacterial process called recombinant DNA technology (Lilly) or complete chemical biosynthesis (Connaught-Novo). Human insulin is reported to be chemically, physically, biologically, and immunologically equivalent to natural human insulin and is used when a highly purified form of insulin is indicated, such as in cases of insulin allergy, for intermittent use (i.e., metabolic testing, pregnancy, surgery, or acute illness), and with many newly diagnosed diabetics. The types of insulin are further described in Table 49-14.

Insulin is measured in units, whereby a unit provides a specific amount of pharmacologic activity per milliliter of liquid. For example, u-100 insulin has 100 units of insulin in 1 ml of liquid. A unit is always constant and is the same for all types of insulin. Insulin is available in various concentrations in the United States, including u-40, u-80, and u-100. The most commonly prescribed concentration is u-100, and this eventually will replace all other concentrations. In

Table 49-14. Types of Insulin

Type	Alternative Names	Appearance	Action Times: Onset	Peak	Duration	Comments
Short- or Rapid-Acting						
Regular (Lilly; Squibb-Novo)	Crystalline Unmodified Clear Rapid	Clear	0.5–1 hr	2–4 hr	4–6 hr	Short-acting insulin is generally used in combination with intermediate-acting insulins or during diabetic ketoacidosis or illness
Humulin R (Lilly)		Clear		1–3 hr	6–8 hr	
Semilente (Lilly; Squibb-Novo)	Demi-Dura Sub Tardum	Cloudy		5–10 hr	5–10 hr	
Intermediate-Acting						
Lente	Modified Isophane	Cloudy	1.5–2 hr	6–10 hr	16–24 hr*	* The effective phase of blood glucose lowering activity seems to pass at 16–18 hr in most persons (Travis et al, 1987)
NPH	Rapitard Retard	Cloudy				
Globin (Lilly; Squibb-Novo)	Protard	Clear			action is longer than rapid-acting but not as long as long-acting	
Humulin N (Lilly)		Cloudy	2 hr		18–24 hr*	
Long-Acting						
PZI	Depotinsulin Retard	Cloudy	4–8 hr	14–24 hr	36+ hr	This long-acting type of insulin is not usually used with children as its action is too long and variable
Ultralente	Extra-dura Extra-Tardum	Cloudy		18–24 hr		

Canada and several other countries, only the u-100 strength insulin is marketed.

Side Effects of Insulin. The most common side effect of insulin is hypoglycemia or lowering of the blood sugar level. Another side effect of insulin is the allergic response or sensitivity, which can occur either locally or systemically.

Local responses include lipodystrophies and sensitivity. Lipodystrophies can be divided into hypertrophy or atrophy of local tissue. Hypertrophy is characterized by thickening of tissue at the site of injection, whereas atrophy refers to the degeneration of subcutaneous fat, causing a hollow or depression. Both are usually caused by either too frequent or too superficial injection into one area and eventually result in poor insulin absorption. Lipoatrophy, in many cases, is thought to be due to a local reaction to the non-insulin substance in the insulin preparation. This reaction is not commonly seen now that purer forms of insulin are available on the market. In fact, by injecting pure pork or human insulin into the depressions, the hollows begin to fill in, thus resolving the problem.

Insulin sensitivity is often identified by burning, stinging, itching, or erythema at the injection site, whereas insulin resistance is characterized by a decreased body response to insulin, usually related to an antibody-mediated reaction. Systemic responses to insulin are extremely rare but may result in urticaria and possibly anaphylactic shock.

Oral Hypoglycemic Agents

Because most children with DM have type I diabetes, they will require insulin injections. However, certain medications in pill and capsule form known as hypoglycemic agents also lower the level of blood sugar. The oral hypoglycemic agents are used to control diabetes in some adult type II patients who produce some endogenous insulin and when diet control alone has been unsuccessful. There are two types of hypoglycemic preparations, including sulfonylureas and biguanides. Sulfonylureas (such as Orinase, Diabinese, Dymelor, Tolinase) primarily stimulate the beta cells of the pancreas to produce more insulin, although their complete mechanism is not clearly understood. Biguanides are thought to help the body cells utilize glucose better. However, various countries have removed many of these drugs from the market owing to increasing reports of lactic acidosis and deaths in patients taking them. The primary nursing role with regard to these pharmaceutical agents is to understand which medication is prescribed, determine the patient's compliance with the medical regimen, and monitor the patient's physiologic and psychologic response to the medication.

Diet

The diabetic diet was one of the earliest forms of diabetes management. However, because this involved starvation regimens and carbohydrate-free diets, adequate nutrition was not possible. With the discovery of insulin in 1921, patients were provided with the opportunity for a nutritionally balanced diet and a prolonged life. In 1950, the Exchange System for meal planning was developed, and although some countries now use a modified version (Choice System), this system is still the most common diabetic teaching tool utilized today.

Young people with diabetes have the same nutritional needs as their nondiabetic counterparts. With diabetes, however, food intake must be balanced with activity and prescribed insulin. Balancing food, insulin, and activity essentially means coordinating nutrition in measured amounts at regular and evenly spaced intervals with the quantity and quality of physical activities and the action patterns of prescribed insulin.

The goals of diet management in children include (1) promotion of normal growth and development; (2) keeping plasma glucose as close to normal as possible in an attempt to prevent both hypoglycemia and hyperglycemia and long-term complications; and (3) improvement or maintenance of the overall health of the patient (American Diabetes Association and American Dietetic Association, 1977). However, health professionals need to remember that one diet prescription cannot meet the needs of everyone, and an individual has the right to an individually designed dietary program which considers both physiologic and psychologic needs. With children, this individual tailoring is especially challenging, as the diet is effective only if it is followed.

Families of children with diabetes need individual dietary counseling that takes into consideration the child's age, level of development, level of activity, likes, dislikes, family eating habits, and numerous other factors. As well, children's diets need to be constantly assessed and changed to keep pace with their physical growth. Parents often find the diet a chronic source of family discontent with problems ranging from the "picky" toddler who refuses to eat anything, to the school-age child who likes sharing and trading his food, to the undisciplined teenager who throws planned diets to the wind in favor of convenience-oriented dietary habits of peers. Parents and their diabetic children need the support, knowledge, and understanding of health professionals and possibly others facing similar dilemmas who realize that lifestyle changes such as diet are extremely difficult and a constant reminder that their child is not "just like any other child."

Good nutrition means sufficient amounts of essential nutritional elements are taken in to meet the needs of the individual at various stages of growth and development. This precise formula often means diets specified in calories or kilojoules (approximately 4.2 kJ = 1 calorie), as all foods give energy values in different amounts. The major components of foods, their energy value, and approximate percentage of the total diabetic diet (because recommendations vary) are presented in Table 49-15.

Exercise

Although exercise has long been recognized as a way to lower insulin requirements in persons with insulin-dependent diabetes mellitus, the recent heightened interest in exercise in general has prompted additional study of the effects of exercise on glucose metabolism for both diabetic and nondiabetic persons. In order to understand the effects of exercise for the child with diabetes, it is important to first review the effects of insulin on normal glucose metabolism.

The Effects of Insulin on Normal Glucose Metabolism. One of the most important functions of insulin is to maintain normal blood levels of glucose. After a meal or sweet snack, when the blood glucose level is high, insulin is the catalyst that causes most of the glucose to be stored in the liver in the form of glycogen. Glycogen is also stored in resting muscle cells. When the circulating blood glucose levels begin to fall between meals, the pancreas decreases its secretion of insulin. As insulin levels decrease, glycogen stored in the liver is converted back into glucose and released into the bloodstream (Guyton, 1987).

The Effects of Exercise on Normal Glucose Metabolism. One of the most significant effects of exercise on normal glucose metabolism is the inhibition of insulin secretion. Decreased insulin levels lead to release of liver glycogen stores. As the glycogen breaks down into glucose molecules it provides energy for the exercising muscles. The body's additional demands for energy are met by *gluconeogenesis* (the pro-

Table 49-15. Components of the Diabetic Diet

Component	Energy Value (calories/gram)	Percentage of Total Diet (Approximate)	Important Teaching for Diabetic Patients
Carbohydrate	4	45*	Comprises sugars and starches. Most should be complex (including breads, pastas, and grains). Restrict use of complex sugars such as jams, honey. Simple sugars, such as those in fruit and milk, need to be included for the growth and development of children More quickly digested simple sugars cause greater and faster increases in blood sugar (i.e., it is preferable to eat fruits in their solid form rather than drink fruit juices)
Protein	4	20 (at least 2 gm/kg)	Must be appropriate for growth needs, nutritional status, and body weight. Attempt to use foods low in fat (e.g., fish, poultry, 2% or skim milk)
Fat	9	30 or less	Should attempt to decrease amounts of food containing visible fats. Attempt to balance between polyunsaturated and saturated fats Foods high in cholesterol need to be restricted (e.g., cheese, egg yolks, cream, and butter)
Alcohol	7		

* Some centers are urging an even higher percentage of carbohydrate (e.g., 50 to 55%)
(Adapted from Skyler, 1983; Travis et al, 1987.)

duction of glucose from proteins and fats). The muscles are able to use the available glucose even though, in the resting state, muscle cells require insulin to transport glucose into the cells. Exercising muscle fibers, for reasons not understood, become highly permeable to glucose even in the absence of insulin (Guyton, 1987).

The Effects of Exercise on Glucose Metabolism in Diabetes Mellitus. There is only one difference in the effects of exercise upon the diabetic individual as compared to the nondiabetic person: *Insulin secretion in persons with type I diabetes is not decreased in response to exercise.* Although the same neurologic and chemical responses that decrease insulin in the exercising nondiabetic subject occur in the exercising diabetic person, they have no effect upon the circulating insulin level because the insulin is (usually) being delivered into the bloodstream from a subcutaneous depot (the last injection) rather than from the pancreas. In fact, exercise, because it increases blood flow, may actually increase the release of insulin from subcutaneous tissues.

When insulin levels remain constant or increase with exercise, the circulating insulin does not allow release of liver glycogen stores to meet metabolic demands for glucose. Therefore, in the diabetic patient, exercise may lead to low plasma levels of glucose and result in *hypoglycemia* (Travis et al, 1987).

Exercise for the child with diabetes, therefore, requires some planning in order to avoid the possibility of hypoglycemia during or following activity.

Severe hypoglycemia can usually be prevented if (1) someone close to the diabetic child (a parent, coach, or team mate) knows how to recognize the hypoglycemic symptoms and provide appropriate treatment, (2) the child eats more food before, during, or possibly after the exercise, or (3) less insulin is taken. The extra food should be carbohydrates (e.g., fruit, bread) or milk and will vary with the length and intensity of the exercise. For children whose exercise is not planned, carrying additional food is a good preventive step; it can be used if and when the need arises. Nurses can also suggest to their patients that performing blood glucose tests might be useful before and after exercise to measure the success of either food or insulin adjustments.

Hypoglycemia may also occur if the uptake of insulin is accelerated by exercise of the limb into which the insulin was injected. When strenuous physical activity can be predicted (e.g., if the child will be participating in a ball game or track meet), the anterior abdominal site can be used, thus eliminating the effects of exercise upon absorption (Gellis and Kagan, 1986).

The opposite problem, ***hyperglycemia*** (increased blood sugar), may also occur during exercise. Sometimes, if the blood sugar level is very high to begin with (>400 mg/dl or >22 mmol/liter) and particularly if ketones are also present, exercise will not have a blood sugar–lowering effect and may in fact increase blood glucose level and ketone production through the processes of gluconeogenesis and hepatic glucose output. This phenomenon is called the Somogyi reflex (Somogyi, 1959). The Somogyi reflex, or rebound hyperglycemia, is simply the body's compensatory action for impaired glucose transport (e.g., insufficient insulin). Its occurrence during exercise is in response to the body's increased need for glucose for energy. Therefore, strenuous exercise should be discouraged until control of blood sugar level has been achieved.

Urine and Blood Glucose Monitoring

Successful management of diabetes appears to be facilitated when patients and their families play an active role in treatment. By monitoring the patient's blood glucose levels through either urine testing or home blood glucose monitoring, the patient can more easily see the effectiveness of treatment and can experience a sense of control.

Urine Testing. Urine testing was the initial method used by patients to monitor their blood glucose level. Essentially, urine testing assesses the percentage of glucose within the volume of urine voided. The patient is usually asked to void twice; however, the value of the two specimens is disputed in the literature. The first voided specimen is most often discarded, as it only indicates the amount of glucose lost in the urine since the previous void. The second voided specimen is used as an indirect assessment of the serum glucose level and reflects the presence of glycosuria during a specific time period. Methods of urine testing and their advantages and disadvantages are summarized in Table 49-16.

Urine testing is often viewed as advantageous because it is inexpensive, noninvasive, and painless. However, there are also many limiting factors in testing urine for glucose, including the following:

1. Renal threshold is variable. The renal threshold is the level that blood glucose must reach before it spills into the urine. This level is usually 180 mg/dl (or 10 mmol/liter). However, this level varies from person to person. Some individuals have a very high renal threshold, whereas others have a low spillover point, making urine tests misleading and uninformative.
2. There is a lag time between blood sugar rise and spilling of the blood glucose into the urine, which ranges from 20 minutes to 2 hours (Burns, 1983).
3. There is often a social stigma attached to handling urine (especially during the teenage years).
4. Urine tests usually do not diagnose blood levels below 180 mg/dl.
5. Urine testing may be inconvenient and frustrating for the patient and the family (particularly in families with very young children). Also, research reveals that urine tests are often performed with less than 50 per cent accuracy (Malone et al, 1976).

Urine can be tested for the presence of ketones as well as glucose. Ketones are produced in the liver as a breakdown product of fat and can be used in the muscle and other tissues as a source of energy. If the body is ineffectively utilizing glucose, fat begins to break down and the byproducts begin to appear first in the blood and then in the urine. A patient should test for the presence of ketones if glucose levels are greater than 2 per cent, during illness (especially during periods of vomiting or diarrhea) or periods of emotional distress, and when insulin doses are adjusted. The presence of ketones can be assessed by using either a separate product for ketones (such as Acetest [Ames] tablets, Ketostix [Ames], or Chemstrip K [Boehringer-Mannheim]) or a combination product that tests for both glucose and ketones in one test (e.g., Ketodiastic [Ames] or Chemstrip GK [Boehringer-Mannheim]). The presence of ketones at any time should be reported to the physician because an excessive build-up leads to ketoacidosis, which can have widespread effects on the body, including diabetic coma and death if not treated.

Blood Testing. Another method of assessing glucose levels is by direct blood glucose measurement (BGM). A variety of methods for home blood glucose monitoring are available on the market. All methods require a drop of blood to be placed on an enzyme-impregnated strip for a specified period of time. When the test is completed, the results may be read either visually or with the use of a reflectance meter. Both methods have become more popular with the increased emphasis on metabolic control and an awareness of the suspected need to attain prolonged normalization of blood sugar level over time.

BGM can be performed by the patient or a family member at home. An adequate sample of capillary blood is obtained using either a simple lancet or a spring-driven lancet (such as Autolet, Autoclix, Hemalit, Monojector) from either the fingertips, earlobes, or toes. The patient can then employ one of the following methods: (1) visual interpretation (utilizing strips with reagent pads which exhibit the glucose oxidase enzyme reactions, such as Dextrostix [Ames], Chemstrips bG [Boehringer-Mannheim], or Visidex [Ames], or (2) a reflectance meter (utilizing the principle of light reflection from a strip). The most common reflectance meters include the Glucometer (Ames), AccuCheck (Boehringer-Mannheim), and Glucoscan II (Lifescan). The market of reflectance meters is rapidly expanding and new, smaller, and more sophisticated products are becoming increasingly available.

Advantages of blood glucose monitoring include the following: (1) the patient can achieve better day-to-day metabolic control through an increased understanding of the pattern of glucose fluctuations; (2) the patient can more accurately diagnose hypoglycemia and hyperglycemia; (3) the results of BGM are immediate and specific, which may lead to increased motivation for the prescribed medical regimen; and (4) the patient's self-confidence, self-esteem, and emotional stability may increase with added responsibility and control over his or her life. BGM is also more expensive, is invasive, and requires more initial commitment on the part of the patient. As well, BGM requires more

Table 49-16. Methods of Urine Testing

Product	Description	Advantages	Disadvantages
Clinitest (Ames)	Copper reduction list 2 drop method (2 drops of urine in 10 drops of water) Offers results from 0–5%	Range of results Less crucial timing Short time sequence Visual chemical reaction	Not glucose-specific Inconvenient
Diastix (Ames)	Glucose oxidase test Dipstick method Offers results from 0–2%	Glucose-specific Convenient Simple	Requires more crucial timing
Chemstrip uG (Boehringer-Mannheim)	Glucose oxidase method Dipstick method Results from 0–5%	Convenient Simple Glucose-specific	Requires longer timing (i.e., 2 minutes)
Tes-tape (Lilly)	Glucose oxidase method Roll of tape in plastic dispenser Dip tape in urine	Convenient Simple Glucose-specific	Requires longer timing (i.e., 2 minutes)

initial teaching, follow-up, and skill on the part of the educator. However, in spite of these apparent disadvantages, research has generally shown that patients who have tried BGM have little technical difficulty in either obtaining blood specimens or analyzing results and prefer this method over urine testing (Miller et al, 1983; Daneman et al, 1985). BGM is especially useful during illness, when the patient is unsure of reactions, for children with threshold problems, for infants who cannot void on demand, for adolescents who have difficulty handling urine, for insulin pump users, and for patients who cannot or *will* not do urine testing (e.g., an uncooperative teenager).

Because of the complexity of nursing diagnoses and strategies for nursing care for insulin-dependent diabetes mellitus, this material will be grouped according to diagnoses and strategies related to (1) metabolic control (2) psychosocial impact, and (3) self-care management.

Major Nursing Diagnoses Related to Metabolic Control

***Altered nutrition: less than body requirements,** related to impaired glucose transport associated with insulin insufficiency*

***Potential for injury,** related to the following complications:*

- hypoglycemia *associated with:*
  - *a. bursts of physical activity without additional food intake*
  - *b. irregular or missed meal times*
  - *c. failure to consume adequate calories to balance prescribed insulin dosage*
  - *d. error in insulin administration: more than the prescribed dose*
- hyperglycemia *associated with relative insulin deficiency, in comparison to body demands for glucose transport elevated by:*
  - *a. infection (which increases metabolism)*
  - *b. physical or mental stress (causing increased glucagon and catecholamine secretion)*
  - *c. exercise (in a client whose blood sugar and ketone levels are already elevated)*
  - *d. insulin excess (resulting in the Somogyi effect or rebound hyperglycemia) (Dickerman and Lucey, 1985)*

***Potential for altered tissue perfusion: systemic,** related to atherosclerotic changes in blood vessels associated with deposition of lipids on the intima of vessels during mobilization of fatty acids in insulin deficiency*

***Altered comfort: paresthesias,** related to peripheral neuropathy associated with:*

- *ischemic changes in nerve function*
- *metabolic alterations in nerve formation*

***Potential for infection,** related to*

- *depressed leukocyte function associated with hyperglycemia*
- *increased susceptibility associated with malnutrition and tissue catabolism*
- *enhancement of the "host medium" associated with readily available blood glucose for metabolism by the pathogen*

***Potential sensory-perceptual alteration: visual,** related to retinal vessel changes associated with insufficient availability of glucose*

***Potential altered patterns of urinary elimination,** related to*

- *infections of the urinary tract*
- *diabetic neuropathy*

Potential for injury: falls, related to
- *orthostatic hypotension associated with neuropathy of the autonomic nervous system*
- *muscular weakness associated with neuropathy in the lower extremities*

Colonic constipation, related to intestinal neuropathy
Potential altered sexual patterns: impotence, related to neurovascular changes

Strategies for Nursing Care Related to Metabolic Control

Strategies for nursing care related to metabolic control are clustered under the following nursing goals: (1) teaching safe administration of insulin, (2) teaching dietary management, (3) maintaining metabolic control during illness and surgery, and (4) decreasing the risk of complications.

Teaching Safe Administration of Insulin

Educating the patient and family in how to administer the insulin injection at the stressful time of diagnosis is difficult and a possible source of frustration. The nurse needs to allow time for the patient and family to overcome the shock of diagnosis but at the same time must encourage them to become involved in the self-care management that will allow them to manage the illness at home. All adult caregivers should be taught how to administer the insulin injection and, if the child is approximately 10 years old, it may be appropriate to teach him or her how to give the injection from the onset of therapy. Young children can be included in parts of the routine at an age-appropriate level.

In order to facilitate the patient and family's learning, the nurse must attempt to create a relaxed atmosphere where teaching can progress at a calm and unhurried pace. The nurse needs to be positive, to be self-confident, and to have adequate and current knowledge about diabetes, insulin, injection techniques, testing techniques, and working with children and families. The family can be reassured that, although the injection will be difficult at first, in time they will be able to incorporate it into their daily routine, although with some families this may take longer than with others.

To provide the families with as much support, supervision, and practice time as possible, teaching of the insulin injection should commence as early in patient teaching as possible. Because the first injection by the parent will be very anxiety-producing, the nurse could initially demonstrate by giving a saline (NaCl, 0.9 per cent) injection to a doll or to the parent, and then reciprocate by allowing the parent to give an injection to the nurse. The nurse should then assist the parents in giving the first injection to the child. If patients or parents are having extreme difficulty in the first session, the nurse may want to divide the teaching session into two parts. Once parents or patients have begun to give injections on their own they will still require frequent reassessment of their technique and ongoing support and encouragement. The nurse needs to always remember that being helpful does not mean being critical and that a calm, reassuring approach will help patients and parents to relax and improve their performance.

Teaching About Insulin

All children require insulin for growth, whether they are diabetic or not. When nondiabetic children experience a growth spurt, their pancreas is able to produce the extra insulin required by the body cells for energy and expansion. However, because diabetic children do not have this built-in control mechanism, they will require increases in both insulin dosage and caloric requirements about every 3 to 4 months to meet their growth needs. Parents who understand their diabetic child's needs during growth spurts can provide additional nutrition and adjust the insulin dose accordingly in order to prevent potential conflict between hunger and glucose control.

Because insulin is a protein and therefore, like all other proteins, it would be inactivated by the gastric juices it cannot be taken orally. Consequently, the usual route of administration is by subcutaneous injection, that is, into the loose space between the fat layer and the underlying muscle (Fig. 49-9). However, regular insulin can be administered either intramuscularly or intravenously in acute situations.

When teaching the patient and the parents how to administer insulin they should first be taught how to administer the type or types of insulin that have been prescribed for them at that particular time. Details concerning insulin adjustment and other insulin preparations can be dealt with at a later time. The patient, family, and nurse need to consider the type of syringe for use, the injection sites, and the actual injection technique. For all insulin administration, the patient needs to be reminded to always check the type of insulin and expiration date before beginning.

Either disposable (plastic) or reusable (glass) syringes may be used to administer insulin. However, only syringes designated especially for insulin administration should be used when giving insulin. There is virtually no dead space between the end of the plunger and the tip of the syringe in insulin syringes, whereas noninsulin syringes (especially glass) may trap air to the 10-unit gradation line. Also, insulin syringes must correspond with the various concentrations of insulin. Therefore for u-100 insulin, u-100 syringes must be

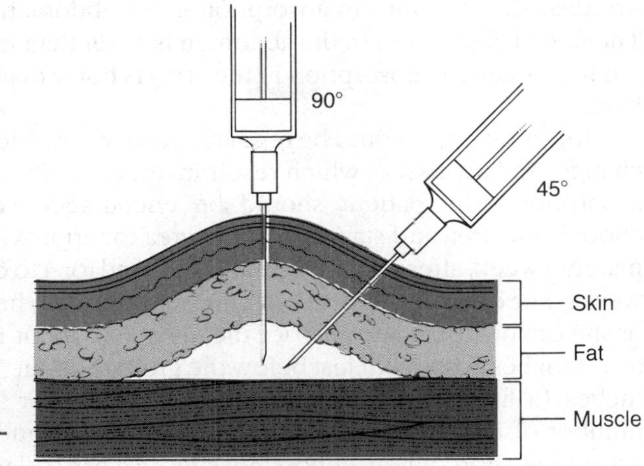

Figure 49-9. Subcutaneous injection of insulin.

used. A low-dosage syringe (0.5 ml), which measures up to 50 units of insulin, is commonly used for children to more accurately measure small dosages. The nurse needs to help the patient and family consider the cost, convenience, ease of reading, handling, and accuracy of measurement when choosing a syringe for daily use.

Because patients with type I diabetes will have a constant need for insulin, they may purchase several bottles at once, which need to be stored. Insulin should be stored in a cool place, avoiding either extreme heat (above 90° F) or freezing, as the protein potency can be altered by extreme temperatures. Insulin is stable for up to 1 year if unopened or up to 3 months opened if stored at room temperature or in the refrigerator. If insulin is stored in the refrigerator, warming it to room temperature before injecting is encouraged because injection of a cold substance is more painful. Patients should also be encouraged to have on hand at all times an extra bottle of both their prescribed insulin and regular short-acting insulin (in case of illness).

Teaching About Injection Sites and Administration Technique. The most common sites for injection of insulin include the outer medial aspect of the upper arms, the abdomen, the medial lateral aspects of the thighs, and the buttocks (Fig. 49-10). The patient should not use the inside of the thighs or the midline of the abdomen or back. When teaching patients how to choose an injection site, the following guidelines may be helpful. Encourage the patient to choose a site that (1) is not painful, (2) is readily accessible for the person giving the shot, (3) has equal absorption, (4) can be pinched up easily, and (5) is large enough to allow several adjacent injections so that the same site is not used too frequently. Insulin is absorbed at different rates in different areas of the body.

Figure 49-10. Injection sites for insulin.

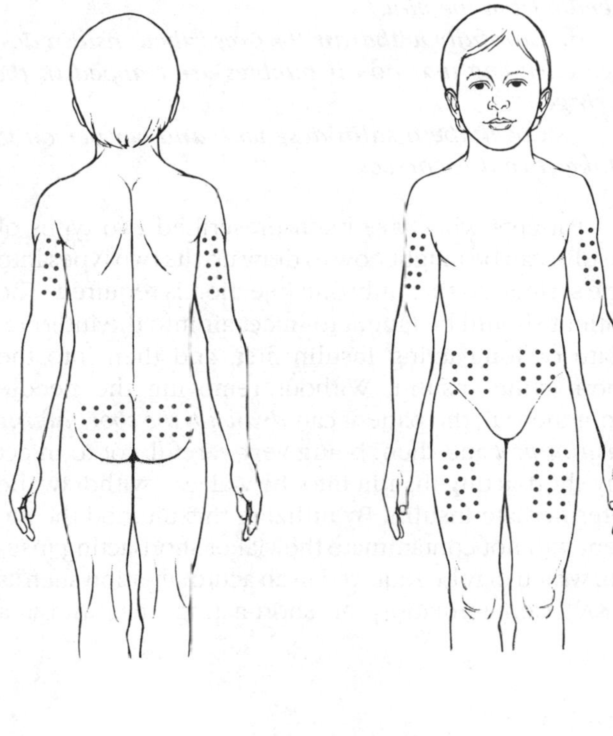

An ideal site for uniform absorption is the abdomen. The rate of absorption in the abdomen is faster than in the legs; likewise, absorption in the arms is faster than in the legs.

Injection sites should be regularly rotated to avoid changes in fatty tissue, which result in altered insulin absorption. The patient should be encouraged to choose one area and stay within that area for approximately a week, after which the area is not used for 4 to 6 weeks. For example, if a patient chooses the thigh, he or she can be instructed to space the injections about 1 to 1½ inches apart from just below the groin to about 3 inches (a fist) above the knee, thus providing for a number of injection sites depending on the age and size of the child. When all possible sites in a particular area have been used, the patient can move on to another site and not return to this area for several weeks. This organized method of site rotation prevents lipodystrophies (an abnormal deposition or metabolism of fat), which are associated with too frequent injections in the same spot.

If the patient is prescribed one type of insulin only, the following steps can be used by the nurse as a guideline when teaching patients and their families how to administer insulin.

1. *Wash hands.*
2. *Gently roll the insulin bottle between hands to thoroughly mix the medication. Do not shake as shaking leads to excess air bubbles in the vial.*
3. *Wipe off the top of the vial with an alcohol swab.*
4. *Draw up the amount of air in the syringe equal to the insulin dosage.*
5. *Inject the air into the insulin vial in order to equalize the pressure in the bottle. Do not remove the needle from the vial.*
6. *Carefully withdraw the prescribed insulin dosage ensuring that no air bubbles are trapped in the syringe.*
7. *Check the insulin dose with another person to make sure it is correct.*

Patients who have been prescribed two types of insulin can be taught how to draw up the two types into one syringe so that only one injection is required. The patient should be taught to inject air into the intermediate or long-acting insulin first, and then into the short-acting insulin. Without removing the needle from the vial, the patient can *draw up the short-acting insulin first* and then, being very careful not to inject any short-acting insulin into the vial, can withdraw the intermediate insulin. By utilizing this method the patient will not contaminate the vial of short-acting insulin, which may be required in an acute situation such as DKA. Contamination of short-acting insulin by a longer-acting variety changes the action of the short-acting insulin, resulting in a less rapid onset of action.

The important point for nurses to stress in patient teaching is that patients be consistent in their method of mixing insulins so that they will not become confused in stressful situations. The importance of checking the acccuracy of the insulin dosage with another

Box 49-3
Sample Portion of Fruit Exchange List

One exchange of fruit contains 10 grams of carbohydrate and 40 calories.

This list shows the kinds and amounts of fruits to use for one Fruit Exchange.

Apple	1 small
Apple Juice or Cider	⅓ cup
Applesauce (unsweetened)	½ cup
Apricots, fresh	2 medium
Apricots, dried	4 halves
Banana	½ small
Berries: Blackberries	½ cup
Blueberries	½ cup
Raspberries	½ cup
Strawberries	¾ cup
Cherries	10 large
Dates	2
Figs, fresh	1
Figs, dried	1
Grapefruit	½
Grapefruit Juice	½ cup
Grapes	12
Grape Juice	¼ cup
Mango	½ small
Melon: Cantaloupe	¼ small
Honeydew	⅛ medium
Watermelon	1 cup
Nectarine	1 small
Orange	1 small
Orange Juice	½ cup
Papaya (fruit)	¾ cup
Peach	1 medium
Pear	1 small
Persimmon, native	1 medium
Pineapple	½ cup
Pineapple Juice	⅓ cup
Plums	2 medium
Prunes	2 medium
Prune Juice	¼ cup
Raisins	2 tablespoons
Tangerine	1 medium
Cranberries	may be used as desired if no sugar is added

(Adapted from American Diabetes Association and American Dietetic Association, 1976.)

Table 49-17. Fiber Content of Foods per 100 Grams

Food	High Fiber (3 g)	Moderate Fiber (1.5 g)	Low Fiber (0.5 g)	Little Fiber (0.2 g)
Bread			Whole wheat bread and crackers	White, cracked wheat, rye, pumpernickel breads
Cereals	All-Bran (4.8 g/cup) Wheat germ (2.5 g/cup)	40% Bran flakes Puffed wheat Raisin bran	Barley, Cheerios, corn flakes, oatmeal, puffed rice, brown rice, Shredded Wheat, Wheaties	Rice Macaroni Noodles Spaghetti
Vegetables	Green peas (canned)	Green and wax beans, dried beans and peas, broccoli, brussel sprouts, cauliflower, mustard greens, green peas, okra, pepper, pumpkin, winter squash	Asparagus, beets, cabbage, carrots, celery, corn, cucumber, eggplant, lettuce, mushrooms, onions, sweet potatoes, white potatoes, tomatoes	
Fruits	Fresh blackberries (4.1 g/¾ C) Dried figs (5.6 g/C) Dried dates (2.3 g/½ C)	Apples, berries except blackberries, figs, pears with skins	Applesauce, apricots, bananas, fruit cocktail, cherries, grapefruit, grapes, mangos, melons, oranges, peaches, pears (without skin), pineapples, plums, prunes, raisins	Juices only

(From Travis et al, 1987)

responsible person should also be emphasized along with the serious effects of overdosing.

Teaching Dietary Management

There are two main approaches to dietary teaching, a strict dietary approach and the "free" dietary approach. As with the overall management of the illness, factors such as professional philosophies, severity of the illness, and financial considerations will influence which approach health professionals will recommend or prescribe. In the more conventionally *strict approach,* formal dietary education centers on "exchange" or "choice" lists. Exchange lists have been developed by the American Diabetes Association and the American Dietetic Association (1976) and consist of six food groups—milk, vegetable, fruit, bread, meat, and fat—which provide a framework for the quantity and quality of food the individual consumes.* Foods are listed in each group with the serving size that represents one exchange (see Box 49-3 for a sample portion of the fruit exchange list). The diet that is based on these exchange lists will specify the number of exchanges in each group that can be eaten at each meal. The patient and family thus have some control and choice in their daily selections. The major advantage of this approach is that it provides strict measurement guidelines for the patient on a recommended caloric intake while giving the patient some flexibility to vary the diet from day to day.

The *"free" approach* to diabetic eating was promoted by those who feared that calorically controlled diets were too restrictive, would foster emotional harm, and would not provide sufficient allowance for a child's growth and development (Heins, 1983). In this approach, specific types and amounts of food are not specified but rather guidelines delineating "do's and don't's" are taught. Parents will require an understanding of the dietary goals, types of food, and eating patterns (e.g., regular intervals and consistency) that will influence their child's dietary well-being. Therefore, dietary instruction is still an important part of the diabetic teaching.

Increasing *dietary fiber* may prove to be an additional method to maintain blood glucose levels. Postprandial blood glucose levels are decreased when the meal includes plant fiber, and it has been suggested that certain plant fibers may even decrease serum cholesterol levels (Gellis and Kagan, 1986). Fruits and vegetables, grains, and legumes are natural sources of plant fiber (Table 49-17).

Travis and colleagues (1987) described two potential problems with high-fiber diets for diabetes control. There is, first, some concern that a high-fiber

* Although the exchange lists have been widely adapted and used, recent research is beginning to demonstrate that there is wide variation in the glycemic response to foods containing identical amounts of carbohydrates (Crapo et al, 1980; Coulston et al, 1980). Jenkins and colleagues (1981), in response to these new findings, developed a glycemic index in order to compare the glycemic responses of different foods. As Skyler (1983) pointed out, most of the relevant research was conducted on nondiabetic subjects and therefore the effects of the research cannot readily be generalized to diabetic subjects. However, a nutritional system based on the *glycemic index* may be a reasonable alternative to the exchange system in the future.

diet may decrease the total caloric intake as foods high in fiber tend to be low in calories. Second, dietary fiber in large amounts may interfere with the absorption of calcium, iron, copper, magnesium, phosphorus, and zinc, as well as certain vitamins. The implications, then, for children on high-fiber diets are for *careful and consistent monitoring of growth and development* to ensure adequate nutritional intake.

An additional implication is the need to *monitor blood sugar levels* more frequently when a high-fiber diet is begun. Because high fiber intake may decrease the amount of insulin needed, the child must be watched for hypoglycemia.

Although consistency and good nutrition are essential to the diabetic child's diet, so are the social aspects, such as eating out, and special events, such as birthday parties, Halloween, and Christmas or other holidays. Eating out is more and more a part of daily living and should be an enjoyable occasion for the diabetic child and family as well. Familiarity with the child's meal plan at home and knowing how to make appropriate choices will facilitate good nutritional habits away from home. In restaurants parents can inquire about the ingredients in unfamiliar entrees and request that certain sauces and dressings be omitted. Guides which translate convenience foods into diabetic exchanges are also available from local diabetic societies. If meals are going to be delayed, the child can eat his or her usual bedtime snack at the regular dinner time and then eat dinner at the regular snack time. During special events, parents need to strike a balance between the rigidity of the diabetic diet and the social well-being of their child. The child should be allowed to have an occasional "treat" but the parents still need to be flexible, creative, well-informed, and supported to manage acceptable alternatives and compromises in many social situations. The child also will learn to understand that the family will not always participate in both the diet and the diabetic regimen. Informing others what the diabetic child can eat or offering to provide the "party dessert" on special occasions often eases the confusion and promotes peer acceptance of diabetic children and their diets.

Artificial Sweeteners. There are a large number of sugar substitutes on the market. These sweeteners can either be nutritive or non-nutritive. Nutritive sweeteners may be carbohydrates, such as lactose and fructose, or alcohols, such as sorbitol, mannitol, or xylitol. These substances contain a few calories but are not a significant problem as long as their use is limited. The newest nutritive sweetener on the market is aspartame (Nutrasweet), a protein substance with very high sweetening power. Therefore, only very small amounts of aspartame are required for sweetening, and the caloric content is insignificant. Despite some concern for potential side effects of aspartame, it has been found quite safe to date (Travis et al, 1987). Non-nutritive chemical sweeteners, including saccharin and cyclamates, have also been used but have been banned in various countries at one time or another owing to uncertainty of their long-term effects on health.

Many of these artificial sweeteners are utilized in dietetic foods. Foods such as candies, syrup, and soda pops are sweetened primarily with aspartame and therefore add little caloric value if used in reasonable amounts. Other dietetic products, however, although carbohydrate reduced, may contain calories from other sources, and their caloric content may be as high or higher than their nondietetic equivalents. Therefore, although dietetic foods may offer variety to the diabetic family, parents need to be cautioned to read their labels carefully to determine the ingredients. Except for water-packed fruits and artificially sweetened soda, few "dietetic" foods justify the expense over standard products.

The diabetic diet is a key element in the management of type I diabetes. The successful diet is one that is nutritious, acceptable, and adhered to by the child and family, and that maintains the balance with insulin and activity to produce near normal plasma glucose levels. Dietary teaching and support must be ongoing for the diabetic child and family. The nurse can play key roles in the initial assessment of the child's and family's nutritional practices, evaluating dietary management and working in collaboration with dietitians to continuously reinforce dietary programs.

Maintaining Metabolic Control During Illness and Surgery

Illness is cause for concern in the child with diabetes because *physical and emotional stressors can lead to hyperglycemia.* (Box 49-4 lists some of the more common stressors.) Infections are often the cause of hyperglycemia and ketosis in young children because of the high frequency of infectious disease in this age group (Travis et al, 1987). The mechanism for hyperglycemia and ketosis begins with the release of the stress hormones (catecholamines, glucagon, cortisol, and growth hormone, which were discussed earlier). The stress hormones activate catabolic enzymes, which mobilize carbohydrate and lipid stores, leading to increased blood levels of sugar and ketones. Hyperglycemia and ketonemia during illness or surgery are monitored by frequent blood or urine (or both) measurements for glucose and ketones, and controlled by adjustments in diet and insulin dosage as needed.

Monitoring for Elevated Glucose and Ketone Levels. Glucose and ketone levels should be measured in blood or urine (or both) every 4 hours during

Box 49-4
Stress Stimuli Producing Hyperglycemia

ILLNESS

A. Infectious
   1. Sepsis
   2. Meningitis
   3. Others
B. Noninfectious
   1. Myocardial infarction
   2. Cerebrovascular accidents

METABOLIC

A. Fasting
B. Hypoglycemia
C. Diabetic ketoacidosis
D. Hypoxia
E. Dehydration

TRAUMA

A. Usual trauma
B. Burns

SURGERY

NONSPECIFIC

A. Fever
B. Hypothermia
C. Pain

PSYCHOLOGIC OR EMOTIONAL

(From Travis et al, 1987.)

an acute illness or other stressful condition. If glucose levels are elevated and ketones are present, the parent(s) should consult the physician. If vomiting occurs, especially more than once, the child should be seen for a more thorough assessment of blood glucose level, electrolyte balance, and hydration.

Adjusting Diet and Insulin. During illness, the child with diabetes may have difficulty tolerating the normally prescribed diet. Adjustments will be needed if the child is nauseated, is vomiting, has diarrhea, or is undergoing surgery. Box 49-5 lists liquid and soft food equivalents for usual portions of fruit, starch, and milk. Another indication for these liquid exchanges may be when the child is febrile. Because fever increases basal metabolism, it increases the body's caloric needs. Calorie-containing liquids can help to maintain more normal blood sugar levels as well as decrease the danger of dehydration. Of course, any calorie-containing liquids must be added to the total calories consumed.

Over-the-counter medications (e.g., antipyretics, analgesics, and cough and cold remedies) may contain concentrated forms of sugar in their syrup formulations. Parents should consult the physician before administering any of these preparations to the child with diabetes.

The family must be alerted that ***the child must always take at least the usual dose of insulin during an illness.*** The ill child who develops hyperglycemia and ketosis will often need supplemental insulin. Typically, regular insulin will be prescribed (Travis et al, 1987). Parents who have become expert at home management of diabetes may be instructed to give the additional insulin at home in response to their detection of increased blood glucose levels. In other instances, the child may be admitted to the hospital until the illness is under control and metabolic balance has been reestablished.

Meeting Metabolic Needs in the Perioperative Period. Because of the unique metabolic needs during the preoperative, intraoperative, and postoperative phases, the child with diabetes who requires surgery will need precise monitoring for blood glucose levels and presence of ketones and for signs and symptoms of hypoglycemia and hyperglycemia. In the preoperative phase control of blood glucose level is a problem because the child must have nothing by mouth (NPO). Although withholding insulin will eliminate the risk of hypoglycemia during surgery, complete lack of insulin increases the chances of hyperglycemia. An insulin-dependent diabetic patient needs some exogenous insulin to prevent tissue catabolism (with resulting hyperglycemia). As noted by Robertson, "current research shows that a continuous insulin supply promotes glucose uptake and glycogenesis, while preventing excessive glucose output and glycogenolysis" (1986, p 30).

The child with diabetes is also at risk for hyperglycemia during the preoperative and immediate postoperative period because epinephrine and cortisol, secreted as a result of the neuroendocrine response to stress, stimulate glycogenolysis and gluconeogenesis. Hyperglycemia is to be avoided because it has been linked to many of the common complications of diabetes mellitus.

Robertson (1986) listed three common preoperative protocols prescribed by physicians for their insulin-dependent diabetic patients: (1) withhold the morning dose of rapid-acting insulin, but administer half the morning dose of intermediate-acting insulin; (2) administer long-acting insulin the night before surgery; (3) give no subcutaneous insulin, but instead administer insulin by intravenous drip. Whatever the prescribed protocol, the nurse must recognize the fine balance required in maintenance of blood glucose levels and monitor the perioperative patient closely for evidence of either hypo- or hyperglycemia.

Box 49-5
Liquid Exchange List, with Carbohydrate Content

FRUIT EXCHANGE: 1 FRUIT EXCHANGE = 10 GRAMS CHO*

8 oz or 1 C Gatorade = 1½ fruits + 130 mg sodium + 24 mg potassium
4 oz or ½ C orange juice or grapefruit juice = 1 fruit
⅓ C apple juice or pineapple juice = 1 fruit
2 oz or ¼ C grape juice or prune juice = 1 fruit
4 oz or ½ C Cran-Apple juice or nectars = 2 fruits
4 oz or ½ C Hi-C or Tang = 1½ fruits
1 C presweetened Kool-Aid, lemonade, or punch = 2½ fruits
1 C Sweet'nLow-flavored drink mix = 1 fruit
3 oz regular soft drink = 1 fruit
1 regular twin Popsicle = 2 fruits
2 tsp sugar = 1 fruit
2 regular hard candies = 1 fruit
5 Lifesavers = 1 fruit

STARCH EXCHANGE: 1 STARCH EXCHANGE = 15 GRAMS CHO*

½ C cooked cereal = 1 starch
½ C mashed potatoes = 1 starch
1 small baked potato = 1 starch
½ C regular Jello = 1 starch
1 C vegetable or cream soup = 1 starch
½ C vanilla ice cream = 1 starch
1½ C V-8 juice = 1 starch

MILK EXCHANGE: 1 MILK EXCHANGE = 12 GRAMS CHO*

8 oz or 1 C (½ pt) whole, skimmed, lowfat, or buttermilk = 1 milk
½ C evaporated milk = 1 milk
⅓ C condensed sweetened milk = 1 milk
8 oz milkshake = 1 milk, 1 starch
8 oz malt = 1 milk, 1 starch, 1 fruit
⅓ C ice milk = ½ milk, 1 fruit
½ C regular vanilla pudding = ½ milk, 2 fruits
½ C regular chocolate or butterscotch pudding = ½ milk, 3 fruits
½ C sugar-free custard mix = 1 milk

FREE FOODS: MAY BE EATEN AS DESIRED

Diet drinks	Broth
Unsweetened Kool-Aid	Sugar-free gelatin
Unsweetened lemonade	Unsweetened Popsicles
Unsweetened tea	Water
Unsweetened coffee	

* CHO = Carbohydrate.
(From Travis et al, 1987.)

Decreasing the Risk of Complications

Although diabetes can now be controlled and diabetic individuals can live a relatively normal life, they are still at risk of developing complications. These complications can be either acute or chronic. Acute complications are related to the day-to-day fluctuations in blood sugar, namely, hypoglycemia (low blood glucose levels) or hyperglycemia (high blood glucose levels). Chronic complications involve degenerative changes of both large and small blood vessels all over the body and are thought by many to be the result of poor metabolic control. The primary role of the nurse in both acute and chronic complications is to help the patient identify the symptoms of the various complications and facilitate understanding and treatment.

Acute Complications. Parents of newly diagnosed diabetic children can be extremely frightened and confused by an unexpected change in the health status of their child. These changes are most often related to fluctuations in serum blood glucose levels. When the blood glucose concentration drops below normal (hypoglycemia), the supply of glucose to the brain is reduced. The body attempts to correct this situation by the production of epinephrine and consequently the person may suddenly begin to feel (e.g., shaky, pale, sweaty, heart thumping) or behave (e.g., drunken-like, loss of consciousness, or convulsions) differently. When the blood glucose levels are elevated above normal, as at the time of diagnosis, the state is called hyperglycemia. The changes in how a person feels and behaves in hyperglycemia usually develop slowly as the blood sugar accumulates. Some people state that they feel quite normal even though their blood sugar is high.

Nurses need to ensure that young patients and their parents, teachers, and other caregivers know how to recognize and treat both hypoglycemia and hyperglycemia (Table 49-18). With this knowledge, those involved should be better prepared and more successful in dealing with either of these acute complications of diabetes.

Because each person may feel and react differently during either hypoglycemic or hyperglycemic reactions, it is important for parents to be aware of the sequence of events leading to their child's reaction. The nurse can then encourage parents to communicate this information to teachers or other caregivers so that they also will feel more comfortable in caring for the child with diabetes in the parent's absence.

In *hypoglycemia,* rapid treatment is of the utmost importance. Brain functioning is dependent upon glucose, and if the hypoglycemic reaction is extremely severe or prolonged, permanent damage, although very rare, may occur. If the patient is alert, he or she can be given one of the oral glucose-containing drinks or candy. If, however, the patient is not alert, the administration of fluids by mouth may cause aspiration and lung complications. In this case, parents may be instructed how to administer glucagon at home, or 50 per cent dextrose can be be administered intravenously in a hospital emergency room. Caution must be exercised in using 50 per cent dextrose in children. The usual pediatric dose is 0.5 gm/kg intravenously immediately. Once the child has regained consciousness he or she should rest and eat some carbohydrate-containing food, such as milk, cheese, peanut butter, or bread, which will be digested slowly to prevent another rapid drop in blood sugar. Severe or frequent hypoglycemic reactions should be reported to the physician. The nurse should also assess the child's routine and health status following a severe reaction or after frequent reactions in an attempt to determine the cause of the reactions so similar occurrences may be prevented.

In *hyperglycemia,* there is a need for the patient and family to reassess the diet, insulin, and exercise patterns. The body must have enough insulin to utilize the blood glucose for energy production. When sufficient insulin is not available, the body begins to break down proteins and fats as alternative sources and, as described previously, diabetic ketoacidosis (DKA) may occur. If the child exhibits these symptoms of ketoacidosis, parents should encourage the child to drink extra sugar-free fluids, stay warm, and refrain from exercise. The parent should contact the physician if DKA symptoms occur or if the child is nauseated and vomiting. In fact, it should be emphasized to take the child to the emergency room if the child vomits more than twice. Table 49-19 details nursing care for the child hospitalized with DKA.

Chronic Complications. The most common chronic complication of diabetes is atherosclerosis or a thickening and degeneration of the walls of both large and small blood vessels of the body. When hypoglycemia results in mobilization of fatty acids, lipids are

Table 49-18. Causes, Symptoms, and Treatment of Hypoglycemia and Hyperglycemia

Hypoglycemia	Hyperglycemia
Causes	
Not enough food Too much insulin More than the usual amount of exercise Insulin absorbed more rapidly than usual	Not enough insulin Too much food Not enough exercise Emotional stress Injury Illness, infection
Symptoms	
Sudden onset Cold perspiration Shaky Hungry Dizzy Mood change Headache Weak Nervous Blurry vision Slurred speech Convulsions, unconsciousness	Increased thirst Increased urination Decreased appetite Dry skin Flushed face Confusion Dullness Blurred vision Nausea and vomiting Acetone breath Coma
Treatment	
Immediately drink half cup orange juice or regular sodapop Take 2 teaspoons sugar or honey Take 3 to 4 Lifesavers or Dextrosol Glucagon subcutaneously or 50% dextrose Follow-up with source of protein for more sustained glucose level	Increase insulin (may introduce regular insulin) Test urine and blood frequently Notify physician

Table 49-19
Nursing Process Plan: The Child with Diabetic Ketoacidosis

By Roxie Foster

Assessment of Physical Function

Nutrition/Metabolism
Elimination
Activity/Exercise

Subjective Assessment

Level of comfort; urinary elimination patterns; presence of hunger, thirst; energy level; usual body weight.

Objective Assessment

Vital signs, mental status, hydration status, breath odor, serum glucose level and urine glucose and acetone levels; serum electrolytes; hematocrit.

Analysis: Nursing Diagnosis 1

Altered fluid and electrolyte balance:
dehydration, *related to osmotic diuresis associated with glycosuria*
metabolic acidosis, *related to*
- *accumulation of keto acids associated with fat metabolism during impaired glucose transport*
- *concomitant loss of bicarbonate with excretion of ketones in the urine*

hyperkalemia, *related to*
- *loss of water in excess of serum electrolytes*
- *release of potassium from the cells in response to acidosis*

hyponatremia, *related to excess glucagon, which is an aldosterone antagonist*
hypophosphatemia, *related to*
- *increased tissue catabolism*
- *impaired cellular uptake*
- *decreased renal reabsorption (Zimmerman and Gildea, 1985)*

Analysis: Nursing Diagnosis 2

Altered nutrition: less than body requirements, *related to hyperglycemia associated with*
- *insufficient insulin for glucose transport*
- *catabolic effects of glucagon and catecholamines, which are stimulated by decreased insulin*

Defining Characteristics for Nursing Diagnoses 1 and 2

Subjective: Report of polydipsia, polyuria, polyphagia, fatigue, headache, stomach cramps, nausea, and vomiting.

Objective: Mental confusion; hyperventilation (Kussmaul respirations); fruity breath odor; low grade fever (if significantly dehydrated); tachycardia; flushed, dry skin; serum pH $<$7.30; blood sugar $>$300 mg/dl; ketonuria; serum sodium $<$136 mEq/L; serum potassium $>$5 mEg/L; serum phosphorus $<$4 mg/dl (may be normal initially); elevated hematocrit; weight loss.

Client Goal/ Evaluation Criteria	Nursing Goals/Strategies (Selected Rationale)*
1. The client will restore fluid and electrolyte balance and resolve hyperglycemia, as evidenced by: a. vital signs and neurologic signs within normal range b. alert and oriented (or usual mental status) c. normal skin turgor, color, and temperature d. moist mucous membranes e. stabilization of weight f. fasting blood sugar 80–120 mg/dl g. absence of abdominal pain, nausea, vomiting h. serum pH 7.35–7.45 i. serum electrolytes and hematocrit within normal limits	For criteria *a* and *b*: *Assess vital signs (pulse, respirations, and blood pressure) and mental status every 15 minutes initially, then every hour until stable.* (Vital signs and mental status will reflect response to treatment. Any decrease in level of consciousness may signal cerebral edema.) For criteria *c* through *e*: *Maintain the intravenous fluid replacement as ordered.* Expect NS to be ordered initially, with $D_5W\frac{1}{2}NS$ when blood sugar drops below 300 mg/dl (Dickerman and Lucey, 1985). (The addition of 5 per cent dextrose will then be needed to prevent hypoglycemia.) *Offer oral fluids if the client is alert and denies nausea (unless ordered NPO).* *Assess hydration status to evaluate response to treatment.* • Accurately record intake and output. (Initial increase in output will signal increased blood volume and adequate kidney perfusion.) • Obtain daily weights (to evaluate fluid replacement.) For criterion *f*: *Expect intravenous insulin orders if the client is significantly dehydrated.* (Dehydration alters tissue perfusion and would lead to slow absorption.) • Before administering insulin, check the dosage in the syringe with another nurse. (Incorrect dosage of insulin is potentially fatal.) • Administer intravenous insulin through a separate line "piggy-backed" into the rehydration fluid. (The dosage will then be independent of rehydration rates [Dickerman and Lucey, 1985].) • Change the syringe or infusion bag every 4 to 5 hours (to prevent insulin adherence to the plastic infusion set) (Dickerman and Lucey, 1985). • Control the insulin dosage with a syringe pump or infusion pump (to prevent accidental error in delivery). *Expect an order for subcutaneous insulin prior to discontinuing intravenous administration* (to prevent marked fluctuations in blood sugar) (Dickerman and Lucey, 1985). *Assist with drawing hourly blood specimens for evaluation of serum glucose and electrolytes.* (Although urine sugar and acetone levels may be checked, these values are significantly less indicative of metabolic status than are serum values.) For criteria *g* through *i*: *Institute use of a cardiac monitor, if this is the nurse's prerogative within the institution.* (Alterations in potassium may cause dysrhythmias.) *If a cardiac monitor is not being used, pay particular attention to the heart rate and rhythm and to the pulse deficit.* (Pulse deficit is the difference between the apical and radial beats and is evidence of ineffective ventricular contractions.)

* These goals and strategies relate to Nursing Diagnoses 1 and 2.

Continued

Table 49-19 (continued)

Nursing Goals/Strategies (Selected Rationale)

Determine that urine output is adequate (i.e., that the oliguria of dehydration has been resolved) before adding potassium to the intravenous infusion. (If urine output is inadequate hyperkalemia may develop rapidly.)

Monitor serum electrolyte levels and alert the physician to significant fluctuations.

Assessment of Emotional/Social Function

See Nursing Process Plan: The Hospitalized Child, Table 31–2.

Assessment of Intellectual-Perceptual Function

Knowledge of Illness
Health Perception/Management

Subjective Assessment

Verbalization of the pathophysiology of diabetes mellitus; of the relationship among diet, insulin, exercise, infection, and hyperglycemia; and of the probable causes of diabetic ketoacidosis in a previously diagnosed diabetic. Verbalization of usual management methods, recent eating patterns, and a typical day's activities.

Objective Assessment

Observation of techniques used for drawing up and administering insulin, and for blood and urine tests. Observation of records kept by child or family of blood and urine test results and of insulin dosages.

Analysis: Nursing Diagnosis 3

Noncompliance with prescribed diabetic protocol, related to

- *inadequate or incorrect information*
- *lack of faith in the protocol*
- *significant changes in activities of daily living imposed by the protocol*
- *lack of adult supervision*
- *nervous overeating*
- *developmental rebellion to "being different"*

Defining Characteristics

Subjective: Evidence of misinformation about or misunderstanding of diabetes and of the prescribed protocol; indication of inconsistent eating practices, insulin administration, and exercise habits. Reports of "eating without even thinking about it when I'm nervous," and of "forgetting" to test blood sugar and urine acetone levels routinely. Comments such as "I use *about* 10 units of insulin most days." Complaints about "not being able to go out with my friends," and questions such as, "Why do I have to have this dumb disease anyway?"

Objective: Inaccurate measurement of insulin dosage and of blood sugar and urine acetone levels. Incomplete record-keeping; written indication of irregular testing of blood and urine.

Client Goals/ Evaluation Criteria	Nursing Goals/Strategies/(Selected Rationale)
3.1. The client will identify the cause of this episode of DKA	*Encourage verbalization of feelings about the illness.* (Expression of emotion often must precede problem solving.) *Facilitate the client's exploration of probable causes of DKA, supplementing needed facts and clarifying misinformation.* Resist identifying the problem as perceived by the nurse. (Important aspects may then be overlooked. Also, the client is more likely to direct energy toward solving a self-identified problem.)
3.2. The client will develop a plan for preventing future episodes of DKA	*Assist the client to explore resources for coping with the identified problem.* *Facilitate the development of options for action.* Suggest options that require the least change in usual habits, e.g., have the child or parent write favorite foods on colored index cards and color code to food groups; then the child can choose cards from the color groups for meals (Billie, 1986). *Let the client choose the options that will formulate the plan, and encourage verbalization of the rationale for the plan.* (It is crucial to compliance that the client "own" the plan and be able to identify the logic involved.) *Collaborate with home care and clinic nurses* (so they can help the client evaluate and redesign the management plan as needed.)

deposited on the intima of blood vessels (Guyton, 1987). Maintenance of normal blood sugar levels is therefore crucial to controlling this complication.

The chief regions affected by large vessel disease are the heart, the brain, and the periphery (especially of the legs and feet). In the heart, patients suffer from narrowing of the coronary arteries and complications due to angina (cramping of the heart tissue) or myocardial infarction (obstruction of the coronary arteries). The brain is subject to several major problems, including cerebral hemorrhage, cerebral thrombosis, and cerebrovascular accidents. Atherosclerosis in the legs and feet leaves this area with a decreased blood supply and thus vulnerable to infection, tissue necrosis, and gangrene.

Although large vessel diseases are among the leading causes of death in adults with diabetes, children with type I diabetes do not usually suffer from large blood vessel damage but more from the small vessel complications. Body regions most affected include the eyes, kidneys, and lower extremities.

Eye. Diabetic retinopathy can be expected to develop in 40 to 60 per cent of all persons who contract diabetes in youth. It often takes many years to develop, and only 5 to 15 per cent will have proliferative changes (Travis et al, 1987). The retina is one of the body's tissues that is dependent upon glucose to supply its energy needs (Guyton, 1987). In periods of hypoglycemia, retinal changes can occur. There are several stages of diabetic retinopathy, which include (1) microaneurysm or small dilations of blood vessels, which can be visualized as red dots in the macular area of the eye; (2) exudates and hemorrhage caused by microaneurysms, which may hemorrhage into the retina or vitreous body; after several weeks these hemorrhages convert into waxy yellowish plaques called exudates; and (3) retinalis proliferans, which is a process of revascularization and rehemorrhaging at the primary hemorrhage site of the disc, which ultimately may be involved in the process of retinal detachment, the primary cause of blindness in diabetes. However, with modern management (e.g., laser treatment) blindness is preventable in the majority of individuals.

Kidney. The kidneys are prone to both infections and nephropathy. Hyperglycemia depresses leukocyte function and provides excellent conditions for bacterial or fungal growth. Diabetics are susceptible to infections throughout the urinary tract system, which can lead to decreased kidney function, pyelonephritis, and damaged renal tissue.

Nephropathy of two types (glomerulosclerosis and tubular nephrosis) occurs almost exclusively in diabetic patients. Kidney damage due to nephropathy is probably irreversible but is thought to be retarded or prevented by good metabolic control. For those with severe renal disease, kidney transplants and mechanical devices may make the future brighter.

Neuropathy. Neuropathy in diabetic subjects is characterized by aching and burning sensations in the lower extremities, loss of sensation, and loss of autonomic function with resulting weakness, postural hypotension, gastrointestinal disturbances, neurogenic bladder, and impotence. The pathophysiology of diabetic neuropathy is thought to involve ischemic changes in the nerves and the vessels supplying the nerves, thereby linking neuropathy to the atherosclerotic process. In addition, altered glucose metabolism results in an accumulation of sorbitol, which may decrease conduction velocity in the nerve pathways and interfere with myelinization of the nerves (Gröer and Shekelton, 1983).

Although it is not clear if diabetic neuropathy is preventable, it seems clear that maintenance of normal blood glucose levels is advisable. If neuropathy does develop, it is usually irreversible and treatment focuses upon palliation of symptoms. Teaching and direct nursing interventions can be instituted to prevent falls related to orthostatic hypotension and gait disturbances associated with weakness and altered sensation. The child and parents should be alert for constipation, possibly requiring changes in diet and exercise patterns, and for urinary retention related to altered innervation to the bladder. (See Chapter 42 for interventions pertinent to urinary retention.) The possibility of impotence should be discussed with the adolescent male who has diabetes so that he does not wrongly attribute erection failure to some "lack of masculinity." Depending upon the young person's values and health beliefs, various methods may be used to compensate for impotence, including helping him to find alternative ways to achieve sexual satisfaction, and a penile implant.

Major Nursing Diagnoses Related to Psychosocial Impact of Diabetes

Altered family process, related to lifestyle changes imposed by the needs of the child with diabetes for
- *monitoring and treatment of the disease*
- *family support to deal with the emotional impact of diabetes*

Potential noncompliance, related to
- *the complexity of the treatment regimen*
- *the lack of immediate rewards for metabolic control*

Potential altered growth and development: emotional/social delay, related to
- *poor self-concept associated with the restrictions of insulin-dependent DM*
- *increased and prolonged dependency upon parents*

Potential altered parenting: overprotection, related to parental anxiety about the possible complications of insulin-dependent DM

Strategies for Nursing Care Related to the Psychosocial Impact of Diabetes

"Your child has diabetes." With these few simple words, a family is often required to change its entire lifestyle. The diagnosis is most often a shock and a highly emotional experience. Parents expect that because their child has always been healthy, he or she will remain that way. They feel secure in the belief that serious health problems only occur in other families, and their first reaction is disbelief. This stage of nonacceptance is normal and is the initial stage of the adaptation process. The stages of adaptation in chronic illness have been characterized by Billie (1981) as : (1) disbelief, (2) developing awareness, (3) reorganization, (4) resolution, (5) identity change, and finally (6) adaptation.

Each child and family will pass through these stages at their own speed. Everyone needs time to overcome the initial impact of the diagnosis and may need substantial help in order to adjust. Most parents feel some relief when they realize their child's illness can be controlled.

The strength of the diagnostic impact on the child will vary greatly with age at the time of diagnosis. School-age children may be particularly impressed with their new "condition" and be challenged by the tasks, routines, and skills in their prescribed therapeutic regime. Adolescents, on the other hand, often feel unfairly victimized and that diabetes is impossible to conquer. These feelings may lead to poor compliance, depression, and low self-esteem.

Patients and parents tend to initially use coping methods that have been successful for them in the past. Some deny what has happened and continue on with their normal lifestyle. Some throw themselves into learning every aspect of management from every available textbook and demand very strict adherence to the therapeutic regimen. Still others become very overprotective and make the child constantly aware of the illness. A further discussion of coping with chronic illness is discussed in Chapter 25.

Facilitating the Family's Adjustment to Diabetes

Nurses can play a key role in facilitating the child's and family's adaptation to the illness. They should strive to be knowledgeable and provide a relaxed and accepting atmosphere. They should stress that the child and family do not have to learn everything at once. Performing a thorough assessment will provide valuable information about how to proceed with the education process and about whether the family can cope with learning more than the survival skills at this time. From the initial assessment, the nurse can also understand the family's social support systems and can include some of these (e.g., grandparents, babysitters, teachers) in the child's treatment.

Nurses should expect that the family will not initially listen, and their early questions may need to be addressed several times. Nurses need to be good listeners and be prepared to discuss the child's and family's frustrations and concerns. When they have difficulty giving the insulin injection or when they stray from the prescribed diet the nurse can help identify the actual problems and shift the focus away from individual guilt. Finally, the nurse can be instrumental in facilitating positive attitudes toward diabetes management and care by emphasizing treatment to maintain health (within the realm of the illness) rather than solely monitoring the illness process.

Promoting Compliance with Treatment

Any individual diagnosed as having diabetes will need to initiate some lifestyle changes. Children diagnosed as having type I diabetes mellitus are often forced to incorporate an imposing regimen (e.g., consisting of insulin injections, a special diet, urine and blood glucose monitoring, and possibly prescribed amounts of exercise) into their daily routine. The complexity of the prescribed regimen and often the nonimmediate rewards provide many opportunities for noncompliance for both the child and the family.

Nearly all physicians caring for a diabetic child will prescribe a specific treatment regimen. The regimen itself may not present an imposing obstacle to the child or the family. However, when the family attempts to integrate the regimen with the problems and demands of the normal activities of "being a child," adherence or compliance often becomes a problem. The following example illustrates the meaning of being "compliant" for a diabetic child.

John is 7 years old and has been diagnosed as having type I diabetes for 1 year. Every morning, John's mother wakes him up at 7 o'clock. He stumbles into the bathroom and "pees." Then his mother hands him a big glass of water so he can "pee" again to get a sample for testing. As usual, he can't find his container to collect the specimen (Jason, his younger brother, must have run off with it). He has to go into Jason's room and find his container. Meanwhile, John's mother is calling from downstairs that it will soon be time for breakfast and tells him to hurry. John finds the container and squeezes out a few drops of urine (when he really doesn't feel like going) and does the urine test. He is supposed to write down the results but someone keeps taking his pencil out of the bathroom. He doesn't have time to look for it because it's time to take his insulin and get dressed. He goes to the kitchen and waits for Mom (who is busy making his special school lunch) to give him his shot. John hates his shot, especially when Mom has forgotten to get the insulin out of the refrigerator and it is cold. It hurts and he feels like crying. Mom throws up her hands and says that there is no time to go through this crying scene again this morning, and John needs to hurry and get dressed or his breakfast will be cold. John saunters upstairs and gets dressed slowly, but he can't find his running shoes and he doesn't feel like looking. While wondering why he has to do all of this when no one even knows he's got diabetes, he spies his favorite comic book and starts to read it instead. Mom suddenly appears at the bedroom door and tells him that if he doesn't come downstairs now, he won't have time to finish all his breakfast before the school bus comes. John knows that he will start to feel "funny" and have one of those reactions in the middle of the morning if he doesn't eat all his breakfast. John runs downstairs and gobbles up as much food as he can, throws on another pair of running shoes that are too small and runs for the school bus that is honking its horn at the front door.

Diabetic children and their parents need the assistance of health professionals in order to promote adherence to the often complex and demanding diabetic regimen. Nurses who are knowledgeable in diabetes and growth and development and experienced in working with children and their families can play an integral part in promoting adherence behavior. In addition to physical parameters, such as blood glucose levels, hemoglobin A_{1C} values, and height and weight measurements, the nurse can further assess the child (or family) in an attempt to determine if they are compliant with the prescribed regimen.

Areas that are most often difficult for families include diet, blood and urine testing, and insulin administration. In all these areas the nurse should attempt to include the child and parents in the decision-making process concerning the timing and frequency of these activities. As well, parents should be encouraged to allow their children to participate in various aspects of the regimen appropriate for their age, interest, and enthusiasm. In testing procedures, parents need to be cautioned not to condemn the child for poor test results but rather to praise his or her efforts and technique. In this way, the child will not be tempted to either hide or falsely report poor results. In children who fear needles or in some adolescents, compliance with taking the insulin shot may also be a problem. For younger children who protest, parents need continued encouragement to persist and often need reinforcement of the child's need for exogenous insulin. In the adolescent, repeated missing of injections might be suggestive of scheduling problems, an expression of frustration or poor self-esteem, or an indication of more serious psychologic problems. For this older child, the support of diabetic peers or psychosocial counseling may be useful. Of all areas of the diabetic regimen, diet provides the most common ground for noncompliance. Nursing interventions designed to promote dietary compliance have been discussed previously in this chapter.

Strauss and colleagues (1984) list characteristics that either deter or enhance a patient's compliance. These include the following:

- degree of difficulty in learning or carrying out a specific regimen;
- the time needed to carry out the regimen;
- whether the regimen causes pain or discomfort;
- the energy required to carry out the regimen;
- whether the regimen is visible to others;
- whether there is stigma attached to the regimen;
- whether the patient perceives that the regimen is effective and efficient;
- whether the regimen causes side effects;
- the cost of the regimen; and
- whether the regimen leads to social isolation.

When all these factors are considered, it is no wonder that children and their families have difficulty following prescribed medical regimens. As health professionals, we may need to try to understand more fully the difficulties patients have in incorporating such regimes as opposed to simply evaluating the patient's and family's compliance.

Promoting Healthy Psychosocial Development

Every child has to deal with accomplishing certain developmental tasks for each age or stage. The child with diabetes has an additional variable that influences normal growth and development. Having diabetes can introduce a number of emotional stresses in a child. The acute onset of symptoms, the initial interaction with a new group of health professionals in either a hospital or an outpatient setting, the concern and worry of parents, and their own feelings of anxiety, worry, and fear are all stress producing. As well, the daily insulin injections, blood or urine testing, and altered diet, which represent the change from a carefree, flexible existence to a more regimented lifestyle, are of concern for the diabetic child and the family. All of these stresses, concerns, and changes require some form of adaptation or coping. The degree of success in the adaptive process depends on many factors, including the age and stage of cognitive development of the child, previous stressful experiences of the child and family, and the amount of social support they receive. The child needs to meet the demands of being both a child and diabetic. Each developmental stage imposes new and different obstacles for the diabetic child. The nurse can play an integral part in promoting both normal growth and development and a healthy adaptation in the diabetic child. See Table 49-20 for a summary of specific concerns that diabetes poses at each stage of growth and development and suggested nursing strategies.

Promoting Healthy Parenting

The diagnosis of diabetes changes the child's life and thus that of the whole family. The child has essentially lost his or her health and both the child and the family will grieve this loss. Diabetes causes anxiety within the family, which may lead to feelings of sorrow, resentment, and hostility. If other family members are also diabetic, there may be tremendous guilt feelings, which may lead to marital problems and family maladjustment.

Nurses can have a key role in enhancing family adaptation. As they perform the assessment of family's motivation and readiness to learn, they can also assess family functioning in areas such as communication patterns, expression of emotions, and support. Nurses should involve both the family and the child in the initial assessment and attempt to establish rapport, alleviate anxiety, and prioritize learning needs. If extreme friction exists between family members they may want to interview client and family separately and attempt to point out anger, guilt, or feelings of stress. If the family problems exceed the nurse's capabilities or knowledge, he or she should immediately seek professional assistance or refer the family for family counseling or psychiatric treatment.

Strategies for Nursing Care Related to Self-Care Management

The teaching needs listed under the nursing diagnosis of knowledge deficit provide, in many ways, a summary of the physical, emotional, and social needs of the child with diabetes and of the family entrusted with home management. Because each of these areas has been addressed previously in this chapter, this section will focus upon the mechanism for effectively teaching the child and family about diabetes, its monitoring, and its control.

Teaching to Support Self-Care Management

In recent years, there has been a shift in health care emphasis, moving from the direct-care model toward self-management. In a chronic illness, such as dia-

Table 49-20. Growth and Development of the Diabetic Child

Developmental Tasks	Specific Concerns Diabetes Poses	Suggested Nursing Strategies
Infancy (0 to 1 Year)		
Development of sense of trust versus mistrust Beginning to view self as separate from mother	Diabetes increases dependence on parent Increased susceptibility to vaginal and perineal infections of non-toilet trained infant owing to moist glucose-laden environment, which is attractive to bacterial growth	Attempt to encourage parents to provide consistency in the quality and quantity of care for their infant (i.e., attempt not to overprotect) Provide support and understanding Explain to parents that fungal infections are more common in glucose-rich environments, which the diabetic child's urine provides. Encourage good hygiene practices and frequent diaper changes
Toddler (1 to 3 Years)		
Development of autonomy and controlling body and environment (mobility, speech, toilet training, pleasure) versus shame and doubt Begins to make some of own choices	Child is dependent on parent for urine and blood samples, injections, and diet Parents have difficulty dealing emotionally with the child's medical regimen, which may lead to tension in the whole family Parents may have difficulty distinguishing between developmental crisis (i.e., temper tantrums) and diabetes complications (i.e., hypoglycemia)	Attempt to help parents learn to deal with tense situations and resistance from child Encourage parents to set limits, agree on these limits, and feel confident with them Encourage parents to allow the child to make some of his or her own choices (i.e., what food to eat or where to inject insulin) Provide parents with understanding and support
Preschooler (3 to 6 Years)		
Development of initiative versus guilt (increases gross motor ability to move freely and language skills and cognitive ability to explore and understand the environment) Begins to understand moral judgments (i.e., "good" and "bad")	Realizes that diabetes makes him or her different from other family members Beginning independence leads to parental fears of things going wrong, and parents may not want to have child out of their sight Urine and blood test results may be interpreted as good or bad and precausal logic (Piaget) will then lead the child to assume that he or she is good or bad	Assist child and parents to acknowledge differences and help child focus on strengths Encourage parents to involve the child in some simple tasks of diabetes management, such as recording results, helping to collect specimens, or preparing insulin for injection Encourage child to express feelings through play, drawings Encourage parents to begin diabetes education using simple concepts and language Provide encouragement and support
School-Age (6 to 12 Years)		
Developing industry versus inferiority Developing cognitive skills, competition with peers, and the rules of the game Child wants to be successful and avoid failure 10- to 12-year-olds begin to play with peers (i.e., team sports and groups) Fine tuning of small motor muscles	Child is often involved in unpredictable activity (may need to alter food intake just before or during activity), which may lead to an increased number of hypoglycemic reactions and the need for frequent diet and insulin changes Children often poor judges of intensity of activities Child interested in the scientific nature of the illness (i.e., important to understand the symptoms of hypo- and hyperglycemia) Parents are attempting to foster the child's independence but at the same time are having much difficulty "letting go" of the diabetes management tasks they have been accustomed to doing School hurdles—school cafeterias, peers, physical education, stress of tests and examinations Manipulative or deceptive behavior to gain attention (urine and blood results)	Encourage the child's independence and acknowledge small successes as children of this age need adult approval Encourage learning through play (exercise is fun and helps in management of diabetes) Teach or reinforce with the child and family how to alter food intake prior to exercise and the scientific basis of hypo- and hyperglycemia Encourage the child to eat snacks prior to and during activities and occasional rest periods Attempt to make diabetes education relevant, enjoyable, and understandable (role playing, school projects) May attempt group education of family members or two small families with children of the same age Parents and child may need to spend time with teachers and school nurse at the beginning of each school year explaining the basics and the child's idiosyncrasies

continued

Table 49-20 *(continued)*

Developmental Tasks	Specific Concerns Diabetes Poses	Suggested Nursing Strategies
School-Age (6 to 12 Years)		
		Provide appropriate support from parents, teachers, health professionals, and peers Encourage parents to allow the children to take over some tasks they are comfortable with Encourage parents to try to understand reasons for manipulative or deceptive behavior so it can be dealt with Suggest diabetic camp where 8- to 12-year-olds can engage in both social and educational activities with peers
Adolescence (12 to 18 Years)		
Transition from childhood to adulthood Sense of identity versus identity diffusion Developing sexual preferences, selecting future life choices, focus of authority shifts from family to peers Self-image (body image) Development of own value system	Diabetes management (i.e., urine or blood testing) is often seen by the adolescent as repulsive and hampering to independence, which may lead to withdrawal or rebellious behavior Physical growth spurt often leads to inappropriate food intake and being either obese or underweight, which may lead to adjustment problems Diabetes causes problems with dependency-independency conflict and ego development (i.e., parents may hassle, peers may reject) Maladjusted family environment may lead to manipulation, repeated hospitalization for insulin reactions or diabetic ketoacidosis Poor self-esteem Isolated from family and health professionals Anxiety about severe reactions causing embarrassment and loss of self-esteem Menstrual periods (in adolescent girls) may lead to hyperglycemia and ketonuria owing to estrogen and progesterone changes	May attempt to form a group of diabetic teenagers to provide peer support Family may need consistent ongoing professional help to identify reasons for maladjustive environment and to rebuild self-esteem, open communication lines, and break down barriers that have been built up Attempt to get adolescent to clarify own values (may need to attempt to work diabetes around the things that are most important to the patient) Approach child and family as equals, set achievable short-term goals, and plan and evaluate objectives together Explain that hypoglycemic reactions rarely cause permanent damage Encourage adolescent to tell peers about diabetes and how they might act in hypoglycemic situation and what they can do Prepare adolescent girls for what may happen to their blood sugar levels during menstrual periods so they will know what to expect and be prepared for possible increases in their insulin dosage

betes, the very nature of the illness necessitates a high level of patient and family responsibility for successful day-to-day management.

Successful management of the diabetic patient ideally requires that the patient and family have a thorough knowledge of the illness and the willingness to monitor the condition themselves. Their major responsibilities will be to make appropriate changes in treatment to keep blood glucose levels controlled. Patient education is the essential first step in motivating successful management. The content of the diabetes teaching program should focus on the needs and capabilities of the learners. Diabetes education can generally be divided into survival skills, health maintenance skills, and health promotion skills (Tupling et al, 1981). Examples of the various content approaches for each skill level are included in Table 49-21. These skill categories can form the basis for a teaching plan.

Chapter 27 details the principles of patient and family education. Table 27-2 lists implications for teaching children of various ages.

Nursing Strategies for Follow-up Care in the Home or Clinic

Obtain a blood sample for determination of HbA_{1C}.

Determine the frequency of transient hypoglycemic reactions, the child's ability to recognize early symptoms, and the effectiveness of glucose replacement in quickly resolving symptoms.

Determine the frequency of hyperglycemia and ketonuria.

Assess developmental level.

Table 49-21. Levels of Diabetic Skills

Survival Skills	Health Maintenance Skills	Health Promotion Skills
Need for insulin	Test blood and urine for glucose and ketones	Use of test results and records to make changes in insulin dose
Differentiate between types of insulin	Keep records	Insulin alteration
Relationship between meals and insulin	Rotate injection sites	Initiate illness regimen
Prepare and administer own insulin	Understand diabetic diet and how to modify during exercise or illness	Ability to modify regimen to maintain good metabolic control
Storage of insulin	How to prevent hypoglycemia	
Foods to avoid	Identification	
How to recognize and treat hypoglycemic reaction	Effect of stress, illness, and exercise	
	Meaning of metabolic control	

Encourage questions and expression of feelings that are stimulated by changing perceptions associated with growth and development.

Assess adequacy of health maintenance and health promotion skills and provide necessary teaching.

Reinforce the child's and family's sense of control and independence in management of this chronic disease.

References

Albisser AM, Liebel BS: The artificial pancreas. *Clin Endocrinol Metab* 1977; 6:457–479.

American Diabetes Association and American Dietetic Association: Exchange list for meal planning. New York, 1976.

American Diabetes Association and American Dietetic Association: A guide for professionals: the effective application of exchange lists for meal planning. New York, 1977.

Aquilino JL, Ely J: Parents and the sexuality of preschool children. *Pediatr Nurs* 1985 Jan/Feb; 11(1):41–46.

Bacon GE, Spencer ML, Hopwood NJ, et al: *A Practical Approach to Pediatric Endocrinology.* 2nd ed. Chicago, Year Book Medical Publishers, 1982.

Baker SW: Psychological management of intersex children. *In* Josso N (ed): *The Intersex Child.* New York, S Karger, 1981.

Billie DA: Tailoring your diabetic patient's care plans to fit his life style. *Nurs 86* 1986; 16(2):54–57.

Billie DA: *Practical Approaches to Patient Teaching.* Boston, Little, Brown and Company, 1981.

Blum A, Hayes TM, Gamble DR: Registry for newly diagnosed diabetic children. *Br Med J* 1975; 3:580.

Bongiovanni AM: Congenital adrenal hyperplasia and related conditions. *In The Metabolic Basis of Inherited Disease.* 4th ed. New York, McGraw-Hill, 1978, 868.

Buckingham BA, Costin G, Roe TF: Hyperthyroidism in children: a reevaluation of treatment. *Am J Dis Child* 1981; 135:112–116.

Bunn HF: Evaluation of glycosylated hemoglobin in diabetic patients. Diabetes 1981; 30:613–617.

Burns EC, Tanner JM, Preece MA, et al: Final height and pubertal development in 55 children with idiopathic growth hormone deficiency, treated for between 2 and 15 years with human growth hormone. *Eur J Pediatr* 1981; 137:155–164.

Burns EM: Diabetes mellitus and pregnancy. *Nurs Clin North Am* 1983; 18(4):673–685.

Christman C, Bennett J: Diabetes: New names, new test, new diet. *Nurs 87* 1987 Jan; 17(1):34–42.

Coody D: Congenital hypothyroidism. *Pediatr Nurs* 1984 Sep/Oct; 10(5):342–345.

Cooper DS: Antithyroid drugs. *N Engl J Med* 1984; 311:1353–1362.

Cornblath M, Schwartz R: *Disorders of Carbohydrate Metabolism in Infancy.* Philadelphia, WB Saunders, 1966.

Coulston A, Greenfield M, Kraemer F, et al: Effect of source of dietary carbohydrate on plasma glucose and insulin responses to test meals in normal subjects. *Am J Clin Nutr* 1980; 33:1279–1282.

Crapo PA, Kolterman OG, Waldeck N, et al: Postprandial hormonal responses to different types of complex carbohydrate in individuals with impaired glucose tolerance. *Am J Clin Nutr* 1980; 33:1723–1728.

Daneman D, Siminerio L, Transue D, et al: The role of self-monitoring of blood glucose in the routine management of children with insulin-dependent diabetes mellitus. *Diabetes Care* 1985; 8(1):1–4.

Davis MS: Variation in patient's compliance with doctor's orders: Analysis of congruence between survey responses and results of empirical investigations. *J Med Educ* 1966; 41:1037–1048.

Dickerman JD, Lucey JF: *Smith's The Critically Ill Child: Diagnosis and Medical Management.* Philadelphia, WB Saunders, 1985.

DiGeorge AM: Disorders of the hypothalamus and pituitary gland. *In* Behrman RE, Vaughan VC III (eds): *Nelson Textbook of Pediatrics.* 13th ed. Philadelphia, WB Saunders, 1987, 1176–1193.

Drash AL, LaPorte RE, Kuller LH, et al: The descriptive epidemiology of insulin-dependent diabetes mellitus in Allegheny County, Pennsylvania. *In* Martin J (ed): *The Etiology and Pathogenesis of Diabetes Mellitus.* New York, Raven Press, 1981, 211.

Drotar D, Owens R, Gotthold J: Personality adjustment of children and adolescents with hypopituitarism. *Child Psychiatr Hum Dev* 1980 Fall; 11(1):59–66.

Ehrlich RM: Diabetes mellitus in childhood. *Clin Endocrinol Metab* 1982; 11(1):195–210.

Erikson E: *Childhood and Society.* 2nd ed. New York, Norton, 1959.

Foley TP: Thyroid disease. *In* Gellis SS, Kagan BM (eds): *Current Pediatric Therapy 12.* Philadelphia, WB Saunders, 1986, 301–306.

Fox RE, Redstone D: Sources of error in glucose determinations in neonatal blood by glucose oxidase methods, including Dextrostix. *Am J Clin Pathol* 1976; 66:658–662.

Frasier SD: *Pediatric Endocrinology.* New York, Grune and Stratton, 1980.

Gellis SS, Kagan BM: *Current Pediatric Therapy 12.* Philadelphia, WB Saunders, 1986.

Gilbert FS, Bailes KL: Sex education in the home: an empirical task analysis. *J Sex Res* 1980; 16(2):148–161.

Gordon M, et al: Psychosocial aspects of constitutional short stature: social competence, behavior problems, self-esteem, and family functioning. *J Pediatr* 1982 Sep; 101(3):477–480.

Grazaitis DM, Sexson WR: Erroneously high Dextrostix values caused by isopropyl alcohol. *Pediatrics* 1980; 66:221–224.

Grew RS, Stabler BS, Williams RW, et al: Facilitating patient understanding in the treatment of growth delay. *Clin Pediatr* 1983 Oct; 22(10):685–690.

Groer MW, Shekelton ME: *Basic Pathophysiology. A Conceptual Approach.* St. Louis, CV Mosby, 1983.

Gutberlet RL, Cornblath M: Neonatal hypoglycemia revisited, 1975. *Pediatrics* 1976; 58:10–17.

Guyton AC: *Human Physiology and Mechanisms of Disease.* Philadelphia; WB Saunders, 1982, 1987.

Habener JF, Potts JT: Biosynthesis of parathyroid hormone. *N Engl J Med* 1978; 229:580–584.

Harris M: The changing prevalence of diabetes. *Diabetes Dateline (The National Diabetes Information Clearinghouse Bulletin)* 1980; 1(5).

Heins JM: Dietary management in diabetes mellitus. *Nurs Clin North Am* 1983; 18(4):631–643.

Hung W, August GP, Glasgow AM: *Pediatric Endocrinology.* New York, Medical Examination Publishing Company, 1983.

Ingelfinger FJ: Debates on diabetes. *N Engl J Med* 1977; 296:1228–1230.

Jackson RL, Guthrie RA: *The Child with Diabetes: Current Concepts.* Kalamazoo, Michigan, The Upjohn Company, 1975.

Jenkins DJA, Wolever TMS, Taylor RH, et al: Glycemic index of foods: A physiological basis for carbohydrate exchange. *Am J Clin Nutr* 1981; 34:362–366.

Job JC, Pierson M (eds): *Pediatric Endocrinology.* New York, John Wiley and Sons, 1981.

Kaplan S: *Clinical Pediatric and Adolescent Endocrinology.* Philadelphia, WB Saunders, 1982.

Kaye R: Research and practice in the treatment of insulin-dependent diabetes: A survey of 53 pediatric diabetologists. *Pediatrics* 1984; 74(6):1079–1085.

Kroc Collaborative Study Group: Blood glucose control and the evolution of diabetic retinopathy and albuminuria. *N Engl J Med* 1984; 311(6):365–371.

Krims M: Observations on children who suffer from dwarfism. *Psychiatr Q* 1968; 42:430–443.

Krueger JA, Ray JC: *Endocrine Problems in Nursing.* St Louis, CV Mosby, 1976.

Kusalic M, Fortin C: Growth hormone treatment in hypopituitary dwarfs. *Can Psychiatr Assoc J* 1975 Aug; 20:325–331.

Kusalic M, Fortin C, Gauthier Y: Psychodynamic aspects of dwarfism. *Can Psychiatr Assoc J* 1972; 17:29–34.

La Franchi SH, Murphey WH, Foley TP: Neonatal hypothyroidism detected by the Northwest Regional Screening Program. *Pediatrics* 1979; 68:180–184.

La Franchi SH: Newbown screening for congenital hypothyroidism. *Pediatr Ann* 1980; 9:390–398.

LaPorte RE, Fishbein HA, Kuller LH, et al: The Pittsburgh insulin-dependent (IDDM) registry: The incidence of insulin-dependent diabetes mellitus in Allegheny County, Pennsylvania (1965–1976). *Diabetes* 1979; 30:297.

Lendrum R, Walker G, Gamble DR: Islet cell antibodies in juvenile diabetes mellitus of recent onset. *Lancet* 1975; 1:880–883.

Lindley M: The small people of Britain. *Nurs Times* 1972; 68:635–636.

Malone JI, Hellrung JM, Malphas EW, et al: Good diabetic control: A study in mass delusion. *J Pediatr* 1976; 88:943.

Mattsson A: Juvenile diabetes: Impacts on life stages and systems. *In* Hamburg BA, et al (eds): *Behavioral and Psychosocial Issues in Diabetes.* Washington, D.C., NIH Publication No. 80-1993, 1979.

Mazur T: Ambiguous genitalia: detection and counseling. *Pediatr Nurs* 1984 Nov/Dec; 9(6):417–421.

Miller P, Stratton C, Tripp J: Blood testing compared with urine testing in the long-term control of diabetes. *Arch Dis Child* 1983; 58:294–297.

Money J, Clark FC, Beck J: Congenital hypothyroidism and IQ increase: a quarter century follow-up. *J Pediatr* 1978; 93:432–435.

Money J, Pollitt E: Studies in the psychology of dwarfism. II. Personality maturation and response to growth hormone treatment in hypopituitary dwarfs. *J Pediatr* 1966; 68:381–390.

National Diabetes Data Group: Classification and diagnosis of diabetes mellitus and other categories of glucose intolerance. *Diabetes* 1979; 28:1039–1057.

Nemchik R: Diabetes today: a whole new world. *RN* 1982; 45(10):31–36.

Notkins AL: The causes of diabetes. *Sci Am* 1979 Nov; 241:62–73.
Okun E, Johnston GP, Boniuk I: *Management of Diabetic Retinopathy.* St. Louis, CV Mosby Company, 1971.
O'Riordan JL, Malan PG, Gould RP: *Essentials of Endocrinology.* Boston, Blackwell Scientific Publications, 1982.
Robertson C: When an insulin-dependent diabetic must be NPO. *Nurs 86* 1986; 16(6):30–31.
Robinson AG: DDAVP in the treatment of central diabetes insipidus. *N Engl J Med* 1976; 294:507–509.
Root AW: *Human Pituitary Growth Hormone.* Springfield, Illinois, Charles C Thomas, 1972.
Sackett DL: The magnitude of compliance and noncompliance. *In* Sackett DL, Haynes RB (eds): *Compliance with Therapeutic Regimens.* Baltimore, Johns Hopkins University Press, 1976.
Schwartz R: Hypoglycemia. *In* Behrman RE, Vaughan VC III (eds): *Nelson Textbook of Pediatrics.* 13th ed. Philadelphia, WB Saunders, 1987, 1264–1272.
Sigurjonsdottir TJ, Hayles AB: Premature pubarche. *Clin Pediatr* 1968; 7:229–232.
Skyler JS: Dietary planning in insulin-dependent diabetes mellitus. *Pediatr Ann* 1983; 12(9):652–657.
Somogyi M: Diabetogenic effects of hyperinsulinism. *Am J Med* 1959; 26:169.
Sperling MA: Diabetes mellitus. *In* Behrman RE, Vaughan VC III (eds): *Nelson Textbook of Pediatrics.* 13th ed. Philadelphia, WB Saunders, 1987, 1248–1264.
Stabler B, et al: Social judgements by children of short stature. *Psycholog Rep* 1980; 46:743–746.
Stern N, Zaiken H: Assessing the child with short stature. *Pediatr Nurs* 1985 Mar/Apr; 11(2):106–110.
Strauss AL, Corbin J, Fagerhaugh S, et al: *Chronic Illness and the Quality of Life.* 2nd ed. St. Louis, CV Mosby Company, 1984.
Travis LB, Brouhard BH, Schreiner BJ: *Diabetes Mellitus in Children and Adolescents.* Philadelphia, WB Saunders, 1987.
Tupling H, Webb K, Harris G, et al: *You've Got to Get Through the Outside Layer.* Sydney, Australia: Diabetes Education and Assessment Programme of the North Shore Hospital of Sydney and The Northern Metropolitan Health Region of the Health Commission of New South Wales, 1981.
U.S. Department of Health, Education and Welfare, PHS National Institutes of Health: Diabetes data, compiled 1977, Publ. No. 79-1468, reprinted August 1979.
Watts NB, Keffer JH: *Practical Endocrine Diagnosis.* Philadelphia, Lea and Febiger, 1982.
Weller-Fahy ER, Berger LW, Troutman WG: Mouthwash: a source of acute ethanol intoxication. *Pediatrics* 1980; 66:302–303.
West R, Belmonte MM, Colley E, et al: Epidemiologic survey of juvenile-onset diabetes in Montreal. *Diabetes* 1979; 28:690.
Winter JSD: Cushing's syndrome in childhood. *In* Gardner LI (ed): *Endocrine and Genetic Diseases of Childhood and Adolescence.* Philadelphia, WB Saunders, 1975, 500.
Zimmerman SS, Gildea JH: *Critical Care Pediatrics.* Philadelphia, WB Saunders, 1985.

Bibliography

Balik B, et al: Diabetes and the school-aged child. *MCN* 1986 Sep/Oct; 11(5):324–330.
Bermel J: How short is too short? *Medica* 1984 Jun; pp 22–26.
Blizzard RM, Sauls HS: Patterns of growth. Human Growth Foundation, 4930 W. 77th St., P.O. Box 20253, Minneapolis, MN 55420, 1976.
Burrows GN, Dussault JH (eds): Guidelines for neonatal thyroid screening programs. *In Neonatal Thyroid Screening.* New York, Raven Press, 1980, 307–310.
Butts DE: Fluid and electrolyte disorders associated with diabetic ketoacidosis and hyperglycemic hyperosmolar nonketotic coma. *Issues Compr Pediatr Nurs* 1987; 10(3):827–836.
Callahan M: Why you should teach your diabetic patients to chart. *Nurs 88* 1988 Mar; 18(3):48–49.
Chase HP, Marlow RA, Dabiere CS, et al: Hypoglycemia and brain development. *Pediatrics* 1973, 52:513–520.
Edwards DR: Initial psychosocial impact of insulin-dependent diabetes mellitus on the pediatric client and family. *Issues Compr Pediatr Nurs* 1987; 10(4):199–207.
Funnell MM, McNitt P: Autonomic neuropathy. Diabetics' hidden foe. *Am J Nurs* 1986 Mar; 86(3):266–270.
Gordon M, Crouthamel C, Post EM, et al: Psychosocial aspects of constitutional short stature: social competence, behavior problems, self-esteem, and family functioning. *J Pediatr* 1982 Sep; 101(3):477–480.
Hallal J: Thyroid disorders. *Am J Nurs* 1977 Mar; 77(3):417–432.
Heins JM, et al: The new look in diabetic diets. *Am J Nurs* 1987 Feb; 87(2):196–198.
Hernandez CMG: Surgery and diabetes. Minimizing the risks. *Am J Nurs* 1987 Jun; 87(6):788–792.
Hurxthal K: Quick! Teach this patient about insulin. *Am J Nurs* 1988 Aug; 88(8):1097–1100.
Hymes JL: How to tell your child about sex. Public Affairs Pamphlet No. 149. New York, Public Affairs Committee, 1974.
Insulin as a nasal spray. *Am J Nurs* 1987 Aug; 87(10):1011.
Johnson S: Facts about precocious puberty. Office of Research & Reporting at the National Institute of Child Health and Human Development, Room A32, Bld. 31, 9000 Rockville Pike, Bethesda, MD 20205, 1983.
Kaplan SA: Disorders of the adrenal cortex. *Pediatr Clin North Am* 1979; 26:65–75.
Loman D, Galgani C: Monitoring diabetic children's blood-glucose levels at home. *MCN* 1984;9(3):192.
Loridan L, Senior B: Cushing's disease in infancy. *J Pediatr* 1969; 75:349–353.
Money J: Psychologic counseling: hermaphroditism. *In* Gardner LI (ed): *Endocrine and Genetic Diseases of Childhood and Adolescence.* 2nd ed. Philadelphia, WB Saunders, 1975.
Money J, Erhardt A: *Man and Woman, Boy and Girl.* Baltimore, Johns Hopkins University Press, 1972.

Money J: *Sex Errors of the Body.* Baltimore, Johns Hopkins University Press, 1969.

Nayle P: *What's Happening to Me?* Secaucus, NJ: Lyle Stuart, 1973.

Owens RP, Root AW: Growth hormone deficiency. Human Growth Foundation, 4930 W. 77th St., P.O. Box 20253, Minneapolis, MN 55420, 1979.

Parks BR, Fischer RG: Growth hormone. *Pediatr Nurs* 1986 Jul/Aug; 12(4):302.

Phifer KG: *Growing Up Small.* Middlebury, VT, Paul S. Ericksson Co, 1979.

Schneier RL, Tenore A: Hypothyroidism and the infant. Arthur Retlaw and Associates, Inc., Suite 2080, 1603 Orrington Avenue, Evanston, IL 60201, 1981.

Short stature and dwarfism . . . why some kids grow up to be small. Human Growth Foundation, Maryland Academy of Science Bldg, 7 W. Mulberry St., Baltimore, MD 21201.

Stabler B, Whitt Jk, Moreault DM, et al: Social judgements by children of short stature. *Psychol Rep* 1980; 46:743–746.

Tyrrell JB, Brooks RM: Cushing's disease. *N Engl J Med* 1978; 298:753–756.

Waxman S: *What Is a Girl? What Is a Boy?* Culver City, CA, Peace Press, 1976.

Zimmerman E, et al: Diabetic camping: Effect on knowledge, attitude, and self-concept. *Issues Compr Pediatr Nurs* 1987; 10(2):99–111.

Nursing Strategies: Altered Metabolic Function

Chapter 50

Eleanor Pask
Claire Smith

There are hundreds of diseases classified as metabolic disorders that affect children in a variety of ways. It would be impossible to attempt in this text to present any great number of them in depth. This chapter identifies the general categories of aminoacidopathies, organic acidopathies, carbohydrate and mineral disorders, and storage diseases and highlights one or two of the more common disorders in each general category. The major emphasis lies in exploring the range of

Nursing Process Plan
NPP: The Family in Need of Genetic Counseling, page 1987

Related Topics
Patterns of inheritance, Chapter 4
Genetic counseling, Chapter 4
Fostering self-esteem, Chapter 16
Impact of chronic illness, Chapter 25
Impact of death and dying, Chapter 26
Mental retardation, Chapter 34

diseases, including the impact on, and implications for, the child's and family's lifestyle. The nurses's role is stressed in the areas of early and ongoing assessment, the provision of guidance, teaching and support appropriate to the child's age and development, and the family's needs. The chapter summarizes the medical and multidisciplinary management of inborn errors of metabolism, necessary to help the child and family achieve and maintain as normal a life as possible.

Metabolic disorders tend to be very complex in nature; the causative defect is usually irreversible, and they present in a range or continuum from the very mild to the extremely profound. Some diseases can now be detected prenatally or in the very early postnatal stages by screening, but the vast majority of inherited metabolic diseases remain undetectable until they present with more overt signs. It is unfortunate that even then, many of these diseases are not accurately diagnosed because of the obscure nature of their presentation and because of the fact that so many of them mimic more readily diagnosed and more common disorders.

The incidence of inborn errors tends to vary not only between countries but also within them. For some diseases, the incidence is not known. Each disease tends to be chronic or lifelong in nature, with many of them necessitating treatment in the form of dietary management, medication, or a combination of both. Sometimes only the control of symptoms, rather than the actual treatment of the disease, can be achieved.

Amino Acid Disorders

The disorders of amino acid metabolism are the classic inborn errors of metabolism (Nyan, 1967). Raine (1979) listed 269 diseases as *inborn errors of metabolism* and concluded that only about 14 per cent of them were known to be associated with a generally acceptable method of treatment. In order to understand the range and complexity of amino acid disorders, it is essential that the nurse have a basic knowledge of protein metabolism.

Normal Protein Metabolism

The metabolic pathways involved in amino acid metabolism are intricate and multiphased. Each step is assisted by a very specific enzyme and, in many cases, by a co-enzyme. If either of these is absent or is decreased in amount or efficiency, the amino acid cannot be metabolized properly. The metabolite that is directly blocked will build up, causing symptoms, or it will be directed through a secondary pathway that may cause pathologic levels of another substance that in turn, produces symptoms.

Proteins are derived almost entirely from animal products and vegetables. In the stomach, the enzyme pepsin splits protein into peptides, peptones, and large polypeptides (Fig. 50-1). In the upper small intestine, pancreatic enzymes, such as trypsin, chymotrypsin, and carboxypeptidase, break these down further to smaller polypeptides and a few amino acids. In the epithelial cells of the small intestine, enzymes called peptidases hydrolyze the polypeptides to amino acids. There are 24 amino acids present in the body. Fifteen of these are nonessential, which means that the body can synthesize them. Nine are essential and must be provided in the diet (Box 50-1).

Box 50-1
Essential Amino Acids and Their Sources

THE NINE ESSENTIAL AMINO ACIDS

Threonine	Valine	Tryptophan
Leucine	Methionine	Isoleucine
Lysine	Phenylalanine	Histidine

- Arginine, cystine, and (perhaps) taurine are essential amino acids for infants of low birth weight.

"COMPLETE PROTEINS": SOURCES OF ESSENTIAL AMINO ACIDS

Animal proteins such as:

Meat	Fish
Eggs	Milk

"INCOMPLETE PROTEINS": SOURCES THAT DO NOT SUPPLY ALL THE ESSENTIAL AMINO ACIDS

Vegetable proteins such as:

Peas	Beans
Cereals	Nuts

(Compiled from Barness, 1987.)

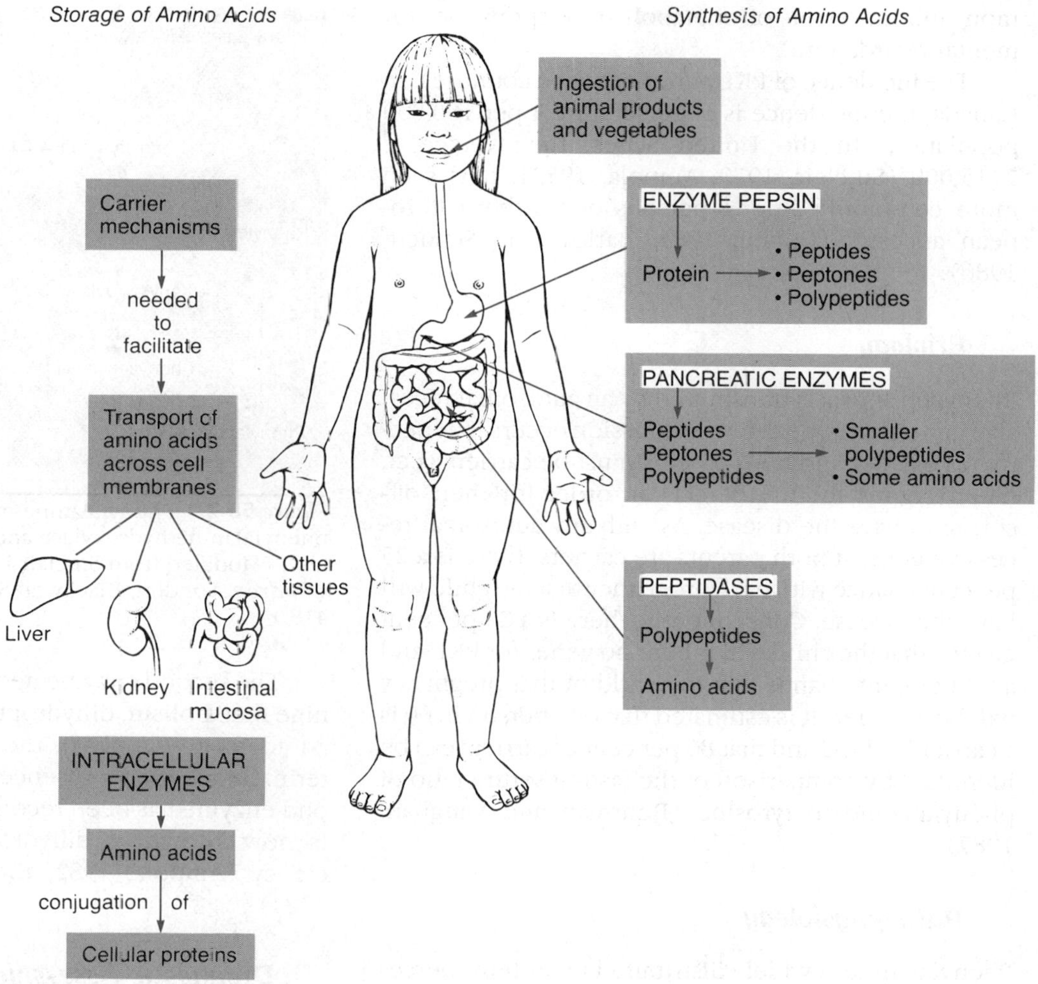

***Figure* 50-1.** Normal protein metabolism.

After a meal, blood amino acid levels rise slightly for 5 to 10 minutes before the amino acids are absorbed by the cells throughout the entire body. Amino acids do not diffuse easily through cell membranes, and their conveyance is facilitated by active transport mechanisms utilizing carriers. Once in the cells, most of the amino acids are conjugated into cellular protein. This means that the actual level of cellular free amino acids remains constant. When plasma concentrations being to drop even slightly, intracellular proteins are reverted to amino acids and are immediately transported out of the cell into the blood stream, where they will be utilized (Guyton, 1987).

This has been a very simplified statement concerning protein metabolism and amino acid production, which is actually a complex process; the reader is referred to a text that deals with anatomy and physiology for in-depth study.

Although a great many rare and obscure inherited metabolic disorders have as their basis a defect in amino acid metabolism, a few prototypes, such as *phenylketonuria* (PKU), because of screening capabilities, relatively high incidence, and the availability of management, are better known than the others. The ultimate measure of the success or failure of treatment of these diseases, classified as inborn errors of metabolism, is the extent to which all aspects of the child's development, growth, and quality of life are improved. Biochemical normalization is only one criterion (Watts, 1982).

Phenylketonuria and maple syrup urine disease (MSUD) are discussed within this section. Nursing diagnoses and strategies specific to these disorders are presented; in-depth coverage of diagnoses and strategies common to metabolic disorders can be found in the nursing care sections beginning on page 1985.

Phenylketonuria

Phenylketonuria is the most common of the amino acidopathies (Sansaricq, 1985). It is a genetically transmitted defect in metabolism of the amino acid phenylalanine. First discovered in 1939, it is the most common inborn error of metabolism responsible for mental retardation.

The incidence of PKU varies between countries. In Canada, the incidence is 1:16,000 or 6.4 per 100,000 population. In the United States, the average is 1:15,000 (Sinclair, 1979; Ampola, 1982). It is seen more commonly among persons of Northern European ancestry (Cohen, 1984; Barlow and Schuett, 1986).

Etiology

Phenylketonuria is transmitted by an autosomal recessive gene; that is, genetic transmission occurs irrespective of gender and both parents must be carriers (i.e., heterozygous for the defect) in order for their offspring to have the disease. As with any autosomal recessive gene, if both parents are carriers, there is a 25 per cent chance with each pregnancy that the child will have the disease. Consequently, there is a 25 per cent chance that the child will inherit no genes for PKU and a 50 per cent chance that the child of that pregnancy will be a carrier. It is estimated that one person in 60 is a carrier for PKU and that 80 per cent of carriers can be identified by comparison of the fasting serum ratio of phenylalanine to tyrosine (Behrman and Vaughan, 1987).

Pathophysiology

Phenylalanine is widely distributed in protein sources and is therefore liberally consumed. Normally, the phenylalanine that is not needed for protein synthesis is converted to tyrosine (Fig. 50-2). Tyrosine, in turn, is important to the synthesis of melanin, thyroxine, and the catecholamines. In order for phenylalanine to be converted to tyrosine, two enzymes must be present. The first is the liver enzyme, phenylalanine hydroxylase. If this enzyme is absent, the degradation of phenylalanine does not occur and *classic PKU* results. If it is present but occurs in insufficient amounts, a *variant of PKU* results, with symptoms related to the proportionate deficiency.

In the absence (or reduction) of phenylalanine hydroxylase, the serum levels of phenylalanine rise to toxic levels. In addition, as shown in Figure 50-2, phenylethylamine, phenylpyruvic acid, and other metabolites are formed. The increase in serum phenylalanine and its metabolites interferes with normal protein metabolism. The major adverse effect of this process is brain damage. Since the brain is still developing within the first year of life, it needs a normal pool of amino acids from which to build tissue and may be irreversibly damaged by blood and cerebrospinal fluid (CSF) that contain distorted patterns of amino acids (Gröer and Shekleton, 1983).

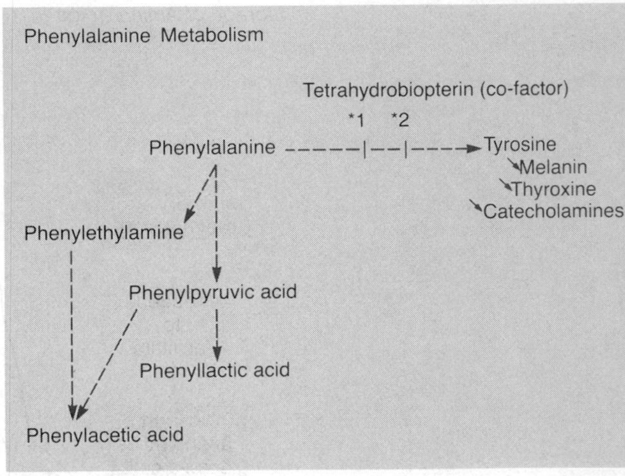

Figure 50-2. Phenylalanine metabolism. Enzymes: phenylalanine hydroxylase and dihydropteridine reductase. (Modified from Sinclair L: *Metabolic Diseases in Children.* London, Blackwell Scientific Publications, 1979, 418.)

The second enzyme needed for normal phenylalanine metabolism, dihydropteridine reductase, insures an adequate supply of the co-factor tetrahydrobiopterin. Reduction or absence in the amount of this second enzyme has been recognized as the cause of what is now known as dihydropteridine reductase deficiency (Ampola, 1982; Bickel et al., 1980; Güttler, 1984).

Diagnostic Assessment

Neonatal screening of newborn babies for inborn errors of metabolism is one of the most exciting advances in pediatric prophylaxis. With the Guthrie test, in which only a few drops of blood are required, the diagnosis of PKU can be made and treatment in the form of a low-phenylalanine formula implemented before irreversible brain damage occurs. The screening, which is a recognized practice in Canada and the United States, should be done anytime from 72 hours to 7 days after birth. Prior to 72 hours, the amount of phenylalanine in the infant's diet has not been sufficient to cause an accumulation. Research has shown that when screening is done within the first 24 hours of life, 16.1 per cent of PKU cases are missed because phenylalanine blood levels are not yet elevated. Screening that was performed between 24 to 48 hours after birth resulted in 2.2 per cent of PKU cases being missed; when screening was done between 48 and 72 hours, 0.3 per cent of cases were missed (Scriver, 1982).

Nurses' responsibility to alert parents, educators, and other health care professionals of the necessity for PKU screening is increasing. Shorter hospital stays, in which the mother may be discharged prior to 72 hours, and an increase in the number of home births are presenting new challenges. Prenatal educators must begin to include information about PKU screening in their parent education programs. Mothers who are planning home deliveries must accept responsibility for requesting the physician or community health nurse to do the screening. For community health nurses to perform PKU screening in the home, it is imperative that the referral be sent to them immediately after the birth of the child.

Clinical Manifestations

Classic PKU

Classic PKU develops in the absence of the enzyme phenylalanine hydroxylase. Infants are normal at birth but begin to show symptoms within the first months of life if untreated. Progressive mental deterioration results; only one child in 20 will have an intelligence quotient (IQ) score greater than 60 by the age of 4 years. It has been estimated that during the first year of life without treatment, a child with PKU loses 50 points on the IQ scale (Rezvani and Auerbach, 1987).

Although brain damage is the most serious effect, other signs and symptoms develop concurrently. Perhaps one of the most classic signs is the musty odor created by the excretion of phenylalanine metabolites in the urine and sweat.

In addition, hypopigmentation of hair, skin, and eyes develop because of the infant's inability to produce melanin. Eczematous skin lesions occur in 25 per cent of untreated children. Seizures also occur in one of every 4 affected children, and 80 per cent go on to show abnormal encephalographic (EEG) results. Behavioral problems develop, and the child becomes hyperactive, agitated, and aggressive (Stanbury et al., 1978). If the child remains untreated, muscular hypertonicity, tremor, microcephaly, prominent maxilla, widened interdental space, enamel hypoplasia, decalcification of the long bones, and decreased rate of growth become evident.

Variants of PKU

Variants have recently become a very important part of the entire PKU spectrum. PKU is not one disease with clearly defined boundaries. It includes variations that are all related to phenylalanine metabolism but that require variations in treatment and affect the patient to different degrees. These variants are becoming increasingly important as knowledge of the disease increases. Table 50-1 compares the levels of enzyme activity in classic PKU and its variants.

Atypical PKU. The enzyme phenylalanine hydroxylase is present but in smaller amounts, as shown in Table 50-1. The children affected by this type of PKU do not have the hypopigmentation of classic PKU; if they remain untreated, a milder degree of mental retardation develops. Since some enzyme activity is present, these children can tolerate a diet higher in phenylalanine (Ampola, 1982; Nyan, 1967).

Benign Persistent PKU. The greater phenylalanine hydroxylase activity in this form of the disease allows the affected child to follow a normal diet and to remain free of special treatment. Careful long-term follow-up of several of these patients revealed entirely normal mental development (Ampola, 1982). Although the child may be relatively free of symptoms, it is extremely important to recognize this variant of PKU, especially in girls, because during pregnancy the fetal level of phenylalanine rises to a level twice that of the mother. Dietary management and medical supervision are essential at that time to prevent mental retardation and other anomalies in the infant.

Transient PKU. This variant occurs in premature neonates. The infant has a higher than normal level of phenylalanine that persists for a few days, although the levels are not sufficiently high to cause any damage. Phenylalanine accumulation in this condition is due to tyrosine accumulation, which in turn is due to the immaturity of tyrosine oxidation in the premature infant. The phenylalanine and tyrosine levels return to normal when the infant's ability to oxidize tyrosine matures (Behrman and Vaughan, 1987).

Dihydropteridine Reductase Deficiency. This variant was previously considered to be a relatively rare form of PKU. A high level of phenylalanine is present shortly after birth. The infants continue to deteriorate neurologically in spite of regular treatment with a low-phenylalanine diet. Special treatment with neurotransmitter precursors, such as 5-hydroxytryptophan, L-dopa and carbidopa, has been beneficial in some cases.

Maternal PKU. In 1957, Dent documented that mentally retarded babies without PKU were born to mothers with PKU. Later Denniston (1966) reported

Table 50-1. Comparison of the Enzyme Activity and Phenylalanine Levels of Phenylketonuria (PKU) and Its Variants

Type of PKU	Phenylalanine Level	Enzyme Activity
Normal	0 mmol/L	Normal
Classic	2.5–3.75 mmol/L	0%
Atypical	1.24 mmol/L	10–15%
Persistent benign	0.125–0.25 mmol/L	35–40%
Transient	>0.625 mmol/L	?
Maternal		
Mother	0.3125 mmol/L	Variable
Baby	0.625 mmol/L	Normal

(Summarized from Güttler, 1984.)

mental retardation among all offspring of several institutionalized women with PKU. Maternal PKU differs from the other types because it is not an autosomal recessive disorder and therefore is not a true variant. It occurs when the mother with either a classical or variant type of PKU has a high level of phenylalanine in her blood. This results in a phenylalanine level for the fetus that is twice that of the mother.

This syndrome presents major problems. Only a few years ago, most women of childbearing age with PKU were mentally retarded and only a few bore children. Now, routine screening and early treatment have resulted in normal intelligence among many females with PKU (Dobson 1977). Given average reproduction rates, however, the frequency of new PKU related mental retardation could return to its former level after only one generation if mothers with PKU are not treated during pregnancy (Kirkman, 1979).

The offspring of mothers with PKU can suffer severe results from continued exposure to high fetal levels of phenylalanine, including microcephaly (75 per cent), congenital anomalies (17 per cent), mental retardation (88 per cent), fetal wastage (23 per cent), and intrauterine growth retardation (30 per cent) (Hanley and Bell, 1982). The defects are in proportion to the degree of elevation of phenylalanine in the maternal blood. In order to minimize the infant's risk of defects, it is recommended that the mother maintain a low-phenylalanine diet prior to conception as well as throughout pregnancy (Barnico and Cullinane, 1985) in order to keep the phenylalanine level at approximately 0.3125 mmol/L. The fetal level can then be maintained at a safe level of 0.625 mmol/L.

Therapeutic Management

Treatment must be initiated within the first weeks of life to prevent brain damage. The objective of treatment of the aminoacidopathies involving essential amino acids is to balance the amino acid needs for normal growth and development against the dangers of amino acid accumulation. In this regard, phenylalanine is an essential amino acid; therefore, enough must be supplied to ensure protein synthesis but accumulation of excess phenylalanine must be prevented.

Dietary treatment ensures a restricted intake of phenylalanine during infancy and early childhood when nervous tissue is still developing. Several low-phenylalanine formulas are available. Breast feeding is also an option, although supplementation with a special formula may be necessary. Lofenalac (for infants) and Phenyl-Free (for older children) are currently the most commonly used formulas. They provide at least 80 to 90 per cent of protein, vitamin, and mineral requirements, and they meet at least 75 per cent of energy needs (Gellis and Kagan, 1986). These formulas have an unpleasant taste, but infants who begin them early in life usually accept them well.

Additional preparations include PKU1, PKU2, Maxamaid XP, and Maxamum XP. These formulas contain no phenylalanine and very little carbohydrate or fat, making supplementation necessary. Because the PKU formulas are designed to prevent phenylalanine accumulation within the body, none of them contains enough phenylalanine to meet body requirements. Measured quantities of milk or regular infant formula must be added to any of these formulas (Gellis and Kagan, 1986). This allows, however, for precise calculation of individual needs.

The initial goal of treatment is to lower the infant's phenylalanine level to prevent neurotoxicity. Then the infant's unique metabolic patterns are determined through frequent serum studies and detailed records of intake. Close follow-up is required and dietary adjustments will be needed throughout infancy and early childhood to allow for growth needs.

Solid foods are begun at the usual time in infants with PKU. The solid foods gradually become the source of needed phenylalanine. It is important, however, that parents and children recognize appropriate sources of this amino acid. Animal proteins, such as meat, fish, eggs, and milk, and some vegetable proteins, such as legumes, grain products, and nuts, contain high levels of phenylalanine and must be avoided. Excellent cookbooks that feature low-phenylalanine foods and formulas are available through therapeutic or special food stores and through PKU treatment centers. These centers are also often a source of supply for special formulas and can offer counseling on financial aid for the low-phenylalanine preparations, which may cost several thousand dollars per year.

Elevations in serum phenylalanine may occur secondary to physical trauma or even from minor illnesses such as influenza or ear infections (Gellis and Kagan, 1986). Parents must be educated to perform early assessment of such conditions and to seek prompt treatment.

Duration of dietary restrictions of phenylalanine is currently at issue. Whereas children previously were treated until 5 to 8 years of age, research is indicating that neurotoxicity may develop beyond this age. Gellis and Kagan (1986) reported that in a 1983 survey of diet termination practices among PKU clinics, 60 of 90 clinics recommended that the PKU diet be continued indefinitely.

Major Nursing Diagnoses for PKU

Altered nutrition: impaired metabolism of phenylalanine, related to inheritance of an autosomal recessive trait

Potential altered growth and development:

brain damage, related to the accumulation of neurotoxic levels of phenylalanine and its metabolites

Potential altered parenting: overprotection, *related to anxiety about brain damage with dietary noncompliance*

Potential disturbance in self-concept: body image, role performance, *related to*
- *eating patterns that differ radically from those of peers*
- *implications for future parenthood: (1) potential for transmitting defective gene to offspring, and (2) potential for fetal injury associated with maternal PKU*

Knowledge deficit: parents (initially); child (later), *related to*
- *normal phenylalanine metabolism and the pathophysiology of PKU*
- *relationship between phenylalanine accumulation and brain damage*
- *dietary treatment*
- *need for close medical follow-up*
- *early signs and symptoms of infection and indications for obtaining medical help*
- *ways to facilitate the child's development despite rigid dietary restrictions*
- *sources of financial, emotional, and informational support for PKU, including genetic counseling.*

Strategies for Nursing Care

Because care of children with metabolic disorders is similar in many ways, the nursing strategies sections in this chapter deal only with the care unique to each disorder. General considerations for psychosocial support of the child and family and for other nursing diagnoses common to all metabolic diseases are covered in the section entitled Nursing Care of Children with Metabolic Disorders (page 1985.).

The major nursing implications for PKU are support of the family during the crisis of diagnosis and early treatment and ongoing teaching during follow-up visits. Perhaps the greatest concern of parents is that accidental noncompliance with the PKU diet will result in brain damage. The parent of an infant has complete control of dietary intake; however, with the increased mobility of the older child, forbidden foods become an increased threat. Messer (1985), a nurse who is the mother of a child with PKU, designed a T-shirt for her toddler son with the words, "Please don't feed me. I'm on a special diet." This reminder to well-meaning neighbors and day care settings allowed the normal parent-child separations that are important to the developmental needs for independence. Messer also described the need to involve her son, now a preschooler, in his dietary management. Box 50-2 contains an excerpt of her strategies.

> Box 50-2
>
> *Managing PKU: A Parent's Perspective*
>
> Our long-term goal is self-management; therefore, Ethan actively participates in dietary control. He helps prepare his "special milk," a phenylalanine-free formula produced by Mead Johnson Laboratories and supplied for a fee by the Public Health Department. He participates in menu planning and weighs his foods before serving. He is also well-versed on which foods have "big," "medium," and "little phe's" (short for phenylalanine). He is incorporating big, medium, and little veggie phe's into his repertoire since, for example, potatoes and broccoli have many more phe's than carrots and green beans. Others, like peas and beans, are in the "super big phe" list of foods, like chicken and peanut butter, that he cannot have.
>
> Ethan also uses a musical calculator for adding his daily phe's and recently has started counting phe's with an abacus we designed together. Colored beads represent exchanges of foods he eats each day. The abacus provides a visual overview of his diet plan. He cannot eat too much of even "little phe" foods unless he eats more "free" foods and/or less of something else. We purchase many of these free foods by mail and use a special wheat starch to bake special foods.
>
> *(From Messer, 1985.)*

The ideal outcome is that the child with phenylketonuria will enjoy normal growth and development and will achieve self-management. Nursing strategies in support of this goal include availability for ongoing support and information through regular follow-up visits in the home or clinic, referral to PKU parent support groups, collaboration with the school nurse or teachers, and referral for genetic counseling.

Nursing Strategies for Follow-up Care in the Home or Clinic

Obtain a blood sample for determination of phenylalanine levels as indicated.

Measure height and weight, and plot on the growth chart; alert the physician if there is failure to maintain the percentile established by the birth weight.

Review the record of dietary intake with the family. Take this opportunity to assess adjustment to the treatment plan; encourage questions and clarify misconceptions.

Assess the child's development, paying particular attention to the sense of autonomy and the self-concept, both of which will be important to eventual self-management.

Support the family's self-management by reinforcing effective techniques, and by asking them to share their expertise with other families.

Maple Syrup Urine Disease

Maple syrup urine disease is an autosomal recessive disorder of metabolism. The genetic defect results in a lack of the enzymes needed for normal metabolism of three essential amino acids, leucine, isoleucine, and valine. When these amino acids are not metabolized normally, they and their corresponding keto acids accumulate in the blood and body tissues, causing the classic maple sugar smell in the urine and resulting in disrupted protein synthesis needed for brain development. If treatment is not initiated within the first week of life, irreversible damage to the central nervous system will result.

Although MSUD is rare, with an incidence of 1 : 350,000, it occurs across ethnic groups and may be the most commonly encountered primary metabolic disease in the intensive care setting (Sansaricq, 1985). Among Pennsylvania Mennonites, however, the incidence has been estimated to be as high as 1 in 176 live births (Cohen, 1984). The nurse generalist should be aware of this disorder because it can be recognized during diaper changes by the classic maple sugar (or burned sugar) smell of the urine, sweat, and ear cerumen. There are severe consequences for the infant if this early sign is missed.

Clinical Manifestations of Classic MSUD

In classic MSUD three essential amino acids—leucine, isoleucine, and valine—as well as their respective keto acids accumulate within the body because of an inborn error in metabolism. This results in profound effects on neurologic tissue. Within the first week of life, the infant begins to feed poorly, starts to vomit, develops a high-pitched cry, and displays altered muscle tone (either hypertonic or hypotonic). As the unmetabolized amino acids continue to accumulate, the infant's condition deteriorates and seizures develop. If untreated, coma and death will follow. Even with vigorous treatment initiated within the first week of life, children may be severely affected with neurologic damage and retardation. Few patients achieve normal physical and intellectual development (Ampola, 1982).

Therapeutic Management

It is imperative, in light of the rapidity of onset and the severity of symptoms of MSUD, that treatment begin as soon as possible. Peritoneal dialysis may be required to clear the amino acids and keto acids from the body quickly. In order to prevent reaccumulation, the infant is fed a diet low in leucine, isoleucine, and valine (the branched chain amino acids, BCAA). MSUD Formula, a preparation without BCAA, is available from Mead Johnson Laboratories. However, because these BCAAs are among the nine essential amino acids, small amounts of them must be added to the diet. The exact amounts must be carefully titrated according to BCAA plasma levels. As the infant grows, foods low in protein, such as fruits, certain vegetables, and cereals, are added to the diet in order to provide the prescribed amount of protein necessary to promote normal growth.

Periods of illness can be especially serious for the child with MSUD. Gluconeogenesis (protein synthesis from stored amino acids and glycerol) is a component of the body's stress response, including the stress of illness. Because enzyme dysfunction in MSUD prevents metabolism of the BCAAs, serum levels of leucine, isoleucine, and valine may rise in response to illness. Early signs of rising BCAA serum levels include irritability, ataxia, and clumsiness in walking (Cohen, 1984).

Parents can become expert in detecting prodromal signs and symptoms of illness in their child if given adequate information and proper reinforcement for their efforts. These prodromal cues include such things as unusual tiredness; lack of interest in eating, play, and other routine activities; flushing of the cheeks; a dulled appearance to the eyes; and general lethargy. If health care professionals are alerted early, the child can sometimes be placed on a treatment regimen (e.g., antibiotic therapy) for the illness before serum levels of BCAA begin to rise.

Intermittent MSUD

In intermittent MSUD, the enzyme activity is approximately 8 to 15 per cent of normal. The infant or child remains symptom-free except during an illness, trauma, or periods of unusually high protein intake when the symptoms mimic those of classical MSUD. At these times, the child requires treatment with a low-protein diet.

Strategies for Nursing Care

Nursing implications and major nursing diagnoses for MSUD are very similar to those for PKU. The nurse's primary roles lie in assessment of MSUD by detecting urine odor during the first week of life, supporting the family during the diagnostic period, and providing ongoing availability for support and information during follow-up visits. The family should be made aware of opportunities for genetic counseling, especially in light of the availability of tests for carrier identification.

Mineral Disorders

There are several disorders associated with the metabolism of minerals. Two diseases involving copper will serve as prototypes, *Wilson disease* and *Menkes disease.* Wilson disease is caused by a defect in copper metabolism and results in the accumulation of *excess* copper in various tissues in the body, including the brain. Menkes disease is associated with *too little* copper in the system. These diseases and symptoms are diverse, but both require extensive lifelong management. Both can result in conditions that range from nearly asymptomatic to profoundly affected, and even death.

Wilson Disease

The nursing care of a patient with Wilson disease is probably as challenging as any nursing can be. There is virtually no body system that remains unaffected, and intense support is needed when the symptoms are at their worst. The initial symptoms may appear anytime from the first to the fifth decade of life. Rarely, however, does evidence of Wilson disease present before a patient is 4 years of age (Rennert, 1986).

Etiology

Wilson disease is an autosomal recessive disease with an incidence of 1 : 200,000. It is slightly more common in males. The cause is thought to be a basic defect in the hepatic synthesis of ceruloplasmin (a protein necessary for copper transport). Normal copper values are between 80 to 120 ug/100 dl, with 95 per cent of the copper being bound to ceruloplasmin.

Clinical Manifestations

In the absence of adequate ceruloplasmin, serum copper levels are low and copper accumulates within the liver, brain, and cornea, leading to the *classic triad of cirrhosis, neurologic abnormalities, and Kayser-Fleischer rings of the cornea.* Renal involvement may occur, leading to a defect of the proximal renal tubules (Behrman and Vaughan, 1987).

The *liver,* which is *the organ predominantly affected in children,* becomes cirrhotic. Hemolytic anemia and jaundice may develop, and severely compromised liver function and liver disease result.

Neurologic manifestations are extremely distressing and may include spasticity, rigidity, drooling of saliva, dysarthria, dysphasia, and painful muscle spasms. In another neurologic form of Wilson disease, although rare in children, the rigidity or spasticity may be replaced by flapping tremors of the wrists and shoulders. These can be extremely disabling, preventing the patient from any self-care. It is important to realize that the mental capacity remains intact, although the patient may have a masklike expressionless face, drool, and experience a variety of communication, personality, and psychiatric problems (Sass-Kortsak et al., 1978).

In the eye, Kayser-Fleischer rings form, with small brown granules appearing in the limbus or border of the cornea. Cataracts have also been reported in some untreated patients (Gellis and Kagan, 1986).

Therapeutic Management

Without treatment, the progression of the disease is relentless. The removal of circulating copper can be accomplished by the administration of chelating agents (Sass-Kortsak and Bearn, 1978). Initially, with treatment, as the copper is freed from the deposits, the symptoms may worsen. Patients and families need a great deal of support during these very early distressing days when things seem to be getting worse instead of better. With continued medication and removal of excess copper through chelation, the symptoms will decrease and the child should be able to return to a normal existence. The presence of residual symptoms depends almost entirely on the degree of damage that occurred to organs prior to diagnosis and the implementation of treatment.

Dietary restriction of copper may also be prescribed to minimize copper deposits within the body. Foods that should be avoided because of their high copper content are liver, nuts, chocolate, cocoa, mushrooms, brain, shellfish, and broccoli (Rennert, 1986).

Strategies for Nursing Care

Nursing care for the child with Wilson disease focuses upon the system or systems involved secondary to the accumulation of copper. Classically, care will be focused upon liver disease. Liver transplant may soon be a considered treatment that will bring new nursing challenges. Detailed nursing interventions specific to each system may be found within the appropriate chapters of this text.

Menkes Disease

Menkes disease (also known as kinky hair or steely hair syndrome) was first recognized by Menkes and his associates (1962). The condition is caused by an X-linked recessive trait affecting only males and is extremely rare. The major defect is the inability to absorb copper from the gastrointestinal tract. There is no defect in the transport of copper or in the binding of copper with ceruloplasmin (its transport mechanism).

Clinical Manifestations

Often a baby with Menkes disease is born prematurely but with weight appropriate for its gestational age. During infancy, the infant feeds slowly, shows poor weight gain, and has a tendency toward hypothermia. By 4 to 6 weeks of age, drowsiness and lethargy may begin insidiously and progressive neurologic deterioration becomes evident. Characteristics of the hair are significant for diagnosis. At birth the hair appears normal but the secondary growth lacks luster, is depigmented, and looks and feels like steel wool (Sass-Kortsak and Bearn, 1978).

Therapeutic Management

Attempted treatment for this disorder involves the parenteral administration of copper to bypass the basic gastrointestinal defect. Parents can be instructed to administer this medication at home. Most of the damage occurring in this disease, however, appears to be prenatal and is irreversible. Severe cerebral degeneration and arterial changes usually lead to death within the first year of life.

Strategies for Nursing Care

Because of the terminal nature of Menkes disease, nursing care involves helping the family deal with the diagnosis and the impending loss of their infant. Nursing strategies include assessment of the family's resources for physical and emotional support, referral to supporting agencies as needed, referral for genetic counseling, and provision of information about the disease and about nursing care for the infant with impairment of neurologic and vascular function. Supporting information can be found in the chapters of this text related to neurologic and cardiovascular impairment; in Chapter 26, Impact of Death and Dying; and Chapter 31, Nursing Care During Hospitalization. (See especially Table 31-2, Nursing Process Plan: The Hospitalized Child.)

Rickets

Rickets is a failure in mineralization of bone resulting in deformities of limbs, retarded bone growth, and shortened stature. Although rickets may occur as a nutritional deficiency of vitamin D or because of inadequate exposure of breast-fed infants to sunlight, vitamin D deficiency is rare among infants and children in industrialized countries because of vitamin supplementation (Behrman and Vaughan, 1987). There exists, however, an increasingly large and diversified list of rachitic conditions that are genetically inherited (Scriver et al., 1982). Vitamin D–resistant rickets (familial hypophosphatemia) and vitamin D–dependent rickets will be presented as prototypes because they are the forms most commonly encountered. The pathophysiology and subsequent treatment for rickets are more easily comprehended if one understands the normal metabolism and function of vitamin D in the body.

Normal Vitamin D Metabolism

As illustrated in Figure 50-3, there are two sources of vitamin D. First, the skin contains 7-dehydrocholesterol, which is converted to vitamin D3 by skin exposure to the ultraviolet rays of the sun. The second source is dietary intake of vitamin D. Ingested vitamin D is absorbed from the intestine along with other fat-soluble vitamins and transported to the liver. In the liver, both ingested and skin-derived vitamin D are converted to an early metabolite, 25-hydroxyvitamin D (25[OH]D). This metabolite is then transported, via binding blood protein (DBP), to the kidney. The kidney relies upon serum levels of calcium, phosphate, and parathyroid hormone (PTH) to determine whether $1,25(OH)_2D$, the most active metabolite of vitamin D, is needed. If either serum calcium or serum phosphate is low or if serum (PTH) is elevated, $1,25(OH)_2D$ is formed. This metabolite is also called *calcitriol.* Calcitriol promotes the absorption of calcium and phosphate in the intestines and promotes the deposition of these minerals in bone tissue.

Etiology and Pathophysiology

Since both phosphate and calcium are involved in formation of bone, the insufficiency of either of these minerals results in rickets (Behrman and Vaughan, 1987). In *vitamin D–resistant rickets* (perhaps more aptly described as *familial hypophosphatemia*), the availability of both of these minerals is decreased. This disease is inherited via an X-linked dominant trait and thus affects some females as well as males. (See Chap-

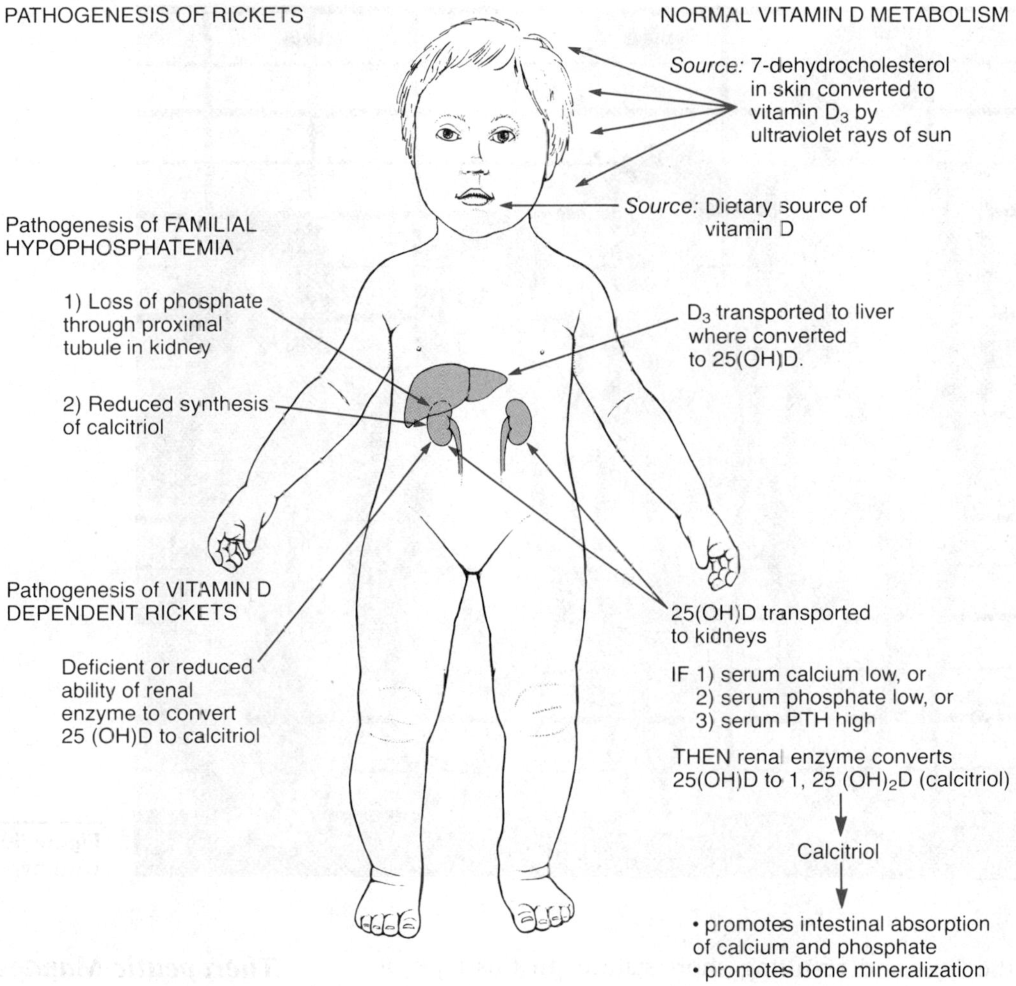
PATHOGENESIS OF RICKETS
NORMAL VITAMIN D METABOLISM
Source: 7-dehydrocholesterol in skin converted to vitamin D_3 by ultraviolet rays of sun
Source: Dietary source of vitamin D
Pathogenesis of FAMILIAL HYPOPHOSPHATEMIA
1) Loss of phosphate through proximal tubule in kidney
2) Reduced synthesis of calcitriol
D_3 transported to liver where converted to 25(OH)D.
Pathogenesis of VITAMIN D DEPENDENT RICKETS
Deficient or reduced ability of renal enzyme to convert 25 (OH)D to calcitriol
25(OH)D transported to kidneys
IF 1) serum calcium low, or
2) serum phosphate low, or
3) serum PTH high
THEN renal enzyme converts 25(OH)D to 1, 25 $(OH)_2D$ (calcitriol)
Calcitriol
• promotes intestinal absorption of calcium and phosphate
• promotes bone mineralization

Figure 50-3. Normal vitamin D metabolism and pathogenesis of common forms and genetic forms of rickets.

ter 4 for a further discussion of X-linked dominant inheritance.) For reasons that remain unclear, in familial hypophosphatemia there is a "renal leak" of phosphate through the proximal tubule, leading to decreased serum phosphate (Gellis and Kagan, 1986). In addition, synthesis of calcitriol (which is usually stimulated by hypophosphatemia) is inadequate (Fig. 50-3). Without sufficient calcitriol, the intestinal absorption of both phosphate and calcium is disrupted.

Vitamin D–dependent rickets is transmitted by autosomal recessive inheritance. The disease is characterized by poor calcium absorption owing either to the defective production of calcitriol or to the vitamin's ineffectiveness at the receptor level. Poor absorption of calcium causes a lowered serum calcium level. Phosphate levels are slightly lower than normal and alkaline phosphatase is consistently elevated (Scriver et al, 1982).

Clinical Manifestations and Diagnostic Assessment

In families with a member affected with *familial hypophosphatemia,* the physician will want to monitor all newborn infants through blood testing, since biochemical changes are evident long before physical symptoms appear. In children without a known family history of this type of rickets, the first signs may appear when the child begins weight bearing at the age of learning to walk. As hypophosphatemia and increased alkaline phosphatase levels develop, the body becomes depleted of phosphate and skeletal growth decreases. Affected children exhibit anterior bowing of

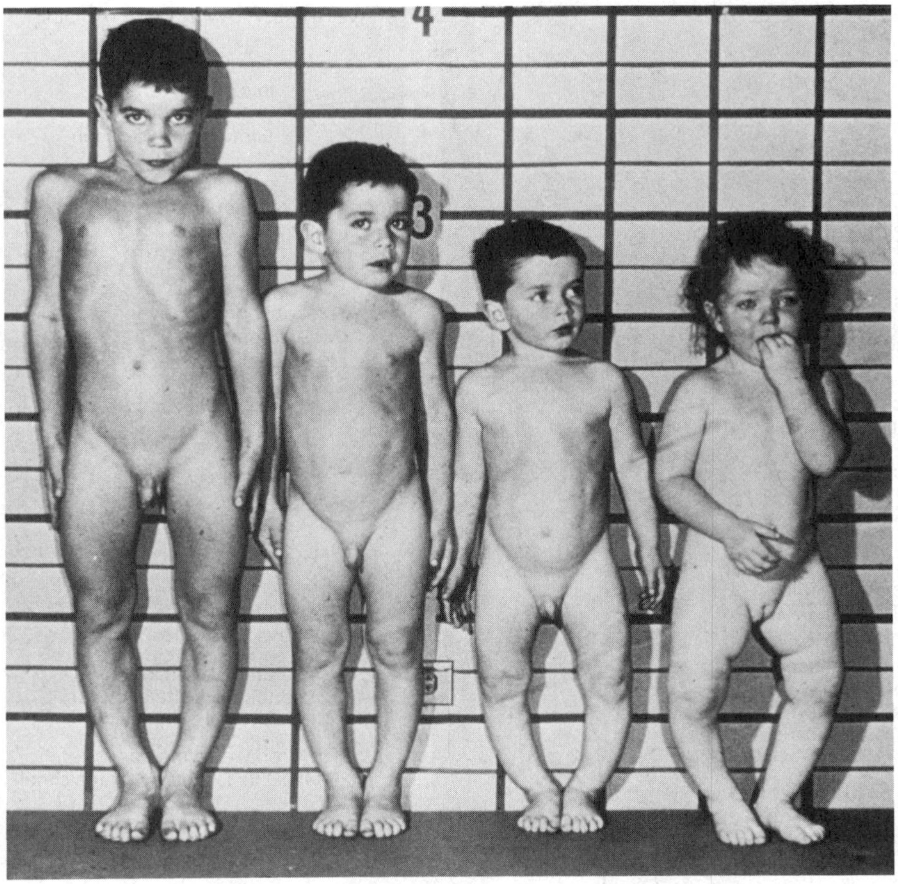

Figure 50-4. Family of four children with hypophosphatemic rickets.

the legs and resulting short stature. In this type of rickets, most of the growth failure occurs in the legs, with the rest of the body appearing relatively normal (Fig. 50-4).

In severely affected children, there may be poor dental development. There may also be skull deformities with frontal bossing, but rachitic rosary deformities (a succession of beadlike prominences along the costal cartilages) and active rickets in the pelvis and spine rarely occur. The aminoaciduria seen in true deficiency rickets is not seen in hypophosphatemic rickets (Scriver et al, 1982).

The symptoms of *Vitamin D–dependent rickets* may appear as early as the third or fourth month of life, usually before 18 months. Growth is retarded, and the infant may appear weak. There may be poor head control and an inability to stand or walk, although these signs of motor retardation may be more pronounced in some children than in others. In some instances, episodes of tetany may occur with hypocalcemic convulsions. Pathologic fractures may also occur, along with other symptoms of bone involvement, such as thickening of the wrists and ankles, beading of the ribs (rachitic rosary), and frontal bossing. Dental hypoplasia may be seen in some children. Mental retardation can occur in the absence of treatment (Ampola, 1982).

Therapeutic Management

Therapy for these two types of rickets follows directly from the metabolic defects discussed. *Familial hypophosphatemia* is treated with oral phosphate supplements and a vitamin D analog. Oral phosphate is usually given every 4 hours at least five times a day because it is quickly excreted in the urine. Diarrhea may occur as an initial side effect of oral phosphate therapy but often improves spontaneously (Behrman and Vaughan, 1987). With early diagnosis and maintenance of therapy, the bowing of long bones in the legs can be minimized; however, some children will still experience short stature (Gellis and Kagan, 1986).

Vitamin D–dependent rickets is treated with large daily doses of vitamin D or with relatively low daily doses of calcitriol. Most children respond well to this form of therapy.

Strategies for Nursing Care

Strategies for nursing care of the child with rickets (of either type) include careful assessment of growth and provision of information to facilitate home management after diagnosis. Measurement of length in infants (or height in toddlers and older children) and recogni-

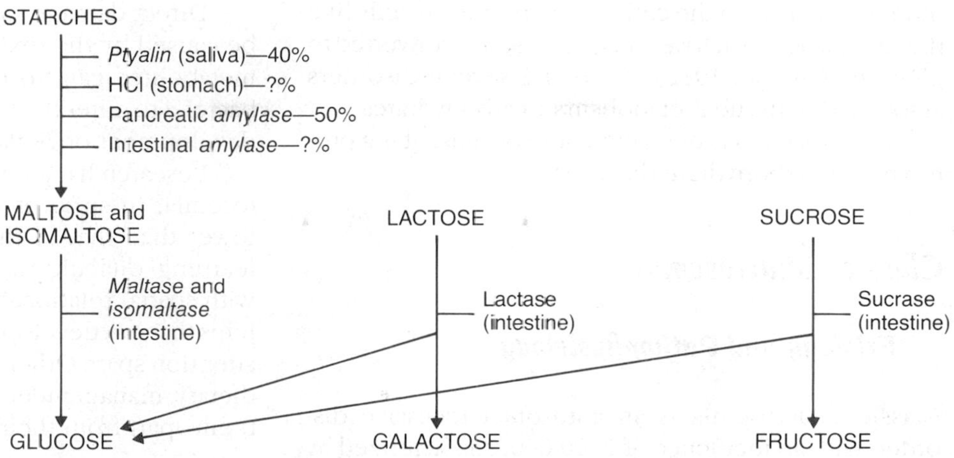

Figure 50-5. Carbohydrate metabolism. (From Guyton AC: *Human Physiology and Mechanisms of Disease.* Philadelphia, WB Saunders, 1982, 512.)

tion of the child's declining pattern on the growth chart may be the first indications of rachitic disease. It is important that this vital part of the nursing assessment not become so routine that the nurse overlooks the critical nature of the child's growth as a diagnostic tool.

Regardless of the type of rickets diagnosed, oral replacement of some form of vitamin D will be involved. Often calcitriol will be the supplement prescribed. In the early weeks of therapy, blood samples will be drawn frequently to help titrate the dosage of calcitriol to prevent hypercalcemia.* The family who is aware of the essential nature of these tests will usually be more tolerant of the inconvenience of repeated clinic visits and of the discomfort of the blood tests.

The nurse can teach the family about the need for adequate calcium in the diet of the child receiving calcitriol. Regardless of the dose of calcitriol, calcium cannot be absorbed unless it is ingested. In children 1 to 10 years of age, the recommended daily allowance (RDA) for calcium is 800 mg; in children 11 to 18 years of age, it is 1200 mg. If calcium intake is a problem because of food preferences, a calcium supplement may be prescribed.

Parents must also be advised against administering or allowing the child to take over-the-counter medications without consulting the physician. Preparations containing magnesium (e.g., some laxatives and antacids) may lead to hypermagnesemia. Vitamin preparations, in addition, should be given only at the direction of the physician, since overdosage of vitamin D must be prevented during calcitriol therapy.

* Hypercalcemia presents with abdominal or flank pain, nausea, vomiting, dry mouth, and hypotonicity of muscles. Stupor, coma, and cardiac arrest may follow.

Carbohydrate Disorders

Intolerance to the dietary disaccharides (sucrose and lactose) and to the hydrolytic products of starch (maltose) results from a deficiency of one or more of the specific intestinal mucosal enzymes responsible for their hydrolysis (Stanbury et al, 1978). Carbohydrates are either polysaccharides or disaccharides, which are combinations of monosaccharides bound together.

Normal Digestion of Carbohydrates

There are three primary sources of carbohydrates: (1) sucrose (sugar cane), a disaccharide; (2) lactose (milk sugar), a disaccharide; and (3) starch (almost all foods, particularly grains), a polysaccharide (Fig. 50-5).

Hydrolysis, or breakdown, of starches begins in the mouth, where the enzyme ptyalin (salivary amylase) is secreted by the parotid glands. The process continues in the stomach with hydrochloric acid and in the small intestine, where intestinal and pancreatic amylase complete the breakdown, until the polysaccharide has become a disaccharide, i.e., sucrose, lactose, maltose, or isomaltose. These are further digested into their constituent monosaccharides (glucose, galactose, and fructose) in the brush borders of the small intestine by their corresponding enzymes (maltase, isomaltase, lactase, and sucrase). The monosaccharides are then immediately absorbed into portal blood. They are taken up by the liver, where they are transported into the cellular cytoplasm by means of a carrier that renders them soluble in the membrane. In the cell, they combine with a phosphate radical in the process of *phosphorylation,* which is aided by enzymes called hexokinases, i.e., glucokinase, galactokinase, and fructokinase. This process tends to capture the monosaccharide in the cell, except in special cells like the liver, where fructose and galactose are converted to glucose (Guyton, 1982). There are several disorders associated with the metabolism of carbohydrates.

Galactosemia is described here because it is a prototype for carbohydrate disorders.

Classic Galactosemia

Etiology and Pathophysiology

Classic galactosemia is an autosomal recessive disorder, with an incidence of 1 : 40,000, characterized by the failure to convert galactose to glucose (Wenger, 1987). This is due to the absence of the enzyme galactose-1-phosphate uridyltransferase. This block results in the cellular accumulation of galactose-1-phosphate, galactose, and galactitol with potentially fatal effects. It has been suggested that accumulation of these galactose products may even be injurious to the fetus in utero (Wenger, 1987). If accumulation continues undetected, damage to the liver (cirrhosis) and to the brain (mental retardation) becomes increasingly severe and irreversible. Cataracts also result.

Clinical Manifestations

The morbidity and mortality resulting from classical galactosemia make prompt recognition of the clinical signs and the institution of immediate treatment imperative. In severe cases, the symptoms begin within the first days of life. In less severe cases, the symptoms may be delayed until the infant is several months of age. In some states, and in Quebec, Canada, routine screening of the newborn for galactosemia is mandatory. In other geographic areas, the move is toward mandatory screening as is done for PKU. It is a very simple test necessitating only a few drops of blood placed on a specially prepared paper mat.

The signs of galactosemia tend to mimic other diseases, with vomiting and diarrhea beginning after feeding a lactose-containing formula. The baby may fail to thrive. However, the development of jaundice that persists beyond the expected period of "physiologic jaundice" provides a more definitive sign. If the child remains untreated, progressive liver damage causes hepatomegaly, hypoglycemia, ascites, or bleeding. When systemic accumulation of galactose occurs, the sugar diffuses freely into the developing lens of the eye and is immediately converted to galactitol, which cannot diffuse out. Osmotic overhydration and swelling occur, and eventually the lens fibers are destroyed (Ampola, 1982). The cataracts that may form can be visualized through slit-lamp examination during the first few weeks of life.

Direct damage to the intestinal mucosal cell may be caused by the toxic accumulation of the abnormal metabolite, galactose-1-phosphate. This may allow bacteria to enter the blood stream with the subsequent development of *Escherichia coli* sepsis.

Research has shown that most children with galactosemia, in spite of vigorous treatment, have an IQ lower than that of their siblings. They tend to have learning difficulties, especially in mathematics and with spatial relationships. Some of the behavior problems that can develop are thought to result from a short attention span. Other problems develop relating to the dietary management, which children often feel sets them apart from their peers.

Therapeutic Management

The implementation of treatment quickly changes the course of disease. Galactose is eliminated from the diet by removing milk and milk products, which contain lactose, and by substituting a soy formula, which is free of lactose. The most commonly used soy formulas are Prosobee (Mead Johnson) and Isomil (Ross). Nutramigen, a casein hydrolysate, may also be used. The most severely affected infant will begin to show improvement almost immediately after starting the galactose-free diet. Vomiting and diarrhea subside, weight gain occurs, liver function improves, and cataracts, if not too advanced, regress (Ampola, 1982). Mental retardation, unfortunately, is not reversible. There does not appear to be any correlation between the time and the severity of onset and the degree of retardation. Very early treatment may help to preserve some of the intellect; however, children with normal intellect may still experience learning disabilities. The symptoms arising from the gastrointestinal defect generally are not seen in the older child. As the child grows, lactose-containing foods are introduced into the diet. Most physicians allow limited and measured amounts of lactose in the form of milk, especially for the older child. The child with galactosemia is never allowed to have milk freely.

Major Nursing Diagnoses for Galactosemia

Altered nutrition: impairment of galactose metabolism, *related to an enzyme deficiency associated with an autosomal recessive trait*

Potential altered growth and development: mental retardation and learning disabilities, *related to neurotoxic properties of the accumulation of galactose and its abnormal metabolites*

Potential for injury: physiologic, *related to liver damage associated with hepatotoxic* *properties of the accumulation of galactose and its abnormal metabolites*

***Potential sensory-perceptual alteration: visual,** related to cataracts associated with the effect of an abnormal metabolite of galactose upon the lens of the eye*

***Potential for infection,** related to bacterial contamination of the blood through intestinal mucosal cells damaged by abnormal galactose metabolism*

***Knowledge deficit: parents (initially), child (later),** related to*
- *etiology and pathophysiology of galactosemia*
- *the need for genetic counseling*
- *galactose-free diet (including soy formula or Nutramigen)*
- *resources, including parent groups*

Strategies for Nursing Care

Nurses can aid in diagnosis of galactosemia by careful assessment and documentation of infant feeding patterns and by promptly referring the family to medical care should classic signs be reported by the parents during the postnatal period. Signs that parents may report include jaundice, feeding difficulties, vomiting, lethargy, and irritability.

As with any of the metabolic disorders, nursing support during the crisis of diagnosis can facilitate the family's adjustment. Ongoing evaluation of the child will provide ample opportunities for the nurse to continue the teaching and informational support begun at the time of diagnosis.

Dietary management can be enhanced if the parents are taught to read labels carefully. Milk solid is a common food additive, and lactose is a common filler for drug preparations (e.g., penicillin). Frequent evaluation is required throughout infancy and childhood to ensure that the diet provides adequate nutrients for optimal growth and development.

If diagnosed and treated early, liver damage and cataracts can usually be prevented. Nursing strategies will include ongoing assessment for hepatomegaly and jaundice, however, as well as attention to the child's visual acuity. The detailed section entitled Nursing Care of Children with Metabolic Disorders (see page 1985) deals with strategies related to mental retardation and learning disabilities, prevention of infection, and family teaching.

Nursing Strategies for Follow-up Care in the Home or Clinic

Obtain blood and urine specimens as indicated for evaluation of dietary compliance.

Measure height and weight, and plot on the growth chart. Alert the physician to evidence of a decrease in percentile status.

Assess for hepatomegaly and jaundice. Test visual acuity according to developmentally appropriate means (see Chapter 15).

Assess development and reinforce parenting that enhances normal development.

Collaborate with the school nurse or teacher to ensure optimum follow-up of learning disabilities, speech problems, and behavioral problems.

Mucopolysaccharide Disorders

Mucopolysaccharides are very complex carbohydrates, characteristically present in connective tissue. Mucopolysaccharides undergo sequential degradation in the lysosomes by specific enzymes. If one or more of these enzymes are deficient, degradation cannot occur and undegraded mucopolysaccharides accumulate in the cell, causing distortion of the cell architecture and interference with cell function. Accumulation of mucopolysaccharides occurs especially in connective tissue, bone, viscera, the heart, the brain, and the spinal cord (Cohen, 1984).

Mucopolysaccharidoses represent the group of disorders resulting from deficiencies of lysosomal enzymes. Taken together, these disorders account for the most common of the rare genetic disorders. All mucopolysaccharidoses are inherited by an autosomal recessive pattern except for *Hunter syndrome,* which has an X-linked recessive pattern. In general, these disorders are all progressive but vary widely in their severity. Coarse facial features are common to all, accounting for the use in the past of the term "gargoylism." There is a wide spectrum of skeletal and joint changes often associated with limitation of movement.

Table 50-2 provides the reader with a summary of some of the more common disorders and their involvement. Only *Hurler syndrome* is presented because it is a prototype for the mucopolysaccharidosis category of diseases.

Hurler Syndrome

Etiology and Pathophysiology

Hurler syndrome is characterized by lack of the enzyme alpha-1-iduronidase. The deficiency of this enzyme leads to accumulation of unmetabolized mucopolysaccharides in body tissues. The disease is transmitted by an autosomal recessive genetic trait.

Table 50-2. Mucopolysaccharidoses

Disease*		Enzyme Defect	Hepatosplenomegaly	Cardiovascular Findings	Ocular Findings	Deafness	Survival
IH Hurler		α-L-Iduronidase	2+ to 3+	2+ to 3+	3+	2+	5–10 years
IH/S Hurler-Scheie Compound		α-L-Iduronidase alleles	+	2+	3+	+/−	20s
IS Scheie		α-L-Iduronidase alleles	+/−	Aortic valve	3+	−	50s
II Hunter		Iduronate sulfatase	2+ to 3+	2+ to 3+	Corneal clouding rare	2+	10–15 years
III Sanfilippo forms (clinically indistinguishable)	A B C	*N*-Sulfamidase *N*-Acetylglucosamidase Acetyl CoA: α-glucosaminide-N-acetyltransferase	+ to 2+	−	−	+	puberty
IV Morquio		Gal-6-sulfate sulfatase	+/−	+	+	+	20–40 years

* All are inherited as autosomal recessive traits except Hunter syndrome, which is X-linked.
+/−, variable; +, minimal; 2+, moderate; 3+, marked.
(Modified from Cohn and Roth, 1983.)

Clinical Manifestations

The major clinical features associated with Hurler syndrome are mental retardation, coarse facies, skeletal and joint deformities, deafness, dwarfism, and corneal clouding (Cohen, 1984) (Fig. 50-6). Hurler syndrome is severe and progressive, leading to death, usually before the age of 10 years.

During the first year of life, the child appears normal; in the second year, however, persistent rhinorrhea, stertorous breathing, and recurrent infections of the respiratory tract and ear often develop. Slit-lamp examination reveals corneal clouding. Physical examination at that time shows lumbar kyphosis, chest deformity (barrel-shaped), and stiff joints. Thereafter, delayed growth becomes quite obvious.

Deterioration of psychomotor development proceeds relentlessly around this time, as does the progressive coarsening of facial features, along with a large head, thickened lips, and hirsutism. An enlarged tongue causes early feeding difficulties. The liver increases in size, causing a protuberant abdomen, which in turn causes discomfort and respiratory embarrassment. Deafness is quite common, and hernias occur in various sites. The skin becomes thickened, causing additional problems if intravenous therapy is required. A communicating hydrocephalus frequently develops.

Repeated respiratory infections and worsening cardiac function often necessitate repeated hospitalizations and are the usual cause of death. Unfortunately, there is no cure for Hurler syndrome; the management and control of symptoms bring only temporary relief (McKusick et al, 1978).

Strategies for Nursing Care

To provide nursing care of the child with Hurler syndrome, a comprehensive plan of care is needed that identifies the problems unique to this child and family and focuses on strategies to deal with involvement of multiple organ systems, alteration of physical and mental growth and development, and ongoing challenges to the family as they attempt to care for this child in the home environment. Because Hurler syndrome is a rare disorder, development of a comprehensive plan of care is beyond the scope of this chapter. The necessary information is available within this text, however, to assist the nurse in developing such a plan.

The child with Hurler syndrome is likely to experience respiratory difficulties, sensory problems (both visual and auditory), alterations in gastrointestinal function ranging from hepatomegaly to feeding difficulties, neurologic dysfunction (notably, hydrocephalus), and cardiovascular disorders. Strategies for nursing care involving these disorders can be found within this unit in the system-specific chapters and in the nursing process plans in those chapters. Chapter 34 presents nursing strategies for care of children who are mentally retarded. Nursing strategies to assist the nurse in support of the child and family are discussed in the nursing strategies section at the end of this chapter (see page 1985) and in the chapters dealing with care of the chronically ill child (see Chapter 25), the terminally ill child (see Chapter 26), and the hospitalized child (see Chapter 31). Table 50-3 on page 1987 provides guidelines for care of the family in need of genetic counseling.

The complex and diversified problems of the child with Hurler syndrome can challenge the nurse's scientific knowledge and skills and the nurse's "art" of therapeutic use of self. Working with a child and family in such great need for professional care, however, can bring immeasurable rewards. The plan of care would do well to include the diagnosis, *family coping: potential for growth.* Professional nursing care can be an effective catalyst for that growth process.

Nursing Care of Children with Metabolic Disorders

The nursing care of children with metabolic disorders is rewarding and challenging. The diseases, in their underlying physiology, presenting symptoms, and course, tend to be complex. Basically, they are all of a chronic nature, with most requiring some form of medication and/or dietary restriction as well as supportive measures necessary during times of exacerbation of the disease.

With each of the diseases, careful and ongoing nursing assessment of both the patient and the family, an ongoing education program structured around the family's needs, involvement of appropriate community resources, the provision of support over a long period of time, and assistance in the parental management of the disease are required.

Major Nursing Diagnoses

Altered family process, related to

- *the impact of diagnosis of an inborn error of metabolism*
- *the need to acquire new knowledge and skills to care for the affected child*
- *the reactions of extended family and friends to the diagnosis*
- *potentially incongruous coping patterns among family members*
- *interruption in the bonding process associated with prolonged and/or frequent hospitalizations*
- *lack of time and energy to provide for needs of all family members associated with the demands of the treatment regimen for the affected child*

Altered growth and development: mental retardation, physical disability, *related to the inborn error of metabolism*

Potential noncompliance with prescribed treatment, *related to child's reluctance to be different from peers*

Potential altered parenting, *related to reluctance to develop and enforce usual rules of behavior for the affected child*

Potential altered growth and development: emotional/social: acting out and other inappropriate behaviors, *related to*

- *ineffective and/or inconsistent discipline*
- *delays in mental and physical development*

Disturbance in self-concept: body image, self-esteem, role performance and personal identity: affected child, *related to*

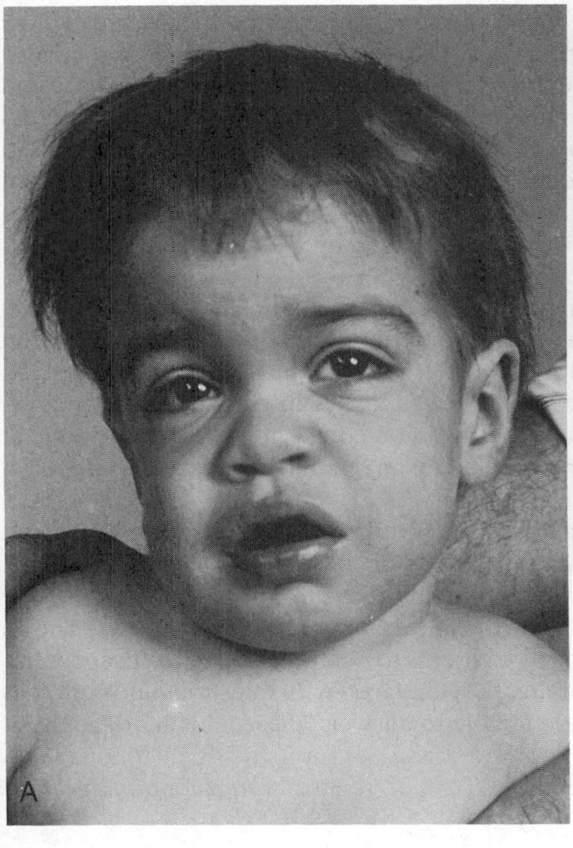

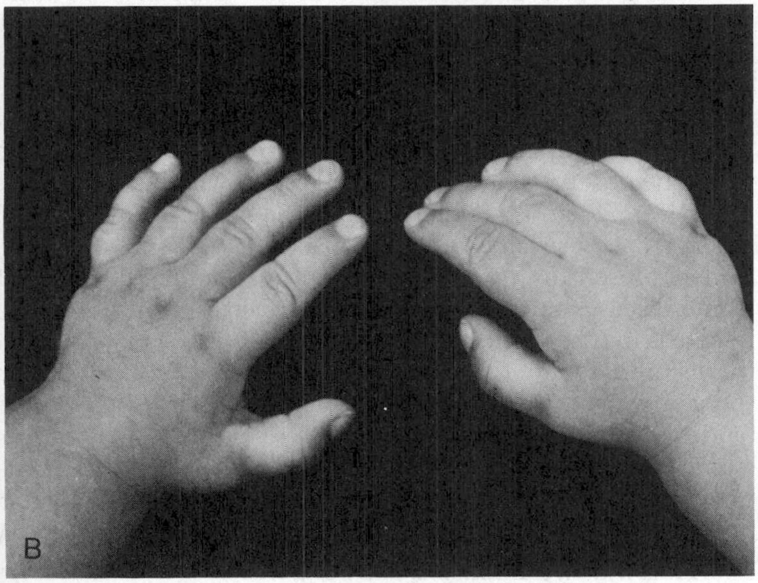

Figure 50-6. Boy with Hurler syndrome, showing coarse facial features *(A)* and joint deformities of the hands *(B)*.

- *treatment regimen that sets the child apart from peers*
- *altered body appearance associated with some inborn errors of metabolism*
- *mental retardation and/or learning disabilities*
- *reactions of significant others, friends, classmates, teachers, etc.*

Powerlessness: parent(s), related to

- *the ever-present burden of the child's illness*
- *lifestyle changes associated with the illness and treatment regimen*

***Knowledge deficit: parent(s), child, siblings,** related to chance of transmission of genetic trait for particular metabolic disorder*

Strategies for Nursing Care

Assisting with Diagnostic Assessment

Parents often compare their child's development with that of normal siblings and/or with normal relatives of the same age. If they find that their child lags behind in meeting developmental milestones, the nurse may be the first to hear the parents' concerns. These concerns should never be dismissed lightly. They may be the first clue to some obscure disorder. A sound knowledge of norms for growth and development is essential to making a careful physical assessment (Chapter 3 deals with principles of development, Unit 2 covers aspects of growth and development for children at various ages, and Chapter 15 details the use of developmental assessment tools.)

Effective physical assessment necessitates that the nurse be observant and be a good listener, with keen interviewing and assessment skills. The nurse is encouraged to use all senses because metabolic disorders present in a variety of ways. For example, in some diseases there are characteristic facial features whereas in others, the skin, hair, hands, or limbs may be visibly different. In still other disorders, a particular odor provides the clue to diagnosis. The child's growth and body proportions are important to observe. In some cases, the limbs may be too short; in others, they may be too long.

Helping the Family Deal with the Lifelong Nature of the Illness

Genetic metabolic disturbances do not go away, no matter how well the disease is treated and managed. They are present until death and in some cases are the cause of death. Ongoing medical management and nursing support are imperative. Additional teaching will be necessary as new forms of treatment are unfolded through research findings. It is often very difficult for parents and patients to "let go" of one form of treatment on which they have become very dependent when a new and perhaps contradictory form of treatment is introduced, even if the latter is easier for the family. All teaching, from the very beginning, should emphasize the possibility that treatment will change with time. It is the physician's responsibility to keep the patient informed, and the nurse should be involved in the teaching, support and evaluation of the patient through the change. It is important to make ongoing, sensitive assessments of the child and the family, and to refer to community resources whenever they will benefit them. There may also be periods of time when the child will require hospitalization because of an exacerbation of the metabolic disease or a secondary disease or for investigational purposes. These bring the well-documented problems of separation and stress associated with hospitalization and must be dealt with through adequate age-appropriate preparation, support, communication, and an awareness of the impact of the event on the child and the family.

Facilitating a Healthy Family Process

The aim of nursing is to develop an ongoing primary nurse relationship with the family, to help family members develop the skills, self-esteem, and confidence necessary to care for their child, and to help the family achieve a lifestyle that is as normal as possible. Parents need to feel comfortable with their infants and to grow with them, just as do the parents of unaffected infants. It is extremely important that parents gain a sound knowledge of the flexibility of normal growth and development patterns as well as the limitations imposed by the infant's disease so that parents can be aware of developmental milestones but not become anxious if their infant fails to keep up with usual developmental standards.

In some of the disorders, such as PKU, the parents' concerns are compounded, because at the time the diagnosis is made, the infant may be asymptomatic. At such a time, there is always an element of uncertainty. Parents are faced with complying with a fairly difficult dietary regimen for an infant who looks and behaves in a normal fashion.

At this time as well, the infant may be hospitalized and the early days of the parent-infant bonding are interrupted. Families have to inform relatives that the new baby has an inborn error of metabolism. This is not easy for parents to comprehend or to accept themselves, and they are faced with questions and concerns they are unable to answer. These days are difficult for

Text continues on page 1992

Table 50-3
Nursing Process Plan: The Family in Need of Genetic Counseling

By Roxie Foster

Assessment to Identify the Need for Genetic Counseling

Physical Function (nutrition-metabolism; elimination; activity/exercise)
Intellectual-Perceptual Function (knowledge of illness, sensory-perception alterations)

Subjective Assessment

Family history of genetic disorders in recent generations; evidence of environmental hazards that could lead to or contribute to genetic disorders; ethnicity; whether proposed marital partner is blood relative (see Box 4-2 for actual assessment questions and Box 4-3 for a protocol for the genetic health history)

Objective Assessment

Variations in anatomic structure or in anatomic or physiologic function; alterations in growth and development (see Box 4-4 for a protocol for physical examination for genetic assessment)

Analysis: Nursing Diagnosis 1

Knowledge deficit, related to lack of information about the potential for a genetic disorder associated with

- a family history of a genetic disorder
- an ethnic predisposition for a genetic disorder
- evidence of significant environmental hazards
- evidence of anomalies in anatomic structure and/or in anatomic or physiologic function
- unexplained delays in growth
- unexplained delays in physical, intellectual, and/or sexual development

Defining Characteristics

Subjective: Family history of genetic disease; any abnormality affecting more than one family member; ethnic predisposition for a genetic disorder; females exposed to radiation, infectious diseases, toxic agents, or potent drugs immediately before or during pregnancy; males planning fatherhood who have been exposed to radiation, toxic agents, or potent drugs

Objective: Major congenital anomalies or the presence of two or more minor anomalies in the same child; unexplained delays in growth or disproportionate growth; unexplained delays in physical, intellectual or sexual development; blindness; deafness

Client Goal/ Evaluation Criteria	Nursing Goals/Strategies (Selected Rationale)
1. The client will have the opportunity to receive needed information in order to make informed choices about family planning as evidenced by:	*Refer the client for genetic counseling.* NOTE: The actual time for referral will depend upon the client's emotional adjustment to the actual or potential diagnosis of a heritable disorder. Often there is a delay of weeks or months between diagnosis and counseling.

Continued

Table 50-3 (continued)

Client Goal/ Evaluation Criteria	Nursing Goals/Strategies (Selected Rationale)
a. being referred for genetic counseling b. verbalizing an understanding of the types of information available through genetic counseling c. verbalizing perceptions of the feasibility of counseling in relation to location and cost	*Explain the purpose and process of genetic counseling* (to clarify the benefits to the family and to reduce anxiety about the process). • Explain that the purpose of genetic counseling is to provide information about the risk of occurrence or recurrence of a genetic abnormality. • Stress that the counselor will provide information that can help the family make their OWN decisions about future pregnancies. (Persons may be fearful of being told not to have children or not to have more children.) • Review the components of the counseling process (as applicable to the type of genetic counseling available). These are likely to be: (1) precounseling assessment, (2) estimation of risk, (3) communication of the diagnosis, recurrence risks and interventions, (4) follow-up visit. (See Chapter 4.) • Discuss with the family, as applicable, the availability of transportation and their ability to pay for counseling. (The nurse should be aware of (1) actual counseling costs [often $70 – 100] and whether a sliding scale for payment is available, and (2) availability and cost of public transportation.) *Encourage questions and verbalization of understanding of the purpose, process, and availability of genetic counseling.* *Identify health care professionals who can provide ongoing support by clarifying genetic information and by listening to feelings and concerns throughout the counseling process.*

Assessment to Identify the Impact of Diagnosis*

Emotional-Social Function (self-perception/self-concept; coping-stress-tolerance patterns; family values/beliefs, role relationships, spiritual health)

Subjective Assessment

Reported symptoms of stress; perceptions of coping ability; whether feeling in control; comfort with decision making

Objective Assessment

Somatic signs of stress; appearance; behavior; significant changes in usual activities of daily living

Analysis: Nursing Diagnosis 2

Ineffective individual coping: temporary impairment of problem-solving abilities, related to the emotional impact of the diagnosis of an actual or potential genetic disorder

Defining Characteristics

Subjective: Comments such as, "I can't think of anything else" or "I don't know how to cope with this"; reported insomnia, feelings of restlessness and anxiety, depression, excessive smoking/use of alcohol/prescription drugs, chronic fatigue, excessive sleeping, forgetfulness, gastrointestinal upsets

Objective: Shortened attention span, easily distracted; weight loss; tired, haggard appearance; lack of vitality in voice, movements, general appearance; "mechanical" aspect to behavior

* The section on emotional-social functionis applicable to care for families throughout the genetic counseling process.

Client Goal/ Evaluation Criteria	**Nursing Goals/Strategies (Selected Rationale)**
2. The client (parent/s, affected child, if not diagnosed in infancy) will become better able to cope with the diagnosis of the anomaly or genetic disorder as evidenced by: a. verbalizing feelings about the diagnosis b. seeking information to help with problem-solving c. identifying resources d. verbalizing planned use of resources	*Encourage expression of feelings about the diagnosis.* • Plan some uninterrupted periods for discussion. • Practice reflective listening (see Chapter 4). • Avoid interjecting personal biases. *Acknowledge each person's right to the feelings expressed.* • Recognize that a diagnosis which seems minor to the nurse (e.g., club foot) may carry quite a different meaning for the family. • Refrain from telling the famly that they are "lucky"; (the conditions of other children are not pertinent to this situation). *Recognize denial as a common defense mechanism in the first weeks after diagnosis.* • Repeat information in simple terms as often as necessary. • Provide written information whenever possible. (Materials that can be read at home can help persons incorporate the reality of the diagnosis and generate questions.) *Recognize grief as a common reaction to diagnosis.* (The parent/s must deal with loss of the expected healthy infant or of the presumed healthy child and must incorporate, instead, the reality of the permanent anomaly or genetic disorder. The affected child, as well, must deal with the loss of formerly perceived health status.) *Facilitate efforts toward problem-focused coping.*† • Help the client to identify family strengths and known resources for emotional, physical and financial support. • Ask if the client has considered how to tell relatives and friends about the diagnosis. Discuss ways to disseminate accurate information. • Discuss with the parent/s age-appropriate ways to tell siblings about the diagnosis. Caution parents that siblings may perceive themselves responsible if they had mixed emotions about the new infant or if normal feelings of sibling rivalry were present between siblings and the affected child. *Assess the need for referral for individual counseling or marital counseling.* (Some individuals will need more in-depth help to cope with the impact of diagnosis and its implications for future life changes. Spouses may react differently and experience discordant coping, disrupted communication patterns, and a potential threat to the marital relationship.)

† Problem-focused coping is the term used by Lazarus and Folkman (1984) to describe strategies directed at "altering environmental pressures, barriers, resources, procedures . . ." and those directed at internal "motivational or cognitive changes such as shifting the level of aspiration, reducing ego involvement, finding alternative channels of gratification, developing new standards of behavior, or learning new skills and procedures" (p 152).

Continued

Table 50-3 (continued)

Analysis: Nursing Diagnosis 3

Spiritual distress, related to
- the attempt to find meaning in the situation
- conflict between religious or spiritual beliefs and the alternatives to giving birth to children with a heritable disorder
- perceived guilt (parent/s) in having transmitted a heritable trait

Defining Characteristics

Subjective: Verbalization of powerlessness, loss of "peace of mind"; questions such as, "Why did this happen to me?"; verbalized anger at God; reported ambivalence in decision-making; verbalized feelings of "being between a rock and a hard place"

Objective: Irritability; tearfulness; distraction; significant changes in usual religious practices; somatic signs of stress

Client Goal/ Evaluation Criteria	Nursing Goals/Strategies (Selected Rationale)
3. The client will experience a renewed sense of inner peace as evidenced by: a. verbalizing feeling less anxious and more at peace b. finding strength in former religious faith c. verbalizing a rationale for decision-making d. appearing less anxious and stressful	*Acknowledge that the loss of "peace of mind" is a normal feeling in this situation.* *Help the client identify appropriate sources of support.* Ask, "Is there a member of the clergy or a special friend who can help you work through the meaning of this in your life?" (Already established, trusting relationships can provide ready support.) *Supplement the support of identified resources as needed to help the client come to terms with personal values and beliefs.* • Assess the meaning of the diagnosis for this client. (Some families see the birth of a child with a congenital anomaly or genetic disorder as a special blessing from God while others may feel they are being punished for real or imagined misdeeds.) • Encourage expression of feelings, guiding persons to discover their own truths. Avoid interjecting personal values. • Validate the normality of expressed feelings by statements such as, "Many parents (or children) tell me they feel that way." • Recognize that the affected child, sibling/s and parent/s may go back through this search for meaning from time to time in the future, especially with the transition between developmental stages.

Assessment of Ability to Make Decisions About Family Planning Based Upon Genetic Counseling

Intellectual-Perceptual Function (Knowledge of Illness)

Subjective Assessment

Verbalized level of understanding of the diagnosed genetic disorder, risks of occurrence or recurrence, availability of screening for carrier status, alternatives to giving birth to children with this heritable trait

Analysis: Nursing Diagnosis 4

Knowledge deficit, related to
- insufficient information present in genetic counseling
- confusion about information presented
- inability to integrate the information associated because of unsettled emotional state

Defining Characteristics

Subjective: States lack of understanding of one or more aspects of the information presented in genetic counseling; verbalizes misinformation; verbalizes feelings that genetic counseling did not help with decision-making; states ongoing feeling of inability to cope with decision making

Client Goal/ Evaluation Criteria

4. The client will receive help to utilize information presented in genetic counseling to facilitate problem solving, as evidenced by:
   a. verbalizing increased understanding of the diagnosis, risks, and/or interventions, as appropriate
   b. discussing alternatives to decrease the risk of occurrence or recurrence

Nursing Goals/Strategies (Selected Rationale)

Assess the reason for the knowledge deficit. (Determine whether due to insufficient information, confusion about the information presented, or unsettling emotions that prevent integration of the information.

Intervene to address the underlying problem.
- Clarify what information was presented (to determine if the client failed to receive the information or failed to comprehend it). Ask the family if they will share with you the written summary of the meeting/s, if one was prepared.
- Refer back to the genetic counselor or to the physician if original information was insufficient to meet the family's needs.
- Discuss the information that was presented to clarify terminology and other aspects about which the client may have questions.
- Refer, as appropriate, for counseling for on-going emotional disturbances.

Evaluate the adequacy of the information to meet the client's needs for problem solving by encouraging the client to discuss the alternatives presented in the counseling sessions.

the family, and a nurse sensitive to the dynamics within the family can help immeasurably in assisting them to develop adaptive attitudes and learning patterns.

Strategies for Teaching. It is wise to remember that the mother and father may be at different stages of acceptance. They may be at different stages in their readiness to learn, and any teaching that is done may have to be repeated and evaluated frequently, leaving adequate time for questions and free discussion. It is better to teach in small increments rather than to try to teach everything at once. Written material can be effective in supplementing the teaching, and ongoing assessment can help the parents accept the fact that their baby or child has a disease for which special care is required. Assessment should help the nurse decide what must be reviewed again (i.e., reinforced) and when and what new information can be introduced.

Although the family must be made aware of the chronic nature of the metabolic illness, the information provided in the first weeks and months following diagnosis should focus upon immediate needs and concerns. It can be overwhelming for a family to think about the increasing complexity of the child's needs in future years. As adjustment is made to the initial impact of the disease, the family can begin to plan for future aspects of care. Family members will give cues of readiness for information needed for longer-range planning; when more information is desired, they will begin to seek help from resources such as the nurse.

Strategies for Family Assessment. Assessment of the family requires as much attention as does the assessment of the baby or child. There is a very strong cultural component underlying the ways in which family members perceive and care for a child's illness. It is imperative that the nurse determine very early in the interaction with the family their traditions and beliefs regarding care of infants and young children within the family. The prescribed care must complement the family's cultural values if there is to be compliance with the treatment regimen.

"Prescribed care," however, does put additional stress on the family. An important nursing strategy is to identify what cultural/social components of the family can provide resources to meet this stress. (See Chapters 1 and 2 for further information on cultural assessment and Chapter 12 for techniques of family assessment.)

Parents can be very helpful in identifying supports that are readily available within the family and community while the nurse can supplement these with appropriate additional resources to provide well-defined services for the family. Home care, infant stimulation programs, parent support groups, and other community and government resources may all play a part in assisting the family on a long- or short-term basis.

Helping the Parents Support Siblings

There is no doubt that the siblings of a child with a metabolic disorder are affected. The effect may be minimal if the symptoms are obscure; however, as the severity of the symptoms increases, so does the effect on the other children. Parents require assistance in interpreting the disease and its treatment to the siblings. Siblings may benefit from their own counseling sessions with the nurse, physician, or other members of the multidisciplinary team. Parents also need help in supporting the siblings and in trying to make the impact of the illness minimal. Honesty, love, and the fostering of each child's individual traits and talents must be ongoing. Siblings, who have in some way been directly involved in learning about and participating in the care of the affected child, will benefit and should have fewer problems dealing with the impact of the illness on their lives.

Teaching Dietary Management

The dietary control required for the management of certain metabolic disorders during infancy is usually not problematic. The infant quickly adjusts to the special-formula diet. The parents, on the other hand, may experience considerable problems around feeding. They must learn to be realistic about the intake and to prevent the manipulation that the young infant can quickly master. Parents and members of the extended family all have preconceived ideas about what and how to feed an infant. The prescribed diet most likely will not conform to their expectations.

Instructions given by health professionals may produce a great deal of anxiety in a parent if they do not allow for any flexibility. Parents may become very anxious if the baby does not eat everything prescribed or if he or she wants more. If a normal infant refuses part of a feeding, it is of no great concern; it is of concern, however, if the child on a reduced-protein intake refuses a feeding. The parents must learn to manage this, to plan to supplement at the next feeding, or to begin to adjust the times of feeding to the infant's hunger patterns. In spite of all attempts, there still may be the odd day when the infant will not eat the prescribed amount; this should not provoke undue alarm or anxiety. It is essential for the parents to think about intake with respect to a 24-hour period rather than to focus on individual feedings.

Parents need help and guidance when they begin to alter the types of foods their baby eats. The introduction of cereal, fruit, or vegetables may cause problems, and parents need guidance from the nurse and the nutritionist. The cultural diversity that will dictate the acceptability or unacceptability of certain foods may prove challenging, but there is nothing to be gained by not integrating culturally acceptable foods into the child's special diet. It is during the first two years that the diet must be most rigidly adhered to, for that is the time during which maximal brain development occurs and irreversible damage can be caused. It should be reassuring for parents, however, that this is the one time in the child's life that they have almost complete control over what the child eats.

Teaching Illness Prevention

All children experience occasional infections or viral illness. For a child affected with a metabolic illness, this can be much more serious. During periods of illness, the diet has to be adjusted to provide additional calories in order to prevent the body from breaking down its own protein (catabolism), which compounds the child's basic problem. Protein restrictions may also be adopted for some children when they are ill.

The decision to send a child to a day care facility or to nursery school is more difficult for parents whose child has a metabolic disorder because of the potential deleterious effects of infection. There are no clear-cut answers for these parents, and it is helpful for them to discuss their concerns openly with the nursing and medical staff. Although children need socialization and play with other children to meet developmental tasks, the parents must decide whether to risk the extra infections that will usually result from the increased contact with other children or to keep the child at home during the preschool years. The nurse can provide information and guidance to facilitate this parental decision. Boxes 7-1 and 7-2 identify criteria for evaluation of day care centers, including health and safety considerations. Many of these same aspects apply to selection of a preschool.

Helping the Family Establish Realistic Expectations for the Affected Child's Growth and Development

All parents have to learn that there is an acceptable range of time during which their infant or child will reach certain milestones. Parents of children affected with any disease must be aware of the expected developmental patterns but remain sensitive to the range. With help and guidance, their child will do his or her best but this effort might not conform with parental expectations. The parents should be encouraged by the staff to develop realistic expectations for their child and not to become disheartened when delays occur. Some parents have a tendency to overcompensate for their affected child, and they may deny developmental lags for which attention is required. The nurse has a very important role in the ongoing assessment of the child and must be alert to discrepancies between what the mother says the child does and what is observed.

There are, depending on the disease and its severity, a great range of growth problems. Some infants and children will achieve normal milestones; others will be profoundly retarded. Support services, such as physiotherapy and occupational therapy, to develop the potential of these children and assist them with the activities of daily living may have to be arranged. Through careful and astute nursing assessment, these services can be introduced in an anticipatory manner and at the appropriate time.

Helping the Child and Family Deal with Mental Retardation

Unfortunately, in many metabolic disorders there is a risk of mental retardation, ranging from the very mildly affected child, who can function with help in the regular school system, to the profoundly damaged child, who may, at some time in life, require care in a facility outside the home. The monitoring of the child's progress throughout all developmental stages is critical. Parents must be helped to be realistic yet to remain hopeful in their expectations. The care of the retarded child depends entirely on the disability, but the overall aim is for all efforts to be coordinated to assist the child to live as normal a life as possible. (See also the discussion of nursing strategies for children with mental retardation in Chapter 34 and Table 51-10, which focuses on promoting a positive self-concept in a child with a handicap.)

Helping the Child and Family Deal with Physical Disability

Many of the metabolic disorders are accompanied by varying degrees of physical disability, again ranging from the mild to the profound. The child requires careful, ongoing assessment. Infant stimulation programs and physiotherapy following a prescribed course will go a long way toward assisting the child to develop his or her maximal physical development. Community resources and supports available to the family must be identified and a referral made whenever necessary.

Helping the Child and Family Achieve Treatment Compliance in the Absence of Symptoms

It might seem strange to the nurse reading this that a section dealing with concerns deals with the absence of symptoms—which, after all, is the ultimate goal of therapy. Sometimes, however, it is easier to continue treatment when one is faced with the overt symptomatology of the disease on a daily basis rather than when either the symptoms have not yet manifested themselves or the disease is well controlled.

With many metabolic disorders, though, a very insidious onset of symptoms, or even an absence of symptoms, may occur in the presence of advanced disease. Such a disease is *cystinuria:* in this instance, a very large staghorn calculus can exist in the calyx of the kidney and the patient may be totally unaware of it until symptoms suddenly develop. In another example, children with well-controlled PKU may be symptom-free on their diet. Children and adults who have metabolic disorders, but who remain free of symptoms, face the problem of having to continue treatment that may involve dietary restriction or having to take medication for prolonged periods of time, or even for their entire life, when they feel and are very well. It is essential that they continue their prescribed therapy, and to do this they need ongoing support, education, encouragement, reassurance, and regular medical and nursing follow-up.

Promoting Healthy Parenting

Many parents, especially mothers of children with chronic illness, have a tendency to be overprotective. It is important that the nurse, in ongoing meetings with the family, be alert to traits of overprotectiveness. Children may grow to resent this. There is a delicate balance to be struck in providing love and care during illness as well as in health while maintaining the support that discipline provides. All children require discipline in the form of guidelines within which they will develop and thrive. The child with a chronic illness who will require lifelong therapy and a regimen of care will require the same form of discipline.

Behavioral guidelines need to be established early in life. This is especially true for children with a chronic illness such as metabolic disease because they can quickly learn to manipulate their parents by using their illness. Although it is difficult for parents, it is important to try to raise the affected child in a family environment that is as "normal" as possible. Parents will often need support for the difficult decisions related to discipline. The nurse's reassurance of the child's developmental need for "rules" can help the parent resolve feelings of guilt for imposing guidelines upon a child who is already burdened by a chronic illness.

Continued observation and assessment of behavioral changes is vital. It is imperative for the family to be open and honest with teachers and other school personnel. As children get older, more people become directly involved in their care. Parents and the health care team will need to expand the educational network so that all involved individuals will have an understanding of the child's illness, thereby reducing the numbers and kinds of problems that the child may encounter.

By the time the child reaches school age, a problem in behavioral management can be manifested in a variety of ways. Acting-out behavior affects not only the child but also the parents and siblings. Ongoing assessment, with early problem identification and resolution, is required for family dynamics and interaction among the members. The nurse working with such families should always keep in mind that it is more difficult to correct a behavioral problem than to prevent one. No matter how difficult it may seem to control a behavioral problem when it arises, it will not become easier to manage as the child gets older.

Helping the Family Make Decisions About Information for the Child's Friends

The socialization of a child throughout the early preschool and school years is of utmost importance. It is an ongoing process. Health care workers are quick to tell parents to raise their affected child as a normal child, but there are a number of restrictions and special problems that must be dealt with and that become more difficult as the child grows. A decision has to be made very early regarding what information about the disease will be given to the family's and child's friends and teachers. A school-age child will begin to feel sensitive about the disease and treatment and may prefer that only certain friends know. This is something that has to be worked out on an individual basis with the child and family. The nurse can be of immeasurable help in discussing different approaches with the child and the parents. Whatever is decided, it is important that a family consensus be reached, that the child and parents feel supported, and that they have the assistance of appropriate community resources whenever necessary.

Helping Parents Deal with Feelings of Powerlessness

Parents have feelings that result from the imposition of their child's disease. They may feel frustrated, angry, or even hostile because they cannot live their lives free of the child's disease and its implications. Frequently, the treatment, the changed lifestyles, or even the child may come between parents. The nurse can help immeasurably by listening to the parents and validating their right to these feelings. Once the frustration is expressed and accepted, the parents can begin to deal with its cause. Parent support groups can be helpful in providing the means for emotional support and for physical assistance in the form of occasional respite care.

Referring the Family for Genetic Counseling

There is always the possibility that families with one affected child may have another before a diagnosis is made, or they may choose to have another child after the diagnosis is made and "take their chances." Many diseases are now identifiable through amniocentesis and chorionic villus sampling, and parents who wish to have additional children should be encouraged to obtain genetic advice regarding prenatal diagnosis. Occasionally, when one child in the family is diagnosed with very obscure symptoms and a later onset of the disease, another child will be diagnosed in the same family through biochemical analysis and screening. The shock of this is compounded for the family, who may then be faced with an unexpected lifelong disease in more than one of their children. The inheritable nature of the disease often causes further distress to the parents, and feelings of guilt and blame pervade the family. Ongoing support, guidance, and teaching are important. Parents need answers, which are not always readily available. They need to discuss their concerns with medical and nursing staff. Repeated teaching is necessary as parents begin to understand and ask questions. There is too much to hear all at once, and nurses must be sensitive to how parents are learning and reacting to what they are told (see Table 50-3).

It is equally important that adolescents be offered the support of genetic counseling and the opportunity to ask their own questions. The risk of recurrence and the risk to offspring must be addressed specifically. The risk varies according to the disease; for example, in PKU there is a high risk whereas in homocystinuria the risk is very low. Prenatal diagnosis is possible for several diseases, and adolescents who contemplate having families will want to know about these options.

References

Ampola MG: *Metabolic Diseases in Pediatric Practice.* Boston, Little, Brown & Co, 1982.

Barlow S, Schuett VE: Hyperphenylalaninemias. *In* Gellis SS, Kagan BM (eds), *Current Pediatric Therapy 12.* Philadelphia, WB Saunders, 1986, 338–342.

Barness LA: Nutrition and nutritional disorders. *In* Behrman RE, Vaughan VC III (eds): *Nelson Textbook of Pediatrics.* Philadelphia, WB Saunders, 1987, 113–154.

Barnico LM, Cullinane MM: Maternal phenylketonuria: An unexpected challenge. *MCN* 10(2):108–110, 1985.

Behrman RE, Vaughan VC III: *Nelson Textbook of Pediatrics.* 13th ed. Philadelphia, WB Saunders, 1987.

Bickel H, Guthrie R, Hammersen G (eds): *Neonatal Screening for Inherited Errors of Metabolism.* New York, Springer-Verlag, 1980.

Cohen FL: Clinical genetics in nursing practice. Philadelphia: Lippincott, 1984.

Cohn RM, Roth CS: *Metabolic Diseases: A Guide to Early Recognition.* Philadelphia, WB Saunders, 1980, 344–350.

Dobson JC, Williamson ML, Azen L, Koch K: Intellectual assessment in 111 four year old children with phenylketonuria. *Pediatrics* 60:822–827, 1977.

Fraser D, Scriver CR: Familiar focus of vitamin D resistant rickets revisited: X-linked hypophosphataemia and autosomal recessive vitamin D dependency. *Am J Clin Nutr* 29:1315–1329, 1974.

Gellis SS, Kagan BM: *Current Pediatric Therapy 12.* Philadelphia, WB Saunders, 1986.

Gröer MW, Shekleton ME: *Basic Pathophysiology* (2nd ed). St. Louis; CV Mosby, 1983.

Güttler F: Phenylketonuria: 50 years since Folling's discovery and still expanding our clinical and biochemical knowledge. *Acta Paediatr Scand* 73:105–116, 1984.

Guyton A: *Human Physiology and Mechanisms of Disease* (4th ed). Philadelphia, WB Saunders, 1987.

Hanley WB, Bell L: Maternal phenylketonuria: Finding and treating before conception (editorial). *Can Med Assoc J* 126:1259–1260, 1982.

Kirkman IN Jr: Projections of mental retardation for P.K.U. (abstr). *Pediatr Res.* 13, 414, 1979.

Lazarus RS, Folkman S: *Stress, Appraisal, and Coping.* New York, Springer Publishing Company, 1984.

McKusick A, Neufield EF, Kelly TE: The mucopolysaccharide storage diseases. In Stanbury JB, Wyngaarden JB, Fredrickson DS (eds). *The Metabolic Basis of Inherited Disease* (4th ed). New York, McGraw-Hill Book Co, 1978, 1282–1307.

Messer SS: PKU: A mother's perspective. *Pediatr Nurs* 11(2):121–123, 1985.

Menkes JH, Alter M, Steigleder GK, Weakley DR, Suna GH: A sex-linked recessive disorder with retardation in growth, peculiar hands and focal cerebral and cerebellar degeneration. *Pediatrics* 29, 764–769, 1962.

Raine DN: Inborn errors of metabolism *In* Brown SF, et al (eds): *Chemical Diagnosis and Disease.* Amsterdam, Elsevier, North Holland Biomedical Press, 1979, 927–1008.

Rennert OM: Hepatolenticular degeneration. *In* Gellis SS, Kagan BM (eds): *Current Pediatric Therapy 12.* Philadelphia, WB Saunders, 1986, 337–338.

Rezvani I, Auerbach VH: Inborn errors of metabolism. *In* Behrman RE, Vaughan VC (eds): *Nelson Textbook of Pediatrics.* 13th ed. Philadelphia: WB Saunders, 1987, 277–305.

Sansaricq, C: Inborn errors of metabolism. *In* Zimmerman SS, Gildea JH (eds): *Critical Care Pediatrics.* Philadelphia, WB Saunders, 1985, 292–309.

Sass-Kortsak A, Bearn AG: Hereditary disorders of copper metabolism. *In* Stanbury JB, Wyngaarden JB, Fredrickson DS (eds): *The Metabolic Basis of Inherited Disease* (4th ed). New York, McGraw-Hill Book Co, 1978, 1098–1126.

Scriver CR: New issues in newborn screening for phenylketonuria and hypoparathyroidism. *Pediatrics* 69:104–106, 1982.

Scriver CR, Fraser D, Kooh SW: Hereditary rickets. In Heath D, Marx SJ (eds): *Butterworth's International Medical*

Reviews. Clinical Endocrinology 2: Calcium Disorders. London, Butterworth, 1982.

Sinclair L: *Metabolic Diseases in Children.* London, Blackwell Scientific Publications, 1979.

Stanbury, JB, Wyngaarden JB, Fredrickson DS (eds): *The Metabolic Basis of Inherited Disease* (4th ed). New York, McGraw-Hill Book Co, 1978.

Watts RWE, Crawford MDA, Gibbs DA (eds): The treatment of inborn errors of metabolism: Introduction and general principles on advances in treatment of inborn errors of metabolism. In *Proceedings of the 2nd Clinical Research Centre Symposium,* Sept., 1981. New York, John Wiley & Sons, 1982.

Wenger D: Defects in metabolism of carbohydrates. *In* Behrman RE, Vaughan VC: *Nelson Textbook of Pediatrics.* 13th ed. Philadelphia, WB Saunders, 1987, 306–338.

Bibliography

Barlow S: Progress in phenylketonuria: Defects in the metabolism of biopterin. *Pediatrics* 65(4), 837–839, 1980.

Bondy P, Rosenberg LE (eds): *Duncan's Diseases of Metabolism: Genetics and Metabolism.* Philadelphia, WB Saunders, 1974.

Cornblath M, Schwartz R: *Disorders of Carbohydrate Metabolism in Infancy* Vol. III. Philadelphia, WB Saunders, 1976.

Deluca HF, Anast C: *Pediatric Diseases Related to Calcium.* New York, Elsevier, 1980.

Dunnigan MG, McIntosh WB, Ford JA, Robertson I: Acquired disorders of vitamin D metabolism. In Heath D, Marx SJ (eds): *Butterworth's International Medical Reviews. Clinical Endocrinology 2: Calcium Disorders.* London, Butterworth, 1982, 125–150.

Galactosaemia in Infancy: A Review of the Problems and Its Dietary Management. Mead Johnson Laboratories, 1976.

Gray M: Intestinal disaccharide deficiencies and glucose galactose malabsorption. *In* Stanbury JB, Wyngaarden JB, Fredrickson, DS (eds): *The Metabolic Basis of Inherited Disease.* (4th ed). New York, McGraw-Hill Book Co, 1978.

Hayes JS, et al: Managing PKU: An update. *MCN* 1987 Mar/Apr; 12(2):119–123.

Irons M, Harvey, LL: Galactosemias. *In* Gellis SS, Kagan BM (eds): *Current Pediatric Therapy 12.* Philadelphia, WB Saunders, 1986, 347–348.

Hanley WB: Revised guidelines for newborn screening for phenylketonuria and hypoparathyroidism. In *Proceedings from Advisory Committee on Inborn Errors of Metabolism.* Toronto, Ministry of Health, Ontario.

Koch R, Blaskovics M, Wenz E, Fishler K, Schaefflev G: Phenylalanaemia and phenylketonuria. *In* Nyan WC (ed). *Heritable Diseases of Amino Acid Metabolism.* New York, John Wiley & Sons, 1974.

Kohn, BA: The differential diagnosis of cataracts in infancy and childhood. *Am J Dis Child* 130:184–192, 1976.

Levy HL: Phenylketonuria. *Pediatr Rev* 7(9)269–275, 1986.

Lott JW: PKU: A nursing update. *J Pediatr Nurs* 1988 Feb; 3(1):29–34.

Marlow DR, Redding B: *Textbook of Pediatric Nursing.* (6th ed.) Philadelphia, WB Saunders, 1987.

McKusick VA: *Heritable Disorders of Connective Tissue* (3rd ed). St. Louis, CV Mosby, 1966.

Scriver CR: Management of maple syrup urine disease in Canada. *CMA J* 115:1005–1112, 1976.

Snyderman SE: Maple syrup urine disease. *In* Nyan WC (ed). *Heritable Diseases of Amino Acid Metabolism.* New York, John Wiley & Sons, 1974, 177–183.

Vaccaro, AM, Mascillo M, Mandara I, et al: Improved isoelectric focussing of normal and variant forms of erythrocyte-1-phosphate uridyl transferase. *Electrophoresis* 3:58–61, 1982.

Nursing Strategies: Sensory and Communication Alterations

Chapter 51

Mabel Hunsberger

Nursing Process Plan
NPP: The Child with an Identified Sensory Impairment, page 2032

Related Topics
Assessing Child Health, Chapter 15
Impact of Chronic Illness, Chapter 25
Administration of Eye Drops and Ear Drops, Chapter 27
Otitis Media, Chapter 38
Foreign Body in the Ear, Chapter 52
Eye Injury, Chapter 52

Human growth and development takes place in a sea of interactive experiences. Formulation of a sense of self, of others, and of the world develops through exchanges involving vision, hearing, touch, taste, smell, and language experiences. The sensory experiences that enable a person to "take in" and "respond to" internal and external stimuli are instrumental in shaping the development of a growing child.

In communication alterations, sensitive adjustment and responsiveness of the environment are required to support optimal development of the child.

Health care to prevent, detect, and manage sensory, speech and language alterations is provided by multidisciplinary teams, including nurses. Although parents provide the major social and developmental support, the nurse can sustain the child and family through counseling, education, assistance with management of technical aspects of care, and facilitating access to community agencies and resources. This chapter discusses the nurse's role in the care of children with vision, hearing, speech, and language alterations.

Alterations in Vision

Infants and children are affected by a variety of visual problems; some can be corrected if identified early, whereas others can only be treated with varying degrees of success. Assessment of visual and physical characteristics of the eye from birth is done to ensure early identification of visual problems. Familiarity with normal developmental characteristics of the immature eye is necessary to make the necessary judgment concerning clinical findings.

Visual Development

Infants' vision is better than was once thought, and visual acuity is now thought to increase significantly between birth and 6 months of age (Nelson, et al, 1984). Careful observation of infant responses and use of assessment techniques such as optokinetic nystagmus, forced preferential looking, and visually evoked potentials have contributed to our understanding of visual development. (Table 51-1 describes assessment techniques.)

Visual Acuity

Visually evoked potential studies indicate that acuity at birth may be in the range of 20/100 – 20/200 and by 6 months of age approximately 20/20 to 20/40 (Nelson, 1984). Visual acuity at birth is thought to be less than 20/20 because of certain immaturities including (1) incomplete myelination of pathways from the retina to the occipital cortex; (2) immaturity of central nervous system synapses; and (3) inability to accommodate the lens. In the first few weeks of life infants gaze around to look at things. They have been found to be interested specifically in the human face. While still in the delivery room, neonates have been noted to be more interested in an object that simulated the human face than in objects that did not have such a pattern (Goble, 1984). Also, sharply contrasting black and white geometric designs seem to be preferred over the more common bunnies and kittens that come in soft shapes and pastel colors (Luddington-Hoe, 1983). According to Field (1982), neonates also discriminate and imitate three facial expressions (happy, sad, and surprised) (Fig. 51-1).

Normal neonates tend to keep their eyes closed much of the time but will respond to illumination and can fixate. Some disconjugate eye movements (eyes not working together) may be noticed at birth. Developmentally the eye is less mature, therefore its function is affected. Developmental variations of the eye are summarized in Table 51-2.

Nurse's Role in Prevention and Early Identification

Genetic and unknown causes are responsible for the majority of cases of congenital blindness in children. A thorough history with a careful eye examination on all well child visits forms a major preventive role of the nurse. A family history of a genetic disease associated with visual loss is significant information that may lead to the early detection of visual impairment in an infant. Also, genetic counseling is an important aspect of prevention of blindness when known genetic diseases that cause blindness are identified in a family history. Prenatal screening for maternal infections that cause blindness (rubella, syphilis), adequate prenatal care to prevent prematurity, and prevention of exposure of premature infants to high levels of oxygen whenever possible are preventive approaches in which the nurse may have responsibility.

Retinopathy of Prematurity (ROP)

The risk for the development of some visual problems can be decreased through some known precautionary measures. Retinopathy of prematurity (ROP) is

Table 51-1. Techniques for Testing Vision in a Young or Retarded Child

Description	Comments
Optokinetic Nystagmus	
Nystagmus is a periodic involuntary movement of the eyes from side to side or up and down. Optokinetic nystagmus is a *visually induced* nystagmus to evaluate vision. A drum with black and white stripes, dots, or pictures is rotated in front of child. A positive response (indicating vision) is the slow movement of the eyes in the direction of the moving drum, followed by a quick return of the eye to its former position (optokinetic nystagmus), done repetitively as the drum turns.	A positive response demonstrates that the child can see, but failure to evoke optokinetic nystagmus (negative response) can either mean poor vision or poor attention. Appropriate for infants from birth to around 3 years of age.
Forced Preferential Looking	
A circle of alternating light and dark stripes (grating) and a gray spot of similar size and brightness are symmetricaly placed in an infant's field of vision. The width of the stripes is gradually reduced until the infant no longer looks preferentially at the grating. The narrowest width of stripe that the infant looks at is then converted into Snellen visual acuity.	Can be used from birth to 2½ years of age. Test is based on the observation that the infant is more likely to look at a figure with black and white stripes than one that is solidly gray. This procedure can be very time-consuming and is still in the experimental stages.
Visually Evoked Potentials (VEP)	
Electrical activity is recorded through scalp electrodes following visual stimulation with single or repeated flashing lights into child's eye, one at a time. It is an electroencephalogram (EEG) of the occipital area.	Child needs to be quiet to avoid electrical interference. A parent can hold the child. Mild sedation may be needed. Because this test does not rely on a motor response from the child, it can be used for brain-damaged children

(From Greenwald, 1983; Nelson, 1984; Kovalesky, 1985.)

Table 51-2. Developmental Variations in Eye Maturation

Structure/Function	Description	Process of Maturation
Sclera	Thin, translucent with a bluish tinge	
Cornea	Proportionately large in the neonate; should appear crystal clear within 1–2 days after birth. Premature infants may have a transient opalescent haze	Reaches adult size by 2 yr of age or sooner. Curvature flattens with age altering refractive characteristics of the eye
Pupils	Small in neonate and difficult to dilate. Pupillary reflexes sluggish at birth	Within a few weeks begin to enlarge. Pupillary reflexes apparent in a few weeks
Lens	Ciliary muscle is immature. Has greater refractive power and this compensates for the short diameter of the globe (hyperopia).	Accommodation developed by 4 mo. With age lens becomes more dense and resistant to change of shape during accommodation
Refraction	Infant eye is hyperopic	Hyperopia increases until age 7, after which it declines
Binocular vision	The ability to fixate on one visual field with both eyes is called binocularity. Binocularity is not present at birth	Binocularity is established by 6 mo of age and probably sooner in many infants
Crying/tears	Lacrimal glands not fully developed at birth but some tearing does occur. Temporary obstruction of lacrimal duct may cause overflow of tears	By 6–8 mo spontaneous canalization of lacrimal duct occurs

(From Greenwald, 1983; Nelson, 1984.)

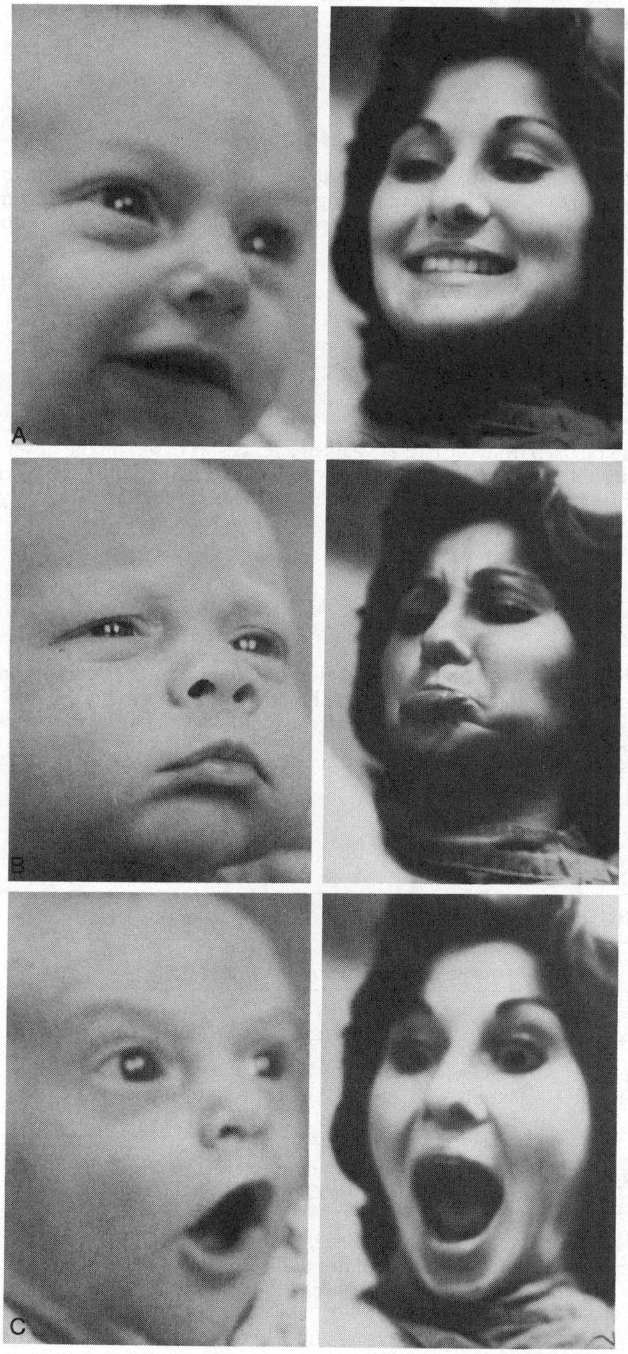

Figure 51-1. Imitation and discrimination by neonates. (From Field JM: Discrimination and imitation of facial expressions by neonates. *Science* 1982 Oct; 218:180.)

thought to be a multifactorial disorder that is associated with, but not limited to, excessive oxygen therapy. Citing research studies to determine the cause of ROP, George and colleagues (1988) listed the following factors as potential causes: immaturity, hyperoxia, hypoxia, blood transfusions, intraventricular hemorrhage, apnea, infection, hypercarbia, hypocarbia, patent ductus arteriosus, prostaglandin synthetase inhibitors, vitamin E deficiency, lactic acidosis, prenatal complications, genetic factors, and possibly even bright lighting in the nursery. Very low birthweight neonates (weighing less than 1500 grams and especially under 1000 grams) are at risk for the development of ROP (Shapiro, 1986). More than 500 infants in the United States are estimated to be blinded each year as a result of ROP (Porat, 1984). The nurse is an important participant in the monitoring of these infants at risk in the neonatal intensive care unit. (See Chapter 38 for further discussion of the risk factors associated with ROP.)

Ophthalmia Neonatorum

The routine use of silver nitrate drops at birth to prevent gonorrheal ophthalmia neonatorum (inflammation of the conjunctiva of the neonate)is controversial. The major objections to this practice are the resultant chemical conjunctivitis that follows its use and its lack of effectiveness against *Chlamydia trachomatis.* Because erythromycin and tetracycline are effective against *Neisseria gonorrhoeae* and against *Chlamydia trachomatis,* these agents are being increasingly recommended for routine use. There is some evidence that erythromycin may be the better choice of the two agents because of its greater effectiveness against *C. trachomatis* (Bernstein et al, 1982).

The nurse administers the eyedrops in most institutions. Understanding of the issues surrounding this debate will allow the nurse to participate actively in decision-making regarding this nursing role.

Eye Injuries

Participation in the prevention of eye injuries is another important role. Anticipatory guidance offered by the nurse should include a discussion of potential dangers associated with rapid developmental advancement. For example, using scissors, chemistry sets, and many self-created toys like sticks and arrows requires teaching and some supervision by parents to prevent eye injuries. Sharp objects, fireworks, chemicals, power tools, and sunlight are potential sources of danger (see Chapter 17 for further discussion of safety teaching).

Nurses can be influential in a variety of ways to promote the health of children's eyes. Promotion of good prenatal care to prevent prematurity and vaginal infections and to advocate immunizations against rubella are important preventive strategies. Nurses can also promote proper care and use of contact lenses and glasses, encourage use of proper lighting for reading, and the practice of good hygiene to prevent eye infection.

Box 51-1
Characteristics of Vision Development

BIRTH TO 2 WEEKS

Eyes blink in response to bright light. Doll's eye reflex present because child is unable to integrate head and eye movements (when examiner rotates infant's head to one side, eyes lag behind). Transitory fixation develops at a distance of approximately 3 feet. Visual acuity 20/100 to 20/200.

1 TO 2 MONTHS

Regards parent's face and watches intently. Follows large moving objects 10–14 in from face through a 90 degree angle (45 degrees from midline), but glances are minimal for moving stimuli beyond 2 ft away.

3 TO 4 MONTHS

Visual following at 6–12 in from face with a combination of head and eye movements through a 180 degree arc. Convergence on near objects now developed. Doll's eye reflex disappears. Watches own hands and feet. Fixates immediately on a 1 in cube brought within 1–2 ft of the eye.

6 TO 7 MONTHS

Ciliary muscle function begins and accommodation-convergence reflex developing. Eyes move together (binocular vision established). Frequent crossing is abnormal and indicates strabismus. Hand-eye coordination developing. Child reaches for anything seen and adjusts own position to see objects. Visual acuity 20/20 to 20/40.*

10 MONTHS

Pats mirror image. Sees tiny objects and reaches for them using fingers and thumb. Follows and watches activities within 10–12 ft.

12 MONTHS

Drops toys and watches them fall. Recognizes familiar people at distance of 20 ft or more.

18 MONTHS

Shows keen interest in pictures. Fixes eyes on small dangling toy at 10 ft. Points to familiar objects. Convergence well established.

2 YEARS

Accommodates well. Recognizes fine details in pictures. Visual acuity 20/20.*

3 YEARS

Attention span fair. Fixation on small pictures or toys approaches 50 sec. Matches letters HOVT in STYCAR test at 10 ft. Visual acuity 20/20 and after 3 yr of age can be assessed by Snellen E chart. (See Chapter 15 for description of STYCAR and Snellen E chart.)

* Estimated visual acuity varies according to the test used. The reported age at which 20/20 vision is achieved ranges from 6 months to 2½ years (Nelson et al, 1984).
(From Johnson, 1978; Stangler et al, 1980; Nelson et al, 1984.)

Visual Problems

Screening programs to detect visual problems begin at birth. Specific vision tests requiring special equipment that can be used for infants are summarized in Table 51-1. Assessment of the development of vision should always be part of well-child examinations. Characteristics of vision development up to age three are summarized in Box 51-1. Techniques used to assess vision according to age are summarized in Box 51-2. (Components of an eye examination and a description of screening techniques are included in Chapter 15.)

In addition to assessing vision during health examinations, the nurse should teach families how to detect a visual problem in their child. The Home Eye Test for Preschoolers is available from the National Society for the Prevention of Blindness.* It contains the Snellen E short eye chart and simple instructions for the parents.

*79 Madison Avenue, New York, NY 10016.

The Committee on the Fetus and Newborn of the American Academy of Pediatrics recommends that a person experienced in recognizing ROP should examine the eyes of all infants born before 36 weeks' gestation, or weighing less than 2000 grams (4 lb, 7 oz) who have received oxygen therapy (Guidelines for Perinatal Care, 1983). Table 51-3 summarizes a recommended time schedule for the first fundus examination and the follow-up.

Screening for refractive errors becomes particularly important as the child approaches the preschool and school-age years. Five per cent of all preschool children have visual problems; 68 per cent of these are refractive errors, 15 per cent are caused by strabismus, 15 per cent by amblyopia, and 2 per cent by other causes (Stangler et al., 1980). Although prevention of these conditions is not possible because they are primarily hereditary, early identification and treatment may prevent or retard loss of vision.

Box 51-2
Techniques of Vision Assessment According to Age

NEONATE

External inspection of eye (check for infection, trauma, and congenital anomalities).
Check for blink response to bright light.
Check for presence of red reflex and pupillary response to light.
Do Hirschberg test for detection of strabismus.
Check for nystagmus* with optokinetic drum† to establish the presence of vision.

6 MONTHS

External inspection of eye as for newborn. (A deviation or anomaly may now be apparent that was not noted in the newborn.)
Test for strabismus: Use cover-uncover test or alternate cover test; Hirschberg test; check whether both eyes follow a light from side to side equally well.
Observe for nystagmus. (Congenital nystagmus is present at birth but is not commonly detected before the age of 2–3 mo.)
Assess visual development (see Table 51-1).
Perform ophthalmoscopic examination.

3 TO 5 YEARS

External inspection of eyes as during infancy. Test for strabismus as described for 6 mo of age. Concerning behavior:
- Frequently rubs eyes
- Brings eyes close to objects
- Frequently squints or frowns in order to see
- Tilts head; shuts or covers one eye
- Complains of itchiness, burning, or a "dusty" feeling in eyes
- Cannot see well (chalkboard, a toy, an object across the room)
- Has abnormal sensitivity to light
- Has more than usual difficulty adapting to low levels of illumination

Visual acuity tested with Snellen E symbol. (Of particular importance is identification of unequal vision caused by amblyopia.) Check for color blindness.
Refer a 3-year-old with visual acuity of 20/50 or less and 4- or 5-year-old with 20/40 or less. (All children should be rescreened on another day before referral.)
Other tests of visual acuity for preschooler:
- STYCAR (letter matching test)
- Allen picture cards

SCHOOL-AGE

Techiques for detection of visual problems similar to that described for 3- to 5-year-olds with the exception that if the letters of the alphabet are learned it is recommended that the standard Snellen alphabet chart be used.
Children 5 years and older should read a majority of the 20/30 line. A two-line difference between eyes warrants referral (Committee on Practice and Ambulatory Medicine, 1986).

* Nystagmus is a rhythmic oscillation of the eyes that normally occurs on lateral gaze.
† An optokinetic drum is a cylinder with stripes or pictures that when twirled within the baby's range of vision normally elicits nystagmus if vision is present.
(Adapted from About Children's Eyes. *Available from National Association for Visually Handicapped. 305 East 24th Street, New York, NY 10010; Stangler, 1980; and Hatfield, 1979.)*

Refractive Errors

In vision, light rays enter the lens and are brought to a single focus on the retina. When the bending of the rays (refraction) and the length of the eyeball are uncoordinated, the image does not fall on a single point on the retina. Reduced acuity and discomfort related to the use of the eye are the two major symptoms of refractive errors (Havener, 1979). While children may not say that they are having trouble seeing, symptoms such as rubbing of the eyes, tearing, red-rimmed eyelids, and squinting should make one suspicious of a refractive error.

The work of the eye—bringing the image into clear focus—involves accommodation and convergence. Accommodation is the focusing mechanism of the eyes that allows a person to see clearly at all distances. As the ciliary muscle contracts, the curvature of the lens and its refractive strength are increased. This results in an increase in the anterior-posterior thickness of the lens. Children with normal eyes usually have excellent accommodative powers (at age 8 years the eye has the maximal potential accommodation) (Goble, 1984).

Convergence of the eyes occurs simultaneously with accommodation in a fixed ratio. Convergence is an increasing inward movement of the eyeballs as an object is brought from a position of distance to closeness. The closer the object is brought to the child's face, the greater the degree of convergence. This re-

Table 51-3. Time Schedule for Fundus Examination in Neonates at Risk for Retinopathy of Prematurity

Gestational Age at Birth	First Exam	Follow-up Exams
<30 wk	6–8 wk	*If no ROP:* Repeat q 3–4 wk, until mature retina, and again in 3–6 mo *If ROP present: Mild*—Re-examine q 2–3 wk until signs of resolution noted. *Severe (Grade 3+)*—Re-examine q 1–2 wk until signs of resolution noted *Resolving RLF:* q 2–4 wk until resolved
30–34 wk	6–7 wk	*If normal:* Repeated in 3–6 mo *If ROP present:* Follow schedule as noted in <30 wk
>34 wk	6 wk	*If normal:* No subsequent exam necessary *If ROP present:* Follow schedule as noted in <30 wk
Anterior chamber hyperemia	Immediate eye exam	
For Detection of Late Complications		
Infants with fully regressed ROP: eye examination q 1–2 yr		
Infants with cicatricial RLF (scarring of the retina): eye examination q 6–12 mo		

(From Porat, 1984.)

flex facilitates focusing of the image at the same position on the retina of each eye, resulting in binocular vision, or fusion of the images. As the object is brought closer to the child's face, constriction of the pupils occurs in addition to convergence.

Measurement of visual acuity is a screening test that can be done easily and quickly to identify refractive errors. The preschool years are an important time to detect these errors to help the child avoid problems in school. The nurse should understand that the eyeball grows as the child grows and that during this time refraction may change significantly. The three types of refractive errors that are most common in children are *hyperopia, myopia, and astigmatism.* Hyperopia increases until around 6 to 7 years of age, after which it decreases gradually until adulthood; myopia usually begins around the preteen years, progresses during the teenage years, then stabilizes (Kovalesky, 1985).

Hyperopia

In hyperopia (farsightedness), there is insufficient refractive power, resulting in poor vision at any distance because the image falls *behind* the retina. Increased accommodative effort brings the focus of the image forward onto the retina. Children are able to accommodate to attain good visual acuity; however, if the hyperopia is great, correction with convex lenses may be required. The constant accommodative effort required for close work causes excessive convergence, which may result in eyestrain and eventually strabismus and amblyopia, to be discussed later. Hyperopia may be corrected by lenses and, if the accommodative-convergence ratio has been normal, the eyes also straighten as a response to the effect of the lenses.

Myopia

In myopia (nearsightedness) an excessive amount of refractive power results in light rays coming to a point of focus in *front* of the retina. The only symptom of myopia is blurred vision for distance. Eyestrain and headaches are not associated with myopia. A child with myopia may be able to read without accommodative effort because near vision requires greater refractive strength than distant vision (Havener, 1979). If myopia is severe, however, the child may have to hold the print close to see it clearly.

Concave lenses readily correct the vision of a myopic child. The problem may become more severe during the early school years; new glasses may be needed every year or two. On the other hand, congenital myopia tends to resolve gradually with age, with a visual acuity of 20/40 by adolescence (Hughes, 1984). These children may or may not need corrective lenses, depending on the severity of the problem.

Astigmatism

In astigmatism the curvature of the cornea is not equal in all directions. The result is that light rays are not focused symmetrically; therefore, the image is blurred and distorted. Eyestrain results from the accommodative effort that is made to bring the image into focus. The problem cannot be compensated by acommodation; it must be corrected with lenses that compensate for the abnormal curvature of the cornea. Astigmatism may coexist with myopia or hyperopia.

Strabismus

In strabismus, the eye muscles lack coordination, resulting in a crossed-eye appearance. The condition occurs in about 2 per cent of all children. The normal infant may at times appear to have strabismus, but it is usually associated with sleepiness. Occasional strabismus should improve from week to week and if by 6 weeks of age (in a full-term infant) it has not resolved, ophthalmic consultation is required. The belief that "most infants have strabismus in the first few weeks of life" is a myth. Constantly evident strabismus is always abnormal (Palmer, 1987). Some children appear to have strabismus because of certain facial features; this is called pseudostrabismus (Fig. 51-2). The features that give a false impression of strabismus are prominent epicanthal folds and a broad, flat nasal bridge.

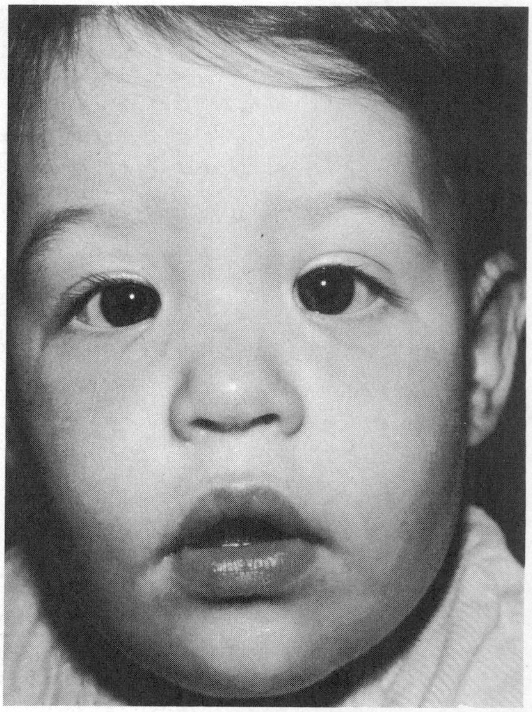

Figure 51-2. Pseudostrabismus. (From Scheie H, Albert D: *Textbook of Ophthalmology*. Philadelphia, WB Saunders, 1977, 337.)

Etiology

About 50 per cent of all children with strabismus have a positive family history for the condition; therefore, any child in a family with a history of strabismus should be closely monitored. Also, the siblings of a child with strabismus should be examined frequently for this defect. The most common cause of strabismus is imbalance of the muscle alignment of the eyes, but other etiologic factors such as brain tumor, infection, retinoblastoma, myasthenia gravis, and cataracts should be considered. Whenever there is any suspicion of strabismus, the child must be referred for further examination.

Any type of misalignment is of concern, and any child who does not see well with each eye should be suspected of having a serious condition (Feman and Reinecke, 1978). Early recognition and treatment are essential to prevent amblyopia. Amblyopia develops when vision is suppressed in the eye that deviates. Without correction, permanent visual loss may occur in the deviated eye.

Pathophysiology

The various terms used to describe strabismus are as follows:

Monocular—one eye is used to fixate and the other deviates. The deviating eye is prone to the development of amblyopia.

Alternating—each eye is alternately used for fixation; vision develops more or less the same in both eyes.

Convergent (esotropia)—eye turns toward the midline (Fig. 51-3).

Divergent (exotropia)—eye turns away from midline.

Nonparalytic (incomitant or nonconcomitant)—all muscles function but not in unison; deviation is the same in all directions of gaze.

Paralytic (comitant or concomitant)—caused by a weakness or paralysis of one or more of the extraocular muscles; the eye appears crossed when turned in the direction of the affected muscle.

Words ending in:
- -tropia: an active, observable misalignment
- -phoria: a latent tendency to misalignment (strabismus becomes evident only during fatigue, illness, or stress)

The two major kinds of strabismus are *nonparalytic* (nonconcomitant) and *paralytic* (comitant).

Nonparalytic strabismus is the most common type in children. The child has difficulty seeing at close range and is likely to squint. Accommodative strabismus is a special type of nonparalytic strabismus that usually develops between 2 and 4 years of age. It has two forms: convergent and divergent. This type of strabismus develops because of a refractive error. Most children normally have a degree of hyperopia (farsightedness) until about 7 years of age. In hyperopia, accommodative effort is required to attain good vision. With accommodation there is normally an accompanying convergence reflex; a fine balance is needed between the accommodative effort and the simultaneous convergence. Generally, the normal hyperopia of childhood is handled through accommodation and an accompanying convergence. If hyperopia is excessive, strabismus can result when the amount of accommodation required for clear vision results in excessive convergence (crossed eyes). Conversely, external deviation (divergence) occurs in myopia; this is less common but may be present at birth.

In paralytic strabismus the child may complain of headache and demonstrate lack of coordination in fine or gross movements. Double vision, or diplopia, is evident by the child's response of closing one eye or tilting the head to avoid seeing a double image.

Strabismus may be obvious or may occur only when the child is ill or tired. Screening tests for strabismus include the cover test and corneal light reflex (Hirschberg test) described in Chapter 15.

Therapeutic Management

The goal of treatment is for the child to attain the best possible vision in each eye and, if possible, equal vision. The ultimate goal is attainment of binocular vision with stereopsis (depth perception); however, in many affected patients this cannot be achieved (Hughes, 1984). The type of treatment varies with the age of the child and type of strabismus. Patching of the good eye is a common method of treatment. This is done to encourage the child to use the deviating eye. In some instances—for example, in the case of accommodative strabismus—the wearing of glasses may correct the deviation.

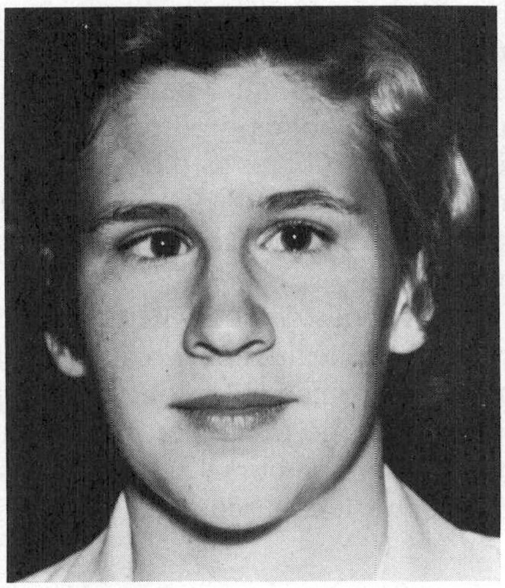

Figure 51-3. Accommodative esotropia, uncorrected. (From Scheie H, Albert D: *Textbook of Ophthalmology.* Philadelphia, WB Saunders, 1977, 337.)

Pharmacologic Therapy

In very young children anticholinesterase drugs (miotics) such as echothiophate iodide (phospholine iodide) and isoflurophate (DFP) are used to correct accommodative esotropia. These drugs are called miotics because one of their actions is to constrict the pupil; however, in the treatment of strabismus they are used because of their action on the ciliary body. They work through a direct chemical action on the ciliary body (i.e., inhibition of cholinesterase). Inhibition of cholinesterase affects the normally fixed relationship between accommodation and convergence. Anticholinesterase causes the ciliary muscle to respond to only a minimal accommodative innervation; that is, fewer impulses are necessary to accomplish a certain amount of accommodation. Miotics make accommodation easier. Consequently, as accommodative innervation is decreased, so is convergence, resulting in correction of the strabismus. Because of certain disadvantages associated with the use of miotics, these agents should be used only in carefully selected cases. Treatment by miotics has the following disadvantages:

- In many children miotics are less effective than glasses.
- In some children miotics cause cysts of the iris (cysts diminish in size when miotics are discontinued). Adding 2.5 per cent Neosynephrine (phenylephrine) eyedrops to the treatment can diminish cyst formation.
- Phospholine iodide is absorbed into the general circulation and has the capacity to lower blood levels of certain enzymes, making the use of succinylcholine unsafe (Goble, 1984).

Because the use of miotic drops will result in a fixed, constricted pupil, it is important that the child wear a Medic Alert bracelet. A bracelet that advises of the use of miotics will be important to the interpretation of neurologic tests for eye function in the case of post-trauma care (Lingua, 1986). Also, drugs used for strabismus interfere with anesthesia containing succinylcholine and should be discontinued 2 to 3 weeks prior to surgery (Kovalesky, 1985).

Eye Exercises

An adjunct to glasses, patching, and medications is the use of eye exercises (orthoptics). Eye exercises should be prescribed by an ophthalmologist; they are useful only in selected cases.

Surgical Correction

Surgical correction is commonly used for congenital strabismus, whenever glasses or miotics cannot correct the problem, and in selected patients for cosmetic reasons. Congenital strabismus is usually corrected before age 12 months. Some ophthalmologists prefer to wait until 18 to 24 months of age, when there is more maturity of the ocular muscles and of the neurologic system. Before surgery is undertaken the stronger eye is patched, to treat any existing amblyopia. Surgery can mechanically straighten an eye, but only patching can stimulate an amblyopic eye to improve vision (Goble, 1984). In most cases strabismus can be corrected with one or two procedures but this varies, and the nurse should consult the surgeon before providing specific information to parents about what to expect as the outcome of surgery.

Major Nursing Diagnoses for Strabismus

Sensory-perceptual alteration: visual, related to incoordination of the eye muscles

Fear/anxiety, related to patching of one or both eyes postoperatively

Disturbance in self-concept: body image, related to reactions of others to a "cross-eyed" appearance

Strategies for Nursing Care

Participating in Early Identification of Strabismus. Early identification of strabismus may be made by performing the cover test and corneal light reflex test, also called the Hirschberg test (see p. 525) during well-child examinations. Early identification and referral can also be initiated by a nurse observing that a child is squinting and showing difficulty with close-range vision. Strabismus may also be suspected when the child complains of frequent headaches or tilts the head to see.

Supporting the Family in Home Management of Strabismus. Nursing interventions for the family include teaching safe use of prescribed eyedrops (see Chapter 28), being understanding of the difficulties in keeping an eye patch on a young child, sharing innovative ways to accomplish this therapy, and encouraging regular eye examinations.

The nurse can help the family carry out the required treatment and ensure that the child has regular eye examinations. Of particular importance is that any child who requires eye patches should be closely followed for decreased vision in the patched eye as a result of the occlusion. In very young children amblyopia can develop in the patched eye in less than 2 weeks.

A frequently encountered problem is the young child's refusal to keep on an eye patch. When patching is required, a pair of clear glasses with a patch occluding the one eye may be more acceptable to a young child. If the condition permits, intermittent patching may be necessary during the first few days. When patching is required postoperatively the child should be introduced to this sensation before surgery by playing games that require having the eyes covered. Arm restraints should also be made available for preoperative experimentation on a doll or favorite stuffed animal.

Reducing Postoperative Fear and Anxiety. Postoperatively the child must be treated as any child with impaired vision. If both eyes are patched he or she must be treated as a blind child; that is, things are placed within easy reach, the environment is described, and the child is told what will be done to him and what he or she is likely to feel before a procedure is begun. The child is allowed to handle things to discover their properties but needs verbal explanations of color. The primary goal is to help the child maintain the usual level of independence even though vision has been temporarily impaired. The surgery is brief and usually the child can be discharged the same day or the following day.

Promoting a Positive Self-Image. During the course of management the nurse is a resource person to the family. The negative effects of strabismus on the child's self-image and personality development can be minimized if attention is given to this potential problem early, beginning at the time of diagnosis. It is disappointing to the child and family when the operation fails to correct the misalignment. It should be explained early that repeated operations may be necessary.

Ongoing communication with the family regarding any difficulty encountered in carrying out the treatment program is an important contribution of the nurse. The child and family should be encouraged to express their thoughts and feelings about the operation and required treatment. The nurse should understand that when the operation is repeated it offers the same likelihood of success as did the original operation (Feman and Reinecke, 1978). Avoid misleading the family into assuming that successful correction will be achieved.

The nurse should decide whether referral of the family to a public health nurse or public agency is needed to meet demands of long-term care. If the child is in school, the treatment plan should be explained to the school nurse and lmitations on the child's school activities discussed.

Nursing Strategies for Follow-up Care in the Home or Clinic

Perform visual screening tests on both eyes (see Chapter 15).

Determine whether prescribed eyedrops are being administered and eye exercises being performed as ordered. Reinforce the importance of these therapies to support the family's motivation to follow through with therapy.

Assess for cysts of the iris of the affected eye if miotic drops are being used. Refer to the physician if a cyst is detected. Assure the child and family that cysts usually diminish with discontinuation of the medication.

Assess the child's body image related to the eyes. Ask the child to draw a picture of himself or herself with friends. With verbal input from the child, assess whether he or she perceives differences between self and friends in appearance and abilities.

Ask the child and family if the strabismus or therapy is adversely affecting schoolwork. Provide a liaison with the school nurse and teacher to be sure they understand the goals and importance of therapeutic measures. Assist them to intervene with the child's classmates to explain about strabismus and its treatment.

Amblyopia

Amblyopia ("lazy eye") is reduction or loss of vision in an eye that is normal on ophthalmoscopic examination (Scheie and Albert, 1977). A commonly accepted diagnostic sign of amblyopia is that visual acuity in the normal eye is at least two Snellen lines better than the acuity in the affected eye. There are various types of amblyopia: strabismic amblyopia, amblyopia ex anopsia, and anisometropic amblyopia.

Pathophysiology

Strabismic Amblyopia

This condition involves the loss of vision in the deviating eye of a child with strabismus. Visual loss occurs because there is an attempt to suppress the double vision experienced by the child with strabismus. The vision in the suppressed eye fails to develop, resulting in loss of vision ranging from a minimal decrease in acuity to severely impaired vision.

Early detection and treatment of strabismus is essential to prevent strabismic amblyopia. Usually by the age of 6 years the brain has developed suppression to a degree that will not readily respond to treatment, and by 8 or 9 years of age reversal of the impairment is considered virtually impossible.

Deprivation and Occlusion Amblyopia

This type of amblyopia can be caused by ptosis (drooping of the upper eyelid), cataracts, and occlusion therapy for strabismic amblyopia. These result in a blockage of the transferal images to the retina. This type is also called *amblyopia ex anopsia.*

Refractive Amblyopia

Amblyopia can also result from dissimilar refractive errors in the two eyes. Hyperopia (farsightedness) is a normal condition until around 6 to 7 years of age. This condition normally requires an accommodative effort by the child to correct the refractive error. When the two eyes are not equally hyperopic, fusion may be impossible because of the differences in the images. The less hyperopic eye may then become the preferred eye because less accommodation is required. Consequently, the other eye (the more hyperopic one) becomes lazy or amblyopic. This is known as *anisometropic amblyopia.* This type of amblyopia can be prevented if discovered and treated early. Glasses are necessary to correct the refractive error and prevent the development of anisometropic amblyopia.

Therapeutic Management

In addition to using glasses to correct any refractive error, patching of the good eye is the basis for treating amblyopia. The patch is usually worn during the waking hours, but some authorities recommend that the child wear the patch 24 hours a day. Careful follow-up is essential to prevent amblyopia of the eye that is being patched. Patching may be required for as long as a year, followed by a period of time during which intermittent patching must be continued. The child and family need reinforcement from the health team for their efforts in complying with the long-term therapy of keeping a young child's eye patched. With early identification and adequate therapy, irreversible loss of vision can be prevented.

Cataract

A cataract is an opacity (clouding) of the crystalline lens of the eye that consists of precipitated lens protein. The lens is a clear flexible disk located behind the pupil and iris. It is normally transparent to allow light to enter the eye and be refracted onto the retina. If a cataract is present light cannot be refracted and visual impairment exists. Cataracts may be unilateral or bilateral, complete or incomplete.

Congenital Cataracts

Cataracts can be congenital or acquired. Congenital cataracts are formed during the sixth or seventh week of fetal life when the lens is being formed. In many instances the presence of congenital cataracts is only one aspect of a complex syndrome.

Fifty per cent of congenital cataracts cannot be attributed to specific causes or associated with other anomalies. Trauma, anoxia, or maternal systemic disease during the first trimester of pregnancy have a definite effect on their development. Infectious conditions (commonly maternal rubella and herpes simplex) or inherited disorders (such as Turner's syndrome or galactosemia) account for approximately 50 per cent of cases.

Acquired Cataracts

Acquired cataracts appear at different times after birth and are usually related to trauma, systemic disease, drug toxicity (steroids, radiation), and infections. Cataracts may also develop secondary to other eye malformations and diseases such as retinopathy of prematurity (retrolental fibroplasia), retinal detachment, retinosis pigmentosa, and uveitis.

Diagnostic Assessment

Assessment and identification of prenatal high-risk populations is an important nursing role in prevention of cataracts. Prenatal factors such as systemic disease or vaginal infections caused by herpes simplex should be identified and treated. Adequate immunization against rubella and early, comprehensive prenatal care are preventive strategies in which the nurse can actively participate. Additionally, genetic counseling should be made available for families with identified familial diseases. Encouraging compliance with medical regimens such as adherence to the prescribed diet when a child has galactosemia can be a factor in retarding the appearance of cataracts.

The sooner cataracts are removed, the better the child's prognosis. Since most cataracts cannot be detected with the unaided eye, checking for the red reflex is an important part of physical assessment (see Chapter 15). Cataracts that lie in the line of vision and produce some visual impairment cause the red reflex to be distorted or impaired. Opacity of the lens blocks the reflected light and is perceived as a dark area or shadow by the examiner. (Calhoun, 1983). Those types of cataracts that affect the anterior portion of the lens can be seen with the naked eye and are frequently noticed by parents. A unilateral cataract results in monocular vision (use of one eye) because binocular cooperation of the two eyes is compromised. Eventually strabismus develops and presents as the first clue to the existing cataract.

When a congenital cataract is suspected, a thorough ophthalmologic examination is indicated. The extent of the cataract can be determined by ultrasonography (B-scan), a nonintrusive, painless diagnostic test that can be done through closed eyelids while the infant is sleeping. The nursing role during the stressful diagnostic period focuses on giving and repeating, if necessary, simple explanations of the diagnostic procedures and the proposed treatment plan. Using terms that the family understands is critical to helping them cope. If surgery is decided upon, the nurse, along with other members of the health team, is responsible for helping the family understand the life-long implications of cataract surgery. There is great emotional and financial stress for these families as they attempt to cope with repeated surgical procedures.

When cataracts are likely to interfere with vision, surgical removal is indicated. The density of the cataract and visual acuity are considerations when determining the need to operate.

Surgical Management

In adults, an incision is made into the eye and the lens is grasped and removed from the eye, leaving its capsule intact (intracapsular approach). In children, this technique is associated with loss of vitreous from the eye and can predispose the child to retinal detachment and corneal edema. The extracapsular approach is preferred for children. The lens is left in place to hold back the vitreous. One disadvantage is that the retained lens capsule becomes opaque, necessitating a second operation (Goble, 1984). New instruments are now available to remove the lens and *some* of the vitreous. This procedure generally does not require a second operation for an opaque capsule but on occasion a characteristic cystlike edema in the macula develops as a complication. Although this edema usually decreases over time, there is no effective treatment and it does interfere with vision while it is present (Goble, 1984). The fitting and wearing of corrective contact lenses or glasses is the next step in management. Infants may be fitted with lenses as early as 3 weeks after surgery.

A newer surgical technique being used for adults is insertion of an intraocular lens, but this is not commonly used for children. Complications of this technique include uveitis and corneal damage (Goble, 1984).

Strategies for Nursing Care

Goals for nursing care include providing information and support for the family in the preoperative period and providing and teaching physical support of the child postoperatively. Strategies to meet these goals are discussed later.

Preoperative preparation of the family includes discussion of eye patches and restraints used in the immediate postoperative period. Explain that vision will not be improved immediately, because corrective lenses are necessary after surgery. Postoperatively, the nurse is involved in physical support of the infant and in teaching the family to carry out the care. An eye shield is used for protection for about a week. If glasses are worn, the eye shield is used only at night and during naptime after the first postoperative day. A combination of antibiotic and steroid drops is given for several weeks to prevent infection and minimize inflammation. Usually, with current surgical techniques activity restriction is minimal. The parents should demonstrate proficiency and ease with administration of eye drops before the infant is discharged from the hospital.

When contact lenses are prescribed, the nurse's teaching includes helping the family learn specific cleaning, insertion, and removal techniques. The nurse also makes sure that the graduated schedule for wearing time is well understood so that corneal damage can be prevented. The importance of close medical follow-up must be stressed to ensure maximum benefits from the cataract surgery and prescribed lenses.

Expected Outcome

The prognosis for visual acuity after cataract surgery varies. The results are often poor because of other ocular defects associated with the cataracts. Visual acuity is also compromised by surgical complications, most commonly secondary glaucoma or, in later years, retinal detachment. The family's desire and ability to help the child wear suitable glasses or contact lenses is another determining factor. The real measure of success following cataract surgery is related to the child's ability to function at an optimal level in his or her environment.

Congenital (Infantile) Glaucoma

Congenital or infantile glaucoma can be of the primary type (inherited as an autosomal recessive disease) or can be associated with other hereditary diseases or syndromes such as Sturge-Weber, Marfan, and Lowe. (See Chapter 4 for a discusssion of patterns of inheritance.) Glaucoma may also develop secondary to trauma, intraocular hemorrhage, inflammation, or intraocular tumor (Martyn, 1987).

Pathophysiology

Glaucoma is a condition characterized by increased intraocular pressure. Intraocular fluid (aqueous) is produced by the ciliary body. It flows between the iris and the lens into the anterior chamber, then into the

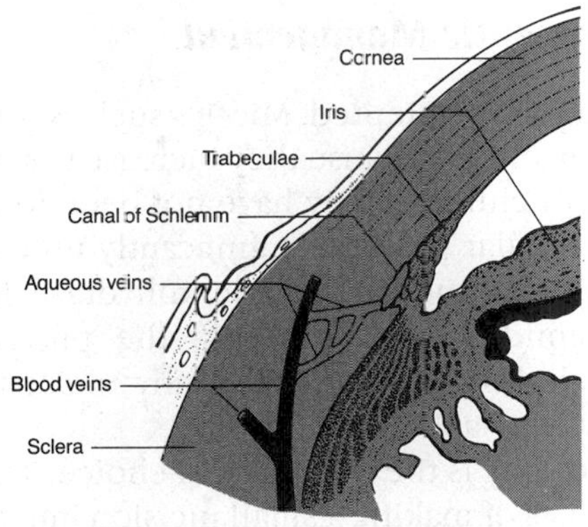

Figure 51-4. Anatomy of the iridocorneal angle, showing the system for outflow of aqueous humor into the conjunctival veins. The iridocorneal angle is that space between the iris and cornea as they approach the canal of Schlemm. (From Guyton AC: *Human Physiology and Mechanisms of Disease,* 3rd ed. Philadelphia, WB Saunders, 1982, 245.)

canal of Schlemm. In glaucoma the outflow of aqueous from the anterior chamber is restricted by a deviation in the angle of the anterior chamber of the eye (Fig. 51-4). Intraocular pressure is increased as a result of aqueous accumulation. As the elastic coating of the eye is stretched by the increased pressure, the globe enlarges and the optic nerve atrophies. Infants with congenital glaucoma have large, cow-like eyes (buphthalmos) as a result of this enlargement.

Clinical Manifestations and Diagnostic Assessment

The nurse needs to be aware of the hereditary factor in identifying the population at high risk for primary congenital glaucoma. Genetic counseling should be available for these families. Early assessment of visual competency is an important component of case finding. The principal signs and symptoms are tearing, photophobia (sensitivity to light), blepharospasm (twitching of the eyelids), corneal clouding (edema), and progressive enlargement of the eye (Martyn, 1984). Frequent rubbing of the eye, accompanied by redness, is also a symptom associated with glaucoma. Furthermore, an infant may burrow his or her head into a pillow to protect the eyes. Identification of these signs necessitates referral for ophthalmologic examination.

Diagnosis before 1 year of age is important to ensure adequate treatment and prevent visual loss. Diagnosis is made by measuring intraocular pressure with a tonometer, an instrument that, when placed on the anesthetized cornea, registers the underlying pressure. Corneal diameters are also measured and complete ophthalmologic examination is carried out. The nurse assists the physician with examinations and provides support to the infant through closeness and gentle touch. The family needs explanations of the various diagnostic tests in easily understood terms.

Therapeutic Management

Medical therapy is limited. Miotics such as pilocarpine are used in adults because they increase the outflow of aqueous. In children they have not been found to reduce intraocular pressure significantly unless a goniotomy is performed. Carbonic anhydrase inhibitors (acetazolamides) will suppress the production of aqueous slightly but not sufficiently to substitute for surgery (Chew and Morin, 1983).

Goniotomy is the treatment of choice. This procedure consists of making a small incision into the tissue obstructing the angle of the anterior chamber. This incision permits flow of aqueous to the canal of Schlemm. Often two or three goniotomies in different locations are required to obtain normal intraocular pressure. Once the pressure is normal, the prognosis for control of glaucoma is good. If corneal clouding is present at birth, however, the prognosis is guarded: only 30 per cent of these children are cured with one or two goniotomies (Goble, 1984).

Strategies for Nursing Care

The major goals of nursing care following surgery for glaucoma in infancy are related to maintaining a low intraocular pressure, reducing the infant's fear and anxiety associated with eye patches, and preparing parents to manage the infant's care at home after discharge. Eye patches are applied postoperatively and the infant should be observed closely for restlessness, which indicates rising intraocular pressure. Strategies to maintain low intraocular pressure are found in the box entitled Postoperative Nursing Care Following Goniotomy. Mydriatic medication is given to maximally dilate the pupil and encourage drainage. Dilating the pupil keeps the eye at rest and facilitates postoperative healing. Frequent tonometric readings of intraocular pressure and measurements of corneal diameters are used to detect increased pressure.

The infant is usually discharged from the hospital on the first or second postoperative day. In preparation for discharge, the nurse instructs the family in proper

Postoperative Nursing Care Following Goniotomy*

Major Nursing Diagnoses	Nursing Goals/Strategies
Potential for Injury: visual, related to increased intraocular pressure following surgery for glaucoma	Assess for evidence of increased intraocular pressure by: • being alert for restlessness that is not relieved by ordinary comfort measures. Institute measures to maintain a low intraocular pressure by: • elevating the head of bed 30 degrees (or as ordered) • comforting the infant to prevent crying (e.g., holding, allowing a pacifier, feeding on demand) • assessing bowel function preoperatively and treating constipation so that the infant will not strain with stool postoperatively • avoiding loud noises that will startle the infant
Fear/Anxiety, related to bilateral eye patches in the immediate postoperative period	Reduce anxiety by: • approaching the infant with a soft voice and speaking before touching • changing the infant's position slowly, speaking soothing words • encouraging parent involvement in care and usual physical contact with the infant
Knowledge Deficit: Parent(s), related to • *instillation of prescribed eyedrops* • *assessment of rising intraocular pressure* • *the need for regular follow-up care*	*Provide information and guidance needed to support home care after discharge.*

* To be used with Table 27-7, Perioperative Nursing Care.

administration of eye medication. Provisions for adequate medical follow-up should be made and discussed with the family. Further surgery may be necessary if intraocular pressure rises again.

Expected Outcome

Surgical correction of glaucoma aims to normalize the intraocular pressure but it does not guarantee 20/20 vision. The earlier the onset of glaucoma, the poorer the visual prognosis. Of children who present with glaucoma at birth, over 50 per cent will be legally blind. Even if intraocular pressure is controlled through surgical intervention, only 35 per cent of cases have visual acuity better than 20/50 (Chew and Morin, 1983). The decrease in vision is caused by optic nerve damage occurring before the pressure was controlled, by opacities such as corneal scars and cataracts, and by amblyopia (Morin and Bryars, 1980). When corneal clouding is noted between 1 and 24 months of age a good prognosis is obtained in 95 per cent of cases with one or two goniotomies (Goble, 1984).

Nursing Strategies for Follow-up Care in the Home or Clinic

Assess the child's apparent level of comfort and question the parents about any unexplained restlessness.

Prepare the infant for tonometric readings by anesthetizing the cornea with drops prescribed by the physician.

Encourage the parents to discuss feelings and concerns about the expected outcome.

Provide early referral to supporting agencies that can teach the parents how to facilitate the infant's normal development despite an existing visual impairment.

Visual Impairment

The term *visual impairment* includes a highly heterogeneous group of conditions. Some people with visual impairment are able to distinguish between light and dark or have good sight for distance but not for peripheral vision (a condition called tunnel vision), while others are totally blind. Visual impairment is classified according to physiologic measurements (visual acuity) as well as functional ability (Alonso et al, 1978; Jan et al, 1977).

Partial Sight. Physiologic measurement: Children with partial sight have vision that cannot be corrected beyond 20/70 in either eye or have a limited field of vision (the widest diameter of visual field being an angle of no greater than 140 degrees).

Functional ability: Vision is considered partial when visual loss interferes with learning processes but still permits the use of print as a chief method of learning.

Blindness. Physiologic measurement: Children with corrected vision in the better eye of not more than 20/200 or a limitation in the visual field (widest diameter of vision being an angle of no more than 20 degrees) are considered blind.

Functional ability: A child is considered blind when other senses (hearing and touch) are relied upon as chief means of task performance and learning.

Promoting Optimal Development. Visually impaired (partially sighted and blind) children must be identified early so that effective treatment programs can be instituted. Early intervention has the potential to prevent developmental delays and life-long maladaptive functioning. While some of these children may show developmental delays, it cannot be assumed that the more limited a child's vision is the greater the developmental delay. Furthermore, depending on how successfully a child can learn through the remaining vision and the other senses, the child's development may not be delayed at all (Alonso et al, 1978).

The term *visual handicap* is usually used to describe the condition in those children with visual impairment who, even after maximum correction, are limited in their ability to learn through the visual channel (Alonso et al, 1978). Most blind children have some remaining (residual) vision that they should be encouraged to use. *Residual vision* is a term used to describe the vision of a child who cannot read print of any size but whose vision is more than only light perception (Jan et al, 1977). Any degree of vision that a child has should be used because the eyes, particularly those of young children, benefit from use.

Visually impaired children have the same needs as other children, but they are met through alternative means. These children need stimulation from their environment and the opportunity to get information and responses from the people around them. These children cannot get information and responses through sight; therefore, experiences must be adapted to support their physical, intellectual, and emotional and social development.

Partial Sight

The dilemma of the partially sighted is best described in the words of a partially sighted child: "It is very hard when you are not really blind or sighted because you are just hanging in the middle" (Jan et al, 1977). Partially sighted children's conditions are often misdiagnosed or remain undiagnosed. Their eyes may look normal, and it is only when the child's development seems to be slow that parents may suspect something is wrong. The behavior and responses of these children are often misinterpreted. For example, when first enrolled in preschool, a partially sighted child may be viewed as clumsy or immature or as a slow learner or a behavior problem because he or she seems uncooperative and inattentive.

Areas in which a partially sighted child needs special help and understanding are related to communication, mobility, spatial perception, and visual fatigue. The partially sighted child is often unsure of how to respond verbally to others. The intent of people's *communication* is often conveyed through facial expression and gestures. Because a partially sighted child's perception is distorted, he or she may be confused as to how to respond. Additional verbal explanations may be required to clarify the exact meaning and intent during conversation.

Mobility and spatial perception are also affected when a child has partial sight. Many of these children walk later and more hesitantly than sighted children. Their depth perception and concept of the body in space may not be developed sufficiently, resulting in clumsiness, falls, and accidents.

Visual fatigue is particularly noticed when a partially sighted child begins school. Teachers, nurses, and parents must recognize that behavior problems may develop because of visual fatigue. As the eyes tire, a child, may become inattentive and irritable. Diagnosis and assessment of the child's vision by an ophthalmologist is essential in order to plan an educational program that best meets the child's needs.

Once the visual capacities have been established, management of the visual disability follows. This includes increasing the retinal image by magnification, increasing the sharpness of the image, or using other senses (auditory or tactile) to compensate for vision loss (Tongue, 1980). A particularly well-accepted visual aid device for preschoolers 4 and 5 years of age is a hand-held prism telescope of six times and eight times magnification; its use is thought to possibly improve self-sufficiency and mobility later in life (Tongue, 1980). Other low-vision aid devices are available through low-vision aid centers. (See Box 51-3.) However, low-vision aid facilities in the United States are primarily located in cities and are fewer in number than service organizations for the blind. (Problems of the Partially Seeing, 1980).

In the past there has been some concern that straining the eyes might result in further loss of vision. Consequently, use of books in Braille was recommended as the major source of learning so that sight would be "saved." Now that it has been determined that using the eyes does not weaken vision, partially sighted children are reading large-print materials, in addition to using a variety of supplemental aids including talking books, tapes and cassettes, magnifiers, telescopes, and closed-circuit television enlarging devices.

The problems of the partially sighted are different from those of the blind. Many of the social and economic rehabilitative services available to the "legally blind" are not available to the partially sighted. The most important aspect of adjustment for the partially sighted child is learning to utilize residual vision fully. With adequate services and devices to supplement their vision, partially sighted children have a chance to participate in their world and reach their maximum potential.

Blindness

Each blind child has individual needs just as any child has; however, ***children who are robbed of one of their most crucial senses have the special need to learn alternate ways of relating to their environment.*** Every area of development is affected by a child's inability to see. The following discussion describes the impact of blindness and appropriate interventions in the areas of (1) developing human attachment, (2) motor development and mobility, (3) language, cognition and learning, (4) play and socialization, (5) independence and self-concept, and (6) perception of space and body image.

Development of Human Attachment

The development of human attachment is basic to a child's growth and serves as the foundation for the parent-child relationship. As noted by Phillips and Hartley (1988), "When infants form affective or emotional ties with their parents, the world has meaning" (p. 202). When a child is blind, the usual facial interplay that is used to express mutual pleasure between the infant and parents must be replaced by an alternate method of communication. The pattern of smiling and the factors that elicit it are different in a blind infant. For the sighted infant the visual stimulus of the human face elicits an automatic smile at 2 to 2½ months of age with a high degree of regularity for which there is no equivalent in the blind baby (Fraiberg, 1974). In a study of seven infants (Fraiberg, 1971; Fraiberg, 1974) it was noted that from the second month on blind babies smiled in response to a familiar voice or sound and increasingly demonstrated a pattern of selective smiling in favor of the mother's voice. However, the smile was not automatic and even the mother's voice did not elicit it regularly. To help parents of a blind baby, the nurse should understand the importance that the smile has in development of a mutually satisfying relationship between parent and infant. Parents can be encouraged to hold their blind infant and to talk, coo,

Box 51-3
Resources for the Visually Impaired

ORGANIZATIONS

American Association of University Affiliated Programs
Suite 406
2033 M Street
Washington, DC 20036
Provides diagnostic, treatment, educational, and consultant services.

American Foundation for the Blind
15 West 16th Street
New york, NY 10011
Publishes *The Journal of Visual Impairment and Blindness.*

Association for the Education of the Visually Handicapped
919 Walnut Street
Philadelphia, PA 19107
Publishes *Education of the Visually Handicapped.*

Canadian National Institute for the Blind
1931 Bayview Avenue
Toronto, Ontario M4G 4C8

Council for Exceptional Children
1920 Association Drive
Reston, VA 22091

National Association for Parents of the Visually Impaired
2011 Hardy Circle
Austin, TX 78657

National Association for the Visually Handicapped
305 East 24th Street
New York, NY 10010

National Society for the Prevention of Blindness, Inc.
79 Madison Avenue
New York, NY 10016

RESOURCES FOR MATERIALS AND CATALOGUES

American Printing House for the Blind, Inc.
1839 Frankfort Avenue
Louisville, KY 40200
Catalogue of large-type materials

National Association for Visually Handicapped
3201 Balboa Street
San Francisco, CA 94121

Library of Congress
Division for the Blind
and Physically Handicapped
Reference Department
1291 Taylor Street N.W.
Washington, DC 20542
Provides for library service to individuals who are unable to read standard print.

Catalog of Optical Aids, Optical Aid Service
New York Association for the Blind
111 East 59th Street
New York, NY 10022

Vision Center
1393 North High Street
Columbus, OH 43201

Touch, Inc.
P.O. Box 1711,
Albany, NY 12201

and sing and play lap games with the baby to help him or her learn to know them and to elicit smiles.

Even when parents and blind infants develop a maximally satisfying relationship, the smile of the blind infant differs from that of the sighted child. Blind babies have a "muted smile" and do not have expressive facial signs that depict various emotions. The absence of these signs may be read as "no affect" and are cause for parents and others to comment that "he looks depressed" or "nothing interests him," (Fraiberg, 1974). The process of developing a satisfying exchange of signals between parents and their blind infant must be recognized by the nurse as a potentially frustrating experience for parents. The nurse has an important responsibility to help parents and blind infants communicate and to provide parents an opportunity to express feelings about the development of their relationship with the infant.

Motor Development and Mobility

Motor development and mobility for a blind infant is another area that requires special intervention from parents. In the sighted child, motor development is enhanced by the child's interest in moving toward the things he or she can see. While auditory experiences in a blind child must replace visual experiences, an important phenomenon regarding a child's response to sound must be recognized. The sighted child reaches for and attains an object at the age of 24 to 28 weeks (Fraiberg, 1966) because the child can see it. However, whether blind or sighted, an infant does not reach for an object he or she *hears* until the last quarter of the first year. Activities of reaching and grasping for and crawling toward an object have a primary role in motor development, but the blind child is dependent on auditory stimulation for self-initiated mobility. Consequently this movement does not occur in the blind child until much later than it does for a sighted child because the sighted child moves toward the object he or she sees. Therefore, the immediate environment of the blind child must provide interesting sounding objects and varied tactile experiences that the child's hands will encounter while randomly moving. A mobile or cradle gym over the crib will provide opportunities for random hand movements to encounter interesting objects and will encourage bringing the hands together at midline (Phillips and Hartley, 1988). At 5 to 8 months, finger foods should be allowed to help perfect grasping. These early experiences with objects provide the blind infant with the necessary stimulation to progress toward a sense of self and object differentiation.

Various stimuli can be used to lure infants to begin to move out into the space around them. Without specific intervention these infants' hands may encounter only each other or the mouth. If mouth and hand activities become fixed at this immature level, these infants are reported to show signs of impending autism (Adelson and Fraiberg, 1972).

Blind babies have been reported to sit and support themselves on their hands and knees at the same time as sighted children, but these activities were not followed by creeping as they were in sighted infants (Fraiberg, 1971). Independent walking for blind children is hampered because they lack the visual model to imitate. A blind baby was described by Adelson and Fraiberg to walk "painstakingly at first, one step at a time, feeling his way repeatedly as he gained familiarity with his old world in a new position." (Adelson and Fraiberg, 1974). The median age for independent walking in blind children reported in their research is 19.25 months, 7 months later than sighted children. If blind babies are given early experience with the interesting possibilities in the space around them and are lured into that space by the familiar voices of their parents and by interesting sounds, they will achieve the developmental task of independent walking, although at a later time than will sighted children.

Achievement of independent walking is encumbered with fears on the part of the child as well as the parents. The children need repeated practice to propel themselves into an experience that provides new sensation; at times they may reach an impasse, when they seem to retreat from their experimentation with walking. Parents, on the other hand, fear that a delay in walking may mean that their child is mentally retarded. Parents need to be prepared for these delays and may need constant encouragement to provide opportunities that will help their blind child learn the skills of mobility.

As the blind child becomes mobile parents are faced with a new dilemma—they fear that he or she will be injured while engaging in normal active play. During the developing years all children need special instructions about dangers, but they should not be prohibited from engaging in normal activities of swinging, biking, sliding, and other recreational activities.

Specific activities must be taught to blind children because they cannot learn by imitation. For example, children's legs and arms may have to be physically manipulated to show them how to skip, hop, or bounce a ball. They can learn how to use play equipment such as a slide and monkey bars by feeling another child's body move or by having someone move their bodies through the motions (Alonso, 1978). While blind children are taught the motions of these physical activities they must also be taught the rules and limitations that will keep them safe.

Successful mobility is one of the most important skills that a blind person acquires. *Early intervention can determine to a large degree how independent a blind person will be in later life.* As a child enters school specific mobility skills can be taught by trained instructors. Blind children are taught to listen for the echo of their breath to tell them when they are about to bump into large objects. Cane technique and guide dogs are invaluable aids to independent movement. Guide dogs are not usually used until the teen years (Jan et al., 1977).

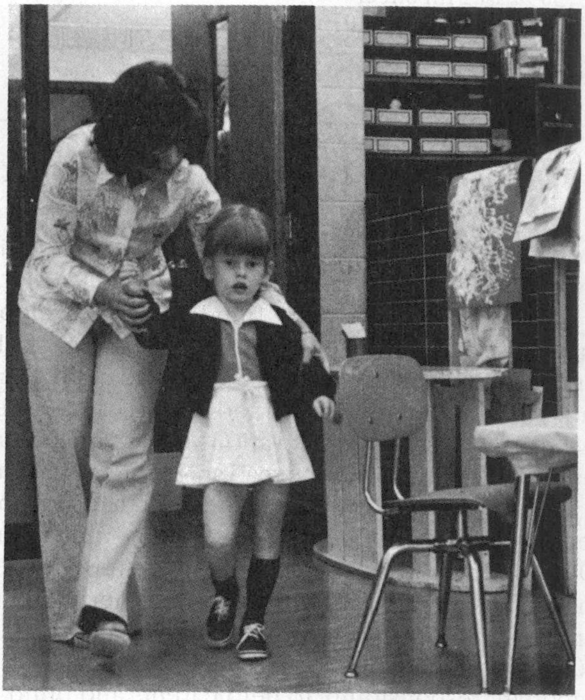

"And now we're coming to the worktable, where Barry is sitting." (From Alonso L, et al: *Mainstreaming preschoolers: children with visual handicaps.* DHEW Publication No (OHDS) 78-3112. Washington, DC, US Govt Printing Office, 1978, 39.)

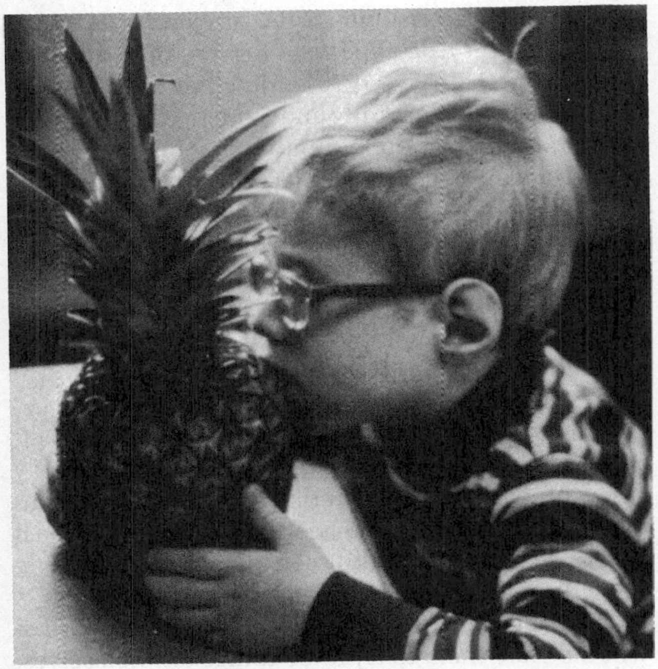

Blind children need the experience of feeling objects. (From Alonso L, et al: *Mainstreaming preschoolers: children with visual handicaps.* DHEW Publication No (OHDS) 78-3112. Washington, DC, US Govt Printing Office, 1978, 37.)

Language, Cognition and Learning

Blindness has a profound impact on the child's abilities in *language, cognition, and learning.* Vocalizations and first words occur during the first year of life at about the same time in a blind child and a sighted child. After this stage, however, language development in a blind child is often delayed, but the degree of visual impairment has not been shown to correlate positively with speech and language difficulties; this indicates that blindness alone is not the decisive factor (Jan et al, 1977).

The family and environment of the blind child greatly influences his or her cognitive and language development. This child must be talked to and the verbalizations should be associated with concrete experiences to enable the child to understand words and concepts. The child needs to handle toys and variously shaped objects while their characteristics are being described.

Blind children must accept verbal descriptions by the sighted of many objects and phenomena that they cannot touch (moon, fire). Therefore, they have an incomplete concept of whatever is being described. Phillips and Hartley (1988) discussed the problem of developing "object concept" as a case where objects fail to exist when they are not being concretely experienced. "The infant lives in a magic world for an extended period of time where people and things mysteriously appear and disappear" (p. 203).

The ability to describe visual concepts verbally while having only partial or inaccurate understanding is called *verbalism. Teaching a blind child from infancy with as many concrete experiences as possible helps the child develop concepts and is an important intervention to promote later academic learning.*

School programs for the visually impaired are varied, ranging from residential schools for the blind to public school programs in which the blind are integrated. Both types of programs require special equipment and devices for the blind student. Academic achievement of blind children who have access to appropriate educational opportunities does not differ from that of sighted children (Chinn, 1979).

Technologic advances are making the printed word more accessible to blind children, but many blind scholars believe that Braille will continue to be a primary method of reading and writing for the blind (Jan et al, 1977). Electronic reading devices in which letters are produced in tactile form are also available. Machines that actually speak the words, talking calculators and tape recordings (with a device that can increase or slow the speed of the recording) can aid the blind student (Jan et al, 1977). In addition to educational materials the blind student may need special help in physical education and sex education, and in music, drama, and art.

Play and Socialization

Blind children's *play and social skills* are profoundly affected by their visual impairment. Infants need toys that will help them establish their ability to affect their environment (Phillips and Hartley, 1988). Toys with 'buttons' to push, cranks to wind, doors to open, etc., give the child a sense of mastery and control. As they become mobile, the active play of young children presents new problems to blind children. In the area of physical activity their ability to learn games through imitation is limited and to compete with peers is diminished. They cannot follow a rolling ball because they cannot see it. Furthermore, because they cannot imitate their peers in actions and behavior, they are unable to gain a sense of being like them.

Blind children need extra help from teachers, other children, and family members during play and socialization experiences. During the toddler and preschool years when a child learns to relate to other children, the blind child must be told about the activity and his or her body must be moved through the activity before the nature of it can be understood. *Visually impaired children benefit from physical contact when being helped to accomplish a task as an alternative to being able to learn by imitation.*

The choice of play materials for the blind child is

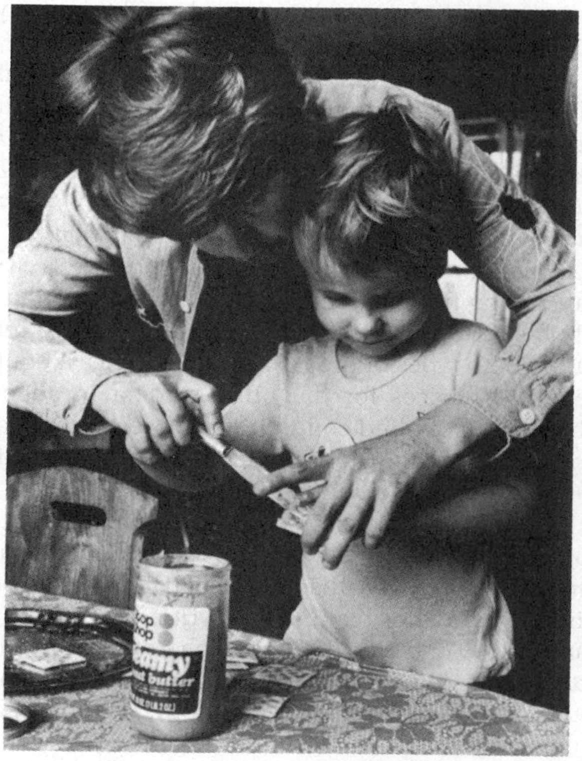

Visually handicapped children often learn best by being "moved" through an activity. (From Alonso L, et al: *Mainstreaming preschoolers: children with visual handicaps.* DHEW Publication No (OHDS) 78-3112. Washington, DC, US Govt Printing Office, 1978, 48.)

based on the guideline that if a child cannot see materials well enough to learn the intended concepts or skills, substitute tactile or auditory material must be provided to teach these things (Jan et al, 1977). *When playing with a blind child, one must talk more than normally about the objects and the activity* so that the child will gain an accurate idea of what constitutes his or her environment. A wide range of textures should be available to the child and their appearance described. During play a blind child is assisted to distinguish various sounds and the direction from which the sounds are coming. The more sensory experiences a blind child has in play, the more opportunity he or she has to take in information to foster normal growth and development.

Self-stimulating mannerisms such as body rocking, eye poking, head rolling, thumb sucking, and other eye, hand, and head movements have been noted in blind children. These are called stereotyped behaviors. These repetitive motor activities vary in frequency, complexity, and intensity. A direct positive correlation with the degree of visual impairment and the frequency of the behaviors has been reported (Jan et al, 1977). Furthermore, these activities seem to intensify with boredom and with excessive stimulation. It has been suggested that self-stimulating behaviors may be done to overstimulate the labyrinth of the inner ear in an effort to compensate for loss of orientation (Siegel and Murphy, 1970). Although the cause of these behaviors is not fully understood, early intervention to provide the opportunity for mobility, exploration, and manipulation of objects is recommended to help the child substitute for them (Jan et al, 1977). That is, blind children need help to "come out" of themselves rather than to escape into their private worlds.

Independence and Self-Concept

Achieving *independence in the activities of daily living* is important for the development of a positive self-concept in all children. Blind children are particularly at risk of losing the opportunity to do things for themselves because they need special help and additional time to learn self-care skills. Being treated as capable people by teachers, friends, and family members is crucial for blind children to develop the initiative that will motivate them to try to do things for themselves. The nurse can aid parents by providing them with hints that they can use to help foster independence as presented in Box 51-4. (See Table 51-10 for additional strategies related to independence and self-concept.)

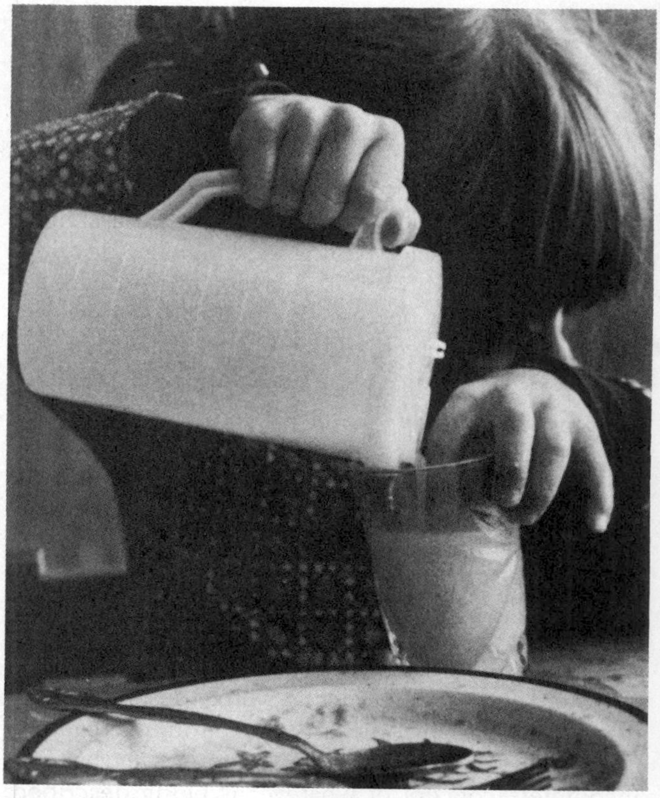

A blind child becomes independent by doing. (From Alonso L, et al: *Mainstreaming preschoolers: children with visual handicaps.* DHEW Publication No (OHDS) 78-3112. Washington, DC, US Govt Printing Office, 1978, 59.)

Box 51-4
Practical Hints to Use in Fostering Independence in a Blind Child

ORIENTATION AND MOBILITY

- To move along a wall, hold arm nearest wall slightly out to the side and forward.
- Hand is in a loosely curved position with the back of the fingers touching the wall to locate openings or obstacles.
- Fingers are curved slightly inward to prevent injury at places such as door frames.
- Explain where you are going when leading a child so that he or she feels more secure.
- Verbally describe the arrangement of desks and furniture so that he or she can become independent more quickly.

MEALTIME AND SNACKS

- Use real dishes—plastic or paper dishes tip and spill easily.
- A dish with a rim and some depth makes it easier for a child to use a scooping maneuver.
- Securing the dish to the table surface eliminates accidental tipping and spilling.
- Placing food in a circle and explaining its position according to the numbers on the clock is useful for children who can tell time.
- Glasses or cups should have a wide base.
- Permit children to pour their own liquids when developmentally able to do so. (Child can grip glass with one hand and place index finger slightly below the rim of the glass to feel when the glass is full.)
- By sitting behind a child in helping him or her learn to use a spoon, one can assist the child with more natural feeding movements.
- In some cases the help of an occupational therapist should be suggested if a child has difficulty in swallowing, chewing, or biting.

DRESSING

- Start with undressing (outerwear, then loose clothing such as T-shirts and sweaters).
- Break tasks down into small steps, explaining each step while the child's hand is over yours as the task is performed.
- Praise the child as each step is learned.
- Tags and special identifying marks on clothes are needed to help a child choose his or her own outfits.

TOILET TRAINING

- A child must be instructed verbally in a step-by-step approach, including where the potty is, how it looks, and its purpose.

(From Mainstreaming Preschoolers: Children with Visual Handicaps. *DHEW Publication No (OHDS) 78-3112. Washington, DC, US Govt Printing Office, 1978.)*

Perception of Space and Body Image

The blind child develops a *body image* through tactile experiences and, once language becomes meaningful, through verbal communication and feedback. The ways a blind child takes in information are inferior to those of the sighted child; consequently, the formation of body image is delayed (Scholl, 1973). Certain activities are thought to aid a child's ability to organize space in relation to his or her own body. For example, bending down, reaching out, and climbing under and over an object assists blind children in developing an idea of where their body fits in relation to the larger space outside it (Barraga, 1973).

A problem of blind children that has been identified as indicating a deficit in body image is the "floppy" posture that some blind children tend to assume. Based on the verbal responses of blind children on tests of body image, Cratty (1971) has identified four stages through which children pass in developing a body image. These are:

Phase I. Awareness of body parts, body planes, and simple movements.

Phase II. Left-right discrimination.

Phase III. Body object relationships; identification of portions of the limbs.

Phase IV. Identification of body parts and body movements of another person.

Body image training as described by Cratty is organized around these four phases.

Development of body image is a central aspect of education of the blind. It cannot be left to chance that children make the connection of how their bodies relate to space. A thorough, systematic effort must be made by the sighted to help blind children learn the dimensions of themselves and their world.

An important nursing intervention consists of providing opportunities for parents to discuss feelings about their infant's response and to explore ways to develop pleasurable interaction patterns. *The nurse's attitude toward the infant may influence the family's ability to interact with their child.* An accepting attitude is conveyed when the nurse touches, holds, and talks to the infant, pointing out normal aspects of development to the parents. Supporting parental attempts to provide sensory stimulation will facilitate early infant attachment.

The special needs of the visually impaired infant dictate use and coordination of a variety of educational and health services. The nurse's role may encompass both coordination of resources and referrals to ensure maximum use of available community resources. Ideally the infant should be enrolled in a structured infant stimulation program to develop age-appropriate skills. Community resources such as the state department of education, division of special education, or rehabilitation services and services for the blind can be consulted for additional help. The goal of habilitation for visually deprived infants, is to emphasize to their parents their likeness to all children and to foster their growth and development. It is not the degree of visual acuity they possess that determines their functional ability but how they use their sight and other senses.

Hearing Impairment

Hearing impairment may be profound, significantly handicapping a child, or so mild that it goes undetected for years. Both the volume (measured in decibels [dB]) and pitch (measured in Hertz [Hz]) of a sound determine whether it is audible to the human ear.

The volume of sound that is required in order for an individual to hear is reported in decibels. This is called the hearing level. Levels of hearing impairment in decibels used to describe severity of hearing loss vary in the literature; however, it is generally agreed that persons with hearing levels exceeding 90 dB are termed "deaf." For educational purposes, however, a *deaf* person is one whose hearing is disabled to a level (usually 70 dB or greater) at which speech through the ear alone, with or without a hearing aid, cannot be understood; a *hard-of-hearing* person is one whose hearing is disabled to a level (usually 35 to 69 dB) that makes it difficult to understand speech through the ear alone, with or without a hearing aid (Moores, 1978). The hard-of-hearing person has sufficient residual hearing to understand speech with the use of a hearing aid, although it is difficult.

For the deaf person vision is the primary mode of language acquisition and communication. The probable handicap that results from the various hearing

Table 51-4. Degree of Handicap and Educational Need According to Hearing Levels

Hearing Level in Decibels (dB) and Degree of Hearing Loss: Children	Adults	Effect of Hearing Loss and Educational Needs
Normal 0–20	0–26	Although this is considered normal hearing, those children in upper limits of this range may be affected. They may show poor language development, have problems in listening, and have reduced ability to hear information needed for academic achievement.
Mild loss 21–35	27–40	Faint and distant speech is heard with difficulty. Child may benefit from a hearing aid and needs special seating and lighting in classroom; may need speechreading instruction.
Moderate loss 36–55	41–55	Understands conversational speech at a distance of 3–5 ft if in face-to-face position. May be limited in vocabulary and exhibit some incorrect speech. Child in the classroom will benefit from special seating and a hearing aid; may need speechreading instruction.
Moderately severe loss 56–70	56–70	Conversation must be loud to be understood. Child has great difficulty participating in classroom discussions. Needs special seating, hearing aid, speechreading instruction, and may need special classes for the hearing impaired to develop speech and language skills.
Severe loss 71–90	71–90	May hear loud voices at a distance of 1 ft from the ear. May be able to distinguish vowels but not consonants. May be able to identify environmental noises. Speech and language is defective. Child required full-time special education hearing aid, and program to develop language and speech.
Profound 91 or more	91 or more	May hear some loud sounds but does so through recognizing vibration rather than tones. Does not rely on hearing as a primary channel for communication. Child requires full-time program with continuous appraisal of needs in regard to communication techniques.

(From Martin, 1978; Stangler, 1980.)

levels in decibels is summarized in Table 51-4. It should be noted that the ranges differ for children and adults. Even slight hearing impairment has the potential to interfere with a child's normal development of speech and language and educational progress.

The summary as provided in this table is only a general guide. It does not take into account important variables that the nurse should always consider when assessing the impact of a hearing impairment. These factors are (1) cause and onset of the hearing loss, (2) type of hearing impairment (see later discussion on types of hearing losses), (3) presence of other impairments (physical, intellectual, emotional), and (4) interactions and relationships within the family (Sweitzer, 1977).

It is important for nurses to realize that a high percentage of children are affected by hearing loss yet it is often a subtle, undetected deficit that can seriously affect the child's development.

By 2 years of age, 1 : 25 children (4 per cent) will have mild to moderate hearing losses secondary to ear disease; in school-age children 7 to 8 per cent have some degree of hearing loss. Severe hearing loss is present in 1 : 1000 infants and 1 : 50 neonates discharged from intensive care nurseries.

Early detection of hearing impairment, regardless of degree, is paramount. By 3 years of age approximately 80 percent of language growth is thought to have taken place (Lennenberg, 1967). Deafness during early childhood, occurring before the acquisition of a functional language base, seriously affects a child in all areas of development. Furthermore, mild hearing loss significantly reduces vocabulary growth, articulation skills, the ability to communicate through spoken language, the use of grammar and syntax, and auditory memory skills (McFarland and Simmons, 1980).

Regular hearing screening therefore becomes a critical feature of health assessment to prevent unnecessary sequelae to hearing deficits. An understanding of the causes and types of hearing impairment provides an important base for the nurse to carry out this responsibility.

Box 51-5
About Decibels and Hertz

Disorders in hearing mean that persons so affected are unable to perceive or translate the sound waves that other people hear.

Sounds are "heard" by means of vibrations, or waves, that travel from the place where the sound originates to the hearer's ear. Different sounds have different cycles, or wave patterns. A wave pattern that completes itself in one second (that is, frequency of 1 cycle per second) is called a Hertz (Hz), after the German physicist Heinrich Rudolf Hertz (1857–1894). The lower the pitch of a sound, the fewer cycles per second; the higher the pitch, the greater the number of cycles.

The decibel (1/10 of a bel) takes its name from Alexander Graham Bell, whose interest in deafness led him to the invention of the telephone. Zero decibel is the least-perceptible sound an average normal human being can hear (in the decibel scale, 0 is not the absence of sound but rather the threshold at which sound can first be perceived). The decibel scale used in measuring hearing ranges from 0 to 110; above that range, at 140 dB, sound produces pain.

(From Bergstrom, 1980.)

Causes

Hearing loss may vary from mild to profound as outlined in Table 51-4. The higher the number in decibels the greater the hearing loss. (See Box 51-5.) Hearing losses are also described according to time of appearance, cause, and pathology involved.

Terms used to differentiate the causes of hearing loss are used inconsistently in the literature. In this discussion *congenital* is used to describe a hearing loss present at birth, whether of genetic or nongenetic origin. *Adventitious* hearing loss refers to a loss that develops after birth and may be due to genetic or nongenetic factors. Genetic-induced disorders that do not result in a hearing impairment until later in life (adventitious) are classified as having a *delayed onset* (e.g., Alport syndrome), while deafness resulting after birth from nongenetic causes is termed *acquired* (Paparella, 1977). A summary of genetic and nongenetic causes of both congenital and adventitious hearing loss is outlined in Box 51-6. Of all cases of congenital deafness 50 per cent are inherited, whereas in adventitious hearing loss environmental factors are of major significance. The nurse's familiarity with the causes of hearing impairment provides a base for taking a pertinent health history.

Types

Types of hearing impairment are categorized as central, peripheral, and functional (nonorganic). *Central disorders* are those within the central nervous system, specifically along the pathway from the brain stem to and including the cortex. *Peripheral impairment* results from lesions outside the central nervous system involving any part of the auditory system from the external ear to the point at which the auditory portion of

Box 51-6
Etiology of Deafness in Children

I. Congenital Deafness
- A. Genetic
  1. Deafness appearing alone due to defects in fetal development (aplasia)
  2. Deafness associated with other conditions (e.g., Waardenburg's syndrome, albinism, hyperpigmentation, visual handicaps)
  3. Chromosomal abnormalities
     Trisomy 13–15
     Trisomy 18
- B. Nongenetic (prenatal and perinatal factors)
  1. Infection (maternal rubella, cytomegalovirus [CMU], toxoplasmosis, herpes simplex, congenital syphilis)
  2. Ototoxic drugs (maternal ingestion of streptomycin, chloroquine, quinine, thalidomide, and possibly excessive use of salicylates)
  3. Metabolic disorders (toxemia, diabetes)
  4. Rh incompatibility
  5. Radiation (first trimester)
  6. Anoxia and birth trauma
  7. Low birth weight

II. Adventitious Deafness
- A. Genetic (delayed onset)
  1. Deafness occurring alone (ostosclerosis)
  2. Deafness occurring with other conditions (Alport's syndrome, Hurler's disease, Paget's disease, von Recklinghausen's disease, sickle cell anemia)
- B. Nongenetic (acquired)
  1. Infection (measles, mumps, chickenpox, influenza, serous otitis media, meningitis)
  2. Ototoxic drugs (kanamycin, streptomycin, gentamicin)
  3. Neoplastic disorders
  4. Trauma (direct injury via skull fracture or head injury or damage resulting from high noise level)
  5. Metabolic disorders (hypothyroidism)

(From Bess, 1977; Carrel, 1977; and Mouney, 1980.)

the eighth cranial nerve synapses within the brain stem (Newby, 1979). *Functional or nonorganic* hearing impairment is a psychologic rather than a physiologic disorder in which "hearing loss" is a defense mechanism to cope with stressful situations. Of these three types central and peripheral are the most prevalent.

Central Disorders

Central hearing impairment involves brain damage that results in the inability to process information. Processing refers to reception, analysis, and integration of auditory material within the central nervous system. The child is unable to interpret the auditory stimulus he or she receives and exhibits complex problems in speech and communication. The inability to express ideas, either spoken or written, is called *expressive aphasia; receptive aphasia* is difficulty in comprehending what one hears or reads (Newby, 1979).

Children with central impairment are easily distracted, have a short attention span, and have reading difficulty when instructed by phonics (Cunningham, 1978). This type of impairment is associated with a history of maternal rubella, diabetes, and pre-eclampsia, and of fetal prematurity and Rh incompatibility. Also, infections (meningitis and encephalitis), trauma, prolonged asphyxia and brain tumors, cysts, and abscesses are among the numerous causes of central impairment. Careful psychologic and educational testing is required because children with auditory imperception (inability to understand the meaning of what is heard) resemble the emotionally disturbed (Cunningham, 1978).

Peripheral Losses

Peripheral losses may be either *conductive* or *sensorineural.* If both conductive and sensorineural losses are present, it is referred to as a mixed loss. These classifications are based on location of the defect.

Conductive Losses. Conductive hearing impairment accounts for most hearing loss in children. There is a dysfunction of the outer (pinna and external auditory canal) or middle (tympanic membrane, eustachian tube, or ossicles) ear that interferes with sound transmission (air conduction). Pinna abnormalities are often associated with abnormalities of the ossicles. Because this often can be surgically corrected early its identification is important.

In conductive hearing loss the inner ear is not affected; therefore, bone conduction is normal and there is no nerve damage. Consequently, these people hear themselves adequately via bone conduction and tend to speak quietly. The speech of others is understood provided they can hear what is said. Conductive hearing losses usually are the same for all frequencies, although high-frequency sounds may be heard better. Hearing levels fluctuate in the child with conductive hearing loss and are usually mild to moderate losses. The child with conductive hearing loss displays a recognizable syndrome of behaviors that include fluctuating attentiveness to the environment, poor language skills, and mild behavior problems.

The transmission of sound is reduced or absent when inner or middle ear pathology obstructs air conduction. Obstruction of the outer ear by cerumen or in some instances a foreign object can cause significant hearing loss. *It is important for the nurse to stress that parents should not use cotton-tipped swabs or a sharp probe to clear the external canal.* When a swab is used, cerumen readily gets pushed deeper into the canal and it may become impacted against the eardrum. Using a probe may cause injury to the external canal or eardrum, resulting in infection. The ear canals may also be occluded because of a defect in development. A missing canal can be constructed or an occluded canal can be corrected by surgery. Most frequently, extensive plastic surgery is required because the eardrum and bones of the middle ear are missing entirely. Other causes of external ear obstructions are growths, swimmer's ear, and trauma.

The most common cause of conductive hearing loss in children is serous otitis media, an infection and inflammation of the middle ear that results in blockage of the eustachian tube and a retracted eardrum. (See Chapter 38 for a discussion of serous otitis media.) Serous otitis media does not necessarily cause pain and the hearing loss rarely exceeds a level of 30 dB; thus, the hearing loss may go undetected. Nursing interventions directed at preventing complications and the recurrence of serous otitis media can reduce the potential for hearing loss to occur. Even though decongestants and antihistamines may be prescribed, these children require follow-up to repeat the otoscopic examination and assess hearing. Furthermore, when a child has had one occurrence of serous otitis media, parents should be advised to seek treatment at the first sign of an upper respiratory infection. An additional preventive measure is to teach the child how to blow the nose properly. Pressing lightly on the nostrils with fingers without pinching prevents mucus from being forced into the orifice of the eustachian tube.

Other middle ear conditions that may produce conductive hearing loss are acute and chronic suppurative otitis media, tumors, and myringitis bullosa (a viral infection of the outer layer of the eardrum resulting in blistering). Screening and auditory tests to detect conductive hearing loss are described later in this section.

Sensorineural Losses. Sensorineural hearing losses are the result of pathology in the inner ear (semicircular canals and cochlea) or along the nerve pathway (auditory nerve) from the inner ear to the brain stem. This loss results in acoustic distortion (difficulty in discriminating speech) and a reduced sensitivity to sound. There is typically better hearing ability for the lower frequencies than for high frequencies. There is an inability to understand what is said because many consonants are high-frequency sounds and cannot be heard; thus, word confusion results. Also, with a sensorineural loss one's own voice is not heard because of the deficit in bone conduction. (We hear our own voices partly through the mechanism of bone conduction [Newby, 1979].) Consequently, with this type of hearing loss one speaks in what others perceive as an excessively loud voice.

Most of the babies who have impaired hearing at birth (congenital) have sensorineural impairment. However, this type of impairment may manifest itself at any time in life (adventitious). Whether congenital or adventitious the cause of the hearing loss may be genetic or nongenetic. The nongenetic factors that adversely affect prenatal and perinatal conditions should be the focus of preventive prenatal and perinatal care. Acquired sensorineural hearing impairment can be prevented by careful management of infections in children, anticipatory guidance to prevent injury, and immunizations against childhood illnesses.

Screening and Diagnostic Assessment

The nurse plays an important part in early identification of hearing impairment. The nurse's focus on thorough history taking (Box 51-7 lists high-risk factors), behavioral observations of the child, a careful physical assessment (Table 51-5), and attentiveness to parents' concerns increases the likelihood that the nurse will detect an existing impairment. Also, the nurse's contact with families in child health settings gives him or

Box 51-7
High-Risk Registry for the Identification of Hearing Impairment

RISK CRITERIA

Family history of childhood hearing impairment.

Congenital perinatal infection (e.g., cytomegalovirus, rubella, herpes, toxoplasmosis, syphilis).

Anatomic malformations involving the head or neck (e.g., dysmorphic appearance including syndromal and nonsyndromal abnormalities, overt or submucous cleft palate, morphologic abnormalities of the pinna).

Birth weight <1500 g.

Hyperbilirubinemia at level exceeding indications for exchange transfusion.

Bacterial meningitis, especially *Haemophilus influenzae.*

Severe asphyxia, which may include infants with Apgar scores of 0 to 3 or those who fail to institute spontaneous respiration by 10 minutes and those with hypotonia persisting to 2 hr of age.

(From American Academy of Pediatrics, 1982.)

Table 51-5. Behavioral Indices and Physical Findings Associated with Hearing Loss

Behavioral Indices

1. Orientation responses
   - Responds more to movement than to sound
   - Turns head and body to sound as if dependent on one ear
   - Responds to spoken sounds only when speaker's face and lips are visible
   - Responds more to changes in facial expression than to words
   - Fails to follow verbal directions
   - Lacks motor or facial response to spoken word
2. Vocalizations and sound production
   - Monotone voice quality and inflection patterns; loud voice
   - Loss of or lack of normal babbling by 7 mo of age; loss pf previously acquired speech a primary indicator
   - Only parts of words vocalized; mispronounces or omits certain words
   - Bangs head or stomps foot to elicit vibratory sensation
   - Uses same sound to express pleasure, annoyance, or need
3. Visual attention
   - Attends closely to facial expression and eyes of the speaker for intent of words
   - Points and uses gestures rather than words to express desires after 15 mo of age
   - Displays marked imitativeness in play
   - Is distracted by gestures and movement when in groups
4. Emotional and social behavior
   - Is shy, timid, and withdrawn in group play
   - Lacks appropriate noises in play with dolls, animals, trucks; no preference for noisy toys
   - Displays intense preoccupation with things rather than people
   - Has puzzled, unhappy, inquiring, and sometimes confused facial expression in group play
   - Is disobedient
   - Has short attention span, hyperactivity, and unusual fatigue
   - Uses tantrums to call attention to self or needs in routine situations
   - Is irritable at not making self understood
   - Appears to daydream or be oblivious to others
   - Displays unpredictable behavioral outbursts

Physical Findings	Significance of Findings
1. White forelock in hairline of forehead	Streak of gray or white hair; indicative of genetic defect (Waardenburg's syndrome) with hearing loss component
2. Heterochromia	A difference of color in portion of same iris: indicative of genetic defect (Waardenburg's syndrome) that has hearing loss component
3. Very bushy eyebrows that almost meet at the nasal bridge	Indicative of congenital defect that has hearing loss component
4. Impacted cerumen in external canal	Leads to a temporary conductive loss
5. Otitis externa	Inflammation of external ear (may result from furuncle or allergy to cleaning solutions used for hearing aid)
6. Pinna abnormalities	Is often associated with abnormal ossicles causing conductive hearing loss
7. Abnormal tympanic membrane	Retraction, bulging, air fluid levels, perforation, scarring all contribute to conductive loss; fluid in ear can lead to labyrinthitis, mastoid disease or cholesteatoma; labyrinthitis can lead to permanent damage to the hairs in the organ of Corti
8. Hypertrophied adenoids	Enlargement of adenoid tissue in posterior nasopharynx; may cause mild conductive loss

Table 51-6. Goals and Strategies for Auditory Screening According to Age*

Goals	Strategies
Neonate	
Identify all hearing losses	1. High-risk register 2. Behavioral responses 3. Crib-O-Gram testing 4. Brain stem evoked response
Birth–3 yr	
1. Identify severe hearing losses that might develop after birth 2. Detect ear conditions that may cause mild hearing losses	1. Follow-up of high-risk children 2. Auditory orientation behavior 3. Brain stem evoked response 4. Assessment of speech and language 5. Tympanometry† (impedance testing) 6. Parents' impression of child's hearing; take concerns seriously
3–5 yr	
1. Detect conductive losses due to otitis media 2. Detect sensorineural losses that might have developed	1. Audiometry (a) Pure-tone screening (b) Non–pure tone screening 2. Assessment of speech and language 3. Tympanometry (impedance testing) 4. Parents' impression of child's hearing and concerns taken seriously
School-age and older	
1. Maintain educationally adequate hearing 2. Detect ear disease	1. Pure-tone audiometry every 2 yr 2. Tympanometry (impedance testing) 3. Parents' and teachers' concerns regarding child's hearing taken seriously 4. Tuning fork

* At each age the ear should be examined with an otoscope.
† For infants under 7 months of age tympanometry is of limited validity.
(From Cunningham, 1978; Downs, 1981.)

her an opportunity to teach parents the normal responses to sound and language development to be expected. The deaf baby often makes normal sounds until 6 to 9 months, at which time vocalization gradually decreases. By the end of the first year the infant is often making only the primitive sound "amah" (Eviator, 1984).

Hearing screening is a nursing responsibility; therefore, an understanding of the various screening techniques is necessary. Hearing impairments can be identified through high-risk registers (see Box 51-7) and various screening techniques appropriate for the age of the child (Table 51-6).

Assessment in the Neonatal Period

In 1973 the Joint Committee on Infant Hearing recommended use of a high-risk register. This is a system to identify those infants that are at risk for hearing impairment. The 1973 criteria were expanded and clarified by the Joint Committee* in 1982 (see Box 51-7).

High-risk factors are identified by reviewing the medical record, asking parents to complete a questionnaire, and examination of the neonate.

It is recommended that all neonates be assessed and those at risk be referred for audiologic evaluation, preferably before age 3 months but not later than age 6 months (American Academy of Pediatrics, 1982). Various behavioral and electrophysiologic methods of testing for hearing impairment also are in use. Table 51-7 describes techniques that are used to follow-up those infants identified by the high-risk register. Although numerous tests are available to identify hearing

* The Joint Committee consisted of representatives from the American Academy of Pediatrics, Academy of Otolaryngology–Head and Neck Surgery, American Nurses Association, and American Speech-Language-Hearing Association.

Table 51-7. Technique to Test Infants and Children at Risk for Hearing Impairment

Description	Use and Implications for Nursing
Crib-O-Gram	
A transducer is attached to the infant's crib to record movements in response to a loud sound. It is relatively inexpensive	Can be used to follow infants identified by high-risk register
Brain Stem Auditory Evoked Potential (BAEP)	
Electrodes are placed on the mid-forehead and mastoid process. As stimuli are pesented, a series of brain wave responses are recorded	Not a routine procedure. Used for selected at-risk populations. A child should be completely relaxed, preferably asleep. Feeding infants immediately before test may suffice. A sedative is often necessary for older infants, toddlers, and preschoolers. School-age children may be able to lie still if adequate explanations are provided
Tympanometry (impedance testing)	
Measures the change in compliance of the ear drum as air pressure in the external canal is varied with an instrument. Reflected sound is measured to evaluate compliance. The instrument used is an electroacoustic impedance audiometer (tympanometer)	Impedance audiometry is especially useful because it requires only minimal cooperation from the child. Impossible to perform, however, if child is squirming. Because of the small ear canals, the test can identify ear pathology *before* hearing loss has occurred
Pure-tone testing	
Electronically generated puretnsof various frequencies and intensities are pesntd hrough the earphones. Child raises hand when sound is heard	Identifies hearing loss after damage has occurred
Play Audiometry	
Involves a play activity such as pictures or a pegboard. The child can be conditioned to put a peg into a board at the sound of a tone	Used for children under age 3 years who may not be able to understand what is expected of them in response to the tone
Behavioral Observation	
In a large, sound-treated room, a sound stimulus is administered. Responses are evaluated according to expected behaviors for age	Used for preverbal children

loss, the nurse should not disregard the value of testing neonates with a bell, which is rung approximately 4 inches from the ear.

During the first 2 months of life responses are generalized and reflexive including the moro reflex, blink reflex, arousal reflex (a sleeping infant response), and cessation reflex (restless or crying infant stops activity). An eyeblink is the most common and reliably observed response to sound in neonates. By 4 months of age, localization efforts are made by a rudimentary head turn and by 7 months a full head turn and eye turn are made toward the sound. By 12 months of age, a response to simple verbal commands is used to assess hearing (Fria, 1983).

Assessment From the Neonatal Period to 3 Years of Age

Once an infant has been identified as high risk, it is essential that he or she be examined regularly to identify hearing loss that may develop at some time after birth. It is recommended that these children have an audiologic evaluation every 3 months through the first year. The nurse can assist parents by helping them understand that although hearing tests are normal, their child is more vulnerable to hearing loss because of the presence of a high-risk factor(s).

The nurse has an important role in screening and detection of hearing problems during all well-child visits. Assessment of hearing development should include an otoscopic examination, assessment of the infant's response to noisemakers (auditory orientation behavior), and an assessment of speech and language development.

The otoscopic examination, including pneumatic otoscopy (described in Chapter 15), uses important techniques for identification of past and present middle ear pathology. These tests must be done by skilled professionals to ensure that hearing losses resulting from ear infections are prevented. When otoscopy is performed in conjunction with tympanometry, ear problems can be detected even earlier. It can be used at any age but is of limited validity in infants under 7 months.

Tympanometry (impedance testing) is an objective measurement of the compliance or mobility of the tympanic membrane in response to air pressure changes in the external auditory canal. Maximum compliance occurs when pressures on either side of the membrane are equal. Even mild disease of the tympanic membrane or middle ear influences the degree of compliance, making this test particularly useful to detect ear pathology *before* it has caused a hearing impairment.

Tympanometry is an efficient, reliable technique that is recommended to be used as a supplement to otoscopic examination and audiometric hearing tests. (See Box 51-8 for a description of tympanometry.)

Assessment From 3 to 5 Years of Age

At this age screening and detection consist of all of the techniques described for birth to 3 years of age. In addition, pure tone audiometric screening must be done to detect any sensorineural loss that may have developed. For this age, pure tone testing using play conditioning techniques is appropriate for the young preschooler; for the 5-year-old the standard pure tone screening is appropriate.

Non–pure tone screening is another technique that can be used to test preschoolers. The child is shown a board of pictures while words are spoken to him or her through earphones. The child is asked to point to the appropriate picture. The first word is spoken at 51 dB and each subsequent word is presented at 4 dB less than the previous one until the 15 dB level is attained (Downs, 1981). When this test is given, differences in language development and word exposure must be taken into consideration. It is more appropriate for most 4- and 5-year-olds than for 3-year-olds.

Assessment of the School-Age Child

The most common method to screen hearing in school-age children is pure-tone audiometry. While the more recent development of impedance audiometry is more effective to detect ear pathology, pure-tone audiometry continues to be the predominant method for screening school-age children. The nurse's responsibility is to maximize its effectiveness by administering the test under optimal conditions. Three important criteria should be met in giving the test: (1) the environment* should be quiet to avoid false-positives; (2) the audiometer should be maintained* in proper working condition; and (3) personnel conducting the test should be properly trained.

The school nurse should supervise the hearing screening program, recognizing its limitations to discover hearing loss and ear pathology in its early stages. Pure-tone audiometry must always be supplemented with serious attention given to the observations and concerns of teachers and parents regarding the hearing of the child. *The purpose of pure-tone audiometry is to identify hearing loss greater than a certain level, whereas impedance audiometry is used to discover the presence of otopathology.* This is an important distinction that is not always made in discussions of auditory screening procedures. Despite the advantages of impedance audiometry it is unlikely to be used in the place of pure-tone screening; therefore, the nurse's responsibility is to upgrade the conditions under which pure-tone audiometry is administered.

Box 51-8
Tympanometry

A tympanometer is an automatic instrument with a probe inserted into the ear canal. (An air-tight cavity is formed between the tip of the probe and the eardrum.)

A pure tone (usually 220 Hz) is then administered through the tip of the probe.

During the test ear canal pressure in the airtight cavity is varied automatically by the tympanometer (± 200 mm H_2O).

As ear canal pressures vary, compliance of the eardrum changes. (Compliance decreases whenever pressures on the two sides of the eardrum are not equal.)

As the ear canal pressures are varied, the sound (220 Hz) is reflected back into the air-tight cavity whenever the eardrum is not free to vibrate. (It vibrates best [is most compliant] when pressure against the two sides of the eardrum are equal.)

When pressures on the two sides of the eardrum are not equal and sound is reflected, the probe tip measures the intensity of the reflected sound in the ear canal. If the tympanic membrane is "stiff," more sound is reflected back; if it is flaccid, sound is absorbed and less is reflected back. Thus, the compliance of the ear is evaluated by measuring the reflected sound in the air-tight portion of the ear canal.

For a normal ear the greatest compliance is attained at 0 pressure.

If ear pathology is present, maximum compliance may be attained at positive or negative pressures. The amount of pressure required (whether positive or negative) to produce maximum compliance is the middle ear pressure.

* American National Standards Institute (ANSI) Specifications 53.1 (1960) and 53.6 (1969) describe criteria for background noise and maintenance, respectively.

A school-age child can cooperate in being assessed by the tuning fork test, in addition to otoscopy, speech and language assessment, impedance audiometry, and pure-tone audiometry. (See Chapter 15 for description of the Weber and Rinne tests.)

At all well-child visits the nurse should inspect the ears and examine the ear with an otoscope. Additionally, the nurse should assess the child for behavioral indications of hearing losses both by direct observation and by asking for pertinent information given by parents. Physical and behavioral findings which may be indicative of a hearing loss were summarized in Table 51-5.

Strategies for Nursing Care

Assisting with Early Detection

Usually parents are the first to notice that something is wrong with their baby's hearing. Delay in diagnosis persists as a serious health care problem. Even *profound* congenital deafness has been reported to be diagnosed at a mean age of 24 months (Coplan, 1987). On the average a full year elapses between the first suspicion and the actual confirmation that a child has a severely handicapping hearing deficit; a child with a mild to moderate hearing loss is often 3 years of age before any concerns are raised and over 4 years old before the hearing loss is confirmed (McFarland and Simmons, 1980). This presents a serious challenge to all health professionals who care for children and especially to nurses, who are often the first to hear the concerns of parents during the process of taking a developmental history. *Nurses thus can make a significant impact on the current problem of delayed intervention by taking concerns of parents seriously and making a referral for audiologic evaluation.*

Helping the Family Adjust to the Child's Handicap

The impact of a hearing impairment on a child is largely affected by how the parents can accept and adapt to the impairment. Not only do parents feel disappointed about the baby's deficit, but also from birth the communication interplay is altered. Parents should be encouraged to interact verbally with their child when in direct line of vision, to permit the child to respond to the stimulation of facial expressions.

Parent involvement is central to the habilitation program, beginning from the moment of diagnosis. They need to learn how the hearing impairment affects normal growth and development and about techniques available to maximize their child's potential. Although the nurse may not be primarily responsible for counseling the parents regarding amplification, communication techniques, and educational methods, the nurse generally functions on a team and should know of the available alternatives. The nurse acts as a resource to the family to discuss any aspect of the habilitation of their child. A list of organizations helpful to the hearing impaired is provided in Box 51-9.

Helping the Family Realize the Impact of Hearing Impairment on the Child

The nurse can prepare parents for the various behaviors of their child and developmental consequences of having a hearing impairment. While a hearing child is highly verbal and readily shares experiences even with strangers, the hearing impaired child may be limited in social skills. With the loss of adequate expressive language there is a tendency to withdraw from social situations. Strangers and peers may not understand the speech of the hearing-impaired child and he or she in turn cannot understand them. The ability to hear en-

Box 51-9
Resources for the Hearing Impaired

Alexander Graham Bell Association for the Deaf, Inc.
3417 Volta Place, N.W.
Washington, DC 20007

Conference of Executives of American Schools for the Deaf
5034 Wisconsin Avenue, N.W.
Washington, DC 20016

Council of Organizations Serving the Deaf
4201 Connecticut Avenue, N.W.
Suite 210
Washington, DC 20008

International Parents Organization
Alexander Graham Bell Association for the Deaf
3417 Volta Place, N.W.
Washington, DC 20007

National Association of the Deaf
814 Thayer Avenue
Silver Spring, MD 20910

National Association of Parents of the Deaf
814 Thayer Avenue
Silver Spring, MD 20910

The American Speech and Hearing Association
9030 Old Georgetown Road
Bethesda, MD 20014

The National Association of Hearing and Speech Action
Suite #201, 814 Thayer Avenue
Silver Spring, MD 20910

ables a child to identify the emotional intent of the words spoken. Hearing children learn what is expected of them from contextual cues and sounds perceived in the environment.

Large groups present a particular problem to hearing-impaired children because they hear only parts of the conversation (for example, in play they may not learn the rules of games well). Their response may be inappropriate to the situation, resulting in teasing by playmates who quickly dissociate them from the activity.

Hearing-impaired children tend to be more active in exploring the environment than hearing children. They want to see and touch everything and desire to touch faces to feel the vibrations of speech. Some people may find this type of behavior intrusive and intolerable. Also loud, unintelligible speech at the wrong time or in the wrong place may embarrass family members. Parents who cannot accept these behaviors may impose social isolation on the whole family or choose the alternative of planning activities whereby the child and one parent are always excluded in family activity. A sense of family unity may never evolve. Furthermore, older siblings may not bring friends home because they fear rejection of the family by their friends.

Helping to Reduce Potential Emotional Problems

Children who have learned to accept their limitation and have made some progress in their developmental skills will have limited emotional problems. Temper tantrums and extremes of destructive behavior and handflapping in response to frustration are often limited in duration. These children may have some difficulty, however, in delaying gratification of needs at times or may become impulsive. Their negative behavior cannot be rewarded with attention from friends and family and with the supplying of their every need. This response to negative behavior encourages a repetition of the behavior and loss of self-esteem. Eventually these children will take on a dependency role and give up trying. Their major drive toward self-reliance may never succeed and their ability to solve problems will be greatly handicapped.

During the early years when the child is developing social conscience about what is improper and what is acceptable behavior, parents must set consistent and firm limits on the child and expect reasonable obedience so he or she can learn socially acceptable behavior. Parents may tend to avoid discipline for the hearing-impaired child because they fear that the child will not understand why the limitation was set. Mild, consistent disapproval with a stern "no" and facial expression of displeasure will enhance the child's understanding of what pleases the parents and will free the child to initiate more social contact. The nurse can help parents determine the normal behavior problems of their child and methods to cope with them. Parents can be encouraged to balance discipline with love and acceptance, which will decrease the child's feelings of rejection. These children need to be reassured that their parents love and accept them.

Methods of Communication

The controversy over the best method of communication is confusing to parents and to professionals. The goal of educators of the hearing impaired in the United States is to assist a child to develop the ability to "speak and understand the spoken word to the highest degree possible" (Moores, 1978). No present-day educators advocate only the use of the manual (sign language and fingerspelling) technique. Two basic methods of communication are used in the United States: oral communication and total communication.

Oral Communication

This method has been predominant until recently. It focuses on the use of residual hearing with amplification and speechreading (lipreading). Proponents of this method believe that it is important for the deaf to be taught to talk and understand speech so that they can communicate in the hearing world of people. Gestures and signs are viewed as an interference to the development of speech and therefore are discouraged. While speech and speechreading is the goal for the hearing impaired, some do not have sufficient residual hearing to distinguish sounds and words that look alike on the lips.

The oral communication method is especially suited for very motivated children and primarily for those who have some residual hearing.

Total Communication

In this approach all techniques of communication are used, including sign language, cued speech, fingerspelling, speechreading, tactile stimulation, and amplification. (See Box 51-10 for a description of various communication techniques.) There is an increasing movement for the use of this method with very young children. This support may be the result of (1) evidence that deaf children with deaf parents are more successful academically than those with hearing parents, (2) the increased acceptance of sign language, (3)dissatisfaction with traditional methods with the profoundly deaf, and (4) strong support from deaf adults who were trained by a rigid oral method (Moores, 1978).

Box 51-10
Communication Techniques for a Child with a Hearing Impairment

Hearing aids include (1) a microphone that picks up sound waves and changes them into electricity, (2) a battery-powered amplifier to increase the strength of the signal coming from the microphone, and (3) a receiver to change the amplified signals back to sound waves. Hearing aid selection with young children requires considerable time devoted to repeated evaluation and trial periods with loaned hearing aids. The various types available include an aid that fits directly in the ear, an ear-level aid that fits behind the ear, a body aid that can be worn in a pocket or attached to clothing, and an aid that is built into the frame of glasses. Hearing aids are binaural (on each ear) or monoaural (on one ear). Binaural aids are more expensive but provide a more natural production of sound. Hearing aids are being fitted in infancy (on children as young as 2 months of age) and are considered important to effect early stimulation of residual hearing.

Auditory training is the process of teaching a child how to listen to spoken language. The emphasis is on listening to natural language, not to separate speech sounds such as vowels and consonants.

Speechreading (also called lipreading) is a concentration on visual clues to decipher the content of the spoken word by watching the lips, tongue, and jaw. Speechreading is difficult because many English sounds require similar formation of the lips. A child's ability to speechread is improved if adequate lighting falls on the speaker's face and if natural speaking is used with normal articulation and complete sentences.

Sign language is a manual form of communication in which an entire concept is communicated by the position, configuration, and movement of the hands.

Fingerspelling is the spelling of a word letter by letter. Letters are represented by hand configurations.

Cued speech is the use of eight hand configurations and four hand placements supplementing natural speech. The hands are placed around the chin, cheek, and neck to give clues to assist in speechreading.

Speech training is the process of teaching a deaf child to speak intelligibly. A child is taught how to regulate his or her voice and articulate correctly.

The nurse can explain to parents that no single method is preferred for all hearing-impaired children, but rather with the guidance of professionals the method is individualized for each child.

The child's type and degree of hearing loss and age of onset are important variables that an audiologist must consider when determining the type of communication technique most suitable for each child. The effect of hearing loss and resultant educational needs are summarized in Table 51-4.

Hearing aids are used to amplify the volume of environmental sounds only. They are helpful when one has good residual hearing. For some children, the sound becomes so grossly distorted when the volume is increased that it may create a barrier to receptive abilities. Knowing the range of sound volume loss as noted on diagnostic audiograms gives the nurse insight into determining the appropriate volume setting that is useful to the child. Significant improvements have been made in the physical appearance and electro-acoustical characteristics of hearing aids. The reader is referred to a recent review for information on the various types available (Gaudry, 1987).

Consistent wearing of the aid is particularly important for a child who is just learning to adjust to wearing it. Testing and changing of the batteries will increase the effectiveness of the aid and the child's social competence. Auditory feedback (a disturbing screech that emanates from the earpiece) occurs when the volume is too high or the ear mold is improperly fitted. The child and family will be taught how to alleviate this problem; however, because the child may not hear the feedback, others have to draw attention to it.

Alterations in Speech and Language

Speech and language skills compose the child's system of communication. Speech is the oral movement of body parts to articulate the thoughts verbally. The cry of a baby is a form of speech in that it communicates a need. Language is a mechanism that communicates thoughts and feelings through oral, written, or gestural methods. Speech and language disorders have a significant influence on the child's social-emotional experiences within the family and community—hence the importance of early recognition and treatment.

Communication disorders result from a wide variety of causes. Although prevalence of communicative disorders is difficult to determine it is estimated that 7 to 10 per cent of the general population has a deficit in one or more aspects of communication (Bax and Hart, 1976). Silva (1980) reported that nearly 8.5 per cent of children have language delays and 3-year-old children have a prevalence rate of 15 per cent for speech problems.

Normal Development and Assessment of Alterations

By the time a child is 4 years old most of the grammatic principles of language have been learned. The critical period for speech and language development has been identified as from 9 to 24 months of age; however, it may even begin before this time (Towne, 1983).

Language development involves two inter-related processes: receptive language (that which one understands) and expressive language (that which one expresses or speaks verbally). Expressive language is consistently less advanced than is receptive language. In other words, children can *understand* more than they can verbalize.

Normal speech and language development requires the presence of:

- Intact hearing from birth (e.g., early and recurring otitis media can diminish hearing)
- An intact nervous system
- The physical structures and physiologic control to accomplish speech (e.g., unrepaired cleft palate can interfere with speech)
- An environment that stimulates the use of verbal skills and verbal exchange

Language can be assessed through directly observing the child's communication in an interaction and through parental reports. Observations are then compared with expected age-appropriate behaviors. Normal speech and language development and signs of problems in development are summarized in Tables 51-8 and 51-9, respectively. A screening tool, the DASE (Denver Articulation Screening Examination), is discussed in Chapter 15 and can be found in Appendix Six.

Deterrents to normal development of speech and language include:

- Hearing loss
- Mental retardation
- Orofacial alterations (cleft palate, tongue thrust, malocclusion)
- Neurologic impairment (i.e., impaired control of muscle affecting speech)
- Bilingualism (may cause a mild delay only)

Table 51-8. Development of Speech and Language

Age at Which Behavior Should Be Established (Months)	Receptive Language Behavior	Expressive Language Behavior
1	Random activity arrested by sound	Random vocalization; primarily vowel sounds
2	Appears to listen to speaker; may smile at speaker	Vocal signs of pleasure; social smile
3	Looks in direction of speaker	Cooing and gurgling; smile in response to speech
4	Responds differentially to angry vs. pleasant voice	Responds vocally to social stimuli
5	Responds to own name	Begins to mimic sounds
6	Recognizes words like "bye-bye," "Mamma," "Daddy"	Protests vocally; squeals with delight
7	Responds with gestures to words such as "up," "come," "bye-bye"	Begins to use wordlike sounds, some jargon
8	Stops activity when own name is called	Imitates sound sequences
9	Stops activity in response to "no"	Imitates intonation pattern of speech
10	Accurately imitates pitch variations	First words appear
11	Responds to simple questions ("where is the dog?") by looking or pointing	Jargon well established
12	Responds with gestures to a variety of verbal requests	Announces awareness of familiar objects by name
15	Recognizes names of various parts of the body	True words heard embedded in jargon, often with gestures
18	Identifies pictures of familiar objects when they are named	Uses words more than gestures to express desires
21	Follows two consecutive, related directions ("pick up your hat and put it on the chair")	Begins combining words ("Daddy car," "Mamma up")
24	Understands more complex sentences ("after we get in the car we'll go to the store")	Refers to self by name

(From Behrman and Vaughan, 1987.)

Table 51-9. Signs of Problems in Language and Speech Development in Preschool Children

1. At 6 mo of age does not turn eyes and head to sound coming from behind or to side
2. At 10 mo does not make some kind of response to his or her name
3. At 15 mo does not understand and respond to "no-no," "bye-bye," and "bottle"
4. At 18 mo is not saying up to 10 single words
5. At 21 mo does not respond to directions (e.g., "sit down," "come here," "stand up")
6. After 24 mo has excessive, inappropriate jargon or echoing
7. At 24 mo does not on request point to body parts (e.g., mouth, nose, eyes, ears)
8. At 24 mo has no z-word phrases
9. At 30 mo has speech that is not intelligible to family members
10. At 36 mo uses no simple sentences
11. At 36 mo has not begun to ask simple questions
12. At 36 mo has speech that is not intelligible to strangers
13. At 3.5 yr of age consistently fails to produce the final consonant (e.g., "ca" for *cat,* "bo" for *bone,* etc.)
14. After 4 yr of age is noticeably dysfluent (stutters)
15. After 7 yr of age has any speech sound errors
16. At any age has noticeable hypernasality or hyponasality, or has a voice that is a monotone, of inappropriate pitch, unduly loud, inaudible, or consistently hoarse

(From Behrman and Vaughan, 1987.)

Problems in Speech and Language Development

Common problems to observe for when assessing speech and language development are problems in articulation, fluency, and voice disorders.

Articulation

Articulation problems make it difficult for speech to be understood. Difficulty in articulation is the most commonly encountered speech problem in children (Towne, 1983). Disorders of articulation comprise four types of problems:

- Substitution (replacement of one sound for another—e.g., wabbit for rabbit)
- Omissions (failure to produce certain sounds—e.g., boo for book)
- Additions (adding an extra syllable or sound—e.g., birtherday for birthday)
- Distortions (inappropriate sound replacing the correct one, such as in the phenomena of lisping)

Sound production is a gradually developing process. By 5 years of age 88 per cent of children are able to pronounce h, w, m, n, ng, f, p, and t correctly. By 6 to 7 years of age 75 per cent of children can produce the sounds th, v, z, zh, and dz; by age 8 development of articulation skills is complete (Levine, 1983).

Fluency

Fluency disorders are defined as a disruption in the rate, rhythm, or general flow of speech. Terms such as stammering and stuttering are used to describe this problem. *Stammering* is the result of involuntary pauses in the formation of words, while *stuttering* is the involuntary repetition of speech sounds. "Stuttering" will be used in this discussion to include both types of dysfluency.

The prevalence of stuttering has been estimated to be 4 per cent in children (Porfert and Rosenfield, 1978). It is more common in males, and approximately 80 per cent of children who stutter "outgrow" it. Health care professionals should, however, recognize that telling parents "not to worry" may in 20 per cent of cases be incorrect information (Rosenfield, 1982).

Most children engage in stuttering behavior at some point during the years they are formulating language skills, most commonly during late toddlerhood or the early preschool years. This behavior is a natural manifestation of the child's concentrated effort to master communication skills and, at best, should be ignored. It is most likely to occur on occasions when the child is tired, experiencing extreme anxiety, or being exposed to overstimulation from his or her environment (Herbert, 1975).

These natural, temporary speech disturbances become a problem only when they become persistent or cause the child extreme distress. Stuttering can become exaggerated when an experience or person (often a parent) draws the child's attention to his or her own speaking. The primary basis for these disturbed speech behaviors is the result of demands on the child to impose conscious control over the involuntary act of forming words (Herber, 1975; Homan, 1977). Thus, a natural behavior is molded, ever so unintentionally, into a behavioral disturbance because of the constant pressures to impose consciousness on an unconscious act by phrases like "Try to say it over again carefully," "Say it this way," and Think about what you are saying!" Once conscious effort is demanded, the stuttering or stammering may become established.

Children with "keyed-up personalities," who demand more than ordinary amounts of sleep, rest, and play, and who are easily over-stimulated or upset are especially at risk to persist in these speech mannerisms if they are brought to the child's attention. Parents who are critical of their child's speech efforts are also more likely to be critical of his or her efforts in other performance areas, making the child more emotionally insecure and more susceptible to development of these speech mannerisms.

The cause of stuttering has not been established but it has been demonstrated that stutterers are fluent (1) when they sing, (2) when they speak during inhalation, (3) when they do not hear themselves speak, and (4) when delayed auditory feedback is provided (i.e., individual hears what he or she has said several milliseconds later) (Rosenfield, 1982).

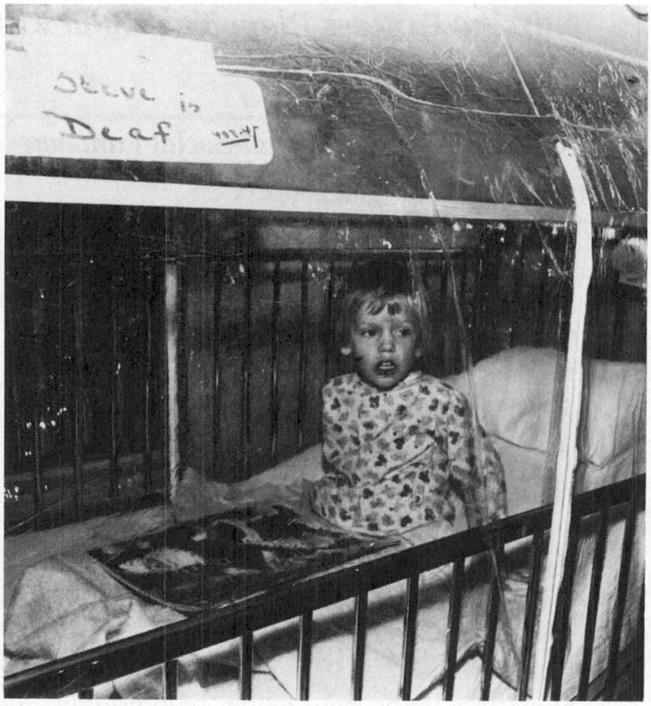

Despite attempts to prepare a sensory-impaired child for hospitalization, a strange environment poses a serious threat to security.

Voice Disorders

Voice disorders may be encountered in children with vocal cord nodules or polyps following chronic shouting or excessive talking (Goldberg, 1984). Voice is assessed for loudness, quality (nasality, hoarseness, breathiness, or harshness), intonation, and pitch. Voice disorders can cause children considerable distress because it sets them apart from peers. This alteration thus requires a referral for speech therapy.

The Sensory-Impaired Child in the Hospital

The sensory-impaired child is particularly dependent on the family at a time of stress. Despite any attempts to prepare a sensory-impaired child for what to expect in the hospital, new people and a strange environment are a threat to security. The stress of hospitalization is best tolerated if parents can be present to assist in orienting the child to the environment and participate in preparing the child for the various hospital events. Nurses are most helpful if they work with the family to learn the special daily care routines and how the child can best relate to others. While this is important for all hospitalized children, it is exceptionally so for those who are sensory-impaired, who use alternate methods of relating to their environment.

Although rooming in by parents is encouraged and beneficial, the nurse should not expect parents to assume full responsibility for the interpretation and explanation of procedures to the child. The nurse should become increasingly adept at communicating effectively with a sensory-impaired child so that parents will feel comfortable to leave for brief periods. Also, if parents are to take an extensive part in the care of their child, the nurse in turn must be prepared to spend adequate time with parents to prepare them for this task. Parents have difficulty knowing what is expected of them regarding the routines and procedures of a hospital and need assistance to understand how they can participate.

Special routines of home must be maintained to provide maximum comfort to a sensory-impaired child. The nurse is responsible for collecting specific data on admission regarding special care needs of a sensory-impaired child such as hearing aids, lenses, self-care skills, and mobility techniques. Also, the level of the impairment and its effect on independent functioning must be ascertained. From this information a care plan must be developed and used by all nurses caring for the child. It is distressing to the child and parents to have to orient each "new" nurse to the child's individual needs.

The nurse who gives nursing care to a sensory-impaired child should make the necessary adaptations that will permit the child to maintain the usual method of communication and foster normal growth and development. Independence in self-care skills such as self-feeding, dressing, bathing, and mobility should be maintained and encouraged, even though for a sensory-impaired child this may require additional patience and time on the nurse's part.

When a procedure is performed, the nurse must carefully assess the implications it may have for the child. For example, the wearing of a mask by health care personnel will cut off an important means of communication for the deaf child and restraint of the hands and arms interferes with one of a blind child's primary methods of taking in the environment. Play with other children should be encouraged to prevent the child from feeling isolated. The help of parents should be elicited to provide a play situation that is suitable to the child's abilities and is similar to the usual play environment. Table 51-10 contains a Nursing Process Plan for sensory-impaired children. This plan is designed to help promote a positive self-concept in the child with a sensory or other physical impairment.

Table 51-10
Nursing Process Plan: The Child with an Identified Sensory Impairment*

By Roxie Foster

Assessment of Emotional-Social Function

Self-perception/Self-concept

Subjective Assessment:

Statements that reflect self-worth, personal competence, and achievement aspirations. Parental patterns related to safety, beliefs and values, social behavior and roles, and self-regulation.

Objective Assessment:

Posture, eye contact, presence of fidgeting, attachment behavior, choice of clothing, choice of activity, physical hygiene.

Analysis: Nursing Diagnosis

Disturbance in self-concept, related to communication by others of nonacceptance associated with "being different"

Defining Characteristics

Subjective: Verbalizes feelings of inferiority, negativity, pessimism; boasts about achievements; declines opportunities for social activities and new experiences.

Objective: Poor attachment behavior; tends to watch rather than participate in group; acting-out behavior; poor impulse control; poor sportsmanship; takes little pride in appearance.

Desired Outcomes/ Evaluation Criteria

1. The client will develop a positive self-concept as evidenced by:
   a. Infant: demonstrating expectation of need gratification from parents and siblings
   b. Toddler: wanting to do things "by myself;" naming body parts
   c. Preschooler: showing pride in gender; seeking new activities and experiences; showing pride in being able to dress self, fixing own breakfast, and so forth
   d. School-age: having and enjoying several friends; showing pride in at least one special ability; showing curiosity about the external world

Nursing Strategies and (Selected Rationale)

Assess self-concept (see evaluation criteria, also Box 16-2).
Assist the family to gain a realistic perspective on the child's handicap.

- Explain the tendency to *generalize* a physical handicap (i.e., to extend it erroneously to include cognitive, emotional, and other physical abilities).
- Encourage family members (and others, as appropriate) to state ways in which *they* are "handicapped"/limited (e.g., poor math ability, poor at sports, uneven facial features). Ask them to list ways in which they compensate for these limitations.
- Clarify with the family the exact ways in which the child is handicapped. Discuss specific strategies to help the child compensate by learning to use full sensory capability with the help of professional instruction, medical therapies, and special equipment; and by developing compensatory sensory skills to access the external world (see strategies throughout this chapter).
- Stress the fact that in all other ways the child has normal needs.
- Discuss the need for routine well-child care, including immunizations and assessment of growth and development.

* The principles in this nursing process plan are appropriate to the enhancement of self-concept in any child with a physical handicap.

e. adolescent: describing physical self in primarily positive ways; indicating interest in heterosexual relationships; discussing realistic plans for the future; viewing self as capable of independence while acknowledging continuing need for love and approval from family	*Initiate strategies to enhance self-concept upon initial family contact and continue this guidance and support throughout the therapeutic relationship.* • Talk with families about their critical role in helping the child value self and abilities. • Ensure that families understand the self-concept goals for each developmental stage and discuss implications for parenting behaviors (see evaluation criteria, Table 13-3 and Table 16-2). • Discuss ways to make the *infant* feel loved, protected, and valued. • Provide reinforcement of appropriate parent bonding whenever possible. • Assist parent/family to recognize infant's positive responses (because sensory deficits may alter such expected behaviors as eye contact, smiling, quieting to a familiar voice, and cooing.) • Discuss importance of allowing *toddler* to do selected things on his or her own. • Acknowledge normal tendency to protect child from potential injury. Discuss ways to balance safety with need for autonomy. • Explain that learning body parts and their functions is important to developing body image. • Urge parents to be truthful and matter-of-fact about ways in which the child's eyes, ears, or other body part, differ from those of other family members. (By neither emphasizing nor ignoring these facts, the child will be able to develop a body image that comfortably incorporates the handicap). • Discuss ways to allow the *preschooler* initiative in choosing playmates from normal as well as other handicapped children; imitating the role of the same-sex parent; self-regulating simple daily activities, e.g., dressing, fixing a sandwich, learning a safe way to cross the street. • Allow the child to experience some frustration and disappointment within a supportive family atmosphere. (Appropriate adveristy can enhance the child's self-concept by increasing faith in ability to overcome the bad times.) • Emphasize the importance to the *school-age* child of identifying and participating in an activity at which he or she can excell, such as swimming or voice lessons for the blind child, or tennis lessons or a computer club for the deaf child; and in peer activities. Social contacts should include children with normal sensory abilities (to normalize social skills). When possible, educate peers about the exact handicap and compensatory mechanisms. (When fear of the unknown is reduced, friendships can be built on the things the children have in common.) Summer camps are available for children with sensory impairments and are an excellent way to enhance peer relationships, independence, and self-worth. • Encourage parents of the school-age child to allow appropriate independence. • Refer families to state and local agencies that provide special programs for the sensory-impaired.

Continued

Table 51-10 *(continued)*

Desired Outcomes/ Evaluation Criteria	Nursing Strategies and (Selected Rationale)
	• Agencies that provide dogs for blind and deaf clients may work with the school-age child. • Teach child to use special telephone equipment (as needed) to summon emergency help. • Counsel family about the importance of allowing the *adolescent* to be as independent as possible. • Encourage the young person to accept a part-time job as school work will permit. • If a driver's license cannot be obtained, teach adolescent to ride public transportation to permit access to activities of interest. • Helping others (e.g., by being a couselor in a summer camp for the sensory-impaired) can be an excellent way for the adolescent to develop feelings of self-worth as well as independence. • Be an advocate for the child (as appropriate) in explaining to the family that fashionable dress is not an adolescent whim but crucial to peer acceptance and self-image. • Encourage siblings or friends to shop with the young person who has a visual impairment. (Parents, although well-meaning, often have a different idea of "fashion".)

References

Adelson E, Fraiberg S: Mouth and hand in the early development of blind infants. *In* Bosma JF: *Third Symposium on Oral Sensation and Perception.* Springfield, IL, Charles C Thomas, 1972.

Adelson E, Fraiberg S: Gross motor development in infants blind from birth. *Child Devel* 1974 Mar; 114.

Alonso L, et al: Mainstreaming preschoolers: children with visual handicaps. US Department of Health, Education and Welfare, Pub No. (OHDS) 78-3112, 1978.

American Academy of Pediatrics, Joint Committee on Infant Hearing: Position Statement 1982. *Pediatrics* 1982 Sep; 70(3):496-497.

American Academy of Pediatrics and American College of Obstetricians and Gynecologists: *Guidelines for Perinatal Care.* 1983.

Barraga N: Utilization of sensory-perceptual abilities. *In* Lowenfeld B (ed): *The Visually Handicapped Child in School.* New York, The John Day Co, 1973.

Bax M, Hart H: Health needs of preschool children. *Arch Dis Child* 1976; 51(2):848-852.

Bax M, Hart H, Jenkins S: Assessment of speech and language development in the young child. *Pediatrics* 1980; 66(3):350-354.

Behrman RE, Vaughan VC III (eds): *Nelson Textbook of Pediatrics.* 13th ed. Philadelphia, WB Saunders, 1987.

Bergstrom L: Causes of reversed hearing loss in early childhood. *Pediatr Ann* 1980 Jan; 13-23.

Bernstein GH, et al: Prophylaxis of neonatal conjunctivitis. An analytic review. *Clin Pediatr* 1982; 21:545-550.

Bess F: *Childhood Deafness.* New York, Grune & Stratton, 1977.

Calhoun JH: Cataracts in children. *Pediatr Clin North Am* 1983 Dec; 30(6):1061-1069.

Carrel R: Epidemiology of hearing loss. *In* Gerber SE: *Audiometry in Infancy.* New York, Grune & Stratton, 1977.

Chew E, Morin JD: Glaucoma in children. *Pediatr Clin North Am* 1983 Dec; 30(6):1043-1059.

Chinn P: *Child Health Maintenance.* St Louis, CV Mosby, 1979.

Committee on Practice and Ambulatory Medicine. *Pediatrics* 1986; 77(6):918-919.

Coplan J: Deafness: ever heard of it? Delayed recognition of permanent hearing loss. *Pediatrics* 1987; 79(2):206-213.

Cratty BJ: *Movement and Spatial Awareness in Blind Children and Youth.* Springfield, IL, Charles C Thomas, 1971.

Cunningham D: Hearing loss. *In* Hoekelman R, et al (eds): *Principles of Pediatrics.* New York, McGraw-Hill, 1978.

Downs M: Early identification of hearing loss. *In* Lass N, et al (eds): *Speech, Language and Hearing.* Philadelphia, WB Saunders, 1981.

Eviator L: Evaluation of hearing in the high-risk infant. *Clin Perinatol* 1984 Feb; 11(1):153-173.

Feman S, Reinecke R: *Handbook of Pediatric Ophthalmology.* New York, Grune & Stratton, 1978.

Field TM: Discrimination and imitation of facial expressions by neonates. *Science* 1982 Oct; 218:179–181.

Fraiberg S, et al: The role of sound in search behavior of a blind infant. *Phychoanalyt Study Child* 1966; XXI, 327.

Fraiberg S, et al: An educational program for blind infants. *J Spec Ed* 1969 Summer; 121.

Fraiberg S: Intervention in infancy: a program for blind infants. *J Am Acad Child Psychiatry* 1971 Jul; 381

Fraiberg S: Blind infants and their mothers: an examination of the sign system. *In* Lewis M, Rosenblum I (eds): *Effect of the Infant on its Caregiver.* New York, John Wiley & Sons, 1974.

Fria TJ: The assessment of hearing and middle ear function in children. *In* Bluestone CD, Stool SE (eds): *Pediatric Otolaryngology.* Vol. 1. Philadelphia, WB Saunders, 1983.

Gaudry F: Hearing aids: a review for the family physician. *Can Fam Physician* 1987; 33:1509–1512.

George DS, et al: The latest on retinopathy of prematurity. *MCN* 1988 Jul/Aug; 13(4):254–258.

Goble JL: *Visual Disorders in the Handicapped Child.* New York, Marcel Dekker, 1984.

Goldberg R: Identifying speech and language delays in children. *Pediatr Nurs* 1984; Jul/Aug 252–259.

Greenwald MJ: Visual development in infancy and childhood. *Pediatr Clin North Am* 30(6) 1983 Dec; 977–993.

Hatfield E: Methods and standards for screening preschool children. *The Sightsaving Review* 1979 Summer.

Havener W: *Synopsis of Ophthalmology,* 5th ed. St Louis, CV Mosby, 1979.

Herbert M: *Problems of Childhood.* Pam Brooks Ltd, 1975.

Homan W: *Child Sense.* New York, Basic Books, 1977.

Hughes J: *Synopsis of Pediatrics,* 6th ed. St Louis, CV Mosby, 1984.

Jan J, et al: *Visual Impairment in Children and Adolescent.* New York, Grune & Stratton, 1977.

Johnson T, et al: *Children Are Different: Developmental Physiology.* 2nd ed. Columbus, OH, Ross Laboratories, 1978.

Kovalesky A: *Nurses' Guide to Children's Eyes.* Orlando, FL, Grune & Stratton, 1985.

Lennenberg E: *Biological Foundation of Language.* New York, John Wiley & Sons, 1967.

Levine MD, et al: *Developmental-Behavioral Pediatrics.* Philadelphia, WB Saunders, 1983.

Lingua RW: The eye. *In* Gellis SS, Kagan BM (eds): *Current Pediatric Therapy 12.* Philadelphia, WB Saunders, 1986, 483–489.

Ludington-Hoe S: What can newborns really see? *Am J Nurs* 1983 Sept; 83:1286–1289.

Martin FN: *Pediatric Audiology.* Englewood Cliffs, NJ, Prentice-Hall, 1978, 38.

Martyn L: Pediatric Ophthalmology. *In* Behrman RE, Vaughn VC (eds): *Textbook of Pediatrics.* Philadelphia, WB Saunders, 1987, 1447–1479.

McFarland W, Simmons F: The importance of early intervention with severe childhood deafness. *Pediatr Ann* 1980 Jan; 6.

Moores D: *Educating the Deaf. Psychology, Principles, and Practices.* New York, Houghton Mifflin, 1978.

Morin JD, Bryars JH: Causes of loss of vision in congenital glaucoma. *Arch Ophthalmo* 1980; 98:1575–1576.

Mouney D: Differential diagnosis of hearing loss in children. *Pediatr Ann* 1980 Jan.

National Association for Visually Handicapped: *Problems of the Partially Seeing.* New York, 1980.

Nelson LB, et al: Developmental aspects in the assessment of visual function in young children. *Pediatrics* 1984 Mar; 73(3):375–381.

Newby H: *Audiology.* Englewood Cliffs, NJ, Prentice-Hall, 1979.

Palmer EA: Strabismus. *In* Hoekelman RA, et al: *Primary Pediatric Care.* St. Louis, CV Mosby, 1987.

Paparella M: Differential diagnosis of childhood deafness. *In* Bess F (ed): *Childhood Deafness.* New York, Grune & Stratton, 1977.

Phillips S, Hartley J: Developmental differences and interventions for blind children. *Pediatr Nurs* 1988 May/Jun; 14(3):201–206.

Porat R: Care of the infant with retinopathy of prematurity. *Clin Perinatol* 1984 Feb; 11(1):123–151.

Porfert AR, Rosenfield DB: Prevalence of stuttering. *J Neurol Neurosurg Psychiatry* 1978; 41:954.

Rosenfield DB: Stuttering. *Curr Prob Pediatr* 1982 Jun; 50(2):4–27.

Scheie H, Albert D: *Textbook of Ophthalmology.* 9th ed. Philadelphia, WB Saunders, 1977.

Scholl G: Understanding and meeting developmental needs. *In* Lowenfeld B (ed): *The Visually Handicapped Child in School.* New York, The John Day Co, 1973.

Shapiro C: Retrolental fibroplasia: what we know and what we don't know. *Neonatal Network* 1986; 4(6):33–45.

Siegel I, Murphy T: Postural Determinants in the Blind. Final Report, US Educational Resources Information Center, ERIC Document FD 048 714, August 1970.

Silva PA: The prevalence, stability and significance of developmental language delay in preschool children. *Dev Med Child Neurol* 1980; 22:768–777.

Stangler S, et al: Screening Growth and Development of Preschool Children: A Guide for Test Selection. New York, McGraw-Hill, 1980.

Sweitzer R: Audiologic evaluation of the infant and young child. *In* Jaffe B: *Hearing Loss in Children: A Comprehensive Text.* Baltimore, University Park Press, 1977.

Tongue A: Low vision examination in children with visual impairment. *J Pediatr Ophthalmol Strabismus* 1980 May/Jun; 175.

Towne C: Disorders of hearing, speech and language. *In* Behrman RE, Vaughan VC (eds): *Textbook of Pediatrics.* Philadelphia, WB Saunders, 1983.

Bibliography

Bellman S: Hearing screening in infancy. *Arch Dis Childh* 1986; 61:637–638.

Biro P, Thompson M: Screening young children for communication disorders. *MCN* 1984; 9(6):410–413.

Bluestone CD, et al: Controversies in screening for middle ear disease and hearing loss in children. *Pediatrics* 1986 Jan; 77(1):57–70.

Desch LW: High technology for handicapped children: A pediatrician's viewpoint. *Pediatrics* 1986 Jan; 77(1):71–87.

Friendly DS: Ophthalmic neonatorum. *Pediatr Clin North Am* 1983 Dec; 30(6):1033–1041.

Gregory HH: *Controversies About Stuttering Therapy*. University Park Press, 1979.

An International Classification of Retinopathy of Prematurity. *Pediatrics* 1984 Jul; 74(1):127–133.

Lumbardino LJ, et al: Evaluating communicative behaviors in infancy. *J Pediatr Health Care* 1987; 1(5):240–246.

Northern JL, Downs MP: *Hearing in Children*. 3rd ed. Baltimore, Williams and Wilkins, 1984.

Reinecke RP: Opthalmic examination of infants and children by the Pediatrician. *Pediatr Clin North Am* 1983 Dec; 30(6):995–1003.

Shannon DA, et al: Hearing screening of high-risk newborns with brainstem auditory evoked potentials: A follow-up study. *Pediatrics* 1984 Jan; 73(1):22–26.

Sullivan L: How effective is preschool vision, hearing, and developmental screening? *Pediatr Nurs* 1988 May/Jun; 14(3):181–183.

Teplin SW: Development of blind infants and children with retrolental fibroplasia: Implications for physicians. *Pediatrics* 1983 Jan; 71(1):6–12.

Thomson LR: Understanding tympanometry. *Pediatr Nurs* 1982; 8(3):193–197.

Nursing Strategies: The Injured Child

Chapter 52

Mabel Hunsberger
Elizabeth Wonnecott

Nursing Process Plan
NPP: The Child with Major Burns, page 2093

Related Topics
Concepts of stress, coping, and illness, Chapter 23
Impact of death and dying, Chapter 26
Procedures adapted to care of children, Chapter 27
Nursing management of pain, Chapter 29
Delivery of blood and blood products, Chapter 40
Head and spinal cord injuries, Chapter 46
Fractures, Chapter 47

The significance of childhood injury is realized when one considers that accidents are the leading cause of death in children. Pediatric nurses and nurses who work in general emergency settings must be aware of the ways in which treatment for trauma in children differs from that for adults. This chapter details a wide range of injury situations, from minor insect bites to life-threatening burns. The sections dealing with age-related differences in structure and function of body systems in preceding chapters provide a base for many of the child-oriented interventions for trauma. The reader is encouraged to review these sections as needed.

Any injury, whether life-threatening or minor, brings a degree of suffering and pain to the child and is distressing for parents. Preventing injury and caring for children and their families, in the event of injury, is a challenge to health care professionals (see Chapter 17 for a discussion of the nurse's role in safety and prevention of injury). Few circumstances demand the extensive knowledge base, quick assessment skills and decision making, and sensitive communication skills that are required to mobilize effective care for the injured child.

Emphasis is placed on immediate, skillful intervention whenever a child is traumatized. Although it is recognized that parents need support and explanations, in the event of injury the goal of saving the child's life with the least possible sequelae is given first attention. The speed and appropriateness of treatment in the first few minutes at an accident scene can determine the quality of life for a child. As soon as the initial emergency has been met, parents are given a full explanation of how the child is and what has been done. When the injury occurs, a nurse must be prepared to make quick decisions based on sound knowledge. When even the quickest of actions cannot reverse the effects of injury, the anguish that parents experience presents an overwhelming challenge to the nurse and other health care professionals who also are sharing the loss.

Principles of Caring for the Injured Child

Incidence and Etiology of Injuries in Children

One out of every three pediatric deaths is due to injury; under 1 year of age injuries account for more deaths than all diseases combined.

The term "injury" as used in this chapter implies that trauma has been inflicted by an agent interrupting the structural integrity of the child. In some circumstances adults are a serious threat to the safety and well-being of children in our society. The care of children who are injured as a result of abusive and neglectful caretakers is addressed in Chapter 35. Recognition of the abused or neglected child is included in this chapter to emphasize that health professionals should regard any injured child with an alertness for signs and clues that could represent abuse or neglect or both. In this chapter, "injury" refers to a wide range of mishaps that befall children, including motor vehicle accidents and auto-pedestrian collisions; burns; near-drowning and drowning; poisonings; eye, ear, nose, and throat injuries; and common childhood events such as frostbite, sun exposure, insect bites, stings, poison ivy exposure, and injuries caused by cuts, scrapes, and punctures.

An injury occurs as a result of the interaction of the host (the person affected), the agent (cause of the injury), and the environment (circumstances of its occurrence). Although most injuries can occur at any age, some occur more frequently at certain developmental stages. Thus, it is evident that the host is a factor in causing injuries. (See Chapter 17 for further discussion of etiologic factors in injury.)

Developmental Differences Affecting Response to Injury

A child cannot be treated as an anatomically smaller adult. There are significant physiologic differences in children, which influence their response to injury. These include airway and breathing, circulation, temperature regulation, and mechanism of injury.

Airway and Breathing

The diameter of a child's airway is proportionately smaller than an adult's, resulting in greater resistance to airflow. Any injury that compromises the airway in a child results in serious reduction in airway diameter with increased effort required to do the work of breathing. The airway is prone to obstruction by blood, vomitus, mucus, or swelling due to injury or infectious disease. Furthermore, in the presence of edema, the greater amount of soft tissue in the neck increases the risk of obstruction.

The smallest diameter of the airway in the child is at the cricoid cartilage and not at the glottis as in the adult. Passage of an endotracheal tube may be complicated by this difference. Because the narrowest point of the child's airway is below the vocal cords at the cricoid cartilage, an uncuffed endotracheal tube is used in children less than 8 years of age. (Standards and Guidelines for Cardiopulmonary Resuscitation [CPR] and Emergency Cardiac Care [ECC], 1986.) In adults and older children, cuffed endotracheal tubes are used to seal the airway.

In infants, the tongue is large in relation to mouth size and is a well-developed organ with strong musculation essential for sucking. This relatively large structure is a common cause of pediatric airway obstruction. When maintaining an airway for a child, the chin-lift/jaw-thrust maneuver should be employed in order to lift the tongue away from the trachea. Hyperextension of the neck should be avoided.

During inspiration, it is normal for an infant or small child to push out the abdomen. Following this, the chest should symmetrically expand as the lungs fill with air. In the event of respiratory distress, the abdomen continues to rise with each inspiration; however, the chest may not rise, and substernal, intercostal, or tracheal in-drawing may be noted. Air is frequently swallowed during periods of respiratory distress, causing gastric distention. This in turn contributes to further distress by reducing diaphragmatic excursion and increasing the work of breathing. Air in the stomach is usually expelled by vomiting and thus, the risk of aspiration is increased. Any increase in the work of breathing may lead to exhaustion and decreased respiratory effort. (For further discussion on respiratory developmental differences, see Table 38-1.)

Circulation

A child's distribution of fluid volume puts him or her at risk for dehydration and electrolyte imbalance. The proportionately greater percentage of fluid in the extracellular space increases risk for rapid loss. Children compensate for blood loss more readily by vasoconstriction and tachycardia. A fall in blood pressure is usually a late indicator of blood or fluid loss that is potentially lethal.

Children are monitored for maintenance of adequate fluid volume by assessing skin color, respirations, pulse, capillary refill, and urinary output, and by watching for inter-related alteration of these signs.

Temperature Regulation

Hypothermia may be either a cause of injury or a result of it. Children have difficulty maintaining their temperature when the body is stressed by illness or injury because of (1) large surface area in relation to weight, (2) less subcutaneous tissue to prevent heat loss, and (3) a large scalp with high blood flow.

When evaluating color and temperature of the extremities, the nurse should recognize that infants may exhibit mottling because of their immature temperature-regulating mechanism.

Mechanism of Injury

It is important to understand that anatomic differences in children result in characteristic types and sequence of injuries.

A child's head provides a prime target for injury. Because of the relatively large size and weight of the head in proportion to the rest of the body, and because children lack well-developed neck muscles and cervical ligaments, their heads are frequently the first point of contact in injuries involving falls or motor vehicle collisions. These differences, coupled with their thin skulls, which afford little protection, increase the potential for brain damage to occur in children. Children with skull fractures are at greater risk for (1) direct brain injury from body fragments and (2) increased intracranial pressure from cerebral bleeds or depressed skull fragments. (See Chapter 46 for further discussion of neurologic differences in children.)

The cervical spine becomes injured during head trauma because of the weight of the child's head, the poorly developed neck muscles, and weak cervical ligaments (Coln, 1985) even though there may be no actual fracture. Because of the child's large head size, cervical injuries tend to occur high in the cervical spine between C-3 and C-5 (Kelley, 1988). The most common mechanism of spinal injury in children is a sudden hyperflexion or hyperextension of the neck combined with a rotational injury. This is the type of injury that is typical in car accidents. Although cervical spine injuries are less common in children than adults, every seriously injured child should be suspected to have a cervical spine injury until proven otherwise. Infants and children may sustain spinal cord injuries without evidence of the injury on radiologic examination. Severe angulation of the spine resulting in cord injury can occur without a disruption of bones and ligaments (ligaments are lax and the cervical spine has a large amount of cartilage).

Because children's chests are quite flexible and they have relatively underdeveloped abdominal and chest wall muscles, they are at risk for injury from blunt, or nonpenetrating, trauma. Blunt trauma is a more frequent cause of chest and abdominal injuries in children than penetrating trauma. Blunt trauma is less obvious (and therefore, more difficult to assess) than the dramatic wounds produced by penetrating objects. For example, punching into soft belly tissues may leave no external bruising but may injure the solid organs of the abdomen. Similarly, during falls onto objects, an internal injury can occur.

Rapid deceleration of a motor vehicle caused by collision or forceful braking may lead to tearing of solid organs. The spleen is most likely to suffer injury in children. Because of the spleen's highly vascular nature, children with splenic laceration or rupture may bleed to death within minutes. Other organs that may be affected are the liver, pancreas, and small bowel.

Children riding in cars who are not restrained by a car seat or seat belt will literally become missiles during a collision. Although head injury is the most common problem resulting from lack of appropriate restraint, chest and abdominal injuries can occur as the child catapults into a dashboard, steering wheel, or the interior walls of the vehicle.

Assessment of the Injured Child

Since the first few minutes may be crucial to the child's survival (and quality of life later on) the nurse must be able to draw on an established body of knowledge and finely honed assessment skills. All nurses who work with critically ill children should have a sound knowledge of developmental differences among pediatric patients within the varied age groups of childhood and differences between pediatric and adult patients.

Primary Survey

Any assessment of a very ill or badly injured child should begin with a quick visual examination of the child. However, the need for a systematic approach to physical assessment cannot be overemphasized. The most common and most effective method of assessment is known as the ABC (*A*irway, *B*reathing, *C*irculation) or primary survey and the head-to-toe or secondary survey. While you are asking yourself if this child "*looks* sick," you can begin to assess the child and simultaneously gather information from the accompanying parent.

If the parent does not offer the information, ask "How does the child in the present condition compare with his or her usual state?" *Pay close attention to the parent who tells you that a child's behavior is significantly altered from normal.* The parent knows the child best. Box 52-1 provides a guide for making effective and rapid primary surveys.

The information obtained from the primary survey should be validated at regular intervals and any changes or trends noted and documented. The basic vital functions *must* be stable before attention is diverted from them to other concerns. For example, a fractured femur may be the more obvious injury but is far less important than assessing for and maintaining an adequate airway.

Medical treatment may be initiated, depending on the findings of the aforementioned assessment. Should time permit, a secondary survey may be carried out in order to obtain more information.

Box 52-1
Guide for Conducting a Rapid Primary Survey

An overall assessment is made immediately regarding level of responsiveness and presence of head and neck trauma. A rapid assessment, following the ABC format, is begun almost simultaneously.

A. Airway:
- Is child maintaining patent airway independently?
- Are there any signs of obstruction?
- Is position of airway facilitating or interfering with air exchange?

B. Breathing:
- Rate of respirations
- Quality of respirations (shallow, stridor, wheezing, grunting, labored)
- Effectiveness of respiratory effort (does chest rise and fall symmetrically)
- Skin color

C. Circulation:
- Rate and quality of pulses (especially apical)
- Capillary refill
- Skin temperature
- Skin color
- Skin turgor

Secondary Survey

The secondary survey involves history-taking and a head-to-toe assessment of the child's condition. A quick assessment is performed as for any physical exam with a focus on fractures, contusions, and lacerations. In a true emergency situation, the child's weight may be estimated, but as soon as possible a real value should be obtained. Accurate weight is essential for determining the rate and amount of intravenous fluid to be administered, dosage of medications that may be given, and parameters for required ventilatory assistance. The child's weight may also be useful in determining the level of toxicity to be anticipated relative to the amount of a noxious substance that has been ingested.

In an emergency, a history and physical assessment are usually done simultaneously. Frequently, a very ill or badly injured child is rushed into the treatment area while the parents are detained at the desk to give information. The parent, understandably, may be extremely distraught and unable to answer questions coherently. The nurse should ask a minimum of questions, and they should be short and simply phrased (Box 52-2 lists the most pertinent areas to include). The nurse may have to repeat or restate questions in order to get the needed information.

Box 52-2
Guide for Rapid History Taking in the Event of Injury

1. History of present illness or injury
2. A description of pain (if present)
3. Pertinent past medical history
4. Current medication
5. Allergies
6. Age
7. Weight (most mothers know this)
8. Immunization history

Assessment for Potential Child Abuse/Neglect

Assessment for an injured child should be approached with an alertness for potential child abuse or neglect. It is essential that health care workers carry an index of suspicion when assessing families in order to avert the disastrous situation of repeated injury by abuse. Indicators of physical abuse, neglect, and psychological maltreatment are discussed in Chapter 35 and summarized in Tables 35-3, 35-5, and 35-6, respectively. Indicators of sexual abuse can be found in Box 35-3.

It is important to remember that adults who abuse their children come from all socioeconomic, religious, and ethnic groups and have various levels of education. Although the lay person may believe child abuse is confined to the less economically advantaged, this may only appear to be so because abused children from lower socioeconomic status may come to the attention of authorities more readily. It is mandatory for the nurse to respond to a beginning suspicion by taking a more thorough history and following up with the appropriate reporting process, irrespective of socioeconomic status of the family.

An important indicator to explore is the inability of parents to give a satisfactory explanation for an injury. For example, if a child with extensive bruising on both front and back of body is reported to have fallen down stairs or if the date of a reported fall does not match the estimated age of a bruise, further data gathering is essential. Also, inconsistent reports are often elicited if the child and parent are interviewed separately. When a story raises a professional's suspicion that a child may have been abused, it is important to keep communication channels open. Box 52-3 provides some basic principles for use in dealing with potentially abusive

Box 52-3
Principles of Interviewing When Assessing the Potentially Abused Child

1. Elicit exact information about the injury including time, place, sequence of events, and who was present.
2. Use open-ended questions (i.e., "How was your child injured?" rather than "Was this injury an accident?").
3. Encourage questions from the parents.
4. Do not approach the family with a judgmental attitude, because rejection and criticism will result in withdrawal by the parent and stop communication.
5. Never *accuse* the parent of abuse. Mandated agencies have the responsibility to investigate and determine whether a child has been abused.
6. Respond to the feelings of the child.
7. Interview parent and child separately when appropriate.

caretakers. (See Chapter 35 for further discussion of the care of the abused child and family.)

Impact of Injury on Child and Family

Children depend on adults to protect them from danger and physical harm, yet many injuries occur because a guardian or caretaker momentarily fails to provide supervision appropriate to the circumstance and the child's developmental level. Lack of information, preoccupation with personal matters, tension between parents, and the time of day are major factors that influence the incidence of injuries.

When a child is injured, a careful analysis of the factors leading to the injury can provide important information in understanding the feelings of the parents. The child's and parents' responses are also affected by the child's age, parent-child relationship, circumstances surrounding the event, and the type and severity of injury.

It is a frightening experience for a child to be injured and then be rapidly taken for emergency care to a threatening environment. A child has difficulty interpreting the extent of the injury but tends to fantasize the worst. Separation from parents, pain and intrusive procedures compound the terror of the experience. Chapters 29 and 31 further discuss the impact of procedures and hospitalization on children.

Regardless of age and situation, stressors for parents include (1) fear and uncertainty about child's prognosis; (2) a degree of guilt and feeling "if only I would have" or "if only I would not have;" (3) an overwhelming concern for the child's immediate condition; and (4) a strong desire to be with their child to alleviate fear and bring comfort. These feelings are magnified in life-threatening situations, but exist even when minor injuries occur.

An injured child often requires intensive care for a period of time. In an intensive care situation, Rothstein (1980) found that parents initially experienced overwhelming shock and disbelief accompanied by a sense of helplessness and guilt. Factors that intensified the state of shock were the child's unstable condition, the complexity of therapy, and the child's physical appearance. After stabilization of the child was apparent, the initial shock experienced by parents was replaced by a phase of "anticipatory waiting." It is during this phase that long-term effects and outcomes are of concern to parents, and they may become demanding of staff, expressing feelings of anger, guilt, and helplessness. Potential stressors for parents of children in intensive care settings as identified by Miles and Carter (1982) are presented in Box 24-2.

When a child is injured, the procedures and immediacy of care that are required to save the child also affect the family's ability to cope with the situation. The threatening appearance of the environment increases the parents' perception of the severity of the child's injury. Although it is necessary to direct all energy to the care of a critically ill child, after the emergency state has resolved attention must be given to the parents (or guardians). An informed parent who is included as much as possible in caring for the child and making decisions about the child's care will be more relaxed and supportive than one who is not. A calm parent usually means a more relaxed and cooperative child. Support of the child and family during acute illness is further discussed in Chapter 24.

Nursing Strategies

An injured child may or may not survive, depending on the type and degree of injury. Survival and quality of life often depend on the accuracy and speed with which care is delivered. Some of the special skills required of the nurse are triage, cardiopulmonary resuscitation (CPR), management of an obstructed airway, transport of the patient, care of the parents, and documentation.

Triage

The word "triage" comes from the French verb meaning "to sort." The concept was first applied to health care in disaster situations in an attempt to ensure that the most seriously ill or injured patients, who *also* stood the best chance of survival if they were promptly treated, were treated first. Triage decisions are made by assessing the severity of a condition and the potential outcome of treatment. The concept of sorting is applied in any situation in which several ill or injured persons must be cared for simultaneously. The emergency room department of a hospital is the most common health care setting where triage is used.

Today, triage represents a complex process of problem solving and planning that involves the entire health care team including the ambulance dispatcher, emergency medical technicians (EMTs), nurses, and physicians. The process depends not only on the needs of the patient but also on the availability of services. Therefore, a critically injured child may be triaged by an EMT as needing immediate transport to a hospital, triaged by the ambulance dispatcher to the nearest facility, triaged by the nurse in the emergency room so that the child is seen immediately by the physician, and triaged after stabilization by transport to an intensive care pediatric facility.

The skills required to perform triage are similar to the assessment skills required by any nurse in any setting. The uniqueness of triage is the speed with which an assessment must be made. The main focus of the subjective assessment is (1) history of the present illness or injury, (2) pertinent past medical history, (3) allergies and medications, and (4) immunization. Objective assessment focuses primarily on (1) general appearance, (2) vital signs, and (3) a localized examination. After an initial assessment is made, a category is assigned, usually ranging from I to IV. This category reflects the severity of the patient's condition.

Cardiopulmonary Resuscitation

Infants and children who require cardiopulmonary resuscitation (CPR) rarely have suffered a *cardiac* arrest in which cardiac pathology is the primary cause (Standards and Guidelines for Cardiopulmonary Resuscitation [CPR] and Emergency Cardiac Care [ECC], Part IV, 1986). A *respiratory* arrest is usually the preceding event. An understanding of how this affects the child's condition is important. First, it means the child has usually been hypoxic for some time. Therefore, the results of a "successful" resuscitation attempt may produce a severely brain-damaged child, or the resuscitative efforts may fail entirely. Second, many events that trigger a respiratory arrest may go unnoticed long enough to cause hypoxia. Recognition of hypoxia in its early phase may make it possible to intercept the need for CPR. Tachycardia, hyperpnea, cyanosis, exertional dyspnea, altered level of consciousness, restlessness, anxiety, and aggressive behavior are changes that the nurse should recognize as signs and symptoms of hypoxia.

Pediatric nurses have an obligation to take courses and maintain proficiency in pediatric basic life support. Nurses who are employed in acute care settings should also be proficient in advanced pediatric life support techniques. Regular mock cardiac arrest drills are an excellent means of practice and review. CPR performance for the infant and child is summarized in Table 52-1 and illustrated in Box 52-4. The American Heart Association has developed, through years of research, the standards that constitute the basic and advanced pediatric life support protocol. Preparation and monitored practice are essential to their safe performance. The reader is referred to Standards and Guidelines for Cardiopulmonary Resuscitation (CPR) and Emergency Cardiac Care (ECC), Parts I to IV, 1986, for further information.

Neonatal resuscitation is a highly specialized activity. Only experienced, well-trained personnel should attempt this, as the size of the infant and the need for expert intervention demands immediate reaction. The most recently developed guidelines can be found in Cropley and Bloom (1987).

Management of an Obstructed Airway

Airway obstruction may be caused by aspirated materials or by infections that cause airway swelling. Children with an infectious cause of obstruction need specific emergency care, and time should not be wasted using airway clearance techniques described here. Attempts to clear an airway are made for (1) a child in whom aspiration is witnessed or strongly suspected, and (2) an unconscious, nonbreathing child whose airway remains obstructed after the usual efforts to open it have been made. Foreign body aspirations is suspected in the presence of acute respiratory distress associated with coughing, gagging or high-pitched noisy breathing (stridor) (Standards and Guidelines for Cardiopulmonary Resuscitation [CPR] and Emergency Cardiac Care [ECC], Part IV, 1986).

Blind finger sweeps should be avoided because a foreign body may be pushed further into the airway. If the aspiration is witnessed or strongly suspected, the child is encouraged to cough and persist with breathing efforts. Manual relief of obstruction is attempted only if the child's efforts are ineffective and/or if increased signs of respiratory difficulty occur.

In the infant under 1 year of age, a combination of back blows and chest thrusts is recommended. The Heimlich maneuver (subdiaphragmatic abdominal thrusts) is used in adults and children over 1 year of age (see Box 52-4). By elevating the diaphragm, air is forced from the lungs. With sufficient air movement,

Text continues on page 2048

Table 52-1. Sequence of Cardiopulmonary Resuscitation (CPR)

Sequence:

	1. Determine unresponsiveness or respiratory difficulty*
	2. Call for help*
	3. Position the victim*
A. { Airway	4. *Open the airway*
B. { Breathing	5. *Determine whether victim is breathing*
	6. *Breathe for the victim*
C. { Circulation	7. *Check the pulse*
	8. Activate the emergency medical service (EMS) system
	9. Perform chest compressions
	10. Coordinate compressions and rescue breathing

Activity	**Infants (under 1 yr of age)**	**Children (1–8 yr of age)**	**Children (over 8 yr of age or adults)**
1. Determine unresponsiveness			
• Assess for head and neck trauma and avoid injury of spinal cord	Flick heels	Gently shake and shout. Call name	Same as for child 1–8 yr of age
• Transport immediately if child is conscious but struggling to breathe			
• Permit child to assume position of comfort during transport			
2. Call for help			
• If rescuer is alone and child is not breathing perform CPR for 1 min, then call for help		(No Variation)	
• If unresponsive or in respiratory difficulty call for help			
3. Position the victim			
• Place victim on back on a firm, flat surface if CPR is necessary		(No Variation)	
• Move carefully if there is head or neck injury			
• Turn child as unit with firm support of head and neck			
4. *Open the airway*			
• After victim is in supine position use a head-tilt chin-lift maneuver. (Hand is placed on victim's forehead to tilt head into a sniffing position; fingers of other hand are placed on bony part of lower jaw and chin is lifted upward)		(No Variation)	
• Head should not be tilted in suspected neck injury			
• Jaw-thrust is used when neck injury is suspected (two or three fingers are placed under each side of the lower jaw at its angle and the jaw is lifted upward. This requires two hands)			
5. *Determine whether victim is breathing*			
• Look, listen, feel, for evidence of respirations for 3–5 sec (look for chest and abdominal movement, listen and feel for exhaled air)		(No Variation)	
• If victim is breathing, rescuer should summon			

Activity	Infants (under 1 yr of age)	Children (1–8 yr of age)	Children (over 8 yr of age or adults)
help and ensure that airway is maintained • If victim is not breathing rescue breathing is initiated			
6. *Breathe for the victim* • Give 2 breaths • Pause between these two breaths to allow for exhalation (each of these 2 breaths should be 1–1.5 seconds in length)	Position: Rescuer's mouth is placed over infant's nose and mouth	Rescuer's mouth is placed over child's mouth. Nose is pinched slightly with fingers of hand doing head-tilt	Same as for child 1–8 yr of age
• For subsequent breaths the rate varies with age • If chest does not rise with breaths adjust head-tilt chin-lift or suspect foreign body aspiration • Volume of breath should be the least amount of pressure that causes chest to rise to avoid gastric distention	Rate: 20 per min	15 per min	12 per min
7. *Check the pulse* If a pulse cannot be palpated chest compressions must be initiated and coordinated with rescue breathing	Brachial (because chubby neck makes carotid less accessible): Brachial is palpated by placing index and middle fingers inside of upper arm between elbow and shoulder	Carotid: Locate Adam's apple, then slide fingers to groove between trachea and neck muscles	Same as for child under 1–8 yr of age
8 Activate the emergency medical service (EMS) system If rescuer cannot activate the EMS system the only option is to continue with CPR			
9. Perform chest compressions • Chest compression must always be accompanied by rescue breathing • Sternum is allowed to return to its normal position between compressions *without removing* fingers (infant) or hand (child/adult) from the sternum • Compression and relaxation phase of each cycle should have equal time	Location: *One fingerbreadth below nipple line on sternum* • Draw an imaginary line joining nipples • Place index finger next on the sternum immediately below the line • Place middle and ring fingers immediately below index finger • Compress chest at level where middle and ring finger are placed (i.e., one finger's width below the imaginary line) • Other hand may be used to support infant's back • Compress 0.5–1 in at a rate of 100 per minute	Location: *One fingerbreadth above costal-sternal notch in sternum* • Locate rib cage with index and middle finger • Follow margin of rib cage to notch where rib cage meets sternum • Place middle finger on notch • Place index finger onto lower end of sternum next to middle finger • Place heel of other hand onto sternum below index finger, with long axis of heel parallel to the sternum • Compress chest (with one hand) 1–1.5 in at a rate of 80–100 per min	Location: (same as for child): • Follow steps as for child but place hand that was used to locate notch on top of hand on sternum so that both hands are parallel • Fingers may be either extended or interlaced but must be kept off chest • Rescuer's elbows are locked into position, arms are straightened, and shoulders are positioned directly over the hands • Each thrust is therefore straight down on the sternum • Compress 1.5–2 in at 80–100 per min
10. Coordinate compressions and rescue breathing When there are two rescuers a pause should be allowed after each five compressions for a ventilation (1.0–1.5 sec per breath)	Ratio of 5:1 compressions: ventilation is maintained for one or two rescuers. Assess after 10 cycles (i.e., approximately 1 min) of compressions and ventilations, and every few minutes thereafter	Same as for infants	One rescuer: Ratio of 15:2 compressions: ventilations (after four cycles of compressions and ventilations [15:2 ratio] pause to reassess) Two rescuers: Ratio of 5:1 compressions: ventilations (assess patient after first minute of CPR and every few minutes thereafter)

* In practice the first three steps occur rapidly and almost simultaneously with airway opening. The A (airway), B (breathing), and C (circulation) of resuscitation provide the guideline for sequence of action.

(From Standards and Guidelines for Cardiopulmonary Resuscitation [CPR] and Emergency Cardiac Care [ECC], 1986. Copyright 1986, American Medical Association.)

Box 52-4

Pediatric Basic Life Support

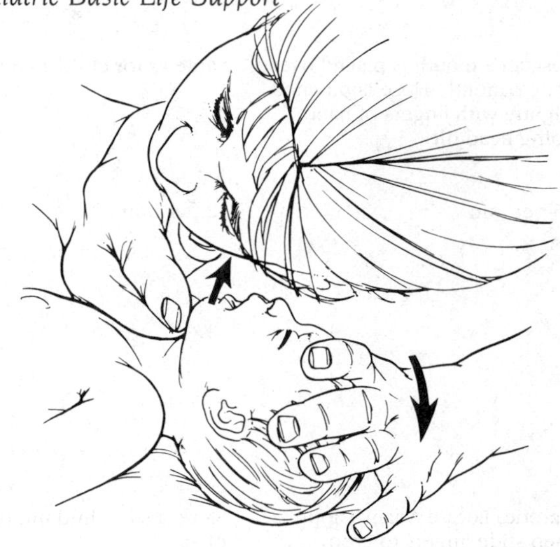

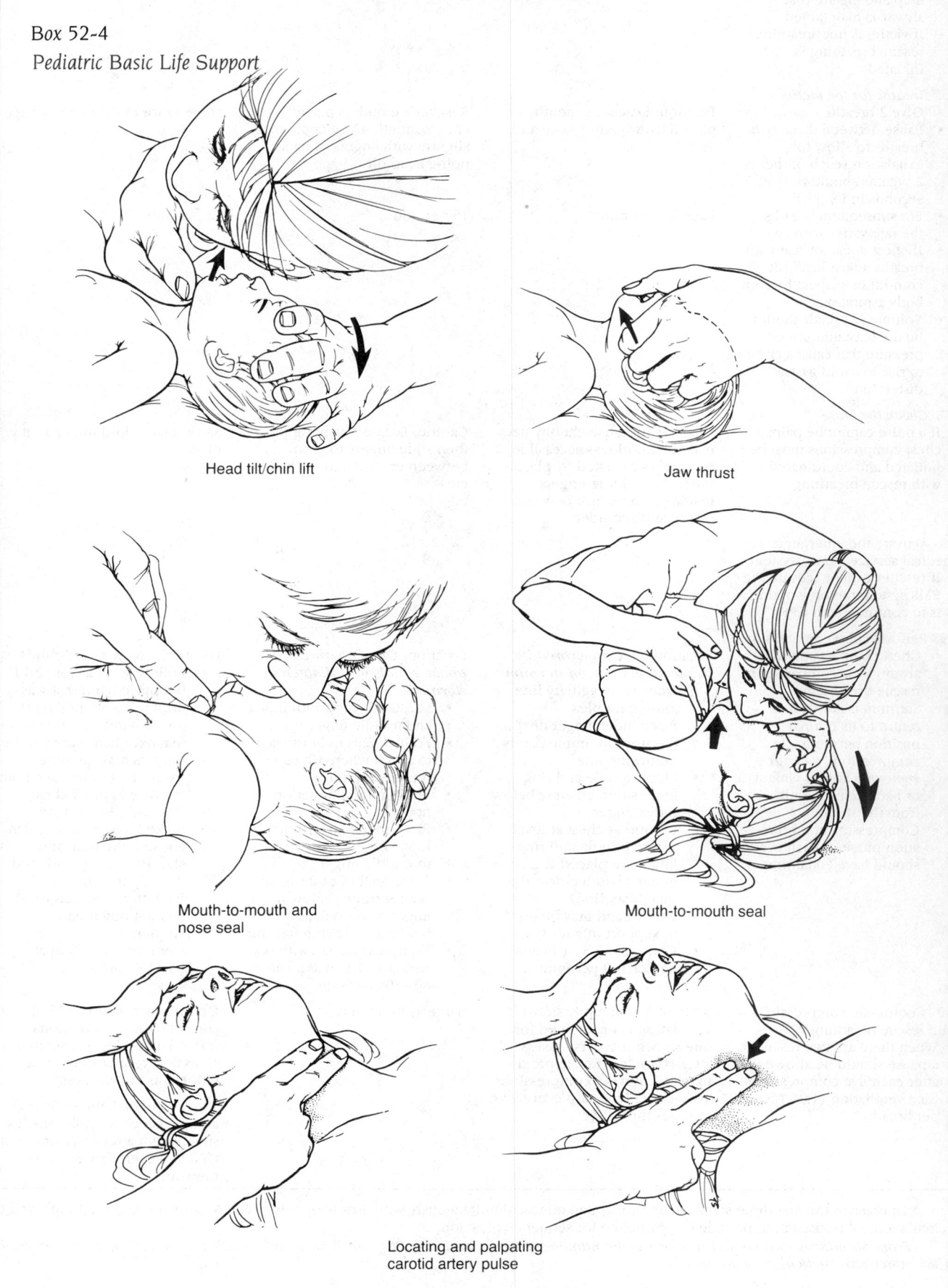

Head tilt/chin lift

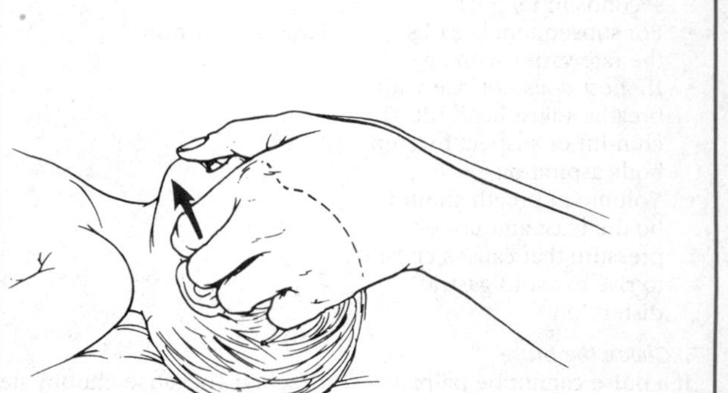

Jaw thrust

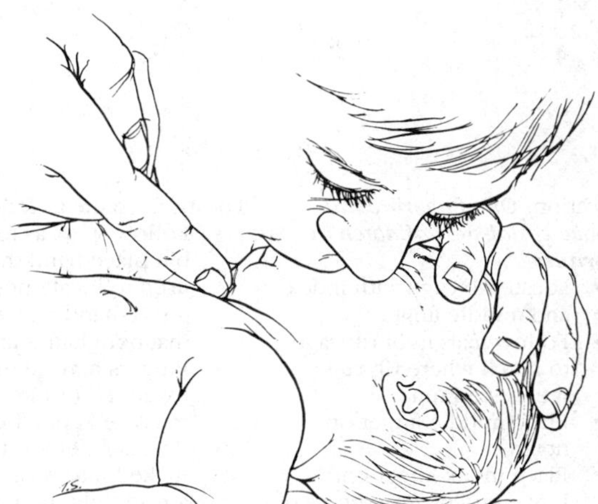

Mouth-to-mouth and
nose seal

Mouth-to-mouth seal

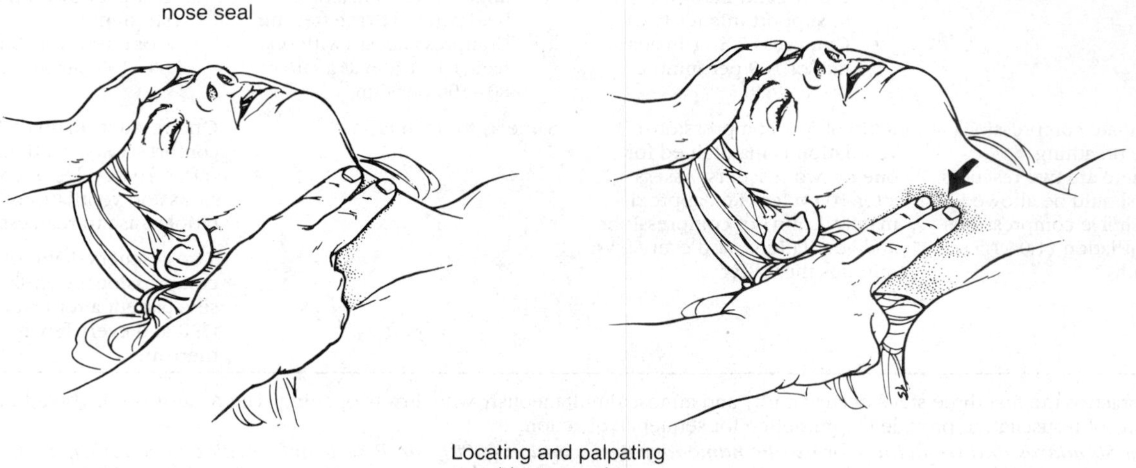

Locating and palpating
carotid artery pulse

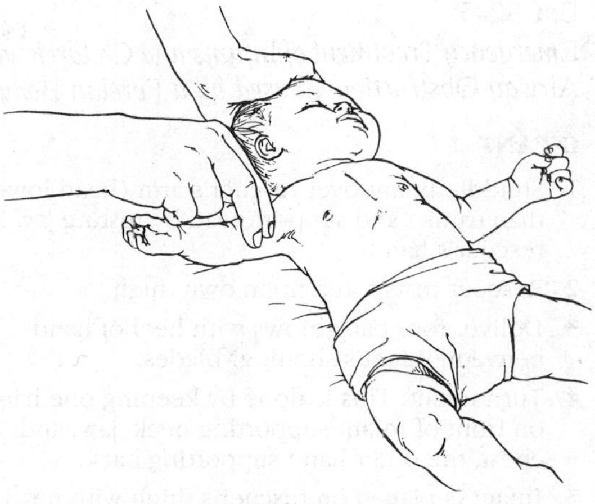

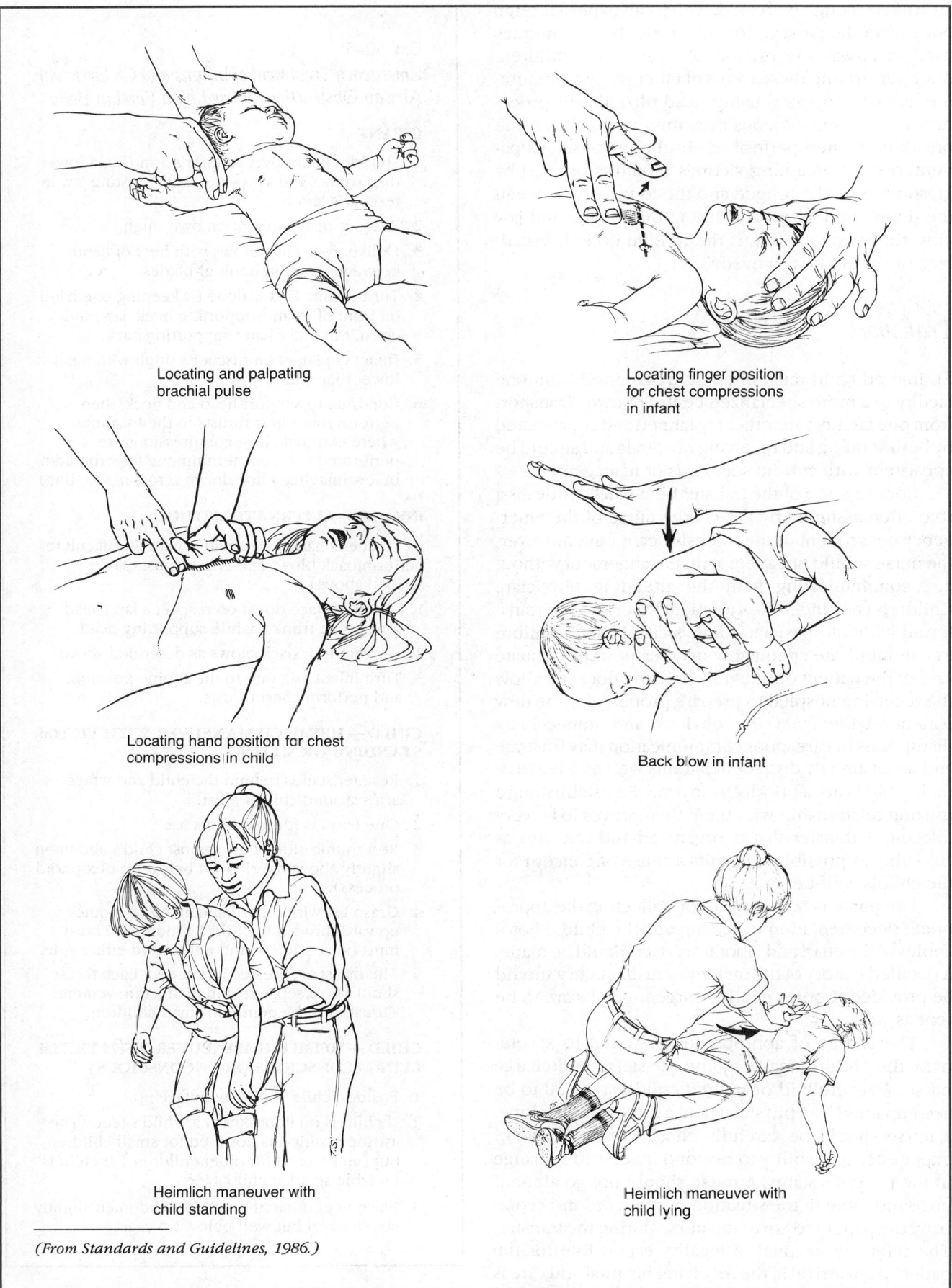

Locating and palpating brachial pulse

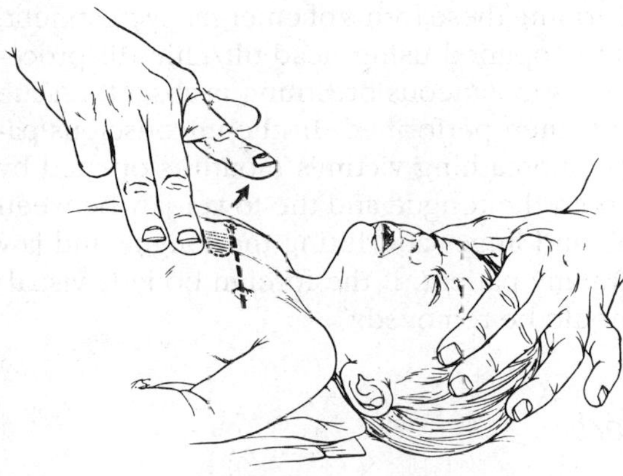

Locating finger position for chest compressions in infant

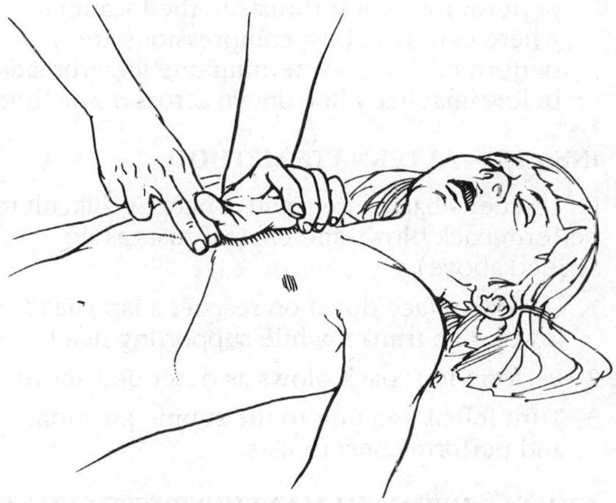

Locating hand position for chest compressions in child

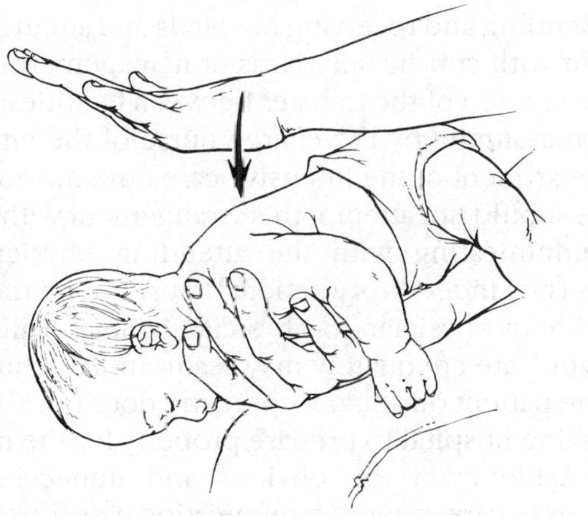

Back blow in infant

Heimlich maneuver with child standing

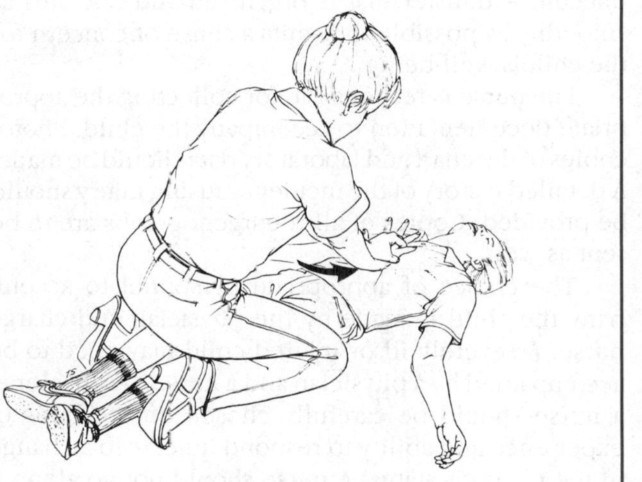

Heimlich maneuver with child lying

(From Standards and Guidelines, 1986.)

an artificial cough is created, which can expel a foreign body from the airway. Box 52-5 describes techniques used in airway obstruction of infants and children. After performing these forms of emergency treatment, the airway is opened using head-tilt/chin-tilt procedures and if spontaneous breathing is absent, rescue breathing is then performed. In the unconscious patient, the nonbreathing victim's mouth is opened by grasping both the tongue and the lower jaw between the thumb and finger and lifting the tongue and jaw upward. In any patient, if the foreign body is visualized, it should be removed.

Transport

An injured child must often be transported from one facility to a more specialized center of care. Transport from one facility to another is planned and coordinated by both sending and receiving hospitals and should be consistent with current standards of management.

Coordination of the transfer between facilities is a role often assumed by the charge nurse of the emergency department or the intensive care unit; however, the nurse should not attempt this arrangement without first communicating with the attending physician. Children (nor indeed *any* patient) must not be transferred without physician-to-physician contact. Failure to communicate adequately may result in inadequate care of the patient during transport and does not allow the receiving hospital to prepare properly for the new patient. Aside from the obvious and unnecessary disruptions in care, poor communication may frustrate and upset already distraught parents who may feel that their child is not a priority to anyone. Re-establishing a trusting relationship with them then proves to be very difficult. A transfer that is organized and operates as smoothly as possible transmits a sense of concern for the child's well-being.

The nurse is responsible for collecting the appropriate documentation to accompany the child. Photocopies of the chart and laboratory data should be made. A detailed history of the incident causing injury should be provided. Copies of all roentgenographs are to be sent as well.

The choice of appropriate personnel to accompany the child is made by the physician and charge nurse. A severely ill or injured child may need to be accompanied by a physician and a nurse. If sent alone, a nurse should be carefully chosen on the basis of experience and ability to respond quickly to a change in the patient's status. A nurse should not go alone if uncomfortable in the situation. Written orders accompany the patient to cover the nurse during the transfer. The referring hospital is legally responsible for the patient until arrival at the receiving hospital and care is

Box 52-5
Emergency Treatment of Infants and Children with Airway Obstruction Caused by a Foreign Body

INFANT

1. Straddle infant over rescuer's arm (head lower than trunk) and support head by resting jaw in rescuer's hand.
2. Rescuer rests forearm on own thigh.
3. Deliver four back blows with heel of hand between infant's shoulder blades.
4. Turn infant. This is done by keeping one hand on front of infant supporting neck, jaw, and chest, the other hand supporting back.
5. Infant is placed on rescuer's thigh with head lower than trunk.
6. Continue to support head and neck, then perform four chest thrusts in the locations where external chest compressions are performed (i.e., on sternum one fingerbreadth below imaginary line drawn across nipple line).

INFANT — ALTERNATE METHOD

(If rescuer's hands are small it may be difficult to perform back blows and chest thrusts as described above)

1. Lay infant face down on rescuer's lap (head lower than trunk), while supporting head.
2. Perform four back blows as described above.
3. Turn infant as a unit to the supine position, and perform chest thrusts.

CHILD — HEIMLICH MANEUVER WITH VICTIM STANDING OR SITTING

1. Rescuer stands behind the child and wraps arms around child's waist.
2. One hand is formed into a fist.
3. Rest thumb side of fist against child's abdomen slightly above navel (well below tip of xiphoid process).
4. Grasp fist with other hand and give a quick upward thrust into child's abdomen. Thrust must be at midline and not toward either side.
5. The thrust is repeated as needed. Each thrust should be a separate and distinct movement. Thrust must be gentle in small children.

CHILD — HEIMLICH MANEUVER WITH VICTIM LYING (CONSCIOUS OR UNCONSCIOUS)

1. Position child supine with face up.
2. If child is on floor, kneel at child's feet. (The astride position is not used for small children but can be used for older children.) If child is on table stand at child's feet.
3. Place heel of hand on child's abdomen slightly above navel but well below rib cage.

4. Place other hand on top of first hand and press into abdomen with an upward thrust. Thrusts must be at midline and not to either side of the abdomen.
5. Thrust is repeated several times as needed. Each thrust should be a separate and distinct movement. Thrust must be gentle in small children.

assumed by that institution. The nurse accompanying the patient practices according to the policies and procedures of his or her employing institution (for example, taking the vital signs every 15 minutes; assessing airway, breathing, and circulation) and documents the assessments.

Some large centers have their own transport teams who will come to the referring facility and assist in stabilization of the patient there; they then take the responsibility for the child's care during transfer. This is done by land ambulance or air transport. Advantages of helicopters include avoiding heavy road traffic and rapid transport with trained personnel to regionalized specialty facilities.

An important task involved in transfer is preparation of the parents. Usually they are in a state of shock and despair over their child's injury. They may feel guilty that the child has been hurt so badly. The child's transfer needs to be presented in a positive way. The expertise of the receiving facility should be stressed to them. Usually the ambulance personnel will allow one parent to accompany the child while the other follows in the family's own vehicle. This has the advantage of providing the receiving facility with someone who can offer detailed information about the child's past medical history and presenting event. If possible, the nurse who has been caring for the child should accompany the child, not only to provide continuity of care but also to give support to the parents. Even though their association may have been brief, the parents may already trust and depend on this nurse.

Care of Parents

Although most busy emergency rooms and intensive care units have "quiet rooms" available for family members of critically ill patients, these rooms are frequently in high demand. Whenever possible, the nurse should find a less distracting area in which to interview a parent. Attempts should be made to stay with the parent(s). A social worker, minister, or volunteer with special training should also be called upon as resources.

Because of the invasive nature of many emergency treatments, parents may or may not be permitted to be with their child, depending on the policy of the institution, the type of treatment being initiated, and the ability of the parents to cope. Pediatric centers generally are supportive of parents' presence during treatment and recognize the benefits for both child and family. If a parent is not able to cope with staying at the child's side, he or she should be supported in the decision to wait in a waiting room. Every effort should be made to keep them informed of the progress of treatment and they should be reunited with their child as soon as possible.

When a child is seriously ill and parents are not permitted in the room while treatment is initiated or if parents arrive later than the child, steps should be taken to prepare them for the child's appearance — for example, many tubes, presence of blood, unresponsiveness, and so forth. Whenever possible, the nurse actually caring for the child should accompany the parents to the room and stay with them to provide support and answer their questions, while continuing to care for their child. Parents are encouraged to touch and talk to their child even if the child is unresponsive.

Documentation

Documentation is essential when dealing with seriously ill or injured children. Because they may be transferred from one unit to another or from one facility to another rapidly, good documentation will provide consistency of care. The importance of this nursing responsibility cannot be overstated. If important data such as vital signs, medications, intravenous fluids, urinary output, and behavioral responses to treatment are not charted accurately important trends may be missed. Also, for those situations in which legal charges are made, nurses may be subpoenaed to give evidence during court proceedings. Specific information that Rund and Rausch (1981) recommend for documentation includes

- Patient identification
- Time of arrival
- Method of arrival
- History of the chief complaint
- Physical findings including the patient's vital signs
- Emergency care given prior to arrival
- Diagnostic and therapeutic orders
- Clinical assessments including results of treatment
- Documentation of tests and procedures done
- Results of procedures and tests
- Diagnostic impression
- Final disposition
- Patient's condition on discharge

- Any instructions given
- Follow-up plan
- Whether or not patient leaves against medical advice

Descriptions of a child's clothing, use of car safety restraints, parental responses to their children, and the child's physical and emotional responses to treatment may also be relevant and, in some cases, may have important legal ramifications.

Common Childhood Injuries

Children who sustain minor injuries may not necessarily seek medical care in a health care setting. Counsel may be sought by telephone to determine the correct course of action to be taken at home. Injuries that are common to children included in this section are cuts, scrapes, and puncture wounds; insect stings and bites; snake and mammalian bites; and injuries caused by environmental exposure including excessive cold (frostbite), and excessive rays of the sun (sunburn). Although some of these injuries are not necessarily life-threatening, hypersensitivity to the agent and inadequate care can have serious consequences. The nurse's telephone counsel and early assessment and management have an impact on the child's recovery. The hurt and discomfort to the child even in minor injuries such as cuts and scrapes should not be overlooked. Children often have had little previous experience with pain. Furthermore, caretakers are anxious about their child's pain and fears and need the support and comfort of an understanding nurse.

Cuts, Scrapes, and Puncture Wounds

Anyone who cares for injured children will soon recognize the dramatic effects that the sight of blood has on a young child. A thorough inspection of the wound is usually made by the child to determine whether it is bleeding. It should be recognized that even though a wound is minor, a child may respond to the sight of blood with terror; therefore, getting a wound cleaned and covered as quickly as possible is important to make the child feel comfortable and safe. Acknowledging the child's fears rather than negating them will also be supportive. The overall goals in the care of these injuries are to (1) reduce the fear of the child, (2) minimize the pain by appropriate and gentle cleansing, (3) control the bleeding, (4) prevent contamination and infection, (5) observe and treat for shock, and (6) assess current immunization status and immunize appropriately. Various types of wounds and their management are summarized in Table 52-2.

Insect Stings and Bites

The incidence of specific bites and stings varies according to geographic areas. Each year approximately 40 to 50 deaths are reported to be caused by insect stings (Mayer, 1985). Children may be affected by having a local reaction of pain and erythema at the site of the sting, or they may have a systemic reaction causing anaphylaxis. Some snakes and spiders are poisonous; however, most are not. Regardless of the type of sting or bite, most are painful and the experience is frightening to a child. A familiarity with the most common and potentially serious bites and stings is necessary for appropriate management and prevention of fatal outcomes (Table 52-3). The allergic reaction is described in greater detail in Chapter 43, page 1568.

Snake Bites

Most of the snakes in the United States are not poisonous. An average of 10 deaths occurring annually in the United States are caused by snake bites—usually by rattlesnakes, cottonmouths, or coral snakes; however, 6000 to 7000 patients receive antiserum (Dreisbach, 1983). Worldwide, deaths are estimated at 30,000 to

Table 52-2. Types of Wounds and First Aid Treatment

Abrasions or Scrapes: Loss of skin surface without penetration. There may be pinhead-sized openings with fluid or blood oozing	Area is washed with soap and water or a mild (nonirritating) antiseptic solution. Small bits of dirt can be picked out with sterile tweezers or wound can be flushed with normal saline. A child's cooperation is gained if they can do some of it themselves as appropriate. A nonadherent dressing is applied for 24 hr
Lacerations: Smooth or jagged cuts penetrating the skin and blood vessels	Area is washed with soap and water or mild antiseptic. If sides can be easily approximated and held together a Steristrip dressing may be used. If it is deep and gaping, sutures are required. To prevent scarring suturing should be done within 6 hr. Facial lacerations may require the expertise of a plastic surgeon for repair
Punctures: Penetration of the skin with a sharp object such as a nail or tooth causing a small hole in the skin (usually produces very little bleeding)	Area is washed with soap and water or mild antiseptic solution. A tetanus booster is administered if the child has not received one in the previous 5-yr period

Table 52-3. Prevention, Identification and Treatment of Insect Bites and Stings

Agent	Identification/Clinical Signs	Prevention	Management
Mosquito bite	Insect penetrates skin to suck blood. During this process the insect's saliva containing a foreign protein is injected. This causes swelling, itchiness, and papules. It can cause an allergic reaction in the hypersensitive	Apply insect repellent when potential for bites is anticipated	Apply cool compresses or give cool bath to reduce swelling. Calamine lotion for itching. Antihistamines if sleep is interrupted.
Hornet, wasp, honey bee (bumble bee), yellow jacket (hymenoptera)	Venom is injected through a stinger. It contains histamine and foreign proteins that cause redness, swelling, tenderness, and itching. Systemic reactions cause generalized edema with possible nausea and vomiting, respiratory difficulty, and shock	Wear shoes and clothing that cover extremities if in area where insects may be present. Avoid insect breeding areas (e.g., flower beds, orchards). Hypersensitive children should be gradually desensitized to minimize future reactions	Carefully remove stinger (Yellow jacket does not leave stinger imbedded). Flick or scrape it away rather than pinching it to avoid squeezing out more venom. Wash with soap and water promptly. Prompt use of epinephrine for anaphylaxis. Application of cool compresses or use of antipruritic lotion may be comforting. A meat tenderizer paste made with a few drops of water is recommended for painful stings. It contains proteolytics that reduce inflammation and edema (Gaunder, 1986)
Ticks and mites	Ticks are brown or gray; mites are colorless, red, or dark and are microscopic. Ticks live on dogs or in the woods. They can carry Rocky Mountain spotted fever, Q fever, and tularemia. Mites, the most common being the chigger, live in tall grass and underbrush. Ticks and mites cause local itching. Chiggers (mites) cause papules that are usually concentrated where clothing is snug. Ticks become partially embedded in the skin and feel like a tiny bump and skin becomes red and swollen. Some ticks (Rocky Mountain wood tick and Eastern dog tick) can cause a flaccid motor paralysis that can be fatal.	Use of insect repellent on clothes and on ankles and legs repels chiggers. Careful inspection of child, clothes, and family dog after an outing in the woods	Mites are treated with antipruritic agents. Starch baths and topical anesthetics for severe pruritus. Ticks are removed as follows: 1. Apply Vaseline, oil, nail polish, or alcohol to suffocate tick, or apply heat (i.e., heated needle) to body of tick causing head to withdraw 2. Remove tick with tweezers 3. Wash area with soap and water. If any part of tick is left in body, tick paralysis may occur
Black widow spider (Venom is neurotoxic causing central nervous system reactions)	Venom is potent and fangs are powerful; therefore they can endanger a child's life. Spider is black with a red spot (hourglass shape) on the ventral side and some red spots on back. Causes a puncture point which is red with edema, pruritus, and swelling around wound. Venom enters bloodstream in 30 min causing dizziness, weakness, tremors, nausea, and vomiting, abdominal rigidity, and cramps with rapid shallow respirations	Do not disturb web, and avoid areas such as wood piles where they thrive	Cleanse wound. IM injection of antivenin for severe cases. Muscle relaxant (calcium gluconate), narcotics, and prolonged warm bath to relieve pain. If treated with antivenin patient should be observed closely for anaphylaxis
Brown recluse spider (venom is coagulotoxic causing localized vasoconstriction)	Found in central and southern US. Yellowish to reddish brown. Has violin-shaped marking on its back. Venom is necrotoxic and causes mild stinging at time of bite. In 2–4 hr pain occurs. Development of an indurated wheal, followed by a star shaped area in 3–4 days and eventually in 7–14 days a deep sloughing ulcer forms	Avoid crushing or entangling them, as it causes them to bite	Administration of corticosteroids may hasten healing of the wound. Tetanus prophylaxis is considered in nonhealing lesions

continued

Table 52-3 *(continued)*

Agent	Identification/Clinical Signs	Prevention	Management
Scorpion	Found mainly in the southwestern US. Venom of some species causes only local reaction, while in others it is neurotoxic. The neurotoxic species causes intense aching pain followed by "pins and needles" sensation. Itching of the nose, mouth, and throat occurs. There is an ascending motor paralysis with convulsions, rapid weak pulse, nausea and vomiting, excessive salivation, thirst, and dysuria.	Wear shoes to avoid stepping on a scorpion	Spread of venom from site of sting can be slowed by applying a temporary tourniquet with momentary releases and cooling with ice packs. The wound should not be excised. Antivenin is available in most countries where the more dangerous species exist. Supportive measures include pain relief, treatment of shock, seizure control. Morphine and its derivatives are contraindicated because they act synergistically with scorpion venom. Deaths occur from scorpion stings, especially in children under 4 yr of age

(From Behrman and Vaughan, 1987; Dreisbach, 1983; Gaunder, 1986; Reece, 1984; Tenebein, 1986.)

40,000 per year. Of all the snake bites that occur in the United States 50 per cent occur in those under 19 years of age (Mayer, 1985). Snakes with poisonous venom are of two families: *Crotalidae* (pit viper) family and *Elapidae* family. Of these, only pit vipers (including rattlesnakes, copperheads, and cottonmouths) and coral snakes reside in the continental United States. Snake venom contains enzymes, proteins, and polypeptides. The venom from pit vipers (rattlesnakes, copperheads, and cottonmouths) causes breakdown of red blood cells and certain proteins, whereas the venom of the coral snake and of other Elapids is neurotoxic. The initial symptoms are immediate burning pain and erythema around the bite. Pit viper venom results in a more pronounced local reaction, whereas coral snake bites have a less pronounced immediate local reaction but have a delayed systemic reaction.

All snake bite victims should be treated as an emergency until established otherwise. Immediate care of a child with a poisonous snake bite is as follows:

1. Reassure and calm the child and parents.
2. Maintain the involved extremity in a dependent position (below the heart) and immobilize as much as possible.
3. Cleanse bite area with soap and water or a mild antiseptic.
4. Apply cool compresses to bite area, but avoid using ice packs.
5. Use of a tourniquet is not recommended (Kinney et al., 1988).
6. Excision and suction outside of a medical facility is used only when transport to medical care exceeds 45 minutes. It should be done by a trained person.

Upon reaching a medical facility, the child is reassessed to determine whether the bite was from a venomous snake. Identification and management of the most common poisonous snake bites are summarized in Table 52-4.

Animal Bites

Household pets can cause serious injury to a child. The most common serious bite is that which is inflicted by a dog. It is important to recognize that fewer than 25 per cent of dog bites involve stray dogs. Therefore, education of children regarding the proper way to handle a family pet or neighborhood dog is of primary importance. Children are attacked on the face and upper extremities because of the usual close range at which they play with an animal (see Chapter 17 for prevention of dog bites).

Dog bite wounds are considered to be highly contaminated and require thorough cleansing, irrigating, debridement, and closure. Primary or secondary closure may be done, depending on the length of time since the injury and the location of the injury. Bites (except of the hand) seen within several hours after injury can be closed after adequate irrigation and debridement. Lacerations of the face may be closed up to 6 to 8 hours after the bite took place. If the bite is potentially disfiguring, then a plastic surgeon is consulted. The need for tetanus prophylaxis is dictated by the child's immunization status and by the severity of the bite.

The most feared complication of animal bites is rabies. An unprovoked attack by an animal should raise

Table 52-4. Poisonous Snake Families

Description of Family	Types of Snakes	Geographic Location	Clinical Manifestations	Management: Field Treatment	Management: Hospital Care
Crotalidae family ("pit viper"): So-called because of its fangs and the two indentations, or pits, between eye and snout. Has a triangle-shaped head and vertical pupils	*Rattlesnake:* has "rattle" or tail plates that are noise-makers *Copperhead (or high-land moccasin):* has hourglass-shaped marking *Cottonmouth (or water moccasin):* has white buccal mucosa and a broad flat head.	All areas of the mainland US. The only poisonous snakes found in Canada Reside from middle New England to northern Florida and from central Illinois to Texas Resides in semiaquatic or aquatic environments (Virginia to Florida and westward to Texas)	Hemotoxic: Local pain, edema, erythema, and ecchymosis in 15–30 min. Severe local reactions. Formation of hemorrhagic bullae with muscle necrosis not unusual. Systemic manifestations include hemolysis, coagulopathy, and circulatory collapse	The snake should be killed and brought to emergency room if it does not delay treatment of the child. Body part should be immobilized and kept dependent (below heart). Incision and suction is not recommended unless transport time to a hospital exceeds 45 min (Moyer, 1985). Cool compresses may be applied but cold ice is avoided to avoid further tissue necrosis.	Supportive therapy. Antivenin therapy according to patient's condition preceded with skin testing. Broad-spectrum antibiotics. Tetanus immunization is evaluated and given if needed. Corticosteroids may be used but their use is controversial
Elapidae family: Includes some of the world's deadliest snakes. Have fangs along with their normal teeth	*Eastern coral* (has bands of red, yellow, and black on its body). *Sonoran coral, cobras* (not in the US.)	Eastern and Sonoran coral are only members of this family that occur naturally in the US	Neurotoxic: Local pain and erythema may be transient or absent when injected with coral snake venom and systemic symptoms may be delayed; therefore, the seriousness of the bite can be overlooked. Also fang marks are not as clearly identifiable as in pit viper. Apprehension, nausea and vomiting, excessive salivation, dysphagia, slurred speech, convulsions, and respiratory paralysis may follow.	Identification of the coral snake bite may be difficult, so the snake should be killed and brought to the emergency room. Extremity is immobilized, patient is kept at rest and transported.	Supportive therapy. Puncture wound is often similar to nonpoisonous snakes, the local reaction is less pronounced than the pit viper, and neurotoxic symptoms develop later; therefore it is more difficult to determine appropriate therapy. Patients with suspected coral snake envenomation are admitted for 48 hr of observation to monitor for late signs of neurotoxicity. Antivenin therapy is administered according to child's condition, preceded by skin testing. In severe circumstances life support may be required

(From Dreisbach, 1983; Reece, 1984; Moyer, 1985; Tenebein, 1986; Behrman and Vaughan, 1987; Kinney et al, 1988).

one's suspicion that the animal is rabid. If the animal is positive for rabies, immunization is begun. (See Chapter 45 for additional information about rabies.) Children who are seriously injured by their family dog need supportive parents and help from professionals to deal with the hurt feelings and anger they harbor toward their previously loved animal. In many cases of serious injury the child and family can no longer keep the dog in their home, even if the incident involved rough or overaggressive play or teasing of the dog.

Human Bites

Human bites occur in young children when they play aggressively or become angry, or in older children when a clenched fist strikes another's teeth. They may also occur as a form of child abuse. Human bites are highly contaminated because of the high number of organisms in saliva and are treated with debridement and irrigation, then left open to permit drainage. Broad spectrum antibodies are used prophylactically for 5 to 7 days.

Injuries Caused by Environmental Exposure

Developmental characteristics of children make them susceptible to injuries resulting from exposure to certain environments. A child's curiosity, lack of understanding of cause and effect relationships, and engrossment in play interfere with a realistic perception of potential danger. Common injuries that result from excessive exposure are frostbite and sunburn.

Frostbite

Frostbite, or tissue freezing, results from exposure to extreme cold. Environmental conditions, including low temperatures, high humidity, and high wind velocity, will increase the rate of heat loss from the body. Children are a high-risk population because most do not comprehend early warning signs of exposure.

There are various degrees of frostbite:

- First-degree frostbite, or a "frost nip," is mild freezing of the epidermis resulting in erythematous skin with edema but no blister formation after rewarming.
- Second-degree frostbite is a partial- or full-thickness injury resulting in erythema with the formation of blisters and bullae after rewarming. Child may experience pain when rewarmed.
- Third-degree frostbite, or deep frostbite, causes necrosis of epidermis, dermis, and subcutaneous tissue; sensation is absent. Child experiences pain on rewarming.
- Fourth-degree frostbite causes complete necrosis with gangrene and possible loss of body part.

Cold causes arteriolar vasoconstriction, resulting in a decreased blood flow and interference with oxygen transport; tissue anoxia is the end result. With tissue freezing, ice crystals form in the interstitial spaces and draw water from surrounding cells. Cell dehydration and the destruction of intracellular structures results.

School nurses working in cold climates can play an important role in the prevention of frostbite. The education of parents, children, and teachers on appropriate outdoor clothing for insulation is essential. Several layers of light clothing under appropriate outerwear provide extra warmth. Children playing outdoors should be instructed to wear two pairs of socks (one pair cotton and one wool), a hood or hat, and mittens or gloves. Clothing layers should not be excessive, to avoid tightness which hinders circulation. Young school-age children should not be allowed to play outside in extremely low temperatures. Older children should be instructed to warm themselves when hands or feet begin to sting.

Blanching of the skin and a stinging sensation are the initial signs of impending frostbite. Numbness will follow and the exposed area will appear white or mottled, feel cold and hard, and be without sensation. Deep frostbite will cause the tissue to blister. The nurse must quickly assess the appearance of the frostbite and institute appropriate first aid measures to prevent further tissue damage. Any child with white or mottled skin after cold exposure should be referred for medical evaluation and further treatment. During school times, treatment for mild frostbite can be managed by the school nurse.

The child should be placed in a warm place, and the affected part rewarmed gradually by blowing on the part or holding warm hands firmly on the area. Rubbing of the area is avoided because it increases tissue damage. For deeper frostbite, it is essential that the part be rapidly rewarmed; slow thawing causes further tissue damage because some refreezing of tissue occurs. Rewarming should continue until circulation has been re-established; that is, a flushed appearance of the skin (Gage and Gage, 1981). Large blisters form within 24 to 48 hours after rewarming. In 5 to 10 days the formation of eschar takes place. A child who is close to medical facilities should be transported at the time of injury, keeping the part frozen. In isolated areas, rapid rewarming in a water bath (90° to 106°F) should be done prior to transport. Because the pain associated with rewarming can be severe, analgesics and sedatives are usually required. It is imperative to avoid refreezing the affected area during transport. Children with severe frostbite will need to be hospitalized and receive long-term treatment similar to that for the burn victim.

Support for the child with mild frostbite should include a discussion as to why it is essential to rewarm the affected part. Stinging sensations may be frightening to children, and it is important for the nurse to explain the normalcy of these sensations. Parents may feel guilty about allowing their child to play outside; therefore, it is important to allow parents to express feelings and then to focus on preventive measures. Siblings should also be included in a discussion of prevention and appropriate first aid measures.

Sunburn

Overexposure to ultraviolet light waves, either from the sun or from the artificial rays of a sunlamp, can result in a burn. Ultraviolet rays are of two types. Ultraviolet A waves cause only minor burning, but play a role in allergic reactions and photosensitivity. Ultraviolet B waves are shorter and cause the more harmful effects known as a sunburn. Glass in windows effectively screens out ultraviolet B but not ultraviolet A waves. Sunburns range from mild to severe. A mild burn is red, tender, and causes mild pain. A more severe burn results in more skin redness, pain, and swelling, and eventually results in blisters. A child with a severe burn has increased pain and cannot tolerate any contact of clothing or bed sheets with the burn. Symptoms of nausea, tachycardia, chills, and fever may accompany a severe burn.

An important role of the nurse is to teach parents and children how to prevent sunburn from overexposure. Burning of the skin can be reduced by allowing the skin's protective responses to develop gradually through a series of short exposures (15 to 20 minutes), and by avoiding the sun altogether between 11 A.M. and 3 P.M., the time of maximum exposure. A program of gradual increases in length of exposure allows time for the skin to produce more melanin resulting in tanned skin. Melanin absorbs incoming rays and protects the skin from further damage. It is therefore important to caution light-skinned children, and especially those with red hair, about the dangers of sun exposure because they are particularly prone to sunburn. Infants and young children require special protection from the sun because of their thin epidermis. Exposure time should be shorter, and clothing that covers extremities and hats should be worn to protect the skin from overexposure.

Although there is less exposure when the sun is hazy, the sun's rays have phenomenal capacity even on cloudy days to cause a burn. Also, it should be remembered that the natural reflection of ultraviolet rays in fresh snow, water, and sand intensifies the effect of the sun.

Protection is also provided by the use of protective agents—topical sunscreens and sun-blockers. Sun screens are recommended to protect the skin from overexposure to ultraviolet rays. The effective ingredient in sunscreens is para-aminobenzoic acid (PABA). Zinc oxide is a sun-blocker that prevents the ultraviolet rays from reaching the skin. Sunscreens and sun-blockers need to be reapplied each time after swimming to be effective unless a waterproof variety is used.

Treatment of sunburn varies according to the severity of the burn. A mild to moderately severe burn is treated with cool tap water or saline compresses for 15 to 20 minutes, three to four times a day. Because the involved skin is often very dry, a moisturizing lotion may be applied. Acetaminophen is recommended to relieve the discomfort of the burn for several days. Severe burns require immediate medical attention because of the complications such as fluid and electrolyte imbalance, infection, and heat exhaustion that can accompany a sunburn. Children with severe sunburns are treated as any other burn victim.

Dental Injuries

Injury to teeth or complete avulsion of a tooth is a common injury during the active childhood years. Boys are more prone to dental injuries of this type than are girls (Abrams and Josell, 1982) probably because of the more aggressive nature of boys' play.

Diagnostic Assessment

Children with dental injuries who are brought to the emergency room usually do not require subsequent hospitalization for their injury. A detailed history of the injury is obtained to rule out head injury. Any injury that produced a loss of consciousness should alert the nurse to perform a neurologic assessment, and hospitalization should be considered. If the child can be discharged, the parents should be instructed in monitoring the child for any signs and symptoms of diminishing neurologic status.

Therapeutic Management

Referral to a dentist for treatment is often the appropriate course of action. When a tooth is avulsed, it is important to preserve the tooth and replant it as quickly as possible. When replantation takes place within 30 minutes, the prognosis is favorable. A tooth can be replanted into the tooth's original socket using the following guidelines (Abrams and Josell, 1982):

1. Hold the tooth by the crown. Avoid touching the root.
2. Rinse the tooth in saline or tap water (cover drain).
3. *Replant the tooth as soon as possible.* Insert into the empty socket.
4. Have patient bite on gauze to stabilize tooth.
5. Have patient seen by a dentist so tooth can be stabilized.
6. If tooth cannot be replanted, have dentist see patient as soon as possible.
7. The best transport medium for avulsed teeth is milk (McTigue, 1988).

Major Nursing Diagnoses for Dental Injury

Potential for aspiration, *related to:*
- *blood*
- *mucus*
- *vomitus*
- *tooth*

Altered comfort: pain, *related to avulsed tooth*

Anxiety, *related to:*
- *injury*
- *unfamiliar environment*

Knowledge deficit, *related to home care of child with a dental injury*

Strategies for Nursing Care

Maintaining Effective Airway. The nurse begins with the ABCs of emergency assessment and ensures that the child has a patent airway. This is particularly important if the tooth cannot be found and/or the child has vomited owing to either distress or potential head injury. Neurologic vital signs are documented as part of the primary assessment and are reassessed until the child is stable. Suction must be available to clear the airway of mucus, blood, and vomitus as required. This is important if the child is unconscious or has a suspected spinal cord injury and is immobilized. If there are no associated injuries, the child may sit up in a chair while being assessed.

Maintaining Comfort. Every effort should be made to provide the child with pain relief. The child's discomfort is enhanced by the fear and anxiety produced by the experience of the accident and the trip to a hospital. The nurse should assess the degree of pain being experienced by the child and request an appropriate medication. Topical local anesthetic agents may suffice, or oral medication such as codeine or acetaminophen can be given. Unless other facial injuries are present, intramuscular or intravenous analgesics are generally not required.

Reducing the Child's and Family's Anxiety. The degree of anxiety experienced by the child and family is associated with the amount of bleeding and number of teeth that are avulsed. Cleaning up the blood from the child's face and hands as quickly as possible is especially important for a young child. A large amount of anxiety experienced has to do with fears associated with losing permanent teeth. Proper care of the avulsed teeth and clear explanations to the child and family about the treatment can reduce some of these fears. A young child may also be fearing reprimand from parents if the accident occurred because of a forbidden activity. A nurse can defuse this fear by encouraging parents and children to talk about what happened and to resolve the feelings associated with the event.

Preparing Child and Family for Discharge. Discharge instructions to the parents should be clear and easy to understand. If follow-up appointments have been made, parents should be given a card stating the dentist's name, address, and phone number and the date and time of the appointment. They should be taught to have the child bite on a wad of moistened gauze if the socket begins to bleed. Pain relief should be reviewed carefully with them. The parents should be encouraged to return to the emergency room or to call the dentist or family doctor if they have concerns after discharge. The risk of further trauma is reduced by restricting the child's activity for one week until the tooth adheres well into the socket.

Epistaxis

Epistaxis in children is usually due to injury rather than pathology. Children with blood dyscrasias may have spontaneous nosebleeds, but healthy children incur them as a result of falls, blows to the face, or trauma. Picking of the nose, insertion of foreign objects, or lack of environmental humidity can be triggers for epistaxis. While a nosebleed can be frightening to both the child and the parents, it is very rarely a life-threatening occurrence.

Diagnostic Assessment

When children with epistaxis are brought to the emergency room, office, or clinic, the nurse remains calm and supportive during her assessment and history taking. Assessing the ABCs is the first important step. The nurse notes rate and quality of respirations, any signs of respiratory distress, pulse rate, and blood pressure, if the child is cooperative. While settling the child, the nurse asks the parents if there was any preceding injury, if the child has had previous episodes of epistaxis and, if so, how long they lasted and what treatment was provided. If the nosebleed is the result of facial trauma, a neurologic assessment is performed as well.

Therapeutic Management

Treatment for epistaxis in children may require no more than firm pressure to the septal cartilage (pinching nostrils) until the bleeding stops. If any facial injuries have been incurred, this should not be done, especially if the nose has been fractured.

If pressure fails to control the epistaxis, more aggressive measures may need to be employed. Once the reason for the bleeding is identified, a vasoconstrictive preparation such as cocaine or phenylephrine is applied or a cauterizing agent like silver nitrate is used to stop the bleeding. The concentration of cocaine should not exceed 4 per cent (2.5 mg/kg/hr). The child should be monitored for about an hour to make sure the bleeding has stopped. If the treatment is unsuccessful a topical thrombin, Gelfoam, or microfibrillar collagen may be tried (Dickerman and Lucey, 1985). More aggressive treatment involves anterior nasal packing made from petrolatum gauze or posterior packing if there is blood trickling down the throat. A patient who receives posterior packing should be admitted for observation, antibiotic therapy, and possibly volume replacement. Severe epistaxis may require volume replacement. Children with coagulation disorders should receive appropriate blood products. In some instances prolonged epistaxis requires fluid replacement and monitoring of the child's hematologic status by blood sampling. Harris (1985) recommends fluid replacement with 5 per cent D_5W in Ringer's lactate solution. A complete blood count (CBC), platelet count, and cross-match may also be required.

Major Nursing Diagnoses for Epistaxis

Potential for aspiration, related to blood in nasopharynx
Potential fluid volume deficit, related to epistaxis
Anxiety, related to:
- *bleeding*
- *unfamiliar environment*

Knowledge deficit, related to first aid treatment of nosebleeds

Strategies for Nursing Care

Maintaining a Patent Airway. The nurse can initiate treatment by settling the child in a comfortable position with the head tilted forward to minimize the amount of blood trickling down the back of the throat. Very young children may feel safer and be more cooperative if seated on a parent's lap. The child should be instructed to spit out blood rather than swallow it; however, small children may be unable to do this. Swallowed blood is irritating and may cause vomiting. The child is positioned to reduce the possibility of aspiration should vomiting occur.

The nurse monitors the child's vital signs and explains the procedures to both parent and child before they are done. Suction equipment and oxygen must be readily available.

Maintaining Fluid Balance. In the event of a very severe or prolonged epistaxis, frequent assessments should be made to identify signs of hypovolemic shock. Changes in vital signs and signs of reduced perfusion (poor capillary refill) are noted and reported to the physician. Careful monitoring of the I.V. is required as for any other child.

Reducing Anxiety Related to the Frightening Experience. Epistaxis is rarely a life-threatening event. If it occurs as the result of trauma, it becomes one of many concerns at that time and is treated along with other injuries. However, it is usually a frightening episode necessitating a quick unanticipated trip to the emergency room. A calm reassuring approach by the nurse will help to alleviate anxiety, promote cooperation, and lessen the negative aspects of the experience. Special attention is given to reducing anxiety by taking blood samples at the same time that intravenous lines are started, to minimize the number of needlesticks the child has to suffer.

Preparing for Discharge and Home Care. If the bleeding is controlled, the child may be discharged from the emergency department. Instructions to the parents should include careful observation for repeat epistaxis, the correct technique for applying nasal pressure, and the avoidance of vigorous nose-blowing or nose-picking in order not to disturb clot formation. Parents are instructed to return with the child if these methods are ineffective in controlling the bleeding.

Instruction cards printed with simple pictures may be useful as teaching aids for parents to take home with them. The nurse might also suggest the use of a humidifier or cold air steamer to add moisture to the air (particularly in the winter) to reduce dryness of the nasal mucous membranes which may contribute to nosebleeds. The nurse should document on the patient's emergency chart any patient teaching that was done with the family and how the family responded to the information.

Injuries Associated with Foreign Bodies

Children are prone to injury from foreign bodies because of their curiosity and drive to taste and manipulate household objects and toys. Although children are known to insert objects into any body orifice, the two types of injury discussed here include foreign body aspiration and foreign body in the ear.

Foreign Body Aspiration

Foreign body aspiration leading to airway obstruction and hypoxia is most common in children under 5 years of age. Items that are frequently aspirated include chunks of hot dogs, candy that is round and hard, peanuts, chunks of dense foods such as carrots or apples, pieces of cereal, and inedible items including coins, deflated balloons, toy car wheels, marbles, or large beads.

Pathophysiology

Most aspirated foreign bodies pass through the larynx and trachea to become lodged in the bronchi. The right main bronchus is a common site for obstruction because it is larger in diameter with greater airflow than the left main bronchus. Also, the right bronchus is shorter and arises from the trachea at a wider angle forming a straighter line of entry.

Obstruction may be partial or complete; a partial obstruction may become complete within seconds. Complete airway obstruction usually occurs in the upper airway and represents an immediate threat to life (Mofenson and Caraccio, 1986). The bronchi can become partially or completely obstructed resulting in different clinical manifestations.

Clinical Manifestations

Initially when a foreign body is aspirated into the respiratory tract, a choking, gagging, or coughing episode occurs. This episode may be followed by an interval of days, hours, or even weeks during which there are no symptoms of respiratory difficulty. Clinical manifestations vary according to the location of the obstruction and the degree of obstruction.

A foreign body in the *larynx* causes an immediate hoarseness, stridor, and aphonia (inability to speak). The site of obstruction becomes inflamed and dyspnea, wheezing, and cyanosis may result followed by complete obstruction requiring emergency treatment.

A *tracheal* foreign body is usually associated with coughing and an asthma-like wheeze. Hoarseness, dyspnea, and cyanosis may also be noted. As the patient coughs, it is possible for the foreign body to be moved from the carina to the glottis where an audible slap can be heard (Conner, 1987). Complete obstruction is a threat because the foreign body could move and become lodged in the subglottis.

A *bronchial* foreign body results in a cough or a wheeze if there is partial airway obstruction. These symptoms occur because air passes around the obstruction during inspiration and expiration. A child with a partial obstruction may be able to ventilate well or be adversely affected causing poor ventilation. With good air exchange, the child breathes and coughs effectively and may be able to speak, but it is not uncommon for hoarseness and stridor to be present. Complete obstruction of the bronchus results in pulmonary changes distal to the obstruction. Because no air bypasses the obstruction, no breath sounds will be heard. If atelectasis or consolidation has developed, bronchial or tubular sounds may be auscultated (Mayer, 1985).

Diagnostic Assessment

A choking child is identified by the severity of clinical signs and symptoms. A child who has an ineffective cough, is unable to make sounds, and has cyanotic lips, nails, and skin must be immediately diagnosed and treated to prevent death. Partial airway obstruction with poor gas exchange is also an emergency and should be managed as a complete obstruction. In the case of obstruction, a child seems to make respiratory efforts which, like the cough, are ineffective. Stridor may still be present, but the child is unable to vocalize at all. If circumoral cyanosis or cyanosis of the nailbeds is present, intervention must be immediate.

In many cases, aspiration of a foreign body is not so obvious. A history of a choking incident, days or weeks prior to admission, or a history of recurrent intractable pneumonia, are reasons to suspect the presence of a foreign body. The health care team clarifies the history with parents or caretakers, and assesses the airway for patency and for the effectiveness of breathing efforts.

Chest and soft tissue roentgenographs are usually ordered to locate the object. These should be taken in the emergency room rather than sending the child to the radiology department, in case the obstruction becomes complete. Radiographic examination shows opaque objects such as a penny but is less useful to identify food matter. Fluoroscopic examination shows a characteristic air-trapping when the obstruction is in the bronchi. The position of the diaphragm is also noted to remain high on the involved side when a foreign body completely obliterates the bronchus.

Therapeutic Management

In some cases the child can be coached to breathe and cough deeply in an effort to expel the object. Mofenson and Greensher (1985) cite examples of children who coughed out the object on the way to the operating room.

If the child is still conscious, the measures developed by the American Heart Association for removal of an aspirated foreign object should be used (see Box 52-5 for management of an obstructed airway).

For the child with an obstruction who becomes unconscious, more aggressive interventions are necessary. Reassessment of the patency of the airway is essential because hypoxia may cause relaxation of the neck muscles and the trachea. Enough relaxation may occur to permit some air to travel around the obstruction until the foreign body can be removed.

Whether the child is conscious or unconscious, visualization and removal of the object may be necessary through direct laryngoscopy or bronchoscopy. Once the object is removed, the bronchoscope is reinserted to look for remaining fragments, to remove secretions for culture, and to assess tissue trauma and/or edema. Children are usually hospitalized postoperatively for a period of observation, and sometimes are given a course of antibiotic therapy. A cool mist tent will help to soothe irritated tissues.

Even if the object is successfully removed, the child must be admitted to the hospital and observed for soft tissue swelling, laryngeal edema, and respiratory difficulty. If a tracheotomy is required, the child should be admitted to intensive care for observation of both respiratory and neurologic stability. An intravenous line is inserted to provide emergency access.

Major Nursing Diagnoses for Foreign Body Aspiration

***Ineffective airway clearance**, related to tracheobronchial obstruction associated with aspiration of a foreign body*
***Anxiety**, related to inability to breathe associated with aspiration of a foreign body*
***Fear**, related to unfamiliar and threatening environment associated with emergency treatment*
***Ineffective family coping: compromised**, related to temporary family disorganization associated with feelings of guilt and anger*
***Knowledge deficit**, related to safety precautions in the home*

Strategies for Nursing Care

Tracheobronchial aspiration of foreign objects represents a serious emergency that nurses who work with children may encounter at any time. Although prevention of such incidents is preferable, knowledge of how to deal with the child who presents with an obstructed airway is essential. Special attention should be paid to the management of the choking child, since early recognition and treatment of respiratory difficulty can prevent a full-blown cardiac arrest. Continued practice for emergency establishment of an airway is achieved through regular mock situations.

Establishing an Airway. The nurse plays a key role in responding quickly to the child's clinical situation. If necessary, an attempt is made to relieve the obstruction, following the guidelines for management of an obstructed airway (see Box 52-5). Notification of the appropriate team member and immediate readiness of equipment facilitate effective management.

Continuous monitoring for respiratory difficulty is instituted and nursing assessments are documented. The nurse remains prepared to assist with emergency procedures at any time should the obstruction become complete or the child become unconscious, or both. Suction equipment and oxygen are kept immediately available.

Maintaining an Airway. Once the object is removed, the child needs to be monitored for secondary obstruction due to laryngeal edema and/or soft tissue swelling or any remaining fragments. The nurse observes the child for signs and symptoms of respiratory distress such as anxiety and restlessness; flaring of the nares; tracheal, substernal, or intercostal in-drawing; and cyanosis. Arterial blood gases may be monitored depending upon the severity of the distress prior to treatment. Cyanosis in children is a late sign of hypoxia and indicates a need for immediate intervention.

The child who has had an emergency tracheotomy needs to be monitored for all the signs and symptoms described earlier. In addition, tracheotomy care is instituted (see Chapter 38 for care of the child with a tracheotomy).

Minimizing Child's Fear and Anxiety. Although monitoring the child's physical status is of utmost importance, the nurse must remember that the child has been exposed to the terror of a life-threatening experience and the unfamiliarity of emergency care, surgery, and possibly the intensive care unit. Using knowledge of growth and development, the nurse prepares the child for treatment (such as tracheotomy care) as completely as possible. The unfamiliar and anxiety-producing environment can be minimized by normalizing the environment. It is helpful to allow the child to wear his or her own pajamas, if possible, after the emergency period is past. The presence of favorite toys, the support of parents and consistency of nursing staff, are strategies used to reduce the child's stress.

Facilitating Resolution of Parental Guilt. Aspiration of a foreign body may make parents feel that they failed to provide adequate supervision for their child. If the aspiration has occurred because a parent *gave* the object to their child, it is particularly distressing for parents to see their child endure such a traumatic experience.

Parents need to be supported during this stressful period. It is therapeutic to allow them to express their feelings of guilt and anger. Involving them in their child's care, if they are receptive to this, is also helpful. Recognizing the strengths of parents and fostering their self-esteem as parents is an important component of the nurse's support to the family.

Reducing Risk of Future Incidents of Foreign Body Aspiration. Nurses who work in parent-child settings or public health are in excellent positions to do patient teaching regarding child safety and child-proofing the home in an effort to prevent aspiration of foreign bodies. Should aspiration occur and necessitate admission to an emergency department, the nurse who cares for the child should review principles of growth and development and safety with the parents before discharge. (See Chapter 17 for a discussion of safety concerning aspiration of a foreign body.) The nurse should assess the need for further follow-up with a public health nurse or a social worker and inform support agencies of the need for assistance.

Nursing Strategies for Follow-up Care in the Home or Clinic

Assess vital signs and breath sounds for evidence of residual pulmonary complications.

Determine if the frightening experience of airway obstruction has resulted in unresolved behavioral changes.

Allow time for parents and child to talk about the experience of airway obstruction, treatment, and recovery.

Assess home environment for adequacy of safety standards and child supervision.

Teach family to change any potentially unsafe practices and environmental hazards that expose the child to risk for future foreign body aspiration.

Foreign Body in the Ear

Foreign bodies of the ear are relatively easy to diagnose and treat (Matlak, 1985). The difficulty is that they may be in place for several days before generating enough of an inflammatory response to alert the parent to seek medical attention. By that time, pain and inflammation contribute to difficulty in examination and removal of the object.

Anything small enough to fit in the external canal may be placed there by a small child. Tiny insects may fly into the ear and become trapped. Because of their potential for causing hearing loss, of great concern are miniature cell batteries used in watches, calculators, and some toys.

Clinical Manifestation and Diagnostic Assessment

Diagnosis is usually based on a history of ear pain and purulent drainage that has not responded to antibiotic therapy (Matlak, 1985). A child's cooperation can usually be gained by explaining that it is important to "look inside your ear to see why it is hurting." If a child cannot be helped to keep the head still or is unduly fearful and uncooperative, examination under general anesthesia may be considered.

Usually the foreign object can be visualized through an otoscope unless excessive purulent drainage is present. Gentle irrigation with suction may help to visualize the eardrum and may even flush out the object.

Therapeutic Management

Small alligator forceps, ear hooks, or wax curettes may be used to remove the item. Care is taken not to push the foreign body further into the ear or perforate the eardrum. Live insects should be killed before removal, especially if they are the biting kind (Matlak, 1985). Agents used for this purpose are mineral oil, alcohol, or lidocaine. A few drops are instilled and in a few minutes the insect can be removed. Topical antibiotics may be administered for minor lacerations or local inflammation of the ear canal. A more serious laceration may require repair. Oral antibiotics are indicated in the event of a perforated eardrum.

In the event of accidental placement of miniature batteries in the ear, early treatment is required. Delay in seeking treatment contributes to deterioration of the battery case, resulting in alkaline burns. Further complications will arise if acetic acid–based eardrops are administered because they provide an external electrolyte bath for the battery. Such an environment promotes leakage of the battery contents and generation of an electrical current. This will eventually cause tissue destruction (Kavanagh and Litovitz, 1986). Removal of a corroding battery must be done carefully: biting or pinching instruments are not used, because they could perforate the casing. Follow-up of the child is arranged to assess healing and to debride necrotic tissue which may slough for a number of weeks (Kavanagh and Litovitz, 1986).

Major Nursing Diagnoses for Foreign Body in the Ear

Fear, related to child's unfamiliarity with equipment procedures used to remove object from ear

Potential for knowledge deficit, related to

lack of recall or lack of experience with instillation of eardrops

Potential for injury, *related to increased risk for foreign body insertion in the ear associated with developmental age and environmental exposure*

Impaired skin integrity: ear canal and/or tympanic membrane, *related to*

- *mechanical removal of a foreign body from the ear*
- *chemical injury associated with leakage of battery fluid from a battery*

Strategies for Nursing Care

The emergency room nurse will obtain a history and try to determine if there is a strong possibility of a foreign body in the ear. She should take the child's vital signs to determine the presence of infection.

Reducing Fear Associated With Treatment. Parents should be given the option of remaining with the child or leaving the room. Whatever decision they make should be supported by the nurse.

The nurse explains in simple terms to the child and parents what to expect during the examination and treatment. Rather than telling a child to "keep your head still," the nurse could suggest to the child that he or she will "help" by holding the child's head during the examination. The child is encouraged to "help" the doctor and nurse by lying as still as possible. Following removal of the object, praise is given to the child for "helping" during the procedure.

Teaching the Family How to Instill Eardrops. The nurse reviews the correct procedure for instilling the prescribed eardrops and the importance of finishing the prescription even though the child may seem much better in a day or two. Correct procedure for instillation of eardrops is presented in Chapter 28.

Reducing Risk of Future Incidents of Foreign Body in the Ear. Principles of home safety and childproofing are reviewed with parents. The young child's curiosity and need to explore presents a special challenge to parents and requires their constant monitoring of a child's play area for hazardous objects. Parents are also encouraged to tell their child *not* to place objects in their body orifices.

Reducing Risk of Damage to Ear Canal and Tympanic Membrane. Parents are provided with eardrops as appropriate to facilitate healing of a damaged ear canal, tympanic membrane, or both. The child is instructed not to place anything in the ears, and if a child is too young to understand, close supervision by parents is required. Follow-up care may be required if the injury is extensive because of the need to debride necrotic tissue. The nurse can assist in follow-up care by giving parents clear explanations about the need to return for assessment of the healing process.

Nursing Strategies for Follow-up Care in the Home or Clinic

Assess tympanic membrane and external ear canal to determine if healing is occurring as expected.

Assess child's hearing to detect hearing loss associated with injury to tympanic membrane.

Determine if entire course of antibiotics was completed as prescribed.

Assess correctness of technique in instillation of eardrops, if treatment regimen is still in progress.

Assess safety of child's environment (especially presence of small objects).

Encourage to continue follow-up visits, if hearing loss exists.

Poisoning

Poisoning affects an estimated 5 to 10 million children annually. Accidental poisoning is the fourth leading cause of death in children ages 1 to 4 years. *Accidental poisoning* accounts for 80 to 85 per cent of poisoning incidents; 15 to 20 per cent of poisonings are *intentional* (Mayer, 1985). The use of drugs in attempted suicide is discussed in Chapter 35.

Epidemiology/Etiology

Although poisoning exposures can occur through oral ingestion, ocular or topical exposure, inhalation, or envenomation, oral ingestion accounts for almost 90 per cent of poisonings. The type of agent ingested varies with the age of the child. Adolescents have a much higher incidence of psychopharmacologic drug ingestion (sedatives, tranquilizers, antidepressants), whereas young children are most frequently affected by ingestion of plants, household detergents and cleaning solutions, or medications such as Tylenol, aspirin, vitamins, or minerals.

The most common age of poisoning in young children is 2 years old and under, with the greatest incidence occurring at 1 year of age (Table 52-5). Children at 1 and 2 years of age become increasingly mobile and curious, seeking to increase their independence; exploration of the environment results in increased contact with many hazards. Furthermore, at this developmental stage, parents are beginning to decrease some of the constant vigilance they kept for their child during infancy.

Table 52-5. Breakdown of Poisoning Cases by the Age of the Victim

Age in Years	1975 (Per cent)*	1983 (Per cent)†
Under 1	6.4	16.9
1	17.0	37.8
2	21.0	13.5
3	14.4	4.5
4	5.4	1.4
5	2.7	1.2
6–17	10.2	6.5
18 and over	20.5	15.6
Not recorded	2.3	2.6

* Data from the Intermountain Regional Poison Control Center, 1975.

† Data from cooperative regional poison control center pilot study, Jan–Feb, 1983, American Association of Poison Control Centers.

(From Mayer, 1985.)

Numerous environmental conditions in a household contribute to poisoning. Family stress can contribute to preoccupation of parents, and subsequently, increase the risk of poisoning. It is also known that poisoning is more common in lower socioeconomic groups and in families with more than one child. Generally, accidental poisoning can be attributed to inappropriate supervision for the age of the child or faulty childproofing of the environment.

Diagnostic Assessment

The initial assessment may be done on the phone or in a clinic, office, or emergency room. The following information should be obtained:

- age, approximate weight, sex of child
- present condition of child
- name of toxic agent
- route of exposure
- how much of agent ingested (or other exposure)
- when incident occurred
- any signs and symptoms present and time of onset
- circumstances of the event

An immediate evaluation of the patient is performed as for any other emergency victim (see Box 52-1):

A—Is the child's *a*irway open and is cervical spine intact?
B—Is the child *b*reathing?
C—Is child's *c*irculatory status established?

Once this has been determined, specific information relative to the poisoning incident is sought. If the initial contact is by phone, sufficient information must be obtained to make a decision about the amount and type of treatment to recommend in the home and whether to instruct the caller to bring the child to an emergency room. In the United States, where syrup of ipecac is used in the home according to instructions given over the phone from a poison control center, emergency room visits have been reduced. In Canada, where provincial health care plans exist, this practice has not been adopted and the child is more commonly brought to the emergency room immediately. Upon arrival to a health care facility, an assessment of the child is made to determine the need for basic life support. Specific information about the poisoning incident is then obtained to determine further management. In severe cases, it may be necessary to immediately establish an airway, provide artificial ventilation, and institute measures to restore circulation. Heart rate, blood pressure, central nervous system status, and hydration are important parameters to assess. Findings on the physical examination that are suggestive of poisoning include altered vital signs, neuromuscular dysfunction, irritation of the eyes or skin, and unusual odors on the breath (Temple, 1985).

When a poisoning occurs, it is also important to gather data concerning the factors that might have contributed to the poisoning. This is usually done after the child is stabilized; in many instances, referral for follow-up is made. Individual factors are assessed including stress in the home, age of the child, status of childproofing in the home, and level of safety education to which the family has been exposed.

Therapeutic Management

Management is based on the history, clinical manifestations, and laboratory reports. The aim of management of all poisonings regardless of agent is to terminate the patient's exposure to a toxic agent or to reduce the potential toxicity. Poison control centers in both the United States and Canada have information on almost all drugs and household products. Management is adapted according to the type of exposure (ocular, topical, inhalation, or ingestion).

Management of Ocular Exposure. First aid care of eyes consists of:

1. Immediately flushing the eye with copious amounts of water, lactated Ringer's, or normal saline
2. Removal of contact lenses
3. Additional irrigation for 10 to 15 minutes

Intravenous saline solution directed through intravenous tubing is a readily available device in the emergency room. In the home the eye can be held open under a *gentle* stream of tepid tap water. All surfaces of the eye should be examined by a physician. Ophthalmologic follow-up is arranged, as these injuries may cause an ulcer that heals very slowly or they may result in the loss of an eye (Reece, 1984).

Management of Topical Exposure. First aid treatment for dermal exposure is to flush the affected area with water followed by a thorough washing. Soap is used to remove oily substances, which are potential systemic toxins (Mayer, 1985). In cases of contamination with pesticides, the child's clothing is removed. Protection by gowning is recommended for health care personnel during this process.

Management of Inhalation Exposure. The first step in management is to move the victim from the locality of exposure to fresh air. Clothing is loosened and an assessment is made to determine the need for intubation and oxygen administration. Early intubation may be necessary because of airway edema, which can ensue rapidly. After emergency treatment, the patient is observed for latent pulmonary symptoms to determine need for respiratory care (see section on the child with burns, later in this chapter).

Management of Ingestions. The majority of poisonings are caused by ingestion. Once the poison has been identified and the patient stabilized through maintenance of an airway, oxygenation, and prevention of shock, care is directed at decontamination of the gastrointestinal tract. Decontamination is accomplished by (1) diluting the toxin, (2) decreasing absorption by gastric evacuation (vomiting or lavage) or local detoxification, and (3) hastening elimination.

Dilution. Dilution is considered only when the toxin acts as an irritant or corrosive. Dilution of the toxin is done in combination with therapy to produce emesis. Dilution without emesis is not recommended, because it may enhance absorption of the drug or force the drug out of the stomach through the pylorus with absorption in the lower gastrointestinal tract. Administration of fluids is encouraged during induction of emesis; water is the preferred diluent. Milk may be administered to reduce the irritating and corrosive effect of an agent.

Decreasing Absorption. *Induction of vomiting* removes a substantial portion of ingested poisons if it is done early on. It is most effective if done within 2 to 4 hours (Temple, 1985). The drug of choice for induction of vomiting is syrup of ipecac. It is *not recommended* when there is altered consciousness, when seizures occur, if the gag reflex is absent, or if the ingested poison is caustic. A rule of thumb is that vomiting is not induced if passing the poisonous substance through the esophagus again will increase the risk of esophageal damage or aspiration of volatile components into the lungs.

The dose of syrup of ipecac is 30 ml for adolescents, 15 ml for children, and 10 ml for infants under 1 year of age. This is followed by 4 to 8 ounces of fluid. Syrup of ipecac, if used appropriately, produces vomiting approximately 90 per cent of the time. Fifty per cent of patients vomit in less than 15 to 20 minutes and 90 per cent in 30 minutes (Mofenson and Caraccio, 1986). If emesis does not occur in 20 to 30 minutes, the ipecac and liquid can be repeated. Ipecac fluid extract, a preparation formerly used, was 14 times more potent than ipecac syrup, but it caused toxicity and overdose in the past because of inappropriate use. This preparation is no longer marketed. Apomorphine is an alternative drug used to induce vomiting if the use of ipecac is unsuccessful. This drug is more likely to produce central nervous system (CNS) depression and results in protracted vomiting more frequently than does syrup of ipecac.

Gastric lavage is indicated when syrup of ipecac or apomorphine has failed to induce emesis. It is also indicated to remove stomach contents in the event of CNS depression, seizures, or altered consciousness, and in circumstances when an ingested poison is rapidly absorbed. Contraindications to treatment by lavage include ingestion of corrosive agents or petroleum distillates and the presence of gastrectomy (Mayer, 1985).

The largest-sized catheter that can be safely used is recommended to ensure that fragments or particles can be removed. The tube is inserted with the same technique as for any other purpose (see section on nasogastric tube insertion in Chapter 41). The child is positioned with the head to one side and slightly lowered, to avoid aspiration in the event of vomiting and to maximize the return of the lavage fluid. In an unconscious patient (or in any patient who cannot adequately protect the airway) intubation precedes placement of a lavage tube to prevent aspiration.

After the lavage tube is in place, the gastric contents are removed; then lavage fluid, usually normal saline, is introduced into the stomach. Gastric washing is accomplished by instilling fluid through the lavage tube (50 to 100 ml at a time). Intermittent suction is used for its removal. Children can receive up to 2 liters at a rate of 1 liter per 5 minutes (Temple, 1985). The process is usually continued until the lavage return is clear. If toxicologic testing is required, it is done on the first lavage fluid returned.

Local detoxification is another method used to interfere with absorption of a toxin. Activated charcoal limits absorption of drugs by absorbing drugs onto its surfaces. It is not itself absorbed by the gastrointestinal mucosa. It is usually given in the dose of 1 gram per kilogram of the child's weight. The activated charcoal is a fine black powder that is premixed to make a black solution. It is given orally or via a nasogastric tube. It should not be given in milk or ice cream. Activated charcoal may be used following the administration of ipecac syrup to bind any remaining poison or prevent further absorption. It should not be used until after vomiting has occurred because it will inactivate the ipecac. Children who are sent home after being treated with activated charcoal should be warned that the stool will be black for a day or two.

Hastening Elimination. Elimination of poison can be hastened by the use of a cathartic lavage. Saline cathartics are preferred. The usual dose is sodium sulfate, 250 mg per kg, as a 20 to 50 per cent solution and magnesium citrate 4 ml per kg (every 1 to 2 hours) as long as bowel sounds are present (Mayer, 1985). Saline cathartics may be used following gastric lavage, emesis, or activated charcoal. They are usually necessary in more complicated cases that require hospitalization.

Poisons already absorbed will be eliminated via the lungs, liver or kidneys. Elimination of absorbed poisons is enhanced by specialized procedures including diuresis, dialysis and hemoperfusion. These techniques are sometimes indicated when a child is brought for treatment several hours after the actual event of poisoning has occurred. While these techniques carry considerable risks, they are instituted when the patient's recovery is threatened.

Most children who are victims of poisonings present with a history of having ingested a toxic substance; however, any child presenting in coma or with strange behavior, unexplained high fever, arrhythmias or seizures should be suspected of a poisoning event. Such children are critically ill and intervention is aimed at making a diagnosis and giving supportive treatment. Pathophysiology and symptomatology vary according to the toxin ingested, but similar nursing diagnoses apply to a variety of poisoning circumstances.

Major Nursing Diagnoses for Poisoning

Potential for injury: multiple organs and systems, related to toxic effects of the poison
Anxiety (parent), related to threat of child's death associated with effects of a poisoning
Fear (child), related to separation from support system during the threatening experience of emergency treatment of a poisoning
Potential for injury: subsequent poisoning, related to parent's inadequate knowledge about child's developmental capabilities

Strategies for Nursing Care

Nursing care of the child varies according to the type of poisoning and number and intrusiveness of emergency treatments required. The single most important role of the nurse is to assist in the stabilization of the patient as described earlier in this chapter. Other areas of concern for the nurse are reduction of the fear and anxiety experienced by the child, preventive teaching concerning the storage of poisons and supervision of children, and removal of the poison to reduce the danger of skin and mucous membrane trauma.

Reducing Physiologic Injury. Poisoning results when a toxic agent comes in contact with a specific area in the body. The nurse can mediate the injury resulting from a toxin by making a rapid assessment and preparing the necessary equipment and materials for immediate removal or dilution of the toxin. Minutes are important; therefore, speed of assessment and initiation of treatment can prevent serious trauma to a child. The nurse is an important team member and familiarity with equipment and procedures is essential for the nurse to achieve in order to prevent unnecessary trauma in poisoning.

Reducing the Child and Family's Fear and Anxiety. A poisoning episode not only requires emergency treatment to save the child, but also emotional support for the parents. They feel devastated and engage in self-blame resulting in threatened feelings as parents. Keeping the parents informed about the status of their child confirms their importance as parents. Anxious feelings of parents about the potential of losing their child are often expressed if they are given the opportunity to do so.

Poisonings often require removal of the toxic agent from the body by using techniques that are frightening to young children. The suddenness of the event, the strangeness of the environment, and the discomfort of the procedures are all factors that nurses regard in planning the care of a poisoned child.

Preventing Future Poisoning Episodes. The nurse has a responsibility to discuss with the family the circumstances surrounding the poisoning episode. If the child is admitted to the hospital, home safety can be discussed during the period of hospitalization or on a home visit after discharge. If the child is discharged home from the emergency room, it is most appropriate to make a public health referral for further assessment.

Nursing Strategies for Follow-up Care in the Home or Clinic

Assess area of contact with toxin (i.e., eye, lungs, skin) to evaluate healing.

Assess function of involved area to detect any complications associated with poisoning.

Determine if emergency room experience and hospitalization has resulted in any persistent behavioral changes in the child.

Assess parental feelings with respect to self-blame.

Assess home environment for safe storage of drugs and chemicals.

Assist family in improvement of home safety as required to prevent poisoning.

Commonly Ingested Poisons

The nurse's role has been discussed with respect to basic principles that apply to most incidents of poisoning. A discussion of some specific types of ingested poisons that occur in children follows.

Salicylate Poisoning

Salicylates are the most common cause of drug poisoning in children. Although there is a trend for aspirin to be used less often to treat children because of its association with Reye syndrome, it continues to be a common drug in most households. Safety packaging has decreased accidental poisoning by 40 to 50 per cent; however, 300 to 400 children die each year of salicylate intoxication (Hughes, 1984). Poisoning may occur as the result of the ingestion of a single dose of aspirin, sodium salicylate, or methyl salicylate (oil of wintergreen). A dose of 4 cc of oil of wintergreen contains the equivalent of approximately 40 baby aspirins; it should be safety stored. Overdose of aspirin can also occur because of repeated small therapeutic doses of aspirin used for the treatment of fever. A child is particularly at risk for overdose when aspirin is given in combination with other medications that contain salicylates such as antihistamine and decongestant compounds.

Pathophysiology

Salicylate ingestion drastically alters acid-base balance, resulting in both respiratory alkalosis and metabolic acidosis. In the first phase of the body's response to a salicylate overdose, stimulation of the respiratory center in the medulla causes hyperventilation, a fall in PCO_2, and *respiratory alkalosis.* Signs of respiratory alkalosis are confusion, loss of consciousness, and eventually respiratory failure. Bicarbonate is excreted in the urine to compensate for respiratory alkalosis; both Na^+ and K^+ are lost with the bicarbonate in the urine.

A second phase occurs as K^+ is lost and depleted. Once K^+ is depleted in the kidney, an exchange of K^+ for H^+ occurs to conserve K^+. This results in acidification of the urine. A "paradoxical aciduria" then occurs in the presence of respiratory alkalosis.

Salicylates inhibit the Kreb cycle, altering carbohydrate and lipid metabolism. The resultant accumulation of ketones and lactic acid accounts for the severe *metabolic acidosis* that results. Young children appear to be especially susceptible to these metabolic effects of salicylates as evidenced by the rapid onset of metabolic acidosis following an initial transitory respiratory alkalosis. Metabolic acidosis also increases the nonionized fraction of salicylic acid. Further penetration of salicylates into the brain thus occurs. The increase of salicylic acid in the brain explains the severe clinical manifestations of salicylate poisoning in children (Gaudreault and Lovejoy, 1985).

Rapid respirations (hyperpnea) during this phase of acid accumulation are in response to acidosis rather than to the primary respiratory drive. Salicylate levels in the plasma escalate because they can no longer be excreted in an acid urine.

Salicylates also affect the process of oxidative phosphorylation—the process whereby oxygen is used by the mitochondria to transfer chemical energy to adenosine triphosphate (ATP). Salicylates cause uncoupling of oxidative phosphorylation (i.e., oxidation is enhanced, but the energy is not synthesized into ATP). The metabolic rate is increased resulting in fever, increased oxygen consumption, and CO_2 production. Altered glucose metabolism may occur with hyperglycemia presenting early and hypoglycemia presenting later.

Hypokalemia and dehydration are also present during the phase of lactic acid accumulation. Renal losses of sodium and potassium accompany organic acid excretion. Simultaneously, there is water loss because of insensible pulmonary loss, sweating and hyperthermia, and an osmotic diuresis that accompanies excretion of organic acids (Hughes, 1984).

Salicylates also inhibit prothrombin formation (secondary to impaired liver function), decrease platelet adhesiveness, increase capillary fragility, decrease platelet levels, and may cause local gastrointestinal irritation. While bleeding can occur in salicylate poisoning, it is generally not a significant clinical problem.

Diagnostic Assessment

The most important means of assessing the status of a child who is suspected to have ingested salicylate is from the history, the clinical signs, and laboratory evaluation.

In most circumstances it is difficult to determine the exact dose ingested. However, some attempt should be made to estimate the dosage. A toxic dose is generally believed to be a single dose that exceeds 200 to 280 mg per kg.

The principal manifestations of salicylate poisoning are hyperpnea and disturbed acid-base balance. Hyperpnea is a frequent sign early in the course of salicylate intoxication. Later manifestations of CNS alterations include CNS depression, vomiting, lethargy, hyperpyrexia, coma, respiratory failure, and circulatory collapse.

Salicylate levels can be estimated by using Phenistix to test urine, separated plasma, or serum. Phenistix cannot be used to test vomitus or lavage fluids because positive results are dependent on acetylsalicyclic acid being changed to salicylic acid. Blood salicylate levels are done to determine toxicity levels, which are essential for appropriate treatment. The Done nomogram (Done, 1960) diagrams the association between serum salicylate concentration and expected severity of the child's condition at certain time intervals, after the ingestion of a single dose of salicylate. In persons with chronic salicylate intoxication, the nomogram should not be used.

Other laboratory assessments include blood gases, serum pH, electrolyte levels, and urine and blood glucose levels. Urine pH and volume is measured hourly in all serious cases. For chronic ingestion abnormal liver function tests and increased creatinine excretion may be significant.

Therapeutic Management

The aim of treatment is to minimize entry of salicylates into the brain. Emergency management begins with efforts to remove the ingested drug from the stomach. Peak gastric absorption occurs within 2 hours of ingestion.

In some instances, the status of the patient interferes with the ability to induce emesis. In patients with altered mental status, gastric lavage is performed. A cuffed endotracheal tube is inserted before lavage to prevent aspiration.

After gastric emptying by lavage or vomiting, activated charcoal is given to decrease salicylate absorption, and magnesium citrate or sulfate is administered to increase gastrointestinal transit (Dickerman and Lucey, 1985).

Fluid therapy is directed at correcting dehydration and promoting elimination of salicylates. If the child is hypotensive, volume expanders may be needed to support circulation. Vitamin K may be administered to correct bleeding tendencies and calcium gluconate to counteract tetany.

Buffering of blood pH by continuous bicarbonate infusion alkalinizes the urine, which in turn promotes salicylate excretion. The presence of hypokalemia interferes with this process because in a state of hypokalemia, potassium is conserved by the kidney and hydrogen ions are excreted in its place. Hydrogen ions in the urine reduce its alkalinity and interfere with salicylate excretion. Alkalinization of urine, however, is not without its hazards including hyponatremia and systemic alkalosis.

Tepid sponging or a cooling mattress may be used for hyperpyrexia. Seizures are usually treated with diazepam followed by phenytoin or phenobarbital if necessary (Gaudreault and Lovejoy, 1985). Peritoneal dialysis, exchange transfusion, hemodialysis, or hemoperfusion may be required in severe cases when the child is unresponsive to therapy.

Major Nursing Diagnoses for Salicylate Poisoning

Potential for injury: physiologic, *related to salicylate-induced alterations of acid-base balance:*
- *stimulation of the respiratory center (respiratory alkalosis)*
- *accumulation of ketones and lactic acid (metabolic acidosis)*

Potential fluid volume deficit, *related to:*
- *insensible pulmonary loss*
- *sweating and hyperthermia*
- *osmotic diuresis associated with organic acid excretion*

Potential hyperthermia, *related to increased metabolic rate*

Anxiety (child and parent), *related to:*
- *perceived threat to self associated with constant monitoring and invasive procedures*
- *discomfort associated with vomiting*
- *unfamiliar equipment and procedures*
- *lack of information about test results and purpose of procedures*

Strategies for Nursing Care

Nursing strategies are based on an ongoing assessment of the patient's condition. Rapid and effective emergency treatment can be facilitated by a nurse who can anticipate the needs of the patient. The nurse plays an active role in carrying out the medical plan of care, as well as in supporting the child and family throughout the experience.

Minimizing Physiologic Injury. Signs of acid-base imbalance (initially respiratory alkalosis and later metabolic acidosis) and signs of hypokalemia are parameters that the nurse monitors, documents, and reports to the physician. Careful monitoring is done during the various phases of salicylate poisoning. Salicylate levels, urine pH and volume, plasma pH, and serum K^+ levels in particular are monitored. The nurse's understanding of the progression of the clinical presentation and recognition and reporting of alterations in acid-base balance are important nursing responsibilities. (See Chapter 30 for indepth discussion of acid-base imbalance.)

Maintaining Fluid Balance. A large part of the nurse's care is focused on accurate administration of fluids and on monitoring the patient's condition accordingly. Hydration is monitored by assessing skin turgor, eyes, fontanelle fullness, and mucous membrane hydration. Because salicylates are more easily eliminated in an alkaline urine the nurse also monitors urinary pH with the goal of maintaining an alkaline urine with a pH of 8 or more.

Vital signs, blood pressure, urine specific gravity, and urinary intake and output are monitored closely. The physician should be notified if urinary output falls below 1 ml/kg/hr. Serum potassium levels are closely monitored and are maintained between 3.5 and 4.5 mEq/l. The nurse monitors urinary output and ensures that it is established before potassium is added to parenteral fluids.

Maintaining Normal Body Temperature. Hyperpyrexia is another condition that the nurse monitors by checking the child's temperature frequently (every 1 to 2 hours according to the child's condition). A tepid water sponge bath or cooling blanket may also be ordered for persistent fever. These interventions are performed with caution and careful monitoring of the child's response to therapy. Rapid changes in temperature can occur; therefore, the temperature of the water or cooling mattress is cool but not cold, and temperature reduction is achieved gradually.

Because these children have the potential to have seizures in association with elevated body temperature, the child is monitored carefully to prevent seizure and protect him or her in the event of a seizure.

Reducing Anxiety of Child and Family. A child who is exposed to the experiences associated with emergency and acute care of salicylate poisoning requires the support of parents and professionals. The anxiety produced by the rapid chain of events is especially overwhelming for young children who are limited in their ability to understand explanations. Keeping parents with the child, whenever possible, is encouraged. Ongoing explanation of both the treatment components and laboratory findings are essential for parents to cope with this experience. Support of the child and family during induction of vomiting is particularly important because of the fear, anxiety, and repulsion associated with vomiting. Young children may feel that the discomfort of vomiting is a way to punish them for taking the aspirin.

Because of the close monitoring required, it is easy for parents to misinterpret testing and evaluation to mean increasing danger with a poor prognosis.

Acetaminophen Poisoning

Acetaminophen (Tylenol) is increasingly used as a substitute for aspirin in the treatment of children. This trend has occurred in response to the identification of an association between the use of aspirin during viral infections and Reye syndrome. Acetaminophen poisoning usually occurs as a result of acute poisoning rather than long-term use of therapeutic doses.

Pathophysiology

Acetaminophen is rapidly absorbed from the gastrointestinal tract with peak plasma concentrations occurring within 1 to 2 hours after ingestion of the tablet form and 30 minutes after the liquid form (Hughes, 1984).

Acetaminophen is metabolized in the liver; therefore, acute overdose can result in hepatic damage. Under normal circumstances, a small fraction of acetaminophen is converted to a reactive metabolite that is toxic to the liver. Normally, the reactive metabolite is detoxified by the hepatic substance glutathione and excreted in the urine. In the event of overdose glutathione can become depleted so that the reactive metabolite binds to cellular protein in the hepatic cell, eventually causing hepatic necrosis.

Hepatic damage is the major cause of morbidity and mortality in acetaminophen poisoning. Children younger than 6 years of age seem to be more resistant to development of hepatotoxicity than older children and adults. Although this mechanism is not understood, it may be associated with the difference in metabolism of acetaminophen.

Clinical Manifestations

Clinical manifestations are frequently nonspecific and delayed. During the first phase (up to 24 hours) there may be some malaise, nausea, vomiting, anorexia, diaphoresis, and pallor. These symptoms may occur within 2 to 4 hours of ingestion or be delayed for 12 to 24 hours. During the next phase (1 to 3 days) there is a latent period with an asymptomatic rise in liver enzymes and bilirubin and prolonged prothrombin time heralding liver damage. Right upper quadrant pain may accompany or follow these signs of hepatic damage. Thereafter, other manifestations of hepatic necrosis are manifested including jaundice, renal failure, clotting disorders, and hepatic encephalopathy. Recovery from even severe hepatic damage is usually complete with no residual abnormalities; however, death may occur as a result of acute hepatic failure if it is not recognized and treated aggressively.

Diagnostic Assessment

Serum acetaminophen levels are obtained to make treatment decisions. The acetaminophen assay is delayed until 4 hours after the ingestion to ensure that peak levels of the drug have been reached. The plasma levels of the drug are plotted on a nomogram developed by Rumack and Matthew (1975) to assess the severity of the poisoning. Baseline liver and renal function tests are also obtained. Initiation of therapy is begun on the basis of the drug level in the plasma. Because therapy begun later than 10 hours after ingestion is not considered to be of any value, it is initiated before liver abnormalities are documented by laboratory tests.

Therapeutic Management

Immediate emptying of the stomach by lavage or emesis induced with syrup of ipecac is performed to lessen absorption of the drug. Activated charcoal effectively adsorbs to acetaminophen but it should not be used if use of the antidote *N*-acetylcysteine (Mucomyst) is anticipated. (Activated charcoal binds the antidote Mucomyst and makes it ineffective.)

Mucomyst protects the liver by acting as a precursor for the production of additional glutathione (Tenenbein, 1986). It is given orally in a carbonated beverage and is diluted to a 20 per cent solution. It is given by gastric tube as an alternate if the oral route is not tolerated. A loading dose of 140 mg/kg is followed by 70 mg/kg every 4 hours, until a total of 18 doses have been given (Hughes, 1984). The intravenous route is recommended by some; however, its use remains controversial (Tenenbein, 1986).

The patient is monitored by assessing liver function, clotting parameters, and renal function. In 3 to 4 days, liver enzymes peak, and thereafter rapidly return to normal.

Strategies for Nursing Care

The most important role of the nurse is to intervene with parents before the incident occurs. Safe storage of acetaminophen should be discussed with parents at the time when it is prescribed for fever in common childhood illness. Especially when it is purchased for the first time, parents should be counseled about the potential danger that it presents.

If a poisoning episode does occur, the nurse must be aware of signs of overdose in order to take a relevant history and to identify the clinical progression from vague symptoms to more serious signs of hepatic toxicity.

An important nursing role is to support the child and family during the treatment and recovery phases of the poisoning. It is especially important to recognize the offensiveness of the antidote *N*-acetylcysteine (Mucomyst 20 per cent solution) and to administer it in a carbonated beverage. In the event it is vomited, it is usually repeated within 1 hour of administration. Sometimes it may be necessary to administer *N*-acetylcysteine by nasogastric tube because of its offensiveness. Soliciting the assistance of parents is often an approach that eases the resistance to its administration.

The patient is frequently monitored with a heart monitor and should have vital signs checked frequently. Assessment and documentation of intake and urinary output and overseeing the collection of blood specimens to monitor liver and renal function tests are important nursing functions.

Plant Ingestion and Exposure

Plants can cause a wide range of toxic symptoms from mild gastrointestinal distress to respiratory distress, convulsions, coma, shock, and cardiotoxicity. See Chapter 17 for a discussion of prevention of plant ingestion. Interested readers are referred to the articles by Fosnot (1979) and Keim (1983) for specific symptomatology of various plant ingestion. In an actual clinical situation, the poison control center provides the information and instructions required for treatment of a specific plant ingestion.

Poison Ivy. Poison ivy is a common plant that grows in woods and fields and can cause a severe dermatitis. Its leaves grow in clusters of three from the same stem, and the edges of the leaves are notched. In autumn and winter, the plant has clusters of white waxy berries. Children should be taught to recognize poison ivy so that they can avoid contact with it.

Poison ivy causes a contact dermatitis consisting of vesicles, papules, and bullae on reddened skin (often in a linear pattern). Lesions usually appear on exposed areas of skin and may appear several hours after contact or not until a few days later. Pruritus, swelling, and burning are commonly associated with the skin lesions. The rash is caused by an irritating oil in the leaves, flowers, stem, and bark. Clothing that has come into contact with the plant should be washed and exposed to sunlight for 48 hours. Even cats and dogs that have touched the plant may cause family members to get the rash. It is, however, not spread from one part of the skin to another by scratching, nor is it spread by the blister fluid to another part of the body or to another person.

Treatment consists of washing the area immediately with mild soap and plenty of water. Other methods used to relieve itching include

- Cool, wet compresses
- Calamine lotion
- Cool starch baths (e.g., Aveeno bath)

Keeping fingernails cleaned and trimmed will discourage the development of an infection in the lesions. The lesions may last 2 to 4 weeks depending on the amount of allergen that has penetrated the skin. (See Chapter 44 for further discussion of poison ivy and other forms of contact dermatitis.)

Vitamins With Iron

The second most common type of accidental ingested medication by children is vitamins (second, that is, to analgesics such as acetaminophen and aspirin). Vitamins are themselves usually harmless; however, many contain iron, making them potentially lethal. Failure to recognize that iron ingestion is potentially lethal results in careless storage and carrying vitamins in a purse. A young child often thinks vitamins are candy because of the enteric coating. Children's chewable vitamins are pleasant in taste and must also be stored safely.

It should be recognized that iron poisoning may be an acute catastrophic life-threatening event. Iron has a corrosive effect on gastrointestinal mucosa and can leave deposits in the liver. Symptoms occur in stages. In the first 1 to 4 hours, the child has gastrointestinal distress such as vomiting, diarrhea, bloody stools, and gastric discomfort. Symptoms subside after 4 to 6 hours and the child remains asymptomatic for 12 to 36 hours. Subsequently, the child can redevelop systemic toxicity resulting in metabolic acidosis, fever, shock, hepatic failure, or later, pyloric stenosis.

Diagnosis is made by trying to ascertain how much elemental iron was ingested and by evaluating clinical symptoms especially the gastrointestinal disturbances. Tests usually performed include serum iron, total iron-binding capacity (TIBC), CBC, and blood glucose. Indicators of potentially serious poisoning include leukocytosis greater than 15,000 cells/mm^3 and blood glucose above 150 mg/100 ml. There is a poor correlation between serum iron levels and clinical symptoms, and severity of toxicity is difficult to determine; however, a serum concentration of greater than 500 μg/dl is generally treated aggressively.

Induction of emesis or removal of iron by lavage constitutes initial management. Chelation therapy with deferoxamine is used in severe intoxication. Deferoxamine is used as an antidote as well as an indicator of severity. With severe overdose, the urine will be pink or red following the administration of deferoxamine but will be clear in smaller overdoses.

Corrosives

Caustics found in toilet and drain cleansers cause severe chemical burns, the degree of severity depending on the concentration of the chemical and the length of time of contact. Children may present with varying degrees of burns around the mouth and of the oral mucosa, throat, and esophagus, which is not visualized. The burns may be red, swollen, and oozing or more severe, with sloughing or erosion of tissue.

Alkali substances have the capability of continuing to cause damage after initial contact. Care must be taken to flood all external areas with large quantities of water. Vomiting should *never* be induced in these cases, as the corrosive may cause additional damage as it again passes through the esophagus. Water is given orally to dilute the substance. Although dilution has not been demonstrated to be of benefit, it is not thought to be harmful as long as small enough quantities are given to avoid stimulus to vomit (Moore, 1986). Endoscopy (flexible or rigid) is done as soon as possible to diagnose esophageal burns, especially circumferential burns (involving an entire diameter of the esophagus). Severe burns causing perforation are accompanied by vascular collapse and shock. Subsequent healing of these lesions can produce strictures in the esophagus. These children should be hospitalized and treated with appropriate therapy which may include steroids, antibiotics, and nasogastric tube feedings. Esophageal stricture and possibly esophageal carcinoma are the two significant long-term problems.

Hydrocarbons

Hydrocarbon ingestion accounts for approximately 5 per cent of all reported accidental ingestion, in children under the age of 5 years (Dickerman and Lucey, 1985). Petroleum distillates such as paint thinner, turpentine, lighter fluid, furniture polish, gasoline, kerosene, and machine oil are commonly ingested substances. Ingestion can cause irritation of mucous membranes with vomiting, diarrhea, and CNS depression. *Aspiration* occurring at the time of ingestion may cause a hydrocarbon pneumonia and acute hemorrhagic necrotizing disease, usually within 24 hours. Secondary respiratory failure is a major problem. Symptoms include respiratory distress, fever, and tachycardia.

The odor of a petroleum distillate can be smelled on the child's breath. Emptying the stomach is a controversial issue, since to induce emesis or lavage increases the possibility of aspiration. On the other hand, to leave the hydrocarbon to be absorbed, increases the likelihood of fatal systemic toxicity. Some advocate removal to reduce toxicity when more than 1 mg/kg of poison has been ingested (Anas et al, 1981) while others do not (Klein and Simon, 1986; Erwin, 1983) because of the increased risk of aspiration. In the unconscious child or if mental status is deteriorating, a cuffed endotracheal tube is inserted followed by lavage. In the alert child syrup of ipecac is generally preferred over gastric lavage if evacuation is required (Klein and Simon, 1986).

Steroids have been generally shown to be ineffective in either preventing the development of pneumonitis or treating it once it is present. The majority of children who ingest hydrocarbons appear to recover fully.

Insecticides

Most incidents of exposure to insecticides result in no symptoms or minor effects; however, severe intoxications with a substance such as organophosphate is a pediatric emergency.

Chlorinated hydrocarbons such as DDT or methoxychlor and organic phosphates such as parathion or malathion act in different ways to produce pathology. Chlorinated hydrocarbons block nerve function, causing increased salivation, vomiting, abdominal pain, tremors, CNS depression, and seizures. Organic phosphates are cholinesterase inhibitors whose ingestion results in mild symptomatology such as headache, dizziness, weakness, and tremor to severe symptomatology including gastrointestinal hyperactivity, respiratory distress, pulmonary edema, miosis, sweating, seizures, coma, neuromuscular paralysis, and in some cases, death.

Treatment is supportive. The effects of organic phosphates are cumulative. Atropine and pralidoxime (2-PAM or Protopam) are specific antidotes for cholinesterase inhibitors. Atropine antagonizes the central and muscarinic cholinergic signs but does *not* reverse muscle weakness; thus, pralidoxime is used for children with respiratory impairment in combination with atropine. If the child's respiratory status deteriorates, intubation and assisted ventilation are required. Airway obstruction may occur even if respirations appear adequate because protective airway reflexes may be lost or because bronchial secretions or malpositioning of the head may obstruct the airway (Mortenson, 1986).

Lead Poisoning

Lead poisoning occurs when abnormal amounts of lead are absorbed in the body. In the late 1960s and early 1970s, 25 to 40 per cent of children in inner city, low-economy housing areas had elevated blood lead levels because of exposure to lead in house paint. It was not until the late 1970s that the addition of lead in paints for houses was banned. Although this ruling has caused a dramatic reduction in the percentage of children that have elevated blood lead levels, the problem of lead poisoning still exists.

Children are exposed to lead through other means such as lead-containing gasoline, lead-contaminated clothing of leadsmelter workers, artists' paint, improperly glazed pottery, and paint chips and putty from old houses painted with lead-containing paint. Children at highest risk are those of lower socioeconomic status who live in older dwellings and who are 1 to 6 years of age, with a peak incidence occurring in spring and summer months. Older children may become lead-poisoned through the practice of gasoline sniffing.

Lead can be absorbed through the skin, lungs, and gastrointestinal tract. Food, air, and water all contain some lead. Pica (an appetite for unusual nonfood substances) is a frequent precipitating factor in lead poisoning, with children ingesting paint chips or putty containing lead.

Pathophysiology and Clinical Manifestations

The amount of lead ingested, the size of the particle, and repeated ingestion over time are factors that contribute to the severity of lead poisoning. Lead accumulates in the body on continued exposure and is excreted much slower than it is absorbed. It has been shown in animal studies that diets high in fat and low in calcium, magnesium, iron, zinc, and copper increase the absorption of lead (Chisolm, 1987). The diets of children in low-income families are often low in calcium and iron, which may be a factor in their susceptibility to lead poisoning.

The major route of absorption of lead in children is the gastrointestinal tract. Lead is deposited in the blood, bone, and soft tissue, but it has an affinity for osseous tissue where it accumulates more than in other tissues. The major toxic effects occur in the bone marrow, the nervous system, and the kidney. Anemia results from the metabolic effect of lead on the formation of red blood cells. Lead affects heme synthesis by blocking the incorporation of iron into the protoporphyrin compound that makes up the heme portion of hemoglobin. This results in an accumulation of "free" erythrocyte protophorphyrins (FEP), which can be measured to provide an indicator of lead exposure.

The most serious complications of lead poisoning are those affecting the central nervous system. There is a wide variation in the effect of lead on the CNS. Acute encephalopathy generally occurs as a result of lead blood levels higher than 80 mg/dl and is manifested by reduced consciousness, seizures, and eventually coma and death (Hughes, 1984). Children who do not exhibit overt lead poisoning manifest more subtle effects. Behavior and learning characteristics such as hyperactivity, cognitive and perceptual-motor difficulties, fine-motor deficits, and attentional difficulties have been reported (Drummond, 1981). In the kidney, lead damages the cells of the proximal tubules with excess excretion of amino acids, glucose, and phosphates in the urine. Early in the course of the disease the damage is reversible with treatment, but with continued lead exposure kidney fibrosis can occur.

Lead intoxication can be acute or chronic. Acute toxicity results in gastrointestinal irritation, renal pathology, and encephalopathy. Symptoms have an abrupt onset and include nausea, abdominal pain, vomiting, diarrhea, black stools, oliguria, seizures, and coma.

Chronic toxicity results in degeneration of nerve and muscle cells, renal pathology, cerebral edema, and bone marrow dysfunction. Symptoms appear insidiously, progressing from hyperirritability, anorexia, lethargy, intermittent gastrointestinal distress, constipation, and weakness to increased nervousness, ataxia, continual vomiting, impaired consciousness, and encephalopathy with seizures and coma.

Diagnostic Assessment

Making a diagnosis on the basis of history and presenting symptoms is difficult, as symptoms appear slowly and are similar to many other conditions. A history of pica is extremely relevant. Pica may be a manifestation of iron-deficiency anemia and other factors such as a low-calcium diet or a glucose-6-phosphate dehydrogenase (G6PD) deficiency. History taking and observations by the nurse will help uncover these deficiencies. Possible recent exposure to lead or lead fumes or recent change of residence should be considered. The possibility that the child has played unsupervised near contaminated sources is also explored.

The most useful tests to identify the risk of lead poisoning are blood lead level and FEP. Blood level of lead alone is not a definitive test, because a considerable amount of lead may be in other body tissues. The FEP test measures the amount of protoporphyrin in red blood cells and provides information about the metabolic effects of lead in the body. Lead poisoning is defined by the Centers for Disease Control to exist when a child has *one* of the following (Needleman, 1984):

1. Two successive venous blood lead levels equal to or greater than 70 μg/dl
2. A venous blood lead level greater than 50 μg/dl and an FEP greater than 250 μg/dl
3. An elevated FEP (109 μg/dl) with an elevated blood lead level (30 μg/dl) and symptoms of headache, lethargy, abdominal pain, and intellectual, behavioral, or motor impairment

Supporting findings are "lead flecks" on abdominal roentgenographs or "lead lines" on long bone roentgenographs.

Therapeutic Management

The goal of treatment is to reduce the amount of lead in the blood tissues. The first line of treatment is to identify and remove the environmental source of lead. Second, the accumulated lead in the body must be reduced. Removal of lead from blood and tissues is accomplished through urinary excretion of lead and deposition of lead into the bones. Children with symptomatic poisoning are usually admitted to the hospital and intravenous fluids are given to maintain urine flow. These children are at risk for cerebral edema; therefore, after urinary flow is established fluids are restricted.

Once urinary flow is well established, chelation therapy is started. Chelation therapy is a treatment that facilitates the formation of a fairly stable, highly soluble compound with lead followed by its excretion through the kidney. Therapy is begun with a drug called British anti-lewisite (BAL) (dimercaprol) and calcium disodium edetate (CaEDTA) by intravenous drip or deep intramuscular injection. A combination of therapy is used because it results in reduced saturation of the drug in the blood, fewer side effects of each drug, and better removal from the brain. The use of CaEDTA reduces lead levels overall, but BAL is more effective in the nervous system.

If a child does not have encephalopathy, then BAL therapy may be discontinued after 48 hours. After 4 to 5 days of CaEDTA therapy, its toxicity increases and the output of lead decreases. Therefore, such therapy is discontinued for 48 to 72 hours, after which chelation is repeated with only CaEDTA for another 5 day course. A chelation course can be reinstituted to reduce the lead level to an excretion ratio of less than 1 (1 μg of lead to 1 mg EDTA. It is desirable to wait 5 to 7 days before beginning a third course of chelation (Piomelli et al, 1984). BAL should not be used for patients with a G6PD deficiency nor in conjunction with iron therapy (Piomelli et al, 1984). Fluid and electrolyte maintenance is important, as is continued monitoring of the child and serial blood studies. The toxic child must be observed for signs of increased intracranial pressure (changing level of consciousness, increased blood pressure, and slow pulse).

Oral D-penicillamine is an effective drug if exposure to lead during its course of administration is definitely curtailed. It is currently classed as an investigational drug for use in lead poisoning (Chisolm, 1987).

Major Nursing Diagnoses for Lead Poisoning

Potential for injury: poisoning, related to exposure to an environment containing lead

Altered comfort: pain, related to painful stimuli associated with injection of BAL and CaEDTA

Altered patterns of urinary elimination, related to renal injury associated with side effects of CaEDTA

Altered tissue perfusion: cerebral, related to:

- *lead toxicity*
- *toxicity of chelating drugs*

Altered family processes, related to situational crises associated with acute and potentially chronic care of a child with lead poisoning

Strategies for Nursing Care

Prevent Continuing Exposure to Lead. The first goal of care is prevention. Control of the environmental sources of lead is a multidisciplinary goal. Nurses can counsel parents to guard against exposure to lead-containing paint chips on old houses as well as alerting them to sources such as snow and ice exposed to automobile exhaust fumes and lead-containing cooking utensils. Early detection of lead poisoning is attempted through a careful history, clinical observation, and screening tests.

Reducing Discomfort Associated With Therapy. Nursing strategies during a course of treatment are focused on the immediate care of the child and long-term concerns of the family. When multiple injections are required the child begins to fear and strongly resist them. Preparation for these injections can bring some comfort to the child, but because of their frequency and painfulness a wide range of approaches is required to reduce the trauma for the child. BAL is available only in oil for intramuscular injection, but CaEDTA is available for intravenous infusion. Intramuscular injection of CaEDTA is extremely painful and it is recommended that it be given with procaine (0.5 per cent) by deep injection (Piomelli et al, 1984). It is drawn up last in the syringe; the syringe is held vertically with the needle pointing down so that the procaine is administered first. Local application of warm soaks to the injected areas should also be offered.

Maintaining Fluid Balance and Renal Flow. Chelation should not be performed in the absence of adequate urine flow. Therefore, urinary output is closely monitored. CaEDTA is a nonmetabolizable drug that is excreted by the kidney (Chisolm, 1987). Impending renal failure and drug toxicity is noted by the appearance of protein in the urine, rising BUN, and serum creatinine. Intake and output is measured and the intravenous infusion is carefully monitored. Urinary output is essential for chelation to take place yet fluid intake is restricted to basal requirements to avoid cerebral edema.

Monitoring for Signs of Encephalopathy. The nurse should observe for signs of encephalopathy associated with toxicity of chelating agents. The side effects of the drugs should be carefully monitored, as some of them are also features of acute lead encephalopathy. Seizure precautions should be taken, and appropriate equipment should be available in the event of respiratory arrest.

Maintaining Family Stability. During acute illness the child's and parents' fear and needs are similar to those in any poisoning. In addition, when parents are told of the possible long-term effects of lead poisoning, they need additional emotional support. Fear for their other children is a concern that needs to be discussed with parents. Helping parents understand how they can help prevent further harm is far more constructive than dwelling on what has already taken place. Other stressors that could hinder the child's or family's adaptation should be identified and managed.

Prognosis

Sequelae associated with lead poisoning are related to the degree and duration of exposure. Manifestations of residual damage in severe encephalopathy may include blindness and hemiparesis. In less severe cases seizure disorders, altered behavior, and a degree of intellectual deficits may occur. These children may not show any residual effects until school-age, when they are noted to be more distractible and have some attentional deficits.

Near-Drowning

Drowning is defined as death from asphyxia while submerged in fresh or salt water, with death occurring within 24 hours. If survival surpasses this crucial period, then the event is referred to as "near-drowning." A child may drown with or without aspiration of fluid into the lungs (death may occur from laryngospasm due to a small amount of water entering the trachea).

Approximately 3200 children under age 4 die annually as a result of drowning (Thompson, 1985). The number of near-drownings is probably much higher. Childhood drownings occur most frequently in swimming pools, although children may drown in bathtubs, hot tubs and whirlpools, roadside ditches, and at the beach. Very young children (about 2 years of age) and adolescents are two age groups that seem to be at greater risk for drowning incidents. In young children this is due to momentary lack of adult supervision. Anyone familiar with toddlers will appreciate the rapidity with which they gravitate to forbidden activity —especially if they perceive that adult attention is momentarily diverted. The potential risk for young adolescents may well be related to drug and/or alcohol consumption leading to impaired judgment. Drowning may also be the result of child abuse or suicide.

Pathophysiology

Factors that influence the prognosis of the near-drowning victim are duration of submersion, temperature of the water, presence and type of pulmonary aspiration, and the age of the child (young children can withstand longer periods of submersion).

Very young children will display the mammalian diving reflex, which results in bradycardia and shunting of blood away from the periphery to the brain and heart (Figure 52-1). Although this unique reflex may be elicited in adult victims, it is more pronounced in very young children and probably contributes significantly to the often miraculous recovery of a child. In order for the reflex to be optimally activated, the water must be colder than 70°F (21°C). Also, facial immersion must occur quite rapidly in order to trigger the vagal stimulation that is essential to the reflex trigger.

When a child is submerged in water, there is a struggle to escape followed by laryngospasm, gasping,

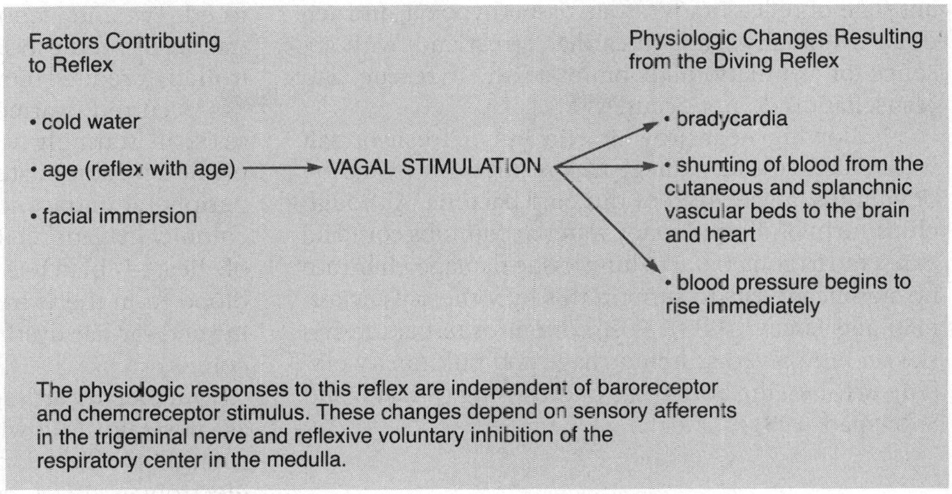

Factors Contributing to Reflex
• cold water
• age (reflex with age)
• facial immersion
VAGAL STIMULATION
Physiologic Changes Resulting from the Diving Reflex
• bradycardia
• shunting of blood from the cutaneous and splanchnic vascular beds to the brain and heart
• blood pressure begins to rise immediately
The physiologic responses to this reflex are independent of baroreceptor and chemoreceptor stimulus. These changes depend on sensory afferents in the trigeminal nerve and reflexive voluntary inhibition of the respiratory center in the medulla.

***Figure* 52-1.** The diving reflex. This reflex operates only in young children. (Based upon Dickerman JD, Lucey JF: *The Critically Ill Child.* 3rd ed. Philadelphia, WB Saunders, 1985.)

and swallowing of water, and often vomiting. When a child reaches the point when a breath must be taken, the following conditions have already developed: arterial hypoxemia, tachycardia, tissue hypoxia, and acidosis (Dickerman and Lucey, 1985). Gasping and the swallowing of water is followed by respiratory arrest and unconsciousness. Loss of consciousness occurs within 3 minutes of submersion. The duration of hypoxia required to cause death is unknown. In water that is very cold (0 to 15°C [32 to 60°F]) children have been known to survive and have normal neurologic function following submersion up to 40 minutes, although full recovery is rare after 20 minutes of submersion (Conn, 1987).

Role of Hypothermia

Children who have been victims of near-drowning and who are admitted with core body temperatures of less than 34°C (93.2°F) demand special resuscitative efforts. It is well known that hypothermia can be useful in lowering the metabolic rate and therefore in reducing oxygen demands by the brain and the core organs.

Unconsciousness occurs when the core body temperature drops below 34°C (93.2°F). Ventricular fibrillation may occur at 28°C (82.4°F) and asystole at 22°C (71.6°F). No cardiovascular activity can be restored as long as the core temperature remains low. Resuscitative efforts must therefore include maintenance of vital functions until rewarming has occurred to a degree at which spontaneous cardiac activity occurs—usually at 29° to 30°C (84.2 to 86°F). This can prolong the resuscitative effort by hours. Initial efforts instituted in the emergency room may be continued in the intensive care unit.

The pathophysiology of drowning in fresh water versus salt water (Table 52-6) is not of such major clinical significance as was once thought. In both types of submersion, arterial hypoxemia develops. The result-

***Table* 52-6.** Comparison of Fresh Water, Salt Water, and Dry Drowning Events

Fresh Water	Salt Water	Dry Drowning
Fresh water is hypotonic compared to blood. Hypotonic fluid is drawn by osmosis into pulmonary vascular beds, causing: 1. Hypervolemia resulting in: • Tachycardia • Elevated BP 2. Hemodilution resulting in: • Decreased hemoglobin and hematocrit; therefore, decreased tissue oxygenation 3. Hemolysis of RBCs and platelets resulting in: • Damaged pulmonary vascular beds causing pulmonary edema • Release of K^+ from RBCs leading to cardiac dysrythmias 4. Surfactant is washed from lungs causing: • Atelectasis and possible pneumothorax	Salt water is 3–4 times more hypertonic than blood. Fluid is pulled from vascular beds by osmosis leading to: 1. Hypovolemia resulting in: • Tachycardia • Decreased BP 2. Hemoconcentration resulting in: • Increased blood viscosity and "sludging" of RBCs in capillary beds leading to decreased availability of oxygen to tissues 3. Pulmonary edema formation resulting in: • Protein-rich substances and fluid being pulled from pulmonary beds into cellular compartments • Decreased ability to breath • Decreased gas exchange • Increased hypoxia	Fatal cerebral hypoxia because of inadequate ventilation which is secondary to laryngospasm or blockage (or both) by mucus or froth (Dickerman, 1985). The drowning event occurs as follows: 1. Small amounts of water enters the larynx or trachea causing instantaneous laryngospasm 2. Thick mucus is produced 3. Foam and froth develop 4. Sometimes (2) & (3) combine to form a mucus plug that further inhibits respiration 5. Death occurs due to brain anoxia

ant state of reflex bradycardia, tissue hypoxia, and acidosis eventually leads to cardiac arrest and, with absence of ventilation, to brain death, if rescue and resuscitation do not occur.

Following near-drowning in either fresh or salt water, further lung damage may result from aspiration of vomitus, algae, sand or dirt, and bacteria. Although chlorine in pools and soapy water in bathtubs could be expected to contribute to lung tissue damage, there are no significant data to support this hypothesis (Dickerman and Lucey, 1985). Postmortem examination has shown intra-alveolar hemorrhage and pulmonary embolism following both types of drowning (Stickler and Snowman, 1981).

Diagnostic Assessment and Therapeutic Management

Initiating treatment for a drowning child must begin immediately upon extraction of the child from the water. CPR is begun immediately and the child is transported by ambulance to an emergency facility. There, acquisition of a detailed history is essential and may be the role of the triage nurse, since all other medical energies will be directed toward resuscitation. Important information includes the child's age and general health, length of submersion (parents will often not be able to give an accurate estimate of time), and any contributing factors such as alcohol and/or drug consumption or history of diabetes or epilepsy.

The primary assessment focuses on the ABCs until they are stable. When assessing for airway and breathing, the rate and pattern of the respiration is noted and recorded. A patent airway is essential. The airway is examined for vomitus, mucus, or aspirated material and suctioned as needed. If there is any reason to suspect cervical spine injury, the airway must be protected with immobilization of the neck and use of the chin-lift technique.

If complete cardiopulmonary arrest has occurred, oxygenation becomes the priority. Before intubating the child, the physician will want to ensure as clean an airway as possible. This is accomplished by suctioning, insertion of an oropharyngeal airway, and ventilation using a bag-valve-mask. The child should be well oxygenated before intubation is attempted. Experienced respiratory technologists, nurses, or physicians may "bag" the child if they are knowledgeable and skilled in the use of the equipment. Once the airway is clean and the child well oxygenated, intubation is performed.

Continuous monitoring, diagnostic studies, laboratory evaluations, and fluid management occur simultaneously. A portable chest roentgenograph is taken, arterial blood gases measured, and vital signs monitored. Two intravenous lines are inserted for administration of medications. Fluid volume is strictly controlled to reduce intracranial pressure. If hypothermia has occurred, warmed fluids can be administered to assist in warming vital organs. This may be accomplished by administering warm intravenous fluids via peripheral intravenous lines, peritoneal lavage, or colonic irrigation. Rapid rewarming by application of heated blankets is contraindicated since cold blood from the extremities may cause rebound cooling and cardiac dysrhythmia as it circulates to the body core.

An electrocardiogram should be obtained as soon as possible following admission. Blood samples should be ordered for baseline values of CBC, serum electrolytes, BUN, creatinine, and glucose levels, as well as arterial blood gases. A urinary catheter is inserted to monitor renal function. A nasogastric tube is inserted to remove swallowed water and debris and to prevent gastric distension due to assisted ventilation.

Medications that are used include oxygen, sodium bicarbonate to counteract acidosis, antibiotics to prevent pulmonary infection, and aminophylline to increase gas exchange by bronchodilation. Short- and long-acting barbiturates or lidocaine may be used to lower intracranial pressure if the need arises (Dickerman and Lucey, 1985).

Major Nursing Diagnoses for Near-Drowning

Ineffective airway clearance*, related to aspiration of water and debris*
Ineffective breathing pattern*, related to cerebral hypoxia from near-drowning episode*
Impaired gas exchange*, related to aspiration of water, debris, and laryngospasm*
Altered tissue perfusion*, related to cerebral, cardiopulmonary, and renal involvement*
Anxiety: parents*, related to uncertainty of outcome*
Potential for injury*, related to knowledge deficit concerning child safety practices to prevent future incidents of water-related injury*
Altered growth and development: self care skills*, related to residual neurologic effects*

Strategies for Nursing Care

Maintaining a Patent Airway. The nurse should assist in achieving and/or maintaining a patent airway by using the chin-lift maneuver, suctioning the trachea, and inserting an oropharyngeal airway if appropriate. In anticipation of the need to intubate, the nurse prepares a pediatric laryngoscope with an appropriately sized blade, a functioning light, and correct tube size.

Once the child is intubated, the nurse is responsible for assessing and maintaining the patency of the tube.

Maintaining an Effective Breathing Pattern. Monitor respirations every 5 minutes for rate and pattern until respirations are stable. If the child is unable to maintain an effective breathing pattern, then mechanical ventilation must be instituted.

Monitoring and Facilitating Gas Exchange. Each time vital signs are taken, the chest is auscultated and findings should be documented. Since near-drowning victims are at risk for developing pulmonary edema, any alterations in breath sounds are reported to the physician. The child is placed in a semi-Fowler's position if possible to maximize diaphragmatic excursion and increase alveolar aeration. Chest physiotherapy is performed by the nurse or physical therapist. The administration of oxygen, at 100 per cent with humidification, is monitored and analyzed by the nurse. Arterial blood gases are reviewed to evaluate the effectiveness of interventions.

Maintaining Tissue Perfusion (Cerebral, Cardiovascular, Renal). The nurse monitors the infusion rate and maintains the intravenous therapy regimen to establish perfusion. If hypothermia is used therapeutically for cerebral edema, the patient's temperature is closely monitored.

Serial monitoring of respirations, heart rate, blood pressure, urinary output, and assessment of intracranial pressure and level of unconsciousness is done every 5 to 15 minutes until stable, at which time monitoring may be reduced to every hour or less often. A urinary catheter is usually inserted to monitor hourly output. All assessments must be accurately documented.

Relieving Parental Anxiety Related to Uncertainty of Outcome. The nurse needs to be supportive of the child's family during this time of crisis and severe stress. They should be encouraged to ask questions and be given accurate, up-to-date information. They should be allowed to see and touch their child as soon as possible, even though this may be emotionally upsetting because of invasive machinery. The nurse prepares them beforehand for the array of equipment and tubes attached to their child. Once the child is transferred to the intensive care unit or to a ward, the parents should be encouraged to participate in their child's daily care if they so desire. Keeping parents informed about the child's condition is an important part of the nurse's supportive role.

Many children survive seemingly insurmountable insults as a result of near-drowning, with remarkable resilience. Often there are no neurologic deficits or they are minimal and seem to resolve with time. Other children suffer deficits ranging from minimal physical disability to profound physical and intellectual impairment. A period of hospitalization on a pediatric ward may be necessary to assess the deficits and institute long-term rehabilitation.

Preventing Water-Related Injury in the Future. Discussions about prevention are inappropriate during the critical phase of care. As the family works through the emotional trauma of this crisis they will often plan ways to avoid future occurrences. Remain alert for "if only" statements. Reinforce appropriate plans for precautions in the future while helping the parents absolve themselves of any unnecessary guilt associated with the present event. In the absence of evidence of plans to rectify a dangerous situation, refer the family for follow-up visits in the home.

Fostering Development of Self-Care Skills and Optimal Communication. If a child suffers neurologic sequelae, a carefully planned rehabilitation program is instituted. During this phase, the nurse assesses the child's progress in gaining optimal self-care skills and plans with the family and professional team to acquire the necessary rehabilitative services. A smooth transition from acute care to rehabilitative services to home is achieved by cooperative planning among the involved disciplines such as occupational therapy, physical therapy, speech therapy, nutritionists, social workers, and a public health nurse. A public health liaison nurse can facilitate the transition by early involvement in care during the acute phase. Within the hospital setting acquisition of special equipment such as a special wheelchair, eating utensils, and simple clothing facilitate optimal achievement of growth and development.

Nursing Strategies for Follow-up Care in the Home or Clinic

Assess vital signs and breath sounds for evidence of residual pulmonary complications.

Assess family's ability to provide specialized care, if any is required.

Assess appropriateness of medical supplies for self-care (if any needed).

Arrange for additional services needed to facilitate child's maximum independence level.

Assess family's knowledge of maintaining child safety around water.

Reinforce the importance of vigilant supervision around bathtubs, beaches, and pools.

Encourage organized swimming lessons as appropriate.

Assess child-parent-sibling interactions for signs of stress associated with near-drowning experience.

Give affirmation to parents for quality of care they are providing for their child.

If the incident results in the death of a child, follow-up visits focus on care of the bereaved family (see Chapter 26 for discussion of care of a family when a child dies).

Child With Multiple Trauma

Multiple trauma involves injury to more than one body system. Multiple trauma most commonly occurs in motor vehicle accidents (MVA), vehicle-pedestrian accidents, child abuse, and falls. Most of the injuries are *blunt* as opposed to *penetrating;* blunt trauma may cause only minimal external evidence of the location and degree of injury. Multiple injuries therefore present a special challenge to the health care team. Since the first 20 minutes of treatment are the most important in terms of stabilization and eventual outcome, the health care professionals who provide this treatment should be highly skilled. Seidel and coworkers (1984) found that most programs for emergency medical technicians and paramedics and for emergency room physicians and nurses are geared to the adult trauma or cardiac victim. Many ambulances do not carry pediatric resuscitation equipment, and general hospitals may have only minimal equipment in limited sizes to care for critically ill children. With these problems in mind, several large teaching centers have established specialized units operated by highly trained personnel to provide optimal care to injured children. The American College of Surgeons recently added an extensive pediatric component to the advanced trauma life support course. The courses offer a clear, simplified approach to trauma management for both adults and children in the first hour following injury. The goal is to provide rapid stabilization of the victim and transfer of the patient as soon as possible to a facility offering specialized care. Nurses who are employed in critical care should be encouraged to take similar courses that have been modified to include nursing interventions so that a coordinated team approach may be developed. Assessment and care of the multiply-injured child is a highly specialized area of study. The reader is referred to emergency and intensive care texts for further information.

The Child with Burns

Claudella Archambeau-Jones
Irving Feller

Few injuries happen as frequently to children or are as traumatic for everyone involved as a severe burn. Few other injuries are as debilitating or require such extended periods of hospitalization and extensive rehabilitation. However, few other catastrophic injuries offer the possibility of full recovery.

Burns and fires are the third leading cause of accidental death in the United States, exceeded only by motor vehicle accidents and falls. For children in the age group 1 to 14 years, burns are the leading cause of accidental death in the home. The highest incidence of burns in children occurs in 1- and 2-year-olds (Fig. 52-2); the incidence is closely related to the amount and adequacy of adult supervision and to the level of emotional stress in the home.

The cause of burns in children varies with age (Table 52-7). For example, 65 per cent of burns to children age 4 and under are scalds, occurring in the home; 62 per cent of burns to children aged 5 and over are by flame. Any child who receives a significant burn must face, after recovery, a long series of rehospitalizations (to adulthood) for reconstruction procedures, both functional and cosmetic. Burned skin that has healed or been grafted does not grow at the same rate as underlying tissue and bone (Feller and Crane, 1970).

Care of the child with burns requires (1) sufficient knowledge and experience to identify the severity of the injury, including the special care required by a child; (2) an understanding of the principles of burn care; and (3) a close monitoring of all aspects of care. The nurse must also give special consideration to the child's place in a family and the family's role in the child's survival and quality of life thereafter.

In thinking of the care required to treat burns, we must first consider the primary body organ system in-

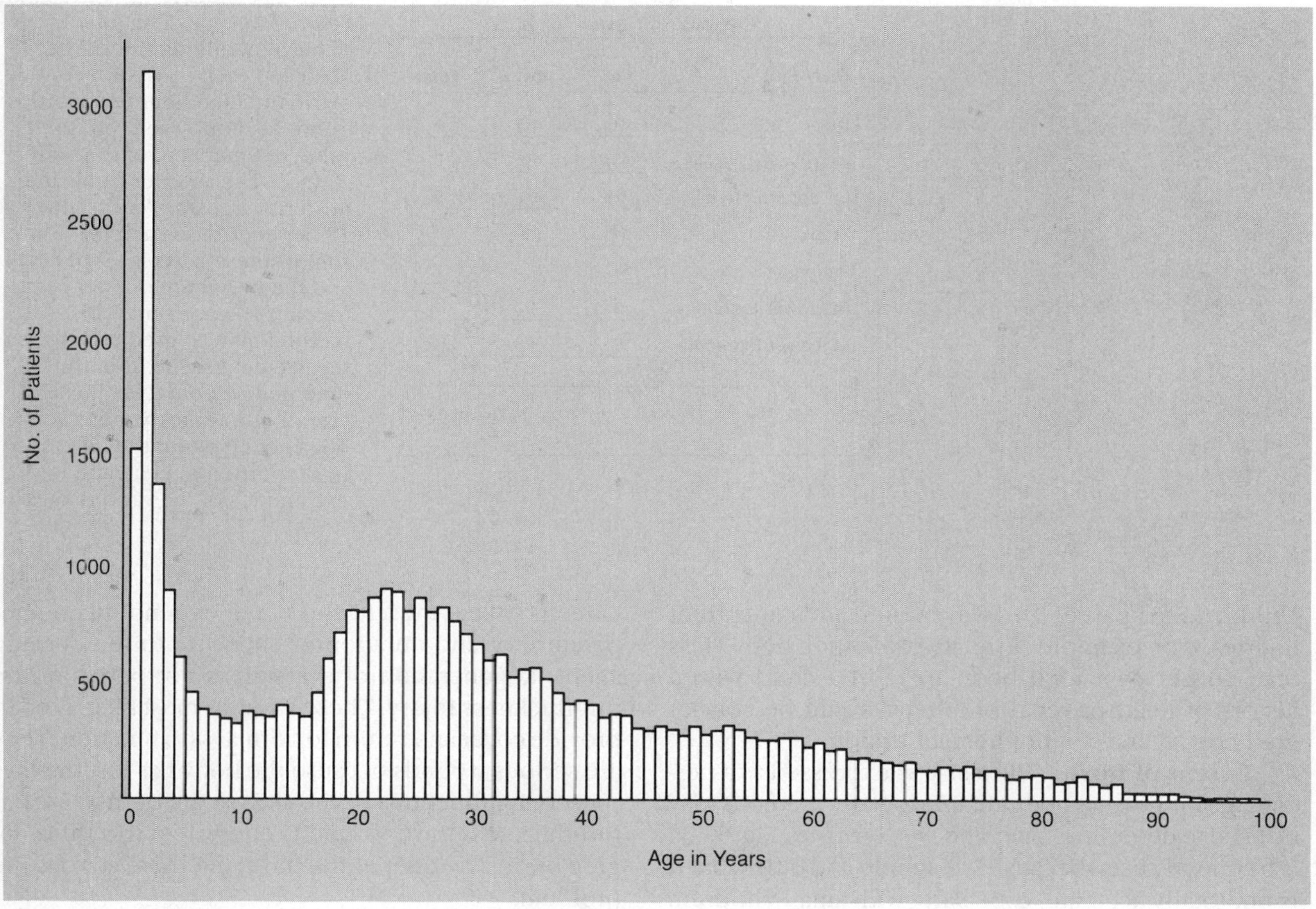

Figure 52-2. Age distribution of victims of severe burns. Thirty per cent of all burns severe enough to require hospitalization in a specialized burn facility occur in children under 16 years of age. N = 38,674. (Data from the NBIE, I. Feller, Director, 1978–1985.)

volved, which is the skin. The skin is the body's largest organ, providing an intact anatomic barrier against infection and loss of body fluids. The skin also helps control body temperature. A vast capillary network is located in the skin, as are nerve endings, hair follicles, and sweat and sebaceous glands. Body image is also related to an intact skin covering.

Table 52-7. Distribution of Burn Accidents by Age Vs Burning Agent (1978–1985)*

	Age	
Burning Agent	0–4 yr	5–15 yr
Flame	14%	62%
Hot liquid	65%	25%
Hot solid	15%	5%
Electrical	2%	3%
Chemical	1%	1%
Radiation	—	—
Other	3%	4%

* Number of subjects studied: 38,674.

(From National Burn Information Exchange, Ann Arbor, MI, I. Feller, MD, Director.)

The skin's functions are either diminished when the skin and its support systems are damaged (when there is a partial-thickness injury) or destroyed (when there is a full-thickness injury). *The trauma of the burn results in a decrease or complete loss of two of the most important functions of the skin: protection against infection and prevention of loss of body fluids.* The nurse's role is to help protect the child until these functions of the skin can be regained. However, once the child has recovered physical function of the skin, the loss of normal appearance, the pleasure-pain sensations, and the change in body appearance can complicate rehabilitation.

Assessing the Severity of the Burn

All burns are not alike. Severity is influenced by five interrelated factors: (1) extent of burn, (2) depth of burn, (3) age of the child, (4) medical history of the

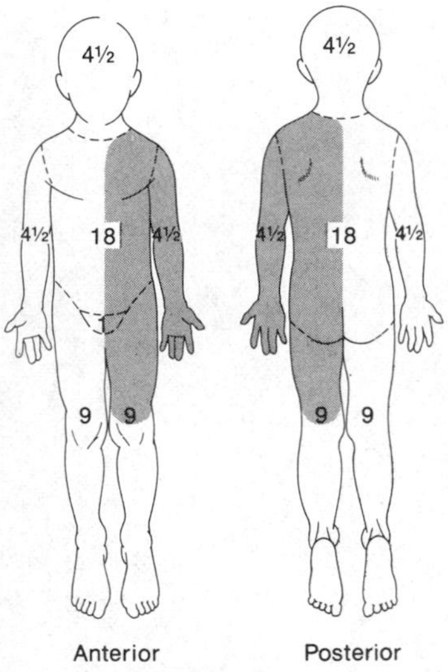

Calculation of Extent of Burn

Body Part	Ant.	Post.	Total
Head	4½	4½	9
Rt. Upper Extremity	4½	4½	9
Lt. Upper Extremity	4½	4½	9
Trunk	18	18	36
Perineum	1		1
Rt. Lower Extremity	9	9	18
Lt. Lower Extremity	9	9	18
			Total 100%

***Figure* 52-3.** Estimation of size of burn by rule of nines. The head and each entire upper extremity (shoulder to fingertips [glove fashion]) are given the value of 9 per cent of the body surface. The anterior trunk and posterior trunk are each valued at 18 per cent, as is each leg. The sum of these parts is 99 per cent and the perineum is 1 per cent, totaling 100 per cent. This method may be used visually at the accident scene or in the emergency room to estimate the size of burn quickly; however, it does not allow for the difference in proportion of head and lower extremities of the various ages.

child, and (5) part of the body injured and concurrent injuries. For example, a relatively minor burn (less than 10 per cent total body area) in a child with a history of heart or renal problems would be considered critical and require hospitalization.

Extent of Burn. Burn size is expressed as a percentage of the total body area. Two basic methods may be used to determine size. The *rule of nines* (Fig. 52-3) is frequently used because it is simple and quick, but it is not totally accurate, especially with small children.

The second method requires use of explanatory figures and tables and is more accurate because it takes into account the change in proportion of the head and lower extremities with age. For example, for an infant the head equals 19 per cent of total body area; in an adult it equals 7 per cent. This method is referred to as the *estimation of size of burn by per cent* (Fig. 52-4). Either way, the palm of the hand of each individual equals 1 per cent of his or her body.

The nurse assessing the extent of the burn must refer to the diagram and to the burn wound to map out the injury accurately. Underestimation may result in inadequate treatment. Overestimation can result in overzealous therapy, especially in a child, in a person with cardiac problems or respiratory injury, or in an older person.

Depth of Burn. The depth of a burn is expressed in terms of full thickness or partial thickness. The term *partial-thickness burn* means that only part of the skin has been damaged or destroyed. Enough epithelial cells remain in hair follicles to grow new skin and sweat glands are left. This type of wound heals by itself if nothing in treatment causes further damage. The partial-thickness burn is equivalent to the first-degree (superficial epidermal injury) burn.

Full-thickness burns are defined as those in which all layers of the skin are destroyed and possibly subcutaneous tissue, muscle and bone, depending on temperature of and duration of exposure to the burning agent. Regeneration of the skin is not possible in a full-thickness injury. These wounds must be grafted to provide cover and return to normal skin function. They are serious wounds because the body has lost the life-preserving functions of the skin in the burned area. A full-thickness burn wound is equivalent to a third-degree burn. The deeper the burn, the more serious the problem.

The skin of the small child is slightly thinner than that of the adult; therefore, a similar insult may result in a more severe injury to the child. The basic principles of evaluation of depth, however, remain the same. Depth of burn is difficult to determine visually. There are signs and symptoms that indicate the level of tissue damaged, but the exact depth of injury can be determined only when spontaneous healing has taken place or granulation tissue has appeared after eschar (dead tissue) removal. Figure 52-5 defines the differences between partial- and full-thickness injuries.

Age of Child. Age is an important factor in determining severity of injury. Children under age 4 have a higher mortality than children of other age groups with similar-size injury (Feller and Crane, 1970). Their smaller body mass represents less "store" of potential fuel for metabolism and healing. Combined with the onslaught of complications, especially infections, this can result in higher mortality; although survival for these age groups has improved dramatically. It should be noted, however, that this improvement has been only in hospitals with specialized burn care and where the treatment plan has an established record of excellence. An average 96 per cent survival rate can be expected for burns of all sizes in children of all ages in the best hospitals. Infants and children up to age 4 respond dramatically to the demands on them during illness,

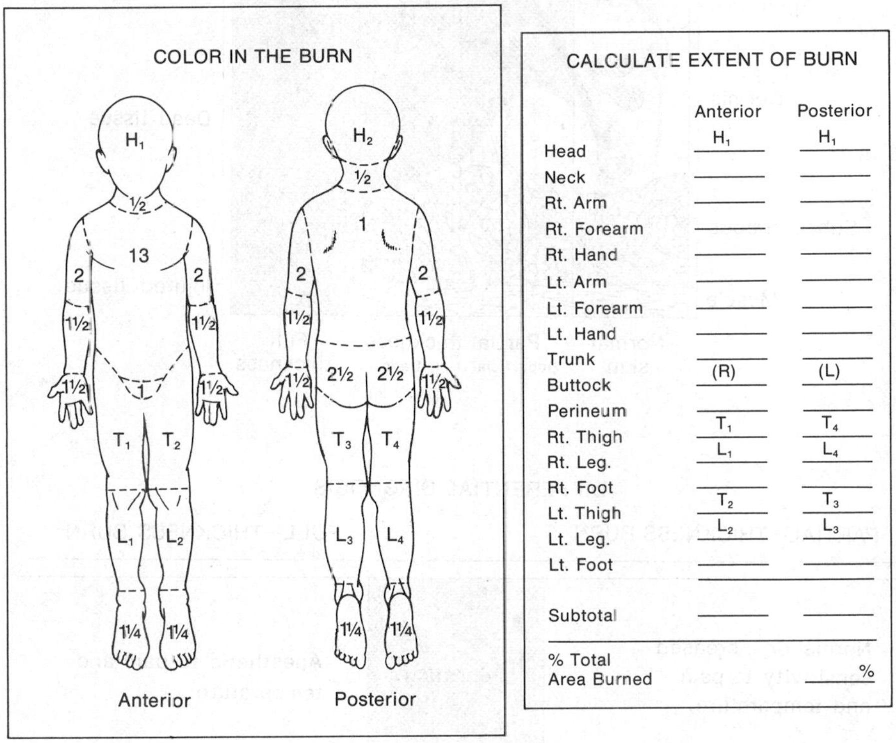

CIRCLE AGE FACTOR

Percentage of Areas Affected by Growth Age	0	1	5	10	15	Adult
H(1 or 2) = ½ of the Head	9½	8½	6½	5½	4½	3½
T(1,2,3, or 4) = ½ of a Thigh	2¾	3¼	4	4¼	4½	4¾
L(1,2,3, or 4) = ½ of a Leg	2½	2½	2¾	3	3¼	3½

Figure 52-4. Estimation of size of burn by per cent. 1. Shade in the diagram to represent the extent of burn, as viewed anteriorly and posteriorly. 2. Circle age closest to that of the patient and use those percentages for the head, thigh, and leg to calculate extent of burn. 3. The percentage of total body surface is printed on the diagram for those areas that do not vary with age. The areas that do vary with age are marked with H (head), T (thigh), and L (leg). The extent of the burn is calculated by adding the percentages of each affected area. If a portion of a body part is burned, an approximate fraction of the percentage should be used. (Redrawn from Feller I, Jones CA: *Emergency Care of the Burn Victim.* National Institute for Burn Medicine, Ann Arbor, MI, 1977.)

and with good care and proper nutrition can do very well. It is important to emphasize that any child with a severe burn should be sent to a specialized burn care facility.

Medical History of Child. The stress of a severe burn will exacerbate any existing disease process, which will in turn increase mortality. In a child, the presence of a major growth-retarding anomaly such as congenital heart disease or failure to thrive complicates the burn. Unknown diseases also may complicate the burn; symptoms of these must be detected and the underlying cause treated simultaneously with the burn.

A dependable history for a child is best taken from the family or from the child's pediatrician. Information to be obtained and prominently recorded includes a history of (1) recent or past illnesses, chronic and severe; (2) dependence on life-sustaining medication; (3) allergies to food or medicine (especially penicillin); (4) symptoms that may indicate latent and undetected diseases; (5) events leading to the injury; and (6) immunization history.

Part of Body Injured and Concurrent Injuries. The part of the body injured is the fifth factor contributing to severity. Burns of the head, neck, and chest lead to increased incidence of pulmonary problems. Burns of the perineum are prone to early infection. These areas are considered critical areas, making the burn affecting them more serious. Circumferential (all the way around) burns of the neck, chest, and extremities contribute to severity. A significant injury sustained in addition to the burn also increases severity (electrical injury, skull fracture, internal injury, or compound fractures). Such injuries must be found and treatment

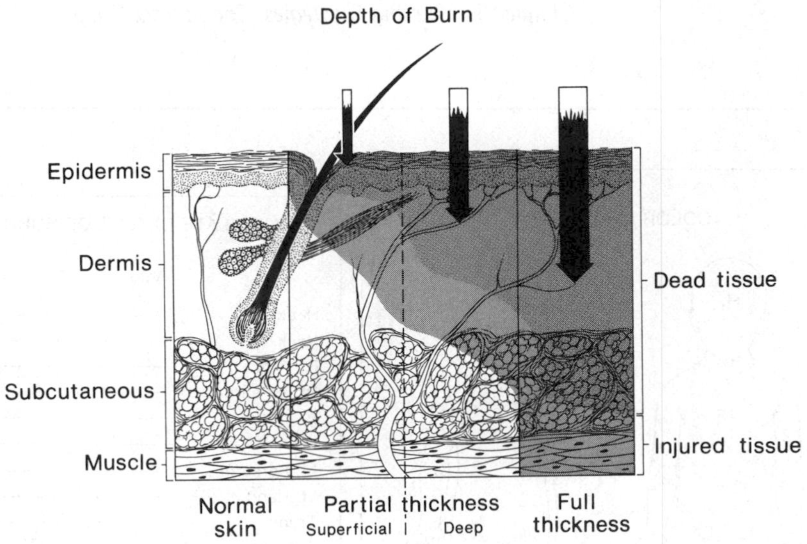

DIFFERENTIAL DIAGNOSIS

PARTIAL–THICKNESS BURN		FULL–THICKNESS BURN
Normal or increased sensitivity to pain and temperature.	Sensation	Anesthetic to pain and temperature.
Large, thick–walled, will usually increase in size.	Blisters	None, or if present, thin–walled and will not increase in size.
Red, will blanch with pressure and refill.	Color	White, brown, black or red. If red, will not blanch with pressure.
Normal or firm.	Texture	Firm or leathery.

***Figure* 52-5.** Differential diagnosis of depth of burn. *Arrows* represent degree of heat or intensity of burning agent and the time of contact with skin. The *darker shaded area* represents dead tissue; the *lighter shaded area,* damaged or injured tissue that will heal with good care. When all tissue (epidermis and dermis) has been destroyed, this is termed full-thickness. Partial-thickness means only part of the skin has been destroyed. Damaged tissue can reheal with good care. (Redrawn from Feller I, Jones CA: *Emergency Care of the Burn Victim.* Ann Arbor, MI, National Institute for Burn Medicine, 1977.)

instituted during first aid procedures. Another factor to note is the ability of the family to care for the child with burns that do not require hospitalization. Without adequate home care, the risk of complications increases.

Diagnosis of Minor and Major Burns

The difference between a minor and a major burn is determined by the aforementioned severity factors in conjunction with general health status and other factors. For example, a 5 per cent full-thickness burn would be serious for an infant or a child with diabetes but may be only minor for a healthy child of the same age, or for an adult. Certain criteria must be met before a minor burn can be treated on an outpatient basis. A child with a major burn must be admitted to specialized care.

Minor Burns. A burn is minor if:

1. The full-thickness and partial-thickness loss is less than 10 per cent total body area

2. The child is at least 4 years old
3. There is no history of chronic or severe illness
4. There are no significant concurrent injuries (e.g., respiratory damage, fractures)
5. The burn does not include the hands, face, feet, or perineum, and/or no circumferential injury exists
6. It is not an electrical injury

Even when a burn is minor, the child is hospitalized if the family cannot cope with home care or there is suspicion of abuse or neglect.

Major Burns. A burn is classified as major if any of the following conditions exist:

1. The wound covers more than 10 per cent total body area
2. The wound is full-thickness
3. The child is less than 4 years old
4. The medical history is positive for chronic or severe illness
5. There are significant concurrent injuries (respiratory damage, fractures, and so forth)
6. There are burns of the face, hands, feet, or perineum, and/or circumferential injury
7. It is an electrical injury

Prognosis in Burns

A major burn requires admission to a hospital providing specialized burn care. This admission must take place as quickly as possible after the burn injury. To ensure proper treatment and a positive outcome, the nurse must be aware of the factors affecting severity and of the hospitals in the area that provide specialized burn care.

The chances for survival of a particular patient can be affected by the size and depth of burn, the child's age, health status and medical history, part of the body injured, and other injuries. Infants and toddlers with 40 per cent total body area burns have a survival rate of 80 per cent, as contrasted with a 13-year-old patient with a similar burn, who has a survival rate of 93 per cent. Figure 52-6 shows survival curves of burned children. These statistics are from hospitals providing specialized burn care. They do not pertain to hospitals that do not offer burn center-level care.

The survival rate is lower when a given area contains all full-thickness burns than when the same area includes both partial-thickness and full-thickness burns. With age and area of burn held constant, the

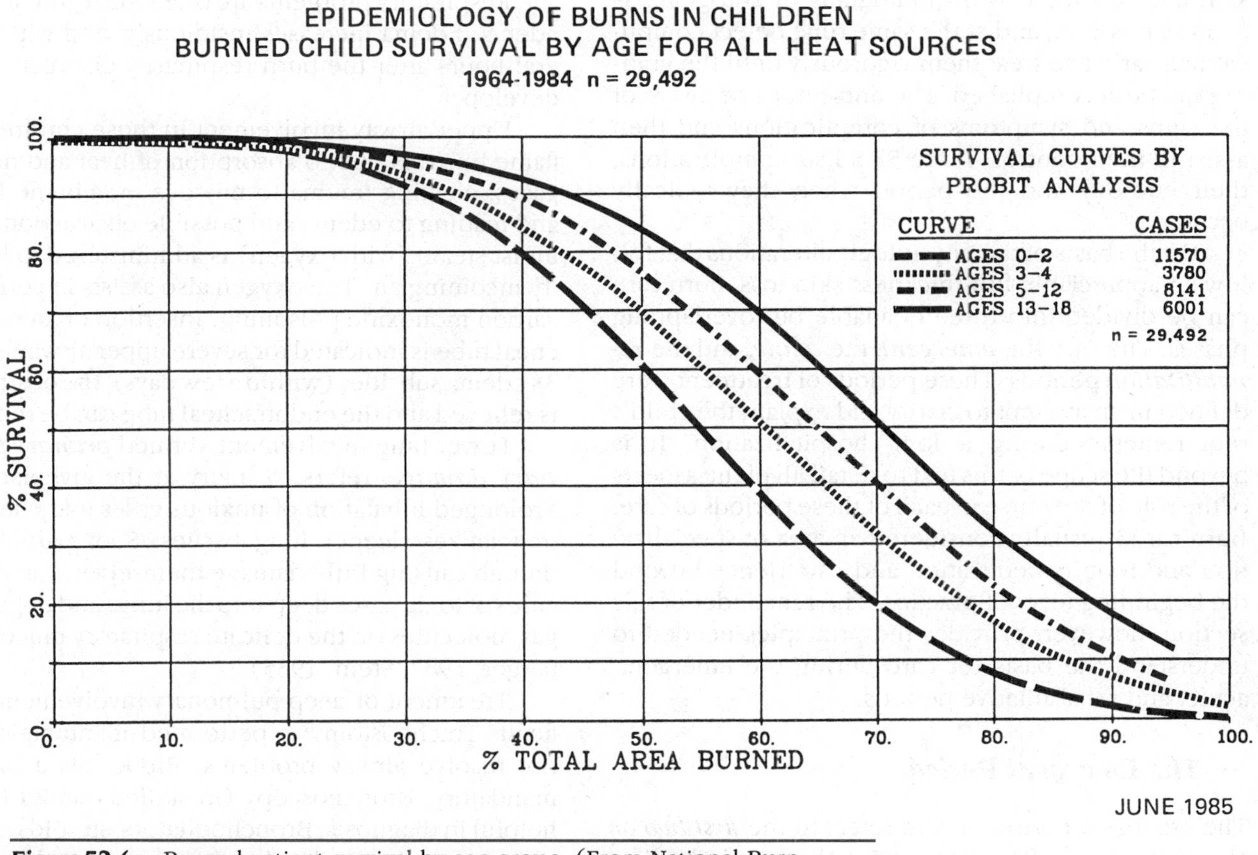

Figure 52-6. Burned patient survival by age group. (From National Burn Information Exchange, I. Feller, MD, Director; Ann Arbor, MI, 1985.)

larger the percentage of body surface area affected by full-thickness burn, the more serious the injury.

Unlike other traumatic injuries, complications are the rule rather than the exception with most severe burns at present, especially in nonspecialized facilities. Typically, a child with a severe burn may have four to six major complications, often at the same time, and one or a combination of several may be fatal. The most common complications seen in burn patients are also the most common causes of death.

Studies conducted by the National Institute for Burn Medicine and the University of Michigan Department of Biostatistics have shown that survival is also related to the hospital in which the patient receives care; survival of children is improved when they are treated in children's hospitals providing specialized burn care (Evaluation of Emergency Medical Services with a National Burn Registry, 1975–1978).

Basic Burn Care: Therapeutic Management and Nursing Strategies

For a full-thickness burn area, only grafting can decrease the negative metabolic processes and reinstitute skin functions. It is necessary to remove the dead skin and replace it with homografts or autografts as soon as possible, and at the same time detect complications early and treat them vigorously until the grafting can be accomplished. The nurse must be aware of the signs and symptoms of complications and then assist in their control. Table 52-8 lists complications, their etiology and the period when they typically occur.

On the basis of the physiologic alterations that follow an appreciable full-thickness skin loss, burn care can be divided into three definable but overlapping phases. They are the *emergent*, the *acute*, and the *rehabilitation* periods. These periods of treatment were defined in an attempt to clarify and explain the child's requirements during a long hospitalization. It is beyond the scope of this text to detail all of the aspects of the role of the nurse in each of these periods of care. Burn care is usually considered an area of specialization and requires education and experience beyond the beginning level of practice. The remainder of this section, however, provides the principles needed to understand the basis for care during the emergent, acute, and rehabilitative periods.

The Emergent Period

The emergent period of care refers to the *first two or three days* immediately following the burn. The life-threatening problems of the burn victim are similar to those of any trauma victim. Therefore, the first principle of care is immediate first aid. Attention should be given to *breathing, bleeding resulting from any concurrent injury*, and *shock*. Once necessary life-saving measures are taken, the treatment should be directed to combating shock through proper fluid therapy and to re-evaluating the respiratory status. Burn wound care is considered only after systemic care is under way.

Respiratory Care. Anticipation of and intervention in respiratory difficulties during the emergent period can reduce the severity of pulmonary complications. Lung involvement may not be apparent immediately post-burn but impending pulmonary problems should be suspected and treated in the case of any or all of the following:

1. The child was burned by flame in an enclosed space and/or forced to breathe products of combustion (explosion, house fire)
2. Blackened oral and nasal mucous membranes or singed nasal hairs or both are present
3. There are burns of the face, neck, or chest, or of all three
4. The child is experiencing obvious respiratory difficulties

Respiratory problems are often the result of airway edema. Edema increases insidiously, and within several hours after the burn respiratory obstruction may develop.

Upper airway involvement in those children with flame burns is due to absorption of heat and noxious gases, creating trauma to mucous membrane linings and leading to edema and possible obstruction. Cold, moist steam (with oxygen) is administered to humidify incoming air. The oxygen also assists in correcting carbon monoxide poisoning. Insertion of an endotracheal tube is indicated for severe upper airway edema. As edema subsides (within a few days), the obstruction is relieved and the endotracheal tube can be removed.

Lower lung involvement, termed *primary pulmonary damage*, refers to injury at the alveolar level. Prolonged inhalation of noxious gases and chemicals traumatizes deeper lung tissues. Soot particles, although causing little damage themselves, carry molecules of toxic gases deep into the lungs and deposit the gas molecules on the delicate respiratory mucosa (Lybarger, 1987; Stein, 1985).

Treatment of deep pulmonary involvement is difficult. Tracheostomy is performed if intubation will not resolve airway problems. Blood gas analysis is mandatory. Bronchoscopy (in skilled hands) may be helpful in diagnosis. Bronchodilators, steroids, and antibiotics may be used in the attempt to open the airways and to reduce the inflammatory process. Pulmonary

Table 52-8. Frequent Complications of Major Burns in Children

Complication	Etiology
Cardiovascular	
Hypovolemia *Occurs:* Emergent phase	Normal inflammatory response to injury. In major burn, fluid shift from vascular to interstitial spaces (3rd spacing) is massive. If untreated it results in hypovolemic shock and death
Hypervolemia *Occurs:* Late emergent phase	Secondary to overzealous fluid therapy or failure to recognize diuretic phase of fluid replacement
Hypertension *Occurs:* May occur during any one or all three phases; but usually seen in late emergent or early acute	Occurs in at least ⅓ of children with severe burns; etiology unclear, but thought to be secondary to stress. May be treated prophylactically in burns of greater tha 40% total body area with drug of physician's choice
Renal	
Oliguria *Occurs:* Emergent or acute phase	Secondary to hypovolemia or hypovolemic shock. Relieved with proper fluid therapy. If fluid therapy delayed or inadequate, leads to anuria and renal failure. May be seen in acute period secondary to septic shock
Hemomyoglobinuria *Occurs:* Emergent phase	Secondary to massive deep full-thickness injury or electrical injury, causing release of myoglobin (muscle protein) and hemoglobin from RBCs. These free globins are then filtered by kidneys and can clog tubules. Sign of this is black urine. Immediate treatment with osmotic diuretic and increased fluids indicated to prevent tubular necrosis or failure
Pulmonary	
Carbon monoxide poisoning *Occurs:* Emergent phase	Byproducts of combustion inhaled by burn victim; treatment with oxygen at the scene relieves symptoms
Upper airway obstruction *Occurs:* Emergent phase	Secondary to absorption of heat and gases by upper airway; results in edema of the airway requiring early intubation. When edema subsides, endotracheal tube can be removed
Primary pulmonary damage *Occurs:* Emergent phase	Secondary to lower airway and lung damage by noxious gases. Requires intubation by endotracheal tube. If unrelieved, then tracheostomy. Further treatment may require antibiotics, aminophylline, cortisone, aerosol antibiotics. Humidified oxygen is indicated for all respiratory involvement
Pulmonary edema *Occurs:* Acute phase	May be secondary to primary pulmonary damage, circumferential chest burn causing decreased chest movement,* overzealous fluid therapy and overload or immobility
Pulmonary embolus *Occurs:* Acute phase	Usually a very late complication. Clot is released when mobility follows enforced immobility. Heparin can be used prophylactically
Bacterial penumonia *Occurs:* Acute phase	Lowered resistance secondary to immobility,* decreased chest movement if circumferential chest burn, inhalation irritation. May be secondary to wound or tracheostomy, sepsis or pooled lung fluids
Sepsis	
Wound infection *Occurs:* Emergent and/or acute phases (If it occurs, infection is often evident by 4 days post trauma)	Infection during emergent phase is usually gram-positive, often staphylococcus, as a result of autocontamination; usually treated prophylactically with penicillin
	Infection during acute phase is frequently from gram-negative organisms, e.g., *Pseudomonas aeruginosa,* secondary to decreased vascular supply to wound, diminished overall immune response and the favorable medium the wound provides—heat, warmth, eschar
	Prevention: A *Pseudomonas aeruginosa* vaccine and a hyperimmune serum have been used successfully since 1963, providing both active and passive coverage, but this remains controversial

continued

Table 52-8 *(continued)*

Complication	Etiology
Sepsis	
Septicemia *Occurs:* Acute phase	Overwhelming systemic infection secondary to unsuccessful treatment of primary wound infection, or due to invading pathogens at indwelling catheter sites (central lines, urinary, etc.) Early detection is essential for proper therapy
Metabolic and Electrolyte Disturbances	
Paralytic ileus (GI) *Occurs:* Emergent phase	Normal response to initial hypovolemic state; usually lasts 2–3 days during which time oral intake is contraindicated. NG tube to intermittent drainage is used to decompress stomach
Weight gain *Occurs:* Emergent phase	Secondary to fluid therapy. Children should gain no more than 10% of normal body weight; above 10% puts child at risk for overload, pulmonary edema, or congestive failure
Weight loss *Occurs:* Acute phase	Secondary to catabolism. Requires high calorie, high protein diet. If greater than 20–30% of total body weight is lost, loss can be fatal
Hypernatremia *Occurs:* Late emergent and acute phases	As fluids return to vascular space at end of emergent period, salt also returns. Fluid therapy is changed to D5W or D10W (salt-poor fluids)
Acid-base imbalance *Occurs:* Late emergent and acute phases	May be secondary to many other complications or result of treatment (e.g., some topical agents)
Adrenal-cortical insufficiency *Occurs:* Emergent and acute phases	Stress response secondary to overwhelming injury; attempt to maintain body equilibrium. Steroids may be indicated (controversial)
Curling's ulcer *Occurs:* Emergent and acute phases	Twice as common in children. Stress response of body to overwhelming injury. Routine use of antacids or Tagamet in burn victims has decreased the incidence. If preventive antacid regimen not followed, GI hemorrhage may result. Once wound is healed, incidence is eliminated
Nervous System	
Personality change *Occurs:* Acute and/or rehabilitation phases	Common in children; may be consequence of stress, fluid or electrolyte imbalance, septicemia, drug therapy. Usually resolved when systemic complications resolve and wound closes, unless there was preburn pathology
Postburn seizures *Occurs:* Acute phase	Same as above; unique complication of children; full recovery is usual
Peripheral neuropathy *Occurs:* Acute or rehabilitation phase	Secondary to immobilization and certain antibiotics. Hearing loss and weakness in limbs (e.g., foot drop) are most frequent
Skin, Bone, Joint	
Scarring and contractures *Occurs:* Acute and rehabilitative phases	Secondary to tissue injury, inflammation and healing. A good prevention program starting on admission involving splinting and activities by OT and PT is essential.
Heterotopic bone (bone growth in abnormal areas) *Occurs:* Acute and rehabilitative phases	Calcium deposits in joint spaces, secondary to fluid and electrolyte disturbances, bed rest, inactivity. Cannot be removed until fully mature (i.e., 1–3 yr postburn)

* Early activity and turning, coughing, and deep breathing exercises are *essential* preventive measures. Escharotomy (incising constricting eschar layer) of circumferential full-thickness burns of chest also indicated.

edema may develop secondary to the injury or to overzealous fluid therapy. Another problem contributing to severe respiratory difficulty is a full-thickness circumferential burn of the chest. The thick eschar acts as a tourniquet and can constrict chest excursion to the point of diminishing air exchange. An escharotomy or release of the eschar is mandatory.

Fluid Therapy. Within a few hours after the burn, loss of circulating fluid causes hypovolemia that, if untreated, can lead to hypovolemic shock and death.

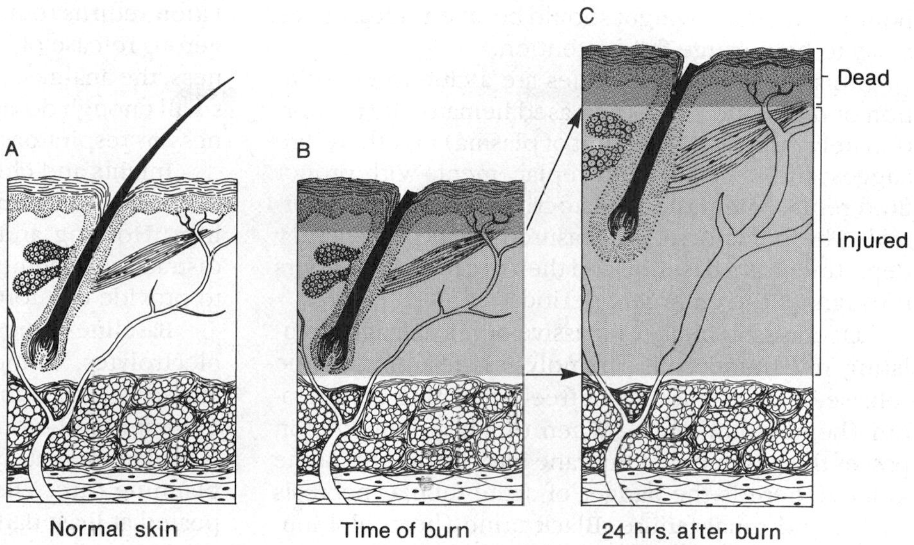

Figure 52-7. Edema formation. Because of the inflammatory process and increased capillary permeability following deep partial- or full-thickness burns, fluids lost from the vascular spaces enter the injured area. *A*, Normal skin; *B*, the depth of the injury at the time of the burn; and *C*, the amount of edema formed in this damaged tissue 24 hours after the burn. (Redrawn from Feller I, Archambeault C: *Nursing the Burned Patient.* Ann Arbor, MI, National Institute for Burn Medicine, 1973.)

Advances in technique of fluid therapy now make it possible to successfully resuscitate even the most severely burned infant. However, fluid overload can be as great a danger as fluid losses and a complication of therapy.

A major burn results in an outer layer of dead tissue and a deeper band or zone of injured or damaged cells (Fig. 52-7). Fluid from injured tissues leaks out of the bloodstream into the interstitial spaces. In the early phase, fluid loss through dead burned tissue (eschar) is insignificant compared with this plasma shift. It is in the zone of damaged tissue that fluid shifts, causing edema within those tissues and depletion of vascular volume (hypovolemia) (Fig. 52-7).

The fluid shift begins immediately after a burn and is profound for the first 24 hours. There is increased capillary permeability in the area of injury, upsetting the delicate balance of interstitial and intravascular fluid. In burns of less than 10 to 20 per cent total body area, depending on age and other severity factors, the child's body can compensate for this fluid shift by saving urine (oliguria) and vasoconstriction (which shunts remaining blood to the vital organs). In larger burns the fluid shift, if untreated, is life-threatening. Intravenous fluids similar to those shifted out of the bloodstream must be given in amounts sufficient to prevent hypovolemic shock, without causing fluid overload and electrolyte imbalance. Paralytic ileus is often seen owing to the hypovolemic state (leading to the shunting of blood away from the bowel) and its presence contraindicates oral fluids.

Fluid lost from the bloodstream in burn shock is composed of water, electrolytes, and albumin and should be replaced in kind. Hartmann's solution (lactated Ringer's) is the fluid of choice because its electrolyte balance is similar to that of the blood. Albumin (human serum) may be added to provide colloid, although investigators who oppose its use during the first 24 hours of fluid therapy believe that the colloid becomes trapped during this time, adding to extravascular fluid retention. Red cell loss related to the burn injury is caused by hemolysis and generally approximates only 10 per cent of the total red cell mass. Whole blood is not necessary to resuscitate the victim of a major burn unless there is significant loss of blood from concurrent injuries. Packed cells may be needed later in care to correct hematocrit or hemoglobin deficiencies due to debridement.

When there is proper fluid replacement, the plasma shift gradually reverses. Within a few days the fluid that has leaked into interstitial spaces returns to the vascular spaces and a profound, spontaneous diuresis occurs, signaling successful treatment. If excessive fluids have been given, the shift back to vascular spaces may cause hypervolemia, congestive heart failure, and pulmonary edema.

Fluid therapy for the burn victim is based on titration. An adequate amount of parenteral fluids to maintain organ perfusion without overloading the circulatory system is determined by measuring urinary output, specific gravity, and other parameters, including vital signs, central venous pressure, hematocrit, hydration, and level of consciousness.

Intravenous replacement fluids also leak into interstitial spaces. Until third-spaced fluids are expelled, no patient should gain more than 10 to 15 per cent of the preburn weight.* In an infant or child with a relatively small circulatory volume, close monitoring of intravenous intake and output is essential. Giving a 30 lb (13 to 14 kg) toddler a liter of fluid is replacing one third to one half of total circulatory volume and represents a weight gain of 7 per cent of the child's normal weight. Vital signs and intake and output are measured

*One liter of fluid weighs 1 kg (2.2 lbs).

hourly and a nude weight should be taken at least once a day to help gauge fluid retention.

Relative hematocrit values are a clue to the dilution of red blood cells. Increased hematocrit (proportionately more RBCs per unit of plasma) may therefore suggest the need for fluid replacement. With proper fluid replacement the hematocrit level returns to normal. The hematocrit is measured in the emergency department as a baseline and then every 12 to 24 hours throughout the emergent period.

Deep tissue injury or massive burns damage circulating red blood cells (hemolysis), resulting in the release of large amounts of free-circulating hemoglobin (hemoglobinemia). When this free hemoglobin passes the basement membrane into the tubules of the kidney, there is the danger of acute tubular necrosis (ATN) and renal failure. Black urine (hemoglobinuria) seen on catheterization or in the immediate postburn period indicates severe hemolysis. An osmotic diuretic is given immediately to flush the tubules. Intravenous intake is temporarily increased until the crisis is over. Obviously, hemoglobinuria will not be detected unless a urinary catheter is inserted early in care.

Monitoring the urinary output is essential in assessing the child's response to trauma. The amount, content, and color of urine is a guide to fluid replacement. The amount of urine measured and recorded each hour is a guide to the amount of fluid to be infused the next hour. Outputs of 1 ml/kg/hr for children up to 30 kg and 30 to 50 ml/hr for larger children or adolescents indicate adequate perfusion of organ systems without systemic overload. Output greater than this *does not* indicate "better" resuscitation but rather warns of potential fluid overload and pulmonary edema.

The emergent period ends when fluid resuscitation is successful. Third-spaced fluids return to the vascular space and are excreted by the kidneys. Fluid therapy is then re-evaluated and discontinued or continued, as indicated, for management of expected or apparent complications such as infection, weight loss, or dehydration.

Other Elements of Care. Other elements of emergent period care include (1) controlling pain, (2) obtaining baseline indices, (3) controlling infection, and (4) treating the wound. Because the principles of wound care are the same during the emergent phase as in the acute phase, its discussion is included in acute period care.

Pain Control. When the child is in burn shock (hypovolemic shock), pain control cannot be achieved with subcutaneous or intramuscular medication because the medication will not be circulated adequately by the depleted blood volume in the periphery—that is, the medication will not provide relief. When circulation returns to normal, there may be a possibly dangerous release of large, pooled dosages. For effectiveness, the analgesic must be given intravenously and in small enough dosages to prevent dulling of consciousness or respiratory centers.

Infants and children should be cuddled and held, while taking precautions to guard catheters and tubings. Holding and rocking the children, along with distraction techniques and security objects, will help to provide comfort.

Baseline Values. Baseline values for all vital signs, electrolytes, hemoglobin, and white cells are obtained, as are a chest roentgenograph, an electrocardiogram, and wound cultures. These should be obtained immediately to serve as a guide to assessing and planning care. Vital signs and laboratory tests are repeated at least daily and more often if indicated.

Infection Control. The burn victim has lost the protective barrier of the skin—invasive infection can threaten the child's life. Septicemia or pneumonia accounts for about 50 per cent of burn fatalities. Burn patients are autocontaminated on admission by the bacteria that normally reside on the skin and in hair follicles and sweat glands, and the normal flora of the gastrointestinal tract. The role of the nurse is to aid in controlling infection, since it cannot be eliminated. Clean or isolation technique is needed to prevent cross-contamination (the spread of bacteria from one patient to another by staff and visitors). Aseptic technique is mandatory for any procedure in which an anatomical barrier is penetrated. Judicious antibiotic use and support of the body's natural immunologic processes further serve to control infection.

Routine tetanus coverage is indicated; it does not need to be given intravenously. Burn wounds provide an excellent medium for growth of *C. tetani* spores.

The Acute Period

The acute period of treatment *begins at the end of the emergent period and lasts until all full-thickness wounds are covered with autografts.* (Autografts are the patient's own skin transferred permanently to cover the wound.) If the burn is only a partial-thickness injury, the acute period is over within 7 to 14 days; the healing is spontaneous and grafts are unnecessary.

During the acute phase there are two main principles of management: The first is to remove the eschar as soon as possible to allow spontaneous healing or covering with autografts or homografts (temporary biologic cover of skin from a donor of the same species). The second is to avoid, as far as possible, the complications that are known to occur with burns.

Complications. Complications of every organ system may be encountered in care of the burned child. The key to successful therapy is anticipation and early detection of complications combined with rigorous therapy. Early detection is accomplished by close monitoring and a knowledge of proper management (basic nursing care) of each organ system. The tedious long-term care required for wound closure is balanced by the need for precise and exacting skill in preventing, detecting, and treating the many possible complications.

The seriously burned patient remains acutely ill for a long time. The patient is not in a chronic state, as this prolonged, difficult period would suggest, but is instead acutely ill, continually in danger of developing complications. The patient may appear to be doing well one day only to be found to have developed a severe complication the next. Only when the full-thickness wound is reduced to less than 20 per cent of the body surface are these dangers past.

Minor Burn Wound Management. Wound management is the main consideration for minor burns. There is generally no need for intravenous fluid therapy or prophylactic antibiotics. However, tetanus toxoid, tetanus antitoxin, or tetanus immune globulin (human) is used in all but small partial-thickness burns, on the basis of history of immunization.

The basic principles of wound management are comfort and cleanliness. A partial-thickness burn is usually painful because pain fibers in the area of tissue damage are irritated. Analgesics should be administered before cleaning the involved surface, but care should be taken to avoid oversedation because some response to pain during cleansing helps nurses judge whether they are causing unnecessary trauma to the tissues. Rough handling of the burned area must be avoided. Partial-thickness wounds can be converted to full-thickness loss when mechanical trauma during cleaning further damages weakened tissues. This can easily occur with infants because their skin is delicate.

After the wound and surrounding areas have been gently but thoroughly cleaned of all debris (foreign matter and dead tissue) with soap and water and after any hairy area has been shaved to a 2-inch margin around the wound, the wound is rinsed thoroughly and a dressing is applied. One layer of a saline- or topical agent–moistened roll bandage is applied directly to the burned area and then covered with a moist Kerlix wrap, followed by a dry one. This will provide a comfortable occlusive dressing. (The type of dressing may be altered according to instructions of the physician in charge of care.)

The child and family are instructed to change this dressing daily by soaking it off with warm tap water, gently cleaning the wound with nonirritating soap and water, and thoroughly rinsing. A new bandage is then applied in the manner just described. Parents should be informed that dressing changes remove exudate and products of infection, allowing the wound to heal spontaneously. Daily dressing changes and cleansing allow for detection of infection. If parental competence in following directions in dressing change is questionable, parents may be instructed to return to the nurse for daily dressing changes and observation of the wound or referral may be made for home care.

Approximately 7 to 14 days are required for healing of a partial-thickness wound; the patient should be followed on an outpatient basis. Appearance of necrotic tissue* or granulation tissue† or both after the necrotic surface is cleaned indicates a full-thickness wound, usually requiring hospital admission for closure with autograft.

The patient or family should be instructed to observe the unburned skin surrounding the wound for early evidence of infection (redness, heat, pain, swelling, or colored drainage) during the daily dressing changes. If any of these are present, a return to the physician is indicated to change topical treatment or start systemic therapy. If cellulitis (intense redness, streaking, swelling, firm infiltration) appears, an immediate return visit is indicated for prescription of the proper antibiotic and hydrotherapy (soaking at home three or four times a day) or hospitalization. In most instances, gram-positive organisms are responsible. Oral antibiotics are usually satisfactory, and more frequent dressing changes with increased soaking periods hasten the control of infection. Oral analgesics are used prior to dressing changes to minimize the child's discomfort during the treatment.

Ointments, other topical medications, and expensive dressings are generally not indicated for minor wound management. There are no known chemicals that can restore vitality to dead tissue, nor do we now know of any that can speed the body's healing process. Many of the substances formerly used to coat burns actually increased the injury by their own chemical action on already weakened tissue. It is not so much what is put on the wound as how the wound is cared for that is important to healing. The attending physician should decide on topical therapy on the basis of the type and location of the wound. Cleanliness is as important as the topical agent used, as long as infection is not present.

Major Burn Wound Management. Care of a burn wound classified as major can be a time-consuming process. Full-thickness wounds cannot heal by themselves; all dead tissue must be removed and the area grafted with the patient's own skin (autografted) for permanent coverage. The same donor site (site

*Necrotic tissue is dead cells that are in contact with living cells.

† Granulation tissue is newly formed tissue that fills in areas where the skin has been destroyed.

from which autografts are taken) may be used every 7 to 10 days if given proper care.

When the full-thickness wound is very large or the child's condition is such that he or she cannot tolerate surgical procedures, homografts (skin from another donor of the same species, such as cadaver skin) or heterografts (pig skin) may be used until autografts can be taken. This temporary skin coverage is rejected by the body. Only a few burn care facilities in the United States today use any of the new skin substitutes, because of the cost and time required for production and because they are usually not necessary.

Daily cleansing and debriding (removing dead tissue) are a time-consuming aspect of burn nursing. Frequently the patient is "tubbed" in a hydrotherapy tub twice daily to assist with this process. Debridement can be accomplished in three ways. One is the *natural* process of proteolytic degradation of tissue by body and bacterial enzymes that loosen tissue. This process is enhanced by dressing changes and gentle cleansing. The second way, *sharp* debridement, is done with a scalpel (as in early tangential excision) or with sharp scissors and pickups; daily sharp debridement may be carried out at the bedside by the nurse or physician. (Early tangential excision is gaining favor among experts.) The third method involves use of *enzymes* such as Travase, which destroy dead tissue. All of these methods may be used in a very large wound.

The human body can heal a partial-thickness wound if proper cleansing is done. In management of full-thickness wounds, bacteria must be controlled that can grow in or on the wound because of the optimal conditions present: body heat, body moisture, and dead tissue. Bacterial growth is controlled by debridement, cleansing, and use of topical agents. The coagulated zone of the burned tissue has no blood supply. This means that neither the body's blood-borne immune defenses nor systemic antibiotics will reach that tissue (Stein, 1985). For this reason topical antimicrobials are used. Topical agents are ordered by the managing physician. Silvadene is a commonly used ointment that is effective against most all organisms. The topical agent should be chosen for its effectiveness against the bacterial population in the wound and its nonantigenic properties.

Debridement removes dead tissue, tubbing dilutes the bacterial population on the wound and softens eschar for debridement while cleansing the body, and topical agents, when used properly, control bacterial growth in the wound. Systemic antibacterial therapy is also necessary.

Use of a dressing for major burns depends on the overall system of care and the condition of the patient's wound. Some burn centers use wet dressings (dressings impregnated with a particular topical agent), as described in the section on minor burns. Others use exposure therapy, which involves allowing the wound to air-dry. Usually exposure is used for minor wounds or for burns in areas that lend themselves to exposure therapy, such as the face or anterior areas of the body. A combination of methods also may be employed. Once the wound is healed, no dressings are required.

As the size of the wound is reduced through debridement and autografting, the patient's chance for survival increases. During wound treatment, nursing care must also deal with prevention of contractures and scar tissue as well as detection and early treatment of complications of other organ systems, as is true with minor burn care.

A physical or occupational therapist should be called in to assist with or direct contracture control. Positioning is essential to future function. Table 52-9 outlines positions to prevent deformity. Nurses cannot be expected to achieve this type of positioning without assistance from physical therapy.

Controlling Pain During Wound Management. Wound debridement through tubbing and other procedures is known to be extremely painful. Contrary to a popular myth, even full-thickness burns are severely painful once debridement and excision of dead tissue begin(Atchison et al, 1986).

It is the nurse who is responsible for the evaluation and alleviation of this pain. Unfortunately, advances in pain control have lagged behind technologic expertise but some researchers, primarily nurses, are attempting to find ways to help children manage the pain of wound care. Elliott and Olson (1983) studied the effects of four types of pain- and stress-management techniques with burned children. The children were taught (1) *attention distraction techniques* such as looking for hidden objects in the room or doing simple mental arithmetic; (2) *relaxation breathing* (e.g., imagining breathing to pump up like a tire and then letting the air out slowly with a hissing noise); (3) *emotive imagery or reinterpretation of the context of pain*, by imagining a situation in which the pain was the result of a heroic situation such as swimming with an injured arm to save a drowning friend, or to imagine floating on a quiet peaceful ocean; and (4) were given *reinforcement* such as smiley faces and small toys for use of these coping techniques. The researchers found that this "package" of pain management strategies substantially reduced the children's distress with hydrotherapy (tubbing), debridement, and dressing changes. It should be noted, however, that pain is usually best managed by a combination of medications and other comfort measures.

Kavanagh (1983), a nurse researcher, proposed strategies to decrease the child's feelings of helplessness and anxiety (which heighten the perception of

Table 52-9. Positioning to Prevent Deformity

Area Burned	Resulting Deformity	Position of Prevention
Neck		
Anterior aspect or circumferential	Flexion contracture of neck	No pillow under head
Posterior aspect (only)	Extensor contracture of neck	Prone—pillow under upper chest to flex cervical spine. Supine—small pillow under neck
Axilla		
Anterior	Adduction and internal rotation	Shoulder joint in abduction (100–130°) and external rotation
Posterior	Adduction and external rotation	Shoulder in forward flexion and 100–130° abduction
Pectoral Region	Shoulder protraction	No pillow. Shoulders abducted and externally rotated
Chest or Abdomen	Kyphosis	As above and hips neutral (*not* flexed)
Lateral trunk	Scoliosis	Supine, affected arm abducted
Elbow		
Anterior surface or circumferential	Flexion and pronation	Arm extended and supinated
Wrist		
Total or flexor surface	Flexion	Splint in 15° extension
Dorsal surface	Extension	Splint in 15° flexion
Hip (includes inguinal and perineal burns)	Internal rotation, flexion and adduction, possible joint subluxation if contracture severe	Neutral rotation and abduction and maintain extension by prone position or *pillow under buttocks*
Knee		
Popliteal surface or circumferential	Flexion	Maintain extension using posterior splints or suspend heels with plastic heel protecting boots. *No pillows* under knees while supine or under ankles while prone
Ankle	Plantar flexion if foot dorsiflexor muscles are weak or their tendons are divided	90° dorsiflexion with splint if possible rather than footboard

pain) by increasing the predictability and controllability of burn wound management. In Kavanagh's studies *predictability* was increased by (1) focusing the child on the event rather than attempting distraction; (2) giving children as much information as possible about what they would feel and see and what would happen, both prior to and during the wound care; and (3) wearing a red apron (or other apparel) only during wound care so that children were not afraid every time they saw the nurse.

Controllability was implemented by encouraging children, from the onset of wound care, to take an active role. For example, they were allowed to make choices about when to start dressing changes and when to rest (within established time limits). Children as young as age 2 were encouraged to help remove dressings, wash wounds, and redress burns. Children aged 5 and over were taught to remove loose eschar and apply medicated gauze to their burns. Before the procedure nurses established what things they would have to do and time limits for procedures the child would do, to eliminate endless negotiating during the wound care. Kavanagh found that, although increased predictability and controllability did not magically eliminate all anger and protests, these behaviors were no longer predominant modes of action and did not interfere with the wound care. Increasing predictability and controllability also dramatically decreased the need for narcotic analgesics and decreased children's pain and anxiety. Further nursing studies have supported Kavanagh's success with these strategies (Lasoff and McEttrick, 1986).

Eland (1987) reported success with musical distraction to reduce pain during tubbing for burn debridement. Children were allowed to choose music for a cassette recorder with earphones. The children stated that listening to music they selected helped to reduce pain sensations. Eland (1987) also reported that the pain of dressing changes was successfully mediated with transcutaneous electrical nerve stimulation (TENS). The small TENS unit can be adjusted by the child to deliver the amount of electrical stimulation that will block pain sensations.

The findings of these researchers have increased

the options for nurses in planning pain management for children during burn wound care. The studies do not indicate whether it is better to use techniques of distraction and stress-management or to involve a child in the procedure or to use a combination of these techniques. Such decisions remain, as always, with the nurse, who must choose from the available options on the basis of knowledge about the pain perceptions and behaviors of an individual child.

Nutrition. The initial insult of the burn injury results in a hypovolemic state, which contributes to a paralytic ileus. Thus the patient is kept NPO for the first 24 to 72 hours, or until normal bowel sounds return. As the gastrointestinal tract returns to normal, the child is progressed to a full diet.

Because of the increased metabolism and catabolism as a result of the burn trauma, the child needs two or three times the normal amount of calories and protein. Caloric increases should be in the form of carbohydrates to spare protein breakdown. Vitamins and trace elements are provided to promote healing, as is iron to control anemia secondary to hemolysis and bleeding during debridement.

The nurse should be aware that burned children are often anorexic and that small, frequent feedings of the child's favorite nutritious foods may be necessary to achieve adequate intake. A list of favorite foods should be included in the care plan and families encouraged to bring in favorite foods from home. Nutrition for children who cannot tolerate oral feedings is provided through a combination of nasogastric feedings and intravenous hyperalimentation until they can again take nourishment orally.

The Rehabilitation Period

Rehabilitation involves returning the child to normal functioning. Fortunately, most children who survive do very well even though they have been through a long and difficult hospitalization. A survey of 250 severely burned patients of all ages treated in the University of Michigan Burn Center revealed that 85 per cent returned to society as well as or better than they were before the accident (Evaluation of Emergency Medical Services with a National Burn Registry, 1975–1978). This study took into consideration both functional and emotional factors. Children with an already good body image responded well to rehabilitation despite physical and cosmetic handicaps. Children who did not "feel good" about themselves prior to the burn accident had more cosmetic and physical problems. Adolescents especially had problems with adjustment, primarily because they were already going through an adjustment phase of their lives and the burn injury only served to compound their problems. With proper intervention, however, their adjustment improved as years passed.

There are two basic considerations during the rehabilitation phase: (1) restoration of function in joint surfaces that were scarred and (2) emotional assistance required by the child. Rehabilitation actually begins in the emergency room and must be kept in mind throughout the child's hospitalization. After the initial discharge, many readmissions may be necessary for reconstructive procedures as well as for emotional assistance and counseling. Children require long-term follow-up through their years of growth so that scarring over joints does not retard normal growth and development.

Working with the child's teacher and classmates also helps smooth re-entry into normal life.

Additional Strategies for Nursing Care

Nursing strategies that are interactive with medical management have been integrated throughout the preceding section on basic burn care. Those strategies are addressed further in Table 52-10, a nursing process plan for the child with major burns. This section presents additional strategies for supportive care of the child and family. Remember that the *burn victim is an accident victim.* The child will have guilt feelings regarding the accident and most likely a fear of death, or at least a fear of the "unknown" concerning the injury and treatment. The shock and pain of the accident, the chaos and rush to the hospital, the unfamiliar surroundings, and new people all produce emotional stress.

Supporting the Child and Family in the Emergent Phase

An attitude showing confidence, genuine interest, and concern is extremely important to the emotional welfare of the child and family. One simple act that provides an anchor in the storm is for the nurse to tell the child his or her name and to explain briefly what to expect of the staff, what sensations will be experienced, and what will be expected of the child. These instructions (a verbal contract) help reduce the inequality and inconsistency in the transition that the child makes from being healthy to being an accident victim to being a patient. Talking to children also allows the nurse to evaluate their sensorium and orientation. The nurse should remember that no burn victim is ever rendered unconscious by the burn itself—a search for an underlying cause is imperative. The following nursing strategies will help children cope with their emotional stress and maintain some control:

1. Give the child your name and call the child by name.
2. Talk *to*, not just *about* the child.
3. State what will be done and why and what the child will feel, hear, and smell.
4. Request the child's cooperation and suggest possible ways of participating.
5. Encourage the child to express feelings, and alter the contract to comply with the child's requests whenever possible.
6. If a parent does not accompany the child, you must, for legal reasons, take the time to notify a parent to get his or her consent for what must be done. Stay with the child during the treatment, acting as a surrogate parent, until a parent arrives. In the parent's absence, assure the child that his or her parents know about the accident and care about the child.

Supporting the Child During Prolonged Hospitalization

Prolonged hospitalization is difficult for any child, but the burned child who must adjust to painful treatments and an altered body image needs special attention. It is important to maintain a consistent plan of care, allowing the child to choose some options when they exist. Never ask children if they want to do something when you know they must do it anyway. The burned child needs to be rocked, cuddled, taught, and disciplined like any other child. Expectations for the child's behavior should be spelled out and maintained.

Maintaining a pleasant, supportive, and loving atmosphere is essential to the child's emotional adjustment. The child should be encouraged to be out of bed as soon as possible and to participate in everyday activities (e.g., playing with toys, continuing with toilet training, eating in a high chair or at the table, and so forth).

The child should be allowed to talk, play, and act out feelings of depression and hostility. The nurse should assess the need for help from other team members such as a social worker, a psychologist, or a play therapist and obtain their help.

Although toddlers are not as affected by their appearance as are older children, they are sensitive to their body intactness and others' reactions to their appearance. To draw attention away from their overwhelming appearance, the nurse can ask parents to supply colorful pajamas and slippers and pretty decorations (jewelry, bows, badges) for the child to wear, and can encourage good general grooming. Studies have also shown that all burned children are more comfortable and feel more "intact" when their dressings are on. Colorful pajamas or gowns can be worn over their dressings.

Supporting the Family

Whether justified or not, parents usually experience extreme guilt and feel acute responsibility for their child's burns. These feelings are compounded by the fact that in many instances the accident could have been prevented if safety precautions or closer adult supervision had been initiated. The same feelings may be experienced by other family members. In addition, there is grave concern for the child's life and about his or her present and future appearance.

In an effort to handle these feelings, some parents may become oversolicitous and lenient with their burned child. Others refuse to look at or touch the child because of his or her appearance and the guilt feelings it produces. Neither reaction is therapeutic or conducive to the child's recovery.

A plan for family teaching should be instituted on admission; the family must have a clear explanation of what must be done and why. They must be prepared for what the child's appearance will be once dressings are applied and when dressings are removed and assisted to accept that treatments that inflict pain are essential to recovery, but that they will be as brief as possible. It should be explained that the consequences of not providing treatment are far worse.

The family should also be prepared for what to expect from the child behaviorally and encouraged to relate to the child in as supportive a fashion as possible. (Frequently the nurse may find a family problem that requires intervention by a social worker or a psychologist.) Enforcement of normal routine, discipline, and expectations (to the extent possible under the circumstances) is comforting and supportive to the child. Parents also benefit from contact with other parents who have recently been through the same ordeal. These contacts are helpful if all parents have been properly oriented. They can be harmful if parents pass along rumors or misinformation. Group time should be allotted on a regular basis for family members to verbalize their feelings and concerns to the nurse or another member of the burn team. Professional assistance for families is frequently required to help the child with a major burn and the family through the long months or years of rehabilitative care. In fact, studies show that this professional intervention is essential.

Impact of Burn Care on Nurses

Burn care of children can be especially difficult for the nurse. To remain calm when confronted by the children's appearance and the discomfort that they must suffer, while attempting to be efficient and effective during burn care activities, is extremely taxing. In ad-

> **Box 52-6**
> *What to Do If a Burn Accident Happens*
>
> **STOP THE DAMAGE!**
>
> - Put out the fire the fastest way you can. Time is critical.
> - Stop child from running.
> - Pull off burned clothes.
> - Wrap the victim in a rug or blanket, if available, and roll to smother flames. Use water, if available, to help extinguish flames.
>
> **IMMEDIATE CARE OF BURNS**
>
> - When a scald burn occurs, flood with cold tap water and remove clothing carefully.
> - If a chemical burn occurs, flood with water and remove clothing.
> - If a large area is burned, wrap the victim in a clean sheet or towel and take him or her immediately to the nearest hospital emergency room.
> - If a small area is burned, wash it with cool water and soap. Do not use ice. Rinse thoroughly, dry gently, and apply a bland ointment (e.g., A & D Ointment). Cover with a sterile gauze bandage.
> - If you have ***any doubt*** about what to do, call your family physician or nearest hospital emergency room and ask for advice.
> - Contact a physician for a tetanus booster if tetanus immunization is not up to date.
>
> **LATER CARE OF MINOR BURNS**
>
> - Cleanse once or twice a day with soap and water; rinse thoroughly and dry. Cover with a thin layer of bland ointment and a sterile dressing.
> - Do not break blisters; they provide a sterile cover over the wound.
> - Watch for any signs of inflammation: redness, pain, heat, or swelling. If they occur, call a doctor or take victim to the nearest hospital emergency room.

dition, the nurse must deal not only with a child who is in pain, but also cope with the fact that she or he inflicts pain during treatments, dressing changes, and when positioning or holding the child. Planning time for interactions with the child that do not involve pain can increase the nurse's sense of role satisfaction. Role satisfaction is also enhanced through effective implementation of pain-reducing strategies (see section on pain reduction).

Nurses caring for the burned child must confront their own feelings and anxieties before they can maintain therapeutic interactions with the child and family. Nurses must learn to respond in a manner that is firm but supportive and recovery-directed. Being well trained and knowledgeable in the intricacies of care relieves some of the nurse's stress and anxiety regarding the physical measures of care and allows the nurse to concentrate on a therapeutic approach. Nurses also need to be aware that a team of specialties is required to meet the patient's many needs; nurses cannot do it alone. They should seek professional outlets (head nurse, social worker, physician) to express the frustrations, dismay, anger, and anxiety created during care of the burned child. Burn care can be rewarding for all involved if properly managed.

Providing Preventive Education

Nurses should take a major role in providing safety education to parents and children. Simple measures can be taken by parents in the home to prevent burn accidents. In addition, every individual should know how to respond if clothing or hair ignites. Likewise, proper immediate first aid for burns should be a part of preventive education so that burns that do occur are not aggravated by inappropriate measures. See Box 52-6.

Table 52-10
Nursing Process Plan: The Child with Major Burns*

by Roxie Foster

Assessment of Physical and Intellectual-Perceptual Function

Activity/Exercise
Elimination
Nutrition/Metabolism
Pain

Subjective Assessment

Report details of the burn incident (i.e., whether inhalation of smoke, materials involved in fire, noxious fumes, falls, or other related trauma), child's medical history, report of pain, appetite, date of last tetanus immunization

Objective Assessment

Respiratory status: Adequacy of airway, gas exchange; excursion; oral and nasal mucous membranes

Integumentary status: Severity of burn (size, depth, age of child, location of burn), concurrent injuries, appearance of wound, catheter sites

Circulatory volume: Intake and output; urine color, specific gravity; vital signs; nude body weight

Gastrointestinal status: Bowel sounds

Musculoskeletal status: Muscle strength and mass, joint mobility

Baseline diagnostic values: Electrolytes, hemoglobin, and hematocrit; chest roentgenograph; total protein, albumin, BUN, glucose, urinalysis

Comfort status: Diaphoresis, muscle tension, facial expression, physical agitation, irritability, sleep patterns, oral intake

Analysis: Nursing Diagnosis 1

Ineffective breathing pattern: airway obstruction, related to upper airway edema associated with
- ***burns of the face, neck, and chest***
- ***thermal injury to the upper airway***

Defining Characteristics

Objective: Shallow breathing, dyspnea, hoarseness, stridor, tachypnea, cyanosis, nasal flaring, restlessness, anxiety, decreased P_{O_2}, increased P_{CO_2}

* Use with Table 31-2, Nursing Process Plan: The Hospitalized Child.

Continued

Table 52-10 (continued)

Client Goal/ Evaluation Criteria	Nursing Goals/Strategies (Selected Rationale)
1. The client will maintain an adequate airway as evidenced by: a. normal rate and depth of respirations for age b. heart rate normal for age c. normal skin color in nonburned areas d. absence of nasal flaring and stridor e. blood gases within normal limits	*Assess for factors predisposing to upper airway edema.* • Burns to the face and neck • Intense heat exposure • Young child (whose small airways obstruct easily) If any of these factors are present intensify surveillence of respiratory competence, especially in the first 8 hr. If hoarseness or stridor present, intubation is indicated *Assess for signs and symptoms associated with upper airway injury:* hemoptysis, singed nasal hairs, sooty tongue or pharynx, hoarseness, carbaceous sputum, redness or edema of pharynx, wheezing, stridor *Assess patency of airway every 15–30 min in the first 8 hr.* • Monitor for tachypnea, tachycardia, rales and rhonchi, pallor, and cyanosis • Assess characteristics of sputum • Monitor reports of blood gases, transcutaneous oxygen monitor or pulse oximeter • Obtain baseline and subsequent chest radiographs as ordered Facilitate air exchange. • Administer 100% humidified oxygen • Elevate head of bed *Calm the frightened child* (crying will further increase airway edema). • Explain all actions to the child in a quiet, reassuring voice • Provide assurance and explanations for parent(s) so they can reassure the child *Alert physician at the first sign of increased respiratory effort* (an endotracheal tube may be inserted at this time).

Analysis: Nursing Diagnosis 2

Ineffective breathing pattern: compromised respiratory excursion, related to
- *constriction of the thorax and abdomen by eschar associated with full-thickness circumferential burns*
- *pain associated with burns to the thorax or abdomen*

Defining Characteristics

Subjective: Verbalization of pain with breathing, irritability, confusion, anxiety

Objective: Decreased or uneven expansion of chest and/or abdomen with inspiration and expiration, tachypnea, pallor, cyanosis, or decreased tidal volume (if intubated)

Client Goal/ Evaluation Criteria	Nursing Goals/Strategies (Selected Rationale)
2. Client will maintain adequate respiratory excursion for effective gas exchange as evidenced by: a. normal rate and depth of respirations b. normal skin color in nonburned areas c. equal breath sounds bilaterally d. arterial or transcutaneous blood oxygen values within normal limits e. normal tidal volume (if intubated)	*Assess for factors predisposing to decreased excursion.* • Full-thickness, circumferential burns of the chest or abdomen (children under age 7 normally use abdominal muscles in breathing) • Burns to the thorax or abdomen which cause pain upon lung expansion *Assess respiratory excursion.* • Observe chest movement, and abdominal movement in young child, with respirations. When injuries allow, one hand can be placed on each side of the chest to feel for equal expansion *Assess for adequate air exchange.* • Auscultate for equal breath sounds (breath sounds are equal when the length of inspiration and expiration are the same in corresponding areas from side to side and when these sounds are equally loud bilaterally) • Assess level of consciousness, i.e., whether agitated, restless • Assess for tachypnea and tachycardia with the child at rest (crying and activity increase respiratory and cardiac rates and create an inappropriate comparison with baselines) • Assess for pallor or duskiness in areas of unburned skin and mucous membranes • Monitor blood gas values • Monitor tidal volume if intubated *Facilitate normal lung excursion.* • Place in semi-Fowler's position or place head of bed on 6 inch shock blocks, or raise the head end of the crib mattress 30° unless this position is contraindicated by other factors. (In this position gravity aids the function of the diaphragm) • Change position every 1–2 hr if the child is not moving spontaneously • Administer prescribed analgesics. Note whether narcotic analgesics depress respirations by counting respirations before and 20–30 min after administration (The child who experiences pain on lung expansion will adopt a pattern of shallow breathing) • Encourage a parent or relative to provide comfort measures appropriate to the child's condition, e.g., holding, rocking, stroking the hair, rubbing a limb, patting the back, singing, reading stories, allowing the child to listen to favorite records or tapes, or hold a security object (Anxiety often results in shallow breathing)

Analysis: Nursing Diagnosis 3

Impaired gas exchange: hypoxemia, related to alveolar damage associated with

- *prolonged inhalation of noxious gases and chemicals*
- *carbon monoxide inhalation*

Continued

Table 52-10 *(continued)*

Analysis: Nursing Diagnosis 3

Defining Characteristics

Subjective: (carbon monoxide inhalation) headache, irritability, restlessness, nausea

Objective: (inhalation of gases) restlessness, irritability, less alert, bronchorrhea, expiratory wheezing, dyspnea, decreased PO_2, increased PCO_2
(carbon monoxide inhalation) vomiting

Client Goal/ Evaluation Criteria	Nursing Goals/Strategies (Selected Rationale)
3. Client will maintain adequate gas exchange as evidenced by: a. absence of restlessness b. absence of unexplained irritability c. usual level of consciousness d. blood gases within normal limits	*Assess for adequate gas exchange.* • Note and chart child's baseline activity and level of consciousness for comparison with later status • Ask the parent to alert you to unusual restlessness, irritability, or change in mental status (Parent may be first to note subtle changes) • Monitor blood gas levels *Alert the physician to changes in oxygenation. Administer oxygen as ordered.* Initially, 100% humidified oxygen will often be administered to counteract the effects of carbon monoxide, a gas present in all fire conditions (Lybarger, 1987) • Continue to monitor gas exchange after oxygen therapy is started (to assess the adequacy of flow) • Check oxygen flow meter and oxygen tubings to make sure the child is receiving humidified oxygen in the amount prescribed *Assist with intubation and mechanical ventilation* if that becomes necessary. *Maintain artificial airway.* • Ensure that the endotracheal tube is well secured • Restrain the child as necessary to prevent accidental extubation or administer sedatives as ordered to decrease anxiety associated with mechanical ventilation • Maintain cuff pressure of the endotracheal tube under 20 mmHg (to prevent tracheal necrosis) (Uncuffed tubes are used on children younger than 10 years because the tracheal cartilage is still soft and the trachea is more prone to necrosis from pressure)

Analysis: Nursing Diagnosis 4

Ineffective airway clearance, related to inadequate removal of damaged tissue from the lower airway associated with damage to cilia

Defining Characteristics

Objective: Nonproductive cough; rales and rhonchi; dyspnea, fatigue; use of accessory muscles in breathing

Client Goal/ Evaluation Criteria	Nursing Goals/Strategies (Selected Rationale)
4. Client will maintain adequate airway clearance as evidenced by: a. sputum production if cough present b. absence of or minimum of adventitious lung sounds c. breathing without effort	*Assess airway clearance.* • Auscultate lungs before and after child coughs • Be alert for clearance of sputum from respiratory tract (Young children rarely expectorate sputum; they swallow it instead. Clearing of loud upper airway rales with coughing is an indication of clearance in this case. Swallowed sputum can also be observed in products of nasogastric suction or in vomitus) • Monitor characteristics of sputum • Observe for use of accessory muscles in breathing (which would indicate increased effort in moving air) *Decrease accumulation and pooling of secretions.* • Ensure that child changes position every 1–2 hr • Liquify secretions by providing humidified oxygen and fluids as ordered *Facilitate clearance of sputum.* • Administer mucolytic treatments via nebulizer, or coordinate these treatments with the respiratory therapist • Gently suction secretions from the mouth and nose of the infant or toddler, especially after respiratory treatments or crying (activities that expand the lungs facilitate mucus clearance) • Encourage the preschooler and older child to breathe deeply and cough to remove mucus • Perform (or assist the respiratory therapist with) chest physiotherapy and postural drainage as ordered *Alert the physician to signs of increasing airway obstruction.*

Analysis: Nursing Diagnosis 5

Potential for infection: pneumonia, related to microorganism invasion of debris-clogged airways

Defining Characteristics

Subjective: Chest pain

Objective: Fever, increased anorexia, lethargy, increasing dyspnea and cyanosis, increased WBC (in bacterial pneumonia), chest roentgenograph indicative of infiltration, positive sputum culture

Continued

Table 52-10 (continued)

Client Goal/ Evaluation Criteria	Nursing Goals/Strategies (Selected Rationale)
5. Client will remain free of pneumonia as evidenced by: a. remaining afebrile b. maintaining or improving respiratory capacity c. absence of unexplained fatigue d. WBC within normal limits e. lungs free of infiltration on chest roentgenography f. negative sputum culture	*Assess for and report signs and symptoms of pneumonia.* • Measure temperature every 4 hr and remain alert for tachypnea and tachycardia • Auscultate for adventitious or diminished breath sounds (diminished breath sounds may also be related to decreased excursion) • Observe sputum for purulent (yellow or green) appearance • Monitor WBC and chest roentgenography reports • Assist with sputum collection for culture and monitor laboratory reports • Observe for unexplained lethargy and fatigue *Decrease the risk of lung infection.* • Practice meticulous handwashing! • Observe established unit precautions for infection control • Ensure that family members and other visitors understand infection control practices • Prevent exposure of the child to persons with a respiratory infection (including health care professionals) • Change disposable oxygen tubing and humidification apparatus every 48–72 hr or according to unit policy (to prevent colonization of these surfaces) • Administer antibiotics as ordered for positive cultures • Establish good pulmonary toilet (turn, cough, and deep breathe; incentive spirometry; chest physical therapy, adequate fluids) • Be alert for signs of infection elsewhere in the body that may be spread to the lungs via the blood • Assess for changes in sensorium (e.g. increasing lethargy) and gastrointestinal disturbances (nausea, diarrhea, abdominal distention) which may indicate an infectious process *Alert physician to signs of infection in respiratory tract or elsewhere.*

Analysis: Nursing Diagnosis 6

Fluid volume deficit: vascular: hypovolemia, related to the shift of intravascular fluid to interstitial spaces associated with increased capillary permeability in injured tissues

Defining Characteristics

Subjective: Thirst

Objective: Decreased urine output; increased specific gravity of urine; increased hematocrit related to hemoconcentration; decreased blood pressure; rapid, thready pulse; decreased peripheral perfusion (decreased peripheral pulses, slow capillary refill time in nailbeds); marked edema surrounding burned tissues; decreased bowel sounds; decreased central venous pressure (CVP) (if central venous line)

Client Goal/ Evaluation Criteria	Nursing Goals/Strategies (Selected Rationale)
6. Client will maintain adequate vascular volume to prevent hypovolemic shock as evidenced by: a. maintaining urine output of 1 ml/kg/hr (children) or 30–50 ml/hr (children > 30 kg) b. heart rate and BP normal for age c. usual mental status d. absence of thirst e. rapid capillary refill in nailbeds f. hematocrit within normal limits g. CVP at 3–10 mmHg h. normal skin perfusion	*Monitor for vascular volume deficit.* • Insert an indwelling catheter (if ordered) and attach to a collection bag designed to measure hourly urine output • Weigh child and calculate expected hourly urine output parameters [e.g., (1 ml)(10 kg) = 10 ml/hr] • Measure and record urine output hourly; then drain urine from hourly collection chamber into larger collection bag • Monitor for tachycardia of 40 points or more above baseline and for hypotension. Measure vital signs under like conditions (BP should be taken with the child in the same position each time. Note: Blood pressure can be misleading in the burned limb in which progressive edema occurs. As the swelling increases the auditory signal diminishes) • Assess capillary refill by depressing nailbeds in the fingers and toes and observing how rapidly color returns • Assess skin perfusion—whether cool, clammy, mottled or warm and dry • Monitor hematocrit levels • Obtain serum chemistries as ordered—Na^+, K^+, Cl, HCO_3, BUN, glucose *Maintain intravenous fluid therapy as ordered.* The intravenous fluid ordered will be carefully selected to replace electrolytes as well as fluid. Colloid (e.g., albumin, fresh frozen plasma) may also be added • Watch glucose levels for infants and toddlers (who have reduced capacity to store and mobilize glucose). If glucose levels drop, dextrose may be added to the IV fluid • Record parenteral intake hourly (it is important to maintain a steady IV rate to prevent volume deficit or overload)

Analysis: Nursing Diagnosis 7

Potential fluid volume excess: vascular: hypervolemia, related to
- *excessive intravenous fluids*
- *reversal of plasma shift without appropriate decrease in intravenous fluid administration*

Defining Characteristics

Objective: Dyspnea, rapid, shallow respirations with presence of rales (crackles), tachycardia, hypertension, gallop heart rhythm, jugular venous distention, restlessness, anxiety, marked decrease in hematocrit

Client Goal/ Evaluation Criteria	Nursing Goals/Strategies (Selected Rationale)
7. Client will not experience hypervolemia as evidenced by: a. clear breath sounds or no increase in adventitious sounds	*Monitor for and report signs and symptoms of hypervolemia.* • Monitor for dyspnea; rales (crackles); tachycardia; clear, frothy sputum; extra heart sounds (S_3, S_4); changes in mental status; and distention of neck veins • Monitor hematocrit values • Monitor chest radiographs

Continued

Table 52-10 (continued)

Client Goal/ Evaluation Criteria	Nursing Goals/Strategies (Selected Rationale)
b. stable pulse and blood pressure c. absence of gallop rhythm (no extra heart sounds) d. absence of distended neck veins e. usual mental status f. hematocrit within normal limits	*Prevent fluid volume overload.* • Maintain intravenous fluids at prescribed rate. Do not increase rate to accommodate for a period of slow infusion without checking with the physician

Analysis: Nursing Diagnosis 8

Altered comfort: pain, related to
- *trauma to sensitive tissues and regenerating nerves during dressing changes and wound debridement*
- *tissue removal at skin graft sites*

Defining Characteristics

Subjective: Crying, verbal report of "hurt" or discomfort

Objective: Diaphoresis, squirming, rigidity, trembling, agitation, irritability, facial expression of discomfort, changes in vital signs, inconsolable infant, anorexia, withdrawal, sleep disturbance (Atchison, Guercio, and Monaco, 1986)

Client Goal/ Evaluation Criteria	Nursing Goals/Strategies (Selected Rationale)
8. Client will experience a minimum amount of pain as evidenced by: a. absence of crying, whimpering b. verbalization of comfort c. physical behaviors appropriate for age (i.e., neither agitated nor lying without movement) d. vital signs within normal limits e. appetite stable f. sleep unaffected by burn wounds	*Assess for pain related to the burn wounds and donor sites.* (Burn pain is known to fluctuate; children may be quite comfortable at rest, but usually experience a great deal of pain with dressing changes and debridement. Donor sites will be very sensitive) • Note crying, whimpering and other vocalizations of pain • Observe the infant and nonverbal child for alteration in normal movements that may indicate pain (either unusual quietness or agitation) • Talk with the preschooler and older child about level of comfort; see Chapter 29 for a discussion of pain assessment instruments • Note changes in vital signs that correspond with other signs and symptoms of pain • Note child's ability for uninterrupted sleep • Ask for the parent's help in evaluating comfort *Relieve unnecessary pain.* • Administer analgesics as needed so that their peak therapeutic action will occur during painful procedures

- Consider distraction techniques (e.g., music via headphones), stress-management techniques (e.g., muscle relaxation), and strategies to maximize predictability and controllability of the procedures for the child (Choose from these strategies on the basis of developmental age, personality, prior coping techniques, and input from the parent and child concerning the likelihood the strategy will be successful)

Analysis: Nursing Diagnosis 9

Potential for infection:
Wound infection, related to
- *loss of protective skin barrier*
- *decreased vascular supply to damaged tissues*
- *diminished immune response*
- *favorable medium for pathogens*

Septicemia, related to uncontained primary infection or invasion of pathogens at indwelling catheter sites

Defining Characteristics

Objective Characteristics of Wound Infection: Fever; redness of skin surrounding burn wounds; purulent drainage; increased WBC; ulceration of the burn wound; deteriorating or pale, waxy granulation tissue; wound culture positive for pathogenic organisms

Objective Characteristics of Sepsis: Fever; lethargy; recurrence or persistence of paralytic ileus after the third postburn day; sudden rise or fall in WBC with an accentuated shift to the left (i.e., increase in mature and immature neutrophils); evidence of infection in burn wound, lungs, urine, IV sites or abdomen (Stein, 1985)

Client Goals/ Evaluation Criteria	Nursing Goals/Strategies (Selected Rationale)
9.1 Client will remain free of wound infection as evidenced by: a. skin around burned area free of erythema b. wound free of purulent exudate and ulceration c. healthy granulation tissue d. WBC within normal limits e. wound culture negative for pathogens	*Monitor and report signs and symptoms of wound infection.* • Inspect the burn wounds daily for erythema, exudate, ulceration and deterioration of granulation tissue; make a detailed record of this assessment • Report the first evidence of erythema at the burn wound perimeter (often the first sign of infection) • Monitor lab reports of WBC • Culture wounds 1–2 times per week or according to unit policy *Prevent wound infection* by meticulous handwashing, aseptic technique, use of chlorine or other disinfecting agent in hydrotherapy tub, debridement of dead tissue, and application of topical antimicrobial agent
9.2 Client will remain free of sepsis as evidenced by: a. remaining afebrile b. absence of lethargy c. return of bowel sounds d. WBC at baseline level e. negative cultures of burn wounds, sputum, urine, central venous catheter sites, and blood	*Monitor and report signs and symptoms of sepsis.* • Record temperature every 4 hr • Observe for lethargy that persists despite rest, sleep, and relief of boredom • Auscultate for bowel sounds every 8 hr • Monitor laboratory reports of cultures of burn wounds, sputum, urine, central venous catheter sites, and blood • Monitor signs and symptoms of infection in burn wounds (see goal 9.1), respiratory tract, genitourinary tract, at sites of IV insertion and the GI tract.

Continued

Table 52-10 (continued)

Client Goal/ Evaluation Criteria	Nursing Goals/Strategies (Selected Rationale)
	Decrease the risk of systemic infection. • Administer prophylactic antibiotics as ordered • Change catheter and connecting tubings every 48–72 hr according to unit policies (to decrease bacterial colonization) • Change oxygen tubings and humidification apparatus every 48–72 hr according to unit policies • Wash and disinfect humidifier units at least every 48 hr (to prevent aerosolization of pathogens) • Wash hands before and after every patient contact • Observe aseptic technique for invasive procedures

Analysis: Nursing Diagnosis 10

Altered nutrition: less than body requirements, related to hypermetabolism associated with the body's need to restore burned tissues

Defining Characteristics

Subjective: Anorexia, verbal refusal of food, report of fatigue

Objective: Weight loss, delay in wound healing, caloric intake less than prescribed for wound healing

Client Goal/ Evaluation Criteria	Nursing Goals/Strategies (Selected Rationale)
10. Client will ingest sufficient calories to compensate for catabolism and to rebuild damaged tissues as evidenced by: a. manitaining/slowly increasing body weight b. possessing energy for activities of daily living c. wound healing d. ingestion of prescribed calories	*Maintain NPO status during the emergent phase.* Hypovolemia during this period contributes to paralytic ileus) • Insert a nasogastric (NG) tube as ordered and maintain it to low suction • Administer antacids or Cimetidine as ordered, clamping the NG tube for 15–20 min after the antacid is inserted. (The child with burns is at increased risk for duodenal ulceration [Curling's ulcer] because of the increased levels of corticosteroids associated with the physiologic response to stress) • Monitor for return of bowel sounds (often by 2nd day) *Encourage oral intake after return of bowel sounds.* • Obtain a detailed history of the child's eating habits and food preferences • Work with the family and the dietitian to provide appetizing meals and snacks • Make small servings of nutritious, protein-rich food available frequently • Monitor urine urea nitrogen. (A positive 4 to 6 grams/24 hours indicates adequate protein intake) • Avoid a power struggle with the child regarding eating; see the section on feeding the hospitalized child in Table 31-2 • Never threaten the child with enteral feeding in an attempt to increase oral intake (the child who needs enteral feeding

should not feel it is a punishment. In some institutions feeding tubes such as the Kao-feed tube are inserted routinely for children with burns greater than 15 to 20% of body surface. This eliminates the struggle over intake and the child's feeling of failure)

Monitor for and report insufficient caloric intake.
- Weigh daily (in emergent phase weight is needed to assess fluid volume, later it is a gauge of adequate intake for healing)
- Keep accurate record of caloric intake (calorie count)
- Monitor activity tolerance

Analysis: Nursing Diagnosis 11

Potential impaired mobility, related to
- *contractures and formation of scar tissue*
- *muscle atrophy associated with significant decrease in physical activity*

Defining Characteristics

Objective: Limitation in range of motion; scarring of burn wounds, which contracts skin and muscle tissue; decreased circumference of muscle mass in limbs; decreased limb strength

Client Goal/ Evaluation Criteria	Nursing Goals/Strategies (Selected Rationale)
11. Client will maintain maximum joint mobility within limitations imposed by the burn injury as evidenced by: a. optimum range of motion in all joints b. minimum of scar tissue c. maintenance of muscle mass	*Prevent contractures.* • Position (with assistance of physical therapist) to prevent deformities (see Table 52-9) • Initiate or assist with an exercise program to maintain muscle strength and joint mobility; enlist help of child and family in performing the exercises several times per day • Encourage play and diversional activities that include limb movement and position changes • Resume exercise to grafted areas as soon as allowed *Minimize scar formation.* • Prevent infection (see goal 9.1) • Utilize fine mesh gauze for dressings (to flatten granulation tissue) • Instruct child and family in use of pressure splints, elastic bandages, or pressure garments to reduce hypertrophy of scar tissue

Assessment of Emotional-Social Function

Self-concept

Subjective Assessment

Verbalization of feelings about self, perception of acceptance by others, feelings of adequacy and ability to perform, projections for the future

Objective Assessment

Affect, posture, social interactions, grooming, behavioral reaction to wounds

Continued

Table 52-10 (continued)

Analysis: Nursing Diagnosis 12

Disturbance in self-concept: body image, related to
- *burn wounds*
- *scars*
- *elasticized apparel to reduce scar formation*

Defining Characteristics

Subjective: Verbalization of fear of (or actual) rejection by others; focus on altered appearance; expression of negative feelings about self or of feelings of hopelessness, helplessness; preoccupation with body changes

Objective: Refusal to look at wounds; refusing visits from friends; change in usual peer interactions; change in usual affect (e.g., becoming quiet, sullen, withdrawn); lack of interest in personal appearance, especially for school-age child or adolescent

Client Goal/ Evaluation Criteria	Nursing Goals/Strategies (Selected Rationale)
12. Client will maintain a positive body image as evidenced by: a. verbalizing positive feelings about self b. verbalizing plans for play, school activities, and so on c. maintaining usual communication patterns and affect d. explaining to others about wounds, scars, and pressure apparel	*Listen and observe for verbal and nonverbal evidence of the child's feelings about changes in appearance. Facilitate a positive body image.* • Encourage family members to talk about and deal with their feelings about the child's appearance (so they can, in turn, be most supportive of the child) • Encourage the child to verbalize feelings about the burns and treatments, and the reactions of others • Explain burn injuries matter-of-factly (a calm and straightforward manner can be reassuring to both child and parent) • Do not contribute to false hopes about plastic surgery (plastic surgery may restore function but can rarely remove all evidence of the burn) • Acknowledge the feelings of grief and sadness expressed by the child and by family members (acknowledgment validates reality and facilitates problem solving) • Encourage contact with extended family and friends during the rehabilitation phase (so child can gradually test a new body image) • Encourage parents to enforce usual rules of conduct and expectations of courtesy (children will feel more secure and maintain more self-esteem if they perceive that adults still find them "capable" of preinjury behavior) • Encourage a visit from a burn "graduate" and/or family • Supply information about burn camps available at major treatment centers • Provide information about school re-entry programs for school-age children

(Based upon Stein, 1985; Atchison et al., 1986; Lybarger, 1987; with contributions from Kris Johnson, RN, Burn Clinician, The Children's Hospital, Denver, Colorado.)

References

Abrams RG, Josell SD: Common oral and dental emergencies and problems. *Pediatr Clin North Am* 1982 Jun; 29(3):681–715.

Atchison N, Guercio P, Monaco C: Pain in the pediatric burn patient: nursing assessment and perception. *Issues Compr Pediatr Nurs* 1986; 9:399–409.

Budassi-Shechy S, Barber J: *Emergency Nursing: Principles and Practice.* St Louis, CV Mosby, 1985.

Chisolm JJ: Increased lead absorption and lead poisoning. *In* Behrman RE, Vaughan VC: *Nelson Textbook of Pediatrics.* 13th ed. Philadelphia, WB Saunders, 1987, 1507–1510.

Coln D: Pediatric trauma. *AORN* 1985 Sep; 42(3):338–342.

Conn AW: Drowning and near-drowning. *In* Behrman RE, Vaughan VC (eds): *Nelson Textbook of Pediatrics.* 13th ed. Philadelphia, WB Saunders, 1987, 220–223.

Conner GH: Foreign bodies of the ear, nose, airway, and esophagus. *In* Hoekelman RA, et al (eds): *Primary Pediatric Care.* St. Louis, Mosby, 1987, 1243–1247.

Cropley C, Bloom R: *Student's Manual for Neonatal Resuscitation.* American Heart Association, 1987.

Dickerman JD, Lucey JF: *Smith's The Critically Ill Child: Diagnosis and Medical Management.* 3rd ed. Philadelphia, WB Saunders, 1985.

Done AK: Nomogram for interpretations of salicylate levels following acute ingestion. *Pediatrics* 1960; 26:800–807.

Drummond AH: Lead poisoning in children. *J School Health* 1981 Jan; 51(1):43–47.

Eland J: Grand Rounds Presentation at The Children's Hospital, Denver, 1987.

Elliott CH, Olson RA: The management of children's distress in response to painful medical treatment for burn injuries. *Behav Res Ther* 1983; 21(6):675–683.

Evaluation of Emergency Medical Services with a National Burn Registry, 1975–1978. Grant #HS-01906-01; HEW, National Center for Health Services Research; University of Michigan School of Public Health, Department of Biostatistics; and National Institute for Burn Medicine.

Feller I, Crane K: National burn information exchange. *Surg Clin North Am* 1970 Dec; 1425.

Fosnot H: Plant-ingestion poisoning from A to Z. *Patient Care* 1979 Jun 30; 86.

Gage AM, Gage AA: Frostbite. *Compr Ther* 1981 Sep; 7(9):25–30.

Gaudreault P, Lovejoy FH: Acute poisoning. *In* Dickerman JD, Lucey JF (eds): *Smith's The Critically Ill Child: Diagnosis and Medical Management.* 3rd ed. Philadelphia, WB Saunders, 1985.

Gaunder BN: Insect bites and stings: managing allergic reactions. *Nurse Pract* 1986 Mar; 11(3):16–28.

Haller JA: Pediatric trauma: the No. 1 killer of children. *JAMA* 1983 Jan 7; 249(1):47.

Harris B: The ABCs on a small scale. *Emerg Med* 1985 Feb 15; 24–32.

Hughes JG, Griffith JF: *Synopsis of Pediatrics.* St Louis, CV Mosby, 1984.

Kavanagh C: A new approach to dressing change in the severely burned child and its effect on burn-related psychopathology. *Heart Lung* 1983 Nov; 12(6):612–619.

Kavanagh KT, Litovitz T: Miniature foreign bodies in auditory and nasal cavities. *JAMA* Mar 21; 255(11):1470–1472.

Keim KA: Preventing and treating plant poisoning in young children. *MCN* 1983 Jul/Aug; 287–289.

Kinney MR, et al: *AACN's Clinical Reference for Critical-Care Nursing.* 2nd ed. New York, McGraw-Hill, 1988.

Lasoff EM, McEttrick MA: Participation versus diversion during dressing change: can nurses' attitudes change? *Iss Compr Pediatr Nurs* 1986; 9:391–398.

Lybarger PM: Inhalation injury in children: Nursing care. *Issues Compr Pediatr Nurs* 1987; 10(1):33–50.

Matlak ME: Foreign bodies. *In* Mayer TA: *Emergency Management of Pediatric Trauma.* Philadelphia, WB Saunders, 1985.

Mayer TA: *Emergency Management of Pediatric Trauma.* Philadelphia, WB Saunders, 1985.

McTigue DJ: Managing traumatic injuries in the young permanent dentition. *In* Pinkham JR: *Pediatric Dentistry: Infancy through Adolescence.* Philadelphia, WB Saunders, 1988.

Miles MS, Carter M: Sources of parental stress in pediatric intensive care units. *Child Health Care* 1982; 11:65–69.

Mofenson HC, Caraccio TR: Benefits/risks of syrup of ipecac. *Pediatrics* 1986 Apr; 77(4):551–552.

Mofenson H, Greensher J: Poisoning—an update. *Clin Pediatr* 1979; 18(3):144–146.

Mofenson HC, Greensher J: Management of the choking child. *Pediatr Clin North Am* 1985; 32(1):183–192.

Moore WR: Caustic ingestions: pathophysiology, diagnosis and treatment. *Clin Pediatr* 1986 Apr; 25(4):192–196.

Mortenson, ML: Management of acute childhood poisonings caused by selected insecticides and herbicides. *Pediatr Clin North Am* 1986; 33:421–445.

Needleman HL: Increased lead absorption and acute lead poisoning. *In* Gellis SS, Kagan BM: *Current Pediatric Therapy, II.* Philadelphia, WB Saunders, 1984.

Piomelli S, et al: Management of childhood lead poisoning. *J Pediatr* 1984 Oct; 105(4):523–532.

Reece RM: *Manual of Emergency Pediatrics.* 3rd ed. Philadelphia, WB Saunders, 1984.

Rothstein P: Psychological stress in families of children in a pediatric intensive care unit. *Pediatr Clin North Am* 1980; 27:613–620.

Rumack BH, Matthew H: Acetaminophen poisoning and toxicity. *Pediatrics* 1975; 55:871–876.

Rund DA, Rausch TS: *Triage.* St Louis, CV Mosby, 1981.

Seidel JS: Emergency medical services and the pediatric patient: are the needs being met? II. *Pediatrics* 1986 Nov; 78(5):808–812.

Standards and Guidelines for Cardiopulmonary Resuscitation (CPR) and Emergency Cardiac Care (ECC). *JAMA* 1986 Jun 6; 255(21):2905–2984.

Stein JM: Burns. *In* Zimmerman SS, Gildea JH (eds): *Critical Care Pediatrics.* Philadelphia, WB Saunders, 1985, 474–483.

Stickler J, Snowman T: A child drowns: a nursing perspective. *MCN* 1981 Sep/Oct; 6:324–328.

Temple AR: Poisoning. *In* Mayer TA: *Emergency Management of Pediatric Trauma.* Philadelphia, WB Saunders, 1985.

Tenenbein M: Pediatric toxicology: current controversies and recent advances. *Curr Prob Pediatr* 1986 Apr; XVI(4):1–233.

Thompson J: Near drowning. *In* Mayer TA: *Emergency Management of Pediatric Trauma.* Philadelphia, WB Saunders, 1985.

Bibliography

Bailey P: Pediatric esophageal foreign body with minimal symptomatology. *Ann Emerg Med* 1983; 12:452–454.

Banner W, Tong TG: Iron poisoning. *Pediatr Clin North Am* 1978 Apr; 33(2):393–410.

Bellucci RJ: Traumatic injuries of the middle ear. *Otolaryngol Clin North Am* 1983 Aug; 16(3):633–650.

Berger L, et al: Injuries from fireworks. *Pediatrics* 1985 May; 5:877–881.

Bergman AB, et al: Changing spectrum of serious child abuse. *Pediatrics* 1986 Jan; 77(1):113–116.

Berkowitz ES, Greenberg C: Child sexual abuse: the role of the NP. *Nurse Pract* 1986; 11:15–22.

Binder L, Anderson WA: Pediatric gastrointestinal foreign body ingestions. *Ann Emerg Med* 1984 Feb; 13:112–117.

Boehnert MT, et al: Advances in clinical toxicology. *Pediatr Clin North Am* 1985 Feb; 32(1):193–212.

Briggs L, Beyda D: Giving pediatric code drugs. No longer a calculated risk. *Nursing 86* 1986 Jul; 16(7):56.

Butler S: Out of the water, but not out of the woods. *RN* 1988 Jun: 26–30.

Cella DF, et al: Depression and stress responses in parents of burned children. *J Pediatr Psychol* 1988; 13(1):87–99.

Culbertson WW: Diagnosis and management of ocular injuries. *Otolaryngol Clin North Am* 1983 Aug; 16(3):563–573.

Donahue A: Beware of the obvious with near-drowning victims. *RN* 1982 Jun; 41–44.

Eichelberger MR, Randolph JG: Pediatric trauma: an algorithm for diagnosis and therapy. *J Trauma* 1983; 23:91–97.

Fikar C: Insect sting treatments. *Pediatrics* 1981 Nov; 68:744.

Fischer RG, Parks BR: Using insect repellents effectively. *Pediatr Nurs* 1986 May/Jun; 12(3):212.

Fuzea LE, et al: Acute poisoning in a children's hospital: a 2-year experience. *Pediatrics* 1986 Feb; 77(2):144–151.

Glass BL: Pediatric trauma units. *AORN* 1985; 42(3):353–356.

Golden H: Action stat! Near-drowning. *Nursing 88* 1988 Jul; 18(7):33.

Haddad LM, Winchester J: *Clinical Management of Poisoning and Overdose.* Philadelphia, WB Saunders, 1987.

Hansen M, et al: Psychological evaluation and support in the pediatric intensive care unit. *Pediatr Ann* 1986 Jan; 15(1).

Harris BM: Management of multiple trauma. *Pediatr Clin North Am* 1985 Feb; 32(1):175–182.

Hirschfeld JJ, Assnel LA: Conservative management of electric burns to the lips of children. *J Maxillofac Surg* 1984; 42(3):197–202.

Honeysett J: Epistaxis. *Nurs Times* 1982 Apr 7; 578–581.

Jacobson MS, et al: Follow-up of adolescent trauma victims: a new model of care. *Pediatrics* 1986; 77(2):236–241.

Josell SD: Traumatic injuries to the dentition and its supporting structures. *Pediatr Clin North Am* 1982; 29(3):717–741.

Kelley SJ: *Pediatric Emergency Nursing.* Norwalk, CT, Appleton & Lange, 1988.

Killam P, Smith K: Getting kids into car seats. *MCN* 1988 Mar/Apr; 13(2):124–126.

Klein BL, Simon JE: Hydrocarbon poisoning. *Pediatr Clin North Am* 1986; 33(2):411–420.

Lee EJ, Jacobson JM: Accident reports: Survey of high school injuries. *Pediatr Nurs* 1987 May/Jun; 13(3):151–154.

Leoni MP: Management of acetaminophen overdose. *Crit Care Nurse* 1985; 5(4):44–47.

McGuigan MA: Treatment of poisoning. *Clin Symp* 1984; 36(5):1–32.

McLoughlin E, Crawford JD: Burns. *Pediatr Clin North Am* 1985; 32(1):61–76.

Maniglia A, Kline S: Maxillofacial trauma in the pediatric age group. *Otolaryngol Clin North Am* 1983; 16(3):717–731.

Maxwell B: Smooth the way for safe emergency transfers. *RN* 1988 Jun: 34–37.

Reece RM, Grodin MA: Recognition of nonaccidental injury. *Pediatr Clin North Am* 1985; 32(1):41–60.

Reynolds EA, Ramenofsky ML: The emotional impact of trauma on toddlers. *MCN* 1988 Mar/Apr; 13(2):106–109.

Rimar JM: Shock in infants and children: Assessment and treatment. *MCN* 1988 Mar/Apr; 13(2):98–105.

Rogers GC, Matyunas NJ: Gastrointestinal decontamination for acute poisoning. *Pediatr Clin North Am* 1986; 33(2):261–286.

Ryan MT: Identifying the sexually abused child. *Pediatr Nurs* 1984; 10(6):419–421.

Saulsbury FT, Hayden GF: Skin conditions simulating child abuse. *Pediatr Emerg Care* 1985; 147–158.

Serra A: Epistaxis. *Nurs Mirror* 1982 Jul 14; vii-ix.

Sneed RC, et al: Spinal cord injury associated with all-terrain vehicle accidents. *Pediatrics* 1986 March; 77(3):271–274.

Snodgrass WR: Salicylate toxicity. *Pediatr Clin North Am* 1986 April; 33(2):381–392.

Spyker DA: Submersion injury: epidemiology, prevention and management. *Pediatr Clin North Am* 1985; 32(1):113–125.

Thomas DO: The ABCs of pediatric emergencies. *RN* 1986; 34–41.

Wall C: The real risk of acetaminophen overdose. *RN* 1985; 48(8):35–38.

Wasserman RL, Ginsburg CM: Caustic substance injuries. *J Pediatr* 1985; 107(2):169–174.

Welch J, Tyler J: Dealing with eye injuries. *RN* 1984 Mar; 53–54.

Nursing Diagnoses Accepted by NANDA *Through* 1988

Appendix One

The nursing diagnoses listed here are those currently accepted by the National Conferences on Nursing Diagnoses (used with permission from North American Nursing Diagnoses Association: *Taxonomy I with Complete Diagnoses.* St. Louis, NANDA). These diagnoses are working documents, with research and revision in progress. National Conferences gather nurses together every 2 years, but research in new categories and for accepted categories is an ongoing priority.

The Eighth National Conference approved 16 new nursing diagnoses in 1988; these are denoted by asterisks.

Diagnosis	**Definition**
Activity intolerance	A state in which an individual has insufficient physiologic or psychologic energy to endure or complete required or desired daily activities.
Activity intolerance, potential	A state in which an individual is at risk of experiencing insufficient physiologic or psychologic energy to endure or complete required or desired daily activities.
Adjustment, impaired	The state in which the individual is unable to modify his or her lifestyle/behavior in a manner consistent with a change in health status.
Airway clearance, ineffective	A state in which an individual is unable to clear secretions or obstructions from the respiratory tract to maintain airway patency.
Anxiety	A vague, uneasy feeling the source of which is often nonspecific or unknown to the individual.
*Aspiration, potential for	The state in which an individual is at risk for entry of gastrointestinal secretions, oropharyngeal secretions, or solids or fluids into tracheobronchial passages.
Body temperature, altered: potential	The state in which the individual is at risk for failure to maintain body temperature within normal range.
Bowel elimination, altered: constipation	A state in which an individual experiences a change in normal bowel habits characterized by decrease in frequency and/or passage of hard, dry stools.
Bowel elimination, altered: diarrhea	A state in which an individual experiences a change in normal bowel habits characterized by the frequent passage of loose, fluid, unformed stools.
Bowel elimination, altered: incontinence	A state in which an individual experiences a change in normal bowel habits characterized by involuntary passage of stool.
*Breastfeeding, ineffective	The state in which a mother, infant, or child experiences dissatisfaction or difficulty with the breastfeeding process.
Breathing pattern, ineffective	The state in which an individual's inhalation and/or exhalation pattern does not enable adequate pulmonary inflation or emptying.
Cardiac output, altered: decreased	A state in which the blood pumped by an individual's heart is sufficiently reduced that it is inadequate to meet the needs of the body's tissues.
Comfort, altered: chronic pain	A state in which the individual experiences pain that continues for more than 6 months in duration.
Comfort, altered: pain	A state in which an individual experiences and reports the presence of severe discomfort or an uncomfortable sensation.
Communication, impaired verbal	The state in which an individual experiences a decreased or absent ability to use or understand language in human interaction.
*Constipation, colonic	The state in which an individual's pattern of elimination is characterized by hard, dry stool that results from a delay in passage of food residue.

continued

Diagnoses	Definition
*Constipation, perceived	The state in which an individual makes a self-diagnosis of constipation and ensures a daily bowel movement through abuse of laxatives, enemas, and suppositories.
*Coping, defensive	The state in which an individual repeatedly projects falsely positive self-evaluation based on a self-protective pattern that defends against underlying perceived threats to positive self-regard.
Coping, family: potential for growth	The family member has effectively managed adaptive tasks involved with the client's health challenge and is exhibiting desire and readiness for enhanced health and growth in regard to self and in relation to client.
Coping, ineffective family: compromised	A usually supportive primary person (family member or close friend) is providing insufficient, ineffective, or compromised support, comfort, assistance, or encouragement which may be needed by the client to manage or master adaptive tasks related to his or her health challenge.
Coping, ineffective family: disabling	The behavior of a significant person (family member or other primary person) disables his or her own capacities and the client's capacities to effectively address tasks essential to either person's adaptation to the health challenge.
Coping, ineffective individual	Ineffective coping is the impairment of adaptive behaviors and problem-solving abilities of a person in meeting life's demands and roles.
*Decisional conflict (specify)	The state of uncertainty about course of action to be taken when choice among competing actions involves risk, loss, or challenge to personal life values.
*Denial, ineffective	The state of a conscious or unconscious attempt to disavow the knowledge or meaning of an event to reduce anxiety/fear to the detriment of health.
*Disuse syndrome, potential	A state in which an individual is at risk for deterioration of body systems as the result of prescribed or unavoidable musculoskeletal inactivity.
Diversional activity deficit	The state in which an individual experiences a decreased stimulation from or interest or engagement in recreational or leisure activities.
*Dysreflexia	The state in which an individual with a spinal cord injury at T7 or above experiences a life-threatening uninhibited sympathetic response of the nervous system to a noxious stimulus.
Family process, altered	The state in which a family that normally functions effectively experiences a dysfunction.
*Fatigue	An overwhelming sustained sense of exhaustion and decreased capacity for physical and mental work.
Fear	Fear is a feeling of dread related to an identifiable source which the person validates.
Fluid volume, altered: excess	The state in which an individual experiences increased fluid retention and edema.
Fluid volume deficit, actual	The state in which an individual experiences vascular, cellular, or intracellular dehydration.
Fluid volume deficit, potential	The state in which an individual is at risk of experiencing vascular, cellular, or intracellular dehydration.
Gas exchange, impaired	The state in which the individual experiences a decreased passage of oxygen and/or carbon dioxide between the alveoli of the lungs and the vascular system.
Grieving, anticipatory	
Grieving, dysfunctional	
Growth and development, altered	The state in which an individual demonstrates deviations in norms from his/her age group.
Health maintenance, altered	Inability to identify, manage, and seek out help to maintain health.
*Health-seeking behaviors (specify)	A state in which an individual in stable health is actively seeking ways to alter personal health habits and/or the environment in order to move toward a higher level of health.

Diagnosis	Definition
Home maintenance management, impaired	The client is unable to independently maintain a safe, growth-promoting immediate environment.
Hopelessness	A subjective state in which an individual sees limited or no alternatives or personal choices available and is unable to mobilize energy on own behalf.
Hyperthermia	A state in which an individual's body temperature is elevated above his/her normal range.
*Hypothermia	The state in which an individual's body temperature is reduced below normal range.
Incontinence, functional	The state in which an individual experiences an involuntary, unpredictable passage of urine.
Incontinence, reflex	The state in which an individual experiences an involuntary loss of urine, occurring at somewhat predictable intervals when a specific bladder volume is reached.
Incontinence, stress	The state in which an individual experiences a loss of urine of less than 50 ml occurring with increased abdominal pressure.
Incontinence, total	The state in which an individual experiences a continuous and unpredictable loss of urine.
Incontinence, urge	The state in which an individual experiences involuntary passage of urine occurring soon after a strong sense of urgency to void.
Infection, potential for	The state in which an individual is at increased risk for being invaded by pathogenic organisms.
Injury, potential for	A state in which the individual is at risk of injury as a result of environmental conditions interacting with the individual's adaptive and defensive resources.
Injury, potential for	
A. Poisoning, potential for	The client has accentuated risk of accidental exposure to or ingestion of drugs or dangerous products in doses sufficient to cause poisoning.
B. Suffocation, potential for	The client has accentuated risk of accidental suffocation (inadequate air is available for inhalation).
C. Trauma, potential for	The client has accentuated risk of accidental tissue injury, e.g., wound, burn, fracture.
Knowledge deficit (specify)	
Mobility, impaired physical	A state in which the individual experiences a limitation of ability for independent physical movement.
Noncompliance (specify)	Noncompliance is a person's informed decision not to adhere to a therapeutic recommendation.
Nutrition, altered: less than body requirements	The state in which an individual experiences an intake of nutrients insufficient to meet metabolic needs.
Nutrition, altered: more than body requirements	
Nutrition, altered: potential for more than body requirements	The state in which an individual is at risk of experiencing an intake of nutrients that exceeds metabolic needs.
Oral mucous membrane, altered	The state in which an individual experiences disruptions in the tissue layers of the oral cavity.
*Parental role conflict	The state in which a parent experiences role confusion and conflict in response to crisis.
Parenting, altered: actual or potential	Parenting is the ability of a nurturing figure(s) to create an environment that promotes the optimal growth and development of another human being. It is important to state as a preface to this diagnosis that adjustment to parenting in general is a normal maturational process that elicits nursing behaviors of prevention of potential problems and health promotion.
Post-trauma response	The state of an individual experiencing a sustained painful response to (an) unexpected extraordinary life event(s).
Powerlessness	The perception that one's own action will not significantly affect an outcome. Powerlessness is a perceived lack of control over a current situation or immediate happening.

continued

Diagnosis	Definition
Rape-trauma syndrome	Rape is forced, violent sexual penetration against the victim's will and without the victim's will and consent. The trauma syndrome that develops from this attack or attempted attack includes an acute phase or disorganization of the victim's lifestyle and a long-term process of reorganization of lifestyle.
Self-care deficit	A state in which the individual experiences an impaired ability to perform or complete feeding, bathing, toileting, dressing, and grooming activities for oneself.
Self-concepts, disturbance in: body image, self-esteem, role performance, personal identity	A disturbance in self-concept is a disruption in the way one perceives one's body image, self-esteem, role performance, and/or personal identity. These four subcomponents, in turn, have their own etiologies and defining characteristics.
*Self-esteem, low: chronic	Longstanding negative self-evaluation/feelings about self or self-capabilities.
*Self-esteem, low: situational	Negative self-evaluation/feelings about self that develop in response to a loss or change in an individual who previously had a positive self-evaluation.
*Self-esteem disturbance	Negative self-evaluation/feelings about self or self-capabilities, which may be directly or indirectly expressed.
Sensory-perceptual alterations: visual, auditory, kinesthetic, gustatory, tactile, olfactory perception	A state in which an individual experiences a change in the amount or patterning of incoming stimuli accompanied by a diminished, exaggerated, distorted, or impaired response to such stimuli.
Sexual dysfunction	The state in which an individual experiences a change in sexual function that is viewed as unsatisfying, unrewarding, or inadequate.
Sexuality, altered patterns	The state in which an individual expresses concern regarding his/her sexuality.
Skin integrity, impaired: actual	A state in which the individual's skin is adversely altered.
Skin integrity, impaired: potential	A state in which the individual's skin is at risk of being adversely altered.
Sleep pattern disturbance	Disruption of sleep time that causes a client discomfort or interferes with the desired lifestyle.
Social interaction, impaired	The state in which an individual participates in an insufficient or excessive quantity or ineffective quality of social exchange.
Social isolation	Condition of aloneness perceived as imposed by others and as a negative or threatening state.
Spiritual distress (distress of the human spirit)	Distress of the human spirit is a disruption in the life principle which pervades a person's entire being and which integrates and transcends one's biologic and psychosocial nature.
Swallowing, impaired	The state in which an individual has decreased ability to voluntarily pass fluids and/or solids from the mouth to the stomach.
Thermoregulation, ineffective	The state in which the individual's temperature fluctuates between hypothermia and hyperthermia.
Thought processes, altered	A state in which an individual experiences a disruption in cognitive operations and activities.
Tissue integrity, impaired	A state in which an individual experiences damage to mucous membrane or corneal, integumentary, or subcutaneous tissue.
Tissue perfusion, altered: cerebral, cardiopulmonary, renal, gastrointestinal, peripheral	The state in which an individual experiences a decrease in nutrition and oxygenation at the cellular level due to a deficit in capillary blood supply.
Unilateral neglect	The state in which an individual is perceptually unaware of and inattentive to one side of the body.
Urinary elimination, altered patterns	The state in which the individual experiences a disturbance in urine elimination.
Urinary retention	The state in which the individual experiences incomplete emptying of the bladder.
Violence, potential for: self-directed or directed at others	A state in which an individual experiences behaviors that can be physically harmful to either the self or others.

* 1988 additions to NANDA nursing diagnoses.

Height, Weight, and Head Circumference for Girls

GIRLS: BIRTH TO 36 MONTHS
PHYSICAL GROWTH
NCHS PERCENTILES*

NAME ______________________ RECORD # ____________

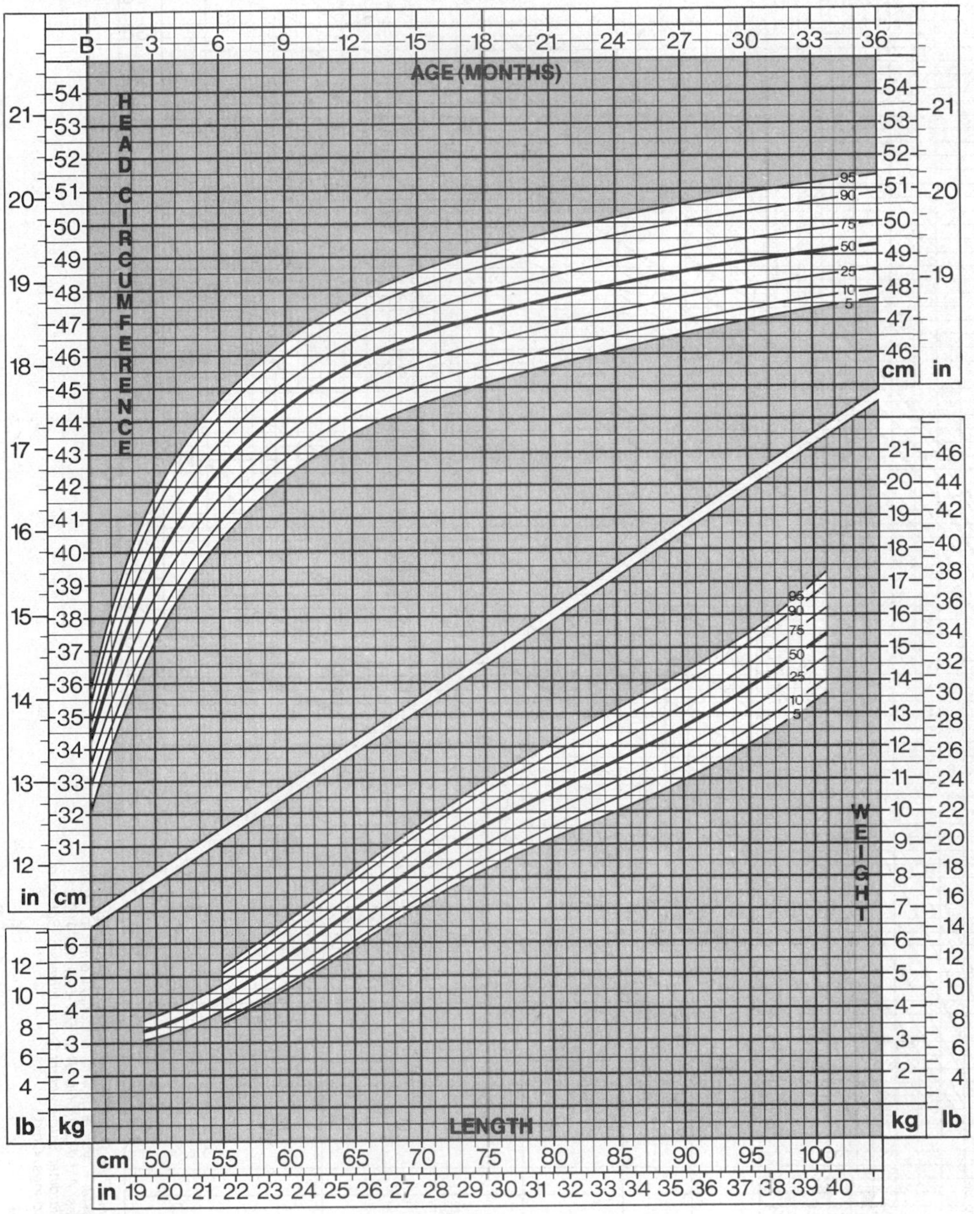

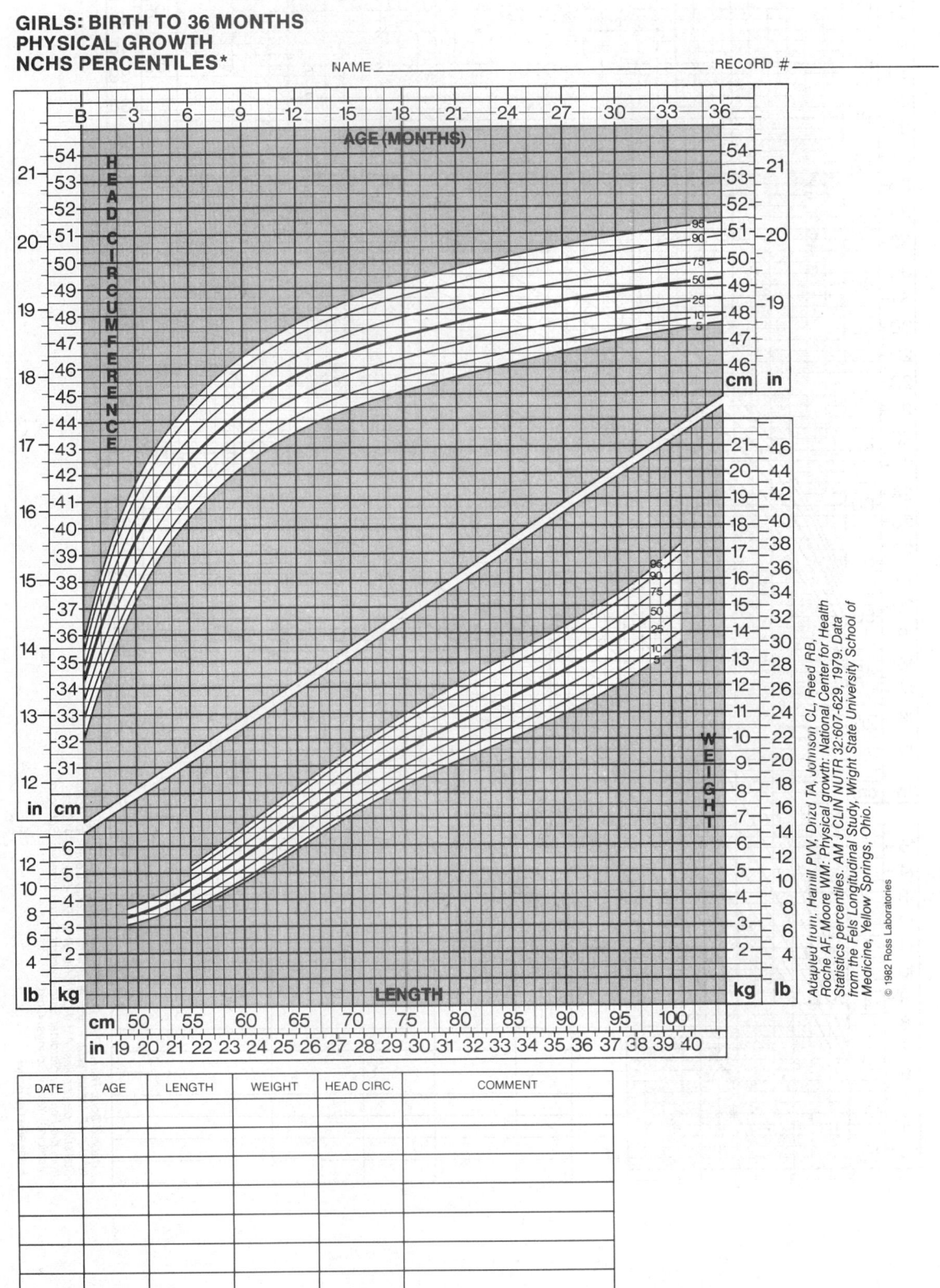

*Adapted from: Hamill PVV, Drizd TA, Johnson CL, Reed RB, Roche AF, Moore WM: Physical growth: National Center for Health Statistics percentiles. AM J CLIN NUTR 32:607-629, 1979. Data from the Fels Longitudinal Study, Wright State University School of Medicine, Yellow Springs, Ohio.

DATE	AGE	LENGTH	WEIGHT	HEAD CIRC.	COMMENT

GIRLS: BIRTH TO 36 MONTHS
PHYSICAL GROWTH
NCHS PERCENTILES*

NAME ______________________ RECORD # ____________

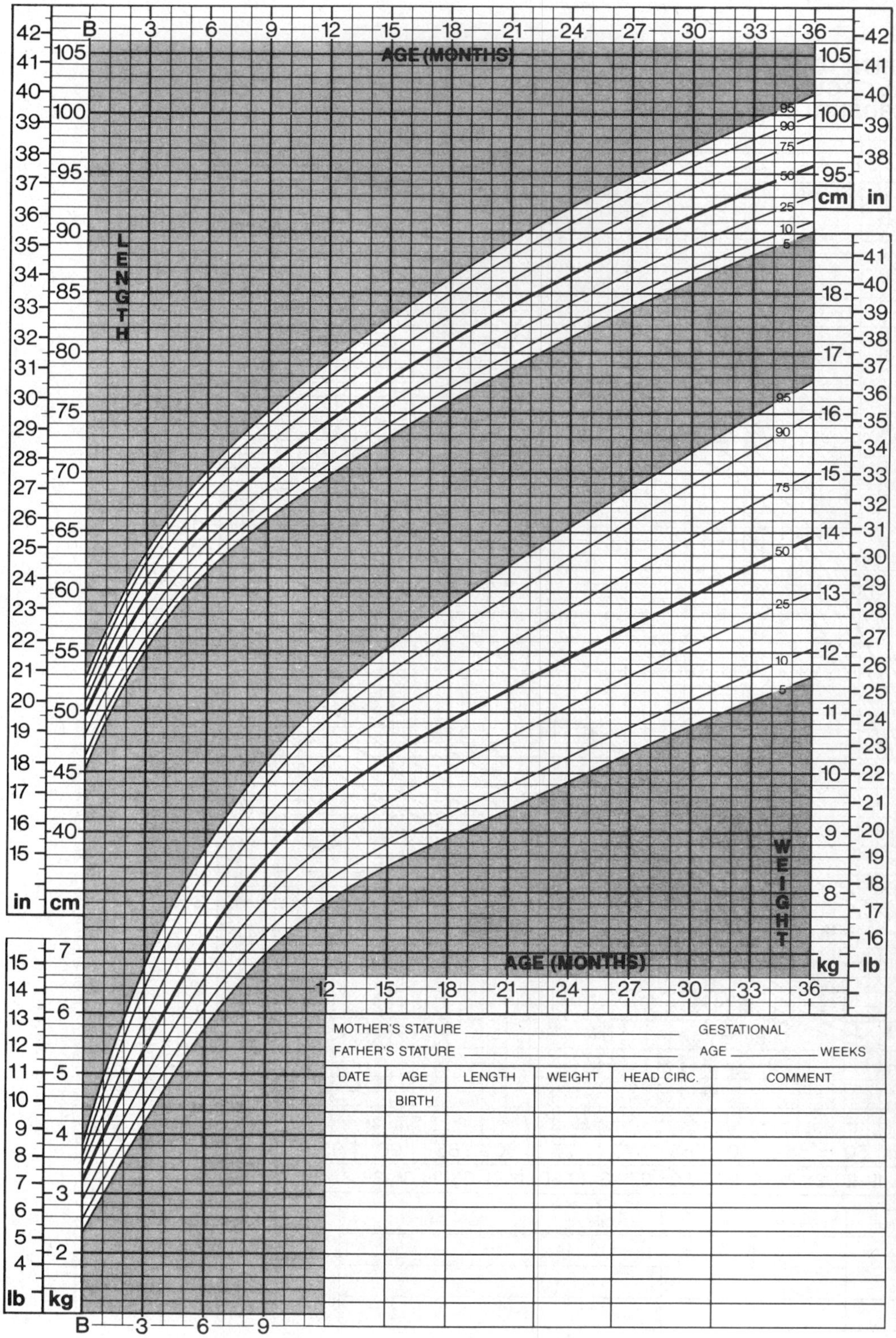

* Adapted from: Hamill PVV, Drizd TA, Johnson CL, Reed RB, Roche AF, Moore WM: Physical growth: National Center for Health Statistics percentiles. AM J CLIN NUTR 32:607-629, 1979. Data from the Fels Longitudinal Study, Wright State University School of Medicine, Yellow Springs, Ohio.

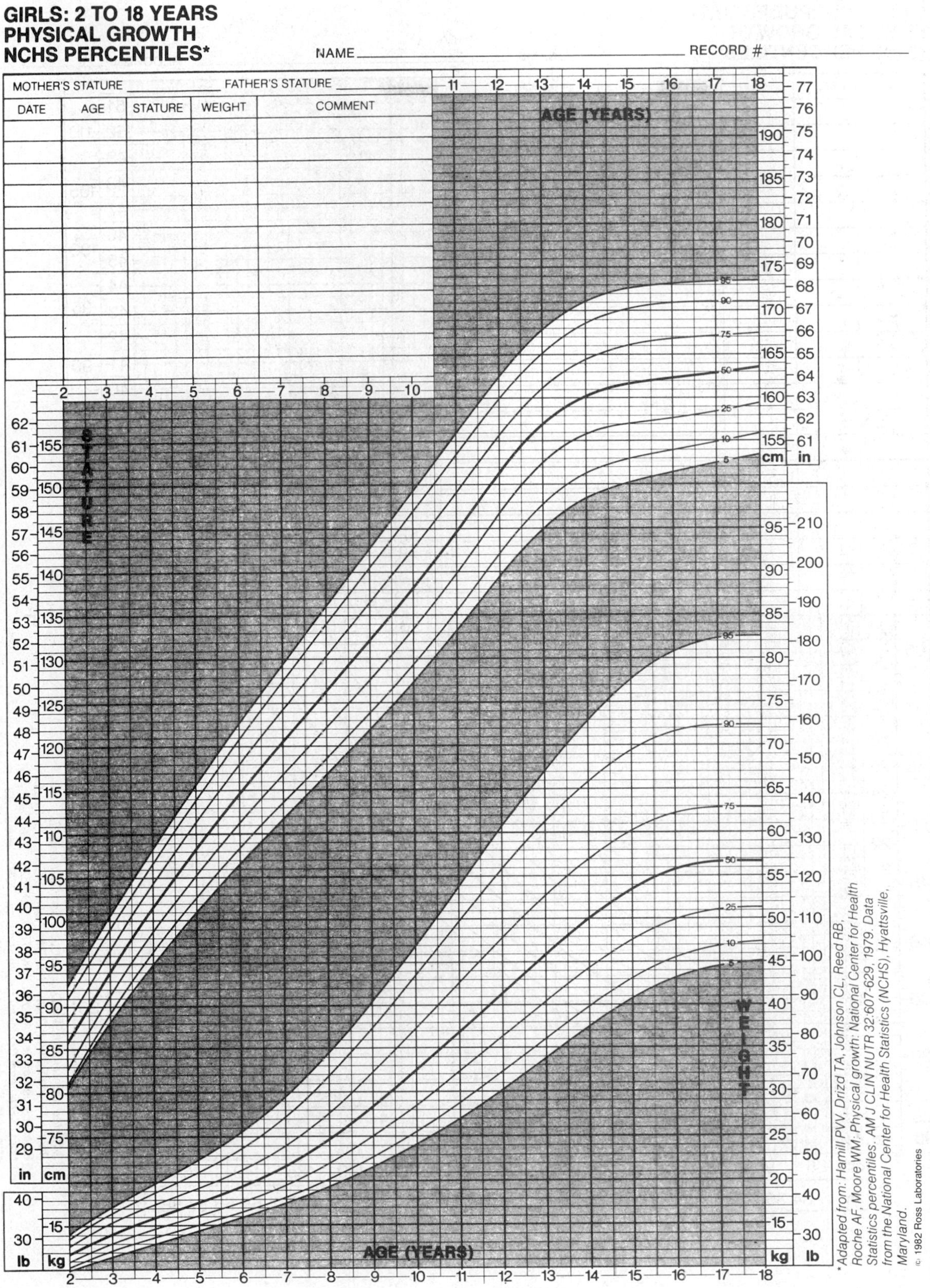
GIRLS: 2 TO 18 YEARS
PHYSICAL GROWTH
NCHS PERCENTILES*
NAME
RECORD #
MOTHER'S STATURE
FATHER'S STATURE
DATE
AGE
STATURE
WEIGHT
COMMENT
AGE (YEARS)
STATURE
WEIGHT
in
cm
lb
kg
*Adapted from: Hamill PVV, Drizd TA, Johnson CL, Reed RB, Roche AF, Moore WM: Physical growth: National Center for Health Statistics percentiles. AM J CLIN NUTR 32:607-629, 1979. Data from the National Center for Health Statistics (NCHS), Hyattsville, Maryland.
© 1982 Ross Laboratories

GIRLS: PREPUBESCENT PHYSICAL GROWTH NCHS PERCENTILES*

NAME____________________ RECORD #__________

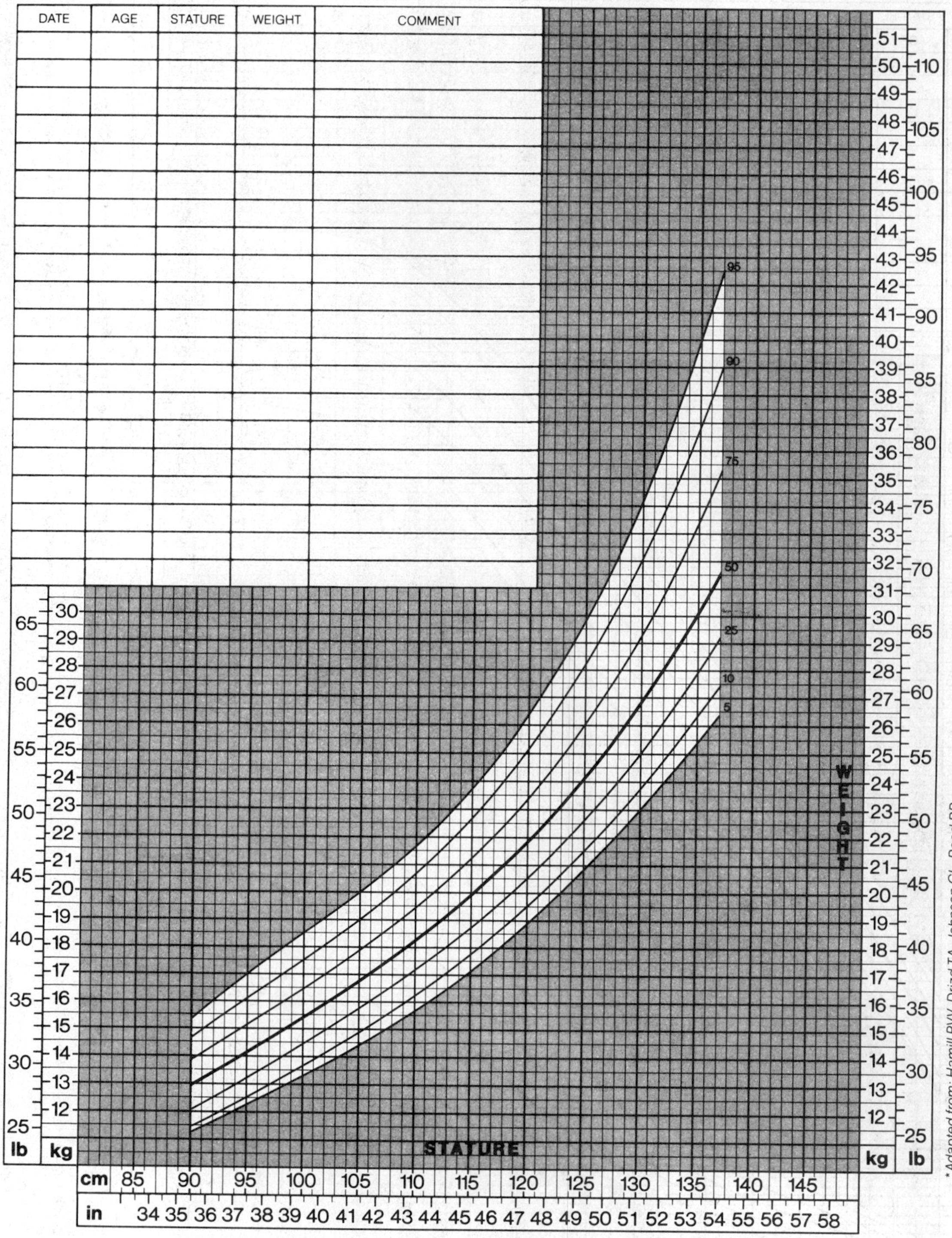

*Adapted from: Hamill PVV, Drizd TA, Johnson CL, Reed RB, Roche AF, Moore WM: Physical growth: National Center for Health Statistics percentiles. AM J CLIN NUTR 32:607-629, 1979. Data from the National Center for Health Statistics (NCHS), Hyattsville, Maryland.

Height, Weight, and Head Circumference for Boys

Appendix Three

**BOYS: BIRTH TO 36 MONTHS
PHYSICAL GROWTH
NCHS PERCENTILES***

NAME ____________________ RECORD # ____________

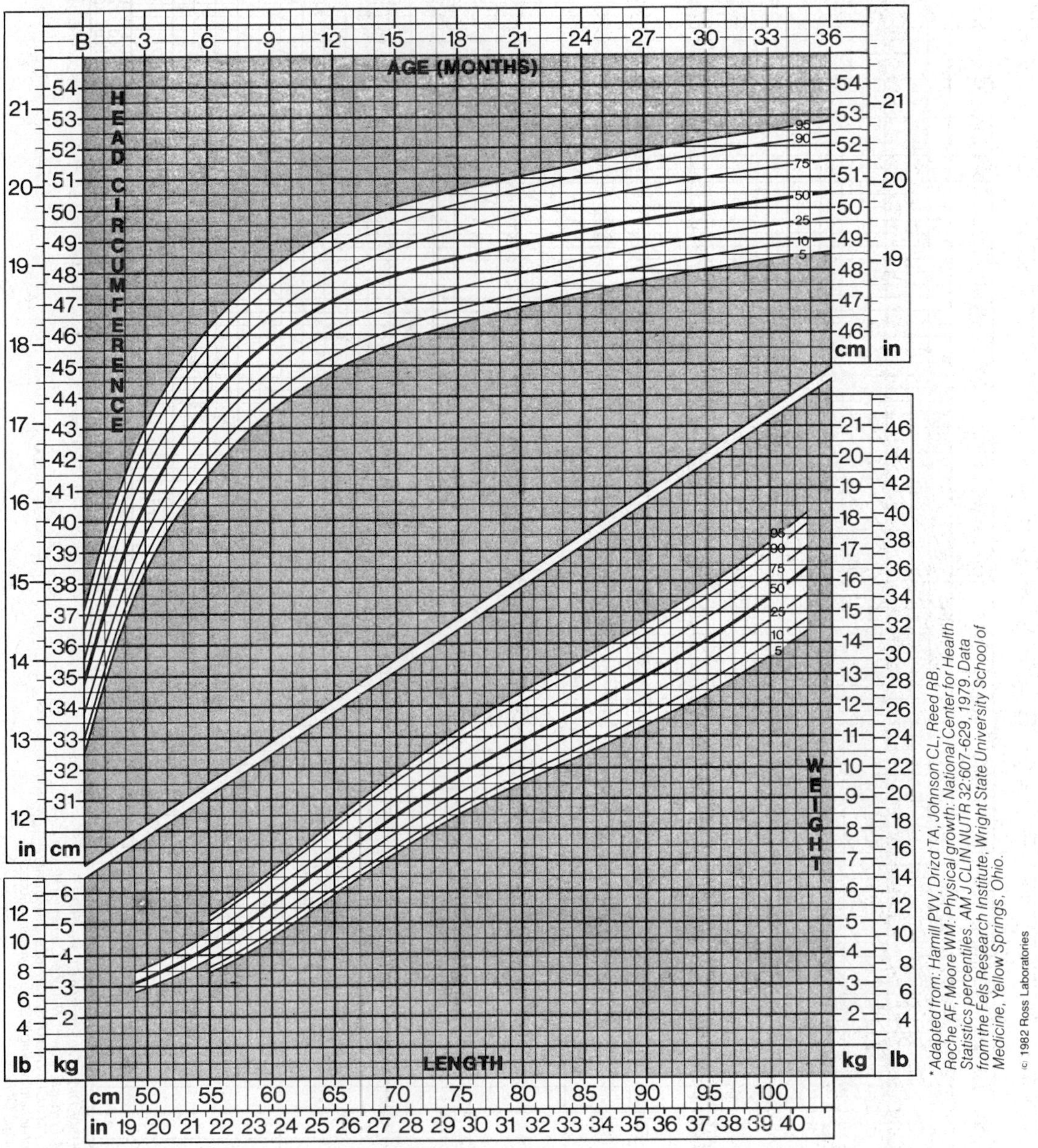

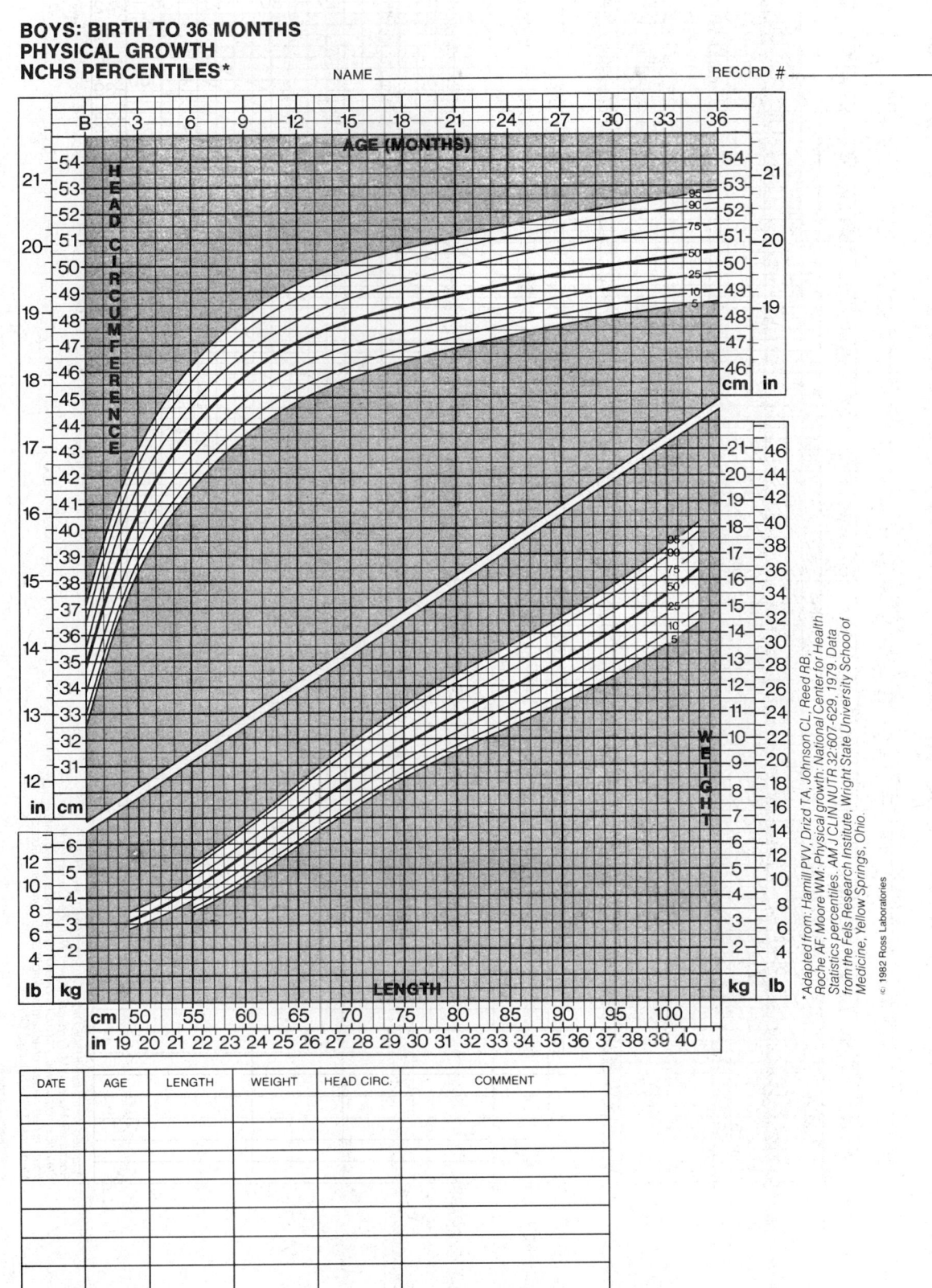

DATE	AGE	LENGTH	WEIGHT	HEAD CIRC.	COMMENT

BOYS: BIRTH TO 36 MONTHS
PHYSICAL GROWTH
NCHS PERCENTILES*

NAME ______________________ RECORD # ____________

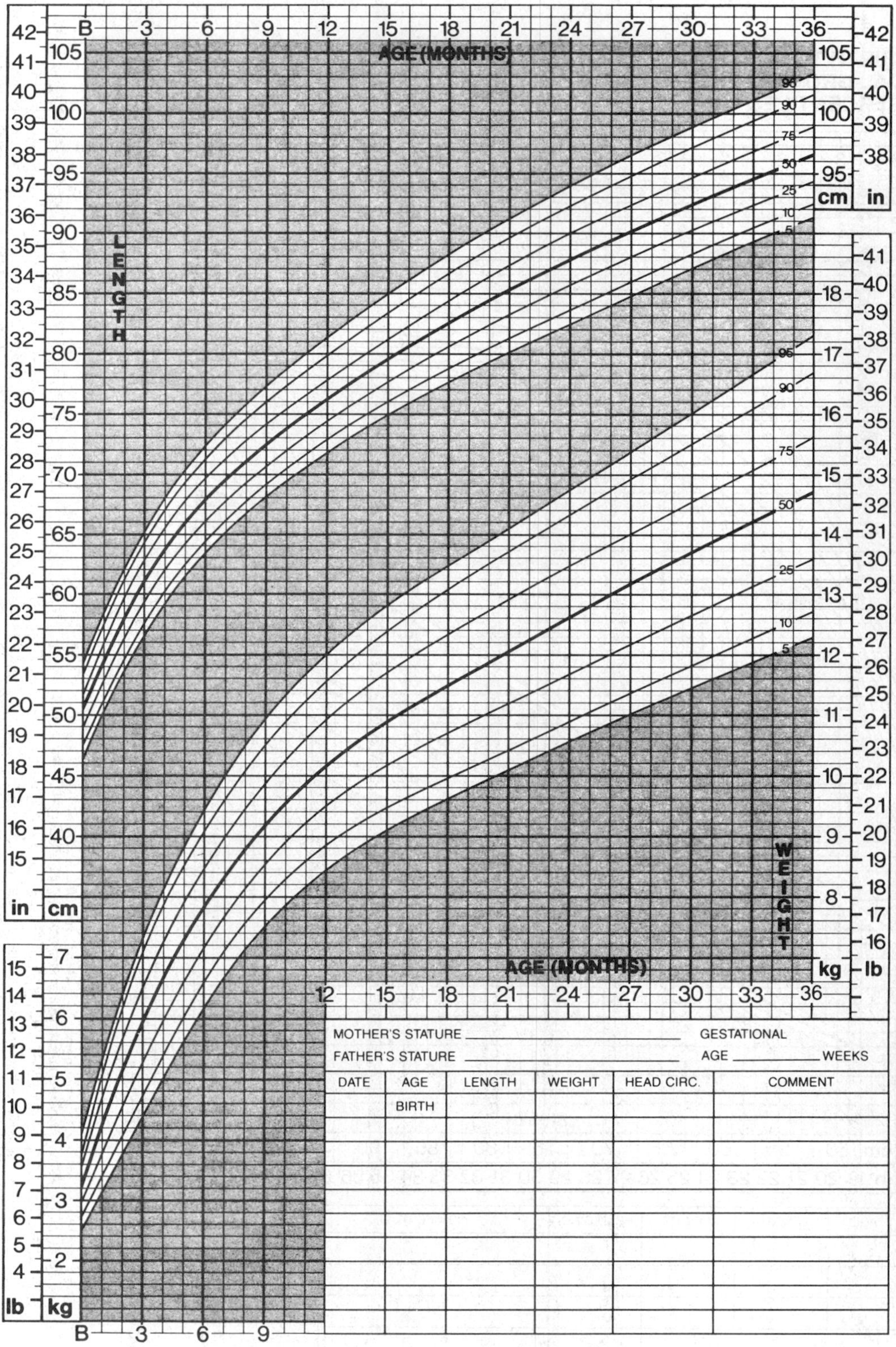

MOTHER'S STATURE ____________ GESTATIONAL
FATHER'S STATURE ____________ AGE ________ WEEKS

DATE	AGE	LENGTH	WEIGHT	HEAD CIRC.	COMMENT
	BIRTH				

*Adapted from: Hamill PVV, Drizd TA, Johnson CL, Reed RB, Roche AF, Moore WM: Physical growth: National Center for Health Statistics percentiles. AM J CLIN NUTR 32:607-629, 1979. Data from the Fels Research Institute, Wright State University School of Medicine, Yellow Springs, Ohio.

BOYS: 2 TO 18 YEARS
PHYSICAL GROWTH
NCHS PERCENTILES*

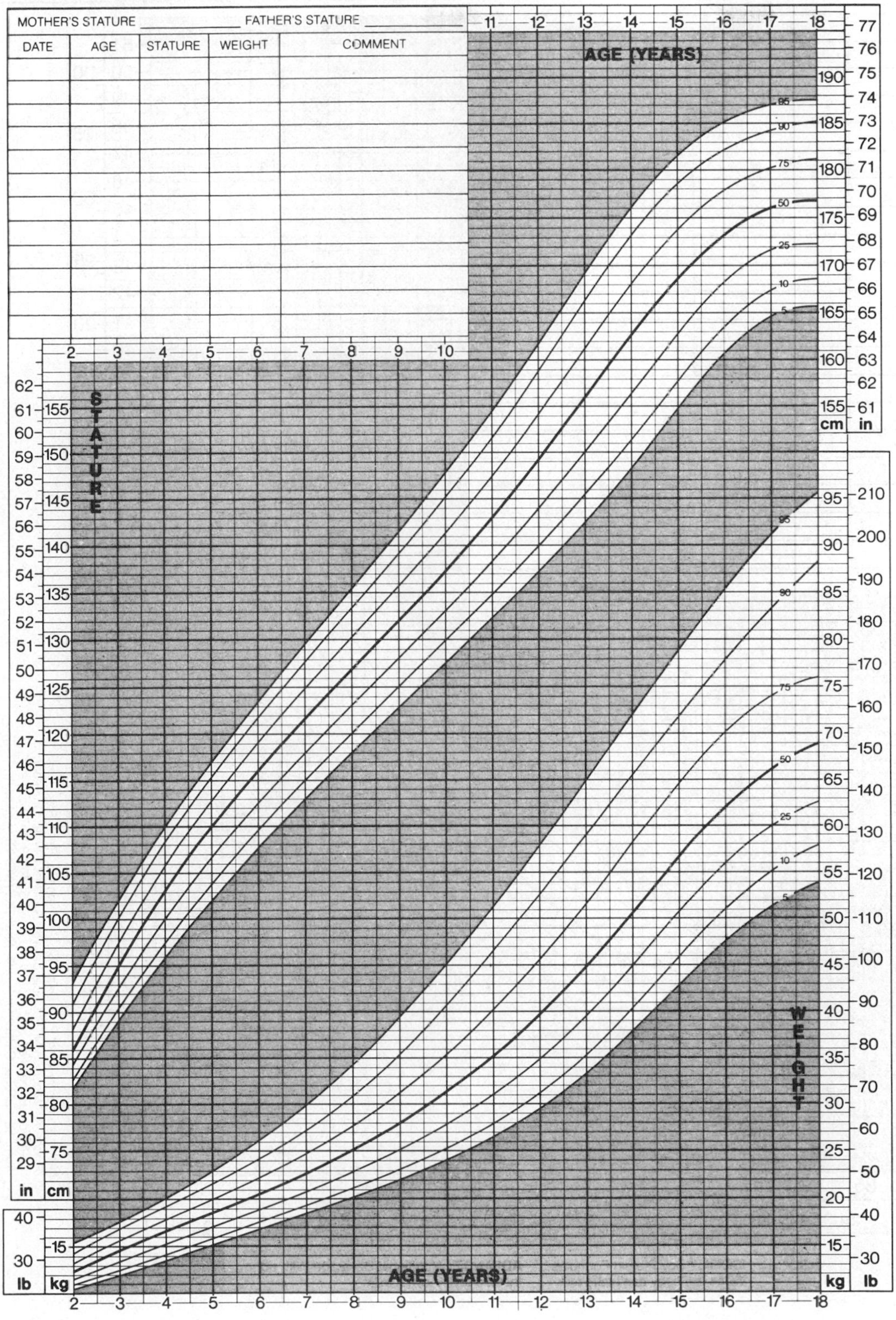

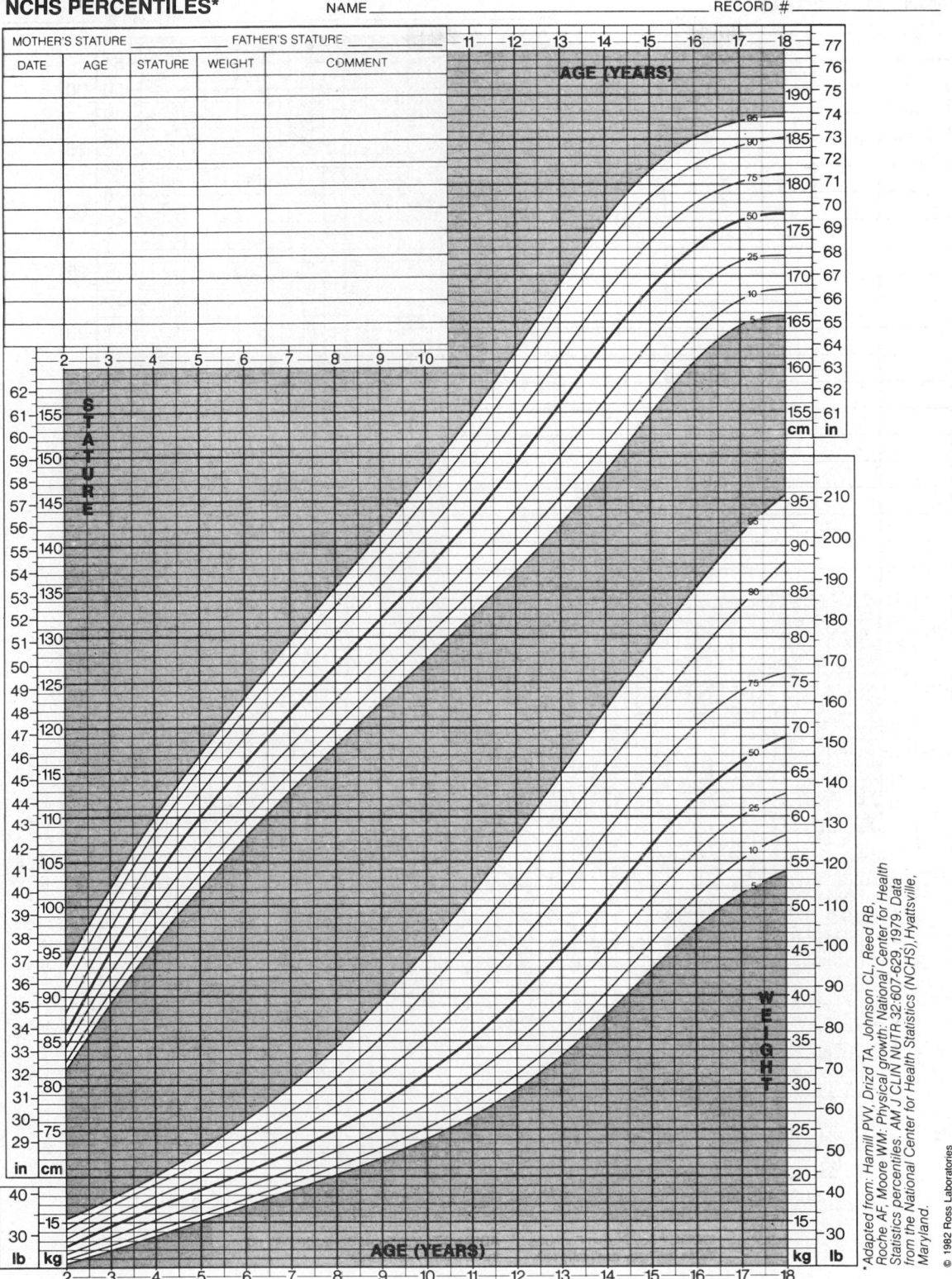

*Adapted from: Hamill PVV, Drizd TA, Johnson CL, Reed RB, Roche AF, Moore WM: Physical growth: National Center for Health Statistics percentiles. AM J CLIN NUTR 32:607-629, 1979. Data from the National Center for Health Statistics (NCHS), Hyattsville, Maryland.

BOYS: PREPUBESCENT PHYSICAL GROWTH NCHS PERCENTILES*

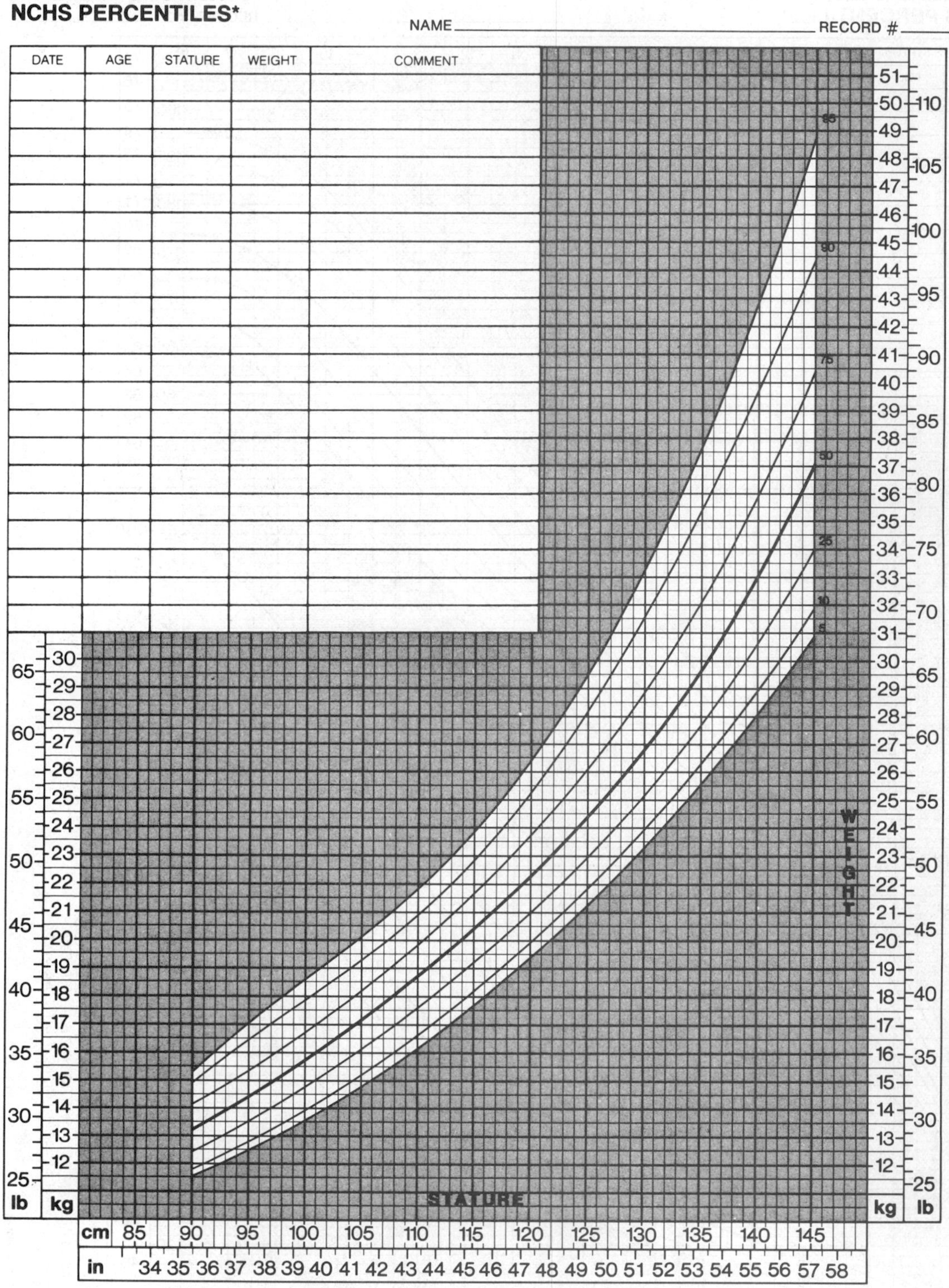

*Adapted from: Hamill PVV, Drizd TA, Johnson CL, Reed RB, Roche AF, Moore WM: Physical growth: National Center for Health Statistics percentiles. AM J CLIN NUTR 32:607-629, 1979. Data from the National Center for Health Statistics (NCHS), Hyattsville, Maryland.

Denver Developmental Screening Test

Appendix Four

DIRECTIONS

DATE ____________________

NAME ____________________

BIRTHDATE ____________________

HOSP. NO. ____________________

1. Try to get child to smile by smiling, talking or waving to him. Do not touch him.
2. When child is playing with toy, pull it away from him. Pass if he resists.
3. Child does not have to be able to tie shoes or button in the back.
4. Move yarn slowly in an arc from one side to the other, about 6″ above child's face. Pass if eyes follow 90° to midline. (Past midline; 180°)
5. Pass if child grasps rattle when it is touched to the backs or tips of fingers.
6. Pass if child continues to look where yarn disappeared or tries to see where it went. Yarn should be dropped quickly from sight from tester's hand without arm movement.
7. Pass if child picks up raisin with any part of thumb and a finger.
8. Pass if child picks up raisin with the ends of thumb and index finger using an over hand approach.

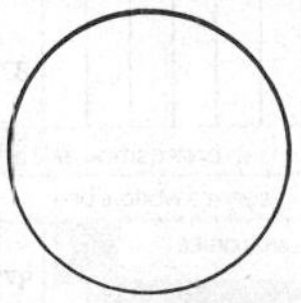

9. Pass any enclosed form. Fail continuous round motions.

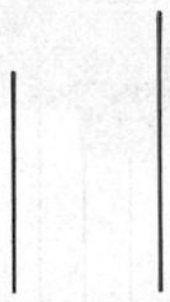

10. Which line is longer? (Not bigger.) Turn paper upside down and repeat. (3/3 or 5/6)

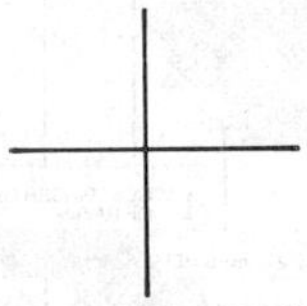

11. Pass any crossing lines.

12. Have child copy first. If failed, demonstrate.

When giving items 9, 11 and 12, do not name the forms. Do not demonstrate 9 and 11.

13. When scoring, each pair (2 arms, 2 legs, etc.) counts as one part.
14. Point to picture and have child name it. (No credit is given for sounds only.)

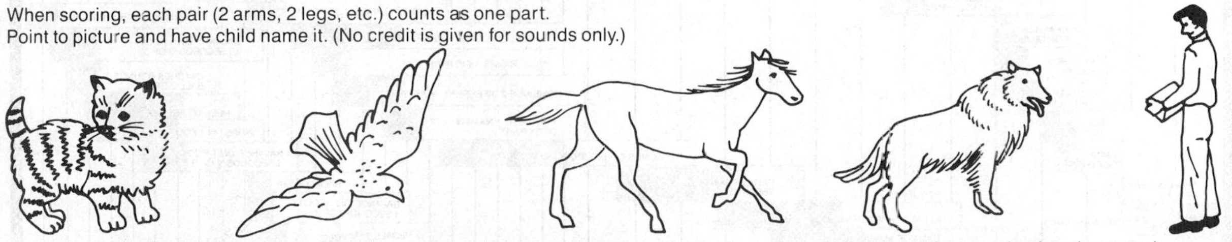

15. Tell child to: Give block to Mommie; put block on table; put block on floor. Pass 2 of 3. (Do not help child by pointing, moving head or eyes.)
16. Ask child: What do you do when you are cold? ..hungry? ..tired? Pass 2 of 3.
17. Tell child to: Put block *on* table; *under* table; *in front* of chair, *behind* chair. Pass 3 of 4. (Do not help child by pointing, moving head or eyes.)
18. Ask child: If fire is hot, ice is ?; Mother is a woman, Dad is a ?; a horse is big, a mouse is ?. Pass 2 of 3.
19. Ask child: What is a ball? ..lake? ..desk? ..house? ..banana? ..curtain? ..ceiling? ..hedge? ..pavement? Pass if defined in terms of use, shape, what it is made of or general category (such as banana is fruit, not just yellow). Pass 6 of 9.
20. Ask child: What is a spoon made of? ..a shoe made of? ..a door made of? (No other objects may be substituted.) Pass 3 of 3.
21. When placed on stomach, child lifts chest off table with support of forearms and/or hands.
22. When child is on back, grasp his hands and pull him to sitting. Pass if head does not hang back.
23. Child may use wall or rail only, not person. May not crawl.
24. Child must throw ball overhand 3 feet to within arm's reach of tester.
25. Child must perform standing broad jump over width of test sheet. (8½ inches)
26. Tell child to walk forward, heel within 1 inch of toe. Tester may demonstrate. Child must walk 4 consecutive steps, 2 out of 3 trials.
27. Bounce ball to child who should stand 3 feet away from tester. Child must catch ball with hands, not arms, 2 out of 3 trials.
28. Tell child to walk backward toe within 1 inch of heel. Tester may demonstrate. Child must walk 4 consecutive steps, 2 out of 3 trials.

DATE AND BEHAVIORAL OBSERVATIONS (how child feels at time of test, relation to tester, attention span, verbal behavior, self-confidence, etc.):

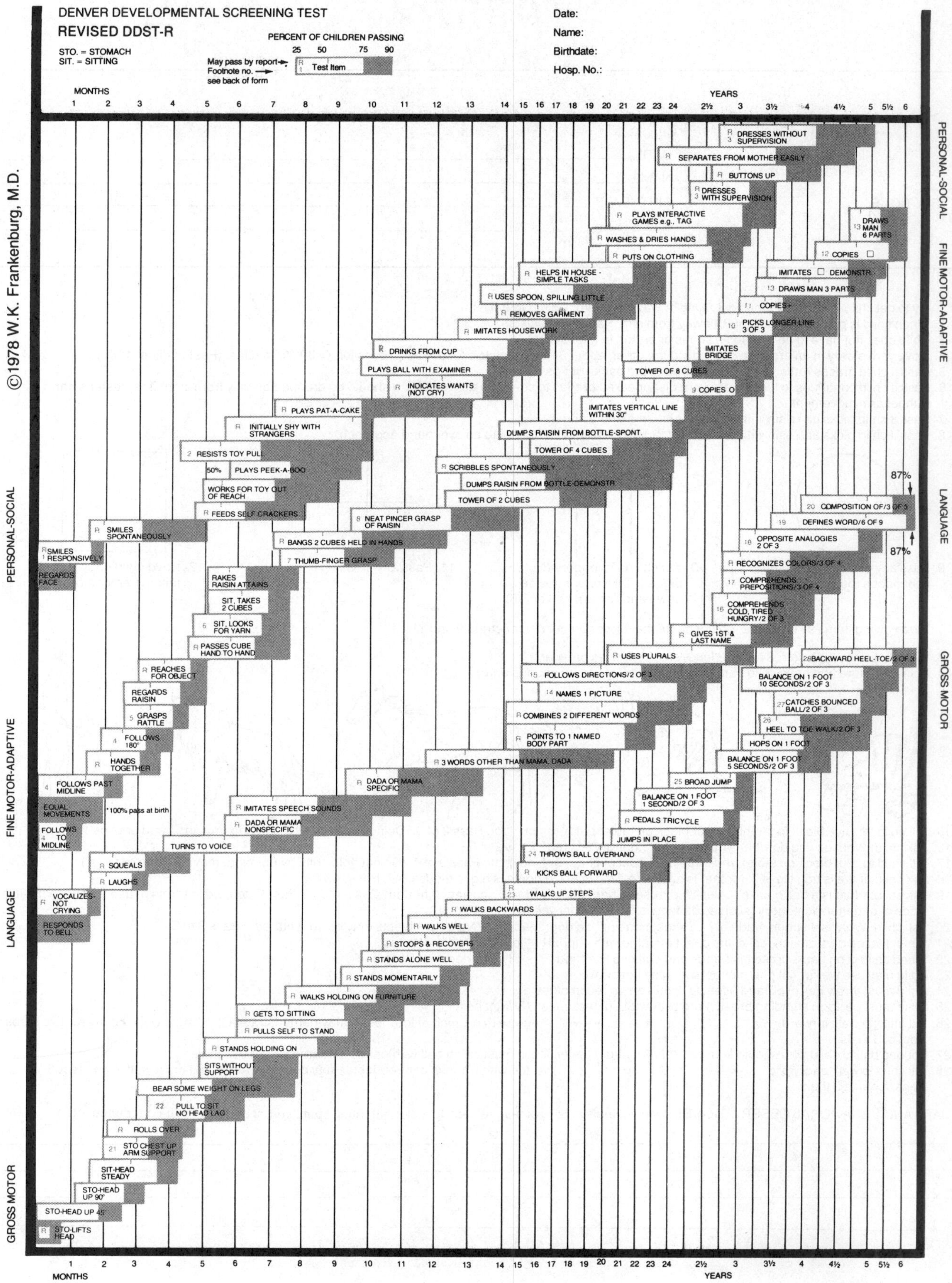
DENVER DEVELOPMENTAL SCREENING TEST
REVISED DDST-R
STO. = STOMACH
SIT. = SITTING
PERCENT OF CHILDREN PASSING
25 50 75 90
May pass by report
Footnote no.
see back of form
Test Item
Date:
Name:
Birthdate:
Hosp. No.:
MONTHS
1 2 3 4 5 6 7 8 9 10 11 12 13 14 15 16 17 18 19 20 21 22 23 24
YEARS
2½ 3 3½ 4 4½ 5 5½ 6
©1978 W.K. Frankenburg, M.D.
PERSONAL-SOCIAL
FINE MOTOR-ADAPTIVE
LANGUAGE
GROSS MOTOR
DRESSES WITHOUT SUPERVISION
SEPARATES FROM MOTHER EASILY
BUTTONS UP
DRESSES WITH SUPERVISION
PLAYS INTERACTIVE GAMES e.g., TAG
WASHES & DRIES HANDS
PUTS ON CLOTHING
HELPS IN HOUSE - SIMPLE TASKS
USES SPOON, SPILLING LITTLE
REMOVES GARMENT
IMITATES HOUSEWORK
DRINKS FROM CUP
PLAYS BALL WITH EXAMINER
INDICATES WANTS (NOT CRY)
PLAYS PAT-A-CAKE
INITIALLY SHY WITH STRANGERS
RESISTS TOY PULL
50% PLAYS PEEK-A-BOO
WORKS FOR TOY OUT OF REACH
FEEDS SELF CRACKERS
SMILES SPONTANEOUSLY
SMILES RESPONSIVELY
REGARDS FACE
DRAWS MAN 6 PARTS
COPIES □
IMITATES □ DEMONSTR.
DRAWS MAN 3 PARTS
COPIES +
PICKS LONGER LINE 3 OF 3
IMITATES BRIDGE
TOWER OF 8 CUBES
COPIES O
IMITATES VERTICAL LINE WITHIN 30°
DUMPS RAISIN FROM BOTTLE-SPONT.
TOWER OF 4 CUBES
SCRIBBLES SPONTANEOUSLY
DUMPS RAISIN FROM BOTTLE-DEMONSTR.
TOWER OF 2 CUBES
NEAT PINCER GRASP OF RAISIN
BANGS 2 CUBES HELD IN HANDS
THUMB-FINGER GRASP
RAKES RAISIN ATTAINS
SIT, TAKES 2 CUBES
SIT, LOOKS FOR YARN
PASSES CUBE HAND TO HAND
REACHES FOR OBJECT
REGARDS RAISIN
GRASPS RATTLE
FOLLOWS 180°
HANDS TOGETHER
FOLLOWS PAST MIDLINE
EQUAL MOVEMENTS
*100% pass at birth
FOLLOWS TO MIDLINE
87%
COMPOSITION OF/3 OF 3
DEFINES WORD/6 OF 9
OPPOSITE ANALOGIES 2 OF 3
RECOGNIZES COLORS/3 OF 4
COMPREHENDS PREPOSITIONS/3 OF 4
COMPREHENDS COLD, TIRED HUNGRY/2 OF 3
GIVES 1ST & LAST NAME
USES PLURALS
FOLLOWS DIRECTIONS/2 OF 3
NAMES 1 PICTURE
COMBINES 2 DIFFERENT WORDS
POINTS TO 1 NAMED BODY PART
3 WORDS OTHER THAN MAMA, DADA
DADA OR MAMA SPECIFIC
IMITATES SPEECH SOUNDS
DADA OR MAMA NONSPECIFIC
TURNS TO VOICE
SQUEALS
LAUGHS
VOCALIZES-NOT CRYING
RESPONDS TO BELL
BACKWARD HEEL-TOE/2 OF 3
BALANCE ON 1 FOOT 10 SECONDS/2 OF 3
CATCHES BOUNCED BALL/2 OF 3
HEEL TO TOE WALK/2 OF 3
HOPS ON 1 FOOT
BALANCE ON 1 FOOT 5 SECONDS/2 OF 3
BROAD JUMP
BALANCE ON 1 FOOT 1 SECOND/2 OF 3
PEDALS TRICYCLE
JUMPS IN PLACE
THROWS BALL OVERHAND
KICKS BALL FORWARD
WALKS UP STEPS
WALKS BACKWARDS
WALKS WELL
STOOPS & RECOVERS
STANDS ALONE WELL
STANDS MOMENTARILY
WALKS HOLDING ON FURNITURE
GETS TO SITTING
PULLS SELF TO STAND
STANDS HOLDING ON
SITS WITHOUT SUPPORT
BEAR SOME WEIGHT ON LEGS
PULL TO SIT NO HEAD LAG
ROLLS OVER
STO CHEST UP ARM SUPPORT
SIT-HEAD STEADY
STO-HEAD UP 90°
STO-HEAD UP 45°
STO-LIFTS HEAD

Home Observation for Measurement of the Environment

Appendix Five

The HOME Manual (Revised 1984 edition) is available from Bettye M. Caldwell and Robert H. Bradley, University of Arkansas at Little Rock, Little Rock, Arkansas. Included here are two inventory forms: infants and toddlers and preschoolers (ages 3 to 6). A HOME Inventory for use with families of children 6 to 10 years of age has also been developed and is being tested for reliability and validity.

The inventory forms shown here are for illustration purposes only; the HOME Manual should be used for actual assessments.

HOME *Inventory for Families of Infants and Toddlers*

Bettye M. Caldwell and Robert H. Bradley

Family Name ______________________ Date __________ Visitor __________

Child's Name ______________________ Birthdate __________ Age ______ Sex ______

Caregiver for visit ______________________ Relationship to child __________

Family Composition ______________________

(Persons living in household, including sex and age of children)

Family Ethnicity __________ Language Spoken __________ Maternal Education __________ Paternal Education __________

Is Mother Employed? __________ Type of work when employed __________ Is Father Employed? __________ Type of work when employed __________

Address ______________________ Phone __________

Current child care arrangements ______________________

Summarize past year's arrangements ______________________

Caregiver for visit ______________________ Other persons present __________

Comments ______________________

____

SUMMARY

Subscale	Score	Lowest Middle	Middle Half	Upper Fourth
I. Emotional and Verbal RESPONSIVITY of Parent		0–6	7–9	10–11
ACCEPTANCE of Child's ...havior		0–4	5–6	7–8
III. C... TeNIZATION of Physical and ...al Environment		0–3	4–5	6
IV. Provisio... PLAY MA... Appropriate ...ALS		0–4	5–7	8–9
V. Parent INVOLV... Child ...ENT with		0–2	3–4	5–6
VI. Opportunities for VA...TY in Daily Stimulation		0–1	2–3	4–5
TOTAL SCORE		0–25	26–36	37–45

For rapid profiling of a family, place an X ...n the box that corresponds to the raw score on each subscale and the total score.

HOME *Inventory**

Place a plus (+) or minus (—) in the box alongside each item if the behavior is observed during the visit or if the parent reports that the conditions or events are characteristic of the home environment. Enter the subtotal and the total on the front side of the Record Sheet.

I. Emotional and Verbal RESPONSIVITY

1. Parent spontaneously vocalized to child twice.	
2. Parent responds verbally to child's verbalizations.	
3. Parent tells child name of object or person during visit.	
4. Parent's speech is distinct and audible.	
5. Parent initiates verbal exchanges with visitor.	
6. Parent converses freely and easily.	
7. Parent permits child to engage in "messy" play.	
8. Parent spontaneously praises child at least twice.	
9. Parent's voice conveys positive feelings toward child.	
10. Parent caresses or kisses child at least once.	
11. Parent responds positively to praise of child offered by visitor.	
Subtotal	

II. ACCEPTANCE of Child's Behavior

12. Parent does not shout at child.	
13. Parent does not express annoyance with or hostility to child.	
14. Parent neither slaps nor spanks child during visit.	
15. No more than one instance of physical punishment during past week.	
16. Parent does not scold or criticize child during visit.	
17. Parent does not interfere or restrict child more than 3 times.	
18. At least ten books are present and visible.	
19. Family has a pet.	
Subtotal	

III. ORGANIZATION of Environment

20. Substitute care is provided by one of three regular substitutes.	
21. Child is taken to grocery store at least once/ week.	
22. Child gets out of house at least four times/ week.	
23. Child is taken regularly to doctor's office or clinic.	
24. Child has a special place for toys and treasures.	
25. Child's play environment is safe.	
Subtotal	

IV. Provision of PLAY MATERIALS

26. Muscle activity toys or equipment.	
27. Push or pull toy.	
28. Stroller or walker, kiddie car, scooter, or tricycle.	
29. Parent provides toys for child during visit.	
30. Learning equipment appropriate to age—cuddly toys or role-playing toys.	
31. Learning facilitators—mobile, table and chairs, high chair, play pen.	
32. Simple eye-hand coordination toys.	
33. Complex eye-hand coordination toys (those permitting combination).	
34. Toys for literature and music.	
Subtotal	

V. Parental INVOLVEMENT with Child

35. Parent keeps child in visual range, looks at often.	
36. Parent talks to child while doing household work.	
37. Parent consciously encourages developmental advance.	
38. Parent invests maturing toys with value via personal attention.	
39. Parent structures child's play periods.	
40. Parent provides toys that challenge child to develop new skills.	
Subtotal	

VI. Opportunities for VARIETY

41. Father provides some care daily.	
42. Parent reads stories to child at least 3 times weekly.	
43. Child eats at least one meal per day with mother and father.	
44. Family visits relatives or receives visits once a month or so.	
45. Child has 3 or more books of his/her own.	
Subtotal	

TOTAL SCORE	

* For complete wording of items, please refer to the Administration Manual.

HOME Inventory for Families of Preschoolers (Three to Six)

Bettye M. Caldwell and Robert H. Bradley

Family Name ______________________ Date __________ Visitor __________

Child's Name ______________________ Birthdate __________ Age ______ Sex ______

Caregiver for visit ______________________ Relationship to child __________

Family Composition ____
(Persons living in household, including sex and age of children)

Family Ethnicity __________ Language Spoken __________ Maternal Education __________ Paternal Education __________

Is Mother Employed? __________ Type of work when employed __________ Is Father Employed? __________ Type of work when employed __________

Address ______________________________________ Phone __________

Current child care arrangements ______________________________

Summarize past year's arrangements ______________________________

Caregiver for visit ______________________ Other persons present __________

SUMMARY

	Subscale	Score	Percentile Range: Lowest Fourth	Middle Half	Upper Fourth
I.	LEARNING STIMULATION		0–2	3–9	10–11
II.	LANGUAGE STIMULATION		0–4	5–6	7
III.	PHYSICAL ENVIRONMENT		0–3	4–6	7
IV.	WARMTH AND AFFECTION		0–3	4–5	6–7
V.	ACADEMIC STIMULATION		0–2	3–4	5
VI.	MODELING		0–1	2–3	4–5
VII.	VARIETY IN EXPERIENCE		0–4	5–7	8–9
VIII.	ACCEPTANCE		0–2	3	4
	TOTAL SCORE		0–29	30–45	46–55

For rapid profiling of a family, place an X in the box that corresponds to the raw score.

HOME *Inventory** (*Preschool*)

Place a plus (+) or minus (—) in the box alongside each item if the behavior is observed during the visit or if the parent reports that the conditions or events are characteristic of the home environment. Enter the subtotals and the total on the front side of the Record Sheet.

I. LEARNING STIMULATION

1. Child has toys which teach color, size, shape.	
2. Child has three or more puzzles.	
3. Child has record player and at least five children's records.	
4. Child has toys permitting free expression.	
5. Child has toys or games requiring refined movements.	
6. Child has toys or games which help teach numbers.	
7. Child has at least 10 children's books.	
8. At least 10 books are visible in the apartment.	
9. Family buys and reads a daily newspaper.	
10. Family subscribes to at least one magazine.	
11. Child is encouraged to learn shapes.	
Subtotal	

II. LANGUAGE STIMULATION

12. Child has toys that help teach the names of animals.	
13. Child is encouraged to learn the alphabet.	
14. Parent teaches child simple verbal manners (please, thank you).	
15. Mother uses correct grammar and pronunciation.	
16. Parent encourages child to talk and takes time to listen.	
17. Parent's voice conveys positive feeling to child.	
18. Child is permitted choice in breakfast or lunch menu.	
Subtotal	

III PHYSICAL ENVIRONMENT

19. Building appears safe.	
20. Outside play environment appears safe.	
21. Interior of apartment not dark or perceptually monotonous.	
22. Neighborhood is esthetically pleasing.	
23. House has 100 square feet of living space per person.	
24. Rooms are not overcrowded with furniture.	
25. House is reasonably clean and minimally cluttered.	
Subtotal	

IV. WARMTH AND AFFECTION

26. Parent holds child close 10–15 minutes per day.	
27. Parent converses with child at least twice during visit.	
28. Parent answers child's questions or requests verbally.	
29. Parent usually responds verbally to child's speech.	
30. Parent praises child's qualities twice during visit.	
31. Parent caresses, kisses, or cuddles child during visit.	
32. Parent helps child demonstrate some achievement during visit.	
Subtotal	

V. ACADEMIC STIMULATION

33. Child is encouraged to learn colors.	
34. Child is encouraged to learn patterned speech (songs, etc.).	
35. Child is encouraged to learn spatial relationships.	
36. Child is encouraged to learn numbers.	
37. Child is encouraged to learn to read a few words.	
Subtotal	

VI. MODELING

38. Some delay of food gratification is expected.	
39. TV is used judiciously.	
40. Parent introduces visitor to child.	
41. Child can express negative feelings without reprisal.	
42. Child can hit parent without harsh reprisal.	
Subtotal	

VII. VARIETY IN EXPERIENCE

43. Child has real or toy musical instrument.	
44. Child is taken on outing by family member at least every other week.	
45. Child has been on trip more than fifty miles during last year.	
46. Child has been taken to a museum during past year.	
47. Parent encourages child to put away toys without help.	
48. Parent uses complex sentence structure and vocabulary.	
49. Child's art work is displayed some place in house.	
50. Child eats at least one meal per day with mother and father.	
51. Parent lets child choose some foods or brands at grocery store.	
Subtotal	

VIII. ACCEPTANCE

52. Parent does not scold or derogate child more than once.	
53. Parent does not use physical restraint during visit.	
54. Parent neither slaps nor spanks child during visit.	
55. No more than one instance of physical punishment during past week.	
Subtotal	

* For complete wording of items, please refer to the Administration Manual.

COMMENTS

Denver Articulation Screening Examination

Appendix Six

DENVER ARTICULATION SCREENING EXAM
for children 2 1/2 to 6 years of age

Instructions: Have child repeat each word after you. Circle the underlined sounds that he pronounces correctly. Total correct sounds is the Raw Score. Use charts on reverse side to score results.

NAME

HOSP. NO.

ADDRESS

Date: ______ Child's Age: ______ Examiner: ______ Raw Score: ______
Percentile: ______ Intelligibility: ______ Result: ______

1. table
2. shirt
3. door
4. trunk
5. jumping
6. zipper
7. grapes
8. flag
9. thumb
10. toothbrush
11. sock
12. vacuum
13. yarn
14. mother
15. twinkle
16. wagon
17. gum
18. house
19. pencil
20. fish
21. leaf
22. carrot

Intelligibility: (circle one)
1. Easy to understand
2. Understandable 1/2 the time.
3. Not understandable
4. Can't evaluate

Comments:

continued

To score DASE words: Note Raw Score for child's performance. Match raw score line (extreme left of chart) with column representing child's age (to the closest previous age group). Where raw score line and age column meet number in that square denotes percentile rank of child's performance when compared to other children that age. Percentiles above heavy line are ABNORMAL percentiles, below heavy line are NORMAL.

PERCENTILE RANK

Raw Score	2.5 yr.	3.0	3.5	4.0	4.5	5.0	5.5	6 years
2	1							
3	2							
4	5							
5	9							
6	16							
7	23							
8	31	2						
9	37	4	1					
10	42	6	2					
11	48	7	4					
12	54	9	6	1	1			
13	58	12	9	2	3	1	1	
14	62	17	11	5	4	2	2	
15	68	23	15	9	5	3	2	
16	75	31	19	12	5	4	3	
17	79	38	25	15	6	6	4	
18	83	46	31	19	8	7	4	
19	86	51	38	24	10	9	5	1
20	89	58	45	30	12	11	7	3
21	92	65	52	36	15	15	9	4
22	94	72	58	43	18	19	12	5
23	96	77	63	50	22	24	15	7
24	97	82	70	58	29	29	20	15
25	99	87	78	66	36	34	26	17
26	99	91	84	75	46	43	34	24
27		94	89	82	57	54	44	34
28		96	94	88	70	68	59	47
29		98	98	94	84	84	77	68
30		100	100	100	100	100	100	100

To Score intelligibility:

	NORMAL	ABNORMAL
2 1/2 years	Understandable 1/2 the time, or, "easy"	Not Understandable
3 years and older	Easy to understand	Understandable 1/2 time Not understandable

Test Result: 1. NORMAL on Dase and Intelligibility = NORMAL

2. ABNORMAL on Dase and/or Intelligibility = ABNORMAL

* If abnormal on initial screening rescreen within 2 weeks. If abnormal again child should be referred for complete speech evaluation.

(Courtesy of William Frankenberg, MD, and Josiah Dodds, PhD, University of Colorado Medical Center.)

Normal Laboratory Values for Children

Appendix Seven

Reference Ranges

Reference ranges are guides for judging health and disease. For many years, the method of defining the normal range was to make a series of measurements in healthy individuals and then calculate the mean and standard deviation of those measurements. By convention the normal range was defined as the mean ± 2 SD. This system does not work in most medical situations because the distribution of measurements does not fit a gaussian distribution. Most biologic measurements are skewed. A more appropriate normal distribution or reference range can be defined as the central 90 per cent (5th to 95th percentiles) of a group of measurements in normal individuals. This listing of reference ranges uses the measured or reasonable estimate of the central 90 per cent of a normal distribution of values. These ranges have proved to be clinically useful in . . . pediatric wards and clinics.

Test and Specimen	Reference Range		Reference Range International Units
Albumin		*g/dL*	*g/L*
Serum	Premature:	3.0–4.2	30–42
	Newborn:	3.6–5.4	36–54
	Infant:	4.0–5.0	40–50
	Thereafter:	3.5–5.0	35–50
CSF	10–30 mg/dL		100–300 mg/L
Urine, *Qualitative*	<20 mg/dL		<200 mg/L
Quantitative	<80 mg/d		<80 mg/d
Ammonia Nitrogen, Resin or Enzymatic		*μg/N/dL*	*μmol/L*
Serum or plasma (Na-heparin)	Newborn	90–150	64–107
	0–2 wk:	79–129	56–92
	> 1 mo:	29–70	21–50
	Thereafter:	15–45	11–32
Urine, 24 hr	500–1200 mg/d		36–86 mmol/d
Amphetamine	Therap. conc. 20–30 ng/mL		150–220 nmol/L
Serum plasma (heparin, EDTA)	Toxic conc.: > 200		> 1500
Amylase (*Beckman; BMD*)			
Serum	Newborn: 5–65 U/L		Same
	>1 yr: 25–125		Same
Urine, timed specimen	1–17 U/hr		Same
Anion Gap [Na − (Cl + CO_2)] Plasma (heparin)	7–16 mmol/L		Same
Anti-Deoxyribonuclease B Titer (Anti-DNAse Titer) Serum	≤ 170 units		Same
Antidiuretic Hormone (hADH, Vasopressin)	*Plasma mOsmol/kg*	*Plasma ADH pg/mL*	*Plasma ADH ng/L*
Plasma (EDTA)	270–280:	<1.5	Same
	280–285:	<2.5	
	285–290:	1–5	
	290–295:	2–7	
	295–300:	4–12	
Anti-Streptolysin-O Titer (ASO titer) Serum	≤166 Todd Units 170–330 Todd Units in school-aged children		

Test and Specimen	Reference Range	Reference Range International Units
Base Excess	*mmol/L*	Same
Whole blood (heparin)	Newborn: (−10)–(−2)	
	Infant: (−7)–(−1)	
	Child: (−4)–(+2)	
	Thereafter: (−3)–(+3)	
Bicarbonate	Arterial: 21–28 mmol/L	Same
Serum	Venous: 22–29	
Bile Acids, Total		
Serum, fasting	0.3–2.3 μg/mL	0.3–2.3 mg/L
Serum, 2 hr postprandial	1.8–3.2 μg/mL	1.8–3.2 mg/L
Feces	120–225 mg/d	120–225 mg/d
Bilirubin	*Premature* / *Full-Term*	
Total Serum	*mg/dL* / *mg/dL*	*μmol/L*
	Cord: <2.0 / <2.0	<34 / <34
	0–1 d: <8.0 / <6.0	<137 / <103
	1–2 d: <12.0 / <8.0	<205 / <137
	2–5 d: <16.0 / <12.0	<274 / <205
	Thereafter: <2.0 / 0.2–1.0	<34 / 3.4–17.1
Total Urine	Negative	Negative
Total Amniotic fluid	28 wk: <0.075 mg/dL (or ΔA_{450} <0.048)	<1.3 μmol/L (or ΔA_{450} <0.048)
	40 wk: <0.025 mg/dL (or ΔA_{450} <0.02)	<0.43 μmol/L (or ΔA_{450} <0.02)
Conjugated (Direct) Serum	0–0.2 mg/dL	0–3.4 μmol/L
Bleeding Time (BT)		
Blood from skin puncture		
Ivy	Normal: 2–7 min	Same
	Borderline: 7–11 min	
Simplate (G-D)	2.75–8 min	
Blood Volume		
Whole blood (heparin)	M: 52–83 mL/kg	M: 0.052–0.083 L/kg
	F: 50–75 mL/kg	F: 0.050–0.075 L/kg
C-Reactive Protein	Cord: 10–350 ng/mL	10–350 μg/L
Serum	Adult: 68–8200	68–8200
Calcium, Ionized (iCa)	*mg/dL*	*mmol/L*
Serum, plasma, or whole blood (heparin)	Cord: 5.0–6.0	1.25–1.50
	Newborn, 3–24 hr: 4.3–5.1	1.07–1.27
	24–48 hr: 4.0–4.7	1.00–1.17
	Thereafter: 4.48–4.92	1.12–1.23
	or 2.24–2.46 mEq/L	1.12–1.23
Calcium, Total	*mg/dL*	*mmol/L*
Serum	Cord: 9.0–11.5	2.25–2.88
	Newborn, 3–24 hr: 9.0–10.6	2.3–2.65
	24–48 hr: 7.0–12.0	1.75–3.0
	4–7 d: 9.0–10.9	2.25–2.73
	Child: 8.8–10.8	2.2–2.70
	Thereafter: 8.4–10.2	2.1–2.55
Urine, 24 hr	*Ca in Diet* / *mg/d*	*mmol/d*
	Ca Free: 5–40	0.13–1.0
	Low to average: 50–150	1.25–3.8
	Average (20 mmol/d): 100–300	2.5–7.5
CSF	2.1–2.7 mEq/L or	1.05–1.35 mmol/L
	4.2–5.4 mg/dL	1.05–1.35 mmol/L
Feces	Avg.: 0.64 g/d	16 mmol/d
Carbamazepine	Therap. conc.: 8–12 μg/mL	34–51 μmol/L
Serum, plasma (heparin, EDTA); collect at trough conc.	Toxic conc.: >15	>63
Carbon Dioxide, Partial Pressure (pCO_2)	*mmHg*	*kPa*
Whole blood (heparin)	Newborn: 27–40	3.6–5.3
	Infant: 27–41	3.6–5.5
	Thereafter, M: 35–48	4.7–6.4
	F: 32–45	4.3–6.0

Test and Specimen	Reference Range	Reference Range International Units
Carbon Dioxide, Total (tCO_2)	*mmol/L*	Same
Serum or plasma (heparin)	Cord: 14–22	
	Premature: 14–27	
	Newborn: 13–22	
	Infant: 20–28	
	Child: 20–28	
	Thereafter: 23–30	
Catecholamines, Fractionated	Norepinephrine,	
Plasma (EDTA-sodium metabisulfite)	Supine: 100–400 pg/mL	591–2364 pmol/L
	Standing: 300–900	1773–5320
	Epinephrine,	
	Supine: <70 pg/mL	<382 pmol/L
	Standing: <100	<546
	Dopamine: <30 pg/mL	<196 pmol/L
	(no postural change)	(no postural change)
Urine, 24 hr	Norepinephrine, *µg/d*	*nmol/d*
	0–1 yr: 0–10	0–59
	1–2 yr: 0–17	0–100
	2–4 yr: 4–29	24–171
	4–7 yr: 8–45	47–266
	7–10 yr: 13–65	77–384
	Thereafter: 15–80	87–473
	Epinephrine, *µg/d*	*nmol/d*
	0–1 yr: 0–2.5	0–13.6
	1–2 yr: 0–3.5	0–19.1
	2–4 yr: 0–6.0	0–32.7
	4–7 yr: 0.2–10	1.1–55
	7–10 yr: 0.5–14	2.7–76
	Thereafter: 0.5–20	2.7–109
	Dopamine, *µg/d*	*nmol/d*
	0–1 yr: 0–85	0–555
	1–2 yr: 10–140	65–914
	2–4 yr: 40–260	261–1697
	Thereafter: 65–400	424–2611
Catecholamines, Total Free	*µg/d*	Same
Urine, 24 hr	0–1 yr: 10–15	
	1–5 yr: 15–40	
	6–15 yr: 20–80	
	Thereafter: 30–100	
Cerebrospinal Fluid Pressure	70–180 mm water	Same
CSF		
Cerebrospinal Fluid Volume	Child: 60–100 mL	0.006–0.10 L
CSF	Adult: 100–160	0.1–0.16
Chloral Hydrate	As Trichloroethanol:	
Serum	Therap. conc.: 2–12 µg/mL	13–80 µmol/L
	Toxic conc.: >20	>134
Chloride	*mmol/L*	
Serum or plasma (heparin)	Cord: 96–104	Same
	Newborn: 97–110	
	Thereafter: 98–106	
CSF	118–132 mmol/L	Same
Urine, 24 hr	*mmol/d*	
	Infant: 2–10	Same
	Child: 15–40	
	Thereafter: 110–250	
	(varies greatly with Cl intake)	
Sweat	*mmol/L*	
	Normal (homozygote): 0–35	Same
	Marginal: 30–60	
	Cystic fibrosis: 60–200	
	Increases by 10 mmol/L during lifetime	
Cholesterol, Total	*mg/dL*	*mmol/L*
Serum or plasma (EDTA or heparin)	Cord: 45–100	1.17–2.59
	Newborn: 53–135	1.37–3.50
	Infant: 70–175	1.81–4.53
	Child: 120–200	3.11–5.18

Table continued on following page

Test and Specimen	Reference Range	Reference Range International Units
Cholesterol, Total		
Serum or plasma (EDTA or heparin) *(Continued)*	Adolescent: 120–210 Adult: 140–310	3.11–5.44 3.63–8.03
	Recommended (desirable) range for adults: 140–250	3.63–6.48
Clotting Time, Lee-White, 37° C		
Whole blood (no anticoagulant)	Glass tubes: 5–8 min (5–15 min at RT) Silicone tubes: about 30 min prolonged	Same
Coagulation Factor Assays		
Plasma (citrate)		
Factor I, see Fibrinogen		
Factor II	0.5–1.5 U/mL or 60–150% of normal	0.5–1.5 kU/L 60–150 AU
Factor IV, see Calcium		
Factor V	0.5–2.0 U/mL or 60–150% of normal	0.5–2.0 kU/L 60–150 AU
Factor VII	65–135% of normal	65–135 AU
Factor VIII	60–145% of normal	60–145 AU
Factor VIII antigen	50–200% of normal	50–200 AU
Factor IX	60–140% of normal	60–140 AU
Factor X	60–130% of normal	60–130 AU
Factor XI	65–135% of normal	65–135 AU
Factor XII	65–150% of normal	65–150 AU
Whole blood (citrate or oxalate)		
Factor XIII (Fibrin Stabilizing Factor, FSF)	Minimal hemostatic level: 0.02–0.05 U/mL or 1–2% of normal	20–50 U/L or 1–2 AU
Complement Components		
Plasma (EDTA)		
Total hemolytic complement activity	75–160 U/mL or >33% of plasma CH_{50}	75–160 kU/mL >0.33 of plasma CH_{50}
Total complement decay rate (functional)	~10–20%	~0.10–0.20 (fraction of decay rate)
	Deficiency: >50%	0.50 (fraction of decay rate)
Copper	*µg/dL*	*µmol/L*
Serum	Birth-6 mo: 20–70 6 yr: 90–190 12 yr: 80–160 Adult, M: 70–140 F: 80–155	3.14–10.99 14.13–29.83 12.56–25.12 10.99–21.98 12.56–24.34
Erythrocytes (heparin)	90–150 µg/dL	14.13–23.55 µmol/L
Urine, 24 hr	15–30 µg/d	0.24–0.47 µmol/d
Coproporphyrin		
Urine, 24 hr	34–234 µg/d	51–351 nmol/d
Feces, 24 hr	<30 µg/g dry wt 400–1200 µg/d	<45 nmol/g dry wt 600–1800 nmol/d
Cortisol	*µg/dL*	*nmol/L*
Serum or plasma (heparin)	Newborn: 1–24 Adults, 0800 hr: 5–23 1600 hr: 3–15 2000 hr: ≤50% of 0800 hr	28–662 138–635 82–413 Fraction of 0800 hr: ≤0.50
Cortisol, Free	*µg/d*	*nmol/d*
Urine, 24 hr	Child: 2–27 Adolescent: 5–55 Adult: 10–100	5.5–74 14–152 27–276
Creatine Kinase (CK, CPK; 30 °C)	*U/L*	
Serum *Total*	Newborn: 68–580 Adult, M: 12–70 F: 10–55	Same
	Ambulatory, M: 25–90 F: 10–70 Higher after exercise	Same
Isoenzymes	Fraction 2 (MB) <5% of total	Fraction of total: <0.05

Test and Specimen	Reference Range	Reference Range International Units
Creatinine	*mg/dL*	*µmol/L*
Serum or plasma	Cord: 0.6–1.2	53–106
Jaffe, kinetic or enzymatic	Newborn: 0.3–1.0	27–88
	Infant: 0.2–0.4	18–35
	Child: 0.3–0.7	27–62
	Adolescent: 0.5–1.0	44–88
	Adult, M: 0.6–1.2	53–106
	F: 0.5–1.1	44–97
Jaffe, manual	0.8–1.5 mg/dL	70–133 µmol/L
Amniotic fluid	After 37 wk gestation: >2.0 mg/dL	After 37 wk gestation: >180 µmol/L
Urine, 24 hr	*mg/kg/d*	*µmol/kg/d*
	Infant: 8–20	71–180
	Child: 8–22	71–195
	Adolescent: 8–30	71–265
	Adult: 14–26	124–230
	or: *mg/d*	*mmol/d*
	M: 800–2000	7–18
	F: 600–1800	5.3–16
Creatinine Clearance (Endogenous) Serum or plasma and urine	Newborn: 40–65 mL/min/1.73 m² <40 yr, M: 97–137 F: 88–128 Decreases ~6.5 mL/min/decade	
Digoxin	*ng/mL*	*nmol/L*
Serum, plasma (heparin, EDTA); collect at least 12 hr after dose	Therap. conc.,	
	CHF: 0.8–1.5	1–1.9
	Arrhythmias: 1.5–2.0	1.9–2.6
	Toxic conc.,	
	Child: >2.5	>3.2
	Adult: >3.0	>3.8
Dihydrotestosterone (DHT)	*ng/dL*	*nmol/L*
Serum	Prepubertal: <3.5	<0.12
	Pubertal: *M* / *F*	*M* / *F*
	stage I: <10 / <10	<0.34 / <0.34
	II: <20 / <15	<0.7 / <0.5
	III: <35 / <25	<1.2 / <0.86
	IV–V: <75 / <25	<2.6 / <0.86
	Adult: 30–85 / 4–22	1.03–2.92 / 0.14–0.76
Eosinophil Count Whole blood (EDTA or heparin); capillary blood	50–350 cells/mm³ (µL)	50–350 × 10⁶ cells/L
Erythrocyte Count (RBC Count)	*millions of cells/mm³ (µL)*	× *10¹² cells/L*
Whole blood (EDTA)	Cord blood: 3.9–5.5	Same
	1–3 d (cap.): 4.0–6.6	
	1 wk: 3.9–6.3	
	2 wk: 3.6–6.2	
	1 mo: 3.0–5.4	
	2 mo: 2.7–4.9	
	3–6 mo: 3.1–4.5	
	0.5–2 yr: 3.7–5.3	
	2–6 yr: 3.9–5.3	
	6–12 yr: 4.0–5.2	
	12–18 yr, M: 4.5–5.3	
	F: 4.1–5.1	
	18–49 yr, M: 4.5–5.9	
	F: 4.0–5.2	
Erythrocyte Sedimentation Rate (ESR)	*mm/hr*	
Whole blood (EDTA)	Child: 0–10	Same
Westergren, modified	Adult: M, <50 yr: 0–15	
	F, <50 yr: 0–20	
Wintrobe	Child: 0–13	
	Adult, M. 0–9	
	F. 0–20	
ZETA	41–54%	41–54 AU
Erythropoietin		
Serum		
RIA	<5–20 mU/mL	<5–20 U/L
Hemagglutination	25–125	25–125
Bioassay	5–18	5–18

Table continued on following page

Test and Specimen	Reference Range		Reference Range International Units
Estradiol		*pg/mL*	*pmol/L*
Serum or plasma (heparin or EDTA)	M, pubertal		
	stage I:	2–8	7–29
	II:	11	40
	III:	>20	>73
	Adult, M:	8–36	29–132
	F, pubertal		
	stage I:	0–23	0–84
	II:	0–66	0–242
	III:	0–105	0–385
	IV:	20–300	73–1101
	Follicular:	10–90	37–330
	Midcycle:	100–500	367–1835
	Luteal:	50–240	184–881
		µg/d	*nmol/d*
Urine, 24 hr	Adult, M:	0–6	0–22
	F:		
	Follicular:	0–3	0–11
	Ovulatory peak:	4–14	15–51
	Luteal:	4–10	15–37
Estrogens, Total		*pg/mL*	*ng/L*
Serum	Child:	<30	Same
	M:	40–115	
	F, cycle—days		
	1–10 d:	61–394	
	11–20 d:	122–437	
	21–30 d:	156–350	
	Prepubertal:	≤40	
		µg/d	*µg/d*
Urine, 24 hr	Child:	<10	Same
	Adult, M:	5–25	
	F, Preovulation:	5–25	
	Ovulation:	28–100	
	Luteal peak:	22–80	
	Pregnancy:	<45,000	
	Postmenopausal:	<10	
Ethanol	Toxic conc.: 50–100 mg/dL		11–22 mmol/L
Whole blood (oxalate), serum	Depression of CNS: >100		>22
Ethosuximide	Therap. conc.: 40–100 µg/mL		280–700 µmol/L
Serum, plasma (heparin, EDTA); collect at trough conc.	Toxic conc.: >150		>1060
Fat, Fecal		*g/d*	*g/d*
Feces, 72 hr	Infant, breast-fed:	<1	Same
	0–6 yr:	<2	
	Adult:	<7	
	Adult (fat-free diet):	<4	
	Coefficient of fat absorption (%)		*Absorbed fraction*
	Infant, breast-fed:	>93	>0.93
	Infant, formula-fed:	>83	>0.83
	>1 yr:	≥95	≥0.95
Fatty Acids, Nonesterified (Free)	Adults: 8–25 mg/dL		0.30–0.90 mmol/L
Serum or plasma (heparin)	Children and obese adults: <31		<1.10
Ferric Chloride Test	Negative		Negative
Urine, fresh random			
Ferritin		*ng/mL*	*µg/L*
Serum	Newborn:	25–200	Same
	1 mo:	200–600	
	2–5 mo:	50–200	
	6 mo–15 yr:	7–140	
	Adult, M:	15–200	
	F:	12–150	
Fibrinogen	Newborn: 125–300 mg/dL		1.25–3.00 g/L
Whole blood (Na citrate)	Adult: 200–400		2.00–4.00
Folate			
Serum	Newborn: 7.0–32 ng/mL		15.9–72.4 nmol/L
	Thereafter: 1.8–9		4.1–20.4
Erythrocytes (EDTA)	150–450 ng/mL cells		340–1020 nmol/L cells

Test and Specimen	Reference Range		Reference Range International Units
Follicle Stimulating Hormone (hFSH)		*mU/mL*	
Serum or plasma (heparin)		*(IRP-2-hMG)*	*IU/L*
	Birth–1 yr, M:	<1–12	Same
	F:	<1–20	
	1–8 yr, M:	<1–6	
	F:	<1–4	
	9–10 yr, M:	<1–10	
	F:	2–8	
	11–12 yr, M:	2–12	
	F:	3–11	
	13–14 yr, M:	3–15	
	F:	3–15	
		mU/mL	*IU/L*
	Adult, M:	4–25	Same
	F,		
	Premenopause:	4–30	Same
	Midcycle peak:	10–90	
	Pregnancy: Low to undetectable		
Galactose			
Serum	Newborn: 0–20 mg/dL		0–1.11 mmol/L
	Thereafter: <5		<0.28
Urine	Newborn: ≤60 mg/dL		≤3.33 mmol/L
	Thereafter: <14 mg/d		<0.08 mmol/d
Glucose		*mg/dL*	*mmol/L*
Serum	Cord:	45–96	2.5–5.3
	Premature:	20–60	1.1–3.3
	Neonate:	30–60	1.7–3.3
	Newborn,		
	1 d:	40–60	2.2–3.3
	>1 d:	50–90	2.8–5.0
	Child:	60–100	3.3–5.5
	Adult:	70–105	3.9–5.8
Whole blood (heparin)	Adult:	65–95	3.6–5.3
CSF	Adult:	40–70	2.2–3.9
Urine			
Quantitative, enzymatic	<0.5 g/d		<2.8 mmol/d
Qualitative	Negative		Negative
Glucose, 2 hr Postprandial	<120 mg/dL		<6.7 mmol/L
Serum	Diabetes: see *Glucose Tolerance Test, Oral*		
Glucose Tolerance Test (GTT), Oral		*mg/dL* Normal / Diabetic	*mmol/L* Normal / Diabetic
Serum	Fasting:	70–105 / >115	3.9–5.8 / >6.4
Dose, Adult: 75 g	60 min:	120–170 / ≥200	6.7–9.4 / ≥11
Child: 1.75 g/kg of ideal weight up to	90 min:	100–140 / ≥200	5.6–7.8 / ≥11
maximum of 75 g	120 min:	70–120 / ≥140	3.9–6.7 / ≥7.8
Growth Hormone (hGH, Somatotropin)		*ng/mL*	*μg/L*
Serum or plasma (EDTA, heparin)	Cord:	10–50	Same
Fasting, at rest	Newborn:	10–40	
	Child:	<5	
	Adult, M:	<5	
	F:	<8	
Hematocrit (HCT, Hct)		*% of packed red cells (V red cells/V whole blood × 100)*	*Volume fraction (V red cells/V whole blood)*
Whole blood (EDTA)	1 d (cap):	48–69	0.48–0.69
Calculated from MCV and	2 d:	48–75	0.48–0.75
RBC (electronic	3 d:	44–72	0.44–0.72
displacement or laser)	2 mo:	28–42	0.28–0.42
	6–12 yr:	35–45	0.35–0.45
	12–18 yr, M:	37–49	0.37–0.49
	F:	36–46	0.36–0.46
	18–49 yr, M:	41–53	0.41–0.53
	F:	36–46	0.36–0.46
Hemoglobin (Hb)		*g/dL*	*mmol/L*
Whole blood (EDTA)	1–3 d (cap):	14.5–22.5	2.25–3.49
	2 mo:	9.0–14.0	1.40–2.17
	6–12 yr:	11.5–15.5	1.78–2.40
	12–18 yr, M:	13.0–16.0	2.02–2.48
	F:	12.0–16.0	1.86–2.48

Table continued on following page

Test and Specimen	Reference Range		Reference Range International Units
Hemoglobin (Hb)			
Whole blood (EDTA)*(Continued)*	18–49 yr, M:	13.5–17.5	2.09–2.71
	F:	12.0–16.0	1.86–2.48
Serum or plasma (heparin, ACD, EDTA)	<10 mg/dL		<1.55 μmol/L
	<3 mg/dL with butterfly set-up and 18 g needle		<0.47 μmol/L with butterfly set-up and 18 g needle
Urine, fresh random	Negative		Negative
Hemoglobin, glycosylated			Fraction of Hb
Whole blood (heparin, EDTA, or oxalate)			
Electrophoresis	5.6–7.5% of total Hb		0.056–0.075
Column	6–9% of total Hb		0.06–0.09
HPLC	HbA_{1a} 1.6% total Hb		0.016
	HbA_{1b} 0.8		0.008
	HbA_{1c} 3.6		0.03–0.06
Hemoglobin A			
Whole blood (EDTA, citrate, or heparin)	>95%		Fraction of Hb: >0.95
Hemoglobin F		*% HbF*	*Mass fraction HbF*
Whole blood (EDTA)	1 d:	63–92	0.62–0.92
Alkali denaturation (White)	5 d:	65–88	0.65–0.88
	3 wk:	55–85	0.55–0.85
	6–9 wk:	31–75	0.31–0.75
	3–4 mo:	<2–59	<0.02–0.59
	6 mo:	<2– 9	<0.02–0.09
	Adult:	<2	<0.02
17-Hydroxyprogesterone (17-OHP)		*ng/mL*	*nmol/L*
Serum	M,		
	Pubertal stage I:	0.1–0.3	0.3–0.9
	Adult:	0.2–1.8	0.6–5.4
	F,		
	Pubertal stage I:	0.2–0.5	0.6–1.5
	Follicular:	0.2–0.8	0.6–2.4
	Luteal:	0.8–3.0	2.4–9.0
	Postmenopausal:	0.04–0.5	0.12–1.5
Immunoglobulin A (IgA)		*mg/dL*	*mg/L*
Serum	Cord:	0–5	0–50
	Newborn:	0–2.2	0–22
	1/2–6 mo:	3–82	30–820
	6 mo–2 yr:	14–108	140–1080
	2–6 yr:	23–190	230–1900
	6–12 yr:	29–270	290–2700
	12–16 yr:	81–232	810–2320
	Thereafter:	60–380	600–3800
Immunoglobulin D (IgD)	Newborn: None detected		None detected
Serum	Thereafter: 0–8 mg/dL		0–0.44 μmol/L
Immunoglobulin E (IgE)	M: 0–230 IU/mL		0–230 kIU/L
Serum	F: 0–170		0–170
Immunoglobulin G (IgG)		*mg/dL*	*g/L*
Serum	Cord:	760–1700	7.6–17
	Newborn:	700–1480	7–14.8
	1/2–6 mo:	300–1000	3–10
	6 mo–2 yr:	500–1200	5–12
	2–6 yr:	500–1300	5–13
	6–12 yr:	700–1650	7–16.5
	12–16 yr:	700–1550	7–15.5
	Adults:	600–1600	6–16
	(higher in blacks)		(higher in blacks)
Immunoglobulin M (IgM)		*mg/dL*	*mg/L*
Serum	Cord:	4–24	40–240
	Newborn:	5–30	50–300
	1/2–6 mo:	15–109	150–1090
	6 mo–2 yr:	43–239	430–2390
	2–6 yr:	50–199	500–1990
	6–12 yr:	50–260	500–2600
	12–16 yr:	45–240	450–2400
	Thereafter:	40–345	400–3450
	Results vary with std. preparation		
Insulin (12 hr Fasting)	Newborn: 3–20 μU/mL		3–20 mU/L
Serum or plasma (no anticoagulant)	Thereafter: 7–24		7–24

Test and Specimen	Reference Range		Reference Range International Units	
Iron		μg/dL	μmol/L	
Serum	Newborn:	100–250	17.90–44.75	
	Infant:	40–100	7.16–17.90	
	Child:	50–120	8.95–21.48	
	Thereafter, M:	50–160	8.95–28.64	
	F:	40–150	7.16–26.85	
	Intoxicated child:	280–2550	50.12–456.5	
	Fatally poisoned child:	>1800	>322.2	
Iron-Binding Capacity, Total (TIBC)	Infant: 100–400 μg/dL		17.90–71.60 μmol/L	
Serum	Thereafter: 250–400		44.75–71.60	
17-Ketogenic Steroids (17-KGS)		mg/d	μmol/d	
Urine, 24 hr	0–1 yr:	<1.0	<3.5	(Conversion based
	1–10 yr:	<5	<17	dehydroepi-
	11–14 yr:	<12	<42	androsterone,
	Thereafter, M:	5–23	17–80	M.W. 288)
	F:	3–15	10–52	
Ketone Bodies				
Serum, random urine *Qualitative*	Negative		Negative	
Serum *Quantitative*	0.5–3.0 mg/dL		5–30 mg/L	
17-Ketosteroids (17-KS), Total		mg/d	μmol/d	
Zimmermann reaction	14 d–2 yr:	<1	<3.5	(Conversion based
Urine, 24 hr	2–6 yr:	<2	<7	on dehydroepi-
	6–10 yr:	1–4	3.5–14	androsterone,
	10–12 yr:	1–6	3.5–21	M.W. 288)
	12–14 yr:	3–10	10–35	
	14–16 yr:	5–12	17–42	
	Thereafter,			
	M, 18–30 yr:	9–22	31–76	
	M, >30 yr:	8–20	28–70	
	F:	6–15	21–52	
	Decreases with age		Decreases with age	
Lactate		mmol/L	mmol/L	
Whole blood (heparin)	Venous:	0.5–2.2	Same	
	Arterial:	0.5–1.6		
	Inpatients,			
	Venous:	0.9–1.7		
	Arterial:	<1.25		
		μg/dL	μmol/L	
Lead	Child:	<30	<1.45	
Whole blood (heparin)	Adult:	<40	<1.93	
	Acceptable for industrial exposure:	<60	<2.90	
	Toxic:	≥100	≥4.83	
Urine, 24 hr	<80 μg/L		<0.39 μmol/L	
Leukocyte Differential Count				
Whole blood (EDTA)		%	Number fraction	
Myelocytes		0	0	
Neutrophils—"bands"		3–5	0.03–0.05	
Neutrophils—"segs"		54–62	0.54–0.62	
Lymphocytes		25–33	0.25–0.33	
Monocytes		3–7	0.03–0.07	
Eosinophils		1–3	0.01–0.03	
Basophils		0–0.75	0–0.0075	
		Cells/mm³ (μL)	× 10⁶ cells/L	
		0	0	
		150–400	150–400	
		3000–5800	3000–5800	
		1500–3000	1500–3000	
		285–500	285–500	
		50–250	50–250	
		15–50	15–50	
Lysergic Acid Diethylamine	After hallucinogenic dose:		After hallucinogenic dose:	
Plasma (EDTA)	0.005–0.009 μg/mL		15.5–27.8 nmol/L	
Urine	0.001–0.050 μg/mL		3.1–155 nmol/L	

Table continued on following page

Test and Specimen	Reference Range		Reference Range International Units	
Magnesium		*mEq/L*	*mmol/L*	
Serum	Newborn, 2–4 d:	1.2–1.8	0.6–0.9	
	5 mo–6 yr:	1.4–1.9	0.7–1.0	
	6–12 yr:	1.4–1.7	0.7–0.8	
	12–20 yr:	1.4–1.8	0.7–0.9	
	Adult:	1.3–2.1	0.6–1.0	
Mean Corpuscular Hemoglobin (MCH)		*pg/cell*	*fmol/cell*	
Whole blood (EDTA)	Birth:	31–37	0.48–0.57	
	1–3 d (cap.):	31–37	0.48–0.57	
	1 wk–1 mo:	28–40	0.43–0.62	
	2 mo:	26–34	0.40–0.53	
	3–6 mo:	25–35	0.39–0.54	
	0.5–2 yr:	23–31	0.36–0.48	
	2–6 yr:	24–30	0.37–0.47	
	6–12 yr:	25–33	0.39–0.51	
	12–18 yr:	25–35	0.39–0.54	
	18–49 yr:	26–34	0.40–0.53	
Mean Corpuscular Hemoglobin Concentration (MCHC)		*% Hb/cell or g Hb/dL RBC*	*mmol Hb/L RBC*	
Whole blood (EDTA)	Birth:	30–36	4.65–5.58	
	1–3 d (cap.):	29–37	4.50–5.74	
	1–2 wk:	28–38	4.34–5.89	
	1–2 mo:	29–37	4.50–5.74	
	3 mo–2 yr:	30–36	4.65–5.58	
	2–18 yr:	31–37	4.81–5.74	
	>18 yr:	31–37	4.81–5.74	
Mean Corpuscular Volume (MCV)		*μm^3*	*fL*	
Whole blood (EDTA)	1–3 d (cap):	95–121	Same	
	0.5–2 yr:	70–86		
	6–12 yr:	77–95		
	12–18 yr, M:	78–98		
	F:	78–102		
	18–49 yr, M:	80–100		
	F:	80–100		
Niacin (Nicotinic Acid)	0.3–1.5 mg/d		2.43–12.17 μmol/d	
Urine, 24 hr				
Occult Blood				
Feces, random	Negative (<2 mL blood/d in ~100–200 g stool)		Negative	
Urine, random	Negative		Negative	
Osmolality				
Serum	Child, Adult: 275–295 mOsmol/kg H_2O			
Urine, random	50–1400 mOsmol/kg H_2O, depending on fluid intake. After 12 hr fluid restriction: >850 mOsmol/kg H_2O			
Urine, 24 hr	≈300–900 mOsmol/kg H_2O			
Osmotic Fragility Test (RBC Fragility)	*% NaCl (g/dl)*	*% Hemolysis*	*NaCl (g/L)*	*Hemolyzed fraction*
Whole blood (heparin)	0.30	97–100	3.0	0.97–1.00
pH 7.4, 20 °C	0.35	90–99	3.5	0.90–0.99
	0.40	50–95	4.0	0.50–0.95
	0.45	5–45	4.5	0.05–0.45
	0.50	0–6	5.0	0.00–0.06
	0.55	0	5.5	0.00
	% NaCl (g/dL)	*% Hemolysis*	*NaCl (g/L)*	*Hemolyzed fraction*
Sterile incubation at 37 °C	0.20	95–100	2.0	0.95–1.00
	0.30	85–100	3.0	0.85–1.00
	0.35	75–100	3.5	0.75–1.00
	0.40	65–100	4.0	0.65–1.00
	0.45	55–95	4.5	0.55–0.95
	0.50	40–85	5.0	0.40–0.85
	0.55	15–70	5.5	0.15–0.70
	0.60	0–40	6.0	0.00–0.40
	0.65	0–10	6.5	0.00–0.10
	0.70	0–5	7.0	0.00–0.05
	0.85	0	8.5	0.00

Test and Specimen	Reference Range		Reference Range International Units
Oxygen, Partial Pressure (pO_2)		*mm Hg*	*kPa*
Whole blood (heparin), arterial	Birth:	8–24	1.1–3.2
	5–10 min:	33–75	4.4–10.0
	30 min:	31–85	4.1–11.3
	>1 hr:	55–80	7.3–10.6
	1 d:	54–95	7.2–12.6
	Thereafter:	83–108	11–14.4
	(Decreases with age)		
Oxygen Saturation			Fraction saturated:
Whole blood (heparin), arterial	Newborn: 40–90%		0.40–0.90
	Thereafter: 95–99%		0.95–0.99
Paraldehyde		*μg/mL*	*μmol/L*
Serum, plasma (heparin, EDTA)	Therap. conc.,		
	Sedation:	10–100	75–750
	Anesthesia:	>200	>1500
	Toxic conc.:	20–40	150–300
	Lethal conc.:	>50	>375
Partial Thromboplastin Time (PTT)			
Whole blood (Na citrate)			
Nonactivated	60–85 s (Platelin)		Same
Activated	25–35 s (differs with method)		
pH			*H^+ concentration:*
Whole blood (heparin), arterial	Premature (48 hr):	7.35–7.50	31–44 nmol/L
	Birth, full term:	7.11–7.36	43–77
	5–10 min:	7.09–7.30	50–81
	30 min:	7.21–7.38	41–61
	>1 hr:	7.26–7.49	32–54
	1 d:	7.29–7.45	35–51
	Thereafter:	7.35–7.45	35–44
	Must be corrected for body temperature		
Urine, random	Newborn/neonate:	5–7	0.1–10 μmol/L
	Thereafter:	4.5–8	0.01–32 μmol/L
	(average ≃ 6)		(average ≃ 1.0 μmol/L)
Stool		7.0–7.5	31–100 nmol/L
Phenacetin	Therap. conc.: 1–20 μg/mL		5.6–110 μmol/L
Plasma (EDTA)	Toxic conc.: 50–250		280–1400
Phenobarbital		*μg/mL*	*μmol/L*
Serum, plasma (heparin, EDTA); collect at trough conc.	Therap. conc.:	15–40	65–170
	Toxic conc.,		
	Slowness, ataxia, nystagmus:	35–80	150–345
	Coma with reflexes:	65–117	280–504
	Coma without reflexes:	>100	>430
Phenylalanine		*mg/dL*	*mmol/L*
Serum	Premature:	2.0–7.5	0.12–0.45
	Newborn:	1.2–3.4	0.07–0.21
	Thereafter:	0.8–1.8	0.05–0.11
		mg/d	*μmol/d*
Urine, 24 hr	10 d–2 wk:	1–2	6–12
	3–12 yr:	4–18	24–110
	Thereafter:	trace–17	trace–103
Phenylpyruvic Acid, Qualitative	Negative by $FeCl_3$ test		Negative by $FeCl_3$ test
Urine, fresh random			
Phenytoin	Therap. conc.: 10–20 μg/mL		40–80 μmol/L
Serum, plasma (heparin, EDTA); collect at steady-state trough conc.	Toxic conc.: >20		>80
Phosphatase, Alkaline (*p*-nitrophenyl phosphate)			
Serum		*U/L*	
SKI method; 30 °C	Infant:	50–155	Same
	Child:	20–150	
	Adult:	20–70	
Bowers and McComb, 30 °C	25–90 U/L		Same

Table continued on following page

Test and Specimen	Reference Range		Reference Range International Units
Phospholipids, Total		*mg/dL*	*g/L*
Serum or plasma (EDTA)	Newborn:	75–170	0.75–1.70
	Infant:	100–275	1.00–2.75
	Child:	180–295	1.80–2.95
	Adult:	125–275	1.25–2.75
Phosphorus, Inorganic		*mg/dL*	*mmol/L*
Serum	Cord:	3.7–8.1	1.2–2.6
	Premature (1 wk):	5.4–10.9	1.7–3.5
	Newborn:	4.3–9.3	1.4–3.0
	Child:	4.5–6.5	1.45–2.1
	Thereafter:	3.0–4.5	0.97–1.45
Plasma Volume	M: 25–43 mL/kg		M: 0.025–0.043 L/kg
Plasma (heparin)	F: 28–45		F: 0.028–0.045
Platelet Count (Thrombocyte Count)		$\times 10^3/mm^3$ *(μL)*	$\times 10^9/L$
Whole blood (EDTA)	Newborn: 84–478		Same
	(After 1 wk, same as adult)		
	Adult: 150–400		
Potassium		*mmol/L*	*mmol/L*
Serum	Newborn:	3.9–5.9	Same
	Infant:	4.1–5.3	
	Child:	3.4–4.7	
	Thereafter:	3.5–5.1	
Plasma (heparin)	3.5–4.5 mmol/L		Same
Urine, 24 hr	2.5–125 mmol/d varies with diet		Same
Progesterone		*ng/mL*	*nmol/L*
Serum	M, Pubertal		
	stage I:	0.11–0.26	0.35–0.83
	Adult:	0.12–0.3	0.38–1
	F, Pubertal stage		
	I:	0–0.3	0–1
	II:	0–0.46	0–1.5
	III:	0–0.6	0–2
	IV:	0.05–13.0	0.16–41
	Follicular:	0.02–0.9	0.06–2.9
	Luteal:	6.0–30.0	19–95
Protein		*g/dL*	*g/L*
Serum, *Total*	Premature:	4.3–7.6	43.0–76.0
	Newborn:	4.6–7.4	46.0–74.0
	Child:	6.2–8.0	62.0–80.0
	Adult, Recumbent:	6.0–7.8	60.0–78.0
	~0.5 g higher in ambulatory patients		~5 g higher in ambulatory patients
Urine, 24 hr *Total*	1–14 mg/dL		10–140 mg/L
	50–80 mg/d (at rest)		50–80 mg/d
	<250 mg/d after intense exercise		<250 mg/d after intense exercise
CSF, *Total Column*	Lumbar: 8–32 mg/dL		80–320 mg/L
Turbidimetry		*mg/dL*	*mg/L*
	Lumbar,		
	Premature:	40–300	400–3000
	Newborn:	45–120	450–1200
	Child:	10–20	100–200
	Adolescent:	15–20	150–200
	Thereafter:	15–45	150–450
Prothrombin Time (PT)			
Whole blood (Na citrate)			
One-stage (Quick)	In general: 11–15 s (varies with type of thromboplastin)		Same
	Newborn: prolonged by 2–3 s		Same
Two-stage modified (Ware and Seegers)	18–22 s		Same

Test and Specimen	Reference Range	Reference Range International Units
RBC Count, see *Erythrocyte Count*		
Red Cell Volume Whole blood (heparin)	M: 20–36 mL/kg F: 19–31	M: 0.020–0.036 L/kg F: 0.019–0.031
Renin (Renin Activity, Plasma; PRA) Plasma (EDTA)	*ng/mL/h* 0–3 yr: <16.6 3–6 yr: < 6.7 6–9 yr: < 4.4 9–12 yr: < 5.9 12–15 yr: < 4.2 15–18 yr: < 4.3 *Normal sodium diet:* Supine: 0.2–2.5 Upright: 0.3–4.3 *Low sodium diet:* Upright 2.9–24	*μg/L/h* Same
Reticulocyte Count Whole blood (EDTA, heparin, or oxalate)	Adults: 0.5–1.5% of erythrocytes or 25,000–75,000/mm³ (μL)	0.005–0.015 (number fraction) 25,000–75,000 × 10⁶/L
Capillary	% 1 d: 0.4–6.0 7 d: <0.1–1.3 1–4 wk: <0.1–1.2 5–6 wk: <0.1–2.4 7–8 wk: 0.1–2.9 9–10 wk: <0.1–2.6 11–12 wk: 0.1–1.3	*Number fraction* 0.004–0.060 <0.001–0.013 <0.001–0.012 <0.001–0.024 0.001–0.029 <0.001–0.026 0.001–0.013
Riboflavin (Vitamin B_2) Urine, random, fasting	*μg/g creatinine* 1–3 yr: 500–900 4–6 yr: 300–600 7–9 yr: 270–500 10–15 yr: 200–400 Adult: 80–269	*μmol/mol creatinine* 150–270 90–180 81–150 60–120 24–81
Salicylates Serum, plasma (heparin, EDTA); collect at trough conc.	Therap. conc.: 15–30 mg/dL Toxic conc.: >30	1.1–2.2 mmol/L >2.2
Sediment Urine, fresh random		
Casts	Hyaline: occasional (0–1) casts/hpf RBC: not seen WBC: not seen Tubular epithelial: not seen Transitional and squamous epithelial: not seen	Same
Cells	RBC: 0–2/hpf WBC, Males: 0–3/hpf Females and children: 0–5/hpf Epithelial: few; more frequent in newborn Bacteria, unspun: no organisms/oil immersion field spun: <20 organisms/hpf	Same
Sedimentation Rate, see *Erythrocyte Sedimentation Rate*		
Sickle Cell Tests *Sodium Metabisulfite* *Dithionite Test* Whole blood (EDTA, heparin, or oxalate)	 Negative Negative	
Sodium Serum or plasma (heparin)	*mmol/L* Newborn: 134–146 Infant: 139–146 Child: 138–145 Thereafter: 136–146	*mmol/L* Same

Table continued on following page

Test and Specimen	Reference Range			Reference Range International Units	
Sodium *(Continued)*					
Urine, 24 hr	Adult:	40–220 (diet-dependent)		Same	
	Full-term, 7–14 d old neonates have Na clearance of ~ 20% of adult values.				
Sweat		10–40 Cystic fibrosis, >70		Same	
Somatomedin C					
Plasma (EDTA)	Vary with laboratory, e.g., Nichols Institute				
		U/mL		*U/L*	
		M	F	M	F
	0–2 yr:	0.10–0.72	0.10–1.7	100–720	100–1700
	3–5 yr:	0.12–1.5	0.15–2.3	120–1500	150–2300
	6–10 yr:	0.19–2.2	0.44–3.6	190–2200	440–3600
	11–12 yr:	0.22–3.6	1.50–6.9	220–3600	150–6900
	13–14 yr:	0.79–5.5	0.81–7.4	790–5500	810–7400
	15–17 yr:	0.76–3.3	0.59–3.1	760–3300	590–3100
	18–64 yr:	0.34–1.9	0.45–2.2	340–1900	450–2200
	Endocrine Sciences				
	Cord:	0.25–0.66		250–660	
	0–1 yr:	0.17–0.62		170–620	
	1–5 yr:	0.14–0.94		140–940	
	6–12 yr:	0.87–2.06		870–2060	
	13–17 yr:	1.35–3.00		1350–3000	
	18–25 yr:	0.92–2.06		920–2060	
	Thereafter:	0.70–2.04		700–2040	
Specific Gravity					
Urine, random	Adult: 1.002–1.030			Same	
	After 12 hr fluid restriction: >1.025				
Urine, 24 hr	1.015–1.025				
Testosterone, Total		*ng/dL*		*nmol/L*	
Serum	Prepubertal,				
	M:	1.6–11.6		0.06–0.40	
	F:	1.6–11.6		0.06–0.40	
	Adult,				
	M:	302–842		10.47–29.19	
	F:	17–57		0.59–1.98	
Theophylline		*μg/mL*		*μmol/L*	
Serum, plasma (heparin, EDTA)	Therap. conc.,				
	Bronchodilator:	8–20		44–110	
	Prem. apnea:	6–13		33–72	
	Toxic conc.:	>20		>110	
Thiamine (Vitamin B_1)					
Serum	0–2.0 μg/dL			0.0–75.4 nmol/L	
		μg/g creatinine		*μmol/mol*	
Urine, acidify with HCl	1–3 yr:	176–200		75–85	
	4–6 yr:	121–400		52–170	
	7–9 yr:	181–350		77–149	
	10–12 yr:	181–300		77–128	
	13–15 yr:	151–250		64–107	
	Thereafter:	66–129		28–55	
Thrombin Time					
Whole blood (Na citrate)	Control time ± 2 s when control is 9–13 s			Same	
Thyroid Stimulating Hormone (hTSH)		*μU/L*		*mU/L*	
Serum or plasma (heparin)	Cord:	3–12		Same	
	Newborn:	3–18			
	Thereafter:	2–10			

Test and Specimen	Reference Range			Reference Range International Units	
Thyroxine, Total (T_4)		*µg/dL*		*nmol/L*	
Serum	Cord:	8–13		103–168	
	Newborn:	11.5–24		148–310	
	(lower in low birth weight infants)				
	Neonate:	9–18		116–232	
	Infant:	7–15		90–194	
	1–5 yr:	7.3–15		94–194	
	5–10 yr:	6.4–13.3		83–172	
	Thereafter:	5–12		65–155	
	Newborn screen (filter paper):	6.2–22		80–284	
Tourniquet Test (Capillary Fragility)	<5–10 petechiae in 2.5 cm circle on forearm (halfway between systolic and diastolic pressure for 5 min); 0–8 petechiae in 6 cm circle (50 torr for 15 min); 10–20 petechiae in 5 cm circle (80 mm Hg)			Same	
Triglycerides (TG)		*mg/dL*		*g/L*	
Serum, after ≥12 hr fast		*M*	*F*	*M*	*F*
	Cord blood:	10–98	10–98	0.10–0.98	0.10–0.98
	0–5 yr:	30–86	32–99	0.30–0.86	0.32–0.99
	6–11 yr:	31–108	35–114	0.31–1.08	0.35–1.14
	12–15 yr:	36–138	41–138	0.36–1.38	0.41–1.38
	16–19 yr:	40–163	40–128	0.40–1.63	0.40–1.28
	20–29 yr:	44–185	40–128	0.44–1.85	0.40–1.28
	Recommended (desirable) levels for adults: Male: 40–160 mg/dL Female: 35–135			*Recommended* (desirable) levels for adults: Male: 0.40–1.60 g/L Female: 0.35–1.35	
Triiodothyronine, Free		*pg/dL*		*pmol/L*	
Serum	Cord:	20–240		0.3–3.7	
	1–3 d:	200–610		3.1–9.4	
	6 wk:	240–560		3.7–8.6	
	Adult (20–50 yr):	230–660		3.5–10.0	
Triiodothyronine, Total (T_3-RIA)		*ng/dL*		*nmol/L*	
Serum	Cord:	30–70		0.46–1.08	
	Newborn:	75–260		1.16–4.00	
	1–5 yr:	100–260		1.54–4.00	
	5–10 yr:	90–240		1.39–3.70	
	10–15 yr:	80–210		1.23–3.23	
	Thereafter:	115–190		1.77–2.93	
Urea Nitrogen		*mg/dL*		*mmol urea/L*	
Serum or plasma	Cord:	21–40		7.5–14.3	
	Premature (1 wk):	3–25		1.1–9	
	Newborn:	3–12		1.1–4.3	
	Infant/Child:	5–18		1.8–6.4	
	Thereafter:	7–18		2.5–6.4	
Uric Acid					
Serum		*mg/dL*		*µmol/L*	
Phosphotungstate	Newborn:	2.0–6.2		119–369	
	Adult, M:	4.5–8.2		268–488	
	F:	3.0–6.5		178–387	
Uricase	Child:	2.0–5.5		119–327	
	Adults, M:	3.5–7.2		208–428	
	F:	2.6–6.0		155–357	
Urine Volume		*mL/d*		*L/d*	
Urine, 24 hr	Newborn:	50–300		0.050–0.300	
	Infant:	350–550		0.350–0.500	
	Child:	500–1000		0.500–1.000	
	Adolescent:	700–1400		0.700–1.400	
	Thereafter, M:	800–1800		0.800–1.800	
	F:	600–1600 (varies with intake and other factors)		0.600–1.600	

Table continued on following page

Test and Specimen	Reference Range		Reference Range International Units
Valproic Acid Serum, plasma (heparin, EDTA); collect at trough conc.	Therap. conc.: 50–100 μg/mL Toxic conc.: >100		350–700 μmol/L >700
Vanillylmandelic Acid (Vanilmandelic Acid) Urine, 24 hr		*mg/d*	*μmol/d*
	Newborn:	<1.0	<5.0
	Infant:	<2.0	<10.1
	Child:	1–3	5–15
	Adolescent:	1–5	5–25
	Thereafter:	2–7	10–35
	or: 1.5–7 μg/mg creatinine		or: 0.86–4 mmol/mol creatinine
Vitamin A Serum		*μg/dL*	*μmol/L*
	Newborn:	35–75	1.22–2.62
	Child:	30–80	1.05–2.79
	Thereafter:	30–65	1.05–2.27
Vitamin B$_1$, see *Thiamine*			
Vitamin B$_2$, see *Riboflavin*			
Vitamin B$_6$ Plasma (EDTA)	3.6–18 ng/mL		14.6–72.8 nmol/L
Vitamin B$_{12}$ Serum	Newborn: 175–800 pg/ml Thereafter: 140–700		129–590 pmol/L 103–517
Vitamin C Plasma (oxalate, heparin, or EDTA)	0.6–2.0 mg/dL		34–113 μmol/L
Vitamin D$_2$, 25-Hydroxy Plasma (heparin)	Summer: 15–80 ng/mL Winter: 14–42		37–200 nmol/L 34–105
Vitamin D$_3$, 1,25-Dihydroxy (Calcitriol) Serum	25–45 pg/mL		60–108 nmol/L
Vitamin E Serum	5.0–20 μg/mL		11.6–46.4 μmol/L
Zinc Serum	70–150 μg/dL		10.7–22.9 μmol/L

From Behrman RE, Vaughan VC III: *Nelson Textbook of Pediatrics.* 13th ed. Philadelphia, WB Saunders, 1987.

Resources for Families

Appendix Eight

Acidemia
Lori Asten, Coordinator
Organic Acidemia Association
1532 South 87th Street
Kansas City, KS 66111
(913)422-7080

Acoustic Neuroma
Virginia Fickel
Acoustic Neuroma Association
P.O. Box 398
Carlisle, PA 17013

Addison Disease
Gertrude Woods, Executive Director
National Addison's Disease Foundation
505 Northern Boulevard, Suite 200
Great Neck, NY 11021
(516)487-4992

Aicardi
Denise Park
Aicardi Newsletter
1502 Woodcliff Road
Baltimore, MD 21228
(301)455-0317

AIDS
American Foundation for AIDS Research
40 West 57th Street, Suite 406
New York, NY 10019
(212)333-3118

Allergies
Allergy Information Center
25 Poynter Drive
Weston, Ontario
Canada M9R 1K8

Alopecia Areata
National Alopecia Areata Foundation
714 C Street
San Rafael, CA 94907
(415)456-4644

Amyotrophic Lateral Sclerosis
Rodney Hauts, President
Amyotrophic Lateral Sclerosis Association
15300 Ventura Boulevard, Suite 315
Sherman Oaks, CA 91403
(818)990-2151

Ankylosing Spondylitis
Jane Bruckel, Executive Director
Ankylosing Spondylitis Association
511 North LaCienega, Suite 216
Los Angeles, CA 90048
(213)652-0609

Aplastic Anemia
Lynn Rauch, Executive Director
Aplastic Anemia Foundation of America
P.O. Box 22689
Baltimore, MD 21203
(301)955-2803

Arthrogryposis
AVES, Arthrogryposis National Support Group
Phoenix Lake Road
P.O. Box 5192
Sonora, CA 95370
(209)533-1468

Ataxia
Myrna Lesinsky, Administrative Assistant
Friedreich's Ataxia Group of America
P.O. Box 11116
Oakland, CA 94611
(415)655-0833

Donna Gruetzmacher, Executive Director
National Ataxia Foundation
600-12 Oaks Center
15500 Wayzata Boulevard
Wayzata, MN 55391
(612)473-7666

Autism
National Society for Autism
1234 Massachusetts Avenue, NW
Washington, DC 20005

Bloom Syndrome
Bloom Syndrome Registry
New York Blood Center
Laboratory of Human Genetics
310 East 67th Street
New York, NY 10021
(212)570-3075

Brain Disorders
Diana Petty, Executive Director
Family Survival Project for Brain-Damaged Adults
44 Page Street, Suite 600
San Francisco, CA 94102
(415)626-6556

Marilyn Spivack, Executive Director
National Head Injury Foundation
333 Turnpike Road
Southboro, MA 01772
(617)879-7473

Association for Brain Tumor Research
2910 West Montrose Avenue
Chicago, IL 60618
(312)286-5571

Charcot-Marie-Tooth Disease
Linda Crabtree, President
Charcot-Marie-Tooth Foundation International
34B Bayview Drive
St. Catherines
Ontario, Canada L2N 4Y6

Howard Shapiro, Ph.D.
Director, Scientific Program
National Foundation for Peroneal Muscular Atrophy
3624 Market Street
Philadelphia, PA 19104
(215)664-6010

Chromosomal Disorders
National Center for Education in Maternal and Child Health
38th and R Streets, NW
Washington, DC 20057
(202)625-8400

Cornelia De Lange Syndrome
Julie Mairano, Director
Cornelia De Lange Syndrome Foundation
60 Dyer Avenue
Collinsville, CT 06022
(800)223-8355

Cri Du Chat Syndrome
Kent Nicholls, Director
5P-Society
11609 Oakmont
Overland Park, KS 66210
(913)469-8900

Cystic Fibrosis
Robert Beall, Executive Vice President
Cystic Fibrosis Foundation
6931 Arlington Road
Bethesda, MD 20814
(301)951-4422

Cystinosis
Jean Hotz, President
Cystinosis Foundation, Inc.
477 15th Street, Suite 200
Oakland, CA 94612
(415)834-7897

Courtesy of Abbey Meyers, National Organization for Rare Disorders, P.O. Box 8923, New Fairfield, Conn. 06812.

Diabetes
American Diabetes Association
National Service Center
1660 Duke Street
Alexandria, VA 22314
(800)232-3472

Dizziness and Balance
Disorders Association of America
1015 NW 22 Avenue
Portland, OR 97210
(503)229-7348

Dwarfism
Peggy Albert, Executive Director
Little People's Research Foundation
St. Joseph Hospital
80 Sr. Pierre Drive
Towson, MD 21204
(301)494-0055

Dysautonomia
Lenore Roseman, Executive Director
Dysautonomia Foundation
370 Lexington Avenue
New York, NY 10017

Dystonia
Nancy Harris, Director of Services
Dystonia Medical Research Foundation
8383 Wilshire Boulevard
Beverly Hills, CA 90211
(213)852-1630

Ectodermal Dysplasia
Mary Kaye Richter, Executive Director
National Foundation for Ectodermal Dysplasia
108 North First Street, Suite 311
Mascoutah, IL 62258
(618)566-2020

Ehlers-Danlos Syndrome
Nancy Hanna, Executive Director
Ehlers-Danlos National Foundation
P.O. Box 1212
Southgate, MI 48195
(313)282-0180

Epidermolysis Bullosa
Arlene Pessar, R.N.
D.E.B.R.A.
Kings County Hospital Center
451 Clarkson, Bldg. E, Room E6101
Brooklyn, NY 11203

Epilepsy
Richard Nugent
Epilepsy Foundation of America
4351 Garden City Drive
Landover, MD 20785
(301)459-3700

Epstein-Barr Virus
Gidget Faubion, President
National Chronic EBV Syndrome Association
P.O. Box 230108
Portland, OR 97223
(503)684-5261

Erythromelalgia
Liz McKinney
Erythromelalgia Association of America
Good Samaritan Hospital Medical Center
1015 NW 22 Avenue
Portland, OR 97210
(503)229-7348

Eye Disease
Eye Research Institute—Retina Foundation
20 Staniford Street
Boston, MA 02114

Facial Reconstruction
National Foundation for Facial Reconstruction
550 1st Avenue
New York, NY 10016

Familial Polyposis
Familial Polyposis Registry
200 Elizabeth Street
10-315 Eaton Building
Toronto, Canada M5G 2C4

Fanconi Anemia
Fanconi Anemia Support Group
2875 Baker Boulevard
Eugene, OR 97403

Gaucher Disease
Jill Talisman, Executive Director
National Gaucher's Foundation
1424 K Street, NW
Washington, DC 20005
(202)393-2777

Genetic Disorders
Greg Weigle, President
Alliance of Genetic Support Groups
38th and R Streets, NW
Washington, DC 20057
(703)281-1211

Gluten Intolerance
Gluten Intolerance Group of North America
Box 23053
Seattle, WA 98102-0353
(206)325-6980

Glycogen Storage Disease
Hollie Arp, President
Association for Glycogen Storage Disease
114 Satinwood Drive
Cheektowaga, NY 14225
(716)684-9765

Growth Disorders
Human Growth Foundation
4720 Montgomery Lane, Suite 909
Bethesda, MD 20814

Guillain-Barré Syndrome
Robert Benson, President
Guillain-Barré Support Group
P.O. Box 262
Wynnewood, PA 19096
(215)642-6855

Hemochromatosis
Dr. Margaret Krikker, President
Hemochromatosis Research Foundation
P.O. Box 8569
Albany, NY 12208
(518)489-0972

Hemophilia
National Hemophilia Foundation
110 Greene Street
The Soho Building, Suite 406
New York, NY 10012
(212)219-8180

Histiocytosis
Jeff Toughill, President
Histiocytosis-X Association
609 New York Road
Glassboro, NJ 08028

Huntington Disease
Dr. Nancy Wexler
Hereditary Disease Foundation
722 West 168th Street, Box 58
New York, NY 10032
(212)960-5667

Gary Wallach, Executive Director
Huntington's Disease Foundation
140 West 22nd Street
New York, NY 10011-2420

Hydrocephalus
James Mazzetti, Executive Director
National Hydrocephalus Foundation
Route 1 River Road
Joliet, IL 60436
(815)467-6548

Ichthyosis
F.I.R.S.T. (Foundation for Ichthyosis and Related Skin Types)
P.O. Box 410453
San Francisco, CA 94103
(415)591-1653

Ileitis and Colitis
National Foundation for Ileitis and Colitis
444 Park Avenue, South
New York, NY 10016
(212)685-3440

Immune Deficiency (Hereditary Immune Deficiencies Only)
Marcia Boyle, President
Immune Deficiency Foundation
P.O. Box 586
Columbia, MD 21045
(301)461-3127

Interstitial Cystitis
Dr. Paula Harbison, President
Interstitial Cystitis Association of America
P.O. Box 151323
San Diego, CA 92115
(714)857-1964

Jaw Joints and Musculoskeletal Disorders
Milton Glass, President
JJAMD
790 Boylston Street, Suite 17-H
Boston, MA 02199
(617)266-2550

Joseph Disease
Rose Marie Silva, Executive Director
International Joseph Disease Foundation
P.O. Box 2550
Livermore, CA 94550

Kidney Disease
American Kidney Fund
6110 Executive Boulevard, Suite 1010
Rockville, MD 20852
(800)638-8299

Klippel-Trenaunay Syndrome
Judy Vessey, Chairperson
Klippel-Trenaunay Support Group
4509 Wooddale Avenue
Edina, MN 55424
(612)925-2596

Laurence-Moon-Biedl Syndrome
Laurence-Moon-Biedl Network
122 Rolling Road
Lexington Park, MD 20653
(301)863-5658

Leukodystrophy
Paula Brazeal, President
United Leukodystrophy Foundation
2304 Highland Drive
Sycamore, IL 60178
(815)895-3211

Lipid Diseases
Harriet Klein, Director
National Lipid Diseases Foundation
1201 Corbin Street
Elizabeth, NJ 07201
(201)527-8000

Lowe Syndrome
Kaye McSpadden, President
Lowe's Syndrome Association, Inc.
222 Lincoln Street
West Lafayette, IN 47906
(317)743-3634

Lupus
Donna DeAngelis, Director
Research and Program Development
Lupus Foundation of America, Inc.
1717 Massachusetts Avenue, NW
Washington, DC 20036
(202)328-4550

Systemic Lupus Erythematosus Foundation
95 Madison Avenue, Room 1402
New York, NY 10016

Malignant Hyperthermia
Suellen Gallamore, Executive Director
Malignant Hyperthermia Association of the United States
P.O. Box 3231
Darien, CT 06820

Maple Syrup Urine Disease
Maple Syrup Urine Disease Parents
24806 SR 119
Goshen, IN 46526
(219)862-2992

Marfan Syndrome
Priscilla Ciccariello, Executive Director
National Marfan Foundation
382 Main Street
Port Washington, NY 11050
(516)883-8712

Meniere Disease
E.A.R. Foundation
Attention: Meniere Network
2000 Church Street
Nashville, TN 32736
(615)329-7807

Mucopolysaccharidosis
Marie Capobianco, President
National Mucopolysaccharidosis Society
17 Kramer Street
Hicksville, NY 11801
(516)931-6338

Leanne Carson-Hanse
Info-Referral Coordinator
Zaine Hansen Mucopolysaccharidosis Foundation
P.O. Box 4768
Arcata, CA 95521

Diane Morris, President
Mucopolysaccharidosis Research Funding Center, Inc.
1215 Maxfield Road
Hartland, MI 48029
(313)363-4412

Multiple Sclerosis
Dr. Steven Rheingold
National Multiple Sclerosis Society
205 East 42nd Street
New York, NY 10017

Myasthenia Gravis
Myasthenia Gravis Foundation
7–11 South Broadway
White Plains, NY 10601

Narcolepsy
William Baird, Executive Director
American Narcolepsy Association
335 Quarry Road
Belmont, CA 94070
(415)591-7979

Neurofibromatosis
Peter Bellerman, Executive Director
National Neurofibromatosis Foundation
141 Fifth Avenue, Suite 7-S
New York, NY 10010

Osteogenesis Imperfecta
Osteogenesis Imperfecta Foundation
P.O. Box 14807
Clearwater, FL 34629-4807
(813)855-7077

Meg Cauffield, President
Osteogenesis Imperfecta-NCA, Inc.
1311 Delaware Avenue, SW
Box 941
Washington, DC 20024
(202)484-0142

Ostomy
United Ostomy Association
2001 West Beverly Boulevard
Los Angeles, CA 90057

Paget Disease
Charlene Waldman, Executive Director
Paget's Disease Foundation
P.O. Box 2772
Brooklyn, NY 11202

Polycystic Kidney Disease
Jean Bacon, Executive Director
Polycystic Kidney Research Foundation
922 Walnut, #411
Kansas City, MO 64106
(816)421-1869

Polyposis
Henry Lyko, Co-Editor
Polyposis Newsletter
2830 NW 55th Avenue, Apt. 1A
Lauderhill, FL 33313
(305)733-2218

Porphyria
Desiree Dodson, Executive Director
American Porphyria Foundation
P.O. Box 11163
Montgomery, AL 36111

Port Wine Stain
National Congenital Port Wine Stain Foundation
125 East 63 Street
New York, NY 10021
(212)755-3820

Pradi-Willi Syndrome
Marge Wett, Executive Director
Prader-Willi Syndrome Association
5515 Malibu Drive
Edina, MN 55436
(612)933-0113

Pseudohypoparathyroidism
Charlotte Foehlich
PHP Self-Help Clearinghouse
104 Northern Parkway West
Plainview, NY 11803

Psoriasis
Gail Zimmerman, Executive Director
National Psoriasis Association
6443 SW Beaverton Highway, Suite 210
Portland, OR 97221
(503)297-1545

Reflex Sympathetic Dystrophy
Audrey Thomas
Reflex Sympathetic Dystrophy Association
P.O. Box 821
Haddonfield, NJ 08033

Retinitis Pigmentosa
Jeanette Felix, Ph.D.
Director of Science
National Retinitis Pigmentosa Foundation
1401 Mt. Royal Avenue, 4th flr.
Baltimore, MD 21217
(301)225-9400

Rett Syndrome
Kathy Hunter, President
International Rett Syndrome Association, Inc.
8511 Rose Marie Drive
Fort Washington, MD 20744
(301)248-7031

Sarcoidosis
Geneva Ausley, Executive Director
Sarcoidosis Family Aid and Research Foundation
760 Clinton Avenue
Newark, NJ 07108
(800)223-6429

Scleroderma
Mark Flapan, Ph.D., President
Scleroderma Federation, Inc.
1725 York Avenue, Suite 29F
New York, NY 10128
(212)427-7040

Nancy Hershey, President
Scleroderma Information Exchange, Inc.
150 Hines Farm Road
Cranston, RI 02920
(401)943-3909

John Barlet, President
Scleroderma International Foundation
704 Gardner Center Road
New Castle, PA 16101

Robert Harrison, Executive Director
United Scleroderma Foundation
P.O. Box 350
Watsonville, CA 95077
(408)728-2202

Sickle Cell Disease
Darnelle Pinkard, Executive Director
Sickle Cell Disease Research Foundation of Texas, Inc.
P.O. Box 8095
Houston, TX 77288-8095
(713)651-8071

Dorothy Boswell, Executive Director
National Association for Sickle Cell Disease, Inc.
4221 Wilshire Boulevard, Suite 360
Los Angeles, CA 90010-3503
(213)936-7205

Sjögren Syndrome
Elaine Harris, President
Sjögren's Syndrome Association, Inc.
29 Gateway Drive
Great Neck, NY 11021
(516)487-2243

Soto Syndrome
Soto Syndrome USA Support Group
2333 W. El Moro
Mesa, AZ 85202
(602)890-1722

Spasmodic Torticollis
National Spasmodic Torticollis Association
905 North Wilson
Royal Oak, MI 48067

Spastic Dysphonia
Midge Kovacs, Editor
Our Voice
799 Broadway, Suite 640
New York, NY 10003
(212)228-8080

Spina Bifida
Spina Bifida Association of Southern Arizona
P.O. Box 57246
Tucson, AZ 85732

Spinal Muscular Atrophy
Audrey Lewis, Executive Director
Families of Spinal Muscular Atrophy
P.O. Box 1465
Highland Park, IL 60035
(312)432-5551

Sturge-Weber Syndrome
Karen Ball
National Foundation for Sturge-Weber Syndrome
3602 South Ouray Circle
Aurora, CO 80013
(303)693-2986

Tay-Sachs Disease
Dale Carre, Executive Director
National Tay-Sachs and Allied Diseases Association
385 Elliot Street
Newton, MA 02164
(617)964-5508

Tourette Syndrome
Dennis Hirshfelder, Executive Director
Tourette Syndrome Association, Inc.
42-40 Bell Boulevard
Bayside, NY 11361
(718)224-2999

Trisomy 18/13
New York Chapter of Trisomy 18/13
2982 South Union Street
Rochester, NY 14624
(716)594-4621

Tuberous Sclerosis
Linda Ham, Executive Director
National Tuberous Sclerosis Association
Box 612
Winfield, IL 60190
(312)668-0787

Turner Syndrome
Lynn Tesch, Executive Director
Turner's Syndrome Society
3539 Tonkawood Road
Minnetonka, MN 55345
(612)938-3118

Drusilla Davis
Turner's Syndrome Support Group of New England
170 Maple Street
Malden, MA 02148
(617)322-4792

Urea-Cycle Disorders
Dr. Emanuel Idelovitch
Association for Children's Urea-Cycle Disorders
11 Bethana Way
Rockville, MD 20850
(301)294-6859

Uveitis
Uveitis Support
16 North Broadway, 2-E
White Plains, NY 10601
(914)686-5968

Vitiligo
Allen Locklin, President
National Vitiligo Foundation, Inc.
P.O. Box 6337
Tyler, TX 75711

Williams Syndrome
Gordon Biescar, President
Williams Syndrome Association
16211 North Greenfield Drive
Spring, TX 77379-7622
(713)376-1626

Wilson Disease
Carol Terry, President
Wilson's Disease Association
P.O. Box 75324
Washington, DC 20013
(703)636-3014

Resources for Home Health Care
Association for Children with Learning Disabilities
4156 Library Road
Pittsburgh, PA 15234

Child Health Affairs
Department of Health and Human Services
5600 Fishers Lane
Rockville, MD 20852

Child Welfare League of America, Inc.
67 Irving Place
New York, NY 10003

La Leche League International
9619 Minneapolis Avenue
Franklin Park, IL 60131

National Easter Seal Society for Crippled Children and Adults
2023 West Ogden Avenue
Chicago, IL 60612

National Foundation—March of Dimes
Box 2000
White Plains, NY 10602

National Institute of Child Health and Human Development
National Institute of Health
9000 Rockville Pike
Bethesda, MD 20014

National Organization for Rare Disorders, Inc.
P.O. Box 8923
New Fairfield, CT 06812

Scouting for Handicapped
Education Relationships Service
Boy Scouts of America
North Brunswick, NJ 08902

Shriner's Hospital for Crippled Children
323 North Michigan Avenue
Chicago, IL 60601

Nutritive Values of Baby Foods

Appendix Nine

Nutritive Value of Baby Foods (Per Serving)

Food	Serving *g*	Energy *kcal*	Pro-Tein *g*	Fat *g*	Carbo-hydrate *g*	Sodium *mg*	Calcium *mg*	Iron *mg*	Vitamin A Value *IU*	Thiamin *mg*	Ribo-flavin *mg*	Niacin *mg*	Ascorbic Acid *mg*
Cereals, precooked, dry and other products													
Barley, added nutrients	15	50	1	0	10	5	95	7	(0)	0.2	0.3	2	0
High protein, added nutrients	15	50	5	1	6	3	95	7	—	0.2	0.3	24.0	0
Mixed, added nutrients	15	40	2	0	9	4	95	7	—	0.2	0.3	22.3	0
Oatmeal, added nutrients	15	50	2	1	9	5	95	7	(0)	0.2	0.3	21.3	0
Rice, added nutrients	15	40	1	0	9	4	95	7	(0)	0.2	0.3	19.7	0
Dinners, canned: cereal, vegetable, meat mixtures (approx. 2–4% protein)													
Beef with vegetables	128	110	7	5	9	40	10	0.7	600	0.04	0.05	2	2
Chicken with vegetables	128	130	8	7	8	35	95	0.8	2200	0.03	0.05	1.5	3
Cottage cheese with pineapple	135	150	8	2	26	200	96	0.3	0	0.05	6	0.4	2
Ham with vegetables	128	110	8	4	10	30	8	0.8	400	0.15	6	1.5	3
Turkey with vegetables	128	120	8	6	9	40	50	0.9	350	0.03	6	2	4
Veal with vegetables	128	90	8	3	9	35	8	1.0	100	0.04	7	2.5	3
Fruits and fruit products with or without thickening, canned													
Applesauce	128	50	0	0	14	2	5	0.1	40	0.01	0.02	0.1	15
Applesauce and apricots	128	80	0	1	18	5.5	5.7	0.1	288	0.01	0.04	0.2	1.5
Bananas (with tapioca or cornstarch added ascorbic acid), strained	128	80	1	0	16		13	0.1	50	0.02	0.02	0.2	15
Bananas and pineapple (with tapioca or cornstarch)	128	70	0	1	16	8.0	20	0.1	45	0.01	0.01	0.1	15
Peaches	128	70	1	1	14	5	6	0.1	300	0.01	0.02	0.7	15
Pears	128	70	1	1	15	3	7	0.1	50	0.02	0.02	0.2	15
Pears and pineapple	128	80	1	1	16	2	7	0.1	45	0.03	0.02	0.2	15
Plums with tapioca, strained	128	90	1	1	19	5	5	0.1	150	0.01	0.02	0.2	1
Prunes with tapioca	135	110	1	1	25	15	7	0.3	300	0.02	0.06	0.4	7
Meats, poultry, and eggs; canned													
Beef:													
Strained	99	90	13	4	0	59	7	1	91	0.01	0.16	3.5	2
Junior	99	100	14	4	1	61	6	1.6	74	0.02	0.20	3.6	2
Chicken junior, strained	99	140	14	9	0	41	8	1	52	0.02	0.16	3.5	2
Egg yolks, strained	94	180	9	16	1	57	79	3.0	542	0.12	0.22	Trace	2
Ham junior	99	120	15	6	1	43	6	1	32	0.01	0.16	2.8	2
Lamb:													
Strained	99	100	14	4	1	51	4	1	99	0.02	0.17	3.3	1
Junior	99	100	15	4	1	54	5	1.6	19	0.01	0.16	3.0	1
Liver, strained	99	90	14.1	3	2	53	4	5.6	25,000	0.05	2.00	7.6	19
Veal:													
Strained	99	0	13	4	1	55	4	1	61	0.03	0.20	4.3	3
Junior	99	100	15	4	0	55	5	1	28	0.01	0.15	4	2
Vegetables, canned													
Beans, green	128	40	2	0	7	1	40	0.7	400	0.02	0.06	0.3	6
Beets, strained	128	40	1	0	10	90	13	0.3	20	0.02	0.03	0.1	3
Carrots	128	40	1	0	8	50	25	0.5	17,000	0.02	0.03	0.4	10
Mixed vegetables, including vegetable soup	128	60	2	1	10	15	14	0.9	7000	0.05	0.04	0.6	3
Peas, strained	128	60	4	1	10	5	14	1.2	600	0.08	0.09	1.2	10
Spinach, creamed	128	70	4	2	9	65	130	1.5	7000	0.02	0.13	0.3	6
Squash	128	40	1	0	8	3	24	0.4	2000	0.02	0.04	0.3	11
Sweet potatoes	135	80	1	0	19	25	16	0.4	6500	0.04	0.03	0.4	11

From various manufacturers.

Index

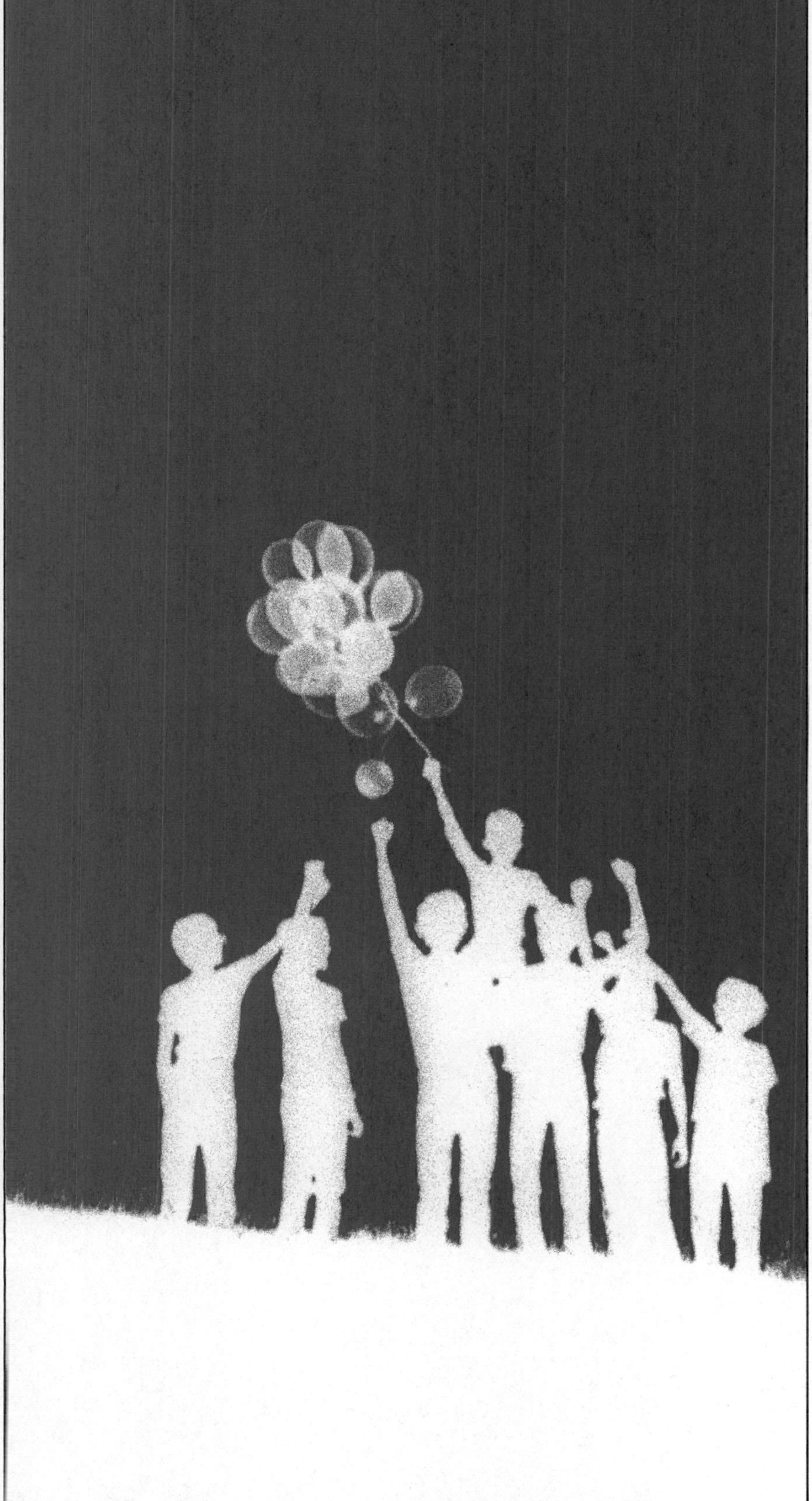

Index

Note: Page numbers in *italics* refer to illustrations; page numbers followed by (t) refer to tables; page numbers followed by (b) refer to boxes.

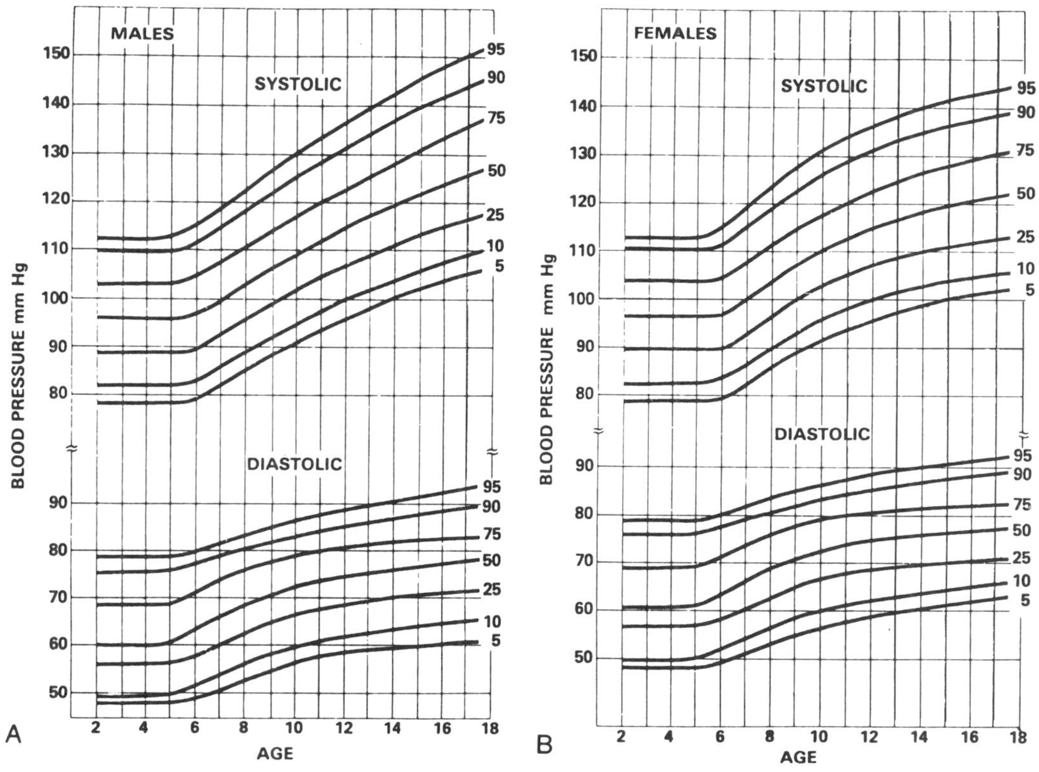

Blood Pressure:

Blood Pressure: Percentiles of blood pressure in seated males (A) and in seated females (B).

From Report of the Task Force on Blood Pressure Control in Children, National Heart, Lung, and Blood Institute. Pediatrics (Suppl) 59:803, 1977. Copyright American Academy of Pediatrics.

***Table* 15-1.** Normal Pulse and Respiratory Rates for Specific Ages*

Age	Pulse (Beats per Minute)	Average Pulse	Respirations (Breaths per Minute)
Neonate	70–170	120	30–40
2 years	80–130	110	25–32
4 years	80–120	100	23–30
6 years	75–115	100	21–26
8 years	70–110	90	20–26
10 years	70–110	90	20–26
12 years	70–110	85	18–22
14 years	65–105	85	18–22
16 years	60–100	85	16–20
18 years	50–90	80	12–24

*These are averages and vary with the sex of the child.

***Table* 18-4.** Range of Average Water Requirements of Children Under Ordinary Conditions

Age	Average Body Weight (kg)	Total Water in 24 Hours (ml)	Water per kg Body Wt in 24 Hours (ml)
3 days	3.0	250–300	80–100
10 days	3.2	400–500	125–150
3 mo	5.4	750–850	140–160
6 mo	7.3	950–1100	130–155
9 mo	8.6	1100–1250	125–145
1 yr	9.5	1150–1300	120–135
2 yr	11.8	1350–1500	115–125
4 yr	16.2	1600–1800	100–110
6 yr	20.0	1800–2000	90–100
10 yr	28.7	2000–2500	70–85
14 yr	45.0	2200–2700	50–60
18 yr	54.0	2200–2700	40–50

(From Behrman and Vaughan, 1987.)

Conversion Factors for Temperature*

Celsius	Fahrenheit	Celsius	Fahrenheit	Celsius	Fahrenheit	Celsius	Fahrenheit
34.0	93.2	36.4	97.5	38.6	101.5	41.0	105.9
34.2	93.6	36.6	97.9	38.8	101.8	41.2	106.1
34.4	93.9	36.8	98.2	39.0	102.0	41.4	106.5
34.6	94.3	37.0	98.6	39.2	102.6	41.6	106.8
34.8	94.6	37.2	99.0	39.4	102.9	41.8	107.2
35.0	95.0	37.4	99.3	39.6	103.3	42.0	107.6
35.2	95.4	37.6	99.7	39.8	103.6	42.2	108.0
35.4	95.7	37.8	100.0	40.0	104.0	42.4	108.3
35.6	96.1	38.0	100.4	40.2	104.4	42.6	108.7
35.8	96.4	38.2	100.8	40.4	104.7	42.8	109.0
36.0	96.8	38.4	101.1	40.6	105.2	43.0	109.4
36.2	97.2			40.8	105.4		

*(°C) x (9/5) + 32 = °F
(°F − 32) x (5/9) = °C
°C = temperature in Celsius (centigrade) degrees
°F = temperature in Fahrenheit degrees